PHYSICAL MEDICINE AND REHABILITATION

ASSOCIATE EDITORS

INTERIM ASSOCIATE EDITORS

MANAGING EDITOR

PHYSICAL MEDICINE AND REHABILITATION

The Complete Approach

Edited by

Martin Grabois, MD

Professor and Chairman
Department of Physical Medicine and Rehabilitation

Susan J. Garrison, MD

Associate Professor
Department of Physical Medicine and Rehabilitation

Karen A. Hart, PhD

Associate Professor
Department of Physical Medicine and Rehabilitation

L. Don Lehmkuhl, PhD

Associate Professor
Department of Physical Medicine and Rehabilitation

Baylor College of Medicine
Houston, Texas

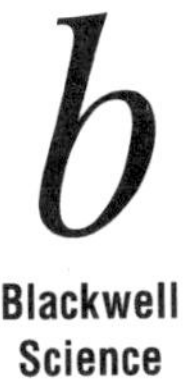

Blackwell
Science

Editorial Offices:
Commerce Place, 350 Main Street, Malden, Massachusetts 02148, USA
Osney Mead, Oxford OX2 0EL, England
25 John Street, London WC1N 2BL, England
23 Ainslie Place, Edinburgh EH3 6AJ, Scotland
54 University Street, Carlton, Victoria 3053, Australia
Other Editorial Offices:
Blackwell Wissenschafts-Verlag GmbH, Kurfürstendamm 57, 10707 Berlin, Germany
Blackwell Science KK, MG Kodenmacho Building, 7-10 Kodenmacho Nihombashi, Chuo-ku, Tokyo 104, Japan

Distributors:
USA
Blackwell Science, Inc.
Commerce Place
350 Main Street
Malden, Massachusetts 02148
(Telephone orders: 800-215-1000 or 781-388-8250; fax orders: 781-388-8270)

Canada
Login Brothers Book Company
324 Saulteaux Crescent
Winnipeg, Manitoba, R3J 3T2
(Telephone orders: 204-224-4068)

Australia
Blackwell Science Pty, Ltd.
54 University Street
Carlton, Victoria 3053
(Telephone orders: 03-9347-0300;
fax orders: 03-9349-3016)

Outside North America and Australia
Blackwell Science, Ltd.
c/o Marston Book Services, Ltd.
P.O. Box 269
Abingdon
Oxon OX14 4YN
England
(Telephone orders: 44-01235-465500;
fax orders: 44-01235-465555)

Acquisitions: Chris Davis
Development: Mike Snider
Production: Irene Herlihy
Manufacturing: Lisa Flanagan
Cover design by Meral Dabcovich, Visual Perspectives
Typeset by Best-set Typesetter Ltd., Hong Kong
Printed and bound by Sheridan Books

Printed in the United States of America
99 00 01 02 5 4 3 2 1

Library of Congress Cataloging-in-Publication Data

Physical medicine and rehabilitation: the complete approach / edited by Martin Grabois . . . [et al.].
p. cm.
Includes bibliographical references and index.
ISBN 0-86542-536-1 (alk. paper)
1. Medicine, Physical. 2. Medical rehabilitation. I. Grabois, Martin.
RM700.P472 2000
615.8′2—dc21 98-17785
CIP

Notice: The indications and dosages of all drugs in this book have been recommended in the medical literature and conform to the practices of the general community. The medications described do not necessarily have specific approval by the Food and Drug Administration for use in the diseases and dosages for which they are recommended. The package insert for each drug should be consulted for use and dosage as approved by the FDA. Because standards for usage change, it is advisable to keep abreast of revised recommendations, particularly those concerning new drugs.

Contents

List of Contributors

Brenda B. Adamovich, PhD
Vice President, Inpatient Division
HealthSouth Rehabilitation Corporation
Birmingham, Alabama

Uma Aggarwal, MD
Rochester General Hospital
Rochester, New York

James C. Agre, MD, PhD
Physiatrist
Howard Young Medical Center
Woodruff, Wisconsin

Michael A. Alexander, MD
Clinical Professor and Chief
Pediatric Rehabilitation
Thomas Jefferson University
Philadelphia, Pennsylvania;
Du Pont Hospital for Children
Wilmington, Delaware

Norman Aliga, MD
Board of Directors
Rehabilitation Medicine Clinic, Inc.;
Assistant Professor
Department of Physical Medicine and Rehabilitation
Rush Medical College
Chicago, Illinois

Neil Alpiner, MD
Director, Department of Physical Medicine and Rehabilitation
Hurley Medical Center
Flint, Michigan

Jill Androwick, OTR/L
Department of Physical Medicine and Rehabilitation
Crozer Chester Medical Center
Chester, Pennsylvania

John R. Bach, MD, FAAPMR, FACCP
Professor and Vice Chairman
Associate Medical Director and Director of Research
Department of Physical Medicine and Rehabilitation
University Hospital
UMDNJ–New Jersey Medical School;
Co-Director, Jerry Lewis Muscular Dystrophy Association Clinic;
Director, Center for Ventilator Management Alternatives
University Hospital
Newark, New Jersey;
Kessler Institute for Rehabilitation
West Orange, New Jersey

Matthew N. Bartels, MD, MPH
Assistant Professor of Clinical Rehabilitation Medicine
Department of Rehabilitation Medicine
Director, Cardiopulmonary Rehabilitation
Director, Human Performance Laboratory
Columbia-Presbyterian Medical Center
New York, New York

Jeffrey R. Basford, MD, PhD
Associate Professor
Department of Physical Medicine and Rehabilitation
Mayo Clinic and Foundation
Rochester, Minnesota

Mary Frances Baxter, MA, OTR, ATP
Assistant Professor
School of Occupational Therapy
Texas Woman's University
Houston, Texas

Carol Beatson, DipOT, NZROT
Approved Driving Instructor (Advanced)
Driver Assessment Service
Auckland, New Zealand

Pelagie M. Beeson, PhD, CCC-SLP
National Center for Neurogenic Communication
Disorders and Department of Speech and Hearing Sciences
The University of Arizona
Tucson, Arizona

Keith Bengtson, MD
Instructor, Mayo Medical School;
Consultant, Mayo Clinic
Rochester, Minnesota

Theresa Frasca Berner, MOT, OTR/L
Rehabilitation Team Leader, Dodd Hall
The Ohio State University Medical Center
Columbus, Ohio

Joseph Bleiberg, PhD
Director, Psychology Services
National Rehabilitation Hospital
Washington, DC

Donna Bloodworth, MD
Department of Physical Medicine and Rehabilitation
Baylor College of Medicine
Houston, Texas

Carol Bodenheimer, MD
Department of Physical Medicine and Rehabilitation
VAMC
Houston, Texas

Richard Bonfiglio, MD
Harmarville Rehabilitation Hospital
Pittsburgh, Pennsylvania

Michael L. Boninger, MD
Assistant Professor and Research Director
Department of Orthopedic Surgery
Division of Physical Medicine and Rehabilitation
University of Pittsburgh Medical Center
Pittsburgh, Pennsylvania

Victoria Anne Brander, MD
Clinical Assistant Professor
Department of Physical Medicine and Rehabilitation;
Director, Arthritis Center
Rehabilitation Institute of Chicago
Northwestern University Medical School
Chicago, Illinois

Valerie Brooke, MEd
Associate Director, Training
Rehabilitation Research and Training Center
on Supported Employment
Virginia Commonwealth University
Richmond, Virginia

Dale R. Broome, MD
Assistant Professor of Radiology
Baylor College of Medicine;
Assistant Chief of Radiology
The Institute for Rehabilitation and Research
Houston, Texas

Laurie A. Browngoehl, MD
Physical Medicine and Rehabilitation
Bala Cynwyd, Pennsylvania

Derek Burnett, MD
Assistant Professor
Department of Physical Medicine and Rehabilitation
Medical College of Virginia
Virginia Commonwealth University
Richmond, Virginia

Stephen P. Burns, MD
Staff Physician, SCI Service
VA Puget Sound Health Care System;
Acting Assistant Professor
Department of Rehabilitation Medicine
University of Washington
Seattle, Washington

Mark H. Bussell, MD, CPO
Medical Director
HealthSouth Cityview Rehabilitation Hospital
Fort Worth, Texas

Diana D. Cardenas, MD
Professor
Department of Rehabilitation Medicine
University of Washington;
Project Director
Northwest Regional Spinal Cord Injury System
Seattle, Washington

John W. Cassidy, MD
Baylor College of Medicine;
Neurobehavioral Healthcare Systems
Houston, Texas

Paul Cauley, CP
University of Michigan Orthotics and Prosthetics Center
Ann Arbor, Michigan

Krystal Chambers, MD, FAAPMR
Georgia Pain Physicians, PC
Marietta, Georgia

Leighton Chan, MD, MPH
Assistant Professor
Department of Rehabilitation Medicine
University of Washington
Seattle, Washington

David Chen, MD
George M. Eisenberg Chair in Spinal Cord Injury Rehabilitation
Director, Spinal Cord Injury Program
Rehabilitation Institute of Chicago;
Assistant Professor
Department of Physical Medicine and Rehabilitation
Northwestern University Medical School
Chicago, Illinois

Martin Childers, DO
Assistant Professor
Department of Physical Medicine and Rehabilitation
University of Missouri–Columbia
Columbia, Missouri

Christopher L. Chong, MD
Assistant Professor of Radiology
Baylor College of Medicine
Houston, Texas

David X. Cifu, MD
Associate Professor and Chairman
Department of Physical Medicine and Rehabilitation;
Medical Director
Rehabilitation and Research Center
Medical College of Virginia
Virginia Commonwealth University
Richmond, Virginia

Gary S. Clark, MD
Clinical Director of Rehabilitation Medicine
CGF Health System;
Clinical Associate Professor
Department of Rehabilitation Medicine
School of Medicine and Biomedical Sciences
State University of New York at Buffalo
Buffalo, New York

Andrew J. Cole, MD, FACSM
Northwest Spine and Sports Physicians, PC;
Medical Director
The Spine Center at Overlake Hospital
Bellevue, Washington;
Clinical Assistant Professor
Department of Rehabilitation Medicine
University of Washington
Seattle, Washington

Miles O. Colwell, MD
Assistant Clinical Professor
Department of Physical Medicine and Rehabilitation
University of Michigan
Ann Arbor, Michigan

Katie Coleman Cornwall, RD
Clinical Dietitian
Kaiser Foundation Rehabilitation Center
Kaiser Foundation Hospital
Vallejo, California

Earl J. Craig, MD
Clinical Assistant Professor
Department of Physical Medicine and Rehabilitation
Indiana University School of Medicine;
Rehabilitation Associates of Indiana
Bloomington, Indiana

Elaine Date, MD
Chief, Physical Medicine and Rehabilitation
Palo Alto VA Health Care System;
Associate Professor
Department of Functional Restoration
Stanford University Medical Center
Palo Alto, California

Alicia J. Davis, CPO
University of Michigan Orthotics and Prosthetics Center
Ann Arbor, Michigan

William J. Dawson, MD
Associate Professor Emeritus of Orthopaedic Surgery
Northwestern University Medical School
Chicago, Illinois

David K. DeDianous, MD
Department of Rehabilitation Medicine
University of Pennsylvania Medical Center
Philadelphia, Pennsylvania

Pedro J. Diaz-Marchan, MD
Assistant Professor of Radiology
Baylor College of Medicine;
Assistant Chief of Radiology
Ben Taub General Hospital
Houston, Texas

Mary L. Dombovy, MD
Associate Professor of Neurology and Rehabilitation
University of Rochester;
Vice President, Integrated Services
Chair, Department of Physical Medicine and Rehabilitation
Unity Health System
Rochester, New York

Jan Dommerholt, MPS, PT
Director of Rehabilitation Services
Pain and Rehabilitation Medicine
Bethesda, Maryland

Susan J. Dreyer, MD
The Emory Spine Center
Assistant Professor of Physical Medicine and Rehabilitation
Assistant Professor of Orthopaedic Surgery
Emory University
Atlanta, Georgia

Stanley H. Ducharme, PhD
Clinical Health Psychologist
Boston Medical Center;
Professor of Rehabilitation Medicine
Assistant Professor of Urology
Boston University School of Medicine
Boston, Massachusetts

Bart Eisfelder, JD
Law Offices of Foland & Wickens PC
Kansas City, Missouri

Timothy R. Elliott, PhD
Department of Physical Medicine and Rehabilitation
University of Alabama at Birmingham
Birmingham, Alabama

Elie Elovic, MD
Clinical Assistant Professor
UMDNJ
Robert Wood Johnson School of Medicine;
Medical Director
Spasticity Clinic;
Associate Medical Director
Center for Head Injuries
JFK Johnson Rehabilitation Institute
Edison, New Jersey

Alberto Esquenazi, MD
Director, Gait and Motion Analysis Laboratory
and Regional Amputee Rehabilitation Center
MossRehab Hospital;
Associate Professor of Rehabilitation Medicine
Temple University School of Medicine
Philadelphia, Pennsylvania

Frank J. E. Falco, MD
Clinical Assistant Professor
Department of Physical Medicine and Rehabilitation
Temple University School of Medicine
Philadelphia, Pennsylvania;
Comprehensive Spine & Sports Medicine, PA
Wilmington, Delaware

Laura Fenwick, CO
Certified Orthotist
Chicago, Illinois

Katherine A. Feuillan, CTRS
Recreational Therapist
Rehabilitation Center of Chicago
Resurrection Medical Center
Chicago, Illinois

Lucretia Fitzpatrick, MD
Department of Physical Medicine and Rehabilitation
Crozer Chester Medical Center
Chester, Pennsylvania

Kathleen D. Francis, MD
Assistant Professor
Clinical Physical Medicine and Rehabilitation
UMDNJ–New Jersey Medical School
Newark, New Jersey;
Attending Physiatrist
Huntington's Disease Clinic
Kessler Institute for Rehabilitation
West Orange, New Jersey

Michael D. Freedman, MD, FACP, FCP
Assistant Professor of Medicine
Johns Hopkins University School of Medicine;
Attending Physician and Director of Clinical Research
The New Childrens Hospital
Baltimore, Maryland

Guy W. Fried, MD
Attending Physician and Outpatient Medical Director
Magee Rehabilitation Hospital;
Assistant Professor
Thomas Jefferson University Hospitals
Philadelphia, Pennsylvania

Karen Mandzak Fried, RN, MSN, CRRN, CCM
Nurse Manager
Comprehensive Acute Rehabilitation Center/Regional Spinal Cord Injury Center
Thomas Jefferson University Hospital;
Clinical Instructor
Thomas Jefferson University College of Health Professionals
Philadelphia, Pennsylvania

Lex Frieden, MA
Professor of Physical Medicine and Rehabilitation and Department of Family and Community Medicine
Baylor College of Medicine;
Senior Vice President, The Institute for Rehabilitation and Research
Director, Independent Living Research Utilization Program
Houston, Texas

Gary S. Friedman, MD
Private Practice
Bartlesville, Oklahoma

Walter R. Frontera, MD, PhD
Earle P. and Ida S. Charlton Associate Professor and Chairman
Department of Physical Medicine and Rehabilitation
Harvard Medical School;
Chief, Department of Physical Medicine and Rehabilitation
Spaulding Rehabilitation Hospital;
Physiatrist-in-Chief, Massachusetts General Hospital
Boston, Massachusetts

Jan Galvin
President
The Galvin Group, LLC
Tucson, Arizona

Susan L. Garber, MA, OTR, FAOTA
Associate Professor
Department of Physical Medicine and Rehabilitation
Baylor College of Medicine
Houston, Texas

Susan J. Garrison, MD
Associate Professor
Department of Physical Medicine and Rehabilitation
Baylor College of Medicine;
Medical Director
Rehabilitation Center
The Methodist Hospital
Houston, Texas

Stephen R. Gaspar, MD
Assistant Professor
Director, Cardiopulmonary Rehabilitation Services
Department of Physical Medicine and Rehabilitation
Temple University School of Medicine
Philadelphia, Pennsylvania

Michael C. Geraci, Jr., MD, PT
Fellowship Program Director and Co-Medical Director
Buffalo Spine and Sports Medicine, PC
Williamsville, New York;
Clinical Assistant Professor
Department of Physical Medicine and Rehabilitation
State University of New York at Buffalo
Buffalo, New York;
College of Osteopathic Medicine
Michigan State University
East Lansing, Michigan

Robert D. Gerwin, MD
Department of Neurology
Johns Hopkins University
Baltimore, Maryland;
Pain and Rehabilitation Medicine, Ltd.
Bethesda, Maryland

Rosamond Gianutsos, PhD, FAAO, CDRS
Head Trauma Vision Rehabilitation Unit
State College of Optometry
State University of New York
New York, New York

Rita M. Glass, EdD
President
Rita Glass Consulting, Inc.
Chicago, Illinois

Steve M. Gnatz, MD, MHA
Professor and Chairman
Department of Physical Medicine and Rehabilitation
University of Missouri–Columbia
Columbia, Missouri

Gary Goldberg, MD
Co-Director, Electrodiagnostic Center
Attending Physiatrist, Drucker Brain Injury Center
Consultant, Stroke Center
MossRehab Hospital;
Associate Professor
Department of Physical Medicine and Rehabilitation
Temple University School of Medicine
Philadelphia, Pennsylvania

Harvey Goldberg, MD
Clinical Assistant Professor
Department of Rehabilitation Medicine
New York University School of Medicine
New York, New York;
Chief, Physical Medicine and Rehabilitation
New York Community Hospital of Brooklyn
Brooklyn, New York

Deborah Goldblum, MS, OTR/L
Department of Physical Medicine and Rehabilitation
Crozer Chester Medical Center
Chester, Pennsylvania

Ellen Grabois, JD, LLM
Assistant Professor
Department of Physical Medicine and Rehabilitation
Baylor College of Medicine
Center for Research on Women with Disabilities
Houston, Texas

Martin Grabois, MD
Professor and Chairman
Department of Physical Medicine and Rehabilitation
Baylor College of Medicine
Houston, Texas

Carl V. Granger, MD
Professor, Department of Rehabilitation Medicine
Director, Center for Functional Assessment Research and the Uniform Date System for Medical Rehabilitation
School of Medicine and Biomedical Sciences
State University of New York at Buffalo
Buffalo, New York

Howard Green, MS
Training Associate
Rehabilitation Research and Training Center on Supported Employment
Virginia Commonwealth University
Richmond, Virginia

Andrew J. Haig, MD
Director, University of Michigan Spine Program
Assistant Professor
Departments of Physical Medicine/Rehabilitation and Surgery
The University of Michigan
Ann Arbor, Michigan;
Clinical Associate Professor
Department of Physical Medicine and Rehabilitation
The Medical College of Wisconsin
Milwaukee, Wisconsin

Steven L. Hendler, MD
Clinical Assistant Professor
Department of Rehabilitation Medicine
University of Kansas Medical Center
Kansas City, Kansas

Stanley A. Herring, MD, FACSM
Clinical Associate Professor
Department of Rehabilitation Medicine
Clinical Associate Professor
Department of Orthopaedics
University of Washington Medical Center;
Puget Sound Sports and Spine Physicians
Seattle, Washington

Kathleen A. Hinderer, MS, MPT, PT
Doctoral Candidate
Division of Kinesiology
University of Michigan
Ann Arbor, Michigan

Steven R. Hinderer, MD, MS, PT
Medical Director of Research and the Clinical Rehabilitation Research Unit
Rehabilitation Institute of Michigan;
Assistant Professor
Department of Physical Medicine and Rehabilitation
Wayne State University School of Medicine
Detroit, Michigan

Fabiane M. Hirsch, MSc, CCC-SLP
National Center for Neurogenic Communication
Disorders and Department of Speech and Hearing Sciences
The University of Arizona
Tucson, Arizona

Margaret L. Ho, MA, CCC/SIP
Supervisor, Speech Pathology
Memorial Sloan-Kettering Cancer Center
New York, New York

Richard Holicky, MA
The Rehabilitation Research and Training Center on Aging with Spinal Cord Injury
Craig Hospital
Englewood, Colorado

Peggy Holmes-Layman, PhD, CTRS
Department of Leisure Studies
Eastern Illinois University
Charleston, Illinois

Lawrence J. Horn, MD
Coghlin Chair and Professor
Department of Physical Medicine and Rehabilitation
Medical College of Ohio
Toledo, Ohio

Carol A. Howland, MPH
Assistant Professor
Department of Physical Medicine and Rehabilitation
Baylor College of Medicine
Houston, Texas

Katherine Inge, PhD, OTR
Project Access Director
Rehabilitation Research and Training Center on Supported Employment
Virginia Commonwealth University
Richmond, Virginia

Sanjiv Jain, MD
Division of Physical Medicine and Rehabilitation
Carle Clinic Association
Urbana, Illinois;
McKinley Health Center
University of Illinois
Urbana/Champaign, Illinois

Suzanne E. Jonas, EdD
Creative Education Foundation;
Program Director
Shallcross Creativity Institute;
President and Founder, Music and Medicine
Maryville, Tennessee;
Faculty, Creative Education Foundation;
Adjunct Faculty
American Holistics Nurses Association Certification Program;
Licensed Mental Health Counsellor
Private Behavioral Medicine Practice

Darryl Kaelin, MD
Clinical Assistant Professor
Department of Physical Medicine and Rehabilitation
Indiana University School of Medicine;
Rehabilitation Associates of Indiana
Bloomington, Indiana

Richard T. Katz, MD
Associate Professor of Clinical Internal Medicine
(Physical Medicine and Rehabilitation Medicine)
St. Louis University School of Medicine
St. Louis, Missouri

W. Ben Kibler, MD, FACSM
Clinical Associate Professor
Department of Physical Medicine and Rehabilitation
Clinical Associate Professor
Department of Family Practice
University of Kentucky;
Medical Director
Lexington Clinic Sports Medicine Center
Lexington, Kentucky

John C. King, MD
Associate Professor
Department of Rehabilitation Medicine
University of Texas Health Sciences Center at San Antonio
San Antonio, Texas

Wade S. Kingery, MD
Assistant Clinical Professor
Division of Physical Medicine and Rehabilitation
Department of Functional Restoration
Stanford Medical School;
Physical Medicine and Rehabilitation Service
Palo Alto Veterans Affairs Health Care System
Palo Alto, California

Andrew E. Kirsteins, MD
Charlotte Institute of Rehabilitation
Charlotte, North Carolina

Dilip S. Kittur, MD
Johns Hopkins University School of Medicine
Baltimore, Maryland

Stephanie A. Kolakowsky-Hayner, MA
Department of Physical Medicine and Rehabilitation
Medical College of Virginia
Virginia Commonwealth University
Richmond, Virginia

Kat Kolaski, MD
Charlotte Institute of Rehabilitation
Charlotte, North Carolina

John Kregel, EdD
Professor of Special Education
Associate Director and Research Director
Rehabilitation Research and Training Center on Supported Employment
Virginia Commonwealth University
Richmond, Virginia

Jeffrey S. Kreutzer, PhD
Department of Physical Medicine and Rehabilitation
Division of Neurological Surgery
Medical College of Virginia
Virginia Commonwealth University
Richmond, Virginia

Thomas A. Krouskop, PhD, PE
Professor
Department of Physical Medicine and Rehabilitation
Baylor College of Medicine
Houston, Texas

Elisabeth Lachmann, MD
Assistant Attending Physiatrist
Department of Rehabilitation Medicine
The New York Presbyterian Hospital–Cornell Campus;
Assistant Professor
Department of Rehabilitation Medicine
Joan and Sanford I. Weill Medical College and Graduate School of Medical Sciences of Cornell University
New York, New York

Christina Yun Lee, MD
Assistant Professor
Department of Physical Medicine and Rehabilitation
Wayne State University;
Rehabilitation Institute of Michigan
Detroit, Michigan

L. Don Lehmkuhl, PhD
Associate Professor
Department of Physical Medicine and Rehabilitation
Baylor College of Medicine
Houston, Texas

Charles E. Levy, MD
Director, Seating and Positioning Clinic
Assistant Professor
Department of Physical Medicine and Rehabilitation
The Ohio State University Medical Center
Columbus, Ohio

Roger E. Levy, MA
Program Specialist
Texas Rehabilitation Commission
Austin, Texas

Maria Lucas, MD
Regional Amputee Rehabilitation Center
MossRehab Hospital
Philadelphia, Pennsylvania

Tom Lunsford, MSE, CO
Lone Star Orthotics
Houston, Texas

Kevin Magee, PhD
Assistant Professor
Department of Physical Medicine and Rehabilitation
Baylor College of Medicine
Houston, Texas

Scott Manley, EdD
The Rehabilitation Research and Training Center on Aging with Spinal Cord Injury
Craig Hospital
Englewood, Colorado

Michèle Masset, PT, ST, Lic. AC
Coordinator, Pelvic Pain Program
Pain and Rehabilitation Medicine
Bethesda, Maryland

Richard S. Materson, MD
Medical Vice-President
Memorial Hermann Healthcare System;
Clinical Professor of Physical Medicine and Rehabilitation
Baylor College of Medicine and
University of Texas Health Science Center
Houston, Texas

James T. McDeavitt, MD
Chairman
Department of Physical Medicine and Rehabilitation
Carolina Medical Center;
Medical Director
Charlotte Institute of Rehabilitation
Charlotte, North Carolina

Marianne McDermott, PT
The Ohio State University Medical Center
Columbus, Ohio

Douglas McGill, MD
Faculty/Attending Physician
Department of Physical Medicine and Rehabilitation
Medical University of South Carolina
Charleston, South Carolina

J. Patrick McGowan, MD
Attending Physiatrist
Columbia HCA Hospitals;
Clinical Assistant Professor
Department of Physical Medicine and Rehabilitation
Medical College of Virginia
Virginia Commonwealth University
Richmond, Virginia

Kevin M. Means, MD
Chief, Physical Medicine and Rehabilitation Service
Medical Director
Falls and Mobility Disorders Program
John L. McClellan Veterans Affairs Medical Center;
Associate Professor and Chairman
Department of Physical Medicine and Rehabilitation
University of Arkansas for Medical Sciences
Little Rock, Arkansas

Robert H. Meier, III, MD
Director of Medical Rehabilitation
O'Hara Regional Center for Rehabilitation
Denver, Colorado

Jay M. Meythaler, MD, JD
Professor
Department of Physical Medicine and Rehabilitation
The University of Alabama School of Medicine
Birmingham, Alabama

Clay Miller, MD, MFA
Instructor, Harvard Medical School;
Consultant, Spaulding Rehabilitation Hospital
Boston, Massachusetts

Wayne J. Miller, PC
Miller, Shpiece & Andrews
Attorneys at Law
Bingham Farms, Michigan;
Adjunct Professor
Wayne State University Law School
Detroit, Michigan

Linda Miner, OTR, CHT
UE Clinical Specialist
Occupational Therapy Division
Department of Physical Medicine and Rehabilitation
University of Michigan
Ann Arbor, Michigan

Patrick Murphy, DO
Department of Physical Medicine and Rehabilitation
Crozer Chester Medical Center
Chester, Pennsylvania

Maureen R. Nelson, MD
Associate Professor
Department of Physical Medicine and Rehabilitation
Department of Pediatrics
Chief, Physical Medicine and Rehabilitation
Texas Children's Hospital
Baylor College of Medicine
Houston, Texas

John J. Nicholas, MD
Professor and Chairman
Department of Physical Medicine and Rehabilitation
Temple University School of Medicine
Philadelphia, Pennsylvania

Richard N. Norris, MD
Medical Director, Arts Medicine Program
North East Rehabilitation Associates
Scranton, Pennsylvania

Margaret A. Nosek, PhD
Professor
Department of Physical Medicine and Rehabilitation
Baylor College of Medicine
Houston, Texas

Terry H. Oh, MD
Consultant
Department of Physical Medicine and Rehabilitation
Mayo Clinic and Mayo Foundation;
Assistant Professor of Physical Medicine and Rehabilitation
Mayo Medical School
Rochester, Minnesota

Jeffrey B. Palmer, MD
Associate Professor
Department of Physical Medicine and Rehabilitation
Department of Otolaryngology–Head and Neck Surgery
Good Samaritan Hospital
Johns Hopkins University
Baltimore, Maryland

Randal A. Palmitier, MD
Grand Rapids Sport & Spine
Orthopaedic Associates
Grand Rapids, Michigan

Inder Perkash, MD
Director, SCI Program
Chief, Physical Medicine and Rehabilitation
Palo Alto VA Health Care System;
Professor
Department of Functional Restoration
Stanford University Medical Center
Palo Alto, California

Joel M. Press, MD, FACSM
Clinical Assistant Professor
Department of Physical Medicine and Rehabilitation
Northwestern University Medical Center;
Director, Sports Rehabilitation Program
Rehabilitation Institute of Chicago
Chicago, Illinois

Gregory Ranlett, PhD
Staff Psychologist
Department of Veterans Affairs Medical Center
Spokane, Washington

Tyrone M. Reyes, MD
Professor
Department of Rehabilitation Medicine
Faculty of Medicine and Surgery
University of Santo Tomas
Manila, Philippines

Elizabeth Rittenberg, MD
Faculty/Attending Physician
Department of Physical Medicine and Rehabilitation
Medical University of South Carolina
Charleston, South Carolina

Keith M. Robinson, MD
Assistant Professor of Rehabilitation Medicine
Vice Chairman, Graduate Medical Education
University of Pennsylvania
Philadelphia, Pennsylvania

Arthur A. Rodriquez, MD
Professor
Department of Rehabilitation Medicine
University of Washington Medical School
Seattle, Washington

Robert D. Rondinelli, MD, PhD
Professor and Chairman
Department of Rehabilitation Medicine
University of Kansas Medical Center
Kansas City, Kansas

David Rosenblum, MD
Medical Director
Spinal Cord Injury and Neuro-Orthopedic Division
Gaylord Hospital
Wallingford, Connecticut;
Clinical Assistant Professor
and Co-Chief of Rehabilitation Medicine
Yale New Haven Hospital
New Haven, Connecticut

E. John Rott, III, MD
Assistant Professor
Department of Pediatrics
Baylor College of Medicine
Houston, Texas

Allen J. Rubin, MD
Associate Professor of Psychiatry and Neurology
Director of Huntington's Disease Program
Allegheny University of the Health Sciences
Philadelphia, Pennsylvania

Michael Saffir, MD
Medical Director
IHC
Stratford, Connecticut;
Senior Attending Physician
Department of Rehabilitation Medicine
St. Francis Hospital
and the Rehabilitation Hospital of Connecticut
Hartford, Connecticut

M. Elizabeth Sandel, MD
Medical Director
Kaiser Foundation Rehabilitation Center
Kaiser Foundation Hospital
Vallejo, California;
Clinical Professor
Department of Physical Medicine and Rehabilitation
University of California, Davis School of Medicine
Davis, California

Staci J. Schwartz, MD
Physical Medicine and Rehabilitation
Geriatric Rehabilitation
Philadelphia, Pennsylvania

Giles R. Scofield, JD
Department of Community Medicine
University of Connecticut School of Medicine
Farmington, Connecticut

Barry L. Seiller, MD
Director of Visual Rehabilitative Services
Visual Fitness Institute
Vernon Hills, Illinois

Kamala Shankar, MD
Assistant Clinical Professor
Department of Physical Medicine and Rehabilitation
University of California at Davis
Davis, California;
Palo Alto VA Health Care System;
Clinical Faculty
Department of Functional Restoration
Stanford University Medical Center
Palo Alto, California

Mark Sherer, PhD, ABPP/Cn
Project Director
TBI Model System of Mississippi;
Director of Neuropsychology
Mississippi Methodist Rehabilitation Center
Jackson, Mississippi

Douglas Slakey, MD
Faculty/Attending Physician
Department of Transplant Surgery
Tulane University
New Orleans, Louisiana

Curtis W. Slipman, MD
Director, Penn Spine Center
Chief, Division of Musculoskeletal Rehabilitation
Assistant Professor of Rehabilitation Medicine
University of Pennsylvania Health System
Philadelphia, Pennsylvania

Charlotte Hoehne Smith, MD
Medical Director
Seton Network and HealthSouth Rehabilitation Hospital
Austin, Texas

Laura Smith, MS
Associate Director, Education and Training Division
CARF—The Rehabilitation Accreditation Commission
Tucson, Arizona

Quentin Smith, MS
Associate Professor
Department of Family and Community Medicine and
Department of Physical Medicine and Rehabilitation
Baylor College of Medicine
Houston, Texas

Kerstin M. Sobus, MD
Medical Director
Child Evaluation and Treatment Center
Altru Health Institute
Grand Forks, North Dakota

Jean Cole Spencer, PhD, OTR, FAOTA
Professor and Doctoral Program Coordinator
School of Occupational Therapy
Texas Woman's University
Houston, Texas

M. Catherine Spires, PT, MS, MD
Assistant Clinical Professor
Department of Physical Medicine and Rehabilitation
University of Michigan
Ann Arbor, Michigan

C. R. Sridhara, MD
Co-Director, Electrodiagnostic Center
MossRehab Hospital;
Associate Chairman
Department of Physical Medicine and Rehabilitation
Albert Einstein Medical Center;
Clinical Associate Professor
Department of Physical Medicine and Rehabilitation
Temple University School of Medicine
Philadelphia, Pennsylvania

Steven A. Stiens, MD
Associate Professor
Department of Rehabilitation Medicine
The University of Washington;
Attending Physician
Spinal Cord Injury Service
Seattle, Washington

Thomas E. Strax, MD
Professor and Chair/Medical Director
JFK Johnson Rehabilitation Institute
Edison, New Jersey

Jay V. Subbarao, MD, MS
Clinical Professor, Physical Medicine and Rehabilitation
Division Chief and Residency Program Director
Loyola University Medical Center
Maywood, Illinois;
Associate Chief of Staff for Rehabilitative Services
Edward Hines Jr. VA Hospital
Hines, Illinois

Irwin Suchoff, OD, DOS
Head Trauma Vision Rehabilitation Unit
State College of Optometry
State University of New York
New York, New York

Mukul Talaty, MS, BME
Research Engineer, Gait and Motion Analysis Laboratory
MossRehab Hospital
Philadelphia, Pennsylvania

Pam Sherron Targett, MEd
Program Manager
Rehabilitation Research and Training Center on Supported Employment
Virginia Commonwealth University
Richmond, Virginia

Richard S. Tunkel, MD
Associate Attending Physiatrist and Director
Rehabilitation Service
Memorial Sloan-Kettering Cancer Center
New York, New York

Gitendra Uswatte, BA
Department of Psychology
University of Alabama at Birmingham
Birmingham, Alabama

Stanley F. Wainapel, MD, MPH
Clinical Director, Rehabilitation Medicine
Montefiore Medical Center;
Associate Professor of Clinical Rehabilitation Medicine
Albert Einstein College of Medicine
Bronx, New York

William C. Walker, MD
Assistant Professor
Department of Physical Medicine and Rehabilitation
Medical College of Virginia
Virginia Commonwealth University
Richmond, Virginia

Patricia Wardius, RPT
Department of Physical Medicine and Rehabilitation
Crozer Chester Medical Center
Chester, Pennsylvania

Mary Warren, MS, OTR
Department of Ophthalmology
Eye Foundation of Kansas City
University of Missouri School of Medicine
Kansas City, Missouri

Lori B. Wasserburger, MD
Active Staff
St. Davids/Columbia Hospital
Austin, Texas

Alfred B. Watson, Jr., MD, MPH, FACR
Professor of Radiology
Professor of Physical Medicine and Rehabilitation
Associate Chairman of Clinical Radiology
Baylor College of Medicine;
Chief of Radiology
Ben Taub General Hospital;
Chief of Radiology
The Institute for Rehabilitation and Research
Houston, Texas

Susan W. Weathers, MD
Assistant Professor of Radiology
Baylor College of Medicine
Houston, Texas

Paul Wehman, PhD
Professor, Department of Physical Medicine and Rehabilitation
Medical College of Virginia;
Director, Rehabilitation Research and Training Center on Supported Employment
Virginia Commonwealth University
Richmond, Virginia

Michael West, PhD
Research Associate
Rehabilitation Research and Training Center on Supported Employment
Virginia Commonwealth University
Richmond, Virginia

Cliff J. Whigham, Jr., DO
Associate Professor of Radiology
Baylor College of Medicine
Houston, Texas

Gale G. Whiteneck, PhD
Director of Research
Craig Hospital
Englewood, Colorado

Denise H. Widmar, CTRS
Recreational Therapist
Rehabilitation Center
The Methodist Hospital
Houston, Texas

Steven L. Wiesner, MD
Chief, Occupational Health Department
Kaiser Permanente East Bay Medical Center
Oakland, California

John Wijtyk, PTA
Department of Physical Medicine and Rehabilitation
Crozer Chester Medical Center
Chester, Pennsylvania

Edward Wikoff, MD
Regional Amputee Rehabilitation Center
MossRehab Hospital
Philadelphia, Pennsylvania

Robert P. Wilder, MD, FACSM
Assistant Professor
Department of Physical Medicine and Rehabilitation
Director, Sports Rehabilitation
Division of Spine and Sports Care
University of Virginia
Charlottesville, Virginia

Wendy Wilkinson
Project Director of the Southwest DETAC (Disability and Business Technical Assistance Center), a Program of ILRU at TIRR;
Principal Investigator on "Legal Protections for People with Disabilities" for the Research and Training Center on Managed Care and Disability;
Clinical Assistant Professor
Department of Physical Medicine and Rehabilitation
Baylor College of Medicine
Houston, Texas

Stuart E. Willick, MD
Fellow
Center for Spine Sports and Occupational Rehabilitation
Rehabilitation Institute of Chicago
Northwestern University Medical Center
Chicago, Illinois

Robert E. Windsor, MD
Clinical Assistant Professor
Department of Physical Medicine and Rehabilitation
Emory University School of Medicine;
Georgia Pain Physicians, PC
Atlanta, Georgia

Leslie Wontorcik, CP
University of Michigan Orthotics and Prosthetics Center
Ann Arbor, Michigan

Yeong-Chi Wu, MD
Associate Professor
Department of Physical Medicine and Rehabilitation
Northwestern University Medical School
Chicago, Illinois

Gary M. Yarkony, MD
Attending Physician
Schwab Rehabilitation Hospital;
Clinical Professor, Section of Orthopaedic Surgery and Rehabilitation Medicine
Department of Surgery
Clinical Professor of Neurology
University of Chicago
Chicago, Illinois

Jeffrey L. Young, MD
Sports Rehabilitation Program
Rehabilitation Institute of Chicago
Chicago, Illinois

Mark A. Young, MD, FACP
Associate Chairman
Department of Physical Medicine and Rehabilitation Medicine
The Maryland Rehabilitation Center;
Attending Physician, Sinai Hospital of Baltimore;
Faculty
Physical Medicine and Rehabilitation Residency Training Program
The Sinai-Johns Hopkins University School of Medicine
Baltimore, Maryland

Mary Ellen Young, PhD, CRC
Assistant Professor
Department of Rehabilitation Counseling
University of Florida
Gainesville, Florida

Ross D. Zafonte, DO
Rehabilitation Institute of Michigan
Detroit, Michigan

Monte F. Zarlingo, MD
Department of Radiology
Baylor College of Medicine
Houston, Texas

Kathryn A. Zidek, MD
Assistant Professor
Department of Physical Medicine and Rehabilitation and Pediatrics
Baylor College of Medicine
Director, Pediatric Rehabilitation
The Institute of Rehabilitation and Research
Houston, Texas

Richard D. Zorowitz, MD
Director of Stroke Rehabilitation
Medical Director, Piersol Rehabilitation Unit
Assistant Professor of Rehabilitation Medicine
University of Pennsylvania
Philadelphia, Pennsylvania

Preface

The purpose of this resource book is to provide the collective wisdom of scientists and clinicians who have experience in identifying problems faced by persons with disabilities and in finding and implementing practical solutions. At major health science centers and community-based facilities around the country, teams of highly qualified professionals representing a wide array of medical, psychosocial, and multicultural disciplines have developed strategies and rehabilitation programs for addressing the complexities of integrating persons with disabilities into the community. The challenges are great. The expertise of health care professionals from many disciplines is necessary for assisting the person with a disability and his or her family in achieving the desired outcome.

The Editors have charged the authors with the task of visualizing the reader of each chapter as a health care professional who has had general medical rehabilitation experience and is seeking more information from a team that specializes in the problem(s) encountered by the patient/client with the specific diagnosis or condition in the chapter.

For the person living with the consequences of a disease or injury that affects functional abilities, "outcome" is not determined solely by the severity of the disabling condition nor by any one intervention. A combination of factors, both in the person and in the environment, has a strong influence on the quality of life that the person leads. The experience of those in the practice of physical medicine and rehabilitation can be a valuable resource for health care professionals who are helping patients and clients engage in appropriate, fulfilling roles.

We hope that you will find the ideas and information contained herein of value in improving the quality of physical medicine and rehabilitation services that you provide.

Martin Grabois, MD
Susan J. Garrison, MD
Karen A. Hart, PhD
L. Don Lehmkuhl, PhD

Introduction

Richard S. Materson

The procedures a physiatrist performs, such as using a reflex hammer to tap a biceps tendon in pursuit of clinical problem solving or taking a history regarding a patient's ability to achieve a daily living activity to prepare a plan of care, are automatic and ingrained in the physiatrist's daily life. Yet have you ever stopped to wonder how this knowledge base of cognitive information, attitudes, and skills came together to form the professional medical specialty called physical medicine and rehabilitation?

Virtually every internist can recount the stories of Sir William Osler. And every surgeon can regale with Mayo or Crile or Halsted episodes. What then are the stories that physiatrists hold dear? Who are their heroes? What unique challenges and obstacles faced the field's founders and its early practitioners? What can be learned from the history of physiatry to better see and prepare for the future?

Today one finds three active major professional societies devoted to the interests of the specialty and of the patients served by physical medicine and rehabilitation practitioners. They are the American Academy of Physical Medicine and Rehabilitation, the American Congress of Rehabilitation Medicine, and the Association of Academic Physiatrists (AAP). These organizations are supplemented by the American Board of Physical Medicine and Rehabilitation, an American Board of Medical Specialties (ABMS)–approved organization, and the American Association of Electrodiagnostic Medicine and its related non-ABMS American Board of Electrodiagnostic Medicine. The American Academy of Physical Medicine and Rehabilitation has an internal subset organization, the Physiatric Association of Spine, Sports, and Occupational Rehabilitation (PASSOR), devoted to the practice of nonsurgical musculoskeletal medicine. There are also related, disease-specific organizations such as the American Academy for Cerebral Palsy and Developmental Medicine. Other groups are subspecialty specific, and include the American Academy of Pain Medicine, the American Academy of Pain Management, the American Pain Society, the International Association for the Study of Pain, the American Back Society, the American Spinal Injury Association, the North American Spine Society, the National Stroke Association, and the National Osteoporosis Foundation. There are a plethora of similar field-related societies to which many physiatrists belong.

As medical physicians, physiatrists are also eligible for membership in their respective county and state medical societies and the American Medical Association (or American Osteopathic Medical Association or National Medical Association). History reveals that the American Medical Association played a major role in the formation and evolution of the specialty.

Each society has evolved over time. Emphasis has changed to fit the needs. Charismatic leaders have come and gone. For today's physiatrists the past is not always well studied. But history must be appreciated if physiatrists are to recognize from where the field has come and where it might aspire to go as a specialty.

THE EARLY YEARS

In the first 20 years of this century there was no medical practitioner called a physiatrist or practicing the specialty of physiatry, nor was there a society related to the interests of physiatry to which physicians could belong. World War I, and the many war-related injuries that benefited from physical measures, led to a change in the situation. The Board of Trustees of the American Medical Association, reacting to the need for physicians experienced in these physical measures, caused the founding of the American Congress of Physical Therapy in September 1921.

> The Congress was intended to provide for a periodic meeting for education and exchange of ideas; it was not intended to become an ongoing organization. Physicians attending the Congress might be considered explorers of the therapeutic aspects of physical agents. Any doctor interested in physical agents, or looking for new methods to improve his practice skills, could attend the Congress; the majority of attendees used physical therapeutics only occasionally. Physicians whose primary emphasis was on use of physical methods for the diagnosis were few in number, were usually located in academic settings, and were engaged in teaching, research, and patient care (1).

During the period 1900 to 1920, ionizing radiation had attracted the interest of some physicians who were also interested in the harnessing of other portions of the electromagnetic spectrum for diagnostic or therapeutic purposes. In 1923 the American College of Radiology and Physiotherapy became the first "physical medicine" society organized. At its subsequent meetings, its name was changed to the American College of Physical Therapy. The organization adopted the *Archives of Physical Therapy, X-ray and Radium* as the official journal. John S. Coulter of Northwestern Medical School in Chicago was elected its third president. In 1930 the word *Congress* was substituted for *College* and the organization became the American Congress of Physical Therapy. In 1945 the name was changed again to the American Congress of Physical Medicine, until 1952 when "and Rehabilitation" was added to the name. In 1967 the name was changed yet again to the American Congress of Rehabilitation Medicine, as its mission and emphasis had evolved. The journal also changed as radiologists developed their own specialty and journals apart from physical medicine. Albert F. Tyler, a professor of radiology at Creighton Medical School in Omaha and a founder of the American Congress of Physical Therapy, was the original owner, editor, and publisher of the journal. In 1930 Tyler transferred ownership by gift to the Congress. The journal's name was changed in 1938 to *Archives of Physical Therapy*, in 1945 to *Archives of Physical Medicine*, and in 1963 to *Archives of Physical Medicine and Rehabilitation*. Disraeli Kobak of Chicago's Cook County Hospital became the editor in 1928 and remained so until he became editor emeritus in 1940.

The Congress and the American Physical Therapy Association amalgamated and formed the American Registry of Physical Therapy Technicians in 1937. Physical therapy became a profession in its own right and later the Congress-supported registry was abandoned and physical therapy became responsible for its own accreditation with its own American Physical Therapy Association. Not until 1945 was the confusion regarding the difference between physical therapists and physical medicine practitioners addressed by the organization's renaming to the American Congress of Physical Medicine. The *Archives* remained the journal of the organization.

The character of a medical society is often reflected in the awards its members establish and the recipients selected. In 1932, the Congress established its Gold Key Award to be given annually in recognition of extraordinary services to the cause of physical therapy. Seven awards were given the first year. The Congress established the John Stanley Coulter Memorial Lecture in 1951; the Sidney and Elizabeth Licht Award for scientific writing in 1980; the Edward W. Lowman, MD, Award for noting those who have contributed to interdisciplinary rehabilitation; and the Distinguished American College of Rehabilitation Member Award in 1989. The names of recipients of the various awards are listed in the introductory section of the annual membership directory of the American Congress of Rehabilitation Medicine.

Returning to the specialty's formation, in the Northeast, particularly the New York area, there were a sizable number of physicians who trained in Central Europe and Scandinavia or who were influenced by practitioners who trained there. In those countries, physical therapeutics and spa therapy were part of the accepted medical armamentarium. These physicians included Benham Snow of Presbyterian Hospital and the College of Physicians and Surgeons, Karl Harpuder at Montefiore Hospital, and George Deaver from New York's Institute of Crippled and Disabled. Frank Krusen, a German physician, was afflicted by acute pulmonary tuberculosis while in a surgical residency at Temple University. He was treated with heliotherapy and was attracted to physical medicine. He initiated the program in physical therapy at Temple University and then moved to the Mayo Clinic in 1936 where he established the first 3-year training program in physical medicine. His first two graduates were Earl Elkins and Robert Bennett in 1939. Also coming from a surgical training background was Miland Knapp of Minneapolis General Hospital whose interest in posttraumatic contractures stimulated his interest in the new field.

Kottke and Knapp (1) recognized 14 pioneers most involved in the formation of the specialty:

John S. Coulter, MD, Northwestern University Medical School

Frank H. Ewerhardt, MD, Washington University of St. Louis Medical School

William Bierman, MD, Mount Sinai Hospital, New York
Frank H. Krusen, MD, Mayo Clinic
Walter J. Zeiter, MD, Cleveland Clinic
Richard Kovacs, MD, New York
Kristian Hansson, MD, Cornell University Medical School
William H. Schmidt, MD, Jefferson Medical College, Philadelphia
Fred B. Moor, MD, College of Medical Evangelists, Los Angeles
Miland E. Knapp, MD, University of Minnesota Medical School, Minneapolis
Disraeli Kobac, MD, Cook County Hospital, Chicago
Nathan H. Polmer, MD, Louisiana State University, New Orleans
Earl C. Elkins, MD, Mayo Clinic, Rochester, MN
Charles O. Molander, MD, Northwestern University Medical School, Chicago

Louis B. Wilson, president of the American Medical Association's Advisory Council of Medical Specialties, became aware of the potential for a new specialty and in 1936 proposed a new certifying board in the field of physical medicine. A specialty was required to have 100 full-time practitioners before it could have its own board, and it was not until 1947 that such a board was realized for physical medicine.

In September 1938, when there were only 42 physicians in the full-time practice of physical therapy, the group that was to evolve as the American Academy of Physical Medicine and Rehabilitation was founded as the Society of Physical Therapy Physicians. The founders were Bierman, Coulter, Kobak, and Krusen. Coulter was elected President pro tempore and Kobak secretary treasurer pro tempore. The society was envisioned as limited in membership to full-time physical therapy physicians with a teaching appointment in a medical school or a departmental directorship. In 1939, forty physicians became charter members. An invitation was required for membership, and until 1944 membership was limited to 100 members. A two-thirds vote was required for election to a membership and 10 written dissents could deny membership. After 1952, all diplomates of the American Board of Physical Medicine and Rehabilitation were invited to join the society.

Fortunately for the field of physical medicine and rehabilitation, an energetic, business-minded academic named Walter J. Zeiter, who was trained by Coulter and Molander at Northwestern University, was available at the start of the Society of Physical Therapy Physicians. Zeiter gave selflessly of his managerial talents, business acumen, and frugality, with success made possible by extraordinary diplomacy. From the founding of the society in 1938 until 1960, he was the executive director. Additionally, he was executive director of the American Congress of Physical Medicine and its American Registry of Physical Therapists (formerly the American Registry of Physical Therapy Technicians). When the American Board of Physical Medicine was founded in 1947, he became chairman until 1953. Through his great skills, the annual membership dues in these postdepression and war years were kept to $5.00 from 1939 to 1956, when the cost doubled to $10.00. In 1941, the income was reported as $503.38 and expenses $182.00! Members paid no registration fees for annual meetings. Instructional sessions for residents and young physicians organized by Earl Elkins cost $2.00 per course in 1946. Physicians taught for free and traveled at their own expense. Zeiter provided direction at little or no cost to the organizations. It is unlikely the field would have enjoyed its developmental success absent this remarkable and capable physician. The Academy Board of Governors honored him in 1961 by establishing the Walter J. Zeiter Lectures, which are to relate to the history of the Academy. In 1968, Frank Krusen delivered the first lecture, titled "The Historical Development in Physical Medicine and Rehabilitation During the Last Forty Years" (2). This lecture remains a masterpiece in the history of physiatry.

In 1954 a motion to change the name of the Academy was passed and in 1956, the new name, American Academy of Physical Medicine and Rehabilitation, became official. The official emblem of the Academy was approved in 1958, utilizing Hippocratic Greek *latrike* (the art and science of medicine), *pharmakon* (the drug of physical object), and *epanorthosis* (restoration), which appear today on the seal.

Like World War I, World War II placed a major demand on this nation's resources. Wounded soldiers required physical measures for treatment and far too few physicians were trained to administer them correctly. Many military physicians were ordered to Rochester, Minnesota for 3 months of training in physical therapy medicine under Krusen and became the so-called 90-day wonders of the field.

The field of physical medicine and rehabilitation would not be the same without the contributions of another post–Pearl Harbor Army Air Corps volunteer, internist Howard A. Rusk of St. Louis, Missouri. Rusk regarded the inactivity of injured soldiers after initial medical treatment as a negative that served as a progenitor for physical and psychological deconditioning. He used overhead aircraft models to train soldiers as effective ground observers, and engaged them in other measured meaningful activities. Rather than prolonged bed rest, he prescribed early ambulation after surgery, ensured aggressive physical therapy, and organized recreation, thereby decreasing the recovery time and returning the troops to the field or other valuable occupations. He noticed a decreased incidence of contractures, skin sores, and muscle wasting and observed maintained strength and endurance with a decreased rate of phlebitis and embolus. His ideas were recognized and adapted locally at first, and then by intervention of Bernard Baruch with President Truman, his methods were ordered put in place throughout the military. When the war ended, Rusk went to New York where he became a professor of rehabilitation medicine at New York University and Bellevue Hospital. He appointed George Deaver as medical director of the clinical program. Together they worked to convince a doubting acute-care medical community of the value of therapeutic activity and the totality of the rehabilitative approach. They overcame the acute-care physicians' resistance by posing rehabilitation medicine as the third phase of medicine following preventive and acute care. Rusk became known as the father of rehabilitation medicine and Deaver as the father of clinical rehabilitation. Rusk founded the World Rehabilitation Foundation and the Institute of Rehabilitation Medicine at New York University, which now bears his name. He wrote "A World to Care For" (3), a classic treatise on the world's need for proper treatment of the physically impaired, and proceeded through his foundation to train a great number of national and international physicians and therapists in his methodologies. He exemplified respect for the capabilities of adequately rehabilitated persons to return to become societal contributors, and elevated the status and acceptability of those persons in an otherwise rather hostile world.

The followers of Rusk championed the idea of multispecialty rehabilitation in an interdisciplinary fashion to enhance self-sufficiency. They were seen as managers and facilitators. Physical medicine physicians, on the other hand, saw themselves as diagnosticians and treating physicians rather than managers. The differences between the two groups heightened in the mid to late 1940s. The fractions finally resolved their differences by action of the ABMS, which acknowledged the combined worth of both approaches and in 1949 inspired the name change from the American Board of Physical Medicine to the American Board of Physical Medicine and Rehabilitation. The Academy's name change followed shortly thereafter.

Poliomyelitis also played a major role in the conversion of the specialty to a civilian rather than military field. Rising from an incidence of 3 to 10 per 100,000 in the early 1940s, summer polio epidemics rose to produce 58,000 cases in 1952. Sister Elizabeth Kenny, an Australian nurse, suggested that she had a better method of treating polio than the classic approach of immobilization and bracing. She demonstrated that the muscle spasms and muscle pain of acute polio could be controlled with therapeutic heat packs named *Kenny packs.* Once these disabling spasms were overcome, cautious therapeutic muscle reeducation prevented overwork fatigue and gave improved outcomes. Knapp and others worked with her in Minnesota to demonstrate the correctness of some of her observations. The National Foundation for Infantile Paralysis established training courses for medical personnel. While some of Kenny's theories were disproved and caused great controversy, it was obvious that the nation needed additional medical manpower to treat disabled civilians as well as veterans. The lessons learned in the military concerning therapeutic activity and combined physical and psychosocial approaches to treatment of the whole person would serve well the disabled population.

In another extraordinary moment for our field, Bernard Baruch, a noted New York philanthropist and financier, elected to honor his physician father and Civil War surgeon, Simon Baruch, who expressed great interest in hydrotherapy when he came to Columbia University's College of Physicians and Surgeons, by supporting the development of this new breed of physical medicine physicians. Appointing Ray Lyman Wilbur, the chancellor of Stanford University, to chair a committee to study the ways in which physical medicine could be most effectively used to treat injured and sick civilians and veterans, Baruch was able to gather together national experts to ponder the field. He wished to establish research and training centers, facilitate research, and promote the establishment of residencies and fellowships. Prominent physiatric leaders served major roles on the Baruch committees. Major grants were given to Columbia University, New York University, and the Medical College of Virginia, and smaller grants were given to MIT, Harvard Medical School, the University of Minnesota Medical School, the University of Southern California School of Medicine, the State University of Iowa College of Medicine, George Washington University School of Medicine in St. Louis, the University of Illinois College of Medicine, George Washington University Medical School, and Marquette University. Ten of 12 schools given the grants eventually developed departments of physical medicine and rehabilitation. Additionally, at least 57 known physiatrists received economic support for training through Baruch Fellowships awarded in the 1940s through mid-1950s. Seventeen Baruch Fellows became heads of academic departments of physical therapy and rehabilitation; others served as chiefs of service at Veterans Administration hospitals or major civilian hospitals. The contributions of this great philanthropist to the field of physical medicine and rehabilitation are beyond estimation.

In 1938 Krusen proposed the term *physiatrist* to identify the physician specializing in physical medicine. Kobak gave the proposal editorial support in the *Archives.* By May 1946, the American Medical Association's Council on Physical Medicine voted to sponsor the term *physiatrist* to designate physicians practicing the specialty. Krusen proposed that the terms be pronounced "fi-zē-′a-trist" and "fi-zē-′a-trē" to eliminate confusion with psychiatry. Only the AAP uses *physiatry* in its name, despite the term being officially accepted by the field. The field rejected the idea that the word be used like "internist" in internal medicine. While any number of physiatrists still *mispronounce* their own name as "fiz-ī-a-trē," putting the accent on the second syllable, this mispronunciation is to be avoided if the term is ever to be commonly used and accepted.

After World War II, there were sufficient numbers of practitioners of physical medicine to become fully recognized as a medical specialty board. The American Board of Physical Medicine was approved by the American Medical Association's Advisory Council for Medical Specialties in 1946 and the first board, consisting of 11 physiatrists, was appointed June 6, 1947. Krusen was the board's first chairman, Zeiter the vice chairman, and Bennett the secretary-treasurer; other members were Coulter, Ewerhardt, Hansson, Huddleston, Kovacs, Schmidt, Strickland, and Watkins. The first examinations were conducted in September 1947. Several physicians were grandfathered into membership, others took the test only to produce a reference standard, and others were seated by the actual results of the examination. A total of 103 physiatrists were thus certified by the American Board of Physical Medicine from its first examination.

Kottke and Knapp (1) described the great contributions to the start of the field by Mary Switzer, who became the director of the Office of Vocational Rehabilitation in 1948. Her tenacity, diplomacy, and understanding of Rusk's concepts led her to the espousal of training grants, fellowship stipends, research sponsorship, and rehabilitation demonstration programs. Coupled with the strong support of the Honorable Hubert Humphrey, then U.S. senator from Minnesota, these programs were promoted and funded, giving additional prominence to the developing field and better serving persons with disability.

THE MIDDLE AND MORE RECENT YEARS

The growth of the specialty was slow at first but rose exponentially after the publication of the reports of the Graduate Medical Education National Advisory Committee (GMENAC) in 1980 and 1982. Most medical specialties were found to have an oversupply, but physiatry, which was predicted to need 4000 physiatrists by 1990, was seriously undersupplied. A great number of high-class-rank students became interested in the field, decreasing the traditionally high percentage of foreign medical graduates and to a lesser extent, women. The Academy became a society heavily populated with physicians under the age of 40 years, meriting significant changes in policy and programs in the early 1980s. In 1950 there were 145 certified diplomates of the board; by the end of the decade, 225 additional persons passed the examinations, for a total of 370. An average of 23 graduates per year became diplomates, compared with 229 new diplomates in 1988. In 1998 over 5400 physicians were members of the Academy, with a correspondingly higher number of diplomates of the American Board of Physical Medicine and Rehabilitation. Since 1993, consistent with ABMS policies, the board status awarded lasts 10 years, with recertification required of all diplomates. In 1956 and 1957 the first complete roster of members of the Academy was published. For the last 30 years, an annual membership directory has been provided, and new diplomates are announced in the *Archives of Physical Medicine and Rehabilitation.*

In 1957 a joint meeting of the Academy and the Congress was held, and proposals to define the different missions and goals of the two organizations emerged. The Academy was to focus more on physiatrists and their education, training, and development. The Academy's responsibilities also included fiscal and policy issues germane to the physiatrist, and they were to be represented in the AMA House of Delegates. The Congress, on the other hand, was responsible for the education of the general practitioner or nonphysiatrist physician regarding rehabilitation; education of members of other nonmedical disciplines; maintenance of the journal; and representation on the section council of the American Medical Association.

At first, the larger Congress subsidized the business activities of the Academy, but as the years passed, that reversed and became a major cause for the functional split of the two organizations in the early 1990s. At first sharing headquarters and executives, the Academy and Congress became more and more dysfunctional as the costs of new headquarters and staff increased, programs became duplicative, and territorial disputes increased. The Academy attempted separate meetings from the Congress in 1968 and 1969 in Chicago. While successful from an educational perspective, the meetings were a business failure as exhibitors wished the larger attendance promoted by joint Academy-Congress meetings. The two organizations reconnected for national annual meetings, but with sequential meetings connected by a single day of joint activities. As the Academy grew, time demands on the program committee made sequential planning ever more difficult, and physiatrists more interested in physical medicine than rehabilitation did not fully appreciate the Congress's leadership in interdisciplinary education. Opening of the Congress membership to nonphysician members in the 1980s, while an advance for interdisciplinary activity and education, caused further divisions as the Academy sought tighter bonds to organized medicine and other physician groups. Competition between some allied health professionals and physiatry began in earnest in the late 1970s and made the relationship between the Academy and the Congress even more testy. The two organizations jointly hired attorney Richard Verville to represent the organizations in Washington, DC, where federal regulation was imposing greater controls over the practice of medicine, important civil rights for persons with disability were evolving, and vocational rehabilitation legislation was being enacted. Verville was a most distinguished and competent leader whose words were respected "on the hill" and who could easily, at first, weather the gulf between the two organizations' political postures. Owing to his leadership, many victories were celebrated and the field influenced legislation far beyond its expected means by numbers alone. With time, the difficulties increased between the physician-dictated interests of the Academy and those of the Congress, which reflected its more extensive membership and perhaps more liberal social agenda.

The Congress had always owned and controlled the *Archives of Physical Medicine and Rehabilitation.* In 1973, agreement was reached to establish an Academy editor and a Congress editor with separate editorial boards and to elect an overall editor. The contributions for more than 22 years of Gerald Herbison as editor in chief and Academy editor continue to be a bright benchmark in academia, and Nicholas Walsh, recently elected to his fourth 1-year term as editor in chief, is following closely in these footsteps of extraordinary excellence. Jeffrey R. Basford succeeded as Academy editor. Current members of the Academy *Archives* editorial board are James Agre, Diana D. Cardenas, Daniel Dumitru, Robert L. Joynt, Noel Rao, and Nicholas Walsh. No mention dare be made of the *Archives* without plaudits for its soft-spoken, mentoring, effective, and diesel engine–reliable managing editor for many years, Marvin A. Schroder. Despite agreements reached in 1986 for the Academy to purchase one-half interest in the *Archives of Physical Medicine and Rehabilitation* for a dollar and considerations that have continued until today, the organizations eventually went their separate ways in 1993. The *Archives* "marriage" still exists as a memory of the once-great interorganizational relationship between the Academy and the Congress, but little else of the relationship survives, with the organizations now housed and administered apart since 1993.

In the 1994 Zeiter lecture, I attempted to repair the rupture between the organizations, pointing out the cost savings by eliminating duplication of effort and by virtue of the size, buying power, and attractiveness to exhibitors of a larger attendance as well as the worth of exposing all physiatrists to interdisciplinary rehabilitation and networking with their nonphysician teammates. A vote in favor of coming back together was achieved at both business meetings, but the die had been cast and now, sadly, the two organizations have irreparably split, with only a modicum of cooperative ventures between them. Searching for a new mission, in the last 2 years the Congress has assumed the mission of promoting research in interdisciplinary medical rehabilitation. Only time will tell the wisdom of the split and the success of the new mission, as large numbers of physiatrists have dropped their Congress membership. However, the Academy continues to grow and offer ever-more innovative and useful programs to its members. A smaller but more goal-directed Congress is in its startup and test time.

In 1967 the Council of Academic Societies was formed as a constituent body of the Association of American Medical Colleges. The Academy was rejected for membership because the majority of its members did not hold academic appointments and the Association was designed for academic medical societies. The AAP was formed in 1967 and held its first meeting in 1968. Since then, with highly capable physician and administrative leadership, it has grown to represent the academic interests of the field, including undergraduate and graduate medical education and continuing medical education, in the academic arena. The Academy still provides the bulk of the general continuing medical education for physiatrists. The AAP has adopted the *American Journal of Physical Medicine* as its official publication, with the incomparable clinician, researcher, and educator Ernest Johnson as its fabled energetic and talented editor. The Appendix provides a list of the AAP's presidents.

In the 1960s the membership of the Academy became restless and voted for nominees from the floor rather than those recommended by the nomination committee. The trend was toward increased influence of academicians in the Academy. The trend continued until the mid-1980s with the election of several private practitioners to the board and later as officers achieving a balance that reflected the rapid growth in the number of practitioners in the Academy and the multiple problems they faced. The influence of leadership from both sources was very beneficial. Successive Academy presidents pressed for greater scientific verification of the field's postulates and the need for research and research funding. The quality and quantity of scientific offerings increased, as represented by the reports at the annual meetings and the number and quality of journal articles submitted. Creston Herold became a reincarnated Walter Zeiter and served as the Academy and Congress executive during these difficult times. His tireless contributions to the organization are fondly remembered by all who worked with him. He retired for health reasons in 1983, a year earlier than his planned retirement.

After Herold retired, Ike Mayeda took over the executive office at a time of heightened altercations between the Congress and Academy. His negotiation background proved invaluable, and he managed to produce an impressive product until the split of the groups became inevitable. Most recently, as of the fall of 1989, Ronald A. Henrichs has served as the Academy executive. He served both the Academy and the Congress until after the annual meeting in San Francisco in 1991, when the Congress left for its own offices and executive management. His background in sound organizational management principles has served the society well, as it has continued to mature in its complex service provision and its budget has increased, yet still requiring ever-vigilant management. Under Henrichs the Academy staff has grown and been compartmentalized into well-functioning subunits dealing with membership, meetings, education, health policy and legislation, member services, and marketing.

Recent officers have held regular strategic planning sessions to tune the Academy to the ever-changing requirements of its members as the practice of medicine evolves from that of the single practitioner to group practice and managed care control of the market. Randall Braddom, Martin Grabois, and James Swenson in particular have been concerned with the realignment of staff and committee structure to achieve a high order of effectiveness in a more limited and prioritized agenda. Richard Harvey deserves special mention as an experienced reasoned voice of leadership in these matters. When Harvey talked, people listened. Sadly Harvey had to turn down the Academy presidency when other demands required his enormous skills, and he could not bask in the presidential glory he so richly deserved. Recently Henrichs was elected to serve as an officer of the Association of Society Executives and through it gain bidirectional influence and knowledge for the Academy.

A rekindling of interest in musculoskeletal medicine and related areas demanded greater attention to physical medicine in lieu of rehabilitation medicine in the 1980s and resulted in mechanisms within the Academy for special interest group development. The extraordinary success of PASSOR, which started in 1992 and now has more than 1000 physiatrist members, attests to the Academy's ability to provide an outlet for its members' interests and also to the creativity and team play of the PASSOR leadership, which could have led a revolt of the membership and further split the field. Jeff and Joel Saal, Joel Press, Robert Windsor, Andrew Cole, Terry Sawchuk, Stuart Weinstein, Peter A. Grant, Richard P. Bonfiglio, Edward Laskowski, Jeffrey Yound, Stan Herring, Lori B. Wasserburger, and Curtis Slipman were the inspired leaders of this organization. Honet and I served as advisors as the organization developed. This type of accommodation to change suggests that the modern Academy is well tuned to the needs of its members and capable leaders have made appropriate and timely decisions.

The requirements of the field in its educational mission must be considered. The American Board of Physical Medicine and Rehabilitation celebrated its fiftieth anniversary in 1997. The history of that organization has been compiled as a special supplement to the *Archives of Physical Medicine and Rehabilitation* (4) under the editorship of Gordon Martin and Joachim L. Opitz, and is mandatory reading for any student interested in the field's history. All of the board's chairmen have been legends in their own time as clinicians, educators, and managers. Each left an imprint on the field as it has matured. Chairs were Frank H. Krusen, 1947 to 1949; Walter J. Zeiter, 1949 to 1953; Robert L. Bennett, 1953 to 1963; Frederic J. Kottke, 1963 to 1969; George H. Koepke, 1969 to 1976; Glen Gullickson, Jr., 1976 to 1981; John F. Ditunno, Jr., 1981 to 1984; B. Stanley Cohen, 1984 to 1988; John L. Melvin, 1988 to 1993; and Joel A. DeLisa, 1993 to present. The board was also served by dedicated and often visionary chief executive officers, namely, Earl C. Elkins, who followed Krusen and Bennett and served from 1952 to 1977. Then Gordon M. Martin served from 1977 to 1992, followed by Joachim L. Opitz from 1992 to 1995. All three were clinical associates of the Mayo Clinic, which supported their voluntary efforts for the field and contributed unlimited expertise and physical facility to examination question writing and to the examination itself. In 1996 after a very intense search, the first nonphysician executive was hired, Mark Raymond, who currently serves the board well. Through the years, physiatrists have volunteered voluminous hours to serve as directors of the board and question writers and guest examiners. No compensation is offered for these efforts, which are truly a labor of love without which the process would be impossible.

In the voluntary private organizational network that guides graduate medical education, the Accreditation Council for Graduate Medical Education has supervisory authority over the Residency Review Committees. These committees have representatives elected from various constituencies including the American Medical Association's Council on Education, the American Board of Physical Medicine and Rehabilitation, and the American Academy of Physical Medicine and Rehabilitation as well as the AAP. The committee is responsible for the authorship of the essentials of an accredited residency in physical medicine and rehabilitation, which are then subject to wide review and a stringent approval process. Once they are approved, the committee ensures that residencies provide the educational materials and experiences necessary to become a physiatrist and successfully produce candidates for examination for board certification. Members are not compensated and only by many hours of devoted service to the field do they accomplish their formidable task. This group, perhaps more than any other, defines the field and is responsible for keeping up with innovations that demand curricular attention balancing the old with the new. Please see the Appendix for a list of Residency Review Committee members and chairs.

The Academy had a great deal of organizational maturing in the 1960s through 1980s as its members expected more educational services. One real hero of this development was Joachim Opitz, a former Academy president, American Board of Physical Medicine and Rehabilitation executive director, academician, and clinician, now retired from the Mayo Clinic. Opitz chaired the Medical Education Committee of the Academy at its inception. He championed the creation of the Academy's learning syllabus for residents and practitioners and saw to its regular update. He was responsible for the development of learning assessment tools for residents and practitioners in the form of medical knowledge assessment tests, which could guide a learner through areas of strengths and weaknesses. His extraordinary energy, diplomacy, tenacity, and skills commanded a great team of contributing writers and educators. The product of their assessments could be used other ways to provide a learners' needs assessment for planning the educational events at the annual meetings. Opitz is clearly one of the unsung heroes of the field, nearly single-handedly bringing meticulous organization and management to the Academy's education efforts. Following Opitz, Robert Weber became the capable leader of the Academy's education ventures, followed most recently by Maury Ellenberg. Gary S. Clark and Andrew Cole are leaders in program planning for the annual meeting. The study guide committee now is chaired by Carolyn Kinney and the self-assessment examination committee, by Ronald S. Taylor.

Research is key to the proof of efficacy and cost-effectiveness of a field's procedures, the gospel of today's managed care. Many Academy presidents have commented regarding the necessity of support for research and research productivity and were themselves able researchers. The earlier presidents expressing research needs began with G. Keith Stillwell, Glenn Gullickson, Jr., Arthur Abramson, Justus F. Lehmann, Carl V. Granger, Ernest W. Johnson, Joseph Goodgold, Fritz Kottke, Joseph C. Honet, William Fowler, Arthur A. Grant, John F. Ditunno, Murray M. Freed, and George H. Kraft. More recent presidents included Myron LaBan, who was schooled by Ernie Johnson and combined an unexcelled clinical private practice with academic leadership and clinical research productivity. With my wife Rosa, I created the Physical Medicine and Rehabilitation Education and Research Foundation with the help of the Texas chairs of physical medicine and rehabilitation departments and members of my private practice group. The foundation was then given to the Academy, the AAP, and the liaison council of physical rehabilitation and medicine societies for management. This foundation was the first such private nonprofit foundation supported by membership in the field. It was managed without cost by us and then Dr and Mrs Barry Smith, until it was turned over to the Academy for management. The foundation has collected considerable sums of money through the generosity of individual physiatrists toward seed research and honoring young investigators and award-worthy research papers. Mark Race now chairs the Management Committee of the Physical Medicine and Rehabilitation Education and Research Foundation. The facilitative and extraordinarily generous contributor role of former Academy and Physical Medicine and Rehabilitation Education and Research Foundation President Barbara deLateur must be noted here. The research theme was especially pursued by later Academy presidents—Joachim Opitz, Ian C. MacLean, Martin Grabois, and Randall Braddom.

Fritz Kottke of Minnesota, Ed Lowman and Howard Rusk of New York, and Justus Lehmann of Seattle were cited by the Academy's legal counsel, Richard Verville, as key to the Academy's early pursuit of public funding for research, as were John Melvin, John Ditunno, James Demopoulos, Thomas Strax, and myself. We concentrated on funding through the Department of Education's Vocational Rehabilitation Acts and its National Institute for Disability and Rehabilitation Research (NIDRR), originally the National Institute for Handicapped Research (NIHR), a name that changed for obvious reasons. We then concentrated on the development of a National Institutes of Health (NIH) research focus, and after much work succeeded in gaining support for the creation of the Center for Medical Rehabilitation Research in the Child Health Institute of the NIH. Former Congress President Marcus Fuhrer is the executive of the Center for Medical Rehabilitation Research. Even more recently, Melvin, Ditunno, deLateur, and Margaret Turk have focused on the Institute of Medicine through the National Academy of Sciences and the Centers for Disease Control and Prevention for additional support. Evidence-based clinical research is the current buzzword. The field of physical medicine must maintain its vigil and constantly encourage and renew its support of basic and clinical research if it is to meet its mission of service to physically impaired individuals.

The practitioners are the body and soul of a medical profession. Services to meet the needs of private practitioners were not always the top priority for a field that was attempting through its academic component to define itself and its credibility. After the 1965 passage of the Medicare Act, progressive federal government regulation of the practice of medicine was at hand. Further, the business community rebelled at ever-increasing health care costs and the percentage of the gross national product consumed by medicine. Exercising their considerable muscle, they created both in- and out-of-government controls on the practice and the rewards for practicing medicine. Not surprisingly, the Academy was looked on by the membership for leadership and political clout. Recognizing this trend, in the mid-1980s, I requested the first strategic planning retreat for the Academy board. This resulted in the reorganization of the Academy board into an accountable governance structure with fiduciary responsibility and safeguards, defined functions for each member of the board, and empowerment and controls for the Academy executive and staff. Myron LaBan, along with Erwin Gonzalez, and later the author and Leon Reinstein, raised the credibility and the importance of the private practitioner within the Academy. They formed a liaison council of physical medicine and rehabilitation societies and initiated attention to local and state community-based issues. Reinstein became an expert on understanding and coping with the Medicare law. The medical practice section of the Academy flourished, providing opinions on the practice of physical medicine and rehabilitation, promoting relationships with allied health practitioners, conducting practice surveys, pressuring for renewed marketing efforts on behalf of physiatry, and responding to coding and administrative issues. With recent reorganization, the Academy has a Practice/Business Services Strategic Management Committee, a Practice Guidelines Committee, a Council of State Society Presidents, and Residents Council, which carries out the practice function. Recent leaders are LaBan, Ronald S. Taylor, Robert B. Goldberg, and Lisa-Ann Gooch, Paul C. Coelho, Scott Abramson, and Martin B. Wice.

Politics plays an ever-increasing role in today's society and physicians neglect their citizenship roles only at their own risk. In 1986, I formalized the heretofore informal political network by founding the Health Policy and

Legislative Committee of the Academy, which I led from its inception until 1993, when leadership was assumed by Bruce M. Gans, who has carried on the functions in a most effective fashion. In 1998 Gans was succeeded by John F. Ditunno, Jr., a stellar veteran of lobbying in Washington. The many hours devoted to policy study and innovation, letter writing, congressional and staff visits, and formal testimony by committee volunteers are a tribute to these men and women who added these chores to their already overflowing plates of activity. Yet the small field of physical medicine and rehabilitation was amazingly successful in influencing legislation because practitioners were most often not asking things for their own benefit, but rather to benefit persons with disability. Despite misadventure in other areas, collaboration between the Academy and the Congress and the AAP continued in the health policy and legislation arena because of the leadership of such individuals as Thomas Strax and Kristjan Ragnarsson, and Honorary Academy members James Liljestrand and Manuel J. Lipson. The glue that made the effort work was the superhuman performance of Academy legal counsel Richard E. Verville, an Academy Distinguished Public Service Awardee. Dick, as he is affectionately known to his colleagues, is a remarkable and gifted lawyer with a profound regard for persons with disability and those who serve them. He has an encyclopedic knowledge of the law and a cadre of congressional leaders and their staff eager to share thoughts with him. He has steered the field on a steady course in obtaining research funding and agency representation. He has championed civil rights for persons with disabilities and led the field's contributions to the passage and refinement of the Americans with Disabilities Act. He assisted me in promotion of the Catastrophic Care Act, which unhappily was rescinded owing to funding deficiencies. He has been active in every nook and cranny of federal and state practice regulation and his law firm can be counted on for sound legal advice for the organization and its members. The Academy has added R. Dawn Brennaman as health policy manager and Lynda M. Leedy to its full-time staff to assist the important functions of this area of responsibility. This staffing finally fulfills the long-held dreams of the original members of the health policy and legislation team for an effective organizational mechanism to be proactive and not simply reactive to legislative issues. Academy members who support these efforts with their dues reap a rich benefit on a regular basis, as do the patients they serve.

A field cannot exist unto itself but is closely intertwined with many other organizations throughout society. Effective representation is an absolute that requires hours of selfless time and creativity given by individual physiatrists on behalf of the field. The Academy has a delegate and alternate delegate to the American Medical Association's House of Delegates, the umbrella organization representing the nation's physicians. From its formation the Academy has enjoyed outstanding representation and has achieved recognition of its issues and support for its policies. In modern times representation was through William Erdman of the University of Pennsylvania. Erdman was a gentleman leader of the first order whose diplomacy and gregarious personality fostered warm relationships for physiatry in both the American Medical Association's House of Delegates and the Council of Medical Specialty Societies as well as the American College of Physicians. Erdman was my mentor, and I served as an alternate delegate while Erdman was delegate and later stepped up to the delegate role in both the Council of Medical Specialty Societies and the American Medical Association. I had the strong support of the Texas delegation, one of the strongest in the House of Delegates. If a resolution was passed in the Texas House of Delegates, the American Medical Association's representatives would tenaciously politic for its adoption as American Medical Association policy. I resigned and Reinstein subsequently took over the American Medical Association's representation and was ably assisted by Gail Gamble of the Mayo Clinic and then Mark Race of Texas. This representation has been most ambitious and successful. Joachim Opitz and John Melvin served as representatives at Council of Medical Specialty Societies followed again by Reinstein. Both Melvin and Reinstein have been elected to higher offices in Council of Medical Specialty Societies, giving additional visibility to physiatry.

Valued representation was also carried out internationally through the International Rehabilitation Medicine Association and International Federation of Physical Medicine and Rehabilitation, which have recently become allied. Flax, Melvin, Grabois, Christopher, Strax, and Reinstein have played major leadership roles.

Communication with the membership is one of the most critical functions of an Academy. Ian MacLean, followed by Claire Wolfe, has used a Shakespearean command of language and great humor and poignant observations in their editorial role in the society's "Physiatrist" newsletter. MacLean also created and inspired the Academy's Web site and authors its electromyography clinical case studies. Use of the Internet was particularly facilitated by former Academy President James Swenson and current President Barry Smith.

The American Academy of Physical Medicine and Rehabilitation has created several awards to honor its most distinguished sons and daughters. The Frank H. Krusen Award is the highest honor bestowed on a person by the Academy, honoring this founding father of our field. The recipients of this gold medal are selected on the basis of their outstanding contributions to the field of physical medicine and rehabilitation in the areas of patient care, research, education, literary contributions, community service, and involvement in the many activities of the Academy. A unanimous vote of the Board of Governors is required. The first award went to Krusen, who was the Academy's fourth president. Only one award was given to a nonphysiatrist and that was to Honorable Hubert H. Humphrey in 1977. Other recipients were Howard A. Rusk, 1973; Sidney Licht, 1974; Frederic J. Kottke, 1979; Arthur S. Abramson, 1980; Justus F. Lehmann, 1983; Ernest W. Johnson, 1984; Joseph Goodgold, 1985; W. Theodore Liberson, 1987; Arthur E. Grant, 1990; Robert C. Darling, 1991; Joachim L. Opitz, 1992; Carl V. Granger, 1993; William M. Fowler, Jr., 1994; John F. Ditunno, Jr., 1995; Joseph C. Honet, 1996; and Myron LaBan, 1997. The winners of this coveted award are indeed the benchmark physiatrists loved, admired, and respected by all who have had the honor of knowing them.

The Walter J. Zeiter Lecture was previously mentioned. The 30 recipients to date were selected by the Awards Committee and approved by vote of the Academy board. Their names are listed in the Appendix. The Academy recognizes distinguished public service of persons whose public service actions have significantly contributed to the growth and development of educational, research, and service activities that directly impact the specialty of physical medicine and rehabilitation, and that benefit the nation's citizens with disabilities. As many as three awards may be given each year upon nomination from the Awards Committee and vote of the Academy Board of Governors. Recipients are listed in the Appendix.

The Academy also awards a Distinguished Service Award to recognize distinguished service to the Academy and the specialty, and to recognize leadership as a clinician, teacher, and mentor. Recipients are physiatrists who have achieved distinction on the basis of their scholarly level of teaching and their outstanding performance in patient care activities, as well as their significant contributions to the Academy and the specialty. Since 1981, as many as three awards have been given per year upon nomination by the Awards Committee and vote of the Board of Governors. The Distinguished Member Award was established in 1994 to honor physiatrist members who have provided invaluable service to the specialty of physical medicine and rehabilitation mainly through participation in physical medicine and rehabilitation–related organizations other than the Academy. One award may be given a year. The Richard and Hinda Rosenthal Foundation Lecture has been awarded since 1983 to honor physicians under the age of 50 who have made notable contributions to clinical achievement in the treatment of lower-back disability. The award consists of a $2000.00 honorarium and an invitation to present the Rosenthal lecture at the Academy's annual meeting. Finally, the Physical Medicine and Rehabilitation Education and Research Foundation Awards are awarded by the foundation at the Academy's annual meeting in the categories of New Investigator Awards and Best Paper Awards. Recipients of these awards represent the best and brightest of the Academy's membership, and are listed in the Appendix.

THE FUTURE

Interdisciplinary teamwork and the leadership skills necessary to make a team function efficiently are the everyday bread-and-butter tools of a well-trained physiatrist. Further, with a knowledge and vocabulary filled with objective measures of daily living skills and quality of life measures, and the tools to achieve the highest levels of both, the physiatrist is unique in skills and experience to bring what the modern medical market demands. Coupled with a knowledge of musculoskeletal and neurologic medicine and practical skills, the physiatrist is first concerned with the preservation and restoration of function and maximization of independence and coping skills. This is what the public wants and needs. The ability to wed modern biotechnology to the needs of persons with disability is highlighted as the year 2000 approaches and a new millennium of unimagined technologic advances begins. The youth of the Academy's membership and the members' great enthusiasm for their clinical task speak well of future success. Physiatrists will be held accountable for as much evidence-based research data as they can derive to test the validity of their armamentarium. They must continue to develop the research infrastructure and person power that will lead to that goal. In addition to public funding, physiatrists will need to support education and research foundations to ensure that the chain of new measures to carry out their tasks is unbroken.

Physiatrists must continue to attract young talented men and women to the field and ensure cultural diversity of their colleagues so that the special needs of the underserved minorities can be met with sensitivity and understanding. The position of the field of physical medicine and rehabilitation in medical school curricula must be expanded sufficiently to expose potential students to the field and to teach others why, when, and how to refer patients to physiatrists. Physiatrists must emphasize the wise economics of function enhancement. They will need to ensure that physiatric services are available across the full continuum of care from preventive through acute diagnostic and treatment services; to rehabilitation services offered in rehabilitation hospitals and units or long-term-care acute hospitals; to the skilled nursing facility; to home care; and to well-ordered ambulatory services as through a comprehensive outpatient rehabilitation facility methodology. Physiatrists must continue to stand up for the benefits of the physiatric approach not only to the U.S. government, but also to all levels of insurance and managed care organizations. They must prepare to assume some risk when that is demanded and warranted and must teach fellow members how to evaluate proposed contracts and relationships. The field of physiatry must not be a well-kept secret but rather marketed effectively.

Physiatrists must not allow society to lose the gains made by Howard Rusk. Social and vocational and avocational successes are indeed still part of the product of organized medical services even if currently rejected from some low-vision businesses and politicians. This means constant vigilance; regular public education; and credible relationships at the local, state, and federal level with health policy makers and with professional colleagues.

Physiatrists must aspire to wellness of the whole person, physically, psychologically, socially, and spiritually. They must be ready to embrace both conventional and unconventional therapies when they are deemed safe and effective and reject those that are unsafe or not cost-effective, keeping in mind societal fiduciary responsibilities.

Physiatrists must support one another in a collegial fashion, competing when they must in an ethical and public service–minded fashion. They must strive for efficiencies in their organizational life, whether in their offices and hospitals or other care environments or in societal relationships. Physiatrists must not have unnecessary duplication of efforts, because that is unaffordable. The professional societies must merge when that is the wise business course to take and do the greatest good with the least cost. Physiatrists must be wise stewards of the public's trust and dollars.

Physiatrists must be spiritual leaders, always using golden rule behavior in their relationships to others and following the wise guidance regarding human relationships derived from the great books and philosophers.

Physiatrists must respect their teachers and support and nourish them, and become great teachers themselves to ensure the propagation of the profession. They must develop and nourish kinship with their professional colleagues in medicine, nursing, and allied health. They must not mistakenly make gains at the expense of others.

Physiatry is a most unusual field. Its practitioners are at once wise and excellent clinicians, and as a group are highly concerned with fellow humans. The ultimate product is enhanced human and societal productivity. In the pages that follow, the reader will learn of the current theories and methodologies to practice this physical medicine and rehabilitation and will be inspired to constructively criticize them and create new and better explanations and methods.

APPENDIX

Presidents of the American Academy of Physical Medicine and Rehabilitation: 1938 to 1998

John S. Coulter, MD
F. H. Ewerhardt, MD
William Bierman, MD
Frank H. Krusen, MD
K. G. Hansson, MD
William H. Schmidt, MD
Fred B. Moor, MD
William D. Paul, MD
Earl C. Elkins, MD
Arthur E. White, MD
Charles O. Molander, MD
Miland E. Knapp, MD
Francis Baker, MD
Walter S. McClellan, MD
Donald L. Rose, MD
Harold Dinken, MD
Ben Boynton, MD
Murray Ferderber, MD
George Wilson, MD
Louis B. Newman, MD
Clarence W. Dail, MD
Ray Piaskoski, MD
Robert W. Boyle, MD
Max K. Newman, MD
Morton Hoberman, MD
Herman L. Rudolph, MD
A. B. C. Knudson, MD
Michael M. Dasco, MD
Robert C. Darling, MD
G. Keith Stillwell, MD
Herman J. Bearzy, MD
Glenn Gullickson, Jr., MD
Arthur S. Abramson, MD
Justus F. Lehmann, MD
Leonard F. Bender, MD
Eugene Moskowitz, MD
Carl V. Granger, MD
Ernest W. Johnson, MD
Joseph Goodgold, MD
Frederic J. Kottke, MD
Joseph C. Honet, MD
William M. Fowler, Jr., MD
John F. Ditunno, Jr., MD
Murray M. Freed, MD
Arthur E. Grant, MD
George H. Kraft, MD
Myron M. LaBan, MD
Richard S. Materson, MD
Joachim L. Opitz, MD
Barbara J. deLateur, MD
Erwin M. Gonzalez, MD
James T. Demopoulos, MD
Ian C. MacLean, MD
Leon Reinstein, MD
Robert P. Christopher, MD
Martin Grabois, MD

Randall L. Braddom, MD
James R. Swenson, MD
Barry Smith, MD

Walter J. Zeiter Lecture Awardees

Frank H. Krusen, MD, 1968
Paul A. Nelson, MD, 1969
Stanley W. Olson, MD, 1970
George H. Koepke, MD, 1971
Sidney Licht, MD, 1972
Frederic J. Kottke, MD, 1973
Donald L. Rose, MD, 1974
Arthur S. Abramson, MD, 1975
Ernest W. Johnson, MD, 1976
Howard A. Rusk, MD, 1977
Rene Cailliet, MD, 1978
Joseph Goodgold, MD, 1979
Edward E. Gordon, MD, 1980
Justus F. Lehmann, MD, 1981
G. Keith Stillwell, MD, 1982
Gerald J. Herbison, MD, 1983
Derrick A. Brewerton, MD, 1984
Sheldon Berrol, MD, 1985
Samuel L. Stover, MD, 1986
John L. Melvin, MD, 1987
Myron M. LaBan, MD, 1988
Joachim L. Opitz, MD, 1989
Joseph C. Honet, MD, 1990
George H. Kraft, MD, 1991
Theodore M. Cole, MD, 1992
Erwin G. Gonzalez, MD, 1993
Richard S. Materson, MD, 1994
Leon Reinstein, MD, 1995
Barbara J. deLateur, MD, 1996
Carl V. Granger, MD, 1997

American Academy of Physical Rehabilitation and Medicine Distinguished Public Service Award

1981

John Duncan
Martin LaVor
J. Paul Thomas

1982

Rep. Arlen Erdahl
Patria Forsythe
Sen. Lowell Weicker

1983

Douglas A. Fenderson

1984

Rep. Joseph D. Early
Frank J. Jirka, MD

1985

Sen. Robert Dole
Sen. Thomas F. Eagleton
Howard A. Rusk, MD

1986

Marilyn Spivack
Martin Spivack, MD

1987

Jerry Lewis
Sen. Claude Pepper
Richard Verville, JD

1988

Charles Hulin, JD
Judith Hulin, JD

1989

Sen. Lloyd Bentsen
Marina Weiss, PhD

1990

Justin Dart, Jr.
Lex Frieden

1991

Sen. Tom Harkin
Rep. Steny H. Hoyer
J. Spencer

1992

Richard S. Materson, MD
William F. Raub, PhD
Alan H. Toppel

1993

Duane F. Alexander, MD
Hon. Doug Walgren

1994

Henry B. Betts, MD
Suzanne R. Sonik
Carolyn C. Zollar, JD

1995

Marcus J. Fuhrer, PhD

John D. Kemp

Rep. John Edward Porter

1996

Judith E. Heumann

B. Caibre McCann, MD

American Academy of Physical Medicine and Rehabilitation Distinguished Service Awardees

Watson D. Parker, Jr., MD, 1995

Murray M. Freed, MD, 1996

Richard and Hinda Rosenthal Foundation Lecturers

Myron M. LaBan, MD, 1983

Jeffrey A. Saal, MD, 1985

Patricia E. Wongsam, MD, 1986

Irina Barkan, MD, 1987

Avital Fast, MD, 1988

Stanley A. Herring, MD, 1989

Joel S. Saal, MD, 1990

Nicholas E. Walsh, MD, 1991

Maury R. Ellenberg, MD, 1992

James Rainville, MD, 1993

Andrew J. Haig, MD, 1994

Joel M. Press, MD, 1995

Paul H. Dreyfuss, MD, 1996

Andrew J. Cole, MD, 1997

American Academy of Physical Medicine and Rehabilitation Distinguished Member Award

Gordon M. Martin, MD, 1994

Joseph C. Honet, MD, 1995

Thomas E. Strax, MD, 1996

Martin Grabois, MD, 1997

Academy Recognition Award for Distinguished Clinicians: 1991 to 1997

Renet Cailliet, MD

Eugene Moskowitz, MD

Joseph Rogoff, MD

William J. Erdman, MD

Ernest W. Johnson, MD

Miland E. Knapp, MD

Edward F. Delagi, MD

Edward W. Lowman, MD

Donald L. Rose, MD

Robert W. Boyle, MD

Robert C. Darling, MD

Arthur A. Rodriguez, MD

John D. Guyton, MD

Edward E. Gordon, MD

Edward M. Krusen, MD

Glenn Gullickson, Jr., MD

Joseph C. Honet, MD

Heinz Lippman, MD

Bruce B. Grynbaum, MD

George H. Koepke, MD

Walter C. Stolov, MD

Leonard F. Bender, MD

Murray M. Freed, MD

Samual S. Sverdlik, MD

Victor Cummings, MD

Jerome W. Gersten, MD

Gariella E. Molnar, MD

Shirley M. McCluer, MD

Matei S. Roussan, MD

Walter J. Treanor, MD

Alfred Ebel, MD

Herman J. Flax, MD

Myron M. LaBan, MD

B. Stanley Cohen, MD

Sherburne W. Heath, Jr., MD

James W. Rae, MD

Leland L. Cross, MD

Franz U. Steinberg, MD

Jerome S. Tobis, MD

Paul J. Corcoran, MD

John F. Ditunno, Jr., MD

Gloria D. Eng, MD

Maury Ellenberg, MD

Dorthea D. Glass, MD

John B. Redford, MD

Joseph Goodgold, MD

Gerald J. Herbison, MD

Inder Perkash, MD

Randall L. Braddom, MD

Phala Helm, MD

F. Patrick Maloney, MD

Physical Medicine and Rehabilitation Education and Research Foundation New Investigator Award: 1984 to 1997

Dennis Dykstra, MD

Robert Rondinelli, MD

Margaret Portwood, MD
Shane Vervoort, MD
Jeffrey Palmer, MD
Gary Goldberg, MD
Keith Robinson, MD
Andrew Haig, MD
Patricia Nance, MD
James K. Richardson, MD
Denise L. Campagnolo, MD
Timothy Dillingham, MD
John Chae, MD
Robert P. Wilder, MD
Lisa P. Gvoic Fugate, MD*
Ralph M. Buschbacher, MD
Anne I. Zeni, DO
Viviane Ugalde, MD*
Thierry H. M. Krivckas, MD
Matthew N. Bartels, MD, MPH*

Physical Medicine and Rehabilitation Education and Research Foundation Best Paper Award: 1990 to 1997

James C. Agre, MD
Thomas R. Lorish, MD
Michael Iee, MD
Nicholas Walsh, MD
Walter R. Fronterra, MD
Andrew J. Gitter, MD
James K. Richardson, MD
Kenneth M. Jaffee, MD
John R. Bach, MD
Gregory Carter, MD
Richard L. Aptaker, DO
Anne I. Zeni, DO
Robert Werner, MD

Presidents of the Association of Academic Physiatrists: 1967 to 1998

William J. Erdman, MD, 1967–1968
Henry B. Betts, MD, 1968–1969
Mieczyslaw Peszcynski, MD, 1969–1970
Murrar Freed, MD, 1970–1971
Nadene Coyne, MD, 1971–1972
Joseph Goodgold, MD, 1972–1973
John F. Ditunno, MD, 1973–1975
Justus F. Lehmann, MD, 1975–1977
Ernest W. Johnson, MD, 1977–1979
George H. Kraft, MD, 1979–1981
Paul J. Corcoran, MD, 1981–1983
Martin Grabois, MD, 1983–1985
John L. Melvin, MD, 1985–1987
Paul E. Kaplan, MD, 1987–1989
Randall L. Braddom, MD, MS, 1989–1991
Joel A. DeLisa, MD, 1991–1993
Bruce M. Gans, MD, 1993–1995
Robert H. Meier, III, MD, 1995–1997
Nicholas E. Walsh, MD, 1997–1999

Presidents of the American Congress of Rehabilitation Medicine: 1923 to 1998

Samuel B. Childs
Curran Pope
John S. Coulter
Disraeli Kobak
James C. Elsom
Frank Walke
Norman T. Titus
Roy W. Fouts
Frank H. Ewerhardt
Gustov Kolischer
Albert F. Tyler
William J. Clark
John S. Hibben
William Bierman
Frederick L. Wahrer
Frank H. Krusen
William H. Schmidt
Nathan H. Polmer
Abraham R. Hollender
Fred B. Moor
Kristian G. Hansson
Miland E. Knapp
Walter S. McClellen
H. Worley Kendall
O. Leonard Huddleston
Earl C. Elkins
Arthur L. Watkins
Robert L. Bennett
Walter M. Solomon
William B. Snow
William D. Paul
Gordan M. Martin
A. B. C Knudson

*Joint Kessler Foundation/Education and Research Foundation Awardee.

Donald L. Rose
Arthur C. Jones
Frederic J. Kottke
Donald A. Covalt
Donald J. Erickson
Jerome S. Tobis
Charles D. Shields
William J. Erdman, II
Lewis A. Leavitt
Edward W. Lowman
Sidney Licht
William A. Spencer
Jerome W. Gerten
Herman J. Flax
Leonard D. Policoff
James W. Rae
Rene Cailliet
John W. Goldschmidt
Henry B. Betts
John E. Affeldt*
June S. Rothberg*
Thomas P. Anderson
William E. Fordyce*
Marcus J. Fuhrer*
Victor Cummings
Sam C. Colachis, Jr.
Alfred J. Szumski
Glen Gullickson
Don A. Olsen
Dorothea D. Glass
John L. Melvin
Leonard Diller*
Dorothy L. Gordon*
William E. Staas, Jr.
Carmella Gonella*
Thodore M. Cole
Robert H. Meier
Thomas E. Strax
Thomas P. Dixon*
Karen A. Hart*
Theodore M. Cole

Residency Review Committee for Physical Medicine and Rehabilitation Members 1954 to present

Robert L. Bennett
Murray Brandstater

*Nonphysiatrist.

Alice Chen
B. Stanley Cohen
Donald A. Covalt
Victor Cummings
Harold Dinken
John F. Ditunno
Marc E. Duerden
Alfred Ebel
Earl C. Elkins*
William J. Erdman
Gerald Felsenthal*
Murray M. Freed
Erwin G. Gonzalez
Arthur M. Grant
Glenn Gullickson, Jr.
Margaret C. Hammond
Catherine N. Hinterbuchner
Thomas F. Hines
Joseph C. Honet*
Ernest W. Johnson
Nancy Kester
A. B. C. Knudson
George F. Koepke
Frederic J. Kottke
Edward M. Krusen
Edward Leveroos
Edward W. Lowman
Gordon M. Martin*
Richard S. Materson*
Malcolm C. McPhee
John L. Melvin
Phyllis Page
Roger Pesch
Leonard D. Policoff
Marc Raymond
James W. Rae
Donald L. Rose
Oscar Selke
Barry S. Smith
Walter M. Solomon
Jay Subbarao
Jerome Tobis
Arthur L. Watkins
Walter J. Zeiter

*Chairs

REFERENCES

1. Kottke FJ, Knapp ME. The development of physiatry before 1950. *Arch Phys Med Rehabil* 1988;69:4–14.
2. Krusen FH. Historical development in physical medicine and rehabilitation during the last forty years. *Arch Phys Med Rehabil* 1969;50:1–5.
3. Rusk HA. *A world to care for.* New York: Random House, 1972.
4. Martin GM, Opitz J, eds. The first 50 years: the American Board of Physical Medicine and Rehabilitation. *Arch Phys Med Rehabil* 1997;78(suppl 2).

BIBLIOGRAPHY

Nelson P, ed. *American Congress of Rehabilitation Medicine: Archives of Physical Medicine and Rehabilitation 50 year cumulative index: volumes 1–50 1920–1969 (including 50-year history).* Chicago, 1970.

Opitz J, ed. Fifty years of physiatry; the forging of the chain. *Arch Phys Med Rehabil* 1988;69:1–3.

Part I.

Overview

Chapter 1

Expanding the Disablement Model

Gale G. Whiteneck
Richard Holicky

A thorough understanding of rehabilitation begins with sound conceptualization not only of its principles, but also of a universally accepted model for describing the consequences of the disablement process. Such a model provides a framework within which to assess rehabilitation outcomes. This model is also necessary for proper documentation and evaluation of broad rehabilitation outcomes in order to demonstrate and improve the impact of the rehabilitation services we provide.

Such conceptualization and measurement is no easy task. Polling rehabilitation specialists for examples of successful outcomes might well result in them citing former clients who, despite significant disabilities, emerged from rehabilitation to become world-class athletes, wealthy business people, recognized scholars, pillars of the community, or simply sensational spouses or parents. Polling long-term survivors of significant disability for examples could produce a list of individuals based on entirely different standards, equally broad in range and subjective in nature. Many definitions of *successful outcome* exist. A perfect world would allow us to use such holistic and all inclusive criteria to evaluate rehabilitation.

However, even though income, academic achievement, athletic accomplishments, and number of children are all quantifiable, they are not the standards used to judge outcome. Instead we lean toward more traditional and universal medical and rehabilitation standards, primarily because we have reliable instruments to measure deficits, skills, and accomplishments acquired during and after rehabilitation. The development of the necessary instruments to measure such concepts as community integration and quality of life, as well as the necessary confidence in them, will facilitate a more global and universal assessment.

WHO MODEL OF DISABLEMENT

The World Health Organization's (WHO) International Classification of Impairments, Disabilities, and Handicaps (ICIDH) (1) is widely accepted and provides a theoretical foundation for discussing rehabilitation outcomes. Though the consequences of disablement are interrelated, they are also quite distinct. The WHO model distinguishes and clarifies the three levels of disablement outcomes as follows:

1. Impairments at the organ level
2. Disabilities at the person level
3. Handicaps at the societal level

The most immediate and basic consequence of disablement is impairment at the level of the individual organ or organ system resulting in "any loss or abnormality of psychological, physiological, or anatomical structure or function" (1). Paralysis, visual losses, profound hearing loss, and amputation are all examples of the wide range of impairments addressed by the ICIDH, and each is assessed with instruments germane to the specific disease, injury, or condition. The American Spinal Injury Association (ASIA) motor scores evaluate the extent of paralysis for spinal cord injury (2), various visual or auditory tools are used to measure sight or hearing impairments, and specific instruments assess speech impairments.

Progressing from the organ level to the person level, impairments can lead to disability, which is defined as "any restriction or lack (resulting from an impairment) of ability to perform an activity in the manner or within the range considered normal for a human being" (1). Disability is measured by the degree of independence with which an individual can perform various activities of daily living (ADLs), or conversely, by the degree those activities involve restrictions or dependencies. Similar disabilities can result from a variety of impairments, just as similar impairments can lead to different disabilities. Rehabilitation professionals rely on a number of instruments to measure disability, including the Functional Independence Measure (FIM) (3).

Outcome measures must also assess how well an individual is able to perform various appropriate roles—worker, family member, volunteer, community official—in society at large. The WHO model labels this as *handicap*, defining it as "a disadvantage for a given individual . . . that limits or prevents the fulfillment of a role that is normal (depending upon age, sex, social and cultural factors) for that individual" (1). The term *handicap* will probably soon yield to a term such as *participation* or *social participation*, in order to better reflect full performance of expected social roles. Relatively few instruments have been developed for the specific purpose of quantifying handicap, two being the Craig Handicap Assessment and Reporting Technique (CHART) (4) and the Community Integration Questionnaire (CIQ) (5). They measure the degree to which an individual is an active, productive member of society, well integrated into family and community life, which is the ideal rehabilitation outcome.

Other classification systems for disablement exist, and it is not unusual for them to employ distinct, sometimes confusing, and occasionally contradictory terminology. The Institute of Medicine and the National Center for Medical Rehabilitation Research use Saad Nagi's suggested terms *functional limitations* in place of *disability* (6). They also use *disability* to describe what the WHO model of disablement refers to as *handicap*. Similarly, the Public Health Service Task Force system defines *impairment* as simply the "organ level," *disability* as the "person level," and *handicap* as the "interaction of environment on person" (7). While various agencies and organizations may use different terminology, the conceptual framework remains quite similar and the disablement process is consistently divided into three basic areas:

1. Organ-system performance
2. Performance of ADLs at the person level
3. Role performance as a member of society

Since the WHO model of disablement is the most widely used and internationally recognized, its terminology is used throughout this chapter.

REHABILITATION OUTCOMES THROUGHOUT THE DISABLEMENT PROCESS

Rehabilitation's charge is to reduce, minimize, and mitigate disablement as much as possible, and this is done in much the same sequential process as disablement itself. Medical interventions and treatments at the organ or organ-system level take center stage during the acute phase. Addressing ADLs in order to maximize functional independence and minimize the disability manifested by a given impairment is accomplished through ADL training, adaptive equipment, and various other rehabilitative therapies. Finally, handicap is minimized as individuals are reintegrated back into their communities and once again assume roles as independent, productive participants (8–12).

It is possible to measure outcomes at each of these levels, and we do so to assess our effectiveness. However, while the overall goal in rehabilitation is to minimize handicap in order to maximize reintegration, the vast majority of outcome assessment work has focused on measuring impairments and disabilities. There are several reasons for this. Both impairment and disability are much easier to measure objectively, as the instruments have been in place for some time and have gained widespread acceptance. Moreover, impairment and disability are far more under the direct control of rehabilitation specialists than are the attitudinal, economic, and social stigma barriers that surround the goal of reducing handicap.

Nonetheless, our goal both professionally and socially is the elimination of these handicapping barriers and the facilitation of full participation in society of people with disabilities. As a result, it becomes both appropriate and necessary to measure outcomes in all three dimensions of the disablement process, and in order for this to happen, a shift in emphasis toward handicap as an equal and appropriate rehabilitation outcome measure is necessary.

GOING BEYOND THE MEDICAL MODEL

As helpful as the WHO model of disablement is in differentiating its three key dimensions, it is not complete. Its reliance on the medical model tends to emphasize the consequences of health conditions without incorporating the context in which they occur. Expansion of the medical model allows rehabilitation to both acknowledge and address the fact that disablement is embedded within the context of both *personal* and *environmental* factors. A more thorough rehabilitative approach recognizes that outcomes are determined not only by *impairment* (organ-system performance) and *disability* (performance of ADLs), but also by environmental factors that act as barriers or facilitators to full participation and by a constellation of personal factors often unique to each individual that also influence outcomes. Disablement must be viewed from a *lifetime perspective*, understanding that it is a dynamic process with ever-changing consequences. In addition, the *subjective perspective* of the individual must be included and considered.

ENVIRONMENTAL FACTORS

Environmental factors can and often do serve as a major contributor to the disablement process, one that can either aid or limit an individual's participation level. In 1993, the WHO called for re-examination of how environmental factors affect ICIDH components (1), as part of its upcoming revision process. The WHO model of disablement has been criticized for its implied causality, which describes disablement as beginning with pathology, which produces impairment, causing disability and culminating in handicap. Unacknowledged in this model is the role of environmental factors, which disability rights activists and organizations point out are equally important as causes of disablement as are disease and trauma. As such, interventions on the environmental level are as important as medical care or rehabilitation treatment (13).

Environmental factors are those characteristics external to an individual that influence, enhance, or restrict that individual's participation level or performance as a member of society. These elements span a broad range, from nature and architecture to culture, politics, or social and legal structures. Examples of environmental barriers include steps without ramps, negative attitudes toward disability, and financial disincentives for returning to work. The Americans with Disabilities Act (ADA) is a good example of an environmental facilitator. What is called for is a system to categorize the major environmental characteristics influential in producing handicap. The major characteristics that provide a foundation for such a system are accessibility, accommodation, resource availability, social support, and equality, as they are all characteristics that are influential in producing handicap (14,15).

Accessibility addresses issues of physical access, including transportation issues and architectural barriers. *Can you get where you want to go?*

Accommodation deals with equipment, services, and modifications of tasks that facilitate full participation in society. This includes places like work, home, and school. *Once you get there, can you do what you want to do?*

Resource availability covers the services made necessary by both impairment and disability, including specialized medical care, personal assistance services, and income security, to name a few. *Are the special needs resulting from your disability met?*

Social support is an attitudinal issue defined by the various social prejudices surrounding disablement, which can come from family members, friends, employers, teachers, neighbors, and other community members. *Are you accepted by those around you?*

Equality focuses on the degree to which policies and regulations of governments produce an equal opportunity for people with disabilities in areas such as discrimination, financial disincentives, legislative mandates, and health care management and rationing. *Are you treated equally with others?*

PERSONAL FACTORS

Just as environmental factors are the *external* influences, personal factors are major *internal* influences on handicap. *Personal factors*—demographics, life experiences, personality, spiritual beliefs, individual style and history of dealing with stress, worldview—are those factors that must be considered throughout the disablement process, as together they can dictate and determine much of an individual's response to disability. Basic personality may be defined as the sum of one's consistent attitudes, values, behavioral patterns, and defense mechanisms, in addition to the consistent manner in which a person perceives, processes, and reacts to the surrounding environment (16). The meaning one assigns to impairment, disability, or handicap can be far more important than any loss of function, loss of independence, or loss of opportunity to participate within the context of the larger society.

Rehabilitation's task is to examine the myriad personal factors involved in the disablement process, in search of those that counseling or psychology can possibly address and modify so as to mitigate their handicapping effects. Demographics must be considered in the formulation of treatment plans and outcome evaluations, as they present a powerful frame of reference from which people view and react to impairment and disability. Past life experiences contribute to the formulation of a worldview and provide a lens through which individuals interpret occurrences in their lives. How people have dealt with adversity, challenge, disappointment, negative events, and obstacles can serve as both predictors of future reactions and reminders of successful responses previously employed. As individuals journey through life, they become their perceptions, and these perceptions drive what they are and what they do. Perceptions are the key to attitude, behavior, motivation, and locus of control. Individuals can alter their histories, modify their present circumstances, and transcend those around them if they can change their perceptions.

Is it possible to refocus this lens in order to enhance outcomes? Counseling has been successful in effecting positive changes in behavior, interpretation of events and the meanings assigned to them, and in the responses individuals make to various events in their lives. Herein lies the rationale for psychology's role in rehabilitation. We need to explore this area and its possibilities and integrate them into the rehabilitation process. By facilitating how people with disabilities employ these personal factors, rehabilitation can have an effect on the final outcome, presently termed *handicap*.

LIFETIME PERSPECTIVE OF DISABLEMENT

The WHO model of disablement must also be expanded to offer greater emphasis to the lifetime nature of many disabling conditions. Such an expanded emphasis will focus on the additional physiologic, functional, and social declines, referring to them as *secondary impairments*, *secondary disabilities*, and *secondary handicaps*. *Secondary impairments* are those medical complications occurring at the organ level following original assessment. Any further declines beyond the original functional losses in the performance of ADLs, or in functional abilities are labeled *secondary disabilities*. *Secondary handicaps* identify any further decreases in social integration, economic self-sufficiency, independence, employment, or productivity that may develop in the time following onset. The primary impairment, disability, or handicap may indeed precipitate secondary impairments, or such secondary impairments could be the result of a new but related secondary disease or injury process (17).

Simply put, disabling conditions are not static (18). Levels of impairment, disability, and handicap are assessed and measured in a timely fashion following the onset of the disablement process, and doing so affords a baseline outcome assessment measure for acute rehabilitation.

The original disabling condition often leads to or results in secondary impairments, secondary disabilities, or secondary handicaps. Or, the primary disabling condition may be a risk factor for other (secondary) conditions, or treatment of the secondary condition is affected or altered by the primary disability (19).

Broad health status measures are needed to track individuals throughout their lifetime, as several organ systems frequently are involved in secondary impairments. Reputable rehabilitation successfully addresses and controls problems and complications during the initial hospitalization, and also addresses and deals with secondary impairments developing years later. In a similar fashion, secondary disabilities and handicaps may develop and increasingly limit ADL performance or social participation.

A variety of concepts and measures can assess general health. Survival, the number of days rehospitalized, the number of physician visits, increased use of durable medical equipment, increases in prescription medications, or other health problems or activity limitations can, together, provide a baseline.

The personal perspective also needs to be honored and included with some type of self-perceived, self-reported health evaluation. Presently the Medical Outcomes Study 36 Item Short-Form Health Survey (SF-36) (20) is the established and widely accepted instrument of choice and is presently available in a 12-item scale. In addition, a more general and global item such as "rate your health on a scale from excellent to poor" could also be included for an overall outcome assessment.

IMPORTANCE OF SUBJECTIVE REALITY

Rehabilitation outcomes are both objective and subjective, but until recently, *measured* outcomes have been almost exclusively objective ones. Needless to say, all the surgeries, treatments, medications, therapies, architectural modifications, and legislation serve little purpose for those who report low subjective well-being. The task of psychosocial rehabilitation is to improve *subjective well-being* and self-esteem, and this takes on added importance as research suggests high subjective well-being is closely related to low levels of handicap (21).

Performance of organ systems or ADLs, and integration back into the community can be measured objectively. No less important are the views of the persons living with disablement. How people view their impairments, disabilities, and handicaps certainly carries as much validity as any muscle test or employment evaluation. The term *perceived health* is used to encompass the sum of all perceived primary and secondary impairments. The term *perceived activity limitations* represents the sum of an individual's perceived primary and secondary disabilities. And in like fashion, an individual's subjective perception of the sum of all primary and secondary handicaps is termed *perceived role limitations*. While similar to the objective measures of impairment, disability, and handicap, these are additional, stand-alone assessments that provide a broader picture of rehabilitation outcomes (22).

Another expansion of the WHO model is needed to include the concept of subjective well-being. In general terms, *subjective well-being* can be defined as the degree to which an individual has positive thoughts about his or her life considered as a whole (21). Therefore, measuring subjective well-being, a synonym for quality of life, would assess not outside observers' perceptions, but the individual's own perceived satisfaction with life.

Spilker (23) argued, with growing support, that quality of life can be conceptualized as a subjective assessment of well-being, composed hierarchically of subjective perceptions in broad domains. Elaborating on the WHO model of disablement, quality of life would be the sum total of perceived well-being in all domains.

AN EXPANDED MODEL OF DISABLEMENT

Figure 1-1 presents a graphic view of a proposed expanded model of disablement. It identifies all the key elements discussed heretofore, and illustrates their interrelationship with each other and over time. Clearly, the progression through the process of health conditions (pathology), impairment, and disability is embedded within and can be

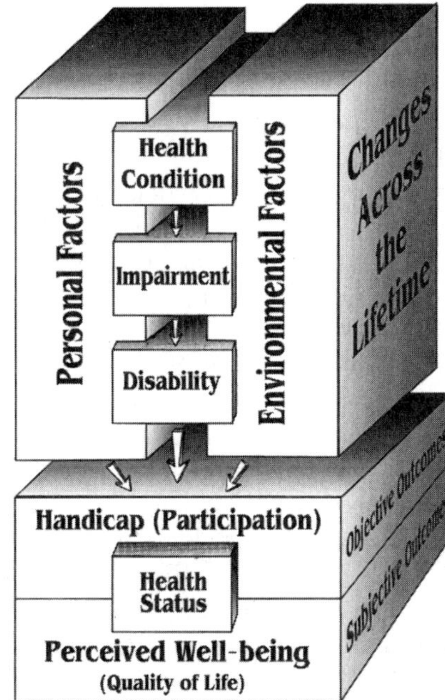

Figure 1-1. An expanded model of disablement.

heavily influenced by both environmental factors and personal factors. The end results of all these elements are handicap and subjective well-being. Immersed within handicap and perceived well-being are health status outcomes, which interact synergistically with the former two outcomes. As such, this expanded model continues to provide objective outcome measures for all those elements measured in the past, while further evolving to include environmental and personal factors, changes over the life span, health status, and valid subjective measurement of key rehabilitation outcomes as well.

RECOMMENDED TOOLS FOR EVALUATING REHABILITATION OUTCOMES

Table 1-1 provides suggestions for evaluating rehabilitation outcomes over the lifetime. It includes the outcome being measured, the specific instrument being used, and a suggested schedule for doing the assessments *over the lifetime.*

Impairments are measured with a variety of instruments specially designed for the specific conditions in question. Examples of such measures are the ASIA/International Medical Society of Paraplegia (IMSOP) motor test and various measures that assess auditory or visual impairments. Such assessments are normally done at the time of initial rehabilitation, as well as periodically thereafter. Disability has been measured with a variety of tools. The FIM (3) is a widely accepted disability assessment tool and employs a seven-point rating scale to measure an individual's degree of independence in performing various ADLs. The FIM is used at the time of initial admission and discharge to provide a baseline outcome, and then periodically throughout the subject's lifetime. Few instruments exist to assess handicap. As a result, CHART (4) was developed as a way to quantify community integration following initial rehabilitation. CHART measures the six domains of handicap identified by WHO—orientation, physical independence, mobility, occupation, social integration, and economic self-sufficiency—in a practical and objective fashion on a 100-point scale normed with the general population (4). CHART is used to assess an individual's level of handicap following disablement, and then periodically over the lifetime.

Table 1-1: Measurement Instruments for Evaluating Rehabilitation Outcomes

Outcome	Measurement	Application
Impairment	Measures germane to specific condition (i.e., ASIA motor scores)	Initial admission and discharge Follow-up at yr 1, 2, 5, 10, and every 5 yr thereafter
Disability	Functional Independence Measure (FIM)	Initial admission and discharge At yr 1, 2, 5, 10, and every 5 yr thereafter
Handicap	Craig Handicap Assessment and Reporting Technique (CHART)	At yr 1, 2, 5, 10, and every 5 yr thereafter
Perceived well-being	Life Satisfaction Index Diener Scale	At yr 1, 2, 5, 10, and every 5 yr thereafter
Health status outcomes	Combination of survival, days rehospitalized, SF-36	At yr 1, 2, 5, 10, and every 5 yr thereafter

ASIA = American Spinal Injury Association; SF-36 = Medical Outcome Study 36 Item Short-Form Health Survey.

Several tools can be used to measure subjective well-being. These range from Flanagan's Quality of Life questionnaire (24) to the Life Satisfaction Index (25) to the Diener Satisfaction with Life Scale (26), which is recommended due to its brevity. A subjective well-being tool is administered after disablement and then periodically thereafter.

The final area that must be included in measuring rehabilitation outcomes is that of health status, which here represents a combination of objective and subjective assessments of health and wellness. The objective dimension of health status is the sum of various indicators of health problems. The SF-36 (20) is used to measure self-reported health status, the subjective dimension. As with handicap and subjective well-being, health status needs to be measured periodically throughout the lifetime. The fact that no instruments are presently used to measure environmental factors or personal factors simply indicates the need to either identify or formulate them in order to measure their influences in the rehabilitation process.

Lifetime rehabilitation costs must also be examined in order to assess the value of a specific system of care. Value can be viewed simplistically as quality rehabilitation for the least number of dollars. Realistically, value can be defined in terms of how well a change in resources yields desired changes in outcomes. Value cannot be adequately assessed in the short term, as is often attempted by comparing functional gain to the cost of a single hospitalization. True value needs to be viewed as the lifetime outcomes compared to lifetime costs. By comparing and evaluating various interventions presently used in policy, environmental, educational, and medical areas, specific interventions can be selected on the basis of value as well as effectiveness in any one of the previously cited dimensions.

CONCLUSION

The time has come to broaden both the conceptualization of the disablement process as well the overall manner in which rehabilitation outcomes are measured. If rehabilitation means minimizing and mitigating disablement as much as possible, then all aspects of that process must be addressed and evaluated. In the past, health care providers have relied solely on the medical model and almost exclusively addressed medical and functional issues. Rehabilitation must go beyond that model in order to deal with all the issues that contribute to or hinder a successful life following disability. One way to accomplish this is by including handicap issues, personal factors, environmental factors, and health status issues. Another is by acknowledging the lifetime, dynamic nature of disablement with continual assessments and tracking of secondary conditions to ensure quality *lifetime* rehabilitation rather than solely focusing on the initial stay. The subjective, perceived aspects of disablement are often as important and powerful as the physical limitations, and must be included and measured. And we must continually use the sum of all these assessments to determine the interventions that provide the best value. This broadening of the concepts will not only ensure quality during initial rehabilitation, but also minimize future complications and maximize quality of life.

REFERENCES

1. World Health Organization. *International classification of impairments, disabilities, and handicaps: a manual of classification relating to the consequences of disease.* Geneva: World Health Organization, 1980.
2. American Spinal Injury Association. *Standards for neurological classification of spinal injury patients.* Chicago: American Spinal Injury Association, 1982.
3. State University of New York at Buffalo, School of Medicine and Biomedical Sciences, Center for Functional Assessment Research, Uniform Data System for Medical Rehabilitation. *Guide for the uniform data set for medical rehabilitation (Adult FIM).* Version 4.0. New York: State University of New York, 1993.
4. Whiteneck GG, Charlifue SW, Gerhart KA, et al. Quantifying handicap: a new measure of long-term rehabilitation outcomes. *Arch Phys Med Rehabil* 1992;73:519–526.
5. Willer B, Rosenthal M, Kreutzer JS, et al. Assessment of community integration following rehabilitation for traumatic brain injury. *J Head Trauma Rehabil* 1993;8:75–87.
6. Pope AM, Tarlov AR, eds. *Disability in America: toward a national agenda for prevention.* Washington: National Press Academy, 1991.
7. National Institutes of Health. *Research plan for the National Center for Medical Rehabilitation Research.* NIH publication no. 93–3509. Bethesda, MD: National Institutes of Health, 1993.
8. Kemp BJ, Vash CL. Productivity after injury in a sample of spinal cord injured persons: a pilot study. *J Chronic Dis* 1971;24:259–275.
9. Carey RG, Posavac EJ. Program evaluation of a physical medicine and rehabilitation unit: a new approach. *Arch Phys Med Rehabil* 1978;59:330–337.
10. Pflueger SS. *Independent living. Emerging issues in rehabilitation.* Washington, DC: Institute for Research Utilization 1977:5, 11.
11. Frey WD. Functional assessment in the '80s. In: Happern AS, Fuhrer MJ, eds. *Functional assessment in rehabilitation.* Baltimore: Brookes, 1984:11–43.
12. Wagner KA. Outcome analysis in comprehensive medical rehabilitation. In: Fuhrer MJ, ed. *Rehabilitation outcomes: analysis and measurement* Baltimore: Brookes, 1987:19–28.
13. Fougeyrollas P. Documenting environmental factors for preventing the handicap creation process: Quebec contributions relating to ICIDH and social participation of people with functional differences. *Disabil Rehabil* 1995;17:145–153.
14. Whiteneck GG, Fougeyrollas P, Gerhart KA. Elaborating the model of disablement. In: Fuhrer MJ, ed. *Assessing medical rehabilitation practices: the promise of outcomes research.* Baltimore, MD: Paul H. Brooks Publishing, 1997.

15. Whiteneck GG. Evaluating outcomes after spinal cord injury: what determines success? 1996 Donald Munro Lecture. *J Spin Cord Med* 1997;20:179–185.

16. Butt L, Lanig I. Stress management. In: Lanig I, Chase T, Butt L, et al, eds. *A practical guide to health promotion after spinal cord injury*. Gaithersburg, MD: Aspen, 1996:140.

17. Whiteneck GG, Menter RR. Where do we go from here? In: Whiteneck GG, Charlifue SW, Gerhart KA, et al. *Aging with spinal cord injury.* New York: Demos, 1993:361–369.

18. Marge M. Health promotion for persons with disabilities: moving beyond rehabilitation. *Am J Health Promotion* 1988;2:29–35.

19. Whiteneck GG. Secondary conditions after spinal cord injury. A presentation at The Conversation on Disability Issues: Secondary Conditions and Aging with a Disability. Syracuse, NY: State University of NY Health Science Center, May 20, 1994.

20. Ware JE, Sherbourne CD. The MOS 36 Item Short-Form Health Survey (SF-36): conceptual framework and item selection. *Med Care* 1992;30:473–481.

21. Fuhrer MJ. The subjective well-being of people with spinal cord injury: relationship to impairment, disability and handicap. *Top Spinal Cord Injury Rehabil* 1996;1:56–71.

22. Whiteneck GG. Measuring what matters: key rehabilitation outcomes. *Arch Phys Rehabil* 1994;75:1073–1076.

23. Spilker B. *Quality of life assessments in clinical trials.* New York: Raven, 1990.

24. Flanagan JC. A research approach to improving our quality of life. *Am Psychol* 1978;2:138–147.

25. Wood V, Wylie ML, Sheafor B. An analysis of a short self-report measure of life satisfaction: correlation with rater judgments. *J Gerontol* 1969;24:465–469.

26. Diener E. Assessing subjective well-being; program and opportunities. *Soc Indicators Res* 1994;31:103–157.

Chapter 2

The Rehabilitation Team

Scott Manley

"There are many objects of great value to men which cannot be obtained by unconnected individuals, but must be obtained if at all, by association." *Daniel Webster*

HISTORICAL OVERVIEW

The marquee of the rehabilitation process is the team approach (1–5). In the continuum of health care, rehabilitation has been the leader in the promotion and development of the team approach. Although the concept of the health care team initially gained momentum in the acute care setting as a result of the increased technology and the multifaceted medical care needs of patients, the utilization of multidisciplinary teams to address increasing specialization and advanced technology became the foundation for the delivery of care within rehabilitation (1–3,6–8).

The Evolving Team

Theodore Brown (3) in an essay entitled "An Historical View of Health Care" described three periods of evolution of the team concept in health care. The first was prior to World War II when there was an increasing recognition that teamwork was a useful alternative to the traditional physician-dominated structure of delivering health care services. The second period was from World War II to the early 1970s. During that period, the use of teams expanded rapidly owing to the increased complexity of medical knowledge and the increased number of new specialists. Teams began working throughout the health care industry to coordinate the efforts of clinicians involved in the treatment of patients. The last period, which began in the 1970s and continues today, involves re-evaluation of the team concept, focusing on two areas: understanding the dynamics involved in the team approach, and evaluating the resource cost/value of the team approach in today's cost-conscious market.

Rehabilitation pioneer Howard Rusk was one of the first to recognize the contribution of the team approach for individuals who were disabled and needed to access multidisciplinary expertise to meet their medical and rehabilitation needs (9,10). Rehabilitation provided an excellent medium for the team concept to grow and today continues to be recognized within the health care continuum for its successful use of a multidisciplinary approach to service delivery.

The multidisciplinary approach began by capitalizing on the expertise of specific disciplines as they worked to assist rehabilitation clients to achieve their optimum levels of functioning (10,11). Multidisciplinary teams involved staff members working individually to assist clients to reach their optimal levels of functioning (10). However, all was not perfect. Although this approach reduced the fragmentation of medical and rehabilitation services to clients, the initial team concept relied heavily on discipline-specific treatments. Individual clinicians tended to work "together separately," failing to maximize the benefits of integrating treatment modalities and failing to fully capitalize on the interactive processes possible between team members. It was only after further development of these early *multi*disciplinary teams that truly *inter*disciplinary teams finally evolved.

The interdisciplinary team recognized that treatment outcomes could be enhanced by promoting an interactive relationship among all disciplines to more effectively coordinate and deliver services to patients and their families (10–12). The interdisciplinary team member works within his or her own sphere of practice but works in coordination with other team members and clients to set and coordinate goals (10). The interdisciplinary process is recognized as a more efficient and effective process within rehabilitation (2,9,11,13,14). Now, in the 1990s further evolution of this highly successful model continues. The newest development: the *trans*disciplinary team (14).

Transdisciplinary team members have a greater appreciation and working knowledge of the role, responsibilities, and expertise of all team members (10). The concept is based on the premise that team members who have a better understanding of the expertise and functions of other team members can work together more effectively and efficiently. This allows for overlapping of treatment approaches and use of two-discipline treating sessions (10). Transdisciplinary teams utilize cross training to enhance the treatment process and increase the effectiveness of all team members in developing and providing services to patients and families (2). Transdisciplinary team members complete client assessments together, involve clients in multidisciplinary cotreatments, and have a greater awareness and understanding of each team member's clinical training and treatment approaches. Transdisciplinary teams are relatively new to rehabilitation and as a result, they have met with resistance because of a lack of research demonstrating their effectiveness and because of individual treatment disciplines' concerns over traditional professional and treatment boundaries (15). However, the increasing cost reduction pressures within health care in general and the high cost of manpower resources within rehabilitation specifically will encourage further development and evaluation of this model as possibly a more cost-effective approach.

OVERVIEW OF RESEARCH ON TEAM EFFECTIVENESS

Although the team process has been viewed as the cornerstone of modern rehabilitation, very little research has been conducted to demonstrate the effectiveness of the team approach (4,8,15,16). Indeed, Halstead (4) argued that despite numerous articles and publications supporting the importance, effectiveness, and efficiency of the health care team, there is little quantitative evidence to support these claims. Most of the articles he reviewed were based on personal experiences; quality research studies that provided objective information were rare (4). Moreover, the seemingly objective information that is available is not all supportive. In a related article on the comprehensive treatment team in rehabilitation, Keith (16) not only acknowledged the difficulty of demonstrating the effectiveness of team functioning but also pointed out that research supporting the "evidence for the superiority of the comprehensive rehabilitation team is not very compelling, with mixed results from several sources."

Both authors made a strong appeal to the rehabilitation field to increase research efforts to evaluate the value of the team approach. Certainly the increasing pressures to provide rehabilitation services at a lower cost and in a more efficient manner—through per diem or capitated reimbursement agreements—will place greater emphasis on evaluating the cost benefits and configuration of rehabilitation teams in the future. Halstead (4) recommended several ways to study the effectiveness of the team approach:

1. Limit study to a homogeneous diagnostic category.
2. Randomly assign subjects into study and control groups.
3. Provide a treatment variable to the study group without altering or denying usual treatment to the control group.
4. Prospectively collect process and outcome data.
5. Periodically and objectively assess psychosocial functional status.
6. Periodically and objectively assess disease, illness status.
7. Follow up for a minimum of 1 year.

Even though rehabilitation as a field has not adequately demonstrated the effectiveness of its own teams, numerous publications in the past 10 years have documented the benefits of team work beyond rehabilitation (3,13,15). Larson and LaFasto, in their book *Teamwork* (13), provide an excellent overview of the characteristics of effective corporate teams and the benefits of utilizing the team approach in the corporate world. The ingredients, organization, and benefits of a team approach cited are very germane to the effectiveness of the team approach in rehabilitation. Larson (13) identifies "four design features that seemed to characterize effectively functioning teams in general: (1) clear roles and accountabilities; (2) an effective communication system; (3) methods for monitoring individual performance and providing feedback; and (4) an emphasis on fact-based judgments." And rehabilitation teams, at least in their intent, work to incorporate all of these features.

In addition to conducting more research on the value and cost-effectiveness of rehabilitation teams, the rehabilitation profession needs to utilize existing resource information on the benefit and organization of high-performance teams within corporate America (13,17). Although rehabilitation has touted the importance of the rehabilitation team in providing quality care to those it serves, the profession has done very little to educate and train staff members on how to develop, maintain, and evaluate rehabilitation teams (6).

TEAM CHALLENGES—IMPACT OF HEALTH CARE REFORM

Rehabilitation as a Growth Industry

"No other time in the history of health care has witnessed such rapid and global changes. Hospitals, health care providers, and patients have all been experiencing a change in the way the health care industry conducts business" (18). Starting with the advent of Medicare's diagnostic-related group (DRG), rehabilitation experienced a phenomenal growth period. DRGs resulted in a proliferation of rehabilitation programs due to the benefits of DRG exemption for rehabilitation facilities (5). Additionally, the DRG exemption allowed rehabilitation programs a level of freedom in the administration and provision of rehabilitation services that was not afforded to acute care providers who were under the scrutiny of the DRG reimbursement process. It comes as no surprise then, that the number of freestanding rehabilitation hospitals increased from 68 to 187 during the period from 1985 to 1994. During the same period, the number of rehabilitation units in acute care hospitals rose from 386 to 884 (19).

The significant growth of rehabilitation during this period allowed an opportunity to further expand the use of "teams," not only within the acute rehabilitation setting, but also in newly developed rehabilitation models in skilled nursing facilities, subacute units, residential care programs, and home rehabilitation programs.

While rehabilitation was undergoing a major transformation, the acute care component of health care was reorganizing in response to concerns about increasing health care costs and the delivery of health care services in the United States. "Health care reform" had been born. Health care providers were under increasing pressures to decrease the length of stay and lower the cost of care for all Americans. Health care costs were perceived as being prohibitive and there was increasing concern for the millions of Americans who were uninsured because of the cost of health care premiums.

During the initial stage of health care reform, rehabilitation continued to expand into other lower-cost markets and explore team models within those markets. However, as health care reform moved into the arena of managed care and as health care delivery itself was changed and reorganized through hospital acquisitions and mergers, the provision of rehabilitation services began to change dramatically. Rehabilitation began to respond to increasing cost pressure, shorter lengths of stays, and the provision of rehabilitation in low-cost settings. These pressures were compounded by changes in referral patterns due to acute care hospital mergers and intensive competition for health maintenance organization (HMO) contracts.

Rehabilitation Grows Leaner

Three major changes associated with health care reform have had major impacts on rehabilitation teams and the delivery of services. First, the consolidation and alignment of acute care services through mergers and acquisitions have significantly altered and will continue to alter referral pathways of patients entering the rehabilitation system. The long-term impact will be varied and difficult to predict. New alignments and relationships may result in increased referral of rehabilitation patients or may significantly alter previously established referral patterns. Patients could be referred earlier in the process with more medical issues for the team to address, or they may be referred to lower-cost rehabilitation programs. Changes like these that have already taken place—as well as those yet to come—profoundly impact and unsettle rehabilitation team members.

A second major change in health care has been the increased use of HMO and preferred provider organization (PPO) insurance products. Many of these have minimally defined benefit programs for rehabilitation that also significantly alter the access to and provision of rehabilitation services.

Finally, the utilization of HMO products has brought about the increased utilization of case managers who provide closer scrutiny of rehabilitation services and provide further control over what and where services are to be provided (5). The impact of these changes has been enormous for rehabilitation and will continue to have a significant effect on the rehabilitation team, including clients and their families.

Some of the effects the rehabilitation team has felt are described here. On one level, rehabilitation programs have been impacted by downsizing, reorganization, and re-engineering—all in an effort to reduce costs and decrease the length of stays. Although the "reduction of length of stay has come to be regarded as a major indication as to both the goal and effectiveness of interventions" (9), there is concern that these shorter lengths of stays have resulted in a greater focus on the motor skills dimension of recovery rather than the equally important aspects of adjustment and adaptation (14). The long-term implications for rehabilitation consumers, their families, employers, and society as a whole have yet to be seen.

Additionally the implementation of product line management, critical pathways, and lower-cost treatment interventions like subacute programs has a major influence on team dynamics, responsibilities, reporting relationships, and treatment delivery methodology. Product line management has streamlined management responsibilities in an effort to improve efficiency and marketing and enhance team integration. The long-term benefit and success of this approach are still being evaluated.

The Impact on Teams

The direct impact on teams varies depending on how service delivery is restructured within an organization. Extensive restructuring could significantly change the dynamics of the team approach. Responding to cost pressures could result in the reduction of staff, increased use of paraprofessionals, and greater emphasis on cross training.

These changes may interfere with the team's ability to meet the moral and instrumental functions of patient care. Moral functions, as defined by Purtilo (14), are activities the team performs for the good of the patient and are well founded in professional ethics related to patient rights, dignity, and the social, psychological, and spiritual needs of patients. Instrumental functions deal with the technical skills and procedures provided in the treatment of patients (14). Instrumental functions include the specialized skills provided by therapists, nurses, and physicians. One of the major concerns with health care reform is the focus on outcomes related to instrumental functions and less attention to outcomes attributed to the moral functions of the team.

The ultimate impact on how teams are constructed could be significant. The team members having a high instrumental value may be more secure than team members whose contribution is basically a moral function (e.g., social workers, rehabilitation counselors, psychologists, chaplains). The increasing pressures to reduce costs could result in those team members being eliminated or reduced in numbers (14). Hopefully, increased attention to outcomes research measuring the benefits of both functions will demonstrate the importance of both in providing quality care.

In the meantime, increasing discussions are emerging about the appropriate scope of practice among rehabilitation therapies (14). Unfortunately, these have increased tensions among team members and their perceived value to the team and have reinforced "territorial" boundaries to preserve discipline-specific role models. Cross training and increased utilization of paraprofessionals have only further escalated tensions among team members. However, for the team to be successful, professional barriers need to be eliminated and trust and collaboration need to be enhanced among team members.

Professional boundaries can be a major stumbling block in allowing team members to accept new role responsibilities, share expertise and experience, and collaborate with team members from different disciplines and educational levels. Professional boundaries within teams have always been an issue in rehabilitation and the current changes may escalate the discord among team members (8,15). If the transition is unsuccessful, dysfunctional teams without a unified goal and lack of trust can negatively impact the quality of services provided, and the broader image of rehabilitation itself.

Altered delivery of care due to decreased lengths of stays or benefit limitations can also create significant ethical dilemmas for team members. Indeed, limitations on lengths of stays, restrictions on type of services, or numbers of treatments authorized can significantly impact the quality of services provided and may stand in the way of successful outcomes. As a result, professional standards, staff morale, and job satisfaction may decline. These ethical and moral dilemmas are an increasing concern and all parties involved need to have an opportunity to openly discuss the ethical impact and the consequences these limitations have on providing quality care to patients and families.

Team's Response: Greater Accountability

More research is needed to evaluate the impact of outcomes based on new treatment models, service delivery systems, and restrictions in medical or rehabilitation benefits. Without research demonstrating the positive or negative implications of new treatment models, the future of rehabilitation will be left in the hands of payers who (in the absence of research that identifies the most cost-effective short- and long-term patient management strategies) will understandably select the lower-cost models.

Another impact from health care reform has been the development of critical pathways for rehabilitation patients. These are timelines documenting crucial steps along a process—whether the process is recovery from a surgical procedure, a college class, or rehabilitation following a stroke or spinal cord injury. Although critical pathways are more common in acute care due to the shorter lengths of stays, they are increasingly being developed and utilized within rehabilitation in an effort to better define treatment pathways and improve efficiency. As critical pathways become more fully developed, they may serve a valuable purpose in assisting the rehabilitation profession to establish an acceptable community standard for medical and rehabilitation management of various disability groups. These standards could then be utilized to educate payers about the importance of establishing benefit provisions that would allow a given individual with a disability to progress through an established care pathway. If prevailing community standards are developed and agreed on, payers are more likely to recognize the standards and select providers that can meet the standards and provide the care in the most cost-efficient manner.

Critical pathways, however, need to be developed across a continuum that includes both the acute and post-acute care needs of patients. During this ongoing developmental phase, team members may be frustrated with certain aspects of critical pathways. Team members may feel pathways are restrictive and do not allow for individual differences among patients and restrict the autonomy of therapists by utilizing a "cookie cutter" approach to treatment. Moreover, current critical pathways address functional gains but do not adequately address the impact of psychosocial variables or progressions throughout the continuum. This can create additional stress for the treatment staff who must account for why the client may not be progressing through the program as expected. Although variances are expected, they may not be accommodated due to benefits that may have restrictive treatment or length of stay provisions. Again, team members are faced with ethical and professional conflicts on how to resolve these issues between patients, payers, and the treatment team.

Critical pathways also need to address the level of resource utilization required for a patient to efficiently progress along a continuum of care. The number of subacute, outpatient, and home-based rehabilitation models has increased so quickly that a concern remains for the continuity of care provided. Most of these new models have less experience with multidisciplinary teams (7).

Treatment teams can no longer keep clients for extended stays to accommodate the psychological, social, financial, or educational needs of patients and families. Once the patient is medically stabilized and able to move to a lower-cost setting, the pressure is on to transfer the patient. The impact on treatment teams is enormous. Relationships established with patients and families are abruptly ended and team members do not receive the same level of job satisfaction experienced by working with patients and families through the entire rehabilitation process.

In response to increasing cost pressures, many rehabilitation programs are incorporating subacute programs within their rehabilitation program to respond to financial constraints and allow team members to continue working with their patients and families. Certainly the financial pressures for lowering costs will continue and reimbursement will become increasingly based on levels of care needed. Rehabilitation teams will be forced to look at ways to improve consistency and communication throughout the rehabilitation continuum and ways to incorporate the subacute model within the rehabilitation continuum.

Although the process throughout the continuum is supposed to be more cost-effective, the impact of passing through several types of rehabilitation programs needs to be evaluated in terms of long-term outcomes. The transition of patients through various treatment models is difficult for patients and team members who have developed a close therapeutic relationship and now need to develop new relationships as they make the transition from a comprehensive treatment program to a subacute or less-intensive setting with a new treatment team. This can make the team's work less satisfying and frustrating if the transition does not involve an in-depth exchange of treatment information, knowledge, and confidence in the program the patient will be entering or lack of feedback regarding the patient's progress.

Consequently, treatment teams will need to develop better models to exchange information. They will need to learn more about the treatment methodologies of each of the team's members in order to improve communications and increase confidence and trust within the team. Many programs are addressing this issue by developing their own subacute or home rehabilitation programs that they believe provide more consistency in treatment approaches through the provision of a continuum of care within one organization. This approach may be particularly helpful in a changing health care system. Indeed, Melvin (7) wrote, "In today's health market the influence of third party payers sometimes thwarts the ability of a facility to provide high quality interdisciplinary care." As a result, "such payers should not be surprised that a fragmented approach results in less satisfactory results in complicated cases."

Health care reform has also caused a closer evaluation of the cost-effectiveness of using the team approach. In the current price competitive market, the use of expensive interdisciplinary teams is being challenged. This also creates additional stress and job security concerns among team members who were indoctrinated with the concept of the rehabilitation team as the cornerstone of the rehabilitation philosophy. Uncertainty about job security and role responsibilities creates a barrier to effective communication and trust among team members. This can lead to further "turf" protection and can mitigate the benefits of using a team approach. Future rehabilitation teams will need to address how this impacts quality of care and develop educational interventions and research protocols if the team approach is to survive.

THE REHABILITATION TEAM OF THE FUTURE

At least in part, the success of rehabilitation in the future will depend on the organization and function of the team. While rehabilitation has relied on the team approach in the past, the future will require the team to organize in a way that is cost efficient and can demonstrate its value to the rehabilitation process (7). Fortunately, increasing research outside the field of rehabilitation has demonstrated the effectiveness of using the team approach in addressing major issues in the corporate world (13).

A Transdisciplinary Focus

Teams of the future will become more *trans*disciplinary in their approach to patient care. Team members will need to become more familiar with the functions and responsibilities of other team members and will need to be cross-trained on the basic functions of other team members. Cross training will occur across all disciplines and will allow treatment teams more flexibility in providing direct patient care to patients and families. Initially, this transition is likely to create major conflicts within professional disciplines, and to create conflicts related to job security and professionalism. The successful rehabilitation team will need to work through these conflicts to evolve into a cohesive unit that is able to deliver services at lower costs and maximize the productivity of all of its members. This becomes especially important in light of the increasing number of specialists in rehabilitation who have added significantly to the composition of the rehabilitation team. The addition of these individuals, unfortunately, has significantly increased the cost of delivering services through the team approach.

The increased cost, however, does not eliminate the need for specialists on the team. Instead, it expands their role to provide the necessary expertise and cross training to other team members who can provide the care more cost-effectively. The use of team rounds and conferences for communication will need to be evaluated for more cost-effective models. Cost constraints may prohibit the luxury of extensive transdisciplinary meetings to develop and review treatment plans. More effective computerized communication systems designed to enhance communication and team interaction, without the need for lengthy meetings, will have to be developed and tested. This will require team members to develop an in-depth understanding of the expertise and knowledge of other team members and to effectively use their own skills to prevent duplication or underutilization of team resources. Reports will become process and outcome oriented utilizing a transdisciplinary approach, eliminating discipline-specific reports. Effective teams will place a higher priority on team goals than on individual or discipline-specific goals. Already, rehabilitation teams have begun reorganizing along product line management with very specific goals and functions. Keith (16) reports that teams involving multiple skills, judgments, and experiences outperform individuals acting alone.

Indeed, the whole will need to become greater than its parts. Teams that work well together bring complementary skills and experiences that exceed those of the individuals on the team (17). "Within teams, there is nothing more important than each team member's commitment to a common purpose and set of related performance goals for which the group holds itself jointly accountable" (17). Without this internal team discipline, the team's potential accomplishments will come up short.

Better Training

Teams of the future will have to be better educated in team organization and dynamics. Unfortunately, very little time is spent in professional training or in on-the-job experiences that build these skills (6). Even though rehabilitation teams are highly touted as a critical component of the rehabilitation process, minimal time is spent in educating team members how to effectively interact and perform as team members. Professional organizations and medical and allied health academic training programs will need to dedicate a larger part of the educational curriculum to a specific introduction relating to the development, organization, and process involved in developing high-performance teams.

Rothberg (6), in writing about the future of the team approach, offers several excellent suggestions for improving the effectiveness of teams:

1. We must teach the various members how to work together and give them sufficient practice time in teamwork.
2. We must ensure that *all* members learn, understand, and respect the knowledge and skills of others.
3. We must develop clearer definitions of the roles and behaviors expected of team participants and lessen ambiguities regarding our expectations of others.
4. We must encourage utilization of the full potential of each member.
5. We need to direct attention to the initiation and maintenance of communication and to the breaking down of the barriers to interdisciplinary communications that are amenable to change—and we should be aware that not all barriers can be razed.
6. We need to attend to the maintenance of the teams—in the same way that organizations need to engage in activities that strengthen their cohesion and offer satisfaction to their personnel.
7. We need to acknowledge that leadership should shift as necessary in terms of the client's paramount needs.
8. We need to ensure that the individual in the leadership role respects the other members, as evidenced by consultation with, listening to, and involvement of them in planning.
9. We need to develop an internal system for demonstrating the accountability of each team member to the group and to the institution in which the team practices.
10. And finally, within each team there needs to be a process to acknowledge conflict as it arises and to deal with it in a manner that strengthens the group and its members.

More Critical Self-evaluation

It will also be crucial for rehabilitation teams of the future to effectively measure outcomes related to the efficiency and effectiveness of treatment interventions over time. The successful team will be able to demonstrate and measure quality throughout the continuum of care and enhance and maintain positive long-term outcomes. Unquestionably, the priority for the effectiveness of tomorrow's teams will shift from short-term outcomes to those that more directly relate to their ability to transition their consumers into the appropriate community settings and their ability to enhance or maintain the goals achieved during the rehabilitation process (20).

More Collaboration and Continuity

Effective teams of the future will develop collaborative relationships that allow the recipient of services to go through a continuum of care based on the most cost-effective resources. This process has already begun with more effective relationships between acute care centers and acute care rehabilitation programs and subsequently with subacute transitional care, home care, and outpatient services. Rehabilitation programs that are successful in integrating the flow of information from one team to another will be the successful rehabilitation teams of the future. The various programs within the continuum of care will need to develop more effective models of working in collaboration to deliver cost-effective treatment. Currently, the continuation is fragmented, in part due to HMOs electing to purchase only parts of an integrated treatment program and utilizing outside providers or in-house staff to provide the remaining components (7). This is particularly evident in capitated health care plans that elect to provide case management, physical, occupational, and psychological services from capitated service agreements in lieu of providing the service from an inpatient or outpatient treatment facility. This results in a fragmented approach without adequate communication between all treatment parties.

CONCLUSION

The challenges for rehabilitation teams in the future are enormous. Fortunately, rehabilitation has developed more experience and expertise in successfully utilizing interdisciplinary teams than have the other areas of health care (5,20). The utilization of teams has prevented the fragmentation of care by specialists working in an independent manner (6). This is one of rehabilitation's greatest assets and cost-effective features. The "aging of America" and chronicity of age-related medical issues make rehabilitation an even more important treatment model for the long-term management of the elderly, versus trying to manage singular episodic medical issues (12).

Rehabilitation can continue to be a leader in demonstrating the benefits of the transdisciplinary team approach and serve as a model for the expanding health care continuum. Improved educational programs on team development in conjunction with better research models on team effectiveness will be critical to establishing the merits of an integrated team approach for the delivery of quality cost-effective care to patients.

REFERENCES

1. Halstead LS, Rintala DH, Kanellos M. The innovative rehabilitation team: an experiment in team building. *Arch Phys Med Rehabil* 1986;67:357–361.
2. Daus C. Seamless rehab—the team approach to spinal cord injury. *Case Rev* 1995;2:64–67.
3. Brown TM. An historical view of health care. In: Agich GJ, ed. *Responsibility in health care.* Boston: D. Reidell, 1982:3–21.
4. Halstead LS. Team care in chronic illness: a critical review of the literature of the past 25 years. *Arch Phys Med Rehabil* 1976;57:507–511.
5. Purtilo RB, Meier RH. Team challenges. *Arch Phys Med Rehabil* 1993;5:327–330.
6. Rothberg JS. The rehabilitation team: future direction. *Arch Phys Med Rehabil* 1981;62:407–410.
7. Melvin JL. Status report on interdisciplinary medical rehabilitation. *Arch Phys Med Rehabil* 1989;70:273–276.
8. Strasser DC, Falconer JA, Martino-Saltzmann D. The rehabilitation team: staff perceptions of the hospital environment, the interdisciplinary team environment, and interprofessional relations. *Arch Phys Med Rehabil* 1994;75:177–182.
9. Diller L. Fostering the interdisciplinary team, fostering research in a society in transition. *Arch Phys Med Rehabil* 1990;71:275–278.
10. Jaffe KB, Walsh PA. The development of the specialty rehabilitation home care team: supporting the creative thought process. *Holistic Nurse Pract* 1993;7:36–41.
11. Melvin JL. Interdisciplinary and multidisciplinary activities and the ACRM. *Arch Phys Med Rehabil* 1980;61:379–380.
12. Fordyce WE. On interdisciplinary peers. *Arch Phys Med Rehabil* 1981;62:51–53.
13. Larson CE, LaFasto FM, eds. *Teamwork.* California: Sage, 1989.
14. Purtilo RB. Managed care: ethical issues for the rehabilitation professions. *Trends Healthcare Law Ethics* 1995;10:105–118.
15. Ducanis AJ, Golin AK. *The interdisciplinary health care team.* Maryland: Aspen Systems, 1979:21–54.
16. Keith RA. The comprehensive treatment team in rehabilitation. *Arch Phys Med Rehabil* 1991;72:269–274.
17. Katzenbach JR, Smith DK. *The wisdom of teams.* New York: HarperCollins, 1994;44:37.
18. Adler SL, Bryk E, Cesta TG, McEachen I. Collaboration: the solution to multidisciplinary care planning. *Orthop Nurs* 1995;14:21–29.
19. DeJong G, Wheatley B, Sulton J. Medical rehabilitation undergoing major shakeup in advanced manage-care markets. In: Elis Rehab Report. Research Triangle Park, NC, 1996:3527–3536.
20. Preston KM. A team approach to rehabilitation. *Home Healthcare Nurse* 1994;8:17–23.

Chapter 3

Ethics and Rehabilitation

Giles R. Scofield

Over the past 50 years, ethics has come to play an increasingly significant role in the practice of medicine, for several reasons (1). For one, advances in medicine and medical technology have dramatically increased medicine's power and expanded the range of options available to patients, families, physicians, and society (2). Second, we have learned that it is both easy to use medicine destructively, instead of constructively, and difficult to know when we are using it for good or for ill (3,4). Happy that we have new choices to make, we simultaneously find ourselves burdened with having to make them (5). The freedom to choose under conditions that are legally, ethically, and empirically complex leaves us anxious about the ambivalent, ambiguous, and uncertain decisions we make as well (6). Unless we allow the so-called technologic imperative to determine how we live and die, it is morally and ethically imperative for us to choose as responsibly, deliberately, and prudently as we can—precisely because these choices are so difficult to make (7).

Although ethics and ethical dilemmas are most commonly associated with acute care medicine, where life-and-death issues arise frequently, ethical issues can and increasingly do arise in any health care setting, making ethics everyone's responsibility, everyone's business (8,9). Medicine's success at postponing death and sustaining life means that persons with disabilities now are found everywhere—at home, work, and school, as well as in health care facilities (10,11). Additionally, because medicine's success at prolonging life has come at considerable cost, cost-containment efforts now under way are likely to challenge the judgment of patients, providers, and society (12,13). For these and other reasons, rehabilitation professionals must exercise ethically responsible judgment (14,15), regardless of where they are (16–20) and regardless of the types of patients they work with (21–24).

Unfortunately, medical ethics cannot make these choices for us, nor should it. It can and does enable and encourage us to make difficult decisions under difficult circumstances, when the law provides some, but limited guidance (25) and when there is genuine conflict and authentic doubt about what we ought to do (26,27). As it turns out, this is easier said than done, for reasons having to do with both the nature of ethics and the nature of the choices we have to make (28,29).

WHAT IS *ETHICS*?

A traditional definition of *ethics* states, "Ethics is the science that deals with conduct, in so far as this is considered as right or wrong, good or bad" (30). Ethics consists of *normative ethics* (actual standards of right and good action), *descriptive ethics* (reports of what people do and believe), and *metaethics* (analyses of the language and concepts used in ethics) (31). Medical ethics, also known as *clinical ethics* (32–34), is an example of normative ethics, in that it concerns itself with prescribed and proscribed behavior, with what people ought and ought not do

(35,36), and with how they ought to go about the business of deciding (37). Ethics attempts to tie the values that underlie *what* we decide with those that underlie *how* we decide (38).

Sources of Guidance

Traditionally, determining what one should or should not do seemed relatively easy, and involved the application of fairly straightforward ethical theories to morally troubling situations (39,40). Moral philosophy and theology once guided conscientious decision making reasonably well; except in the eyes of nostalgic sentimentalists, those days are long gone (28,41,42). It is no longer clear that traditional ways of thinking about right and wrong can and do produce good and prevent bad results (28,43). Because of the legacy of medicine in the first half of the twentieth century (44,45), deciding morally requires knowing the value and the limitations of dominant ethical theories.

Schools of Thought and the Elusive "Ought"

Given the history of moral thought and the complex intricacies of the numerous schools of thought that currently exist, it is not possible to do more than discuss the most general aspects of the most influential ethical theories (46). We would find more conflict than resolution.

One dispute among ethicists is whether it is better to reason from the clouds down or from the ground up, that is, deductively or inductively. Another is whether it is better to adhere to principles regardless of the consequences, or to produce the right consequences regardless of the means. In truth, there is something to be said for paying attention to ideas and to reality, to ends and to means. The "art" of moral reasoning, however, requires balancing these different ways of figuring out what we ought to do. To see how and why this is so, we need to take a brief look at ethical theory.

Deontologists

Deontologists believe that individuals should adhere to certain principles, regardless of the consequences that befall them or others. What makes something right or wrong is whether it is done in good faith for the right reasons, that is, according to an accepted principle or rule. There is not nothing to this perspective. That we should not lie, not wrongfully take a life, or not wrongfully deprive someone of liberty are maxims few of us would question. Related to this approach is the belief that we should not use individuals as the means to an end, our own or someone else's, a belief that most people would endorse.

For all that deontology has to offer, it has a few problems. One is that it leaves unanswered what we should do when forced to choose between two equally valid principles. If, for example, my telling the truth will jeopardize someone else's life or freedom, what should I do? More concretely, if a psychiatrist has reason to believe that my patient is going to harm another person, should he or she maintain a confidence, even though someone may be harmed as a result, or breach it even though someone may be detained and feel betrayed as a result? Not only can and do individuals feel torn by such conflicts, so can entire societies. The abortion debate, for example, can be seen as a kind of moral gridlock created by one group's insistence that we always protect life, and another's that we always respect liberty.

For all its value, deontology can be a bit prohibitive. It is better at telling us what we should not do than it is at telling us what we ought to do. And, it suggests that the world is (or should be) neater and tidier than it in fact is. For example, since all research involving human subjects requires using people as the means to an end, strict adherence to deontology would seem to prohibit research altogether, which may explain why researchers tend to favor the Helsinki Code over the Nuremberg Code. Thus, while deontology offers a lot that is of value, it is not entirely coherent or always practical.

Consequentialists

Consequentialists, also known as utilitarians, believe that what makes a decision right or wrong depends on whether the consequences are good or not. The goal here is to attain the greatest possible balance of good over evil, or the least possible harm in the pursuit of good. In contrast to deontology, what matters is not adherence to some supposedly intrinsic valid rule of right or wrong, but acting in ways that produce intrinsically good as opposed to bad consequences.

Just as few people would say that fundamental values do not matter, few people would say that consequences do not matter, which explains why consequentialism has it followers. Valuable though it is, consequentialism also has its problems. For one thing, it suggests that balancing goods is easy, as if the world consisted of apples alone, and not apples and oranges, or worse yet, apples and asparagus. Is it always so clear that we should fund one type of research instead of another? Add a new wing instead of more comfortable beds? These choices do not announce themselves, as if we had nothing to do with this balancing act. We do the balancing, and the decision about what, why, and how we balance some goods against others depends on values we bring to the analysis.

Even if we can—and we often do—accept the give and take that comes of allocating scarce resources on a grand scale, what do we do when the global decisions have a local impact on identified lives? It is all well and good to talk about the need to set limits, until the nightly news shows us someone whose life is shortened by our decision not to provide some type of care. How does one balance the need to set limits against the value of human life, or individual liberty? Does, for example, the fact that it makes no sense to render medically futile care to patients mean that we must deny them not only such care, but also the right to participate in the decision-making process? Does, for another example, the need to increase the supply of organs for transplantation purposes mean that we should loosen the rules around consent?

Like deontology, consequentialism is valuable in many respects, but troubled and even troubling in others.

It Is Not the What, but the How

While the incoherence of both deontology and consequentialism has spawned a good number of suggested solutions—phenomenology, existentialism, feminism, and virtue theory—if anything, the dizzying array of theories has made it only more difficult to know what to do. One response to this state of affairs has been the suggestion that we could avoid difficulty if we reasoned from the ground up instead of from the clouds down. Casuists suggest that it is reality, not abstract theory, that matters. To anyone who has ever listened to an ethicist or a philosopher, this theory sounds pretty attractive. Just get enough facts, understand what is going on in a situation, and what we ought to do will emerge. Because clinicians and just about everybody else are grounded in reality, casuistry seems to offer a lot.

In fact, casuistry does offer a lot, but it too has its limitations. In any given case, which facts count for what? When do we have enough facts? Anyone who has ever been on the horns of a dilemma can think of times when more facts made things less, not more clear. And anyone who has ever made a tough decision has encountered instances when they later found out something that they wish they had known earlier. Finally, the right kind of enough facts does not cause the answer to our dilemma to emerge through spontaneous generation. We decide what to do on the basis of what we know, and on the basis of what value we place on what we know. And unless we choose as we do just because we feel like it, this means that we are using something more than facts to understand what we ought to do. So, just as one cannot divorce theory from reality, one cannot divorce reality from theory, which means that casuistry, like everything else, answers some questions—and raises many others.

While there is something to be said for thinking both from the top down and from the ground up, some have suggested that the method lies elsewhere, in pragmatism or neopragmatism. Pragmatism accepts the notion that no one school of thought—be it deontologic, consequential, or something else—can or does hold the answers to what we "ought" to do. Yet it adheres to the belief that we can develop a method for discerning right from wrong, good from evil—that sensible people, if they put their heads together, can figure out what works and what does not.

While pragmatism is an understandable response to the realization that no one school of thought has a monopoly on moral truth, it is difficult to know whether it is a sophomoric or a sophisticated response to the situation in which we find ourselves. If there is something to what differing perspectives have to offer, then what seems to be the most sensible solution might be nothing other than the solution offered up by the most dominant member of the community. Thus, pragmatism has been criticized for its inability and seeming unwillingness to address the extent to which issues of power may affect moral deliberation.

Reflective Equilibrium, Postmodernism, and Beyond

The current state of ethics suggests that we need to pay attention to what we think and to how we think, but that conventional ethics has its limits in both departments. To some, this means that what we need to do is engage in "reflective equilibrium," in which we make considered judgments based on an array of considerations, judgments that we are free to revise at a latter point in time. Instead of slavish adherence to linear thinking or noncontradictory coherentism, we need to be more eclectic in what we decide and more relaxed about how things fit together. Basically, this means that instead of fighting about who is right and who is wrong, we need to decide what is valuable (and what is not) and make considered judgments, that is, choices that seem good enough for now, even though we might revise them a bit later. Instead of expecting coherence in the here and now, we should just plug along until we finally get it right. Although reflective equilibrium sounds like a sensible solution to the problem of living in a world that is as diverse as ours has turned out to be, it seems to do a better job of describing the problem than at fashioning a solution (47).

At this juncture, it is worth pointing out that conventional ethics seems to be as wedded to one view of what ethics must be as it is fearful of another view of what ethics might be. Because conventional ethics is a product of the age of reason, it reflects the belief that we can "know" the basis on which moral thinking rests, and rely on a sound method for knowing right from wrong. Simply stated, there must be a foundation and a method, or else there is only the abyss and chaos. In the minds of some, this suggests that conventional ethics is the product of "cartesian anxiety," the insistence that we must have something to rest our decisions on and the fear of what it might mean if everything amounted to nothing.

This is where postmodernism steps in. Contrary to popular belief, postmodernism is not antimodernism. It does not reject all that has come before it, but, like neopragmatism and reflective equilibrium, it agrees that we find ourselves in a world that is diverse and a bit incoherent. The difference is that postmodernism tolerates diversity and incoherence even if they turn out to be a permanent state of affairs (as opposed to the temporary condition that neopragmatism and reflective equilibrium take them to be). Interestingly, postmodernism tends to view excessive reliance on ethical theory as a kind of crutch that handicaps us, and prevents us from exercising critical judgment. Postmodernism suggests that we need to learn how to "walk without banisters," that is, to exercise the greatest degree of independent judgment we can within the limitations of human knowledge. It also suggests the virtues of tolerance and dialogue are the means by which moral "strangers" come to understand one another and to live and work amicably despite their differences (43).

The postmodern perspective is based on the belief that conventional ethics, far from avoiding nihilism, produces it. That is to say, by picking everything apart, conventional ethics creates the situation it abhors, and yet resists the realization that there is no such thing as moral knowledge, in the scientific sense, but only differing interpretations of right and wrong. And because in a world of many plausible interpretations, we cannot dismiss the possibility that dominant interpretations are not the result of reason, but of power, conventional ethics allows its belief in reason to mask the workings of power, thereby opening up the very abyss it professes to wish to avoid.

Suffice it to say that the gap that separates postmodernism from conventional ethics, while not that far, is quite deep. Nonetheless, it is possible to see the bridge that links the one with the other. That bridge is philosophical hermeneutics.

Hermeneutics is a fancy word for understanding and interpreting the world. It takes as its starting point not that we are "knowing" beings, but that we are interpretive beings. Instead of coming from nowhere, we come from somewhere. As interpretive beings, we struggle to understand others and understand the situations in which we find ourselves, which we can only do if we first understand ourselves and the perspective we bring to a situation. What is interesting about hermeneutics is that it not only acknowledges that as interpretive beings we have prejudices, but also takes as its starting point that the exercise of discerning judgment requires examining ourselves as well as the situation we confront. To the extent that philosophy is nothing more than disguised interpretation, philosophical hermeneutics seems to be the next stage in our moral development.

Interestingly, whether one follows conventional or postmodern wisdom, all roads seem to be leading to conversation, as the means by which we can make sense of ourselves, of one another, and of the world in which we find ourselves. The only difference is that conventional ethicists believe that there can be something such as an ideal speech situation, whereas the hermeneuticist believes that all conversations are historically situated. Finally, because hermeneutics acknowledges the reality of nihilism and issues of power, it is believed to stand a better chance of exorcising that demon than do theories that act as if power is not an issue. Instead of eliminating uncertainty from our lives, we need to learn to cope with it by understanding ourselves and others through conversation. Ironically, the hermeneutic message, which seems odd to conventional ethicists, sounds familiar to anyone involved in physical medicine and rehabilitation.

What to do? How to do it?

Although the current state of medical ethics may make it seem that ethics has less definitive guidance to offer than is wanted, in fact ethics offers what is needed to make complex decisions under conditions of empirical and moral uncertainty, the very conditions under which rehabilitation medicine is practiced.

At bottom, three fundamental values underlie medical ethics, regardless of what perspective one has. These are 1) respect for persons, 2) beneficence, and 3) justice (48). Respect for persons incorporates two separate, but related values: 1) that persons should be regarded as autonomous agents, and 2) that persons with diminished capacity are entitled to special protection. In short, persons are to be respected and protected. Beneficence also incorporates two separate, but related values: 1) to do no harm, and 2) to maximize the potential benefits and minimize the potential harms in any given situation, a delicate balancing act given the tension that exists between paternalism and autonomy in the rehabilitation setting. Justice implies the obligation to treat similarly situated persons similarly, and to promote fairness generally.

Integrally related to these substantive values is the informed consent doctrine (37,49). The informed consent doctrine enables clinicians and patients to negotiate what they wish to do in instances where medicine lacks an objectively definitive answer for one course of action, and in which the patient's reasonable subjective preferences deserve respect. This balances respect for the clinician's judgment in technical matters with respect for the intrinsic values of self-determination and creative self-agency that justify allowing patients to participate meaningfully in and to direct decisions affecting them (50). Thus seen, the informed consent doctrine is not an impediment to the practice of medicine, but vital to decision making under uncertain circumstances (26,51–57).

While it is not possible to catalogue all of the values that underlie the informed consent process, they certainly include 1) encouraging respect for the patient's human dignity; 2) promoting professional self-awareness; 3) discouraging deceit, coercion, manipulation, and overreaching; 4) promoting shared decision making; and 5) educating the persons involved in and affected by medical decision making (38). Because of the fundamental role that informed consent plays in medical decision making, and the misperceptions clinicians often have about it, it is worth elaborating briefly on each of these points.

Respect for a patient's human dignity involves respecting the patient for the person he or she is (58), and integrating the patient's values into decisions that set and pursue the goals of rehabilitation (59). It also requires being attentive to the nonphysical as well as the physical aspects of what it means to be a human being (60,61), and treating the patient as an essential partner to the therapeutic relationship and to decisions made within the context of that relationship (62). In short, taking persons seriously requires taking patients seriously.

Professionals can understand patients better by understanding themselves better also. Professional self-awareness concerns itself with understanding one's attitudes and beliefs about what it means to be a professional or a patient, as well as what it may mean to say that a patient is hateful (63,64) or undesirable (65). It also requires understanding what one's own beliefs are concerning what it means for a patient to be disabled, diseased, or dying. Self-understanding enhances the understanding one has of others.

Rational, shared decision making speaks to the desirability of setting and pursuing the goals of treatment realistically and collaboratively, in a manner that values what the patient and the physician bring to the physician-patient relationship. Patients are less likely to understand or to become personally invested in treatment goals that are imposed on them instead of formulated with them. When patients and families play a central role in the decision-making process, they are less likely to undermine the goals of treatment, and more likely to complement the interdisciplinary team approach to rehabilitation (66).

To the extent that we value voluntary, shared decision making, clinicians must eschew decision-making strategies that are coercive, deceptive, or otherwise prevent patients from choosing as seems best to them (31,50). While few clinicians are likely to resort to the use of force or the threat of using force in order to "get" patients to decide matters a certain way, avoiding coercion also requires attending to the inherently coercive nature of institutionalized treatment, especially in the context of institutionalized long-term care (67,68). Similarly, while few clinicians are likely to engage in outright deceit in order to secure a patient's consent, the subtle creation of false hopes and unreasonable expectations within the clinic, and the not-too-subtle misrepresentations made in the context of marketing health care services must be guarded against (69,70).

Manipulation is a generic label applied to forms of influence that are neither persuasive nor coercive. In medical decision making, manipulation commonly takes the form of informational manipulation, in which information is packaged and presented in a manner that alters the patient's understanding of a situation and, correspondingly, steers or motivates him or her to be inclined to accept the recommendation of the clinician. While it is impossible to package and present information in order to make decisions that are absolutely free of extraneous influence, attending to the how and the what of information presentation can reduce the extent to which manipulation occurs.

Because education is essential to the rehabilitation model, its importance in the informed consent process is likely to be self-evident to many rehabilitation professionals (71,72). Educating those involved in and affected by clinical decision making requires involving in the decision-making process those individuals whose participation and understanding are essential to the patient's successful rehabilitation and reintegration into society. Educating the patient and the patient's family enables them to understand what the patient's disability consists of, and what achievements and limitations they can reasonably expect to encounter. This should enable them to manage and cope better with the vicissitudes of the rehabilitation process, the progress, setbacks, and plateaus that come of living with a disability, and equip them to cope intellectually and emotionally with the situation in which they find themselves.

Education involves more than the patient and the patient's family. Because education has as much to do with learning as with teaching, it also concerns the provider's obligation to learn about the patient, in order to better assist the patient to live with a disability. Finally, educating third-party payors and those who will work with and around the patient can smooth the patient's reintegration into society when the patient is discharged.

If clinicians keep these values and purposes in mind as they work with patients, they are likely to be able to identify, address, and discuss ethical dilemmas in a manner that is structured enough and fluid enough to enable them to conduct themselves comfortably under the dynamic, fluid, and often uncertain conditions they encounter in the rehabilitation context. Having discussed the what and the how of ethical decision making, I now address some specific issues that come up frequently within the practice of physical medicine and rehabilitation.

COMMON ISSUES

Admission/Placement

Because the number of individuals in need of rehabilitation exceeds the resources—personnel, facilities and equipment, money, and time—that can be dedicated to this aspect of patient care, admitting patients to rehabilitation programs and discharging them properly remain chronic problems (73,74). Although their proximity to these issues makes rehabilitation professionals especially concerned with the ethical dilemmas that the gap between demand and supply creates for them (75), in truth, the dilemmas they encounter are similar to those encountered by others whose decisions about allocating scarce resources affect the quality and even the length of life enjoyed by patients, most notably in the area of solid organ transplantation (76,77).

Ideally, admission decisions are supposed to reflect the application of objective, medical criteria to the evaluation of particular patients in light of their diagnosis and prognosis. In fact, it does not always work out that way. Even if the criteria employed are objective, they may not be applied accurately and fairly. Additionally, subjective concerns and biases can and do influence decisions about which patients merit admission and which do not (78). Although medical professionals are expected to properly exercise discretion in this area, the limits of proper discretion remain contested (79,80).

Of particular concern in a health care system that manifests financial diversity but not universal access is the likelihood that patients who are equally qualified from the medical perspective may be treated differently for financial reasons. In one sense, it makes little sense to expend funds for rehabilitation if the funding needed to make rehabilitation succeed upon discharge is lacking. On the other hand, it is troubling to deny patients the opportunity for meaningful rehabilitation simply because society and its health care system fail them. For those patients for whom the necessary funding is absent or fragmented, those in charge of admissions and discharge planning need to be creative and inventive (81).

Compliance/Noncompliance

Because how well patients do depends on how well they take care of themselves, compliance and noncompliance are important concerns for rehabilitation professionals (82). Because self-care is a long-term prospect for persons with a chronic disability, addressing noncompliance enhances the quality and length of a patient's life, and reduces the ways in which noncompliance wastes time, money, and resources. As it turns out, noncompliance is a multifactored phenomenon, making the problem of noncompliance more complex than is commonly imagined to be the case (83).

For one thing, compliance and noncompliance are ill-defined and hard to measure (84). Also, the expectation of compliance depends on a number of factors, such as the patient's physical, cognitive, and emotional state (85), and the patient's education, resources, and environment (86). To the extent that providers fail to communicate clearly, consistently, and effectively, compliance also can be inhibited (87,88). Finally, to a large extent, what is regarded as noncompliance from the physician's perspective is nothing other than the patient's decision about what he or she is willing to do in order to have an acceptable quality of life (89).

Simply put, just as there is no one way to live as an able-bodied person, there is no one way to live as a person with a disability. Not everyone with a disability needs to be a paralympian. If we are to live in the world of difference that disability creates, we must tolerate difference within and among the members of all communities, including the community of persons with disabilities.

For all these reasons, the educational model of informed consent found within the rehabilitation context is important, both because it enhances the patient's understanding of the goals of treatment and because it enhances the provider's understanding of what the patient values (90,91). Informed consent does not eliminate the problem of noncompliance—nothing can or should eliminate the diversity of lifestyle choices. But it can enable individuals whose beliefs differ to understand one another better despite their differences. Whether the advent of managed care and cost-containment measures limits or curtails the long-term cost-effectiveness of education for the sake of achieving short-term gains remains to be seen (92).

Cost-Containment Measures

Utilization review, managed care, and the increased use of cost-containment measures challenge rehabilitation medicine (93–95) as they do medicine generally (96–98). The challenge is to continue to provide a meaningful level of care with increasingly restricted resources (99–101) to patients who have traditionally been underserved by the health care system (102) and disfavored by the insurance industry (103–106). Restrictive payment systems and capitation are likely to introduce conflicts of interest into the physician-patient relationship (107–109), some of which may be resolved in ways that risk legal liability as state and federal governments prosecute fraud and abuse (110).

At the clinical level, managed care's emphasis on definitive outcomes and its interest in efficient procedures are likely to frustrate rehabilitation's emphasis on care as opposed to cure, and for a treatment process that enables patients to attain and sustain a meaningful quality of life (111–115). This reflects what happens when disability care is judged according to acute care expectations. To the extent that acute care endorses a "normal" outcome that is essentially cured, largely devoid of residual impairment or morbidity, with function fully restored, rehabilitation never can and never will meet those expectations unless it stops being rehabilitative (116). Until our expectations of medicine change, such that we can and do reconcile the different perspectives that acute care and rehabilitative medicine bring to the table, the disabled and rehabilitation providers will be judged according to standards that create not simply false, but inappropriate expectations for patients and providers alike.

While the development of integrated systems of care is likely to benefit persons who are poorly served by fragmented systems, capitation and the tendency of insurers to be averse to persons with a chronic illness or disability are as likely to work to the disadvantage of persons with disabilities (117,118). Whether managed care adversely impacts the delivery of rehabilitation and the education of physiatrists remains to be seen (119,120). All told, this makes it more important and more difficult for institutions to provide care in a manner that reconciles the ethics of care with the ethics of business (121–123).

Confidentiality

We value confidentiality for two reasons (124). First, confidentiality is intrinsically good, in that maintaining confidences demonstrates respect for an individual's right to determine how information concerning himself or herself is disseminated. Confidentiality also serves an instrumental function, in that patients are more inclined to seek out treatment from and be candid with their providers if they believe that information shared in the clinical encounter will be kept confidential. For these reasons, the general rule is that confidential information concerning a patient may not and should not be disclosed to others without the patient's consent (31–33).

As with any such general rule, there are difficulties in fulfilling the expectation of privacy (125). Within medical institutions, a vast array of individuals need to have access to information concerning a patient in order for them to be able to do their jobs. The sheer number of persons who have access to otherwise confidential information because of their need to know has led some to wonder whether confidentiality, within medicine, is a decrepit concept (126). Such concerns are heightened within rehabilitation medicine, where the concept of the interdisciplinary team requires the sharing of confidential information. Finally, the introduction of the computers into medical practice raises practical questions about how the integrity of confidential information can be protected (127,128).

As troubling as it is to maintain confidentiality is the recognition of situations in which providers are under a duty to reveal otherwise confidential information (129). In many states, for example, the law requires health care professionals to report injuries and wounds caused by weapons such as knives and guns. The states commonly impose other sorts of requirements concerning instances of abuse and neglect, or instances in which an individual has a communicable disease, acquired immunodeficiency syndrome (AIDS) being an especially prominent concern for many persons (130,131). Similarly, the law in many states imposes the requirement to take some action when there is a reasonable basis to believe that a patient poses a danger to third parties. Finally, there remains the difficulty of dealing with a patient whose ability to function within the community is sufficiently impaired that, for example, his or her driving privileges need to be curtailed (132).

One as-yet-unexplored aspect of confidentiality concerns the reintegration of patients into school or employment. While persons with disabilities are as entitled as others are to the assurance that confidential information concerning them will be maintained, this need must be balanced against the disclosure of the kind and amount of information that others need to know in order for the integration process to go forward. The dilemmas here exist on several levels.

First, while the disclosure of information concerning a patient, together with the sort of education that can enable others to appreciate its significance, ideally should enable persons to return to school or employment, it may have the opposite effect. Second, as persons with disabilities leave institutions where the practice of maintaining confidentiality is routine, and move into settings where it is not, they may lose some of the protections that they would be afforded within the medical community (133). This suggests that the delicate balance between maintaining confidences and properly sharing information is likely to create novel tensions as persons with disabilities move beyond the clinical setting.

Research

Research involving human subjects is important for the advancement of medical knowledge, and risky in that it subjects human beings to what may turn out to have been unwarranted risk. Balancing the end of advancing knowledge against the means employed toward that end makes research one of the most morally perilous aspects of medical science. The Nuremberg Code of Ethics and the subsequent Helsinki Code of Ethics attest to the ethical significance of experimentation involving human subjects (134). Repeated instances in which experimentation involving human subjects has exceeded the limits of proper conduct attest to the persistent need for concern in this area, and of the seeming inability of external controls to adequately protect human subjects involved in research (135–137).

Within the United States, research involving human subjects is subject to regulations promulgated by the Food and Drug Administration and by the National Institutes of Health, and overseen at the clinical level through institutional review boards (138). In order to approve a research protocol, an institutional review board must 1) ensure that the risk to human subjects is minimized; 2) determine that the risk to the human subjects is minimal in relation to the anticipated benefits, if any, to the human subjects and to the importance of the knowledge that may reasonably be expected to result; 3) determine that the selection of subjects is equitable; 4) provide for the proper monitoring of the data; 5) ensure that each subject gives adequate informed consent and that the informed consent is properly documented; and 6) provide adequate protection for the privacy of the human subjects and the confidentiality of the data (139). For consent to be adequate, the circumstances under which consent is sought must afford the subject sufficient opportunity to consider whether or not to participate, and minimize the possibility of coercion or undue influence. Special rules provide additional protection to subjects of experimentation who are or may be particularly vulnerable, such as children and prisoners.

Of particular interest to those who are interested in cerebral resuscitation and spinal cord preservation are recently issued regulations that enable informed consent to be waived when it involves "emergency research" (140–142). Of additional concern are the conflicts of interest created by the fact that researchers and their institutions are able to benefit financially from research and the corporatization of research generally (143).

Limiting Life

Medicine's ability to extend life makes it possible for individuals to choose whether, and if so, for how long, they wish to be sustained by life-sustaining technology. (144,145). Generally speaking, patients have the right to refuse treatment, including life-sustaining treatment (146). The difficulties have to do with determining whether, when, and how this is to occur within the fluid and uncertain conditions of the rehabilitation context (147).

The right to refuse treatment is not limited to patients who are terminally ill, but extends also to individuals who are chronically ill or disabled, which would include persons with tetraplegia (148–152), persons with traumatic brain injury (153,154), and burn patients. The right to refuse treatment includes the right to refuse treatment whether it is regarded as extraordinary or ordinary, advanced or basic, optional or obligatory. This means that patients have the right to refuse ventilators, cardiopulmonary resuscitation (155,156), and feeding tubes. Finally, decisions to forgo treatment are as legally and ethically permissible regardless of whether the choice is to withhold or to withdraw treatment. While it can be more difficult psychologically to withdraw than to withhold treatment, the one decision is as legal as the other.

In order to effect such a decision, it is first necessary to determine whether the patient is competent and has the requisite decisional capacity to refuse treatment, a task that can be made difficult because of the variability in assessments of competency (157,158) and the difficulty in judging the presence or absence of neurobehavioral (159,160) and emotional problems (161). It can be especially difficult to assess whether the patient has sufficient knowledge of and insight into his or her condition when the request to refuse treatment is made relatively soon after injury (162).

If the patient is incompetent, a decision to forgo treatment is made through the process of surrogate decision making, in which a duly authorized person "speaks for" the patient (163). Although the legal requirements for surrogate decision making vary somewhat from one state to the next (164), generally speaking, a surrogate may authorize a decision to forgo life-sustaining treatment based on one of three factors (165,166): 1) clear and convincing evidence of the patient's actual wish to halt treatment, based on statements the patient made while competent; 2) substituted judgment, in which all that is known about the patient is used to determine what the patient in all likelihood would say if asked; and 3) best interests, in which the objective determination is that continued treatment would not serve this patient's best interests (167,168). In addition to the difficulties that can be encountered in ascertaining, interpreting, and fulfilling the wishes of a once-competent patient, there is the difficulty of integrating quality of life considerations into these decisions in a manner that reflects the patient's subjective values and that does not project others' beliefs about disability onto the disabled (169–171).

The ongoing controversy about a patient's right to refuse treatment has been complicated by two additional developments: medical futility and physician-assisted suicide. The medical futility debate concerns itself with whether patients may be denied treatment even if they wish it. The physician-assisted suicide debate has to do with whether patients may demand that physicians write a prescription for life-ending medication.

Because there is no right to treatment and supposedly there is no harm done when a patient is denied treatment that would be medically futile, there is a burgeoning controversy about whether patients have any interest in decisions concerning medically futile treatment. For example, some argue that persons with irreversible, incurable conditions, such as patients in a persistent vegetative state, should not be resuscitated regardless of their own prior or their surrogate's current preferences, and that it may be wrong altogether to render any life-sustaining treatment to such persons. This debate has been complicated by the fact that no definition of medical futility has been reached; by the fact that there is evidence that physicians do not and cannot make futility assessments objectively, fairly, and accurately; and by a limited number of cases that have refused to uphold a physician's right to unilaterally forgo medically futile care. Of interest to persons with disabilities is the concern that decisions about medically futile treatment may, and in all likelihood will, fall disproportionately on them. As pressures to limit the costs associated with health care mount, the debate about medically futile treatment is likely to become increasingly significant.

Physician-assisted suicide is distinguishable from decisions to forgo life-sustaining treatment in that the intent of the person and the manner of death differ. A decision to allow a patient to die naturally is not the same as a decision to enable a patient to die as the result of a drug overdose. The legalization of physician-assisted suicide has been debated for many years. Now that the U.S. Supreme Court has ruled that the constitution does not require the legalization of physician-assisted suicide, the issue will move to the legislative arena. At that juncture, the unanswered question will become whether the constitution prohibits the legalization of physician-assisted suicide.

Discrimination

The emergence of the disabilities rights movement as a credible political force (172) suggests that it is only a matter of time before the issue of what it means to discriminate against someone on account of his or her disability is forthrightly addressed. Within the United States, the Americans with Disabilities Act provides some protection against discrimination in the context of housing, employment, education, and access to public facilities. Interestingly, and perhaps tellingly, the Americans with Disabilities Act does not extend to decisions about whether to provide or withhold treatment, or to decisions about whether to underwrite or pay for health care, even though such decisions are of obvious significance to individuals whose quality and length of life depend on the extent and manner of treatment that they receive (173).

For the time being, it is difficult to know what society will make of this issue. To be sure, a health care system that is dedicated to curing patients with acute conditions is less concerned about persons with chronic, incurable conditions. Similarly, what the insurance industry regards as the sound actuarial practice of not paying for chronic conditions and "custodial" care means that "valid" insurance practice is not good for persons who are "invalids," that is, the disabled. What this really means is that the survival of the private financing of health care makes it incumbent upon insurers to avoid or limit the financial risks of insuring persons with chronic conditions. Simply stated, the survival of artificially created persons (corporations) depends on their ability to avoid financing the care of artificially sustained persons (the disabled). Given the extent to which American society believes that the free market can and will make every problem go away, and to which it disfavors persons with disabilities, to understand the situation is to see how intractable it is. For persons with disabilities to receive decent care, Americans will have to forsake what they favor and embrace what they shun. You do not need a degree in psychiatry to appreciate how difficult this is likely to be (174).

Now that we see the problem, let us see how it plays itself out. If one believes that every decision to limit care discriminates against persons with disabilities, then it would seem impossible to ever limit anyone's care. This turns the Americans with Disabilities Act into the Universal Access to Care Guarantee Act, something that Congress never intended, even if it should have. If, on the other hand, one believes that decisions to limit care cannot possibly be discriminatory, then one denies the possibility (much less the established reality) that prejudicial attitudes and beliefs about persons with disabilities affect decisions about housing, employment, and access to facilities as well as health care.

It obviously makes no more sense to believe that every decision is discriminatory than it does to believe that no decision can be. By the same token, if what is wrong with the current system is that it allows providers to deny care indiscriminately, forcing them to provide care indiscriminately is no solution. The real problem seems to lie in our inability and unwillingness to make difficult choices about who does and who does not receive treatment. Instead we delegate these choices to the invisible workings of the marketplace, in the vain and unproven hope that things will turn out right.

Simply put, we are afraid of making the sorts of choices we must make if we are to discriminate among persons with disabilities without discriminating against them. The situation has more to do with emotion than with reason, because we dread the prospect of having to care for everyone as much as the prospect of caring for some, but not for others. Fear about what it *might* mean—as opposed to what it *would* mean (175)—were health care decisions subjected to antidiscrimination claims probably explains why the desire to subject health care decision making to such review is dismissed as an impossibility (176,177), and as the overzealous perspective of disability rights extremists (178). Because we believe ourselves to be caught between two unpalatable possibilities—of never denying care or of cavalierly doing so—we are paralyzed from exercising responsible judgment. Fear of the unknown, the root of all prejudice, makes us so afraid of doing the wrong thing that we cannot bring ourselves to do what would be the right thing.

Instead of succumbing to the dread of actually choosing, or finding false comfort in the illusion that the market chooses just fine, we must face the real burden of choice. The first step in that process requires admitting that individuals can and do hold prejudicial attitudes and beliefs about persons with disabilities (179–184). Unless we wish to indulge in the wishful notion that these beliefs are compartmentalized or neutralized, we cannot dismiss the possibility that they can and sometimes do improperly influence a decision maker's discretion. Yet, that insight cuts both ways. It is just as wrong to limit treatment on the belief that no one would want to live "like that," as it is to compel treatment because of the belief that no one would not want to live "like that." The reality is that few people choose to have a catastrophe befall them, and that people respond to catastrophic injury differently. Unless we believe that people should respond uniformly to being disabled, we need to enable and allow them to make that choice, provisional and fluctuating though it may be, in terms of who they wish to be and not as seems best to others.

If that is so, then the task lies in distinguishing those decisions that are discriminating from those that are discriminatory. While that is easier said than done, it is better attempted than not. In fact, if one returns to the earlier discussion of reflective equilibrium, and of the values that guide the informed consent process, it is easy to see why it is important to pay close attention to how we decide—because we cannot know for certain what we ought to do. Ironically, in order for us to get it right when it comes to persons with disabilities, *we* need to learn how to "walk without banisters."

To the extent that the informed consent doctrine enables and encourages us to discuss matters we might prefer not to, and requires us to make decisions visibly instead of invisibly, it makes it possible for us to make decisions under conditions of uncertainty, as attentive to the prospects of being correct as to the possibilities of being in error. Once we accept the fact that human beings make decisions about human beings—that these are not decisions made for and about us by some external guidance—we can go about the business of making them in a manner that is morally attentive to what is at stake. While making these decisions in a less than forthright manner has its appeal, ultimately everyone is best served if these choices are made openly and honestly, especially if we are concerned about the possibility of inflicting unwarranted suffering or unwarranted death on persons with disabilities.

CONCLUSIONS

In the end, ethics is everyone's responsibility, for the simple reason that choosing is something that we—not the system—do. It would probably be easier for all of us if we knew that the answers we give today would be correct tomorrow, or if we could hand these decisions over to some invisible force, whether that is some ethical theory or the invisible hand of the marketplace. It just does not work that way. Instead of dreading what it might be like to make these decisions, we must come to know what it is like to make them if we are to be as morally attentive as we say we would like to be. If there is one thing more fearful than fear itself, it is what happens when we choose on the basis of ignorance instead of knowledge.

Making our way through the world with an attitude of reflective equilibrium can link, instead of separate, the able-bodied and the disabled, and tie what we think to how we think. Whether the uncertainty of choosing leads us to build walls that separate, or bridges that connect us to one another is for us to choose.

To be sure, the burden of choice is enormous; but so too are the perils of acting as if we do not choose, or of delegating the burden of choice to others. If the ethics of rehabilitation teaches us anything, it is not only that we can, but also that we must, find the heart and the courage to choose under conditions of doubt. While there is every reason to believe that we can and should make these decisions openly and responsibly, only time will tell whether we have the will to so.

REFERENCES

1. Institute of Medicine. *Society's choices: social and ethical decision making in biomedicine.* Washington, DC: National Academy Press, 1995.
2. Veatch RM. *Death, dying and the biological revolution: our last quest for responsibility.* New Haven, CT: Yale University Press, 1989.
3. Bauman Z. *Modernity and the holocaust.* Ithaca, NY: Cornell University Press, 1992.
4. Scofield GR. Lost and not yet found. *HEC Forum* 1996;8:372–391.
5. Calabresi G, Bobbitt P. *Tragic choices.* New York: WW Norton, 1978.
6. Bauman Z. *Modernity and ambivalence.* Ithaca: Cornell University Press, 1991.
7. Jonas H. *The imperative of responsibility: in search of an ethics for the technological age.* Chicago: University of Chicago Press, 1984.
8. Jennings B, Callahan D, Caplan AL. Ethical challenges of chronic illness. *Hastings Cent Rep* 1988;18(1):1–16.
9. Caplan AL, Callahan D, Haas J. Ethical and policy issues in rehabilitation medicine. *Hastings Cent Rep* 1987;17(2):1–20.
10. Banja J. Rehabilitation medicine. In: Reich W. ed. *Encyclopedia of bioethics.* New York: Macmillan, 1995;2201–2206.
11. The Hastings Center. The technological tether: an introduction to ethical and social issues in high-tech home care. *Hastings Cent Rep* 1994;24(suppl):S1–S28.
12. Meier RH. Recent developments in rehabilitation giving rise to important new (and old) ethical issues and concerns. *Am J Phys Med Rehabil* 1988;67:7–11.
13. Rubin SE, Millard RP. Ethical principles and American public policy on disability. *J Rehab* 1991;57:13–16.
14. Haas J. Ethics in rehabilitation medicine. *Arch Phys Med Rehabil* 1986;67:270–271.
15. Pearson L. Ethics and rehabilitation. *SCI Nurs* 1989;6(3):48–51.
16. Kaiser JM, Brown J. Ethical dilemmas in private rehabilitation. *J Rehabil* 1988;54(4):27–30.
17. Wong HD, Millard RP. Ethical dilemmas encountered by independent living service providers. *J Rehab* 1992;58:10–15.
18. Patterson JB. Ethics and rehabilitation supervision. *J Rehabil* 1989;55(4):44–49.
19. Cook CA, Semmler CJ. Ethical dilemmas in driver education. *Am J Occup Ther* 1991;45:517–522.
20. Hotes LS, Johnson JA, Sicilian L. Long-term care, rehabilitation, and legal and ethical considerations in the management of neuromuscular disease with respiratory dysfunction. *Clin Chest Med* 1994;15:783–795.

21. Groce NE, Zola IK. Multiculturalism, chronic illness and disability. *Pediatrics* 1993;91:1048–1055.

22. Matthews DJ, Meier RH. Bartholome W. Ethical issues encountered in pediatric rehabilitation. *Pediatrician* 1990;17:108–114.

23. Bach JR, Barnett V. Ethical considerations in the management of individuals with severe neuromuscular disorders. *Am J Phys Med Rehabil* 1994;73:134–140.

24. Anzalone ME. Occupational therapy in neonatology: what is our ethical response? *Am J Occup Ther* 1994;48:563–566.

25. Hazard GC. Law, morals, and ethics. *So Ill Univ Law J* 1995;19:447–458.

26. Scofield GR. Ethical considerations in rehabilitation medicine. *Arch Phys Med Rehabil* 1993;74:341–346.

27. Holzman IR, Stillo JV. Cases and doubts. *Mt Sinai J Med* 1995;62:112–115.

28. Engelhardt HT. *The foundations of bioethics.* New York: Oxford University Press, 1996.

29. Engelhardt HT. Medical ethics for the 21st century. *J Am Coll Cardiol* 1991;18:303–307.

30. Dewey J, Tufts JH. *Ethics.* New York: Henry Holt, 1932:8.

31. Beauchamp TL, Childress JF. *Principles of biomedical ethics.* New York: Oxford University Press, 1994.

32. Lo B. *Resolving ethical dilemmas: a guide for clinicians.* Baltimore: Williams & Wilkins, 1995.

33. Jonsen AR, Siegler M, Winslade WJ. *Clinical ethics.* New York: McGraw-Hill, 1992.

34. Beauchamp TL, McCullough LB. *Medical ethics: the moral responsibilities of physicians.* Englewood Cliffs, NJ: Prentice-Hall, 1984.

35. Pellegrino ED. Clinical ethics: biomedical ethics at the bedside. *JAMA* 1988;260:837–839.

36. Raz J. *Practical reasons and norms.* Princeton, NJ: Princeton University Press, 1990.

37. Faden R, Beauchamp TL, King NMP. *A history and theory of informed consent.* New York: Oxford University Press, 1986.

38. Katz J, Capron AM. *Catastrophic diseases: who decides what?* New Brunswick, NJ: Transaction Books, 1982.

39. Calabresi G. *Ideals, beliefs, attitudes and the law.* Syracuse, NY: Syracuse University Press, 1985:87–114.

40. Ramsey P. *Ethics at the edges of life.* New Haven, CT: Yale University Press, 1978.

41. Arras JD, Steinbock B. *Ethical issues in modern medicine.* Mountainview, CA: Mayfield Publishing, 1995:1–39.

42. Pellegrino ED. The metamorphosis of medical ethics. *JAMA* 1993;269:1158–1162.

43. Engelhardt HT. *Bioethics and secular humanism: the search for a common morality.* London: SCM Press, 1991.

44. Burt RA. The suppressed legacy of Nuremberg. *Hastings Cent Rep* 1996;26(5):30–33.

45. Jonas H. *Mortality and morality: the search for the good after Auschwitz.* Evanston, IL: Northwestern University Press, 1996.

46. Brillhart BA. Ethics in rehabilitation nursing. *Rehabil Nurs* 1995;20:44–47.

47. Horkheimer M. *Eclipse of reason.* New York: Continuum Press, 1996.

48. National Commission for the Protection of Human Subjects in Biomedical and Behavioral Research. *The Belmont report: ethical guidelines for the protection of human subjects of research.* Washington, DC: U.S. Government Printing Office, 1979.

49. Katz J. Legal and ethical issues of consent in health care. In: Reich W, ed. *Encyclopedia of bioethics.* New York: Macmillan, 1995:1256–1265.

50. President's Commission for the Study of Ethical Problems in Medicine and Biomedical and Behavioral Research. *Making health care decisions.* Washington, DC: U.S. Government Printing Office, 1982.

51. Brody H. Transparency: informed consent in primary care. *Hastings Cent Rep* 1989;19:5–9.

52. Laine C, Davidoff F. Patient-centered medicine: a professional evolution. (The patient-physician relationship.) *JAMA* 1996;275:152–156.

53. Quill TE, Brody H. Physician recommendations and patient autonomy: finding a balance between physician power and patient choice. *Ann Intern Med* 1996;125:763–769.

54. Caplan AL. Informed consent and provider-patient relationships in rehabilitation medicine. *Arch Phys Med Rehabil* 1988;69:312–317.

55. Szasz TS, Hollender MH. The basic models of the doctor-patient relationship. *Arch Intern Med* 1956;97:585–592.

56. Katz J. Why doctors don't disclose uncertainty. *Hastings Cent Rep* 1984;14:35–44.

57. Fox RC. *Experiment perilous: physicians and patients facing the unknown.* Glencoe, IL: Free Press, 1959.

58. Spelman EV. On treating persons as persons. *Ethics* 1978;88:150–161.

59. Meier RH, Purtilo RB. Ethical issues and the patient-provider relationship. *Am J Phys Med Rehabil* 1994;73:365–366.

60. Barnard D. Healing the damaged self: identity, intimacy, and meaning in the lives of the chronically ill. *Perspect Biol Med* 1990;33:535–546.

61. Zola IK. Denial of emotional needs to people with handicaps. *Arch Phys Med Rehabil* 982;63:63–67.

62. Haas JF. Ethical considerations of goal setting for patient care in rehabilitation medicine. *Am J Phys Med Rehabil* 1993;72:228–232.

63. Groves JE. Taking care of the hateful patient. *N Engl J Med* 1978;298:883–887.

64. Gans JS. Hate in the rehabilitation setting. *Arch Phys Med Rehabil* 1983;64;176–179.

65. Papper S. The undesirable patient. *J Chronic Dis* 1970;22:777–779.

66. Purtilo RB. Ethical issues in team work: the context of rehabilitation. *Arch Phys Med Rehabil* 1988;69:318–322.

67. Agich GJ. *Autonomy and long-term care.* New York: Oxford University Press, 1993.

68. Lidz CW, Fischer L, Arnold RM. *The erosion of autonomy in long-term care.* New York: Oxford University Press, 1992.

69. Banja JD. Deception in advertising and marketing: ethical implications in rehabilitation. *Arch Phys Med Rehabil* 1994;75:1015–1018.

70. Patterson JB. The client as customer: achieving service quality and customer satisfaction in rehabilitation. *J Rehabil* 1992;58(4): 16–21.

71. Anderson T. Educational frame of reference: an additional model for rehabilitation medicine. *Arch Phys Med Rehabil* 1978;59:203–206.

72. Anderson T. An alternative frame of reference for rehabilitation: the helping process versus the medical model. *Arch Phys Med Rehabil* 1975;56:101–104.

73. Haas JF. Admission to rehabilitation centers: selection of patients. *Arch Phys Med Rehabil* 1988;69:329–322.

74. Caplan AL. The ethics of gatekeeping in rehabilitation medicine. *J Head Rehabil Trauma* 1996;12: 29–36.

75. Callahan D. Allocating health care resources: the vexing case of rehabilitation. *Am J Phys Med Rehabil* 1993;72:101–105.

76. Fox RC, Swats J. *The courage to fail.* Chicago: University of Chicago Press, 1978.

77. Annas GJ. Prostitute, poet, and playboy: rationing schemes for organ transplantation. *Am J Public Health* 1985;75:187–189.

78. Dougherty CJ. Values in rehabilitation: happiness, freedom, and fairness. *J Rehabil* 1991;57(1):7–12.

79. Hadorn D. The problem of discrimination in health care priority setting. *JAMA* 1992;268:1454–1459.

80. Scofield GR. Medical futility judgments: discriminating or discriminatory? *Seton Hall Law Rev* 1995;25:927–948.

81. Johnson K, Tracy P, Riccio SN, Grant T. Collaborative admission and discharge planning for the individual with high tetraplegia and ventilator dependency. *Top Spinal Cord Injury Rehabil* 1997;2(3):1–10.

82. Scofield GR. The problem of (non-)compliance: is it patients or patience? *HEC Forum* 1995;7:150–165.

83. Eraker SA, Kirscht J, Becker MH. Understanding and improving patient compliance. *Ann Intern Med* 1984;100:258–268.

84. Rudd P. In search of the gold standard for compliance measurement. *Arch Intern Med* 1979;139:627–628.

85. Ley P. Cognitive variables and noncompliance. *J Compliance Health Care* 1986;1:171–188.

86. Garrity TF. Medical compliance and the clinician-patient relationship: a review. *Soc Sci Med* 1981;15:215–222.

87. Francis V, Korsch BM, Morris MJ. Gaps in doctor-patient communication: patients' response to medical advice. *N Engl J Med* 1969;280:535–540.

88. Haney CA, Colson AC. Ethical responsibility in physician-patient communication. *Ethics Sci Med* 1980;7:27–36.

89. Veatch RM. Voluntary risks to health: the ethical issues. *JAMA* 1980;243:50–55.

90. Coy JA. Autonomy-based informed consent: ethical implications for patient noncompliance. *Phys Ther* 1989;69:826–833.

91. Bone RC. The bottom line in asthma management is patient education. *Am J Med* 1993;94:561–563.

92. Morreim H. Lifestyles of the risky and infamous: from managed care to managed lives. *Hastings Cent Rep* 1995;26(5):5–12.

93. Purtilo RB. Managed care: ethical issues for the rehabilitation professions. *Trends Health Care Law Ethics* 1995;10(1–2):105–108.

94. Leri JE. The psychological, political, and economic realities of brain injury rehabilitation in the 1990's. *Brain Injury* 1995;9: 533–542.

95. Wheatley B, DeJong G, Sutton JP. Managed care and the transformation of the medical rehabilitation industry. *Health Care Manage Rev* 1997;22(3):25–39.

96. AMA Council on Ethical and Judicial Affairs. Ethical issues in managed care. *JAMA* 1995;273:330–335.

97. Emanuel E, Dubler NN. Preserving the physician-patient relationship in the era of managed care. *JAMA* 1995;273:323–329.

98. Institute of Medicine. *Controlling costs and changing patient care? The role of utilization management.* Washington, DC: National Academy Press, 1989.

99. Kane JT, Gallagher AJ, Davis DM. Diagnostic related groups: their impact on an inpatient rehabilitation program. *Arch Phys Med Rehabil* 1987;68:833–836.

100. Batavia AI, DeJong G. Prospective payment for medical rehabilitation. *Arch Phys Med Rehabil* 1988;69:377–380.

101. Evans RL, Hendricks RD, Bishop DS, et al. Prospective payment

for rehabilitation: effects on hospital readmission, home care, and placement. *Arch Phys Med Rehabil* 1990;71:291–294.

102. Alexcis LMB, Corea J, Kennell DL. Implications of health care financing, delivery, and benefit design for persons with disabilities. In: Weiner JM, Clauser SB, Kennell DL, eds. *Persons with disabilities: issues in health care financing and service delivery.* Washington, DC: Brookings Institution, 1996:95–116.

103. Kinney ED, Steinmetz SK. Notes from the insurance underground: how the chronically ill cope. *J Health Polit Policy Law* 1994;19:633–642.

104. Enteen R. People with MS view health insurance ills. *Inside MS* 1993;11(1):5–6.

105. Parette HP, Van Biervliet A. Rehabilitation assistive technology issues for infants and young children with disabilities: a preliminary examination. *J Rehabil* 1991;57(3):27–36.

106. MacManus MA, Newacheck P. Health insurance differentials among minority children with chronic conditions and the role of federal agencies and private foundations in improving financial access. *Pediatrics* 1993;91:1040–1047.

107. Berenson RA. Capitation and conflict of interest. *Health Affairs* 1986;5:141–146.

108. Morriem H. The ethics of incentives in managed care. *Trends Health Care Law Ethics* 1995;10(1–2):56–62.

109. Rodwin MA. Conflicts in managed care. *N Engl J Med* 1995;332:604–607.

110. Rodwin MA. *Medicine, money and morals.* New York: Oxford University Press, 1993.

111. Sutton J, DeJong G, Wilkerson D. Function-based payment model for inpatient medical rehabilitation: an evaluation. *Arch Phys Med Rehabil* 1996;77:693–701.

112. Wilkerson D, Batavia A, DeJong G. Use of functional status measures in payment for medical rehabilitation services. *Arch Phys Med Rehabil* 1992;73:111–120.

113. Kane RL. Looking for physical therapy outcomes. *Phys Ther* 1994;74(5):56–60.

114. Banja JD, Johnston MV. Outcomes evaluation in TBI rehabilitation. Part III. Ethical perspectives and social policy. *Arch Phys Med Rehabil* 1994;75:SC-19–26.

115. Purtilo RB, Meier RH. Regulatory constraints and patient empowerment. *Am J Phys Med Rehabil* 1993; 72:327–330.

116. Whiteneck GG. Evaluating outcome after spinal cord injury: what determines success? *J Spinal Cord Injury Med* 1997;20:179–185.

117. Tanenbaum SJ, Hurley RE. Disability and the managed care frenzy: a cautionary note. *Health Affairs* 1995;14:213–219.

118. Greenwood RJ, McMillan TM, Brooks DN, et al. Effects of case management after severe head injury. *BMJ* 1994;308:1199–1205.

119. Haffey WJ, Welsh JH. Subacute care: evolution in search of value. *Arch Phys Med Rehabil* 1995;76:SC-2–4.

120. Hogan PF, Dobson A, Haynie B, et al. Physical medicine and rehabilitation workforce study: the supply and demand for physiatrists. *Arch Phys Med Rehabil* 1996;77:95–99.

121. Friedman E. Managed care and managing ethics. *Healthcare Forum J* 1996;336:9–15.

122. Ross JW. Ethical decision making in managed care environments. *Bioethics Forum* 1994;10(4):22–26.

123. Woodstock Theological Center. *Ethical considerations in the business aspects of health care.* Washington, DC: Georgetown University Press, 1995.

124. Winslade WJ. Confidentiality. In: Reich W, ed. *Encyclopedia of bioethics.* New York: Macmillan, 1995:451–459.

125. Weiss BD. Confidentiality expectations of patients, physicians, and medical students. *JAMA* 1982;247:2695–2697.

126. Siegler M. Confidentiality in medicine—a decrepit concept. *N Engl J Med* 1982;307:1518–1521.

127. Gostin LO, Turek-Brezina J, Powers M, et al. Privacy and security of information in a new health care system. *JAMA* 1993;270:2487–2493.

128. Institute of Medicine. *Health data in the information age: use, disclosure, and privacy.* Washington, DC: National Academy Press, 1994.

129. Furrow BR, Greaney TL, Johnson SH, et al. *Health law.* Minneapolis: West Publishing, 1995;241–249.

130. Strax TE. Ethical issues of treating patients with AIDS in a rehabilitation setting. *Am J Phys Med Rehabil* 1994;73:293–295.

131. Ingenito EF, Gershkoff AM, Staas WE, Coyne FR, Rehabilitation of patients with human immunodeficiency virus (HIV): patient confidentiality versus treatment team right to know. *Am J Phys Med Rehabil* 1990;69:330–332.

132. Drachman DM. Who may drive? Who may not? Who decides? *Ann Neurol* 1988;24:787–788.

133. Anfield RN. Americans with Disabilities Act of 1990: a primer of Title I provisions for occupational health care professionals. *J Occup Med* 1992;34:503–509.

134. President's Commission for the Study of Ethical Problems in Medicine and Biomedical and Behavioral Research. *Compensating for research injuries.* Washington, DC: U.S. Government Printing Office, 1982;25–43.

135. Hotopf M, Wessley S, Noah N. Are ethical committees reliable? *J R Soc Med* 1995;88:31–33.

136. National Research Council, Institute of Medicine. *The Arctic Aeromedical Laboratory's thyroid function study.* Washington, DC: National Academy Press, 1996.

137. Advisory Committee on Human Radiation Experiments. *Final report.* Washington, DC: U.S. Government Printing Office, 1996.

138. Levine R. *Ethics and the regulation of clinical research.* New Haven, CT: Yale University Press, 1986.

139. Code of Federal Regulations. Vol. 45, section 46.111(a).

140. Lurie KG, Benditt D. Regulated to death: the matter of informed consent for human experimentation in emergency resuscitation research *Pacing Clin Electrophysiol.* 1995;18:1443–1447.

141. *Fed Reg* 1996;61:51531–51533.

142. Safar P. Resuscitation medicine research: quo vadis? *Ann Emerg Med* 1996;27:542–552.

143. Spece RG, Shine DS, Buchanan AE. *Conflicts of interest in clinical practice and research.* New York: Oxford University Press, 1996.

144. President's Commission for the Study of Ethical Problems in Medicine and Biomedical and Behavioral Research. *Deciding to forego life-sustaining treatment.* Washington, DC: U.S. Government Printing Office, 1982.

145. Weir R. *Abating treatment with critically ill patients: ethical and legal limits to the medical prolongation of life.* New York: Oxford University Press, 1989.

146. Meisel A. *The right to die.* New York: Wiley, 1995.

147. Reidy K, Crozier KS. Refusing treatment during rehabilitation: a model for conflict resolution. *West J Med* 1991;154:622–623.

148. Maynard FM. The choice to end life as a ventilator-dependent quadriplegic. *Arch Phys Med Rehabil* 1987;68:862–864.

149. Longmore PK. The strange death of David Rivlin. *West J Med* 1991;154;615–616.

150. Batavia AI. A disability rights-independent living perspective on euthanasia. *West J Med* 1991;154:616–617.

151. Maynard FM. Responding to requests for ventilator removal from patients with quadriplegia. *West J Med* 1991;154:617–619.

152. Powell T, Lowenstein B. Refusing life-sustaining treatment after catastrophic injury: ethical implications. *J Law Med Ethics* 1996; 24:54–61.

153. Dresser R. Still troubled: in re Martin. *Hastings Cent Rep* 1996;26(4):21–22.

154. Beresford HR. Moral, ethical, and legal issues raised by catastrophic brain injury. In: Levin HS, Benton AL, Muizelaar J, Eisenberg HM, eds. *Catastrophic brain injury.* New York: Oxford University Press, 1996:153–173.

155. Rusin MJ. Communicating with families of rehabilitation patients about "do not resuscitate" decisions. *Arch Phys Med Rehabil* 1992;73:922–925.

156. Banja JD, Bilsky GS. Discussing cardiopulmonary resuscitation with elderly rehabilitation patients. *Am J Phys Med Rehabil* 1993;72:168–171.

157. Appelbaum PS. Assessing patients' capacities to consent to treatment. *N Engl J Med* 1988; 319:1635–1638.

158. Markson LJ, Kern DC, Annas GJ, Glantz LH. Physician assessment of patient competence. *J Am Geriatr Soc* 1994;42:1074–1080.

159. Freedman M, Stuss DT, Gordon M. Assessment of competency: the role of neurobehavioral deficits. *Ann Intern Med* 1991;115:203–208.

160. Callahan CD, Haggulund KJ. Comparing neuropsychological and psychiatric evaluation of competency in rehabilitation: a case example. *Arch Phys Med Rehabil* 1995;76:909–912.

161. Sullivan MD, Youngner SJ. Depression, competence, and the right to refuse lifesaving medical treatment. *Am J Psychiatry* 1994; 151:971–978.

162. Patterson DR, Miller-Perrin C, McCormick TR, Hudson LD. When life support is questioned early in the care of patients with cervical-level quadriplegia. *N Engl J Med* 1993;328:506–509.

163. Council on Ethical and Judicial Affairs. Decisions near the end of life. *JAMA* 1992;267:2229–2233.

164. David Orentlicher. Advance medical directives. *JAMA* 1990; 263:2365–2367.

165. Weir RF, Gostin L. Decisions to abate life-sustaining treatment for nonautonomous patients. *JAMA* 1990;264:274–281.

166. Stebnicki MA. Ethical dilemmas in adult guardianship and substitute decision-making: considerations for rehabilitation professionals. *J Rehabil* 1994; 60(2):23–27.

167. King NMP. *Making sense of advance directives.* Washington, DC: Georgetown University Press, 1996.

168. Cantor NL. *Advance directives and the pursuit of death with dignity.* Bloomington, IN: University of Indiana Press, 1993.

169. Pearlman RA, Jonson A. The use of quality-of-life considerations in medical decision making. *J Am Geriatr Soc* 1985;33:344–350.

170. Kottke FJ. Philosophic considerations of quality of life for the disabled. *Arch Phys Med Rehabil* 1982;63:60–62.

171. Freed MM. Quality of life: the physician's dilemma. *Arch Phys Med Rehabil* 1984;65:109–111.

172. Rodwin MA. Patient accountability and quality of care: lessons from medical consumerism and the patients' rights, women's

health, and disability rights movements. *Am J Law Med* 1994;20:147–168.

173. Dennis RE, Williams W, Giangreco MF, Cloninger CJ. Quality of life as context for planning and evaluation of services for people with disabilities. *Exceptional Child* 1993;59: 499–512.

174. Orentlicher D. Rationing and the Americans with Disabilities Act. *JAMA* 1994;271:1903–1904.

175. Miaow M. *Making all the difference: inclusion, exclusion and American law.* Cambridge, MA: Harvard University Press, 1990.

176. Crossley MA. Medical futility and disability discrimination. *Iowa Law Rev* 1995;81: 179–259.

177. Orentlicher D. Destructuring disability: rationing of health care and unfair discrimination against the sick. *Harv Civ Rts -Civ Lib Law Rev* 1991;31:49–83.

178. Schneiderian LJ, Jacker N. *Wrong medicine: doctors, patients, and futile treatment.* Baltimore: Johns Hopkins University Press, 1996.

179. Gething L. Perceptions of disability of persons with cerebral palsy, their close relatives and able bodied persons. *Soc Sci Med* 1985;30:561–565.

180. Gething L. Generality versus specificity of attitudes towards people with disabilities. *Br J Med Psychol* 1991;64:55–64.

181. Gething L. Judgments by health professionals of personal characteristics of people with a visible physical disability. *Soc Sci Med* 1992;34:809–815.

182. Gething L. Attitudes to people with disabilities. *Med J Aust* 1992;157:725–726.

183. Gerhart KA, Koziol-McLain J, Lowenstein SR, Whiteneck GG. Quality of life following spinal cord injury: knowledge and attitudes of emergency care providers. *Ann Emerg Med* 1994;23:807–812.

184. Gerhart KA. Quality of life: the danger of differing perceptions. *Top Spinal Cord Inj Rehabil* 1997;2(3):78–84.

Chapter 4

The Legal Aspects of Physical Medicine and Rehabilitation

Ellen Grabois
Richard Bonfiglio

Howard Rusk said that the purpose of rehabilitative care was to restore and maintain patients in a high quality of health and life (1). Frederic Kottke emphasized that restoring the functional capacity of patients with chronic disease or physical disability is to enable them to participate in the community at an optimal level of function (2). Rehabilitation therefore is the maintenance of a stable living environment and the achievement of productivity (3). Rehabilitation goals include reestablishing emotional well-being, preserving residual function, preventing disabling complications, and developing compensatory functional capacities needed for carrying out daily activities (4).

Many people influence the treatment of rehabilitation patients. Rehabilitation practice teaches patients and their families to maintain and enhance functional capabilities despite residual impairments. Patients may want to make their own decisions as to their treatment, because they know best about their preferences, lifestyle, habits, and support systems. And family members may want to help design the treatment program because they will assume a special burden of providing ongoing care for the patient (3,5).

The practice of rehabilitation medicine has unique aspects. The duration of treatment may be extended, patients have to deal with many professionals, and there are issues of mental and physical capacity (4). Yet, in the practice of medicine in the United States, patients, families, and physicians in rehabilitation must deal with certain legal issues (6): What are the rights of patients and what are the rights of families? How do these rights intersect and when do they conflict?

Additionally, since many patients receiving rehabilitative care have experienced catastrophic injuries and illnesses, litigation frequently results, especially when others may have contributed to the condition. Therefore, meeting the needs of rehabilitation patients includes the provision of adequate documentation of the person's remaining abilities and the need for any ongoing assistance. Documentation of the needs for ongoing daily care, medical and rehabilitative follow-up, adaptive equipment, and daily supplies and of potential secondary complications is important. Additionally, physicians in rehabilitative medicine may need to provide testimony regarding a patient's ongoing care needs. Accurate testimony can facilitate the provision of appropriate economic awards that will fund the ongoing needs of these patients.

INFORMED CONSENT

In the United States, historically, the legal rule has been that physicians must obtain their patients' consent before they are legally entitled to commence treatment. The rule grew out of the time-honored concept that the nonconsensual and unprivileged touching of another person's body is a battery, and also on the fact that it was the custom of surgeons not to operate on their patients without their consent. This professional custom was probably based on the need for the patient's cooperation if surgery were to be performed, especially before anesthetics were available. In the early twentieth century, a simple interchange between physician and patient passed for a valid consent. But in the 1950s, the term *informed consent* was coined. The doctrine of informed consent cautioned physicians that they had an affirmative duty to disclose information about the risks of treatment, and if the duty was not filled, any breach constituted negligence (7). In the famous case of *Natanson v Kline* (8), a woman suffered burns to her thorax from radiation therapy after a mastectomy. The patient had consented to treatment, but the physician had not informed her as to the risks of treatment. The court ruled that it was necessary for physicians to make a reasonable disclosure of the dangers within their knowledge that were incident to the treatment they proposed to administer.

The central goals of the doctrine of informed consent are twofold. The first goal is that of patient autonomy, or self-determination in the control of one's own body. This is effectuated by allowing patients to make their own decisions about health care based on their own values. The core notion is the primacy of individual choice (9). The legal basis for autonomy in health care decisions is the 1914 case of *Schloendorff v Society of New York Hospitals* (10), in which a famous American jurist, Justice Cardozo, stated that every man and woman of adult years who is of sound mind has the right to determine what shall be done with his or her body.

The second goal of informed consent is that patients be enabled to exercise their autonomy rationally and intelligently. In order to do so, they must be given the information needed for making rational and intelligent decisions about their health care (9,11).

The rehabilitation physician not only should strive to educate patients about the clinician's goals for the patient's rehabilitation process, but also should frequently elicit from the patient and family members their preference regarding therapies, goal setting, and time frames for treatment.

Informed consent is defined as the willing acceptance of a medical intervention by a patient after adequate disclosure by the physician of the nature of the intervention, its risks and benefits, as well as of alternatives with their risks and benefits (12). It is a process, not a single event, of collaborative decision making in which the physician and patient, perhaps more than once, discuss the therapeutic options available. Whether the information is provided orally or in a consent form, or both, the goal is not to warn the patient, but to provide enough information to permit intelligent decision making. Physicians are not prohibited from giving advice to their patients, and many patients want the advice. The only restriction is that the advice not be coercive (9).

The doctrine of informed consent imposes on physicians two duties. These are the duty to inform and the duty to obtain consent. They are actionable, in the United States, as separate legal causes of action. The source of these duties is the fiduciary nature of the physician-patient relationship. The heavy dependence of the patient on the physician for well-being means that this is not an arm's-length transaction (transaction negotiated by unrelated parties, each acting in his or her self-interest) (9).

The informed consent doctrine has five elements that are fundamental: disclosure, comprehension, voluntariness, competence, and consent (13). In the United States, the disclosure element is measured by two different standards. In other words, the adequacy of the physician's disclosure is measured by a fact finder who must evaluate if the duty of disclosure was fulfilled. These two standards are the 1) reasonable person standard and 2) the professional or reasonable physician standard. Under the professional standard, a physician is required to disclose the kind and degree of information that a reasonable prudent physician, under like circumstances, would disclose. This requires expert witness evidence. Under the reasonable person standard, a physician is required to disclose the information that a reasonable patient would find material in deciding about the treatment in question (9). The standard one follows would depend on what standard was adopted in a particular jurisdiction or state in the United States.

The element of consent is more than an assent. Consent indicates an assent that is legally effective. To be effective, the patient's permission must be voluntary. Therefore, the permission must be freely given and without duress and undue influence. To give consent, the patient must be competent to give his or her permission for treatment. Competent adults must have the capacity to consent. They must be able to share in the decision making and have the ability to appreciate the nature, extent, and probable consequences of the physician's conduct to which consent is given. The patient should be able to comprehend or understand the information the physician is providing, but the physician is not necessarily required to ensure that the patient understands the information he or she has been given (9).

There are situations in which informed consent is not required in the United States. In emergencies, the physician may render treatment without the informed consent of the patient; if the patient waives the rights to be informed, the duty is dispensed with. If the patient is incompetent, informed consent is not necessary. And if the physician decides that the patient will be harmed by disclosing information to him or her, then the therapeutic privilege exception applies (9).

Patients undergoing rehabilitation are frequently faced with difficult lifestyle determinations. Health care providers must avoid making these decisions for patients with disabilities. The rehabilitative effort should be geared toward enhancing independence. Incumbent in this process is providing adequate information to patients and families and then allowing them to make decisions (14,15).

As an example, many rehabilitation patients have mobility limitations. The rehabilitation process includes an inherent risk when the boundaries of these mobility limitations are being explored. For instance, an individual with traumatic brain injury who has the ability to ambulate, but with impaired balance and judgment, is at risk for falling. The use of physical or chemical restraints in such situations has been a common practice. Rehabilitation physicians should carefully weigh treatment options in such cases and use the minimum restraint appropriate for the situation. Adequate explanation to patients and family members is imperative. An ongoing dialogue can reduce the potential for conflict in such situations (16,17).

COMPETENCE TO MAKE MEDICAL DECISIONS

Closely linked with the patient's right to be informed about the medical treatment he or she is about to undergo, and the right, in the United States, for patients to refuse all treatment, is the necessity that the patient who consents to treatment be competent. The underlying principles of informed consent include the idea that the patient who is competent is autonomous, and that the incompetent patient must be protected by means other than informed consent (18).

In the United States, all individuals are presumed by the law to be competent. Incompetence refers to a *legal status*. Although the court system may depend on information provided by clinicians, the determination of incompetence is ultimately a legal decision, not a medical one. A person may be legally incompetent either as a result of a judicial determination or by virtue of being a minor. There are many kinds of incompetence to enter into a contract. Here we refer to *incompetence* as an inability to have a decision-making capacity to consent to medical treatment. *Decision-making capacity* or *decision-making incapacity* have often been shortened to the terms *capacity* and *incapacity*. Therefore, *competence* and *capacity* are terms often used interchangeably, although their meanings are different. Capacity to make a decision is necessary, or the patient could attain the legal status of incompetence (9).

Competence is a prerequisite to a patient's making a legally binding decision about medical treatment. The consequence of incompetence is a disenfranchisement or loss of a right or power to control one's own life. A patient's lack of decision-making capacity suspends a physician's obligation to obtain the patient's consent to treatment. The patient's decisions about medical care need not be honored by the physician. Incompetence can be general or specific. A general adjudication by a court of incompetence renders a person incompetent for all purposes. An adjudication of specific incompetence renders one incompetent for only limited purposes (9).

A guardian should be appointed to exercise authority over the incompetent's affairs. If a rehabilitation patient clinically appears to be incompetent, an effort should be made to have the legal system identify a guardian. A guardian who takes care of financial affairs is termed *guardian of the estate*. The guardian over personal matters is a *guardian of the person*. A family member can be appointed guardian. If a decision has to be made, for instance, to continue or to forgo life-sustaining treatment for an incompetent, the guardian of the person would make that decision (9).

When a patient is totally incapable of making a reasoned decision about medical treatment or lacks the ability to understand the information conveyed, to evaluate the options, or to communicate a decision, a court in the United States will likely rule that a patient is incompetent (19). However, until a patient has been determined by a court to be incompetent, the physician cannot automatically assume that there is no need to seek the patient's consent to treatment.

What triggers an inquiry into the competency status of a patient? The physician should first observe if the patient has the core skills to make a medical decision such as attention and concentration, linguistic abilities, memory, and executive skills, including problem solving and judgment. Beyond the core skills, a physician should look at the patient's ability to recognize that a decision must be made, the patient must be able to examine the pros and cons of his or her options, and the patient must be able to communicate his or her decision (19). A physician should look at the patient's demeanor, difficulty in communicating, and the patient's medical condition (9). Generally, competence is not questioned until a patient refuses to consent to treatment. Of course, a disagreement with the physician's recommendation is no basis for a finding of incompetence (20).

Once competence is called into question, most commentators agree that competence can vary over time and determining competence involves a process. Competence is competence to do a task and there can be variation in the kind of decision the patient has to make. It may depend on the complexity of information necessary to make the decision. The patient has to understand the diagnosis, treatment alternatives, and his or her physician's recommendations. The patient must bring his or her own set of values to the decision. The minimal standard in competence is one in which the patient must express a preference. Beyond the minimal standard, one must focus not on the content of the patient's decision, but on the process that leads to a decision (20).

Two American authors (21) proposed a construct of competence to consent to medical treatment. The construct contains three parts: understanding, deliberation, and decision. *Understanding* means that the patient must understand the relevant information necessary to reach a decision regarding treatment. *Deliberation* means that a patient must be able to integrate, analyze, and process treatment information. *Decision* means that a patient must be able to formulate and express a decision based on his or her understanding and deliberation of the treatment information (21). In *In re Conroy* (22), the Supreme Court of New Jersey said a patient may be incompetent because he or she lacks the ability to understand the information conveyed, to evaluate the options, or to communicate a decision.

The Fourth Circuit Court of Appeals (23) in the United States has held that the standard for a trial court to consider competence to consent to medical treatment should involve two parts. One is that the court should evaluate whether the patient follows a rational process in his or her decision, and the other is whether the patient can give rational reasons for the choice he or she has made. The competence to consent to medical treatment, according to the case *Miller v Rhode Island Hospital* (24) is not the same as legal competence to make decisions. A person's ability to make legal transactions is not necessarily equivalent to the ability to make medical decisions. Looking at one's capacity should be done by looking at the particular circumstances of each case.

All states or all jurisdictions in the United States have statutorily prescribed procedures for adjudicating incompetence and appointing a guardian of the person. It is not clear from the state statutes whether they are intended to be the exclusive means for medical decision making for individuals unable to do so for themselves. Is an adjudication of incompetence in a court the only way to name a surrogate decision maker? Unless there is a statute or case law to the contrary, some jurisdictions permit physicians to turn to family members to make decisions on behalf of incompetent patients. This is a clinically designated surrogate. If there are close family members such as a spouse, adult children, or parents who are willing to exercise rights on behalf of patients, they are often picked by the physician. Generally, but not always, family members are very concerned about the good of the patient, and family members are said to be in the best position to know the patient's own feelings and desires. If the patient has no family, a trusted friend may be suitable as a surrogate (9).

Rehabilitation physicians should recognize that family members may have perspectives and preferences regarding patient care that may differ from the rehabilitation professionals. Additionally, there may be conflicts between family members regarding goals of treatment. Family members may have an inadequate understanding of the potential for recovery and may have inflated expectations of the rehabilitation process. Appropriate and timely communication between the rehabilitation team and the family can reduce the potential for conflict regarding treatment measures and outcome. Patient and family input regarding the nature and scope of treatment, the goals of rehabilitation, and the time course of its provision is a basic tenet of rehabilitation (14).

THE RIGHT TO REFUSE TREATMENT AND THE RIGHT TO TREATMENT WITHDRAWAL: COMPETENT AND INCOMPETENT PATIENTS

In the United States, a competent patient has the right to refuse the medical treatment that his or her physician has recommended. Patients must consent to medical treatment, or the physician, as we have said, may be liable for committing battery. Medical decisions are usually made on a continuing basis, depending on the patient's condition (9), and this is especially true in rehabilitation. Therefore, the available options are constantly changing, and the rehabilitation physician must carry on a therapeutic conversation with the patient and family on a continual basis.

In the law, the right to refuse treatment springs from the concerns of the courts in the United States for human dignity, self-determination, and unwanted infringement of bodily integrity. These concerns have led the courts to draw on two sources to justify the right of competent patients to refuse unwanted medical treatment. One is the common law or case law developed in the United States. In the *Schloendorff* (10) case mentioned earlier, the court held that a human being of adult years and of sound mind has the right to determine what should be done with his or her own body. After the physician complies with the doctrine of informed consent, the individual patient has the right to behave and act as he or she deems fit. This is a privacy, autonomy, and self-determination issue. In the famous cases in New Jersey of *In re Quinlan* (25) and *In re Conroy* (22), the New Jersey Supreme Court cited the common law right to refuse treatment, and said that this right must be free of all restraint or interference of others. The patient is the final arbiter of what to do about any medical treatment.

Not only do the courts in the United States rely on the common law right to refuse treatment, but also they look to the U.S. Constitution. The U.S. Supreme Court has recognized a right of personal privacy that exists in the penumbras of specific guarantees in the Bill of Rights. This right is not explicit in the Constitution, but in *In re Quinlan* (25), it was applied to the patient, Karen Ann Quinlan, who was in a persistent vegetative state. Quinlan had the right of privacy and, as a patient, she could decline medical treatment. Yet this right of privacy to decline medical treatment is not absolute. It must be measured by the courts against countervailing societal interests, including the preservation of life, the prevention of suicide, the safeguarding of the integrity of the medical profession, and the protection of innocent third parties.

An important case in the United States concerning the right to refuse medical treatment is *Cruzan v Director, Missouri Department of Health* (26). In that case, Chief Justice Rehnquist of the U.S. Supreme Court recognized that a competent individual generally possesses the right to refuse treatment as a logical corollary to the doctrine of informed consent. Under the Fourteenth Amendment to the U.S. Constitution, no state may deprive any person of life, liberty, or property, without due process of law, and a competent person has a constitutionally protected liberty interest in refusing unwanted medical treatment. This liberty interest has to be balanced against relevant state interests.

How do the courts handle the withdrawal of life-sustaining treatment of incompetent patients? Incompetent patients are those in a persistent vegetative state, those who are suffering from dementia, those who are terminally ill and comatose, and patients lacking the ability to understand and evaluate the information conveyed by the physician because they are mentally ill, mentally deficient, of an advanced age, or chronically ill. In the *Cruzan* (26) case, the patient was in a persistent vegetative state, and the state courts in Missouri held that the evidence presented by her guardians that Nancy Cruzan wanted to terminate her life-sustaining treatment was not clear and convincing. On appeal, the U.S. Supreme Court agreed that Missouri could require the standard of clear and convincing evidence to safeguard against any abuses of surrogate decision makers.

When surrogate decision makers such as family members or guardians make decisions to refuse or terminate treatment for incompetent patients, the courts in the United States recognize two standards: the substituted judgment standard and the best interests standard. The substituted judgment standard attempts to determine what treatment alternative an incompetent patient would choose if he or she were competent and cognizant of the information relevant to the current treatment situation. In the *Quinlan* (25) case, the court held that the guardian and family of Karen Ann Quinlan, who was in a persistent vegetative state, had to render their best judgment as to whether she would exercise her right to terminate treatment under the existing circumstances. The standard requires the surrogate to make decisions in accordance with the patient's subjective preferences. If the patient's preferences are not clear, this standard may present difficulties.

Another standard applied to surrogate decision making is the best interests standard. This is patient centered and asks the surrogate to decide according to what will confer the greatest net benefit on the patient (27). It is a more objective standard. The surrogate tries to determine the probable benefits of available treatments to the patient, the possible burdens of the treatment, and the relative balance of the benefits and burdens (28). This standard is not preferred over the substituted judgment standard. It is too paternalistic and too vague. The best interests standard is often used in cases concerning minors (9).

What is the role of family members in the refusal or termination of medical treatment? Close relatives usually know what the patient has previously said about his or her preferences for care. Family members may be able to intuit what they believe the patient would want. And relatives may be presumed to act in the best interests of the incompetent patient. Of course family members can be inappropriate as surrogate decision makers. A family member may not have the patient's best interests at heart. Some surrogates have an approach where they may not be willing to listen to other points of view, or may not appreciate potential conflicts of interest (29). In rehabilitation, the role of the surrogate decision maker can be extremely important, and if the surrogate is a family member, his or her cooperation in the rehabilitation process is a great help and support for the patient. Certain state legislatures in the United States have passed family consent laws that empower enumerated relatives, in a stated priority order, to make medical decisions on behalf of an incapacitated person who has no advance directive. These laws explicitly confer immunity against criminal and civil liability for physicians and other health care professionals who withdraw or withhold medical interventions in accordance with the decisions. The statutes provide a clear process for effectuating the decisional rights already extant under federal and state constitutional interpretations and common law principles of bodily integrity. Typically, the statutes direct turning first to a court-appointed guardian, if there is one, then to the patient's spouse, then to an adult child, and then to either parent (30).

ADVANCE DIRECTIVES

One way for patients to make clear their wishes concerning medical decisions when they may be at a stage of incompetency is to execute an advance directive. Advance directives, in the United States, are vehicles for people to control postcompetence medical interventions. The object of an advance directive is to permit an individual to prescribe personal preferences, in advance, and so to maintain a measure of autonomy even after incompetency. Norman Cantor (31) called this "prospective autonomy."

By formulating advance instructions, a declarant can seek to shape future medical handling according to his or her own values. An advance directive may also designate an agent who will ultimately be responsible for implementing a declarant's instructions or, in the absence of discernible instructions, for making medical decisions on behalf of the incompetent patient. Such a person is known as the health care agent, representative, surrogate, attorney-in-fact, or proxy (31).

Written advance directives allow persons to project their preferences into the future for consideration by those responsible for their care when they themselves are incapable of expressing preferences. Advance directives have explicit legal validity in nearly every state in the United States (12). In the *Cruzan* (26) case, the U.S. Supreme Court stated that competent persons have a constitutionally protected "liberty interest" in refusing unwanted medical treatment, and this interest is not extinguished after mental capacity is lost. The Supreme Court did uphold a Missouri statute, in the *Cruzan* (26) case, requiring "clear and convincing" evidence of an incapacitated person's wishes. This implies the utility and legitimacy of advance directives. Of course, the idea of advance directives has been familiar and accepted in ethics and in the law for several decades in the United States (12).

Advance directives can take several forms. These include natural death acts or "death with dignity acts" or "medical treatment decision acts." They are statutes passed by state legislatures in the United States. These acts affirm a person's right to make decisions regarding terminal care, and provide directions about how the right can be effected after the loss of decision-making capacity. They usually contain a model document, called a *directive to physicians*. The patient can sign the directive and it can be given to a physician (12). Various topics are covered by specific provisions in natural death acts and can include personalized instructions, proxy appointments, an immunity clause for physicians who carry out patient directives, terminal condition diagnosis, permission and prohibition of withdrawing or withholding of artificial feeding and hydration, whether a declaration is part of one's medical record, and others. Many states in their statutes limit abatement of treatment to patients with terminal conditions in which death is imminent. A few states also allow abatement of treatment for patients who are irreversibly comatose or in a persistent vegetative state. These directives to physicians are a form of living wills.

Living wills are documents recording an individual's preferences and values concerning medical treatment—including the withholding or withdrawal of life-sustaining procedures—in the event a person loses capacity to make health care decisions. Living wills can be in a less formal, less legalistic form such as a model document from organizations in the United States such as Concern for Dying or the Hemlock Society. The individual directs that he or she be allowed to die in the event that he or she cannot take part in decisions for the future, and there is no reasonable expectation for recovery. Living wills can also be composed by the individual in a personalized fashion and can expand on specific instructions for specific medical outcomes. Sometimes, individuals will include instructions for treatment or abatement of treatment for a wider range of conditions including comas, persistent vegetative states, and other critical illnesses. In some states, these personalized living wills are given legal standing equivalent to the directives to physicians (12).

It is impossible for a living will to anticipate all the complex circumstances that arise. The language in the living will may be vague. A better alternative to living wills is the durable power of attorney for health care (DPOA-HC). For decades, individuals in the United States have been able to designate a representative with the legal authority to execute binding financial transactions on his or her behalf. The scope of the authority granted can be as broad or as narrow as the grantor chooses. Every state has adopted legislation allowing designation of a durable power of attorney. And a majority of states now specifically authorize execution of a durable power of attorney for health care decisions. In the *Cruzan* (26) case, Justice Sandra Day O'Connor endorsed the wisdom of state statutes that specifically authorize medical treatment decisions by surrogates under a durable power of attorney. These statutes authorize individuals to appoint another person, an attorney-in-fact, to act as their agent to make all health care decisions after they become incapacitated (12). A durable power of attorney for health care can be helpful even if one has executed a living will or a directive to physicians. They avoid court proceedings, possible delays in receiving needed medical treatment, and the emotional and financial stress on family and friends (20).

All living wills, including directives to physicians, and durable powers of attorney for health care documents may be revised by the maker or revoked at any time.

In many cases, individuals who execute these advance directives that appoint a proxy or surrogate to make medical decisions for them will choose a family member. Family members are often the best persons to implement health care decisions because they are in the most advantageous position to know the patient's values, and what the patient would decide in circumstances about which the patient did not express preference. Of course some patients do not have family members who are available or willing to make medical decisions. It is not uncommon, also, for family members to have ulterior motives that may affect their treatment decisions.

There are also situations in which physicians fail to adhere to advance directives because of opposition of family members when there is an incompetent, moribund patient. Physicians do not like to contest a surrounding family's instructions, and this can be a disruptive element in any situation. Family opposition can be grounded in the family members' beliefs that they understand the patient's real wishes, or the family may want to substitute their views for the patient's ill-considered instructions. Yet the patient's wishes in the advance directive should prevail (31).

These decisions are further complicated by the recognition that healthy individuals frequently report not being interested in potentially lifesaving measures, like the use of a ventilator. However, when actually faced with death, individuals often change their mind (32).

Few Americans have actually executed advance directives (33–35). A federal law in the United States, the Patient Self-Determination Act may help this problem (36). All health care institutions are required, as of 1991, to provide each patient with written information about his or her rights under state law to make decisions concerning medical care, including the right to accept or refuse medical or surgical treatment, and the right to formulate advance directives. Health care providers are further required to document in the individual's medical record whether or not the individual has executed an advance directive (37).

RIGHT TO CONFIDENTIALITY

One right of the patient that may be overlooked is that of confidentiality. Confidentiality is a relationship between two or more persons in which one person exposes himself or herself in some way to the other or discloses personal information to the other. Confidentiality assumes that there is a relationship of trust between the persons. That which is confidential is shared, and it is trust in another that ensures confidentiality (38). Confidentiality is not synonymous with the concept of privacy. Privacy is a concept that refers to self-regarding concerns, and a person's privacy is something that can be preserved by not granting access to others or by not disclosing one's thoughts and feelings (39). In the United States, case law holds that physicians have a fiduciary duty to their patients. This fiduciary obligation imposes the duties of good faith and fair dealing on the physician. Both the patient and the physician know that the patient will rely on the judgment and expertise of the physician (40). The physician, as a fiduciary, must place the interests and well-being of the patient above his or her own.

The introduction of a trusting relationship between physician and patient means that the patient relies not only on the physician's skills, but also on his or her discretion. Patients enter into a contractual relationship with their physicians for treatment, but there is an implied condition in the contract that the physician warrants that any confidential information gained through the relationship will not be released without the patient's consent (40).

What other mechanisms exist to ensure confidentiality for the information that the patient reveals? One is ethical and professional codes that affirm the importance of confidentiality. The physician is bound by the Hippocratic Oath not to divulge what he or she sees and hears in the course of his or her profession (41), and the American Medical Association's Code of Medical Ethics (16) states that the information disclosed to a physician during the course of the relationship between physician and patient is confidential to the greatest possible degree. The patient should feel free to make the disclosure of information to the physician in order that the physician may effectively provide needed services. The World Medical Association has made the statement that maintaining medical secrecy to protect the privacy of the individual as the basis for the confidential relationship between patient and his or her physician is vitally important (42).

Not only do professional and ethical codes protect patient confidentiality, but also many jurisdictions in the United States have physician-patient testimonial privilege statutes that protect patient confidentiality. Privilege statutes exist to protect communications between the physician and patient, and relate to the rules of evidence in a particular jurisdiction or state. There is a general rule that all relevant facts may be inquired into in a court of law, but the privilege statute is an exception to the general rule (43). Physicians may invoke the privilege and they do not have to testify in court proceedings so that they may protect the confidential relationship they have with patients. This protects the patient from unauthorized disclosure. Without a privilege statute, a professional may be charged with contempt of court if he or she chooses not to testify. Patients have sued their physicians for breach of confidentiality when the patient feels the physician has disclosed something the patient does not want disclosed (44). The first privilege statute was passed in New York State in 1828 (45). Today, a majority of states have statutes or rules of evidence recognizing the privilege.

In addition to professional and ethical codes and privilege statutes that protect patient confidentiality, courts in many jurisdictions hold that they have a public policy which requires all communications between physicians and patients to be kept confidential. The courts will defer to the public policy embodied in their physician-patient privilege statutes that protect confidentiality, and will look at the duty the physician has to his or her patient that requires confidentiality (46).

MANAGED CARE CONTRACTING

Types of Managed Care Organizations

Managed care organizations (MCOs) arrange for the provision of defined medical, hospital, and other health care services to be provided to beneficiaries or subscribers of a payor, where the providers and the MCO, among other duties, undertake mechanisms to control unnecessary and costly utilization and agree to compensation at a certain rate or formula. Some major types of MCOs are health maintenance organizations (HMOs), preferred provider organizations (PPOs), and physician hospital organizations (PHOs) (47).

HMOs include three types of models: staff model, group model, and independent practice associations (IPAs). The staff model employs physicians and other professionals; the group model contracts with large medical groups; and the IPA contracts with individual practice associations or organizations comprised of individually practicing physicians and/or medical groups formed for the purpose of contacting with MCOs. With the staff and group model HMOs, the HMO typically owns clinical facilities and hospitals. In the IPA model, there is typically no ownership of its own facilities. Care is managed through utilization management and control procedures (i.e., preauthorization of services) (47).

PPOs are generally for-profit corporations or mutual-benefit nonprofit corporations. The PPO typically contracts with and does not employ provider members in a network where the members agree to provide services to beneficiaries at a negotiated rate of payment. The PPO also contracts with payors or may be the payor itself, and the PPO network providers provide services to payor beneficiaries in return for a negotiated payment of the payor (47). The PPO may have point-of-service (POS) options in which beneficiaries may have some flexibility in choosing a provider or service outside the network without referral. Care is managed through utilization review (48).

PHOs are entities with physician and hospital ownership and/or control, whose primary purpose is to negotiate, manage, and monitor managed care contracts for the physician and hospital participants. PHOs develop systems for utilization review and quality assurance. PHOs can be nonprofit taxable organizations or for-profit entities. Models include a single hospital and a single physician organization, or a single hospital and multiple physician organizations (49).

Recent innovations in MCOs include exclusive provider organizations (EPOs) which combine HMO and PPO concepts, and potentially may control costs. An EPO limits the enrollees' selection of physicians to a particular network, but it does not usually reimburse the physicians on a prepaid basis. EPOs will use gatekeeper physicians to manage the enrollees' medical care. Multiple option plans permit employers to offer employees choices of health care coverage, and place all employees in a single-risk pool that spreads the risk and mitigates the effects of "adverse selection." Management service organizations (MSOs) are organizations that negotiate, manage, and monitor managed care contracts on behalf of physician and hospital participants and others, and develop appropriate utilization review and quality assurance programs, credentialing procedures, and information systems to monitor the billing and claims. These organizations may also provide administrative services for physician offices, accounting, marketing, and employment of nonphysical personnel. An integrated delivery system (IDS) is an organization or group of organizations that are affiliated and provide both physician and hospital services to patients (49).

Contracting with Managed Care Organizations

When rehabilitation and other providers consider contracting with an MCO, they are usually given an agreement by the MCO. The provider must identify those important issues in the agreement that the MCO or payor is willing to negotiate. Before the provider initiates negotiations, he or she should consider evaluating the ability of the MCO to adequately perform. The provider should look at the financial statements of the MCO, the MCO's licensing agency, who are the other contracting providers, the MCO's market position and marketing strategy, the management and administrative depth of the MCO, and the MCO's demographics, such as number of enrolled or covered lives, key employer groups offering the MCO's plans, the extent of the network in the area, and the age and marital status of the enrolled or covered lives. The physician should ask about the plan's general management style, utilization review policies, payment practices, and the overall level of satisfaction of participating providers (47,48).

There are certain contract issues that rehabilitation providers should be aware of when contracting with MCOs. The first is compensation. If payments are made on a capitation or per diem basis, the payment rates or schedules should be specified in the agreement or incorporated by reference into the agreement. The rates should not be subject to unilateral change by the plan, but should be subject to renegotiation by the plan and the provider. The provider should look at the demographic profile of the patient population, the amount of the regular capitation payments, how the reserve or withheld funds are calculated and collected, any minimum enrollment guarantees, and the possible need of an actuarial study of whether payments are reasonable and financially viable. The provider must consider the risk reserve pool terms such as the purposes of the pool, the share in the risk for providers of any significant financial loss, financial incentives to control utilization, when the risk reserve pool is distributed, and whether the method of allocation of the risk pool is equitable. Other compensation considerations with a capitation contract include whether stop-loss insurance should be purchased by providers to protect them from losses due to intensive treatment of particular patients, what the fund withholds for outside providers, what adjustments to enrollments are allowed, who pays for services to persons retroactively enrolled or retroactively disenrolled, and a determination of whether payments are tied to the collection of premiums (i.e., is the provider at risk for collections?) (47).

With noncapitated payment mechanisms (i.e., payments made on the basis of fee-for-service), the fee schedule should be specified in the contract or incorporated by reference into the contract. The schedule should not be subject to unilateral amendment by the plan. Physician participants should be given the opportunity to terminate the contract on relatively short notice in the event of changes in payment timing or amount. Payment should be made within a specified period of time after the claim has been submitted, generally within 30 or 60 days. Negotiation of a set late payment penalty is advisable. The provider should also look for clauses in the contract when there are limitations on the acceptance of the contract rates as payment in full, that is, when there is a coordination of benefits (the patient has multiple insurance coverage), if there are copayment and deductible obligations of patients, and if there are noncovered services for which providers may seek the right to make full charge. Participants must also evaluate the feasibility of the contract if there is a "most favored nation" clause, which compels the provider to offer the MCO or payor the lowest rate given to any payor (48).

Rehabilitation providers considering managed care plans should also look at what the covered services are and who the covered patients are. Services to be provided by the provider are typically defined as *covered services*. This term should be clearly defined and limited to those services in fact offered by the provider as of the date of the contract and covered by the payor. Evaluate the eligibility authorization and coverage verification procedures. Determine whether the contract clearly specifies which services may be subcontracted and which ancillary services are to be provided; whether the authorization/verification procedures should be written or oral; what the liability is for erroneous determinations; and whether the provider's obligation to perform a service is subject to the availability of the services, to the verification of eligibility and coverage, and to utilization review requirements (47).

Rehabilitation providers should look at the term of the contract that the MCO provides, and the termination procedures. Typically a term is 1 year, but if it is longer, the provider should do a review if renegotiation of the terms is permitted. The contract should provide "without cause" termination rights, and if there are "for cause" termination rights, the provider should evaluate the notice length and the events constituting cause. MCO contracts typically include ongoing obligations after termination. Providers should attempt to limit the period and obligations after termination, and seek a favorable payment formula for posttermination services (47).

A significant component of MCO activity is its utilization review and quality assurance plans which evaluate the necessity and quality of provider services. The MCO plans are not always detailed in the contract, and are often not provided until after the agreement is executed. Providers should look for a right to review and approve all plans before being bound to comply. Providers need to know whether authorization and review procedures comply with applicable law, whether there are circumstances under which retrospective review is permitted, and whether there are penalties for errors found as a result of reviews. Provider appeal procedures should also be evaluated (47).

Rehabilitation providers must also consider, in contracting with MCOs, what the malpractice and other insurance requirements are, what the dispute resolution procedures are, what the patient grievance procedures are, what record confidentiality and maintenance requirements are, and what the contractual indemnities are. If the provider is obligated to give indemnity, consider having an attorney and one's insurance carrier review these clauses. Providers should not agree to contract provisions that attempt to shift all of the responsibility for medical care decisions to them. Such provisions may void malpractice insurance coverage, and should be reciprocal (48).

The provider seeking to increase volume would find an exclusivity clause extremely attractive in MCO contracts, because of the potential for significant volume increases. However, these types of provisions can give rise to potential antitrust challenges if the payor physician group is a dominant player in the market.

EMPLOYMENT CONTRACTS

Rehabilitation physicians may also enter into a variety of employment contracts. Facility-based physicians may have an employment contract with the facility. Physicians joining a group practice will usually have a contract outlining the relationship. Although there are many potential terms in these contracts, there are some common elements. The physician's compensation will generally be described. The physician should be aware of the difference between net and gross receipts. Physician payment reductions for expenses including billing should be delineated. The expectations of the physician should also be delineated. Especially if the physician's role includes administrative responsibilities, the physician should be certain that the reimbursement adequately covers the time involved. Physician employment contracts frequently contain a "covenant not to compete." Although when beginning a practice all parties tend to be optimistic about the relationship, over time things do not always work as anticipated. The physician should feel comfortable with the terms of the covenant not to compete, since it may limit the physician's ability to practice, especially without relocating in the event that the employment situation does not work.

Review of the proposed contract with an attorney representing the interests of the physician is generally prudent. The physician may not be aware of the complexities of the terminology or specific meaning to the words used in a legal context. Additionally, the contract generally replaces any agreements made prior to its signing. Many promises may be made during negotiations; only those provisions covered in the contract are binding.

DOCUMENTATION ISSUES

Developing practice habits that include precise, accurate, and thorough documentation facilitates rehabilitative care. Since physicians cannot choose which documentation is utilized in legal proceedings, all written communications should be provided in a way that would not be problematic if scrutinized during legal proceedings. Therefore, accurate information regarding patient needs and limitations, the rehabilitation process, and the results of treatment is essential to the care of rehabilitation patients. Descriptions of potential conflicts between patients, families, and rehabilitation caregivers should be appropriately documented, especially without any derogatory or inflammatory language.

Documentation content is also improved when the information is provided in a clear and concise manner. Handwritten material must be readable. Errors should be corrected according to facility policy. Rendering mistakes in documentation unreadable can lead to the implication that the error contains information that the physician does not want the reader to see. Only facility-approved abbreviations should be used.

Sensitive patient information particularly regarding lifestyle choices should be handled carefully. Information that a patient shares in confidence with a physician should be carefully considered regarding its medical value prior to inclusion in the medical record.

Since rehabilitation care is most often provided in a team setting, review of the documentation of other team members is important to ensure a consistent team philosophy. Team conference reporting should help to explore and resolve any apparent conflicts between team members. Reports by clinicians still in training should also be regularly reviewed for consistency.

Rehabilitation care is improved when adequate time has been taken in obtaining historical information. Since rehabilitation patients have often already received extensive treatment prior to the inpatient rehabilitation stay, review of available information can facilitate ongoing care. However, the rehabilitation physician must recognize that errors are often inadvertently entered into patients' medical records and may be promulgated if historical information is not verified. Use of a format for patient questioning may facilitate its thoroughness.

A thorough physical examination is also essential to the rehabilitative effort. Adequate documentation of the results is important. Since progress in rehabilitation is generally gradual, periodic reassessment of physical findings is important. As an example, when dealing with a patient with chronic pain, it is impossible to measure or even verify the existence of the patient's primary symptom and limitation, pain. The rehabilitation physician must depend on clinical skills including an understanding of the pathophysiology of potentially contributing medical conditions. When patients with chronic pain limit their functional performance, the physician must determine whether this is based on medical limitations or patient motivation. Appropriate rehabilitation strategies can then be used to enhance outcome.

Medical documentation is frequently used for making compensation decisions (50). Rehabilitation patients' receipt of appropriate compensation and even medical care is often dependent on adequate documentation of their abilities and limitations. Establishing a causal link between the inciting episode and ongoing symptoms and limitations is essential to such compensation decisions. These decisions can be complicated when multiple episodes of potential injury have occurred or when there has been an insidious onset of disability. The physician's role is to provide sufficient documentation so that an appropriate adjudication can be made. Physicians do not need to become unduly burdened into assuming such decision making.

Rehabilitation physicians should avoid inflammatory medical record entries, especially as conflicts arise in the provision of services. Accurate descriptions of recommended services and of decisions made by patients or family members are needed.

TESTIMONY

Rehabilitation clinicians are frequently requested to provide medical testimony regarding patients for whom care has been provided. Provision of this testimony should be viewed as one more aspect of medical care. Accurate testimony regarding the patient's current medical condition is often needed so that appropriate compensation can be provided. The believability of a rehabilitation physician's testimony can be enhanced by appropriate documentation and an adequate delivery style. Being prepared for testimony is essential. Reviewing all available medical records, especially reports of opposing physicians, is essential. Understanding the key issues in the legal case is also important. The attorney requesting the physician's testimony can generally delineate these issues. The physician should recognize the role being served. Usually as a treating clinician, the physician provides information based on the facts of the case. As an expert witness, the physician is also asked to provide expert opinions. The goal of the testifying physician should always be to provide accurate information and opinions, but in an efficient manner. Providing opinions that are not well founded or on the edge of the clinician's expertise can significantly complicate and prolong the testimony experience. For newly trained physicians, as with other areas of practice, it is generally preferable to observe another clinician providing testimony, prior to having to perform this service. Recognizing common questions and appropriate responses is thus facilitated. The attorney requesting the physician's testimony may also be able to provide insight regarding the opposing attorney's style of questioning. Some attorneys utilize an argumentative style. Others are repetitious or circumloquitious. Some seem to attempt to catch the witness in incongruities.

The rehabilitation physician should be prepared to review the facts of the case. Future care needs and the prognosis for patients with catastrophic injuries or illnesses are common areas of questioning. The physician may also be asked to review a life care plan that delineates the ongoing needs of a patient with a significant disability. The life care plan includes projected future medical, rehabilitative, and daily care needs including physician visits, nursing care, therapies, adaptive equipment and supplies, medications, and potential future complications. The physician will be particularly questioned regarding the medical necessity and appropriateness of the items listed. The physician may also be requested to project a life expectancy for the patient, since this is important in determining the extent of future needs in the damages part of the case. Depending on the nature of the litigation, there may also be questions regarding whether or not the patient has reached maximal medical improvement and the extent of permanent impairment (51,52). The patient's medical prognosis for returning to work may also be questioned.

Questions regarding the physician's education, training, and experience in the appropriate areas are also likely. The physician may also be questioned regarding the costs of services. The physician should make every effort to provide consistent testimony regardless of the requesting party. The physician should provide factual information and opinions based on training and experience, but attempt to refrain from injecting his or her own bias based on personal philosophy regarding pain, work, and ambiguities in diagnosis, management, and prognosis (53,54). Testimony should be limited to the area of practice of the physician.

Testimony may be provided via deposition or in a courtroom setting. Depositions are usually done for the convenience of the clinician and are therefore done at the physician's office. The deposition may be either for discovery purposes or in lieu of courtroom testimony. The purpose of a discovery deposition is to determine all of the physician's opinions regarding the case. The evidentiary deposition takes the place of the physician actually appearing at trial. The deposition is usually recorded by a court stenographer and additionally may be videotaped.

CONCLUSIONS

Treating rehabilitation patients, especially following catastrophic illnesses or injuries, requires an understanding of the legal implications. Adequately informing patients and family members of treatment options and anticipated outcomes is inherent in the rehabilitation process, as such information facilitates independence and community reentry. Rehabilitation physicians need to recognize the legal aspects of competence decisions. Physicians are bound legally and ethically to maintain patient confidentiality. Appropriate physician documentation facilitates the rehabilitation effort. Rehabilitation physicians should be prepared to provide medical testimony when needed.

REFERENCES

1. Rusk HA. The 1977 Walter Zeiter Lecture. Rehabilitation medicine: knowledge in search of understanding. *Arch Phys Med Rehabil* 1978;59(4):156–160.
2. Kottke FJ. Future focus of rehabilitation medicine. *Arch Phys Med Rehabil* 1980;61(1):1–6.
3. Haas J. Ethical considerations of goal setting for patients care in rehabilitation medicine. *Am J Phys Med Rehabil* 1993;72:228–232.
4. Caplan AL, Callahan D, Haas J. Ethical & policy issues in rehabilitation medicine. *Hastings Cent Rep* 1987; (August Special Suppl): 1–20.
5. Cooper J, Vernon S. *Disability and the law.* London: Jessica Kingsley, 1996.
6. Romano JL. *Legal rights of the catastrophically ill and injured: a family guide.* 2nd ed. Philadelphia, 1998.
7. Appelbaum PS, Lidz CW, Meisel A. *Informed consent; legal theory and clinical practice.* New York: Oxford University Press, 1987.
8. *Natanson v Kline,* 350 P2d 1093 (Kan 1960).
9. Meisel A. *The right to die.* New York: Wiley, 1989.
10. *Schloendorff v Socy of New York Hosp.* 211 NY 125, 105 NE 92 (1914).
11. Venesy BA. A clinician's guide to decision making capacity and ethically sound medical decisions. *Am J Phys Med Rehabil* 1994;74:S41–S48.
12. Jonsen AR, Siegler M, Winslade WJ. *Clinical ethics; a practical approach to ethical decisions in clinical medicine.* New York: McGraw-Hill, 1982.
13. Veatch RM. *Medical ethics.* Boston: Jones & Bartlett, 1989.
14. Commission on Accreditation of Rehabilitation Facilities. *Standard manual for organizations serving people with disabilities.* 1998.
15. Kapp MB. Proxy decision making in Alzheimer disease research: durable powers of attorney, guardianship, and other alternatives. *Alzheimer Dis Associ Disord* 1994;8(4):28–37.
16. *Code of medical ethics: current opinions with annotations.* Chicago: American Medical Association, 1996.
17. Cope DN. Legal and ethical issues in the psychopharmacologic treatment of traumatic brain injury. *J Head Trauma Rehabil* 1989;4:13–20.
18. Appelbaum PS, Roth LH. Clinical issues in the assessment of competency to consent to psychiatric hospitalization. *Am J Psychiatry* 1981;138:1462–1467.
19. Callahan CD, Hagglund K. Comparing neuropsychological and psychiatric evaluation of competency in rehabilitation: a case example. *Arch Phys Med Rehabil* 1995;76: 909–912.
20. Buchanan AE, Brock DW. *Deciding for others: the ethics of surrogate decision making.* New York: Cambridge University Press, 1989.

21. Tepper AM, Elwork A. Competence to consent to treatment as a psychological construct. *Law Hum Behav* 1984;8:205–223.

22. *In re Conroy*, 98 NJ 321, 486 A2d 1209 (1985).

23. *U.S. v Charters*, 829 F2d 479 (4th Cir 1987).

24. *Miller v Rhode Island Hosp.*, 625 A2d 778 (RI 1993).

25. *In re Quinlan*, 70 NJ 10, 355 A2d 647 (1976).

26. *Cruzan v Director, Missouri Dept. of Health*, 497 US 261 (1990)

27. Dresser R. Life, death, and incompetent patients: conceptual infirmities and hidden values in the law. *Ariz Law Rev* 1986;28:373–405.

28. Weir RF, Gostin L. Decisions to abate life-sustaining treatment for nonautonomous patients; ethical standards and legal liability for physicians after *Cruzan*. *JAMA* 1990;264:1846–1853.

29. Lo B. Caring for incompetent patients: is there a physician on the case? *Law Med Health Care* 1989;17:214–221.

30. Areen J. The legal status of consent obtained from families of adult patients to withhold or withdraw treatment. *JAMA* 1987;258: 229–235.

31. Cantor NL. *Advance directives and the pursuit of death with dignity.* Bloomington: Indiana University Press, 1993.

32. Hotes LS, Johnson JA, Sicilian L. Long-term care, rehabilitation, and legal and ethical considerations in the management of neuromuscular disease with respiratory dysfunction. *Clin Chest Med* 1994;15: 783–795.

33. Terry M, Zweig S. Prevalence of advance directives and do-not-resuscitate orders in community nursing facilities. *Arch Fam Med* 1994;3:141–145.

34. Wenger NS, Halpern J. The physician's role in completing advance directives: ensuring patients' capacity to make healthcare dicisions in advance. *J Clin Ethics* 1994;5:320–323.

35. Teno JM, Lynn J, Phillips RS, et al. Do formal advance directives affect resuscitation decisions and the use of resources for seriously ill patients? *J Clin Ethics* 1994; 5:23–30.

36. 42 USC Sec 1395 cc (f) (West Supp 1996).

37. Banja JD, Bilsky GS. Discussing cardiopulmonary resuscitation with elderly rehabilitation patients. *Am J Phys Med Rehabil* 1993;74: S12–S24.

38. Winslade W, Ross J. Privacy, confidentiality and autonomy in psychotherapy. *Nebraska Law Rev* 1985;64:578–636.

39. Winslade W. Confidentiality of medical records. *J Legal Med* 1982;3:497–533.

40. *Hammonds v Aetna Casualty & Surety Co.*, 243 F Supp 793 (ND Ohio 1965).

41. Gellman R. Prescribing privacy: the uncertain role of the physician in the protection of privacy. *North Car Law Rev* 1984;62:255–294 (quoting 1 Hippocrates 164–165 (W. Jones trans. 1923).

42. Thompson I. Nature of confidentiality. *J Med Ethics* 1979;5:57–64.

43. Slovenko R. Psychiatry and a second look at the medical privilege. *Wayne Law Rev* 1960;6: 175–203.

44. *Doe v Roe*, 93 Misc 2d 201, 400 NYS 2d 668 (1977).

45. Hayden D. Should there be a psychotherapist privilege in military courts-martial? *Mil Law Rev* 1989;123:31–107.

46. *MacDonald v Clinger*, 84 AD 2d 482, 446 NYS 2d 801 (1982).

47. Miller WJ, Miller JN. Managed care contracting. *PLI/Comm* 1993;669:547–556.

48. McCandlish TW. Representing physicians in the development of managed care plans. *ALI-ABA* 1991;C653:139–163.

49. Demuro PR. Medical group development, PHOs, MSOs, medical foundations, and fully integrated delivery systems. *PLI/Comm* 1994;700:81–189.

50. Bonfiglio RP, Bonfiglio RL. Pearls of industrial rehabilitation medicine. *Phys Med Rehabil Clin N Am* 1996;7:601–617.

51. *Guides to the evaluation of permanent impairment.* 4th ed. Chicago: American Medical Association, 1993.

52. Frymoyer JW, Haldeman S, Andersson GBJ. Impairment rating—the United States perspective. In: *Occupational low back pain: assessment, treatment and prevention.* St. Louis: Mosby, 1991,279–295.

53. Tait RC, Margolis RB, Krause SJ, Liebowitz E. Compensation status and symptoms reported by patients with chronic pain. *Arch Phys Med Rehabil* 1988;69:1027–1029.

54. Dworkin RH, Handlin DS, Richlin DM, et al. Unraveling the effects of compensation, litigation, and employment in treatment response in chronic pain. *Pain* 1985;23:49–59.

Part II.

Assessment, Evaluation, and Diagnostic Approach

Chapter 5

Clinical Evaluation

Guy W. Fried
Karen Mandzak Fried

The clinical evaluation in medicine is the cornerstone of all clinical impressions and ultimately is the basis for diagnoses and treatments. In physical medicine and rehabilitation, the clinical evaluation goes one step further by encompassing the patient's needs, desires, and functional strengths and weaknesses. The unique perspective in rehabilitation medicine is to go beyond the diagnosis of disease to look at the impact of disease on function. The same disease entity may have very different impacts given different scenarios. For example, a young sports enthusiast with a traumatic transfemoral amputation will have different rehabilitation issues than will an elderly widow with the same impairment due to peripheral vascular disease. Rehabilitation goals must be individualized. The young sports enthusiast's goal may be to return to active sports and work. The elderly widow may have a goal of reaching independence with activities of daily living and ambulation within the community.

The clinical evaluation must have the broad perspective of the whole person and not just a myopic view of a single organ or system. It includes assessment of the role of the patient within the family and community. The evaluation may incorporate the expertise of various disciplines, including but not limited to physiatry, physical therapy, occupational therapy, speech therapy, vocational counseling, therapeutic recreation, case management, psychology, and rehabilitation nursing. It is during the clinical evaluation that the patient's needs, treatments, and goals are determined. In rehabilitation medicine the clinical evaluation is an ongoing, interactive process extending beyond the initial assessment. Important details regarding the physical examination and functional abilities are not necessarily entirely forthcoming at the initial evaluation, and are often revealed over time.

To develop a clear understanding of the impact that a disease has on a patient's life, it is important that the clinician be able to distinguish between impairment, disability, and handicap. (See Chapter 2 for further discussion.) Briefly, according to the World Health Organization (WHO), an *impairment* is any loss or abnormality of psychological function or physical structure or function. A *disability* is any restriction (resulting from an impairment) in performing an activity in the manner or within the range considered normal. WHO defines *handicap* as a disadvantage for a given individual resulting from an impairment or disability that limits or prevents the fulfillment of a role that is normal for that individual. Understanding the patient's impairment, disability, and handicap enables the treatment team to minimize the impact of a disease entity (1).

The comprehensiveness of the history and physical examination is partially determined by its purpose. It may differ depending on the setting, whether it is an inpatient admission, consultation, outpatient evaluation, independent medical examination, or evaluation at a specific treatment clinic. Although this chapter describes the different parts of the clinical evaluation in a particular order, each clinician will develop an individual style and order of gathering information (2–6).

HISTORY

The patient's history is broken down into the separate components of chief complaint, history of present illness, past medical history, family history, functional history, social history, habits, allergies, medications, and a focused review of systems.

The patient history is obtained by reviewing prior records and interviewing the patient. It is useful to speak to the patient and family, or significant others, together to get a complete history of all of the patient's functions and roles. It may be necessary to speak to caregivers such as nurses, home health aides, and employers to get the most complete picture.

The chief complaint is a logical starting point of an evaluation. It represents the prime reason the patient is seeking help. Whenever possible, it is expressed in the patient's own words. The chief complaint often conveys more than just disease symptomatology. It may imply disability or handicap and the subsequent loss associated with the clinical symptoms.

To obtain the history of the present illness, the physician uses the art of interview to elucidate various problems and the pertinent chronologic milestones. The physician must listen carefully and guide the process. The patient should be allowed to express the history and symptoms in his or her own words. Frequently, the patient will use medical terms such as "spasm" and "weakness" to describe symptoms; these words will have a different meaning to the physician. Encourage the patient to describe and define what he or she means. The present illness and the symptoms should be organized in a chronologic narrative account, described in terms of onset, setting, manifestations, and impact on the patient's life. The description should include the location, quality, severity, duration, onset, timing, modifying features, and associated signs and symptoms of each problem. The history of prior successful and unsuccessful treatments is beneficial for development of a treatment plan. It helps the physician to know whether the disease process or functional difficulties are progressing or improving. Pertinent data such as laboratory results should be included. A review of pertinent absent signs and symptoms is helpful in defining the history of the present illness.

A thorough past medical and surgical history allows the physician to further characterize the effect of past conditions on the present level of function. A special focus on neurologic, cardiopulmonary, musculoskeletal, and cognitive abilities clarifies the patient's functional limitations, which in turn aid in the determination of the recovery potential and functional prognosis. Methods for treating and coping with prior disorders should be reviewed, as they will help organize treatment strategies.

A history of previous neurologic disorders has a tremendous impact on future function. Identification of congenital, progressive, or a recent isolated event is significant because prior disorders can influence strength, sensation, tone, or cognition. Previous neurologic problems may negatively impact on the new, but unrelated, present problem due to a cumulative damage effect.

A previous history of cardiopulmonary disorders may influence a patient's physical reserves. The patient with a new disability will consume more energy to accomplish the same tasks. A detailed past medical history of cardiac and pulmonary disorders allows the physician to determine current and potential functional limitations. The rehabilitation prescription and precautions are tailored to meet specific goals within safe parameters.

Musculoskeletal disorders are extremely common. Frequently, limitations are caused by pain, joint immobility, and weakness. Comorbidities such as amputation may determine a baseline functional status. Any new problem will be compounded by previous musculoskeletal disorders.

A history of psychiatric or cognitive disorders frequently affects functional capability by impacting on a patient's emotional and intellectual capacity to handle a new problem. Physical illness or impairment may precipitate previous emotional problems, a schizophrenic episode, or depression. A patient with memory deficits may find it difficult to learn the new information and techniques that are necessary for successful rehabilitation.

A family history of medical disorders will provide the practitioner with a better sense of the family unit. The age and health of each immediate family member should be questioned and documented. This will help give clues to the patient's potential health problems. In addition, the practitioner will gain valuable information regarding how the family has coped with illness or impairment. The physician should ask specifically about diabetes, heart disease, hypertension, stroke, arthritis, alcoholism, or mental illness, as these diseases may have a familial pattern.

Current and prior use of medications, including prescription and nonprescription drugs, as well as information about allergic responses must be carefully documented. It is helpful to know how long, how much, how often, and why the patient takes the medication. Many medications have potential side effects and interactions. Medications commonly affect function in such areas as mental alertness, fatigue, gastrointestinal and bladder function, tone changes, and pain. The physiatrist may become quite adept at adjusting medication usage to make the side effect least offensive or perhaps even desirable. For example, the antidepressant amitriptyline can produce the potentially desired side effects of better sleep, weight gain, and a decrease in urinary detrusor hyperactivity. Any allergic response to any medication must be clarified. A patient has to describe the "allergic" response in order to evaluate the best course of action for further treatment.

In summary, the clinical history must include a broad review of symptoms. The physiatric review of symptoms includes the general medical review of systems plus an expanded review of those systems, but with a fundamental emphasis.

FUNCTIONAL REVIEW OF SYSTEMS

In addition to an assessment of physical impairments and functional problems, the review of systems can also be used to explore broader issues in the patient's life, such as advance directives. Specific questions about resuscitation in the event of an emergency, including the use of cardiopulmonary resuscitation, intubation/ventilators, feeding tubes, and antibiotics should be asked during this process in order to fully incorporate the patient's wishes into the plan of care.

Neurologic Symptoms

A neurologic review of systems includes queries on thought processes, memory, weakness, tremor, paresthesias, syncope, seizures, pain, coordination, vertigo, and falls. Ask if pain, weakness, or coordination limits ambulation distances. Does the patient find it difficult to remember names, directions, or times to take medicines? Is there a history of falls? If so, what were the circumstances? Was it because of weakness, syncope, or vertigo? Does the patient have spasticity? How does this impact on function?

Respiratory Symptoms

The respiratory review of systems elicits details regarding cough, pain, sputum (color, consistency, quantity), hemoptysis, and dyspnea. Is oxygen used? If so, how much and for which activities? How many pillows does the patient use for sleep? Is there any history of exposure to asbestos, industrial smoke, or dust? Does the patient have a history of smoking? If so, how much and for how long (packs versus years)?

Cardiovascular Symptoms

A cardiovascular review of systems includes queries about angina, dyspnea, claudication, palpitations, orthopnea, edema, hypertension, and murmurs. The results of past electrocardiograms or cardiac testing are reviewed. It is important to ask if any activities are limited by chest pain or calf aching, or if the patient gets dizzy when first standing up.

Musculoskeletal Symptoms

The musculoskeletal review of systems is critical in rehabilitation medicine and often is the underlying reason for physiatric referral. The patient should be questioned about muscle weakness, joint stiffness, swelling, erythema, and pain. How is the patient's function and mobility affected by these factors? Does the patient use any special techniques, medications, or equipment to accomplish functional tasks?

Head and Neck Symptoms

The review of the head and neck should include questions about swallowing, vision, hearing, smelling, and headache. Does the patient have any double vision? When was the last time vision was checked? How do disturbances in these functions affect the patient's daily life?

Communication Impairments

Clearly, while interviewing a patient, the examiner is indirectly evaluating the patient's ability to communicate effectively. More specifically, the interviewer must delve into the limitations and abilities the patient has with speaking, listening, writing, and reading. It must be ascertained whether the patient has difficulty finding words, or being understood by others. Questions should identify any difficulty with voice volume, difficulty with thought expression (verbal or written), or difficulty hearing. Other important information includes whether the patient uses a hearing aid, understands what others say, reads and recalls what is read, or is able to write and/or type.

Eating Impairments

The review of eating impairments assesses whether the patient can eat independently, can open boxes or cut food, and can chew and swallow safely. Is there a history of choking? If so, is this with solids or liquids? Eating difficulties may be reflected indirectly by weight loss or loss of appetite. Additionally, it must be kept in mind that any change in weight or appetite may be a manifestation of depression.

Grooming Impairments

The examiner should determine whether the patient is able to groom and present himself or herself. These tasks include brushing teeth, inserting dentures, combing hair, applying makeup and deodorant, and showering. Equally important is reviewing whether the patient has lost the desire to groom and present himself or herself.

Toileting Impairments

Toileting functions are frequently taken for granted or not discussed. These functions are regarded as private, and difficulties may lead to shame, depression, and isolation (7). The practitioner must obtain this information from the patient with specific questions, as the patient may gloss over difficulties. Toileting difficulties can have extremely disabling features and psychologically devastating results for adults. A rehabilitation review of systems with a functional emphasis focuses on continence of the bowel and bladder, urgency, and frequency. Can the patient volitionally start and stop a urine stream? How frequent are bowel movements compared with the historical baseline? Can the patient independently use appliances such as urinary catheters or ostomies? If not, who cares for these appliances? How is feminine hygiene managed?

Dressing Impairments

The physician should inquire whether or not the patient can dress independently. If not, how much assistance is needed? What does the patient usually wear, both indoors and outdoors? Can the patient manage buttons, zippers, snaps, and shoelaces?

Mobility Impairments

The most elementary level of mobility is bed mobility. It is important to know whether the patient can turn in the bed, roll, sit up, and maintain balance. Does the patient ever get "stuck" in any position? The patient's ability to transfer to and from the bed to a wheelchair, a shower chair, the floor, or a car should be addressed. Any information about falls must be evaluated further. Skin problems are often related to mobility deficits and should be explored further.

For the patient who uses a wheelchair, the physician should assess mobility, the patient's ability to wheel on a flat surface, uneven outdoor terrain, ramps, and carpet. How far can the patient manually propel the wheelchair, and how much time does it take to achieve that distance? Is a power wheelchair in use? If so, for what indications?

Ambulation

The patient should be questioned about the need for assistance to ambulate, including the physical assistance of another person. A history of falls should be explored further. Does the patient use ambulation aides, such as a straight cane, quadripod cane, or walker? Is there any difficulty with stairs, carpets, ramps, or public transportation?

Motor Vehicle Use

Does the patient drive or have a valid driver's license? Are there any driving violations or accidents? What distances or limitations does the patient have with driving? Does the patient have driving restrictions regarding distance or night driving?

The review of the patient's symptoms and impairments with a functional emphasis provides the basis for a patient profile. Additional information on psychological, social, vocational, family, and lifestyle issues completes the profile.

Psychological, Social, Vocational, Family, and Lifestyle Issues

A psychological review reveals the patient's past abilities to cope with life's stresses. While responding to these questions, the patient's cognitive ability should also be assessed. By clarifying the patient's psychological and cognitive profile, the physician can direct any therapeutic approach to maximize the patient's likelihood of successful adjustment. Each patient has a specific coping style in response to challenges or losses. Patients may have a recurrence of past psychiatric disorders when placed in a stressful situation. It is important to ascertain whether there is any history of depression, suicide, thought disorder, or sleep disorder, in response to stress. Failure to account for previous psychiatric history may complicate the rehabilitation program or undermine goals and treatment interventions.

Understanding the patient's habits, desires and motivations, and lifestyle facilitates program planning, and helps the team to set attainable goals. What leisure activities does the patient enjoy? How important are sexuality and spirituality? These interests can be incorporated into the patient's goals and therefore become motivational agents.

It is important to explore the patient's work history. Work requirements should be defined, in terms of physical and cognitive function, as well as time commitment. Does the patient desire a return to work? Are work modifications possible? What education level is required for a patient to attain a vocational goal? Chapter 18 on vocational assessment provides an in-depth discussion of these issues.

The social history is quite broad, covering areas such as living situation; family support systems; habits such as smoking, alcohol, or drug use; and financial status. A review of insurance coverage is necessary to guide the rehabilitation team in setting treatment goals and time frames. In addition, insurance coverage will influence decisions about equipment and ongoing services. Litigation may influence the patient's financial and insurance status. What is the patient's role in the family? Who is available to the patient for financial, emotional, or physical support?

PHYSICAL EXAMINATION

The rehabilitation physical examination embodies the basic general medical examination but with a specific focus on areas that impact function. The physical examination consists of an assessment of all the body systems with an emphasis on the neuromuscular areas. The following are the key areas of the physical examination.

General Appearance

As an overview, the physician first assesses the patient's general appearance and affect. Vital signs should be recorded. Positional blood pressure recordings may be indicated, for instance, in the patient with a history of falls or dizziness. Often, assessments of mobility and function can be made before the "official" physical examination begins, by observing the patient arising from a waiting-room chair and ambulating to the examination room.

Skin

Skin disorders are commonly encountered in the rehabilitation population. This can be a manifestation of underlying diseases, such as lupus or peripheral vascular disease, or a result of physical limitations, such as pressure sores from a lack of sensation or from immobility. It is critically important to examine the patient fully undressed and in good light. The intragluteal, perineal, and ischial areas must be examined for skin breakdown from stool, urine, and sweat. These areas can be overlooked by health care workers in the spirit of modesty or misguided efficiency. It is necessary to examine any areas of pressure or skin overlying a bony prominence. The feet, especially the posterior part of the heels and between the toes, should be examined for any areas of skin breakdown due to recumbency or peripheral vascular disorders.

Head

The head should be inspected for any signs of past or present trauma. Palpation can be done to ascertain evidence of prior surgery or shunts. Two salivary glands can be palpated—the parotid gland and the submandibular gland. The opening of the glands may be visible in the mouth. The superficial temporal artery may be visible and palpable just anterior to the ear. This may be tender in the patient with temporal arteritis. Vision should be checked for disturbances. If charts are unavailable, newsprint can be held at a distance and compared with the acuity of the examiner. Check for funduscopic evidence of diabetes mellitus or hypertension. Check that the eyelids close adequately.

Ears

Hearing can be tested easily with the ticking of a watch. Any abnormality should be addressed further with an audiogram. It is useful to assess whether a hearing aid can compensate for some of the loss. Poor hearing can contribute to inadequate teaching, or even misdiagnosis.

Throat

Check for signs of erythema, candidiasis, poor oral hygiene, or inadequate denture fitting. There should be a general examination of the neck, including examination of the thyroid and the carotid arteries.

Chest and Respiratory Assessment

The chest should be inspected for symmetric inspiration and expiration while also observing for restrictions that may be due to structural abnormalities such as kyphoscoliosis.

Male patients should be inspected for signs of gynecomastia. The breasts and axillae should be inspected and palpated for symmetry and masses. Changes in skin texture or evidence of drainage should be investigated further. Axillary, subscapular, and submandibular lymph nodes should be evaluated. If a patient has chest tubes or tracheostomy tubes, the incision site should be inspected and palpated for tenderness, erythema, and drainage. If the patient has a tracheostomy, one should be familiar with the types used, such as cuffed or cuffless, solid or fenestrated. The amount of pulmonary secretions should be quantified. The current program to manage secretions should also be reviewed. Auscultation will yield vital information about the patient's respiratory ability.

Cardiovascular Assessment

Cardiovascular disease can be a limiting determinant for function. Auscultation will provide information regarding murmurs or carotid bruits. Internal jugular vein distention is useful as a reliable measure of right atrial pressures. More sophisticated testing may be indicated if cardiac impairment is expected to impact the rehabilitation program.

Peripheral arterial disease should be evaluated with palpation of the carotid, radial, femoral, dorsal pedis, and posterior tibialis pulses for symmetry and strength. It is useful to have a bedside Doppler machine available for checking weak pulses, especially in the patient with a history of peripheral vascular disease or amputation. Peripheral vascular states must be closely followed in any patient considered for orthoses or prostheses. Braces should not impede blood flow or cause irritation. The peripheral vascular assessment should include palpation of the abdomen for evidence of abdominal aortic aneurysm.

Gastrointestinal and Genitourinary Assessment

The rectal and genital areas may be examined generally but must have a more focused examination if there are any difficulties with bowel or bladder elimination, incontinence, or impotence. It is essential to inspect the skin for maceration or genital infection, and the urethra for signs of damage from indwelling or intermittent catheterization. In male patients, the prostate should be checked for texture and symmetry. The bulbocavernosus response should be assessed by squeezing the clitoris or glans penis with one hand while feeling with a finger in the rectum for a reflex contraction. Anal wink reflex is checked with a perianal pinprick while watching for an anal contraction. Both indicate an intact bulbocavernosus reflex. The physician should check for rectal tone as well as carefully distinguish between a volitional anal contraction and a Valsalva maneuver. Stool should be tested for blood.

Musculoskeletal Assessment

Musculoskeletal disorders are extremely common in rehabilitation and frequently are the source of functional deficits. The examiner must proceed in an orderly fashion, evaluating the regions individually and as part of a whole. A suggested order of examination is inspection, palpation, active range of motion, passive range of motion, joint stability, and muscular strength.

Inspection of the body looking for joint symmetry, swelling, edema, scoliosis, kyphosis, leg-length discrepancy, and atrophy of muscle is helpful. If a peripheral polyneuropathy is suspected, the distal parts of the hands and feet should be evaluated to assess muscle atrophy. Inspect for hair loss, skin texture, and regional diaphoresis in the patient suspected to have a sympathetic nervous disorder. If radiculopathy is suspected, the physician should include bilateral limb circumferential measurements.

To fully evaluate joints for disease or trauma, the physician must assess active, assisted, and passive range of motion. To test active range of motion, the examiner has the patient move the joint in a particular plane through the full possible range of motion. The examiner tests active assisted range of motion by assisting the patient in performing a tolerable range of motion. To test passive range of motion, the examiner moves the joint to the greatest tolerable range of motion (8). Figures 5-1 to 5-24 demonstrate range of motion quantified by joint plane and degree. The angles of the joint are measured by a goniometer, which has two flexible arms attached to a protractor. The apex of the goniometer is placed over the center of the joint and the two arms are placed over the corresponding bones, allowing a number representing degrees to be read. Additionally, the examiner should note any perceived cause of limitation, such as pain or a structural abnormality (9,10).

There are specialized physical maneuvers to test movements of the joint in several planes as well as the integrity of the joint and particular ligaments. Although the specific tests are out of the realm of this chapter, this topic is covered in other chapters. If joint instability is documented, radiographs may be indicated.

Multiple factors, including cooperation, the ability to understand directions, pain, joint disease, age, gender, and fatigue, contribute to performance on manual muscle testing. Muscle grades are described as absent to normal on a 0 to 5 scale. Grade 0 or 1 (trace) muscle contraction is determined by careful observation and palpation of the muscle and tendon. Grade 2 (poor) muscle strength is when contraction yields a full range of joint motion in a gravity-eliminated position. Grade 3 (fair) is when muscle contraction moves a joint through full range of motion against gravity. Grade 4 (good) is when a muscle can resist a moderate amount of resistance against gravity, whereas a grade 5 (normal) muscle can resist a maximal effort.

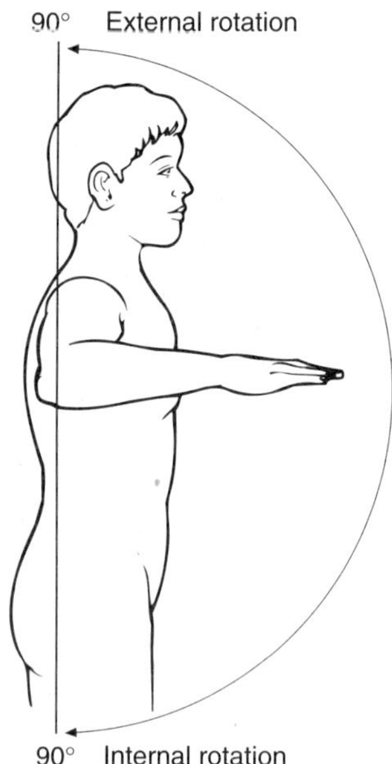

Figure 5-2. Shoulder external rotation/internal rotation.

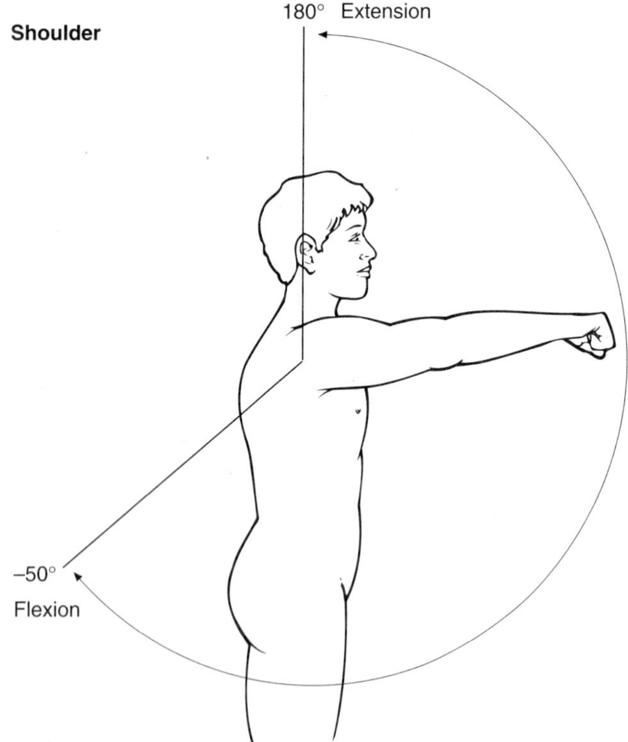

Figure 5-1. Shoulder flexion/extension.

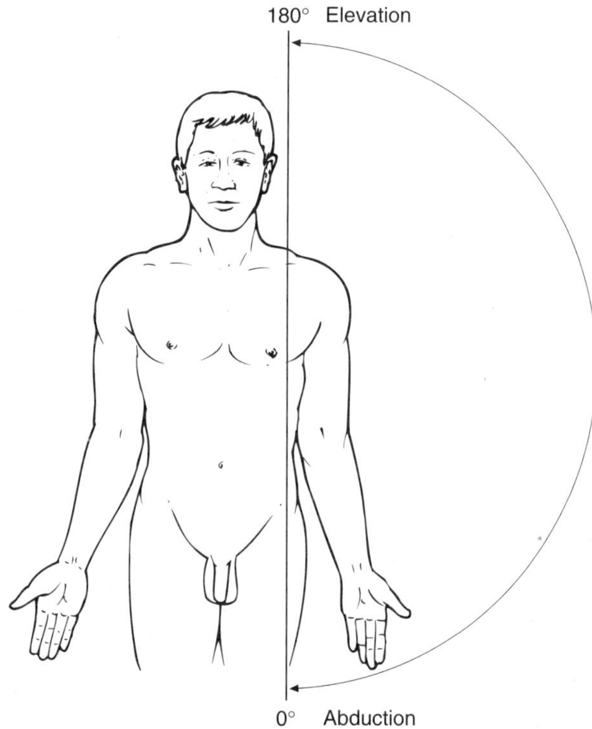

Figure 5-3. Shoulder abduction.

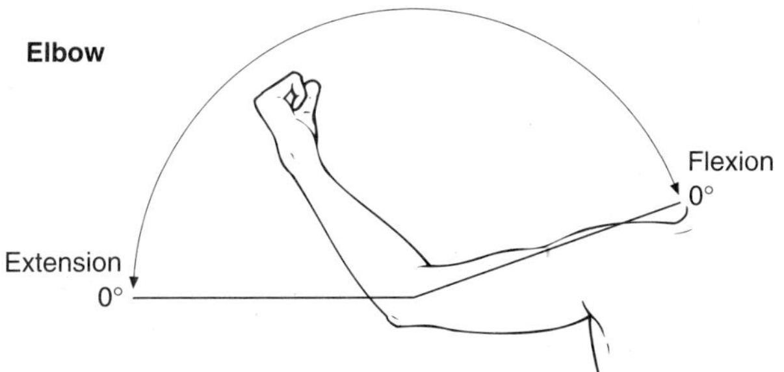

Figure 5-4. Elbow extension/flexion.

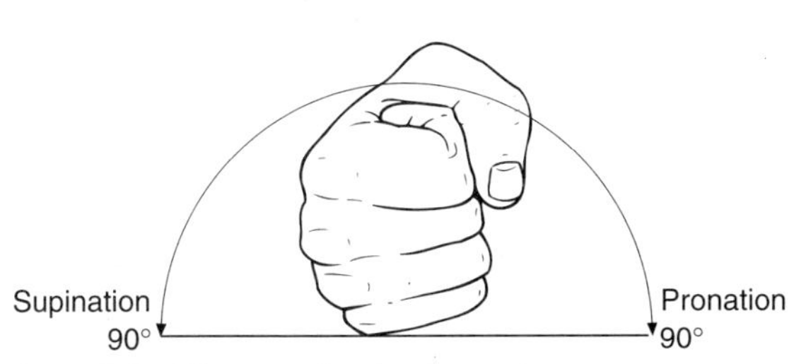

Figure 5-5. Elbow supination/pronation.

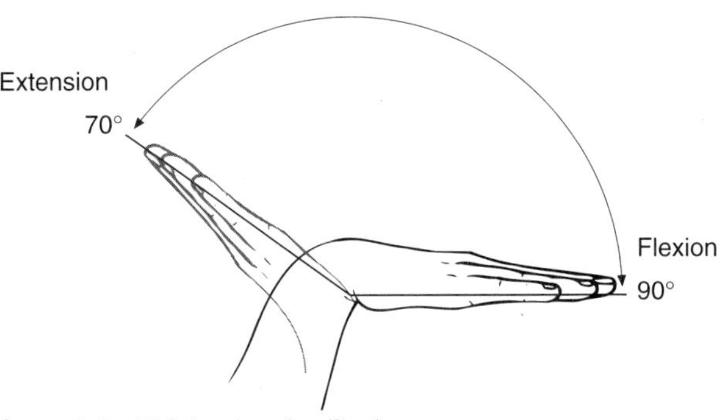

Figure 5-6. Wrist extension/flexion.

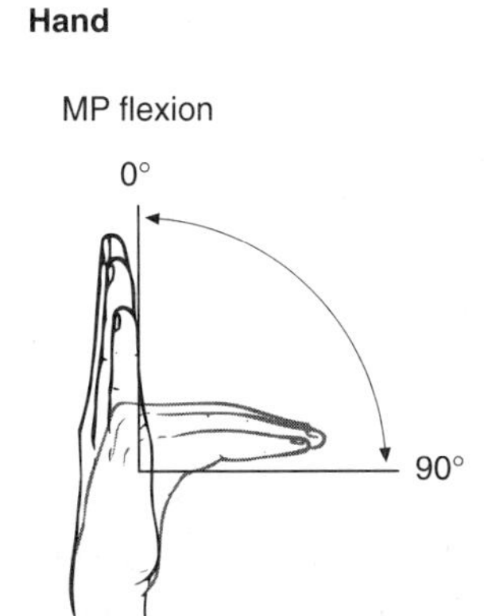

Figure 5-7. Metaphalangeal flexion.

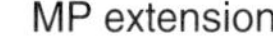

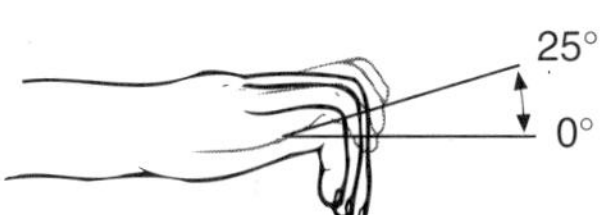

Figure 5-8. Metaphalangeal extension.

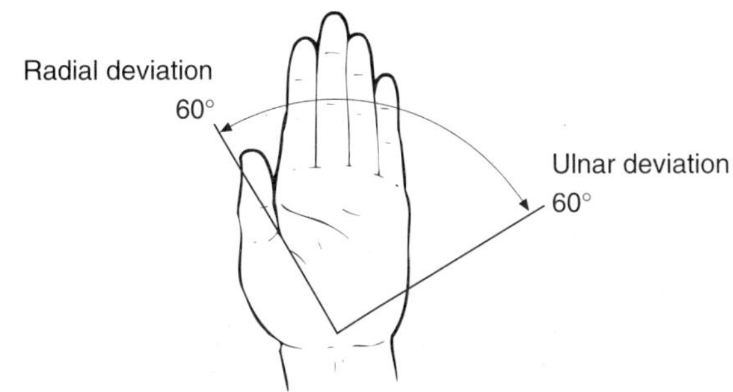

Figure 5-9. Wrist radial and ulnar deviation.

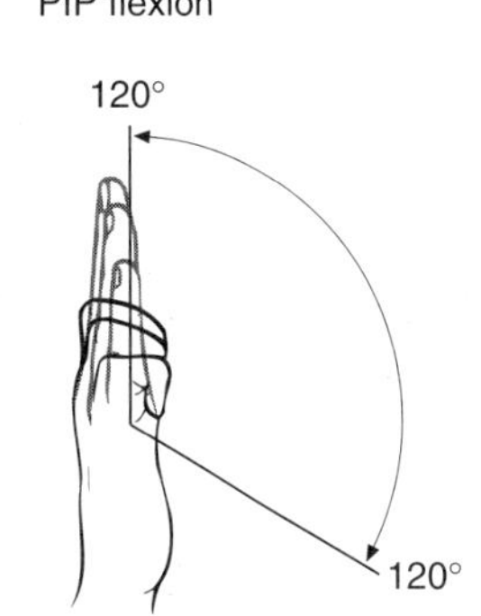

Figure 5-10. Proximal interphalangeal flexion.

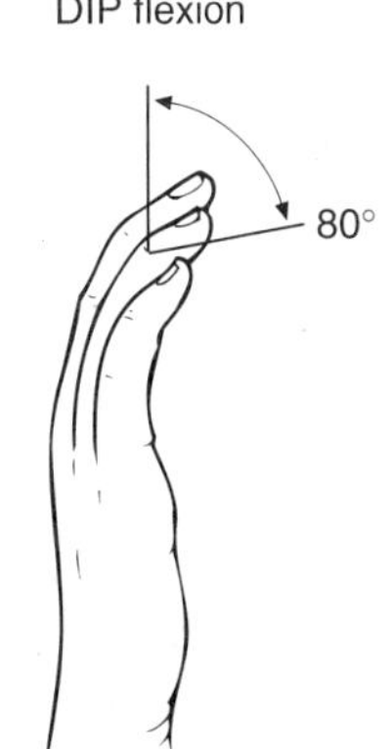

Figure 5-11. Distal interphalangeal flexion.

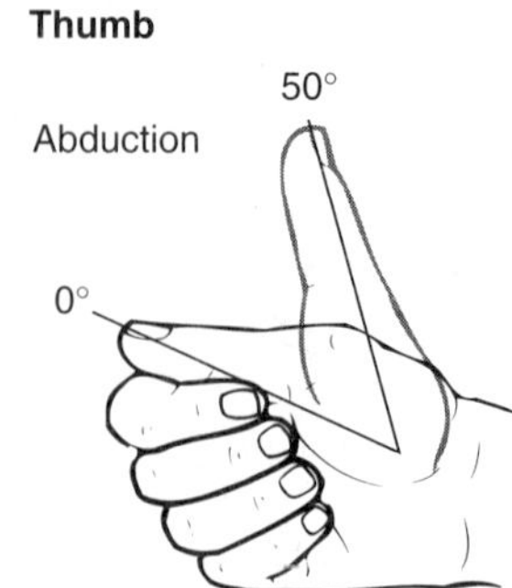

Figure 5-12. Thumb abduction.

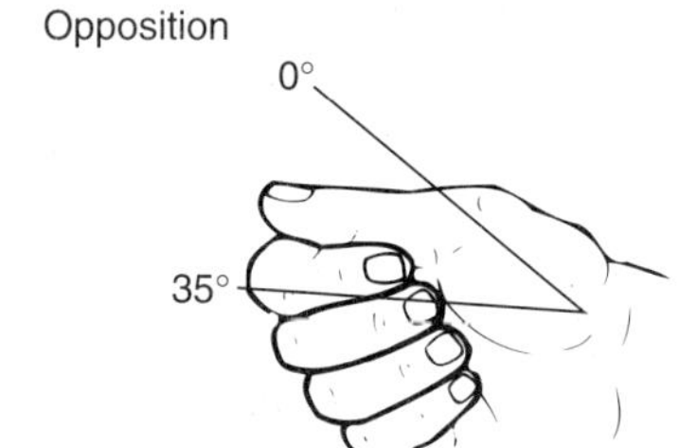

Figure 5-13. Thumb opposition.

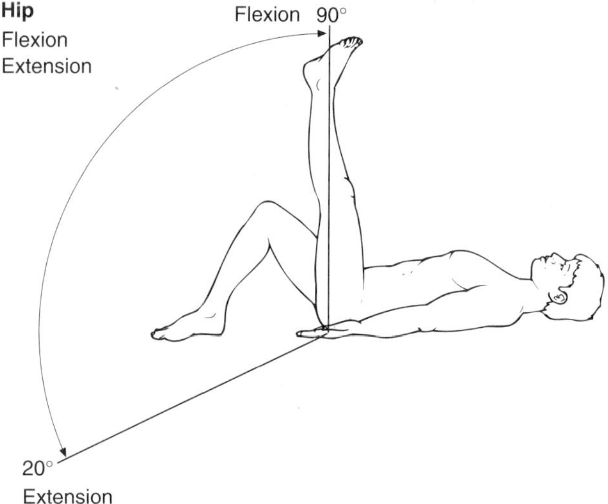

Figure 5-14. Hip extension/flexion.

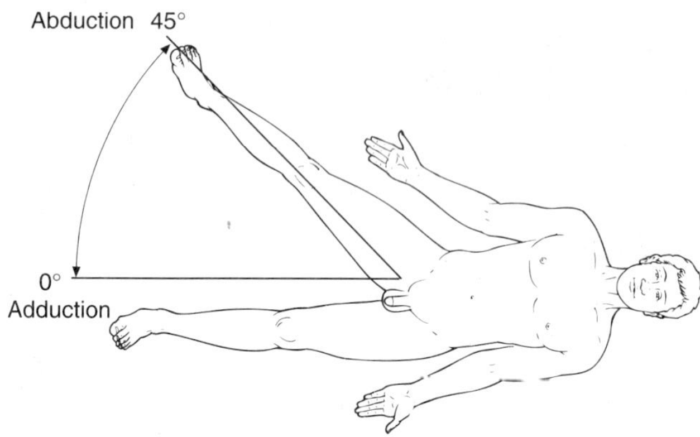

Figure 5-15. Hip abduction.

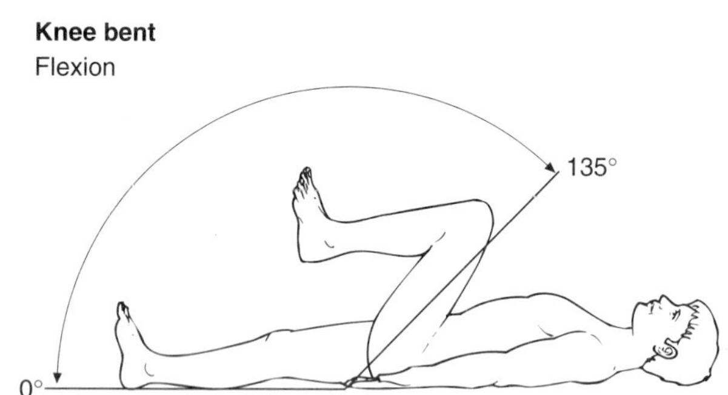

Figure 5-16. Hip flexion with knee bent.

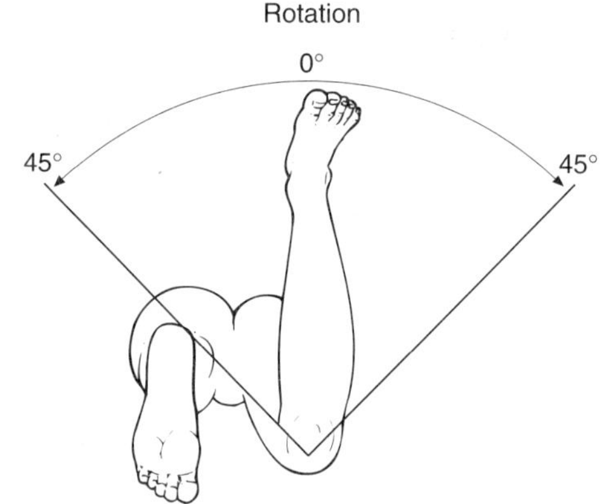

Figure 5-17. Hip internal/external rotation.

In addition to joint range of motion and manual muscle testing procedures, the classic Haymaker diagrams of radicular patterns and peripheral nerve distributions must be familiar to all physiatrists (11) (Figs. 5-25 and 5-26). Numbness in a particular area may be caused by damage in one of several different peripheral and central pathways. The clues given by sensory loss must be correlated with the other physical findings in order to isolate and diagnose a neurologic lesion.

Neurologic Assessment

The neurologic examination and the musculoskeletal examination are usually the most important components of the physical examination in the rehabilitative clinical assessment. Although the neurological examination is being described here separately, in practice it is frequently integrated within the rest of the physical examination. For example, the cranial nerves are usually tested during the head, ear, nose, and throat examination.

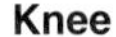

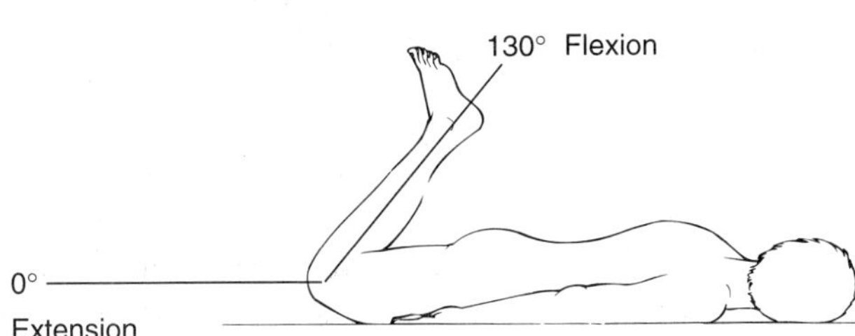

Figure 5-18. Knee flexion.

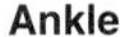

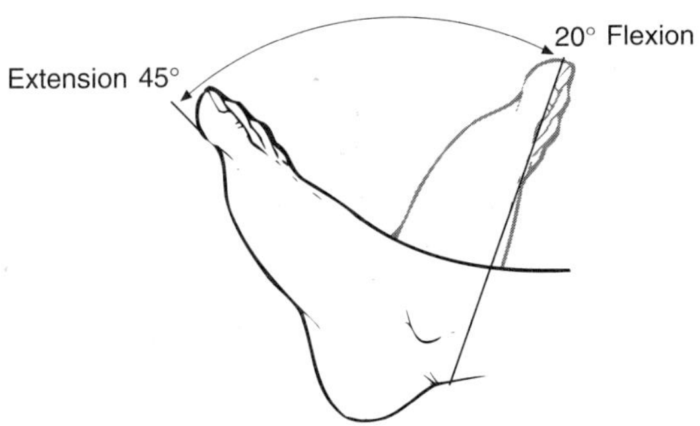

Figure 5-19. Ankle extension/flexion.

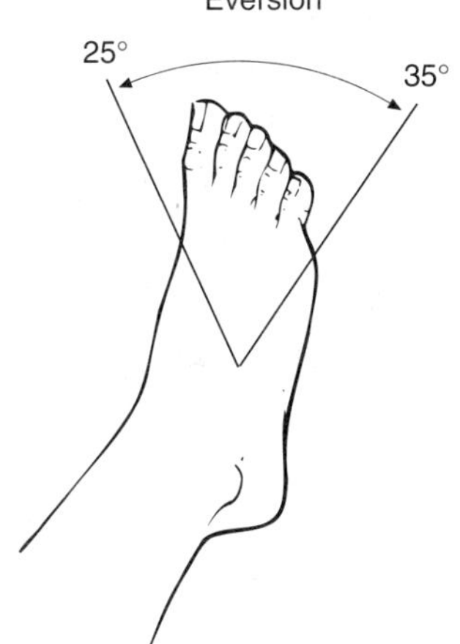

Figure 5-20. Ankle eversion.

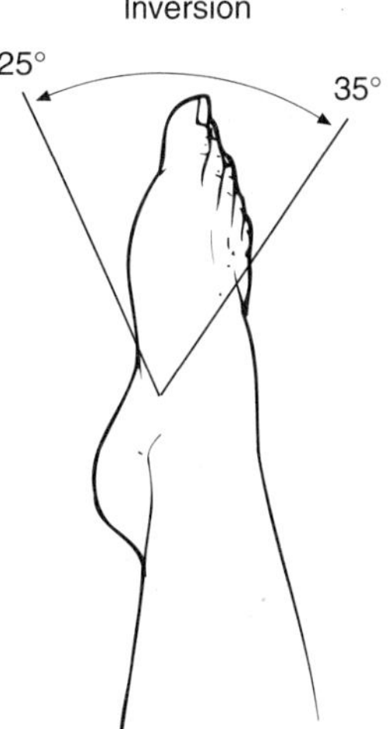

Figure 5-21. Ankle inversion.

Neck

Rotation

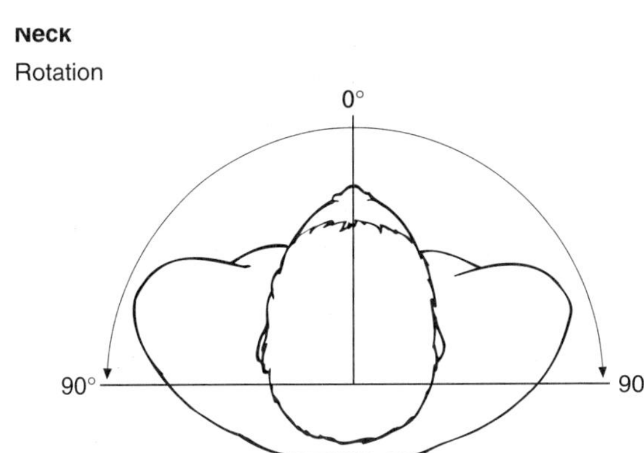

Figure 5-22. Neck rotation.

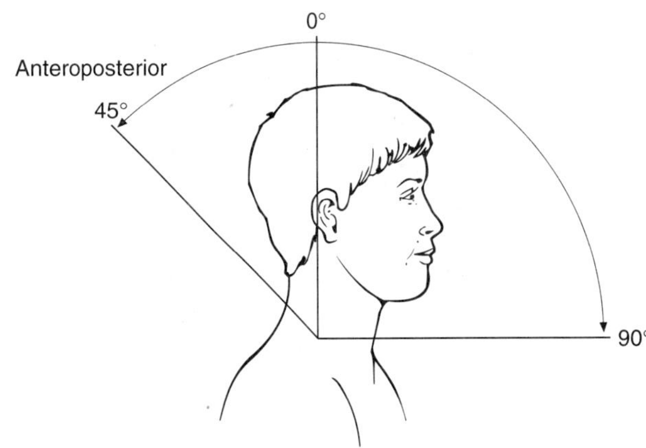

Figure 5-23. Neck flexion/extension.

It is important to formally test the patient's mental status including orientation, short-term memory, long-term memory, and abstractions. The patient's level of consciousness, whether normal or abnormal, should be noted and described. Orientation should be checked by having the patient state his or her full name and the date, day, and place. Attention can be tested utilizing a digit span test. This is performed by having the patient repeat random digits that are spoken by the examiner. For example, numbers such as 1-3-9 are given to the patient and then asked to be repeated. Recall of a span of seven digits is considered normal, this being the same number of digits in a telephone number. Alternatively, the patient can be given digits and asked to repeat them in reverse order. In this example, if the patient is given the numbers 1-3-9, he or she is expected to respond with the reverse order, 9-3-1. Reversing a sequence of numbers is a little more difficult and an ability to repeat five digits in reverse order is considered to be normal (12).

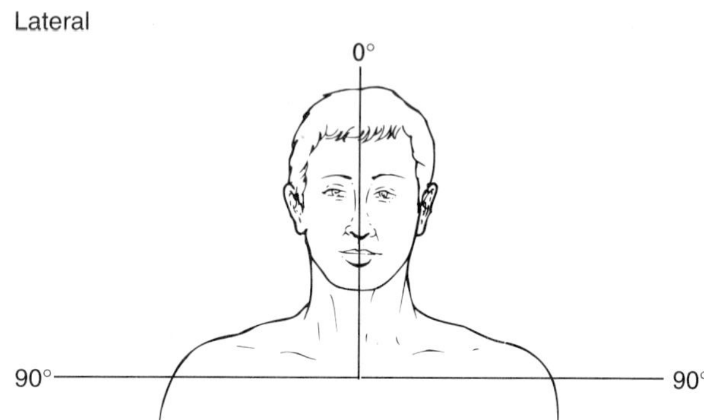

Figure 5-24. Neck lateral rotation.

The short-term memory is tested by asking the patient to remember three objects. Five minutes later, the patient is asked to repeat these objects. If the patient forgets, he or she can be reminded and tested again in an additional 5 minutes. Intermediate-term memory skills can also be assessed by asking the patient to recall the three objects later in the examination. The ability of the patient to calculate can be tested by "serial sevens," asking the patient to subtract 7 from 100 in a successive fashion (i.e., 93, 86, etc). The number of errors the patient makes should be recorded.

To test abstract thinking, the patient may be asked to explain the meaning of common proverbs. Answers may reveal concrete thinking. For example, when a patient is asked to explain the meaning of "People who live in glass houses shouldn't throw stones," they may respond with an explanation regarding the dangers of broken glass.

As another test of thinking, the patient is asked how two objects are alike, such as a table and a chair, piano and violin, or a cat and a mouse. Once again, the examiner should note whether the response is concrete or abstract.

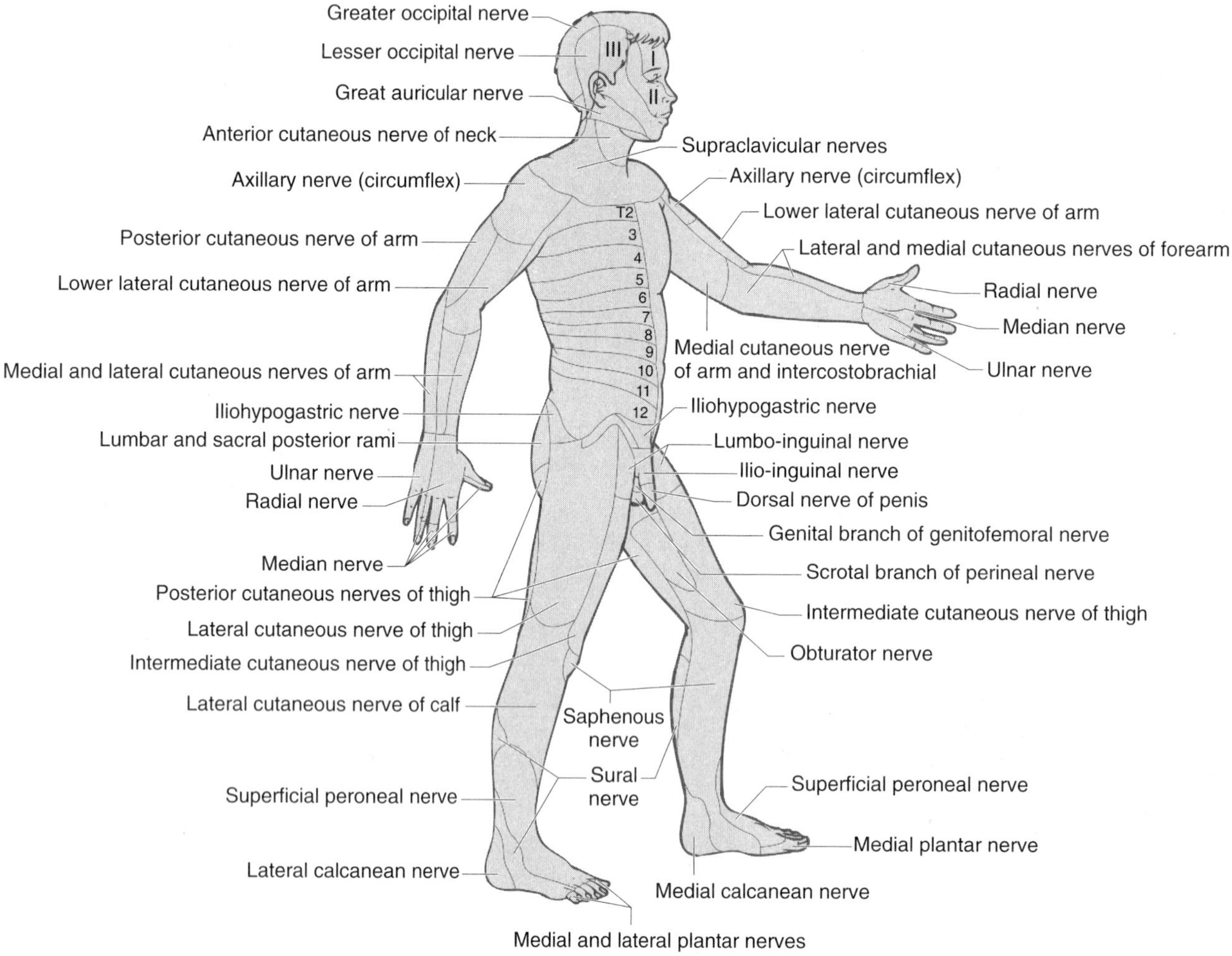

Greater occipital nerve
Lesser occipital nerve
Great auricular nerve
Anterior cutaneous nerve of neck
Axillary nerve (circumflex)
Posterior cutaneous nerve of arm
Lower lateral cutaneous nerve of arm
Medial and lateral cutaneous nerves of arm
Iliohypogastric nerve
Lumbar and sacral posterior rami
Ulnar nerve
Radial nerve
Median nerve
Posterior cutaneous nerves of thigh
Lateral cutaneous nerve of thigh
Intermediate cutaneous nerve of thigh
Lateral cutaneous nerve of calf
Superficial peroneal nerve
Lateral calcanean nerve
III
I
II
T2
3
4
5
6
7
8
9
10
11
12
Supraclavicular nerves
Axillary nerve (circumflex)
Lower lateral cutaneous nerve of arm
Lateral and medial cutaneous nerves of forearm
Radial nerve
Median nerve
Medial cutaneous nerve of arm and intercostobrachial
Ulnar nerve
Iliohypogastric nerve
Lumbo-inguinal nerve
Ilio-inguinal nerve
Dorsal nerve of penis
Genital branch of genitofemoral nerve
Scrotal branch of perineal nerve
Intermediate cutaneous nerve of thigh
Obturator nerve
Saphenous nerve
Sural nerve
Superficial peroneal nerve
Medial plantar nerve
Medial calcanean nerve
Medial and lateral plantar nerves

Figure 5-25. Peripheral nerve territory (side view).

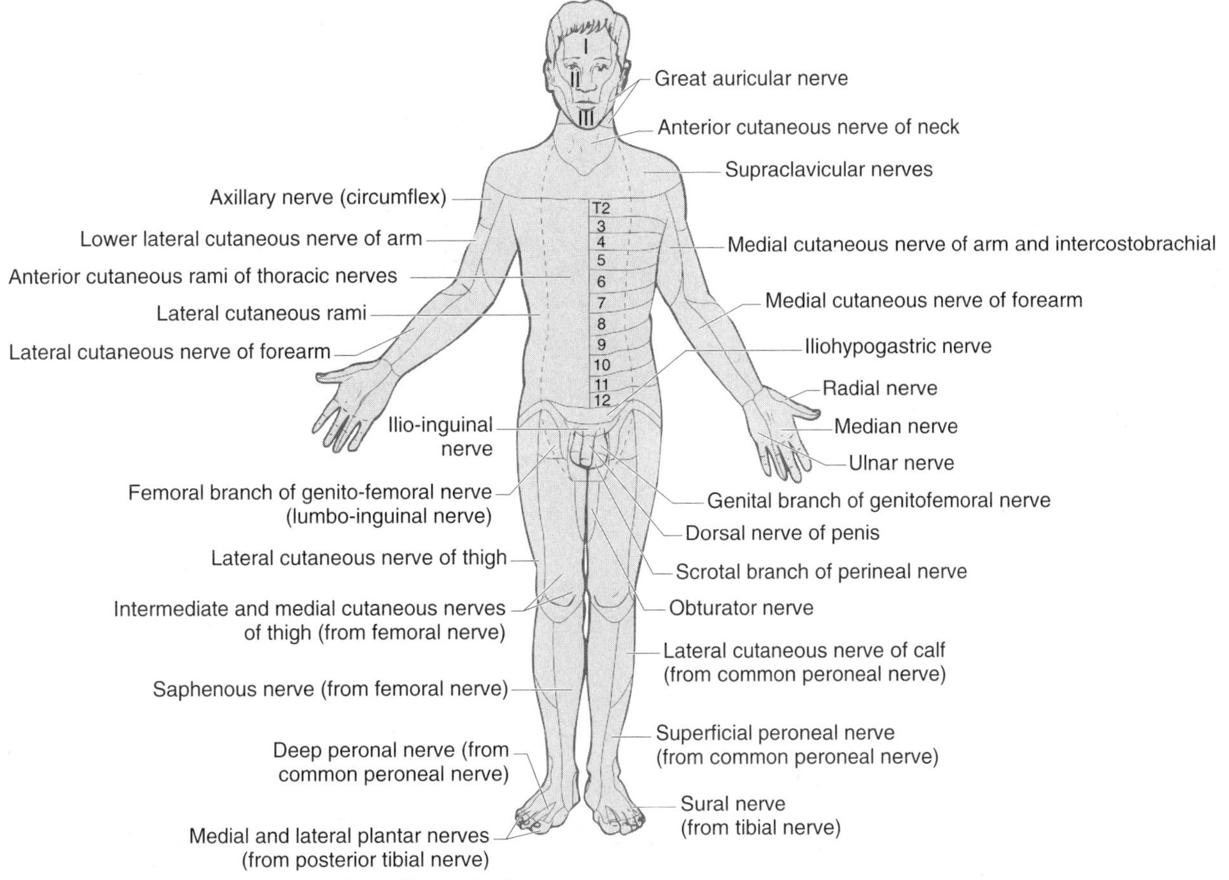

Figure 5-26. Peripheral nerve territory (front view).

Judgment can be tested by asking the patient to respond to a sample scenario, such as a fire in a movie theater, or a lost library book.

Speech function is tested informally throughout the entire clinical examination. As noted in other chapters, abnormal language function is important in defining a neurologic disorder. Specific tests of listening, reading, speaking, and writing should be administered.

A good cranial nerve examination is often overlooked. Cranial nerve impairments have a significant impact on overall function (12). Table 5-1 provides guidelines for the cranial nerve assessment (13–15).

The deep tendon reflexes commonly tested include the biceps (C5–C6), brachial radialis (C5–C6), triceps (C7–C8), finger flexors (C8–T1), quadriceps (L2–L4), medial hamstring (L4, S1), gastrocnemius (S1–S2), and bulbocavernosus (S2–S4). Deep tendon reflexes are graded 0 to 4: Grade 2 is considered normal; grade 3, brisk; and a grade 4, to signify clonus. The examiner should note the symmetry of the reflexes. Pathologic reflexes such as the Babinski sign, indicative of corticospinal disease, are usually checked at this point in the examination. The Babinski sign is elicited by stroking the outer edge of the sole, leading to extension of the great toe with spreading of the small toes. If the response is equivocal, consider assessing the Oppenheim or Chaddock reflex. The Oppenheim reflex is elicited by a firm stroke on the medial aspect of the tibia leading to extension of the great toe. The Chaddock reflex is induced by stroking the dorsal lateral part of the foot and checking for great toe extension.

Superficial reflexes can be helpful in isolating a lesion. The epigastric (T7–T9), abdominal (T10–T12), cremasteric (L1–L2), gluteal (L4–L5), and anal wink (S2–S4) reflexes should be tested when a neurologic impairment is suspected at a related spinal level.

Muscle tone should be tested for cogwheeling, rigidity, spasticity, and hypotonicity. Spasticity is the velocity-dependent increase in tone. The increased tone may not be exhibited at a slow velocity but when the muscle is rapidly stretched, the spasticity will cause the muscle to contract. This is indicative of an abnormality in the corticospinal tract. Rigidity is a form of hypertonia found in parkinsonism and other extrapyramidal diseases. It is present even when the muscle is at rest. There is increased resistance to passive movements, giving a feel of being fairly even as in the "lead pipe" or the "cogwheel" variety, which exhibits a ratchety effect (16).

Table 5-1: Cranial Nerve Assessment			
Cranial Nerve		**Function**	**Method of Assessment**
I	Olfactory	Odor Identification	Make sure nasal passages are patent. The patient's eyes should be closed. Each nostril should be tested while the other nostril is occluded.
II	Optic	Visual	Evaluation is by direct inspection of the optic fundus as well as testing visual acuity and perceptual fields. The optic fundus should be inspected with an ophthalmoscope, which can pick up evidence of systematic processes, such as diabetes, hypertension, and peripheral vascular disease. Both visual fields can be tested by having the patient cover one eye and then fix his or her vision on the examiner's nose at a distance of 2–3 ft. The examiner's finger can be brought in and out of the visual field while the patient identifies when he or she sees it. Visual acuity can be ascertained with a standard chart. Visual field deficits associated with lesions of the optic pathways are illustrated in Figure 5-27 (13).
III, IV, VI	Oculomotor, trochlear, abducens	Extraocular movements and pupillary reaction	The oculomotor nerve innervates all the orbital muscles except for the superior oblique and lateral rectus. To test the nerve, ask the patient to move the eyes upward, downward, and inward. The fourth cranial nerve supplies the superior oblique muscle and the sixth cranial nerve supplies the lateral rectus. These muscles work in opposition to move the eye in a lateral downward gaze. Figure 5-28 (14) demonstrates the actions of each muscle, presuming that each is acting alone.
V	Trigeminal	Mastication	To test this function, palpate the temporal and masseter muscles.
VII	Facial	Facial movement	The corneal reflex tests the response to a wisp of cotton against the cornea, watching for eye blinking. The electronic analogue to this is the blink reflex (15). The patient's face should be inspected for asymmetry. To test, the patient should be asked to show the teeth, raise the eyebrows, and tightly close the eyes.
VIII	Acoustic-vestibular	Hearing	The auditory nerve is tested by evaluating the cochlear and vestibular branches. The cochlear nerve is tested by evaluating the patient's hearing. This can be grossly tested by whispering in either ear of the patient. In addition, Rinne and Weber tests should also be performed. The vestibular portion is evaluated by the patient doing a finger-to-nose motion. Nystagmus is also characteristic of vestibular disease. To test for nystagmus, ask the patient to move the eyes in an extreme deviation.

Table 5-1: (*Continued*)

Cranial Nerve		Function	Method of Assessment
			Nystagmus is characterized by a sustained motion consisting of a fast jerk to the side of deviation, then followed by a slow jerk back to the midline.
IX, X	Glossopharyngeal, vagus	Pharyngeal movement	These nerves are tested by observing pharyngeal movements when the patient says "Ah," looking for the soft palate and uvula to be symmetrically pulled up. The gag reflex is evaluated by touching the back of the pharynx, which induces the protective contraction of the palatal muscles.
XI	Spinal accessory	Shoulder motion	This nerve innervates the trapezius and Sternocleidomastoid muscles. Test the strength of the trapezius muscle by having the patient shrug the shoulders. To test the sternocleidomastoid, hold the opposite side of the chin when the patient turns the head.
XII	Hypoglossal	Tongue motion	To test, ask the patient to stick out and move the tongue. Unilateral weakness can be detected by deviation of the tongue to one side on protrusion. The tongue will deviate to the side of the weakness.

Coordination should be tested with the finger-to-nose and the heel-to-shin maneuvers. Coordination is also tested with rapid alternating movements.

Apraxia is the inability to perform a purposeful action that cannot be accounted for by a deficit in strength or sensation. Apraxia is a motor-planning deficit. The patient may exhibit the desired action automatically but not be able to perform it upon command. A motor-planning deficit may impact on complex motor tasks, such as dressing, walking, and speaking.

The sensory examination should include position sense and vibration, as well as responses to pinprick, touch, and temperature stimuli. Deep sensation can be tested by squeezing the muscles and joints. Graphesthesia (the ability to identify a letter written on the palm of the patient), stereognosis (the ability to recognize a familiar object placed in the patient's hand), and double simultaneous stimulation test cortical sensation. Cortical sensation may also be tested with the two-point discrimination test.

Gait assessment is a part of the physical examination. This aspect of the evaluation is discussed fully in other chapters.

SPECIAL CONSIDERATIONS IN THE PEDIATRIC POPULATION

Although the evaluation of a child has many similarities to that of an adult, several unique features must be mentioned. The pediatric rehabilitation history should focus on developmental as well as functional aspects. The history is usually taken from the caregiver for younger children, whereas older children can actively participate (17).

Many childhood disabilities are caused by prenatal or perinatal difficulties. A detailed history of maternal health, including diabetes and drug and alcohol use, should be obtained. Questions should be asked regarding gestation and labor complications, as they may affect the child. Prematurity may also lead to developmental delays. Apgar scores at birth may be the first sign of a disability or a disorder. One should also take a history of any feeding difficulties. The child's height, weight, and head circumference should be plotted along a growth and development chart, as this can provide information regarding the child's overall health (18). Prematurity with a low birth weight has been associated with diplegic cerebral palsy, whereas high-birth-weight children may have had a traumatic delivery and potential injury to the central nervous system (19).

It is critical to understand the normal developmental milestones in order to recognize developmental deviations and identify potential disability. The Gesell Development Schedule measures developmental states by evaluating gross motor, fine motor, adaptive, language, and personal-social abilities (20). This helps to define whether an impairment is localized only to the neuromuscular realm or whether it effects other areas as well. Many developmental tests rely heavily on motor abilities from which they infer a

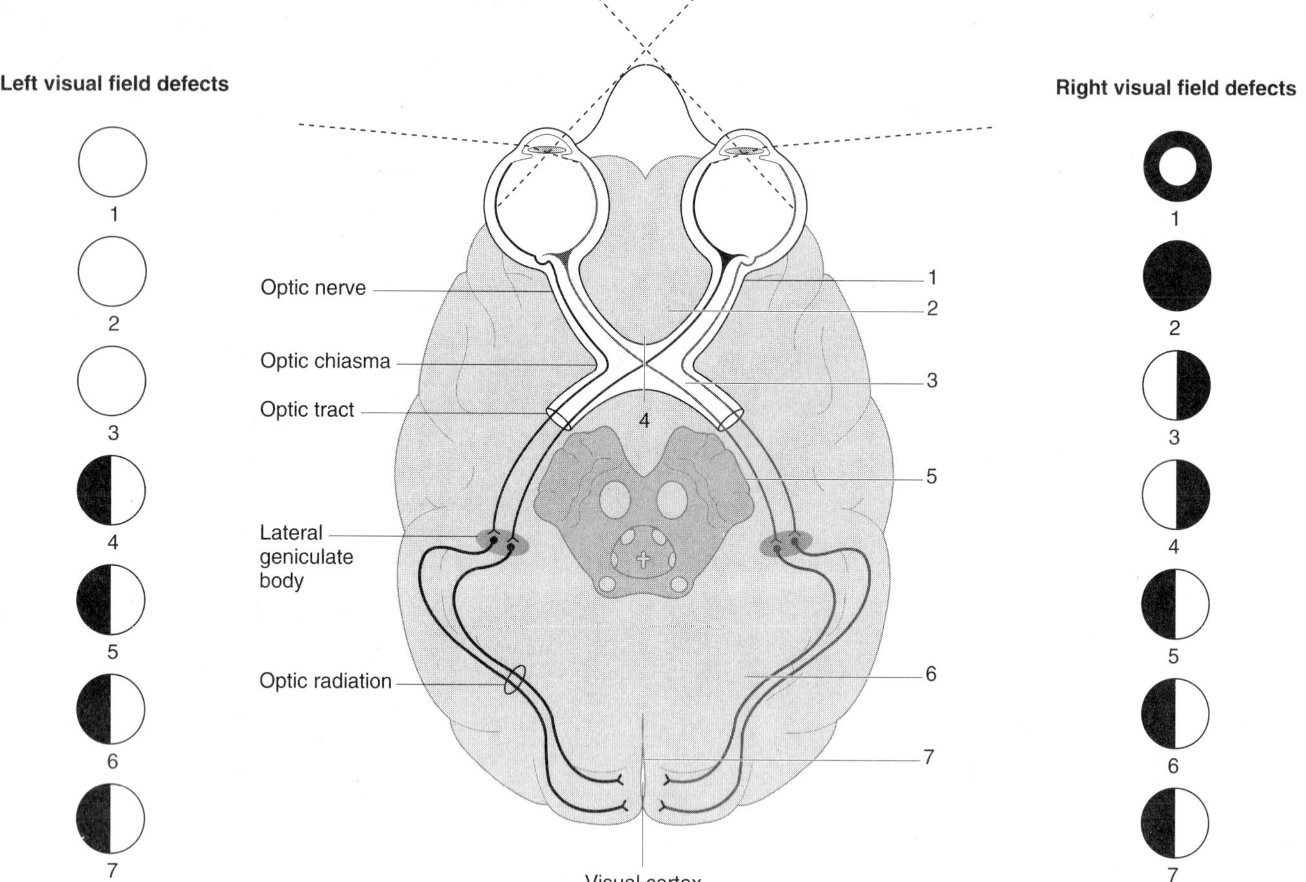

Figure 5-27. Visual field defects from lesions of the optic pathway.

correlation to intellect. These tests have some limitations when applied to the disabled population (21).

Further insight into the functional impact of a disability is gathered throughout the psychosocial history, school history, and family history. This can help identify some of the behavioral and intellectual strengths and weaknesses.

The physical examination must be performed in an environment where the child is comfortable and trusting. Observation of the child is frequently the most informative part of data collection during the clinical evaluation. The infant can be examined on the parent's lap or while playing with toys. The examiner may be able to engage the younger child in a game of peekaboo or the older child in conversation. The examination proceeds from interactive play to actual physical handling. Hands-on testing of muscle tone and range of motion, and visualization of the optic fundi and ears should be reserved for later in the examination.

Examination of the child focuses on neuromuscular testing, reflexes, tone, active motion, coordination, and strength (22). A thorough knowledge of primitive reflexes and their timing is important. The reflexes are evaluated for asymmetry, failure to develop, or failure to extinguish. A reflex abnormality can be one of the first indications of damage to the motor control center of the cortex (23). An infant's muscle tone shows a great deal of variability and must be tested when the infant is cooperative. Flexor tone dominates in the first few months. Injuries to the central nervous system may be present with hypertonicity or hypotonicity. Muscle tightness and decreased range of motion may give clues to possible weakness. Sensory testing can be challenging in children, but helpful information may be obtained by observing the reaction of the child or infant to bilateral pin or touch stimulation.

SPECIAL CONSIDERATIONS IN THE GERIATRIC PATIENT

The last few decades have seen a dramatic increase in the geriatric population and accordingly, an increase in the prevalence of disabilities. The population older than 65 years has grown at a rate of 3.5 times the overall population since 1900 (24). More than 20% of the elderly are disabled by one or more specific conditions. About 80% of

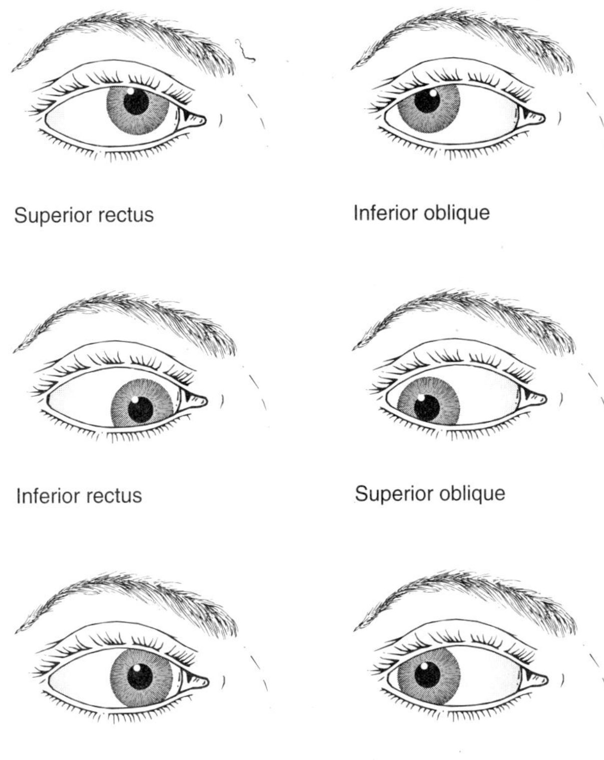

Figure 5-28. Action of the extraocular muscles of the right eye, assuming that each muscle acts alone.

U.S. citizens over 65 years old exhibit at least one chronic illness (25). Musculoskeletal disease such as degenerative joint disease, osteoporosis, fracture, cerebral vascular accidents, Parkinson's disease, and Alzheimer's disease, to name a few, are more prevalent in the geriatric population.

In the elderly, common neurologic changes include increased reaction time, decreased memory, decreased position sense, and gait abnormalities. As the patient ages, there is an accumulation of disease processes—all of which have an impact on function.

The eyes and ears change significantly with aging. Visual acuity remains stable until about age 50, then it diminishes gradually until age 70, when it starts to diminish more rapidly (6).

The aging population is more likely to develop skin conditions. Although they are not lethal, they do affect the quality of life. Persons over 70 years old have a 66% prevalence rate of skin conditions requiring the care of a physician. Many of the problems with aging and skin are believed to be a cumulative result of ultraviolet radiation exposure (26).

The geriatric population has an increased risk of developing pressure ulcers. One study compared sacral pressure on mattresses in the young and elderly populations. Pressure measurements included mean pressure over time and the occurrence of impulse pressure. Impulse pressure is the measure of a pressure recorded at two second intervals expressed as the total pressure that would be applied per bed occupation hour. In elderly persons, both mean pressure and pressure impulses were increased as compared with younger subjects (26). These factors are the reasons why the elderly have a higher risk of developing pressure ulcers.

Pathologic changes associated with normal aging lead to musculoskeletal degeneration beginning in early adulthood. There is an increase in the number, size, and mass of muscle fibers, leading to a decrease in muscular strength and endurance. It has been demonstrated that isometric, isokinetic, and isotonic strengths peek in the third decade and then decrease in each successive decade. In an aging person there is a loss of chondroitin sulfate and water from the nucleus pulposus, leading to decreased flexibility of the disk between the vertebral bodies of the spinal column and decreased disk height (27). In the study of cadaver spinal joint dissections in the fifth decade of life, all individuals had some osteophytes and by the ninth decade all had high grade osteophytes. These changes lead to decreased range of motion of the spine, which may impact on a variety of functional abilities (28). In the aging population, the majority of degenerative changes occur in the lower extremities. Hypertrophic cartilage ossifies and may form peripheral osteophytes in the leg joints. In the knee, the medial and lateral menisci serve as shock absorbers during weight bearing. The aging articular cartilage loses its elasticity and is more susceptible to tears. This can lead to pain and stiffness, especially with rising in the morning or prolonged activity.

Osteoporosis occurs with aging and can be a leading cause of functional impairment. Peak bone mass occurs at approximately age 30. In men and premenopausal women, there is a 0.3% to 0.5% decrease in mass per year. In postmenopausal women, the rate of bone loss increases to 1% to 3% per year (29). Osteoporosis can lead to fractures, especially in the vertebrae, distal part of the forearm, and proximal part of the femur. Disability may also greatly increase osteoporosis. Garland (30) found that most bone loss occurs early after a spinal cord injury. Within the first 4 months after an injury, there is a 27% decrease in bone mineral density of the distal part of the femur and the percentage increases to 63% by 16 months.

The cardiovascular reserve decreases with aging. The maximal obtainable heart rate at age 20 is 200 beats/min. This gradually declines to 160 beats/min at age 70. The aging process also affects the respiratory system. There is a reduction in compliance of the chest wall with decreased elasticity, loss of muscle bulk, and stiffening of the costovertebral joints. This decreases the gas exchange (31). Maximal oxygen consumption in the aged can be increased by fitness training (32). The typical rehabilitation prescription for the elderly is at a slower pace but allows aerobic conditioning. Aging leads to a decrease in bladder capacity as well as increased uninhibited detrucer contractions. This may increase the likelihood of infection or incontinence.

It is a commonly held belief that some complications later in life can be attributed to a congenital or early acquired disability. Older persons with a long-standing neurologic disease may experience increased vulnerability to respiratory complications. Patients with spina bifida may experience neurologic deteriorations secondary to shunt failure, Arnold-Chiari malformations, or tethering of the spinal cord. Clinically this may present as a progressive upper- or lower-motor neuron symptom or a change in bowel or bladder function. The ability to walk may be lost later in life due to earlier neurologic or orthopedic problems. Patients with spinal cord injuries who have been treated with bowel evacuation programs 1 to 2 times per week may find that this program is no longer effective. Patients with a long history of polio may develop postpolio syndrome, experiencing the constellation of weakness, fatigue, and joint and muscle pain. A slight decrease in strength or joint range of motion may profoundly impact function in these patients (33).

PATIENT SUMMARY AND PRESCRIPTION

After the physician performs the history and physical examination, a summary listing the salient features should be written to allow effective communication with the other team members. The summary should briefly include the medical and surgical problems, as well as the impairments and functional deficits. The list of problems helps organize the treatment plan. A treatment plan can then be written, and identify which discipline should address specific deficits. The time frame should be estimated. The treatment plan includes identifying and prioritizing goals that can be accomplished on an inpatient basis versus long-term goals that can be accomplished on an outpatient basis.

The following is a sample summary statement:

> DW is a 42-year-old right-handed male carpenter with a past medical history significant for hypertension and diabetes mellitus. He was in his usual state of good health until 2 weeks ago when he fell from a roof, sustaining a T4 compression fracture and T4 complete paraplegia. The patient underwent Harrington rod placement and is deemed orthopedically stable while in a clamshell (thoracic-lumbar-sacral) orthosis. The patient's current medical history is significant for episodic autonomic dysreflexia.
>
> Physical impairments upon examination include lower-extremity flaccid paralysis, normal sensation to T4 with absent sensation below, low rectal tone, positive bulbocavernosus reflex, and no volitional anal contraction.
>
> The patient has an indwelling Foley catheter and severe constipation. He has a grade II sacral decubitus. He has not yet been out of bed for more than an hour each day. He is independent in his feeding but requires assistance for his activities of daily living. He presently needs assistance for wheelchair mobility.
>
> Socially, the patient is divorced and lives alone in a two-floor home with the bedroom and bathroom on the second floor. He works as a self-employed carpenter.

Medical Surgical Problems

1. T4 compression fracture—orthopedically stable after Harrington rod placement with clamshell orthosis
2. Diabetes mellitus, sugar levels under fair control
3. Autonomic dysreflexia

Rehabilitation Problems

1. Functional deficits—dependent mobility level, assistance for activities of daily living, inability to drive
2. Flaccid paralysis
3. Sacral decubitus
4. Neurogenic bladder
5. Neurogenic bowel with constipation
6. Adjustment to disability
7. Sexuality concerns
8. Inaccessible housing
9. Skin breakdown
10. Blood pressure management

Precautions

The clamshell brace should be worn when the patient is out of bed. While he is out of the brace and in bed, the head of the bed should be at less than a 30-degree elevation. The patient needs to be logrolled, in bed, while out of the brace. It is important to assess for signs and symptoms of autonomic dysreflexia, hyperglycemia, and hypoglycemia.

Plan

1. Physical therapy: Assess and improve deficits in bed mobility, wheelchair mobility, transfers, balance, and endurance and strengthening. Teach patient and caregivers range of motion and how to don and doff the clamshell brace.
2. Occupational therapy: Evaluate activities of daily living; have patient attend classes for adaptive equipment and homemaking; have patient perform upper-extremity strengthening and endurance exercises.
3. Psychology: Work with patient on his adjustment to disability.
4. Therapeutic recreation: Have patient work on outdoor wheelchair skills and participate in community activities.
5. Nursing: Initiate and teach bowel and bladder routine, how to do skin checks with mirrors. Provide patient and caregiver education. Reinforce activities of range of motion, bed mobility, and activities of

daily living in coordination with occupational and physical therapy. Please give patient instruction about hyperglycemia, hypoglycemia, and autonomic dysreflexia.

6. Vocational rehabilitation: Evaluate return to work activities. Investigate federal or state offices of vocational rehabilitation to help fund the altering of the patient's job to working as a carpenter at a wheelchair level.

Estimated Length of Stay

4 weeks. (This amount of time allows the goals to be obtained, to get back to independent living. The patient would continue outpatient therapy after this.)

Goals

As an inpatient, the patient should achieve independent wheelchair mobility, minimal assistance with rolls, moderate assistance with clamshell orthosis management, minimal assistance with activities of daily living (due to clamshell brace), moderate assistance with the bowel routine, and minimal assistance for skin checks. Since the patient lives alone, family, friends, or caregivers will need to be trained to assist with his care. A first-floor living situation is desirable; however, if this cannot be achieved, alternative levels of care may need to be pursued.

Long-Term Goals

1. Independent advanced wheelchair mobility
2. Independent bowel and bladder routine
3. Return to work

The patient's summary and prescription provide the treatment team with an overview of the impairments and goals. The goals must be discussed with the patient to verify an agreeable set of achievements that are realistic and attainable. The rehabilitation prescription and summary are the culmination of the clinical evaluation, incorporating all information from the history and physical examination and leading to treatment.

REFERENCES

1. World Health Organization. *International classification by impairments, disabilities and handicaps: a manual of classification relating to the consequences of disease.* Geneva: World Health Organization, 1980.
2. DeGowin EL, DeGowin RL. *Bedside diagnostic examination.* 6th ed. New York: Macmillan, 1994.
3. Ericson RP, McPhee MC. Clinical evaluation. In: Delisa JA, Gans BM, eds. *Rehabilitation medicine: principles and practice.* Philadelphia: JB Lippincott, 1993:51–95.
4. McPeak LA. Physiatric history and examination. In: Braddom RL, ed. *Physical medicine and rehabilitation.* Philadelphia: WB Saunders, 1996:3–42.
5. Stolov WC, Hays RM. Evaluation of the patient. In: Kottle FS, Lehmann JF, eds. *Krusen's handbook of physical medicine and rehabilitation.* 4th ed. Philadelphia: WB Saunders, 1990: 1–19.
6. Bates B. *A guide to physical examination.* 2nd ed. Philadelphia: JB Lippincott, 1979.
7. Ouslander JG, Morishita L, Blaustein J, et al. Clinical, functional and psychosocial characteristics of an incontinent nursing home population. *J Gerentol* 1987;42:631–637.
8. Greenberger NJ, Hinthorn DR. *History taking and physical examination: essentials and clinical correlates.* St. Louis: Mosby, 1993: 352–355.
9. Daniels L, Worthingham C. *Muscle testing: techniques of manual evaluation.* 5th ed. Philadelphia: WB Saunders, 1986.
10. Hollingshead WH, Jenkins DB. *Functional anatomy of the limbs and back.* 6th ed. Philadelphia: WB Saunders, 1991.
11. Haymaker W, Woodall B. *Peripheral nerve injuries: principles of diagnosis.* 2nd ed. Philadelphia: WB Saunders, 1945:42–43.
12. Mancall EL. Examination of the nervous system. In: Mancall EL, ed. *Alpers and Mancall's essentials of the neurologic examination.* 2nd ed. Philadelphia: FA Davis, 1991: 1–33.
13. Snell RS, Smith MS. *Clinical anatomy for emergency medicine.* St. Louis: Mosby, 1993:265.
14. Snell RS. *Clinical anatomy for medical students.* 4th ed. Boston: Little, Brown, 1992:840.
15. Kimura J, Delisa JA, Hallett M. *Cranial nerve testing: an AAEE workshop.* Rochester, MN: American Association of Electiodiagnostic Medicine, 1984.
16. Guberman A. *An introduction to clinical neurology: pathophysiology, diagnosis and treatment.* Boston: Little, Brown, 1994.
17. Molnar GE, ed. *Pediatric rehabilitation.* 2nd ed. Baltimore: Williams & Wilkins, 1992.
18. Barness LA. The pediatric history and examination. In: Ocki FA, ed. *Principle and practice of pediatrics.* Philadelphia: JB Lippincott, 1994:29–34.
19. Fenichel GM. *Neonatal neurology.* New York: Churchill Livingstone, 1980.

20. Gessell A. *Gessell Development Schedule*. New York: Psychological Corporation, 1940.

21. Chintz SZ, Feder CZ. Psychological assessment. In: Molnar GE, ed. *Pediatric rehabilitation*. 2nd ed. Baltimore: Williams & Wilkins, 1992:55–58.

22. Johnson EW. Examination for muscle weakness in infants and small children. *JAMA* 1958;16: 1306–1313.

23. Pidcock FS, Christensen JR. General and neuromuscular rehabilitation in children. In: O'Young B, Young MA, eds. *PM&R Secrets*. Philadelphia: Hanley and Belfus, 1996:402–407.

24. Gershoff AM, Cifu DX, Means KM. Geriatric rehabilitation. 1. Social, attitudinal and economic factors. *Arch Phys Med Rehabil* 1993; 74(5S):402–406.

25. Betts H. In: Brody SJ, Pawlson LG, eds. *Aging and rehabilitation; the state of the practice*. New York: Springer, 1990:31.

26. Yarkony GM. Aging skin, pressure ulcerations, and spinal cord injury. In: Whiteneck GG, ed. *Aging with spinal cord injury*. New York: Demos, 1993:41–43.

27. Eaters RL, Sie IH, Adkins RH. The musculoskeletal systems. In: Whiteneck GG, ed. *Aging with spinal cord injury*. New York: Demos, 1993:53–54.

28. Nathan H. Osteophytes of the vertebral column. An anatomical study of their development according to age, race, and sex with consideration as to their etiology and significance. *J Bone Joint Surg* 1962;44:243.

29. Heaney RP. Prevention of age related osteoporosis in women. In: Avioli LC, ed. *The osteoporotic syndrome*. New York: Grune & Straton, 1983.

30. Garland DE, Steward CA, Adkins RH, et al. Osteoporosis following spinal cord injury. *J Orthop Res* 1992;10:371–378.

31. Ragnarrson KT. The cardiovascular system. In: Whiteneck GG, ed. *Aging with spinal cord injury*. New York: Demos, 1993:77.

32. Cifu DX, Means KM, Currie DM, Gershkoff AM. Geriatric rehabilitation. 2. Diagnosis and management of acquired disabling disorders. *Arch Phys Med Rehabil* 1993;74(5S):406–412.

33. Currie DM, Gershkoff AM, Cifu DX. Geriatric rehabilitation. Three mid- and late-life effects of early-life disabilities. *Arch Phys Med Rehabil* 1993;74:5414.

Chapter 6

Diagnostic Imaging for the Physiatrist: Introduction and Chest, Gastrointestinal, and Musculoskeletal Imaging

Alfred B. Watson, Jr.
Christopher L. Chong
Monte F. Zarlingo

Diagnostic imaging is a key component of the total care of physically impaired patients. It is essential in determining the cause of and the treatment regimen for disease processes in these patients. By choosing the proper imaging modality, one can increase the likelihood of making the proper diagnosis and developing a specific and effective plan of therapy, which is crucial in alleviating symptoms and producing a satisfactory outcome. This is the first of three chapters on imaging of the following organ systems: respiratory, gastrointestinal (GI), genitourinary, musculoskeletal, and nervous systems. In addition, interventional radiologic procedures are discussed.

The technical personnel performing diagnostic imaging studies in a rehabilitation facility must be very attentive, patient, and compassionate. Extreme care must be exercised while transferring patients from the wheelchair or stretcher onto the diagnostic imaging equipment. The use of mechanical patient lifters or roller transfer devices is greatly recommended, for the protection of both patients and employees.

Once patients reach the diagnostic imaging room, they cannot be left unattended. Radiographic tables generally are not equipped to restrain the mentally or physically impaired, and personnel need to be present to monitor the patients and to prevent injury.

When possible, the radiology staff should encourage that radiographs be obtained utilizing stationary equipment within the department instead of portable x-ray equipment at the patient's bedside. Portable equipment is very limited, capable of only low kilovolt peak output (approximately 100 kVp) and amperage (approximately 100 mA). The reduced kilovolt peak and amperage capabilities require an increase in exposure time to obtain an adequately exposed film. Increased exposure time reduces the radiographic resolution (detail) because of the motion artifact produced by breathing or other physiologic movement. Fixed x-ray equipment in the radiology department is capable of high kilovolt peak (120–145 kVp) and high amperage (300–500 mA) values, requiring less exposure time, thereby decreasing patient motion artifact and improving the image quality.

CHEST IMAGING

All the respiratory problems found in the general population are also found in physically impaired patients, in whom the more frequently encountered ones are atelectasis, alveolar consolidation, and pneumothorax. There is also an increased incidence of diaphragmatic excursion abnormalities.

Atelectasis

Atelectasis represents a loss of lung volume, ranging from involvement of small pulmonary subdivisions to complete lobar collapse. There are numerous types of atelectasis; however, in the physically impaired patient, obstructive and compressive atelectases are the most frequently encountered.

Obstructive atelectasis (lobar or segmental collapse) is usually secondary to a mucous plug. One of the hallmarks of mucous plug atelectasis is "wandering opacification" of the lungs. The mucous plug shifts from one major bronchi to another in a matter of days, resulting in wandering atelectasis.

Common causes of compressive atelectasis in the physically impaired patient are pneumothorax and paresis/paralysis of the diaphragm. Pneumothorax can be spontaneous, iatrogenic (central line placement), or post-traumatic (rib fracture).

The predominant radiographic findings of lobar collapse are opacification (or increased tissue density) of the lung and shift of the interlobar fissure. Secondary signs include elevation of the hemidiaphragm, shift of the mediastinum (heart, hilum, or trachea), crowding of the pulmonary vasculature, ipsilateral rib narrowing, and hyperlucency of the unaffected lung.

Atelectasis is transient and clears once the cause is determined and treated.

Lung Consolidation (Air Space Disease)

Lung consolidation (air space disease) is filling of the alveoli with fluids. The fluid may be transudative (edema) or exudative (pus, blood, tumor). The two most common causes of air space disease in physically impaired patients are edema and infection (pneumonia).

Cerebral injury–induced neurogenic pulmonary edema is usually seen in the acute and potentially subacute phase. Air space edema results from an increased permeability and an associated capillary leak of fluid into the alveoli, unlike the edema seen with congestive heart failure due to increased hydrostatic pressure. Freundlich and Bragg (1) described the radiographic differentiation of the two types of pulmonary edema. They (1) stated that the findings of hydrostatic pulmonary edema on portable chest radiographs include an "abnormal right costophrenic angle containing edematous septal (Kerley B) lines, subpleural edema and/or a pleural effusion." Patients with neurogenic pulmonary edema frequently have a "normal right costophrenic angle and the presence of air bronchograms" (1).

Patients on assisted ventilation and those with endotracheal tubes or tracheostomies are at increased risk of infection. This is primarily due to the stasis of respiratory secretions that results from impaired diaphragmatic motion, decreased mucociliary movement, impaired cough reflex, and lack of patient mobility.

Physically impaired patients are also at increased risk for aspiration pneumonia. Aspiration of gastric contents causes both consolidation and atelectasis on the lungs. The most frequent segments involved are the superior and posterior segments of the lower lobes and the posterior segments of the upper lobes. The aspirated fluid induces a consolidation pneumonitis that is slow to respond to treatment.

Pneumothorax

Pneumothorax can be diagnosed on a chest radiograph. The radiographic findings of a pneumothorax include a thin line (<1 mm, representing the lateral aspect of the visceral pleura) that parallels the contour of the thoracic cage, absence of lung markings lateral to this line, air along the diaphragm, air along the mediastinal structures, and a "deep sulcus sign" (Fig. 6-1). In the supine patient, pneumothorax may be best visualized at the diaphragm (highest anatomic part of the thorax in the supine patient); the diaphragm is clearly defined secondary to the lucent adjacent air (Fig. 6-2). This is called *anterior pneumothorax.*

A true pneumothorax must be differentiated from a pseudopneumothorax caused by skinfolds. The skin in the debilitated patient may fold on itself when the patient is placed on the imaging table, and is seen on the chest x-ray film as a white line. The hallmarks of skinfolds are a wider

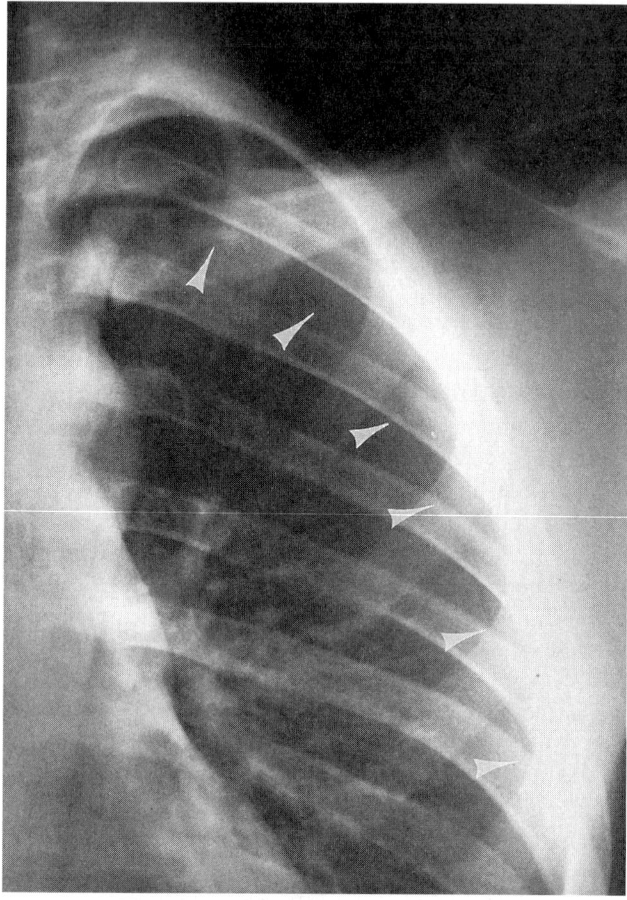

Figure 6-1. Pneumothorax. Note the thin visceral pleural line (white arrows) follows the curved contour of the thorax, and the absence of lung markings lateral to the pleural line.

"pleural" line that is more dense medially, lung markings lateral to the line, and a line that does not follow the contour of the thorax cage (Fig. 6-3). Occasionally, the line extends outside the thoracic cage, which is not possible with a pneumothorax.

Evaluation for Diaphragmatic Paralysis and Motion

The normal movement of the diaphragm during respiration is relatively symmetric; movement of the two hemidiaphragms normally differs by less than 1 cm. The usual excursion of the diaphragm is generally 3 cm to 6 or 7 cm. However, excursion of less than 3 cm can be seen in 14% to 23% of normal patients (2).

Fluoroscopy or double-exposure films of the lower part of the chest and upper part of the abdomen can be obtained during inspiration and expiration. Fluoroscopy enables real-time observation of diaphragmatic excursion during inspiration and expiration. The Hitzenberger sniff test is accomplished by imaging the patient while he or she inhales quickly through the nose with the mouth closed. The sniff should result in downward movement of the diaphragm. As normal diaphragmatic movement may be less than 3 cm, incorporating the Hitzenberger sniff test can be extremely helpful in differentiating normal versus diaphragmatic paralysis in physically impaired patients. In patients with diaphragmatic paralysis, there will be ipsilateral passive (paradoxical) upward movement of the diaphragm during sniffing (2).

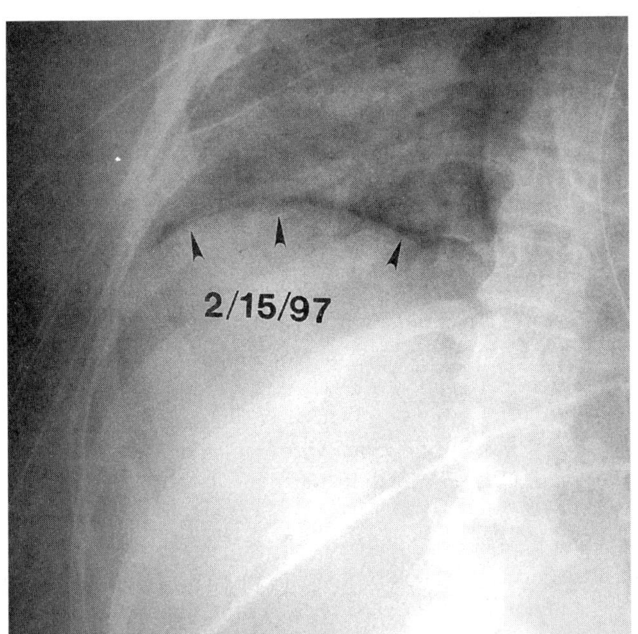

A

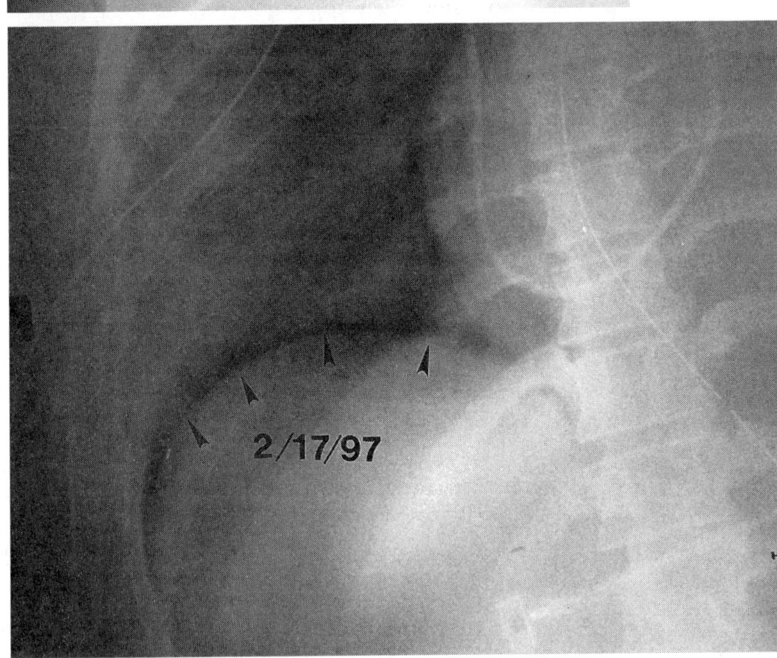

B

Figure 6-2. Anterior pneumothorax. *A–C.* Air from the pneumothorax causes progressive accentuation of the superior diaphragm surface (black arrows) in the supine patient with time (2/15/97 to 2/21/97).

Figure 6-2. *Continued.*

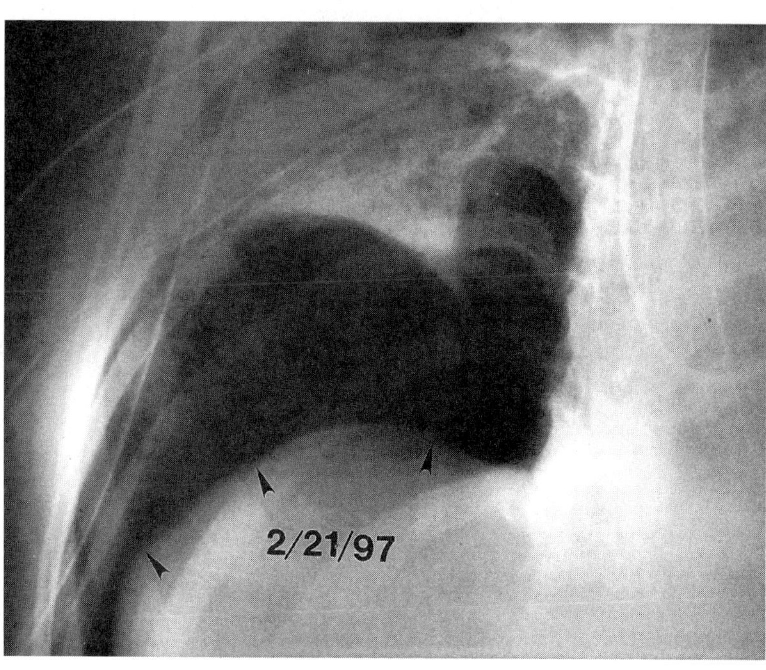

Diaphragmatic motion can also be evaluated in the supine patient by exposing a single radiograph twice, during maximum inspiration and expiration. Then one can determine the excursion of the diaphragm by comparing the two diaphragmatic levels. To keep from overexposing the radiograph, the technician utilizes normal kilovolt peak values but only 50% of the normal amperage for each of the two exposure.

GASTROINTESTINAL RADIOLOGY

Diagnostic imaging in the physically impaired involves assessing all aspects of the GI tract. However, the radiologist is most involved with evaluating the swallowing function.

Oral Pharynx and Esophagus

The radiologist, in conjunction with the speech therapist and physical therapist, evaluates a patient's ability to initiate and complete swallowing and to determine whether the patient is aspirating or choking. The study called the *dynamic barium swallow* can be used to assess the patient's ability to tolerate dietary progression from liquids to solids. The patient sits in a special chair that provides stabilization via Velcro straps or sheets and is located within the fluoroscopy unit (a C-arm or routine fluoroscopy table at 90 degrees), providing a true lateral view of the oral pharynx. The patient is observed by fluoroscopy and the examination is recorded on videotape as oral intake progresses from liquid to purees to solids. Barium is mixed with the various substances, enabling evaluation of the act of swallowing. Pooling of the substances, laryngeal penetration, or frank aspiration can be identified. Videotape recording provides a dynamic review. An excellent and complete discussion of swallowing function and imaging is found in Jones and Donner's textbook (3).

Stomach

The fundus is the most dependent (posterior) portion of the stomach when the patient lies in the supine position. A "pseudotumor" in the left upper quadrant of the abdomen in supine patients is produced by fluid collecting in the gastric fundus and is confirmed as it disappears when the patient is placed in the prone position. Contents in this location can persist for days (Fig. 6-4) if the patient is left supine and not turned onto his or her side. Thus, barium, nutrients, and medicine given by mouth or oral gastric tubes will probably pool in the fundus for an indefinite time and may not be absorbed in a timely manner.

Although placement of a Dobhoff tube in the duodenum can provide a means to directly administer medications and nutrients into the duodenum, thereby aiding absorption, gastric secretions will continue to be produced and are retained in the stomach, and the tube may increase the risk of reflux. Placement of a Dobhoff tube can be performed under fluoroscopic guidance.

Occasionally, physically impaired patients will develop stress ulcers of the stomach and duodenum; these can be diagnosed by upper GI or flexible endoscopy.

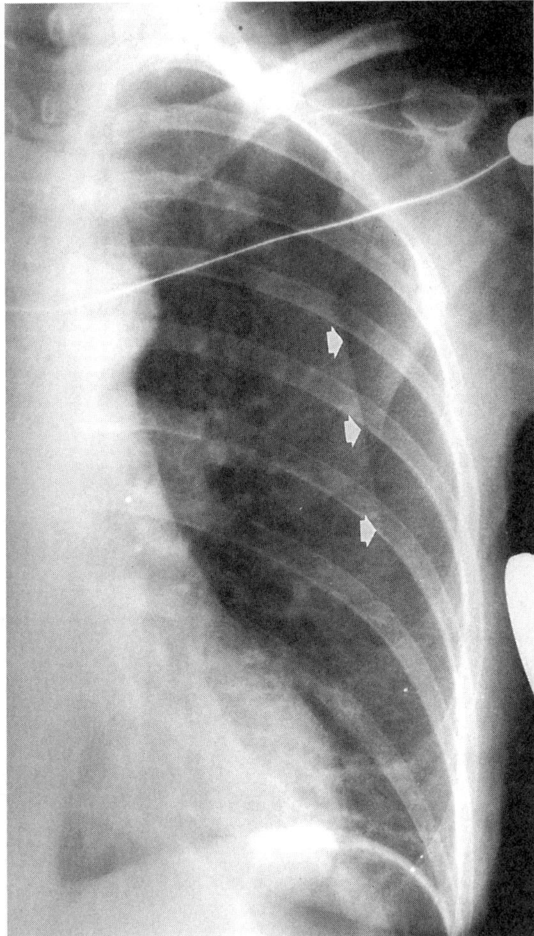

Figure 6-3. Skinfold (white arrows) simulating pneumothorax. Note the "wider" pleural line, which is straight and does not follow the contour of the thorax, and the lung marking lateral to the line.

Colon

A major problem of physically impaired patients is constipation. Severe impaction can result in mechanical obstruction of both the colon and the small bowel. Treatment of constipation includes routine cathartics and cleansing enemas. Occasionally, a therapeutic enema utilizing water-soluble contrast in a 50:50 mixture with water can alleviate the obstruction. The patient should be well hydrated for this procedure, as the contrast material can increase fluid absorption of the bowel, resulting in intravascular fluid depletion.

Colonic disease processes run the gamut of those found in the general population, including volvulus, polyps, cancer, and diverticulitis. Performing a barium enema on a paraplegic or quadriplegic can be difficult. Use of a single-contrast technique is frequently recommended because of the patient's physical limitations. Double-contrast examinations require a great deal of patient mobility, which may not be possible in certain patients. In addition, use of the "retaining donut apparatus" (in which the patient's buttocks is placed in the center of a restraining ring) will assist in keeping the barium and bowel contents contained in a localized area. The balloon on the enema tip is inflated and kept in contact with the anus, reducing the leakage of bowel contents and barium during the study. If barium studies are not diagnostic, endoscopy is recommended to evaluate the colon.

MUSCULOSKELETAL IMAGING

This section covers the basic imaging modalities of the musculoskeletal system and the indications for each, as well as more specific topics pertinent to rehabilitative medicine. Emphasis is placed on the variety of modalities that are available and their applicability for specific clinical problems.

General Considerations

Plain film radiography is still the "workhorse" in the imaging of osseous structures. It remains the initial step in routine imaging for tumors, fractures, infection, degenerative changes, and osteoporosis. More specialized and technologically advanced studies can help in making the diagnosis, but they are always compared to the initial plain films. The soft tissues also can be assessed fairly well, especially for joint effusions, subcutaneous air, foreign bodies, calcification, muscle atrophy and hypertrophy, and edema.

Plain film tomography is useful in detecting small areas of calcification or ossification and to assess for fractures and fracture healing, but has been supplanted by computed tomography (CT).

CT provides a more detailed evaluation of both the osseous structures and the adjacent soft tissues. Images are generally acquired in the axial plane, but reconstructions can be performed in any plane desired, affording a three-dimensional assessment. The fine detail of the cortex and medullary cavity of bone can be evaluated. Abnormal fluid collections from trauma, infection, or tumor are well depicted and joint cartilage, synovium, and internal structures can be imaged (arthrography). Fractures and other posttraumatic sequelae are better elucidated. Imaging after intravenous administration of iodinated contrast material helps to diagnose infection, and possibly to evaluate tumors. Specialized software is available for densitometry.

Sonography is a relatively new imaging modality in the musculoskeletal armamentarium. Sonographic imaging of the shoulder and wrist have had varying degrees of success, and remain highly operator dependent. However, studies have shown its utility in diagnosing abnormalities in the rotator cuff and in the wrist. Ultrasound can be used for detecting soft-tissue abscesses and also has had success in identifying

Figure 6-4. *A.* Pooling of gastric contents in the stomach (S) of an 18-month-old patient with prune-belly syndrome. Oral barium was given on 2/20/97. *B–D.* Follow-up kidney-ureter-bladder films (2/24/97, 3/3/97, and 3/13/97) show stasis of barium in the fundus for 3 weeks. The patient was not turned and had no gastric outlet obstruction.

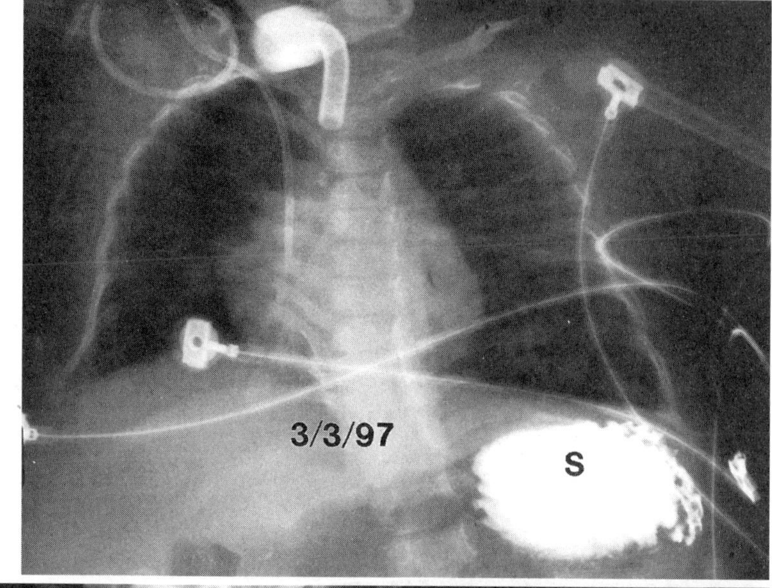

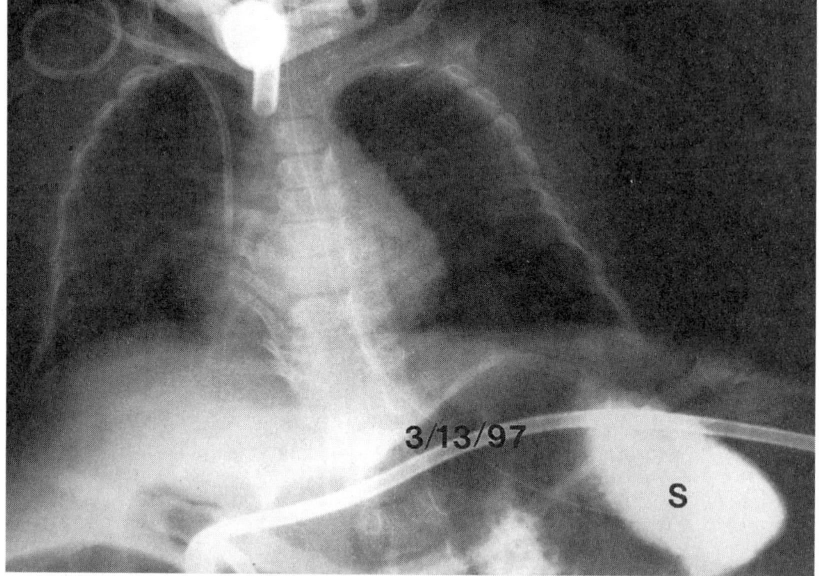

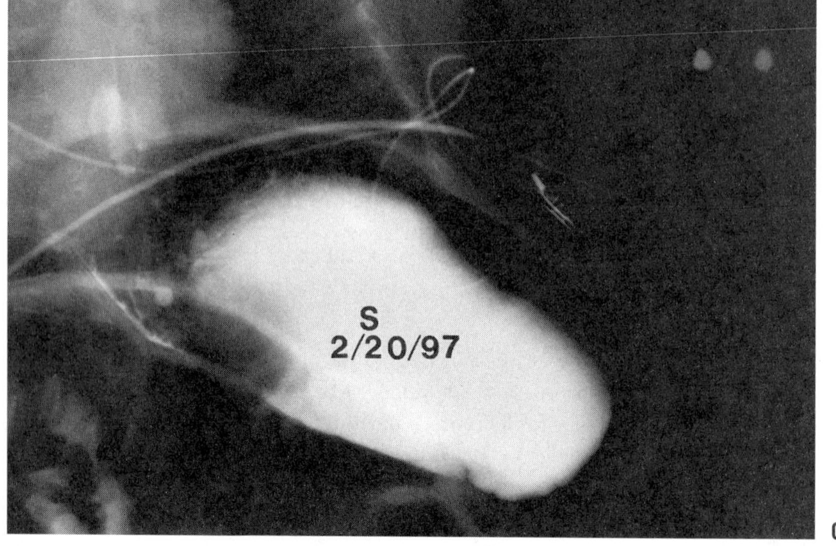

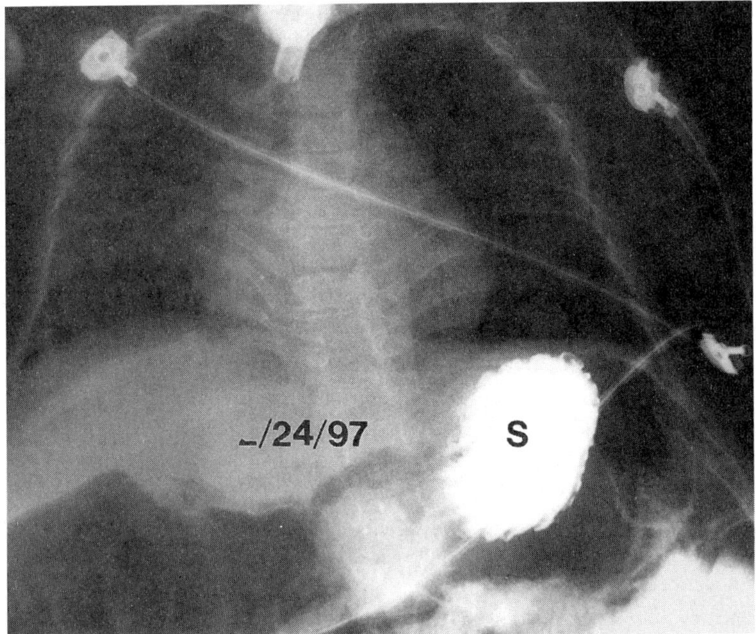

D

Figure 6-4. *Continued.*

retained foreign bodies in the soft tissues, such as those consisting of glass, plastic, and wood.

Magnetic resonance imaging (MRI) produces differential contrast of varying tissues based on their interaction with radiowave pulses. The soft-tissue contrast inherent to MRI and the capability for multiplanar imaging make it the modality of choice for evaluating subtle areas of inflammation and infection. It is also the optimal study for noninvasive imaging of most joints for internal derangement, being especially efficacious in the shoulder and knee joints. Magnetic resonance (MR) arthrography combines the contrast of fluid injected into a joint with the inherent contrast of MRI to increase the sensitivity of diagnosing ligamentous, tendinous, and cartilaginous abnormalities. Intravenous administration of heavy-metal contrast agents (gadolinium) can increase the sensitivity and specificity when evaluating for infection or neoplasm.

Contrast arthrography is still occasionally performed to diagnose abnormalities of the tendons, ligaments, joint capsule, and cartilage, but it has been replaced by noninvasive, three-dimensional MRI.

Osseous Abnormalities

Osteoporosis

Regional or diffuse osteoporosis can occur in the setting of immobilization, paralysis, or disuse (4) and is a result of the predominance of bone resorption over bone formation (5). Radiographically, one sees focal, patchy, or diffuse demineralization of the bone, with loss of cortex and accentuation of stress (primary) trabeculae. The radiographic counterpart of this process is termed *osteopenia.* Weakened bone is susceptible to fracture with ordinary or mildly traumatic stressors. If the bone becomes very weak, spontaneous fractures may occur, or fractures may result from contractures, altered patterns of ambulation, or even aggressive physical therapy (6).

Fractures

Plain film radiography is still the best initial examination for the diagnosis of acute fractures and for assessment of fracture healing. The size and type of fracture can be seen with two orthogonal views. In equivocal cases, CT may delineate a subtle fracture. Nuclear scintigraphy will show increased uptake of the radioisotope in areas of subtle fracture; this is especially helpful in the osteoporotic patient in whom the fracture may not be visible on plain films. In the elderly or patients who may have decreased perfusion and osteoporosis, the sensitivity of bone scans increases when performed 48 to 72 hours following the acute event.

MRI is very sensitive in detecting fractures or bony contusions that are occult on conventional radiographs and that may lead to fracture, but is cost prohibitive except when management concerns outweigh those for cost, such as in the high-performance athlete.

For following the progression of fractures, abnormal healing is usually well demonstrated on plain films. Excessive callus formation is produced in the healing phase as a result of continued motion at the fracture site. Partial or delayed union is also usually seen on x-ray films. Synostosis and soft-tissue calcification can also be seen (7). If there is concern for delayed union or nonunion and neither is seen on plain films, CT with thin-section acquisition and three-dimensional reconstruction may be beneficial.

Orthopedic Hardware

Conventional radiographs are sufficient for assessing hardware in the vast majority of patients. Location, alignment, and integrity of internal and external fixation devices and prostheses are best evaluated on plain films. Plain films can also be used to screen for complications of hardware, such as fracture, loosening, heterotopic bone formation, and infection (8–10).

CT can be effective in the preoperative setting as it can aid in determining the approach, the type of reconstruction, and the type of prosthesis to use. It may also provide additional information postoperatively but can be compromised by the beam hardening and "streak artifact" that occur from the photons interacting with the metallic hardware. CT techniques can be modified in patients with retained hardware, enabling imaging for a specific problem. Stainless-steel hardware is not usually amenable to MRI, mostly owing to significant artifact. There is also a minimal potential for strong magnetic field interaction with the hardware. Patients with newer nonferromagnetic hardware such as implants made of titanium can be safely placed in the magnet, but significant artifact may be produced and render the images suboptimal or even nondiagnostic.

Osteomyelitis

Osteomyelitis (11) can have a variable appearance on plain films, depending on the age of the patient, the mode of infection, and the route of spread. Cortical erosion, lucency, and destruction are seen with both hematogenous and direct invasion. Proliferation can occur in response to the infectious process, as can periostitis, producing sclerosing osteomyelitis. The nidus and fistula (sinus tract) formation associated with this process are best seen on CT scans (Fig. 6-5). There is usually soft-tissue edema. The findings are nonspecific, and early infection may not be apparent on conventional films (12,13).

Nuclear scintigraphy can be used to identify infections that are radiographically occult. Three-phase bone scans can differentiate between soft-tissue and bone involvement, and leukocyte-labeled imaging can be more specific for infection.

MRI is extremely sensitive to soft-tissue and osseous abnormalities. However, abnormal signal on fluid-sensitive T2-weighted scans is nonspecific, and the expense of the examination precludes its employment as a routine test for osteomyelitis.

Joint Abnormalities

Arthritis

Osteoarthritis, inflammatory arthritides, and posttraumatic degeneration can be diagnosed on plain films. These processes present with findings amenable to plain film diagnosis, such as joint space narrowing, osteophytes, sclerosis, geode formation, osteopenia, soft-tissue edema, and erosions (14).

CT is of limited value in the diagnosis of osteoarthritis, but can be useful in detecting loose bodies. It also provides better contrast resolution than do conventional films.

MRI may help to distinguish between the various types of joint disease, being sensitive for marrow, cartilage, synovial, and ligamentous abnormalities that may be occult on plain films. In general, although MRI is much more sensitive for earlier changes of arthritis, conventional radiographs remain a sensitive and cost-effective means of assessment.

Articular Cartilage Damage

Plain radiographs should be the first imaging modality used in evaluating a joint. The signs of cartilage damage are mostly indirect, and include calcification in the cartilage and soft tissues, subchondral sclerosis and cysts, osteophyte formation, and joint space narrowing (15). Weight-bearing views will accentuate joint space narrowing.

CT can detect secondary osseous changes earlier than plain radiographs can, but provides no direct visualization of the cartilage. Arthrography or CT-arthrography can be used to assess the cartilage volume and identify defects in the articular surface.

MRI directly visualizes the articular cartilage and may be the optimal modality for detecting focal erosions, contour irregularities, and thinning. In one cadaveric study, injection of saline solution to simulate effusion enabled detection of chondral defects as small as 3 mm (16). The excellent soft-tissue contrast of MRI allows for detection of associated abnormalities such as osteochondral fractures, chondromalacia patellae, degenerative osteoarthritis, and synovitis (17). Newer sequences are being developed and show promise for monitoring the progression or regression of articular cartilage degradation during treatment.

Capsular Abnormalities

Patients who sustain recurrent dislocations or in whom there is concern for joint subluxation and capsular laxity can be diagnosed with conventional or stress plain film imaging as well as with CT or MRI arthrography. This is especially true for the glenohumeral joint. The "drooping shoulder" sign refers to inferior subluxation of the humeral head relative to the glenoid. This is seen with capsular laxity or with large effusions (usually hemorrhage) that distend the capsule. Over 50% of patients with paralysis will develop shoulder capsule laxity due to significant muscle atrophy (18).

Adhesive capsulitis can be confirmed with arthrography by the decreased volume of contrast material that can be injected into a fibrosed, contracted capsule (19). This is most marked in the glenohumeral joint, and the fibrotic process likely accounts for the high association between adhesive capsulitis and neurologic injury.

Synovitis can result in periarticular soft-tissue prominence and adjacent bony erosion on plain films. In the acute phase, it will be manifested by the appearance of edema in and along the capsule and the joint on MRI

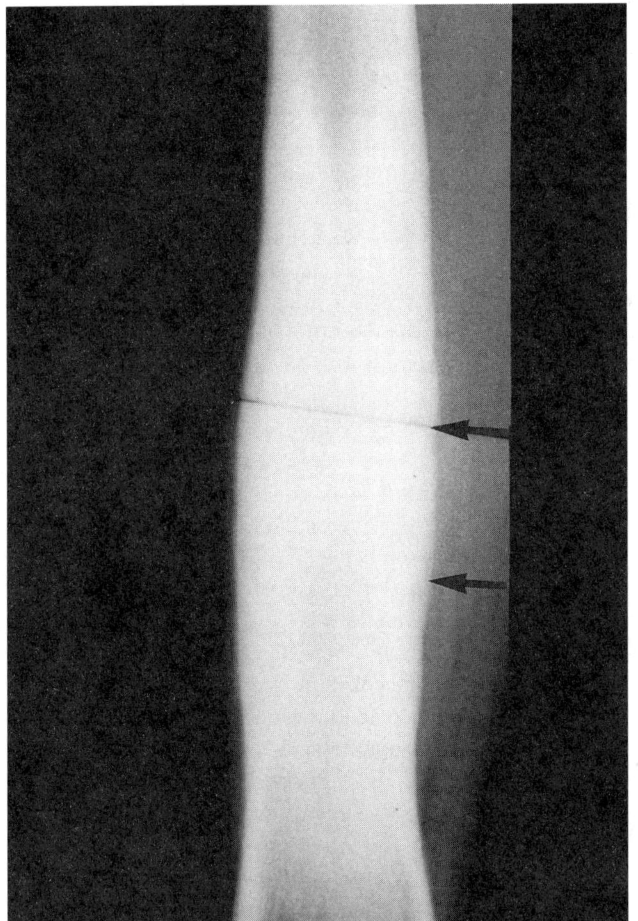

A

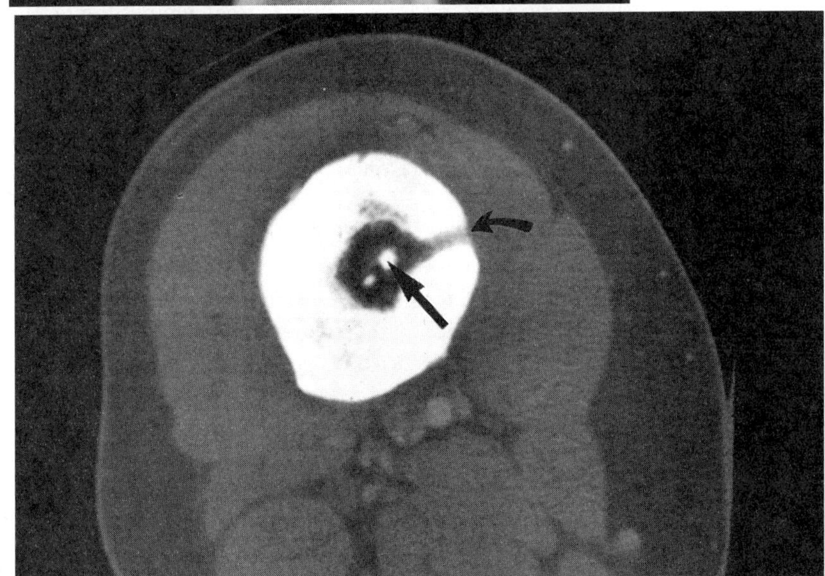

B

Figure 6-5. A 40-year-old patient with pain and fever secondary to chronic sclerosing osteomyelitis. *A.* A Conventional radiograph demonstrates an area of sclerosis in the tibia (*arrows*). *B.* An axial unenhanced CT scan demonstrates a sequestrum (*arrow*) and a sinus tract draining out to the soft tissues (*curved arrow*).

scans. Intravenous contrast material will enhance the areas of inflammation on both CT and MRI scans, but this is nonspecific.

Neuroarthropathy

Alteration of the osseous and soft-tissue structures in neuropathy may be attributable to repeated trauma in conjunction with sympathetic nerve dysfunction. Loss of the normal, neurally mediated reflex results in loss of vasoconstriction and secondary hyperemia (20,21). Impaired sensation, weakened bone, and hyperemia result in soft-tissue swelling, joint effusion, and bone destruction.

Radiographic manifestations of neuropathy can be destructive or resorptive. Destructive neuropathy includes destruction, debris, disruption of articular surfaces, and displacement or dislocation. The bone density is preserved. The resorptive form presents with loss of mineralization and lacks the significant destruction of cortex that produces the fragmentation and dislocation (22). Both forms can occur separately or together.

Conventional radiography is sensitive for detecting both the destructive and the resorptive form of a neuropathic joint. Magnification radiography can help in subtle cases. CT may detect small debris not seen on routine x-ray films and enables assessment of the soft tissues. Preoperatively, the level of involvement can be identified to establish a level for amputation.

Distinguishing a neuropathic joint from vascular and infectious arthropathy can be difficult. Nuclear scintigraphy can be quite useful when infection is a concern. Neuropathic joints have an increased risk of secondary infection, and leukocyte-labeled imaging or gallium scans can aid in distinguishing between the two. In diabetic patients, the small-vessel disease that accompanies the neuropathy can be evaluated with angiography, segmental Doppler analysis, and triphasic bone scans. The goal of these studies is to establish the appropriate level for amputation prior to surgery (23).

Soft-Tissue Abnormalities

Inflammation and Infection

Localized infections (24) are often the result of skin breakdown over pressure points, a common problem in the paralyzed or debilitated patient. Bony protuberances such as the trochanters of the femur and the tuberosities of the ischium are typical sites of involvement. The sacroiliac joints also tend to be involved, which has been attributed in part to chronic pelvic sepsis with resultant osseous contamination.

One of the earliest manifestations of infection (24) is edematous obscuration of fascial planes. Edema of the soft tissues seen on x-ray films generally correlates with clinical findings. If there is concern for myofascitis or abscess, MRI is the most sensitive modality for assessing infection and inflammation; it will also better delineate the extent of involvement (Fig. 6-6). However, the cost must be considered, and contrast-enhanced CT is a sensitive alternative. Sonography can localize abnormal fluid collections, and is especially useful for drainage of abscesses. Nuclear scintigraphy includes leukocyte labeling, gallium, and triphasic bone scans.

Heterotopic Ossification

Heterotopic ossification is the deposition of periarticular bone. It occurs following various insults or injuries, most commonly in patients with spinal cord injury (in 16%–53% of them) (25). The joints most frequently involved are the hips, knees, and shoulders, though any joint below the spinal lesion may be affected (26) (Fig. 6-7). It is also frequently seen in burn patients and in patients who have had total hip arthroplasty.

The elbow is most commonly involved after thermal injury, with the hip in children and the shoulder in adults less often affected. Patients who have had full-thickness burns to the upper extremities involving 20% or more of the total body surface area are most vulnerable to the development of heterotopic ossification (27).

Patients who are going to develop heterotopic bone typically will have changes within 2 to 6 months after injury, with the earliest development within 1 month. In children the presentation may be delayed up to 1 year or longer (28).

The exact etiology of heterotopic ossification is unknown, though it is postulated that cells of mesenchymal origin located in the soft tissues are transformed into osteoblasts secondary to trauma. The cells lay down matrix in the connective tissue between muscle fascicles; the osteoid is then calcified and ossified (29). On plain radiographs, poorly defined periarticular radiodense areas without trabeculation are seen initially. Eventually, these areas merge with adjacent bone, forming irregular conglomerates with trabeculation. Once fully matured, bony bridges may form across the joint, causing ankylosis. Spontaneous resorption occurs infrequently, and is more common in children (30). Symptoms vary from no clinical symptomatology, to pain, swelling, warmth, and restricted joint motion. When symptomatic, heterotopic ossification may be confused with deep venous thrombosis or infection. Laboratory evaluation may not be helpful, though the bone fraction of alkaline phosphatase is often elevated.

Because of the varied clinical presentations, radiologic evaluation is beneficial in making the proper diagnosis. Very early in the disease, plain radiographs may appear normal. Bone scintigraphy is more sensitive in the early phase; scans may be positive as much as 2 weeks before findings are evident on plain film radiographs. If early heterotopic ossification is suspected, triphasic bone scanning is recommended. During the active phase of heterotopic ossification, radioisotope uptake is increased in all three phases of scanning. Occasionally, the uptake will be increased during the first two phases and normal in the last phase. If surgery is performed prior to full maturation of the new bone, the rate of recurrence is high (31). Therefore, serial bone scans can be used to monitor the maturation of the bony excrescence.

Surgery is more successful once uptake and activity have decreased and are equal to those of normal bone.

CT has also been used to evaluate ectopic bone. The emergence of heterotopic ossification is heralded on CT scans by the appearance of soft-tissue densities of lower attenuation than muscle. As the disease progresses, these areas develop calcific density consistent with the radiographic and scintigraphic appearance. However, these low-density areas adjacent to areas of ossification may persist on follow-up scans for long periods of time.

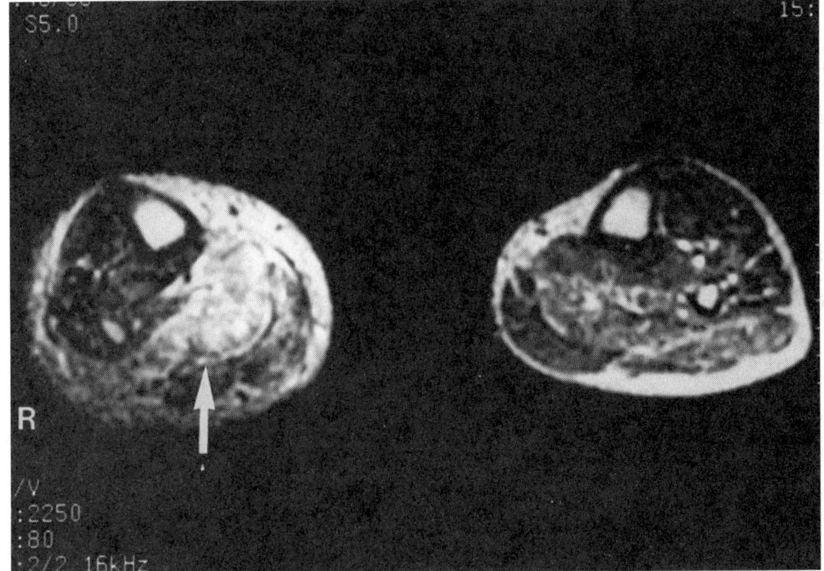

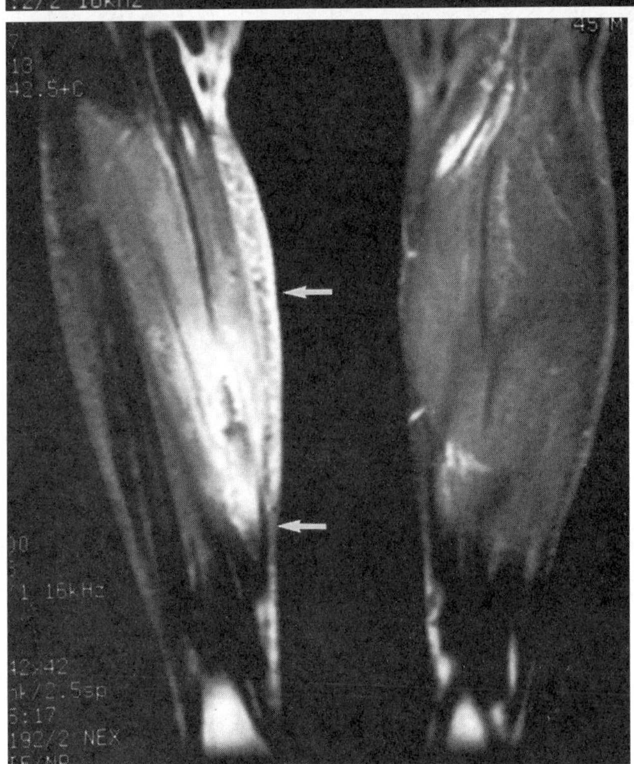

Figure 6-6. A 45-year-old diabetic with fever, and calf pain and swelling. *A.* A T2-weighted axial scan of both extremities demonstrates an increased signal intensity within the right gastrocnemius muscle (*arrow*), consistent with edema or infection. *B.* An inversion recovery sequence scan in the coronal plane depicts the superior and inferior extent of the involvement (*arrows*). The patient had myofascitis secondary to staphylococcal infection.

MRI has been used infrequently in the evaluation of heterotopic ossification. Little, if any, additional information is obtained in comparison to conventional and nuclear imaging.

Imaging of Specific Joints

Temporomandibular Joint

Degenerative and posttraumatic pathology and internal derangement can be evaluated by MRI, which images the disk and adjacent structures of the temporomandibular joint (32). Static and dynamic images can detect disk subluxation and dislocation, degenerative disease of the mandibular condyle, and disruption of the ligamentous structures. Joint mobility can be evaluated by plain film radiography or tomography with the mouth in the open and closed positions. Arthrography is rarely performed.

Shoulder

Anterior and posterior dislocation and luxatio erecta are diagnosed on plain films. Lateral and other special views

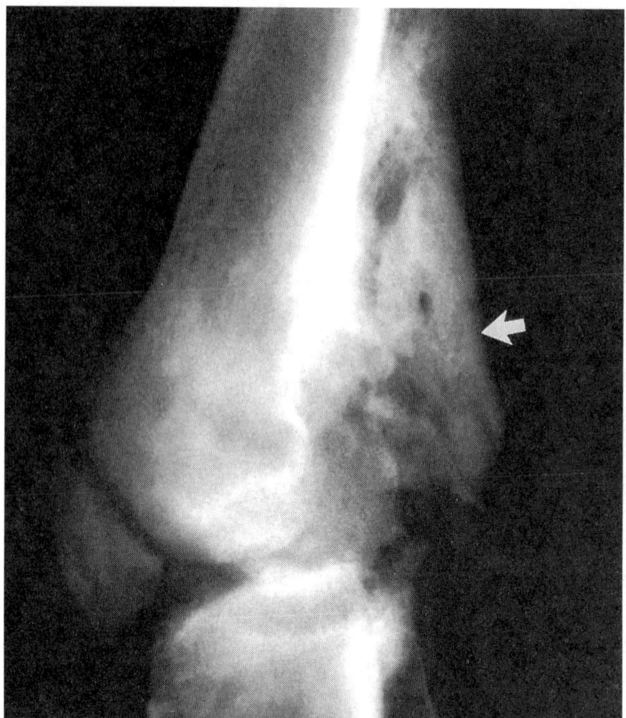

Figure 6-7. Lateral radiography of the knee in a 31-year-old quadriplegic. Heterotopic ossification courses along the posterior aspect of the knee (*arrow*).

(scapular "Y" view or axillary view) help detect subtle dislocations. The sequelae to dislocation, such as impaction fractures, are likewise present on x-ray films, or can be confirmed with CT in difficult cases. The classic "high-riding humeral head" can tip one off to a rotator cuff abnormality.

Capsular abnormalities are best addressed with MRI or with arthrography; the latter can be in conjunction with fluoroscopic imaging, CT, or MRI. Adhesive capsulitis is confirmed not only by resistance to the injection of contrast material into the joint, but also by marked decreased joint volume (19). Capsular laxity or instability requires either a joint effusion or injection of contrast material to demonstrate the capacious joint and to assess the glenohumeral ligaments and the glenoid labrum for abnormality. Abnormal insertion of the ligaments or tears of the labrum can predispose to repeated glenohumeral dislocations (33).

The glenoid labrum is best depicted with MRI. Usually, routine fluid-sensitive MRI is adequate enough for the diagnosis of labral tears; however, MR arthrography may be required. Evaluation for superior labral, anterior-posterior (SLAP) lesions may require an infusion of contrast material into the joint.

Sonography has been gaining in popularity for assessing rotator cuff pathology. In experienced hands, ultrasound can be sensitive for detecting tears, depending on their location. However, MRI is the gold standard in evaluating the rotator cuff. Conventional plain film arthrography is adequate for confirming complete tears of the rotator cuff, but only detects those partial tears amenable to contrast material imbibition (inferior surface tears). Partial tears and tendinosis are best seen with MRI. Not only is atrophy of the rotator cuff muscles best demonstrated on MRI, but also potential underlying causes, such as ganglion cysts in the supraspinous recess or in the spinoglenoid notch, are detectable, owing to the intrinsic differential in soft-tissue signal intensity and to three-dimensional imaging. Isolated atrophy of the teres minor muscle can occur with impingement of a branch of the axillary nerve in the quadrilateral space. Pain is aggravated with abduction and external rotation; however, the diagnosis may not be confirmed unless impingement of the posterior humeral circumflex artery is demonstrated on angiograms when the humerus is in this position (34).

Biceps dislocation can be confirmed with CT, though tendinopathy and tears are best imaged with MRI. Calcific tendinitis can be difficult to diagnose with MRI, and plain film correlation for gross calcification is beneficial.

Acromioclavicular joint degenerative changes are detectable on plain films and CT and MRI scans. The coracoclavicular and coracohumeral ligaments, configuration of the acromion, and potential associated rotator cuff pathology are only demonstrated by MRI.

Elbow

Osseous injuries at the elbow (35) are usually detected with conventional radiographs. Subtle fractures or areas of contusion within the humerus, radius, and ulna can be identified with nuclear scintigraphy. CT can aid in detecting subtle fracture lines. If there is persistent pain and high suspicion for occult fracture, MRI is beneficial.

Joint-related or articulator injuries can be assessed with arthrography. CT or plain film tomography in conjunction with an arthrogram can increase the sensitivity for detecting cartilaginous and capsular abnormalities.

If imaging is desired for evaluating epicondylitis (pitcher's or tennis elbow), capsular disruptions, early osteonecrosis, defects in the articular cartilage, or any soft-tissue pathology (bursae, ligaments, tendons, muscles, and nerves), then MRI is the modality of choice. Ulnar, radial, and median nerve entrapment syndromes are also best imaged with MRI.

Wrist and Hand

The clinical presentation and physical findings can be important factors in determining not only which radiographic modality to use, but also which specific protocol to chose for each examination. If there is a desire to evaluate the ligamentous anatomy and its pathology, MRI is advantageous, though arthrography still has a role. The carpal ligaments can be visualized with MRI. The triangular fibrocartilage can be evaluated with a tricompartmental arthrogram of the wrist (36) or with MRI (37).

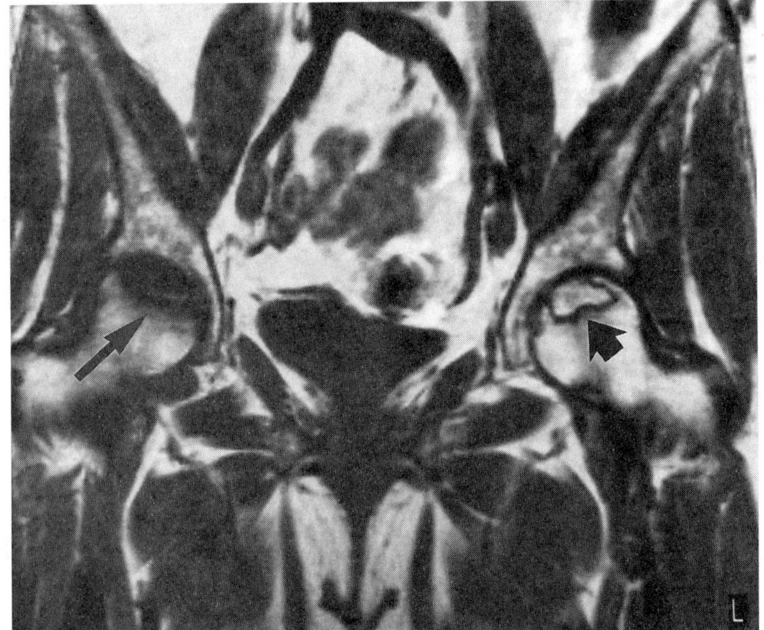

Figure 6-8. A 62-year-old patient with bilateral hip pain. T1-weighted coronal MRI shows avascular necrosis of both femoral heads. In the right hip, there is mainly sclerosis, as evidenced by low signal intensity in the femoral head due to loss of normal marrow signal (*arrow*). The left femur is in an earlier phase (*wide arrow*).

Subluxations of the distal radioulnar joint are best assessed via CT, if plain films are inconclusive. Triangular fibrocartilage disruption or degenerative or posttraumatic changes have been evaluated with arthrography, though MRI is more frequently used. The sensitivity and specificity of MRI have been very high (approaching 100%), especially when the thicker ulnar margin is involved.

The most sensitive imaging modality for carpal tunnel syndrome is MRI. The nerve itself and bone or soft-tissue abnormalities that may cause compression of the nerve can be identified. The patient with classic symptoms rarely needs imaging, but for those with atypical symptoms, MRI can be performed (38); it is also useful in checking the patient following decompressive surgery.

Soft-tissue and osseous tumors are rare in the wrist and hand. One of the most common abnormalities is a ganglion cyst. If this cannot be diagnosed clinically, MRI can confirm the benign cystic nature of this lesion, and likely its origin, and possibly play a role in predicting the long-term effects of the process (38).

Hip

Initial plain film screening for hip symptoms can demonstrate degenerative changes and large joint effusions. Cortical irregularities from infection and tumor can be visualized when there is fairly extensive involvement. Late-stage avascular necrosis will present as sclerosis and a heterogeneous appearance, subchondral lucency, or fragmentation of the femoral head (39,40).

However, many of the pathologic entities in the hip can be occult on x-ray films. In these instances, MRI is the most sensitive modality overall, allowing detection of joint effusion, bony abnormalities, and soft-tissue pathology (Fig. 6-8). Nuclear scintigraphy can demonstrate isotope uptake at sites of fractures, osteonecrosis, arthritis, and infection; however, it is nonspecific. CT can demonstrate joint subluxations and subtle fractures, but is not very helpful in the assessment of the status of the marrow, the joint capsule, or the articular cartilage.

MRI has the advantage of being very sensitive for demonstrating marrow edema, fractures, joint effusions, cartilaginous changes, articular surface abnormalities, osteonecrosis (41), and transient osteoporosis. Sequences can be designed to answer a specific question, thereby improving the sensitivity and specificity of the examination while limiting the number of sequences and thus increasing cost-effectiveness.

Pediatric conditions such as developmental dysplasia, traumatic epiphyseal slip, slipped capital femoral epiphysis, and Legg-Perthes disease can be assessed with plain films or sonography. In problem cases, MRI and the ability to evaluate the joint in three dimensions can be beneficial (39).

Pigmented villonodular synovitis has typical findings on MRI that correspond to the hemosiderin deposition found histologically (42,43). Likewise, synovial osteochondromatosis demonstrates characteristic signal intensity on MRI (44).

Knee

Arthritic changes and tumors in the knee are usually detectable on x-ray films. For persistent symptoms, CT and MRI can identify subtle joint changes and fractures that may not be visible on plain films. Loose bodies can be seen on x-ray films if there is sufficient calcification; otherwise CT and MRI are superior for locating small fracture fragments.

Occasionally arthrography is performed to assess for meniscal pathology, but it has been essentially replaced by MRI. Intra-articular contrast studies are still performed; however, they may be more beneficial when in conjunction with MRI, rather than plain films or CT.

When there is suspicion for internal derangement, that is, meniscal tears, ligamentous injury, articular cartilage abnormalities, trabecular injury or edema, synovial processes, patellar chondromalacia or dislocation, and retinacular tears, MRI is far superior. Intra-articular injection of contrast material is generally not required, and the routine sequences provide an excellent view of the anatomy and pathology of the knee joint. Clinical history can determine whether special sequences may be of benefit. For example, three-dimensional volume gradient-echo acquisitions enable optimal imaging of the patellar cartilage; the short tau inversion recovery (STIR) sequence improves the sensitivity for detecting subtle marrow edema, tumors, and infections.

The tendons of the knee are also well suited to MRI. The patella and quadriceps mechanism, the tendons of the pes anserinus, and the popliteus tendon can be evaluated for tears or inflammation.

MRI is also better for depicting the soft-tissue structures around the knee. Bursitis, synovial cysts, Baker cysts, popliteal artery entrapment syndrome or aneurysms, and popliteal vein varices can be identified with the various sequences and orthogonal imaging that MRI provides (45–47).

Ankle and Foot

As in any other joint, fractures and dislocations of the ankle and foot are initially evaluated with routine x-ray films. CT can be useful for subtle abnormalities; when there is persistent pain and negative findings on plain films, CT can provide a better look at the fracture, and thin cuts with three-dimensional reconstructions can aid in surgical planning.

The tendons and ligaments are best evaluated with MRI. Achilles tears or tendinopathy, disruption of the posterior tibial tendon, or pathology of the peroneal tendons can be identified with the proper image sequences and orientation. Direct visualization of the tendons helps differentiate tendonitis from rupture (48–51).

Avascular necrosis and osteochondral injury that is occult to plain films and CT can be identified on MRI with T2-weighted or STIR images. Subtle fractures are identified by the appearance of marrow edema and frank infiltration of fluid into a fracture line. Osteochondral injury can also be staged (52).

Sinus tarsi syndrome is most often secondary to trauma, especially with lateral ligamentous injury. MRI is the modality of choice for making the diagnosis, being confirmed by the presence of abnormal fluid in the sinus, in the region where the interosseous ligament normally courses (53).

The diagnosis of tarsal tunnel syndrome can be difficult to make. Impingement of the posterior tibial nerve in the medial (flexor) tunnel can be posttraumatic or due to an intrinsic mass in the confines of the fibro-osseous tunnel that runs from the medial malleolus to the navicular. MRI enables identification of focal lesions as well as compressive fibrosis that may result from previous trauma (54) (Fig. 6-9).

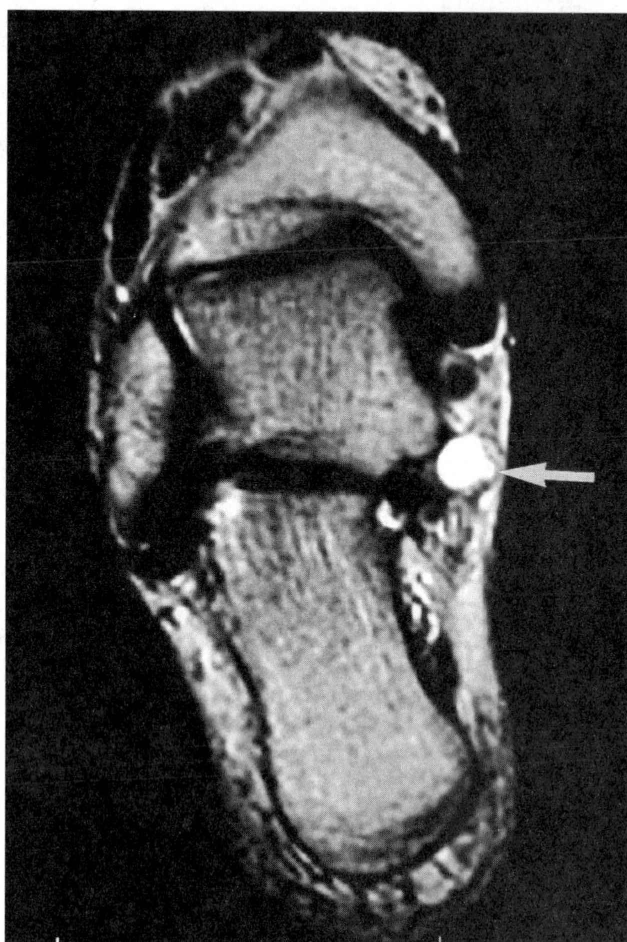

Figure 6-9. A 38-year-old patient with posterior tibial nerve symptoms. A high-signal-intensity ganglion cyst (*arrow*) within the tarsal tunnel was compressing the nerve.

If not grossly confirmed on plain films, tarsal coalitions are best assessed with CT. MRI does not appear to offer much advantage over CT for evaluating either fibrous or osseous coalition (50).

Ankle instability due to ligamentous disruption can be diagnosed on stress x-ray films and by measuring the distances of the ankle mortise. With MRI, the ligaments can be evaluated directly. Acute tears and chronic fibrosis can be seen when the ligaments are adequately visualized. However, this is not always the case. The oblique course of most ligaments in the ankle may require tailored image planes and sequences to increase the likelihood of diagnosing pathology. These can be performed if there is forehand knowledge of suspected ligamentous abnormality.

REFERENCES

1. Freundlich IM, Bragg DB. *A radiologic approach to diseases of the chest.* Baltimore: Williams & Wilkins, 1992.
2. Felson B. *Chest roentgenology.* Philadelphia: WB Saunders, 1973.
3. Jones B, Donner MW. *Normal and abnormal swallowing, imaging in diagnosis and therapy.* New York: Springer, 1991.
4. Albright F, Burnett CH, Cope O, Parsons W. Acute atrophy of bone (osteoporosis) simulating hyperparathyroidism. *J Clin Endocrinol* 1941;1:711–716.
5. Eichenholtz N. Management of long-bone fractures in paraplegic patients. *J Bone Joint Surg [Am]* 1963;45A:299–310.
6. Handelsman JE. Spontaneous fractures in spina bifida. *J Bone Joint Surg [Br]* 1972;54:381.
7. Resnick D, Goergen TG, Niwayama G. Physical injury. In: Resnick D, Niwayama G, eds. *Diagnosis of bone and joint disorders.* 2nd ed. Philadelphia: WB Saunders, 1988:2756–3008.
8. Griffiths HJ, Priest DR, Kushner D. Total hip replacement and other orthopedic hip procedures. *Radiol Clin North Am* 1995;33:267–287.
9. Warren Weissman BN, Simmons BP, Thomas WH. Replacement of "other" joints. *Radiol Clin North Am* 1995;33:355–373.
10. Chew FS, Pappas CN. Radiology of devices for fracture treatment in the extremities. *Radiol Clin North Am* 1995;33:375–390.
11. Resnick D, Niwayama G. Osteomyelitis, septic arthritis, and soft tissue infection: the mechanisms and situations. In: Resnick D, Niwayama G, eds. *Diagnosis of bone and joint disorders.* 2nd ed. Philadelphia: WB Saunders, 1988:2525–2618.
12. Jaffe HL. *Metabolic, degenerative and inflammatory diseases of bones and joints.* Philadelphia: Lea & Febiger, 1972.
13. Butt WP. The radiology of infection. *Clin Orthop* 1973;96:20–30.
14. Weissman BN, ed. Imaging of arthropathies. *Radiol Clin North Am* 1996:34.
15. Hodler J, Resnick D. Current status of imaging of articular cartilage. *Skel Radiol* 1996;25: 703–709.
16. Chandani V, Ho C, Chu P, et al. Knee hyaline cartilage evaluated with MR imaging: a cadaveric study involving multiple imaging sequences and intra-articular injection of gadolinium and saline solution. *Radiology* 1991;178: 557–561.
17. Chan WP, Lang P, Genant HK. *MRI of the musculoskeletal system.* Philadelphia: WB Saunders, 1994.
18. Fitzgerald-Finch OP, Gibson II. Subluxation of the shoulder in hemiplegia. *Age Aging* 1975;4(1):16–18.
19. Bruckner FE, Nye CJS. Prospective study of adhesive capsulitis of the shoulder ("frozen shoulder") in a high risk population. *Q J Med* 1981;198:191–204.
20. Brower AC, Allman RM. Neuropathic osteoarthropathy. *Orthop Rev* 1985;14:81–88.
21. Thomasson JL, Sundaram M. The diabetic foot: radiographic appearances. *Orthopedics* 1985;8:668–677.
22. Kraft E, Spyropoulos E, Finby N. Neurogenic disorders of the foot in diabetes mellitus. *AJR* 1975;124: 17–24.
23. Zlatkin MB, Pathri M, Sartoris DJ, Resnick D. The diabetic foot. *Radiol Clin North Am* 1987;25: 1095–1105.
24. Resnick D. Neuromuscular disorders. In: Resnick D, Niwayama G, eds. *Diagnosis of bone and joint disorders.* 2nd ed. Philadelphia: WB Saunders, 1988:3115–3153.
25. Nichols JJ. Ectopic bone formation in patients with spinal cord injury. *Arch Phys Med Rehabil* 1973;54: 354–359.
26. Sinaki M, ed. *Basic clinical rehabilitation medicine.* 2nd ed. St. Louis: Mosby, 1993.
27. Delisa J, ed. *Rehabilitation Medicine, principle and practice.* Philadelphia: JB Lippincott, 1988.
28. Resnick D, ed. *Diagnosis of bone and joint disorders.* 3rd ed. Philadelphia: WB Saunders, 1995.
29. Collier BD Jr, Fogelman I, Rosenthall L, eds. *Skeletal nuclear medicine.* St. Louis: Mosby–Year Book, 1996.
30. Garland DE, Shimoyama ST, Lugo C, et al. Spinal cord insults and heterotopic ossification in the pediatric population. *Clin Orthop* 1989;245:303–310.
31. Bressler EL, Marn CS, Gore RM, et al. Evaluation of ectopic bone by CT. *AJR* 1987;148:931–935.
32. Stoller DW, Jacobson RL. The temporomandibular joint. In: Stoller DW, ed. *MRI in orthopedics and sports medicine.* 2nd ed. Philadelphia: Lippincott-Raven, 1997: 995–1022.
33. Stoller DW. MR arthrography of the glenohumeral joint. *Radiol Clin North Am* 1997;35:97–116.
34. Helms CA. The shoulder. In: Higgins CB, Hricak H, Helms CA, eds. *Magnetic resonance of the body.* 3rd ed. New York: Lippincott-Raven, 1997:1153–1174.
35. Fritz RC, Steinbach LS, Tirman PFJ, Martinez S. MR imaging of the elbow: an update. *Radiol Clin North Am* 1997;35:117–144.
36. Levinsohn EM, Rosen ID, Palmer AK. Wrist arthrography: the value of the three-compartment injection method. *Radiol N Y* 1991;179: 231–239.
37. Metz VM, Schratter M, Dock WI, et al. Age-associated changes of the triangular fibrocartilage of the wrist: evaluation of the diagnostic performance of MR imaging. *Radiology* 1992;84:217–220.
38. Smith DK. The hand and wrist. In: Higgins CB, Hricak H, Helms CA, eds. *Magnetic resonance of the*

body. 3rd ed. New York: Lippincott-Raven, 1997:1175–1217.

39. Major NM, Helms CA. The hip. In: Higgins CB, Hricak H, Helms CA, eds. *Magnetic resonance of the body.* 3rd ed. New York: Lippincott-Raven, 1997:1087–1101.

40. Berquist TH. Pelvis, hips, thighs. In: Berquist TH, ed. *MRI of the musculoskeletal system.* 3rd ed. Philadelphia: Lippincott-Raven, 1996:197–284.

41. Mitchell D, Rao V, Dalinka M. Femoral head avascular necrosis: correlation of MR imaging, radiographic staging, radionuclide imaging, and clinical findings. *Radiology* 1987;162:709–715.

42. Jelinek J, Kransdorf M, Utz J. Imaging of pigmented villonodular synovitis with emphasis on MR imaging. *AJR* 1989;152:337–342.

43. Kottal R, Vogler J, Matamoros A, et al. Pigmented villonodular synovitis: a report of MR imaging in two cases. *Radiology* 1987;163:551–553.

44. Hermann G, Abdelwahab IF, Klein M, et al. Synovial osteochondromatosis. *Skel Radiol* 95;24:298–300.

45. Munk PL, Janzen DL, Helms CA. The knee. In: Higgins CB, Hricak H, Helms CA, eds. *Magnetic resonance of the body.* 3rd ed. New York: Lippincott-Raven, 1997: 1103–1131.

46. Mink JH, Reicher MA, Crues JV, Deutsch AL. *MRI of the knee.* 2nd ed. New York: Raven, 1993.

47. Berquist TH. Knee. In: Berquist TH, ed. *MRI of the musculoskeletal system.* 3rd ed. Philadelphia: Lippincott-Raven, 1996: 285–410.

48. Beltran J, ed. The ankle and foot. *Magn Reson Imaging Clin N Am* 1994;2(1).

49. Berqist TH. Foot, calf, and ankle. In: Berquist TH, ed. *MRI of the musculoskeletal system.* 3rd ed. Philadelphia: Lippincott-Raven, 1996:411–516.

50. Helms CA. The foot and ankle. In: Higgins CB, Hricak H, Helms CA, eds. *Magnetic resonance of the body.* 3rd ed. New York: Lippincott-Raven, 1997:1239–1255.

51. Rosenberg ZS, Cheung Y, Jahss MH, et al. Rupture of posterior tibial tendons: CT and MR imaging with surgical correlation. *Radiology* 1988;196:229–236.

52. De Smet A, Fisher D, Burnstein M, et al. Value of MR imaging in staging osteochondral lesions of the talus (osteochondritis dissecans): results in 14 patients. *AJR* 1990;154:555–558.

53. Beltran J. Sinus tarsi syndrome. *Magn Reson Imaging Clin N Am* 1994;2:59–65.

54. Finkel JE. Tarsal tunnel syndrome. *Magn Reson Imaging Clin N Am* 1994;2:67–78.

Chapter 7

Diagnostic Imaging for the Physiatrist: Urinary Tract Imaging and Interventional Radiologic Management of the Rehabilitation Patient

Dale R. Broome
Cliff J. Whigham, Jr.

IMAGING OF THE URINARY TRACT

Overview of Imaging Modalities

Acute and chronic neuromuscular disorders can often lead to significant urologic complications that require diagnostic imaging. Most complications arise in patients with a neurogenic bladder resulting in urinary stasis and high intravesical pressure, which usually requires intermittent catheterization. A variety of imaging modalities are available to the physiatrist to diagnose urinary tract abnormalities. It is important to understand the diagnostic capabilities of the various modalities and to order imaging studies in an appropriate sequence in consultation with a radiologist.

Plain film radiography of the abdomen remains one of the most useful and least expensive examinations to image the urinary tract. Approximately 85% to 90% of urinary calculi are calcified and visible on the supine abdominal [kidney-ureter-bladder (KUB)] radiograph. Oblique films are obtained to confirm the intrarenal location of renal calculi. Abnormal collections of gas within the urinary tract as seen with emphysematous pyelonephritis and cystitis can also be identified on the abdominal film. Nephrotomography of the abdomen can be performed without intravenous contrast material, primarily to confirm the presence of smaller renal calculi when supine and oblique films are inconclusive.

Intraveous Urography

The intravenous urogram (IVU) or intravenous pyelogram (IVP) is the primary diagnostic imaging study of the urinary tract because it can demonstrate most urinary tract disorders including urinary stones, upper urinary tract obstruction and injuries, and sequelae of recurrent infection and reflux nephropathy. Nephrotomography is frequently incorporated into the IVU study because it allows better visualization of the kidneys. This is particularly useful in the neuromuscular patients with a significant amount of retained stool and in those patients older than 50 years because they have a high incidence of unsuspected renal neoplasms. Prior to the examination, serum creatinine levels should be measured and the patient should be fasting for 6 to 8 hours. Many institutions administer an oral cathartic such as castor oil, bisacodyl, X-prep, or Dulcolax 12 to 18 hours prior to the examination. On the morning of the examination, an additional suppository may be helpful to further cleanse the sedentary or bedridden patient.

The principal complications of IVU are related to the iodinated contrast agent administered intravenously during the examination. The first potential complication is an idiosyncratic or anaphylactoid reaction. Reactions to the contrast agent can be classified as mild (nausea, mild vomiting, sneezing, heat sensation, or mild urticaria), moderate (severe vomiting, faintness, mild hypotension, diffuse urticaria, mild bronchospasm, dyspnea, facial edema, bradycardia, or tachycardia), or severe (severe bronchospasm or laryngospasm, hypotensive shock, loss of consciousness, sustained cardiac dysrhythmias, pulmonary edema, cardiac arrest, or death). The incidence of severe reactions is 0.05% to 0.10% with traditional ionic contrast agents but can be reduced by a factor of 4 to 12 with the use of newer nonionic contrast agents (1,2).

To minimize the risk of a reaction, several precautions should be taken. Patients with a history of a previous reaction to contrast material, severe allergies, asthma, or atopy should receive a nonionic contrast agent and premedication. Commonly used premedications include corticosteroids (32 mg of methylprednisolone or 50 mg of prednisone orally) administered 12 hours and 2 hours before injection of the contrast material. Additionally histamine antagonists can be administered—50 mg of diphenhydramine and either 300 mg of cimetidine or 50 mg of ranitidine, each given orally 1 hour prior to the examination (3). If the patient previously had a severe reaction, intravenous iodinated contrast material should be avoided and alternative imaging studies should be performed.

Renal failure is another potential complication to the use of iodinated contrast agents. This is a nonidiosyncratic or chemotoxic reaction that is related to the dose and concentration of contrast material administered. Contrast material–induced nephropathy is usually transient and resolves in 7 to 10 days. Patients who are at particular risk for this complication include those with class IV congestive heart failure, diabetics with preexisting renal insufficiency or on metformin (Glucophage), and possibly patients with multiple myeloma. Metformin should be discontinued 48 hours before and can be reinstituted 48 hours after contrast agent administration. Most radiologists avoid the use of intravenous contrast agents when the serum creatinine level is higher than 2.0 mg/dL. Patients with renal insufficiency or multiple myeloma should be vigorously hydrated prior to the examination. Patients with preexisting renal insufficiency may also be given mannitol, 25 g in 500 mL of D51/2NS infused during and just after contrast injection, to induce diuresis, or they can undergo dialysis immediately after the examination.

Other Imaging Modalities

Ultrasonography is primarily used as a screening examination to assess for upper urinary tract obstruction and to evaluate incidental renal masses noted on the IVU.

Computed tomography (CT) is most frequently performed with intravenous contrast material, although a nonenhanced study can be used to detect urinary calculi. CT is the preferred examination for the initial assessment of acute renal traumatic injuries. It is also invaluable for the detection of abscesses and for the assessment of masses arising from or adjacent to the urinary tract. As with IVU, the complications of CT pertain to the use of intravenous contrast material, discussed in the previous section.

Nuclear medicine renal scans performed most commonly with technetium 99m–diethylenetriamine pentaacetic acid (^{99m}Tc-DTPA) or MAG3 can be used to quantitate the differential glomerular filtration rates of the kidneys and also to demonstrate ureteral obstruction when iodinated contrast material cannot be given. A furosemide (Lasix) washout study can be performed with this examination to distinguish the dilated, obstructed upper urinary tract from the dilated, nonobstructed upper urinary tract.

The lower urinary tract is most frequently imaged by directly injecting an iodinated contrast agent into the urethra and bladder through a catheter. Cystography is primarily used to detect a postsurgical or posttraumatic bladder leak and to confirm the presence of bladder stones. Voiding cystourethrography (VCUG) is used primarily for the detection of mechanical or functional bladder obstructions (including neurogenic bladders) and for the detection of vesicoureteral reflux (VUR) (particularly in patients with urinary tract infections, neurogenic bladders, or IVU signs of reflux nephropathy). The retrograde urethrogram (RUG) is utilized to detect urethral injuries from trauma or catheterization and to detect urethral strictures, false passages, and diverticula.

Inflammatory Disorders of the Urinary Tract and Reflux Nephropathy

Urinary Tract Infections

Urinary tract infections most commonly arise in patients with a neuromuscular disorder and associated neurogenic bladder. Although once the leading cause of death in spinal cord injury (SCI) patients, urosepsis mortality rates have significantly decreased with the use of intermittent catheterization and improvements in antibiotic therapy. Most adult urinary tract infections do not require imaging unless they are complicated or recurrent. Patients with known urinary tract stones, diabetes mellitus, and urinary obstruction are especially at risk for complicated infections.

Lower urinary tract infections rarely require diagnostic imaging unless there is concern for an associated infected stone or obstruction of the bladder or urethra. Voiding cystography can confirm all of these conditions; however, RUG will better delineate the cause of urethral obstruction. Although cystitis does not typically require imaging, signs of chronic cystitis including diffuse or nodular wall thickening can be detected with IVU, cystography, and CT. Emphysematous cystitis is an unusual form of chronic cystitis that is usually seen in patients with poorly controlled diabetes but can occur in patients with chronic bladder outlet obstruction or neurogenic bladder. It can be easily diagnosed with radiography because air is identified in the bladder wall. Epididymo-orchitis is an important lower genitourinary tract infection that may require imaging. Sometimes it can be confused clinically with testicular torsion in the patient presenting with acute scrotum pain and swelling. Both scrotal sonography with color Doppler evaluation and nuclear medicine scrotal scintigraphy are useful diagnostic examinations to distinguish these two entities.

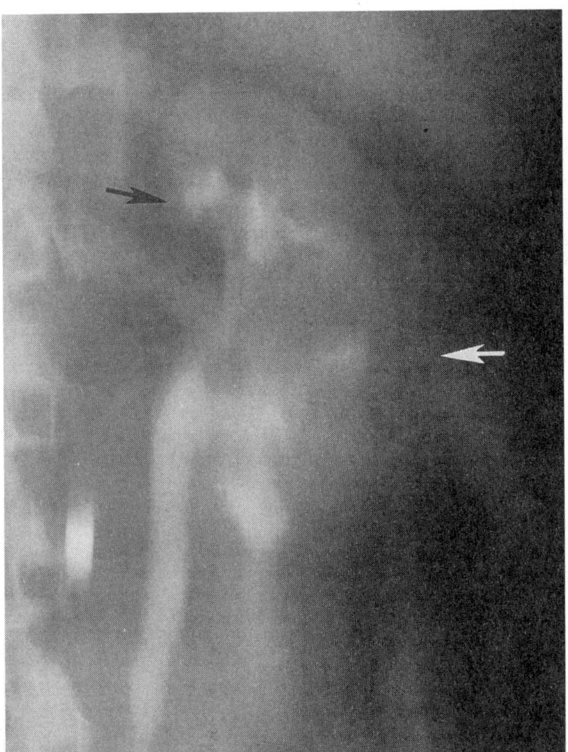

Figure 7-1. Chronic atrophic pyelonephritis changes on an intravenous urogram in a paraplegic with a history of vesicoureteral reflux and repeated episodes of pyelonephritis. The kidney is small and shows numerous areas of focal cortical scarring (*arrows*) with associated dilated underlying calyces.

IVU is useful in the initial work-up of upper urinary tract infections to detect any associated stones or obstruction. IVU can also demonstrate signs of chronic upper tract infections including parenchymal scarring (Fig. 7-1), papillary necrosis, and ureteritis cystica. Complicated upper urinary tract infections should be suspected in patients who do not respond to antibiotic therapy or who have suspected obstruction. Sonography is a useful screening examination because it can detect pyonephrosis and most renal and perinephric abscesses. On ultrasound scans pyonephrosis appears as hydronephrosis with echogenic debris within the collecting system (Fig. 7-2). Pyonephrosis can also be suggested on CT and IVU images when hydronephrosis and obstruction are noted in the clinical setting of pyelonephritis. Although ultrasonography can detect most renal and perinephric abscesses, CT is usually necessary to assess the full extent of these abscesses and to more accurately assess the cause of any associated obstruction. CT can also detect small abscesses or areas of acute focal bacterial nephritis (formerly called lobar nephronia) that may be occult on ultrasound scans. Renal and perinephric abscesses typically appear as masses of variable echogenicity on ultrasound and water density on CT scans (Fig. 7-3).

Vesicoureteral Reflux and Reflux Nephropathy

Chronic atrophic pyelonephritis is thought to be due to long-standing VUR and is better termed *reflux nephropathy*. Most cases develop idiopathically in early childhood, but patients with neurogenic bladders can acquire it secondarily. VUR will develop in as many as 30% of meningomyelocele patients (4) and 16% of SCI patients (5). Because reflux nephropathy is a significant cause of renal failure in these patients, early detection with VCUG or radionuclide cystography is essential. The latter is often favored in children because of the lower gonadal radiation dose. VUR is graded from 1 to 5: grade 1—ureteral reflux without dilatation; grade 2—reflux to the kidney without dilatation; grade 3—reflux to the kidney with mild dilatation; grade 4—reflux to the kidney with moderate dilatation and tortuousity; and grade 5—severe dilatation with calyceal clubbing (Fig. 7-4) (6). In patients with long-standing grade 4 or 5 VUR, focal scarring with varying degrees of hydronephrosis and hydroureter without a mechanical obstruction can be seen on IVU, CT, and ultrasound images. The scarring is most notable in the interpolar regions where there is focal cortical thinning overlying the dilated calyx (see Fig. 7-1).

Urinary Tract Calculi

Patients with neuromuscular disorders are particularly predisposed to calculi formation because of several factors: hypercalciuria, infection, urinary stasis, and a foreign body nidus. Hypercalciuria is exacerbated in the nonambulatory SCI patient, especially in the first 3 years (7). Patients with neurogenic bladders are at particular risk because of the urinary stasis that necessitates repeated catheterization, which can lead to infection or introduction of a nidus. Approximately 8% of all SCI patients develop renal calculi (8). Approximately 98% of these stones are composed of struvite (magnesium ammonium phosphate) and apatite (calcium carbonate and phosphate) (9). They tend to form in alkaline urine produced by urease-forming organisms such as *Proteus*, *Klebsiella*, and *Pseudomonas* species. Although struvite itself is not opaque, these stones attract calcium deposits (apatite component) and become slightly to moderately opaque on radiography. They can be single or multiple, unilateral or bilateral. When left untreated, they can progress to a staghorn appearance, filling the renal pelvis and infundibula. The remaining 2% of stones in SCI patients are calcium oxalate stones, which are slightly more opaque and not typically infected. Fifty percent of bladder stones associated with indwelling catheters are composed of struvite. The remainder are composed of a mixture of calcium oxalate and calcium phosphate or pure calcium phosphate (10).

Diagnostic Imaging Findings

Approximately 85% to 90% of urinary calculi are sufficiently calcified to be visible on the abdominal film (KUB).

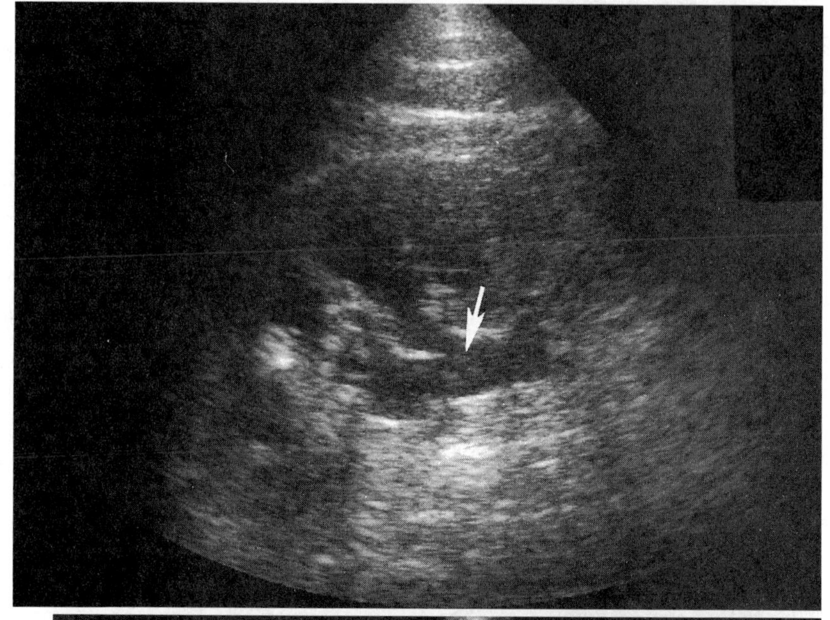

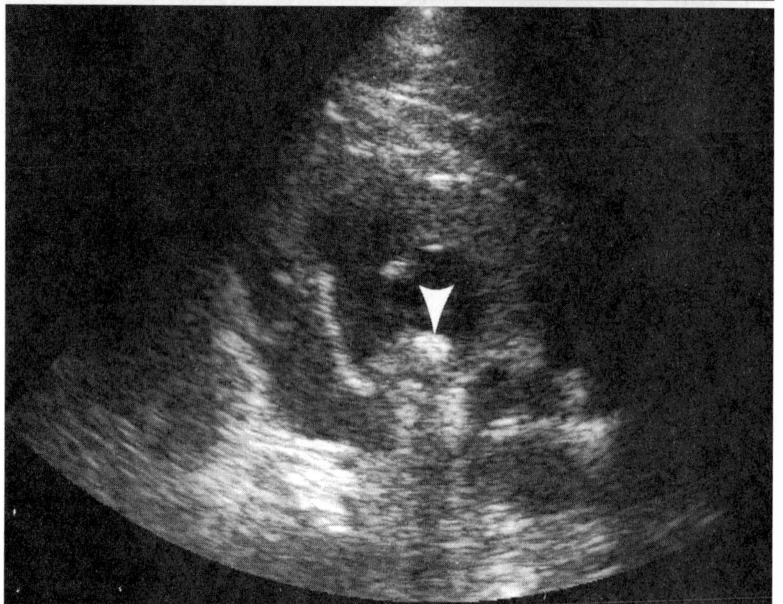

Figure 7-2. Pyonephrosis and renal calculi on a sonogram spinal cord injury of a patient. Note the moderate hydronephrosis with mildly echogenic debris/pus (*arrow*) (*A*) and the more echogenic shadowing calculi (*arrowhead*) (*B*).

They can usually be localized within the kidney, proximal ureter, bladder, and urethra on supine and oblique radiographs of the abdomen and pelvis (Fig. 7-5). Distal ureteral stones are more difficult to see because they can be obscured by the underlying bony sacrum or confused with adjacent pelvic calcified phleboliths. Less common types of stones such as uric acid stones (nonopaque) and cystine stones (slightly radiopaque) are more difficult to visualize on radiographs. Nephrotomography prior to IVU (and for that matter CT) can allow better detection of small calculi (<5 mm) if this is of significant clinical concern. IVU can localize the vast majority of urinary calculi and demonstrate the calcification within the urinary tract. Once contrast material fills the urinary tract, the calculi may appear of similar density to the contrast material or slightly less opaque. When a stone partially obstructs the ureter, there is typically columnation of contrast material above the stone. With more severe obstruction there is hydroureter and hydronephrosis, an increasingly dense appearance on the nephrogram, and delayed excretion of contrast material.

When IVU cannot be performed because of a previous severe reaction to contrast material or renal insufficiency, alternative examinations can be performed. The least invasive is ultrasonography, which is usually performed in combination with a KUB radiograph. Sonography is very sensitive (96%) for detecting renal stones, including nonopaque uric acid stones (11). They appear as echogenic, shadowing foci within the central part of the

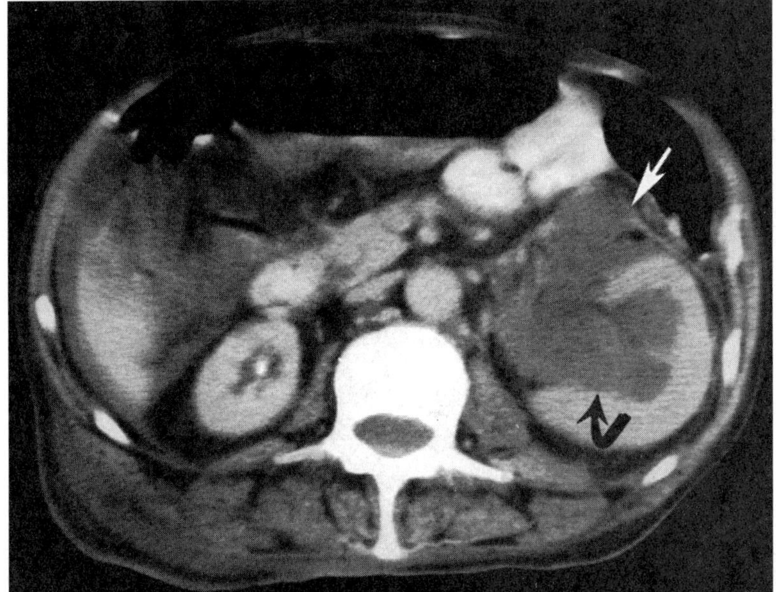

A

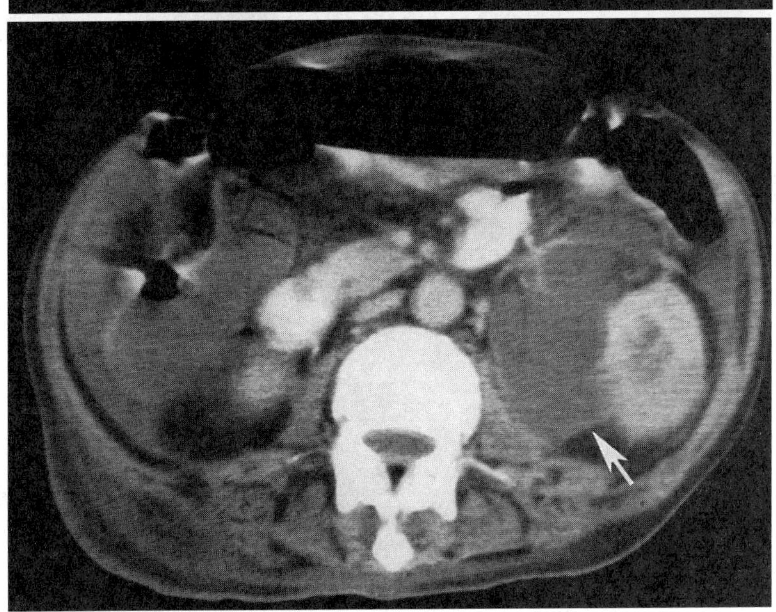

B

Figure 7-3. Large perinephric abscess that resulted from urine extravasation due to an obstructing distal ureteral stone. *A.* CT demonstrates moderate hydronephrosis (*curved arrow*) and the water-density perinephric abscess (*arrow*). *B.* CT demonstrates the inferior extension of the abscess (*arrow*).

kidney (see Fig. 7-2). However, small stones and stones located at the ureteropelvic junction may be difficult to see. Ureteral stones are even more difficult to detect unless they are lodged at the ureterovesical junction, where they can frequently be seen by scanning over the bladder. Ultrasonography is particularly useful to detect the presence of hydronephrosis and hydroureter; however, this is frequently absent with partial or early ureteral obstructions. More recently, nonenhanced spiral CT was shown to be extremely sensitive (97%) for the detection of ureteral stones (12). Retrograde pyelography performed at the time of cystoscopy is more invasive but will detect almost all stones. This is often performed when ureteral stent placement or retrograde stone retrieval is anticipated. Cystography or ultrasonography can be used to confirm the presence and location of bladder calculi; however, cystoscopy is the most definitive method of diagnosis. Small stones can also be retrieved cystoscopically.

Urinary Tract Obstruction and Renal Failure

Renal failure is perhaps the most significant urologic complication in patients with neuromuscular diseases because it can lead to the patient's demise. Prior to use of urinary catheterization, renal failure was the most frequent cause of death in SCI patients (13). Owing to advances in treatment and monitoring of patients with neurogenic bladder, renal failure now represents only 3% to 15% of all causes of death in SCI patients (14,15). The principal goal of radiologic imaging in patients with renal failure is to detect postrenal causes of the failure such as urinary tract obstruction or reflux nephropathy. Urinary obstruction can result from a mechanical obstruction such as benign pros-

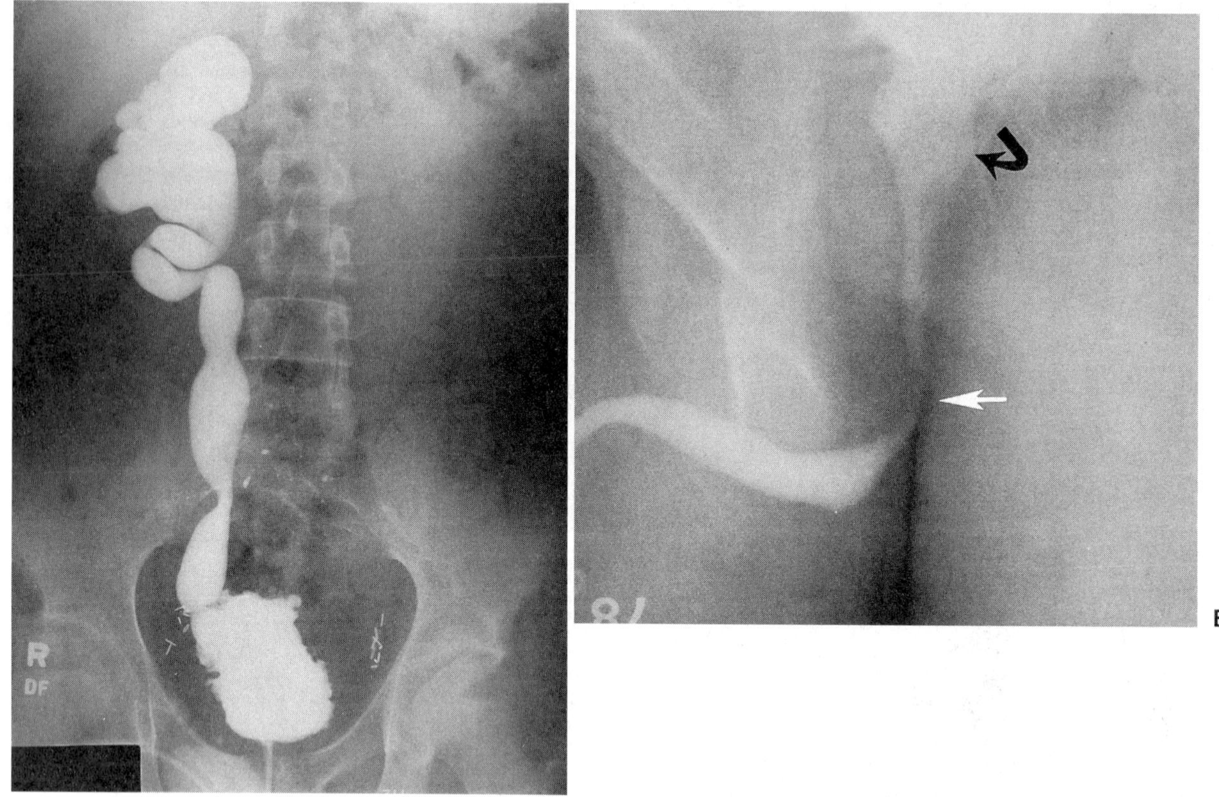

Figure 7-4. Long-standing detrusor hyperreflexia and detrusor-sphincteric dyssynergy in a spinal cord injury patient. *A.* Voiding cystourethrography (VCUG) demonstrates grade 5 vesicoureteral reflux and a small spastic bladder with a pinecone shape. *B.* VCUG also demonstrates a dilated posterior urethra and bladder neck (*curved arrow*) and poor relaxation of the external sphincter (*arrow*).

tatic hyperplasia, a ureteral stone, urothelial tumor, or urethral stricture. Many neuromuscular disease patients have a functional bladder obstruction that lacks a fixed point of narrowing but has a significant pressure gradient between the bladder and the urethra.

Upper Urinary Tract Obstruction

The principal imaging signs of upper urinary tract obstruction are hydrocalycosis, hydronephrosis, and hydroureter. It is important to realize that these signs are not specific for urinary tract obstruction and can be seen with causes of nonobstructive dilatation such as VUR (see Fig. 7-4), infection, pregnancy, previous severe obstructions, and congenital abnormalities (prune-belly syndrome, megaloureter). Also approximately 30% of all SCI patients will have mild nonobstructive ureterectasis and pyelectasis (or "silent hydronephrosis") demonstrated by IVU (16). This usually results from a sustained elevated intravesical pressure higher than 37 mm Hg, which leads to diminished ureteral peristalsis (17). In many cases this is reversible with proper bladder drainage therapy.

Ultrasonography is the most useful imaging study to screen for obstruction in the setting of renal insufficiency. Not only can it detect hydronephrosis in most patients with obstruction, but also it can detect signs of intrinsic renal disease such as cortical thinning and increased cortical echogenicity. However, in the setting of acute obstruction, hydronephrosis may not yet be detectable with sonography. IVU is particularly useful for the evaluation of acute upper urinary tract obstruction. IVU can also be used in the setting of mild (creatinine < 2.0 mg/dL) chronic renal insufficiency or for the routine surveillance of patients with neurogenic bladders. Some authors (16) alternatively proposed using renal scintigraphy in combination with abdominal radiography (to exclude calculi) for surveillance of patients with neurogenic bladder. Renal scintigraphy not only can detect obstruction but also can provide a more quantitative assessment of renal function (glomerular filtration rate, creatinine clearance rate, and estimated renal plasma flow) with a lower radiation dose to the patient, which is particularly important in children. Renal scintigraphy with furosemide washout can more accurately distinguish the nonobstructive dilated upper urinary tract from the obstructed upper urinary tract. This technique involves radionuclide imaging with ^{99m}Tc-labeled MAG3 or DTPA and computerized time-activity assessment of the kidneys prior to and following the intravenous administration of furosemide. Following diuresis, the nonobstructed,

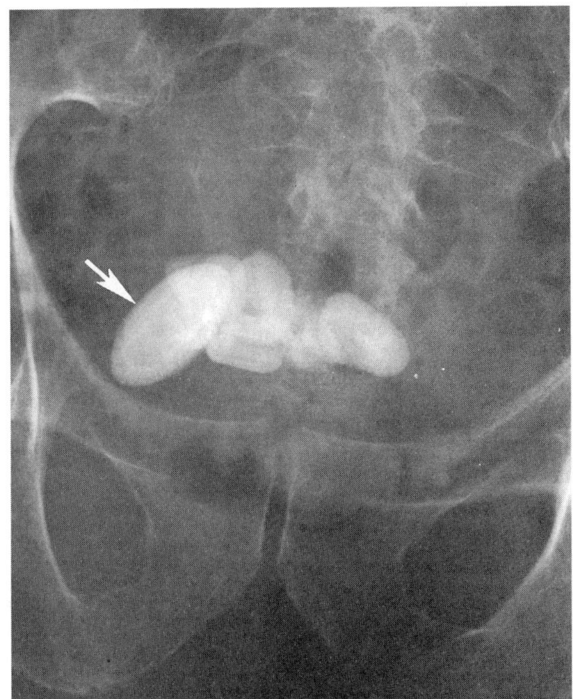

Figure 7-5. Numerous smooth, oval, bladder calculi on an abdominal radiograph. Many of these stones show a laminated appearance (*arrow*).

dilated system will show prompt washout and a drop in the time-activity curve compared to the obstructed system, which shows only minimal or no washout of the radionuclide.

Imaging studies can be used to grade the severity of hydronephrosis as mild, moderate, or severe. Mild hydronephrosis can be seen as an anechoic region splaying the central echo complex on the sonogram and as dilatation of the renal pelvis on IVU. With moderate hydronephrosis, branching anechoic, dilated calyces or hydrocalyces can be seen to extend from the renal pelvis (see Fig. 7-2). Severe hydronephrosis appears as severe dilatation of the renal pelvis and calyces and associated parenchymal atrophy. Additionally, with acute obstruction IVU will show mild renal enlargement, an increasingly dense appearance on the nephrogram, delayed excretion of contrast material, and occasionally pyelosinus extravasation of contrast material. Only minimal to moderate upper tract dilatation is typically seen. With chronic obstruction the kidneys are small to normal in size. On nephrograms, in the setting of moderate chronic obstruction, the kidneys appear normal, and in the setting of severe obstruction, they may not be visualized or may be faintly visualized. With pyelography, delayed films as late as 24 hours may be necessary for visualization. Hydroureter associated with ureteral obstructions is best detected with IVU or renal scintigraphy and is poorly seen with ultrasonography because of overlying bowel gas.

Lower Urinary Tract Obstruction and Neurogenic Bladder

The most common cause of lower urinary tract obstruction in patients with neuromuscular disorders is a neurogenic bladder. The physiology of micturition and classification of bladder dysfunctions are discussed in more detail in Chapter 51. Micturition is primarily a spinal cord reflex mediated through the spinal micturition center at the S2–S4 cord level located near the conus medullaris at the T12–L1 vertebral level. Parasympathetic efferent nerves arising from this center are primarily responsible for contraction of the detrusor smooth muscle and relaxation of the smooth muscle in the bladder neck or "internal sphincter." Higher centers within the cerebral cortex and pontomesencephalic gray matter can have facilitatory or inhibitory influences on micturition by allowing contraction and relaxation of the striated muscle within the external sphincter in the urogenital diaphragm. Most neurologic bladder dysfunctions can be diagnosed from the clinical history, physical examination, and urodynamic studies. Radiologic imaging with cystourethrography can be performed to confirm the diagnosis but is primarily performed to exclude certain mechanical causes of obstruction (enlarged prostate, posterior urethral valve, strictures), to confirm the presence and location of bladder stones, and to detect associated VUR. However, urethral strictures are better evaluated with RUG.

Depending on the level or site of neurologic insult or injury, various types of voiding dysfunction can occur and have distinct cystourethrographic findings. Suprapontine lesions (due to strokes, brain trauma, Alzheimer dementia, Parkinson disease, or multiple sclerosis) can result in loss of volitional control of bladder function, which is predominantly inhibitory to the micturition reflex. Because the spinal level reflex is still preserved, the result is overactivity of this reflex or detrusor hyperreflexia. The cystourethrographic findings of detrusor hyperreflexia consist of involuntary intermittent detrusor contractions; rounding of the bladder; mucosal serrations, especially along the posterior bladder wall; and a small bladder capacity. Bladder trabeculations are seen occasionally with long-standing detrusor hyperreflexia.

With spinal cord insults at or above the T12 level, the cortical inhibition and the pontine coordination of micturition are lost, resulting in both detrusor hyperreflexia and detrusor-sphincter dyssynergy. This can be seen with spinal cord injuries and spinal multiple sclerosis, and occasionally is related to disk disease. During VCUG, the bladder contracts, the bladder neck relaxes, but the external urethral sphincter contracts instead of relaxes. The result is a dilated posterior urethra and bladder neck. The bladder often shows trabeculation, wall thickening, and diverticula with long-standing disease. In severe cases the bladder shape can resemble a Christmas tree or pine cone (see Fig. 7-4). Because high pressures are generated within the bladder, VUR commonly occurs. Reflux can occur even into the prostate, ejaculatory ducts, seminal vesicles, and vas deferens. Patients with spinal cord injuries or lesions above the T6 level can also manifest signs of bladder neck dysfunction, which is often associated with autonomic dysreflexia. In this condition the bladder neck remains contracted during VCUG.

Injuries or lesions localized at or below the sacral micturition center below the T12 vertebral level (involving the conus medullaris, cauda equina, or peripheral nerves) result in detrusor areflexia, also known as an atonic or flaccid bladder. This can result from spinal trauma, spinal dysraphism, diabetes or alcoholic neuropathies, tumors, and surgical injury during abdominoperineal resection or radical hysterectomy. Detrusor areflexia can also be seen in SCI patients during the initial stage of spinal shock, which can last from several weeks to 3 months. Cystourethrography demonstrates a dilated bladder typically with a smooth contour. In patients with untreated chronic detrusor areflexia, bladder wall thickening, trabeculation, and diverticula can be visible by cystourethrography. With training, patients can void with abdominal straining or use the Credé method, but there is usually a significant postvoid residual. VUR can also be seen.

Traumatic Injuries of the Urinary Tract

Most injuries to the urinary tract related to blunt or penetrating trauma are diagnosed prior to referral of the patient to the physiatrist. Many of these patients have had multisystem injuries, often including brain or spinal cord injuries. Conservative nonsurgical management is preferred for many urinary tract injuries, and follow-up imaging studies are often necessary during the patient's rehabilitation process. For this reason the physiatrist should be aware of the common urinary tract injuries and their radiologic evaluation.

Renal injuries are most commonly caused by blunt trauma and almost always present with hematuria. Penetrating injuries usually result from a gunshot wound or stab wound. Acute renal injuries are best evaluated with CT with intravenous contrast material. IVU or CT examinations may be used for follow-up of those injuries that are managed conservatively. Minor injuries comprise approximately 85% of renal injuries and rarely require surgical intervention. These include renal contusions, small subcapsular or perinephric hematomas, small cortical lacerations, or small infarcts. On CT scans the renal contusion may appear normal or show focal or diffuse renal swelling with decreased enhancement. Small lacerations can appear as a linear or curvilinear nonenhancing area, often with a small associated perinephric or subcapsular hyperdense hematoma. Intermediate injuries represent 10% of renal injuries and occasionally require surgery. These include large lacerations that extend through the capsule to the renal sinus and vascular injuries to segmental renal arteries. Laceration can extend into the collecting system and cause extravasation of contrast material as well as large perinephric hematomas. When the renal fragments are distracted, this is referred to as a *renal fracture*. Severe injuries represent 5% of renal injuries and almost always require surgery. These include vascular pedicle injuries, avulsions of the ureteropelvic junction, and multiple deep lacerations that threaten renal viability or cause persistent bleeding.

Bladder injuries from blunt trauma are best evaluated using cystography, which can detect 85% to 100% of all bladder injuries (18,19). The IVU findings will often be falsely negative. Bladder contusions are the most common bladder injury but appear normal cystographically. Intraperitoneal bladder rupture represents one-third of major bladder injuries and often results from a seat belt or steering wheel injury in a person with a dilated bladder. On cystography, contrast material is extravasated from the dome of the bladder and fills the peritoneal cavity, outlining the abdominal viscera. Extraperitoneal bladder ruptures represent 60% of all major bladder injuries and are much more strongly associated with pelvic fractures. On cystography, contrast material extends into the extraperitoneal spaces and does not outline bowel. Five percent of major bladder injuries will have a combined intraperitoneal and extraperitoneal leak.

Urethral injuries from blunt trauma almost always occur in male patients. Most are posterior urethral injuries, which are often associated with pelvic fractures. The patients typically present with blood in the urethral meatus, an inability to void, and a nonpalpable or "high-riding" prostate. Prior to catheterization, the urethra should be evaluated by RUG, which can be used to classify posterior urethral injuries: type I—involving stretching and narrowing of an intact urethra from a hematoma in the prostatic fossa, which elevates the bladder; type II—with urethral disruption and contrast material extravasation into the true pelvis above the urogenital diaphragm; and type III—with disruption of the membranous (and often bulbous) urethra at the level of the urogenital diaphragm and contrast material extravasation into the pelvis and perineum (20). The injuries are further classified as partial (if contrast material enters the bladder) or complete (if contrast material cannot enter the bladder). Patients with type I injuries may be catheterized, but the bladder in patients with type II or III injuries is drained via a suprapubic catheter and not by a urethral catheter. Type II and III injuries typically require surgery, which is most often performed in a delayed fashion. Preoperative urethrograms usually demonstrate a short (<2 cm) stricture at the site of injury. Prior to delayed urethroplasty the urethra is evaluated with both RUG and VCUG via the suprapubic catheter. Following surgical repair the incidence of stricture formation is still quite high and follow-up RUG is often necessary.

Anterior urethral injuries commonly result from straddle injuries and rarely are associated with pelvic fractures. With minor injuries the hematoma is confined to the shaft of the penis. With more severe injuries the hematoma extends beyond the Buck fascia to involve the perineum, scrotum, and anterior abdominal wall. RUG shows extravasation of contrast material from the bulbous urethra. The injuries may be partial or complete, depending on whether there is filling of the proximal urethra. Urethral catheterization should generally not be performed, and suprapubic urinary diversion is required until the time of urethroplasty. Posttraumatic stricture formation is not uncommon, especially in the setting of complete transections.

Iatrogenic urethral injuries most commonly result from urethral instrumentation, indwelling catheters, or surgical procedures (bladder neck resection, urethral sphincterotomy, prostatectomy, abdominoperineal resection, and circumcision). The anterior urethral injuries are best evaluated with RUG; however, for complete evaluation of the posterior urethra both RUG and VCUG may be required. The vast majority of iatrogenic urethral complications occur in males. The two most frequently injured sites from catheterization or instrumentation include the penoscrotal junction and the membranous urethra. In a study of VCUG performed in 154 male SCI patients, 49 (32%) had urethral abnormalities (21). The most commonly encountered urethral injuries were diverticula, usually at the penoscrotal junction or the membranous urethra and occasionally at the fossa navicularis. In fact, these were pseudodiverticula that resulted from focal overdistention injuries to the urethra, and therefore lacked a true epithelial lining. RUG typically shows a small (≤3 cm) area of concentric dilatation of the urethra. Prior to the development of a diverticulum within the membranous urethra, RUG can demonstrate the "spiral sign," which represents extravasated contrast material within the rings of the external sphincter muscle (Fig. 7-6). A second type of diverticulum, called the *perineal diverticulum*, can develop at the penoscrotal junction in patients who have had bilateral partial or total ischiectomy. The urethra is subjected to chronic weight-bearing pressure because the attachments of the triangular ligament to the inferior pubic rami have been severed.

Other urethral complications that can be seen in the catheterized patient include the ragged urethra, urethral strictures, pressure necrosis, and false passages. RUG shows the ragged urethra as having an irregular mucosal contour that is related to multiple episodes of minor urethral trauma from repeated catheterization. Urethral strictures can result from scarring due to urethral laceration during catheterization or associated urethritis. Urethrography will demonstrate focal, multifocal, or diffuse areas of narrowing that can occur in any urethral segment, but most frequently at the penoscrotal junction and membranous urethra. On VCUG the urethra proximal to the stricture appears dilated and can give rise to pseudodiverticula, fistulas, and filling of an abscess. Pressure necrosis is a mucosal erosion that occurs at the penoscrotal junction of the urethra from an improperly positioned, chronically indwelling Foley catheter. With urethrography a small collection of extraluminal contrast material is seen along the undersurface of the urethra at this site. Pressure necrosis can progress to fistula and scrotal abscess formation. Urethral false passages are usually iatrogenic, created by inad-

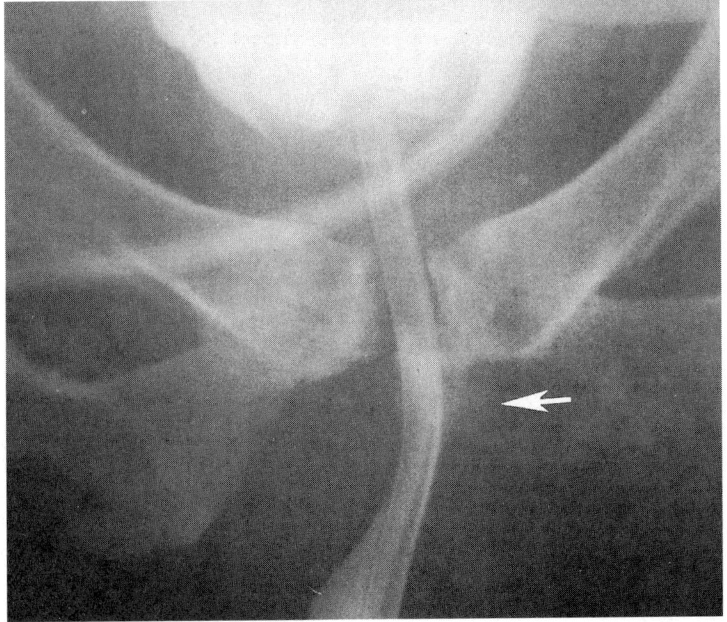

Figure 7-6. A catheter-induced membranous urethral injury producing the spiral sign on a voiding cystourethrogram. The spiral sign is a precursor to an iatrogenic diverticulum. Note the spiral collection of contrast material within the external sphincter (*arrow*).

vertently advancing a catheter or instrument through a small tear in the mucosa. Patients receiving intermittent catheterization and particularly those with strictures or diverticula are prone to false passage formation. The RUG best illustrates the false passage, which often has a ragged contour.

Conclusions

Although neuromuscular disorders do not primarily affect the urinary tract, significant urologic complications can occur in patients with these disorders. Urinary tract infections, stones, obstruction, and VUR are the principal complications of the urinary stasis and high intravesical pressures encountered with the neurogenic bladder. Uroradiologic imaging with IVU, ultrasonography, CT, scintigraphy, and cystourethrography is often necessary to diagnose these conditions and their complications.

THE INTERVENTIONAL RADIOLOGIC MANAGEMENT OF THE REHABILITATION PATIENT

Interventional radiology has made tremendous advances, mostly due to catheter and guide wire technology. Guidance by imaging has improved with state-of-the-art angiographic equipment, digital fluoroscopy, and high-resolution ultrasound equipment. Procedures that are being performed today were virtually unheard of in the past few decades. Almost all community-based hospitals have radiologists with interventional training. Acute care facilities and tertiary referral centers certainly possess the necessary equipment, specialists, and support personnel to assist the physiatrist in the diagnosis, management, and treatment of these specialized patients. Generally, the interventional radiologist can perform the interventional procedures in a timely manner with the least invasive techniques. This portion of the chapter focuses on thromboembolization prophylaxis, nutritional support, urinary tract interventions, and injection procedures for the diagnosis, management, and treatment of the rehabilitation patient.

Venous Thromboembolic Management and Prophylaxis

Venous thromboembolic disease remains a major and common complication in hospitalized and physically impaired patients, especially in the postoperative period. Pulmonary thromboembolism and deep venous thrombosis are responsible for over 1 million hospital admissions in the United States each year (22). In addition, pulmonary embolism occurs in over 600,000 patients every year in the United States and results in a 5% mortality rate in patients undergoing surgery (23). Conventional anticoagulation may fall short as effective therapy for deep venous thrombosis or against pulmonary embolism. Therefore, vena caval interruption offers an effective adjunct in therapy. Currently, a vena caval filter is the preferred mechanical device for caval interruption because of the ease of percutaneous insertion and proven efficacy (24).

Risk factors associated with pulmonary embolism include prolonged immobilization, recent surgery, cerebrovascular accident, recent myocardial infarction, hypercoagulable states, major trauma, and malignancy. Approximately 90% of pulmonary emboli originate from thrombi within the deep venous system of the legs and pelvis (25). Venous thrombosis proximal to the popliteal vein carries as much as a 40% risk of embolization (26). It is estimated that 20% of calf vein thromboses are complicated by proximal propagation (27). High-risk rehabilitation patients include those with traumatic brain injuries or SCIs, those who have had a cerebrovascular accident with paralysis, and patients undergoing neurosurgical procedures. Prophylactic regimens against deep venous thrombosis and pulmonary embolism may fail in up to 10% of these patients (28). Much controversy exists concerning the most appropriate and effective means of prophylaxis for deep vein thrombosis and pulmonary embolism. Accepted prophylactic treatment regimens include low-dose heparin, low-molecular-weight heparin, sequential compression devices, and vena caval filter insertion.

There are several problems associated with pharmacologic and compression device prophylaxis. Up to 14% of high-risk trauma patients cannot be given anticoagulants because of the severity of their injuries (29). Sequential compression devices also may not be practical in severely traumatized patients and cannot be used in patients with extensive coexisting lower-extremity fractures. In addition, these measures may fail to prevent deep venous thrombosis up to 33% of the time (30,31).

Low-molecular-weight heparin may offer an advantage in the thromboprophylaxis of rehabilitation patients. Two studies (32,33) showed a decreased incidence of hemorrhagic complications with low-molecular-weight heparin. A retrospective study of 105 SCI patients (34) found low-molecular-weight heparin to be the safest and most effective agent for prophylaxis, reporting no clinical evidence of pulmonary embolus, and bleeding problems in only 3 patients.

The incidence of pulmonary embolism in SCI patients may be as high as 5% despite thromboprophylaxis (35). Patients with paraplegia or quadriplegia may remain at risk for pulmonary embolism long after the time of the initial injury. In a study of 111 patients with SCI, 83 patients (75%) had pulmonary embolus after discharge from the acute care facility (36). The incidence of pulmonary embolism associated with acute stroke is difficult to determine. The mean time of onset of pulmonary embolism following acute stroke is 20 days, with a range of 3 to 120 days (37). Therefore, pharmacologic thromboembolism prophylaxis may not be practical in protecting against pulmonary embolism in the chronic care of SCI or stroke patients.

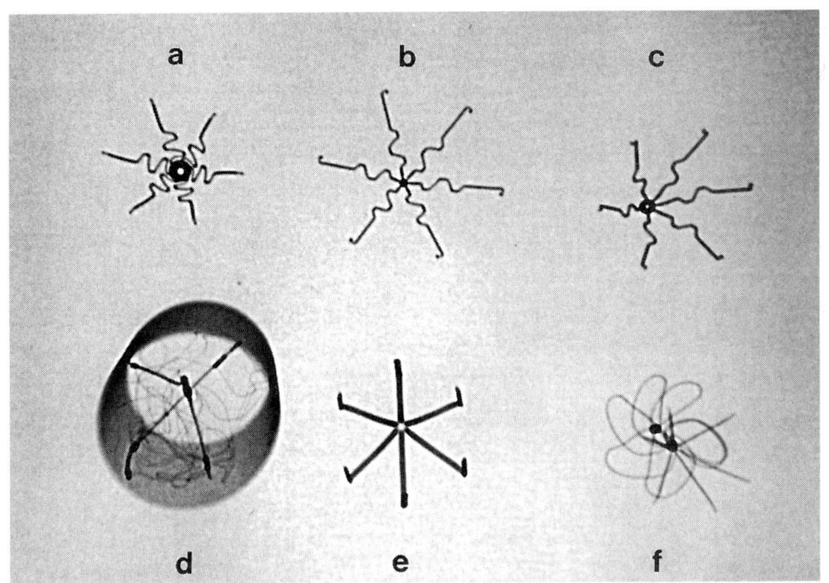

Figure 7-7. "End on" radiographic view of the six different inferior vena caval filters currently approved by the Food and Drug Administration: the stainless-steel 24Fr Greenfield (*a*), the titanium 12Fr Greenfield (*b*), the stainless-steel 12Fr Greenfield (*c*), the Bird's Nest Filter (*d*), the LGM Vena Tech filter (*e*), and the Simon Nitinol filter (*f*).

Inferior vena caval filtration offers an attractive alternative to these other modalities in selected high-risk rehabilitation patients. Currently, six different filters are approved by the Food and Drug Administration (FDA) for use in the United States (Fig. 7-7). The first implantable device was the Mobin-Uddin umbrella introduced in 1967 and modified and placed percutaneously by Rizk and Amplatz in 1973 (38). This was an effective device for protection against pulmonary emboli, but proved to have an unacceptable caval thrombosis rate. In 1973, the Greenfield filter was introduced and initially placed surgically. In 1984, Tadavarthy et al (39) first described percutaneous placement. Apparent shortcomings including a high incidence of insertion-site thrombosis associated with percutaneous insertion of the Greenfield filter led to the development of other filters and delivery systems such as the Bird's Nest Filter, LGM Vena Tech filter, and the titanium Greenfield filter in the 1980s. The Simon Nitinol filter was introduced in 1990 and has the smallest introduction system. The most recent addition in 1995 was the "over the wire" 12Fr stainless-steel Greenfield filter.

The 24Fr stainless-steel Greenfield filter remains the "gold standard" by which all other filters are judged. However, its large introduction sheath size has rendered it mostly obsolete. It is associated with a recurrent pulmonary embolism rate of 4% and a caval thrombosis rate of 4% (40). The 12Fr titanium Greenfield filter with its ease of introduction has replaced the older and larger version. The recurrent pulmonary embolism rate remains low, at 3.7% (41). The caval thrombosis rate is similar to that for the 24Fr stainless-steel Greenfield filter. As mentioned earlier, the newest filter in the Greenfield family is the 12Fr "over the wire" stainless-steel filter. With the advantage of being able to be placed over the wire, the problem of filter tilt should be diminished. A tilted filter may offer less protection against recurrent pulmonary embolus. The LGM Vena Tech filter, a device similar to the Greenfield filter, received FDA clearance for use in the United States without any significant American clinical trials being performed. It is commonly used in Europe and has a reported recurrent pulmonary embolism rate of 2% to 3% (42). However, the caval thrombosis rate ranges from 5% to 22% (42,43). The Vena Tech filter has one of the smaller introduction sheaths, 10Fr. The Simon Nitinol filter is a unique design with a two-tiered filter surface. It is made of a nickel-titanium alloy with a thermal memory. It has the smallest introducer sheath, 7Fr. It may also be placed by an arm approach from the antecubital veins. The recurrent pulmonary embolism rate is 1% to 2% but the caval thrombosis rate may be 7% (44). All of the above filters are recommended for use in inferior vena cavas 28 mm or smaller. The Bird's Nest Filter has a different design and can be placed in a cava as large as 40 mm. It has an advantage of being flexible and can be placed in patients with anatomic variations (Fig. 7-8). The sheath size is 12Fr and the filter can be used to trap partially adherent caval thrombus. The recurrent pulmonary embolism rate is 2.7% (45) but the caval thrombosis rate may be higher, from 2.9% to 14.6% (45,46).

Prophylactic vena caval filter insertion offers an added protection in certain patients at high risk for pulmonary embolism. In several series involving a total of 417 high-risk patients who received a prophylactic vena caval filter, only 3 patients (0.7%) had pulmonary emboli (47). However, the cost of filter placement for prophylaxis may not justify use of this treatment modality. The risks, benefits, and costs must be evaluated in relation to the cost of hospitalization of the high-risk patient who has a fatal or

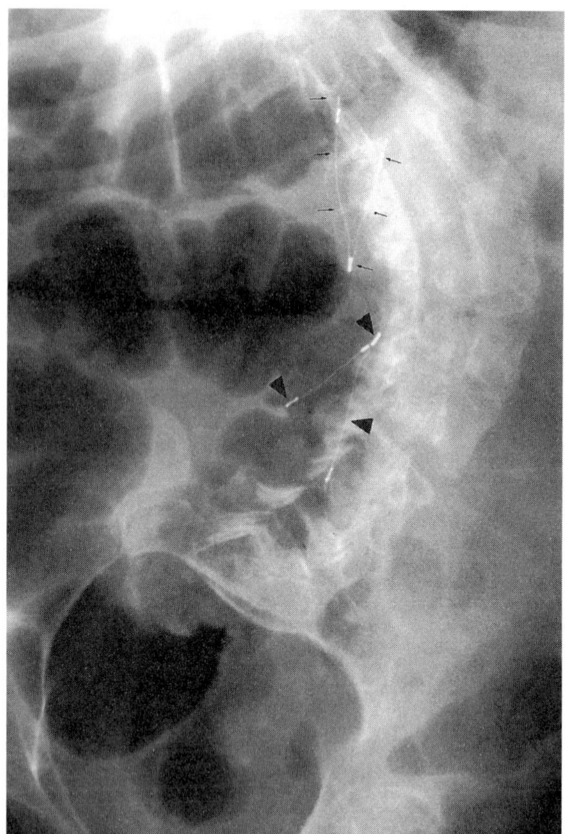

Figure 7-8. Patient with severe spinal deformity secondary to scoliosis. The Bird's Nest Filter was placed due to the flexibility inherent in its design. A more rigid filter, such as one of the other five types, might not conform to the angular deformity of the spine. Note the superior anchoring struts (*small arrows*) and the inferior struts (*arrowhead*). The tiny connecting wires between the two sets of struts forming the nest are barely visible.

nonfatal pulmonary embolism. The physiatrist should evaluate each patient on an individual basis to determine which prophylaxis regimen is best.

Nutritional Support

Nutritional support in the patient undergoing rehabilitation can be divided into those patients requiring total parenteral nutrition (TPN) and those patients with swallowing disorders from strokes or central nervous system disorders who require percutaneous gastrostomy. Each is discussed with regard to the radiologic guidance for placement.

Traditionally, tunneled catheter and implantable subcutaneous ports were placed by surgeons in the operating suite. However, now placement of central venous catheters can be performed safely and expeditiously in the interventional radiology department (48–50). Infection rates, ease of insertion, catheter maintenance surveillance, and complication rates equal those associated with surgical placement. For patients without extremity access, radiologic guidance can aid in placement directly into the inferior vena cava (51) or through the liver into the inferior vena cava (52).

Guidance using either ultrasound or direct fluoroscopic visualization helps to avoid fracturing or misplacement of catheters (53). With such guidance, patients requiring TPN can have a tunneled catheter such as a Hickman or Broviac catheter placed through the subclavian or jugular vein. Implantable subcutaneous ports can be introduced from a chest approach or from an arm approach. The interventional radiologist also can manage these patients, attend to complications, and ultimately remove catheters when they are no longer necessary.

Percutaneous radiologic gastrostomy or gastrojejunostomy as performed by the interventional radiologist under fluoroscopic guidance is usually an easy procedure with a very high technical success rate. The typical patient population includes patients with esophageal obstruction, those with central nervous system disorders such as strokes and head injuries, and persons with neurologic disorders causing aspiration. The radiologic technique was first described in 1983 (54,55).

The radiologic technique for placement of tubes is usually very safe with low complication rates. First, the left lobe of the liver and spleen are mapped out with the use of ultrasonography. The stomach is then inflated with room air via nasogastric tube. Then the anterior wall of the stomach is affixed to the anterior abdominal wall through the use of T-fasteners. This prevents displacement of the stomach much like a gastropexy. The stomach is then punctured equidistant between the greater and lesser curvatures and a 12Fr or 14Fr gastrostomy tube is then placed. The T-fasteners are removed in 1 to 2 weeks, which allows the stomach time to form a fibrous adhesion to the anterior abdominal wall. A simple gastrostomy tube (Fig. 7-9) or a gastrojejunostomy tube can be placed. A gastrojejunostomy tube, however, will require a more expensive diet to be delivered.

Modification of the above procedure can be accomplished with placement of a gastric button through a mature tract at a later date. This device is less conspicuous and has advantages in patients receiving physical therapy.

The success rate in radiologic placement of gastrostomy tubes is very high, 98.0% to 99.4% (55,56). The major and minor complication rates are approximately 5% for each category and in general are as low or lower than the rates associated with surgical or endoscopic techniques (57). Fluoroscopically guided gastrostomy tube placement is also the least invasive of the three techniques and is the most cost-effective, not requiring endoscopy or operating room time.

Urinary Tract Manipulations

Urinary tract diversion and decompression play an important role in the management of the rehabilitation patient.

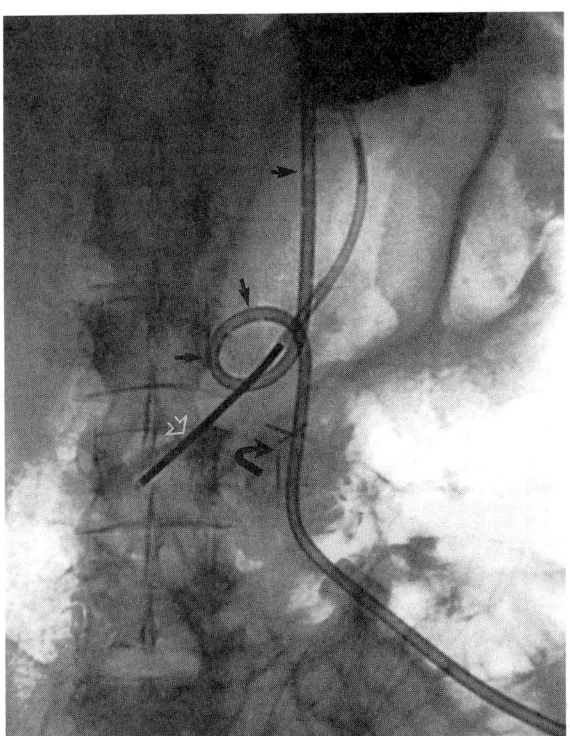

Figure 7-9. Percutaneous gastrostomy tube (*small black arrows*) placed in a patient who had a cerebrovascular accident and swallowing disorder. Note the T-fastener (*curved arrow*) which holds the anterior wall of the stomach to the abdominal wall. The feeding tube (*open white arrow*) enables air insufflation of the stomach prior to T-fastener and tube placement.

From a simple procedure such as suprapubic catheterization to more complex stone debulking procedures, interventional radiologists remain at the forefront of patient management. With the advent of state-of-the-art imaging guidance, and catheter and guide wire technology, the percutaneous nephrostomy procedure, first described in 1955, has become a domain of the interventional radiologist.

Indications for percutaneous nephrostomy in the rehabilitation patient include rapid decompression of the hydronephrotic kidney in the septic patient, stone manipulation and debulking procedures performed in conjunction with the urologist, and functional dynamic studies of the chronically obstructed kidney. A percutaneous nephrostomy is best performed under guidance with ultrasonography or fluoroscopy. An opaque caliceal stone or staghorn stone also can serve as a target for puncture. The actual procedure is usually straightforward. A catheter (usually an 8Fr or 10Fr locking catheter) is placed through a lower-pole or mid-pole calyx. Complex stones may require upper-pole or intercostal approaches. Complication rates of simple nephrostomies are low. The mortality rate is lower than that seen with surgical creation of an opening. The rate of major complications such as hemorrhage requiring transfusion and selective embolization is less than 3% (59).

Percutaneous nephrostomy and extracorporeal shock wave lithotripsy (ESWL) have virtually eliminated the need for open surgical lithotomy in the management of stone disease (60). Stone burden will dictate whether ESWL or percutaneous nephrostolithotomy (PCNL) will be most effective. Stones 2 to 3 cm in size usually require PCNL for removal (61). Planning the tract angle and access approach to stones requires interaction between the interventional radiologist and the urologist (Fig. 7-10). The goal of ESWL or PCNL is to render the patient stone free. At times a combination of ESWL and PCNL is required.

Urinary obstruction and stasis predispose to calculus formation. Patients with stones within a caliceal diverticulum pose a particular challenge to the interventional radiologist. ESWL usually will not work as the outflow path for fragments is usually narrowed. Usually PCNL is required to adequately treat caliceal stones. Outlet obstruction such as seen in patients with a neurogenic bladder, which results in urinary stasis and therefore predisposes to calculi formation, also poses a particular problem. The risk for renal deterioration and renal cause–specific death in patients with a neurogenic bladder and staghorn calculi is 25% higher than the risk in patients with normal voiding mechanisms (62). Therefore, an aggressive approach to render neurogenic bladder patients stone free is suggested.

Injection Techniques

The interventional radiologist can aid in the management of rehabilitation patients with chronic pain through the use of diagnostic and therapeutic injection techniques. These techniques include but are not limited to epidural injection of anesthetics and steroids, injections to perform diskography, and facet injections to help diagnose sources of chronic pain and perform diagnostic arthrography.

Epidural injection of corticosteroids to relieve low-back pain has been used since the early 1950s. Usually inflammation is the main cause of sciatica, one of the most incapacitating and difficult-to-treat benign pains, and related back pain. Much controversy exists concerning the benefit of epidural corticosteroids in patients with chronic low-back pain. There may be a correlation with the duration of symptoms: One study (63) examining 108 patients in whom methylprednisolone was injected in the epidural or intrathecal space showed a 75% response rate in those who had symptoms for less than 4 weeks. However, patients with symptoms for longer than 6 weeks only had a response rate of 43% (63). Another investigation (64) reported a short-term success rate of 87% and relief of pain for up to 6 months in 34% of patients. A randomized British study (65), however, showed that patients who received injections of steroids, saline solution, or local

Figure 7-10. Patient with long-standing urinary infection and staghorn calculus of the left kidney. *A.* Note the laminated appearance (*arrowheads*) of the stone. *B.* A late-excretion-phase excretory urogram shows the central staghorn, which is not obstructing (*arrow*). *C.* An angiographic catheter has been placed through a mid-pole calyx (*white arrowheads*) to provide access in the operating room for tract dilation and percutaneous nephrostolithotomy.

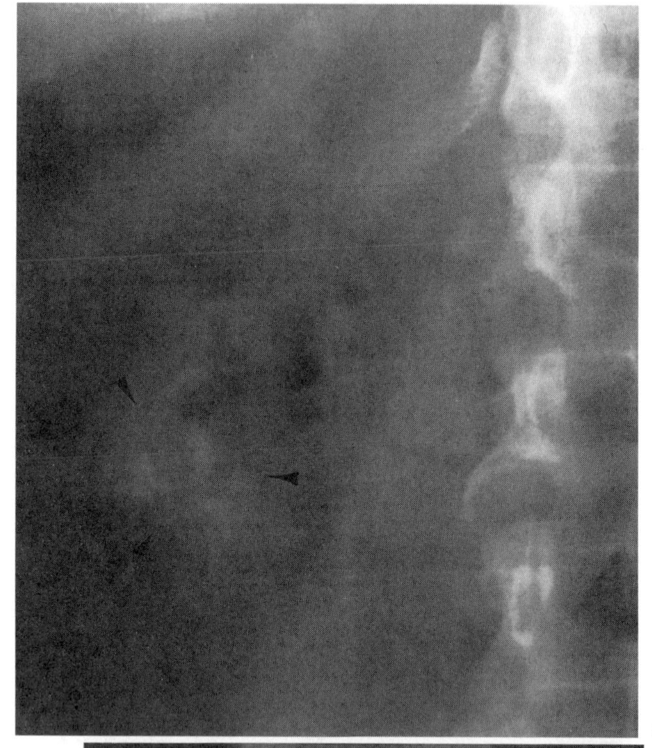

A

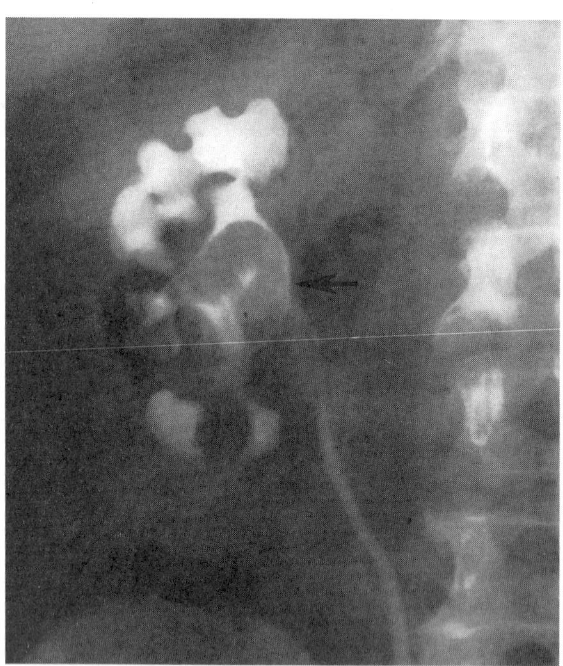

B

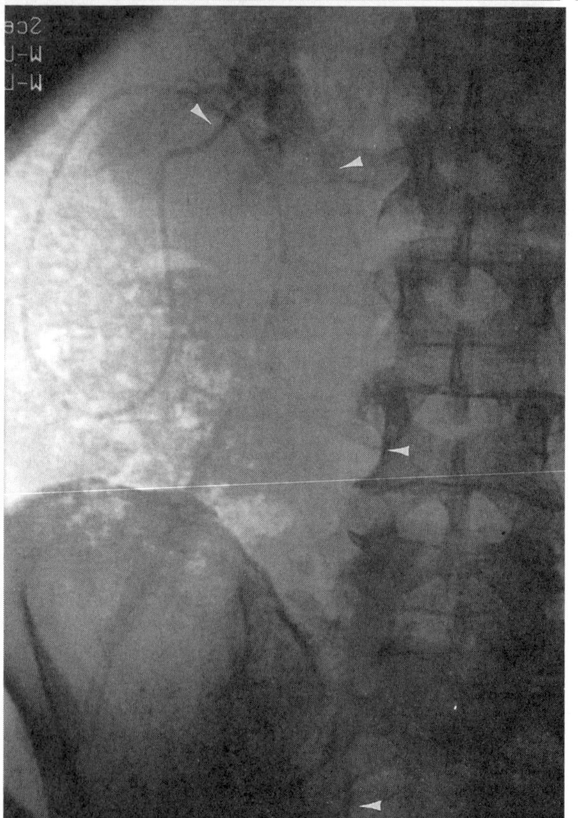

C

anesthetic or no injection at all, just needle placement, improved at about the same rate. The authors concluded that the epidural injections administered achieved effects partially as a placebo and partially by virtue of the natural history of the acute sciatic syndrome.

There has been a revival of diskography in the evaluation of lumbar disk disease. However, with the advent of magnetic resonance imaging (MRI) and its exquisite evaluation of the lumbar region of the spine, diskography still only plays a relatively minor role. Probably its main role is as a clinical test in patients with multilevel disk disease. Injection at different levels will help determine the diseased disk that reproduces the patient's symptoms (66). This will help in operative planning.

Occasionally, the lumbar apophyseal facet joints may be the source of low-back pain and sciatica, instead of the intervertebral disk. Several theories may explain the role of the facet joints in low-back pain. The articular capsule of the facet joint is richly innervated, the medial aspect of the joint is in contact with the intervertebral foramen and the lumbar nerve root, and the posterior ramus of the spinal nerve passes in close proximity to the lateral border of the capsule (67). An easy way to ascertain the role of the facets in lumbar pain is to inject them with a local anesthetic or steroids. Arthrography should also be performed to confirm the intra-articular position of the needle.

Other injection techniques include injection of the sacroiliac joint to relieve pain. The lower portion of the sacroiliac joint is synovial and occasionally injection with anesthetics or steroids provides some pain relief (Fig. 7-11). Arthrography of peripheral joints still has a role in patients with chronic joint pain but has largely been replaced by MRI. Rotator cuff tear of the shoulder can easily be diagnosed by arthrography, but MRI is just as reliable, better visualizes a partial tear, and is able to evaluate "blind areas" to arthrography such as the glenoid labrum. MRI of the knee, ankle, wrist, and elbow has become common and arthrography of these joints is rarely performed now.

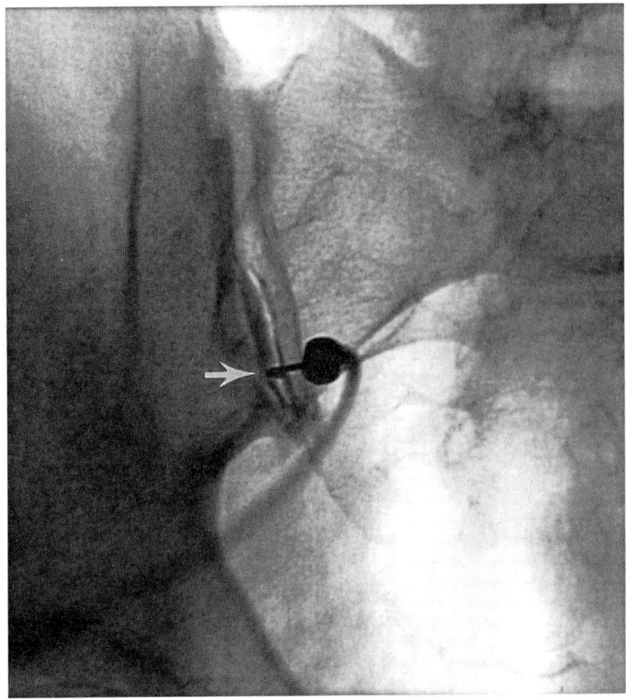

Figure 7-11. Patient with chronic back and sacroiliac (SI) joint pain from a motor vehicle accident. SI joint injection was requested as a trial to see if the SI joint was the source of pain. A needle (*white arrow*) placed in the lower portion of the SI joint reproduced the pain exactly. Following needle placement, a mixture of long-acting steroid and anesthetic was instilled and provided relief of pain for 4 months.

REFERENCES

1. Palmer FJ. The R.A.C.R. survey of intravenous contrast media reactions: final report. *Australas Radiol* 1988;32:426–428.
2. Katayama H, Yamaguchi K, Kosuka T, et al. Adverse reactions to ionic and nonionic contrast: a report from the Japanese Committee on the Safety of Contrast Media. *Radiology* 1990;175:621–628.
3. Cohan RH, Dunnick NR, Bashore TM. Treatment of reactions to radiographic contrast material. *AJR* 1988;151:263–270.
4. Kaplan WE. Management of the urinary tract in myelomeningocele. *Prog Urol* 1988;2:121–124.
5. Dykstra DD, Price MM. Vesicoureteral reflux in patients with spinal cord injury: a long term follow-up. *Arch Phys Med Rehabil* 1988;69:747.
6. Duckett JW, Bellinger MF. A plea for standardized grading of vesicoureteral reflux. *Eur Urol* 1982;8:74–77.
7. Comarr AE. Long-term survey of incidence of renal calculosis in paraplegia. *J Urol* 1955;74:447–452.
8. DeVivo MJ, Fine PR, Cutter GR, et al. Risk of renal calculi in spinal cord injury patients. *J Urol* 1984;131:857–859.
9. Comarr AE, Kawaichi GK, Bors E. Renal calculosis of patients with traumatic cord lesions. *J Urol* 1962;87:647–656.

10. Otnes B. Correlation between causes and composition of urinary stones. *Scand J Urol Nephrol* 1983;17:93–98.

11. Middleton WD, Dodd WJ, Lawson TL, et al. Renal calculi: sensitivity for detection with ultrasound. *Radiology* 1988;167:239–244.

12. Smith RC, Verga M, McCarthy SM, Rosenfield AF. Diagnosis of acute flank pain: value of unenhanced helical CT. *AJR* 1996;166: 97–101.

13. Hackler RH. A 25-year prospective mortality study in the spinal cord injured patient: comparison with the long-term living paraplegic. *J Urol* 1977;117:486–488.

14. Geisler WO, Jousse AT, Wynne-Jones M, Breithaupt D. Survival in traumatic spinal cord injury. *Paraplegia* 1983;21:364–373.

15. DeVivo MJ, Fine PR, Stover SL. Cause of death following spinal cord injury. *Arch Phys Med Rehabil* 1984;65:622.

16. Kuhlemeier KV, Lloyd LK, Stover SL. Clinical significance of minimal changes on intravenous urography after spinal cord injury. *Br J Urol* 1986;58:256–260.

17. Butler ED Jr, Friedland GW, Gowan DE. A radiological study of the effect of elevated intravesical pressures on ureteral calibre and peristalsis in patients with neurogenic bladder dysfunction. *Clin Radiol* 1971;22:198–204.

18. Carroll PR, McAninch JW. Major bladder trauma: the accuracy of cystography. *J Urol* 1983;130: 887–888.

19. Cass AS. Bladder trauma in multiple injured patient. *J Urol* 1976; 115:667–669.

20. Colapinto V, McCallum RW. Injury to the male posterior urethra in fractured pelvis: a new classification. *J Urol* 1977;118:575–580.

21. Calenoff L, Foley MJ, Hendrix RW. Evaluation of the urethra in males with spinal cord injury. *Radiology* 1982;142:71–76.

22. Goldhaber SZ. The guide to cardiology: pulmonary embolism. *CVR&R* 1992;32–41.

23. Sabiston DC Jr. The diagnosis and treatment of pulmonary thromboembolism. In: Najavian JS, Delaney JP, eds. *Advances in vascular surgery.* Chicago: Year Book Medical, 1983:219–230.

24. Becker DM, Philbrick JT, Selby JB. Inferior vena cava filters; indications, safety and effectiveness. *Arch Interv Med* 1992;152: 1985–1994.

25. Risius B, Graor RA. Fibrinolytic therapy in pulmonary thromboembolic disease. *Semin Int Radiol* 1985;2:338–348.

26. Moser KM, LeMoine JR. Is embolic risk conditioned by location of deep venous thrombosis? *Ann Intern Med* 1981;94:439.

27. Kakkar VV, Corrigan TP, Fossard DP, et al. Prevention of fatal postoperative pulmonary embolism by low doses of heparin. *Lancet* 1975;2:45.

28. Dennis JW, Menant SS, Von Thron J, et al. Efficacy of deep venous thrombosis prophylaxis in trauma patients and identification of high-risk groups. *J Trauma* 1993;35: 132–139.

29. Shackford SR, Davis JW, Hollingsworth-Fridlund P, et al. Venous thromboembolism in patients with major trauma. *Am J Surg* 1990;159:365–369.

30. Knudson MM, Collins JA, Goodman SB, et al. Thromboembolism following multiple trauma. *J Trauma* 1992;32:2–11.

31. Green D, Rossi EC, Yao JS, et al. Deep vein thrombosis in spinal cord injury: effect of prophylaxis with calf compression, aspirin, and dipyridamole. *Paraplegia* 1982;20:227–234.

32. Hirsh J, Levine MN. Low molecular weight heparin. *Blood* 1992;79: 1–17.

33. Green D, Lee MY, Lim AC, et al. Prevention of thromboembolism after spinal cord injury using low-molecular weight heparin. *Ann Intern Med* 1990;113: 571–574.

34. Harris S, Chen D, Green D. Enoxaparin for thromboembolism prophylaxis in spinal injury. *Am J Phys Med Rehabil* 1996;75:326–327.

35. Green D, Chen D, Chmiel JS, et al. Prevention of thromboembolism in spinal cord injury: role of low molecular weight heparin. *Arch Phys Med Rehabil* 1994;75:290–292.

36. Wilson JT, Rogers FB, Wald SL, et al. Prophylactic vena cava filter insertion in patients with traumatic spinal cord injury: preliminary results. *Neurosurgery* 1994;35: 234–239.

37. Wiljdicks EFM, Scott JP. Pulmonary embolism associated with acute stroke. *Mayo Clin Proc* 1997;72:297–300.

38. Rizk GK, Amplatz K. A percutaneous method of introducing the caval umbrella. *AJR* 1973;117: 903–909.

39. Tadavarthy SM, Castaneda-Zuniga WR, Salomonowitz E, et al. Kimray-Greenfield vena cava filter: percutaneous introduction. *Radiology* 1984;151:525–526.

40. Greenfield LJ, Michna BA. Twelve-year clinical experience with the Greenfield vena caval filter. *Surgery* 1988;104:706–712.

41. Greenfield LJ, Cho KJ, Proctor B, et al. Results of a multicenter study of the modified hook-titanium Greenfield filter. *J Vasc Surg* 1991;14:253–257.

42. Ricco JB, Crochet D, Sebilotte P, et al. Percutaneous transvenous caval interruption with the "LGM" filter: early results of a multicenter trial. *Ann Vasc Surg* 3:242–247.

43. Millward SF, Marsh JI, Peterson RA, et al. LGM (Vena Tech) vena cava filter: clinical experience in 64 patients. *J Vasc Intern Radiol* 1991;2:429–433.

44. Simon M, Athanasoulis CA, Kim D, et al. Simon Nitinol inferior vena caval filter: initial clinical experience. *Radiology* 1989;172:99–103.

45. Roehm JOF, Johnsrude IS, Barth MH, et al. The Bird's Nest inferior vena cava filter: progress report. *Radiology* 1988;168:745–749.

46. Mohan CR, Holballah JJ, Sharp WJ, et al. Comparative efficacy and complications of vena caval filters.

J Vasc Surg 1995;21:235–246.

47. Rogers FB, Shackford SR, Ricci MA, et al. Routine prophylactic vena cava filter insertion in severely injured trauma patients decreases the incidence of pulmonary embolism. *J Am Coll Surg* 1995;180:641–647.

48. Lameris JS, Post PJM, Zonderland HM, et al. Percutaneous placement of Hickman catheter: comparison of sonographically guided and blind techniques. *AJR* 1990;155:1097–1099.

49. Kahn ML, Barboza RB, Kling GA, et al. Initial experience with percutaneous placement of the PAS port implantable venous access device. *J Vasc Interv Radiol* 1992;3:459–461.

50. Mauro MA, Jaques RF. Radiologic placement of long-term central venous catheter: a review. *J Vasc Interv Radiol* 1993;4:127–137.

51. Denny DF, Greenwood LH, Morse SS, et al. Inferior vena cava: translumbar catheterization for central venous access. *Radiology* 1989;170:1013–1014.

52. Kaufman JA, Greenfield AJ, Fitzpatrick GF. Transhepatic cannulation of the inferior vena cava. *J Vasc Interv Radiol* 1991;2:331–334.

53. Hinke DH, Zandt-Stastney DA, Goodman LR, et al. Pinch-off syndrome: a complication of implantable subclavian venous access devices. *Radiology* 1990;177:353–356.

54. Wills JS, Oglesby JT. Percutaneous gastrostomy. *Radiology* 1983;149:449–453.

55. Ho CS. Percutaneous gastrostomy for jejunal feeding. *Radiology* 1983;149:595–596.

56. Ryan JM, Hahn PF, Boland GW, et al. Percutaneous gastrostomy with T-fastener gastropexy: results of 316 consecutive procedures. *Radiology* 1997;203:496–500.

57. Ho SC, Yeung EY. Percutaneous gastrostomy and transgastric jejunostromy. *AJR* 1992;158:251–257.

58. Goodwin WE, Casey WC, Woolf W. Percutaneous trocar nephrostomy in hydronephrosis. *JAMA* 1955;157:891–894.

59. Lee WJ, Patel U, Patel S, et al. Emergency percutaneous nephrostomy: results and complication. *J Vasc Interv Radiol* 1994;5:135–139.

60. Segura JW. Surgical management of urinary calculi. *Semin Nephrol* 1990;10:53–63.

61. Segura JW. Percutaneous nephrolithotomy: technique, indications and complications. *AUA Update Series* 1993;12:154–159.

62. Teichman JMH, Long RD, Hulbert JC. Long term renal fate and prognosis after staghorn calculus management. *J Urol* 1995;153:1403–1407.

63. Ryan MD, Taylor TK. Management of lumbar nerve-root pain by intrathecal and epidural injections of depot methylprednisolone acetate. *Med J Aust* 1981;2:532–534.

64. White AH, Derby R, Wynne G. Epidural injections for the diagnosis and treatment of low back pain. *Spine* 1980;5:78–86.

65. Klenerman L, Greenwood R, Davenport HT, et al. Lumbar epidural injections in the treatment of sciatica. *Br J Rheumatol* 1984;23:35–38.

66. Milette PC, Melanson D. A reappraisal of lumbar discography. *J Can Assoc Radiol* 1982;33:176–182.

67. Dory MA. Arthrography of the lumbar facet joints. *Radiology* 1981;140:23–27.

Chapter 8

Neuroradiology

Susan W. Weathers
Pedro J. Diaz-Marchan

DIAGNOSTIC AND THERAPEUTIC RADIOLOGY: TECHNIQUES AND THEIR LIMITATIONS

Nearly everything in the varied armamentarium of the modern radiologist has a role in the evaluation and treatment of diseases of the spine and central nervous system. Familiarity with the capabilities and limitations of current imaging techniques helps the physiatrist select the examination that is most appropriate for the clinical problem and anticipate logistical difficulties unique to physical medicine patients. It also contributes to an understanding of the degree of certainty of the information provided, the expected benefits of a therapeutic radiologic procedure, and the risks involved.

Diagnostic Techniques

Plain Film and Tomography

Although seldom used for the brain, plain film remains a useful starting point for the spine. Its low cost and convenience, the variety of projections obtainable, and the ease of examining large portions of the spine make it an excellent screening tool. It also provides information about previous surgical intervention that may be important in deciding which modality should be used for further evaluation and in interpreting subsequent studies. Polytomography is a plain film technique that is available in most facilities and is useful for examining areas that are obscured by overlying structures. However, it is time-consuming and requires prolonged patient cooperation. The patient must be placed and held in the positions required for each projection. Flexion-extension plain films or fluoroscopy (to which video-recording devices may be connected) are valuable in the assessment of spinal motion and stability. For the brain, however, computed tomography (CT) and magnetic resonance imaging (MRI) have replaced plain films except for a few specific indications, such as screening for suspected metallic foreign bodies prior to MRI (1,2).

Computed Tomography

CT is often a very useful initial procedure in the diagnosis of brain disorders. It is now widely available not only on a routine basis but also for emergencies and can provide critical information relatively quickly. A routine slice takes about 2 seconds or less to acquire, making it possible to obtain diagnostic information on patients who cannot remain still throughout the entire duration of the examination. Monitoring equipment and ventilators usually can be easily accommodated in the CT suite. Some institutions have the added capability of xenon CT, which is used to quantitate cerebral blood flow. After a baseline CT scan is obtained, the patient inhales stable xenon gas while another set of images is acquired. The difference in densities between the two sets of images is used to calculate regional blood flow. The technique may be useful in patients with acute head trauma to predict areas of the brain that are not viable and can be resected, and in stroke patients to select those who are most likely to benefit from thrombolytic therapy.

For spine imaging the spiral capability of many modern CT scanners makes it practical to obtain 1-mm-thick axial images that provide excellent bone detail and can be reformatted in coronal and sagittal projections. With the spiral technique, the scanner, instead of producing one slice at a time, rotates the x-ray tube continually as the patient couch moves, generating a helical set of data for short segments of the spine. These data are then used to make typical axial "slices." Patients must be able to cooperate by remaining still for periods of 30 seconds or longer. Reformatting the images in sagittal or coronal planes is performed after the patient leaves, and requires additional computer and technologist time, adding expense to a moderately costly examination. However, because of the superiority of the images and the ease of acquiring them, CT has largely replaced conventional tomography of the spine.

CT has certain limitations in addition to the relative problem of patient motion. Beam-hardening artifacts occur when very radiopaque objects are imaged, producing the familiar star pattern seen around metal objects, such as bullet fragments, aneurysm clips, and spinal rods. The same problem occurs at bone interfaces with soft tissues, creating the streak artifacts that limit the diagnostic usefulness of CT for temporal lobe and brain stem disease, although recent technologic advances have reduced this problem somewhat. Similarly, soft tissues within the spinal canal, including the spinal cord, hematomas, tumors, and abscesses, are not well seen with CT because of the dense surrounding bone.

Intravenous iodinated contrast material may be required in some CT examinations to demonstrate pathology such as tumors and abscesses. Relative contraindications to the use of such contrast media include a history of an allergic reaction to the agent, renal insufficiency, current use of the antihyperglycemic medication metformin hydrochloride (Glucophage), pregnancy, multiple myeloma, and congestive heart failure. The newer, nonionic contrast agents, which are safer and better tolerated than their predecessors, are expensive and for this reason have not universally replaced older agents.

Magnetic Resonance Imaging

MRI is generally the most expensive noninterventional radiological examination, but nevertheless is often the preferred modality for evaluation of the brain, spine, and spinal canal. Compared to CT, MRI provides superior soft-tissue contrast and lacks the beam-hardening limitation of CT. With the advent of MRI, it is now possible to visualize well the soft tissues in the spinal canal. Like CT, MRI provides direct visualization of the intervertebral disks, but MRI is also capable of demonstrating the disk morphology and its hydration, which can be important in spondylosis and infection (3). MRI can also be useful in evaluating the spine itself because of its sensitivity to changes in the marrow. Although it cannot demonstrate disruptions in the trabeculae and cortices with the clarity of CT, its sensitivity to edema and fat content in the marrow may help in the detection of occult fractures (4), infection, and benign or malignant marrow-replacing diseases. More recently, MRI has been used to look for evidence of ligament injury in acute spine trauma (4).

Nevertheless, MRI has some significant limitations. Safety in the magnet environment is an important concern. Considerations center around possible malfunction of an implanted device, movement of a foreign body causing damage to a vital structure, and possible thermal injury to the patient (5). Currently it is contraindicated to examine patients with functional electronic devices such as pacemakers, implanted defibrillators, cochlear implants, bone growth stimulators, implanted drug infusion pumps, and neurostimulators. Rapidly changing magnetic gradients in the scanner induce electric currents in the wires of the devices, interfering with their function (6,7). Cerebral aneurysm clips and ferromagnetic foreign bodies in or near the brain, spinal cord, or orbit can be moved by the magnetic field, with disastrous consequences (1,8,9). Some stapes prostheses move under experimental conditions and theoretically could be dislodged by the magnetic field. Some halo vests have been designated as MRI compatible and can be accommodated in the magnet, but electric arcing has been observed in a noncompatible halo vest. External fixators used for extremity fractures may be strongly attracted by the magnetic field.

The presence of metallic foreign bodies is not necessarily a contraindication to MRI, however. Silver surgical clips, for example, are not ferromagnetic and do not move or cause artifacts during scanning. Some devices, such as certain vena caval filters and heart valves, are deflected by a magnetic field under experimental conditions but are either well embedded or are expected to move under physiologic conditions. Heating of metallic implants is a potential problem but has seldom necessitated termination of an examination. Implants often cause local artifacts in the images, but frequently the images still provide useful information in the area of interest (Fig. 8-1). However, it is important that the radiologist be aware of the hardware so that pulse sequences that magnify the artifact problem can be avoided (Fig. 8-2).

Other limitations of MRI are related to the patient's condition. Each set of MRIs typically takes several minutes to acquire, sometimes as long as 15 minutes or more, during which time the patient must remain motionless. A single examination typically takes longer than 30 minutes; if more than one area is requested, the study may last well over 1 hour. The length of time spent supine on a stretcher in a waiting room and then on a minimally padded examination table may be a concern for patients who are at risk for developing decubitus ulcers. Also, most patients, even those with normal mental status and atten-

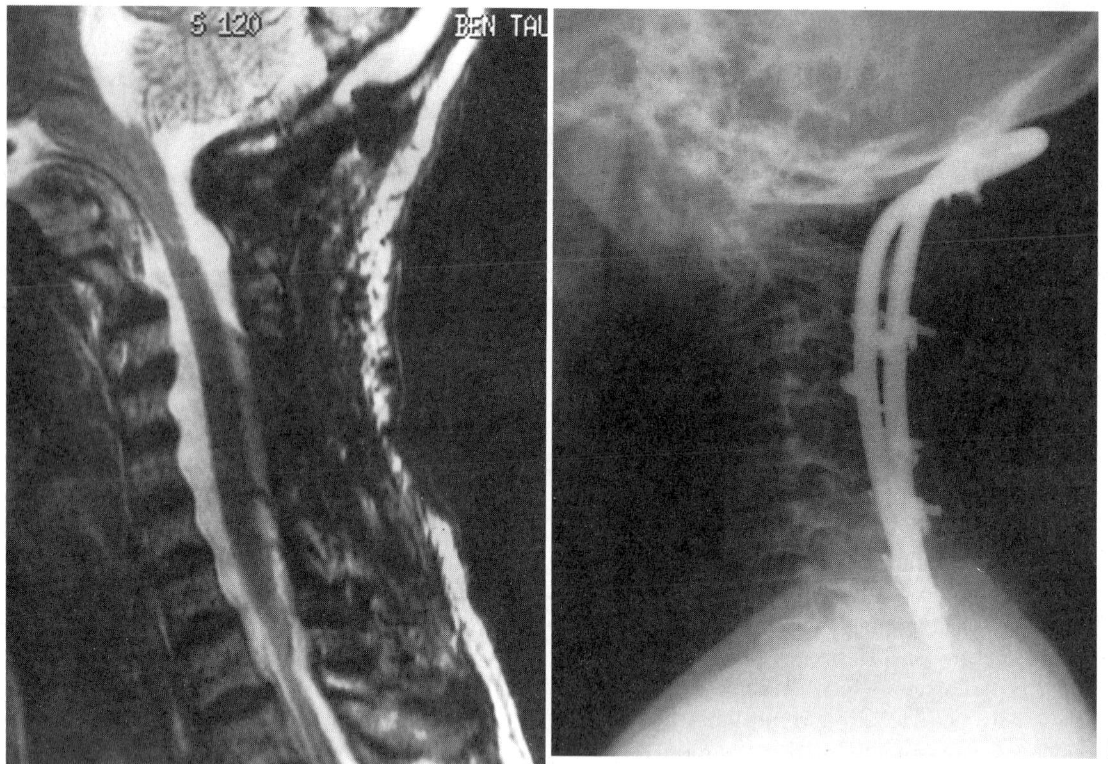

Figure 8-1. MRI and hardware compatibility. Diagnostic information can often be obtained with MRI (*A*) despite the presence of surgical hardware (*B*). This patient is also in a halo vest. See also Figure 8-6A.

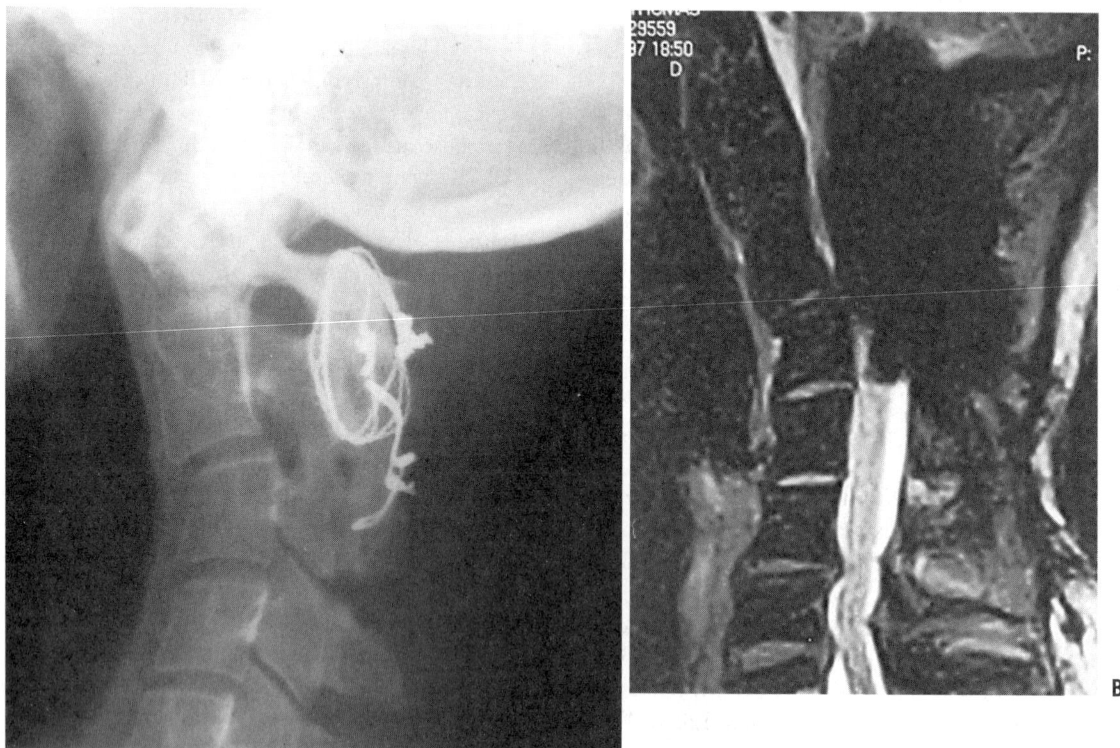

Figure 8-2. Hardware artifacts on MRI. Unaware of the presence of surgical wires (*A*), the radiologist instructed the technologist to use the department's usual cervical spinal protocol. This included pulse sequences that exacerbate the problem of artifacts from ferromagnetic metal (*B*), obscuring the region of interest. See also Figure 8-5.

tion span, have difficulty lying still this long. Involuntary spasms frequently degrade images, even when the part of the body being examined is remote from the moving limb. Sedation can be helpful but carries some risk because of the difficulty of observing patients closely inside the bore of the magnet. Special MRI-compatible monitoring equipment is required. Similarly, to examine ventilator-dependent patients, the imaging facility must have MRI-compatible ventilators. The close confines of the bore of most scanners places limits on patient size and is intolerable to claustrophobic patients. While the latter can usually be examined with sedation, so-called "open" magnets may be the best alternative for both of these groups. Intravenous contrast material for magnetic resonance (MR) scanning is not chemically related to that used for CT and is generally associated with fewer instances of allergic reaction. It is not toxic to the kidneys but should be used cautiously for patients with renal insufficiency, liver failure, or sickle cell disease.

MR angiography, which uses special pulse sequences to take advantage of the sensitivity of MR to motion, provides images that resemble angiograms but do not involve injections of contrast material and do not expose patients to the risks of conventional angiography. With computer postprocessing, vessels of interest can be isolated from overlapping vessels and rotated 180 degrees for viewing in multiple projections. The technique is useful as a screening examination in the evaluation of extracranial carotid artery stenosis but has a tendency to overestimate the degree of stenosis present and cannot clearly demonstrate ulcerations. Intracranially it is most useful for the larger arteries: the distal internal carotid, proximal cerebral, vertebral, basilar, and posterior and anterior communicating arteries. Smaller branches are not well seen, so the technique's usefulness for detecting small arteriovenous malformations (AVMs) and vasculitis is quite limited. It can be helpful in screening for asymptomatic berry aneurysms; sensitivities of 85% or higher have been reported for detecting 5-mm aneurysms (10). MR venography has contributed greatly to the evaluation of dural sinus thrombosis. Because the scanning technique is slightly different from that used for MR arteriography, it is necessary to communicate in advance to the radiologist whether arteries or veins are the vessels of interest.

Doppler Ultrasonography

Duplex scanning, which combines ultrasound imaging and Doppler spectrum analysis, is a useful screening examination in the evaluation of atherosclerotic disease of the common carotid artery bifurcation (11). While still a subject of controversy, current practice involves screening patients with ultrasound and referring those with moderate or severe stenosis for evaluation by angiography. This is based on the finding that symptomatic patients with 70% stenosis or greater and asymptomatic patients with at least 60% stenosis are likely to benefit from carotid endarterectomy (12,13). In this regard, Doppler is useful in identifying patients who may benefit from surgery and should be evaluated by angiography, or equally important, identifying those who should be spared the risks and expense of the more invasive procedure (14). With conventional arteriography as the gold standard, accuracy rates mostly of 90% or better have been reported (15) for duplex scanning. However, in a multicenter validation study, Howard et al (16) found sensitivity rates ranging from 18% to 90% among their centers and noted that duplex scanning is dependent on the equipment, sonographer, and interpreter. They questioned whether "publication bias" selected good results to appear in the previous literature, and cautioned against generalizing results among laboratories. Srinivasan et al (15) also emphasized caution in the use of ultrasound as the basis of clinical decisions for patients with carotid atherosclerosis.

Angiography

Conventional angiography remains the definitive examination for vascular diseases such as atherosclerotic cerebrovascular disease, traumatic arterial injury, berry aneurysms, vasculitis, cerebral and spinal AVMs, and vascular tumors. However, because of the significant risk of stroke, reported as 0.3% to 4.0% in recent series (14,17,18), the procedure should be undertaken only when the information provided will determine the choice of therapy and the patient is not opposed to the proposed therapy. Other risks include sensitivity to contrast material or local anesthetic, hemorrhage, vascular injury, and deterioration of renal function (usually only if baseline function is compromised or the patient is diabetic or dehydrated). In most institutions, routine arteriography can be performed on a "day-surgery" basis. Laboratory tests of renal function and clotting parameters are performed in advance, and medication for contrast sensitivity, if necessary, is begun the day prior to the examination. The patient arrives fasting, remains in observation for several hours after the procedure, and must be driven home by someone else.

Myelography

Myelography, frequently followed immediately by CT, is now usually a second choice or supplementary examination in the evaluation of diseases of the spine or canal contents. It is an alternative for patients for whom MRI is contraindicated or whose MRI is suboptimal or inconclusive. In the case of spinal AVMs, for which the definitive test is arteriography, myelography is a very useful intermediate step when AVM is suspected on MRI. Because spinal angiography carries a moderate risk and is both expensive and tedious, myelographic confirmation of the presence of dilated vessels is desirable before undertaking angiography to localize the specific feeding arteries and draining veins. However, this role of myelography may soon be replaced by MR angiography. To investigate suspected nerve root

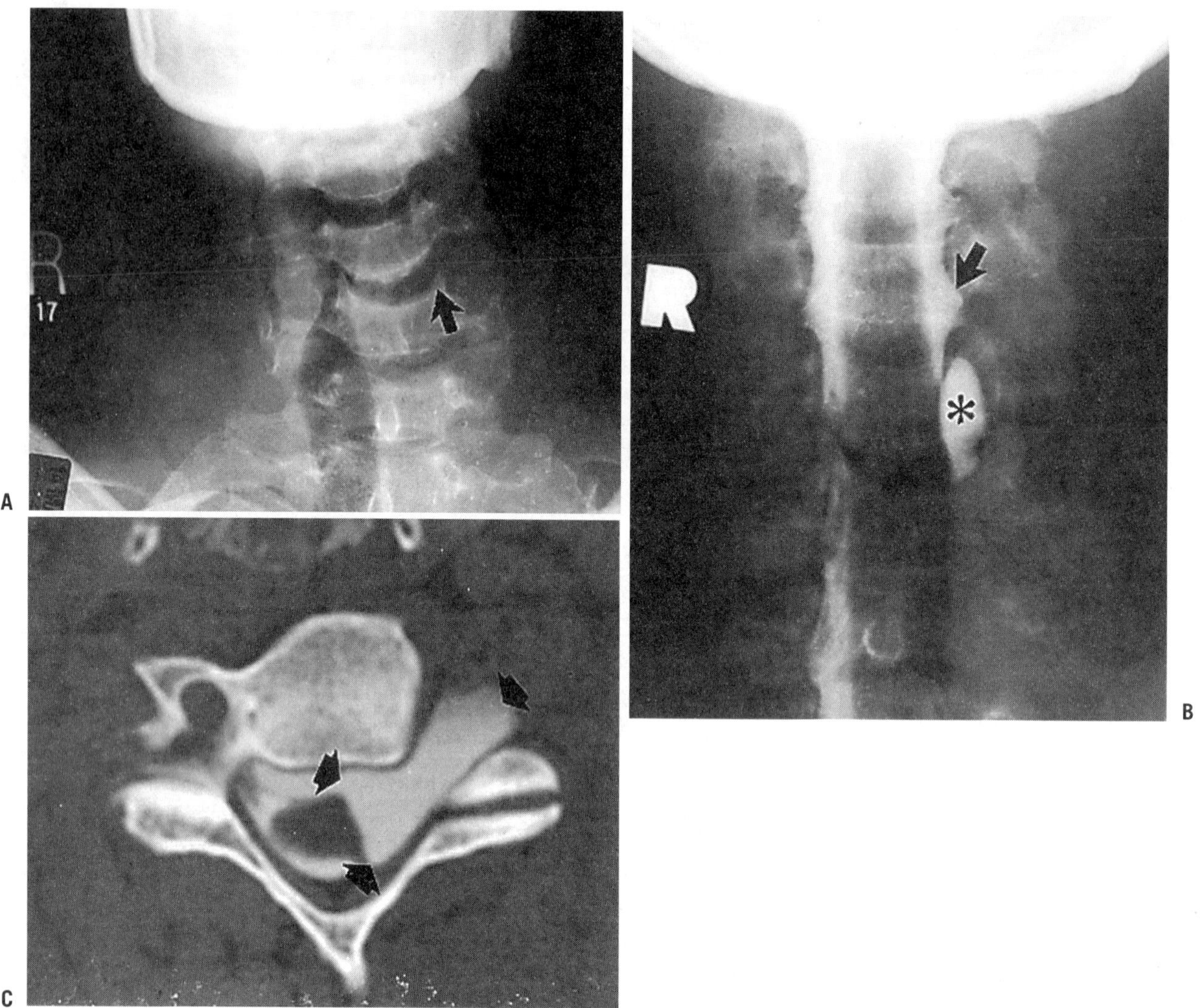

Figure 8-3. Nerve root avulsion. *A.* Lateral flexion injury of the cervical region of the spine with widening of the C5–C6 disk space (*arrow*) and distraction of the facet joint, indicating disruption of the annulus and joint capsule. *B.* Anteroposterior cervical myelogram showing incomplete opacification of a pseudomeningocele (*asterisk*) and absence of the C6 nerve root. Compare with a normal C5 root (*arrow*). *C.* Pseudomeningocele (*arrowheads*) and absence of nerve root on a postmyelographic CT scan.

avulsion, myelography has traditionally provided the optimal demonstration (Fig. 8-3); however, MR "myelography," which uses coronal images and techniques to make cerebrospinal fluid (CSF) appear very white, may also supplant conventional myelography as the software required for this technique becomes more widely available. Myelography is probably also the most reliable examination for evaluating arachnoiditis, but therapy should dictate whether an invasive procedure is justified for this diagnosis. In the evaluation of spondylosis, the combination of myelography and CT is sometimes preferred over MRI in preoperative planning because of superior bone depiction and fewer artifacts.

Myelography has certain risks as well as technical limitations. Although rare, there is the risk of infection, specifically meningitis or epidural abscess, and bleeding. Significant hemorrhage can occur, usually in the setting of clotting disorders, and can cause cauda equina compression. Seizures and focal neurologic deficits due to the presence of water-soluble contrast material in the CSF have been reported, although the incidence with newer contrast agents is extremely low. The prone position required for the examination may be impossible for patients who have contractures or require mechanical ventilation. Lack of a lordotic curve in the cervical portion of the spine makes it very difficult to concentrate the contrast material in that region. For these patients, examination may have to be limited to intrathecal injection of contrast material followed by CT. Extensive fusion, ankylosing spondylitis, and severe arachnoiditis create technical difficulties related to the injection of contrast material into the subarachnoid space. The contrast material used for myelography is like that given intravenously for CT and has the same contraindications. Myelography is generally available on a day-surgery basis requiring the same planning as described for angiography. In addition, medications that can potentiate seizures, most notably phenothiazines and other neuroleptics, should be withheld for 48 hours prior to and after the procedure.

Other Diagnostic Techniques

A few other diagnostic modalities deserve mention. Although ultrasonography (other than Doppler imaging) has very limited application in neuroradiology because of the bony barriers, neurosurgeons use this tool intraoperatively to examine the spinal cord for the extent of tumor or syrinx (19–22). Some radiologists found it useful to look for a syrinx in spinal cord injury patients who have a laminectomy window (23).

Percutaneous fine-needle aspiration of a vertebral body or disk is a procedure that can be performed under fluoroscopic or CT guidance for the purpose of diagnosing spinal infection or neoplasm. There is usually very little morbidity associated with this procedure, although at the thoracic level it is possible to cause a pneumothorax. The introduction of infection into the spine is a potential complication, particularly when the procedure is undertaken to differentiate the radiographically similar Charcot spine and chronic diskitis.

Diskography, which involves fluoroscopically guided injection of a small amount of contrast material into the nucleus pulposus, remains a controversial procedure (24). In a normal disk the contrast material remains in the center of the disk, but in a degenerated disk it tracks outward along fissures in the annulus. Diskography is no longer needed to demonstrate herniations, which can be seen by CT and MRI, or simply to show disk degeneration, which can be appreciated on MRI. Now, however, advocates of the procedure consider its value to be in confirming the diskogenic origin of a patient's pain and in localizing the offending disk or disks (24–26). An invasive procedure with the risk of diskitis and osteomyelitis, it is only justifiable for patients in whom conservative management has failed and who are potential candidates for spinal fusion. The most important part of the examination is not the images themselves but the response of the patient to questions about pain during the procedure. When the injection of contrast material reproduces the patient's symptoms, spinal fusion at the symptomatic level is proposed. The question that is still debated is whether diskography improves the outcome of treatment for spinal pain (24).

Therapeutic Techniques

Intravascular

Therapeutic intervention by neuroradiologists is a burgeoning field (27). In the brain and spinal cord, embolization techniques are becoming more refined and safer. Preoperative embolization of AVMs and vascular tumors is believed to minimize surgical blood loss. Temporary occlusion of the internal carotid artery gives information about the patient's ability to tolerate ligation of the artery if necessary, for example, in en bloc resection of a large skull-base mass. Arteriovenous fistulas, AVMs, and berry aneurysms in some patients can now be treated definitively by the interventional neuroradiologist. Angioplasty, which has been performed on peripheral arteries for many years, is currently an experimental procedure for proximal internal carotid stenosis. Studies are under way to determine whether it can match the safety and effectiveness of carotid endarterectomy. The technique is also being applied to intracranial and vertebral artery stenosis, for which there has been no widely accepted alternative to medical therapy, and to vasospasm after subarachnoid hemorrhage. In patients with acute stroke or dural sinus thrombosis, investigators have successfully recanalized thrombosed vessels by means of infusion of thrombolytic substances directly into the clot. Currently trials are under way to improve the selection of patients who are most likely to benefit from this procedure. Xenon CT and diffusion-perfusion MRI, which are not widely available, may be useful for estimating the extent of ischemic but salvageable brain. The risks and preparations associated with these vascular procedures are similar to those described for diagnostic angiography, but often general anesthesia and postprocedure observation in an intensive care unit are also required.

Spinal

In the spine therapeutic intervention by radiologists includes injections of corticosteroids and local anesthetics into facet joints (28,29), around exiting nerve roots, and in the epidural space at the lumbar level. These may simultaneously confirm the source of a patient's pain and provide temporary relief, but frequently the symptoms return after several weeks or months. Patients undergoing epidural injection must be monitored after the procedure for urinary retention, lower-extremity weakness, and ascending paralysis including respiratory arrest.

SPINE

Trauma

Acute

In acute spinal trauma with neurologic deficit, the role of imaging is threefold: to investigate the cause of spinal cord or root injury, to evaluate the stability of the spine, and to help predict recovery. Ideally, the initial examination consists of a series of plain film radiographs of the area of interest: anteroposterior (AP) and lateral views for all levels and an odontoid view for cervical spinal trauma. These are scrutinized for fractures, subluxation, and indirect signs of injury such as soft-tissue swelling, angulation, and inconsistent alignment of all of the parts of the vertebrae. Plain films remain the best screening examination, but the clinician must keep in mind that a significant proportion of injuries may be missed initially (30,31) and that it is worthwhile to obtain follow-up films, including oblique and flexion-extension views, for patients who remain symptomatic. If it is not possible to obtain an adequate spinal series, which must include visualization of C7–T1 levels on the lateral view and an AP view of the odontoid, or if injury is detected, CT is typically the next step as it provides more accurate and complete characterization of the fracture. CT can clearly demonstrate bone fragments in the spinal canal or neural foramina that may need to be removed. The demonstration of facet dislocation or fracture of the transverse processes should alert the clinician to the possibility of vertebral artery injury (32). Injuries that are difficult to see on plain films but relatively easy to see on CT scans include those at the craniocervical junction, such as fractures of the occipital condyles, rotary atlantoaxial dislocation, and Jefferson (C1 burst) fractures (32). On the other hand, Pech et al (33) demonstrated that even with high-resolution imaging techniques and reformatted images, CT may not be reliable for visualizing pedicle and lateral mass fractures. MRI can contribute information about the cause of neurologic injury when plain films and CT show no fracture or dislocation. It can easily demonstrate cord or cauda equina compression due to acute disk herniation and epidural hematoma (either of which can occur even without significant antecedent trauma) (32). Similarly it can reveal underlying cervical spinal stenosis that can result in cord injury without fracture or ligament disruption. In the case of nerve root deficits, MRI can show acute disk herniation or a pseudomeningocele associated with nerve root avulsion.

An unstable spinal injury is one that can cause progressive spinal deformity or increasing cord damage. In evaluating spinal stability after trauma, Denis (34) proposed a three-column concept of the spine consisting of the anterior longitudinal ligament and anterior two-thirds of the disk, the posterior third of the disk and posterior longitudinal ligament, and the posterior elements with their capsules and ligaments. When two adjacent columns have been disrupted, the spine is unstable and surgical intervention is usually recommended. Plain film indicators of instability include the following: vertebral body displacement of more than 2 mm, widening of the distance between spinous processes, widening of the facet joints, increased interpedicular distance on the AP view, and disruption of the posterior vertebral body cortex (35). As the middle column is the key to stability and disruptions of the posterior vertebral body cortex may be difficult to see on plain films alone, CT is very helpful. On the other hand, ligament disruption in the absence of fracture may not be readily apparent on CT scans. Plain film flexion-extension views are inexpensive and provide a functional demonstration of stability. However, muscle spasm at the time of injury may give a false impression of stability; re-evaluation after several weeks may be required. MRI has been used to detect edema in acutely injured patients around structures that are important for stability, in particular, the supraspinous, interspinous, capsular, and longitudinal ligaments. This information is indirect evidence of ligamentous injury. Discontinuity of the anterior and posterior longitudinal ligaments, the interspinous ligaments, the ligamenta flava, and the intervertebral disks can also be directly visualized on MRI (Fig. 8-4) (4,32,36). Occasionally the presence of occult fractures is suggested by changes in marrow signal intensity (4). MRI equipment that is not widely available provides dynamic motion

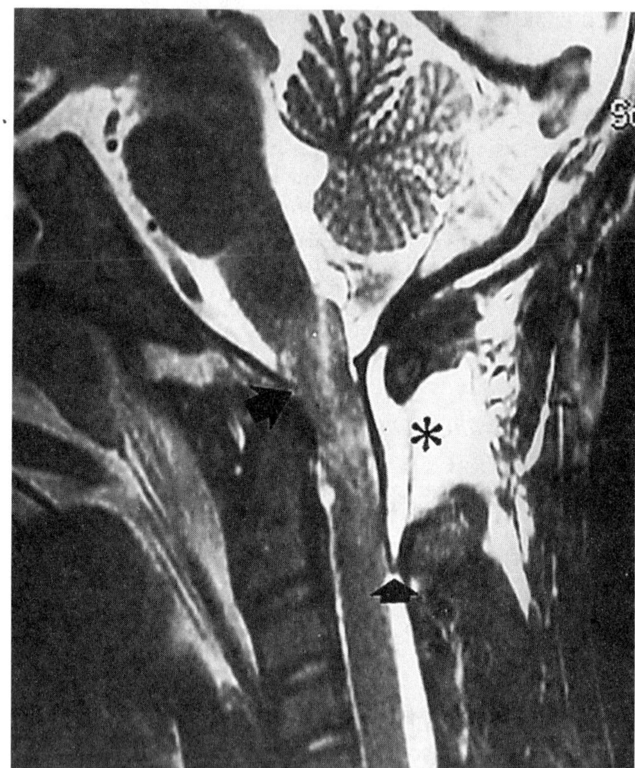

Figure 8-4. Ligament disruption and cord contusion. T2-weighted sagittal MRI of a 9-year-old who sustained a C1–C2 distraction injury and occipitoatlantal dislocation in an automobile accident. Disruptions of the posterior longitudinal ligament (*arrow*) and ligamentum flavum (*arrowhead*) are visible. Note also the marked separation of the posterior arch of C1 and spinous process of C2 and the marked edema in between (*asterisk*). Hyperintensity in the cord indicates edema.

imaging, which demonstrates the effect of spine motion on the cord (37).

The demonstration of injury to the spinal cord itself essentially requires MRI; CT is extremely limited by comparison. The MRI appearance of the cord in the acute phase of injury correlates with the prognosis (4,38,39). In particular, MRI performed within 72 hours of injury increases the accuracy of predicting outcome at 1 year compared with clinical evaluation alone (40). If the spinal cord shows only focal enlargement but no abnormal signal intensity, good recovery can be expected. Patients with cord edema as suggested by hyperintensity on T2-weighted images have an intermediate prognosis (see Fig. 8-4). Evidence of hemorrhage correlates with poor recovery after 1 year.

Chronic

In the more chronic phases of spinal injury, imaging is used to evaluate fracture or fusion healing, to re-evaluate the nature of injury to the cord, and to detect complications involving the spine or the cord. In the early months following spinal fusion, it can be very difficult to appreciate the progress of healing. Plain films and polytomography are recommended as the most cost-effective and reproducible methods for following fracture healing (37,41). Karasick (41) begins with a baseline examination in the immediate postoperative period, then again at 8 weeks, and obtains flexion-extension views at 3 months. Evidence of bone bridging and lack of motion on flexion-extension views is indicative of arthrodesis. Cancellous graft incorporation is usually complete by 6 months, whereas cortical grafts take longer and initially become weaker in the first 6 months due to bone resorption preceding osteoblastic activity (41). Graft incorporation is seen as new bone formation at the margins of grafted bone and a uniform appearance at the graft-vertebra interface. CT may be used on an individual basis to evaluate fusion, but discontinuity between the graft and vertebra does not necessarily equate with functional failure (37). Flexion-extension views, either static (plain films) or dynamic (fluoroscopy with spot films or video recording), demonstrate the functional integrity of the fusion. Optimally these are obtained with the patient's physiatrist or neurosurgeon supervising the examination to encourage maximum spinal movement up to but not beyond the patient's pain or neurologic threshold. Passive flexion-extension is not recommended. In a well-healed graft, typically after several years, the plug becomes so well incorporated into the trabecular pattern of the vertebra as to be scarcely recognizable. A posterior fusion, in which bone fragments have been laid on a soft-tissue bed, may appear as fragments for many months. Serial examinations may show progressive resorption of the fragments in a failed graft. At times the fragments unite in a bony strut, but close scrutiny of the CT images is required to determine whether the strut actually crosses a joint. A mature posterior fusion, on the other hand, appears as a solid mass of bone that is continuous from one level to the next.

In addition to pseudarthrosis, early complications of the graft itself include extrusion of the strut, subsidence of the graft, and infection (37,41). Anterior extrusion of the strut may be associated with dysphagia and posterior extrusion, with cord compression. The latter is best evaluated with MRI or CT-myelography. Graft subsidence may result in kyphosis, which is evident on plain films or tomograms. Suspected infection should be investigated with MRI. Hardware complications, which can be seen on plain films or CT scans, include protruding or misplaced screws; fractures of plates, screws, or rods; screw migration; and impingement by wires on the spinal cord (Fig. 8-5). Complications due to soft-tissue scarring following spinal surgery include epidural fibrosis and arachnoiditis. These are discussed in the section on degenerative spinal disease.

Patients with spinal injuries may develop delayed graft problems or other complications of the vertebral column that require radiologic evaluation. Graft fracture is visible on plain films, polytomograms, or CT scans. Overgrowth of bone grafts resulting in spinal stenosis is best seen on CT scans. Spondylosis may occur anywhere but is particularly prone to affect disk levels immediately above or below a fusion. While CT, CT-myelography, and MRI are all useful in the evaluation of degenerative disk disease, the additional superiority of MRI in the detection of syringomyelia is a distinct advantage because of the similarity of the presenting symptoms in these two conditions and the need to differentiate them. Two other spinal complications that at times can be difficult to distinguish are diskitis/osteomyelitis and neuropathic changes. Both can show loss of disk height, disruption of the vertebral endplates, and bone destruction on plain films, CT scans, and MRIs. The presence of inflammatory changes in the surrounding soft tissues is very helpful for diagnosing infection, but fluoroscopy-guided fine-needle aspiration to obtain material for culture may be required to differentiate these conditions.

To visualize the nature of the chronic pathologic changes in traumatic spinal cord injury, MRI is indispensable. Spinal cord atrophy is visible in most cases. A transected segment of the cord appears amorphous; the cord margins are virtually impossible to follow from intact cord across the transection to another segment of intact cord. Adhesions between the cord and the meninges are present when the cord appears kinked, tethered, or adherent to the dura. It may be important clinically to distinguish between a spinal cord cyst or syrinx and myelomalacia because of possible potential benefit from a decompressive procedure in the former. While the most accurate determination is provided by intraoperative ultrasound imaging, MRI offers the most reliable noninvasive evaluation. A cystic cavity appears as a well-defined area that has signal intensities like those of CSF, whereas myelomalacia does not follow

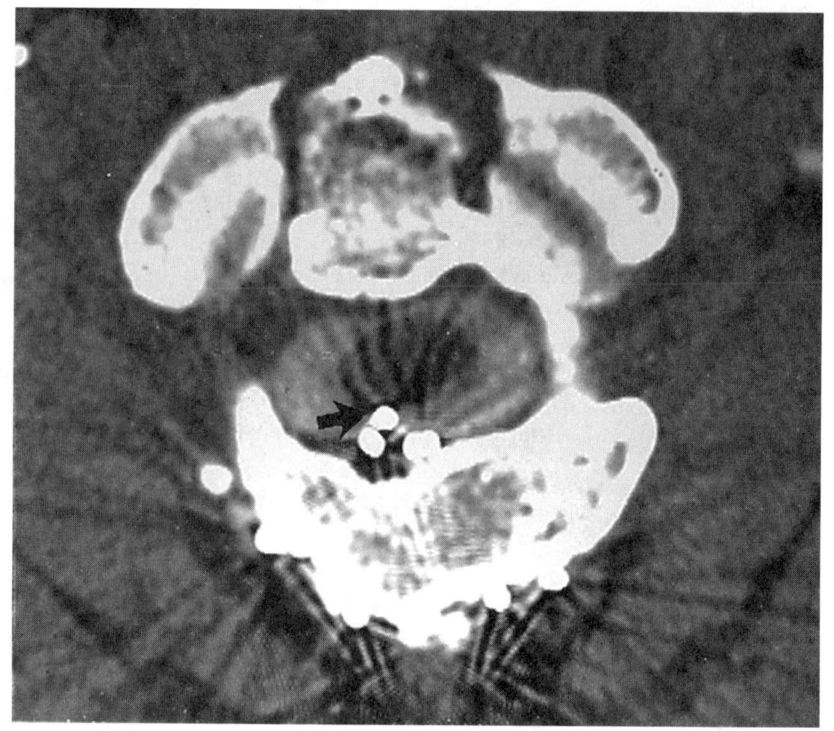

Figure 8-5. Complication of surgical wire. In this postmyelographic CT scan, surgical wire (*arrow*) is seen impinging on the posterior surface of the spinal cord in a patient who presented with paresthesias and the Lhermitte sign 11 years after a posterior fusion for an odontoid fracture. This is the same patient as in Figure 8-2.

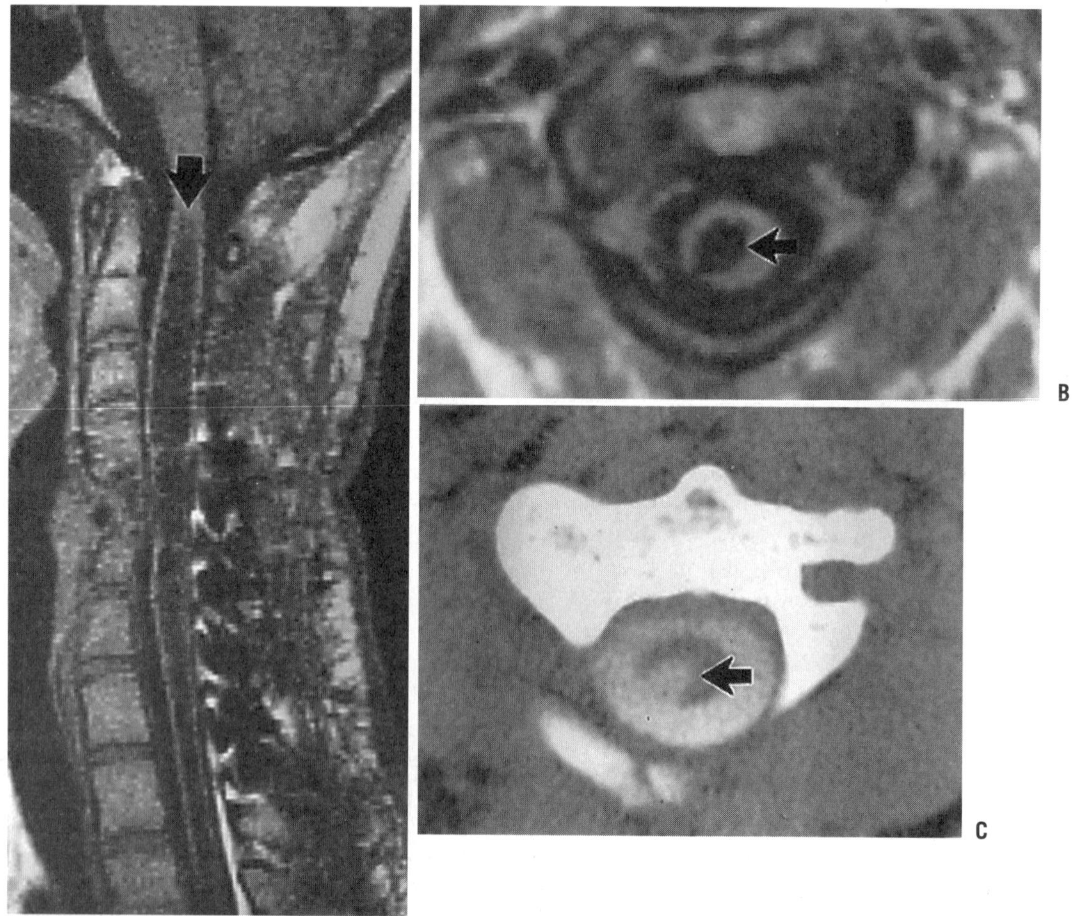

Figure 8-6. Syrinx. *A*, *B*. T1-weighted MRIs showing a syrinx (*arrows*) that developed after a C5 fracture and spinal cord injury. The syrinx eventually extended over the entire length of the spinal cord. Surgical wires in the posterior elements create minor artifacts in *A*. *C*. CT-myelogram in a patient who could not undergo MRI. Contrast material penetrates into the syrinx cavity (*arrow*).

CSF signal intensity on all images (4). Overlap between the appearances of these conditions may reflect the coexistence of the two conditions or the possibility that a cyst may develop from myelomalacia.

A cystic cavity that has dissected superiorly or inferiorly from the level of the original cord injury creating an elongated fluid-containing space is known as a *syrinx*. MRI is the optimal technique for detecting and following syringomyelia (Fig. 8-6A, B), but if MRI is contraindicated, the radiologist can substitute CT-myelography, in which contrast material injected into the subarachnoid space can be detected in the syrinx cavity usually after several hours (Fig. 8-6C). Asano et al (42), reporting on a small number of subjects, advocated relying on the MRI appearance of the cavity to select patients for surgery. The patients who are most likely to benefit from decompression are those with a high-pressure syrinx, which correlates with a "flow void," an area of decreased signal intensity due to motion of fluid within the cavity.

Nontraumatic Spinal Cord Disease

Physiatrists may come in contact with patients who have a variety of nontraumatic diseases of the spinal cord of neoplastic, postradiation, inflammatory, demyelinating, or ischemic etiology. Plain films may give clues of underlying neurologic disease by demonstrating scoliosis or spinal canal widening in the case of spinal cord tumors. Regular monitoring of the spine with plain films is important for detecting the development of spinal deformity, which should be anticipated in children who have received radiotherapy to the spine and in all patients who have undergone extensive laminectomies (43). Since the majority of patients followed for more than 1 year after tumor resection have pain and since spinal instability and osteoarthritis are among the causes, plain films are useful in the initial evaluation of these patients (43). CT may reveal fat in a limited number of tumors but is of limited usefulness for tumor detection unless combined with myelography. MRI is by far the most important modality for the evaluation of all intrinsic spinal cord lesions.

Spinal cord neoplasms typically appear on MRI as solid or cystic masses that expand the cord and usually show contrast enhancement. Some may show evidence of recent or old hemorrhage and many are associated with syringohydromyelia (Fig. 8-7A). Fischer and Brotchi (43) recommended MRI in the first few days following tumor resection, at 6 months, and thereafter depending on tumor histology and extent of surgery. Focal atrophy of the cord and resolution of the syrinx are expected (Fig. 8-7B). Enhancement of the tumor bed in the early postoperative period may be seen, but later raises the suspicion of tumor recurrence, especially if there has been an interval without enhancement (43). On the other hand, if the cord has been irradiated, enhancement may indicate radiation myelopathy. Differentiating these two conditions requires follow-up examination demonstrating resolution in the case of radiation myelopathy. In addition, MRI may reveal adhesions tethering the cord to the dura at the operative site. Hyperintensity of irradiated vertebrae on T1-weighted images is expected and reflects the replacement of marrow by fat.

Inflammatory diseases, such as Lyme disease, sarcoidosis, and acute-phase multiple sclerosis, appear as focal areas of hyperintensity in the cord on T2-weighted images and show patchy enhancement after contrast injection. The cord may show focal enlargement. The findings are nonspecific but reflect the activity of the disease and suggest an inflammatory rather than a neoplastic process. Chronic plaques in multiple sclerosis appear hyperintense on T2-weighted images but do not enhance. Spinal cord infarction may also show T2 hyperintensity but is less likely to show focal cord enlargement or enhancement if imaged acutely.

Degenerative Spinal Disease

The term *spondylosis* refers to a constellation of abnormalities that develop in response to degeneration of the intervertebral disk. One of the earliest changes that may be seen by MRI is a decrease in the signal intensity of the disk on T2-weighted images, which is thought to correlate with desiccation of the disk. Fissures may form in the disk, allowing material from the nucleus pulposus, annulus fibrosis, and cartilaginous end-plate to migrate out from the center in either a radial direction or a superior-inferior direction. If herniation occurs through the end-plate of an adjacent vertebral body, it is visible on MRI or plain film as a Schmorl node. If it migrates in a radial direction completely through the annulus fibrosis, it is considered herniated (Fig. 8-8). In the spinal canal, it is visible on MRI as a focal anterior extradural mass usually connected to the disk, although a fragment may be somewhat remote from the disk without apparent connection, a so-called free disk fragment or sequestered disk. With myelography one sees a focal anterior or anterolateral indentation on the thecal sac, usually at disk level. The adjacent nerve root may be displaced or its dural sleeve, if compressed, may not fill with contrast material and so appear "cutoff." When a fissure disrupts the inner layers of the annulus but the outer layers remain intact, CT or MRI demonstrates a focal but broad change in the contour of the disk. The variety of terms—such as *bulging*, *protruding*, *herniated*, and *extruded*—used to describe the changes seen in degenerated disks can be confusing (44–46). For the most part, this lack of semantic uniformity reflects the continuum of the process of disk material migration outward through a fissure and the lack of radiographic precision in determining the integrity of the outermost fibers of the annulus.

Frequently a degenerating disk extends beyond the vertebral body margins in all directions. Since the outer layers of the annulus contain the Sharpey fibers, which

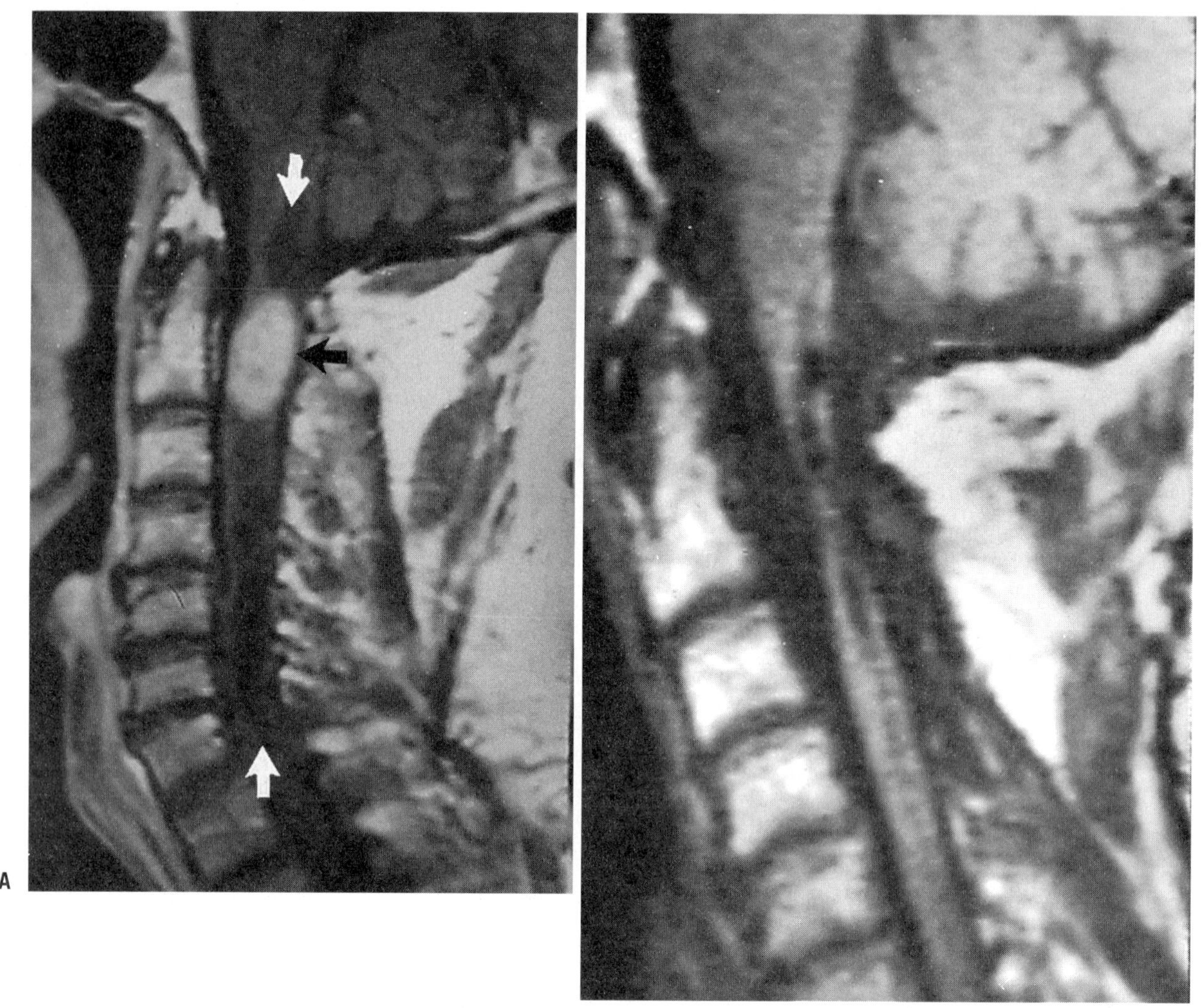

Figure 8-7. Ependymoma. *A*. Sagittal T1-weighted postcontrast MRI showing an enhancing ependymoma at C2 (*arrow*) with a syrinx extending superiorly and inferiorly (*white arrows*). *B*. The postoperative scan shows focal atrophy at the level of tumor resection and collapse of the syrinx.

insert into the periosteum of the vertebral body, chronic elevation of these fibers causes new bone formation, or osteophytes, at the end-plate margins. The bulging annulus with its osteophytes may encroach on the neural foramen or spinal canal. In addition, as the disk height decreases, the facet joints sublux slightly, their articular surfaces sliding past each other. This telescoping of the facet joints decreases the size of the neural foramen. It also causes buckling of the ligamentum flavum in the foramen and induces hypertrophic changes in the facet joints, all of which further encroach on the cross-sectional area of the foramen. Similarly, a bulging annulus, buckled ligamenta flava, and hypertrophic facet joints encroach on the space in the spinal canal, resulting in compression of the spinal cord or cauda equina (Fig. 8-9). Lumbar nerve roots that have been compressed chronically become stretched and appear redundant on myelograms or MRI (Fig. 8-10) (47,48). These situations are known as *foraminal* or *canal stenosis*.

Recurrent or chronic pain following back surgery may be due to a number of causes including facet fracture (49), fusion failure (discussed in the section on spinal trauma), facet joint disease, infection, recurrent disk herniation, and epidural or arachnoid fibrosis (50). Facet fracture may be suspected on bone scan and confirmed by CT. Facet joint degenerative disease can be detected on plain films or more easily on CT scans as osteophytes, joint space narrowing or subluxation, or subchondral cysts. Determination that the patient's pain originates from the joint may require fluoroscopic injection of anesthetic. Diskitis and osteomyelitis can complicate diskectomy and are most easily confirmed with MRI. The earliest changes seen include hypointensity of the adjacent vertebral body marrow and inflammatory changes of the surrounding soft tissues. Subsequently there may be loss of disk height, disruption of the end-plates, and hyperintensity of the disk on T2-weighted images (Fig. 8-11).

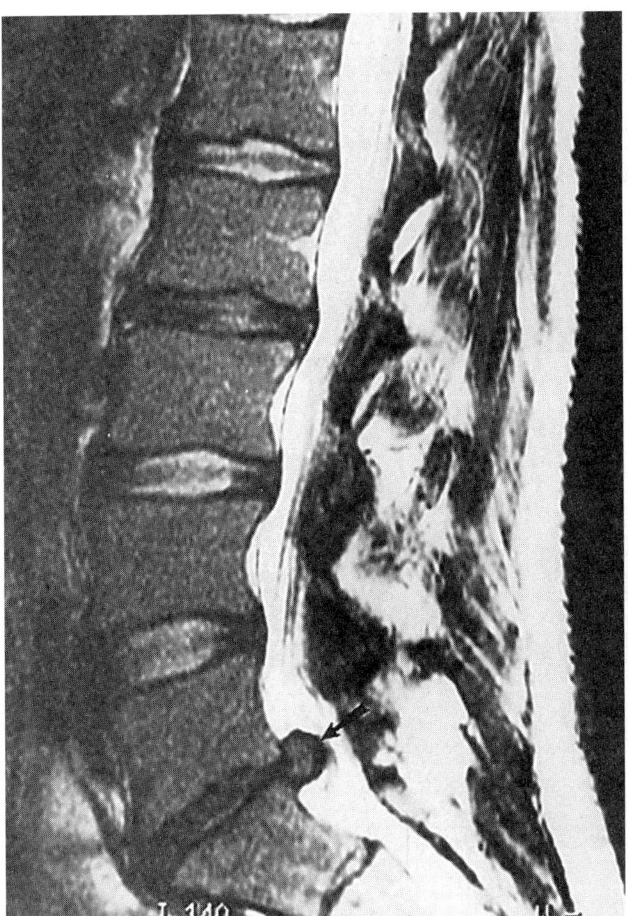

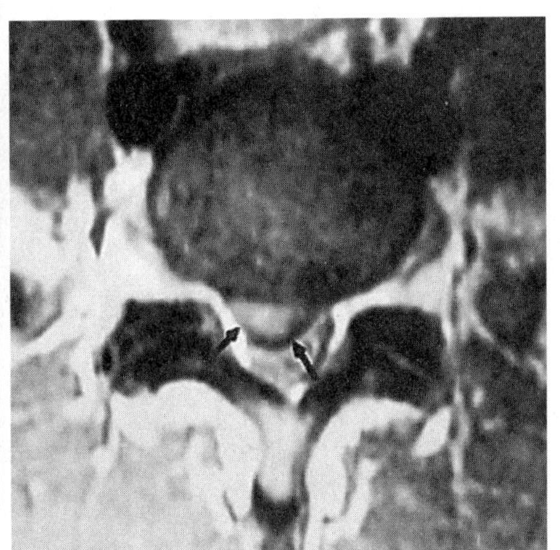

Figure 8-8. Disk herniation. T2-weighted sagittal (*A*) and axial (*B*) MRIs showing a herniated disk at L5–S1 (*arrows*). Note the focality of the disk protrusion on the axial image. Early degenerative change of the L2–L3 disk (*arrowhead*) is evident in the decreased signal intensity and disk height.

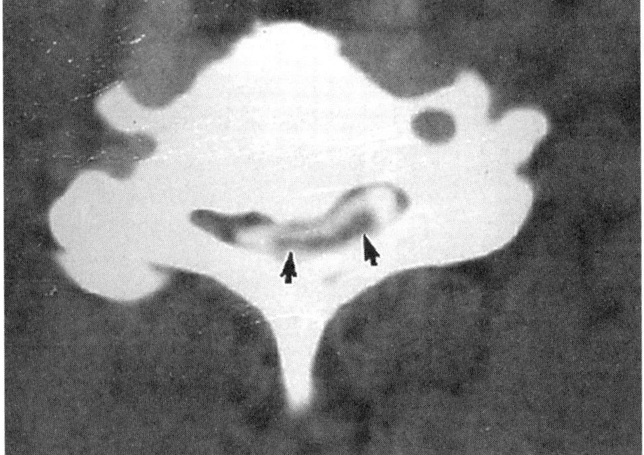

Figure 8-9. Spinal stenosis with cord compression. Postmyelographic cervical spine CT scan showing marked spinal cord atrophy (*arrows*) because of longstanding cord compression. The patient has severe spinal stenosis due to the combination of a congenitally small canal and posterior hypertrophic changes of the vertebral body.

Scar tissue is thought to be the source of radiculopathy due to tethering of adjacent nerve roots. The signal intensity of the fibrosis differs from that of the normal epidural fat but tends to obscure the margins of the nerve root and disk. Intravenous contrast material, which enhances scar tissue, helps to define the relationship of the nerve root to the scar tissue and to differentiate recurrent disk herniation from scar (50). Arachnoiditis may also complicate extensive spinal surgery or trauma. The presence of arachnoiditis can be suspected on MRIs when nerve roots appear clumped or adherent to the thecal sac. However, these features as well as deformity of the thecal sac are easier to appreciate with myelography (Fig. 8-12). In severe cases the thecal sac is so constricted that the flow of contrast material in the subarachnoid space is blocked.

In the condition known as *spondylolysis*, the portion of the lamina between the superior and inferior facet joints (the pars interarticularis) is disrupted. Although occasionally attributed to an identifiable traumatic incident, the defect is generally considered to reflect a chronic stress fracture and typically is surrounded by abundant fibrous tissue. It occurs most often at the L5–S1 and L4–L5 levels and can be the source of low-back pain. It can be seen on lateral or oblique radiographs (Fig. 8-13A, B), CT, or less reliably MRI (51). When it is bilateral, the lack of

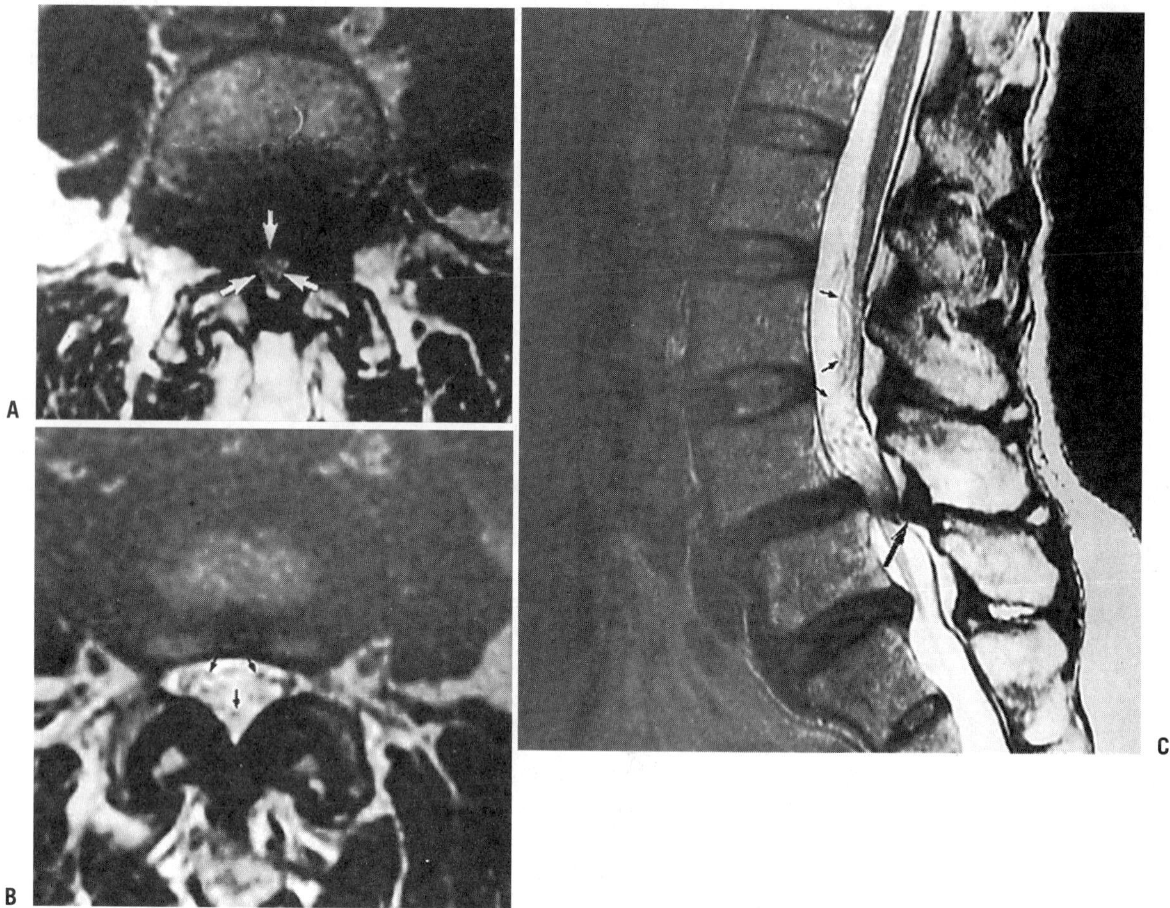

Figure 8-10. Spinal stenosis with cauda equina compression. T2-weighted MRIs of the lumbar region of the spine. *A.* The axial image shows severe stenosis of the spinal canal. No cerebrospinal fluid (CSF) can be seen surrounding the compressed nerve roots (*arrows*). *B.* Compare to the normal-size canal at a higher level showing punctate nerve roots (*arrows* indicating a few roots) bathed in white CSF. *C.* The sagittal image shows that the stenosis is due to spondylolisthesis, a bulging annulus, and thickened (probably buckled) ligamenta flava (*large arrow*). The chronic stenosis has resulted in stretching and elongation of the nerve roots, which appear serpiginous above the stenosis (*small arrows*). Note also degenerative changes of the L5–S1 disk, which shows decreased signal intensity and a circumferential annular bulge.

continuity between one level of facet joints and the next lower level allows the affected vertebra to slip forward (spondylolisthesis), since the intervertebral disk and spinal ligaments do not resist horizontal shear forces well. This anterior displacement causes narrowing of the neural foramina and stretching of the exiting nerve roots and may also cause compression of the cauda equina (Fig. 8-13C).

BRAIN

CT and MRI play a crucial role in evaluating the brain. CT is utilized primarily in the acute setting to delineate the extent and location of life-threatening intracranial pathology. Once these situations are excluded, MRI becomes the imaging study of choice due to its greater sensitivity and multiplanar capabilities. This section reviews the CT and MRI appearance of intracranial hemorrhage, traumatic and nontraumatic injuries, cerebrovascular accidents, and multiple sclerosis.

Intracranial Hemorrhage

Acute (0–3 days) intracranial hematomas appear hyperdense on CT scans with respect to the brain parenchyma. This appearance is due to the increased concentration of hemoglobin in intact red blood cells (Fig. 8-14A). During the subacute stage (4–21 days), as red blood cells are lysed and the hemoglobin is reabsorbed, the hematomas become progressively isodense (Fig. 8-14B). If intravenous contrast material is given at this time, peripheral enhancement may occur as a result of perivascular inflammation and vascular proliferation. In the chronic stage (>21 days), if enough tissue damage has occurred, a hypodense focus similar in density to CSF will remain (Fig. 8-14C) (52).

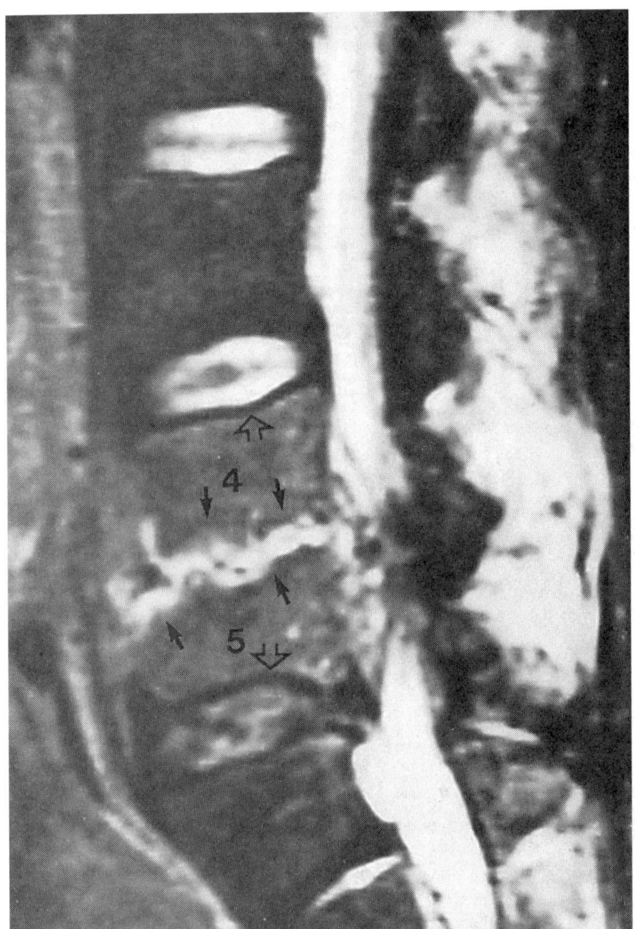

A

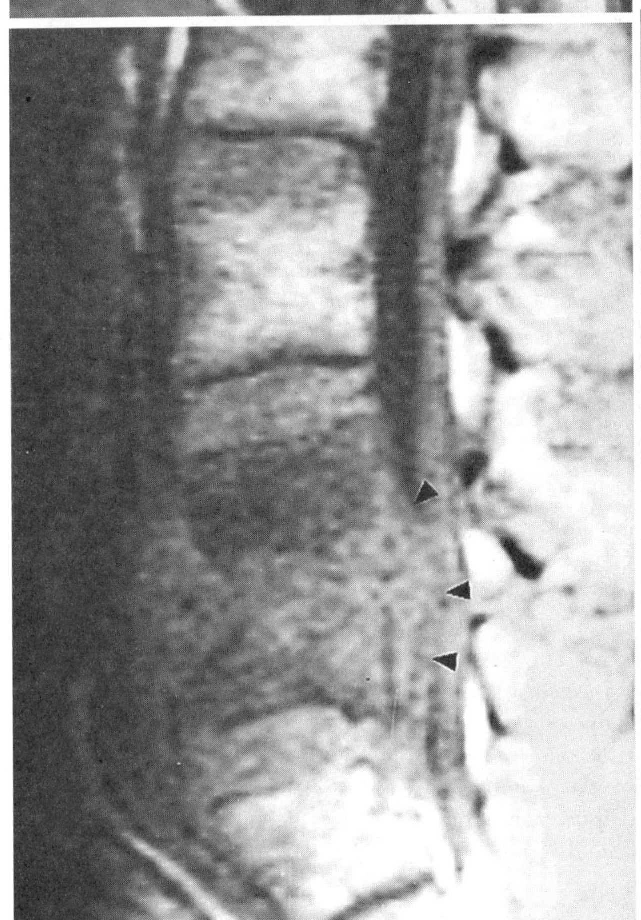

B

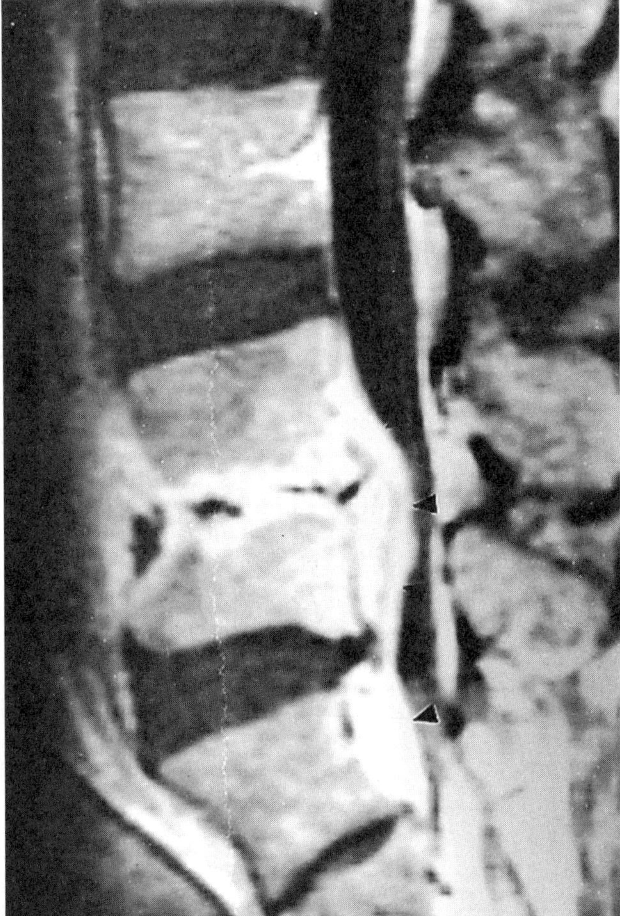

C

Figure 8-11. Advanced diskitis with osteomyelitis. T2-weighted (*A*) and T1-weighted precontrast (*B*) MRIs show marked loss of the height of the L4–L5 disk. The end-plates (*black arrows*) appear irregular and have been destroyed. Compare with normal end-plates (*open arrows*). Signal intensity of the L4 and L5 marrow is decreased in *B* and subtly increased in *A*. Soft-tissue inflammation appears as a mass anteriorly and posteriorly (*arrowheads*) that enhances after administration of a contrast agent (*C*). Note also the marrow enhancement in the L4 and L5 vertebral bodies.

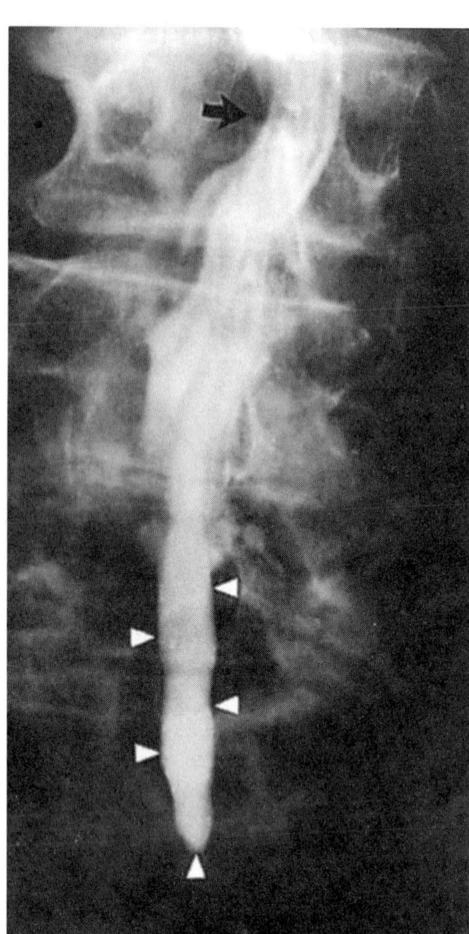

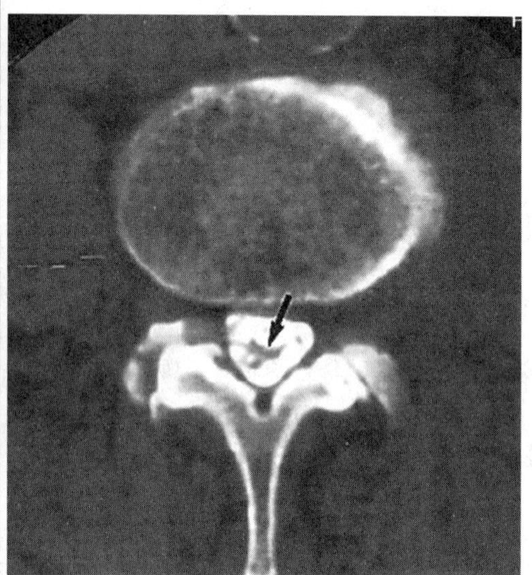

A B

Figure 8-12. Arachnoiditis. *A.* From L4–L5 distally the thecal sac appears featureless on this myelogram (*white arrowheads*). No nerve roots or nerve root sleeves can be identified. The sac is also somewhat constricted. Incidentally, the large defect on the left (*black arrow*) is due to a disk herniation. *B.* On the CT-myelogram most of the nerve roots are clumped together centrally (*arrow*).

The appearance of extravasated blood on MRI is more complex. It is dependent on the strength of the magnetic field, the pulse sequences used, and the presence of hemoglobin degradation products such as oxyhemoglobin, deoxyhemoglobin, methemoglobin, and hemosiderin. Table 8-1 summarizes the signal intensities on both T1- and T2-weighted images and the main hemoglobin degradation product responsible for the MRI appearance (Fig. 8-15) (53–57).

Head Trauma

Excluding scalp injuries and fractures, traumatic injuries are classified as intra- or extra-axial. Intra-axial lesions are located within the brain parenchyma and include contusions and diffuse axonal injuries. Extra-axial injuries are located outside the pia mater, including epidural, subdural, subarachnoid, and intraventricular spaces (58–60).

Contusions

Acute contusions are cortical-based injuries, the result of acceleration or deceleration forces and the direct impact of the brain against the calvarium. The most frequent locations are the anterior aspects of the frontal and temporal lobes (Fig. 8-16). They are usually hemorrhagic, reflecting the increased vascularity of the cerebral cortex with respect to the white matter. During the subacute and chronic phases, removal of irreversibly damaged brain tissue will result in areas of encephalomacia similar in CT density and MRI signal to the CSF (58–62).

Diffuse Axonal Injury

Diffuse axonal injuries are axonal shearing insults that result from rotational and acceleration or deceleration forces on the white matter tracts. Lesions are most commonly seen at the subcortical gray-white matter interface, in the corpus callosum and internal and external capsules, and along the dorsolateral aspect of the midbrain (Fig. 8-17A). They are usually associated with severe loss of consciousness at the moment of impact. Much of the damage is microscopic and therefore not detected by CT or MRI. If lesions are hemorrhagic and large enough, they can be seen acutely on CT scans as linear or ovoid foci of hyperdensity. In the subacute phase, foci of increased signal on both T1- and T2-weighted MRIs are observed due to the

Table 8-1: Temporal Description of Hematomas at 1.5-T Magnetic Resonance

STAGE	TIME	PRESUMED HEMOGLOBIN STATE	PREDOMINANT T1 APPEARANCE*	PREDOMINANT T2 APPEARANCE*
Hyperacute	<24 hr	Oxyhemoglombin	→ ↑	↑
Acute	1–7 day	Deoxyhemoglobin	→ ↑	↓
Early subacute	1–2 wk	Intracellular methemoglobin	↑	↓
Late subacute	2–4 wk	Extracellular methemoglobin	↑	↑
Chronic	>1 mo–years	Hemosiderin	↓	↑

* Arrows indicate the signal intensity compared to gray matter: ↑ = increased; ↓ = decreased.

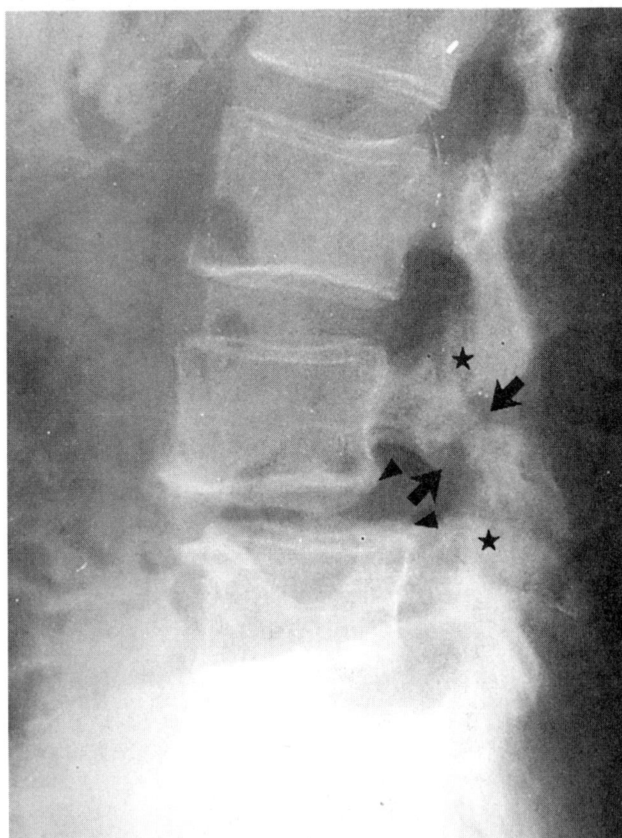

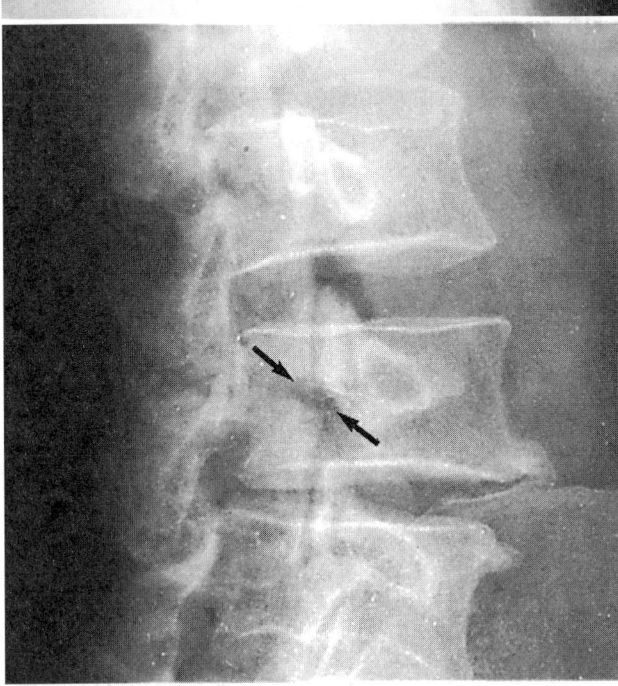

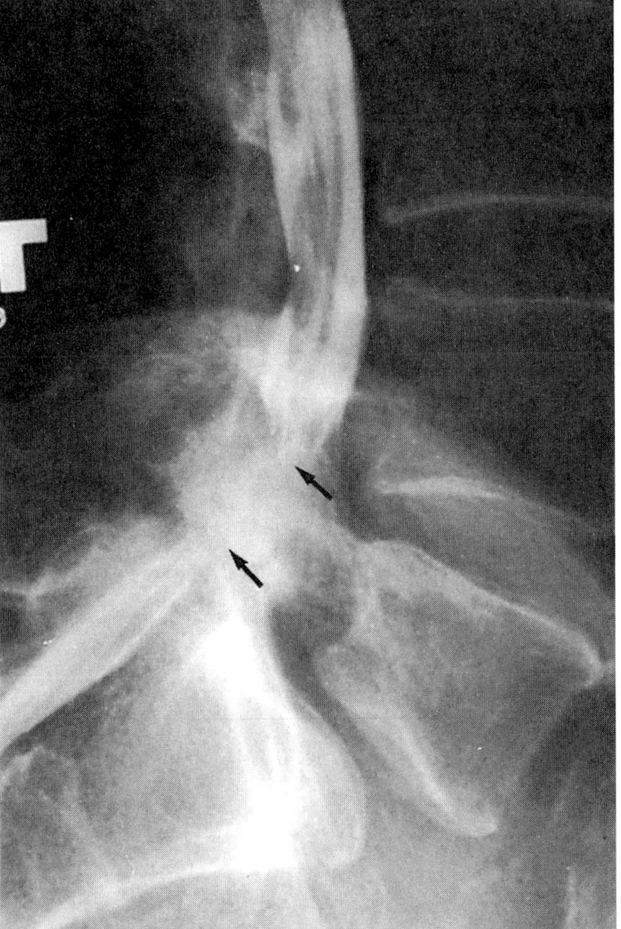

Figure 8-13. Spondylolysis with spondylolisthesis. Lateral (*A*) and oblique (*B*) radiographs show a defect in the L4 pars interarticularis (*arrows*). This defect interrupts the continuity between facet joints (*stars*). Grade I spondylolisthesis is evident in *A* (*arrowheads*). *C*. The myelogram of a patient with grade II spondylolisthesis at L5–S1 shows a subtotal block to the passage of contrast material (*arrows*).

Figure 8-14. Temporal progression of acute intracranial hematoma in a hypertensive patient. *A*. Axial CT scan without contrast material at the level of the putamen shows an acute hyperdense hematoma. *B*. Two weeks later, the hematoma is progressively becoming isodense with respect to the gray matter. *C*. One year later, a cavitated focus similar in density to the cerebrospinal fluid remains. Note the compensatory dilatation of the frontal horn of the lateral ventricle (*arrow*).

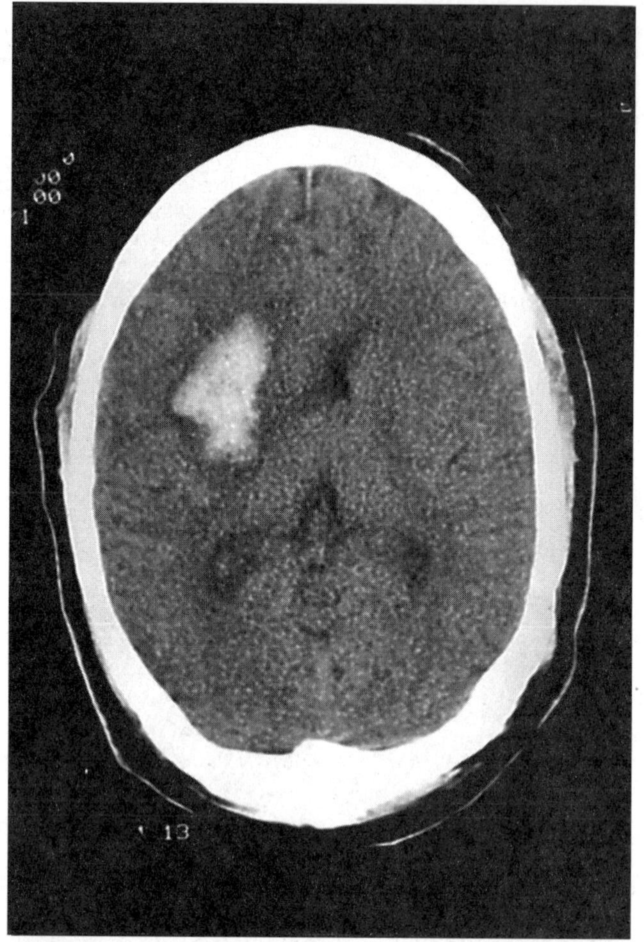

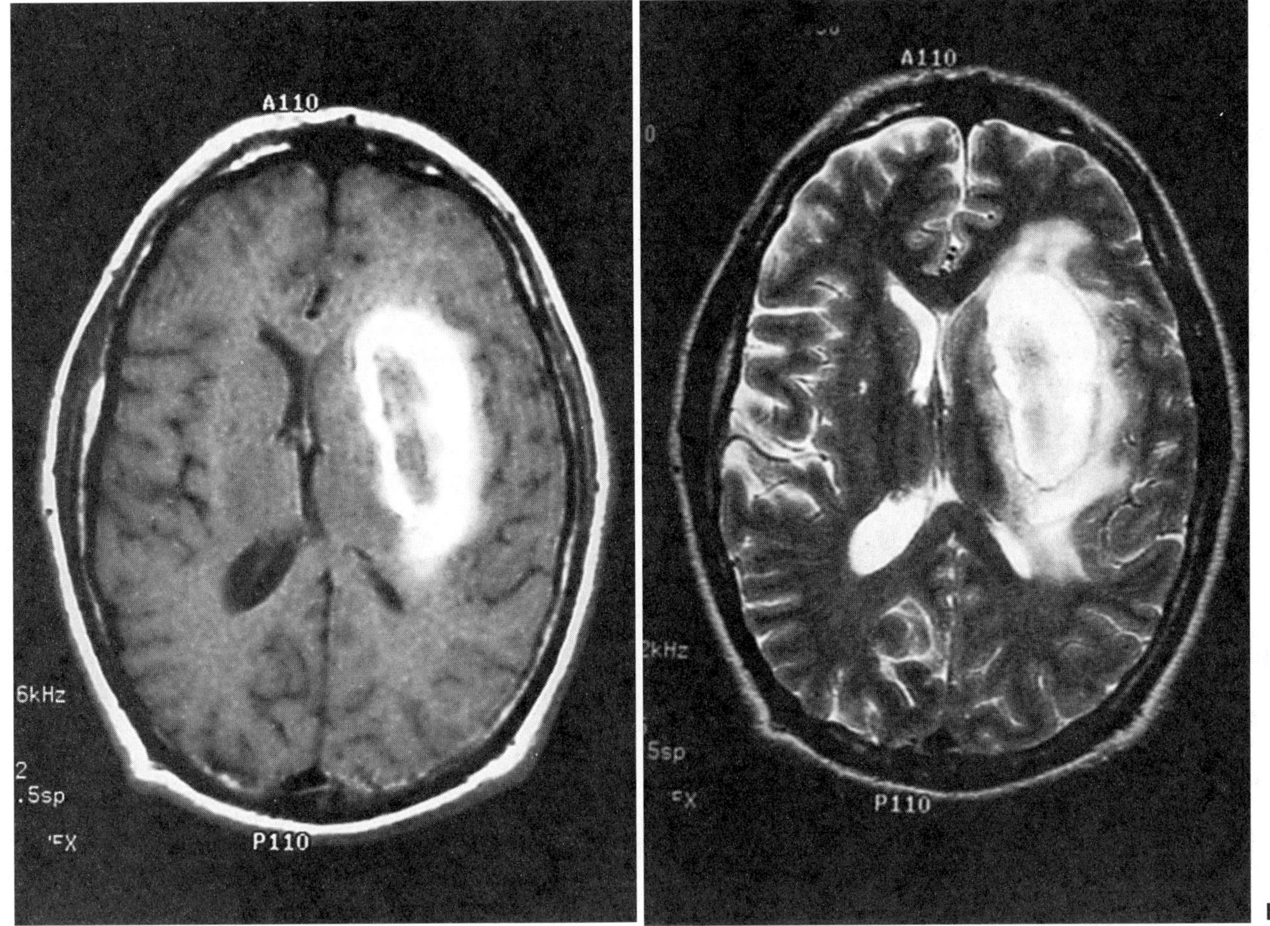

Figure 8-15. Left-putamen subacute hematoma. *A, B.* Axial T1- and T2-weighted images, respectively. The hematoma is predominantly hyperintense on both images, owing to the presence of extracellular methemoglobin.

presence of extracellular methemoglobin (Fig. 8-17B). Residual hemosiderin in the chronic phase is identified as hypointense foci on T2-weighted and gradient-echo sequences (53). Both CT and MRI can detect brain atrophy and compensatory ventricular enlargements (58–62).

Epidural Hematoma

Epidural hematomas (EDHs) occur as blood accumulates in the epidural space, stripping the dura away from the inner table of the skull. Ninety percent of EDHs are the result of a fracture that leads to injury of a meningeal artery. These hematomas are commonly found along the temporal and parietal convexities. The remaining 10% of EDHs are the result of a ruptured venous sinus and therefore are located in the posterior fossa or at the vertex. EDHs appear on CT scans as biconvex, lens-shaped collections that are prevented from spreading by the calvarial sutures and may extend across the midline (Fig. 8-18). Both of these features differentiate them from subdural collections. Acute EDHs are rarely imaged on MRI due to the usual emergent nature of the clinical situation. Their appearance on T1- or T2-weighted images is dependent on the predominant blood degradation product at the time of imaging (53,58–62).

Subdural Hematoma

Unlike EDHs, subdural hematomas (SDHs) are venous in origin and result from laceration of a bridging vein by rapid acceleration or deceleration forces. Blood accumulates in the potential space between the inner meningeal layer of the dura and the underlying arachnoid. On CT scans, acute SDHs appear as hyperdense crescentic collections closely related to the cerebral surface (Fig. 8-19). They are not limited by the calvarial sutures but are prevented from crossing the midline by the falx and tentorium. In the subacute and chronic phases, the hematoma becomes progressively hypodense until eventually its density is similar to that of CSF. MRI is not commonly used in the acute setting, but when used in the subacute or chronic stages, it can be helpful in detecting small hematomas. Their appearance on the T1- and T2-weighted images is also dependent on the predominant blood degradation product (53,58–62).

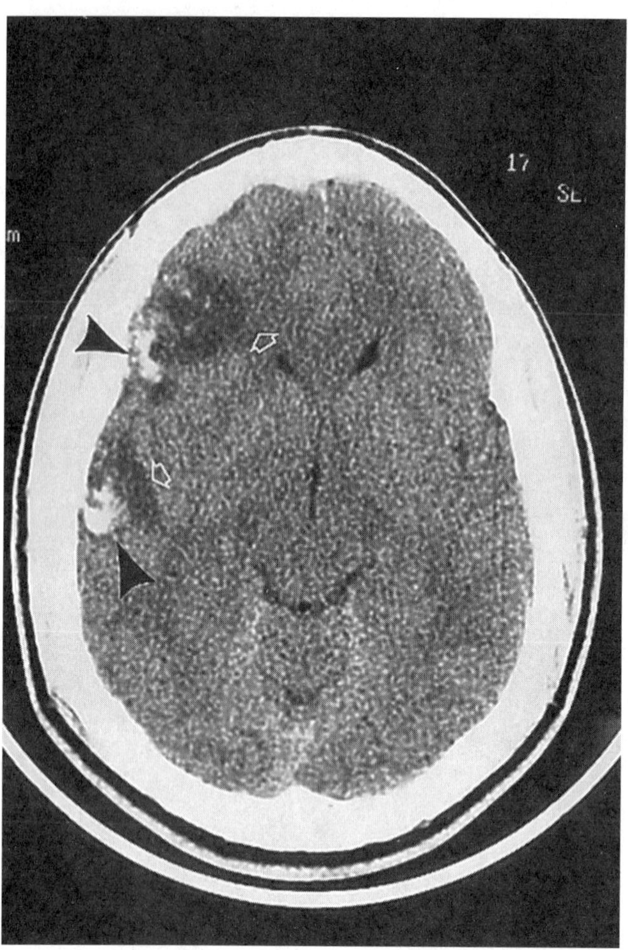

Figure 8-16. Contusions. Axial CT scan without contrast material shows focal hyperdense cortical-based hemorrhagic contusions in the right frontal and temporal lobes (*black arrowheads*). Hypodense areas adjacent to the hematomas represent associated edema (*open white arrows*).

Figure 8-17. Midbrain shearing injury. *A*. Nonenhanced axial CT scan shows a hyperdense focus along the dorsolateral aspect of the midbrain (*arrowhead*). *B*. Coronal T1-weighted MRI a week later shows the hemorrhage as a hyperintense focus (*arrow*).

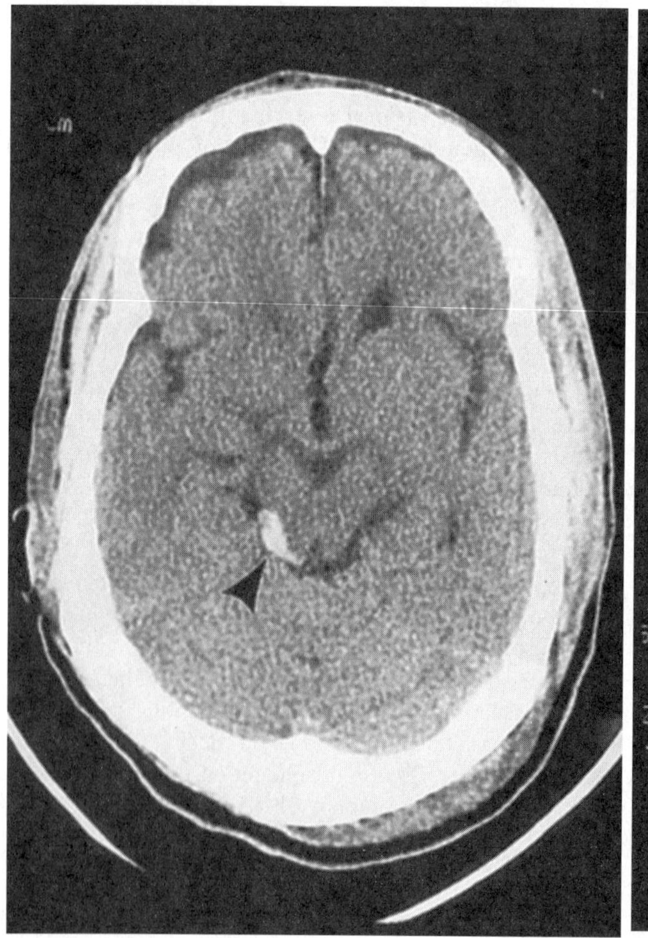

A

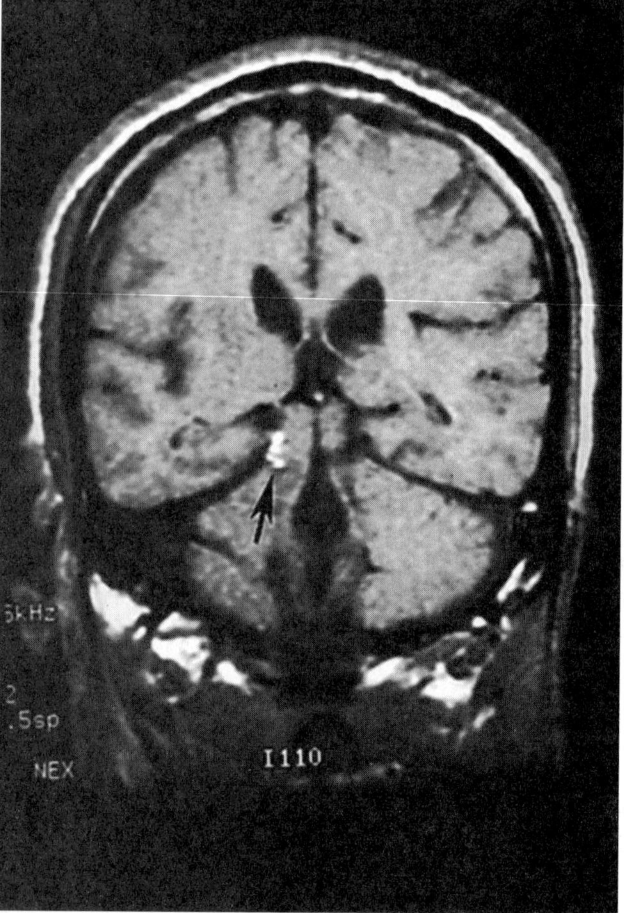

B

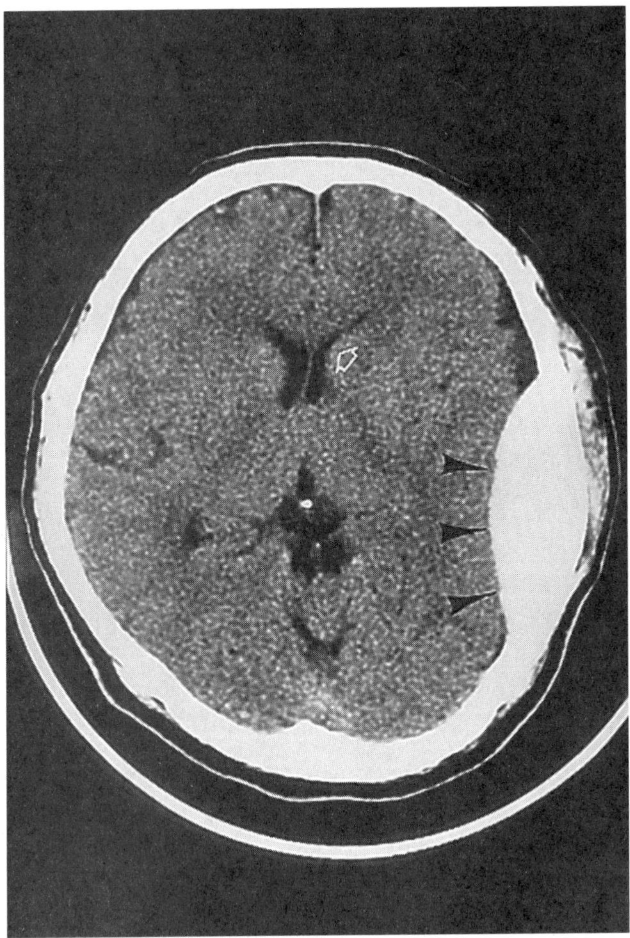

Figure 8-18. Epidural hematoma. Non-contrast-enhanced axial CT scan of a left temporal epidural hematoma (*solid black arrows*). Note the mild mass effect on the frontal horn of the lateral ventricle (*open white arrow*).

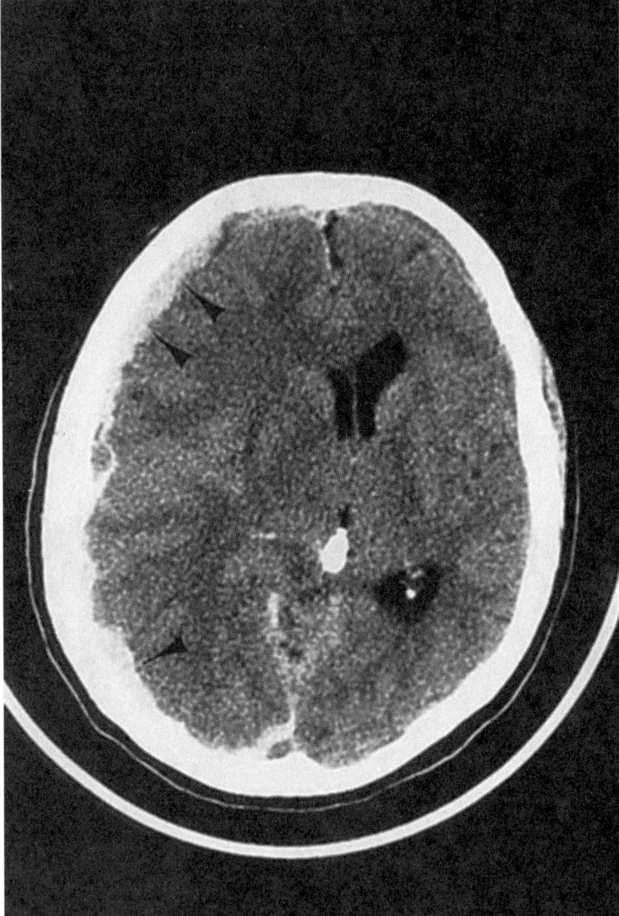

Figure 8-19. Subdural hematoma. Non-contrast-enhanced axial CT scan shows a large right hemispheric subdural hematoma resulting in a midline shift (*solid black arrows*).

Subarachnoid and Intraventricular Hemorrhage

Acute subarachnoid hemorrhage and intraventricular hemorrhage are usually associated with other posttraumatic injuries. If acute subarachoid hemorrhage occurs as an isolated finding, even in the clinical setting of trauma, cerebral angiography is often required to exclude the presence of a ruptured aneurysm. Acute subarachnoid blood on CT scans appears as linear hyperdense foci along the sulci or within the cisternal spaces. Acute intraventricular blood is readily detected as well, frequently seen in the supine patient as it layers within the occipital horns of the lateral ventricles. In spite of recent technologic advances, MRI is still not sensitive enough in the detection of acute subarachnoid hemorrhage (63,64). In the chronic setting, however, hypointense hemosiderin deposits can be seen, especially if gradient-echo techniques are used (53,60).

There are secondary effects of craniocerebral trauma that may, at times, be of greater clinical relevance than the primary insult. Most are the result of increased intracranial pressure and include displacements (referred to as *herniations*), direct vascular injuries, infarcts, hydrocephalus, and compression of cranial nerves and brain parenchyma (65).

Diffuse Brain Swelling

Diffuse brain swelling after head trauma can occur secondary to diffuse edema and/or a reactive increase in blood volume. It can occur as an isolated phenomenon or associated with other intracranial injuries. Diffuse effacement of the sulci and subarachnoid cisterns as well as loss of tissue contrast at the gray-white matter interfaces of the cortex and basal ganglia are seen (Fig. 8-20) (66,67).

Nontraumatic Intracranial Hemorrhage

Nontraumatic intracranial hemorrhage is frequently due to uncontrolled arterial hypertension, ruptured aneurysm, or vascular malformations. Other etiologic factors include embolic vascular insult, tumors, blood dyscrasias,

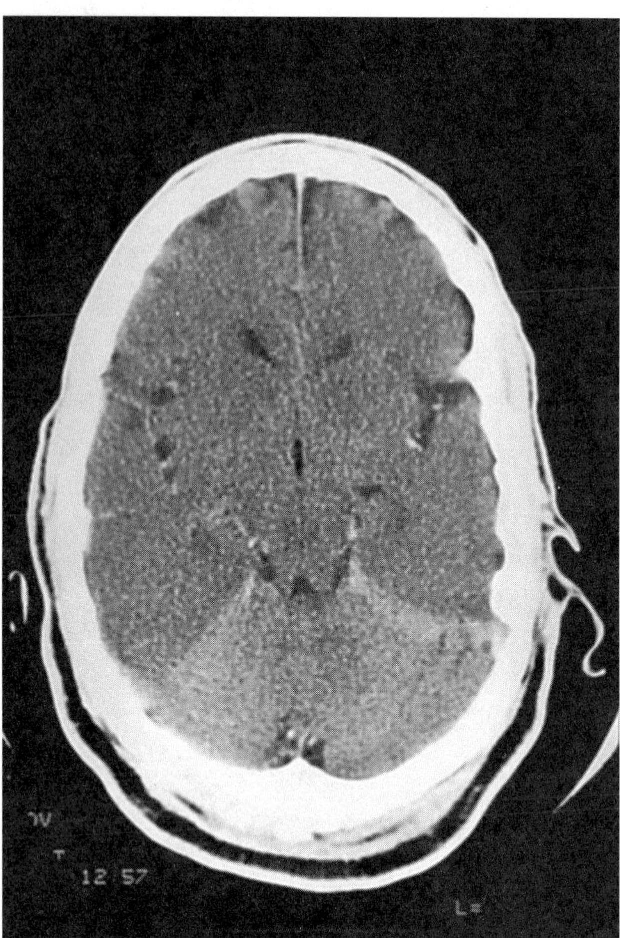

Figure 8-20. Diffuse brain swelling. Postcontrast axial CT scan shows diffuse low density throughout both cerebral hemispheres compared with the cerebellum. Note the diffuse effacement of the gray-white matter interface.

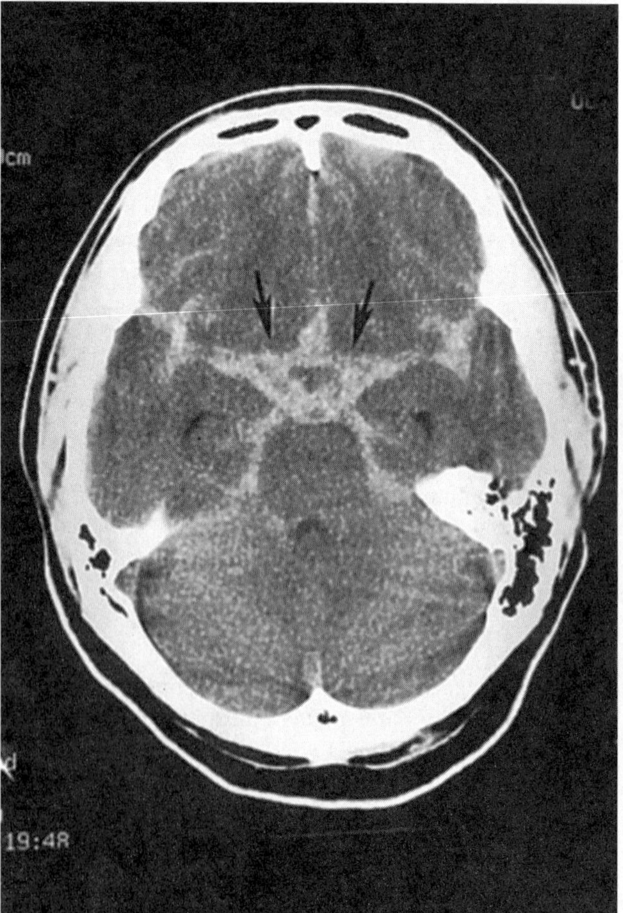

A

Figure 8-21. Acute subarachnoid hemorrhage due to a ruptured aneurysm. *A.* Non-contrast-enhanced axial CT scan shows diffuse acute subarachnoid blood throughout the basal cisterns (*solid black arrows*). *B.* Lateral angiogram of the left internal carotid artery shows a posterior communicating artery aneurysm projecting posteriorly (*solid white arrow*).

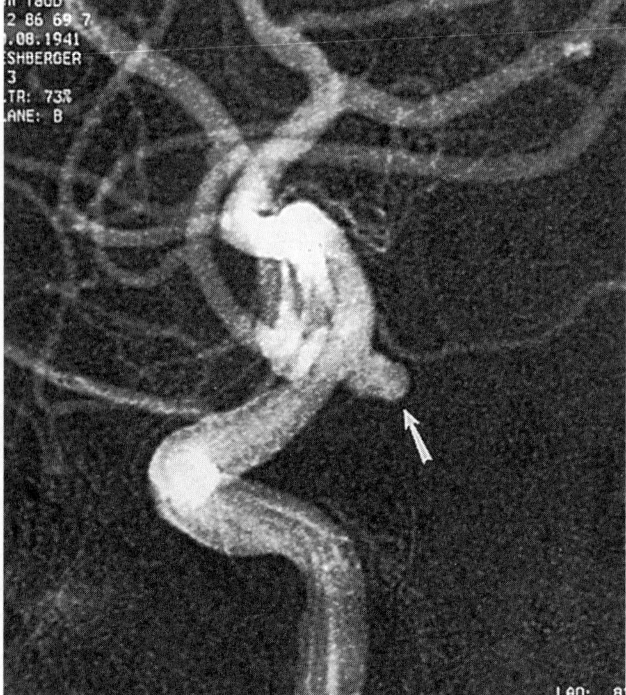

B

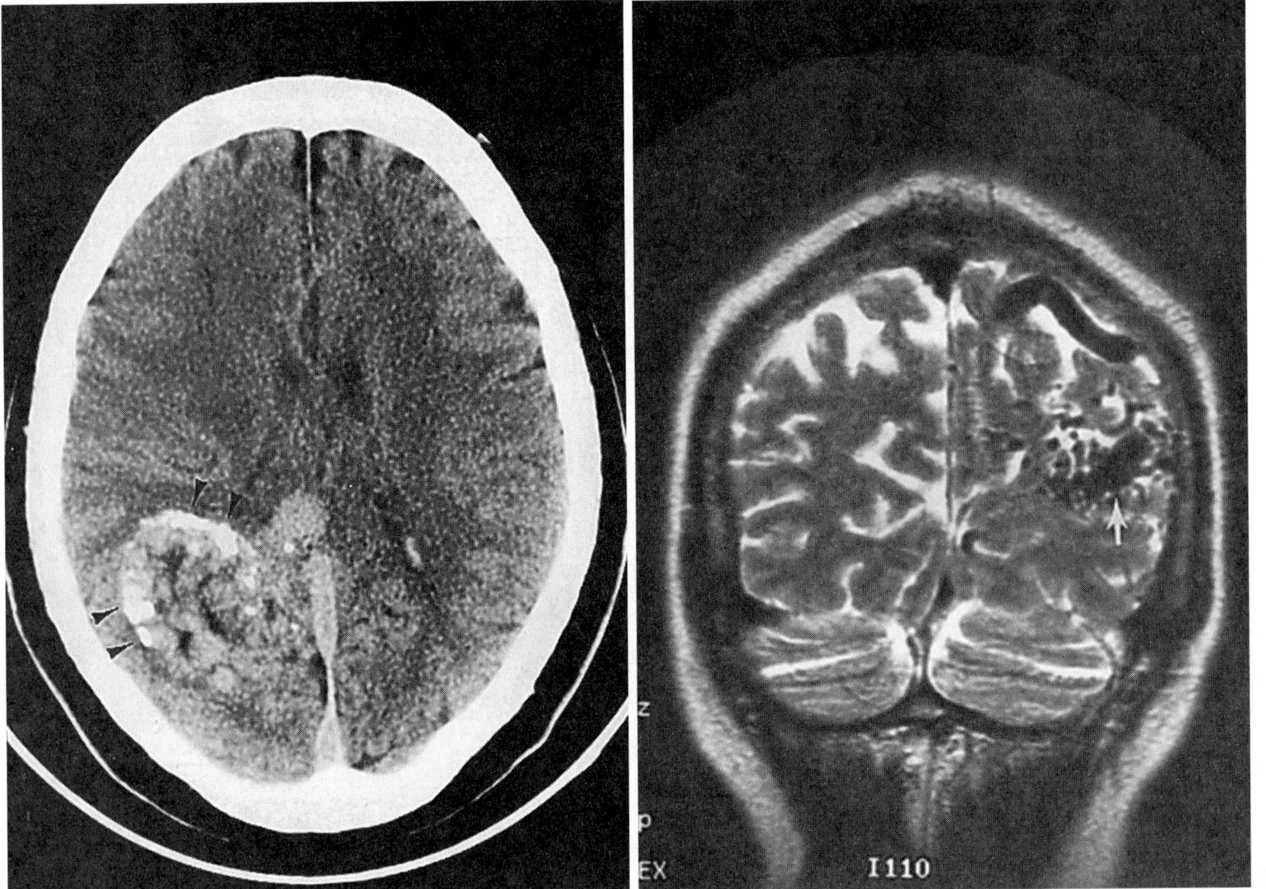

Figure 8-22. Unruptured arteriovenous malformation. *A*. Nonenhanced axial CT scan shows a mildly hyperdense arteriovenous malformation in the right occipital lobe. Hyperdense peripheral foci are consistent with calcifications (*solid black arrows*). *B*. Coronal T2-weighted image in a different patient shows the nidus of the malformation as areas devoid of signal (*solid white arrow*). The elongated structure along the superior surface of the brain represents the patent draining vein.

anticoagulants, vasculitis, drug abuse, and amyloid angiopathy (68).

Hypertension

Spontaneous intracranial hemorrhage in the hypertensive patient most commonly occurs in the putamen (>50%) (see Fig. 8-14A). Other locations include the thalamus, pons, dentate region of the cerebellum, and the subcortical white matter. Rupture of the small perforating arterioles supplying these regions, either simultaneously or in succession, results in intraparenchymal hematomas. These can be small or massive and in certain cases can rupture into the ventricular system, leading to acute hydrocephalus (68,69).

Intracranial Aneurysms

Intracranial aneurysms are the result of structural abnormalities involving the intracerebral vessels. These lesions most commonly occur at the circle of Willis in the anterior and posterior communicating arteries, the middle cerebral artery bifurcation, and the basilar tip. Other locations include the posterior inferior cerebellar artery and the cavernous and supraclinoid segments of the internal carotid artery (70).

Most patients, after complaining of the "worst headache of their lives," show acute subarachnoid hemorrhage on CT scans (Fig. 8-21A). The hemorrhage can be localized or diffuse and associated with intraventricular hemorrhage. After the acute ictus (1–3 days), vasospasm may occur, sometimes leading to vascular ischemic insults and significant morbidity. Cerebral angiography is the gold standard in detecting aneurysms and providing surgeons and endovascular therapists with the information necessary for treatment (Fig. 8-21B). MR angiography and CT-angiography are increasingly playing noninvasive roles in the evaluation of these patients (70–74).

Vascular Malformations

These congenital lesions include AVMs, cavernous angiomas, venous malformations, and capillary telangiectasias (75,76).

Figure 8-23. Cavernous angioma with MRI evidence of old hemorrhage. *A*. Axial CT scan without contrast shows a round, mildly hyperdense focus in the right frontal lobe (*solid black arrowhead*). *B*. The lesion on this axial T2-weighted image is centrally hyperintense due to the presence of methemoglobin. The peripheral hypointense rim is due to hemosiderin. *C*. The lesion becomes more conspicuous on the gradient-echo image.

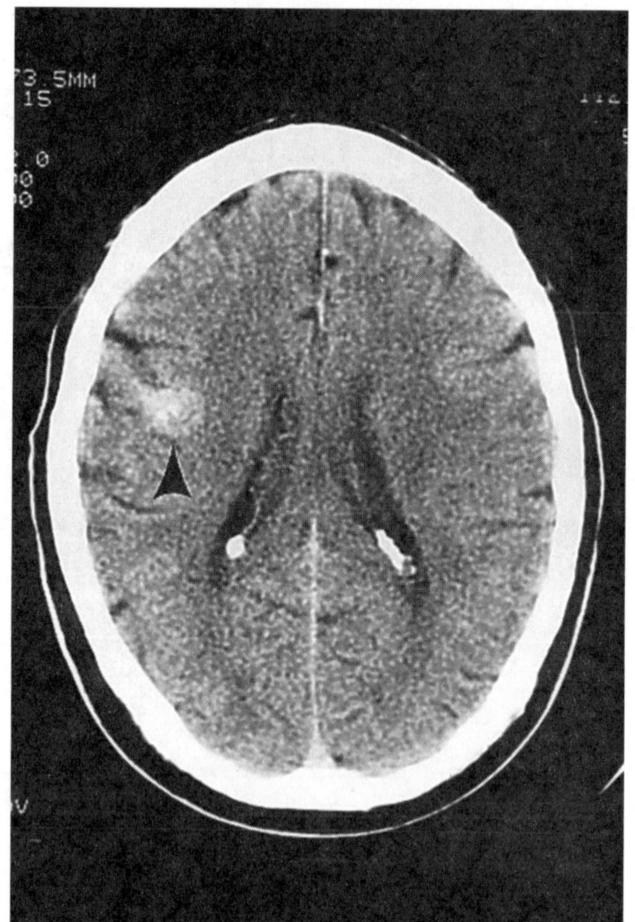

A

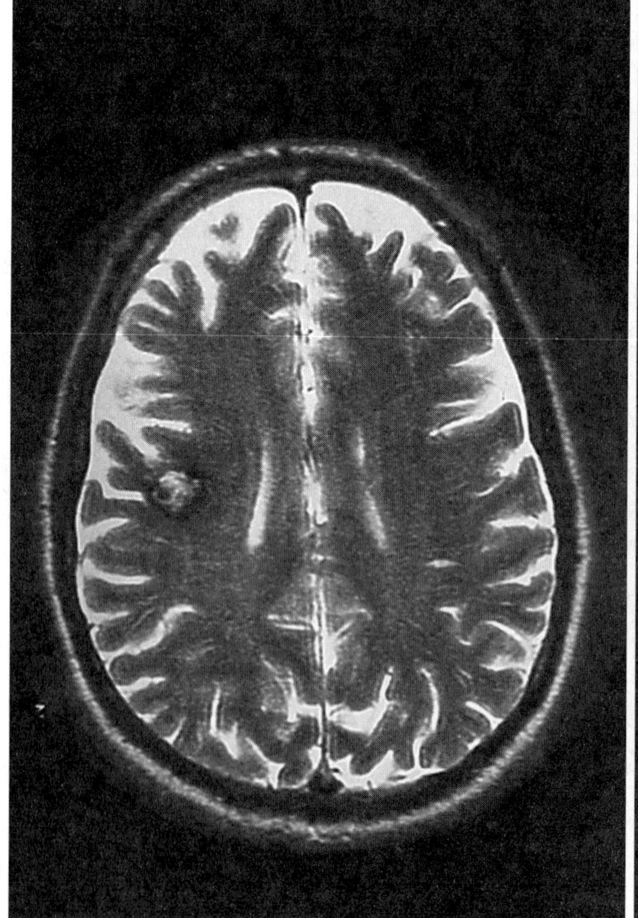

B

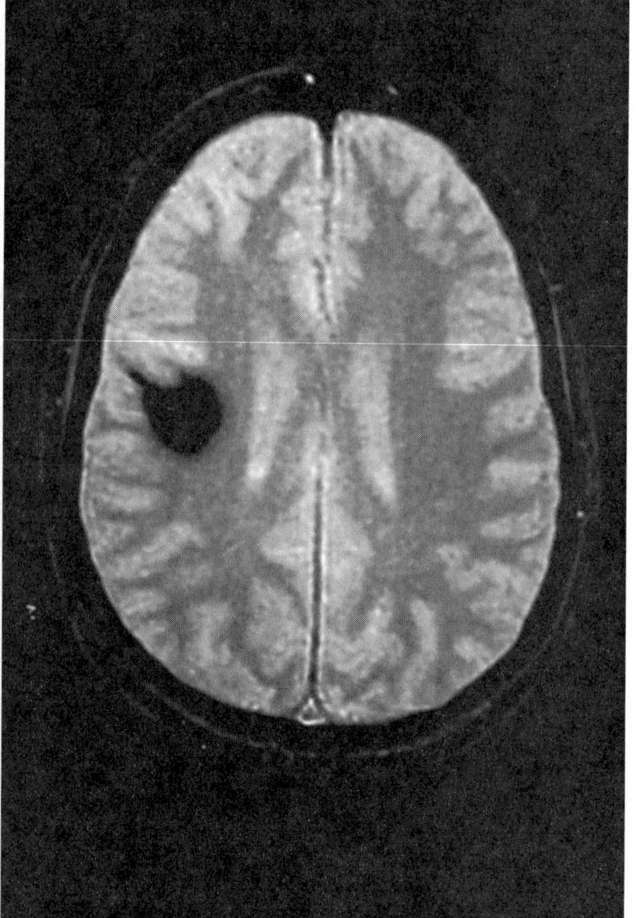

C

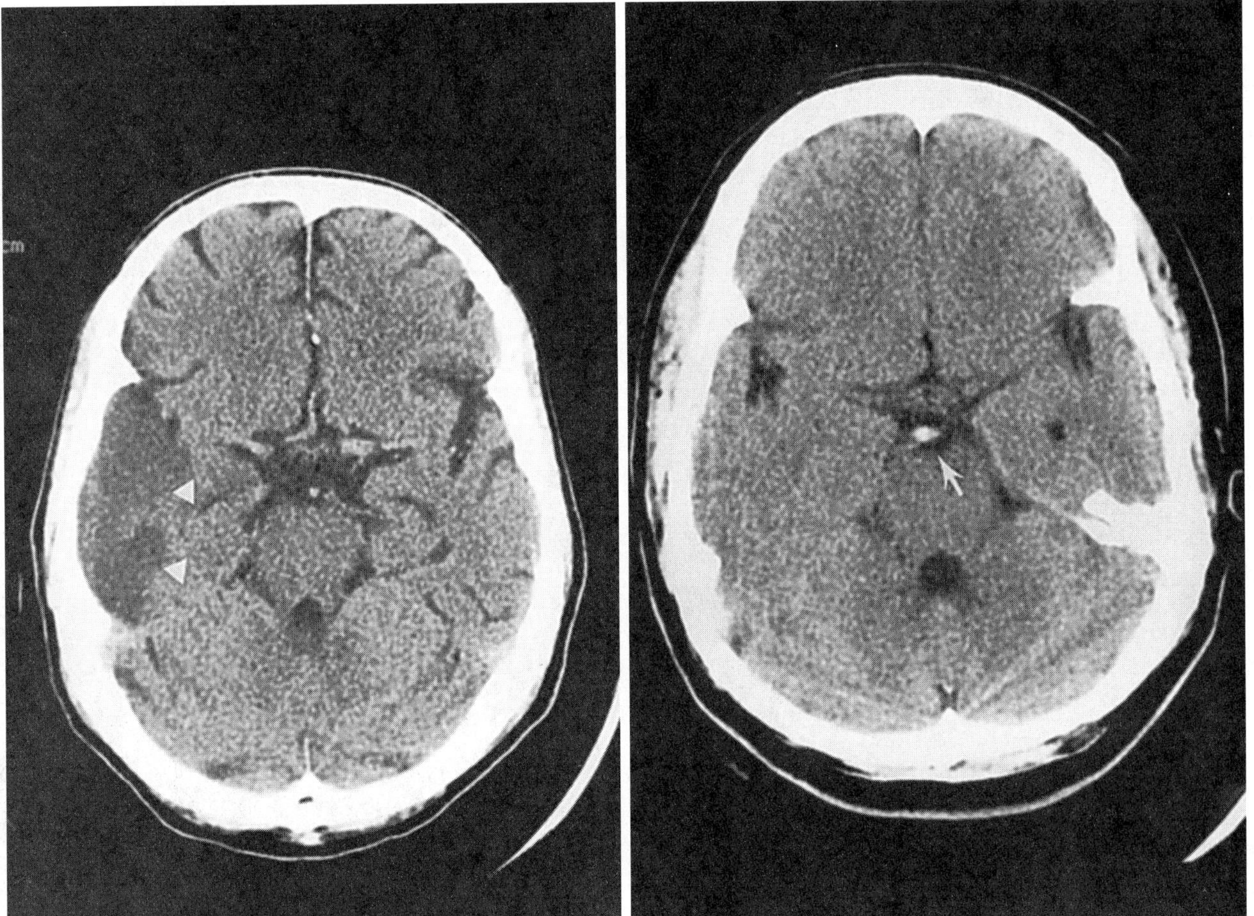

Figure 8-24. Acute ischemic insults on axial CT scans without contrast in two different patients. *A*. Cortical-based hypodensity is seen in the right temporal lobe (*white arrowheads*). *B*. Acute thrombus within the basilar artery 8 hours after the ictus (*solid white arrow*).

AVMs have four components, including an arterial feeder, arterial collaterals, a nidus, and venous outflow. If unruptured and large enough, the nidus can be visualized on an unenhanced CT scan as a tangle of vessels associated with enlarged feeding arteries and enlarged draining veins (Fig. 8-22A). On MRI these components will be seen as serpiginous structures devoid of signal on all MRI sequences (Fig. 8-22B). Cerebral angiography is still the gold standard for precisely delineating the vascular anatomy for both the neurosurgeon and the endovascular therapist. Ruptured AVMs will exhibit different patterns on CT and MRI, depending on the size of the hematoma, the associated mass effect, and the chronologic status of the extravasated blood.

Cavernous angiomas are thin-walled vascular channels separated by septations. Nearly all of them show evidence of acute or chronic hemorrhage. They are often not detected by conventional angiography. If not obscured by the associated hemorrhage, cavernous angiomas on CT scans are usually oval or round foci of moderately increased density without mass effect that exhibit variable degrees of enhancement following injection of contrast material. The complex nature of the hemoglobin degradation products within the lesion on MRI results in areas of high and low signal on T1- and T2-weighted images described as having a "popcorn" appearance. Gradient-echo techniques are helpful in detecting cavernous angiomas due to their greater sensitivity in detecting hemosiderin (Fig. 8-23).

Venous malformations are the result of occlusion or abnormal development of normal medullary veins or their tributaries. They are usually incidental findings but controversy still exists regarding whether they can rupture and lead to intracranial hemorrhage. On CT scans and MRIs, dilated veins are seen converging into an enlarged vein, which then drains peripherally into a venous sinus or into the periventricular region.

Capillary telangiectasias are small malformations composed of dilated capillaries usually located in the pons. Hemorrhage and thrombosis are extremely rare in these otherwise incidental lesions.

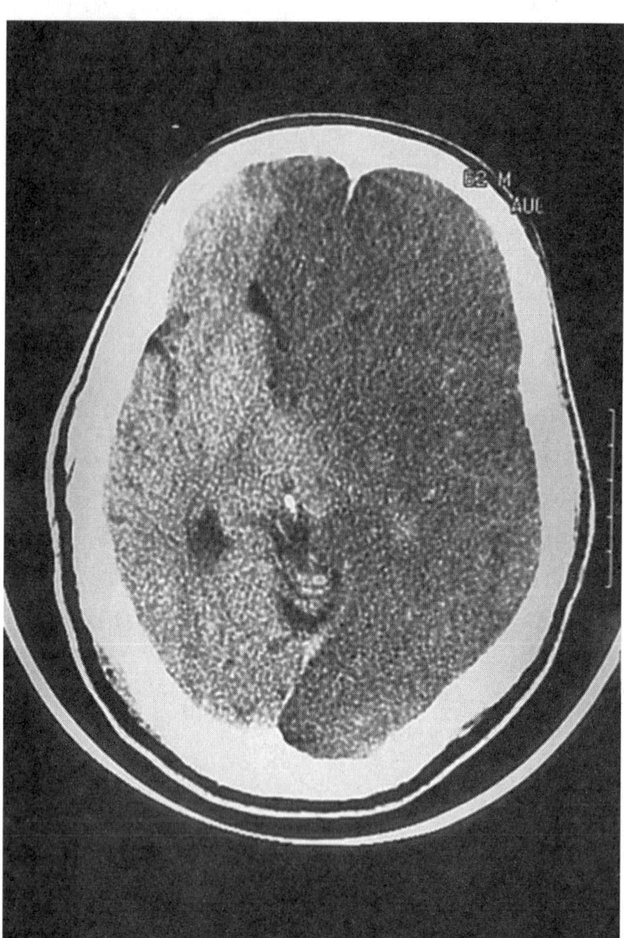

Figure 8-25. Axial CT scan 4 days after acute occlusion of the left internal carotid artery. The left cerebral hemisphere is diffusely hypodense. The mass effect and midline shift are significant, additionally compromising the left posterior cerebral and right anterior cerebral vascular territories.

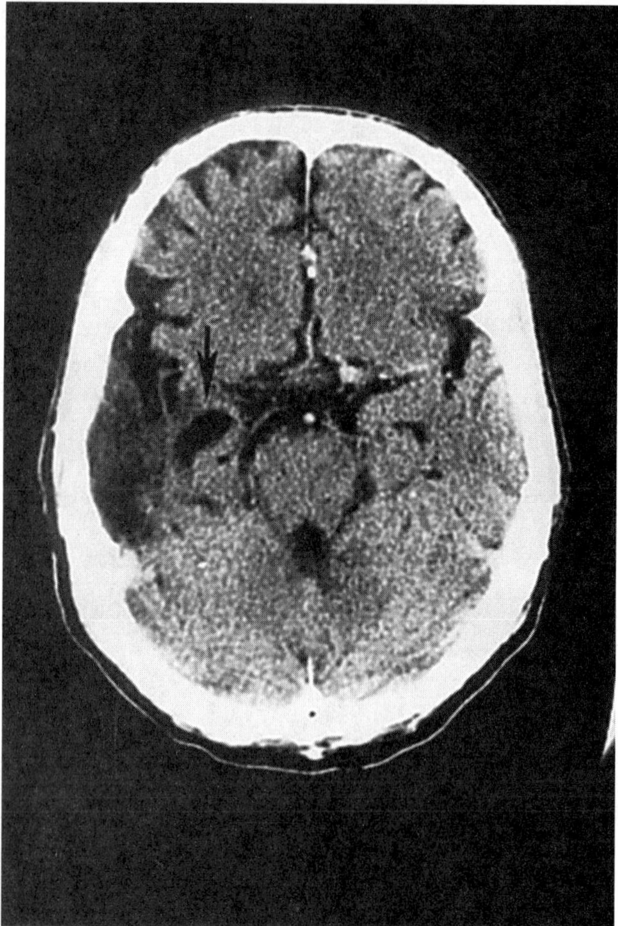

Figure 8-26. Follow-up axial CT scan of the same patient as in Figure 8-11A shows a hypodense area similar in density to cerebrospinal fluid, indicative of an old infarction. Note the compensatory dilatation of the temporal horn of the right lateral ventricle (*solid black arrow*).

Cerebrovascular Disease

The appearance of cortical vascular insults on CT scans and MRIs is dependent on the age and size of the lesion and the occurrence of associated hemorrhage. During the first 24 to 48 hours, small nonhemorrhagic lesions may not be visualized on CT scans. Larger vascular occlusions may produce loss of the gray-white matter interface due to cytotoxic edema (Fig. 8-24A). Occasionally, the acute hyperdense thrombus is identified within the middle cerebral and basilar arteries (Fig. 8-24B). Maximum mass effect associated with large infarcts occurs 3 to 5 days after the ictus. It may lead to vasogenic edema that if extensive enough, may result in herniation and death (Fig. 8-25). As the mass effect subsides, gyriform cortical enhancement on a CT scan with contrast appears in the subacute stage (7–21 days). This is due to reactive hyperemia, neovascular processes, and luxury perfusion. In the chronic stage (>3 weeks), atrophy and cystic changes are seen, representing the healing process of gliosis and liquefaction of dead brain tissue (Fig. 8-26). Enhancement surrounding this area may persist for up to 6 months (77).

MRI is more sensitive than CT in detecting vascular insults, determining their extent, and evaluating for the presence of hemorrhage. Within the first 24 hours, gyral swelling can be detected on T1-weighted MRI and increased gray matter signal, on T2-weighted images. Vascular enhancement can also be seen, indicative of the abnormal accumulation of contrast material in the ischemic or infarcted territory (Fig. 8-27). Following the period of maximum mass effect (3–5 days), gyriform parenchymal enhancement begins as part of the reparative process. During the subacute phase (4–21 days), parenchymal signal abnormalities become more obvious on T1- (hypointense) and T2-weighted images (hyperintense). Radiographic resolution proceeds thereafter, manifested by a decrease in the degree of enhancement and mass effect. Parenchymal loss, ventricular enlargement, and atrophy are seen in the chronic stage (78,79). If hemorrhage is

A

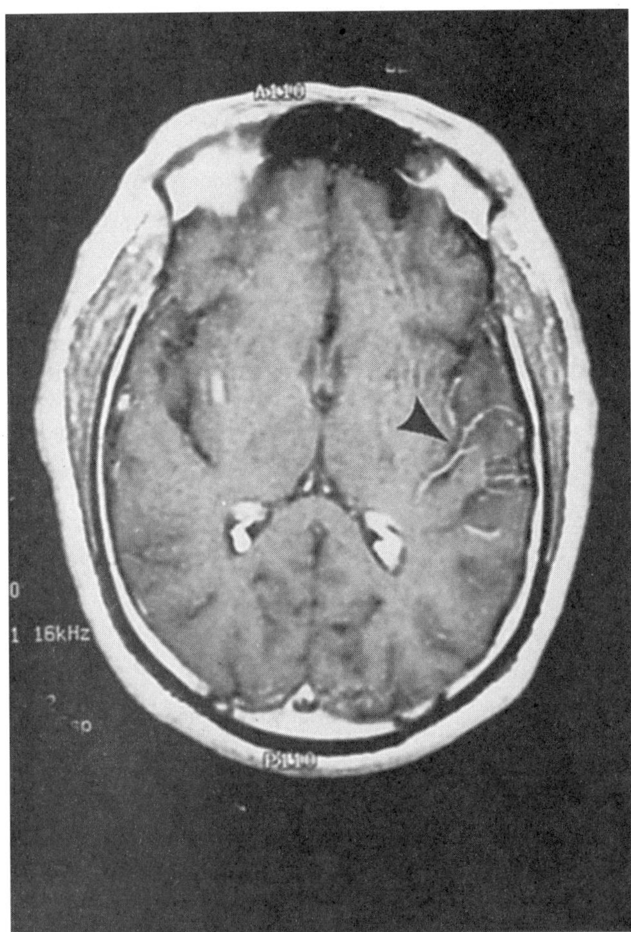

B

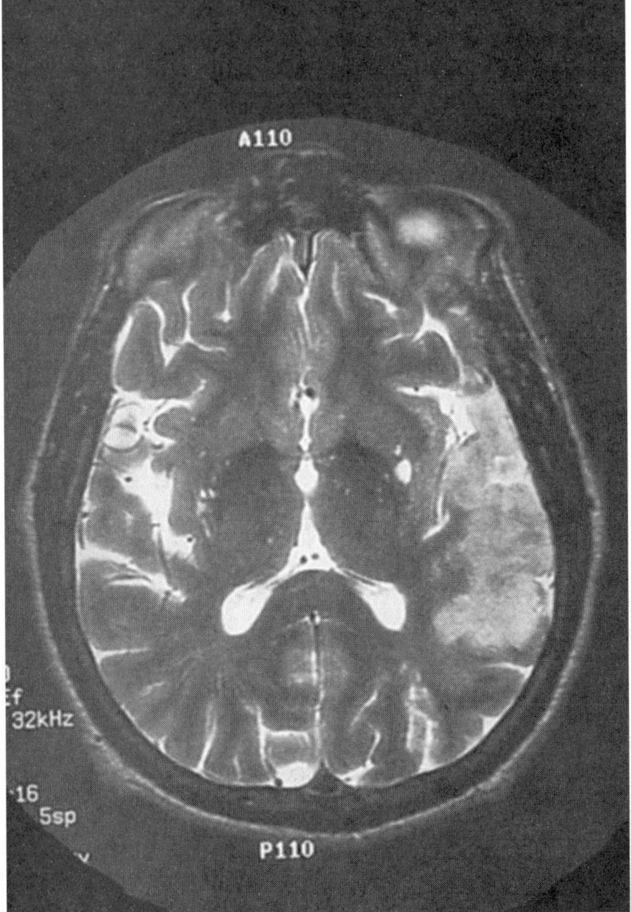

Figure 8-27. Acute ischemic insult on MRI. *A.* Postcontrast axial T1-weighted image shows stagnation of contrast material in the left sylvian fissure (*solid arrowhead*). *B.* Axial T2-weighted image in the same patient demonstrates increased signal in the underlying temporal lobe.

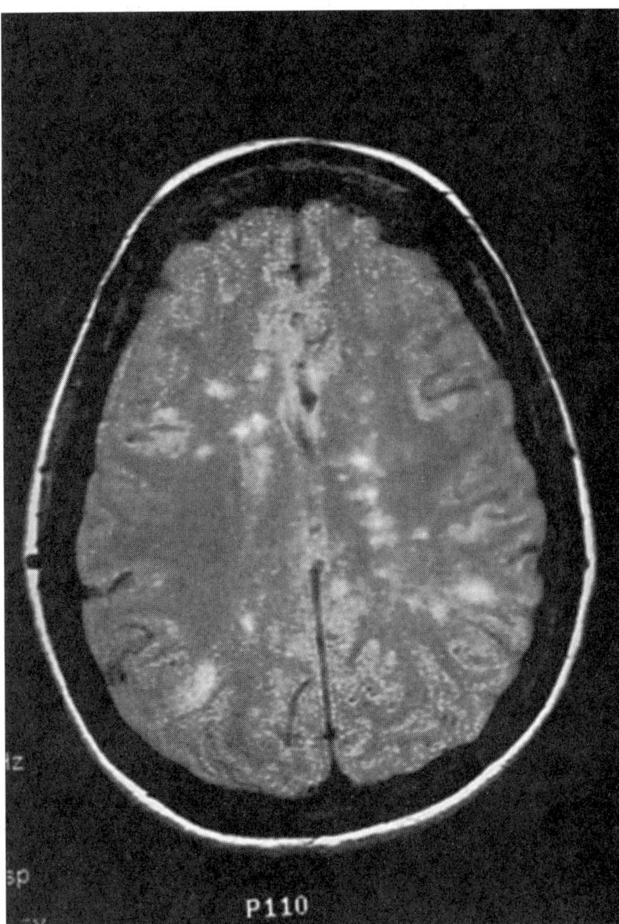

Figure 8-28. Non-contrast-enhanced axial spin density image demonstrates foci of increased signal predominantly in the periventricular white matter. This pattern is strongly suspicious for multiple sclerosis.

present, MRI will display the same signal changes as seen with traumatic injuries, owing to the presence of hemoglobin degradation products.

Lacunar lesions are round or oval insults located in regions of the brain supplied by small penetrating arterioles. These generally occur in the basal ganglia, deep white matter, thalamus, and brain stem. In the acute setting the CT scan may appear normal. In later stages it may show small focal areas of decreased density. MRI is more sensitive than CT in the detection of these insults. Findings on MRI include small foci of decreased intensity on T1- and increased intensity on T2-weighted images.

White Matter Diseases

Diseases of the white matter are divided into dysmyelinating and demyelinating categories. Dysmyelinating disorders refer to the leukodystrophies, in which abnormal myelin is formed as the result of an enzymatic deficiency. In demyelinating diseases, such as multiple sclerosis, normal myelin is slowly destroyed. Demylination can also occur secondary to vascular, infectious, or toxic insults.

MRI is the imaging study of choice for multiple sclerosis. Plaques are detected as oval or elongated foci of increased signal on T2-weighted images and more recently on the new FLAIR sequences, in the periventricular white matter (Fig. 8-28) (80–83). Other locations include the corpus callosum and brain stem. Contrast enhancement can be seen in the acute phase. Occasionally acute lesions may resemble neoplasms or abscesses (80–84).

REFERENCES

1. Kelly WM, Paglen PG, Pearson JA, et al. Ferromagnetism of intraocular foreign body causes unilateral blindness after MR study. *AJNR* 1986;7:243–245.
2. Williams S, Char DH, Dillon WP, et al. Ferrous intraocular foreign bodies and magnetic resonanace imaging. *Am J Ophthalmol* 1988;105:398–401.
3. Modic MT, Pavlicek W, Weinstein MA, et al. Magnetic resonance imaging of intervertebral disk disease: clinical and pulse sequence considerations. *Radiology* 1984;152:103–111.
4. Pathria MN, Petersilge CA. Spinal trauma. *Radiol Clin North Am* 1991;29:847–865.
5. Shellock FG, Morisoli S, Kanal E. MR procedures and biomedical implants, materials, and devices: 1993 update. *Radiology* 1993; 189:587–599.
6. Pavlicek W, Geisinger M, Castle L, et al. The effects of nuclear magnetic resonance on patients with cardiac pacemakers. *Radiology* 1983;147:149–153.
7. Shellock FG, Kanal E, SMRI Safety Committee. Policies, guidelines, and recommendations for MR imaging safety and patient management. *J Magn Reson Imaging* 1991;1:97–101.
8. Klucznik RP, Carrier DA, Pyka R, Haid RW. Placement of a ferromagnetic intracerebral aneurysm clip in a magnetic field with a fatal outcome. *Radiology* 1993;187: 855–856.
9. Kanal E, Shellock FG, Lewin JS. Aneurysm clip testing for ferromagnetic properties: clip variability issues. *Radiology* 1996;200:576–578.
10. Atlas SW, Sheppard L, Goldberg HI, et al. Intracranial aneurysms: detection and characterization with MR angiography with use of an advanced postprocessing technique in a blinded-reader study. *Radiology* 1997;203:807–814.
11. Derdeyn CP, Powers WJ, Moran CJ, et al. Role of Doppler US in screening for carotid atherosclerotic disease. *Radiology* 1995;197:635–643.
12. North American Symptomatic Carotid Endarterectomy Trial Collaborators. Beneficial effect of carotid endarterectomy in symptomatic patients with high-grade carotid stenosis. *N Engl J Med* 1991;325:445–453.
13. Executive Committee for the Asymptomatic Carotid Atherosclerosis Study. Endarterectomy for asymptomatic carotid artery stenosis. *JAMA* 1995;273: 1421–1428.
14. Davies KN, Humphrey PR. Complications of cerebral angiography in patients with symptomatic carotid territory ischaemia screened by carotid ultrasound. *J Neurol Neurosurg Psychiatry* 1993;56:967–972.
15. Srinivasan J, Mayberg MR, Weiss DG, Eskridge J. Duplex accuracy compared with angiography in the Veterans Affairs Cooperative Studies Trial for Symptomatic Carotid Stenosis. *Neurosurgery* 1995;36:648–653.
16. Howard G, Chambless LE, Baker WH, et al. A multicenter validation study of Doppler ultrasound versus angiography. *J Stroke Cerebrovasc Dis* 1991;1:166–173.
17. Waugh JR, Sacharias N. Arteriographic complications in the DSA era. *Radiology* 1992;182:243–246.
18. Heiserman JE, Dean BL, Hodak JA, et al. Neurologic complications of cerebral angiography. *AJNR* 1994;15:1401–1407.
19. Raghavendra BN, Epstein FJ, McCleary L. Intramedullary spinal cord tumors in children: localization by intraoperative sonography. *AJNR* 1984;5:395–397.
20. Knake JE, Chandler WF, McGillicuddy JE, et al. Intraoperative sonography of intraspinal tumors:

initial experience. *AJNR* 1983;4:1199–1201.

21. Quencer RM, Morse BMM, Green BA, et al. Intraoperative spinal sonography: adjunct to metrizamide CT in the assessment and surgical decompression of posttraumatic spinal cord cysts. *AJNR* 1984;5:71–79.

22. Gebarski SS, Maynard FW, Gabrielsen TO, et al. Posttraumatic progressive myelopathy: clinical and radiologic correlation employing MR imaging, delayed CT metrizamide myelography, and intraoperative sonography. *Radiology* 1985;157:379–385.

23. Braun IF, Raghavendra BN, Kricheff II. Spinal cord imaging using real-time high resolution ultrasound. *Radiology* 1983;147: 459–465.

24. Lebwohl NH. Diskography for the diagnosis of radiculopathy without nerve root compression. *AJNR* 1995;16:1614–1615.

25. Milette PC, Fontaine S, Lepanto L, Breton G. Radiating pain to the lower extremities caused by lumbar disk rupture without spinal nerve root involvement. *AJNR* 1995; 16:1605–1613.

26. The Executive Committee of the North American Spine Society. Position statement on discography. *Spine* 1988;13:1343.

27. Barnwell SL. Interventional neuroradiology. *West J Med* 1993; 158:162–170.

28. Dory MA. Arthrography of the lumbar facet joints. *Radiology* 1981;140:23–27.

29. Carrera GF. Lumbar facet joint injection in low back pain and sciatica: preliminary results. *Radiology* 1980;137:665–667.

30. Reid DC, Henderson R, Saboe L, Miller JDR. Etiology and clinical course of missed spine fractures. *J Trauma* 1987;27: 980–986.

31. Davis JW, Phreaner DL, Hoyt DB, Mackersie RC. The etiology of missed cervical spine injuries. *J Trauma* 1993;34:342–346.

32. El-Khoury GY, Kathol MH, Daniel WW. Imaging of acute injuries of the cervical spine: value of plain radiography, CT, and MR imaging. *AJR* 1995;164:43–50.

33. Pech P, Kilgore DP, Pojunas KW, Haughton VM. Cervical spinal fractures: CT detection. *Radiology* 1985;157:117–120.

34. Denis F. The three-column spine and its significance in the classification of acute thoracolumbar spinal injuries. *Spine* 1983;8: 817–831.

35. Daffner RH. Vertebral stability and instability. In: Daffner RH. *Imaging of vertebral trauma*. Philadelphia: Lippincott–Raven, 1996:223–236.

36. Kliewer MA, Gray L, Paver J, et al. Acute spinal ligament disruption: MR imaging with anatomic correlation. *Magn Reson Imaging* 1993;3:855–861.

37. Yeakley JW, Harris JH Jr. Imaging of spinal fusions. In: Cotler JM, Cotler HB, eds. *Spinal fusion: science and technique*. New York: Springer-Verlag, 1990:335–347.

38. Flanders AE, Schaefer DM, Doan HT, et al. Acute cervical spine trauma: correlation of MR imaging findings with degree of neurologic deficit. *Radiology* 1990; 177: 25–33.

39. Silberstein M, Tress BM, Hennessy O. Prediction of neurologic outcome in acute spinal cord injury: the role of CT and MR. *AJNR* 1992;18:1597–1608.

40. Flanders AE, Spettell CM, Tartaglino LM, et al. Forecasting motor recovery after cervical spinal cord injury: value of MR imaging. *Radiology* 1996;201:649–655.

41. Karasick D. Anterior cervical spine fusion: struts, plugs, and plates. *Skel Radiol* 1993;22:85–94.

42. Asano M, Fujiwara K, Yonenobu K, Hiroshima K. Post-traumatic syringomyelia. *Spine* 1996;21: 1446–1453.

43. Fischer G, Brotchi J. Results. In: Fischer G, Brotchi J. *Intramedullary spinal cord tumors*. New York: Thieme, 1996:85–104.

44. Czervionke LF. Lumbar intervertebral disc disease. *Neuroimaging Clin N Am* 1993;3:465–485.

45. Takahashi M, Shimomura O, Sakae T. Comparison of magnetic resonance imaging with myelography and computed tomography-myelography in the diagnosis of lumbar disc herniation. *Neuroimaging Clin N Am* 1993;3:487–498.

46. Masaryk TJ, Ross JS, Modic MT, et al. High-resolution MR imaging of sequestered lumbar intervertebral disks. *AJNR* 1988;9:351–358.

47. Duncan AW, Kido DK. Serpentine cauda equina nerve roots. *Radiology* 1981;139:109–111.

48. Hacker DA, Latchaw RE, Yock DH Jr, et al. Redundant lumbar nerve root syndrome: myelographic features. *Radiology* 1982;143: 457–461.

49. Rothman SLG, Glenn WV Jr, Kerber CW. Postoperative fractures of lumbar articular facets: occult cause of radiculopathy. *AJR* 1985;145:779–784.

50. Bundschuh CV. Imaging of the postoperative lumbosacral spine. *Neuroimaging Clin N Am* 1993;3:499–516.

51. Rauch RA, Jinkins JR. Lumbosacral spondylolisthesis associated with spondylolysis. *Neuroimaging Clin N Am* 1993; 3:543–555.

52. Cohen WA, Hayman LA. Computed tomography of intracranial hemorrhage. *Neuroimaging Clin N Am* 1992;2:75–87.

53. Bradley WG. MRI of intracranial hemorrhage. *Radiology* 1993;189: 15.

54. Zimmerman RD, Heier LA, Snow RB, et al. Acute intracranial hemorrhage: intensity changes on sequential MR scans at 0.5T. *AJNR* 1988;9:47–57.

55. Gomori JM, Grossman RI. Mechanisms responsible for the MRI appearance and evolution of intracranial hemorrhage. *Radiographics* 1988;8:427–440.

56. Hardy PA, Kucharczyk E, Henkelman RM. Cause of signal loss in

MRI images of old hemorrhagic lesions. *Radiology* 1990;174: 549–555.

57. Hayman LA, Taber KH, Ford JJ, Bryan RN. Mechanisms of MR signal alteration by acute intracerebral blood: old concepts and new theories. *AJNR* 1991;12:899–907.

58. Cornelius RS, et al. Traumatic intracranial hemorrhage. *Neuroimaging Clin N Am* 1991; 1:433–441.

59. Diaz-Marchan PJ, et al. Computed tomography of closed head trauma. In: Narayan RK, Wilberger JE, Povlishock JT, eds. *Neurotrauma.* McGraw Hill, 1996:137–149.

60. Gentry LR. Primary neuronal injuries. *Neuroimaging Clin N Am* 1991;1:411–432.

61. Gentry LR, et al. Traumatic brain stem injury. MR imaging. *Radiology* 1989;171:177–187.

62. Sackett J. Overview of diagnostic imaging and classification of intracranial injuries. *Neuroimaging Clin N Am* 1991;1:381–386.

63. Atlas SW. MR imaging is highly sensitive for acute subarachnoid hemorrhage ... not! *Radiology* 1993;186:319.

64. Ogawa T, et al. MR imaging is highly sensitive for acute subarachnoid hemorrhage ... not! Reply. *Radiology* 1993;186:323.

65. Osborn AG. Secondary effects of intracranial trauma. *Neuroimaging Clin N Am* 1991;1:461–474.

66. Bird CR, Drayer BP, Gilles FH. Pathophysiology of "reverse" edema in global cerebral ischemia. *AJNR* 1989;10:95–98.

67. Lobato RD, Sarabia R, Cordobes F, et al. Posttraumatic brain swelling. *J Neurosurg* 1988;68:417–423.

68. Hayman LA, Taber KH, eds. Non traumatic intracranial hemorrhage. *Neuroimaging Clin N Am* 1992; 2:1–250.

69. Gokaslan ZL, Narayan RK. Intracranial hemorrhage in the hypertensive patient. *Neuroimaging Clin N Am* 1992;2:171–186.

70. Osborn AG. Intracranial aneurysms. In: Osborn AG. *Diagnostic neuroradiology.* St Louis: Mosby–Year Book, 1991:248–281.

71. Wilcock DJ, Jaspan T, Holland I, et al. Comparison of magnetic resonance angiography with conventional angiography in the detection of intracranial aneurysms in patients presenting with subarachnoid hemorrhage. *Clin Radiol* 1996;51:330.

72. Ronkainen A, et al. Intracranial aneurysms: MR angiographic screening in 400 asymptomatic individuals with increased family risk. *Radiology* 1995;195:35.

73. Wilms G, Guffins M, Gyspeerdts, et al. Spiral CT of intracranial aneurysms: correlation with digital subtraction and magnetic resonance angiography. *Neuroradiology* 1996;38:320.

74. Hope JKA, Wilson JL, Thomson FJ. Three dimensional CT angiography in the detection and characterization of intracranial berry aneurysms. *AJNR* 1996;17:439.

75. Osborn AG. Intracranial vascular malformations. In: Osborn AG. *Diagnostic neuroradiology.* St. Louis: Mosby–Year Book, 1991:284–329.

76. Hoang T, Hasso AN. Intracranial vascular malformations. *Neuroimaging Clin N Am* 1994;4: 823–847.

77. Weintergarten K. Computed tomography of cerebral infarction. *Neuroimaging Clin N Am* 1992;2: 409–419.

78. Crain MR, Yuh WTC, Greene GM, et al. Cerebral ischemia: evaluation with contrast enhanced MR imaging. *AJNR* 1991;12:631–639.

79. Yuh WTC, Crain MR. Magnetic resonance imaging of acute cerebral ischemia. *Neuroimaging Clin N Am* 1992;2:421–439.

80. Simon JH. Neuroimaging of multiple sclerosis. *Neuroimaging Clin N Am* 1993;3:229–246.

81. Horowitz AL, Kaplan ED, Grewe G, et al. The ovoid lesion: a new MR observation in patients with multiple sclerosis. *AJNR* 1989;10: 303–305.

82. Gean-Marton AD, Vezina LG, Marton KI, et al. Abnormal corpus callosum: a sensitive and specific indicator of multiple sclerosis. *Radiology* 1991;180:215–221.

83. Rovaris M, et al. Sensitivity and reproducibility of fast FLAIR, FSE and Tgse sequences for the MRI assessment of brain lesion load in multiple sclerosis: a preliminary study. *J Neuroimaging* 1997;7: 98–102.

84. Dagher AP, Smirniotopoulus J. Tumefactive demyelinating lesions. *Neuroradiology* 1996;38:560–565.

Chapter 9

Clinical Neurophysiology of the Peripheral Nervous System: Electromyography and Nerve Conduction Studies

Gary Goldberg
C. R. Sridhara

Neurophysiologic assessment of the peripheral nervous system is an important component of the complete evaluation of the patient with suspected neuromuscular impairment and related disability. The neurophysiologic evaluation provides objective information about the diagnosis; localization, nature, and severity of the pathology; prognosis; and effectiveness of treatment. The chapter reviews the basic principles involved in the neurophysiologic evaluation of the peripheral nervous system, briefly examines some technical issues involved in recording neurophysiologic signals from the intact human subject, and reviews the principles and methods involved in performing nerve conduction studies (NCSs) and electromyography (EMG) and in interpreting the results. The approach taken is to emphasize an understanding of an underlying conceptual framework and basic principles rather than to provide all the details the reader will require to successfully perform electrodiagnostic studies in clinical practice. Some specific recommendations for recording and interpretation of potentials are included. For a comprehensive examination of the details, the interested reader is referred to some of the excellent specialized textbooks (1–22), book chapters (23–31), and journal articles (32–34) that deal specifically with various aspects of electrodiagnostic medicine. Textbooks that present principles of electrodiagnostic medicine through detailed reviews of actual cases are especially instructive (16,20). Additional books (35–43) and review articles (44–50) that deal with various aspects of pertinent basic neuroscience provide background information relevant to clinical neuromuscular physiology. References that address conditions of the peripheral nerve (51–53), muscle (54,55), and nerve injuries and their repair (56–60) should also be consulted for supplementary information related to these specific pathologies affecting the motor unit. Another excellent educational resource is the American Association of Electrodiagnostic Medicine (AAEM), which maintains a large inventory of printed materials as well as instructional videotapes. The educational catalog is available directly from the AAEM (421 First Avenue S. W., Suite 300 East, Rochester, MN 55902) or on the World Wide Web (http://www.aaem.net/). Furthermore, nothing can substitute for direct supervision and instruction by a knowledgeable electrodiagnostician in the context of an apprenticeship in electrodiagnostic medicine, either during residency training or during a fellowship.

BASIC PRINCIPLES

Neuromuscular signals are products of rapid, controlled changes in the difference in electrical potential across nerve and muscle cell membranes. These membranes are lipid bilayers about 6 to 8 nm thick that serve as water seals and form critical boundaries between the inside and the outside of the cell. The nerve cell membrane is referred to as the *neurolemma* while the muscle cell membrane is referred to as the *sarcolemma*. Rapid changes in transmembrane potential are made possible through the action of *ion channels* allow-

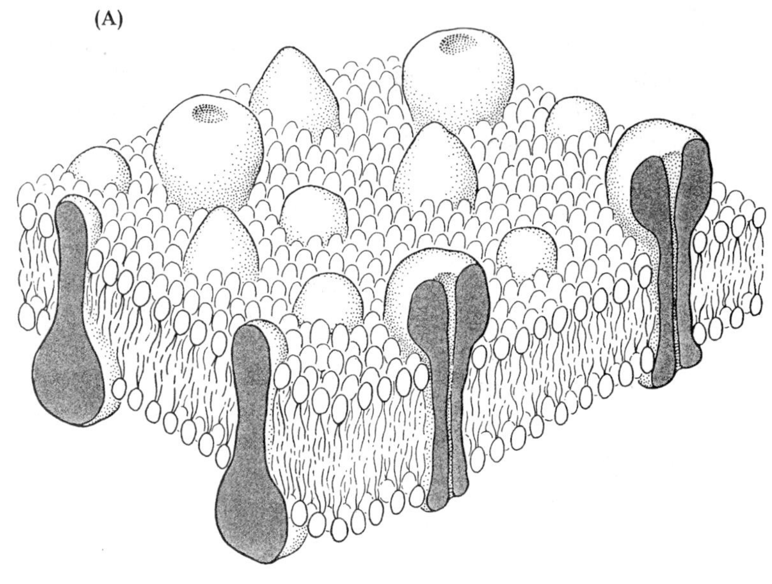

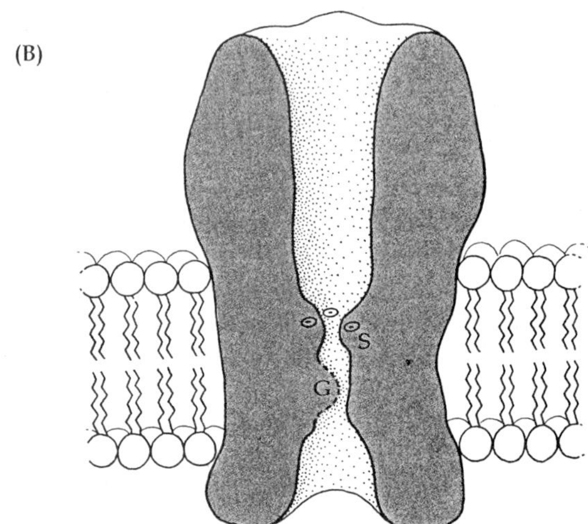

Figure 9-1. Illustration of the cellular membrane and cross-section of an ion channel. *A.* The cell membrane is composed of a lipid bilayer in which a large variety of proteins are embedded. Some of these proteins traverse the membrane and serve as conduits through the membrane for the controlled passage of specific substances. *B.* Schematic diagram of an ion channel with a water-filled inner pore, selectivity filter (S), and channel gate (G). The filter restricts the ion flow to certain ion species according to charge and size. The gate has a probability of opening that may be responsive to transmembrane potential (as in the voltage-dependent channels), the binding of a particular transmitter at a receptor site at the outer end of the channel (as in the acetylcholine-dependent channel in the postsynaptic membrane of the neuromuscular junction), or some other specific condition. (Reproduced by permission from Nicholls JG, Martin AR, Wallace BG. *From neuron to brain. A cellular and molecular approach to the function of the nervous system.* Sunderland, MA: Sinauer Associates, 1992:30.)

ing controlled movement of hydrated ions in and out of the cell. The ion channels are a class of proteins embedded in the lipid bilayer of the cell membrane that serve as ion-conducting pores traversing the membrane (Fig. 9-1). Different ion channels are selective for different ion species. These "channel proteins" may undergo conformational changes under specific triggering circumstances that can then alter their likelihood of allowing different ion species to pass through the membrane. The process whereby the ion channel dynamically changes its ability to pass ions through the membrane is called *gating*. Large ionic currents that flow briefly across cell membranes underlie the rapid changes in transmembrane potential. Such changes are necessary for development of the action potential (AP) and the wave-like transmission of the AP along the length of the membrane. It is this phenomenon of controlled transient changes in transmembrane ionic conductance mediated by dynamic transformation of ionic channel proteins that underlies neuromuscular signaling. Therefore, a great deal of attention in basic cellular neurobiology has focused on the molecular structure and genetics of channel proteins (45,46).

Two types of forces acting on ions influence their movement or diffusion across membranes and through the intracellular and extracellular spaces:

1. Chemical/thermodynamic forces causing ions to diffuse from areas of high concentration toward areas of low concentration (i.e., along a chemical concentration gradient)
2. Electromotive forces that push ions from areas in which the net charge concentration is of the same

polarity as that of the ion, toward areas where the net charge concentration is of opposite polarity as that of the ion (e.g., cations, which are positively charged, move from areas of net positive-charge concentration toward areas of net negative- or relatively less positive-charge concentration)

The net effect of these two forces produces an "electrochemical" potential gradient which is the driving force that determines the direction and rate of ionic movement across the membrane. The actual flow of ions of a particular type across the membrane also depends on the membrane conductance for that type, which in turn depends on the relative concentration of ion-specific channels in the membrane.

There is a fundamental asymmetry in the concentration of negatively charged proteins between the inside and the outside of the cell. These proteins, restricted to the inside of the cell, constitute the cell's internal machinery and structure. The concentration asymmetry across the cell membrane creates a concentration gradient for water such that water molecules tend to be driven into the cell. *Osmosis* is the movement of water along its concentration gradient and *osmotic pressure* is the pressure that builds up when water cannot move along its concentration gradient due to the impermeability of the membrane. The pressure that develops when water moves into a closed space because of osmosis and causes it to swell is called *oncotic pressure.* If the cell membrane were completely permeable to water, then water would rush into the cell, increasing the intracellular volume and oncotic pressure until the cell expands to the point of membrane rupture and cellular explosion. If the cell membrane were a complete water seal, then the buildup of osmotic pressure would cause implosion of the cell. The cell must have a way to efficiently deal with this "water problem." Somehow it must allow movement of water in and out of the cell in a controlled manner. It does not deal directly with this problem by pumping water out but instead controls water equilibrium indirectly by controlling the flow of hydrated cations. These cations are primarily sodium (Na) and potassium (K), which have different and controlled membrane permeabilities. Controlling the relative concentrations of different cation types inside and outside the membrane, and controlling the movement of these cations between the inside and outside of the cell, allows the cell to solve the "water problem."

There is a fundamental asymmetry in ionic concentrations across the plasma membrane. The concentration of Na ions inside the cell is much lower than the concentration of Na ions outside the cell, while the concentration of K ions inside the cell is significantly higher than the concentration of K ions outside the cell. This asymmetry is maintained by the fact that the cell membrane is only partially permeable to ions and in its resting state, it is much more permeable to K than it is to Na (about 25–100 times more permeable to K). The asymmetry is also dynamically maintained by the action of the electrogenic "active" Na-K transport pump in the cell membrane that pumps three Na ions out of the cell for every two K ions pumped into the cell. The pump is active and consumes metabolic energy provided by adenosine triphosphate (ATP) in order to move the cations *against* their electrochemical gradients. The Na ion is smaller than the K ion but is more heavily hydrated. More water travels with the Na ion than the K ion. Thus, the cell is able to produce a net movement of water out of the cell and therefore can control water equilibrium, cell volume, and osmotic pressure across the membrane.

The end result of this activity is the net separation of electrical charge across the cell membrane such that the cell, at rest, has an excess of positive charges on the outside of the membrane and an excess of negative charges on the inside of the membrane. The charge separation is maintained by the lipid bilayer of the membrane, which acts as a barrier to the diffusion of both ions and water molecules, giving rise to an electrical potential difference across the membrane: the *resting transmembrane potential.* In most neurons and muscle cells, the fluid inside the cell is about *60 to 90 millivolts (mV) negative* with respect to the fluid outside the cell. However, it is important to recognize that this "resting" potential is actually actively maintained by an energy-dependent mechanism present in the membrane. Any disturbance affecting membrane function can significantly alter the stability of the processes involved in maintaining this baseline transmembrane potential.

In electrical component terms, the overall membrane with the lipid bilayer and penetrating ion channels in parallel between the intracellular and extracellular spaces can be viewed as a "leaky" capacitor, a capacitor formed by the insulating lipid bilayer with a current-passing parallel resistance. Since the density of the channel proteins is relatively low, the capacitor portion of the membrane occupies about 100 times the area of all the ion channels in the membrane combined. The capacitor has the capacity to store charge and acts as a charge reservoir (61,62). Because a capacitor is able to store charge, it is also able to sustain a voltage difference across it. The *capacitance* of a capacitor is a measure of its capacity to store charge and is defined in terms of the amount of charge stored per unit of voltage applied across the capacitor. A capacitor acts as an infinite resistance to a nonvarying (i.e., "direct current" or DC) signal but allows some passage of a varying (i.e., "alternating current" or AC) signal. The impedance (i.e., frequency-dependence resistance) to the passage of the signal varies inversely with the frequency of the signal—that is, the more rapidly the signal varies, the better it is transmitted across the capacitor. The capacitor thus allows high-frequency components of a signal through but blocks low-frequency components of the signal. A shunting capacitance allows only the low-frequency components of the signal to be transmitted beyond the shunt since the higher-frequency components will be shunted away. Thus,

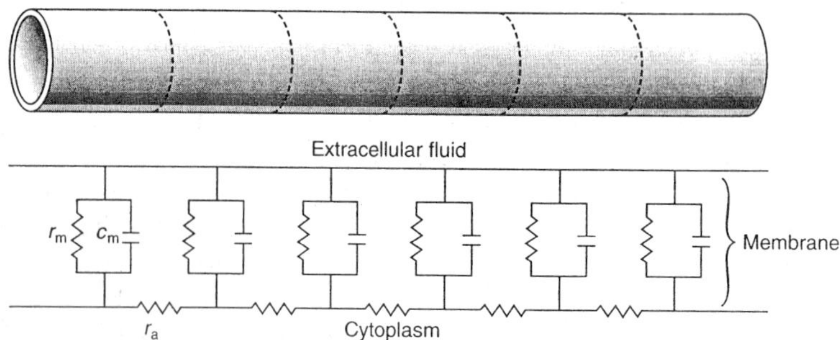

Figure 9-2. Lumped electrical component model of the passive "cable" properties of the axon. Each unit length of the membrane has a resistance (r_m) and a parallel capacitance (c_m) associated with it. These are interconnected by resistors (r_a) which indicate the internal axial resistance associated with the cytoplasm of the axon. (Reproduced by permission from Kandel ER, Schwartz JH, Jessell TM. *Principles of neural science.* 3rd ed. New York: Elsevier, 1991:98.)

the effect of the membrane capacitance is to shunt high-frequency current fluctuations out into the extracellular fluid and to "smooth out" a transient potential that is being transmitted along the length of the membrane. The higher the membrane capacitance, the more the transmitted potential will be slowed down and smoothed out. This is an important point for understanding limits on the rate of transmission of the AP along the membrane. An electrical circuit model of the passive "cable" properties of the axonal membrane is shown in Figure 9-2.

Passive Membrane Properties and Conduction Velocity of the Action Potential

The effect of the membrane capacitance is to slow down the response to a sudden change in current passed along the membrane. If a pulse of current is injected into an axon, the resulting voltage change shows a gradual upward deflection as the membrane capacitance is charged and then a slow downward deflection as the membrane capacitance discharges (Fig. 9-3). The degree to which the change in voltage is slowed down depends on how long it takes to "charge up" the membrane capacitance. This delay is determined by the membrane *time constant*, T_m, which is a product of the membrane resistance, R_m, and the membrane capacitance, C_m.

$$T_m = R_m C_m$$

If a pulse of current is injected into the axon, there is leakage of current out through the membrane down the length of the axon and the voltage is attenuated and actually decays exponentially with distance from the site of stimulation. The current that is injected into the cell can distribute itself either by flowing along the length of the axon against the intracellular resistance to axial conduction of current through the axon, or by flowing out of the axon through the "leaky" cell membrane. Since current will always take the path of least resistance, it will divide according to the ratio of the membrane resistance, R_m, to the internal resistance of the axon, R_a. The voltage produced at the membrane falls off exponentially with dis-

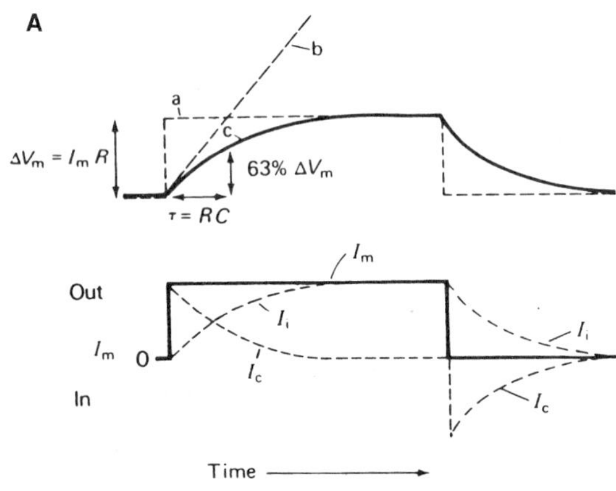

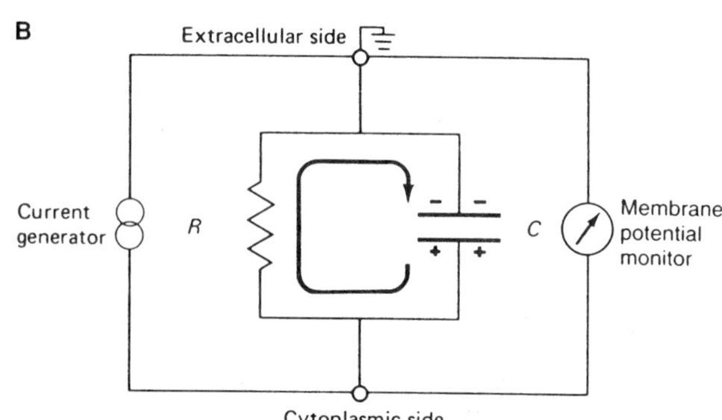

Figure 9-3. Effect of transmembrane capacitance of the rate of development of voltage change across the membrane when a pulse of current is injected across the membrane. Note that the larger the membrane time constant (τ), the longer it takes the voltage to rise. (Reproduced by permission from Kandel ER, Schwartz JH, Jessell TM. *Principles of neural science.* 3rd ed. New York: Elsevier, 1991:98.)

A

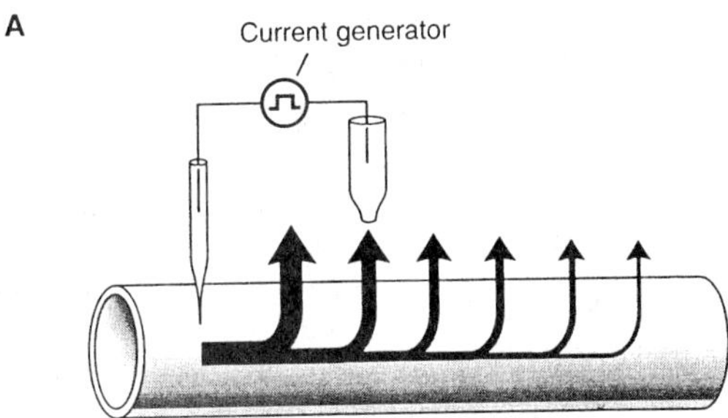

B

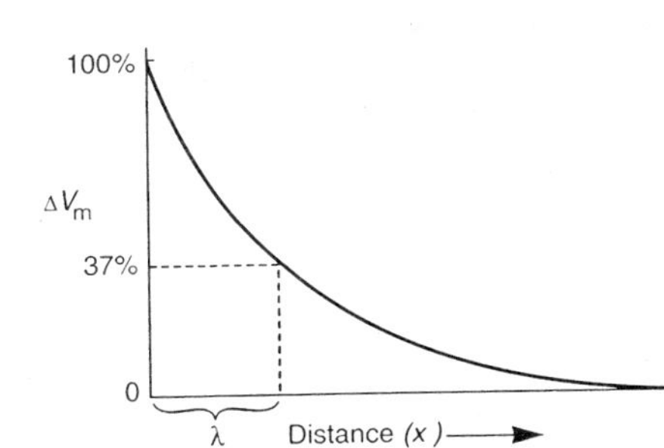

Figure 9-4. Passive transmission of current down the axon when a pulse of intracellular current is applied. Current is injected at one point and then the peak voltage is measured at different points along the length of the axon at increasing distances from the point of current injection. The voltage drops off exponentially the farther away from the point of injection one goes. Note that the larger the length constant (λ), the farther down the axon the current spreads from the site where it is injected. (Reproduced by permission from Kandel ER, Schwartz JH, Jessell TM. *Principles of neural science.* 3rd ed. New York: Elsevier, 1991;99.)

tance from the site of injection and the rate at which it falls with distance is determined by the ratio of R_m to R_a, the square root of which is the *length constant* of the axon or λ (Fig. 9-4).

$$\lambda = \sqrt{(R_m/R_a)}$$

Thus, the higher the membrane resistance, or the lower the internal resistance along the inside of the axon, the less quickly the voltage falls away as one moves away from the site of stimulation and the more efficiently energy is transmitted along the membrane. This passive conduction of current along the length of the axon is extremely important in the conduction of the AP. Once the membrane has been depolarized to the threshold level at any point along the axon, the AP is generated at that site. This activity is conducted in both directions from the site of excitation by local-circuit *passive* current flows called *eddy currents* that result from potential differences between the active region and the immediately adjacent inactive regions. Once the depolarization of the membrane due to the eddy currents in the adjacent region of membrane reaches threshold, it too produces an AP. This activity is then transmitted to its adjacent region by the local-circuit passive flow of current, the cycle repeats itself, and the AP is conducted as a wave-like phenomenon down the length of the membrane. The speed with which excitation of one part of the membrane leads to transmitted excitation and activation of an immediately adjacent piece of membrane determines the speed of conduction of the AP. Conduction speed is limited by delays due to the *passive* properties of the membrane, namely, its resistance, and its capacitance, as well as the axial resistance to current flow. These factors control the pattern and amplitude of the local passive spread of current along the axon and through the membrane.

The ability to excite the axon as well as its ability to conduct an AP rapidly is related to the diameter of the axon. The larger the diameter of the axon, the more cross-sectional area there is for flow of current and the lower the axial resistance to current flow. Since axial resistance to current flow is lower in the larger-diameter axon, the length constant, λ, is larger and the local-circuit current flows show relatively larger currents in the axial direction as compared to the transmembrane direction. This leads to a lower current threshold for stimulation, since a greater amount of current enters the larger axon so it is depolarized more effectively by a given stimulating current than is a smaller axon. The larger axon is said to have a lower "input impedance" and a lower excitatory threshold. Thus, large-diameter axons are generally low-threshold axons. The addition of the myelin sheath layered around the membrane effectively increases membrane resistance, reduces the membrane capacitance, and thus further lowers the excitation current required to activate the axon. The larger-diameter, myelinated axons that have the lowest thresholds therefore are most readily excited by an external stimulus current.

The conduction of the AP down the length of the axon is limited by the rate at which the local-circuit currents carry the activity from the activated region of the membrane to the adjacent inactive region of the membrane (Fig. 9-5). The rate of passive spread of current is determined by the product of the axial resistance, R_a, and the membrane capacitance, C_m. If this product is reduced, then the rate of passive spread of current will increase for a constant R_m and the AP will propagate at higher velocity.

Thus, passive conduction of axial current and therefore the conduction velocity of the AP can be optimized in one of three ways:

1. Reducing the axial resistance, R_a (usually by increasing the diameter and thus the cross-sectional area of the axon)
2. Reducing the membrane capacitance, C_m
3. Increasing the membrane resistance, R_m

Information transmission along a nerve is determined by three different issues: the number of conducting elements (i.e., axons), which determines the number of independent channels of information transmission in the

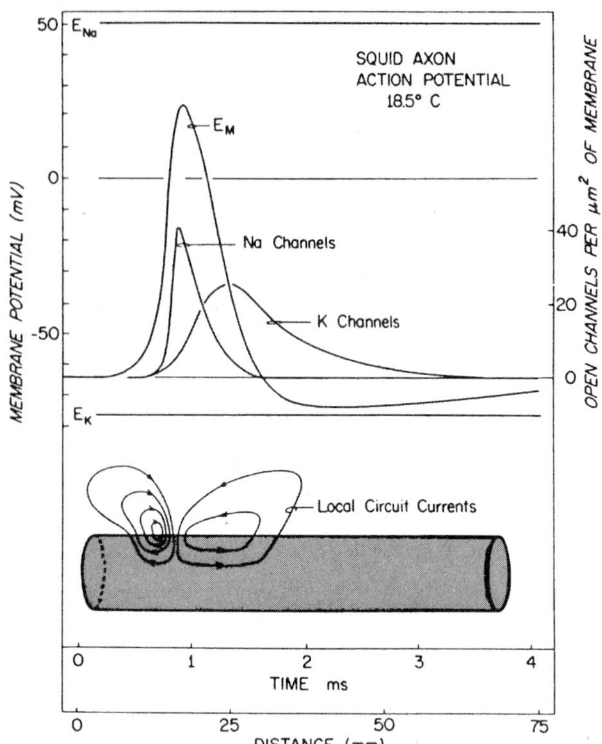

Figure 9-5. Conduction of the action potential (AP) along the giant squid axon by local passive (i.e., subthreshold) current flows. E_M is the transmembrane potential. The Na channels open rapidly but for a brief period of time associated with the rapid rise of E_M. The closure of the Na channels and the delayed opening of the K channels leads to the return of the potential to the resting level. The prolonged duration of opening of the K channels leads to a period after the potential during which the membrane is hyperpolarized and refractory to activation. The local current flows are responsible for the continuous wave-like conduction of the AP. (Reproduced by permission from Hille B. Introduction to the physiology of excitable cells. In: Patton HD, Fuchs AF, Hille B, et al, eds. *Textbook of physiology.* 21st ed. Philadelphia: WB Saunders, 1989:1–80.)

nerve; the speed at which the elements conduct; and the upper frequency of repetitive activation that the axon can sustain. This has obvious functional implications for the organism. Two distinct mechanisms have evolved to attempt to maximize conduction velocity. One strategy that has been used in evolution, especially in invertebrates, is to increase the diameter of the axon. Since the axial resistance decreases in proportion to the square of the axon diameter (i.e., in proportion to the cross-sectional area of the axon) and the membrane capacitance increases in direct proportion to the diameter, the net effect is to decrease the product of R_a and C_m. However, this strategy eventually leads to problems with packing sufficient numbers of axons (i.e., independent channels) into a limited space available for the nerve and increases the metabolic demands required to materially support and maintain such large axons. In turn, these are limited by the distances across which metabolic substrates like oxygen and glucose are able to diffuse from adjacent microcapillaries. Safety factors are limited because important functions must rely on the intact transmission of information along a single large axon (e.g., the squid "giant" axon).

The second mechanism for increasing the conduction velocity is through the process of *myelination.* Myelin is a lipid and thus serves as an electrical insulator. Myelin is formed by a specialized cell called the *Schwann cell.* One Schwann cell is wrapped around each internodal segment of the axon. The effect of adding myelin is to increase the thickness of the axonal membrane by as much as 100 times. The effect of increasing the thickness of the membrane is to decrease its capacitance since the capacitance of a parallel plate capacitor is inversely related to the thickness of the insulator between the plates. Thus, membrane capacitance gets smaller. At the same time, wrapping myelin around the membrane effectively increases the electrical resistance of the membrane. Thus, the leakage of current out through the membrane is reduced and the membrane is effectively "sealed" by the myelin sheath formed by the Schwann cell along the length of the internode.

The myelin, however, does not allow for an adequate flow of current across the membrane to permit the regeneration of the AP and the amplitude of the AP slowly attenuates along the length of the myelinated internodal segment. For this reason, the myelin is interrupted every 1 to 2 mm by the *nodes of Ranvier,* where there is a short length of exposed membrane in which there is a high density of voltage-gated Na channels to optimize the process of regenerating the AP. The density of voltage-gated Na channels in the nodal membrane is 5000 to 12,000 channels per square micrometer of membrane as compared to 35 to 500 channels per square micrometer of membrane in unmyelinated axons. The AP that is transmitted rapidly along the internode because of the low capacitance of the myelinated membrane slows down as it crosses the relatively high-capacitance unmyelinated node. There is also a brief delay associated with the ion channel activation process that reconstitutes the AP at the node. Thus, the transmission is characterized by bursts of rapid conduction alternating with short intervals of slowed conduction associated with active revival of the AP at the unmyelinated nodes. The axon is thus spatially "digitized" and the process is broken up into component processes of passive transmission along internodal segments of membrane and active regeneration of the AP at the nodes, with the different regions of the axon each optimized for these functions. The AP effectively leaps down the axon from node to node, a process referred to as *saltatory conduction.* At any point in time, the excitation associated with the AP will actually span several contiguous nodes along the fiber.

While myelin has been an important evolutionary innovation and advance, its loss or physical deformation under pathologic conditions can produce a devastating effect on the transmission of APs because *the internodal membrane underneath the myelin sheath does not contain voltage-gated Na channels* and therefore cannot actively conduct the AP (50). As the AP goes from a myelinated region of axon to a demyelinated stretch of axon without voltage-gated Na channels, it encounters a region of high membrane capacitance and low membrane resistance. For this region, the current generated at the node must flow for a longer period of time and the local-circuit current flow does not spread as far because it is flowing into a segment of axon that, because of its low membrane resistance, has a short length constant. These two factors combine to significantly *slow down*, *attenuate*, and in some instances, actually *block* the conduction of the AP. The major effect of myelin disruption is significant slowing of transmission of the AP across the myelin-impaired segment. However, if the amplitude of the depolarization drops down *below the threshold level* by the time the wave of depolarization is passively conducted to the next excitable region of the membrane containing a concentration of voltage-gated Na channels capable of reconstituting the AP (see next section), the AP will *not* regenerate and its conduction will be completely halted at that point. This circumstance is referred to as *conduction block*, and is the most significant functional consequence of myelin disruption.

Generation of the Action Potential

The ability of the membrane to sustain and conduct an AP depends on the opening of voltage-gated Na channels. Some of the properties of voltage-gated Na channels are listed in Table 9-1. The voltage-gated Na channel is a channel whose probability of opening *increases* as the membrane depolarizes. As the membrane becomes depolarized (i.e., less negative internally), more voltage-gated Na channels open and there is increased flow of Na into the cell. This creates a regenerative feedback loop in which flow of Na into the cell leads to further depolarization of the membrane, which opens more voltage-gated Na channels, which allows more Na to flow into the cell, further depolarizing the membrane, and so on. Furthermore, the relationship between Na channel opening and membrane potential is nonlinear. When the membrane has depolarized to the critical threshold level, this process rapidly accelerates, producing an explosive rise in the transmembrane potential from the threshold level up toward the Na equilibrium potential, which is around +55 mV. At the peak of the AP, the membrane is locally much more permeable to Na than it is to either K or chloride (Cl) ions, a complete reversal of the resting situation. However, this sudden local increase in Na permeability is transient; the phenomenon is both spatially and temporally constrained.

Table 9-1: Properties of Voltage-Gated Sodium Channels

1. Relatively low concentration in the membrane (1/100 of area).
2. Large transient Na^+ currents can be passed when channels open with membrane depolarization.
3. Channels are open in an all-or-none fashion. When the channels are open, a pulse of current that is variable in duration but constant in amplitude flows.
4. Voltage-gated potassium, sodium, and calcium channels are encoded in one gene family and may involve a single, voltage-sensitive gating mechanism within the channel proteins.
5. In unmyelinated axons, voltage-gated sodium channels are distributed evenly throughout the membrane with a density of 35–500 channels/μm^2 of membrane area, while in myelinated axons, they are distributed in higher concentrations at the nodes of Ranvier with a density of 5000–12,000 channels/μm^2 of membrane area and are found to be extremely sparse or absent in the internodal membrane underlying the myelin sheath.

There are at least two different processes that bring this explosive rise in transmembrane potential under control and reduce the potential back down to its resting level. First, as the depolarization of the membrane continues, the voltage-gated Na channels begin to *inactivate* or turn off. The second process that helps to control the depolarization and to repolarize the membrane is the delayed opening of voltage-gated K channels. As these channels begin to open, the K efflux increases and together with the decrease in the Na influx associated with the inactivation of the Na channels, produces a net efflux of positive ions from the cell, which continues until the resting membrane potential is reestablished. There is actually a short period of "overshoot" of this repolarizing process during which the membrane is transiently "hyperpolarized" (i.e., becomes more negative internally than the resting membrane potential). This "afterpolarization" is critically important because it produces a short period of postexcitatory inhibition during which the membrane is relatively resistant or refractory to excitation. This then prevents the reexcitation of the membrane, maintains the directional conduction of the AP, and avoids the problem of rapidly repeated "backfiring" of the AP. Of interest in this regard is the fact that the *nodal membrane* at the node of Ranvier in myelinated fibers contains high concentrations of voltage-gated Na channels to support the generation of the AP but does not contain voltage-gated K channels to fully support the repolarization process that restores the resting membrane potential and transiently hyperpolarizes the membrane immediately following the AP (44,49). While the nodal membrane is optimized for the regeneration of the AP, it is also somewhat at risk under pathologic conditions for the generation of ectopic activity and abnormal reexcitation because of a relative lack of postexcitatory refractoriness.

Synaptic Transmission at the Neuromuscular Junction

APs in muscle fibers normally originate at the end-plate, a region of the sarcolemma that is specialized to receive the neurotransmitter acetylcholine (ACh) through a concentration of nicotinic-type ACh receptors (AChRs) on the postsynaptic membrane in the end-plate zone directly across from the presynaptic terminal. As the motor axon approaches the end-plate area, it loses its myelin sheath and splits into several fine branches. These fine branches then form multiple grape-like varicosities called *synaptic boutons*, where transmitter is stored in vesicles and released. The postsynaptic membrane is heavily folded into junctional folds. It is separated from the distal membrane of the presynaptic boutons by an extracellular space called the *synaptic cleft*. In the presynaptic boutons are regions of the presynaptic membrane where the machinery for the release of transmitter is concentrated. These presynaptic *active zones* contain three components: the vesicles in which the ACh is concentrated, membrane specialized for the release of the contents of the vesicles into the synaptic cleft, and voltage-gated calcium (Ca) channels in the outer membrane of the presynaptic terminal. Across the synaptic cleft from the active zones are high concentrations of AChRs at the crests of the junctional folds. The general structure of the neuromuscular junction is shown in Figure 9-6.

Small, incoherent releases of "quanta" of ACh are constantly occurring as vesicles fuse with the presynaptic membrane and their contents are randomly dumped into the synaptic cleft. These small pulses of released ACh arrive at the postsynaptic membrane and activate the AChRs, producing small postsynaptic excitatory potentials called *miniature end-plate potentials* (MEPPs). The amplitude of the MEPP reflects the actual amount of ACh in each quanta. When recorded by an EMG electrode in the muscle, the constant random activity of the MEPPs at the neuromuscular junction can be heard on the loudspeaker as a high-frequency, hissing, "sea-shell" noise.

When an AP travels down the motor fiber and depolarizes the presynaptic terminal, the voltage-sensitive Ca channels in the presynaptic terminal are activated. These channels open up and allow Ca ions to flow into the active zone of the presynaptic terminal. The transiently increased Ca concentration inside the active zone then triggers a large coordinated movement of synaptic vesicles toward the presynaptic membrane. The synaptic vesicles are then absorbed into the presynaptic membrane with synchronized release of their contents into the synaptic cleft. The released Ach then diffuses across the synaptic cleft to the region of the postsynaptic membrane where it activates the high concentration of AChRs on the crests of the junctional folds. The AChRs are coupled to nonselective ion channels traversing the postsynaptic sarcolemma that open when ACh links to the receptor sites. When these pores open, Na ions rush into the cell, depolarizing the membrane, and an excitatory postsynaptic potential is produced, called the *end-plate potential* (EPP). The EPPs can be recorded when an intramuscular EMG electrode is adjacent to the end-plate region. They are identified as short-duration, rapid but irregular discharges often with an initial negative deflection. The EPP is well above the threshold level and large enough to trigger an AP in the muscle fiber.

The amplitude of the EPP reflects the number of quanta that are released in the coherent pulse of ACh coming from the presynaptic terminal. The EPP amplitude can be increased significantly following high-frequency activation of the junction, as would occur when the motor unit is firing rapidly during muscular exercise. This occurs because of a buildup of Ca current into the presynaptic terminal that facilitates the release of greater numbers of quanta associated with each EPP. This transient rise in EPP amplitude, called *posttetanic facilitation*, gradually resolves, with the EPP amplitude returning to baseline over the course of 2 to 3 minutes following less than 10 seconds of *tetanization* (high-frequency activation of the junction). If the period of tetanization of the junction is longer, lasting over a minute, then the posttetanic facilitation is followed by a prolonged period of *reduction* of the EPP amplitude, called *posttetanic depression*, presumably due to an exhaustion of the mobilized and available supply of ACh in the presynaptic terminal. This posttetanic period of reduced EPP amplitude can last for several minutes.

The muscle fiber AP is generated when the currents produced by the opening of the ACh channels are coupled to adjacent voltage-gated Na channels in the sarcolemma surrounding the end-plate region. The end-plates are concentrated in a region of the muscle near the middle, the *motor point*, where the motor nerve enters the muscle. The muscle fiber AP is transmitted from this region in either direction to both ends of the muscle.

The sarcolemma surrounding the muscle fiber has a system of deep invaginations that allows the AP to be conducted down into the depths of the fiber. These tubular penetrations from the surface down into the depths of the fiber are termed the *T tubules*. This system of channels into the midst of the fiber ensures that the excitation on the surface is conducted down into the region within the fiber called the *sarcoplasmic reticulum* (SR) that surrounds the contractile regions. The SR contains a reservoir of Ca ions whose high concentration is maintained when the fiber is at rest by an active metabolic pumping mechanism. The spreading depolarization of the AP conducted into the SR through the T-tubule system releases Ca from the SR into the intracellular space of the sarcomere where the linked contractile proteins, myosin and actin, are located. Ca ions flow into the sarcomere and, together with the presence of ATP, permit the formation of cross-bridges between the actin and myosin filaments and rotation of the myosin

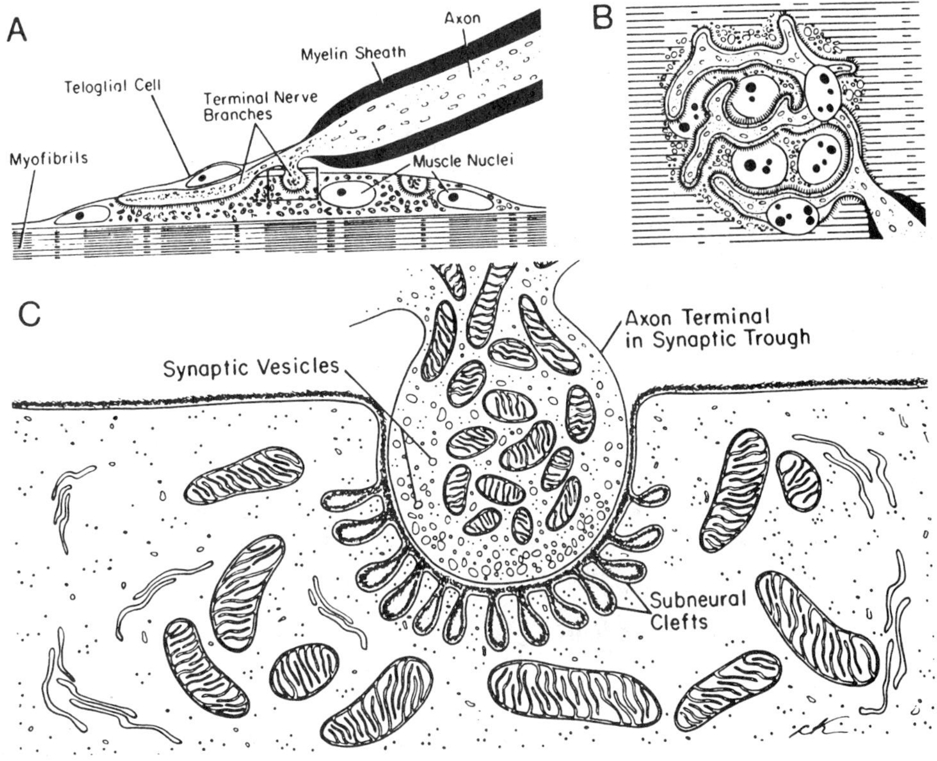

D

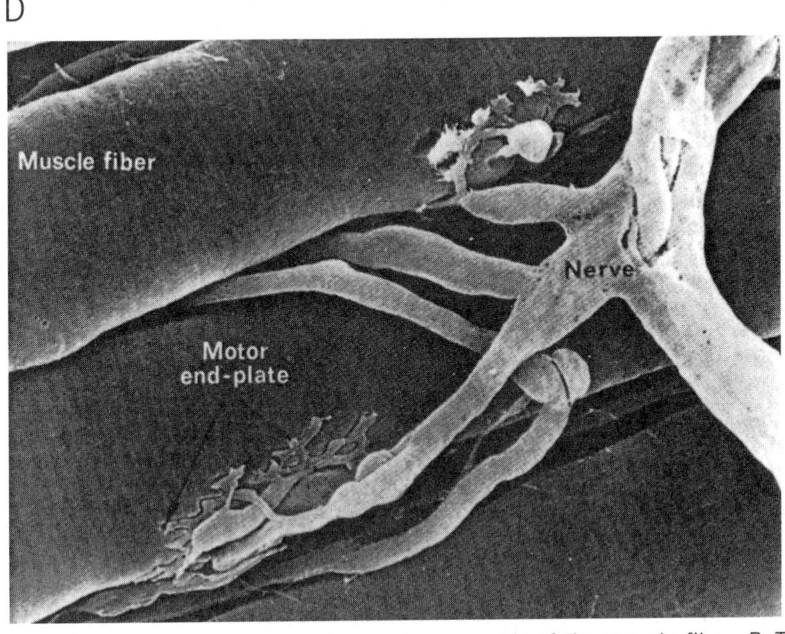

Figure 9-6. *A.* Structure of the neuromuscular junction in the long axis of the muscle fiber. *B.* The surface view looking down from above in the light microscope. *C.* Electron microscope view of a section through the neuromuscular junction in the region shown in the small rectangle in *A.* Note the mitochondria and synaptic vesicles in the axon terminal that lies in the synaptic trough within the muscle. Also note the heavily folded postsynaptic membrane and the multiple subneural clefts. (A–C: Reproduced by permission from Bloom W, Fawcett DW. *A textbook of histology.* 11th ed. Philadelphia: WB Saunders, 1986:290.) *D.* A photomicrograph of the connection between the nerve terminals and the muscle fiber with demonstration of the structure of the neuromuscular junction or "motor end-plate." (Reproduced by permission from Bloom W, Fawcett DW. *A textbook of histology.* 11th ed. Philadelphia: WB Saunders, 1986:291.)

heads (or cross-bridges). This causes the thin actin filaments to move over the thick myosin filaments and toward the center of the sarcomere, thus dynamically reducing the length of the sarcomere. After the myosin head has fully rotated, it dissociates from the actin filament, returns to its original relaxed position, and then reattaches. The cyclical process of attachment, rotation, and detachment of the myosin heads continues as long as Ca and ATP are present in the myofibril in sufficient concentration. During a single twitch, a single cross-bridge may go through the attachment-detachment cycle many times. When the AP depolarization is completed, Ca is pumped back into the SR and out of the sarcomere, and relaxation occurs because cross-bridge attachment can no longer occur. This process, whereby the electrical excitation of the muscle fiber is coupled to the brief contraction of the fiber and the generation of the twitch, is termed *excitation-contraction coupling*. Further details of the sequence of events involved in excitation-contraction coupling are provided in Table 9-2.

Table 9-2: Sequence of Events in Muscular Contraction

Excitation-Contraction Coupling

1. The sarcolemma depolarizes with conduction of muscle fiber action potential.
2. Internal fibers depolarize through transmission along T-tubule system.
3. Ca^{2+} is released from sarcoplasmic reticulum.
4. Ca^{2+} diffuses into sarcomeres.

Contraction

5. Ca^{2+} binds to troponin.
6. Troponin-Ca^{2+} complex removes tropomyosin blockage of actin-binding sites.
7. Myosin heads containing high-energy myosin-ADP-Pi complex attach to actin-binding sites and form cross-bridges between thick and thin filaments.
8. Conformational energy-releasing changes in high-energy myosin heads cause them to swivel, producing relative motion of the thick and thin filaments, releasing ADP and Pi and returning the myosin head to its low-energy state.
9. A new ATP molecule binds to myosin head, allowing release of the head from actin-binding site.
10. The ATP splits to ADP and Pi, producing a high-energy myosin-ADP-Pi complex.
11. Return to step 7 with repeating of cycle of steps 7 through 10 as long as actin-binding sites remain available for attachment.

Relaxation

12. Ca^{2+} is pumped back into sarcoplasmic reticulum.
13. Ca^{2+} around thin filaments diffuses back toward sarcoplasmic reticulum.
14. Ca^{2+} is released from troponin-Ca^{2+} complex.
15. Troponin permits return to tropomyosin to the blocking position.
16. Myosin-actin cross-bridges break with addition of ATP to the myosin head but new cross-bridges cannot form as the actin-binding sites are no longer available due to blocking action of tropomyosin.

Pi = inorganic phosphate.

Volume Conduction and the Extracellular Recording of the Action Potential

The recording of the electrical activity by electrodes placed at a distance from the structure transmitting an AP (e.g., a muscle fiber) is made possible by the induction of currents in the extracellular space through the activation of the physiologic source, a process termed *volume conduction* (63). What is actually recorded at a distance from the source depends on a variety of factors. These factors include the electrical properties of the extracellular fluid, the geometry of the volume conductor (i.e., the structure of the tissue surrounding the physiologic source places "boundary conditions" on the distribution of current induced by the physiologic source), and the position of the recording electrodes with respect to the source. When there are multiple discrete sources active simultaneously in the volume conductor, as with the APs generated by the set of muscle fibers in a single motor unit, the electrode records a linear sum of the potential contributed by each individual source. The currents produced in the volume conductor by each source summate. Thus, there is a process of *temporal summation* whereby there is a summation of the potentials contributed from multiple sources owing to the relative temporal synchrony of their activation, and there is a process of *spatial summation* whereby there is summation of the potentials contributed from multiple sources owing to their relative spatial proximity to the recording electrode (64).

The path through extracellular fluid will have both an electrical resistance and a shunt capacitance. This will produce an attenuation as well as a delay and smoothing (i.e., a relative attenuation of the high-frequency components of the signal) of the recorded waveform as compared to that actually produced at the source itself. This change in the shape of the recorded potential can be identified by carefully listening to the sounds produced by the audio amplifier of the EMG machine. The motor unit action potential (MUAP) that is undistorted, retaining its high-frequency content, will have a loud, sharp, popping, crisp sound. The potential that has been relatively smoothed with attenuation of high-frequency content will have a soft, dull, thudding, muffled sound. This change in sound is heard, for example, when an electrode is moved close to and then away from a motor unit potential source. As the electrode moves in close to "focus" on the active muscle fibers in the normal motor unit, the sound becomes sharper and a crisper "pop" is heard with each contraction of the unit. Visually, the MUAP waveform has a greater amplitude with a shorter rise time and duration. As the electrode moves away from the active muscle fibers in the unit, the sound becomes a duller, muffled "thud" and visually, the MUAP waveform has a lower amplitude, a longer rise time, and a broader duration. These changes are illustrated in Figure 9-7.

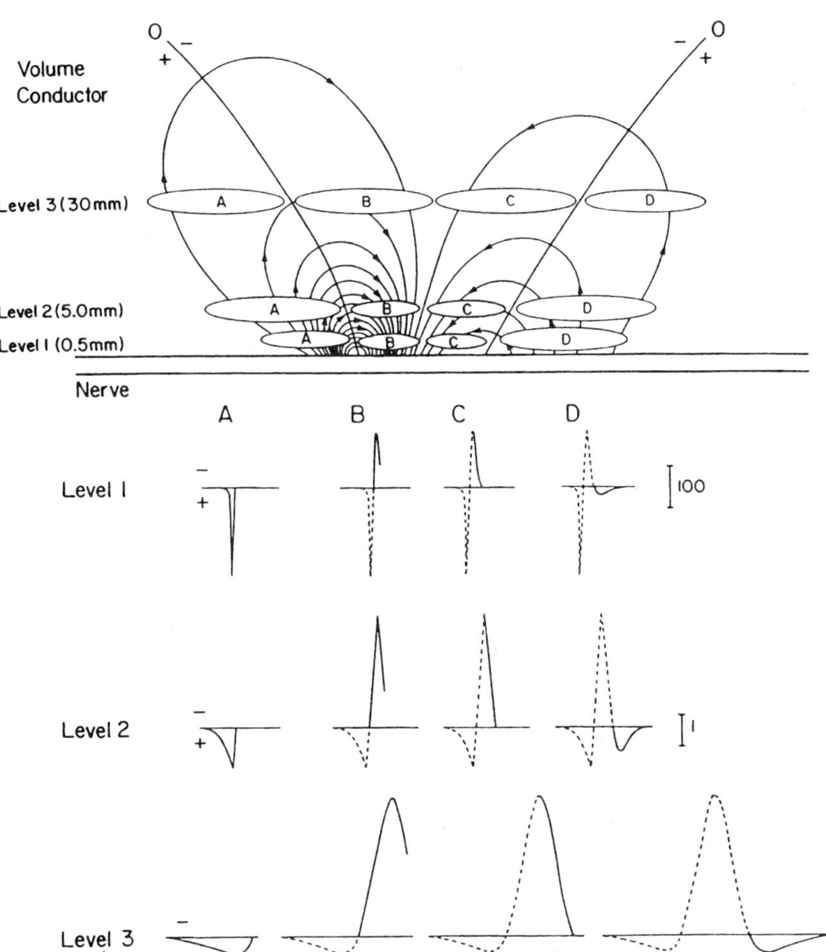

Figure 9-7. Effects of recording an action potential at a distance from the source. Computer-simulated field distribution surrounding an action potential propagation from the right to the left. Waveforms show the effects of recording the potential at increasing distances away from the source in a volume conductor. (Reproduced by permission from Dumitru D. Volume conduction. Theory and application. In: Dumitru D, ed. *Clinical electrophysiology.* Philadelphia: Hanley & Belfus, 1989:665–681.)

The degree of attenuation and distortion of the waveform will be directly related to the distance between the source and the recording electrode. The greater the distance between the electrode and the source, the greater the attenuation and smoothing of the potential. This distance affects the rise time and spike duration of the recorded AP. The closer the electrode is to the contracting fiber, the shorter the rise time, and the louder and sharper the sound associated with the AP on the loudspeaker. The electromyographer can use this change in sound to minimize the rise time and maximize the amplitude of the MUAP by "focusing" on a particular MUAP being recorded from the muscle.

Furthermore, the shape and structure of the AP recorded from an extracellular electrode are related to the pattern of current flows induced in the extracellular fluid at different phases of the AP transmission:

1. When the AP is approaching the electrode position, extracellular current is flowing out of the membrane region adjacent to the electrode and toward the current zone of membrane excitation. The electrode thus sees positive charges flowing toward it and becomes relatively positively charged compared to a distant "neutral" reference point; a positive deflection of the voltage recorded at the electrode is noted.
2. When the AP is directly under the electrode position, a large amount of current is now flowing from the electrode location down into the adjacent zone of membrane excitation where the rapid inward flows of Na ions are occurring. At this point, the electrode sees a flow of positive charges flowing away from it and into the membrane and becomes relatively negatively charged; a large negative deflection of the voltage is recorded at the electrode.
3. When the AP has gone past the electrode position, the slower currents of repolarization of the membrane are occurring as flow of positive charges now occurs from the depolarizing region of membrane out into the zone of membrane excitation, which has now gone down the fiber past the electrode. The electrode thus sees a slower second positive deflection of the voltage recorded.

The AP transmitted down the fiber adjacent to the electrode thus induces a positive-negative-positive *triphasic*

Table 9-3: Elements of the Electrodiagnostic Recording System

Analog Components
1. Electrodes
2. Preamplifier
3. Amplifier
4. Cathode-ray tube display
5. Stimulator
6. Audio amplifier/loudspeaker
7. Calibration circuit
8. Time base/triggering circuitry
9. Front panel controls
10. Footswitch

Elements related to the digital-processing aspects of the system
1. Microprocessor
2. Floating-point processor
3. Read-only memory (ROM)
4. Random-access memory (RAM)
5. Digital storage devices: hard disk, floppy disks, tape drive
6. Keyboard
7. Analog-to-digital converter
8. Printer
9. Software: operating system and instrument system software
10. Front panel display lights
11. System clock
12. Day clock under battery power
13. Control bus
14. Input/output circuits for digital interfacing
15. Control panel
16. Computer monitor

Table 9-4: Advantages of Microprocessor-Based Control of Electrodiagnostic Recording System

1. Complete flexibility in the operation of the instrument by implementing the features of the machine in software
2. Ability to add updates and to modularize the system features
3. Ability to provide flexible displays that include tables of parameters
4. Ability to perform flexible signal processing such as averaging, spectral analysis, interference pattern analysis, etc.
5. Ability to do quantitative EMG analysis, e.g., for motor unit potential assessment
6. Ability to do automatic parameter measurement
7. Ability to integrate flexible report generation capability
8. Ability to store data readily for subsequent analyses and recall
9. Ability to store recording parameters and do automatic setup of recording protocols
10. Ability to do statistical comparisons to normative data

waveform in the extracellular recording electrode. This type of waveform is usually associated with the recording of a fibrillation potential.

Note that if the AP is initiated from a site on the fiber adjacent to the recording electrode (e.g., when the electrode is located over the motor point of the muscle), then the initial phase when the AP is traveling down the fiber from a point distant toward the electrode does not occur and the electrode "sees" an initial negative deflection followed by a positive deflection as the AP moves away: a *negative-positive biphasic* waveform. This waveform structure is usually seen with recording of the EPP and with a normal compound muscle action potential (CMAP), with the active electrode properly placed directly over the motor point of the muscle.

If, for some reason, the AP is transmitted down the fiber toward the electrode but stops conducting at a point prior to the arrival of the AP, the electrode will see an initial positive deflection associated with the phase of conduction of the AP toward it. This position deflection is followed by a slow negative variation and movement back toward the baseline as the currents associated with the conduction of the AP diffuse out into the surrounding region. This occurs as the AP suddenly stops conducting and the eddy currents induced by the AP gradually dissipate through the surrounding volume conductor. This *positive-negative biphasic* structure resembles the waveform seen with recording of the positive sharp wave (PSW).

ELECTRODIAGNOSTIC INSTRUMENTATION

Knowledge of the EMG instrument and the principles of how it works is important for safely obtaining technically acceptable recordings (65–70). The basic elements of the electrodiagnostic recording system are shown in Table 9-3. The various advantages of the digital, microprocessor-based EMG instrument over the analog EMG instrument are listed in Table 9-4.

Electrodes

The electrodes are the critical link in the EMG system. The electrical activity produced by the relevant anatomic structures is transmitted through volume conduction via the patient's body and is converted into an electrical signal. The signal is transmitted to the instrument through the electrodes. The different features of the electrode determine exactly how this transduction occurs and how accurately the physiologic process is captured and represented by the instrument. Various electrode factors affecting the recorded potentials are listed in Table 9-5.

Note that the effects of electrode polarization and increased impedance of the electrode-patient interface (related to poor contact between the patient and the electrode) can lead to highly unstable, large, slow potential

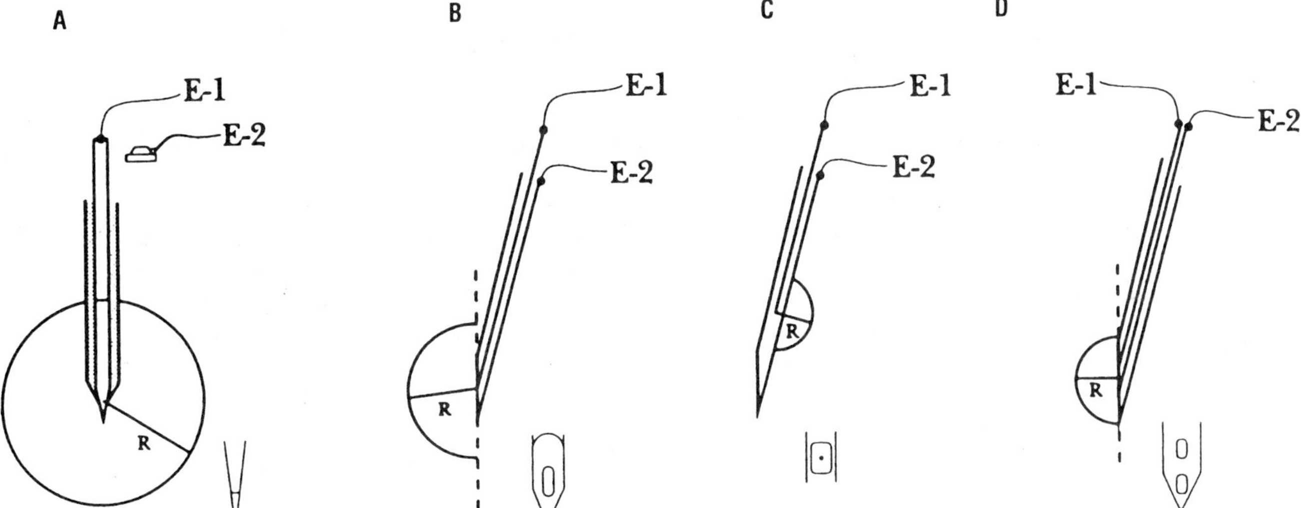

Figure 9-8. Different types of intramuscular recording electrodes and their recording areas. *A.* Monopolar needle electrode showing a spherical recording zone and the need for a surface reference electrode in addition to a ground. *B.* A standard concentric electrode where the cannula is used as the reference. This electrode also needs a separate ground. *C.* Single-fiber electrode has a side window with a small recording surface that is insulated from the cannula. The cannula serves as a reference. *D.* Bipolar concentric needle electrode has two separate wires and recording surfaces within the cannula. The cannula serves as the ground while the two central wires and their associated recording surfaces serve as the active and reference recording electrodes. (Reproduced by permission from Dumitru D. *Electrodiagnostic medicine.* Philadelphia: Hanley & Belfus, 1995:70.)

Table 9-5: Factors Influencing Amplitude and Shape of the Recorded Potentials

1. Surface area of the recording surface of the electrode relative to the size and volume distribution of the physiologically active structures
2. Electrical properties of the metal-electrolyte interface
3. The effect of volume conduction through intervening tissues, including how the electrical properties of the volume conductor vary in space—especially important with surface electrodes where the skin impedance may become a factor
4. The relative temporal synchrony with which structures become physiologically activated and their spatial distribution in the tissue with respect to the positioning of the recording electrode(s)
5. Geometric configuration and location of the different recording electrodes: active, reference, and ground

variations that can be produced with slight movement of the electrodes or their cables. These potentials can be an important source of slowly varying "movement" artifact in the EMG signal. These effects can be reduced by taking care to reduce the skin impedance, to properly affix surface electrodes to the skin, to avoid traction on the cable, and to ensure that the preamplifier is close to the recording site (i.e., cables are relatively short). It is also important to have a high input impedance relative to the potential swings of impedance that may occur at the electrode-patient interface. Use of a recessed electrode surface where the recording surface "floats" on a bead of conductive gel can reduce the artifact introduced when the metal recording surface moves with respect to the underlying skin. Shielded electrode cables can also reduce the pickup of stray interference. Care should be taken to clean the skin perspiration, to avoid the formation of a low-resistance path between the surface recording electrodes, stimulating electrodes, and the ground electrode. The use of a conductive electrode gel reduces the impedance of the interface, improves the quality of the recording, and also reduces the amount of current required to stimulate nerves percutaneously, thus improving patient tolerance and reducing stimulus artifact. The quality of the recording can be improved by lightly abrading the skin to reduce the high impedance of the stratum corneum at the skin's surface. Occasionally, it will be necessary to use subdermal needles instead of surface electrodes to allow "near-nerve" recording or stimulation when large amounts of subcutaneous fat or edema fluid introduce increased resistance between the surface electrodes and the underlying neuromuscular structures.

A variety of different intramuscular recording electrodes are shown in Figure 9-8. The simplest recording electrode is the monopolar needle introduced by Jasper and Ballem in 1949 (71). It can be in a sterilizable, reusable, or a single-use, presterilized, disposable form. The electrode is a stainless-steel wire tempered for strength and point stability that is coated with the electrical insulator Teflon, except for the tip. Stainless steel has relatively poor electrical properties for recording purposes but has satisfactory mechanical properties and is relatively inert.

The monopolar needle must be used with a surface reference electrode that is placed close to the site of insertion, to avoid recording distant EMG signals from the reference site. The advantages of the monopolar needle include a simple, relatively inexpensive construction and an omnidirectional pickup because of the spatial symmetry of the recording tip. Insertion and movement of the electrode in the muscle are better tolerated because of the small diameter and the reduction in friction of the shaft of the needle due to the Teflon coating. Difficulties include standardization of the area of the bare tip. Measuring electrode impedance can indirectly assess the area of the bared tip: The higher the impedance, the smaller the recording surface area. The coating is also susceptible to damage with repeated use. Requiring a separate reference electrode in addition to a ground electrode adds a potential source of variation as well as inconvenience. The larger the recording surface of the tip of the electrode, the larger the area from which it samples and averages its input, the lower the electrode impedance and the smaller and more smoothed-out are the recorded potentials. The recording surface area typically ranges from 0.15 to 0.20 mm^2. Compared to concentric electrodes, the monopolar needles tend to sample from a larger region of the muscle, are less directional in their pickup, have a larger recording area, are better tolerated by the patients, and are less selective in focusing on individual MUAPs.

The concentric or coaxial electrode, introduced by Adrian and Bronk in 1929 (72), is composed of a stainless-steel hollow cannula with an insulated wire running within the lumen. The active recording surface is the bared wire surface where it emerges from the beveled tip of the needle. The bare stainless-steel cannula is the reference electrode. A separate ground electrode is required but not a separate reference electrode. The exposed surface area of the active inner conductor ranges from 0.030 to 0.080 mm^2 depending on the manufacturer of the electrode. The advantages of the concentric needle include the more closely standardized exposed surface area of the active electrode and the fixed location of the reference electrode with respect to the active electrode. For this reason, the concentric electrode has been used more extensively in quantitative analysis of the motor unit potential. The more restrictive pickup area and the directional selectivity of the recording surface can be helpful in isolating individual MUAPs from the background. Disadvantages include less tolerance for the use of this electrode compared to the monopolar electrode, an inability to widely sample the muscle when looking for evidence of membrane instability, and the possibility of doing more tissue damage with an electrode with a diameter wider than that of the monopolar needle.

The bipolar electrode is similar to the concentric electrode except that two wires are placed inside the lumen of the cannula and serve as both the active and the reference electrode. The cannula serves as the ground electrode. This is the best electrode for selectively isolating individual MUAPs, even under conditions in which a moderate contraction is occurring. The impedances of the active and reference electrodes are closely matched. It is least susceptible to artifact because of the closeness of the active and reference electrodes. No additional electrodes are required, and the electrode is completely self-contained. Disadvantages include the facts that the electrode has a high impedance, and that the amplitudes of the units recorded are small with respect to the thermal noise background. The active and reference electrodes can "short out" with a low-impedance pathway between them because they are so close together. Larger-diameter cannulae must be used to accommodate the two internal insulated wires and therefore patient tolerance is lower.

The advantages and disadvantages of the different needle electrodes suggest the need to choose the electrode most appropriate to the particular clinical situation. The electromyographer should be adept at using the different available electrode types while being aware of how the configuration of the recording surface will influence signal parameters as well as the interpretation of the signal.

Preamplifier and Amplifier System

After the electrode and its cables, the next components of the system that critically influence the quality of the recording are the preamplifier and amplifier. The purposes of these parts of the system are to register the signal detected by the electrode and to amplify the voltage of the signal so that subsequent processing can be performed. The amplifier and preamplifier should be able to reproduce the signal detected at the electrode with high fidelity, and together with the filters, be able to selectively amplify the physiologic signal and reject or attenuate artifactual signals and noise.

For reasons noted already, the input impedance of the preamplifier should be very high (up to over 100 MΩ) with a shunt capacitance of 10 to 100 pF. The input impedance of the preamplifier should be many times that of the electrode to minimize the effect of attenuation of the signal due to voltage drop over the electrode impedance. This is especially important for single-fiber EMG where the surface area of the electrode is very small and impedance of the electrode is thus high.

The preamplifier is a *differential amplifier*. It amplifies the difference between two signals and rejects any element of the signal that is commonly recorded on the two inputs. This is why physiologic recordings require an active, a reference, and a ground electrode. The differential amplifier amplifies the difference of the potential seen between the active and the ground electrode, and the potential seen between the reference and the ground electrode. Because the body is a relatively good conductor, any interference potentials picked up from external sources such as the adjacent power lines in the walls of the room or the fluorescent lamps overhead will appear almost uniformly over the entire surface of the body. These interference potentials should be very close to identical at two closely spaced recording sites on the body. This common-mode signal is rejected by the differential amplifier. This signal is often larger than the physiologic signals of interest and it is the differential amplification feature of the preamplifier that is most important in discriminating the physiologic differential signal from the large common-mode interference signals. The overall ability to discriminate the differential signal from the common-mode signal will also depend on a close matching of electrode impedances for both the active and the reference electrode, although the effects of moderate differences in electrode impedance can be "swamped out" by very large, well-matched input impedances of the preamplifier.

Ideally, the amplification system would amplify only the elements of the signal of interest and would reject artifactual signals contaminating the target signal. The signal of interest can be separated from the contaminants if the artifactual signals have frequencies that are at least partially outside of the frequency range of the target signal. This is done by intentionally limiting amplification only to the frequency spectrum of the waves being studied by using filters. For example, most of the signal above 10,000 Hz in the recording is related to amplifier noise rather than to the EMG. Therefore, the amplification of signals above 10,000 Hz can be reduced using a low-pass filter with a cutoff frequency of 10,000 Hz. Similarly, most of the signal below about 20 Hz is due to movement artifact and baseline wander. This unwanted part of the signal can be omitted by using a high-pass filter that will attenuate slowly varying components of the signal with frequencies below 20 Hz. On the other hand, the CMAP contains significant power in frequencies below 20 Hz and will be significantly attenuated and distorted with a low-pass filter set at 20 Hz. Therefore, the low-end cutoff frequency for the high-pass filter must be set to a much lower frequency, usually around 1 Hz, for the recording of this potential. Thus, one can choose filter settings to maximize the separation of the signal from artifactual signals as long as the frequency spectrum of the signal does not significantly overlap with that of the artifactual signals. Each type of potential has a different spectrum of frequencies that require different filter settings to avoid distortion of the signal. Recommended filter settings for recording different types of potentials are shown in Table 9-6.

Table 9-6: Recommended Cutoff Frequency Settings for Bandpass Filters

Signal to Be Recorded	Low Cutoff Frequency (Hz)	High Cutoff Frequency (Hz)
Sensory nerve action potential	20	2,000
Compound muscle action potential	1	10,000
Needle electromyography	20	10,000

Stimulation Circuitry, the Stimulator, and the Control of Stimulus Artifact

One of the practical issues in performing NCSs is the control of the size of the *stimulus artifact* (73). The EMG instrument contains an electrically isolated, ground-free output circuit to limit the stimulus artifact transmitted to the amplifier input. With stimulus isolation, the common ground path between the stimulator and the amplifier is interrupted. The isolation can be achieved through the use of a transformer. A transformer is composed of two adjacent coils of wire or inductors—a primary and a secondary coil. These coils share a common magnetic field and the passage of current through the primary coil induces a current in the secondary coil by the process of electromagnetic induction. It is the current in the second groundless coil that is used to stimulate the patient. Because there is no direct electrical current path between the first coil and the second coil, the potential artifact pathway through a common ground is broken. A more recent solution is the use of *optical isolation* where the common ground pathway is broken by a transparent insulator through which the signal is transmitted as a beam of light.

In actual practice, it is not possible to achieve total isolation of the stimulus from the ground, because of unequal capacitance of each of the output terminals to the ground. The isolator is not able to eliminate the shock artifact component that is directed through the patient to the ground. Ways to limit this are to be sure to have a good low-impedance contact at the ground electrode, to place the ground electrode between the stimulus site and the recording electrodes, and to be sure that the stimulator cable is kept well away from the ground wire and the recording electrode wires so as to limit capacitive coupling between the wires. Locating the stimulus electrodes so that they are equidistant from the ground and recording electrodes can also help to reduce the stimulus artifact. Care must be taken to avoid allowing a current path between a stimulus electrode and either the ground electrode or the recording electrodes through a low-resistance bridge, a bridge of either electrode paste, excessive skin perspiration, or moisturizing skin cream.

The EMG stimulator circuit provides rectangular pulses with an adjustable duration and amplitude. Both of these parameters can be independently adjusted upward to increase the total stimulus energy. Increasing the duration rather than the amplitude appears to be more effective in selectively stimulating the low-threshold axons in the peripheral nerve, as would be preferable in inducing the H-reflex, for example. A typical technique for finding the supramaximal level of stimulation of the nerve and avoiding excessive stimulation is to slowly increase the stimulus amplitude while holding the duration constant. Further increasing the duration will help obtain a maximal response if it has not been achieved when the maximal stimulus amplitude in the available range has been applied. The different populations of axons in the nerve will have different excitation thresholds, with the lower thresholds being found in the myelinated axons with the largest diameter. The stimulus current is distributed in accordance with the laws of volume conduction that also govern the distribution of the currents induced by the physiologic generator. Only a fraction of the current applied actually reaches the nerve and produces the excitation. The goal of good technique is to maximize this fraction so that distribution of current via volume conduction through the body outside of the region of the targeted nerve is limited. The amount of current required to reach maximal stimulus levels will vary according to the location of the nerve trunk with respect to the body surface, the placement and separation of the stimulus electrodes on the skin, and the impedance of the intervening tissues. It is thus important to reduce the skin impedance at the site of the stimulating electrodes in order to limit the amount of current required to stimulate the nerve. This also can help to control the size of the stimulus artifact. Another way in which the stimulus artifact is suppressed is through the differential amplification of the preamplifier where the artifact should be processed as a common-mode signal. As long as both the active and reference electrode "see" the same artifactual signal, it should be strongly reduced by differential amplification. However, if one of the recording electrodes is placed so that it is much closer to the stimulating site than the other, there will be a different distribution of the artifact to the two recording electrodes and the artifact will not be as readily suppressed by differential amplification. Another way to reduce stimulus artifact is to rotate the stimulator so that the distribution of the stimulus current is such that the recording electrodes are placed near a zero-crossing point for the bipolar field produced by the stimulation current. Another approach is to average together stimulation trials during which the polarity of the stimulus is alternated.

Using Signal Averaging to Eliminate Noise and Interference

A common means of extracting a small biologic signal from a noisy background is to use signal averaging. This approach works as long as the noise source is uncorrelated with the biologic source and the stimulus frequency is in no way synchronized to a major frequency contained within the noise source. Averaging simply involves adding together ensembles of signals obtained with repeated applications of a stimulus, for example, when recording a sensory nerve action potential (SNAP). Artifact or system fluctuations that are synchronized with the stimulus will not be eliminated by averaging and should be avoided. The stimulus rate should not divide equally into the power line frequency. Averagers are often provided with an artifact rejection capability that rejects a sweep that goes outside of a preset amplitude range within a particular range of time with respect to the stimulus onset. Such variation of amplitude outside of the range is indicative of a grossly artifactual potential that would cause a large-amplitude distortion of the averaged signal. Averagers will often allow for viewing of the accumulated averaged waveform or the input waveform and will display the number of sweeps accumulated in the average as well as the number rejected. It can be set to automatically terminate the averaging process after a particular number of sweeps have been accepted.

Avoiding Electrical Hazards and Patient Safety Issues

One must always keep in mind the fundamental restriction placed on the activity of the physician—"Above all, do not harm"—when using electrodiagnostic equipment. There are significant, potentially harmful effects of placing equipment powered from a plug in the wall, in contact with a patient. The probability of injury is reduced to a minimum level through various design features incorporated into modern machines that must meet stringent safety codes to allow them to be used in clinical environments (66,69). However, it is incumbent on the physician operating the equipment to ensure that the equipment continuously measures up to safety standards and that the equipment is used in a working environment in which maximum safety for the patient is ensured.

The problem of leakage current passing through the patient to ground is reduced by having a third wire ground in the power line circuit. If this grounding of the power source is lost, then larger leakage currents may flow. Such problems could include a broken grounding pin or ground wire in the power cord, poor ground connections inside the equipment, reduced contact in the power socket, the use of adapters that defeat the grounding capability, or faulty wiring and poor establishment of ground in the wiring of the building in which the EMG is being performed. The integrity of the ground contact and the grounding of the building must be examined with regularity, and clearly, all equipment used in this capacity must meet basic electrical safety codes such as those published by the Underwriters Laboratory (UL). The operation of equipment without UL rating may result in loss of insurance coverage in the case of injury related to the operation of the equipment. One should always check the equipment for the UL sticker, usually placed on the rear or underside of the machine where its power requirements and serial number have been stamped. One must be aware of the potential risks involved in operating equipment in areas in which the provision of electrical power does not meet the basic specifications of hospital-grade electrical power supply. The Joint Commission for the Accreditation of Healthcare Organizations (JCAHO) requires a regular schedule of safety inspections in which grounding is tested, leakage currents are measured, and the equipment is inspected for potential safety hazards. The outlets and wiring in the laboratory should also be checked at least on an annual basis. Records documenting these safety inspections should be maintained in the laboratory and made available for JCAHO inspection.

CLINICAL CONSIDERATIONS

The electrodiagnostic examination should always be viewed as an extension of the history and physical examination as they relate to evaluation of the muscular system, peripheral nervous system, and segmental spinal cord structures. The electrodiagnostician is consulted to provide focused information that addresses a clinical question regarding the function of the peripheral nerve and muscle. The evaluation should begin with a careful, focused clinical history and physical examination that delineates the clinical problem so that the electrodiagnostic study can be constructed to shed light on this specific problem. Referral forms should allow the referring physician to indicate the nature of the information that is being sought from the study. It is not cost-effective or appropriate to blindly study every nerve and muscle exhaustively. The study must be planned to zero in on testing that is directly relevant to the patient's presentation and promises to maximally enlighten the diagnostic assessment process. This process involves the generation of various hypotheses regarding the patient's pathology and the selective use of elements of the electrodiagnostic examination to specifically test these hypotheses and differentiate between them. The examination is thus a highly interactive exercise in medical diagnosis during which data are gathered, evaluated, and used "on-line" to make any necessary adjustments to the hypotheses being entertained, which then in turn shape the subsequent selection of electrodiagnostic studies. As such, electrodiagnosis is a medical procedure that can only legitimately be performed or directly supervised by physicians with specialized training in neuromusculoskeletal diagnostic skills.

Table 9-7: Clinical Applications of Nerve Conduction Studies

1. To obtain objective information about disease affecting the motor units in the presence of clinical weakness
2. To obtain objective information about disease affecting the peripheral sensory fibers in the presence of a clinical alteration of sensation or when a sensory nerve impairment is suspected but the clinical sensory examination results are equivocal or unreliable
3. To identify, localize, and characterize sites of nerve compression and/or ischemia and to help to classify the type (neurapraxia versus axonotmesis versus neurotmesis) and severity of the nerve injury:
   a. To assess for the presence of conduction block
   b. To detect slowing of conduction across a site of injury
   c. To measure conduction distal and proximal to a site of injury
   d. To determine whether there has been secondary wallerian degeneration of the distal axons following nerve injury
4. To differentiate primary neuropathic from primary myopathic disorders in patients presenting with clinical weakness
5. To differentiate peripheral nerve disease processes affecting myelin structure and function (myelinopathies) from those affecting the structure and integrity of the peripheral nerve axon (axonopathies)
6. To delineate patterns of spatial distribution of abnormal peripheral nerve function, e.g., to differentiate a generalized peripheral neuropathy from focal nerve compression
7. To detect the presence of a subclinical disease entity, e.g., in family members of clinically identified patients with familial forms of polyneuropathy
8. To identify the presence of anomalous peripheral neuromuscular anatomy in the presence of clinical pathology where clinical findings are not readily explained without assuming the presence of anomalous peripheral innervation
9. To detect and distinguish defects of neuromuscular transmission

NERVE CONDUCTION STUDIES

The skills involved in proficient performance of NCSs can only be adequately acquired through hands-on experience under the supervision of an experienced electromyographer. The specifics of the techniques, especially for the less frequently performed tests, can also vary somewhat from laboratory to laboratory. This chapter focuses on the general principles that guide and inform the practice of performing and interpreting NCSs without getting into the details of studies on individual nerves. Specific information about nerve conduction techniques along with normal values for nerve conduction parameters can be obtained in several of the references provided in the bibliography (8,9,15,17,19,22,25,26,28). Some of the clinical applications of NCSs are listed in Table 9-7.

Two Different Types of Nerve Conduction Study

1. Sensory conduction study: Stimulate a nerve at one point and record an SNAP at some other point. With the antidromic technique, a mixed or cutaneous nerve is stimulated at a proximal site while the SNAP is recorded from electrodes placed over a cutaneous branch at a more distal site. With the orthodromic technique, a cutaneous nerve branch is stimulated distally and recording electrodes pick up the SNAP from either a cutaneous or a mixed nerve at a more proximal site. Sensory studies are useful

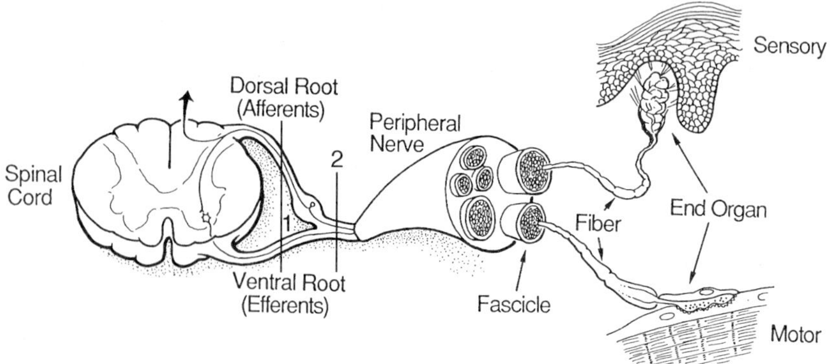

Figure 9-9. Architecture of the peripheral nerve showing central and peripheral connections. A lesion at site 1 is termed *preganglionic* and is associated with attenuation of motor action potentials due to wallerian degeneration of the distal axon that has been separated from its cell body, while the sensory action potentials remain relatively intact, owing to a relative lack of wallerian degeneration of the distal sensory fibers that have not been separated from their cell body in the dorsal root ganglion. A lesion at site 2 is termed *postganglionic* and is associated with wallerian degeneration of both sensory and motor fibers with a similar reduction in amplitude of the compound muscle action potential and the sensory nerve action potential. (Modified from Terzis JK, Smith KL. *The peripheral nerve. Structure function and reconstruction.* New York: Raven, 1990: 2.)

in distinguishing between *preganglionic* and *postganglionic* lesions. Preganglionic damage leaves the cell body of the primary sensory neuron intact in the dorsal root ganglion, and distal extension continues to function normally, giving a relatively normal sensory nerve conduction in the setting of a clinical sensory deficit. Postganglionic disorders produce damage to the cell body or the distal axon and lead to abnormal sensory nerve conduction if the damage is severe enough to be detected with these methods (Fig. 9-9).

2. Motor conduction study: Stimulate a peripheral nerve proximal to its point of innervation of the target muscle and then record the CMAP from recording electrodes placed on the target muscle innervated by the stimulated nerve. The results of this study may be affected by a process that affects the motor units including the anterior horn cell, the peripheral motor fiber (including the Schwann cells that produce the internodal myelin), the neuromuscular junction, and the muscle cells. Note that the motor studies cannot distinguish between preganglionic and postganglionic lesion localization the way the sensory studies can, since the nerve cell body for the motor unit, the anterior horn cell, is located intra-axially. Thus any lesion of the peripheral nerve, whether proximal or distal, will produce potential problems with the motor axon. Therefore, dissociation between motor and sensory conduction study results can be helpful in localization although this can also be seen in some pathologic processes that tend to be more selective for one (i.e., motor or sensory) over the other.

The peripheral nerve consists of large populations of axons that are not homogeneous in terms of their diameter and degree of myelination. Thus, the conduction characteristics of the different axons within a peripheral nerve will vary widely and the resulting *compound* potentials produced with whole nerve excitation will reflect the summated activity produced by the activation of each of the individual axons comprising the nerve. A mixed nerve trunk will contain both sensory and motor fiber axon types. The motor fibers will generally be either extrafusal α motor neurons innervating nonspindle muscle fibers (with a larger axonal diameter and faster conduction velocity) or intrafusal γ motor neurons innervating the muscle fibers that are contiguous with the muscle spindles (with a smaller axonal diameter and slower conduction velocity). Afferent fibers in a mixed nerve will consist of both cutaneous and muscle sensory fibers. There will also be both myelinated and unmyelinated afferents. Myelinated cutaneous afferent fiber groups are classified as A-alpha, A-beta, and A-delta. Unmyelinated axons are designated *C fibers*. Muscle afferents have also been classified as types I, II, III, and IV, which roughly correspond to A-alpha through C, respectively, in terms of their structural characteristics. The largest myelinated afferent fibers in a mixed nerve tend to be the Ia primary spindle afferents and the Ib Golgi tendon organ afferents. The limb proprioception afferents are the A-alpha fibers while the cutaneous afferents are the A-beta, A-delta, and C fibers. Cutaneous mechanoreceptors tend to be connected through A-beta fibers while mechanical, thermal, and polymodal nociceptors tend to be wired in through the A-delta and C fibers.

Stimulation Technique

Electrical current is applied between an anode (positively charged electrode) and a cathode (negatively charged electrode). Positively charged ions are pulled toward the cathode, thus depolarizing the membrane under the cathode and bringing the axons toward threshold for generation of the AP. Hyperpolarization can occur under the anode, leading to so-called *anodal block*, although the practical importance of this issue is not clear. For this reason, the bipolar stimulating electrodes should be placed with the cathode oriented in the direction in which the induced APs are to be conducted (e.g., toward the recording electrodes in the case of a simple motor conduction study). Most nerves can be stimulated to a supramaximal level using percutaneous stimulation. However, when there is significant peripheral edema or subcutaneous adipose tissue, it may be necessary to use a subdermal needle electrode placed subcutaneously close to the nerve. Smaller stimulus currents are generally required when needle stimulation is employed. With a monopolar stimulation technique, the needle becomes the cathode while the anode may be a surface electrode placed close by or another needle electrode placed along the length of the nerve.

To ensure that there is no selective activation of fibers related to technique, a supramaximal stimulus intensity should be used. The response to supramaximal stimulation should be relatively stable. If the stimulus is turned up too high, the waveform of the evoked CMAP will change as other adjacent nerves begin to be stimulated. An excessively high stimulus intensity, besides causing unnecessary discomfort for the patient, can also lead to a false shortening of latencies because of current spread and activation of the nerve at a site distal to the site of contact of the stimulus electrodes. In addition, an excessively large stimulus intensity will lead to difficulties with a large stimulus artifact, which can obscure and distort the recording. Ideally, the stimulus artifact is short in duration and there is a flat baseline reestablished between the time of the stimulation and the time at which the recorded response begins to appear. Methods for controlling stimulus artifact and factors affecting the stimulus artifact were discussed in the previous section. The electromyographer must avoid errors that result from submaximal stimulation of the nerve but must also avoid problems related to excessive stimulation above the supramaximal level. When supramaximal stimulation is used for a motor conduction study and the latency is measured to the onset of the CMAP, the measure is one that applies to the largest, fastest-conducting fibers in the population—that is, those that "get there first."

Recording Technique

Surface electrodes are generally used to record the CMAP and SNAP. Pairs of disk electrodes are placed on the skin, using a small amount of conductive gel to ensure good electrical contact, and then are taped to the skin to hold them in place. Ring electrodes consisting of an adjustable loop of coiled wire are convenient for recording SNAPs from the digits. Subdermal needle electrodes placed perpendicular to the sensory nerve can significantly reduce the signal-to-noise ratio and may be helpful particularly for recording SNAPs in the distal part of the lower extremity when the surface recording technique produces a marginal result requiring averaging to identify the SNAP. This may also be necessary when peripheral edema or excessive subcutaneous adipose tissue presents an electrical impedance barrier to recording the potentials. The display gain should be adjusted so that the full range of the display is used without saturating the display range. When the signal is digitized and displayed under software control, the display gain and time scale can be adjusted without having to stimulate the patient again. In this case, the gain can be increased to check the location of the onset and peak of the evoked response and then decreased again to measure the amplitude of the response.

Various problems in the recording system can lead to erroneous results. Damaged electrodes or cables can lead to faulty and distorted recordings and exaggerated motion artifact. An improperly connected ground electrode can lead to 60-cycle interference and an enlarged stimulus artifact. Waveform distortion can also occur with inappropriate filter settings or the insertion of a 60-Hz notch filter. Inaccurate readings can result from a system that is not properly calibrated so that checks of both amplitude and time calibration of the display should be performed regularly.

The compound AP is characterized with specific measures:

1. Latency. The latency is the time between the stimulation of the nerve and a key discrete feature of the responses, either the onset or a particular peak. The onset latency reflects the conduction of the fastest fibers in the nerve. Generally, the onset latency is more readily interpreted than the peak latency. Many people, however, continue to use the peak latency in sensory studies because of difficulty in clearly identifying the onset latency of the SNAP.
2. Amplitude. Amplitude reflects the number of active elements contributing to the response as well as their degree of synchrony or coherence. A number of technical factors, including the distance from the source to the recording electrodes and the resistance of the intervening tissues, can also affect amplitude. Amplitude can be measured from negative peak to positive peak or from baseline to the negative peak. The latter measure is more readily interpretable and less likely to be affected by interactions between different phases of the component APs via phase cancellation.
3. Duration and shape. The duration of the compound AP is a measure of the degree of temporal synchrony in the components contributing to the response. Duration reflects the range of conduction velocities of the fibers in the nerve population: the difference between the fastest and the slowest fibers contributing to the response. The degree of asynchrony produced by this difference is referred to as *temporal dispersion*. The greater the degree of asyn-

chrony, the wider the potential. The spread between APs conducted in the fastest fibers and those conducted in the slowest fibers increases with increasing distance between the stimulating and the recording electrodes. Pathologic conditions that alter conduction velocities of some of the fibers in the population will produce increased asynchrony and may also alter the overall shape of the response. The response may lose its biphasic structure and become "polyphasic" if there is segmentation of the distribution of conduction velocities within the nerve fiber population as the result of an inhomogeneous pathologic process.

Motor Nerve Conduction Study Technique

To record the CMAP, an active electrode is placed over the motor point in the middle of the muscle while a reference electrode is placed over the tendon or a nearby joint. When the active electrode is accurately placed, the muscle fiber APs take their origin from the neuromuscular junctions concentrated at the motor point directly beneath the active electrode, and the electrode "sees" only movement of the APs spreading through the muscle moving away from the site directly beneath it. When this occurs, a biphasic (negative-positive deflection) response is recorded. When an initial positivity is seen, this means there is an initial phase in which the electrode "sees" APs being conducted *toward* its location. This could result from placement away from the motor point or from volume-conducted activity from other adjacent muscles as may be seen when there is anomalous innervation of muscle or when the stimulus current has spread to other nerves that activate muscles away from the recording site. Since the physiologic amplifier is arranged so that a negative deflection on the G1 grid results in an upward deflection, the negative-positive biphasic CMAP should be displayed as an upward-downward deflection. If the reverse occurs, the possibility of an accidental reversal of the connections of the recording electrodes should be considered. The amplifier filters should be set up with a relatively wide band of recording, usually about 1 Hz to 10 kHz.

The CMAP is characterized in terms of measured parameters including amplitude (baseline to peak), onset latency, and duration (25). The waveform structure is noted and the area under the curve can be electronically measured. The onset latency measures the time taken from the stimulus onset to the initial recording of the muscle response. This consists of two major components: the nerve conduction time and the synaptic delay time at the neuromuscular junction. When the nerve is stimulated at a proximal and a distal location and the onset latencies are subtracted, the result is the difference in the nerve conduction times. The motor conduction velocity of the fastest fibers in the population is then estimated by measuring the distance between the two points of stimulation and dividing this distance by the latency difference. The latency from the distal stimulation to the CMAP onset is called the *distal motor latency*. The *terminal latency* is the difference between the measured distal motor latency and the latency that is calculated given the distance from the distal stimulation site to the recording site and the computed conduction velocity of the nerve between the proximal and distal stimulation sites. Separating the sites of stimulation improves the accuracy and stability of the computed conduction velocity by making potential measurement errors small compared to the total measurement. If the study is being used to identify a focal lesion, it is better isolated and identified by using small segmental examinations at levels above, below, and through the level of the suspected nerve lesion. The basic technique for motor conduction studies is shown schematically in Figure 9-10.

Sensory Nerve Conduction Study Technique

The recording of the SNAP is technically more demanding than the recording of the CMAP because the SNAP has a much lower amplitude (in the microvolt as opposed to the millivolt range) and may be obscured with low signal-to-noise ratio conditions (28). The SNAP is particularly difficult to record at times in the lower limb of elderly individuals. The CMAP from distal muscles can interfere with the recording of the SNAP when one is using antidromic techniques in the hand. Care must be taken to avoid excessive activation of adjacent motor fibers by using a lower stimulus intensity or duration, and the recording electrodes should be positioned so as to minimize interference from adjacent muscles. The fingers should be kept separated from each other when recording the SNAP in the distal end of the upper extremity. Higher amplifier gains must be used to record the SNAP and internal amplifier noise can obscure the potential. Amplifier noise can be limited by decreasing the band of high frequencies passed through the amplifier filter. Since amplifier noise is generally high frequency, it can be limited by reducing the upper filter cutoff frequency to about 2 kHz. Since the SNAP has little low-frequency content, the lower filter cutoff can be increased to about 20 Hz.

Since the SNAP is a compound *nerve* AP, one can estimate the conduction velocity of the fastest-conducting fibers by measuring the distance between the stimulation site and the recording site and dividing this by the onset latency of the SNAP. The onset latency of the SNAP is generally used for antidromic recording methods. Both onset and peak latencies have been used for orthodromic recording techniques where the amplitude of the AP is often lower and the onset latency is more difficult to define. The interpretation of the peak latency is somewhat more problematic because of its dependence on the distance between the stimulation and recording sites, and the conduction velocity computed using peak measurements is more difficult to interpret in terms of which fibers in the nerve are actually conducting with this velocity. When one is using a "bipolar" recording technique in which electrodes are placed along

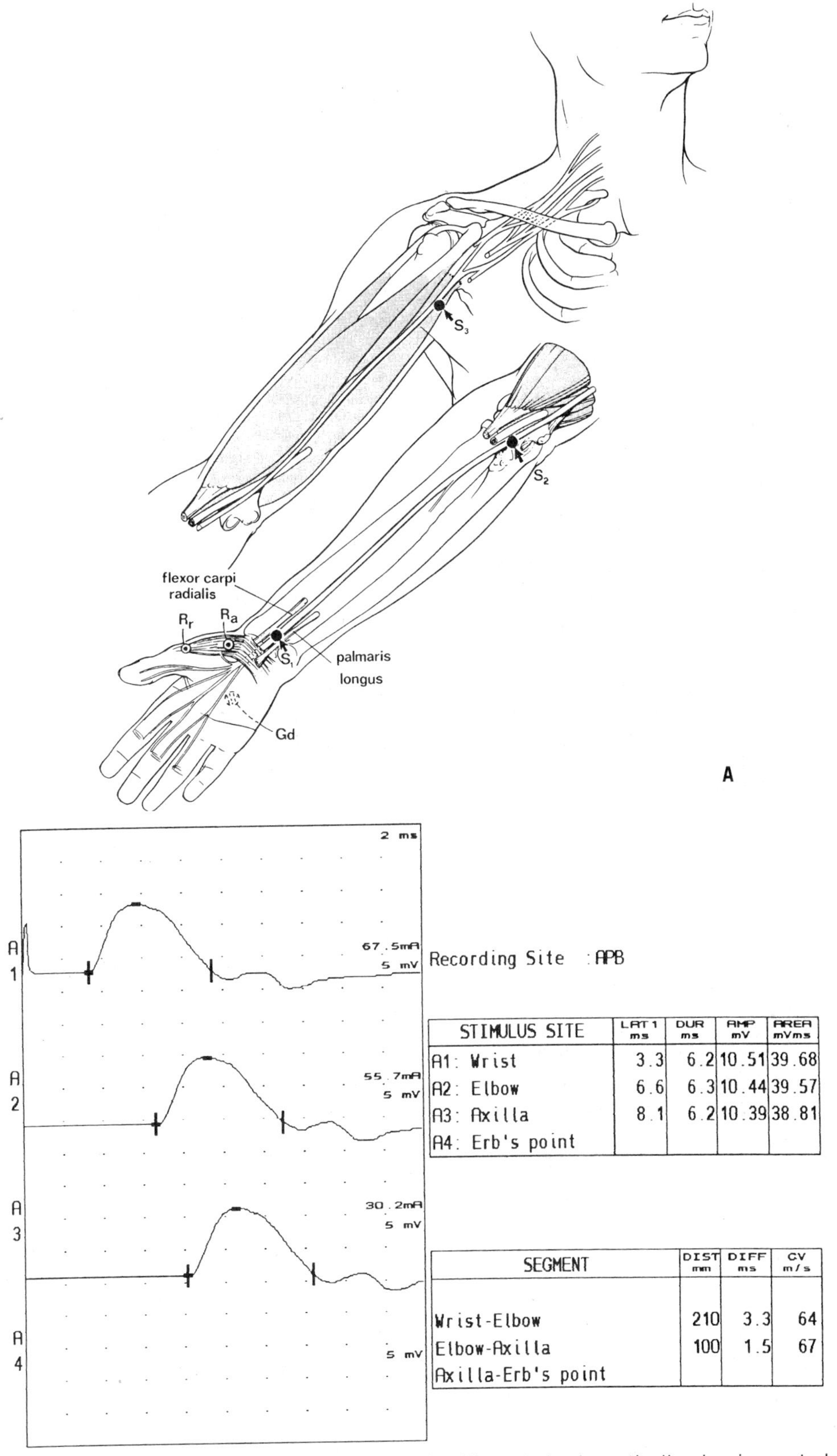

STIMULUS SITE	LAT 1 ms	DUR ms	AMP mV	AREA mVms
A1: Wrist	3.3	6.2	10.51	39.68
A2: Elbow	6.6	6.3	10.44	39.57
A3: Axilla	8.1	6.2	10.39	38.81
A4: Erb's point				

SEGMENT	DIST mm	DIFF ms	CV m/s
Wrist-Elbow	210	3.3	64
Elbow-Axilla	100	1.5	67
Axilla-Erb's point			

Figure 9-10. *A.* Basic technique for motor nerve conduction studies illustrated schematically, showing a study of the median nerve as an example. Stimulation of the median nerve is performed at the wrist, elbow, and proximal region of the arm. Recording electrodes are placed over the abductor pollicis brevis. Gd = ground; Ra = active recording electrode; Rr = reference recording electrode. (Reproduced by permission from Liveson JA, Ma DM. *Laboratory reference for clinical neurophysiology.* Philadelphia: FA Davis, 1992:84). *B.* Median nerve compound muscle action potentials recorded from the abductor pollicis brevis with stimulation at the wrist (*top*), elbow (*middle*), and axilla (*bottom*). Two horizontal amplitude markers and two vertical latency markers are noted on each trace. Onset latencies, durations, and baseline-to-peak amplitudes are noted in the upper table on the right. Segmental conduction velocities are shown in the table at the bottom right.

the length of the nerve, a biphasic negative-positive potential is recorded, a result predicated by the proximity of the active and reference electrodes to the nerve and to each other. If the reference electrode is placed farther away from the active electrode or at a relatively remote site, this becomes a "monopolar" recording. An initial positivity is now observed in the response, reflecting the fact that the active electrode now "sees" the approach of the AP along the nerve quite differently than does the distant reference electrode—the SNAP now has a positive-negative-positive triphasic structure. Amplitude of the SNAP is usually measured baseline to peak or from the first negative peak to the subsequent positive peak. This latter measurement may be more sensitive to "phase cancellation" effects that will depend on the spacing of the two recording electrodes. The maximum amplitude is obtained when the electrodes are spaced so that the negativity associated with the AP is completed under the active electrode before it begins to significantly influence the reference electrode. Given a lower limit on the duration of the negative phase of about 0.6 msec and a conduction velocity of 60 m/sec, the spatial extent of the negative phase is about 36 mm. Thus, bipolar electrodes should be spaced more than 36 mm apart. When the electrodes are spaced closer together, the amplitude of the potential begins to fall off. If they are spaced farther apart than 45 to 50 mm, "far-field" components that relate to the complicated path the AP takes through the volume conductor on its way to the recording site begin to appear. The basic technique for sensory nerve conduction is shown in Figure 9-11.

Several potential sources of error in the performance of NCSs are listed in Table 9-8 [see also article by Kimura (74) for further detailed examination of sources of error].

Table 9-8: Sources of Error in Performing Nerve Conduction Studies

- Recognizing anomalous anatomy
  - Martin-Gruber anastomosis
  - Accessory peroneal nerve
  - Ulnar hand
  - Others
- Stimulation errors
  - Too weak
  - Too strong
  - Too little distance between stimulation sites
  - Too much distance between stimulation sites
  - Wrong site
  - Wrong way (polarity reversal)
  - Check using collision technique
- Recording errors
  - Wrong placement
  - Damaged electrodes/wires/contacts
  - Electrolyte "bridging"
  - Excessive tissue impedance
- Measurement errors
- Instrument errors
  - Filters
  - Gain
  - Time base
- Prepotentials and volume-conducted "far-field" potentials
- Temporal dispersion effects
  - Sensory versus motor conduction study effects
- Phase cancellation

Influence of Subject Factors and Normal Physiologic Variation

Conduction velocities in newborns are approximately half those of adults and are even slower in premature infants (75). The conduction velocity reaches approximately 80% of the adult values by the age of 1 year and reaches the adult values by the ages of 3 to 5 years. Conduction velocity in the legs tends to decline slightly during the growth phase while conduction velocity in the arms tends to increase slightly. Conduction velocity tends to stay relatively stable with increasing age in carefully screened healthy adults, although earlier studies have recorded a steady decline in conduction velocity. Values obtained in studies of the effects of normal aging may vary because of differences in technique (e.g., in the control of temperature) as well as differences in the care with which conditions known to influence nerve function have been ruled out in the test populations. The effects of aging are also found to be different in different nerves because of the relative susceptibility of the nerves to the effects of lifelong trauma at common entrapment sites. Recent studies that applied strict criteria in identifying subjects without clinical evidence of peripheral nerve impairment suggested that the effects of aging on nerve conduction may not be as great as was once thought (76,77). While conduction velocity is somewhat slower and motor and sensory amplitudes tend to be lower, especially in the lower limbs, compared to a young population, many of the parameters stay reasonably stable between the ages of 60 and 90+ years. It appears that the range of normal variability of nerve conduction parameters tends to increase with age so that the amount of deviation from the mean value that is sufficient to allow the measurement to be judged abnormal is generally greater in the elderly than in a younger population. For some parameters, like the amplitude of the SNAP recorded from the fingers, the effect of gender is stronger than the effect of age (76).

Motor conduction velocities in the tibial and peroneal nerves are significantly lower than those in the median and ulnar nerves. Sural nerve and superficial peroneal nerve sensory conduction velocities also tend to be slower than the median, ulnar, and radial sensory conduction velocities. A number of factors may contribute to these differences.

Conduction of the AP depends on changes in conformation of the ionic channel proteins in the membranes of the excitable cells, as discussed at the beginning of this chapter. These conformational changes are exquisitely sensitive to changes in temperature and this must be taken

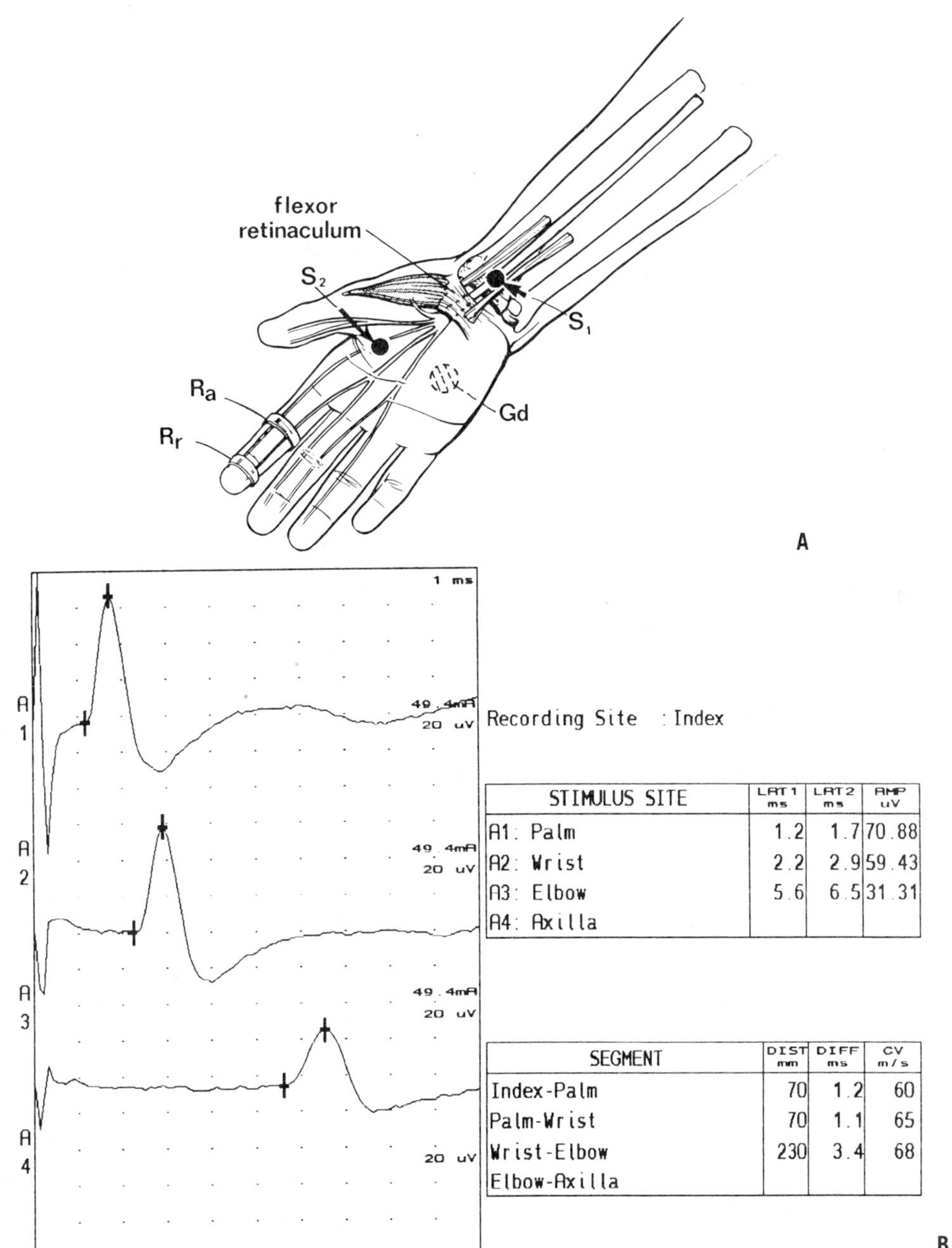

STIMULUS SITE	LAT1 ms	LAT2 ms	AMP uV
A1: Palm	1.2	1.7	70.88
A2: Wrist	2.2	2.9	59.43
A3: Elbow	5.6	6.5	31.31
A4: Axilla			

SEGMENT	DIST mm	DIFF ms	CV m/s
Index-Palm	70	1.2	60
Palm-Wrist	70	1.1	65
Wrist-Elbow	230	3.4	68
Elbow-Axilla			

Figure 9-11. *A.* Basic technique for sensory nerve conduction studies illustrated schematically, showing an antidromic study of the median nerve as an example. Stimulation of the median nerve is performed in the palm, wrist, and elbow (not shown). Ring electrodes are placed around the index finger to record the sensory nerve action potentials. Gd = ground; Ra= active recording electrode; Rr = reference recording electrode. (Reproduced by permission from Liveson JA, Ma DM. *Laboratory reference for clinical neurophysiology.* Philadelphia: FA Davis, 1992:120.) *B.* Normal median sensory nerve action potentials recorded with stimulation in the palm (*top*), wrist (*middle*), and elbow (*bottom*). Onset and peak latencies as well as the baseline-to-peak amplitudes are shown in the first two columns of the upper table on the right. Segmental conduction velocities are shown in the table at the bottom right. *C.* Abnormal median sensory nerve action potentials showing focal slowing of conduction across the wrist segment. This finding is indicative of a focal median mononeuropathy at the wrist. The clinical entity most commonly associated with these findings is carpal tunnel syndrome.

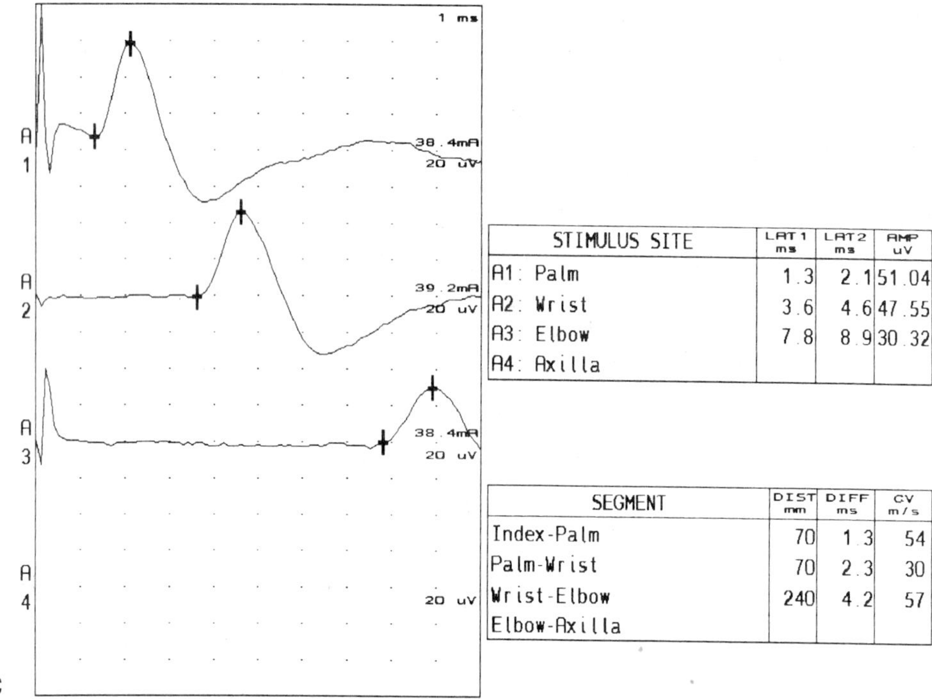

STIMULUS SITE	LAT1 ms	LAT2 ms	AMP uV
A1: Palm	1.3	2.1	51.04
A2: Wrist	3.6	4.6	47.55
A3: Elbow	7.8	8.9	30.32
A4: Axilla			

SEGMENT	DIST mm	DIFF ms	CV m/s
Index-Palm	70	1.3	54
Palm-Wrist	70	2.3	30
Wrist-Elbow	240	4.2	57
Elbow-Axilla			

Figure 9-11. *Continued*

into account when performing NCSs and interpreting the findings (78). Velocity increases with increasing temperature by 2.0 to 2.5 m/sec per Celsius degree between 29°C and 38°C. The distal latencies increase with decreasing temperature by 0.2 to 0.3 msec per Celsius degree. Skin temperature can be checked with a metal-encased thermistor or with an infrared probe. The limb should be warmed using an infrared lamp or immersion in warm water when the skin temperature drops below 32°C in the hand or 30°C in the foot. Temperature correction using an adjustment factor is problematic since the adjustment factors have been derived from studies of normal individuals and may not be valid for patients with neuromuscular or vascular pathology.

Conduction velocities tend to be lower in the legs in taller individuals, although arm length and height tend to have relatively little influence on nerve conduction velocities in the arms (79). The reason for this difference between the upper and lower limbs is not well understood. One could speculate that the lower limbs are relatively elongated as compared to the arms and that this break in vertical body symmetry could be associated with a relative elongation of the nerves in the lower limbs, which increases with increasing height. This relative elongation of the nerves could result in reduced axon diameters or changes in the distribution of myelin on the nerves, or both.

Classification of Nerve Injury

The response of the peripheral nerve to injury should be understood in terms of the pathology of the relevant structures of the peripheral nerve. The components of the peripheral nerve are identified in Figure 9-12. A variety of different processes can induce pathologic changes in the peripheral nerve and affect its ability to conduct. Here we look specifically at the response of the nerve to mechanical trauma.

Seddon described three major categories of traumatic nerve injury (80).

Neurapraxia or type I injury: focal demyelination or myelin distortion producing localized slowing of conduction and conduction block. Degeneration of axons does *not* occur and repair occurs through remyelination of the damaged segment, a relatively rapid process.

Axonotmesis or type II injury: significant damage to axons leading to wallerian degeneration of damaged axons distal to the site of injury. All connective tissue sheaths and the supporting structure of the nerve remain intact. This lesion leaves the ultrastructural component of the nerve "in continuity" as might occur with a crush injury. Recovery occurs through axonal regeneration down the intact connective tissue channels.

Neurotmesis or type III injury: significant damage not only to axons but also to the supportive connective tissue structure of the nerve so that the "guideposts" for axonal regeneration have been disrupted. In this case, spontaneous recovery is unlikely to occur to any significant extent without surgical repair of the connective tissue structure of the nerve.

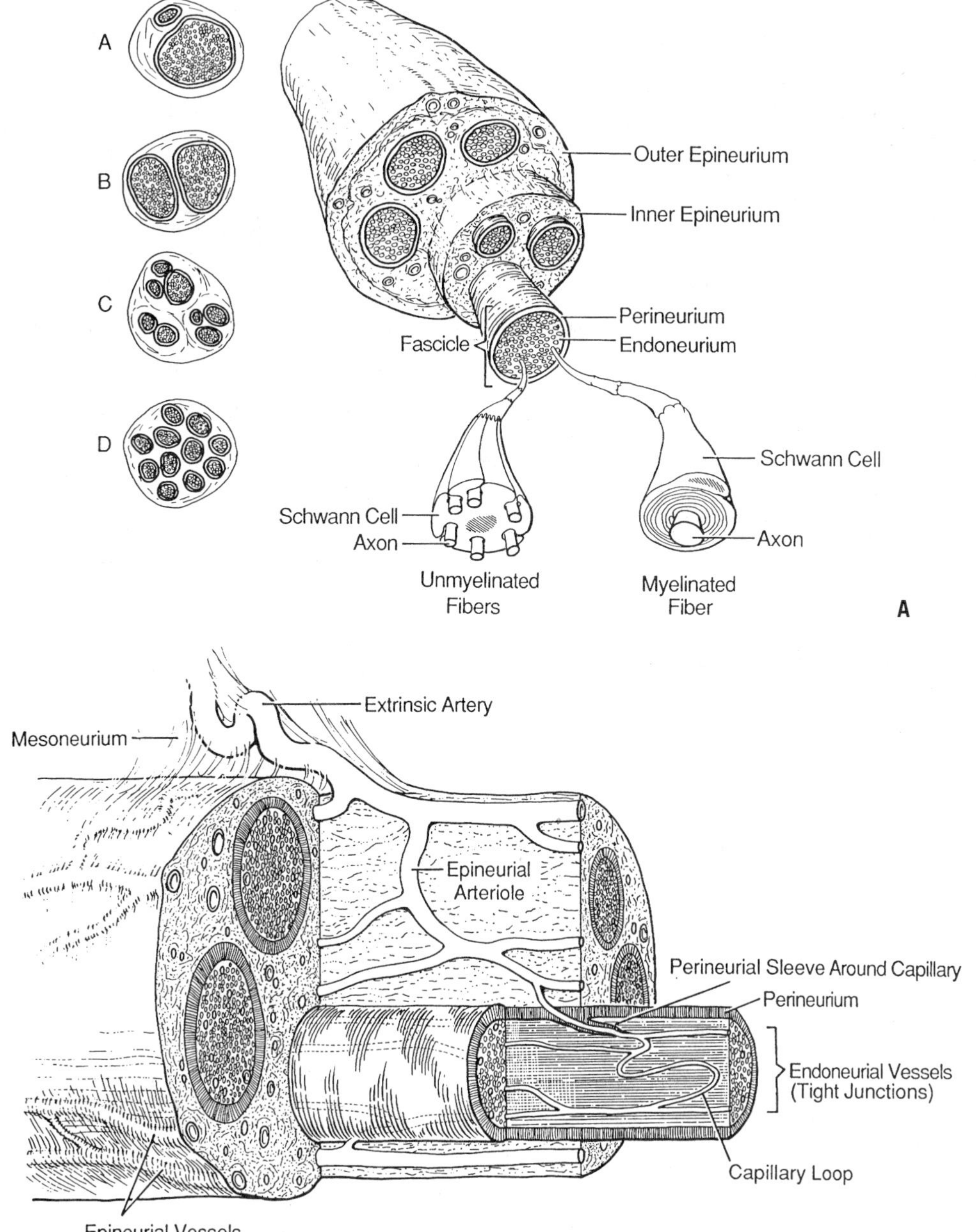

Figure 9-12. *A.* A schematic diagram of peripheral nerve architecture showing the connective tissue elements: endoneurium, perineurium, and epineurium. Individual fascicles may contain a mixture of both myelinated and unmyelinated axons, although some fascicles may hold a preponderance of one type or the other. The cross-sectional structure of the nerve may be monofascicular (A), oligofascicular (B), grouped polyfascicular (C), or ungrouped polyfascicular (D). *B.* A schematic diagram of the peripheral nerve vascular system that shows the arterial supply entering the nerve via the mesoneurium to form a richly anastomosing plexus of vessels in the epineurium. (Reproduced by permission from Terzis JK, Smith KL. *The peripheral nerve. Structure function and reconstruction.* New York: Raven, 1990:16,19.)

An alternate scheme for classifying nerve injury proposed by Sunderland (81) is shown schematically in Figure 9-13.

In understanding the electrodiagnostic evaluation of a nerve injury, it is extremely important to recognize that the response to injury is dynamic and that the interpretation will depend critically on the time frame with respect to the injury event since the studies constitute a "snapshot" of the injury-response process at a particular point in time. A schematic summary of the data that can be gathered from motor conduction studies and needle EMG is illustrated in Figure 9-14. Electrodiagnostic studies can be used to assess the extent and nature of the injury as well as to evaluate the recovery process, prognosis, and response to treatment.

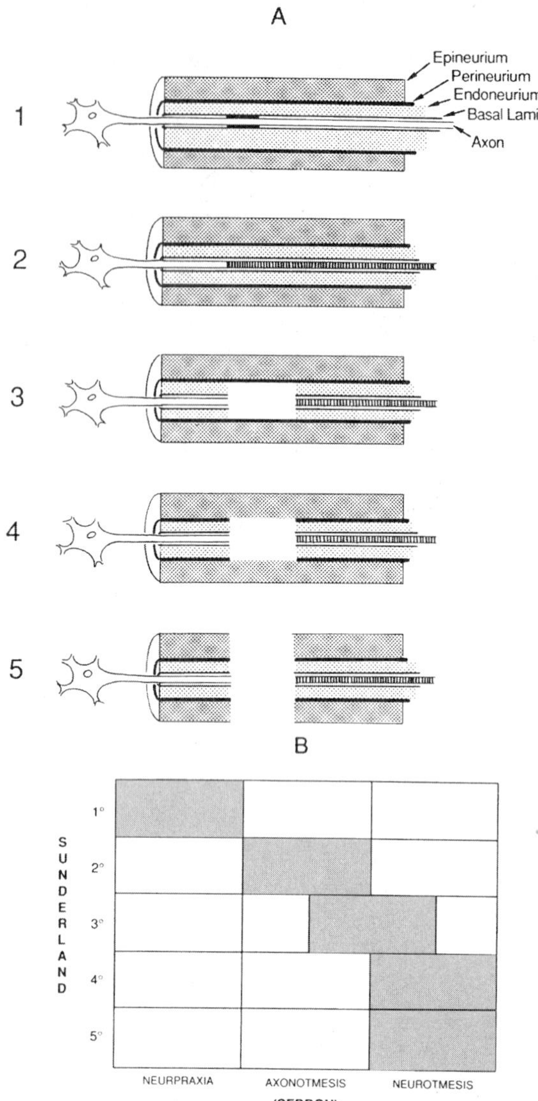

Figure 9-13. Degrees of nerve injury severity according to Sunderland's classification:

1. First degree—local conduction blockade with minimal change in structure. Prognosis: rapid full recovery.
2. Second degree—axonal disruption with secondary wallerian degeneration. Basal lamina remains intact. Prognosis: recovery but more prolonged time course requiring axonal regeneration. Likelihood of crossing over to another "channel" is low.
3. Third degree—axonal and endoneurial disruption. Prognosis: *intra*fascicular cross-overs during regeneration resulting in mild to moderate dysfunction.
4. Fourth degree—axonal, endoneurial, and perineurial disruption. Prognosis: *inter*fascicular cross-overs during regeneration resulting in moderate to severe dysfunction.
5. Fifth degree—complete structural disruption including axonal, endoneurial, perineurial, and epineurial discontinuity. Prognosis: no return unless the nerve undergoes microsurgical reconstruction.

(Reproduced by permission from Terzis JK, Smith KL. *The peripheral nerve. Structure function and reconstruction.* New York: Raven, 1990:40.)

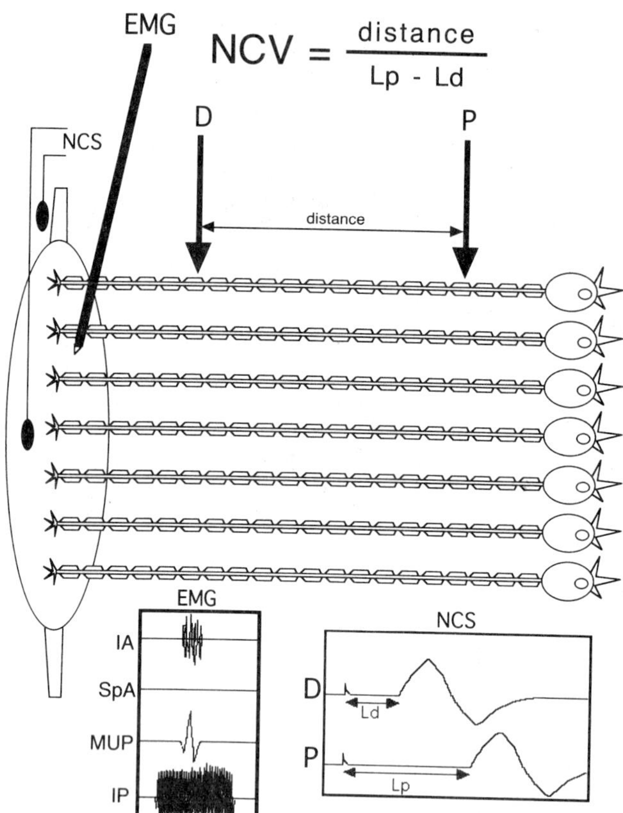

Figure 9-14. Schematic illustration of the data that can be gathered from a combination of motor nerve conduction studies (NCS) and needle electromyography (EMG) with reference to the basic structure of the myelinated motor nerve fibers. The nerve is stimulated at point D and at point P and the compound muscle action potential is recorded following stimulation at each site. The onset latencies are measured, the distance between stimulation sites is measured, and the nerve conduction velocity (NCV) is computed. In needle EMG, the potentials associated with needle movement are recorded (insertional activity); the spontaneous activity at rest is recorded; the shape, duration, and size of the motor unit action potentials are noted; and the interference pattern with maximum voluntary contraction is recorded. Lp = proximal latency; Ld = distal latency; D = distal site of stimulation; P = proximal site of stimulation; IA = insertional activity; SpA = spontaneous activity; MUP = motor unit potentials; IP = interference pattern.

Effects of Myelin Disruption

The first section of this chapter examined the effect of myelination on the conduction of the AP. Isolated myelin damage to a nerve fiber produces focal slowing of conduction across the damaged segment or conduction block, depending on the length of the axon continuously affected and the severity of the myelin damage. In motor conduction studies, stimulation above the level of the lesion shows a prolonged latency or reduced amplitude of the response or both, while stimulation below the level of the lesion shows normal latency and amplitude throughout the recovery process since the nerve structure remains intact distal to the lesion site. Thus, the amplitude of the response with stimulation below the level of the lesion is often larger than the amplitude with stimulation above the level of the lesion, reflecting the presence of conduction block as well as increased dispersion produced by the lesion. A difference in the structure of the waveform with stimulation above the lesion as compared to stimulation below the lesion may also be due to phase cancellation in the response related to an increased dispersion of the conduction times for different fibers. A drop in amplitude of the response could reflect increased temporal dispersion or it may be due to conduction block at the lesion site. If the demyelinating process is relatively homogeneous in its distribution throughout the fiber population, then the effect on the population will be relatively uniform, producing increased temporal dispersion with decreased amplitude and increased duration of the response, but the overall structure of the response will generally maintain a biphasic shape. This is what is generally observed in the inherited myelinopathies (see Fig. 9-15A). If, on the other hand, the segmental demyelination of different axonal populations is "patchy" so that the process distributes inhomogeneously across the fiber population, then there may be segmentation of the conduction velocity distribution in the nerve.

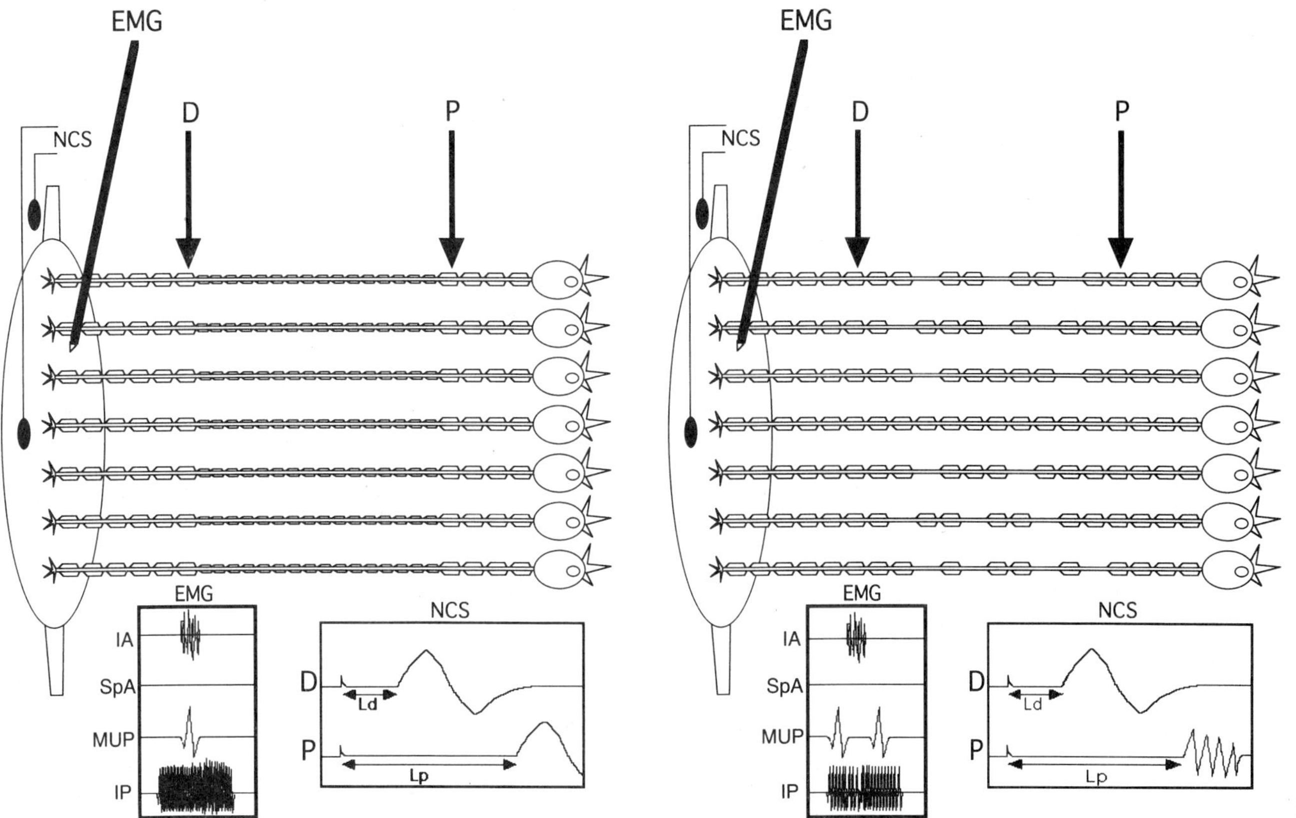

Figure 9-15. Nerve conduction study (NCS) and electromyographic (EMG) findings with demyelinating lesions. *A.* The effects of a homogeneous demyelinating lesion on NCS/EMG studies. There is focal slowing across the lesion without major dispersion of the response of stimulation proximal to the lesion. *B.* The effects of a heterogeneous demyelinating partial lesion on NCS/EMG studies. There is focal slowing across the lesion and the appearance of a polyphasic compound muscle action potential due to significant dispersion effects following stimulation proximal to the lesion. *C.* The subacute effects of a demyelinating severe lesion on NCS/EMG studies showing severe conduction block *without* evidence of distal axonal degeneration. There is no response following stimulation proximal to the lesion due to conduction block at the level of the lesion. Note the similarity between this picture and that seen in Figure 10-16A. Often there is secondary axonal degeneration when there has been a severe demyelinating process. In this case abnormal spontaneous activity is seen in the muscle.

Figure 9-15. *Continued*

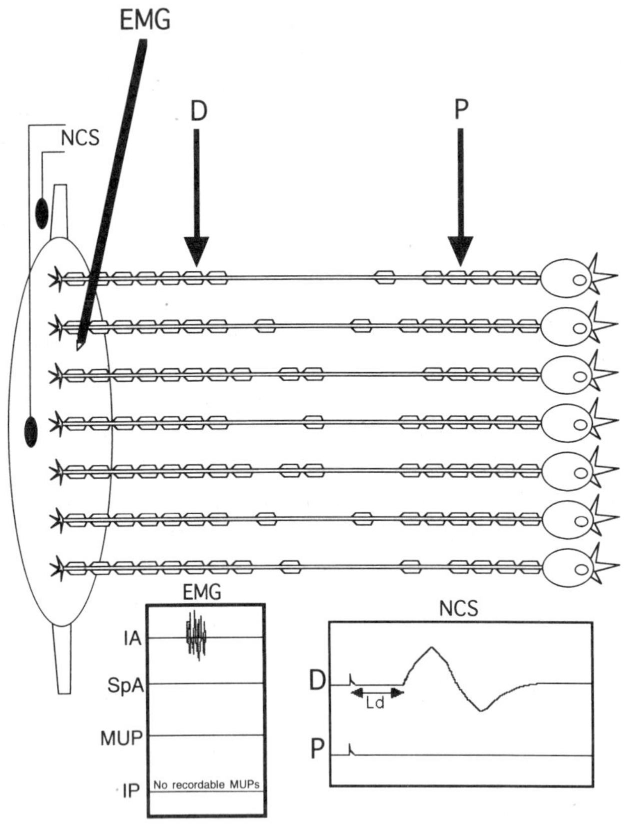

This will lead to a nonuniform dispersion and loss of the smooth and continuous activation of the muscle. The resultant effect is a discontinuous activation of the muscle and a "polyphasic" structure of the CMAP (see Fig. 9-15B). In pure demyelinating lesions, there is no distal axonal degeneration, and no effects on the EMG associated with the denervation of muscle fibers are detected (see Fig. 9-15C), although the nerve conduction findings cannot be distinguished from those of a severe localized axonal injury studied within the first few hours (Fig. 9-16A).

Effects of Axonal Injury

When the axonal component of the nerve is significantly damaged, the distal segment of the axon undergoes wallerian degeneration and the axon no longer conducts. This can take 3 to 5 days to occur. The corresponding evolution of electrodiagnostic findings in a complete injury to all of the axons of the nerve is shown in Figure 9-16. Loss of axons from the nerve distal to the site of injury produces a progressive drop in the amplitude of the CMAP in response to nerve stimulation distal to the lesion. When there is a partial axonotmetic injury, the amplitude of the response with stimulation distal to the injury is reduced to the same extent as the amplitude of the response proximal to the injury when the study is performed several days after the injury (Fig. 9-17). Distal degeneration of axons should eventually be associated with the appearance of abnormal spontaneous potentials in the EMG evaluation of the affected muscles innervated by the injured nerve. This fact emphasizes the importance of integrating information obtained from the NCSs with that obtained from needle EMG to obtain a complete picture.

In most cases encountered clinically, there may be a complicated mix of both demyelination and axonal degeneration. In general, when there is axonal degeneration, the effect is one of reduced amplitude of the evoked response without a significant increase in latency, although latency can increase when there is a significant selective loss of the fast-conducting fibers. Reduced amplitude can be due to an actual loss of axons but can also be seen with conduction block in structurally preserved axons. If there is diffuse nonselective axonal injury, then there is a significant drop in amplitude before the latency begins to increase. If the amplitude of the response is not reduced below 50% of normal, a decrease in conduction velocity to below 80% of the minimal normal conduction velocity indicates the presence of significant myelin loss.

F-Wave

By using setups for performing motor conduction studies, it is possible to look at waves that appear well after the initial response of the muscle, the so-called *M-wave*. These "late responses" can be studied by reducing the sweep speed of the display and looking for discrete waveforms that arise well after the initial muscle contraction is complete. When a supramaximal stimulus is applied to a peripheral mixed nerve, a coherent volley of APs travels away in both directions from the point of stimulation. In the motor fibers, the distally conducted volley activates the distal muscle to produce the CMAP, the M-wave. The proximally conducting volley travels up the nerve and into the motor nucleus in the anterolateral gray matter of the spinal cord. In this area, it activates a small proportion of the motor neurons by raising their excitation to above threshold and thus producing a "backfiring" of this small group of cells in the nucleus. These APs then are conducted back down the nerve out to the muscle and activate the muscle at a point in time well beyond the M-wave. This late response is called the *F-wave* and can be elicited from all muscles used in standard motor conduction studies. The ability to record the F-wave is facilitated by slight voluntary contraction of the muscle from which the signal is being recorded. The relative latency of this late F-wave and that of the M-wave depends on where the nerve is stimulated along the length of the limb. The more distal the point of stimulation, the earlier the M-wave and the later the F-wave. A sample normal F-wave and the pathway involved in the production of a tibial nerve F-wave with stimulation at the ankle are shown in Figure 9-18A. The F-wave latency is measured as the shortest latency for the onset of the F-wave in a fixed number of stimulation trials, usually around 16. The F-wave latency is most useful for demonstrating the presence of a mild peripheral neuropathy at an early stage because it samples a long segment of the nerve. F-waves also tend to be more sensitive in diagnosing neuropathies that are more likely to involve proximal segments of the nerve. In addition, F-wave latency may be helpful in demonstrating isolated proximal lesions as can be seen, for example, in early acute inflammatory demyelinating

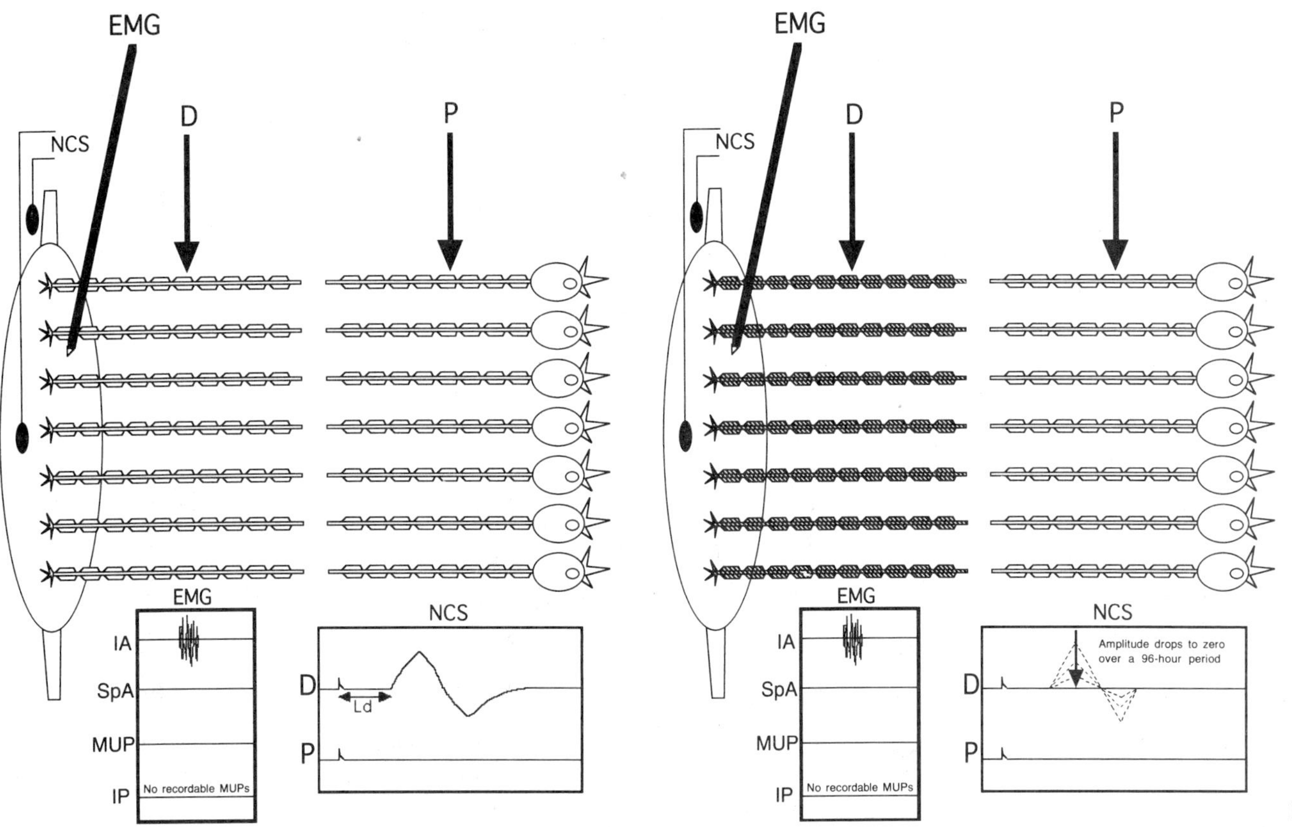

Figure 9-16. EMG/NCS findings during evolution of a complete axonotmetic lesion. *A.* The effects of a complete axonotmetic lesion within the first 24 hours. The fibers distal to the lesion continue to conduct normally but there is no response to stimulation proximal to the lesion. The situation at this point in time is indistinguishable from a severe focal demyelinating lesion producing conduction block. *B.* The effects of a complete axonotmetic lesion after the first 96 hours. The disconnected motor fibers distal to the lesion increasingly fail to conduct and the amplitude of the compound motor action potential following stimulation distal to the lesion steadily drops. *C.* The effects of a complete axonotmetic lesion after the first 14 days, showing the appearance of abnormal spontaneous potentials in the muscle reflecting the onset of muscle fibrillation. *D.* The effects of a complete axonotmetic lesion with axonal regeneration and initial reinnervation of the muscle, demonstrating the appearance of newly formed highly polyphasic, low-amplitude, long-duration motor unit action potentials. *E.* With time, the distal processes of the reinnervation motor fibers remyelinate and mature with increasing synchronization of activation of the motor unit. The motor unit action potential remains polyphasic but the amplitude increases and the duration decreases.

Figure 9-16. *Continued*

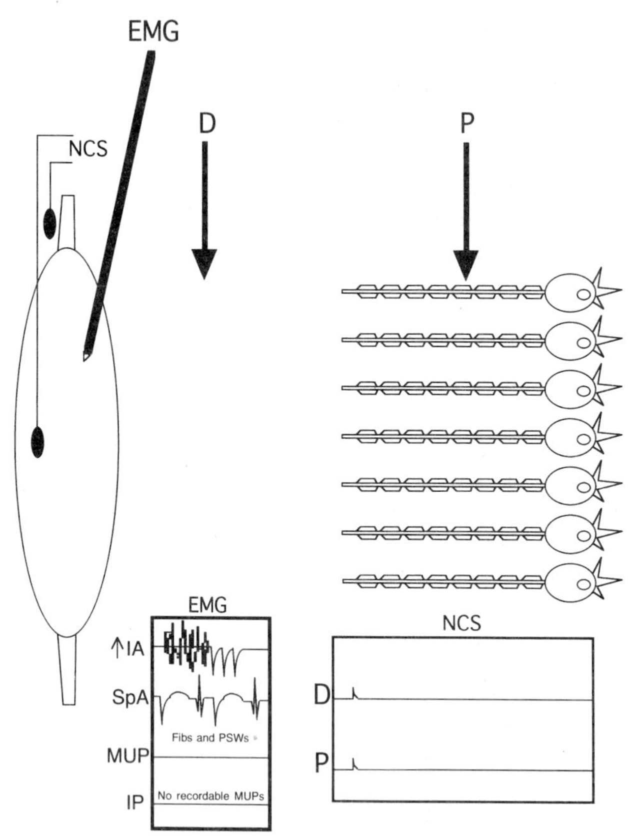

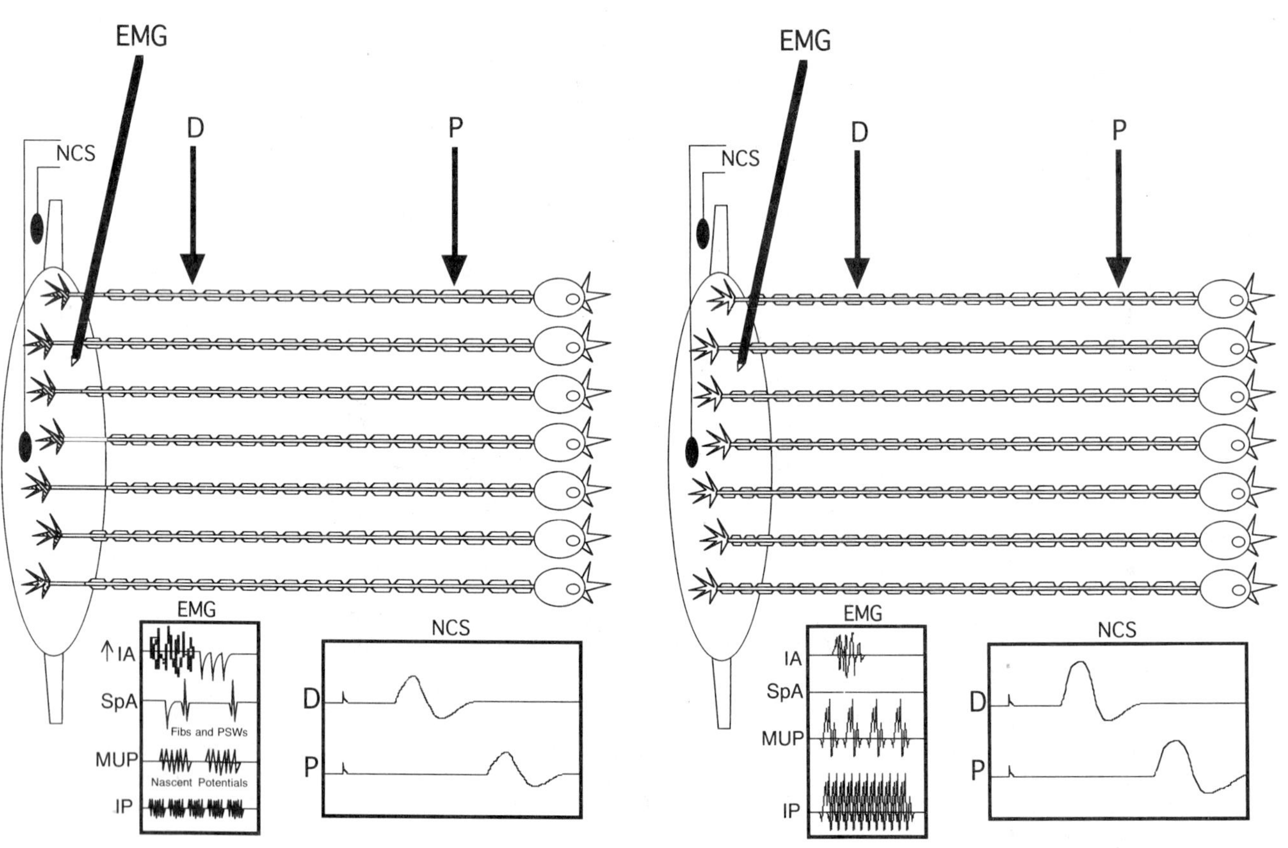

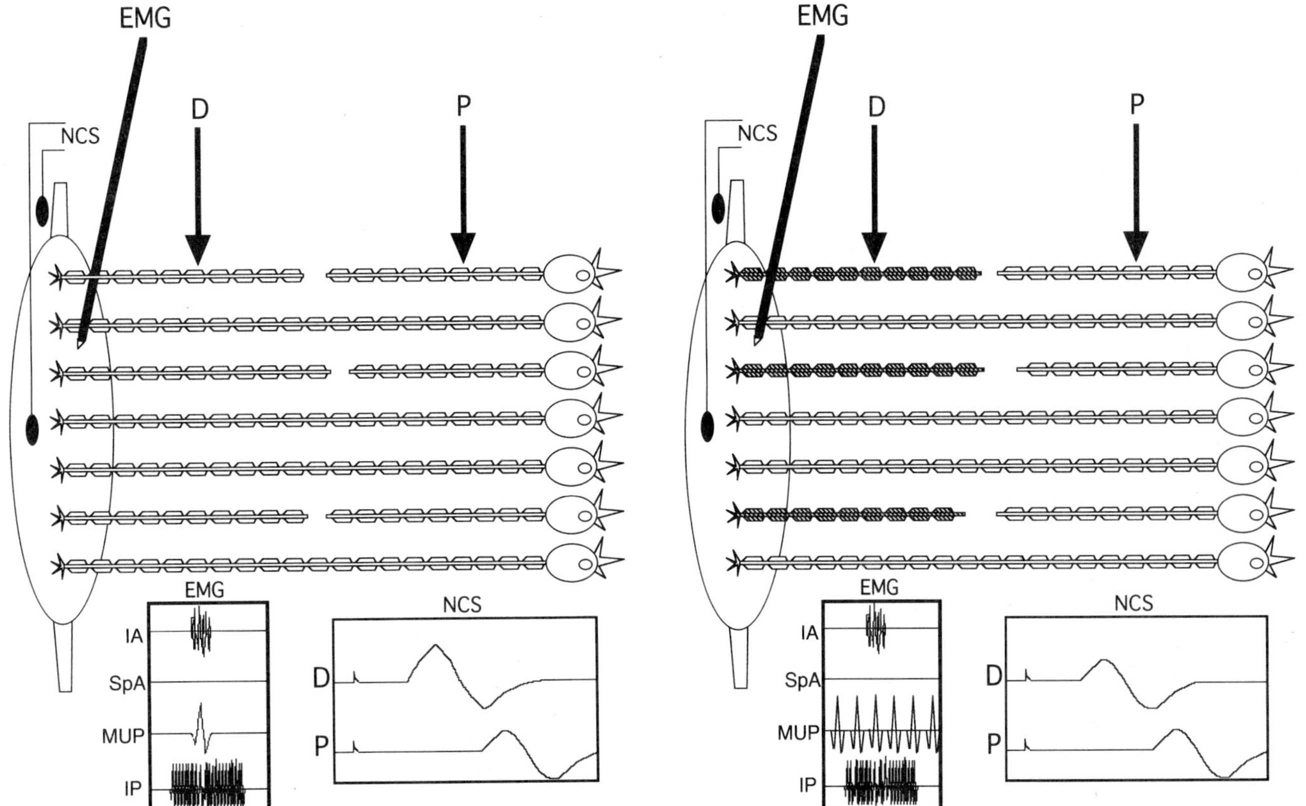

Figure 9-17. EMG/NCS findings during evolution of a partial axonotmetic lesion. *A.* The effects of a partial axonotmetic lesion in the first 24 hours. The distal fiber segments continue to conduct normally for a short period. Motor unit recruitment is reduced and recruitment frequency is increased. *B.* The effects of a partial axonotmetic lesion after the first 96 hours. The damaged distal fiber segments no longer conduct and the amplitude of the compound motor action potential with stimulation distal to the lesion falls off proportionate to the number of injured fibers in the nerve. It is still too early to see abnormal spontaneous potentials. *C.* Subacute effects of a partial axonotmetic lesion showing the effects of peripheral motor fiber sprouting and motor unit enlargement actively in process. The motor unit action potentials now have a polyphasic structure corresponding to the active remodeling of the motor unit with the formation of new sprouts and the activation of newly innervated muscle fibers acquired by the sprouts. *D.* Late effects of a partial axonotmetic lesion showing the effects of peripheral motor fiber sprouting and motor unit enlargement after maturation of the sprouting process and more synchronous activation of the enlarged motor unit. Motor unit action potentials are significantly increased in amplitude and may or may not be increased in duration depending on the degree of synchrony achieved.

polyradiculoneuritis (i.e., Guillain-Barré syndrome). If the pathology is partial in its involvement, is isolated to the root level, or is not associated with a major degree of focal demyelination of the root, the long expanse of normal nerve in the conducting pathway can effectively dilute the effect of the local slowing at the site of injury. In this situation, the F-wave latency is not abnormally prolonged but the trial-to-trial variation of F-wave latency or the *chronodispersion* within the F-wave itself may be increased. In the presence of normal peripheral nerve conduction, a prolonged F-wave latency is relatively specific for slowing at a proximal level of the nerve, but is not especially sensitive in diagnosing the presence of isolated proximal pathology. It is more sensitive when attempting to diagnose a diffusely distributed peripheral neuropathy that produces some degree of slowing along the entire pathway evaluated by the F-wave latency.

H-Reflex

In the adult subject, another late response, the Hoffman or H-reflex, can be recorded from a limited number of muscles and distinguished from the F-wave in terms of the conditions that maximally elicit the response. The H-reflex can only be recorded reliably in the normal adult from the calf muscles with stimulation of the tibial nerve and from the flexor carpi radialis with stimulation of the median nerve. While the F-wave is best elicited by a maximal stimulus to the nerve that excites all of the motor fibers together, the H-reflex is best produced by a submaximal stimulus of long duration that is more likely to selectively activate the low-threshold Ia afferent fibers to a greater degree than efferent motor fibers or other cutaneous afferents. With stimulation of the tibial nerve at the popliteal crease behind the knee and with recording electrodes placed over the medial gastrocnemius and soleus, for

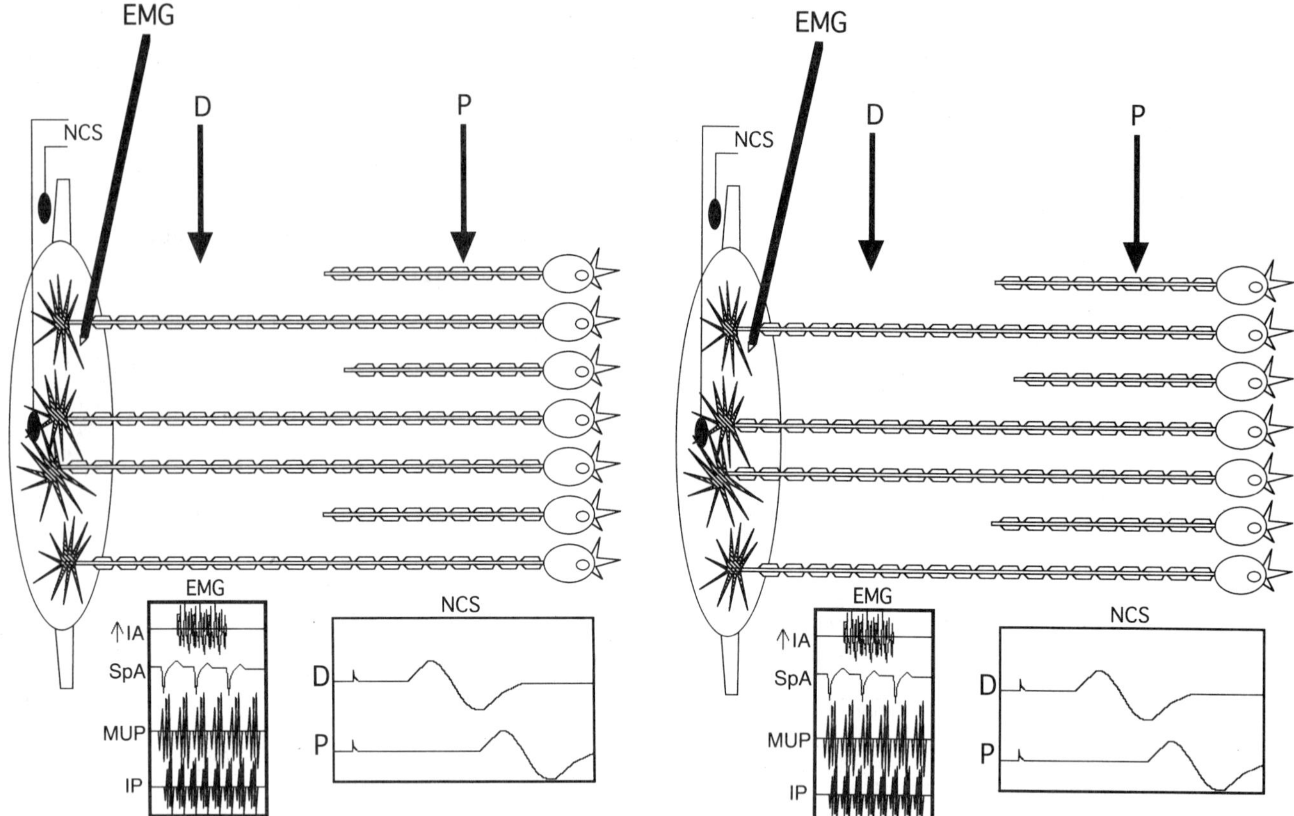

Figure 9-17. *Continued.*

example, the H-reflex is first elicited as the stimulus intensity is slowly increased and then is extinguished as the stimulus intensity is increased further, with the subsequent appearance of the F-wave at higher stimulus levels. The H-reflex is thought to be an electrical equivalent of the deep tendon reflex at the Achilles tendon, with activation of a monosynaptic reflex arc primarily through muscle spindle stretch-sensitive afferents. A similar waveform can be elicited when the tendon is tapped with an adapted tendon hammer; when contact with the tendon is made, the trace on the EMG machine is triggered. The amplitude of the H-reflex is variable, depending on the degree of background voluntary activation of the muscle. The H-reflex latency is thus the more useful derived measure and can be used as a test for S1 radiculopathy, where it may be especially helpful when the pathology is unilateral and the side contralateral to the injury can be used as a control value. A side-to-side latency difference of more than 1.5 msec can indicate an abnormality. In individuals older than 60 years, this upper limit is increased to 1.8 msec (82). An example recording of an H-reflex and the relevant pathway involved are shown in Figure 9-18B and 19-18C.

Repetitive Stimulation Studies to Investigate Neuromuscular Junction Pathology

When there is clinical muscular weakness or a complaint of fatigue that appears to be significantly modified, either downward or upward, by exercise, the possibility of neuromuscular junction pathology must be considered. Junctional transmission pathophysiology can be directly investigated and detected using electrodiagnostic methods that involve a modification of the motor conduction study method in which the nerve is repetitively stimulated and time-dependent sequential changes in the amplitude of the CMAP are documented. The effect of sustained isometric exercise on the amplitude of the CMAP can also reveal abnormalities of neuromuscular transmission. Normally, repetitive stimulation at a rate under 5 Hz should not have any major progressive effect on the amplitude of the CMAP recorded with each successive stimulus delivered. Likewise, a brief period of exercise should not significantly alter the amplitude of the CMAP subsequently recorded with repetitive stimulation. A decrement in amplitude, if seen, should be less than 10%. However, in the presence of neuromuscular junction pathology, significant effects of exercise on neuromuscular transmission can be systematically investigated using neurophysiologic protocols that involve repetitive stimulation performed before and after sustained muscular exercise.

The junctional disorders can be divided into three categories based on where in the neuromuscular junction the interference with synaptic transmission takes place: presynaptic, postsynaptic, and synaptic cleft. Presynaptic conditions result from pathology that is localized to the mechanisms involved in ACh synthesis and release from the nerve terminal. Postsynaptic conditions result from pathology that alters the function of the AChRs and the specialized muscle fiber membrane of the end-plate region. Synaptic cleft disorders result from alteration in ACh metabolism and concentration in the synaptic space. This would include the effect of anticholinesterase drugs. Examples of conditions and agents that produce presynaptic, postsynaptic, and synaptic cleft neuromuscular junction disorders are listed in Table 9-9. The structure and physiology of the neuromuscular junction have been reviewed already.

One well-studied postsynaptic condition is myasthenia gravis (47). It is a relatively rare condition, but one for which the pathophysiologic mechanism is reasonably well worked out. The key clinical finding is exercise-induced fatigue that is most commonly reported in external ocular muscles, face, jaw, bulbar, and proximal limb muscles. Symptoms are often worse in the evening when patients are tired, and patients may present with isolated cranial nerve involvement. The disease involves an autoimmune response to the postsynaptic membrane of the neuromuscular junction associated with a reduction in the numbers of postsynaptic AChRs. Thus, while the presynaptic

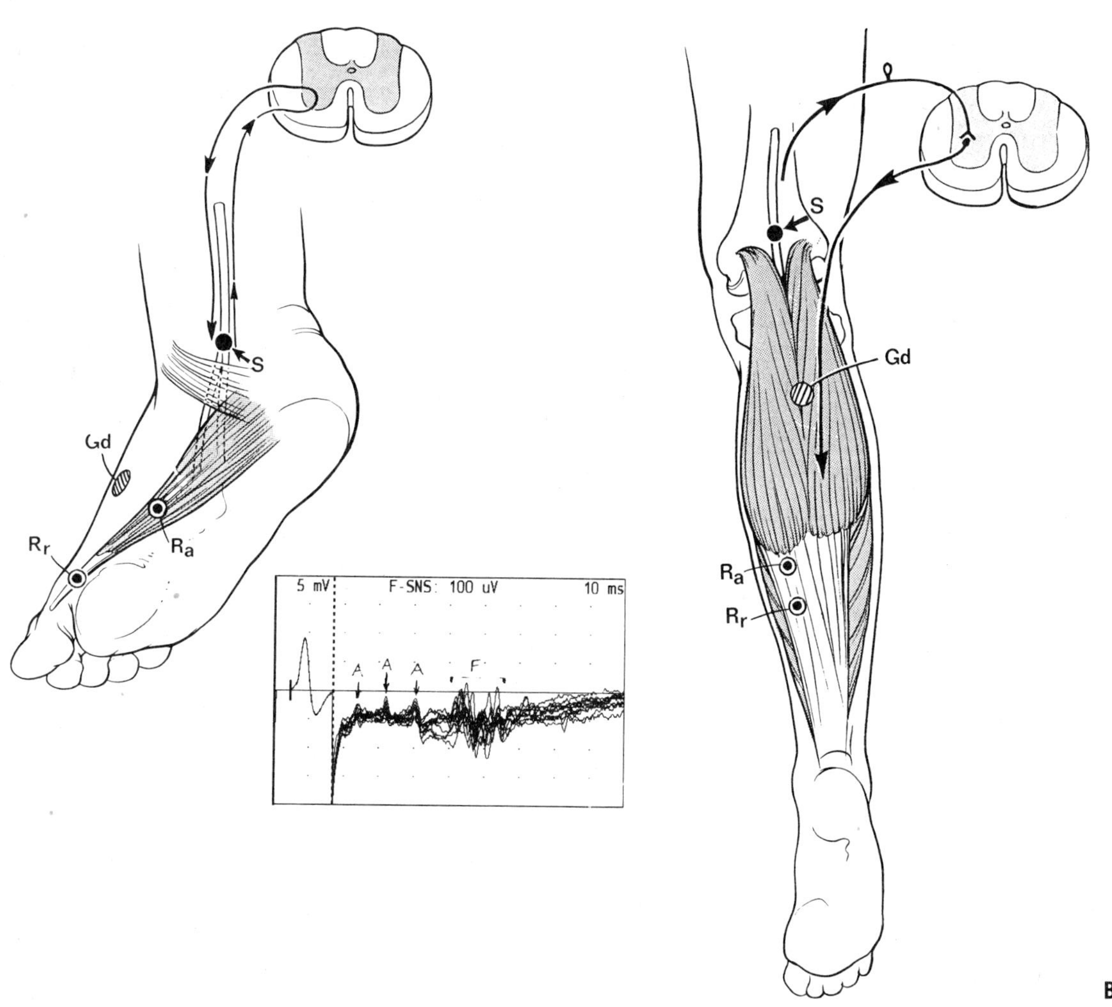

Figure 9-18. *A.* Demonstration of the pathway and technique for recording the F-wave with stimulation of the tibial nerve at the ankle and recording from the abductor hallucis. The *inset* shows an abnormal tibial F-wave study from a patient with sarcoid-related polyneuropathy. Multiple axonal reflex or "A-waves" are seen reflecting axonal branching or ephaptic interaxonal transmission. The F-wave also has increased chronodispersion. The M-wave is the wave to the left of the *vertical dashed line. B.* Demonstration of the pathway and technique for recording the H-reflex with stimulation of the tibial nerve at the popliteal fossa and recording from electrodes placed over the soleus muscle. Gd = ground electrode; Ra = active recording electrode; Rr = reference recording electrode; S = site of stimulation. *C.* Recording of the H-reflex showing multiple traces with increasing stimulus current. Note the early appearance of the H-wave on the right side of the traces with the subsequent appearance of the M-wave. As the M-wave increases in amplitude with increasing stimulus current, the H-reflex amplitude drops back down. *Vertical markers* are placed at the onset latencies for the M-wave and the H-wave. The amplitude graphs show the steady rise in amplitude of the M-wave and the rise and fall of the amplitude of the H-reflex.

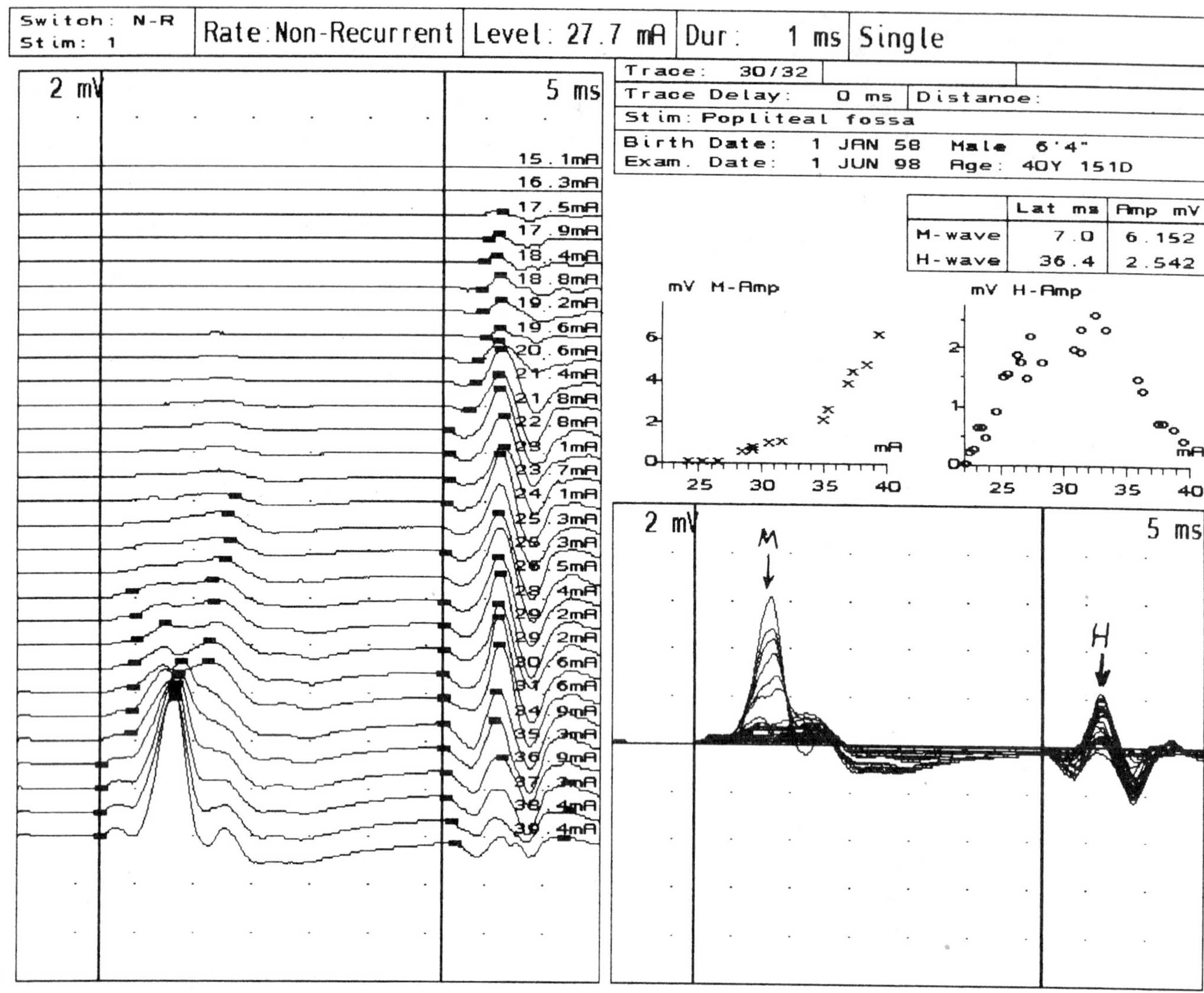

C

Figure 9-18. *Continued*

release of ACh is normal, the postsynaptic response and the depolarization of the postsynaptic membrane that normally follows the depolarization of the presynaptic membrane are abnormal. The postsynaptic depolarization may be inadequate to bring the postsynaptic membrane to threshold with the failure to produce a postsynaptic muscle fiber AP (a phenomenon called *blocking*). In addition, the postsynaptic depolarization reaches threshold with a much greater degree of variability in the delay between presynaptic activation and the production of the postsynaptically generated AP (sometimes referred to as *increased jitter*). These phenomena can be detected directly using single-fiber EMG (83). In addition, with repeated activation of the junctions following repetitive peripheral nerve stimulation at a rate of three stimulations per second, there is a tendency for the reduced population of available AChRs to become saturated, with fewer and fewer AChRs available to respond to the ACh that has been released. This leads to a progressive increase in the number of neuromuscular junctions that "block" with each successive impulse. The result is a progressive reduction or *decrement* in the amplitude of the CMAP as an increasing number of neuromuscular junctions fail to transmit. This "decremental response" in the amplitude of successive CMAPs with repetitive nerve stimulation is the major electrodiagnostic finding in myasthenia gravis. The effect of exercise is to temporarily "repair" the decrement through the facilitated presynaptic release of ACh resulting from enhanced Ca ion flow into the presynaptic terminal associated with posttetanic facilitation. One to 3 minutes later, in the period of posttetanic depression, when the facilitation effect is over and there is a relative reduction in ACh release from the presynaptic terminal, the decrement reappears and is enhanced. These effects can also be partially reduced through the administration of medications like the anticholinesterase inhibitors, which facilitate the action of ACh by antagonizing the breakdown of ACh in the synaptic cleft. This corresponds clinically to the so-called Tensilon

Table 9-9: Examples of Conditions and Agents Producing Neuromuscular Junction Dysfunction
Presynaptic
Lambert-Eaton myasthenic syndrome
Botulism
Tetanus
Tick paralysis
Familial infantile myasthenia
Tetrodotoxin
Ciguatoxin
ω-Conotoxin
Magnesium poisoning
Postsynaptic
Myasthenia gravis
Transient neonatal autoimmune myasthenia gravis
Slow-channel syndrome
Congenital end-plate acetylcholinesterase receptor deficiency
d-Tubocurarine
Succinylcholine
Nicotine
α-Bungarotoxin
α-Conotoxin
Synaptic cleft
Anticholinesterase drugs
Edrophonium chloride
Pyridostigmine bromide
Neostigmine bromide
Organophosphate poisoning
Acetylcholinesterase deficiency

test where the clinical deficit is temporarily reduced through the intravenous administration of edrophonium, a rapid-acting cholinesterase inhibitor. The yield of the electrodiagnostic testing can be increased by warming the muscles and by sampling multiple muscles, especially proximal ones using setups involving the accessory nerve or the facial nerve.

In Lambert-Eaton myasthenic syndrome (LEMS) (84), a rare presynaptic condition associated with malignancy, the defect involves impairment of the presynaptic release of ACh, possibly through an autoimmune process that attacks voltage-sensitive Ca channels in the membrane of the presynaptic nerve terminal (85). Clinically, patients present with proximal muscle weakness without prominent wasting and the deep tendon reflexes are found to be suppressed but can be readily elicited after the muscles have been exercised. Patients may also complain of symptoms referable to dysfunction of the autonomic nervous system. In LEMS, the short-term effect of tetanizing the neuromuscular junction through sustained isometric contraction is to greatly facilitate neuromuscular junction transmission with a resulting dramatic increase in the amplitude of the CMAP immediately after exercise. Prior to exercise, the baseline amplitude of the CMAP is generally reduced. Immediately following exercise, the amplitude of the CMAP may increase by 50% to 1000% or better.

While these conditions are quite rare, if they are clinically suspected, they may be readily detected when the appropriate electrodiagnostic methods are applied. Examples of repetitive stimulation studies in myasthenia gravis and LEMS patients are shown in Figure 9-19. Some potential sources of error that can confound the results of repetitive stimulation testing are listed in Table 9-10. Single-fiber EMG, although a more arduous method requiring a specialized setup, tends to have a higher sensitivity for diagnosing neuromuscular junction pathophysiology as compared to repetitive stimulation techniques (83).

ELECTROMYOGRAPHY

The Motor Unit

The motor unit is the "final common pathway" of voluntary movement—the quantal element of motor function. One cannot voluntarily activate subgroups of the muscle fibers innervated in a motor unit under normal physiologic conditions. The clinical EMG examination involves the examination of physiologic events in the muscle during different conditions, and involves examination of the physiology of motor unit activation and motor unit recruitment during voluntary contraction of the muscle. The structure of the motor unit is schematically illustrated in Figure 9-20.

The motor unit has a natural tree-like anatomic structure, with a dividing of the peripheral motor fiber when it enters the muscle into individual terminal branches, each of which innervates a single muscle fiber. In the mature human neuromuscular system, each muscle fiber is innervated by only one peripheral nerve motor fiber. This means that each peripheral motor nerve fiber innervates and controls the contraction of a unique and nonoverlapping set of muscle fibers in the muscle.

The motor neurons innervating a particular muscle are arranged in nuclear clusters called *motor nuclei* in the anterior horn of the spinal cord at the segmental level. The total population of motor neurons innervating a particular muscle is sometimes called the *motor neuron pool.*

The metabolic characteristics of the muscle fibers in a muscle tend to be nonuniform and can be categorized into different types [e.g., slow oxidative (SO), fast oxidative-glycolytic (FOG), fast glycolytic (FG)] that are randomly distributed throughout the muscle. The metabolic characteristics determine the twitch tension, and the rate of development of tension with each activation of the motor unit. They also determine the extent to which the motor unit fatigues with repetitive firing of the motor unit. The metabolic characteristics of the muscle fibers in a particular motor unit are uniform and are determined and controlled by the characteristics of the motor neuron innervating the muscle fibers.

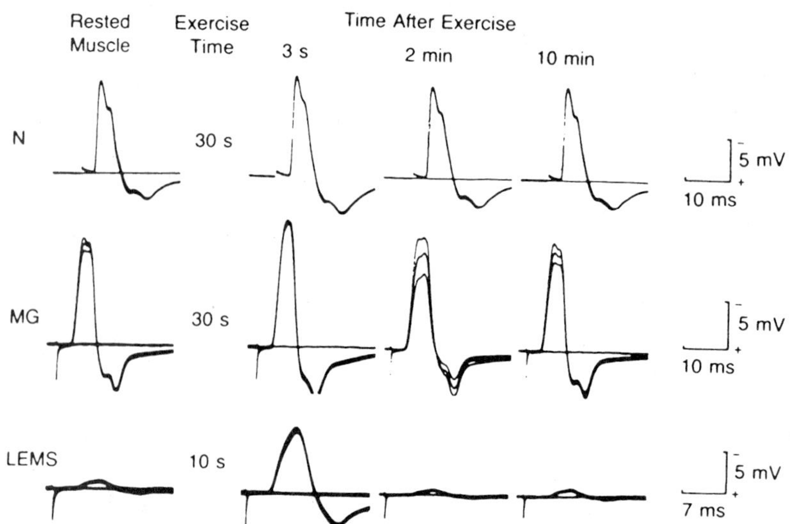

Figure 9-19. Demonstration of repetitive stimulation effects in a normal subject (*N*), a patient with myasthenia gravis (*MG*), and a patient with Lambert-Eaton myasthenic syndrome (*LEMS*). In the normal subject, there is no decrement in amplitude with multiple stimulation and the effects of exercise and rest are not very significant. However, in the patient with MG, the decrement at rest is initially repaired immediately after 30 seconds of exercise and then becomes much more marked 2 minutes after the exercise, with posttetanic exhaustion effects. The most remarkable finding in the LEMS patient is the massive but transient facilitatory effect of a short burst of exercise on the amplitude of the compound muscle action potential. (Modified from Lambert EH, Rooke ED, Eaton LM, Hodgson CH. Myasthenic syndrome occasionally associated with bronchial neoplasm. Neurophysiologic studies. In: Viets HR, ed. *Myasthenia gravis.* Springfield, IL: Charles C Thomas, 1961:362–410.)

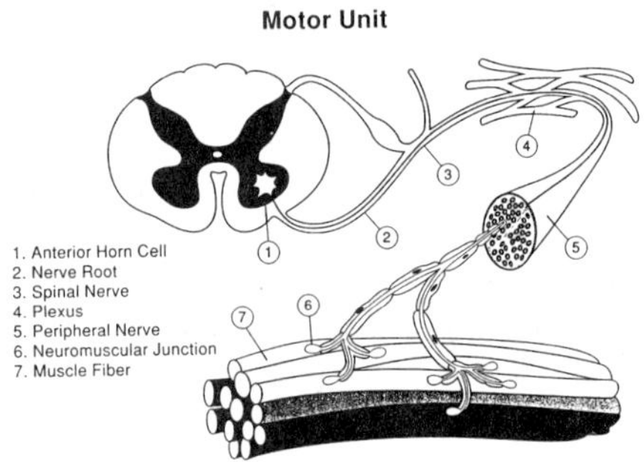

Figure 9-20. Schematic drawing of the motor unit and its structural components. (Reproduced by permission from Dumitru D. *Electrodiagnostic medicine.* Philadelphia: Hanley & Belfus, 1995.)

Size of the Motor Unit and the "Size Principle"

The size of the motor unit is the number of muscle fibers innervated by the axon of the individual motor neuron. Average motor unit size can vary significantly from muscle to muscle. The size of the motor unit is roughly related to the size of the cell body of the motor neuron and the corresponding diameter of the motor axon. Larger motor units have larger motor neuron cell bodies and axons with a larger diameter. Smaller units tend to be SO units with slowly developing, low-amplitude twitch tensions. The SO muscle fibers are able to produce energy substrates through oxidative metabolism and are thus resistant to fatigue. These units are important for the prolonged generation of low-level tension as would be used in prolonged standing. SO motor units depend on increased capillary blood flow to deliver oxygen and glucose in maintaining the ongoing contraction. Larger units tend to be FG units with relatively fast-developing, large twitch tensions that rely on glycolytic pathways and are susceptible to fatigue. They are important for fast, short-lived, high-level bursts of tension as would be used in a sprint. Intermediate-size units tend to be FOG units, which are a hybrid of the SO and the FG units. These units have the ability to generate intermediate-level tensions and are relatively resistant to fatigue but not as resistant as the SO units. The general mix of different motor unit types can vary significantly from muscle to muscle.

The "size principle" states that motor units are recruited in an orderly way and that the order of recruitment is such that smaller units, which are usually of the SO type, are recruited before the larger units, which are of the FOG and FG types. This also means that low-level contractions can be sustained for long periods of time without being subject to fatigue while high-level contractions in which the FOG and FG units are recruited cannot be sustained.

The motor unit organizes voluntary muscular contractions through the controlled synchronous contractions of groups of fibers in the muscle. The upper motor neuron and segmental interneurons form a control network that controls activation of the motor neurons in the different motor neuron pools that innervate the muscles of the moving limb. Each anterior horn cell receives large num-

Table 9-10: Sources of Error in Performing Repetitive Stimulation Studies

1. Change of stimulator contact resistance associated with stimulus-induced movement changes the amount of stimulus current that reaches the nerve and results in an artifactual reduction in amplitude of the compound muscle action potential. A stimulator block should be securely taped over the nerve, and limb movement should be limited by carefully restraining the limb.
2. Limb movement can change the position and contact of the recording electrodes placed over the muscle. For this reason, again, the limb should be carefully restrained and the recording electrodes should be in good stable contact with the skin over the motor point of the responding muscle. If available, adhesive electrodes that are securely attached to the skin over the muscle are preferred.
3. If the distal extent of the limb is cool, this can reduce or abolish the decrement. Studies in the upper limb should be done after the limb has been warmed to 34°C.
4. A significant decrement may not be seen in a distal muscle. If the distal examination shows no significant decrement, repeat the study on a more proximal muscle like the trapezius or deltoid.
5. The diagnosis may not be established because of a lack of sensitivity of the repetitive stimulation techniques. If the clinical index of suspicion is high and the results of the repetitive stimulation studies are normal or equivocal, use single-fiber electromyography.

Source: Adapted from Binnie CD, Cooper R, Fowler CJ, et al, eds. *Clinical neurophysiology. EMG, nerve conduction and evoked potentials.* Oxford: Butterworth-Heinemann, 1995:203.

bers of synaptic inputs from three sources. It receives input directly from upper motor neurons projecting down to the segment from above (suprasegmental inputs). There is also direct input from sensory neurons transmitting from peripheral receptors (e.g., Ia afferents in the monosynaptic muscle stretch reflex arc). The third input is from interneurons that transmit both inhibitory and excitatory drive to the motor unit based on integration of activity at the spinal segmental level. All of this input is integrated in the dendritic tree and cell body of the motor neuron and controls the firing pattern of the motor unit. Production of an AP at the cell body of the motor neuron normally initiates a highly predictable and controllable sequence of events. The AP is transmitted down the peripheral motor fiber and into the terminal branches. There is transmission across the neuromuscular junctions, and a relatively synchronous electrical activation of all of the muscle fibers in the motor unit. This produces a mechanical "twitch" of tension in the muscle via electromechanical coupling in the muscle fibers. Tension in the muscle can be graded upward in two major ways. First, the activated motor neurons can be fired more rapidly, leading to an increasing overlap of the twitches produced by each individual twitch contraction and therefore a graded buildup of tension in the motor unit. This is called *firing frequency modulation.* Second, more motor neurons from the available motor neuron pool can be activated. This is called *motor unit recruitment.*

Approach to Localization

The EMG examination is useful for localizing the site of a lesion affecting the motor unit (86). To determine whether the damage is at the peripheral nerve, plexus, or root level, it is important to use a directed, deductive process. Different muscles that have the same root innervation but through different peripheral nerves are studied, as well as muscles that have the same peripheral nerve innervation from different roots. One looks for consistent involvement within a particular peripheral nerve or root distribution. When an abnormal muscle is identified, a different muscle with the same peripheral nerve innervation from a different root level is examined. Another muscle with the same root level innervation by way of a different peripheral nerve should also be examined. The approach to lesion localization can be viewed as an exercise in deductive reasoning, working from a knowledge base of peripheral neuromuscular anatomy and root level innervation of limb muscles. To be successful, the electromyographer must have a solid working knowledge of the relevant neuromuscular anatomy and innervation patterns as well as an awareness of common patterns of anomalous anatomic structure within the plexus and peripheral nerve branching patterns.

Recurrent Elements of the Clinical EMG Examination

The clinical EMG examination consists of repeated application of the following steps to different muscles:

1. Insertion of the intramuscular electrode and verification of its location through activation of the targeted muscle, whenever possible, using kinesiologic principles.
2. The search for spontaneous activity in the resting muscle: examination of the muscle at rest by moving the electrode through different regions of the muscle to sample the activity while the muscle is completely relaxed. Abnormal spontaneous activity must be distinguished from normal spontaneous activity seen near the neuromuscular junction and from normal motor unit activation. At each penetration of the muscle, the electrode should be moved in very short intervals along a track, then brought back out of the muscle tissue into the subcutaneous tissue and reentered into the muscle angled in different directions in order to adequately sample different regions of the muscle without requiring different skin penetrations. The central

region of the muscle near the motor point contains the highest concentration of neuromuscular junctions and should be avoided in order to limit confusion between abnormal spontaneous potentials and normal EPPs. Abnormal spontaneous activity may be seen in the muscle without electrode movement or it may be seen only after the electrode has been moved, resulting in a provocative mechanical irritation of the muscle fiber membrane. Thus, electrode movement can be viewed as a way to provoke the presence of abnormal spontaneous activity in the muscle. It is a challenge to the muscle fiber membrane to see how readily it is able to reestablish a stable baseline after being mechanically irritated. Normally a series of "injury" potentials are produced when the needle is moved in the muscle. These recurrent potentials quickly subside once the needle is no longer moving. This *insertional activity* should not last more than 300 msec after the needle stops moving.

3. Characterization of the MUAPs by isolating individual MUAPs while recording with low-level contraction of the muscle. The electrode is positioned to maximize the amplitude and minimize the rise time of the targeted MUAP, thus ensuring the closest approach to the muscle fibers activated through the firing of the unit. This can be guided by listening to the sound of the unit on the loudspeaker.

   Characterization of the MUAP occurs through measured parameters: amplitude, duration, and number of phases. Recruitment measures include recruitment and onset frequencies.

   When the patient performs a slowly graded increase in contraction of the muscle being examined, new motor units are steadily activated and added to the active group. With a steady tension in the normal muscle, a motor unit begins firing at somewhere between 6 and 14 Hz depending on the muscle (87,88). The lowest stable initial firing rate of a newly recruited unit is called the *onset frequency* and its inverse, the interspike interval between MUAPs at onset, is called the *onset interval*. The firing frequency of the MUAP then starts to increase until the next unit is recruited. The *recruitment frequency* is the firing rate of a unit at the point at which the next unit is recruited, with its inverse being the *recruitment interval*. In normal muscle, recruitment frequencies can vary from about 10 Hz in the multifidus to 29 Hz in the orbicularis oris (87). These definitions are illustrated graphically in Figure 9-21.

   The MUAP should also be examined for the stability of its parameters as it fires repetitively—for example, does the amplitude or shape of the MUAP vary? The MUAP can be examined using a triggering capability and a delayed display. The trigger level is adjusted so that triggering occurs only on the spike of the MUAP of interest. Some machines will have a more sophisticated "window" triggering capability that allows one to set a lower and upper limit for a trigger window on the peak of the MUAP of interest. Some machines will allow repeated occurrences of the isolated MUAP to be averaged together prior to the measurement of parameters. However, recurrent firing of the same MUAP should be viewed in a raster display to evaluate the variability of the morphology of the MUAP and to check that the averaging takes place on multiple occurrences of the same MUAP.

4. Characterization of the interference pattern (IP) produced when the patient is exerting a maximal effort to contract the muscle. This is an assessment of the maximum number of motor units available in the motor neuron pool innervating the muscle. A normal IP is termed *full* and indicates a complete obliteration of the baseline by the superposition of a large number of simultaneously contracting motor units. A *reduced* IP may be identified as indicating a *moderate* level of recruitment when the baseline is intermittently flat and unbroken by the recruitment of motor units. A further reduction in recruitment allows individual MUAPs to be identified without interference from overlapping MUAPs and this may be termed a *discrete* IP. Maximal voluntary contraction resulting in the rapid firing of an individual motor unit is referred to as a *single-unit IP*. Reduced recruitment may be due to at least three different possible factors:

   1. Loss of motor units in the pool. This is associated with an increase in recruitment frequency.
   2. Inability to activate units in the pool due to an upper motor neuron problem. The motor unit firing pattern and the recruitment of motor units are irregular.
   3. Reduced voluntary effort that results in a submaximal activation of the motor unit pool. The recruitment frequency is normal.

   In the presence of a myopathic process, recruitment may be termed *increased* when there is rapid development of a full IP even with a minimal contraction of the muscle.

The elements of the needle EMG examination are shown schematically in Figure 9-22.

Normal Spontaneous Activity

Normal insertional activity is related to the direct damage produced in muscle fibers when the electrode is advanced through the muscle. If the electrical properties of the membrane are stable, then the effects of the movement of

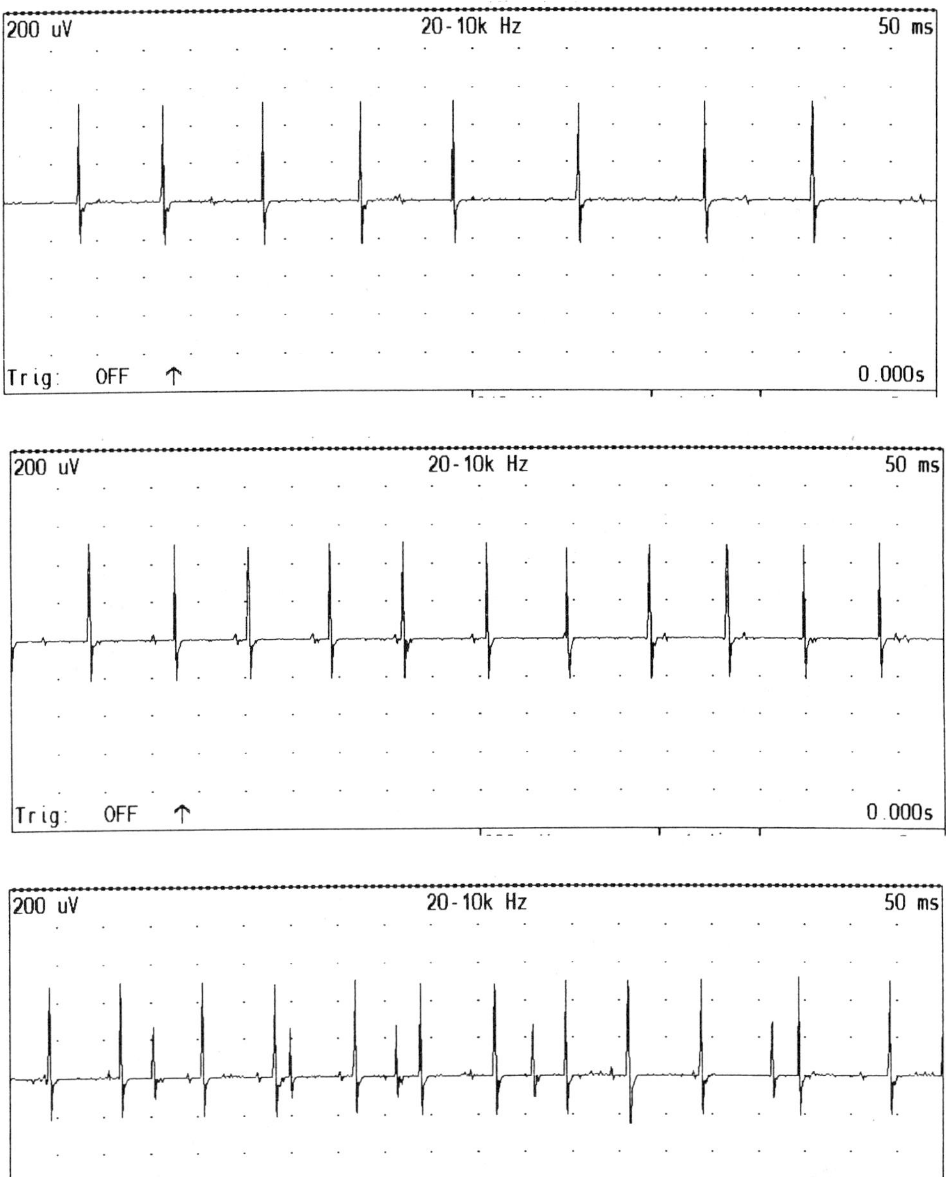

Figure 9-21. Definition of the onset and recruitment frequencies. *Top trace.* Single motor unit potential begins to fire at 8 Hz in the first dorsal interosseous muscle. This is the onset frequency. *Middle trace.* As the muscle tension is graded up, the firing rate of the motor unit potential increases steadily. Here it has increased to 11 Hz. *Bottom trace.* At this point, a second motor unit potential appears. The firing rate of the original potential when the second appears is 12 Hz. This is the recruitment frequency.

the needle rapidly subside within 300 msec. The value of insertional activity is that it indicates when the needle is actually moving through muscle tissue. It will not be seen when the needle is advanced through tissue in which the cells do not have excitable membranes. Severely decreased insertional activity indicates that the needle is not in the muscle but rather is in subcutaneous fat or in an intermuscular plane. Decreased or absent insertional activity can also be noted when the muscle has undergone neurogenic atrophy seen with prolonged severe denervation. In this case, the excitable muscle tissue has been replaced with nonexcitable fat and fibrous connective tissue. Similar replacement of muscle tissue can be seen in advanced degenerative myopathy.

A nonmoving electrode sitting in quiescent normal muscle, located away from the motor point, should record complete electrical silence.

Normal activity recorded during the examination for spontaneous activity can include MUAPs if the muscle is not completely relaxed, and potentials that arise at the

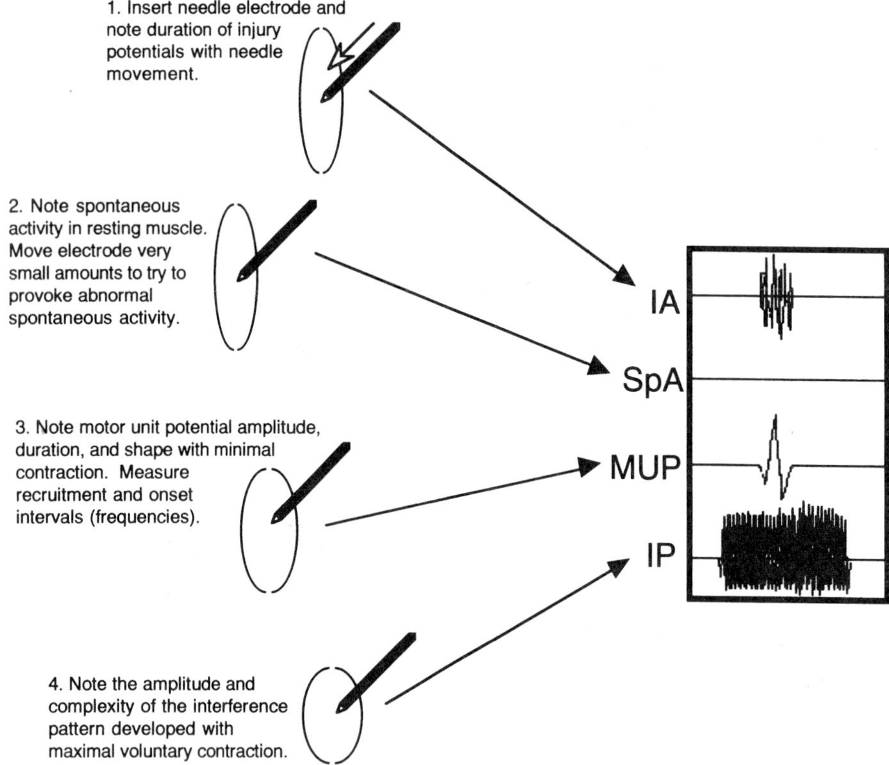

1. Insert needle electrode and note duration of injury potentials with needle movement.
2. Note spontaneous activity in resting muscle. Move electrode very small amounts to try to provoke abnormal spontaneous activity.
3. Note motor unit potential amplitude, duration, and shape with minimal contraction. Measure recruitment and onset intervals (frequencies).
4. Note the amplitude and complexity of the interference pattern developed with maximal voluntary contraction.
IA
SpA
MUP
IP

Figure 9-22. A schematic illustration of the four elements of the electromyographic examination.

neuromuscular junction including EPPs and end-plate noise (MEPPs). These potentials recorded in normal muscle must be accurately differentiated from the abnormal spontaneous activity reviewed in the next section. Electrode noise and artifactual electrode potentials generated by a faulty needle EMG electrode (see Fig. 9-23H) must also be recognized and differentiated from abnormal spontaneous potentials.

Abnormal Spontaneous Activity

Abnormal Individual Muscle Fiber Contractions—Fibrillation Potentials and Positive Sharp Waves

These potentials may be seen in both neuropathic and myopathic processes. They must be carefully differentiated from potentials normally seen in the vicinity of the end-plate zone. Single muscle fiber action potentials (SFAPs) are associated with spontaneous contraction or *fibrillation* of the muscle fiber. These spontaneous contractions of single muscle fibers occur because the muscle membrane has become electrically leaky and the resting membrane potential is unstable, allowing the occurrence of spontaneous depolarization. When the resting membrane potential spontaneously drifts up toward the threshold level, the fiber fires an AP and contracts. This event is always indicative of some form of pathology whose end point has produced electrical instability of the muscle fiber membrane. Normally, the only time a muscle fiber should contract is when it is activated from the junctional region by the innervating motor fiber. Individual muscle fibers should not fire spontaneously unless some form of pathology is present.

Evidence of muscle fiber fibrillation comes in two major forms, which appear to be different waveforms that are reflections of the same underlying phenomenon. The two major forms are the "spike" form of the potential and the "positive wave" form. The spike form of the SFAP has come to be known as the *fibrillation potential* (FP). This is somewhat misleading in that it implies that this is the only way that a muscle fiber fibrillation can be identified. In fact, there is a spectrum of forms that can be seen that range from the triphasic spike form to the positive sharp wave (PSW) form. It is not unusual to see a spike form gradually convert into two adjacent positive forms, with a deepening of the positive phases of the triphasic spike and a gradual loss of the interposed negative spike. The underlying pathophysiologic process that explains this transformation and the equivalence of the forms is not well understood.

The spike form of the SFAP, or FP, is a triphasic positive-negative-positive waveform with a dominant negative spike. It has a similar general appearance to a normal MUAP. However, the FP is generally of shorter duration than the MUAP (usually < 5 msec) and the amplitude is generally lower (approximately 50–1000 μV). The amplitude of the FP tends to decrease with the chronicity of the disease process, with the muscle fibers decreasing in size as they atrophy. FPs appear to be normally conducted SFAPs. It is thought that the positive form, or PSW, occurs when the muscle fiber membrane has deteriorated to the point where it is no longer conducting APs through different scattered segments. In this case, the conduction of an SFAP is suddenly blocked in the vicinity of the recording electrode and there is a gradual return of the potential to the baseline after an initial positive deflection, seen as the potential approaches the electrode.

When abnormal spontaneous activity is due to denervation, there is a delay between nerve injury and the appearance of FPs and PSWs associated with the period of time that it takes for the distal component of the nerve to undergo wallerian degeneration and for the changes in the muscle fiber in response to denervation to occur. This time period is roughly proportional to the length of the fiber that is undergoing degeneration. The time period for abnormal spontaneous activity to appear is roughly 7 to 14 days but may be up to 3 weeks when distal extremity muscles are being examined after a root level injury.

The appearance and amount of abnormal spontaneous fiber activity can be roughly quantified and related to the time course of the particular pathologic process being examined. For example, abnormal spontaneous fiber activity may begin to disappear at the point at which a muscle is being reinnervated. SFAPs can also be seen in myopathy either due to secondary involvement of peripheral nerve terminals in degenerating or inflamed muscle or due to direct damage to the muscle fiber cell membrane as may occur as the result of inflammatory infiltrates in polymyositis.

FPs must be carefully differentiated from normal EPPs and MUAPs. FPs tend to fire with regular rates at relatively low frequencies (1–20 impulses/sec) while EPPs tend to fire irregularly at higher frequencies (5–50 impulses/sec). While FPs tend to have an initial positive deflection and a triphasic structure, EPPs tend to have an initial negative deflection with a biphasic structure. A provocative maneuver to elicit FPs is to warm the muscle. No visible muscle movement or contraction occurs in association with a muscle fiber fibrillation.

The quantification scheme for the abnormal spontaneous activity is as follows:

1+: persistent but unsustained single trains in at least two muscle regions

2+: occasional abnormal potentials seen at rest in no less than three sites

3+: sustained abnormal potentials seen at rest in all locations examined

4+: abundant abnormal potentials seen at rest in all locations so that the potentials practically obliterate the baseline

Abnormal Motor Unit Contraction—Fasciculation Potentials

These are spontaneous, single discharges of the motor unit. They correspond to visible twitches in the muscle. The slower the firing rate, the more likely it is related to a pathologic process. The pathologic significance of the fasciculation potential is determined by whether or not it is accompanied by the appearance of other abnormal spontaneous potentials or significant changes in MUAP characteristics. Fasciculation potentials may be seen in motor neuron disease, peripheral neuropathy, and radiculopathy, and can also be seen in benign idiopathic conditions.

Abnormal Recurrent Muscle Fiber Group Contraction—Complex Repetitive Discharges

This relatively nonspecific abnormality presents as high-frequency, repetitive firing of a complex waveform that has a machine-like sound on audio. The firing rate tends to be high and relatively stable. These discharges are characterized by abrupt onset and cessation. The complex repetitive discharge is thought to be related to an ephaptic circuit formed within abnormal muscle and activated by a spontaneously discharging pacemaker cell that sustains the firing of the circuit and is reexcited by a reentrant process whereby the circuit of activation returns to the original pacemaker cell. This abnormality can be seen in Duchenne muscular dystrophy, spinal muscular atrophy, and Charcot-Marie-Tooth disease. It can also be seen in chronic neuropathy, radiculopathy, and inflammatory myopathies.

Myotonic Discharges

This sustained run of spike potentials or PSWs is seen at rest and begins at high frequency and then slowly drops in frequency, producing a so-called dive-bomber sound on audio. Waxing and waning of the firing frequency can also be seen, with the amplitude of the spike generally falling as the frequency decreases, thus giving a sound that resembles that of a chain saw in use. These potentials are often evoked by needle movement or by percussion of the muscle or voluntary contraction. Myotonic discharges are classically associated with myotonic dystrophy but can be seen in other conditions in which clinical myotonia is present. They may also be seen in hyperkalemic periodic paralysis.

Abnormal Rhythmic Motor Unit Contraction—Myokymia

Spontaneous rhythmic bursting of a motor unit associated with vermicular ("worm-like") movements under the skin is the characteristic feature of myokymia. Bursts of discharges from a single motor unit containing 2 to 10 spikes firing at up to 40 discharges per second and recurring with intervals of 0.1 to 10.0 seconds are seen in the involved muscle (89). These bursts probably are due to ectopic generation of APs in demyelinated segments of a nerve fiber. Myokymia involving the face muscles is most commonly seen in patients with brain stem gliomas or multiple sclerosis. Myokymia in the limb muscles is most often related to

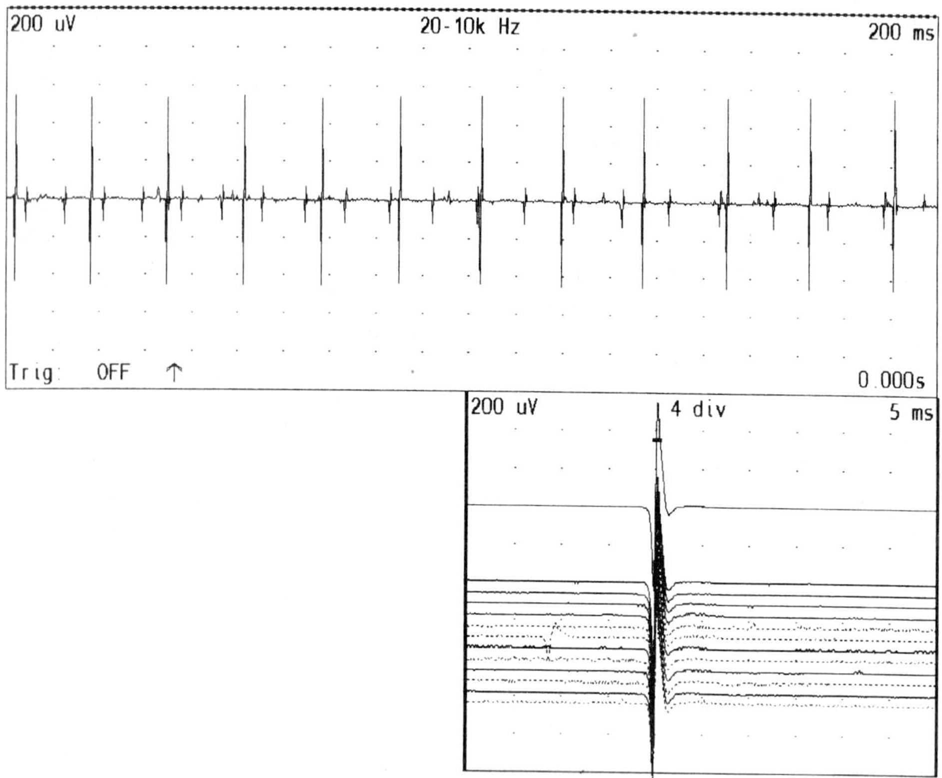

Figure 9-23. Examples of abnormal spontaneous activity. *A.* Single muscle fiber action potential—spike form, also known as fibrillation potentials. Note the narrow duration and slow, regular firing rate that tends to distinguish this potential from a motor unit potential. A motor unit cannot fire steadily at this low a rate under normal voluntary control. On the audio, multiple potentials of this form sound like light rain on a tin roof. *B.* Single muscle fiber action potential—positive wave form, also known as positive sharp waves. *C.* Fasciculation potentials recorded from a patient with amyotrophic lateral sclerosis. Note the low firing rates and the highly irregular recurrence of the potential. (Reproduced by permission from Brown WF. *The physiological and technical basis of electromyography.* Boston: Butterworth, 1984.) *D.* Three examples of complex repetitive discharges. Note the highly regularized internal structure of the discharge and the regular firing rate. On the audio, the sound associated with the discharges has a machine-like quality like a motorcycle or chain saw. It is characterized by fitful and sudden stops and starts. *E.* Myotonic discharges. These potentials have slowly waxing and waning frequencies and amplitudes, and sound like a "dive-bomber" on the audio. (Reproduced by permission from Binnie CD, Cooper R, Fowler CJ, et al. *Clinical neurophysiology. EMG, nerve conduction and evoked potentials.* Oxford: Butterworth-Heinemann, 1995:86.) *F.* Myokymic discharges recorded from patients with radiation plexopathy. There are regular recurrent bursts of motor unit action potentials with variable numbers of potentials in each burst. (Reproduced by permission from Albers JW, Allen AA, Bastron JD, et al. Limb myokymia. *Muscle Nerve* 1981;4:494–504.) *G.* Neuromyotonic discharges found in a patient with Isaacs syndrome or stiff-man syndrome. (Reproduced by permission from Daube JR. *AAEM minimonograph #11. Needle examination in electromyography.* Rochester, MN: American Association of Electrodiagnostic Medicine. 1979.) *H.* Sawtooth electrode artifact. This is an artifact that can be seen when recording from a faulty electrode and must be distinguished from a pathologic discharge.

chronic inflammatory polyradiculoneuritis or radiation neuritis or plexitis.

Abnormal High-Frequency Motor Unit Contraction—Neuromyotonia

This rare finding is associated with sustained whole muscle contraction in which motor units show spontaneous, involuntary, continuous high-frequency discharge activity. Firing rates are greater than 150 Hz and bursts of activity may last from 0.5 to 2.0 seconds. The amplitude of the potentials gradually wanes during a burst. Neuromyotonia is associated with stiff-man syndrome, also know as Isaacs syndrome. It may be viewed as an exaggerated form of myokymia where the bursts have higher firing rates and last for longer intervals, producing sustained muscle contractions rather than intermittent, rhythmic contractions.

Examples of abnormal spontaneous potentials are illustrated in Figure 9-23.

Motor Unit Action Potentials

The MUAP is the electrophysiologic correlate of the contraction of the motor unit and is a *compound muscle fiber action potential* in which the individual SFAPs synchronously

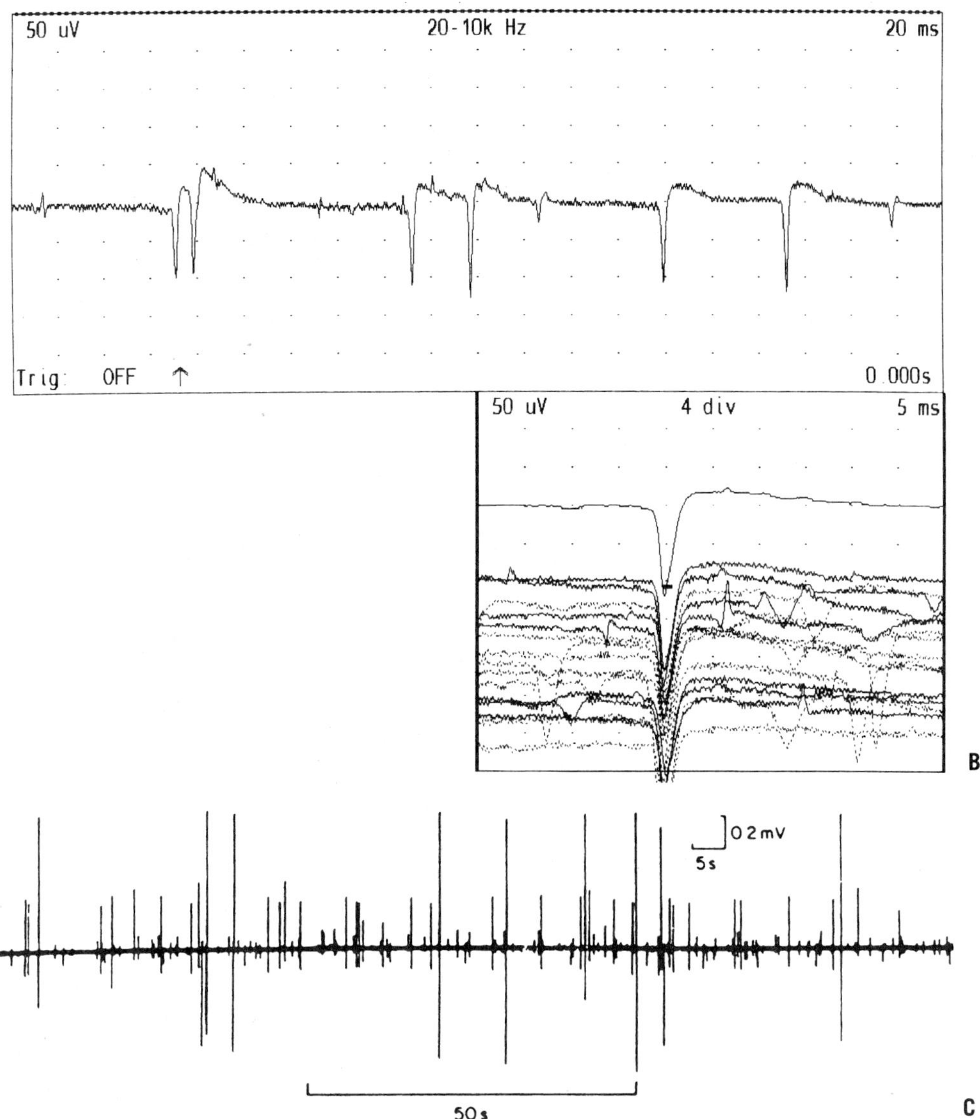

Figure 9-23. *Continued*

generated in the muscle fibers of the unit overlap in time and are summated at the recording electrode. The actual shape and configuration of the MUAP depend critically on the location of the electrode with respect to the active muscle fibers in the unit, and a small movement of the needle can generate a very different appearance of the MUAP from the same motor unit. The parameters of a motor unit potential are illustrated in Figure 9-24.

The following points are important in the interpretation of MUAP parameters:

1. The appearance of the MUAP is dominated by the fibers in the unit that are closest to the recording electrode. The amplitude of the SFAP falls off with the square of the distance as one moves away from the electrode. When the electrode is close to active fibers in the unit, the rise time is short and the MUAP has a sharp cracking "pop." However, small movements of the electrode may lead to large changes in MUAP amplitude and configuration. It is important to first "focus" the MUAP by moving the electrode into a stable position with respect to the active fibers in the unit and then "hold" the unit while sampling it for measurement of its parameters. In order to avoid overlap and interference with too many other units, the patient should be generating a low-level contraction of the muscle. Note that this implies a sampling bias toward units that tend to be recruited early in the recruitment process.
2. Fibers that are farther away from the electrode will contribute more to duration than to amplitude since one of the effects of the volume conduction capacitance is to increase the effective duration of the SFAP as one moves away from the fiber. The closest 1 to 20 fibers within a 1-mm radius, along with the relative spatial density of active fibers around the electrode, will determine the amplitude of the

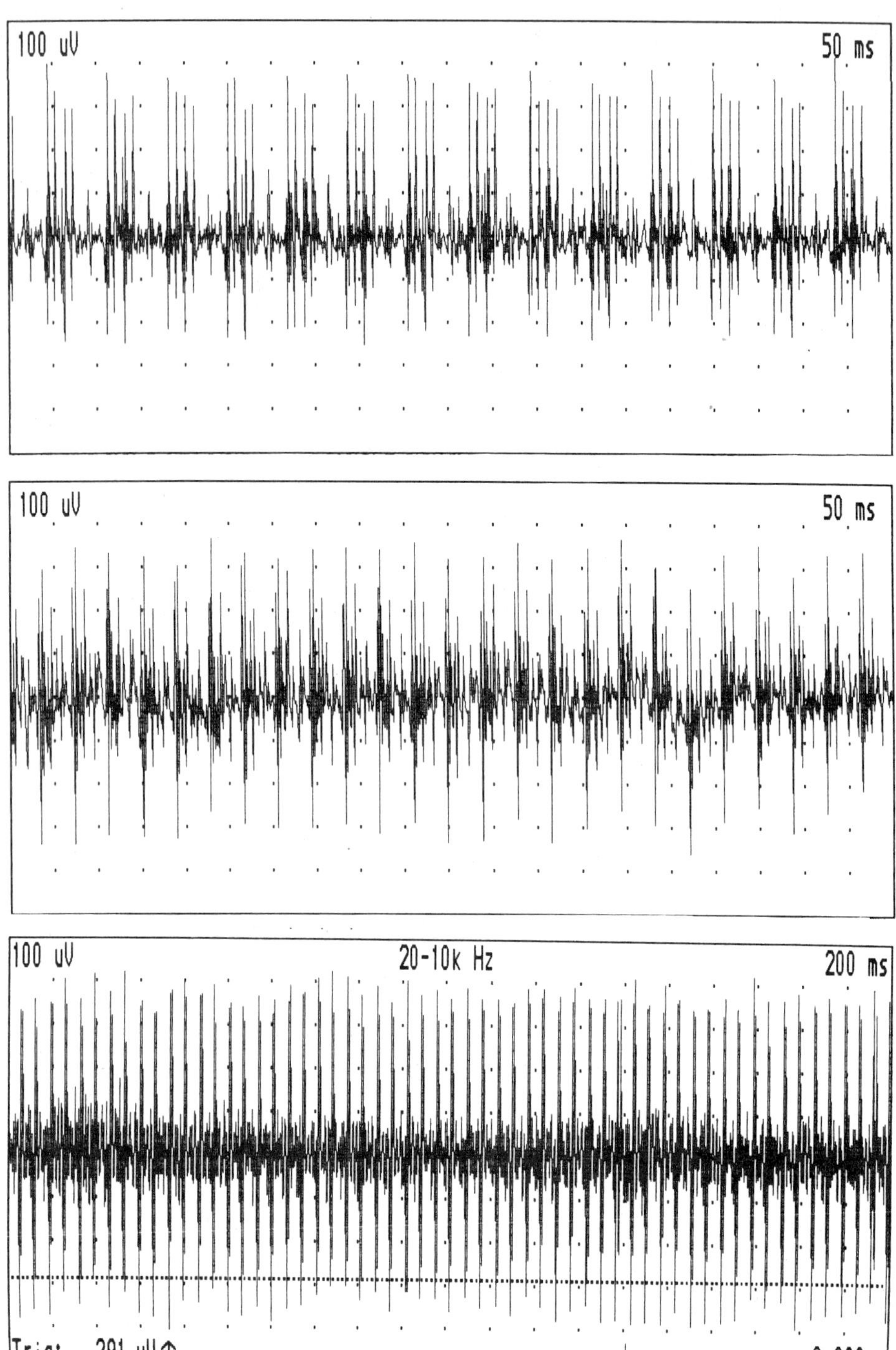

Figure 9-23. *Continued*

MUAP. Many more fibers in the unit distributed throughout the muscle will contribute to the recording primarily by adding to duration, because of the effects of temporal dispersion. The temporal dispersion is produced by the combination of capacitive delays due to volume conduction from the muscle fiber to the electrode and conduction delays associated with transmission in the terminal branches of the motor nerve fiber. A schematic illustration of the recording of a normal MUAP is shown is Figure 9-25A.

3. Temperature effects must be considered (78). Cooling increases the MUAP duration 10% to 30% per Celsius degree and decreases MUAP amplitude up to 50% per Celsius degree. Polyphasia increases significantly with decreasing temperature because of a differential slowing of conduction in the terminal

Figure 9-23. *Continued.*

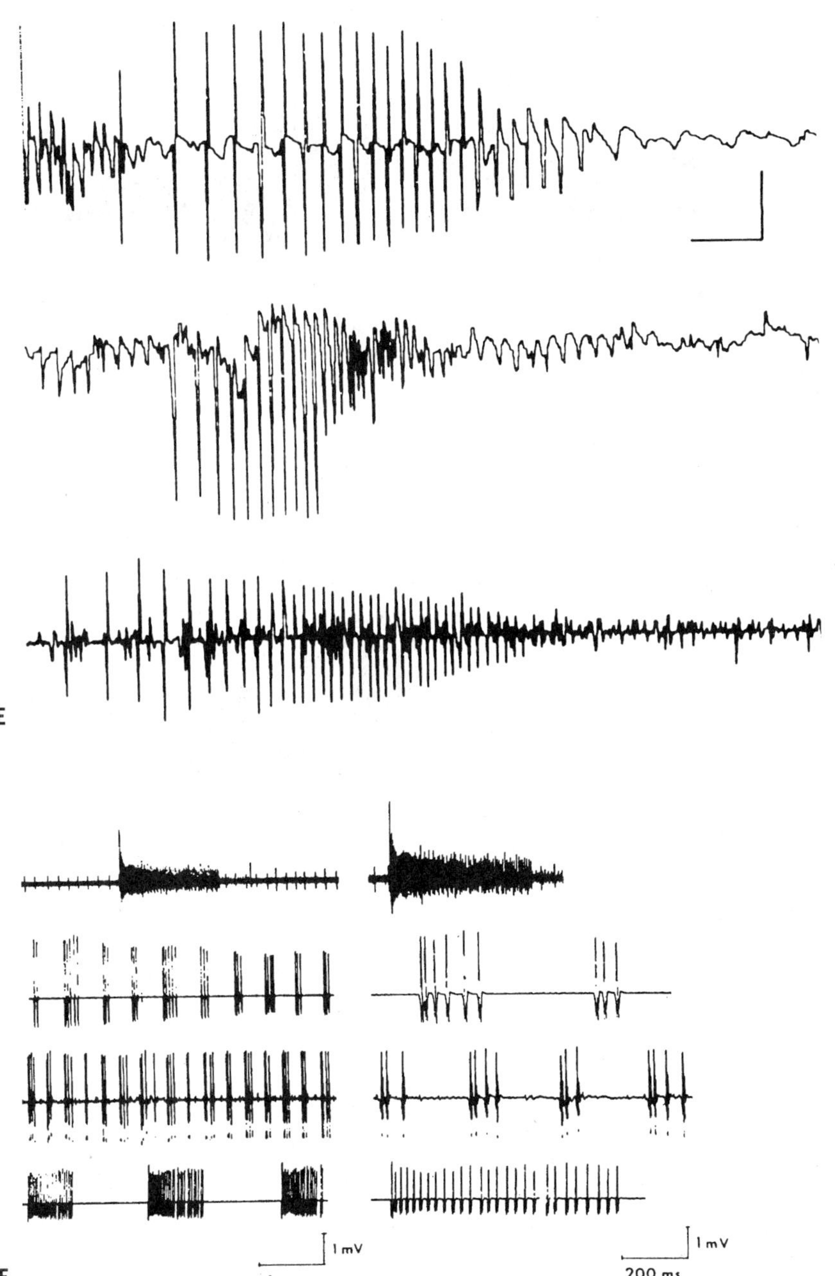

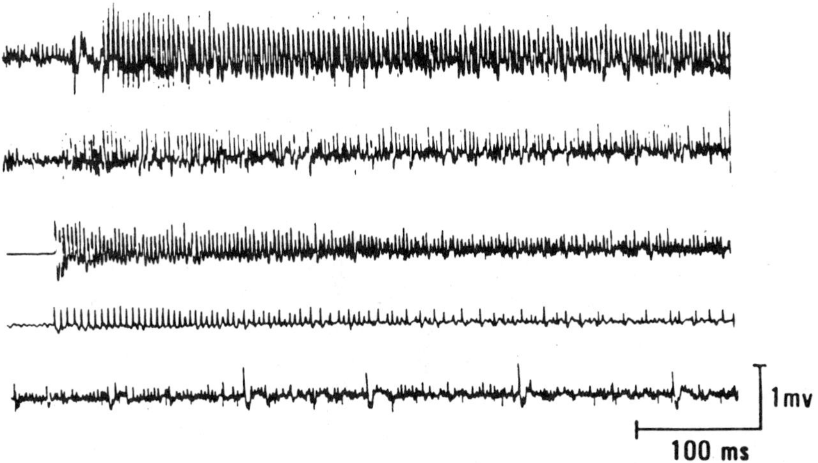

Figure 9-23. *Continued.*

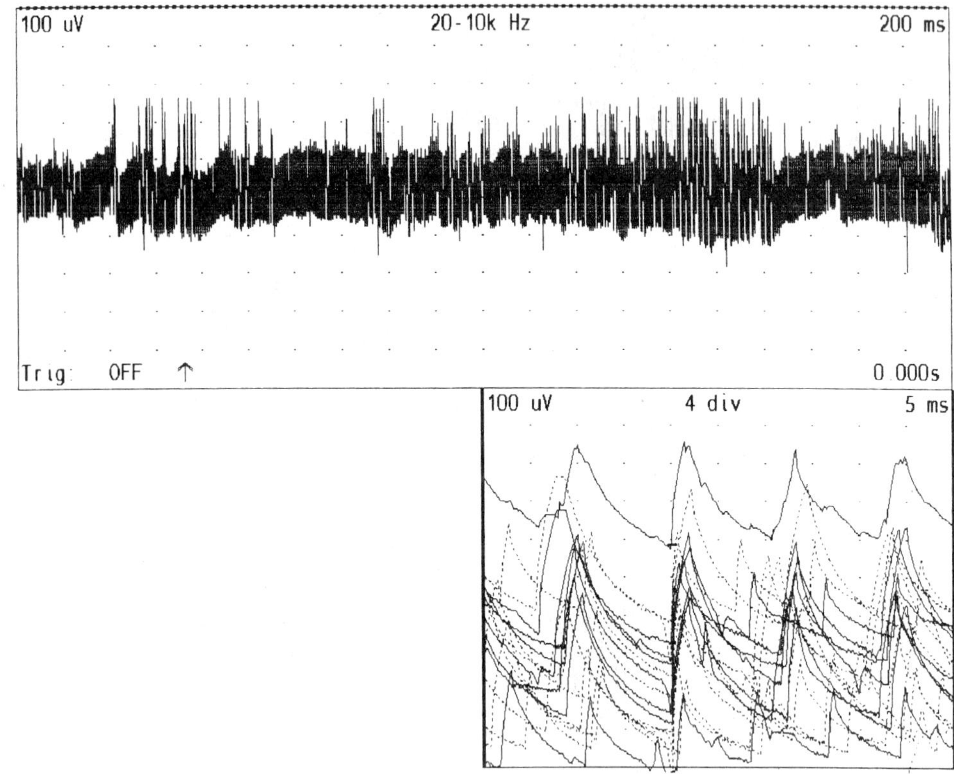

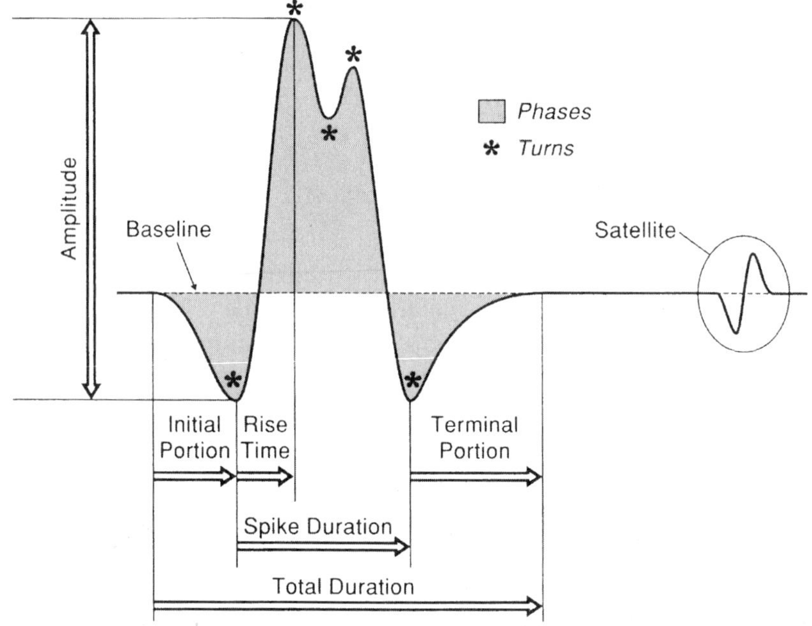

Figure 9-24. Parameters of the motor unit action potential. (Reproduced by permission from Dumitru D. *Electrodiagnostic medicine.* Philadelphia: Hanley & Belfus, 1995:53.)

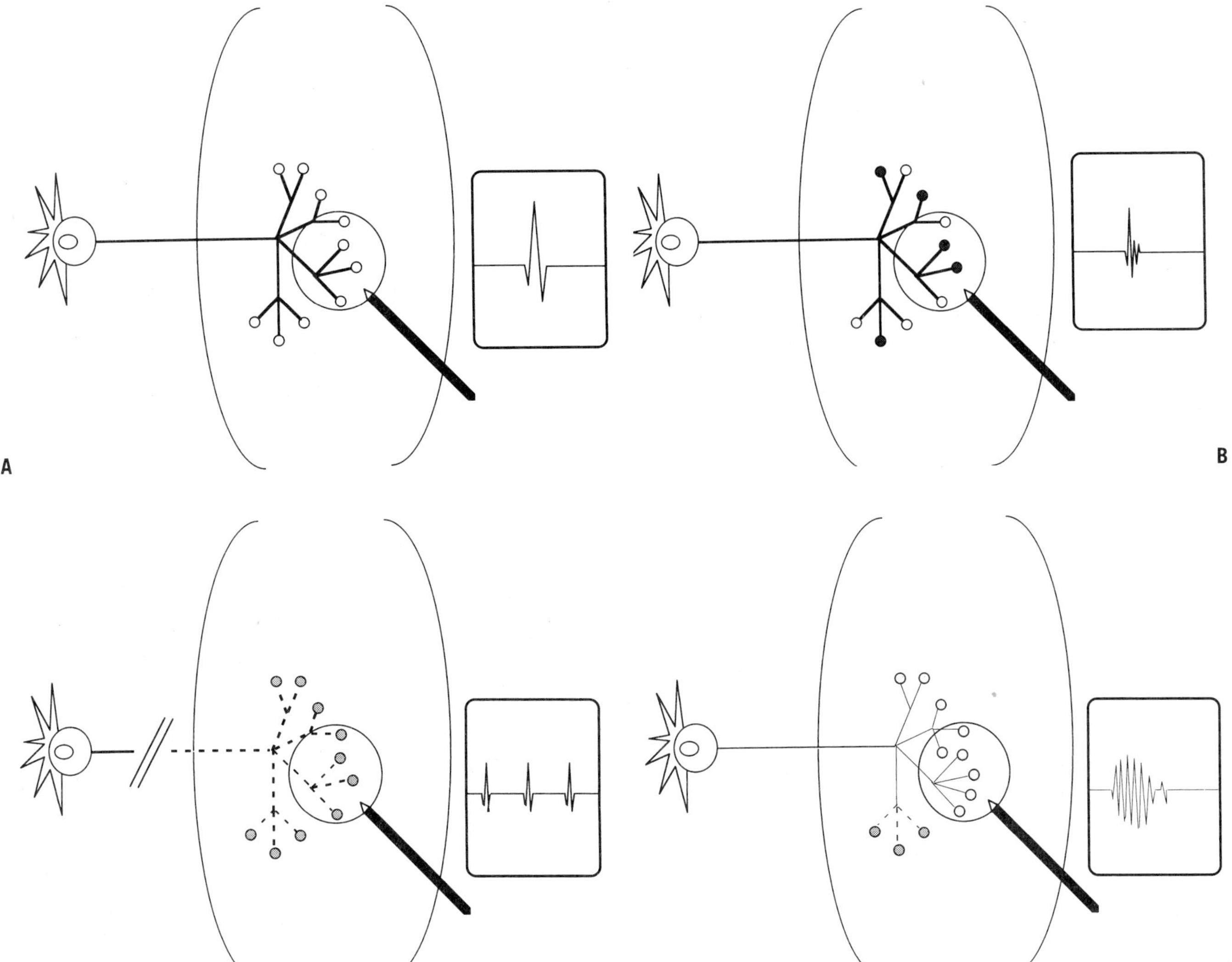

Figure 9-25. Needle EMG findings under different circumstances. *A.* Recording of a normal motor unit action potential (MUAP). *B.* Recording of an abnormal MUAP in the presence of myopathy. Note the random dropout of muscle fibers from the motor unit, which reduces the number of fibers in the unit that contribute to the recording of the MUAP. The MUAP is low in amplitude and brief in duration and may also be polyphasic. *C.* Acute severe neuropathic process. There are no recordable MUAPs and single muscle fiber action potentials (spike form) are seen at rest in the muscle. *D.* Recovery from an acute severe neuropathic process. There is the de novo formation of new motor units in the muscle heralded by the appearance of low-amplitude, long-duration, highly complex polyphasic MUAPs known as *nascent potentials. E.* Recovery from a subtotal neuropathic process at a subacute phase. There is motor fiber sprouting from the remaining intact motor fibers to innervate denervated muscle fibers. These sprouts remain unmyelinated initially and conduct relatively slowly, leading to asynchronous activation of the individual muscle fibers. This results in a polyphasic MUAP. *F.* Recovery from a subtotal neuropathic process at a chronic phase. The motor fiber sprouts have now matured and the enlarged motor unit activates more synchronously, leading to the appearance of a large, triphasic MUAP that may be mildly increased in duration. These units may be up to tens of millivolts in amplitude and are sometimes called *giant* MUAPs.

branches and a desynchronization of muscle fiber activation.

4. MUAP parameter values vary from muscle to muscle because of the variation of motor unit size and distribution between muscles. These parameters also change significantly with age and are affected by the type of recording electrode used.
5. MUAP parameters change in systematic ways that differentiate between primary myopathic and neuropathic processes as well as different stages of recovery from a neuropathic process. In myopathies, MUAPs tend to have short durations and low amplitudes and can be polyphasic. These changes are mainly the result of muscle fiber dropout (see Fig. 9-25B). In a severe neuropathic process, one may only see abnormal spontaneous activity and no recruited MUAPs (see Fig. 9-25C). In subacute, subtotal neuropathic injuries or neuropathies, MUAPs tend to

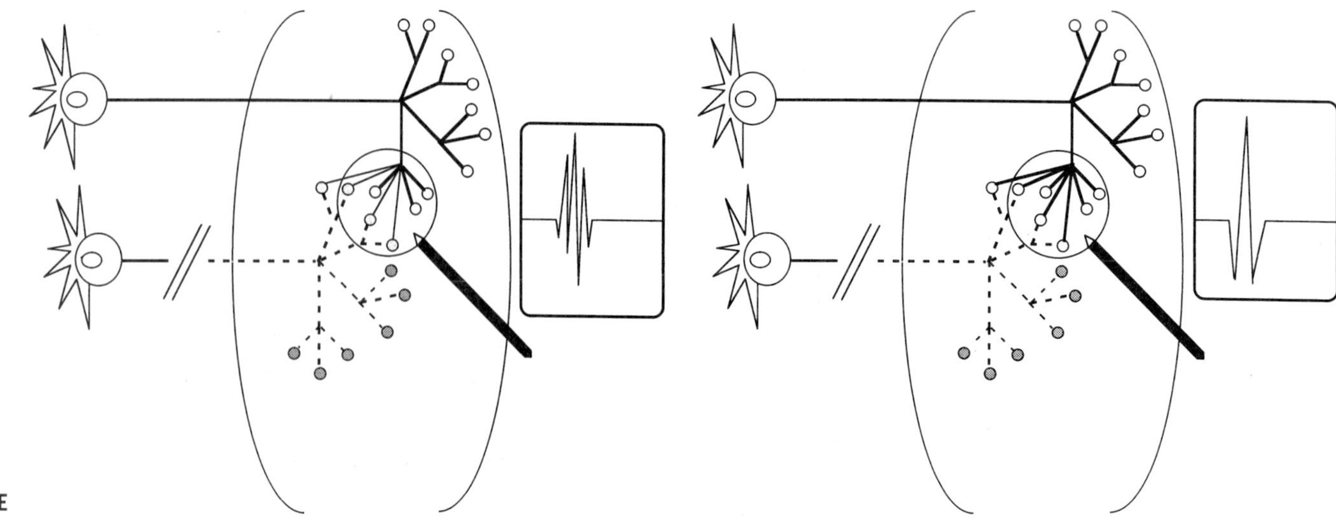

Figure 9-25. *Continued.*

have longer durations and polyphasic structure due to increased temporal dispersion within the unit because of the relatively asynchronous activation of the muscle fibers of the remodeling motor unit by immature motor fiber sprouts (see Fig. 9-25E). An increase in the amplitude of the MUAP can be seen in the chronic phase of a neuropathic process as the motor fiber sprouts mature, conducting more quickly and reliably, and activation of the muscle fibers in the motor unit becomes more synchronous (see Fig. 9-25F). The increase in MUAP amplitude is also related to increased fiber density for the muscle fibers innervated in the same motor unit.

Amplitude

MUAP amplitude is usually measured peak to peak from the maximum negative to the maximum positive extremes. Normal values for monopolar needle electrodes vary with both age and muscle. Amplitudes tend to be somewhat larger with increasing age. Generally, the amplitudes vary from a few hundred microvolts to several thousand microvolts for the monopolar recording electrode and up to a few thousand microvolts when using a concentric needle. The amplitude is related to the number of active fibers located in a small neighborhood of the electrode. Amplitude will decrease when the number of active fibers decreases or when the spatial density of the motor unit muscle fibers decreases. The amplitude will increase when the number of muscle fibers in the unit close to the electrode increases or when the spatial density of active fibers in a motor unit increases. When motor nerve fibers generate collateral sprouts and the unit enlarges after chronic partial denervation, fibers from an individual unit tend to be "bunched" together in a muscle rather than randomly distributed throughout the muscle as they are normally. The process of compensatory sprouting of motor fibers associated with motor unit remodeling after partial denervation leads to a significant increase in the amplitude and duration of the MUAP. As the process of collateral sprouting progresses and the sprouts mature, there is a corresponding reduction and decreased dispersion in terminal branch latencies. As a result, the activation of the muscle fibers in the motor unit becomes more synchronous. The MUAP amplitude progressively increases and the duration decreases as the synchronization of muscle fiber activation improves. Sometimes, the MUAPs that are found under these conditions are called *giant MUAPs* (see Fig. 9–25F). Such units are typically seen in partially denervated muscles after a period of time has elapsed, during which the motor unit remodeling process has been completed.

Conversely, in conditions in which the muscle fibers are primarily damaged, there is dropout of muscle fibers from the motor unit and the total number of active muscle fibers contributing to the MUAP decreases. In this case, the MUAP will decrease in amplitude and may also decrease in duration. The MUAP may still have a polyphasic structure secondary to spatial dispersion of fiber activation either related to abnormal muscle fiber splitting or due to scattered and random loss of muscle fibers. These changes are illustrated in Figure 9-25B.

Rise Time

The rise time is the interval from the peak of the initial positive deflection to that of the initial major negative deflection of the MUAP. This measure decreases as the needle comes closer to the active muscle fibers and the sound of the unit changes from a dull thud to a sharp crack. An MUAP that is to be accepted for quantitative study should be close enough to the recording electrode to have a rise time of 500 μsec or less. The MUAP can often be focused to the point where the rise time is decreased to 100 to 200 μsec.

Duration

The duration of the MUAP measured from the initial break from baseline to the return to baseline is determined by the degree of temporal dispersion in the activation of the different muscle fibers contained within the motor unit. MUAP durations can normally vary from 5 to 18 msec, with significant changes in range depending on the age of the subject as well as the muscle being studied. Duration generally increases with increasing age. For example, the durations of MUAPs recorded from the biceps brachii using a concentric electrode vary from 6.4 to 8.2 msec for ages 0 to 4 years through to 11.1 to 14.4 msec for ages 70 to 79 years (90). The duration reflects the number and spatial distribution of the fibers of the motor unit in the muscle relative to the position of the electrode, as well as the relative uniformity of conduction speed in the terminal branches of the motor axon. The duration increases as the degree of asynchrony of activation of the muscle fibers in a motor unit increases.

Polyphasia

Polyphasia relates to the configuration or structure of the MUAP waveform and refers to the number of different phases that can be distinguished in the waveform. One can define polyphasia in terms of baseline crossings with complete reversal in polarity in adjacent phases, or one may define polyphasia in terms of slope reversals, or *serrations*. The definition of polyphasia using the concept of serrations is probably a more useful one since many pathologic processes may add serrations to the MUAP without necessarily adding complete polarity reversals. Increased polyphasic structure indicates increased temporal dispersion within the motor unit and temporal segmentation of muscle fiber activation, as would be seen when some of the terminals are immature because they are part of a reinnervation process. The initial MUAPs in a recently reinnervated muscle are low in amplitude and long in duration and tend to be highly polyphasic and complex (see Fig. 9-25D). These are sometimes referred to as *nascent potentials* since they herald the "rebirth" of motor units in the muscle. These should be distinguished from larger-amplitude polyphasic MUAPs in a partially denervated muscle in which collateral sprouting of motor nerve fibers is occurring. Single muscle fibers may be innervated by a highly immature fiber terminal and show activation well after the bulk of the muscle fibers in the unit have activated. This leads to the appearance of a *satellite* or *linked potential* that comes well after the main part of the MUAP. Up to 20% of MUAPs in normal muscle can be polyphasic and the number of polyphasic MUAPs normally seen in a muscle increases with age.

Waveform Stability

The stability of the amplitude and the waveform of the repetitively discharging MUAP help to examine the reliability of the neuromuscular junctions in the unit. If some junctions are unstable and are intermittently "blocking," then the amplitude and configuration of the MUAP will vary depending on which of the fibers in the unit has fired reliably and which fibers are intermittently dropping out because of intermittent failure at the neuromuscular junction. This phenomenon can be seen in primary disease of the neuromuscular junction as well as in the presence of immature motor fiber sprouts, for example, during reinnervation.

Partial Axonal Disruption—Discrete Insult Followed by a Period of Recovery

When a nerve is partially damaged and is allowed to recover, a particular sequence of events occurs in the structure and function of the motor unit as the neuromuscular system responds and adapts to the injury. Initially, recruitment is reduced and at a later point, fibrillations and PSWs may appear in the affected muscle.

Denervated muscle fibers may undergo atrophy, thus increasing fiber density for the remaining motor units, and an increase in amplitude may be seen early on as a result. Remaining motor nerve fibers begin to reinnervate the denervated muscle fibers through a process of collateral sprouting. This is associated with an increased amplitude of the MUAP, increased duration, and polyphasia due to the increased temporal dispersion in the terminal branches of the motor nerve. Abnormal FPs and PSWs begin to disappear as the sprouting process proceeds and the muscle fibers are reinnervated.

As the sprouted motor unit's terminal branches mature, the MUAPs become increasingly large in amplitude but less polyphasic and less broad in duration. There is greater synchrony of muscle fiber activation and a larger number of activated muscle fibers, both factors contributing to an increase in MUAP amplitude.

The amount of change observed is related to the degree to which the muscle has been denervated. As the percentage of lost motor neurons increases, more muscle fibers have to be innervated by fewer remaining viable motor neurons in the available pool. The result is an increase in the number of muscle fibers associated with the enlarged motor units and a greater degree of "clustering" or "grouping" of the muscle fibers innervated by individual motor nerve fibers. This clustering corresponds to *fiber-type grouping*, seen in chronically denervated muscle, and to the loss of the normal interspersed mosaic pattern of fiber-type distribution seen on histologic section of chronically denervated muscle. Persisting abnormal spontaneous activity may or may not be present, depending on how successful the reinnervation process has been in reestablishing neural contact with denervated muscle fibers and stabilizing the resting membrane potential. When axonal injury is severe enough, parts of the muscle are reinnervated through de novo formation of new motor units when

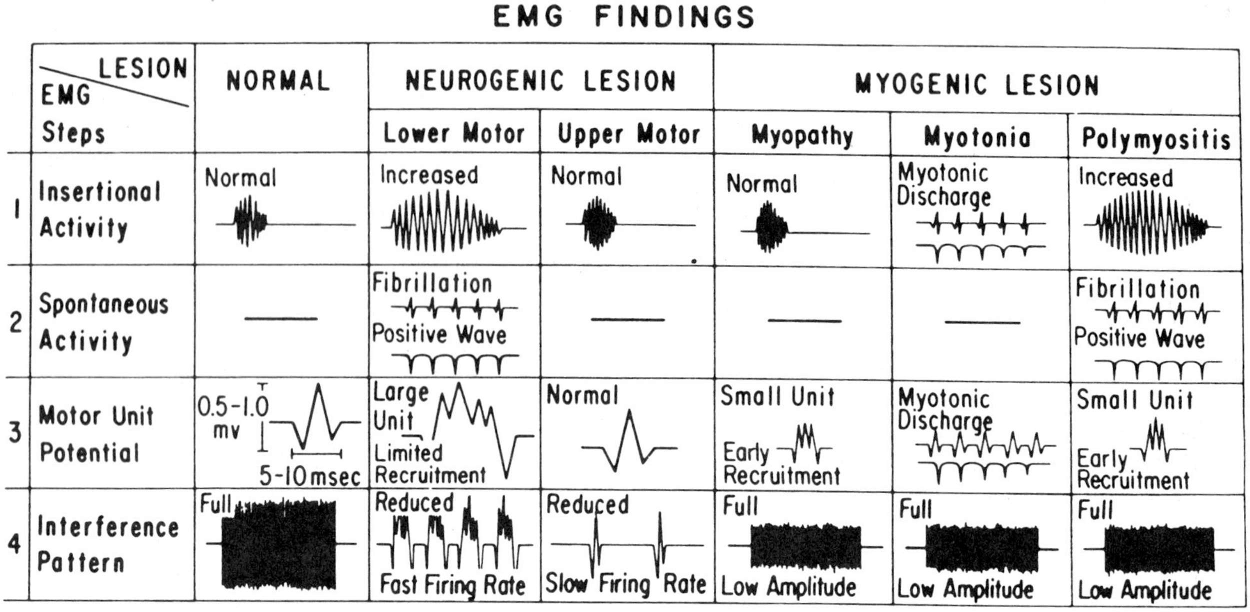

EMG FINDINGS

	LESION / EMG Steps	NORMAL	NEUROGENIC LESION		MYOGENIC LESION		
			Lower Motor	Upper Motor	Myopathy	Myotonia	Polymyositis
1	Insertional Activity	Normal	Increased	Normal	Normal	Myotonic Discharge	Increased
2	Spontaneous Activity	—	Fibrillation Positive Wave	—	—	—	Fibrillation Positive Wave
3	Motor Unit Potential	0.5-1.0 mv 5-10 msec	Large Unit Limited Recruitment	Normal	Small Unit Early Recruitment	Myotonic Discharge	Small Unit Early Recruitment
4	Interference Pattern	Full	Reduced Fast Firing Rate	Reduced Slow Firing Rate	Full Low Amplitude	Full Low Amplitude	Full Low Amplitude

Figure 9-26. Electrodiagnostic features that differentiate between neuropathic and myopathic pathologies. (Reproduced by permission from Kimura J. *Electrodiagnosis in diseases of nerve and muscle. Principles and practice.* 2nd ed. Philadelphia: FA Davis, 1989:252.)

regenerating motor nerve fibers reenter the muscle. This is associated with the appearance of nascent potentials, mentioned earlier. To some extent, the processes of collateral sprouting and that of de novo reestablishment of motor units compete with each other to reinnervate the muscle fibers.

Lower Motor Neuron Versus Myopathic Pathology

MUAP parameters tend to diverge in systematic ways, depending on whether the pathology is primary neuropathic or primary myopathic in nature. As noted earlier, chronic neuropathic involvement producing partial axonal loss in a nerve will eventually be associated with sprouting of motor nerve fibers and an enlargement of amplitude and duration of the MUAP. In contrast, in myopathy, there is a progressive dropout of muscle fibers from the motor unit, leading to an impoverishment of the MUAP with a decrease in the amplitude and duration. Disorders of neuromuscular junction transmission such as myasthenia gravis, myasthenic syndrome, and botulism can also show these typical changes in which the MUAP loses both amplitude and duration compared to normal.

Lower motor neuron and myopathic/neuromuscular junction pathologies can also be differentiated through divergent changes in the recruitment patterns observed. Recruitment is reduced in diseases of the lower motor neuron since there is a reduction in the total number of motor units available for recruitment from the motor neuron pool. To maintain tension, the recruited units must fire at abnormally high rates. Recruitment frequencies are increased because firing frequency modulation must compensate for a lack of ability to intensify tension through the additional recruitment of motor units (91). In myopathy, there is also an increase in recruitment frequency compared to normal, but usually to a lesser degree than is seen in neuropathic pathology, and a reduced motor unit twitch tension due to dropout of muscle fibers. Thus, many more units must be recruited and fired at maximal rates in order to sustain a tension similar to that observed in normal muscle. Therefore, slight contraction of the muscle is associated with rapid recruitment of large numbers of motor units. This gives rise to a full IP (generally with reduced amplitude) at less than maximal contraction. When the myopathy is advanced and there is a loss of muscle fibers that has outstripped the available motor units, one may actually see decreased recruitment patterns because of loss of whole motor units as a result of advanced degeneration of the muscle fibers. Divergent findings differentiating neuropathic and myopathic pathologies are illustrated schematically in Figure 9-26.

REPORTING OF ELECTRODIAGNOSTIC FINDINGS

The electromyographer is providing a critical service both to the patient and to the referring physician who is looking for important information that will help in clinical decision making. The challenge to the electromyographer is to clearly determine the clinical questions to be addressed and the specific hypotheses to be tested, to design a study that gathers data to either support or refute specific hypotheses, and then to synthesize the results of the study in a way that can be communicated with simplicity and relevance. The test results should be made meaningful, useful, and accessible to the referring physician, who can then act on the results appropriately. Comparison of results obtained in the patient with normal reference values must be done with care and attention paid to relevant statistical principles (92,93).

With regard to the EMG part of the examination, the electromyographer must be able to justify the selection of muscles that were studied, formulate the pattern of abnormality in terms of potential causes, and integrate the results obtained on the EMG examination with those that were obtained with the NCSs. The two major components of the test are clearly complementary in nature. An attempt should be made to identify, where possible, the pathology, its localization and nature, its severity, temporal phase of activity, degree of progression, and prognosis. The significance and value of the test can be greatly enhanced and communication with referral sources served by providing a clearly stated report of the result. Overinterpretation of the results and speculation beyond the available findings should be avoided. Ultimately, the results of the EMG examination must be interpreted in the context of the clinical presentation of the patient and correlated with all other clinical and laboratory information that has been gathered.

REFERENCES

1. Aminoff MJ, ed. *Electrodiagnosis in clinical neurology.* 3rd ed. New York: Churchill Livingstone, 1992.
2. Aminoff MJ. *Electromyography in clinical practice. Clinical and electrodiagnostic aspects of neuromuscular disease.* 3rd ed. New York: Churchill Livingstone, 1998.
3. Binnie CD, Cooper R, Fowler CJ, et al, eds. *Clinical neurophysiology. EMG, nerve conduction and evoked potentials.* Oxford: Butterworth-Heinemann, 1995.
4. Brown WF, Bolton CF. *Clinical electromyography.* 2nd ed. Boston: Butterworth-Heinemann, 1993.
5. Brown WF. *The physiological and technical basis of electromyography. Boston*: Butterworths, 1984.
6. Chu-Andrews J, Johnson RJ. *Electrodiagnosis: an anatomical and clinical approach.* New York: JB Lippincott, 1986.
7. Daube JR, ed. *Clinical neurophysiology.* Philadelphia: FA Davis, 1996.
8. Delisa JA, Mackenzie K, Baren EM. *Manual of nerve conduction velocity and somatosensory evoked potentials.* 2nd ed. New York: Raven, 1987.
9. Dumitru D. *Electrodiagnostic medicine.* Philadelphia: Hanley & Belfus, 1995.
10. Geiringer SR. *Anatomic localization for needle electromyography.* Philadelphia: Hanley & Belfus, 1994.
11. Goodgold J, Eberstein A. *Electrodiagnosis of neuromuscular diseases.* 3rd ed. Baltimore: Williams & Wilkins, 1983.
12. Johnson EW, Pease WS, eds. *Practical electromyography.* 3rd ed. Baltimore: Williams & Wilkins, 1997.
13. Jones HR Jr, Bolton CF, Harper CM. *Pediatric clinical electromyography.* Philadelphia: Lippincott–Raven, 1996.
14. Kimura J. *Electrodiagnosis in diseases of nerve and muscle: principles and practice.* 2nd ed. Philadelphia: FA Davis, 1989.
15. Liveson JA, Ma DM. *Laboratory reference for clinical neurophysiology.* Philadelphia: FA Davis, 1992.
16. Liveson JA. *Peripheral neurology. Case studies in electrodiagnosis.* 2nd ed. Philadelphia; FA Davis, 1991.
17. Ma D. *Nerve conduction handbook.* Philadelphia: FA Davis, 1983.
18. Oh SJ. *Electromyography. Neuromuscular transmission studies.* Baltimore: Williams & Wilkins, 1988.
19. Oh SJ. *Clinical electromyography. Nerve conduction studies.* 2nd ed. Baltimore: Williams & Wilkins, 1993.
20. Oh SJ. *Principles of clinical electromyography. Case studies.* Baltimore: Williams & Wilkins, 1998.
21. Preston DC, Shapiro BE. *Electromyography and neuromuscular disorders. Clinical-electrophysiologic correlations.* Boston: Butterworth-Heinemann, 1997.
22. Sethi RK, *Thompson LL. The electromyographer's handbook.* 2nd ed. Boston: Little, Brown, 1989.
23. Ball RD. Electrodiagnostic evaluation of the peripheral nervous system. In: DeLisa JA, ed. *Rehabilitation medicine. Principles and practice.* Philadelphia: JB Lippincott, 1988: 196–227.
24. Daube JR. Assessing the motor unit with needle electromyography. In: Daube JR, ed. *Clinical neurophysiology.* Philadelphia: FA Davis, 1996:257–281.
25. Daube JR. Compound muscle action potentials. In: Daube JR, ed. *Clinical neurophysiology.* Philadelphia: FA Davis, 1996:199–234.
26. Daube JR. Nerve conduction studies. In: Aminoff MJ, ed. *Electrodiagnosis in clinical neurology.* 3rd ed. New York: Churchill Livingstone, 1992:283–326.
27. Dumitru D. Electrodiagnostic medicine. I. Basic aspects. In:

Braddom RL, ed. *Physical medicine and rehabilitation.* Philadelphia: WB Saunders, 1995:104–131.

28. Evans BD. Nerve action potentials. In: Daube JR, ed. *Clinical neurophysiology.* Philadelphia: FA Davis, 1996:147–156.

29. Falco FJE, Goldberg G. *Electrodiagnostic testing. In: Windsor RE, Lox DM, eds. Soft tissue injuries: diagnosis and treatment.* Philadelphia: Hanley & Belfus, 1998:293–319.

30. Robinson LR. Electrodiagnostic medicine. II. Clinical evaluation and findings. In: Braddom RL, ed. *Physical medicine and rehabilitation.* Philadelphia: WB Saunders, 1995:132–152.

31. Stolp-Smith KA. Electrodiagnostic medicine. III. Case studies. In: Braddom RL, ed. *Physical medicine and rehabilitation.* Philadelphia: WB Saunders, 1995:153–176.

32. Dumitru D, ed. Clinical electrophysiology. *State Art Rev Phys Med Rehabil* 1989;3:665–840.

33. MacLean IC, ed. Electromyography: a guide for the referring physician. *Phys Med Rehabil Clin N Am* 1990;1:1–233.

34. Robinson LR, ed. New developments in electrodiagnostic medicine. *Phys Med Rehabil Clin N Am* 1994;5:397–661.

35. Hille B. *Ionic channels of excitable membranes.* 2nd ed. Sunderland, MA: Sinauer Associates, 1992.

36. Junge D. *Nerve and muscle excitation.* Sunderland, MA: Sinauer Associates, 1981.

37. Kandel ER, Schwartz JH, Jessell TM, eds. *Principles of neural science.* 3rd ed. New York: Elsevier, 1991.

38. Katz B. *Nerve, muscle and synapse.* New York: McGraw-Hill, 1966.

39. Nicholls JG, Martin AR, Wallace BG. *From neuron to brain. A cellular and molecular approach to the function of the nervous system.* 3rd ed. Sunderland, MA: Sinauer Associates, 1992.

40. Patton HD, Fuchs AF, Hille B, et al, eds. *Textbook of physiology. Vol. 1. Excitable cells and neurophysiology.* 21st ed. Philadelphia: WB Saunders, 1989.

41. Prosser CL. *Adaptational biology. Molecules to organisms.* New York: John Wiley, 1986.

42. Schmidt-Neilsen K. Animal physiology. *Adaptation and environment.* 4th ed. Cambridge: Cambridge University Press, 1990.

43. Sumner AJ, ed. *The physiology of peripheral nerve disease.* Philadelphia: WB Saunders, 1980.

44. Black JA, Kocsis JD, Waxman SG. Ion channel organization of the myelinated fiber. *Trends Neurosci* 1990;13:48–54.

45. Catterall WA. Structure and function of voltage-sensitive ion channels. *Science* 1988; 242:50–61.

46. Catterall WA. The molecular basis of neuronal excitability. *Science* 1984;223:653–661.

47. Drachman D. Myasthenia gravis. *N Engl J Med* 1994;330: 1797–1810.

48. Hodgkin AL. Chance and design in electrophysiology. An informal account of certain experiments in nerve carried out between 1934 and 1952. *J Physiol (Lond)* 1976;263:1–21.

49. Waxman SG, Foster RE. Ionic channel distribution and heterogeneity of the axon membrane in myelinated fibers. *Brain Res Rev* 1980;2:205–234.

50. Waxman SG, Ritchie JM. Organization of ion channels in the myelinated nerve fiber. *Science* 1985;228:1502–1507.

51. Dyck PJ, Thomas PK, Griffin JW, et al, eds. *Peripheral neuropathy.* 3rd ed. Philadelphia: WB Saunders, 1993.

52. Dawson DM, Hallett M, Millender LH. *Entrapment neuropathies.* 2nd ed. Boston: Little, Brown, 1990.

53. Layzer RB. *Neuromuscular manifestations of systemic disease.* Philadelphia: FA Davis, 1985.

54. Engel AG, Franzini-Armstrong C, eds. *Myology. Basic and clinical.* 2nd ed. New York: McGraw-Hill, 1994.

55. Brooke MH. *A clinician's view of neuromuscular diseases.* Baltimore: Williams & Wilkins, 1986.

56. Kline DG, Hudson AR. *Nerve injuries. Operative results for major nerve injuries, entrapments and tumors.* Philadelphia: WB Saunders, 1995.

57. Omer GE Jr, Spinner M, Van Beek AL, eds. *Management of peripheral nerve problems.* 2nd ed. Philadelphia: WB Saunders, 1998.

58. Sunderland S. *Nerve and nerve injuries.* 2nd ed. Edinburgh: Churchill Livingstone, 1978.

59. Sunderland S. *Nerve injuries and their repair. A critical appraisal.* Edinburgh: Churchill Livingstone, 1991.

60. Terzis JK, Smith KL. *The peripheral nerve. Structure, function and reconstruction.* New York: Raven, 1990.

61. Barry DT. AAEM minimonograph #36. Basic concepts of electricity and electronics in clinical electromyography. *Muscle Nerve* 1991;14:937–946.

62. Lagerlund TD. Electricity and electronics in clinical neurophysiology. In: Daube JR, ed. *Clinical neurophysiology.* Philadelphia: FA Davis, 1996:3–17.

63. Dumitru D, DeLisa JA. Volume conduction. *Muscle Nerve* 1991;14:605–624.

64. Stegeman DF, de Weerd JP, Eijkman EG. A volume conductor study of compound action potentials of nerves in situ: the forward problem. *Biol Cybern* 1979;33:97–111.

65. Geddes LA, Baker LE. *Principles of applied biomedical instrumentation.* 3rd ed. New York: John Wiley, 1989.

66. Cadwell JA, Villarreal RA. Electrophysiologic equipment and electrical safety. In: Aminoff MJ, ed. *Electrodiagnosis in clinical neurology*. 3rd ed. New York: Churchill Livingstone, 1992:17–39.

67. Gitter A, Stolov W. AAEM minimonograph #16. Instrumentation and measurement in electrodiagnostic medicine—part I and part II. *Muscle Nerve* 1995;18: 799–811, 812–824.

68. Gitter A. Advances in electrodiagnostic instruments. Principles and applications of digital signal processing. *Phys Med Rehabil Clin N Am* 1994;5:397–419.

69. Lagerlund TD. Electrical safety in the laboratory and hospital. In: Daube JR, ed. *Clinical neurophysiology*. Philadelphia: FA Davis, 1996:18–28.

70. Reiner S, Rogoff JB. Instrumentation. In: Johnson EW, ed. *Practical electromyography*. 2nd ed. Baltimore: Williams & Wilkins, 1988:498–559.

71. Jasper H, Ballem G. Unipolar electromyograms of normal and denervated human muscle. J *Neurophysiol* 1949;12:231–244.

72. Adrian ED, Bronk DW. The discharge of impulses in motor fibers. II. The frequency of discharge in reflex and voluntary contractions. *J Physiol (Lond)* 1929;67: 119–151.

73. McGill KC, Cummins KL, Dorfman LJ, et al. On the nature and elimination of stimulus artifact in nerve signals evoked and recorded using surface electrodes. *IEEE Trans Biomed Eng* 1982;29: 129–137.

74. Kimura J. Principles and pitfalls of nerve conduction studies. *Ann Neurol* 1984;16:415–429.

75. Baer RD, Johnson EW. Motor nerve conduction velocities in normal children. Arch Phys Med Rehabil 1965;46:698–704.

76. Falco FJE, Hennessey WJ, Braddom RL, et al. Standardized nerve conduction studies in the upper limb of the healthy elderly. *Am J Phys Med Rehabil* 1992;71:263–271.

77. Falco FJE, Hennessey WJ, Goldberg G, et al. Standardized nerve conduction studies in the lower limb of the healthy elderly. *Am J Phys Med Rehabil* 1994;73:168–174.

78. Denys EH. AAEM minimonograph #14. The influence of temperature in clinical neurophysiology. *Muscle Nerve* 1991;14:795–811.

79. Campbell WW, Ward LC, Swift TR. Nerve conduction varies inversely with height. *Muscle Nerve* 1981;4:520–523.

80. Seddon H. Three types of nerve injury. *Brain* 1943;66:237–288.

81. Sunderland S. A classification of peripheral nerve injuries producing loss of function. *Brain* 1951;74:491–516.

82. Falco FJE, Hennessey WJ, Goldberg G, et al. H-reflex latency in the healthy elderly. *Muscle Nerve* 1994;17:161–167.

83. Sanders DB, Stålberg EV: AAEM minimonograph #25. Single-fiber electromyography. *Muscle Nerve* 1996;19:1069–1083.

84. Lambert EH, Eaton LM, Rooke ED. Defect of neuromuscular conduction associated with malignant neoplasm. *Am J Physiol* 1956;187:612–613.

85. Lennon VA, Kryzer TJ, Griesmann GE, et al. Calcium-channel antibodies in the Lambert-Eaton syndrome and other paraneoplastic syndromes. *N Eng J Med* 1995;332:1467–1474.

86. Kraft GH. An approach to electrodiagnostic medicine. The power of needle electromyography. *Phys Med Rehabil Clin N Am* 1994;5: 495–508.

87. Petajan JH, Philip BA. Frequency control of motor unit action potentials. *Electroencephalogr Clin Neurophysiol* 1969;27: 66–72.

88. Petajan JH. AAEM minimonograph #3. Motor unit recruitment. *Muscle Nerve* 1991;14:489–502.

89. Albers JW, Allen AA, Bastron JD, et al. Limb myokymia. *Muscle Nerve* 1981;4:494–504.

90. Buchthal F, Rosenfalck P. Action potential parameters in different human muscles. *Acta Psychiatr Neurol Scand* 1955;30:125–131.

91. Petajan JH. Clinical electromyographic studies of diseases of the motor unit. *Electroencephalogr Clin Neurophysiol* 1974;36: 395–401.

92. Robinson LR, Rubner DE. Statistical considerations for the development and use of reference values as applied to nerve conduction studies. *Phys Med Rehabil Clin N Am* 1994;5:531–540.

93. Dorfman LJ, Robinson LR. AAEM minimonograph #47. Normative data in electrodiagnostic medicine. *Muscle Nerve* 1997;20:4–14.

Chapter 10

Clinical Neurophysiology of the Central Nervous System: Evoked Potentials and Other Neurophysiologic Techniques

Gary Goldberg

This chapter begins by laying down the philosophical perspective that motivates the physiologic approach to central nervous system (CNS) function in rehabilitation. The rehabilitation specialist is frequently called on to evaluate and treat patients with disability arising from impairments affecting the CNS. There are basically three ways to assess such impairment noninvasively in the living human subject: observing the behavioral impact, imaging the pathology, and evaluating the physiologic dysfunction. Of these three perspectives, the two that relate most directly to the functional impact of the pathology are behavioral and physiologic assessment. Imaging the structures can certainly provide important information about the nature and localization of the pathology, but unless one is imaging the functional activation of the tissues, it has limited implications for the capacity to function. In many ways, physiologic investigation and behavioral assessment of the impact of CNS pathology are complementary. The study of behavior is no less a science than the study of physiology. The great advantage of behavioral assessment is that it can be done effectively by a keen and well-trained observer without the need for a tremendous amount of technology. The disadvantage is that it is a level up from the direct observation of the function of the involved tissues and is limited by the quality of the interaction between the observer and the observed, being an inherently subjective dyadic process filtered through the consciousness of both the subject and the observer. This disadvantage can be a problem when the subject may be attempting to intentionally or unintentionally deceive the observer. Furthermore, various difficulties attributable to the observer can limit the quality and validity of the information obtained. The behavioral assessment is also limited when the subject is unable to respond to verbal inquiries about internal events (e.g., "Can you hear this?") because of the unavailability of a functioning language system that is able to communicate introspective reports. This limitation occurs, for example, in the unresponsive or minimally conscious subject as well as the subject who has not yet acquired expressive language. Thus, the great advantage of the physiologic perspective is that it allows direct objective observation of the functioning CNS tissues in response to stimuli or in the process of generating responses. In the case of certain short-latency sensory evoked potential studies such as the brain stem auditory evoked potential (BAEP), one can achieve a relatively robust investigation of the physiologic anatomy that is relatively insensitive to the subjective state. The major disadvantage of the physiologic approach is that it is highly dependent on technology and technique. Physiologic observations such as the sensory evoked potentials must be performed in highly specific ways under highly controlled circumstances in order to limit interference by artifactual signal and in order to extract the physiologic signal of interest from a noisy background. These studies must be performed with extreme care by highly trained personnel, to avoid misinterpretation or significant contamination of the data obtained.

This chapter examines the neurophysiologic methods used to evaluate the function of the CNS. Neurophysiologic methods applied to the CNS most often involve the measurement of electrical signals that are the manifestation of central processes involved in the registration and processing of external stimuli. These methods can provide an alternative physiologic "window" on the behavioral manifestations of clinical conditions affecting the CNS. They may be used to diagnose, monitor, and prognosticate based on objective, reproducible, and quantifiable measures derived from the electrical signals. Neurophysiologic methods, reviewed in Chapter 9 and developed to assess conduction and transmission along peripheral nerve pathways, can be extended, with a variety of special considerations and caveats, to the study of the transmission through central sensory afferent and motor efferent pathways. The extension of the orthodromic sensory nerve conduction study into the CNS is known as a *sensory evoked potential.* Rather than obtaining a compound action potential, or *afferent neurogram*, recording over a proximal point of a stimulated peripheral nerve, the recording point is moved more proximal to locations on the skin overlying the brain and, in the case of the somatosensory evoked potential (SEP), the spinal cord. The evoked potential signal is extracted from electric potential fluctuations detectable on the skin, specifically by electroencephalography (EEG) and electrospinography (ESG), that reflect ongoing operation of these CNS structures. The sensory evoked potential paradigm involves repeated stimulation of a special sensory organ (e.g., the retina or cochlea) or peripheral nerve with a well-defined discrete stimulus. The types of stimuli that can be employed for the common sensory modalities tested are listed in Table 10-1. This process of stimulation is directly linked to the recording and extraction of the electrical responses evoked by this stimulus from central structures including the relevant regions of the brain and spinal cord. In this way, various latencies can be identified and measured along segments of the afferent pathway, and the presence or absence of components generated by specific structures or "generators" in the pathway can be checked. The sensory evoked potential is therefore effectively a "continuity check" of a specific afferent pathway through the CNS traced from the periphery to the responding central spinal cord and brain areas. Some of the various advantages and disadvantages of sensory evoked potential techniques are listed in Table 10-2.

The extension of the motor conduction study into the CNS is known as a *motor evoked potential.* This more recent and less widely applied technique involves the transcranial stimulation of regions of the primary motor cortex. This stimulation can be accomplished electrically but, for reasons to be discussed in a later section, is most commonly accomplished with large, rapidly changing magnetic fields produced by specialized stimulators that induce stimulus currents within the motor cortex. These stimulus currents then excite cortical neurons that give rise to efferent fibers projecting into the corticospinal tract. A synchronous volley of action potentials is thus generated within the corticospinal tract and conveyed down to the spinal segment. This efferent volley then excites a population of motor neurons to which the corticospinal fibers project. Synchronous excitation of motor neurons in the spinal cord then results in a muscle contraction in the limb. With surface electrodes placed over the contracting muscle, a

Table 10-1: Stimuli Used in Sensory Evoked Potentials

Modality	Selected Stimuli Types
Visual	Flash (e.g., provided by an activated array of red light-emitting diodes) Shifting black-and-white checkerboard pattern (e.g., on television monitor) Spatial grating
Auditory	Clicks (rarefaction or condensation) Tone pips
Somatosensory	Electrical stimulus (current or voltage pulse) to: Peripheral mixed nerve Cutaneous nerve Skin in a particular dermatome Mechanical tap Muscle stretch Thermal pulse (e.g., with infrared laser)

Table 10-2: Advantages and Disadvantages of Evoked Potentials

Advantages
- Reliable clinical tests that yield valid reproducible results with clinical relevance
- Provide an objective, quantitative extension of the clinical examination
- Objective measure of physiologic function within a particular sensory system
- Can detect abnormalities that may be clinically undetectable otherwise
- Can be used to localize the anatomic level of damage
- Can be used to assess prognosis
- Can be used to monitor the integrity of a pathway (e.g., as in intraoperative monitoring)
- Totally noninvasive and can be repeated serially to evaluate physiologic change over time
- Can be performed by a well-trained technologist under direct physician supervision

Disadvantages
- Prone to artifact
- Can be technically challenging
- Require either a cooperative subject or sedation to limit movement and electromyographic artifact
- Have been subject to overuse or misuse by inadequately qualified personnel
- Do not provide specific etiologic information

compound muscle action potential can be readily recorded exactly as it would be recorded with stimulation of the peripheral nerve in a motor conduction study. In this way, latencies can be derived for transmission from the cortex out to the muscle in the limb, and problems affecting transmission in efferent systems in the CNS can be detected. If the same magnetic stimulation technique is used to activate spinal nerve roots directly, the latency of this peripheral conduction time can be subtracted out, leaving a latency that reflects a conduction time along the central neuraxis from the cortical level down to the segmental spinal level via the corticospinal tract.

This chapter initially examines some of the basic principles involved in recording these potentials and then moves on to look at specific sensory evoked potential paradigms including the visual, auditory, and somatosensory testing techniques. Since these are the methods most commonly employed clinically, the chapter focuses primarily on their performance and clinical application. The chapter then concludes by looking in a more cursory fashion at a number of other neurophysiologic methods for evaluating function in the CNS, including the motor evoked potential. For a more thorough treatment of the subject and for more detailed information regarding these methods, the interested reader is referred to a number of excellent texts (1–6).

BASIC PRINCIPLES

The basic principles involved in the recording of sensory evoked potentials are quite different from those involved in the recording of motor evoked potentials, which are addressed separately.

Sensory Evoked Potentials

The basic issue in the recording of sensory evoked potentials is how one can reliably extract a signal of low amplitude (0.1–20.0 μV) from a background mix of normal EEG (or ESG), electromyographic (EMG), and various artifactual signals that range up to hundreds of microvolts in amplitude. This is really one of the most technically challenging aspects of recording sensory evoked potentials and one to which a great deal of technique development and technologic sophistication has been applied. While it may be possible and necessary to reduce the amplitude of the background EMG activity through relaxation of the subject and, if needed, light sedation, physiologic background related to the ongoing activity of the brain and spinal cord will continue unaltered. The generally utilized means of extracting the tiny evoked potential signal from the background that swamps it out is *signal averaging*. Averaging permits a powerful amplification of the signal-to-noise ratio when the signal can be time-locked to a recurring event with which it is reliably correlated, while the noise remains uncorrelated to the stimulus train. Since one of the main sources of noise is the electric power lines, care must be taken to be sure that the stimulus rate is not an integral factor of the line frequency. Thus, in a North American laboratory where the line frequency is 60 Hz, the stimulus rate must not be an integer that divides evenly into 60 or there will be the chance of phase locking between the stimulus and the line frequency, resulting in the appearance of a 60-Hz contaminating artifact in the average signal.

The recurring event in the sensory evoked potential paradigm is the point in time at which the stimulus is applied. The stimulus is applied repetitively and *sweeps* or epochs of digitized data points are acquired over an interval that is time-locked to the point of stimulus application. Most often the sweep is a fixed interval of time that immediately follows the application of the stimulus. However, prestimulus and poststimulus delays can also be used to move the position of stimulus application with respect to the interval across which the sweep data are collected. The process is generally accomplished in the modern electrodiagnostic system through computer-based real-time signal acquisition and processing techniques. The computer acquires each sweep and adds the new data into an accumulating average signal that is maintained in memory. A condition can be imposed between the acquisition of the sweep and the addition of the new data into the average, to check the sweep for evidence of artifact and reject the sweep if this evidence is found. This is referred to as an *artifact rejection* filtering method. Most often the condition relates to a swing of amplitude during the sweep that goes beyond a carefully selected preestablished amplitude range. A large fluctuation in amplitude is automatically assumed to be an indication of an artifact in the sweep. The average signal can be displayed on the monitor as it is being acquired and updated. The input signals can also be directly inspected. The averaging process can be manually paused when evidence of artifact is seen in the input data stream. The averaging process can be terminated once the appearance of the evoked potential signal has been adequately defined and stabilized. Usually a preset number of sweeps is automatically acquired and averaged, with the number of sweeps chosen to ensure that an adequate extraction of the evoked potential signal can be accomplished. With certain assumptions about the characteristics of the noise, the signal-to-noise ratio can be shown to improve in direct relationship to the square root of the number of sweeps in the average. This would indicate that the greatest improvement in the definition of the signal would occur in the initial stages of the acquisition, following which the improvement would continue but at a slower and slower rate. At some point, a trade-off is reached between the advantage of any further improvement that could be achieved by continuing the process and the extended period of time that would be required to achieve this improvement.

The evoked potential signal voltage reflects a difference in potential between two electrodes that are inserted into the two differential amplifier inputs, I1 and I2, with respect to a common ground electrode. There is no clear value in identifying one of the electrodes as active and the other as reference since both electrodes can be either at different times in the recording epoch. However, in the display of the signal, it is important to know how relative positivity versus negativity of I1 versus I2 is reflected in the deflection of the displayed signal. This is the issue of polarity convention, which can be quite confusing for the uninitiated when one enters the world of evoked potential signal review. In EMG, the convention is that a relative negativity of the I1 input is reflected in an upward deflection. For the display of evoked potential waveforms, there is, unfortunately, no standard convention that applies in terms of whether an upward deflection reflects a relative positivity or negativity of the I1 electrode. To avoid confusion, it is best to use the predominant approach in the relevant literature that has been used for each of the sensory modalities employed, as follows:

1. Positivity in the occipital region with respect to the vertex region of the head is reflected in an upward deflection for visual evoked potentials.
2. Positivity at the vertex with respect to the earlobes or mastoid regions is reflected in an upward deflection for auditory evoked potentials.
3. Negativity at the parietal scalp with respect to the frontal areas or other distantly placed electrodes is reflected in an upward deflection for SEPs.

Thus, the SEPs use the same polarity convention as EMG while the visual and auditory evoked potentials use an opposite convention.

The evoked potential signal is a variation of voltage over time drawn as a graph of voltage versus time that is viewed as a series of waves termed *components*. The peaks of each of the components are labeled in specific ways that vary according to the sensory modality being used. For the visual evoked potentials and the SEPs, the most frequently employed method of component nomenclature is through identifying the component with a combination of the letter "N" (for "negative") or "P" (for "positive"), which designates the polarity of the component, followed by a number indicating the normal median latency of the component in milliseconds. In the case of the BAEP, the six initial vertex-positive components are named in sequence with Roman numerals I to VI. Ideally, each component, or peak, of the evoked potential waveform can be associated with a particular physiologic generator. Sometimes this degree of correlation between the physiology and anatomy can be approached, as in the BAEP, through clinicopathologic correlation and comparative animal studies. More often, the situation is far more complex, owing to the overlap of activity generated by different structures in a pathway. Measures that can be obtained from the evoked potential waveform include latencies from the stimulus to individual components (i.e., absolute component latencies), latencies between components (often called *interpeak latencies*), and component amplitudes defined as either the amplitude above or below a baseline value or the amplitude between specific positive and negative peaks. In general, amplitude measurements have limited usefulness and must be made relative to some comparative reference such as the identical component on the opposite side obtained from the same subject. This is usually done by computing an amplitude ratio. Amplitudes tend to be much more variable than latencies and also may require special statistical treatment because they are often not normally distributed.

Electrode application technique involves two issues: (1) obtaining a low-impedance electrical connection to the skin, and (2) proper electrode positioning with the guidance of the International 10–20 System (7) for locating EEG electrodes on the scalp (Fig. 10-1). Electrodes may be gold or silver-silver chloride surface electrode cups that are held to the scalp with a thick, adhesive conductive paste, or subdermal needle electrodes may be employed. The use of subdermal needle electrodes should be avoided in the intensive care unit because of the risk of infection and also

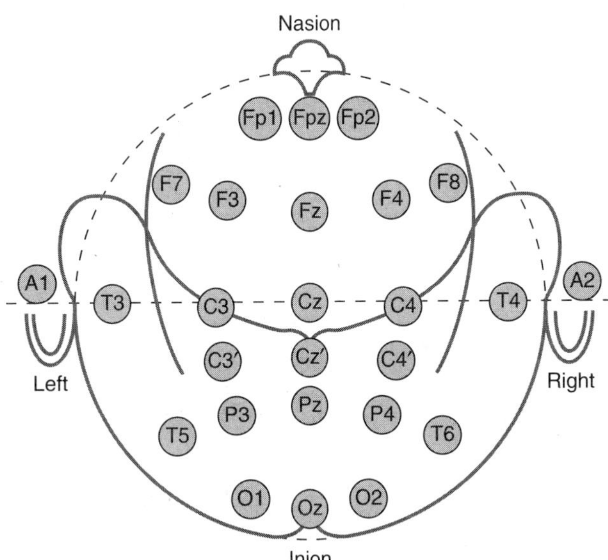

Figure 10-1. The International 10–20 System for locating electrode placement sites on the scalp: A=earlobe; C=central; F=frontal; Fp=frontopolar; P=parietal; T=temporal; O=occipital. The mastoid sites are not shown but are designated M1 and M2. Placements on the right side of the head have even numbers, while placements on the left side have odd numbers. Placements in the midline are denoted by "z." Note that the C3′, Cz′, and C4′ sites that are used in recording the somatosensory evoked potential are placed 2 cm posterior to the corresponding standard sites, C3, Cz, and C4, respectively. This is to ensure their placement posterior to the central sulcus and over the somatosensory cortex.

during intraoperative monitoring because of their tendency to loosen and dislodge. In recording evoked potentials with surface electrodes, it is important to abrade the skin prior to applying the electrode in order to minimize the impedance of the electrode contact with the skin. This can be done by lightly rubbing the skin with a cotton-tipped applicator soaked with skin preparation solution containing an abrasive and degreasing agent or with a pre-soaked skin preparation pad. An alternative technique is to lightly rub the skin with a piece of fine-grain sandpaper followed by an acetone swab to degrease the area. The electrode impedance can be checked after the electrodes have been affixed to the skin and should generally be under 10 kΩ and ideally under 5 kΩ.

Recording of the sensory evoked potentials requires high-quality low-noise physiologic differential amplifiers with high input impedances and high common-mode rejection ability. Often a preamplification phase is employed in the electrode switching box in order to provide initial amplification and to maximize the input factors. The clarity and definition of the evoked potential waveforms can also be improved somewhat with careful selection of filter settings. Suggested recording bandpasses for different evoked potential studies are shown in Table 10-3. A list of the stimulation and recording parameters and conditions that must be selected for each evoked potential study is provided in Table 10-4.

Another important issue in the interpretation of the sensory evoked potential is the need to clearly establish the presence of an adequate input to the CNS before interpretation of the CNS signals can be performed. One should attempt to obtain evidence that peripheral or caudal structures have been sufficiently activated before concluding that a particular central or rostral structure has failed to respond to its input. So, for example, one needs to establish that an afferent neurogram is recordable from the peripheral nervous system in the somatosensory evoked potential before concluding that the absence of a cortical response reflects pathology at the cortical level. If there is a severe peripheral nerve lesion proximal to the site of stimulation that is blocking conduction in the activated peripheral pathway, this could clearly explain the absence of the cortical response without there actually being any problem localized to the cortical level. Similarly, if the components of the BAEP are all absent, there is little that can be concluded about brain stem transmission since one cannot be sure that an adequate activation of the peripheral mechanism and auditory nerve has occurred. This issue is addressed in more detail in subsequent sections of the chapter.

Motor Evoked Potentials

The initial technique for the transcranial stimulation of the motor cortex was described by Merton and Morton in 1980 (8) who used a high-voltage electrical pulse applied through electrodes affixed to the scalp. A painless, safe, and much better-tolerated method for the transcranial stimulation of motor cortex was subsequently developed by Barker et al (9) who used transcranial magnetic field stimulation to induce excitatory electric currents in the underlying motor cortex, thus eliciting synchronous activation of a population of pyramidal cells sending axons into the corticospinal tract. The resulting activation of the motor neurons at the segmental level elicits a compound muscle

Table 10-3: Recording Bandpass Filter Settings for Different Evoked Potential Studies

Evoked Potential	Low Cutoff Setting	High Cutoff Setting
Visual evoked potential	1 Hz	300 Hz
Brain stem auditory evoked potential	100 Hz	3000 Hz
Somatosensory evoked potential		
Afferent neurogram	30 Hz	3000 Hz
Erb point / midclavicular	30 Hz	3000 Hz
Cervical spine / lumbar spine	10 Hz	3000 Hz
Cortical	1 Hz	3000 Hz

Table 10-4: Stimulation / Recording Parameters and Conditions for Evoked Potentials

- Stimulus parameters
  - Stimulus form and modality
  - Repetition rate
  - Duration
  - Intensity
  - Stimulus conditions / parameters for multiple sequential stimuli (for use in P3 recording)
- Amplification parameters for each recording channel
  - Amplifier sensitivity
  - Bandpass filter settings (high-cut and low-cut frequencies)
- Averaging parameters
  - Sweep duration
  - Number of digitized points in sweep or sampling rate
  - Prestimulus and poststimulus delays (optional)
  - Rejection filter settings
  - Number of sweeps to acquire
  - Number of channels to record
  - Electrode montage selection for I1 and I2 amplifier inputs and ground
- Electrode setup
  - Recording electrode site locations and placements
  - Ground electrode site location and placement
  - Stimulating electrode site location and placement (for somatosensory modality)

action potential from the peripheral muscle that can readily be measured without the need for averaging through surface electrodes placed over the activated limb muscle. The excitation of the motor cortex produced and the resulting efferent volley are powerful enough to cause some of the spinal motor neurons to fire repetitively, producing a more sustained response than that seen with a single supramaximal stimulation of the peripheral nerve. The amplitude of the peripheral muscle response depends on whether or not there is baseline voluntary activation of the muscle. When the muscle is lightly contracted, the threshold for excitation of the motor cortex becomes significantly lower and a larger response can be elicited. This observation is presumably related to tonic subthreshold excitation of the motor neuron pool at the spinal segment level, making it easier to excite the prefacilitated motor neurons to the threshold level for firing an action potential. The compound muscle action potential is recorded just as it would be in a standard motor nerve conduction study. For upper-limb studies, a 50-msec sweep time is adequate while for lower-limb studies, a 100-msec sweep time is used. The degree to which the muscle is relaxed can be monitored by using a high-gain, free-running display of the EMG signal recorded from the same electrodes used to record the elicited potential. To avoid the problem of facilitation during low-level baseline contraction influencing the recording, there should be complete relaxation of the muscle prior to performing the transcranial stimulation. The configuration of the stimulus coil can influence the spatial distribution of the magnetic field and the induced current. For basic activation of the cortex, a small circular coil can be used. However, for more focal activation of a specific region of the motor cortex, a figure-of-eight coil can be used where two small circular coils wound in opposite directions are configured immediately adjacent to each other. There is a high concentration of the magnetic field under the region at which the two circular coils overlap and the intensity of the magnetic field drops off quickly as one moves out from that point. Single transcranial stimuli are generally sufficient for performing a standard clinical study and can be safely applied. Because there is often significant intertrial variability, two to three replications of the stimulation should be repeated with the elicited muscle responses superimposed. Rapidly repeated transcranial magnetic stimulation has been used in research settings but is not recommended for clinical application because of the risk of producing seizures in normal subjects (10).

Dependent Factors

The major objective of the clinical neurophysiologic approach to CNS disorders is to provide information about the underlying pathophysiologic process. However, it is important to recognize that a number of other factors can influence the component structure of the signal. These can be divided into factors related to the stimulus and factors related to the subject. Stimulus factors will vary somewhat with the different sensory modality but generally include the physical features of the stimulus, including its intensity and the rate at which the stimulus is applied. Subject-dependent issues include the normal range of variation in evoked potential measures attributable to age, gender, brain and body size, body temperature, and medications. These issues are addressed separately for each of the different major sensory modalities.

VISUAL EVOKED POTENTIALS

Stimulus Factors

The physiologic evaluation of vision and the investigation of the physiologic anatomy of the visual system can be accomplished using the visual evoked potential paradigm. It has been known for many years that specific EEG changes occur in response to changes in visual input. These include the suppression of the α rhythm over the posterior head regions when the eyes open, as well as typically small perturbations associated with photic driving produced by stroboscopic stimulation. The major issue in visual stimulation is whether the driving stimulus factor is a luminance variation such as a bright flash of light or a visual pattern stimulation such as the sudden shift of a checkerboard pattern. In the latter, the total luminance, or light amplitude, of the stimulus stays constant. In the former, it does not. There are at least three major advantages to the constant-luminance pattern-shift stimulus:

1. There is significantly less inherent variation in the structure of the response between individuals and better test-retest reproducibility within subjects.
2. There are evoked potential parameters that are significantly more stable and sensitive to the presence of conduction impairments in the visual pathway.
3. By varying the size of the different components of the stimulus pattern and looking at how the evoked response varies with these changes, a measure of visual acuity can be approached.

The major disadvantage is that in order to be able to use the pattern-shift stimulus, the subject must be awake, alert, and sufficiently attentive to the stimulus so as to maintain an optimal stable focusing of the pattern on the retina. When this is possible, then, clearly, the pattern-shift stimulus is preferred. When this is not possible, then the flash stimulus is the only available option and a significant sacrifice in the utility of the study must be made. This is the case, for example, in infants or in unconscious or uncooperative subjects. The flash visual evoked potential has clinical utility in addressing the question of whether or not the pathway from the retina to the visual cortex remains intact and as such, is more qualitative in nature than quantitative.

For the pattern-shift stimulus, a number of different methods for producing the stimulus have been devised, but the one most commonly used and generally most flexible is the display of the pattern on a television monitor, with the pattern generation and switching controlled by pattern-generating electronic circuitry. This permits flexible control over such parameters as pattern structure, location, check size, stimulus field size, and rate of pattern-shift. The control over luminance can occur through the brightness control of the monitor and the control over contrast can be similarly adjusted. The disadvantage of this flexibility is that all of these stimulus parameters can have significant influence on the evoked potential measures. Therefore, they must be carefully controlled so as not to vary significantly from one test to the next, or between the control test used to establish normal values and the patient test.

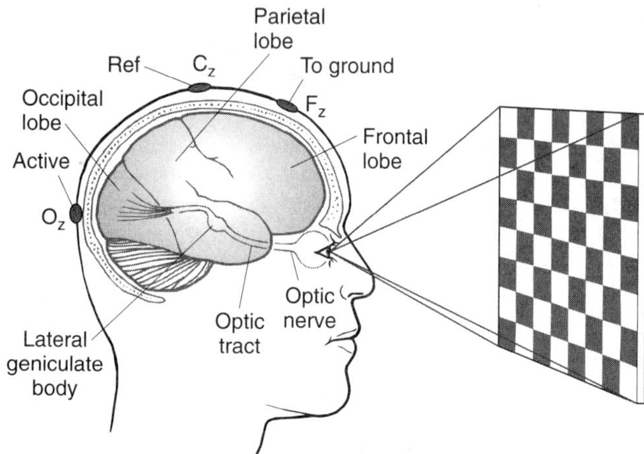

Figure 10-2. General recording setup for the pattern-shift visual evoked potential showing the subject positioned in front of a television monitor on which the pattern is displayed. The recording is obtained from a midoccipital (Oz) electrode with reference to the vertex (Cz), using the midfrontal (Fz) electrode as a ground. Improved resolution of the scalp field requires the use of additional recording sites. (Modified from Liveson JA, Ma DM. *Laboratory reference for clinical neurophysiology*. Philadelphia: FA Davis, 1992: 333.)

Subject Factors

Age-related increases in the P100 latency appear in subjects after age 60. The increase amounts to between 2 and 5 msec per decade (11,12). Variations in the amount of slowing reported are most likely related to differences in stimulus selection, since there is a more rapid increase in P100 latency for smaller check sizes (13). The P100 latency is normally slightly shorter, on average, in women than in men (14). However, this difference may be explained by differences in brain size and corresponding differences in the length of the visual pathway as opposed to differences in gender (15).

Technique

Care should be taken to ensure that conditions of optimal visual acuity are used. A patient should wear corrective lenses for the performance of the test and should not be studied after taking any medication or eyedrops that interfere with pupillary or lens control. The eyes should be studied one at a time with the opposite eye occluded with an eye patch.

The general setup for recording the pattern-shift visual evoked potential (PSVEP) is shown in Figure 10-2. The pattern-shift cortical response is generally a triphasic waveform that has a negative-positive-negative structure when recorded from an electrode over the midoccipital location (Oz) with respect to the vertex (Cz). A normal bilateral PSVEP study is shown in Figure 10-3. Clinical interpretation is based primarily on latency and secondarily on amplitude comparisons. The major latency measure is that of the primary positive peak, the P100. The recording setup should be chosen so as to maximize the registration of the P100 component. In most subjects, the P100 is maximum at around the level of the inion over the back of the head and reverses to a negativity at the vertex and frontal regions, with the reversal occurring between the midline parietal (Pz) and the Cz sites. Thus, a bipolar variation with one electrode located midoccipitally and the other located at the midfrontal (Fz) or Cz sites will produce a maximum amplitude for the P100 component. The Cz vertex site is probably a better choice because the peak negativity seen at the frontal area around the time of the peak positivity occipitally can sometimes be phase delayed, thus leading to a bilobed difference waveform in the Oz-Fz lead. In some subjects, the voltage distribution on the scalp may show a maximum positivity that is shifted anterior up to the Pz site and may have a low amplitude at the Oz site. Such variations may relate to interindividual variability in the location of the calcarine cortex (i.e., primary visual cortex) with respect to the scalp landmarks and need to be kept in mind when the standard Oz-Cz lead does not demonstrate a clear cortical waveform. To register such variants and not make an erroneous interpretation that the visual response is absent if not seen in the Oz-Cz recording, it has been recommended that additional recordings be obtained from the Pz and Cz sites with reference to the relatively inactive earlobe site (3). Another possible variation is the shifting of the peak positivity of the P100 laterally on the scalp to the left or right of the midline. In this case, the P100 may be absent in the occipital midline but clearly present with normal latency either to the right or left of the midline. When multiple recording channels are available, one can consider recording with four channels that include the Oz, Pz, left occipital, and right occipital sites referenced to a common, relatively indifferent site such as the earlobe. The left occipital and right occipital sites can be located at a standard distance of 5 cm to the left and right of the Oz site.

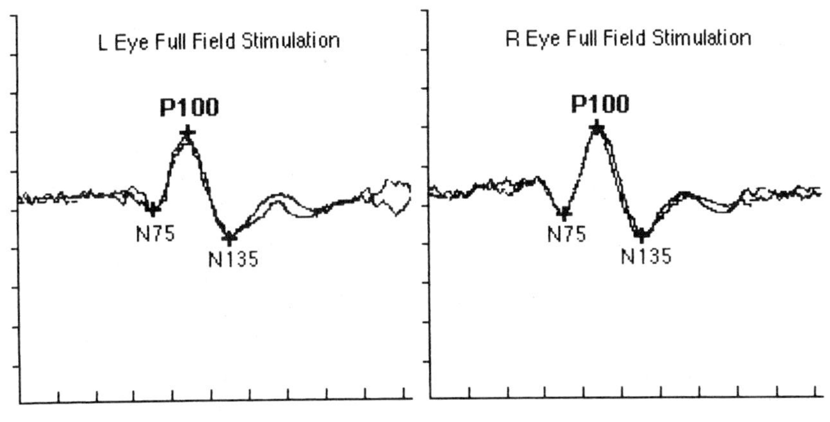

PSVEP - Full Field

LEFT EYE		RIGHT EYE	
Latencies			
N75	72.00	N75	75.00
P100	102.0	P100	105.0
N135	133.8	N135	135.0
Inter-Ocular Latency Difference:		3.0	
Amplitudes			
N75-P100	5.94	N75-P100	6.34
P100-N135	8.06	P100-N135	7.81

Figure 10-3. A bilateral normal pattern-shift visual evoked potential (PSVEP) waveform.Recordings were obtained from the midoccipital electrode (Oz) to the vertex (Cz). Stimulation was performed with a black-and-white checkerboard pattern where each check subtended an angle of 20 minutes of arc with a full screen stimulus of 15 degrees of arc. The major waveform peaks are marked. Note the triphasic structure of the cortical response with a major positive peak at a latency of approximately 100 msec. There is a 10% (30-msec) prestimulus period. Positive deflection at the Oz site relative to the Cz site is displayed upward. Vertical scale: 3 μV/division. Horizontal scale: 20 msec/division.

The maximum amplitude of the PSVEP occurs when the check size subtends between 15 and 30 minutes of arc, with the total field size subtending about 15 degrees of arc. The subject is positioned a meter from the monitor screen and the size of the checks is adjusted so as to obtain a visual angle between 15 and 30 minutes of arc. The visual angle subtended by a check is a function of the distance of the eye to the pattern and the width of the check. It is calculated by first dividing the width of the check by 2 and then dividing this by the distance to the screen measured in the same units as the width of the check. Using a calculator or trigonometric tables, one then uses the inverse tangent function to find the angle for which the tangent has this value. This angle is then multiplied by 2 to give the total visual angle subtended.

The subject is then set up with the eye patch on one eye and instructed to maintain gaze on a dot in the center of the screen display. Background illumination is reduced. The stimulation should start with the pattern shifting at a rate of about two shifts per second. If the subject's gaze wanders during the study, the amplitude of the P100 will begin to fall off in proportion to the time during which the pattern is not registered on the retina due to diverted gaze. The subject should be closely monitored by the technologist and regularly encouraged to maintain an attentive focus on the displayed pattern.

The averaging process should continue until a clear demonstration of the waveform is apparent. This is frequently accomplished after 100 to 150 sweeps have been acquired. Duplicate averages should be obtained and superimposed on the display in order to document the degree to which the structure is reproducible. If the components are not clearly identified or a significant amount of variability is encountered, multiple duplications may be needed. If the cortical waveform cannot be identified, there may be a problem with acuity. The check size is enlarged and the attempt to record the PSVEP is repeated. The absence of a cortical response could also be related to a primary retinal problem. To investigate this possibility, a pattern-shift or flash-evoked electroretinogram (ERG) can be recorded using a specialized electrode made from a thin strip of gold foil that slips between the lower eyelid and the globe of the eye using a temple site as a reference (16). The absence of a PSVEP at the cortical level in the presence of a normal ERG indicates a retrobulbar problem in the visual pathway. The absence of both the PSVEP and the ERG indicates either some type of technical problem with the recording system or a primary retinal problem.

Interpretation

Interpretation of the PSVEP must be done in the context of an understanding of the anatomic connections between the retinal fields and the primary visual cortex. Given that the eyes are tested one at a time with a full-field stimulation, both the nasal and temporal hemiretinas are stimulated. The nasal hemiretina maps to the visual cortex of the hemisphere contralateral to the eye being stimulated, with its fibers crossing in the optic chiasm. The temporal hemiretina maps to the visual cortex of the hemisphere ipsilateral to the eye. Its fibers do not cross at the optic chiasm. Thus, with full-field stimulation of one eye, *input to both hemispheres is generated*. Therefore, a lesion affecting the visual pathway on one side posterior to the optic chiasm does not generally produce a distinct abnormality of the PSVEP recorded in the occipital midline. Therefore, with full-field monocular stimulation, when an abnormality is noted in the cortical PSVEP with stimulation of only one of the eyes, it correlates with a unilateral lesion that is anterior to the optic chiasm on the same side as the abnormality. When abnormalities are noted in both eyes, then the abnormality is bilateral but may be located anywhere from the retina back through to the visual cortex. A large asymmetry in the abnormality tends to correlate more closely with a prechiasmal involvement of the optic nerves rather than bilateral retrochiasmal lesions.

Delays in the latency of the P100 component correlate with demyelinating lesions, whereas axonal injury or retinal dysfunction typically results in a loss of amplitude without necessarily altering the latency. Latency abnormalities due to delays of the P100 component are most often an indication of a demyelinating lesion of the optic pathway and the absolute latency of the P100 component is a reliable indicator of such an abnormality when it is delayed beyond 3 standard deviations above the mean normal value. The interocular latency difference is also a reliable and more sensitive indicator of a relative abnormality affecting one eye more than the other, since the interocular latency difference for the P100 is normally less than 8 to 10 msec. Latency delays are more reliable than changes in the amplitude of the cortical PSVEP. The most reliable amplitude abnormalities are those that are unilateral and the contralateral response can be used as a control. When a bilateral amplitude abnormality occurs without a latency abnormality, however, care must be taken to be sure that this is not due to a technical problem with the recording of the response, such as an undetected abnormality of visual acuity, poor fixation of the pattern, nystagmus that does not allow for pattern stabilization on the retina, or a patient who is falling asleep and closing the eyes during the study. Most often, when conduction defects are produced in the optic nerve, latency differences develop initially and often before the appearance of an amplitude abnormality. Studies of patients with multiple sclerosis indicate that latency abnormalities of the P100 are a very sensitive indication of demyelination of the optic fibers (17). When the P100 was normal, the clinical examination of visual function never showed an abnormality, while in a significant number of patients with pathology demonstrated by an abnormal P100 latency, a detailed neuro-ophthalmologic evaluation was normal. The main limitation of the PSVEP is that it shows physiologic impairment without being able to distinguish between different underlying etiologic mechanisms. The abnormal findings of the PSVEP must be carefully correlated with the clinical evaluation of the patient and with other laboratory investigations that can help to differentiate between possible specific disease processes underlying the abnormality.

Clinical Applications

There are a variety of situations in which the visual evoked potential has been applied to the diagnosis of different disease processes. The major clinical indication for the performance of PSVEP studies is in the diagnosis of optic neuritis or multiple sclerosis. When the PSVEP is recorded together with the pattern-shift ERG, the most common finding is a normal ERG with a delayed PSVEP. If the impairment is long-standing with the secondary development of optic atrophy and degeneration of the retinal ganglion cells, the ERG may also become abnormal (18). While magnetic resonance imaging (MRI) has become the preferred screening study for the diagnosis of multiple sclerosis, in selected patients in whom the possibility of optic tract involvement is being considered based on clinical evaluation, the PSVEP remains more sensitive than MRI for picking up an isolated optic nerve lesion (19). Some of the clinical applications of the PSVEP that have been described are listed in Table 10-5. The interested reader is referred to the relevant chapters of the textbooks edited by Chiappa (3) and Aminoff (1) for additional information and detail regarding visual evoked potentials and their clinical applications.

BRAIN STEM AUDITORY EVOKED POTENTIALS

In the first 10 msec after the monaural application of an acoustic stimulus (e.g., a rarefaction click), there is a sequence of waves of current in the brain that reflect the sequential activation of different structures in the auditory pathway ranging from the cochlear nerve through the pontomedullary, pontine, and midbrain elements of the pathway. These waves are volume conducted to the surface of the scalp and appear there as low-amplitude far fields with broad distribution centered at the vertex. When a recording is made from an electrode placed at the vertex and one placed on the ipsilateral earlobe, a series of positive and negative waves are registered as the result of this activation of the brain stem auditory pathway. This study

Table 10-5: Clinical Applications of the Visual Evoked Potential
Diagnosis in adults Optic neuritis Multiple sclerosis Pseudotumor cerebri Tumors (e.g., meningiomas, craniopharyngiomas, chiasmal gliomas) Brain trauma Parkinsonism Spinocerebellar degeneration Vitamin deficiencies Cortical blindness Loss of vision associated with conversion disorder Malingering Coma assessment Optic neuropathy/atrophy Special applications in pediatrics Estimation of visual acuity Amblyopia Neonatal asphyxia Neurodegenerative disease Hydrocephalus Monitoring for neurotoxic effects of medication (e.g., desferoxamine) Congenital malformations Other applications Intraoperative monitoring (e.g., during pituitary tumor excision)

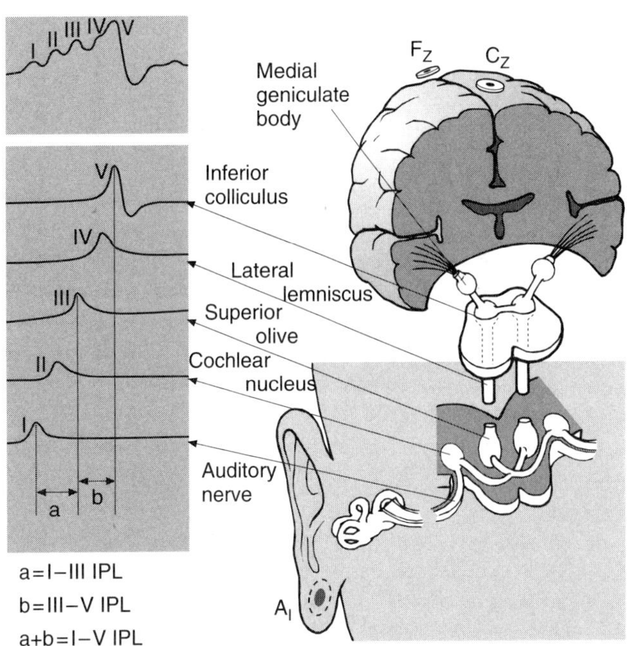

Figure 10-4. Source generation of the brain stem auditory evoked potential (BAEP). Note the origin of wave I from the auditory nerve, wave II from the cochlear nucleus, wave III from the superior olive, wave IV from the lateral lemniscus, and wave V from the inferior colliculus. Wave IV may be generated within the medial geniculate nucleus of the thalamus. The BAEP is recorded from the vertex (Cz) with respect to the ipsilateral earlobe (A1). A ground electrode is placed at the midfrontal site (Fz). IPL = interpeak latency. (Modified from Liveson JA, Ma DM. *Laboratory reference for clinical neurophysiology.* Philadelphia: FA Davis, 1992: 325.)

is called the *brain stem auditory evoked potential* (BAEP). The generation of the BAEP is illustrated in Figure 10-4. As noted, these signals are, by convention, plotted with vertex-positive deflection upward. The sequence of vertex-positive waves is identified with Roman numerals as waves I through IV. A set of normal bilateral BAEP signals is shown in Figure 10-5. Based on clinicopathologic correlation and animal studies, wave I corresponds to activation of the acoustic nerve, wave III reflects activation in the vicinity of the superior olive in the midpons, and wave V reflects activation of the inferior colliculus at the level of the midbrain. The interpeak latencies between these three waves reflect neural conduction through specific segments of the pathway. The I–III interpeak latency reflects conduction in the lower pontine component of the pathway, while the III–V interpeak latency reflects conduction in the upper pontine component of the pathway. The I–V interpeak latency is a measure of conduction from the point of activation of the acoustic nerve and its entry at the pontomedullary junction, up to the midbrain at the top of the brain stem. This conduction latency is sometimes called the *brain stem transit time.*

Stimulus Factors

The stimulus is most often a brief 100-μsec click provided through earphones where the diaphragm is either pulsed inward toward the ear to produce a condensation click, or pulsed outward away from the ear to produce a rarefaction click. The use of rarefaction clicks has been recommended for routine BAEP applications (20). Occasionally, alternating polarity must be used to minimize the stimulus artifact. Changes in the intensity of the click lead to significant changes in the latency and amplitude of all the waves of the BAEP. The intensity of the click is measured in units of decibels (dB) above a reference level, defined as normal hearing threshold from behavioral audiometry in a group of normal adult subjects. The abbreviation for these units is *dB nHL.* Amplitude falls off and the component latencies increase with decreasing click intensity or loudness. All the waves shift by about the same amount so that the interpeak latencies are less affected than the absolute wave latencies. This finding is important since it is difficult to control the stimulus intensity exactly because of a variety of factors that affect the conduction of the acoustic stimulus to the basilar membrane of the cochlea. For the purpose of lesion localization using the BAEP, the absolute latencies are practically useless for this reason. The interpeak latencies, however, are found

Figure 10-5. Normal two-channel brain stem auditory evoked potential (BAEP) signals. *A*. With left ear stimulation. *B*. With right ear stimulation. Note the absence of the wave I component when the earlobe contralateral to the applied stimulation is used as a reference. A relative positivity at the Cz electrode is displayed upward. Vertical scale: 0.18 μV/division. Horizontal scale: 1 msec/division.

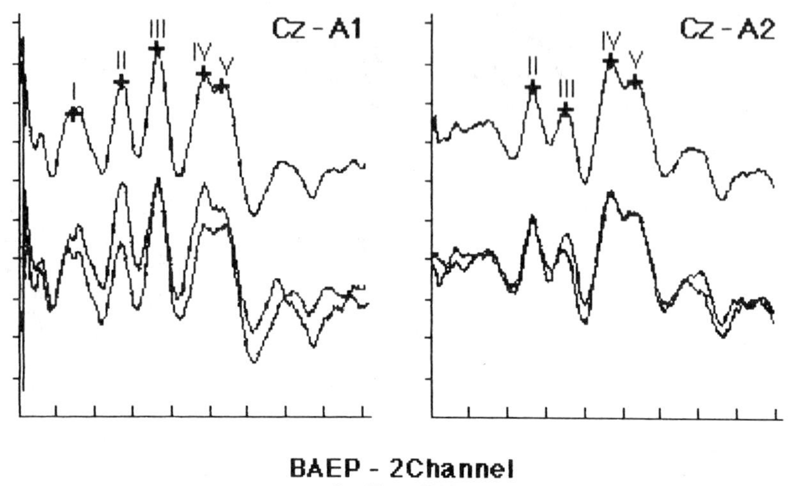

BAEP - 2Channel
L. Ear Stim.

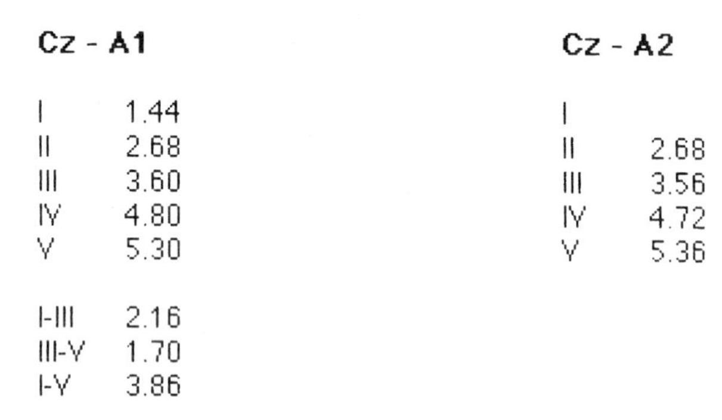

Cz - A1		Cz - A2	
I	1.44	I	
II	2.68	II	2.68
III	3.60	III	3.56
IV	4.80	IV	4.72
V	5.30	V	5.36
I-III	2.16		
III-V	1.70		
I-V	3.86		

A

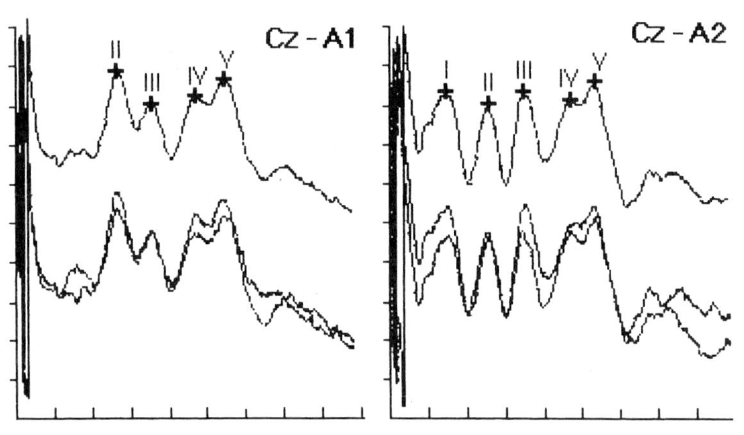

BAEP - 2Channel
R. Ear Stim.

Cz - A1		Cz - A2	
I		I	1.52
II	2.64	II	2.58
III	3.54	III	3.52
IV	4.70	IV	4.72
V	5.44	V	5.34
		I-III	2.00
		III-V	1.82
		I-V	3.82

B

to be quite reliable and stable. If the stimulus intensity is at least 75 dB nHL, then all the waves of the BAEP should be clearly defined. At lower stimulus intensities, component amplitudes begin to drop off, with the wave I, II and IV components disappearing initially, then the wave III component, and finally the wave V component. The wave V component is the one component that remains recognizable down to the lowest levels of stimulation. For this reason, it is the latency of the wave V component that can be tracked down with decreasing stimulus intensity to the point at which it finally disappears. This point is used to define an evoked response production threshold that appears about 20 to 30 dB above the behavioral hearing threshold. The definition of this threshold and the variation of the latency of the wave V component with decreasing click intensity at levels above this threshold form the basic elements of evoked response audiometry (see below).

The effect of increasing click rate is an increased absolute latency of all components of the BAEP as well as a decreased component amplitude. The wave I, III, and V components tend to be more robust and less affected in terms of amplitude or recognizability by the increasing click rate. Abnormalities identified at lower stimulus rates can sometimes be exaggerated as the click rate is increased. The question of whether or not abnormalities may appear only at the higher stimulus rates remains controversial. The choice of a click rate of 11.1 clicks/sec ensures there will be no chance of phase-locking with line frequency during the averaging process. For evoked response audiometry, a higher rate of 31.1 clicks/sec can be employed since the only wave of interest in this circumstance is the wave V component, which is relatively resistant to the effects of an increased stimulus rate at this level.

Subject Factors

The brain stem produces responses that are relatively unaffected by most pharmacologic agents. In fact, normal BAEPs can be recorded in the presence of cerebral electrical silence induced by medications like the barbiturates. The interpeak latencies are particularly independent of effects of most CNS depressants. An associated hypothermia, however, can lead to mildly prolonged interpeak latencies and must be recognized as a possible influencing factor. Hyperthermia can have mild opposite effects.

The BAEP undergoes a remarkable maturational process before the age of 2, with interpeak latencies being prolonged and not reaching stable adult-level values until around this age. The maturational changes in BAEP morphology and component latency are especially noticeable in the premature infant in whom significant changes in component structure and interpeak latencies are occurring as a function of conceptual age. The maximum rate of change of the interpeak latencies as a function of increasing age occurs at around 32 to 34 weeks and then this gradually slows down beyond this point (21). Up to the age of 6 months, the absolute latency of wave I is also prolonged compared to adult levels because of the prematurity of the peripheral auditory mechanism and acoustic nerve. These rapidly changing maturational effects necessitate the use of age-specific normal values when testing premature infants, newborns, and children under the age of 18 months. The effects of advanced age on the BAEP have been found to be relatively minor and studies that showed some effect were not able to clearly demonstrate that hearing function as revealed through behavioral audiometry was normal in the older control subjects (22).

Female subjects have been found to have significantly shorter III–V and I–V interpeak latencies compared with males. The amplitude of the BAEP also tends to be greater in females than males. Most authorities believe that this observation relates to differences in head and brain stem size. For the purposes of establishing normal adult values, it is best to maintain normative data separately for males and females (20). The effects of peripheral hearing disorders is considered later in the section on evoked response audiometry. There are no changes in the BAEP associated with changes in level of consciousness, attentional focus, or sleep.

Technique

The basic setup for recording auditory evoked potentials is shown in Figure 10-6. For the two-channel BAEP study, electrodes are placed at the vertex (Cz) and on each earlobe (A1 on the left and A2 on the right). A ground electrode is placed at the midfrontal or midforehead site (Fz or Fpz). At times, when the wave I component cannot be clearly identified, a subdermal EEG electrode can be substituted for the earlobe electrode and placed in the external auditory canal. The two channels obtained are Cz with respect to the earlobe on the stimulated side, and Cz with respect to the earlobe on the opposite side. The test is performed with the subject lying supine, with towels placed under the neck and a pillow under the head to minimize muscle contraction in the neck. The room should be darkened and quiet. The subject is encouraged to relax, close the eyes, allow the jaw to drop loosely open (in order to relax facial muscles and muscles of mastication), and fall into a light sleep. If the patient is unable to relax and there is excessive EMG artifact noted on the inputs, a mild hypnotic/sedative medication can be used, although care will have to be taken to be sure that the patient does not drive home after the study. Another way to encourage sleep and relaxation is to have the subject come in for the study in the morning after staying up until the early morning hours and taking no stimulants including caffeine at breakfast.

The earphones are placed on the patient and the click intensity, rate, and polarity are selected for the side to be tested. Masking white noise is applied to the opposite ear in order to prevent it from generating a response to the applied click stimuli. Both ears are tested separately. The patient is positioned, as just described, and

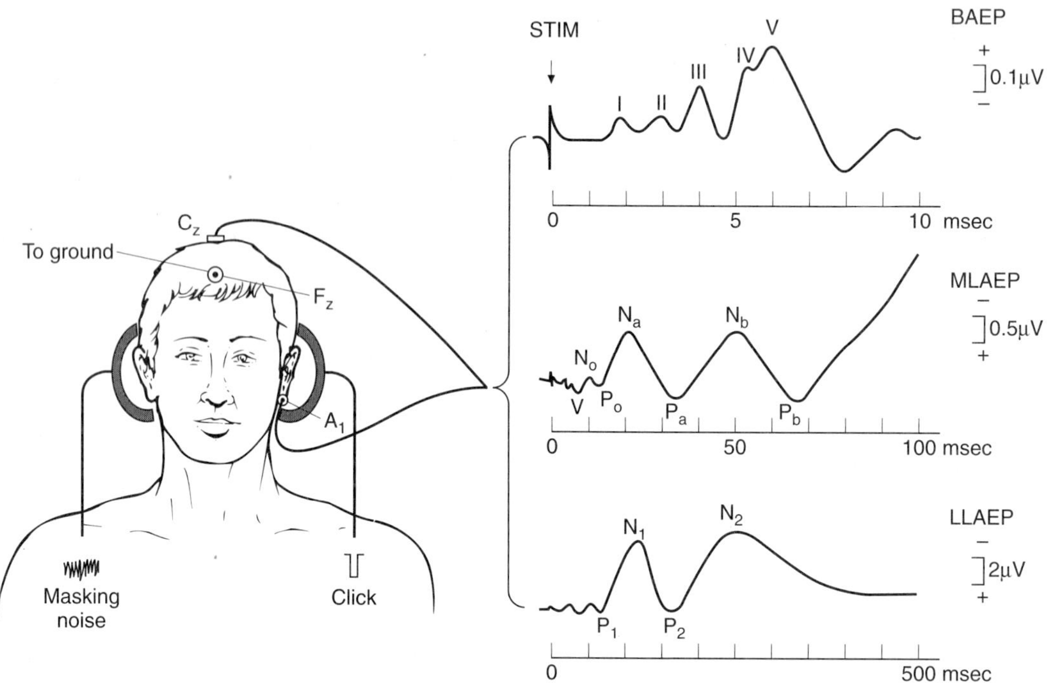

Figure 10-6. Basic setup for recording auditory evoked potentials. Note that the earlobe electrodes A1 and A2 serve as reference sites for the vertex (Cz) electrode. Different components of the auditory evoked potential can be seen, depending on the recording parameters and the sweep duration. BAEP = brain stem auditory evoked potential; MLAEP = middle latency auditory evoked potential; LLAEP = long latency auditory evoked potential. (Modified from Misulis KE. *Spehlmann's evoked potential primer: visual, auditory, and somatosensory evoked potentials in clinical diagnosis.* 2nd ed. Boston: Butterworth-Heinemann, 1994: 118.)

settled in, and the test is started. Initially, the stimulation is started and the input signals are monitored for a short period of time before the averaging is initiated. This allows for a period of accommodation to the stimulation and also allows for a check of the input signals to be sure that the EMG artifact is under good control and the signal remains generally within amplitude range. The degree of EMG artifact can also be evaluated by turning up the sound to the audio amplifier and listening for surface EMG activity on the monitors. If the artifactual activity is excessive, the patient may need to be repositioned, the headphone position adjusted, or some other problem causing the patient to be unable to relax the head and facial muscles identified and addressed (e.g., the patient needs to use the bathroom). The averaging is continued until approximately 2000 trials have been accepted into the average. Again, the study should be repeated at least once in order to document the reproducibility of the waveform structure. The study should be repeated until the degree of variability of the signal is clearly defined by the superposition of multiple trials. Once the study has been brought to a satisfactory conclusion for one ear, the other ear is tested in similar fashion.

Interpretation

The major challenge in interpreting the BAEP is to clearly identify each of the components in the waveform and to determine whether or not a particular component is present or absent. There is a significant amount of inherent interindividual variability in the component structure of the BAEP. Wave V is the most prominent peak in the waveform after around 5.5 msec. It is defined also by a negative trough that immediately follows it. If wave V is absent but wave IV remains, this trough is generally not present and the signal comes directly back down to baseline after the wave IV peak. The wave IV and V components are often fused together in a single bifid component. The wave IV component may be absent. Since wave V is the most resistant component to decreased click intensity, its presence can sometimes be confirmed by repeating the study with a significantly reduced click intensity. Wave II appears between wave I and wave III usually about halfway between unless abnormalities are present. If it is not clear which wave is wave III, the stimulus intensity can be reduced, which will tend to leave wave III alone since this wave and wave V are the only two components that remain present in the waveform at reduced stimulus intensities.

Clinical Applications

A variety of clinical applications of the BAEP have been identified. These include those in the areas of diagnosis, prognosis, and intraoperative monitoring. A list of some of these identified applications is given in Table 10-6.

Diagnostic

The BAEP study has proved useful because of the close relationship between identified anatomic structures in the brain stem auditory pathway and specific BAEP components. Furthermore, the BAEP is relatively robust and unlikely to be affected by factors other than local pathology affecting conduction in the brain stem auditory pathway. It can be used in the context of evoked response audiometry to differentiate between conductive and sensorineural hearing impairments and it can be used to localize abnormalities affecting brain stem conduction in CNS disorders. The BAEP is very sensitive in the early detection of acoustic neuroma and other tumors of the cerebellopontine angle, where a variety of abnormalities can be seen. The BAEP is also useful for detecting the presence of demyelinating disease localized to the upper brain stem. This would include multiple sclerosis most commonly, but also conditions such as central pontine myelinolysis and the leukodystrophies. The BAEP is also useful in assessing the status of the brain stem under conditions of suspected brain death where one may see preservation of wave I and II but absence of all other components. However, if one sees no components at all, then no definite conclusions can be drawn regarding the brain stem pathway. This finding is likely to correspond to significant damage of the auditory nerve, but without evidence of activation of this input structure (i.e., without the presence of the wave I component at least), one cannot infer that the brain stem received a stimulus sufficient to generate subsequent responses. Therefore, the lack of subsequent components in the response cannot be used to generate inferences about transmission through the brain stem auditory pathways. This is actually a generally important principle in the interpretation of the BAEP and emphasizes the importance of being sure that an adequate registration of wave I can be demonstrated.

The BAEP has been used to assess patients with the sequelae of concussion that have been termed the *postconcussion syndrome.* In studying 27 patients, Rowe and Carlson (23) found that 3 patients had clearly prolonged interpeak latencies and that the patient group as a whole had prolonged mean interpeak latencies for the I–III, III–V, and I–V intervals compared to control subjects, even though not all individual patients had significant abnormalities. Benna et al (24) also found a significant percentage of abnormalities of the BAEP in patients with postconcussion syndrome. The clinical value of BAEP testing in patients with this problem remains somewhat unclear since the yield of significant abnormalities for individual patients is not particularly high, even though group means show abnormalities for patients with this condition taken as a whole.

Table 10-6: Clinical Applications of the Brain Stem Auditory Evoked Potential

- Diagnosis in adults
  - Acoustic neuroma / cerebellopontine-angle tumors
  - Multiple sclerosis
  - Central pontine myelinolysis
  - Leukodystrophy
  - Friedreich ataxia
  - Spinocerebellar / brain stem degeneration and ataxias
  - Brain stem tumors (e.g., glioma, pinealoma)
  - Brain stem hemorrhage / infarction
  - Coma assessment
  - Brain death evaluation
  - Postconcussion syndrome
  - Hearing impairment (investigated with evoked response or "objective" audiometry)
- Special applications in pediatrics
  - Brain stem gliomas
  - Neurodegenerative disorders
  - Central nervous system malformations
  - Developmental disorders
  - Coma prognosis
  - Hydrocephalus
  - Screening for hearing impairment in at-risk infants
  - Meningitis
  - Monitoring for neurotoxic effects of medication (e.g., aminoglycosides)
- Other applications
  - Intraoperative monitoring (e.g., posterior fossa tumor excision)

Prognostic

The BAEP has been applied to the assessment of prognosis following severe anoxic and traumatic encephalopathies producing coma. While significant abnormality of the BAEP is clearly an indicator of a poor prognosis, the presence of normal BAEPs does not imply a uniformly good prognosis. This is particularly the case in anoxic encephalopathy in which the BAEP may indicate retained conduction through the brain stem in spite of severe cerebral dysfunction. Patients in a persistent vegetative state, in fact, can often have normal BAEPs. Thus, it appears that the BAEP has a better utility as a negative prognostic indicator than as a positive prognostic indicator in this situation. In a study of patients in a minimally conscious state primarily due to severe traumatic brain injury, the BAEP had a high sensitivity but low specificity for predicting recovery from this state (25).

Intraoperative Monitoring

The BAEP has utility in monitoring the integrity of the acoustic nerve, auditory function, and the integrity of the brain stem during surgical intervention in the posterior fossa. Changes in the BAEP have been shown to occur following specific operative maneuvers, and restoration of baseline BAEP appearance following corrective surgical or anesthesiologic action reflects reversal of the neurophysiologic impairment of the affected structures. The relative preservation of hearing function postoperatively, however, does not always correlate directly with the preservation of the BAEP documented during the procedure.

Evoked Response Audiometry

As noted earlier, there are systematic changes that normally occur in the structure of the BAEP as the click intensity is gradually reduced. The wave that is most resistant to the effects of reduced intensity is wave V. It is therefore possible to identify the relationship between the latency of the wave V component and click intensity down to levels close to the behavioral hearing threshold. This relationship is normally hyperbolic, with wave V latency steadily increasing with decreasing click intensity. The relationship can be documented as a graph of wave V latency versus click intensity.

Evoked response audiometry involves the performance of BAEPs generated with an intensity series, that is, with clicks applied at sequentially reduced intensities. A typical intensity series in an infant undergoing a screening examination might include studies performed at 70, 50, and 35 dB nHL. A good approach would involve adjusting the stimulus intensities used in the series until one is able to define two closely spaced intensities in the series where wave V is clearly present at the higher intensity but absent at the lower intensity. A normal evoked response audiometry study in a newborn is shown in Figure 10-7A.

Different types of abnormalities can be identified with evoked response audiometry. The first abnormality is an elevation of the threshold at which wave V can first be seen. This corresponds to an elevation of the behavioral hearing threshold. The second type of abnormality is a systematic shift in the latency-intensity curve from its normal position. If the curve is shifted upward but remains parallel to the normal curve, consistent with a similar increase in wave V latency at each level of stimulation, the test indicates the presence of a conductive hearing loss. The conductive impairment introduces a constant delay into the system so that the wave V latency is similarly displaced outward at each level of stimulation. In the presence of a sensorineural deficit, on the other hand, the slope of the curve is also shifted up so that wave V latency may be near normal at the high intensities but increases disproportionately with decreasing click intensity. With a sensorineural impairment, there is an abnormality that is partially correctable at high intensities but rapidly becomes apparent as intensity decreases, so that the wave V latency is nearly normal at high intensities but quickly increases as the intensity of the stimulus decreases. An example of an abnormal study in a 6-month-old infant is shown in Figure 10-7B. In both conductive and sensorineural hearing impairment, the wave V threshold is often found to be elevated.

Evoked response audiometry thus provides important objective information about the function of the peripheral auditory mechanism that would otherwise be very difficult to obtain in a patient for whom behavioral audiometry could not be performed. This is particularly important for the developing child, where an undetected bilateral hearing impairment can lead to significant delays in language acquisition. If the hearing impairment is not detected and corrected with a program of aural rehabilitation and augmentation until after the age of about 3, then the child will not develop normal language expression. Thus, the ability to identify correctable hearing impairment in infants using evoked response audiometry can have a major moderating influence on the impact of this problem on language development. Whether such screening should be done universally or only with infants who are identified as having significant risk factors for hearing impairment remains a point of debate conditioned primarily by the costs associated with universal screening using this methodology. For further information on the application of BAEPs in pediatrics to this and other problems, the interested reader is referred to the excellent book chapter by Picton et al (26). For a more thorough discussion of the general clinical applications of auditory evoked potentials with projection of trends for the future see the recent article by Thornton (27), the book chapter by Stockard et al (20), and the relevant sections of the book edited by Chiappa (3).

SOMATOSENSORY EVOKED POTENTIALS

By far the most useful and most frequently applied type of evoked potential for patients encountered in physical medicine and rehabilitation is the somatosensory evoked potential (SEP). The most common technique for producing a stimulus for the SEP involves stimulation with a pulse of electrical current applied percutaneously to a peripheral nerve or directly to the skin as in the dermatomal SEP. More physiologic stimulation techniques such as a mechanical skin tap or a muscle stretch have been reported in research studies but have not been generally incorporated into clinical laboratories. The electrical stimulation of a mixed nerve at submaximal levels produces a selective activation of the low-threshold afferents, the large, myelinated fibers that include the type Ia muscle spindle afferents and the group II cutaneous afferents. These afferents are also the fastest-conducting afferents and their arrival at proximal levels predominates in the activation of proximal structures in the pathway. When a cutaneous nerve is stimulated, the group II cutaneous afferents predominate. Transmission through the spinal cord occurs primarily through the dorsal columns when this type of stimulation is used, since the large myelinated afferents will tend to travel with this system. Conditions that involve the spinal cord but spare the dorsal columns may often leave the SEP intact. On the other hand, conditions that selectively damage the dorsal columns will significantly affect the SEP even though the remainder of the spinal cord continues to function well.

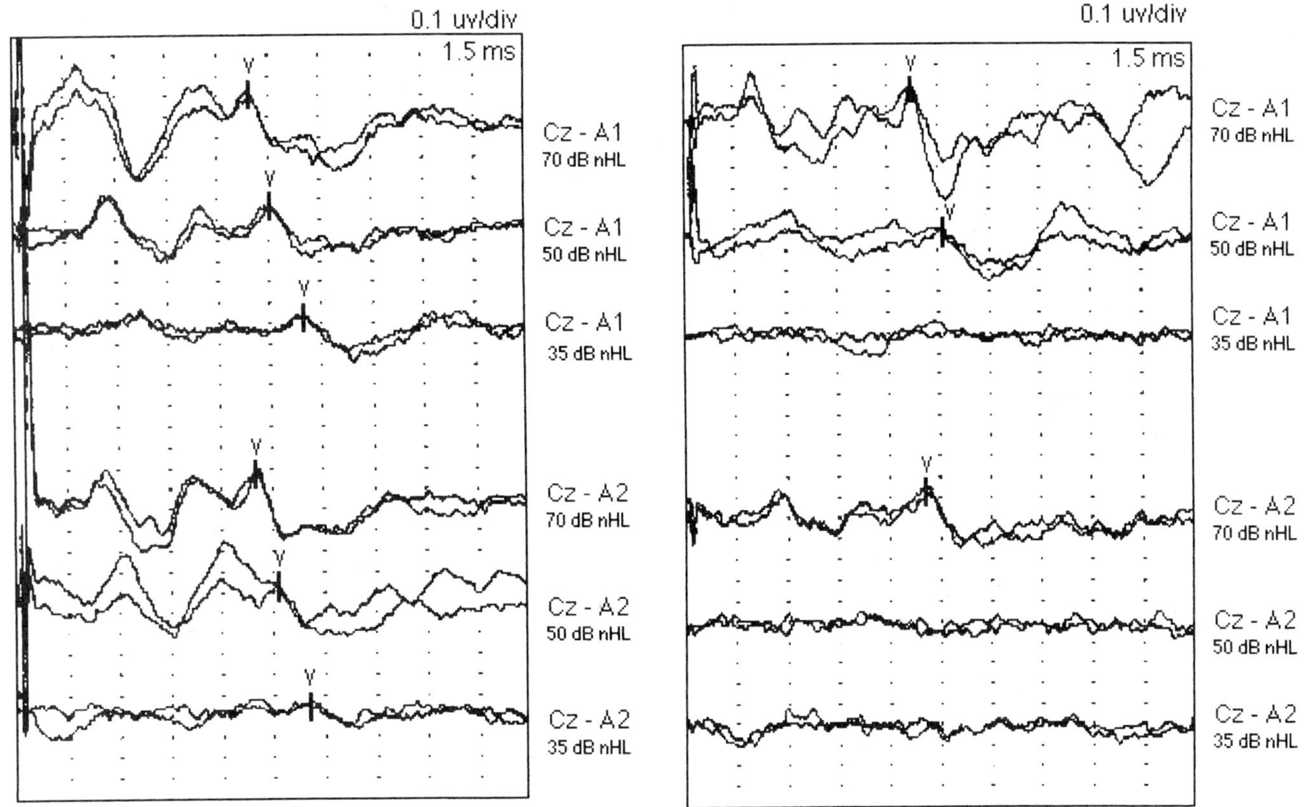

Figure 10-7. Evoked response audiometry. *A.* A normal evoked response audiometry examination of both ears of a newborn. Rarefaction clicks are applied at a rate of 31.1 clicks sec and intensities of 70, 50, and 35 dB nHL are used. The left ear is tested first (*top three traces*), and then the right ear is tested (*bottom three traces*). The recording sites and stimulus intensities are indicated to the right of the traces. Note the increase in wave V latency and gradual decrease in amplitude with decreasing stimulus intensity. Wave V can be seen clearly, however, down to 35 dB nHL. *B.* An abnormal evoked response audiometry examination of both ears of a 6-month-old infant with a history of premature birth and neonatal sepsis treated with antibiotics. The patient's mother felt the infant was not responding normally to her voice. Findings are consistent with an asymmetric bilateral sensorineural impairment. The wave V component is bilaterally absent at 35 dB nHL and can only be seen with left ear stimulation at 50 dB nHL. Auditory augmentation and aural rehabilitation were recommended for this child based on this examination. Because of the asymmetry of the response structure, it was recommended that auditory amplification be applied to the left ear. Vertical scale: 0.1 μv/division. Horizontal scale: 1.5 msec/division.

Stimulus Factors

The SEP waveform latencies remain quite stable across a range of stimulus intensities. As long as a visible twitch is noted in the innervated muscle, the stimulus intensity is adequate to produce the SEP waveforms and increasing the stimulus intensity further does not significantly further enhance the responses. Stimulation above this level may risk the occlusion of stimulus-produced action potentials, spread of current to activate other adjacent structures, problems with stimulus artifact, and an increase in EMG artifact because of patient discomfort. A recommended level of at least three times the sensory threshold has also been put forward but is probably not as useful with mixed-nerve studies as it is with cutaneous nerve studies where there is no muscle twitch to be registered.

Studies of stimulus rate show that the amplitude of major components of the response decreases with increasing stimulus rate. Thus, the choice of stimulus rate is a compromise between an adequate definition and amplitude of the key components of the SEP and the speed with which the study can be performed. Higher rates of stimulation are also associated with greater patient discomfort. Greater waveform distortion at higher rates occurs in the lower-limb studies as compared to the upper-limb studies and suggests that lower stimulation rates should be used when performing lower-limb SEPs.

While some authors have recommended techniques that use bilateral simultaneous stimulation, the use of unilateral stimulation is preferred in evaluating for lateralized abnormalities.

Subject Factors

Relatively few studies have looked at aging effects on the SEP. Hume et al (28) examined the effects of age on the interpeak latency between the neck and the cortical peaks, also known as the *central somatosensory conduction time* (CSCT), to be discussed later. They found no significant change in this measure from 10 to 49 years but then noted an abrupt increase of about 0.3 msec between the fifth and sixth decades. Beyond that point, the measure remained stable. The central somatosensory interpeak latencies gradually decrease over time during maturation as the latency of the cortical response steadily decreases until the adult levels are reached at around 6 to 8 years. The interpeak latency between the Erb point potential and cervical spine response stays fairly stable during maturation. The overall morphology of the evoked responses also gradually changes during early maturation. The cortical components are broader and lower in amplitude in children than they are in adults. In young infants, these components may not be clearly discernible, especially following stimulation of the tibial nerve at the ankle. This finding underscores the need to perform serial follow-up studies in young infants when a cortical component cannot be identified in the initial studies. In this situation it becomes important to determine whether or not the observed lack of identifiable SEP components at the cortex is related to a normal maturational variation or to the presence of pathology.

There is a steady decrease in the duration of the cortical waves with increasing age, suggesting greater coherence in the cortical activity. Components recorded at subcortical levels tend to be of higher amplitude and complexity in young children than those recorded at these levels in adults. The SEP waveform morphology in children approaches that of adults by the time the child is 5 to 8 years old.

The absolute latencies of components of the SEP are related to the length of the pathway between the peripheral site of stimulation and the point at which the recording is obtained. The pathway length is clearly related to body size. If absolute latencies are used rather than interpeak latencies for the upper-limb studies, the difference in body size contributes significantly to the variability of the values and the sensitivity of the measures is thus reduced. However, if the central latencies proximal to the recording at the Erb point are measured as interpeak latencies for the upper-limb studies, most of the additional variability due to differences in body size is reduced to tolerable levels. The effects of body size are significantly greater for lower-limb studies where a correction for height can be made for both the absolute latencies of the components as well as the conduction time from the lumbar spine to the cerebral cortex. The effects of changes in body temperature are also significantly greater for absolute latencies, which tend to increase with lowering of temperature. However, central interpeak latencies are relatively insensitive to physiologic changes in temperature.

The short-latency SEP components are remarkably resistant to the effects of medications and changes in central state. Therapeutic coma induction with phenobarbital does not produce a significant variation of the latencies of the short-latency SEP components or the central interpeak latencies, although the long-latency SEP components may have significant reductions in amplitude and increases in latency.

Technique

The major challenges in the performance of the SEP are to 1) control artifact due to EMG signal from muscles near the recording electrodes, and 2) control stimulus artifact. The upper-limb studies can be done with the patient sitting in a comfortable padded chair or lying supine on a comfortable examination table. Pillows should be placed under the head and a towel roll under the back of the neck to relax the muscles of the head and neck. The upper limbs can also be propped up on pillows to relax the arm and shoulder musculature. The lower-limb studies should be done when possible with the patient lying prone on a comfortable examination table, with the head turned to one side and the arms allowed to hang over the edges of the table. Pillows are placed under the hips to help flex the lumbar spine and relax the paraspinal muscles, much as is done in the needle EMG examination of the paraspinal muscles.

Needle EEG subdermal electrodes or EEG surface cup electrodes can be used to record the SEP signals. The surface electrodes should be applied, as reviewed earlier, with careful preparation of the skin to reduce skin impedance. Recording electrodes, stimulus electrodes, and the ground electrode should all be applied following careful skin preparation to minimize the skin impedance. Skin impedances associated with EEG needle electrodes may be somewhat higher than those associated with surface electrodes because of the smaller recording surface. Needle electrodes should be handled very carefully to avoid risk of infection. Infection-control guidelines are most readily met with disposable subdermal electrodes. Reusable electrodes should be properly sterilized and stored if this option is selected.

The amplifier gains are adjusted to give maximum range of amplitude without excessive activation of the artifact rejection filter. The filters are set according to guidelines in Table 10-3. The sweep duration should be set to between 40 and 50 msec for upper-limb studies and between 60 and 100 msec for lower-limb studies. The number of sweeps to gather for the averages should be set at 1000, although under some circumstances, an adequate definition of the waveforms can be obtained after 500 sweeps have been added to the average. As always, the studies should be replicated with superposition of the signals from each replication in order to document the variability of the waveform structure.

A stimulus duration of 200 μsec can be used, although a longer duration of up to 1 msec may be more effective in activating the low-threshold afferents. The stimulus rate for upper-limb studies should be around 3.1 stimuli/sec since rates higher than 5 stimuli/sec lead to significant problems with component resolution and latency changes. The stimulus rate for lower-limb studies should be around 2.1 stimuli/sec. The left and right limbs should always be tested separately.

The approach to the control of stimulus artifact is similar to that discussed in Chapter 9 with regard to technique for nerve conduction studies. A stimulus isolation technique must be used. The skin impedance associated with the ground electrode should be carefully checked and should be under 7 kΩ. The ground electrode should be positioned between the stimulation site and all of the recording sites. If the stimulus current is excessively high, this should be addressed. The stimulus electrode sites should be carefully prepared to allow an adequate stimulation of the peripheral structure with a minimum amount of current. The stimulus site should be adjusted if necessary. If the problem is due to excessive subcutaneous tissue intervening between the skin and the underlying nerve, consideration should be given to the use of subdermal needle electrodes for delivery of the stimuli. Sometimes rotating the position of the stimulus bar electrode with respect to the position of the recording electrodes can reduce or neutralize the stimulus artifact. Adjustment of the low cutoff filter setting can sometimes reduce the amplitude of the stimulus artifact, although care must be taken to avoid causing significant changes in the evoked response signal. Various schemes to suppress the stimulus artifact such as the use of an alternating polarity stimulus are usually not very helpful.

Mixed Nerve

The technique that gives the most satisfactory SEP studies involves stimulation of major mixed-nerve trunks. The stimulating electrodes, most often a pair of electrodes embedded in a plastic bar, are carefully positioned immediately over the nerve to be stimulated. The stimulus intensity is gradually increased until a brief muscle twitch is visible in the muscles innervated by the nerve distal to the point of stimulation. Care should be taken not to over-stimulate the nerve as this can cause blocking of the afferent fibers, spread to other nerves, increased likelihood of a troublesome stimulus artifact, and also increased EMG artifact due to patient discomfort.

Median Nerve

One of the most common upper-limb SEP studies involves stimulation of the median nerve at the wrist. A ground electrode that works well is a strip of malleable metal in a sleeve of cloth that can be adjusted to fit around the forearm and maintained with a Velcro closure. The skin should be carefully prepared under the ground electrode just as it is for all of the other electrodes that make contact with the skin in order to ensure a low skin impedance. A typical four-channel study with median nerve stimulation would involve the following:

1. The recording of a peripheral nerve afferent neurogram from electrodes placed over the median nerve at the elbow. The I1 electrode is placed over the nerve in the anterior antecubital area and the I2 electrode is placed over the medial epicondyle of the humerus or the olecranon. With the electrodes properly located, this recording should show a clear triphasic positive-negative-positive potential reflecting conduction of the volley induced by the wrist stimulation through the median nerve at the level of the elbow. The prominent negative component should have a peak latency of around 5 msec. This component is the *N5*.
2. The recording of an afferent neurogram from the brachial plexus with an electrode placed at the Erb point in the supraclavicular fossa. The Erb point is defined as the point behind the posterior edge of the clavicle at the angle between the clavicle and the posterior border of the sternocleidomastoid muscle. The I1 electrode is placed at the Erb point ipsilateral to the stimulated median nerve. The I2 electrode is placed at the contralateral Erb point. This reference site should be relatively quiet at the time during which conduction of the afferent volley is passing through the brachial plexus on the stimulated side. The other advantage of using this reference site is that it is simple to just reverse the two electrodes between the I1 and I2 inputs for this channel when studying the opposite side. This recording should show a prominent negative peak at around 9 msec, reflecting passage of the volley through the brachial plexus region. This component is termed the *Erb point potential* (EP) or the *N9*. The exact latency of the peak depends on the length of the arm. A peripheral conduction velocity can be estimated by measuring the distance between the elbow electrode and the Erb point electrode and dividing this by the difference in latency between the negative peak recorded at the elbow and that recorded at the Erb point.
3. The recording of a cervical spine response from an electrode placed over the posterior midline of the neck at the level of the second cervical vertebra. This can be located about 2 to 3 cm below the base of the skull at a point just below the hairline. The I2 electrode is placed at the frontal midline (Fz). Other authors (29) suggested an anterior cervical reference for this recording to provide for better localization of the recording to the cervical spinal cord. This signal shows a prominent negative peak at around 13 msec, the *N13* component. The N13 component reflects activation at the cervicomedullary junction near to where the dorsal

column nuclei are located. Sometimes a small peak precedes the main negative peak and occurs with a latency of about 11 msec. This is the *N11* component. The N11 component may reflect a root entry potential.

4. The recording of a cortical response from the contralateral primary somatosensory cortex. The I1 electrode is placed at a point 2 cm behind the lateral central electrode location from the International 10–20 System (C3 or C4) over the side of the head opposite to the median nerve being stimulated. The I2 electrode can be the Fz electrode already placed for step 3 above. Alternatively, the I2 electrode can be the central electrode on the opposite side of the head so that this channel measures the *difference* in potential between homologous central sites over the two hemispheres when unilateral stimulation is performed. A sequence of waves is seen in this recording that typically begins with a large negative deflection peaking at around 19 msec. This is the *N19* component.

This basic setup for the four-channel median SEP is illustrated in Figure 10-8 and the signals obtained in a normal bilateral four-channel study are shown in Figure 10-9.

Some authors advocate the use of at least one channel that links a "cephalic" scalp electrode to a "noncephalic" reference such as the contralateral Erb point or shoulder. This is meant to serve as a check on the relatively infrequent situation in which the major negative peak of the response at the cortex, the N19, cannot be clearly seen because of a lack of difference in potential on the scalp between the central and frontal cephalic electrodes. This situation can occur occasionally because of an anterior spread of the parietal negativity that defines the N19 component. However, the noncephalic reference recording is often difficult to record accurately owing to large amounts of EMG artifact that also make the recording difficult to interpret. It is recommended that this recording be performed initially with the bipolar cephalic lead, but if the N19 is not clearly registered with this lead, consideration should be given to performance of the study with a cephalic site at the lateral central electrode referenced to a noncephalic site. The noncephalic site could be the contralateral Erb point site, which should already have an electrode placed.

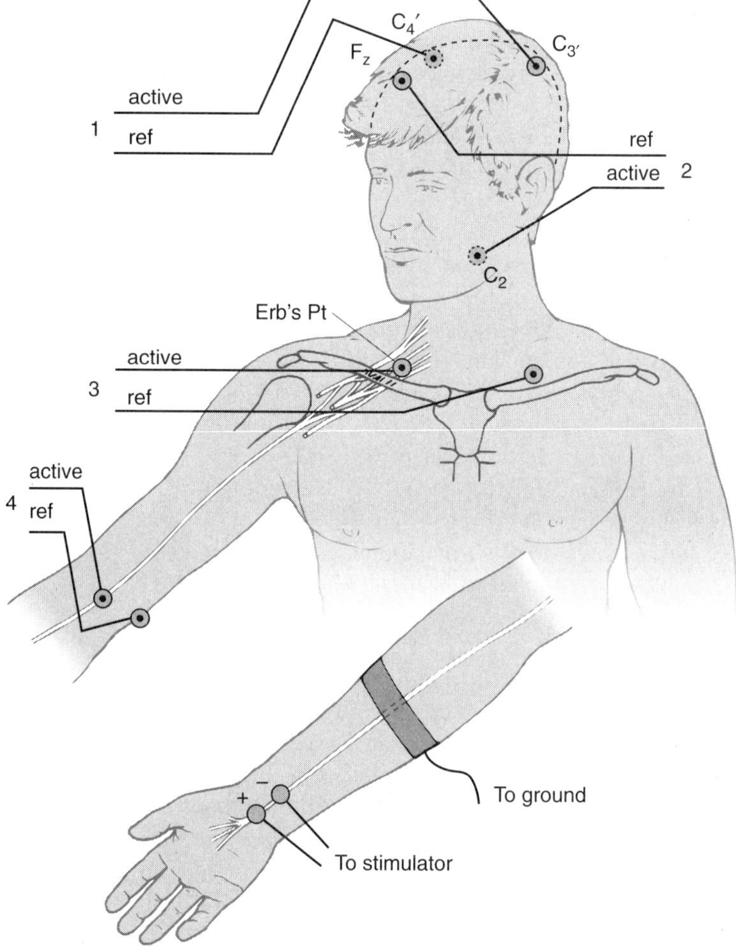

Figure 10-8. Basic setup for recording the four-channel median nerve somatosensory evoked potential. (Modified from Liveson JA, Ma DM. *Laboratory reference for clinical neurophysiology.* Philadelphia: FA Davis, 1992: 279.)

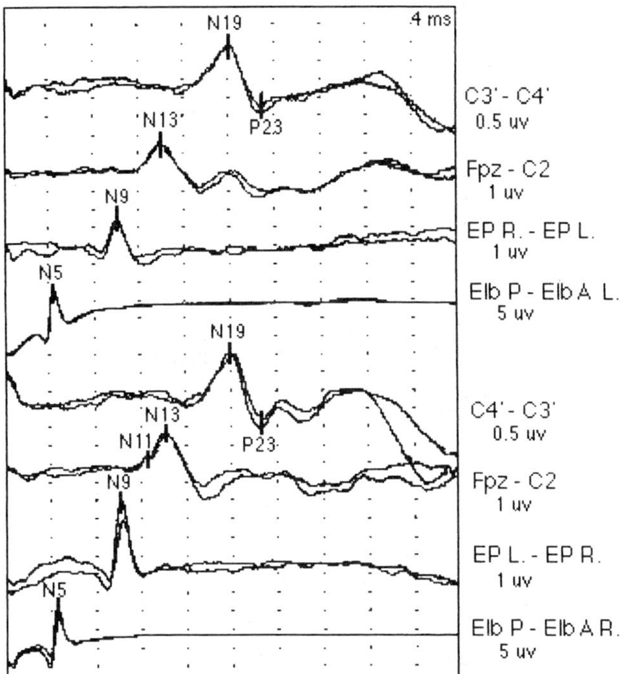

Figure 10-9. Normal bilateral four-channel study of the median nerve somatosensory evoked potential. The recording sites and vertical scale values for each channel are indicated to the right of the traces. The top four sets of traces were recorded following stimulation of the left median nerve. The bottom four sets of traces were recorded following stimulation of the right median nerve. Major components are marked on each set of traces. Note the steady progression in latency of the major negative deflection as one proceeds proximally from the site of stimulation. Note the symmetry of latency and amplitude comparing the responses to the two sides. Abbreviations are as in the International 10–20 System for scalp site identification. Also: C2 = posterior neck midline at the level of the C2 vertebral body; EPR = right Erb point; EPL = left Erb point; Elb P = posterior aspect of the elbow; Elb A = anterior aspect of the elbow overlying the median nerve at this level. A relative negative deflection at the second electrode for each channel is displayed upward. Horizontal scale: 4 msec/division.

Absolute peak latencies can be defined for all of the major components identified above. In addition, various component amplitudes and amplitude ratios can also be defined. Interpeak latencies can be measured between major components identified for stimulation on one side. These include the N5-EP, EP-N13, and the N13–N19 interpeak latencies. The last interpeak latency between the major negative peak at the cervical spine and that at the cortex has been termed the *central somatosensory conduction time* (CSCT) and reflects conduction across the central neuraxis from the base of the brain stem up to the cortical level. It has a mean value of about 5.5 msec with a standard deviation of 0.42 msec (3). The upper limit for the CSCT is about 6.8 msec if one uses mean plus 3 standard deviations as a criterion. There is an upper limit on the side-to-side difference for this measure of 1.1 msec. The CSCT can be very useful as a measure of conduction delay in the somatosensory pathway produced by lesions affecting transmission in the pathway at any point in the central neuraxis above the cervicomedullary junction (30).

A very similar setup to this can be used to record an SEP associated with stimulation of the ulnar nerve at the wrist. The stimulating electrodes need to be positioned medially at the distal part of the forearm over the ulnar nerve to elicit the appropriate activation of the ulnar nerve. The recording of the peripheral nerve afferent neurogram also requires that the electrode sites described in step 1 be placed over the ulnar nerve as it passes around the elbow in the antecubital tunnel.

Tibial Nerve

The most technically satisfactory study among those available for the lower-limb SEP is that in which stimulation is applied to the tibial nerve at the ankle. The major advantage of this study is that it allows an evaluation of conduction along the length of the spinal cord and can be usefully applied to the assessment of the functional integrity of the spinal cord below the cervical level. This study then complements the upper-limb investigation in the sense that the upper-limb studies are limited to the evaluation of spinal cord conduction at the cervical levels above the point of cervical root entry. A ground electrode similar to that described for the median nerve study is wrapped around the foreleg after preparation of the skin to reduce skin impedance. A typical four-channel study with tibial nerve stimulation at the ankle would involve the following:

1. The recording of a peripheral nerve afferent neurogram from electrodes placed over the tibial nerve at the knee. The I1 electrode is placed over the trunk of the nerve in the posterior popliteal fossa and the I2 electrode is placed over the fibular head or over the patella anteriorly. When electrodes are placed properly, this recording should normally show a clear triphasic positive-negative-positive potential with a negative peak latency of around 8 msec. This is the *N8* component.
2. A potential obtained from the lower spinal cord with the placement of an electrode over the spinous process of the L1 or T12 vertebra in the posterior midline. The I2 electrode is placed over the contralateral iliac crest. This recording is often difficult to obtain because of the small amplitude of the response at this level and the EMG artifact from the surrounding paraspinal muscles. The quality of the recording can sometimes be improved by using a modified monopolar EMG needle electrode where

the Teflon coating has been stripped off for the distal 10 mm to expose a larger recording surface. This electrode is inserted down into the interspinous ligament between the T12 and L1 spinous processes and replaces the surface electrode at this level. When the potential is identified, there is an isolated negative deflection that is seen at a latency of around 22 msec. This is sometimes termed the *lumbar potential* (LP) or the *N22*.

3. The recording of a primary cortical response obtained from an electrode placed 2 cm posterior to the vertex site (Cz) overlying the foot region of the primary somatosensory cortex. The I2 electrode is placed at the midfrontal site. This recording shows a series of positive-negative waves with the initial positive deflection having a peak latency of around 37 msec. This is the *P37* component.
4. A second bipolar cephalic recording obtained between the lateral central sites. The I1 electrode is placed 2 cm posterior to the contralateral central site (either C4 or C3) and the I2 electrode is placed 2 cm posterior to the ipsilateral site on the opposite side of the head (either C3 or C4). When the ipsilateral central site is referenced to the contralateral central site, a series of positive-negative waves is also seen that is similar to those observed in the channel described in step 3 above.

It is important to have the two cephalic bipolar recordings in order to carefully identify the presence of the cortical response, which is usually seen best in the Cz-Fz bipolar recording but may sometimes only be seen adequately in the bipolar lateral central recording due to the orientation of the dipole vector for the primary cortical response. Generally, the posterior region of the head behind the central sulcus tends to become positive with respect to the midline frontal region so that the initial cortical response is actually a large positive deflection, the P37. The ipsilateral central region also becomes relatively positive with respect to the contralateral central region. Thus, when a bipolar recording is obtained with a central electrode placed ipsilaterally referenced to an electrode placed in a similar position over the opposite side of the head, the initial cortical component is also a positive deflection. Since the convention for SEP is negative deflection going upward, the initial cortical response in the tibial SEP is a large downward deflection. This basic setup for the four-channel tibial SEP is illustrated in Figure 10-10 and a set of signals obtained in a bilateral normal four-channel study following stimulation of the tibial nerves at the ankle is shown in Figure 10-11.

If additional recording channels are available, a cervical spine response can also be recorded with an electrode placed over the fifth cervical vertebra in the posterior midline of the neck with reference to the Fz site. However, this response is often very small and difficult to resolve reliably. When it is important to obtain this response, a modified EMG monopolar needle electrode, similar to that which can be used at the lumbar level as described earlier, can be used at the cervical spine level to try to get closer to the source of the conducted potential in the dorsal columns of the cervical spine.

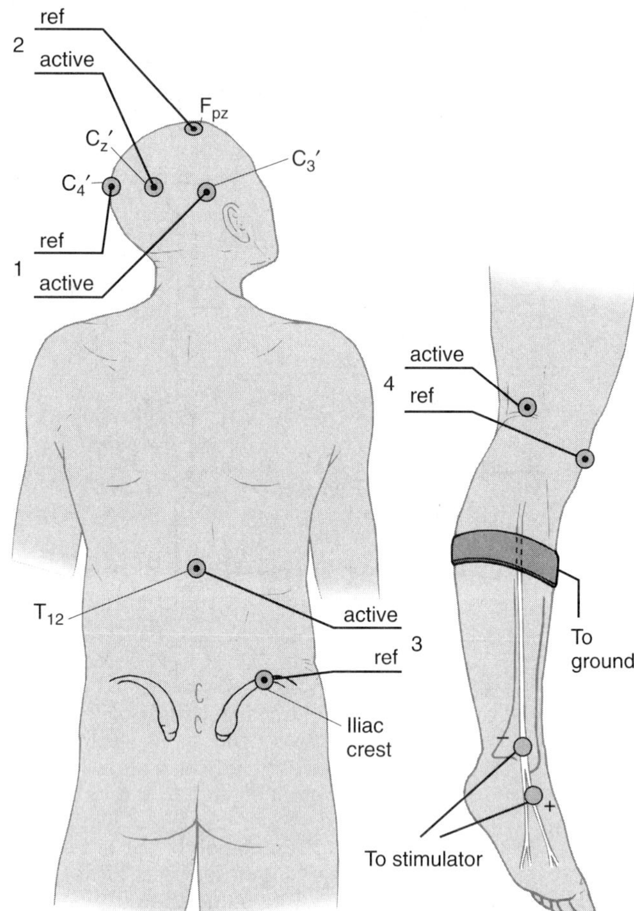

Figure 10-10. Basic setup for recording the four-channel tibial nerve somatosensory evoked potential. (Modified from Liveson JA, Ma DM. *Laboratory reference for clinical neurophysiology*. Philadelphia: FA Davis, 1992: 291.)

Absolute peak latencies for all of the major components can be measured for the tibial nerve SEP. In addition, various interpeak latencies can also be defined including that from the N8 to the LP, and from LP to the P27. The absolute latency of the P37, the conduction time from the knee to the lumbar spine, and the conduction time from the lumbar spine to the cortex vary linearly as a function of height (3). Therefore the height should be recorded when performing the lower-limb study in order to increase the sensitivity of the measures.

Cutaneous Nerve

Any cutaneous nerve that is accessible to activation by percutaneous stimulation can be used for an SEP study. The

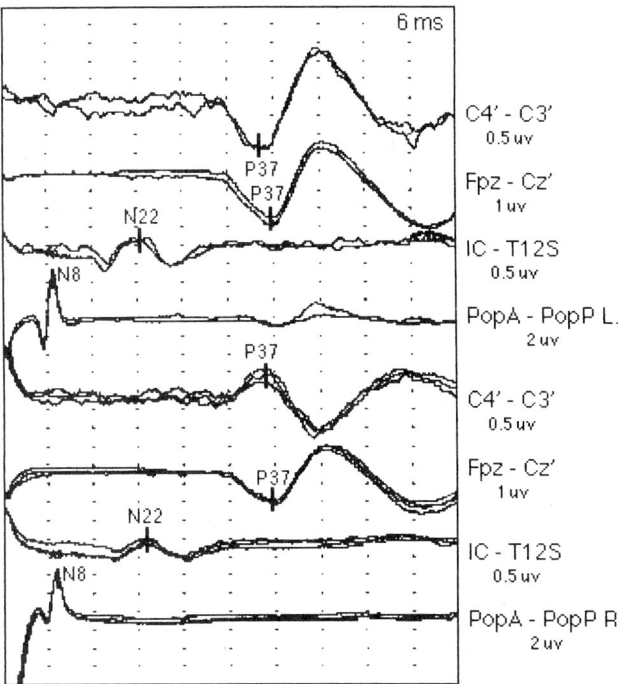

Figure 10-11. Normal four-channel study of the tibial nerve somatosensory evoked potential. The recording sites and vertical scale values for each channel are indicated to the right of the traces. The top four sets of traces were recorded following stimulation of the left tibial nerve at the ankle. The bottom four sets of traces were recorded following stimulation of the right tibial nerve. Major components are marked on each set of traces. Note the symmetry of latency and amplitude for major components comparing the responses to the two sides. Abbreviations are as in the International 10–20 System for scalp site identification. Also: IC = iliac crest; T12S = over the level of the T12 vertebra in the posterior midline of the back; PopA = anterior aspect of the knee; PopP = posterior aspect of the popliteal fossa overlying the tibial nerve at this level; L = left; R = right. A relative negative deflection at the second electrode for each channel is displayed upward. Horizontal scale: 6 msec/division.

cortical responses are readily recorded but are slightly delayed compared to studies using mixed-nerve stimulation. The cortical responses following cutaneous nerve stimulation are also about half of the amplitude of the SEP cortical responses seen with mixed-nerve stimulation. With cutaneous nerve stimulation, it is also significantly more difficult to record the spinal potentials because of their reduced amplitudes. The major advantage of the use of cutaneous nerves as opposed to mixed nerves is that a more precise and limited transmission through root levels can be achieved, making this approach somewhat more useful in the evaluation of radiculopathies (31). Available cutaneous nerves and their associated spinal root levels are

Table 10-7: Cutaneous Nerves and Associated Spinal Root Levels

Nerve	Root Level(s)
Cervical segments (upper limb)	
Lateral antebrachial cutaneous	C5, C6
Superficial radial	C6
Digital nerves to middle finger	C7
Digital nerves to little finger	C8
Medial antebrachial cutaneous	T1
Lumbosacral segments (lower limb / perineum)	
Lateral femoral cutaneous	L2, L3
Saphenous	L3, L4
Superficial peroneal	L4, L5
Sural	S1, S2
Pudendal	S3, S4

listed in Table 10-7. However, from a technical standpoint, the major improvement in SEP amplitude and the reduction in intersubject variability achieved with mixed-nerve studies when compared to cutaneous nerve studies indicates that they are significantly more useful for routine clinical application (32).

Dermatomal

To be more specific in the activation of fibers that traverse individual nerve roots, dermatomal stimulation of the skin can be used to elicit the SEP. For example, the L5 dermatome can be tested with stimulation on the dorsum of the foot between the first and second toes. The S1 dermatome can be tested with stimulation applied to the skin on the lateral side of the fifth metatarsophalangeal joint. The spread of activation to adjacent or overlapping dermatomal segments can be avoided by minimizing the amount of current required to activate the dermatome and produce a clearly recordable SEP. This can be done by adjusting the current level until it is approximately 2.5 times the sensory detection threshold. Normative data for these techniques in the L5 and S1 dermatomes have been published (33). Chiappa and Cros (34) caution that there is significant normal variability in the SEP parameters using these techniques and so they should be used with extreme care, especially in individuals who have no other defined test abnormalities. Dumitru and Dreyfuss (35) performed a prospective study of dermatomal SEPs on 20 patients with clearly demonstrated focal nerve root compression at either the L5 or S1 levels using a variety of strict criteria. Sensitivities for the correlation of the dermatomal SEP abnormalities with nerve root compromise were found to be disappointingly low and the clinical utility of these studies in patients with root compression was questioned. Further studies will need to be done to more clearly demonstrate the value of dermatomal SEPs in this situation before they can be recommended as a justifiable clinical investigation of isolated nerve root damage. There remains the possibility that dermatomal SEP studies may be of value in investigating patients with lumbar spinal stenosis in which sensory involvement of multiple roots may be expected (36).

Paraspinal

A technique has been described whereby an electrical stimulus is applied bilaterally to the paraspinal muscles at different levels along the vertebral column in order to isolate input to the spinal cord through a relatively short pathway at a specific spinal level (37). Input occurs through activation of cutaneous fibers in the dorsal root rami as well as Ia afferents from the paraspinal muscles. Stimulus intensity is increased until a small visible muscle twitch is noted in the paraspinal muscles. With this technique, conduction times between different spinal cord levels can be measured and focal slowing of spinal conduction can be localized to a particular region of the spinal cord.

Pain-Related Systems

As noted, the standard techniques for performing SEP studies with electrical stimulation selectively examine the dorsal column–medial lemniscal somatosensory system. Isolated involvement of the spinothalamic system is not readily examined with these methods. Attempts have been made to perform studies that evaluate the long-latency SEP components generated in response to painful thermal stimulation generated by infrared laser pulses (38,39). The technique shows significant variability depending on attentional and arousal factors that can be difficult to control (40). For this and other reasons, this technique has not received very much in the way of general clinical acceptance and validation. At present, it remains a clinical research tool for investigating central conduction in the nociceptively driven somatosensory systems. The SEP does not yet have demonstrated clinical utility for the direct investigation of conduction in pain-related somatosensory systems.

Interpretation

Abnormalities of the SEP can be divided into changes in component or interpeak latencies, changes in component amplitude, or loss of specific components. Peripheral nerve myelinopathies would be expected to produce increases in absolute latencies due to increased peripheral delays in conduction. If such abnormalities extend into the CNS, then central interpeak latencies may also be prolonged. Central demyelinating pathology tends to produce increases in central interpeak latencies as its primary effect. The effects of axonal loss lesions, for example, due to ischemic lesions, would be expected to produce loss of component amplitude rather than latency changes, or the complete loss of an expected central component. An amplitude difference between the two sides of more than 2.5 times can be considered suggestive of a unilateral lesion, although an isolated interside amplitude comparison abnormality cannot be considered as certain an indicator of abnormality as a significant latency change or the complete absence of a component. In terms of interside latency comparisons, this can be a useful and sensitive indication of a unilateral lesion or of asymmetric pathology. For example, a significant difference in latencies between the two sides for a particular absolute or interpeak latency can be seen in the presence of a small demyelinating plaque due to multiple sclerosis that is small enough only to affect transmission in fibers from one limb while sparing those from the opposite side.

Clinical Applications

There are a large number of clinical conditions to which SEP testing has been applied. The SEP offers a view of the physiologic anatomy at multiple levels of the dorsal column/lemniscal system. The abnormalities demonstrated by the SEP are etiologically nonspecific, and the specific pathology producing the observed impairment must be approached through the full integration of the SEP findings with information from the clinical assessment and other investigations. The pathway traversed by the SEPs covers the peripheral nervous system, the spinal roots, the spinal cord, and the central neuraxis. Therefore, the SEPs can be applied to evaluate conditions affecting the peripheral nervous system including the spinal roots, as well as impairment affecting the large-fiber sensory tracts of the CNS. A detailed understanding of the relevant neuroanatomy and related pathophysiologic principles is critical for an effective interpretation of the findings.

Diagnostic

The SEP study has been applied to the diagnosis of a large variety of clinical conditions. Some of these are listed in Table 10-8 and are considered in the following sections.

Peripheral Nervous System

The primary methods of neurophysiologic investigation of the peripheral nervous system include nerve conduction studies and EMG, the studies examined in Chapter 9. However, detection of peripheral nerve conditions can be facilitated by the application of the SEP under certain conditions. The application of SEP methods to conditions involving the peripheral nervous system was recently reviewed (41). When peripheral nerve conduction is so severely affected that conduction parameters cannot be reliably recorded with standard methods, the SEP can help to assess peripheral conduction. Focal nerve entrapments or entrapments at a proximal level or proximal nerve injuries affecting sensory fiber conduction can be investigated with SEPs. In suspected acute inflammatory demyelinating polyradiculoneuritis (i.e., Guillain-Barré syndrome), when the peripheral nerve conductions and F-waves are normal, the SEP can demonstrate significant proximal showing of conduction.

Table 10-8: Clinical Applications of the Somatosensory Evoked Potential
Diagnosis in adults
Peripheral nervous system
Peripheral neuropathy
Acute inflammatory polyradiculoneuritis (Guillain-Barré syndrome)
Plexopathy
Thoracic outlet syndrome
Radiculopathy
Spinal stenosis
Central nervous system
Multiple sclerosis
Myelopathy
Spinocerebellar degenerations / ataxias
Hereditary spastic paraparesis
Tumors
Hemorrhagic / ischemic lesions
Anoxic encephalopathy
Traumatic encephalopathy
Spinal cord trauma
Coma assessment
Brain death evaluation
Conversion disorder with anesthesia or weakness
Myoclonic epilepsy
HIV-related CNS pathology
Radiotherapy-related CNS effects
Motor neuron disease
Vitamin deficiencies
Impotence and neurourologic dysfunction (using pudendal nerve stimulation)
Special applications in pediatrics
Neurodegenerative disorders (e.g., leukodystrophies, adrenomyeloneuropathy, etc)
Coma assessment
HIV-related encephalopathy
Perinatal asphyxia
Other applications
Intraoperative monitoring (e.g., spinal scoliosis surgery)

HIV = human immunodeficiency virus.

The SEP, together with sensory nerve conduction studies, can be used to investigate plexus injuries where it is important to differentiate a partial root injury from a complete root avulsion in terms of planning management as well as assessing prognosis for recovery (42). This approach is also helpful in defining to what extent the injury is localizable to a postganglionic versus a preganglionic site and whether or not there remains any evidence of axonal continuity through to the CNS from the periphery.

The ulnar SEP has been shown by some investigators to have some value in the assessment of neurogenic thoracic outlet syndrome (TOS) in patients with positive neurologic signs. In nonneurogenic TOS, the value of the SEP is more controversial, with some investigators claiming that the ulnar SEP is more sensitive than conventional EMG and nerve conduction studies in the detection of significant abnormalities, even in patients who do not have clinical neurologic findings (41).

The mixed-nerve SEP is generally not very sensitive in the detection of radiculopathy. The application of the dermatomal and segmental SEP to the detection of radiculopathy has been noted already. The application of SEP methods to the diagnosis of radiculopathy remains somewhat controversial. To date, there have been no clear demonstrations of impressive utility of SEP methods in the diagnosis of radiculopathy. However, there may be a role for the evaluation of spinal root function in the presence of cervical or lumbar spinal stenosis in which multiple roots may be affected and in which there may be a concomitant myelopathy.

Central Nervous System

SEPs can be used to evaluate patients suspected to have multiple sclerosis, although the application of MRI to this situation has changed the relative utility of these studies for the diagnosis of multiple sclerosis. The SEP can help to establish the diagnosis by demonstrating the presence of multiple lesions when these may not be clinically evident. For example, in a patient with acute visual complaints but minimal limb complaints, a significant SEP abnormality in the median or tibial nerve study can help to document the presence of multiple lesions in the CNS at spatially distinct sites. This would make the diagnosis of multiple sclerosis more likely than with an isolated involvement of the optic nerve. SEPs can be used to assess conduction in the spinal cord at different levels in the process of evaluating for the presence of a myelopathy. Several other conditions of the CNS to which SEP testing has been applied are listed in Table 10-7.

Prognostic

SEPs have an important role in the evaluation of prognosis in patients who present with coma due to brain trauma or anoxic-ischemic encephalopathy. The bilateral absence of the cortical responses remains an important predictor of a poor or limited outcome. The preservation of bilaterally normal SEP cortical responses suggests a much better prognosis for functional improvement, though the degree of residual disability cannot be precisely predicted. Overall, the median nerve SEP appears to be a better predictor of outcome in the minimally conscious patient than the BAEP (25). The application of SEPs in coma assessment in adults should be differentiated from the application of these methods for similar purposes in children, although in children, as in adults, the bilateral absence of the primary cortical SEP components is highly predictive of a poor outcome in both traumatic and atraumatic coma (43). The SEP can also be used to assist with the confirmation of a diagnosis of brain death (44,45).

Intraoperative Monitoring

The SEP technique has been applied effectively to the problem of monitoring spinal cord function during spinal surgery. The most common application is to monitor spinal cord function while the spine is being distracted and instrumented for the treatment of scoliosis. This is especially important when an aggressive approach to correcting a large curvature is being planned. The use of SEP monitoring has made the more difficult "wake-up test," where the anesthesia is lightened and the patient is asked to move the legs, less necessary. The major problem with the wake-up test is that it can only be done once or twice during a procedure and is effectively a brief snapshot of spinal function during the procedure. The advantage of SEP monitoring is that it provides continuous information about the status of the spinal cord throughout the procedure. When an abnormality is noted to develop, the monitoring neurophysiologist informs the surgeon, who can then take evasive action to preserve spinal cord function (46). The preservation of normal SEPs throughout the procedure does not guarantee, however, that there may not be a significant postoperative neurologic deficit that presumably spares the dorsal columns (47).

The use of SEP monitoring of spinal cord function has also been applied to other procedures in which a significant risk to the spinal cord may occur. These include other forms of spine surgery as well as surgery requiring aortic cross-clamping, such as aortic aneurysm repair, that can result in spinal cord ischemia. SEPs can also be applied to monitor cortical function and proximal peripheral nerve conduction. Intraoperative SEPs have also been used to identify the position of the central sulcus since there is a polarity reversal that can be identified in the cortical SEP as one moves the recording electrode from posterior to the central sulcus to a position anterior to it. Monitoring with SEPs has been applied during thalamotomy, cerebrovascular surgery (e.g., carotid endarterectomy), brachial plexus repairs, pelvic surgery, and hip replacement surgery.

Further Information on Clinical Applications of Somatosensory Evoked Potentials

The application of SEP techniques to clinical evaluation continues to evolve and there is an active research literature dealing with this issue. For a recent review of the current situation with regard to the clinical application of SEPs, the reader is referred to the article by Aminoff and Eisen (48). An examination of current controversies and a view of what the future may hold for SEP application has been published by Mauguiere (49).

OTHER CLINICAL NEUROPHYSIOLOGY PARADIGMS

A number of additional recording and testing paradigms for investigating function in the CNS under a variety of different conditions are briefly discussed in the next sections.

Motor Evoked Potentials

The technique and application of motor evoked potentials have been examined in some detail in previous sections of the chapter. In this section, we look specifically at clinical applications of the motor evoked potential. Motor evoked potential abnormality types include the following:

1. Prolonged onset latency
2. Reduction in amplitude or absence of the motor response to brain stimulation
3. Abnormal waveform of the muscle response
4. Abnormal trial-to-trial variability in the amplitude and shape of the muscle response

Prolongation of latency is most often due to a central demyelinating lesion. The amplitude of the response may be reduced as the result of degeneration or blockade of corticospinal fibers. Some of the clinical conditions and situations in which the motor evoked potential has been applied are listed in Table 10-9. The basic setup for stimulating the motor cortex and the cervical spine region using the magnetic coil is shown in Figure 10-12. The evoked compound muscle action potential is recorded from a peripheral muscle such as the abductor digiti minimi. Normal motor evoked potential recordings obtained after multiple magnetic stimulation of the hand region of the primary motor cortex and the cervical spine region are shown in Figure 10-13. The interval required for the efferent volley to travel in the corticospinal tract from the cortex to the cervical spinal segment level, the central motor conduction time, can be estimated using this approach. For further information on motor evoked potentials and their clinical application, the interested reader is referred to the book chapters by Murray (50) and Cros and Chiappa (51).

Cognitive Event-Related Potentials

The evoked potential components of long latency that reflect cognitive functions are called the *cognitive* or *endogenous event-related potentials* (ERPs). A variety of these responses correspond to different paradigms. The common factor is that these components are more responsive to internal state issues such as attention, and active cognitive processing of external stimuli, than they are to the physical properties of the stimuli. This is therefore quite the opposite of what has been described above for the short-latency sensory evoked potentials, which have also been referred to as the exogenous ERPs since they are more dependent on exogenous stimulus-related factors than on internal processing. Some examples of the endogenous ERPs are the so-called P3 or P300 component, the movement-related cortical potential (MRCP), and the contingent negative variation (CNV).

Table 10-9: Clinical Applications of the Motor Evoked Potential

Diagnosis
Multiple sclerosis
Motor neuron disease
Cervical spondylosis
Hereditary spastic paraparesis
Myelopathy / spinal cord injury
Spinocerebellar degenerations / ataxias
Movement disorders (e.g., parkinsonism)
Cerebrovascular disease
Hereditary motor and sensory neuropathy
Conversion disorder with weakness
Functional weakness
Other applications
Intraoperative monitoring of the corticospinal pathway
Evaluation of prognosis for motor recovery in stroke

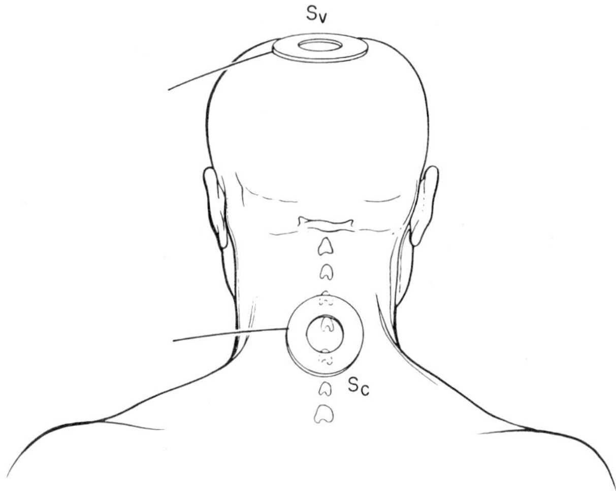

Figure 10-12. Basic setup for measuring the central motor conduction time (CMCT) by stimulating the motor cortex with placement of the stimulator coil at the vertex (Sv) and the cervical spinal cord (Sc). The activation of the motor fibers results from direct electrical current stimulation induced by a brief but very strong magnetic field produced by passing a very high current for a short period of time through a circular coil embedded in the stimulator. For more localized cortical activation, a double-circle figure-of-eight coil can be used. The recordings are obtained from surface electrodes placed over a peripheral limb muscle such as the abductor digiti minimi. (Reproduced by permission from Liveson JA, Ma DM. *Laboratory reference for clinical neurophysiology.* Philadelphia: FA Davis, 1992: 358.)

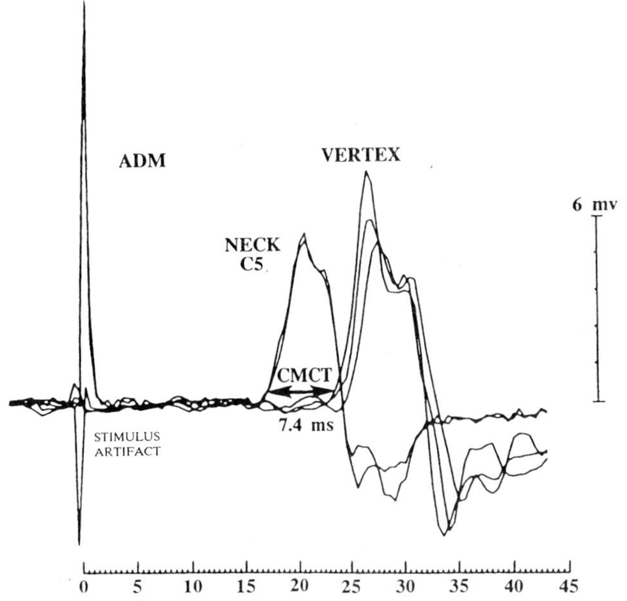

Figure 10-13. Normal motor evoked potential studies recording compound muscle action potentials from the abductor digiti minimi (ADM) following magnetic stimulation of the motor cortex and cervical spine/nerve roots. The central motor conduction time (CMCT) is the difference in onset latencies between these two compound muscle action potentials. The stimulus that occurred at the point of the artifact was delivered during a low-level voluntary contraction of the target muscle. Calibrations are noted in milliseconds on the horizontal scale and millivolts on the vertical scale. The 6-mV mark is for the response from cortical stimulation. The calibration bar is 3.1 mV for the neck stimulation. (Reproduced by permission from Cros D, Chiappa KH. Motor evoked potentials. In: Chiappa KH, ed. *Evoked potentials in clinical medicine.* 3rd ed. Philadelphia: Lippincott–Raven, 1997: 488.)

The P3 component is elicited by a rare target stimulus that is buried randomly in a train of common nontarget stimuli. Usually a sequence of auditory tone pips is used, with the target and nontarget tone pips having different frequencies. The target stimuli are embedded randomly in the train of stimuli with a sequential probability of 10% to 20%. The sweeps that follow the target stimuli are averaged separately from those that follow the nontarget stimuli. The P3 component is a large positive wave with a median peak latency of about 300 msec that is seen only in the averaged signals generated in response to the target stimuli. It reflects the activation of an orienting, attentionally modulated system that responds selectively to the presentation of the target stimuli but not the nontarget "distracters."

The MRCP is a series of slowly varying components that develop over an interval of many hundreds of milliseconds that precedes the overt appearance of a self-initiated voluntary movement. The initial component is a slowly developing negative ramp centered on the vertex that begins rising away from the baseline over 1200 msec before the appearance of the movement. Within a few hundred milliseconds of the onset of a finger or thumb movement, the negative potential begins to accelerate in amplitude and reaches a peak over the vertex and contralateral central scalp region overlying the primary motor cortex, just prior to the appearance of EMG signal in the activated forearm and hand muscles.

The CNV is a slow negative potential shift that is seen in the period between a warning stimulus (e.g., "get set!") and the subsequent imperative stimulus (e.g., "go!") to which a response must occur. The CNV is a brain response that reflects the learning of a temporal contingency rule between the warning and the imperative stimulus that allows the arrival of the imperative stimulus to be anticipated. All of these ERPs require special setups, amplification parameters, and recording programs to permit their performance. They have primarily been used for research studies and have as yet had limited clinical utility. However, the fact that they can be used to investigate the active cognitive processing capacity of the brain suggests that they may be of some value in assessing patients with memory impairment, attentional problems, and a variety of other information-processing difficulties that can significantly limit their ability to perform in functional contexts. For further information and detail regarding the endogenous ERPs and their clinical applications, the interested reader is referred to the book chapters by Oken (52) and Goodin (53).

Electronystagmography and Posturography

Investigation of patients with problems with balance and dysequilibrium can include an investigation of vestibular function as well as the capacity of the brain to integrate visual, kinesthetic, and vestibular information in the process of maintaining stable upright posture. Vestibular function, as reflected in the relationships between dynamic head position and eye movements, can be investigated using standardized protocols for electronystagmography, to document eye movement behaviors during different provocative procedures.

The general purpose of these tests of integrative function related to the vestibular system, kinesthesis, and vision is to evaluate the functional impact of CNS damage on the capacity to maintain quiet standing balance. The outcome of this testing is a picture of which sensory and motor systems have been impaired to produce the balance problem and what type of difficulty the patient is having with integrating relevant information for the support of quiet standing. This information can then be applied to the problem of developing a specific rehabilitation program that emerges from this detailed understanding of the basis of the dysequilibrium. For further details regarding electronystagmography and posturography, the interested reader is referred to the book chapter by Cyr (54).

Polysomnography

One of the most important functions of the CNS is the regulation of the sleep-wake cycle. Disturbances affecting sleep can also significantly exacerbate concomitant conditions and sleep disorders can be associated with a variety of conditions affecting the CNS. Many of the problems that are encountered in physical medicine and rehabilitation have an associated sleep disturbance. Sleep disorders can occur in patients with traumatic brain injury or cerebrovascular disorders as well as in the presence of various forms of neuropathic and myofascial pain, such as fibromyalgia. In many cases, recognizing and addressing the sleep disorders with which patients present can be beneficial to their overall situation. Polysomnography is the application of multichannel neurophysiologic and cardiorespiratory physiologic recording to the study of sleep disturbance. It includes assessment of the EEG signal during sleep, and evaluation of various indicators of autonomic function and breathing during sleep. A polysomnographic investigation can provide more detailed information regarding the specific nature of the sleep disturbance that is affecting patient function and can direct the physician to better treatment for the identified problems with sleep hygiene. For further details regarding polysomnography, the interested reader is referred to the recent article by Chesson et al (55) and the book chapter by Guilleminault (56).

CONCLUSIONS

In many ways, physiology is the basic science of rehabilitation, with its concern for examining and understanding the dynamic biologic underpinnings of the function and performance of the whole organism. Clinical neurophysiology can provide valuable and unique insights into the pathophysiology underlying clinical disorders affecting the CNS. These studies may also be applied to assess the pathophysiologic correlates of impaired function in patients with CNS lesions. The methods must be thoughtfully selected as well as performed, and the results interpreted with great care. The studies are generally not pathognomonic. In most instances, direct indication of the nature of the underlying pathology is not provided but its pathophysiologic manifestation is, thus the need to carefully integrate the results with the complete clinical picture. Their greatest utility and future promise for physical medicine and rehabilitation may be in the area of assessing prognosis for functional recovery in conditions that produce impairment of the CNS, and gaining a better understanding of the physiologic underpinnings of the recovery process. Thus, these methods may serve not only the purposes of clinical investigation, but also the needs of research inquiry into questions of concern to clinical rehabilitation neuroscience.

REFERENCES

1. Amino MJ, ed. *Electrodiagnosis in clinical neurology.* 3rd ed. New York: Churchill Livingstone, 1992.
2. Binnie CD, Cooper R, Fowler CJ, et al, eds. *Clinical neurophysiology. EMG, nerve conduction and evoked potentials.* Oxford: Butterworth-Heinemann, 1995.
3. Chiappa KH, ed. *Evoked potentials in clinical medicine.* 3rd ed. Philadelphia: Lippincott–Raven, 1997.
4. Misulis KE. *Spehlmann's evoked potential primer. Visual, auditory and somatosensory evoked potentials in clinical diagnosis.* 2nd ed. Boston: Butterworth-Heinemann, 1994.
5. Delisa JA, Mackenzie K, Baren EM. *Manual of nerve conduction velocity and somatosensory evoked potentials.* 2nd ed. New York: Raven, 1987.
6. Dumitru D. *Electrodiagnostic medicine.* Philadelphia: Hanley & Belfus, 1995.
7. Jasper HH. The ten-twenty electrode system of the International Federation. *Electroencephalogr Clin Neurophysiol* 1958;10:371–375.
8. Merton PA, Morton HB. Stimulation of the cerebral cortex in the intact human subject. *Nature* 1980;285:227.
9. Barker AT, Freeston IL, Jalinous R. Noninvasive magnetic stimulation of the human motor cortex. *Lancet* 1985;2:1106–1107.
10. Wasserman EM, Cohen LG, Flitman S, et al. Seizures in healthy people with repeated "safe" trains of transcranial magnetic stimuli. *Lancet* 1996;347:825–826.
11. Stockard JJ, Hughes JF, Sharbrough FW. Visually evoked potentials to electronic pattern reversal. Latency variations with gender, age and technical factors. *Am J EEG Technol* 1979;19:171–204.
12. Allison T, Hume AL, Wood CC, Goff WR. Developmental and aging changes in somatosensory, auditory and visual evoked potentials. *Electroencephalogr Clin Neurophysiol* 1984;58:14–24.
13. Sokol S, Moskowitz A, Towle VL. Age-related changes in the latency of the visual evoked potential. Influence of check size. *Electroencephalogr Clin Neurophysiol* 1981;51:559–562.
14. Allison T, Wood CC, Goff WR. Brain stem auditory, pattern-reversal visual, and short-latency somatosensory evoked potentials. Latencies in relation to age, sex, brain and body size. *Electroencephalogr Clin Neurophysiol* 1983;55:619–636.
15. Guthkelch AN, Bursick D, Sclabassi RJ. The relationship of the latency of the P100 to gender and head size. *Electroencephalogr Clin Neurophysiol* 1987;68:219–222.
16. Tan CT, King PJL, Chiappa KH. Pattern ERG. Effects of reference electrode site, stimulus mode and check size. *Electroencephalogr Clin Neurophysiol* 1989;74:11–18.
17. Brooks EB, Chiappa KH. A comparison of clinical neuro-ophthalmological findings and pattern shift visual evoked potentials in multiple sclerosis. In: Courjon J, Mauguiere F, Revol M, eds. *Clinical applications of evoked potentials in neurology.* New York: Raven, 1982;453–457.
18. Celesia GC, Kaufman D, Cone S. Simultaneous recording of pattern electroretinography and visual evoked potentials in multiple sclerosis. *Arch Neurol* 1986;43:1247–1252.
19. Farlow MR, Markland ON, Edwards MK, et al. Multiple sclerosis. Magnetic resonance imaging, evoked responses, and spinal fluid electrophoresis. *Neurology* 1986;36:828–831.
20. Stockard JJ, Pope-Stockard JE, Sharbrough FW. Brainstem auditory evoked potentials in neurology. Methodology, interpretation, and clinical application. In: Aminoff MJ, ed. *Electrodiagnosis in clinical neurology.* 3rd ed. New York: Churchill Livingstone, 1992:503–536.
21. Starr A, Amlie RN, Martin WH, Sanders S. Development of auditory function in newborn infants revealed by auditory brainstem potentials. *Pediatrics* 1977;60:831–839.
22. Rowe MJ III. Normal variability of the brain-stem auditory evoked response in young and old adult subjects. *Electroencephalogr Clin Neurophysiol* 1978;44:459–470.
23. Rowe MJ III, Carlson C. Brainstem auditory evoked potentials in post-concussion dizziness. *Arch Neurol* 1980;37:679–683.
24. Benna P, Bergamasco B, Bianco C, et al. Brainstem auditory evoked potentials in postconcussion syndrome. *Ital J Neurol Sci* 1982;4:281–287.
25. Goldberg G, Karazim E. Application of evoked potentials to the prediction of discharge status in minimally responsive patients. A pilot study. *J Head Trauma Rehabil* 1998;13:51–68.
26. Picton TW, Taylor MJ, Durieux-Smith A. Brainstem auditory evoked potentials in pediatrics. In: Aminoff MJ, ed. *Electrodiagnosis in clinical neurology.* 3rd ed. New York: Churchill Livingstone, 1992:537–569.
27. Thornton AR. Auditory evoked potentials. Clinical applications and future trends. *Electroencephalogr Clin Neurophysiol Suppl* 1996;46:15–46.
28. Hume AL, Cant BR, Shaw NA, et al. Central somatosensory conduction time from 10 to 79 years. *Electroencephalogr Clin Neurophysiol* 1982;54:49–54.
29. Mauguiere F, Restuccia D. Inadequacy of the forehead reference montage for detecting abnormalities of the spinal N13 SEP in cervical cord lesions. *Electroencephalogr Clin Neurophysiol* 1991;79:448–456.
30. Cant BR, Shaw NA. Central somatosensory conduction time. Method and clinical applications. In: Cracco RQ, Bodis-Wollner I, eds. *Frontiers of clinical neuroscience. Evoked potentials.* New York: Alan R. Liss, 1986:58–67.

31. Eisen A. SEP in the evaluation of disorders of the peripheral nervous system. In: Cracco RQ, Bodis-Wollner I, eds. *Frontiers of clinical neuroscience. Evoked potentials.* New York: Alan R. Liss, 1986: 409–417.

32. Pelosi L, Cracco JB, Cracco RQ. Conduction characteristics of somatosensory evoked potentials to peroneal, tibial and sural nerve stimulation in man. *Electroencephalogr Clin Neurophysiol* 1987;68:287–294.

33. Slimp JC, Rubner DE, Snowden ML, et al. Dermatomal somatosensory evoked potentials. Cervical, thoracic and lumbosacral levels. *Electroencephalogr Clin Neurophysiol* 1992;84:55–70.

34. Chiappa KH, Cros D. Dermatomal somatosensory evoked potentials. In: Chiappa KH, ed. *Evoked potentials in clinical medicine.* 3rd ed. Philadelphia: Lippincott–Raven, 1997:471–475.

35. Dumitru D, Dreyfuss P. Dermatomal/segmental somatosensory evoked potential evaluation of L5/S1 unilateral/unilevel radiculopathies. *Muscle Nerve* 1996;19:442–449.

36. Snowden ML, Haselkorn JK, Kraft GH, et al. Dermatomal somatosensory evoked potentials in the diagnosis of lumbosacral spinal stenosis. Comparison with imaging studies. *Muscle Nerve* 1992;15:1036–1044.

37. Goodridge A, Eisen A, Hoirch M. Paraspinal stimulation to elicit somatosensory evoked potentials. An approach to physiological localization of spinal lesions. *Electroencephalogr Clin Neurophysiol* 1987;68:268–276.

38. Carmon A, Mor J, Goldberg J. Evoked cerebral responses to noxious thermal stimuli in humans. *Exp Brain Res* 1976;25:103–107.

39. Kakigi R, Shibasaki H, Ikeda A. Pain-related somatosensory evoked potentials following CO_2 laser stimulation in man. *Electroencephalogr Clin Neurophysiol* 1989;74:139–146.

40. Beydoun A, Morrow TJ, Shen JF, et al. Variability of laser-evoked potentials. Attention, arousal and lateralized differences. *Electroencephalogr Clin Neurophysiol* 1993;88:173–181.

41. Yiannikas C. Short-latency somatosensory evoked potentials in peripheral nerve lesions, plexopathies and radiculopathies. In: Chiappa KH, ed. *Evoked potentials in clinical medicine.* 3rd ed. Philadelphia: Lippincott–Raven, 1997:425–451.

42. Jones SJ, Wynn Parry CB, Landi A. Diagnosis of brachial plexus traction lesions by sensory nerve action potentials and somatosensory evoked potentials. *Injury* 1981;12:376–382.

43. Levy SB. Somatosensory evoked potentials in pediatrics. In: Chiappa KH, ed. *Evoked potentials in clinical medicine.* 3rd ed. Philadelphia: Lippincott–Raven, 1997:453–469.

44. Belsh JM, Chokroverty S. Short-latency somatosensory evoked potentials in brain-dead patients. *Electroencephalogr Clin Neurophysiol* 1987;68:75–78.

45. Chatrian G-E. Electrophysiologic evaluation of brain death. A critical appraisal. In: Aminoff MJ, ed. *Electrodiagnosis in clinical neurology.* 3rd ed. New York: Churchill Livingstone, 1992:737–793.

46. Daube J. Intraoperative monitoring by evoked potentials for spinal cord surgery: the pros. *Electroencephalogr Clin Neurophysiol* 1989;73:374–377.

47. Lesser RP, Baudzens P, Luders H, et al. Postoperative neurologic deficits may occur despite unchanged intraoperative somatosensory evoked potentials. *Ann Neurol* 1986;19:22–25.

48. Aminoff MJ, Eisen AA. AAEM minimonograph #19. Somatosensory evoked potentials. *Muscle Nerve* 1998;21:277–290.

49. Mauguiere F. Clinical utility of somatosensory evoked potentials (SEPs): present debates and future trends. *Electroencephalogr Clin Neurophysiol Suppl* 1996;46:27–33.

50. Murray NMF. Motor evoked potentials. In: Aminoff MJ, ed. *Electrodiagnosis in clinical neurology.* 3rd ed. New York: Churchill Livingstone, 1992:605–626.

51. Cros D, Chiappa KH. Motor evoked potentials. In: Chiappa KH, ed. *Evoked potentials in clinical medicine.* 3rd ed. Philadelphia: Lippincott–Raven, 1997:477–507.

52. Oken BS. Endogenous event-related potentials. In: Chiappa KH, ed. *Evoked potentials in clinical medicine.* 3rd ed. Philadelphia: Lippincott–Raven, 1997:529–563.

53. Goodin DS. Event-related (endogenous) potentials. In: Aminoff MJ, ed. *Electrodiagnosis in clinical neurology.* 3rd ed. New York: Churchill Livingstone, 1992:627–648.

54. Cyr DG. Electronystagmography and posturography. In: Aminoff MJ, ed. *Electrodiagnosis in clinical neurology.* 3rd ed. New York: Churchill Livingstone, 1992:683–709.

55. Chesson AL Jr, Ferber RA, Fry JM, et al. The indications for polysomnography and related procedures. *Sleep* 1997;20:423–487.

56. Guilleminault C. The polysomnographic evaluation of sleep disorders. In: Aminoff MJ, ed. *Electrodiagnosis in clinical neurology.* 3rd ed. New York: Churchill Livingstone, 1992:711–736.

Chapter 11

Functional Evaluation and Outcome Measurement

Gary S. Clark
Carl V. Granger

With the evolution of the U.S. health care system toward managed care and the increasing focus on cost containment and the cost-effectiveness of health care interventions, there is a corresponding need to accurately and objectively document the benefit and value of rehabilitation efforts. The primary mission of rehabilitation medicine is to restore and improve function. While improvements in an individual's level of function can be described in a narrative fashion, this does not provide the objectivity or consistency needed to track serial changes over time, or to compare results among groups of individuals. This has led to the development of the discipline and science of functional assessment, to provide a means of objectively documenting and quantitatively measuring the level of function of persons with disability. Use of functional rating scales has also facilitated comparisons between individuals and groups of individuals to better analyze functional outcomes with various forms of rehabilitation, with determination of cost-effectiveness and efficiency.

DEFINITIONS

Functional assessment is a method for describing a person's abilities and limitations, in order to measure performance of activities necessary for daily living (1). These daily living activities can include personal care skills (e.g., grooming, bathing, dressing, toileting, mobility), maintaining one's personal environment (e.g., homemaking, shopping), and engaging in leisure activities, vocational pursuits, social interactions, and other desired behaviors. According to Lawton (2), functional assessment includes "any systematic attempt to measure objectively the level at which a person is functioning in any of a variety of areas such as physical health, quality of self-maintenance, quality of role activity, intellectual status, social activity, attitude toward the world and self, and emotional status."

The traditional medical model combines an accurate diagnosis with an understanding of the underlying pathophysiologic processes of organ dysfunction to determine the need for and the type of treatment. In rehabilitation, the focus is expanded to consider the impact on the person as a whole, including impairments resulting from the underlying illness or injury, and consequent disability and handicap. Functional assessment enables accurate "diagnosis" of the functional loss, thereby facilitating the development of appropriate and effective rehabilitation. Serial assessment of function at various intervals over time makes it possible to identify and measure changes in functional status in an individual, or groups of individuals, and provides a basis for describing the functional outcomes resulting from rehabilitation. Analysis of functional outcomes provides an indicator of a rehabilitation program's effectiveness in reversing functional loss, which is the cornerstone of program evaluation (3). Program evaluation is defined by the Commission on Accreditation of Rehabilitation Facilities (CARF) as a systematic procedure for measuring the outcomes of care, and represents a method of measuring the effectiveness and efficiency of rehabilitation services (4). The standard for evaluating rehabilitation outcomes is the degree to which the program results in practical improvement in an individual's function (i.e., relevant to his or her needs, enabling independence in desired activities), which is sustained after completion of treatment and return to the community (5). Program evaluation is considered a component of quality assessment and improvement, with other components including utilization review, risk management, infection control, and documentation (6). The Joint Commission on Accreditation of Healthcare Organizations (JCAHO) characterizes quality assessment and quality improvement as "ongoing activities designed to objectively and systematically evaluate the quality of patient care and services, pursue opportunities to improve patient care and services, and resolve identified problems."(7)

PURPOSES AND BENEFITS OF FUNCTIONAL EVALUATION

Interest in evaluating function in American medical rehabilitation settings has evolved over the past 30 years, since the first major structured functional assessment instrument (PULSES Profile) was published by Moskowitz and McCann in 1957 (8). Benefits of functional assessment have been described as including consideration of all areas of function to obtain a more complete picture, documentation of evidence to support the clinical impression, facilitation of communication, ability to evaluate results of treatment, and provision of a tool to monitor results of treatment (2). Donaldson et al (9) summarized the objectives of a functional assessment instrument as follows:

1. Objective description of functional status at a given point in time
2. Serial repetition allowing detection of changed functional status
3. Data collected through observation relevant to and useful in monitoring the treatment program
4. Enhancement of communication among treatment team members and between referral agencies and
5. Comparable clinical observations compatible with research questions

Functional assessment is useful for the management of individual patients, and is necessary for program evaluation. The clinician who is knowledgeable in the diagnosis of pathologic conditions and impairment states and also proficient in using functional assessment is able to integrate a patient's medical status with his or her ability to perform functional tasks and fulfill social roles. This composite profile of the whole person allows more accurate, orderly, and complete identification of the person's problems and areas of need. From this, interventions and long-range coordination strategies (e.g., case management and critical pathways) can be developed to maximize personal independence and subjective well-being (3).

It is possible to compare changes in status over periods of time for an individual or a group of individuals by assessing function at appropriate intervals. In this manner, outcomes of professional interventions of health care, rehabilitation, education, or psychological and social counseling may be described and monitored. Once outcomes become measurable, then, presumably, they become manageable.

Granger (10) noted multiple uses and applications for functional assessment:

1. Planning treatment
   a. Systematically developing a patient problem list that includes limitations in functioning
2. Determining the effectiveness and efficiency of treatment
   a. Determining clinical care changes in patients or clients by comparing measures of function before and after treatment interventions
   b. Determining the benefits of clinical care by analyzing cost benefits and cost-effectiveness
   c. Reviewing the necessity of given levels of care and alternative levels of care, to justify costs
3. Maintaining continuity of care
   a. Tracking patients through a system of care in order to determine the strengths and weaknesses of the system
   b. Facilitating case management in order to ensure that a program of care is addressing issues that are most likely to maximize the quality of life for the disabled person
4. Developing treatment resources
   a. Relating the needs of a defined population through assessment and analysis of function measured from samples of individuals representative of that population
   b. Performing manpower studies that can relate the needs for various numbers and kinds of health care personnel to levels of severity of disability in the patients being served
   c. Prioritizing the needs should it become necessary to ration scarce resources
5. Improving treatment resources
   a. Performing program evaluation, quality assurance, and medical care audit studies in order to detect deficiencies in care and then to improve care
   b. Establishing comparability of groups of patients for research studies and policy planning

Under the impetus of CARF, medical rehabilitation facilities began to use certain common data elements to implement models of program evaluation. Program evaluation was designed to present patient care outcomes in ways that would permit analysis for determining optimal as well as less than optimal practices. Based on this analysis, facilities can adjust treatment procedures to improve outcomes on a continuing basis. To measure outcomes, the functional status of patients must be assessed on admission, as well as at discharge and follow-up after completion of the rehabilitation plan. For this effort to be successful, reliable, valid, feasible, and meaningful methods of functional assessment are necessary.

CONCEPTUAL MODEL FOR FUNCTIONAL ASSESSMENT

The traditional "medical model" tends to focus on disease characteristics (etiology, pathology, manifestations) and their cure. This creates a dilemma for patients with chronic ("incurable" by definition) conditions who need "care" rather than "cure" (10,11). With improved survival rates for previously fatal diseases (e.g., myocardial infarction, stroke, cancer) and increasing longevity, the incidence and prevalence of chronic conditions (often multiple in an individual) have risen significantly. Functional limitations in an individual with an acute illness are usually transient and resolve with appropriate treatment of the underlying illness. Losses of function related to a chronic disease (and particularly multiple chronic diseases) are typically more persistent, and may even be progressive, but are also potentially reversible with appropriate timing and type of intervention (12). There is no direct relationship between a particular disease and the degree of functional limitation that may result; on the other hand, a single disease process may cause multiple disabilities (e.g., a stroke may result in impairments in language, self-care ability, mobility, and/or continence) (13). This lack of correlation between medical diagnoses and resulting functional disability was the basis for exemption of comprehensive medical rehabilitation hospitals and units from prospective payment based on diagnosis related groups (DRGs). Considerable attention has focused on the development of more appropriate models that would accurately predict costs and outcomes of rehabilitation programs focused on reversal of functional disability. Figure 11-1 illustrates the relationship between the effectiveness of rehabilitation (i.e., the amount of improvement in function) and the efficiency of the rehabilitation program, which is calculated by dividing effectiveness by the cost of care (e.g., length of stay in the rehabilitation program) (1).

Granger (10) developed a synthesized version of Nagi's (14) and Wood's (15) "disability model" which incorporates the medical model in the context of impairment, disability, and handicap, and illustrates the role of functional assessment in identifying unmet needs and related intervention strategies (Fig. 11-2). Functional assessment provides the tool by which the clinician can comprehensively view disease and its impact on function, and plan appropriate interventions and mobilization of resources to

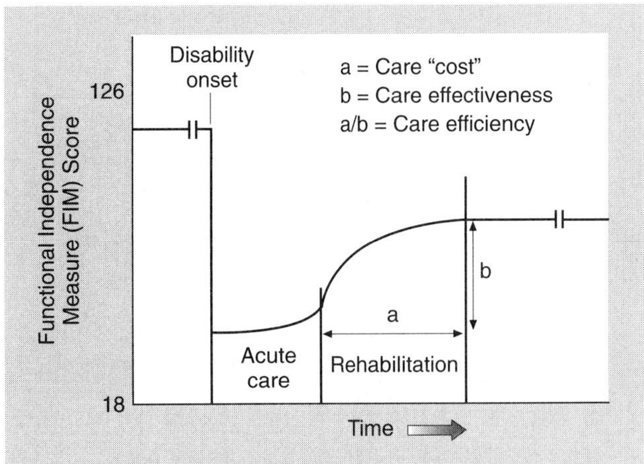

Figure 11-1. The relationship between effectiveness and efficiency in medical rehabilitation. (Redrawn with permission from Toole JF, Good DC, eds. *Imaging in neurologic rehabilitation.* New York: Demos Vermande, 1996:41–50. Copyright © 1996, Demos Vermande.)

address identified needs (medical, restorative, psychosocial, environmental, and supportive) (10).

The major goal of rehabilitation is to improve the functional skills of individuals with disability, thereby enabling them to perform desired activities (life skills) and helping to restore their quality of daily living (QODL). QODL is a concept distinct from quality of life, as it focuses on the functional nature of daily living, is more amenable to empiric investigation, and is analogous to the rehabilitation concept of activities of daily living (ADLs). Granger defined QODL as the "ever-changing balance between one's choices, options, and expectations versus the physical, cognitive, and emotional demands of daily living" (1). Figure 11-3 proposes that an individual's fulfillment and QODL are the result of balancing functional opportunities (on the left) and functional requirements or demands (on the right). Functional opportunities are expressed as the individual's choices, options, and expectations, while functional requirements are expressed in physical, cognitive, and emotional terms. To achieve fulfillment and to maximize the QODL there must be a balance between improved opportunities through individual health and functioning (on the left) and the reduction or removal of life's barriers causing constraints (on the right). While these functional opportunities and requirements (demands) are not directly quantifiable, the contributing factors (in the domains of health and functioning, and barriers) can be measured using a variety of scales, including functional assessment scales (3). This model of challenges to QODL is based on Maslow's research on human motivation (16), and incorporates his industrial psychological beliefs that health and functioning result from the individual's being presented with life's work in the form of barriers and sys-

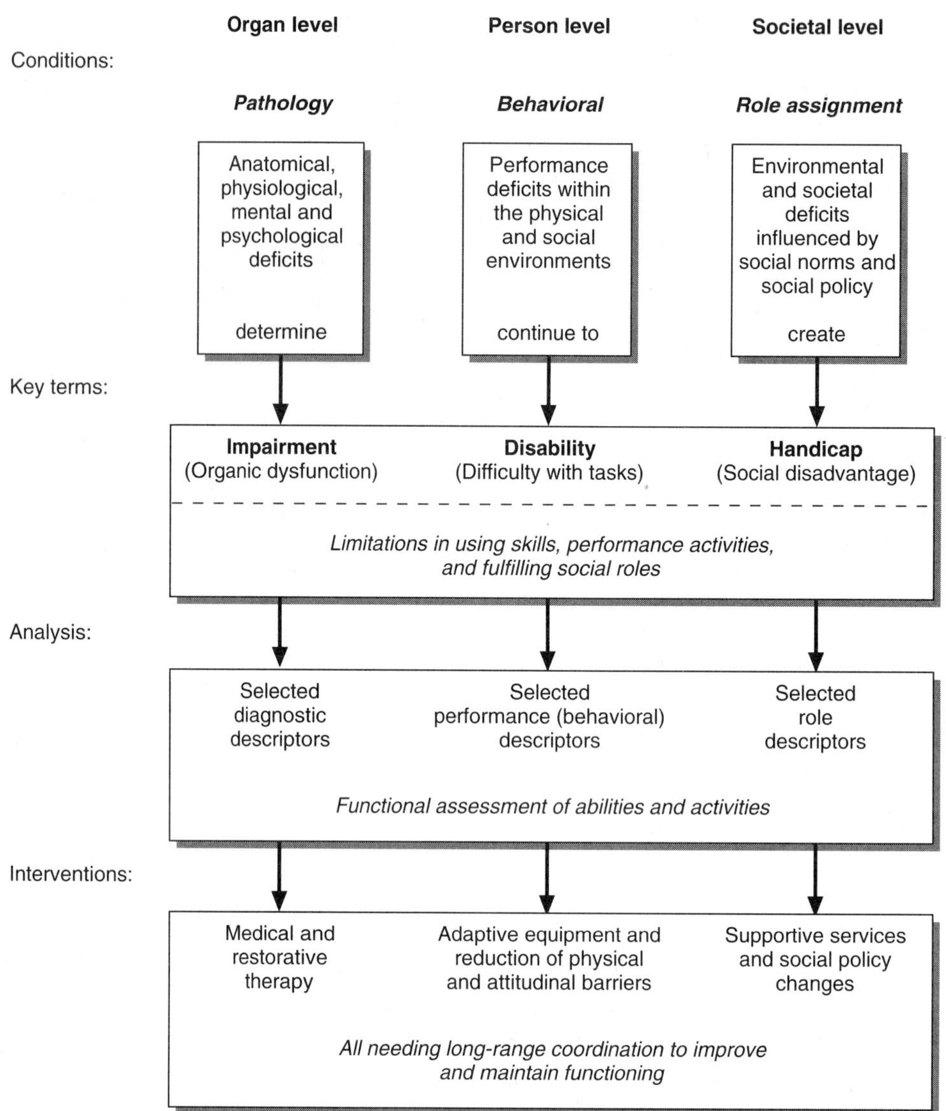

Figure 11-2. A conceptual model for functional assessment. Graphic formulation of the International Classification of Impairments, Disabilities, and Handicaps, developed by Wood (15) and the concepts of Nagi (14). (Redrawn with permission from Granger CV, Gresham GE, eds. *Functional assessment in rehabilitation medicine.* Baltimore: Williams & Wilkins, 1984:14–25. Copyright © 1984, Williams & Wilkins Co.)

tematically overcoming them (1). The model further reflects Maslow's hierarchical beliefs by viewing the individual with a disability as meeting progressively higher needs of function (from basic physical needs to issues of security, social interaction, and self-esteem) through medical rehabilitation. The goal of developing such a conceptual theoretical model is to translate the concepts into measurement systems, and to implement those systems into clinical practice through research (1).

PRINCIPLES OF MEASUREMENT

There have been numerous criticisms of the quality of measurement and evaluation procedures in rehabilitation, most commonly citing inadequate attention to the basic technical properties of developed scales (e.g., validity, reliability, scalability, standardization) (3,17,18). Other concerns relate to insufficient documentation (necessary for interrater reliability), and the frequent pattern of a measurement scale developed for a particular purpose within one facility and then exported for use in other settings or populations without adequate testing. In a collaborative effort to develop standardized guidelines for the development and application of assessment procedures, an interdisciplinary task force on measurement and evaluation was formed by the American Congress of Rehabilitation Medicine, culminating in publication of "Measurement Standards for Interdisciplinary Medical Rehabilitation" as a supplement to the *Archives of Physical Medicine and Rehabilitation* in 1992

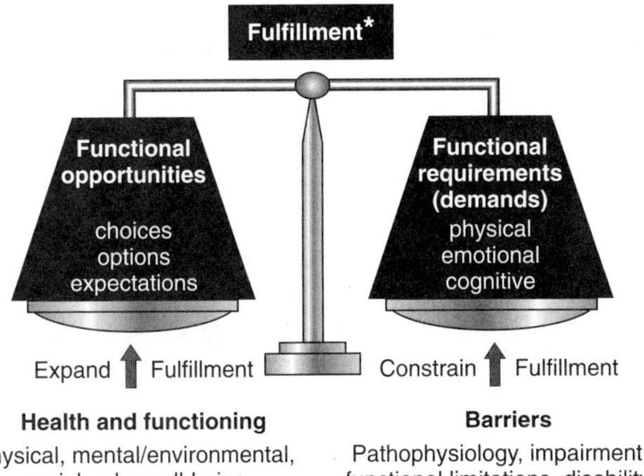

*Fulfillment = balance between Health and Functioning versus Barriers

Figure 11-3. Challenges to quality of daily living (Redrawn with permission from Toole JF, Good DC, eds. *Imaging in neurologic rehabilitation.* New York: Demos Vermande, 1996:41–50. Copyright © 1996, Demos Vermande.)

(17). These standards are intended to guide the development, choice, use, and interpretation of assessment instruments in clinical and research settings. They are applicable to the assessment of impairments (e.g., specific anatomic, physiologic, and psychological functional limitations) as well as disability, societal limitations (handicap), and QODL (3). Following is a brief summary of relevant measurement principles.

Validity

Validity is the property of measuring what one intends to measure, and includes consideration of the appropriateness, meaningfulness, and usefulness of an instrument, and inferences made from it (3). It is considered the "paramount criterion" regarding selection of an appropriate measure (17). Validation always relates to a specified application (e.g., purpose, setting, patient population), and requires linking a concept with operations involved in the assessment procedure, with subsequent collection of evidence to support logical inferences made from it (18). There are three primary and interrelated types of validity: content validity, criterion-referenced validity, and construct validity.

Content Validity

Content validity is the simplest form of validity, and refers to the degree to which a test includes a representative sample of items critical or relevant to the domain of interest (17). For a functional assessment instrument to have content validity, for example, it must include components that address various aspects of function, such as self-care and mobility. Consensus of a panel of experts, combining clinical experience and past research, is the most common basis for determining content validity. *Face validity*, or sensibility, reflects the personal opinion of the individual either taking or administering the test as to whether it measures what it is intended to, and does not significantly contribute to a determination of validity of the test (19).

Criterion-Referenced Validity

Criterion-referenced validity refers to the extent to which a scale is related to a relevant outcome or other external criterion (e.g., a "gold standard"). For an instrument to be clinically useful, it should be able to predict certain important events outside of itself (18). *Concurrent validity* involves prediction of some important event or criterion occurring at the same time, and serves as a form of proxy. An example would be use of a telephone interview in lieu of an on-site or in-person functional assessment (20). Related concepts include *sensitivity* (the ability to correctly identify the specified problem or characteristic) and *specificity* (the ability to avoid false-positive labeling). *Predictive validity* is the degree to which a test can accurately forecast a future occurrence or outcome. Ability to predict outcomes after rehabilitation is the acid test for functional assessment instruments.

Construct Validity

The most difficult, yet most valuable form of validity is construct validity, which examines the degree to which an instrument conforms to its underlying theoretical constructs. Since many clinically important constructs (concepts) are not directly measurable (e.g., memory, functional independence), attempts are made to establish construct validity by studying relationships between various relevant parameters. Attention is focused on whether the instrument consistently produces a pattern of converging or predictive relationships as expected (*convergent validity*), distinguishes from irrelevant or confounding factors (*divergent or discriminant validity*), and can be applied in differing circumstances (e.g., setting, population, etc.) to demonstrate *generalizability* beyond a narrow application (18). The interdisciplinary measurement standards specify that 1) a measure should have evidence of content, criterion, and construct validity, with all three at least addressed; 2) statements about validity should refer to the particular situations, purposes, or populations for which the measure is to be used; 3) the use of subscores or composite scores also requires evidence of their validity; and 4) measures used as criteria should be described accurately and the reasons for their selection stated (17).

Reliability

All measures are subject to error, and reliability refers to the degree to which a measure is free from random error, or provides reproducible results. Since it is not possible to render measures entirely free of error, the amount of error should be estimated and taken into account (21). Clinical applications of instruments require high, or at least specified, levels of reliability (even more so when applied to individual patients, as opposed to groups) (22). The reliability of an instrument is usually quantified in terms of the degree to which consistent results are produced when it is properly administered under similar circumstances. *Agreement*, which is related but not equivalent to reliability, is defined as the extent to which identical measurements are made, and is calculated using different statistical techniques (19). Reliability is a necessary, but not sufficient, condition for establishing validity. There are a number of methods for estimating reliability. *Interrater reliability* refers to the degree to which different trained raters achieve the same results, and is crucial for an instrument to be able to be used in multiple settings. *Test-retest reliability*, or stability over time, is the consistency of findings on serial evaluation. This characteristic is critical for analyzing changes occurring over time, to ensure that they represent true changes in a patient's condition. Another concept affecting reliability is *internal consistency*, which refers to correlations of predictive ability among similar items on a scale, and between individual items and the scale as a whole. Otherwise, adding unrelated items within a scale may produce a meaningless value that does not predict well, even though a number of the items added may individually be highly correlated with the outcome of interest. Factor analysis and Rasch analysis can be used to identify items that do fit well together in terms of predictive ability (3). The interdisciplinary measurement standards specify that 1) reports of the use of measures in rehabilitation should be accompanied by numeric estimates of reliability, the population(s) used, and the method of determining reliability of scores; 2) the developers of measures have the primary responsibility for establishing initial reliability estimates for the populations to which the measure is to be applied; and 3) if scores are separated into subscores or aggregated into summative or other combinations of scores, estimates of reliability and errors of measurement should be reported for these subscores and combinations.

Norms and Scaling

The clinical use and interpretation of functional assessment measures are facilitated by a context of "normal" for comparing or contrasting results, as well as a scaling method to transform raw data into more meaningful or interpretable scores.

Norms

The application of most measures, particularly functional assessment instruments, necessitates comparison of the individual(s) being tested with a reference group. An obvious focus in rehabilitation is on the progress of a disabled person toward what is considered normal function. Norms from a general reference population are essential for this process, particularly if there are any concerns regarding degree or prevalence of age-adjusted and gender-adjusted functional limitations. Another common correlation is the progress (i.e., functional improvement) over time of a particular patient compared to that of similar patients. The issue is response to treatment (outcome) based on a "bench mark" comparison, to determine if modification of the treatment program is indicated. Utilization review, quality improvement, and program evaluation all imply comparison of patient progress with the progress of similar patients in other facilities (5). Related to these concepts is the evolving interest in establishing practice guidelines throughout health care, and the expectations of predicted outcomes on the part of third-party payers (22). Considerable normative data on progress in rehabilitation programs have been published, overall as well as for specific disability categories (23–28). There is also increasing attention to establishing normative data for rehabilitation outcomes for patients within various age groups (29) and in differing treatment settings (30), as well as identifying gender-specific characteristics (31).

Scaling

Most empirical instruments use a variety of scaling techniques to convert raw data scores into a more meaningful or easily interpretable derived score. Raw scores in and of themselves are typically either meaningless or very difficult to translate into clinically relevant information. However, both raw and derived scores are subject to being misconstrued; the scaling method used accordingly should facilitate appropriate score interpretation (17). *Unidimensionality* is a fundamental issue in scaling. A set of raw scores encompassing multiple dimensions is by definition internally heterogeneous (inconsistent) and should not be added together as if a single dimension is being measured. However, certain statistical techniques (Rasch analysis, factor analysis) can be useful in analyzing the dimensions implied by a pattern of raw rating scores (32). The four basic levels of measurement data include nominal, ordinal, interval, and ratio. Nominal and ordinal scales are used to classify discrete measures, because the scores produced fall into discrete categories or levels, while interval and ratio scales classify continuous measures, as the scores can range anywhere along a continuum (19). A *nominal scale* is used to categorize data (e.g., people, objects) lacking a rank order into different groups based on a specific variable. An example would be grouping patients with and those without diabetes. Ordinal scales have a logical hierarchy of categories that are mutually exclusive and discrete, although equality of intervals between each category cannot be assumed. Ordinal scales are the most frequently used level of measurement in the clinical setting, with examples including the manual muscle test scale (33) and the Functional Independence Measure (FIM instrument) (34). Unlike nominal and ordinal scales, *interval scales* are continuous, with sequential units numerically equidistant between points. Interval data are typically generated from quantitative processes (e.g., latent trait analysis), rather than by clinical observation. Examples include temperature (in degrees Celsius) and joint range of motion (in degrees). Finally, a *ratio scale* represents a form of interval scale where the zero point reflects a total absence of the quantity being measured. Force of muscle contraction scores obtained on a quantitative muscle strength testing device represent an example of a ratio scale. While interval and ratio scales are more sophisticated, nominal and ordinal scales are more commonly used because they are easier to create. Significant controversy has developed regarding the appropriate role and use of ordinal versus interval scaling, particularly in the field of functional assessment, with some suggesting that all ordinal or imperfectly interval scales be abandoned (35). However, well-established nonparametric statistical techniques are available to test the validity of inferences made from ordinal scales (36). The interdisciplinary measurement standards specify that 1) whenever possible, the reference group for comparing patient performance should be explicitly stated; 2) when possible, empirically derived norms should supplement clinical experience in uses of measures involving inferences relative to a comparison group; 3) when normative populations are used, their characteristics and the circumstances under which the data were collected should be clearly described in publications, including the representativeness of such populations; and 4) scales used for reporting scores should be clearly described in publications, including reasons for choosing the scaling method when new or nonstandard scaling methods are used (17).

Purpose of Testing

After determining the level of measurement, the purpose for testing must be considered. Tests are generally either screening in nature, or provide an in-depth assessment of specific variables.

Screening Tests

Applications of screening instruments include differentiating between "normal" individuals and those suspected to have the condition or characteristic of concern, identifying individuals who require further assessment, and superficially evaluating a number of broad categories (19). Screening tests are designed to be brief, with items selected to achieve the desired level of sensitivity and specificity for sampling a broad range of behaviors, traits, or characteristics. However, the limited number of specific behaviors sampled results in a higher proportion of false-positive results. Accordingly, screening instruments should be used with caution as a basis for diagnosis, placement or treatment planning decisions. An example of a screening tool for dementia is the Mini-Mental State Exam (37). Ideally, the screening tool should be refined to the point of being able to administer it by phone or by a layperson, or even by self-report (38).

Assessment Tests

Assessment tests may be used to evaluate specific behaviors in greater depth, to obtain additional information to facilitate treatment interventions, to determine placement into specialized programs, or to monitor progress or status via periodic measurements (19). Advantages of assessment tests include a lower frequency of false-positive findings, more accurate evaluation based on a representative set of behaviors, and the ability to apply results for diagnosis, placement or treatment planning. They are limited, however, by the needs for extended time for testing and for specially trained personnel to administer, score, and interpret results. Ideally, comprehensive assessment instruments should be keyed to thresholds with clinical significance, and be capable of measuring increments of function that reflect meaningful improvement or deterioration (39). An example of an in-depth assessment tool is the Sickness Impact Profile (39).

Practicality

For a functional assessment instrument to be useful clinically, it must be practical: easy and efficient to administer, inexpensive, and with clear and concise instructions and clearly defined scoring criteria. The qualifications and training needs of the tester should be clearly delineated, as well as the required time to administer the test. The test duration and level of difficulty should be appropriate to the attention span and anticipated capabilities of the population to be tested (19).

Limitations of Testing

A number of additional factors need to be considered in deciding what type of functional assessment instrument to use, in what patient population to use it, for what purpose it is to be used, and how the data collected will be analyzed and applied. A critical decision involves what source to collect data from: the patient, a family member, or a professional caregiver. The choice of informant can markedly influence testing results (40). Another caution relates to whether the functional ability to be measured reflects a patient's capacity to perform, versus that person's actual performance. Significant cognitive and social components affecting performance-based functional assessment have been documented, and can greatly influence results and interpretation (41–43). Interpretation of assessment test results must also factor in potential influences based on ethnicity or social class, and age-cohort characteristics. Built into a number of assessment instruments are underlying assumptions (value judgments) regarding inclusion or exclusion of items, and relative weighting of items for aggregation (44). Many scales are limited in the range of potential scores, with ceiling or floor effects that also may affect appropriate interpretation (45).

Not only do the goals and rationale for choosing a specific functional instrument need to be taken into account, but equally important and commonly overlooked are the training, experience, skills, and perspective of the person performing the assessment and interpreting the results. An example of a well-developed and structured support system to address these methodologic concerns is the Uniform Data System for Medical Rehabilitation (UDSMR), which provides licensed software and a system of services to subscribing facilities (training and credentialing for clinicians and administrators, data collection and analysis with validation, internal reporting capabilities, and quarterly aggregate reports of facility, regional, and national data.) (34).

CURRENT FUNCTIONAL EVALUATION SCALES

Several comprehensive reviews on the evolution of functional assessment instruments, with detailed descriptions of the various scales, are available (41–46).

Activities of Daily Living Scales

Well-known early ADL scales, used less frequently now, include the PULSES Profile (8), the Katz Index of ADL (47), and the Kenny Self-Care Evaluation (48). The PULSES Profile is a global scale that provides a measure of general functional performance, including overall mobility and self-care ability, as well as medical status and psychosocial factors. The scale rates physical condition (P), upper limbs (U), lower limbs (L), sensory status (S), excretory management (E), and psychosocial status (S), with scoring ranging from 6 (fully independent, medically stable) to 24 (dependent, requiring extensive medical/nursing care). Developed from studies of geriatric patients with various disabilities, the Katz Index of ADL rates six areas of ADL: bathing, dressing, toileting, transfers, continence, and feeding. Each area is rated as independent or not, with functional status graded from A (totally independent) to G (totally dependent). While the Katz Index has practical utility, it is mainly a descriptive, not a quantitative, instrument. The Kenny Self-Care Evaluation rates patients from 0 (dependent) to 4 (independent) in six categories of self-care: bed activities, transfers, locomotion, dressing, personal hygiene, and feeding. With scores ranging from 0 to 24, this scale has proved to be one of the most sensitive to change in functional ability (49).

One of the best known and most frequently used functional assessment instruments in the Barthel Index (50), which rates 10 aspects of function (using different relative weights for each variable based on the authors' clinical experience) with scores ranging from 0 (totally dependent) to 100 (fully independent). A number of variations of the Barthel Index have been published, including the Granger three-level modification (51), Granger four-level modification (52), zero to 20-point scoring modification (53), and Shah modification (54). The original Barthel Index, as well as various adapted versions, has been extensively studied, with documentation of high degrees of validity and reliability, sensitivity to changes in function over time, and ability to use across many types of physical disability (44–46).

More recently developed functional assessment instruments include the FIM instrument, the Patient Evaluation and Conference Systems (PECS), and the Level of Rehabilitation Scale (LORS). The FIM instrument (Fig. 11-4) was developed as a minimum uniform data set by a national task force jointly sponsored by the American Congress of Rehabilitation Medicine and the American Academy of Physical Medicine and Rehabilitation, with grant support from the National Institute on Disability and Rehabilitation Research, using a professional consensus process (34). The FIM instrument consists of 18 categories of function (subgrouped under self-care, sphincter control, mobility, locomotion, communication, and social cognition), each scored on an ordinal scale from 1 (dependent) to 7 (independent). The FIM instrument is the most commonly used functional measure in medical rehabilitation, and has undergone extensive testing of validity and reliability, as well as sensitivity to changes in function over time, across multiple disability categories (46). The PECS system (55) was also developed by a multidisciplinary team, using a scoring range of 1 (dependent) to 7 (independent) for 76 separate functional performance areas (medical, physical, psychological, social, and vocational categories), as well as rehabilitation team goals, providing feedback on frequency of goal achievement by patients. PECS has been evaluated as an outcome measure for a number of disability categories (46). The Functional Life Scale (FLS) (56) was developed to be used primarily in a community setting, as it contains 44 items in five categories (cognition, self-care, home activities, community activities and social interaction), with ratings from 0 to 4. The LORS (57) was adapted from the FLS, and has also been studied in a variety of disability populations (46). Subsequent adaptations of the instrument have been published, with development of the LORS American Data System (LADS) (58). Table 11-1 compares selected features of several ADL scales.

Instrumental Activities of Daily Living Scales

Several scales have been developed to assess function beyond personal care skills, such as various homemaking and "community survival" skills (e.g., using a telephone, preparing meals, cleaning, doing laundry, shopping, managing money) (44). Three such instruments, developed in geriatric care settings, include the Functional Health Status (59), the Older Americans Resources and Services Multidimensional Functional Assessment Questionnaire (OARS MFAQ) (60), and the Philadelphia Geriatric Center Instrumental Activities of Daily Living (61). All three have documented reliability and validity, and are most appropriate to administer in a community setting (44). These instrumental

FIM™ instrument

Functional Independence Measure

LEVELS		
	7 Complete Independence (Timely, Safely) 6 Modified Independence (Device)	**NO HELPER**
	Modified Dependence 5 Supervision (Subject = 100%+) 4 Minimal Assist (Subject = 75%+) 3 Moderate Assist (Subject = 50%+) **Complete Dependence** 2 Maximal Assist (Subject = 25%+) 1 Total Assist (Subject = less than 25%)	**HELPER**

	ADMISSION	DISCHARGE	FOLLOW-UP
Self-Care			
A. Eating			
B. Grooming			
C. Bathing			
D. Dressing - Upper Body			
E. Dressing - Lower Body			
F. Toileting			
Sphincter Control			
G. Bladder Management			
H. Bowel Management			
Transfers			
I. Bed, Chair, Wheelchair			
J. Toilet			
K. Tub, Shower			
Locomotion	W Walk C Wheelchair B Both	W Walk C Wheelchair B Both	W Walk C Wheelchair B Both
L. Walk/Wheelchair			
M. Stairs			
Motor Subtotal Score			
Communication			
N. Comprehension	A Auditory V Visual B Both	A Auditory V Visual B Both	A Auditory V Visual B Both
O. Expression	V Vocal N Nonvocal B Both	V Vocal N Nonvocal B Both	V Vocal N Nonvocal B Both
Social Cognition			
P. Social Interaction			
Q. Problem Solving			
R. Memory			
Cognitive Subtotal Score			
TOTAL FIM Score			

NOTE: Leave no blanks; enter 1 if patient not testable due to risk

Figure 11-4. Functional Independence Measure. (Reprinted with permission of Uniform Data System for Medical Rehabilitation, a Division of U B Foundation Activities, Inc. *Guide for the Uniform Data Set for Medical Rehabilitation (including the FIM™ instrument)*, Version 5.0 Buffalo, NY 14214: State University of New York at Buffalo; 1996.)

Table 11-1: Selected Measures of Activities of Daily Living (ADLs)

Scale	Description and Type of Scale	Reliability, Validity, and Sensitivity	Time and Administration	Comments
Barthel Index (BI) (50)	Ordinal scale with total scores ranging from 0 (totally dependent)–100 (independent); 10 weighted items: feeding, bathing, grooming, dressing, bladder control, bowel control, toileting, chair/bed transfer, mobility, and stair climbing	Well-documented reliability and validity; not sensitive to minor changes at higher levels of ADL functioning	Clinician observation: <40 min; appropriate for screening, formal assessment, monitoring, maintenance	Widely accepted scale for disability; strong reliability and validity
Index of Independence in ADL	Dichotomous rating in hierarchical order of dependency: bathing, dressing, toileting, transfer, continence, and feeding; cases ranked from A (independent in all 6 items) to G (dependent in all 6 items)	Documented reliability and validity; limited range of activities assessed; not as sensitive to change as BI or other instruments	Clinician observation: <20 min; appropriate for screening, formal assessment, monitoring, maintenance	Widely accepted scale, especially in geriatrics; assesses some basic skills but not walking and climbing stairs
Kenny Self-Care Evaluation (48)	Ordinal scale with 17 specific activities under 6 major categories: bed activities, transfers, locomotion, personal hygiene, dressing, and feeding; measured on 5-point scale, 0 = dependence–4 = independence; range of total scores: 0–24	Documented reliability and validity; reasonable sensitivity	Clinician observation or judgment: >30 min; appropriate for formal assessment, monitoring, maintenance	Range of inclusive categories, geared to rehabilitation assessment; ratings can be subjective
Functional Independence Measure (FIM) (34)	Ordinal scale with 18 items, 7-level scale with scores running from 18–126; areas of evaluation include self-care, sphincter control, transfers, locomotion, communication, and social cognition	Well-documented reliability and validity; able to detect minor changes with 7 levels; physical and cognitive components able to detect increments of change; can be converted into two Rasch-derived measures	Clinician observation: <20 min; appropriate for screening, formal assessment, monitoring, maintenance, and program evaluation	Widely accepted in medical rehabilitation, including international; proven measure of ADL and social cognition; standardized interobserver reliability by credentialing of clinicians; extensive training materials
Level of Rehabilitation Scale (LORS) (57) and LORS American Data	Five interval subscales assessing ADL, mobility, communications, cognitive ability	Documented reliability and validity; specific to physical and cognitive measures in	Clinical observation: 10 min per subscale, >60 min total; appropriate for screening, monitoring,	Measures broad functional outcome categories; provides separate scores for subscales; does not measure bladder or

Table 11-1: (*Continued*)

Scale	Description and Type of Scale	Reliability, Validity, and Sensitivity	Time and Administration	Comments
System (LADS) (LORS/LADS) (58)	and memory, measured on 5-point scale from 0 = unable to perform activity–4 = able to perform	medical rehabilitation setting	maintenance, and program evaluation	bowel incontinence
Patient Evaluation and Conference System (PECS) (55)	Ordinal scale with 115 items in a 6-step scale ranging from total dependence to total independence; major headings include medicine, nursing, physical mobility, ADL, communication, medications, device utilization, pay, neuropsychology, social issues, therapeutic recreation, procedures, nutrition, pain, pulmonary	Documented reliability and validity; broad range of categories relating to medical rehabilitation services	Discipline-specific evaluations: <60 min for most disciplines; appropriate for formal assessment, monitoring, maintenance, and program evaluation	Extensive number of items evaluated; focuses on long-term needs and program evaluation; an ADL subscale has been Rasch-analyzed

Reproduced with permission from Braddom RL, ed. *Physical medicine and rehabilitation.* Philadelphia: WB Saunders, 1996:239–253.

activities of daily living (IADL) scales are described in greater detail in Table 11-2.

Quality of Life Scales

In contrast to the relatively discrete items included in most ADL and IADL scales, the domains involved in assessing "quality of life" are less well defined or categorized. Components of a quality of life evaluation could include social roles and interactions, physical as well as intellectual functioning, perception of health status, and general satisfaction with life (3). Most such scales, rather than being criterion referenced, ask the individual to compare himself or herself with (the recollection or perception of) his or her previous "healthy" state. The relevance of these types of scales to people with chronic or permanent disabilities has yet to be established. Two examples of quality of life instruments are the MOS 36-Item Short Form Survey (SF36) (62) and the Sickness Impact Profile (SIP) (39,63), described in greater detail in Table 11-3.

FUNCTIONAL ASSESSMENT IN VARIOUS SETTINGS AND POPULATIONS

With the expanding scope of rehabilitation into multiple levels of care and settings (e.g., skilled nursing facility, outpatient clinic, home-based programs), there is increasing interest in the applicability and validity of functional assessment instruments, as well as feasibility of tracking individual patients through various health care settings and levels. The FIM instrument was originally developed for inpatient settings in rehabilitation hospitals or hospital-based rehabilitation units (referred to as "acute" or comprehensive medical rehabilitation), but has also been used in skilled nursing facility (nursing home) based rehabilitation programs (referred to as "subacute" rehabilitation) (4) and in home-based rehabilitation programs (46).

A functional assessment instrument designed specifically for use in medical rehabilitation outpatient settings is the LIFEware Medical Rehabilitation Follow Along (MRFA instrument) which was developed using Rasch analysis (64). The MRFA instrument includes musculoskeletal, neurologic, multiple sclerosis, cardiac, and pulmonary forms, and has been tested for reliability (65) and validity (64,66). The various forms cover physical functioning, pain experience, affective well-being, and cognitive functioning. Rasch analysis was used to construct nonredundant, unidimensional, linear, equal-interval measures that reflect the QODL for individuals with disability, and can assist in screening to identify early functional difficulties to prevent secondary complications (46). LIFEware uti-

Table 11-2: Selected Measures of Instrumental Activities of Daily Living (ADLs)

Scale	Description and Type of Scale	Reliability, Validity, and Sensitivity	Time and Administration	Comments
Functional Health Status (59)	Guttman scale containing 25 questions indicating ascending dependency; questions include out-of-home activities such as going to the movies, waking half a mile, and doing heavy work	Documented reliability and validity	Interviewer: <30 min; appropriate for maintenance in community setting	Simple scale design with general functioning questions; limited utility with disabled population; difficult to validate in an institutional setting
Older Americans Resources and Services Multidimensional Functional Assessment Questionnaire (OARS MFAQ) (40)	Multidimensional assessment tool containing 105 questions in 5 domains: social resources, economic resources, mental health, physical health, and ADLs	Documented reliability and validity	Interviewer: >10 min; appropriate for maintenance in the community	Measures broad base of information necessary for independent living; complex domains assessed
Philadelphia Geriatric Center Instrumental Activities of Daily Living (41)	Guttman scale includes questions on use of telephone, walking, shopping, food preparation, housekeeping, laundry, public transportation, and medicine	Documented reliability and validity	Time: <30 min	Strength: measures broad base of information necessary for independent living

Reproduced with permission from Braddom RL, ed. *Physical medicine and rehabilitation.* Philadelphia: WB Saunders, 1996:239–253.

lizes internet technology to collect assessment data and to report patient progress and outcomes. This unique methodology allows ready access to information for clinicians at a reasonable cost.

A variety of functional assessment instruments have been studied in specific disability populations, including patients with stroke (67–71), traumatic brain injury (72–74), spinal cord injury (75,76), and amputation (77). Others have also evaluated function in home settings (78–80).

Functional assessment of pediatric disabled individuals has also been the subject of significant research effort. In 1987 the FIM instrument was adapted for use with children by a multidisciplinary team of physicians, nurses, and therapists, resulting in the Functional Independence Measure for Children, or WeeFIM instrument (81). The WeeFIM instrument is a measure of functional abilities and the need for assistance associated with disabling conditions in children 6 months to 7 years old, and can also be used with children beyond age 7 in the presence of delays in functional development (3). Like its parent, it is a minimum data set that measures severity of disability, contains 18 items organized in six domains (self-care, transfers, locomotion, sphincter control, communication, and social cognition), with each item scored on a seven-level ordinal scale ranging from complete or modified independence to modified and complete dependence, and is supported by an extensive and growing national database with bench mark values for comparative reporting of progress and outcomes. The WeeFIM System offers the opportunity to use a single assessment system across a spectrum of settings (inpatient, outpatient, home and school). Reliability studies have shown robust intrarater and interrater correlations (82).

Another comprehensive pediatric assessment instrument in common use clinically is the Pediatric Evaluation

Table 11-3: Selected Measures of Quality of Life

Scale	Description and Type of Scale	Reliability, Validity, and Sensitivity	Time and Administration	Comments
MOS 36-Item Short Form Survey (SF-36) (62)	Assesses 8 health domains including physical and social activities, mental health, general health perceptions, vitality, and discomfort	Documented reliability and validity	Interviewer in person or phone: <30 min; appropriate for maintenance in community setting	Items well standardized; widely used in community; utility for following persons with disability not known
Sickness Impact Profile (SIP) (39,63)	Subscales evaluate the following areas: ambulation, self-care, emotions, communications, alertness, habits, home and recreation, vocation, and social interactions	Adequate reliability and validity	Interviewer in person or phone: <30 min; appropriate for maintenance in community setting	Comprehensive evaluation; behavioral rather than subjective health items; focus on community life; utility for following persons with disability not known

of Disability Inventory (PEDI), which consists of 197 functional skill items together with 20 complex functional items for which caregiver assistance and modifications are assessed (83). The PEDI evaluates function in self-care, mobility, and social function domains, and was developed using the Rasch rating scale methodology (32). It has been standardized on a normative sample of nondisabled children, and validated on a sample of children with a wide range of motor and cognitive disabilities (84).

FUTURE DIRECTIONS

What are the advantages of a database, what are its uses, and how can it be applied to improve the rehabilitation of patients over the long run? Databases store information for subsequent analyses by both clinicians and research experts. Ongoing databases allow data to accumulate, which is particularly advantageous for studying patterns of care and ways in which they may change over time. One key advantage of accumulated data is that the sample size at any point in time is large enough for statistical interpretation and generalization of the results. Statistical research often depends on the availability of large sample sizes to reach a substantive conclusion about health care outcomes.

The measurement of functional changes over time has received considerable attention in the statistical literature due to the complicated nature of repeated measure statistics. Despite this, the application of good measurement principles to the FIM instrument have resulted in tools that investigators can have confidence in using over time with little measurement error. The UDSMR System can be used with considerable statistical power and measurement confidence to provide unique insights into the long-term care of patients in medical rehabilitation.

Since inception of the UDSMR System in 1987, admission and discharge data have been collected on over two million medical rehabilitation patients with a variety of diagnoses. About one-third of these cases also have follow-up records. Thus, the collection of comparable data from clinical sites across the country is an ongoing activity. We learn by having a common language for comparing and contrasting. The unique uniformity of data allows direct comparisons with confidence in the FIM item, subscale, domain, and total scores across the population of the UDSMR data. Continuing accumulation of data from many treatment sites within a single database facilitates a variety of comparisons, including within-site, across-site, across-region, national, and even international. Besides contributing to the larger database, clinical sites are able to keep their own data in a readily accessible form for in-house data analysis and research efforts. Thus, facilities may examine their outcomes at any time and compare with those of the region and nation. These comparisons provide a basis for critical evaluation and planning for any one site at any single point in time and across time from admission to discharge to follow-up (program evaluation).

The next development is using the database to track trends in rehabilitative care from year to year. As the reporting is by type of impairment, facilities may use the data to focus in detail on individual patient groups to make comparisons with regional and national trends. The most remarkable trend over the past 6 or more years has been the drop in the average length of stay in rehabilitation (23–28). Also, there has been a concurrent reduction in the interval from admission to an acute hospital to admission to a rehabilitation setting (the so-called quicker and sicker phenomenon). According to the data, there has been no perceptible change (as yet) in such national average outcomes as level of function at discharge or in discharge destination. However, it is important to continue to monitor for any decrement in the quality of rehabilitation services (as reflected in outcomes) associated with increasingly shorter lengths of stay.

Data trends should be monitored for changes in the following (85):

1. Patient characteristics as in distribution by age and gender
2. Case mix by diagnostic categories (impairment type)
3. Case mix by severity
4. Number of patients treated
5. Length of stay
6. Functional status at admission, discharge, and follow-up
7. Time from onset of rehabilitation admission
8. Duration, effectiveness, and efficiency of rehabilitation
9. Charges/costs per patient
10. Frequency of program interruptions
11. Discharge patterns
12. The intensity, modalities, and types of clinicians involved with treatment

With the advent of rehabilitation in subacute units and in home care, there is a growing tendency for rehabilitation to occur, not in just one setting, but through a continuum in a variety of settings. Thus, in tracking outcomes we need to incorporate methods for following the pathways of individual patients when their rehabilitation takes place in more than one venue. The development of UDSMR databases for subacute facilities, home care, outpatients, and other sites, as well as in the area of pediatrics using the WeeFIM instrument, allows for a broad perspective on meeting the needs of patients from birth through old age. The advantages of uniformity and matching measuring tools such as the FIM and WeeFIM instruments allow for a unique opportunity to develop secondary prevention models by linking WeeFIM databases to adult databases to study lifetime outcomes. In addition, when connections may be made between the UDSMR and other national data sets, then ever-more detailed studies may become available.

In other developments, the predictive power of the FIM instrument is being used for models of Function-Related Groups (FIM-FRGs) through the work of Stineman et al (86–88). The appearance of FIM-FRGs signals the next step in putting the national database to work for improving rehabilitative care: efficiency pattern matrices. This tool allows the clinician to view a plot of the distribution between two outcome variables (such as change in FIM score against length of stay). When a group of patients of similar age and severity of disability at admission are displayed, one may readily locate in the matrix those cases that match the expected value and those that either exceed it or did not meet it. "High"- or "low"-achieving patients may be identified and the reasons for the outcomes investigated. Finally, there is interest in reducing excessive variation in practice unless the evidence justifies that variation. Development of standards ultimately gives impetus to a shift in the basis of assessment from authority to scientific data. The UDSMR database offers an opportunity to seek and to find regions of the country where the best practices prevail.

In 1985, Granger (89) predicted that by the year 2000:

> All healthcare workers will be using standardized terminology to describe the problems consequent to chronic disease and we will be employing systematic computerized methods for tracking individuals' functional abilities and their unmet needs over time. Medical rehabilitation programs will be mandated into the healthcare plans of individuals disabled by accident or disease. However, authorization for payment by third parties will entail requirements for (a) an organized system of care with a comprehensive plan of management, (b) a functional prognosis in terms of probabilities for therapeutic gains in terms of quality of life, (c) efficient delivery of services, and (d) documentation of outcomes through periodic assessments of functional status in order to determine the most favorable benefit/cost ratios.

As standardized functional assessment instruments evolve to better approximate the clinical situation, they will be used increasingly as a basis for predicting outcomes of care, and will contribute significantly to decision making in the health care arena. Further, functional assessment will facilitate comparisons of effectiveness and efficiency of alternative therapeutic interventions and settings, resulting in predictable relationships between "doses" of specific rehabilitation treatments and the consequent "response" of the patient (3).

REFERENCES

1. Fiedler RC, Granger CV. The relationship between functional assessment and outcome. In: Toole JF, Good DC, eds. *Imaging in neurologic rehabilitation.* New York: Demos Vermande, 1996:41–50.
2. Lawton MP. The functional assessment of elderly people. *J Am Geriatr Soc* 1971;19:465–481.

3. Granger CV, Kelly-Hayes M, Johnston M, et al. Quality and outcome measures for medial rehabilitation. In: Braddom RL, ed. *Physical medicine and rehabilitation.* Philadelphia: WB Saunders, 1996:239–253.

4. Commission on Accreditation of Rehabilitation Facilities (CARF). *Program evaluation: a guide to utilization.* Tucson: CARF, 1982.

5. Johnston MV, Wilkerson DL, Maney M. Evaluation of the quality and outcomes of medical rehabilitation programs. In: DeLisa JA, ed. *Rehabilitation medicine: principles and practice.* 2nd ed. Philadelphia: JB Lippincott, 1993:240–268.

6. Gonnella C. Program evaluation. In: Fletcher GF, Banja JD, Jann BB, Wolf SL, eds. *Rehabilitation medicine: contemporary clinical perspectives.* Philadelphia: Lea & Febiger, 1992:243–268.

7. Joint Commission on Accreditation of Healthcare Organization (JCAHO). *1983 Accreditation manual for hospitals.* Oakbrook Terrace, IL: JCAHO, 1992:234.

8. Moscowitz E, McCann CB. Classification of disability in the chronically ill and aging. *J Chronic Dis* 1957;5:342–346.

9. Donaldson SW, Wagner CC, Gresham GE. A unified ADL form. *Arch Phys Med Rehabil* 1973;54:175–179.

10. Granger CV. A conceptual model for functional assessment. In: Granger CV, Gresham GE, eds. *Functional assessment in rehabilitation medicine.* Baltimore: Williams & Wilkins, 1984:14–25.

11. World Health Organization. *International classification of impairments, disabilities, and handicaps.* Geneva: World Health Organization, 1980.

12. Clark GS, Siebens H. Rehabilitation of the geriatric patient. In: DeLisa JA, ed. *Rehabilitation medicine: principles and practice.* 2nd ed. Philadelphia: JB Lippincott, 1993:642–665.

13. Clark GS. Functional assessment in the elderly. In: Williams TF, ed. *Rehabilitation in the aging.* New York: Raven, 1984:111–124.

14. Nagi SZ. *Disability and rehabilitation.* Columbus: Ohio State University Press, 1965.

15. Wood PHN. The language of disablement: a glossary relating to disease and its consequences. *Int Rehabil Med* 1980;2:86–92.

16. Maslow AH. *Motivation and personality.* New York: Harper & Row, 1954.

17. Johnston MV, Keith RA, Hinderer SR. Measurement standards for interdisciplinary medical rehabilitation. *Arch Phys Med Rehabil* 1992;73:S3–S23.

18. Johnston MV, Keith RA. Measurement standards for medical rehabilitation and clinical applications. *Phys Med Rehabil Clin North Am* 1993;4:425–449.

19. Hinderer SR, Hinderer KA. Objective measurement in rehabilitation: theory and application. In: DeLisa JA, ed. *Rehabilitation medicine: principles and practice.* 2nd ed. Philadelphia: JB Lippincott, 1993:96–121.

20. Smith PM, Bennett Illig S, Fielder RC, et al. Intermodal agreement of follow-up telephone functional assessment using the Functional Independence Measure in patients with stroke. *Arch Phys Med Rehabil* 1996;77:431–435.

21. Kraemer HC. *Evaluating medical tests: qualitative and objective guidelines.* Newbury Park, CA: Sage, 1992.

22. Committee to Advise the Public Health Service on Clinical Practice Guidelines, Institute of Medicine. *Clinical practice guidelines.* Washington, DC: National Academy, 1990.

23. Granger CV, Hamilton BB. UDS report: the Uniform Data System for Medical Rehabilitation: report of first admissions for 1990. *Am J Phys Med Rehabil* 1992;71: 108–113.

24. Granger CV, Hamilton BB. The Uniform Data System for Medical Rehabilitation: report of first admissions for 1991. *Am J Phys Med Rehabil* 1993;72:33–38.

25. Granger CV, Hamilton BB. The Uniform Data System for Medical Rehabilitation: report of first admissions for 1992. *Am J Phys Med Rehabil* 1994;73:51–55.

26. Granger CV, Ottenbacher KJ, Fiedler RC. The Uniform Data System for Medical Rehabilitation: report of first admissions for 1993. *Am J Phys Med Rehabil* 1995;74:62–66.

27. Fiedler RC, Granger CV, Ottenbacher KJ. The Uniform Data System for Medical Rehabilitation: report of first admissions for 1994. *Am J Phys Med Rehabil* 1996;75:125–129.

28. Fiedler RC, Granger CV. Uniform Data System for Medical Rehabilitation: report of first admissions for 1995. *Am J Phys Med Rehabil* 1997;776:76–81.

29. Pollak N, Rheault W, Stoecker JL. Reliability and validity of the FIM for persons aged 80 years and above from a multilevel continuing care retirement community. *Arch Phys Med Rehabil* 1996;77:1056–1061.

30. Baker JG, Granger CV, Fiedler RC. A brief outpatient functional assessment measure: validity using Rasch measures. *Am J Phys Med Rehabil* 1997;76:8–13.

31. Duran LJ, Fisher AG. Male and female performance on the assessment of motor and process skills. *Arch Phys Med Rehabil* 1996;77:1019–1024.

32. Wright BD, Masters G. *Rating scale analysis.* Chicago: MESA, 1982.

33. Daniels L, Worthingham C. *Muscle testing: techniques of manual examination*, 4th ed. Philadelphia: WB Saunders, 1980.

34. *Guide for the Uniform Data Set for Medical Rehabilitation (Adult FIM™)*, Version 4.0. Buffalo, NY: State University of New York at Buffalo, 1993.

35. Merbitz C, Morris J, Grip JC. Ordinal scales and foundations of

misinference. *Arch Phys Med Rehabil* 1989;70:308–312.

36. Johnston MV. Statistical approaches to ordinal measures. *Arch Phys Med Rehabil* 1989;70: 861.

37. Folstein MF, Folstein SE, McHugh PR. Mini-Mental State: a practical method for grading the cognitive state of patients for the clinician. *J Psychiatr Res* 1975;12:189–198.

38. Kane RA. Instruments to assess functional status. In: Cassel CK, Riesenberg DE, Sorensen LB, Walsh JR, eds. *Geriatric medicine*, 2nd ed. New York: Springer, 1990:55–65.

39. Bergner M, Bobbitt RA, Pollard WE, et al. Sickness Impact Profile: validation of a health status measure. *Med Care* 1976;14: 57–67.

40. Rubenstein LZ, Schairer C, Wieland GD, Kane R. Systematic biases in functional status assessment of elderly adults: effects of different data sources. *J Gerontol* 1984;39:686–691.

41. Kaplan CP, Corrigan JD. The relationship between cognition and functional independence in adults with traumatic brain injury. *Arch Phys Med Rehabil* 1994;75: 643–647.

42. Kelly-Hayes M, Jett A, Wolf PA, et al. Functional limitations and disability among elders in the Framingham study. *Am J Public Health* 1992;82:841–845.

43. Nagi S. Disability concepts revisited. In: Sussman MB, ed. *Sociology and rehabilitation*. Washington, DC: American Sociological Association, 1965:100–113.

44. Kane RA, Kane RL. *Assessing the elderly: a practical guide to measurement*. Lexington, MA: Lexington Books, 1981.

45. Gresham GE, Labi MLC. Functional assessment instruments currently available for documenting outcomes in rehabilitation medicine. In: Granger CV, Gresham GE, eds. *Functional assessment in rehabilitation medicine*. Baltimore: Williams & Wilkins, 1984:65–85.

46. Gresham GE, Dittmar SS. Instruments used to assess function and measure outcomes in physical rehabilitation. In: Dittmar SS, Gresham GE, eds. *Functional assessment and outcome measures for the rehabilitation health professional*. Gaithersburg, MD: Aspen, 1997:27–30.

47. Katz S, Ford AB, Moscowitz RW, et al. Studies of illness in the aged. *JAMA* 1967;185:914–919.

48. Schoening HA, Anderegg L, Bergstrom D, et al. Numerical scoring of self-care status of patients. *Arch Phys Med Rehabil* 1965;46:689–697.

49. Clark GS, Granger CV. Functional outcome measurements. In: O'Young B, Young MA, Stiens SA, eds. *PM&R Secrets*. Philadelphia: Hanley & Belfus, 1996:4–8.

50. Mahoney FL, Barthel DW. Functional evaluation: Barthel Index. *Md State Med J* 1965;14:61–65.

51. Granger CV, Albrecht GL, Hamilton BB. Outcome of comprehensive medical rehabilitation: measurement by PULSES Profile and the Barthel Index. *Arch Phys Med Rehabil* 1979;60:145–154.

52. Fortinsky RH, Granger CV, Seltzer GB. The use of functional assessment in understanding home care needs. *Med Care* 1981;19:489–497.

53. Collin C, Wade DT, Davies S, Horne V. The Barthel ADL Index: a reliability study. *Int Disabil Studies* 1988;10:61–63.

54. Shah S, Vanclay F, Cooper B. Efficiency, effectiveness and duration of stroke rehabilitation. *Stroke* 1990;21:241–246.

55. Harvey RF, Jellinek HM. Functional performance assessment: a program approach. *Arch Phys Med Rehabil* 1981;62:456–460.

56. Sarno JE, Sarno MT, Levita E. The functional life scale. *Arch Phys Med Rehabil* 1973;54:214–220.

57. Carey RG, Posavac EJ. Program evaluation of a physical medicine and rehabilitation unit: a new approach. *Arch Phys Med Rehabil* 1978;59:330–337.

58. Gonnella C. Program evaluation. In: Fletcher GF, Banja JD, Jann BB, Wolf SL, eds. *Rehabilitation medicine: contemporary clinical perspectives*. Philadelphia: Lea & Febiger, 1992:243–268.

59. Rosow I, Breslau N. A Guttman health scale for the aged. *J Gerontol* 1966;21:556–559.

60. Duke University Center for the Study of Aging and Human Development. *Multidimensional functional assessment: the OARS methodology*. Durham, NC: Duke, 1978.

61. Lawton MP. The functional assessment of elderly people. *J Am Geriatr Soc* 1971;6:465–480.

62. Ware JE, Sherbourne CD. The MOS 36-Item Short Form Survey (SF-36): conceptual framework and item selection. *Med Care* 1992;30:473–483.

63. Carter WB, Bobbitt RA, Bergner M, Gilson BS. Validation of an interval scaling: the Sickness Impact Profile. *Health Serv Res* 1976;11: 515–528.

64. Baker JG, Granger CV, Fiedler RC. A brief outpatient functional assessment measure: validity using Rasch measures. *Am J Phys Med Rehabil* 1997;76:8–13.

65. Granger CV, Ottenbacher KJ, Baker JG, Sehgal A. Reliability of a brief outpatient functional outcome assessment measure. *Am J Phys Med Rehabil* 1995;74:469–475.

66. Baker JG, Granger CV, Ottenbacher KJ. Validity of a brief outpatient functional assessment measure. *Am J Phys Med Rehabil* 1996;75:356–363.

67. Pedersen PM, Jorgensen HS, Nakayama H, et al. Comprehensive assessment of activities of daily living in stroke: the Copenhagen Stroke Study. *Arch Phys Med Rehabil* 1997;78:161–165.

68. Chae J, Zorowitz RD, Johnston MV. Functional outcome of hemorrhagic and nonhemorrhagic stroke patients after in-patient rehabilitation: a matched comparison. *Am J Phys Med Rehabil* 1996;76:177–182.

69. Mauthe RW, Haaf DC, Hayn P, Krall JM. Predicting discharge destination of stroke patients using a mathematical model based on six items from the Functional Independence Measure. *Arch Phys Med Rehabil* 1996;77:10–13.

70. Chae J, Johnston M, Kim H, Zorowitz R. Admission motor impairment as a predictor of physical disability after stroke rehabilitation. *Am J Phys Med Rehabil* 1995;74:218–223.

71. Granger CV, Clark GS. Functional status and outcomes of stroke rehabilitation. *Top Geriatr Rehabil* 1994;9:72–84.

72. Cifu DX, Kreutzer JS, Marwitz JH, et al. Functional outcomes of older adults with traumatic brain injury: a prospective, multicenter analysis. *Arch Phys Med Rehabil* 1996;77:883–888.

73. Whitlock JA Jr, Hamilton BB. Functional outcome after rehabilitation for severe traumatic brain injury. *Arch Phys Med Rehabil* 1995;76:1103–1112.

74. Cowen TD, Meythaler JM, DeVivo MJ, et al. Influence of early variables in traumatic brain injury on Functional Independence Measure scores and rehabilitation length of stay and charges. *Arch Phys Med Rehabil* 1995;76:797–803.

75. Heinemann AW, Kirk P, Hastie BA, et al. Relationships between disability measures and nursing effort during medical rehabilitation for patients with traumatic brain and spinal cord injury. *Arch Phys Med Rehabil* 1997;78:143–149.

76. McKinley WO, Conti-Wyneken AR, Vokac CW, Cifu DX. Rehabilitative functional outcome of patients with neoplastic spinal cord compression. *Arch Phys Med Rehabil* 1996;77:892–895.

77. Melchiorre PJ, Findley T, Boda W. Functional outcome and comorbidity indexes in the rehabilitation of the traumatic versus the vascular unilateral lower limb amputee. *Am J Phys Med Rehabil* 1996;75:9–14.

78. Grimby G, Andren E, Holmgren E, et al. Structure of a combination of Functional Independence Measure and instrumental activity measure items in community-living persons: a study of individuals with cerebral palsy and spina bifida. *Arch Phys Med Rehabil* 1996;77:1109–1114.

79. Priebe MM, Rintala DH. Functional assessment in a community setting. *Top Stroke Rehabil* 1994;1:16–29.

80. Post MWM, de Bruin A, de Witte L, Schrijvers A. The SIP68: a measure of health-related functional status in rehabilitation medicine. *Arch Phys Med Rehabil* 1996;77:440–445.

81. *Guide for the Uniform Data Set for Medical Rehabilitation for Children (WeeFIM®).* Version 4.0-inpatient/outpatient. Buffalo: State University of New York at Buffalo, 1993.

82. Ottenbacher KJ, Msall ME, Lyon NR, et al. Interrater agreement and stability on the functional independence measure for children (WeeFIM® instrument): use in children with developmental disabilities. *Arch Phys Med Rehabil* 1997;78:1309–1315.

83. Haley SM, Coster WJ, Ludlow LH, et al. *Pediatric Evaluation of Disability Inventory: development, standardization and administration manual.* Boston: PEDI Research Group, New England Medical Center Hospitals, 1992.

84. Haley SM, Ludlow LH, Coster WJ. Pediatric Evaluation of Disability Inventory: clinical interpretation of summary scores using Rasch rating scale methodology. *Phys Med Rehabil Clin North Am* 1993;4:529–540.

85. Forer S. How to make program evaluation work for you. *Neurorehabilitation* 1992;2:52–71.

86. Stineman MG, Hamilton BB, Goin JE, et al. Functional gain and length of stay for major rehabilitation impairment categories: patterns revealed by Function Related Groups. *Am J Phys Med Rehabil* 1996;75:68–78.

87. Stineman MG, Shea JA, Jette A, et al. The Functional Independence Measure: tests of scaling assumptions, structure, and reliability across 20 diverse impairment categories. *Arch Phys Med Rehabil* 1996;77:1101–1108.

88. Stineman MG, Hamilton BB, Granger CV, et al. Four methods for characterizing disability in the formation of Function Related Groups. *Arch Phys Med Rehabil* 1994;75:1277–1283.

89. Granger CV. Medical rehabilitation: predicting needs and measuring outcomes for quality of life. In: Gaitz CM, Niederehe G, Wilson NL, eds. *Aging 2000: our health care destiny.* Vol. 2: *Psychosocial and policy issues.* New York: Springer, 1985:255.

Chapter 12

Normal and Pathologic Gait Analysis

Alberto Esquenazi
Mukul Talaty

INTRODUCTION TO GAIT

Walking requires much balance and coordination, yet most people can perform this complicated task without even thinking about it. The fundamental objective of bipedal human locomotion is to move safely and efficiently from one point to another. In a simplistic way, walking has been described as "controlled falling." But bipedal human gait is a complex task. Not only do the feet have to move across the ground, but the knees, hips, spine, arms, shoulders, and head all move in synchrony to keep the system in balance and to achieve forward advancement. This involves cyclic motions of the trunk and extremities. Gait can be described as an interplay between the two extremities: one in touch with the ground, producing sequential restraint and propulsion, and the other swinging freely and carrying with it the forward momentum of the body. It is quite proper, therefore, to designate the human gait as a dynamic equilibrium, that is, one in which equilibrium is constantly lost and recovered. However, cycle-to-cycle variations of movements are slight (1,2). Despite these complexities, gait patterns are highly repeatable both within a subject and between subjects.

Walking is accomplished in a similar manner by all healthy adults and most children 8 years and older, because everyone has the same basic anatomic and physiologic makeup. However, the inherent differences in body proportions, level of coordination, motivation, and other factors make each individual's gait pattern unique. Walking is performed in a subconscious manner in most circumstances. Under some conditions (e.g., slippery, irregular, or less than ideally illuminated surfaces) walking requires a concerted effort, making use of the ample physiologic reserve mechanisms of the neuromuscular system. When injuries to this system occur, the reserves are limited and walking even on level surfaces requires considerably more attention and effort.

The history of the human race indicates that walking was an essential function to survive in a nomadic society. Even in the modern sedentary society, walking continues to be an essential activity that promotes fitness, learning, and socialization. A child with limited mobility will have less opportunity to interact with other children and the environment, and thus to learn. In patients with dementia, an inability to walk increases the probability for internment in a nursing home. Thus, ambulation disorders are a vital focus of rehabilitation medicine and its role in promoting independent living.

Historical documentation confirms that attempts were made to investigate human walking since the time of Aristotle. The modern quantitative study of human locomotion dates back to 1836 with the observational studies of the Weber brothers. Murray (3) was the first to use photography to analyze movements of the body, using light marking strips on the dark-clad subject. Later Muybridge (4) contributed to the understanding of gait with his sequential photographs, first of horses and then of walking and running men. Bernstein (5) performed detailed photographic studies of the movements that occur during normal human locomotion and with this, initiated the study of kinematics. In 1947, Schwartz made the first quantitative studies of the forces generated at the floor-foot interface during gait. Later, electromyographic (EMG) recordings were made possible with the development of amplifier technology. Inman and the group at the University of California Biomechanics Laboratory (6) refined the simultaneous recording of multiple muscle group activity during normal ambulation.

Recently, within the context of clinical rehabilitation, orthopedic surgery, and sports and industrial medicine, there has been an increase in interest in the quantitative assessment of gait and human kinesiology. This has been advanced in part because of the ease with which computers can analyze massive amounts of data obtained simultaneously from a variety of sources (e.g., force transducers, foot switches, EMG amplifiers, electrogoniometers, motion analysis systems). These specialized transducers transform a physical variable, such as movement or muscle potential, into an electrical signal that can be converted to a digital signal, recorded by a computer, displayed against dependent variables such as time and distance, and easily and efficiently saved for future reference. These data can then be subjected to a process of analysis in which derived information (velocities, accelerations, joint moments, powers, and mechanical energy) is calculated. (Under certain conditions internal muscle forces can be estimated as well.) The desire to quantify function and the rapid progress in computer technology have promoted the proliferation of gait analysis laboratories in many centers.

For gait analysis to be useful in the clinical evaluation of patients, certain criteria must be fulfilled. The measured parameters must correlate with the functional capacity of the patient; supply additional, more relevant information than the clinical examination; be accurate and repeatable; result from a test that does not alter the natural performance of the patient; and be interpreted by experienced clinicians familiar with the scope of the test protocol, instrumentation, and limitations of the equipment. This last criterion implies that the clinician be familiar with the subtleties and complex interactions of normal gait, as well as with the technology, to effectively diagnose and address the problems of pathologic gait.

NCRMAL LOCOMOTION

The three fundamental goals of human ambulation are to move from one place to another and to do so as safely and as efficiently as possible (7). To accomplish these, four basic motor issues are simultaneously addressed: 1) the generation of mechanical energy for controlled forward progression, 2) absorption of mechanical energy to minimize shock or to control the forward progression of the body, 3) support of the upper body on the lower limb during the stance phase, and 4) control of the foot trajectory to ensure appropriate articulation with the support surface during the stance phase and foot clearance during the swing phase.

Three functional properties of locomotion give rise to the natural redundancy or flexibility humans have in generating patterns of walking:

- A range of step or stride lengths and base widths that contribute to diverse energy-efficient gaits
- A range of stable and recoverable upright postures
- An ability to change direction and rhythm

Together these properties provide a range of adaptations, a result of the natural redundancy of the neuromuscular system, that allow navigation of different environmental surfaces (e.g., inclines, elevations).

Identification of the numerous simultaneous events that occur during walking is imperative to understand gait. The basic terms and definitions used to describe the components and events of the gait cycle (6,7) can be based on the timing of reciprocal floor contacts. A single sequence of functions by one limb is called a *gait cycle*. Each gait cycle has two basic components (Table 12-1): The *stance phase* designates the duration of foot contact with the ground and the *swing phase* is the period during which the foot is in the air for limb advancement. The stance phase can be subdivided into five subphases: 1) *initial contact*, 2) *loading response*, 3) *mid-stance*, 4) *terminal stance*, and 5) *pre-*

Table 12-1: Phases of the Gait Cycle

Phase	Description
Stance Phase	
Initial contact	The instant the foot contacts the ground
Loading response	From flat foot position until the opposite foot is off the ground for swing
Mid-stance	From the time the opposite foot is lifted until the ipsilateral tibia is vertical
Terminal stance	From heel rise until the opposite foot contacts the ground (contralateral initial contact)
Pre-swing	From initial contact of the opposite foot and ends with ipsilateral toe-off
Swing Phase	
Initial swing	Begins with lift-off of the foot from the floor and ends when the foot is aligned with the opposite foot
Mid-swing	Begins when the foot is aligned with the opposite foot and ends when the tibia is vertical
Terminal swing	Begins when the tibia is vertical and ends when the foot contacts the ground (initial contact)

swing. The swing phase can be divided into three functional subphases: 1) *initial swing*, 2) *mid-swing*, and 3) *terminal swing* (8,9). The weight of the body is transferred from one limb to the other during the period of double support, while the swing phase achieves advancement of the limb (Fig. 12-1).

Alternatively the stance phase can be subdivided into three periods according to floor contact patterns. The beginning and the end of the stance phase mark the *double support* period during which both feet are in contact with the floor. *Single-limb support* begins when the opposite foot is lifted for the swing phase. The broad normal distribution of the floor contact period during the gait cycle is 40% for the swing phase, 60% for stance phase, with approximately 10% for each double support time. These proportions apply to normal subjects walking at self-selected comfortable speeds. However, they will vary greatly with changes in walking velocity. For example, walking more slowly will reduce single-limb support time and increase double support time. With increasing *cadence* (number of steps/min), the double support period steadily decreases, and disappears during running.

The *step period* is the time measured from an event in one foot to the subsequent occurrence of the same event in the other foot. There are two steps in each stride or gait cycle. The *stride period* can be defined as the time from initial contact of one foot until the next initial contact for the same foot and is normally equal for left and right strides. *Stride length* is the distance covered during one stride. The stride period is often normalized to the full gait cycle for the purpose of averaging gait parameters over several strides both within and between subjects. The step period is useful for identifying and measuring asymmetry between the two sides of the body, especially in pathologic conditions. *Step length* is the distance covered during one step. The step length and the step time are fairly symmetric for both legs in normal individuals. These are all important parameters when evaluating pathologic gait.

Walking speed is defined as the average horizontal speed of the body along the plane of progression (distance/time). Under normal conditions, comfortable walking speed corresponds to the speed at which the energy cost per unit of distance is minimum. Individuals with abnormal gait patterns who have a normal cardiopulmonary mechanism and nutritional status do not ordinarily expend more energy per minute than able-bodied persons, although the energy required per unit of distance increases (10). Energy efficiency is dependent on controlled functional joint mobility and the precise timing and intensity of coordinated muscle action. The result of abnormal biomechanics is increased energy cost, usually with a compensatory decrease in walking speed. Many mechanisms serve to minimize the energy expenditure of normal walking.

The kinematics (geometry of motion without regard to the forces that cause it) of the gait cycle are organized to minimize the movement of the body's center of gravity in both the vertical and horizontal planes, resulting in energy-efficient movement. The average total displacement of the center of gravity in a stride is less than 5 cm in normal subjects. Impairments of the gait mechanism can result in decreased energy efficiency due to increased excursions of the center of gravity. Saunders et al (11) identified six key factors (determinants of gait) that minimize the excursion of the center of gravity and help produce forward progression with the least expenditure of energy. These determinants, listed in Table 12-2, are coordinated patterns of motion between the various lower-extremity segments and the muscles that move them. These patterns have evolved over thousands of years, since the inception of bipedal locomotion.

Specific mechanisms, not entirely independent of the above-named six determinants, are used during both the swing and the stance phase of normal ambulation to produce limb clearance and advancement. Knowledge of these events is important because they permit a clear understanding of the biomechanical causes of problems encountered during gait.

The clearance mechanisms for the swinging limb require specific coordinated events to lift the foot off the ground. These include knee flexion during the pre-swing phase, coordinated hip and knee flexion during early- to mid-swing phases, and ankle dorsiflexion in mid- to late-swing phase. These events are critical for the swing phase to occur. The presence of two of these three events is indispensable to achieve limb clearance. Pelvis stabilization is also critical and is achieved by the hip abductors, which control the amount of pelvic drop (tilt) in the swing phase.

Table 12-2: Determinants of Gait

Pelvic rotation (in the horizontal plane)	The swinging hip moves forward faster than the stance hip.
Pelvic tilt (in the frontal plane)	The pelvis on the side of the swinging leg is lowered. This is controlled by activity in the hip abductors of the stance limb.
Early knee flexion	This is 15 degrees during the first part of stance.
Weight transfer (from the heel to flat foot)	Weight transfer is associated with controlled plantarflexion during the first part of stance.
Late knee flexion	This is 30 to 40 degrees during the last part of the stance phase.
Lateral displacement of the pelvis	Lateral displacement occurs toward the stance limb.

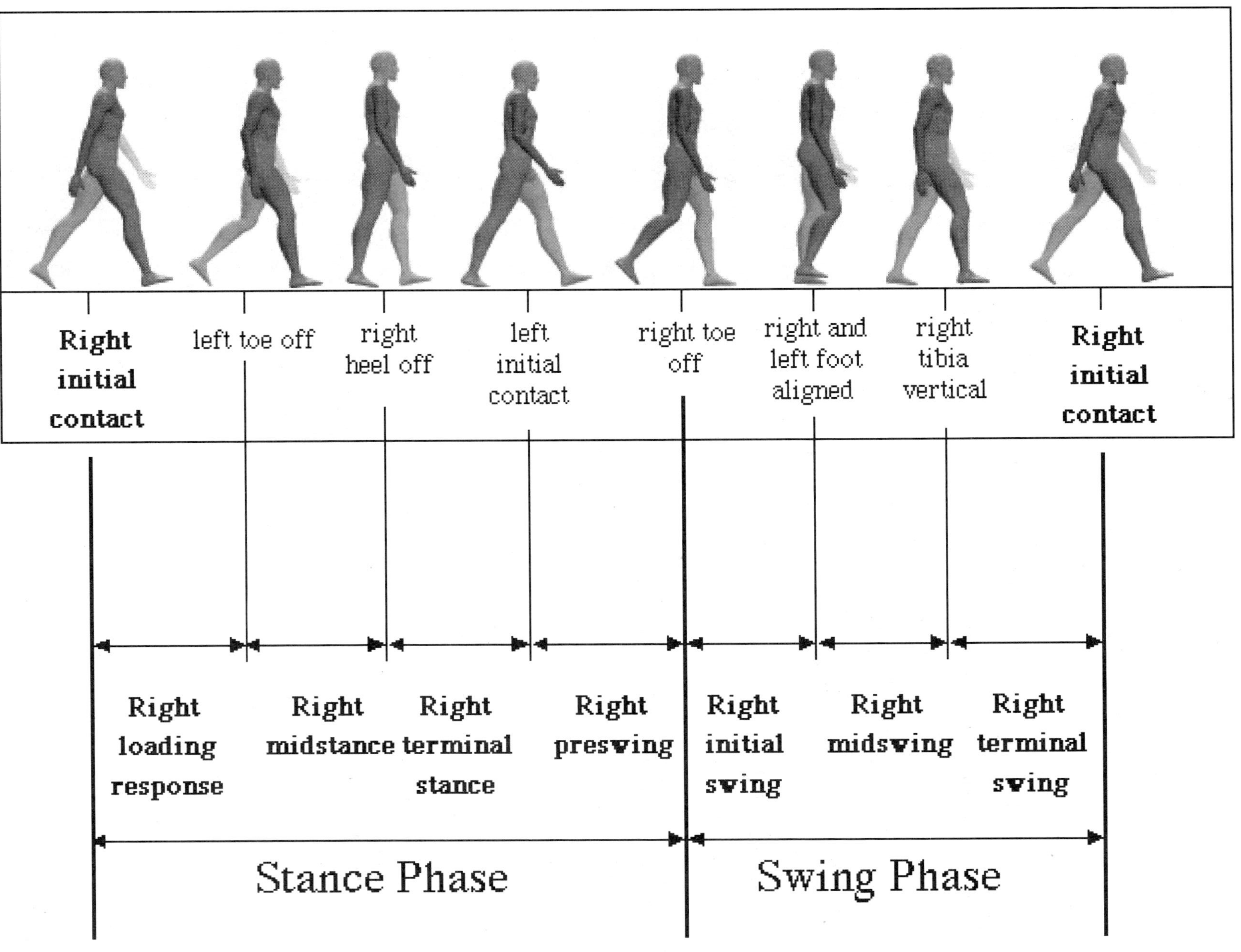

Figure 12-1. Gait cycle. The series of postures illustrates the gait cycle. Events used to demarcate specific epochs in the gait cycle are provided immediately below the figures, while the specific epochs of the gait cycle are denoted in bold.

To further ensure limb clearance while optimizing energy efficiency, the stance limb has several mechanisms to provide sufficient clearance for the swinging limb. These include mid-stance ankle dorsiflexion control (to prevent excessive forward rotation of the tibia through the forces exerted by the ankle plantarflexors), mid- to terminal-stance knee extension, and terminal-stance heel rise (ankle plantarflexion).

To achieve the most efficient gait while maximizing step length, optimal limb advancement must occur. For step length to be the longest, the swing limb must have hip flexion occurring in combination with terminal-swing knee extension while the stance limb permits stance ankle dorsiflexion (controlled forward progression of the tibia), terminal-stance heel rise (ankle plantarflexion) with weight transfer to the metatarsal heads (rollover), and terminal-stance knee and hip extension. It is also imperative that tilt and internal rotation of the pelvis take place.

QUANTITATIVE GAIT ANALYSIS

Clinicians routinely perform an informal visual analysis of gait. Careful, systematic visualization can yield some useful descriptive information, especially if slow-motion video technology is used, although there are many limitations. The speed and complexity of the mechanisms, combined with the deviations and possible compensations that occur with pathologic gait, limit a visual-based qualitative analysis of gait. Such an analysis does not provide quantitative information (7). Fortunately, there are a great many tools available to increase the ability to observe and quantify many of these mechanisms.

Gait can be studied through the collection of a wide range of information in the laboratory. The three primary components of quantitative gait analysis that can be recorded are 1) poly-EMG or dynamic EMG (analysis of muscle activity and identification of the period and relative intensity of muscle function), 2) kinetics (analysis of forces or loads that cause motion), and 3) kinematics (temporal and stride measures and motion analysis). Walking is an interplay of these factors (Fig. 12-2).

Electromyographic Activation Patterns in Human Gait

In normal locomotion the gravitational forces are carefully controlled by opposing muscular forces (see Fig. 12-2) to yield a smooth and energy-efficient movement pattern. The efficiency of this interaction depends on a highly coordinated sequence of the timing and strength of the muscle contractions. Because of the redundant relationship between muscles and the joints they span, there is no

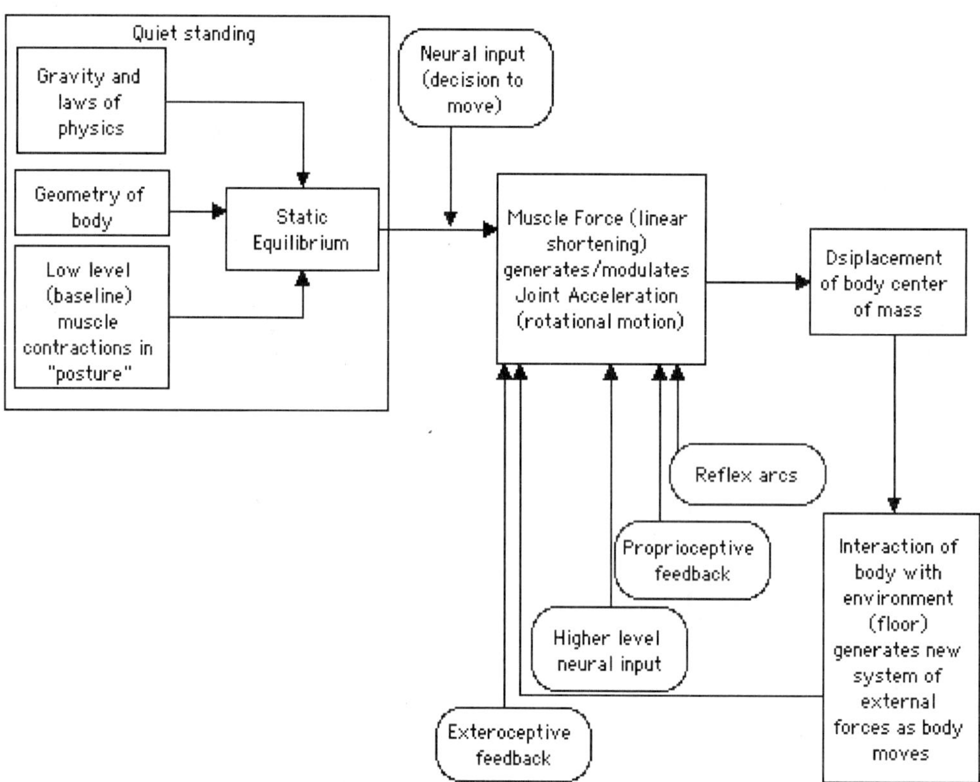

Figure 12-2. Walking model. Walking is mediated by a complex set of factors and inputs. This flowchart attempts to show some of the major contributors that precede walking as well as those that influence the dynamic process during walking.

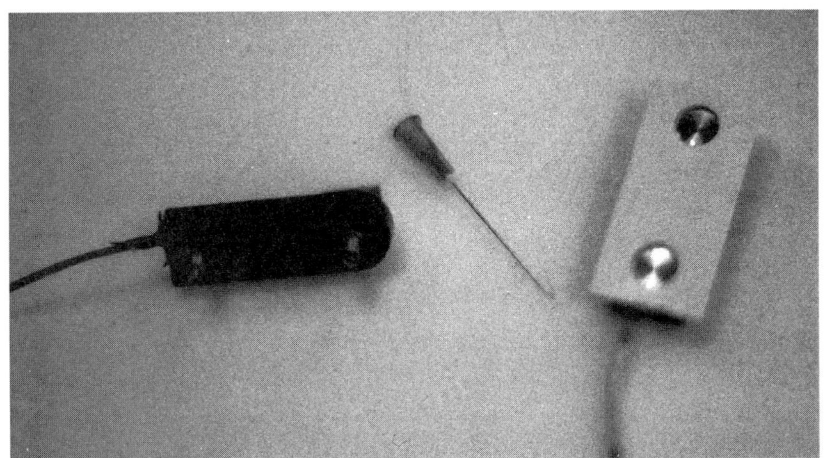

Figure 12-3. Electromyographic electrodes. The shell containing signal conditioning electronics (internal) and the attachment springs (external) for a wire electrode (*left*), the needle and wire electrode (thin wire emerging from the needle base) used to insert it in deep muscles (*middle*), and a surface electrode with double-sided tape used to affix to the skin with cutout for electrode gel (*right*).

unique association between a particular movement and the pattern of muscle forces producing movement. Therefore, the cause of an aberrant movement cannot be uniquely traced to a muscle based on the movement itself. The activity of the muscles that are capable of producing the noticed effect needs to be measured. EMG recordings provide information about the timing, duration, and relative strength of muscle activation. The EMG signal can be used as an accurate indicator of neurologic control over muscle activation. Superficial muscles can be studied using bipolar surface electrodes secured with double-sided tape (Fig. 12-3). For deep muscles or to differentiate between adjacent muscles, indwelling fine-wire electrodes are inserted through a hypodermic needle (see Fig. 12-3). The wires are coated with Teflon, except at the tips from where the muscle electrical potentials are recorded.

Patient EMG profiles can be compared to the means and standard deviations of tabulated normative data to identify how the timing deviates from normal. It is critical to be aware that EMG patterns are highly sensitive to walking speed. It is incorrect and potentially misleading to compare the recording of a patient with a slow gait to that of an able-bodied control population walking at a higher velocity with natural cadence. In addition to timing, an estimate of which is shown in Table 12-3 for 22 muscles, amplitude of the EMG signal may provide valuable information for making clinical decisions. A particular muscle may be overactive or underactive during a given portion of the cycle. Such deviations should be carefully correlated with patient kinematics. When interpreting dynamic-EMG data, it is important to distinguish cause and effect. For example, ankle inversion can be caused by one or more of the several muscles that can invert the ankle. This includes the tibialis anterior, tibialis posterior, gastrocnemius, soleus, and extensor hallucis longus (EHL). Each muscle alone, or in combination with one or more of the others, can produce ankle inversion. Determining which muscles are active during the observed abnormal ankle inversion posture may uncover a potential treatment strategy. If there is a clinical correlation between the EMG pattern and the observed kinematics, then a fairly confident diagnostic conclusion can be drawn regarding the cause of an observed gait deviation.

Kinetics

Kinetic analysis deals with the forces produced during walking. A reaction force acts under the entire surface of the foot. To understand the origin of the ground reaction forces (GRFs) and their effect on gait, one should be familiar with Newton's third law of motion, which specifies that for every action force there is an equal and opposite reaction force. In our laboratory the component of the total force in the sagittal and frontal planes is displayed using laser optics in real time and superimposed on the image of the walking subject (Fig. 12-4) (12).

GRFs are generally recorded using a triaxial force plate. Force plates measure the total force (a vector summation of all the components) assumed to be acting at a focal point (the center of pressure) under the foot. A force plate is a "sophisticated scale" that can measure vertical as well as shear forces in the anterior-posterior and medial-lateral directions. The *vertical force* is similar to the body weight registered on a scale. Anterior-posterior shear is the back-and-forth "push" against the floor. These are also sometimes referred to as *propulsion* and *breaking forces*. Recall how it is particularly difficult to build up speed while standing on ice; this is because the propulsive force normally generated by plantarflexion cannot be transmitted to the ground due to the lack of friction. Therefore, although one may generate a sufficient plantarflexion moment, it cannot be transmitted to the floor and consequently, the "equal and opposite reaction" (recall Newton's third law) produced by the floor (which moves the body) is reduced. There are also analogous forces in the medial-lateral direction, often referred to as *mediolateral shear forces*. Together, the forces in the three directions comprise the total force.

Preferably two platforms placed adjacent to each other are used so that the total force under each foot can

Table 12-3: Dynamic Electromyography During Normal-Velocity Walking

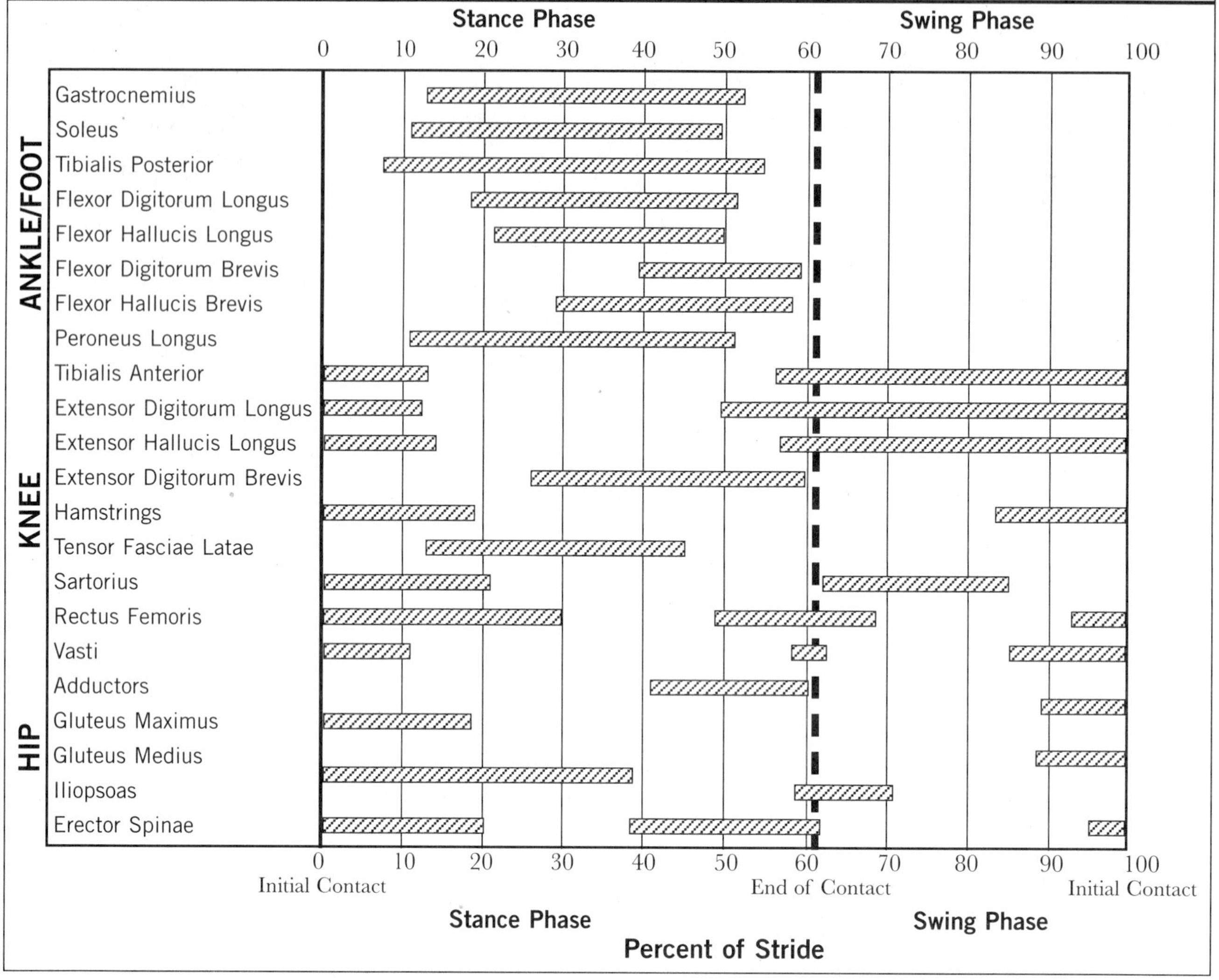

Stance Phase — Swing Phase

0 10 20 30 40 50 60 70 80 90 100

ANKLE/FOOT

- Gastrocnemius
- Soleus
- Tibialis Posterior
- Flexor Digitorum Longus
- Flexor Hallucis Longus
- Flexor Digitorum Brevis
- Flexor Hallucis Brevis
- Peroneus Longus
- Tibialis Anterior
- Extensor Digitorum Longus
- Extensor Hallucis Longus
- Extensor Digitorum Brevis

KNEE

- Hamstrings
- Tensor Fasciae Latae
- Sartorius
- Rectus Femoris
- Vasti

HIP

- Adductors
- Gluteus Maximus
- Gluteus Medius
- Iliopsoas
- Erector Spinae

0 (Initial Contact) 10 20 30 40 50 60 (End of Contact) 70 80 90 100 (Initial Contact)

Stance Phase — Swing Phase

Percent of Stride

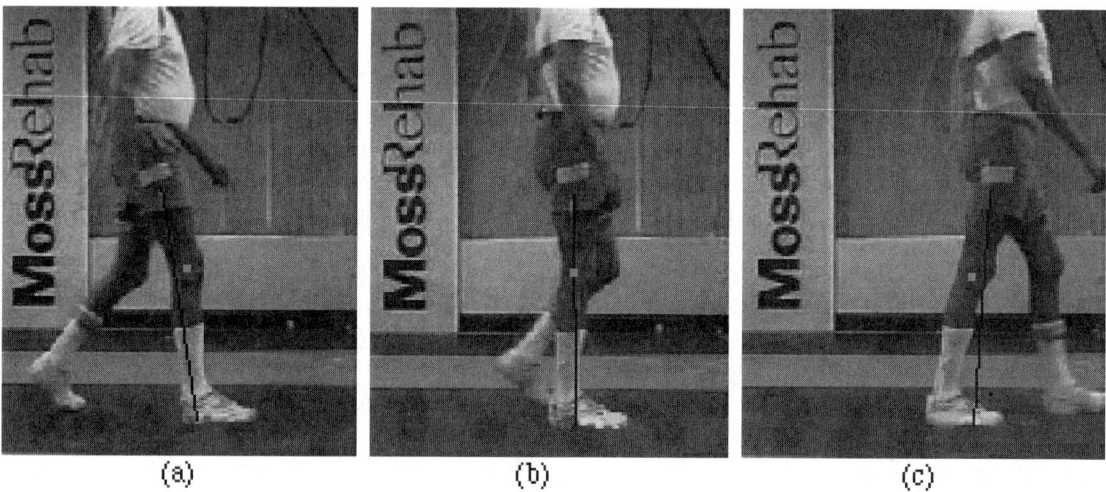

Figure 12-4. Force-line visualization. This series of pictures demonstrates the force-line visualization system, developed at the MossRehab gait laboratory, to estimate stance-phase joint moments. This method offers the advantage of not having to use instrumentation on the subject. The frames taken from video of the subject show how the force-line position changes with respect to the knee center (*bright circle*). *A.* The force line is posterior to the knee center and so the sagittal knee moment is a flexor one. *B.* The line passes through the knee center; the sagittal moment due to the force is roughly zero. *C.* The line is anterior to the knee center; the sagittal moment is an extensor one.

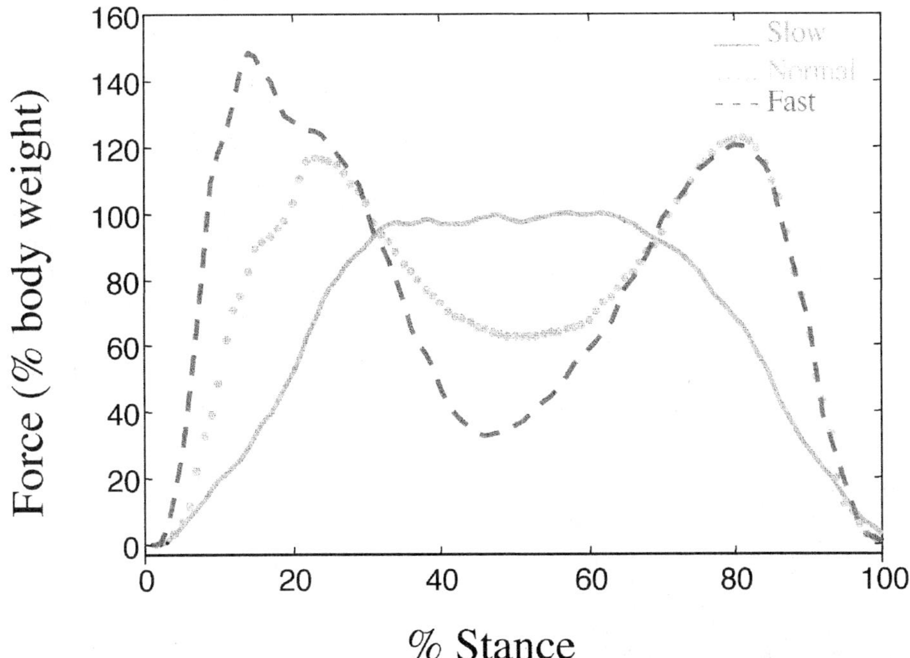

Figure 12-5. Normal force-plate data. For the stance phase, the vertical component of the ground reaction force is shown for three different walking speeds. Note how as walking speed increases, and more acceleration is generated, the vertical force exceeds the body weight. This is the "dynamic effect" of acceleration, which is seen as force.

be recorded independently and simultaneously. In most instances, the force platforms are placed in the midpoint of the walkway used for evaluation so that steady-state walking parameters are measured. The reaction forces are plotted as a function of time or are normalized as a percentage of the stride time. For comparison to standard values, the measured GRFs should be routinely normalized and reported as a percent of body mass (Fig. 12-5).

It is useful to know the *magnitude* of the total force for comparing profiles, and the *location* of that total force for computing joint moments and powers (see the end of the section on kinematics). The product of the magnitude of the GRF under each foot and its location with respect to a given joint center (hip, knee, ankle) are major factors that determine the moments, or torque produced by the external force about that joint. This moment characterizes the direction and magnitude of the tendency of the external force to produce joint rotation (flexion/extension, abduction/adduction, internal/external rotation). Internal forces, generated primarily by muscles and to a lesser degree by tendons, ligaments, and the geometry of the joint articulation (bony contact), act to control the rotation of the joints caused by this external force. These concepts are explained in more detail in the section on kinematics.

Whereas force plates measure the sum or total force acting under the entire foot, it is sometimes useful to measure discrete components of that force acting over specific areas of the foot, or the distribution of pressure. The characteristics of the contact surface may have profound effects on the gait pattern. A given force acting over an area produces larger pressures than the same force distributed over a large area. Pressure is defined as a force acting over a certain area. Mathematically, pressure = force/area. The forces generated at the point of contact with the floor (floor-foot or -shoe interface) can be measured with force platforms as just described. Measurement of the forces as they occur inside the shoe necessitates the use of devices that can be placed inside the footwear without disturbing the foot-shoe interface. Ultrathin mylar pressure sensors such as those produced by TekScan are very useful for this purpose. Figure 12-6 shows an actual pressure distribution measured with such a sensor. Height and color of the contour lines are used to designate absolute values of average pressure acting at a finite area of the foot. These devices have clinical value, particularly in the assessment of the insensate or painful foot and in the evaluation and fitting of customized ankle-foot or foot orthotics.

Kinematics

A kinematic analysis refers to the time and space aspects of the patterns of motion, regardless of what forces are required to produce those motions.

Temporal and Spatial Descriptive Measures

A relatively simple and summarized (integrated) method is used to quantify some useful gait parameters. Temporal-spatial footfall patterns are the end product of the total integrated locomotor movement. To characterize gait, basic variables concerning the temporal-spatial sequencing of the stance and swing phases can be measured by determining the distances and timing involved in the floor contacts of the feet. Several techniques are available and include the use of ink and paper, foot switches, instrumented walkways, and other more sophisticated systems that require patient instrumentation. Our laboratory uses the electronic Gait Mat (Fig. 12-7) (13). The mat, measuring 4 m in length, contains over 10,000 electronic switches that record foot contact and generates a timed "electronic footprint" without the need of applying any instrumentation to the subject. A printout that provides calculated data about walking velocity, cadence, and stance and swing times for each foot, as well as stride lengths, step lengths, and the width of the base of support is generated (Fig. 12-8) (9,11). By comparing the timing parameters with normative data matched for gender, age, and walking velocity, a clear determination of the level of dysfunction can be made. When the parameters of the two legs are compared, measures of symmetry can be obtained to determine the extent of unilateral impairment.

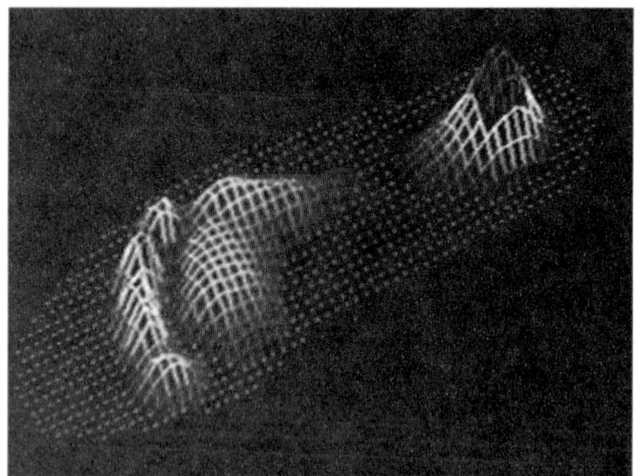

Figure 12-6. Three-dimensional view of F scan foot forces and sensors. In this view, the pressure distribution under the foot is shown as a snapshot in time. The height of the peaks corresponds to the magnitude of the pressure levels. Other views may make use of contour lines and color schemes to display pressure magnitudes and gradients. Usually a continually changing trace is recorded as a patient walks with the sensor in the shoe.

Motion Analysis

Motion analysis refers to a quantitative description of the motion of body segments without regard for the forces generating it. Current state-of-the-art techniques involve imaging of markers placed on the body. A camera is generally used to track the markers on the body as the subject moves through a predetermined field of view and then computerized mathematical triangulation is performed to calculate three-dimensional (3-D) motion. Earlier techniques included photographic and cinematographic analyses. Other techniques include the use of accelerometers and electrogoniometers.

Most modern systems involve the use of high-speed video recording or a specialized optoelectronic apparatus in which passive or active optical sources (e.g., infrared-reflecting or emitting diodes) attached to the subject serve as markers. Cameras or detectors track each marker as it

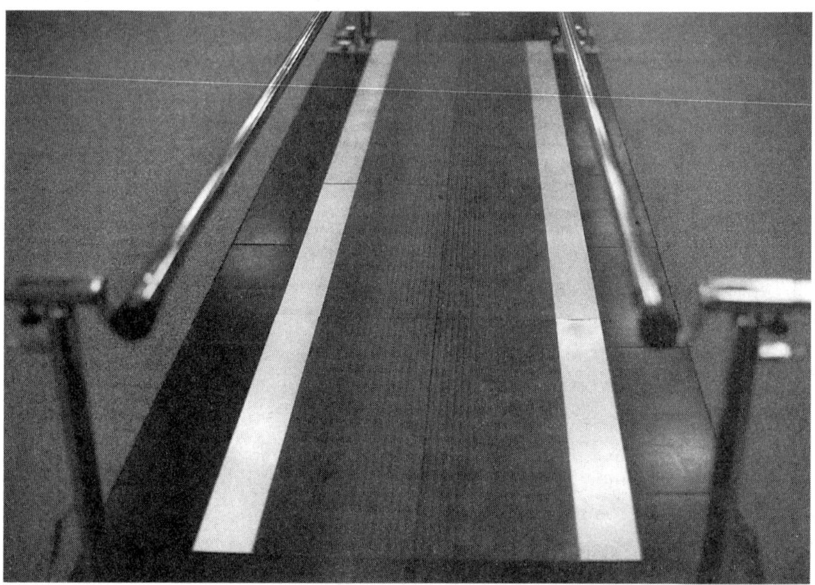

Figure 12-7. The Gait Mat, a series of 10,000 switches, used to measure temporal-spatial footfall parameters. Notice the sensors are flush with the floor and run between the parallel bars along a segment of the 10-m-long walkway.

moves with the subject. When two or more cameras or detectors identify the same marker, 3-D coordinates can be generated by mathematical triangulation, in a manner analogous to how the human eyes and brain use input from both eyes to perceive depth in the field of vision. Video and passive optoelectronic systems are unique in their capacity to record with minimal instrumentation applied to the subject (passive systems). All markers placed on a subject are "illuminated" by an external power source, and are thus tracked by the detector (camera). Automatic marker identification and digitization are reliable if the markers do not cross. However, conversion into quantitative data can require some manual intervention for marker identification. Manual digitization/tracking of the raw data can be error prone and on occasions time-consuming (9,14). Other problems with passive systems include the limited sampling rate with video and the need for enhanced lighting with high-speed video cameras. With active optoelectronic systems, each marker is self-illuminated (hence, the designation "active") and no post-collection marker identification is needed. The synchronization of time between marker illumination and detection uniquely identifies each light-emitting diode (14) as each marker is "on" at a slightly different (on the order of microseconds) instant in time. A disadvantage of the active system is the connection wires required to power each marker. The wires can be arranged in such a way that they are less encumbering and may be combined with telemetry transmitters to reduce the clutter and entangling; however, the wires often hinder high-velocity motion.

Once the marker trajectories are available as 3-D data, they can be processed and displayed as a function of time or as a percent of the stride period. Joint angles, linear and angular velocities, and accelerations are some of the commonly calculated parameters. When combined with anthropometric measures and kinetic (force) data, joint moments and powers as well as mechanical energy and energy transfer can be calculated. The physical meaning behind the values for these parameters should be clearly understood if they are to provide any diagnostic information.

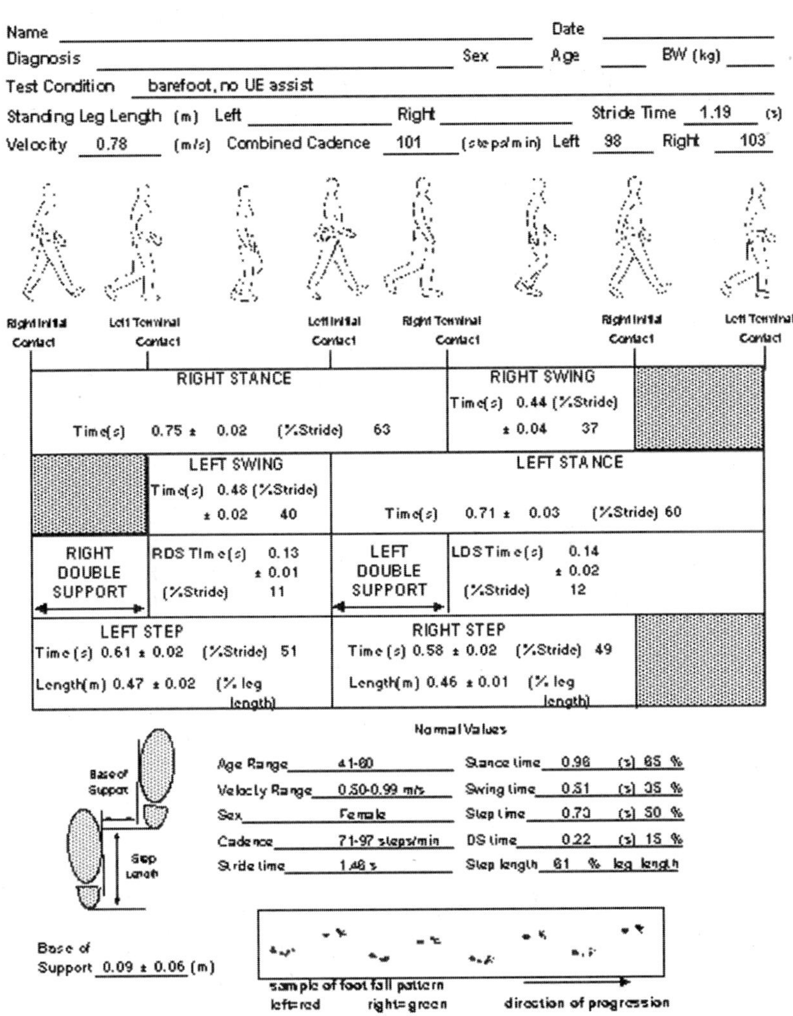

MossRehab Gait & Motion Analysis Laboratory

Name ______ Date ______
Diagnosis ______ Sex ___ Age ___ BW (kg) ___
Test Condition barefoot, no UE assist
Standing Leg Length (m) Left ______ Right ______ Stride Time 1.19 (s)
Velocity 0.78 (m/s) Combined Cadence 101 (steps/min) Left 98 Right 103

Right Initial Contact — Left Terminal Contact — Left Initial Contact — Right Terminal Contact — Right Initial Contact — Left Terminal Contact

RIGHT STANCE: Time(s) 0.75 ± 0.02 (%Stride) 63
RIGHT SWING: Time(s) 0.44 (%Stride) ± 0.04 37

LEFT SWING: Time(s) 0.48 (%Stride) ± 0.02 40
LEFT STANCE: Time(s) 0.71 ± 0.03 (%Stride) 60

RIGHT DOUBLE SUPPORT: RDS Time(s) 0.13 ± 0.01 (%Stride) 11
LEFT DOUBLE SUPPORT: LDS Time(s) 0.14 ± 0.02 (%Stride) 12

LEFT STEP: Time (s) 0.61 ± 0.02 (%Stride) 51; Length(m) 0.47 ± 0.02 (% leg length)
RIGHT STEP: Time (s) 0.58 ± 0.02 (%Stride) 49; Length(m) 0.46 ± 0.01 (% leg length)

Normal Values

Base of Support — Step Length

Age Range	41-60	Stance time	0.96 (s) 65 %
Velocity Range	0.50-0.99 m/s	Swing time	0.51 (s) 35 %
Sex	Female	Step time	0.73 (s) 50 %
Cadence	71-97 steps/min	DS time	0.22 (s) 15 %
Stride time	1.48 s	Step length	61 % leg length

Base of Support 0.09 ± 0.06 (m)

sample of foot fall pattern left=red right=green

direction of progression

Figure 12-8. Gait Mat data report. A sample of the report sent out with each Gait Mat recording. This report provides information about many important temporal-spatial parameters including step and swing timing and lengths, as well as about symmetry, in a convenient semigraphical format. Patient data can also be compared to gender-, age-, and walking speed–matched normalized normal data, as shown at the bottom right of the form.

The product of a force acting at a distance is defined as a *moment* (or *torque*). Imagine a 5-lb weight hanging on a yardstick. If we hold the stick at one end and hang the weight 1 inch from where we are holding it, we will exert much less effort (force) to keep the stick level than if the 5-lb weight were at the other end of the stick. In this example, the moment arm (distance from force to the wrist joint center) was increased. Alternatively, we could have kept the location of the weight the same, but changed the weight to a 50-lb weight. This would also have increased the amount of effort required to keep the stick horizontal. The same factors are at work in the lower-extremity joints during gait.

The GRF, which is a reflection of the body weight and the acceleration of the body, produces moments about the ankle, knee, hip, and spine that must be countered and controlled by the muscles (Fig. 12-9). For example, the GRF can produce a moment that tends to drive the knee into flexion or extension or that does not affect the knee (if the line of action of the force passes right through the center of knee joint rotation). Note, for a system in motion (or more correctly, one that is accelerating—as the body is at all times during even slow and "constant"-speed gait), the product of force multiplied by distance is only an estimate of the total moment (although it is a significant part that must be stabilized).

The other components are due to the products of the accelerations and masses of individual lower-limb segments. This phenomenon can be clarified by recalling the force felt when taking a turn in a car. How much force you produce on the arm rest as you take a right turn depends on how fast (related to acceleration) you are turning, how much you weigh (mass), and how that mass is distributed. Whereas the product of force and distance only provides an estimate of the total moment, the product of mass and acceleration contributes a relatively small component to the total. During the stance phase of normal-speed walking, the error caused by omitting the mass acceleration products is roughly 1% for the ankle, 5% for the knee, and 8% for the hip. While it should not be forgotten that the force-distance product provides only an estimate, it provides a fairly accurate, quick, and simple basis from which to make comparisons and decisions, when its limitations are realized.

CLINICAL APPLICATIONS

Gait is the first aspect of most physical examinations. The patient's walking pattern is observed as he or she enters the examination room. Findings from this visual inspection may be useful in eliciting symptoms and guiding the physical examination. Gait analysis can be used to evaluate the dynamic basis for an observed gait deviation. Gait analysis and accurate clinical diagnosis can be used to select appropriate interventions and to guide a gait retraining program.

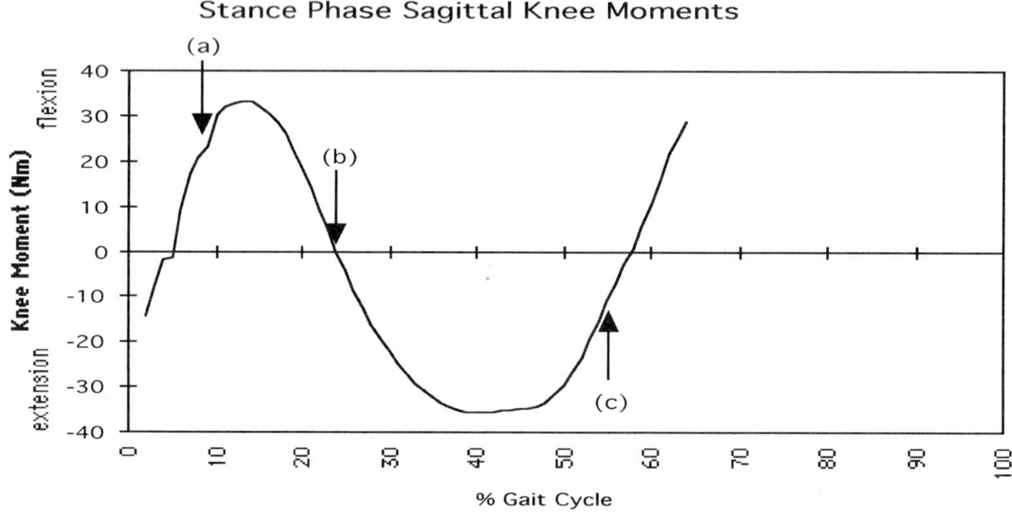

Figure 12-9. Estimating moments from the force line. The actual calculated knee moment from fully instrumented analysis. One of the main advantages of the force line is that it allows estimation of this calculated joint moment without having to use instrumentation on the subject. A comparison to calculated moments from a fully instrumented analysis corroborated in value of the force-line estimation technique in determining polarity and relative magnitude of the joint moment. Areas on the curve labeled (a), (b), and (c) correspond to Figure 13-5A, B, and C. Simple measurements of the height of the line and the perpendicular distance from the knee center can be made to obtain a more quantitative estimate of the moment. However, this method still is capable of providing only an approximation because additional forces and moments produced due to the acceleration of limb segments cannot be accounted for, and so swing-phase moments cannot be estimated either. Please see the CD-ROM due out with this book for a video clip with more details.

It is also a valuable aid to objectively assess the impact of various treatment interventions and to develop objective criteria for selecting different long-term management options. Evaluation can be performed prior to and following a therapeutic intervention, to help assess the effectiveness of a treatment. As noted, the first step is to determine the basis for the gait deviation.

In patients with a pathologic gait, it is imperative to differentiate an obligatory or primary deviation from a compensatory one. This allows treatment to be targeted at the correct level, and allows treatment interventions to be most effective and efficient. For example, the presence of hallux hyperextension during gait can be the result of compensation for insufficient ankle dorsiflexion provided by the tibialis anterior or of an obligatory reflexive toe extension posture. This differentiation can be best accomplished through gait analysis, interpreted by an experienced clinician. Gait analysis is a useful and at times indispensable tool to gather information with which to uncover the underlying functional deficits and to subsequently plan the most efficient treatment options.

Interventions typically include the following:

1. Specific stretching and strengthening exercises to a given muscle group or joint.
2. Systemic or local pharmacologic intervention (e.g., diagnostic nerve blocks, chemodenervation). For chronic neurologic impairment, gait analysis together with selective nerve and motor point blocks can be used to differentiate fixed contractures (static deformity) from muscular overactivity or spasticity (dynamic deformity).
3. Application or modification of an orthosis; use of a special shoe, lift, or wedge; or realignment of a prosthesis.
4. Use of a walking aid and selecting its optimal application (e.g., cane or walker and which hand to hold).

Evaluation may sometimes be directed toward the development of rational criteria for specific surgical interventions such as tendon releases and transfers. For example, a spastic equinovarus posture can result from several distinct dynamic patterns (i.e., overactivity of gastrocnemius-soleus and tibialis anterior or tibialis posterior or EHL) that can be differentiated with gait analysis and dynamic EMG. In all cases, gait analysis is useful to determine a felicitous course of action, as well as to evaluate the results after intervention.

A clear knowledge of factors that gives rise to pathologic gait make it easier to understand the basis for observed deviations and potential treatment interventions. Pathologic gait can result from a variety of clinical conditions, and can be broken down into three major classes of etiologies: joint and soft-tissue pathology (arthritis or soft-tissue contractures), structural (musculoskeletal deformities such as limb amputation), and neurologic disorders (pathology of the peripheral and/or central nervous system).

PATHOLOGIC GAIT

The three functional goals of locomotion (to move from one place to another, to move safely, and to move efficiently) are frequently compromised in the patient with pathologic gait. Patients often have problems with ambulation because of inefficient movement strategies, decreased safety, and the presence of pain due to abnormal limb postures. The compensatory movements necessary for ambulation produce abnormal exaggerated displacement of the center of gravity, resulting in increased energy expenditure. Pain, instability, impaired balance, sensory deficits, weakness, inadequate limb clearance, and limb deformities all contribute to increased anxiety regarding ambulation, frequent loss of balance, and possible falls.

When a patient with a complex multifactorial gait dysfunction presents for management, gait analysis should be utilized to better understand the nature and source of the problem. In many laboratories the initial method of gait analysis involves the measurement of spatial and temporal parameters and video recording. A high-quality video that can be reviewed in slow motion with clear freeze frame can be extremely valuable to a well-trained eye. A special effects generator can allow a split-screen image with frontal and sagittal views simultaneously. After initial evaluation of the patient's gait pattern, objective kinematic, kinetic, and EMG data are obtained when necessary.

A comparison of normal gait patterns to those exhibited by individuals with pathology demonstrates differences in temporal, kinetic, and kinematic factors and muscle activity patterns. Although differences exist from patient to patient based on their pathology and ability to compensate, some generalizations can be made. These include a decrease in walking velocity with asymmetric stance and swing phases and decreased weight bearing for the involved limb.

From a functional perspective, gait deficiencies can be categorized with respect to the gait cycle. During the stance phase, an abnormal base of support (e.g., ankle instability), knee instability (e.g., knee buckling or hyperextension), and hip instability (e.g., hip flexion or adduction) may make walking unsafe, inefficient, and frequently painful. During the swing phase, inadequate limb clearance (e.g., toe drag) and impairment of limb advancement (e.g., limited hip and/or knee flexion and ankle dorsiflexion) may interfere with safety and energy efficiency.

It is useful to identify during which subphase of the gait cycle (i.e., initial or terminal stance) and where in the body (i.e., ankle or hip) the primary abnormal behavior is noted. The results will point to the source of the problem. Determining if this is an obligatory (primary) problem or a compensation is paramount, as this will determine the best treatment approach. In addition, knowing the appropriate available interventions and obtaining a thorough medical, cognitive, and social history of the patient are necessary to determine the most appropriate treatment course.

Abnormalities of gait caused by muscle weakness can be addressed through muscle strengthening exercises or by the use of orthotic devices, or by both approaches. Gait analysis should permit minimization of the orthotic intervention and optimization of its alignment. In the patient with limited joint range of motion such as ankle equinus, appropriate accommodation can be achieved with a shoe heel lift. Gait analysis can be used to optimize the shoe modification and achieve more appropriate biomechanics during walking. Patients who use a lower-limb prosthesis often benefit from gait analysis to evaluate the effects of the prosthetic alignment, the height, and the settings at the knee and ankle. With this information one can determine what modifications should be made to enhance the settings.

Surgery to address gait dysfunction should be considered only after a careful gait analysis, including dynamic poly-EMG, is completed, to determine which muscles require intervention. This is particularly important for patients with spastic hemiplegia or diplegia such as that caused by cerebrovascular accident, craniocerebral trauma, or static encephalopathy. It is also used for other conditions that may result in muscle imbalance, such as muscular dystrophy, spina bifida, and spinal cord injury.

GAIT DYSFUNCTION CATEGORIZATION

Stance-phase dysfunction can be categorized into three groups:

1. Abnormal base of support: equinus or equinovarus, ankle valgus with or without equinus, toe flexion, hallux extension (hitchhiker's great toe);
2. Limb instability: excessive ankle dorsiflexion during stance, flexed or hyperextended knee (although it may be a compensatory response to avoid limb instability like that seen with excessive uncontrolled knee flexion, excessive hyperextension and painful hyperextension may be inherently unstable), valgus or varus knee, adducted hip, flexed hip;
3. Trunk instability: as seen with hip abductor or extensor weakness.

Swing-phase dysfunction involves two groups:

1. Impaired limb clearance: drop foot, stiff knee, limited hip flexion, adducted hip;
2. Limb advancement: stiff knee, limited hip flexion or contralateral extension, adducted hips.

Abnormal Base of Support

Equinovarus Foot Deformity

This abnormal posture is most frequently seen in the lower limb after an upper- or lower-motor-neuron injury. The deformity may also be the result of ankle immobilization, fractures, or surgery. The foot and ankle are in a toe-down and frequently turned-in position and toe curling may coexist. The patient complains of pain over the lateral border of the foot during weight bearing. The concept of an abnormal or unstable base of support can be explained in a comparison with a person using shoes with wide heels or shoes with narrow, high heels. During gait, contact with the ground occurs first with the forefoot; weight is borne primarily on the anterior and lateral border of the foot and may be concentrated in the area of the fifth metatarsal. Toe flexion may be present, particularly in patients with neurologic injuries or with a plantarflexion contracture. Limited dorsiflexion during mid-stance prevents forward progression of the tibia over the stationary foot, increasing pressure over the metatarsals, promoting ankle instability, and causing knee hyperextension. Compensatory hip flexion may occur. An ankle equinus posture during late stance and pre-swing interferes with rollover, push-off, and forward propulsion. During the swing phase, sustained plantarflexion and inversion of the foot may result in a limb clearance problem that may necessitate compensation. The presence of an inadequate base of support results in instability of the whole body and correction of the problem is essential, even for limited ambulation.

For the patient with residual of a neurologic injury, an imbalance between muscles, including the tibialis anterior, tibialis posterior, long toe flexors, gastrocnemius, soleus, EHL, and peroneus longus, can potentially contribute to this deformity. Clinical examination combined with kinetics, kinematics, and dynamic EMG recordings will elucidate the cause of the deformity. Dynamic EMG often demonstrates prolonged activation of the gastrocnemius-soleus complex and the long toe flexors as the most frequent cause of plantarflexion. Inversion is the result of abnormal activity in the tibialis posterior or anterior muscles, combined with the gastrocnemius-soleus group and sometimes the EHL. In some patients, ankle inversion may result from a lack of activity in the peroneal group during the stance phase. When it is difficult to differentiate between the contributions of the tibialis anterior and tibialis posterior to the varus deformity, a diagnostic tibial nerve block with lidocaine should be performed. If the deformity is corrected, then the tibialis posterior is the offending muscle.

Equinovalgus Foot

Equinovalgus foot can be caused by a number of different problems including limited ankle dorsiflexion (particularly in the child or young adult), upper- or lower-motor-neuron injury, bony and ligamentous injuries, surgery, and prolonged immobilization with loss of range of motion. The foot and ankle are turned out and toe flexion may be present as well. The patient may complain of pain over the medial aspect of the foot (first metatarsal). During gait, contact with the ground occurs with the forefoot and weight is borne primarily on the medial aspect of the foot. This position is maintained or worsened during the stance phase and interferes with weight bearing. If present, limited dorsiflexion prevents forward progression of the tibia over the stationary foot and increases the valgus posture, the result of a compensatory mechanism at the subtalar joint. If the deformity is severe, a leg-length discrepancy may be evident and ankle and subtalar joint pain is reported. Knee hyperextension can be seen during early stance and lack of push-off and forward propulsion may be seen during terminal stance and per-swing. During the swing phase, sustained plantarflexion of the foot may result in a limb clearance problem unless proximal mechanisms of compensation such as increased hip and knee flexion are used.

Muscles that can potentially contribute to valgus include the peroneus longus, peroneus brevis, tibialis anterior, tibialis posterior, gastrocnemius, soleus, and the long toe flexors. Combined with clinical and radiographic examination, dynamic EMG recordings at a minimum from these muscles provide greater detail in understanding the cause of the deformity. The EMG recordings may demonstrate prolonged activation of the peroneus longus or brevis. In some cases, a lack of activity in the tibialis anterior or posterior may be the cause of the problem. Joint instability and ligamentous laxity can also be present. If the deformity is muscular in nature and due to an upper-motor-neuron injury, it may be difficult to differentiate between the valgus contribution of the peroneus longus and peroneus brevis; for this, a diagnostic lidocaine motor point block to one of them could be performed.

Flexion Deformity of the Toes

The toes are held in flexion during the stance phase. Likely causes are neurologic injuries, reflex sympathetic dystrophy, prolonged immobilization, and contractures. Ankle equinus and varus may accompany this abnormal foot posture. When wearing shoes, the patient complains of pain at the tip of the toes and also over the dorsum of the phalangeal joints. Callus formation that interferes with weight bearing is frequently seen. The patient will alter walking to gradually load the limb and shorten the step length and stance time on the affected side. There is interference with push-off and forward propulsion during terminal stance and pre-swing. Frequently the patient will use corn pads or the shoe is stretched in the toe box area in an attempt to relieve pressure.

Muscles that frequently contribute to this deformity are the flexor digitorum longus (FDL) and flexor hallucis longus (FHL). Equinus deformity may also contribute to this deformity, as shortening of the toe flexors may be more evident when the ankle is dorsiflexed (tenodesis effect). Clinical examination combined with kinetics and dynamic EMG recordings can be helpful in sorting out the cause of the deformity. In patients with spasticity, the recordings likely will demonstrate prolonged or out-of-phase activation of the FDL and FHL and may demonstrate abnormal activation of the gastrocnemius-soleus or lack of activation of the toe extensors.

Hitchhiker's Great Toe

This deformity is a notable problem in patients with upper-motor-neuron complication. The great toe is held in extension during the stance and frequently during the swing phase. Equinus and varus posture of the ankle may accompany this deformity. When wearing shoes, the patient complains of pain at the dorsum and the tip of the big toe, and during the weight-bearing phase of the gait cycle, under the first metatarsal head. During gait, toe extension is maintained during early stance and mid-stance, interfering with weight bearing. The patient will shorten the limb stance time of the affected limb and there is interference with push-off and forward propulsion during terminal stance and pre-swing. During the swing phase, there may be sustained hallux extension. Frequently the shoe is cut out in the toe box area in an attempt to relieve the pain produced by pressure.

Muscles that frequently contribute to this deformity are the EHL and lack of FHL. Dynamic EMG recordings combined with clinical examination are helpful to elucidate the source of the deformity and whether its nature is obligatory or compensatory in nature. EMG recordings should be obtained at a minimum from the EHL and FHL, tibialis anterior and posterior, gastrocnemius, and soleus. The recordings likely will demonstrate prolonged or out-of-phase activation of the EHL and may demonstrate abnormal activation of the tibialis anterior and gastrocnemius-soleus group. In some patients, a lack of activity of the FHL may be encountered.

In the population with acquired neurologic pathology, the clinical pattern of abnormality usually will be common to both legs. At times the biomechanical cause of the deformity may be different. Figure 12-10 demonstrates bilateral EMG recordings of the tibialis anterior and posterior in a patient with symmetric bilateral equinovarus deformity. The recordings show significant activation of the left tibialis anterior and minimal activation of the left tibialis posterior during passive eversion of the foot by the clinical examiner. The pattern is reversed for the right leg, with increased activation of the tibialis posterior being observed. These findings are critical, as treatment interventions will differ based on the source of the problem.

Figure 12-10. Bilateral electromyographic recordings of tibialis anterior and tibialis posterior in a patient with symmetric bilateral equinovarus deformity (*A*). During the first 1.5 to 2.0 seconds of the recordings shown, the foot was passively everted by the clinical examiner. The recordings (*B*) show significant activation of the left tibialis anterior and minimal activation of the left tibialis posterior during this time period. The pattern is reversed for the right leg, with increased activation of the tibialis posterior being observed.

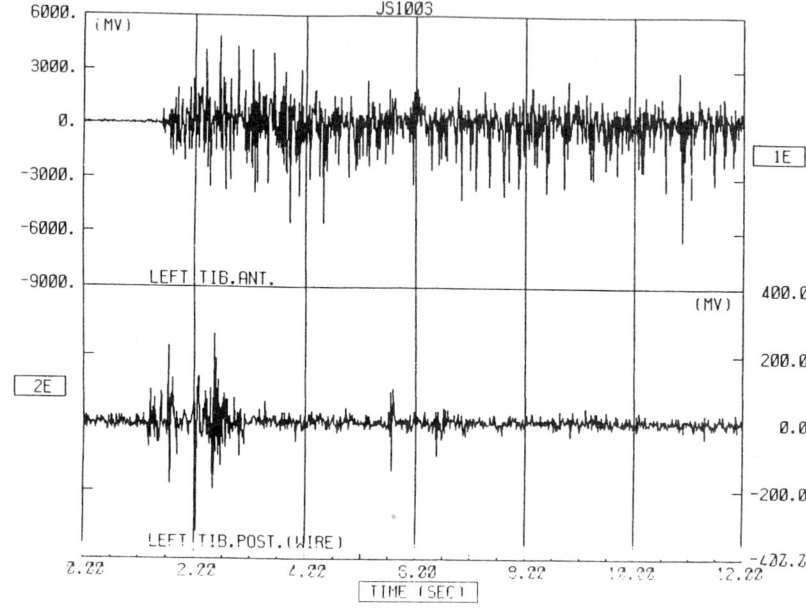

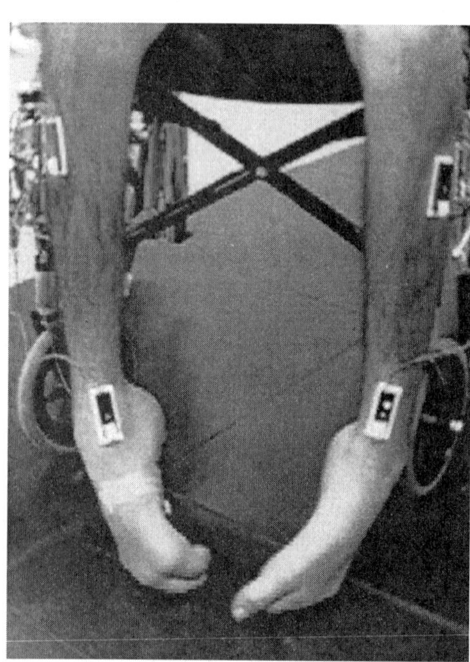

A

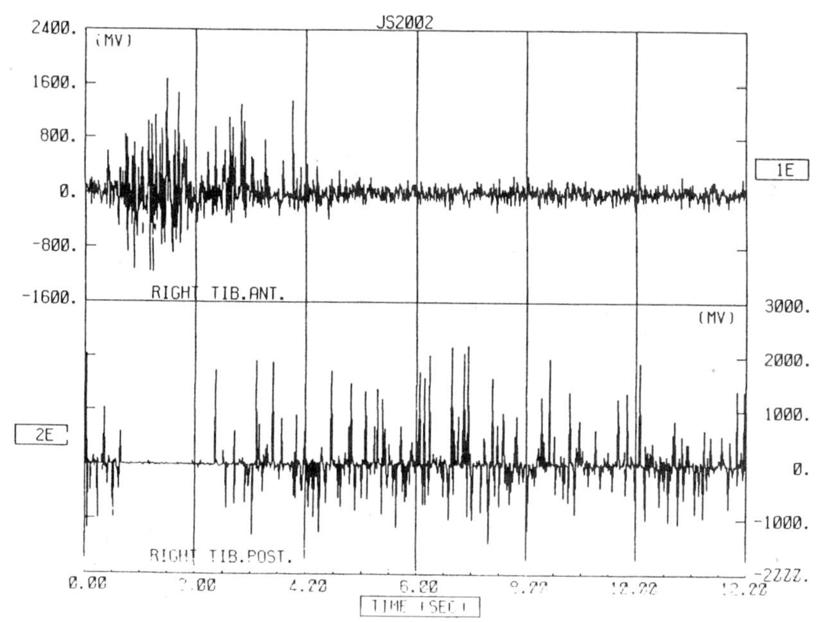

B

Limb Instability

Limb instability can produce knee collapse or hyperextension. This may occur when normal knee flexion during the early-stance phase is combined with quadriceps weakness, as may be seen in persons with knee extensor weakness, lower-motor-neuron syndrome, or quadriceps tendon rupture. It may also be observed in the early phase of recovery after upper-motor-neuron injury when flaccidity and weakness affect the involved limb. The patient may not produce the normally expected, full knee extension during either the swing or the stance phase, further compromising limb stability. A flexed knee during the stance phase requires compensatory ipsilateral hip flexion and contralateral knee and hip flexion that results in a crouched gait. This results in a marked increase in energy consumption and muscle fatigue and pain. If knee buckling occurs, the patient may require the upper extremity for support. The lack of full knee extension during terminal swing limits limb advancement and reduces step length.

Drop-off Gait

This deviation is caused by excessive untimely forward progression of the tibia in the mid- to late-stance phase. This is usually the result of insufficient calf musculature, which controls the forward progression of the tibia over the stationary foot. The patient may be noted to have premature knee flexion with a resulting contralateral reduction in step length, delayed ipsilateral heel-off, and rollover. However, the patient may mask the early knee flexion with prolonged quadriceps activation during the stance phase to stabilize the knee, and this may actually result in delayed ipsilateral knee flexion. Such a compensation may result in overuse syndrome of the knee extensor mechanism. If knee buckling occurs with fatigue, the patient may require the upper extremities for support.

Muscles that can potentially contribute to drop-off gait include the gastrocnemius-soleus and quadriceps. Manual muscle testing of the ankle plantarflexors, kinetic and kinematic data, and dynamic EMG recordings may be necessary to understand the cause of the deformity. Recordings may demonstrate abnormal prolonged activation of the rectus femoris and other quadriceps. Overactivation of the hip extensors may promote knee stability during stance phase.

Knee Hyperextension

Compensation for knee weakness is a potential cause of the opposite gait deviation, knee hyperextension. Knee hyperextension may also be present in the stance phase as a result of a plantarflexion contracture, ankle equinus produced by increased activity of the gastrocnemius-soleus group, or spasticity of the plantarflexor group. Marked weakness of this muscle group can produce drop-off gait for which the patient may compensate through knee hyperextension. Spasticity of the knee extensors and forward trunk flexion may be another cause for knee hyperextension during the stance phase. In the patient with forward trunk flexion, the force line is moved anterior to the knee joint center (Fig. 12-11). This abnormal posture of the knee prevents adequate contralateral limb advancement, resulting in decreased step length.

Muscles that can force the knee into hyperextension include the gluteus maximus, iliopsoas, quadriceps, and gastrocnemius-soleus with equinus posture. Manual muscle testing, kinetic and kinematic evaluation, dynamic EMG recordings, and measurements of ankle, knee, and hip ranges of motion may be indicated to discern the cause of the deformity. Dynamic poly-EMG of the quadriceps demonstrates prolonged, shortened, or out-of-phase activities. Occasionally, increased activity of the knee flexors, the hip extensors, and the ankle plantarflexors during the stance phase is also seen.

Trunk Instability

Excessive Hip Flexion

Excessive hip flexion during the stance phase is a less common gait deviation. It is characterized by sustained hip flexion that interferes with limb positioning during gait. During the stance phase, excessive hip flexion interferes with contralateral limb advancement and results in a shortened step length. Trunk instability can result from hip extensor weakness; limited hip extension as compensation for knee extensor weakness and ankle plantarflexor posture; and hip flexor spasticity. Hip hiking and contralateral trunk lean may compensate for decreased limb advancement and swing-phase clearance problems. Possible causes include degenerative changes of the hip joint, bony deformities such as heterotopic ossification, knee extensor weakness and ankle plantarflexor posture, hip flexion contractures, and flexor spasticity. For trunk instability due to flexor spasticity, the potentially contributing muscles include the iliopsoas, pectineus, rectus femoris, gluteus maximus, hip adductors, and gluteus medius.

Dynamic EMG should be obtained at a minimum from the muscles previously mentioned and the hamstrings. Recordings may demonstrate overactivity of the iliopsoas and the hip adductor musculature or imbalance between the hip flexor and extensor muscle groups as the main cause of this problem. Degenerative joint disease or heterotopic bone formation should be ruled out.

Hip Adduction

Hip adduction may occur during the swing phase and interfere with limb clearance and advancement. This deviation results in a narrow base of support (feet together) during stance with potential impairment of balance. Hip adduction and associated mechanisms can interfere with a patient's hygiene, dressing, toileting, and sexuality. Muscles that potentially contribute to this deformity include the hip adductors, hip abductors, iliopsoas, pectineus, and sartorius. Kinetic and kinematic studies and dynamic EMG recordings are necessary to understand the cause of the deformity. EMG should be obtained at a minimum from the muscles previously mentioned, along with the medial hamstrings and gluteus maximus. Recordings may demonstrate imbalance between the hip abductor and adductor muscle groups or demonstrate overactivity in the hip adductor musculature as the main cause of this problem. Decreased activity may be present in the hip flexors and extensors.

Since many patients may compensate for hip flexion weakness by using the hip adductors to advance the limb during the swing phase, the clinician needs to be certain that elimination or reduction of adductor activity does not render the patient nonambulatory. A temporary diagnostic obturator nerve block may provide critical information on this issue.

Limb Clearance and Advancement

Limb clearance and advancement occur during the swing phase of gait and are vital precursors for proper limb positioning so the leg can accept the body weight. When limb clearance is inadequate, limb advancement is usually compromised. Impaired limb clearance may cause a patient to trip and fall, particularly when walking on uneven,

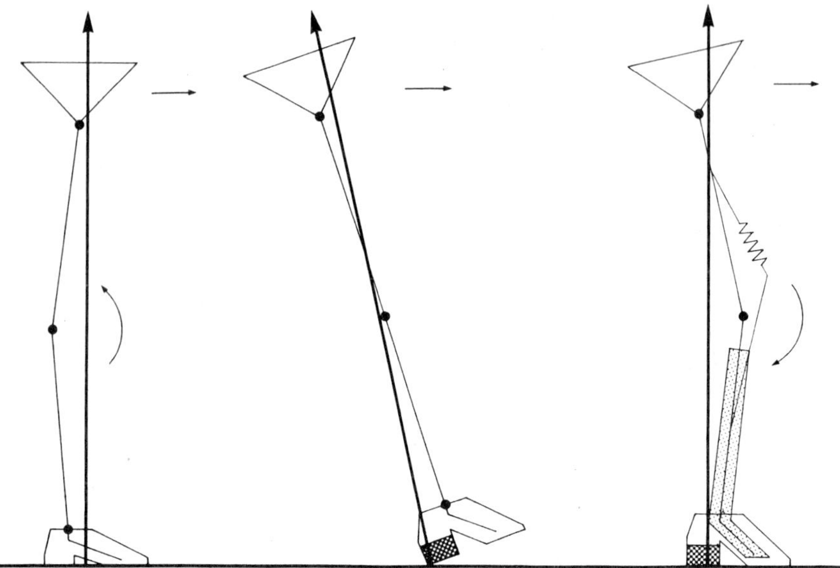

Figure 12-11. Effect of heel lift or ankle-foot orthosis in combination with a heel lift to control knee hyperextension. In the *left* illustration, the force (*thick arrow*) is shown passing anteriorly to the knee center, pushing the knee into extension. In the *middle*, a heel lift is shown to move the force posterior to the knee and thus keep it in flexion. On the *right*, an ankle-foot orthosis is shown (dotted box surrounding foot and shank combined with the spring on the anterior of the thigh) to keep the knee in flexion without allowing excessive and unstable flexion in late stance, by pulling the knee toward extension and by prohibiting the shank from rotating too far forward.

inclined, or carpeted surfaces. In the patient with residual of stroke or brain injury, the most common causes of limb clearance problems are lack of adequate hip flexion, knee flexion, and ankle dorsiflexion. Both total joint displacement and synchronization of motion between the involved joints are essential for adequate limb clearance. The clinician needs to recognize the importance of coordinated lower-limb motion during the swing phase of gait. For the amputee and wearer of an orthotic appliance, excessive ankle plantarflexion or knee friction may be to blame.

Stiff Knee Gait

Stiff knee gait is most commonly seen in the patient with spastic hemiplegia. Use of a locked transfemoral prosthesis or a locked knee brace is another cause of this gait deviation. In the stiff knee gait pattern, the knee is kept extended in the swing phase, instead of flexing up to the approximate normal 60 degrees of flexion. At times a reduced arc of motion for the knee may be present but it may be delayed in relationship to the gait cycle. The patient's inability to flex the knee adequately results in an increased moment of inertia. The moment of inertia is a measure of the effort needed to swing the leg about the hip, and it is based on the distribution of the mass of the leg. If the leg is extended, there is more mass located at a greater distance from the point of rotation (the hip), and this increases the energy required to initiate the swing phase of the involved limb (15). During the swing phase, the patient will utilize compensatory mechanisms for limb clearance. These include trunk and ipsilateral hip and contralateral limb compensatory motions. Even if the ankle-foot system has an appropriate dorsiflexed position, the lack of adequate limb clearance may result in a foot drag, causing whole-body instability. When this problem is evident in the early-swing phase, it can be corrected only by generating sufficient knee or hip flexion or by increasing the contralateral limb length with a shoe lift, or in the case of a prosthetic limb, by shortening the device. When the foot drags, friction with the floor may reduce limb advancement as well.

Muscles that can potentially contribute to stiff knee gait include the iliopsoas, quadriceps, hamstrings, and hip extensors. In addition, if the ankle is in equinus position or the hip has a flexion deformity (which puts the hip flexors at a mechanical and physiologic disadvantage), the necessary flexion moment for the hip and knee may be reduced or absent. Kinetic, kinematic, and dynamic EMG data are necessary to understand the cause of the deformity. EMG should be obtained at a minimum from the muscles previously noted. One explanation for the problem of stiff knee gait pattern that dynamic EMG helps to clarify is whether increased muscular activity is present in the quadriceps muscles as a group or whether there is preferential activity in part of the quadriceps such as the rectus femoris and vastus intermedius, with or without hamstring co-contraction. Lack of momentum associated with slow walking speed, spastic equinus, and a lack of hip flexion generated by a weak iliopsoas or spastic hip extensors (gluteus maximus or hamstrings) are other possible causes for stiff knee gait.

Increased Hip Adduction

Increased hip adduction can interfere with ipsilateral and contralateral limb advancement and with other activities of daily living such as dressing and hygiene. Overactivity of the adductor musculature and imbalance of the abductor and adductor muscle groups are the main causes of this problem. Since many hemiplegic patients use the adductors to compensate for reduced hip flexion in limb advancement, the clinician needs to be certain that elimination or reduction of adductor activities does not render the patient nonambulatory.

Inadequate Hip Flexion

Inadequate hip flexion is another cause of abnormal limb clearance. This problem effectively prevents physiologic "shortening" of the limb, producing a swing-phase toe drag. Compensatory techniques such as hip external rotation to promote the use of the adductors to advance the limb should be attempted. The use of a shoe lift to cause functional lengthening of the contralateral limb, or the use of a thigh corset with a waist belt to reduce lengthening of the affected limb by gravity in combination with circumduction, can be tried. With the existing technology, electrical stimulation applied directly to the iliopsoas has many problems but may be useful. Stimulation of the hamstrings or the sural nerve of the foot to elicit a flexor withdrawal has been attempted for research purposes, with improvement in some patients.

Drop Foot

Drop foot refers to the lack of ankle dorsiflexion during the swing phase. This may result in impairment of limb clearance unless appropriate compensation is afforded in other anatomic segments such as the knee and hip or by the contralateral limb. The frequent cause of this problem is lack of activation of the tibialis anterior. This may be secondary to a peroneal nerve injury, loss of strength such as that seen in residual of polio, imbalance between ankle plantarflexors and dorsiflexors, or out-of-phase activation of the tibialis anterior in the swing phase of locomotion.

Limb advancement during the swing phase is reduced by the presence of ankle plantarflexion, knee flexion, or hip flexion deformities. Ankle plantarflexion deformities may interfere with contralateral limb advancement. This relates to the inability to move the center of gravity over the stance limb and will necessitate a compensatory mechanism such as knee flexion or the application of a heel lift.

Other Causes

Another common gait deviation in the neurologic and the amputee populations is incomplete knee extension during the late-swing and early-stance phases, resulting from hamstring spasticity, contracture, or in the case of the amputee, excessive resistance to knee extension. This problem interferes with ipsilateral limb advancement resulting in a shortened step length, as the knee is flexed and is not able to easily "reach" the ground. Contralateral limb clearance may also be affected, as a decrease in functional height occurs during the stance phase for the involved limb, requiring increased hip and knee flexion for the uninvolved limb to avoid foot drag.

Pelvic retraction affecting the involved limb during the gait cycle interferes with limb advancement, resulting in a shortened step. Hip flexion deformity affects advancement of the contralateral limb, resulting in a shortened step.

MANAGEMENT OF SPECIFIC GAIT DYSFUNCTIONS

In our laboratory we have developed simple flowcharts to better understand and follow the specific issues that affect the patient with a particular gait problem. Samples of this work are included here. The full process of gait analysis and the thought process that go into assessing a situation, selecting suitable diagnostic techniques, understanding confounding factors, assessing data, and making a treatment decision are broken down in an attempt to clarify the rationale behind each step.

Clinical Feature of the Problem

Equinovarus in terminal swing and stance

Potential Issues

Abnormal base of support, poor balance, unstable gait, inability to transfer full weight bearing to affected limb

Penalties and Manifestations

- Difficulty with balance, impairs weight bearing, decreases weight acceptance, increases loading phase, decreases unloading phase time
- Increases pressure over the lateral portion of the foot, ankle instability, decreased weight bearing in the heel
- Pain on loading, shortens stance time, genu varum and recurvatum thrust
- Interferes with smooth forward progression of the center of gravity, increases vertical displacement of center of gravity, produces a functional leg-length discrepancy, and increases energy consumption
- Interferes with transfers to different surfaces; shortened contralateral step length

Analysis and Differential Diagnosis

- Rule out ankle bony deformity, fracture, and heterotopic ossification.
- Rule out soft-tissue contracture (static) and dynamic deformity (spasticity).
- When possible, determine specific muscle causing the deformity, that is, gastrocnemius, soleus, tibialis anterior, tibialis posterior, EHL, flexor digitorum communis (FDC), and peroneus longus.

Diagnostic Work-up

- Gait analysis

  EMG of gastrocnemius, soleus, tibialis anterior, tibialis posterior, EHL, FDC, peroneus longus

  3-D motion analysis to quantify ankle equinus and if possible ankle varus

  GRF analysis to quantify anterior-posterior, medial-lateral shear and vertical forces
- Passive and active range of motion while in bed, sitting, and standing
- Sensory examination, including proprioception
- Motor control, especially of the proximal joints
- Rule out ataxia (trunk versus limb)
- Standing balance if possible; if not, kneeling balance
- Determine limb advancement capability while standing or kneeling
- Temporary diagnostic percutaneous tibial nerve block to differentiate static and dynamic deformity; may unmask gait potential, if previous surgery has been done
- X-ray studies to rule out bony abnormality (heterotopic ossification, fracture, subluxation, or dislocation)

Findings

- EMG demonstrates gastrocnemius and/or soleus to have abnormal activation (out of phase) in swing phase or throughout the gait cycle.
- Activation of tibialis anterior is increased during swing or abnormal during stance phase.
- Activation of FHL and FDC is increased during swing or abnormal during stance phase.
- Activation of tibialis posterior is abnormal in swing or prolonged in stance phase.
- Activation of EHL is increased in swing or abnormal in stance phase, most commonly to supplement tibialis anterior or because of increased tone.
- Activation of peroneus longus is increased in stance or abnormal in swing phase.
- GRF analysis demonstrates abnormal medial-lateral and anterior-posterior shear forces and reduction in loading phase and peak vertical force.
- Temporary diagnostic percutaneous tibial nerve block results in increased ankle dorsiflexion, indicating a dynamic deformity (spasticity) without contracture. One can expect an increase in ankle dorsiflexion strength.
- If varus persists during the swing phase, the most likely cause is the tibialis anterior or extensor hallucis longus.
- No significant change in range of motion after a block indicates a static deformity (contracture).

Treatment Options

An ankle-foot orthosis or molded ankle-foot orthosis can be used to control the equinus and with appropriate components, the inversion and toe flexion. If ankle clonus is present, articulated braces should not be used, but instead a rigid device can be used. If the deformity is dynamic in origin, a percutaneous motor point block with phenol should be considered if injury occurred in last 6 to 12 months, followed by aggressive stretching of ankle plantarflexors and strengthening of ankle dorsiflexors. If the deformity is static in origin, Achilles tendon lengthening or intramuscular lengthening is indicated. Toe flexor release and transfer to the oscalcis is commonly done to avoid forefoot and toe flexion. Split anterior tibialis tendon transfer (SPLATT) is considered if inversion is present and caused by the tibialis anterior. If inversion is caused preferentially by tibialis posterior, a release of this muscle is indicated. If the tibialis posterior is found to be active during swing, a tendon transfer to produce ankle dorsiflexion is recommended. EHL lengthening or transfer may be necessary.

Clinical Feature of Problem

Knee flexion (buckling) in the stance phase

Potential Issues

Limb instability, poor balance, unstable gait, inability to transfer full weight bearing to affected limb

Penalties and Manifestations

- Difficulty with balance, impaired weight bearing, decreased weight acceptance, increased loading phase
- Shortened stance time, may be genu recurvatum
- Interferes with smooth forward progression of the center of gravity, increases vertical displacement of center of gravity, increases energy consumption
- Interferes with ability to transfer to different surfaces, shortens contralateral step length

Analysis and Differential Diagnosis

- Rule out knee joint ligamentous and meniscus injury and patellar tendon rupture.

- Rule out flexion contracture, femoral nerve injury, and other causes for loss of knee extensor power.
- Rule out calf weakness.

Diagnostic Work-up

- Gait analysis

  EMG of quadriceps, hamstrings, and ankle plantarflexors

  3-D motion analysis to quantify knee position

  GRF analysis to quantify vertical loading-unloading, anterior-posterior, and medial-lateral shear forces
- Passive and active range of motion
- Sensory examination, including proprioception
- X-ray studies to rule out bony abnormality
- EMG and nerve conduction velocity studies to rule out nerve injury and radiculopathy

Findings

- EMG demonstrates lack of quadriceps activation or hamstrings overactivation (out of phase) in the late-swing and early-stance phases or throughout the gait cycle. The gastrocnemius is not appropriately active during stance to control excessive forward progression of the tibia.
- Hip extensors demonstrate decreased activation during the stance phase.
- Forward flexion of the trunk during the stance phase is documented, and may be accompanied by knee hyperextension. GRF analysis demonstrates a prolonged and reduced loading phase and peak vertical force.

Treatment Options

The patient should avoid shoes with heels. An articulated ankle-foot orthosis or molded ankle-foot orthosis with limited dorsiflexion to −5 degrees of plantarflexion and free plantarflexion can be used to control the excessive forward progression of the tibia, position the force line anterior to the knee joint, and control the knee flexion moment in early stance. Note solutions that unload knee extensors may benefit from knee extensor strengthening (16). A knee-ankle-foot or thosis with an articulated ankle with settings as mentioned and offset knee joints can be used if the knee and ankle weakness is severe. If a static flexion deformity of the knee is present, a knee-ankle-foot or thosis with single-axis knee and drop locks is recommended. Alternatively, a distal hamstring release may be considered so the patient may use a brace without a knee lock. If the hamstring strength is grade 4/5 or better, a transfer of the hamstrings to the quadriceps should be considered, to provide increased knee stability in the stance phase.

CONCLUSIONS

Gait dysfunctions are usually multifactorial in origin. Appropriate intervention requires a clear understanding of normal locomotion and of the biomechanics and underlying pathophysiology of gait deviations. Gait analysis, combined with sound clinical judgment, can elucidate the factors involved in pathologic gait and aid in the selection of appropriate treatment interventions. Other applications of gait and movement analysis, such as in sports, the workplace, the evaluation of leg-length discrepancy, and mechanical imbalance, are increasing the utility of this assessment tool.

REFERENCES

1. Winter DA. Pathologic gait diagnosis with computer-averaged electromyographic profiles. *Arch Phys Med Rehabil* 1984;65:393–398.
2. Winter DA. *The biomechanics and motor control of human gait.* Waterloo, Ontario, Canada: Waterloo University Press, 1987.
3. Murray MP, Drought AB, Kory RC. Walking patterns of normal men. J Bone Joint Surg 1964;46A:335–360.
4. Muybridge E. Animals in motion. 5th ed. London: Chapman and Hall, 1925.
5. Bernstein N. The technique of the study of movements. In: Conrady Gr, Farfel V, Slonim A, eds. *Textbook of the physiology of work.* Moscow, 1934:1–26.
6. Inman VT, Ralston HJ, Todd F. *Human walking.* Baltimore: Williams & Wilkins, 1981.
7. Cappozzo A. Gait analysis methodology. *Hum Mov Sci* 1984;3:27–50.
8. Bampton S. *A guide to the visual examination of pathological gait.* Philadelphia: Temple University-Moss Rehabilitation Hospital, Rehabilitation Research and Training Center No. 8, 1979.
9. Esquenazi A, Hirai B. Assessment of gait and orthotic prescription. *Phys Med Rehabil Clin N Am* 1991;2:473–485.
10. Cotes J, Meade F. The energy expenditure and mechanical energy demand in walking. *Ergonomics* 1960;3:97–119.
11. Saunders JB, Inman VT, Eberhart HD. The major determinants in normal and pathological gait. *J Bone Joint Surg [Am]* 1953;35:543–558.
12. Cook TM. Cozzens BA, Kenosian H. *A technique for force-line, visualization.* Philadelphia: Moss Reha-

bilitation Hospital, Rehabilitation Engineering Center No. 2, March 1979.

13. Taylor DR. An instrumented Gait Mat. In: *Proceedings of the International Conference on Rehabilitation Engineering.* Toronto: RESNA, 1980;278–279.

14. Rowell D, Mann RW. Human movement analysis. *Soma* 1989;3:3–20.

15. Skinner HB, French HG, Dlabel TA, et al. Correlation of gait analysis and clinical evaluation of polycentric total knee arthroplasty. *Orthopedics* 1983;6:576–579.

16. Esquenazi A, Wikoff E, Hirai B, et al. Effects of a plantar flexed plastic molded ankle foot orthosis on gait pattern and lower limb muscle strength. In: *Proceedings, VI World Congress.* International Society for Prosthetics and Orthotics. Kobe, Japan: ISPO, 1989:208.

Chapter 13

Assessment of Communication

Richard D. Zorowitz
Brenda B. Adamovich

Man has been fascinated with the origins and development of language for thousands of years. The use of names is regarded as characteristic of the first man: "G-d had formed every wild beast and every bird of heaven out of the ground. He brought them to the man to see what he would name each one. Whatever the man called each living thing would remain its name." Even Biblical civilization was developed upon one language: "The entire earth had one language with uniform words." However, the same authority attributed to the development of a single language is credited with its demise as a result of the building of the Tower of Babel: "Come, let us descend and confuse their speech, so that one person will not understand another's speech."

The first secular ideas regarding the origin of language were published in Plato's *Cratylus*: "Everything has a right name of its own, which comes by nature, and that a name is not whatever people call a thing by agreement, just a piece of their voice applied to the thing, but that there is kind of inherent correctness in names, which is the same for all men, both Greeks and Barbarians." However, Herder (1744–1803) is credited with laying the foundations of the science of language in his essay *Uber den Ürsprung der Sprache* (1772). He attempted to refute the hypothesis of the divine origins of language by showing that man had developed language with the powers of reason. Max Müller (1823–1900) (1) and William Dwight Whitney (1827–1894) (2) further emphasized the human character of language, but facetiously hypothesized that language emanated from onomatopoeia, involuntary ejaculations and interjections of speech, and sounds associated with communal physical effort. Charles Darwin, in his *Descent of Man* (1871), challenged the prevailing belief of language as a distinctly human trait by contending that animal cries are not a difference of kind, but only of degree of articulation.

Just as it is important to understand the evolution of normal speech and language, it is more important to identify problems in these areas. As early as approximately 1700 BC, people with speech-language disorders have been documented: "He is speechless. He is silent in sadness, without speaking, like one suffering with feebleness" (3). The field of speech-language pathology, whose history extends back to the time of Herodotus (4) and Hippocrates (5), addresses many of the aspects of expression and comprehension of language. As a result, the domain of the speech-language pathologist can be divided into several areas: speech-language disorders (aphasia, apraxia, dysarthria, cognitive-communication impairment), audiology, and augmentative communication. The present chapter surveys the evaluation of the first two areas, while Chapter 42 discusses treatment strategies of all three areas.

SPEECH-LANGUAGE DISORDERS

Differential Diagnosis

Classification of speech-language disorders begins with a conversational interaction with the patient. Although

Table 13-1: Speaking with a Person with Speech-Language Disorder
1. Maintain eye contact with the person.
2. Speak directly to the person, not to a companion, even if the patient has an interpreter. Use the first person, not the third person.
3. Speak slowly and simply in a normal tone of voice. Most people with speech-language disorders are *not* deaf.
4. Give the person adequate time and opportunity to express himself or herself.
5. Listen more carefully than you usually do.
6. Focus on *what* the person is saying, and not *how* he or she is saying it.
7. Never fill in a word or complete a sentence unless you are asked.
8. Ask the person to repeat or rephrase something you do not understand.
9. Put the person first, not the disability.

Adapted from Van Riper C, Emerick L. *Speech correction: an introduction to speech pathology and audiology.* Englewood Cliffs, NJ: Prentice-Hall, 1990.

formal diagnostic tools may be helpful in detailing the nature of the problem, clinicians can begin to describe impairments in speech and language by engaging the patient in normal conversation. Questions should be posed in an open-ended manner, such as having the patient describe the nature of the illness or his or her family, so that the patient gives the clinician an example of his or her speech patterns. This may require the presence of a family member in order to confirm the information. Questions requiring a "yes" or "no" or single-word answer are discouraged. Also, other methods used to converse with people with speech-language disorders should be incorporated into the encounter (Table 13-1).

While listening to the patient, the examiner should be formulating the nature of the impairment in terms of two types of problems: impaired content or impaired acoustic features. *Impaired content* refers to alterations in the language aspects of communication. Such abnormalities may occur at the syllabic or word level (e.g., substitutions or word finding), or at the sentence level (e.g., omission of functors, substitution of descriptions of objects). The content of speech may be disjointed, tangential, vague, irrelevant, or confabulatory. Facial or body gestures may be absent or dissociated from the content of speech. Speech intonation may be blunted or absent. Language disorders are classified as *aphasias* or *cognitive-communication impairments.*

On the other hand, *impaired acoustic features* refer to alterations in the production of speech. The patient with an acoustic impairment may exhibit problems in articulation, phonation, or resonance. Voice volume may be decreased, and breath control may be impaired. Motor speech disorders are classified as *dysarthrias* or *apraxias.*

Aphasia

Aphasia is defined as a "loss of the ability to utilize language, disproportionate to the impairment of other intellectual functions, manifested by reduced available vocabulary, auditory comprehension, and reading and writing abilities" (6). It is a multimodal loss, involving each element to a varying degree, that is not attributable to dementia, sensory loss, or motor dysfunction. The elements of language affected in aphasia include *fluency*, *comprehension*, and *repetition.*

Classification

Traditionally, aphasia syndromes were classified into a dichotomy of "expressive" versus "receptive" (7,8). The scheme was produced on the notion that "expressive" or "motor" aphasias occurred as a result of a lesion in or around the Broca area in the inferior frontal lobe. Similarly, "receptive" or "sensory" aphasias were thought to be due to lesions in or around the Wernicke area in the superior temporal lobe. However, it is well known that anterior lesions may produce impairments of comprehension and posterior lesions may cause problems with verbal expression. More recently, aphasias resulting from subcortical lesions have been described (9–11).

In the 1960s and 1970s, Geschwind (12,13) proposed a modification in the classification scheme of aphasias. The new dichotomy was based on "fluency," or rate of speech. *Fluent* speech can be produced at normal to rapid rates, while *nonfluent* speech tends to be sparse with labored production. Characteristics of fluent and nonfluent aphasias are compared in Table 13-2.

Aphasias may be described by a variety of abnormalities of speech production. *Agrammatism* is the absence of grammatical elements during speech attempts. *Paraphasia* refers to substitutions of syllables or consonants with words ("literal") or of the words themselves ("verbal" or "semantic"). *Anomia* denotes difficulty at producing nouns. *Echolalia* consists of repetition of an utterance that does not require repetition. *Circumlocution* refers to descriptions or associated words related to a word that cannot be retrieved. A *neologism* is a word well articulated but mostly contrived or incomprehensible. *Jargon* consists of well-articulated but mostly incomprehensible language. *Stereotypes* refers to the repetition of nonsensical syllables (e.g., "no, no, no") during attempts at communication.

A classification of aphasia is found in Table 13-3. Although the clinician may attempt to classify an aphasia into one of the categories listed, many aphasias cannot be classified as such because the relationships between modalities may be unclear. As a result, it may be appropriate to diagnose an aphasia as *fluent* or *nonfluent* alone.

Global aphasias cannot be categorized as fluent or nonfluent, but must be classified by themselves. Global aphasias severely affect all modalities. On the one hand, a subject with a global aphasia may be mute, utter grunts or

Table 13-2: Characteristics of Fluent and Nonfluent Aphasias		
Parameter	**Nonfluent Aphasia**	**Fluent Aphasia**
Rate	Slow, labored	Normal or rapid
Content and delivery	Telegraphic; absence or reduction of functors	Vague or general delivery; more functors than content words
Articulation	Accurate or with substitutions; usually accompanied by struggle	Accurate or with substitutions; without struggle, but moving toward target word
Paraphasias	Usually related to target word	Usually unrelated to target word
Auditory comprehension	Varied, but usually better than speech	Varied, but usually worse than speech
Awareness	Good	Poor to good
Affect	Appropriate or depressed	Euphoric or agitated, but may be appropriate

Table 13-3: Classification of Aphasias				
	Comp	**Rep**	**Neuroanatomic Lesion**	**Characteristics**
Nonfluent				
Broca	(+)	(–)	Third convolution of left frontal lobe; extending to inferior portion of precentral gyrus	Telegraphic, dysgrammatic expression; often associated with apraxia; paraphasic and articulatory errors or struggle; relatively intact comprehension except on abstract concepts
Transcortical motor	(+)	(+)	Anterior or superior to Broca area; subcortical region deep to Broca area	Limited language output, but some fluent utterances; reduced initiation and organization; fair naming; preserved repetition, possibly echolalia
Transcortical mixed	(+)	(+)	Borderzone of the frontal, temporal, and parietal areas	Poor initiation and comprehension; echolalia present
Fluent				
Wernicke	(–)	(–)	Posterior portion of first left temporal gyrus	Normal or rapid rate; decreased nouns and verbs; paraphasic or neologistic substitutions; paragrammatism; poor comprehension
Conduction	(+)	(–)	Arcuate fasciculus; deep to supramarginal gyrus insula	Normal or rapid rate; literal paraphasias with targeting; relatively preserved auditory comprehension; impaired repetition of low-probability phrases
Anomic	(+)	(+)	Left angular gyrus; left temporoparietal lobe; basal portion of posterior temporal lobe	Decreased output of nouns; word-finding difficulties; sometimes presence of alexia and agraphia
Transcortical sensory	(–)	(+)	Left angular gyrus; left posteroinferior temporal lobe; isolates perisylvian speech structures from posterior brain	Fluent neologistic output; poor auditory comprehension; preserved repetition
Global	(–)	(–)	Left perisylvian region	Fluent: total neologistic or jargon output; nonfluent: rare vocalizations or verbal stereotypes; poor comprehension and repetition

other incomprehensible vocalizations, or express one or more verbal stereotypes or syllables. On the other hand, another subject may have a normal or rapid output of paraphasias, neologisms, or jargon that is so incomprehensible that the listener cannot understand the context of the output. In both cases, however, the subject comprehends no or little verbal or written speech, and cannot repeat or name on confrontation.

Evaluation

An evaluation of aphasias can be undertaken to determine the presence and severity of the aphasia, the patient's baseline abilities, the effectiveness of treatment, or the prognosis, or to explore research issues. The ideal aphasia battery should address the latest, theoretically important items and be adequately standardized and validated (14). The test should differentiate all clinically relevant types of aphasia. It should also discriminate between normal, aphasic, and nonaphasic brain-damaged subjects. The subtests should include the full spectrum of language abilities: spontaneous speech, comprehension of spoken language, repetition, confrontational naming, reading and writing, praxis, and calculations. Several of the most commonly used aphasia batteries are described here.

Minnesota Test for Differential Diagnosis of Aphasia (MTDDA)

This comprehensive test battery has been in existence longer than all the other test batteries. It contains 505 items in 46 subtests. The subtests are distributed among five sections: auditory, visual and reading, speech and language, visuomotor and writing, and numerical relationships and arithmetic processes. The method of scoring varies among subtests. Most utilize plus-minus or correct-incorrect scoring (15).

Boston Diagnostic Aphasia Examination (BDAE)

This examination is a comprehensive assessment that identifies and quantitates strengths and weaknesses in all areas of language. Expository speech is rated along six 7-point scales: melodic line, phrase length, articulatory agility, grammatical form, paraphasia in running speech, and word finding. Auditory comprehension is assessed through word recognition, body part identification, and responses to commands and yes-no questions. Oral expression is evaluated by oral agility, automatic speech, recitation, repetition, reading, word fluency, and naming. Reading comprehension is analyzed through four subtests. Related tests include the Boston Naming Test (BNT) (16) and several perceptual tests. Administration of the entire BDAE takes several hours (17).

Western Aphasia Battery (WAB)

This battery is largely based on the BDAE but can be administered in 1 hour. Expressive abilities are tested using spontaneous speech, comprehension, repetition, and naming. Auditory comprehension is evaluated using yes-no questions, or pointing to a visual representation of an auditory stimulus. Naming is tested using visual confrontation. Reading and writing are assessed using screen tests, and subtests are given only when the subject fails the screen tests. Other parameters tested include word fluency, sentence completion, responsive speech, praxis, construction, and calculation. A language quotient based on oral and written language subscores has been used to follow recovery (18–20).

Porch Index of Communicative Abilities (PICA)

The PICA uses 10 common objects as stimuli for 18 subtests addressing three response modalities: verbal, gestural, and graphic. Areas of testing include naming, use of an object, matching, reading, completing sentences, repeating, writing, and construction. Subtests are scored on a scale of 1 to 16 in five dimensions: accuracy, responsiveness, completeness, promptness, and efficiency. The index requires approximately 90 minutes to complete. It has been widely accepted in clinical, research, and medicolegal applications (21).

Neurosensory Center Comprehensive Examination of Aphasia (NCCEA)

The NCCEA differs from previous aphasia batteries in that it does not attempt to classify aphasias. It contains 20 subtests to assess language abilities and four control tests to assess visual and tactile functions. The subtests comprise the following categories: visual naming, description of usage of objects, tactile naming, sentence and digit repetition, digit reversal, word fluency, sentence construction, auditory comprehension, reading and writing, and articulation. Spontaneous speech is not formally tested. Some subtests are not administered if the patient passes screening tests. Some subtests have a low “ceiling” that is unsuitable for testing subjects with mild aphasia. This test is used to follow recovery (22).

Functional Communication Profile (FCP)

This evaluation was designed to rate the ability of a subject to communicate in functional situations rather than during formal testing. Testing is performed in the areas of movement, speaking, understanding, reading, writing, and calculation. Scoring is based on a percentage of estimated premorbid ability. The profile takes about 30 minutes to complete, and can be used to monitor recovery (23,24).

Communicative Abilities in Daily Living (CADL)

This test assesses the ability of a subject to communicate through verbal or nonverbal means in functional situations. Sixty-eight items in 10 categories are rated, such as visiting a doctor, shopping, or making a telephone call. Scoring is based on a correct, adequate, or incorrect response. The CADL is helpful in assessing improvements in communication in subjects who may have reached a plateau on other batteries (25).

Token Test

The Token test assesses comprehension using small tokens of five colors, two sizes, and two shapes. The subject is asked to follow commands of progressive length and complexity related to the tokens. It can differentiate among normal, aphasic, and nonaphasic brain-injured subjects. It can detect subtle comprehension impairments but cannot measure severity of aphasia. The related Reporter test is an expressive equivalent of the Token test in which subjects are asked to verbally report manipulations performed on the tokens (26).

Revised Token Test (RTT)

This test applies standardized administration procedures and multidimensional scoring and minor changes in stimuli to the Token test. The test contains 10 sections with 10 commands per section. Subtests I through IV are constructed similar to parts I through IV in the original Token test. The remaining six subtests are expansions of the original part V items, which include prepositions and spatial relationships and conditional clauses (27).

Supplemental Tests

Screening examinations include the Sklar Aphasia Scale (SAS) (28), Aphasia Language Performance Scales (AIPS) (29), Bedside Evaluation Screening Test (BEST) (30), Brief Test of Head Injury (BTHI) (31), Aphasia Screening Test (32), and the Frenchay Aphasia Screeing Test (FAST) (33).

Auditory comprehension tests include the Auditory Comprehension Test for Sentences (ACTS) (34) and The Functional Auditory Comprehension Task (FACT) (35).

Reading comprehension tests include the Reading Comprehension Battery for Aphasia (36).

Language Production tests include the BNT (16).

Pantomime tests include the Pantomime Recognition Test (37) and the Assessment of Nonverbal Communication (38).

Functional assessment tests include the FCP (23) and the Functional Independence Measure (FIM) (39).

Apraxia

Apraxia is defined as "an articulatory disorder resulting from impairment, as a result of brain damage, of the capacity to program the positioning of speech muscles and the sequencing of muscle movements for the volitional production of phonemes" (6). There usually is no significant weakness, slowness, or incoordination of muscles during reflex or automatic acts. Alterations in the intonation, rhythm, and stress of speech, known as *prosody*, may be associated with apraxic subjects, sometimes in compensation for the impairment. A comparison of the characteristics of apraxia and dysarthria is found in Table 13-4.

Classification

There are two accepted types of apraxia with respect to oral musculature. *Oral apraxia* is an apraxia of nonverbal oral postures. Impairments may be seen in single movements (e.g., sticking out tongue) or with multiple tasks (e.g., sticking out tongue, licking lips, and protruding lips). *Verbal apraxia*, or *apraxia of speech (AOS)*, refers to apraxia when applied to the production of speech. AOS is generally associated with lesions of the third convolution of the left frontal lobe, but also has been reported in association with lesions of the left inferior parietal, superior temporal, inferior frontal, and subcortical regions.

Not all clinicians agree with the concept of apraxia as unpredictable. AOS has been described as a phonologic disorder extending from aphasia that occurs in predictable, recognizable patterns within linguistic and morphologic constraints (40). As a result, two apraxic subgroups of aphasia have been proposed (41): *afferent motor aphasia*, the inability to use kinesthetic information in repetition or spontaneous speech attributed to damage of the facial

Table 13-4: Differential Diagnosis of Apraxia and Dysarthria

	Apraxia	Dysarthria
Oral-peripheral examination	Dysfunction when requested to perform voluntary movements; vegetative functions (i.e., sucking, chewing) adequate	Slow, weak, uncoordinated muscles; vegetative functions impaired
Articulation	Complication a. Transpositions, reversals b. Perseverative and anticipatory errors	Simplification a. Distortions b. Substitutions c. Fewer distortions, more substitutions, intrusive additions
	Errors inconsistent; errors proportional to word complexity; fewer errors in spontaneous performance	Errors consistent; errors consistent with neurologic record; more errors in final position; severity related to neuromuscular involvement
Repeated utterance	Gropes or struggles for correct performance, but may achieve correct performance with repeated attempts	Same performance
Rate	Performance improves at faster rate; slow, labored speech with disturbances of prosody	Performance deteriorates at faster rates; slow rate of speech
Response to stimulation	Best performance if given several chances to match presented model	Best response if specific articulatory gestures demonstrated

Adapted from Haynes WO, Pindzola RH, Emerick LL. *Diagnosis and evaluation in speech pathology.* 4th ed. Englewood Cliffs, NJ: Prentice-Hall, 1992.

region of the sensory cortex; and *efferent motor aphasia*, the traditional definition of AOS.

Evaluation

The diagnosis of AOS is usually clinical. Four pronounced characteristics have been listed to make a definitive diagnosis (42): effortful trial and error, groping articulatory movement, and attempts and self-correction; dysprosody unrelieved by extended periods of normal rhythm, stress, and intonation; articulatory inconsistency on repeated productions of the same utterance; and obvious difficulty initiating utterances. However, because aphasias usually are associated with apraxias, the task of diagnosis becomes more difficult.

Few formal instruments are available to assess the presence of apraxia. The Motor Speech Evaluation tests vowel production, diadochokinesis, repetition of words and sentences of progressive phonemic complexity, counting, and verbal description, but must be correlated with other testing data to ensure a correct diagnosis (43). The Apraxia Battery for Adults (ABA) provides qualitative and quantitative information in making a diagnosis. The six subtests include repetition of progressively difficult phonemic combinations, repetition of progressively difficult words, presence of limb and oral apraxia by imitation, perseveration of language, degree of improvement during a three-trial repetition of multisyllabic words, and presence of articulatory characteristics associated with AOS through spontaneous speech and reading.

Dysarthria

Dysarthria is defined as a "speech disorder resulting from disturbances in muscular control—weakness, slowness, or incoordination—of the speech mechanism due to damage to the central or peripheral nervous system. The term encompasses coexisting neurogenic disorders of several or all of the basic processes of speech: respiration, phonation, resonance, articulation, and prosody" (6). A comparison of the characteristics of dysarthria and apraxia is found in Table 13-4.

Understanding of the abnormalities of human speech requires a brief summary of the processes required to produce speech. *Respiration* actually refers to ventilation. *Inhalation* is the active process that moves air into the lungs, using the diaphragm, costal elevator, serratus, and other muscles. *Exhalation* is the process that allows air to pass between the vocal cords to produce speech. Exhalation may be passive, through relaxation of the diaphragm, or active, using abdominal or intercostal muscles. *Phonation* involves modification of exhaled air, either by altering the subglottic air pressure or by altering the length and tension of the vocal cords. *Resonation* refers to the modification of raw vocal tone through changes in the tension of the pharyngeal wall or in the position of the jaw, tongue, lips, soft palate, or larynx. *Articulation* is the coordinated action of the lips, jaw, tongue, and soft palate to produce meaningful sounds. *Prosody* is the rhythm and intonation of speech.

Classification

A number of systems for classifying dysarthrias have been proposed. Clinicians have attempted to systematize dysarthrias by neurophysiology (44), by medical diagnosis (45), and by neuroanatomic site (46,47). However, the most comprehensive classification scheme breaks dysarthrias into seven types, as listed in Table 13-5 (48,49). In developing this scheme, each type of dysarthria was found to have unique characteristics in terms of pitch, loudness, vocal quality, respiration, prosody, articulation, and general impression when rated across 38 dimensions. However, single features such as imprecise articulation or hypernasality may not be adequate to make a specific diagnosis.

Evaluation

The diagnosis of dysarthria usually is made clinically. The clinician must evaluate each of the components required to produce speech. Numbers of words produced per breath, pitch characteristics, nasality, and articulatory precision are only several of the perceptual measures that assist in the diagnosis. The Assessment in Intelligibility of Dysarthric Speech (AIDS) (50) provides a large number of well-designed stimuli with which speech intelligibility may be evaluated, but two people are required to administer it. The Frenchay Dysarthria Assessment (51) combines elements of a formal oral-motor examination with a functional speech assessment, but lacks sensitivity in diagnosing more moderate degrees of impairment. The Motor Speech Evaluation may assist in differentiating dysarthria from ataxia, and was described earlier.

Instrumentation may assist in the diagnosis of certain types of dysarthria. A *pneumotachometer* uses a differential pressure transducer that measures subglottic air pressure. *Fiberoptic laryngoscopy* or *fluoroscopy* may be used to visualize oral, pharyngeal, or velopharyngeal structures at rest or during specific maneuvers.

Cognitive-Communication Impairment

Cognitive-communicative impairments is defined by the American Speech-Language-Hearing Association (52) as

> those communicative disorders that result from deficits in linguistic and non-linguistic cognitive processes: Language deficits can be outward manifestations of underlying impairments in cognitive processes, such as attention, perception, and/or memory; inflexibility, impulsivity, disorganized thinking; difficulty processing complex information; problems with learning new information; inefficient retrieval of stored information; ineffective problem solving or judgment; inappropriate social behavior (pragmatics); impaired executive functioning. Cognitive-communicative impairments result in disabilities and handicaps that affect an individual's ability to function effectively in all aspects of life including the

Table 13-5: Classification of Dysarthrias			
Type	**Neuropathic Location (examples)**	**Neuromuscular Deficit**	**Characteristics**
Flaccid	Lower motor neuron (bulbar palsy)	Muscular weakness; hypotonia	Marked hypernasality, often with nasal emissions; continuous breathiness; audible inspiration
Spastic	Upper motor neuron (pseudobulbar palsy)	Reduced range, force, speed; hypertonia	Very imprecise articulation; slow rate; low pitch; harsh strained-strangled voice
Ataxic	Cerebellum (cerebellar ataxia)	Inaccurate range, timing, direction; reduced speed; hypotonia	Excess and equal stress; phoneme and interval prolongation; dysrhythmia of speech and syllable repetition; slow rate; some excess loudness variation
Hypokinetic	Extrapyramidal system (parkinsonism)	Variable speed of repetitive movements; movement arrest, rigidity	Monopitch, monoloudness, reduced overall loudness; variable rate; short rushes; reduced range of speech; some inappropriate silences
Hyperkinetic 1. Quick	Extrapyramidal system (a. Chorea; b. Myoclonus; c. Tourette syndrome)	Quick, unsustained, random, involuntary movements	a. Highly variable pattern of imprecise articulation; episodes of hypernasality; sudden variations in loudness b. Rhythmic hypernasality; rhythmic phonatory interruption c. Sudden tic-like grunts, barks, coprolalia
2. Slow	(a. Athetosis; b. Dyskinesias; c. Dystonias)	Sustained, distorted movements and postures; slowness; variable hypertonias	a. Distinctive deviations unreported b. Distinctive deviations unreported c. Prolongation of phonemes, intervals; unsteady rate, loudness
3. Tremors	(Organic voice tremor)	Involuntary, rhythmic, purposeless oscillatory movements	Rhythmic alterations in pitch, loudness; voice stoppages
Mixed	Multiple motor systems (a. Amyotrophic lateral sclerosis; b. Multiple sclerosis; c. Wilson disease)	Muscular weakness; reduced range, speed	a. Grossly defective articulation; extremely slow, laborious rate; marked hypernasality; severe harshness, strain-strangled voice; nearly complete disruption of prosody b. Impaired control of loudness; harshness c. Reduced stress; monopitch; monoloudness; similar to hypokinetic except no short rushes of speech

Adapted from Rosenbek JC, LaPointe LL. The dysarthrias: description, diagnosis, and treatment. In: Johns DF, ed. *Clinical management of neurogenic communicative disorders*. 2nd ed. Boston: Little, Brown, 1985.

home, community, school, and workplace. *Pragmatics* refers to "a system of rules that clarify the use of language in terms of situation or social context" (53). The characteristics of cognitive-communication impairment are listed in Table 13-6.

Classification

Cognitive-communication impairments occur primarily with three conditions: right hemispheric dysfunction (RHD), dementia, and traumatic brain injury (TBI). Focal lesions can occur with all three conditions, resulting in speech, language, voice, hearing, fluency, or swallowing impairments similar to those that occur following stroke. However, the widespread, diffuse brain damage that generally occurs results in generalized cognitive impairments. Cognitive-communicative impairments result from impaired attention, information processing, and cognition. Specific cognitive processes that cause impaired communication include perception, discrimination, organization, recall, and reasoning. The ability to communicate or exchange information between individuals requires intrinsic relationships among cognition, language, attention, and information processing. In subjects with RHD, many of the listed characteristics are found. Subjects who fail to recognize affective cues may mistakenly be considered rude or indifferent. Subjects who cannot take turns or maintain topics in conversation may be labeled as difficult. Subjects who cannot interpret humor or abstract concepts might be construed as apathetic or depressed.

Dementia occurs with conditions such as Alzheimer disease, multi-infarct dementia, Parkinson disease, Huntington disease, and Pick disease. Dementia usually can be classified as *cortical* and *subcortical* (54). Subjects

Table 13-6: Characteristics of Cognitive-Communication Impairment

Impairment	Symptoms
Linguistic-pragmatic	Impaired initiation of conversation Impaired narrative coherence Increased embellishments, irrelevancies Impaired topic maintenance Impaired turn taking Impaired processing Impaired language organization Impaired expression or comprehension of abstract concepts Impaired prosody Impaired recall, comprehension, or repetition of prosodic or affective material Impaired appreciation of humor
Nonverbal	Altered affect Emotional lability Impaired eye contact Impaired gestures Indifference Denial Motor impersistence
Visual-perceptual	Hemi-inattention or neglect Impaired perception of objects, faces Altered spatial relationships
Cognitive	Impaired orientation Impaired problem solving Impaired visual-verbal memory Impaired verbal integration Impaired mathematical computation Impaired attention, concentration Impaired reasoning and judgment Impaired insight Impaired daily planning (executive functioning)

Adapted from Morganstein S, Smith MC. Aphasia and right-hemisphere disorders. In: Gordon WA, ed. *Advances in stroke rehabilitation.* Boston: Andover Medical, 1993.

with cortical dementia tend to have problems with aphasia, amnesia, agnosias, and acalculia. Speech and response times usually are normal, although they tend to deteriorate in end-stage dementia. On the other hand, subjects with subcortical dementias have difficulties with verbal recall and problem solving. Processing times are usually delayed, and speech is dysarthric. Over time, dementia progresses until communication is largely neologistic and echolalic. Subsequently, meaningful output disappears and the subject becomes mute.

Cognitive-communicative impairments are most frequently used to describe the deficits that occur following TBI. Adamovich and Henderson (55) suggested a hierarchy of cognitive skills based on research with TBI patients, including perception, discrimination, organization, recall, and high-level problem solving (convergent thinking, deductive thinking, inductive reasoning, divergent thinking, and multiprocess reasoning).

The establishment of unrealistic individual goals and aspirations due to a denial of deficits may be attributed to attentional disturbances such that the head-injured individual does not attend to existing mental and physical problems that result in difficulty completing activities of daily living.

Cognitive impairments can cause disabilities in social interactions and interpersonal or pragmatic communication. A disability in pragmatic communication can result from cognitive impairments that cause an inability to comprehend subtlety in language as in metaphorical and figurative use and a reduced ability to draw conclusions and to give coherence to a narrative. Mildly impaired head-injured patients have impairments in executive functioning or metacognitive skills, making them appear unusual to others in the community. *Executive functioning* refers to the ability to formulate goals, develop plans, and effectively execute a plan (56). Executive or metacognitive skills include self-awareness in goal setting, planning, self-directing/initiating, self-inhibiting, self-monitoring, self-evaluating, and flexible problem solving (57). A person who lacks these skills appears to be egocentric, rude, impulsive, disinhibited, stubborn, denying, or incoherent.

Lezak (56) emphasized that various personality impairments after TBI cause social difficulties. The severity and type of problems are related to the nature of the injury, and categorized as 1) impaired capacity for social perceptiveness, resulting in self-centered behavior in which both empathy and self-reflective attitudes are greatly diminished; 2) impaired capacity for self-regulation leading to impulsivity and impatience; 3) social dependency, resulting in difficulties in planning and organizing; and 4) emotional lability and depression.

Ylkvisaker and Szekeres (58) attributed reduced social skills to 1) poor awareness and perception of social and communication events; 2) inadequate retrieval of rules of social interactions; 3) reduced ability to take alternative perspectives; 4) disorganization at the level of introducing, maintaining, and terminating topics of conversation; and 5) disinhibition and weak self-monitoring of verbal and nonverbal behavior that may result in repetition of information, making inappropriate and offensive remarks, and demonstrating poor comprehension for spoken utterances.

The ability to return to work or school is often used as an index of outcome following TBI because survivors are often young adults of work or school age with an average life span.

Wehman et al (59) suggested that key barriers to employability relate to cognitive issues such as new learning, memory, and impaired self-awareness. People lose jobs because of poor social or interpersonal skills, not because of deficient task performance. Haffey and Lewis (60) listed barriers to job placement and retention following TBI, including cognitive-communicative disorders, emotional and social behaviorial control problems, psychomotor and cognitive processing slowness, and inadequate interpersonal and social skills.

Evaluation

For a long time, the diagnosis of cognitive-communication impairment required a large number of formal tests, improvised questions, and conversational interactions. Portions of the BDAE might be combined with informal inquiries to explain metaphors, proverbs, or punchlines of fables or jokes in order to produce an evaluation.

Recently, several formal evaluations of cognitive-communication impairment have appeared. The RIC Evaluation of Communication Problems in Right Hemisphere Dysfunction (RICE) is the first formal assessment of RHD (61), and evaluates the following areas: attention, including focus, impulse control, facial recognition, and left hemiattention; orientation; perception of space, facial contours, emotion, environmental sounds, melody, and prosody; pragmatics, including affective language, contextual cues, intonation, and expression; visual memory; and integration, including problem solving, metaphoric interpretation, humor, organization, and comprehension of conversation. The Mini Inventory of Right Brain Injury (MIRBI) screens subjects for the following symptoms (62): visual and language processing, emotion and affect, general behavior and neuropsychological integrity, memory, orientation, and nonverbal processing. The Adult Conversational Analysis Tool (A-CAT) (63) complements other batteries to analyze various components of conversation, such as organization of ideas, vocal intonation, responsive listening, and eye contact. The Arizona Battery for Communication Disorders in Dementia (ABCD) relates memory to communication, and consists of 16 subtests. Four subtests—story retelling, delayed; word learning, free recall; word learning, total recall; and recognition—may be used to screen patients with Alzheimer disease.

Scales of Cognition after Traumatic Brain Injury (SCATBI) (64) is a new diagnostic test for adolescents and adults that was designed to provide clinicians with cognitive information that can be directly applied to treatment. The test consists of five scales made up of a series of smaller tests or "testlets," which are collections of similar items designed to measure a common trait. Items generally progress from easier to more difficult tasks.

Perception refers to the integration and interpretation of information received at the sense organs based on an internal or stored representation of the stimulus. *Discrimination* refers to the ability to differentiate two or more stimuli. *Organization* refers to the ability to deal with discrete actions or components that must be grouped or sequenced according to the priority of each component, using a learned strategy. General organizational skills include categorization, closure, and sequencing. Memory deficits occur due to ineffective encoding of information, inadequate storage of information, difficulty retrieving information using recognition, cued recall or free recall, or a lack of strategies to deal with interferences.

Reasoning and *problem solving* require the generation of responses based on relevant information to formulate a solution to a problem that must then be checked or tested as to the appropriateness of the solution. Such high-level thought processing includes the following:

1. *Convergent thinking*, which refers to the recognition and analysis of relevant and missing information in visually or aurally presented sentences, paragraphs, conversations, and stories to identify the central theme or main point. For example, if presented with the statements "Jack opened the door to his home and was greeted by a houseful of people. The room was decorated with crepe paper and balloons and on the table sat a cake with candles," the individual should identify the central theme as being a surprise birthday party for Jack.
2. *Deductive reasoning*, which refers to the drawing of conclusions regarding a given situation based on premises or general principles, in a step-by-step manner. For example, given the following facts, "It does not open things, it is made of metal, it becomes hot, and it is not used in the preparation of food," the individual should be able to select the correct item: can opener, iron, toaster, blender, or coffee maker.
3. *Inductive reasoning*, which involves the formulation of a solution based on details that lead to, but do not necessarily support, a standard conclusion. Inductive reasoning tasks include the formulation of antonyms and synonyms; analogous thinking; the recognition of cause-and-effect relationships; and open-ended problem solving, including story completion tasks.
4. *Divergent thinking*, which involves the generation of unique abstract concepts or hypotheses that deviate from standard concepts or ideas. Divergent thinking tasks include the recognition and interpretation of homographs, idioms, absurdities, proverbs, similes and metaphors, poetry, fables, puns, jokes, and riddles.

The most commonly used neuropsychological tests to obtain measurements of cognitive impairments are summarized in Table 13-7. Several tests are often combined to form test batteries; however, if test batteries are too lengthy, fatigue and impaired concentration interfere with performance and may invalidate results (65).

The *SCATBI* is a diagnostic test for adolescents and adults (64) designed to assess cognitive-linguistic status after closed head injury and to describe the extent of changes during and following rehabilitation. This test was constructed to measure performance on five scales, each repre-

Table 13-7: Instruments Available to Measure Cognitive Processes: Attention/Orientation, Perception/Discrimination, Memory, and Organization, and Reasoning

	Tests
Tests Measuring Skills	
Attention/orientation	Digit Span (WAIS-R) (Wechsler, 1981) Galveston Orientation and Amnesia Test (GOAT) (Levin et al., 1975) Glasgow Coma Scale (GCS) (Jennett and Teasdale, 1974) Paced Auditory Serial Addition (PASA) (Levin, 1983) Symbol Digit Modalities Test: Written & Oral (Smith, 1968, 1973) Trail Making Test, A&B (Reitan and Davison, 1958, 1974) Wisconsin Card Sorting Test (WCST) (Nelson, 1976)
Perception/discrimination	Color Form Sorting Test (Goldstein and Scheerer, 1945) Developmental Test of Visual Perception (Frostig, 1963) Facial Recognition Test (Benton, desHamsher, Varney, and Spreen, 1983) G-F-W Test of Auditory Discrimination and Sound Symbol Tests (Goldman, 1974) Southern California Figure-Ground Visual Perception Test (Ayres, 1966)
Memory	Auditory-Verbal Learning Task (Rey, 1990) Benton Visual Retention Test (Benton, 1974) Controlled Word Association Test (Benton Hamsher, 1976) Denman Neuropsychology Memory Scale (DNMS) (Denman, 1984) Facial Recognition Test (Benton, Deshamsher, Varney, and Spreen, 1983) G-F-W Auditory Memory Test (Goldman, Fristoe, and Woodcock, 1974) Memory for Designs Test (Graham-Kendall, 1960) Paced Auditory Serial Addition Task (PASAT) (Gronwall, 1977) Post Traumatic Amnesia (PTA) (Teasdale and Jennett, 1974) Revised Benton Visual Retention Test (RBVRT) (Benton, 1974) Randt Memory Test (RMT) (Randt, Brown, and Osborne, 1980) Rey-Osterrieth Complex Figure (Osterrieth, 1944) Rivermead Behavioral Memory Test (Wilson, Cockburn, and Baddeley, 1985) Selective Reminding Test (Buschke and Fuld, 1974) Symbol Digit Modalities Test (Smith, 1982) Tactual Performance Test (Halstead, 1947; Reitan and Davidson, 1974) Visual Retention Test (Benton, 1974, 1992) Wechsler Memory Scale (WMS) (Wechsler and Stone, 1945) Word Fluency Test (Borkowski, Benton, and Spreen, 1967)
Organization and reasoning	Auditory Verbal Learning (Rey, 1964) Category Test (Halstead, 1947) Controlled Oral Word Association Test (COWAT) (Malec et al., 1993) Detroit Tests of Learning Aptitude (Baker and Leland, 1935) Hooper Visual Organization Test (Hooper, 1958) Hooper Test of Visual Organization (Hooper, 1966) Paired Associates Test (Inglis, 1994) Raven's Progressive Matrices (Raven, 1960) Rey-Osterrieth Complex Figure Test (Osterrieth, 1944) Ross Test of Higher Cognitive Processes (Ross and Ross, 1976) Wisconsin Card Sorting Test (WCST) (Nelson, 1976) Wisconsin Card Sorting Test (Grant and Berg, 1948; Heaton, 1981)
Test batteries designed to measure several cognitive processes	Detroit Test of Learning Aptitude (Baker and Leland, 1935) Neurobehavioral Rating Scale (NRS) (Levin, 1987) Orientation Group Monitoring System (OGMS) (Jackson, Mysin, and Corrigan, 1989) Ross Test of Higher Cognitive Processes (Ross and Ross, 1976) Scales of Cognitive Abilities After Traumatic Brain Injury (SCATBI) (Adamovich and Henderson, 1992) Wechsler Adult Intelligence Scale (WAISR) (Wechsler, 1981)
Instruments available to measure social adjustment, severity of injury, personalities and behavior, and independence	

Table 13-7: (*Continued*)

	Tests
Personality and behavior	Brief Psychiatric Rating Scale (BPRS) (Overall and Gorham, 1962) Minnesota Multiphasic Personality Inventory (MMPI, 1992)
Independence	Disability Rating Scale (DRS) (Rappaport et al., 1982) Functional Independence Measure (FIM) (State University of New York at Buffalo, 1993) Glasgow Outcome Scale (GOS) (Jennett and Bond, 1975) Glasgow Assessment Schedule (GAS) (Livingston and Livingston, 1985)
Social adjustment	The Katz Adjustment Scale (Katz and Lyerly, 1963) The Katz Adjustment Scale—Relatives Form (KAS-R) (Katz and Lyerly, 1963) Social Adjustment Scale—Self Report (SAS-SR) (Weissman, 1975)
Severity of injury	Glasgow Coma Scale (GCS) (Teasdale and Jennett, 1974) Post-Traumatic Amnesia (PTA) (Russell, 1932) Rancho Los Amigos Scale of Cognitive Function (Hagen, 1982)

senting a general area of cognitive ability that may be impaired after closed head injury and is ultimately necessary to function in day-to-day living. The five scales are perception and discrimination, orientation, organization, recall, and reasoning. Each scale is made up of a series of small tests, or "testlets" (66). Testlets are collections of similar items designed to measure a common trait or subdomain. In general, individual items within each testlet were designed to exhibit a slight progression in difficulty from easier to more difficult. The cognitive rehabilitation treatment hierarchy based on the hierarchy of cognitive processes in the SCATBI satisfies theories of instruction and general learning as stated by Collins et al (67) and Bruner (68).

Subtle cognitive deficits of high-level clients often become apparent during group interactions. Unfamiliar situations are particularly stressful. Specific behaviors that emerge include the following:

1. Inability to understand the point of view of others
2. Rigidity in modifying an opinion
3. Difficulty recognizing the main point of a conversation
4. Inability to question or clarify in an attempt to gain additional information necessary to form an appropriate conclusion
5. Difficulty taking turns
6. Difficulty giving and receiving feedback
7. Concern for self-goals, causing difficulty accepting group decisions
8. Presentation of too little or excessive information
9. Difficulty switching from one topic to another
10. Lack of self-esteem and self-appraisal
11. Inability to connect short-term goals and long-term goals, such that the individuals fail to see the relevancy of therapy tasks or group activities to their life in general
12. Establishment of unrealistic individual goals and aspirations due to a denial of deficits

Higher-level attention deficits tend to result in more pragmatic and interactive or interpersonal disruptions. Attentional disturbances experienced by persons with closed head injury functioning at a higher cognitive level may result in behavior that appears to be egocentric, rude, impulsive, disinhibited, denying, and lacking in coherence (i.e., information conveyed both verbally and graphically is out of sequence). Conversations tend to turn on and off, with frequent, off-the-track interjections. The off-the-track interjections often become new topics, leaving the previous topic abandoned and incomplete. Distractibility also interferes with task completion. The performance of high-level head-injured persons deteriorates when distractions occur or if they are given too much information or stimulation, causing them to become overwhelmed and unable to proceed effectively.

AUDIOLOGY

Hearing is the first stage in the process of comprehension. While this may be an obvious statement, the impact of hearing is poorly appreciated until a hearing loss actually is experienced. In the normal population, hearing loss may result in depression and social isolation. In the subject with a neurologic impairment, a hearing deficit may compound problems in auditory processing, thereby significantly hindering a positive functional outcome. Because of the ramifications of hearing loss, it is incumbent on the clinician to understand the physiology, pathophysiology, diagnosis, and treatment options for hearing loss.

Anatomy and Physiology

The hearing mechanism consists of three major portions: the *outer ear*, the *middle ear*, and the *inner ear*. The *outer ear* contains the auricle and auditory canal. The *auricle* assists in funneling sounds into the ear; if it were not present, it would only affect hearing sensitivity by 5 to 6 decibels. The *auditory canal* is a narrow tube covered by cilia, which secrete cerumen to protect the outer-ear structures from foreign bodies. The *tympanic membrane* vibrates in synchronization to sounds that enter the canal.

The *middle ear* contains the *ossicular chain*, which converts acoustic energy into mechanical energy. The chain consists of three bones: the *malleus (hammer)*, the *incus (anvil)*, and the *stapes (stirrup)*. The *eustachian tube* connects the middle ear with the nasopharynx, and serves to equilibrate pressures on both sides of the tympanic membrane. The middle ear also contains two muscles, the *tensor tympani* and the *stapedius*, which protect the hearing mechanism from damage by tightening the tympanic membrane during loud noises.

The *inner ear* articulates with the middle ear at the *oval window*, from which energy is transmitted via the tympanic membrane. Energy is converted into fluid waves, which enter the *cochlea*. The cochlea contains *hair cells* connected to specialized nerve endings that are activated in response to specific pitches. In addition, there are three *semicircular canals* that provide vestibular input in three planes. The cochlea and semicircular canals are connected by the *vestibule*. The nerve impulses travel to the central nervous system through *cranial nerve VIII*.

Pathophysiology

The type of hearing loss depends on the location of the impairment. A *conductive* hearing loss results from abnormalities in the outer or middle ear. Subjects with conductive hearing loss usually can discriminate speech normally, but require louder volumes to compensate for the conductive deficit. Conditions resulting in conductive hearing loss include cerumen impaction, foreign body, tympanic membrane perforation, otitis media, otosclerosis, or ossicular discontinuity.

Sensorineural hearing loss results from abnormalities in the inner ear or associated neural pathways. Subjects with sensorineural hearing loss usually have reduced speech discrimination. Conditions resulting in sensorineural hearing loss include drug ototoxicity, childhood diseases (e.g., mumps, measles, chickenpox, diphtheria, scarlet fever, whooping cough), prolonged exposure to excess noise, presbycusis (hearing loss with advancing age), acoustic neuroma, and cortical lesions (e.g., aphasia, auditory agnosia). A *mixed* hearing loss occurs if components of both conductive and sensorineural hearing losses are present.

Evaluation

Audiometric screenings may be accomplished with *pure-tone air conduction audiometry* (PTACA) or *speech audiometry* (SA). A complete audiometric evaluation (CAE) may also include *pure-tone bone conduction audiometry* (PTBCA), *speech discrimination assessment* (SDA), and *impedance testing*. If needed, more elaborate testing can be performed to localize the site of the lesion.

PTACA tests the intensity of audible frequencies ranging from 125 to 8000 Hz. It provides information on the degree and configuration of hearing loss, but cannot specifically locate a site of lesion. SA tests the softest levels at which 25 to 50 two-syllable words can be comprehended. A *speech reception threshold* (SRT), defined as the hearing level at which a subject repeats 50% of the words accurately, may be calculated from the results.

PTBCA tests the integrity of the middle ear by determining thresholds at which sound vibrations between 250 and 4000 Hz applied to the mastoid process can be heard. SDA analyzes the ability to understand 25 to 50 one-syllable words when presented at normal volumes. Impedance testing measures the mobility of the tympanic membrane, the resistance of the ossicular chain to air pressure, and the reflex action of the stapedius muscle.

More specialized tests can be performed if the subject cannot respond appropriately to conventional tests or if precise location of a lesion site is required. Tests of *brain stem auditory evoked potential* (BAEP) assess cortical responses to a "click," and are sensitive in the diagnosis of acoustic neuroma. *Electrocochleography* measures electrophysiologic activity beginning in the cochlea and may augment information obtained by BAEP testing. Other tests can be performed to assess the presence of loudness recruitment, which is a cochlear sign, or abnormal auditory adaptation, which is a neural sign.

REFERENCES

1. Müller FM. *Lectures on the science of language*. London: Longman, 1891.
2. Whitney WD. *Language and the study of language*. New York: Scribner, 1867.
3. Breasted JH. *The Edwin Smith sugical papyrus*. Chicago: University of Chicago Press, 1930.
4. Herodotus. *Herodotus II*. 4th ed. Book IV, Vol. 3. London: S & R Bentley, 54.
5. Hippocrates; Jones WHS, trans. *The sacred disease*. Vol. 2, XVII. London: Heinemann, 1923.
6. Wertz RT. Neuropathologies of speech and language: an introduction to patient management. In: Johns DF, ed. *Clinical management of neurogenic communicative disorders*. 2nd ed. Boston: Little, Brown, 1985:23.
7. Head H. *Aphasia and kindred disorders of speech*. New York: Macmillan, 1926.
8. Brain WR. *Speech disorders*. London: Butterworths, 1961.

9. Mohr JP, Watters W, Duncan G. Thalamic hemorrhage and aphasia. *Brain Lang* 1975;2:3–17.

10. Naeser MA, Alexander M, Helm-Estabrooks N, et al. Aphasia with predominantly subcortical sites. *Arch Neurol* 1982;29:2–14.

11. Gorelick P, Hier D, Benevento L, et al. Aphasia after left thalamic infarction. *Arch Neurol* 1984;41: 1296–1298.

12. Geschwind N. Anatomical understanding of the aphasias. In: Benton AL, ed. *Contribution to clinical neuropsychology.* Chicago: Aldine, 1969.

13. Geschwind N. Current concepts: aphasia. *N Engl J Med* 1971;284: 654–656.

14. Kirk A, Kertesz A. Assessment of aphasia. *Phys Med Rehabil STAR* 1992;6:433–450.

15. Schuell HM. *Differential diagnosis of aphasis with the Minnesota Test (second edition, revised by Sefer, J.W.).* Minneapolis: University of Minnesota Press, 1973:15.

16. Kaplan E, Goodglass H, Weintraub S. *The Boston Naming Test. Philadelphia*: Lea & Febiger, 1983.

17. Goodglass H, Kaplan E. *Assessment of aphasia and related disorders.* 2nd ed. Philadelphia: Lea & Febiger, 1983.

18. Kertesz A, Poole E. The aphasia quotient: the taxonomic approach to measurement of aphasic disability. *Can J Neurol Sci* 1974;11: 7–16.

19. Kertesz A. *The Western Aphasia Battery.* New York: Grune & Stratton, 1982.

20. Shewan CM, Kertesz A. Reliability and validity characteristics of the Western Aphasia Battery (WAB). *J Speech Hear Disord* 1984;45: 308–324.

21. Porch BE. *The Porch Index of Communicative Ability.* Palo Alto: Consulting Psychologists Press, 1981.

22. Spreen O, Benton AL. *Neurosensory Center Comprehensive Examination for Aphasia.* 2nd ed. Victoria, BC, Canada: University of Victoria, Neuropsychology Laboratory, 1977.

23. Sarno MT. *The Functional Communication Profile: manual of directions.* New York: New York University Medical Center, Institute of Rehabilitation Medicine, 1969.

24. Sarno MT, Buonaguro A, Levita E. Gender and recovery from aphasia after stroke. *J Nerv Ment Dis* 1985;173:605–609.

25. Holland AL. *Communicative Abilities in Daily Living: Manual.* Baltimore: University Park Press, 1980.

26. De Renzi E. The Token Test and the Reporter's Test: a measure of verbal input and a measure of verbal output. In: Sarno MT, Hook O, eds. *Aphasia: assessment and treatment.* New York: Masson, 1980.

27. McNeil MR, Prescott TE. *Revised Token Test.* Baltimore: University Park Press, 1978.

28. Sklar M. Sklar Aphasia Scale. *Rev. ed.* Los Angeles: Western Psychological Services, 1973.

29. Keenan JS, Brassell EG. *Aphasia Language Performance Scales.* Murfreesboro, TN: Pinnacle Press, 1975.

30. Fitch-West J, Sands ES. *Bedside Evaluation Screening Test.* Rockville, MD: Aspen, 1987.

31. Helm-Estabrooks N, Hotz G. *Brief Test of Head Injury (BTHI).* Chicago: Riverside, 1990.

32. Whurr R. *An Aphasia Screening Test.* Teading, UK: University of Reading, 1974.

33. Enderby P, Wood V, Wade D. *Frenchay Aphasia Screening Test.* Windson, UK: Nelson, 1987.

34. Shewan CM. *Auditory Comprehension Test for Sentences.* Chicago: Biolinguistics Clinical Institutes, 1979.

35. LaPointe LL, Horner J. The Functional Auditory Comprehension Task (FACT): protocol and test format. *FLASHA* 1978:27–33.

36. LaPoint LL, Horner J. *Reading Comprehension Battery for Aphasia.* Chicago: Riverside, 1979.

37. Varney NR, Benton AL. *Pantomime Recognition Test.* Iowa City: Benton Laboratory of Neuropsychology, 1978.

38. Duffy RJ, Duffy JR. *Assessment of Nonverbal Communication.* Tigard, OR: CC Publications, 1984.

39. State University of New York at Buffalo, Research Foundation. *Guide for Use of the Uniform Data Set for Medical Rehabilitation*: Functional Independence Measure. Buffalo: Research Foundation, 1990.

40. Martin D. Some objections to the term, "apraxia of speech." *J Speech Hear Disord* 1974;39: 53–64.

41. Luria AR. *Higher cortical functions in man.* New York: Basic Books, 1980.

42. Wertz RT, LaPointe LL, Rosenbek JC. *Apraxia of speech in adults: the disorder and its management.* New York: Grune & Stratton, 1984.

43. Dabul B. *Apraxia Battery for Adults.* Tigard, OR: CC Publications, 1979.

44. Peacher WG. Speech disorders in World War II. VII. Treatment of dysarthria. *J Nerv Ment Disord* 1947;106:66.

45. Morley DE. The rehabilitation of adults with dysarthric speech. *J Speech Hear Disord* 1955;20:58.

46. Grewel F. Classification of dysanthrias. *Acta Psychiatr Neurol Scand* 1957;32:325.

47. Canter GJ. Neuromotor pathologies of speech. *Am J Phys Med* 1967;46:659.

48. Darley FL, Aronson AE, Brown JE. Differential diagnostic patterns of dysarthria. *J Speech Hear Disord* 1969;12:246–269.

49. Darley FL, Aronson AE, Brown JE. Clusters of deviant speech dimen-

sion in the dysarthrias. *J Speech Hear Disord* 1969;12:462–496.

50. Yorkston KM, Beukelman DR. *Assessment of Intelligibility of Dysarthric Speech.* Austin, TX: PRO-ED, 1982.

51. Enderby P. *The Frenchay Dysarthria Assessment.* San Diego: College-Hill, 1983.

52. American Speech-Language-Hearing Association, Task Force on Cognitive-Communicative Impairments. Working draft of the role of speech-language pathologists in the habilitation and rehabilitation of cognitively impaired individuals. American Speech-Language-Hearing Associations, 1987.

53. Sohlberg MM, Mateer CA. *Introduction to cognitive rehabilitation: theory and practice.* New York: Guilford, 1989.

54. Bayles KA, Kaszniak A. *Communication and cognition in normal aging and dementia.* Boston: College-Hill, 1987.

55. Adamovich BB, Henderson JA, Auerbach S. *Cognitive rehabilitation of closed head injured patients.* San Diego: College-Hill, 1985.

56. Lezak MD. The problem of assessing executive functions. *Int J Psychol* 1982;17:281–297.

57. Ylvisaker M. Cognitive and psychosocial outcome following head injury in children. In: Hoff JT, Anderson TE, Cole TM, eds. *Mild to moderate head injury.* London; Blackwell Scientific, 1989.

58. Ylkvisaker M, Szekeres HK. Topics in cognitive rehabilitation therapy. In: Ylvisaker M, Gobble E, eds. *Community re-entry for head injured adults.* Boston: Little, Brown, 1987:174–175.

59. Wehman P, Kreutzer J, West M, et al. Employment outcomes of persons following traumatic brain injury: pre-injury, post-injury and supported employment. *Brain Injury* 1989;3:397–412.

60. Haffey WJ, Lewis FD. Programming for occupational outcome following traumatic brain injury. *Rehabil Psychol* 1989;34:147–159.

61. Burns MS, Halper AS, Mogil SI. *Clinical management of right hemisphere dysfunction.* Gaithersburg, MD: Aspen Systems, 1985.

62. Pimental PA, Kingsbury NA, eds. *Neuropsychological aspects of right brain injury.* Austin, TX: PRO-ED, 1989.

63. Kennedy MRT, Burton W, Peterson C. *Adult Conversational Analysis Tool.* Downey, CA: Communication Disorders Department, Ranchos Los Amigos Medical Center, 1990.

64. Adamovich BLB, Henderson J. *Scales of Cognitive Ability for Traumatic Brain Injury* (SCATBI). Chicago: Riverside, 1992.

65. Bond MR, Brooks DN. Understanding the process of recovery as a basis for the investigation of rehabilitation for the brain injured. *Scand J Rehabil Med* 1976;8: 127–133.

66. Thissen D, Steinberg L, Mooney JA. Trace line for testlets: a use of multiple-categorical-response models. *J Educ Measure* 1989:26.

67. Collins A, Brown JS, Newman SE. Cognitive apprenticeship: teaching the crafts of reading, writing and mathematics. In: Resnick LB, ed. *Knowing, learning, and instruction: essays in honor of Robert Glaser.* Hillsdale, NJ: Erlbaum, 1989.

68. Bruner JS. *Toward a theory of instruction.* Cambridge: Belknap, 1966.

Chapter 14

Swallowing Disorders

Jeffrey B. Palmer

Swallowing is an essential biologic function that begins in utero and continues throughout life. Difficulty with swallowing (or dysphagia) is common in elderly and disabled individuals, and may lead to serious sequelae including dehydration, starvation, aspiration pneumonia, and airway obstruction. Disorders that cause an impairment in swallowing, such as stroke, cancer, and connective tissue disease, are commonly treated by comprehensive rehabilitation. Management of impaired swallowing often requires an integrated, multidisciplinary approach to diagnosis and treatment. For these reasons, among others, management of dysphagia is an important part of rehabilitation medicine. This chapter reviews the physiology of normal and abnormal swallowing, and discusses the rehabilitation approach to patient evaluation, including the history, physical examination, and diagnostic studies.

PHYSIOLOGY

Normal Swallowing

The key structures of swallowing reside in the oral cavity, pharynx, larynx, and esophagus (Fig. 14-1). For convenience, the process of swallowing is commonly divided into oral, pharyngeal, and esophageal phases, based on the anatomic location of the food being swallowed (1–3). Thus, food is prepared for swallowing and propelled into the pharynx during the oral phase. It is propelled through the upper esophageal sphincter (UES) and into the esophagus during the pharyngeal phase. In the esophageal phase, the bolus is propelled down the esophagus, through the lower esophageal sphincter (LES), and into the stomach. However, this phase model applies anatomic terminology to a physiologic process. In reality, the phases are not always sequential. Indeed, they may overlap or occur out of sequence.

Oral Phase

The oral phase includes both preparatory behaviors (which soften foods and mix them with saliva) and propulsive behaviors (which transport food through the faucial pillars and into the oropharynx). The first event in the oral phase is ingestion, in which food enters the mouth by one of several mechanisms (such as biting, licking, suckling, or manual placement). In stage I transport, food is propelled from the anterior part of the oral cavity to the molar region; it moves from the oral cavity to the pharynx during stage II transport (4). Liquids may be transported through the oral cavity and into the oropharynx in one smooth, continuous motion. Solid foods, however, require additional processing. During mastication (including chewing and mixing with saliva), food is pushed between the upper and lower molars by the tongue and crushed during cyclical opening and closing of the jaws. The physical consistency of the food is monitored continuously by mechanoreceptors in the periodontal ligament and palate. When a portion of the food is softened enough for swallowing, the tongue segregates it from the remaining oral

Figure 14-1. Lateral and posterior views of the pharynx. *A.* The structures in the sagittal plane: the tongue (T), uvula (u), epiglottis (*upper arrow*), hyoid bone (h), laryngeal vestibule (ve), vocal folds (false, *short arrow*; true, *arrowhead*), arytenoid mass (a), cricoid cartilage (*lower arrow*), and trachea (t). *B.* The structures in the anterior wall of the pharynx as viewed from the posterior aspect. The midposterior pharyngeal raphe and the posterior portion of the proximal cervical esophagus have been sectioned and each side drawn laterally to expose the structures. On the right side, the mucosa has been stripped to demonstrate the underlying muscles, while on the left side the mucosa remains intact. This drawing shows the contours of the valleculae and pyriform sinuses and demonstrates the relationship of the valleculae to the base of the tongue and epiglottis. (Reproduced by permission from Donner MW, Bosma JF, Robertson DL. Anatomy and physiology of the pharynx. *Gastrointest Radiol* 1985; 10:196–212.)

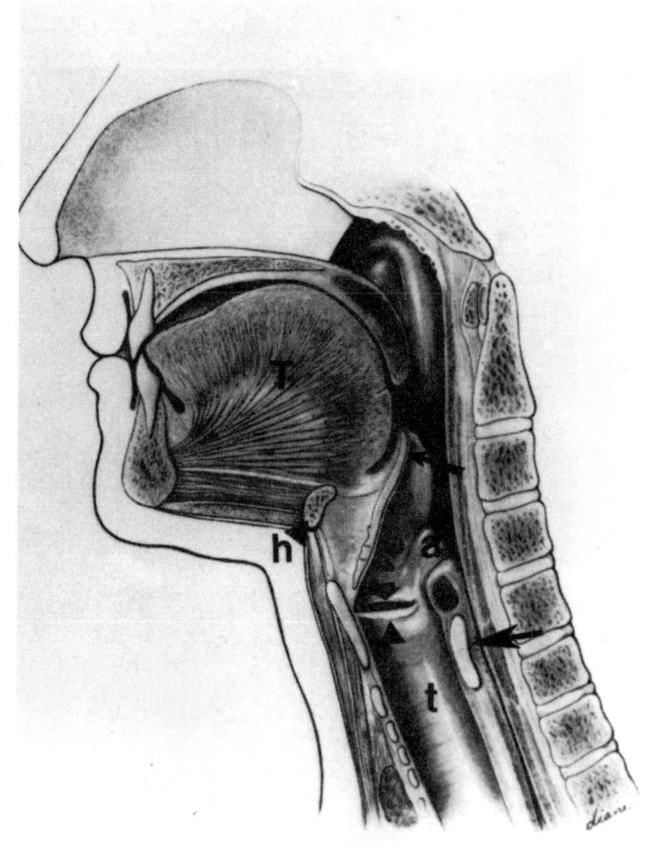

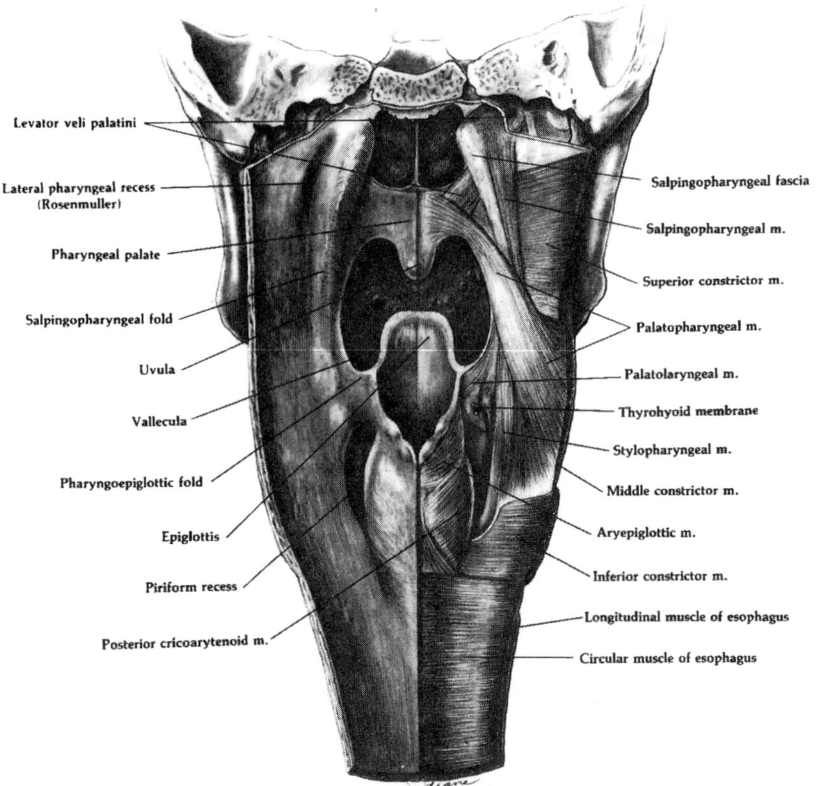

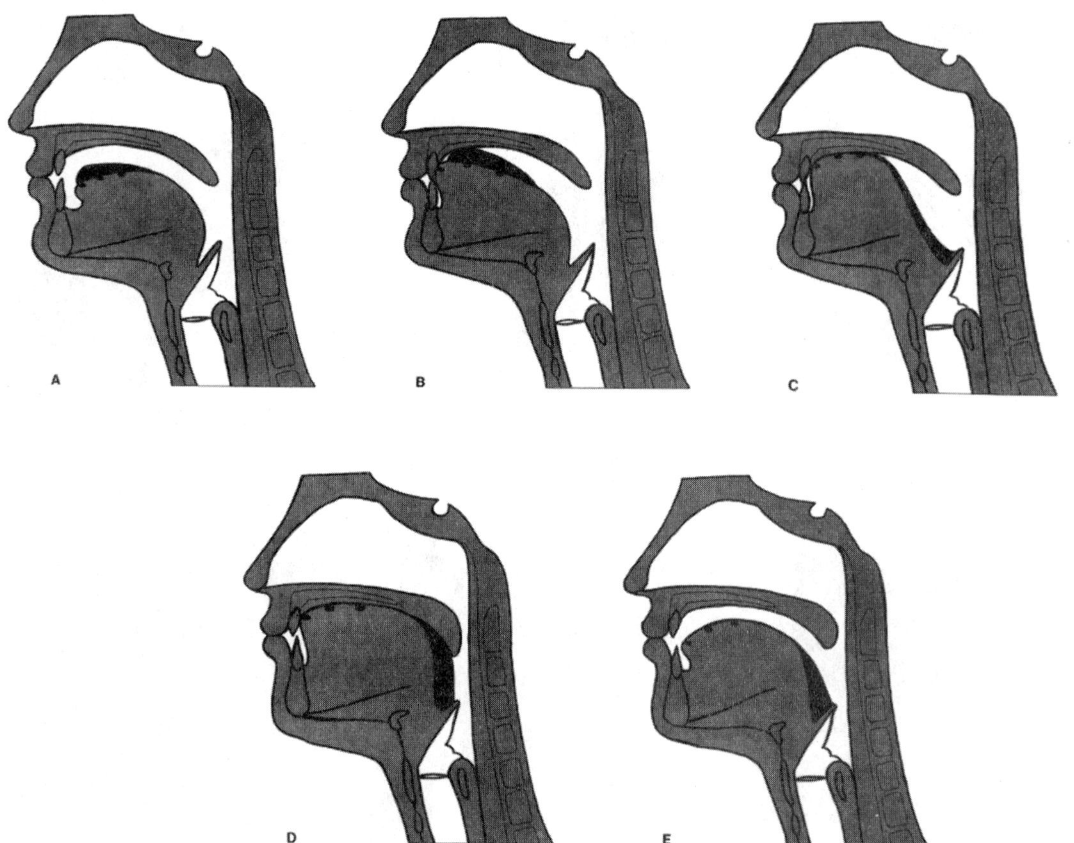

Figure 14-2. Stage II transport as seen in the lateral projection. These drawings show selected frames of a normal subject eating solid food combined with barium, recorded by videofluorography. Three small radiopaque markers were glued to the surface of the tongue to highlight its movement. *A.* A quantity of food (shown in *black*) has been softened and mixed with saliva, and is sitting on the dorsum of the tongue. *B.* The jaws close, and the tongue tip moves upward and forward, contacting the hard palate anteriorly. *C.* The tongue moves upward while the jaws remain closed. The area of tongue-palate contact expands posteriorly, pushing food into the oropharynx. *D.* The tongue continues to move upward as the mouth opens. The area of tongue-palate contact continues to increase as a portion of the food collects in the valleculae (the space between the epiglottis and the back of the tongue). *E.* The jaw reaches its maximum downward position (maximum gape) and the tongue drops away from the palate. A portion of food remains in the valleculae. (Illustration by Jianmin Liu, MD.)

contents, and propels it into the oropharynx. At the onset of stage II transport, the tongue pushes upward and forward, contacting the hard palate anteriorly (Fig. 14-2). The tongue surface continues to move upward, expanding the area of tongue-palate contact from the front of the palate toward the back, and propelling the prepared portion of food through the faucial pillars and into the oropharynx. This prepared portion may remain in the oropharynx for many additional chewing cycles, and stage II transport may be repeated several times before the pharyngeal phase is initiated (5).

Pharyngeal Phase

When the pharyngeal phase of swallowing begins, there is a rapid, overlapping sequence of events (Fig. 14-3). Respiration ceases temporarily. The soft palate presses against the lateral and posterior pharyngeal walls, closing off the nasopharynx. The true vocal folds close tightly, to prevent aspiration. The larynx is pulled forward under the base of the tongue, and the epiglottis tilts back, deflecting the bolus away from the laryngeal aditus (opening). The tongue pushes the bolus back and down into the hypopharynx. The UES opens, allowing the bolus to pass into the esophagus. The pharyngeal constrictor muscles contract sequentially from top to bottom, clearing the remaining material from the pharynx. After the bolus enters the esophagus, respiration resumes, and the pharyngeal and laryngeal structures return to their original anatomic position (1).

The UES is held closed between swallows by tonic contraction of the cricopharyngeus muscle (6). This tonic contraction is necessary to prevent air from entering the esophagus during the inspiratory phase of breathing. The mechanism of UES opening is a complex, active process. When a pharyngeal swallow is initiated, the cricopharyngeus muscle relaxes for about a second, allowing the

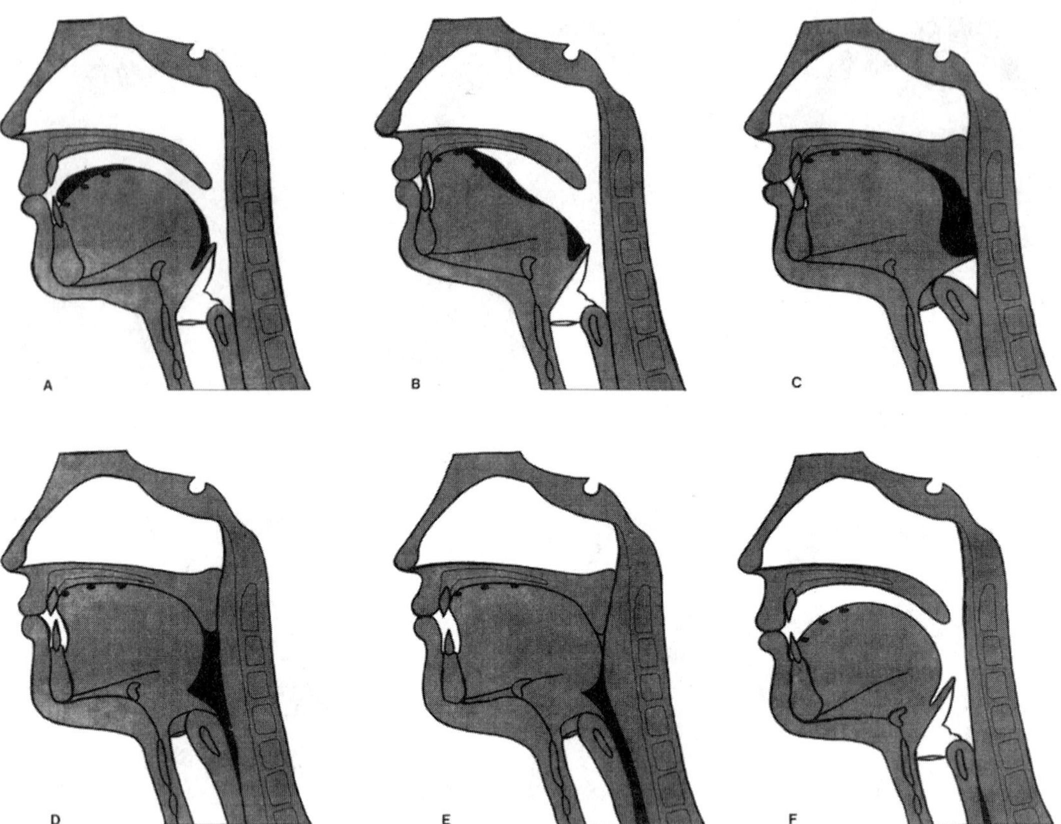

Figure 14-3. A swallow in the lateral projection. *A.* A quantity of food (shown in *black*) is sitting on the dorsum of the tongue. An additional portion of the food is already in the valleculae; it was propelled there during a prior stage II transport cycle, as shown in Figure 14-2. *B.* The jaws close, and the tongue tip moves upward and forward, contacting the hard palate anteriorly. *C.* The tongue continues moving upward while the jaws remain closed. The area of tongue-palate contact expands posteriorly, pushing additional food into the oropharynx. This bolus joins the small portion already in the valleculae. The soft palate and larynx begin to elevate, and the epiglottis begins to tilt. *D.* The jaws begin to open as the tongue pushes back into the pharynx, pushing the bolus downward through the hypopharynx. The hyoid bone and larynx are pulled upward and forward, opening the upper esophageal sphincter. *E.* The jaw reaches maximum gape as the tongue continues pushing backward and the bolus passes through the upper esophageal sphincter. The posterior pharyngeal wall pushes forward to contact the posterior surface of the tongue, clearing the pharynx of residue. *F.* The tongue drops away from the palate, the larynx and nasopharynx open, and the upper esophageal sphincter closes as the bolus passes down the esophagus. (Illustration by Jianmin Liu, MD.)

sphincter to open. The hyoid bone and larynx are pulled forward and upward by contraction of the suprahyoid and thyrohyoid muscles. This pulls the cricoid cartilage and the attached anterior pharyngeal wall away from the posterior pharyngeal wall and underlying vertebral column, opening the pharyngoesophageal sphincter (7). Some additional impetus for sphincter opening is provided by the pressure of the descending bolus. The key concept is that opening of the pharyngoesophageal sphincter is primarily an active process, dependent on contraction of the suprahyoid and thyrohyoid muscles (5). In this way it differs from the classic concept of the anatomic sphincter, which is a circular band of muscle that is tonically active; when it relaxes, it is simply pushed open by the pressure of the passing bolus.

Esophageal Phase

The bolus moves down the esophagus, through the LES, and into the stomach during the esophageal phase (2). Immediately following the pharyngeal phase there is a primary peristaltic wave in the esophagus that begins at the pharyngoesophageal junction and propagates downward to the LES. Peristalsis consists of a wave of relaxation followed by a wave of contraction that propels the bolus through the esophagus. When subjects swallow in the upright position, gravity also assists esophageal transport. The LES is closed between swallows, but relaxes during the esophageal phase. It is pushed open by the pressure of the descending bolus. If the subject swallows again during esophageal peristalsis, the primary peristaltic wave is interrupted and starts again at the top of the esophagus.

A critical role of the LES is prevention of gastroesophageal reflux. The stomach is well protected against damage by its highly acidic contents. The epithelium of the esophagus, however, is not so protected, and exposure to gastric acid may cause esophagitis, ulceration, and subsequent fibrosis. Gastroesophageal reflux and its sequelae are prevented (or limited) by contraction of the LES and UES, and by secondary peristalsis, a propagated propulsive wave in the esophagus that is elicited by localized esophageal distention. It occurs in the absence of pharyngeal swallow, while primary esophageal peristalsis, by definition, always follows immediately after the pharyngeal phase of swallowing.

Abnormal Swallowing

Swallowing has two basic purposes. The first, and most obvious, is transport of food from the oral cavity to the stomach. The second is protection of the airway; swallowing clears the pharynx and prevents inappropriate material from entering the larynx, trachea, and lungs. Disorders of swallowing, regardless of etiology, may jeopardize airway integrity, cause failure of transport, or do both (8).

A number of structural disorders cause swallowing impairment. These may mimic physiologic disorders, since their effects (failure of transport or airway protection) are similar. Consequently, a high index of suspicion is necessary to avoid misdiagnosis. Transport functions are commonly disrupted by structural disorders. Obstruction of the foodway by a mass or stricture may prevent bolus transport via a direct mechanical effect. Surgical excision of foodway structures may impair or prevent bolus propulsion. Stiffness or fixation of foodway structures (due to fibrosis or infiltration) may also impair bolus transport by altering muscle contractility. Airway protection may be compromised by fixation or surgical alteration of the larynx, tongue, or suprahyoid muscles. Passageway obstruction may secondarily affect airway protection if a large bolus accumulates adjacent to the laryngeal aditus (3).

Oral Phase

Oral phase abnormalities include the inability to prepare food for swallowing (by forming a swallow-safe bolus) and the inability to transfer food to the oropharynx (3). Anatomic lesions of the tongue (such as partial glossectomy) may cause functional abnormalities including retention of food in the buccal recesses, failure of oral transport, or uncontrolled flow of liquids into the pharynx under the influence of gravity. These same functional abnormalities may be seen in patients with weakness or incoordination of the tongue. There are many possible causes, including cerebral or brain stem infarction (9), intracranial hemorrhage, brain tumor, motor neuron disease, and primary muscle disease (such as polymyositis) (10). Spasticity of the tongue in pseudobulbar palsy may obstruct oral transport.

Pharyngeal Phase

Aspiration of microscopic quantities is a physiologic event, but aspiration of larger quantities is uncommon in normal individuals. Aspiration can occur before, during, or after swallowing. If the onset of pharyngeal swallowing is substantially delayed after oral propulsion, liquid may be aspirated into the trachea through a wide-open larynx. Solid food may be inhaled and obstruct the airway, with potentially lethal consequences (11). Delayed onset of swallowing is common with a wide range of disorders including stroke, radiation fibrosis, and muscle disease, and following head and neck surgery (3). Aspiration during the swallow may occur if laryngeal closure is delayed or incomplete due to laryngeal tumor, vocal cord paralysis, supraglottic laryngectomy, or cerebral dysfunction. Following the swallow, food retained in the pharynx may be aspirated as the patient inhales air.

The clinical consequences of aspiration are highly variable. Some patients sustain serious illness (such as aspiration pneumonia) in response to aspiration, while others suffer no ill effects (12). The risk of illness due to aspiration depends on several factors. One factor is the depth of aspiration; that is, whether the material merely enters the subglottic portion of the larynx or actually passes down into the distal airways and lung. A second factor is the nature of the aspirated material. Aspiration of solid food may be disastrous if it obstructs the airway. Acids are much more harmful to the lung than alkali, so stomach contents are particularly hazardous. A third factor is the amount of material aspirated; a tiny amount is usually well tolerated. Finally, the physiologic response to aspiration is critical. Pneumonia is unlikely if prompt, effective coughing clears the larynx and trachea. However, airway protection reflexes are often impaired in individuals with dysphagia due to central nervous system dysfunction. Aspiration that fails to elicit coughing (so-called silent aspiration) often leads to respiratory sequelae (13).

Normal subjects occasionally retain small amounts of food in the pharyngeal recesses after swallowing (5). However, excessive retention of food in the pharynx after swallowing may be produced by obstruction of the foodway (as in pharyngeal webs or strictures) or by weakness or incoordination of the pharynx. Pharyngeal weakness may be caused by a reduction in the driving force of the tongue or a weakness of the pharyngeal constrictor muscles due to nerve or muscle disease. Unilateral constrictor palsy usually results from lower motor neuron (LMN) dysfunction subsequent to lesions of the nucleus ambiguus, such as the lateral medullary syndrome of Wallenberg. Pharyngeal retention may also occur in patients with struc-

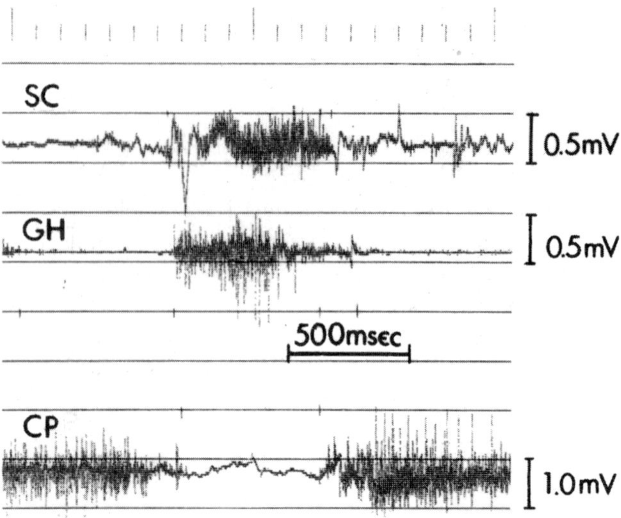

Figure 14-4. Myoelectric activity during a swallow of water, simultaneously recorded in the superior constrictor (SC), geniohyoid (GH, one of the suprahyoid muscles), and cricopharyngeus (CP) muscles, using hooked fine-wire electrodes. The CP muscle is tonically active before and after swallowing, because it helps to hold the upper esophageal sphincter closed, and relaxes for about 1 second during a swallow. The SC and GH muscles relax between swallows but contract phasically during the swallow. (Reproduced by permission from Palmer JB, Tanaka E, Siebens AA. Electromyography of the pharyngeal musculature: technical considerations. *Arch Phys Med Rehabil* 1989;70:283–287.)

tural deficits including partial glossectomy, pharyngotomy, or supraglottic laryngectomy (3,8).

Impaired opening of the UES is another cause of pharyngeal retention after swallowing (8). Functional narrowing of the UES may be caused by a reduction in anterior motion of the larynx during a swallow, or by the presence of a posterior pharyngeal "bar" defect that impinges on the lumen (Fig. 14-4). The physiologic basis for this bar defect has been presumed to be sustained contraction (failure of relaxation) of the cricopharyngeus muscle during swallowing. Indeed, this is the basis for performing a therapeutic cricopharyngeal myotomy, a surgical procedure in which the cricopharyngeus muscle is disrupted to reduce the resistance to pharyngeal outflow. However, sustained contraction of the cricopharyngeus muscle has never been verified with electromyography (EMG), and the role of myotomy remains uncertain.

Esophageal Phase

Esophageal disorders are common in the elderly (2,10). The esophagus has two critical functions: transport of food from the pharynx to the stomach, and prevention of gastroesophageal reflux. Impairment of esophageal transport may be caused by anatomic obstruction, derangement of esophageal peristalsis, or dysfunction of the gastroesophageal sphincter. Patients may experience pain, difficulty swallowing, or regurgitation of food from the esophagus back into the pharynx. Gastroesophageal reflux disease can have serious sequelae. Ulceration and scarring of the esophageal mucosa by stomach acid can cause strictures, with resultant esophageal obstruction. Dysphagia for solid foods suggests a mechanical obstruction, whereas dysphagia for both solids and liquids suggests a motility disorder. If refluxed material is regurgitated into the pharynx, it can be aspirated. Serious respiratory complications may ensue, since the larynx and lungs are highly vulnerable to gastric acid. Intermittent dysphagia may be due to esophageal spasm. Progressive dysphagia may be caused by achalasia. This disease causes loss of esophageal contractility and stenosis of the LES. Progressive obstruction of the esophagus may be caused by esophageal cancer, a disease with high morbidity and mortality.

CLINICAL EVALUATION

Dysphagia may be caused by a wide spectrum of disorders, including neurologic disease, neoplasia, connective tissue disease, trauma, infection, or iatrogenic illness, so it may be necessary to obtain a wide range of historical information to make an etiologic diagnosis. Here I focus on the elements of medical history, physical examination, and diagnostic studies that are most relevant to dysphagia rehabilitation.

History

The medical history is the most important component of the rehabilitation evaluation for dysphagia. It includes medical data pertaining to the etiologic diagnosis, functional data pertaining to analysis of disability, and psychosocial data pertaining to the impact of the dysphagia on social function. The history of present illness should include a precise description of the patient's complaints. Important details include the sensation of food sticking in the throat or chest (sometimes called "true" dysphagia), coughing or choking during or after meals, pain during swallowing (odynophagia), slow rate of eating, change in dietary habits, drooling, difficulty swallowing saliva, changes in voice or speech, the sensation of a lump in the throat (also called globus sensation), and any differences between eating solid foods and drinking liquids. Some patients may describe difficulties with a particular subset of solid or liquid foods. An important point is difficulty with nocturnal drooling or choking; awakening during the night with choking, coughing, and difficulty clearing saliva is associated with severe dysphagia. The past medical history should make note particularly of stroke, neurologic disease, cancer, radiation therapy, head and neck surgery, connective tissue disorders, or respiratory disease. Current medications should be listed, because several of these, including benzodiazepines and anticholinergic drugs, can hamper swallowing. The review of systems should note complaints of dyspnea, cough, sensory loss, weakness, dental problems, or symptoms referable to gastroesophageal reflux disease. The latter include heartburn and regurgitation of acidic, bitter, or solid food (undigested or partially digested).

Social history is essential to the rehabilitation evaluation, and should include information on psychological adjustment as well as the impact of the swallowing problem on the family, social relationships, and vocation. This aspect of the dysphagia evaluation is often overlooked. In fact, dysphagia may have profound effects on social function. In society, much of the social interaction is structured around meals and food consumption. Many families have the bulk of their interpersonal contact during meals. Interaction among friends, colleagues, and business associates is often linked to having cocktails, hor d'oeuvres, dinner, coffee, or dessert together. The inability to participate in these activities profoundly limits an individual's opportunities for human contact and participation in critical vocational and avocational activities. The ultimate goal of the rehabilitation program is to enable the individual to resume social roles, thus minimizing the handicap. Doing so requires an understanding of his or her social roles, and what they demand of the individual. Two patients with the same structural or physiologic impairment of swallowing may have radically different rehabilitation plans, depending on their essential social activities. For example, a retired individual may need an aggressive program of exercise and therapy that would be inappropriate for an individual who is employed full-time. The latter individual may prefer to return to work with a gastrostomy feeding tube in place, rather than taking the time for an elaborate program of therapeutic feeding.

Physical Examination

Examining the dysphagic patient requires 1) a general physical examination, 2) screening examination of mental status, 3) special attention to the anatomic structures and physiologic processes related to swallowing and feeding, and 4) observation of trial swallows. The general appearance of the patient may offer important clues regarding ability to swallow. Note whether the patient exhibits drooling; frequent coughing or expectorating; posturing of the head, neck, jaw, or tongue; or respiratory distress. Some dysphagic patients will expectorate frequently or use a tissue to remove saliva from the oral cavity. The general physical examination should include a brief assessment of major body systems, including the respiratory, cardiovascular, gastrointestinal, musculoskeletal, and neurologic systems. Depending on the differential diagnosis of the underlying disorder, these or other body systems may require comprehensive physical examination.

Cognitive and communicative skills should be assessed carefully in dysphagic patients. There is a high rate of cognitive and linguistic dysfunction in patients with disorders of feeding and swallowing (14). The screening examination of mental status should include a brief assessment of orientation, memory, attention, and the patient's ability to follow verbal and gestural commands. It is important to note if the patient is impulsive, confused, or uncooperative or has severe perceptual deficits (such as left-sided hemi-inattention) because these factors may affect the ability to participate in a structured dysphagia rehabilitation program. The cognitively impaired patient may need close supervision during a therapeutic feeding program to prevent aspiration or airway obstruction. Speech must be examined carefully, because dysphonia and dysarthria are often associated with dysphagia. Dysphonia is of particular importance, because its presence may be predictive of aspiration.

In examining structure related to swallowing, the head and neck are examined for evidence of inflammation or structural abnormalities, including masses or abnormal curvature of the spine. The anterior region of the neck is palpated gently. The hyoid bone and thyroid and cricoid cartilages are manipulated and should be mobile. The mandible should move freely. Jaw opening should be smooth and symmetric, with a full range of motion for opening as well as anteroposterior motion. The oral cavity is inspected (and palpated as necessary) for dentition, mucosal lesions, and retained food or secretions. Respiration is examined for rate and rhythm of breathing, use of accessory muscles, and presence of stridor. The oral cavity and lips should be closed comfortably during tidal breathing.

On neurologic examination, the cranial nerves deserve special attention. Pupillary responses, visual fields, extraocular movements, and facial muscle strength should be evaluated. The motor component of the trigeminal nerve (cranial nerve V) is assessed by checking facial sensation, strength and bulk in the jaw-closing (masseter and temporalis) and jaw-opening (suprahyoid) muscles, and the jaw jerk reflex. Hearing should be present bilaterally (cranial nerve VIII). The palate should be symmetric at rest and should elevate symmetrically during phonation. The gag reflex is tested bilaterally with an applicator stick; the soft palate and pharynx should contract symmetrically. The gag reflex, however, is a poor parameter for testing the ability to swallow, and is not a substitute for thorough examination of swallowing, per se. Absence of the gag reflex does not correlate with presence of aspiration (15). In patients with unilateral weakness of the pharynx due to LMN dysfunction (as in lesions of the nucleus ambiguus or vagus nerve), the soft palate and posterior pharyngeal wall may pull to the strong side during phonation or gagging; this is known as the *curtain sign*, because lateral motion of the pharyngeal wall resembles a curtain pulling to one side. The strength of the tongue is assessed by protrusion in the midline and by lateralization to each side. The tongue, in contrast to the palate, moves preferentially to the strong side when there is unilateral weakness.

An essential, but often neglected part of the examination of the dysphagic patient is trial swallows. One can no more evaluate a dysphagic patient without examining test swallows than one can evaluate a gait disorder without watching the patient walk. Even in severely dysphagic patients, there is minimal risk of medical sequelae if the patient aspirates a few milliliters of tap water. Initially, the patient is observed swallowing a small sip of water. If the patient is able to swallow a sip of water without difficulty, it is appropriate to test swallowing with a larger amount of water, or with foods of other consistencies. The swallow should begin promptly after ingestion. The hyoid bone and larynx should elevate briskly, and a strong contraction of the suprahyoid muscles should be noted. It is often useful to palpate the hyoid bone and laryngeal cartilages during swallowing, to verify that they are elevating. The oral cavity should be checked to ensure that food is not retained there. Coughing or choking during or immediately after swallowing is suggestive of aspiration. A change in voice quality immediately after swallowing is suggestive of either aspiration or retention of liquid in the hypopharynx. These clinical signs of aspiration or pharyngeal retention, however, are not highly accurate. Some dysphagic individuals experience "silent" aspiration, that is, aspiration without prompt reflexive coughing or throat clearing. In these individuals, the absence of coughing after a test swallow may be wrongly interpreted as indicating that there is no aspiration (13).

Videofluorographic Swallowing Study

The videofluorographic swallowing study (VFSS) is an essential component of dysphagia evaluation and management. Videofluorography is videotape recording of a fluoroscopic procedure. During VFSS, the patient is observed eating and drinking foods of a variety of consistencies. Motions of the jaws, tongue, palate, pharynx, larynx, and esophagus are recorded. The foods are made radiopaque by adding barium, so the processes of mastication, oral food transport, and swallowing can be visualized (16,17). VFSS is a powerful tool for the assessment of dysphagic individuals, and has little risk. VFSS is tolerated well by patients, and the radiation dose is small (18).

Indications

The purpose of the VFSS is not simply to determine whether a patient is aspirating. Rather, its purpose is twofold: first, to identify abnormalities of swallowing, and second, to determine the circumstances under which the patient can swallow safely. VFSS is indicated in any patient who complains of dysphagia when there is a need to visualize the foodway for a description of structural defects and pathophysiology, or to establish a method of safe alimentation and hydration. The history and physical examination are valuable for determining whether there is a problem related to feeding or swallowing, and for establishing essential information regarding the detailed symptomatology, function of related body systems, and other data related to etiology. The physical examination, however, does not reveal the actual events occurring in the oral cavity, pharynx, larynx, and esophagus during a swallow (19). Abnormalities of structure and swallowing are frequently missed on physical examination. These include diverticula, webs, and strictures of the pharynx and esophagus; failure of laryngeal closure and epiglottic tilt; aspiration; impaired opening of the UES or LES; pharyngeal retention after swallowing; and esophageal dysmotility. VFSS is therefore necessary for most patients presenting with dysphagia. There are occasional exceptions. This is particularly true for patients believed to have transient dysphagia due to a well-documented acute medical condition, such as viral pharyngitis or acute cerebral infarction. When such a patient complains of mild dysphagia, there are no symptoms or signs of aspiration, and there is no history of respiratory problems, it is probably reasonable to manage the patient empirically. If the dysphagia persists, or there is any evidence of airway compromise, VFSS is essential. Thus, VFSS is necessary in patients who experience frequent coughing or choking during meals, drooling or difficulty handling secretions, odynophagia, or recurrent aspiration pneumonia.

Equipment and Supplies

Standard videofluoroscopy equipment is generally suitable for the VFSS. The study should be taped with a videotape cassette recorder. VHS equipment is typically sufficient for this purpose, but super-VHS provides optimal resolution. A video timer (e.g., VC-436, Thalner Electronics, Ann Arbor, MI) is used to put the precise time in hundredths of a second directly on the screen for each frame of videotape. Foods of several consistencies (20) including thin, thick, and "ultra-thick" liquids, pudding, a puree, and a solid food are prepared in advance (Table 14-1). I suggest using standardized foods; I use apple juice, apricot nectar, pudding, chicken salad sandwich spread, and a graham cracker, respectively. If the patient complains of difficulty swallowing a specific food, it is helpful to have a sample of that food available. Also needed are supplies of barium powder and barium paste. These can be mixed with the foods as needed in the radiology suite. Several implements should be available for feeding. These include a teaspoon, straw, cup, and syringe with flexible tubing. A glossectomy spoon may be helpful in selected patients. The examination chair should have a headrest and an adjustable back.

Method of Examination

I strongly recommend using a formal protocol for VFSS. In the Good Samaritan Hospital in Baltimore, I have used a structured VFSS protocol for several years, and it has

Table 14-1: Food Categories

Category	Examples*
Thin liquids	Apple juice, soda pop, water
Thick liquids	Apricot nectar, tomato juice, milk shakes
Ultra-thick liquids	"Slushie," pudding, custard, yogurt
Puree	Chicken salad sandwich spread, mashed potatoes
Solid	Graham cracker

* The first item in each category is the standard test food. The category of a particular food may vary depending on its manner of preparation.

Table 14-2: Standard Sequence for Videofluorography

- Lateral projection, patient sitting upright in usual position of comfort
  - Speech sample
  - Command swallow: 5 mL of thin liquid from a spoon
  - Drink thin liquid from a cup (patient controls rate and volume)
  - Command swallow: 5 mL of thick liquid from a spoon
  - Drink thick liquid from a cup (patient controls rate and volume)
  - Eat 1 tsp of chicken salad sandwich spread with barium
  - Eat a small piece of graham cracker with barium paste
  - Modifications and other foods as appropriate
- Posteroanterior projection, patient sitting upright (with neck slightly extended if possible)
  - Visualize larynx during phonation
  - Command swallow: thick liquid or barium paste
  - Modifications or other foods as appropriate
  - Additional swallows as needed for imaging the esophagus

contributed greatly to the development of the dysphagia rehabilitation program (16). The structured approach has resulted in more efficient use of time, better quality of care, more consistent data collection, and improved reporting. The protocol includes a standard sequence but allows for modifications (Table 14-2).

The patient is positioned initially in the lateral projection. The x-ray image intensifier is adjusted to show the patient from the lips anteriorly to the spine posteriorly, and from the nasal cavity superiorly to the upper esophagus inferiorly (at least 5 cm below the vocal folds). Before feeding, I inspect for structural abnormalities, and ask the patient to repeat a standard phrase, such as "The mom got the Pamper for the baby Suzie." This should reveal good apposition of the soft palate to the posterior pharyngeal wall. I then ask the patient to take a teaspoon of thin liquid barium in the mouth, hold it, and swallow on command. This "command swallow" shows the patient's ability to control the bolus in the oral cavity as well as the swallow itself. Next, the patient drinks thin liquid from a cup. The patient is permitted to control the rate of drinking and the bolus size. (A straw is used if the patient cannot handle a cup.) If there is difficulty with bolus control, the patient is next given thick liquids, first from a spoon and then from a cup, and may subsequently be given a teaspoon of "ultra-thick" liquid or pudding. When the liquids and pudding are completed, we feed the patient a teaspoon of the chicken spread, and finally a small piece of graham cracker with barium paste. During these recordings in the lateral projection, structural abnormalities of the oral cavity, pharynx, larynx, and cervical portion of the esophagus are carefully noted. The examiner checks for the adequacy and timing of mastication, oral bolus formation, and propulsion; elevation of the soft palate, hyoid bone, and larynx; epiglottic tilt; posterior thrust of the tongue; contraction of the pharynx; and opening of the UES. If all goes well, the patient is next positioned in a posteroanterior projection. The larynx is visualized while the patient phonates, to check for symmetry of motion of the vocal folds. The patient then does a command swallow with liquid barium or barium paste.

Recordings are checked for structural defects, symmetry of pharyngeal constriction, and opening of the UES. Esophageal disorders are common and may coexist with oral and pharyngeal disorders of swallowing. The optimal VFSS will include at least a limited evaluation of esophageal function, but complete esophagography requires a somewhat different approach.

If aspiration and/or excessive pharyngeal retention are noted, an attempt is made to determine the proximate cause of the abnormality, based on the principles of pathophysiology discussed earlier. A variety of therapeutic and compensatory modifications of feeding and swallowing may be tested, and fluoroscopy provides immediate feedback regarding the efficacy of each maneuver. A number of these modifications are known to be effective, but the response of individual patients is variable and somewhat unpredictable, so an empirical approach is necessary (17).

A comprehensive discussion of therapeutic and compensatory modifications of feeding and swallowing is beyond the scope of this chapter, but several are listed in Table 14-3. Several common maneuvers are useful for reducing aspiration and laryngeal penetration. For a patient with aspiration due to delayed laryngeal closure, instruction to inhale and hold the breath prior to swallowing (supraglottic swallow) may reduce or eliminate the aspiration. Flexing the neck before swallowing typically improves bolus control in the posterior part of the oral cavity and reduces premature transport of liquids into the pharynx. This may also result in reduced aspiration (21). Some impulsive patients tend to eat and drink very quickly, thereby overloading the oral cavity and pharynx and causing overflow aspiration. For these patients, instructions

Table 14-3: Therapeutic and Compensatory Maneuvers

Posture of body
  Sitting in usual position of comfort
  Sitting upright
  Reclining
Position of head and neck
  Upright (neutral position)
  Neck flexion or extension
  Neck rotation
Respiratory and phonatory maneuvers
  Cough, clear throat, or phonate after swallowing
  Supraglottic swallow
  Plug or apply valve to tracheostomy cannula
  Apply nose clips
Mendelssohn maneuver
Clearance maneuvers: multiple swallows, clearing liquid swallow (alternating consistencies)
Modify volume of bolus
Delivery system: spoon, cup, straw, syringe with tube, glossectomy spoon
Modify food consistency, e.g., thicken liquids

and supervision to slow the rate of ingestion may be beneficial.

Other approaches may be useful for patients with excessive pharyngeal retention after swallowing. For some patients with retention of solid food after swallowing, drinking a small amount of liquid after eating a few bites may wash the residue out of the pharynx. In patients with unilateral weakness of the pharyngeal constrictor muscles (as in lateral medullary syndrome), turning the head toward the weak side may close off that side and direct the bolus toward the strong side of the pharynx, resulting in improved pharyngeal clearance (22,23). Patients with impaired opening of the UES may be able to hold the sphincter open more effectively using the Mendelssohn maneuver. In this maneuver, the patient is taught to hold the larynx in an elevated position during swallowing, by voluntarily contracting the suprahyoid muscles while laryngeal rise is maximal. The Mendelssohn maneuver results in prolonged opening of the UES in some individuals, reducing pharyngeal residue (24).

An important issue is what to do when the patient aspirates. Some examiners respond to even a minimal amount of aspiration by discontinuing the VFSS. This undermines the purpose of the study. Indeed, the most useful portion of the VFSS is testing the efficacy of maneuvers designed to reduce aspiration. This cannot be done if the VFSS is halted at the first sign of aspiration. There are rare circumstances in which the VFSS should be halted, however. The following are absolute contraindications to continuing the VFSS: 1) total or near-total obstruction of the airway or foodway by solid or semisolid food, 2) laryngospasm (with one exception: the VFSS may continue if the patient has a tracheostomy cannula), 3) bronchospasm, 4) aspiration of stomach contents, 5) complete absence of laryngeal protection mechanisms (laryngeal elevation, glottic closure, epiglottic tilt, and reflex cough), and 6) any other true medical emergency (such as cardiac or respiratory arrest). In addition there are several relative contraindications to continuing the VFSS: 1) Aspiration is observed in a patient with a history of recurrent aspiration pneumonia or severe respiratory disease, 2) silent aspiration (i.e., without reflex cough) is observed, 3) a large quantity of solid food is retained in the pharynx after swallowing, and 4) maneuvers to reduce aspiration are ineffective (16).

Interpretation and Report

The VFSS report should summarize the major functional components of swallowing, report occurrences of aspiration and/or pharyngeal retention, and describe the effects of therapeutic and compensatory maneuvers that are tested during the study. A structural or pathophysiologic diagnosis is given, further diagnostic studies may be suggested, and if appropriate, detailed recommendations are provided for developing a therapeutic feeding program. This may include instructions regarding positioning of the patient, method of feeding, choice of food consistencies, need for supervision, and use of compensatory maneuvers.

Other Diagnostic Studies

Endoscopy

Laryngoscopy is the method of choice for assessing the structure and function of the larynx. Fiberoptic laryngoscopy is a simple office procedure that is well tolerated by patients and has few complications. It provides the opportunity to directly visualize the pharyngeal and laryngeal mucosa for structural lesions (inflammation, ulceration, or tumor) and to evaluate the motion of the vocal folds. A formal protocol for fiberoptic endoscopic examination of swallowing (FEES) (25) may be useful in patients for whom VFSS is impractical, such as immobilized nursing home patients. A limitation of the FEES is that it cannot actually show the motions of the pharynx and larynx during the pharyngeal phase of a swallow, because the pharynx and larynx are closed, leaving only a potential space. The onset of swallow can be visualized, however, and the larynx can be inspected immediately after swallowing for aspirated material. Endoscopy of the esophagus (esophagoscopy) is critical for identification and biopsy of structural mucosal lesions, such as inflammation or neoplasm, and has a fundamental role in evaluating esophageal dysphagia or odynophagia. Endoscopy may be coupled with dilatation for patients with esophageal strictures.

Esophageal Manometry

Manometry of the esophagus is important in the evaluation of patients with esophageal dysphagia, noncardiac chest pain, and gastroesophageal reflux disease. Manometry is particularly helpful for detecting and differentiating disorders of esophageal motility, such as achalasia, spasm, defective peristalsis, and scleroderma. A thin, flexible manometry catheter is swallowed into the esophagus through the nose or mouth. The catheter has several pressure transducers positioned at variable distances from its lower end. The upper end is attached to a multichannel physiologic recorder. The manometry catheter is anchored in the esophagus with the pressure transducers at a fixed distance from the LES. Pressures are recorded continuously in all transducers while the patient swallows. In a normal recording, pressure drops in the LES at the onset of swallowing, and this is followed immediately by a wave of high pressure that begins in the upper esophagus and progresses downward to the LES. In dysphagic patients, manometric findings may include abnormally high or low pressures in the body of the esophagus and/or LES, incoordin-ation of esophageal peristalsis, or nonperistaltic contractions after the swallow. Manometry of the pharynx and UES is more difficult, and prone to errors because the pharynx moves briskly relative to the catheter during swallowing. These inaccuracies may be reduced by simultaneously recording pressure (via manometry) and motion (via videofluorography). This combined approach reveals subtleties of pharyngeal function and dysfunction that are not detectable with either technique alone (26).

Electromyography

EMG has several roles in the management of patients with dysphagia (27). Kinesiologic EMG studies reveal the coordination of specific muscles during the swallowing process (Fig. 14-5). It is essential in detecting and differentiating among neuromuscular diseases that may cause dysphagia, such as polymyositis, muscular dystrophy, and motor neuron disease. EMG of the laryngeal and pharyngeal musculature is useful for detecting LMN dysfunction affecting these muscles (28). EMG biofeedback may be useful for teaching patients volitional control of selected muscles, particularly the suprahyoid muscles. These muscles are important in elevating the larynx and opening the UES; this is the basis for the Mendelssohn maneuver. Some patients have difficulty learning to control the suprahyoid muscles. Surface EMG may help these patients to gain voluntary muscle control and have a role in swallowing rehabilitation.

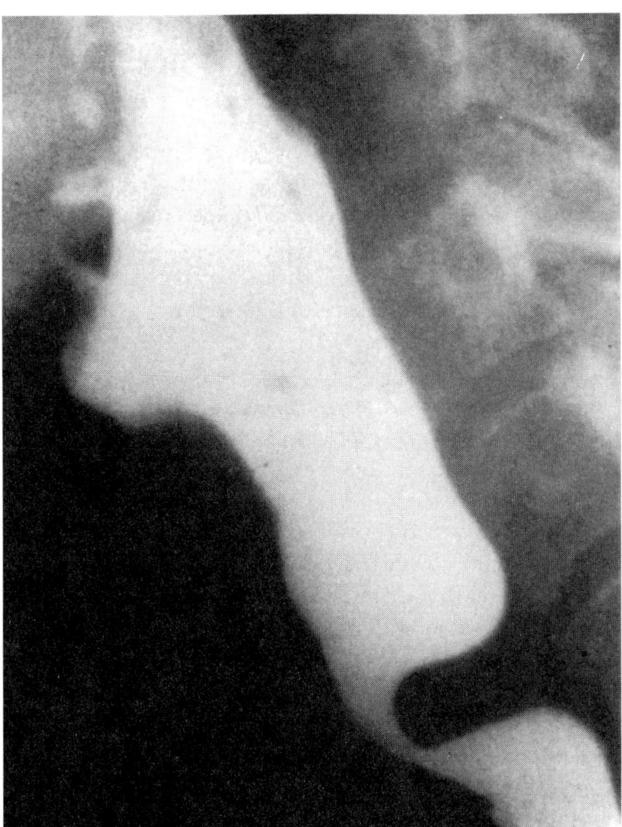

Figure 14-5. Cricopharyngeal prominence. A lateral still-frame print from a cinepharyngogram demonstrates marked cricopharyngeal prominence during passage of a large bolus, with luminal compromise of about 80%. Despite this, the patient's dysphagia responded to dilatation. Note that it is unnecessary to give such a patient a solid bolus (and may be potentially dangerous!). (Reproduced by permission from Jones B, Donner MW, eds. *Normal and abnormal swallowing: imaging in diagnosis and therapy.* New York: Springer-Verlag 1991:66.)

SPECIAL CONSIDERATIONS

Tracheostomy and Ventilator Dependency

Many dysphagic patients have associated respiratory and communication impairments that necessitate use of a tracheostomy or mechanical ventilation (29). A tracheostomy may actually simplify the care of the dysphagic patient because it provides access for tracheal suctioning after aspiration. The cuff on a tracheostomy tube may reduce the quantity of aspiration by partially obstructing flow around the tube. The presence of a cuffed tracheostomy tube (or endotracheal tube) does not entirely prevent aspiration, however. Patients with cuffed tubes may develop severe aspiration pneumonia. Coughing and phonating are impaired in the patient with a tracheostomy tube (cuffed or cuffless) because the tracheal stoma prevents the development of the high subglottal pressure that is essential for effective coughing. On the other hand, a unidirectional tracheostomy speaking valve may restore the ability to cough. The valve permits inspiratory airflow (but not expiratory flow) into the trachea through the tube. Expiratory airflow is directed upward, around the tracheostomy tube and through the larynx, restoring the ability to phonate as well as cough.

Mechanical ventilation does not prevent swallowing. A cuffed tracheostomy tube prevents airflow through the larynx, however, eliminating phonation. With a cuffless tracheostomy tube, many ventilator-dependent patients can learn to speak. Many have difficulty coordinating breathing and swallowing, but this skill can be taught. The evaluation and management of swallowing in ventilator-dependent patients requires an understanding of the dynamics of the upper aerodigestive tract, and should be coordinated with the management of speaking and breathing.

Pediatric Dysphagia

Children with disorders affecting feeding and swallowing present a special set of problems to the rehabilitation team. Their assessment requires an understanding of not only the normal feeding process, but also the development of feeding and swallowing functions. The pharyngeal anatomy of the newborn differs fundamentally from that of the adult, in that the larynx is located high in the neck. The epiglottis is in direct contact with the soft palate, as it is in all other mammals (4). This soft-tissue contact helps to prevent aspiration while the infant is suckling, but contact is broken during swallowing when the epiglottis inverts and the larynx and pharynx contract. During the first few years of life, the larynx migrates downward in the neck, drawing the epiglottis away from the soft palate. Older children and adults lack velar-epiglottic contact and the resulting airway protective mechanism.

At birth, infants have a limited repertoire of oral behavior; they are unable to articulate speech, feed only by suckling, and are unable to eat soft solid foods. During the first years of life, the upper aerodigestive tract mechanism matures, and children develop sophisticated oral proficiencies, including the ability to articulate speech, drink from a cup, and eat solid foods (30). Treating developmentally disabled individuals requires a knowledge of this developmental sequence. Another factor complicating the treatment of dysphagic children is the importance of limiting their exposure to ionizing radiation, which makes it more difficult to perform VFSSs. When there is serious risk of aspiration, however, the VFSS remains essential (31).

CASE STUDIES

Case 1

A 45-year-old African-American man was admitted to the hospital on 8/27/96, complaining of dysphagia of several hours' duration, accompanied by headache, nausea, dizziness, and left-sided paresthesias. He had difficulty with accumulated saliva in the mouth. Past medical history was significant for untreated hypertension. Physical examination revealed an obese man with dysarthria, right Horner syndrome, infranuclear right facial palsy, weakness of the soft palate on the right, excessive saliva in the oral cavity, loss of left-sided pain and temperature sensation, mild ataxia, and minimal left hemiparesis. Electrocardiography revealed left ventricular hypertrophy. Computed tomography (CT) revealed bilateral subcortical and pontine infarctions. A speech-language pathologist evaluated the patient on 8/28/96 and reported that he was unable to swallow his own saliva. There was no laryngeal elevation on attempts to swallow thin liquid. Dysphonia was noted with a mildly hoarse and wet voice quality. Fiberoptic laryngoscopy on 8/30/96 revealed pooling of secretions in the right pyriform sinus, reduced motion of the right vocal fold during phonation. A percutaneous feeding gastrostomy tube was inserted on 9/4/96.

A VFSS was done on 9/5/96. Sitting upright with his head in anatomic position, the patient was aphagic; the bolus was transported normally through the oral cavity and into the pharynx, but there was no pharyngeal phase. Material accumulated in the hypopharynx until he coughed it out. When he turned his head toward the right before swallowing, the bolus was directed to the left and there was some pharyngeal contraction (but on the left side only). With the head turned leftward, a small quantity of barium entered the esophagus, and there was only minimal aspiration followed by prompt coughing. Next the patient drank from a straw while keeping his head turned to the right. Under these conditions, he had a brisk pharyngeal swallow, good opening of the pharyngoesophageal sphincter, no aspiration, and only minimal retention of barium in the hypopharynx after swallowing.

The assessment was bulbar palsy due to multiple cerebral and brain stem infarctions. The unilateral weakness of intrinsic laryngeal, palatal, and pharyngeal muscles is indicative of a lateral medullary lesion involving the nucleus ambiguous, even though a medullary lesion was not seen on imaging. Risk of aspiration pneumonia was considered low because the cough reflex was intact after aspiration. The patient was advised to continue taking liquids by straw with his head turned to the right. When seen by his primary care physician on 11/19/96, he was taking liquids by mouth without difficulty but was still unable to swallow solid foods. No respiratory dysfunction was noted. The patient elected not to return for a follow-up visit, because his dysphagia was improving.

Case 2

An 82-year-old white woman was admitted to the hospital on 11/20/96 for comprehensive rehabilitation following an acute right cerebral infarction. She complained of dysphagia, left facial droop, and left-sided weakness. She exhibited frequent coughing during meals. Past medical history was significant for a subdural hematoma (evacuated in 1993), morbid obesity, obstructive sleep apnea, hypertension, type II diabetes mellitus, chronic obstructive pulmonary disease, bilateral mastectomies for breast cancer, and coronary artery disease. Physical examination revealed a morbidly obese, elderly woman with supranuclear left-sided facial palsy, mild left hemiparesis, and reduced sensitivity of the gag reflex on the left (normal on the right) but normal contraction of the pharynx and palate during gagging. On trial swallows, the patient demonstrated good oral control but had intermittent coughing with a variety of food consistencies. CT of the brain revealed an old left-sided pontine infarction and generalized cerebral atrophy.

VFSS was performed on 11/27/96 and revealed abnormal swallowing. There was minimal glottic aspiration when the patient drank thin liquids, and this was followed by prompt and effective reflex coughing. With thick liquids, there was only supraglottic laryngeal penetration. She did not have aspiration or laryngeal penetration with soft solid foods, but the onset of the pharyngeal phase of swallowing was markedly delayed after the bolus of chewed solid food entered the pharynx. There was minimal retention in the pharyngeal recesses after swallowing, and this was uniform across the various food consistencies. Flexing the neck prior to swallowing caused no change. When the patient performed a supraglottic swallow (taking a breath and holding it before swallowing), there was no aspiration or laryngeal penetration.

The assessment was neurogenic dysphagia due to stroke, with impaired pharyngeal swallow initiation and minimal aspiration. The risk for aspiration pneumonia was considered low, because of the strong cough response following aspiration. It was recommended that the patient consume a mechanical soft diet with thick liquids during meals. The speech-language pathologist worked with the patient in swallowing therapy, teaching her to use the supraglottic swallow when drinking thin liquids. On discharge from the hospital 12/5/96, the patient was eating a mechanical soft diet, but continued to experience occasional coughing during meals.

ACKNOWLEDGMENTS

I am grateful to the faculty and staff of the Johns Hopkins University-Good Samaritan Hospital Swallowing Rehabilitation Program and the Johns Hopkins Swallowing Center for their assistance and support. Jianmin Liu, MD, provided invaluable assistance with preparing the illustrations and Sara Palmer, PhD, made thoughtful comments on the manuscript. This work was supported in part by a FIRST award R29-DC01575 from the National Institutes of Health/National Institute on Deafness and Other Communication Disorders.

REFERENCES

1. Dodds WJ, Stewart ET, Logemann JA. Physiology and radiology of the normal oral and pharyngeal phases of swallowing. *AJR* 1990;154: 953–963.
2. Gelfand DW, Richter JE, eds. *Dysphagia: diagnosis and treatment.* New York: Igaku-Shoin, 1989.
3. Logemann JA. *Evaluation and treatment of swallowing disorders.* San Diego: College-Hill, 1983.
4. Hiiemae KM, Crompton AW. Mastication, food transport, and swallowing. In: Hildebrand M, Bramble DM, Liem KF, Wake DB, eds. *Functional vertebrate morphology.* Cambridge: Harvard University Press, 1984:262–290.
5. Palmer JB, Rudin NJ, Lara G, Crompton AW. Coordination of mastication and swallowing. *Dysphagia* 1992;7:187–200.
6. Palmer JB, Tanaka E, Siebens AA. Electromyography of the pharyngeal musculature: technical considerations. *Arch Phys Med Rehabil* 1989;70:283–287.
7. Cook IJ, Dodds WJ, Dantas RO, et al. Opening mechanisms of the human upper esophageal sphincter. *Am J Physiol* 1989;257: G748–G759.
8. Dodds WJ, Stewart ET, Logemann JA. Radiologic assessment of the abnormal oral and pharyngeal phases of swallowing. *AJR* 1990; 154:965–974.
9. Palmer JB, DuChane AS. Rehabilitation of swallowing disorders due to stroke. *Phys Med Rehabil Clin North Am* 1991;2:529–546.
10. Palmer JB, DuChane AS. Rehabilitation of swallowing disorders in the elderly. In: Felsenthal G, Garrison SJ, Steinberg FU, eds. *Rehabilitation of the aging and older patient.* Baltimore: Williams & Wilkins, 1994:275–287.
11. Feinberg MJ, Ekberg O. Deglutition after near-fatal choking episode: radiologic evaluation. *Radiology* 1990;176:637–640.
12. Holas MA, DePippo KL, Reding MJ. Aspiration and relative risk of medical complications following stroke. *Arch Neurol* 1994;51: 1051–1053.
13. Horner J, Massey EW. Silent aspiration following stroke. *Neurology* 1988;38:317–319.
14. Martin BJW, Corlew MM. The incidence of communication disorders in dysphagic patients. *J Speech Hear Disord* 1990;55: 28–32.
15. Leder SB. Videofluoroscopic evaluation of aspiration with visual examination of the gag reflex and velar movement. *Dysphagia* 1997;12:21–23.
16. Palmer JB, Kuhlemeier KV, Tippett DC, Lynch C. A protocol for the videofluorographic swallowing study. *Dysphagia* 1993;8:209–214.
17. Logemann JA. *Manual for the videofluorographic study of swallowing.* Boston: College-Hill Press, 1986.
18. Beck TJ, Gayler BW. Radiation in video-recorded fluoroscopy. In: Jones B, Donner MW, eds. *Normal*

and abnormal swallowing: imaging in diagnosis and therapy. New York: Springer-Verlag, 1991:1–6.

19. Linden PL, Siebens AA. Dysphagia: predicting laryngeal penetration. *Arch Phys Med Rehabil* 1983;64:281–284.

20. Dantas RO, Kern MK, Massey BT, et al. Effect of swallowed bolus variables on oral and pharyngeal phases of swallowing. *Am J Physiol* 1990;258:G675–G681.

21. Rasley A, Logemann JA, Kahrilas PJ, et al. Prevention of barium aspiration during videofluoroscopic swallowing studies: the value of change in posture. *AJR* 1993;160: 1005–1009.

22. Logemann JA, Kahrilas PJ, Kobara M, et al. The benefit of head rotation on pharyngoesophageal dysphagia. *Arch Phys Med Rehabil* 1989;70:767–771.

23. Robbins J, Levine R. Swallowing after lateral medullary syndrome plus. *Clin Comm Disord* 1993;3: 45-55.

24. Kahrilas PJ, Logemann JA, Krugler C, Flanagan E. Volitional augmentation of upper esophageal sphincter opening during swallowing. *Am J Physiol* 1991;260:G450–G456.

25. Langmore SE, Schatz K, Olsen N. Fiberoptic endoscopic examination of swallowing safety: a new procedure. *Dysphagia* 1988;2:216–219.

26. McConnel FMS, Cerenko D, Hersh T, Weil LJ. Evaluation of pharyngeal dysphagia with manofluorography. *Dysphagia* 1988;2:187–195.

27. Palmer JB. Electromyography of the muscles of oropharyngeal swallowing: basic concepts. *Dysphagia* 1989;3:192–198.

28. Palmer JB, Holloway AM, Tanaka E. Detecting lower motor neuron dysfunction of the pharynx and larynx with electromyography. *Arch Phys Med Rehabil* 1991;72:237–242.

29. Tippett DC, Siebens AA. Using ventilators for speaking and swallowing. *Dysphagia* 1991;6:94–99.

30. Gisel EG. Chewing cycles in 2- to 8-year-old normal children: a developmental profile. *Am J Occup Ther* 1988;42:40–46.

31. Mirrett PL, Riski JE, Glascott J, Johnson V. Videofluoroscopic assessment of dysphagia in children with severe spastic cerebral palsy. *Dysphagia* 1994;9:174–179.

Chapter 15

Nutritional Management

Katie Coleman Cornwall
M. Elizabeth Sandel

Rehabilitation as a process is focused on the improvement of function. Toward this goal, the nutrition services agenda needs to focus on correcting as many existing nutritional deficits as possible, especially those that prevent optimization of function, and preventing any new deficits that would result from rehabilitation schedules and continued institutionalization. Appropriate delivery of nutrients to the patient must be coordinated with other rehabilitation priorities. The patient's recovery may also be hampered by a recurrence of nutritionally related diseases that affect the patient's primary diagnoses; therefore, proper education and correction of detrimental dietary habits may also be a goal.

SCREENING AND NUTRITIONAL ASSESSMENT

Although the average length of stay in most acute care facilities has decreased dramatically in the last 10 years, the dietitian in the rehabilitation setting has the opportunity to develop nutritional care plans that improve the patient's function during hospitalization. Conversely, because the average stay in rehabilitation may be as long as 4 to 6 weeks, a patient's nutritional status could become compromised if not for ongoing regularly scheduled re-evaluations. It is this valuable, long-term re-evaluation process that separates nutritional therapy for the rehabilitation patient from nutritional therapy in the acute setting.

Table 15-1 outlines the basic guidelines for determination of ideal body weight, nutrient needs, water and electrolyte needs, and indices of nutritional depletion for patients in acute or rehabilitation settings.

Not all patients in this population present, simply by virtue of their diagnoses, nutritional risk. To determine an appropriate care plan and nutritional therapy, each patient must be screened for nutritional risk. Each patient should also be evaluated for any goals relative to his or her functional status. There are patients for whom nutrition does not play a significant role in the rehabilitation process. These patients will be routinely and continually evaluated for any changes that would require nutrition intervention.

The evaluation should include the identification of steps required for the prevention of further morbidity. These are as follows:

- Nutrition screening: determination of nutritional risk
- Development of nutritional goals: correction of nutritional deficits and improvement and normalization of diet
- Prevention of further morbidity
- Continued evaluation for changes in status

This comprehensive approach to patient care is achievable within the patient's average length of stay. It is therapeutic, adjunctive, and preventative.

All patients must be evaluated with a systematic procedure that identifies not only their nutritional risk, but also the role nutrition will play in their rehabilitation. Risk

Table 15-1: Nutrition Assessment

Determining Ideal Body Weight (IBW)

Men: 106 lb (47.7 kg) for first 5 feet,
6 lb (2.7 kg) for each additional inch

Women: 100 lb (45 kg) for first 5 feet,
5 lb (2.25 kg) for each additional inch

Adjustments:
1. Quadriplegic: 10%–20% decrease in IBW
2. Paraplegic: 5%–10% decrease in IBW
3. Amputees: See Table 15-5

Calculating Nutrient Needs

CALORIES:

Harris-Benedict equations

Men: BEE = 66 + 13.7(W) + 5(H) − 6.8(A)

Women: BEE = 655 + 9.6(W) + 1.7(h) − 4.7(A)

where *W = weight (kg), H = height (cm), A = age (yr), BEE = basal energy expenditure*

Factors for the stress/activity level of each patient should be considered for final needs:

Activity	*Stress*
1.2—Bed rest	1.2—Minor surgery
1.3—Out of bed (sedentary)	1.35—Skeleton trauma
1.4—Light—moderate	1.5—Cancer
	1.6—Major sepsis
	2.1—Severe burn

PROTEIN:

Minimum protein requirement	0.45 g/kg of IBW
Maintenance	0.8 g/kg of IBW
Mild Trauma	1.5 g/kg of IBW
Severe Trauma	2.0 g/kg of IBW

Assessment of Water and Electrolyte Requirements

WATER: Methods to determine requirements

- 1500 mL/m²
- 1500 mL for the first 20 kg + 20 mL/kg over 20 kg
- 30–40 mL/kg (average-size adult)
- 30–40 mL/kg: 18–64 years old
  30 mL/kg: 55–65 years old
  25 mL/kg: >65 years old
- Recommended daily allowance 1 mL/kcal
- 1 mL/kcal + 100 mL/g of nitrogen

FLUID NEEDS:

Fluid needs are similar as for most patients. In the presence of syndrome of inappropriate antidiuretic hormoner, fluids would need to be restricted. In patients with central fevers, an additional 500–1500 mL of fluid may be required. Patients with diabetes insipidus have increased urine output and are at risk for dehydration if fluid is not appropriately increased.

Indices of Nutritional Depletion

	Mild Depletion	*Moderate Depletion*	*Severe Depletion*
Total Lymphocyte Count	1200–1500	800–1200	<800
Albumin	2.8–3.5	2.1–2.7	<2.1
% IBW	80%–90%	70%–80%	<70%
% Weight loss/6 mo	5%–15%	15%–25%	25%

Table 15-2: Rehabilitation Nutritional Assessment Screening Tool: Diagnoses Requiring Assessment of Nutritional Risk

Acquired immunodeficiency syndrome
Aspiration pneumonia
Burns
Cancer
Decubitus ulcer/nonhealing wound
Dysphagia
Gastrointestinal disorders: Crohn's disease, irritable bowel disorder, malabsorption, ulcerative colitis
Liver failure/hepatitis/cirrhosis
Malnutrition/failure to thrive
Multiple trauma/fractures
Pancreatitis
Renal failure
Ventilator dependency

factors must be identified and become the focus for nutritional goals in the rehabilitation setting. Criteria for nutritional risk include the following:

- Admitting and secondary diagnoses: Certain diagnoses place a patient at nutritional risk (Table 15-2).
- Previous hospital admissions: Patients who have been in another health care setting are at greater risk for depletion.
- Body weight as compared to normal values or to usual body weight: Patients who are less than 90% of ideal body weight or who have had a 10% weight decrease in less than a month are at greater risk for depletion.
- Dysphagia.
- Low serum albumin level (<3.5 g/dL).
- Need for alternate route of nutrition support.
- Age older than 80 years or younger than 14 years.
- Pressure sores.
- Previous history of poor oral intake for more than 3 days.

The nutrition care plan should incorporate any identified risks and correction strategies and outcomes must be measurable. The following case is illustrative.

Case Study

A 53-year old woman had a stroke and was hospitalized and transferred to a skilled nursing facility where she developed a stage III pressure sore. She is 5 foot 7 inches tall and weighs 90.9 kg (202 lb), 153% of the ideal body weight. She is diabetic and taking insulin. She has been receiving 1800 calories via gastric tube feeding.

This patient represents a high nutrition care priority and should be assessed for caloric requirements, appropriateness of feeding schedule, and need for ongoing evaluation within the first 24 hours after admission.

Rehabilitation Goals

1. Successful transition to oral feedings with sufficient calories to prevent further deficits
2. Determination of degree of depletion (albumin)
3. Correction of any nutritional deficits
4. Wound healing with appropriate caloric intake
5. Prevention of disruption of therapies due to feeding schedule
6. Education of patient and family concerning the diabetic diet for improved glucose control in anticipation of transition to oral feedings.

ENTERAL NUTRITION SUPPORT

Many patients are unable to consume adequate nutrition by mouth for any number of reasons. They may be a candidate for a feeding tube. When the patient has a functioning gut, enteral nutrition is *always* preferable over parenteral nutrition. The indications and contraindications for feeding by tube and the routes of enteral feeding are listed in Table 15-3.

Patients requiring an alternative means of nutrition support in the acute care setting are frequently placed on continuous 20 to 24-hour feedings. This is hardly compatible with many rehabilitation schedules. If at all possible, patients should be transitioned to intermittent bolus feedings.

Before a transition is made, the patient's tolerance to the current enteral feeding schedule should be reviewed. Contraindications to bolus feedings would be 1) a history of delayed gastric emptying; 2) a history of poor tolerance to a large volume or a high rate of feeding as indicated by high gastric residuals; and 3) a history of aspiration, although this may not be an absolute contraindication. (If a proper feeding positioning is adhered to and bolus size is increased slowly, bolus feedings can still be accomplished.)

Controversy exists regarding the imperative for jejunal feedings if the patient has a history of recurrent aspiration pneumonia (1). If at all possible, gastric tubes should be placed. Recommendations for jejunal feedings rarely suggest rates higher than 150 mL/hr. To meet the caloric needs of most patients, continuous feedings will be necessary if a jejunal tube is utilized. This is not only disruptive to therapy schedules, but also burdensome for care providers after discharge.

Selection of an appropriate formula need not be a complicated matter. Table 15-4 provides descriptions of the generic formulas. In patients with healthy gastrointestinal systems, an isotonic, 1-kcal/mL formula containing fiber is sufficient. To reduce the total volume of feeding needed and further minimize the risk of aspiration, the

Table 15-3: Enteral Nutrition Support in Rehabilitation

Potential indications for tube feeding
- Hypermetabolic state (trauma)
- Anorexia nervosa
- Depression
- Protein-calorie malnutrition
- Burns
- Dysphagia
- Decreased level of awareness

Contraindications for tube feeding
- Intestinal obstruction
- Paralytic ileus
- Gastrointestinal hemorrhage
- Intractable vomiting or diarrhea

Routes of enteral feeding

The route of tube feeding should be based on the patient's individual needs and abilities.
- Nasogastric—This is the most common, from nose to stomach.
- Nasoduodenal—Extends from the nose, through the pylorus into the duodenum.
- Nasojejunal—Extends from the nose through the pylorus into the jejunum. It is usually placed radioscopically.
- Tube enterostomy—Surgically placed in the operating room.
- Gastrostomy—Placed directly into the stomach. Tube sizes and pliability differ.
- Jejunostomy—Several types are seen, including needle catheter, direct tube, and creation of a jejunal stoma that can be intermittently catheterized.
- Percutaneous endoscopic gastrostomy (PEG)—Under endoscopic guidance, a feeding tube is percutaneously placed in the stomach and secured.

practitioner may be tempted to order a nutrient-dense formula. However, the precaution here is the hyperosmolality of these products, and the total amount of free water in these products is usually less than that in isocaloric products. For example, a 1.5-cal/mL product is typically 78% free water, so that in 1 liter of formula, there is 780 mL of free water. The minimum fluid requirement for most patients is 1 mL/kcal. A patient would need 220 mL of additional water for every 1000 mL of formula.

These high-calorie formulas do not require a lower total volume compared to 1-kcal/mL products. For example, an isocaloric formula would provide 84% to 85% free water. So for every 1000 kcal, an additional 150 mL of free water is needed, resulting in a total volume of 1150 mL to provide 1000 kcal. A 1.5-kcal/mL product provides 1000 kcal in 670 mL, of which 522 mL is free water. Such a product would require an additional 478 mL of free water, resulting in a total volume of 1148 mL. The total volume needed to provide the same number of calories and free water is essentially the same in the calorically dense product, as in the isocalorie product.

For an example, a patient requires 1500 cal and 1500 mL of free water. He will need the following: EvenFiber-Cal 1 kcal/mL of 85% free water. 1500 mL of formula + 225 mL of water = 1725 mL 375 mL of formula with 60 mL of water four times per day total volume 435 mL per feeding HyperCal 1.5 kcal/mL of 78% free water. 1000 mL of formula + 720 mL of water = 1720 mL 250 mL of formula with 180 mL of water four times a day total 430 mL of volume per feeding.

One possible way to take advantage of the higher-calorie product is that extra fluid could be given at night or at different intervals when one would normally not give formula. Patients with diabetes who are placed on hypercaloric formulas will need close monitoring of their blood glucose level and this caution should be noted in the medical record and the physician should be informed.

Administration of Enteral Feedings

As a practical rule in tube feeding administration, one should not change the rate and the volume of a feeding at the same time. Bolus feedings may be started out at full strength, but it is recommended that initial bolus volumes be small and calculated using the volume that the patient tolerated for the previous feeding schedule.

As with any feeding regimen, flexibility is important. The feasibility of feeding schedules should be discussed with nursing staff. For some patients, the optimum regimen can be attained within 24 hours of initiation of bolus feedings.

The keys to successful transition are as follows:

- Monitor carefully. Nurses should note any adverse effects and cease progression if tolerance is poor.
- Write specific orders (Fig. 15-1).
- Involve the patient when possible. The patient should be informed of changes in the regimen and be encouraged to inform staff of any symptoms of intolerance (e.g., bloating, distention, nausea, diaphoresis, cramping).
- Do not rush the transition. A combination of bolus feedings and continuous feedings at night can be implemented during the transition.

Patients requiring more than 2000 cal/day can present a scheduling problem for bolus feedings. It is difficult in these situations to avoid nighttime feedings. A possible regimen in this instance could be 500 mL of 1-kcal/mL formula with 80 mL of water five times per day at 5:00 AM, noon, 3:00 PM, and 9:00 PM. The fifth feeding could be either in the middle of the morning or in the middle of the night. This requires balancing rehabilitation schedules to prevent nutritional compromise.

Table 15-4: Generic Description of House Formulas	
Isotonic with fiber	Isotonic, lactose free, containing fiber 1 cal/mL. For tube feedings. Examples: Jevity, Ultracal, Nutren with fiber.
Isotonic	Isotonic, lactose free, low residue, no sucrose, 1 cal/mL. For tube feeding or oral use. Examples: Isocal, Osmolite, Nutren without fiber.
Blenderized	Whole foods, isotonic, lactose free, no sucrose, 1 cal/mL. For tube feeding only. Examples: Vitaneed, Complete Modified.
Oral supplements	Palatable oral supplements, lactose free, low residue, hypertonic available as 1 cal/mL and 1.5 cal/mL. May also be used as tube feeding. Examples: Ensure, Sustacal, Ensure Plus, Sustacal HC, Resource Plus.
Fiber enriched	Fiber enriched, lactose free, hypertonic, 1 cal/mL. Suited for oral supplementation or use as tube feeding. Examples: Enrich, Sustacal with fiber.
Pulmonary	Special high-fat formula to reduce CO_2 production, lactose free, low residue, hypertonic, 1.5 cal/mL. For oral or tube feeding. Example: Pulmocare.
Elemental high nitrogen	Elemental high protein for impaired gut function. Low residue, hypertonic, 1 cal/mL. For tube feeding only. Examples: Criticare HN, Vivonex HN.
Modulars	Carbohydrate, protein, lipid. Available for oral or tube feeding supplementation. Examples: Polycose, Promod, MCT oil.
Specialty	Renal and hepatic tube feeding formulas available for short-term use with acutely ill patients.
Diabetic	Diabetic low carbohydrate, high fiber, isotonic, 1 cal/mL. Formula used for tube feeding or orally. Example: Glucerna.
Clear liquid supplement	Palatable supplements for patients on clear liquid diets for more than 3 days. Examples: SLD, Citrotein, Critrisource.

Transition to Oral Feedings

When a dysphagia therapist has determined that the patient is safe to attempt oral intake, communication between the patient, family, therapists, nursing, physician, and the dietitian is critical.

Objective Measurement

Objective measurement of calorie and fluid intake is vital. Meaningless records such as "ate 85% of meal" are unacceptable and should never be used as a basis for decreasing enteral support. Records of the percent of specified foods ingested must be kept to truly judge a patient's intake.

Consideration of Patient's Nutritional Status

Before decreasing feedings, the patient's nutritional status is vital. The nutritionist must obtain accurate measurements of weight and albumin level, and a history of weight changes. In some patients, nutritional status will not be compromised by decreasing feedings for 1 to 2 days to increase appetite. However, those with low weight or excessive weight loss, wound healing, poor endurance, or increased needs should be given the appropriate calories determined during goal setting. Obesity is not necessarily a reason to limit calories during this transition.

Patient Food Preferences

The patient may be capable of eating sufficiently to meet needs, but a dislike of institutional food limits the intake. If this is the case, and there is no other apparent reason why the patient is not meeting the calorie needs orally, it is recommended that during a therapeutic pass when the patient is able to eat familiar foods, the family be given a food record to complete. If it is documented that the patient would be able to take adequate nutrition at home, then feedings would not need to be planned for discharge.

Discharge Plans

Families and caregivers should always be involved in feeding decisions. How capable will the caregiver be to provide foods of the appropriate consistency? Will the caregiver be able to feed the patient? Is the caregiver capable of administering tube feedings and caring for the equipment? Does the caregiver have appropriate resources or contact persons if problems occur?

Case Study

An 85-year-old patient had a cerebrovascular accident. She was transferred from an extended care facility where she, received continuous gastrostomy-tube feedings for 18 hours. Her weight has been stable. Her diet progressed to a mechanical soft diet with semithick liquids. She needs to be fed and each meal takes approximately 45 minutes, but she *can* take adequate amounts orally. Her granddaughter will be taking her into her home and caring for her. The granddaughter is 30 years old and has a 3-year-old and a 6-year-old child and is expecting a third. She is very willing to do what she can for her grandmother. Because the patient can orally consume an adequate number of calories, Medicare will not cover the cost of enteral feedings.

DOCTOR'S ORDER SHEET

DOCTOR	SERVICE **Rehab Services**

ORDERED DATE	ORDERED HOUR	TUBE FEEDING ORDERS	✓ BY
		ALLERGIES: ______	
		☐ 1. Dietary Consult. "To assess caloric and fluid needs."	
		FORMULA SELECTION: ☐ Isotonic 1.0 kcal/mL (e.g., Osmolite, Isocal)	
		☐ Isotonic with fiber 1.0 kcal/mL (e.g., Ultracal, Jevity, Vitaneed) ☐ Hypertonic 1.5 kcal/mL (e.g., Resource Plus, Ensure Plus, Sustacal HC)	
		☐ Elemental 1.0 kcal/mL (e.g., Criticare, Vital, Vivonix) ☐ Other ______	
		ADMINISTRATION	
		☐ Bolus Feeding: Begin 120 mL four times a day (06, 12, 17, 21). If tolerated for 12 hours,	
		advance each bolus in 120 mL increments until ______ ML qid is reached. Flush tube with at least 30 mL of water before and after each feeding.	
		☐ 2. FLUSH FEEDING TUBE WITH ______ mL WATER Q ____ HOURS, or WITH EACH FEEDING.	
		☐ 3. If feeding tube in the stomach, check residual q______ hrs. If > ______ (100–150), hold feeding X ______ hrs.	
		☐ 4. Lab: CBC, albumin, creatinine, fasting blood sugar, NA^+, K^+. Initially, then q week:	
		☐ 5. Daily input and output. Baseline height and weight.	
		☐ 6. Record weight: ☐ daily ☐ qod ☐ weekly.	
		☐ 7. Elevate head of bed ______ degrees during feedings and 1 hour after each bolus feeding.	
		☐ 8. Assess for nausea, vomiting, bloating, changes in bowel habits, diarrhea, edema, and, if present, notify physician.	
DATE	TIME	PHYSICIAN'S SIGNATURE	

Figure 15-1. Example of an order sheet.

Recommendations

1. Discontinue continuous feedings.
2. Begin the transition to bolus feedings.
3. Educate the granddaughter in this procedure and about the mechanical soft diet with semithick liquids.
4. Provide the granddaughter with information on solid-food calorie, protein, and fluid equivalents for one can of tube feeding.
5. Consider reliance primarily on oral intake, but with the ability to use enteral feedings as a supplement.

Case Study

A 5-year-old patient with a brain injury who is making the transition to a mechanical soft diet with semithick liquids. He continued to require supplemental bolus feedings of a pediatric formula because although he "eats 100%" of his meals, what he actually ate did not meet his needs. He was a finicky eater, and as with many children, food became a battleground. Since switching to solid foods, he lost 0.9 kg (2 lb). The option of continuing the tube feeding after discharge was discussed with the family, who felt that he would eat better once home. On an overnight home pass, the gastrostomy tube was flushed, but the patient did not receive any formula. Food records indicated that the patient met 85% of his needs orally. The decision was made to continue supplemental feedings during the hospital stay, but that these would not be continued at home, if possible. He was referred to a continuity-of-care dietitian for home follow-up. Food records kept by the family were reviewed and it was subsequently determined that oral intake was adequate. The gastrostomy tube was subsequently removed.

DYSPHAGIA

Disturbances in the ability to adequately pass food from the oral cavity to the stomach have been described elsewhere in this text. This chapter deals with the application of the diet for dysphagia. The goal of food management for these patients is to create palatability and variety and to promote the patient's independence within the limitations imposed.

It is extremely important that dysphagia therapists communicate to the dietitian what a patient's *specific* deficits are, so that meals will be individually tailored. General dysphagia diet guidelines often will not take subtle differences in patients into consideration. Without this communication between the therapist and the dietitian, a patient's diet could be overly restricted or be more liberal than the therapist had intended. Clear communication and understanding of the different consistencies of diets by dysphagia therapists is essential. The entire health care team and the physician must be involved in this aspect of care. Each facility needs to agree on nomenclature and the extent of restriction for each dysphagia level. This communication of specific problems is essential if the dietitian is to educate families and care providers about modified diets. At this printing, the American Dietetics Association's practice group for Dietetics in Physical Medicine and Rehabilitation is developing the National Dysphagia Diet.

General Dysphagia Modifications

Puree

These foods, by definition, have been not only blended, but also strained. They are perhaps the biggest challenge to the food service and to the home care provider. During preparation, care needs to be taken not to dilute food products and lose nutrients. It is very difficult to provide adequate calories and protein with this diet. Supplementation with fortified liquid supplements is almost always necessary. This diet is indicated when a patient has limited oral motor skills or pharyngeal dysfunction.

Finely Ground, Chopped

This level frequently includes foods that require some, but limited ability to masticate, limited oral motor skills, and delayed swallow or gag. Usually, food has some "mouth feel" but chewing would not be essential. Whole foods are usually still restricted at this level. Liquid supplements and fortified foods are frequently required to meet nutrient needs.

Mechanical Soft Diet

This diet is perhaps the level that has the most variation from institution to institution The patient should have grinding and lateral oral motor skills. Meats are usually still ground, minced, or diced. Whole, tender, but not fresh fruits and vegetables are usually permitted. Foods that break apart or that do not form a bolus are usually restricted. This level could also be appropriate for patients who have adequate oral motor skills and swallowing ability, but who are impulsive.

Soft Diet

This level, too, will vary widely in the foods permitted. In most cases, foods are still tender and well cooked. With a few exceptions, raw fruits and vegetables are excluded. Crunchy foods, rice, thinly sliced meats, and dry cereals may be permitted.

Regular Diet

There are no restrictions. Patients should be able to adequately chew, form a bolus, and swallow safely. Patients who are impulsive require supervision if permitted this diet. It is imperative that all staff be educated regarding each facility's specific guidelines. This should be included in orientations of new therapists.

Thickened Liquids

Dehydration in patients requiring thickened liquids is of major concern. Although products that are used to thicken liquids do not impart a flavor, they may alter the perception of taste in a liquid because the liquid stays on the taste buds for a longer period of time than if it were not thickened. Beverages served in paper cups, styrofoam, or plastic will frequently take on the taste of the cup and this taste will be accentuated by the thickener. Beverages are frequently more acceptable if served cold in a glass. Care providers must be instructed not to add ice to beverages. Pitchers of appropriately thickened water should be placed at the bedside for patients who do not require supervision.

Standard fluid requirements are 1 mL/cal. The needs increase for patients with fever. Prevention of constipation requires adequate fluid intake. Early physical signs of dehydration are confusion, lethargy, dry skin, decreased urine output, fatigue, and dry mucous membranes. Decline in performance during therapies may be a signal of early dehydration. Accurate intake and output records should be kept daily, by both the dietitian and the nurse. These records should be kept not only in a care facility, but also at home. Care providers must know the patient's fluid intake goal. Dehydration need not come as a surprise.

General orders to "push fluids" are frequently not sufficient. Physician orders may need to include specific fluid goals per shift. These may be met by incorporating fluids as part of the medication schedule. Fluid administration can also be included in nursing protocols and standards of care for dysphagic patients.

The ability to take adequate nutrients does not coincide with adequate hydration. It should also be remembered that liquid nutritional supplements are only 84% to 85% fluid and extra free fluid needs to be given.

Case Study

A 46-year-old man was admitted to the acute rehabilitation facility, having had multiple strokes. He was at 150% of the ideal body weight, but lost 10% of his usual weight during acute hospitalization. He had a history of dehydration requiring intravenous fluid replacement. He tolerated semithick liquids. He took a nutritional supplement with meals. He enjoyed eating. Calorie count records and intake and output records indicated that although he enjoyed eating, he frequently fell asleep during meals. He refused to drink thickened liquids. He drank nectars, but this was insufficient to meet his fluid needs of 2200 mL/day. To prevent recurrent dehydration, a gastric tube was placed. The family was instructed concerning fluid administration and supplemental enteral feeds.

HEAD INJURY

In the acute phase of injury, patients with severe traumatic brain injury experience increased protein turnover. Despite high calorie and protein intakes to meet assessed needs, it may not be possible to achieve nitrogen balance during the acute phase (2–3 weeks after surgery). Patients in the acute phase are hypermetabolic and catabolic. The percent of calories derived from protein is as high as 30% (normal, 10%–15%) (2). This increased need often lasts for the duration of coma (3). Calorie needs can vary from 1.1 times to 2.0 times the basal energy expenditure. Increased posturing and tone may increase the metabolic need in vegetative patients months after injury (4). Brooke and Barbour (5) reported that brain injury patients admitted to a rehabilitation unit were on average at 85% of their ideal body weight; one-third had low albumin levels.

Close monitoring of weight is important. Albumin, prealbumin, and transferrin levels are important to monitor for appropriateness of calories provided. These indicators have their limitations, however, in the presence of other factors. Transferrin levels can be falsely elevated in the setting of iron-deficiency anemia. Prealbumin values may be falsely elevated in patients taking steroids or who are volume depleted. Initial measurements of albumin will not be a good predictor of nutritional status because of its long half-life. However, measurements should be repeated 2 weeks after injury. Protein needs are 1.5 to 2.0 g/kg of body weight (see Table 16-1). As with any trauma patient, other factors such as wounds, agitation, fever, restlessness, ventilator dependency, and infection will influence needs. After this period of increased need, there is frequently a decline in metabolic rate, resulting in weight gain. Appropriate management of this gain will frequently need to involve the family and behavioral medicine staff (6).

The location of the brain injury is important in identifying potential nutrition issues:

- Brain stem injury and cranial nerve injury that are involved in swallowing can result in dysphagia.
- Cranial nerve damage can also result in changes in sense of taste or smell.
- Hypothalamic injury may impact the satiety control, which could lead to hyperphagia. Injury in this part of the brain could also result in the syndrome of inappropriate antidiuretic hormone or diabetes insipidus.
- Cerebellar damage may affect equilibrium and result in nausea with positional changes.
- Frontal lobe damage can lead to emotional lability and outbursts that interfere with oral intake. Hyperphagia can also occur.

Cognitive ability directly affects a patient's ability to take in adequate nutrition (7). Patients with a cognitive level I to III according to Ranchos Los Amigos criteria (8) will require enteral nutrition support. Because of agitation and confusion, patients with level IV cognition should have a dysphagia evaluation, and although they may not have organic dysphagia, they may not cognitively be able to orally take in adequate nutrition and may require adjunctive enteral feeding. Patients at level V may be relatively successful with oral feedings alone. Patients with level VI cognition are frequently independent in feeding.

Patients in the chronic phase of recovery may not be able to regulate food intake (in some cases, hyperphagia). The precise mechanism for this is unclear. Education concerning appropriate nutrition for weight management needs to be part of postdischarge education. Extended care and residential facilities should consider this when planning menus.

GUILLAIN-BARRÉ SYNDROME

During the acute phase of Guillain-Barré syndrome (at least 2–4 weeks) the patient is hypercatabolic and hypermetabolic. Prevention of waiting of respiratory skeletal muscles is clearly important. This is one of the main causes of death of patients with adult respiratory distress syndrome (9). Patients need 40 to 46 kcal/kg of body weight and 2.0 to 2.5 g of protein per kilogram of body weight to achieve positive nitrogen balance. During rehabilitation, an assessment of any existing depletion must be determined and a high-calorie, high-protein diet may be needed for repletion.

AMPUTATION

Nutritional assessment of the amputee must be based on accurate height and weight. This must be done by measurement, not estimation. Comparison of current weight to previous weight must take into consideration the estimated weight of the lost limb (Table 15-5) (10). Accurate assessment of the level of amputation is important.

Determination of the calorie requirements postoperatively needs to take into consideration the adjusted weight as above, with additional calories for surgery and wound healing (see Table 15-1).

Once wound healing has taken place and the patient is in active rehabilitation or living in the community, calorie needs are based on estimated activity level. These may be difficult to assess. The higher the level of amputation of the lower extremity, the greater the energy expended in walking (11). The loss of the knee joint is significant in increasing the energy cost of walking. Likewise, the longer the stump is after a below-the-knee amputation, the less energy is expended in walking. Bilateral above-the-knee amputation in a patient over 50 years old may result in a prohibitive level of energy expenditure for locomotion (12).

Body mass index has been adapted for use with the amputee. Himes (13) described a method for this calculation. For people who can be weighed, an estimate of the total body weight (Wt_E) including missing limb segments may be calculated:

$$Wt_E = Wt_O/(1-P)$$

where Wt_O is the observed body weight and P is the proportion of total body weight represented by the missing limb segments, shown in Table 16-5. This estimated weight might then be used to calculate body mass index, which is weight (in kilograms) divided by height squared (in square meters). Accurate estimation of ideal body weight and calorie needs is particularly important and relevant for the diabetic, tube-fed, or pediatric patient. In the diabetic patient, the appropriate number of calories is the cornerstone of glucose control. In patients who have had an amputation secondary to diabetic neuropathy and a history of poor glucose control, a calculation of carbohydrate needs is essential.

Table 15-5: How to Determine Ideal Weight of Adults Who Have One or More Limbs Amputated

Amputation above knee of 1 leg = Ideal weight–	18.5%
Amputation above knee of 2 legs = Ideal weight–	37%
Amputation below knee of 1 leg = Ideal weight–	7.1%
Amputation below knee of 2 legs = Ideal weight–	14.2%
Amputation of 1 foot – Ideal weight–	1.8%
Amputation of 2 feet = Ideal weight–	3.6%
Amputation of entire arm = Ideal weight–	6.5%
Amputation of 2 entire arms = Ideal weight–	13%
Amputation below elbow in 1 arm = Ideal weight–	3.1%
Amputation below elbow in 2 arms = Ideal weight–	6.2%
Amputation of 1 hand = Ideal weight–	0.8%
Amputation of 2 hands = Ideal weight–	1.6%

Source: Adapted from Brunnstom S. Clinical kinesiology 3rd ed. Philadelphia: FA Davis, 1981: 284.

WEIGHT MANAGEMENT

Ideal body weights are summarized in Table 15-1. Obesity is a chronic disease. It can impair function and mobility, and is not ameliorated quickly. Prudent weight loss means 0.45 to 0.90 kg (1–2 lb) per week, achieved with no less than a 500-cal/day deficit. Within the rehabilitation setting, realistic approaches are as follows:

1. Patient education concerning eating habits. The rehabilitation patient is learning a host of new adaptive behaviors and it is reasonable to begin nutritional training as well.
2. Adaptation to smaller portions, lower fat intake, and regular meal times.
3. Emphasis on the impact weight has on physical limitations and development of a desire to manage weight.
4. In diabetic patients, glucose may sometimes be controlled with an appropriate diet. Frequently, patients who either have been noncompliant or have a nutrition knowledge deficit will see significant improvement in glucose control while they are in a controlled environment. The physician, the dietitian, and diabetic educator should share this improvement with the patient, to motivate the patient for further compliance.
5. Family education. This is of utmost importance for continued weight management.

It must be remembered that merely being overweight is not an indication that there is no nutritional depletion. Any approach to weight management needs to be with the patient's expressed agreement and should not be imposed on the patient. Overeating is frequently a direct result of food restriction. The goal, as with other therapies, is that changes in behaviors will continue after discharge to aid in the recovery process.

STROKE

The prevalence of malnutrition in the stroke population is estimated at 49% to 60% (14). Finestone et al (14) and Newmark et al (15) noted that malnutrition, independent of low albumin levels, affects functional outcomes. The mechanism for this effect on outcome is unclear, although factors such as depressed glycogen levels, reduced muscle mass, altered muscle function (16), and immune dysfunction leading to increased susceptibility to infection may limit a stroke patient's ability to progress. Possible causes for malnutrition in stroke patients include dysphagia, paresis or paralysis of the extremities, disorientation, depression, apraxia, agnosia, neglect, and adverse effects of medications (14). Additionally, malnutrition may reflect poor prior health. The usual methods for calculating macronutrient needs apply (see Table 16-1). The imperative is to identify patients with malnutrition and provide timely intervention.

Stroke patents also frequently present with existing hyperlipidemia, hypertension, diabetes, and obesity. Medical nutrition therapy for these diseases must be weighed against the degree of depletion when one determines the strictness of the diet. While a long-term goal may be correction of diet habits that contributed to these diseases, the immediate goal for successful rehabilitation outcome is correction of the malnutrition. While weight loss for obese patients may improve mobility, it is not an acceptable goal in the presence of malnutrition.

PRESSURE ULCERS

Any person who is immobilized is at risk for pressure ulcers. Persons with spinal cord injury (SCI) and the elderly are two high-risk groups (17–20). Protein-calorie–malnourished patients and vitamin-deficient patients are also at risk (21,22). Maintaining adequate protein, calorie, and fluid intake to prevent negative nitrogen balance and dehydration is essential (23,24).

Protein should be provided at 1.5 to 2.0 g/kg of weight. The major source of calories should come from carbohydrates. In diabetic patients, however, careful attention needs to be paid to good glucose control, as hyperglycemia can impair wound healing. The number of calories should not be lowered to improve blood glucose levels. Medical therapy must be responsive.

The role of zinc and vitamin C in wound healing continues to be controversial. Excess zinc, while necessary for protein synthesis, can interfere with macrophage function and may only be appropriate for zinc-deficient patients (25,26).

SPINAL CORD INJURY

In the acute phase of SCI, nitrogen balance becomes negative almost immediately (27). The Harris-Benedict equations are adequate for assessing calorie needs in the presence of stress factors (see Table 15-1). However, indirect calorimetry is preferred if available. For protein requirements, the ratio of nonprotein calories to nitrogen should equal 150 : 1. Gastrointestinal function may be either hypoactive or hyperactive (28).

In the stable phase, the patient may be in a hypometabolic state and a decline in weight (increased proportion of body fat), energy expenditure, and calorie requirements is related to the level of SCI and muscle atrophy (29).

SCI patients are at increased risk for pressure ulcers due to decreased mobility and frequently poor intake. Sixty percent of quadriplegics and 52% of paraplegics may develop pressure ulcers (30,31). Reasons for poor intake include anorexia, facial trauma, depression, cervical collars, halo vests, and mechanical ventilation. Attention must be paid to ensure adequate protein consumption, 1.5 to 2.0 g/kg of ideal body weight, and to maintain adequate vitamin C intake.

Hypercalciuria due to immobilization results in a loss of bone calcium. Limiting dietary calcium does not appear to be effective in decreasing the serum calcium level and may further contribute to the development of osteoporosis. Adequate fluid intake of 2 to 3 L/day is important for the prevention of renal calculi due to increased urinary calcium excretion. Regular catheterization plays a role as well (32).

Constipation is frequently a problem in SCI patients. Adequate fluid intake is important, coupled with a high fiber intake and an appropriate bowel program. Weight management also plays an important role for these patients and their caregivers.

CONCLUSIONS

Patient receiving rehabilitation services or in programs in rehabilitation environments may be similar to patients in acute care settings in terms of their nutritional needs. However, rehabilitation populations sometimes require the practitioner to consider additional assessment and treatment issues. This may be a result of the aftermath of trauma and acute care treatments, or of the demands of activity and exercise on metabolic and biochemical systems. In addition, various subpopulations of patients in rehabilitation may have other special needs. Finally, the coordination of rehabilitative care and feeding to provide sufficient intake is a unique challenge for rehabilitation professionals caring for these patients.

REFERENCES

1. Lazarus BA, Murphy JB, Culpepper L. Aspiration associated with long-term gastric versus jejunal feeding: critical analysis of literature. *Arch Phys Med Rehabil* 1990;71:46–53.
2. Clifton GL, Robertson CS, Grossman RG, et al. The metabolic response to severe head injury. *J Neurosurg* 1984;60:687–695.
3. Annis K, Ott L, Kearney P. Nutritional support of the severe head-injured patient. *JPEN J Parenter Enter Nutr* 1991;6:239–244.
4. Sandel ME, Norcross ED, Ross SR, et al. Protein metabolism after severe brain injury. *Arch Phys Med Rehabil* 1990;71:764–765.
5. Brooke M, Barbour PC. Assessment of nutritional status during rehabilitation after brain injury. *Arch Phys Med Rehabil* 1986;67:634.
6. Henson M, DeCastro JM, Stringer AY, Johnson C. Food intake by brain injured humans who are in the chronic phase of recovery. *Brain Inj* 1993;7:169–178.
7. Yorkston K. The relationship between speech and swallowing disorders in head injured patients. *J Head Trauma Rehabil* 1989;4:1–4.
8. Hagen C, Malkmus D, Durham P. Levels of cognitive functioning. In: Rehabilitation of the head injured adult: comprehensive physical management. Downey, CA: Professional Staff Association of Rancho Los Amigos Hospital, 1979.
9. Roubenoff RA, Borel CO, Hanley DF. Hypermetabolism and hypercatabolism in Guillain-Barré syndrome. *JPEN J Parenter Enter Nutr* 1992;16:464–472.
10. Kautz Osterkamp L. Current perspective on assessment of human body proportions of relevance to amputees. *J Am Diet Assoc* 1995;95:215–218.
11. Gonzalez E, Corcoran P, Reyes R. Energy expenditure in below-the-knee amputees: correlation with stump length. *Arch Phys Med Rehabil* 1974;55:111–119.
12. McCollough N, Jennings J, Sarmiento A. Bilateral below-the-knee amputation in patients over fifty years of age. *J Bone Joint Surg [Am]* 1972;54:1217–1223.
13. Himes J. New equation to estimate body mass index in amputees. *J Am Diet Assoc* 1995;6:646.
14. Finestone HM, Greene-Finestone LS, Wilson ES, Teasell RW. Prolonged length of stay and reduced functional improvement rate in malnourished stroke rehabilitation patients. *Arch Phys Med Rehabil* 1996;77:340–345.
15. Newmark SR, Sublett D, Block J, Geller R. Nutritional assessment in a rehabilitation unit. *Arch Phys Med Rehabil* 1981;62:279–282.
16. Lopes J, McRussel D, Whitwell J, Jeejeebhoy KN. Skeletal muscle function in malnutrition. *J Clin Nutr* 1982;36:602–610.
17. Allman RM. Pressure ulcers among the elderly. *N Engl J Med* 1989;320:850–853.
18. Yarkony GM. Aging skin, pressure ulcerations, and spinal cord injury. In: Whiteneck GG, ed. *Aging with spinal cord injury.* New York: Demos, 1993:39–52.
19. Kligman AM, Grove GL, Balin AK. Aging of human skin. In: Finch CE, Schneider EL, eds. *Handbook of the biology of aging.* New York: Van Nostrand Reinhold, 1985.
20. Young JR, Burns PE, Bowen AM, McCutchen R. *Spinal cord injury statistics.* Phoenix: Good Samaritan Medical Center, 1982.
21. Mulholland JH, Tui C, Wright AM, et al. Protein metabolism and bed sores. *Ann Surg* 1943;118:1015–1023.
22. Pinchcofsky-Devis GD, Kaminski MU Jr. Correlation of pressure sores and nutritional status. *J Am Geriatr Soc* 1986;34:435–440.
23. Silane M, Oot-giromini B. Systemic and other factors that affect wound healing. In: Eaglstein WH, ed. *New directions in wound healing.* Princeton: ER Squibb, 1990.
24. Constantian MB, Jackson HS. Biology and care of the pressure ulcer wound. In: Constantian M, ed. *Pressure ulcers: principles and techniques of management.* Boston: Little, Brown, 1980:69–100.
25. Williams CM, Lines CM, McKay EC. Iron and zinc status in multiple sclerosis patients with pressure sores. *Eur J Clin Nutr* 1988;42:321–328.
26. Norris JR, Reynolds RE. The effect of oral zinc sulfate on decubitus ulcers. *J Am Geriatr Soc* 1971;19:793–797.
27. Kaufman HH, Rowlands BJ, Stein DK, et al. General metabolism in patients with acute paraplegia and quadriplegia. *Neurosurgery* 1985;16:309–313.
28. Gordon EE, Vanderwalde H. Energy requirements in paraplegic ambulation. *Arch Phys Med Rehabil* 1953;37:276–285.
29. Claus-Walker J, Halstead LS. Metabolic and endocrine changes in spinal cord injury. II. Partial decentralization of the autonomic nervous system. *Arch Phys Med Rehabil* 1982;63:576–580.

30. Rodriguez GP, Claus-Walker J. Biochemical changes in skin composition in spinal cord injury: a possible contribution to decubitus ulcers. *Paraplegia* 1988;26:302–309.

31. Richardson RR, Meyer PR. Prevalence and incidence of pressure sores in acute spinal cord injuries. *Paraplegia* 1981;19:235–247.

32. Chantraine A. Actual concept of osteoporosis in paraplegia. *Paraplegia* 1978;16:51–58.

Chapter 16

Psychological Assessment in the Rehabilitation Setting

Gregory Ranlett
Joseph Bleiberg

Psychological assessment often is viewed as synonymous with psychological testing. In reality, psychological assessment may or may not include psychological testing, and psychological testing rarely is the sole source of data in a psychological assessment. Psychological assessment includes a wide range of data sources, such as interviews with the patient and family, naturalistic behavioral observations, the patient's life history, self-report behavioral and mood rating scales, rating scales completed by the patient's family and therapists, standardized tests of specific cognitive functions, standardized measures of personality and psychopathology, and behavioral and mood diaries kept by a patient or caregiver.

The wide range of data sources available still is not enough to produce a psychological assessment. The essential remaining ingredient is a well-trained psychologist who can utilize data from multiple sources and integrate it with the patient's current life circumstances and challenges, and then use such an integrated view to explain the patient's current psychological state, diagnose any psychological or psychiatric disorders and recommend appropriate treatments, and most importantly, attempt to predict the patient's reactions to future events. As noted by Sweet et al (1), the psychologist must understand the patient within the context of his or her social and cultural environment, family system, medical and psychological history, and vocational and educational attainments and aspirations.

This chapter discusses the application of psychological assessment to specific issues and patient populations frequently encountered in the rehabilitation setting. Appropriate assessment instruments and formats also are reviewed.

ASSESSMENT PROCEDURES

The Psychological Interview

Regardless of the patient's specific illness or disability, psychological assessment always should attempt to include interviews of the patient, the patient's treatment team, and the patient's family and significant others. The interviews have several purposes: to assess the patient's current emotional adjustment; to assess the patient's understanding of the nature of the injury or illness and its prognosis; to evaluate the availability and quality of family and social support; to understand the patient's style of coping by examining current coping strategies as well as how the patient has managed personal crises in his or her past; to identify factors that may produce idiosyncratic or maladaptive responses to injury or illness (e.g., a history of childhood physical abuse); to assess the patient's perception of and reaction to the rehabilitation hospital and his or her treatment team; and to assess the treatment team's reaction to the patient, particularly to see if the patient is stimulating negative, countertherapeutic reactions within any members of the treatment team (2). Such interviews provide the psychologist with the overall context within which psychological testing or rating scale data are analyzed.

In some cases, the above-mentioned interview procedures are all that are necessary to proceed with an effective diagnosis and intervention. Just as psychiatrists and other mental health practitioners formulate a diagnosis and treatment plan without psychological testing, so can and does the psychologist. However, in many cases, the psychologist can use psychological tests to substantially enhance the usefulness and power of the interview-based assessment. One of the main benefits of psychological testing is that it provides a *quantified* measure of a wide range of mental functions and thus is useful for documenting a patient's improvement or deterioration, supporting eligibility for entitlements and insurance such as Social Security Disability Income and Worker's Compensation, and demonstrating damages in personal injury legal actions. Another benefit of psychological testing is that it permits comparing the patient's level of performance with that of known reference groups, usually in the form of "norms." Comparison to normative groups is useful for setting appropriate rehabilitation goals and expectations, and can be essential for return to school or work questions.

The initial psychological interview sets the tone for the patient's future reaction to psychological services, and to some degree, to all rehabilitation services. The psychological interview is an opportunity to communicate to the patient that the rehabilitation team cares not only about the patient's physical and cognitive performance, but also about how the patient feels and how he or she will integrate the consequences of the current illness or injury into a revised sense of self, with appropriate and adaptive expectations and goals for the future.

Another function of the interview is to establish rapport. Rehabilitation patients typically do not arrive at the rehabilitation hospital asking to see a psychologist or requesting mental health services. The initial interview is an opportunity for the psychologist to destigmatize psychological services and allow the patient to see that the psychological issues that he or she is facing are "normal" and do not imply that he or she is "crazy." We have found that framing psychological services within a sports psychology model, which emphasizes performance enhancement and does not rest on assumptions of psychopathology, often helps patients to view psychological services as a way to enhance achievement of their *own* rehabilitation goals, in essence, an enhancement of their empowerment. Should psychopathologic factors emerge, they can be addressed within a sports psychology model as impediments to performance enhancement.

The psychologist also uses the interview to derive information useful for selection of the psychological tests (if any) to use for further assessment, and to determine the optimal timing for psychological testing. Doing so can involve a careful balancing of factors. For example, patients with severe physical injuries such as spinal cord injury may view their intelligence, personality, and other elements of their internal mental life as the only things about them that were *not* injured, which may lead them to view the psychologist as an adversary challenging the integrity of exactly those functions they believe to have been spared. The psychologist thus must balance the benefits gained from psychological testing against the potential harm of injuring the patient's self-esteem, as, for example, might be the case when assessing a spinal cord–injured patient for cognitive impairment secondary to concurrent mild brain injury. This dilemma is intensified by two factors. The first is the importance of the patient's self-esteem to his or her participation in the rehabilitation process, and therefore to its very success. The second is the importance of information about cognitive ability and personality to the rehabilitation team. Since so much of rehabilitation is based on the patient's ability to learn and retain information, and to maintain productive interpersonal relationships with the rehabilitation team, cognitive deficits and personality disorders need to be identified and accommodated as soon as possible, hopefully before they result in therapeutic impasses or ruptured patient-staff relationships (3).

Test Interpretation Issues

Rehabilitation patients frequently have sensory and motor impairments that were not present in the normative and standardization samples for most psychological tests. It thus is not particularly meaningful, for example, to use normative data for the Digit Symbol subtest of the Wechsler Adult Intelligence Scale (4) in a patient with a hemiparesis of the dominant hand: The patient will be performing with his or her nondominant hand while the normative group performed with their dominant hand. Similarly, the hypochondriasis scale of the Minnesota Multiphasic Personality Inventory (MMPI) (5) was normed using medically healthy subjects, such that substantial concerns regarding physical health may be signs of hypochondriasis or somatization. However, patients in a rehabilitation hospital typically have multiple physical disorders and physical and mental (e.g., brain injury) malfunctions, such that what was a pathologic level of somatic complaints in the normative group may be an entirely accurate reflection of the physical and mental state in rehabilitation patients. In essence, as Elliott and Umlauf noted, the interpretation of psychological test results of rehabilitation patients cannot be based on uncritical application of normative data (6). This limitation in the use of psychological testing further reinforces the importance of the psychologist using historical data from the patient and family and using the previously discussed interview procedures. Moreover, it also underscores the importance of the psychologist's experience and training in rehabilitation issues.

Measures of Psychopathology and Maladjustment

The most common test for assessing psychological adjustment and psychopathology is the MMPI (5). The MMPI was developed in the 1940s primarily for screening psychiatric patients. Although there have been few normative studies done with disabled populations, this test is among the most widely used in the field of behavioral health (7). The current version of this test is the MMPI II, which consists of 560 statements to which the patient responds as being true or false about himself or herself. The MMPI II requires a sixth-grade reading level and normative data beginning at age 15. The pencil and paper version can be difficult for individuals with limited upper-extremity capacity, and alternative versions that use a tape-recorded presentation and computerized administration are available. As a last resort, the MMPI II can be read to the patient, with the examiner recording the patient's responses, though it should be understood that the results likely will be distorted if the patient experiences shame or embarrassment in answering sensitive questions in the presence of another person.

Psychological adjustment can also be assessed using the Millon Clinical Multiaxial Inventory-II (MCMI-II) (8), which is noteworthy in that it can provide diagnostic information congruent with the *Diagnostic and Statistical Manual of Mental Disorders* (DSM-III-R) (9). The more recent MCMI-III coincides with DSM IV criteria (10). The primary strength of the MCMI scales lies in the fact that they can be linked theoretically to standardized diagnostic entities. A related weakness is the MCMI's orientation toward the detection of pathology, which might produce an overly pathologic view of rehabilitation patients. This is important because no normative data exist to help guide the use of the MCMI in the rehabilitation setting (6).

The Millon Behavioral Health Inventory (MBHI) can be quite useful in rehabilitation settings because it measures patients' attitudes toward health and health care providers (11). The MBHI can help the rehabilitation team better understand how health attitudes and personality factors are likely to influence the patient's participation in the rehabilitation process. By virtue of identifying health attitudes held by the patient, the MCMI permits the rehabilitation team to anticipate and prevent trouble spots.

Depression inventories include a number of self-report screening measures, including the Beck Depression Inventory (BDI) (12), the Zung Depression Scale (13), and the Hamilton Rating Scale (14). The main advantage of these scales is that they are quite brief. However, the brevity and clear focus on depression makes the scales transparent to the patient and thus highly vulnerable to the patient "guiding" his or her own score. Moreover, because these scales focus only on depression, they cannot identify additional psychological comorbidities, such as anxiety disorders.

Measures of Personality

The clinical and theoretical literature has not covered measures of "normal" personality as extensively as they have measures of psychopathology such as the MMPI and MCMI. As noted by Elliott and Umlauf (6), there has been a "preoccupation with aberrant behaviors culminating in or subsequent to disability," but very little attention given to the use of nonpathologic personality instruments in rehabilitation settings.

The Sixteen Personality Factor Questionnaire—Form E (16PF) has been studied in rehabilitation settings and has extensive normative data for individuals with a wide array of physical impairments (15). Its use in rehabilitation settings has been discussed in some detail (16,17). The 16PF measures 16 primary normal personality characteristics and five second-order dimensions. It is based on Cattell's factor analytic description of personality (18). Research supports the basic structure and psychometric adequacy of 16PF for use with the physically disabled (6). The Neuroticism, Extroversion and Openness Personality Inventory (NEO-PI) (19) is a measure of trait aspects of personality that is based on the five-factor model of personality (20). The five factors are extroversion, neuroticism, openness to experience, conscientiousness, and agreeableness. The NEO-PI has not been systematically studied in rehabilitation settings, even though it has been well received as a research instrument.

Common social-cognitive measures of personality include the Locus of Control (LOC) scales, which measure the extent to which patients believe they have control over the impact of illness or disease. LOC is easily measured with a brief questionnaire (21). The 18-item Multidimensional Health LOC scale is most applicable to rehabilitation settings (22). This is a well-researched rating scale, with adequate normative data. Another social-cognitive measure is the Problem Solving Inventory (PSI), a measure of self-appraised problem-solving ability (23). It assesses the degree to which individuals perceive a high degree of confidence in their ability to solve everyday problems, their ability to regulate emotional reactions to problems, and their general tendency to approach rather than avoid problems. The PSI has been correlated in meaningful directions with several variables pertinent to rehabilitation. High scores showed a positive correlation with lower depression and less psychosocial impairment secondary to disability among 90 spinal cord–injured patients (24). The PSI's emphasis on social learning makes it especially relevant in rehabilitation settings, where patients with lower scores may benefit from cognitive-behavioral interventions to enhance their problem-solving ability (25).

Intelligence and Academic Achievement Tests

The primary uses of intelligence and academic achievement tests are to assist in vocational and academic planning or as part of a neuropsychological examination of patients with known or suspected brain dysfunction. The most common tests in this category are the Wechsler Adult Intelligence Scale—Revised (WAIS-R) (4), the Wide Range Achievement Test III (WRAT-III) (26), and the Peabody Individual Achievement Test—Revised (PIAT-R) (27).

The WAIS-R typically takes between 1 and 2 hours to administer and includes 11 subtests measuring verbal and performance intelligence. The verbal subtests all utilize a format where the examiner orally presents questions to the patient. The performance subtests, with only one exception, use a format of the patient manually manipulating the test materials. Sensory and upper-extremity motor deficits can confound WAIS-R scores and no norms for such handicaps exist. When one is working with patients who have sensory or motor impairments, it is necessary to be cautious when applying norms, or to use alternative tests that are not confounded by the patient's sensory-motor impairments. For example, the Ravens Progressive Matrices (28), a multiple-choice test of visual-spatial reasoning, requires no upper-extremity function and thereby can serve as an alternative to the WAIS-R performance subtests.

Neuropsychological Tests

Neuropsychological tests were devised originally to assist in neurologic diagnosis, primarily to address questions regarding the presence or absence of brain lesions and lesion localization. The neurodiagnostic procedures of the 1950s, such as pneumoencephalography and cerebral angiography, were relatively low-yield but high-morbidity procedures and neuropsychological assessment offered an accurate and risk-free procedure to assist in diagnosis and to identify behavioral consequences of neurosurgical interventions. The major "neuropsychological laboratories" of the 1950s and 1960s were within academic neurosurgical departments and combined clinical diagnosis with research.

The Halstead Reitan Neuropsychological Test Battery (HRB) is the most frequently used neuropsychological test battery in the United States (29,30). The HRB has been the focus of dozens of validation studies across multiple neurologic and psychiatric populations, and it provides an objective and quantitative evaluation of a wide range of neuropsychological functions. The HRB is a "fixed" battery in that the same tests always are given to each patient, regardless of the presenting problem or referral question. Different configurations of scores on the various tests of the HRB can be "mapped" to different neurobehavioral syndromes and lesion characteristics and locations. Most importantly, configuration analysis can support the differential diagnosis because some configurations can be identified as nonneurologic or as internally inconsistent.

Unfortunately, the comprehensiveness of the HRB also is the cause of several limitations to its use. The HRB requires approximately 7 hours for administration, which makes it expensive, difficult to schedule within acute inpatient rehabilitation, and beyond the stamina of many patients. During early stages of recovery from brain injury, when recovery of function typically is rapid, the patient may be quite different by the time the neuropsychological report has returned from dictation and is placed in the medical record, making the HRB a poor cost-benefit choice. Moreover, when brain impairment is moderately severe, the behavioral manifestations generally are readily apparent and easy to elicit and quantify using shorter and less comprehensive procedures. Thus, while the HRB is the "gold standard," there are situations where it is not economical or efficient.

A different, more qualitative and subjective approach to neuropsychological assessment was constructed in the former Soviet Union by Luria (31,32). Luria's examination procedures were based on his theory of brain function, and he used a flexible approach to test selection, such that any given patient's evaluation may include tests different from those administered to another patient. The test procedures used by Luria were of a "pass-fail" type, not yielding a gradation of scores. In place of the quantitative analysis used in the HRB, Luria emphasized qualitative analysis through discovering the cognitive processes by which patients completed or failed his tests. The essence of his examination procedure was for the examiner to systematically manipulate the requirements of a test to determine the underlying reasons for failure and to identify those task modifications that enabled the patient to successfully perform the task. Such identification and analysis of the factors that impair and the factors that assist performance present substantial advantages for rehabilitation. Luria's approach was developed into a standardized test battery—the Luria-Nebraska Neuropsychological Battery (LNNB) (33). However, the LLNB bears little resemblance to Luria's qualitative and individualized approach. Another approach to neuropsychological assessment is the Boston Process Approach developed by Kaplan (34) and Millburg et al (35). Kaplan's process approach combines features of the quantitative (HRB) and qualitative (Luria) approaches just noted.

While the argument between the advocates of the qualitative and the quantitative approaches continues, the two approaches are not mutually incompatible and many practitioners simply combine both. Moreover, specific choices regarding test selection are not nearly as important as the psychologist's ability to translate examination findings into conclusions and recommendations that reflect sound neuroscience and that enhance the patient's care.

Communication of Psychological Information

One of the most important functions of the psychologist is to communicate the results of psychological assessment. Communicating the results of psychological assessments often is complicated by the diversity of "consumers" for that information. In addition to the obvious need of communicating with the patient, in many cases there is the need to communicate with the patient's family and with the rehabilitation team, which may include physicians, rehabilitation nurses, therapists (e.g., physical, occupational, recreational, respiratory, nutritional), speech-language pathologists, vocational rehabilitation specialists, biomedical engineers, and social workers. Moreover, since rehabilitation patients often are involved in legal actions such as those involving workers' compensation, automobile or other liability insurance, and disability insurance claims, the patient's attorney or the insurance company case-manager often also becomes a consumer. An essential component of assessment, therefore, is for the psychologist to clarify his or her communication responsibilities and obligations, preferably in advance of delivering any services. The diversity of potential clients raises the possibility of the psychologist entering into dual relationships; an event that invariably has negative consequences and that is considered a violation of the American Psychological Association's code of ethics.

Communication of psychological information also is difficult because the typical rehabilitation team has not been constructed on the basis of delivering mental health services, and team members view their mission as *physical* rehabilitation. Indeed, patients themselves may wonder why a psychologist is necessary to what they perceive as a purely physical process of rehabilitation. When such teams request psychological consultation, it often is for situations where behavioral and emotional issues are impeding or preventing satisfactory physical rehabilitation. Thus, it is important for the psychologist to communicate psychological information in a manner whereby the connection to physical rehabilitation is direct and explicit. In some cases, the connection is clear (e.g., the patient is too depressed to get out of bed and participate in therapies), but in other cases, especially when character or personality disorders are causing disturbed interpersonal relationships between the patient and the team, communication must be done with great thoughtfulness and sensitivity to the capacity of team members to address their own emotional reactions to the patient [e.g., the patient is an avoidant personality who does not form positive relationships, the therapists interpret the patient's lack of response to them as a rejection of their enthusiastic desire to be helpful and therapeutic, and some or all of the therapists respond to feeling rejected by concluding that the patient "is not motivated" and therefore not worthy of their treatment, or develop an outright dislike for the patient, even to the point of hatred, or develop disguised reactions such as increased fatigue or illness (2)].

One classic problem noted throughout the literature is the tendency for rehabilitation staff to "overpathologize" rehabilitation patients. For instance, Caplan (36) found that rehabilitation professionals may assign depressive symptoms to patients who are not actually depressed. This may be especially likely in patients who are relatively resistant to treatment. Alternatively, staff may overidentify with the patient, assuming that since they themselves would be depressed if they suffered a given disability, the patient must necessarily be so as well (37). In fact, major psychological reactions (severe depression, for instance) occur only in a minority of acutely impaired individuals (38). As noted by Trexler and Fordyce (39), rates of depression in rehabilitation patients mirror those found in other types of inpatients and outpatients.

The task of communicating psychological assessment information, thus, at times may include carefully and sensitively assisting members of the rehabilitation to become aware of how their own psychological reactions are influencing their perception of, and behavior toward, the patient.

ASSESSMENT OF SPECIFIC POPULATIONS

Brain-Injured Patients

Psychologists performing neuropsychological assessment must have adequate clinical neuropsychological experience and training. Standards for the training of neuropsychologists now exist, and the American Board of Clinical Neuropsychology awards a diploma in clinical neuropsychology based on academic training, postdoctoral experience and training, and written and oral examinations. Clinical neuropsychologists are expected to have a working knowledge of clinical neuroscience and cognitive neuroscience, as well as general training in clinical psychology. By today's standards it is considered incompetent to simply give a neuropsychological test and report that the patient is in the brain-damaged or normal range. It is expected that a neuropsychological assessment will integrate the patient's premorbid cognitive capacities and neurobehavioral status with the injury or illness in question, and examine critically whether the patient's neuropsychological status is reasonable given the existing medical information. For example, in examining a patient hospitalized for rehabilitation following a recent cerebrovascular accident (CVA) in the middle cerebral artery distribution, it is essential for the neuropsychologist to discriminate between patients who have had the CVA in otherwise healthy brains versus patients who have an underlying dementia in addition to the CVA.

Another important factor for the assessment of brain injury is timing. Many traumatic brain injury patients, especially in the early stages of recovery, are unable to tolerate or cooperate with lengthy neuropsychological test batteries. Giving 10 different neuropsychological tests to a severely inattentive patient results in measurements of his or her inattentiveness 10 times, no matter what the different neuropsychological tests are designed to measure. It obviously is more cost-effective to measure such a patient's inattentiveness only once, and then, when inattentiveness is resolved or meaningfully improved, to begin more comprehensive assessment.

It also is important to assess various factors that mediate the relationship between traumatic brain injury patients' cognitive abilities on the one hand, and how these abilities are expressed in real life performances on the other hand. These include mood and psychological adjustment, personality and coping style, capacity for accurate self-appraisal, willingness to use compensatory procedures, and interpersonal and social skills. All these factors influence rehabilitation outcomes, and understanding them can help enormously in the development of treatment interventions (40).

Geriatric Patients

Normal aging involves multiple challenges, including altered role status resulting from retirement, changes in family roles, loss of friends and family, increasing frequency of medical conditions, and changes in cognitive functioning. Older adults may also find themselves with fewer resources to cope with the stresses of aging, and be increasingly vulnerable to despair (41). It is not clear whether depression or anxiety disorders are more prevalent among older than younger adults, but research has shown that the incidence of suicide increases in older adults (42–43). Mittenberg et al (44) also found that older adults perform relatively poorly on neuropsychological measures of frontal lobe functioning, including reduced mental flexibility, abstract reasoning, and initiative. Older adults also are less efficient in developing problem-solving strategies, and have trouble generating alternative solutions when their initial strategies fail (45).

Significant neurobehavioral syndromes can result from stroke, affecting new learning and memory, the ability to generalize new learning to other settings and circumstances, communication, spatial-perceptual skills, and the capacity for self-regulation of behavior and affect. Stroke patients exhibit neurobehavioral syndromes—disturbances directly related to brain dysfunction—that can affect the full repertoire of human abilities, since stroke can affect any part of the brain [for a comprehensive discussion, see works by Lishman (46), Mesulam (47), and Strub and Black (48)]. Ullman (49), for instance, found that deficits in orientation, memory, judgment, and all aspects of cognitive functioning are the primary cause of poor rehabilitation outcomes for stroke patients. Moreover, geriatric stroke patients often have concurrent diseases or dementing illnesses, or both.

Mood disorders are also common among stroke patients, with depression being the more prevalent diagnosis. The identification of depression in stroke patients is critical for at least three reasons: First, it is common, and can often be treated successfully; second, it is often manifested in a loss of motivation, a reduction of energy, and heightened fatigue, all of which can reduce a patient's involvement in the rehabilitation process; and third, the failure to diagnose depression can result in the patient's failure to achieve goals that are within her or his capacity. Depression, then, is a mediating variable, limiting the potential success of rehabilitation (50).

Not surprisingly, all of these sequelae of stroke can make it more difficult to perform psychological assessment. Yet assessment is critical to distinguish between the behaviors and psychological states that are related simply to normal aging and those that resulted from the stroke, and to understand the relationship between these two sets of factors. Indeed, some of the aspects of normal aging may become problematic only in a nonfamiliar and nonpredictable environment, such as the rehabilitation setting.

Therefore, assessment of geriatric stroke patients should be multidimensional. It should include formal neuropsychological evaluation (to determine cognitive deficits), the assessment of psychological adjustment (to detect possible anxiety or depression), trait and social-cognitive measures of personality (which can help determine premorbid personality functioning), and the observation of functioning in real life situations (to see how well patients can acquire new skills, utilize compensatory strategies, and generalize learning to new situations). Data from these various sources represent different but overlapping aspects of functioning, and together help clarify the overall clinical picture.

Patients with Chronic Pain

Acute pain usually is managed through medical treatment of the underlying causes and through administration of analgesic medications. Treatment of chronic pain focuses on reducing suffering and enhancing functional performance and quality of life, even when pain reduction is not achieved. The assessment and treatment of chronic pain increasingly has involved psychologists, stimulated in part by Fordyce's landmark book on behavioral treatment of chronic pain (51). The Commission on Accreditation of Rehabilitation Facilities (CARF) now mandates that a chronic pain management program includes a psychologist or psychiatrist as part of its core team.

Psychological assessment of the chronic pain patient focuses on identifying behaviors, beliefs, and emotions that can exacerbate the experience of pain, particularly the component of suffering. These factors may be reactive to the pain disorder (e.g., a depression that develops in response to the pain disorder) or they may initially be independent comorbidities (e.g., a long-standing depression that exacerbates the pain disorder). The assessment also focuses on the differential diagnosis to rule out conversion disorder, hypochondriasis, somatization disorder, and factitious disorder. Also addressed are the ways in which the pain has altered the patient's physical, social, and recreational activities, work-related activities, and self-image. The ultimate goal of the assessment is to identify ways to reduce the patient's suffering, increase his or her functional capacity, and improve quality of life.

CONCLUSIONS

Three main conclusions can be derived from this brief overview of psychological assessment within physical medicine and rehabilitation settings: 1) Psychological testing, by itself, hardly constitutes a competent psychological assessment, and extremely useful psychological assessments often will include no psychological testing. 2) Psychological assessments need to be customized for different rehabilitation patient populations. 3) The timing of psychological assessment is a crucial factor to maintaining optimal cost-benefit ratios.

REFERENCES

1. Sweet JJ. Psychological evaluation and testing services in medical settings. In: Sweet JJ, Rozensky RH, Tovian SM, eds. *Handbook of clinical psychology in medical settings.* New York: Plenum, 1991: 291–313.
2. Gans J. Facilitating staff interaction in rehabilitation. In: Caplan B, ed. *Rehabilitation psychology desk reference.* Rockville, MD: Aspen, 1987:185–213.
3. Bleiberg J, Merbitz C. Learning goals during initial rehabilitation hospitalization. *Arch Phys Med Rehabil* 1983;64:448–450.
4. Wechsler D. *WAIS-R manual.* New York: Psychological Corporation, 1981.
5. Hathaway SR, McKinley JC. *The Minnesota Multiphasic Personality Inventory manual (revised).* New York: Psychological Corporation, 1951.
6. Elliott TR, Umlauf RL. Measurement of personality and psychopathology following acquired physical disability. In: Cushman L, Scherer MJ, eds. *Psychological assessment in medical rehabilitation.* Washington, DC: American Psychological Association, 1995: 325–358.
7. Piotrowsky C, Lubin B. Assessment practices of health psychologists: survey of APA division 38 clinicians. *Prof Psychol Res Pract* 1990;21:99–106.
8. Millon T. *Manual for the MCMI-II.* 2nd ed. Minneapolis: National Computer Systems, 1987.
9. American Psychiatric Association. *Diagnostic and statistical manual of mental disorders.* 3rd rev. ed. Washington, DC: Author, 1987.
10. American Psychiatric Association. *Diagnostic and statistical manual of mental disorders.* 4th ed. Washington, DC: Author, 1994.
11. Millon T, Green CJ, Meagher RB Jr. *Millon Behavioral Health Inventory manual.* 3rd ed. Minneapolis: National Computer Systems, 1982.
12. Beck A, Ward CH, Mendleson M, et al. An inventory for measuring depression. *Arch Gen Psychiatry* 1961;4:561–571.
13. Zung WW. Self-rating depression scale in an outpatient clinic. Further validation of the SDS. *Arch Gen Psychiatry* 1965;13: 508–515.
14. Hamilton M. Development of a rating scale for primary depressive illness. *Br J Soc Clin Psychol* 1967;6:278–296.
15. Eber HW, Cattell RB, Institute for Personality and Ability Testing Staff. *Manual for Form E of the 16PF.* Champaign, IL: Institute for Personality and Ability Testing, 1985.
16. Bolton B, Brookings JB. Prediction of job satisfactoriness for workers with severe handicaps from aptitudes, personality, and training ratings. *J Business Psychol* 1993;7:359–366.
17. Brookings JB, Bolton B, Young G. Employability assessment of persons with disabilities: research, instruments, and applications. *Assess Rehab Exceptionality* 1994;1:259–275.
18. Cattell R, Eber HW, Tatsuoka MN. *Handbook for the 16PF.* Champaign, IL: Institute for Personality and Ability Testing, 1985.
19. Costa PT, McCrae R. *The NEO Personality Inventory: manual.* Odessa, FL: Psychological Assessment Resources, 1995.
20. Digman JM. Personality structure: emergence of the five factor model. *Annu Rev Psychol* 1990; 41:417–440.
21. Rotter JB. Generalized expectancies for internal versus external control of reinforcements. *Psychol Monogr Gen Appl* 1996;80:1–28.
22. Wallston KA, Wallston BS, Devellis R. Development of the Multidimensional Health Locus of Control (MHLC) scales. *Health Educ Monogr* 1978;6:160–170.
23. Heppner PP. *The problem-solving inventory: manual.* Palo Alto, CA: Psychologists Press, 1988.
24. Elliott TR, Witty TE, Herrick SM, Hoffman JT. Negotiating reality after physical loss: hope, depression, and disability. *J Pers Soc Psychol* 1991;61:608–613.
25. Nezu A, Perri M. Social problem-solving therapy for unipolar depression: an initial dismantling investigation. *J Consult Clin Psychol* 1989;57:408–413.
26. Wilkinson GS. *WRAT3: Wide-Range Achievement Test administration manual.* Wilmington, DE: Wide Range, 1993.
27. Dunn L, Markwardt FC. *Peabody Individual Achievement Test manual.* Circle Pines, MN: American Guidance Service, 1970.
28. Raven JC. *Guide to the standard progressive matrices.* London: AK Lewis, 1960.
29. Reitan RM. Theoretical and methodological bases of the

Halstead-Reitan Neuropsychological Test Battery. In: Grant I, Adams K, eds. *Neuropsychological assessment of neuropsychiatric disorders.* New York: Oxford, 1986:3–42.

30. Reitan RM, Wolfson D. *The Halstead-Reitan Neuropsychological Test Battery: theory and clinical interpretation.* Tucson, AZ: Neuropsychology Press, 1993.

31. Luria AR. *The working brain.* New York: Basic Books, 1973.

32. Luria AR. *Higher cortical functions in man.* New York: Basic Books, 1980.

33. Golden C, Hammeke AD, Purisch TA. *Luria Nebraska Neuropsychological Test Battery: forms I and II.* Los Angeles: Western Psychological Services, 1985.

34. Kaplan E. A process approach to neuropsychological assessment. In: Boll T, Bryant B, eds. *Clinical neuropsychology and brain function: research, measurement, and practice.* Washington, DC: American Psychological Association, 1988: 125–169.

35. Millburg WP, Hebben N, Kaplan E. The Boston Process Approach to neuropsychological assessment. In: Grant I, Adams K, eds. *Neuropsychological assessment of neuropsychiatric disorders.* New York: Oxford, 1986:65–86.

36. Caplan B. Staff and patient perception of patient mood. *Rehabil Psychol* 1983;28:67–78.

37. Wills T. Perceptions of clients by professional helpers. *Psychol Bull* 1978;85:968–1000.

38. Davidoff G, Roth E, Thomas P, et al. Depression among acute spinal cord injury patients: a study utilizing the Zung Self-Rating Depression Scale. *Rehabil Psychol* 1990; 35:171–180.

39. Trexler LE, Fordyce DJ. Psychological perspectives on rehabilitation: contemporary assessment and intervention strategies. In: Braddom RL, Buschbacher RM, Dumitru D, et al, eds. *Physical medicine and rehabilitation.* Philadelphia: WB Saunders, 1996: 66–81.

40. Diller L, Gordon WA. Interventions for cognitive deficits in brain-injured adults. *J Consult Clin Psychol* 1981;49:822–834.

41. Berezin MA, et al. The elderly person. In: Nicholi AM, ed. *The new Harvard guide to psychiatry.* Cambridge, MA: Belknap Press, 1988:665–680.

42. Trezona RR. Assessment and treatment of depression in the older rehabilitation patient. In: Hartke RJ, ed. *Psychological aspects of geriatric rehabilitation.* The Rehabilitation Institute of Chicago publication series. Gaithersburg, MD: Aspen Press, 1991:187–210.

43. Stoudemire A, Blazer DG. Depression in the elderly. In: Beckman EE, Leber WR, eds. *Handbook of depression.* Homewood, IL: Dorsey Press, 1985:556–586.

44. Mittenberg W, Seidenberg M, O'Leary DS, DiGiulio DV. Changes in cerebral functioning associated with normal aging. *J Clin Exp Neuropsychol* 1989;11:918–932.

45. Van Gorp W, Mahler M. Subcortical features of normal aging. In: Cummings J, ed. *Subcortical dementia.* New York: Oxford University Press, 1990:231–250.

46. Lishman WA. *Organic psychology: the psychological consequences of cerebral disorder.* London: Blackwell Scientific, 1978.

47. Mesulam M. *Principles of behavioral neurology.* Philadelphia: FA Davis, 1985.

48. Strub RL, Black FW. *Neurobehavioral disorders: a clinical approach.* Philadelphia: FA Davis, 1988.

49. Ullman M. *Behavioral changes in patients following strokes.* Springfield, IL: Charles Thomas, 1962.

50. Garmoe W, Newman A, Bleiberg J. Neuropsychologic aspects of normal aging and stroke rehabilitation. In: Ozer MN, Materson RS, Caplan LR, eds. *Management of persons with stroke.* Boston: Mosby, 1994:219–250.

51. Fordyce, WE. *Behavioral methods for chronic pain and illness.* St. Louis: Mosby, 1976.

Chapter 17

Disability Evaluation

Robert D. Rondinelli
Richard T. Katz
Steven L. Hendler
Bart E. Eisfelder

The evaluation and treatment of impairment and disability are central to the practice of physiatry. However, there has been a relative paucity of direct and formal training within our field regarding the practices and procedures of medical impairment rating and disability determination. Certification programs are emerging within the American Academy of Physical Medicine and Rehabilitation (1) and elsewhere, and disability evaluation is playing an increasingly important role in the physiatric practice, particularly in those settings receiving musculoskeletal emphasis. Practice opportunities within the field of disability evaluation are also facing increasing competition from other specialty fields. The physiatrist must rapidly acquire a familiarity, expertise, and comfort level with all aspects of disability evaluation in order to proceed competently, confidently, and competitively in this increasingly attractive arena of patient evaluation and care.

This chapter has several key purposes. The first is to provide the physiatrist with an overview of the various major disability systems within the United States with respect to definitions, entitlement, benefits, and their respective roles for the physiatrist as disability examiner. The second is to familiarize the physiatrist with the application of the American Medical Association's Guides to the Evaluation of Permanent Impairment, 4th ed. (2) (hereafter referred to as AMA *Guides*) to the practice of musculoskeletal impairment rating. The third purpose is to illustrate the role and relationship of work fitness determinations to the process of disability evaluation. The fourth is to highlight the disability-related processes of independent medical evaluation and life care planning that the physiatrist can be expected to undertake. The fifth is to address the complex issue of chronic pain as it relates to disability evaluation. Finally, due to the frequent litiginous nature of disability ratings, the medicolegal ramifications of the physiatrist as disability examiner are discussed.

UNITED STATES DISABILITY SYSTEMS

Tort Law

Over the years, state and federal governments have enacted legislation intended to grant various benefits to employees who are injured as a result of their employment. Tort liability has its origins in the English system of "Common Law" in which the claimant seeking redress for civil wrongdoings could file suit. A *tort*, by definition, is a "breech of duty that gives rise to an action for damages" (3). Historically, the claimant was required to bring a civil suit against his or her employer alleging and proving negligence or some fault of the employer that directly resulted in harm or damage to the employee. Many such claims were barred because of theories that the employee had assumed the risk of injury in accepting employment, that the employee had been comparatively negligent in contributing to his or her injury, or that a third party had contributed to the resulting injury. Most often, persons were denied benefits because the employer was determined not at fault, or because the employee was, in part, at fault for his or her own injury. As a result of inadequacies with the tort claim system, the workers' compensation law was enacted throughout the United States.

There are four requisite components of a tort claim. It must be shown that

A legal duty existed

There was a breech of that legal duty

There was proximate or direct cause

There was harm or damage as a result

At present, tort claims are less a creature of statute than the workers' compensation system (see below). In a tort claim, the physician is given much more latitude in determining the extent or effect of an injury on a claimant's life. Tort claims often arise out of injuries to a person by virtue of automobile accidents, medical malpractice, or defective products. While the criteria for recovery will often vary from state to state, the physician will generally be asked to provide an opinion as to the extent of impairment or disability, and how that impairment or disability may affect the claimant's life in terms of work and social activities.

Workers' Compensation

Entitlement

The U.S. workers' compensation system is a state-based system of compensation, first established in Wisconsin in 1911. A comprehensive plan exists for all 50 states as well as the District of Columbia and the trust territories of Puerto Rico and the Virgin Islands (2). The workers' compensation system is compulsory in all states except Texas, South Carolina, and New Jersey (4). Significant differences exist between the plans for the various states; however, they all have adopted a "no-fault" system whereby an employee suffering injury, accident, or occupational disease arising out of and in the course and scope of employment may recover benefits from the employer without having to prove that the employer was at fault. In exchange, the injured employee gives up the right to sue the employer for damages due to occupational causes. The key phrases "injury, accidents or occupational disease" and "arising out of and in the course and scope of employment" have been used and variously defined from state to state, and generally must be proved in order to recover benefits under workers' compensation.

Injury has been defined generally as a change to the body pathology caused by either accident, repetitive use or trauma, or occupational disease.

Accident refers to the event(s) caused by the employment and resulting in injury.

Occupational disease has been defined as a disease peculiar to and arising out of employment that subjects the employee to a hazard to which the public is not generally exposed.

Arising out of generally refers to the method of injury—did the condition arise out of or was it causally related to the work being performed?

In the course and scope of refers more to the time of occurrence—was the employee performing duties required by the employer at a time and place when those duties should have been performed?

Definitions

Workers' compensation generally recognizes four categories of disability (5) as follows:

1. *Temporary total disability* renders an employee completely incapable of returning to work and earning wages on a temporary basis. Where it exists, the employee is expected to make some recovery. The employee must be evaluated by a physician who provides work restrictions during the time period and to the extent that they remove the employee from any gainful occupation.
2. *Temporary partial disability* renders an employee partially incapable of performing work on a temporary basis, while under a physician's care and restrictions that remove the injured worker from some part of the job, as well as precluding a portion of the preinjury earning capacity.
3. *Permanent total disability* renders an employee completely and totally incapable of ongoing or future gainful employment. In such cases, restrictions placed on the injured worker by the physician or vocational expert after the "healing period" is completed, preclude ever returning to *any* gainful employment. Most states do not require or preclude recovery if the person can perform some job, even of a menial nature.
4. *Permanent partial disability* renders an employee partially incapable of gainful employment at their preinjury wage earning capacity, or precludes an employee from doing all that he or she could do prior to the injury whether or not a wage loss occurred.

Benefits

Benefits also vary from state to state. In general, benefits are provided in the event of death; or for medical costs associated with treatment; or for wage losses due to temporary total disability, temporary partial disability, and permanent total or partial disability (6). Some states discuss wage-loss benefits in terms of "impairment" of a permanent nature. Others provide a concept of "work disability." Criteria may vary according to a concept of functional loss, which is readily evaluated by a physician utilizing a guide such as the AMA *Guides*. Alternatively, a wage-loss concept that requires the expertise of a vocational expert may be employed. In some cases a combination of the two approaches is used. For example, Kansas has a general bodily impairment recovery that is based solely on "functional impairment" assessed by a physician using the AMA *Guides*, and a "work disability" that considers the impairment and its putative impact on task loss and wage loss (7). Missouri, a neighboring state to Kansas, utilizes the term *disability*; however, in most instances, Missouri relies solely on a physician's opinion expressed in terms of disability, and reserves formal vocational considerations of wage and task loss for only the most serious cases (8).

Most states provide various death benefits if death follows as a result of a work-related accident. Benefits generally include funeral benefits and ongoing compensation to the surviving spouse and children. Utilizing Missouri again as an example, death benefits are paid to the widow(er) at the same rate that temporary total disabilities are paid and continue until that widow(er) remarries or is deceased. If children are minors, they are likewise entitled to benefits that are divided according to agreement or judicial interpretation. Such benefits may continue until age 18 or longer, if certain conditions preclude independent wage-earning apply (9).

Nearly all states allow for medical benefits to cure or relieve the effects of a work-related condition, and typically provide for 100% of associated medical bills. States may vary as to who controls the selection of the treating physician. Both Kansas and Missouri allow for the employer to select and designate the treating physician. Unauthorized medical expenses are the obligation of the injured employee; however, Kansas has a maximum allowance of $500 for unauthorized medical expenses (10) whereas Missouri has no such allowance. Some states have fee schedules that set limits on physician charges and utilize Physicians' Current Procedural Terminology (CPT) codes; others have a "reasonable and customary" clause using an internal database to determine physician charges.

Many states utilize a wage-loss theory to compute temporary total or partial benefits calculated as two-thirds of the average weekly wage an employee earned prior to injury, not to exceed the maximum cap set by statute.

Losses due to permanent total or partial disability may be compensated either according to a "functional impairment" model or a "work disability" model. In Missouri, for example, the disability model applies (11). If the injury is to the body as a whole (i.e., not a scheduled injury), an employee who is partially disabled is entitled to 400 weeks compensation × the percentage of disability × the maximum rate of disability, which is set by statute (as of 7/1/96–6/30/97 at $268.72/wk). To illustrate, and assuming the employee's preinjury compensation was at or above the maximal weekly rate, a 10% permanent disability to the body as a whole due to back injury is computed as 400 weeks × 10% × $268.72/wk or a lump sum payment of $10,748.80. If preinjury compensation was less than maximum, the entitlement is reduced proportionally. In Kansas, the functional impairment model applies (7). The body as a whole is considered to be worth 415 weeks. Thirty weeks are allotted for temporary total disability during the healing period, of which 15 may be reduced from the total disability payout. The employee is then entitled to the remaining weeks × the percentage of impairment × the maximum rate (as of 7/1/93–6/30/95 at $313.00/wk). To illustrate, if a 10% impairment determination for the above injury in Kansas is rendered after 30 weeks of temporary total disability payments have been made, a final award would be determined as follows: 415 – 15 weeks (no credit for the first 15 weeks allowed), which results in 400 weeks. The remaining disability is computed as 400 weeks × 10% × $313.00/wk or a lump sum payment of $12,520.00.

In addition to "whole body" criteria, nearly every state has a "scheduled" injury classification. By statute, certain parts of the body are listed on a schedule according to the number of weeks of value assigned for their total loss. For example, the Missouri schedule for loss of the arm at the shoulder is 232 weeks and the disabled individual is entitled to the percentage of loss at the shoulder (% of 232 weeks) × the maximum rate for permanent disability (11). Kansas likewise has a schedule of injuries, and the shoulder, by comparison, is worth 225 weeks (12). Some states like Kansas allow reduction of temporary total payments from the schedule before computing final benefits. Assuming 20 weeks of compensation for a shoulder injury, the Kansas employee would be entitled to 225 weeks less 20 weeks of compensation × the percentage of impairment × the maximum rate of compensation.

Many states have a cap on benefits. In Kansas (as of 7/1/93) medical benefits are unlimited; death benefits are capped at $200,000; permanent total benefits are capped at $125,000, and permanent partial benefits at $50,000 (13). Missouri has no such caps.

It is vital that each physiatrist study the workers' compensation statutes in his or her individual state or jurisdiction and become familiar with them. Summaries of state-by-state benefits are available (14,15).

Jurisdictional Variations

The basis to invoke workers' compensation varies from state to state; however, most states employ one or more of the following:

1. The most common basis for jurisdiction is place of accident; that is, jurisdiction is invoked if the injury occurred within a given state.
2. Jurisdiction may be invoked if the employee's principal place of employment (where <50% of his or her time is spent) is located within a given state. In cases such as over-the-road trucking, the principal place of employment may be where the greatest percentage of time is spent.
3. The third jurisdictional ground is based on which locale the contract of hire was entered.

Second Injury Fund

Many states have enacted a Second Injury Fund to encourage the employment of individuals with preexisting disabilities. The criteria for recovery from the Fund varies from state to state. Furthermore, the enactment of the Americans with Disabilities Act (ADA) has reduced or eliminated the impact of the Fund in many states. For example, Kansas abolished the Fund in 1994. Prior to that time, if an employer hired an individual with a preexisting work-related disability due to injury, the employer could recover from the Second Injury Fund under the following two scenarios: If disability or death resulted from the second injury, which in all likelihood "would not have occurred but for" the preexisting disability, the employer could recover all benefits payable from the Fund. However, if the second injury would have occurrred whether or not the preexisting disability was present, and the ensuing disability is contributed to by preexisting disability, the employer could recover that percentage of benefits apportioned to the preexisting disability from the Fund (16).

In Missouri, the right to recover from the Second Injury Fund rests with the employee. If the employee has a preexisting permanent partial disability, whether from a compensable injury or otherwise, and experiences subsequent compensable injury with resultant permanent disability, he or she may be entitled to benefits from the Fund if the overall disability is greater than that which is solely attributable to the second injury. Under that scenario, the employer pays only for benefits due to the last injury, had there been no preexisting injury. The overall disability is then determined and an apportionment of preexisting and subsequent disability made. The balance due to the employee from the Fund is the additive difference after preexisting disability has been factored out (17).

The Physiatrist's Role

The physiatrist may be contacted directly by the employer, employer's attorney, or the claimant or claimant's attorney in order to direct medical diagnostic and therapeutic care. Under the workers' compensation law the physician is generally responsible for completing the eight steps in the evaluation and treatment process listed in Table 17-1.

The physiatrist must render a formal *diagnosis* and address the *severity* of the condition in question.

Causality refers to an association that can be drawn within medical probability between a causal event and its potential effect. An event is considered *medically probable* if the physician's estimated likelihood of occurrence is greater than 50%; or else it is considered *medically possible* if the likelihood is estimated to be less than or equal to 50%. In addressing causality, the physiatrist must determine within medical probability whether or not a causal event took place that could give rise to the claimant's condition, the claimant has the condition, and the causal event gave rise to the condition in question.

Table 17-1: Eight Steps as Responsibilities of the Physician under Workers' Compensation

1. Diagnosis and severity
2. Causality
3. Necessary tests/treatments completed
4. Additional tests/treatments needed
5. Maximum medical improvement reached (>6 mo)
6. Impairment rating
7. Apportionment
8. Restrictions

The physiatrist is responsible to identify *necessary tests and treatment* that have already been completed. Furthermore, he or she must ensure completion of any *additional tests and treatment* needed.

Maximum medical improvement (MMI) is believed to occur when the medical condition has resolved or else becomes stable to the degree that there is no ongoing or future progress anticipated toward resolution of the condition. MMI is believed to occur when a sufficient healing period has elapsed but no specific time frame is given. The AMA *Guides* (2) formerly recognized 6 months as a necessary and sufficient healing period but duration of healing is no longer specified. The physiatrist may gauge the adequacy of the healing period and MMI end point from a functional perspective—that is, to continue treatment as long as further progress toward functional recovery appears tenable. When MMI is reached, the physiatrist may need to address the future medical stability of the condition (e.g., worsening or deterioration over time in association with the normal aging process would not necessarily preclude MMI), and the ongoing and future medical needs to maintain MMI (see Life Care Planning/Future Medical Needs).

Impairment rating is a process that must be carried out on request and according to the AMA *Guides* or other accepted rating systems as specified by state or jurisdictional law. The AMA *Guides* is currently mandated or recommended in 29 (55%) of 53 Workers' compensation jurisdictions; not mandated or recommended but frequently used in 11 (21%) jurisdictions; and not mandated or recommended or frequently used in 13 (24%) jurisdictions (2). The physiatrist must become familiar with the laws applicable to his or her jurisdiction and follow prescribed guidelines and procedures. For purposes of this discussion, the impairment rating procedure according to the AMA *Guides* is described in detail (see Impairment Rating Guidelines).

Apportionment is necessary in cases of recurrent injury or where permanent aggravation to a preexisting condition applies. The impairment rating thereby derived is a composite rating of resulting and preexisting conditions. In such cases, the physiatrist must asssign a portion of the final rating to the current condition in question and a portion to the preexisting conditions to account for their presence and possible progression over time without an associated or aggravating new injury (18).

During the *healing period*, the physiatrist must determine whether the injured party is capable of *limited* or *modified duty* or whether *temporary total disability* applies. The physiatrist must specify what conditions of modified duty apply in terms of permissible hours and physical *restrictions* imposed at the workplace; the duration for which restrictions are in effect (usually until date of follow-up); and estimated time of recovery until MMI is achieved. The determination of work disability and applicable work restrictions is discussed in further detail in Work Fitness and Disability Evaluation.

Social Security Disability

Definition and Entitlement

The Social Security Administration (SSA) defines disability as "the inability to engage in any substantial gainful activity by reason of any medically determinable physical or mental impairments which can be expected to result in death or which has lasted or can be expected to last for a continuous period of not less than 12 months" (19). "Substantial gainful activity" in this context includes former occupation and all other occupations appropriate to the individual's age, education, and employment experience.

Eligibility is determined by nonmedical and medical means. Nonmedical eligibility requires that the applicant demonstrate a history of having actively worked for at least 5 of the preceding 10 years, that they have remained unemployed for at least 6 months previously, and that their current income is less than $300 per month.

After determining nonmedical eligibility, the SSA refers the applicant's case to the State Disability Determination Service (DDS) to determine medical eligibility. The preferred source of information by the DDS is prior medical records and reports from treating physicians; where such information is incomplete or lacking, a physician consultative examination may be ordered.

The SSA publishes its own guideline for disability evaluation, titled *Disability Evaluation Under Social Security (Listing of Impairments)* (19), which is updated annually. Physicians providing consultative examinations for the DDS must become familiar with the content and application of the guideline, which delineates the specific pertinent findings for determining the presence of impairment, and the components of the physical examination required to validate that impairment criteria have been met. The conceptual underpinning of this methodology is that objective findings must be present on examination or diagnostic testing, to justify impairment determination. The DDS recently placed new emphasis on functional assessment and recognizes the ability to sit, stand, lift, carry, and so on as objective criteria (Roseburrough T. Written communication, 1996).

Benefits

Social Security Disability Insurance (SSDI), also known as Title II, provides cash benefits to participants in the Federal Insurance Contribution Act (FICA) who qualify from an impairment point of view. Supplemental Security Income (SSI) provides cash benefits to those who have a requisite impairment, who have not worked an adequate period of time to qualify for SSDI, and who demonstrate financial need according to a "means test." The two programs serve more than 4 million Americans annually, with 7 million new applicants every year (Bastable J, Robert D. Written communication, 1996).

The Physiatrist's Role

The physiatrist's role is to identify the SSI claimant's extent and severity of impairment(s) and to make a brief functional assessment persuant to same. The DDS will request examination of specific areas, which the physiatrist must identifiably address in the report. The SSA requires, on an annual basis, that a certain number of its active beneficiaries have their cases reviewed. In such cases, the physiatrist must address those areas on which the disability determination was originally made. Additionally, recipients of SSDI (see below) undergo periodic review of eligibility; in such cases the physiatrist may be asked to assess impairment as well.

The physiatric report should include a thorough and sufficient history and physical examination, and should address the resulting impairment(s) in question following the guideline terminology as closely as possible. Comments may include rationale for the assessment that is not otherwise obvious, or any qualifications to the impairment determination. For example, certain determinations may suggest or require x-ray evidence that may be unavailable at the time of evaluation. The physiatrist is not expected or requested to determine presence or absence of disability, or eligibility for benefits; consequently, conclusions or opinions about these issues should be omitted from the report.

After a physician assessment of impairment is rendered, it is reviewed by the DDS team, which includes a physician, vocational counselor, and administrator, in order that a disability determination can be made.

Feberal Employees' Compensation Act/Longshore and Harbor Workers' Compensation Act

The Federal Employees' Compensation Act (FECA) was enacted in 1916 to provide federal compensation for work-related disability. It covers more than 3 million federal civilian employees, as well as some nonfederal employees such as state and local law enforcement personnel and employees of the Civil Air Patrol. The Longshore and

Harbor Workers' Compensation Act (LHWCA) was similarly enacted in 1927. It covers approximately 500,000 longshore workers for disability arising from occupational causes occurring on navigable waterways of the United States, and also applies to some employees of military bases. Both programs are no-fault workers' compensation systems under federal administration by the Department of Labor (20).

Federal Employers' Liability Act

The Federal Employers' Liability Act (FELA) was enacted in 1908 to provide protection to federal employees of the railroad industry. At that time the railroads were the largest employer in the United States and rail work was an exceptionally hazardous occupation. Prior to passage of the act, injured employees could attempt to seek redress under tort law as described above. Under FELA, employer defenses were limited and liability for workplace injuries was increased. Today, FELA covers nearly all railroads providing interstate service including most commuter railroads and more than 260,000 federal employees (20).

Under FELA, and in contrast to the no-fault systems described above, injured workers must either negotiate a settlement or else file lawsuit against the railroad for personal losses. If a lawsuit is filed under FELA, the injured party must show negligence on the part of the employer. However, recovery for damages suffered can be proportionately reduced to the extent that employee contributory negligence is shown to occur. FELA allows the injured party to recover economic damages such as medical expenses and lost wages. FELA also provides compensation for noneconomic damages due to pain and suffering. Such damages are generally not awarded under workers' compensation. Under FELA, injured employees may also be eligible for retirement benefits, sickness benefits, and disability annuities (20).

Department of Veterans Affairs

Definition and Entitlement

The Department of Veterans Affairs defines total disability "when there is present any impairment of mind or body which is sufficient to render it impossible for the average person to follow a substantially gainful occupation" (21). Total disability may be temporary, or permanent provided it is reasonably certain that such disability will continue throughout the life of the disabled person (21). Examples of permanent total disability include the permanent loss of the use of both hands, of both feet, of one hand and one foot, or of the sight of both eyes, or becoming permanently helpless or permanently bedridden. Other total disability ratings are scheduled according to the various bodily systems comprising a *Schedule for Rating Disabilities* (22). For purposes of compensation, a total disability rating may be assigned where the scheduled rating is less than total, but sufficient to preclude substantial gainful employment according to the rating agency. That is, provided that if there is only one scheduled rating, it meets or exceeds 60%, or if there are two or more scheduled ratings, at least one meets or exceeds 40%, and their combined value meets or exceeds 70% (22). Finally, veterans who fail to meet the above percentage criteria, but who are judged unable to secure and follow substantial gainful employment by reason of a *service-connected* disability are still eligible for total disability compensation and pension status (22).

Service-connected entitlement exists if the veteran becomes disabled as a result of injury or illness (including aggravation of a preexisting and underlying condition) while in active service and in the line of duty (21). Non-service-connected entitlement exists for disabilities that can be shown to arise after the course of active service.

Benefits

Benefits for eligible veterans include a pension compensation in the form of monthly payments directly to the veteran because of service-connected disability, or to a spouse, child, or parent of the veteran because of service-connected death (21). Additional benefits are provided in the form of hospitalization and medical care, orthotic and prosthetic devices, durable medical equipment, and allowances for adaptive modifications to the home or motor vehicle in appropriate cases.

The Physiatrist's Role

In order to validate a disability claim, the Department of Veterans Affairs will authorize and require a complete physical examination in most cases. Medical evidence including hospital records and physician reports from nonmilitary sources may be accepted in support of a claim, and may satisfy the requirement for disability determinations in some cases, in lieu of the "examination." In cases where improvement of a disabling condition might be expected, periodic physician re-examination is required to verify the accuracy of a current disability rating.

The basis of disability evaluations is the determination of the ability of the body as a whole, or of an organ or system of the body to function under ordinary conditions of daily life including employment. The rating physician must refer to the above-mentioned *Schedule* which provides comprehensive guidelines for rating the musculoskeletal and other organ systems. Physician evaluation must include a determination of "lack of usefulness" of the body, body part, or system, particularly in activities of self-support. Consequently, the physiatrist can be expected to furnish an opinion supported by medical data concerning the etiology, anatomy, pathology, laboratory aspects, and prognosis of the condition in question, as well as a full description of the effects of the condition on the person's ordinary activity (22).

Private Disability Insurance

It is estimated that 40 million Americans are covered by some type of private long-term disability insurance, the majority through their workplace (Bastable J, Robert D. Written communication, 1996). In such insurance plans, the definitions and provisions of disability are determined not by law but by contractual language (23). Although there are many similarities among policies, every disability evaluation performed by a physician for the adjudication of private insurance claims may differ to some degree.

The employee who becomes disabled is initially covered under short-term disability for a certain number of days (often 90 days) before long-term disability takes over. Long-term disability policies may be *group policies*, which are often sold to companies, or *individual policies*. Group policies generally provide coverage for *any occupation*. This often translates as follows—a person who is injured will be paid disability if he or she cannot perform the requirements of the particular job for a certain period (often 2 years). After this period, the person will only continue to be paid disability benefits if he or she cannot perform the job requirements of "any occupation." These definitions are variably interpreted by employer and insurer.

An individual policy often provides greater protection, as it may provide benefits if the disabled person can no longer perform the particular duties of his or her own occupation. As a rule, most disability policies do not pay more than 60% of the employee's full salary, to maintain an incentive to return to work. Policies may add certain riders which include protection for cost-of-living adjustments.

In general, the physiatrist must determine disability according to criteria of impairment set forth by the private insurer. Additionally, private insurance disability evaluations may include assessment of functional capacity (i.e., lifting, carrying, push/pull, sitting, standing, etc.), and often, a determination of whether or not additional rehabilitation will favorably impact on the claimant's impairment and disability.

IMPAIRMENT RATING GUIDELINES

Using the American Medical Association's *Guides*

The AMA *Guides* was created in 1971 for the purpose of providing physicians with a standard framework of reference concerning the evaluation and reporting about impairments affecting any human organ system. It has undergone four separate revisions and updating such that the fourth edition (2) is the currently accepted edition recommended by the AMA. Historically, the musculoskeletal system has received the greatest amount of attention and detail, with almost 40% of the current text devoted to this system. A full and detailed discussion of impairment rating of all organ systems falls outside the scope and purpose of this chapter, and the physiatrist who incorporates impairment rating and disability determinations into practice will need to become intimately familiar with all sections of the AMA *Guides*. However, many of the concepts and methodologic approaches central to the AMA *Guides* are best illustrated through a brief orientation to impairment rating of the musculoskeletal system, and can readily be applied to other systems when the need arises.

The Anatomic Model

Regional Units of the Whole Person

For the musculoskeletal system the body as a whole is divided into four separate regions (upper extremity, lower extremity, spine, and pelvis), each with its own respective units and subunits (Table 17-2). According to the *anatomic model*, impairments to the spine and pelvis are awarded directly to the "whole person" whereas impairments affecting the extremities are awarded in terms of percentage loss to that extremity. Impairment to the upper extremity can be converted to the whole person by multiplying by a factor of 0.6 (i.e., 100% upper-extremity impairment equals 60% whole person) and lower-extremity conversion is made by multiplying by a factor of 0.4 (i.e., 100% lower-extremity impairment equals 40% whole person).

Upper-Extremity Impairment Rating

When rating the upper extremity, the AMA *Guides* (2) has adopted a system endorsed by leading hand surgery societies. Three key parameters provide the mainstays of upper-extremity impairment rating: amputation, ankylosis and range-of-motion (ROM), and sensation of the digits. Impairments are compared to amputations at various levels. For example, 100% amputation of the upper extremity equals 60% of whole person impairment. One hundred percent loss of the hand equals a 90% loss of the upper extremity, and a complete loss of the thumb equals a 40% loss of the hand.

When ROM and ankylosis are considered, only active range is measured using standard goniometric techniques. Range must be assessed in each of the cardinal directions of movement of the thumb, digits, wrist, elbow, and shoulder.

Sensation is assessed with two-point discrimination as the preferred modality. When two-point discrimination of a digit is assessed, discrimination of more than 15 mm is considered a total sensory loss; 7 to 15 mm, partial sensory loss; and less than 6 mm is normal. The AMA *Guides* defines complete sensory loss of a limb or its portion as equivalent to 50% of the value for amputation of the limb or its portion.

As the upper extremity may have more than one impairment, the concept of "combining" impairments applies (see section Adding and Combining Impairments). Hand impairments are combined, and then combined with other upper-extremity impairments to give impairment ratings for the upper extremity. These can be converted to

Table 17-2: Regional Impairments of the Musculoskeletal System

Whole Person Conversion Factor	Region	Unit	Subunit	Impairment Criteria: Range of Motion Ankylosis	Amputation	Sensory	Other
0.6	Upper extremity						
		Shoulder		+	+	−	+
		Elbow		+	+	−	+
		Wrist		+	+	−	+
		Hand		+	+	+	+
			Thumb	+	+	+	+
			Index	+	+	+	+
			Middle	+	+	+	+
			Ring	+	+	+	+
			Little	+	+	−	+
0.4	Lower extremity						
		Hip		+	+	−	+
		Knee		+	+	−	+
		Ankle		+	+	−	+
		Foot		+	+	−	+
			Hind foot	+	+	−	+
			Mid foot	+	+	−	+
			Forefoot	+	+	−	+
			Great toe	+	+	−	+
			Lesser toes	+	+	−	+
1.0	Spine						
		Cervical		+	−	−	+
		Thoracic		+	−	−	+
		Lumbar		+	−	−	+
		Sacral		+	−	−	+
1.0	Pelvis			−	+	−	+

"whole person" impairments using appropriate tables in the AMA *Guides*.

Strength is generally not assessed unless there is an injury of the peripheral nervous system, as it is believed to be highly effort dependent on the part of the patient. Hand strength can be assessed with a Jamar dynamometer and a pinch strength gauge. Validity of the dynamometer can be improved by testing strength in different positions on the device, as well as noting values as the patient rapidly exchanges the dynamometer from side to side.

Peripheral nervous system disorders of the upper extremity are based first on the anatomic structure involved: root, plexus, or nerve. The impairment rater must assess the severity of sensory deficit or pain impairment, as well as the weakness in key innervated muscles. The motor and sensory values are combined utilizing schedules within the AMA *Guides*. Reflex sympathetic dystrophy (more recently renamed "complex regional pain syndrome") is rated according to the degree of sensory loss, pain, motor weakness, and loss of ROM.

It is also recognized that many impairments are inadequately addressed utilizing the criteria above, and so separate schedules have been included in the AMA *Guides*. These include joint crepitation, synovial hypertrophy, digit lateral deviation, digit rotational deformity, persistent joint subluxation, joint instability, wrist/elbow deviations, carpal instability, arthroplasty, intrinsic muscle tightness, constrictive tenosynovitis, and extensor tendon subluxation at the metacarpophalangeal joint. There is also a separate schedule for vascular disorders of the upper extremity.

Lower-Extremity Impairment Rating

The AMA *Guides* offers nine categories with which the physiatrist can assess impairment in the lower extremity. Again, amputation is a "yardstick" by which other impairments are compared. A total amputation of the lower extremity is equivalent to a 40% impairment of the whole person. A great-toe amputation is equivalent to a 17% of the foot, 12% of the lower extremity, or 5% of the whole person. Schedules are provided for leg-length discrepancy, gait derangement, muscle atrophy secondary to fracture, neurologic weakness, loss of ROM or ankylosis, nerve injuries, and arthritis—as assessed by loss of joint space on standing film. Diagnosis-related estimates (DREs) of impairment are provided for fractures, joint replacements, and instabilities.

Spinal Impairment Rating

The major anatomic criterion for impairment of the spine is loss of ROM of the cervical (flexion/extension, lateral flexion, rotation), thoracic (flexion/extension, rotation), and lumbosacral (flexion/extension, lateral flexion) regions. Previous editions of the AMA *Guides* utilized the ROM model, which is very complex and tedious. According to the fourth edition (2), it is considered an alternative method of rating spinal impairment when the DRE model (see below) would be inappropriate (almost never). According to the ROM model, the examiner is expected to make multiple measurements of spinal motion, preferably with two inclinometers. Measurements need to be repeated until three readings conform to certain reliability criteria—a daunting task in patients who may be in pain or who are less than optimally cooperative with the examiner. In addition, the ROM model also includes a diagnosis-related component, as well as adjustments for fractures, disk or soft-tissue injury, operative interventions, spondylolysis and spondylolisthesis, spinal stenosis, fracture, instability, and dislocation. These may then need to be combined with any neurologic impairment that is present. All in all, the ROM model is not a tenable system of rating spinal impairment.

Diagnosis-Related Estimates Model

The most recent edition of the AMA *Guides* offers an alternative approach to the assessment of impairment affecting the spine, replacing ROM estimates with *diagnosis-related estimates* (DREs) of impairment. This is the preferred method of rating impairment of the spine. The DRE model is also referred to as the *injury* model because it is predicated on obtaining a history of losses to the spine that are directly attributable to injury as opposed to the normal developmental and aging processes. The DRE model is constructed with eight levels of impairment for the cervicothoracic, thoracolumbar, and lumbosacral regional units. The accepted differentiators of severity of impairment are objective and specific findings include evidence of vertebral body, transverse process, or posterior element fracture, radiculopathy, instability, or myelopathic changes. Instability, also known as "loss of motion segment integrity," can be assessed on flexion-extension films. Translational instability and angular motion instability criteria are outlined in the guides, but these criteria are not universally accepted. The impairments in the eight categories vary from 0% to 75% of the whole person in the cervicothoracic and lumbosacral regions of the spine, and 0% to 70% of the whole person in the thoracic region.

Adding and Combining Impairments

Impairments within a regional unit, or between regional units can be combined according to the following formula, such that the cumulative impairment never exceeds 100% of the value of the unit or whole person respectively:

$$C = A + B(100 - A)$$

where C is the combined impairment, A is the larger of two values being combined, and B is the smaller of the two values (2). In the special case of the upper extremity, some impairments (of the same type) are added directly (i.e., loss of ROM in multiple digits of the hand), whereas others (of more than one type) are combined (i.e., impairments due to loss of ROM and sensation in the digits). In general, impairments within a functional unit are combined or added at the smallest (distal) subunit, before converting and combining into the next larger (proximal) subunit.

WORK FITNESS AND DISABILITY EVALUATION

Limitations of the American Medical Association's *Guides*

The relationship between impairment ratings and disability determinations remains a source of confusion and debate among physicians (24–30). Problems have included lack of universally accepted rating criteria (18,31–34) and lack of uniformity of application and timing of ratings (24,27,29). The resulting inconsistencies and confusion have been a source of embarassment to physicians (26) and the process has been likened to "educated guesswork" (25). The reliability of commonly accepted anthropometric techniques applicable to impairment rating is questionable (35). For example, conflicting estimates of the reliability of surface inclinometry have been put forward (36,37). The validity of impairment ratings as predictors of ensuing disability remains highly questionable (38), and there is a paucity of empirical data linking medical impairment to real life disability (39). The very process of impairment rating may even contribute to a counter-therapeutic disability conviction in some cases (40).

In its present form, the AMA *Guides* fails to rise substantially above its predecessors and retains many of the shortcomings inherent to the process of impairment rating in general. It is predicated on the conceptual flaw that impairment can be considered an objective medical construct, in contrast to disability which is assessed by "nonmedical means" (41). The interaction between impairment and disability remains complex and poorly understood, and may not be revealed through the conventional approach to physical testing to determine strength, flexibility, or other physical capacities (42). Furthermore, the authority of the AMA *Guides* rests on the subjective opinons of a panel of recognized experts, whose validation is derived by consensus (2) rather than science.

Normally, as has been shown already, medically determined physical impairments and associated disability compensations are derived independently of the impaired individual's capacity to work. An additional critical problem arises when the physician is asked to help determine the percentage by which the "industrial use" of the body is reduced by physical impairment, in cases of compensable injury. Although information concerning the nature and extent of medical impairment is generally believed to be essential to this determination, there is no formula or direct means whereby knowledge of the medical condition can be combined with nonmedical factors (i.e., age, occupation, training, and experience) to predict employability or work-related disability from impairment in a given case (2). *Employability* refers to the individual's capacity to travel to and from work, to be at work, and to carry out assignments and perform physical tasks during the course of the day and in exchange for wages (43). Knowledge concerning medical impairment is not always necessary and certainly not sufficient criterion for determining employability, and the physiatrist making such determinations must be aware of and should also consider criteria and perspectives offered by the ADA.

The Americans with Disabilities Act

The ADA was signed into law on July 26, 1992. Provisions governing employment under the ADA are listed in Title 1 and apply to businesses in the private sector with 25 or more employees. The ADA defines disability as "(A) A physical or mental impairment that substantially limits one or more of the major life activities of the individual; (B) A record of such an impairment; or (C) Being regarded as having such an impairment" (44). This definition is broad and inclusive, and is not dependent on a physician's statement for determination or recognition of disability.

According to the ADA, an employment position can be operationally defined in terms of its *essential functions*—those duties of the position which are fundamental to its existence. Failure of the employee to perform the essential functions of a job would result in termination for cause. The essential functions are typically listed in a *job description*, which should be available from the employer on request. Work disability is relative to the disabled individual's residual physical capacity to perform the essential functions of the position in question with or without *reasonable accommodation*. Accommodation involves modification of the job or workplace in order to enable the disabled employee to better perform the essential functions, and is judged reasonable according to considerations of cost and logistic feasibility to the employer. In cases where reasonable accommodation can be shown to pose *undue hardship* on the employer, or *direct threat* to the health and safety of the disabled individual or immediate coworkers, the ADA requirements are exempted (45).

At present, workers' compensation law and the ADA are separate and parallel systems whose concepts and statutory requirements remain to be integrated. However, the physiatrist can apply these concepts in order to generate ADA-compatible return-to-work determinations, by specifically addressing the essential functions and employer willingness to accommodate in specific cases.

Functional Capacity Evaluation

Functional capacity evaluation (FCE) involves the systematic measurement of a worker's ability to safely and dependably perform job-related tasks (46). It is carried out in a supervised therapeutic setting in which a variety of job-related tasks and material handling can be simulated or duplicated, while adhering to standards of safety, practicality, and reproducibility of results. An FCE can be individualized according to the worker's job description to assess performance ability relative to each specific task demand, or it can be applied more generally to determine the worker's maximum dependable ability according to work categories specified by the U.S. Department of Labor (47) as listed in Table 17-3. Basic components of the FCE are listed in Table 17-4. FCE includes assessment of performance effort and validity. FCE can provide useful, empirically based data to support the physiatrist's decisions regarding return-to-work transition at the appropriate level (48). However, application of FCE is limited in cases where the injured worker self-inhibits and thereby invalidates test results, or in situations where the insurance carrier is reluctant to authorize obtainment of an FCE.

Fitness for Duty

Determination of *fitness for duty* involves assessment of job risk according to essential functions, personal risk to the worker and coworkers in terms of direct threat, and legal risk involved in matching job risk to personal risk (43). Assessment of job risk may include determination of the

Table 17-3: U.S. Department of Labor Categories of Physical Demand

1. Sedentary: lifting ≤10 lb occasionally; sitting 6 out of 8 hr/day
2. Light: lifting ≤20 lb occasionally; ≤10 lb frequently; significant standing/walking, 6 out of 8 hr/day; pushing/pulling, arm/leg controls
3. Medium: lifting ≤50 lb occasionally; ≤20 lb frequently; on feet 6 out of 8 hr/day
4. Heavy: lifting ≤100 lb occasionally; ≤50 lb frequently; standing/walking 6 out of 8 hr/day
5. Very heavy: lifting >100 lb occasionally; >50 lb frequently; standing/walking continuous

Table 17-4: Components of Functional Capacity Evaluation

1. Strength
2. Flexibility
3. Endurance
4. Ability to lift, carry, push/pull
5. Ability to bend, crawl, sit, stand, walk
6. Determination of safety on ladders, steps, and around unprotected heights
7. Frequency of each task
   Occasional: ≤33% of the time
   Frequent: 34–66% of the day
   Constant/frequent: 67%+ of the day

"fit" between the worker and the work environment. Overlap between essential task demands and demonstrated functional capacities can be assessed according to FCE, as noted already. Personal risk assessment may include examination of the individual's previous work experience and vocational potential, as well as the employer's willingness and ability to accommodate. A vocational analyst can be helpful in addressing these issues and concerns. Establishing direct threat is the responsibility of the employer, who must be able to demonstrate a high probability of substantial bodily harm to the impaired individual or coworkers. This demonstration may be based, in part, on objective medical evidence, which the physiatrist is expected to provide. Reasonable accommodation is a process whereby job, personal, and legal risk can potentially be minimized. Under the ADA it is the employer's responsibility to accommodate the impaired but otherwise-qualified individual in order to aid his or her performance of the essential functions of the job, provided that doing so does not create undue hardship. It is not the responsibility of the physiatrist to determine the essential functions of the job, to devise accommodation, or to determine reasonableness of any proposed accommodation.

When making fitness for duty recommendations, the physiatrist can rely on his or her clinical judgment and the FCE. Generally, the physiatrist cannot be found negligent if the worker is reinjured in the workplace unless the physician makes false statements in reports, or recommendations are made recklessly.

INDEPENDENT MEDICAL EXAMINATION AND REPORTING REQUIREMENTS

Scope and Purpose

The *independent medical examination* (IME) is commonly requested by attorneys, insurance adjusters, or case managers for the purpose of assessing treatment and care given to a patient and to determine the need for ongoing or future care. In workers' compensation claims, an IME may be requested to determine if MMI has been achieved, and if it has, to provide an assessment of impairment or disability; determine if temporary or permanent; and to render an opinion as to *causation* and *apportionment.* An administrative law judge adjudicating workers' compensation claims frequently requests an IME for these purposes, and typically does so when resolving a dispute between claimant/plaintiff attorney and the employer/insurance adjustor.

The Physiatrist's Role

IMEs (also known as *third-party examinations*) are performed by physicians not directly involved in the ongoing care of the individual being examined. They are commonly (but not always) part of an adversarial process and, therefore, should be regarded more as a medicolegal examination than a strictly medical assessment. The physiatrist is often forced to adopt a role as "physician detective" or "double agent" and should be comfortable with the ethical and moral implications of this distinction from the traditional physician-patient relationship. Several of the legal implications and nuances of this relationship are discussed in the section Rating Versus Treating Physician.

Because the IME is generally a medicolegal function, careful attention must be paid to the entire process of physician involvement. Office staff involved in scheduling or interacting with IME requesters must recognize and account for the additional time required and allotted to the examination and records review.

A review of available records of diagnostic evaluation and treatment is critical to the IME process. The examining physician may take on the role of detective, especially in highly adversarial situations where records may contain strong clues as to the basis of the dispute. It remains debatable whether the physician examiner should review records (often a time-consuming process) before or after interviewing and examining the patient. Proponents of reviewing prior to examination argue that the information gained will help direct the history and physical examination and therefore, render a more complete and efficient evaluation. Those in favor of reviewing records after seeing the patient argue that the records may inadvertently prejudice the examiner, thus decreasing the objectivity of the examination. Additionally, they argue that there can be a high no-show rate among IME referrals and that previewing such records may be time-consuming and costly. One option is to afford a nurse-clinician (if available) the opportunity to perform a cursory review of records prior to examination and cue the physiatrist to important issues that may not have arisen in the process of the patient interview.

For medicolegal reasons, the physician should make clear to the patient that the evaluation is an IME only, and that the physician will not in any way be assuming care for the patient. This may be important for the litigious patient who claims that the physician became a caregiver and "abandoned" the patient. All patients should be required to sign a disclosure waiver prior to the IME.

Every attempt should be made to minimize adversarial contact during and after the examination. An explanation of the purpose of the visit is helpful and a description of the process may also help put the patient at ease. The patient may prefer to have someone accompany him or her during the examination and this should be allowed whenever possible. Occasionally, an attorney may accompany the patient, but unless a court order requires an attorney's presence, allowing one into the examination room is entirely at the discretion of the physiatrist. In any event, any adult person present other than the patient should be advised that his or her role is strictly to observe, and not to distract or attempt to influence the examiner.

The history and physical examination should be performed in sufficient detail, allowing the patient adequate time to tell the story in his or her own way. This helps create a sense of caring on the part of the physiatrist, who can then go back and efficiently complete elements of the database as needed. Consideration of the patient's concerns such as pain or discomfort, while always important, may need to be verbalized to reinforce the physiatrist's concern for the patient's well-being. The physiatrist should avoid the appearance of being rushed, as this may contribute to a common postexamination complaint that the physician did not spend enough time with the patient or did not perform a thorough examination. The IME, unlike the typical patient-physician interaction, is concluded after the physical examination. In most instances, the referring party will request that the findings not be reviewed directly with the patient.

The IME report will typically address a series of questions similar to those presented earlier for the workers' compensation examiner (see Table 17-1) as part of the examination and report (49).

The IME report, like other medical reports, is a legal document. The potentially adversarial nature of the process dictates the increased likelihood of legal proceedings; consequently, extra care should be taken to ensure a thorough, detailed, and well-organized report of findings. Sources of information should be clear; this is particularly true if the patient's history conflicts with records reviewed. The report may be reviewed by persons with varied, and nonmedical backgrounds (i.e., jurors); consequently, the report should be structured for ease of reading with attention on such details as paragraph length and topic headings. Similarly, the report should be reviewed both for content accuracy and process accuracy such as spelling, syntax, and punctuation. Poor attention to process detail may create the impression that similar poor attention was paid to content details of the history and examination. The laws and regulations governing distribution of third-party examination reports vary from state to state, and may differ from those governing other medical documents.

The IME process raises several issues of concern to the physiatrist. Unlike most patient encounters, under the process of IME the customer and patient are rarely the same. The patient's needs may be prioritized at or below those of the referring agent. Furthermore, the IME process only rarely allows for follow-up, and recommendations made at the time of the original IME may not be implemented—a source of frustration to the physician. The legal system often demands definitive answers to medically complex, and sometimes ambiguous questions. IMEs are more likely to result in depositions or courtroom testimony than are other forms of consultation. The physiatrist contemplating including IMEs into practice should carefully consider these issues and be comfortable with them before undertaking IMEs.

LIFE CARE PLANNING/FUTURE MEDICAL NEEDS

When planning the lifelong care needs and associated costs for an individual who is chronically ill or disabled, a *life care plan* (LCP) may be constructed (50). An LCP estimates what services likely will be needed in the future in order to meet the expected needs of the injured party. The LCP may be either *direct* or *indirect* in nature. A direct plan involves outlining those goods and services needed to optimize medical status, recapture the highest level of function, and compensate for extra needs of day-to-day living as a result of disability. The indirect plan focuses on lost income and lost economic opportunities resulting from a disability.

LCPs are most frequently requested by attorneys and insurance companies, and may be used in cases of civil litigation or workers' compensation to help assess the financial costs of damages incurred in an accident or injury. The planning process will vary according to the specific needs of the requesting party, and may range from a simple description of typical needs and associated costs according to a literature review, to detailed case-specific reporting requirements.

There are no specific training or credentialing requirements for participation in LCPs, and physicians, psychologists, physical and occupational therapists, vocational counselors, and economists may all contribute meaningfully. The physiatrist, by virtue of training and experience in long-term care and the evaluation and treatment of medical impairments and disabilities, is ideally suited to oversee the direct LCP. Vocational specialists may be needed for the indirect LCP. Economists may also be involved for purposes of creating economic models for cost-of-living adjustments and to determine how much money would need to be set aside and invested now to meet the patient's outlined future care needs—a concept known as *reduction for present value.*

When constructing an LCP, the physiatrist first must determine the extent and sequelae of the person's physical and cognitive impairments (Table 17-5). This may require serial observations over the course of evaluating the patient in order to derive increasingly accurate estimates of a person's prognosis for improvement. In children, the

Table 17-5: Steps in the Formation of a Life Care Plan

1. Determine the extent and sequelae of the individual's physical and cognitive impairments
2. Estimate prognosis
3. Estimate the need for and benefit of further medical and rehabilitative interventions
4. Calculate the costs of future personal needs (e.g., wheelchairs, orthopedic equipment, home furnishings and modifications, medical supplies, and recreational equipment)

natural recovery of neurologic impairment is further complicated by ongoing developmental issues such as gross motor skills, fine motor and adaptive skills, personal/social skills, speech and language skills, and cognitive and emotional development. With this knowledge, one can develop a cogent plan to assess the needs and benefits of future medical treatments and rehabilitative interventions (e.g., physical, occupational, and speech therapy).

Often, because of various tort issues, the physiatrist may be asked to calculate the costs of these potential interventions and personal needs. This readily can be performed with a systematic approach outlined in Table 17-6 (51–54). The initial step in formulating these costs is to estimate the life expectancy of the child or adult, which has been a source of considerable debate. This can be readily performed based on review of survival literature in various diagnostic groups such as spinal cord injury (55–57) or cerebral palsy (58).

Second, the physiatrist must estimate the need, duration of need, and costs for a wide variety of hardware items and services. Examples of such devices include wheelchairs, seating systems, orthopedic aids, orthotics and prosthetics, home furnishings, architectural modifications, aids for independent function, drugs, supplies, and leisure time equipment. The patient's future home or facility care costs can similarily be approximated by planning for the appropriate level of care (e.g., home aid, skilled care within the home, or nursing facility). The life care costs must include services rendered by physical, occupational, and speech therapists, and other educational and psychological services if they are not readily available. Finally, the costs of future medical and surgical care, and the costs of potential future medical complications and procedures must be appraised.

Finally, after the total cost of an LCP is calculated in present dollars, a financial adjustment must be made to account for future interest rates and inflation. Such calculations need to account for the increasing costs of health care versus the consumer price index, return on investments, estimations of the present value of goods versus future costs (the discount rate), and taxes on investments. Economic modeling of these items is considered within the purview of an economist and is generally not carried out by the physician.

Table 17-6: Estimating Future Costs in a Life Care Plan

1. Estimate life expectancy
2. Estimate costs of yearly services: evaluations by caregivers, therapy services, hardware needs (e.g., wheelchairs, orthotic and prosthetic devices/equipment, maintenance, aids to independence), home modification and furnishings, architectural changes, drugs and supplies, home or facility care, transportation, leisure time and/or recreational equipment, future medical/surgical care, costs of potential complications
3. Financial adjustments of estimated costs for future interest rates and inflation (generally within the expertise of an economist)

PAIN AND DISABILITY

An in-depth discussion of the evaluation and treatment of acute and chronic pain is beyond the scope of this section and is dealt with in Chapters 57 and 58, respectively, to which the reader is referred. However, the relationship between pain and disability raises issues of added complexity including subjectivity of patient (and disability examiner), validity of presentation, reliability of physical findings, and implications of symptom magnification and self-inhibition due to pain on impairment rating and work disability derived. Consequently, these issues deserve additional attention and discussion at this point.

Definition and Classification

Pain has been defined by the International Association for the Study of Pain as "an unpleasant sensory and emotional experience associated with actual or potential tissue damage, or described in terms of such damage" (59). Alternatively, pain has been described as a "complex experience, embracing physical, mental, social, and behavioral processes, which compromises the quality of life of many individuals" (60).

Pain has been classified according to a "biopsychosocial" model of four categories: acute, recurrent acute (e.g., trigeminal neuralgia), cancer-related, and chronic (benign or nonmalignant). The first three categories of pain tend to be characterized by a tight linkage of pain and suffering to a nociceptive focus, and by a limited tendency, in general, for learned pain behavior to arise from the painful experience. In chronic pain situations, by contrast, the linkage between pain and suffering and an underlying nociceptor is thought to be loose, and most likely does not reflect a state of impending or ongoing tissue damage or injury. Furthermore, there is ample opportunity for learned behavior and social reinforcement to arise out of the painful experience over time.

Psychiatric Diagnoses/Terminology

The *Diagnostic and Statistical Manual of Mental Disorders* (DSM-IV) (61) recognizes at least eight separate diagnoses associated with acute and chronic pain, which are listed and described briefly in Appendix I. The physiatrist should be able to render or obtain an appropriate diagnosis, where applicable, in order to recognize, effectively treat, and hopefully minimize psychological barriers to recovery that may foster or promote disability. Furthermore, such information can assist in the assessment and rendering of an impairment rating in situations where the validity of presentation is suspect.

Personality disorders may also significantly complicate the management, rehabilitation, and rating of chronic pain patients. DSM-IV recognizes that it is often useful to group these axis II diagnoses into clusters A, B, and C. The cluster B group comprises patients of particular challenge in a chronic pain setting. These patients may have traits of antisocial, borderline, histrionic, and narcissistic personality disorders. They may be highly emotional, erratic, demanding, and superficially charming until crossed. One of the hallmarks of this group is their difficulty in maintaining long-term relationships on the job, in marriage, with family, and so on. They may show a lack of empathy ranging from insensitivity to amoral disregard of others, instability, grandiosity, immaturity, and emotional fragility (62,63).

In addition to pain-related diagnoses, there are several psychiatric comorbidities of interest. *Anxiety* is the most common affect in acute pain states and *depression* is the most common in chronic pain conditions (64). Individuals suffering from chronic low-back pain are virtually certain to exhibit one or more psychiatric comorbidities (e.g., major depression, substance abuse, anxiety disorder) (65). In most cases the psychiatric diagnoses were established prior to the onset of back pain. Consequently, psychiatric comorbidities may contribute to the development of physical impairment or disability. Furthermore, they are likely to be disabling in and of themselves, and particularly so in patients with limited inherent coping skills.

It is often debated whether psychiatric conditions such as depression, anxiety, and personality changes precede or follow the chronic painful disability. While the "pain personality" has been variably affirmed and refuted (66), there is now emerging evidence that indeed the psychiatric issues preceded the disability (65,67,68).

Symptom magnification refers to the tendency to exhibit pain behavior or associated disability that is clearly excessive in proportion to any observable underlying pathology (69). It is a feature common to many of the pain-related psychiatric conditions listed in Appendix I. In contrast to malingering, it is likely to be an unconscious phenomenon, and thereby driven by factors other than overt manipulation for secondary gain (70). It is a useful term to describe and document the presence of inconsistencies on physical examination due to overreaction and self-inhibition, as well as the perceptual discrepancies reflected by the observed pain behavior versus the stated pain level in some cases. It does not require physician judgment regarding motivation or intent and is thereby free of pejorative connotations that might otherwise reflect physician bias and subjectivity.

The physiatrist, although lacking formal psychiatric training in most cases, can improve on his or her clinical detection of psychiatric problems during the clinical interview by considering the following questions:

1. Is somatization present? Does the patient have low libido, undiagnosed medical complaints, a spouse with antisocial personality traits, history of alcohol or drug abuse, marital problems, or a history of domestic violence?
2. How hard is the patient working to try to get better? Don't work harder than the patient!
3. Are antisocial traits present? Is there a history of failure in the basic issues in life—marriage, school, job, history of arrests, fights, etc? Are drugs or alcohol a chronic problem?
4. How are you reacting to the patient? If you are internally becoming angry with a patient's behavior, this may be a clue that the patient represents "cluster B" and generates similar angry feelings in others.

Finally, use a screening questionnaire such as the PRIME MD. This simple-to-use intake interview schedule provides a brief and effective method of screening for three very important diagnoses: somatization, depression, and substance abuse. Additionally, it requires little physician time or experience to administer effectively (see Appendix II) (71–73).

Pain and Impairment Rating

Impairment rating for painful conditions becomes problematic when there is no clear objective evidence for end-organ damage or where clinically significant symptom magnification is evident. The experience of pain, even severe and persistent, is thought to be a widespread and common experience (74), and the relationship of pain to impairment and disability remains poorly understood.

The administrative approach to pain and disability determinations varies according to the system involved. The SSA and Veterans' Administration systems recognize pain only insofar as it can be directly related to underlying physical impairment. The workers' compensation approach varies from state to state but is generally designed to compensate those injuries for which physical impairment can be demonstrated in a straightforward fashion. Pain, in the absence of significant physical findings, tends to be similarly discounted. For those systems and jurisdictions where the AMA *Guides* is applicable, the physiatrist may choose to restrict ratings for pain to those conditions where an associated end-organ abnormality or dysfunction is objectively demonstrated. Alternatively, in situations where functional limitations due to pain appear evident, and the presentation appears valid and reproducible, the physiatrist can award additional impairment according to his or her own estimate of severity and degree of functional loss. Some additional suggestions and guidelines that may assist in this estimation are as follows.

For painful conditions affecting organ systems other than the neurologic and musculoskeletal systems (e.g., cardiac, respiratory, gastrointestinal), ratings for functional losses should be rendered according to the categorical descriptors provided and for which objective differentiators between categories are listed. However, within a given category, there may exist a range of permissible impairment according to the physician's estimate of severity, and for which pain severity may be an appropriate differentiator. For example, the AMA *Guides* recognizes impairment of the lower extremities due to peripheral vascular disease and severity of claudication (2). Five classes of severity are listed according to subjective and objective differentiators. Within each class, variations in impairment from 9% to 29% are listed, and it is the purview of the rating physician to weight the final impairment according to his or her subjective estimate of the severity of pain in any given case.

Chronic pain affecting the neurologic and musculoskeletal systems must be stable and must interfere with activities of daily living (ADLs) in order to receive consideration for rating (2). A *4 × 4 pain grid* is a useful descriptive tool to enable the patient to categorize the pain according to frequency (intermittent = <25%; occasional = 25%–50%; frequent = 51%–75%; constant = >75% awake hours) and intensity (minimal, slight, moderate, marked) in terms of interference and effects on ADLs, sleep, socialization, and medication, respectively.

A number of tools are available to assist in determining validity and reliability of presentation. These include the *pain drawing*, which enables the patient to graphically identify his or her perceived location(s) of pain in relation to an anatomic model. Quantified pain drawings correlate mainly with a tendency to somatize and to display pain behavior (75). Patients with widespread pain as noted on the pain drawing have higher levels of disability (76).

The physiatrist should be familiar with the "Waddell signs" in low-back pain (superficial/nonanatomic tenderness, provocation response to sham maneuvers, inconsistencies with distraction, nonanatomic numbness and/or weakness, and overreaction to examiner) (77) and recognize that positive signs are suggestive of symptom magnification. Another useful examination technique is the "forced choice paradigm" (78) for assessing reliability of sensory numbness. For example, during the assessment of hand numbness, if the examiner forces the patient to guess which of two fingers is being touched, he or she should guess correctly about 50% of the time. Patients who self-invalidate will score correctly considerably less than 50% of the time.

A number of formal psychological tests are available to assist in the identification of psychological barriers to recovery that may foster and enhance disability. These include the Minnesota Multiphasic Personality Inventory (MMPI), Cornell Medical Index Health Questionnaire, McGill Pain Questionnaire (79), Beck and Zung Depression indices, Beck Anxiety Scale, and Westhaven-Yale Multidimensional Pain Inventory (WHYMPI) (76). The MMPI has a long history of detection of invalid presentation and malingering through an elevated F scale. The WHYMPI is useful to assess impact of pain on overall functioning and adequacy of coping and adaptive skills.

The assessment of strength and reproducibility of effort has been carried out using the Jamar dynamometer (80–82) and isokinetic ergometers (83). The "coefficient of variation" (COV; defined as the variance divided by the mean) (84) has been used in assessing maximal effort. The COV is considered normal if equal to or less than 10% for males and 12% for females (85); larger values may be indicative of submaximal effort due to pain and self-inhibition. Although the COV may be useful as a research tool to determine sincerity of effort in normal subjects (86), its application to determine compliance during FCEs with symptomatic patients remains suspect (83,87).

Application of the above-mentioned tests and examination techniques may help the physiatrist to effectively identify and document the presence of symptom magnification and physiologic inconsistencies, and to uncover the potential dimensions of psychological dysfunction that may account for such observations. Such information should be appropriately and objectively weighed by the physiatrist without undue penalization of the patient who is guilty of such displays, and without imputing judgment regarding possible malingering or other dimensions of patient malintent. The final impairment rating should reflect these considerations while remaining sensitive to the possibility that pain and suffering may be disabling in the absence of a demonstrable pain generator.

THE PHYSIATRIST AS A DISABILITY WITNESS

Preparing for Deposition and Courtroom Testimony

In situations where the physiatrist is required to provide testimony as either a treating or an independent examining witness, questioning may take place in the form of deposition or courtroom examination. Deposition is an oral examination taken outside the courtroom. Generally, those present include all representing attorneys, a court reporter, and the physician. On occasion, the injured party or the employer representative may likewise be present. Testimony obtained at deposition can be used to impeach (discredit) the witness if he or she testifies differently at the time of trial. Often, in cases of compensible injury, the deposition takes the place of the physician's live appearance at trial.

Objections entered at the time of deposition are not ruled on at that time because a judge is not present. In most cases the physician will answer the question even though objections are made. If the physician testifies at a trial before a court, the additional party will be the judge trying the case. In that case, once objections are entered, the judge will rule before the physician responds.

In preparing for deposition or courtroom testimony, it may be important for the physiatrist to meet with the attorney presenting the physician's testimony to discuss the procedure as well as the questions to be asked, especially hypotheticals or opinions dealing with causation or extent of disability. The attorney will often elicit the foundation testimony such as the physiatrist's teaching, training, and experience. Once that is obtained, the questions then turn to the examination including details of the history provided, the physical examination, and the ultimate conclusions derived. Either by way of hypothetical or direct questioning, the attorney proffering the physiatrist's testimony will then ask for opinions about causation, presence, and extent of disability.

Whether the physiatrist testifies live or by deposition, the physiatrist should remember that he or she is offering his or her best medical opinion as to the questions asked. Most states require that opinion testimony be given with a qualification that it be based on the physician's teaching, training, and experience and with reasonable medical certainty or probability.

Providing Expert Witness Testimony

The physiatrist's role in disability evaluations generally results in classification as an *expert witness*. By that, the physician has more expertise in the medical field than the judge or attorney, and the testimony aids the court in determining various legal issues such as causation and extent of disability. In most cases the opposing sides will each have an expert witness. The judge determines the facts and ultimate outcome based on, among other factors, the credibility given to the various expert witnesses. Factors such as impartiality, reputation, teaching, training and experience, details of examination findings, and explanation of those findings will be considered by the judge in deciding which witness is more credible.

Often, a physiatrist will testify in different cases for an injured employee or for an employer. This can show impartiality but can also create problems for the testifying physician. For example, a contrary position registered by the physiatrist in a prior case can be used to impeach or discredit subsequent testimony by that physician. Such information, if shared with the attorney in a predeposition or pretrial conference, may proactively assist the attorney in dealing with potential inconsistencies and embarrassment.

The attorney and physician must tailor the testimony so as to educate the judge. It is important that when technical medical terms are used, the attorney elicit and the physician provide an explanation in a way that is understandable to a judge or jury, and convert medical terminology into nonmedical language.

Often in the litigation process, especially in testimony, a physician is asked whether he or she is being paid for testimony provided. Obviously, the physician will bill for services; however, the physiatrist should remember that he or she not being paid for the opinion, but for the time spent in evaluating and providing the opinion.

Rating Versus Treating Physician

In the testifying process the physiatrist should clarify his or her role (85). This should be elicited by the questioning attorney. If the physiatrist is the treating physician, there is a physician-patient relationship. Under that scenario, the physician owes a duty of care to the patient and to protect confidentiality. Even if the physician is selected by the employer, as authorized in approximately half of the states, the physician still owes a duty of confidentiality and maintains a physician-patient relationship to the injured employee. At the outset, the treating physiatrist should obtain a signed release of medical information from the injured employee to the employer by way of office notes, reports, and personal consultations with the employer or the employer's representatives.

If the physiatrist is serving as an independent medical examiner, there is some question as to that physician's actual role. That physician is an expert witness for the party retaining him or her for the purpose of providing expertise in a given instance. At the outset, the physiatrist must clarify his or her role with the injured employee and inform the employee that there is no physician-patient relationship, since the physiatrist is not the treating physician. The patient needs to be so informed, and it is recommended that the physiatrist obtain a signed document from the injured party acknowledging this disclaimer and limited relationship.

Notwithstanding the limited role of an independent medical examiner, if a condition is discovered that poses an adverse consequence or increased risk to the injured party, the physiatrist should notify at least the engaging party and injured party of that condition. Furthermore, whether or not the condition is related specifically to the illness or injury in question, the physiatrist should recommend that the patient seek independent medical consultation from a personal physician for that condition. For example, during the course of examination for a routine back injury, the physiatrist might discover the presence of a neoplasm (e.g., myeloma) not directly related to the history of back injury. In that case the physiatrist should call the presence of the neoplasm to the attention of the party engaging the physician's services, and recommend that the information be shared with all interested parties, or alternatively, that the physician be allowed to inform the injured party directly of the condition. The physiatrist might also opt to render a separate and limited report to all interested parties detailing incidental findings that might warrant further independent investigation.

APPENDIX I. PSYCHIATRIC DIAGNOSES ASSOCIATED WITH CHRONIC PAIN AND DISABILITY

Somatization disorder (DSM 300.81)—also known as Briquet syndrome. This syndrome is characterized by a history of multiple physical complaints beginning before age 30, persisting over several years, and resulting in treatment sought and significant disability in social, occupational, and/or other important areas of functioning. The criteria to be met include four pain symptoms from different sites or functions, two gastrointestinal symptoms other than pain, one sexual symptom of dysfunction other than pain, and one pseudoneurologic symptom other than pain. In addition, after appropriate investigation, each of the symptoms cannot be fully explained and the associated complaints and disability are out of proportion to what is expected on the basis of any objective findings. The symptoms are not intentionally produced or feigned (as in factitious disorder or malingering).

Undifferentiated somatoform disorder (DSM 300.81)—a condition characterized by one or more physical complaints (e.g., fatigue, loss of appetite, gastrointestinal complaints) that either lack a full and satisfactory explanation after appropriate investigation, or produce complaints and disability out of proportion to what is expected on the basis of objective findings. In addition, symptoms must persist at least 6 months; are significantly disabling in social, occupational, and/or other important areas of functioning; are not satisfactorily accounted for by another mental disorder; and are not intentionally produced or feigned.

Conversion disorder (DSM 300.11)—a condition characterized by one or more symptoms affecting voluntary motor or sensory function suggestive of a neurologic or other medical condition, where psychological factors are implicated because conflict or other stressors precede the onset or exacerbation of symptoms. Furthermore, the symptoms are not intentionally produced or feigned; they cannot be fully explained after appropriate investigation; they result in significant disability in social, occupational, and/or other important areas of functioning; and they are not better accounted for by another mental disorder.

Pain disorder (DSM 307.80)—pain at one or more anatomic sites being the predominant clinical presentation, with associated distress which produces significant disability in social, occupational, and/or other important areas of functioning. Furthermore, psychological factors are judged to have an important contributory role in the onset, severity, exacerbation, or maintenance of the pain. Symptoms are not intentionally produced or feigned, and are not better accounted for by a mood, anxiety, or psychotic disorder and do not meet the criteria for dyspareunia.

Hypochondriasis (DSM 300.7)—a preoccupation with fears of having a serious disease based on the individual's misinterpretation of bodily symptoms, which persists despite appropriate medical evaluation and reassurance. The belief is not of delusional intensity (as in delusional disorder, somatic type) and is not restricted to a circumscribed concern about appearance (as in body dysmorphic disorder). The preoccupation persists for at least 6 months; is significantly disabling in social, occupational, or other important areas of functioning; and is not better accounted for by generalized anxiety disorder, obsessive-compulsive disorder, panic disorder, a major depressive episode, separation anxiety, or other somatoform disorder.

Factitious disorder (DSM 300.19)—intentional production or feigning of physical or psychological signs or symptoms. The motivation for pain behavior is to assume the sick role where obvious external incentives (e.g., economic or other secondary gain) are not evident. Clues to the presence of fictitious disorder include proven exaggeration of symptoms by the patient; invariable relapse following improvement; worsening of findings by self-manipulation; an exceptional willingness to undergo invasive procedures; patient forecasts exacerbations; patient resists communication efforts with prior physicians and caregivers; patient strongly resists psychiatric consultation; patient or family member works in a health-related field; and patient exhibits poor continuity of care or has been treated in multiple medical settings (64).

Malingering (V65.2)—the essential feature being the intentional production of false or grossly exaggerated physical or psychological symptoms, motivated by external incentives and secondary gain. Malingering may be suspected if any combination of the following is noted: medicolegal context of presentation, marked discrepancy between claimed distress and disability and objective findings, lack of cooperation during diagnostic evaluation and poor compliance with prescribed treatment regimen, and presence of antisocial personality disorder.

Substance dependence and abuse—a maladaptive pattern of substance use leading to clinically significant impairment or distress manifested by three or more of the following criteria occurring within a 12-month interval:

Tolerance, as defined by the need for markedly increased amounts of the substance to achieve the desired effect or else a markedly diminished effect seen with continued use of a given amount of substance.

Withdrawal, as manifested by either the characteristic withdrawal syndrome or the same (or closely related) substance being taken to relieve or avoid withdrawal symptoms

Taking the substance in larger amounts over a longer period than was intended

Persistent desire for substance use

Significant time spent in activity necessary to obtain the substance

Reduction in other important social, occupational, or recreational activities

Continuation of substance use despite educational efforts regarding adverse consequences of substance use

Substance abuse is manifested by recurrent substance use resulting in a failure to fulfill major role obligations at work, school, or home; use in physically hazardous situations; recurrent substance-related legal problems; and continued use despite having persistent or recurrent social or interpersonal problems caused or exacerbated by the effects of the substance.

APPENDIX II: PRIME-MD: PRIMARY CARE EVALUATION OF MENTAL DISORDERS

- During the *past month* have you *often* been bothered by:

		Yes	No
1.	Stomach pain	☐	☐
2.	Back pain	☐	☐
3.	Pain in your arms, legs, or joints (knees, hips, etc.)	☐	☐
4.	Menstrual pain or problems	☐	☐
5.	Pain or problems during sexual intercourse	☐	☐
6.	Headaches	☐	☐
7.	Chest pain	☐	☐
8.	Dizziness	☐	☐
9.	Fainting spells	☐	☐
10.	Feeling your heart pound or race	☐	☐
11.	Shortness of breath	☐	☐
12.	Constipation, loose bowels, or diarrhea	☐	☐
13.	Nausea, gas, or indigestion	☐	☐
14.	Feeling tired or having low energy	☐	☐
15.	Trouble sleeping	☐	☐
16.	Your eating being out of control	☐	☐
17.	Little interest or pleasure in doing things	☐	☐
18.	Feeling down, depressed, or hopeless	☐	☐
19.	"Nerves" or feeling anxious or on edge	☐	☐
20	Worrying about a lot of different things	☐	☐

- During the *past month*:
  21. Have you had an anxiety attack (suddenly feeling fear or panic)? ☐ Yes ☐ No
  22. Have you thought you should cut down on your drinking of alcohol? ☐ Yes ☐ No
  23. Has anyone complained about your drinking? ☐ Yes ☐ No
  24. Have you felt guilty or upset about your drinking? ☐ Yes ☐ No
  25. Was there ever a single day in which you had 5 or more drinks of beer, wine, or liquor? ☐ Yes ☐ No
- Overall, would you say your health is:
  ☐ Excellent ☐ Very Good ☐Good ☐ Fair ☐ Poor

REFERENCES

1. Disability evaluation. American Academy of Physical Medicine and Rehabilitation Certificate Program. Chicago: American Academy of Physical Medicine and Rehabilitation, 1996.
2. American Medical Association. *Guides to the evaluation of permanent impairment.* 4th ed. Milwaukee: American Medical Association, 1993.
3. Ranavaya MI. Impairment, disability and compensation in the United States. An overview. *Disability* 1996;5:1–20.
4. Elisburg D. Workers' compensation. In: Demeter SL, Andersson GB, Smith GM, eds. *Disability evaluation.* St. Louis: Mosby, 1996:36–44.
5. Kemp JD, Pope MH. Workers' compensation. In: Pope MH, Andersson GB, Frymoyer JW, et al., eds. *Occupational low back pain: assessment, treatment, and prevention.* St. Louis: Mosby-Year Book, 1991:296–304.
6. Steinberg FM. Workers' compensation—legal issues. In: Kasdan ML, ed. *Occupational hand & upper extremity injuries & diseases.* Philadelphia: Hanley & Belfus, 1991:515–525.
7. Kansas statute 44KSA510. Kansas Statutes Annotated compiled and edited by Office of Reviser of Statutes of Kansas Norman J. Furse, Reviser, under authority of KSA 77-151. Printed and bound by Division of Printing, Department of Administration, Division of Labor and Industries, Topeka, Kansas.
8. Revised Missouri statute 287 R.S.Mo. 1993 Vernon's Annotated Missouri Statutes sections 285–287, Labor and Industrial Relations, Vol. 15, West Publishing Company, St. Paul, Minnesota.
9. Revised Missouri statute 287.240 R.S.Mo. 1993 Vernon's Annotated Missouri Statutes sections 285–287, Labor and Industrial Relations, Vol. 15, West Publishing Company, St. Paul, Minnesota.
10. Kansas statute 44KSA510C. Kansas Statutes Annotated compiled and edited by Office of Reviser of Statutes of Kansas Norman J. Furse, Reviser, under authority of KSA 77-151. Printed and bound by Division of Printing, Department of Administration, Division of Labor and Industries, Topeka, Kansas.
11. Revised Missouri statute 287.190 R.S.Mo. 1993 Vernon's Annotated Missouri Statutes sections 285–287, Labor and Industrial Relations, Vol. 15, West Publishing Company, St. Paul, Minnesota.

12. Kansas statute 44KSA510D. Kansas Statutes Annotated compiled and edited by Office of Reviser of Statutes of Kansas Norman J. Furse, Reviser, under authority of KSA 77-151. Printed and bound by Division of Printing, Department of Administration, Division of Labor and Industries, Topeka, Kansas.

13. Kansas statute 44KSA510Y. Kansas Statutes Annotated compiled and edited by Office of Reviser of Statutes of Kansas Norman J. Furse, Reviser, under authority of KSA 77-151. Printed and bound by Division of Printing, Department of Administration, Division of Labor and Industries, Topeka, Kansas.

14. Croft C. Something more important than money-vocational rehabilitation in workers' compensation cases. *Alaska Law Rev* 1986;3(1):49–124.

15. Bonner WF, Guest DM, Barlow RA, et al. Acute industrial rehabilitation. *Phys Med Rehabil Clin North Am* 1992;3:513–530.

16. Kansas statute 44KSA566. Kansas Statutes Annotated compiled and edited by Office of Reviser of Statutes of Kansas Norman J. Furse, Reviser, under authority of KSA 77-151. Printed and bound by Division of Printing, Department of Administration, Division of Labor and Industries, Topeka, Kansas.

17. Revised Missouri statute 287.220 R.S.Mo. 1993 Vernon's Annotated Missouri Statutes sections 285–287, Labor and Industrial Relations, Vol. 15, West Publishing Company, St. Paul, Minnesota.

18. McBride ED. *Disability evaluation and principles of treatment of compensible injuries.* 6th ed. Philadelphia: JB Lippincott, 1963.

19. *Disability evaluation under Social Security.* Washington, DC: U.S. Dept. of Health and Human Services. Social Security Administration, September 1994. SSA publication no. 64-039, ICN No. 468600.

20. Federal Employers' Liability Act. Issues associated with changing how railroad work-related injuries are compensated. Gaithersburg, MD: U.S. General Accounting Office, August 1996. GAO/RCED-96-199.

21. Veterans Benefits Administration Department of Veterans Affairs. *Book B—Adjudication.* CFR 38:3. Austin, TX: Jonathan Publishing, 1991.

22. Veterans Benefits Administration Department of Veterans Affairs. *Book C—Schedule for Rating Disabilities.* CFR 38:4. Austin, TX: Jonathan Publishing, 1992.

23. *Employee benefits in small private establishments.* Washington, DC: U.S. Department of Labor, 1994:20–34.

24. Brand RA, Lehmann TR. Low-back impairment rating practices of orthopedic surgeons. *Spine* 1983;8:75–78.

25. Burd JG. The educated guess: doctors and permanent partial disability percentage. *J Tenn Med Assoc* 1980;73:441.

26. Carey TS, Hadler NM. The role of the primary physician in disability determination for Social Security Insurance and Workers' Compensation. *Ann Intern Med* 1986;104:706–710.

27. Clark WL, Haldeman S, Johnson P, et al. Back impairment and disability determination. Another attempt at objective, reliable rating. *Spine* 1988;13:332–341.

28. Clark WL, Haldeman S. The development of guideline factors for the evaluation of disability in neck and back injuries. *Spine* 1993;18:1736–1745.

29. Greenwood JG. Low-back impairment-rating practices of orthopaedic surgeons and neurosurgeons in West Virginia. *Spine* 1985;10:773–776.

30. Luck J, Florence D. A brief history and comparative analysis of disability systems and impairment rating guides. *Orthop Clin North Am* 1988;19:839–844.

31. American Academy of Orthopedic Surgeons. *Manual for orthopedic surgeons in evaluating permanent physical impairment.* Chicago: American Academy of Orthopedic Surgeons, 1975.

32. Kessler HH. *Disability determination and evaluation.* Philadelphia: Lea & Febiger, 1970.

33. Rice CO. *Calculation of industrial disability of the extremities and the back.* 2nd edition. Springfield, IL: Charles C Thomas, 1968.

34. Smith WC. *Principles of disability evaluation.* Philadelphia: JB Lippincott, 1959.

35. Bennett KA, Osborne RH. Interobserver measurement reliability in anthropometry. *Hum Biol* 1986;58:751–759.

36. Keely J, Mayer T, Cox R, et al. Quantification of lumbar function. Part 5. Reliability of range of motion measures in the sagittal plane and an in vivo torso rotation measurement technique. *Spine* 1986;11:31–35.

37. Rondinelli R, Murphy J, Esler A, et al. Estimation of normal lumbar flexion with surface inclinometry: a comparison of three methods. *Am J Phys Med Rehabil* 1992;71:219–224.

38. Rondinelli R, Dunn W, Hassanein KM, et al. A simulation of hand impairments: effects on upper extremity function and implications towards medical impairment rating and disability determinations. *Arch Phys Med Rehabil* 1997;78:1358–1363.

39. Gloss DS, Wardle MG. Reliability and validity of American Medical Association's guide to ratings of permanent impairment. *JAMA* 1982;248:2292–2296.

40. Hadler NM. If you have to prove you are ill, you can't get well. The object lesson of fibromyalgia. *Spine* 1996;21:2397–2400.

41. Pryor ES. Flawed promises: a critical evaluation of the American Medical Association Guides to the Evaluation of Permanent Impairment. *Harv Law Rev* 1990;103:964–976.

42. Stieg RL. The futility of physical testing in the assessment of disability. *Am Pain Soc J* 1994;3(3):187–190.

43. Johns RE Jr, Elegante JM, Teynor PD, et al. Fitness for duty. In: Demeter SL, Andersson GB, Smith GM, eds. *Disability evaluation.* St. Louis: Mosby, 1996;592–604.

44. Americans with Disabilities Act. Part III. Department of Justice. 28 CFR Part 36 Nondiscrimination on the Basis of Disability by Public Accommodations and in Commercial Facilities; Final Rule. *Federal Register* 1991;56(144): 35548.

45. Bell C. Overview of the Americans with Disabilities Act and the Family and Medical Leave Act. In: Demeter SL, Andersson GB, Smith GM, eds. *Disability evaluation.* St. Louis: Mosby, 1996:582–591.

46. Matheson LN. Functional capacity evaluation. In: Demeter SL, Andersson GB, Smith GM, eds. *Disability evaluation.* St. Louis: Mosby, 1996:168–188.

47. Appendix A. Physical demands. In: *Dictionary of Occupational Titles.* Washington, DC: U.S. Department of Labor, Employment and Training Administration, 1981:465–466.

48. Scheer SJ, Wickstrom RJ. Vocational capacity with low back pain impairment. In: Scheer SJ, ed. *Medical perspectives in vocational assessment of impaired workers.* Gaithersburg, MD: Aspen, 1991:19–63.

49. Scheer SJ. The role of the physician in disability management: In: Shrey DE, Lacerte M, eds. *Principles and practices of disability management in industry.* Winter Park, FL: GR Press, 1995:175–205.

50. Deutsch PM, Weed OR, Kitchen JA, Sluis A. *Life care planning for the spinal cord injured: a step-by-step guide.* Orland: PMD Press, 1989.

51. Bush GW. Calculating the cost of long-term living: a four-step process. *J Head Trauma Rehabil* 1990;5:47–56.

52. Deutsch PM. Discharge planning: structuring the home environment. In: Deutsch PM, Fralish KB. eds. *Innovations in head injury rehabilitation.* New York: Matthew Bender, 1989.

53. Dussault W. How to keep setttlement funds and maintain government benefits. In: *The head injury case: what the trial lawyer needs to know.* Southborough, MA: National Head Injury Foundation, 1989:688–726.

54. Zasler CP. Primer for the rehabilitation professional on the life care planning process. *Neuro Rehabil* 1996;7:79–93.

55. DeVivo MJ. Life expectancy and causes of death for persons with spinal cord injury. In: Apple DF, Hudson LA, eds. *Spinal cord injury: the model.* Atlanta: Fenley Communications, 1990:66–71.

56. DeVivo MJ, Stover SL. Long-term survival and causes of death. In: Stover DL, DeLisa JA, Whiteneck GG, eds. *Spinal cord injury: clinical outcomes from the model systems.* Gaithersburg, MD: Aspen, 1995:289–316.

57. Kennedy EJ. *Spinal cord injury: the facts and figures.* Birmingham: University of Alabama Press, 1986:57–60.

58. Katz RT. Life care planning for the child with cerebral palsy. *J Missouri Bar Assoc* 1996;52:365–372.

59. Merskey H, Bogduk N, eds. Classification of chronic pain: description of chronic pain syndrome and definitions of pain terms. 2nd ed. Seattle: IASP Press, 1994:210.

60. U.S. Department of Health and Human Services. *Report of the Commission on the Evaluation of Pain.* Washington, DC: Social Security Administration Office of Disability, 1987. Publication no. 64-031.

61. American Psychiatric Association. *Diagnostic and statistical manual of mental disorders.* 4th ed. Washington, DC: American Psychiatric Association, 1994.

62. DeLong K, Smith G, Grange J. Does that "difficult" patient have a personality disorder? *Emerg Med* 1996;28:75–96.

63. Oldham J. Personality disorders: current perspectives. *JAMA* 1994;272:1770–1776.

64. Eisendrath SJ. Psychiatric aspects of chronic pain. *Neurology* 1995;45(suppl 9):S26–S34.

65. Polatin PB, Kinney RK, Gatchel RJ, et al. Psychiatric illness and chronic low back pain. *Spine* 1993;18:66–71.

66. Gamsa A. Role of psychological factors in chronic pain. *Pain* 1994;57:5–29.

67. Mannion AF, Dolan P, Adams MA. Psychological questionnaires: do "abnormal" scores precede or follow first-time low back pain? *Spine* 1996;21:2603–2611.

68. Hazard RG, Haugh LD, Reid S, et al. Early prediction of chronic disability after occupational low back injury. *Spine* 1996;21: 945–951.

69. Matheson LN. Symptom magnification syndrome structured interview: rationale and procedure. *J Occup Rehabil* 1991;1:43–56.

70. Voiss DV. Occupational injury: fact, fantasy or fraud? *Neurol Clin* 1995;13:431–446.

71. Glass RM. Mental disorders: quality of life and inequality of insurance coverage. *JAMA* 1995;274:1557. Editorial.

72. Spitzer RL, Williams JB, Kroenke K, et al. Utility of a new procedure for diagnosing mental disorders in primary care: PRIME-MD 1000 study. *JAMA* 1994;272: 1749–1756.

73. Spitzer RL, Kroenke K, Linzer M, et al. Health-related quality of life in primary care patients with mental disorders: results from the PRIME-MD 1000 study. *JAMA* 1995;274:1511–1517.

74. Ford CV. Dimensions of somatization and hypochondriasis. *Neurol Clin* 1995;13:241–253.

75. Ohlund C, Eek C, Palmblad S, et al. Quantified pain drawing in subacute low back pain. *Spine* 1996;21:1021–1031.

76. Tait RC. Psychological factors in the assessment of disability among patients with chronic pain. *J Back Musculoskel Rehabil* 1993;3:20–47.

77. Waddell G, McCulloch JA, Kummel E, Venner RM. Nonorganic physical signs in low back pain. *Spine* 1980;5:117–125.

78. Binder LM. Forced-choice testing provides evidence of malingering. *Arch Phys Med Rehabil* 1992;73:377–380.

79. Melzack R. Short form McGill Pain Questionnaire. *Pain* 1987;30:191–197.

80. Stokes HM. The seriously uninjured hand-weakness of grip. *J Occup Med* 1983;25:683–684.

81. Smith GA, Nelson RC, Sadoff SJ, Sadoff AM. Assessing sincerity of effort in maximal grip strength tests. *Am J Phys Med Rehabil* 1989;68:73–80.

82. Chengalur SN, Smith GA, Nelson RC, Sadoff AM. Assessing sincerity of effort in maximal grip strength tests. *Am J Phys Med Rehabil* 1990;69:148–153.

83. Simonsen JC. Coefficient of variation as a measure of subject effort. *Arch Phys Med Rehabil* 1995;76:516–520.

84. Matheson LN. How do you know that he tried his best? The reliability crisis in industrial rehabilitation. *Indust Rehabil Q* 1988;1(1):11–17.

85. King JW, Berryhill BH. Assessing maximum effort in upper-extremity functional testing. *Work* 1991;1(3):65–76.

86. Hazard RG, Reid S, Fenwick J, Reeves V. Isokinetic trunk and lifting strength measurements: variability as an indicator of effort. *Spine* 1988;13:54–57.

87. Newton M, Waddell G. Trunk strength testing with iso-machines. Part 1. Review of a decade of scientific evidence. *Spine* 1993;18:801–811.

88. Sullivan MD, Loeser JD. The diagnosis of disability. Treating and rating disability in a pain clinic. *Arch Intern Med* 1992;152:1829–1835.

Chapter 18

Vocational Assessment: Translating Functional Recovery into Real-World Possibilities

Mary Ellen Young

THE QUESTION OF EMPLOYABILITY

A man with a spinal cord injury who has done heavy labor all his life will most likely not be able to return to his previous employment activities. A young adult with cerebral palsy facing high school graduation ponders her career and vocational choices. Each has a basic question, "Will I be able to work?" and "If so, doing what?" The answer to the question of employability depends on knowing and understanding each person as a whole being—including medical status, educational level, vocational skills and aptitudes, interests, work history, and work habits—as well as knowing about his or her environment—urban or rural geographic area, local job market, access to transportation, educational and work site accessibility, and family and cultural supports. Successful employment is achieved by a careful matching of the person with the environment, the attributes of the individual with the demands of the workplace.

The Meaning of Work

Understanding disability in our society requires understanding the value placed on both paid employment and unpaid productive activity. The ability to fulfill the social role of a productive person is a central element of our familial, educational, political, and cultural milieu. Using definitions from the World Health Organization, for someone whose "impairment" (psychological, physiologic, or anatomic loss or abnormality) leads to "disability" (restriction of ability to perform an activity), the result may be a "handicap" (that which limits or prevents fulfillment of a role that would be considered normal for that person) (1). For many adults with disabilities, this handicap is defined by a loss of a significant social role in our culture, that of worker.

Productivity Versus Employment

Much emphasis in America is put on paid employment, but the concept of productivity provides a broader view. *Work* may be defined as activity that is of benefit to others and may be paid or unpaid (2). *Productivity* may be defined as being engaged in an activity that is of benefit to others and may encompass paid employment, educational activities, homemaking and child care activities, and volunteer work. Obtaining and maintaining paid employment has been the standard by which vocational rehabilitation efforts have been judged, but recent efforts have been made to recognize and acknowledge the contribution of other productive activities (3).

Who Decides?

The determination of *employability* requires the gathering of data from a number of sources—medical service providers, educators, former employers, family members, and most especially, the individual with a disability. Each of these resources contributes to the understanding of the individual's employment potential, but none can make the decision for the individual as to whether he or she wants to pursue employment. This decision rests ultimately with the individual (4).

The second party to the "Who decides?" question, however, is the employer who is making the employment decision. Employers have the power to make positive or negative employment decisions when faced with an applicant with a disability. Employers also make job retention decisions (5). As a result of the open employment market in the United States, employers have tremendous power to make decisions affecting the lives of persons with disabilities. As we near the end of the twentieth century, we are participating in a revolution in the way people with disabilities are perceived as workers—a revolution prompted by legislation such as the Americans with Disabilities Act (ADA) and by the disability rights movement. The continual education of employers as to the *abilities* of persons with disabilities, and the legal prohibition on discrimination based on disability alone are essential factors in increasing their employment opportunities.

Employability Criteria

What else makes one person employable and another not? The ADA provides some legal language that helps us understand the concept of employability—a person must be able to perform the essential functions of the job; that is, the person must be able to do the key components of any given position, with or without job modifications or assistive technology. Employers are not required to hire persons with disabilities who cannot do the job. Likewise, persons with disabilities have to meet the educational and experience requirements of the job. Within these parameters, employers cannot discriminate against persons with disabilities in their hiring practices. The Equal Employment Opportunities Commission is charged with reviewing ADA employment complaints and resolving the situations or recommending legal actions. Beyond the legal requirements faced by potential employers, other elements of employability include the employee's work behaviors and attitudes that are critical to job retention. A person with a disability must be able to get to work on time, be regular in attendance, get along with coworkers, and respond appropriately to supervision. A person with a disability must also have the endurance to tolerate full or partial workdays.

Vocational Assessment

A comprehensive vocational assessment examines not only the person's ability to do the job, but also his or her global work behaviors and tolerances. The terms *vocational assessment* and *vocational evaluation* are used to describe the process of determining the employability of a person with a disability. Vocational evaluation is sometimes seen as a more formal testing process. In this chapter, the term *vocational assessment* is used to describe the comprehensive process of determining the employment potential of a person with a disability, including formalized testing. Vocational assessment is usually a time-limited, discrete process that is a part of the vocational rehabilitation process.

PURPOSE OF VOCATIONAL ASSESSMENT

Power (6) defined vocational assessment as "a comprehensive, intradisciplinary process of evaluating an individual's physical, mental, and emotional abilities, limitations, and tolerance in order to identify an optimal outcome." Thus, the primary purpose of a vocational assessment is to answer the basic question of employability, along with providing information to answer the "Doing what?" question. Other reasons for the assessment often dictate what is done in the assessment and how the assessment data are interpreted.

Disability Determination

Vocational assessments may be conducted for the purpose of determining whether the individual has a vocational handicap. This type of assessment is likely to focus on the individual's impairment and functional limitations and how those limitations negatively impact the capacity to enter or return to the workforce. Often this type of assessment is concerned with meeting eligibility criteria for certain programs, such as in applications for Social Security disability determinations, vocational rehabilitation eligibility, workers' compensation, or long-term disability (7). Sometimes a vocational assessment is requested in personal injury litigation as the financial impact of the individual's vocational loss is to be determined (8).

Educational and Vocational Planning

Another purpose of a vocational assessment is for educational and vocational planning. This type of assessment is more likely to focus on identifying the individual's strengths and developing strategies for overcoming and accommodating a person's limitations. Such an assessment is crucial for planning an individualized vocational rehabilitation program. One critical factor is understanding the individual's career maturity and career development (9). Vocational counseling for someone who has never held a job is different from that for someone with a work history.

Referral Questions and Background Information

The vocational evaluator needs to know the purpose of the assessment, to have an idea of the specific questions from the client or the referral source to be answered by the assessment, and to have as much background information on the medical condition, functional limitations, and recovery prognosis as possible. Assessment for disability determination may be at odds with assessment for educational or vocational planning, since one focuses on limitations and problems and the other on strengths and compensatory strategies. Most assessments combine elements of both types, but it is critical that the written report reflects the information needed to respond to the referral questions.

TIMING OF VOCATIONAL ASSESSMENT

The optimal timing of vocational services has been a point of debate in rehabilitation literature and practice (10,11). Some have advocated early intervention, with vocational counseling beginning shortly after illness or injury (11,12). This approach has the advantage of addressing vocational questions early in the recovery process and planning therapies and services that will promote return to work options. Others have advocated waiting until maximum medical improvement has been achieved, which would provide a clearer picture of the individual's vocational limitations (10). There does appear to be a consensus that many people have "fallen through the cracks" in the system over the years, not using vocational services until years after the onset of their disability. Vocational rehabilitation efforts that begin years after recovery from injury or illness often are hindered by significant disincentives such as financial benefits or family needs.

Vocational Readiness

While cogent arguments can be made for both early and later referral for rehabilitation services, the consensus seems to be that there is a point of optimal timing for vocational intervention for each individual. Clinicians speak of the concept of *vocational readiness*. This can be defined as the time at which persons with disabilities express concern over the vocational future, begin asking questions about how the illness or injury will affect their career choices, or initiate some work or educational activities. It is at this point of readiness, which may vary from client to client, that a plan for vocational assessment and vocational services needs to be laid out. Some efforts have been made to further define and quantify readiness in order to make more appropriate referrals for vocational assessment (13).

Career and Life Planning

While adults who acquire disabilities may face their vocational rehabilitation with a background of a significant work history, many who are born with their disabilities or acquire them as children or young adults have never entered the workforce, made a vocational decision, looked for a job, or completed training for a career. The challenge in dealing with young people with disabilities entering the workforce for the first time is to recognize the developmental aspects of career decision making and to engage in life planning as well as rehabilitation planning. Facilitating a smooth transition from school to work is crucial to young adults with disabilities (14). A timely vocational assessment is one key to a successful transition.

VOCATIONAL ASSESSMENT TECHNIQUES

Vocational assessment has roots in the industrial revolution and the application of psychological measurement to the aptitudes and skills of job applicants. To increase worker productivity, testing tools and techniques were developed in the early twentieth century to help predict which applicants would perform best at which jobs (15). Such testing was used during World War I and World War II, when masses of servicemen were tested before being assigned to various military jobs. After World War II, as large numbers of returning veterans were provided assistance in obtaining employment, data gathered through vocational testing were then applied to the civilian workforce (6,16). World War II was also the first time when large numbers of injured veterans were provided vocational rehabilitation services, so the testing techniques developed for military and civilian employment were adapted for determining the skills of workers with disabilities (17).

Different approaches may be used, either alone or in combination, during a vocational assessment (17). The first assessment approach used was the psychological testing approach, in which the job-related tests used for matching military and civilian workers with jobs were used to test workers with disabilities. Other approaches that have proved useful have included work samples, situational assessments, and job trials (18), as well as physical capacity and work tolerance evaluations (8).

Psychological Testing Approach

The psychological testing approach makes an assumption that there are underlying factors that are common to many jobs, such as finger and manual dexterity, perceptual abilities, general intelligence, or verbal and numerical skills. If one identifies the job factors, identifies the level of each factor required by each job, and measures those same factors or worker traits in the individual, it is assumed that one can then match the worker to the job with some precision. There are numerous tests and test batteries that measure individual factors related to the world of work, including interest, achievement, aptitude, and personality tests (15). These tests are usually norm referenced to the general population or to workers in a particular job. Many of these tests have proved useful in assessing persons with disabilities and matching their skills, abilities, and interests with job requirements (6).

Situational Assessment Approach

The problem with the psychological testing approach is that it gives the vocational counselor very little information about how the individual will perform in a more realistic work setting. Situational assessment is used to assess employability through short-term placement in real or simulated job activities (6). The goal of the situational assessment is not to determine whether the individual can do a particular job, but rather to evaluate the person's global work behaviors and skills such as attendance, punctuality, endurance, ability to get along with coworkers, and supervisory relationships. Global rating scales are completed and behavior that would cause problems on the job is documented (19).

Work Sample Approach

The problem with using situational assessment to make vocational recommendations is that there is no standardization of the assessment experience. There is limited opportunity for comparison of one person's skills with those of another and no frame of reference for interpreting the results of the assessment except for the personal experience of the evaluator (6). These limitations prompted the development of the work sample approach as another way to measure skills and aptitudes to be used in both vocational counseling and vocational rehabilitation for persons with disabilities (18). A work sample is a simulation of the tasks of an actual job, using the tools, materials, and procedures that would be used in a particular industry. The setup, administration, and scoring of the work sample are standardized so that meaningful comparisons can be made between the individual being tested and a normative group, either the general population, employed workers, or other people with disabilities (20). More standardized behavioral rating scales are usually included with work samples as well.

Job Trial Approach

Neither situational assessments nor work samples are capable of completely and satisfactorily answering the question, "Can this person do this job?" Thus, whenever possible, job trials are used to assess whether a client will be successful in a particular occupation. A job trial is the placement of an individual in a real situation for a short period of time for the purpose of determining whether that person can do that specific job (18). Job trials and situational assessments may look similar, but the assessment goals are very different. Job trials are used to confirm the feasibility of the chosen vocational objective, to indicate potential problem areas, to identify needed accommodations or modifications, or to rule that occupation out of consideration. As with situational assessment, there is little standardization or normative referencing, but the evaluative criteria are the real-world criteria of actual job performance. Situational assessments and job trials are recommended for clients who do not perform well on standardized measures or who have complex diagnoses such as brain injury (21).

Physical Capacity and Work Tolerance Approach

The physical capacity to tolerate work or to perform the physical demands of a job is sometimes assessed more specifically (8). Measurement devices for systematically assessing physical capacities and work tolerance are available (22). Special techniques have been developed to evaluate physical capacity and work tolerance for particular conditions such as heart and circulatory problems (23–27), burns (28), upper-extremity impairment (29), and low-back problems (30,31). Physical capacities and work tolerance may also be observed during work samples, situational assessments, or job tryouts. Information on the individual's physical capacities and work tolerance is used in developing a vocational profile and in determining the range of jobs open to the individual.

VOCATIONAL ASSESSMENT TOOLS

A vocational evaluator has many tools to assist the person with a disability in making informed vocational choices. Many of these tools and techniques can also be used for career and vocational guidance in the general population, that is, persons without disabilities. The vocational evaluator should follow standardized procedures, except when modifications are necessary in the testing conditions to accommodate the disability. Accommodations may include arrangements for physical accessibility (e.g., elevated table), modifications in instructions (e.g., oral versus written), and modifications in the task itself (e.g., extended time to complete items). Procedures that do not follow standardized instructions must be documented and taken into consideration when interpreting information.

Vocational Interview

The vocational interview is usually the starting place for the vocational assessment (6). In addition to necessary medical and psychological information, the client will be asked about his or her work history, educational background, and family and economic situation. Each area of inquiry is important to developing the picture of the client as a worker, identifying potential strengths, limitations, and problems to be addressed in the assessment. Based on the referral information, the referral questions, and the expressed needs and interests of the client, the evaluator should develop an evaluation plan, explaining what is to be done at each step to the client, along with the purpose of each part of the evaluation.

Interest Tests

A client's vocational choices should be based on his or her interests. Interest testing is one way to examine a person's interest patterns in comparison to other people in general or other workers in specific occupations (6). A number of standardized interest inventories are available. Most persons with disabilities who are undecided in their career interests are able to take these untimed, exploratory tests. If the individual has difficulty reading, several picture inventories will provide similar information (Fig. 18-1).

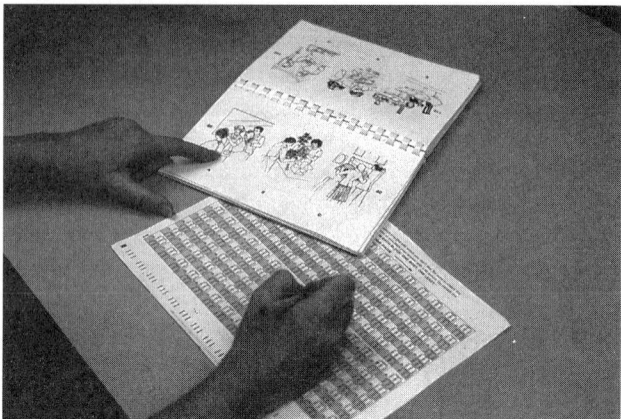

Figure 18-1. Picture interest inventory. (*Photograph by Wayne G. Alfred.*)

Aptitude and Achievement Tests

Standardized intelligence, aptitude, and achievement tests are frequently used in vocational assessments (6). The General Aptitude Test Battery (GATB) from the U.S. Department of Labor is frequently used and is the prototype for other commercial testing systems (20). The subtests of the GATB measure nine areas—general intelligence, verbal and numerical reasoning, spatial aptitude, form perception, clerical perception, motor coordination, finger dexterity, and manual dexterity. The GATB and similar batteries are examples of assessment systems employing the psychological testing approach. Scores are used to develop a worker trait profile that is then compared (manually or using computer systems) with profiles of jobs or groups of jobs. Other instruments measure one specific aptitude like finger dexterity, manual dexterity, or spatial perception (Figs. 18-2 and 18-3).

Work Sample and Computerized Assessment Systems

Work sample systems have been on the market for several decades. Work samples have been developed to measure abilities in diverse areas such as bookkeeping, clerical work, reception-related tasks, assembly work, drafting, electronics and soldering, masonry, plumbing, small-engine repair, and cosmetology (20). Several developers of commercial vocational assessment systems have assembled their components into standardized packages, some computerized for ease of administration, scoring, and interpretation (Figs. 18-4 and 18-5).

Personality Inventories

Personality testing is sometimes included in vocational assessments to assist in matching the temperaments of the individual with the requirements of the job (6). Job-related factors might include ability to work with others contrasted with ability to work alone, or tolerance for routine structure activity compared with flexibility and adaptability to varied tasks. More formalized psychological tests (intelligence tests and personality inventories) are usually administered by psychologists for diagnostic and treatment purposes that are not related to vocational goal setting. The results of these tests may be taken into consideration for vocational planning by the vocational evaluator.

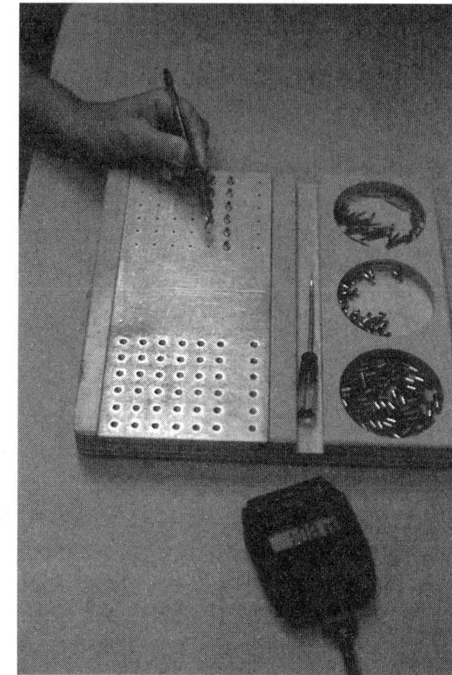

Figure 18-2. Test of finger dexterity. (*Photograph by Wayne G. Alfred.*)

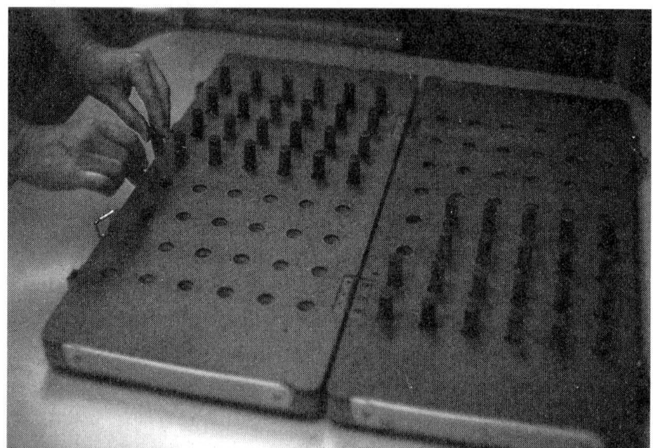

Figure 18-3. Manual dexterity test. (*Photograph by Wayne G. Alfred.*)

Occupational Information Resources

Once all testing has been completed, scored, and interpreted, the next step in the vocational assessment process is to use occupational information resources to determine the range of vocational options and to assist the client, through the vocational counseling process, in identifying a vocational objective and developing an employment plan.

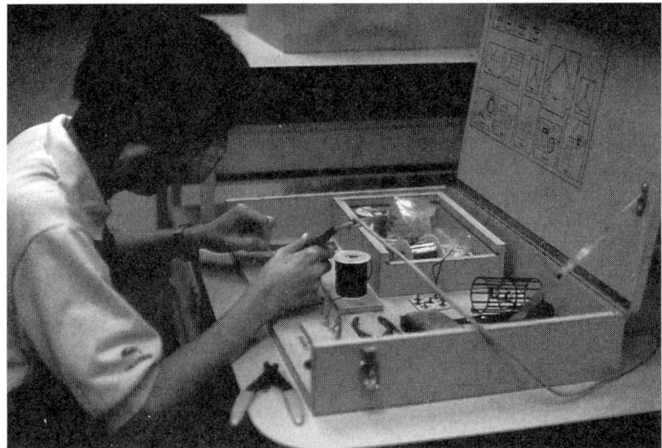

Figure 18-4. Work sample in electronics. (*Photograph by Wayne G. Alfred.*)

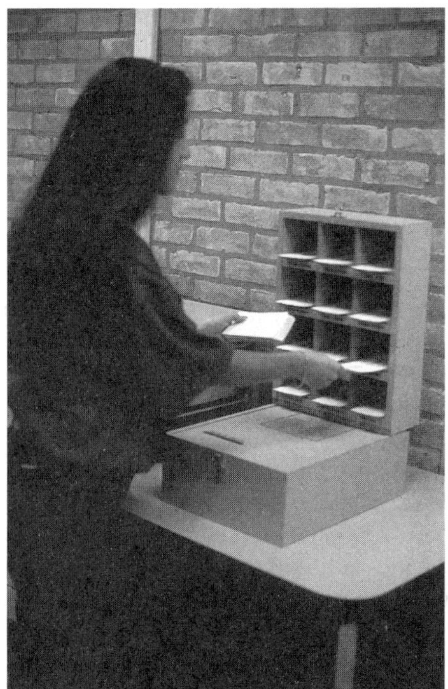

Figure 18-5. Mail-sorting work sample. (*Photograph by Wayne G. Alfred.*)

The *Dictionary of Occupational Titles* (DOT) (32) is a comprehensive listing of over 60,000 jobs that exist in the U.S. national economy. Each job is assigned a unique nine-digit number reflecting that job's position within specified occupational categories, divisions, and groups and its relationship to data, people, and things. The DOT contains a brief description of each job and provides some additional relevant data about the job requirements. What is most useful about the DOT, however, is that the nine-digit number is used in a number of other occupational information resources that categorize job information, allowing a cross-referencing, or "cross walk" with other sources of

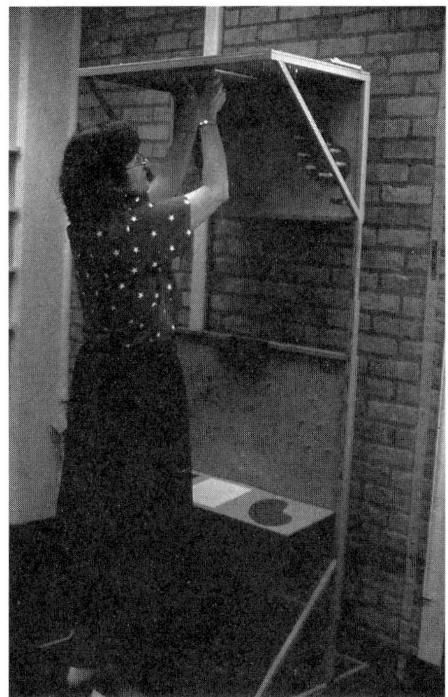

Figure 18-6. Work sample designed to assess overhead reaching ability. (*Photograph by Wayne G. Alfred.*)

vocational information. These other sources include the *Occupational Outlook Handbook* (33), *The Enhanced Guide for Occupational Exploration* (34), *The Classification of Jobs* (35), and *The Revised Handbook for Analyzing Jobs* (36).

Physical Capacity Assessment

Vocational assessment usually incorporates information on physical capacity assessment, either from a physician, an occupational therapist, or a physical therapist or from testing during the assessment (37). Work-related physical capacities include lifting, walking, standing, reaching, handling, fingering, feeling, stooping, bending, crawling, climbing, and balancing as well as sensory capacities such as hearing, talking, and seeing. The vocational evaluator will make use of reports from other specialists, but may use some standardized physiologic measurements or tasks to determine what the client is capable of doing (Figs. 18-6 and 18-7). Where physical capacities are limited by the nature of the disability, the evaluator should take care to test the client within the limitations set by the physician.

Transferrable Skills Analysis

If a person with a disability has a prior work history, then his or her previous jobs may be used to determine "transferrable skills," that is, those aptitudes and abilities that are not affected by the disability. These transferrable skills, adjusted for functional limitations based on the disability, may be the basis for vocational recommendations without formalized testing.

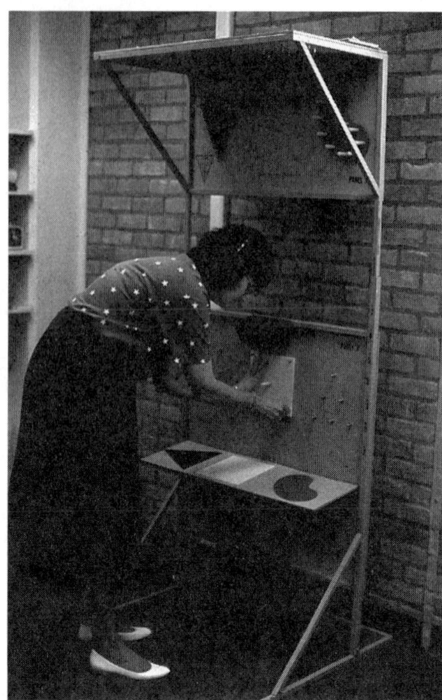

Figure 18-7. The same work sample used to assess ability to bend. (*Photograph by Wayne G. Alfred.*)

Behavioral Assessment and Work Adjustment

A critical part of any vocational assessment is the observation of the client's work-related behavior. The evaluator pays particular attention to behavioral factors such as attendance, punctuality, response to supervision, interaction with others, and grooming, as well as the client's ability to follow instructions, maintain physical stamina, maintain concentration, and work under pressure. Checklists (19) are used to describe and rate behavior. The objective is to identify behavioral problems that may affect the individual's ability to get or keep a job as well as to identify positive work behaviors that may contribute to job success. Individuals with behavioral problems or limitations can be referred to programs specializing in work adjustment to improve their opportunities for obtaining and retaining employment.

Job Analysis and Job Matching

Using the information obtained through the review of medical records, testing, transferrable skills analysis, and behavioral observations, the vocational evaluator is able to develop a vocational profile of the client. This profile may be used to determine the feasibility of a wide range of occupations or may be used to examine the requirements of a specific job (38). Occasionally, the evaluator will be called on to conduct an analysis of a specific job and to determine whether the skills and abilities of the client match or correspond to the job requirements. Some programs use computer databases to provide job matching for use in vocational counseling (20).

INTERPRETING VOCATIONAL ASSESSMENT DATA

The interpretation of vocational assessment data poses significant challenges because of the limitations inherent in standardized testing and the dilemma of transforming clinical data into *real-world* applicability (6). Normative data must be used appropriately to make recommendations and the validity and reliability of measurements must be taken into consideration. Recommendations must be based on current labor market information as well as employment options in the client's community.

Normative Data

As with any type of psychometric testing, standardized testing used in the vocational assessment should have adequate and well-defined normative groups with which to compare and interpret client scores (6). In vocational rehabilitation, the question of norms is particularly complex, because the selection of the normative group may very well determine the feasibility of vocational alternatives. For instance, some instruments use *employed worker* norms, comparing the client to workers in a particular industry. This is the most competitive normative group, people who have been screened, hired, and trained for a specific occupation and who have achieved some degree of experience in the job. The most frequently used normative group, however, is the *general population.* This group is usually composed of individuals representing a wide variety of abilities. Thus, the comparison of the client's abilities is to people in general. The use of both employed worker and general population normative data has been criticized as being too restrictive for persons with disabilities and as eliminating some persons from the workforce whose scores are not "competitive," yet who have shown the ability to work in a wide variety of occupations. Sometimes comparisons are made to others with similar disabilities to increase the opportunities for positive rather than negative vocational recommendations with particular types of disability. While this may boost the chances for positive feedback and more vocational possibilities to explore, it also defeats the purpose of an assessment geared to predict realistic, competitive outcomes.

Validity and Reliability

As with normative data, the psychometric properties of validity and reliability must be taken into consideration in the selection of assessment instruments and measurements and in the interpretation of test results (6). The tests used in the psychological testing approach have been criticized for not appearing to be related to the world of work and thus for not having much face validity for the client, one factor that led to the development of work samples. But questions of construct and concurrent as well as predictive validity plague many of the assessment systems and instruments on the market. Each instrument must also be judged on its reliability, both its internal consistency and test-retest reliability. Interrater reliability is also crucial, so that the interpretation and scoring of each instrument are not based on the subjective opinion of the evaluator.

Assessing the Labor Market

Because of the real-world criteria required as the basis of realistic vocational recommendations, the interpretation of vocational assessment results and the development of vocational recommendations must be based on an accurate assessment of the jobs available in the client's geographic area and local labor market (6,39). Vocational evaluators and rehabilitation counselors are aware of local labor trends and often have contacts with employers in the area who have hired persons with disabilities in the past. Sometimes in cases requiring vocational expert testimony, vocational evaluators are asked to estimate the number of jobs in the local or national economy that a particular client would be able to do. Labor market surveys are an important part of this assessment.

Job-Seeking Skills

One final assessment that should be included as part of a comprehensive vocational assessment is the examination of the client's job-seeking skills. Persons with disabilities who have significant work experience may be well versed in job-seeking skills. More likely, however, is the situation in which the person with limited or no job-seeking experience will need assistance in the following areas: a) developing a resume, b) identifying job leads, c) filling out job applications, and d) interviewing for jobs. Persons with disabilities have faced discrimination in the workplace but are now protected by the ADA and should be taught their rights under the act. By evaluating previous job-seeking experiences, the vocational evaluator may make recommendations for training in job-seeking skills necessary to achieve vocational goals.

PUTTING IT ALL TOGETHER

A vocational evaluator reports data in several different ways. It is very important to provide feedback to the client both during testing and in a follow-up interview after all tests have been scored. Every client has a right to know what the results are and what the vocational evaluator's recommendations are. A formal staff meeting will usually be held with the client, the person who made the referral for the assessment, and members of the clinical team who may be working with the client in the future. Often it is desirable to involve family members in the decision-making process as well. In client meetings, it is important to focus not just on deficits and problems, but also on strengths noted in the assessment as well as strategies to be used to compensate for any problems identified.

The vocational evaluator also prepares a written report making recommendations to be used in developing a vocational rehabilitation plan. The report should include the client's vocational objectives, areas of strength, problem areas, and specific recommendations for addressing the problems that present barriers to employment. These recommendations are supported by summaries of information from interviews, medical record reviews, testing, and behavioral observations. The written vocational assessment report may also be used as the basis for expert witness testimony in cases involving litigation.

EMPLOYMENT OPTIONS

In making recommendations for vocational planning and career goals, the vocational evaluator must take into consideration the level of support that may be necessary for the client to succeed in achieving his or her vocational objectives. *Competitive employment* (either full-time or part-time) is recommended when the client is able to compete in the labor market (i.e., to do the job at the degree of speed and accuracy of other, nondisabled workers) with or without accommodations or job modifications. *Sheltered work* is traditionally recommended when the client cannot compete in terms of production speed or accuracy or when work behaviors substantially interfere with the client's ability to retain employment. Sheltered work is usually performed in workshops employing many persons with disabilities. Competitive production standards (either piece rate or speed and accuracy) may not be attainable by the workers, but they are paid for what they are able to produce.

The concept of *supported work* has been developed as an alternative to segregating persons with disabilities into sheltered workshops (40,41). The philosophy of supported work is that persons with severe disabilities who have not succeeded in traditional vocational rehabilitation programs may be employable in a competitive environment if enough support is provided by supervisors, coworkers, family members, or job coaches. Supported work programs use either short-term or long-term job coaching, in which a vocational specialist provides intensive services at the work site, gradually "fading" as the worker becomes competitive in the job. Evidence of the effectiveness of supported work for some persons with disabilities is emerging, but opportunities are currently limited because of lack of funding and limited availability of supported employment programs (40–45).

If the person with the disability undergoing the vocational assessment is not ready or able to pursue vocational objectives, recommendations may be made for other productive activities, including volunteer work, homemaking, or educational pursuits, either instead of or in addition to paid employment.

ROLE OF THE VOCATIONAL EVALUATOR ON THE REHABILITATION TEAM

The vocational evaluator is an important part of the rehabilitation team. Early in the rehabilitation process the evaluator may be useful in answering employment-related questions and in talking with employers (11,12). The vocational evaluator will work with the vocational rehabilitation counselor in determining when vocational assessment should take place and what the referral questions are. The evaluator's recommendations will provide the basis for vocational counseling, rehabilitation planning, and job placement. Vocational evaluators usually have either a bachelor's degree in rehabilitation services or a master's degree in rehabilitation counseling, vocational evaluation, or a related field with specialized training in psychometrics and the development, administration, scoring, and interpretation of vocational assessment instruments (46). Service providers with the credentials of Certified Rehabilitation Counselor (CRC) or Certified Vocational Evaluator (CVE) have met the educational and experience criteria necessary to conduct valid assessments. States may also license individuals to administer tests used in vocational assessment.

DIAGNOSIS VERSUS PROGNOSIS

Vocational assessment is a process by which a diagnostic "snapshot" is taken of a particular individual with a disability, and taking into consideration the attributes of the individual and the characteristics of the labor market that he or she wishes to enter, recommendations are made for services that will help him or her achieve specified career goals. One mistake sometimes made is to assume that this snapshot is static and will not change over time. Persons with disabilities may experience additional medical recovery, may experience changes in their family or social circumstances, may develop different vocational interests, or may simply develop a higher degree of career maturity. While information from a vocational assessment is useful in determining a prognosis for return to work, it is not an infallible prediction, and additional information may be needed in the future to assist the individual in making sound vocational choices.

Often a person's fulfillment of his or her hopes and dreams rests on the results obtained during the assessment. Vocational assessment provides a realistic basis for decision making and expenditure of limited rehabilitation resources. This crucial part of the rehabilitation process should not be ignored or diminished in importance. It is often the opportunity to open doors for persons with severe disabilities. With so many societal changes, including technologic developments, new and expanded models for services, legal protections against discrimination in the workplace, and elimination of physical and attitudinal barriers, persons with disabilities should have every opportunity to participate in the workforce and thus be productive members of society.

REFERENCES

1. World Health Organization. *International classification of impairments, disabilities, and handicaps.* Geneva: World Health Organization, 1980.
2. Special Task Force to the Secretary of Health, Education, and Welfare. *Work in America.* Cambridge, MA: MIT Press, 1973.
3. Young ME, Alfred WG, Rintala DH, et al. Vocational status of persons with spinal cord injury living in the community. *Rehabil Couns Bull* 1994;37:229–243.
4. Aitken RCB, Cornes P. To work or not to work: that is the question. *Br J Indust Med* 1990;47:436–441.
5. Louis Harris and Associates. *The ICD survey II: employing disabled Americans.* New York: Louis Harris and Associates, 1987.
6. Power PW. *A guide to vocational assessment.* Baltimore: University Park Press, 1984.
7. Coudroglou A, Poole DL. *Disability, work, and social policy.* New York: Springer, 1984.
8. Deutsch PM, Sawyer HW. *A guide to rehabilitation.* 5th ed. New York: Matthew Bender, 1990.
9. Vandergoot D. *Placement and career development in rehabilitation.* Parker RM, ed. *Rehabilitation counseling: basics and beyond.* Austin, TX: Pro-Ed, 1987: 121–156.
10. Alfred WG, Fuhrer MJ, Rossi CD. Vocational development following severe spinal cord injury: a longitudinal study. *Arch Phys Med Rehabil* 1987;68: 854–857.
11. Sawyer HW, Saxon JP, Mitchell ME. Vocational assessment of acute care patients. *Vocational Eval Work Adjustment Bull* 1984;17(3):90–94.
12. Spencer JC, Young ME, Rintala D, Bates S. Socialization to the culture of a rehabilitation hospital: an ethnographic study. *Am J Occup Ther* 1995;49:53–62.
13. Mysiw WJ, Corrigan JD, Hunt M, et al. Vocational evaluation of traumatic brain injury patients using the Functional Assessment Inventory. *Brain Inj* 1989;3: 27–34.
14. Agran M, Morgan RL. Current transition assessment practices. *Res Dev Disabil* 1991;12(2):113–126.
15. Anastasi A. *Psychological testing.* 5th ed. New York: Macmillan, 1982.

16. Pruitt WA. *Vocational evaluation.* 2nd ed. Menomonie, WI: Walt Pruitt Associates, 1986.

17. Rubin SE, Roessler RT. *Foundations of the vocational rehabilitation process.* 3rd ed. Austin, TX: Pro-Ed, 1987.

18. Nadolsky JM. *Development of a model for vocational evaluation of the disadvantaged.* Auburn, AL: Department of Vocational and Adult Education, School of Education, Auburn University, 1971.

19. Botterbusch KF. *Revised MDC Behavior Identification Form.* Menomonie, WI: Materials Development Center, University of Wisconsin-Stout, 1984.

20. Botterbusch KF. *Vocational assessment and evaluation systems: a comparison.* Menomonie, WI: Materials Development Center, University of Wisconsin-Stout, 1987.

21. Fraser RT. Vocational evaluation. *J Head Trauma Rehabil* 1991;6:46–58.

22. Powell DM, Zimmer CA, Antoine MM, et al. Computer analysis of the performance of the BTE Work Simulator. *J Burn Care Rehabil* 1991;12:250–256.

23. Emery CF. Components of cardiac rehabilitation other than exercise. *Semin Respir Med* 1993;14:139–147.

24. Landes J, Rod JL. Return-to-work evaluation after coronary events. Special emphasis on simulated work activity. *Sports Med* 1992;13:365–375.

25. Picard MH, Dennis C, Schwartz RG, et al. Cost-benefit analysis of early return to work after uncomplicated acute myocardial infarction. *Am J Cardiol* 1989;63:1308–1314.

26. Dennis C, Houston-Miller N, Schwartz RG, et al. Early return to work after uncomplicated myocardial infarction. Results of a randomized trial. *JAMA* 1988;260:214–220.

27. Sheldahl LM, Wilke NA, Tristani FE. Exercise prescription for return to work. *J Cardpulm Rehabil* 1985;5:567–575.

28. Zeller J, Sturm G, Cruse CW. Patients with burns are successful in work hardening program. *J Burn Care Rehabil* 1993;14(suppl II):189–196.

29. Blair SJ, McCormick E, Bear-Lehman J, et al Evaluation of impairment of the upper extremity. *Clin Orthop* 1987;221:42–58.

30. Milhous RL, Haugh LD, Frymoyer JW, et al. Determinants of vocational disability in patients with low back pain. *Arch Phys Med Rehabil* 1989;70:589–593.

31. Burke SA, Harms-Constas CK, Aden PS. Return to work/work retention outcomes of a functional restoration program: a multi-center, prospective study with a comparison group. *Spine* 1994;19:1880–1886.

32. U.S. Department of Labor. *Dictionary of occupational titles.* 4th ed. Indianapolis, IN: JIST Works, 1991.

33. U.S. Department of Labor. *Occupational outlook handbook.* 1994–95 ed. Indianapolis, IN: JIST Works, 1994.

34. Maze M, Mayall D, eds. *The enhanced guide for occupational exploration—descriptions for the 2500 most important jobs.* Indianapolis, IN: JIST Works, 1991.

35. Field JE, Field TF. *The classification of jobs.* 4th ed. Athens, GA: Elliott & Fitzpatrick, 1992.

36. U.S. Department of Labor. *The revised handbook for analyzing jobs.* Indianapolis, IN: JIST Works, 1991.

37. Noyes FR, Mooar LA, Barber SD. The assessment of work-related activities and limitations in knee disorders. *Am J Sports Med* 1991;19:178–188.

38. Sobush DC, Kuhne K, Harbers T. Resources for vocational planning applied to the job title of physical therapist. *Phys Ther* 1985;65:1524–1527.

39. Biefang S, Potthoff P. Assessment methods for rehabilitation. *Int J Rehabil Res* 1995;18:201–213.

40. Barrett J, Lavin D. *The industrial work model: a guide for developing transitional and supported employment.* Menomonie, WI: Materials Development Center, University of Wisconsin-Stout, 1987.

41. Botterbusch KF. *Understanding community based employment and follow-up services.* Menomonie, WI: Research and Training Center, 1989.

42. Thomas DF, Menz FE. *Head Injury Re-entry Project (Project HIRe).* Menomonie, WI: Research and Training Center, University of Wisconsin-Stout, 1990.

43. Corthell DW, Boone L, eds. *Marketing: an approach to placement.* Menomonie, WI: Research and Training Center, University of Wisconsin-Stout, 1982.

44. Wehman P, Sherron P, Kregel J, et al. Return to work for persons following severe traumatic brain injury: supported employment outcomes after five years. *Am J Phys Med Rehabil* 1993;72:355–363.

45. Wehman P, Kreutzer J, Wood W, et al. Helping traumatically brain injured patients return to work with supported employment: three case studies. *Arch Phys Med Rehabil* 1989;70:109–113.

46. Corthell DW, Griswold PP, eds. The use of vocational evaluation in VR. Menomonie, WI: Research and Training Center, University of Wisconsin-Stout, 1987.

Chapter 19

Assessment of Visual Impairment Following Adult Acquired Brain Injury

Barry L. Seiller
Mary Warren

TYPE AND SIGNIFICANCE OF VISUAL IMPAIRMENT FOLLOWING BRAIN INJURY

After traumatic brain injury, brain tumors, cerebrovascular accident, multiple sclerosis, or postconcussion syndrome, patients may experience a variety of visual impairments that can result in both overt and insidious symptoms. It has been estimated that between 40% and 75% of persons surviving head trauma and stroke require some form of rehabilitation of visual impairments (1–4). The impact of visual deficits may be further complicated by the injured person not being aware of a change in vision (5) and therefore not attempting to compensate for the deficit. Also, because visual perception is a subjective experience, the person may have difficulty articulating his or her difficulties and relating them to an impairment in vision (3,5). The person may also have developed a compensatory strategy as a result of the impairment that interferes with his or her ability to compensate in other areas of visual functioning and that may confuse both the person and the rehabilitation team. However, if the visual impairment can be correctly and promptly diagnosed and appropriate therapeutic intervention prescribed, the patient's rehabilitation course may be improved and the medical outcome enhanced (2).

The severity or number of visual problems do not appear to be related to the severity of the brain injury. While moderate to severe brain injury can understandably cause significant visual problems, it is now postulated that even mild brain injuries can disrupt the overall speed, efficiency, and integration of mental and central nervous function. There may be severe cognitive and behavioral impairments causing headaches, dizziness, memory difficulties, delay in return to work, inability to drive, and emotional instability (6). Symptoms may be a combination of organic and psychological factors (7). Because of the need for a uniform diagnosis, a specific definition of mild traumatic brain injury was recently established (8). Some authors reported that whiplash and cervical strain can cause visual dysfunctions without a documented traumatic brain injury (9).

Visual impairment following brain injury occurs primarily as a result of changes in four areas of visual function: visual acuity, visual field, oculomotor control, and central visual processing (10). Diminishment of visual acuity can occur secondary to brain injury (11,12) or as a result of an unrelated condition occurring simultaneously with the neurologic insult. Vision loss is the third leading cause of disability in older adults, ranking only behind cardiovascular disease and arthritis (13). An estimated 25% of adults over the age of 80 have a visual impairment so significant that they are no longer able to read standard-size print (14,15). Age-related diseases such as macular degeneration, glaucoma, and diabetic retinopathy comprise the major cause of irreversible vision loss in older adults (16). Wainapel et al (15) found that 6.8% of persons admitted to a rehabilitation unit for treatment of another physical impairment also had a significant vision loss that affected functional performance and interfered with the rehabilitation process. According to these same authors (15), "vision loss was encountered more often than such typical RM [rehabilitation medicine] diagnoses as paraplegia/quadriplegia, Parkinson disease, peripheral neuropathy or rheumatoid arthritis." Conditions associated with head trauma such as optic nerve injury, retinal detachment, vitreal hemorrhage, cataract, and reduced accommodative function can cause a reduction in visual acuity. Some of these conditions can result in significant, permanent, and uncorrectable vision loss that requires intervention from professionals specializing in low-vision rehabilitation. A reduction in contrast sensitivity function (the ability to distinguish between subtle gradations of contrast between objects) is associated with multiple sclerosis (17) and posterior cortical lesions (18–20). Bulens et al (20) reported that 62% of subjects with ischemic lesions affecting the posterior visual pathways demonstrated reduced contrast sensitivity function. Reduced contrast sensitivity function can result in difficulty completing a variety of daily living tasks involving the detection of low-contrast features, including facial recognition, identifying curbs and steps, filling a glass with water, and driving under cloudy or rainy conditions (21,22).

Homonymous hemianopsia is the most common visual impairment observed following brain injury (23). Visual field deficits, depending on the extent of the vision loss, can have a significant impact on the person's mobility, reading, writing, and performance of a variety of daily living tasks including driving (12,23).

Impairment of oculomotor control is frequently associated with traumatic brain injury. A recent review reported that only 13% of persons with a primary diagnosis of head trauma have associated cranial nerve lesions (6). However, an estimated 75% of patients experience some reduction of oculomotor control secondary to brain stem injury and disruption of central neural control (4). Diplopia and perceptual instability are frequent complaints voiced by the patient with oculomotor impairment (24–27). These conditions can have a detrimental effect on postural control and mobility, eye-hand coordination, and reading and other near-vision tasks (25,27).

Changes in the processing of visual input by the central nervous system invariably accompany any insult to the brain because all four lobes in both hemispheres, the brain stem, and the cerebellum are involved in the integration of visual information (28,29). Diminishment of visual attention perhaps has the greatest impact on visual-perceptual processing because if, and how, one attends to something determines whether further perceptual analysis will be completed, as well as the quality of that analysis. Brain injury can result in a variety of deficiencies in visual attention. These can include 1) difficulty arousing and sustaining attention, which is associated with brain stem injuries (28); 2) difficulty directing attention toward one side, known as hemi-inattention or neglect and which is associated with right-hemisphere injuries (29–31); 3) difficulty attending to visual detail, which is associated with posterior temporal lesions (32,33); 4) difficulty attending globally to the environment, which is associated with right parietal lesions (32,34); 5) difficulty shifting attention between tasks (29); and 6) difficulty eliciting the emotional arousal for attention, resulting in indifference, which is associated with cingulate lesions (28). Alteration of visual attention can impact on the higher-level perceptual skills that require visual attention, including pattern recognition, visual memory, and complex visual processing (35).

PRIMARY DISCIPLINES INVOLVED IN REHABILITATION OF VISUAL IMPAIRMENT FOLLOWING BRAIN INJURY

In order for survivors of acquired brain injury to benefit from visual rehabilitation interventions, an interdisciplinary effort is required (36). A number of disciplines, including ophthalmology, optometry, and occupational therapy, may assume responsibility for different aspects of the evaluation and treatment of visual impairment. To understand how these disciplines work together to rehabilitate the patient, it is necessary to recognize the differences between the professions and their unique qualifications and contributions to the rehabilitation process. It is especially important to distinguish between ophthalmology and optometry, as either physician can serve as the primary eye care specialist and evaluate, prescribe, or implement treatment recommendations. There is often confusion, and sometimes controversy, as to the role that each should play in the rehabilitation process.

Ophthalmology

Ophthalmologists are medically trained physicians who specialize in the diagnosis and treatment of ocular disease. Assessment completed by the ophthalmologist concentrates on determining the presence of pathology and structural dysfunction of the eye and its neuromuscular control, often at the expense of addressing cognitive and functional problems. Academic requirements include 4 years of undergraduate education, 4 years of medical school, 1 year of hospital internship, 3 years of ophthalmology residency, and often 1 to 2 years of fellowship training in a specialty area. Neuro-ophthalmologists complete an additional 1 to 2 years studying the relationship between the central nervous system and the eye. Ophthalmologists are licensed by the state to prescribe all types of medications and perform surgical procedures. As traditionally accepted members of the medical team, they typically possess hospital privileges, enabling them to be involved in a patient's case during the acute stage of rehabilitation. As a physician, the ophthalmologist may also be a member of the patient's medical insurance plan.

Optometry

Optometrists are health care professionals specializing in the diagnosis and treatment of ocular *refractive* disorders. An optometric examination typically concentrates on determining whether the patient requires correction of an ocular defect with glasses, contact lenses, prisms, or patches. Ocular pathology may be encountered in the course of the examination. If the optometrist believes that the condition warrants advanced medical or surgical care, he or she will usually refer the patient to a primary care physician or an ophthalmologist. Academic requirements include 4 years of undergraduate education, 4 years of optometry school, and optional postgraduate specialty training. Optometrists are licensed by the state to use diagnostic eyedrops and prescribe specific medications. Optometrists may choose to specialize in an aspect of rehabilitation. Specialties in optometry include 1) behavioral optometry, which addresses how vision relates to and governs cognitive processes, movement, and postural control; 2) neuro-optometry, which is concerned with how these functions are affected following traumatic brain injury or stroke; and 3) developmental optometry, which is behavioral optometry as it relates to children, especially those with learning disabilities.

Occupational Therapy

Occupational therapists are health care professionals who work with persons with disabilities to enable them to complete necessary daily living activities and attain a satisfying and productive lifestyle. In evaluating the patient with visual impairment, the occupational therapist concentrates on how the impairment has affected the functional ability of the patient. Emphasis is on the patient's ability to compensate for the deficit in completing daily living activities such as reading, writing, eating, grooming, home management, meal preparation, management of finances, vocational responsibilities, mobility in the environment, and driving. Academic requirements include a bachelor or masters of science degree in occupational therapy from an accredited university, 6 to 9 months of fieldwork in a specific area of disability, and successful completion of a national certification examination.

EVALUATION SETTINGS

Whether an ophthalmologist or optometrist examines the patient with brain injury is dependent on numerous circumstances. The small number of practitioners involved in this field, the timing of the examination phase, and the accessibility to physicians are frequently limiting factors. Contrary to previous thinking, the eye care practitioner should be consulted to perform an eye examination as soon as visual impairment is suspected. Otherwise, many correctable vision impairments may be allowed to go untreated during the patient's rehabilitation process, compromising the benefits gained from rehabilitation (36).

Eye examinations can be completed during any of the three primary phases of rehabilitation: acute, subacute, and chronic.

Acute Rehabilitation Setting

The acute rehabilitation phase is initiated when the patient is medically stable but still in an acute hospital setting, such as the intensive care unit or emergency room. Examination of the patient is usually completed by an ophthalmologist who has hospital staff privileges. The attending primary care physician or neurosurgeon will consult with the ophthalmologist in examining the patient for the integrity of the visual system. Even though the hospital may have a well-equipped eye examination room, the physical limitations of the patient at this stage may dictate completion of a bedside examination using a penlight and a direct ophthalmoscope. It is not unusual for the patient to be uncooperative or noncommunicative while having concomitant multiple medical problems. These medical problems can be responsible for findings such as nystagmus or abnormal pupillary responses. The ocular examination should be directed toward revealing any vision-threatening conditions such as globe perforation, orbital fracture, optic nerve or retinal injury, or reduction in gross visual acuity.

Subacute Rehabilitation Setting

In the subacute rehabilitation phase, the patient has been moved to either a general hospital room or a rehabilitation unit. The patient is referred for evaluation by either the attending primary care physician, a consulting neurologist or physiatrist, or a member of the rehabilitation team. Because it is unusual for an optometrist to have staff privileges in a hospital, an ophthalmologist is typically consulted. Portable equipment can be brought to the patient's room or the patient can be transported to an eye examination room in the hospital. At this stage, the patient is usually cooperative enough to allow a more comprehensive examination of near and far visual acuity, pupillary responses, extraocular motility, the retina (dilated or undilated), gross visual field, and intraocular pressure. The examination may require special modifications for patients who are confined to bed (37).

Chronic Rehabilitation Setting

In the long-term rehabilitation phase, the patient is either an inpatient in a long-term rehabilitation facility or receiving outpatient rehabilitation services. The examination will take place either in the rehabilitation facility or in the eye practitioner's office. An optometrist or an ophthalmologist may complete the examination. Specialized equipment can be used to examine the entire visual system including refractive error and visual field deficit. The patient may be referred by the primary care physician, neurologist, physiatrist, attorney, insurance representative, family member, or a member of the rehabilitation team.

EVALUATION PROTOCOL FOR OPHTHALMOLOGY AND OPTOMETRY

After obtaining the patient's consent, the eye practitioner should review the history and date of the patient's event in preparation for the examination. Personal history and insurance information should be recorded. The patient and family need to be questioned about previous ocular or medical evaluations. The practitioner usually will interact with other medical professionals involved in the case to determine whether any specific referring situation exists. The patient and family or companion should be asked to complete a questionnaire listing the patient's symptoms, abilities, and goals and objectives if treatment is applicable. The companion should be quizzed about his or her objective observations of the patient's conditions. All medical tests, radiological examinations, and medications should be recorded.

Any evaluation of the visual system should begin with an ocular health assessment. Trauma to the head can cause concomitant injury to the face and orbit. Direct and indirect force can disrupt the ocular-visual process. A thorough external and internal examination of the globe and adnexa is essential. Orbital fractures can result in damage to the extraocular muscles and optic nerve.

Changes in visual function following brain injury occur primarily as result of changes in four areas: 1) visual pathway integrity, 2) ocular motility, 3) sensory fusion status, and 4) visual processing. Each area should be assessed with the knowledge that they are integrated and are not isolated areas.

Visual Pathway Assessment

Visual Acuity

Visual acuity has been, and probably will continue to be, the cornerstone of a functional visual assessment. The standard of vision testing is the Snellen chart, developed in 1862. This test is accurate, reproducible, and easily interpreted by physicians and patients. However, it has its limitations, since it measures the eye's resolving power using high-contrast targets in a darkened room. This highly specific and restricted environment is rarely encountered in daily living tasks. The Snellen-type acuity charts are currently used to measure ocular health, as a tool for refraction, and as a standard for determining eligibility to operate motor vehicles (38). Besides distance visual acuity, near vision is typically tested to evaluate reading vision (39).

Contrast Sensitivity

Contrast sensitivity is the ability to discern subtle differences in shades of gray. In recent years, contrast sensitivity testing has been considered an important adjunct to, if not a replacement for, visual acuity (40). Snellen acuity testing evaluates the eye's ability to resolve fine detail at high contrast but may not adequately describe its ability to see low-contrast patterns, faces, road signs, or objects. In a person with normal vision, visual acuity and contrast sensitivity may vary in the same fashion. In addition to identifying visual defects due to optical factors, contrast sensitivity may be used to evaluate the quality of contrast perception at the level of the retina or brain. The quality of contrast perception is measured by the use of a repeated series of light and dark bars called sine-wave gratings, presented on computer-controlled video displays, optical projectors, and photographic plates (38,41).

Optokinetic Nystagmus

The optokinetic nystagmus test is an objective method of assessing visual acuity that can be used with patients who have difficulty in communicating. The responsive nystagmoid-like movements of the eye are assessed when stimulated by viewing a series of rapidly moving, similar targets, all traveling in the same direction (42).

Refractive Errors

An examination for any refractive disorder is an important part of the ocular evaluation. Proper corrective lenses may improve both distance and near visual acuity and contrast sensitivity. If the vision cannot be improved by these methods, either it is damaged or there is a functional loss. The patient may have had an undetermined preexisting refractive problem or one that has been caused or exacerbated by trauma. The eye practitioner may improve the patient's visual abilities by prescribing glasses that help compensate for a special problem that has been uncovered by the examination. This would include distance or near-vision glasses or bifocals if appropriate. The glasses can also serve as a mechanism to incorporate special lenses such as prisms or mirrors.

Visual Evoked Potentials

Visual evoked potentials (VEPs) are graded electrical signals generated within the brain in response to visual stimulation. VEPs are also known as visual evoked responses (VERs) and visual evoked cortical potentials (VECPs). Evaluating these electrical patterns can detect abnormalities of the optic nerve, chiasm, optic tracts, lateral geniculate nucleus, optic radiations, and occipital cortex (43). As an objective assessment of visual function, this evaluation can confirm psychogenic vision loss and assist in the medical diagnoses of nonverbal patients (44). Available in hospitals and some physician's offices, it has become a standard clinical test of visual function. Electroretinograms (ERGs) and electro-oculograms (EOGs) are also electrophysiologic tests of the visual system, but are concerned only with electrical activity within the eye.

Visual Fields

Visual field testing is one of the most important, but often neglected, aspects of visual assessment. A fully conscious, articulate patient may not be aware of visual field defects (5). The site of the insult along the optic pathway determines the nature of the visual field loss. Prechiasmal optic nerve lesions result in visual field disturbances restricted to the affected eye. Chiasmal lesions result in variable field loss patterns. Postchiasmal lesions (optic tract, radiations, cerebral cortex) produce homonymous hemianopsia or quadrantanopsia. They can be congruous or incongruous, left or right sided, or superior or inferior in nature (45). When visual field loss is not pattern specific or does not correlate with clinical findings, functional vision loss should be considered. This type of visual field loss may be seen with frank malingering for secondary gain or with a conversion reaction or hysteria (46).

Ocular Motility

The development of binocular vision depends on both motor and sensory components. The motor component deals with control of eye movements regulated by the oculomotor system. These consist of movements caused by the extrinsic and intrinsic muscles, fixational ability, pursuits, saccades, accommodation, and pupillary changes. Each part can be measured and recorded indirectly (subjectively) or directly (objectively).

Ocular Motility Assessment

In brain injury, the oculomotor system can be damaged at any level. However, it is the very complexity of the oculomotor system that allows for the precise diagnosis and treatment of the motility defect. Changes in eye movements may provide an important measure of recovery or deterioration during the acute illness, and ocular misalignment may have profound effects on the long-term rehabilitative process (6).

Extrinsic or Extraocular Muscles

This requires assessment of function of the six extraocular muscles (medial, lateral, inferior, and superior recti, superior and inferior oblique muscles), the ocular motor cranial nerves, and supranuclear function. There may be direct damage to the muscles or restriction of their movement associated with orbital fractures. Nuclear disorders affect the function of extraocular muscles in various positions of gaze:

- Abducens nerve (VI) injury results in paralysis of lateral or outward movement of the eye. This results in inward turning of the eye and horizontal double vision.
- Oculomotor nerve (III) lesions result in the inability to rotate the eye upward, downward, or inward and may also result in drooping of the upper eyelid. The iris may be dilated and nonreactive and accommodation may be paralyzed.
- Trochlear nerve (IV) damage results in paralysis of the superior oblique muscle and may cause vertical diplopia and a compensatory head position.

The pathology may be specific to one nerve or a combination of nerves. Supranuclear disorders limit the voluntary ability to move either eye in a particular direction of gaze (up, down, right, or left).

Fixation

Fixation is the maintenance of an object of conscious regard on the foveal portion of the retina. Fixation is controlled by pursuit and saccadic movements (24).

Pursuits

Pursuits are involuntary, parallel, slow-tracking movements of an eye fixing on a moving target. The neuropathway is from the occipital lobe to the midbrain-pons and on to the nuclei of cranial nerves III, IV, and VI (42).

Saccades

Saccades are fast, abrupt shifts in fixations. Vision is interrupted during the shifts to eliminate any sensation of movement. The neuropathway is from the frontal lobe to the midbrain-pons and on to the nuclei of the cranial nerves III, IV, and VI (42). With brain trauma, saccades and pursuits may be affected individually or in combination.

Vergences

Vergences are disjunctive or nonparallel binocular movements in which the eyes move in opposite directions. These may be either convergence (inward) or divergence (outward). Pursuits and saccades are conjunctive movements with the eyes moving in the same directions. The near reflex, consisting of centrally controlled convergence, accommodation, and pupillary constriction, may be disrupted in brain injury (2). No single nucleus for controlling vergence has been identified in humans, but it is known that lesions in the pretectal midbrain rostral to the third nerve nucleus may cause paralysis of convergence (6,47). Divergence is an active, nonvoluntary process and not just relaxation of convergence. Lesions in the area of the nucleus of cranial nerve VI can produce paralysis of divergence (6,48).

Intrinsic Ocular Muscles

These consist of the ciliary muscles and the sphincter and dilator muscles of the iris. Injury to this system can result in difficulty establishing, maintaining, and changing focus. Evaluation of this area includes assessment of accommodation and pupil diameter.

Accommodation

Accommodation is the ability to focus at near distances. Accommodation is controlled by the ciliary muscles, which weaken with age and are affected by direct trauma, brain trauma, and medications. Pathologic conditions that affect the crystalline lens, the ciliary muscle, or cranial nerve III can cause accommodative insufficiency or loss.

Pupil Diameter

The diameter of the pupil is determined by the balance of innervation between the autonomically innervated sphincter and radially arranged dilator muscles. The pupilloconstrictor (parasympathetic) fibers arise in the midbrain and join the oculomotor nerve by way of the short ciliary nerves in order to innervate the iris. They are also accompanied by fibers that innervate the ciliary body. The pupillodilator (sympathetic) fibers arise in the hypothalamus and reach the eye as the long ciliary nerve (48). The size and reaction of the pupil can be affected by age, direct trauma to the globe and optic nerve, brain injury, or medication.

Sensory Fusion Function Assessment

Evaluation of the motor and sensory functions of the visual system is essential for the rehabilitation of the brain-injured patient (24). The system of saccades, pursuits, accommodation, and vergences is principally motoric and dysfunction of any part of this system will cause problems in ocular alignment. There must be sensory input in order for visual functioning, fusion of the two images, and subsequent binocularity to occur (42). A single image is indicative of correspondence. Simultaneous stimulation of noncorresponding retinal elements induces visualization of the points in two directions, or diplopia (double vision). If ocular alignment is disrupted, diplopia may result. Sensory fusion is the unification of corresponding retinal images into a single construct. The separation of the two eyes produces slightly different, horizontally disparate images that are fused by the sensory system to produce a three-dimensional construct (stereopsis). Stereopsis is the ability to visualize the third dimension of depth, which increases the ability to locate objects in space. While easily measured, it can be lost from interruption of sensory fusion functions. Brain-injured patients with fusion and without diplopia commonly have no depth perception (24).

Visual Processing Assessment

The complex visual processing component of the examination is typically performed by the eye care practitioner who, unless specially trained, may be unfamiliar with the patient's cognitive functions and interactions. The occupational therapist, however, is trained to recognize symptoms that may arise from processing dysfunctions and relate them to their affects on the patient's functional ability.

EVALUATION PROTOCOL FOR OCCUPATIONAL THERAPY

The occupational therapist's primary responsibility on the rehabilitation team is to provide treatment interventions designed to compensate for the patient's disability so that the activities of daily living necessary for an independent, productive, and satisfying lifestyle can be performed. In working with a patient who has visual impairment, the therapist's goal in assessment is to determine how the visual impairment interferes with functional adaptation. Whether a patient has a visual deficit that requires therapeutic intervention depends on the life demands of the patient. For example, the demands placed on visual processing for a 19-year-old college student majoring in architecture are quite different from those of an 85-year-old living in a nursing home. In terms of therapeutic intervention, the patient is considered to have a visual deficit if his or her ability to obtain or process visual information has been altered in such a way as to prevent the completion of a necessary activity of daily living. Not all patients with visual impairments will require special remediation efforts.

Because the occupational therapist addresses the patient's ability to perform basic daily living skills, he or she is often the first member of the rehabilitation team to observe that the patient may be experiencing a visual impairment that interferes with function. This frequently places the occupational therapist in the position of recommending further evaluation by an eye care specialist (the ophthalmologist or optometrist). In order to make an appropriate referral, the occupational therapist completes a basic screening of visual function for the purpose of identifying deficiencies that may affect functional performance. The screening assessment may be organized around the concept that visual perceptual processing is organized in a hierarchy of skill levels (35). The foundation in the perceptual hierarchy consists of visual acuity, visual field, and oculomotor function; these are followed in order by visual attention, visual scanning, pattern recognition, and visual memory, culminating in complex visual processing, which enables vision to be used in cognitive processing.

The assessment begins with a basic visual screening to determine if the foundation skills have been affected. A reading card with graduated sizes of print may be used to determine if visual acuity is diminished, a gross assessment of visual field can be completed using a confrontation technique, and oculomotor function can be measured by observing ocular alignment and by observing the patient execute smooth pursuit (tracking) and saccadic eye movements. A deficiency in any of these areas warrants immediate request for an eye examination by the eye care specialist.

Impairments of visual attention and visual scanning are measured together by assessing the patient's ability to initiate a symmetric, organized, efficient, and effective scanning pattern in both personal and extrapersonal space

(35,49). The Behavioral Inattention Test (BIT) (50) can be used to provide a quick screening of visual attention and scanning. The BIT is a standardized test battery that provides a valid and reliable measurement of deficits in visual attention, with a strong correlation to deficits in functional activities (51,52). The Scanboard test developed by Warren (49) can be used to identify deficient scanning strategies in extrapersonal space.

Evaluations that involve a matching component are most often used to assess pattern recognition. A computerized test called Match (Lifesciences software) and created by Gianutsos and Matheson (10) provides an objective assessment of the patient's accuracy and response times for matches where the critical feature of the stimuli varies between the left side, right side, and center. Disruption of higher-level perceptual skills, such as visual memory and complex visual processing, is difficult to accurately distinguish from deficits in other cognitive functions. These high-level visual perceptual skills are also strongly influenced by the presence of deficits in lower-level perceptual skills such as visual field, visual scanning, and attention (53). While standardized tests that measure complex visual processing can be used to affirm the presence of neurologic impairment in the cortical areas that process visual information, they do not necessarily provide information that is useful in determining whether treatment intervention is needed or in designing successful treatment strategies (54). Therefore, its often more useful to measure the patient's ability to complete complex visual processing by observing his or her performance of functional activities that require this level of processing, for example, paying bills, preparing a meal with several dishes, or shopping.

The final aspect of the screening process, and the one that may provide the best indication that the patient has a visual impairment, is careful listening to the patient's complaints about his or her vision and observation of the patient's performance when completing various activities. A list of significant complaints and clinical observations for each area of the visual assessment is provided in Table 19-1. Recording these complaints and observations and comparing them to those observed by other members of the rehabilitation team can assist in making a timely referral to the eye care specialist and can also assist the eye care specialist in selecting appropriate evaluations to measure the patient's visual performance.

CONCLUSIONS

Eye care practitioners typically have not been considered as part of the rehabilitation team. However, given the frequency of visual symptomatology that results from brain injury, they should be integrated as part of an interdisciplinary team. Rehabilitation specialists such as occupational therapists must observe their patient's visual processing systems, coordinate referral to the eye care physician specializing in rehabilitation, and ensure that all recommendations are followed. Ideally these recommendations will be integrated into an overall treatment program. Significant issues need to be addressed in order to implement

Table 19-1: Patient Complaints and Clinical Observations Indicating Visual Impairment

Decreased acuity/contrast
- Print looks fuzzy or blurry; unable to bring print into focus
- Complains that print is too small or too faint to read
- Complains of inability to recognize faces
- Misses curbs, steps, or other objects with low-contrast features
- Requests additional light to perform a task
- Uses hands to guide self around an object
- Unable to accurately distinguish colors of similar hue such as dark blue and black

Oculomotor dysfunction
- Complains of double vision, blurring vision, or shadow when viewing objects
- Complains of blurring when changing focus from near object to distant object and vice versa
- Assumes a consistent, deliberate head position when viewing objects
- Complains print swirling on a page of print after a period of sustained focus
- Complains of difficulty concentrating on tasks requiring sustained focus at a near focal distance
- Eyes appear to turn in or out when viewing objects

Visual field deficit
- Collides with obstacles consistently on one side in an unfamiliar environment
- Complains of disorientation when riding in a car
- Transposes or misread numbers
- Omits or misread letters on one side of words
- Abbreviates scan toward one side when reading a page of print, omitting words on the page
- Complains of being unable to follow events on TV when viewing shows with action

Visual inattention
- Only comments on objects or visual details on one side of a visual scene
- Fails to search environment for relevant information needed to complete a task
- Fails to check work for errors when completing a complex task
- Hesitant to shift eyes across midline when scanning
- Unable to maintain concentration on task requiring attention to visual detail
- Reduced effort in performing tasks

this approach. These include education to recognize symptoms, assistance in therapeutic intervention, availability of interested and educated eye care practitioners, logistics of service and equipment availability, and coding, billing, and reimbursement. The role and interaction of each health care practitioner involved in visual rehabilitation depends on the degree to which these issues are addressed.

REFERENCES

1. Cohen AH, Rein LD. The effect of head trauma on the visual system. The doctor of optometry as a member of the rehabilitation team. *J Am Optom Assoc* 1992;63:530–536.
2. Schlageter K, Gray B, Hall K, et al. Incidence and treatment of visual function in traumatic brain injury. *Brain Inj* 1993;7:439–448.
3. Gianutsos R, Ramsey G, Perlin R. Rehabilitative optometric services for survivors of acquired brain injury. *Arch Phys Med Rehabil* 1988;69:573–578.
4. Ron S, Najenson T, Hary D, Pryworkin W. Eye movements on brain damaged patients. *Scand J Rehabil Med* 1978;10:39–44.
5. Levine D. Unawareness of visual and sensorimotor deficits: a hypothesis. *Brain Cogn* 1990;13:233–281.
6. Baker RS, Epstein AD. Ocular motor abnormalities from head trauma. *Surv Ophthalmol* 1991;35:245–266.
7. Colohan AT, Dacey RG, Alves WM, et al. Neurologic and neurosurgical implications of mild head injury. *J Head Trauma Rehabil* 1986;1(2):13–21.
8. Kay T, Harrington D, Adams R, et al. Definition of mild traumatic brain injury. *J Head Trauma Rehabil* 1993;8:86–87.
9. Hellerstein LF, Freed S. Rehabilitative optometric management of a traumatic brain injury patient. *J Behav Optom* 1994;5:143–148.
10. Gianutsos R, Matheson P. The rehabilitation of visual perceptual disorders attributable to brain injury. In: Meier MJ, Benton AL, Diller L, eds. *Neuropsychological rehabilitation.* New York: Guilford, 1987:202–241.
11. Sergent J. Inferences from unilateral brain damage about normal hemispheric functions in visual pattern recognition. *Psychol Bull* 1984;96:99–115.
12. Zihl J. Rehabilitation of visual impairments in patients with brain damage. In: Kooijam AC, Looijestijn PL, Welling JA, van der Wildt GJ, eds. *Low vision research and new developments in rehabilitation.* Amsterdam: IOS Press, 1994:287–295.
13. LaPlante MP. Prevalence of conditions causing need for assistance in activities of daily living. In: *Data on disability from the National Health Interview Survey, 1983–1985—information use report.* Washington, DC: U.S. National Institute on Disability and Rehabilitation Research, 1988: 212–215.
14. Fletcher DC, Shindell S, Hindman T, Schaffrath M. Low vision rehabilitation: finding capable people behind damaged eyeballs. *West J Med* 1991;154:554–556.
15. Wainapel SF, Kwon YS, Fazzari PJ. Severe visual impairment on a rehabilitation unit: incidence and implications. *Arch Phys Med Rehabil* 1989;70:439–441.
16. DeSylvia DA. Low vision and aging. *Optom Vis Sci* 1990;67:319–322.
17. Regan D, Silver R, Murray TJ. Visual acuity and contrast sensitivity in multiple sclerosis—hidden visual loss. *Brain* 1977;100:563–579.
18. Hess RF, Pointer JS. Spatial and temporal contrast sensitivity in hemianopia: a comparative study of the sighted and blind hemifields. *Brain* 1989;112:871–894.
19. Bodis-Wollner I, Diamond SP. The measurement of spatial contrast sensitivity in cases of blurred vision associated with cerebral lesions. *Brain* 1976;99:695–710.
20. Bulens C, Meerwaldt JD, van der Wildt GJ, Keemink CJ. Spatial contrast sensitivity in unilateral cerebral ischaemic lesion involving the posterior visual pathway. *Brain* 1989;112:507–520.
21. Warren M, Lampert J. Considerations in addressing the daily living needs in older persons with low vision. *Ophthalmol Clin North Am* 1994;7:187–196.
22. Colenbrander A. The basic low vision evaluation. *Ophthalmol Clin North Am* 1994;7:151–162.
23. Zihl J. Visual scanning behavior in patients with homonymous hemianopia. *Neuropsychologia* 1995;33:287–303.
24. Neger RE. The evaluation of diplopia in head trauma. *J Head Trauma Rehabil* 1989;4(2):27–34.
25. Padula WV, Shapiro JB, Jasin P. Head injury causing post trauma vision syndrome. *N Engl J Optom* 1988;41:16–21.
26. Bogousslavsky J, Meienberg O. Eye-movement disorders in brain stem and cerebellar stroke. *Arch Neurol* 1987;44:141–148.
27. Kerkhoff G, Stogerer E. Recovery of fusional convergence after systematic practice. *Brain Inj* 1994;8:15–22.
28. Mesulam MM. A cortical network for directed attention and unilateral neglect. *Ann Neurol* 1981;10:309–325.
29. Posner MI, Peterson SE, Fox PT, Raichle ME. Localization of cognitive operations in the human brain. *Science* 1988;240:1627–1631.
30. Corbetta M, Miezin FM, Shulman GL, Petersen SE. A PET study of

visuospatial attention. *J Neurosci* 1993;13:1202–1226.

31. Spiers PA, Schomer DL, Blume HW, et al. Visual neglect during intracarotid amobarbital testing. *Neurology* 1990;40:1600–1606.

32. Palmer T, Tzeng OJL. Cerebral asymmetry in visual attention. *Brain Cogn* 1990;13:46–58.

33. Mishkin M, Ungerleider LG, Macko KA. Object vision and spatial vision: two cortical pathways. *Trends Neurosci* 1983;6:414–417.

34. Gross CG, Graziano MSA. Multiple representations of space in the brain. *Neuroscientist* 1995;1(1):43–49.

35. Warren M. A hierarchical model for evaluation and treatment of visual perceptual dysfunction in adult acquired brain injury: parts 1 & 2. *Am J Occup Ther* 1993;47:42–66.

36. Gianutsos R, Ramsey G. Enabling rehabilitation optometrists to help survivors of acquired brain injury. *J Vision Rehabil* 1988;2:37–58.

37. Falk NS, Aksionoff EB. The primary care optometrist evaluation of the traumatic brain injury patient. *J Am Optom Assoc* 1992;63:547–552.

38. Ginsburg A. The evaluation of contact lenses and refractive surgery using contrast sensitivity. In: *Contact lenses: CLAO guide to basic science & clinical practice update #2*. Orlando: Grune & Stratton, 1987;56:1–17.

39. Rubin GS. Assessment of visual function in eyes with vision loss. *Ophthalmol Clin North Am* 1989;2:357–367.

40. Campbell FW. Why do we measure contrast sensitivity? *Behav Brain Res* 1983;10:87–97.

41. Koch DD. Glare and contrast sensitivity for the clinician. *Ophthalmol Clin North Am* 1989;2:415–429.

42. Griffin JR. Efficient visual skills. In: *Binocular anomalies*. 2nd ed. Boston: Butterworth–Heinemann, 1982:345.

43. Skarf B. Clinical use of visual evoked potentials. *Ophthalmol Clin North Am* 1989;2:499–518.

44. Sherman J. How to maximize the potential of VEP's. *Rev Optom* 1995;132(5):77–81.

45. Gottlieb DD, Freeman P, Williams M. Clinical research and statistical analysis of a visual field awareness system. *J Am Optom Assoc* 1992;63:581–588.

46. Slavin ML. Functional vision loss. Focal points. *Clin Modules Ophthalmol* 1991;9(2):1–12.

47. Cohen M, Grosswasser Z, Barchadski R, Appel A. Convergence insufficiency in brain-injured patients. *Brain Inj* 1989;3:187–189.

48. Adams RA, Victor M. Disorders of pupillary movement and ocular function. In: *Principles of neurology*. 5th ed. New York: McGraw-Hill, 1993:225–246.

49. Warren M. Identification of visual scanning deficits in adults after cerebrovascular accident. *Am J Occup Ther* 1991;44:391–399.

50. Wilson B, Cockburn J, Halligan P. Development of a behavioral test of visuospatial neglect. *Arch Phys Med Rehabil* 1987;68:98–102.

51. Hartman-Maeir A, Katz N. Validity of the behavioral inattention test (bit): relationships with functional tasks. *Am J Occup Ther* 1995;46:507–516.

52. Chen Sea MJ, Henderson A, Cermak SA. Patterns of visual spatial inattention and their functional significance in stroke patients. *Arch Phys Med Rehabil* 1993;74:355–360.

53. Locher PJ, Bigelow DL. Visual exploratory activity of hemiplegic patients viewing the motor-free visual perception test. *Percept Mot Skills* 1983;57:91–100.

54. Toglia JP. Visual perception of objects: an approach to assessment and intervention. *Am J Occup Ther* 1989;43:587–596.

Chapter 20

Cardiopulmonary Assessment

Matthew N. Bartels

CARDIOPULMONARY HISTORY AND PHYSICAL EXAMINATION

The cardiopulmonary history and physical examination are important parts of the evaluation of the patient with cardiopulmonary disease who is to undergo cardiac or pulmonary rehabilitation. The history often will reveal very important issues to be addressed and will give the treating physiatrist the information needed to develop and direct a rehabilitation program. As the patient establishes a relationship of trust with the physician, concerns and goals can be discussed more openly. This can allow the patient and physician to establish mutual goals, resulting in improved compliance. The family or caregivers can often substantiate or give additional information, especially concerning functional limitations and disability, family dynamics, and the effect of the cardiopulmonary illness on the patient's performance of his or her role in the community. This historical information can help to limit further diagnostic testing and can help with the interpretation of the results obtained.

The History

As with all medical history taking, the cardiopulmonary history should include an evaluation of the symptoms and prior medical care. A complete review of systems should be performed and a complete medical history should be obtained to rule out any other compounding factors in the patient's medical condition. It is not uncommon for a systemic medical illness to manifest primarily through cardiac or pulmonary illness. Examples of these include thyroid and rheumatologic conditions. There are also many noncardiopulmonary manifestations of heart and lung disease that should not be overlooked. Table 20-1 provides examples of these types of complications. Concurrent illnesses and disabilities also need to be taken into account when designing the rehabilitation program. In the disabled population, arthritis, amputations, stroke, and neuropathies are common. The functional history, occupational history, social history, and personal habits should be verified to ensure a realistic goal for the eventual rehabilitation outcome. A 50-year-old patient who was sedate, overweight, and unemployed does not have the same anticipated recovery as the active 50-year-old who jogged 3 miles a day. Also, the patient in an urban setting who lives in a fifth-floor walk-up apartment and has developed emphysema has a different rehabilitation problem than the nursing home resident who is confined to a wheelchair. A history of cooperation of the family and other caregivers in aiding the patient allows discussion of any adaptations and alterations in the patient's and family's life that may need to be made. Important historical considerations are noted in Table 20-2.

In taking the cardiopulmonary history, the clinician needs to direct special attention to the nature of the symptoms at rest and during activity and the effect of the symptoms on activities. Visual and verbal cues such as evidence of depression, anxiety, evasiveness, denial, and the relation-

Table 20-1: Cardiopulmonary Complications

Cardiac	Pulmonary
Embolic events	Polycythemia
Stroke	Cachexia
Renal failure	Cancer
Cardiac cachexia	Pulmonary hypertension
Pulmonary hypertension	

Table 20-2: Issues to Address in the History of a Patient with Cardiopulmonary Disease

- Family history
  - Premature coronary artery disease (before age 55 in a first-degree relative)
  - Family history of familial hypercholesterolemia or hyperlipidemia
  - Family history of sudden death
  - Family history of arrhythmias
  - Family history of pulmonary disease
  - Family history of chronic obstructive pulmonary disease
- Social history
  - Cigarette use, cigar/pipe use
  - Sedentary lifestyle
  - Alcohol abuse history
- Symptom history
  - Chest pain: duration, location, character, precipitating and relieving factors, radiation
  - Shortness of breath: duration, precipitating and relieving factors, day or night, position
  - Dizziness/light-headedness
  - Syncope
  - Presence of nausea/vomiting, anorexia, weight loss
  - Cyanosis/pallor
  - Palpitations
  - Edema
  - Cough
  - Hemoptysis
  - Fatigue
- Functional history
  - Prior level of activity
  - Present level of activity
  - Exercise tolerance level
  - Level of activity required at home and at work
  - Stability of level of function
  - Extent and rate of activities performed
- Patient goals
  - Vocational plans
  - Leisure activities
  - Emotional adaptation to the cardiac condition
- Medications
- Complete review of systems and past medical history

ship between the patient and caregiver can add important data that will help in designing the appropriate program. The best approach to the new patient is an open-minded one, never assuming that the past evaluations are correct and complete. The several important components specific to the cardiopulmonary history are discussed in textbooks on the physical examination and those specific to both cardiac and pulmonary disease. Some of the more common findings are discussed here.

Dyspnea

Shortness of breath (SOB) is one of the central symptoms in a patient with cardiopulmonary disease. The history of dyspnea needs to be complete to enable the physician to make a good assessment of the cardiac status of the patient. The history can also allow for a reasonable assessment of exercise tolerance of the patient in the community.

The distinction between acute and subacute SOB is important to make, as an acute onset of SOB often indicates a pulmonary rather than a cardiac etiology for the dyspnea. Pulmonary causes of SOB include pulmonary embolus, pneumothorax, bronchospasm, and aspiration. Flash pulmonary edema is one of the few purely cardiac causes of acute SOB. Subacute SOB can be caused by both pulmonary and cardiac factors, including pneumonia and cardiac conditions such as angina, idiopathic subaortic stenosis (IHSS), and valvular disease. Table 20-3 lists some of the causes of dyspnea. Exertional dyspnea also has a legion of causes that often can be differentiated with careful history taking, limiting the amount of work-up a patient will face and allowing an appropriate program of rehabilitation to be designed.

Chest Pain

Chest pain, tightness, and burning are the classic symptoms reported by a patient with coronary artery disease (CAD). Table 20-4 outlines some of the features distinguishing cardiac from noncardiac causes of chest pain. Of particular interest to the physiatrist are the possible precipitating factors for chest pain, as these will assist in the design of a therapy program that relates to the patient's functional limitations.

Physical Examination

The cardiac and pulmonary examination is an important part of the diagnostic evaluation of the cardiopulmonary patient as well as all patients being considered for rehabilitation. The basics of the cardiopulmonary examination are found in numerous texts and review articles. It is important to remember that the patient may have noncardiopulmonary findings related to underlying cardiac or pulmonary disease. For example, conditions such as ankylosing spondylitis are associated with aortic valve disease or conduction defects; patients with Down syndrome may have associated cardiac abnormalities;

Table 20-3: Causes of Dyspnea

Disorder	Site of Pathology	Pathophysiology
Airflow limitation	Lung	Mechanical limitation to ventilation
Restriction (intrinsic)	Lung	Poor lung compliance
Restriction (extrinsic)	Chest wall	Poor chest wall compliance
Valvular disease	Heart	Limited cardiac output
Coronary disease	Heart	Coronary insufficiency
Heart failure	Heart	Limited cardiac output
Anemia	Blood	Limited oxygen-carrying capacity
Peripheral circulation	Peripheral vessels	Inadequate oxygen supply to metabolically active tissues
Obesity	Adipose tissue	Increased work of movement Respiratory restriction if severe
Psychogenic	Emotional	Hyperventilation
Deconditioning	Multiple organ systems	Loss of ability to effectively distribute systemic blood flow
Malingering	Emotional	Inconsistent results
Acute pulmonary disease	Lungs	Increased V/Q mismatch

myasthenia gravis and other neuromuscular diseases are often related to cardiomyopathy or pulmonary restrictive disease.

Conclusions

Although the cardiopulmonary history and examination are important in the detection of cardiac and pulmonary disease and in the determination of prognosis, the new imaging and testing techniques available offer the best assessment of the patient's true cardiopulmonary status. Still, the detection of patients at risk for complications in a cardiopulmonary rehabilitation program can often be started in the physiatrist's office. The basic history and physical examination are crucial to developing the appropriate treatment plan. This is especially true in this era of cost concerns, so that patients with subtle findings can get limited appropriate testing, leading to a diagnosis and treatment best suited to their condition.

ASSESSMENT OF CARDIAC FUNCTION

Cardiac Exercise Tolerance Testing

In the post-myocardial infarction (MI) or at-risk CAD patient, cardiac stress testing has become the hallmark for ischemic risk stratification and diagnosis. The use of graded exercise testing in the assessment of functional capacity and for prognosis goes back to at least 1964 (1). The accuracy and the sophistication of the testing have advanced significantly since then. Cardiac stress testing is now used in the evaluation of syncope, in patients with congestive heart failure (CHF), and to evaluate for risk of arrhythmias. Besides the classic exercise treadmill test, there are many newer techniques for cardiac evaluation, such as signal-averaged electrocardiography (ECG), electrophysiologic testing, and pharmacologic and radionuclide stress testing. These tests can be applied to patients with physical disabilities, broadening the scope of patients who can be tested and allowing the physiatrist to better assess the cardiac status of all patients. The techniques vary in the methods of application of cardiac stress and in the

Table 20-4: Cardiac Versus Noncardiac Chest Pain

Cardiac Pain Symptoms	Noncardiac Pain Symptoms
Pain quality	
Constricting/squeezing	Dull aching
Visceral quality	Sharp, stabbing, piercing, knife-like
Burning	Muscular
Heaviness	
Pain location	
Substernal	Left submammary area, apex of heart
Across precordium	Superficial tissues of the left side of the chest
Neck	Right lower part of the chest
One or both shoulders, arms	Very discrete localization possible
Intrascapular region	
One or both forearms, hands	
Epigastrium	
Pain duration	
Angina, 2–10 min	<20 sec
Infarction, >20 min to 24 hr	Persistent without change for >24–48 hr
Precipitating and aggravating factors	
Exercise, particularly with hurrying	After the completion of exercise
Excitement	With specific body positions, chest wall movement and respiration
Cold temperature exposure	With direct palpation of the chest wall
Stressful stimuli	Spontaneous
Postprandially, after a heavy meal	Head and neck movement
	During fasting, with cold liquids
Relieving factors	
Rest	Antacids
Nitroglycerin	Food
	Nonsteroidal analgesia

Table 20-5: Indications for Exercise Stress Testing

Clear indication
1. Men with atypical symptoms for diagnosis
2. Prognosis and cardiac risk assessment in patients with
   a. Chronic stable angina
   b. Myocardial infarction
3. Symptomatic exercise-induced arrhythmias
4. Evaluation after coronary revascularization procedure

May be indicated
1. Women with typical or atypical symptoms for diagnosis
2. Functional capacity evaluation in patients with CAD or CHF to monitor cardiovascular therapy
3. Evaluation of patients with variant angina
4. Annual follow-up of patients with known CAD
5. Evaluation of selected asymptomatic men over 40:
   a. Special occupations (pilots, firemen, police officers, bus/truck drivers, railroad engineers)
   b. Men with two or more CAD risk factors who will enter a vigorous exercise training program

Probably not indicated
1. Patients with isolated PVCs and no evidence of CAD
2. Multiple serial testing during a cardiac rehabilitation program
3. Diagnosis of CAD in patients with pre-excitation, with LBBB, or on digitalis therapy
4. Young to middle-aged men and women who are asymptomatic with:
   a. No atherosclerotic risk factors, or
   b. Noncardiac chest discomfort

Indications for patients with valvular heart disease
1. Evaluation of functional capacity in selected patients
2. Blood pressure evaluation of hypertensive patients who plan to pursue vigorous dynamic or static exercise

CAD = coronary artery disease; CHF = congestive heart failure; PVCs = premature ventricular contractions; LBBB = left bundle branch block.

evaluation of the response of the myocardium. The sensitivity and the specificity of these new tests are the same or better than those of classic stress testing. The following sections discuss the classic method of exercise testing and the variants.

Exercise Stress Testing

Although other more modern tests are now used to diagnose cardiac ischemia, the exercise stress test is still the most commonly used test to perform cardiac risk stratification and to determine functional capacity. The American Heart Association (AHA) and American College of Cardiology (ACC) Exercise Task Force in 1986 determined the indications for exercise stress testing based on the existing literature, dividing patients into the following categories:

Table 20-6: Contraindications to Exercise Testing

Absolute cardiac contraindications
1. Unstable angina with recent chest pain
2. Untreated life-threatening cardiac arrhythmias
3. Uncompensated congestive heart failure
4. Advanced atrioventricular block
5. Acute myocarditis or pericarditis
6. Critical aortic stenosis
7. Severe hypertrophic obstructive cardiomyopathy
8. Uncontrolled hypertension
9. Acute myocardial Infarction
10. Active endocarditis

Absolute noncardiac contraindications to exercise testing
1. Severe physical handicap or disability
2. Acute pulmonary embolus or pulmonary infarction
3. Acute systemic illness

Relative contraindications
1. Less serious noncardiac test
2. Significant pulmonary hypertension
3. Significant arterial hypertension
4. Tachyarrhythmias or bradyarrhythmias
5. Moderate valvular heart disease
6. Myocardial heart disease
7. Electrolyte abnormalities
8. Left main coronary obstruction
9. Hypertrophic cardiomyopathy
10. Psychiatric disease

those for whom testing is clearly indicated, patients for whom testing may be indicated, and those for whom testing probably is not indicated (Table 20-5) (2). There are also contraindications to exercise stress testing (Table 20-6). Some of the noncardiac contraindications can be overcome with the newer techniques of applying cardiac stress or recording the responses. The cardiac factors cannot be overcome by any means (3).

Exercise Physiology

The basic principle of the exercise stress test is to exercise to increase the physiologic demand on the myocardium and increase the myocardial oxygen demand (VO_2). This can provoke ischemic changes on the ECG. The exercise stress test can also be used to determine the maximum heart rate (MHR) that an individual can achieve. The normal physiologic responses to cardiac stress testing are as follows:

1. Anticipation of exercise leads to an acceleration of ventricular rate, increase in alveolar ventilation, and increased venous return. The net effect is increased resting cardiac output.
2. In early exercise, cardiac output increases due to augmented stroke volume via the Frank-Starling mechanism.
3. In late exercise, cardiac output is increased primarily through an increase in ventricular rate (4).

4. During strenuous exercise, sympathetic discharge is at maximum and parasympathetic stimulation is at minimum.
5. With exercise, systolic blood pressure (BP), systemic systolic BP, mean arterial pressure (MAP), and pulse pressure increase.
6. Cardiac output increases four to six times normal at maximal exercise.
7. After exercise, hemodynamics return to baseline within minutes of cessation of exercise. Oxygen (O_2) debt (total O_2 uptake in excess of the resting O_2 uptake during recovery) is resolved.

As a rule, the true MHR for an individual can only be determined through an exercise stress test; however, an estimation of the maximum achievable heart rate can be calculated by using the formula: MHR = 220 − age (in years) of patient. This estimation of MHR has a standard deviation of 10 to 12 beats/min (5).

Exercise Protocols

The two main types of exercise are isotonic (dynamic) and isometric (static) exercise. Exercise protocols are normally designed to be 6 to 10 minutes in duration in order to achieve a sufficient level of myocardial VO_2 to be of diagnostic and prognostic use (5). Usually protocols include a warm-up period of low-intensity exercise, and end with a cool-down period of suitable length to allow normal recovery. The exercise protocol needs to be tailored to the individual patient and is adapted to test patients with very limited reserve as well as patients with excellent aerobic conditioning. Sometimes a protocol may be designed to test a patient at a certain intensity of exercise to assess minimal qualifications for certain industrial tasks or sports programs (6).

Preparation

Although the techniques of stress testing may vary slightly from laboratory to laboratory, there are some basic rules that generally apply. Patients should not eat for at least 3 hours before a stress test, and should have no caffeinated beverages for up to 24 hours before the stress test. Patients should wear comfortable loose-fitting clothes and comfortable walking shoes. A 12-lead ECG is obtained before the start of the test and a limited physical examination is performed. Usually the ECG is obtained with torso electrodes while the patient is supine and then erect, to ensure that there are no changes on the ECG solely based on positional changes. The patient is taught how to walk on the treadmill. Vital signs and the ECG are recorded before, after, and at each stage of the test. Every minute during the first 5 to 10 minutes of the recovery, the ECG and vital signs are also recorded. The patient can be either in the supine or in the seated position during the recovery.

Table 20-7: Bruce Protocol

Stage*	Grade (%)	Speed (MPH)	Time (min)	Total Time
Warm-up 1	0	1.7	3	NA
Warm-up 2	5	1.7	3	NA
1	10	1.7	3	3
2	12	2.5	3	6
3	14	3.4	3	9
4	16	4.2	3	12
5	18	5.0	3+	15+

*For each stage, both the grade and the speed are increased every 3 minutes. NA = not applicable.

Treadmill Protocols

The most commonly used and one of the best treadmill protocols is the Bruce protocol (7,8), which is outlined in Table 20-7. The Bruce protocol is divided into 3-minute subsections which start with two warm-up stages, one with the treadmill speed at 1.7 mph and the ramp grade at 0%, followed by one at the same speed and the ramp grade at 5%. The patient stays at each stage for 3 minutes to achieve steady state before attempting the next level. The limitations in this protocol are in the large increases in VO_2 (5 METs) between stages and the additional cost of energy in running during stage 3 and higher (6). In order to overcome some of these limitations, especially in patients with disability or limited cardiac reserve, some other protocols are available.

The Naughton, Weber, and Balke-Ware protocols use 1- to 2-minute stages which have 1-MET increments and can sometimes be better tolerated by patients with CHF, deconditioning, or other causes of limited exercise tolerance. The Cornell protocol is a modification of the Bruce protocol with increments in 2-minute stages, allowing a better estimate of ST-segment and heart rate measurements (9). Table 20-8 compares some of the more commonly used protocols.

Ramp Protocols

The goal of ramp protocols is to assess cardiovascular fitness. As opposed to the treadmill protocols, the patient never achieves a steady state and the rate of work continually increases. The estimates of VO_2 are more precise than with standard treadmill testing. The protocols are executed by starting the patient at a slow treadmill speed, and then increasing it to a good stride. The angle of incline is steadily increased every 10 to 60 seconds until at 6 to 10 minutes, the patient's calculated functional capacity is reached (10). An equation (11) by which the VO_2 may be estimated in a treadmill test is:

$$VO_2(\text{mL } O_2/\text{kg}/\text{min}) = (\text{mph} \times 2.68) + (1.8 \times 26.82 \times \text{mph} \times \text{grade} \div 100) + 3.5$$

Table 20-8: Comparison of Exercise Tolerance Testing

	Bruce	Cornell	Weber	Balke-Ware	Naughton
Time of stages	3 min	2 min	2 min	1 min	2 min
MET level	2–16	2–16	1–10	4–16	2–7 to 2 mph 3–16 at 3 mph 4–16 at 3.4 mph
Step changes	2 MET steps from 2 to 7 MET 3 MET steps from 7 to >16 MET	2 MET	1 MET	1/2 MET	1 MET
Changes grade	Yes	Yes	Yes	Yes	Yes
Range of grade	0%–20%	0%–18%	0%–15%	1%–26%	0%–17.5% at 2 mph 0%–32.5% at 3 mph 0%–26% at 4 mph
Step changes	5% from 0% to 10% 2% from 10% to 20%	5% from 0% to 10% 1% from 10% to 18%	3.5% from 0% to 10.5% (2 mph) 2.5% from 7.5% to 15% (3 mph) 14% fixed at 3.4 mph	1% from 1% to 26%	3.5% from 0% to 17.5% (2 mph) 2.5% from 0% to 32.5% (3 mph) 2% from 2% to 26% (3.4 mph)
Changes speed	Yes	Yes	Yes	No	No
Range of speed	1.7–5.5 mph	1.7–5.0 mph	1.0–3.4 mph	Constant 3.3 mph	2, 3, or 4 mph
Step changes	0.8 mph	0.4 mph	0.5 mph		
NYHA functional classes tested	Normal, I, II, III	Normal, I, II, III	Normal, I, II, III, IV	Normal, I, II, mild III	Normal, I, II, III

Finally, in all exercise treadmill tests, it is important that the patient does not hold the handrail, as functional capacity can be overestimated by as much as 20% and the VO_2 is decreased (12).

Interpretation of Results

Electrocardiographic Criteria

The normal lead placement in cardiac stress testing is based on the modified 12-lead system. The bipolar lead group is useful in functional cardiac stress testing for rehabilitation programs, as a limited amount of information regarding ischemia is sought.

The hallmark of ischemia on the exercise cardiogram is ST-segment depression of 2 mm or more in one lead (12). Not all ST-segment depression is of cardiac origin, and causes can include left ventricular hypertrophy (LVH) and ventricular pre-excitation (Table 20-9) (12).

Table 20-9: Causes of ST-Segment Depression

Cardiac Causes	Noncardiac Causes
Cardiomyopathy	Severe aortic stenosis
Digitalis	Severe hypertension
Left ventricular hypertrophy	Anemia
Mitral valve prolapse	Hypokalemia
Intraventricular conduction delay	Sudden excessive exercise
Pre-excitation	Glucose load
Supraventricular tachyarrhythmias	Hyperventilation
	Severe volume overload

ST-segment elevation, upsloping ST segments, and variation of the R-wave amplitude are also seen in patients during exercise stress testing. ST-segment elevation in a lead with an abnormal Q wave can be seen in patients with poor left ventricular function (13). ST-segment elevation in these Q-wave leads is not a marker of cardiac ischemia (14). In the absence of a previous MI or Q wave, ST-segment elevation is a marker of high-grade stenosis or coronary vasospasm causing transmural ischemia. It is a rare finding, seen in only approximately 1% of patients.

Upsloping ST segment are normal findings on the ECG during maximum exercise. The finding of a slowly upsloping ST segment after a >1.5-mm ST-segment depression is an indicator of probable ischemia (15). The changes in R-wave amplitude during exercise are relatively nonspecific. When the R wave meets the criteria for LVH, the ST-segment response is not usable for a diagnosis of ischemia, and in post-MI patients, loss of the R wave in a lead reduces the prognostic use of that particular lead for ischemic changes.

Nonelectrocardiographic Criteria

In addition to the ECG, there are many other clinical factors to observe during the performance of the exercise stress test. The BP, postexercise systolic BP, and symptoms of chest discomfort are also important indicators in a stress test. The items of information that are particularly useful

Table 20-10: Nonischemic Causes of a Fall in Systolic Blood Pressure

Cardiomyopathy
Cardiac arrhythmias
Vasovagal reaction
Left ventricular outflow tract obstruction
Antihypertensive drugs
Hypovolemia
Prolonged vigorous exercise

to the physiatrist are the maximal work capacity, the rate-pressure product, and the heart rate response. Each of these is briefly considered.

The BP during normal exercise increases progressively to a peak of 160 to 220 mm Hg. In older patients, the BPs are in the higher range due to poorly compliant vascular systems (5,7,8). The diastolic BP does not change significantly in normal patients; if changes are present, they may be an indicator of ischemia. In patients with pump failure or three-vessel or left main coronary disease, the BP may not increase above 120 mmHg, or may even decrease. In the presence of CAD, this can be evidence of significant coronary ischemia (7,8). The nonischemic causes of decreases in systolic BP during exercise testing are outlined in Table 20-10.

After exercise, there should be a gradual decline in the systolic BP. According to some reports in the literature, when the ratio of the systolic BP at 3 minutes after exercise to the peak exercise systolic BP is >0.9, there may be a greater extent of myocardial ischemia with an associated risk of more extensive cardiac damage (16). Healthy normal adults may have an episode of profound postexercise hypotension that is not due to CAD. In one study, up to 3.1% of subjects younger than 55 years and 0.3% of subjects older than 55 years had postexertional hypotension (17). In follow-up, none of these subjects had a cardiac event in 4 years.

In some patients, chest pain may be the only indicator of ischemia, and the ECG may remain normal. In most cases, the chest pain will start after the onset of ST-segment depression, and diastolic BP may increase (18). The presence of pain with no ECG changes is often an indication for thallium scintigraphy.

The maximal work capacity can be determined in the stress test and is an important prognostic measurement. It also determines the maximal work that can be performed by the patient during a rehabilitation program (19–21). A limited exercise capacity in a patient with known cardiac disease is associated with an increased risk of cardiac events and worse prognosis. The best estimate of functional capacity is the amount of work performed or the level reached on a given protocol. The exercise impairment is determined by comparing the patient's performance to a table of normal levels adjusted for age, which is available in the literature specific to the exercise protocol employed (22). If serial tests of exercise capacity are to be performed, the patient needs to follow the exact same protocol, preferably administered by the same testing team, as small variations can easily occur, owing to technical factors.

The other quantitative variable that can be determined during an exercise test is the rate-pressure product. The rate-pressure product increases progressively with exercise, and the peak value can be used as an estimate of maximum cardiovascular performance. In normal patients, the peak value is in the range of 20 to 35 mm Hg × beats/min × 10^{-3}. In patients with CAD, the peak value does not usually exceed 25 mm Hg × beats/min × 10^{-3}, and many factors including deconditioning and pulmonary disease can limit the rate-pressure product (12).

Alternative Cardiac Stress Testing

Recently, there have been numerous additions to the armamentarium of procedures that are available for cardiac stress testing. These new variations can be roughly divided into two areas: those that apply the cardiac stress in a different way and those that measure the effects of cardiac stress in a different way. The new techniques of applying a cardiac stress allow for the testing of disabled and debilitated individuals, and overcome anxiety, poor patient effort, peripheral vascular disease, as well as orthopedic and neurologic limitations. The new techniques of detecting cardiac ischemia have the benefits of allowing testing in patients who previously had obstacles to assessment, such as those with left bundle branch block, and those who had atypical findings on standard ECG test. These two new variations in techniques can be combined or used separately in selected patients.

Bicycle Ergometry

The most common variation to the treadmill protocols is bicycle ergometry, which offers several advantages. The patient's chest and arms remain relatively stable, allowing for better ECG and BP recording during the test. The influence of the patient's weight is also less, and a bicycle will often take up less room in the laboratory. With bicycle ergometry, the test can be done with the patient supine, which may be an advantage in some patients. There are also some disadvantages, including a decreased ability to gradually increase the patient's effort, compared to a treadmill where gradually increasing the incline is easy to do. These are also patients who have difficulty with pedaling a bicycle due to either incoordination or fatigue (23). During testing on a bicycle ergometer, the rate-pressure product and systolic BP are higher at a given level of submaximal O_2 consumption. The maximum myocardial consumption, however, is approximately 10% higher during the treadmill test (24). See Table 20-11 for a comparison of testing protocols.

Table 20-11: Pros and Cons of Alternative Test Devices

Test	Bicycle Ergometry	Upper-Extremity Ergometry	Treadmill	Pharmacologic Agents
Advantages	Has good correlation with treadmill testing Thorax and arms remain stable Less effect of patient body weight	Useful for patients with orthopedic, vascular, or neurologic conditions who cannot perform leg exercise	Readily available Well standardized Multiple protocols available Can be used for ramp protocols	Can be used in all patients, even the most deconditioned or impaired Good reliability Well standardized
Disadvantages	Patient may not be able to learn to bicycle Myocardial VO_2 6%–25% less than in treadmill exercise Greater cardiac stress (rate-pressure product) for a given myocardial VO_2 Bicycle takes space in the lab	Less increase in cardiac output than in treadmill testing Greater rate-pressure product increase than in treadmill testing	Overweight, orthopedic, neurologic, vascular, or arthritic patients may not be able to reach acceptable exercise levels	Not physiologic Some risks involved, depending on the agent Invasive Need to have special imaging equipment and and properly equipped and staffed lab

Upper-Arm Ergometry

This form of cardiac stress test has been commonly used in patients who have orthopedic, vascular, or neurologic disabilities that do not permit them to perform the standard treadmill test (25). In the disabled population, these patients are represented by lower-limb amputees, paraplegics, and patients with arthritis or other orthopedic conditions. Because of the poor sensitivity of ECG recording alone with upper-extremity ergometry, the test is usually performed with thallium-201 scintigraphy (26). The physiology of upper-extremity ergometry is different from that seen with treadmill exercise testing. The rate-pressure product is elevated more in upper-extremity ergometry, because of a greater increase in the systolic BP than in the heart rate. This effect is thought to be due to the increase in vascular tone seen in the nonexercising vascular beds. There is also less of an increase in cardiac output in subjects during upper-extremity ergometry than during treadmill exercise testing (27). The advantages of the upper-extremity ergometry test are predominantly in the disabled population. The test is an easy adaptation of the standard stress test, and only requires the purchase of an upper-extremity ergometer to be used in any laboratory that can perform thallium testing. The test physiology is also appropriate for patients who are disabled and wheelchair bound or using extensive upper-extremity effort to ambulate with assistive devices. This can help in risk stratification and in the design of a cardiac rehabilitation program in the disabled population. The disadvantages of the test include the need for the somewhat invasive thallium-201 imaging (discussed later), the altered physiology of arm ergometry, and the degree of upper-extremity exercise conditioning prior to the test, which may limit the amount of stress that can be generated in some patient populations.

Pharmacologic Stress Testing

Among the most common and perhaps the best types of cardiac testing available for patients with physical impairments are the pharmacologic stress tests. The earliest tests performed with pharmacologic agents were limited to the use of dipyridamole, but in recent years other agents have been added to the armamentarium and have gained acceptance. The general benefit of using these agents for cardiac stress testing is that a patient can be tested regardless of his or her ability to perform adequate levels of exercise. The usual protocols call for a form of cardiac imaging and follow distinct protocols. Three main agents are profiled briefly: dipyridamole, dobutamine, and adenosine.

Dipyridamole

Dipyridamole has been well studied as a pharmacologic agent to induce cardiac stress, most often used in conjunction with thallium-201 scintigraphy (28,29). It has been used for detection of CAD, cardiac risk stratification, and perioperative risk evaluation. Protocols for the use of thallium-201 scintigraphy with dipyridamole and the simultaneous application of isometric handgrip or low-level exercise to increase the accuracy of the test have been proposed (30,31). This test in particularly useful in patients who are unable to exercise. In more recent developments, dipyridamole was used in combination with new imaging techniques, including two-dimensional echocardiography and magnetic resonance imaging (MRI) (32–35).

The mechanism of action of dipyridamole is via its activity as a coronary artery vasodilator, especially of the smaller arterioles (36). Although the mechanism has not been clearly elucidated, the coronary blood vessels appear to dilate through an increase in plasma adenosine (37). In research, dipyridamole was shown to block the transmembrane uptake and transport of adenosine in myocardial cells, and to inhibit adenosine deaminase, preventing the conversion of adenosine to adenine. There is also an increase in the accumulation of cyclic adenosine monophosphate (cAMP) in vascular cells through the inhibition of phosphodiesterase, causing further vasodilation. Dipyridamole can be administered by mouth or intravenously. It is excreted in the biliary tract after being formed into its glucuronide conjugate and undergoes reabsorption via enterohepatic circulation. An administered dose has a half-life of 10 hours (37).

The develpment of ischemia in the cardiac vessels is through differential vasodilation of the cardiac arteries and arterioles. Normal vessels will dilate and cause a decrease in the vascular resistance of the coronary bed with a subsequent increase in coronary blood flow. In normal coronary arteries, this increase in blood flow can be as much as four to five times the normal resting blood flow and is known as the *pharmacologic vasodilator reserve* (38–40). In areas of significant CAD, the distal vessels already have a degree of vasodilatation, causing a resultant decrease in vasodilator reserve so that a dose of dipyridamole can result in a perfusion maldistribution, described in some portions of the cardiac literature as *cardiac steal.* If the absolute perfusion of the subendocardium is lower than that at rest, the resulting ischemia is caused by the loss of sufficient pressure over the stenotic segment due to vasodilation and a pressure decrease in the normal vessels. This is called *subendocardial steal, endocardial-epicardial steal, vertical steal,* or *intracoronary steal* by different authors in the literature (41–44). *Classic steal* can occur when in the presence of collateral vessels, there is a loss of perfusion pressure at the head of the collaterals due to vasodilation of the donor artery, with more flow going to the natural distribution of that artery (45). Using the fact that any differential between vessel blood flow greater than 2:1 can be seen by thallium-201 imaging, one can detect the heterogeneity of blood flow created by inducing steal with dipyridamole (40).

The other pharmacologic effects on cardiovascular physiology are small. There is a small increase in rate-pressure product due to some systemic vasodilation, but dipyridamole is a relatively selective coronary vasodilator (28,29,46,47). There may be a mild reflex increase in heart rate due to the small systemic decrease in BP, with a small increase in cardiac output. This results in a small increase in myocardial VO_2; however, the primary induction of ischemia is via the creation of subendocardial ischemia by the steal mechanisms just described.

There are both cardiac and noncardiac side effects to dipyridamole, with the noncardiac side effects being far more common. The potential cardiac side effects include MI, ST-segment depression, angina, and arrhythmias. The noncardiac side effects are mostly attributable to the systemic vasodilation induced by dipyridamole, and include headaches, nausea, flushing, dizziness, dyspepsia, and epigastric pain (48). The noncardiac side effects are usually transient and usually do not require treatment. A rare but alarming side effect of dipyridamole testing is bronchospasm after intravenous administration. Intravenous aminophylline administration rapidly reverses the bronchospasm, by blocking the adenosine receptors and negating the effect of dipyridamole (49,50). In episodes of severe cardiac side effects, a combination of aminophylline and nitroglycerin may be required. The interaction of xanthine compounds and dipyridamole must be kept in mind when considering patients for pharmacologic stress testing, as patients taking theophylline cannot undergo dipyridamole testing, and all caffeine-containing compounds should be avoided prior to testing.

All of the alternative techniques to thallium-201 cardiac imaging rely on detecting wall motion abnormalities. Since dipyridamole is better at causing flow maldistribution, which is best seen with thallium-201 imaging, the lack of increase in the double product yields a marked decrease in sensitivities, even with high-dose protocols. Thus, dipyridamole is best used with thallium-201 imaging rather than with MRI, echocardiography, or radionuclide ventriculography.

Adenosine

Adenosine is a powerful vasodilator and causes its effects via two types of receptors in blood vessels: a vascular smooth muscle receptor and an endothelial cell receptor (51). Since both dipyridamole and adenosine work similarly in the cardiac circulation, their effects are similar. The major benefit to the use of adenosine via intravenous administration is that it has a rapid onset of action and a brief half-life of 10 to 30 seconds (52). This short duration of action allows for repeated measurements, an advantage over dipyridamole. Adenosine raises coronary blood flow by a factor of 4.4 times, to near the maximum coronary blood flow reserve. Adenosine's other effects are to cause systemic vasodilation, depress sinoatrial node activity, decrease atrioventricular node conduction, decrease atrial and ventricular contractility, decrease platelet aggregation, increase cerebral blood flow, and stimulate respiration. The side effects of adenosine are due to these multiple effects. Many patients experience these side effects, but most are transient, and only a few patients require an infusion of aminophylline to reverse the action of adenosine. Protocols for the administration of adenosine for cardiac testing in conjunction with thallium-210 scintigraphy have been established (53,54).

The use of imaging techniques other than thallium-201 scintigraphy with adenosine share the same benefits and limitations as those with dipyridamole. The high incidence of side effects can limit its use in some patients who do not tolerate the side effects well. The most alarming side effects are transient heart block and sinoatrial node suppression, which can lead to a profound hypotension in some patients. This possibility would make a physician reluctant to use this test in an individual with high-degree heart block or sinoatrial node dysfunction.

Dobutamine

The mechanism of action of dobutamine, a synthetic catecholamine, is via the β_1-, β_2-, and α_1-adrenergic receptors. Dobutamine has strong β_1, moderate β_2, and mild α_1 activity (55,56). In the heart, β_1 stimulation leads to increased inotropy and chronotropy while α_1 stimulation causes only a mild increase in inotropy and β_2 stimulation yields moderate coronary vasodilation. Thus, intravenous dobutamine causes increased stroke volume and cardiac output, increasing the double product. Dobutamine also increases the stroke volume and ejection fraction, resulting in a decreased end-systolic volume, decreasing wall stress and myocardial O_2 consumption. The BP usually remains relatively constant with dobutamine infusion, as β_2 stimulation decreases systemic vascular resistance and sympathetic tone decreases due to the increased cardiac output. The half-life of dobutamine via infusion is usually about 2 minutes. The onset of action usually occurs at about 2 minutes, with a peak effect at about 10 minutes (57). The drug is metabolized via catechol-O-transferase and the metabolites are excreted by the kidneys.

The side effects of dobutamine include tachycardia, arrhythmias, headaches, tremors, and anxiety. The cardiac side effects are usually only seen with high doses and they usually rapidly resolve after the termination of the infusion. If needed, β blockers can be given to overcome the side effects (58).

The rationale for the use of dobutamine as a pharmacologic stressor lies in the ability it has to raise the rate-pressure product by raising both inotropy and chronotropy. Dobutamine has been shown to be relatively safe in patients with CAD, even in the peri-MI period (59,60). At moderate doses, it has powerful inotropy with only mild chronotropy, arrhythmogenicity, and systemic vascular effects. The myocardial VO_2 increases due to the increase in the double product, and ischemia is thought to be due to the coronary steal phenomenon when diseased arteries cannot dilate to increase blood flow as the double product increases.

Dobutamine with echocardiography has good sensitivity and specificity in the detection of CAD (58). In a direct comparison, echocardiography with dobutamine was more sensitive and specific than echocardiography with dipyridamole (61). This can be easily understood in view of the fact that dobutamine increases the double product and can thus increase ischemia more. MRI with dobutamine also is of use in the detection of ischemia in CAD, and the mild chronotropy of dobutamine has the advantage of making the scan times somewhat shorter (62).

The final resolution of the issue of the best agent to use for cardiac stress testing still must be decided on an individual basis. The variety of agents described have their advantages, and offer the ability to test the severely disabled or deconditioned patient who might be encountered in a physiatric practice.

Echocardiographic Stress Testing

Exercise echocardiography is one of the commonly used techniques in exercise tolerance testing. There are three basic assumptions that underlie the use of echocardiography in stress testing: 1) Induction of ischemia will result in an area of left ventricular dyssynergy, 2) these regional wall motion abnormalities are specific for ischemia, and 3) changes in wall motion can be accurately seen on two-dimensional echocardiograms (63). The evidence for the first two assumptions has been long-standing, and the improvement in technique and the addition of digital echocardiography have now also made the third assumption true (64). The exercise can be performed either on a treadmill or with a bicycle ergometer. The use of treadmill testing is limited to scanning before and after exercise only, while testing on the bicycle can allow for continuous monitoring and the detection of transient ischemic changes (65,66). One report showed increased sensitivity with lower specificity for the bicycle versus the treadmill (67).

Exercise echocardiography with the newer techniques and digital imaging has a diagnostic sensitivity and specificity on the order of 74% to 97% and 64% to 100%, respectively. This compares favorably with the results of stress ECG (63). Comparisons between the findings on ECG, radionuclide ventriculography, and thallium-201 scanning during exercise with a treadmill and that on a bicycle ergometer demonstrated that the diagnosis with scintigraphy is more accurate than that done by ECG alone (68,69). The test is particularly useful in situations where the stress ECG is ambiguous or not diagnostic, in women who have a high likelihood of a false-positive result, and in those with abnormalities on the resting ECG. The indications for echocardiographic stress testing are listed in Table 20-12. The advantage of being a noninvasive test, with no radiation exposure and no increased risk to the patient, makes the stress echocardiogram a viable alternative to ECG in cardiac stress testing.

Thallium-201 Stress Testing

Thallium-201 perfusion scintigraphy is a widely accepted modality for the detection of ischemia in CAD. It has proved to be more accurate than stress echocardiography alone (70,71). Most commonly, imaging is performed in conjunction with a treadmill test (72). It is also used with dipyridamole and adenosine pharmacologic stress testing (29,40). Comparisons between the findings on ECG, radionuclide ventriculography, and thallium-201 scanning

Table 20-12: Indications for Exercise Echocardiography
Prior nondiagnostic stress test
High likelihood of a false-positive result or stress ECG, i.e., women or those taking digitalis
Conduction or repolarization abnormalities on rest ECG
High pretest likelihood of disease where the test is to determine the extent and/or location of ischemia
In order to assess physiologic significance of a lesion and effect of therapy
After myocardial infarction for prognostic information

ECG = electrocardiography.

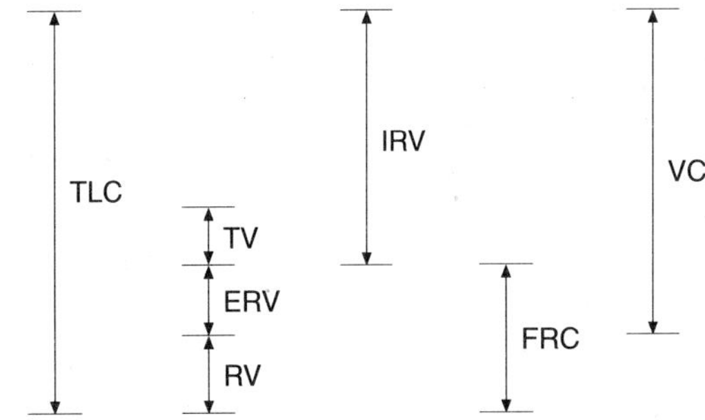

Figure 20-1. Schematic diagram of lung volumes. TLC = total lung capacity; TV = tidal volume; ERV = expiratory reserve volume; RV = residual volume; FRC = functional reserve capacity; IRV = inspiratory reserve volume; VC = vital capacity.

during exercise with a treadmill and a bicycle ergometer demonstrated that the diagnosis with scintigraphy is more accurate than that done by ECG alone (68,69).

The physiologic basis behind the use of thallium-201 scintigraphy is the uptake of thallium 201 in the cardiac myocyte via the Na^+, K^+-ATPase pump. The first-pass extraction is 85%, and it is continuously exchanged (73). This means that images taken early and late after injection provide different pathophysiologic data: 1) Immediate images give information about regional myocardial blood flow, and 2) delayed images (2–24 hours) show distribution of the potassium pool and thus myocardial viability (46). These principles are used in the stress test, as an area of ischemia with a more than 50% drop in blood flow will appear as an area of decreased uptake in the original image, and then will appear with normal uptake after a delay. Using this fact that any differential between vessel blood flow greater than 2:1 can be seen by thallium-201 imaging, one can detect the heterogeneity of blood flow created (40). The late redistribution, at 24 hours, can be an indicator of viable, but underperfused ("hibernating") myocardium that may be rescued with revascularization (12).

Thallium-201 testing offers the advantages of the ability to image all patients regardless of habitus, and is able to be done in patients in whom echocardiography cannot be performed. It also can be used with both exercise and pharmacologic testing. The disadvantages to thallium-201 testing lie in the fact that the test is invasive, with the injection of a radioactive agent with a long half-life, and the need for expensive and complex imaging equipment (12). Recent advances that have increased the sensitivity and specificity of thallium-201 scanning are the use of single-photon emission computed tomography scintigraphy with its inherent three-dimensional imaging (72).

Other Cardiac Imaging Techniques for Stress Testing

Technical advances in cardiac imaging have led to the introduction of stress MRI, technetium-99m Sestamibi stress imaging, gated radionuclide angiography, positron emission tomography, and other techniques to attempt to increase the ability to quantify exercise tolerance and cardiac risk (74). Each of these techniques has its advantages and disadvantages, with the establishment of standards and the assessment of relative cost still ongoing. For the time being, stress echocardiography, stress and pharmacologic thallium imaging, and the standard stress test are the most economical and readily available tests. For the practicing physiatrist interested in the assessment of patients for cardiac rehabilitation, it is important to use a familiar test that is readily available in the community. Looking to the future, some of the new imaging techniques may provide the ideal mix of cost, accuracy, noninvasiveness, and convenience.

ASSESSMENT OF PULMONARY FUNCTION

Tests of the Mechanics of Breathing

Static Lung Volumes

The basic tests for the function of the lungs involve the measurement of the static lung volumes (Fig. 20-1):

Total lung capacity (TLC)—the volume of air in the lungs at full inspiration. The limit to inspiration comes from the elastic recoil of the lungs, and maintenance of the volume depends on the compliance of the lungs and chest wall and the strength of the muscles of inspiration. Full inspiration normally only occurs with sneezing, coughing, and yawning.

Vital capacity (VC)—volume change of air through the mouth between full inspiration and full expiration. Inspiration is affected by the distensibility (compliance) of the lungs (intraparenchymal) and the chest wall (extraparenchymal), while expiration is affected by bronchial and obstructive diseases and chest wall disease. VC can be decreased by either the loss of inspiratory reserve or an increase in the volume of residual air. Table 20-13 presents causes of both.

Table 20-13: Lung Pathology	
Loss of Inspiratory Reserve	**Increase in the Residual Volume**
Intrinsic	Intrinsic
Lung fibrosis	Bronchial obstruction
Obliteration of alveoli	Airway collapse
Pulmonary edema	
Extrinsic	Extrinsic
Chest wall rigidity	Respiratory muscle weakness
Respiratory muscle weakness	Chest wall rigidity
Chest wall restriction from bracing	

Expired vital capacity (EVC)—volume of air exhaled without force from the lungs after a complete inspiration.

Inspired vital capacity (IVC)—volume of air inspired into lungs after a full expiration.

Forced expired vital capacity (FVC)—maximum volume that can be expired from the lungs after a maximal forced expiration.

Forced expiratory volume (FEV)—the maximum volume that can be exhaled from the lungs after a full inspiration. It is usually reported over a time interval.

Forced expiratory volume in 1 second (FEV_1)—the FEV over 1 second. This is the most commonly reported value, and is severely limited in airway obstruction.

Maximum breathing capacity (MBC)—maximum volume of air that a subject can expire in 1 minute when breathing as rapidly and as deeply as possible.

Maximal voluntary ventilation (MVV)—measurement of the MBC over 15 seconds.

Residual volume (RV)—volume of air in the lungs after a full expiration. As a person ages, the chest wall becomes more rigid and the lungs loose some elasticity so that the RV increases with age at the expense of the VC. RV should not exceed 37% of the TLC (75), and when high values are seen, they often are the result of airflow obstruction, and more rarely, muscle weakness.

Functional reserve capacity (FRC)—volume of air in the chest at the end of a tidal breath when the respiratory muscles are at their most relaxed. The FRC is maintained by the balance of the elastic recoil of the lung and the chest wall. It can be affected by position (e.g., in supine position it will decrease as the abdominal viscera will rise into the chest to decrease the FRC) and by pathologic conditions. In chronic obstructive pulmonary disease (COPD), the FRC is increased by the trapping of air, and in neuromuscular diseases affecting the chest wall, it is increased due to the inability to forcefully exhale.

Expiratory reserve volume (ERV)—the volume that can be exhaled from the FRC to the RV. This volume can be reduced by any condition that limits active exhalation. The ERV is decreased in pregnancy and in obesity by the effects of those conditions on the diaphragm, and in conditions with expiratory muscle weakness.

Inspiratory reserve volume (IRV)—the volume that can be inhaled from the FRC to the TLC. The IRV can be reduced in pregnancy and in obesity by the influence of the abdominal volume in limiting diaphragm excursion, and in conditions with chest wall restriction caused by either muscle weakness or chest wall rigidity.

Tidal volume (TV)—the volume of a regular nonforced breath at rest.

Measurement of Static Volumes

Three different parameters are measured to determine the static volume of the lungs: expired and inspired volumes (measured by spirometry), thoracic gas volumes, and the volume of the thoracic cage. In clinical practice, static lung volumes are usually best determined by spirometry, at measurements of the other parameters require better patient compliance and are usually difficult to do. Thoracic gas volumes can be measured with body plethysmography in a sealed tank where the subject breathes against a plethysmograph, and the ratio of the volumes in the chest and in the sealed tank is determined. The volume of the thoracic cage is measured by use of radiographs or fluoroscopy of the chest.

Spirometry is done in either an open or a closed system. Usually the open system is used, even though there are greater inaccuracies, because of convenience and the ability to do the tests rapidly. Closed-circuit spirometry is done by having the subject breath a mixture of an insoluble gas at a known dilution. After equilibration, the FRC can be readily calculated. It usually takes approximately 5 minutes to reach equilibrium in normal individuals, but can take far longer in those with obstructive conditions, somewhat limiting the clinical utility of the test. The machine is not portable and has a high associated cost. Ventilatory capacity measured through a bellows spirometer has the advantages of portability, low cost, reproducibility, speed, and low complexity. The bellows spirometer is best used to determine FEV_1, FEV, and VC, which are the most important values for clinical practice. The patient is usually in a seated position, with a nose clip and an oral mouthpiece in place. The subject then is asked to perform the tests for VC and FEV_1 three times in a row. The best test results are reported. If the subject has a bout of coughing while doing the test, then the FEV_1 is done separately, as the coughing can cause a reactive bronchospasm that will alter the results.

Table 20-14: Causes of Alterations in Lung Compliance	
Increased Compliance	**Decreased Compliance**
Intrinsic	Intrinsic
Decreased elastic recoil	Alveolar obliteration
Loss of alveolar walls	Increased alveolar stiffness
	Increased alveolar wall thickness
	Decreased surfactant
Extrinsic	Extrinsic
Flail chest	Chest wall stiffness
Multiple rib fractures	Chest wall deformity
	Chest wall bracing

Lung Compliance

Compliance of the lungs is the elasticity and distensibility of the lungs with change in volume for a given pressure. The elasticity of the lungs can be either increased or decreased in a number of conditions, as seen in Table 20-14.

Airway Resistance

Airway resistance is the pressure required to allow for airflow along the airways of the lung. It is usually approximately 90% of the total pulmonary resistance. The airway resistance is described by the simple relationship of resistance = pressure/flow, and it is usually measured in centimeters of water per liter per second. Airway resistance is determined by multiple factors, including diameter of the airway, flow velocity, turbulence of airflow, and the density and viscosity of the respired gases. It is usually measured in a closed box in order to obtain the differences between alveolar and external thoracic pressures. Technically measurement of this is demanding as small differences in technique can cause significant alterations in the acquired traces.

Tissue Resistance

Tissue resistance is classically described as being 10% of the total pulmonary resistance (76). Tissue resistance has a greater contribution at large lung volumes, and in conditions such as pulmonary fibrosis in which the quantity of interstitial lung tissue is increased. The tissue resistance is indirectly determined by subtracting the airway resistance from the total pulmonary resistance. It is usually not determined clinically, but it is helpful to keep in mind that tissue factors can increase pulmonary resistance in certain medical conditions.

Work of Breathing

The work of breathing is the amount of muscular effort required to allow normal breathing. In normal situations, there are three contributors to the work of breathing:

1. Elastic recoil of the lungs and chest wall (at end inspiration)
2. Airway resistance and tissue resistance (at end inspiration)
3. Inertia of the testing system and of the respired gases (this is usually minimal)

Expiration is usually passive and is secondary to the elastic recoil of the lung tissues, and with effort or airway obstruction, the abdominal muscles can help to increase VC by the reduction of end-expiratory volumes.

Tests of Gas Transfer

It is through the exchange of gases in the alveoli that the excretion of carbon dioxide (CO_2) and the absorption of O_2 is achieved. The normal values for pCO_2 pressure are maintained close to 40 mm Hg in the healthy individual, and O_2 saturation is usually maintained at a level of higher than 95%. The tests of arterial blood gases can help to determine the physiologic alterations in disease states, and can determine the compromises to pulmonary ventilation and gas exchange. Some basic principles related to gas exchange are reviewed briefly.

Respiratory Quotient

The respiratory quotient (RQ) is the ratio of CO_2 output to O_2 consumption at a cellular level. In a state where carbohydrates are the only substrates, the RQ is 1. With the use of fats and fatty acids as an energy source, there is less CO_2 produced for every mole of O_2 consumed, at a ratio of approximately 0.7. Proteins have an RQ of approximately 0.8. In the basal state, the resting RQ is normally about 0.8, but falls with fasting as fats and fatty acids become the primary sources of energy.

Respiratory Exchange Ratio

The respiratory exchange ratio (R) is the ratio of CO_2 output to O_2 consumption that is applied to the measurement of pulmonary gas exchange in the measurement of expired gases. It is affected in the short term by variations in cardiac output, metabolic rate, and pulmonary function. The R is proportional to the RQ when an individual achieves a steady state, and is usually difficult to achieve well in a standard testing situation. However, with a stepped testing protocol, approximations of steady state are achievable and useful data can be obtained. Hyperventilation and breath holding can cause rapid alterations in the value of R due to the ability of the body to store more CO_2 than O_2 in the tissues and blood.

Dissociation Curves for CO_2 and O_2

Dissociation curves are plots of partial pressures of gases versus the saturation of the gas in the blood. Standard

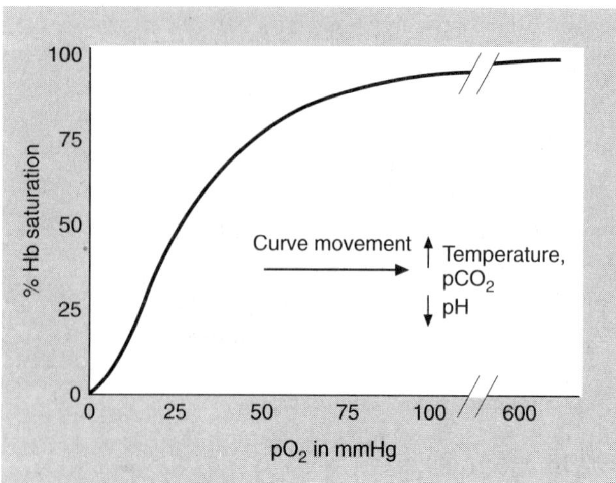

Figure 20-2. The absorption of oxygen. Hb = hemoglobin.

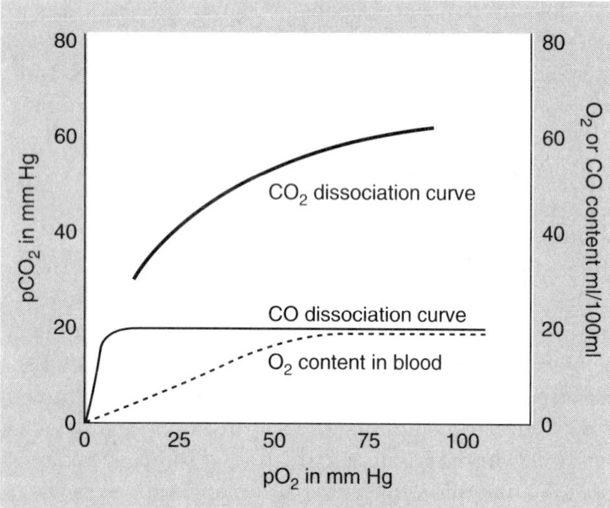

Figure 20-3. The absorption of carbon dioxide.

physiology textbooks provide a good review of the mechanisms of CO_2 and O_2 absorption in the blood. The basic curves for the absorption of O_2 and CO_2 are provided in Figures 20-2 and 20-3. It is with the educated use of these basic principles and a good understanding of the O_2 and CO_2 curves that rational estimation of pulmonary capacity can be achieved. There are a few basic principles to recall about the O_2 dissociation curve. The O_2-carrying capacity of the plasma in an individual breathing room air is only 0.3 mL/100 mL of plasma, rising to 2.0 mL/100 mL of plasma at 100% O_2. At a normal hematocrit, the O_2-carrying capacity of the blood is 20 mL of O_2/100 mL of blood (1.39 mL of O_2/g of hemoglobin) (76). The O_2 saturation drops rapidly after the O_2 tension drops below 60 mm Hg (90%), with the O_2 saturation only 50% at an O_2 tension of 25%. This translates into the need for close observation during testing and rehabilitation, and severely limited exercise tolerance and exercise reserve at even mildly decreased O_2 saturations.

With CO_2, it is important to recall two important features of the saturation curve. Pulmonary CO_2 exchange is governed by the carriage of CO_2 as bicarbonate or bound to carbaminohemoglobin. The dissociation curve for CO_2 is linear at around the normal range of alveolar pCO_2. This translates into an ability to continue to release significant amounts of CO_2 with alveolar hyperventilation without a corresponding rise in O_2 pressure (pO_2), since the O_2-carrying capacity is very much saturated at normal alveolar pO_2. Also, the capacity to take up CO_2 is very large, and even under severe metabolic demands, the venous pCO_2 is only 4 mm Hg or so above the arterial pCO_2, while the corresponding pO_2 may be different by as much as 40 to 50 mm Hg. Clinically, this is illustrated by the hypoventilation present in individuals with chronic CO_2 retention. They have already saturated their CO_2-carrying capacity and may be at risk for respiratory acidosis with fatigue, increased metabolic demand, or overexertion (75).

The interpretation of blood gas values is covered in detail in medical, pulmonary, and physiology textbooks. The essential principles regarding blood gas analysis are that an elevation of the pCO_2 is an indication of ventilatory failure, and can be seen in conditions of severe restrictive disease (kyphoscoliosis), diseases of muscle failure (neuromuscular conditions or paralysis), and severe obstructive disease (emphysema). In an acute state, the elevation of pCO_2 is an emergency requiring assisted ventilation, but in a chronic state, it may be well tolerated. These patients are at risk of acute failure with any increase in metabolic demand. Chronic CO_2 elevation appears to occur when resting minute ventilation would have to be greater than 12 L/min to maintain a normal pCO_2 (77,78). Low arterial pO_2 is usually a reflection of one of two situations: low inspired pO_2 (e.g., at a high altitude) or conditions that impair alveolar gas exchange or alveolar ventilation with a subsequent ventilation-perfusion mismatch. Respiratory drive is normally increased significantly at an arterial pO_2 below 60 mm Hg. With long-standing disease, pO_2 may fall as low as 50 mm Hg and be well tolerated. The result is that individuals with chronic lung disease may have normal to low pO_2 with either normal, low, or high pCO_2, depending on the nature of the disorder. A useful outline for interpretation of blood gas abnormalities is given in Table 20-15.

Pulmonary Gas Exchange

Actual pulmonary gas exchange is determined by measuring either the uptake of gases that are inert and rare, or the uptake of carbon monoxide (CO). The evaluation of pulmonary function can be performed with either single or multiple breath tests. A gas used for gas exchange testing should be unreactive chemically with the blood and reach equilibrium in the period of time required for the blood to

Table 20-15: Interpretations of Blood Gas Abnormalities

	$pO_2 \leftrightarrow$	Decreased pO_2
Increased pCO_2	COPD	COPD Central hypoventilation
Decreased pCO_2	Hyperventilation Anxiety	Ventilation-perfusion mismatch Respiratory failure
Unchanged pCO_2	Normal	Alveolar process Pneumonia

COPD = chronic obstructive pulmonary disease.

pass through the capillary bed of the alveoli. A gas that is useful for testing the diffusing capacity of the lung is CO, which binds so rapidly with the hemoglobin in the blood that it is only limited by the rate at which it can diffuse. Diffusion equilibrium is never reached with CO, so that partial pressures cannot be determined, but it can reflect the ability of the hemoglobin to transfer O_2 between the blood and the inspired air.

Breath-holding and rebreathing tests of pulmonary gas exchange are used to evaluate the efficiency of gas transport from inspired air to the tissues in diseased lungs. For these tests, respiratory mass spectrometers assess the mixture of gases in small samples as they are collected from the patient. The basic breath-holding test involves the subject inspiring a known volume of gas, followed by analysis of expired air at set intervals of time. Three factors account for the change in expired gas concentrations over time:

1. Dilution within the lung volume
2. Solution in the lung tissue
3. Uptake and removal by the pulmonary blood

Often the system is closed with a rebreather, to allow the subject to rebreath the mixed alveolar gas and allow for equilibration. Three types of gases are used for this testing: insoluble gases, which allow for the study of diffusion of gas into the alveolar volume; CO, for the study of diffusion of gases over the alveolar membrane; and soluble inert gases, to measure the pulmonary blood flow and pulmonary tissue volume.

Inert Gases

The most commonly used gases for inert gas testing are helium, neon, and argon. In the normal lung, equilibration occurs within 3 to 4 seconds. A slow equilibrium, which may take up to minutes, is characteristic of chronic airflow obstruction, as is seen with emphysema. The nitrogen washout technique can also be used, and is performed by having the subject breath pure O_2 while the falling concentrations of N_2 are measured. Normal curves are established, and a prolonged washout is consistent with obstructive disease. There are several standardized techniques for the performance of the nitrogen washout test, a discussion of which is beyond the scope of this text (79–81). The single-breath nitrogen test also uses similar principles, and is used in epidemiology to detect pulmonary disease. Since it is of limited clinical use, it is not discussed further.

Carbon Monoxide

The CO test measures the ability to deliver gases between the hemoglobin and the inspired air across the alveolar membrane and capillaries. Measurement of the removal of trace amounts of CO from inspired air can be used to test the integrity of the function of the entire lung. The most commonly performed test of CO in the lung is the single-breath CO uptake test. This was first developed in the beginning of the century, and was standardized in the 1950s (82–84). Because the normal range is very narrow (only 25% of the predicted mean value), this test is used commonly as a screening test of pulmonary function and provides good quantitative values reflecting the gas exchange capabilities of the lung.

Normal CO uptake requires the function of the lungs and circulation to be intact in four areas: normal hemoglobin concentration, normal pulmonary capillaries, normal surface area and thickness of alveoli, and normal airway function. Disease processes affecting any or all of these will lead to a decreased diffusion capacity on the CO uptake test. In the presence of normal hemoglobin, normal lung volumes, and normal airways, the CO test can clearly demonstrate abnormalities at the level of the alveoli.

The procedure to perform the CO uptake test is relatively simple. The patient exhales to the RV and then inhales a mixture of air, 10% helium, and 0.3% CO to 10% less than the TLC. The breath is held for 10 seconds, and then exhaled. The first 0.7 liter is discarded, and the next 0.6 liter is captured as a representative sample of the alveolar air (75). The analysis of this sample relies on the fact that helium, as an inert gas, is essentially not absorbed, while the CO is taken up at any capillary surface at which it is in close proximity to hemoglobin. The uptake of CO is then determined as a ratio of the apparent dilution of the CO compared to the apparent dilution of the helium. This treatment of the lung assumes the lung to be a single well-mixed gas exchange system. Commonly, this value is termed the *diffusion capacity of the lung*, and is abbreviated as the DL_{CO}. The name is really a misnomer and can be deceptive unless it is recognized to be the value that reflects the gas transfer ability of the lung as a whole [called the *transfer factor* for CO (TL_{CO}) in physiology literature] and is independent from, but dependent on, the actual alveolar capillary diffusion capacity. The normal value is roughly 25 mL/min/mm Hg, with approximately 18 to 19 mL/min/mm Hg being the bottom range

Table 20-16: Alterations in the Diffusion Capacity of the Lung (DL_{CO}) and Physiologic Correlation

	DL_{CO}	Membrane Diffusion	Alveolar Blood Volume	Hematocrit
Physiologic state				
Exercise	↑	↔	↑	↔
Lying down	↑	↔	↑	↔
↑ Sympathetic tone	↑	↔	↑	↔
Polycythemia	↑	↔	↔	↑
Hypoxia	↑	↔	↔	↑
Cold shower	↑	↔	↑	↔
Goodpasture syndrome	↑	↔	↔	↑
Hyperkinetic cardiac states	↑	↔	↑	↔
Minimally raised pulmonary venous pressures	↑	↔	↑	↔
Moderately raised pulmonary venous pressure	↔	↓	↑	↔
Severely raised pulmonary venous pressure	↓	↓	↓	↔
Postprandial	↓	↔	↓	↔
Erect posture	↓	↔	↓	↔
Valsalva maneuver	↓	↔	↓	↔
Cigarette smoking	↓	↔	↓	↔
Age	↓	↓	↔	↔
Expiration	↓	↓	↔	↔
Anemia	↓	↔	↔	↓
Medical condition				
Asthma	↔ or ↑	↔ or ↑	↔	↔
Bronchitis	↔ or ↓	↔	↔	↔
Emphysema	↔ or ↓	↓	↓	↔ or ↑
Diffuse infiltrates	↓	↓	↓	↔
Restrictive disease (intrinsic)	↓	↓	↔	↔
Restrictive disease (extrinsic)	↓	↓	↔	↔
Loss of lung tissue	↓	↔ or ↓	↔ or ↓	↔
Low cardiac output	↓	↔		
Pulmonary edema	↓	↓	↓	↔

↑ = increased; ↓ = decreased; ↔ = unchanged.

for normal. The clinician should be familiar with the normal values of his or her own laboratory.

The causes of a low DL_{CO} are numerous. Table 20-16 reviews some of the various conditions associated with abnormal DL_{CO}, along with the area of lung function that causes the abnormality. Low DL_{CO} can be seen in several states including loss of lung tissue, thickening of the alveolar membranes or capillaries, decrease in the volume of the blood in the alveolar capillaries, decreased hematocrit or hemoglobin concentration, and regional ventilation-perfusion mismatch. Increases in DL_{CO} can be seen in states with an excess of hemoglobin in the lungs, either through polycythemia, pulmonary congestion (mild), or extravasation of blood into the alveoli as seen with Goodpasture syndrome. In normal individuals, the DL_{CO} may vary by about 5%. Exercise can increase DL_{CO} by up to 25% (85) and lying supine can increase the DL_{CO} by increasing the filling of the apical segments of the lung (86). The judicious use of the DL_{CO} in pulmonary evaluation can help with the design of a rehabilitation program, as it helps to elucidate the cause of the gas exchange abnormality.

Exercise Tolerance Testing

In the rehabilitation of the patient with pulmonary disease, the pulmonary exercise test is the most important portion of the evaluation. Most of the testing discussed up to this point is principally concerned with determining the pathophysiology of the pulmonary disease process, and as such is critical in the medical management of the patient, but the pulmonary stress test is most important in the determination of the patient's actual ability to perform exercise. The functional data obtained with this test can be used to determine the tolerable workload for the patient, and with reference to the tables of metabolic energy requirements presented elsewhere in the text, can help to outline the physical limitations that may be present and may be adapted for. These compensatory techniques and treatments are addressed more fully in Chapter 80. The techniques, interpretation, and uses of pulmonary exercise testing are discussed here.

As in cardiac exercise testing, there are a number of protocols that can be followed. For details of the exact administration of these tests, the reader is referred to several textbooks devoted to cardiac and pulmonary stress testing (5,87). The principles that govern cardiac stress testing apply as well to pulmonary stress testing, and the position of the subject, the muscle groups used, and type of exercise affect $\dot{V}O_2$ as described in Chapter 79 and earlier in this chapter. These are briefly outlined in Table 20-17. A cycle ergometer is often easier to use for pulmonary testing, as it is easier to use a mouthpiece for gas testing, and pulse oximetry may be easier. Also, an ergometer is readily adapted for testing in the supine position for individuals who cannot tolerate the erect position. It is the availability of equipment, the needs of the patient, and the standards of the laboratory that determine the exact nature of the test performed. For most patients, a treadmill test is easily done and well tolerated, providing data specific to a functional activity that all patients must perform anyway, ambulation. The protocols used are maximal with incremental increases in exertion, following the protocols outlined earlier in the cardiac stress testing section, following one of the protocols outlined there. For treadmill

Table 20-17: Physiology of Pulmonary Exercise Compared to Upright Treadmill Exercise

Type of Exercise	VO_2	Systolic/Diastolic Blood Pressure	Myocardial VO_2
Isometric	↑	↑↑/↑↑	↑
Isotonic	↔	↔/↔	↔
Supine	↓	↔/↔	↓
Erect	↔	↔/↔	↔
Upper extremity	↑	↑/↑	↑
Lower extremity	↔	↔/↔	↔
Treadmill	↔	↔/↔	↔
Ergometer	↔ or ↓	↔/↔	↔ or ↓

↑ = increased; ↑↑ = very increased; ↓ = decreased; ↔ = unchanged.

testing, either the Bruce protocol with increased exertion every 3 minutes or the Balke protocol with incremental increases every minute is commonly used. The Jones protocol is a cycle ergometry protocol that has incremental increases every minute. The details of these and other protocols are outlined in Table 20-8. The contraindications and the indications for stopping exercise testing are the same as with cardiac stress testing. A unique variable that may be added to functional pulmonary stress testing is the addition of supplemental O_2 to allow for the maintenance of adequate pO_2 during testing (> 90%).

Blood gas analysis of O_2 and CO_2 during exercise should demonstrate that the pCO_2 and pO_2 remain in normal ranges during mild to moderate exercise. To maintain this constant level of blood gases, CO_2 is kept close to its normal values by the control of breathing, which allows the elimination of CO_2 at a rate consistent with its formation. The dead space of ventilation is approximately 150 to 180 mL/breath, with another 30 to 60 mL/breath for the wasted ventilation associated with the upright position. Patients who have an abnormal pCO_2 with low to moderate exercise demonstrate one of several abnormalities. They can have disturbed pulmonary gas exchange, or a low pCO_2 due to hyperventilation caused by hypoxia, lactic acidosis, or anxiety. In patients with severe COPD, there may be ventilatory failure with a subsequent elevation of pCO_2. Anemia, with hemoglobin below 50% of normal, will cause a relatively hypoxic state with subsequent hyperventilation and declining pCO_2 (88). When exercise is performed at a high level, the patient will begin to go into anaerobic exercise and there will be peripheral tissue hypoxia with the generation of lactic acidosis. The lactate production begins to rise sharply at approximately 50% of maximal oxygen uptake (VO_2max). This point in the curve is known as the *anaerobic threshold*, when lactate production creates a rise in the blood lactate level. This corresponds to a rise in the respiratory rate and output of CO_2 during exercise. The anaerobic threshold is most accurately determined with the use of a breath-to-breath analysis of expired gases. The achievement of equilibrium in a stepped exercise takes approximately 2 minutes, so observations to determine the anaerobic threshold by stress testing are best done with protocols with steps of that length or longer.

Arterial oxygenation also remains steady, with oxygen saturation remaining constant or rising slightly during exercise. Standard pulse oximetry is used to monitor O_2 saturations during exercise, and may show a significant fall in patients with severe chronic lung disease or with emphysema or fibrosing alveolitis. The O_2 saturation may also drop precipitously during exercise in patients with large intrapulmonary vascular shunts. It is the hallmark of these shunts that they do not respond to supplemental O_2 administration. The symptom index used during the exercise test is the Borg or modified Borg scale, both of which are shown in Chapter 79. Interpretations of the abnormalities encountered during pulmonary exercise stress testing are listed in Table 20-18.

The simplest of the exercise tests for the evaluation of functional pulmonary exercise tolerance is the 12- or 6-minute walk test. This test has the benefits of ease of administration, safety, and reproducibility and is a time-honored and readily accepted test of exercise tolerance in patients with pulmonary disease. The test is administered in a flat indoor hallway or walkway with no obstacles and no distractions. The subject walks as quickly as he or she can for exactly 12 minutes. The subject is instructed to hurry at a speed that is as rapid as possible without causing exhaustion. At the end of the time, the exact distance is measured, and the average speed is calculated. There is a practice effect, and patients can increase performance by 5% on repeat testing. The test may have pauses in it as long as the total distance is measured accurately (89). In patients with pure respiratory disease, a shorter variation of the test, 6 minutes, is as acceptable as the 12-minute test, and is easier to administer (90,91). A limitation of the 6- and 12-minute walk tests in practice is the presence of other conditions (e.g., orthopedic, neurologic) that may impede the ability to walk at full speed. Substitutes for severely disabled patients can include raising a leg in time to a metronome and supine ergometry. Standardizations for these alternatives are not well established however, which limits their utility.

Disability Assessment Through Pulmonary Function Testing

The assessment of disability through pulmonary function testing is essentially the determination of an estimate of functional capacity. Through the combination of the tests discussed earlier, including the spirometric measures, the estimation of DL_{CO}, the determination of VO_2max, and the estimate of exercise tolerance by the 6- or 12-minute walk tests, an estimate can be made of the functional capacity of the individual. Fitness is best described by the

Table 20-18: Effects of Physiologic Conditions on the Intrepretation of Pulmonary Testing		
Abnormality	**Physiologic Abnormality**	**Gas Exchange**
Obesity	Increased work with activity	Rapid alveolar-arterial pO_2 fall with exercise
Peripheral vascular disease	Claudication limits exercise	Low VO_2max Low anaerobic threshold
Pulmonary vascular disease	Impaired pulmonary blood flow	Decreased oxygen uptake at maximum work Low anaerobic threshold Rapid pulse at low exercise
Anemia	Low oxygen-carrying capacity	Low VO_2max Low anaerobic threshold Rapid pulse at low exercise
Chronic obstructive pulmonary disease	Restricted expiratory phase of breathing Decreased alveolar ventilation	Low VO_2max Low anaerobic threshold Rapid pulse at low exercise Submaximal heart rate achieved
Restrictive lung disease (intrinsic)	Poor diffusion capacity Poor pulmonary compliance	Low VO_2max Low anaerobic threshold Tachypnea Low pulmonary reserve High alveolar-arterial pO_2 difference
Restrictive lung disease (extrinsic)	Poor pulmonary compliance	Low VO_2max Low anaerobic threshold Tachypnea Low pulmonary reserve Submaximal heart rate achieved
Asthma	Restricted expiratory phase of breathing Decreased alveolar ventilation In exercise-induced asthma, peak flows drop 5–10 min into exercise	Most findings normal when not symptomatic, resemble obstructive with acute attack
Ventricular failure	Compromised pulmonary blood flow	Low VO_2max Low anaerobic threshold Tachypnea Exaggerated heart rate response to exercise
Ischemic heart disease	Chest pain/cardiac ischemia Can precipitate ventricular failure	Often normal Can appear like mild ventricular failure Can have inability to raise blood pressure
Metabolic acidosis	Metabolic acidosis Low bicarbonate	Normal diffusion Exaggerated response of ventilation to exercise

VO_2max, and an estimate of the ability to perform activities can be made using the tables of metabolic equivalents that are readily available. The determination of the level of disability is made using standards that have been set by numerous organizations. The American Medical Association uses VO_2max, FVC, FEV_1, and FEV_1/FVC ratio, and the extent of dyspnea established according to its tables, to classify the degree of impairment from class 1 (no impairment) to 4 (severe impairment) (Table 20-19) (92). The European Society for Clinical Respiratory Physiology recommends a disability rating based solely on the VO_2max. By their scale, 100% disability is the inability to achieve a level of more than 2 METs during exercise (93). The American Thoracic Society uses the FVC, FEV_1, FEV_1/FVC ratio, and the DL_{CO}, and assesses disability as none, mild, moderate, or severe (Table 20-20) (94). The Social Security Administration uses spirometry (FVC, FEV_1, and FEV_1/FVC ratio), arterial blood gas analysis, DL_{CO}, and VO_2max to assess impairment. The tables are too elaborate to present in their entirety here, but are adjusted for age, height, and condition; the interested clinician can obtain the documents from the U.S. Government Printing Office (95).

Because the correlations of spirometric values (FVC, FEV_1, and FEV_1/FVC ratio), arterial blood gas values, and DL_{CO} with actual function are poor, a more useful assessment is often obtained through the VO_2max. The Occupational Safety and Health Administration (OSHA) has

Table 20-19: American Medical Association's Disability Guidelines

Impairment	Dyspnea	FVC, FEV_1, and FEV_1/FVC ratio	VO_2max
Class 1 (no impairment) 0%–5%	None	Normal (>95% confidence level for age for all measures)	>25 mL/kg/min
Class 2 (mild impairment) 10%–25%	Dyspnea with exertion, uphill, or on stairs; can keep up with a peer on the level	60%–95% of predicted normal for age for all measures	20–25 mL/kg/min
Class 3 (moderate impairment) 30%–45%	Dyspnea on level ground when walking with a peer; dyspnea on climbing one flight	50%–60% FVC 40%–60% FEV_1 40%–60% FEV_1/FVC	15–20 mL/kg/min
Class 4 (severe impairment) 50%–100%	Dyspnea walking more than 100 m, or even at rest	<50% FVC <40% FEV_1 <40% FEV_1/FVC	<15 mL/kg/min

Table 20-20: American Thoracic Society's Disability Guidelines

Disability Level	FVC	FEV_1	FEV_1/FVC	DL_{CO}
Normal	≥80%	≤80%	≥75%	≥80%
Mild	60%–79%	60%–79%	60%–74%	60%–79%
Moderate	51%–59%	41%–59%	41–59%	41%–59%
Severe	≤50%	≤40%	≤40%	≤40%

assessed the difficulty of tasks as a percentage of the VO_2max required for the task and as a function of the time it took to do the task. The use of these types of estimates in disease is not standardized, but can be helpful in assessing the ability of a patient to perform activities. Task-specific testing is of use, and the effects of training can increase the capacity for work after a rehabilitation program. This is addressed fully in Chapter 80.

Respiratory Monitoring During Sleep

With the recognition of sleep apnea as a cause of morbidity and mortality, the assessment of respiration during sleep is being performed and encountered more frequently (96). The condition is primarily encountered in individuals with obesity and upper-airway obstruction. It is a cause of fatigue, and can be seen in the disabled population, with the tendency to obesity. The hallmark of the sleep apneic episode is a continuation of respiratory movements with no air movement. The patient suffers from O_2 desaturation at this time, and often partially wakes in order to take a breath. Clinically, the patients are usually loud snorers, have daytime somnolence, are obese, are depressed, and may have right ventricular failure out of proportion to any lung disease that is seen.

Testing for this condition is done during monitored sleep. Complete polysomnography includes electroencephalography to monitor REM sleep, O_2 saturation monitoring, surface electromyographic monitoring, and video observation. Limited testing can also be done to observe only for apnea and O_2 desaturation. Abnormality is defined as more than 10 episodes of apnea (> 10 seconds) or hypopnea (> 50% decrease in respiratory excursion) per hour over a 7-hour night (97), or five or more desaturations per hour of 4% or more (98). The treatments include nasal continuous positive airway pressure and are discussed in Chapter 80.

Other Experimental Measures of Lung Function

Other testing techniques are used for diagnostic purposes, but more frequently are done in a research setting. There are texts and references specializing in pulmonary assessment that can provide a complete review of these types of studies.

REFERENCES

1. Torkelson LO. Rehabilitation of the patient with acute myocardial infarction. *J Chronic Dis* 1964;17: 685–704.
2. Schlant RC, Blonquist CG, Brandenburg RO. Guidelines for exercise stress testing: a report of the Joint American College of Cardiology-American Heart Association Task Force on Assessment of Cardiovascular Procedures (Subcommittee on Exercise Testing).

Circulation 1986;74(suppl III): 653A–667A.

3. Fletcher GF, Froelicher VF, Hartley LH. Exercise standards—a statement for health professionals. *AHA* 1990;82:2286–2322.

4. Flamm SD, Taki J, Moore R, et al. Redistribution of regional and organ blood volume and effect on cardiac function in relation to upright exercise intensity in healthy human subjects. *Circulation* 1990;18:1550–1559.

5. Froelicher VF, Marcondes GD. *Manual of exercise testing.* Chicago: Year Book Medical, 1989.

6. Chaitman B. Exercise stress testing. In: Braunwald E, ed. *Heart disease, a textbook of cardiovascular medicine.* Philadelphia: WB Saunders, 1992:161–179.

7. Froelicher VF. *Exercise and the heart. Clinical concepts.* Chicago: Year Book Medical, 1987.

8. Ellestad MH. *Stress testing, principles and practice.* 3rd ed. Philadelphia: FA Davis, 1986.

9. Okin PM, Klingfeld P. Effect of exercise protocol and lead selection on the accuracy of heart rate adjusted indices of ST-segment depression for the detection of three vessel coronary artery disease. *J Electrocardiol* 1989;22:187–194.

10. Myers J, Walsh D, Buchanan N, Froelicher VF. Can maximal cardiopulmonary capacity be recognized by a plateau in oxygen uptake? *Chest* 1989;96:1312–1316.

11. Blair SN, Gibbons LW, Painter P, et al. *Guidelines for exercise testing and prescriptions.* 3rd ed. Philadelphia: Lea & Febiger, 1986.

12. Zaret BL, Wackers FJ, Soufer R. Nuclear cardiology. In: Braunwald, E, ed. *Heart disease, a textbook of cardiovascular medicine.* Philadelphia: WB Saunders 1992:276–311.

13. Bruce RA, Fischer LD, Pettinger M, et al. ST segment elevation with exercise: a marker for poor ventricular function and poor prognosis. Coronary Artery Surgery Study (CASS) confirmation of Seattle Heart Watch results. *Circulation* 1988;77:897–905.

14. Haines DE, Beller GA, Watson DD, et al. Exercised induced ST segment elevation 2-weeks after uncomplicated myocardial infarction: contributing factors and prognostic significance. *J Am Coll Cardiol* 1987;9:996–1003.

15. Chaitman BR. The changing role of the exercise electrocardiogram as a diagnostic and prognostic test in chronic ischemic heart disease. *J Am Coll Cardiol* 1986;8:1195–1210.

16. Acanfora D, DeCaprio L, Cuomo S, et al. Diagnostic value of the ratio of recovery of systolic BP for the detection of coronary artery disease. *Circulation* 1988;77: 1306–1310.

17. Fleg JL, Lakatta EG. Prevalence and significance of postexercise hypotension in apparently healthy subjects. *Am J Cardiol* 1986;57: 1380–1384.

18. McCance AJ, Forfar JC. Selective enhancement of the cardiac sympathetic response to exercise by anginal chest pain in humans. *Circulation* 1989;80:1642–1651.

19. Bogaty P, Dagenais GR, Cantin B, et al. Prognosis in patients with a strongly positive exercise electrocardiogram. *Am J Cardiol* 1989; 64:1284–1288.

20. Mark DB, Hlatky MA, Harrel FE, et al. Exercise treadmill score for predicting prognosis in coronary artery disease. *Ann Intern Med* 1987; 106:793–800.

21. Weiner DA, Ryan TJ, McCabe CH, et al. Prognostic importance of a clinical profile and exercise test in medically treated patients with coronary artery disease. *J Am Coll Cardiol* 1984;3:722–729.

22. Wasserman K, Hansen JE, Sue DY, Whipp BJ. *Principles of exercise testing and interpretation.* Philadelphia: Lea & Febiger, 1987. Alternative stress methods for the diagnosis of coronary artery disease.

23. Niemeyer MG, van der Wall EE, Dihaene EG, et al. *Neth J Med* 1992;41:284–294.

24. Niederberger M, Bruce RA, Kusumi F, Whitkanak S. Disparities in ventilatory and circulatory responses to bicycle and treadmill exercise. *Br Heart J* 1974;36: 377–382.

25. Balady GJ, Weiner DA, Rothendler JA, et al. Arm exercise thallium imaging testing for the detection of coronary artery disease. *J Am Coll Cardiol* 1987;9:84–88.

26. Balady GJ, Weiner DA, McCabe CH, et al. Value of arm exercise testing in detecting coronary artery disease. *Am J Cardiol* 1985;55: 37–39.

27. Astrand PO, Ekblom B, Messin R, et al. Intra-arterial blood pressure during exercise with different muscle groups. *J Appl Physiol* 1965;20:253–260.

28. Albro PC, Gould KL, Westcott RJ, et al. Noninvasive assessment of coronary stenoses by myocardial imaging during pharmacologic vasodilation. III. Clinical trial. *Am J Cardiol* 1978;42:751–760.

29. Leppo JA. Dipyridamole-thallium-201 imaging: the lazy man's stress test. *J Nucl Med* 1989;30:281–287.

30. Brown BG, Josephson MA, Peterson RB, et al. Intravenous dipyridamole combined with isometric handgrip for near maximal acute increase in coronary flow in patients with coronary artery disease. *Am J Cardiol* 1981;48: 1077–1085.

31. Casale PN, Guiney TE, Strauss HW, Boucher Ca. Simultaneous low level treadmill exercise and intravenous dipyridamole stress thallium imaging. *Am J Cardiol* 1988;62:799–802.

32. Picano E, Disante A, Masini M, et al. Dipyridamole echocardiography test in effort angina pectoris. *Am J Cardiol* 1985;56:452–456.

33. Picano E. Dipyridamole-echocardiography test: historical background and physiologic basis. *Eur Heart J* 1989;10:365–376.

34. Pennell DJ, Underwood SR, Longmore DB. Detection of coronary artery disease using MR imaging with dipyridamole infusion. *J Comput Assist Tomogr* 1990;14:167–170.

35. Cates CU, Kronenberg MW, Collins HW, Sandler MP. Dipyridamole radionuclide ventriculography: a test with high specificity for severe coronary artery disease. *J Am Coll Cardiol* 1989;13: 841–851.

36. Elliot EC. The effect of Persantine on coronary flow and cardiac dynamics. *Can Med Assoc J* 1961;85:469–476.

37. Fitzgerald GA. Dipyridamole. *N Engl J Med* 1987;316:1247–1257.

38. Hoffman JIE. Maximal coronary flow and the concept of coronary vascular reserve. *Circulation* 1984;70:153–164.

39. Dole WP. Autoregulation of the coronary circulation. *Prog Cardiovasc Dis* 1987;29:293–323.

40. Gould KL. Noninvasive assessment of coronary stenoses by myocardial perfusion imaging during pharmacologic coronary vasodilation. I. Physiologic basis and experimental vasodilation. *Am J Cardiol* 1978; 41:267–278.

41. Gould KL, Westcott RJ, Albro PC, Hamilton GW. Noninvasive assessment of coronary stenoses by myocardial imaging during pharmacologic coronary vasodilation. II. Clinical methodology and feasibility. *Am J Cardiol* 1978;41:279–287.

42. Meerdink DJ, Okada RD, Leppo JA. The effect of dipyridamole on transmural blood flow gradients. *Chest* 1989;96:400–405.

43. Gould KL. Assessing coronary stenosis severity—a recurrent clinical need. *J Am Cardiol* 1986;8: 91–94. Editorial.

44. Braunwald E, Sobel BE. Coronary blood flow and myocardial ischemia. In: Braunwald E, ed. *Heart disease, a textbook of cardiovascular medicine.* Philadelphia: WB Saunders 1992:1161–1199.

45. Gould KL. Coronary steal; is it clinically important? *Chest* 1989;96:227–229. Editorial.

46. Zhu YY, Lee W, Botvinick E, et al. The clinical and pathophysiologic implications of pain, ST abnormalities, and scintigraphic changes during dipyridamole infusion: their relationships to the peripheral hemodynamic response. *Am Heart J* 1988;116:1071–1080.

47. Beer SG, Heo J, Iskandrian AS. Dipyridamole thallium imaging. *Am J Cardiol* 1991;67:18D–26D.

48. Ranhosky A, Kemperthorne-Rawson J, the Intravenous Dipyridamole-Thallium Imaging Study Group. The safety of intravenous dipyridamole thallium myocardial perfusion imaging. *Circulation* 1990;81:1205–1209.

49. Alfonso S. Inhibition of coronary vasodilating action of dipyridamole and adenosine by aminophylline in the dog. *Circ Res* 1970;26:742–752.

50. Fredholm BB, Persson CG. Xanthine derivatives as adenosine receptor antagonists. *Eur J Pharmacol* 1982;81:673–676.

51. Belardinelli L, Linden J, Berne RM. The cardiac effects of adenosine. *Prog Cardiovasc Dis* 1989; 32:73–97.

52. Wilson RF, Wyche K, Christensen BV, et al. Effects of adenosine on human coronary arterial circulation. *Circulation* 1990;82:1595–1606.

53. Biaggione I, Olafsson B, Robertson RM, et al. Cardiovascular and respiratory effects of adenosine in conscious man. Evidence for chemoreceptor activation. *Circ Res* 1987;61:779–786.

54. Coyne EP, Belveder DA, Vande Streek PR, et al. Thallium-201 scintigriaphy after intravenous infusion of adenosine compared with exercise thallium testing in the diagnosis of coronary artery disease. *J Am Coll Cardiol* 1991;67:1190–1194.

55. Tuttle RR, Mills J. Dobutamine: development of a new catecholamine to selectively increase cardiac contractility. *Circ Res* 1975;36:185–196.

56. Ruffolo RR Jr. The Pharmacology of dobutamine. *Am J Med Sci* 1987;294:244–248.

57. Kates RE, Leier CV. Dobutamine pharmacokinetics in severe heart failure. *Clin Pharmacol Ther* 1978;24:537–541.

58. Cohen JL, Greene TO, Ottenweiler J, et al. Dobutamine digital echocardiography for detecting coronary artery disease. *Am J Cardiol* 1991;67:131–138.

59. Willerson JT, Hutton I, Watson JT, et al. Influence of dobutamine on regional myocardial blood flow and ventricular performance during acute and chronic ischemia in dogs. *Circulation* 1976;53:828–833.

60. Cillespie TA, Ambos HD, Sobel BE, Roberts R. Effects of dobutamine in patients with acute myocardial infarction. *Am J Cardiol* 1977;39:588–594.

61. Previtali M, Lanzarini L, Ferrarion M, et al. Dobutamine versus dipyridamole echocardiography for detecting coronary artery disease. *Circulation* 1991;83(suppl III):III-27–31.

62. Pennel DJ, Underwood SR. Stress magnetic resonance imaging in coronary artery disease. In: van der Wall EE, de Roos A, eds. *Magnetic resonance in coronary artery disease.* Boston: Kluwer Academic, 1990:217–239.

63. Ryan T, Feigenbaum H. Exercise echocardiography. *Am J Cardiol* 1992;69:82H–89H.

64. Feigenbaum H. Exercise echocardiography. *J Am Soc Echocardiogr* 1988;1:161–166.

65. Heng MK, Simard M, Lake R, Udhoji VH. Exercise two dimensional echocardiography for the diagnosis of coronary artery disease. *Am J Cardiol* 1984;54: 502–507.

66. Duchak J, Ryan T, Sawada SG, et al. Bicycle stress echocardiography for the detection of coronary artery disease. *J Am Soc Echocardiogr* 1990;3:225. Abstract.

67. Sawada SG, Ryan T, Fineberg NS, et al. Exercise echocardiographic detection of coronary artery disease in women. *J Am Coll Cardiol* 1989;67:1213–1218.

68. Borer JS, Kent KM, Bacharach SL, et al. Sensitivity, specificity and predictive accuracy of radionuclide cineangiography during exercise in patients with coronary artery disease: comparison with electrocardiography. *Circulation* 1979;60:572–580.

69. Beller GA, Gibsen RS. Sensitivity, specificity, and prognostic significance of non invasive testing for occult or known coronary disease. *Prog Cardiovasc Dis* 1987;241–270.

70. Iskandrian AS, Wasserman LA, Anderson GS, et al. Merits of stress thallium-201 myocardial perfusion imaging in patients with inconclusive exercise electrocardiograms: correlation with coronary arteriograms. *Am J Cardiol* 1980;46:553–558.

71. Ritchie L, Trobaugh GB, Hamilton GW, et al. Myocardial imaging with thallium-201 at rest and during exercise: comparison with coronary arteriography and resting and stress electrocardiography. *Circulation* 1977;56:66–71.

72. Mahmarian JJ, Verani MS. Exercise thallium-201 perfusion scintigraphy in the assessment of coronary artery disease. *Am J Cardiol* 1991;67:2D–11D.

73. Weich HF, Strauss HW, Pitt B. The extraction of thallium-201 by the myocardium. *Circulation* 1977;56:188.

74. Skorton DJ, Schlelbert HR, Wolf GL, Marcus ML. Relative merits of imaging techniques. In: Braunwald E, ed. *Heart disease, a textbook of cardiovascular medicine.* Philadelphia: WB Saunders 1992:342–350.

75. Laszlo G. Testing the mechanics of breathing. In: *Pulmonary function: a guide for clinicians.* New York: Cambidge University Press, 1994.

76. Cotes JE. *Lung function: assessment and application in medicine.* 5th ed. Boston: Blackwell Scientific, 1993.

77. Robin ED, O'Neill RP. The fighter versus the non-fighter: control of ventilation in chronic lung disease. *Arch Environ Health* 1983;72:125–127.

78. Begin P, Grassino A. Inspiratory muscle dysfunction and chronic hypercapnea in chronic obstructive pulmonary disease. *Am Rev Respir Dis* 1983;143:905–912.

79. Cournand A, Baldwin E, Darling RC, Richards DW. Studies on intrapulmonary mixture of gases. IV: the significance of pulmonary emptying rate and a simplified open circuit measurement of residual air. *J Clin Invest* 1941;20:681–689.

80. Becklake MR. A new index of the intrapulmonary mixture of inspired air. *Thorax* 1952;7:111–116.

81. Prowse K, Cumming G. Effects of lung volume and disease on the lung nitrogen decay curve. *J Appl Physiol* 1973;34:23-33.

82. Krogh A, Krogh M. Rate of diffusion of CO into the lungs of man. *Stand Arch Physiol* 1909;23:236–237.

83. Ogilvie CM, Forster RE, Blakemore WS, Morton JW. A standardized breath-holding technique for the clinical measurement of the diffusing capacity of the lung for carbon monoxide. *J Clin Invest* 1957;36:1–17.

84. McGrath MW, Thompson ML. The effect of age, body size and lung volume change on alveolar capillary permeability and diffusing capacity in man. *J Physiol* 1959;146:572–582.

85. Kendrick AH, Cullen T, Green H, et al. Measurement of single breath carbon monoxide transfer factor (diffusion capacity) during progressive exercise. *Bull Eur Physiopathol Respir* 1986;22:365–370.

86. Stam H, Kreuzer FJA, Versprille A. Effect of lung volume and positional change on pulmonary diffusing capacity with its components. *J Appl Physiol* 1991;71:1477–1488.

87. Wasserman K, Hansen JE, Seu DY, et al. *Principals of exercise testing and interpretation.* 2nd ed. Philadelphia: Lea & Febiger, 1994.

88. Cotes JE, Dabbs JM, Elwood PC, et al. Iron deficiency anemia: its effect on transfer factor for the lung and ventilation and card frequency during submaximal exercise. *Clin Sci* 1972;42:325–335.

89. McGavin CR, Gupta SP, McHardy GJR. Twelve minute walking test for the assessment of disability in chronic bronchitis. *BMJ* 1976;242:241–243.

90. Butland RJA, Pang JA, Gross ER, et al. Two, six and twelve minute walks compared. *BMJ* 1982;248:1607–1608.

91. Guyatt GH, Sullivan MJ, Thompson PJ, et al. The 6-minute walk: a new measure of exercise capacity in patients with chronic heart failure. *Can Med Assoc J* 1985;132:919–923.

92. American Medical Association. *American Medical Association guides to the evaluation of permanent impairment.* 2nd ed. Chicago: American Medical Association, 1984:85–101.

93. Coles JE, Chinn DJ, Reed JW, et al. Experience of standardised method for assessing respiratory disability. *Eur Respir J* 1994;7:875–880.

94. Haas F, Axen F. *Pulmonary therapy and rehabilitation: principles and practice.* 2nd ed. Baltimore: Williams & Wilkins, 1991:111.

95. U.S. Department of Health and Human Services. *Disability evaluation under Social Security.* Washington, DC: U.S. Government Printing Office, 1986:28–34. SSA publication no. 05-10089.

96. Guilleminault C, Tilkian A, Dement WC. The sleep apnea syndromes. *Ann Rev Med* 1976;27:465–484.

97. Whytew KF, Allen MB, Jeffrey AA, et al. Clinical features of the sleep apnea/hypopnea syndrome. *Q J Med* 1989;267:659–666.

98. Douglas NJ, Thomas S, Jan MA. Clinical value of polysomnography. *Lancet* 1992;339:347–350.

Part III.

Therapeutic Interventions

Chapter 21

Physical Medicine and Rehabilitation Consultation and Prescription Writing

Martin Grabois
Donna Bloodworth
Carol Bodenheimer

The concept for this chapter was conceived out of a realization that consultation, establishment of goals, and prescription writing are fundamental to the field of physical medicine and rehabilitation. However, the literature, both scientific articles and book chapters on the topic, are sparse and anecdotal. Most of the information utilized to educate trainees on these subjects is conveyed by bedside teaching, lectures, and handouts and is not noted in the literature.

The goals of this chapter are to provide an overview of the subject, but more importantly, specific and detailed information on appropriate consultation, goal setting, and prescription writing in physical medicine and rehabilitation. In accomplishing this task, the issues of who does the consultations, sets goals, and writes prescriptions are addressed. Additionally, why they are done, how they are done, and when they should be done are discussed.

The resources utilized to write this chapter are contained in chapters in traditional textbooks of physical medicine and rehabilitation including those by Krusen et al (1), Rusk (2), Delisa (3) and Braddom (4); in handouts passed down through the years (with the original references unknown); and in lectures at Baylor College of Medicine Department of Physical Medicine and Rehabilitation and in grand rounds on the subject.

THE REHABILITATION TEAM

Determining the health care professional who is best able to perform consultations, set goals, and prescribe the treatment program depends on educational background, experience, legal requirements, and the medical or team model utilized. Currie and Marburger (5) noted that the person with a disability needs someone to act as a case manager to help bring all the caregivers together as a team. They further stated that this person should be a professional who understands individual problems and the possible interaction between them. Obviously having an understanding of medical rehabilitation, resources available, and team management skills is necessary.

While physicians have the medical skills, knowledge, and legal authority to evaluate, set goals, and prescribe treatment, many lack training in rehabilitation (5). Allied health professionals have extensive knowledge and skills within their own discipline, many with excellent team skills; however, they may not be familiar with other disciplines and lack extensive medical training (5). The physiatrist or other physician with extensive rehabilitation training and experience is one of the health care professionals who has the combination of medical and rehabilitation training, legal authority, and knowledge of allied health care professional and team skills necessary to be the case manager.

While a case manager is usually not necessary for the patient with a limited and straightforward disability, for the patient with a more complex problem, the physiatrist or similarly trained individual brings together the unique combination of knowledge and skills necessary to manage the patient and lead the team (5). However, that individual does not perform the task alone or in isolation.

Comprehensive medical rehabilitation often requires the interaction of multiple caregivers to provide the breadth of services needed for people with physical impairment (5–7). The primary goal of these multiple caregivers and their interaction is communication of the patient's need and coordination of their efforts in a synergetic manner (8). In essence, the physiatrist or other medical specialist with rehabilitation training is the one who often provides the communication by consultation and prescription writing, to provide adequate services from a multitude of rehabilitation health care professionals.

The form that consultation, goal setting, and prescription writing will take is based on four general styles of interaction between physicians and other rehabilitation health care providers (8). The *medical model* (Fig. 21-1) basically is appropriate for the simple, limited, and straightforward rehabilitation problem (e.g., acute low-back pain) (8). The physician in isolation evaluates, sets goals, and prescribes or provides therapy. If services of another discipline are desired, the appropriate professional is consulted and given either specific or general requests for assistance to meet the needs of the patient, as prescribed by the attending physician, and then provides direct feedback to that attending physician of any additional needs or modifications of the request.

The *multidisciplinary model* keeps the attending physician at the center of the process of evaluating, setting goals, and establishing the prescription. However, now multiple therapists are often involved (Fig. 21-2) and there may be interactions with each other if the physician sees the need for such interactions (8). King and Titus (8) noted that this mode typically is an attending physician–controlled team in which most interactions are between consultants and the primary attending physician. Discussions between other health care professionals are held to a minimum or at best directed by the attending physician when necessary. This model is currently utilized by many comprehensive rehabilitation programs.

In the *interdisciplinary model* or *case manager model*, the case manager orchestrates the team, with the attending physician and all other health care professionals and the patient as equal members of the team (Fig. 21-3). Note that the case manager can be any member of the team and sometimes the case manager changes depending on the needs of the patient. While this model offers the advantages of increased communication and equality of team members, it is more time-consuming and thus more expensive to follow than are the other models. Additionally, the physician may be uncomfortable with the team decision-making process because the physician is often the one who has to assume the medicolegal responsibility of the team's action and plans.

The more recently developed *transitional disciplinary team model* is a variant of the multidisciplinary and interdisciplinary models where communication and cross evaluation and treatment between disciplines are allowed and encouraged. While it can be considered a separate model, more often it is integrated into other models for its cost-effectiveness in providing needed services without members of each of the separate allied health care professions present or participating.

Thus, the way the process of consultation, goal setting, and prescription writing is carried out depends on the model of team interaction. For this chapter the multi-

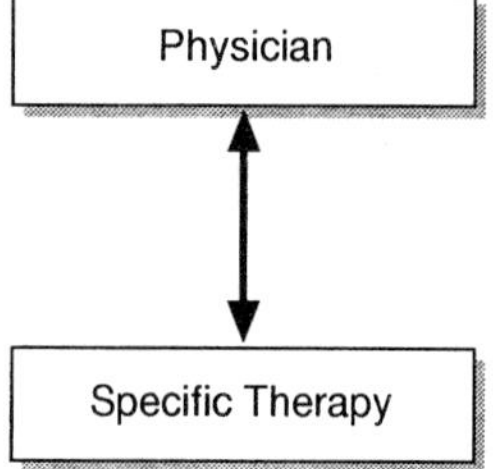

Figure 21-1. Medical model.

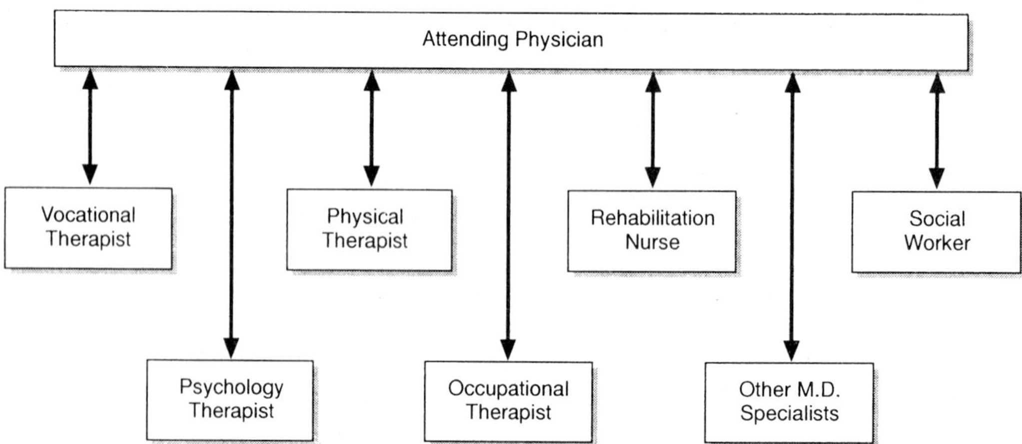

Figure 21-2. Multidisciplinary model.

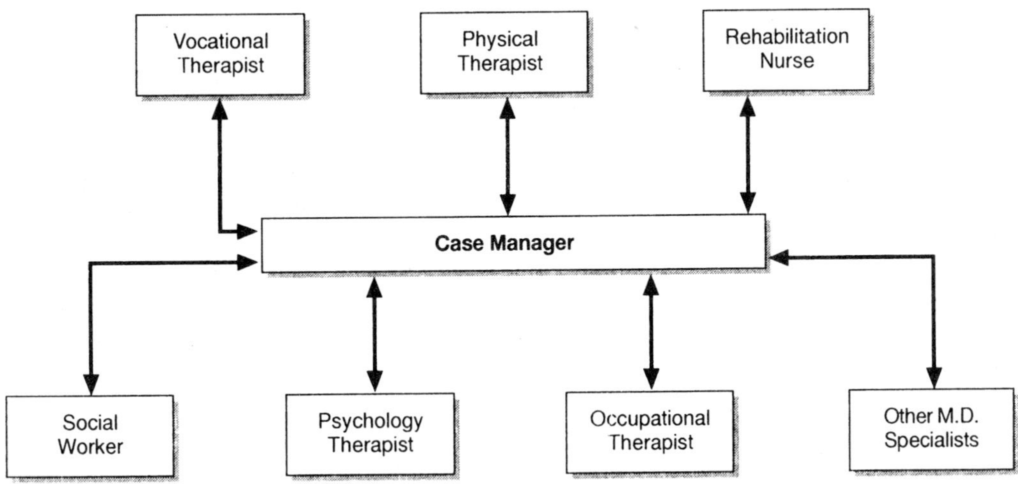

Figure 21-3. Case manager model.

disiplinary model is emphasized, with comparisons and contrasts with other models of care.

Obviously, evaluation is the initial step in deciding on goals and a treatment program. For most of the team models, the physician will provide the initial and broadest evaluation, with other team members providing more detailed evaluation of specific problems within their area of expertise. The specific evaluations by team members amplify and supplement the general evaluation (5). Differences in findings are forwarded to the team leader and discussed by the team, and goals and treatment plans are modified as necessary. The evaluation should identify the medical diagnosis, the impairment, the disability, and the handicap in order to identify a problem list and then establish appropriate goals.

For each problem a goal should be developed, leading to the improvement in the quality of life of the individual being evaluated and treated. The physician's goals tend to be more general and long term, while those of the individual therapist include one or more specific short-term goals (5). Goals should be stated in terms of functional significance or change and their influence on the individual's impairment, disability, and handicap.

It is important not to forget the patient's goals (5). The patient's contributions to the process include describing social and vocational desires as well as the resources available to fulfill those desires.

The role of the individual team member in prescribing treatment again depends on the team model chosen. Essentially in the medical model, the physician prescribes and the therapist treats (9). Thus, the prescription needs to be complete and specific. However, to minimize the potential negative impact on professional credibility and problem-solving expertise, request for feedback should be specifically included. This model is usually used in the traditional outpatient setting (5,10–25). Team members who are unwilling to follow a specific treatment and are unwilling to communicate with the physician should not be tolerated. General orders requesting "evaluation and treatment" from less-knowledgeable physicians tend to promote such practices (8).

In the traditional medical model, the physician may elect to treat the patient with medication, simple modalities, and home exercise programs, without using additional team members. However, without the benefit of a therapist who interacts frequently with the patient and reports problems regularly, more frequent evaluations may be necessary to ensure compliance and progress (8).

In the multidisciplinary team model, similar guidelines for prescriptions are utilized except there is significantly more input from team members, often in a team conference setting. Priorities of goals and treatment are more easily discussed verbally than in written form and the setting does not require statement of the next visit, desired frequency of visits, and mechanism of follow-up therapy reports (4).

In the interdisciplinary team model, territory is relinquished by all and embraced by all, although in the end, specific tasks and interventions are assigned by the group to the individual team members who have the greatest expertise in the area of need (4). The comprehensive treatment plan is not developed solely by the admitting physician, and specific interventions are decided by mutual consensus among all the team members. In this setting, general orders are usually accepted but may be counterproductive to the educational process of the physician, the medical supervision of the patient, and the collective group synergism that can enhance creative problem solving (5).

With clinical pathways and practice parameters, the goals and prescription of therapy may be determined in advance by the team, following a set sequence of events. However, not every patient fits in the predetermined pathways and modification of the program is essential if there is a difference or additional need determined by the evaluation process.

COMPONENTS, OBJECTIVES, AND RESPONSIBILITIES OF PHYSICAL MEDICINE AND REHABILITATION CONSULTATION

Rehabilitation textbooks and the literature, and even seasoned attending physicians, are not necessarily in agreement with an explanation of what a physical medicine and rehabilitation consultation is, what its content and objectives are. A literature review did not reveal a definition or characterization of the "physical medicine and rehabilitation consultation." Therefore, here we blended information from parallel readings that define consultation, qualify the essential components of a consultation, define physical medicine and rehabilitation, and review the philosophy of physical medicine and rehabilitation, to define a physical medicine and rehabilitation consultation and characterize its objectives and responsibilities.

A succinct definition of *consultation* is provided in *Krusen's Handbook of Physical Medicine and Rehabilitation*, in the context of explaining the role of the social worker as a rehabilitation team member. The textbook explains that "consultation involves giving of expert advice, information or insights related to the treatment of a patient" (26). Borrowing this definition, a physical medicine and rehabilitation consultation should provide expert advice, information, or insights related to the *physiatric* treatment of a patient.

Defining *physiatric treatment* is complex, but unique features of this medical specialty distinguish it from all other medical fields. Halstead (27) explained that "traditionally, the central concern of rehabilitation has been the restoration of function so that a person can perform to his or her fullest physical, emotional, social, and vocational potential." In short, rehabilitation physicians are *function doctors*. The physiatric history and physical examination focus on functional abilities at a personal and at a social level (28–30). In daily practice the physiatrist distinguishes himself or herself from all other medical practitioners by assessing not only the patient's disease diagnosis, but also the patient's impairments, disabilities, and handicaps (28–30). The physiatric history and physical examination (Table 21-1) identify the individual's *impairments, disabilities,* and *handicaps*, as defined by the World Health Organization (Table 21-2) (28–30). Like routine medical histories and physical examinations, the physiatrist's evaluation also verifies the disease diagnosis. Lastly, physiatric treatment implies the implementation of a multidisciplinary team to maximize the function of the patient with a chronic

Table 21-1: Physiatric History and Physical Examination
Historic questions
Prior level of independence in the home
Prior level of independence in the community
Prior use of assistive devices
Resistance to use of assistive devices and why
Prior assistance with personal or household tasks
Rate of decline if functional level has diminished
Prior therapeutic interventions and efficacy
Employment and household and social responsibilities
Architectural features and barriers of current abode
Household members and their physical abilities
Current questions
Current level of independence or assistance for mobility
Current level of independence or assistance for personal tasks
Current level of independence or assistance for household tasks
Current use of assistive devices for mobility, self-care, or household activities
Current knowledge of these devices or therapies available to improve function
Current therapeutic activities
Current understanding of symptoms and diagnostic condition
Beliefs about the resolution of symptoms and diagnosis condition
Beliefs about the anticipated household and social responsibilities with or after diagnoses
Physical examination
Mobility, including in bed and for transitions
Self-care ability during examination
Range of motion of large and small joints
Strength of large and small muscle groups
Dexterity and coordination
Sensory perception, including sight, hearing, and smell
Other cranial nerve integrity, including coordinated motions for speech and swallow
Observations of the distracted patient

Table 21-2: Abbreviated Definitions After the World Health Organization

Disease	A pathologic condition of the body
Impairment	A loss of normal anatomic, physiologic, or psychological status
Disability	A loss of normal function; inability to perform a task
Handicap	A loss of normal social function; inability to perform a role

impairment, disability, or handicap through comprehensive, coordinated care (27). Thus, physiatric assessment and treatment address functional issues.

A practicable definition of physical medicine and rehabilitation consultation includes the performance of a history and physical examination to identify anticipated or permanent impairments, disabilities, and handicaps. It also includes 1) providing advice and information about assistive devices, 2) coordinating multidisciplinary services to minimize further functional morbidity, and 3) coordinating multidisciplinary services to compensate and maximize function. Lastly, the consultation includes predicting functional prognosis, and anticipating the patient's needs for equipment and caregivers.

MEDICAL CONSULTATION

In the literature, physician authors define *consultation* practically in terms of a medical service that is provided, whereas administrative authors define *consultation* legally in terms of the component features on which charges are based. Physician authors also describe effective interview and communication techniques as regards to consultations, as well as the ethical standards that direct the physician's interaction with the patient. Yesner's definition of consultation describes the medical service rendered (26): Consultation "is the giving of expert advice, information or insights related to the patient of the patient." In *Current Procedural Terminology* (CPT), the American Medical Association (AMA) offers a legal and administrative definition of consultation and standardizes the components of a consultation for the purposes of equitable charging (31):

> Consulting is a type of service provided by a physician whose opinion or advice regarding the diagnosing or treatment options is requested by another physician or other appropriate source. . . . The consultant's opinion and any services that were ordered or performed must be documented in the patient's medical record and communicated to the requesting physician or other appropriate source.

In CPT, the AMA elaborates on the required contents of consultations of variable complexity, from focused consultation to comprehensive consultation. It describes proper documentation of consultation; the documentation of information is a rote process once learned. However, the art and ethical aspects of consultation deserve discourse.

Yesner's definition that consultation is the giving of advice begs the question, the giving of advice to whom? The literature indicates that the consultant disseminates advice and information to two parties: the referring physician and the patient. The CPT definition of consultation notes that this service is requested by another physician, and that the consultant should return recommendations to the referring physician. However, British articles and guidelines published by the American Association of Electrodiagnostic Medicine (AAEM) noted that the patient is the primary person receiving service (32–34). The AAEM wrote that "the consultant has an ethical duty to consider the interests of the patient first" (32).

The patient is the most important person receiving the consultant's service and opinion. In the treatment of the patient, the literature stresses courteous and clear communication. Several articles, primarily from the British literature, described effective interview techniques that improve the ability of the physician to obtain information from the patient and to communicate an opinion to the patient. According to Fallowfield (33), the referred patient values communication with the physician as much or more than specific expertise. Fallowfield (33) summarized Ley's survey work from 1988 that revealed a 38% dissatisfaction rate with medical communication. Dissatisfaction leads to poor understanding, recall, and compliance with medical advice, and dissatisfaction increases the risk of litigation (33). Rather, summarizing the work of Korsch in 1968, Fallowfield (33) remarked that "patient satisfaction with communication during a consultation correlated highly with satisfaction of other aspects of the doctor/patient interaction." To improve communication during a consultation, Fallowfield (33) encouraged the establishment of eye contact, greeting the patient by name as well as introducing oneself, starting the history taking with open-ended questions, and not interrupting the patient's recounting. Fallowfield (33) noted that in a 1984 study by Beckman and Frankel, physicians interrupted their patient's initial statement within 18 seconds. In a complementary article about improving consulting skills, Havelock (34) instructed that during any consultation, there are two experts: the patient, "an expert about his or her bodily feelings," and the physician, with medical expertise. Successful communication with the patient is a primary goal of the consultation process.

As regards giving advice, a consultation fails, according to Fallowfield (33), if the patient leaves the consultation without a clearer picture of what is wrong, what the physician is going to do, and what has to be done with respect to tests, medications, or therapy. To communicate successfully with the patient, the physician must relay information in nonmedical, layman's terms, must encourage the patient to ask questions, and must not rush the patient (32–34). According to Benett (35), encouraging the patient to write and bring a list of concerns and questions about his or her condition significantly improves the likelihood that the physician will address all the patient's questions. To increase the patient's understanding and comfort during consultation, Fallowfield (33) suggested providing preprinted information, asking the patient to repeat what he or she understands about the diagnosis and treatment plan, and asking the patient to bring a close companion in the event that information will provoke anxiety. Physicians can learn interviewing and consulting skills to elicit a greater quantity as well as improved quality of information, but without spending more time, according to Evans and Sweet (36). The available literature emphasizes that effective communication skills affect patient satisfaction with the physician consultant, and improve understanding and compliance with treatment recommendations.

Consultation also involves giving expert advice, information, and insight to the referring physician. As the AAEM guidelines state, referrals to consultants come primarily from other physicians (32). Devor et al (37) cited a definition of *medical consultation* as a "deliberation between physicians on case or treatment." They (37) explained that "because of busy schedules, advances in communication technology, and the volume of consultation, the process of consultation has evolved from a meeting of physicians at the bedside to independent patient interactions separated by time and space." Successful consulting involves scheduling and completing the consultation in a timely manner, and conveying recommendations in a prompt fashion. As regards relaying information, Devor et al (37) noted that physicians preferred and most commonly used verbal communication to communicate to other physicians. These authors (37) instructed that residents who learn to contact the referring physician personally not only will offer better patient care but also will improve their future practice by mastering this skill. Depending on the consultant's relationship with the referring physician, the consulting physician may initiate treatments, but it is proper to return recommendations to the referring physician and allow that physician to discuss treatment options with the patient. Devor et al (37) did note, however, that consultants who write their own orders improve compliance with recommendations. The art of consultation as it relates to the referring physician succeeds if the interaction is prompt, pertinent, and personal.

The available literature not only defines consultation and describes the features of a successful consultation, it also outlines the consulting physician's ethical and legal responsibilities when providing consultation (32). The foremost ethical duty of the physician is again the interest of the patient; these interests include practicing competently and respecting the patient's autonomy, confidentiality, and welfare (32). The AAEM (32) explained that competent practice requires the physician to participate in regular continuing education, and to provide care consistent with the prevailing standard of care. To paraphrase the AAEM guidelines (32), competent practice also dictates that the physician prepare and catalog records of adequate detail, and that the physician comply with reasonable requests from insurance and compensation agencies, within the constraints of patient confidentiality. The AAEM guidelines (32) noted that a physician should not condone unsavory or impaired practice by another physician. Short (38) considered it unprofessional to deride a physician to a peer or to a patient or to undermine a patient's confidence in the primary physician. However, the consultant also has ethical responsibilities to the patient.

In addition to the interpersonal aspects of the physician's interaction with the patient, there are legal aspects of the interaction. The AAEM (32) noted that the physician may accept or decline to give a consultation, but the physician may not decline based on discriminatory criteria. Legitimate reasons to decline a referral include conflicts of interest, time constraints, and limitations of expertise. The physician must disclose and resolve conflicts of interest with the patient prior to initiating the service, or must decline consulting on the case (32). A physician should have the patient's consent to proceed with a consultation; however, while the patient may withdraw this consent at any time, the physician must complete the consultation once he or she has agreed to evaluate the patient (32). The physician must handle the patient's case and records confidentially, and avoid publicizing any detail that would identify the patient (32). The physician must confer with the patient honestly. Short (38) discussed dealing honestly with patients. When the patient's diagnosis or prognosis is poor, being honest allows the physician to review the truth at the rate that the patient requests it (38). Based on the work of Savage and Armstrong in 1990, Short (38) also recommended a *directing form* of consultation. The *directing form* of consultation is in contrast to a *sharing form*, which encourages the patient to make a choice among treatment options (38). Short (38) commented that patients seek "an element of direction from their medical advisors." In addition to effective communication techniques, obvious legal and ethical principles of competence, consent, confidentiality, honesty, and disclosure guide the physician's interaction with the patient.

Consultation is a medical service that involves the written or verbal deliberation between physicians regarding the evaluation or treatment of a patient. What once was an interaction at the bedside of the patient is now more likely to be a service that the consulting physician provides seeing the patient alone. Consultation involves giving expert advise, information, or insight about the diagnosis or treatment of a patient both to the individual referred and to the primary physician. Gathering information, the consulting physician will be more successful if he or she interviews the patient in a courteous and engaging manner.

Disseminating information, the physician will be more successful if he or she speaks plainly, calmly, reassuringly, and truthfully. At all times, the physician maintains professional decorum and ethical propriety.

PHYSICAL MEDICINE AND REHABILITATION CONSULTATION

Physicians and allied health professionals in any discipline benefit from understanding the qualities and requirements of effective consultation. Each medical and allied health specialty studies, understands, and assesses the human patient from a unique vantage point. Physicians in physical medicine and rehabilitation consider the function of the person and the modulation and compensation of symptoms, and consultation reflects these considerations.

In history and in practice, the field of physical medicine and rehabilitation distinguishes itself from other medical specialties by its focus on human function and its recognition and utilization of nonmedicinal therapeutics. Krusen did not publish the first physical medicine textbook until 1941, and Krusen, Coulter, and Zeiter did not incorporate the American Board of Physical Medicine until 1947 (39), but medical history describes physiatric applications prior to the early twentieth century. DeLisa et al (39) described therapeutic uses of electrical current antecedent to this century. The use of various physical modalities, and of physical and occupational therapy increased early in this century (39). Kottke et al (40) identified a trend away from convalescence and the application of rehabilitation to restore function in the era between the World Wars. Howard Rusk demonstrated in 1943 that rehabilitation, as opposed to convalescence, was necessary to restore soldiers' fitness for duty (40). Concurrently, in civilian hospitals, physicians were departing from the tradition of prolonged bed rest prescribed after abdominal surgery, and patients were benefiting from early ambulation (40). Rusk referred to rehabilitation as "the third phase of medical care," with the first phase being preventive and the second phase being curative medicine and surgery (40). Not a curative medical art, the specialty physical medicine and rehabilitation provides patients options of treatment to improve and compensate function, and to modulate symptoms.

Because physiatrists attend to the function of the patient, they assess and treat not only the disease process but also any impairment, disability, and handicap resulting from the disease. Physical medicine and rehabilitation textbooks commonly cite the World Health Organization definitions of *impairment, disability*, and *handicap* (see Table 21-2) (28,29,41). Stolov (30) and Kirby (41) explained the ramifications and subtleties of impairment, disability, and handicap. Paraphrasing Stolov (30), one should note that *no* one-to-one correlation exists between disease and disability. Disease may, in fact, not yield disability, even if impairment exists; disability may resolve although disease and impairment remain. Therefore, when the physiatrist encounters a new patient, consults on a referred patient, or discusses the care of a typical patient as in grand rounds or panel discussions, the physiatrist should comment on the disease process in the context of the impairment, disease, and handicap that the disease imparts. The physiatrist should then outline a plan of care to resolve or compensate disability and handicap when these sequelae exist.

The tool by which the physiatrist discerns impairment, disability, and handicap is the physiatric history and physical examination, which converge on function (see Table 21-1). Interviewing the patient, the physiatrist must investigate past function, rate of functional decline, and current functional ability to discern the disability. The physiatrist must also investigate the topography of the habitation and vocation to which the person will return. To discern handicap, the physiatrist must question the patient's current personal and social responsibilities and obligations. The physician must know to what degree family members or reliable companions can supervise or physically assist the patient with a temporary or permanent disability and handicap. Existing textbooks detail the neurologic assessment, the calculation of range of motion, and the determination of the patient's ability to care for himself or herself and move in the environment (28,30,41,42). These same sources catalog questions that elicit details about functional history (28,30,41,42). The physiatrist uses the history and physical examination to assess how the patient's disease affects the patient's function.

In the role of a consultant, the physiatrist attends to the functional sequelae of the referred patient's disease processes. Engaging the patient with eye contact and open-ended questions, the physiatrist gathers and assimilates information on the patient's history, which eventually focuses on questions about past and current function, assistive devices, and functional stability or rate of decline of function. Answers to questions about current and anticipated responsibilities or environments provide the physiatrist with long-term goals for the patient's treatment program. Treating the patient with courtesy and respect, the physiatrist performs the physical examination, which may include a neurologic assessment, an evaluation of joint motion, and an assessment of ability to complete self-care. The physician should allow the patient an opportunity to add other information that he or she considers important and to ask questions. The physiatrist then assimilates these data and arrives at a differential diagnosis, if this is requested, but more importantly determines the patient's impairments that result from the symptomatology, and disabilities and handicaps that are temporary or permanent as a result of the disease and its associated impairments.

The facility of the physiatrist with the differential diagnoses of symptom complexes is requisite when evaluating the patient. The physiatrist's anticipation of the natural

Table 21-3: Relativity of Impairments, Disability, and Handicap over Time with Respect to the Diagnosis of Radicular Low-Back Pain

	Temporary	Permanent	Anticipated	Interventions
Impairment	Pain, weakness, sensory loss and "clumsiness" Signs of myelopathy Stiffness Decreased flexibility	Residual pain, weakness, and sensory loss or none	Similar Frustration, depression with prolonged symptoms Adverse medication reactions or none	Pain medication Dynamic lumbar stabilization Modalities for pain relief Psychological support and prolonged symptoms
Disability	Self-care dysfunction Ambulation dysfunction Pain limiting sitting or activity movements	Weakness, pain, or sensory loss limiting sitting, standing, ambulation, or functional range for self-care or none	Similar	Assistive devices Flexibility and strengthening program Back conservation education Environmental adaptation (workstation)
Handicap	Limitations for jobs or household or parenting responsibilities with lifting, carrying, sitting, standing, or stooping	Some restrictions or limitations for job requirements, or avocational pursuits or none	Similar	Vocational retraining

history of a disease process allows him or her to predict the transience or permanence of the disability and handicap associated with the symptoms of the disease.

The resources a physiatrist accesses and coordinates include members of the multidisciplinary team of allied health care providers whose services or skills modulate, compensate, or remediate the patient's impairment, disability, and handicap. Other authors (28,29) have described these rehabilitation team members elsewhere. The physiatrist, in consultation, will recommend medicinal and therapeutic modalities to begin to compensate or ameliorate temporary, permanent, and anticipated impairment, disability, and handicap that result from the disease (Table 21-3).

THE NEED FOR PHYSIATRIC CONSULTATION

Other medical specialists continue to need the assistance of physiatrists to utilize and coordinate rehabilitation modalities and personnel. A study of house officers found that while 98% of house staff referred patients to physical therapy, 46% felt inadequately prepared to do so (43). Brogan (44) found that physicians underestimated the need of their patients for physiatric intervention. Davidoff et al (45) found that a referral to physical therapy by a nonphysiatric physician underestimated significantly the need for more comprehensive rehabilitation services. Additionally, the narrative of the consultation request by the nonphysiatrist did not suggest the perception of a need for more complex services, and only a physiatric evaluation revealed the need (20). Finestone (46) found that rheumatology residents requesting physical medicine and rehabilitation services did so in general terms, that is, requesting evaluation and treatment. Wrigley et al (47) found that receiving a physical medicine and rehabilitation consultation correlated with a greater likelihood of a patient with traumatic brain injury receiving more comprehensive rehabilitation services. Criticism of Davidoff's and Wrigley's studies (45,47) might include that physiatric providers would be biased to demonstrate physiatric need; however, this tendency is balanced by the ethical requirement that a physician not exploit the patient and that the physician practice in the best interest of the patient. Wrigley et al (47) wrote that "rehabilitation is the process by which biologic, psychological and social functions are restored or developed after damage, thereby allowing a person to regain personal autonomy and achieve an independent, noninstitutional lifestyle." They continued that "a referral to rehab . . . should reflect a purposeful, goal-oriented transition from the acute care setting to the most formal rehabilitation environment needed for the patient."

According to Gonzalez et al (48), consultation continues to be the principal clinical activity in which physiatrists are involved. As regards preparing residents to perform as consultants, an interesting study of internists by Devor et al (37) suggested methods for preparing residents as consultants. In this study former residents were surveyed as to what diagnoses they received excessive training in and what diagnoses they frequently encountered in practice but had been underexposed to in residency, and the diagnoses for which training and frequency of encounter in practice were proportional. The researchers' work finds recommendations to increase exposure to diagnoses for which there was inadequate training. Interestingly, the research led to recommendations *not* to alter other training, even to diagnoses for which training was excessive. Rehabilitation, as a medical specialty, is practiced largely in the realm of consultation; physiatrists can borrow work from other specialties to learn how to better prepare residents for this consulting role.

Physiatric consultation has been found to increase the patient's access to other services that may be beneficial. In a study of patients with acquired immunodeficiency syndrome (AIDS), physiatric referral led to increased diagnoses, namely of painful neuropathies, and referral for modalities and therapeutics (48). O'Dell (49), however, was careful to note that further research should address the efficacy of these interventions and the value of early rehabilitation. Physical medicine and rehabilitation consultation with rheumatology patients, as reviewed by Finestone (46), led to physical therapy referral for 92% of the patients, physical therapy and occupational therapy in half of the patients, and orthotics prescription for 89% of the patients. Echoing O'Dell, Finestone (46) questioned subsequent outcome as regards to quality of life, degree of independence, and alleviation of pain. Physiatric consultation facilitates diagnoses in some processes and promotes referral of the patient for orthotic and therapeutic services.

The need for physiatric consultation, as the literature reveals, is twofold. First, nonphysiatric colleagues perceive that they are underprepared to request rehabilitation therapeutics. Studies (37) revealed that nonphysiatric colleagues ordering rehabilitation therapeutics and allied rehabilitative services do so in a general way, and that patients receive more comprehensive service when a physiatric specialist evaluates the patient. Second, evaluation by the physiatric specialist increases the patient's likelihood of being referred for useful functional services, such as orthotic evaluation and occupational therapy.

Appendices I through III are sample rehabilitation consultation outlines.

THE PRESCRIPTION

Why Write a Prescription?

Essentially, a prescription is the ultimate form of communication from the physician to the patient and other clinicians involved in the patient's care. It allows the physician to present to the patient, at the end of an evaluation and examination, a diagnosis and a plan of action. Patients and referring physicians have come to expect that a medical consultation or visit will result in either a "prescription" of further tests to confirm a diagnosis or a prescription that will treat the patient's problem. In our modern medical era, both patients and physicians associate a prescription for treatment with a medication. As practitioners, we bemoan the great number of patients who come to our offices wanting a "quick fix" in the form of a pill. A complete rehabilitation prescription is our opportunity as physiatrists to demonstrate to patients that we have seriously considered their condition and rendered a professional opinion as to the appropriate treatment. A copy of the rehabilitation prescription should become a part of the patient's chart, documenting the level of complexity of physician services rendered.

A prescription, in its essence, is a means of communicating to other clinicians. In the example of a medication, the communication is with a pharmacist. However, the same parameters for describing a prescription hold true for a therapy prescription. "The prescription order . . . represents a summary of the physician's diagnosis and treatment of the patient's illness. It brings into focus, on one slip of paper, the diagnostic acuteness and therapeutic proficiency of the physician with instructions for the palliation or restoration of the patient's health" (50). Therefore, the therapy prescription must convey the essential diagnostic as well as treatments information.

A clearly written prescription informs other clinicians (and the patient) of the predicated outcome of the treatment. Engaging the patient early in the treatment course as to the expected goals of a therapy program assists the patient in developing realistic short-term and long-term goals in conjunction with the treatment team. A statement of expected goals of a treatment plan at the outset allows the team to determine when discharge from a specific level of care (e.g., inpatient acute, subacute, or outpatient rehabilitation) is indicated.

Specifics of Prescription Order Writing

Prescription writing is a daily part of physiatric practice. The American Council of Graduate Medicine Education (ACGME) criteria for residency educational objectives (51) include "the training program must provide opportunity for the graduate . . . to write adequately detailed prescriptions based on factual goals for physiatric management." The American Board of Physical Medicine and Rehabilitation (52) also recognizes the importance of prescription writing by stating "the resident must develop . . . measurable competencies in . . . prescription for orthotics, prosthetics, wheelchair and ambulatory devices, . . . prescriptions with specific details appropriate to the patient for therapeutic modalities and therapeutic exercises performed by physical therapists and occupational therapists." While writing a prescription is considered a critical part of physiatric practice, there is no broad consensus on what constitutes an appropriate prescription.

Prescriptions ought to be written in clear, concise language (50). Physiatrists who work with a specific group

Appendix I: Patient Evaluation in Rehabilitation

- I. Historical
  - A. Chief complaint
  - B. Present illness
  - C. Past medical history
  - D. Review by systems
  - E. Psychosocial inventory
    - 1. Personal psychological status
      - a. Personality
        - (1) Preillness
        - (2) Effect of illness
      - b. Intelligence
        - (1) Native
        - (2) Impairment
      - c. Mental status
        - (1) Sensorium
        - (2) Orientation
        - (3) Memory
        - (4) Emotional tone
        - (5) Behavior
        - (6) Insight
    - 2. Family status
      - a. Parents
      - b. Spouse
      - c. Siblings
      - d. Offspring
    - 3. Community
      - a. Location
      - b. Size
      - c. Industries
      - d. Resources
      - e. Obstacles
    - 4. Financial status
      - a. Income
      - b. Family resources
      - c. Community or agency aid or service
  - F. Vocational inventory
    - 1. Education
    - 2. Vocational interests
    - 3. Vocational training
    - 4. Vocational experience
- II. Physical examination
  - A. General medical
  - B. Musculoskeletal evaluation
    - 1. Posture
    - 2. Habitus
    - 3. Reflexes
      - a. Cranial
      - b. Spinal
    - 4. Mobility
      - a. Range of joint motion—test and record
      - b. Muscular strength—manual muscle test
      - c. Abnormal muscular status
        - (1) Flaccidity
        - (2) Spasticity
        - (3) Rigidity
        - (4) Contractures
      - d. Abnormal movements
        - (1) Athetoid
        - (2) Choreiform
        - (3) Dystonic
        - (4) Fasciculation
        - (5) Tremor
          - (a) Parkinsonism
          - (b) Intention
        - (6) Coordination
  - C. Sensation
    - 1. Superficial
      - a. Pain
      - b. Light touch
      - c. Temperative
      - d. Two-point discrimination
    - 2. Deep
      - a. Pain
      - b. Position
      - c. Vibration
      - d. Stereognosis
  - D. Speech and communication
    - 1. Expressive
    - 2. Receptive
    - 3. Cognitive
  - E. Performance
    - 1. Gait
    - 2. Manual dexterity
    - 3. Activities of daily living
- III. Laboratory studies
  - A. Chemical
    - 1. Blood
    - 2. Urine
    - 3. Other
  - B. Morphologic
    - 1. Hematology
    - 2. Pathology
  - C. Roentgenologic
    - 1. Postural
    - 2. Mobility
    - 3. Cinefluorographic
  - D. Electromyographic
    - 1. Nerve conduction
  - E. Circulatory
  - F. Ergographic
- IV. Special evaluation for rehabilitation
  - A. Clinical psychology
    - 1. Personality
    - 2. Intelligence
    - 3. Interests
    - 4. Aptitudes
  - B. Vocational counseling
    - 1. Vocational education
    - 2. Vocational interests
    - 3. Vocational aptitudes
  - C. Speech pathology
    - 1. Schuell
    - 2. Eisenson
    - 3. Bender Gestalt
  - D. Activities of daily living—evaluation

Appendix II: Physical Medicine and Rehabilitation Consultation

I. Premorbid function
   A. General state of health
   B. Relative independence in activities of daily living (ADLs)
   C. Living arrangement—alone? family? architectural barriers? meals? finances? medical care?

II. Present illness
   A. What happened to patient
   B. Medical, surgical care
   C. Complications
   D. Incidental or associated medical problems discovered or developed

Why has a consultation from physical medicine and rehabilitation been requested?

III. Current status—details of physical examination and current history
   A. Pain—describe
   B. Limitations of movement—Why? What structures?
   C. Weakness
   D. Cardiorespiratory
   E. Skin—breakdown (decubiti), wound healing
   F. Urinary—continent? catheter?
   G. Bowel
   H. Neurologic—including communication if applicable
   I. Psychological—orientation, insight into present status, affect, etc.
   J. Social status only if different from I-C above

IV. Objectives—potential goals that the patient could and wants to accomplish. Is this a short-term problem of physical restoration or a major rehabilitation case? The overall goal of rehabilitation is to help the patient achieve this optimum level of physical, social, emotional, and vocational performance. With this as a guide, try to determine what the patient's potential might be in each area:
   A. Physical
      1. ADLs—eating, dressing, grooming, household
      2. Transfers—bed to standing, bed to wheelchair to toilet to auto, etc.
      3. Ambulation—ambulative aides and type, stairs and curbs, wheelchair, bed bound, prosthetic/orthotic devices, endurance
      4. Review applicable systems under III above
   B. Social—review as per under I-C above. Can patient benefit from public health nurse referral?
   C. Psychological—Are your goals those of the patients? How will mental status in each of its ramifications bear on attainment of potential?
   D. Vocational—is there any work potential? Is referral to DVR indicated?

V. Methods and time required
   A. What equipment will patient need? How can it be obtained?
   B. Special x-ray, laboratory, etc. Consultations needed? Review per III.
   C. Any factors in overall management of patient that attending physician is not aware of? Requires finesse in presentation to and misinterpretation of motives.
   D. Are the potential goals or objectives such that the patient will never realize a sufficient level of function, and discharge to a nursing home is inevitable?

Then..................

   E. If not, briefly state rehabilitative procedures and try to estimate time required.
   F. Transfer to physical medicine and rehabilitation may be suggested if an extensive program is anticipated.

VI. Write a set of orders
   A. Physical therapy
   B. Occupational therapy
   C. Braces, prosthetics, wheelchair, ambulation aids
   D. Psychology—social service—vocational rehabilitation—speech pathology—etc.

Appendix III: The Rehabilitation Work-up

This outline only indicates and stresses those areas where the student should expand beyond this current practice. The usual standard work-up material still applies.

History

Chief complaint

History of present illness	To include in addition to the development of the disease, the patient's statements with regard to premorbid physical functioning and current physical functioning as expressed by the degree of independence and dependence in the performance of the activities of daily living (ADLs), i.e., ambulation spectrum, transfers, driving, rating, personal hygiene.
Review of symptoms	In addition to routine review, study should also be geared to physical reserve for participating in a rehabilitation program.
Past medical history	Search routinely and specifically with regard to number and response to previous medical stresses.

Social history

1. Determine the current social situation for social impact of illness on:
   A. Vocational and recreational activities and responsibilities
   B. Family relationships
   C. Economic resources
   D. Environmental resources (physical characteristics of home)
2. Determine previous social adjustment
   A. Socioeconomic status of family of origin and immediate family
   B. Experiences of childhood and adolescence
   C. Level of success, maturity, and responsibility achieved as an adult and in school, work, marriage

Vocational history

1. Chronology of employment, duties, length of stay, income, reason for leaving, stability of most recent or current work
2. Education and special training or licenses
3. Current vocational plans

Physical examination

1. Routine aspects, including assessment of physical reserve for rehabilitation
2. Neurologic examination
3. Muscle function examination
4. Range of motion examination
5. Functional neuromuscular examination (observation of patient performance in ADLs)
6. Mental status examination (details of evaluation of intellectual deficit in symbolic, perceptual, memory, quality control, and emotional organic function—details of evaluation of psychological response to illness)

Impression

1. Diagnosis
2. Statement of status of global disability (medical, psychological, social, and vocational)

Plan

1. Immediate diagnostic and medical treatment needs; long-term anticipated medical needs
2. Goal of physical restoration expressed in functional ADL terms
3. Plan and direction of social disposition after hospitalization
4. Plan and direction of vocational disposition
5. Estimated length of time to achieve above goals
6. Possible problems—medical, psychological, or environmental—that may impede or delay goal achievement

of therapists may be in the habit of using abbreviations and "standard" protocols. Care must be exercised to avoid jargon or diagnostic terms that are open to interpretation, particularly in the outpatient setting where the prescribing physiatrist and the treating therapist may not have a common set of expectations or clinical language. This is especially true with less common abbreviations or abbreviations that may refer to more than one clinical entity.

The physiatrist should be familiar with the licensing provisions for various therapists and associated health care providers. When the physician is working within a multidisciplinary team setting (or interdisciplinary team setting), the team may assist in determining which interventions will be handled by the different health care providers on the team. However, who may provide specific types of therapeutic interventions can vary from jurisdiction to jurisdiction. Again, the physician must be knowledgeable regarding who can provide different therapies as determined by state law and licensing requirements, insurance regulations, institutional guidelines or procedures, and customs. Again, especially for the physician who may be prescribing for outpatient services, knowledge of the local provider network and skills is critical to ensuring a beneficial outcome from the prescribed therapy.

Anatomy of a Prescription

As mentioned, there is no broad consensus on the details of what constitutes an appropriate prescription. Martin and Gamble (53) stated there are five "essential" parts to a prescription: diagnosis, modalities, follow-up, cautions, and home care. Currie and Marburger (5) stated that a prescription must have five items: diagnosis, goals, discipline of treating therapist, precautions, and date of re-evaluation. They further stated that a prescription may have seven items: estimated length of stay, evaluation instruments, modalities, frequency, duration, discharge criteria, and treatment plan (54).

In reviewing the components of a physiatric prescription, certain parts form a "backbone" or template from which any detailed prescription will flow. Table 21-4 presents a template of basic components that should be included in any prescription. A detailed review of what information or instructions need to be included to "flesh out" a prescription is contained in the following paragraphs. Modifications to this basic prescription form for the inpatient or outpatient setting are also noted.

Demographic information needs to be included in the prescription to assist the therapists or treatment team in identifying the patient and for the more mundane reasons of billing or verification of insurance. Demographic information also is important to the treatment team with regard to potential roles and responsibilities (i.e., functional tasks) of the patient based on age, gender, or ethnic background. This statement is not meant to imply that stereotypes or prejudices should determine what role we assist patients in attaining, but rather that alerting the treatment team to evaluate age-, gender-, or ethnic group–specific roles with a patient assists all of the team in providing the treatment plan most sensitive to the patient's desires and needs. This issue is trivial in cognitively intact patients without communication difficulties who can easily express to the treating team the functional skills that hold meaning and importance to them. It, however, becomes more important in the patient with cognitive deficits or communication difficulties. In these latter circumstances, awareness of basic demographic information allows the team to begin exploring these functional roles with the patient and the family.

Table 21-4: Anatomy of a Prescription

Demographic information	Physician name and contact information
Diagnosis	Date of onset of impairment
Precautions	Date of follow-up appointment with physician
Treatment goals Treating therapies requested, e.g., occupational, physical, play, and speech therapy, therapeutic and vocational recreation Specifics of therapy requested, e.g., mode of exercise (aerobic, strength training), modality and intensity of exercise, frequency and duration of individual sessions, duration of total treatment, follow-up instructions	

The diagnosis should include the major relevant physical findings as well as underlying medical conditions. In patients with multiple medical problems, this portion of the prescription may be lengthy. The physician must exercise judgment as to which historical diagnoses are important for the treatment team. For example, a diagnosis of hypothyroidism in a patient now stable on medicine may not be relevant to the therapists, but a diagnosis of gouty arthritis, or a diagnosis of hypertension now stable with medication, would be very relevant for any therapist using a physical modality. The diagnosis portion of the prescription is critical in assisting the therapy staff in performing a thorough evaluation of the patient as well.

When listing a diagnosis for a patient, it is useful to identify the patient's impairments, disabilities, and handicaps, as defined by the World Health Organization. Detailing the impairment, disability, or handicap assists in the next step of designing a therapeutic intervention to address each item. Table 21-3 and Appendices IV to VII are examples of detailed prescriptions for specific common medical conditions frequently treated by physiatrists. These detailed examples of prescriptions use the World Health Organization's impairment, disability, and handicap definitions as a distinct axis for construction of a prescription (54).

The date of onset of the diagnosis is necessary in the prescription as well. Most physicians list the date of onset for the disease process, a concept borrowed from the medical model. However, the date of onset of the impairment being treated is generally most relevant for the treating team in determining the duration of therapy needed. Therefore, it is recommended to use the date of onset of the primary impairment being treated as the date of onset. The date of onset of the disorder will help the physiatrist in determining the appropriate goals for the treatments presented. It allows the therapist to evaluate changes in the patient's symptoms or recovery over time. It also provides some guidance in predicting the patient's progress during therapy. An understanding of the chronicle of the disorder being treated is critical to the entire treatment team. It will

Appendix IV: Relativity of Impairment, Disability, and Handicap over Time with Respect to the Diagnosis of Osteoporosis with Dorsal Compression Fractures

	Temporary	Permanent	Anticipated	Interventions
Impairment	Pain Ileus Atelectasis Adverse drug effects	Pain, possible Loss of height Kyphosis, scoliosis Restrictive lung disease	Same Same Same Same Adverse drug effects	TENS Extension brace Thoracic extension Exercise Pain medications Bowel care Bone loss preventive medication
Disability	Pain with bed mobility Pain with self-care Pain with transfers Pain with ambulation	Pain or loss of functional range of motion for mobility and self-care	Same	Back conversation Exercise TENS, bracing Long-handled equipment Ambulation assistive devices
Handicap	Inability to complete housework Inability to prepare meals Vocational, avocational interference	Similar	Similar	Work simplification Family and social assistance Modified work environment duration or responsibilities

TENS = transcutaneous electrical nerve stimulation.

Appendix V: Relativity of Impairment, Disability, and Handicap over Time with Respect to the Diagnosis of Metabolic or Postoperative Encephalopathy

	Temporary	Permanent	Anticipated	Interventions
Impairment	Obtundation, disorientation Immobility vs unsafe activity Malpositioning Bowel immobility Urinary stasis Atelectasis Skin breakdown Orthostasis and deconditioning	Confusion, executive dysfunction Balance deficit Contracture Scarring, loss of tissue integrity	Similar	Minimize sedation Mobilize to a chair or structure brief activity Preventive splinting Bowel program Urinary drainage Turning and positioning
Disability	Dysphagia or altered feeding status Impaired communication Dependent or minimal self-care and mobility, or unsafe activity Poor endurance for activity	Residual dysphagia or impulsively with feeding Confusion, disorientation Impaired pathfinding or problem solving Decreased self-care or mobility because of cognitive deficits	Similar	Swallowing and oromotor therapy Cognitive assessment and therapy Various memory and planning aids Assistive devices for balance safety supervisory personnel Paced strength and endurance activity
Handicap	Vocational inability Household role dysfunction	Impaired memory or judgment for household or vocational role	Similar	Transfer of responsibility for key or monetary decisions Transfer of responsibility for complex tasks

Appendix VI: Relativity of Impairment, Disability and Handicap over Time with Respect to Diagnosis of Fractured Hip

	Temporary	Permanent	Anticipated	Interventions
Impairment	Postoperative pain Bowel immobility Orthostasis Cardiac deconditioning Surgical incision Atelectasis Urinary stasis Muscle weakness due to surgical incision	Residual pain, decreased flexibility, scar tissue formation, or none	High-risk skin breakdown or none Reconditioning hip musculature Exercises	Pain medication Bowel and bladder program Cardiac
Disability	Inability to perform self-care Inability to transfer safely Inability to ambulate Pain with limb movement	Pain or loss of range of motion limiting ability to perform self-care or for ambulation or none	Same Concerns regarding sexual functioning	Gait training with assistive devices, assistive devices for self-care, toileting, and safe transfers Counseling regarding sexuality
Handicap	Inability to perform household routine (housework, cooking, laundry) Barriers to returning to prior vocational activities Barriers to returning to prior avocational activities	Similar	Similar Concerns regarding sexual functioning	Modified work and home environment Family and social assistance Counseling of significant other regarding sexuality

affect the goals set and the time it may take to achieve those goals.

A statement of precautions is useful for communicating information critical for patient safety to the therapy staff. These precautions should include any added risks the patient may present during a therapy treatment. Again, physiatrists used to working with a small group of therapists may be in the habit of limiting the types of precautions they convey or of using protocols to determine the necessary precautions. Particularly in the outpatient setting, where the physician's and therapist's primary means of communication is the prescription, an explicit listing of precautions is critical.

There are many commonly used precautions such as weight-bearing status of a fractured limb or postsurgical joint. Specific precautions for identifying the patient with a high risk of falling, or in the hospital setting, a patient prone to wandering should be detailed. Cardiac precautions need to state the phase of cardiac rehabilitation the patient is in or to include a target heart rate from an exercise stress test, if applicable. If a patient has been started on a new medication with unusual side effects or side effects likely to be exacerbated by exercise, such as orthostasis, a precaution to alert the treating therapist improves patient safety.

Determining treatment goals is the most difficult task facing a physiatrist writing a prescription. The rationale for using the impairment, disability, and handicap model outlined in the examples in this chapter is the way this framework clarifies the appropriate goals. For each functional problem listed, the outcome that will result in an improved quality of life is the appropriate goal. In general, physicians' goals tend to focus on this level, that is, improving the quality of life or the ultimate outcome desired (4). The treating therapist then works within the broad and long-term goals set out in the prescription to determine the necessary steps and short-term goals. Since the overall goal is to improve the quality of life of the patient, discussion of the goals with the patient is a critical step in the process.

As the patient progresses through therapy sessions, or even during the evaluation process, varying members of the treatment team may become aware of problems that were not addressed by the initial prescription. Since communication between clinicians and coordination of clinical efforts is the hallmark of the rehabilitative process, every member of the treatment team is responsible to bring such problems to the attention of the entire team (8). In the inpatient setting, this occurs both during informal communications between treating therapists or a treating therapist

Appendix VII: Relativity of Impairment, Disability, and Handicap over Time with Respect to Diagnosis of Below-Knee (or Transtibial) Amputation

	Temporary	Permanent	Anticipated	Interventions
Impairment	Postoperative pain Bowel immobility Orthostasis Deconditioning Surgical incision Residual limb edema Atelectasis Urinary stasis Knee contracture Balance dysfunction	Transtibial amputation Peripheral neuropathy Phantom limb pain Scar tissue formation Balance dysfunction	High risk of contralateral limb loss	Pain medication Bowel and bladder program Reconditioning Ultrasound and stretching to hamstrings Stump wrapping Balance training Lower-limb strengthening
Disability	Inability to perform self-care Inability to transfer safely Inability to ambulate Pain with limb in dependent position Inability to care for residual limb	Pain limiting ability to perform self-care or for ambulation Loss of range of motion limiting ability to perform self-care or for ambulation Balance limiting ability to perform self-care or for ambulation or none	Same Concerns regarding sexual functioning or none	Gait training with assistive devices Wheelchair management Assistive devices for self-care, toileting, and safe transfers Counseling regarding sexuality
Handicap	Inability to perform household routine (housework, cooking, laundry) Barriers to returning prior avocational activities	Similar or none	Similar Concerns regarding sexual functioning	Modified work and home environment Transportation/automobile modifications Family and social assistance Counseling of significant other regarding sexuality

and the physician, and during formal treatment team meetings. Since the abilities of many patients evolve during the rehabilitation process, the physician writing the prescription and the therapist receiving the prescription should expect the treatment goals in some patients to evolve as well. In the inpatient setting, this flow of information within the team is supported with many informal and formal structures. However, in the outpatient setting, the treating therapist needs to communicate any newly identified problems to the treating physician. Most therapists provide physicians with copies of the initial evaluations, therapy notes, and summaries of treatment, including progress toward the goals. It is incumbent on physicians to read these notes and follow up on any newly identified problems as indicated.

The discipline of the therapist to whom the prescription is directed should be stated clearly. The details of the therapy being prescribed are then delineated. Such details may include the mode of therapeutic exercises or therapy treatments such as "water-based exercise program" or "supportive group counseling." The intensity of therapeutic exercise or a specific physical modality should be included when relevant. The frequency and duration of individual sessions as well as the total duration of treatment should be included in all therapy prescriptions. Follow-up instructions are the final item that needs to be included in a prescription. Especially in the outpatient setting, the prescription should state when the patient is to be seen by the physician. This allows the treating therapist to ensure that any necessary communications with the physician occur prior to the follow-up visit. Also this date will be helpful in the circumstance when a therapist must halt therapy.

CONCLUSIONS

An understanding of the rehabilitation process, combined with an appropriate and complete rehabilitation consultation and prescription, is the foundation for providing appropriate evaluation and treatment of a patient with a disability.

REFERENCES

1. Krusen FH, Kottke FJ, Ellowood PM. *Handbook of physical medicine and rehabilitation.* Philadelphia: WB Saunders, 1996.

2. Rusk HA. Preventive medicine, curative medicine—then rehabilitation. *New Physician* 1964;12: 165–167.

3. Delisa JA, ed. *Rehabilitation medicine: principles and practice.* 2nd ed. Philadelphia: JB Lippincott, 1993.

4. Braddom RL. *Physical medicine and rehabilitation.* Philadelphia: WB Saunders, 1966.

5. Currie DM, Marburger RA. Writing therapy referrals and treatment plans and the interdisciplinary team. In: Delisa JA, ed. *Rehabilitation medicine: principles and practice.* 2nd ed. Philadelphia: JB Lippincott, 1993:145–157.

6. Keith RA. The comprehensive treatment team in rehabilitation. *Arch Phys Med Rehabil* 1991;72: 269–274.

7. Nevlud GN. The team approach: current trends and issues in rehabilitation. *Tex J Audiol Speech Pathol* 1990;16:21–23.

8. King JC, Titus MND. Prescriptions, referrals and the rehabilitation Team. In: Delisa JA, ed. *Rehabilitation medicine: principles and practice.* 2nd ed. Philadelphia: JB Lippincott, 1993:227–239.

9. Darling LA, Ogg HL. Basic requirements for initiating an interdisciplinary process. *Phys Ther* 1984;64:1684–1686.

10. Schultz IL, Texidor MS. The interdisciplinary approach: an exercise in futility or a song of praise? *Med Psychother* 1991;4:1–8.

11. Porilo RB. Ethical issues in teamwork: the content of rehabilitation. *Arch Phys Med Rehabil* 1988;69: 318–322.

12. Halstead LS. Team care in chronic illness: critical review of literature of past 25 years. *Arch Phys Med Rehabil* 1976;57:501–511.

13. Melvin JL. Status report on interdisciplinary medical rehabilitation. *Arch Phys Med Rehabil* 1989;70: 273–276.

14. Deutsch PM, Falsih KB. *Innovations in head injury rehabilitation.* New York: Mathew Bender, 1989.

15. Rothberg JS. The rehabilitation team: future directions. *Arch Phys Med Rehabil* 1981;62:407–410.

16. Given B, Simmons S. The interdisciplinary health-care team: fact or fiction? *Nurs Forum* 1977;16: 165–183.

17. Walton RE, Dutton JM. The management of interdepartmental conflict: a model and review. *Admin Sci Q* 1969;14:73–84.

18. Melvin J. Interdisciplinary and multi-disciplinary activities and the ACRM. *Arch Phys Med Rehabil* 1980;61:379–380.

19. Gaston EH. Developing a motivating organizational climate for effective team functioning. *Hosp Commun Psychiatry* 1980;31: 407–417.

20. Longest BB. *Management practices for the health professional.* 4th ed. Norwalk, CT: Appleton & Lange, 1990.

21. Anderson TP. An alternative frame of reference for rehabilitation: the helping process versus the medical model. *Arch Phys Med Rehabil* 1975;56:101–104.

22. Becker MC, Abrams KS, Onder J. Goal setting: a joint patient-staff method. *Arch Phys Med Rehabil* 1974;55:87–89.

23. Halstead LS, Rintala DH, Kanellos M, et al. The innovative rehabilitation team: an experiment in team building. *Arch Phys Med Rehabil* 1986;67:357–361.

24. Tollison CD. Preface. In: Tollison CD, ed. *Handbook of chronic pain management.* Baltimore: Williams & Wilkins, 1989:1–4.

25. Mazur H, Beeston JJ, Yerxa EJ. Clinical interdisciplinary health team care: an educational experiment. *J Med Educ* 1979;54:703–713.

26. Yesner HJ. Psychosocial diagnosis and social services—one aspect of the rehabilitation process. In: Kottke FJ, Stillwell GK, Lehmann JF, eds. *Krusen's handbook of physical medicine and rehabilitation.* Philadelphia: WB Saunders, 1982:151–162.

27. Halstead LS. Philosophy of rehabilitation medicine. In: Halstead LS, Grabois M, eds. *Medical rehabilitation.* New York: Raven, 1985:1–5.

28. McPeak LA. Physiatric history and physical. In: Braddom RL, ed. *Physical medicine and rehabilitation.* Philadelphia: WB Saunders, 1996:3–42.

29. Erickson RP, McPhee MC. Clinical evaluation. In: Delisa JA, ed. *Rehabilitation medicine.* Philadelphia: JB Lippincott, 1988:25–65.

30. Stolov WC. Evaluation of the patient. In: Kottke FJ, Stillwell GK, Lehmann JF, eds. *Krusen's handbook of physical medicine and rehabilitation.* Philadelphia: WB Saunders, 1982:1–18.

31. American Medical Association. *Current procedural terminology.* Washington, DC: American Medicine Association, 1993.

32. American Association of Electrodiagnostic Medicine. Guidelines for ethical behavior relating to clinical practice issues in electrodiagnostic medicine. *Muscle Nerve* 1994;17: 965–967.

33. Fallowfield L. The ideal consultation. *Br J Hosp Med* 1992;47: 364–367.

34. Havelock P. Improving consultation skills. *Practitioner* 1991;235:495–498.

35. Benett I. Can the use of lists improve the proportion of concerns addressed in the consultation? *Diabet Med* 1995;12:452–454.

36. Evans BJ, Sweet B. Consulting-skills training to improve medical

students' diagnostic efficiency. *Arch Med* 1993;68:170–171.

37. Devor M, Renvall M, Ramsdell J. Practice patterns and the adequacy of residency training in consultation medicine. *J Gen Intern Med* 1993;8:554–560.

38. Short D. Principles of patient management. *Br J Hosp Med* 1993; 50:480–483.

39. Delisa JA, Martin GM, Currie DM. Rehabilitation medicine: past, present and future. In: Delisa JA, Gans BM, eds. *Rehabilitation medicine: principles and practice.* 2nd ed. Philadelphia: JB Lippincott, 1993:3–27.

40. Kottke FJ, Lehmann JF, Stillwell GK. Preface. In: Kottke FJ, Lehmann JF, Stillwell GK, eds. *Krusen's handbook of physical medicine and rehabilitation.* Philadelphia: WB Saunders, 1982:xi–xix.

41. Kirby RL. Impairment, disability and handicap. In: Delisa JA, Gans BM, eds. *Rehabilitation medicine: principles and practice.* 2nd ed. Philadelphia: JB Lippincott, 1993:40–50.

42. Erickson RP, McPhee MC. Clinical evaluation. In: Delisa JA, ed. *Rehabilitation medicine: principles and practice.* 2nd ed. Philadelphia: JB Lippincott, 1993:51–95.

43. Stanton PE, Fox FK, Frangos KM, et al. Assessment of resident physicians' knowledge of physical therapy. *Phys Ther* 1985;65:27–30.

44. Brogan DR. Rehabilitation service needs: physician's perception and referrals. *Arch Phys Med Rehabil* 1981;62:215–219.

45. Davidoff G, Stolp-Smith KA, Waring WP, et al. Patterns of referral to a university hospital consultation service: failure to accurately predict need for physiatric services. *Arch Phys Med Rehabil* 1988;69:449–450.

46. Finestone HM. Rheumatology rehabilitation: the role of a physical medicine and rehabilitation liaison consultation service. *Am J Phys Med Rehabil* 1992;71:191–192.

47. Wrigley JM, Yoels WC, Webb CR, et al. Social and physical factors in the referral of people with traumatic brain injury. *Arch Phys Med Rehabil* 1994;75:149–155.

48. Gonzalez EG, Honet JC, LaBan MM. Physiatric practice characteristics: report of a membership survey. *Arch Phys Med Rehabil* 1988;69:52–56.

49. O'Dell MW. Rehabilitation medicine consultation in persons hospitalized with AIDS. *Am J Phys Med Rehabil* 1993;72:90–96.

50. Swinyard EA. Appendix I, principles of prescription order writing and patient compliance instruction. In: Goodman, Gillman, eds. *The pharmacologic basis of therapeutics.* 8th ed. New York: Macmillan, 1980.

51. Policies and procedures for residency education in physical medicine and rehabilitation. In: *Graduate medical education directory 1996.* Minneapolis: Am Board of PMR, 1996:1–6.

52. *The American Board of Physical Medicine and Rehabilitation Booklet of Information.* Revised. Rochester, MN: American Board of Physical Medicine and Rehabilitation, July 1992.

53. Martin, Gamble. Prescription writing in physical medicine and rehabilitation. In: Kottke FJ, Stillwell GK, Lehman JF, eds. *Krusen's handbook of physical medicine and rehabilitation.* Philadelphia: WB Saunders, 1982:9–17.

54. Zimmermann KZ, Brown RD. Rehabilitation technology prescription: determinations of failure and elements of success in advances in rehabilitation technology. *Phys Med Rehabil State Art Rev* 1997;11:1–12.

Chapter 22

Drugs Used in Rehabilitation

Richard D. Zorowitz
Keith M. Robinson

The basis of allopathic medicine is to treat disease by "producing a second condition that is incompatible with or antagonistic to the first" (1). Often, pharmacologic interventions are employed to provide the milieu in which pathologic conditions can be remedied. Even in osteopathic medicine, in which the body "makes use of its own remedies against infections and other toxic conditions" (1), clinicians may use the therapeutic measures of conventional medicine in addition to manual medicine in appropriately treating a patient.

The practice of physical medicine and rehabilitation depends on the expertise of allied health professionals to decrease impairment and improve function. However, the physiatrist often is called on to supplement treatments with medications that complement and expedite the rehabilitation process. In doing so, the physiatrist should incorporate four principles into the choosing of drugs for a given medical condition. First and foremost, the most appropriate drugs should be chosen as first-line therapies for any condition. Second, medications that encourage patient compliance (i.e., daily or twice-daily regimens) should be chosen, especially when patients have deficits that physically or cognitively impair the reliable administration of such medications. Third, cost should be considered, especially when the patient has no health insurance plan that subsidizes prescription expenses. Finally, regimens should be reassessed periodically to eliminate medications that are no longer necessary.

This chapter is organized by conditions, rather than classes of medications, that the physiatrist encounters in daily practice. This approach is more practical since medications may have multiple purposes in the treatment of patients with assorted impairments and disabilities. Most of the conditions listed are specific to patients with neuromuscular and musculoskeletal conditions. However, some conditions are more generalized to patients seen in a primary care practice. While this review does not discuss medications for every medical condition, it nonetheless will enable the physiatrist to become knowledgeable in the treatment options for common conditions he or she will encounter.

HYPERTENSION

Hypertension is defined as a systolic blood pressure 140 mm Hg or higher or a diastolic blood pressure of 90 mm Hg or higher, or both. The prevalence of hypertension increases with age, is greater in African-Americans than in whites, and is greater in less educated people than in more educated people. In younger adults, hypertension is more prevalent in men than in women, but becomes more prevalent in women as age increases. Hypertension is more common in the southeastern United States, thereby resulting in a higher incidence of complications, such as stroke, coronary artery disease, and renal disease (2). The relationship between blood pressure and medical comorbidities is graded, independent, predictive, and etiologically consistent. At every level of increasing diastolic blood pressure, the risks are greater with increasing systolic blood pressure. In middle-aged and elderly patients, even isolated systolic hypertension is a risk factor for cardiovascular disease.

Table 22-1 lists the classification scheme of blood pressure in adults based on its impact on risk (3). Stage 1 hypertension is the most common form in adults and is therefore responsible for a majority of the morbidity, disability, and mortality attributable to hypertension. The risks of cardiovascular disease at any level of hypertension are significantly increased when patients experience cardiac (left ventricular hypertrophy or dysfunction), cerebrovascular, peripheral vascular, renal, or retinal disease. All stages of hypertension should be treated with lifestyle modifications or medications.

Lifestyle modifications include weight reduction, moderation of alcohol intake, physical activity, moderation of sodium intake, and increases in potassium and calcium intake. A weight loss as little as 4.5 kg (10 lb) may result in significant reductions in blood pressure (4). Weight reduction can enhance the effect of antihypertensive medications and can significantly reduce the risk of cardiovascular disease. Cessation of cigarette smoking will reduce the risk of cardiovascular disease. Excessive alcohol intake can raise blood pressure and make antihypertensive medications less effective (5). Regular aerobic physical activity (i.e., moderate activity 30–45 minutes in duration 3–5 times per week) may reduce systolic blood pressure at least 10 mm Hg (6). Reductions in sodium intake to less than 6 mg of sodium chloride per day may be adequate to control blood pressure in stage 1 hypertensive patients. Adequate intake of potassium (7) may protect against hypertension. Adequate calcium intake may lower the blood pressure of some patients (8). Magnesium also may affect blood pressure, but there is currently no substantiating evidence of efficacy. Moderation in intake of lipids or caffeine may be indicated in certain individuals. Stress management through the use of biofeedback techniques may be helpful, but the literature does not support it for prevention or therapy (9).

Treatment of high blood pressure with medications (Tables 22-2 and 22-3) clearly reduces the risk of cardiovascular mortality and morbidity (10,11). Reduction of diastolic blood pressure by 5 to 6 mm Hg reduces the risk of stroke by 42% and of cardiovascular disease by 20% to 25%. Therefore, if blood pressure exceeds 140/90 mm Hg during a 3- to 6-month period despite attempts to modify unhealthy lifestyles, antihypertensive therapy should be started, especially if there is target-organ disease or other risk factors of cardiovascular disease. However, drug therapy should be started well before the development of target-organ disease (12).

In stage 1 or 2 hypertensive patients, monotherapy with diuretics or β-blockers is indicated since they reduce cardiovascular morbidity and mortality (13). While alternative drugs, such as angiotensin-converting enzyme (ACE) inhibitors, α_1-blockers, and αβ-blockers, are equally effective in reducing blood pressure, no long-term controlled studies have demonstrated their efficacy in reducing cardiovascular morbidity and mortality. These drugs should be reserved for circumstances when diuretics and β-blockers have not been effective. If the response of monotherapy is inadequate, drug dosages may be maximized, another drug may be substituted, or a second agent from a different antihypertensive class may be added.

Table 22-1: Classification of Blood Pressure in Adults Age 18 Years and Older

Classification	Systolic (mm Hg)	Diastolic (mm Hg)
Normal	<130	<85
High normal	130–139	85–89
Mild (stage 1)	140–159	90–99
Moderate (stage 2)	160–179	100–109
Severe (stage 3)	180–209	110–119
Very severe (stage 4)	≥210	≥120

Source: Adapted from The Sixth Report of the Joint National Committee on Detection, Evaluation, and Treatment of High Blood Pressure (JNC VI). *Arch Intern Med* 1997;157:2413–2446.

Table 22-2: Classification of Initial Antihypertensive Agents

- Diuretics
  - Thiazides and related agents
  - Loop diuretics
  - Potassium sparing
- Adrenergic inhibitors
  - β-Blockers
  - β-Blockers with intrinsic sympathomimetic activity
  - αβ-Blockers
  - α_1-Blockers
- Angiotensin-converting enzyme (ACE) inhibitors
- Calcium antagonists
- Dihydropyridines

Table 22-3: Classification of Supplemental Antihypertensive Agents

- Centrally acting α_2-agonists (clonidine, guanabenz, guanfacine, methyldopa)
- Peripheral acting adrenergic antagonists (hydralazine, minoxidil)
- Direct vasodilators

In stage 3 or 4 hypertensive patients, it may be necessary to begin therapy with more than one agent. Patients with a diastolic blood pressure higher than 120 mm Hg may require hospitalization with parenteral administration of agents. In cases of hypertensive emergency or crisis, blood pressure should be reduced over 30 minutes to several hours to prevent myocardial or cerebral hypoperfusion. Agents such as sublingual nifedipine should be avoided, because these can cause rapid, uncontrolled decreases in blood pressure that are difficult, if not impossible, to reverse.

Patients with hypertension and comorbid conditions may require specific classes of antihypertensive therapy (3). Patients with renal insufficiency should receive an ACE inhibitor, although they should be monitored carefully if the serum creatinine concentration is 3 mg/dL or higher. Patients with diabetes may receive ACE inhibitors, α-blockers, calcium channel antagonists, and low-dose diuretics because these drugs have fewer side effects regarding glucose homeostasis, lipid levels, and renal function. Patients with dyslipidemia may receive low-dose diuretics, α-blockers, ACE inhibitors, angiotensin II receptor antagonists, calcium channel antagonists, and central adrenergic agonists, as they have clinically neutral effects on serum lipids and lipoproteins. The β-blockers transiently may increase serum triglyceride and decrease high-density lipoprotein levels, and high-dose diuretics also may increase plasma cholesterol, triglyceride, and low-density lipoprotein levels in the short term. Patients with asthma or chronic obstructive pulmonary disease should not receive β-blockers or αβ-blockers, as symptoms may be exacerbated. ACE inhibitors may be used safely, but if an ACE inhibitor–associated cough occurs, angiotensin II receptor antagonists may be given alternatively. Patients with gout should not receive thiazide diuretics because these can cause hyperuricemia.

DIABETES MELLITUS

Diabetes mellitus is "a group of metabolic diseases characterized by hyperglycemia resulting from defects in insulin secretion, insulin action, or both" (14). Diabetes may result from a number of etiologies: autoimmune destruction of pancreatic beta cells, deficient action of insulin on target tissues, and inadequate insulin secretion. Symptoms of diabetes range from polyuria, polydipsia, and polyphagia to weight loss, blurry vision, impaired growth, and susceptibility to infection. Diabetes can be life-threatening and can be manifested by ketoacidosis or nonketotic hyperosmolarity. The long-term complications of diabetes affect the eyes, kidneys, nerves, heart, and blood vessels.

Diabetes mellitus can be classified into several types. *Type 1 diabetes* refers to hyperglycemia due to beta cell destruction, resulting in absolute insulin deficiency. Type 1 diabetes usually results from some autoimmune mechanism, but idiopathic forms have been identified. Ketoacidosis is more common in type 1 diabetics. *Type 2 diabetes* represents a range of disease from a degree of insulin resistance with relative insulin deficiency to a degree of secretory deficit with insulin resistance. Type 2 diabetes occurs most commonly, with the most common mechanism resulting from insulin resistance with a secretory deficit. *Other types* of diabetes include genetic defects of beta cell function, genetic deficits in insulin action, diseases of the exocrine pancreas, endocrinopathies, and drug- or chemical-induced diabetes.

Diabetes mellitus may be diagnosed in three ways: 1) a plasma glucose concentration higher than 200 mg/dL (11.1 mmol/L) without regard to postprandial time associated with symptoms of polyuria, polydipsia, and unexplained weight loss; 2) a plasma glucose concentration higher than 126 mg/dL (7.0 mmol/L) associated with a fast of at least 8 hours; and 3) a plasma glucose level higher than 200 mg/dL (11.1 mmol/L) measured at least 2 hours after intake of the equivalent of 75 g of anhydrous glucose (15). Intermediate forms of diabetes may be diagnosed when the fasting plasma glucose concentration is between 110 and 126 mg/dL, or when the plasma glucose concentration is between 140 and 200 mg/dL at least 2 hours after a 75-g load of anhydrous glucose is given.

The general principle of treating diabetes mellitus is to reduce the plasma glucose concentration to prevent ketoacidosis and nonketotic hyperglycemia, to alleviate acute symptoms, to reduce serum lipid concentration, and to prevent long-term complications. Serum glucose concentrations should be targeted at 80 to 120 mg/dL preprandially, and 100 to 140 mg/dL at bedtime. Treatment should focus on multiple factors, including exercise; weight control when indicated; use of insulin or antihyperglycemic agents; and comorbid conditions including hypertension, smoking, and dyslipidemia.

Insulin

Insulin is manufactured from beef or pork pancreas, or is synthesized using recombinant DNA technology or chemical modification of pork insulin. Insulin is available in rapid-, short-, intermediate-, and long-acting forms that may be administered separately or in combination. Concentrations include 100 or 500 U/mL, but also may be formulated as 10 U/mL for infants. Insulin species or types should not be mixed without the approval of the prescribing physician or the patient. Human insulin should be given if the type of insulin a patient normally uses is not known. Human insulin also should be used in patients who are allergic or have immune resistance to animal insulins, those who use insulin intermittently, and women who are pregnant or are considering pregnancy. Dosing usually is proportional to insulin response as well as caloric intake and exercise regimens. Insulin may be given subcutaneously or by continuous subcutaneous infusion.

Table 22-4: Antihyperglycemic Medications

	Duration of Action (hr)	Daily Dose (mg/day)
Sulfonylureas		
Acetohexamide	12–18	500–750
Chlorpropamide	24–72	250–375
Glipizide	10–16	10–20
Glyburide	18–24	5–20
Tolazamide	12–24	250–500
Tolbutamide	6–12	1000–2000
Metformin	6–17	1000–2650
Acarbose	14–24	75–300

Antihyperglycemic Agents

The antihyperglycemic agents used in the United States are listed in Table 22-4. Most of the commonly used antihyperglycemic agents are sulfonylureas. The hypoglycemic activity of sulfur-containing compounds is related to the sulfonamide group, which stimulates the release of insulin by increasing beta cell sensitivity to glucose (16). They also may inhibit the release of glucagon (17).

Metformin is an antihyperglycemic not related to sulfonylurea medications. Metformin decreases hepatic glucose production and increases glucose intake, but does not cause clinical hypoglycemia (18). It does not affect pancreatic insulin production and requires the presence of insulin to be effective. Metformin can be used concurrently with a sulfonylurea, and can be used as monotherapy when endogenous secretion of insulin is adequate. Adverse effects include nausea, vomiting, diarrhea, and decreased vitamin B_{12} and folate absorption. Doses range between 500 mg twice a day and 850 mg three times a day.

Acarbose is an oral α-glucosidase inhibitor that has a high affinity for pancreatic amylase and α-glucosidases on the brush border of intestinal cells (19). It delays the absorption of glucose by interfering with the hydrolysis of dietary disaccharides. Acarbose decreases postprandial serum glucose concentrations and glycosylated hemoglobin with little effect on serum C-peptide and lipid concentrations. Adverse effects include flatulence, cramps, abdominal distention, and diarrhea. Acarbose must be taken before meals to be effective. Doses range from 25 to 50 mg three times a day for patients weighing less than 60 kg, and up to 100 mg three times a day for heavier patients.

SEIZURES

Anticonvulsants commonly are used for seizure prophylaxis during early recovery from acquired traumatic and non-traumatic brain injury, and for the suppression of seizure activity in patients with witnessed or reported behavior or abnormal electrical activity on an electroencephalogram (EEG) consistent with seizure activity. They also are used in the management of neuropathic pain (20–24) and behavioral difficulties after brain injuries (25–27). The latter indications are discussed in the appropriate sections of this chapter.

In patients with severe traumatic brain injuries who have no obvious structural changes, diffuse neural injury, or dural disruption, the incidence of posttraumatic seizures is low beyond the first week after the injury occurred (28). Seizure prophylaxis often is provided only through the first posttraumatic week, but in certain cases is discontinued no later than 6 months after injury. However, seizure prophylaxis is continued for at least 1 year in patients following traumatic brain injuries with dural disruption, hemorrhagic lesions, or history of heavy alcohol use, all of which increase the risk of abnormal epileptogenic foci. Seizure prophylaxis usually is not indicated in patients with post-concussive syndromes or mild traumatic brain injuries (22–24).

The goal of anticonvulsant therapy is to prevent or suppress seizure activity using the minimal dose of medication, preferably with monotherapy. The most commonly used agents for seizure treatment and prophylaxis include carbamazepine, phenytoin, valproic acid, gabapentin, and phenobarbital. Carbamazepine is less disruptive of intellectual processing and may stabilize disruptive behaviors in some brain-injured patients when compared to phenytoin and phenobarbital (29). However, carbamazepine can be sedating in elderly patients and can cause bone marrow suppression. As a result, blood cell counts must be regularly monitored. Phenytoin can be sedating and impairs balance because of a dose-related ataxia. Phenobarbital and its derivatives are also universally sedating and should be avoided whenever possible. Valproic acid still is recommended as a first-line monotherapy for absence seizures and myoclonic activity but is increasingly used as first-line treatment and adjunctive prophylaxis for primary, partial, secondary, and mixed forms of generalized seizures. Valproic acid is comparable to carbamazepine with respect to sedation. Gabapentin increasingly is being used as monotherapy and combination therapy in patients with complex partial seizures and secondary generalized seizures, when other anticonvulsants have failed to control seizure activity (24,30–32). A summary of information on the commonly used anticonvulsants is provided in Table 22-5.

If the patient is seizure free after 1 year or more, one may begin to taper the medications after EEG studies are performed. A slow medication taper of at least 6 weeks' duration is necessary because of the long half-lives of many of these medications. An EEG may be repeated 3 months after completion of the taper to assess the risk of seizure recurrence. If seizures recur after completion of the medication taper, the patient probably will require lifetime medical intervention unless extenuating circumstances are identified.

Anticonvulsant medications often are substituted for each other to minimize the adverse effects on conscious-

Table 22-5: Anticonvulsants

Agent	Dose	Mechanism of Action	Therapeutic Uses	Side Effects/Cautions	Caveats
Carbamazepine	100 mg bid to start. Increase by 100 mg bid every 3 days or sooner until therapeutic levels are achieved. Check levels at doses of 200 mg bid or higher. Maximal doses: 1200 mg daily for chronic pain; up to 4800 mg daily for seizure, given as tid or qid regimen.	GABA-agonist; α_2-adrenergic agonist; stabilizes sodium channels on neurons	Seizure prophylaxis and treatment; aggression/agitation; mania; chronic pain	Sedation; dizziness; ataxia; nausea; vomiting; rash; blurred vision; delirium, diplopia; headache; marrow suppression; exfoliative dermatitis	Although generally not as interfering with cognitive function, decreased motor reaction time and visual-motor speed are reported. A therapeutic dose by laboratory studies is not essential to achieve control of agitation or aggression, or chronic pain. Levels will increase when concurrently used with cimetidine or erythromycin; may also interfere with warfarin metabolism.
Gabapentin	Start at 100 mg tid for chronic pain, and 200 mg tid for seizures. Monitor levels starting at 200 mg tid. Maximal dose is 1500 mg daily for chronic pain and up to 2400 mg or higher for seizure. Consult a neurologist for higher dosing.	GABA-agonist	Seizure treatment; chronic pain	Sedation; fatigue; ataxia; memory loss	Serum levels may decrease when used concurrently with magnesium- or aluminum-containing laxatives.
Phenytoin	Start at 100 mg bid. Check levels after 3 days and increase by 100 mg weekly until there is a therapeutic response, or levels are therapeutic. Maximal dose is 600 mg daily given as bid or tid regimen.	Neuron membrane stabilization probably via promoting sodium efflux, thus reducing membrane sodium gradient	Seizure prophylaxis and treatment; chronic pain	Sedation; ataxia; nystagmus; hyperplasia of gums; long half-life (up to 40 hr)	Abrupt withdrawal may precipitate seizures. Serum concentrations may increase with concurrent use of cimetidine and warfarin.
Phenobarbital	Start at 30 mg at bedtime and increased by 30 mg weekly. Monitor levels closely. Maximal dose is 180 mg daily.	Nonselective central nervous system suppressant	Seizure prophylaxis and treatment	Sedation, especially when used concurrently with other sedating psychotropic agents; respiratory depression; nausea; vomiting; headache	Habit forming. Lowers plasma levels of warfarin; enhanced metabolism of exogenous steroids and probably of phenytoin as well.

Table 22-5: (*Continued*)

Agent	Dose	Mechanism of Action	Therapeutic Uses	Side Effects/Cautions	Caveats
					Its serum levels are increased by concomitant use of valproic acid; MAO inhibitors can prolong its effect.
Valproic Acid	Start at 250 mg daily. Increase 250 mg no sooner than every 3 days to maximal daily dose of 1500–3000 mg daily, given as tid regimen. Check plasma level with every dose increase.	Increases brain levels of GABA through catabolic inhibition, anabolic activation, and postsynaptic activation	Seizure treatment; aggression/agitation	Nausea; abdominal pain; anxiety; depression; hair loss; tremor; ataxia; rash; insomnia; headaches; marrow suppression; hepatitis; pancreatitis	A therapeutic dose by laboratory studies is not essential to achieve control of agitation or aggression. Levels may increase when concurrently used with cimetidine and salicylates; levels may decrease when concurrently used with carbamazepine.
Topiramate	Start with 50 mg at bedtime. Increase by 50 mg weekly, given as bid regimen. Maximal dosage 400 mg day.	Unknown; possible mechanisms: 1) sodium channel–blocking action; 2) GABA-agonist; 3) Kainate/AMPA subtype of glutamate receptor antagonist	Prophylaxis and treatment of partial-onset seizures with or without secondary generalization	Somnolence; dizziness; ataxia; speech disorders; psychomotor slowing; nystagmus; paresthesias; kidney stones; decreased hepatic function	Levels may decrease when concurrently used with phenytoin, carbamazepine, or valproic acid. Serum digoxin and valproic acid levels may decrease with concurrent topiramate usage.
Lamotrigine	Start with 25 mg every other day. Increase by 25–50 mg/day every 1 to 2 wk in two divided doses. Maximal dosage: 700 mg/day as monotherapy; 200 mg/day as adjunctive therapy.	Unknown; possible mechanism: sodium channel–blocking action	Adjunctive therapy in partial seizures	Rash; Stevens-Johnson syndrome; toxic epidermal necrolysis; dizziness; ataxia; somnolence; headache; diplopia, blurred vision; nausea; vomiting	Value of plasma concentration monitoring has not been established. Levels may decrease when used concurrently with phenytoin, or carbamazepine. Levels may increase when used concurrently with valproic acid. Valproic acid levels may decrease when used concurrently with lamotrigine.

GABA = γ-aminobutyric acid; MAO = monoamine oxidase; AMPA = γ-amino-3-hydroxy-5-methyl-4-isoxazole propionate.

ness or cognition. For example, many brain-injured patients initially are treated with phenytoin or phenobarbital, but then are converted to treatment with carbamazepine. To avoid toxic effects, the dose of the substitute drug should be slowly increased until a therapeutic level is achieved, before the initial drug is gradually tapered. Therapeutic serum levels of the substitute drug may be difficult to achieve since both medications compete for the same serum carrier protein. Thus, plasma levels of the substitute drug must be closely monitored during taper of the initial drug, and adjustments made accordingly. A phenytoin taper may be initiated when carbamazepine levels are in the low therapeutic range, in an effort to avoid carbamazepine toxicity during the phenytoin taper (24).

PSYCHOTIC, AFFECTIVE, AND BEHAVIORAL DISORDERS

Psychotropic agents comprise a variety of medications including neuroleptics, hypnotic/sedatives, antidepressants, psychostimulants, and other behavior-influencing drugs. These agents are used to treat an array of behavioral disturbances, cognitive impairments, and affective disorders frequently encountered in brain-injured patients.

Neuroleptics

Neuroleptics must be used cautiously because of their potential negative influences on cognitive functioning (29). Dopaminergic overstimulation is thought to be central to the pathophysiology of traumatic brain injury. However, this line of thinking is based on extrapolation from animal (33) and human studies (34) in which nonproductive behaviors occurred after administration of these agents.

Neuroleptic agents traditionally have been used to suppress psychotic symptoms, such as hallucinations, delusions, and paranoia, in patients with psychiatric or neurologic diseases (35,36). They also are frequently used to dampen severe agitation, delirium, and aggression when the patient is at risk of self-injury (e.g., hallucinogenic suicidal ideations) or compromise of optimal care (e.g., interfering with enteral nutritional support) (37). The "potency" of these agents is defined by their specificity of interaction with dopaminergic receptors. For example, haloperidol is considered a high-potency neuroleptic agent with relatively exclusive and rapid dopaminergic affinity. It may be the best choice for short-term control of acute agitation because it is rapidly acting and nonsedating, and can be administered orally or parenterally, but more likely may augment extrapyramidal signs (38). Chlorpromazine and thioridazine are lower-potency agents since they interact with dopaminergic, cholinergic, and serotonergic receptors, and may be useful for its sedating effects. Regardless, the use of neuroleptics to control agitation and delirium is considered second-line therapy after short-acting benzodiazepines (discussed later), but neuroleptics are useful when benzodiazepines are too sedating or disinhibiting of disturbing behaviors.

The principles for the administration of neuroleptics are simple. First, they may be given to brain-injured patients when no other pharmacologic or behavioral treatments are effective. Second, the minimal possible dosage needed to dampen the target behavior should be used. Third, clinicians must periodically weigh the postulated risks of disrupting neural recovery with the benefits of enhancing participation with behavioral management and structured, procedural learning (25,26). For example, an agitated or delirious hospitalized patient may be given a standing dose of haloperidol, 0.5 mg orally or parenterally every 12 hours, with a dose of 0.5 mg parenterally every 6 to 8 hours as needed. Every 24 hours, the standing dose can be readjusted or converted to an oral dose based on the amount and effectiveness of the medication during the 24-hour period (39).

Antidepressants

The use of antidepressant medications is widespread in rehabilitation practices. Reactions of loss are a part of the adaptation process that occurs with functional disability. When these adjustment behaviors interfere with daily activities and the disabled individual struggles to redefine his or her sense of control, clinical depression may be present and may require treatment. Antidepressants also are used in the treatment of sleep disorders, agitation and disinhibitive behaviors, and anxiety and panic disorders (26,37). Antidepressants can be categorized according to what neurotransmitter system is being activated primarily, and this influences the clinician's choice of agent, as summarized in Table 22-6.

Tricyclic antidepressants activate the noradrenergic and serotonergic systems by presynaptic inhibition of neurotransmitter reuptake. These agents can be categorized according to their anticholinergic side effect profiles. Amitriptyline and imipramine are the oldest tricyclic antidepressants and have been studied in the greatest detail. They have become the standard drugs for comparison of sedation and anticholinergic effects. Until the development of selective serotonergic reuptake inhibitors (SSRIs), these noradrenergic agents were used as first-line treatment of depression. In some patient groups, they may still be used as first-line treatment. For example, depressed patients having chronic pain syndromes associated with sleep disorders may be prescribed a relatively sedating tricyclic antidepressant that may help to treat the depression, the pain syndrome, and the sleep problem. For such patients who find amitriptyline too sedating, less sedating drugs such as nortriptyline can be tried. It is advised always to start with the lowest possible bedtime dose (e.g., 10–25 mg of amitriptyline or nortriptyline at bedtime), even in younger patients, as a test dose for several days to see if the drug is tolerated. Subsequently, the dose must be increased gradually with close monitoring of target symptoms, until a

Table 22-6: Antidepressants				
Agent	**Mechanism of Action**	**Therapeutic Uses**	**Side Effects/ Cautions**	**Caveats**
Tricyclics Amitriptyline Nortriptyline Imipramine Doxepin Desipramine	Noradrenergic and serotonergic agonist, muscarinic and histaminic blockers	Chronic pain, depression, disinhibition, aggression	Primarily anticholinergic including delirium; sedation; constipation; dry mouth; cardiac conduction deficits; orthostasis; sexual dysfunction; weight gain; urinary retention.	Maximal does of amitriptyline to treat agitation rarely exceeds 75 mg daily. Abrupt discontinuation is not recommended. Dose ranges for amitriptyline, imipramine, doxepin, and desipramine are comparable (10–200 mg), and for nortriptyline are less (10–150 mg)
SSRIs Trazodone Nefazodone	 SSRI SSRI	Sleep disorders, chronic pain, depression	Priapism; sedation.	Although primarily an SSRI, they are also mediated by α-adrenergic (agonist) and histaminic (blocker) systems. Most commonly used to treat agitation in doses ranging from 25–400 mg daily. Nefazodone has more noradrenergic activity.
Fluoxetine Sertraline Paroxetine	SSRI SSRI SSRI	Depression, disinhibition, aggression, chronic pain	Anxiety; sexual dysfunction; weight loss; nausea; headache; insomnia; anorgasmia. Concurrent use of fluoxetine and paroxetine with tricyclics will increase plasma levels of the latter.	Initial anxiety may subside after 1–2 wk of exposure. When changing from fluoxetine to an MAO inhibitor, at least a 5-wk "wash out" is necessary; at least a 2-wk "wash out" for sertraline and paroxetine.
Bupropion	—	Depression	Agitation; seizures.	—
Venlafaxine	—	Depression	Same as for SSRIs; also diastolic hypertension.	—
MAO inhibitors (e.g., phenelzine, tranylcypromine)	—	Depression	Many drug-drug interactions leading to hypertensive crises, including levodopa and sympathomimetic agents (e.g., pseudoephedrine, tyramine-rich foods).	Abrupt discontinuation is not recommended. At least a 2-wk "wash out" period is necessary after stopping a psychostimulant to treat depression; at least a 1-wk "wash out" after stopping a tricyclic agent. Consulting a psychiatrist is recommended prior to using these agents.

SSRI = selective serotonergic reuptake inhibitor; MAO = monoamine oxidase.

maximal dosage, therapeutic effect, or side effect is observed. Twice-daily dosing schedules should be considered when higher doses are used, or when side effects develop. Measurements of serum drug levels of these tricyclic antidepressants are useful as doses are increased more than 50 mg daily. If not tolerated, the drug should be rapidly tapered (40–42).

Trazodone is another, relatively selective, presynaptic serotonin reuptake blocker that has minimal anticholinergic side effects (except orthostasis). Similar to amitriptyline, its sedating qualities sometime are advantageous to treat insomnia, sleep disorders associated with depression, and chronic pain syndromes. Its lack of cardiac toxicity is more appealing to elderly patients. The risk of priapism should be considered seriously when using trazodone in male patients. Nefazodone is similar to trazodone except it has more noradrenergic activity (43,44).

Recently, SSRIs such as fluoxetine, sertraline, and paroxetine have emerged as first-line pharmacologic treatments of depression, especially of mild to moderate severity (35,36,45). The serotonergic side effects (e.g., nausea, nervousness, headache, sleep disturbances, tremor, diarrhea) have been presented as more tolerable than the anticholinergic side effects associated with tricyclic antidepressants (e.g., dry mouth, sedation, orthostasis, constipation, urinary retention, weight gain, cardiac conduction block). Anorgasmia continues to be a disturbing side effect of SSRIs. Their general lack of cardiovascular side effects makes SSRIs safer for use in patients with cardiac conduction defects and autonomic instability (46–49). While comparative studies among SSRIs are few, paroxetine is thought to have a more rapid onset of action. Fluoxetine is associated with more side effects, especially gastrointestinal ones. The efficacy among SSRIs and between SSRIs and tricyclic antidepressants is comparable (49,50).

Second-line antidepressants include bupropion, venlafaxine, and monoamine oxidase (MAO) inhibitors. Bupropion weakly blocks dopamine, but its major mechanism of action is unknown. It is particularly nonsedating, nonorthostatic, and nonarrhythmogenic. However, it can cause agitation or dose-related seizures. It should not be used with other dopaminergic agents such as levodopa and bromocriptine. Venlafaxine is chemically related to bupropion, strongly inhibits the reuptake of norepinephrine and serotonin, and weakly inhibits the reuptake of dopamine. Its side effect profile resembles that of SSRIs, and includes dose-related diastolic hypertension (51,52). MAO inhibitors may precipitate hypertensive crises when combined with foods containing tyramine (e.g., aged cheeses, red wine), sympathomimetic amines (e.g., pseudoephedrine), and dopaminergic agents. They should not be used in patients who are noncompliant to taking medications.

Antidepressants also are used to treat nonmalignant neurogenic and musculoskeletal chronic pain syndromes (20,21,50,53–56). Antidepressants are helpful in treating overlapping features of depression and chronic pain, such as sleep disorders. Moreover, depression can present clinically with amplified somatic symptoms. While it can be viewed as an appropriate affective response to ongoing disabling chronic pain, depression may evolve into having "a life of its own" that deserves aggressive pharmacologic intervention (54).

Finally, antidepressants, particularly tricyclic agents and trazodone, are used to treat aggression, attentional disorders, and disinhibitive behaviors in brain-injured patients (25,26,37). The sedating effects of amitriptyline and trazodone can facilitate a therapeutic effect that is useful in reorienting and regulating sleep-wake cycles, thus eliminating one contributing component of behavioral obstreperousness. SSRIs can be used empirically when these and other agents fail. Antidepressant agents should be considered when patients exhibit depressive features or when agents such as propranolol and psychostimulants are ineffective or not tolerated.

Anticonvulsants

Anticonvulsants are effective agents in treating selected patients with aggression, mania, and disinhibition associated with frontal lobe injury (25–27,37). Carbamazepine may control episodic dyscontrol associated with temporal lobe seizures. It also can dampen aggressive behaviors associated with limbic system dysfunction when high therapeutic serum levels are attained. Carbamazepine is frequently used as adjunctive therapy for the refractory behaviors associated with mania, for depression in bipolar disease, and for the psychotic behaviors of schizophrenic disorders. Valproic acid also can be used to treat aggression, but should be considered after carbamazepine and propranolol have been tried. Valproic acid more commonly has been used to stabilize hypomanic or manic behaviors associated with bipolar disease, and has been generalized for stabilizing disinhibited and antisocial behaviors in brain-injured patients (25–27).

Psychostimulants

Psychostimulants are being used increasingly in patients with acquired brain injuries who demonstrate deficits in selective and sustained attention, depression, or poor initiation for functional activities. Methylphenidate, a short-acting agent, has been used for over 20 years to treat attentional deficit hyperkinetic disorder (ADHD) in children. These children are distractable owing to perceived difficulties in selectively engaging target stimuli while disengaging contextual stimuli. Further, these children also may have difficulty sustaining their attention selectively for long enough periods of time to process and complete target tasks. These basic deficits in attention are thought to contribute to a breakdown of all higher-level cognitive functions including memory, language, visual perception, and executive functions. Methylphenidate is thought to enhance attentional functions through dopaminergic and noradrenergic neurotransmitter systems, especially in the frontal and prefrontal lobes (25,57).

During the 1980s, clinicians began to use methylphenidate in adult brain injury populations that demonstrated attentional deficit syndromes similar to ADHD, deficits in arousal and initiation, frontal lobe syndromes, and depression (25,58). In adult patients younger than 40 years, appetite suppression and insomnia can usually be avoided if the daily dose is kept to less than 40 mg given in two or three divided doses. In adult patients, tachycardia and hypertension must be closely monitored, even at lower doses. In elderly patients with cerebrovascular disease and parkinsonism, poor initiation may be indistinguishable from depression. The use of methylphenidate to treat both syndromes should be considered, especially when other antidepressant agents are contraindicated (e.g., tricyclic antidepressants in patients with cardiac conduction deficits) or not tolerated.

Further, a positive clinical response to methylphenidate should be observed as early as 2 or 3 days after the first dose is given, as compared to at least 1 week for tricyclic antidepressants and SSRIs (58). When methylphenidate is not tolerated, pemoline or dextroamphetamine should be considered. Long-acting forms of these agents are available and usually contribute to their longer durations of clinical response (57,58). Pemoline is approved exclusively for ADHD. Acute hepatic failure associated with pemoline use developed in a small number of patients, and jaundice was observed no sooner than 6 months after therapy was initiated. However, some observed dark urine and a prodrome of malaise, anorexia, and other gastrointestinal symptoms before this (59). The clinical application of these psychostimulants in adult populations is summarized in Table 22-7.

β-Blockers

Lipophilic β-blockers are recommended as second-line and chronic treatment for aggression, severe agitation, and disinhibition in brain-injured patients. These include propranolol, metoprolol, and nadolol. Propranolol is the oldest of the β-blockers and is the most lipophilic. Treatment must be initiated with the lowest possible dose, then increased slowly until the desired effect is attained or side effects are reported. However, a desired therapeutic effect may not occur for as long as 8 weeks after a steady dose is achieved. The starting dose of propranolol is 20 mg three times a day in patients without cardiovascular or pulmonary diseases. Propranolol can be increased by 60 mg every 3 to 5 days when the resting heart rate is over 50 beats/min and the resting systolic blood pressure is over 90 mm Hg. In patients at risk for or demonstrating side effects, propranolol should be started at 20 mg daily and increased by 20 mg every 3 to 5 days. Therapeutic daily doses range between 200 and 800 mg, but may be as high 1000 mg. β-Blockers should never be abruptly stopped (25,26,37,39). A trial of these agents for behavioral control should not be

Table 22-7: Psychostimulants

Agent	Dose	Side Effects/Cautions	Caveats
Methylphenidate	Start at 2.5–5.0 mg po bid at 8 AM (breakfast) and at noon (lunch). Increase by 2.5–5.0 mg increments until therapeutic effect or side effects to a daily dose of 20 mg. If tolerated, but not optimal effect, increase by 5 mg weekly until a maximal daily dose of 40 mg in 2 divided doses.	Insomnia, appetite suppression, headache, tachycardia, hypertension, anxiety, hyperirritability, elevated plasma levels of phenytoin and tricyclic antidepressants when used concurrently. Also lowers seizure threshold, psychotic symptoms, dyskinesias, oculogyric crisis, nystagmus, tics/Tourette syndrome, abdominal pain, hyperacusis.	If tolerance develops on maximal doses, then stop for 2 wk, then restart another trial. Tachycardia and hypertension can be more pronounced during exercise. Many of these side effects are alleviated by lowering the dose, or adjusting the dosing schedule. Abrupt discontinuation is not recommended in brain-injured patients.
Dextroamphetamine sulfate	Start at 5–10 mg daily at 8 AM. Increase by 5 mg every 48 hr until therapeutic effect or toxicity to maximal dose of 40 mg daily.	Same as methylphenidate.	Long-acting preparation allows once-daily dosing.
Pemoline	Check baseline liver function parameters. Start at 18.75 mg daily at 8 AM. Increase by 18.75 mg weekly until therapeutic effect or toxicity to maximal dose of 75 mg daily.	Acute hepatic failure. Otherwise, same as methylphenidate.	Long-acting preparation allows once-daily dosing. Do not use in patients with abnormal liver function.

considered a failure until the patient has been on a stable dose for at least 8 weeks.

Adverse effects include worsening of target symptoms, psychotic symptoms, bradycardia, hypotension, sexual dysfunction, depression, and lethargy. Side effects of peripheral β-blockade become less noticeable at daily doses over 120 mg. These agents are contraindicated in patients with persistent angina, congestive heart failure, cardiac conduction deficits, hypothyroidism, asthma, or chronic obstructive pulmonary disease. They should be used cautiously in diabetic patients since the β-adrenergic response to hypoglycemia will be blunted.

Bromocriptine

Bromocriptine mesylate, a D_2 dopamine receptor agonist, is gaining popularity in the treatment of brain-injured patients with deficits in arousal, attention, and motivation, especially when dysfunction of dopaminergic pathways among the upper brain stem, basal ganglia, and prefrontal lobe (mesolimbic/mesocortical tracts) is suspected. Dosing may begin at 1.25 mg two or three times a day with food and may be increased by 1.25 mg weekly to a maximal daily dose of 90 mg in three divided doses (60–63). Arousal, attention, and functional activities should be monitored closely. Commonly reported side effects include sedation, nausea, involuntary motor activity, constipation, hypertension, and hypotension. A dose-related delirium can last several weeks after discontinuation of the drug. Liver and renal function should be monitored when bromocriptine is used for extended periods.

Anxiolytic and Sedative Agents

Anxiety and sleep disturbances (insomnia, depression associated, pain associated) are ubiquitous among hospitalized patients. Anticipating disability for the short or long term can create enough anxiety that learning ability is impaired and participation in a therapeutic program is suboptimal. Interrupted sleep will translate into poor functional performance. The increased pressure on care providers for shortening hospital lengths of stay may be encouraging the use of anxiolytic and sedative agents in order to optimize patients' performances during inpatient rehabilitation. However, even in low dosages, these agents continue to have negative side effects. alone or synergistically with other agents (e.g., narcotic analgesics). Thus, anxiety and sleep disorders must be treated with these agents only when the clinical presentation is extreme, and behavioral and interpersonal approaches have failed.

The reasons for anxiety and sleep difficulties must be explored with the patient prior to committing to one of these agents. For example, specific precipitants such as pain must be considered and treated appropriately. For patients who have been hospitalized longer than 1 week, these agents can be useful for re-establishing disrupted sleep-wake cycles. Long-acting benzodiazepines (e.g., diazepam, flurazepam), chlordiazepoxide, and chlorazepate are not considered first-line treatments for anxiety and sleep disorders, especially in elderly patients. Short-acting benzodiazepines (e.g., lorazepam, temazepam), chloral hydrate, and zolpidem are preferred since their sedating effects usually wear off by morning (36,64,65). Further, it is not unusual to treat patients who have used long-acting agents as therapy for anxiety for many years. In these cases, the specific anxiolytic agent should be restarted, or the possibility of inducting a withdrawal syndrome exists (hyperautonomia, delirium, seizures) (66). Psychiatric consultation may help to verify the diagnosis of an anxiety disorder, and for consideration of alternative medications such as a long-acting benzodiazepine or buspirone (42).

Many clinicians and patients use antihistamines such as diphenhydramine to treat insomnia. However, daytime somnolence with delirium, interference with sleep, and impairment of driving performance are reported, especially in elderly patients (65,67). Chloral hydrate is a safe alternative in the elderly as long as it is used for no more than 2 or 3 consecutive nights, in order to avoid tolerance and physical dependence. Zolpidem, a recently introduced short-acting, nonbenzodiazepine hypnotic agent, uses a variety of γ-aminobutyric acid (GABA) receptors. Although it is less disruptive of stage 3 or 4 or "restorative" sleep, it does have dose-related side effects similar to those of other comparable benzodiazepines (64). However, as clinicians gain more experience with zolpidem, it is emerging as a preferred agent to treat insomnia. Regardless, use of short-acting, sleep-facilitating agents should be limited to only when they are absolutely necessary, and should be limited to three used per week over 3 or 4 consecutive weeks, in an effort to minimize tolerance to and dependence on these agents (65).

Panic disorders generally should not be treated with these agents unless absolutely necessary. Standing doses of tricyclic antidepressants and SSRIs are considered first-line treatment for panic disorders. Alprazolam often is recommended as needed as a "rescue" medication superimposing daily doses of antidepressants to treat panic disorders (36,68).

Short-acting benzodiazepines, specifically parenteral lorazepam (0.5–1.0 mg every 8 hours, and 1–2 mg as needed every hour for rapid sedation to a maximal dose of 2 mg three times a day or 6 mg over 24 hours), has been recommended as first-line treatment for aggression, agitation, mania, and delirium when the behaviors displayed are considered dangerous to the patient or others. Once these behaviors are controlled, the choice to convert to a standing oral dose of lorazepam or to a low-dose neuroleptic agent, such as haloperidol, must be made. For patients who demonstrate a significant amount of anxiety in their clinical presentations, lorazepam should be continued. However, patients should be monitored for excessive sedation, disinhibition, amplification of difficult behaviors, and ineffectiveness. In patients displaying these signs, a low-dose neuroleptic agent such as haloperidol should be used (39).

Benzodiazepines also have been used as analgesic agents. However, the literature argues against their use as either first-line or adjuvant analgesics, except for acute muscle spasm, chronic pain with a prominent anxiety component, and "lancinating" neuropathic pain. In these cases, clonazepam (originally used as an anticonvulsant) and alprazolam are the preferred agents (69).

Benzodiazepines and other sedative agents are used ubiquitously in hospitalized elderly patients. Regardless, they are a major offending risk factor for delirium and falls causing fractures. They should be used cautiously in patients over 60 years old. The lowest measurable dose should be given, and doses should be increased slowly.

PAIN AND INFLAMMATION

The International Association for the Study of Pain defines pain as an "unpleasant sensory or emotional experience associated with actual or potential tissue damage, or described in terms of such damage" (70). Acute pain usually is characterized by some combination of tissue damage, pain, and anxiety. It is associated with some nociceptor stimulation and is expected to be transitory in duration. On the other hand, chronic pain may be a syndrome unto itself, usually persists after tissue healing has been completed, and usually serves no purpose since associated diseases or injuries have resolved. Chronic pain may be associated with helplessness, hopelessness, and meaninglessness (71).

The mechanisms of chronic pain are varied and may or may not be associated with peripheral stimulation. Sometimes the peripheral nociceptors respond normally to chronic stimulation (e.g., osteoarthritis). Other types of pain (e.g., neuropathic pain) result from abnormalities in the peripheral or central nervous system without any peripheral stimulation. Cancer pain (which can be acute or chronic) has a wide variety of causes, including visceral, soft-tissue, infectious, pleural, or gastric factors.

A multitude of pain medications are available for both acute and chronic pain (Table 22-8). When one is selecting a pain medication, two goals should be taken into consideration. First, the medication should relieve pain, which is the main presenting symptom. Second, the medication should slow or arrest the cause of the pain. The pain medications described in this section are listed in a "ladder" from acetaminophen to narcotics. Other medications that can be used for soft-tissue or nerve pain are included to complete the discussion.

Table 22-8: Classification of Pain Medications

Primary analgesics
Acetaminophen
Aspirin and salicylates
Nonsteroidal anti-inflammatory drugs (NSAIDs)
Synthetic narcotic analogues
Narcotics
Secondary analgesics
Antidepressants
Anticonvulsants
Muscle relaxants
Corticosteroids
Other drugs

Acetaminophen

Acetaminophen is an over-the-counter analgesic commonly used for pain relief. Acetaminophen produces pain relief by raising the pain threshold. It does not produce any anti-inflammatory effect and is indicated for the relief of minor pain associated with common conditions such as headache, toothache, musculoskeletal aches, arthritis, and menstrual cramps. Overdosage of acetaminophen can result in fatal hepatonecrosis. However, fatality from acetaminophen usually is uncommon in overdoses of less than 15 g.

Aspirin and Salicylates

The name *aspirin* is derived from the German word for the compound, *a*cetyl*spir*säure ("*Spirea*," the genus of plant from which it was obtained, and "*Säure*," the German word for *acid*). Aspirin comes from cinchona or willow bark and dates back to the eighteenth century. Aspirin is effective because of its ability to inhibit prostaglandin synthesis by blocking the enzyme cyclooxygenase, which catalyzes the conversion of arachidonic acid to endoperoxide compounds. Aspirin also inhibits granulocyte adherence to damaged vasculature, stabilizes lysosomes, and inhibits polymorphonuclear leukocyte and macrophage migration, thereby reducing the inflammatory response.

Aspirin is one of the most commonly prescribed drugs for relieving mild to moderate pain of various origins. Aspirin may be combined with other analgesics, and is available in a multitude of over-the-counter products. The optimal analgesic dose is less than the 650-mg oral dose commonly used. The average anti-inflammatory dose of 4 g/day usually is tolerated by most patients. The average dose for children is 50 to 75 mg/kg/day.

The side effects of aspirin usually involve the gastrointestinal and nervous systems. The gastrointestinal side effects include gastric upset, gastric or duodenal ulcers, upper gastrointestinal bleeding, and vomiting. The central nervous system effects include tinnitus, decreased hearing, and vertigo. Other side effects include respiratory alkalosis followed by metabolic acidosis, and hyperuricemia. However, salicylates are thought to be generally less offensive in inducing reported side effects (49,72–75).

Nonsteroidal Anti-inflammatory Drugs

While aspirin and other salicylates are effective in treating the arthritides and other painful conditions, adverse effects such as gastric irritation spurred the search for alternative drugs with safer profiles. The discovery of phenylbutazone in 1949 created a new class of drugs with aspirin-like properties known as *nonsteroidal anti-inflammatory drugs* (NSAIDs). The NSAIDs are grouped into several chemical classes, as shown in Table 22-9.

The pharmacodynamics of NSAIDs is similar to that of aspirin in that they generally inhibit the biosynthesis of prostaglandins. However, unlike aspirin, they are reversible inhibitors of cyclooxygenase. In addition, certain drugs such as indomethacin and diclofenac reduce the production of both prostaglandins and leukotrienes. Like aspirin, the NSAIDs have inflammatory properties associated with the decreased release of mediators from granulocytes, basophils, and mast cells. The NSAIDs reverse vasodilation by decreasing the sensitivity of blood vessels to bradykinin and histamine and affecting lymphokine production from T lymphocytes.

Most NSAIDs are indicated for patients with rheumatoid arthritis, osteoarthritis, and ankylosing spondylitis. They also are used to treat a variety of inflammatory disorders including acute soft-tissue traumatic injuries, disk herniations, and repetitive strain or overuse injuries. Several of the NSAIDs have received approval by the Food and Drug Administration (FDA) for special indications. *Indomethacin* is not recommended as a general analgesic, but is indicated for extra-articular inflammatory conditions such as pericarditis, pleurisy, Bartter syndrome, acute gout, patent ductus arteriosus, and heterotopic ossification. *Phenylbutazone* is indicated for acute gouty arthritis and superficial thrombophlebitis, but drugs such as indomethacin may be safer for these indications. *Ketorolac* is used primarily as an analgesic; it has been used successfully to replace morphine sulfate in treating mild to moderate postsurgical pain. An ophthalmic preparation also is available for certain inflammatory conditions.

The side effects of NSAIDs may be multisystemic in nature. Gastrointestinal adverse effects are most common and include abdominal pain, dyspepsia, nausea, vomiting, diarrhea, and peptic ulcers. They may be reduced using misoprostol, a prostaglandin E_1 analogue that increases the secretion of gastric mucosal protective factors and probably inhibits gastric acid secretion at some doses. With the exception of ibuprofen or tolmetin, NSAIDs may potentiate the effects of antihyperglycemic drugs or warfarin. Other side effects of NSAIDs may include prolonged bleeding time, thrombocytopenia, agranulocytosis, liver toxicity, peripheral edema, and toxic epidermal necrolysis.

Some NSAIDs have been responsible for nephrotic syndrome, renovascular insufficiency, and acute renal failure. The mechanism involves inhibition of the conversion of arachidonic acid to prostaglandins and thromboxanes, resulting in compromised glomerular filtration, renal blood flow, electrolyte exchange, and water resorption. Renal side effects usually occur insidiously and are not correlated with dosage or duration of use. Intestitial nephritis with a peripheral and urinary eosinophilia rarely occurs. Renal side effects are reversible with withdrawal of the offending agent. The potential for renovascular insufficiency requires close observation in older adults, especially those with existing comorbidities that compromise renal perfusion (e.g., congestive heart failure, dehydration, cirrhosis, peripheral vascular disease, coronary artery disease, diabetes mellitus, and hypertension). When indicated, serum blood urea nitrogen (BUN), creatinine, calcium, and phosphorus levels should be monitored.

Corticosteroids

Corticosteroids play a significant role in alleviating pain since they have potent anti-inflammatory properties. They block leukotriene synthesis as well as prostaglandin synthesis. Corticosteroids are effective in reducing pain caused by nerve compression and ectopic neuronal activity (76). A list of corticosteroids and their potencies and half-lives is provided in Table 22-10.

Systemic corticosteroids suppress the pituitary-hypothalamic-adrenocortical system that normally induces cortisol secretion during physiologic and psychological stress. In patients repeatedly treated with systemic steroids (e.g., those with multiple sclerosis), the pituitary-hypothalamic-adrenocortical system will be suppressed and corticosteroid receptors will be less responsive. This may be one mechanism that influences not only the variability of responsive-

Table 22-9: Classification of Nonsteroidal Anti-inflammatory Drugs

Class	Example
Proprionic acid derivatives	Ibuprofen
Pyrrolealkanoic acid derivatives	Tolmetin
Phenylalkanoic acid derivatives	Flurbiprofen
Indole derivatives	Indomethacin
Pyrazolone derivatives	Phenylbutazone
Phenylacetic acid derivatives	Diclofenac
Fenamates	Meclofenamic acid
Oxicams	Piroxicam
Naphthylacetic acid prodrug	Nabumetone

Table 22-10: Corticosteroid Potencies and Half-Lives

Name	Potency (Relative Standard to Hydrocortisone)	Half-Life (hr)
Cortisone	0.8	8–12
Hydrocortisone	1	8–12
Prednisone	4	18–36
Prednisolone	4	18–36
Triamcinolone	5	18–36
Methylprednisolone	5	18–36
Dexamethasone	20–30	36–54
Betamethasone	20–30	36–54

ness of patients with multiple sclerosis to systemic steroids during subsequent treatments of exacerbations, but also the unmasking or worsening of cognitive and behavioral difficulties caused by steroids (77).

In patients who are treated with less than 10 mg of prednisone or equivalent for autoimmune and inflammatory disorders (e.g., chronic inflammatory demyelinating polyneuropathy, rheumatoid arthritis, asthma, inflammatory bowel diseases), an acute illness or major surgery may require increasing the dose of steroids for "stress" coverage. For minor illnesses and surgical procedures, prednisone at 25 mg daily for 3 days is recommended. Patients with moderately stressful illnesses or procedures may require prednisone at 50 to 75 mg daily for 3 days. With prolonged illnesses or major procedures, hydrocortisone at 100 to 150 mg daily for 3 days is recommended. After the "stress" period has passed, a gradual taper to baseline steroid dose then should occur (78).

The use of rapid tapering courses of corticosteroids is a common first-line treatment of acute spinal disk herniation. When they are used for less than 2 weeks, side effects are unusual. However, chronically ill patients who take more than 10 mg of prednisone or equivalent for prolonged periods of time (e.g., those with rheumatoid arthritis, polymyalgia rheumatica, cerebral aneurysm clipping to treat arteriovenous malformation, brain tumors, or organ transplantation) often experience side effects. These side effects include glucose intolerance via decreased peripheral glucose utilization and increased gluconeogenesis; osteopenia via osteoblastic inhibition and osteoclastic stimulation; gastric ulceration; myopathy with proximal weakness; cataracts; avascular necrosis; and immune compromise. "Stress" steroid coverage similarly is necessary to replace normal physiologic responses in patients who are receiving long-term corticosteroid therapy. When one is attempting to discontinue steroids in a long-term user, a slow taper is necessary to allow the pituitary-hypothalamic-adrenocortical system to re-establish homeostasis (73).

Since the early 1990s, the use of parenteral high-dose methylprednisolone for 24 hours has become a common treatment for acute traumatic spinal cord injury. Treatment should be initiated within 8 hours of injury. Short-term and long-term neurologic recovery is reported to be enhanced; however, it is unclear whether this translates into functional recovery (79).

Intra-articular and periarticular corticosteroid injections are useful in patients who do not tolerate systemic steroids, who do not respond to conservative treatments, or who have focal joint or periarticular soft-tissue inflammation with intolerable pain that interferes with functional movement. Their use is controversial, however, because of their deleterious effects on collagen, resulting in a reduction of its tensile strength. Steroids also may interfere with collagen repair by slowing fibroblastic metabolic activity. Many clinicians would consider intra-articular steroid injections only sparingly, and do not support the use of periarticular steroid injections for the treatment of acute traumatic or repetitive overuse injuries. One common approach for intra-articular injection is to mix steroids with 1% or 2% lidocaine in as much as a 1 : 1 ratio, with the volume determined by the size of the joint space to be injected. In the event that soft-tissue injections become necessary, a higher ratio of local anesthetic to steroid is recommended to try to minimize local adverse effects (e.g., subcutaneous atrophy, depigmentation, striae, telangiectasia) (74). Many preparations of injectable steroids including triamcinolone hexacetonide (5 mg/mL) and betamethasone sodium (6 mg/mL) are available.

Intraspinal corticosteroid injections are becoming increasingly common in physiatric practice for the symptomatic treatment of patients with neck and back pain due to degenerative disk and facet disease for whom conservative or surgical treatments have failed. For these indications, clinicians usually intend to inject steroids into the lower lumbar and upper sacral epidural or intrathecal spaces. However, there is no guarantee that the steroid suspension will stay confined to these spaces, because there is potential access to the subdural and subarachnoid spaces through the arachnoid villi that juxtapose the membranes of the epidural space. There also may be diffusion of the suspension from higher or lower levels across the epidural and intrathecal spaces. Serious but rare complications from epidural and intrathecal injections include death from septic meningitis, arachnoiditis with nerve root traction and constriction resulting in progressive pain, paraparesis, and loss of bowel and bladder control. However, adverse events can be minimized by the use of videofluorographic guidance to direct steroids into the interspinous ligaments and subdural and subarachnoid spaces, the use of transforaminal selective nerve root epidural injections at multiple segmental levels, and the use of newer steroid preparations.

The proposed therapeutic mechanism of epidural steroid injection on selective nerve roots is the reduction of chemical inflammation at or near nerve roots, in response to mechanical impingement from degenerative disease. Additionally, videofluorographically guided injections into facet joints and nerve roots at multiple spinal segmental levels are sometimes performed in tandem to treat patients who have back pain from multiple pain-generating inflammatory sources. It is unclear whether the therapeutic mechanisms of multiple, segmental facet joint injections is a reduction of chemical inflammation inside the joint capsule itself, local extravasation of the steroid suspension into adjacent epidural space, or diffusion of the steroid into posterior sensory afferent-rich ligamentous structures due to facet joint capsular rupture (80–82).

Low-Affinity Opioid Receptor Drugs

For many years, there were no analgesic medications between the classes of NSAIDs and narcotics. Recently, *tramadol* was approved as a synthetic analogue of codeine that has a low affinity for opiate receptors and thus has not been classified as a controlled substance (83). Tramadol has selectivity for μ narcotic receptors but is 10-fold less potent than codeine, 60-fold less potent than propoxyphene, 1000-fold less potent than methadone, and 6000-fold less potent than morphine (84). The analgesic activity of tramadol is attributed to both the parent drug and the *O*-desmethyl (M1) metabolite, which has two to four times the analgesic potency of the parent compound.

Tramadol can be used orally, intramuscularly, intravenously, or epidurally. Oral doses range up to 50 to 100 mg four times a day. Intramuscular doses of 50 or 100 mg may be given in single injections. Intravenous tramadol may be given as intermittent or continuous infusions. One double-blind, placebo-controlled trial in 35 patients undergoing major gynecologic surgery demonstrated 60% less need for supplemental tramadol when a continuous tramadol infusion of 15 mg/hr was compared with intermittent administration of 150 mg (85). Tramadol also may be self-administered [patient-controlled analgesia (PCA)] for postoperative pain. Epidural administration of tramadol has been used in patients after abdominal surgery (86).

Tramadol may be used for acute and chronic pain conditions. Aside from postoperative pain, tramadol has been used to treat ureteral calculi (87), labor pain (88), dental pain (89), and cardiac pain (90). Tramadol also has been used to treat cancer pain (91), neuropathic pain, primary fibrosis, and osteitis deformans (92).

The side effects of tramadol may affect the central nervous, gastrointestinal, and cardiovascular systems. Central nervous system effects include irritation, sedation, central stimulation headache, weakness, euphoria, dysphoria, and seizures. Gastrointestinal effects include nausea, vomiting, constipation, and alterations in appetite. Tramadol also may cause tachycardia, dry mouth, diaphoresis, and allergic skin reactions.

Opioid Analgesics

Opioid analgesics are drugs that bind to opioid receptors and are reversed by naloxone (93). There are at least three specific types of opioid receptors, μ, κ, and δ, and these have been subclassified: μ_1 and μ_2; κ_1, κ_2, and κ_3; and δ_1 and δ_2. All receptor sites produce analgesia when activated (94). The μ receptors may cause respiratory depression, miosis, euphoria, and reduced gastrointestinal motility. The κ receptors may produce dysphoria, psychotomimetic effects, miosis, and respiratory depression. Opioid receptors are found particularly in the periaqueductal gray matter and throughout the spinal cord. More recently, they also were found in the peripheral nervous system (95).

Opioid analgesics are classified according to their interactions with the various receptor subtypes. *Pure agonists* increase the analgesic effect in a log-linear relationship to the dose, without any apparent ceiling effect until analgesia or adverse effects (such as somnolence, cognitive impairment, myoclonus, or ventilatory depression) occur. *Antagonists* interfere with the actions of pure agonists, but do not have any intrinsic analgesic properties of their own. Antagonists may compete with pure agonists for receptor sites (*competitive*) or may block the effects of pure agonists by some other mechanism (*noncompetitive*). *Mixed agonist-antagonists* produce agonist effects at one receptor site while producing antagonist effects at other receptor sites. These medications tend to have a ceiling effect for analgesia. *Partial agonists* have low intrinsic activity at receptor sites, thus producing a ceiling effect at less than the maximal analgesic levels produced by pure agonists. Examples of various opioid analgesics are listed in Table 22-11. The relative potency of each opioid analgesic compared with a 10-mg intramuscular or 30-mg oral dose of morphine is listed in Table 22-12.

The use of opioid analgesics is based on a comprehensive evaluation of the pain problem. They can be used as part of a plan that treats the underlying cause of pain, and can be used concurrently with other appropriate medications, rehabilitation services, and psychological support. Patients should be evaluated frequently and should be prepared to modify treatment plans as adverse effects or inadequate pain relief occur. Opioid analgesics are indicated for moderate to severe cancer pain, and in short-term use for pain caused by burns, trauma, surgery, or other procedures. They may be used for conditions causing acute recurrent pain, such as sickle cell anemia, hemophilia, or pancreatitis, but are considered controversial for use in conditions such as recurrent refractory headache (96), dysmenorrhea, chronic nonmalignant pain (97), and neuropathic pain (98).

The choice of opioid analgesic depends on the type and intensity of pain to be treated. Pain from procedures

Table 22-11: Classification of Opioid Analgesics
Pure agonists (short half-life)
Codeine
Dihydrocodeine
Dextropropoxyphene
Fentanyl
Heroin
Meperidine
Morphine
Oxycodone
Oxymorphone
Phenazocine
Pure agonists (long half-life)
Methadone
Levorphanol
Partial agonists
Buprenorphine
Mixed agonist-antagonists
Butorphanol
Meptazinol
Nalbuphine
Pentazocine

Table 22-12: Relative Potency of Opioid Analgesics as Compared with Morphine

Drug	IM Dosage (mg)	PO Dosage (mg)
Morphine	10	30
Butorphenol	1 (transnasal)	—
Buprenorphine	0.4	0.8
Codeine	130	200
Fentanyl	0.1 (transdermal)	—
Heroin	5	60
Hydromorphone	1.5	7.5
Levorphanol	2	4
Meperidine	75	300
Methadone	10	20
Nalbuphine	10	—
Oxycodone	15	30
Oxymorphone	1	10
Pentazocine	35	100
Phenazocine	—	6
Propoxyphene	—	100

IM = intramuscular; PO = oral.

or surgeries usually can be treated with pure agonists such as morphine, fentanyl, hydromorphone, and meperidine. Parenteral, epidural, intrathecal, intramuscular, or rectal routes may be used if the patient is dysphagic or requires localized administration. Sublingual buprenorphine also can be used if the patient is alert.

Treatment of chronic pain depends on its intensity, the availability of specific opioid analgesics, the risk of adverse effects, and comorbidities. Patients with moderate pain may be given acetaminophen or aspirin plus codeine, dihydrocodeine, hydrocodone, oxycodone, or dextropropoxyphene (99). Patients with severe pain may be treated with morphine, hydromorphone, oxycodone, oxymorphone, fentanyl, methadone, or levorphanol. Dosing may be titrated with short-acting opioid analgesics, as they require shorter periods to reach steady-state serum concentrations. Controlled-release or long-acting opioid analgesics then may be substituted. Several opioid analgesics or routes of administration may be tried before a drug is identified as effective and well tolerated. Dosages should be adjusted in patients with renal impairment so as to prevent an accumulation of drug and metabolites.

Patients with continuous or frequent pain should receive opioid analgesics on a fixed schedule not only to relieve pain, but also to prevent pain. Controlled-release or long-acting formulations are more convenient to use when 24-hour dosing is required. Patients receiving 24-hour dosing should be offered a *rescue* dose when pain breaks through the fixed schedule. The rescue dose may equal 5% to 15% of the 24-hour baseline dose. Likewise, PCA may be offered in parenteral or intrathecal forms. Using PCA, the patient may self-administer boluses of opioid analgesic at fixed intervals with or without a continuous infusion of drug. Patients using PCA should be cognitively intact in order that the opioid is dispensed appropriately in response to pain.

Successful treatment with opioid analgesics should reflect relief of pain with minimal adverse effects. The most common adverse effect associated with opioid analgesics is constipation (100). Constipation is so common that prophylaxis with a combination of a stool softener (e.g., docusate) and bowel stimulant (e.g., senna, casanthranol, bisacodyl, phenolphthalein) should be given in conjunction with the opioid analgesic. Nausea and vomiting may occur as a result of stimulation of the medullary chemoreceptor trigger zone. Sedation, cognitive impairment, and ventilatory depression require emergent reduction of dosing or administration of naloxone, or both. Myoclonus occurs as a result of accumulation of a metabolite of meperidine. Physical addiction usually can be prevented if opioid analgesics are tapered rather than abruptly discontinued. However, psychological addiction should be suspected if patients lose control over their use or continue their use despite serious adverse effects.

Other Analgesics

A number of drugs may be used for analgesia although they primarily have indications in other conditions. These *secondary analgesics* usually have no role in treating acute pain but primarily are used for conditions of chronic pain.

Antidepressants are especially useful in patients with trigeminal or postherpetic neuralgias, diabetic neuropathies, migraine headaches, fibromyalgias, or chronic regional pain syndromes. Many of these patients may become depressed owing to the unabating pain they experience. The analgesic effect of antidepressants usually is independent from the antidepressant effect since changes in mood occur after the onset of pain and require dosages smaller than those required to treat depression. Analgesia is thought to be due to increased central nervous system levels of norepinephrine caused by the reuptake inhibition of these drugs. Antidepressants may not abolish pain, but they can be effective agents to reduce pain to a level that allows increased function (55). Amitriptyline is the most commonly used medication in this class, usually starting at a dose of 10 mg at bedtime, and slowly titrating the dose as tolerated. If anticholinergic side effects become intolerable, less noradrenergic or more serotonergic agents such as nortriptyline, desipramine, doxepin, trazodone, or SSRIs may be systematically substituted (65). Specific SSRI antidepressants are gaining more acceptance and use for treating chronic pain (50,53,55).

Anticonvulsants also have a role in chronic pain that is "burning" or "shooting" in nature. They often are used alone or as adjuvant therapy for the management of chronic neuropathic pain such as post-stroke central pain, migraine headache, trigeminal neuralgia, and diabetic neuropathy (20,21,56,101). Carbamazepine, phenytoin, and gabapentin have been used both as monotherapy and as adjuvant treatment with agents that are mediated through other neurotransmitter systems (e.g., narcotic analgesics, tricyclic antidepressants). Valproic acid is preferred only as adjuvant treatment. Carbamazepine is the best studied anticonvulsant for the treatment of trigeminal neuralgia. Gabapentin is increasingly being used with some success for many types of neuropathic pain.

Muscle relaxants and *antispasticity drugs* may relieve pain when caused by hypertonicity of muscle, but can be sedating and weakening. Baclofen is indicated for multiple sclerosis and spinal spasticity, while dantrolene and tizanidine are the favored drugs for cerebral spasticity. Botulinum toxin and phenol blocks can be used when pain of spastic origin appears in localized areas.

Capsaicin is the most pungent ingredient contained in the red pepper and has been used throughout history as a medication to cure symptoms such as pain, itching, and constipation (102). Capsaicin acts by selectively activating type C unmyelinated neurons in an antidromic direction, resulting in the release of substance P and *N*-methyl-D-aspartic acid (NMDA) at the periphery (103). Following this first exposure, nerve fibers no longer are activated by capsaicin or other stimuli known to activate them (104). Traditionally, capsaicin has been used to relieve pain through single local application. However, more recently, repeated local applications have been used for postmastectomy pain (105), postherpetic (106) and trigeminal (107) neuralgias, diabetic neuropathy (108), and complex regional pain syndrome (109). Concentrations such as 0.050% to 0.075% are required for sufficient desensitization. Side effects are local and include burning sensations.

Other drugs include clonidine, mexiletine, and flecainide. *Clonidine* is an α_2-antagonist that acts on potassium channels similar to those opened by opioid μ-agonists. Side effects include orthostatic hypotension and sedation. *Mexiletine* and *flecainide* are antiarrhythmic agents that have membrane-stabilizing properties. These drugs are used in patients with neuropathic pain resistant to other medications.

SPASTICITY

Spasticity is defined as "a motor disorder characterized by a velocity-dependent increase in tonic stretch reflexes with exaggerated tendon jerks, resulting from hyperexcitability of the stretch reflex, as one component of the upper motor neuron syndrome (110). Spasticity is characterized by exaggerated myotatic reflexes due to the loss of reciprocal inhibition mediated by Ia afferents. The hypertonicity associated with spasticity originally was thought to be due to the same mechansim but is now thought to be due to the loss of nonreciprocal inhibition mediated by Ib afferents (111).

Figure 22-1 illustrates the mechanisms involved in spasticity that form the basis for treatment. GABA usually suppresses the tonic stretch and myotatic reflexes by presynaptic inhibition onto Ia afferents. Amino acids provide excitatory input into the spinal cord through the corticospinal, rubrospinal, reticulospinal, and vestibulospinal tracts, resulting in increased muscle stretch reflexes. Disruption of these pathways during traumatic spinal cord or brain injury and stroke may account for the phenomenon of "spinal shock." Noradrenergic and serotonergic inputs to the spinal cord through the reticulospinal tract are thought to suppress myotatic and muscle stretch reflexes, but the mechanisms that produce this are poorly understood.

Medications used to treat spasticity may be divided into *systemic* and *focal* drugs. Systemic medications include baclofen, dantrolene, diazepam, clonidine, and tizanidine. Focal medications include phenol, denatured alcohol, and botulinum toxin.

Baclofen

Baclofen is a GABA-B agonist that inhibits the influx of calcium into presynaptic terminals. It also may exert direct action on the polarization state of the neuron membrane. Baclofen has a half-life of approximately 3.5 hours. It is indicated for multiple sclerosis and spasticity of spinal origin, but no studies have proved its efficacy for cerebral spasticity. Side effects may include transient drowsiness, dizziness, weakness, and fatigue. Dosing begins at 5 mg orally three times a day, and can be titrated by 15 mg every 3 or 4 days. Likewise, baclofen should be weaned at approximately the same rate since abrupt withdrawal can

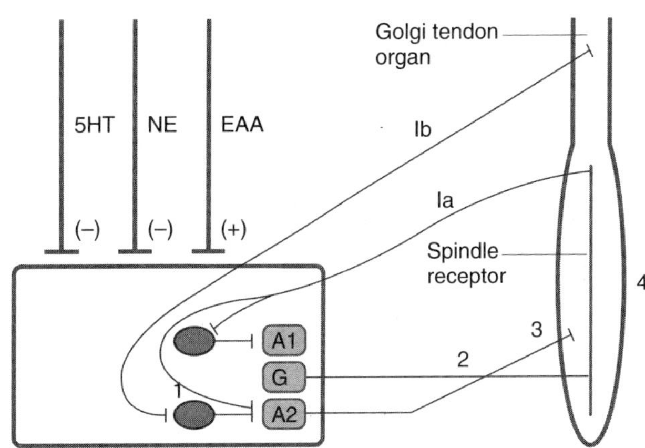

Figure 22-1. Mechanisms of spasticity medications. Neurotransmitter pathways: 5HT = 5-hydroxytriptamine; NE = norepinephrine; EAA = excitatory amino acids. Spinal cord neurons: A1 = antagonist motor neuron; G = α motor neuron; A2 = agonist motor neuron. Sites of action: 1 = interneurons (baclofen, diazepam, tizanidine, clonidine); 2 = peripheral nerve (phenol, denatured alcohol); 3 = neuromuscular junction (botulinum toxin); 4 = muscle (dantrolene).

cause seizures. There are no specific dosing recommendations for geriatric patients.

More recently, baclofen has been administered intrathecally through the use of a microchip-controlled pump (112,113). A test dose of baclofen usually is administered via lumbar puncture prior to implantation of the pump, to determine the efficacy of the drug. If the test dose is effective, the pump is implanted subdermally in the abdomen, and a catheter is threaded through the subcutaneous space into the cerebrospinal fluid in the lower thoracic and upper lumbar regions. This allows baclofen to be infused around the spinal cord, thus bypassing the blood-brain barrier. Doses may range from 25 μg/day or less to over 200 μg/day. The pump is filled by transdermal puncture every few weeks or months as needed. Intrathecal baclofen is highly effective treatment for spasticity of spinal origin (114,115), and has been used in patients with multiple sclerosis and traumatic brain injury (116,117). Studies currently are in progress for use in stroke survivors. Intrathecal morphine has been shown to be similarly effective (118).

Dantrolene

Dantrolene reduces spasticity by inhibiting the influx of calcium into the sarcoplasmic reticulum of muscle (119). It reduces phasic stretch reflexes more than tonic stretch reflexes and affects fast muscle fibers more than slow muscle fibers. The half-life of dantrolene is approximately 8.7 hours. Dantrolene is the drug of choice for cerebral spasticity and can be a useful adjunct for spinal spasticity. Patients with chronic obstructive pulmonary disease and impaired cardiac function (especially due to myocardial disease) should not use dantrolene. The side effects include drowsiness, dizziness, weakness, malaise, fatigue, and diarrhea. Hepatotoxicity can occur at a rate of approximately 1%. Dosing can begin at 25 mg orally every day and can be titrated 25 mg every 3 or 4 days. Weaning should occur at the same rate to prevent rebound spasticity. No special recommendations have been made for geriatric patients.

Diazepam

Diazepam is a GABA-A agonist that exerts an indirect mimetic effect only when GABA transmission is functional (120,121). The half-life of diazepam is approximately 27 to 37 hours, but its primary metabolite has a longer half-life. Diazepam has been used successfully for spasticity of spinal origin, but usually is unsuitable for patients with cerebral spasticity. The side effects include drowsiness, fatigue, and ataxia. Dosing can range up to 10 mg three or four times a day. The recommended geriatric starting dose ranges between 2.0 and 2.5 mg orally every day.

Clonidine

Clonidine is an α_2-adrenergic agonist whose mechanism of action is unknown (122,123). Its half-life is approximately 12 to 16 hours. Clonidine has been used with fair success for spinal spasticity, but its success for cerebral spasticity is unknown. The side effects include dry mouth, drowsiness, dizziness, constipation, sedation, nausea and vomiting, and hypotension. Dosing begins at 0.1 mg orally twice a day, and can be titrated to 0.2 to 0.6 mg orally twice a day (maximum, 2.4 mg/day). With transdermal clonidine, the dose can range from the 0.1-mg patch to two 0.3-mg patches per week. No recommendations have been made for geriatric patients.

Tizanidine

Tizanidine was approved for use by the FDA in February 1997 (124,125). Tizanidine is an imidazoline derivative that is a central α_2-receptor agonist. It may facilitate glycine action, and decreases the release of excitatory amino acids, leading to an inhibition of spinal motor neurons (126). Its peak effect occurs in 1 to 2 hours, and lasts between 3 and 6 hours. Tizanidine has an efficacy equivalent to that of baclofen for spinal spasticity, and is better tolerated for cerebral spasticity than is baclofen or diazepam. The side effects include hypotension, psychosis, and renal impairment. Hepatotoxicity may occur at the same rate as that of dantrolene. Dosing begins at 2 mg once or twice a day and should be increased gradually in 2- to 4-mg increments. The total daily dose should not exceed 36 mg.

Local Injection

Focal treatment of spasticity may be accomplished through chemical neurolysis. Agents such as *phenol* (127,128) and *denatured alcohol* (129,130) produce protein coagulation and necrosis, which destroys neurons. Phenol (2%–6% aqueous solution) and denatured alcohol may be administered on peripheral nerves or at the neuromuscular junction (i.e., motor point). Both agents may be titrated according to response. They act immediately upon injection and the effects usually last between 3 and 6 months. Spasticity recurs usually because contact with the denervated muscle is re-established by collateral sprouting of the affected nerves.

Botulinum toxin also has been used in the treatment of various types of spasticity. Botulinum toxin is absorbed into presynaptic terminals and prevents the release of acetylcholine into the neuromuscular junction. Its action begins approximately 24 to 72 hours after injection, reaches its maximum effect in approximately 6 weeks, and usually lasts about 12 weeks. The side effects include weakness in adjacent muscles and formation of antibodies against the toxin, especially when injections are repeated less than 12 weeks apart. Botulinum toxin is indicated for use for blepharospasm and strabismus, but has been used in off-label trials for cervical dystonia and spasmodic torticollis, spasticity of spinal and cerebral origins, cricopharyngeal dysfunction, achalasia, anal achalasia, and various plastic surgery procedures (e.g., "crow's feet").

BLADDER MEDICATIONS

The bladder receives innervation from both the autonomic and the somatic nervous system (Fig. 22-2). *Parasympathetic* stimulation through the pelvic nerve and sacral micturition center (levels S2–S4) causes detrusor contraction, funneling of the bladder neck, and opening of the internal sphincter. Afferent fibers are responsible for the sensation of distention and urge of voiding. *Sympathetic* outflow is mediated through the hypogastric nerve (levels T11-L2). α-Adrenergic stimulation impedes urinary outflow by contracting the internal sphincter. β-Adrenergic stimulation causes relaxation of the detrusor. Afferent fibers transmit pain, temperature, and tactile sensation. *Somatic* excitation causes contraction of the striated external sphincter as well as other voluntary muscles in the pelvic floor. Neuroanatomy of the genitourinary system is discussed in further detail in Chapter 51.

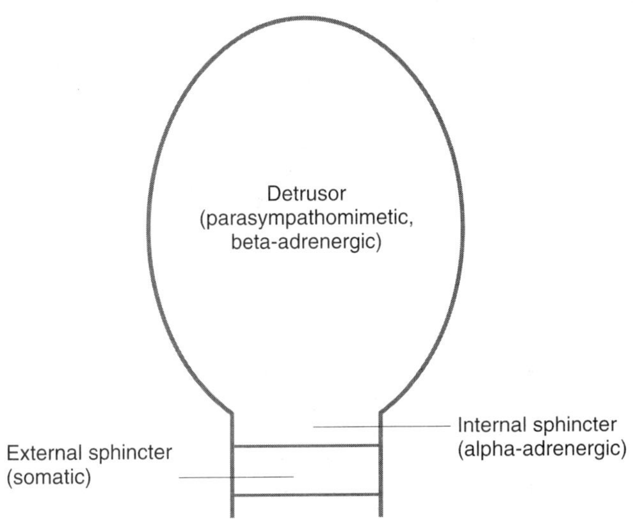

Figure 22-2. Bladder neuroanatomy.

Neuropharmacologic management of the bladder can effectively eliminate the symptoms of urinary frequency, urgency, and incontinence. Management of the bladder can be divided into two categories: *failure to empty* and *failure to fill.* Failure to empty the bladder occurs when the hypotonic or atonic detrusor cannot effectively contrast, or when the internal or external sphincter does not synergistically relax when the detrusor contracts. Failure to fill the bladder occurs when the hypertonic detrusor contracts spontaneously, or when the internal or external sphincter is not contracted at rest. Medications used to treat the bladder that does not adequately fill are listed in Table 22-13, and medications used to treat the bladder that does not adequately empty are listed in Table 22-14. Prior to beginning any medications to modify bladder behavior, it is incumbent on the clinician to complete an evaluation that includes a urinalysis and urine culture, postvoid residual measurements, and urodynamic studies where necessary.

BOWEL MEDICATIONS

Constipation is ubiquitous in immobilized patients. It is not uncommon for patients to enter rehabilitation settings without having had a bowel movement for several days. These patients have variable experiences with oral caloric intake, hydration, and exposure to medications that discourage defecation (e.g., anticholinergic agents, narcotic analgesics). Sleep-wake cycles also have often been disrupted in hospitalized patients, and the usual behavioral and environmental cues that facilitate bowel evacuation are missing.

The general principles of bowel programs include optimizing hydration (in the range of 2 liters daily for maintenance), using natural substances to encourage evacuation (e.g., caffeinated beverages, prune juice, apricot

Table 22-13: Medications to Aid Bladder Filling

Anatomic Component	Drug	Action	Side Effects	Dosing
Hypertonic detrusor	Oxybutinin	Anticholinergic	Dry mouth, constipation, tachycardia, mydriasis, gastroesophageal reflux	2.5 mg tid, up to 20 mg/day
	Propantheline	Anticholinergic	Same as oxybutinin	15 mg tid–qid, up to 180 mg/day
	Hyoscyamine	Anticholinergic	Same as oxybutinin	0.125–0.250 mg q4h, up to 2.5 mg/day; 0.375–0.750 mg q12h (extended release)
	Flavoxate	Anticholinergic	Same as oxybutinin	100–200 mg tid–qid
	Amitriptyline (tricyclic antidepressant)	Anticholinergic	Same as oxybutinin	10 mg qhs, follow serum levels
Hypotonic/atonic internal sphincter	Ephedrine	α Sympathomimetic	Hypertension, insomnia, anxiety	Up to 25–50 mg qid

Table 22-14: Medications to Aid Bladder Emptying

Anatomic Component	Drug	Action	Side Effects	Dosing
Hypotonic detrusor	Bethanechol	Cholinomimetic	Flushing, headache, salivation, sweating, nausea, vomiting, diarrhea, bronchospasm, visual accommodation difficulties	10 mg qid, up to 150 mg/day
Hypertonic/dyssynergic internal sphincter	Prazosin	α-Adrenolytic	Orthostatic hypotension, reflex tachycardia, impotence	1 mg qhs, up to 10 mg qhs
	Terazosin	α-Adrenolytic	Same as prazosin	—
	Oxazosin	α-Adrenolytic	Same as prazosin	—
Hypertonic external sphincter	Baclofen	Antispasticity	Drowsiness, dizziness, weakness, ataxia, nausea	5 mg bid–tid, up to 40–50 mg qid
	Dantrolene	Antispasticity	Drowsiness, weakness, hepatotoxicity	25 mg bid, up to 100 mg qid
	Tizanidine	Antispasticity	Drowsiness, weakness, hepatotoxicity	1–2 mg bid, up to 8 my qid

nectar), and creating as natural a pattern and setting as possible to facilitate bowel evacuation. For example, private use of a bedside commode or toilet and planning bowel evacuation after a meal to capitalize on the gastrocolic reflex should be ordered as part of a prescription. Encouraging resumption of regular bowel habits that simulates the patient's prehospital pattern is essential. Constipation-inducing medications should be minimized whenever possible. Digital stimulation is another essential component of the program for the neurogenic bowel.

The essential ingredients required for an effective bowel program include fiber, stool softeners, and laxatives. Dietary intake of fiber found in whole grains, fruit, vegetables, and beans causes stool to retain water, resulting in bulkier, more uniform, and pliable stool during evacuation. Fiber supplementation also decreases colonic transit time but does not expedite immediate evacuation. For example, psyllium, up to 20 to 30 g daily in two or three divided doses, can be added to maintenance programs when dietary intake of fiber is insufficient. Each tablespoon should be taken with at least 8 oz of water, fruit juice, or milk to avoid intestinal obstruction (131–134). The side effects include transient abdominal bloating and flatulence, especially if psyllium is taken without water. If bloating persists, the dose should be reduced by one-half.

The combination of fiber and stool softeners is recommended as the fist-line approach to prevent constipation (134,135). Stool softeners such as docusate sodium are lubricating agents that wet the surface of the stool. They allow water and fat to penetrate the fecal mass and soften the stool by lowering its surface tension. They are sometimes referred to as emollient laxatives, but they are not bowel irritants. They can stimulate sodium and water secretion into the bowel and decrease jejunal water absorption from the bowel by 80%. They also may potentiate the actions of other medications by facilitating their gastrointestinal and hepatic uptakes. Their use in specific combination with some laxatives has been associated with liver toxicity (135). Docusate sodium has been combined with casanthranol, a mild stimulant laxative that provides gentle peristaltic stimulation.

Lubricant laxatives, such as mineral oil, are discouraged. They may be absorbed by the stool if a stool softener is being used concurrently. They can also interfere with the absorption of fat-soluble vitamins and medications. If they are refluxed, a lipid pneumonia aspiration can result (131,133,134).

Stimulant laxatives and cathartics act by a variety of mechanisms that allow a more immediate bowel evacuation. They can be added incrementally as single agents when diet, fiber supplements, and stool softeners are producing less than optimal results during a maintenance bowel program. Senna derivatives are naturally occurring glycosides that increase intraluminal fluids by modifying membrane electrolyte transport, and augment peristalsis by myenteric plexus stimulation. Senna derivatives should be given up to 8 hours prior to the desired time of evacuation. Oral polyphenolic derivatives (e.g., bisacodyl) have similar mechanisms of action and dosing schedules as senna derivatives. Dose-related side effects of orally administered stimulant laxatives and cathartics include abdominal cramping, diarrhea, electrolyte imbalance, and dehydration. Chronic use of these agents can result in tolerance, dictating the use of agents with other mechanisms of action. Rectal polyphenolic stimulant cathartics administered via suppositories should be considered when the side effects of oral stimulants are not tolerated, and when more immediate bowel evacuation is necessary. For maintenance bowel programs, they can be used intermittently to facilitate complete evacuation when the results of orally administered agents are unsatisfactory. In conjunction with digital stimulation, they are often useful in the early stages of bowel training, but usually are needed intermittently in later stages. In some cases, they are required as part of the maintenance bowel program. However, they are rectal and colonic mucosal irritants when used chronically. After rectal administration of a stimulant laxative and cathartic, bowel evacuation should occur within 1 hour (134).

Saline cathartics and laxatives are salts, commonly magnesium (e.g., magnesium hydroxide) or sodium (e.g., sodium phosphate/biphosphate). Orally administered saline laxatives draw fluid into the small-bowel lumen, with subsequent mixing of digested materials and peristaltic stimulation. They also stimulate secretion of cholecystokinin, which accelerates the bowel transit time. Rectally administered saline laxatives work similarly in the rectum and colon. Results should occur in no less than 6 hours, usually sooner. Saline cathartics are not usually recommended for maintenance bowel programs, unless other agents are ineffective. They are especially useful for ensuring complete bowel evacuation, prior to initiating a maintenance bowel program with less aggressive agents, as discussed already. Abdominal cramping and watery stool should be expected. Dehydration and electrolyte imbalances can occur with repeated use (133,134).

Hyperosmolar, nonabsorbable, disaccharide cathartics and laxatives (e.g., lactulose, glycerin, sorbitol) draw fluid primarily into the colon after being metabolized by bowel bacteria into short-chain amino acids. They are irritating to the bowel mucosa, and can cause cramping and flatulence. Chronic use can induce dehydration and electrolyte abnormalities. Concurrent use of antacids may inhibit their cathartic effect. Lactulose and sorbitol are administered orally, with results expected within several hours. Glycerin is usually administered rectally, with results expected within 1 hour or less. Glycerin suppositories are considered a more gentle alternative to bisacodyl suppositories (133,134).

Finally, cisapride is an agent that interacts with 5-hydroxytryptamine-4 receptors. It also facilitates the local release of acetylcholine from postganglionic neurons within the myenteric plexus, thus stimulating small- and large-bowel peristalsis. It is used for intractable constipation (e.g., diabetic autonomic neuropathy) when other agents have failed. Systemic side effects include ventricular arrhythmias and headache. The starting dose is 5 mg, three times daily, taken 15 minutes before meals or at bedtime. The maximal dose is 20 mg, four times daily (136,137).

ANTICOAGULATION

Antiplatelet and anticoagulant medications are used for a wide variety of indications. In the hyperacute setting, thrombolytic agents may be used to dissolve thromboses that affect vessels in the brain, heart, or extremities. These agents, such as tissue-type plasminogen activator, streptokinase, and urokinase, are beyond the scope of this discussion. However, in the acute and rehabilitation environments, anticoagulants and antiplatelet agents may be used in patients with venous thromboembolism, atrial fibrillation, valvular heart disease, mechanical or biologic heart valves, coronary artery disease, saphenous vein or internal mammary artery bypass grafts, or cerebrovascular disease. These same agents may be used to prevent venous thromboembolism in patients with stroke, joint replacements, or other conditions that render the patient immobile. Aspirin has not been shown to reduce the risk of preeclampsia and low-weight births due to placental insufficiency (138). Proper knowledge and use of these medications is important to prevent complications from their underusage (e.g., venous thromboembolism, stroke) as well as their overusage (e.g., hemorrhage). The discussion of these medications progresses from antiplatelet agents to anticoagulants.

Aspirin

Aspirin was discussed earlier in this chapter as a pain medication. It works similarly as an antiplatelet agent by acetylating cyclooxygenase on platelets, resulting in a significant reduction in platelet thromboxane A_2 and prostacyclin levels. On the other hand, platelets and vascular endothelium process prostaglandin H_2 to produce thromboxane A_2 and prostacyclin, respectively (139). Since thromboxane A_2 causes platelet aggregation and vasoconstriction and prostacyclin inhibits platelet aggregation and causes vasodilation, aspirin potentially can be either thrombogenic or antithrombogenic. Although studies have demonstrated a dose-related suppression of thromboxane A_2 and prostacyclin with doses of aspirin as low as 20 mg, the importance of thromboxane A_2 and prostacyclin on the clinical efficacy of aspirin remains unclear (140).

Aspirin is an effective treatment in preventing thromboembolism in patients with cerebrovascular or cardiovascular disease. An update of the Antiplatelet Trialists' Collaboration confirmed the effectiveness of aspirin in preventing thromboembolism in patients with arterial disease (141). Aspirin was effective at doses as low as 75 mg/day in randomized clinical trials (142,143) or 30 mg/day (144) in a less rigorous trial. The addition of 100 mg of aspirin per day to warfarin treatment in patients with mechanical (145) prosthetic valves can help prevent systemic embolism and vascular death (146). Aspirin has limited benefit in preventing recurrent stroke in patients with nonvalvular atrial fibrillation, but can be used in younger patients without other comorbidities (147). Aspirin also is less efficacious than other anticoagulants in preventing venous thromboembolism. Overall, aspirin is indicated in patients with stable angina, unstable angina, acute myocardial infarction, transient ischemic attack, thrombotic stroke, or peripheral arterial disease. The benefits of preventing ischemic stroke far outweigh the potential for cerebral hemorrhage in high-risk patients.

Dipyridamole

Dipyridamole is a pyrimidine derivative whose mechanism of action is not fully understood. It may stimulate prostacyclin synthesis, potentiate the platelet inhibitory action of prostacyclin, inhibit phosphodiesterase to raise cyclic adenosine monophosphate levels, and block adenosine uptake into red blood cells (148). Dipyridamole lengthens abnormally shortened platelet survival times in a dose-dependent manner. It does not affect prothrombin time (PT) or partial thromboplastin time when administered with anticoagulant agents, such as heparin or warfarin.

Dipyridamole originally was not thought to be efficacious as an antiplatelet agent when used alone for any indication (149). However, recent studies show that dipyridamole adds benefit to aspirin when used to prevent stroke (150), prevents the spread of peripheral vascular disease (151), protects the myocardium during percutaneous coronary angioplasty (152), and prevents thromboembolism in patients with mechanical heart valves (153). Dipyridamole does not secondarily prevent myocardial infarction (154) or thrombosis of coronary artery bypass grafts (154a).

Dipyridamole may be taken in doses of 75 to 100 mg four times daily in conjunction with warfarin. The side effects include gastrointestinal distress, dizziness, headache, and rash, and are usually transient. Rarely, a coronary "steal" phenomenon is observed.

Ticlopidine

Ticlopidine is a thienopyridine derivative that inhibits platelet aggregation by blocking the interaction between fibrinogen and the platelet membrane glycoprotein receptor GP IIb/IIIa (155). The antiplatelet effect of ticlopidine begins 24 to 48 hours following its administration owing to significant contributions by its metabolites (156), but requires a minimum of 3 to 5 days to achieve maximal prolongation of bleeding time. Similarly, the antiplatelet effects persist up to 10 days following discontinuation and are dependent on platelet survival time (157).

Ticlopidine was effective as secondary prophylaxis for transient ischemic attack (158), stroke (159), unstable angina (160), and intermittent claudication (161) and after coronary artery bypass graft surgery (162) in randomized clinical trials. Ticlopidine is more effective than aspirin in treating patients with transient ischemic attack and minor stroke, but is not more effective in preventing stroke, myocardial infarction, and death combined (158).

The dose of ticlopidine is 250 mg twice daily. Its most common side effect is diarrhea, which occurs in up to 20% of patients. The most serious adverse effect is neutropenia, which occurs in 2.4% of patients and is most severe in 0.85% of patients (158,159). Neutropenia usually occurs within the first 3 months of therapy and is reversible when ticlopidine is stopped. White blood cell counts should be determined every 2 weeks during the first 3 months of ticlopidine therapy.

Clopidogrel

Clopidogrel is a thienopyridine derivative whose activity in animal models is greater than that of ticlopidine (163). Like ticlopidine, clopidogrel irreversibly inhibits platelet activation by inhibiting the binding of adenosine diphosphate to its receptor on the cell membrane, thus preventing the activation of the GP IIb/IIIa complex, which is the major fibrinogen receptor. Clopidogrel has a dose-related effect that prolongs bleeding up to 1.5 to 1.7 times baseline levels (164).

Clopidogrel carries the same indications as ticlopidine. In the major randomized clinical trial with aspirin, clopidogrel demonstrated relative-risk reductions of 7.3% and 23.8% for stroke and peripheral vascular disease, respectively, but demonstrated a relative-risk increase of 3.7% for myocardial infarction (165). However, when patients with a history of myocardial infarction were included, clopidogrel exhibited a relative-risk reduction of 7.4%.

The dose of clopidogrel is 75 mg/day. The most common side effects include diarrhea, upper gastrointestinal discomfort, and rash. The incidence of neutropenia (0.10%) is equal to that of aspirin treatment (0.17%).

Heparin

Heparin is the anticoagulant of choice when rapid intravenous anticoagulation is required. It is a glycosaminoglycan composed of chains of alternating D-glucosamine and uronic acid residues. Its major mechanism is the inactivation of coagulation factors IIa (thrombin), Xa, and IXa by changes in antithrombin III mediated by interactions with antithrombins I and II (166). Heparin molecules vary in size, anticoagulant activity, and pharmacokinetic properties. Only one-third of heparin molecules have antithrombin III–mediated anticoagulant activity, which is influenced by the chain length of the molecule.

Heparin is indicated for the prevention and treatment of venous thromboembolism in a number of medical conditions (167). It is effective for the early treatment of unstable angina and acute myocardial infarction (168), and in patients who have undergone coronary angioplasty, coronary stent placement, or surgery utilizing cardiac bypass (169). Clinical trials support the use of heparin in patients who have had vascular surgery and in some patients with disseminated intravascular thrombosis (170).

The anticoagulant effect of heparin usually is monitored using the activated partial thromboplastin time (APTT). There may be variability in APTT with given dosages of heparin, owing to fluctuations in plasma heparin concentrations. Sick patients may experience elevated levels of factor VIII as a result of the acute-phase reaction response resulting in reduced APTT in relation to heparin levels. While clinicians generally define the therapeutic range of heparin as an APTT ratio of 1.5 (ratio of measured to control values), different reagents used to process the test may be associated with a wide variation in

APTT. As a result, APTT reagents should be calibrated to a heparin level of 0.2 to 0.4 U/mL.

Heparin is dosed according to amount and route of administration, depending on the indication. Prevention of venous thrombosis usually requires low doses such as 5000 units subcutaneously two or three times per day. Efficacy may be increased by adjusting the dose of subcutaneous heparin to an APTT ratio up to 1.1 to 1.2 after hip surgery (171), and up to 1.5 after spinal cord injury (172). The dose of intravenous heparin given as treatment for other conditions is usually determined using nomograms based on weight or other parameters. Continuous infusions may be preceded by a weight-based bolus, depending on the algorithm.

Heparin therapy may be hampered by numerous side effects. The major complication of heparin is bleeding. Long-term heparin usage has been associated with osteoporosis resulting in rib fractures, vertebral collapse, and osteopenia of thoracolumbar vertebrae. However, these adverse effects have been described only in case reports or series (173). Heparin-induced thrombocytopenia (HIT) is a well-known complication that can be manifested by a reversible nonimmune thrombocytopenia, and an IgG-mediated immune thrombocytopenia. HIT may be accompanied by arterial or venous thrombotic phenomenon, inflammatory or pulmonary reactions, or skin rash or necrosis. Less commonly, heparin may cause hypoaldosteronism, hypersensitivity reactions, or priapism.

Low-Molecular-Weight Heparins

Low-molecular-weight heparins (LMWHs) are a class of anticoagulants used more commonly in Europe that are derived from the depolymerization of heparin into chains approximately one-third of the size of standard heparin molecules. LMWHs demonstrate a progressive loss of the ability to catalyze thrombin inhibition, improved pharmacokinetic properties due to decreased protein binding, and decreased platelet interactions, which may be responsible for reduced bleeding diatheses and incidence of HIT. Because different LMWH preparations are made using different depolymerization methods, each type of LMWH is not necessarily interchangeable with another.

LMWHs have longer half-life and more predictable anticoagulant response than does standard heparin. As a result, LMWHs may be administered as a standard dose without the need for laboratory monitoring. LMWHs are more effective in preventing deep venous thrombosis than are subcutaneous heparin (174), adjusted-dose heparin (175), oral anticoagulants (176), dextran (177), and aspirin after hip and knee surgery. LMWHs also are effective in preventing venous thrombosis in patients with strokes (178), spinal cord injuries (179), or other medical conditions (180). However, LMWHs are not effective in reducing unfavorable outcomes 3 months after stroke (181). The side effects are similar to those of heparin, although the incidence of side effects using an LMWH is lower than that of standard heparin.

Warfarin

Warfarin, a 4-hydroxy compound, is the most widely used oral anticoagulant agent in North America (182). Warfarin interferes with the cyclical interconversion of vitamin K and vitamin K epoxide by inhibiting vitamin K epoxide reductase and possibly vitamin K reductase. As a result of this reaction, vitamin KH_2 is depleted and the associated coagulation factors (prothrombin, VII, IX, and X) are not carboxylated. Additionally, the regulatory proteins C and S also are not carboxylated and cannot become activated anticoagulation proteins.

Warfarin is indicated for numerous medical conditions requiring anticoagulation. It is effective in the primary and secondary prophylaxis of venous thromboembolism; of systemic thromboembolism in patients with tissue or prosthetic heart valves (183), atrial fibrillation (184,185), or mitral valve stenosis (186); of acute myocardial infarction in patients with peripheral vascular disease; and of stroke and death in patients with myocardial infarction or significant precerebral or intracerebral stenosis. Warfarin also is used in the treatment of deep vein thrombosis and pulmonary embolism (187).

Warfarin dosing is monitored using the PT test. During the first few days of warfarin therapy, the PT reflects the depression of factor VII. Subsequently, depletion of prothrombin and factor X contribute to the PT result. Reagents used to measure PT are rated by the International Sensitivity Index (ISI), which reflects their responsiveness to the anticoagulation effects of warfarin. The ISI of thromboplastin reagents used in the United States varies between 1.4 and 2.8 (188). As a result, PT ratios may reflect different degrees of anticoagulation although numeric values are equal between laboratories.

To standardize PT ratios, a calibration model was adopted in 1982, thereby converting the PT ratio by raising it to a power of the ISI. The resulting value, known as the *international standardized ratio* (INR), is recognized in most laboratories across North America. However, there are potential problems with the INR system: 1) The INR is not accurate during the initial days of warfarin therapy since only factor VII (and possibly factor X) is depleted during this time. 2) The INR becomes less accurate using reagents with high ISI values. 3) The INR is less accurate when automatic clot detectors are used. 4) The INR may be incorrect if the ISI for a new batch of reagent is reported incorrectly. 5) The INR may be calculated incorrectly because of inappropriate control plasma to calculate the PT ratio (182). Despite these potential flaws, the American College of Chest Physicians recommends an INR of 2.0 to 3.0 for all indications except mechanical heart valves and acute myocardial infarction, for which an INR of 2.5 to 3.5 is recommended.

The major complication of warfarin therapy is bleeding. The risk of hemorrhage is increased when the patient is over 65 years old; has a history of stroke or gastrointestinal bleed; has atrial fibrillation or significant comorbid conditions such as renal insufficiency or anemia; and concomitantly is taking aspirin (182). The risk of bleeding can be reduced if the INR is reduced from a range of 3.0 to 4.5 to a range of 2.0 to 3.0 (183). The most serious nonhemorrhagic side effect of warfarin is skin necrosis, which may be associated with protein C or S deficiencies (189,190).

HETEROTOPIC OSSIFICATION

Heterotopic ossification, also known as *myositis ossificans*, is the formation of mature trabecular bone in sites where it is not normally present (191). Most cases of heterotopic ossificaton are asymptomatic, but symptoms of warmth, edema, and erythema may be observed (192). Serum alkaline phosphatase levels may be elevated abnormally due to active osteoblastic activity. Heterotopic ossification usually is diagnosed by the appearance of ectopic bone on a radiograph. However, the triple-phase bone scan, which provides information on dynamic blood flow, blood pooling, and accumulation of radionuclide in bone, may provide evidence of bone formation up to 4 to 6 weeks before its appearance on a radiograph (193).

Heterotopic ossification is associated with numerous conditions. It can occur after many types of surgery, most commonly total hip arthroplasty. Other procedures associated with heterotopic ossification formation are knee (194) and shoulder (195) arthroplasty, breast implantation (196), and laparotomy (197). Heterotopic ossification may be observed after neurologic insults such as traumatic spinal cord or brain injury or long-term coma. It is less likely seen after the occurrence of encephalitis, meningitis, myelitis, tetanus, tumor, epidural abscess, and subarachnoid hemorrhage. After severe burns, heterotopic ossification can occur in proximity to any large joint, including the elbows, hips, and knees and in the hands. In most cases, the condition occurs in areas underlying the burns, but has been observed in joints remote to the burn process. Heterotopic ossification also may occur in muscles or joints after localized trauma.

The only treatment of heterotopic ossification to date is surgical resection. Surgery is indicated for patients with significant symptoms such as pain, limited range of joint motion, and entrapment of tissues such as peripheral nerve. Surgical resection often fails as the recurrence rate of heterotopic ossification is high. As a result, it is incumbent on the clinician to judge the risk of heterotopic ossification formation in high-risk patients and attempt prophylactic measures. The three prophylactic measures include radiation, NSAIDs, and diphosphonates.

Radiation

Local radiation for the prevention of heterotopic ossificaton is used largely after hip surgery. Radiation should be administered within the first few days after surgery, when the transformation of inducible osteoprogenitor cells is thought to occur. However, radiation may cause decreased fixation of porous-coated joint prostheses and pseudoarthrosis around the surgical site.

Nonsteroidal Anti-iflammatory Drugs

The use of indomethacin (198), ibuprofen (199), or diclofenac (200) decreases the incidence and severity of heterotopic ossification after hip surgery, but has not been shown to be efficacious after acetabular fracture (201). NSAIDs may decrease the formation of osteoblastic cells because of decreased prostaglandin synthesis. No dosage of indomethacin or ibuprofen has been recommended for heterotopic ossification. However, in other indications, the dose of indomethacin may range up to 150 mg/day in three or four divided doses. The maximal dose of ibuprofen for other indications is 800 mg four times per day. The recommended dose of diclofenac is 50 mg three times per day. The side effects of NSAIDs were discussed earlier in this chapter.

Etidronate

Etidronate is a diphosphonate that inhibits the growth of hydroxyapatite crystals, thus delaying the mineralization of osteoid into trabecular bone (202). Etidronate does not affect mature heterotopic ossification. It is indicated for the prevention and treatment of heterotopic ossification only after hip surgery or spinal cord injury. Etidronate should be given as 20 mg/kg/day 1 month prior to surgery and 3 months following surgery. In spinal cord injury patients, etidronate is given 20 mg/kg/day for 2 weeks, then 10 mg/kg/day for 10 weeks. If given chronically, etidronate may retard mineralization of bone and may cause nephrotic syndrome and fracture.

REFERENCES

1. *Stedman's medical dictionary.* Baltimore: Williams & Wilkins, 1995.
2. Roccella EJ, Lenfant C. Regional and racial differences among stroke victims in the United States. *Clin Cardiol* 1989;12:IV-18–IV-22.
3. The Sixth Report of the Joint National Committee for Prevention, Detection, Evaluation, and Treatment of High Blood Pressure (JNC VI). *Arch Intern Med* 1997;157:2413–2446.
4. Schotte DE, Stunkard AJ. The effects of weight reduction on blood pressure in 301 obese patients. *Arch Intern Med* 1990;150:1701–1704.
5. World Hypertension League. Alcohol and hypertension—implications for management: a consensus statement by the World Hypertension League. *J*

Hum Hypertens 1991;5:1854–1856.

6. World Hypertension League. Physical exercise in the management of hypertension: a consensus statement by the World Hypertension League. *J Hypertens* 1991;9:283–287.

7. Whelton PK, He J, Cutler JA, et al. Effects of oral potassium on blood pressure. Meta-analysis of randomized controlled clinical trials. *JAMA* 1997;277:1624–1632.

8. Cutler JA, Brittain E. Calcium and blood pressure: an epidemiologic perspective. *Am J Hypertens* 1990;3:137S–146S.

9. Trials of Hypertension Prevention Collaborative Research Group. The effects of nonpharmacologic interventions on blood pressure of persons with high normal levels: results of the Trials of Hypertension Prevention, phase I. *JAMA* 1992;267:1213–1220.

10. Collins R, Peto R, MacMahon S, et al. Blood pressure, stroke, and coronary heart disease, part 2, short-term reductions in blood pressure: overview of randomised drug trials in their epidemiological context. *Lancet* 1990;335:827–838.

11. MacMahon S, Peto R, Cutler J, et al. Blood pressure, stroke, and coronary heart disease, part 1, prolonged differences in blood pressure: prospective observational studies corrected for the regression dilution bias. *Lancet* 1990;335:765–774.

12. Hypertension Detection and Follow-up Program Cooperative Group. The effect of treatment on mortality in "mild" hypertension: results of the Hypertension Detection and Follow-up Program. *N Engl J Med* 1982; 307:976–980.

13. Alderman MH. Which antihypertensive drugs first—and why! *JAMA* 1992;267:2786–2787.

14. American Diabetes Association. Clinical practice recommendations 1998. Report of the Expert Committee on the Diagnosis and Classification of Diabetes Mellitus. *Diabetes Care* 1998;21:S5–S19.

15. World Health Organization. Diabetes mellitus: report of a WHO study group. *World Health Organ Tech Rep Ser* 1985:727.

16. Grodsky GM, Epstein GH, Fanska R, Karam JH. Pancreatic action of the sulfonyl-ureas. *Fed Proc* 1977;36:2714–2719.

17. Samols E, Tyler JM, Miahe P. Suppression of pancreatic glucagon release by the hypoglycaemic sulphonylureas. *Lancet* 1969;1:174–176.

18. Metformin for non-insulin-dependent diabetes mellitus. *Med Lett Drug Ther* 1995;37: 41–42.

19. Acarbose for diabetes mellitus. *Med Lett Drug Ther* 1996;38:9–10.

20. Bowsher D. The management of central post-stroke pain. *Postgrad Med J* 1995;71:598–604.

21. Bowsher D. Pathophysiology of herpetic neuralgia: towards a rational treatment. *Neurology* 1995;45(suppl 8):556–557.

22. Dugan EM, Howell JM. Post traumatic seizures. *Emerg Med Clin North Am* 1994;12:1081–1087.

23. Willmore LJ. Post-traumatic epilepsy. *Neurol Clin* 1992;10: 869–878.

24. Yablon SA. Post-traumatic seizures. *Arch Phys Med Rehabil* 1993;74:983–1001.

25. Gaultieri CT. Pharmacotherapy and the neurobehavioral sequelae of traumatic brain injury. *Brain Inj* 1988;2:101–129.

26. Rowland TR, DePalma RL. Current neuropharmacologic interventions for the management of brain injury agitation. *Neurorehabilitation* 1995;5: 219–232.

27. Valproate for bipolar disorder. *Med Lett Drug Ther* 1994;36: 74–75.

28. Temkin NR, Dikmen SS, Wilensky AJ, et al. A randomized, double-blind study of phenytoin for the prevention of post-traumatic seizures. *N Engl J Med* 1990; 323:497–502.

29. Goldstein LB. Common drugs may influence motor recovery after stroke. The Sygen in Acute Stroke Study Investigators. *Neurology* 1995;45:865–871.

30. Fromm GH. Gabapentin: discussion. *Epilepsia* 1994;35:S77–S80.

31. Leiderman DB. Gabapentin as add-on therapy for refractory partial epilepsy: results of five placebo-controlled trials. *Epilepsia* 1994;35:S74–S76.

32. Prevey ML, Delaney RC, Cramer JA, et al. Effect of valproate on cognitive functioning. *Arch Neurol* 1996;53:1008–1016.

33. Feeney DM, Gonzalez A, Law WA. Amphetamine, haloperidol and experience interact to affect rate of recovery after motor cortex injury. *Science* 1982; 217:855–857.

34. Killian GA, Holzman PS, Davis JM, et al. Effects of psychotropic medication on selected cognitive and perceptual measures. *J Abnorm Psychol* 1984;93:58–70.

35. Drugs for psychiatric disorders. *Med Lett Drug Ther* 1991;33: 43–50.

36. Drugs for psychiatric disorders. *Med Lett Drug Ther* 1994;36: 89–96.

37. Mysiw WJ, Sandel ME. The agitated brain injured patient. Part 2: pathophysiology and treatment. *Arch Phys Med Rehabil* 1997;78:213–220.

38. Seneff MG, Mathews RA. Use of haloperidol infusions to control delirium in critically ill adults. *Ann Pharmacol* 1995;29:690–693.

39. Yudofsky SC, Silver JM, Hales RE. Pharmacologic management of aggression in the elderly. *J Clin Psychol* 1990;51(10 suppl):22–28.

40. Drugs for psychiatric disorders. *Med Lett Drug Ther* 1980;22: 77–84.

41. Drugs for psychiatric disorders. *Med Lett Drug Ther* 1983;25: 45–52.

42. Drugs for psychiatric disorders. *Med Lett Drug Ther* 1989;31: 13–20.

43. Trazodone (Desyrel): a new nontricyclic antidepressant. *Med Lett Drug Ther* 1982;24:47–48.

44. Nefazodone for depression. *Med Lett Drug Ther* 1995;37:33–35.

45. Paroxetine for treatment of depression. *Med Lett Drug Ther* 1993;35:24–25.

46. Fluoxetine for depression. *Med Lett Drug Ther* 1988;30:45–47.

47. Fluoxetine (Prozac) revisited. *Med Lett Drug Ther* 1990;32: 83–85.

48. Sertraline for treatment of depression. *Med Lett Drug Ther* 1992;34:47–48.

49. Choice of an antidepressant. *Med Lett Drug Ther* 1993;35: 25–26.

50. Finley PR. Selective serotonin reuptake inhibitors: pharmacologic profiles and potential therapeutic distinctions. *Ann Pharmacol* 1994;28:1359–1369.

51. Bupropion for depression. *Med Lett Drug Ther* 1989;31:97–98.

52. Venlafaxine—a new antidepressant. *Med Lett Drug Ther* 1994; 36:49–50.

53. Godfrey RG. A guide to the understanding and use of tricyclic antidepressants in the overall management of fibromyalgia and other chronic pain syndromes. *Arch Intern Med* 1996;156:1047–1052.

54. Smith GR. The epidemiology and treatment of depression when it coexists with somatoform disorders, somatization, or pain. *Gen Hosp Psychiatry* 1992;14:265–272.

55. Watson PN. Antidepressant drugs as adjuvant analgesics. *J Pain Symptom Manage* 1994;9: 392–405.

56. Philipp M, Fickinger M. Psychotropic drugs in the management of chronic pain syndromes. *Pharmacopsychiatry* 1993;26: 221–226.

57. Methylphenidate and other drugs for treatment of hyperactive children. *Med Lett Drug Ther* 1977;19:53–55.

58. Frierson RL, Wey JJ, Tabler JB. Psycho-stimulants for depression in the medically ill. *Am Fam Physician* 1991;43:163–170.

59. Pizzuti D. Reference 03-4735-R18. Abbott Park, IL: Abbott Laboratories, Pharmaceutical Products Division, December 1996. Letter.

60. Dobkin BH, Hanlon R. Dopamine agonist treatment of antegrade amnesia from a mediobasal forebrain injury. *Ann Neurol* 1993;33:313–316.

61. Powell JH, al-Adawi S, Morgan J, Greenwood RJ. Motivational deficits after brain injury: effects of bromocriptine in 11 patients. *J Neurol Neurosurg Psychiatry* 1996;60:416–412.

62. Muller U, von Cramon DY. The therapeutic potential of bromocriptine in neuropsychological rehabilitation of patients with acquired brain damage. *Prog Neuropsychopharmacol Biol Psychiatry* 1994;18:1103–1120.

63. Pulaski KH, Emmett L. The combined intervention of therapy and bromocriptine mesylate to improve functional performance after brain injury. *Am J Occup Ther* 1994;48: 263–270.

64. Zolpidem for insomnia. *Med Lett Drug Ther* 1993;35:35–36.

65. Kupfer DJ, Reynolds CF. Insomnia. *N Engl J Med* 1997;336: 341–346.

66. Choice of benzodiazepines. *Med Lett Drug Ther* 1981;23:41–43.

67. Hypnotic drugs. *Med Lett Drug Ther* 1996;38:59–61.

68. Alprazolam for panic disorder. *Med Lett Drug Ther* 1991;33: 30–31.

69. Reddy S, Patt RB. The benzodiazepines as adjuvant analgesics. *J Pain Symptom Manage* 1994;9:510–514.

70. Bushnell TG, Justins DM. Choosing the right analgesic. A guide to selection. *Drugs* 1993;46: 394–408.

71. Melzack R, Wall P. *The challenge of pain.* rev. ed. New York: Basic Books, 1982.

72. Corwin HL, Bonvente JV. Renal insufficiency associated with nonsteroidal antiinflammatory agents. *Am J Kidney Dis* 1984;4:147–152.

73. Dillin W, Uppal G. Analysis of medications used in the treatment of cervical disk degeneration. *Orthop Clin North Am* 1992;23:421–433.

74. Kellett J. Acute soft tissue injuries—a review of the literature. *Med Sci Sports Exerc* 1986;18:489–500.

75. Ketoprofen. *Med Lett Drug Ther* 1986;28:61–62.

76. Hanks GW, Justins DM. Cancer pain: management. *Lancet* 1992;339:1031–1036.

77. Holsboer F, Grasser A, Friess E, Wiedemann K. Steroid effects on central neurons and implications for psychiatric and neurological disorders. *Ann NY Acad Sci* 1994;746:345–361.

78. Lamberts SWJ, Bruining HA, deJong FH. Corticosteroid therapy in severe illness. *N Engl J Med* 1997;337:1285–1292.

79. Drugs for acute spinal cord injury. *Med Lett Drug Ther* 1993;35:72–73.

80. Jeffries B. Epidural steroid injections. *Spine State Art Rev* 1988;2:419–426.

81. Nelson DA. Dangers from methylprednisolone acetate

therapy by intraspinal injection. *Arch Neurol* 1988;45:804–806.

82. Raymond J, Dumas JM. Intraarticular facet block: diagnostic test or therapeutic procedure? *Radiology* 1984;151:333–336.

83. Lewis KS, Han NH. Tramadol: a new centrally acting analgesic. *Am J Health Syst Pharm* 1997;54:643–652.

84. Raffa RB, Friderichs E, Reimann W, et al. Opioid and nonopioid components independently contribute to the mechanism of action of tramadol, an "atypical" opioid analgesic. *J Pharmacol Exp Ther* 1992;260: 275–285.

85. Churbasik M, Buzina M, Schulte-Monting J, et al. Intravenous tramadol in post-operative pain—comparison of intermittent dose regimens with and without maintenance infusion. *Eur J Anaesthesiol* 1992;9:23–28.

86. Delilkan AE, Vijayan R. Epidural tramadol for postoperative pain relief. *Anaesthesia* 1993;48: 328–331.

87. Stankov G, Schmeider G, Zerle G, et al. Double-blind study with dipyrone versus tramadol and butylscopolamine in acute renal colic pain. *World J Urol* 1994; 12:155–161.

88. Prasertsawat PO, Herabutya Y, Chaturachinda K. Obstetric analgesia: comparison between tramadol, morphine, and pethidine. *Curr Ther Res* 1986;40: 1022–1028.

89. Sunshine A. New clinical experience with tramadol. *Drugs* 1994;47(suppl 1):8–18.

90. Bettig G, Kropp J. Analgetische wirkung von tramadol beim akuten myocardinfarkt. *Therapiewoche* 1980;30:5561–5566.

91. Osipova NA, Novikov GA, Beresnev VA, et al. Analgesic effect of tramadol in cancer patients with chronic pain: a comparison with prolonged-action morphine sulfate. *Curr Ther Res* 1991;50:812–821.

92. Rauck RL, Ruoff GE, McMillen JI. Comparison of tramadol and acetaminophen with codeine for long-term pain management in elderly patients. *Curr Ther Res* 1994;55:1417–1431.

93. Cherny NI. Opioid analgesics. Comparative features and prescribing guidelines. *Drugs* 1996;51:713–737.

94. Jaffe JH, Martin WR. Opioid analgesics and antagonists. In: Gilman AG, Rall TW, Nies AS, et al, eds. *The pharmacological basis of therapeutics.* 8th ed. New York: Pergamon, 1990: 485–521.

95. Pasternak GW. Pharmacological mechanisms of opioid analgesics. *Clin Neuropharmacol* 1993;16:1–18.

96. Ziegler DK. Opiate and opioid use in patients with refractory headache. *Cephalalgia* 1994; 14:5–10.

97. Zenz M, Strumpf M, Tryba M. Long-term oral opioid therapy in patients with chronic nonmalignant pain. *J Pain Symptom Manage* 1992;7:69–77.

98. Portenoy RK, Foley KM, Inturrisi CE. The nature of opioid responsiveness and its implications for neuropathic pain: new hypotheses derived from studies of opioid infusions. *Pain* 1990;43: 273–286.

99. World Health Organization. *Cancer pain relief and palliative care.* Geneva: World Health Organization, 1990.

100. Portenoy RK. Management of common opioid side effects during long-term therapy of cancer pain. *Ann Acad Med Singapore* 1994;23:160–170.

101. McQuay H, Carroll D, Jadad AR, et al. Anticonvulsant drugs for management of pain: a systematic review. *BMJ* 1995;311: 1047–1052.

102. Fusco BM, Giacovazzo M. Peppers and pain. The promise of capsaicin. *Drugs* 1997;53: 909–914.

103. Geppetti P, Tramontana M, Evangelista S, et al. Differential effect on neuropeptide release of different concentrations of hydrogen ions on afferent and intrinsic neurons of the rat stomach. *Gastroenterology* 1991;101:1505–1511.

104. Janeso G, Kiraly E, Janeso-Gabor A, et al. Direct evidence for an axonal site of action of capsaicin. *Naunyn Schmiedebergs Arch Pharmacol* 1980; 313:91–94.

105. Watson CPN, Evans RJ, Watt VR. The post-mastectomy pain syndrome and the effect of topical capsaicin. *Pain* 1989; 38:177–186.

106. Watson CPN, Evans RJ, Watt VR. Post-herpetic neuralgia and topical capsaicin. *Pain* 1988; 33:333–340.

107. Fusco BM, Alessandri M. Effect of topical application of capsaicin in trigeminal neuralgia. *Anesth Analg* 1992;74:375–377.

108. Ross DR, Varipapa RJ. Treatment of painful diabetic neuropathy with topical capsaicin. *N Engl J Med* 1989;321:474–475.

109. Cheshire WP, Snyder CR. Treatment of reflex sympathetic dystrophy with topical capsaicin. Case report. *Pain* 1990;42: 307–311.

110. Lance JW. Symposium synopsis. In: Feldman RG, Young RR, Koella WP, eds. *Spasticity: disordered motor control.* Chicago: Year Book, 1980:485–494.

111. Delawaide PJ, Pennisi G. Tizanidine and electrophysiologic analysis of spinal control mechanisms in humans with spasticity. *Neurology* 1994;44:S21–S27.

112. Ochs GA. Intrathecal baclofen. *Baillieres Clin Neurol* 1993;2:73–86.

113. Stewart-Wynne EG, Silbert PL, Buffery S, et al. Intrathecal baclofen for severe spasticity: five years experience. *Clin Exp Neurol* 1991;28:244–255.

114. Abel NA, Smith RA. Intrathecal baclofen for treatment of

intractable spinal spasticity. *Arch Phys Med Rehabil* 1994; 75:54–58.

115. Coffey JR, Cahill D, Steers W, et al. Intrathecal baclofen for intractable spasticity of spinal origin: results of a long-term multicenter trial. *J Neurosurg* 1993;78:225–232.

116. Saltuari L, Kronenberg M, Marosi MJ, et al. Long-term intrathecal baclofen treatment in supraspinal spasticity. *Acta Neurol (Napoli)* 1992;14:195–207.

117. Albright AL, Barron WB, Fasick MP, et al. Continuous intrathecal baclofen infusion for spasticity of cerebral origin. *JAMA* 1993;270:2475–2477.

118. Erickson DL, Blacklock JB, Michaelson M, et al. Control of spasticity by implantable continuous flow morphine pump. *Neurology* 1985;16:215–217.

119. Katrak PH, Cole AM, Poulos CJ, McCauley JC. Objective assessment of spasticity, strength, and function with early exhibition of dantrolene sodium after cerebrovascular accident: a randomized double-blind study. *Arch Phys Med Rehabil* 1992;73:4–9.

120. Cook JB, Nathan PW. On the site of action of diazepam in spasticity in man. *J Neurol Sci* 1967;5:33–37.

121. Verrier M, Ashby P, MacLeod S. Diazepam effect on reflex activity in patients with complete spinal lesions and in those with other causes of spasticity. *Arch Phys Med Rehabil* 1977;58: 148–153.

122. Yablon SA, Sipski ML. Effect of transdermal clonidine on spinal spasticity. *Am J Phys Med Rehabil* 1993;72:154–157.

123. Sandford PR, Spengler SE, Sawasky KB. Clonidine in the treatment of brainstem spasticity. Case report. *Am J Phys Med Rehabil* 1992;71:301–303.

124. Tizanidine for spasticity. *Med Lett Drug Ther* 1997;39:62–63.

125. Wallace JD. Summary of the combined clinical analysis of controlled clinical trials with tizanidine. *Neurology* 1994; 44(suppl 9):S60–S68.

126. Roberts RC, Part NJ, Pokorny R, et al. Pharmacokinetics and pharmacodynamics of tizanidine. *Neurology* 1994;44(suppl 9):S29–S31.

127. Wood KM. The use of phenol as a neurolytic agent. *Pain* 1978; 5:205–229.

128. Nathan PW. Intrathecal phenol to relieve spasticity in paraplegia. *Lancet* 1959;2:1099–1102.

129. Herz DA, Looman JE, Tiberio A, et al. The management of paralytic spasticity. *Neurosurgery* 1990;26:300–305.

130. Pelissier J, Viel E, Enjalbert M, et al. Chemical neurolysis using alcohol (alcoholization) in the treatment of spasticity in the hemiplegic. *Cah Anesthesiol* 1993;41:139–143.

131. Camilleri M, Thompson WG, Fleshman JW, Pemberton JH. Clinical management of intractable constipation. *Ann Intern Med* 1994;121:520–528.

132. Ewald GA, McKenzie CR. Constipation. In: *Manual of Therapeutics.* 28th ed. Boston: Little, Brown, 1995:338–339.

133. Romero Y, Evans JM, Fleming KC, Phillips SF. Constipation and fecal incontinence in the elderly population. *Mayo Clin Proc* 1996;71:81–92.

134. Stiens SA, Bergman SB, Goetz LL. Neurogenic bowel dysfunction after spinal cord injury: clinical evaluation and rehabilitative management. *Arch Phys Med Rehabil* 1997;78:S86–S102.

135. Safety of stool softeners. *Med Lett Drug Ther* 1977;19:45–46.

136. Gardner VY, Beckwith JV, Heyneman CA. Cisapride for the treatment of chronic idiopathic constipation. *Ann Pharmacol* 1995;29:1161–1163.

137. Cisapride for nocturnal heartburn. *Med Lett Drug Ther* 1994;36:11–13.

138. CLASP (Collaborative Low-Dose Aspirin Study in Pregnancy) Collaborative Group. CLASP: a randomized trial for the prevention and treatment of pre-eclampsia among 9364 pregnant women. *Lancet* 1994;343:619–629.

139. Preston FE, Whipps S, Jackson CA, et al. Inhibition of prostacyclin and platelet thromboxane A_2 after low-dose aspirin. *N Engl J Med* 1981;304:76–79.

140. Lorenz RL, Boehlig B, Uedelhoven WM, et al. Superior antiplatelet action of alternative day pulsed dosing. *Am J Cardiol* 1989;64:1185–1188.

141. Antiplatelet Trialists' Collaboration. Collaborative overview of randomized trials of antiplatelet therapy: I. Prevention of death, myocardial infarction, and stroke by prolonged antiplatelet therapy in various categories of patients. *BMJ* 1994;308:81–106.

142. Juul-Miller S, Edvardsson N, Jahnmatz B, et al. Double-blind trial of aspirin in primary prevention of myocardial infarction in patients with stable chronic angina pectoris. *Lancet* 1992; 340:1421–1425.

143. Lindblad B, Persson NH, Iakolander R, et al. Does low-dose acetylsalicylic acid prevent stroke after carotid surgery? A double-blind, placebo-controlled randomized trial. *Stroke* 1993; 24:1125 1128.

144. The Dutch TIA Trial Study Group. A comparison of two doses of aspirin (30 mg vs. 283 mg a day) in patients after a transient ischemic attack or minor ischemic stroke. *N Engl J Med* 1991;325:1261–1266.

145. Hirsh J, Dalen JE, Fuster V, et al. Aspirin and other platelet-active drugs. The relationship between dose, effectiveness, and side effects. *Chest* 1995;108(suppl 4):247S–257S.

146. Trupie AGG, Gent M, Laupacis A, et al. A comparison of aspirin with placebo in patients treated with warfarin after heart-valve replacement. *N Engl J Med* 1993;329:524–529.

147. Albers GW. Atrial fibrillation and stroke: three new studies, three remaining questions. *Arch Intern Med* 1994;154:1443–1448.

148. Schafer AI. Antiplatelet therapy. *Am J Med* 1996;101:199–209.

149. FitzGerald GA. Dipyridamole. *N Engl J Med* 1987;316:1247–1257.

150. Diener HC, Cunha L, Forbes C, et al. European Stroke Prevention Study. 2. Dipyridamole and acetylsalicylic acid in the secondary prevention of stroke. *J Neurol Sci* 1996;143(1–2):1–13.

151. Hess H, Mietaschk A, Deichsel G. Drug-induced inhibition of platelet function delays progression of peripheral occlusive arterial disease: a prospective double-blind angiographically controlled trial. *Lancet* 1985; 1:415–419.

152. Strauer BE, Heidland UE, Heintzen MP, Schwartzkoff B. Pharmacologic myocardial protection during percutaneous transluminal coronary angioplasty by intracoronary application of dipyridamole: impact on hemodynamic function and left ventricular performance. *J Am Coll Cardiol* 1996;28(5):1119–1126.

153. Stein PD, Alpert JS, Dalen JE, et al. Antithrombotic therapy in patients with mechanical and biological prosthetic heart valves. *Chest* 1998;114(5): 602S–610S.

154. Klimt CR, Knatterud GL, Stamler J, Meier P. Persantine-aspirin reinfarction study. II: secondary coronary prevention with persantine and aspirin. *J Am Coll Cardiol* 1986;7:251–269.

154a. Mulder BJ, van der Doef RM, van der Wall EE, et al. Effect of various antithrombotic regimens (aspirin, aspirin plus dipyridamole, anticoagulants) on the functional status of patients and grafts one year after coronary artery bypass grafting. *Eur Heart J* 1994;15:1129–1134.

155. DiMinno G, Cerbone AM, Mattoili PL, et al. Functionally thrombosthenic state in normal platelets following the administration of ticlopidine. *J Clin Invest* 1985;75:328–338.

156. Saltiel E, Ward A. Ticlopidine. A review of its pharmacodynamic and pharmacokinetic properties and therapeutic properties and therapeutic efficacy in platelet dependent disease states. *Drugs* 1987;34:222–226.

157. McTavish D, Faulds D, Goa KL. Ticlopidine: an updated review of its pharmacology and therapeutic use in platelet-dependent disorders. *Drugs* 1990;40:238–259.

158. Hass WK, Easton JD, Adams HP, et al. A randomized trial comparing ticlopidine hydrochloride with aspirin for the prevention of stroke in high-risk patients. *N Engl J Med* 1989;321:501–507.

159. Gent M, Blakeley JA, Easton JD, et al. The Canadian-American Ticlopidine Study (CATS) in thromboembolic stroke. *Lancet* 1989;2:1215–1220.

160. Balsano F, Rizzon P, Violi F, et al. Antiplatelet treatment in ticlopidine in unstable angina: a controlled multicenter clinical trial. *Circulation* 1990;82:17–26.

161. Janzon L, Bergqvist D, Boberg A, et al. Ticlopidine in the treatment of intermittent claudications: a 21-month double-blind trial. *J Lab Clin Med* 1989;114: 84–91.

162. Limet R, David JL, Magotteaux P, et al. Prevention of aorta-coronary bypass graft occlusion: beneficial effect of ticlopidine on early and late patency rate of venous coronary bypass grafts: a double-blind study. *J Thorac Cardiovasc Surg* 1987;94:773–783.

163. Herbert JM, Frechel D, Vallee E, et al. Clopidogrel, a novel antiplatelet and antithrombotic agent. *Cardiovasc Drug Rev* 1993;11:180–198.

164. Boneu B, Destelle G. Platelet anti-aggregating activity and tolerance of clopidogrel in atherosclerotic patients. *Thromb Haemost* 1996;76:939–943.

165. CAPRIE Steering Committee. A randomised, blinded trial of clopidogrel versus aspirin in patients at risk of ischemic events (CAPRIE). *Lancet* 1996;348:1329–1339.

166. Bjork I, Lindahl U. Mechanism of the anticoagulant action of heparin. *Mol Cell Biochem* 1982;48:161–182.

167. Clagett GP, Anderson FA, Heit J, et al. Prevention of venous thromboembolism. *Chest* 1995; 108(suppl 4):312S–334S.

168. Caims JA, Lewis D, Meade TW, et al. Antithrombotic agents in coronary artery disease. *Chest* 1995;108(suppl 4):380S–400S.

169. Popma JJ, Weitz J, Bittl JA, et al. Antithrombotic therapy in patients undergoing coronary angioplasty. *Chest* 1998;114(5): 728S–741S.

170. Jackson MR, Clagett GP. Antithrombotic therapy in peripheral arterial occlusive disease. *Chest* 1995;114(5): 666S–682S.

171. Taberner DA, Poller L, Thomson JM, et al. Randomized study of adjusted versus fixed low dose heparin prophylaxis of deep vein thrombosis in hip surgery. *Br J Surg* 1989;76:933–935.

172. Green D, Lee MY, Ito VY, et al. Fixed- vs. adjusted-dose heparin in the prophylaxis of thromboembolism in spinal cord injury. *JAMA* 1988;260:1255–1258.

173. Hirsh J, Warkentin TE, Raschke R, et al. Heparin and low-molecular weight heparin: mechanisms of action, pharmacokinetics, dosing considerations, monitor-ing, efficacy, and safety. *Chest* 1998;114(5):489S–510S.

174. Eriksson BI, Kalebo P, Anthimyr BA, et al. Prevention of deep vein thrombosis and pulmonary embolism after total hip replacement. *J Bone Joint Surg [Am]* 1991;73:484–493.

175. Leyvraz PF, Bachmann F, Bohnet J, et al. Thromboem-

bolic prophylaxis in total hip replacement: a comparison between the low molecular weight heparinoid lomoparin and heparin-dihydroergotamine. *Br J Surg* 1992;79:911–914.

176. RD Heparin Arthroplasty Group. RD heparin compared with warfarin for prevention of venous thromboembolic disease following total hip or knee arthroplasty. *J Bone Joint Surg [Am]* 1994;76:1174–1185.

177. Borris LC, Hauch O, Jorgensen LN, et al. Low-molecular weight heparin (enoxaparin) vs. dextran 70: the prevention of postoperative deep vein thrombosis after total hip replacement. *Arch Intern Med* 1991;151:1621–1624.

178. Turpie AGG, Levine MN, Hirsh J, et al. A double-blind randomized trial of ORG 10172 low molecular weight heparinoid in the prevention of deep vein thrombosis in thrombotic stroke. *Lancet* 1987;1:523–526.

179. Green D, Lee MY, Lim AC, et al. Prevention of thromboembolism after spinal cord injury using low molecular weight heparin. *Ann Intern Med* 1990;113:571–574.

180. Dahan R, Houlbert D, Caulin C, et al. Prevention of deep vein thrombosis in elderly medical patients by a low molecular weight heparin: a randomized double-blind trial. *Haemostasis* 1986;16:150–164.

181. Publications Committee for the Trial of ORG 10172 in Acute Stroke Treatment (TOAST) Investigators. Low molecular weight heparinoid, ORG 10172 (danaparoid), and outcome after acute ischemic stroke. A randomized controlled trial. *JAMA* 1998;279:1265–1272.

182. Hirsh J, Dalen JE, Deykin D, et al. Oral anticoagulants. Mechanism of action, clinical effectiveness, and optimal therapeutic range. *Chest* 1995;108(suppl 4):231S–246S.

183. Altman R, Rouvier J, Gurfinkel E, et al. Comparison of two levels of anticoagulant therapy in patients with substitute heart valves. *J Thorac Cardiovasc Surg* 1991;101:427–431.

184. The Stroke Prevention in Atrial Fibrillation Investigators. The Stroke Prevention in Atrial Fibrillation study: final results. *Circulation* 1991;84:527–539.

185. Stroke Prevention in Atrial Fibrillation Investigators. Warfarin versus aspirin for prevention of thromboembolism in atrial fibrillation: Stroke Prevention in Atrial Fibrillation II study. *Lancet* 1994;343:687–691.

186. Levine HJ, Pauker SG, Eckman MH. Antithrombotic therapy in valvular heart disease. *Chest* 1995;108(suppl 4):360S–370S.

187. Hull R, Delmore T, Carter C, et al. Adjusted subcutaneous heparin versus warfarin sodium in the long-term treatment of venous thrombosis. *N Engl J Med* 1982;306:189–194.

188. Bussey HI, Force RW, Bianco TM, et al. Reliance on prothrombin time ratios causes significant errors in anticoagulation therapy. *Arch Intern Med* 1992;152:278–282.

189. Samarna M, Horellon HM, Soria J, et al. Successful progressive anticoagulation in a severe protein C deficiency and previous skin necrosis at the initiation of oral anticoagulation treatment. *Thromb Haemost* 1984;51:332–333.

190. Grimando V, Gueissaz F, Hanert J, et al. Necrosis of skin induced by coumarin in a patient deficient in protein S. *BMJ* 1989;298:233–234.

191. Sawyer JA, Myers MA, Rosier RN, Puzas E. Heterotopic ossification: clinical and cellular aspects. *Calcif Tissue Int* 1991;49:208–215.

192. Rossier AB, Bussat P, Infante F, et al. Current facts on paraosteo-arthropathy (POA). *Paraplegia* 1973;11:36–78.

193. Freed JH, Hahn H, Menter R, Dillon T. The use of the three-phase bone scan in the early diagnosis of heterotopic ossification (HO) and in the evaluation of didronel therapy. *Paraplegia* 1982;20:208–216.

194. McClelland SJ, Rudolf LM. Myositis ossificans following porous-ingrowth total knee replacement. *Orthop Res* 1986;15:223–227.

195. Kjaersgaard-Andersen P, Frich LH, Sojbjerg JO, Sneppen O. Heterotopic bone formation following total shoulder arthroplasty. *J Arthroplasty* 1989;4:99–104.

196. Peters WJ, Pritzker KP. Massive heterotopic ossification in breast implant capsules. *Aesth Plastic Surg* 1985;9:43–45.

197. Myers MA, Minton JP. Heterotopic ossification within the small bowel mesentery. *Arch Surg* 1989;124:982–983.

198. Schmidt SA, Kjaesgaard-Andersen P, Pederson NW, et al. The use of indomethacin to prevent the formation of heterotopic bone after total hip replacement. *J Bone Joint Surg [Am]* 1988;77:834–838.

199. Elmstedt E, Lindholm TS, Nilsson OS, Tornkvist H. Effect of ibuprofen on heterotopic ossification after hip replacement. *Act Orthop Scand* 1985;56:25–27.

200. Sell S, Willms R, Kusswetter W. Heterotopic ossificans—a prospective comparison of two prophylactic methods. *J Bone Joint Surg [Br]* 1997;79:170. Abstract.

201. Matta JM, Siebenrock KA. Does indomethacin reduce heterotopic bone formation after operations for acetabular fractures? A prospective randomised study. *J Bone Joint Surg [Br]* 1997;79:959–963.

202. Fliesch HA, Russell RGG, Bisaz S, et al. The inhibitory effect of phosphonates on the formation of calcium phosphate crystals in vitro and on aortic and kidney calcification in vivo. *Eur J Clin Invest* 1970;1:12–18.

Chapter 23

The Physical Agents

Jeffrey R. Basford

This chapter reviews the strengths, weaknesses, and rationale of the physical agents. The discussion begins with the superficial and cooling agents, progresses to hydrotherapy, and then addresses the diathermies and electrical therapies. Less established modalities such as pulsed electromagnetic fields and microelectrical stimulation are considered more briefly. The laboratory effects of these agents are well established, but their use in the clinic is often more subjective than one would wish.

SUPERFICIAL HEAT AND COLD

Heat and cold have profound effects on the body. Temperature elevations of only a few degrees can alter blood flow, increase collagen extensibility, lessen joint viscosity, alter nerve conduction, and increase enzymatic activity (1). Decreases of the same amount produce the opposite effects: lessened extensibility, increased viscosity, slowed nerve conduction, and reduced metabolic activity. Temperatures above 45°C or below 15°C are uncomfortable over even limited areas and those only a few degrees higher or near 0°C may cause injury.

Each of the most common heating and cooling agents has unique attributes. Nevertheless, to add or remove heat from the body, all use one of three mechanisms: conduction (e.g., hot packs), convection (e.g., hydrotherapy), or conversion (e.g., radiant heat, ultrasound). As a result, these agents share many indications and safety concerns (Tables 23-1–23-4).

Hot Packs

Hot packs (often simply called Hydrocollator packs) consist of segmented canvas sacks filled with a hydroscopic substance (e.g., silica dioxide) which, when soaked in water, absorbs several times its weight in water. The packs are immersed in water baths at 70–80°C (Fig. 23-1) and when needed are taken from the baths. Once excess water is drained off, the packs are placed in an insulating cover or wrapped in several layers of toweling and placed on (not under) the patient. Packs can maintain therapeutic temperatures for 30 minutes and have the advantages of reliability, low cost, good patient acceptance, and the possibility of home use. Disadvantages include their weight, the need for specific patient positioning, and the requirement for a large supply of towels.

Kenny packs are wool cloths soaked in 60°C water and spun in a drum to extract most of the water before use. These packs cool rapidly and are applied and removed at intervals of a few minutes, to provide a cyclic heating effect. Use is now rare, probably because of the close supervision they require and a failure to generalize their use much beyond the pain and muscle spasms associated with poliomyelitis.

Heat Lamps

Heat lamps provide a superficial heating alternative to hot packs. Specifically designed infrared (IR) lamps with tungsten or quartz heating elements are often used in the clinic, but incandescent bulbs (which radiate most of their energy

Table 23-1: Indications for Therapeutic Heat
Chronic or subacute injury
Pain
Muscle spasm
Hematoma resolution
Diffuse musculoskeletal pain
Tension myalgia
Fibromyalgia
Fibrositis
Contractures
Degenerative arthritis
Tenosynovitis
"Bursitis"
Collagen vascular disease*
Production of hyperemia
Acceleration of metabolic processes
Superficial thrombophlebitis
Induction of reflex vasodilatation

*Role of heat in the inflammatory arthropathies is unclear.

Table 23-2: Contraindications for Therapeutic Heat
Acute inflammation, trauma, or hemorrhage
Bleeding dyscrasias
Insensitivity/inability to respond
Impaired thermal regulation[a]
Malignancy[b]
Ischemia
Edema
Atrophic skin or scars

[a] Systemic heating.
[b] Localized hyperthermia may be used, at times as an adjunct to radiation and chemotherapy.

Table 23-3: Indications for Therapeutic Cold
Acute trauma
Edema
Hemorrhage
Analgesia
Subacute musculoskeletal pain
Muscle spasm
Bursitis
Muscle attachment pain
Reduction of metabolic activity
Adjunct to muscle re-education

Table 23-4: Contraindications to Therapeutic Cold
Cold intolerance
Severe cold pressor response
Raynaud phenomenon or disease
Cold allergy
Insensitivity/inability to respond
Ischemia

Table 23-5: Reported Applications for Transcutaneous Electrical Nerve Stimulation
Acute pain
Posttraumatic
Postsurgical
First stage of childbirth
Chronic and subacute pain
Low-back and neck pain
Osteoarthritis
Rheumatoid arthritis
Neurogenic pain
Brachioplexitis
Diabetic neuropathy
Postherpetic neuralgia
Peripheral nerve injury
Phantom limb pain
Sympathetically medicated pain
Ischemic pain
Raynaud disease
Dental procedures

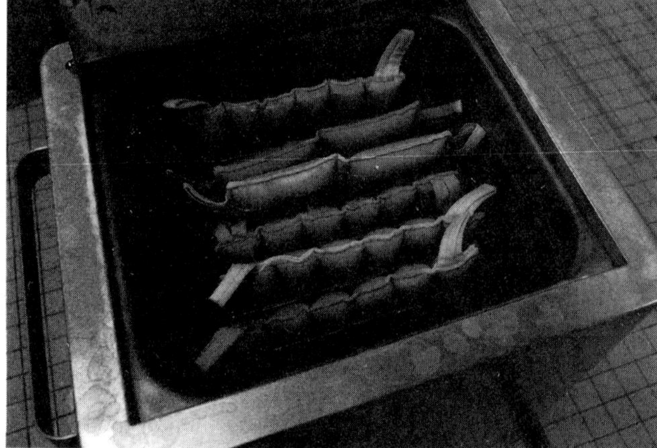

Figure 23-1. Hot packs are kept in racks in 70 to 80°C water baths until needed for treatment. As is true for most of these baths, the bath in this figure is constructed of stainless steel, has a hinged lid, and contains more than one type of pack. Hot packs have a life of several years and baths have been in continuous use for as many as 30 years.

as heat) are inexpensive, work as well, and may be used at home.

Heating rates and maximum temperatures are controlled by adjusting the distance between the lamp and the patient. Specifics vary with the lamp. The classically described "$1/r^2$" relationship (r = distance between the skin and the source) is appropriate for point sources such as incandescent light bulbs. However, an "1/r" relationship may be more appropriate for elongated heating elements such as some quartz and tungsten filaments. In practice, the patient-source distance is often about 50 cm and is ultimately determined by the heating intensity desired and patient tolerance. The advantages of heat lamps include ease of use and a lesser need for supplies (e.g., towels, covers) compared to hot packs. Hot packs and heat lamps both provide superficial heating. As "moist" heat has little or no physiologic advantage over "dry" heat, the choice is ultimately dictated by patient and therapist preference.

Safety

The general safety issues of Table 23-2 apply to hot packs and heat lamps. Patients should be instructed to lie *under* and not on hot packs (as well as most heating pads). Burns can occur with both agents and chronic use of superficial heat may cause a mottled skin pigment alteration known as *erythema ab igne*.

Paraffin Baths

Paraffin baths consist of reservoirs filled with a 1 : 7 mixture of mineral oil and paraffin. The baths are maintained at temperatures between 52 and 54°C, which keep the mixture liquefied but are unlikely to produce burns in normal usage.

Treatments usually involve one of two approaches: dipping or immersion. Dipping is the most common and involves putting the distal part of an extremity (usually a hand) into the bath, removing it, pausing briefly to allow the paraffin to solidify, and then repeating the process. Typically, 10 dips are performed, and the extremity is wrapped in a layer of plastic and then placed within an insulating mitt. At the end of about 20 minutes the paraffin is stripped off and returned to the reservoir. The second approach, immersion, involves dipping the extremity in the bath, removing it long enough to permit the paraffin to solidify, and then immersing the dipped portion in the bath for an additional 20 to 30 minutes.

Each approach produces maximal skin temperatures of about 47°C. With the dipping method, however, skin temperatures fall within a few degrees of baseline at the end of 30 minutes and increases in subcutaneous and intramuscluar temperatures are restricted to about 3 and 1°C, respectively. Immersion results in more vigorous heating: Skin temperatures are maintained at about 41.5°C and subcutaneous and intramuscular temperatures are about 2°C higher than with dipping (2).

Indications

Paraffin baths are often used to treat hand contractures due to rheumatoid arthritis, scleroderma, or burns. Most treatments involve the dipping and immersion methods just outlined. Occasionally the feet will be treated or the paraffin will be layered on a sensitive or awkward area with a brush in an approach that otherwise mimics the dipping method. Home units are available and baths can be done at home by the patients. Treatments are messy and, for many, hot water soaks are as effective and far easier.

Precautions

The precautions common to all heating agents apply to paraffin (see Table 23-2). In addition, paraffin baths are, in essence, hot oil. As such, fire is a risk. Burns are possible and temperatures should be monitored with a thermometer. (As a rule of thumb, if there isn't a rim of congealed wax at the edges of a bath, the temperature may be too high.)

Cryotherapy

Chilling the skin with an agent such as ice produces a series of sensations, beginning with a feeling of "coldness" and then progressing through the stages of burning, aching, and numbness. Skin temperature initially drops rapidly, then slows its decline, and at 10 minutes reaches equilibrium 12 to 16°C below its beginning value. Subcutaneous temperatures decline more slowly but will fall by 3 to 5°C over the same period. Intramuscular temperatures fall more slowly yet, and while perhaps dropping a degree or less at 10 minutes, may ultimately fall by 6 to 16°C with prolonged cooling (3–5). Studies by Hollander and Horvath (6–8) in the late 1940s showed that superficial cold and heat had paradoxical effects: the former increasing intra-articular temperatures and the latter decreasing them. More recent work supported more intuitive results: Intra-articular knee temperatures decrease 6°C over a 3-hour period of cooling with ice chips (9). Cooling is limited to superficial agents and characteristics such as obesity moderate its effects.

An initial period of vasoconstriction accompanies cooling, and may or may not be followed by the cyclic cutaneous digital vasodilation described when tissue temperature falls below about 15°C (10–12). Vasoconstriction occurs within 5 minutes of packing a knee in ice and can produce 30% decreases in soft tissue as well as 20% decreases in skeletal blood flow after 25 minutes of cooling (11). Cold raises pain thresholds (13), decreases enzymatic activity (1), increases tissue viscosity, slows nerve conduction (5), and lessens muscle tone and spasticity (4,14). Consensual vasoconstriction and increased gastrointestinal mobility may occur following cooling of a different extremity or the abdominal wall (15).

A variety of vaporizing sprays, chemical ice packs, and refrigerated cuffs (Fig. 23-2) can produce therapeutic

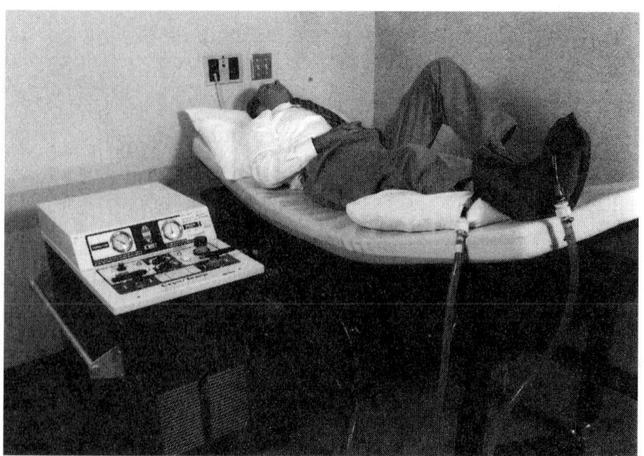

Figure 23-2. Ice, due to its high heat capacity, low cost, and easy availability, is the mainstay of cryotherapy. Nevertheless, alternatives such a vapocoolant sprays and refrigerated units are common in therapy departments. This picture demonstrates a compressive boot filled with circulating chilled water, which might be used in the treatment of an acute ankle sprain.

cooling. Nevertheless, ice and cold water remain the mainstays of treatment due to their convenience, high cooling capacity (i.e., specific heat), and low cost.

Application

Ice packs are typically wrapped in dry or moist toweling (to slow cooling and increase comfort) and applied for 20 to 25 minutes. Ice massage, on the other hand, produces intense, vigorous cooling over smaller areas (e.g., greater trochanter, lateral epicondyle). In this latter case, application often involves peeling back the sides of a cup that was filled with water and frozen, and then rubbing the exposed ice over the treatment site with smooth strokes until numbness occurs (about 7–10 minutes). Iced whirlpools and slushes also provide vigorous cooling and can create quite intense analgesia. Covering exposed untreated areas of the hands or feet with insulating mitts or booties may improve patient tolerance. The average person finds temperatures below 15°C uncomfortable and the more vigorous ice treatments are reserved for the most motivated patients.

Vapocoolant sprays (less flammable and less environmentally dubious alternatives have replaced earlier agents) and vaporized liquid nitrogen produce abrupt temperature changes of as much as 20°C (9). These sprays can produce local analgesia and are used for the "spray and stretch" techniques popularized by Travell (16). Other cooling agents including commercial gels, circulator cuffs, and packs are available (see Fig. 23-2). Frozen orange juice containers and packages of frozen peas, which after being struck on a flat surface easily conform to the body, are handy for home use.

Indications

Ice is almost universal in the treatment of acute musculoskeletal trauma. While there has been concern that cooling produces a reactive edema and might exacerbate an injury, recent research showed that reactive vasodilation does not occur during treatment (12) and that blood flow and metabolism are reduced by cooling (11). In addition, cooling may slow surgical graft deterioration and improve neovascularization (17). It is interesting, however, that clinical studies of the postsurgical knee (18,19) and cesarean section (20) did not find cryotherapy beneficial.

The relative benefits of heat and cold in the treatment of rheumatoid joints are arguable. Research findings support the idea that superficial cooling lowers joint temperatures, increases joint stiffness, and lowers intraarticular enzymatic activity within the joints of rheumatoid arthritics (9,21). On the other hand, warming improves comfort, lessens viscosity, and increases enzymatic activity. The implications remain poorly understood, but gentle warming remains a mainstay in the treatment of the subacute rheumatoid joint.

Safety

Cold (see Table 23-4) shares many of the precautions of heat. In addition, specific cold effects such as frostnip and frostbite must be avoided. Pressor responses, consensual vasoconstriction, Raynaud phenomenon, cold allergy, and cold urticaria are also concerns.

HYDROTHERAPY

Hydrotherapy uses water to heat or cool the body. Whirlpool baths and Hubbard tanks use pumps to agitate the water, while sitz baths and contrast baths achieve their effects without turbulence. This section discusses these forms of hydrotherapy as well as the less common alternatives of water exercise and balneotherapy.

Whirlpool Baths and Hubbard Tanks

Whirlpool baths and Hubbard tanks use agitated water to provide convective heating or cooling, massage, and gentle debridement. Tanks vary in size from several-thousand-liter Hubbard tanks to small whirlpools designed to treat a single extremity (Figs. 23-3 and 23-4). Handheld shower heads and small water jets are also used for vigorous, localized irrigation and debridement.

Whirlpools and Hubbard tanks are well suited for wound and burn treatments in which the warm, gently agitated water permits comfortable solvent action and debridement. Temperatures between 33 and 38°C are usually chosen (with higher temperatures chosen as more of the body is immersed) and once the patient is in the bath, agitation is gently increased to assist with debridement and removal of adherent dressings. "Sterile" procedures should be followed with specific cleaning protocols

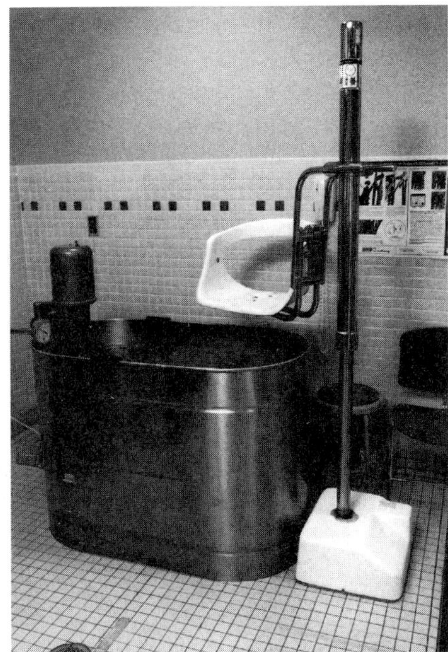

Figure 23-3. Whirlpools are available in many shapes and sizes. The size of this bath is typical. Its stainless-steel construction ensures durability and easy cleaning. The hydraulic lift facilitates transfers into and out of the bath.

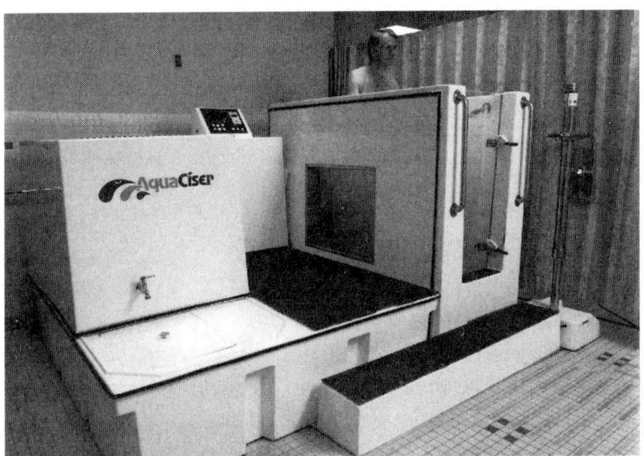

Figure 23-4. Hydrotherapy units can be complex and cost tens of thousands of dollars. This unit has a door that permits easy entry, contains a treadmill, and maintains its own supply of heated water. The transparent side window and front door allow the therapist to observe the patient's performance.

before and after each wound or burn treatment. Large wounds, exposed organs, or discomfort dictate that sodium chloride (NaCl) should be added to the water to approximate normal saline solution (10 kg might be needed for a Hubbard tank!) and lessen the chances of hemolysis, water intoxication, and pain. Gentle detergents, povidone-iodine, and a variety of dermatologic agents may also be added to the water as desired.

Whirlpools and Hubbard tanks are also used to help mobilize joints following cast removal, and as an adjunct in the treatment of the contractures and discomfort of rheumatoid arthritis; tension and fibromyalgia; and muscle spasm. Temperatures may range from 36 to 38°C when large portions of the body are submerged, to as much as 43 or 45°C for limited areas. Temperatures above 39°C should be avoided in Hubbard tanks to avoid systemic hyperthermia. As agitated water heats convectively, remember that heating intensity is higher than would be expected from the water temperature alone. Debilitated patients with wounds are often frightened of hydrotherapy. They should be reassured that treatment is usually surprisingly pleasant and warned if plinths and hoists will be used.

Contrast Baths

Contrast baths alternate heat and cold in the hopes of increasing reflex hyperemia and producing neurologic desensitization (21). These baths are most often used for patients with rheumatoid arthritis and sympathetically mediated pain (reflex sympathetic dystrophy). Rheumatoid arthritics frequently benefit from these treatments but may find simple warm soaks easier and as effective.

Two baths are used. One typically at 43°C and the other at 16°C. Treatment begins with soaking the hands or feet in the warm bath for 10 minutes and then alternating four sets of 1- to 4-minute cold soaks with 6- to 10-minute warm soaks. Patients with sympathetically mediated pain may find beginning with less extreme temperatures more tolerable. In any event, contrast baths serve as an adjunct to an overall treatment plan.

Sitz Baths

Sitz baths are widely used to lessen pain and speed anorectal healing. This practice has support. One study involving normal subjects, as well as those with anorectal fistulas and hemorrhoids, found that sitting in water between 40 and 50°C lowered anal pressures and lessened sphincter activity (22). Effects became more pronounced as temperatures increased but were not found in a study of normal subjects evaluated at 40°C (23).

Water-Based Exercise

Water-based exercises are popular for rheumatoid arthritis and musculoskeletal pain, but benefits may be equivocal. For example, patients with osteoarthritis of the hip who exercised twice a week in water in addition to a home exercise program showed no more improvement than did those who followed the home program alone (24). Another study that compared land- and water-based anterior cruciate ligament reconstruction rehabilitation programs (25) found mixed results: The land-based group gained strength more rapidly; the water-based group felt better and had less effusion.

Edema

The classical Greeks, as well as physicians in the eighteenth century, used water immersion to treat edema (26). Recent findings support this tradition and show that immersion increases renal salt and water loss in normal subjects as well as those with cirrhosis and the nephrotic syndrome (26). Neutral temperatures (33–36°C) would seem the most appropriate.

Spa Therapy (Balneotherapy)

Water has a role in myth and religion for healing, and springs with unusual attributes of warmth, gas content, or mineral concentration have been visited for centuries (26,27). Faith in "water cures" has faded with time and improvements in medicine. Today, "spa therapy" is a curiosity in North America (despite the former prominence of Warm Springs, GA, Hot Springs, AR, Saratoga, NY, and Banff, Canada). In Europe, however, acceptance remains stronger and insurance programs may still fund spa visits.

Physiologic Effects

If the solute content of water is ignored, the physiologic effects of spa therapy should be the same as those of otherwise identical hydrotherapy. Skin does not permit significant penetration of mineral or gas solutes and unique effects seem less likely when the skin is intact. Effects seem more credible if the skin barrier is damaged; for example, serum bromine and rubidium concentrations are elevated in psoriatics after bathing in the mineral-rich waters of the Dead Sea (28). Despite this, the presence of these elements, as well as atmospheric gases (nitrogen, carbon dioxide, and methane), hydrogen sulfide (27), calcium, magnesium, and trace elements such as cobalt and zinc (29) in the waters of spas remains of unclear significance.

Applications

Rheumatoid Arthritis

Rheumatoid arthritis is a common balneotherapy application that has been evaluated. One blinded study, for example, examined the effectiveness of mineral-rich hot packs in comparison with identical packs whose mineral contents had been reduced a hundredfold by repeated rinsing. Grip strength, morning stiffness, and perception of disease severity improved significantly in the group treated with the "active" packs compared to the control group (30). Another study, marred by incomplete blinding, found that programs involving daily Dead Sea or sulfur baths was more effective than similar treatment without these baths (31).

Musculoskeletal Pain

Low-back and mechanical joint pain have also been evaluated. One controlled study, for example, investigated the relative benefits of balneotherapy, water jet massage, and underwater traction on low-back pain. Analgesic consumption and pain scores at the end of treatment, and on follow-up, were lower in the treated subjects than in the control subjects (32). As all treatment groups improved similarly, the question of what is ascribable to water properties is unanswered. Studies of chronic low-back pain found significantly less pain in balneotherapy groups than in unblinded controls subjects (33,34).

Safety

Hydrotherapy requires the same precautions as any heat or cold modality (see Tables 23-2 and 23-4). In addition, immersion and the potential of systemic temperature changes raise the risks of drowning and hyperthermia or hypothermia.

Cardiovascular Risk

While caution seems reasonable, heart disease and cardiovascular stress may be overrated fears. Thus, Finnish patients who have had heart attacks resume sauna bathing within a year without an increased risk of recurrence (35,36). Similarly a study of men with stable heart disease found that 15 minutes in a 40°C hot tub resulted in no electrocardiographic ischemic changes and lower systolic and diastolic blood pressures than the clinically accepted levels seen during stationary bicycle exercise (37). The risk in spinal cord injury patients is also of concern. A study of six quadriplegic and four paraplegic individuals found that 15 minutes of bathing in a sauna at 85°C increased heart rates and elevated oral temperatures almost 2.5°C (38). This study found no significant changes in supine systolic blood pressure, but orthostatism seems a concern.

Infection

Tap water is amazingly sterile and its diluting effect probably contributes to the infrequency of hydrotherapy-associated infection. Nevertheless, bacteria such as *Pseudomonas aeruginosa* frequently colonize hydrotherapy facilities. These facilities should be built to prevent water supply contamination (e.g., antisiphon faucets), and the staff should follow careful cleaning protocols between hydrotherapy sessions, each evening as well as before and after treatment of patients with wounds or skin infections.

Reproduction

Systemic temperature elevations may contribute to infertility and fetal central nervous system deficits. For example, one study found that the relative risk of a neural tube deficit in the children of 23,000 women using hot tubs and saunas during early pregnancy increased by 2.6 to 2.9 over that of women not exposed (39). Data are limited but sperm counts may decrease following isolated or repeated sauna exposures (40). Care seems reasonable, but risks remain unclear.

DIATHERMY

Ultrasound

Ultrasound (US) is simply sound at frequencies above the 17,000- to 20,000-Hz limit of human hearing. While sound has physiologic effects over a wide range of frequencies, the majority of therapeutic US occurs between 0.8 and 3 MHz: Sound at lower frequencies is difficult to focus; sound at higher frequencies attenuates too rapidly to permit reasonable depths of penetration. US machines are designed to deliver US in one of two modes. The first, continuous-wave (CW) US uses a continuous waveform to heat tissue. Comfort and thermal effects usually restrict CW treatment intensities to less than 2.0 to 2.5 W/cm^2. Pulsed US, on the other hand, permits higher instantaneous intensities and is designed to circumvent the heating limitations of CW US by alternating brief bursts of US at intensities perhaps three to four times higher than those in the CW setting with periods of no signal. The goal of pulsed US is the production of nonthermal effects such as cavitation (oscillation or collapse of US-generated bubbles) and streaming (US-induced movement), which become prominent at intensities higher than those possible with CW US. While most of the established effects of US have a thermal basis, many believe nonthermal phenomena have therapeutic benefits also.

Treatment

US treatment requires selection of a number of parameters: waveform (CW or pulsed), intensity, and duration (typically 7–10 minutes). In most cases, the applicator (Fig. 23-5) is moved in smooth overlapping sweeps or circles at rates of a few centimeters per second over areas of about 100 cm^2. Less often, irregular surfaces (such as the ankle) may be immersed in water and the applicator moved over them at a short distance. In either case the skin should be cleansed before treatment and a coupling agent is needed. In the first, the "direct contact" mode, the coupling agent is a commercial gel or mineral oil; in the second approach, "degassed" water (i.e., water that has been allowed to sit and lose its gas content) is used because the gases in tap water will form bubbles and attenuate the beam. The direct contact method is usually preferred.

US machines vary but typically include a way to adjust the power output, a way to select the waveform (pulsed, CW), and a timer. US frequencies are stable and usually remain within 5% of the manufacturer's specifications. Output powers may vary significantly during a session and over time and require regular calibration (41–43).

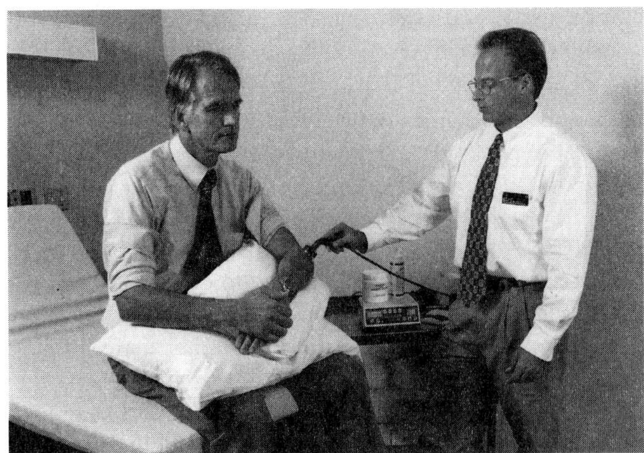

Figure 23-5. Ultrasound units may be quite compact. Note that a therapist must be present at all times and that the applicator must be kept in constant movement. Acoustic coupling is essential. The cylindrical container contains a commercial coupling gel that is often used during conventional ultrasound treatment. Phonophoresis is controversial, but the opaque white jar contains a hydrocortisone-gel mixture which could be used if hydrocortisone phonophoresis was desired.

Applications

Tendinitis and Bursitis

Even though tendinitis and bursitis are common US indications, support from clinical trials for US treatment is mixed. For example, controlled and uncontrolled studies found that 1-MHz US between 1.2 and 3.0 W/cm^2 improves range of motion (ROM) and reduces pain alone and in conjunction with cortisone injections (44–46). On the other hand, controlled studies of lateral epicondylitis (47), rotator cuff tendinitis (48), and subacromial bursitis (46) found that US combined with exercise is either not beneficial or no more effective than oral anti-inflammatories in gaining ROM. Additional studies also found that US is not always more effective than placebo in the treatment of lateral epicondylitis, subacromial bursitis, and facial pain (49–51). Unfortunately, small sample sizes, incomplete blinding, inadequate controls, and varying treatment approaches limit evaluation.

Contractures

Lehman et al (52–54) found that US is the only agent that significantly heats the deep tissues of the hip joint. In addition, this group found that US in conjunction with prolonged stretching persisting after heating is discontinued increased the ROM of contracted hips and shoulders (52–54). US is also used to improve the ROM in the setting of burn contractures. However, a large component of these contractures can be superficial and while one study found no benefit from US (55), interpretation is difficult as the study was small and involved stretching after US.

Osteoarthritis

US also is a frequent adjunct to strengthening, stretching, and education in the treatment of degenerative spine and joint diseases. Goals are reduced pain, increased ROM, reduction of muscle spasm, and pain relief. Benefits in 70% of subjects may be claimed (56) but optimal regimens and even effectiveness are difficult to evaluate owing to small study sizes, differing treatment approaches, and variable blinding.

Soft-Tissue Wound and Fracture Healing

Wound healing is notoriously difficult to evaluate. Nevertheless, many feel that US, either through heating (and the associated increased metabolic and enzymatic activity) or through nonthermal effects (e.g., streaming and cavitation increasing tissue permeability), accelerates wound healing. Laboratory findings offer some support (57) but clinical results are mixed. One controlled study, for example, found that pulsed low-intensity 3.28-MHz US did not improve the healing of decubitus ulcers in nursing home patients (58). On the other hand, another study using a similar low-intensity pulsed US regimen along with ultraviolet (UV) light found treatment more effective than standard nursing care for similar wounds (59). Lower-extremity venous stasis ulcers are common: Unfortunately, positive (60,61) and negative (62) effects are reported following US treatment.

US's ability to accelerate the healing of bony injuries was established by the early 1980s (63,64) and has been approved by the Food and Drug Administration for the treatment of some fractures (64). Intensities tend to be low and a recent blinded controlled study found that 30-mW/cm^2, pulsed, 1.5-MHz US accelerated the healing of both closed and grade 1 open fractures (65). US is not often used in physical therapy clinics for this purpose, and healing is delayed in about 5% to 10% of fractures (64).

Other Indications

US is used for many other applications. Among these—but with far less substantiation—are lymphedema (66), postherpetic neuralgia (67–69), plantar warts (70–72), keloids (73), and "inflammation" (74,75).

Phonophoresis

Phonophoresis is a US technique in which medications such as corticosteroids, analgesics, and anesthetics are mixed in the coupling agent in the hope that they will be "driven" by the US through the skin into deeper tissues. Penetration to depths of several centimeters has been reported (76,77), but many find the concept arguable in that substances may not always pass through the skin and once past the epidermis, may be dispersed by the subcutaneous circulation. Whether phonophoresis is more beneficial than US alone is unclear. Both no and significant effects are reported (78–81), but the studies were small, blinding was ambiguous, and comparisons to local injection or oral administration of the same medication were lacking.

Safety

US produces intense localized heating and the concerns outlined in Table 23-2 are pertinent. In addition, US can produce nonthermal effects—standing waves, streaming, and cavitation—which have their own risks. Standing waves, for example, can place nonuniform stresses in tissue but are easily avoided by constantly moving the sound head during treatment. Tissue damage from cavitation and streaming is controlled by using accepted treatment intensities, constantly moving the sound head, and avoiding fluid-filled cavities such as the gravid uterus and the eyes. Treatment directly over the spine, brain, and laminectomy sites as well as the heart, ischemic areas, and implanted devices is avoided. While US over metal may produce no more of a temperature elevation than would occur in its absence (82–84), it seems possible that some geometries might produce localized temperature assymetries.

Effectiveness

There are legitimate questions about US dosage and efficacy for many of its most common indications. Meta-analysis might provide an objective evaluation but this approach is also limited by the variability of study designs, parameters, and quality. For example, one meta-analytic attempt to study the effect of US on musculoskeletal pain (85) found that fewer than 5% of almost 300 studies met its analysis criteria. This study found no benefit from US. However, as acute and chronic conditions were pooled with pulsed and CW waveforms, the meaningfulness of this finding is unclear.

Electromagnetic Fields

Although short-wave (SWD) and microwave diathermy (MWD) are discussed separately here, these waves occupy adjacent positions in the electromagnetic spectrum and share common properties. In particular, each heats conversively with a combination of the electrical currents it generates in the tissue as well as by the increased vibration its field imposes on the tissue's molecules.

Short-Wave Diathermy

The Federal Communications Commission (FCC) restricts the industrial, scientific, and medical (ISM) use of the short-wave spectrum to 13.56, 27.12, and 40.68 MHz. [Wavelengths (22, 11, and 7 m, respectively) even in this "short-wave" portion of the spectrum are not "short."] In the United States, most SWD machines operate at 27.12 MHz.

Biophysics

The depth of SWD heating depends on the composition of the tissue and the characteristics of radiowaves. For example, even though all these wavelengths are too long to be focused by these devices, higher frequencies attenuate more rapidly in tissue than do lower frequencies. Thus, SWD at 27.12 MHz heats more deeply than does 40.68-MHz SWD or MWD at the still higher frequencies of 915 and 2456 MHz. Heating localization also depends on the coupling of the waves to the patient. Inductively coupled SWD units use magnetically induced eddy currents to heat tissue. These currents are largest in low-impedance water-rich tissues and muscle heating is emphasized. Capacitively coupled units, on the other hand, use electrical fields to heat tissue. Here the same field is present in all the tissues between the plates, and maximal heating occurs in higher-impedance water-poor tissues such as fat (86). At clinically relevant energies, SWD can raise subcutaneous fat temperatures 15°C and muscle temperatures 4 to 6°C at 4 to 5-cm depths (87).

A variety of applicators are available. Various inductive applicators such as drums, cables, and pads as well as capacitive plates and rectal and vaginal probes have had periods of preference. Today inductive applicators (Fig. 23-6) and capacitive plates are common in the treatment of musculoskeletal conditions. Rectal and vaginal probes were used to treat prostatitis (88), pelvic inflammatory disease, and pelvic floor myalgia. Nevertheless, despite their ability to raise pelvic temperatures 5 to 6°C, patient resistance and antibiotics have made their once common use rare.

Safety

SWD requires precautions in addition to those due to heat (see Table 23-2) alone. In particular, SWD preferentially heats water and metal and it is important to keep the treatment area free of metal and the patient dry (note the toweling in Fig. 23-6). Rigorous documentation is limited but pacemakers, implanted devices, contact lenses, and the menstruating or gravid uterus should not be exposed to SWD. Many believe that SWD does not heat metallic surgical clips significantly. This may be true, but experimental work shows that juxtaposed 1-cm wires in 90-MHz fields can elevate tissue temperatures 3 to 4°C over that which would occur in their absence (89). Thus, many adopt the rule of "no metal" when using SWD. The effect of diathermy on active bony growth plates is poorly known and treatment of these areas is typically avoided in the skeletally immature.

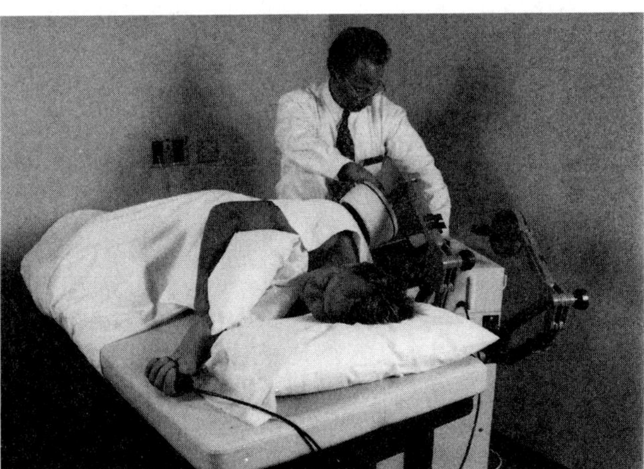

Figure 23-6. Short-wave diathermy (SWD) using an inductive applicator. Note that the patient is being treated on a wooden table, is draped with a towel to absorb moisture, and is carefully positioned. (The switch in the patient's hand is an emergency cutoff switch and alarm.) A round capacitive plate (not in use) is attached to the arm on the right side of the picture.

Microwave Diathermy

The MWD frequencies (915 and 2456 MHz) approved by the FCC for ISM use are 20 to 40 times higher than those of SWD. The corresponding wavelengths (33 and 12 cm) are about the same size as MWD applicators, and as a result, MWD has the advantage of being easily focused. Due to their high frequencies, microwaves are rapidly attenuated in water and tissue. As an example, 915-MHz MWD may increase subcutaneous fat temperatures 10 to 12°C while underlying muscles might be elevated only 3 to 5°C (90).

MWD was widely used to treat superficial joints and tissues such as the shoulder. Today, except for specialized usages such as hyperthermia to potentiate the tumoricidal effects of radiation and chemotherapy (89), MWD has been replaced with SWD and US.

Pulsed Electromagnetic

SWD and MWD can be delivered in a pulsed mode. Average energies may be the same as for the CW mode, but are often much lower to avoid heating and promote nonthermal effects. Although nonthermal applications are gaining prominence (see below), conventional treatment still emphasizes tissue heating.

Interest in low-intensity pulsed fields is growing for many reasons. For example, cells and tissues produced electrical fields (and currents) that are altered by injury and healing (91). In addition, intracellular calcium concentrations, cell metabolism, and receptor and messenger behaviors are altered by low-intensity electromagnetic fields (92). Furthermore, brief intense fields increase cell permeability (93). Unfortunately clinical extensions are difficult to establish and acceptance, beyond the treatment of bony fractures, remains slow.

General Safety Issues of Electromagnetic

SWD and MWD exposures are quantified in American National Standards Institute guidelines (94) that permit the determination of permissible exposure limits for industrial and medical workers. There guidelines are frequency dependent. Thus, at 27.12 MHz, time-averaged SWD exposure of therapists should be less than 1 mW/cm^2. The same guidelines for MWD at 915 and 2456 MHz restrict exposures to 3 and 5 mW/cm^2, respectively. Inductively coupled devices have broader fields than do capacitive devices. Nevertheless, intensities fall rapidly and are usually lower than 10 mW/cm^2 50 to 60 cm from an applicator (95,96). Therapists typically are only intermittently within a meter of SWD or MWD machines during operation and seem safe within these guidelines.

Epidemiologic evidence seems to supports the workplace safety of SWD and MWD. Thus, while one study reported increased miscarriage rates in women exposed to MWD (97), others found no alterations in miscarriage frequency, congenital malformations, or sex ratios in the children of exposed therapists (97–99). Prudence still dictates minimizing unnecessary exposure.

ELECTRICAL STIMULATION

Although the ancient Greeks knew that certain rays, eels, and catfish could produce numbness (100), electricity did not play a significant role in medicine until recently. In the eighteenth and nineteenth centuries, however, rapid improvements in the understanding of electricity were accompanied by an enthusiastic reception of "electrical" treatments (e.g., electrostatic baths, spark treatments, and galvanic muscle stimulation) by the public (100,101). Benefits were minimal and the excesses of this period probably contribute to the skepticism of this approach that persists today. This section outlines the applications of electricity to analgesia, wound healing, and iontophoresis.

Analgesia

Melzack and Wall's "gate control theory" of pain (102), published in the 1960s, postulated that nociceptive signals can be blocked in the substantia gelatinosa of the spinal cord by nonpainful afferent sensory signals. Electrical stimulation could easily provide these signals and after successful trials, use of transcutaneous electrical nerve stimulation (TENS) became widespread.

TENS use has grown even though TENS analgesia is not completely explained by the gate control theory (e.g., sensory neuropathy can be painless and analgesia may start after treatment begins and may persist after stimulation is stopped). As a result, alternative explanations such as those involving central nervous system endorphins have been advanced for at least some TENS approaches.

Technique

TENS units are small and fit in a pocket or on a belt without difficulty. All contain a battery, a signal generator, and one or more sets of electrodes. Output currents are less than 100 mA. Pulse frequencies range from a few hertz to 200 Hz, with pulse widths between 10 μsec and a few hundred microseconds. Biphasic waveforms are usually chosen to avoid electrolysis and iontophoretic effects. Although a variety of waveforms (e.g., ramped, continuous, burst) are available, there is little evidence that one is clearly more effective than another.

Many begin treatment over the painful area or trigger point with the barely perceptible settings of "convention" or "high TENS" at 40 to 80 Hz. If initial trials are not successful, higher-amplitude and lower-frequency (4–8 Hz) "low TENS" may be tried as well as electrode placement over an afferent nerve, distal to or contralateral to the painful area. Acupuncture or auricular theory points may also be used (103–105). Electrode placement and parameter choices are ultimately determined by the preferences of the patient and therapist.

TENS units are expensive to purchase ($800–1000) or to rent ($80–100/mo). Benefits, on the other hand, are difficult to establish and often diminish with time. As a result, effectiveness should be evaluated carefully in a few sessions—and, if possible, in an overnight trial. If beneficial, the same model should be rented and purchase considered if significant benefits persist for more than a few months. In practice, about half the patients evaluating TENS may find it helpful initially and perhaps less than half of those may find useful analgesia persisting after a few months of use.

Application

Pain is subjective and difficult to measure. TENS studies reflect this and in addition, assessment of treatment success is made more difficult owing to differences in the conditions examined, electrode placement, and stimulation parameters. Success rates vary widely and even in well-designed studies range from no better than placebo to 90%.

Some general statements are possible, however. For example, investigators in the 1970s and 1980s tended to find that TENS treatment of postoperative, obstetric, and acute pain produced reductions in pain and analgesic use of about 80% (106). Effectiveness was most marked for milder pain (e.g., the first, rather than second, stage of labor) and lessened with time (106). Chronic pain seemed to respond more variably, with benefits ranging from placebo levels to 75% to 80%. Psychogenic pain seemed particularly unresponsive (106).

More recent studies report similar, but less pronounced, TENS benefits. For example, TENS use following arthrography (107) and surgery (108) may result in less need for analgesia but may have no benefit on postanesthesia respiratory function (109) or ischemic pain (110). The more recent studies also found psychogenic and chronic pain to be relatively refractory, with several reporting that TENS is either ineffective or adds nothing to low-back pain therapy programs involving exercise, manipulation, corsets, or massage (111–113). Although one study found high-intensity TENS beneficial for low-back pain (114), others found TENS no more effective than naproxen in knee osteoarthritis (115) or dysmenorrhea (116). Findings are difficult to quantify; however, a retrospective review of long-term TENS users supports the idea that a small subset of individuals benefit from protracted TENS use (117).

Safety

Serious problems are rare. Contact dermatitis and the stinging that occurs when an electrode partially detaches (and concentrates current flow) are the most common complaints. These problems are usually easily solved with hypoallergenic electrodes and repositioning. Cardiac pacemakers are usually not influenced by TENS. Nevertheless, caution seems to dictate avoiding TENS use in patients with pacemakers, or dysrhythmias or over the carotid sinus and anterior upper part of the neck. Treatment near the pregnant uterus is avoided, but as is true for many precautions, danger has not been established.

Wound Healing

Interest in electrical stimulation of wound healing was awakened in the late 1960s and 1970s by the report of Wolcott et al (118) that low-intensity direct-current accelerated ischemic wound healing. This study aroused interest but due to poor controls, puzzling methodology, and difficulties in patient selection, was difficult to replicate. Research continued (119) but low-intensity direct-current stimulation did not gain general acceptance.

Due to the availability of TENS, low-frequency pulsed waveforms are particularly common. For example, studies found that a variety of waveforms, intensities, and techniques (application over, near to, distant from acupuncture points) can relieve pain, improve healing, and elevate temperatures in the distal part of limbs in people with diabetic neuropathy and scleroderma (120,121). Studies with pulsed electromagnetic fields (already used to treat bony nonunions) (122,123) as well as some with low current intensities ($\mu A/cm^2$) and others with voltages of 100 to 500 V also found benefits (124–129). Unfortunately, concerns about study size, differing approaches, and blinding slow generalization to clinical treatment.

Iontophoresis

Iontophoresis uses electrical fields to drive charged or electrically polarized substances (e.g., salicylates, acetic acid) through the epidermis. Much of the penetration probably occurs at sweat glands and sites of skin breakdown (130). Penetration is variable (131,132) and how much of a substance is actually delivered to the treated tissue rather than the blood remains contentious.

Technique

Iontophoretic equipment (Fig. 23-7) consists of a direct-current power source, two electrodes, and moistened pads that are placed between the electrodes and the skin. The pads (Fig. 23-8) may be moistened with normal saline solution and a 1% solution of the chosen agent is placed on the pad under the electrode of the same polarity. Electrical fields, which are proportional to the voltage, provide the driving force. Currents are usually limited to produce intensities of 0.1 to 0.5 mA/cm^2 and are proportional to the active material delivered.

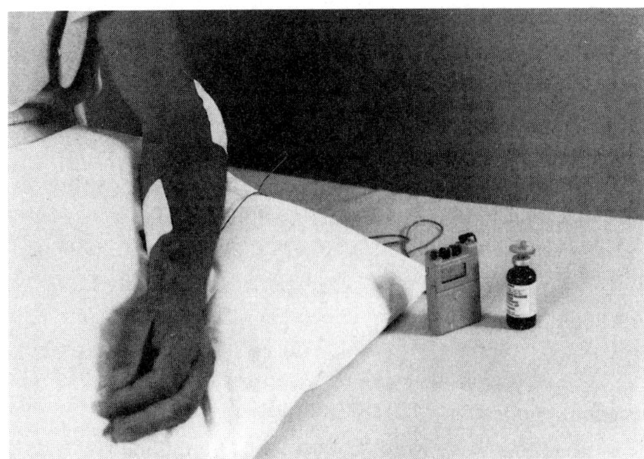

Figure 23-7. Iontophoresis. Note the adjustable battery-powered current source and the vial containing the active substance. In this figure the treatment site is the lateral epicondyle. The medication is applied to the gauze of the electrode at this site. The polarity is chosen to match the charge or polarity of the medication. The electrode on the volar aspect of the forearm is needed to complete the circuit.

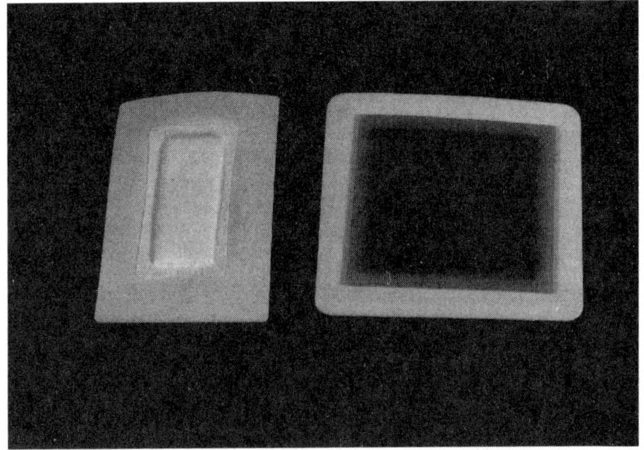

Figure 23-8. Iontophoretic electrodes. Note the gauze on the smaller active electrode and the larger surface area of the inactive electrode.

Indications

Iontophoresis is an accepted treatment of hyperhidrosis. The mechanism of action is unclear, but success rates of 90% are achieved with tap water alone and may persist for weeks (130,131,133). Typically the hands or feet are placed in water, and the circuit adjusted to deliver 10 to 30 mA. Tooth hypersensitivity has also been treated successfully with sodium fluoride (134). Iontophoretic antibiotic delivery is possible but has not become common. Other uses such as salicylates for postsurgical pain, iodine for scar tissue reduction, acetic acid for calcific tendinitis, zinc for ischemic ulcers, and lidocaine for local anesthesia are reported (106) but effectiveness is not established.

ULTRAVIOLET THERAPY

The UV spectrum can be divided in several ways. The nonmedical scientific literature often breaks it into near (300–400 μm) and far (200–300 μm) UV light. The biomedical literature, on the other hand, emphasizes a three-part classification [UV-A (0.315–0.400 μm), UV-B (0.290–0.315 μm), and UV-C (0.20–0.29 μm)], which tends to mirror biologic activity. UV-A penetrates deeply but produces minimal biologic effects. UV-B produces sunburn and skin erythema (at rates a thousand times higher than UV-A) and is primarily responsible for mutagenic and carcinogenic effects on DNA; UV-C is germicidal.

UV is used in wound treatment to kill bacteria and accelerate healing. Motile bacteria are killed and neovascularization is reported around the margins of UV-treated wounds (135); healing acceleration is questionable (136).

Treatment

Broad-spectrum "hot quartz" sources were once common, but were bulky and difficult to use. Safer and more convenient handheld "cold quartz" lamps that produce UV-C radiation in a narrow band at 0.254 μm next became available and supplanted these earlier devices.

Exposure times are quantified for *each* UV source in terms of the dose that produces a minimal erythema within several hours of exposure of untanned (typically volar forearm) skin. This dose (usually requiring between 5 and 20 seconds) is defined as 1 MED (minimal erythemal dose). Treatment with 2.5 MEDs produces a more severe erythema that may last several days; 5 MEDs produces edema and desquamation and 10 MEDs will cause blistering (135).

Initial exposures begin with 1 to 2 MEDs and are usually kept to lower than 5 MEDs to avoid tissue destruction (133). Treatments involved shielding the surrounding intact tissue and holding the lamp over a cleansed wound. Special probes, however, permit treatment of fistulas, cavities, and undermined wounds. Despite limited use now, this agent has had in the past, and may again have, a significant role in medicine.

Safety

The chief concerns of UV (sunburn, cataracts, and retinal damage) are avoided by shielding the therapist and patient (except for the area treated) and wearing protective goggles during treatment. Systemic (e.g., tetracycline) and topical (e.g., green soap) photosensitizing medications, scars, atrophic skin, and fair skin are additional issues that must be considered.

VIBRATION

Vibration and tapping are often used for "neuromuscular facilitation" following stroke and upper motor neuron injuries. Tapping is often sufficient but a variety of vibrators are used. Some believe that frequencies of about 150 Hz and vibratory amplitudes of about 1.5 mm are the most effective (137,138). Effects can be quite marked and vibratory facilitation is a common component of stroke rehabilitation at many centers.

Vibration has analgesic effects and some studies find 100- to 200-Hz vibration as beneficial as TENS and aspirin for musculoskeletal pain (139). Vibration is also reported to accelerate wound healing (140). While intriguing, work in this area is limited and poorly controlled.

LOW-INTENSITY LASER THERAPY

Low-power lasers have been promoted for more than 25 years as a safe and effective way to produce analgesia and speed healing. Marked effects are found in the laboratory (often at powers <1 mW) for a variety of processes such as cell metabolism, protein production, and DNA synthesis. Unfortunately, results in animal and human trials have been less convincing. Over the years powers have crept up into the 30- to 100-mW range, laser choice has converged to the red (0.633 μm) or IR (0.904–0.930 μm) region, and study quality has improved. This approach has yet to receive Food and Drug Administration approval for any indication. While some investigators find laser therapy beneficial in the treatment of numerous musculoskeletal, neurologic, and wound-healing conditions, others find no effect (141).

ALTERNATIVE THERAPIES

The usage of physical agents is not stagnant. Hyperthermia, MWD, and UV were common in the past and are now rare. Stimulation with low-intensity pulsed electrical, electromagnetic, and US fields is gaining attention and is used to accelerate fracture healing. Newer (at times "rediscovered") concepts, such as microstimulation, magnetotherapy, and laser therapy, frequently seem preposterous—and often may be. Nevertheless, each has characteristics that make clinical effects at least possible. Thus, the enthusiasm of the convert should be met with skepticism, but the mind should be kept open to new ideas subjected to controlled and replicated studies.

REFERENCES

1. Harris ED, McCroskery PA. The influence of temperature and fibril stability on degradation of cartilage collagen by rheumatoid synovial collagenase. *N Engl J Med* 1974;290:1–6.
2. Abramson DI, Tuck S, Chu LSW, Agustin C. Effect of paraffin bath and hot fomentations on local

tissue temperatures. *Arch Phys Med Rehabil* 1964;45:87–94.

3. Lehmann JF, de Lateur BJ. Diathermy and superficial heat and cold therapy. In: Kottke FJ, Stillwell GK, Lehmann JF, eds. *Krusen's handbook of physical medicine and rehabilitation.* 3rd ed. Philadelphia: WB Saunders, 1982:275–350.
4. Hartviksen K. Ice therapy in spasticity. *Acta Neurol Scand* 1962;38:79–84.
5. Abramson DI, Chu LSW, Tuck S Jr, et al. Effect of tissue temperature and blood flow on motor nerve conduction velocity. *JAMA* 1966;198:1082–1088.
6. Hollander JL, Horvath SM. The influence of physical therapy procedures on the intra-articular temperature of normal and arthritis subjects. *Am J Med Sci* 1949;218:543–548.
7. Horvath SM, Hollander JL. Intra-articular temperature as a measure of joint reaction. *J Clin Invest* 1949;28:469–473.
8. Hollander JL, Horvath SM. Changes in temperature produced by diseases and by physical therapy (preliminary report). *Arch Phys Med Rehabil* 1949;30:437–440.
9. Oosterveld FGJ, Rasker JJ. Effects of local heat and cold treatment of surface and articular temperature of arthritic knees. *Arthritis Rheum* 1994;37:1578–1582.
10. Guyton AC, Hall JE. Body temperature, temperature regulation and fever. In: *Textbook of medical physiology.* 9th ed. Philadelphia: WB Saunders, 1996:911–922.
11. Ho SSW, Illgen RL, Meyer RW, et al. Comparison of various icing times in decreasing bone metabolism and blood flow in the knee. *Am J Sports Med* 1995;23:74–76.
12. Taber C, Contryman K, Fahrenbruch J, et al. Measurement of reactive vasodilation during cold gel pack application to nontraumatized ankles. *Phys Ther* 1992;72:294–299.
13. Curkovic B, Vitulic V, Babic-Naglic D, Durrigl T. The influence of heat and cold on the pain threshold in rheumatoid arthritis. *Z Rheumatol* 1993;52:289–291.
14. Miglietta O. Action of cold on spasticity. *Am J Phys Med* 1973;52:198–205.
15. Bisgard JD, Nye D. The influence of hot and cold application upon gastric and intestinal motor activity. *Surg Gynecol Obstet* 1940; 71:172–180.
16. Travell J. Ethyl chloride spray for painful muscle spasm. *Arch Phys Med Rehabil* 1952;33:291–298.
17. Hirase Y. Postoperative cooling enhances composite graft survival in nasal-alar and finger tip reconstruction. *Br J Plast Surg* 1993; 46:707–711.
18. Whitelaw GP, DeMuth KA, Demos HA, et al. The use of the cryo/cuff versus ice and elastic wrap in the postoperative care of knee arthroscopy patients. *Am J Knee Surg* 1995;8:28–30.
19. Daniel DM, Stone ML, Arendt DL. The effect of cold therapy on pain, swelling, and range of motion after anterior cruciate ligament reconstructive surgery. *Arthroscopy* 1994;10:530–533.
20. Amin-Hanjani S, Corcoran J, Chatwani A. Cold therapy in the management of postoperative cesarean section pain. *J Obstet Gynecol* 1992;167:108–109.
21. Woodmansey A, Collins DH, Ernst MM. Vascular reactions to the contrast bath in health and in rheumatoid arthritis. *Lancet* 1938;2:1350–1353.
22. Shafik A. Role of warm-water bath in anorectal conditions. The "thermosphincteric reflex." *J Clin Gastroenterol* 1993;16:304–308.
23. Pinho M, Correa JCO, Furtado A, Ramos JR. Do hot baths promote anal sphincter relaxation? *Dis Colon Rectum* 1993;36:273–274.
24. Green J, McKenna F, Redfern EJ, Chamberlain MA. Home exercises are as effective as outpatient hydrotherapy for osteoarthritis of the hip. *Br J Rheumatol* 1993;32:812–815.
25. Tovin BJ, Wolf, SL, Greenfield BH, et al. Comparison of the effects of exercise in water and on land on the rehabilitation of patients with intra-articular anterior cruciate ligament reconstructions. *Phys Ther* 1994;74:710–719.
26. Adler AJ. Water immersion: lessons from antiquity to modern times. *Contrib Nephrol* 1993; 102:171–186.
27. Forster MM. Mineral springs and miracles. *Can Fam Physician* 1994;40:729–737.
28. Sukenik S, Giryes H, Halevy S, et al. Treatment of psoriatic arthritis at the Dead Sea. *J Rheumatol* 1994;21:1305–1309.
29. Rishler M, Brostovski Y, Yaron M. Effect of spa therapy in Tiberias on patients with ankylosing spondylitis. *Clin Rheumatol* 1995;14:21–25.
30. Sukenik S, Buskila D, Neumann L, Kleiner-Baungarten A. Mud pack therapy in rheumatoid arthritis. *Clin Rheumatol* 1992; 11:243–247.
31. Sukenik S, Neumann L, Flusser, D, Kleiner-Baumgarten A. Balneotherapy for rheumatoid arthritis at the Dead Sea. *Isr J Med Sci* 1995;31:210–214.
32. Konrad K, Tatrai T, Hunka A, et al. Controlled trial of balneotherapy in treatment of low back pain. *Ann Rheum Dis* 1992;51: 820–822.
33. Constant F, Coloin JF, Guillemin F, Boulange M. Effectiveness of spa therapy in chronic low back pain: a randomized clinical trial. *J Rheumatol* 1995;22:1315–1320.
34. Guillemin F, Constant F, Collin JE, Boulange M. Short and long-term effect of spa therapy in chronic low back pain. *Br J Rheumatol* 1994;33:148–151.

35. Luurila OJ. Cardiac arrhythmias, sudden death and the Finnish sauna bath. *Adv Cardiol* 1978; 25:73–81.

36. Romo J. Factors related to sudden death in acute ischemic heart disease: a community study in Helsinki. *Acta Med Scand Suppl* 1972;547:1–92.

37. Allison TG, Miller TD, Squires RW, Gau GT. Cardiovascular responses to immersion in a hot tub in comparison with exercise in male subjects with coronary artery disease. *Mayo Clin Proc* 1993;68:19–25.

38. Gerner HJ, Engel P, Gass GC, et al. The effects of sauna on tetraplegic and paraplegic subjects. *Paraplegia* 1992;30:410–419.

39. Pleet H, Graham JM Jr, Smith DW. Central nervous system and facial defects associated with maternal hypothermia at four to 14 weeks' gestation. *Pediatrics* 1981;67:785–789.

40. Kauppinen K, Vuori I. Man in the sauna. *Ann Clin Res* 1986;4: 173–185.

41. Stewart HF, Harris GR, Herman BA, et al. Survey of use and performance of ultrasonic therapy equipment in Pinellas County, Florida. *Phys Ther* 1974;54: 707–714.

42. Coakley WT. Biophysical effects of ultrasound at therapeutic intensities. *Physiotherapy* 1978;64:166–169.

43. Allen KGR, Battye CK. Performance of ultrasonic therapy instruments. *Physiotherapy* 1978;64:174–179.

44. Echternach JL. Ultrasound: an adjunct treatment for shoulder disabilities. *Phys Ther* 1965;45: 865–869.

45. Coodley EL. Bursitis and post-traumatic lesions: management with combined use of ultrasound and intra-articular hydrocortisone. *Am Practit* 1960;11:181–188.

46. Downing DS, Weinstein A. Ultrasound therapy of subacromial bursitis: a double blind trial. *Phys Ther* 1986;66:194–199.

47. Haker E, Lundeberg T. Pulsed ultrasound treatment in lateral epicondylagia. *Scand J Rehabil Med* 1991;23:115–118.

48. Nykanen M. Pulsed ultrasound treatment of the painful shoulder. A randomized, double-blind, placebo controlled study. *Scand J Rehabil Med* 1995;27:105–108.

49. Dijs H, Mortier G, Driessens M, et al. A retrospective study of the conservative treatment of tennis-elbow. *Acta Belg Med Phys* 1990;13:73–77.

50. Lundeberg T, Abrahamsson P, Haker E. A comparative study of continuous ultrasound and rest in epicondyalgia. *Scand J Rehabil Med* 1988;20;99–101.

51. Taube S, Ylipaavaliniemi P, Kononen M, Sunden B. The effect of pulsed ultrasound on myofacial pain: a placebo controlled study. *Proc Finn Dent Soc* 1988;84:241–246.

52. Lehmann JF, Erickson DJ, Martin GM, Krusen FH. Comparison of ultrasonic and microwave diathermy in the physical treatment of periarthritis of the shoulder. *Arch Phys Med Rehabil* 1954;35:627–634.

53. Lehmann JF, Fordyce WE, Rathbun LA, et al. Clinical evaluation of a new approach in the treatment of contracture associated with hip fracture after internal fixation. *Arch Phys Med Rehabil* 1961;42:95.

54. Lehmann JF, McMillan JA, Brunner GD, Blumberg JB. Comparative study of the efficiency of short-wave, microwave, and ultrasonic diathermy in heating the hip joint. *Arch Phys Med Rehabil* 1959;40:510–512.

55. Ward RS, Hayes-Lundy C, Reddy R, et al. Evaluation of topical therapeutic ultrasound to improve response to physical therapy and lessen scar contracture after burn injury. *J Burn Care Rehabil* 1994;15:74–79.

56. Aldes JH, Jadeson WJ. Ultrasonic therapy in the treatment of hypertrophic arthritis in elderly patients. *Ann West Med Surg* 1952;6:545–550.

57. Young S, Dyson M. Effect of therapeutic ultrasound on the healing of full-thickness excised skin lesions. *Ultrasonics* 1990;28: 175–180.

58. ter Riet G, Kessels AGH, Knipschild P. Randomized clinical trial of ultrasound treatment for pressure ulcers. *BMJ* 1995;310: 1040–1041.

59. Nussbaum EL, Biemann I, Mustard B. Comparison of ultrasound/ultraviolet-C and laser for treatment of pressure ulcers in patients with spinal cord injury. *Phys Ther* 1994;74:812–823.

60. Dyson M, Frank C, Suckling J. Stimulation of healing of varicose ulcers by ultrasound. *Ultrasonics* 1987;25:232–236.

61. Callam M, Harper D, Dale J, et al. A controlled trial of weekly ultrasound therapy in chronic leg ulceration. *Lancet* 1987;25:204–206.

62. Eriksson SV, Luneberg T, Malm M. A placebo controlled trial of ultrasound therapy in chronic leg ulceration. *Scand J Rehabil Med* 1991;23:211–213.

63. Duarte LR. The stimulation of bone growth by ultrasound. *Arch Orthop Trauma Surg* 1983;101: 153–159.

64. Einhorn TA. Current concepts review: enhancement of fracture-healing. *J Bone Joint Surg [Am]* 1995;77:940–956.

65. Heckman JD, Ryaby JP, McCabe J, et al. Acceleration of tibial fracture-healing by non-invasive, low intensity pulsed ultrasound. *J Bone Joint Surg [Am]* 1994;76: 26–34.

66. Balzarini A, Pirovano C, Diazzi G, et al. Ultrasound therapy of chronic arm lymphedema after surgical treatment of breast cancer. *Lymphology* 1993;26: 128–134.

67. Garrett AS, Garrett M. Ultrasound therapy for herpes zoster pain. *J Coll Gen Pract* 1982;32:709–710.

68. Jones RJ. Treatment of acute herpes zoster using ultrasonic therapy: report on a series of twelve patients. *Physiotherapy* 1984;70:94–95.

69. Payne C. Ultrasound for post herpetic neuralgia: a study to investigate the results of treatment. *Physiotherapy* 1984;70:96–97.

70. Cherup N, Urben J, Bender LF. The treatment of plantar warts with ultrasound. *Arch Phys Med Rehabil* 1963;44:602–604.

71. Vaughn DT. Direct method versus underwater method in the treatment of plantar warts with ultrasound. A comparative study. *Phys Ther* 1973;53:396–397.

72. Braatz JH, McAlistar BR, Broaddus MD. Ultrasound and plantar warts: a double blind study. *Mil Med* 1974;139:199–201.

73. Wright ET, Haase KH. Keloids and ultrasound. *Arch Phys Med Rehabil* 1971;52:280–281.

74. Hashishi I, Hai HK, Havey W, et al. Reduction of postoperative pain and swelling by ultrasound treatment: a placebo effect. *Pain* 1988;33:303–311.

75. Grant A, Sleep J, McIntosh J, Ashurts H. Ultrasound and pulsed electromagnetic energy treatment for perineal trauma: a randomized placebo-controlled trial. *Br J Obstet Gynaecol* 1989;96:434–439.

76. Griffin JE, Touchstone JC, Liu A. Ultrasonic movement of cortisol into pig tissue: II. Movement into paravertebral nerve. *Am J Phys Med* 1965;44:20–25.

77. Novak EJ. Experimental transmission of lidocaine through intact skin by ultrasound. *Arch Phys Med Rehabil* 1964;45:231–232.

78. Goddard DJ, Revell PA, Cason J, et al. Ultrasound has no anti-inflammatory effect. *Ann Rheum Dis* 1983;42:582–584.

79. Moll MJ. A new approach to pain: lidocaine and Decadron with ultrasound. *Med Serv Dig* 1979;29:8–11.

80. Wanet G, Dehon N. Etude clinique de l'ultrasonophorese avec un topique associant phenylbutazone et alpha-chymotrypsine. *J Belge Rhumatol Med Phys* 1976;31:49–58.

81. El-Hadidi T, El-Garf A. Double-blind study comparing the use of Voltaren Emulgel versus regular gel during ultrasonic sessions in the treatment of localized traumatic and rheumatic painful conditions. *J Int Med Res* 1991;19:219–227.

82. Brunner GD, Lehmann JF, McMillan JA, et al. Can ultrasound be used in the presence of surgical metal implants: an experimental approach. *Phys Ther* 1958;38:823–824.

83. Gersten JW. Effect of metallic objects of temperature rises produced in tissue by ultrasound. *Am J Phys Med* 1958;37:75–82.

84. Skoubo-Kristensen E, Sommer J. Ultrasound influence on internal fixation with a rigid plate in dogs. *Arch Phys Med Rehabil* 1982;63:371–373.

85. Gam AN, Johannsen F. Ultrasound therapy in musculoskeletal disorders: a meta-analysis. *Pain* 1995;63:85–91.

86. Kantor G. Evaluation and survey of microwave and radio frequency applicators. *J Microw Power Electromagn Energy* 1981;16:135–150.

87. Lehmann JF, deLateur BJ, Stonebridge JB. Selective heating by shortwave diathermy with a helical coil. *Arch Phys Med Rehabil* 1969;50:117–123.

88. Zanetic F, Markovic B, Starcevic LJ. Kratkotalasna terapija kao komplementarna terapija hronicnog prostatitisa. *Med Arh* 1981;35:157–159.

89. Lee ER, Sullivan DM, Kapp DS. Potential hazards of radioactive electromagnetic hyperthermia in the presence of multiple metallic surgical clips. *Int J Hyperthermia* 1992;8:809–817.

90. DeLateur BJ, Lehmann JF, Stonebridge JB, et al. Muscle heating in human subjects with 915 MHz: microwave contact applicator. *Arch Phys Med Rehabil* 1970;51:147–151.

91. Marcer M, Musatti G, Bassett CAL. Results of pulsed electromagnetic fields (PEMEFs) in ununited fractures after external skeletal fixation. *Clin Orthop* 1984;190:260–265.

92. Stuchly MA, Repacholi MH, Lecuyer DW, Mann RD. Exposure to the operator and patient during short wave diathermy treatments. *Health Phys* 1982;42:341–366.

93. Albanese R, Blaschak J, Medina R, Penn J. Ultrashort electromagnetic signals: biophysical questions, safety issues, and medical opportunities. *Aviat Space Environ Med* 1994;65(suppl 5):A116–A120.

94. American National Standards Institute, Inc. *Safety levels with respect to human exposure to radio frequency electromagnetic fields, 300 kHz to 100 GHz.* Washington, DC: American National Standards Institute, 1982.

95. Martin CJ, McCallum HM, Heaton B. An evaluation of radio frequency exposure from therapeutic diathermy equipment in the light of current recommendations. *Clin Phys Physiol Meas* 1990;11:53–63.

96. Witters DM, Kantor G. An evaluation of microwave diathermy applicators using free space electric field mapping. *Phys Med Biol* 1981;26:1099–1114.

97. Ouellet-Hellstrom R, Stewart WF. Miscarriages among female physical therapists who report using radio- and microwave-frequency electromagnetic radiation. *Am J Epidemiol* 1993;138:775–786.

98. Larsen AI. Congenital malformations and exposure to high-frequency electromagnetic radiation among Danish physiotherapists. *Scand J Work Environ Health* 1991;17:318–323.

99. Guberane E, Campana A, Faval P, et al. Gender ratio of offspring and exposure to short-wave radiation among female physiothera-

pists. *Scand J Work Environ Health* 1994;20:345–348.

100. Kane K, Taub A. A history of local electrical analgesia. *Pain* 1975;1:125–128.

101. Geddes LA. A short history of the electrical stimulation of excitable tissue including electrotherapeutic applications. *Physiologist* 1984;27(suppl):515–547.

102. Melzack R, Wall PD. Pain mechanism: a new theory. *Science* 1965;150:971–979.

103. Melzack R, Stillwell DM, Fox EJ. Trigger points and acupuncture points for pain: correlations and implications. *Pain* 1977;3: 3–23.

104. Oleson TD, Kroening RJ, Bresler DE. An experimental evaluation of auricular diagnosis: the somatotopic mapping of musculoskeletal pain at ear acupuncture points. *Pain* 1980;8:217–229.

105. Noling LB, Clelland JA, Jackson JR, Knowles CJ. Effect of transcutaneous electrical nerve stimulation at auricular points on experimental cutaneous pain threshold [published erratum appears in *Phys Ther* 1988;68: 1145]. *Phys Ther* 1988;68:328–332.

106. Basford JR. Physical agents. In: DeLisa JA, Gans BM, Currie DM, et al, eds. *Rehabilitation medicine.* 2nd ed. Philadelphia: JB Lippincott, 1993:404–425.

107. Morgan B, Jones AR, Mulcahy KA, et al. Transcutaneous electric nerve stimulation (TENS) during distension shoulder arthrography—a controlled trial. *Pain* 1996;64:265–267.

108. Rainov NG, Heidecke V, Albertz C, Burkert W. Transcutaneous electrical nerve stimulation (TENS) for acute postoperative pain after spinal surgery. *Eur J Pain* 1994;15:44–49.

109. Forster EL, Kramer JF, Lucy SD, et al. Effect of TENS on pain, medications, and pulmonary function following coronary artery bypass graft surgery. *Chest* 1994;106:1343–1348.

110. Walsh DM, Liggett C, Baxter D, Allen JM. A double-blind investigation of the hypoalgesic effects of transcutaneous electrical nerve stimulation upon experimentally induced ischaemic pain. *Pain* 1995;61:39–45.

111. Pope MH, Phillips RB, Haugh LD, et al. A prospective randomized three-week trial of spinal manipulation, transcutaneous muscle stimulation, massage and corset in the treatment of subacute low back pain. *Spine* 1994;19:2571–2577.

112. Deyo RA, Walsh NE, Martin DC, et al. A controlled trial of transcutaneous electrical nerve stimulation (TENS) and exercise for chronic low back pain. *N Engl J Med* 1990;322:1627–1634.

113. Herman E, Williams R, Stratford P, et al. A randomized controlled trial of transcutaneous electrical nerve stimulation (CEDETRON) to determine its benefits in a rehabilitation program for acute occupational low back pain. *Spine* 1994;19:561–568.

114. Marchand S, Charest J, Li J, et al. Is TENS purely a placebo effect? A controlled study on chronic low back pain. *Pain* 1993;54:99–106.

115. Lewis B, Lewis D, Cumming G. The comparative analgesic efficacy of transcutaneous electrical nerve stimulation and a non-steroidal anti-inflammatory drug for painful osteoarthritis. *Br J Rheumatol* 1994;33:455–460.

116. Milsom I, Hedner N, Mannheimer C. A comparative study of the effect of high-intensity transcutaneous nerve stimulation and oral naproxen on intrauterine pressure and menstrual pain in patients with primary dysmenorrhea. *Am J Obstet Gynecol* 1994;170:123–129.

117. Fishbain DA, Chabal C, Abbott A, et al. Transcutaneous electrical nerve stimulation (TENS) treatment outcome in long-term users. *Clin J Pain* 1996;12:201–214.

118. Wolcott LE, Wheeler PC, Hardwick HM, Rowley BA. Accelerated healing of skin ulcers by electrotherapy: preliminary clinical results. *South Med J* 1969;62:795–801.

119. Gault WR, Gatens PF Jr. Use of low intensity direct current in management of ischemic skin ulcers. *Phys Ther* 1976;56:265–268.

120. Vodovnik L, Karba R, Treatment of chronic wounds by means of electric and electromagnetic fields. Part 1. Literature review. *Med Biol Eng Comput* 1992;30: 257–266.

121. Kaada B, Vasodilatation induced by transcutaneous nerve stimulation in peripheral ischemia (Raynaud's phenomenon and diabetic neuropathy). *Eur Heart J* 1982;3:303–341.

122. Brighton CT. Treatment of nonunion of the tibia with constant direct current (1980 Fitts Lecture, AAST). *J Trauma* 1981;21:189–195.

123. Mammi GI, Rocchi R, Cadossi R, et al. The electrical stimulation of tibial osteotomies. *Clin Orthop* 1993;288:246–253.

124. Kloth LC, Feedar JA, Gentzkow GD. Pulsed electrical stimulation accelerates healing of chronic dermal ulcers. In: *Transactions of the 11th annual meeting of the bioelectrical repair and growth society. September 29–October 2, 1991.* Dresher, PA: BRAGS, 1991:4.

125. Gentzkow GD, Miller KH, Kause JD. Dermapulse for the treatment of decubitus ulcers: a baseline controlled trial. In: *Transactions of the 11th annual meeting of the bioelectrical repair and growth society. September 29–October 2, 1993.* Dresher, PA: BRAGS, 1991:5.

126. Salzberg CA, Cooper-Vastola SA. The effects of non-thermal pulsed electromagnetic energy on wound healing of pressure ulcers in spinal cord-injured patients: a randomized double-blind study. *Ostomy Wound Manage* 1995;41: 42–51.

127. Feeder JA, Kloth LC, Gentzkow GD. Chronic dermal ulcer healing

enhanced with monophasic pulsed electrical stimulation. *Phys Ther* 1991;71:639–649.

128. Mulder GD. Treatment of open-skin wounds with electric stimulation. *Arch Phys Med Rehabil* 1991;72:375–377.

129. Griffin JW, Tooms RE, Mendius RA, et al. Efficacy of high voltage pulsed current for healing of pressure ulcers in patients with spinal cord injury. *Phys Ther* 1991;71:433–444.

130. Hill AC, Baker GF, Jansen GT. Mechanisms of action of iontophoresis in the treatment of palmar hyperhidrosis. *Cutis* 1981;28:69–70, 72.

131. O'Malley EP, Oseter YT. Influence of some physical chemical factors on iontophoresis using radio isotopes. *Arch Phys Med Rehabil* 1955;36:310–316.

132. Chantraine A, Ludy JP, Berger D. Is cortisone iontophoresis possible? *Arch Phys Med Rehabil* 1986;67:38–40.

133. Peterson JL, Read SI, Rodman OG. A new device in the treatment of hyperhidrosis by iontophoresis. *Cutis* 1982;29:82–83, 87–89.

134. Carlo GT, Ciancio SG, Seyrek SK. An evaluation of iontophoretic application of fluoride for tooth desenstitization. *J Am Dent Assoc* 1982;105:452–454.

135. Basford JR. Ultraviolet therapy. In: Kottke FJ, Lehmann JF, eds. *Krusen's handbook of physical medicine and rehabilitation.* 4th ed. Philadelphia: WB Saunders. 1990:368–374.

136. Basford JR, Hallman HO, Sheffied CG, Mackey GL. Comparison of cold quartz ultraviolet, low-energy laser, and occlusion in wound healing in a swine model. *Arch Phys Med Rehabil* 1986;67:151–154.

137. Bishop B. Vibratory stimulation: part I. Neurophysiology of motor response evoked by vibratory stimulation. *Phys Ther* 1974;54:1273–1282.

138. Bishop B. Vibratory stimulation: part III. Possible applications of vibration in treatment of motor dysfunctions. *Phys Ther* 1975;55:139–143.

139. Lundeberg T. The pain suppressive effect of vibratory stimulation and transcutaneous electrical nerve stimulation (TENS) as compared to aspirin. *Brain Res* 1984;294:201–209.

140. Leduc A, Lievens P, Dewald J. The influence of multi-directional vibrations on wound healing and on regeneration of blood and lymph vessels. *Lymphology* 1981;14:179–185.

141. Basford JR. Low intensity laser therapy: still not an established clinical tool. *Lasers Surg Med* 1995;16:331–342.

Chapter 24

Physical Modalities

Earl J. Craig
Darryl Kaelin

The "laying on of hands" for the diagnosis and treatment of illness has always been a special part of the physician-patient relationship. As direct extensions of this contact, traction, manipulation, and massage have been commonly used treatment modalities for painful disorders. This chapter addresses the theory and practical use of traction, manipulation, and massage in the aggressive, nonoperative management of musculoskeletal disorders. Although these modalities are used for dysfunction of the extremities, attention is directed toward spinal disorders, as the majority of treatment and the preponderance of literature are focused there.

The problem of neck and low-back pain has reached epidemic proportions in the industrialized nations. Approximately 80% of all people will have one or more episodes of back pain in the course of their lives, and about 50% will have one or more episodes of neck pain (1–3). Moreover, the costs for surgical methods of treatment have escalated, driving the medical field to search for more effective and less costly conservative options. Only a few studies showed that either traction or manipulation causes anatomic changes in the vertebral column. Though the methods used in most clinical trials were flawed, few can argue that these physical modalities do not provide at least subjective short-term relief of neck and low-back symptoms. The Agency for Health Care Policy and Research (AHCPR) guidelines recently included manipulation as an effective strategy for the initial treatment of acute low-back pain (4). However, it remains unclear whether reduction in symptoms is secondary to neurophysiologic or mechanical changes. The scarcity of positive long-term outcomes has led to the greatest criticisms of these modalities for their role in the nonoperative treatment of spinal disorders. The failure to transfer responsibility of treatment and improvement to the patient is another shortcoming cited. Patient education, home exercise programs, and portable home traction units are used to facilitate treatment and address many of these concerns.

Prior to prescription of any modality, a physician must ask what he or she is treating. Only in making an accurate diagnosis can the underlying cause of pain and dysfunction be targeted. Accurate diagnoses help direct specific treatment and rehabilitation programs aimed at efficient and cost-effective recovery.

TRACTION

Traction is the application of forces in direct opposition to each other. The components of applied forces not directly opposed may create shear or compression (Figure 24-1). As a treatment modality, traction is used to produce a separation between two adjacent body parts. It can be utilized to stretch soft tissue, separate joint spaces, or change the angle or alignment between bony structures (5). Patient position and the magnitude and angle of the applied force are important factors to isolate the involved structures and produce the desired effect. For joint dislocation, a single application of traction may be successful to create realign-

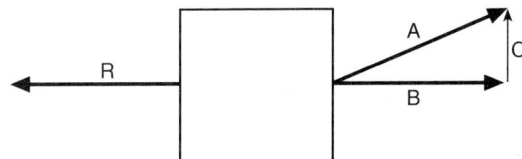

Figure 24-1. Tension-traction diagram. A = applied force; B = component of force creating traction; C = component of force creating shear or compression; R = reaction force.

ment. More commonly, traction is one component of a more complex rehabilitation treatment plan designed to reduce pain and improve function. To date most studies designed to evaluate the efficacy of traction for back and neck pain were methodologically flawed and did not allow clear conclusions. A study by van der Heijden et al (6) reviewed randomized control trials to assess the efficacy of traction for patients with neck and back pain. Only 3 of the 17 studies were deemed of sufficient quality to be analyzed and none of these showed favorable results in support of traction (6). There are no indications, however, that traction is an ineffective modality for such conditions, and it continues to be widely used with beneficial effects.

History

In ancient times, traction techniques were utilized to relieve pain and treat fractures and dislocations. Hippocrates described traction for spinal disorders with a goal of correcting scoliosis and kyphosis (6,7). A resurgence of interest in the biomechanical and clinical effects of traction began in the 1950s, led by Cyriax, Lehmann, Crue, and Judovich (8–14). In the 1960s, Colachis and Strohm (15–17) attempted to identify the relationships between traction force, angle, and duration on vertebral separation, thought to be the primary generator of symptom relief. The last two decades have seen even more investigation into the clinical application of various types of traction units, and the effect of traction forces on intervertebral disk pressure (18–22). Today, traction continues to play a vital role in the acute management of spinal trauma, fractures, and burns (5,23).

Indications

Traction of the extremities has been prescribed to maintain alignment, lessen deformities, expand joint spaces before surgery, and decrease muscle spasm and pain. It may also promote mobilization and rest to a diseased or injured body part, and promote pain-free exercise. Traction to the lower extremities of patients with painful osteoarthritis appears to provide additional pain relief as compared to hydrotherapy alone (24). Hamilton Russell traction, a form of vectored skin traction, is still used on femoral fractures for purposes of preoperative immobilization and pain relief. In the pediatric population, a modified form of Neufeld skeletal traction has been described for treating children with femoral or pelvic fractures. It allows for mobilization of the patient to a sitting position and earlier discharge from the hospital while remaining in traction (25). Overhead traction facilitates closed reduction of untreated congenitally dislocated hips in young children, thus reducing the risk of avascular necrosis (26,27). It appears to be more effective for partial dislocations (type A and B) than for complete dislocations (type C) (28).

Proximal interphalangeal joint fractures can severely affect hand functioning. A dynamic in-line traction system has been described that unloads the joint throughout its range of motion, thus reducing pain and allowing for early active therapy, improved joint nutrition, contouring, and healing (29).

Traction has been prescribed to reduce pain in several spinal disorders including nerve root compression from disk herniation, disk degeneration, or foraminal stenosis (7,11,18,30–32). It has been applied to the treatment of nonspecific low-back pain with some success (8,33). Soft-tissue injury and myofascial pain are generally less responsive to traction techniques, which if administered in a sustained fashion, can actually worsen symptoms. Short, intermittent schedules are usually more productive in this setting.

Because clinical research has been unable to consistently show clear indications and favorable outcomes, practice has been driven more by biomechanical and anatomic effects. Traction has been shown to 1) enlarge intervertebral foramina (15–17,34,35), 2) separate apophyseal joints (15–17,34,35), 3) stretch muscles and ligaments (34), 4) tighten the posterior longitudinal ligament to exert a centrifugal force on the adjacent annulus fibrosis (5), and 5) enlarge the intervertebral space (15,34). It is theorized that this separation may produce a suction effect on the disk, thus improving the blood supply and nutrition to the disk (22,36). Traction is potentially useful for any condition that could benefit from these anatomic changes (Table 24-1). These effects appear predominantly in the cervical and lumbar regions of the spine, with a lesser impact on the thoracic portion.

Types of Spinal Traction

Spinal traction can be divided into cervical (Figs. 24-2 and 24-3) and lumbar (Fig. 24-4) traction. The benefits in the thoracic and sacral regions of the spine are limited, although manual traction recently was shown to be an accurate predictor of the minimal surgical correction expected from Harrington rod placement in patients with juvenile or adolescent idiopathic scoliosis (37).

Manual traction can be delivered by a therapist (30,38–40) or self-administered through autotraction (18,20,41,42). Autotraction utilizes a special bench that is angled and rotated to place the patient in the least painful position. The patient then applies traction by pulling with his or her own arms. Simplified systems impose direct mechanical traction through a series of pulleys and weights

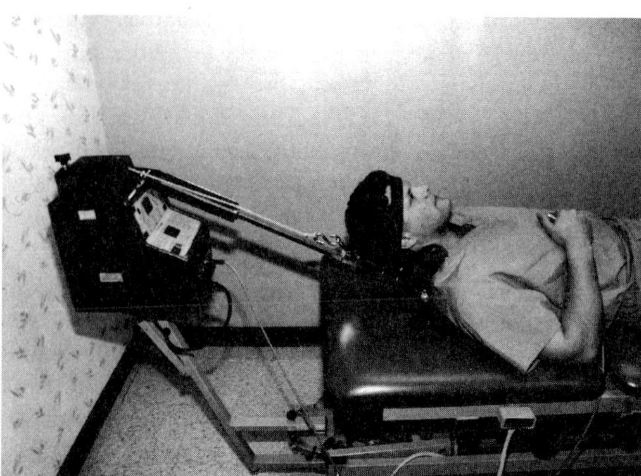

Figure 24-2. Saunders cervical traction unit provides intermittent or sustained traction in multiple head and neck positions without causing encroachment on the chin and temporomandibular joints. (This device is marketed by the Chattanooga Corporation.)

Table 24-1: Theoretical and Observed Changes with Axial Spine Traction
Diminution of disk protrusion
Reduction of cervical disk space pressure
Enlargement of intervertebral foramen
Opening up of the intervertebral disk space
Separation of the intervertebral joints
Stretching of tight painful capsule
Release of entrapped synovial membrane
Freeing of adherent nerve roots
Production of central vacuum to reduce herniated disk
Production of posterior longitudinal ligament tension to reduce herniated disk
Relaxation of muscle spasm

Source: Reproduced by permission From White AA, Panjabi MM. *Clinical biomechanics of the spine.* 2nd ed. Philadelphia: JB Lippincott, 1990:432.

(see Fig. 24-3). Gravitational lumbar traction and inversion traction use the patient's own weight to provide the force of distraction. Gravitational lumbar traction suspends the trunk through a vest secured around the lower part of the rib cage and anchored to the top of the bed. The patient is tilted into a near-vertical position so that the free weight of the lower body (40% of body weight) creates a traction force on the lumbar portion of the spine (43). Inversion traction utilizes suspension boots or a device in which the patient is supported on the anterior part of the thighs and is able to hang inverted in a hip- and knee-flexed position (43). More commonly, motorized traction units utilize split traction tables to reduce the effects of friction and more easily separate the lower body from the stabilized upper body (see Fig. 24-4).

Continuous traction utilizes low distraction forces over several hours (5). In the past, many patients were hospitalized for acute low-back pain and placed in continuous traction. This was not proved to be effective and is no longer considered standard care. It has been replaced by short-term bed rest.

Sustained traction uses greater forces than continuous traction but is maintained only over a period of 20 to 60 minutes (5). Sustained lumbar traction is most effective if a split table is used to reduce the effects of friction. Occasionally, this method has been cited as evoking post traction pain. Theoretically, this phenomenon is the result of a rapid rise in intervertebral disk pressure and soft-tissue irritation following cessation of traction.

Intermittent traction utilizes a mechanical device that alternately applies and releases traction every few seconds. Traction is applied for 10 to 60 seconds and rest periods vary from 5 to 15 seconds. The on-off cycle is repeated every 15 to 25 minutes (16,17,34). Larger distraction forces are utilized in patients with soft-tissue and myofascial pain who can better tolerate this method.

Cervical Traction

It appears that most forms of cervical traction are capable of providing beneficial effects in patients with neck pain. There are some indications, however, that intermittent traction may reduce pain and increase flexibility to a greater degree (44). In the acute setting, cervical traction is used to help reduce locked facets in the cervical region of the spine following trauma. Surgical exploration suggests that despite this reduction, associated soft tissues may still produce cord compression and surgery is still indicated in this category of patients (45).

Colachis and Strohm (15) studied the degree of posterior and vertebral separation at various angles with patients in a supine position. They reported the greatest separation at 24 degrees of flexion (15). The amount of force needed to provide adequate vertebral separation has been estimated to be between 25 and 45 lb (11). Jackson (36) advocated that cervical traction should begin with 15 to 20 lb and gradually be increased to 35 to 40 lb as tolerated over a period of several treatments. He also suggested that a 30-minute period of intermittent traction be applied daily for 3 to 6 days, followed by sessions three times weekly for 2 weeks (36). Although the majority of separation occurs in the first several seconds after traction, the maximum separation occurs anteriorly at C4–C5 after 25 minutes and posteriorly at C5–C7 after 20 minutes (17). Radiologic evidence of this distraction is lost within several minutes of the patient resuming an active standing posture (17). Clinically, a study of 31 prolapsed disks showed that an intervertebral separation could be obtained with cervical traction. This same study revealed a correlation between the reduction in intervertebral disk pressure and

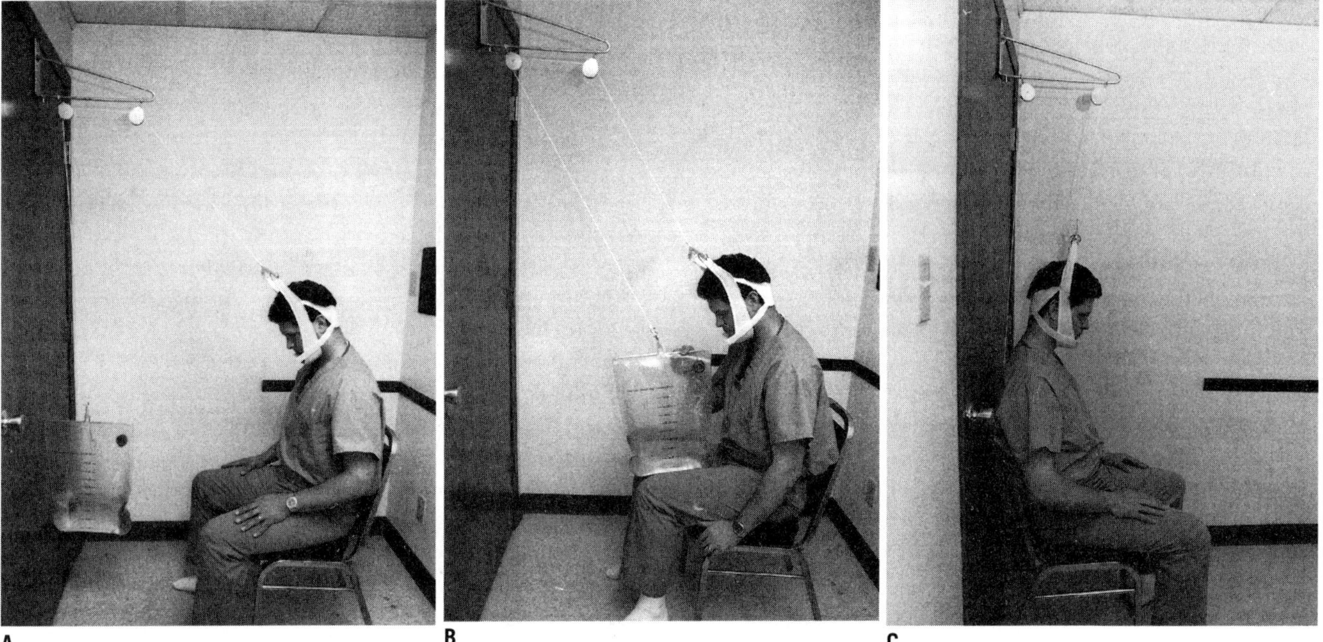

A B C

Figure 24-3. Seated home cervical traction unit. *A.* The pulley device applies force through the slightly flexed cervical region of the spine. *B.* Intermittent traction can be applied by supporting the weight and releasing the rope tension. *C.* A more neutral position can be achieved by placing the chair close to the door and facing away from the unit. Extension of the neck is not generally recommended with seated traction.

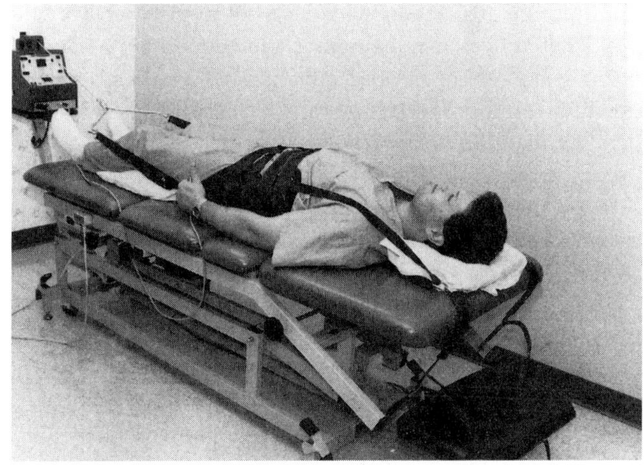

A

Figure 24-4. Motorized lumbar traction. *A.* In the supine position. *B.* With 70 degrees of knee flexion. *C.* In the prone position. Notice the lower (pelvic) belt applies the distraction force while the upper (thoracic) belt stabilizes the patient's trunk. A handheld shut-off mechanism should be available for safety.

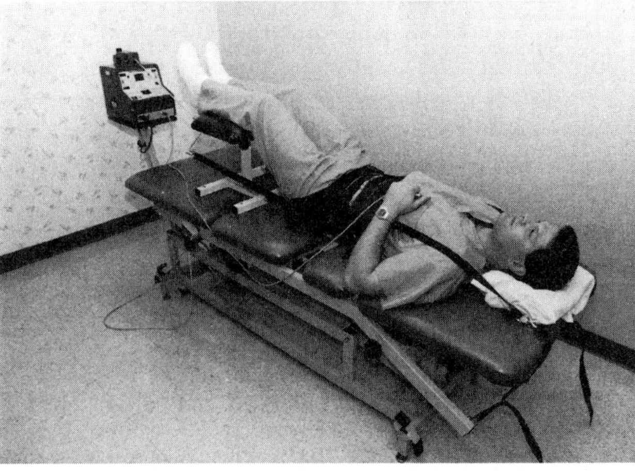

B

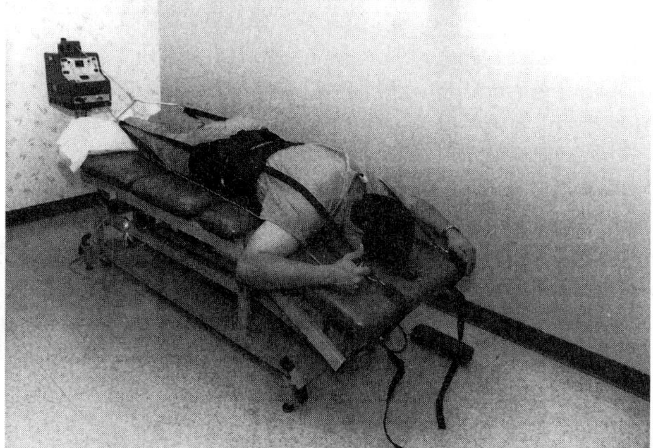

C

elongation of the intervertebral space (46). Intermittent cervical traction produces significantly improved blood flow to the neck and shoulder musculature. In patients obtaining relief from traction, surface electromyography (EMG) shows an increased recruitment of myoelectrical signals (47). A significant increase in cervical lordosis was measured in 35 nonrandomized patients 3 months following treatment with daily extension-compression cervical traction combined with chiropractic manipulation, as compared to those receiving manipulation alone or no treatment (48). This transformation to a more normal configuration may prove beneficial in patients slow to regain cervical lordosis after acute whiplash (extension-flexion) injuries (48).

Evidence supports the use of cervical traction in the supine as compared to the sitting position. The advantages include 1) greater posterior intervertebral separation, 2) increased patient relaxation, 3) decreased muscle guarding, 4) increased stability, 5) less force required to overcome head weight, 6) diminished anterior anatomic curve of the cervical region, and 7) easier ability to align the neck in proper position (49). When benefit has clearly been established and the patient is comfortable in the self-application of traction, a home unit may be obtained for daily use. Home traction units are now available for both the sitting and the supine position (see Fig. 24-3).

Lumbar Traction

Lumbar traction creates several anatomic changes previously described (see Table 24-1). In lumbar radiculopathy, traction forces create expansion of the neuroforamina that theoretically reduces pressure on the adjacent exiting nerve root (50). It should be noted, however, that other nonvertebral musculoskeletal structures are being distracted as well, since patient stature increases by as much as 9 mm after 25 minutes of lumbar traction (51). Significantly larger forces are required compared to those used for cervical traction (9,13,33). It is generally accepted that a force equivalent to 30% to 50% of the patient's body weight is needed to produce anatomic changes (34). One hundred pounds of traction force produces both anterior and posterior vertebral separation, most prominently at the L4–L5 segmental level, followed by L3–L4 and L5–S1 interspaces (34). Both computed tomography (CT) and epidurography have demonstrated a strong correlation between the reduction in the size of a disk herniation and improvement in clinical findings (52,53).

Lumbar traction can be performed using continuous, sustained, or intermittent methods. Of the 10 types of lumbar traction described in the literature, most therapists utilize bilateral, sustained, or intermittent mechanical traction (54). Unilateral lumbar traction has been theorized to be superior to bilateral lumbar traction in certain patients with protective scoliosis who would otherwise be unable to tolerate bilateral traction. Although the theory behind this treatment seems sound, very little unilateral lumbar traction is used clinically because of problems with patient positioning and adaptability of available equipment. Saunders (55) described a useful and more effective way of applying unilateral traction with conventional bilateral systems.

Autotraction was first proposed by Lind in 1974 (56). In 1984, Natchev (57) developed a simplified version of the technique. The table is divided into two movable parts that can be tilted or rotated, or both, by the therapist in order to find the position of most comfort. The patient then provides the traction force by pulling vigorously on a bar at the head of the table for a period of 3 to 6 seconds. After a 1-minute period of rest, the procedure is repeated over a 30- to 60-minute session. Within this time, the therapist moves the spine toward the former painful position, helping to restore mobility of the spine without inducing pain. When autotraction was compared to passive lumbar traction, favorable responses were more than three times greater in the autotraction group and persisted for 3 months in 63% of the responders (20). Benefit from autotraction was shown to be a strong predictor of good outcomes in patients with a herniated lumbar disk who went on to have surgical correction (58). Unfortunately, the complexity and time commitment required of the therapist to perform autotraction have limited its clinical usefulness.

Research has yet to define the most effective force, duration, or frequency of lumbar traction. Higher forces produce greater anatomic change but must be delivered intermittently and remain poorly tolerated by the patient (9). Flexion of the lumbar spinal region allows for greater patient comfort and relaxation (5). Vertebral separation can be maximized with the flexed to 70 degrees and a traction angle of 18 degrees from the horizontal (34).

One of the more recent additions to the various forms of lumbar traction therapy is termed *vertebral axial decompression*. With this method, the patient lies prone on a special motorized table, stabilizing the upper body by holding on to a set of handgrips (Fig. 24-5). The distraction force is intermittent in nature and produced through a pelvic harness. One study measured intervertebral disk pressure through a percutaneous pressure transducer and found that tensions between 50 and 100 lb could produce negative intervertebral disk pressures of up to −160 mm Hg (22). Negative pressures theoretically could facilitate disk rehydration, nutritional transfer, and fibroblast migration, thus promoting healing and repair of the annulus fibrosus. No large-sample clinical investigations have been published, but multiple case studies (50,52,55) revealed considerable efficacy of lumbar traction in the treatment of lumbar disk herniation, degenerative disk disease, and facet joint arthropathy.

Many studies assessing the efficacy of lumbar traction lacked a strong experimental design. Beurskens et al (59) conducted one of only a few randomized controlled studies comparing high-dose traction (30%–50% of total body weight) to sham traction (<20% of total body weight)

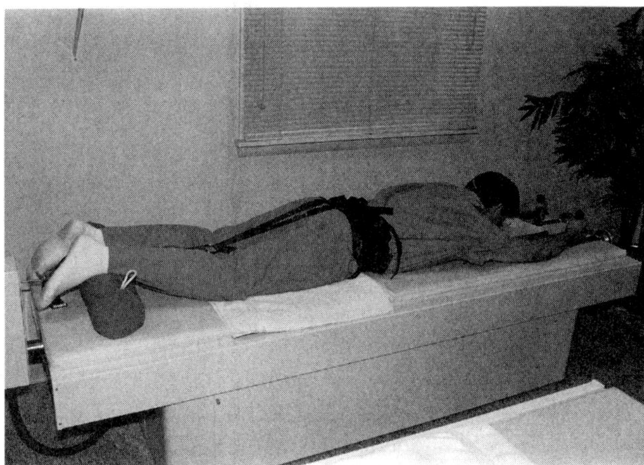

Figure 24-5. Vertebral axial decompression table. With the patient prone and holding onto the handles, the distraction forces are applied through the pelvic harness.

Table 24-2: Contraindications to Traction

General traction
Osteomyelitis or diskitis
Malignancy
Unstable fracture
Osteoporosis
Uncontrolled hypertension
Severe cardiovascular disease
Cervical traction
Central disk herniation
Hypermobility
Rheumatoid arthritis of the cervical spinal region
Carotid or vertebral artery disease
Lumbar traction
Pregnancy
Cauda equina compression
Aortic aneurism
Caution in peptic ulcer disease and gastroesophageal reflux disease
Hemorrhoids
Vertebral axial decompression
Shoulder pain
Shoulder instability
Hand weakness
Arthritis of the hand
Inability to lie prone

for 151 patients with a 6-week history of nonspecific low-back pain. Treatment was given over a 6-week period. There were no statistical differences between groups on all outcome measures (59).

Contraindications and Risks

As with any physical modality, traction is not without its negative side effects (Table 24-2). Frazer (33) reported an "untoward sequelae" rate of only 6 per 25,000 treatments with lumbar traction. The incidence for cervical traction is unpublished. In particular, lumbar inversion traction produces several adverse side effects including an increase in systolic and diastolic blood pressures, decreased heart rate, periorbital and pharyngeal petechiae, and subjective complaints of persistent blurred vision and headaches (60). Lumbar traction can decrease inspiratory vital capacity and tidal volume, while increasing respiratory rate. Patients with pulmonary disease should be observed closely for signs of respiratory distress during the first few treatments (61).

LaBan et al (62) observed that rarely, cervical traction can act as a progenitor of lumbar radicular pain. It is theorized that axial tension produced through traction forces on the dura can be transmitted to lumbar nerve roots already tethered by anatomic variants or associated degenerative changes in the lumbar region of the spine (62). Cervical traction should be discontinued whenever patients complain of increased pain in the soft tissues of the neck, persistent headache, light-headedness, dizziness, nausea, or worsening of temporomandibular joint dysfunction.

Traction of any kind is absolutely contraindicated in the presence of cord compression, diskitis, osteomyelitis, or osteoporosis. It should not be performed in patients with malignancy, rheumatoid arthritis, tuberculosis, uncontrolled hypertension, or cardiovascular disease or during pregnancy (5,63). Cervical traction should be used cautiously in patients with significant carotid or vertebral artery disease. Because lumbar traction can increase intra-abdominal pressure, physicians should prescribe it for persons with peptic ulcer disease, hiatal hernia, aortic aneurysm, or hemorrhoids only when absolutely necessary. Patients with nerve root entrapment causing neurogenic bladder should not undergo lumbar traction (see Table 24-2) (5).

Vertebral axial decompression is contraindicated in patients with shoulder pain, a history of shoulder subluxation or dislocation, decreased grip strength, arthritis of the hands, or an inability to lie prone.

Practice Guidelines

Theoretically, any patient with degeneration, protrusion, or herniation of a disk, neuroforaminal narrowing, painful facet joints, or even periaxial muscle spasm could benefit from a trial of traction. When implementing a treatment plan that includes traction, both the physician and therapist must have a clear understanding of the patient's medical and surgical history, as well as how the patient's anatomy correlates with the symptom complex. They must also have a working knowledge of the properties of collagen and the principles of thermal modalities in order to best control the elasticity of surrounding connective tissue. Clear communication is vital in selecting the correct timing and mode of traction. Experience has shown that disk protrusions are usually treated more effectively with sustained traction, while myofascial pain and degenerative disk disease respond well to intermittent traction (43).

For cervical traction, the first question in evaluating the patient is to determine whether a seated or supine position will be used. Although both positions are commonly utilized, research reveals that the supine position provides greater relaxation and vertebral separation (49). Placement of the head harness is also very important. Caution should be taken to ensure that pull is exerted to a greater degree at the occiput rather than at the chin. This ensures that a lower force is imposed on the temporomandibular joint. While research supports the use of cervical traction with the neck in flexion, comfort and the diagnosis may indicate that the patient should maintain a more neutral position (15). Though most patients cannot tolerate cervical forces over 10 to 15 lb initially, consensus indicates 20 to 30 lb is required before anatomic separation can exist.

With lumbar traction, a split table is necessary to eliminate the effects of friction and reduce restrictive forces. The use of a heavy-duty, nonslip traction harness is essential in promoting patient security and relaxation. Care should be taken to remove all slack in the harness before the split table is released. Placement of the pelvic harness is probably the most important determinant of the amount of spinal flexion achieved (43). Lumbar traction can be administered effectively in the prone or supine position. Physically, the prone position encourages more normal lumbar lordosis. Prone traction can be especially useful in the patient with disk protrusion and moderate to severe pain and muscle guarding. Although it may be impossible to place the patient in a position of normal lordosis initially, the therapist will want to work toward the goal of normal posture as treatment progresses and pain diminishes. Early on, pillows can be placed below the abdomen to promote lumbar flexion. Additionally, other modalities can be applied directly to the low back and traction can follow without moving the patient (43). Theoretically, if the intervertebral disk pressure decreases during traction, it will likely increase again after it is released. Shorter periods of traction (<10 minutes) have not been noted to elicit posttraction discomfort as frequently as prolonged sessions (43). Often, a patient with a herniated disk will have a flattened lumbar lordosis and reactive lateral scoliosis. As pain subsides, careful attention should be paid to correcting any abnormal posture that may exist. Between treatments, or once discharged from a therapy program, the patient should be instructed to avoid positions or activities that would increase intervertebral disk pressure (64,65).

Conclusions

Considerable controversy exists with regard to the various techniques currently employed to treat patients with low-back pain and sciatica associated with herniated disk and degenerative disk disease. One of the more promising noninterventional methods for relieving pressure on vital structures of the cervical or lumbar region is distraction of the vertebrae by a mechanical force applied along the axis of the spinal column. Although the theory of traction is based on sound biomechanical principles, the anatomic changes that occur are short-lived. Neurophysiologic changes occurring after traction have yet to be proved. Many studies support the use of traction for cervical and lumbar spinal disorders. Unfortunately, most were methodologically flawed. To date, the research has yet to identify clear indications for traction or determine the most effective magnitude, duration, frequency, or angle of traction for clinical use. Further randomized investigations are justified in this ever-growing field of the aggressive, nonoperative management of neck and low-back pain.

MANIPULATION

Manipulation, as used in this chapter, refers to a modality in which a practitioner passively, often forcefully, moves a bone in an attempt to improve range of motion or alignment of a joint, or both. This definition includes spinal manipulation, joint mobilization, and muscle energy techniques. The goals are often decreased pain and improved function.

History

Remains from ancient Egypt, ancient Rome, and Thailand, 2000 BC, show evidence of the use of the art of manipulation. Hippocrates (460–380 BC) described the placement of localized force over the spine along with the use of steam heat and traction for the treatment of lumbar kyphosis. Hippocrates also described other manual techniques to include massage, sitting on a patient to provide long-term pressure, and use of feet and other devices, such as padded boards, to apply localized forces (66).

Beginning in the seventeenth century, bone setters in Europe were documented using manipulation techniques. The techniques were passed on from generation to generation as a family profession. Manipulation of the spine and extremities was performed to relocate a bone that was out of place. Limited anatomic knowledge was available to help define the techniques of the bone setters. They reportedly were most successful in treating joint stiffness and pain caused by immobilization and disuse after joint or soft-tissue injury. Successful treatment of joint derangement after meniscus injury, subluxation of the small joints of the hands and feet, and pain in the cervical, thoracic, and lumbosacral regions has also been reported (67).

Andrew Taylor Still (1828–1917) founded the school of osteopathy in 1892 on the premises that the body had the ability to fight off all diseases and that all disease was the product of mechanical pressure on nerves and vessels of the vertebral spine (67,68). This mechanical pressure was believed to be caused by dislocated vertebral bones, malalignment of soft tissues, or contracted muscles in the back. Still termed the mechanical pressure on the nerves and vessels the *osteopathic lesion*. This lesion became the basis of his treatment protocol. Osteopathic medical schools have integrated the science taught in allopathic medical schools along with the techniques of manipulation. Manipulation is now taught to be used as an adjunct to nutrition, medication, and surgery.

Daniel David Palmer (1845–1914) founded the chiropractic school in 1897 with the premise that most disease was due to subluxed vertebrae interfering with the function of the spinal nerves (67,68). Palmer described realigning a subluxed vertebra by using the spinous and transverse processes as lever arms. Included in his reports is the successful treatment of deafness in one of his first patients by adjustment of a cervical vertebra. Many chiropractors recognize that the majority of diseases are not effectively treated with manipulation and now focus treatment to those with vertebral dysfunction.

General

Despite its longevity, manipulation as a method of treatment is not well received by traditional Western medicine. A survey conducted by Cherkin et al (69) showed that of the physicians who responded, more than 80% believed physical therapy was effective in the treatment of low-back pain, but less than half believed spinal manipulation was effective in the treatment of acute or chronic low-back pain. Manipulation's lack of acceptance by traditional medicine is often attributed to the lack of scientific explanation and research (70,71). The randomized studies performed to prove the benefits of manipulation did not universally show statistical significance (72–78). Cassidy et al (79) reported a randomized controlled trial which showed an immediate improvement in range of motion and a decrease in pain with manipulation. Long-term follow-up was not part of the study. Koes et al (70) performed a randomized study to evaluate the efficacy of manual therapy and physiotherapy. Treatment with analgesics, education, and rest, as well as placebo of detuned short-wave or ultrasound treatment, was also compared to the manual therapy. Although this study utilized a randomized treatment design and suggested manual therapy was better in the treatment of low-back pain than the other options, the treatment regimen for each subgroup was not standardized and varied with each individual practitioner (70). Several attempts to evaluate the effectiveness of spinal manipulation by literature review have been reported (80–82). Di Fabio (80) reviewed the literature on the efficacy of manual therapy and reported "there was a paucity of valid explanatory research in all areas and a particular absence of controlled trials involving manual therapy applied to the peripheral joints." The available research does suggest that a patient with acute (<1 month) trunk/perivertebral low-back pain would likely benefit from manipulation (80). Koes et al (81) evaluated 35 randomized clinical trials and scored them on a 17-category, 100-point scale. No trial had a score higher than 56. Twenty-three of the 35 studies reported positive results from spinal manipulation. Koes et al (81) concluded that the results from manipulation were promising, but that more research with improved methods is needed. Anderson et al (82) reviewed 23 randomized controlled trials, scored them on a 135-point scale, and applied meta-analysis. The scores of the reviewed studies ranged from 9 to 73. In a review of 58 articles, including 25 controlled trials, Skekelle et al (83) concluded that spinal manipulation is of short-term benefit in acute uncomplicated low-back pain, but data are insufficient to determine the efficacy in chronic low-back pain. The majority of studies compared manipulation with alternative treatments; few compared manipulation to no treatment. In addition to the limited objective data in support of manipulation, catastrophic complications, such as fracture and paraplegia, occur on rare occasion and strengthen the case against the use of manipulation (84–86). Even so, manipulation as a method of treatment continues to become more accepted, but continued growth in acceptance requires the demonstration of effectiveness in a scientific manner (87,88). Eisenberg et al (89) reported that one in three persons who responded to a telephone interview admitted to using unconventional therapy such as manipulation or acupuncture. The estimated expenditure for unconventional treatment in the United States in 1990 was $13.7 billion. Physical therapists and some physicians have recently begun to learn the techniques and utilize this modality (71,90). Atchison et al (91) reported widespread interest in learning manipulation techniques by residents in the physical medicine and rehabilitation specialty. Manipulation techniques are now taught in schools of osteopathy, chiropractic, physical therapy, and some medical residency programs as well as via weekend seminars, videotapes, and textbooks.

Some proponents for manipulation insist that it has the ability to cure most any disease process. On the other hand, opponents believe its adds nothing to treatment. The truth appears to lie somewhere between the two extremes. Continued scientific evaluation, to include clinical and bench research, is needed to help determine which diagnoses warrant treatment with manipulation (75,91–93). Manipulation of the cervical, thoracic, and lumbosacral regions of the spine for pain of musculoskeletal origin are currently the most accepted treatments.

Several schools of thought have developed over the past 100 years regarding the specific function of manipulation as well as the proper technique. Despite the similarities, the premise and techniques of the different schools vary. Chiropractic techniques focus on relief of nerve root pressure in the spine only and recommend manipulation of a single vertebra. Cyriax also focused on the relief of nerve root pressure in the spine, but taught general manipulation with the addition of traction. Maitland taught manipulation of spine and extremities for pain relief by graded oscillations in the direction of pain but within the pain-free range, and Maigne recommended movement in the direction opposite to that which produced pain (94). Osteopaths have many specific techniques to improve joint mobility in the spine and extremities. Kaltenborn taught techniques to treat stiffness and improve joint mobility in both the spine and extremities but based his treatment on the use of arthrokinematic principles (68).

A number of manipulation techniques have been described, including direct and indirect, cyclic and sustained loading, specific and general thrust, oscillation, and muscle energy techniques. Although providing descriptions of specific manipulation techniques is beyond the scope of this chapter, it is important to understand the basic concepts used in manipulation. Manipulative techniques move a joint, often passively, through its range of motion to and through a physiologic tissue barrier (resistance) with the goal of realignment of the joint and improved motion of the periarticular tissues. Positioning of the practitioner and the patient is important for the effectiveness and safety of each technique. The direction, localization, and application of forces are determined by the technique chosen (95).

Joint Motion

Joints have a normal orientation, defined by the articular surfaces, that allows for pain-free, static and dynamic function. The movement of joints is directed by articular surfaces and limited by bone and soft tissues. The study of the movement of bone is called *osteokinematics* and the study of movement in the joint between the articular cartilage is called *arthrokinematics*. Osteokinematic motions are described in terms of spin and swing of a particular bone on another bone. *Spin* is a pure rotation around a mechanical axis and *swing* is any movement that is not pure spin. Arthrokinematic motions are described by glide, angular movement, circumduction, and rotation of one articular cartilage with respect to another. Arthrokinematics and osteokinematics describe the same motion from different points of reference. Each joint has the potential for translation and rotation about each of the three axes (X, Y, Z) of three-dimensional space, giving six potential movements. Each potential direction of movement is termed a *degree of freedom* (96).

Each joint has a range of motion that is utilized during active range of motion and an accessory range of motion or joint play that exists outside the active range but within the range allowed by the periarticular tissues. The accessory range of motion is available only during passive motion. Although the accessory range of motion is not used during voluntary motor activity, it is required for pain-free range of motion during both active and passive movement. Manipulation utilizes the accessory range of motion to improve joint alignment, increase periarticular extensibility, facilitate pain-free movement, and maximize active and passive range of motion (67).

Tissues Properties

Tissues such as the tendons and ligaments that make up the joint capsule have elastic and plastic properties which should be understood by practitioners of manipulation. This concept is best explained utilizing the stress-strain diagram. Stress is equal to the applied force divided by the cross-sectional area of the tissue. Strain is the change in length of the tissue divided by the original length of that same tissue. Figure 24-6 is a stress-strain diagram. When the strain, change in length, caused by an applied load disappears with the removal of the load, the material is behaving elastically (segment A–B). The largest stress for which a material acts elastically is termed the *elastic limit* (stress EL). Stress applied over the elastic limit causes deformation outside of the linear range. This nonlinear region is termed the *plastic range* (beyond point B). Once the tissue is stressed into the plastic range and the stress is removed, stress and strain decrease in a linear fashion parallel to the elastic portion of the original curve—resulting in a new resting length (segment C–D). The change in resting length indicates that a "permanent" set or plastic deformation has occurred (A to D). This plastic deformation is the goal of stretching and manipulation techniques. The change in length is both stress dependent (force) and time and temperature dependent. The force-dependent portion of strain is termed *slip* and the time- and temperature-dependent portion is termed *creep*. Reloading a material that previously underwent plastic deformation causes the material to follow a loading curve similar to the previous unloading curve until the plastic range is once

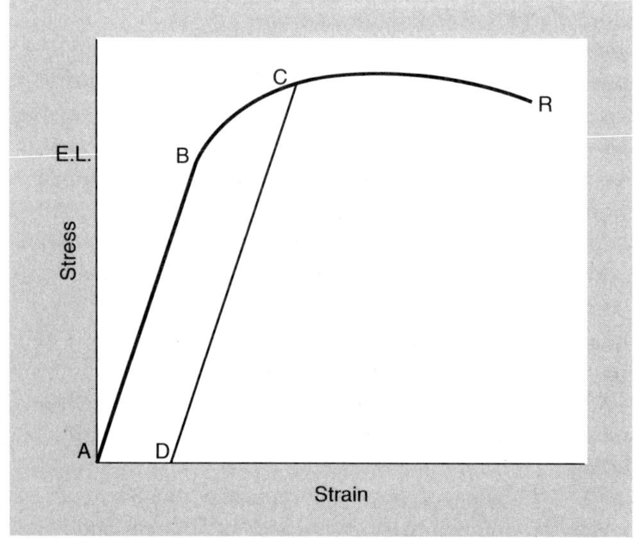

Figure 24-6. Stress-strain diagram. Segment A–B is the linear or elastic range. Segment B–C is in the plastic range. Segment A–D is plastic deformation or change in resting length. E.L. = elastic limit (stress at which material stops acting elastic); R = point of rupture.

again reached. Excessive loading can cause rupture (point R). Repetitive loading can cause rupture of the material at a stress much less than the static breaking strength. This is termed *fatigue*. The goal of manipulation, as well as stretching exercise, is to apply a force that causes the periarticular tissues to deform into the plastic region, thus increasing tissue length without reaching the point of rupture. Notice that increased time and temperature facilitate the use of force via creep (96,97).

Evaluation

Prior to applying a manipulation technique, the patient should undergo a complete evaluation to include the history and physical examination. The history should include the onset, location, radiation, quality, course, and intensity of the pain as well as a list of exacerbating and relieving factors. In addition, the precipitating event should be reviewed in a detailed fashion and previous pain or injury should be evaluated. The history should also include the patient's report of changes in strength, sensation, and function.

With the pain and dysfunction defined, the physical examination is performed to help further delineate the causative lesion and to evaluate for limitation of range, asymmetry of motion, reproduction of pain, and abnormal control of motion when the patient performs active motion. Range of motion may be limited by structural abnormalities or pain. The cause of the limitation should be documented. The position or motion that reproduces the pain should also be documented. Deviation from normal motion, such as rotation or side bending during forward flexion, should be noted. Asymmetry may also be noted by comparing an affected joint with an unaffected joint on the opposite side (95).

Passive range of motion can reveal positions of pain, limitation of range of motion, laxity, or disruption of joint structures. Deep palpation, starting in an area free of pain, can be used to evaluate muscle tone, tissue thickness, areas of tenderness, and location of positional faults. More specifically, a procedure called *passive intervertebral motion testing* of the vertebral spine uses digital palpation on a facet joint or interspinous space to classify the joint motion available into one of six categories on the Passive Intervertebral Motion (PIVM) grading scale (Table 24-3). Joints receiving a grade 1 or 2 may benefit from manipulation (95,96).

The practitioner uses the collected information to determine whether manipulation is safe and warranted and which technique should be utilized. A single treatable lesion that explains all the patient's symptoms should be sought.

Effects

Manipulation has been used for centuries for the treatment of multiple disorders, but few scientifically sound studies have been conducted to document its efficacy. Rather, justification for using manipulation as a treatment modality is based on the unconfirmed results of the individual practitioner and the theoretical benefits that are believed to be possible. These theories include mechanical, neurophysiologic, and psychological effects (67,95).

Table 24-3: Grading of Passive Intervertebral Motion (PIVM)

Grade	Description	Criteria
0	Ankylosed	No detectable movement within the segment
1	Extremely hypomobile	Decrease in expected range and significant resistance to motion
2	Slightly hypomobile	Limitation in expected range and some resistance to motion
3	Normal	Expected range with uniform resistance through range
4	Slightly hypermobile	Some increase in range and less than expected resistance
5	Extremely hypermobile	Excessive range with eventual soft-tissue limitation
6	Unstable	Excessive range without soft-tissue limitation

Mechanical

Manipulation of a joint allows the soft tissues of the joint capsule, including the ligaments, to regain lost flexibility and the ability to stretch. The myofascial tissues surrounding the joints are also thought to gain flexibility. Formation of intra-articular and extra-articular adhesions occurs after a variety of injuries and periods of immobilization. Manipulation is believed to rupture the abnormal cross-links between the fibers of these adhesions, resulting in improved joint motion (89,98).

A minor alignment abnormality of articular surfaces is called a *positional fault*. A positional fault can result in abnormal stress on articular surfaces as well as limit motion and produce pain. The increased stress can result in damage to the articular cartilage. A positional fault can occur between facet joints of the vertebral spine as well as in the joints of the extremities. Restoration of proper alignment, with elimination of a positional fault, is a theoretical mechanical effect of manipulation. The purpose of manipulation is often the correction of a positional fault to produce subsequent improvement in range of motion and reduce pain.

Some practitioners attempt treatment of intervertebral disk herniations with manipulation. The hypothesis is that during spinal manipulation, sufficient negative pressure develops in the disk to draw the material back into the intervertebral space. Once again, no scientific data exist to substantiate this hypothesis. Manipulation can also be used to release a trapped intracapsular meniscus. This structure, present in the facet joint of the vertebra, can cause locking of the two joint structures with subsequent pain and limitation of motion.

Twomey (99) reported in a 1992 review that the theories pertaining to adjusting joint subluxations, restoring bony alignment, and reducing herniated disk material have no factual basis and the success of manipulation is simply because collagen, muscle, and bone require movement of joints to maintain the health of the tissues. The effects of immobilization on soft tissues are well documented and will not be repeated here (100–102).

Neurophysiologic

The activation of mechanoreceptors during manipulation and stretching of the periarticular tissues is hypothesized to have an inhibitory effect on the presynaptic cells of the substantia gelatinosa. According to the Melzak and Wall's "gate control theory," this inhibitory effect depresses nociceptive activity (103,104). Wyke (105) postulated that the perception of pain from a spinal lesion is inversely proportional to the mechanoreceptor activity in an embryologic-related spinal tissue. Stretch during manipulation activates type III mechanoreceptors, which are thought to have a direct reflex inhibitory effect on associated musculature, causing relaxation of the associated muscles (105–107). The activation of mechanoreceptors may also improve proprioceptive input and thus improve posture and kinematics (108).

A positional fault can cause the abnormal opposition of joint surfaces. The opposition of these surfaces is believed to cause increased tone in periarticular muscle through an overreaction of the associated γ motor neuron. The γ motor neuron causes the muscle fibers to be hypersensitive and with time, they become shortened. The shortened and hypersensitive muscles in turn increase the pressure on the opposed joint surfaces. This cycle is believed to be broken by the movement of the affected joint and stretching of affected tissues during manipulation.

Psychological

Pain often has an emotional component. This emotional factor can often be assessed when performing the history and physical examination. From a purely psychological standpoint, the laying of hands on a person often will have a calming effect as well as a placebo effect.

Indications and Contraindications

The indications for manipulation are pain and limitation of function secondary to a joint or soft-tissue lesion that has caused malalignment or limitation of motion. This modality is most often applied to the vertebral spine, but can be used for extremity joints. As mentioned already, catastrophic complications have occurred following manipulation. The avoidance of these complications is aided by carefully choosing patients. Patients with hemophilia, osteoporosis, acutely inflamed joints, recent fracture, or acute radiculopathy are at risk for complications that outweighs the benefits of manipulation. Manipulation has the potential to spread local infection or malignancy, damage the epiphyseal plate in a child, worsen spinal cord compression, or decrease cranial blood flow in a patient with vertebral artery insufficiency. Patients with long-standing rheumatoid arthritis or Down syndrome are at increased risk for odontoid subluxation. Table 24-4 lists contraindications that are intended to guide the clinician but are not intended to replace clinical judgment (107).

Table 24-4: Contraindications to Manipulation
Local infection
Local malignancy
Acute or subacute fracture
Spinal cord compression, including cauda equina
Vertebral artery insufficiency
Acutely inflamed joints
Rheumatoid arthritis or Down syndrome (increased risk of odontoid subluxation)
Spondylolisthesis with symptoms
Acute radiculopathy
Children prior to closure of the epiphyseal plates
Joint instability
Last trimester of pregnancy
Bleeding disorder (genetic, acquired, or iatrogenic)
Osteoporosis
Acute whiplash injury

Conclusions

Manipulation should be considered a modality that is added to a complete treatment plan. Careful evaluation of patients is required to determine which patients would benefit from this modality (93). Treatments to help facilitate the action of the manipulation include stretching programs, to help the patient maintain range of motion, and strengthening programs and improvements in posture, to help the patient maintain the alignment gained with manipulation.

Further research is warranted to help prove the efficacy of manipulation and further define the indications for the various treatments.

MASSAGE

Massage, as used in this chapter, is a modality in which manual stimulation is applied superficially to affect the skin, muscles, ligaments, tendons, or other soft tissues, as well as the flow of venous blood and lymph from a region of the body. The stimulation can be one of many forms, including stroke, friction, vibration, percussion, kneading, stretching, and compression.

History

Massage, like manipulation, is an ancient art with written descriptions that date back to 2000 BC. Historic medical literature from Ancient Egypt, Persia, and Japan all show references to massage. Hippocrates (460–377 BC) specifically described the benefits of massage (109).

The modern version of massage is believed to have been introduced to the West via a French translation of an ancient Chinese book, *The Cong-Fou of the Tao-Tse.* The French terms for the massage strokes continue to be used throughout much of the modern world. Per Henrick Ling (1776–1839) from Sweden is credited with organizing and describing massage techniques that became known as the *Swedish massage* and served as the basis for the "standard" massage (110,111).

General

Much like manipulation, massage has little objective research to support its use and has yet to be fully embraced by the mainstream of modern medical science. In the last century, the massage community has worked to ensure quality among its practitioners by regulating schools and establishing national organizations. The American Massage Therapy Association (AMTA) was founded in 1943 and has chapters in all 50 states and 20 countries. Membership is around 25,000. AMTA publishes the *Massage Therapy Journal.* AMTA accredits training programs via its Commission on Massage Training Accreditation/Approval. Three hundred hours of training in therapy, 100 hours of course work on anatomy and physiology, and 100 hours of other course contents are required.

Massage can be subcategorized as Swedish massage, sports massage, reflexology, and shiatsu and acupressure.

Classic massage developed from Swedish massage and consists of a series of motions to include pétrissage, kneading, friction, stroking, and effleurage (112).

Pétrissage is the application of firm but gentle pressure in a rhythmic fashion while gently grasping the underlying tissues within their own contours and lifting and squeezing them. The skin should move with the fingers. Movement is accomplished by gliding of the hands and occurs in a centripetal pattern.

Kneading lifts, squeezes, and moves larger amounts of tissue than pétrissage, but in a similar fashion. The centripetal pattern and the rhythmic application of pressure are similar, but in kneading the circular pattern is performed with each of the two hands working in opposite directions.

Friction massage is carried out with the fingers or ball of the thumb applying pressure in a slow circular pattern. It is used on small areas with scar tissue. Friction massage should be started lightly, with pressure advanced as tolerated.

Stroking and effleurage, glide or stroke, can be either superficial or deep. Superficial stroking can be in centripetal or centrifugal patterns with only the lightest touch to maintain contact. Deep stroking should be performed in the direction of lymph or venous drainage and requires application of firm pressure.

Tapotement is the technique of applying light "chops" in series with the ulnar border of the hand.

Sports massage is massage therapy that focuses on the muscles. Knowledge of the individual sports and the muscles used in the sport is integral to sports massage (113–120). Some high-profile athletes use massage to prepare them to compete. Callaghan (117) reported the results of a literature review in 1993 stating that although the subjective reports suggest massage is beneficial to athletes, little agreement is documented in the literature on the efficacy of massage and more study is required. Benefits of sports massage are reported to be improvement in performance and limitation of injuries. Sports massage was an integral part of the Summer Olympic Games in Atlanta in 1996. Medical services included 120 massage therapists who were chosen to assist during the games.

Reflexology is a massage system based on a series of points in the hands and feet that are believed to correspond to a reflex pattern in all areas of the body. Treatment consists of compression of the feet or hands by firm pressure from the thumbs of the practitioner. The treatments are concentrated over the areas of tenderness (110,121).

Shiatsu and *acupressure* are both massage techniques that utilize pressure applied by fingers over predetermined points. The pressure points used in acupressure are derived using the same theories and meridians as those of acupuncture. These meridians are based on theoretical energy-flow lines in the body. Shiatsu, on the other hand, is derived from traditional Japanese massage, called *Anma,* with a more anatomic and physiologic basis (110).

Short treatments are reported to be more beneficial than prolonged treatments. The amount of pressure applied, use of powders or oils, rhythm of application, and duration and frequency of treatment are also important variables in the use of the massage as a therapeutic modality (109). Specific programs have been developed for pediatric massage (122–125) and geriatric massage, as well as pet massage.

Effects

The theoretical mechanical effects of massage include improved circulation, breakdown of soft-tissue adhesions, and activation of the peripheral nervous system. Arterial flow, venous return, and lymphatic flow are all theoretically improved with massage (126,127). The improvement in the peripheral circulation includes improvement in the local circulation with subsequent improvement in local nutrition and removal of waste products. This helps to decrease aches in muscles and to facilitate healing. Improvements of edema and induration are also seen with improved circulation. The breakdown of soft-tissue adhesions, such as fibrosis or scar tissue, improves flexibility of the joints, ligaments, and tendons. Activation of the peripheral nervous system is thought to help via the gate control theory of Melzak and Wall and the inhibition of overactive proprioceptors (103,104,110,111,113,114, 128,129).

Ironson et al (130) reported that therapeutic massage enhanced the cytotoxic capacity of the immune system in individuals infected with the human immunodeficiency virus (HIV). Clinical implications for HIV-positive patients and other patients are not yet determined.

As mentioned already, the laying of hands on a patient has a placebo and a calming effect, which adds to the mechanical and physiologic effects.

Indications

Although some research has been completed, current indications for massage are based on clinical experience and theory. Massage as a modality to facilitate other medical treatment is indicated in many causes of pain and limited function. Massage can be used with manipulation and other modalities for the treatment of limited motion of joints or other structures caused by fibrosis. Treatment of trigger points and myofascial pain has been documented (131–133). Massage can be used effectively to mobilize the fluid causing edema or lymphedema. Treatment of lymphedema is important in the postmastectomy patient and self-massage or professional massage is a proven treatment (134–138). The pain and spasm in individuals with upper motor neuron injuries can be decreased with massage. Massage has been used successfully in the treatment of neuromas, postherpetic neuralgia, and reflex sympathetic dystrophy. Finally, massage can be used to treat the stress and tension that occur with everyday life. In addition to the more traditional uses of massage, sports massage is becoming more popular. Massage can be used to help athletes prepare for competition as well as to "cool down" after competition. Table 24-5 lists the indications for massage (139). The avoidance of complications is aided by carefully choosing patients. Massage has the potential to worsen inflammatory or traumatic arthritis, bursitis, phlebitis, and entrapment neuropathies; can cause the spread of local infection or malignancy; and can cause bleeding in patients with hemophilia or anticoagulation. Table 24-6 lists contraindications and is intended to guide the clinician but is not intended to replace clinical judgment. Massage should at no time cause pain, ecchymosis, or swelling (98,140).

Table 24-5: Indications for Massage
Contracture of joints
Fibrosis of ligaments or muscles
Hypertonicity
Muscle cramps
Strains and sprains
Tendonitis/tenosynovitis
Edema
Lymphedema
Neuroma
Postherpetic neuralgia
Stress/tension

Table 24-6: Contraindications to Massage
Local malignancy
Local infection (cellulitis)
Calcification of soft tissues
Inflammatory arthritis (rheumatic, gout, infective)
Traumatic arthritis
Bursitis
Entrapment neuropathy
Phlebitis or lymphangitis
Open wound
Bleeding disorder (genetic, acquired, or iatrogenic)

CONCLUSIONS

As direct extensions of the contact between physicians and patients, traction, manipulation, and massage have been commonly used treatment modalities for painful disorders. Although described in ancient literature, these techniques have only begun to gain general acceptance in the last 50 years. The preponderance of studies presented in the literature are methodologically flawed and current clinical practice is based on subjective experience and limited biomechanical studies focused on the anatomic changes created.

Traction is the application of forces in direct opposition to one another to create a separation in joint spaces. Traction can be applied to the cervical or lumbar region of the spine. It can be administered manually or mechanically via weights and pulleys or motorized systems. It may be applied in a sustained or intermittent fashion. Manipulation is the passive, often forceful, movement of a joint in an attempt to improve range of motion and correct anatomic alignment. Manipulation techniques include direct and indirect, cyclic and sustained loading, specific and general thrust, oscillation, and muscle energy techniques. Massage is the superficial application of manual stimulation to affect the skin, muscle, ligaments, tendons, or other soft tissues and the circulation of blood and lymph. Massage techniques include stroke, friction, vibration, percussion, kneading, stretching, and compression.

Each of these forms of treatment appears to have some temporary anatomic, physiologic, and psychological effects. The hypotheses behind these changes, however, remain unproved. Sound clinical studies into the effective application of traction, manipulation, and massage are still needed before they can be considered standard components in the treatment program for painful musculoskeletal disorders.

REFERENCES

1. Frymoyer JW. Back pain and sciatica. *N Engl J Med* 1988; 381:291–300.
2. Kelsey JL, White AA. Epidemiology and impact of low back pain. *Spine* 1980;5:133–142.
3. Kelsey JL. *Epidemiology of musculoskeletal disorders.* New York: Oxford University Press, 1982: 145–167.
4. Bigos S, Bowyer O, Braen G, et al. *Acute low back problems in adults. Clinical practice guideline, quick reference guide NO. 14.* Rockville, MD: U.S. Department of Health and Human Services, Public Health Service, Agency for Health Care Policy and Research, December 1994. AHCPR publication no. 95-0643.
5. Hinterbuchner C. Traction. In: Basmajian JB, ed. *Manipulation, traction and massage.* Baltimore: Williams & Wilkins, 1985:172–201.
6. van der Heijden GJ, Beurskens AJ, Koes BW, et al. The efficacy of traction for back and neck pain: a systematic, blinded review of randomized clinical trial methods. *Phys Ther* 1995;75: 73–104.
7. Hoehler FK, Tobis JS, Buerger AA. Spinal manipulation for low back pain. *JAMA* 1981;245: 1835–1838.
8. Crue BL, Todd EM. Importance of flexion in cervical traction for radiculitis. *USAF Med J* 1957;8: 374–380.
9. Crisp EJ, Cyriax J, Christie BJ. Discussion of the treatment of backache by traction. *Proc R Soc Med (Sect Phys Med)* 1995;48: 805–814.
10. Lehmann JF, Brunner GD. A device for the application of heavy lumbar traction; its mechanical affects. *Arch Phy Med Rehabil* 1958;39:696–700.
11. Judovich BD. Herniated cervical disks: a new form of traction therapy. *Am J Surg* 1952;84: 646–656.
12. Judovich BD. Lumbar traction therapy and dissipated force factors. *Lancet* 1954;74:411.
13. Judovich BD. Lumbar traction therapy—elimination of physical factors that prevent lumbar stretch. *JAMA* 1955;159: 549–550.
14. Judovich BD, Nobel GR. Traction therapy: a study of resistance forces. *Am J Surg* 1957;93:108.
15. Colachis SC Jr, Strohm BR. A study of tractive forces and angle of pull on vertebral interspaces in the cervical spine. *Arch Phys Med Rehabil* 1965;46:820–830.
16. Colichis SC Jr, Strohm BR. Cervical traction: relationship of traction time to varied tractive force with constant angle of pull. *Arch Phys Med Rehabil* 1965;46:815–819.
17. Colichis SC Jr, Strohm BR. Effects of duration of intermittent cervical traction on vertebral separation. *Arch Phys Med Rehabil* 1966;47:353–359.
18. Gillstrom P, Ehrmberg A. Long-term results of autotraction in the treatment of lumbego and sciatica. *Arch Orthop Trauma Surg* 1985;104:294–298.
19. Rogoff JB. Motorized intermittent traction. In: Basmajian JB. ed. *Manipulation, traction and massage.* Baltimore: Williams & Wilkins, 1985:201–207.
20. Tesio L, Merlo A. Autotraction versus passive traction: an open controlled study in lumbar disk herniation. *Arch Phys Med Rehabil* 1993;74:871–876.
21. Anderson GB, Schultz AB, Nachemson AL. Intravertebral disk pressures during traction. *Scand J Rehabil Med Suppl* 1983;9:88–91.
22. Ramos G, Martin W. Effects of vertebral axial decompression in intradiskal pressure. *J Neurosurg* 1994;81:350–353.
23. Larson DL, Evans EB. Skeletal suspension and traction in the treatment of burns. *Ann Surg* 1968;168:981.
24. Sheviaridze GL, Gridor-eva VD. Traction of the lower extremities in treating and rehabilitating osteoarthritis patients. *Vopr Kurortol Fizioter Lech Fiz Kult* 1995;5:19–21.
25. Newton PO, Mabarak SJ. The use of modified Neufeld's skeletal traction in children and adolescents. *J Pediatr Orthop* 1995;15: 467–469.
26. Daoud A, Saighi-Bououina A. Congenital dislocation of the hip in the older child. The effectiveness of overhead traction. *J Bone Joint Surg Am* 1996;78:30–40.
27. Gumanski R, Miodonski W, Ostrowski M, et al. Treatment outcome for displastic hip after overhead traction. *Chir Narzadow Ruc-hu Ortop Pol* 1995;60: 491–494.
28. Suzuki S, Kashiwagi N, Kasahara Y, et al. Avascular necrosis and the Pablik harness. The incidence of avascular necrosis in three types of congenital dislocation of the hip as classified by ultrasound. *J Bone Joint Surg [Br]* 1996;78:631–635.

29. Murray KA, McIntyre FH. Active traction splinting for proximal interphalangeal joint injuries. *Ann Plast Surg* 1995;35:15–18.

30. Naigne R. *Orthopaedic medicine: a new approach to vertebral manipulations.* Springfield, IL: Thomas, 1972.

31. Nayak NN. Cervical traction: prescription patterns. *Arch Phys Med Rehabil* 1993;74:1268. Abstract.

32. Cyriax J. Conservative treatment of lumbar disk lesions. *Physiotherapy* 1964;50:300–303.

33. Frazer EH. The use of traction in backache. *Med J Aust* 1954;41: 694–697.

34. Colachis SC Jr, Strohm BR. Effects of intermittent traction on separation of lumbar vertebrae. *Arch Phys Med Rehabil* 1969;50:251–258.

35. Wong AMK, Leong CP, Chen C. The traction angle and cervical intervertebral separation. *Spine* 1992;17:136–138.

36. Jackson R. *The cervical syndrome.* Springfield, IL: Thomas, 1958.

37. Souzacos PK, Souzacos PN, Bevis AE. Scoliosis elasticity assessed by manual traction: 49 juvenile and adolescent idiopathic cases. *Acta Orthop Scand* 1996;67:169–172.

38. Cyriax J, Russell G. *Textbook of orthopaedic medicine.* Vol II: *treatment by manipulation, massage and injection.* London: Bailliere Tindall, 1980.

39. Greenman PE. *Principals of manual medicine.* Baltimore: Williams & Wilkins, 1989.

40. Grieve GP. *Mobilisation of the spine: a primary handbook of clinical method.* New York: Churchill Livingstone, 1991.

41. Gillstrom P, Ericson K, Hindmarsh T. Autotraction in lumbar disk herniation. *Arch Orthop Trauma Surg* 1985;104: 207–210.

42. Gillstrom P, Ericson K, Hindmarsh T. Computed tomography examination of the influence of autotraction on herniation of the lumbar disk. *Arch Orthop Trauma Surg* 1985;104:289–293.

43. Saunders HD. Mechanical agents: traction. In: Scully RM, ed. *Physical therapy.* Philadelphia: JB Lippincott, 1989:901–908.

44. Zylbergold RS, Piper MC. Cervical spine disorders. A comparison of three types of traction, cervical. *Spine* 1985;10:867–871.

45. Moraes AC, Serdeira A, Pereiva Filho A, et al. Soft tissue injury associated with traumatic locked facets in the cervical spine. *Paraplegia* 1995;33:434–436.

46. Chen YG, Li SB, Huang CD. Biomechanics of traction for treatment of lumbar disk prolapse. *Chin Med J* 1994;74:40–42.

47. Nanno M. Effects of intermittent cervical traction on muscle pain. Flowmetric and electromyographic studies of the cervical paraspinal muscles. *J Nippon Med Sch* 1994;61:137–147.

48. Harrison DD, Jackson BL, Troyanovich J, et al. The efficacy of cervical extension-compression traction combined with diversified manipulation and drop table adjustments in the rehabilitation of cervical lordosis: a pilot study. *J Manipulative Physiol Ther* 1994;17:454–464.

49. Deets D, Hands KL, Hopp SS. Cervical traction. A comparison of sitting and supine positions. *Phys Ther* 1977;57:255–261.

50. Creighton DS. Positional distraction, a radiological confirmation. *J Manual Manipulative Ther* 1993;1:83–86.

51. Bridger RS, Ossey S, Fourie G. Effect of lumbar traction on stature. *Spine* 1990;15: 522–524.

52. Gupta RC, Ramaro SV. Epidurography in reduction of lumbar disk prolapse by traction. *Arch Phys Med Rehabil* 1978;59:322–327.

53. Pio A, Rendina M, Benazzio F, et al. Computed tomography changes after conservative treatment for lumbar disk herniation *Acta Radiol* 1994;35:415–419.

54. Pellechecchia GL. Lumbar traction: a review of the literature. *J Orthop Sports Phys Ther* 1994; 20:262–267.

55. Saunders HD. Unilateral lumbar traction. *Phys Ther* 1981;61: 221–225.

56. Lind GAM. Autotraction treatment of low back pain and sciatica. Thesis. University of Linköping, Sweden, 1974.

57. Natchev E. *Manual on autotraction for low back Pain.* Stockholm: Folksam Scientific Council, 1984:1–319.

58. Barrios C, Ahmeb M, Arrotegrei J, et al. Clinical factors predicting outcome after surgery for herniated lumbar disks: an epidemiological multivariant analysis. *J Spinal Disord* 1990;3:205–209.

59. Beurskens AJ, deVet HC, Kocke AJ, et al. Efficacy of traction for non-specific low back pain: a randomised clinical trial. *Lancet* 1995;346:1596–1600.

60. Gianakopoulos G, Waylonis TW, Grant PA, et al. Inversion devices: role in producing lumbar distraction. *Arch Phys Med Rehabil* 1985;66:100–102.

61. Quain MB, Tecklin JS. Lumbar traction: its effect on restoration. *Phys Ther* 1985;65:1343–1346.

62. LaBan MM, Macy JA, Meerschaert JR. Intermittent cervical traction: a progenitor of lumbar radicular pain. *Arch Phys Med Rehabil* 1992;73:295–296.

63. Yates DAH. Indications and contra-indications for spinal traction. *Physiotherapy* 1972;58: 55–57.

64. Nachemson A. The load of lumbar disks in different positions of the body. *Clin Orthop* 1966;45:107–122.

65. Nachemson A, Elsftrom G. Intravital dynamic pressure measurements in lumbar disks. A study of common movements, maneuvers and exercises. *Scand J Rehabil Med* 1971;2:1.

66. Harris JD. History and development of manipulation and mobilization. In: Basmajian JV, ed. *Manipulation, traction and massage*. Baltimore: Williams & Wilkins, 1985:3–21.

67. Bourdillon JF, Day EA, eds. *Spinal manipulation*. Norwalk, CT: William Heinemann Medical, 1987:1–40.

68. Barak T, Rosen E, Sofer R. Mobility: passive orthopaedic manual therapy. In: Gould JA, Davies GJ, eds. *Orthopaedic and sports physical therapy*. St. Louis: Mosby, 1985:212–227.

69. Cherkin DC, Deyo RA, Wheeler K, Ciol MA. Physician views about treating low back pain. The results of a national survey. *Spine* 1995;20:1–10.

70. Koes BW, Bouter LM, Van Mameren H, et al. A randomized clinical trial of manual therapy and physiotherapy for persistent back and neck complaints: subgroup analysis and relationship between outcome measures. *J Manipulative Physiol Ther* 1993;16:211–219.

71. Farrell JP, Jensen GM. Manual therapy: a critical assessment of role in the profession of physical therapy. *Phys Ther* 1992;72: 843–852.

72. Blomberg S, Hallin G, Grann K, et al. Manual therapy with steroid injections—a new approach to treatment of low back pain. A controlled multicenter trial with an evaluation by orthopedic surgeons. *Spine* 1994;19:569–577.

73. Nilsson N. A randomized controlled trial of the effect of spinal manipulation in the treatment of cervicogenic headache. *J Manipulative Physiol Ther* 1995;18: 435–440.

74. Sheer SJ, Radack KL, O'Brien DR. Randomized controlled trials in industrial low back pain relating to return to work. Part 1. Acute interventions. *Arch Phys Med Rehabil* 1995;76:966–973.

75. Nilsson N, Christensen HW, Hartvigsen J. Lasting changes in passive range of motion after spinal manipulation: a randomized, blind, controlled trial. *J Manipulative Physiol Ther* 1996;19:165–168.

76. Boline PD, Kassak K, Bronfort G, et al. Spinal manipulation vs. amitriptyline for the treatment of chronic tension-type headaches: a randomized clinical trial. *J Manipulative Physiol Ther* 1995;18:148–154.

77. Hsieh CY, Phillips RB, Adams AH, Pope MH. Functional outcomes of low back pain: comparison of four treatment groups in a randomized controlled trial. *J Manipulative Physiol Ther* 1992;15:4–9.

78. Pope MH, Phillips RB, Haugh LD, et al. A prospective, randomized three week trial of spinal manipulation, transcutaneous muscle stimulation, massage and corset in the treatment of subacute low back pain. *Spine* 1994;19:2571–2577.

79. Cassidy JD, Lopes AA, Yong-Hing K. The immediate effect of manipulation versus mobilization on pain and range of motion in the cervical spine: a randomized controlled trial. *J Manipulative Physiol Ther* 1992;15:570–575.

80. Di Fabio RP. Efficacy of manual therapy. *Phys Ther* 1992;72: 853–864.

81. Koes BW, Assendelft WJJ, van der Heijden MG, et al. Spinal manipulation and mobilization for back and neck pain: a blinded review. *BMJ* 1991;303: 1298–1303.

82. Skekelle PG, Adams AH, Chassin MR, et al. Spinal manipulation for low-back pain. *Ann Intern Med* 1992;117:590–598.

83. Anderson R, Meeker WC, Wirick BE, et al. A meta-analysis of clinical trials of spinal manipulation. *J Manipulative Physiol Ther* 1992;15:181–194.

84. Senstad O, Leboeuf-Yde C, Borchgrevink CF. Side-effects of chiropractic manipulation: types, frequency, discomfort and course. *Scand J Prim Health Care* 1996;14:50–53.

85. Assendelft WJ, Bouter SM, Knipschild PG. Complications of spinal manipulation: a comprehensive review of the literature. *J Fam Pract* 1996;42:475–480.

86. Crowther ER. Missed cervical spine fractures: the importance of reviewing radiographs in chiropractic practice. *J Manipulative Physiol Ther* 1995;18:29–33.

87. Fitzgerald GK, McClure PW, Beattie P, Riddle DL. Issues in determing effectiveness of manual therapy. *Phys Ther* 1994;74:227–233.

88. Lowry F. "Scientific" chiropractors hope to improve status of chiropractic within scientific community. *Can Med Assoc J* 1995;152:402–404.

89. Eisenberg DM, Kessler RC, Foster C, et al. Unconventional medicine in the United States. Prevalence, costs, and patterns of use. *N Engl J Med* 1993;328:246–252.

90. Fisher P, Ward A. Complementary medicine in Europe. *BMJ* 1994; 309:107–111.

91. Atchison JW, Newman RL, Klim GV. Interest in manual medicine among residents in physical medicine and rehabilitation. The need for increased instruction. *Am J Phys Med Rehabil* 1995;74: 439–443.

92. Koes BW, Bouter LM, van der Heijden GJ. Methodological quality of randomized clinical trials on treatment efficacy in low back pain. *Spine* 1995;20: 228–235.

93. Shekelle PG, Hurwitz EL, Coulter I, et al. The appropriateness of chiropractic spinal manipulation for low back pain: a pilot study. *J Manipulative Physiol Ther* 1995;18:265–270.

94. Koury MJ, Scarpelli E. A manual therapy approach to evaluation and treatment of a patient with chronic lumbar nerve root irritation. *Phys Ther* 1994;74: 548–560.

95. Nyberg R. Role of physical therapists in spinal manipulation. In: Basmajian JV, ed. *Manipulation, traction and massage*. Baltimore: Williams & Wilkins, 1985:22–45.

96. Edmond SL, ed. *Manipulation and mobilization: extremity and spinal techniques.* St. Louis: Mosby 1993:1–21.

97. Beer FP, Johnston ER, eds. *Mechanics of materials.* New York: McGraw-Hill, 1981:17–41.

98. Geiringer SR, deLateur BJ. Physiatric therapeutics. 3. Traction, manipulation and massage. *Arch Phys Med Rehabil* 1990;71(4-S):S264–S262.

99. Twomey LT. A rationale for the treatment of back pain and joint pain by manual therapy. *Phys Ther* 1992;72:885–892.

100. Amiel D, Wallace CD, Harwood FL. The effects of immobilization on the maturation of the anterior cruciate ligament of the rabbit knee. *Iowa Orthop J* 1994;14: 134–140.

101. Harwood FL, Amiel D. Differential metabolic responses of periarticular ligaments and tendon to joint immobilization. *J Applied Physiol* 1992;72:1687–1691.

102. Kannus P, Jozsa L, Kvist M, et al. The effect of immobilization on myotendinous junction: an ultrastructural, histochemical and immunohistochemical study. *Acta Physiol Scand* 1992;144: 387–394.

103. Melzack R, Wall PD. Pain mechanisms: a new theory. *Science* 1965;150:971–977.

104. Melzack R. The gate control theory 25 years later: new perspectives in phantom limb pain. In: Bond MR, Charlton JE, Woolf CJ, eds. *Proceedings of the VIth World Congress on Pain.* Amsterdam: Elsevier, 1991:9–21.

105. Wyke B. Neurological aspects of low back pain. In: Jayson M, ed. *The lumbar spine and back pain.* New York: Grune & Stratton, 1987:56–99.

106. Paris SV. *The spine course notebook.* Atlanta: Institute Press, 1979:21–30.

107. Brunner P, Khan K. *Principles and treatment in clinical sports medicine.* New York: McGraw-Hill, 1993:116–118.

108. Pickar JG, McLain RF. Responses of mechanosensitive afferents to manipulation of the lumbar facet in the cat. *Spine* 1995;20: 2379–2385.

109. Ginsburg F, Famaey JP. A double-blind study of topical massage with rado-salil ointment in mechanical low back pain. *J Int Med Res* 1987;15(3):148–153.

110. Tappan FM, ed. *Healing massage techniques: holistic, classic, and emerging methods.* Norwalk, CT: Appleton & Lange, 1988:3–33, 183, 255.

111. Fritz S, ed. *Mosby's fundamentals of therapeutic massage.* St. Louis: Mosby Lifeline, 1995: 3–102.

112. Hofkosh JM. Classical massage. In: Basmajian JV, ed. *Manipulation, traction and massage.* Baltimore: Williams & Wilkins, 1985: 263–269.

113. Goats GC. Massage—the scientific basis of an ancient art: part 1. *Br J Sports Med* 1994;28: 149–152.

114. Goats GC. Massage—the scientific basis of an ancient art: part 2. *Br J Sports Med* 1994;28: 153–156.

115. Smith LL, Keating MN, Holbert D, et al. The effects of athletic massage on delayed onset muscle soreness, creatine kinase, and neutrophil count: a preliminary report. *J Orthop Sports Phys Ther* 1994;19:93–99.

116. Tiidus PM, Shoemaker JK. Effleurage massage, muscle blood flow and long term post-exercise strength recovery. *Int J Sports Med* 1995;16:478–483.

117. Callaghan MJ. The role of massage in the management of the athlete: a review. *Br J Sports Med* 1993;27:28–33.

118. Rodenberg JB, Steenbeek D, Schiereck P, Bar PR. Warm-up, stretching and massage diminish harmful effects of eccentric exercise. *Int J Sports Med* 1994;15: 414–419.

119. Weber MD, Servedio FJ, Woodall WR. The effects of three modalities on delayed onset muscle soreness. *J Orthop Sports Phys Ther* 1994;20:236–242.

120. Cafarelli E, Flint F. The role of massage in preparation for and recovery from exercise. An overview. *Sports Med* 1992;14: 1–9.

121. Lynn J. Using complementary therapies: reflexology. *Prof Nurse* 1996;11:321–322.

122. Field T. Massage therapy for infants and children. *J Dev Behav Pediatr* 1995;16: 105–111.

123. Scafidi FA, Field T, Schanberg SM. Factors that predict which preterm infants benefit most from massage therapy. *J Dev Behav Pediatr* 1993;14:176–180.

124. Field T, Morrow C, Valdeon C, et al. Massage reduces anxiety in child and adolescent psychiatric patients. *J Am Acad Child Adolesc Psychiatry* 1992;31: 125–131.

125. Scafidi FA, et al. Effect of tactile/kinesthetic stimulation on the clinical course and sleep/wake state of preterm neonates. *Infant Behav Dev* 1986;9:91–105.

126. Goats GC, Keir KA. Connective tissue massage. *Br J Sports Med* 1991;25:131–133.

127. Sullivan SJ, Williams LR, Seaborne DE, Morelli M. Effects of massage on alpha motoneuron excitability. *Phys Ther* 1991;71: 555–560.

128. Wakim KG. Physiologic effects of massage. In: Basmajian JV, ed. *Manipulation, traction and massage.* Baltimore: Williams & Wilkins, 1985:256–262.

129. Longworth JC. Psychophysiological effects of slow stroke back massage in normotensive females. *Adv Nurs Sci* 1982;4: 44–61.

130. Ironson G, Field T, Scafidi F, et al. Massage therapy is associated with enhancement of the immune

system's cytotoxic capacity. *Int J Neurosci* 1996;84:205–217.

131. Travell JG, Simons DG, eds. *Myofascial pain and dysfunction: the trigger point manual.* Baltimore: Williams & Wilkins, 1983.

132. Danneskiold-Samsoe B, Christiansen E, Anderson RB. Myofascial pain and the role of myoglobin. *Scand J Rheumatol* 1986;15:174–178.

133. Puustjarvi K, Airaksinen O, Pontinen PJ. The effects of massage in patients with chronic tension headache. *Acupunct Electrother Res* 1990;15:159–162.

134. Kirshbaum M. Using massage in the relief of lymphedema. *Prof Nurse* 1996;11:230–232.

135. Bunce IH, Mirolo BR, Hennessy JM, et al. Post-mastectomy treatment and measurement. *Med J Aust* 1994;161:125–128.

136. Brennan MJ, Weitz J. Lymphedema 30 years after radical mastecomy. *Am J Phys Med Rehabil* 1992;71:12–14.

137. Swedborg I. Effectiveness of combined methods of physiotherapy for post-mastectomy lymphoedema. *Scand J Rehabil Med* 1980;12:77–85.

138. Zanolla R, Monzeglio C, Balzarini A, Martino G. Evaluation of the results of three different methods of postmastectomy lymphedema treatment. *J Surg Oncol* 1994;26:210–213.

139. Cyriax JH. Clinical applications of massage. In: Basmajian JV, ed. *Manipulation traction and massage.* Baltimore: Williams & Wilkins, 1985:270–288.

140. Yeo TC, Choo MH, Tay MB. Massive haematoma from digital massage in an anticoagulated patient: a case report. *Singapore Med J* 1994;35:319–320.

Chapter 25

Injection Techniques

Curtis W. Slipman
Randal A. Palmitier
David K. DeDianous

Injections performed by the interventional physiatrist fall into two broad categories: axial and peripheral. Axial, or spinal, injections tend to be more technically difficult to perform because of the deep location and small size of the target structures. As such, these procedures typically require fluoroscopic guidance and specialized training if they are to be performed with precision. The superficial and palpable location of most peripheral injection sites, on the other hand, makes simultaneous imaging unnecessary, but the precise performance of these injections is no less important.

Both axial and peripheral injections can be done for diagnostic or therapeutic purposes, but in either case, accurate needle placement is key. A diagnostic block involves the injection of local anesthetic to confirm the nociceptive source and assist in determining whether a patient will respond to a subsequent therapeutic procedure. A diagnostic injection requires absolute precision to avoid making an erroneous diagnosis. Only enough local anesthetic should be used to ensure anesthesia of the target structure while leaving the surrounding structures unaffected. Use of excessive volumes of local anesthetic could lead to spurious results. For example, a diagnostic zygapophyseal injection could inadvertently anesthetize the exiting nerve root or sinuvertebral nerve if overflow of anesthetic occurs. Either scenario would lead to a false-positive result. Therapeutic injections involve instillation of corticosteroid into or around the painful structure to reduce inflammation. Although a misplaced therapeutic injection would not necessarily affect the working diagnosis, it may preclude a successful nonsurgical outcome. For instance, unnecessary arthroscopic surgery may be the result of a subacromial injection that is mistakenly placed in the subcutaneous soft tissues. In short, accuracy of injection is critical if quality outcomes are to be achieved.

The goal of this chapter is to provide the clinician with the information needed to improve the ability to deliver and prescribe diagnostic and therapeutic injections and as a consequence enhance nonsurgical and surgical patient care.

PERIPHERAL INJECTIONS

Peripheral corticosteroid injections are relatively safe procedures that are useful both diagnostically and therapeutically. Most peripheral procedures are easy to learn and can be mastered quickly. Exceptions include those involving the small joints and tendons of the hand and foot, and the deep joints such as the hip and pelvis, which require fluoroscopic guidance (1,2).

General Guidelines

Corticosteroid injections can be performed in joints, bursae, entheses, and muscles, as well as in peritendinous and ligamentous locations (3,4). They are indicated for soft-tissue and joint inflammatory conditions unresponsive to other conservative treatments including rest, nonsteroidal anti-inflammatory drugs (NSAIDs), and physical therapy. They may also be indicated for systemic conditions where oral therapy is contraindicated, such as renal failure, cardiac failure, and peptic ulcer disease. Injection therapy should typically be thought of as an adjunct to a comprehensive rehabilitation program (4–7). Table 25-1 lists some of the conditions that are amenable to corticosteroid injection.

It should be noted that corticosteroid injection of osteoarthritic joints remains controversial, as there may only be a minimal component of inflammation. A recent study showed that in the case of knee osteoarthritis, intra-articular steroids are most effective if there is enough effusion to allow joint aspiration (3,8). Nonetheless, many patients with osteoarthritic joints lacking a large effusion will have long-term relief with intra-articular injection.

Table 25-1: Conditions Frequently Treated by Local Corticosteroid Injections

- Synovitis
  - Adult and juvenile rheumatoid arthritis
  - Seronegative spondyloarthropathies
  - Crystal-induced arthropathies
  - Knee synovitis following hip arthroplasty
  - Knee trauma
- Osteoarthritis
  - Knee, shoulder, and hip
  - First metacarpophalangeal, carpometacarpal, metatarsophalangeal joints
  - Acromioclavicular joints
  - Lumbar facet arthropathy
  - Sacroiliac joint dysfunction
- Fibrositis
- Bursitis
  - Subacromial, coracoid, olecranon, trochanteric, anserine, prepatellar, infrapatellar, calcaneal, retrocalcaneal, ischial
- Adhesive capsulitis
- Tenosynovitis and tendinitis
  - Supraspinatus, bicipital, wrist extensor, de Quervain, flexor carpi radialis and ulnaris, digital flexor, semimembranosus
- Carpal, Guyon, and tarsal tunnel syndromes
- Radiculitis
- Costochondritis
- Tietze syndrome
- Dupuytren contracture
- Shoulder-hand syndrome
- Popliteal and antecubital cysts
- Plantar fasciitis
- Ganglion cyst
- Temporomandibular joint syndrome

Source: Adapted from Gray RG, Gottlieb NL. Intra-articular corticosteroids. An updated assessment. *Clin Orthop* 1983;177:235–263.

Therefore, some authors proposed a therapeutic trial be used to select appropriate patients, as opposed to trying to predict outcome prior to injection (2,3,7,9).

Contraindications

Absolute contraindications to injection include infectious arthritis, bacteremia, periarticular cellulitis or ulceration, bacterial endocarditis, adjacent osteochondral fracture, joint prosthesis, adjacent osteomyelitis, and uncontrolled coagulopathy. No more than three injections should be given in a weight-bearing joint in a given year. Relative contraindications include anticoagulant therapy, joint instability, osteoarthritis without effusion, poorly controlled diabetes, lack of response to prior injections, adjacent skin abrasion, internal derangement of the knee, hemarthrosis, decubitus ulcer, and other chronic foci of infection (1,3,4,6,7,9–11).

Potential Complications

When the injection is done properly, the prevalence of complications is very low (Table 25-2). The most common complication, steroid flare, represents a true crystal-induced arthritis (1,4,6,7,12,13). The mechanism is uncertain but the flare is likely caused by the crystalline structure of the steroid itself. It tends to occur more frequently with short-acting preparations such as hydrocortisone and prednisolone acetate (3). The patient usually experiences the onset of symptoms 6 to 12 hours after injection and symptoms typically last from 12 to 72 hours. Steroid flare is best treated with NSAIDs and ice (6). If symptoms persist beyond 72 hours, infection must be ruled out (1).

The risk of steroid arthropathy in weight-bearing joints has been based largely on subprimate animal studies and anecdotal cases (1,6,7,14). Development of Charcot

Table 25-2: Potential Complications of Local Corticosteroid Injection

Complication	Prevalence (%)
Postinjection flare	2–5
Steroid arthropathy of weight-bearing joints	0.8
Tendon rupture	<1
Facial flushing	<1
Skin atrophy, depigmentation	<1
Infection	<0.00006
Transient paresis of injected extremity	Rare
Hypersensitivity reaction	Rare
Asymptomatic pericapsular calcification of interphalangeal joints	43

Source: Adapted from Gray RG, Gottlieb NL. Intra-articular corticosteroids. An updated assessment. *Clin Orthop* 1983;177:235–263.

joints has also been proposed as a possible side effect due to steroid-induced analgesia allowing increased joint abuse (4,6,14). It is generally accepted, however, that joint deterioration from repeat injections cannot be readily distinguished from the natural progression of osteoarthritis itself (6,13).

The incidence of tendon or ligament rupture after corticosteroid injection is rare. Intra-articular injection, however, can reduce the tensile strength of the anterior cruciate ligament (ACL) in primates for up to 15 months (1,14). An increased incidence of tendon or ligament failure is noted with concomitant oral steroid use, frequent injection, inadequate rest after an injection of a weight-bearing joint, periarticular soft-tissue injection, direct intratendinous or ligamentous injection, or injection of an inappropriately high dose of corticosteroid (1,6).

Local cutaneous side effects including depigmentation, scarring, and skin depression secondary to subcutaneous fat or muscle atrophy are unsightly and may persist for a number of years. These side effects may be unavoidable in some patients but occur more frequently when the corticosteroid is injected subcutaneously. They may be partially avoided by using less concentrated preparations and injecting at a depth greater than 5 mm when possible (1,3,6,13).

Systemic absorption of corticosteroid may lead to facial flushing (especially with triamcinolone acetonide), transient hyperglycemia in diabetics (with short-acting preparations), and rarely, Cushing syndrome, pancreatitis, and abnormal uterine bleeding (3,4,6,7,13).

Technical Considerations

Many different techniques have been described. A recent survey of British rheumatologists illustrated that the approach to joint and soft-tissue injections varies even among clinicians within the same specialty (15). There also continues to be debate regarding the proper skin preparation prior to needle insertion. Crawley et al (16) found no significant difference in needle contamination between skin preparation with a single swipe of alcohol and cleansing with chlorhexidine.

We recommend strict adherence to aseptic technique. The skin should be cleansed with three povidone-iodine (Betadine) swabs and patted dry or swiped with alcohol prior to needle insertion (3,4,6,9,11,12,17). The skin can be anesthetized with local anesthetic or ethyl chloride spray for patient comfort (4,6). A 21- to 25-gauge needle should be used for injection. Once in the joint, the needle should move freely (6). There should be little resistance to injection. If resistance is encountered, the needle should be repositioned to avoid intratendinous or intraligamentous injection. The plunger of the syringe should be slightly withdrawn just prior to injection to rule out inadvertent intravascular needle placement (11).

Corticosteroid Preparations and Dosages

Several corticosteroid preparations are now available. These preparations vary in potency, concentration, and duration of effect (1,6,13,17). The relative potency of a preparation is based on the degree of hypothalamic-pituitary-adrenal axis suppression, not its anti-inflammatory effect (6,13). The duration of effect correlates inversely with the water solubility of the suspension (Table 25-3). Intermediate and long-acting preparations will continue to have an anti-inflammatory effect for 8 to 14 days, respectively, but have a relatively slow onset of action when compared to the short-acting preparations (6). For this reason, we prefer preparations that include a mixture of short- and long-acting medications such as betamethasone sodium phosphate and acetate suspension (Celestone Soluspan) (4,7). Although the choice of corticosteroid should be based on the presenting problem (i.e., a short-acting preparation for a self-limiting condition such as bursitis), most clinicians settle on one or two preparations that based on their experience, give the most benefit with few side effects (7).

Mixing a short-acting local anesthetic (1%–2% procaine or lidocaine without epinephrine) with the corticosteroid provides the patient with immediate pain relief and is helpful diagnostically (2,6,10). Such a mixture also dilutes the corticosteroid, thus reducing the chance of steroid flare, cutaneous atrophy, and tendon weakening (2,6,7,17). The clinician should avoid mixing corticosteroid with local anesthetics containing preservatives such as parabens, to prevent the increased risk of steroid flare due to the precipitation of steroid crystals (1,6,7). Some clinicians prefer to inject the corticosteroid suspension first and then remove the syringe and inject the local anesthetic from a separate syringe while keeping the needle within the joint. Flushing the needle in this way theoretically prevents pericapsular calcifications that can arise from corticosteroid deposition during needle withdrawal (7).

There is no consensus regarding the amount of corticosteroid that should be injected in the various joints and soft tissues. Common dosages for common sites are listed in Table 25-3. In general, the volume of corticosteroid used for large joints is 1 to 2 mL; medium joints, 0.5 to 1.0 mL; and small joints, 0.1 to 0.5 mL. One-half to 2 mL of local anesthetic is added, depending on the size of the joint or soft-tissue area to be injected (6,7).

The following recommendations are offered to minimize potential side effects during peripheral injections (2,4,5,7,17,18).

- Use aseptic technique.
- Limit the number of injections to three per year, especially in weight-bearing joints.
- Know the surrounding anatomy to avoid intravascular, intratendinous or ligamentous, and intraneural injection.

Table 25-3: Corticosteroid Preparations and Relative Potency

Corticosteroid	Small Joints	Large Joints	Available Strengths	Common Dosages (mg)	
				Relative Potency*	Tendon Sheaths and Bursae
Short-acting					
Cortisone acetate	10–25	50–125	50 mg/mL	0.8	20–50
Hydrocortisone acetate	8–20	40–100	25 mg/mL	1	8–40
Intermediate-acting					
Prednisolone tebutate (Hydeltra-T.B.A.)	2–5	10–25	20 mg/mL	4	4–10
Triamcinolone acetonide	10–25			4–10	2–5
(Kenalog-10)			10 mg/mL	2.5	
(Kenalog-40)			40 mg/mL	10.5	
Triamcinolone hexacetonide (Aristospan)	2–5	10–25	20 mg/mL	2.5	4–10
Triamcinolone diacetate (Aristocort)	2–5	10–25	40 mg/mL	5	4–10
Methylprednisolone acetate (Depo-Medrol)	2–5	10–25			4–10
			20 mg/mL	5	
			40 mg/mL	10	
			80 mg/mL	20	
Long-acting					
Dexamethasone sodium phosphate (Decadron, Hexadrol)	0.8–1.0	2–4	4 mg/mL	8	1.5–3.0
Dexamethasone acetate (Decadron-LA)	0.8–1.0	2–4	8 mg/mL	16	1.5–3.0
Betamethasone sodium phosphate and acetate suspension (Celestone Soluspan)	0.8–1.0	2–4	6 mg/mL	10	1.5–3.0

* Compared with 5 mg of prednisone.

Source: Adapted from Owen DS. Aspiration and injection of joints and soft tissues. In: Kelly WN, Harris ED Jr, Ruddy S, et al, eds. *Textbook of rheumatology.* 3rd ed. New York: WB Saunders, 1989: 621–636; Pfenninger JL. Injections of joints and soft tissue: part I. General guidelines. *Am Fam Physician* 1991;44:1196–1202.

- Select the appropriate steroid dose based on joint size and disease process.
- Rest the extremity after injection—4 to 5 days for the non-weight-bearing joint and 2 to 3 weeks for weight-bearing joints. Withhold injection in patients who cannot or will not rest the extremity.
- Avoid repeat injection if prior injections have been ineffective.
- Avoid articular cartilage contact.

Diagnostic Peripheral Blocks

Diagnostic blocks have a more limited role peripherally than axially. As stated previously, the superficial and palpable location of most peripheral pain generators makes diagnosis through clinical examination more straightforward. Also, the lack of complexity of peripheral joint function and pain referral patterns makes the risk of misdiagnosis less likely. The shoulder region and hip joint are exceptions to this generalization, however.

Shoulder injury now ranks as one of the leading causes of musculoskeletal disability. Being a four-joint complex, the difficulty in identifying the pain generator in the shoulder can rival that of the spine. Therefore, the diagnostic and therapeutic algorithm should be equally specific and precise. Diagnostic injections should be used prior to indiscriminant injection of corticosteroid into the subacromial space when the etiology of pain is still in question. Potential pain generators in the shoulder region include the rotator cuff, subacromial bursa, acromioclavicular (AC) joint, glenohumeral joint, bicipital tendon, suprascapular nerve, subscapular bursa, and sternoclavicular joint. Other entities can refer pain to the shoulder region, including carpal tunnel syndrome and cervical spinal or brachial plexus pathology. Therefore, diagnostic blocks are useful not only to pinpoint the pain generator with a positive block, but also to redirect attention to a more remote site of pathology with a negative block. As in the case of diagnostic axial injections, diagnostic shoulder blocks can simultaneously reduce the number of unnecessary and unsuccessful corticosteroid injections while providing the confidence to both clinician and patient that a given therapeutic injection is appropriate even after a negative first trial. The end result is more successful nonsurgical treatment and improved surgical outcomes.

Diagnostic blocks are useful in the hip, because the pain from hip disease is frequently difficult to differentiate from axial pathology such as spinal stenosis and sacroiliac syndrome. Significant hip and spinal disease will sometimes coexist, in which case diagnostic blocks are helpful in identifying the primary pain generator. Unlike the shoulder where fluoroscopic guidance is as yet rarely used during injection procedures, the deep location of the hip necessitates fluoroscopic guidance and the use of contrast material to confirm proper placement of the injectant.

The interventional physiatrist should consider diagnostic injection in any peripheral location where the specific diagnosis has not otherwise been confirmed. Such an approach will enhance nonsurgical intervention. Our approach to diagnostic blocks is elucidated in the axial injection section of this chapter.

The Shoulder Region

Glenohumeral Joint

Intra-articular injection in the shoulder is used for treatment of rheumatoid arthritis, osteoarthritis, and adhesive capsulitis. Anterior, posterior, and anterior-superior approaches have been described.

Anterior Approach

This approach is most easily performed with the patient seated and the shoulder externally rotated. A 20- to 22-gauge needle is directed dorsally and slightly superiorly and laterally. The needle should pass unobstructed into the joint space. If bone is encountered, the needle is withdrawn and repositioned appropriately. Injection medial to the coracoid process may result in inadvertent damage to the brachial plexus, subclavian artery, subclavian vein, or lung (3,4,7,9,12,18,19).

Posterior Approach

The posterior approach provides ready access to the joint but no bony landmarks are available. The patient should have the shoulder internally rotated to open the posterior joint space. The needle is inserted 2 to 3 cm inferior to the posterolateral corner of the acromion and directed anteriorly in the direction of the coracoid process. Again, the needle should pass unobstructed into the joint space (3,4,9,11,14,18).

Anterior-Superior Approach

The anterior aspect of the acromion is used as a bony landmark in this approach. A 22-gauge, 1.5-inch needle is directed inferiorly into the joint. When resistance is felt at the tip of the needle, the shoulder is gently and passively rotated in an internal-external manner. If there is any movement at the tip of the needle with this maneuver, the needle is slightly retracted, the joint is aspirated, and then the injectant injected (17).

Subacromial Space

Injection of the subacromial space is one of the more commonly performed peripheral injection procedures. Diagnostic subacromial injection will be positive when the pain generator is the rotator cuff or subacromial bursa itself, but will be negative if the source of pain is the glenohumeral joint, acromioclavicular joint, bicipital tendon, or a more remote site referring pain to the subacromial region. Diagnostic injection of the subacromial space is also helpful in differentiating rotator cuff weakness due to pain inhibition from true weakness due to a rotator cuff tear. Therapeutic injection is indicated not only in patients with rotator cuff or subacromial bursa inflammation, but also in patients who need relief from the pain of adhesive capsulitis. Therapeutic injection is indicated in the elderly patient with a rotator cuff tear who may not be a surgical candidate.

Three approaches to injection have been described: anterior, lateral, and posterolateral. All are relatively simple and effective. We find the posterolateral approach to be the easiest and least painful in most situations. The anterior approach may be difficult if there is an anterior acromial osteophyte or hooked acromion (20,21). The lateral approach is difficult if not impossible in the obese or muscular patient in whom the lateral edge of the acromion may not be palpable (20).

Posterolateral Approach

The patient is placed in a seated position on the examination table with the hands resting in the lap. The skin is prepared over the often visible and palpable indentation beneath the posterolateral edge of the acromion. The thumb of the palpating hand is slipped firmly under the inferior edge of the posterolateral part of the acromion, with the palm of the palpating hand above the shoulder and the fingers placed anteriorly in the supraclavicular fossa. A 1.5-inch, 20- to 25-gauge needle is inserted just beneath the palpating thumb (1.0–1.5 cm below the inferior border of the acromion) and oriented toward the sternoclavicular joint to pass beneath the acromion and above the supraspinatus tendon. If resistance is encountered during injection, the needle should be repositioned to prevent direct injection into the rotator cuff tendon (17,20,21). Traction can be applied to the arm to facilitate injection, but is rarely needed if adequate patient relaxation is achieved. In the case of a diagnostic block, active range of motion and impingement tests should be reevaluated for the expected 80% reduction in symptoms. Rotator cuff strength is reassessed if a diagnostic block is being used to differentiate between pain-inhibitory weakness and cuff tear.

Acromioclavicular Joint

Isolated AC pain is sometimes difficult to differentiate from rotator cuff tendonitis since impingement testing will reproduce pain in either situation. It is not uncommon for the problems to coexist along with a biceps tendonitis in the so-called impingement syndrome. Direct palpation of the AC joint and horizontal adduction are typically the most provocative factors in an isolated AC joint problem, but diagnostic blocks may be necessary to confirm the diagnosis.

It is easiest to insert the needle and palpate this joint at its posterior superior border. Since the joint has an oblique orientation that varies from person to person, an x-ray study of the shoulder is helpful in planning the path of needle insertion. A 22- to 25-gauge needle is directed anteriorly and inferiorly through the posterior superior aspect of the joint until there is a slight loss of resistance. There should be only moderate resistance to injection if the needle is properly placed. One to 1.5 mL of injectant can be used. In the case of a diagnostic injection, horizontal adduction and extremes of flexion should be significantly less painful after injection (4,7,11,17,21,22).

Long Head of the Biceps Tendon

As stated earlier, biceps tendonitis can occur in impingement syndrome but can also present as an isolated pathology. Pain is experienced in the anterior region of the shoulder and is exacerbated by impingement testing, recruitment of the biceps muscle, and direct palpation. Diagnostic block may be needed to confirm the site of pathology.

This is not an easy structure to insert a needle into with precision. The patient is seated with the elbow flexed to 90 degrees and the forearm supinated. With the arm externally rotated 20 to 30 degrees, the bicipital groove and tendon can be palpated anteriorly. A 23- to 25-gauge needle is inserted just proximal to the site of maximal tenderness and advanced into the bicipital groove in a proximal to distal direction until resistance from the tendon is encountered. The needle is then slightly withdrawn and reoriented more parallel to the tendon. Injection is made along the tendon and if properly placed, there is little resistance to injection and a palpable fullness along the tendon sheath (2,4,7,17,18,19,21). The clinician must take great care to avoid injection into the tendon itself because tendon rupture could result.

Suprascapular Nerve

Suprascapular nerve injury or impingement at the scapular notch can cause nonradiating pain above the scapular spine or shoulder pain secondary to weakness of the supraspinatus and infraspinatus muscles with resultant impingement. If the electromyography (EMG) findings are negative, this uncommon cause of shoulder pain can be difficult to diagnose without the use of diagnostic blocks. It has been shown to respond to therapeutic injection, but frequently requires surgical intervention.

With the patient prone, the needle is advanced just superior to the scapular spine at the junction between the middle and lateral thirds. The needle is advanced anteriorly until bone of the supraspinatous fossa is encountered. The needle is then redirected superiorly to lie within the suprascapular notch. One milliliter of 1% lidocaine is injected for diagnostic purposes and 2 to 3 mL of corticosteroid is used for a therapeutic injection.

Subscapular Bursa

Inflammation of the subscapular bursa can result in pain along the medial scapular border and snapping scapula syndrome. This entity must be differentiated from typical myofascial pain and referred pain from cervical diskogenic disease or radiculopathy. A diagnostic block can be helpful in this regard.

The patient is positioned prone on the examination table and the skin is prepared along the length of the medial scapular border. Positioning the ipsilateral arm such that the back of the patient's hand rests on the back at the level of the beltline will tip the medial scapular border to provide easy access for bursal injection. A 3.5-inch, 22- to 25-gauge needle is inserted parallel to the plane of the scapula at the junction between the proximal and distal thirds of the medial scapular border. The needle is advanced to a point that would place the tip of the needle beneath the midpoint of the scapular spine. Five to 10 mL of a short-acting local anesthetic is injected for diagnostic purposes, and if the diagnostic block proves positive, 2 to 3 mL of corticosteroid is used for a therapeutic injection. Care must be taken to keep the needle in the scapular plane during advancement to avoid pneumothorax.

Sternoclavicular Joint

The proximal part of the clavicle meets the superior aspect of the manubrium to form the sternoclavicular joint. The joint can become painful with any change in the mechanics of the AC articulation or after direct trauma to the anterior chest wall, which can result in subluxation of the sternoclavicular joint. Pain is experienced in the ipsilateral anterior chest wall and along the length of the clavicle. Symptoms typically coexist, and are sometimes confused, with AC synovitis.

The patient is positioned supine on the table with the ipsilateral arm abducted to 90 degrees and externally rotated to open the sternoclavicular articulation. The joint is entered anteriorly at the superior border of the manubrium where there is often a palpable depression. The needle is inserted in a cephalad to caudad direction.

There should be minimal resistance to injection. One to 1.5 mL of either local anesthetic or a mixture of local anesthetic and corticosteroid are injected.

The Elbow Region

Injection in the elbow is most commonly undertaken for treatment of symptoms emanating from the epicondylar regions. Both lateral and medial common extensor tendon pathology (lateral and medial epicondylitis) respond well to instillation of corticosteroid. It is not uncommon, however, for lateral symptoms to be caused by radiohumeral synovitis and for cervical pathology to refer symptoms to the elbow region. Again, if the diagnosis is in doubt, diagnostic block should be considered.

Radiohumeral Joint

This joint is best approached from the posterolateral aspect with the patient supine, the elbow in full extension, and the forearm pronated. If synovitis exists, a palpable outpouching of the joint capsule will be present. The skin is prepared in the usual manner and a 25-gauge needle is inserted perpendicular to the palpable joint space. One to 1.5 mL of injectant can be used (2,3,4,7,9,11,18,23).

Lateral Epicondyle

The injection is performed with the patient seated, the elbow flexed and pronated, and the hand resting on the lap. The point of maximal tenderness is identified. Injection is administered using a 23- to 25-gauge needle. The area is infiltrated by alternately injecting and withdrawing and redirecting the needle until the entire area is bathed, including the common extensor tendon insertion and radial collateral ligament. If paresthesias are experienced during needle placement or at any point during the injection, the needle should be repositioned to avoid injection into the radial nerve. It is not uncommon, however, for the patient to have referred symptoms along the extensor muscle mass to the wrist during injection. Every effort should be made to keep the needle tip below the dermis during injection to avoid the side effect of cutaneous atrophy (2,4,7,11,14,17,18,23).

Medial Epicondyle

A technique similar to that described for the lateral epicondyle is used, but the patient is best positioned supine with the shoulder abducted and externally rotated and the elbow partially flexed. Prior to injection in this position, however, the clinician should rule out ulnar subluxation as the ulnar nerve could then be subluxed into the injection site. During the injection procedure, the needle should remain medial and anterior to the epicondyle and never reach the posterior border of the epicondyle near the ulnar groove. Again the entire anterior and medial area should be bathed with injectant, paying particular attention to the pronator teres tendon, which is commonly the primary pain generator (4,18,21,23).

The Wrist Region

Carpal Joints

The wrist is a complex of many small joints, most of which interconnect, allowing symptom relief from a single injection site. The injection is carried out dorsally just distal to the radius and just lateral to the border of the anatomic snuff box (extensor pollicis longus tendon). The joint space can be made more accessible through slight passive flexion (20–30 degrees). A 24- to 26-gauge needle is inserted perpendicular to the skin and to a depth of 1 to 2 cm. If bone is contacted, the needle should be withdrawn and repositioned more radially (2,4,7,9,18).

de Quervain Tenosynovitis

Injection for this condition is directed into the common tendon sheath of the abductor pollicis longus and extensor pollicis brevis. The most tender area in the region of the radial styloid is identified with Finkelstein's test and palpation. The patient abducts the thumb so the tendon becomes obvious. A 23- to 25-gauge needle is introduced about 1 cm distal to the area of maximal tenderness and directed toward the site of tenderness at a 45-degree angle. The needle is slightly withdrawn after making contact with the tendon. There should be minimal to no resistance to injection and proper placement is confirmed by a visible swelling along the sheath with injection (7,17,18,23–26). Failure of injection may be due to anatomic variants where the extensor pollicis brevis and abductor pollicis longus are located in separate compartments (25).

First Carpometacarpal Joint

To facilitate entry into the joint, the thumb is flexed into the palm of the hand (4,7,23). A dorsal approach is commonly used, taking care to avoid the radial artery and superficial radial nerve. Two techniques have been described. With the first method, the proximal margin of the first metacarpal bone is palpated within the anatomic snuff box. The needle is inserted between the long extensor and long abductor tendons, avoiding the radial artery. The tip is directed toward the base of the little finger and inserted to a depth of about 1 cm (23). With the second method, a mark is made at the base of the first metacarpal bone radial to the border of the snuff box. A 22- to 25-gauge needle is inserted at the mark and directed toward the base of the fourth metacarpal. This keeps the needle away from the radial artery (4,7).

Carpal Tunnel

Generally patients with pain from carpal tunnel syndrome respond better to injection than do those with numbness only (17,27). Although therapeutic injection can provide long-lasting relief of carpal tunnel symptoms, especially in patients with traumatic or pregnancy-induced symptoms, injection is also helpful in predicting surgical outcome. A positive response to injection tends to suggest a favorable response to surgical release.

The flexor retinaculum is 2 to 3 cm long and nearly the same width. It is attached laterally to the tuberosity of the scaphoid and to both lips of the groove of the trapezium. Medially it attaches to the hook of the hamate and the pisiform bone (27). Injection can be made either medial or lateral to the palmaris longus tendon. The medial approach is considered the safest, considering the anatomy of the wrist and the location of the median nerve.

Ulnar (Medial) Approach

The wrist is positioned in neutral or slight flexion. A 25-gauge needle is inserted just ulnar to the palmaris longus tendon (or in line with the fourth ray, if the palmaris longus tendon is absent) at the distal wrist crease. The needle is directed at a 30- to 45-degree angle toward the tip of the middle finger. Increased resistance is encountered when the needle reaches the transverse carpal ligament. If paresthesias are felt by the patient during needle insertion, the needle is withdrawn and directed more superficially. There should be minimal resistance to injection. The patient should feel the gradual onset of numbness in the distribution of the median nerve if the injection was properly placed.

Radial (Lateral) Approach

The needle is inserted just medial to the palmaris longus tendon and lateral to the tendon of the flexor carpi radialis at the level of the distal wrist crease. The needle is directed at a 30- to 45-degree angle toward the tip of the middle finger (2,4,9,11,18).

Kay et al (28) described an alternative approach. Their review of 250 patients revealed no median nerve injuries. The needle is inserted just distal to the distal wrist crease in line with the fourth ray. The needle is directed radially and down at a 45-degree angle to ensure the tip of the needle lies deep to the median nerve. The tip is purposefully embedded in one of the flexor tendons or its synovium. Proper position is demonstrated by movement of the needle when the fingers are flexed and extended. The needle is then slightly withdrawn until no movement is noted with finger flexion. The fingers are then fully extended and the steroid is injected (28).

The Hand Region

Digital Flexor Tendon Sheaths

Stenosing tenosynovitis of the finger flexor tendons, trigger finger, is due to thickening of the digital flexor tendon sheaths with associated nodular thickening of the tendon. This occurs just proximal to the digital fibrous sheath (26) and adjacent to the metacarpophalangeal joint. The main pathology usually lies over the head of the metacarpals in the palm, with a localized swelling palpated over the area (7).

A 23- to 25-gauge needle is inserted at a 45-degree angle over the palmar aspect of the metacarpal head, and then directed proximally almost parallel to the skin to enter the tendon sheath. Correct placement is confirmed by lack of resistance with injection (4,7,23,26). Alternative methods involve directing the needle 30 to 45 degrees distally into the tendon sheaths (29,30).

Another method described by Liu and Canoso (29) to avoid intratendinous injection involves insertion of a butterfly needle just distal to the distal palmar crease and angled toward the tendon at 45 degrees. The needle is slowly advanced by 2-mm increments, checking position by having the patient flex and extend the interphalangeal joint. Tendon contact is confirmed when reciprocal movement of the needle occurs with finger movement. The needle is then slowly withdrawn at 1-mm increments until movement stops. The injectant is then infused into the sheath (29).

Metacarpophalangeal and Interphalangeal Joints

Injection into these joints may be difficult to perform owing to their small size. It is not necessary for the needle to be directly interposed between the articular surfaces to get a positive result. Synovitis usually causes the synovium to bulge dorsally. The metacarpophalangeal joint can be palpated just distal to the knuckle. A 25-gauge needle is inserted on either the radial or the ulnar side just under the extensor tendon mechanism. Slight flexion may make it easier to enter the joint. If the needle is inserted too laterally, the digital nerve, artery, or vein could be damaged. It is unusual to obtain synovial fluid from these joints (4,7,9,11,18).

The Pelvic Region

Hip Joint

Diagnostic injection into the hip joint is helpful in differentiating pain due to hip osteoarthritis from that caused by spinal stenosis or sacroiliac syndrome. Since these problems can coexist, diagnostic block can help determine which is the primary pain generator. Therapeutic injection is reserved for patients with severe osteoarthritis who are not yet ready for hip replacement or who are poor surgical candidates.

Injection into the hip joint is very difficult to perform without the use of simultaneous imaging, as synovial fluid can rarely be aspirated to confirm intra-articular needle placement. A number of techniques have been described to confirm proper needle placement (6,7), but we recommend the use of fluoroscopy to avoid a misplaced injection.

With the patient supine on the fluoroscopy table, the femoral pulse and ilioinguinal ligament are identified. A 3.5-inch, 20- to 22-gauge spinal needle is inserted 2 to

3 cm lateral to the femoral artery and 2 cm distal to the inguinal ligament. The needle is advanced at a 60-degree angle under fluoroscopic guidance, targeting the physiologic neck of the femur. When bone is contacted, the needle is slightly withdrawn and intra-articular placement is confirmed by injecting 1 to 2 mL of contrast material to outline the hip joint capsule. Three to 5 mL of local anesthetic is then injected for diagnostic purposes and 3 mL of corticosteroid is used for a therapeutic procedure (4,6,7,9,18).

Greater Trochanteric Bursa

The greater trochanteric bursa is located just superior to the greater trochanter of the femur. With the patient in the lateral decubitus position, the area of maximal tenderness is identified with palpation. A 1.5- to 3.5-inch, 22-gauge needle is inserted perpendicular to the skin and advanced until bone is contacted. The needle is then withdrawn slightly and 3 mL of injectant is placed. The needle is once again withdrawn slightly and another 2 mL is injected more superficially. It is also useful to inject inferior and superior to the trochanter if the patient has diffuse tenderness, since more than one bursa may be involved (6,7).

Piriformis

The piriformis muscle arises from inside the pelvis and over the front of the sacrum, the gluteal surface of the ilium, and anterior capsule of the sacroiliac joint. It runs laterally through the sciatic notch to become tendinous, inserting on the greater trochanter of the femur. The belly of the muscle crosses over the sciatic nerve (31,32). In 15% of the population it has two bellies. In these cases, the sciatic nerve either passes between the two bellies as one nerve, or divides into two trunks that interdigitate with the two muscle bellies (31). The injection into the muscle should be at the point of maximal tenderness (31–33).

Injection into the piriformis muscle belly has traditionally been performed without the use of fluoroscopy (31,32). To confirm proper needle placement and avoid vital structures, however, we recommend fluoroscopic guidance during injection. Blind medial, paravaginal, and vaginal approaches are included in this discussion for completeness.

Fluoroscopically Guided Injection

The patient is placed prone on the fluoroscopy table. A 20- to 22-gauge, 3.5-inch spinal needle is inserted over the inferior aspect of the sacroiliac joint and guided to the lateral inferior border of the joint where bone is contacted. The needle is then slightly withdrawn and redirected just under the ilium. At this point, the needle tip will lie in the belly of the piriformis superior and posterior to the sciatic nerve. Radiographic contrast dye is injected to confirm needle placement prior to injection.

Medial Approach

The patient is positioned in the lateral decubitus position with the affected side up and the legs flexed at the hips and knees. The index finger of the clinician's nondominant hand is inserted into the rectum or vagina to palpate the lateral edge of the sacrum high in the sciatic notch. The piriformis is palpable just lateral to this point and should be very tender. A 6-inch, 20-gauge needle is inserted perpendicular to the skin at a point on the buttock overlying the palpating finger. The needle is advanced to stop 2 to 3 cm short of the tip of the finger, which is confirmed by repeatedly wiggling the needle hub as it is advanced. The injection is then completed (31–34). It is suggested that a small test dose of local anesthetic be injected first, and some time be allowed to elapse before the final injection, to confirm that the needle is not near the sciatic nerve (31,32).

Paravaginal Approach

The muscle belly is palpated vaginally. The needle is then introduced from the perineum medial to the ischial tuberosity and advanced along the vagina into the muscle (32).

Vaginal Approach

Injection is performed from the lateral fornix of the vagina, similar to the approach for a paracervical block (32).

Pubic Symphysis

The symphysis pubis is an amphiarthrodial joint composed of the two pubic bones and a thick fibrocartilaginous disk. The disk has a transverse anterior width of 5 to 6 mm, and an anteroposterior width of 10 to 15 mm. The central raphe of the disk is the target structure for injection.

With the patient supine, the pubic hair overlying the symphysis is shaved and the area prepared in the usual manner. The patient is instructed to relax the abdominal muscles to allow the margins of the pubic symphysis to be palpated. A 1.5-inch, 19-gauge needle is inserted into the center of the pubic symphysis in an anteroposterior direction and advanced approximately 1 inch. Loss of needle resistance is felt as the needle tip enters the central soft portion of the symphysis pubis. With correct needle placement, injection should flow freely without resistance. Proper needle placement in the central raphe and advancement of no more than 1 inch will avoid complications, which include injury to the spermatic cord and penetration into the bladder (35).

The Knee Region

Knee Joint

A variety of medial and lateral approaches have been described. The superior medial and superior lateral approaches are considered optimal for both aspiration and injection (6,20). The superior lateral approach avoids the saphenous nerve and does not require insertion through muscle, which may cause more bleeding (4,6). Proponents of the superior medial approach believe there is more potential space between the patella and femur than with the lateral approach (6,9).

Superior Lateral Approach

The patient is supine with the knee extended. The quadriceps must be relaxed. An 18- to 21-gauge needle is inserted 1 cm superior and lateral to the patella. The needle is directed distally and posteriorly at a 45-degree angle under the patella. While advancing the needle, negative pressure should be applied until fluid enters the syringe. Medial pressure may also be helpful to cause pooling of the fluid in the area of aspiration (2,4,6,14,18).

Superior Medial Approach

This approach is similar to the superior lateral technique but with the needle inserted just superior to the medial patella (3,7,9,11).

The joint can be entered from a direct medial or direct lateral approach as well. In either case, the needle is inserted beneath the midpoint of the patella and directed posteriorly and inferiorly (19).

Inferior Approach

This is the preferred method for injection into the nondistended joint. Usually, joint fluid cannot be aspirated efficiently by this route. The patient is seated with the knee flexed at 90 degrees. A 22-gauge, 1.5-inch needle is inserted below the inferior pole of the patella, 1 cm medial or lateral to the patellar tendon. A sulcus may be palpable at this location. The needle is directed posteriorly and superiorly toward the intercondylar notch of the femur until the joint is entered. No bony contact is made. This method is thought to be less painful, cause less chondral damage, and reduce the risk of ACL injection (2,3,6,7,11,36).

Transpatellar Tendon Approach

Injection by this approach is also done with the knee flexed 90 degrees. The needle is then passed through the patellar tendon and through the infrapatellar fat pad, entering the knee joint adjacent to the ACL. This approach may be less painful, but the tip of the needle may come to rest in the fat pad or ACL. Injection into the fat pad may be very painful, while injection into the ACL may weaken the ligament, making it more susceptible to rupture (36).

Pes Anserine Bursa

The pes anserine bursa is interposed between the tibial attachment of the medial collateral ligament and the pes anserinous tendon (a conjoined tendon consisting of the insertions of the sartorius, gracilis, and semitendinosus tendons on the tibia). The patient is seated with the knee flexed to 90 degrees. A 22- to 25-gauge needle is inserted through the area of maximal tenderness until the tibial surface is reached. The needle is then slightly withdrawn and the injection completed.

Prepatellar Bursa

The prepatellar bursa is superficial to the superior aspect of the patella. The patient lies supine with the knee extended. Pressure is applied over the patella to force any fluid superiorly, making needle placement easier. Fluid is aspirated with a 20-gauge, 1.5-inch needle prior to injection (4,18,29).

The Foot and Ankle Region

Tibiotalar Joint

The anteromedial approach is recommended. Local anesthesia is advisable because of the tight ankle mortise and joint capsule (6). The patient is supine or sitting with the foot in neutral position. The joint is identified by palpating the talus while the patient plantar flexes and dorsiflexes the foot. A 20- to 22-gauge, 1.5-inch needle is inserted just medial to the tibialis tendon and lateral to the lateral malleolus (approximately 1 cm). The needle is advanced posteriorly to enter the joint space without striking bone (2,4,6,7,9,19).

Subtalar Joint

In extremely arthritic joints, verification of needle placement with contrast material and fluoroscopy may be needed. The patient is supine with the ankle in the neutral position. The skin is marked just inferior to the tip of the lateral malleolus and anterior to the Achilles tendon. A 22-gauge needle is inserted perpendicular to the skin and advanced medially into the joint. If bone is contacted, the needle is withdrawn and repositioned. Because needle positioning may be difficult, the use of local anesthetic prior to injection is advised (4,6,7).

Metatarsophalangeal and Interphalangeal Joints

These techniques are similar to those used in the hand, but many prefer to insert the needle more dorsally. For the first metatarsophalangeal joint, many clinicians prefer the dorsomedial approach. Gentle longitudinal traction on the phalanx may be useful (4,6,7,9).

Calcaneal Bursa

The lateral approach is less painful than the plantar approach. A 22-gauge needle is inserted perpendicular to the plantar surface of the midcalcaneal region and advanced until bone is contacted. The needle is withdrawn slightly, and the injection is completed at the area of maximal tenderness (7,18).

Trigger Point Injections

A trigger point is a tender nodule or taut band that refers pain when palpated. The goal of injection is to inactivate the hyperirritable area and interrupt the pain cycle through counterirritation of the active focus. Injections may be done with a local anesthetic, steroid, or saline solution (37). Dry needling or direct sustained pressure to the area may also be effective. Garvey et al (38) studied trigger points after back strain and found that using vapocoolant spray followed by acupressure or using acupuncture by itself was as effective as injection.

Many techniques are described, but generally a 25-gauge needle is inserted into the palpable nodule or taut band. A small amount of fluid (0.1–0.5 mL) is injected after a twitch response is obtained. The area is needled and infiltrated until the twitch response is no longer obtainable. Injection may be combined with passive stretching of the area with or without use of vapocoolant spray or other modalities. This postinjection regimen is used to inactivate remaining irritative foci and aid in restoring normal muscle resting length (37).

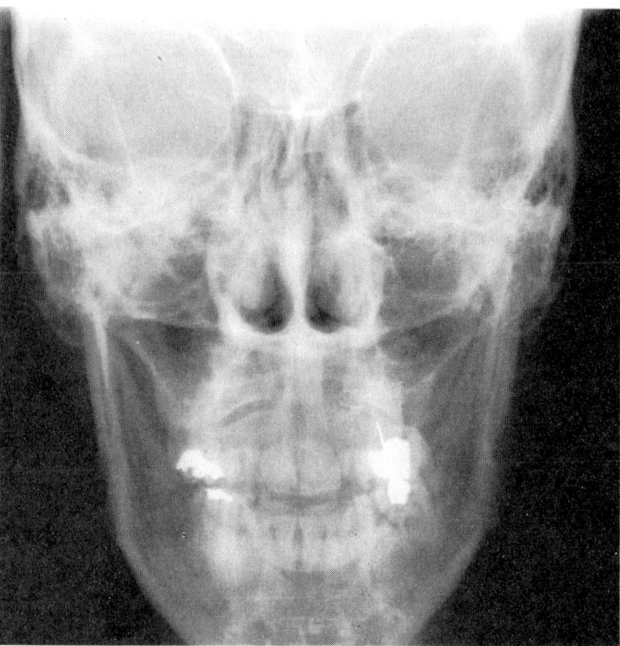

Figure 25-1. Diagnostic atlantoaxial joint block in a 30-year-old white man. This procedure demonstrated that his right-sided occipital pain, with radiation to the vertex, was emanating from the C1–C2 joint.

AXIAL INJECTIONS

General Considerations

Physiatrists are currently performing an array of fluoroscopically guided injection procedures used to assess or treat specific spinal structures including the occipitoatlantal joint, atlantoaxial joint (Fig. 25-1), facet joint, sacroiliac joint, pseudoarticulations (Fig. 25-2), spondylolitic defects, disk nucleus, piriformis muscle, epidural space, nerve root, medial branch of the dorsal ramus, and sympathetic chain.

Prior to recommending these sophisticated invasive procedures to a patient, the clinician must follow two guiding principles: Spinal injections should only be suggested when absolutely necessary and should follow a rational basis of implementation. If these concepts are adhered to, unnecessary procedures will be avoided and appropriate therapeutic intervention will not be abandoned early. At the Penn Spine Center we achieve this goal through the following process. All possible causes for the given pain presentation are considered and then prioritized based on their respective probability of occurrence. A diagnostic or treatment algorithm is developed from this differential diagnosis. If the diagnosis cannot be confirmed with noninvasive tools, then diagnostic blocks may be required. Injection procedures are then performed in a manner that allows for the efficient evaluation of potential etiologies. After a working diagnosis is made, a therapeutic algorithm should be devised to incorporate all nonsurgical and surgical possibilities. It should also include termination points in treatment as discontinuation of formal therapeutic intervention is a legitimate step in certain instances. Forgetting this latter element could lead the patient to seek unneces-

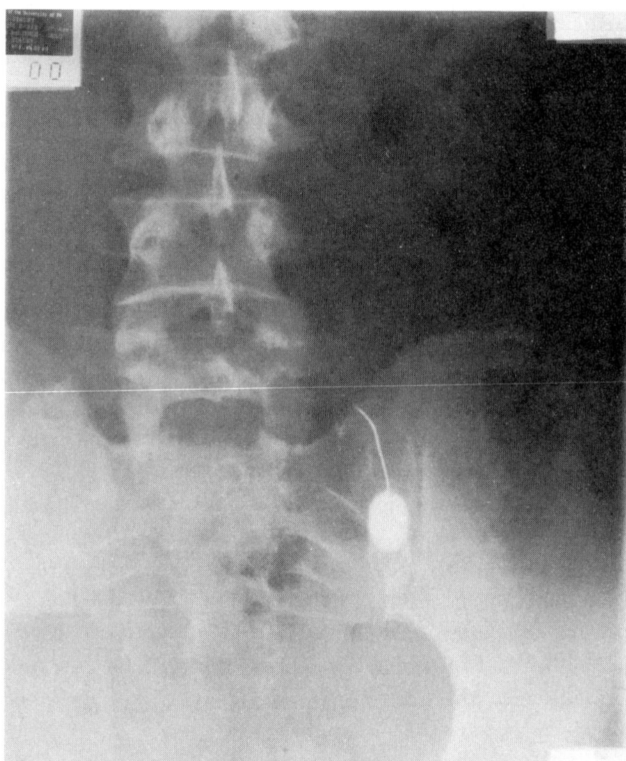

Figure 25-2. Diagnostic injection demonstrated that this false joint caused low-back pain for 3 years in a 26-year-old woman.

sary medical advice, with potentially disastrous consequences. For example, an 86-year-old man with poor cardiac function and classic symptoms of neurogenic claudication involving the L4 nerve root, negative straight-leg-raise response, weakness in the proximal and distal L4 muscles, and magnetic resonance imaging (MRI) result revealing grade II degenerative spondylolisthesis with severe ipsilateral foraminal stenosis at L4–L5, would be a candidate for L4 selective nerve root block (SNRB) but would not be a candidate for surgery. For this patient, the therapeutic algorithm would include a therapeutic block, but if it fails, there are no other reasonable measures that would offer a cure.

It cannot be overemphasized that each of these procedures must be performed as part of a comprehensive rehabilitation program and integrated into a sound diagnostic and therapeutic algorithm. In this way, similar patients with identical diagnoses receive nearly identical care.

Diagnostic Axial Blocks

A structured process should be implemented for the performance of diagnostic blocks. At the Penn Spine Center, the purpose of a diagnostic block is explained to the patient at least twice. This prevents the potential confusion and disappointment that can arise from a patient anticipating long-term relief from a procedure that is only meant to provide diagnostic information. Each patient completes a visual analogue scale (VAS) and pain drawing immediately prior to and 30 minutes after the procedure (Fig. 25-3). In this way, a determination of whether the diagnostic block results were positive or negative can be made that day. We never depend on a follow-up visit to assess the results of a diagnostic block, since memory of pain intensity is notoriously unreliable (39).

An independently trained medical professional administers the preassessments and postassessments to ensure objectivity. A threshold of 80% pain reduction on the VAS defines a positive block. Others have used thresholds as low as 50% (40) and as high as 90% (41). Often the patient must undergo provocative testing to demonstrate adequate pain relief from the procedure. For example, the patient with neurogenic claudication must demonstrate the ability to ambulate pain free for a longer distance than would have been possible prior to the procedure. Obviously, questioning that individual about the pain while he

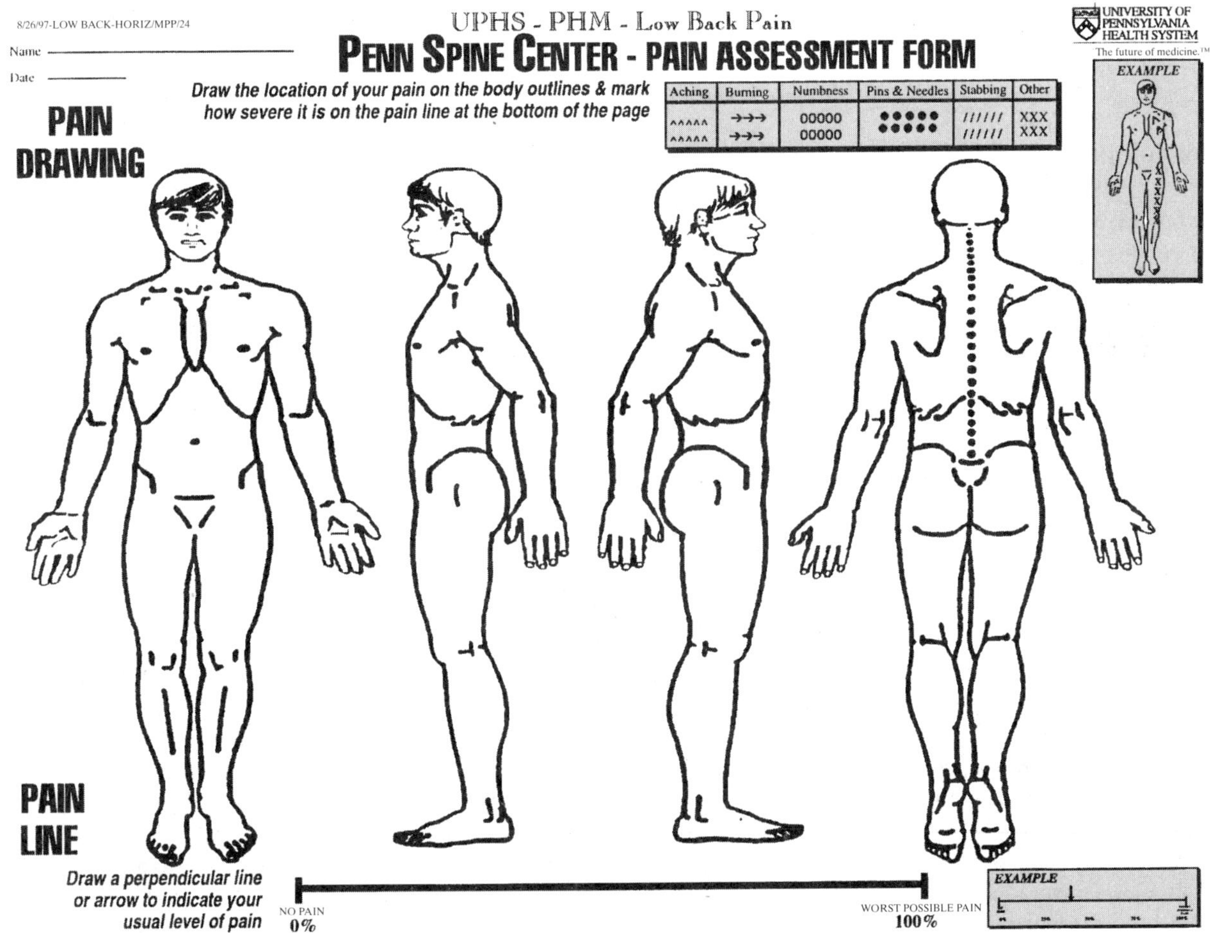
8/26/97-LOW BACK-HORIZ/MPP/24

UPHS - PHM - Low Back Pain

PENN SPINE CENTER - PAIN ASSESSMENT FORM

UNIVERSITY OF PENNSYLVANIA HEALTH SYSTEM
The future of medicine.™

Name ______________

Date ______

PAIN DRAWING

Draw the location of your pain on the body outlines & mark how severe it is on the pain line at the bottom of the page

Aching	Burning	Numbness	Pins & Needles	Stabbing	Other
^^^^^	→→→	00000	•••••	//////	XXX
^^^^^	→→→	00000	•••••	//////	XXX

EXAMPLE

PAIN LINE

Draw a perpendicular line or arrow to indicate your usual level of pain

NO PAIN 0%

WORST POSSIBLE PAIN 100%

EXAMPLE

Figure 25-3. Penn Spine Center pain assessment form.

or she is sitting in a chair after the procedure could lead to a false-positive result.

Diagnostic blocks should only be performed when the information is not available by other means and the result of the block would alter the therapeutic plan. For example, a diagnostic L5 SNRB would be indicated in an individual with lateral thigh and pretibial pain who has normal results from the physical examination, normal electrodiagnostic findings, and normal imaging results. The information obtained from such a test may lead to a new path in the diagnostic or therapeutic algorithm. If the block were positive, that individual would undergo a therapeutic L5 SNRB to treat L5 radiculitis. If the block were negative, the next step in the algorithm would be followed. An epidural injection may be indicated if the patient has pain while sitting, has relief while standing, and avoids flexion or rotational maneuvers due to pain. Diagnostic sacroiliac joint block may be indicated to assess the possibility of sclerotomally referred pain from sacroiliac syndrome if the patient reports pain while standing, has relief while sitting, and has positive responses to provocative maneuvers (42–44). In contrast, the same patient with weakness in the gluteus medius, hamstrings, and extensor hallucis longus, positive straight-leg-raise response, and an MRI revealing an ipsilateral posterolateral protrusion at the L4–L5 level would not require diagnostic block at all. This patient would instead be a candidate for therapeutic L5 SNRB as a first step, since the diagnosis of L5 radiculopathy is readily apparent.

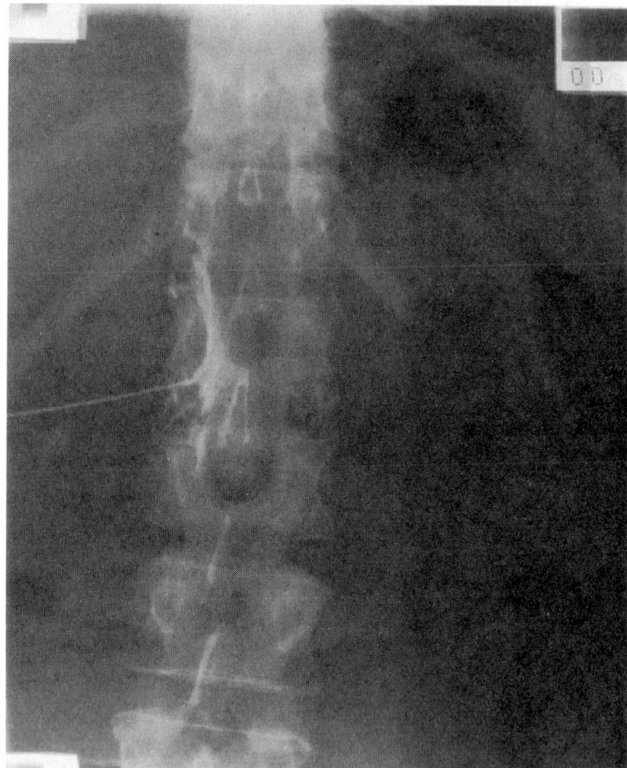

Figure 25-4. L1 transforaminal epidural injection. The contrast agent highlights the medial border of the pedicle and epidural space, with minimal presence extraforaminally along the route of the exiting nerve root.

Epidural Injection

Delivering medication to the epidural space requires an access route. Patient size and prior surgical history will dictate whether a translaminar, transforaminal, or caudal approach is used.

Overweight patients are best approached with one of the two former techniques. Caudal injections depend on palpating bony landmarks. If too much adipose tissue resides between the fingertips and the sacral cornu, the procedure will be painful for the patient and frustrating for the clinician. For those who have undergone prior lumbar surgery, the translaminar approach is usually inappropriate. When a translaminar injection is used, the therapeutic agent is delivered dorsal to scar tissue, but the target site, typically the dorsal root ganglion (DRG), resides ventral to the scar mass, and the agent cannot travel through this mass of tissue to exert its beneficial effect. These patients are best served with a transforaminal technique, bilateral if necessary. In this manner, the injectant is delivered ventral to the scar tissue. Depending on needle placement and bevel orientation, the injectant can be delivered to the nerve root, epidural space, or both (Fig. 25-4). Performing an L5 transforaminal epidural injection on individuals who have a fusion incorporating the L5–S1 segment, have a collapsed L5–S1 disk space, and are overweight may be impossible. In such patients, a caudal or sacral transforaminal approach is the best alternative.

Translaminar Epidural

A seated, lateral decubitus, or prone position can be used, but only the latter two are convenient for fluoroscopic applications. After proper positioning and skin preparation, 1.0 to 1.5 mL of 1% lidocaine is infused along the anticipated track of the needle. An 18- to 20-gauge Tuohy needle is advanced in the midline of the desired level. Before the epidural space is reached, the stylet is removed. A 5.0-mL glass syringe filled with normal saline solution is attached. The needle tip is incrementally advanced, with pressure simultaneously applied to the plunger. When a sudden drop in resistance is encountered, the epidural space has been entered. A contrast agent, 1.0 to 2.0 mL, is infused to demonstrate proper flow. Thereafter, 2.0 to 3.0 mL of betamethasone sodium phosphate (Celestone) and 5.0 to 7.0 mL of 1.0% lidocaine is instilled.

For the cervical, upper thoracic, and lumbar regions of the spine, the above approach is applicable. For the lower half of the thoracic region, beginning at the T5–T6 interspace, a paramedian approach is necessary due to the steep incline of the thoracic spinous processes. For this approach the Tuohy needle enters the skin approximately 1.0 cm lateral to the midline at a 45-degree cephalocaudal angle and 15 to 20 degrees ipsilateral to the midline.

Caudal Epidural

Entry to the epidural space through the sacral hiatus is easy in thin individuals and extremely difficult in the obese. For the latter individual, a translaminar or transforaminal epidural approach is preferable. With the patient resting in the prone position and after sterile preparation, the sacral cornua are identified. Right-handed operators should approach the patient from the patient's left. The long finger of the operator's left hand is placed on the right cornu and the index finger on the left. The sacral hiatus is located between these two landmarks. After local anesthetic is infused, a 22- to 25-gauge, 3.0-inch spinal needle is advanced at a 45-degree angle to the horizontal plane. Once the sacrococcygeal ligament is reached, the hub of the needle is dropped to rest parallel with the horizontal plane and advanced slightly. With fluoroscopic control, the needle tip can be advanced to the inferior edge of S2. If the needle tip is advanced beyond this site, dural puncture may result.

Typically, 1.0 to 3.0 mL of contrast medium will demonstrate appropriate flow (Figs. 25-5 and 25-6). Thereafter, 2.0 to 3.0 mL of betamethasone sodium phosphate and 5.0 mL of lidocaine are instilled. This represents sufficient volume to easily reach the level of the L3 vertebral body.

Selective Nerve Root Block/Transforaminal Epidural

Cervical

The patient is placed in the supine position. The entire trunk is rotated as a unit, creating an oblique view of the anterior-posterior (AP)–oriented x-ray beam. A bolster is placed under the posterior part of the shoulder and upper part of the back, which allows the patient to maintain position. Performing upper cervical root blocks requires a body position closer to AP, while a more lateral position is necessary for performing lower cervical root blocks. A thin pillow is placed under the occiput, and the head is then rotated toward the contralateral shoulder. Proper positioning is achieved when the superior articular process becomes just visible as a distinct structure located at the most lateral portion of the neural foramen. A skin wheal is raised just lateral to the base of the superior articular process. The needle is incrementally advanced under fluoroscopic guidance until the base of the articular process is reached. The caudal aspect of the foramen is targeted since the cervical roots leave the foramen at this location (Fig. 25-7). Three sequential steps are then followed. The needle is slightly withdrawn, the needle tip is oriented to a more lateral location by directing the hub dorsally, and finally the needle tip is advanced 1 to 2 mm. If needle advancement is limited to 2 mm, a dural puncture can safely be avoided, except when performing a C3 SNRB in women. The depth of the neural foramen in the latter instance has been reported to be as little as 1 mm (45). If a transforaminal injection is desired, the needle tip can be slightly withdrawn and advanced superiorly, above the exiting root, to end at the same depth previously reached (Fig. 25-8).

Specific guidelines concerning injection volumes have not been devised. In general, we use 0.5 mL of 2% lidocaine during diagnostic blocks. For therapeutic injection, we infuse 1.0 to 2.5 mL of betamethasone sodium phosphate followed by 0.5 to 1.0 mL of lidocaine.

Complications specific to cervical SNRB include advancing the needle through the foramen, causing a dural puncture or even impaling the spinal cord. Factors that predispose to these complications include using a 3.5-inch needle rather than a 1.5-inch needle because of a muscular, obese, or short neck; raising the skin wheal medially, thereby advancing the needle in a medial to lateral direction; and patient motion during injection. Retrospective and prospective studies demonstrated the safety of this procedure, as well as lumbar SNRB, provided an experienced spine physician is involved (46).

Thoracic

SNRB in the thoracic region is analogous to the technique in the lumbar region with the addition of two specific issues. First, if the skin wheal is raised too laterally, the needle will be advanced into the pleural cavity. Therefore, it is safest to err with a starting point that is too medial. Second, if the needle is advanced too ventrally when performing a left upper thoracic SNRB, the aorta may be entered. If it is too difficult to position the needle at the level of the pedicle, another approach can be used. A medial intercostal nerve block can be performed. When the needle is positioned properly, a nerve root block or transforaminal epidural can be accomplished (Fig. 25-9).

Specific guidelines concerning injection volumes have not been devised. In general, we use 1.0 mL of 2% lidocaine during diagnostic blocks, unless epidural flow is observed during the injection of 1.0 mL of contrast material. In that instance, 0.5 mL of local anesthetic is instilled to prevent anesthetization of structures other than the nerve root. For therapeutic injection, we infuse 1.0 to 3.0 mL of betamethasone followed by 0.5 to 1.0 mL of lidocaine.

Lumbar

The patient is placed in the prone position with the x-ray beam oriented obliquely. For all nerves, except L5, concentrating on the spatial relationship of three structures is the key to a successful block. The transverse process will be difficult to visualize as it becomes superimposed on the ipsilateral pedicle during rotation of the x-ray beam.

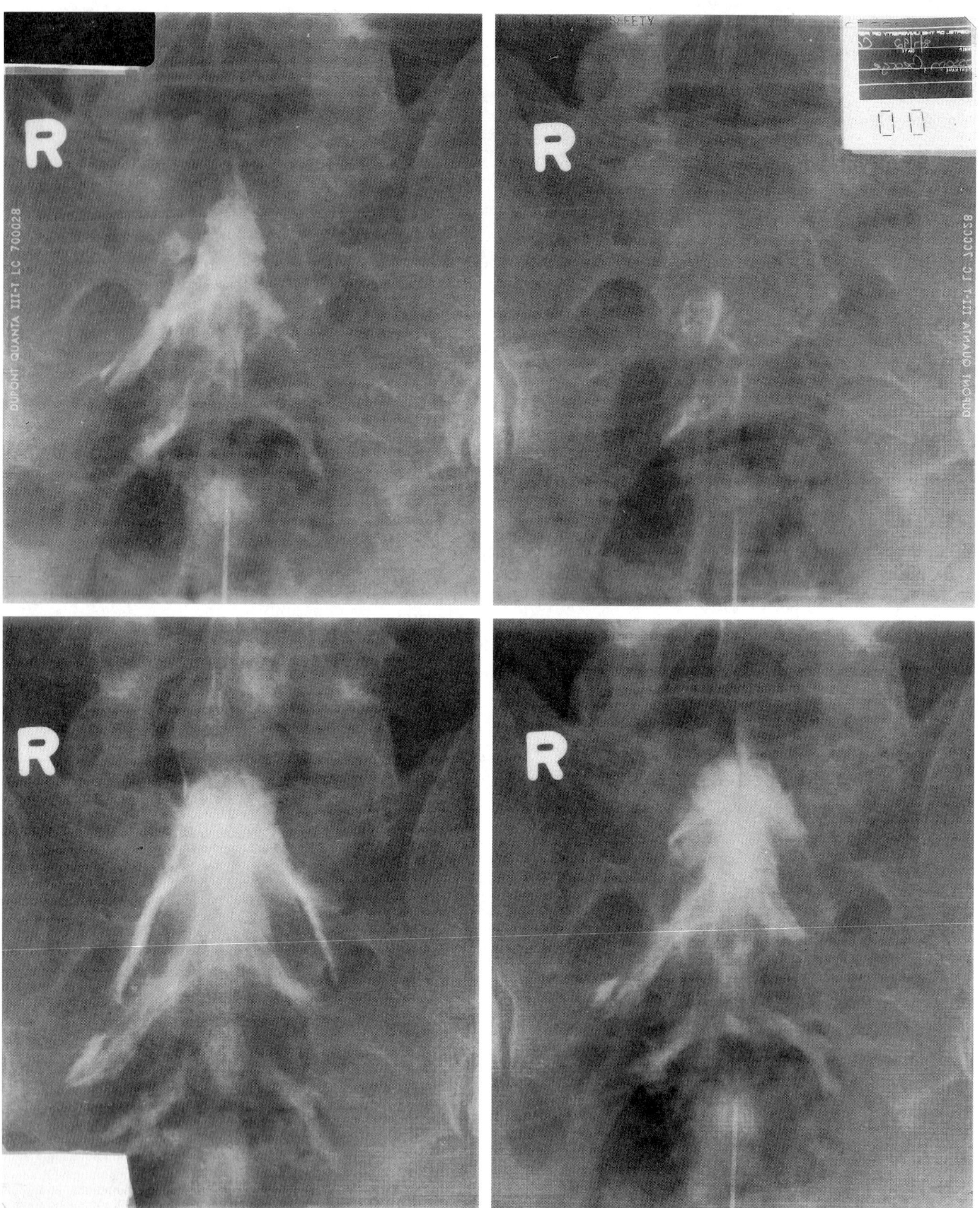

Figure 25-5. Sequential posterior-anterior images demonstrating dispersal of 1 to 2 mL of contrast medium infused into the epidural space by the caudal route.

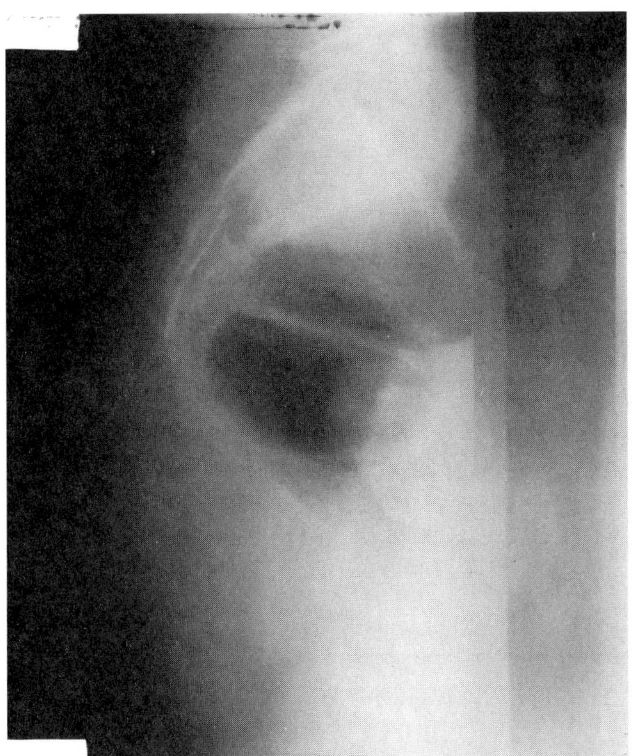

Figure 25-6. Lateral view of a caudal block with contrast filling the epidural space.

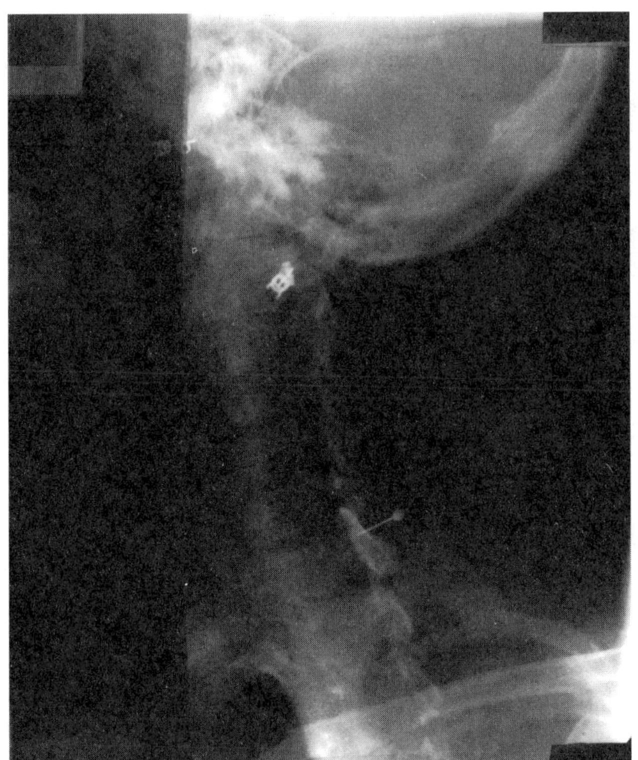

Figure 25-7. C7 selective nerve root block. Contrast is limited to the perineural sheath without any flow into the epidural space.

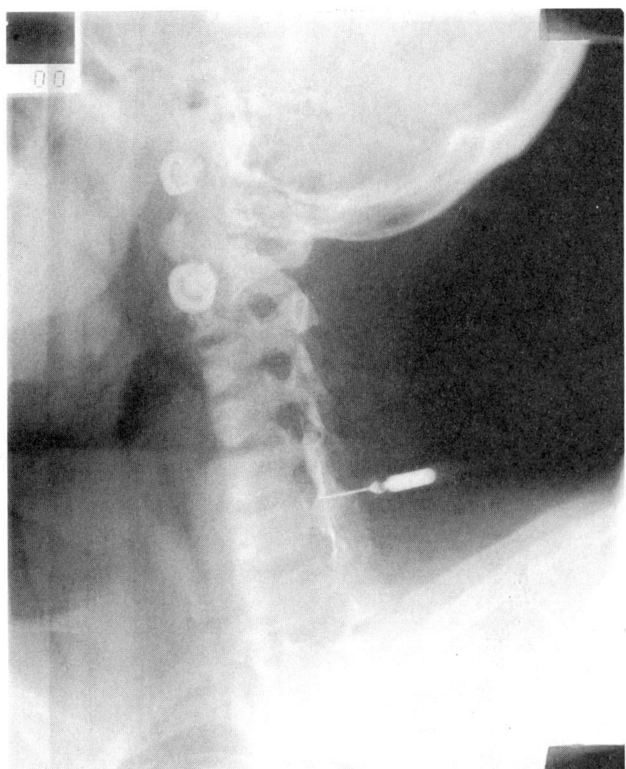

Figure 25-8. C6 transforaminal epidural injection. Contrast outlines the epidural space with no enhancement of the exiting nerve root.

Usually the inferior edge of the transverse process can be identified. Sometimes this will require real-time imaging as the gantry changes from an AP to its oblique terminal position. The starting point for the injection should be just caudal to the inferior edge of the transverse process. If the skin wheal is too caudal, then the needle may hit the flare of the inferior edge of the vertebral body, for example, the L3 vertebral body when performing an L3 SNRB. The superior facet arising from the inferior vertebral body (L4 during an L3 SNRB) should be superimposed on the medial edge of the pedicle. At this location the pedicle will appear oblong. A skin wheal is raised where the two points in the horizontal and vertical axes cross. The location in the vertical axis is just inferior to the transverse process and in the horizontal, at the midpoint of the pedicle. This site is targeted because the lumbar roots hug their respective pedicle as they exit the foramen. The needle is advanced in a bull's-eye manner until a change in tissue density is appreciated or the hub reaches skin (Fig. 25-10). Attaining this tactile ability requires experience; therefore, novices should expect to prod the root. When the change in density is appreciated, the needle tip will be "locked" in position. If the clamp is removed and the needle tip strays, the needle has not been advanced enough. If this transpired because the hub has reached skin, then another smaller-diameter and longer needle should be inserted through the initial needle (Fig. 25-11). After the second

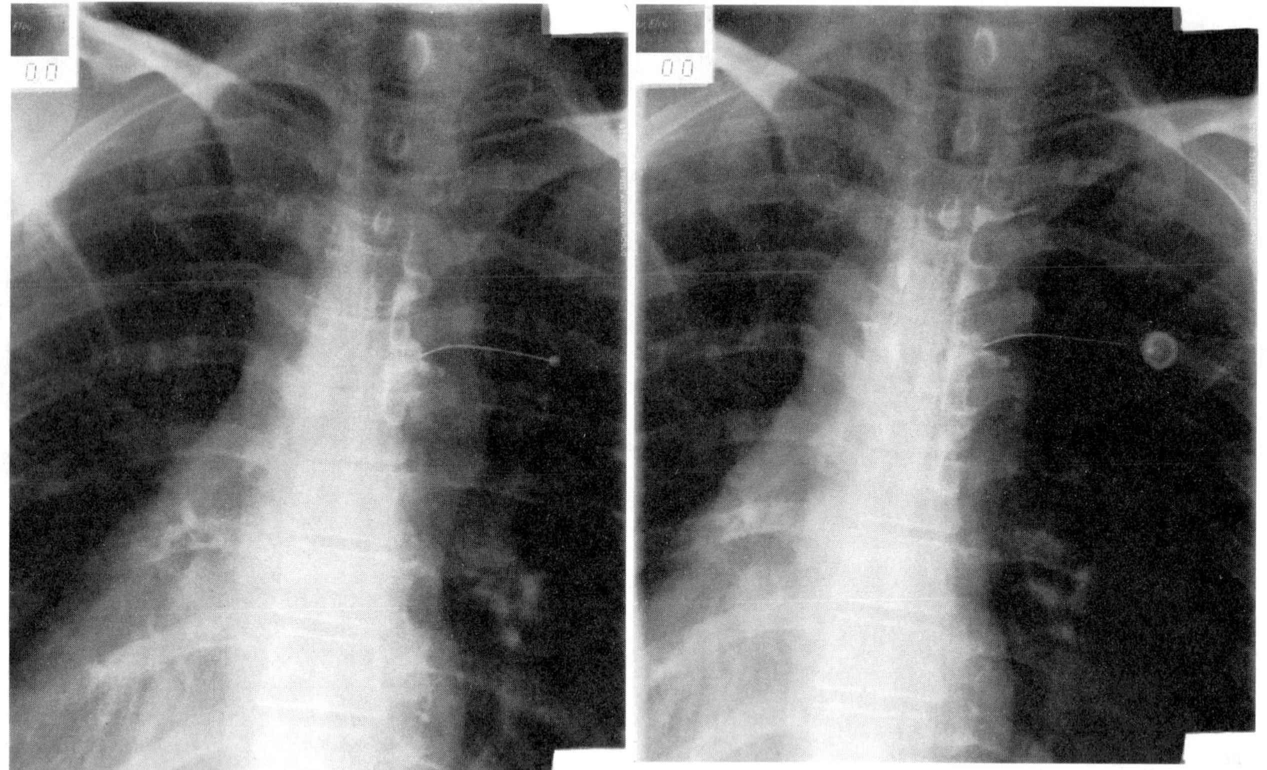

Figure 25-9. Anterior-posterior view of a T5 transforaminal epidural. *A.* Contrast material (0.3 mL) flows unilaterally and outlines three contiguous segments. *B.* Contrast material (0.6 mL) flows bilaterally and outlines five contiguous segments.

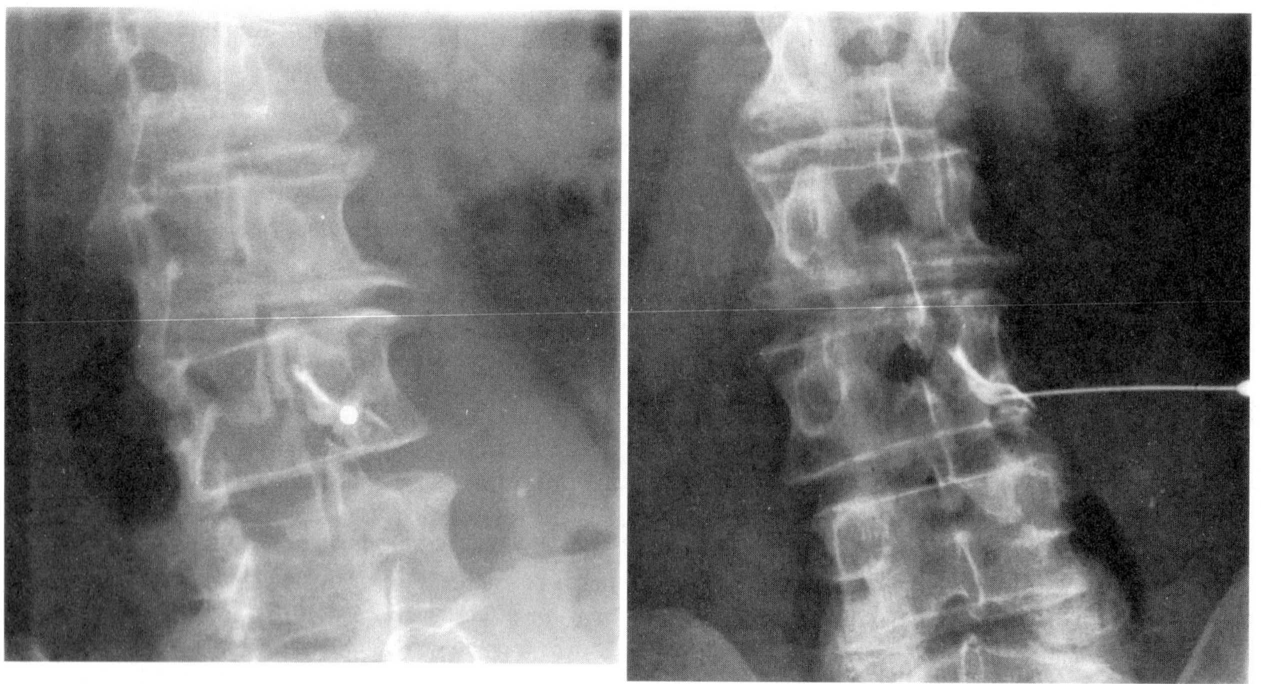

Figure 25-10. L3 selective nerve root block. *A.* Oblique view demonstrating the appropriate gantry angle for advancing a 22-gauge needle to rest just under the L3 pedicle. Note how the needle tip cannot be visualized in this "bull's-eye" shot. *B.* Anterior-posterior view demonstrating the needle tip resting at the 6-o'clock position of the L3 pedicle.

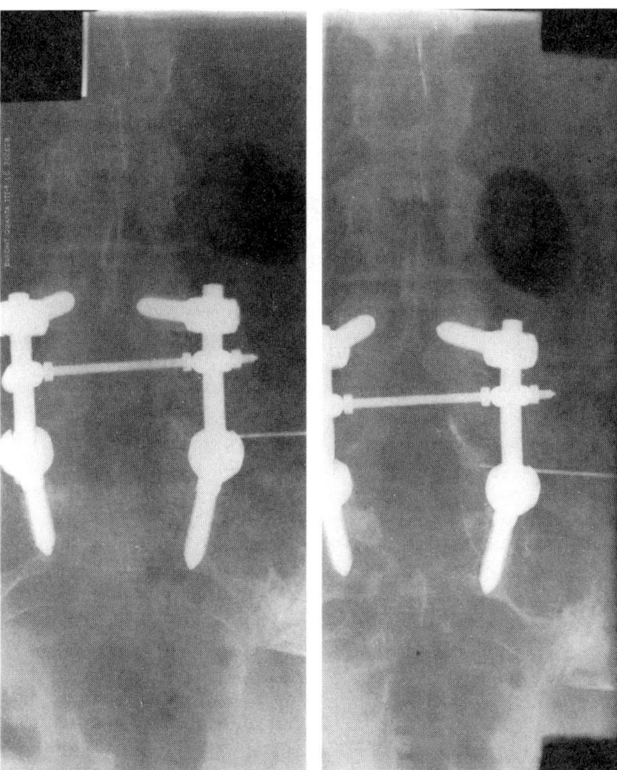

Figure 25-11. Anterior-posterior view of an L5 selective nerve root block employing a two-needle technique.

needle is inserted, the clamp and fluoroscope are used to orient the guide (first) needle into proper position. One should make sure the advancing needle does not advance into tissue before the guide needle is oriented; therefore, the advancing needle is too deep, it will curve away from the target during attempts to push it through. Once the needle is "locked," the gantry is oriented to obtain a posterior-anterior (PA) view. The needle is then advanced until it rests at the 6-o'clock position of the pedicle.

For L5 SNRB the location of pelvic structures must be considered. Direct, straight-shot access to the foramen may not be possible. This may occur if the patient has a transitional L5 vertebra, steeply inclined pelvis, large L5 transverse process, collapsed disk space, L5–S1 fusion, or spondylolisthesis. In these instances, advanced skills are requisite to complete the procedure. One- or two-needle techniques are available (Fig. 25-12).

To begin the single-needle technique, a skin wheal is raised at a point immediately lateral to the edge of the iliac crest and just inferior to the L5 transverse process. The needle tip is brought to rest just medial to the iliac crest. This will create tension in the needle. With the bevel facing medially, the needle is advanced with pressure applied at the interface between the needle and the iliac crest. This will create a dynamic curve, allowing the needle to reach the target. If the superior facet is approximated, precluding further needle advancement, a small aliquot of local anesthetic (0.1 mL of 1% lidocaine) is injected. Pressure is then directed toward the needle tip, creating a structural curve. The needle is slightly withdrawn, rotated 180 degrees, advanced deep enough to rest ventral to the superior articular process, rotated 180 degrees, and then advanced to the neural foramen. In this manner the needle will have curved around the superior facet.

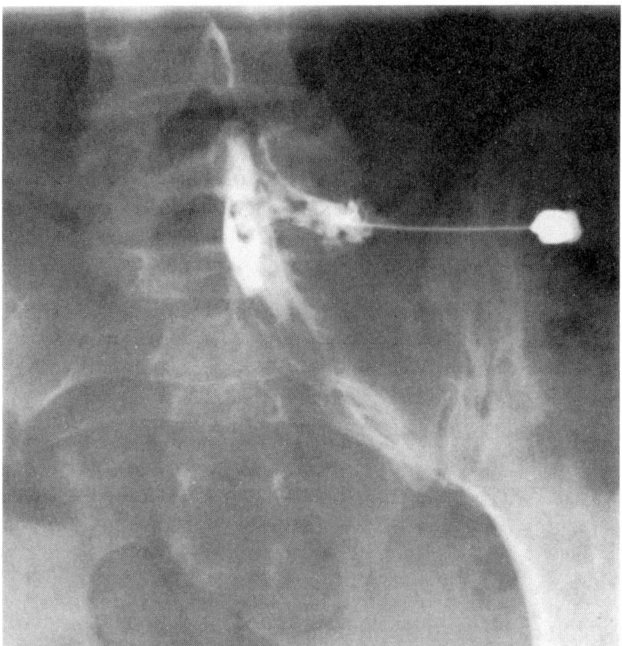

Figure 25-12. L5 transforaminal epidural. One milliliter of contrast outlines the L5 nerve root, midline epidural space, and ipsilateral S1 nerve root.

Instead of using the superior facet as a fulcrum for bending the needle, a second needle can be advanced through the first (guide)—the two-needle technique. A gentle curve in the second needle is created prior to placing it in the guide needle. The guide needle is slightly withdrawn and the second needle is advanced just beyond the bevel of the guide. While holding the advancing needle in place, the clinician gradually withdraws the guide needle. This process allows the curve to develop. The second needle is then advanced to the target location. When this technique is used, the clinician must be certain he or she is not placing the advancing needle in a position that is too ventral. Iliac artery or peritoneal puncture may ensue with inadvertent ventral needle placement.

A completely different approach for an L5 SNRB may be necessary when there is partial or full sacralization of L5. In this instance, a neural foramen similar to that found in the sacrum may be present. Unlike the approach for a sacral nerve root block, a skin wheal is raised lateral and inferior to the foramen. After the depth is gauged by advancing the needle tip to the periosteum, a caudal to cephalad and lateral to medial direction is used.

For a sacral nerve root block, the skin wheal is raised lateral and superior to the foramen. The needle is advanced parallel with the x-ray beam until periosteum is reached. A small amount of local anesthetic (0.2–0.4 mL of 1% lidocaine) can be injected quickly. This will anesthetize nearby periosteum, allowing needle advancement with minimal discomfort. For diagnostic injections this step should be avoided lest a false-positive result occur. The needle is slightly withdrawn and reoriented such that the tip will move medially and inferiorly.

As with other axial injections, except for diskography, the primary purpose of infusing contrast material is to establish proper needle position. For SNRB, additional information may be obtained as some consider the pattern of contrast flow to be diagnostic or helpful in surgical planning (47–50).

Typically, 1.0 mL of local anesthetic is instilled for a diagnostic injection; however, volumes ranging from 1.0 to 3.0 mL have been used (47,50). One should expect a high percentage of false-positive blocks when volumes larger than 1.0 mL are used.

Zygapophyseal Joint Injection

Cervical

A lateral or posterior approach can be used. The former carries a greater risk of dural or vertebral artery puncture and spinal cord impalement. These injections and, in particular, the lateral joint approach, should not be performed by novices, unless under direct supervision of an experienced physician.

For a lateral approach, the patient should be resting in the lateral position. The patient should understand the importance of keeping the shoulders relaxed or the clinician's view will be obstructed. Once the joint is identified, the patient is gently and slowly rolled to determine which is the ipsilateral joint space. This process is the critical portion of the procedure. One should never assume that an obviously visible and clear joint space is located on the ipsilateral side. Often it is the contralateral joint. A skin wheal is raised at the dorsal aspect of the joint, in order to steer clear of the vertebral artery, and just superior to the inferior aspect of the inferior articular process. The needle is advanced incrementally under fluoroscopic guidance until it abuts periosteum (Figs. 25-13 to 25-17). The needle tip is reoriented to a slightly more inferior location and advanced into the joint. During therapeutic injections, a small aliquot of local anesthetic (0.1 mL of 1% lidocaine) can be injected prior to advancement of the needle into the joint.

The posterior approach can be used for C3–C4 to C6–C7 joints. In contrast to the lateral approach, penetration of the vertebral artery is unlikely as this requires advancing the needle through the anterior capsule. This technique requires the patient to rest in the prone position. A slight tilt of the imaging beam is typically necessary to identify the joint. A skin wheal is raised just inferior to the joint and the needle advanced to the target.

We typically infuse 0.10 to 0.15 mL of contrast medium for confirmation of needle placement. Diagnostic injections are completed with 0.5 mL of 2% lidocaine or 0.25%, 0.50%, or 0.75% bupivacaine (Sensorcaine). Therapeutic injections include a combination of 0.8 mL of betamethasone sodium phosphate and 0.2 mL of 1% or 2% lidocaine.

Thoracic

A skin wheal is raised at the mid aspect of the pedicle two segments below the joint level to be treated, for example, T8 for a T6–T7 joint block. The needle is kept at a 60-degree angle to the skin and advanced in a cephalad direction. During periodic fluoroscopic imaging, the needle is maintained within the midpoint of the interpedicular column. The medial and lateral boundaries of this column are delineated by an imaginary line connecting the medial and lateral aspects of the pedicle above and below the joint of interest, respectively. After periosteum is reached, the beam is rotated from PA view toward the lateral. Once the joint is clearly visualized, the needle tip can be advanced through its most cephalad aspect.

We typically infuse 0.2 to 0.3 mL of contrast medium for confirmation of needle placement. Diagnostic injections are completed with 0.5 mL of 2% lidocaine or 0.25%, 0.50%, or 0.75% bupivacaine. Therapeutic injections include a combination of 0.8 mL of betamethasone sodium phosphate and 0.2 mL of 1% or 2% lidocaine.

Lumbar

After the joint is brought into view by rotating the x-ray beam, a skin wheal is raised medial to the most inferior edge of the joint. Under simultaneous fluoroscopic imaging the needle is rapidly advanced. The tip should be brought to rest on the lateral edge of the inferior facet. A slight dynamic bend should be created during needle positioning. A slight tension in the needle will be appreciated. This tension can be used to quickly pierce the joint capsule. The needle is slightly withdrawn and the tip will spring across the edge of the inferior facet to rest on the joint. Advancing the needle 1 or 2 mm more will place it intra-articularly (Fig. 25-18). Bogduk et al (51) advocated using the midportion of the joint as the target, but this site tends to be more difficult for novices.

We typically infuse 0.2 to 0.4 mL of a contrast agent for confirmation of needle placement. Diagnostic injections are completed with 0.75 to 1.00 mL of 2% lidocaine or 0.25%, 0.50%, 0.75 bupivacaine. Therapeutic injections include a combination of 0.5 to 0.8 mL of betamethasone sodium phosphate and 0.2 to 0.5 mL of 1% or 2% lidocaine.

Sacroiliac Joint Block

With the patient resting prone, a true lateral image of the joint should be obtained first. This occurs when the dorsal and ventral aspects of the facet joint are superimposed. The C-arm is then rotated 0 to 15 degrees, directing the

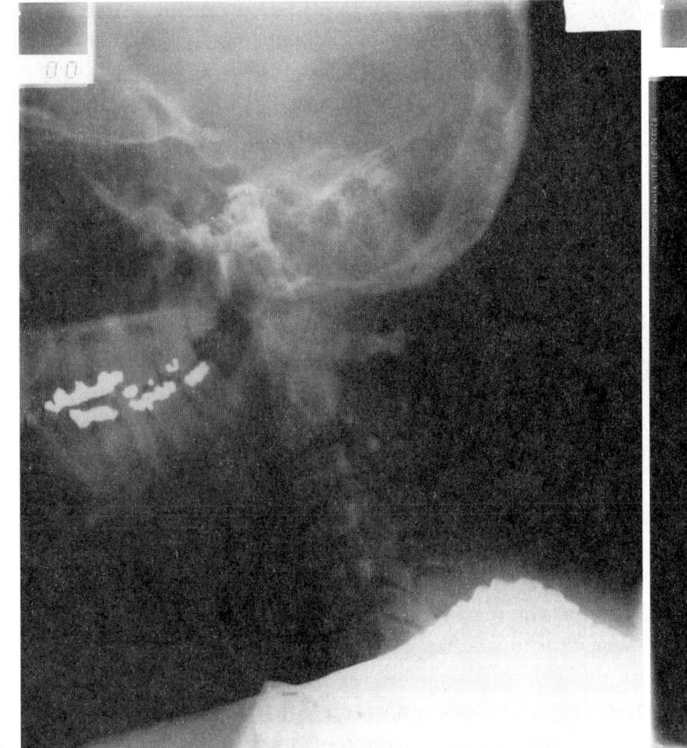

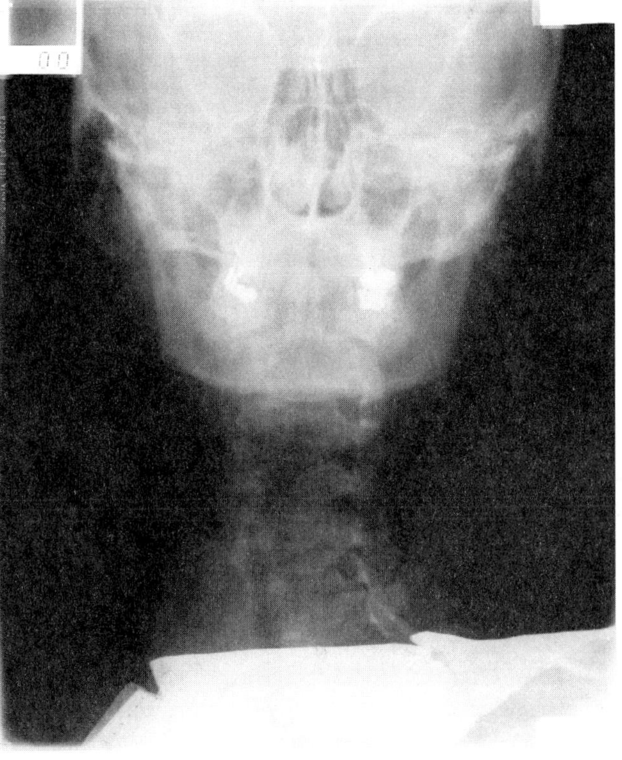

Figure 25-13. C2–C3 facet joint block. *A*. Lateral view revealing contrast (0.1 mL) filling the inferior and superior recesses. *B*. Contrast (0.2 mL) filling the inferior and superior recesses. *C*. Anterior-posterior view of contrast outlining the C2–C3 facet joint.

x-ray beam in a contralateral to ipsilateral direction. When the medial joint line, which always represents the dorsal component, begins to separate from the lateral joint line, beam rotation is halted. A small lucent area at the most caudal aspect of the joint will be seen. This represents the final target. A skin wheal is raised 1 to 3 mm medial to this point. A 22-gauge or narrower, 3.5-inch needle is advanced until the periosteum of the lateral edge of the sacrum is abutted. If a therapeutic injection is being performed, 0.1 to 0.3 mL of lidocaine can be slowly

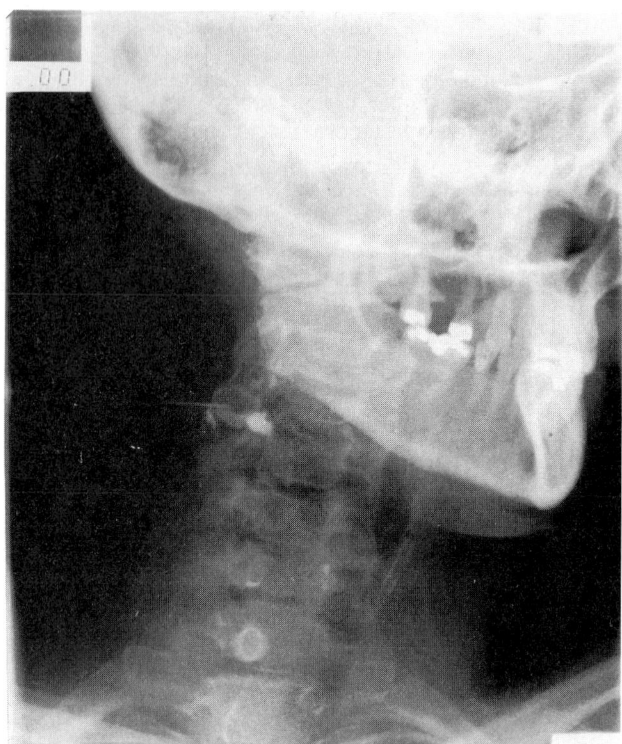

Figure 25-14. Anterior-posterior view of a C2–C3 facet joint block. The *arrow* demonstrates diverticulum or expansion of the inferior recess.

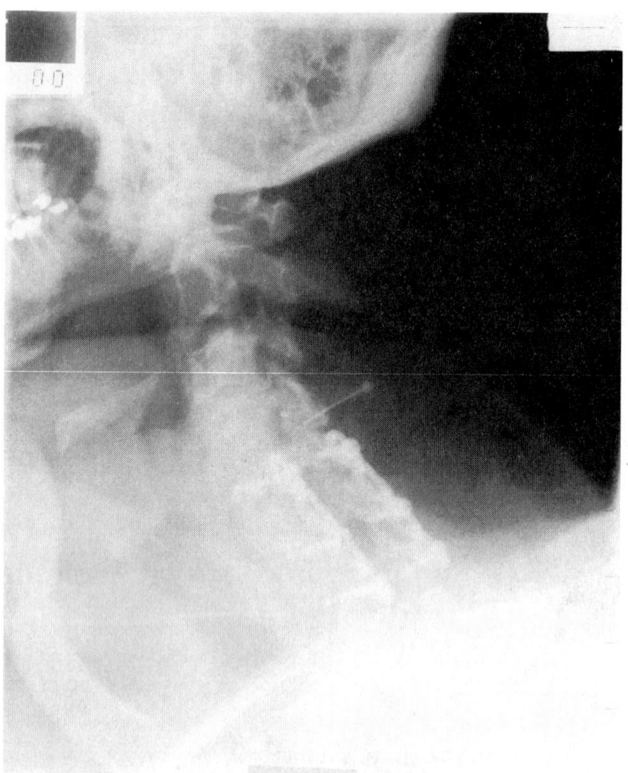

Figure 25-15. Diagnostic C4–C5 facet joint block in a 45-year-old woman with a C5–C7 fusion. Chronic neck and periscapular pain was emanating from this joint.

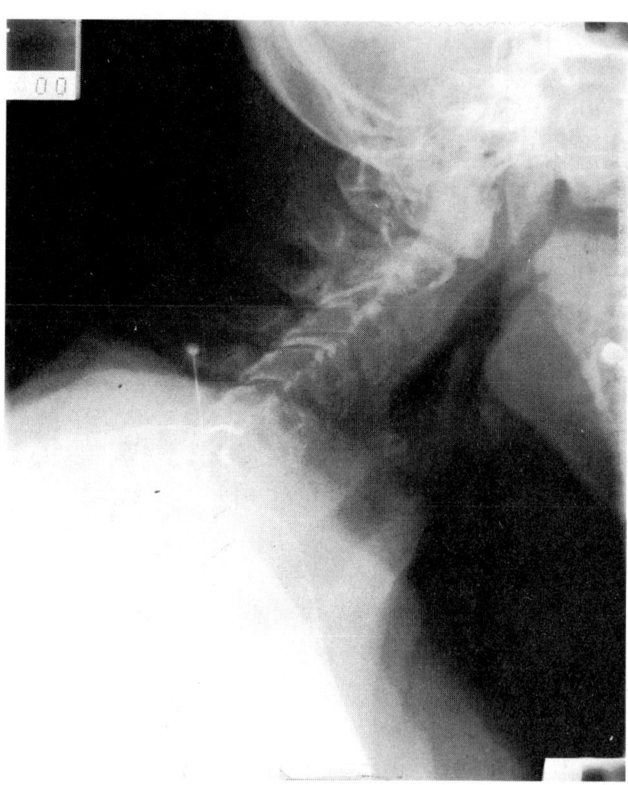

Figure 25-16. C5–C6 facet joint block. Compare the cephalocaudal inclination of this needle with that in Figures 25-14 and 25-15. Note the increased angle of inclination required as one performs injections in progressively lower cervical joints. This is not a consequence of joint orientation but rather a result of the relationship between the supraclavicular fossa and the cervical region of the spine.

infiltrated. The needle is withdrawn 0.5 to 1.0 cm before it is advanced directly into the mid portion of the previously identified lucency. Shwarzer et al (52) advocated a technique in which a skin wheal is raised inferior to the target with the needle advancement to the ileum. No more than 0.5 mL of contrast material is required to demonstrate an arthrographic, synovial, or combined pattern (Fig. 25-19); however, larger volumes may be needed to demonstrate an anomaly or abnormality. Preliminary study suggests a maximal volume of 2.0 mL be used (53) but some authors suggest up to 5.0 mL is reasonable (54). Reacquiring a lateral view may be necessary as it will reveal an arthrographic pattern not easily seen from the AP perspective. Moving the beam in a counterclockwise manner will provide an oblique view (Fig. 25-20). Synovial patterns are easier to appreciate with this view.

Synovial tears and diverticula commonly occur and the former have been associated with symptom relief following a diagnostic block (52). The possibility of a synovial tear has important implications about the validity of the result of a diagnostic block, since it is unclear into which structure(s) the local anesthetic was ultimately deposited. A

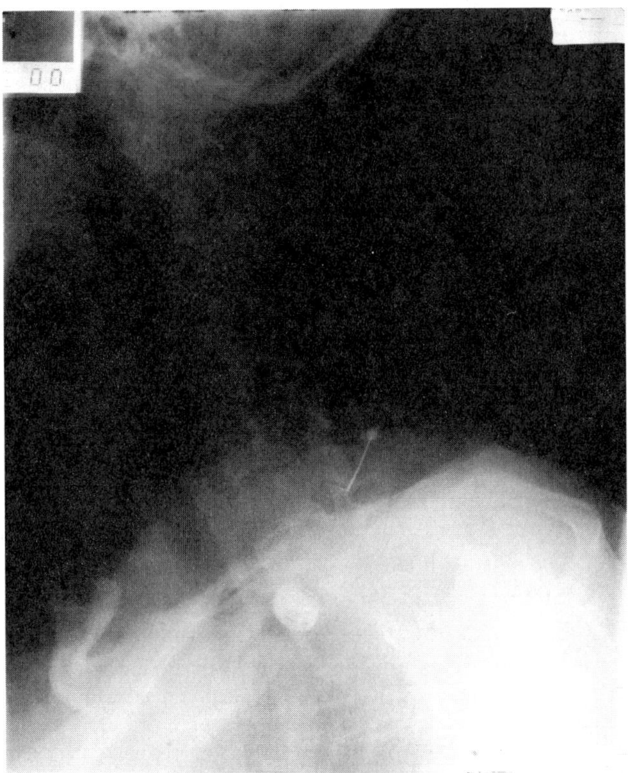

Figure 25-17. C7–T1 facet joint block.

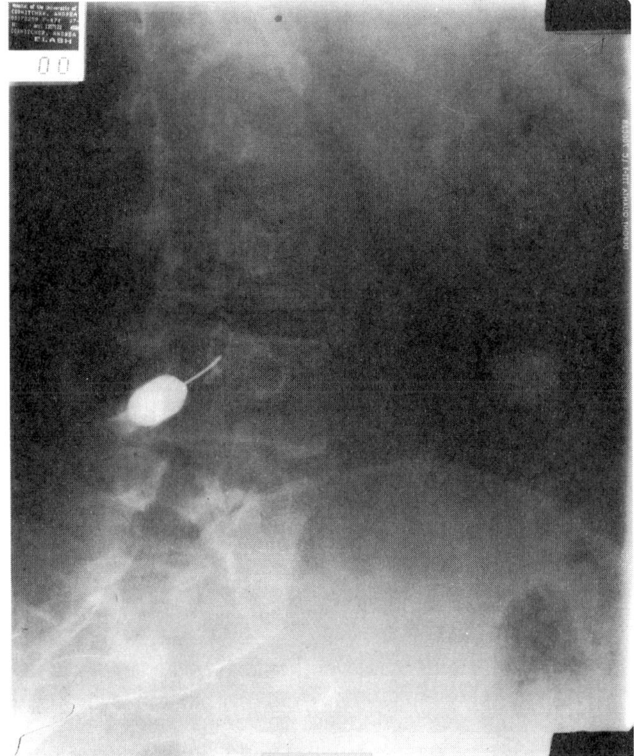

Figure 25-18. L3–L4 facet joint block.

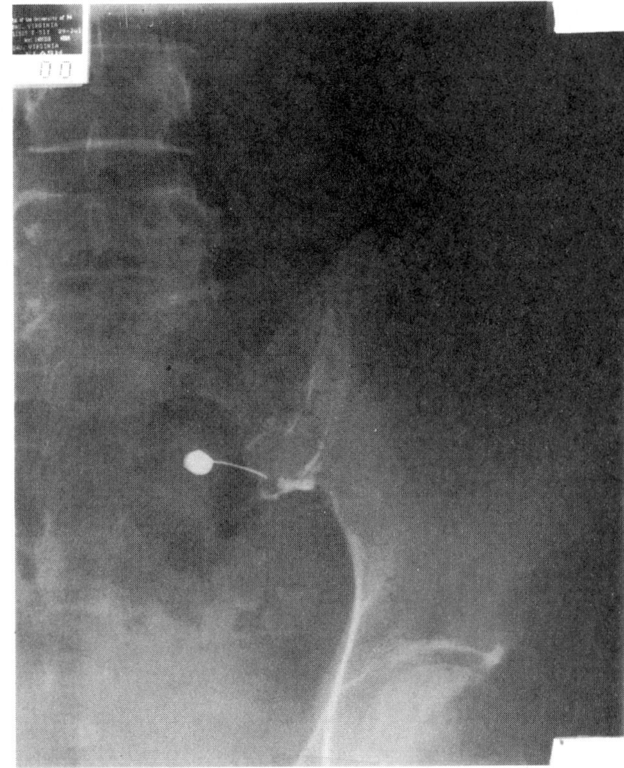

Figure 25-19. Anterior-posterior view of a sacroiliac joint block.

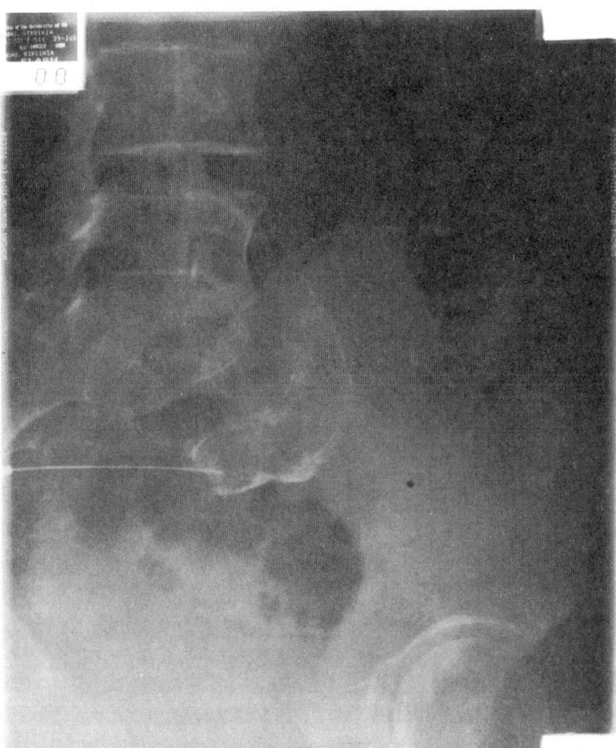

Figure 25-20. Oblique or "en-face" view of a sacroiliac joint block. Note the classic auricular pattern.

combination of contrast material and local anesthetic can be injected after the initial aliquot of contrast material has been given, to prevent this potentially confounding event from transpiring. If continuous fluoroscopic imaging is employed, injection can be discontinued if contrast material leaks into surrounding tissue.

Lumbar Sympathetic Block

Numerous techniques have been offered to anesthetize the sympathetic chain. Our preference is to have the patient rest prone, the involved side prepared using a sterile technique, and the patient rotated approximately 20 to 40 degrees. Typically, the transverse process is figuratively divided in half at this location. The medial 50% is superimposed on its respective vertebra, while the lateral 50% is beyond the lateral border of its respective vertebra. With a caudal to cephalad approach, the inferior edge of the midpoint of the L2 transverse process is approached. A small aliquot, 0.5 mL, of local anesthetic is distributed about the periosteum. The needle is then repositioned such that it slips under the transverse process, but superior to the exiting nerve root. The needle is simultaneously oriented lateral to medial. Once the vertebral body is reached, the needle can be advanced in small increments ventrally to rest in the plane of the sympathetic chain. Just ventral to the ventral aspect of the vertebral body is the peritoneum. Consequently, small incremental needle advancements are used once the needle tip has advanced beyond the junction of the dorsal two-thirds and ventral one-third of the vertebral body as viewed in the lateral plane.

After proper needle placement is attained, 1 to 3 mL of contrast material is infused. It should track superiorly and inferiorly along the plane of the sympathetic chain. Usually 10 mL of 1% lidocaine will be sufficient to obtain adequate blockade.

Diskography

Diskography involves demonstrating nuclear morphology by injecting a contrast agent into the central portion of the disk with the simultaneous recording of pain provocation. Abnormal-appearing nucleograms alone are insufficient to identify a painful disk. Correlation between the quality, location, and intensity of pain with the nucleogram findings is required.

Interpretation of the radiographic image is straightforward. Only rents that extend into the periphery of the annulus are considered abnormal and potential pain generators. This concept is based on anatomic studies demonstrating that the outer one-third of the annulus is the only innervated portion of the disk (55–59).

Ensuring accuracy in the interpretation of pain production can be the most difficult aspect of diskography. The patient must be alert, be able to articulate the quality and location of the pain produced, and be able to compare the injection-induced pain to the normal pain. All patients must be apprised of their role in this procedure just before contrast material is injected, regardless of the extent of preprocedural explanations.

Questions have been raised about diskogram interpretation. As recently as 1995, the Agency for Health Care Policy and Research concluded that diskogram interpretation is equivocal (60). This judgment was unfounded and subsequently critiqued (61). The 1990 study by Walsh et al (62) unequivocally demonstrated the reliability of this test.

Diskography can be performed in the cervical, thoracic, lumbar, and coccygeal regions of the spine. A paucity of literature discussing indications for cervical, thoracic, or coccygeal diskography is available (63–66).

In general, diskography is performed for patients who have chronic, intractable, axial pain that has dramatically impaired their quality of life. Several in-depth publications have identified the broader indications for lumbar diskography (67–70). It is recommended for the following:

1. Patients with chronic and intractable low-back pain (69)
2. Patients with radicular pain, positive tension signs, and equivocal imaging studies—particularly for the previously operated spine (67,69)

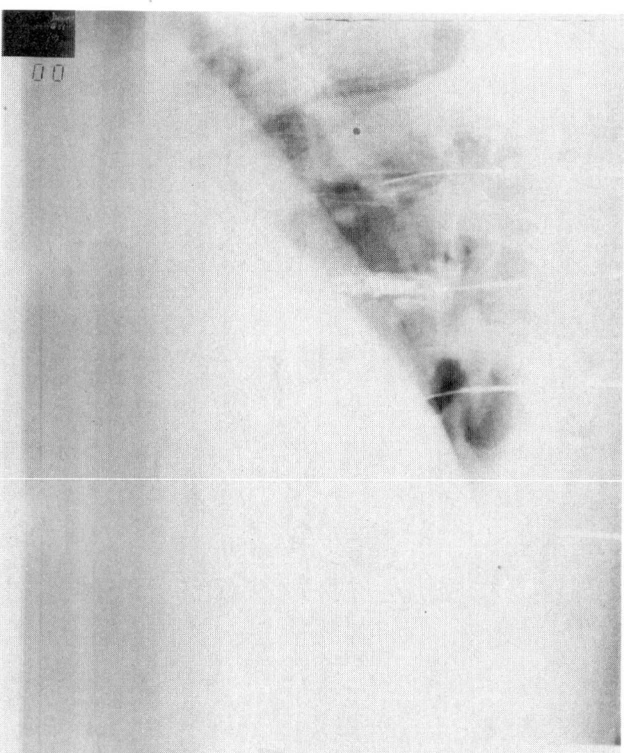

Figure 25-21. Lateral four-level thoracic diskogram performed on a 36-year-old man who had undergone a four-level laminectomy with residual back pain. The plain diskograms are only partially readable. These films can no longer be regenerated; therefore, information concerning the T8–T9 and T9–T10 disks is permanently lost. The anterior-posterior view was overexposed and unreadable.

3. To evaluate disks adjacent to an impending fusion level for spondylolisthesis, pseudarthrosis, and segmental instability (68–70)
4. Prior to chemonucleolysis or minimally invasive spine surgery (69).

All patients who undergo diskography should have an immediate postprocedure computed tomography (CT) study. Disko-CT provides valuable information, including demonstration of the site of injection, nuclear versus annular lesion site; the extent and distribution of annular disruption; epidural flow of contrast material, thereby revealing a herniation; and previously missed osseous lesions, such as spondylolysis (Figs. 25-21 and 25-22).

Cervical

Performance of this technique demands precise needle control, refined tactile perception, and an advanced ability to translate two-dimensional radiography into three-dimensional mental images. These criteria must be met if complications are to be avoided. Spine physicians can develop these skills by performing a minimum of 100 lumbar disk injections and thousands of other spine injections.

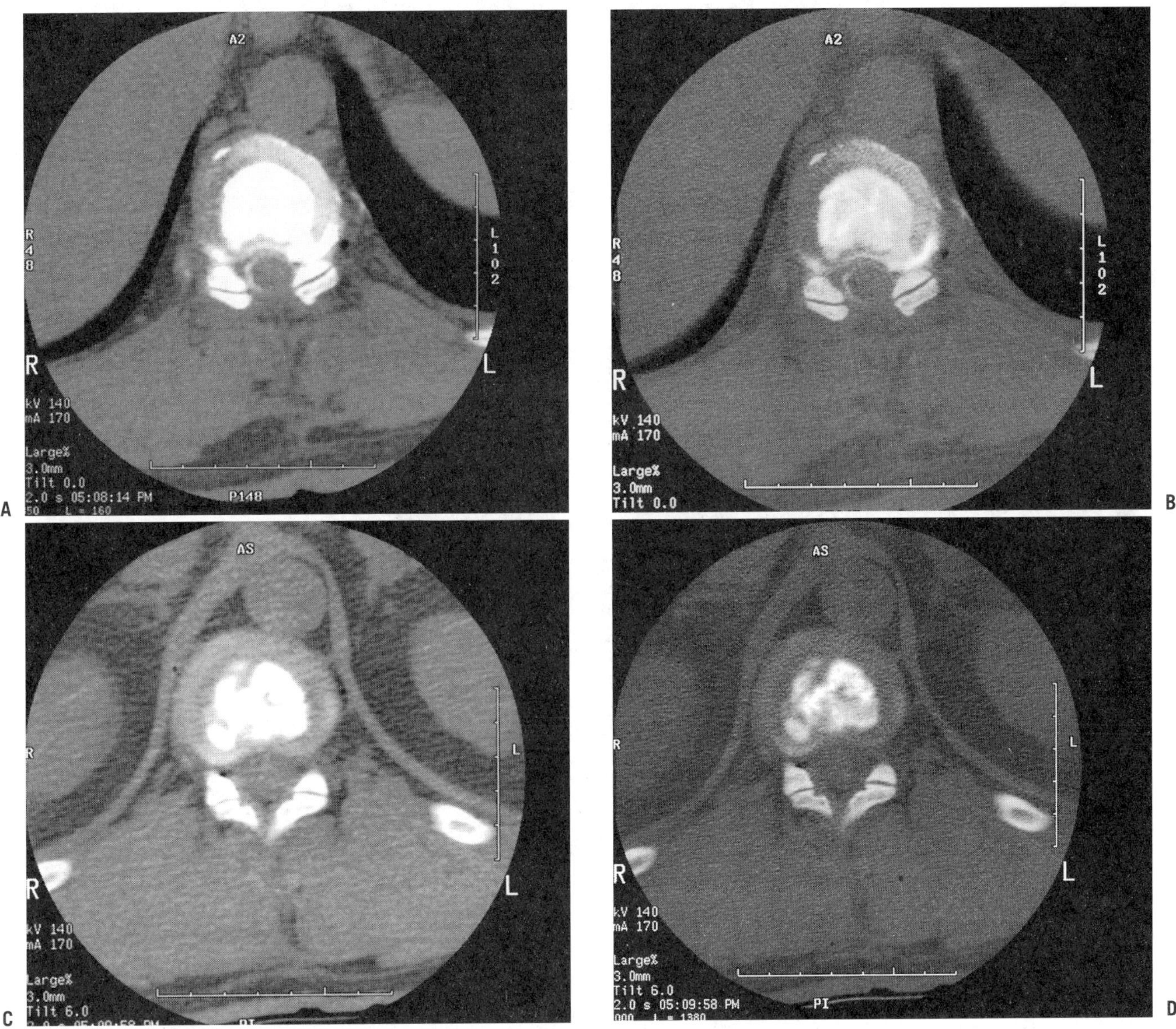

Figure 25-22. Computed tomography (CT) scan of the thoracic diskogram demonstrated in Figure 25-21. The information lost on the plain films is obtainable from the CT scan. This case demonstrates one of the reasons why CT should be performed after every diskogram—to preserve information. *A.* Soft-tissue windows of the symptomatic T9–T10 disk. A left posterolateral protrusion allows contrast flow to fill the ipsilateral foramen and epidural space. *B.* Bone window of the symptomatic T9–T10 disk. *C.* Soft-tissue window of the asymptomatic T11–T12 disk. *D.* Bone window of the asymptomatic T11–T12 disk.

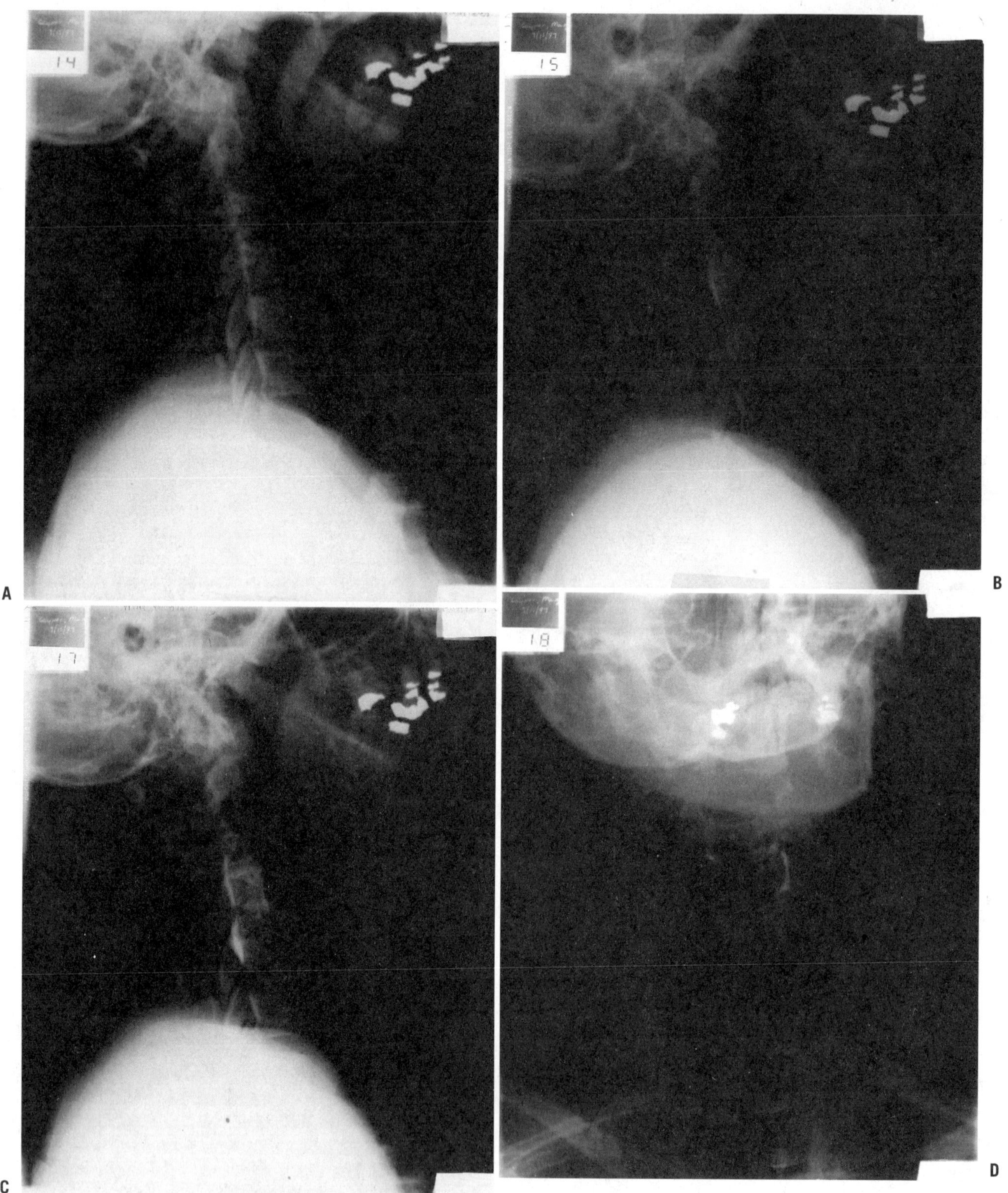

Figure 25-23. Lateral cervical diskogram in a 32-year-old woman with neck and periscapular pain for 4 years. *A.* Needles are properly positioned in this plane within the C3–C4, C4–C5, and C5–C6 disks. *B.* Lateral view of contrast injected into the nucleus of the C3–C4 disk. Contrast material fills the entire disk and extends into the epidural space. *C.* Lateral view of contrast injected into the C4–C5 disk. Contrast material extravasates from the nucleus into the epidural space. *D.* Anterior-posterior view after injection into the C3–C4 followed by C4–C5 disks. Note how contrast extends to the lateral margins of the disks at both levels, revealing a confluent annular tear connecting the nucleus to the outer limits of the annulus. *E.* Lateral view of contrast injected into the C5–C6 disk. Contrast material is located within the nucleus and extends into the epidural space. All three levels demonstrated concordant pain.

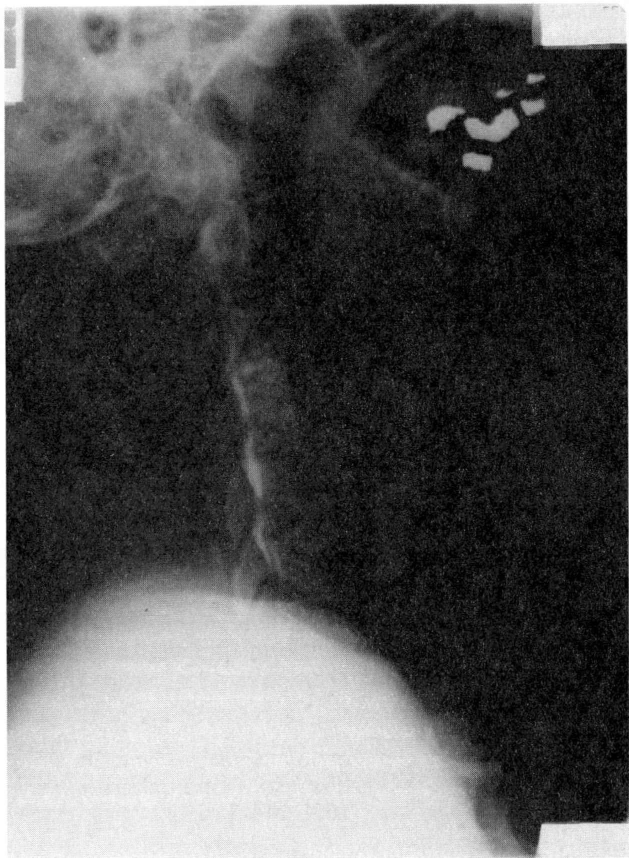

E

Figure 25-23. *Continued.*

After the patient is placed in the supine position, the right side of the neck is prepared using a sterile technique. Since the esophagus lies in the left paracervical region, inadvertent puncture will be minimized. With gentle pressure applied with the nondominant hand, the trachea is mobilized to the left, while the carotid is displaced to the right or is fixed in place by the index finger. The ventral disk space is now easily appreciated with mild pressure exerted by the long finger. The dominant hand then advances the 22- to 25-gauge, 3.5-inch needle to the outer annulus. Rotating the C-arm from the AP to the lateral perspective will confirm accurate needle placement. Any advancement of the needle beyond this location requires repeat lateral spot views. In comparison to the lumbar nuclei, cervical nuclei are much smaller; therefore, midline target sites are used for the lateral and AP views. This size differential also translates to much smaller injection volumes. In most instances, 0.3 to 0.5 mL of contrast material is infused (Fig. 25-23). When pain provocation occurs, local anesthetic or steroid or both can be instilled.

Thoracic

As for cervical diskography, only experienced diskographers should attempt this technique. The patient is placed in the prone position and the side contralateral to the site of pain is prepared using a sterile technique. A slight oblique view, approximately 20 degrees, is required. A 22- to 25-gauge, 3.5-inch needle is advanced just lateral to the interpedicular line, but medial to the costovertebral articulation. In a manner similar to cervical disk injection, the needle is advanced such that a midline end point is reached in the lateral and AP views. The needle should be advanced in small increments and viewed in both planes before this target site is reached.

Lumbar

Lumbar diskography can be accomplished in three ways, representing a combination of two techniques and two approaches:

1. Posterolateral approach with the patient resting in the prone-oblique position. A right-sided entrance site is typically employed, thereby requiring that the patient rest on the left side. The right hip is flexed and slightly abducted, while the right knee is flexed. Pillows are placed under the distal medial aspect of the thigh to support the right leg. This leg position relaxes the right L5 nerve root, thereby minimizing the chance of needle contact during an attempt to enter the L5–S1 disk. A bolster is placed under the left flank, which will slightly tilt the pelvis and open the entrance to the L5–S1 disk.
2. Posterolateral approach with the patient prone. In contrast to the aforementioned posterolateral approach, this technique requires biplanar imaging with each advance of the needle.
3. Transdural approach with the patient prone. A paramedian needle entrance point is used. Extra care is taken when aligning the guide needle, as the second needle will pierce the dural membrane twice prior to entering the disk space. If alignment is not accurate, repeat attempts to advance the needle will be required, with each trial causing not one, but two dural punctures. Therefore, the risk of headache, nerve root injury, meningitis, and meningocele formation is theoretically increased. Consequently, a transdural approach should be reserved for instances in which the L5–S1 disk cannot be entered with the two other techniques.

Before the patient is positioned for this test, an evaluation is required to determine which technique and approach should be used. Factors influencing this decision include patient size, patient compliance, disk space height, pelvic configuration, presence of transitional segments, and prior diskectomy or fusion. Once this determination is made, the procedure is re-explained to the patient. A sterile field is then created. A two-needle technique is used in each instance. The introduce or guide needle does not enter the disk space, to obviate placement of skin flora into the nucleus. A curved two-needle technique is often needed for the posterolateral approach, with the patient resting obliquely. In this case, the second needle is given a gentle curve, allowing it to slip around the right S1 superior articular process and under the exiting L5 nerve root (55–58, 62, 67–70).

CONCLUSIONS

A vast array of diagnostic and therapeutic injections is available to the musculoskeletal physiatrist. To be performed proficiently, some procedures require little advanced training and no specialized equipment. Others are very technically demanding and require precision and expertise to avoid serious or even life-threatening complications. Well-trained musculoskeletal practitioners should be familiar with the techniques described here and understand the rationale behind proper prescription of these procedures, even if they do not intend to perform the procedures themselves. Proper use and delivery of diagnostic and therapeutic injections will improve nonoperative care, reduce unnecessary procedures, and enhance operative outcomes.

REFERENCES

1. Pfenninger JL. Injections of joints and soft tissue: part I. General guidelines. *Am Fam Physician* 1991;44:1196–1202.
2. Wilke WS, Tuggle CJ. Optimal techniques for intra-articular and periarticular joint injections. *Mod Med* 1988;56:58–72.
3. Nicholas JJ. Articular and soft-tissue injections. *Phys Med Rehabil Clin N Am* 1996;7:643–658.
4. Zuckerman JD, Meislin RJ, Rothberg M. Injections for joint and soft tissue disorders: when and how to use them. *Geriatrics* 1990;45:45–52,55.
5. Kerlan RK, Glousman RE. Injections and techniques in athletic medicine. *Clin Sports Med* 1989;8:541–560.
6. Millard RS, Dillingham MF. Peripheral joint injections. Lower extremity. *Phys Med Rehabil Clin N Am* 1995;6:841–849.
7. Owen DS. Aspiration and injection of joints and soft tissues. *In*: Kelly WN, Harris ED Jr, Ruddy S, et al, eds. *Textbook of rheumatology*. 3rd ed. New York: WB Saunders, 1989:621–636.
8. Gaffney K, Ledingham J, Perry JD. Intra-articular triamcinolone hexacetonide in knee osteoarthritis: factors influencing the clinical response. *Ann Rheum Dis* 1995;54:379–381.
9. Samuelson CO, Cannon GW, Ward JR. Arthrocentesis. *J Fam Pract* 1985;20:179–184.
10. Birrer RB. Aspiration and corticosteroid injection. Practical pointers for safe relief. *Phys Sports Med* 1992;20:57–71.
11. Nicholas JJ. Joint and soft tissue injection techniques. *In*: Braddom RL, ed. *Physical medicine and rehabilitation*. Philadelphia: WB Saunders, 1996:503–513.
12. Doherty M. Soft tissue injections in the surgery. *Practitioner* 1989;233:1305.
13. Gray RG, Gottlieb NL. Intra-articular corticosteroids. An updated assessment. *Clin Orthop* 1983;177:235–263.
14. Brown J. Injections and aspirations. *Br J Clin Pract* 1987;41:641–644.
15. Haslock I, Macfarlane D, Speed C. Intra-articular and soft tissue injections: a survey of current practice. *Br J Rheumatol* 1995;34:449–452.
16. Cawley PJ, Morris IM. A study to compare the efficacy of two methods of skin preparation prior to joint injection. *Br J Rheumatol* 1992;31:847–848.
17. Micheo WF, Rodriguez RA, Amy E. Joint and soft-tissue injections of the upper extremity. *Phys Med Rehabil Clin N Am* 1995;6:823–840.
18. Pfenninger JL. Injections of joints and soft tissue: part II. Guidelines for specific joints. *Am Fam Physician* 1991;44:1690–1701.
19. Williams P, Gumpel M. Aspiration and injection of joints (1). *BMJ* 1980;281:990–992.
20. Bach BR, Bush-Joseph C. Subacromial space injections: a tool for evaluating shoulder pain. *Phys Sports Med* 1992;20:93–97.
21. Rowe CR. Injection technique for shoulder and elbow. *Orthop Clin North Am* 1988;19:773–777.
22. Woodburne RT, Burkel WE. *Essentials of human anatomy*, 8th ed. New York: Oxford University Press, 1988:144–145.
23. Williams P, Gumpel M. Aspiration and injection of joints (2). *BMJ* 1980;281:1048–1050.
24. Anderson BC, Manthey R, Brouns MC. Treatment of de Quervain's tenosynovitis with corticosteroids. *Arthritis Rheum* 1991;34:793–798.
25. Harvey FJ, Harvey PM, Horsley MW. de Quervain's disease: surgical or nonsurgical treatment. *J Hand Surg* 1990;15A:83–87.
26. Janecki CJ. Extraarticular steroid injection for hand and wrist disorders. *Postgrad Med* 1980;66:173–181.
27. Green DP. Diagnostic and therapeutic value of carpal tunnel injection. *J Hand Surg* 1984;9A:850–854.
28. Kay NRM, Marshall PD. A safe, reliable method of carpal tunnel injection. *J Hand Surg* 1992;17A:1160–1161.
29. Liu N, Canoso JJ. Dynamic injection of the digital flexor tendon sheaths. *Rheum Dis* 1990;49:327–328.

30. Neustadt DH. Local corticosteroid injection therapy in soft tissue rheumatic conditions of the hand and wrist. *Arthritis Rheum* 1991;34:923–926.

31. Pace JB, Nagle D. Piriform syndrome. *West J Med* 1976;124: 435–439.

32. Wyant GM. Chronic pain syndromes and their treatment. III. The piriformis syndrome. *Can Anaesth Soc J* 1979;26:305–308.

33. Yong-Hing K. Surgical techniques. *In*: Kirkaldy-Willis WH, Burton CV, eds. *Managing low back pain.* 3rd ed. New York: Churchill Livingstone, 1992:375.

34. Barton PM. Piriformis syndrome: a rational approach to management. *Pain* 1991;47:345–352.

35. Holt MA, Keene JS, Graf BK, Helwig DC. Treatment of osteitis pubis in athletes. Results of corticosteroid injections. *Am J Sports Med* 1995;23:601–606.

36. Cohn BT, Shapiro PS. An effective technique for corticosteroid injection into the knee joint. *Orthop Rev* 1993;22:1341–1342.

37. Fischer AA. Local injections in pain management. Trigger point needling with infiltration and somatic blocks. *Phys Med Rehabil Clin N Am* 1995;6:851–870.

38. Garvey TA, Marks MR, Wiesel SW. A prospective, randomized, double-blind evaluation of trigger-point injection therapy for low-back pain. *Spine* 1989;14:962–964.

39. Porzelius J. Memory for pain after nerve-block injections. *Clin J Pain* 1995;11:112–120.

40. Derby R, Kine G, Saal JA, et al. Response to steroid and duration of radicular pain as predictors of surgical outcome. *Spine* 1992;6: S176–S183.

41. Dreyfuss P, Michaelsen DC, Pauza K. The value of medical history and physical examination in diagnosing sacroiliac joint pain. *Spine* 1996;21:2594–2602.

42. Slipman CW, Sterenfeld EB, Chou LH, et al. The predictive value of provocative sacroiliac joint stress maneuvers in the diagnosis of sacroiliac joint syndrome. *Arch Phys Med Rehabil* (submitted for publication).

43. Dreyfus P, Michaelsen DC, Pauza K. The value of medical history and physical examination in diagnosing sacroiliac joint pain. *Spine* 1996;21:2594–2602.

44. Maigne J, Aivaliklis A, Pfefer F. Results of sacroiliac joint double block and value of sacroiliac pain provocation tests in 54 patients with low back pain. *Spine* 1996;21:1889–1892.

45. Ebraheim NA, An HS, Xu R, et al. The quantitative anatomy of the cervical nerve root groove and the intervertebral foramen. *Spine* 1996;21:1619–1623.

46. Huston CW, Slipman CW, Meyers JS, et al. Side effects and complications of fluoroscopically guided nerve root injections. *Arch Phys Med Rehabil* 1996;77:937.

47. Tajima T, Furukawa K, Kuramochi E. Selective lumbosacral radiculography and block. *Spine* 1980;1: 68–77.

48. Kikuchi S, Hasue M. Combined contrast studies in lumbar spine disease: myelography (peridurography) and nerve root infiltration. *Spine* 1988;13:1327–1331.

49. Krempen JF, Smith BS. Nerve root injection: a method for evaluating the etiology of sciatica. *J Bone Joint Surg [Am]* 1974;56:1435–1444.

50. Macnab I. Negative disc exploration: an analysis of the causes of nerve root involvement in sixty-eight patients. *J Bone Joint Surg [Am]* 1971;53:5891–5903.

51. Bogduk N, Aprill C, Derby R. Diagnostic blocks of spinal synovial joints. In: White AH, Schofferman JA, eds. *Spine care. Diagnosis and conservative treatment.* Vol 1. St. Louis: Mosby-Year Book, Inc.

52. Shwarzer AC, Aprill CN, Bogduk N. The sacroiliac joint in chronic low back pain. *Spine* 1995;20: 31–37.

53. Fortin JD, Dwyer AP, West S, Pier J. Sacroiliac joint: pain referral maps upon applying a new injection/arthrography technique: part 1. Asymptomatic volunteers. *Spine* 1994;19:1475–1482.

54. Hendrix RW, Lin PP, Kane WJ. Simplified aspiration or injection technique for the sacroiliac joint. *J Bone Joint Surg [Am]* 1982;64: 1249–1252.

55. Bogduk N. The innervation of the lumbar spine. *Spine* 1983;8:286.

56. Bogduk N, Twomey LT. *Clinical anatomy of the lumbar spine.* New York: Churchill Livingstone, 1991:161.

57. Hirsch C, Ingelmark BE, Miller M. The anatomical basis for low back pain. *Acta Orthop Scand* 1963;33: 1–17.

58. Jackson HC, Winkelmann RK, Bickel WH. Nerve endings in the human lumbar spinal column and related structures. *J Bone Joint Surg [Am]* 1966;48:1272–1281.

59. Malinsky J. The ontogenetic development of nerve terminations in the intervertebral discs of man. *Acta Anat* 1959;38:96–113.

60. Bigos S, Bowyer O, Broon G, et al. *Acute low back problems in adults. Clinical practice guideline No. 14.* Rockurlle, MD: U.S. Department of Health and Human Services, 1994. AHCPR publication no. 95-0642.

61. Slipman CW. Discography. *In*: Gonzalex EG, Materson RS, eds. *The nonsurgical management of acute low back pain.* New York: Demos Vermande, 1998;35–45.

62. Walsh TR, Weinstein JN, Spratt KF, et al. Lumbar discography in normal subjects: a controlled, prospective study. *J Bone Joint Surg [Am]* 1990;7:1081–1088.

63. Maigne JY, Guedj S, Straus C. Idiopathic coccydynia: lateral roentgenograms in the sitting position and coccygeal discography. *Spine* 1994;19: 930–934.

64. Schellhas KP, Pollei SR, Dorwart RH. Thoracic discography: a safe

and reliable technique. *Spine* 1994;19:2103–2109.

65. Gill K. Point of view. *Spine* 1994;19:2109.

66. Whitecloud TS, Seago RA. Cervical discogenic syndrome. Results of operative intervention in patients with positive discography. *Spine* 1987;12:313–317.

67. Bernard TN Jr. Using computed tomography/discography and enhanced magnetic resonance imaging to distinguish between scar tissue and recurrent lumbar disc herniation. *Spine* 1994;24: 2826–2832.

68. Errico TJ. The role of discography in the 1980's. *Radiology* 1988; 162:285, Letter.

69. Guyer RD, Ohnmeiss DD. Contemporary concepts in spine care. Lumbar discography. Position statement from the North American Spine Society and Therapeutic Committee. *Spine* 1995;18:2048–2059.

70. Murtagh FR, Arrington JA. Computer tomographically guided discography as a determinant of normal disc level before fusion. *Spine* 1992;17:826–830.

Chapter 26

Exercise in Physical Medicine and Rehabilitation

Walter R. Frontera

SCOPE

Exercise is one of the most frequently used therapeutic modalities in the habilitation or rehabilitation of patients. Understanding the principles of muscle actions and the associated physiologic reactions is of fundamental importance to designing appropriate exercise interventions for patients with a wide variety of impairments and disabilities. The physiology of exercise and its therapeutic effectiveness have received significant attention in the scientific literature during the last two decades. In this chapter, I review relevant concepts and definitions, discuss the determinants of exercise performance, explain the acute adaptations in various systems of the human body to exercise, analyze the fundamental elements of an exercise prescription, and discuss the adaptations to strength and endurance exercise training programs.

BASIC CONCEPTS AND DEFINITIONS

The use of proper terminology in exercise physiology and rehabilitation is of utmost importance to promote better communication among professionals in the field (1,2). Here I review the basic concepts and definitions commonly used when studying the role of exercise in the prevention, treatment, and rehabilitation of human disease.

Physical Concepts

Exercise can be defined as any and all activity involving generation of force by the activated muscle(s). Three physical concepts are frequently used to quantify exercise and describe human performance (1,2). *Force* [measured in newtons (N)] is defined as that which changes or tends to change the state of rest or motion in matter; force = mass × acceleration. A force may produce either linear displacement or rotation of a joint about its axis. The product of force and the perpendicular distance from the line of action of the force and the axis of rotation of a joint is known as *torque* [measured in newton-meters (Nm)]. *Work* [measured in joules (J)] is defined as force expressed through a distance with no consideration for time and is comparable to heat and energy; work = force × distance. Finally, *power* [measured in watts (W)] is the rate of performing work; power = force × velocity, and time is a critical factor.

Types of Skeletal Muscle Actions

The active state of skeletal muscle is characterized by an *attempt* to shorten the longitudinal axis of the muscle cells when activated. The term *contraction* is frequently used to describe muscle actions but it may be misleading because shortening, as contraction is usually defined, does not occur with all types of muscle actions. Depending on the force generated by the contractile elements and the forces applied externally, an active muscle may maintain its length, shorten, or lengthen. Based on this definition, muscle actions can be divided into static (isometric) and dynamic (isotonic, isokinetic) categories (Table 26-1, Fig. 26-1) (1). Dynamic actions, in turn, can be classified as concentric or eccentric.

Table 26-1: Types of Skeletal Muscle Actions

Static (isometric, no work or power)
Dynamic (isotonic, isokinetic)
Concentric (shortening, positive work)
Eccentric (lengthening, negative work)

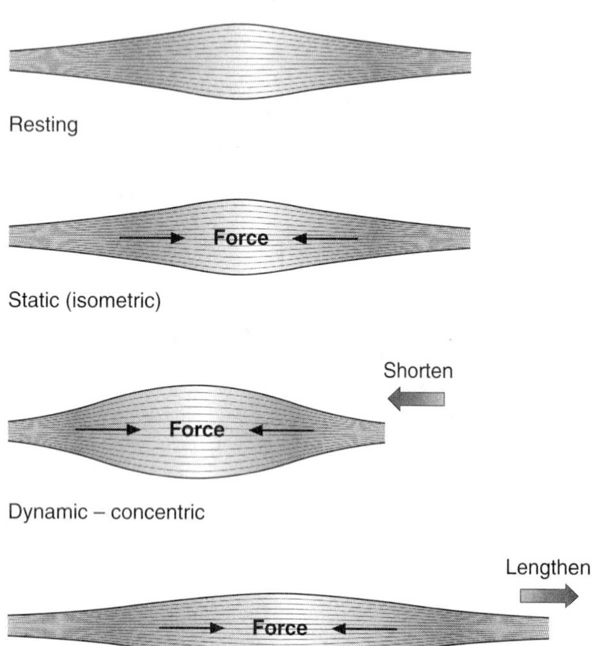

Figure 26-1. The basic types of muscle actions (see text for explanation). (Modified by permission from Knuttgen HG, Kraemer WJ. Terminology and measurement in exercise performance. *J Appl Sports Sci Res* 1987;1:1–10.)

When the activation of a muscle does not result in shortening and no change in the position of a joint can be detected, the muscle action is called *static*. During static actions, force is generated without displacement. Thus no work is done and no external power is produced. This situation occurs when the bony attachments of the muscle are fixed or when the external forces are of the same magnitude and act in the opposite direction as those developed by the muscle.

A *dynamic* action involves movement and consists of either a concentric or an eccentric action. During a dynamic concentric action (commonly known as an *isotonic contraction*), muscle shortens and the bony attachments move closer to each other. The term *isotonic* is not accurate because it implies constant force, a condition not present in common human muscle actions, partly due to the fact that the force generated by muscle fibers varies with its length, which in turn changes at different joint angles. During dynamic concentric actions, force is generated, work is done, and various levels of external power production can be achieved depending on the velocity of movement. This type of action is also known as *positive work* because displacement occurs in the direction of the forces generated by the muscle fibers.

Eccentric or lengthening muscle actions are characterized by external forces that move the bony attachments farther apart. Because displacement occurs in the opposite direction to the forces generated by muscle cells, this type of action is known as *negative work*. Eccentric actions generate more force than do concentric actions (Fig. 26-2) independent of the speed of movement (3–5). Also, at any given exercise level, energy consumption is lower during eccentric actions (see Fig. 26-2).

Isokinetic actions constitute a special type of dynamic (concentric or eccentric) action that results in body movements at a constant velocity as controlled by an ergometer. This is an artificial situation that can only be simulated in the laboratory.

Finally, it should be noted that most of the daily activities performed in the natural environment, such as walking and jumping, involve a sequence or combination of static and dynamic concentric and eccentric actions. In fact, concentric and eccentric actions can occur simultaneously in antagonistic muscles such as the elbow flexors and extensors.

MUSCLE FIBER TYPES

The diversity of muscle fibers is one of the fundamental properties of the neuromuscular system (6). Muscle fibers have been classified into different types according to their mechanical, histochemical, metabolic, and biochemical characteristics (7). A frequently used classification divides muscle cells into type I (slow, fatigue resistant, oxidative), type IIA (fast, fatigue resistant, oxidative-glycolytic), and type IIB (fast, fatigable, glycolytic). Recent studies showed that human type IIB fibers may correspond to the type IIX fibers identified in animals (8,9).

In recent years, it has become evident that the above classification does not reflect the true biologic diversity of fibers in human skeletal muscles. The fiber-type composition of muscle must be viewed as a continuum rather than discrete groups (10,11). This continuum is defined by the presence of different isoforms of the contractile (myosin heavy and light chains) and regulatory (troponin and tropomyosin) muscle proteins (12,13) whose expression is controlled at the gene level (14). Further, studies in single muscle fibers obtained with the percutaneous muscle biopsy technique showed that more than one isoform can be expressed simultaneously in the same fiber (15,16). In other words, a single hybrid fiber may coexpress myosin heavy-chain types I and IIA (type I/IIA) or IIA and IIB

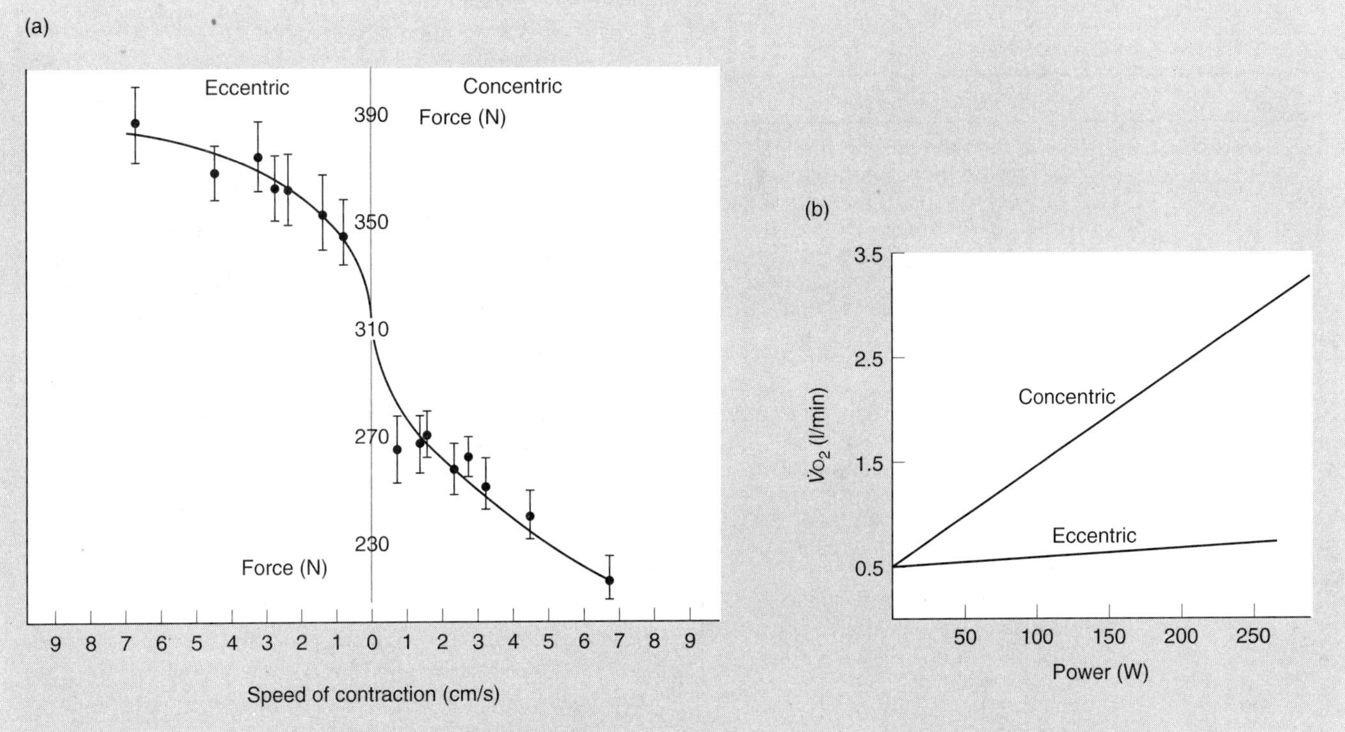

Figure 26-2. *a.* The force-velocity relationship of skeletal muscle showing higher forces during eccentric actions at all speeds. (Reproduced by permission from Komi PV. The musculoskeletal system. In: Dirix A, Knuttgen HG, Tittel K, eds. *The Olympic book of sports medicine.* Boston: Blackwell Science, 1988:25.) *b.* Relationship between oxygen uptake ($\dot{V}O_2$) and power output during concentric and eccentric muscle actions. (Modified by permission from Komi PV. The musculoskeletal system. In: Dirix A, Knuttgen HG, Tittel K, eds. *The Olympic book of sports medicine.* Boston: Blackwell Science, 1988:26.)

(type IIA/B). These fibers can be identified with techniques such as protein electrophoresis but may not be identified correctly using standard histochemical staining techniques.

Muscle fiber-type composition is a dynamic property and fibers may change their isoform composition in response to various stimuli such as electrical stimulation, bed rest, and exercise training (6,14,17–20). These stimuli may act to activate or inactivate genes responsible for the synthesis of a particular isoform (18). Isoform composition is a major determinant of the contractile properties of the muscle cell (15,16) and muscle function correlates with fiber-type composition. Knowledge of the prevalence of the different fiber types and their contractile and biochemical properties is fundamental to understanding both the acute responses to an exercise bout and the adaptations to exercise training.

ACUTE PHYSIOLOGIC ADAPTATIONS TO EXERCISE

During exercise, energy expenditure and force production for movement are made possible by a well-coordinated series of adaptations in various organs and systems of the body (Table 26-2). Understanding these adaptations is essential to evaluate the functional status of a patient and to formulate an exercise prescription for rehabilitation. In general, the responses to an acute bout of endurance exercise are similar to those seen in a heavy-resistance training session. Exceptions to this statement will be noted. A more comprehensive discussion of the physiologic adaptations discussed here can be found in various textbooks on the subject (21–24). Some differences between children and adults in the hemodynamic and respiratory responses are presented in Table 26-3 (25).

Metabolic and Endocrine Responses

Energy production during exercise is achieved by mobilization of the adenosine triphosphate (ATP)–phosphocreatine (PCr) stores in the muscle cell and activation of the glycolytic and oxidative metabolic pathways. The nature and time sequence of these adaptations are closely related to the intensity and duration of the exercise. In general, high-intensity, very-short-duration (<10 seconds) exercise depends on the ATP-PCr stores available in the muscle fiber (11,26–29). For exercise of longer duration, up to 2 minutes, glycolysis (anaerobic metabolism) becomes the main source of energy. Under these conditions, various

Table 26-2: Acute Physiologic Responses to Exercise

System	Nature of the Response
Energy production	Mobilization of phosphocreatine–adenosine triphosphate stores and activation of glycolytic and oxidative pathways
Fuel supply	Mainly carbohydrate and fat with a small contribution from proteins
Endocrine	Increases in enzymes favoring lipolysis, glycogenolysis, and gluconeogenesis; reduction in insulin
Circulatory	Increase in systolic blood pressure, no change in diastolic blood pressure, vasodilation in active muscles, vasoconstriction in splanchnic region and inactive muscles, reduced peripheral resistance
Cardiac	Increases in heart rate, stroke volume, cardiac output, coronary blood flow, and myocardial O_2 consumption
Pulmonary	Increases in respiratory rate, tidal volume, minute ventilation, and pulmonary blood flow; improved ventilation-perfusion ratio
Thermoregulatory	Increased skin circulation, evaporation of sweat, reduction in urine production, production of enzymes to conserve body fluids

metabolites (including Pi, H^+, lactic acid) may accumulate, altering the intracellular and extracellular environment of the muscle fiber, limiting its capacity to generate force, and resulting in fatigue. After 2 minutes. oxidative (aerobic) pathways predominate and prevent metabolite accumulation. Thus, muscle actions can be repeated many times as long as the demands for oxygen are met. Also, during repeated sprints, aerobic metabolism makes an important contribution to energy supply during the recovery period. It is important to point out that there may be significant overlap between systems and more than one system can be active simultaneously. Further, during predominately aerobic exercise, there may be instances when the intensity of the exercise increases (e.g., the final sprint of the 10,000-m race), and the glycolytic pathways are reactivated.

To support the energy production by the metabolic machinery of the muscle cell, fuels are supplied from different sources. The most important sources are the carbohydrate (glycogen) and triglyceride stores in muscle, the triglyceride stores in subcutaneous fat tissue, the liver glycogen stores, and the lactate produced during exercise (30–33). The intensity and duration of the exercise are, once again, major determinants of the selection of fuel (34). In general, exercise of high intensity and short duration utilizes glycogen (glycogenolysis) stores in muscle and in the liver. When the exercise is of relatively long duration and low intensity, free fatty acids released from the breakdown of triglycerides become the predominant fuel for the production of energy. It should be noted that varying the composition of the diet affects the relative availability of fats versus carbohydrates during exercise (35,36). Finally,

Table 26-3: Hemodynamic and Respiratory Characteristics of Children's Responses to Exercise

Function	Typical for Children (Compared with Adults)
Hemodynamic	
Submaximal heart rate	Higher, especially in first decade
Maximal heart rate	Higher
Submaximal and maximal stroke volume	Lower
Cardiac output at given $\dot{V}O_2$	Somewhat lower
Difference in O_2 concentration between arterial and venous blood at given $\dot{V}O_2$	Somewhat higher
Blood flow to active muscles	Higher
Submaximal and maximal systolic and diastolic blood pressure	Lower
Respiratory	
Ventilation at given $\dot{V}O_2$	Higher
Respiratory rate	Higher
Tidal volume/vital capacity	Lower

Source: Modified by permission from Bar-Or O. Importance of differences between children and adults for exercise testing and exercise prescription. In: Skinner JS, ed. *Exercise testing and exercise prescription for special cases.* Philadelphia: Lea & Febiger, 1987:52.

$\dot{V}O_2$ = oxygen uptake.

amino acids from protein metabolism may contribute between 5% and 10% of the total energy expended during exercise (37,38).

The hormonal response to exercise is coordinated mainly to facilitate fuel mobilization for energy production and to maintain fluid homeostasis (32,39,40). The levels of several hormones including epinephrine, norepinephrine, growth hormone, cortisol, and glucagon increase during exercise. At the same time, insulin concentration in plasma decreases (41). These changes serve to promote the breakdown of muscle glycogen, increase blood glucose (from the breakdown of liver glycogen, and the new synthesis of glucose from other substrates), and increase lipolysis and mobilization of free fatty acids (42). On the other hand, activation of the renin-angiotensin-aldosterone axis and release of antidiuretic hormone serve to maintain the blood volume by retaining sodium and water, respectively.

Circulation and Oxygen Delivery

To supply the necessary nutrients to and remove the waste products from the active muscle cell, significant adaptations occur in the circulatory system (43,44). Increased blood flow in the active muscles is achieved by vasodilation of their vascular beds and redistribution of blood flow from the splanchnic organs (spleen, kidney, and liver) and inactive muscles to the active regions (45–47). Factors associated with vasodilation and opening of muscle capillaries are substances released from the active cells (i.e., K^+, adenosine, H^+, and others) and the influence of the autonomic nervous system.

Blood pressure (BP) is the product of cardiac output (blood flow) and total peripheral resistance. Aerobic exercise is characterized by an increase in systolic blood pressure (SBP) (largely due to an increase in cardiac output), a constant or slight increase in diastolic blood pressure (DBP), and a reduction in peripheral resistance (48). Exercise with heavy resistance (weight lifting), on the other hand, may produce very large increases (320/250 mg Hg during the double-leg press) in both SBP and DBP (49). This is caused by simultaneous increases in both peripheral resistance and cardiac output.

The amount of muscle mass active during exercise is an important determinant of the circulatory responses to exercise. At a given level of power output, arm exercise produces a higher BP and peripheral resistance compared to leg exercise. This response is mostly related to the amount of active muscle mass rather than to the type of muscle action (static versus dynamic) (50,51). Also, vascular resistance is greater in the arms and in the legs during combined arm-leg exercise than is the resistance in the arms or legs when each is exercised separately (52). In other words, oxygen supply to one large group of exercising muscles (legs) may be limited by vasoconstriction or by a fall in arterial pressure when another large group of muscles is exercising simultaneously (53,54).

In addition to the hemodynamic changes resulting in increased blood flow, oxygen extraction by muscle cells is enhanced during exercise (55). Unloading of oxygen from hemoglobin is facilitated by the low pH, high carbon dioxide, and higher temperature prevalent in exercising muscles. Also muscle myoglobin lowers the concentration of free oxygen in the sarcoplasm and facilitates its diffusion from the red blood cell to the myocyte (56). These changes augment the difference in oxygen concentration between arterial and venous blood (a-vO_2 diff) mainly by lowering venous oxygen content with little changes in arterial blood oxygen content (57,58). It is interesting that tissue hypoxia during exercise is a stimulus for the production of growth factors that may result in new capillary formation (59).

Cardiac Adaptations

The goal of the cardiac response to the exercise stimulus is the production of a higher cardiac output (60). This is achieved by an increase in both heart rate and stroke volume (61,62). Cardiac output increases approximately 5 L/min for every 1-L/min increase in oxygen consumption. During mild exercise, heart rate increases due to a reduction in parasympathetic stimulation, while at higher intensities sympathetic stimulation predominates (63,64). At a given power output, heart rate will be higher when exercising with a smaller muscle mass (arms) because a higher force per unit of muscle produces more metabolic byproducts and feedback to the cardiovascular center in the medulla. However, maximal heart rate (heart rate during maximal exercise) will be higher when exercising with the legs because a larger muscle mass is activated and generates more power.

Stroke volume increases mainly during mild to moderate exercise but remains stable with increasing intensity (65). A reduction in peripheral resistance facilitates muscle blood flow and enhances venous return, contributing to the increase in stroke volume. Significant adaptations in the heart that result in an enhanced stroke volume during exercise include a fall in end-systolic volume, an increase in peak filling rate, and an enhanced myocardial contractility (65). During exercise with a small muscle mass, stroke volume is relatively low because of high peripheral resistance, which reduces venous return to the heart. A distinction has to be made between exercise in the supine and in the upright positions. In the former position, initial stroke volume is higher and the elevation usually seen with exercise is small, when compared to the upright position.

Finally, the major determinants of myocardial oxygen consumption (contractility, heart rate, and wall tension) increase with exercise. Thus, coronary blood flow increases in a linear fashion to supply the needed oxygen (66,67). A very high correlation exists between both myocardial oxygen consumption and coronary blood flow and the product of heart rate (HR) and SBP (double product = HR × SBP) (67).

Pulmonary Adaptations

The pulmonary system also adapts to the exercise stimulus (68,69). Ventilation increases with the onset of exercise. At low-power outputs, this increase in ventilation is mostly due to a rise in tidal volume while at higher levels, the ventilatory rate becomes the predominant factor. The time spent in inspiration during each cycle also increases. Ventilation can rise from a resting value of approximately 6 to 10 liters of air per minute to 100 to 125 L/min in untrained subjects and 150 to 200 L/min in well-trained athletes. Changes in ventilation are accompanied by increases in mean pulmonary arterial pressure, increases in pulmonary blood flow, and improvements in the ventilation-perfusion ratio. Thus, venous blood circulates through well-ventilated areas to ensure complete gas exchange (removal of carbon dioxide and oxygen uptake) in a shorter period of time. It is interesting to note that at high-power outputs, well-trained athletes show exercise-induced arterial hypoxemia, suggesting that diffusion of gases in the lung may be limiting maximal exercise performance (70,71). An associated limiting factor may be stress failure of pulmonary capillaries (72).

Maximal Oxygen Uptake

The maximal oxygen uptake ($\dot{V}O_2max$) is the amount of oxygen that can be transported in the blood and utilized in the muscles during maximal exercise while breathing air at sea level (57,73–75). Physiologically, $\dot{V}O_2max$ is the product of cardiac output and the arteriovenous oxygen difference, integrating central and peripheral organs and systems responsible for supplying oxygen to active muscles (Fig. 26-3) (76).

The transport of oxygen from the atmosphere to the mitochondria is dependent on the coordination of various physiologic processes including lung ventilation, oxygen diffusion across the alveolar-capillary membrane, oxygen binding to hemoglobin and circulation in the blood, diffusion from the capillaries to the mitochondria in muscle, and incorporation as the final electron acceptor in the electron transport chain (73). Under different conditions, $\dot{V}O_2max$ may be limited by different physiologic factors (55,77–80). Also, different diseases interfere with one or more of the determinants of $\dot{V}O_2max$ (see Fig. 26-1), limiting the capacity of the patient to exercise.

Thermoregulation

Muscle actions liberate heat, which must be dissipated to maintain core temperature. The ability to regulate internal body temperature has provided organisms with a certain independence from the environment (81,82). During exercise, blood vessels in the skin dilate and blood is diverted to the body's surface where heat can be transferred to the environment (43). However, if diversion of blood is significant, stroke volume may be compromised. Evaporation of sweat is the predominant mechanism used during exercise to avoid hyperthermia. High air temperature, high relative humidity, low air velocity, and radiation from the sun all make evaporation and thermoregulation more difficult. Ingestion of glucose-electrolyte drinks can improve exercise performance even when the amount of glucose is small. Performance may also be enhanced, albeit to a lesser degree, by ingestion of water (83).

THE EXERCISE PRESCRIPTION

When exercise is indicated for preventive, therapeutic, or rehabilitative purposes, a specific prescription is of fundamental importance. It is not sufficient to recommend any kind of exercise for all patients. A drug prescription requires the name of the drug, the dose, the frequency of administration, and the duration of treatment; similarly, an exercise prescription requires a detailed description of its components. The four major components of an exercise prescription are the type of activity, the frequency of exercise (number of sessions per week), the duration of each exercise session (for strength training the number of sets and repetitions per set are given), and the relative intensity of the effort. Typical exercise prescriptions for developing strength and cardiovascular endurance are presented in Table 26-4.

Elements of a Prescription for Strength Conditioning

The most important characteristic of a strength training program is that it has to be *progressive* in nature (84,85). In other words, the training load (intensity) must be adjusted as the strength increases. Adjustments may be made every 1 to 2 weeks.

Both weight resistance and accommodating resistance (isokinetic) devices effectively increase strength and muscle mass, but the weight-training regimen may be more effective for increasing muscle mass (86,87). The inclusion of eccentric actions seems to be necessary to optimize the effects of training (88). Thus, exercises should include concentric and eccentric muscle actions. For example, when one is training the elbow flexors or knee extensors, the weight has to be lifted and lowered as part of the same repetition. A split routine (dividing the exercise in two groups and doing each group on separate days of the week) seems to be as effective as doing all exercises the same day (89). It is interesting that muscular strength can be maintained with reduced training frequency (90). Thus, once a desired level of strength has been achieved, the number of training sessions per week can be reduced to one or two without losing strength. Finally, the training has to be specific for the task (91,92). In other words, the task has to be analyzed in terms of its static and dynamic components, joint angle, velocity of movement, and metabolic requirements and the training must simulate these requirements.

It is worth considering the nature of the stimulus for increases in strength and muscle hypertrophy. Evidence

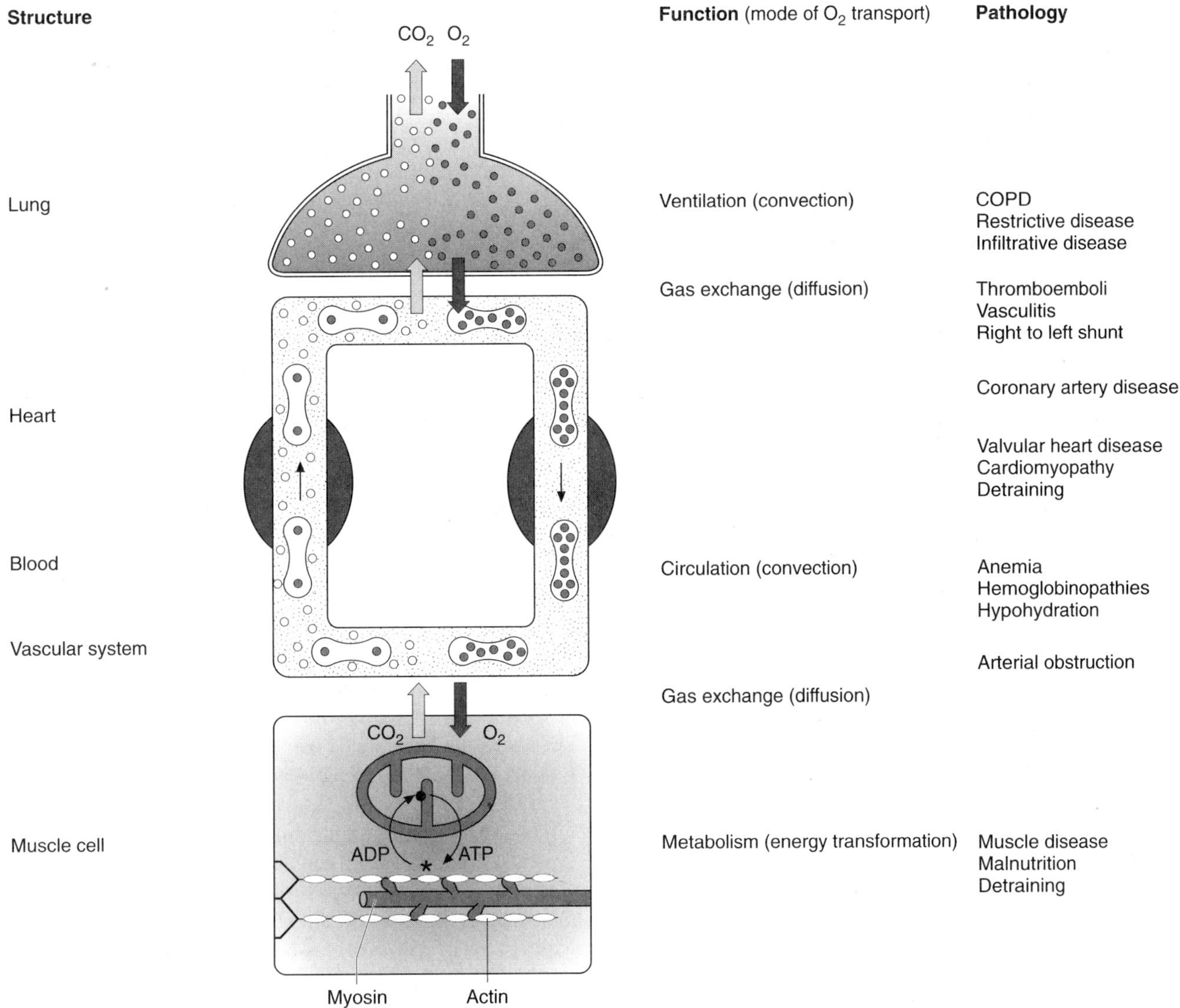

Figure 26-3. Structural and functional aspects of the oxygen transport system. Pathologic conditions that may limit the performance of the system are also included. COPD = chronic obstructive pulmonary disease. (Modified by permission from Billeter R, Hoppeler H. Muscular basis of strength. In: Komi PV, ed. *Strength and power in sport.* Boston: Blackwell Science, 1992:56.)

suggests that mechanical overloading is required for adaptations to occur (93). In addition, various hormones that may stimulate protein synthesis are released during and after exercise (94). Factors related to the metabolic cost of exercise and fatigue may also be involved in stimulating strength gain and muscle hypertrophy (95–97). These factors may interact in response to strength training.

Elements of a Prescription for Endurance or Aerobic Conditioning

The elements of a prescription to develop endurance or aerobic capacity are similar to those just described; the type, frequency, duration, and intensity must be clearly defined (98,99). However, it should be noted that the prescription to improve fitness levels may be different from that for obtaining health benefits. The latter objective may be more relevant to many of the patient populations in the rehabilitation setting.

In general, the type of exercise must be one that activates large muscle groups for relatively long periods of time. Examples of such activities include walking, swimming, cross-country skiing, rowing, dancing, cycling, and games like tennis (if played appropriately). The recommended frequency is three to five training sessions per week and the recommended duration is 15 to 60 minutes of continuous exercise. Finally, the intensity should be from 40% to 85% of the $\dot{V}O_2$max or 55% to 90% of the maximal heart rate. Lower intensities may be more appro-

Table 26-4: Typical Exercise Prescription[a] for Developing Strength and Endurance[b]

Component	Strength	Endurance
Type	Dynamic (free weights, variable resistance, concentric and eccentric actions)	Walking, cycling, rowing, swimming, dancing, cross-country skiing
Frequency	2–3 times/wk	3–5 times/wk
Duration	—	15–60 min
Sets and repetitions	1–3 sets, 8–12 repetitions/set	—
Intensity	60%–80% 1 RM	55%–90% maximal heart rate (measured or age-adjusted) 40–85% $\dot{V}O_2max$
Rest intervals	Variable Seconds between repetitions Minutes between sets	Continuous (interval training possible)

RM = repetition maximum; $\dot{V}O_2max$ = maximum oxygen consumption.

[a] This description does not include circuit-weight-training programs characterized by low resistance (40%–60% 1RM) and a larger number of repetitions (15–30).

[b] All training sessions should start with a 10-min warm-up period and flexibility exercises and finish with a 10-min cool-down period.

priate during the initial stages of the training program, in older populations, and in patients with diseases such as arthritis. This combination of elements seems to produce the expected benefits without the risks and side effects of a prescription for higher-intensity, longer-duration, and more-frequent exercise (100).

In a rehabilitation gymnasium, several pieces of equipment can be used to develop aerobic capacity; examples include the stationary bicycle, a rowing machine, a treadmill, and an arm ergometer. The adaptations will be both central and peripheral (54) and to a certain extent, specific to the apparatus used.

ADAPTATIONS TO STRENGTH CONDITIONING

A Definition of Strength

Strength can be defined as the maximal force (or torque) generated by a muscle or a group of muscles at a specified velocity (1).

Adaptations to Strength Training

Strength conditioning or training produces significant adaptations (Table 26-5, Fig. 26-4) in the structure and function of the adult neuromuscular system in men and women (92,101–109). Also, many recent studies documented the benefits and safety of strength training in children (110–115) and older adults (116–118).

Muscle strength gains and hypertrophy are the two crucial adaptations to strength training (119). In humans, muscle hypertrophy results from an enlargement of individual muscle fibers without an absolute increase in their number, although the results of some animal studies suggest that hyperplasia may also contribute to the observed increases in muscle size. Relative changes in strength are usually larger than the changes in size, suggesting that the central nervous system contributes to the gains in strength. Other observations supporting the neural adaptation hypothesis are the rapid (in days) increase in muscle strength; the changes in muscle strength in the absence of hypertrophy; the changes in voluntary strength but not in force produced by electrically stimulating the muscle; the gains in strength in the untrained limb after contralateral training; the specificity of the adaptations to the angle, speed of training, and type of muscle action (eccentric versus concentric); and the alterations in the electromyogram (EMG) recorded after training (88,92,112,113,120–122). Finally, adaptations to training with eccentric actions are associated with greater neural adaptations and muscle hypertrophy than are adaptations to training with concentric actions (88).

Several studies (101,102) showed that the metabolic machinery of the cell and the fuel supply systems adapt differently to the stimuli of strength training than to the stimuli of endurance training (see Table 26-5). It is worth noting that important structures related to force transduction such as tendons, ligaments, and bone also adapt to strength training with an increase in tissue strength in the former two and an elevation of mineral content in the latter.

In general, the vascular and cardiopulmonary systems do not show the favorable adaptations seen with endurance training. Thus, with the exception of circuit weight training, which is characterized by low resistance and a high number of repetitions with short rest intervals between repetitions, the effects of strength training of $\dot{V}O_2max$ are minimal. It should be noted, however, that favorable outcomes include an improved serum lipid profile (increased high-density and decreased low-density lipoprotein levels), a decrease in body fat, and in some instances, a reduction in BP when the form of training is similar to circuit weight training (123).

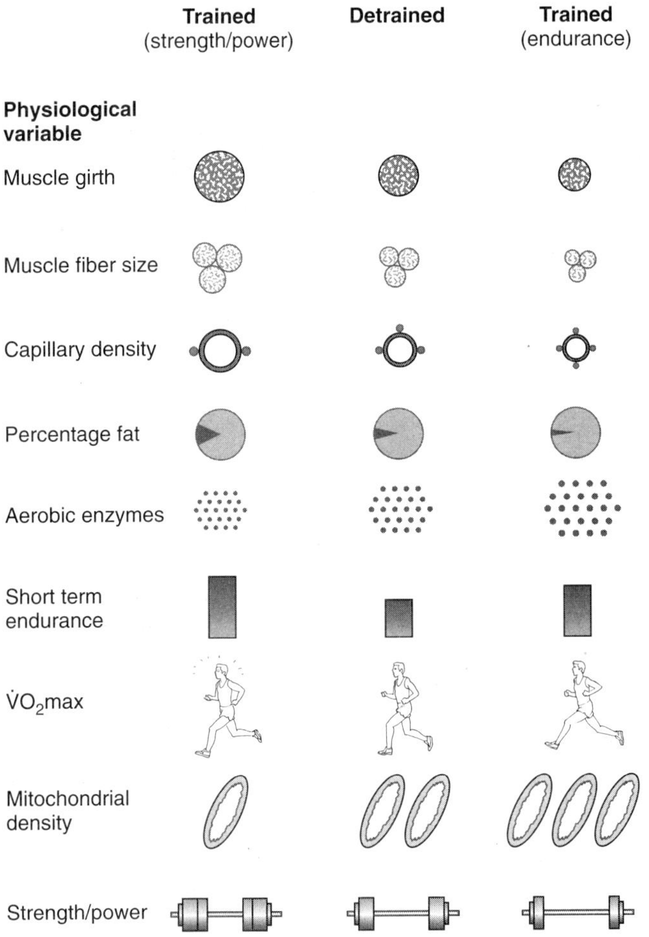

	Trained (strength/power)	Detrained	Trained (endurance)
Physiological variable			
Muscle girth			
Muscle fiber size			
Capillary density			
Percentage fat			
Aerobic enzymes			
Short term endurance			
$\dot{V}O_2$max			
Mitochondrial density			
Strength/power			

Figure 26-4. A schematic description of the changes in various physiologic variables with strength training, detraining, and endurance training. (Reproduced by permission from Fleck SJ, Kraemer WJ. *Designing resistance training programs.* 1st Ed. Champaign, IL: Human Kinetics, 1987:184.)

Table 26-5: Adaptations to a Typical Strength Training Program

Variable	Adaptations
Strength	Significant increases (1%–3% day)
Fiber size	Increase in myofibril area and number; Hypertrophy of various fiber types
Fiber number	Documented in animal models, unknown in humans
Mitochondrial volume density	Decrease
ATP-PCr enzymes (CK, MK)	Increase
Glycolytic enzymes	Increase in PFK, no change in LDH
Muscle fuel stores	
ATP and PCr	Increase
Glycogen	Increase
Triglycerides	Not known
Capillary density	Decrease in power lifters
Maximal integrated EMG	Increase activation of prime movers and synergists
Motor unit synchronization	Increase
Reflex potentiation	Increase
Connective tissue	Increase absolute amount in muscle
Ligament strength	Increase
Tendon strength	Increase
Bone mineral content	Increase
Body composition	Decrease in percent body fat; increase in lean body mass
Lipid profile	Increased HDL, decreased LDL
Blood pressure	No change in resting; decrease during training
$\dot{V}O_2$max	No change unless circuit weight training used

Source: Modified from Fleck SJ, Kraemer WJ. Resistance training: physiological responses and adaptations (part 2 of 4). *Phys Sportsmed* 1988;16:108–124; (part 3 of 4). *Phys Sportsmed* 1988;16:63–74.

ATP = adenosine triphosphate; PCr = phosphocreatine; EMG = electromyogram; $\dot{V}O_2$max = maximum oxygen consumption; PFK = phosphofructokinase; LDH = lactate dehydrogenase; HDL = high-density lipoprotein; LDL = low-density lipoprotein.

ADAPTATIONS TO ANAEROBIC OR SPRINT TRAINING

A Definition

Sprint training is characterized by a high-intensity effort sustained for a short period of time (124). Such training involves supramaximal exercise that exceeds the capacity of the musculature to derive energy via oxidative phosphorylation. Thus, energy must be produced by glycogenolysis and utilization of ATP and PCr stores (125). From a metabolic point of view, strength training can be considered a type of anaerobic training.

Adaptations to Anaerobic Training

A higher prevalence of fast twitch oxidative (IIA) fibers (125–128) and larger type II fibers are observed after sprint training in women (129). Sprinters show a decreased number of fibers expressing myosin heavy-chain isoform I and a concomitant increase in fibers expressing myosin heavy-chain isoform IIA after a period of intensive strength and interval training (130).

Anaerobic training also changes the metabolic machinery of the cell. The activities of some enzymes involved in the ATP-PCr and glycolytic systems including creatine kinase, myokinase, phosphofructokinase, and lactate dehydrogenase (125,126,129) increase after sprint training. In addition, the magnitude of ATP depletion during sprinting is reduced, reflecting an improved balance between hydrolysis and synthesis of ATP (131).

Other reported adaptations to anaerobic training include (21) improvements in skill and coordination for performing at higher intensities, increases in peak and mean power during "all-out" sprint tests (131), enhancement of the muscle's aerobic capacity (132), and improvements in muscle buffering capacity (133), which may delay the onset of fatigue and result in higher peak lactate concentrations during anaerobic exercise (125).

ADAPTATIONS TO ENDURANC E OR AEROBIC TRAINING

A Definition of Endurance

Endurance can be defined as the time that a person can maintain either a static force or a power level involving a combination of concentric or eccentric muscular actions. A patient's endurance for a specific exercise intensity depends on how much energy is needed to successfully perform the task relative to the patient's maximal capacity. When aerobic activities are analyzed, this level of exercise intensity is commonly expressed as a percent of $\dot{V}O_2max$.

Adaptations to Endurance Training

Several biochemical and physiologic adaptations are responsible for the increase in both endurance and aerobic capacity or $\dot{V}O_2max$ seen after regular aerobic or endurance exercise training (Table 26-6, see Fig. 26-4) (134).

At the muscle fiber level, endurance exercise training induces the expression of the slow isoforms of the contractile and regulatory proteins (19,135,136). The number and size of mitochondria, the principal site of energy production during this type of exercise, increase with training, especially in the subsarcolemma region of the cell or closer to the capillaries (137–140). This is accompanied by an increase in the activity of the mitochondrial enzymes involved in the oxidation of fat and carbohydrate (141–143). Together, these changes improve the efficiency of oxidative metabolism, which results in greater oxygen extraction at the muscle cell level and a higher a-vO_2 diff.

From the point of view of substrate utilization, exercise at the same power output results in a greater reliance on fatty acid oxidation (predominantly intramuscular triglycerides), lower utilization of glycogen stores, lower production of lactate, and smaller increases in ADP, inorganic phosphate, and creatine due to conservation of high-energy phosphates after training (124,137,143–150). The hormonal response to exercise after training is characterized by a reduction in the cathecolamine and growth hormone levels to a constant-load exercise stimulus (151).

Blood flow to the muscle is improved by several mechanisms. The number of capillaries supplying the muscle fibers increases 5% to 15% (140,152). Angiogenesis may be stimulated by angiogenic growth factors released during exercise, probably due to local hypoxia (59). The increased capillary density enhances the exchange of gases, heat, nutrients, and waste products. In addition, regular endurance exercise increases the capacity for vasodilation in active limbs and also enables the trained individual to utilize a larger fraction of maximal vascular conductance than the sedentary subject (48,153). Blood volume expands and although the red blood cell count is also augmented, hematocrit declines because of the relatively larger

Table 26-6: Adaptations to Endurance or Aerobic Training

SYSTEM	NATURE OF THE ADAPTATION
Energy production	Increase in number and size of mitochondria; increased activity of oxidative enzymes; smaller decrease in PCr and ATP, smaller rise in Pi, creatine, and ADP; lower lactate production
Fuel supply	Greater glycogen and fat content, slower glycogen depletion, greater reliance on fat
Endocrine	Increased number of glucose transporter; decrease in hormonal levels at a given power output level
Circulatory	Increased capillarization of muscles; increase in vascular conductance; expanded blood volume, increase in RBC count, lower hematocrit
Cardiac	At rest and similar submaximal power output levels: lower HR, higher SV, and same Q; at maximal levels: same or lower HR, higher SV, and higher Q
Respiratory	At rest and similar submaximal power output levels: small reduction in VR, similar TV, and slightly reduced $\hat{VE}$; at maximal levels: higher VR, increased TV, higher VE, and higher gas diffusion
Thermoregulation	Increased sweating rate, reduced rate of glycogen use, reduced cardiovascular response at same power level, better maintenance of body fluid balance

PCr = phosphocreatine; ATP = adenosine triphosphate; Pi = inorganic phosphate; ADP = adenosine diphosphate; RBC = red blood cell; HR = heart rate; SV = stroke volume; Q = cardiac output; VR = ventilatory rate; TV = tidal volume; $\hat{VE}$ = minute ventilation.

increase in plasma volume (154,155). Finally, resting SBP and DBP generally decrease after training in people with mild to moderate hypertension (123,156).

The most important adaptation in the heart is the increase in stroke volume. This is mainly due to the expansion of blood volume mentioned earlier, which is evident 1 week after the start of the training program and can be measured at rest and during submaximal and maximal exercise (154). The expansion of plasma volume results in a larger venous return, an increase in end-diastolic volume (157), a larger ejection fraction, and consequently a larger stroke volume. After endurance training, the heart rate declines at rest and during submaximal exercise, and is either slightly lower or does not change during maximal exercise (158). When the two determinants of cardiac output (heart rate and stroke volume) are combined, cardiac output remains unchanged at rest and during submaximal exercise but increases during maximal exercise. Maximal cardiac output is 14 to 16 $L \cdot min^{-1}$ in untrained people, 20 to 25 $L \cdot min^{-1}$ in trained subjects, and 40 $L \cdot min^{-1}$ in well-trained athletes. With endurance (and strength) training, left ventricular chamber dimensions and left ventricular wall thickness increase. Endurance athletes have larger and thicker left ventricles relative to their body mass (159–162).

The pulmonary system shows some adaptations to endurance training (21). At rest and similar submaximal exercise levels, tidal volume is unchanged. On the other hand, the ventilatory rate is usually lowered. As a result, ventilation is slightly reduced at both levels. Maximal values for tidal volume, ventilatory rate, and ventilation are increased after training. In addition, gas exchange in the alveoli (i.e., pulmonary diffusion) increases with training.

It should be obvious that with all the adaptations in the various systems and components of the oxygen transport chain, the integrated response, the $\dot{V}O_2max$, increases (163). Oxygen consumption at rest and the amount of oxygen required for any activity does not change with training. However, since the maximal oxygen uptake is higher after training, a given submaximal level represents a lower percentage of the maximal capacity. Of particular importance is the fact that after training, individuals can perform at a higher percentage of the $\dot{V}O_2max$ for extended periods of time without reaching the point at which lactate begins to accumulate (150). High-intensity, but submaximal, training in endurance athletes results in a higher muscle buffering capacity (164) in the absence of changes in $\dot{V}O_2max$. Thus, endurance can be improved without alterations in aerobic power.

FLEXIBILITY TRAINING

A Definition of Flexibility

Flexibility can be defined as the ability to move a joint smoothly throughout a full range of motion (165). Flexibility can be limited by neurologic or muscular mechanisms, articular dysfunction, and skin or subcutaneous tissue constraints (166).

Training Alternatives and Adaptations

Developing flexibility may be important for the prevention of injuries and enhancement of neuromuscular performance (165–167). Techniques to improve flexibility include the ballistic stretch, static stretch, and the proprioceptive neuromuscular facilitation (PNF) stretch (166–168). The ballistic stretch makes use of fast repetitive bouncing motions. The static stretch involves stretching slowly to the point of discomfort and holding the position for 10 to 60 seconds. The stretching force may be provided by gravity, passively applied manipulation, or the application of weights. The PNF techniques include the *contract relax* (CR) and the *contract relax agonist contract* (CRAC). In the former, the muscles to be stretched are first maximally contracted (static action for 5–10 seconds) and then stretched as in the static stretch technique. In the latter, the stretch is accompanied by a contraction of the antagonist. During the first few days after injury, static stretching is recommended because ballistic or PNF techniques may produce further injury. Later in recovery, heat and stretching can be used to increase elongation of passive elements within the muscle (169), and PNF techniques can be used to increase flexibility (167).

The PNF techniques produce the greatest absolute gains in range of motion when compared to the static stretching and ballistic training methods. Training three to five times a week results in significant improvements in flexibility (170,171). Training once a week is enough to maintain improved flexibility (170). The importance of proper warm-up before flexibility exercises has been emphasized by some authors (165,167).

REFERENCES

1. Knuttgen HG, Kraemer WJ. Terminology and measurement in exercise performance. *J Appl Sports Sci Res* 1987;1:1–10.
2. Knuttgen HG. Force, work, power, and exercise. *Med Sci Sports* 1978;10:227–228.
3. Komi PV. The musculoskeletal system. In: Dirix A, Knuttgen HG, Tittel K, eds. *The Olympic book of sports medicine*. Boston: Blackwell Science, 1988:15–39.
4. Komi PV. Measurement of the force-velocity relationship in human muscle under concentric and eccentric contractions. In: *Medicine and sport*. Vol 8. *Biomechanics III*. Basel: Karger, 1973:224–229.
5. Asmussen E. Positive and negative muscular work. *Acta Physiol Scand* 1952;28:364.

6. Pette D, Staron RS. The molecular diversity of mammalian muscle fibers. *News Physiol Sci* 1993;8:153–157.

7. Barnard R, Edgerton VR, Furukawa T, Peter JB. Histochemical, biochemical, and contractile properties of white, red, and intermediate fibers. *Am J Physiol* 1971;220:410–414.

8. Ennion S, Sant'Ana Pereira J, Sargeant AJ, et al. Characterization of human skeletal muscle fibers according to the myosin heavy chain they express. *J Muscle Res Cell Motil* 1994;16: 35–43.

9. Smerdu V, Karsch-Mizrachi I, Campione M, et al. Type IIx myosin heavy chain transcripts are expressed in type IIb fibers of human skeletal muscle. *Am J Physiol* 1994;267:C1723–C1728.

10. Billeter R, Heizmann CW, Howald H, Jenny E. Analysis of myosin light and heavy chain types in single human skeletal muscle fibers. *Eur J Biochem* 1981;116: 389–395.

11. Sant'Ana Pereira JAA, Sargent AJ, Rademaker ACHJ, et al. Myosin heavy chain isoform expression and high energy phosphate content in human muscle fibres at rest and post-exercise. *J Physiol* 1996;496:583–588.

12. Billeter R, Heizmann CW, Reist U, et al. α- and β-Tropomyosin in typed single fibers of human skeletal muscle. *FEBS Lett* 1981;132:133–136.

13. Schiaffino S, Reggiani C. Myosin isoforms in mammalian skeletal muscle. *J Appl Physiol* 1994;77: 493–501.

14. Moss RL, Diffee GM, Greaser ML. Contractile properties of skeletal muscle fibers in relation to myofibrillar protein isoforms. *Rev Physiol Biochem Pharmacol* 1995;126:1–63.

15. Larsson L, Salviati G. A technique for studies of the contractile apparatus in single human muscle fibre segments obtained by percutaneous biopsy. *Acta Physiol Scand* 1992;146:485–495.

16. Larsson L, Moss RL. Maximum velocity of shortening in relation to myosin isoform composition in single fibres from human skeletal muscles. *J Physiol* 1993;472: 595–614.

17. Larsson L, Li X, Berg HE, Frontera WR. Effects of removal of weight-bearing function on contractility and myosin isoform composition in single human skeletal muscle cells. *Eur J Physiol* 1996;432:320–328.

18. Goldspink G, Scutt A, Loughna PT, et al. Gene expression in skeletal muscle in response to stretch and force generation. *Am J Physiol* 1992;262:R356–R363.

19. Klitgaard H, Bergman O, Betto R, et al. Co-existence of myosin heavy chain I and IIA isoforms in human skeletal muscle fibres with endurance training. *Eur J Physiol* 1990;416:470–472.

20. Andersen JL, Schiaffino S. Mismatch between myosin heavy chain mRNA and protein distribution in human skeletal muscle fibers. *Am J Physiol* 1997;272: C1881–C1889.

21. Wilmore JH, Costill DL. *Physiology of sport and exercise.* Champaign, IL: Human Kinetics, 1994.

22. McArdle WD, Katch FI, Katch VL. *Essentials of exercise physiology.* Philadelphia: Lea & Febiger, 1994.

23. Brooks GA, Fahey TD, White TP. *Exercise physiology: human bioenergetics and its applications.* Mountain View: Mayfield Publishing, 1996.

24. Rowell LB. *Human cardiovascular control.* New York: Oxford University Press, 1993.

25. Bar-Or O. Importance of differences between children and adults for exercise testing and exercise prescription. In: Skinner JS, ed. *Exercise testing and exercise prescription for special cases.* Philadelphia: Lea & Febiger, 1987:49–65.

26. Withers RT, Sherman WM, Clark DG, et al. Muscle metabolism during 30, 60 and 90s of maximal cycling on an air-braked ergometer. *Eur J Appl Physiol* 1991;63:354–362.

27. Bodin K, Esbjornsson M, Jansson E. Alactic ATP turnover rate during a 30-s cycle sprint in females and males. *Clin Sci (Colch)* 1994 (suppl);87:205.

28. Bogdanis GC, Nevill ME, Boobis LH, et al. Recovery of power output and muscle metabolites following 30s of maximal sprint cycling in man. *J Physiol* 1995;482:467–480.

29. Bogdanis GC, Nevill ME, Boobis LH, Lakomy HKA. Contribution of phosphocreatine and aerobic metabolism to energy supply during repeated sprint exercise. *J Appl Physiol* 1996;80:876–884.

30. Coggan AR, Coyle EF. Carbohydrate ingestion during prolonged exercise: effects on metabolism and performance. *Exerc Sports Sci Rev* 1991;19:1–40.

31. Vollestäd NK, Blom PCS. Effect of varying exercise intensity on glycogen depletion in human muscle fibers. *Acta Physiol Scand* 1988;125:395–405.

32. Gorski J. Muscle triglyceride metabolism during exercise. *Can J Physiol Pharmacol* 1992;70: 123–131.

33. Péronnet F, Burelle Y, Massicotte D, et al. Respective oxidation of ^{13}C-labeled lactate and glucose ingested simutaneously during exercise. *J Appl Physiol* 1997; 82:440–446.

34. Romijn JA, Coyle EF, Sidossis LS, et al. Regulations of endogenous fat and carbohydrate metabolism in relation to exercise intensity and duration. *Am J Physiol* 1993;265:E380–E391.

35. Evans WJ, Hughes VA. Dietary carbohydrates and endurance exercise. *Am J Clin Nutr* 1985; 41:1146–1154.

36. Muoio DM, Leddy JJ, Horvath PJ, et al. Effect of dietary fat on metabolic adjustments to maximal VO_2 and endurance in runners. *Med Sci Sports Exerc* 1994;26:81–88.

37. Brooks GA. Amino acid and protein metabolism during exercise and recovery. *Med Sci Sports Exerc* 1987;19:S150–S156.

38. Graham TE, MacLean DA. Ammonia and amino acid metabolism in human skeletal muscle during exercise. *Can J Physiol Pharmacol* 1992;70:132–141.

39. Galbo H. Autonomic neuroendocrine responses to exercise. *Scand J Sports Sci* 1986;8:3–17.

40. Jansson E, Hjemdahl P, Kaijser L. Epinephrine-induced changes in muscle carbohydrate metabolism during exercise in male subjects. *J Appl Physiol* 1986;60: 1466–1470.

41. Kjaer M, Kiens B, Hargraves M, Richter EA. Influence of active muscle mass on glucose homeostasis during exercise. *J Appl Physiol* 1991;71:552–557.

42. Kjaer M, Engfred K, Fernandes A, et al. Regulation of hepatic glucose production during exercise in humans: role of sympathoadrenergic activity. *Am J Physiol* 1993;265:E275–E283.

43. Rowell LB. Human cardiovascular adjustments to exercise and thermal stress. *Physiol Rev* 1974;54:75–159.

44. Andersen P, Saltin B. Maximal perfusion of skeletal muscle in man. *J Physiol* 1985;366:233–249.

45. Flamm SD, Taki J, Moore R, et al. Redistribution of regional and organ blood volume and effect on cardiac function in relation to upright exercise intensity in healthy subjects. *Circulation* 1990;81:1550–1559.

46. Laub M, Hvid-Jacobsen K, Hovind P, et al. Spleen emptying and venous hematocrit in humans during exercise. *J Appl Physiol* 1993;74:1024–1026.

47. Rowell LB. Muscle blood flow in humans: how high can it go? *Med Sci Sports Exerc* 1988;20: S97–S103.

48. Snell PG, Martin WH, Buckey JC, Blomqvist CG. Maximal vascular leg conductance in trained and untrained men. *J Appl Physiol* 1987;62:606–610.

49. MacDougall JD, Tuxen D, Sales DG, et al. Arterial blood pressure response to heavy resistance exercise. *J Appl Physiol* 1985; 58:758–790.

50. Lewis SF, Snell PG, Taylor WF, et al. Role of muscle mass and mode of contraction in circulatory responses to exercise. *J Appl Physiol* 1985;58:146–151.

51. Blomqvist CG, Lewis SF, Taylor WF, Graham RM. Similarity of the hemodynamic responses to static and dynamic exercise of small muscle groups. *Circ Res* 1981;48(suppl I):I87–I92.

52. Reybrouck T, Heigenhauser GF, Faulkner JA. Limitations to maximum oxygen uptake in arm, leg, and combined arm-leg ergometry. *J Appl Physiol* 1975;38:774–779.

53. Secher NH, Clausen JP, Klausen K, et al. Central and regional circulatory effects of adding arm exercise to leg exercise. *Acta Physiol Scand* 1977;100:288–297.

54. Klausen K, Secher NH, Clausen JP, et al. Central and regional circulatory adaptations to one-leg training. *J Appl Physiol* 1982;52: 976–983.

55. Roca J, Hogan MC, Story D, et al. Evidence for tissue diffusion limitation of VO_{2max} in normal humans. *J Appl Physiol* 1989; 67:291–299.

56. Honig CR, Connett RJ, Gayeski TEJ. O_2 transport and its interaction with metabolism: a systems view of aerobic capacity. *Med Sci Sports Exerc* 1992;24:47–53.

57. Richardson RS, Knight DR, Poole DC, et al. Determinants of maximal exercise VO_2 during single leg knee-extensor exercise in humans. *Am J Physiol* 1995; 268:H1453–H1461.

58. Grassi B, Poole DC, Richardson RS, et al. Muscle O_2 uptake kinetics in humans: implications for metabolic control. *J Appl Physiol* 1996;80:988–998.

59. Breen EC, Johnson EC, Wagner H, et al. Angiogenic growth factor mRNA responses in muscle to a single bout of exercise. *J Appl Physiol* 1996;81:355–361.

60. Strange S, Secher NH, Pawelczyk JA, et al. Neural control of cardiovascular responses and of ventilation during dynamic exercise in man. *J Physiol* 1993;470: 693–704.

61. Eriksen M, Waaler BA, Walloe L, Wesche J. Dynamics and dimensions of cardiac output changes in humans at the onset and at the end of moderate rhythmic exercise. *J Physiol* 1990;426: 423–437.

62. Mier CM, Domenick MA, Turner NS, Wilmore JH. Changes in stroke volume and maximal aerobic capacity with increased blood volume in men and women. *J Appl Physiol* 1996;80: 1180–1186.

63. Ekblom BA, Kilbom A, Soltysiak J. Physical training bradycardia and autonomic nervous system. *Scand J Clin Lab Invest* 1973; 32:249–256.

64. Maciel BC, Gallo L Jr, Marin Neto JA, et al. Autonomic nervous control of the heart rate during dynamic exercise in normal man. *Clin Sci (Colch)* 1986;71:457–460.

65. Nonogi H, Hess OM, Ritter M, Krayenbuehl HP. Diastolic properties of the normal left ventricle during supine exercise. *Br Heart J* 1988;60:30–38.

66. Lowell Stone H, Liang IYS. Cardiovascular response and control during exercise. *Am Rev Respir Dis* 1984;129:S13–S16.

67. Jorgensen CR, Gobel FL, Taylor HL, Wang Y. Myocardial blood flow and oxygen consumption during exercise. *Ann N Y Acad Sci* 1977;301:213–223.

68. Dempsey JA, Johnson BD, Saupe KW, Adaptations and limitations in the pulmonary system during exercise. *Chest* 1990;97:81S–87S.

69. Sliwinski P, Yan S, Gauthier AP, Macklem PT. Influence of global

inspiratory muscle fatigue on breathing during exercise. *J Appl Physiol* 1996;80:1270–1278.

70. Dempsey JA, Hanson PG, Henderson KS. Exercise-induced arterial hypoxaemia in healthy human subjects at sea level. *J Physiol* 1984;355:161–175.

71. Powers SK, Lawler J, Dempsey JA, et al. Effects of incomplete pulmonary gas exchange on VO_{2max}. *J Appl Physiol* 1989;66: 2491–2495.

72. West JB, Mathieu-Costello O. Stress failure of pulmonary capillaries as a limiting factor for maximal exercise. *Eur J Appl Physiol* 1995;70:99–108.

73. Wagner PD. Determinants of maximal oxygen transport and utilization. *Annu Rev Physiol* 1996;58:21–50.

74. Saltin B, Strange S. Maximal oxygen upyake: "old" and "new" arguments for a cardiovascular limitation. *Med Sci Sports Exerc* 1992;24:30–37.

75. Lindstedt SL, Wells DJ, Jones JH, et al. Limitations to aerobic performance in mammals: interaction of structure and demand. *Int J Sports Med* 1998;9:210–217.

76. Billeter R, Hoppeler H. Muscular basis of strength. In: Komi PV, ed. *Strength and power in sport.* Boston: Blackwell Science, 1992:39–63.

77. di Prampero P, Ferretti G. Factors limiting maximal oxygen consumption in humans. *Respir Physiol* 1990;80:113–128.

78. Schaffartzik W, Barton ED, Poole DC, et al. Effect of reduced hemoglobin concentration on leg oxygen uptake during maximal exercise in humans. *J Appl Physiol* 1993;75:491–498.

79. Boutellier U, Piwko P. The respiratory system as an exercise limiting factor in normal sedentary subjects. *Eur J Appl Physiol* 1992;64:145–152.

80. Boutellier U, Buchel R, Kundert A, Spengler C. The respiratory system as an exercise limiting factor in normal trained subjects. *Eur J Appl Physiol* 1992;65: 347–353.

81. Nadel ER. Temperature regulation and hyperthermia during exercise. *Clin Chest Med* 1984;5:13–20.

82. Nadel ER. Recent advances in temperature regulation during exercise in humans. *Fed Proc* 1985;44:2286–2292.

83. Maughan RJ, Bethell LR, Leiper JB. Effects of ingested fluids on exercise capacity and on cardiovascular and metabolic responses to prolonged exercise in man. *Exp Physiol* 1996;81:847–859.

84. DeLorme TL. Restoration of muscle power by heavy resistance exercise. *J Bone Joint Surg* 1945;27:645–667.

85. DeLorme TL, Watkins AL. Technics of progressive resistance exercise. *Arch Phys Med* 1948;29:263–273.

86. Coté C, Simoneau JA, Lagassé P, et al. Isokinetic strength training protocols: do they induce skeletal muscle fiber hypertrophy? *Arch Phys Med Rehabil* 1988;69:281–285.

87. O'Hagan FT, Sale DG, MacDougall JD, Garner SH. Comparative effectiveness of accommodating and weight resistance training modes. *Med Sci Sports Exerc* 1995;27:1210–1219.

88. Hortobagyi T, Hill JP, Houmard JA, et al. Adaptive responses to muscle lengthening and shortening in humans. *J Appl Physiol* 1996;80:765–772.

89. Calder AW, Chilibeck PD, Webber CE, Sale DG. Comparison of whole and split weight training routines in young women. *Can J Appl Physiol* 1994;19:185–199.

90. Graves JE, Pollock ML, Leggett SH, et al. Effect of reduced training frequency on muscular strength. *Int J Sports Med* 1988;9:316–319.

91. DeLateur BJ, Lehmann J, Stonebridge J, Warren CG. Isotonic vs. isometric exercises: a double shift, transfer-of-training study. *Arch Phys Med Rehabil* 1972;53:212–217.

92. Jones DA, Rutherford OM, Parker DF. Physiological changes in skeletal muscle as a result of strength training. *Q J Exp Physiol* 1989;74:233–256.

93. Booth FW, Tseng BS. Olympic goal: molecular and cellular approaches to understanding muscle adaptation. *News Physiol Sci* 1993;8:165–169.

94. Kraemer WJ. Endocrine responses and adaptation to strength training. In: Komi PV, ed. *Strength and power in sport.* Oxford: Blackwell, 1992:291–304.

95. DeLateur BJ, Lehmann JF, Fordyce WE. A test of the DeLorme axiom. *Arch Phys Med Rehabil* 1968;49:245–248.

96. Carey Smith R, Rutherford OM. The role of metabolites in strength training. I. A comparison of eccentric and concentric contractions. *Eur J Appl Physiol* 1995;71:332–336.

97. Schott J, McCully K, Rutherford OM. The role of metabolites in strength training. II. Short versus long isometric contractions. *Eur J Appl Physiol* 1995;71:332–336.

98. American College of Sports Medicine. Position stand: the recommended quantity and quality of exercise for developing and maintaining cardiorespiratory and muscular fitness in healthy adults. *Med Sci Sports Exerc* 1990;22:265–274.

99. World Hypertension League. Physical exercise in the management of hypertension: a consensus statement by the World Hypertension League. *J Hypertens* 1991;9:283–287.

100. Vuori I. Exercise prescription in medical practice. *Ann Clin Res* 1988;20:84–93.

101. Fleck SJ, Kraemer WJ. Resistance training: physiological responses and adaptations (part 2 of 4). *Phys Sportsmed* 1988;16:108–124.

102. Fleck SJ, Kraemer WJ. Resistance training: physiological

responses and adaptations (part 3 of 4). *Phys Sportsmed* 1988;16:63–74.

103. Fleck SJ, Kraemer WJ. *Designing resistance training programs.* 1st Ed. Champaign, IL: Human Kinetics, 1987:184.

104. McDonagh MJN, Davies CTM. Adaptive response of mammalian skeletal muscle to exercise with high loads. *Eur J Appl Physiol* 1984;52:139–155.

105. Howald H. Malleability of the motor system: training for maximizing power output. *J Exp Biol* 1985;115:365–373.

106. Taylor NAS, Wilkinson JG. Exercise-induced skeletal msucle growth: hypertrophy or hyperplasia? *Sports Med* 1986;3:190–200.

107. MacDougall JD. Morphological changes in human skeletal muscle following strength training and immobilization. In: Jones NL, McCartney N, McComas AJ, eds. *Human muscle power.* Champaign, IL: Human Kinetics, 1986:269–284.

108. Lillegard WA, Terrio JD. Appropriate strength training. *Med Clin North Am* 1994;78:457–477.

109. Staron RS, Karapondo DL, Kraemer WJ, et al. Skeletal muscle adaptation during early phase of heavy-resistance training in men and women. *J Appl Physiol* 1994;76:1247–1255.

110. Siegel JA, Camaione DN, Manfredi TG. The effects of upper body resistance training on prepubescent children. *Pediatr Exerc Sci* 1989;1:145–154.

111. Kraemer WJ, Fry AC, Frykman PN, et al. Resistance training and youth. *Pediatr Exerc Sci* 1989;1:336–350.

112. Ramsay JA, Blimkie CJR, Smith K, et al. Strength training effects in prepubescent boys. *Med Sci Sports Exerc* 1990;22:605–614.

113. Blimkie CJR. Resistance training during pre- and early puberty: efficacy, trainability, mechanisms, and persistence. *Can J Sport Sci* 1992;17:264–279.

114. Faigenbaum AD, Zaichkowsky LD, Westcott WL, et al. The effects of a twice-a-week strength training program on children. *Pediatr Exerc Sci* 1993;5:339–346.

115. Ozmun JC, Mikesky AE, Surburg PR. Neuromuscular adaptations following prepubescent strength training. *Med Sci Sports Exerc* 1994;26:510–514.

116. Frontera WR, Meredith CN, O'Reilly KP, et al. Strength conditioning in older men: skeletal muscle hypertrophy and improved function. *J Appl Physiol* 1988; 64:1038–1044.

117. Nelson ME, Fiatarone MA, Morganti CM, et al. Effects of high-intensity strength training on multiple risk factors for osteoporotic fractures. *JAMA* 1994; 272:1909–1914.

118. Lexell J, Downham DY, Larsson Y, et al. Heavy-resistance training in older Scandinavian men and women: short- and long-term effects on arm and leg muscles. *Scand J Med Sci Sports* 1995; 5:329–341.

119. Staron RS, Leonardi MJ, Karapondo DL, et al. Strength and skeletal muscle adaptations in heavy-resistance-trained women after detraining and retraining. *J Appl Physiol* 1991;70:631–640.

120. Hakkinen K, Komi PV. Effect of explosive type strength training on electromyographic and force production characteristics of leg extensor muscles during concentric and various stretch-shortening cycle exercise. *Scand J Sports Sci* 1985;7:65–76.

121. Kanehisa H, Miyashita M. Specificity of velocity in strength training. *Eur J Appl Physiol* 1983;52:104–106.

122. Davies CTM, Dooley P, McDonagh MJN, White MJ. Adaptation of mechanical properties of muscle to high force training in man. *J Physiol* 1985;365:277–284.

123. American College of Sports Medicine. Physical activity, physical fitness, and hypertension. *Med Sci Sports Exerc* 1993;25:i–x.

124. Abernethy PJ, Thayer R, Taylor AW. Acute and chronic responses of skeletal muscle to endurance and sprint exercise: a review. *Sports Med* 1990;10:365–389.

125. Jacobs I, Esbjörnsson M, Sylvén C, et al. Sprint training effects on muscle myoglobin, enzymes, fiber types, and blood lactate. *Med Sci Sports Exerc* 1987;19: 368–374.

126. Costill DL, Coyle EF, Fink WF, et al. Adaptations in skeletal muscle following strength training. *J Appl Physiol* 1979;46:96–99.

127. Jansson E, Esbjörnsson M, Holm I, Jacobs I. Increase in the proportion of fast-twitch muscle fibres by sprint training in males. *Acta Physiol Scand* 1990;140: 359–363.

128. Esbjörnsson M, Hellsten-Westing Y, Balsom PD, et al. Muscle fibre type changes with sprint training: effect of training pattern. *Acta Physiol Scand* 1993;149:245–246.

129. Esbjörnsson M, Holm I, Sylvén C, Jansson E. Different responses of skeletal muscle following sprint training in men and women. *Eur J Appl Physiol* 1996;74:375–383.

130. Andersen JL, Klitgaard H, Saltin B. Influence of intensive training on myosin heavy chain isoforms in single fibres from m. vastus lateralis of sprinters. *Acta Physiol Scand Suppl* 1992;608:108(P1. 30).

131. Stathis CG, Febbraio MA, Carey MF, Snow RJ. Influence of sprint training on human skeletal muscle purine nucleotide metabolism. *J Appl Physiol* 1994;76: 1802–1809.

132. Tabata I, Nishimura K, Kouzaki M, et al. Effects of moderate-intensity endurance and high-intensity intermittent training on anaerobic capacity and VO_{2max}. *Med Sci Sports Exerc* 1996;28: 1327–1330.

133. Sharp RL, Costill DL, Fink WJ, King DS. Effects of eight weeks of bicycle ergometry sprint training on human muscle buffer capacity. *Int J Sports Med* 1986;7:13–17.

134. American Heart Association. Statement on exercise: benefits and recommendations for physical activity programs for all Americans: a statement for health professionals by the Committee on Exercise and Cardiac Rehabilitation of the Council on Clinical Cardiology, American Heart Association. *Circulation* 1992;86:340–344.

135. Schantz PG, Dhoot GK. Coexistence of slow and fast isoforms of contractile and regulatory proteins in human skeletal muscle fibres induced by endurance training. *Acta Physiol Scand* 1987;131:147–154.

136. Baumann H, Jaggi M, Soland F, et al. Exercise training induces transitions of myosin isoform subunits within histochemically typed human muscle fibres. *Pflugers Arch* 1987;409:349–360.

137. Holloszy JO, Coyle EF. Adaptations of skeletal muscle to endurance exercise and their metabolic consequences. *J Appl Physiol* 1984;56:831–839.

138. Howald H. Training induced morphological and functional changes in skeletal muscle. *Int J Sports Med* 1982;3:1–12.

139. Howald H, Hoppeler H, Claasen H, et al. Influences of endurance training on the ultrastructural composition of the different muscle fiber types in humans. *Pflugers Arch* 1985;403:369–376.

140. Rosler K, Conley KE, Howald H, et al. Specificity of leg power changes to velocities used in bicycle endurance training. *J Appl Physiol* 1986;61:30–36.

141. Gollnick PD, Saltin B. Hypothesis: significance of skeletal muscle oxidative enzyme enhancement with endurance training. *Clin Physiol* 1982;2:1–12.

142. Costill DL, Fink WJ, Ivy JL, et al. Lipid metabolism in skeletal muscle of endurance-trained males and females. *J Appl Physiol* 1979;28:251–255.

143. Spina RJ, Chi MMY, Hopkins MG, et al. Mitochondrial enzymes increase in muscle in response to 7–10 days of cycle exercise. *J Appl Physiol* 1996;80:2250–2254.

144. Martin WH. Effect of endurance training on fatty acid metabolism during whole body exercise. *Med Sci Sports Exerc* 1997;29:635–639.

145. Hurley BF, Hagberg JM, Allen WK, et al. Effect of training on blood lactate levels during submaximal exercise. *J Appl Physiol* 1984;56:1260–1264.

146. Turcotte LP, Richter EA, Kiens B. Increased plasma FFA uptake and oxidation during prolonged exercise in trained vs. untrained humans. *Am J Physiol* 1992;262:E791–E799.

147. Favier RJ, Constable SH, Chen M, Holloszy JO. Endurance exercise training reduces lactate production. *J Appl Physiol* 1986;61:885–889.

148. Kiens B. Effect of endurance training on fatty acid metabolism: local adaptations. *Med Sci Sports Exerc* 1997;29:640–645.

149. Henriksson J. Training-induced adaptations of skeletal muscle and metabolism during submaximal exercise. *J Physiol* 1977;270:661–675.

150. McRae HS, Dennis SC, Bosch AN, Noakes TD. Effects of training on lactate production and removal during progressive exercise in humans. *J Appl Physiol* 1992;72:1649–1656.

151. Weltman A, Weltman JY, Womack CJ, et al. Exercise training decreases the growth hormone (GH) response to acute constant-load exercise. *Med Sci Sports Exerc* 1997;29:669–676.

152. Ingjer F. Capillary supply and mitochondrial content of different skeletal muscle fiber types in untrained and endurance trained men: a histochemical and ultrastructural study. *Eur J Appl Physiol* 1979;40:197–209.

153. Martin WH III, Montgomery J, Snell PG, et al. Cardiovascular adaptations to intense swim training in sedentary middle-aged men and women. *Circulation* 1987;75:323–330.

154. Hopper MK, Coggan AR, Coyle EF. Exercise stroke volume relative to plasma-volume expansion. *J Appl Physiol* 1988;64:404–408.

155. Green HJ, Sutton JR, Coates G, et al. Response of red cell and plasma volume to prolonged training in humans. *J Appl Physiol* 1991;70:1810–1815.

156. Tipton CM. Exercise, training, and hypertension. *Exerc Sports Sci Rev* 1991;19:447–505.

157. Gledhill N, Cox D, Jamnik R. Endurance athletes' stroke volume does not plateau: major advantage is diastolic function. *Med Sci Sports Exerc* 1994;26:1116–1121.

158. Astrand PO. Exercise physiology and its role in disease prevention and in rehabilitation. *Arch Phys Med Rehabil* 1987;68:305–309.

159. Landry F, Bouchard C, Dumesnil J. Cardiac dimension changes with endurance training. *JAMA* 1985;254:77–80.

160. Milliken MC, Stray-Gundersen J, Peshock RM, et al. Left ventricular mass as determined by magnetic resonance imaging in male endurance athletes. *Am J Cardiol* 1988;62:301–305.

161. Ehsani AA, Ogawa T, Miller TR, et al. Exercise training improves left ventricular systolic function in older men. *Circulation* 1991;83:96–103.

162. Urhausen A, Kindermann W. One- and two-dimensional echocardiography in body builders and endurance-trained subjects. *Int J Sports Med* 1989;10:139–144.

163. Kohrt WM, Malley MT, Coggan AR, et al. Effects of gender, age, and fitness level on response on VO_2max to training in 60–71 yr olds. *J Appl Physiol* 1991;71:2004–2011.

164. Weston AR, Myburgh KH, Lindsay FH, et al. Skeletal muscle buffering capacity and endurance performance after high-intensity

interval training by well-trained cyclists. *Eur J Appl Physiol* 1997;75:7–13.

165. Shellock FG, Prentice WE. Warming-up and stretching for improved physical performance and prevention of sports-related injuries. *Sports Med* 1985;2: 267–278.

166. Hutton RS. Neuromuscular basis of stretching exercises. In: Komi PV, ed. *Strength and power in sport.* Boston: Blackwell Science, 1992:29–38.

167. Stanish WD, McVicar SF. Flexibility in injury prevention. In: Renströn PAFH, ed. *Basic principles of prevention and care.* Boston: Blackwell Science, 1993:262–276.

168. Sady SP, Wortman M, Blanke D. Flexibility training: ballistic, static or propioceptive neuromuscular facilitation? *Arch Phys Med Rehabil* 1982;63:261–263.

169. Wiktorsson-Moller M, Oberg B, Ekstrand J, Gillquist J. Effects of warming-up, massage, and stretching on range of motion and muscle strength in the lower extremity. *Am J Sports Med* 1983;11:249–252.

170. Etnyre BR, Lee EJ. Comments on proprioceptive neuromuscular facilitation stretching techniques. *Res Q Exerc Sport* 1987;58: 184–188.

171. Wallin D, Ekblom B, Grahn R, Nordenborg T. Improvement of muscle flexibility: a comparison between two techniques. *Am J Sports Med* 1985;13:263–268.

Chapter 27

Family Intervention After Traumatic Brain Injury

Stephanie A. Kolakowsky-Hayner
Jeffrey S. Kreutzer

Practitioners typically attend to patients' problems and needs during the early course of treatment. However, the focus may necessarily shift to the needs, concerns, and problems of family members. The shift in focus toward family members' needs relates to two factors. First, injury may impair patients' awareness of difficulties, ability to participate in therapy, and ability to express themselves. In contrast, caregivers are often capable of vocalizing their needs, patients' needs, and opinions pertaining to the quality of care. Second, family members often take over long-term caregiving responsibilities, replacing the role of rehabilitation professionals.

Interdisciplinary treatment team members must take into account a variety of issues when addressing family concerns in the context of rehabilitation. The coping skills of individual family members and their emotional health play an important role in rehabilitation outcomes. Caregivers' interest, willingness, and ability to participate in the treatment process varies based on the quality of familial relationships before and after the injury. Caregivers often misinterpret the long-term effects of injury. Unfortunately, preconceived stereotypes of persons with disabilities may lead to family conflicts and unrealistic treatment goals. It is the responsibility of the rehabilitation team to dispel any and all misinformation. Rehabilitation specialists must also address practical considerations including length of stay, availability of specialized family intervention, and family resources such as insurance coverage for mental health services as well as the commitment of the organization and individual staff to provide holistic rehabilitation.

Family intervention should ideally follow a methodical and complete assessment (1). However, the need for family intervention may instantaneously originate during a developing crisis. In the case of crisis, a variety of concerns must be addressed to prevent retrogression, regardless of whether or not a full assessment has been completed. For example, during a family conference, the patient's mother insists that the rehabilitation staff is demanding "too much" from her daughter and that she would like to have the daughter transferred to a different program, while the father insists the program is not pushing his daughter hard enough. Family therapy may be initiated early during treatment to fully explain the necessity and course of treatment, and quell conflicts between the parents that may hinder treatment.

This chapter furnishes an overview of family intervention strategies. It considers the full extent of issues relevant in hospital and community settings. Some strategies simply require common sense and caring. Others may require involvement of licensed mental health professionals. Each case should be considered independently and within the context of the treatment teams' resources.

Although a thorough discussion of family intervention would require an entire book, we simply focus on the most advantageous techniques and the most frequently encountered and salient concerns. Readers who desire more information are encouraged to read the works of Hosack and Rocchio (2), Maitz and Sachs (3), Serio et al (4), Williams and Kay (5), and Witol et al (6).

FAMILY INTERVENTION TECHNIQUES

Professionals in the fields of psychology, social work, and psychiatry have developed an abundance of information illustrating intervention with families in mental health settings. Many of these interventions have been adapted for the brain injury population (3,7–12). Considering typical brain injury sequelae, the psychosocial characteristics of patients, and the rehabilitation environment, seven principal techniques have been applied and found useful: family education, family support groups, social support networks, family advocacy, family therapy, marital therapy, and sexual counseling.

Family Education

Family education provides family members with a wealth of information pertaining to postinjury changes in the patient, including personality, intellectual, psychomotor, perceptual, and neurologic changes, and furnishes recommendations regarding rehabilitation options. In addition, family education can provide the names of support and advocacy groups. Family education specialists also discuss the availability of treatment and estimates of the cost.

The need for information often causes the family to feel overwhelmed or confused and ranks among the highest needs of family members (4,13–16). Family education helps to attenuate the confusion. Similarly, family education prepares family members for the overall treatment process and provides reasonable expectations regarding rehabilitation outcome. Professionals should ensure that all information is understandable and relevant to each situation. Approaches to family education may include the following:

- Developing a resource library (17) including professional journal articles, booklets, and other materials written particularly for injured persons and their families
- Providing families with information on professional meetings and conferences
- Supplying families with the names and numbers of local brain injury associations or support groups affiliated with the Brain Injury Association

Additionally, information may be obtained through use of the Internet. With access to a computer, a modem, and an Internet service provider, family members can access a wealth of free information. Resources on the Internet include the following:

- Search engines. Using resources like Yahoo, Infoseek, or Excite, readers can type in a word or phrase. The engine generates a list of relevant Web sites for exploration.
- Web sites developed by organizations (including rehabilitation providers, advocacy groups, health care organizations, and pharmaceutical companies) that provide free information about brain injury to visitors.
- Vendors of audiovisual materials and books, including book stores. Visitors can type in a topic, book title, or author, search a company database for materials, and order books and audiovisual materials on-line for home delivery.
- Bulletin boards. Readers can review questions and answers, and using e-mail, post information including announcements, or ask questions.
- List servers. These provide a means of sharing ideas, requesting information, discussing issues, and announcing events on-line with people who have similar interests. Subscribing members can easily send an identical e-mail message to all the subscribers of a list simply by sending one message to the list server address. All subscribing members receive the e-mail message. Several brain injury list servers have been established for professionals and consumers.

Although family education is beneficial in most cases, transition from a structured hospital environment to an unstructured home setting, the stress of current therapeutic needs, physical distance of services, and lack of outpatient programs may affect family members' ability to retain the information provided in these educational sessions. A more structured rehabilitation program can be provided with a case management approach in which a caseworker organizes all information among medical staff as well as between the medical staff and the family. The caseworker should also ensure that the information presented is in lay terms, avoiding all technical jargon, so as not to further confuse the family.

Family Support Groups

Family support groups provide emotional support, a source of education, and social networking for the caregivers and patients alike. Professionals facilitating the groups often furnish educational material based on extensive knowledge of the medical, therapeutic, emotional, and physical needs of persons with brain injury. In the beginning stages, professionals typically facilitate the groups; later, the members of the group assume leadership roles. Rehabilitation professionals should continue to supervise the groups to ensure that meetings are productive, assist with personality conflicts, and caution against heightened or diminished expectations based on others' experiences.

Rehabilitation professionals often facilitate family support groups, including immediate and extended family members of persons with brain injury, and occasionally the persons with brain injury themselves. However, only one semicontrolled study on the efficacy of family intervention (18) has been published to date, and opinions differ regarding the inclusion of patients in family support groups. One opinion suggests that patients should not be included in family support groups because the interests and concerns of family members and patients are too divergent. Differing interests and concerns often cause unnecessary tension between the individual and the family. Regardless of the increased conflict, the other opinion suggests including patients in family support groups because the large representation of both family members and patients provides a forum for additional suggestions with balanced opinions. Family support groups often have common characteristics, including the following:

- Experienced family members share knowledge with less experienced members of the group.
- Participants are more responsive, less aggressive, and more likely to accept advice from other brain injury survivors and their family members than from professionals.
- Participants exhibit a variety of conversational styles.
- Participants have an easier time developing social bonds among group members due to an abundance of commonly shared experiences.

Feelings of mutual assistance, support, and reassurance, coupled with limited financial strain, make family support groups advantageous to other clinical techniques. Group members ultimately provide continuous support to other members even outside the group setting.

Social Support Networks

Speck and Attenave (19) and Rueveni (20) developed social network interventions to help family members of persons with mental illness avoid and better deal with conflicts. Social support networks provide immediate and extended family members, coworkers, friends, and acquaintances with a vehicle for problem identification, problem solving, and solution implementation. Social support networks often exhibit group cohesion, a sense of kinship, and responsibility for treatment outcome.

There is a need to develop a social support network for persons with brain injury and their families (7,21–24). According to Kozloff (22), persons recovering from a traumatic brain injury rely much more on fewer people relative to before the injury, owing to a decrease in social support from extended family and friends. Lezak (25) also reported an increase in conflict between immediate and extended family with regard to care issues.

Rogers and Kreutzer (24) implemented such network interventions with persons with brain injury. These groups also included a professional facilitator, rehabilitation professionals, multiple persons with brain injury, their immediate and extended families, and other acquaintances. Interventions primarily included the following:

- Introduction of relatives and acquaintances
- Development of a support network
- Problem-solving tasks
- An educational component
- Grieving sessions recounting preinjury relations

Social support networks often encourage discussion of feelings and provide suggestions to alleviate the guilt caregivers often experience about overburdening relatives with requests for support (25). Network members commonly share respite care and other resources, which provides a stronger support structure than that of one family trying to obtain services alone. Family networks typically require two to three meetings facilitated by a professional, prior to group cohesion. Group meetings only need to occur every 3 to 6 months to maintain the network system and if necessary, meetings can be called more frequently. Although difficult to arrange, interim meetings often provide a tremendous amount of support not otherwise available.

Family Advocacy

Essential services for persons with brain injury are not offered in many communities. The lack of service has led to caregivers' spending significant time at home caring for the patient or traveling long distances to obtain services, and has commanded the need for family advocacy. Family advocacy includes teaching professionals in related disciplines about the special needs of persons with brain injury, aiding in cost-effectiveness. Family advocacy limits the amount of time caregivers are compelled to stay at home. Additionally, advocacy alleviates the amount of time family members must expend locating services.

Family advocacy is often provided by rehabilitation professionals such as social workers, psychologists, and case managers; family networks; local support groups; and the Brain Injury Association. Family advocacy incorporates changing services to meet the needs of persons with head injury, helping families to take full advantage of the resources available to them, and developing services not readily available. When an advocate is obtaining services for a person with brain injury, the responsibilities are extensive and include the following:

- Identifying which services are essential
- Providing families with information regarding service options
- Locating an existing service or one that will require minimum modification to meet the needs of the patient and the family members
- Assisting in the modeling and implementation of new services
- Recommending traditional rehabilitation services and social and recreational activities necessary to community integration
- Evaluating the system to ensure a positive outcome and any additional need
- Providing reassurance to families once a decision about care has been made

- Facilitating cost assessment
- Obtaining third-party payment

Wehman and colleagues' (26–28) supported employment model of vocational rehabilitation represents the benefits of family advocacy. The research suggests that rehabilitation programs need to supplement supported employment with additional services, including recreational therapy, family therapy, marital therapy, and other support groups and networks (26,27). The supported employment model focuses fundamentally on postemployment supervision and intervention. The model is extremely cost-effective. Additionally, the employment model enables caregivers to work outside the home and ultimately diminishes family stress.

Many school systems are ignorant of the special needs of children with brain injury (29–31). Therefore, advocacy is extremely important for children with brain injury and their families. The following are responsibilities of the advocate:

- Prepare information for teachers and schools regarding brain injury.
- Arrange individualized education programs.
- Set up social support networks including other school-age children with brain injuries and their families.
- Evaluate programs.
- Encourage families about program successes.

Families are more likely to trust the advocate's evaluation and encouragement than information provided by staff in the schools, even when the staff has good intentions.

Family Therapy

There are many pressures and changes imposed on families and their support networks following traumatic brain injury. Family therapy techniques are designed to facilitate community integration after brain injury (12,32–35). Family therapy is an interactive system (36,37), structured around the family, including the person with the injury, the immediate family, and in some cases, extended family members who frequently interact with the patient.

Family therapy involves identifying behavior patterns within the family, increasing adaptive behaviors, and curbing maladaptive behaviors. Therapists should be sensitive to and account for cultural, religious, and ethnic issues that may arise (38,39). Family therapists, typically a social worker, psychologist, or other rehabilitation professional, focus on the following:

- Grief reduction
- Stress reduction
- Problem solving
- Communication
- Social skills
- Decreasing feelings of helplessness
- Reassigning family responsibilities
- Restructuring the family into a cohesive team

Therapy is tailored to meet the specific needs of the patient, change as the individual changes, and provide ongoing education. Therapy must also address common concerns associated with traumatic brain injury including false hopes and fears regarding outcome, lack of available community services, and permanent changes in personality following brain injury that are usually the most distressing (25) to family members.

Therapists also help families to recognize and accept their own limitations with regard to satisfying all the needs of the patient. It is the responsibility of the therapist to reassure the family that recovery is a long-term process and can become time-consuming. For example, during therapy, if the patient's wife indicates that she no longer has time to spend with her friends and is beginning to resent the patient, the therapist should suggest alternatives to spending all of her time with the patient (e.g., asking another relative to spend a few hours per week with the patient). Similarly, Mr. Jones may express concern regarding mounting medical or rehabilitation bills from his son's brain injury, and lack of financial support from the insurance company. Therapists should advocate for third-party payment and seek additional funding sources as well as auxiliary service providers. When the efforts of the therapist and family do not culminate in a positive outcome, the therapist should still reassure family members and continually praise their efforts.

Family therapy should include anyone related to the caregiving process. Family therapy allows families to act out possible conflicts occurring in their everyday lives (10), with all family members offering their individual perspectives on the predicament. Listening to individual accounts provides the therapist with a more impartial view of the situation. Acting out family conflicts also reduces the likelihood of placing blame.

Family therapy often proves most beneficial for children. Reassuring noninjured siblings that they are still loved and encouraging them to ask questions regarding changes in the family structure can help to avert feelings of neglect. Questions also provide a means for ongoing education to lessen confusion. Reduced self-esteem is also common in children of persons with brain injury and may cause misdirected anger and uncharacteristic yelling. The therapist must reassure the child that the anger is indeed a result of the injury and not a result of how the parent feels toward the child. Overall, therapy provides an outlet for the child's feelings as well as an educational forum.

Similarly, the parents are subjected to significant stress when their child's brain is injured. The stress of the situation often causes conflict between the parents. The child can again become the victim. A child with a brain injury must deal not only with the regular conflicts that arise within a family, but also with conflicts resulting from arguments over treatment options. If the child is consistently becoming the victim of the parents' arguments, the therapist must focus on teaching them problem-solving skills based on what is best for the child. A six-step method of problem solving (40) has proved effective in an assortment of circumstances (41):

- Identify the conflict.
- Generate a variety of possible solutions to the problem.
- Discuss pros and cons of all solutions.
- Pick the best solution.
- Decide how to apply the solution.
- Review the efficacy of the solution. (Repeat steps if necessary.)

Parents must learn to compromise for the child's sake. However, family members should keep in mind that conflicts are a natural and inevitable part of all relationships. The belief that all conflicts are avoidable can have negative consequences and actually increase conflict. Therapists should teach families constructive conflict resolution strategies.

Marital Therapy

Marital therapy is similar to family therapy in that a licensed professional such as a psychologist, psychiatrist, or social worker typically provides it. However, marital therapy attends solely to the couple. Marital therapy may also be beneficial to other couples who are not married but in an intimate relationship. The therapist should make certain that both partners realize that any form of change will require comprehensive treatment and time. The therapist must do the following:

- Have the couple identify why they chose to be married to each other, refreshing positive feelings about the relationship.
- Inquire about any preinjury difficulties the couple may have had.
- Discuss goals that were set before the injury and how they may have changed.
- Ask the couple to determine new goals or discuss any postinjury goals they have already set.
- Encourage the couple to accept responsibility for their problems and for finding and implementing solutions.
- Inform the couple that problems will most likely occur again, and that the eventual objective is long-term happiness.

Marriage is a voluntary commitment, and is intended to last for life (42). Both individuals within a marriage are independent of each other, yet they depend on each other exclusively, without interference from other family members. Additionally, marriage typifies a goal-oriented compromise. Spouses of injured persons must deal with a variety of changes relative to before the injury (43–46). For instance, spouses often encounter lack of emotional support, lack of financial support, and changes in personality and behavior, making the injured person seem like a "stranger" relative to before the injury, including violent and abusive behavior (7), childishness, irritability, restlessness, and emotional instability (47). Additionally, after a brain injury, couples tend to become socially isolated and rely less on people outside the relationship (22,25).

Spouses of persons with brain injury often stick with their mate throughout the early stages of recovery—typically owing to social pressures and feelings of guilt (25). Nonetheless, personality changes and other injury-related stressors often result in divorce about the time of community reintegration. However, no research findings imply an increase in divorce rates among couples with brain injury when compared with normal couples.

After a brain injury, the uninjured spouse may be required to take on the injured spouse's chores and obligations as well as his or her own. Conflicts frequently arise over assignment of household obligations. For example, a wife who has not worked a day since she was married 10 years ago, has not had any experience with the household finances, and probably has not been involved in her son's sporting events, must now return to the workforce and become the sole source of income for the household, balance the checkbook and pay the bills, and take her son to football practice. Additionally, spouses often encounter a great amount of difficulty obtaining rehabilitation and support services that are relatively close in location, and affordable. Research has indicated a lack of effective vocational rehabilitation programs (48,49). Successful vocational rehabilitation programs can help relieve emotional and monetary stresses caused by the difficulty in obtaining employment.

The therapist is responsible for determining which of the new responsibilities is causing the uninjured spouse the most stress, and for providing potential solutions. In addition to reports from the uninjured spouse, the clinician should gain a better perspective by interviewing children, extended family, and close friends. Individual sessions may be scheduled with the uninjured spouse prior to the initiation of couples therapy, if the injured spouse is severely impaired. During these sessions, the clinician and spouse should set rehabilitation goals, provide education, recommend strategies to reduce stress, and develop behavior management programs. The therapist should act as a mediator for the couple and should ensure that both husband and wife are heard without interference or criticism from their partner.

Sexual Counseling

Sexual counseling should be thought of as an integral part of the rehabilitation process. Sexual counseling is often conducted as a part of marital therapy; however, sexual counseling may be conducted with injured persons without partners, with unwed couples, and as an educational forum for extended family and caregivers. Research suggests that sexual dysfunction and problems relating to sexuality are prevalent after brain injury (25,50–55). Rehabilitation efforts aimed at enhancing sexual functioning and satisfaction are essential to recovery of self-esteem and should be weighed as heavily as physical, cognitive, avocational, and vocational interventions.

FAMILY REACTIONS TO BRAIN INJURY

A variety of behavioral responses are typically exhibited by patients and family members after brain injury. Clinicians should reassure patients and family members that these responses are quite normal for anyone experiencing a tragic event and extended negative outcomes. The following describes such behavioral responses and provides suggestions for intervention strategies.

Anger

Anger is a common reaction to brain injury. Typically, 63% of wives and 45% of mothers of adults with brain injury report feelings of anger (7). Anger is commonly the result of disappointment, directly related to the patient's unusual behavior. Patients often act out in an aggressive manner, causing family members to withdraw affection. Anger may also materialize slowly over time, with prolonged stress and diminishing patience. In addition, caregivers may become disappointed with the availability and quality of rehabilitation services. Anger often leads to reduced affection or punishment and can easily encourage further aggression from the patient.

In order to properly address anger within the context of therapy, clinicians should do the following:

- Ensure that the injured person and family members are able to recognize and label their own feelings.
- Supply simple labels rather than professional jargon.
- Teach appropriate problem-solving skills and coping techniques.
- Effectively elicit descriptions of the injured person's and family's feelings by asking careful questions during interviews and counseling sessions.
- Facilitate adjustment by reassuring the injured person and family members that feelings of anger emerge naturally in similar situations.
- Teach family members and patients to express anger constructively.
- Suggest alternatives to alleviate frustration (e.g., exercise).

Blame

Similar to anger, blame is caused by frustration difficulties stemming from the brain injury. Family members may try to identify the culprit. Blame may be misplaced on the injured person, other family members, doctors, case managers, insurance companies, and community leaders, when services are unavailable or when there is disappointment with the recovery rates. Blame can be extremely detrimental to the family as a whole. Family members must continue to provide cooperation, support, and assistance throughout the recovery process.

Blame may be most harmful when immediate family members begin to blame each other for the patient's problems. For example, a mother blames the husband for impeding their daughter's recovery by coddling her. Similarly, a child may blame his or her mother because she divorced the injured father when he became verbally abusive after the injury. Furthermore, patients often become scapegoats, owing to their bizarre or disturbing behavior. For example, a wife may leave her injured husband when she can no longer go out in public with him because of his incessant swearing following brain damage. Similarly, parents may blame their child for preexisting marital problems.

Families should be encouraged to adopt practical alternatives to avoid the negative aftermath of blaming. Clinicians can help family members alleviate blaming behavior by teaching them the following:

- To adopt more effective problem-solving methods
- To recognize that blame serves to exacerbate rather than mitigate problems
- To identify alternative sources of funding, local rehabilitation providers, and support programs
- To appeal the insurance company's decision to deny coverage for rehabilitation services
- About the normal injury-related psychological and physiologic changes

Guilt

Guilt is a direct result of both anger and blame. Typically, each emotion influences the severity of the others. When anger is directed toward oneself, guilt is the result. For instance, family members may become angry with themselves, and blame themselves for the patient's initial injury, bizarre behavior, lack of progress, or lack of appropriate rehabilitation resources. Phrases such as "I should have" or "I could have" are telltale signs that the family member is experiencing guilt.

Guilt is a widespread response to anger and blame after a severe injury. Clinicians should address guilt promptly so that it does not deteriorate into depression. Depression can be very detrimental to a family member's participation in the treatment effort. By caring for themselves, family members can more effectively address the needs of the patient, as well as others. When addressing guilt, the clinician should do the following:

- Help family members identify and label their feelings.
- Provide reassurance that family members are reacting normally to a very abnormal situation.

- Indicate that guilt has no practical value and is typically self-defeating.
- Review the benefits of the family's ongoing support.
- Discuss the frustrations and difficulties inherent in helping a severely injured person.
- Provide encouragement that caregivers are doing the best they can and reassurance that they have done all anyone could ask of them.
- Provide continual education and allow the family time to process new information.

Aggressive Behavior

Aggressive behavior may be the most detrimental reaction to traumatic brain injury. Aggressive behavior typically increases over time and family members become detached and unwilling to provide support (25,56). Family members may also begin to feel guilt due to conflicting feelings of anger and sympathy. Additionally, family members may begin blaming everyday problems on the aggressive patient. In turn, when support is withdrawn, patients are likely to feel rejected and may become more hostile.

Clinicians may recommend a variety of strategies for reducing aggressive behaviors and the negative consequences that accompany such behaviors. For example, use of family members as cotherapists, assertiveness training, and behavior management has been successful at curtailing aggressive behaviors (57). In extreme cases, clinicians may also need to resort to psychopharmacologic interventions (58).

The following are behavior management techniques that are useful for reducing aggressive behaviors after brain injury:

- Teach families to identify potential aggressive situations.
- Educate family members on typical warning signs of anger and aggression.
- Train family members to utilize appropriate coping strategies.
- Teach patients and family members that if the strategies are not working in a particular situation, they should remove themselves from that situation.

Denial

Denial is often the healthy expression of anxiety and occurs as a result of family members' unwillingness to accept the competencies and limitations of the person with the brain injury. Denial allows family members to have a much more optimistic outlook on the recovery process. It can be the result of confusion associated with disagreements among treatment team members, or of providing the family members with too much information at once. Lastly, denial is most prevalent when the family is excluded from the treatment-planning process. Ignorance about the treatment fosters denial.

Direct denial may be exhibited when family members openly disagree with the rehabilitation staff regarding prognosis and treatment planning. Direct denial often occurs in the early stages of recovery, when the family tends to be more optimistic than the rehabilitation staff. On the other hand, denial may be expressed indirectly. For example, a mother may begin to question the treatment progress, and ask to have her injured son moved to another treatment facility "that will do some good for her son." Such a case would be considered "doctor shopping," in which the family continually dismisses the opinions of the rehabilitation staff and moves from one rehabilitation center to another until they find the answers for which they are looking.

Clinicians should take heed at acknowledging and addressing denial to avoid a pursuit of unrealistic goals and wasting of limited rehabilitation resources. A number of effective techniques are available to clinicians for diminishing denial. For example:

- Provide ongoing family education.
- Include family members in treatment planning.
- Provide family support (e.g., refer to social support groups and networks).
- Allow family members time to understand the wealth of new information that has been given to them.
- Provide the family with clear and consistent information.
- Avoid technical jargon.
- Convey a sense of sympathy and caring.
- Highlight positive aspects of recovery.
- Provide detailed examples for each situation.
- Encourage questions and paraphrasing.
- Review and provide family members with written information for later reference.
- Maintain regular communication with family members.
- Clear up conflicting viewpoints and opinions among family members and among staff members.
- Develop constructive forums that promote consensus (e.g., case conferences, treatment team meetings).

CONCLUSIONS AND IMPLICATIONS

A plethora of negative changes occur after brain injury. It is imperative that family interventions address the needs and concerns of family members and patients. The opportune time to commence family intervention is early during the recovery process. Here, professionals may have their best chance to furnish many family support services including family education, family advocacy, marital and family therapy, social support groups, social networks, and sexual counseling.

Currently there is a tremendous need for adequate services for families of persons with brain injuries. The prevailing focus of rehabilitation centers is on the individual needs of patients and integration into the community rather than the critical needs of the family. Additionally, the reductions in length of stay and lack of adequate insurance coverage make it increasingly difficult for rehabilitation professionals to provide ample family interventions. Further research and training are necessary to authenticate the significance of family interventions.

ACKNOWLEDGMENTS

This work was partly supported by grants G0087C0219 and H133P2006 from the National Institute on Disability and Rehabilitation Research, U.S. Department of Education.

REFERENCES

1. Sander A, Kreutzer J. A holistic approach to family assessment after brain injury. In: Rosenthal M, Griffith E, Kreutzer J, Pentland B, eds. *Rehabilitation of the adult and child with traumatic brain injury.* 3rd ed. Philadelphia: FA Davis, (in press).
2. Hosack KR, Rocchio CA. Serving families of persons with severe brain injury in an era of managed care. *J Head Trauma Rehabil* 1995;10:57–65.
3. Maitz EA, Sachs PR. Treating families of individuals with traumatic brain injury from a family systems perspective. *J Head Trauma Rehabil* 1995;10:1–11.
4. Serio C, Kreutzer J, Gervasio A. Predicting family needs after traumatic brain injury: implications for intervention. *J Head Trauma Rehabil* 1995;10:32–45.
5. Williams JM, Kay T. *Head injury: a family matter.* Baltimore: Paul H. Brookes, 1990.
6. Witol A, Sander A, Kreutzer J. A longitudinal analysis of family needs following traumatic brain injury. *Neurorehabilitation* 1996;7:175–187.
7. Mauss-Clum N, Ryan M. Brain injury and the family. *J Neurosurg Nurs* 1981;13:165–169.
8. Lehr E. *Psychological management of traumatic brain injuries in children and adults.* Rockville, MD: Aspen, 1990.
9. Lezak MD. Brain damage is a family affair. *J Clin Exp Neuropsychol* 1988;10:111–123.
10. Minuchin S. *Families and family therapy.* Cambridge: Harvard University Press, 1974.
11. Muir C, Rosenthal M, Diehl L. Methods of family intervention. In: Rosenthal M, Griffith ER, Bond M, Miller J, eds. *Rehabilitation of the adult and child with traumatic brain injury.* 2nd ed. Philadelphia: FA Davis, 1990:433–447.
12. Rosenthal M, Young T. Effective family intervention after traumatic brain injury. *J Head Trauma Rehabil* 1988;3:42–51.
13. Leske J. Needs of relatives of critically ill patients: a follow-up. *Heart Lung* 1986;15:189–193.
14. Norris LD, Grove SK. Investigation of selected psychosocial needs of family members of critically ill adult patients. *Heart Lung* 1986;15:194–199.
15. Serio C, Kreutzer J, Witol A. Family needs after traumatic brain injury: a factor analytic study of the Family Needs Questionnaire. *Brain Inj* 1997;11:1–9.
16. Rosenthal M, Hutchins BF. Interdisciplinary family education in head injury rehabilitation. In: Williams JM, Kay T, eds. *Head injury: a family matter.* Baltimore: Paul H. Brookes, 1990:273–282.
17. Eisner J, Kreutzer JS. A family information system for education following traumatic brain injury. *Brain Inj* 1989;3:79–90.
18. Smith LP, Godfrey HPD. *Family support programs and rehabilitation: a cognitive-behavioral approach to traumatic brain injury.* New York: Plenum, 1995.
19. Speck R, Attenave C. *Family networks.* New York: Pantheon Books, 1973.
20. Rueveni U. *Networking families in crisis.* New York: Human Science Press, 1979.
21. Jacobs HE. The Los Angeles Head Injury survey: procedures and initial findings. *Arch Phys Med Rehabil* 1988;69:425–431.
22. Kozloff R. Networks of social support and the outcome from severe head injury. *J Head Trauma Rehabil* 1987;2:14–23.
23. Panting A, Merry PH. The long-term rehabilitation of severe head injuries with particular reference to the need for social and medical support for the patient's family *Rehabilitation (Stattg)* 1972;38:33–37.
24. Rogers PM, Kreutzer JS. Family crises following head injury: a network intervention strategy. *J Neurosurg Nurs* 1984;16:343–346.
25. Lezak MD. Living with the characterologically altered brain-injured patient. *J Clin Psychiatry* 1978;39:111–123.
26. Wehman P, Kreutzer J, Sale P, et al. Cognitive impairment and remediation: implications for employment following traumatic brain injury. *J Head Trauma Rehabil* 1989;4:66–75.
27. Wehman P, Kreutzer J, Stonnington H, et al. Supported employment for persons with traumatic brain injury: a preliminary report. *J Head Trauma Rehabil* 1988;3:82–94.

28. Wehman P, Kreutzer J, Wood W, et al. Helping traumatically brain injured patients return to work with supported employment: three case studies. *Arch Phys Med Rehabil* 1989;70:109–113.

29. Waaland PK, Kreutzer JS. Family response to childhood traumatic brain injury. *J Head Trauma Rehabil* 1988;3:51–63.

30. Waaland P, Burns C, Cockrell J. Evaluation of needs of high and low income families following pediatric brain injury. *Brain Inj* 1993;7:35–146.

31. Waaland PK. Family response to childhood brain injury. In: Kreutzer J, Wehman P, eds. *Community integration following traumatic brain injury*. Baltimore: Paul H. Brookes, 1990:225–248.

32. Rosenthal M, Greckler C. Family therapy issues in neuropsychology. In: Wedding D, Horton AM, Webster J, eds. *The neuropsychology handbook*. 1st ed. New York: Springer, 1986:325–344.

33. Rosenthal M, Greckler C. Family therapy issues in neuropsychology. In: Horton AM, Wedding D,Webster J, eds. *The neuropsychology handbook*. 2nd ed. New York: Springer, 1997:47–72.

34. Sachs PR. *Treating families of brain-injury survivors*. New York: Springer, 1991.

35. Zarski JJ, Hall DE, DePompei R. Closed head injury patients: a family therapy approach to the rehabilitation process. *Am J Fam Ther* 1987;15:62–68.

36. Satir V. Family systems and approaches to family therapy. In: Erickson G, Hogan T, eds. *Family therapy: an introduction to theory and technique*. Monterey, CA: Wadsworth, 1972:211–221.

37. Terkelsen K. Toward a theory of the family life cycle. In: Carter E, McGoldrick M, eds. *The family life cycle: a framework for family therapy*. New York: Gardner, 1980:21–52.

38. Kay T, Cavallo MM. Evolutions: research and clinical perspectives on families. In: Williams JM, Kay T, eds. *Head injury: a family matter*. Baltimore: Paul H. Brookes, 1990:121–150.

39. Cavallo MM, Saucedo C. Traumatic brain injury in families from culturally diverse populations. *J Head Trauma Rehabil* 1995;10: 66–77.

40. Gordon T. *Parent effectiveness training*. New York: New American Library, 1975.

41. Goldfried M, Davison G. *Clinical behavior therapy*. New York: Holt, Rinehart, & Winston, 1976.

42. Jackson DD. Family rules: marital quid pro quo. In: Erickson G, Hogan T, eds. *Family therapy: an introduction to theory and technique*. Monterey, CA: Wadsworth, 1972:76–85.

43. Peters LC, Stambrook M, Moore AD, Esses L. Psychosocial sequelae of closed head injury. Effects on the marital relationship. *Brain Inj* 1990;4:39–47.

44. Peters LC, Stambrook M, Moore AD, et al. Differential effects of spinal cord injury and head injury on marital adjustment. *Brain Inj* 1992;6:461–467.

45. Rosenbaum M, Najenson T. Changes in life patterns and symptoms of low mood reported by wives of severely brain-injured soldiers. *J Consult Clin Psychol* 1976;44:881–888.

46. Willer BS, Allen KM, Liss M, Zicht MS. Problems and coping strategies of individuals with traumatic brain injury and their sppouses. *Arch Phys Med Rehabil* 1991;72:460–464.

47. Thomsen IV. The patient with severe head injury and his family. *Scand J Rehabil Med* 1974;6: 180–183.

48. Ben-Yishay Y, Silver SM, Piasetsky E, Rattok J. Relationship between employability and vocational outcome after intensive holistic cognitive rehabilitation. *J Head Trauma Rehabil* 1987;2:35–48.

49. Fawber H, Wachter J. Job placements: a treatment component of the vocational rehabilitation process. *J Head Trauma Rehabil* 1987;2:27–33.

50. Blackerby WF. A treatment model for sexuality disturbance following brain injury. *J Head Trauma Rehabil* 1990;5:73–82.

51. Davis DL, Schneider LK. Ramifications of traumatic brain injury for sexuality. *J Head Trauma Rehabil* 1990;5:31–37.

52. Graden FH, Bontke CF, Hoffman M. Sexual functioning and marital adjustment after traumatic brain injury. *J Head Trauma Rehabil* 1990;5:52–59.

53. Kreutzer JS, Zasler ND. Psychosexual consequences of traumatic brain injury: methodology and preliminary findings. *Brain Inj* 1989;3:177–186.

54. Zasler ND, Horn LJ. Rehabilitative management of sexual dysfunction. *J Head Trauma Rehabil* 1990;5:14–24.

55. Zasler ND, Kreutzer JS. Family and sexuality. In: Williams JM, Kay T, eds. *Head injury: a family matter*. Baltimore: Paul H. Brookes, 1990:253–270.

56. Brooks DN, Campsie L, Symington C, et al. The five year outcome of severe blunt head injury: a relative's view. *J Neurol Neurosurg Psychiatry* 1986;49:764–770.

57. McKinley W, Hickox A. How can families help in the rehabilitation of the head injured? *J Head Trauma Rehabil* 1988;3:64–72.

58. Matthies B, Kreutzer J, West D. *The behavior management handbook: a practical approach to patients with neurological disorders*. San Antonio, TX: Therapy Skill Builders, 1997.

Chapter 28

Retraining the Neuromuscular System: Biofeedback and Neuromuscular Electrical Stimulation

William C. Walker

TREATMENT PRINCIPLES

Neuromuscular Impairment

The full extent of impairment must be defined prior to embarking on a rehabilitative treatment program. Either upper or lower motor neuron lesions can cause neuromuscular impairment, and while every patient needs to be evaluated individually, some general statements apply. Lower motor neuron lesions typically result in lost motor power (strength), endurance, or sensation, and secondarily lost joint motion or stability. Upper motor neuron lesions additionally can cause spasticity and lost motor control, and can be complicated by nonneuromuscular deficits such as aphasia, memory loss, poor attention, neglect, visual perceptual problems, and apraxia when cerebral structures are involved.

Treatment goals should be established simultaneously for each impairment and each functional deficit. Rehabilitation goals generally fall within one of three categories: prevention, restoration, and compensation (e.g., substitution).

Preventative Rehabilitation

Neuromuscular lesions create weakness and immobility that limit the physiologic stretching normally encountered by the soft tissues during daily activities. Soft-tissue shortening and contractures ensue (1), leading to altered biomechanics and excessive effort of movement, in turn further hindering mobility. When inactivity limits muscle contractions to less than 20% of their maximal tension, disuse atrophy will develop, further exacerbating the weakness caused by upper or lower motor neuron lesions. A preventative program should be initiated early to maintain the basic components of neuromuscular function and prevent the downward spiral of weakness and lost range of motion. Traditional preventative treatment strategies include positioning, splinting, range of motion exercises, generalized mobility, and frequent inspection and protection of sensory impaired areas. Strengthening exercises should also be performed on nonimpaired muscle groups.

Restorative Rehabilitation

Whenever possible, every effort should be made to restore all physiologic parameters that have deviated from normal, including strength, sensation, and motor control. I consider reduction of impairment to be the hallmark of "retraining" the neuromuscular system. The rehabilitation treatments most often advocated for reduction of neuromuscular impairments are therapeutic exercise and electrotherapy, so these modalities will receive the bulk of attention in this chapter. Other restorative treatments, such as surgery and pharmacology, are not purely rehabilitative and are not discussed in this chapter.

Compensatory Rehabilitation

Many neuromuscular impairments can be neither prevented nor significantly reduced. An extreme example is leg paresis following complete cervical spinal cord injury, for which traditional rehabilitation goals concentrate on compensating for the absent leg strength and lessening the secondary mobility problem (the disability). When significant physiologic improvement cannot be expected within a reasonable time frame, compensatory or substitutive treatments should be introduced as soon as possible. Orthotic devices and adaptive equipment can often compensate for joint instability, weakness, spasticity, lost sensory feedback, or poor balance. Their judicious use can facilitate daily activities even when profound impairment exists, and should be considered an integral part of the rehabilitation process. Functional electrical stimulation (FES) is a recently developed technology that can also be employed. Other compensatory treatment strategies include teaching substitution patterns and alternative functional techniques. An example is teaching one-handed dressing and bathing techniques to the hemiplegic patient lacking functional motor recovery of one upper extremity.

Comprehensive Neuromuscular Rehabilitation

The objective of comprehensive rehabilitation is to maximize an individual's entire functional status (e.g., minimize disability). The comprehensive neuromuscular rehabilitation program utilizes prevention strategies, compensatory strategies, and restorative treatments, and integrates all of these together to maximize neuromuscular function. Other nonneuromuscular aspects of disability (e.g., cardiac disease, cognitive impairment) are addressed as well. A holistic approach with attention to daily activity training, impairments of other body systems, and psychosocial issues is paramount for an optimal outcome. When all facets of the comprehensive neuromuscular rehabilitation program are well integrated, the result is an earlier and more efficient return to a healthy lifestyle. Table 28-1 summarizes the subcomponents of comprehensive neuromuscular rehabilitation.

Table 28-1: Rehabilitative Treatment of Neuromuscular Impairment

Program Type	Treatment Options
Prevention	Positioning, splinting, therapeutic exercise, maintaining mobility, electrical stimulation of denervated muscle
Restoration	Therapeutic exercise, muscle re-education, neuromuscular electrical strimulation
Compensation	Orthotics, gait aids, adaptive equipment, alternative functional techniques, functional electrical stimulation
Comprehensive	Combines all of the above; addresses all aspects of disability, functional deficits, and impairment

BASICS OF THERAPEUTIC EXERCISE

Strength

Traditional resistive strengthening exercises identify the weak muscular movements and use resistance against those movements. For example, for a peroneal nerve lesion causing footdrop, resistive exercises are developed for the ankle dorsiflexors and evertors. Knowledge of functional anatomy allows one to devise resistive strengthening exercises to any muscle group in the body.

Resistance exercise promotes muscle fiber hypertrophy, a metabolic adaptive response that is largely responsible for clinical strength gains (2). The rate and extent of hypertrophy are proportional to the resistance the muscle must overcome (3). Additionally, neural adaptation is believed to contribute to strength gains, especially in the first 2 weeks of resistive training (4). One possible mechanism of neural adaptation is improved synchronization of motor unit firing (5). Another possible mechanism is the nervous system "learning" to activate muscles more efficiently, for example, improved neural drive (6).

Exercise intensity must be greater than the existing capacity in order to achieve a training effect; for example, overload is required for improved performance (7). Application of high resistance maximizes strength gains, and the number of repetitions need not be high as long as muscular fatigue is reached. A weight that can only be lifted for 1 to 10 repetitions is recommended, with the individual only able to lift it slowly through the full range (3). At least three sets should be performed with rest breaks in between, and sessions should be performed at least twice a week.

When exercise intensity is overzealous, and too near the maximal attainable tension, damage can occur due to the overworking of the muscle. Weakened muscle, or muscle unaccustomed to training, is particularly susceptible to overwork-induced damage (8), probably because it is already functioning closer to its maximal limits. Thus, the beneficial effects of strength training occur only at an intensity within a therapeutic "window," below which no overload and no training will occur and above which muscle damage will occur (Fig. 28-1).

Endurance

If resistance is lowered (to <50% of maximal force capacity) and more repetitions are used, muscle biochemical adaptations differ. Increased oxidative capacity more than muscle hypertrophy results, particularly in type I fibers, leading to improved muscular endurance (e.g., resistance to fatigue) (9). To train most effectively for muscular endurance, low resistance and a high number of repetitions should be used, as opposed to the high-resistance, low-repetition program recommended for absolute strength (3). Notably, however, a high degree of transfer of training exists if exercise is of a similar nature and continues to the

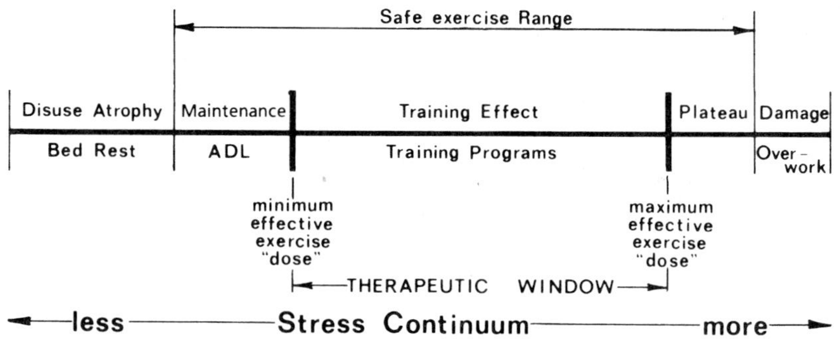

Figure 28-1. Therapeutic window for exercise training. Below a certain level of activity, disuse weakness and atrophy will occur. Exercise that is too intense can cause muscle damage. Strength training dosed within the therapeutic window promotes muscle hypertrophy and strength gains. ADL = activity of daily living. (Reproduced by permission from Maloney FP, Burks JS, Ringel SP, eds. *Interdisciplinary rehabilitation of multiple sclerosis and neuromuscular disorders.* New York: JB Lippincott, 1985:230.)

point of muscular fatigue (10). So when simplicity is important, an intermediate program can be utilized to train simultaneously for strength and endurance.

Velocity

Resistance training at a particular speed (angular joint velocity) improves performance most effectively for that speed only, although significant crossover into other speeds does occur (2). Since muscles are required to contract at a variety of speeds during functional activities, resistance training at different speeds is desirable. A complete strengthening program would include varying speeds of both concentric and eccentric training, as well as isometric exercises.

Flexibility

Range of motion can usually be maintained with standard positioning, splinting, and range of motion exercises, although some patients, particularly those with spasticity from upper motor neuron lesions or with pain or coexisting connective tissue disease, need more aggressive programs. If a particular segment of the neuromuscular system is primarily impaired, range of motion exercises should be concentrated on that segment. If the patient is completely incapacitated, then range of motion of all involved joints should be performed at least once a day. Overall mobility also should be maintained when feasible, by having the patient perform bed to chair activities and simple daily activities when standing and ambulation are precluded.

Mild continuous stretching for at least 20 minutes is more beneficial than stronger, brief stretching exercises (11). Splinting provides even longer durations of mild stretching and should be done for all joints at high risk to lose functional motion. If weakness is less than good, passive or active assisted motion exercises should be performed by a therapist or trained individual.

THERAPEUTIC EXERCISE FOR LOWER MOTOR NEURON LESIONS

Widespread Neuromuscular Diseases (Polio as Model)

The beneficial effects of therapeutic exercises for systemic neuromuscular disease have been repeatedly demonstrated, especially with low-intensity strengthening programs (12). Aerobic training, although less well studied, likewise improved overall function without causing loss of strength in a group of postpolio subjects (13).

Despite positive reports, therapeutic exercise must be undertaken with caution in patients with neuromuscular disease, because damage caused by overwork can occur with intensities that elicit a training effect in normal muscle. Anecdotal evidence that muscle activity or exercise for neuromuscular disease can lead to a loss of muscle strength has been reported since the poliomyelitis epidemic of the 1940s and 1950s (14). This impression has been substantiated by clinical pathologic evidence (12). If the intensity of the exercise is too great or the number of motor units too few, damage will occur (15). Thus, the therapeutic "window" where muscle can be exercised to promote gains in strength and endurance, while simultaneously preventing disuse atrophy and avoiding overwork-induced damage, is much smaller when neuromuscular disease is present (16) (Fig. 28-2).

When neuromuscular disease is severe, daily functional activities may even be taxing to the weakened muscle, and the adaptive response may be a catabolic one. The patient should limit activities until fair to good muscle power is achieved without complaints of fatigue (12). Daily activities should be thought of as strengthening exercises themselves, and structured as such with appropriate rest breaks to keep the "dose" within the therapeutic window. As recovery proceeds, very-low-resistance and nonfatiguing (e.g., submaximal) strengthening and endurance exercises are added. The optimal frequency is not known, but frequent (daily or twice-daily) sessions of low resistance and

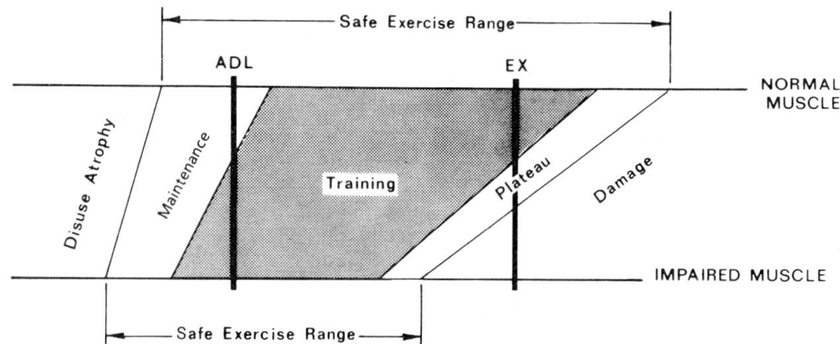

Figure 28-2. Therapeutic window for strength training in neuromuscular disease. In neuromuscular disease. the therapeutic window for strengthening is much narrower than normal, and muscle is much more susceptible to overwork damage. In very severe disease, the window may be completely closed. EX = exercise; ADL = activity of daily living. (Reproduced by permission from Maloney FP, Burks JS, Ringel SP, eds. *Interdisciplinary rehabilitation of multiple sclerosis and neuromuscular disorders.* New York: JB Lippincott, 1985:233.)

nonfatiguing repetitions is more desirable than higher-intensity and less-frequent training sessions. There is evidence, based on the work of Dickenson et al (17), that weakened muscle gains maximum performance when a strengthening program is preceded by endurance training. Thus, resistance initially should be kept significantly less than 50% of the muscle's maximum capacity and repetitions may be high but not to the point of muscular exhaustion. A typical starting point is applied weight that allows the patient to perform 30 repetitions with moderate effort and to do two to four sets. As strength improves, resistance should increase. If excessive fatigue develops or a decrease in motor power is noted, exercise should be scaled back or temporarily discontinued. While it is normal to feel a transient muscle fatigue from moderately heavy work, this must be distinguished from the prolonged, persistent decrease in muscle strength and endurance following excessive exercise of weakened muscles. In short, subjective methods are used to ensure that the individual is exercising somewhat hard but not excessively hard.

Peripheral Nerve, Plexus, and Root Lesions

Peripheral nerve, plexus, and root injuries physiologically manifest as demyelination (nerve conduction slowing), conduction block, axonal loss with denervation, or some combination of each. Resolution of these physiologic abnormalities, through remyelination, conduction block resolution, axonal regeneration, and muscle reinnervation, is necessary for complete (or nearly complete) recovery. These recovery processes are neither expedited nor facilitated by therapeutic exercise (12). Rather, exercise maintains the musculoskeletal system in the optimal "ready" state and paces the recovery process by maximizing the strength and endurance of the operational motor units and muscle fibers. As more motor units become functional via nerve regeneration or resolution of conduction block, the intensity of the strengthening exercises can increase. Strengthening exercises should continue well beyond the time when nerve regrowth has completed or conduction block has resolved, in order to maximally train all potentially available muscle fibers.

The specific prescription for strengthening exercises depends on the extent of axonal loss or conduction block. In completely denervated muscle (or total conduction block), there are no functioning motor units, so active resistive strengthening will not be feasible. In nearly complete partial axonal lesions, resistive exercises may not lead to clinically significant strength gains, and may even lead to harmful effects if the intensity is too high. Apparently, below a critical level of remaining motor units, there is no benefit to exposing muscle to higher forces; that is, there is no therapeutic window for strengthening exercises (12). In less-severe partial axonal injuries, strengthening exercises are safe and effective within certain guidelines. These guidelines are similar to those discussed for systemic neuromuscular disease.

Progressive Neuromuscular Disease (Hereditary Myopathy as Model)

Studies of therapeutic exercise of dystrophic muscles in humans (myopathies) have shown mixed results (18–21). Overall, the data from animal and human studies suggest that submaximal exercise is not harmful and may be helpful in maintaining maximal mobility if the patient does not exercise to marked fatigue. If properly supervised, active resistance exercise programs do not result in overwork-induced weakness, and the susceptibility to overwork-induced weakness depends on the severity of disease (22). Hassan (23) concluded that exercise consisting of brief periods of low- or high-intensity activity can improve strength for patients with minimal to moderate weakness, but that exercise programs have no effect on the strength of muscles that are already severely weakened. Aerobic and endurance training programs have not been adequately studied in patients with myopathies. Regular daily physical activity should be maintained as long as possible.

CENTRAL NERVOUS SYSTEM FACTORS IN THERAPEUTIC EXERCISE

Upper motor neuron lesions directly injure the central nervous system (CNS) control centers and pathways, resulting in weakness from the decreased numbers of motor units recruited and abnormal synergistic patterns. CNS factors are also important in lower motor neuron lesions, because upper motor neuron centers and pathways are necessary to access the injured peripheral neuromuscular structures.

Motor Control

The CNS role in exercise is complicated. Under usual conditions, CNS pathways are organized not in terms of individual muscle function, but rather in terms of motions or combinations of motions (24). The CNS control centers organize and direct these motions, in turn giving rise to purposeful movements and activities. Motor control is built on interactions between the basic reflexes, the sensory inputs, the cortical motor centers (and associated motor centers), and the subcortical movement centers. Motor control is learned and acquired by repetition and reinforcement and is extinguished by nonuse and reinforcement of other patterns (25). Through learning, complex motor patterns can become "hardwired" into subcortical centers as "engrams," no longer requiring willed cortical signals for each subcomponent of movement. Speed, coordination, direction, precision, and smoothness can continue to improve with practice.

Synergies

In the hierarchically organized brain theory, higher centers have dominance over lower centers. In systems theory, movement is the net result of many different areas (systems) interacting, with each system having a degree of CNS influence that can be enhanced or diminished depending on the task to be accomplished (26). Synergies, or motor patterns, are seen as the basic building block of movement in the systems theory (24), and are defined as a fixed set of muscles contracting with a preset sequence and time of contraction. There are an infinite number of movement combinations possible, allowing a great deal of flexibility in motor control. However, a rapid response time is needed for many movements, such as balance reactions, emphasizing the need for the brain to organize movement into quick response groups.

Many therapists advocate training basic "subtask skills" (e.g., combinations of synergy patterns) that are coordinated together into functional whole tasks (24). An example is to work on half a gait cycle by moving the stance hip from the full backward to the full forward position during opposite leg swing and ending with weight shift to the swing leg (27). As progress advances, the emphasis shifts to whole-task training. The synergies can be further modified and shaped by reversing the direction of the subtask skill and starting and stopping at various points, helping to establish flexibility, which is important during interactions with the ever-changing environment (24).

Neurofacilitative Therapy (Overflow Strengthening)

Neurofacilitative exercise programs have been advocated by Knott and Voss (28), Rood (29), Bobath (30), Brunnestrom (31), and Sullivan (32), among others, as an alternative to traditional exercise in the treatment of upper motor neuron lesions. The most common clinical practice is to incorporate elements of the various methods into treatment (33). The most widely used method is neurodevelopmental treatment, originally developed by Bobath for cerebral palsy (30).

Neurofacilitative treatment is based on the theory that reflex and voluntary motor responses are not discrete entities, and that manipulation of the former can shape and influence the latter (34). The therapist uses a series of facilitation and synergy patterns in an effort to get muscle strengthening, neuromuscular re-education, and overflow from the stronger muscle groups to the weaker muscle groups (32). The weaker muscles are allowed to work with the stronger muscles and not in isolation, leading to so-called overflow strengthening. Other sensory inputs can be used as inhibitory influences to block unwanted spasticity, reflexes, and synergies. By using both facilitating and inhibitory techniques, the therapist shapes the response, ultimately developing a variety of movement and postural responses. The final goal is to reinforce these responses until they become automatic and are incorporated into functional activities.

Controlled studies comparing a specific neurofacilitative treatment with traditional physical therapy have been performed primarily in the pediatric population, and meta-analysis showed no difference in outcome (35). One small randomized study in an adult population demonstrated no advantage of neurodevelopmental treatment, with results actually favoring the conventional-therapy group (36). The cost-effectiveness of neurofacilitative treatment, a very labor-intensive form of therapy, has clearly not been demonstrated.

Dynamic Responses

Advanced motor control involves integrating movements into dynamic responses, the capability to respond to a variety of environmental changes. Clinically, dynamic movements can be practiced with ball activities. Punching, catching, throwing, and kicking activities with weighted balls as well as regular balls will change force and speed requirements, teaching the patient to adapt responses for ever-changing environmental demands. Treadmills also help patients adapt their motion to the environmental changes and make anticipatory responses (24).

Learning

Learning motor control requires that proper technique be reinforced and improper technique be extinguished

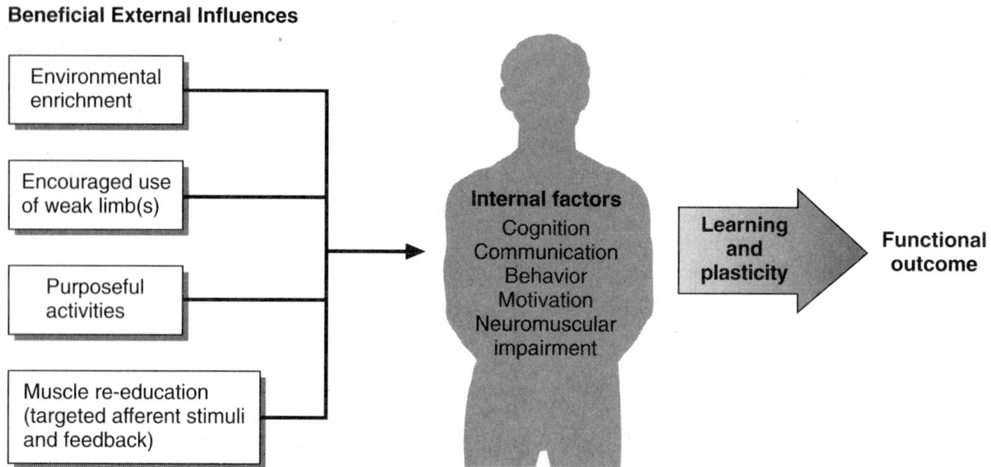

Figure 28-3. Theory of neuromuscular retraining. Application of external influences can improve functional outcome through learning and plasticity. The degree of improvement depends not only on the types of influences, but also on the nature of the preexisting internal factors, including the severity of neuromuscular impairment.

through feedback. The therapist initially supplies most of the feedback, but as higher levels of functioning and movements are attained, this responsibility shifts to the patient, and self-criticism is important. Other key elements in learning are repetition, exposure to environmental conditions, and motivation. Motivation is enhanced using therapeutic interventions that are meaningful to the patient, such as goal-oriented functional activities (2). Figure 28-3 depicts how learning is influenced by a variety of external and internal factors.

Functional Activity Training

Functional activity training directly addresses function and disability. In comprehensive rehabilitation, training activities specific for all affected mobility and daily living activities should be included. Richards (37) provided evidence for the clinical efficacy of functional training in acute stroke patients, demonstrating improved gait velocity using a task-specific physical therapy program compared with conventional physical therapy techniques. Repetitive training of a particular functional activity probably has a broader beneficial effect as well. For instance, repetitive stair-climbing activities performed by patients with a femoral nerve injury not only will best maximize the ability to climb stairs, but also will train the quadriceps and other leg muscles to enhance other lower-extremity functions as well.

To prevent overwork-induced injury, functionally directed exercise should be started judiciously when weakness is present, and activities should be appropriate for the muscle grade. When the muscle grade is 2, activities requiring antigravity movement of that muscle should be avoided, and exercises allowing the patient to work the muscle in gravity-free positions should be developed first.

MUSCLE RE-EDUCATION

Muscle re-education refers to treatments, excluding traditional strengthening and motion exercises, employed to regain lost motor control of body position and movements. Most muscle re-education techniques involve the application of targeted environmental stimuli to generate an afferent signal, with the goal of providing feedback and shaping the efferent motor response. Afferent neural pathways, in addition to efferent pathways and central control centers, play a major role in motor control. In fact, interrupting afferent fibers at the dorsal roots causes paralysis in animal models, even though efferent pathways are intact (38).

In a broad sense, muscle re-education encompasses all therapist-patient treatment interactions (i.e., demonstration of movement, passive movements, active assisted contractions, facilitatory techniques, corrective responses, inhibitory techniques, and translation of motor control into functional activities). Specific muscle re-education techniques include the use of stroking, tapping, touching, and icing or passive trunk and limb positioning for proprioceptive feedback (24). These techniques are often integrated with synergy techniques to comprise the main methods of the neurofacilitative therapy approaches mentioned earlier. Electrical stimulation and electromyographic biofeedback (EMG-BF) are "high-tech" re-education techniques and are discussed later. Table 28-2 lists muscle re-education techniques.

Muscle re-education relies on the theory that structured inputs can trigger quiescent pathways and reorganize the neurologic system in order to shape (facilitate or inhibit) a given motor response. Neural plasticity, the ability of the nervous system to reorganize in response to environmental changes, is present during human development and is presumed to occur after CNS injury (25). It is

Table 28-2: Muscle Re-education Techniques

General	Specific
Demonstration	Stroking
Passive movements	Tapping
Active assisted movements	Touching
Facilitation	Icing
Correction	Synergy positioning
Inhibition	Postural positioning
	Neuromuscular electrical stimulation
	Electromyography biofeedback

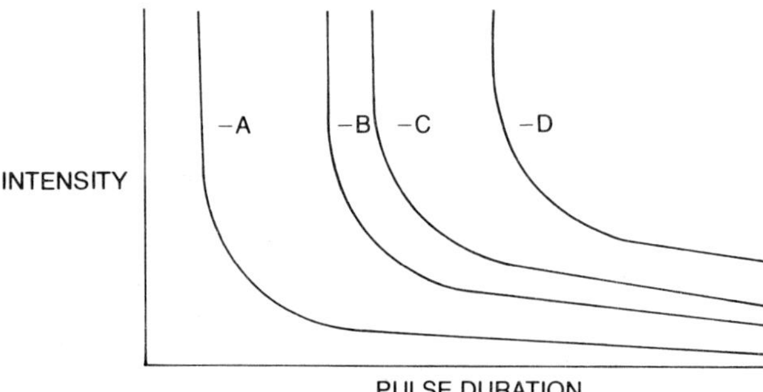

Figure 28-4. Strength duration curve. Plot of time versus intensity of current to excite (A) large-diameter myelinated motor and sensory nerve fibers (A-alpha), (B) small-diameter myelinated sensory nerve fibers (A-delta), (C) small-diameter myelinated nerve fibers (C-fibers), and (D) denervated muscle. (Reproduced by permission from Wolf SL. *Electrotherapy.* New York: Churchill Livingstone, 1981:14.)

well accepted that uninjured brain structures are capable of reorganizing to perform functions previously performed by injured structures. Several animal and human studies documented the influence that manipulation of the environment can have on motor recovery after head injury (39–43). More controversial is the clinical efficacy of specific muscle re-education techniques, which have yet to be validated with controlled studies.

BASICS OF ELECTRICAL STIMULATION

Electrical stimulation has long been advocated for use in various aspects of neuromuscular rehabilitation. The first reported medical treatment dates back to 1744 when Christian Gottlieb Kratzenstein claimed to have restored function to a paralyzed small finger of a female patient by applying electricity for less that one-fourth of an hour (44). The various applications currently available are summarized in Table 28-3.

Theoretically, impaired internal neuromuscular pathways can be circumvented by providing externally generated nerve action potentials distal to the impaired segment. An electrical stimulus applied to the skin can depolarize nearby nerve tissue, generating a propagating action potential that can depolarize muscle or trigger afferent pathways. Muscle contraction can also be elicited by direct electrical stimulation over the motor point of the muscle belly. Since muscle membrane has a much higher excitation threshold than do nerve axons (Fig. 28-4), as long as the muscle is innervated, contraction occurs through terminal motor neuron depolarization rather than direct muscle membrane depolarization (45).

Electrically generated muscle contractions have motor unit firing patterns that differ from the orderly recruitment progression seen during voluntary muscle contraction. Electrical current densities are higher closest to the active electrode, so superficial axons (nearby axons) will be preferentially recruited, regardless of their fiber-type makeup (46). Large neurons are more electrically excitable

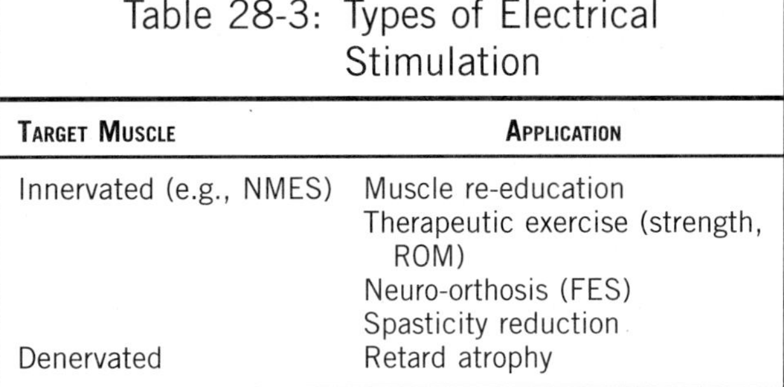

Table 28-3: Types of Electrical Stimulation

Target Muscle	Application
Innervated (e.g., NMES)	Muscle re-education Therapeutic exercise (strength, ROM) Neuro-orthosis (FES) Spasticity reduction
Denervated	Retard atrophy

NMES = neuromuscular electrical stimulation; ROM = range of motion; FES = functional electrical stimulation.

than smaller ones (see Fig. 28-4), so fatigable type II fibers are recruited initially, rather than fatigue-resistant type I fibers as seen with voluntary contraction (45). With increasing stimulation intensity, there is further recruitment of heterogeneous units near the electrode and of low-threshold (large-diameter axon) units that are farther away.

All electrically recruited motor units fire in synchrony (at the frequency of the electrical pulse), resulting in a muscle contractile force that is higher than that of a comparable number of voluntarily firing motor units. Voluntary motor units fire asynchronously (each at their own autonomous rate), which is suboptimal for force generation but is preventative against fatigue. Thus, electrically stimulated muscle is more fatigue sensitive. If electrically overstimulated, the motor units begin to fatigue and tension in the muscle will begin to decrease unless the stimulus intensity is increased to recruit additional motor units (47). Excessive muscle fatigue can be minimized by limiting the frequency at which the stimulus is applied and limiting the duration of the contraction. For repeated contractions, an intermittent "off-time" from electrical stimulation increases the likelihood that subsequent muscle contractions will be sufficiently strong (45).

In theory, a short pulse duration (0.01–0.05 msec) can preferentially activate larger motor neurons in lieu of the small pain-conducting fibers, which have a higher excitation threshold (see Fig. 28-4), thereby minimizing pain perception during muscle contraction (45). However, since axons closest to the electrodes will be exposed to a greater current density, it is difficult to activate enough large axons to cause muscle contraction without also activating some superficial small axons. Clinically the ability to select motor neurons of a given size or type with cutaneously applied electrical stimulation is unpredictable (45).

NEUROMUSCULAR ELECTRICAL STIMULATION

Neuromuscular electrical stimulation (NMES) refers to the application of electrical current in CNS rehabilitation (e.g., for upper motor neuron injuries or innervated muscle). The current is delivered by a stimulator as a train of "pulses" either directly to the paretic muscle(s) or to the associated peripheral nerve(s). The electrical pulses are characterized by their waveform, phase duration, pulse frequency, and amplitude, and can be interrupted by periodic off time. Figure 28-5 demonstrates NMES of the wrist extensors using a bipolar electrode configuration.

Application Parameters

Electrodes

NMES electrodes can be set up in monopolar or bipolar configurations. In the monopolar configuration, an individual muscle contraction is generated with placement of the active electrode (cathode or negative polarity) over a motor point (Fig. 28-6) and a second larger reference electrode (anode or positive pole) distally, often over the tendinous portion of the muscle. A bipolar configuration employs two electrodes of the same size, both over the target muscle, and is more commonly used in NMES. Close spacing of electrodes encourages superficial passage of current, whereas spacing of electrodes farther apart promotes deeper penetration of current (48). With either configuration, the surface electrode should generally be no smaller than a dime to avoid concentration of current, sensory discomfort, and possible burns. Larger electrodes will be effective in generating torque from large muscles or groups of muscles that contract together (48).

Electrodes are of three basic types: surface, percutaneous intramuscular, and implantable radiofrequency controlled. Surface electrodes require stimulations 10 times the intensity used for intramuscular or implanted electrodes because of higher impedance (49). The surface electrode is applied conductively to skin with either electrode gel or semirigid gel-type material, and is held in place with either an elastic strap or adhesive tape.

The advantages of surface electrodes are ease of application and removeability. Disadvantages include poor repeatability because of day to day variation in their placement (50), poor selectivity (47), the need to don and doff electrodes, undesirable sensations, unwanted reflexes, and skin irritation (51). Surface electrodes are indicated when NMES use is anticipated to be temporary (i.e., exercise training, neuromuscular re-education, or feasibility planning for chronic FES use).

For chronic NMES, percutaneous electrodes offer several advantages: improved repeatability, improved selectivity, access to anatomically deep muscles, and low current requirements (51). However, several technical limitations of percutaneous electrodes exist: breakage and movement of electrode leads, irritation and infection of skin exit sites, and frailness of external cables and connectors (52). Implantable NMES devices have recently been developed to address the shortcomings of surface and percutaneous systems (51,53). Implanted electrodes are not widely used

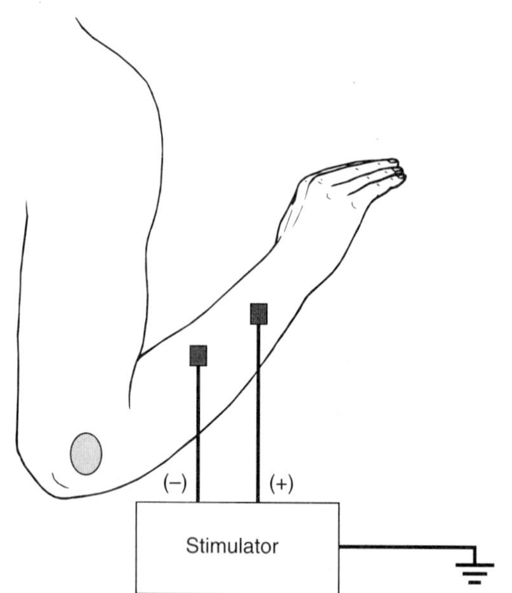

Figure 28-5. Neuromuscular electrical stimulation of wrist extensors using surface electrodes with a bipolar configuration.

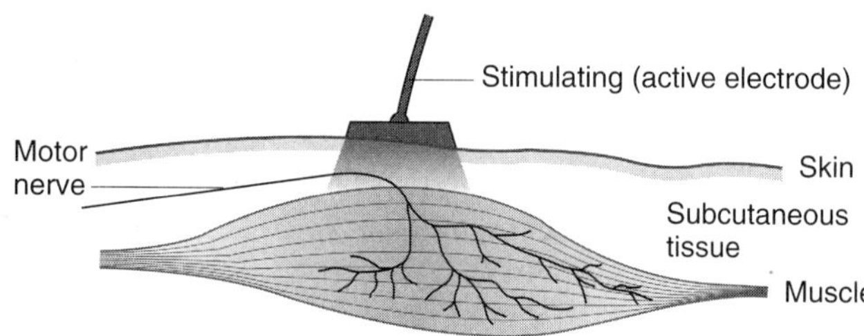

Figure 28-6. Motor point. (Adapted from Low J, Reed A. *Electrotherapy explained.* Oxford: Butterworth–Heinemann, 1994:57.)

clinically, although they have been advocated by many for FES, and their use in the future is anticipated to increase.

Waveforms

NMES units traditionally use either symmetric or asymmetric biphasic square waveform pulses, with current flowing back and forth between the two electrodes. The symmetric waveform dictates current flows equally "hard and fast" in both phases, thus allowing both electrodes to act as active electrodes, and is preferred for stimulation of large muscle groups (49). The asymmetric waveform permits selective activation of smaller muscles by allowing the clinician to identify the anode and cathode, and choose the most effective direction of current flow for depolarization (49). The stimulating phase of the asymmetric waveform acts much as a monophasic current would, with the balancing phase merely reducing the likelihood of untoward polar effects. Tissue irritants can accumulate under one of the electrodes if the asymmetric wave is unbalanced, with an accumulation of charge and associated burning or itching sensations (45). The asymmetric waveform is more comfortable than the symmetric waveform (54,55).

Amplitude

Amplitude and pulse duration determine the intensity of the electrical pulse. The pulse duration is usually set empirically, and the amplitude is adjusted to achieve the desired clinical effect. It is possible to stimulate large-diameter sensory axons at low amplitudes without evoking any muscle contraction. The earliest sensory awareness of the electrical stimulation is referred to as *sensory threshold amplitude.* Likewise, contraction of one or a few axons is known as *contraction threshold.* Stronger contraction is achieved by increasing the amplitude further, resulting in depolarization of more axons, recruitment of more motor units, and increased muscle contractile force. Maximal contractile force is achieved when all axons of a given nerve (or motor point) are depolarized. Increasing the amplitude further to supramaximal intensity can increase pain without adding any clinical benefit.

Phase Duration

The phase duration, like the amplitude, directly determines stimulus intensity and can be adjusted to achieve the desired clinical effect. As stated earlier, a short phase duration may provide some degree of selectivity in depolarizing motor axons in lieu of pain-conduction axons and may also help limit electrically induced fatigue. There is a minimal pulse duration below which the nerve cannot be depolarized regardless of amplitude (0.05–0.10 msec for surface stimulation of innervated muscle). A phase duration of 0.3 msec is widely used clinically for surface electrodes, based on research indicating effective muscle contraction with minimal pain at this duration (56,57).

Frequency (Pulse Rate)

The pulse rate must reach tetanic frequency (usually begins at 20–35 Hz in innervated muscle) in order to achieve a smooth, nontwitching contraction (58). As pulse rate increases, however, the muscle becomes more fatigable. The minimum frequency that achieves tetany is usually the best compromise (59), and clinically frequencies from 20 to 50 Hz are used.

Duty Cycle

Regardless of the frequency chosen, if the pulse train continues without interruption for more than several seconds, neuromuscular fatigue will result. Intermittent off-times from stimulation will allow continued stimulation. The ratio of on-time to off-time is known as the *duty cycle.* A commonly used duty cycle for exercise training is 1 : 3, with 4 to 6 seconds of cyclic on-time followed by 12 to 18 seconds of off-time (58). Packman-Braun's study (60) indicated the best duty cycle to begin with in patients with hemiparesis is 1 : 5. As muscle strength and endurance improve, the ratio of on- to off-times may be decreased, approaching 1 : 1. When NMES is used for functional movements (FES), the sequence of muscular activation will determine the on- and off-times, so duty cycle is not applicable.

Ramp Time

Ramp time allows a gradual increase in pulse intensity to soften the start of a train of pulses, typically over 1.5 to 3.0 seconds. This helps the patient adjust to the stimulus, and to better tolerate high-intensity stimulation as used in exercise training. Ramp time also helps prevent a sudden high-intensity electrical pulse from exacerbating spasticity. When stimulation is used for functional movements, rapid or instantaneous force is needed, so ramp time is not appropriate.

Contraindications

A seizure disorder and the presence of a demand-type cardiac pacemaker are absolute containdications to NMES (58). Placement near the vagus or phrenic nerve, close to an incision, or over a scar is contraindicated, as is placement in the abdominal, perineal, or lumbar region during pregnancy (49). Obesity can impede the stimulation from reaching necessary intensity at the neuromuscular target when surface electrodes are used.

Applications

Muscle Re-education

NMES can be adjusted to a purely sensory level and used in a fashion analogous to facilitation techniques that involve light stroking, tapping, or touch. Current amplitude is adjusted to sensory threshold to evoke the earliest feeling of light touch or tapping but allowing no visible or palpable muscle contraction (49). Using NMES at a higher intensity capable of evoking muscle contraction, several researchers documented improvements in motor control (61–64). Liberson noted that after use of a functional peroneal nerve stimulator for footdrop was discontinued, improvements in dorsiflexion and gait persisted. Gracanin (64) theorized that NMES helps to establish a more-normal pattern of movement that can be integrated by supraspinal mechanisms and that its repetitive nature assists the CNS in adapting this new pattern as the motor engram of choice. And in the case where traditional active strengthening exercises are prohibited by absence of motor control, NMES may be one way to "jump-start" the system.

Several steps are involved in the process of NMES-facilitated muscle re-education and the cooperation of the patient is imperative. The therapist should first carefully demonstrate to the patient the expected movement, and then passively move the patient's limb while the patient observes. After gaining a clear understanding of what movement is expected, the patient is encouraged to actively contract the muscles. NMES is then used to initiate movement, complete the arc of motion, or sustain the contraction. Intensity is adjusted for the desired response, but is always submaximal. Short sessions of 15 minutes or less, preferably several times a day, are recommended (58). The patient should attempt to perform the desired movement or contraction together with the stimulation. The therapist can also add other facilitating techniques. Once the patient achieves voluntary control of target movements, the given muscles can be strengthened either in traditional fashion or through neurofacilitative techniques. Ultimately the progression of muscle education involves translation of the target movements into functional activities.

Therapeutic Exercise

NMES has improved strength and range of motion in several studies (65–69), indicating that it can substitute for traditional therapeutic exercise. Extremely vigorous application is needed for strengthening effects. Baker (58) recommended 4 to 6 hours per day of maximal (or near-maximal) intensity stimulation, which may be broken into several sessions per day, and lasting for at least 4 to 6 weeks. For range of motion programs he recommended 1 to 2 hours daily to gain motion and 30 minutes daily for maintenance, adjusting intensity to generate a moderate contraction through the full range of motion. Typical range of motion settings are a 2-second ramp-on time, 4-second plateau, and 12-second rest period (58). Given the high dosing requirements of NMES for exercise, particularly strengthening, NMES can be justified only when other less-expensive and less-noxious forms of therapeutic exercise are not feasible.

Orthotic Substitution (Functional Electrical Stimulation)

FES is the use of NMES to enhance the function of paralyzed or weak muscles, often eliminating or reducing the need for traditional bracing. Surface, percutaneous, and implanted electrodes have been used. FES, as first demonstrated by Liberson et al (70) in 1961, consisted of a peroneal nerve stimulator whose signal was interrupted by a foot switch during heel contact to treat hemiparetic footdrop (Fig. 28-7). Several other investigators reported on the successful treatment of hemiparetic patients with peroneal stimulators (71–73). According to Merletti et al (74), an appropriate candidate for a peroneal stimulator has a responsible mental state, good learning ability, upper motor neuron weakness, adequate protective sensation in the leg, near-normal passive range of motion of the leg, less than severe spasticity, ability to walk with or without a cane, and toe drag while walking.

Technologic breakthroughs have led to the application of FES for other more complicated upper motor neuron deficits. Multichannel units allow stimulation to be applied to the gluteal and quadriceps muscles to enhance stability during the stance phase of gait in patients with

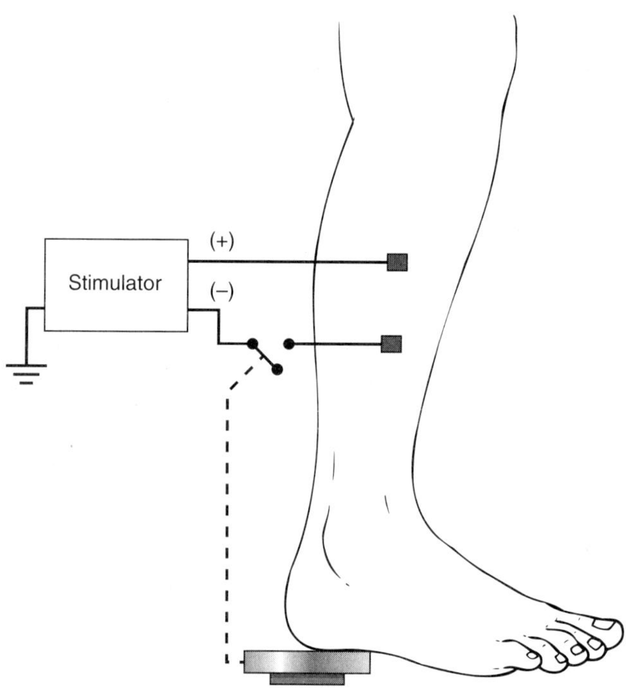

Figure 28-7. Peroneal (tibialis anterior) functional electrical stimulation with heel switch cut-off for correction of footdrop. The tibialis anterior is stimulated using surface electrodes during the swing phase, and stimulation is disrupted during heel contact via a switch. Percutaneous or implantable electrodes can also be substituted for long-term use.

either hemiplegia or quadriplegia. Plantarflexors and hamstring muscles can also be facilitated during the brief push-off and late-swing phases of the gait cycle. Control circuits and modulating circuits allow for timed coordination of multiple separate muscle group contractions and reproduction of a vast array of functional movements including ambulation. Upper-extremity movements, although much more complex than lower-extremity movements, have also been demonstrated with FES (74–76).

The need to have functionally innervated muscle fibers has obfuscated the use of FES for lower motor neuron lesions. FES is likewise contraindicated in myopathic disease and generally avoided in progressive diseases. Other physiologic limitations include obesity, joint contracture, joint instability, and uncontrollable spasticity (46).

Prior to beginning FES, the patient should build up endurance in the target muscles to minimize any preexisting disuse atrophy. This is typically accomplished by an NMES strengthening program. For FES gait training, balance should be sufficient to stand with a gait aid and minimal assistance, and target muscles should be able to consistently generate strong contractions for over 30 minutes.

Spasticity Management

Research has demonstrated beneficial effects of NMES on spasticity reduction (77,78). Muscles that are antagonistic to the spastic muscles are stimulated to counterbalance the spastic position and for reciprocal inhibition. Long ramp-on times, long on-times, and long off-times are recommended (58), and intensity should be just high enough to break the spastic positioning. NMES should only be considered as an adjunct to traditional spasticity treatments.

Efficacy

Stroke Recovery

Despite numerous uncontrolled trials, there is an absence of double-blind, randomized, controlled trials evaluating the efficacy of NMES in patients with hemiplegia from stroke. Glanz et al (79) pooled data from unblinded randomized trails and concluded that NMES improved muscle strength recovery after stroke. Whether this was an effect of maximizing strength of residual motor neurons or a result of re-education of a quiescent pathway was not discussed. Glanz et al did acknowledge that although motor force improved, it does not necessarily follow that functional benefit is derived. Unfortunately, the studies Glanz et al included did not have common functional indices with which to make comparisons.

Footdrop Neuro-orthosis in Hemiparesis

For footdrop due to upper motor neuron injury, FES of the peroneal nerve (or tibialis anterior muscle) is intended to replace the traditional ankle-foot orthosis (AFO) and provide a more physiologic gait pattern (see Fig. 28-7). Waters et al (72) reported that a peroneal stimulator may dramatically stimulate a hip and knee flexion synergy as well as safely dorsiflex the foot. This "multijoint" effect, according to Waters et al (72), can change a patient who is only a laborious room-distance ambulator into an independent household ambulator. Despite the reported benefits, peroneal FES has not been shown in a controlled comparison to achieve gait function superior to that achieved by the less costly and less complex AFO.

Upper Extremity

Using control subjects, investigators studied the efficacy of NMES for wrist extensors and for the recovery of tenodesis grasp in persons with C5 and C6 quadriplegia. Kohlmeyer et al (80) found to benefit with electrical stimulation, used either alone or in combination with EMG-BF. Upper-extremity FES is considered in the research stages only, as current technology is insufficient to reliably reproduce the highly complex upper-extremity functional movements (58).

Paraplegic Ambulation

In 1987 Marsolais and Kobetic (81) first reported on the application of a patterned FES to various leg and hip muscles to produce a walking-like motion in persons with paraplegia. The technology for FES-assisted ambulation in such patients has since advanced. In April 1994 the Food and Drug Administration approved for marketing the first microcomputer-controlled functional neuromuscular stimulation device called the Parastep System. The computer-controlled electrical stimulator is activated by a walker with handgrip-mounted control switches and sends current to surface electrodes placed over leg muscles. Other paraplegic systems use percutaneous wires or implantable electrodes as opposed to surface skin electrodes.

FES for paraplegic ambulation has many drawbacks. Sophisticated multichannel stance-phase stimulators are not highly reliable, and sudden failure and serious injury remain concerns (82). FES-assisted ambulation utilizes extraordinarily high amounts of energy (83), restricting its use primarily for selective exercise training only. Hybrid systems, combining some type of passive mechanical orthosis with a modified FES system, have been developed in an attempt to lower energy costs (84,85). However, the modest reduction in energy consumption and the added disadvantage of a cumbersome mechanical orthosis has precluded the widespread clinical use of hybrid systems, and technologic development remains an active area of research interest (86).

ELECTRICAL STIMULATION OF DENERVATED MUSCLE

After denervation, muscle fibers progressively become atrophic and lose their physiologic integrity. If not reinnervated within 2 years, fibers become completely replaced by connective tissue. Electrical stimulation of denervated muscle attempts to exercise the muscle and maintain fibers in a viable state until reinnervated by collateral axons from surviving motor neurons or by axons regenerating across the lesion site.

The potential benefits of electrical stimulation of denervated muscle were first reported by Reid in 1841 (87). The use of electrical treatment of peripheral nerve injuries grew during World War II with the development of a clinical stimulator capable of exciting both denervated and partially innervated muscles (88). Since the early 1940s numerous investigators have studied the effect of electrical stimulation on denervated muscle in animals and in humans, producing varying results.

Application Parameters for Stimulation of Denervated Muscle

After denervation, the electrical stimulus must directly depolarize the muscle membrane in order to evoke a muscle contraction. Because muscle is significantly less excitable than nerve tissue (see Fig. 28-4), pulse durations much longer than those used for NMES will be required. Pulse durations of 10 msec or longer, also known as *galvanic stimulation*, are needed to stimulate denervated muscle. Many clinically available NMES stimulators are not capable of generating pulses of this duration (76). Once an appropriate pulse duration is established, amplitude is adjusted to elicit a maximal contraction. Maximal contractions are necessary to prevent atrophy in denervated muscle (89), although stimulation intensity of this magnitude is often poorly tolerated by patients because of pain (12).

The frequency used to stimulate denervated muscle can be lower than that used in NMES, because tetany occurs at lower frequencies in denervated muscle. Several investigators showed a benefit of stimulation at 25 cycles per second (90,91). A monopolar electrode configuration is usually used with the active reference placed over the motor point of the denervated muscle and the reference electrode placed over a distant body part. A small (1–2 cm^2) active electrode is used for specificity and generating a larger current density. A larger electrode is used for the reference to minimize current flow there. Alternatively, a bipolar configuration can be used (92).

Efficacy of Electrical Stimulation of Denervated Muscle

The efficacy of electrical stimulation of denervated muscle is controversial. The Gutmans' classic study (93) showed that electrical stimulation was effective in retarding atrophy in denervated muscle of rabbits. Other animal studies confirmed this, but showed there were no beneficial effects beyond retarding atrophy (89,94,95). Still others found no benefit at all in animal models (96), and even found that electrical stimulation may actually hinder terminal sprouting of motor axons (97–99). Comparison of the many studies is difficult because the effectiveness seems to depend on many factors including the type of current, duration of stimulus, current amplitude, number of stimuli per second, type of contraction, length and frequency of treatment sessions, time between treatment sessions, and telapsed time between denervation and initiation of stimulation.

In humans, although few controlled studies have been done, electrical stimulation appears to retard atrophy but does not enhance regeneration (100). To effectively retard atrophy, stimulation must be of sufficient current intensity, pulse duration, and frequency to achieve tetanic contraction for several seconds and should be repeated several times daily (12). A linear relationship between the number of treatment periods and maintenance of mass has been described (90). Treatment should begin as soon as possible after the injury and should continue to 4 to 6 weeks beyond the projected time for reinnervation to occur. Thus, the treatment schedule and intensity requirements make electrical stimulation of denervated muscle largely impractical.

ELECTROMYOGRAPHIC BIOFEEDBACK

EMG-BF for neuromuscular re-education was first reported in 1960 (101). The premise, as with other re-education techniques, is that undamaged, yet subliminal pathways can be recruited and assume the function of pathways that have been irreversibly damaged (102). The technique allows subjects to gain conscious control over a voluntary but latent neurofunction by alerting them, with an auditory or visual clue, that their efforts have activated a targeted neuromuscular pathway (Fig. 28-8).

Application

EMG-BF amplifies the electrical signals generated by muscle contraction and visually displays them on a monitor. An integrated electromyographic value can also be used and connected to various forms of audio signals preset at certain thresholds. Using these feedback signals, the patient is trained to either reduce or enhance selected muscle activity. Enhancement of activity is usually the goal when training a muscle for motor control, but reduction of muscle contraction is also important in spastic antagonist muscles.

Clinical applications are broad and varied, but realistic appraisal of recovery potential is mandatory. EMG-BF is not useful when no motor restoration is expected, such as with the leg muscles of a patient with complete injury of the cervical spiral cord. The patient must also have sufficient vision to see the visual display, audition and reception to hear and comprehend simple directions, and

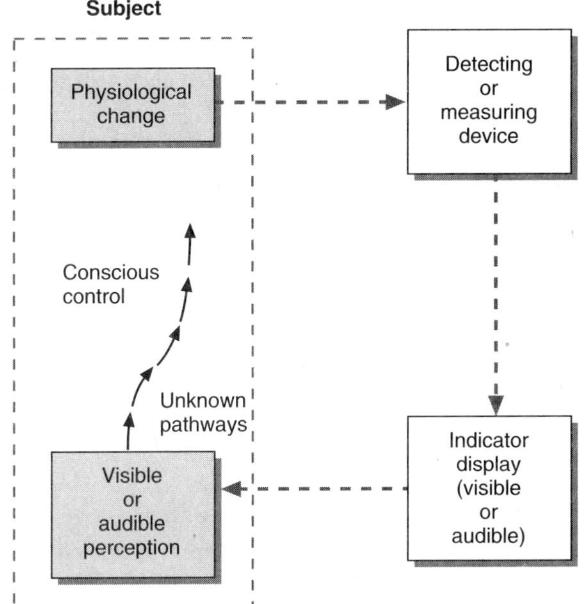

Figure 28-8. Biofeedback theory. (Adapted from Low J, Reed A. *Electrotherapy explained.* Oxford: Butterworth–Heinemann, 1994:135.)

expressive abilities and motor planning skills to respond to basic instructions (103).

Before EMG-BF is started, functional goals must be determined and factors affecting the goals examined (i.e., spasticity, synergies, weakness, or joint limitations). The functional goals is then divided into subtasks, with each subtask analyzed in terms of muscle activity changes needed. Electrodes are applied to the muscles to give the patient feedback on whether they are turned on or off, and hopefully to teach the patient to modify the motor response. EMG-BF should be incorporated into functional activities as soon as possible.

The number of EMG-BF sessions required to produce observable changes varies greatly and frequency is determined subjectively. The primary factors affecting frequency and length of treatment sessions are the ability of the patient to assimilate the learned motor skills and the patient's distractibility and mental and physical fatigue (103). Selected patients may even be able to progress to use of home units for independent treatment.

Efficacy

Hemiparesis

Numerous studies have been conducted on the efficacy of EMG-BF in stroke rehabilitation, with much controversy still existing. Even the better randomized studies (104–106) are flawed by small sample sizes, failure to account for spontaneous recovery, inadequate controls, and lack of functional outcome measures. The meta-analysis by Schleenbaker and Mainous (107) of selected studies indicated a significant improvement in functional outcome with EMG-BF of both the upper and lower extremity. The majority of the included studies were conducted more than 3 months after stroke occurred, at a time when the majority of spontaneous neurologic recovery can be assumed to have occurred (108). This meta-analysis has been criticized on several grounds, particularly the inclusion of studies with matched (nonrandomized) control subjects (102).

Attempting to correct for the methodologic shortcomings in Schleenbaker and Mainous's study, Glanz et al (102) performed a meta-analysis including only randomized controlled trails, and found no significant improvement in range of motion of paretic joints. The range of motion end point was chosen because the investigators believed it represented a valid physiologic measurement of a basic fundamental of neuromuscular function and was frequently measured by other investigators. In conclusion, until larger studies of high quality and randomized design are forthcoming, the efficacy of EMG-BF for hemiparesis after stroke will be debated, as will the optimal timing and cost-effectiveness of this very resource-intensive form of treatment.

Spinal Cord Injury

EMG-BF has also been investigated in patients with spinal cord injury to assist with motor recovery near the zone of injury. In a trial of C6 spinal cord injury subjects, Brucker and Bulaeva (109) reported significant increases in electromyographic activity in the triceps muscles. However, no evidence of increased strength or functional gains was reported and no control subjects were used. In the study with control subjects by Kohlmeyer et al (80), where both NMES and EMG-BF were used on wrist extensors, no benefit was found with EMG-BF. Clearly, further randomized trials are needed to substantiate any potential functional benefits of EMG-BF for spinal cord injury.

REFERENCES

1. Kottke FJ, Pauley DL, Ptak RA. The rationale for prolonged stretching for the correction of shortening of connective tissue. *Arch Phys Med Rehabil* 1966;47:345–352.

2. Darling RC. Exercise. In: Downing JA, Darling RC, eds. *Physiological basis of rehabilitation medicine.* Philadelphia: WB Saunders, 1971:167–184.

3. DeLateur BJ. Strength and local muscle endurance. *Phys Med Rehabil Clin N Am* 1994;5:269–294.

4. McDonagh MJN, Hayward CM, Davies CTM. Isometric training in human elbow flexors. *J Bone Joint Surg [Br]* 1983;65:355–358.

5. Milner-Brown HS, Stein RB, Lee RG. Synchronization of human

motor units: possible roles of exercise and supraspinal reflexes. *Electroencephalogr Clin Neurophysiol* 1975;38:245–254.

6. Moritani T, DeVries HA. Neural factors versus hypertrophy in the time course of muscle strength gain. *Am J Phys Med* 1979;58: 115–130.

7. DeLorme TL. Restoration of muscle power by heavy-resistance exercises. *J Bone Joint Surg* 1945;27:645–666.

8. Ebbeling CB, Clarkson PM. Exercise-induced muscle damage and adaptation. *Sports Med* 1989;7:207–234.

9. Karpovich PC, Cohan PH, Ikai M. Study of endurance of various muscle groups. *Res Q Am Assoc Health Phys Educ* 1964;35 (suppl):393–397.

10. DeLateur BJ, Lehman JF, Fordyce WE. A test of the DeLorme axiom. *Arch Phys Med Rehabil* 1968;49:245–248.

11. DeLateur BJ. Flexibility. *Phys Med Rehabil Clin N Am* 1994;5:295-307.

12. Herbison GJ, Jaweed M, Ditunno JF. Exercise therapy in peripheral neuropathies. *Arch Phys Med Rehabil* 1983;64:201–204.

13. Ernstoff B, Wetterqvist H, Kvist H, Grimby G. Endurance training effect on individuals with postpoliomyelitis. *Arch Phys Med Rehabil* 1996;77:843–848.

14. Bennett RL, Knowlton GC. Overwork weakness in partially denervated skeletal muscle. *Clin Orthop* 1958;12:22.

15. Herbison GJ, Jaweed MM, Ditunno JF, Scott CM. Effect of overwork during reinnervation of rat muscle. *Exp Neurol* 1973;41: 1–14.

16. Hallum A. Neuromuscular diseases. In: Umphred DA, ed. *Neurological rehabilitation.* 3rd ed. St. Louis: Mosby, 1995:375–420.

17. Dickenson AL, Jackson CGR, Layne DL, Ringel Sp. The effect of different sequences of high and low intensity resistance exercises on muscular performance and cellular change. *Med Sci Sports Exerc* 1983;15:154–155.

18. Vignos PJ, Watkins MP. The effect of exercise in muscular dystrophy. *JAMA* 1966;197:843–848.

19. Fowler WM, Gardner GW, Kazerunian HH, Lauvstad WA. The effect of exercise on serum enzymes. *Arch Phys Med Rehabil* 1968;49:554–565.

20. Johnson EW, Braddom R. Overwork weakness in facioscapulohumeral muscular dystrophy. *Arch Phys Med Rehabil* 1971;52:333–336.

21. DeLateur BJ, Gianconi RM. Effect on maximal strength of submaximal exercise in Duchenne muscular dystrophy. *Am J Phys Med* 1979;58:26–36.

22. Vignos PJ. Physical models of rehabilitation in neuromuscular disease. *Muscle Nerve* 1983;6: 323–338.

23. Hasson SM. Progressive and degenerative neuromuscular disease and severe muscular atrophy. In: Hasson SM, ed. *Clinical exercise physiology.* St. Louis: Mosby, 1994:178–198.

24. Winkler PA. Head injury. In: Umphred DA, ed. *Neurological rehabilitation.* 3rd ed. St. Louis: Mosby, 1995.

25. Kottke FJ. The neurophysiology of motor function. In: Kottke FJ, Lehmann JF. *Krusen's handbook of physical medicine and rehabilitation.* 4th ed. Philadelphia: WB Saunders, 1990:234–269.

26. Bernstein N. *Coordination and regulation of movements.* New York: Pergamon Press, 1967.

27. Winstein CJ, Gardner ER, McNeal DR, et al. Standing balance training: effect on balance and locomotion in hemiparetic adults. *Arch Phys Med Rehabil* 1989;70:755–762.

28. Knott M, Voss D. *Proprioceptive neuromuscular facilitation.* Philadelphia: Harper & Row, 1968.

29. Rood MS. Neurophysiological mechanisms utilized in the treatment of neuromuscular dysfunction. *Am J Occup Ther* 1956;10: 220–224.

30. Bobath B. *Adult hemiplegia: evaluation and treatment.* 2nd ed. London: Heinman Medical Books, 1978.

31. Brunnestrom S. *Movement therapy in hemiplegia.* New York: Harper & Row, 1970.

32. Sullivan P. *An integrated approach to therapeutic exercise.* Reston: Reston Publishing, 1982.

33. Lorish TR, Sandish KJ, Rothe EJ, Noll SF. Stroke rehabilitation: rehabilitation evaluation and management. *Arch Phys Med Rehabil* 1994;75S:S47–S51.

34. Badke MB, DiFabio RP. Facilitation: new theoretical perspective and clinical approach. In: Basmajian JV, Wolf SL, eds. *Therapeutic exercise.* Baltimore: Williams & Wilkins, 1990:77–92.

35. Palisano RJ. Research on the effectiveness of neurodevelopmental treatment. *Pediatr Phys Ther* 1991;3:143–147.

36. Brunham S, Snow CJ. The effectiveness of neurodevelopmental treatment in adults with neurological conditions: a single subject study. *Physiother Theory Pract* 1992;8:215–222.

37. Richards CL, Malouin F, Wood-Dauphinee S, et al. Task-specific physical therapy for optimization of gait recovery in acute stroke patients. *Arch Phys Med Rehabil* 1993;74:612–620.

38. Bachy-Rita P. Sensory substitution: the basis for a new therapy. In: Bachy-Rita P. *New directions in rehabilitation medicine: retraining neuromuscular function with EMG sensory feedback therapy.* Miami: Cordis Corp., 1981:10.

39. Wolf SL, Lecraw DE, Barton LA, Jann BB. Forced use of hemiplegic upper extremities to reverse the effect of learned nonuse among stroke and head-injured patients. *Exp Neurol* 1989;104:125–132.

40. Taub E, Millwe NE, Novack TA, et al. Technique to improve chronic motor deficit after stroke. *Arch Phys Med Rehabil* 1993; 74:347–354.

41. Tower SS. Pyramidal lesion in the monkey. *Brain* 1940;63:36–90.

42. Black P, Markowitz RS, Cionci SN. Recovery of motor function after lesions in the motor cortex of monkey. In: Porter R, Fitzsimmons DW, eds. *Outcome of severe damage to the central nervous system.* Ciba Foundation Symposium 34. New York: Elsevier, 1975:65–83.

43. Mitchell DE, Cynader M, Movshon JA. Recovery from the effects of monocular deprivation in kittens. *J Comp Neurol* 1977;176:53–63.

44. Licht S. History of electrotherapy. In: Stillwell GR, ed. *Therapeutic electricity and ultraviolet radiation.* Baltimore: Williams & Wilkins, 1983:6.

45. Kukulka CG. Principles of neuromuscular excitation. In: Gersh MR, ed. *Electrotherapy in rehabilitation.* Philadelphia: FA Davis, 1992:3–25.

46. Basford JR. Electrical therapy. In: Kottke FJ, Lehmann JF, eds. *Krusen's handbook of physical medicine and rehabilitation.* 4th ed. Philadelphia: WB Saunders, 1990.

47. Benton LA, et al. *Functional electrical stimulation: a practical clinical guide.* Downy, CA: Rancho Los Amigos Engineering Center, 1981.

48. DeVahl J. Neuromuscular electrical stimulation in rehabilitation. In: Gersh MR, ed. *Electrotherapy in rehabilitation.* Philadelphia: FA Davis, 1992:218–268.

49. Patterson RR. Instrumentation for electrotherapy. In: Stillwell GK, ed. *Therapeutic electricity and ultraviolet radiation.* 3rd ed. Baltimore: Williams & Wilkins, 1983:65–108.

50. Gardner ER, Triolo RJ, Betz RR. Repeatability of isometric strength and endurance of the electrically stimulated quadriceps in children with spinal cord injuries. *Phys Ther* 1989;69: 369. Abstract.

51. Triolo RJ, Biere C, Uhlir J, et al. Implanted functional neuromuscular stimulation systems for individuals with cervical spinal cord injuries: clinical case reports. *Arch Phys Med Rehabil* 1996;77:1119–1128.

52. Smith BT, Betz RR, Mulcahey MJ, Triolo RJ. Reliability of percutaneous intramuscular electrodes for upper extremity functional neuromuscular stimulation in adolescents with tetraplegia. *Arch Phys Med Rehabil* 1994;75:939–945.

53. Smith B, Peckham PH, Roscoe DD, et al. An externally powered, multichannel implantable stimulator for versatile control of parelyzed muscle. *IEEE Trans Biomed Eng* 1987;34:499–508.

54. Baker LL, Bowman BR, McNeal DR. Effects of waveform on comfort during neuromuscular electrical stimulation. *Clin Orthop* 1988;233:75–85.

55. McNeal DR, Baker LL. Effects of joint angle, electrodes and waveform on electrical stimulation of the quadriceps and hamstrings. *Ann Biomed Eng* 1988;16:299–310.

56. Bowman BR, Baker LL. Effects of waveform parameters on comfort during transcutaneous neuromuscular electrical stimulation. *Ann Biomed Eng* 1985;13:59–74.

57. Gracanin F, Trnkoczy A. Optimal stimulus parameters for minimum pain in the chronic stimulation of innervated muscle. *Arch Phys Med Rehabil* 1975;56:243–249.

58. Baker LL. Neuromuscular electrical stimulation in the restoration of purposeful limb movements. In: Wolf SL, ed. *Electrotherapy.* New York: Churchill Livingstone, 1981:25–48.

59. Jones DA, Bigland-Ritchie B, Edwards RHT. Excitation frequency and muscle fatigue, mechanical responses during voluntary and stimulated contraction. *Exp Neurol* 1979;64:401–413.

60. Packman-Braun R. Relationship between functional electrical stimulation duty cycle and fatigue in wrist extensor muscles of patients with hemiparesis. *Phys Ther* 1988;68:51–56.

61. Baker LL, Parker K. Neuromuscular electrical stimulation of the muscles surrounding the shoulder. *Phys Ther* 1986;6:1930–1937.

62. Baker LL, Yeh C, Wilson D, Waters RL. Electrical stimulation of wrist and fingers for hemiplegic patients. *Phys Ther* 1979;59:1495–1499.

63. Carnstam B, Larsson LE, Prevec TS. Improvement of gait following functional electrical stimulation. *Scand J Rehabil Med* 1977;9:7–13.

64. Gracanin F. Functional electrical stimulation in control of motor output and movements. In: Cobb WA, VanDuijn H, eds. *Contemporary clinical neurophysiology (EEG suppl).* Amsterdam: Elsevier, 1978:355.

65. Bowman BR, Baker LL, Waters RL. Positional feedback and electrical stimulation: an automated approach for the hemiplegic wrist. *Arch Phys Med Rehabil* 1979;60:497–502.

66. Merletti R, Zelaschi F, Latella D, et al. A controlled study of muscle force recovery in hemiparetic patients during treatment with functional electrical stimulation. *Scand J Rehabil Med* 1978;10:147–154.

67. Winchester P, Montgomery J, Bowman B, Hislop H. Effects of feedback stimulation training and cyclical electrical stimulation on knee extension in hemiparetic patients. *Phys Ther* 1983;63: 1096–1103.

68. Levin M. Relief of hemiparetic by TENS is associated with improvement in voluntary and motor functions. *Electroencephalogr Clin Neurophysiol* 1992;85:31–42.

69. Waters RC, McNeal DR, Tasto J. Peroneal nerve conduction velocity after chronic electrical stimulation. *Arch Phys Med Rehabil* 1975;56:240–243.

70. Liberson WT, Holmquest HJ, Scott D, Dow ML. Functional electrotherapy: stimulation of the peroneal nerve synchronized with the swing phase of the gait of hemiplegic patients. *Arch Phys Med Rehabil* 1961;42:101–105.

71. Merletti R, Andina A, Galonte M, Furlan I. Clinical experience of electronic peroneal stimulators in 50 hemiparetic patients. *Scand J Rehabil Med* 1979;11:111–121.

72. Waters RL, McNeal DR, Perry J. Experimental correction of foot drop by electrical stimulation of the peroneal nerve. *J Bone Joint Surg [AM]* 1975;57:1047–1054.

73. Hambret FT. Neural prostheses. *Annu Rev Biophys Bioeng* 1979;8:239–267.

74. Merletti R, Acimovic R, Grobolnik S, Cvilak G. Electrophysiological orthosis for the upper extremity in hemiplegia; feasibility study. *Arch Phys Med Rehabil* 1975;56:507–513.

75. Long C, Masciarelli VD. An electrophysiologic splint for the hand. *Arch Phys Med Rehabil* 1963;44:499–503.

76. Rebersek S, Vodovnik L. Proportionally controlled functional electrical stimulation of the hand. *Arch Phys Med Rehabil* 1973;54:378–382.

77. Lee WJ, McGovern JP, Duvall NE. Continuous tetanizing (low voltage) currents for relief of spasm: a clinical study of twenty-seven spinal cord injured patients: *Arch Phys Med Rehabil* 1956;31:766.

78. Mooney V, Wilemon WK, McNeal DR. Stimulator reduces spastic activity. *JAMA* 1969;207:2199–2200.

79. Glanz M, Klawansky S, Stason W, et al. Functional electrostimulation in poststroke rehabilitation: a meta-analysis of the randomized controlled trials. *Arch Phys Med Rehabil* 1996;77:549–553.

80. Kohlmeyer KM, Hill JP, Yarkony GM, Jaeger RJ. Electrical stimulation and biofeedback effect on recovery of tenodesis grasp: a controlled study. *Arch Phys Med Rehabil* 1996;77:702–706.

81. Marsolais EB, Kobetic R. Functional electrical stimulation for walking in paraplegia. *J Bone Joint Surg [Am]* 1987;69:728–733.

82. Jacobs SR, Jaweed MM, Herbison GT, Stillwell GK. Electrical stimulation of muscle. In: Stillwell GK, ed. *Therapeutic electricity and ultraviolet radiation.* 3rd ed. Baltimore: Williams & Wilkins, 1983:124–173.

83. Marsolias EB, Edwards BG. Energy costs of walking and standing with functional neuromuscular stimulation and long leg braces. *Arch Phys Med Rehabil* 1988;69:243–249.

84. Solomonow M, Baratta R, Hirokawa S, et al. The RGO generation II: muscle stimulation powered orthosis as a practical walking system for thoracic paraplegics. *Orthopedics* 1989;12: 1309–1315.

85. Hirokawa S, Grimm M, Le T, et al. Energy consumption in paraplegic ambulation using the reciprocating gait orthosis and electrical stimulation of the thigh muscles. *Arch Phys Med Rehabil* 1990;71:687–694.

86. Kagaya H, Shimada Y, Sato K, et al. An electrical knee lock system for functional electrical stimulation. *Arch Phys Med Rehabil* 1996;77:870–873.

87. Reid J. On the relation between muscular contractibility and the nervous system. *Lond Edinb Mon J Med Sci* 1841;1:320.

88. Shriber WJ. *A manual of electrotherapy.* Philadelphia: Lea & Febiger, 1975:144, 178.

89. Wehrmacher WH, Thompson JD, Hines HM. Effect of electrical stimulation on denervated skeletal muscle. *Arch Phys Med Rehabil* 1945;26:261.

90. Solandt DV, DeLury DB, Hunter J. Effect of electrical stimulation on atrophy of denervated skeletal muscle. *Arch Neurol Psychiatry* 1943;49:802–807.

91. Kosman AJ, Osborne SL, Ivy AC. Importance of current form and frequency in electrical stimulation of muscles. *Arch Phys Med* 1948;29:559–562.

92. Cummings JP. Electrical stimulation of denervated muscle. In: Gersh MR, ed. *Electrotherapy in rehabilitation.* Philadelphia: FA Davis, 1992;269–290.

93. Gutman E, Gutman L. Effect of electrotherapy on denervated muscles in rabbits. *Lancet* 1942;1:169–170.

94. Kosman AJ. Osborne SL, Ivy AC. The effect of electrical stimulation upon the course of atrophy and recovery of the gastrocnemius muscle of the rat. *Am J Phys* 1946;145:447–451.

95. Kosman AJ, Osborne SL, Ivy AC. The influence of duration and frequency of treatment in electrical stimulation of paralyzed muscle. *Arch Phys Med* 1947;28:12–17.

96. Pollock LJ, Arieff AJ, Sherman IC, et al. Electrotherapy in experimentally induced lesions of peripheral nerves. *Arch Phys Med Rehabil* 1951;32:377–387.

97. Brown MC, Holland RL. A central role for denervated tissues in causing nerve sprouting. *Nature* 1979;282:724–726.

98. Brown MC. Sprouting of motor nerves in adult muscles: a recapitulation of ontogeny. *Trends Neurosci* 1984;7:10–14.

99. Sanes JR, Covault J. Axon guidance during reinnervation of skeletal muscle. *Trends Neurosci* 1985;8:523.

100. Herbison GJ, Graziani V. Anatomy and physiology of nerve and muscle. *Arch Phys Med Rehabil* 1995;76S:S3–S9.

101. Marcinacci A, Horande M. Electromyogram in neuromuscular reeducation. *Bull L A Neurol Soc* 1960;25:57–71.

102. Glanz M, Klawansky S, Stason W, et al. Biofeedback therapy in poststroke rehabilitation: a meta-analysis of the randomized controlled trials. *Arch Phys Med Rehabil* 1995;76:508–515.

103. LeCraw DE, Wolf SL. Electromyographic biofeedback for neuromuscular relaxation and re-education. In: Gersh MR, ed. *Electrotherapy in rehabilitation.* Philadelphia: FA Davis, 1992:291–327.

104. Basmajian JV, Kukulka C, Narayan M, Takeve K. Biofeedback treatment of footdrop after stroke compared with standard rehabilitation technique: effects in voluntary control and strength. *Arch Phys Med Rehabil* 1975; 56:231–239.

105. Hurd WW, Pegram V, Nepomuceno C. Comparison of actual and simulated EMG feedback in the treatment of hemiplegic patients. *Am J Phys Med* 1980; 59:73–82.

106. Cozean CD, Pease WS, Hubbell SL. Biofeedback and functional electrical stimulation in stroke rehabilitation. *Arch Phys Med Rehabil* 1988;69:401–405.

107. Schleenbaker RE, Mainous AG. Electromyographic biofeedback for neuromuscular reeducation in the hemiplegic stroke patient: a meta-analysis. *Arch Phys Med Rehabil* 1993;74:1301–1304.

108. Kelly-Hayes M, Wolf PA, Kase CS, et al. Time course of functional recovery after stroke: the Framingham study. *J Neurorehabil* 1989;3:65–70.

109. Brucker BS, Bulaeva NV. Biofeedback effect on electromyography responses in patients with spinal cord injury. *Arch Phys Med Rehabil* 1996; 77:133–137.

Chapter 29

Upper-Limb Orthoses

Tom Lunsford

Upper-limb orthoses are distinct from other orthoses because of their complexity. There are many simultaneous joint motions to be considered for mobilization or immobilization [i.e., nine interphalangeal (IP), five metacarpal-phalangeal (MCP), wrist, forearm, elbow, and three shoulder joints], very short levers (this translates to high forces, high pressures, and skin intolerance), and very little soft-tissue padding for bands and other components. Orthotic design for the upper limb must give equal focus to mechanical efficiency and precision of fit, since comfort is critical for acceptance. Therefore, the small segments, limitations in soft-tissue padding, and multiplicity of joint motion create high demands, which only a skilled orthotist with both a keen problem-solving sense and finely tuned fabrication skills can meet (1).

Upper-limb orthoses are more likely to be accepted by patients if there is a well-defined therapeutic purpose or if the orthosis provides function that cannot be accomplished by any other means (e.g., substitution). Since the best upper-limb orthosis lacks the mechanical versatility to grasp objects that vary widely in size, shape, and weight with equal ease, upper-limb orthotic design tends to be optimized for a specific purpose. Combine this mechanical shortcoming with impaired sensation, reduced skin friction, and poor subcutaneous contouring and one can see that patients have to produce greater prehension force than that required by the normal hand for routine activities. Add to this the inescapable fact that an upper-limb orthosis is conspicuous and advertises the disability. In spite of these limitations, upper-limb orthoses offer appealing advantages to a limb left impaired by paralysis, deformity, or pain.

To the uninitiated, upper-limb orthotics seems widely diversified and hopelessly unorganized. This is probably the result of the enormous versatility of the upper limb. With lower-limb orthotic management the goals are generally directed to alleviating deviations while walking or running. The task of walking or running is defined by specific repeatable phases, but no such organized definition is available to describe upper-limb function. The upper limb is involved with so many activities that identifying a specific goal or function is difficult. Occupational therapists talk of "activities of daily living," which provides an abbreviated list of functional goals. Add treatment objectives to the functional goals and a lucid organization seems impossible.

Upper-limb orthoses can be organized categorically by pathology (e.g., spinal injury, arthritis, trauma, brain injury) or arthrosegmentally according to the joint encompassed (e.g., shoulder, elbow, wrist, hand, fingers) or by treatment objective (e.g., promote healing, direct growth, prevent deformity, correct deformity, enhance function). Other possible categories are "static" and "dynamic." Under each of these categories, it is convenient to further group upper-limb orthoses as either "therapeutic" or "functional." For example, a *static therapeutic upper-limb orthosis* would be a short opponens (static hand) orthosis. The purpose of this orthosis is to preserve the architecture of the hand (i.e., palmar arch and thumb in opposition).

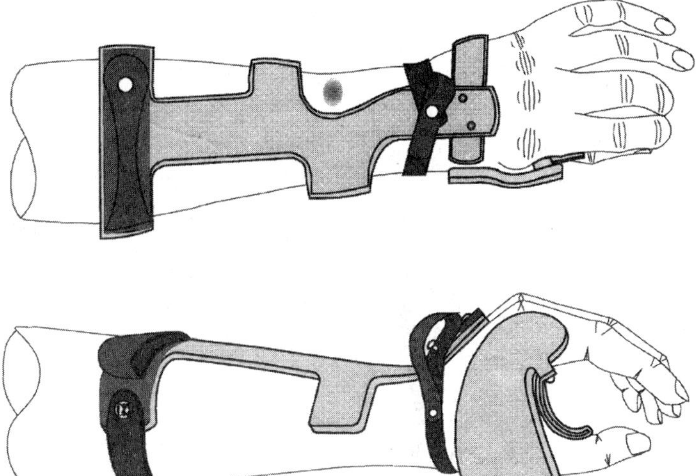

Figure 29-1. Static wrist-hand orthosis.

However, this same orthosis becomes a *static functional upper-limb orthosis* when attachments for eating, reading, page turning, shaving, grooming, and so on, are added.

A separate category includes the temporary upper-limb orthoses made from low-temperature thermoplastics. This group of upper-limb orthoses can be fit immediately after surgery or trauma. The orthoses are designed using paper patterns, the material used is a relatively low-temperature thermoplastic that is heated in hot water, and the orthosis is formed directly on the patient's limb.

STATIC-THERAPEUTIC

The orthoses chosen to represent this category are the static wrist-hand orthosis, static hand orthosis, elbow orthosis, shoulder-elbow orthosis, and shoulder-elbow-wrist orthosis. Several specific therapeutic attachments to these are described. Although there are many other static orthoses used occasionally for therapeutic purposes, space limitations do not permit a listing and description of all custom-designed and fabricated orthoses.

Static Wrist-Hand Orthosis

Clinical Application

The static wrist-hand orthosis (Fig. 29-1) supports the wrist joint, maintains the functional architecture of the hand, and prevents wrist-hand deformities. Occasionally the static wrist-hand orthosis is used as a platform for other therapeutic attachments (e.g., MCP extension stop, IP extension assist, thumb extension assist).

Patient Population

Patients with severe weakness or paralysis of the wrist and hand musculature are appropriate candidates for the static wrist-hand orthosis. Without proper support, these patients are at risk of developing the "claw hand" deformity and overstretching weak muscles (Fig. 29-2). For example, tetraplegics (also known as *quadriplegics**) exhibit the above weakness and can benefit from a static wrist-hand orthosis to preserve the functional posture of their hand and wrist (see Figs. 29-1 and 29-2). This is important if they become a candidate for a functional wrist-hand orthosis, to preclude encumbering contracture or deformities. It also is important to prevent overstretching of the weakened musculature so that maximum functional potential is preserved. In the case of spinal cord injury, the static wrist-hand orthosis is indicated as a positional orthosis for persons with tetraplegia resulting from injury to spinal cord segments C1 through C5 with zero wrist extensors and an "intrinsic minus" hand.

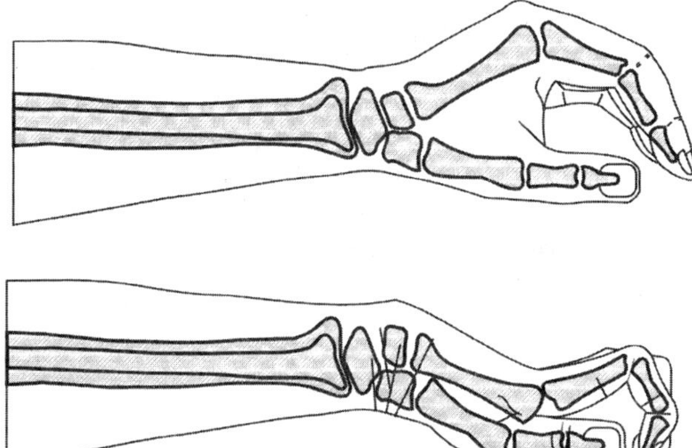

Figure 29-2. Claw hand deformity (wrist flexed, metacarpal-phalangeal joints hyperextended, and thumb extended and abducted).

*In 1993 the American Spinal Injury Association suggested use of the prefix *tetra* over *quadri* since *tetra* is Greek and *quadri* is Latin. This prefix change was consistent with the Greek prefix *para* as used in *paraplegia*.

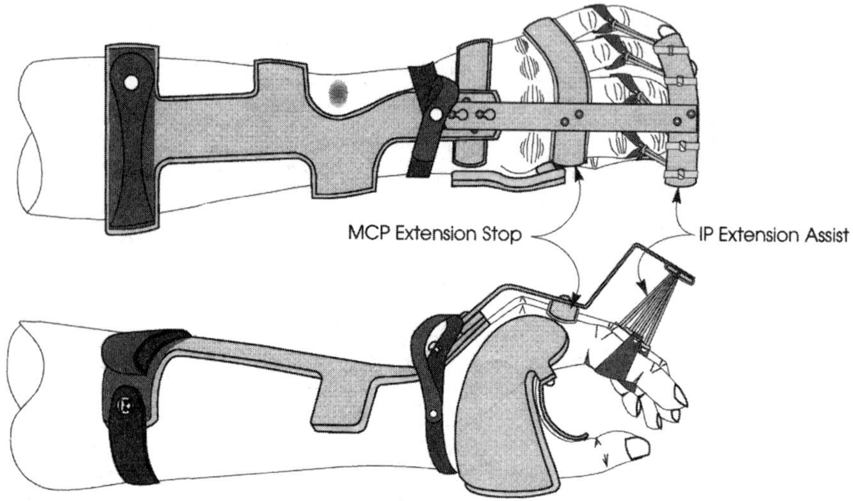

Figure 29-3. Static wrist-hand orthosis with metacarpal-phalangeal (MCP) extension stop and interphalangeal (IP) extension assist.

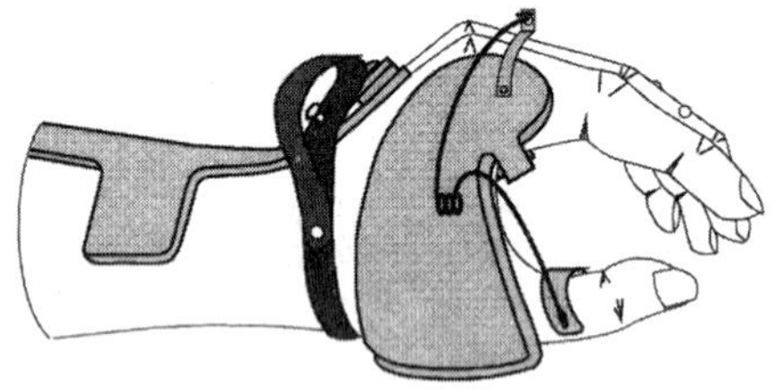
Figure 29-4. Swivel thumb attached to static wrist-hand orthosis.

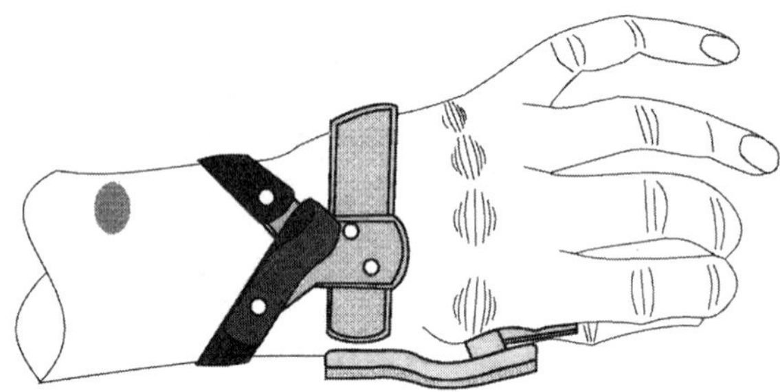

Attachments

Two of the most common attachments used with the static wrist-hand orthosis are the MCP extension stop and the IP extension assist (Fig. 29-3). If there is a loss of range in flexion at the MCP joints and a loss of range in extension at the proximal IP joints, then these two attachments can help prevent a claw hand deformity by preventing hyperextension of the MCP joints while simultaneously encouraging extension of the IP joints of the second through fifth fingers. Both of these attachments can be mounted on the same outrigger bar. This outrigger bar has two keyholes that facilitate installation and removal of the assembly.

The thumb can be maintained in opposition with a limited range of motion by the addition of a "swivel thumb" (Fig. 29-4). The swivel thumb acts as a carpal-metacarpal (CM) abduction/flexion assist for the thumb and consists of a custom-contoured metal band over the proximal phalanx of the thumb that is secured to the radial extension of the palmar piece with a simple cantilevered wire spring (see Fig. 29-4).

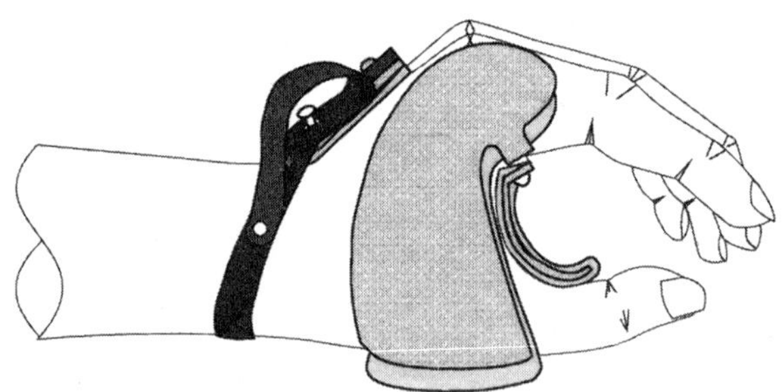
Figure 29-5. Static hand orthosis.

Static Hand Orthosis

Clinical Application

The static hand orthosis (Fig. 29-5) maintains the functional position of the hand and prevents deformities of the hand. When the functional position of the hand is achieved, the palmar arch will be maintained by the fourth and fifth digits being depressed volarly and the thumb will be prevented from excessive adduction and extension. Occasionally the static hand orthosis is used as a platform for other therapeutic attachments. All the attachments described for the static wrist-hand orthosis can also be used with the static hand orthosis. For example, consider a patient with a radial nerve injury in the forearm. In this patient, it would be desirable to add an MCP extension stop with an IP extension assist while simultaneously maintaining the palmar arch.

Patient Population

Patients with weakness or paralysis of the intrinsic musculature of the hand are appropriate candidates for the static hand orthosis. Without this orthosis the patients are at risk of developing a flat hand with the thumb CM joint in extension. Tetraplegics can develop this deformity by placing their hands on a lapboard for extended periods of time. The patient with tetraplegia caused by a lesion or injury at the C7 neurosegmental level exhibits this weakness and can benefit from a static-therapeutic hand orthosis.

Elbow Orthosis

Clinical Application

Elbow orthoses designed for reducing soft-tissue contracture must be custom-designed and fabricated with structural plastic (e.g., polypropylene) bands, totally contacting flexible plastic (e.g., polyethylene) cuffs and straps, and incorporate at least one of a variety of mechanisms for increasing the range of motion.

It is preferable to apply low-magnitude, long-duration forces when attempting to reduce an elbow flexion or extension contracture (Fig. 29-6). Particular attention must be given to mechanical and anatomic elbow joint alignment and the arm and forearm must be restricted to pure single-axis rotation with minimum translation, to avoid joint compression, tension, subluxation, or dislocation. The contracture-reduction force must be gradually increased therapeutically (see Fig. 29-6; slowly lengthen or shorten the turnbuckle*) so the soft-tissue collagen adhesions responsible for the contracture can undergo microtears without causing trauma to the joint. The bands and cuffs should be placed near the elbow joint so the levers of the three-point contracture-reduction-force system are maximized, correction forces are minimized, and skin pressure is within tolerance. The edges of the bands and cuffs should be flared to avoid excessive edge pressure and shear. The therapeutic strategy should be to tease the tissues into lengthening without provoking an antagonistic response, without causing permanent red marks on the skin, and without creating internal bruising.

An alternative to the turnbuckle is a *constant force–variable displacement* mechanism acting at the elbow joint to stretch the soft tissues. It is preferable for the force to be adjustable so that it can be set at a low value initially and gradually increased.

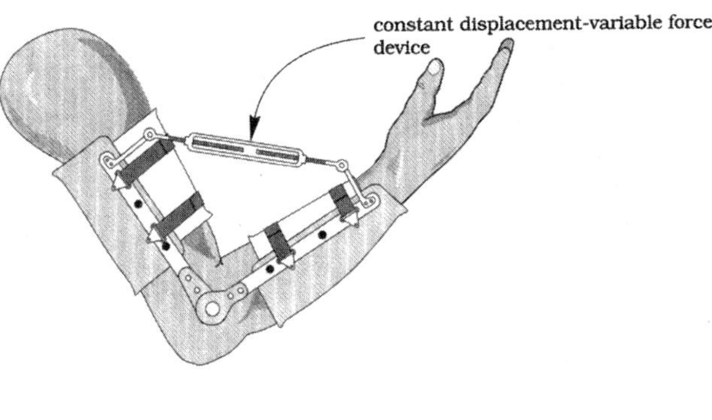

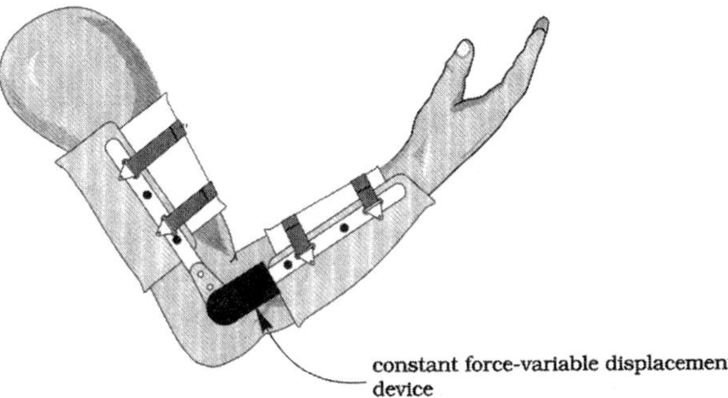

Figure 29-6. Elbow orthosis (contracture-reduction application).

Patient Population

Elbow orthoses are used for the reduction of soft-tissue contractures of the elbow that are responsible for functional limitations. The need to reduce elbow flexion or extension contracture applies to many disease and condition categories. However, the largest population affected are individuals with spinal cord injury who heavily depend on full range of motion of their elbow for alleviating ischial sitting pressure, propelling a manual wheelchair, and approximating their hand to their face.

Other individuals with tight elbows include patients who have been immobilized following trauma or surgery and risk range of motion limitations without orthotic intervention.

Shoulder-Elbow Orthosis

Clinical Application

It may be necessary to support a painful shoulder or traumatized brachial plexus with an orthosis. In many cases a conventional arm sling will suffice if there is not excessive force on the base of the neck and the duration of use will be short. However, for long-term use a sling has very little functional potential and is insufficient to meet therapeutic and functional demands. The abduction splint, if properly anchored on the hip, can be a successful alternative. A better answer was developed at Rancho Los Amigos Medical Center (Downey, CA). It is a dynamic arm and shoulder support called the *gunslinger* (Fig. 29-7). The patient's arm is strapped to a forearm trough, which is mechanically coupled to a plastic interface anchored on

---

*The turnbuckle is a constant displacement–variable force device that requires frequent adjustments to optimize the reduction. If consistent patient access and management are not possible, the reduction is minimal.

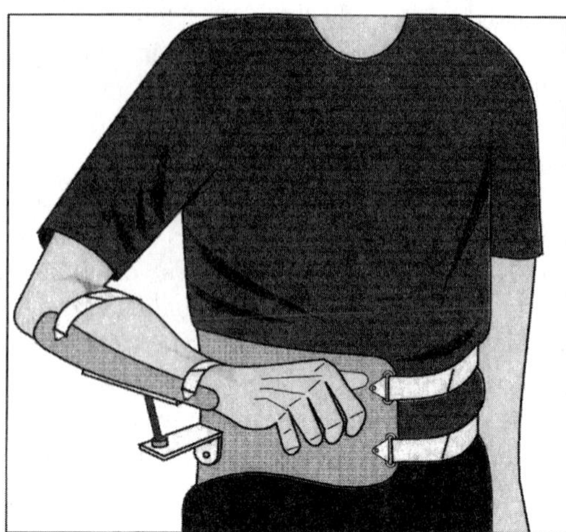

Figure 29-7. Gunslinger shoulder-elbow orthosis.

the patient's pelvis (iliac crest). The coupling between the forearm trough and iliac cap can be customized to permit a variety of motions including internal and external rotation, flexion extension, and horizontal flexion and extension at the glenohumeral joint, and flexion and extension at the elbow joint. The arm and hand are held in a cosmetically pleasing pose, and the hand is available for use, enabling early recovery while allowing limited functional activities. The gunslinger shoulder-elbow orthosis is easy to put on and take off, and can support the full weight of the arm.

Patient Population

The patient with an injured brachial plexus can benefit from the application of the gunslinger shoulder-elbow orthosis both for the prevention of further stretch injury during the healing process and for positioning of the hand in a useful location for functional activities. The iliac cap and arm trough can be concealed with a long-sleeve shirt, making the orthosis more cosmetically acceptable.

Shoulder-Elbow-Wrist Orthosis

Clinical Application

Shoulder and elbow orthoses are frequently used to protect soft tissues or to prevent contracture of soft tissues. Occasionally these orthoses are used to correct an existing deformity.

The specific design depends on the therapeutic nature of the prescription. Interim shoulder-elbow-wrist orthoses, which are used to relieve pain or to promote healing, are frequently custom-fit to the patient from prefabricated kits or assemblies. The hardware is usually very adjustable so that a few sizes can be made to fit most individuals.

The shoulder-elbow-wrist orthoses used for the long term are custom-designed and fabricated with carefully selected structural and biomechanical components. The bands and joints are not adjustable and only the straps can accommodate physical changes in the patient.

The shoulder-elbow-wrist orthosis depicted in Figure 29-8 transmits the weight of the upper limb to the ipsilateral side of the pelvis and the system is stabilized with trunk straps. This type of shoulder-elbow-wrist orthosis is often used for patients with an axillary burn (2), the objective being to provide as much contact as possible while keeping the glenohumeral joint in maximum abduction. The anatomic elbow joint may be restricted or left with free motion. Generally, the wrist is supported in extension to protect the associated soft tissues against the forces of gravity.

The disadvantage of prefabricated and custom-fit versus custom-designed and fabricated shoulder-elbow-wrist orthoses is that the prefabricated custom-fit orthoses require more follow-up to guard against excessive pressure or shear. This is especially true if the patient has sensory impairment where the biomechanical forces are being applied. Also, the prefabricated and custom-fit orthoses have to be adjusted if the patient has episodes of edema, whereas the custom-fabricated device can be designed to counter edema with total contacting bands and cuffs that are adjustable with straps.

The orthosis shown in Figure 29-8 is also known as the *airplane orthosis*, owing to the obvious appearance when it is used bilaterally. An alternative name for this orthosis is the *shoulder stabilizer*. By external rotation of the glenohumeral joint with the shoulder-elbow-wrist orthosis (see Fig. 29-8), the internal rotators are stretched and the tension on the deltoid and rotator cuff is relieved (this is often the desired posture after shoulder surgery).

It is possible to design the shoulder-elbow-wrist orthosis with maximum mobility for therapeutic purposes. Full range of abduction-adduction, flexion-extension, internal-external, and horizontal flexion-extension motions at the glenohumeral joint can be incorporated into the orthosis by careful selection of the subaxillary mechanical joints utilized. This permits postoperative rehabilitation without removing the orthosis.

Patient Population

The airplane shoulder-elbow-wrist orthosis is an excellent orthosis to prescribe after rotator cuff repairs, after anterior or posterior capsular repairs, after manipulation, and in conjunction with Bankart procedures. This orthosis is also frequently prescribed for axillary burns to prevent contracture, and alternatively, to help reduce soft-tissue contractures resulting from a variety of causes (e.g., long-term immobility).

STATIC-FUNCTIONAL

Clinical Application

The static wrist-hand orthosis and hand orthosis previously described were purely therapeutic. However, they can be

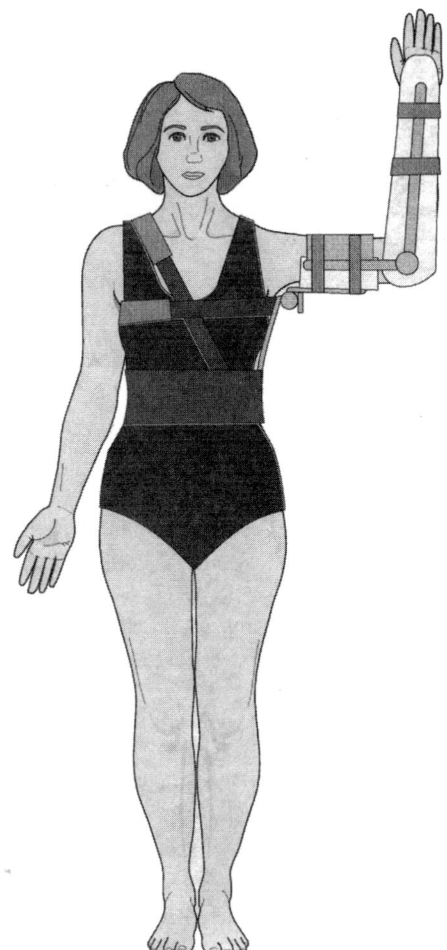

Figure 29-8. Shoulder-elbow-wrist orthosis.

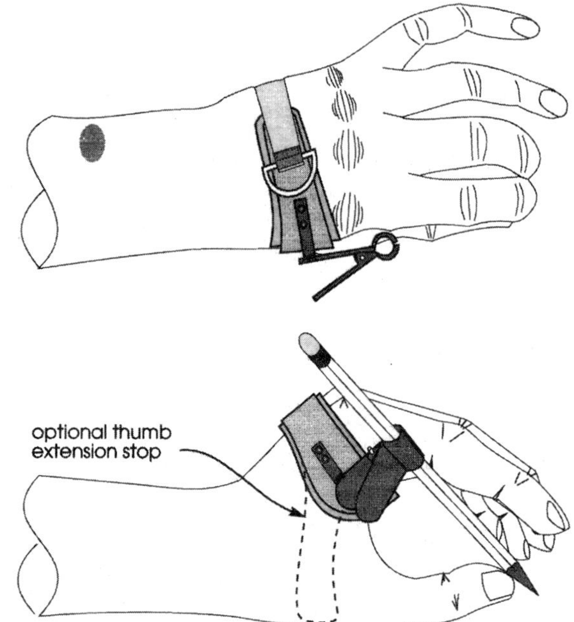

Figure 29-9. Static hand orthosis with "butterfly" writing clip.

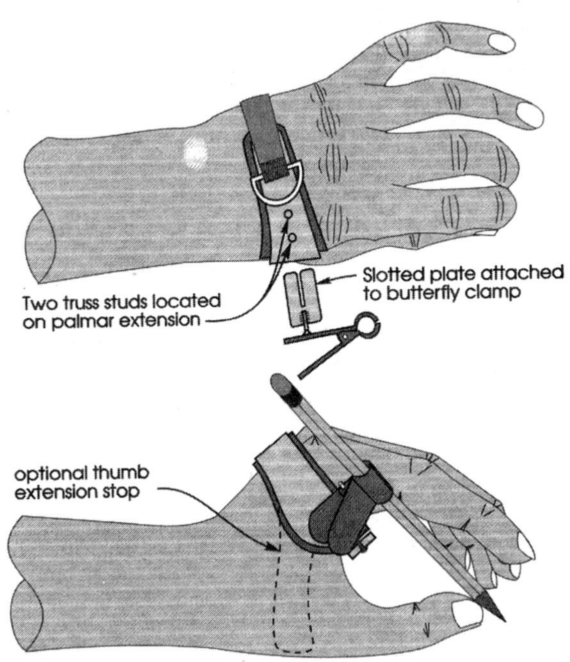

Figure 29-10. Static hand orthosis with truss stud attachment.

modified to provide functional activities by attaching clips and pockets that can hold utensils, writing devices, page turners, and so on. The static hand orthosis shown in Figure 29-9 has a butterfly type of clamp attached to the radial extension that can be used to clasp the shaft of a writing device. An alternative to the clamp is the truss stud configuration on the palmar extension of the palmar side (Fig. 29-10). Utensils and other attachments are adapted with a slotted plate that can be secured to the truss studs on the palmar side of the orthosis. A simple hand orthosis can be modified with an aluminum rod to create an ulnar page turner (Fig. 29-11). The rubber end of an eyedropper is used on the end of the aluminum rod for friction to facilitate page turning or depressing the keys on a computer keyboard. The devices that can be attached to a hand orthosis or wrist-hand orthosis include toothbrushes, razors, combs, brushes, hygiene aids, eating utensils, arts and crafts implements, and instruments unique to the injured individual's work environment.

Patient Population

Adapting the static hand orthosis or wrist-hand orthosis in this fashion is usually done when rigid deformities exist in the hand and finger joints and supple prehension is not feasible, precluding use of a more functional dynamic wrist-hand orthosis. Some individuals with spinal cord injury and residual tetraplegia lose the flexibility of their fingers and hands over time and become candidates for the hand orthosis or wrist-hand orthosis with a variety of attachments.

DYNAMIC-THERAPEUTIC

Wrist-Action Wrist-Hand Orthosis

Clinical Application

The wrist-action wrist-hand orthosis functions as a positional and therapeutic orthosis (3). As with the static wrist-hand orthosis, it maintains the functional position of the hand and prevents wrist and hand deformities (Fig. 29-12). Its therapeutic function is to protect and assist weak wrist extensors with mechanical wrist motion stops. Sometimes the wrist-action wrist-hand orthosis is used with a rubber band and pulley arrangement to assist wrist extension (Fig. 29-13). Also, if necessary, the previously described MCP extension stop and IP extension assist can be added (see Fig. 29-3). The protection and strengthening of weak muscles are achieved by limiting wrist motion, while the functional position of the hand is maintained by the orthosis. Again, preventing overstretching of the weakened musculature while allowing a safe range of motion is the main goal of this design.

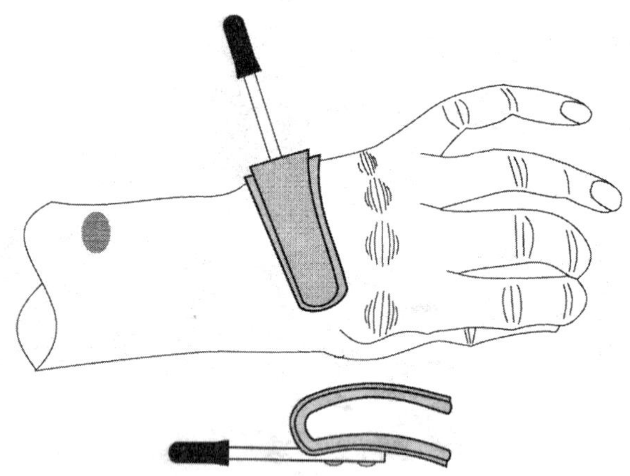

Figure 29-11. Static hand orthosis with ulnar page turner.

Patient Population

Patients with weak (grade 2, poor, to grade 3, fair) wrist extensors and paralyzed hand muscles, or patients who have potential for return of wrist extensor musculature are appropriate candidates for a wrist-action wrist-hand orthosis. For patients with wrist extensors of poor to fair strength or those with grade 3+ (fair+) wrist extensors with limited endurance, a wrist-action wrist-hand orthosis with extension assist is indicated (see Fig. 29-13). The wrist-action wrist-hand orthosis has a hinge at the wrist allowing active extension and gravity-assisted flexion. A flexion stop (see Figs. 29-12 and 29-13) is used to prevent prolonged stretching of the extensors, which can cause further weakness. A rubber band can be used to assist weak extensors

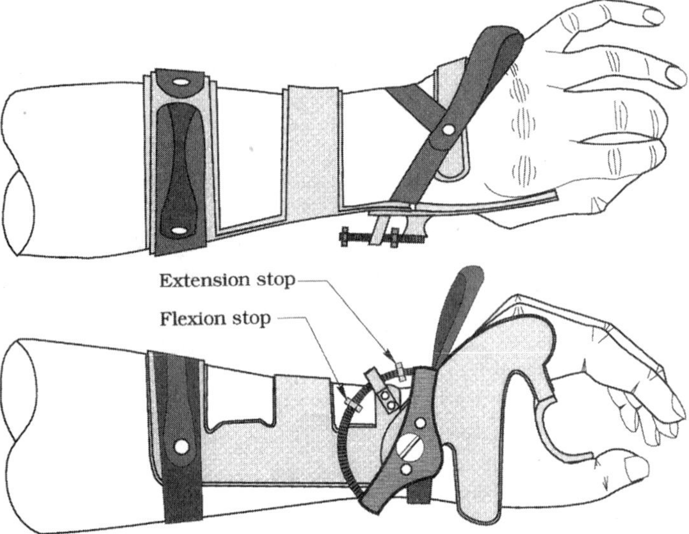

Figure 29-12. Wrist-action wrist-hand orthosis.

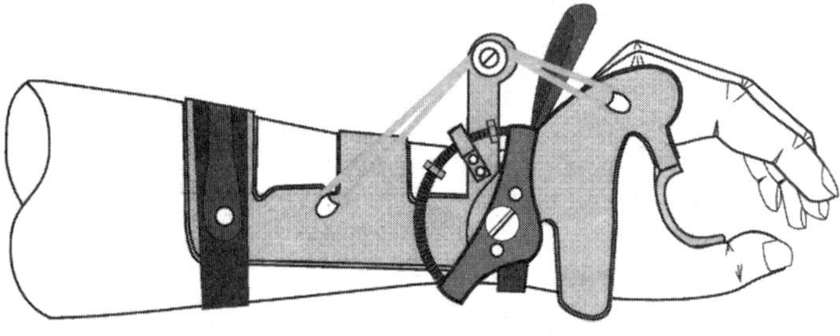

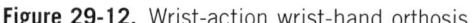

Figure 29-13. Wrist-action wrist-hand orthosis with wrist extension assist.

(see Fig. 29-13). Progress usually is made by locking the wrist joint when muscle strength is less than fair (grade 3) and loosening the wrist joint for periods of specific therapy. When wrist extensors are grade 3+ (fair+) or better with good endurance, static positioning is discontinued during the day, allowing more advanced functional training. Positioning at night is continued until it is determined that functional hand position is maintained and no loss of range of motion or stretching is occurring.

Elbow Orthosis

Clinical Application

Elbow orthoses are frequently used immediately after trauma or surgery (Fig. 29-14). Usually a three-point force system is used in conjunction with a hydraulic lock of the semiliquid tissues surrounding the fragments, to maintain the fracture fragments as a single unit during the healing process. In the past, this was done with a cast. A cast, however, does not allow normal joint motion, the fit eventually loosens, and the fragments may migrate, thereby complicating the pathology. The advantage of a well-fitting, custom-designed, and fabricated elbow orthosis over a cast is that the former is much lighter, is more comfortable, allows hygiene, and provides optimum control at the fracture site. As the patient gains or loses weight, the cuffs and straps opposing the bands can be loosened or tightened to maintain control. Many mechanical elbow joints are currently available for use on a custom-made elbow orthosis, and permit limited and adjustable range of motions at the elbow for controlled mobility without sacrificing vital bone fixation.

Patient Population

Elbow orthoses are indicated after removal of a cast, postoperatively as an adjunct to internal fixation, for management of elbow dislocation, and for strains, sprains, and muscle trauma. The design of an elbow orthosis depends on the specific application. Postsurgical or posttrauma devices often are of the "off-the-shelf" variety. However, these devices are used for a relatively short period during which the intensity of the therapeutic intervention has to be balanced with comfort. Therefore, they tend to have soft cuffs with multiple straps and an adjustable mechanical elbow joint (see Fig. 29-14).

The therapeutic strategy in the case of a fracture is to promote callus formation and simultaneously permit a safe and painless range of motion to stimulate metabolism and to avoid the nuisance of an iatrogenic joint contracture.

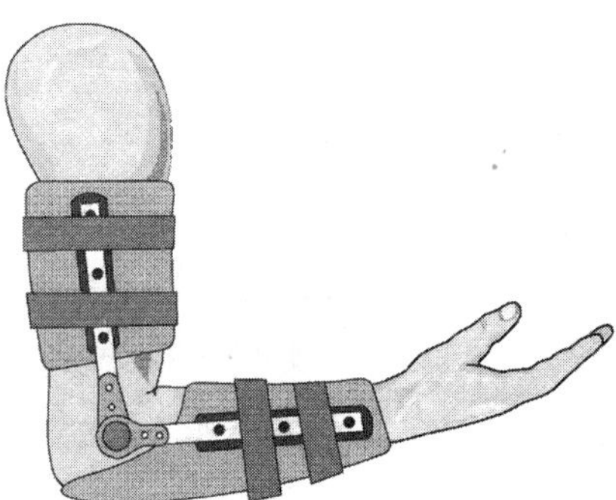

Figure 29-14. Elbow orthosis (postsurgical application).

DYNAMIC-FUNCTIONAL

Ratchet Wrist-Hand Orthosis

Clinical Application

The ratchet wrist-hand orthosis is a functional prehension orthosis (Fig. 29-15) that enables the patient to grasp and release objects by utilizing external power (2). The ratchet wrist-hand orthosis is manually controlled and substitutes for finger flexor and extensor muscles that are less than grade 3 (fair) in strength. The wrist is stabilized for function, but the position can be changed for different activities. A thumb post is used to maintain abduction and to position the thumb in alignment with the finger pads. A finger-piece assembly is provided to maintain the index and long fingers in position for pinch. A ratchet system is employed so that the hand can be closed in discrete increments. Pinch is achieved by applying distally directed force on the proximal end of the ratchet bar (black knob) or by using the patient's own chin, other arm, or any stationary object to flex the second and third fingers toward the thumb to form a three-jaw chuck. When the ratchet disk is tapped, the ratchet lock is released and spring-assisted opening of the hand occurs.

The ratchet wrist-hand orthosis allows the patient increased independence in a variety of functional activities without needing multiple pieces of adaptive equipment (Fig. 29-16). Following a carefully organized and sequenced

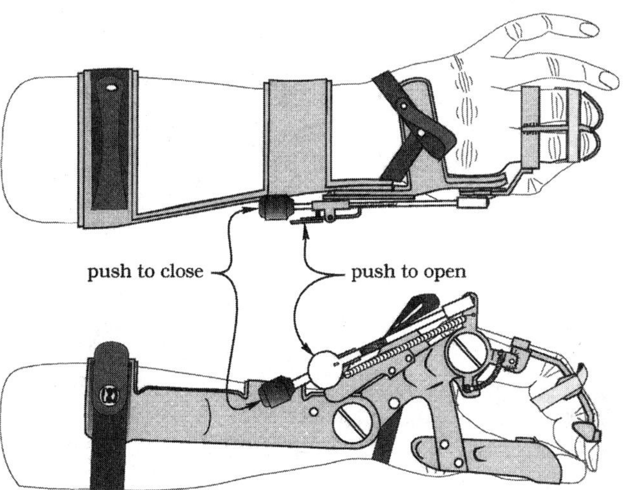

Figure 29-15. Ratchet wrist-hand orthosis.

Figure 29-16. Pen spring applications.

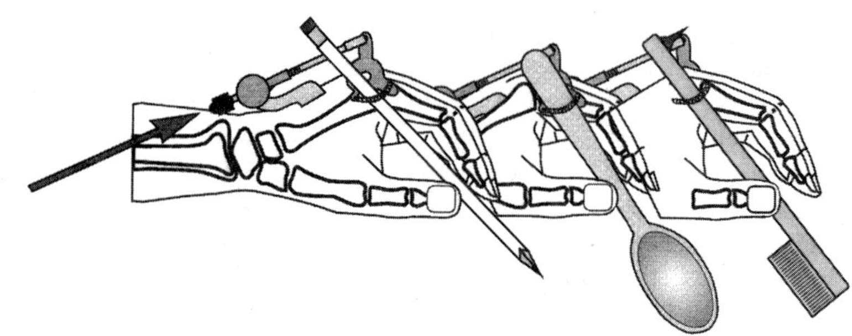

training program, a patient with C5 tetraplegia may attain independence in feeding, light hygiene (application of makeup, shaving, and hair grooming), desktop activities (e.g., writing and typing), and donning and doffing the orthosis. More complex desk tasks (writing, typing) are feasible using a well-organized desk arrangement. By using gross motion to close the hand, the patient can achieve a functional three-point pinch.

Patient Population

The ratchet wrist-hand orthosis is appropriate for patients with paralysis or severe weakness of the hand and wrist musculature. Some functional proximal strength is required to use the ratchet wrist-hand orthosis. For optimal use the patient should have at least grade 3+ (fair+) strength in shoulder flexion, abduction, external rotation, and internal rotation. However, patients with weaker proximal muscles may be able to use the ratchet wrist-hand orthosis along with a mobile arm support. Other considerations that should be evaluated are endurance, range of motion limitations, spasticity, sensation, and the patient's motivation and social support. Patients with shoulder and elbow control (i.e., functional C5 tetraplegia) are appropriate candidates for the ratchet wrist-hand orthosis.

Wrist-Driven Wrist-Hand Orthosis

Clinical Application

The wrist-driven wrist-hand orthosis (flexor hinge wrist-hand orthosis) is a dynamic prehension orthosis utilizing a transfer of power from the wrist extensors to the fingers (Fig. 29-17). Active wrist extension provides grasp and gravity-assisted wrist flexion enables the patient to open the hand.

The proximal and distal IP joints of the second and third fingers are immobilized along with the CM and MCP joints of the thumb. Active wrist extension results in the fingers' approximating the posted thumb. Conversely, passive (gravity-assisted) wrist flexion causes the hand to open (i.e., MCP extension). An adjustable actuating lever system at the wrist joint allows the user to fine-tune the wrist joint angle at which prehension occurs. It may be desirable for the prehension to occur when the wrist is in 30 degrees of extension for writing or drawing on a flat surface. However, for picking up small objects, it is preferable for the wrist to be set in flexion. This variability of wrist joint angle is necessary if maximum prehensile force is to be achieved for the specific activity being pursued. As with the ratchet wrist-hand orthosis, the wrist-driven wrist-hand orthosis replaces the need for multiple assistive devices.

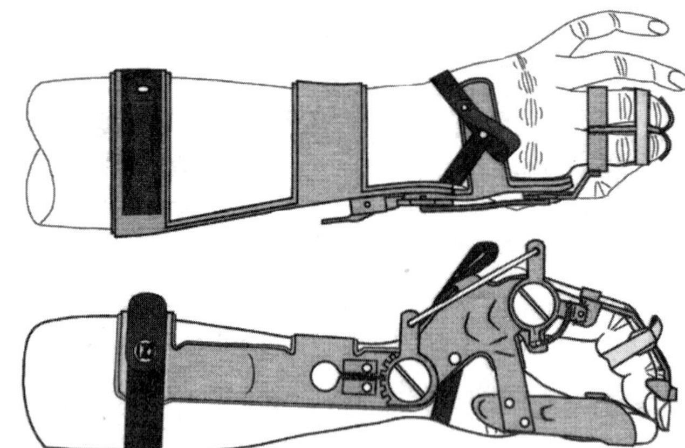

Figure 29-17. Wrist-driven wrist-hand orthosis.

Patient Population

The wrist-driven wrist-hand orthosis is an appropriate orthosis for the patient with paralysis or severe weakness of the hand. Wrist extensor strength must be at least grade 3+ (fair+) and proximal strength must be functional. For patients with wrist extensor strength of less than grade 3+ who are improving or with grade 3+ (fair+) strength with poor endurance, a rubber band wrist extension assist is indicated. Candidates for the wrist-driven wrist-hand orthosis are patients with C5 functional level with some return of C6 functional level (wrist extensors), C6, or C7 tetraplegia. By using active wrist extension, a patient can achieve functional three-point pinch.

When function in the extrinsic muscles begins to get return, the patient becomes a candidate for a wrist-driven wrist-hand orthosis. In general, if patients use their orthoses for function throughout the day, they will gain wrist strength and consequently improved prehension.

Mobile Arm Support

Clinical Application

Mobile arm support (MAS) is a shoulder-elbow orthosis that supports the weight of the arm and provides assistance to the shoulder and elbow motions through a linkage of mechanical joints (Fig. 29-18). This orthosis performs a wide range of useful purposes. A properly installed and adjusted MAS enables patients to perform self-care and vocational and recreational activities and can decrease the patient's dependency on the family or hospital personnel.

MASs are therapeutic in that they can be adjusted to complement weak muscles so they can function while being protected and strengthened. Joint range of motion can be maintained with the use of a MAS. The MAS can also provide considerable psychological value by enabling patients to do meaningful activities in spite of severe disability.

The MAS can provide assistance for shoulder and elbow motions by the following:

1. Using gravitational forces, and occasionally tension from rubber bands or springs, to substitute for or supplement loss of strength in shoulder and elbow musculature. For example, the inclined plane of an MAS may assist weak elbow extension, and the elastic mechanism assists shoulder elevation.
2. Supporting the weight of the arm so that weak muscles can move the arm over a useful range of motion.

The basic components of the MAS are the wheelchair mounting bracket, the proximal arm, the distal arm, and the forearm trough (Fig. 29-19). The elevating proximal arm is an available option with an elevating feature to counterbalance the weight of the patient's arm (see Fig. 29-19). Also, an optional standard wheelchair mounting

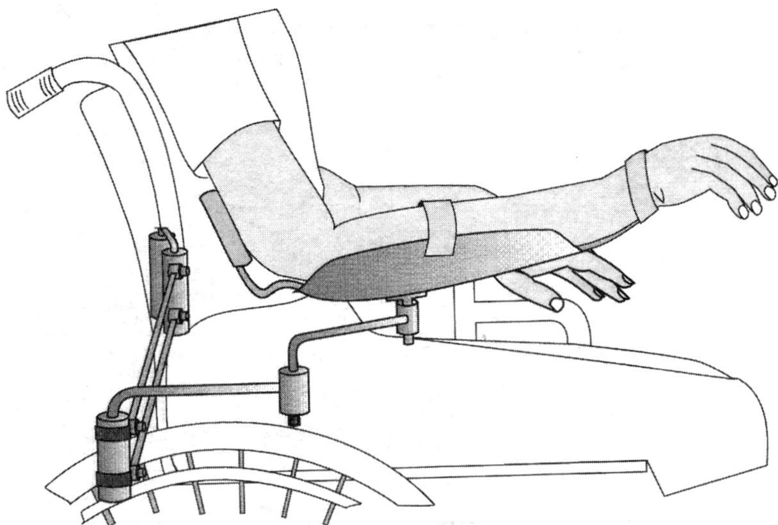

Figure 29-18. Mobile arm support with elevating proximal arm.

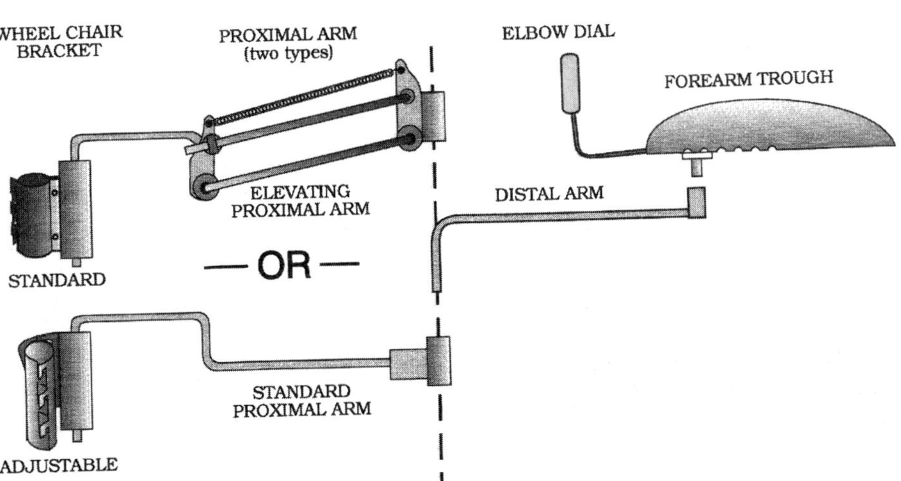

Figure 29-19. Mobile arm support components and proximal arm options.

bracket is available with a pivot type of adjustment for tilting the axis of the proximal arm (see Fig. 29-19).

Patient Population

The MAS can increase upper-limb function for patients who have severe arm paralysis due to such disabilities as muscular dystrophy, poliomyelitis, cervical spinal cord lesion, Guillain-Barré syndrome, and amyotrophic lateral sclerosis.

Patients should have sufficient muscle weakness or limited endurance to warrant use of the support. The deltoid, elbow flexors, and external rotators are the most significant muscles to evaluate because of their importance in arm function. The criteria for MAS use are as follows:

1. Absent or weak elbow flexion (poor to fair)
2. Absent or weak shoulder flexion and abduction (poor to fair)
3. Absent or weak external rotation (poor to fair)
4. Limited endurance for sustained upper-limb activity

The patient must have adequate muscular strength to move the MAS. The neck, trunk, shoulder girdle, shoulder, and elbow may serve alone or in combination as power sources.

An exact minimum strength to power an MAS is difficult to formulate. The patient's basic coordination may be as important as the amount of muscle strength present. To have control over the lapboard range in the planes of horizontal motion at the elbow and at the shoulder, it is essential that the patient have some controlling muscles in both the elbow and the shoulder.

The patient with at least poor muscle strength, especially in the shoulder girdle, shoulder, elbow, or trunk, will operate the MAS more effectively and do more with it, and the MAS will be much easier to adjust and to stabilize for function. Some hand function widens the scope of available activities, but is not always a necessity. Lack of grasp may be substituted for by the wrist-driven wrist-hand orthosis or the ratchet wrist-hand orthosis. This is common for persons with tetraplegia for whom the MAS is indicated.

Elbow Orthosis

Clinical Application

Elbow orthoses designed to assist normal motion in functional activities are definitive in nature and should be custom-designed and fabricated with the highest-quality components and materials, and fit to provide durable function for many years. Functional elbow orthoses usually incorporate an elastic device with a locking mechanism to assist elbow flexion with multiple angular lock points (Fig. 29-20). The user initiates elbow flexion using residual musculature and/or body mechanics, and the elastic device (e.g., spiral spring) assists the flexion until one of the flexion stops is reached. A release on the stop permits the elbow to either advance to a new greater angle or fall back into extension.

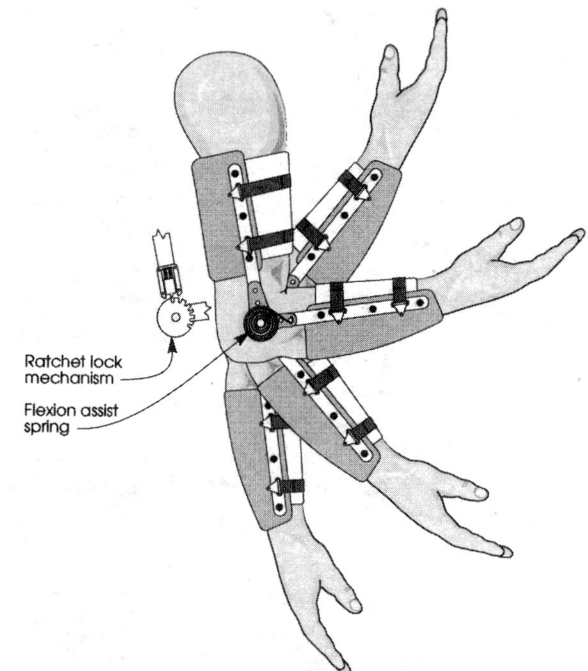

Figure 29-20. Elbow orthosis (flexion assist).

Patient Population

Individuals with selective loss of elbow flexion secondary to a brachial plexus injury or congenital deficit are appropriate candidates for the elbow orthosis with elbow flexion assist. Bilateral applications are more likely to be successful than unilateral ones. If the activity desired by the individual requires use of both the normal side and the impaired side, a successful outcome is more likely.

LOW-TEMPERATURE THERMOPLASTIC ORTHOSES

Because of their ease of fabrication, these upper-limb orthoses have proved to meet the need for a quickly available device in the clinical setting. However, because of a combination of the hand-forming technique used to produce them and the poor mechanical properties of the material, these orthoses are not well suited for long-term use when intimacy of fit is closely related to function.

These upper-limb orthoses are generally fabricated from low-temperature thermoplastics such as Orthoplast, Formsplint, and Plastazote (4,5). Orthoplast can be formed in water heated to 140 to 170°F. Higher-temperature thermoplastics, such as nyloplex, kydex, and vinyl, can be used but a plaster mold of the patient's forearm, wrist, and/or hand should be made to avoid burning the patient. Also, the higher-temperature materials cannot be cut with scissors; a power tool such as a bandsaw must be used.

A large variety of both static and dynamic upper-

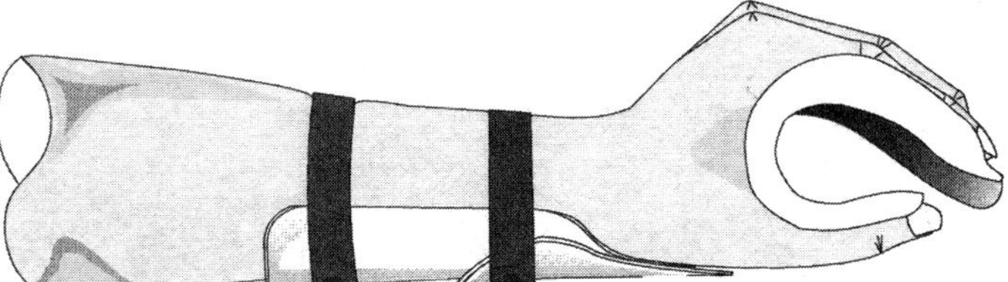

Figure 29-21. Resting wrist-hand orthosis.

limb orthoses have been designed. The static orthoses may be protective, supportive, or corrective. Protective designs are intended to protect weak muscles from being stretched and therefore prevent further weakness. By "supportive," the orthoses are intended to support a joint or an arch in substitution for weak muscles. Supportive can mean "immobilize" such as the case with a painful arthritic joint. Corrective designs may force the involved joint into a correct or near-correct alignment. The use of static orthoses must include concern for swelling and long-term immobility. Therapy should include a regimen of activities where the patient is encouraged to use the limb as often as possible.

The main advantages of the low-temperature thermoplastic orthoses are that they can be fitted early after trauma or injury and they are light in weight. For example, to prevent a deformity and position a limb in a functional position, it may be necessary to fit the patient within hours after the injury occurred. The disadvantages in using these materials are that they do not have sufficient stiffness to hold their form and hand forming results in limited intimacy of fit.

Dynamic upper-limb orthoses must be designed to provide specific forces with correct direction, often utilizing outriggers attached to the body of the main orthosis. The use of mechanical joints in parallel with the anatomic joints can decrease joint adhesions, maintain joint function, and prevent ankylosis of the joint. A large percentage of patients fitted with a low-temperature dynamic orthosis are treated in acute hospitals following surgery or trauma to the forearm and hand, and subsequently are treated as outpatients and in rehabilitation centers.

The pearls of wisdom most often employed are as follows:

1. It is much easier to prevent joint stiffness than it is to overcome one once it has occurred.
2. A static or dynamic upper-limb orthosis that fits everyone fits no one.

Resting Wrist-Hand Orthosis

The resting wrist-hand orthosis (Fig. 29-21) is designed to maintain the arches of the hand, keep the thumb abducted and flexed, and maintain the wrist in a functional position (30 degrees). This orthosis is made by placing the patient's limb on a piece of paper and drawing a pattern that encompasses the tips of the fingers. It is expanded at the

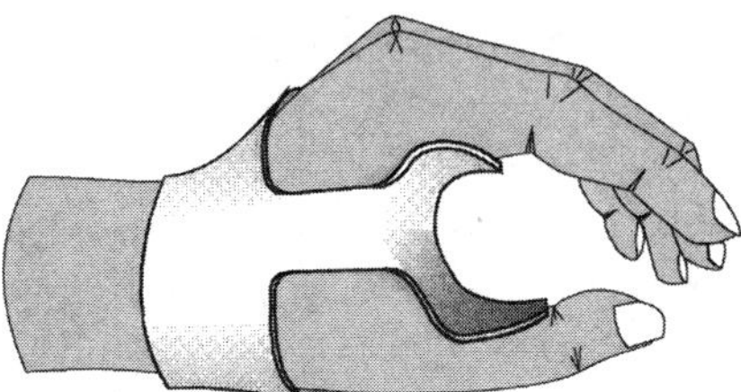

Figure 29-22. Hand orthosis with thumb adduction stop (C-bar).

forearm for a wraparound, and is slotted so that the thumb can be separated from the other fingers. If the affected side cannot be straightened for the drawing of the pattern, then the unaffected side can be used and then the pattern is reversed. When drawing the pattern, one must allow extra width for padding. The pertinent joints and landmarks are noted. There are many popular patterns published that can be used as a guide in the fabrication. Scissors or tin snips can be used to cut the chosen material (e.g., Orthoplast). Heating the cut line with a heat gun facilitates the cutting. Orthoplast is heated in a long, shallow pan of hot water until it is "rubbery." It is wiped dry, and then molded over the patient's limb and secured with an elastic bandage wrap. After the orthosis cools, the straps can be added by placing rivets, using contact cement, or sandwiching them between pieces of Orthoplast and securing with a solvent.

Although the resting wrist-hand orthosis is most often used to preserve the architecture of the hand and wrist on a patient with paralyzed musculature, it can also be used to reduce hypertonicity by abducting the fingers. This modification requires angular ridges between the digits and extra straps.

Finger separators can be designed and fabricated such that the fingers are placed in abduction to decrease spasticity.

The dorsal static resting orthosis can be fabricated to decrease flexor tone and synergy can be facilitated by tactile stimulation of the volar aspect of the forearm.

Hand Orthosis with Thumb Adduction Stop

This upper-limb orthosis is used to position the thumb in opposition and maintain the thumb web space, leaving the hand in a functional position for use (Fig. 29-22). If the dorsal and palmar extensions are formed snugly and with curvature for the palmar arch, then the orthosis can be worn without straps.

Patterns for this orthosis should be custom-designed by placing a flexible piece of paper around the appropriate portion of the patient's hand and sketching the pattern in place. The hand part is formed first and then the thumb web component can be formed. The thumb web component must allow IP flexion of the thumb and flexion of the second MCP joint.

Hand Orthosis with Metacarpal-Phalangeal Extension Stop

Intrinsic weakness of the hand can leave the hand in a resting posture that encourages MCP hyperextension. If the source of the weakness is believed to resolve and the potential for function is good, then the hand orthosis with an MCP extension stop is desired (Fig. 29-23). An oval piece of Orthoplast is heated and wrapped around the dorsum of the patient's hand distal to the wrist and proximal to the proximal IP joints. A cutout is made in the pattern to avoid pressure on the MCP joints. A rectangular piece of Orthoplast is formed into a "tootsie roll" shape and wrapped under the palmar aspect of the hand and secured to the ulnar and radial sides of the oval. The design requires no straps if snugly fabricated.

This orthosis is used when a median and radial nerve injury causes weakening of the transverse arch. If the curvature is formed into the palmar roll, then the palmar arch is preserved.

Dynamic Dorsal Wrist-Hand Orthosis

This orthosis consists of three main components (Fig. 29-24): the dorsal forearm piece, the palmar piece, and the MCP extension assist. The forearm and palmar pieces are connected with a rubber band, which assists wrist extension. For this feature to be effective, a large forearm strap is required to prevent distal migration of the forearm piece.

The dorsum of the forearm piece provides a base of support for the wire outrigger to which the rubber band for MCP extension is attached. One rubber band is usually sufficient to extend the MCP joint of the second through fifth digits and is attached to the ends of the palmar phalangeal bar. The wire outrigger can be shaped to fine-tune the extension torque.

This orthosis is designed and fabricated in the same fashion described previously. The patterns should be custom-designed and the material heated to the appropriate temperature and formed on the patient. Again, the small pads holding the hooks for the rubber bands are secured with a solvent (Carbona) or contact cement.

General

The edges of the upper-limb orthoses made from low-temperature thermoplastic, such as Orthoplast, can be folded over to create a rounded, smooth finish. Reinforcing strips can be made the same way and attached to certain weak areas (such as the wrist area) of the orthosis with solvent or contact cement. Instead of rolls of plastic, it may be desirable to create small corrugations by forming a small rectangular piece of plastic around a cylindrical object and then attaching to the main body of the orthosis where reinforcement is desired.

There are hundreds of designs of low-temperature plastic upper-limb orthoses. Only a few have been described here to give the reader a general idea of their potential. The designer is limited by his or her imagination and to a certain degree by the poor mechanical properties and bulk of the low-temperature thermoplastic materials.

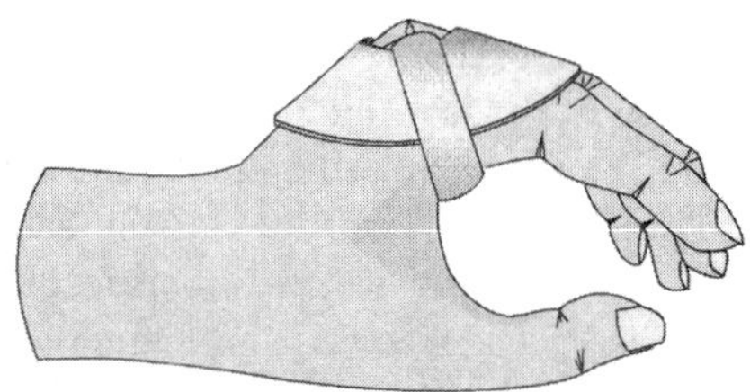

Figure 29-23. Hand orthosis with metacarpal-phalangeal extension stop (lumbrical bar).

TEAM APPROACH TO ORTHOTIC MANAGEMENT

It has been shown that patient acceptance of the orthosis can be high when there is a well-organized team approach to orthotic management (2). Both the orthotist and the occupational therapist have a vital role in ensuring successful orthotic management. The occupational therapist eval-

Figure 29-24. Dorsal wrist-hand orthosis with wrist extension assist and metacarpal-phalangeal extension assist.

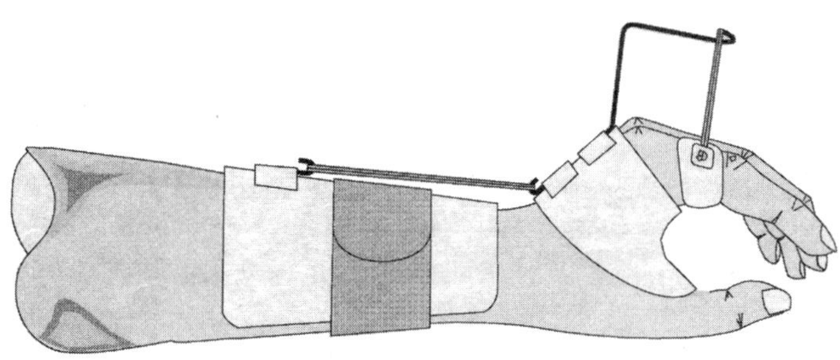

uates the need for orthoses, recommends them, and trains the patient in their use. The orthotist's role is to design, fabricate, and ensure an optimal fit.

To best meet the patient's orthotic needs, a team clinic is suggested. During this clinic, the orthotist, occupational therapist, and physician meet with the patient. The goals of the team clinic are as follows:

1. To ensure a correct fit and re-evaluate the fit over time as the patient's hand contours and functional needs may change
2. To facilitate the patient's compliance by incorporating his or her feedback to the team discussion and by educating the patient to the fit and function of the orthosis
3. To provide ongoing "hands-on" training of both orthotic and occupational therapy students and staff
4. To provide a setting for routine dialogue between the orthotist, the therapist, the physician, and the patient
5. To facilitate brainstorming of solutions to specific problems so that optimal and consensus outcomes are achieved

The benefits of such a clinic can best be illustrated by an example. A patient presented after a month of using his wrist-driven wrist-hand orthosis. The patient was able to use the wrist-driven wrist-hand orthosis for hygiene and grooming and for tabletop activities. A problem occurred when the patient was ready to begin self-catheterization. He was unable to hold the plastic tube tightly enough to insert it into the urethra. The nurse presented the problem at the team clinic and after discussion the team decided to compromise some finger opening for a tighter pinch by having the orthotist shorten the tenodesis bar and having the therapist provide additional training.

TRAINING

To gain maximum use of the orthosis, the patient must be thoroughly trained. The occupational therapy training process involves the following steps (2):

1. Education. The patient is instructed in the purpose and function of the orthosis. This learning is facilitated by the therapist as well as by a peer who is successfully using the same orthosis.
2. Exploration and experimentation. Before starting with functional tasks, the therapist puts the orthosis on the patient and the patient gets to "feel it out," open it, move it; and examine it. Step-by-step instructions are given. At this time the patient observes, but is not expected to attempt donning the orthosis. The patient is encouraged to experiment with the orthosis and become familiar with the mechanical principles before objects or activities are introduced.
3. Prefunctional training. This step involves practicing grasp, hold, placement, and release of objects of various sizes, shapes, textures, and weights.
4. Functional activities. The sequence usually begins with passive maintenance of pinch while the patient performs some activity. Typing, prewriting, and feeding oneself finger food (e.g., carrot sticks) are often used as initial activities. Training the patient to use the orthosis for feeding is graded initially by providing the setup for cutting meat, opening containers, and placement of utensils.
5. Donning and doffing. This task is taught only after the patient achieves some proficiency using the orthosis, as it is a more advanced skill and may be frustrating to the patient. Training in removing the orthosis is done first because it is easier than donning the orthosis.
6. Advanced functional training. This area includes fine-motor skills such as activities using bilateral wrist-driven wrist-hand orthoses or ratchet wrist-hand orthoses. This training is done selectively only with patients who are very skilled in using one orthosis and who have a specific functional need.
7. Follow-up. After the patient leaves the rehabilitation facility, his or her orthotic needs must be re-evaluated periodically for maintenance of proper fit and optimal function.

REFERENCES

1. Perry J. Prescription principles. In: *Atlas of orthotics.* St. Louis: CV Mosby, 1975.
2. Wilson DJ, McKenzie MW, Barber LM, Watson KL. *Spinal cord injury—a treatment guide for occupational therapists.* Revised ed. Thorofare, NJ: Slack, 1984.
3. Baumgarten JM. Upper extremity adaptations for the person with tetraplegia. In: *Spinal cord injury.* New York: Churchill Livingstone, 1985:219–242.
4. Malick MH. *Manual on static hand splinting.* 5th ed. Pittsburgh: Harmarville Rehabilitation Center, 1976.
5. Malick MH. *Manual on dynamic hand splinting with thermoplastic materials.* Pittsburgh: Harmarville Rehabilitation Center, 1974.

Chapter 30

Lower-Limb Orthotics

Mark H. Bussell
Laura Fenwick

The lower limb is wonderfully designed for efficient gait. Once it is affected by trauma or disease, the purpose of the clinical team is to recommend the best lower-limb orthosis to protect the limb, prevent deformity, and return function. Lower-limb orthoses serve many purposes. They increase the load-bearing capabilities of the limb for ambulation or protect the limb in non-weight-bearing situations. These purposes are achieved through basic biomechanical principles. This chapter will outline the biomechanical principles involved in lower-limb orthoses. The orthoses will be categorized according to type and function. Throughout the chapter, examples for given disabilities will be used.

Lower-limb orthoses may be used temporarily, during recovery from an injury or illness, or definitively for permanent disability. Temporary orthoses are often simple, low-cost, noncustom designs. Definitive orthoses may need to be custom made to create the most comfortable, functional device. An orthotist certified by the American Board for Certification (ABC) in Orthotics and Prosthetics is highly qualified to custom fit or custom fabricate any orthosis. A certified orthotist evaluates patients for the use of orthoses. The orthotist designs, fabricates, fits, and modifies all types of orthoses. The ABC is prepared to recommend certified practitioners and laboratories around the country (1).

Orthoses are known by many names. Generally, the most appropriate name is *orthosis*, the person fitting the orthosis is an *orthotist*, and orthotists study *orthotics*. For example, foot orthotics is the study of foot orthoses.

Specifically, each orthosis can be named for the area of the body it encompasses. Lower-limb orthoses are named as follows:

HKAFO	hip knee ankle foot orthosis
HO	hip orthosis
KAFO	knee ankle foot orthosis
KO	knee orthosis
AFO	ankle foot orthosis
FO	foot orthosis

This terminology is generic and was created by a task force of the American Academy of Orthopedic Surgeons (AAOS). Their system for naming orthoses was published in the Atlas of Orthotics in 1975 (2). Certain eponyms are commonly used and widely recognized; however, generic terminology will primarily be used in this text.

The area of the body encompassed and the control afforded across that area categorize orthoses. For example, a knee orthosis is so named because it controls motion across the knee joint. The knee orthosis may be static, holding all motion across the knee, or dynamic. A dynamic knee orthosis may allow motion in one plane, while controlling motion in other planes. There are some frequently used terms for motion control, also created by the task force for the AAOS (2). These terms are as follows:

Free — Allow motion.

Assist — Application of an external force for the purpose of increasing the range, velocity, or force of a motion.

Resist — Application of an external force for the

purpose of decreasing the range, velocity, or force of a motion.

Stop — Inclusion of a static unit to deter an undesired motion in one direction.

Variable — A unit that can be adjusted without making a structural change.

BIOMECHANICAL PRINCIPLES

Three-Point Pressure System

A *three-point pressure system* (3) is the most basic of orthotic principles. This set of opposing forces prevents joint motion in a given direction. Two sets of opposite three-point force systems would limit all motion in a given plane. Three-point pressure systems can be defined for the sagittal and coronal planes. Most orthoses can be identified as having multiple three-point pressure systems at work to control motion.

Circumferential Pressure

Circumferential pressure (3) is applied to the lower limb in many orthoses. The simplest example is an elastic knee sleeve, which squeezes the structures of the limb and may actually increase intracavitary pressure in the limb, lending increased stability. Fracture orthoses use circumferential compression to align and heal fractures.

Axial Load

To best reduce the vertical or *axial load* on a limb, non-weight-bearing with crutches is most successful (3). To attempt axial load reduction while still allowing ambulation, an axial load–reducing orthosis is indicated. Axial unloading orthoses are specially designed to reduce the forces through a specific body segment. They function by transferring weight from more proximal segments of the limb through the orthosis to the floor. A KAFO may be specially designed to transmit the body weight from the pelvis and thigh tissues through the plastic and metal of the orthosis to the ground, reducing the forces on the knee, ankle, and foot. One such axial unloading KAFO is called an "ischial containment" KAFO (4), borrowing its proximal brim design from prosthetic modification principles. A specially designed AFO may transmit the load from the knee and calf structures through the AFO to the ground. One such device is called a patellar tendon bearing orthosis (5), and also borrows proximal brim design from prosthetics. The percentage of body weight transmitted through the orthosis depends on many factors, including orthosis style and gait pattern. Axial unloading orthoses can be identified as containing three-point pressure systems and circumferential pressure to effect the desired control.

Translation Control

The most common site of aberrant translation in the lower limb is at the knee in the sagittal plane (3). In the absence of normal function of the anterior cruciate ligament, a positive anterior drawer shows impairment in translational stability. Orthotically, a KO attempts to reduce this translational instability through shear pressure on the limb. Multiple points of pressure can be defined in the functional KO to reduce translational instability.

Floor Reaction

Floor reaction is a term to describe the forces acting on the limb during ambulation (3). The floor reaction line is an imaginary line passing from the contact point of the lower limb on the floor to the center of mass of the person walking. For the double support phase of the gait cycle, the floor reaction line moves between the feet. In the stance phase of gait, the limb must generate enough force to counteract the forces tending to buckle the limb, and to enable progression through the cycle. At each phase of the gait cycle the floor reaction line can be described as it passes anterior or posterior to the joint axis of the ankle, knee, or hip. For example, at heel strike, the floor reaction line passes posterior to the knee. This represents a flexion moment on the knee at this point, which must be counteracted by the extensors of the knee to prevent the knee from flexing. Lower-limb orthoses substitute for absent musculature and attempt to return the normal components of the gait cycle. They attempt to alter the floor reaction line or reduce the moment on the limb at a given point in the gait cycle. Floor reaction is an important ingredient of any ambulatory orthosis. The proper use of floor reaction forces will offer the patient stability, thus improving confidence and adding value to the orthotic management.

Serial Correction

Contractures and deformities of the lower limb may correct with the application of slow, constant stretch (3). Correction can be achieved through the progressive use of corrective orthoses or casts. When casts are used for serial correction, new casts are applied once to twice a week until full correction is achieved. When orthoses are used for serial correction, dial locks, ratchet locks, or spring-loaded joints perform the correction. Upon full correction, new orthoses that best represent the corrected limb may need to be fabricated. The objective of serial correction is to improve alignment of the limb, which can improve standing balance and energy costs of standing and walking.

EVALUATION

An evaluation of the lower limb must be completed prior to the recommendation of any orthosis. Evaluation of the patient's range of motion and muscle strength at the foot and ankle, knee, and hip is mandatory. An assessment of upper-limb strength and sitting and standing balance should also be included as these are also important to improving functional ambulation. Observational gait analysis is the final determinant in making an orthotic recommendation. If available, a gait analysis laboratory is of great benefit for evaluation and recommendation.

MOTION CONTROL

Recommendation of lower-limb orthoses can be simplified if one looks at the body in segments and considers orthoses in their component parts. There are three planes of motion available to the limb at the hip, knee, and ankle. Othoses are typically capable of allowing sagittal plane motion, and they block out coronal and transverse plane motion. However, if the patient has ligamentous laxity in the coronal or transverse plane, it will be exhibited within the orthosis. While an orthosis may stabilize the limb in the sagittal plane, it may not prevent the limb from exhibiting poor alignment within the orthosis. There are specific design criteria for alignment correction in the coronal plane (6). There are also specific design criteria to correct transverse plane alignment (7). All three planes should be evaluated for the use of these principles within any orthosis.

Ankle Control

To recommend the appropriate ankle joint control on a lower-limb orthosis, one must consider the patient's motor strength at the ankle, as well as the deforming forces acting on the weakened ankle. In an AFO, an anterior stop replaces weak plantar flexion by stopping unopposed dorsiflexion. A posterior stop replaces weak dorsiflexion and prevents equinus in swing phase. In the coronal plane, total contact and three-point pressure systems can prevent valgus and varus deformities. Transverse plane deviation at the ankle presents itself as an internal or external rotation deformity. Axial unloading AFOs with a combination of pressure systems can reduce transverse plane deformities.

Knee Control

At the knee, an extension stop is used to prevent hyperextension due to weakened posterior ligaments. A ring lock may be used for flexion instability due to weakened knee extensors. Coronal instability at the knee can be controlled with a KAFO or KO. Either orthosis must have trimlines that describe a three-point pressure system for varum/valgum control. Transverse plane deformity at the knee can result from inadequate ligaments as in an ACL deficiency, or as a result of severe muscle weakness. Although many KOs purport to control transverse plane abnormalities, it is usually necessary to use the leverage of a KAFO with axial unloading design features to gain transverse plane control.

Hip Control

A hip joint that is free moving holds hip coronal and transverse plane motion. In this way weakened hip transverse rotators and weak hip abductors or adductors are stabilized. A ring lock may be used on the hip joint to prevent flexion. This lock is used in the presence of weakened hip extensors.

Although each body segment can be evaluated individually for motion control, orthoses should also be evaluated as complete devices with an impact on the entire body in gait.

ORTHOSES

HKAFO

HKAFOs are required when there is complete lower-limb paralysis. In order for a person to stand in HKAFOs with such paralysis, the person must have sitting balance and must not have contractures. From a patient's perspective, HKAFOs are large, cumbersome devices, so compliance can be difficult. To increase the possibility that these expensive devices will actually be used, one can narrow the field of prospective patients. Obesity, contractures, severe spasticity, low cognitive state, lack of motivation, poor support network, and lack of sitting balance are all characteristics that rule out HKAFO use (8). If the patient has all of the appropriate characteristics for use, there are orthotic options within the HKAFO category. Static HKAFOs, which are locked at the hip, knee, and ankle, are used for standing, swivel-type ambulation or crutch ambulation. Parapodium-type HKAFOs, swivel walkers, and standard HKAFOs all fit into this parameter. Reciprocal gait orthoses are dynamic at the hip, while locked at the knee and ankle. Reciprocal gait orthoses can be used for standing and walking. A third type of HKAFO, with free hip joint but locked knee and ankle, can be used for standing and walking when the primary disability at the hip is excessive adduction or rotation, but active hip flexion/extension is present.

HO

HOs are so named for their control of the hip joint. Motion control at the hip may be needed in any of the three planes of available motion. Common disabilities requiring hip joint control are cerebral palsy and hip replacement surgery. Children with lower-limb disability from cerebral palsy may present with unopposed adduction and internal rotation at the hip, and an HO can be used nocturnally to maintain neutral alignment and prevent dislocation (9).

HOs may be fitted after hip replacement surgery, after a dislocation, or to prevent one. They are limited in their motion control of the hip joint. These orthoses offer limited rotation control and can easily be overpowered in the other two planes. If true rotation control is required, an HKAFO is needed. HOs for postoperative hip replacement surgery are usually set in 15 to 20 degrees of abduction with a 70-degree flexion stop. With this setting, internal rotation of the hip is somewhat restricted. Most dislocations occur with hip flexion, internal rotation, and adduction. The patient must be well educated in the use of the orthosis, and cautioned that it is merely a reminder not to move in the restricted planes of motion (10).

KAFO

KAFOs control motion at the knee, ankle, and foot. Typically, some hip joint active range of motion is present when KAFOs are used. A "spreader bar" can be added to lock a pair of KAFOs together. In this way, the user can be trained in "swing-to" and "swing-through" type ambulation. Bilateral KAFOs are typically used secondary to spinal cord injury when paraplegia or paraparesis is present (11). Unilateral KAFOs can be used for a variety of purposes, including ligamentous laxities that lead to genu varum or valgum, flexion, or extension instability of the knee.

Functional uses of a KAFO include training in standing balance, weight shifting for ambulation, and ambulation. If locks are used, locking and unlocking the knee joint is also part of training. To unlock a ring lock, the patient must bend at the waist so that the hand can reach the lock and raise it above the level of the joint. A spring-loaded retainer can be used with this type of joint to hold the lock in place after it has been raised. These retainers are often used, as one KAFO has two locks to unlock and it is very difficult for the patient to independently unlock the joints, keep them unlocked, and reach for a chair to sit down.

The dial lock mechanism is used to reduce contracture at the knee, or to allow the knee to lock with a flexion contracture. The mechanism includes a dial adjustable knee lock that can be set in varying degrees of knee flexion. Proximal to the dial lock mechanism, there is a ring lock that allows flexion and extension of the knee for sitting and locks for standing. A spring-loaded retainer can be added to this ring lock as well.

The lever lock mechanism is a cam lock with a bail mechanism. It can be spring loaded for locking or locked with an elastic strap. It thus locks automatically on full extension of the knee and is unlocked by lifting the bail. The bail can be removed, and a trigger mechanism can be added proximally on the orthosis to unlock the joint.

KO

KOs are so named as they encompass and control motion at the knee. KOs can be static or dynamic. Static KOs are typically used to maintain full extension and to protect the joint surfaces, ligaments, and muscle structures of the knee. Dynamic KOs are used to stabilize these structures in gait. KOs can be defined by type of use. The three basic uses are prophylactic, rehabilitative, and functional.

Prophylactic KOs are used to prevent injury to the knee as they are worn. A lateral knee guard that is strapped or taped to the knee is such a device. Intended to protect the knee from ligament injury during football or other game play, these orthoses have *not* been found to be useful (12).

Rehabilitative KOs are those used after injury or surgery to the knee, during recovery. These orthoses tend to be static, bulky devices. However, if one considers the length of time worn, the desired functional outcome, and the need for increasing movement over time to best enable functional recovery, then a device capable of change over time is indicated. A dial lock rehab KO is capable of such change.

Functional KOs are also used after injury or surgery, but by definition, are those that replace function to the knee. The definitions of rehabilitative and functional KOs cross over in that the same orthosis could be used during rehabilitation and functionally or definitively. Functional KOs are less bulky, more cosmetic, more often custom made, and more expensive than rehabilitative KOs. Conservative management of knee ligament injuries can be effective using functional/rehabilitative KOs in concert with therapy.

KOs can also be categorized by motion control. In this way, a static KO is distinguished from a free motion KO. A hinged KO holds motion in the coronal plane, and usually has a stop at full extension with free flexion. With these controls, some manufacturers claim that transverse plane motion control is afforded in the devices, although this claim is not supported in the literature. It is more appropriate to use a KAFO or even HKAFO for true transverse plane control of the lower limb.

AFO

AFOs are so named for the control provided at the ankle and foot. However, it must be noted that immobilizing the ankle influences the stability of the knee in gait. To recommend the appropriate ankle joint control on a lower-limb orthosis, one must consider the patient's motor strength at the ankle and knee. Consider this sagittal plane example. An AFO with an anterior stop acts like plantar flexors to stabilize the knee. A knee extension moment is created from foot flat to toe off when walking with such an orthosis. This increases knee stability, but could potentially cause hyperextension without proper alignment at the foot and ankle. A posterior stop replaces weak dorsiflexion and prevents equinus in swing phase. A posterior stop can cause a knee flexion moment at heel strike, and could cause the knee to buckle if there is flexion instability and the orthosis is malaligned with excessive flexion. The best AFO is one that can balance the floor reaction forces to the patient's advantage in the gait cycle, reducing deforming forces and allowing normal ones.

There are a wide variety of AFO styles, but they can basically be separated into metal, plastic, and hybrid metal and plastic styles. Any orthosis that crosses the ankle is technically an AFO, so the supramalleolar orthosis is an

AFO, although it only provides subtalar and midtarsal support and allows full talocrural joint motion. AFOs can be static or dynamic. An AFO can provide control in one, two, or all three planes. In order to afford triplanar control, the orthosis must use axial unloading principles.

Although there have been many styles of metal orthoses, there are only a few that are commonly used today. There are three very good reasons to choose a metal orthosis as opposed to a plastic style. Fluctuating edema can be readily accommodated in a metal orthosis. An insensate limb can be fitted in a metal orthosis, which does not contact the limb at the ankle, and can be fabricated with a soft leather shoe with soft inner lining to avoid skin irritation. A metal orthosis with a double-action ankle joint is intended for rehabilitative use. The ankle joint control can be easily modified to provide the changing needs as motor control is gained. One could argue that plastic orthoses can be used for all of these purposes. In the case of fluctuating edema, a total contact orthosis with anterior panel might well contol edema in the limb, while the metal orthosis simply allows it to occur uninterrupted. For insensate limbs, a fully lined orthosis that is carefully fitted may well protect and prevent further deformity. This practice requires the patient to comply with vigilant observation of his or her limb for any signs of irritation. During rehabilitation, a plastic AFO can be fabricated with the joints in place, but not activated. In this way the plastic AFO is a solid ankle at the beginning of rehabilitation, and an articulated AFO as knee control and ankle motion are achieved. Patient preference is also a consideration in the choice of plastic or metal orthoses.

Hybrid AFOs are those which have metal ankle joints, usually double action, with laminated or plastic calf and foot sections. These orthoses can be fabricated to be extremely rigid and are the best style to achieve axial unloading (13).

CONCLUSION

The best orthotic management is accomplished by a team that includes the prescribing doctor, the orthotist, the physical therapist, and the patient. This team works for the common goal of improving function, maintaining structural alignment, and thus improving ambulation. The prevention of joint contractures is of utmost importance throughout the acute, rehabilitative, and long-term care of the patient. The maintenance of structural alignment of the knee, ankle, and foot at all phases of rehabilitation facilitates the functional orthotic management. The orthosis must be more than functional, however. Most importantly, it must control the structural needs of the patient, then meet as many functional goals as possible. Of course, the orthosis must be comfortable. The most comfortable orthoses are those that achieve appropriate alignment and maintain alignment with the most efficient set of forces possible. Further, the orthosis must be cosmetic as well. The most functional device may be discarded if it is unappealing or uncomfortable. The best orthosis blends value, comfort, structural alignment, function, and cosmesis into an acceptable package.

REFERENCES

1. Perry J. Fundamentals. In: *Gait analysis: normal and pathological function.* Thorofare, NJ: SLACK, 1992:1–49.
2. American Academy of Orthopedic Surgeons. *Atlas of orthotics*, 1975, 1985, 1997.
3. Bowker P, Condie DN, Bader DL, Pratt KJ, eds. *Biomechanical basis of orthotic management.* Oxford: Butterworth-Heinemann,1993.
4. McCullough NC, III: Biomechanical analysis systems of orthotic prescription. In: *Atlas of orthotics.* St. Louis: Mosby, 1975.
5. Titus BR. A patellar-tendon-bearing orthosis. *Orthot Prosthet* 1975; 29:35–40.
6. Carlson MJ, Berghund G. An effective orthotic design for controlling the unstable subtalar joint. *Orthot Prosthet* 1979;33:39.
7. Nielsen JP, Fish D. OOS-1 basic seminar in lower extremity pathomechanics and rotational control orthotics. Seminar sponsored by Oregon Orthotic Systems Inc., 1988–1995.
8. Douglas R, Larson PF, D'Ambrosia R, McCall R. The LSU reciprocation-gait orthosis. *Orthpedics* 1983:6.
9. Furvis JM, et al. Preliminary experience with the Scottish Rite Hospital abjection orthosis for Legg-Prethes disease. *Clin Orthoped* 1980;150:49–53.
10. Lima D, Magmis R, Paprosky WG. Team management of hip revision patients using a post-op hip orthosis. *J Prosthet Orthot* 1994: 6.
11. Waters RL, Miller L. A physiological rational for orthotic prescription in paraplegia. *Clin Prosthet Orthot* 1987;11:66–73.
12. Teitz CC, Hermanson BK. Evaluation of the use of braces to prevent injury to the knee in collegiate football players. *JBJS* 1987;69A:2–8.
13. Andrews BJ, et al. Hybrid FES orthosis incorporating closed loop control and sensory feedback. *J Biomed Eng* 1988;10:189–195.

Chapter 31

Upper-Extremity Amputation and Prosthetic Rehabilitation

M. Catherine Spires
Linda Miner
Miles O. Colwell

Amputation is an ancient surgical procedure used to save life or to preserve body parts. It can be a devastating loss, particularly when it involves the dominant hand or both upper extremities. Over 12,000 persons experience a major upper-extremity or hand amputation in the United States annually (1). Upper-extremity amputations constitute less than 20% of all amputations performed in the United States. Trauma is the number one cause of transhumeral to fingertip amputations (2,3). More than 90% of upper-extremity limb losses result from accidents, usually industrial accidents. This is in contrast to lower-extremity amputations, which usually result from systemic disease, such as diabetes mellitus or peripheral vascular disease.

Lower-extremity amputation occurs typically in the older individual with chronic medical problems, usually during the fifth through seventh decades, while upper-extremity loss occurs primarily in healthy young men between the ages 20 and 40 years (1–4). Because of the youth and good health of the upper-limb amputee, these individuals comprise a larger percentage of the disabled community than the 20% incidence of upper-extremity amputation would suggest. The person with upper-extremity loss will live longer than the lower-extremity counterpart, imposing heavy costs on the individual and society as a whole.

Amputation is not merely the loss of a body part. Limb loss impacts a person's body image, self-perception, physical identity, career, and psychosocial functioning. In some cultures, amputation is performed as a punishment for criminal behavior, consequently carrying a powerful negative social stigma regardless of the etiology. Though less dramatic in American culture, amputees frequently experience negative interpersonal reactions from others and are often isolated from other people.

Rehabilitation is not simply a matter of replacing missing body parts. Because amputation impacts the person at all levels of psychosocial and physical functioning, successful prosthetic restoration and rehabilitation must address the individual's physical and psychosocial well-being. If these areas are effectively addressed, the individual who has had an upper-extremity amputation will return to a productive and satisfying life.

The principles of upper-extremity prosthetic restoration and rehabilitation differ from those of lower-limb prosthetic restoration. While an upper-extremity prosthesis, like the lower-limb prosthesis, replaces some of the lost gross movements, modern technology does not approach the sophistication of the intact human upper extremity and hand. The upper extremity's specialized functions of precise fine-motor control and the multimodality sensation, including proprioceptive feedback, have yet to be achieved. Since lower-extremity function is less complex, prosthetic design focuses primarily on gross motor activities, such as walking and standing.

One of the earliest known upper-limb prostheses dates back to the second Punic Wars of the second century BC (218–201 BC). Marcus Sergius, a Roman general who lost his arm in battle, held his shield using an iron prosthetic hand during combat (per account by Pliny).

During the following centuries, a variety of devices were used to replace the upper extremity. By the sixteenth century, Ambroise Paré, a French military surgeon, designed the forerunner of today's modern upper-extremity prosthesis. His design allowed the amputee to passively position the hand and lock it into place. Though a locksmith could duplicate his design, it was expensive. As a result, Paré's design was only available to the wealthy. The commoner managed without a prosthesis or used a leather socket with a stationary hook.

In the nineteenth century, Peter Baliff, a dentist, designed the first body-powered prosthesis, which used proximal muscle force to produce a weak prosthetic grasp and release. Though originally designed for the below-elbow (BE) amputee, it was soon modified for the above-elbow (AE) amputee using a chest lever to control the AE prosthesis. During this same period, Comte de Beaufort developed the double spring hook, the forerunner of today's hook terminal device (TD).

The twentieth century brought major changes in upper-extremity prosthetics. The injuries during the world wars, as well as the thalidomide tragedy of the late 1950s, accelerated the pace of prosthetic technology and research. After decades of research, the myoelectric prostheses became a reality. These prostheses remain the most successful externally powered prostheses ever developed. Though modern prostheses are not as elegant and complex as the human upper extremity and hand, the current generation of upper-extremity amputees lead full and productive lives because of the advances of prosthetic technology and research (e.g., improved fitting and suspension techniques, new lightweight durable materials, and more sophisticated body-powered and externally powered components).

Prosthetic technology changes rapidly. It is impossible for a text of this type to keep pace with the rapid changes and availability of new technology. However, the basic principles of prosthetic restoration and rehabilitation after upper-extremity amputation change little. This chapter focuses on these basic principles. If the physiatrist and other rehabilitation team members follow these fundamental principles, the upper-extremity amputee will achieve the optimal prosthetic restoration and function possible with today's advanced technology. As in any field of medicine, this text cannot substitute for the clinician's need to study ongoing research and to learn from one's patients and their experience.

The basic surgical principles of amputation are reviewed. Obviously, a trained surgeon is the appropriate professional to perform amputations. However, the physiatrist, and other rehabilitation team members, need to understand the surgical principles of limb amputation. The informed rehabilitation specialist is able to discuss the prosthetic and rehabilitation implications of various surgical procedures. Collaboration between the surgeon, physiatrist, patient, prosthetist, therapists, and other rehabilitation team members guarantees that the patient receives optimal surgical and rehabilitation care. This chapter is written to assist the surgical and rehabilitation team in their efforts to collaborate and maximize the patient's functional outcome. An overview of surgical principles is presented first, followed by a presentation of prosthetic restoration and rehabilitation.

SURGICAL PRINCIPLES

General Principles

Upper-extremity amputation is performed infrequently. As a result, few surgeons have the opportunity to work with upper-extremity amputees. Surgeons often consult with physiatrists to advise them regarding the prosthetic and rehabilitation implications of surgical decisions. Collaboration between the surgical and rehabilitation team guarantees that the patient will experience the best surgical and functional outcome.

Many consider amputation a surgical failure: "The limb could not be 'saved'." However, amputation does not equate to failure. New surgical techniques and prosthetic technology make it possible for amputation to be a part of an overall plan of upper-extremity reconstruction, not simply a surgery of last resort. Obviously, if amputation is not necessary, it should not be done. But when it is the best option for the patient, amputation can be the basis of upper-limb reconstruction and the first step in upper-extremity rehabilitation. Approaching the amputation as a reconstructive procedure facilitates achieving a painless, cosmetic, and functional limb. This reconstructive approach, coupled with a patient-oriented approach, focuses the medical team's efforts on achieving a positive functional outcome as defined by the individual's needs.

The goal of successful rehabilitation is an individual who can assume autonomy and responsibility for all aspects of his or her life. The patient's attitude, as well as the attitude of the surgical and rehabilitation team, is key to achieving this goal. The patient needs to know that a multidisciplinary coordinated effort is being made to optimize upper-extremity repair and reconstruction.

In general, there are two types of amputation. The *open* amputation, also called a *guillotine amputation*, is indicated when severe infection or sepsis is present. The amputation wound is not closed; treatment is directed at resolution of the infection. Definitive closure is performed once the infection has resolved. The second type, the *closed* or *definitive amputation*, involves primary closure of the amputation site. Definitive closure is indicated if the limb is not infected and wound healing is a reasonable expectation.

Typically, the surgical incision is best placed in a transverse position, with anterior and posterior skin flaps of equal length. With this technique, the surgical scar will be at the end of the residual limb where it will not be in contact with the prosthetic socket. Scar formation on the posterior or anterior surface of the residual limb causes pain from the mechanical pressure of the prosthetic socket. Like other amputations, "dog ears," soft-tissue projections from the medial or lateral end of the surgical incision, are undesirable.

Often plastic procedures, such as placement of skin grafts or flaps, are required to preserve length and function. The choice of the type of graft or flap depends on the specific surgical needs and available viable tissue. Length is a crucial issue for amputations about the shoulder and below the elbow. Split-thickness skin grafts can effectively preserve needed length (5).

Bone section should be a clean cut across the level, with rough surfaces smoothed. The shaping of the bone must be compatible with future prosthetic use and socket fitting. In the case of disarticulation, cartilage surfaces are preserved. The articular cartilage provides a weight-bearing surface, and in children, prevents bony overgrowth at the distal end of the residual limb.

The muscle and tendons are divided distal to the site of bone sectioning. Except for in digits, a myoplasty is typically performed. Muscles, at their normal resting length, are sewn to their antagonists to secure them together. A myodesis, which secures the tendon and muscle to the bone, is another option. If the distal musculature and tendons are not secured, they will retract proximally. If this occurs, the patient is not able to use these muscles to control the residual limb or use these muscles for future myoelectric control sites.

Neuromas are an inevitable consequence of surgical sectioning of a peripheral nerve. During amputation, nerve division must be done carefully. The involved nerves should be isolated, gentle traction should be applied, and then the nerves sharply sectioned 2 to 4 cm proximal to the osteotomy site (4). Once the nerve is sectioned, traction is relieved, allowing the nerve to retract into proximal tissues. This technique allows the neuroma to develop deep in soft tissues, where irritation from scarring or pressure is less likely to occur. Meticulous surgical techniques will ensure that neuromas form away from areas of potential irritation caused by the prosthetic socket or components. Neuromas that develop in flexion crease regions trigger acute and chronic neurogenic pain.

Lastly, closure should be meticulous. Closure should be done in such a way as to avoid the development of adherent scar, redundant tissue, or an irregularly shaped residual limb. Especially in the AE amputee, redundant tissue should be avoided. Excess soft tissue makes prosthetic socket fitting and prosthetic control difficult.

Characteristics of a residual upper extremity suitable for prosthetic fitting include a cylindrical limb with a well-placed scar, good skin coverage, adequate soft-tissue coverage, and intact sensation. Ideally, the patient should be pain free. If this is not feasible, pain should be sufficiently controlled so that the person is able to tolerate the prosthesis.

In summary, the goals of surgical amputation are to 1) preserve functional length of the extremity, 2) preserve useful sensation, 3) prevent symptomatic neuromas or pain syndromes, 4) prevent adjacent joint contractures, 5) minimize recovery time, and 6) achieve early prosthetic fitting to facilitate return to work, activities of daily living (ADLs), recreation, and socialization (6).

Lastly, the development of sophisticated microsurgery techniques makes upper-limb replantation and reconstruction feasible. In some situations of traumatic limb loss, replantation is an option; replantation of the proximal part of the arm is less successful than BE replantation. Kleinert and others (7–9) suggested that the lower success rate is secondary to warm ischemia affecting a greater muscle mass. Additionally, reinnervation must occur over a much longer segment in proximal replantation. If replantation is performed, it is most successful in the very young patient whose injuries do not preclude skeletal and neurovascular reattachment (10). Functional neurologic recovery is best in children. Since replantation is not without risk, the patient's overall status, the duration of limb ischemia, and the likelihood of metabolic replantation toxemia must be considered (11).

Selection of Amputation Site

The level of amputation is dictated by the site of trauma, tumor, or pathology. Though there is limited control over the etiology and its effects, the surgeon may have some choice of the amputation level. The surgeon must choose the most distal amputation site that will allow satisfactory healing, prosthetic restoration, and rehabilitation. Judicious selection of the surgical level, implementation of appropriate amputation techniques, and careful tissue management will have a long-lasting positive influence on future prosthetic restoration, rehabilitation, and lifestyle.

Anatomically, there are many levels of amputation, including partial hand, wrist disarticulation (WD), BE (also called a transradial) amputation, AE (or transhumeral) amputation, shoulder disarticulation (SD), and forequarter (FQ) amputation (Fig. 31-1).

Partial Hand Amputations

The hand is a very complex and intricate element of the human upper extremity. Object manipulation, precision pinch, and power grasp are the primary functions of the hand. Precision pinch requires, at minimum, two opposing digits. Not only must the digits be capable of motion, but they must also have functional sensation. Pinch can be subdivided into three basic types: tip-to-tip pinch, three-digit pinch, and lateral pinch. In the normal hand, the thumb opposing the index and long fingers, also called the *radial tripod*, creates a precise pinch.

Power grasp is the action of holding something

Figure 31-1. The various anatomic levels of an upper-extremity amputation.

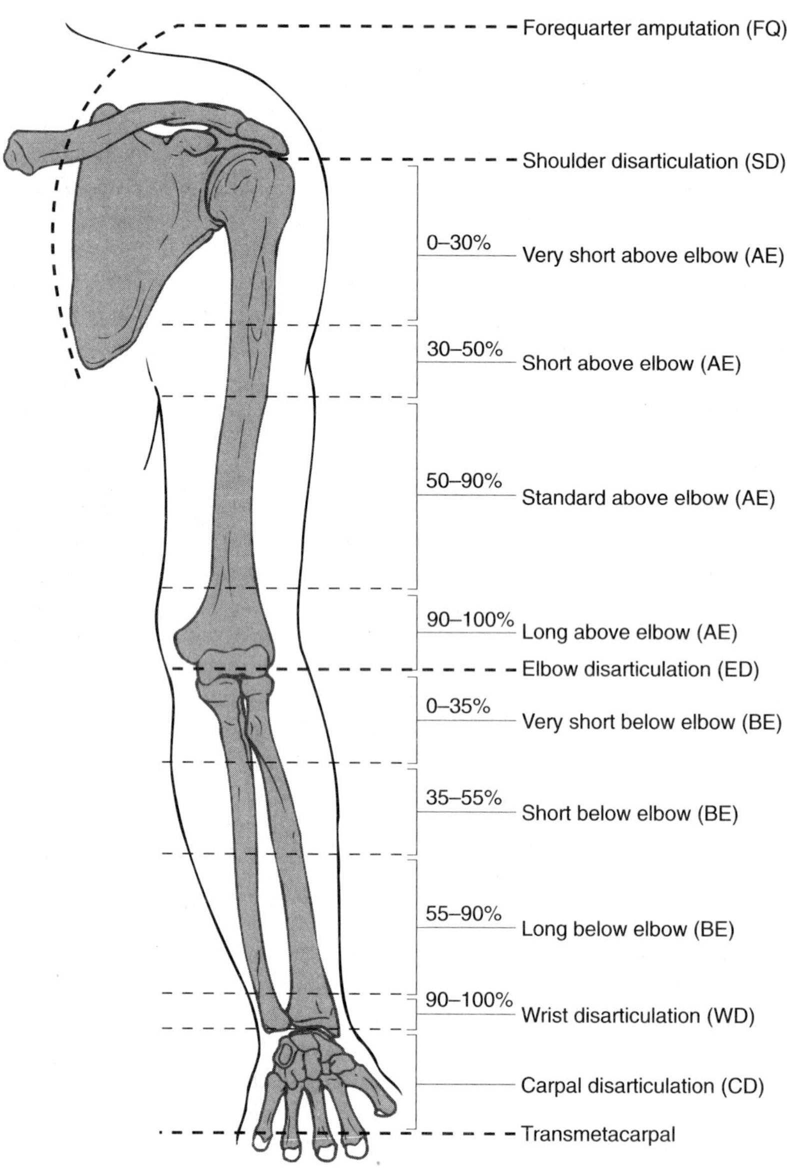

securely against the palm of the hand. The prerequisites for a power grasp are sufficient hand width, at least three metacarpal heads, and mobile metacarpophalangeal (MCP) and interphalangeal (IP) joints. The thumb and index finger facilitate control and strengthen grasp, but the middle, ring, and small fingers are also considered key elements. The fifth finger, or so-called small digit, superficially seems unimportant but it prevents the object slipping away from the palm by creating an ulnar cup. It is essential for gripping tools. The index finger provides 50% of the stability and 20% of the strength of the power grasp (6).

The most common type of upper-extremity amputation is the fingertip amputation. Some propose grafting while others propose conservative treatment if the amputation is distal to the distal interphalangeal (DIP) joint. Primary suture or closure by secondary intention is acceptable and prevents the morbidity associated with skin grafting. However with bone exposure, one must shorten the bone or cover using a flap (12). If the amputation is through the IP joint, the condyles are usually shaped to improve cosmesis. Of adults with a fingertip injury and pulp loss, 30% to 50% have cold intolerance or aberration of sensibility regardless of the technique used (6).

The flexors and extensors of the hand are treated differently than other upper-extremity muscles. Generally, myodesis or myoplasty is advised when sectioning muscles and tendons. In the hand, however, the flexor and extensor tendons are divided and allowed to retract. These tendons are not sewn together. This prevents the development of a finger flexor condition, known as *quadriga.* Amputation through the middle phalanx distal to the flexor digitorum sublimis (FDS) preserves functional flexion of the middle phalanx. However, if the FDS insertion cannot be preserved, amputation through the proximal interphalangeal (PIP) joint is usually performed.

With loss of the long or ring finger at the level of the MCP joint, or the presence of a very short digital residuum, small objects can fall out of the hand. If the individual cannot voluntarily flex the digital remnant, or the amputation is at the level of the MCP joint, a ray deletion or transposition may increase function and improve cosmesis. If transposition is not possible, then deletion with closure of the central defect creates a functional and cosmetic hand.

Ray amputations are often done electively to minimize disability from a previous injury to a digit. This is usually not done at the time of trauma because the patient needs to determine if a digit stump is useful or not. If the index finger is very short and cannot be used for pinch, the remnant may interfere with the individual pinching between the thumb and the middle finger. Since the index finger provides stability to the power grip, significant effort is made to preserve the length and sensation of the index finger, particularly in manual laborers. Resection of the index ray can reduce grip strength by 20%, but can markedly improve cosmesis (13).

Though the underlying pathology primarily dictates the level of amputation, the patient's lifestyle and occupation also impact this decision. The jeweler who has lost an index finger at the MCP joint requires preservation of a precise pinch, or if not possible, hand reconstruction to restore precise pinch. This may require resection of the index ray to prevent it from mechanically interfering with opposition of the thumb and long finger. However, digit loss at the same level in a construction worker dictates a different approach. In this case, preservation of the ray of the index finger preserves power grip by preserving palmar width and stability.

The thumb provides 40% to 50% of hand function and 30% of upper-extremity function. It is important for power and precision grasp. Length, sensation, and stability of the thumb for opposition are high priorities. When indicated, skin grafting can preserve length, allowing sufficient residuum for pinch and grip. The precise length needed to preserve thumb function is controversial, but a minimum length of 2 cm has been proposed (14). Distraction, bone grafting, and phalangealization of the first web space are options available to lengthen the thumb remnant. It is important to remember that the replanted thumb, as well as the reconstructed thumb, will not necessarily have normal function (15). If pollicization is required, the index finger is the best digit to use (16).

For multiple-digit amputation, it is important to remember that rudimentary grasp requires a cleft between two opposing poles that are rotated to be opposite to each other or can be adducted together (parallel adduction).

Wrist Disarticulation

In the past, WD gained popularity because it preserves the articular surface of the distal radioulnar joint and maximal forearm supination and pronation. WD provides a tolerant end-bearing surface. The shape of the distal end is conducive to a self-suspending socket, though additional straps may be required for heavy work (17).

WD has disadvantages, however. The broad distal socket required to accommodate the residual styloid processes makes fabricating an aesthetically acceptable prosthesis difficult. The styloid prominences can be reduced at the time of disarticulation but some of the advantage of the wide distal residual limb for a self-suspending socket is lost. The addition of a prosthetic wrist unit, which allows for an interchange of TDs such as hands and hooks on the prosthesis, can make the artificial limb longer than the intact arm. This is more obvious with a prosthetic hand than with a hook. Extra length reduces cosmesis and interferes with midline hand to mouth activities. Consequently, the selection of wrist units and TDs is limited. Additionally, if a person's goal is to use a myoelectric prosthesis, disarticulation is a poor choice because myoelectric units also add length to the prosthetic forearm. A long transradial amputation would be a better choice if the patient is a candidate for a myoelectric prosthesis.

Transradial or Below-Elbow Amputation

For transradial or BE amputation, the forearm is divided into three lengths: the distal, middle, and proximal thirds. It is important to conserve all possible length of the limb (18), with a minimum of 10 cm below the lateral epicondyle of the humerus being preferred. Individuals with a very short forearm remnant have difficulty tolerating the weight of a BE prosthesis. However, it is worthwhile to save even 4 to 5 cm of the limb if the brachialis is intact and the biceps brachii can be divided and transferred to the ulna, to add control and facilitate prosthetic fitting (19). The radius and ulna are typically sectioned at the same length. The elbow joint should be saved whenever feasible. Natural flexion and extension are preserved and one less prosthetic joint is required. Many authors contend that preservation of the elbow cannot be overemphasized (1).

A longer residuum provides a greater lever arm and consequently greater forearm strength and power. Greater forearm rotation is preserved. An amputation at 2 cm or more proximal to the wrist allows more room for prosthetic components (1,20). At this level, approximately 70% to 80% of natural pronation and supination are preserved. As the forearm length decreases to 60% or shorter, there is rapid loss of rotation until no natural pronation or supination is preserved. Without natural forearm supination and pronation, a method of rotating the forearm must be incorporated in the prosthesis.

Elbow Disarticulation

Elbow disarticulation (ED) has several advantages. Preservation of the humeral condylar flares facilitates prosthetic suspension. Because the humeral condyles fit snugly into the prosthetic socket, humeral rotation is efficiently transmitted to the prosthesis. ED provides a longer lever arm than an AE amputation does. Additionally, the distal end is pressure tolerant since the articular cartilage is preserved.

Cosmesis is the primary disadvantage of ED. The distal end of the prosthesis is bulky. Fewer prosthetic elbows are available. At this level, outside locking elbow hinges are required but they can damage clothing and reduce cosmesis. Myoelectric elbow units, such as the Utah arm, also create an abnormally long prosthetic arm. To avoid this length differential, it is possible to fit the patient with a hybrid prosthesis fabricated with both body-powered and electronic components.

Transhumeral Amputation

Amputation through the humerus can be done at several levels. The transcondylar amputation, like ED, preserves the condylar flares which can transmit humeral rotation to the prosthesis. Like ED, an external hinge elbow joint is required, since other elbow units make the prosthetic limb abnormally long. The remaining humeral condyles require a socket with a wide distal end, detracting from the overall appearance of the prosthesis.

A residual limb that is at least 10 cm long, measuring from the axillary fold, is preferred according to many sources. The greater the upper-limb loss, the less humeral rotation is preserved. Designing the prosthesis with an internal locking prosthetic elbow joint with a turntable for internal and external rotation (21) offsets this loss to some degree.

Shoulder Disarticulation and Forequarter Amputation

Amputations at this level are uncommon. Tumor is the primary cause (22), while major trauma is the second most frequent cause. Less than 3% of traumatic upper-extremity amputations occur at this level (23). Traumatic amputation at this level is frequently secondary to avulsion forces.

Congenital deficiency occurs infrequently at this level. Like congenital deficiency at other levels, these limbs rarely need revision. Congenital limb absence often involves the additional problem of bony malformations and vestiges of missing portions of the limb; therefore, prosthetic fitting is often more challenging. A full understanding of the anatomy and function of the congenitally deficient limb is key for proper prosthesis selection and fitting, especially if surgical revision is being considered.

Cosmesis is a major problem (Fig. 31-2). If the scapula can be retained, disfigurement is less than that with a FQ limb loss. Though amputation through the surgical neck of the humerus is functionally equivalent to SD, retention of the surgical neck preserves shoulder fullness, width, and contours. Not only is this aesthetically more pleasing, but also the shoulder contours provide a more stable purchase for the prosthetic socket. Additionally, the shoulder contour significantly affects the fit of clothing. This is particularly important for women's clothing, such as bras and other undergarments. The contour and symmetry of the female breast are relatively preserved because the pectoralis major insertion is not disrupted as with SD. Lastly, if the deltoid remains, it potentially can be used as a site for myoelectric control.

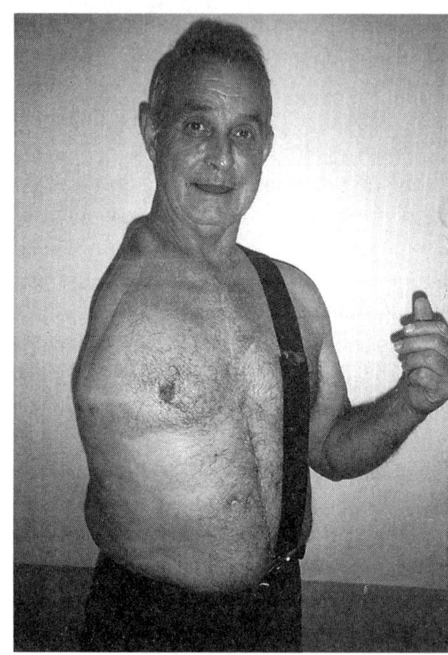

Figure 31-2. Forequarter amputation results in the loss of the normal shoulder contour and profile.

At this level, the upper-extremity residuum provides minimal function. The more proximal an amputation is, the less functional are the available prostheses. Clinically, it is observed that the more proximal the upper-extremity amputation is, the higher the prosthetic rejection rate is. Clinical experience suggests that externally powered prostheses are rejected less frequently than body-powered prostheses. The externally powered hand is more cosmetic and more functional than the mechanical hand or hook (24,25). However, these prostheses are heavy. Because these prostheses are expensive, many funding agencies will not finance an externally powered prostheses at this level of amputation.

Juvenile Amputees

Though the surgical principles of pediatric amputation are similar to those for the adult, there are two major distinctions: A disarticulation is preferred to a transdiaphyseal section and more heroic efforts are indicated to conserve length (26). In children, epiphyseal preservation is important. The growth potential of the distal epiphyses is greater than that of the proximal radial and ulnar epiphyses, while in the humerus, the proximal epiphysis has greater growth potential.

Disarticulation allows for undisturbed epiphyseal bone growth, preserving longitudinal growth. Disarticulation also prevents the development of bony overgrowth at the terminal bone. Since bony prominences (e.g., condyles) become less prominent with age, disarticulation does not present the same cosmetic problems that are seen in adults.

In children, bony overgrowth at the site of a traumatic amputation is the most common postamputation complication. Occurring in about 10% to 30% of pediatric metaphyseal or diaphyseal transections, bony overgrowth is most common in children less than 12 years old (27). Disarticulation prevents this complication.

The earliest sign of bony overgrowth is the development of an adventitious bursa between the distal end of the transected bone and the soft tissues. Typically an advancing bony spike develops, irritating the bursa and local tissues. Not only pain develops, but also local infection can occur. Terminal bone overgrowth occurs most often after humeral transection, followed by fibular, tibial, and femoral transections (27,28).

Studies have shown that bony overgrowth is additive appositional bone growth from the distal end of the transected bone. Epiphysiodesis does not control the problem since the bony overgrowth is not the result of epiphyseal growth. In fact, epiphysiodesis will unnecessarily shorten the residual limb, potentially causing further functional and cosmetic loss. Interestingly, bony overgrowth typically stops with skeletal maturity (29).

Bony overgrowth occurs primarily in children who have had a surgical or traumatic amputation. Children with a congenitally deficient limb, particularly those with amniotic band syndrome (30,31), may develop bony overgrowth. This problem is also seen in adults whose amputations are secondary to an electrical injury (32,33).

If prosthetic modification cannot control the problems associated with bony overgrowth, surgical resection remains the most effective option (34). Resection is required in about 10% of children (34).

OVERVIEW OF PROSTHETICS FOR THE UPPER EXTREMITY

Prostheses can be categorized in many ways: exoskeletal versus endoskeletal design, passive versus active, body-powered versus externally powered, and by anatomic level. Prostheses can also be identified by the stage of prosthetic restoration and rehabilitation.

The prosthesis with a rigid external structure is called an *exoskeletal prosthesis*. This type of prosthesis is more durable than the endoskeletal prosthesis, which has a rigid internal structure but a soft exterior. The hard external layer of the exoskeletal prosthesis allows this prosthesis to withstand contact with hard or sharp surfaces. The

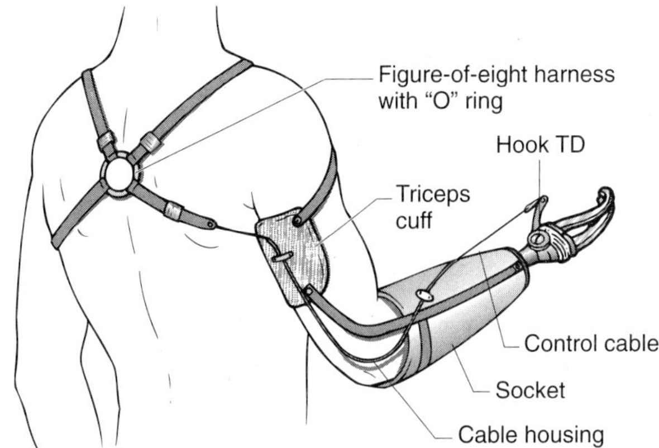

Figure 31-3. Illustration of a typical body-powered, or conventional, cable-controlled below-elbow prosthesis with a hook terminal device (TD).

endoskeletal prosthesis has a soft removable outer cover, which allows easy access to the prosthetic components. Though endoskeletal designs often weigh less, exoskeletal prostheses are typically prescribed because of superior durability.

Some prostheses provide no active function, passively replacing the missing body part. The appearance resembles the missing limb. These prostheses are chosen for cosmesis and their relative light weight. Highly sophisticated and nearly perfect anatomic replicas of the missing limb are available but are very expensive.

Prostheses are also classified by power source, that is, body-powered versus externally powered prostheses. The body-powered prosthesis uses a system of straps and cables to transfer energy of one body part to the prosthesis to perform a specific motion (Fig. 31-3). For example, the AE amputee uses scapular and humeral motion to operate a prosthetic elbow and hand. Externally powered systems rely on an external source of energy to operate the prosthesis. The most frequently used externally powered prosthesis employs the myoelectric control system, but other systems exist, including electric switch controls. Myoelectric prostheses use the electrical potential of a muscle to voluntarily operate components of the prosthesis, for example, to open and close a prosthetic hand (Fig. 31-4).

Prostheses are also identified by the stage of rehabilitation: the temporary and the definitive prosthesis. The temporary prosthesis, also called a *preparatory* or *provisional prosthesis*, is used while the residual limb volume is stabilizing and the individual is learning how to use a prosthesis. This period also allows the amputee to determine which prosthetic components and options are most appropriate. A preparatory prosthesis can be very simple. For example, materials used to make the temporary socket can range from casting materials to sophisticated thermoplastics. Though the provisional or preparatory prosthesis is made with the same attention to fit and function as the definitive prosthesis, the materials of the temporary prosthesis are

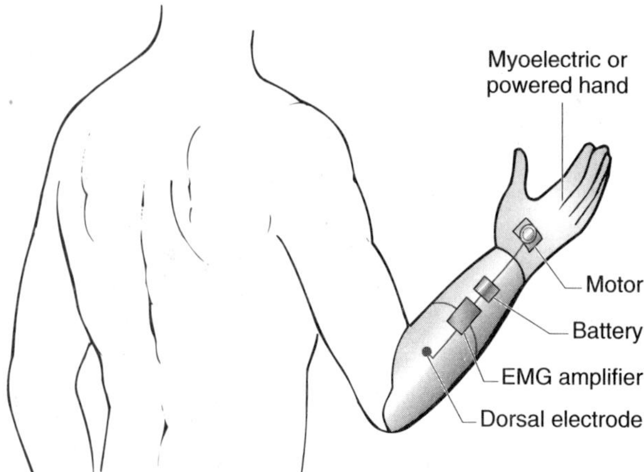

Figure 31-4. A typical myoelectrically controlled below-elbow prosthesis with a hand terminal device. EMG = electromyograph.

not as durable as those of the definitive prosthesis. The preparatory prosthesis is modified periodically to meet the amputee's advancing skill and to accommodate changes in the residual limb volume and shape. At this phase of rehabilitation, the final design of the prosthesis is still evolving.

The definitive prosthesis is the final or permanent prosthesis prescribed and fabricated for the individual. It is prescribed after the residual limb volume has stabilized and when the patient is experienced using a prosthesis and the patient and the rehabilitation team have determined the most appropriate prosthetic design.

The Principle of Early Prosthetic Fitting

The most important development in the last 15 years of upper-extremity prosthetics is the realization that upper-extremity amputees need to be fitted for a prosthesis early. Malone et al (35) found that patients fitted within 30 days of upper-extremity amputation, sometimes called "Malone's golden period," demonstrate the greatest success in prosthetic acceptance and use. Previous to these observations, most patients were fitted with an upper-extremity prosthesis 3 to 6 months after surgery, or even later. The rejection rate was as high as 50%. Fitting a prosthesis within 4 weeks of upper-extremity amputation dramatically improves the long-term outcome. Some (36) centers report success rates as high as 90%.

Early prosthetic fitting preserves bimanual upper-extremity patterns, increasing prosthetic acceptance and use. Minimizing the time period between loss of bilateral upper-extremity activity and the return of bilateral function through prosthetic restoration maximizes success. If prosthetic fitting is delayed, patients quickly learn to be "one handed" and forfeit the use of a prosthesis. They do activities with one hand or expect others to perform two-handed activities for them. Some will avoid bimanual activities alltogether. The goal of independence is jeopardized.

Patients can be fitted while still in the operating room or fitted early (i.e., within the first 2 weeks) after amputation. The techniques of immediate or early fitting remain underutilized, even though studies of both techniques have demonstrated high acceptance rates without jeopardizing wound healing (36–38). Early fitting appears to be the single most important variable predicting successful prosthetic use.

Preparatory Prostheses

The *immediate postoperative prosthesis fitting technique* is available, but it is used infrequently. While still in the operating room, the patient is fitted with an immediate postoperative prosthesis made of a rigid dressing with minimal, but functional prosthetic components attached. The socket can be applied once the surgical incision is closed. Initially, the incision is dressed with a light layer of bandages, and plaster or fiberglass is used to form a socket on the patient's residual limb. The immediate postoperative prosthesis functions as the final wound dressing.

Immediate postoperative fitting has many advantages, including controlling postoperative edema and pain. Reducing postoperative edema minimizes postoperative pain and phantom pain. The immediate postoperative prosthesis conditions and shapes the residual limb, preparing it for future prosthetic fitting. Additionally, the immediate postoperative prosthesis allows the occupational therapist (OT) to begin training almost immediately. It is important that prosthetic training does not begin before the surgeon agrees. In some cases, the surgeon may allow the OT to begin training within the first 24 hours of surgery, whereas others prefer waiting several days. As a result, the amputee experiences the immediate usefulness of the residual limb and the prosthesis.

While immediate postoperative fitting sounds ideal, it requires an experienced, multidisciplinary, surgical and prosthetic rehabilitation team, available to fit the prosthesis in the operating or recovery room and to ensure that the fit is correct to prevent tissue damage and risk further limb loss. Most amputations are the result of trauma, however, and there is limited time to assemble an experienced multidisciplinary team.

Early fitting of a temporary prosthesis is more common than the immediate fitting approach. Once sutures are removed, about 1 to 2 weeks after surgery, fitting is begun. Though early fitting occurs during Malone's golden period, some (36) question whether use of the early fitting technique results in as much acceptance as use of the immediate fitting approach. However, many investigators (35,37–41) found no appreciable difference between the success rate of prosthetic use between the two prosthetic fitting techniques.

Many of the same advantages of immediate postoperative fitting are also seen with early prosthetic fitting. Bimanual activities are preserved and prosthetic acceptance is high. However, the early fitting approach has additional advantages, including allowing a longer time for the incised tissues to heal and allowing the prosthetist more time to design and fabricate an individualized prosthesis and use a greater variety of prosthetic components.

The bilateral upper-extremity amputee must receive a prosthesis early. Without a prosthesis, the amputee is dependent in virtually all aspects of everyday life. The earlier a prosthesis is issued, the earlier training in hygiene, feeding, and self-care can begin. Immediate or early fitting helps to decrease dependency and reduces some of the negative psychological and social impact of bilateral amputation. Though for somewhat different reasons, both the unilateral and the bilateral upper-extremity amputee should be fit early.

The preparatory or provisional prosthesis may be a body-powered, myoelectrically controlled, or a combination or hybrid system. This stage of wearing the preparatory prosthesis is a distinct step in prosthetic restoration and rehabilitation; it involves an evaluation to determine the most appropriate prosthetic design for the individual. During this period, the amputee "test drives" the various prosthetic designs and develops realistic expectations about what a prosthesis can and cannot do. The individual experiences firsthand the advantages and disadvantages of various sockets, suspension systems, elbow and wrist units, hands, and other terminal devices. Unfortunately, some funding agencies do not finance a temporary prosthesis and will only pay for a permanent prosthesis. As a result, the amputee's financial situation may not allow for an evaluation of various prosthetic designs.

Definitive Prostheses

The final or definitive prosthesis represents the culmination of all the experience and information gained during the preparatory phase. The definitive prosthesis is the permanent one, the prosthesis the person is "going to live with" (Fig. 31-5). Test driving various provisional designs ensures that no major oversights occur in the design of the permanent prosthesis. Like the provisional prosthesis, the definitive prosthesis can be body powered, myoelectric, or a hybrid of both. The permanent prosthesis, which must withstand all types of activities over the long term, is constructed with more durable materials than is the provisional prosthesis.

Upper-Extremity Prosthetic Control Systems

The body-powered prosthesis, also called a *mechanical prosthesis*, is the conventional upper-extremity prosthesis. Estimates indicate that 90% of upper-extremity amputees who use a prosthesis use a body-powered system at least part time. Amputees prefer this system because it is relatively inexpensive, durable, reliable, and functional. This system provides some sensory feedback via the cables and harness control systems (42). Many prefer the speed of operation and accuracy of body-powered prostheses. Because they do not require external sources of power, there are no batteries to recharge or replace. However, many do not like the appearance of body-powered prostheses. In general, they are less aesthetic and do not have "the high-tech" appeal of the myoelectric system. A body-powered prosthesis has a weaker grip than the myoelectric one, but it is more durable for manual work such as lifting (43–45).

The myoelectric system is the externally powered system of choice and is the preference of many amputees. It harnesses the electrical potential of a contracting muscle to operate the prosthesis (Fig. 31-6). These prostheses require minimal proximal muscle control and can be used in all planes of motion (e.g., overhead reaching). Compared to body-powered prostheses, myoelectric prostheses provide a stronger, graded grasp. Though more expensive than body-powered prostheses, they are often more cosmetic since many do not require a harness for suspension. However, some myoelectric TDs, such as the Greifer hook, are bulky and robot-looking. This appearance is unacceptable to some (Fig. 31-7).

Myoelectric prostheses are expensive. They are comparatively fragile devices and frequently break down. Greater technical skill is needed to repair and maintain these systems. Unlike the body-powered prostheses, myoelectric systems do not tolerate many environmental factors, such as dust and moisture. They are not as durable or as well suited as body-powered prostheses for manual labor. Because the weight of the prosthesis is not transferred to more proximal body parts, as in the body-powered systems, myoelectric prostheses create more pressure at the point of suspension, the distal part of the limb. Additionally, they feel heavier to the user.

Precise criteria for determining the ideal control system for each person do not exist. The patient's lifestyle, needs, funding source, and personal preference dominate the choice. Frequently, amputees own both a body-powered and a myoelectric prosthesis and then wear the prosthesis most appropriate for a particular situation. For example, the construction worker may use a body-powered system on the job, but wear a myoelectric prosthesis at social events (46). Recently, hybrid systems, with both body-powered and myoelectric components, have become more popular, since these systems can provide the advantage of both body power and myoelectric power.

In summary, a typical prosthetic restoration and rehabilitation schedule has several stages. Initially, the amputee is fitted with a prosthesis in the immediate or early postamputation period. Over the next 2 to 6 weeks, fitting and training with a preparatory body-powered prosthesis occur. Once trained, and after prosthetic needs are determined, the amputee is fitted with a definitive body-powered prosthesis. Typically, the amputee is ready for a definitive body-powered prosthesis approximately 6 to 12 weeks after amputation. As a general rule, a person is fitted with a body-powered prosthesis first. Once the individual is successfully using the body-powered prosthesis, he or she is evaluated for the more expensive myoelectric system.

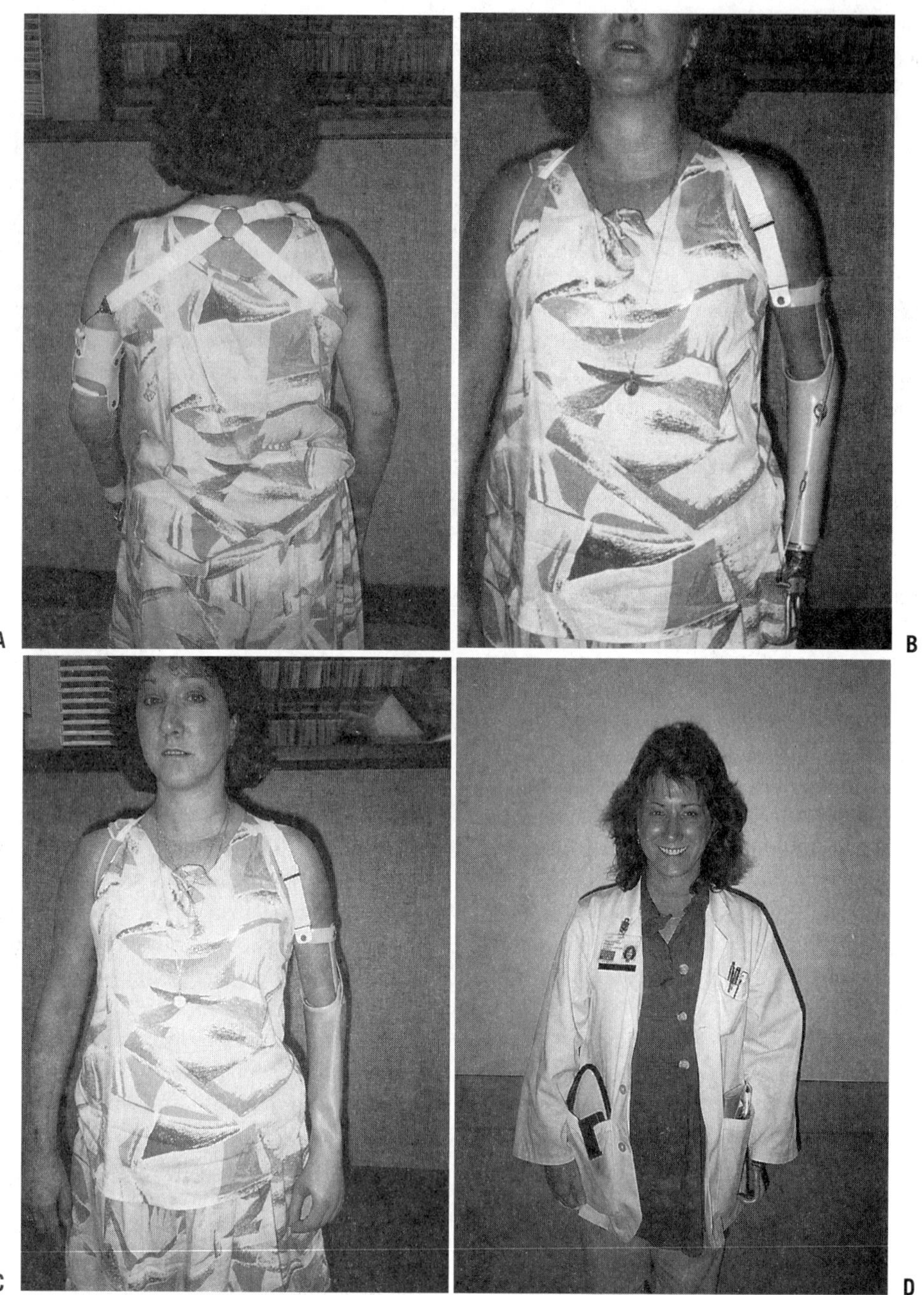

Figure 31-5. The amputee is fitted with a prosthesis in stages. *A.* First, a preparatory or provisional prosthesis is fabricated. After a period of prosthetic training and use, the individual is fitted with a definitive body-powered prosthesis. *B.* Definitive left below-elbow prosthesis with a hook but without a cosmetic cover. *C.* The same prosthesis with cosmetic glove and hand. *D.* The definitive prosthesis used for everyday activities.

In some cases, the preparatory myoelectric fitting phase may begin prior to the completion of the definitive body-powered prosthesis phase. Approximately 4 to 6 months after surgery, the amputee completes the final steps of myoelectric prosthesis training.

Harness

The harness provides suspension and a way to control the active parts of the prosthesis. The type of socket and the intimacy of the fit between the socket and the residual limb also provide suspension. The harness is composed of a collection of strategically placed straps around the shoulder or thorax to transmit the force of proximal body motion to the prosthetic components. The straps, which are typically made of Dacron, must be carefully placed and fitted so that body power is efficiently transmitted to the active prosthetic components.

A cable system is secured proximally on the harness

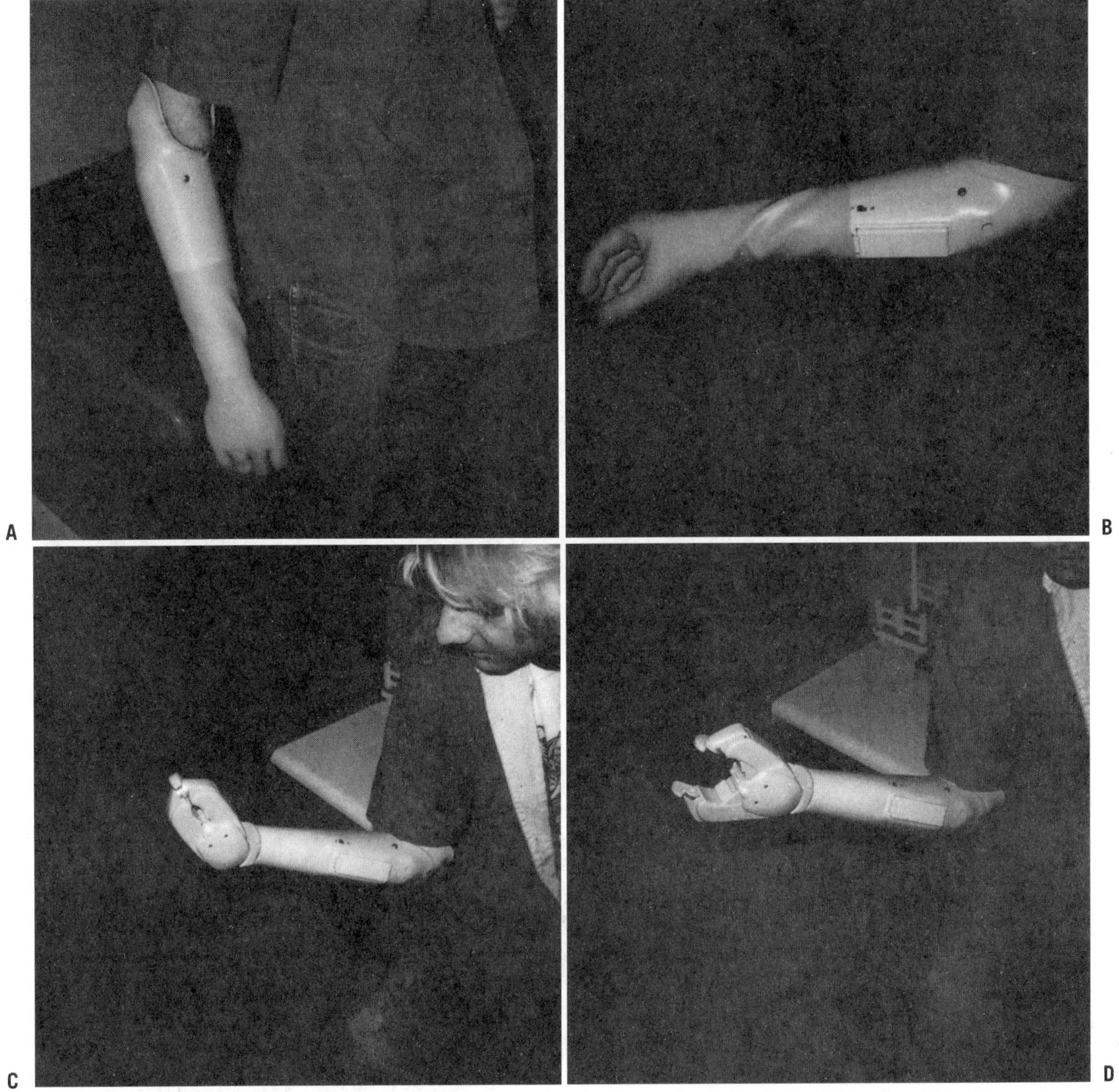

Figure 31-6. Myoelectric prosthesis with a wrist rotator, prosthetic hand, and polyvinyl chloride glove. The rectangular compartment on the medial aspect of the forearm contains the battery that powers the prosthesis.

and terminates on the TD. There are two basic types: the single control system, which typically operates the TD for the BE amputee; and the dual control system required by the AE amputee. The amputee transmits muscle tension along the stainless-steel cables of the prosthesis to perform the desired motion. For example, in the BE amputee, the cable terminates on the TD. The OT trains the patient to perform coordinated movements of arm flexion and shoulder abduction to operate the TD. The body-powered AE prosthesis uses the same principles but requires a second cable to control the elbow unit.

PROSTHESES BY LEVEL OF AMPUTATION

Partial Hand Prosthesis

A partial hand prosthesis or orthosis is useful only if it increases function with minimal impairment of sensation and residual hand function or if it improves cosmesis. Typically, a prosthesis is not required to improve function if two or more digits remain. With two remaining digits, a person is able to adduct or oppose one finger to the other. If opposition is not possible with the remaining digits, a rotation osteotomy may be considered in an attempt to

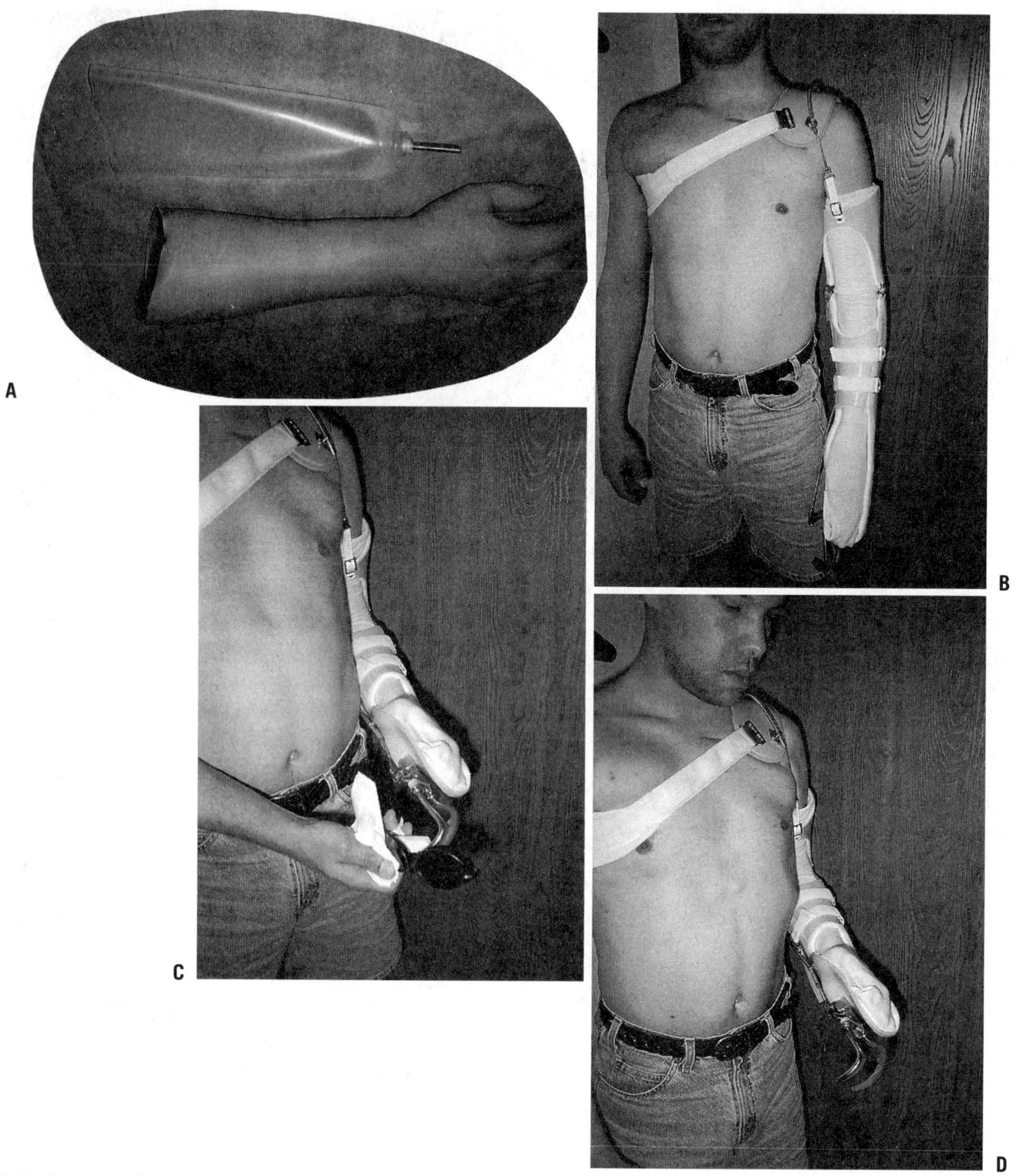

Figure 31-7. Self-contained myoelectrically powered prosthesis with a wrist rotator and Greifer hook. On the medial aspect of the prosthetic forearm there is a panel to access the battery. A functional arm orthosis. A hook is present on the palm of the hand, as would be needed after a partial hand amputation. Because of the flail upper extremity, chest expansion activates the hook. However, a partial hand amputee would use arm muscles to activate the hook.

create opposition. If only the thumb remains, an orthosis that provides a surface for opposition can be fabricated.

A partial hand amputation weakens grasp. Grasp strength can be improved by fitting the person with a prosthesis with a hook, for example, to assist heavy lifting or other work. The prosthesis is cable driven and the hook protrudes from the palmar surface of the hand. This provides a fine tweezer-like grasp but covers part of the sensate residual hand. In addition, this prosthesis is difficult to use overhead (see Fig. 31-7). Because of its appearance, many patients do not accept the partial hand body-powered prosthesis with a hook.

Cosmesis is the number one concern for some individuals with this level of amputation. Personal preference

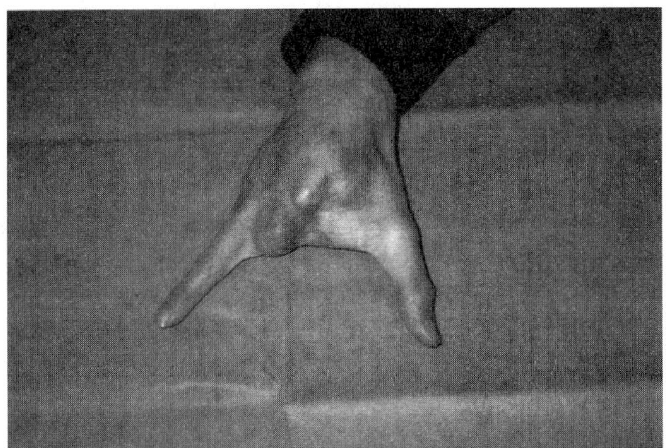

A

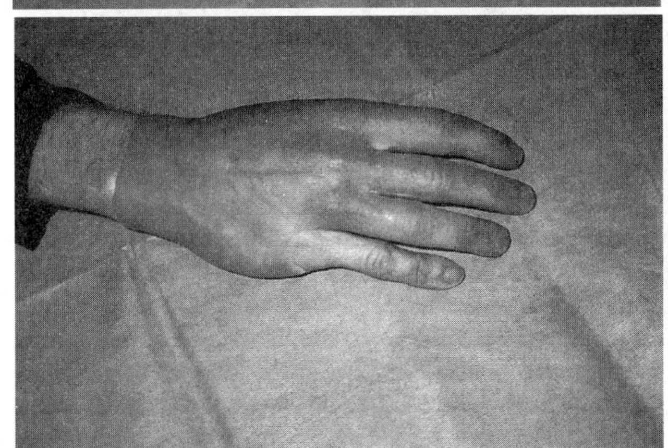

B

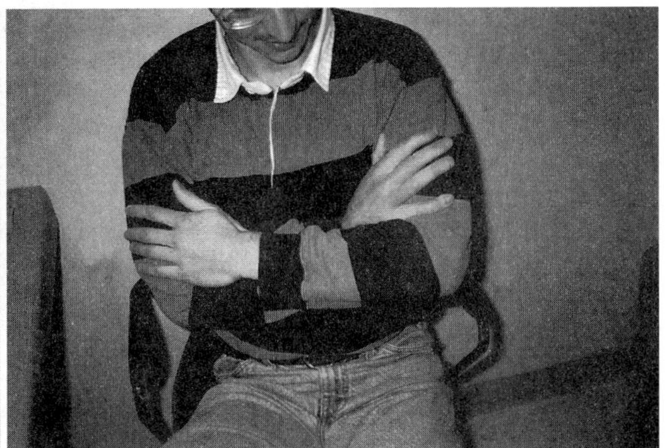

C

Figure 31-8. For this individual with a partial hand amputation, a cosmetic prosthesis creates a very natural-appearing limb.

or vocational demands may require a very natural-appearing passive prosthesis (Fig. 31-8). Because the intact human hand changes color with position, activity, or ambient temperature, a prosthesis cannot perfectly replicate the human hand. A passive hand improves appearance while allowing the person to use the hand for limited pushing or as a gross assist.

Cosmetic gloves to cover the TD of a prosthesis are available. Though some very expensive gloves are near-perfect replicas of the hand, the cost and quality of cosmetic gloves vary. Most cosmetic gloves provide satisfactory cosmesis and are fairly inexpensive. Cosmetic gloves must be cared for properly to preserve their appearance. They are also easily torn, stained, and damaged.

Terminal Devices

The TD is the most distal component of an upper-extremity prosthesis. A TD is either active or passive. A passive TD is usually very light and has no moving parts. However, some passive TDs are function specific; for example, designed to hold a golf club (Figs. 31-9 and 31-10) (47).

The typical active prehension TD is a hook, hand, or specialized device or tool with moveable parts (Fig. 31-11). The opening width of the TD must be compatible with the ability to handle common objects. TDs can be voluntary opening (VO) or voluntary closing (VC). The hook TD has two "fingers," one stationary and one moveable. The amputee activates the hook using either a body-powered or myoelectric control system.

A variety of hooks are available, but the most frequently prescribed VO hook is the Hosmer-Dorrance No. 5 with neoprene grips. The tension of a VO TD opens the fingers against resistance (i.e., rubber bands), and it is this resistant force that holds an object if there is no cable tension produced.

The VC TD creates more exact tension to hold an object because the tension created in the cable results from voluntary muscle contraction rather than the elastic action of a spring or other elastic materials. As a result, the VC hook has the advantage of providing graded prehension and provides a stronger grip, as much as 20 to 25 lb (9.00–11.25 kg) of force.

Many hook designs and sizes, ranging from infant to adult, are available to meet the demands of the individual amputee (see Fig. 31-11). The VC TD, though more analogous to the human hand, is less popular than the VO TD. The rehabilitation team needs to assist the individual in selecting the most appropriate TD.

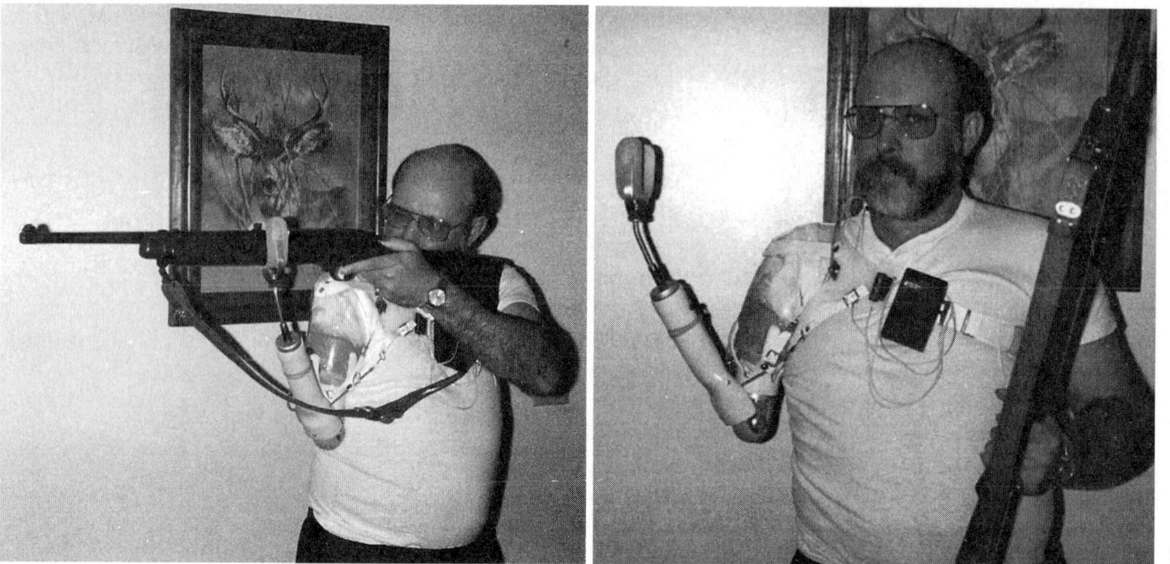
Figure 31-9. *A, B.* This specialized rifle-holding terminal device allows this individual to participate in recreational target shooting. This prosthesis is a preparatory short above-elbow prosthesis.

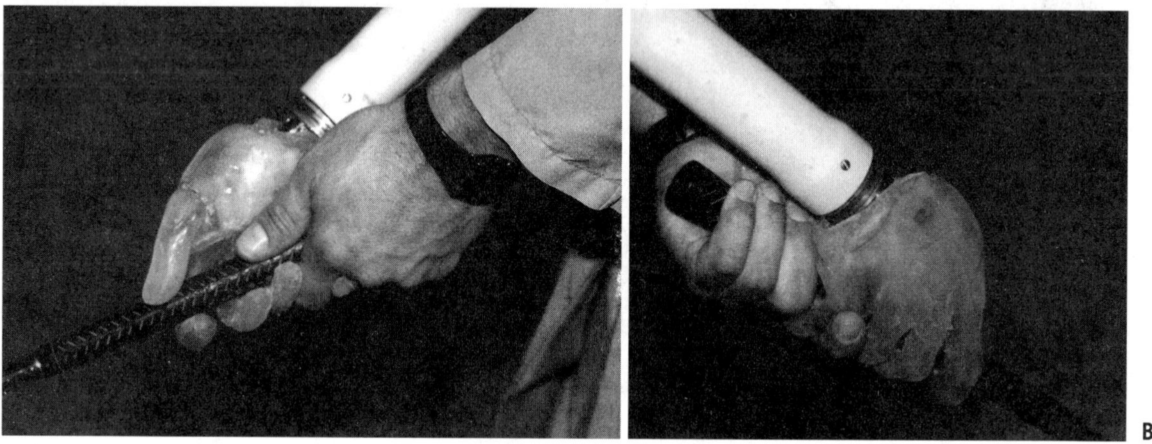
Figure 31-10. *A, B.* This terminal device is made specifically for holding a golf club.

In the conventional body-powered prosthesis, the number of rubber bands located at the base of the hook fingers determines the grip force of the TD. One rubber band is equivalent to approximately 1 lb (0.45 kg) of pinch between the two hook fingers. By producing tension on the cable, the amputee is able to open or close the hook (Fig. 31-12). Though a hook is more functional, the amputee may reject it for social and cosmetic reasons.

Prosthetic hands are bulkier and more difficult to use than hooks. Hook TDs provide a more precise grip. The mechanical hand, which is bodypowered, provides only 3 lb of grip force while a myoelectric hand can provide 25 lb (11.25 kg). However, both hands appear the same if a cosmetic glove is worn over the TD.

Because of the advantages and disadvantages of the hook and the hand, most patients prefer a prosthesis design that allows them to change the TD depending on the situation, for example, cutting the lawn versus going to a wedding. If the individual intends to vary the TD, a quick disconnect wrist is preferred over a friction wrist, which is screwed onto the prosthesis.

Below-Elbow Prosthesis

For UE amputation the elbow is the point of reference, that is, AE or BE amputation. This terminology is easy to understand and readily conveys the same information to the physician, the therapist, and prosthetist. One can readily generalize about the upper-extremity function remaining, the function lost, and the basic prosthetic components needed. However, terms such as *transradial* and *transhumeral* are more accurate anatomic descriptions and are consistent with terms used for other common levels of

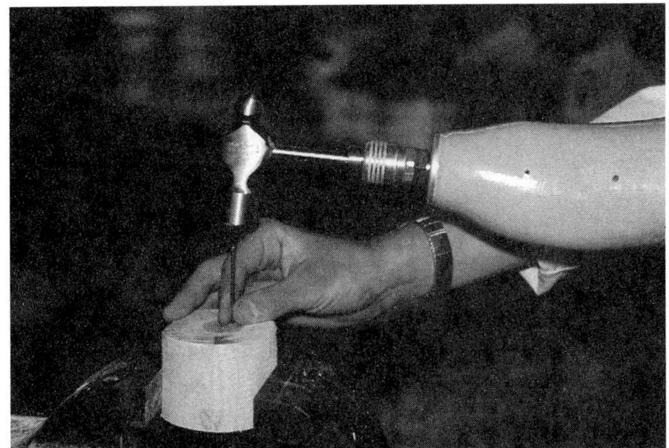

A

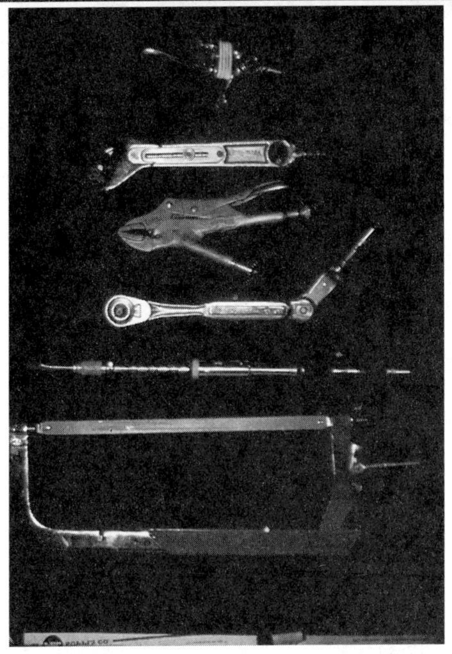

B

Figure 31-11. A variety of tools that are also terminal devices.

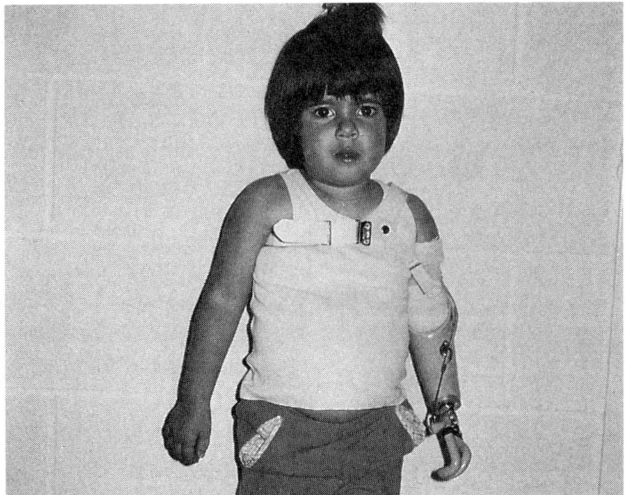

A

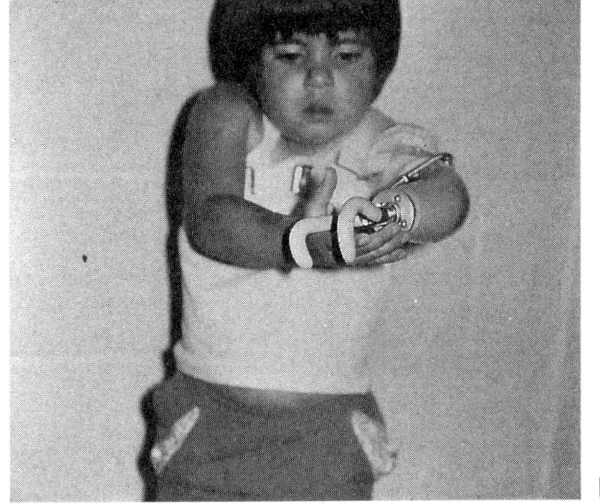

B

Figure 31-12. This child demonstrates how to use humeral flexion to open the terminal device of the body-powered below-elbow prosthesis.

amputation, such as WD and transmetacarpal amputation. Though the terms *transradial* and *transhumeral* are preferred, the terms *above elbow (AE)* and *below elbow (BE)* are well established in the professional literature.

With the loss of the wrist, and possibly forearm rotation, the BE amputee needs a wrist substitute. Three basic types of wrist units are available for conventional prostheses. The first two types provide pronation and supination but not wrist flexion and extension. The amputee must position the wrist unit in the desired position of pronation or supination. The variable friction wrist unit adjusts for variable rotation friction, that is, from loose to tight. Most individuals prefer the quick-change wrist units because the amputee can change the TD quickly.

The third type, the wrist flexion unit, provides not only variable friction for wrist rotation but also wrist flexion. This is an important option for the bilateral amputee, or the person with a nonfunctional contralateral limb, who is dependent on the prosthesis to do midline activities, such as dressing. In the bilateral amputee, this unit is placed on the dominant upper-extremity prosthesis. Unilateral amputees rarely require this type.

These three units fulfill the basic purpose of a wrist unit; that is, they act as a site for attaching and positioning the TD. The wrist units available for the forearm after WD are considerably thinner than the standard wrist unit but typically do not lend to a quick interchange of TDs.

There are three basic types of elbow hinges: the flexible hinges, the rigid hinges, and step-up hinges. In the presence of a long residual forearm, flexible elbow hinges allow natural forearm rotation. Rigid hinges impede this motion. However, because functional pronation and supination motions are lost as the residual forearm becomes shorter, flexible hinges become unnecessary. Rigid hinges are a better option for the shorter residual forearm because more forearm stability is needed.

The individual with a very short limb after transradial amputation can benefit from step-up hinges since

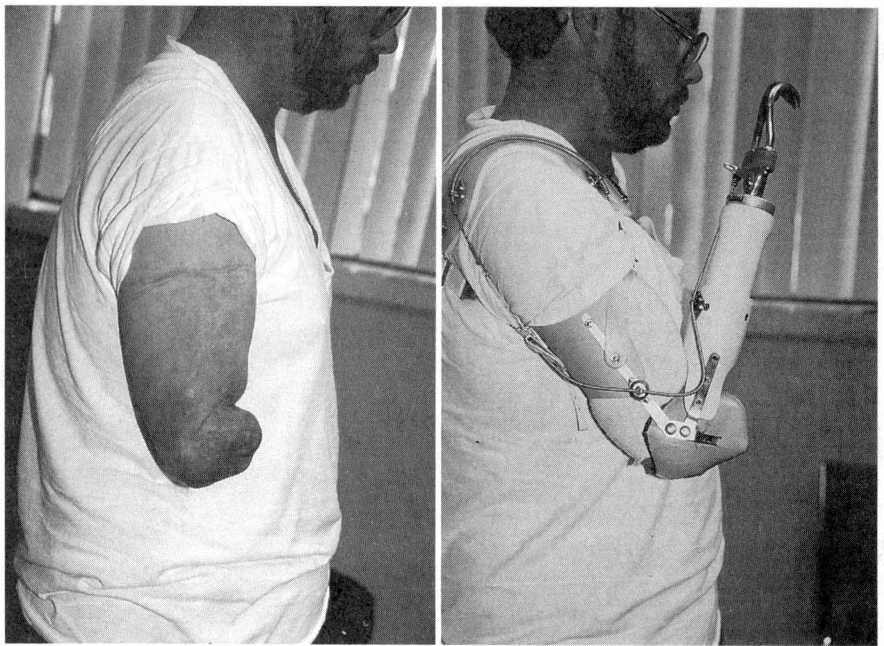

Figure 31-13. A step-up elbow amplifies the amount of natural elbow flexion in the individual with a very short limb after below-elbow amputation.

anatomic elbow flexion is usually limited to less than 90 degrees. These hinges amplify the range of motion (ROM) at the elbow in a ratio of 1:2. For instance, 50 degrees of elbow flexion results in approximately 100 degrees of prosthetic flexion. The step-up hinge design requires that the socket be a separate unit from the prosthetic forearm (split socket design) (Fig. 31-13). Unfortunately, though flexion is increased, the lever arm force is reduced approximately 50%. The force applied to the volar surface of the residual forearm is high and many patients do not tolerate the pressure. This system is preferred for the amputee with a very short residual forearm with limited ROM for whom increased ROM is more important than strength. These hinges can be very useful, particularly for the bilateral upper-extremity amputee.

The distal inner socket in *the long BE*, or *transradial prosthesis*, characteristically is flat to capture the natural pronation and supination of the forearm and to transmit this motion to the TD. The triceps cuff transfers the forces between the socket and the shoulder harness. The Muenster-type socket often is used in the case of the *short BE amputation*. It reduces the amount of suspension needed; however, a cable system is still required to operate the TD.

Two basic types of harnesses are available for the patient who underwent transradial amputation: the figure-of-eight harness and the shoulder harness with a chest strap. Because the figure-of-eight harness allows for the widest range of activities with the least restriction, it is the most common harness used by unilateral and bilateral upper-extremity amputees. It is the harness of choice for women because there is no chest strap to interfere with clothing. A figure-of-nine harness affords more freedom of motion and is an excellent choice for a BE prosthesis, but usually requires supracondylar suspension as well.

Elbow Disarticulation Prosthesis

The person who has undergone ED needs mechanical replacement of elbow flexion and extension. There is little room for a standard prosthetic elbow, however. To avoid making the prosthesis too long when compared to the intact upper extremity, an external locking elbow joint is required rather than the standard internal locking joint. These units are less cosmetic and easily damage clothing. However, ED can be a valuable option for the bilateral amputee who must use a residual limb for self-care. ED is preferred in children to avoid the complication of bony overgrowth associated with diaphyseal amputations.

Because an ED prosthesis requires the individual to control both elbow and TD functions, a dual type of shoulder harness is needed. Humeral rotation, preserved by disarticulation, is captured by configuring the internal distal socket with an oval shape and achieving an intimate socket-limb interface in the region of the humeral condyles. Only about 50% of available humeral rotation is transmitted to the prosthesis, however.

The physical characteristics of the residual limb influence the socket design prescribed. For this level of amputation, there are basically three options available: socket with a fenestration or window, a screw-in type of socket, or a socket with supracondylar wedges. Sockets with pneumatic bladders are available. Though used infrequently, pneumatic bladders are an option for the person

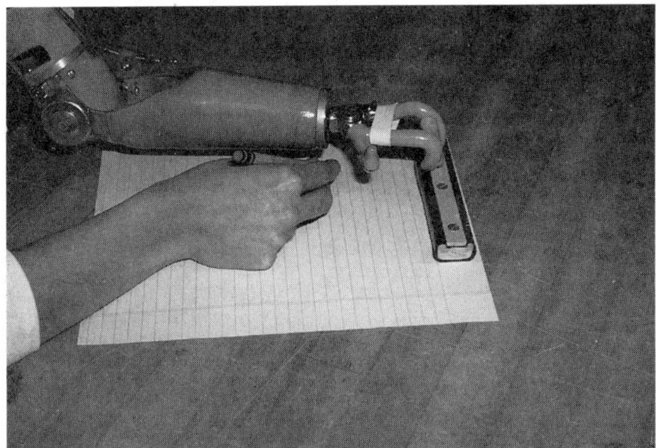

Figure 31-14. An example of an above-elbow prosthesis being used as a functional assist. Note the internal locking elbow unit with an externally attached forearm lift assist (spring loaded).

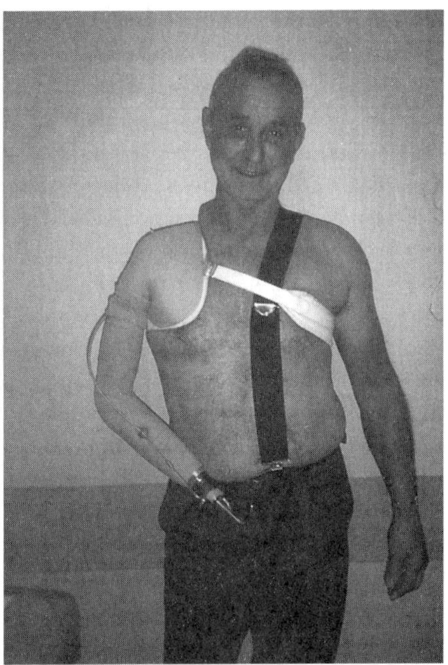

Figure 31-15. Forequarter body-powered prosthesis. The prosthetic components include a chest strap, detachable shoulder cap, single-control terminal device cable, passive locking elbow, quick-change wrist, and hook terminal device.

with a bulbous distal limb or whose limb volume varies significantly.

Sockets with flexible inner liners, like those used for lower-extremity prostheses, are popular among upper-extremity amputees. They are cooler than the standard hard socket. Made of moldable plastics, these liners are thin and accommodate changes in limb shape and volume that occur with muscle contraction. Many amputees find these more comfortable than other sockets.

Above-Elbow Prosthesis

The shorter the remaining humerus is, the more the patient loses rotation, power, and leverage. An amputation at or below the distal third of the humerus affords the amputee many of the advantages of ED, but supracondylar suspension and rotation control are lost. Though scapular motion provides some control, humeral motion provides primary control for the transhumeral prosthesis. A figure-of-eight harness with dual-control design is the most popular system.

Transhumeral amputation that is performed at least 5 cm proximal to the elbow leaves a limb that can accommodate an internal or inside locking elbow unit (Fig. 31-14). The turntable multiple locking elbow unit, which is the most common unit used by the AE amputee, has 11 locking positions. It provides 5 to 135 degrees of flexion, whereas the elbow unit used in a disarticulation prosthesis has only seven positions, or fewer if it is a heavy-duty design. With a body-powered prosthesis, if the elbow is unlocked, pulling the cable flexes the elbow. If however the elbow is locked, a pull on the main cable operates the TD (48).

A residual limb of less than 10 cm after transhumeral amputation can be fitted with an AE prosthesis but often requires a forearm spring lift assist incorporated into the elbow unit. The most proximal transhumeral amputation that results in a functional limb is performed at approximately 5 cm distal to the axillary fold. A shorter residuum is unable to control the prosthetic socket effectively (49).

Hybrids of myoelectric and body-powered systems are very valuable for the AE amputee. A body-powered elbow with a myoelectric hand is a common choice. The myoelectric hand, with its stronger grip and graded control, is valuable for the person whose work or avocation involves a lot of holding and stabilizing objects. The myoelectric elbow with a body-powered TD affords more sensory feedback for the patient who needs feedback regarding TD function.

Shoulder Disarticulation and Forequarter Prostheses

At this level of amputation the majority of upperextremity function is lost. The patient has little residuum to operate a prosthesis. More mechanical replacement is required to compensate for the lost hand, wrist, elbow, and shoulder function (Fig. 31-15). In general, the individual needs a TD, wrist rotator, elbow flexion-extension unit, and a locking turntable. Passive shoulder positioning is required. Not surprisingly, the prosthetic rejection rate is highest among these patients. For some persons, this level of prosthetic replacement represents overgadgetization, that is, more technology than they find functional or tolerable. These individuals often opt for a simple passive prosthesis for aesthetic reasons. Others choose no prosthesis at all.

Depending on the shoulder profile remaining, stabilizing a prosthesis can be difficult. Sockets are fabricated using plastic laminates. Control of perspiration is more problematic than with more distal amputations. The prosthetist is challenged to achieve an intimate socket-limb interface to suspend the prosthesis while providing sufficient ventilation. Moisture-absorbing material placed or worn under the socket (e.g., cotton T-shirt) helps to control perspiration. Antiperspirants that control excess perspiration and need only to be used once or twice weekly are available commercially. The weight of the prosthetic arm creates high pressure over bony prominences. During socket fabrication, sufficient relief must be provided in these areas to avoid pain and skin breakdown.

Some individuals benefit from a prosthetic shoulder joint while others prefer a bulkhead design. With the bulkhead design, the prosthetic humerus is attached directly to the socket and no shoulder motion is provided. Omitting the shoulder unit reduces the weight of the prosthesis, making it very attractive to some amputees. At this level, a lightweight endoskeletal prosthesis is also an option.

Currently, shoulder units require passive positioning. Basic types include the single-axis joint that allows only shoulder abduction, the double-axis unit that provides shoulder flexion and abduction, and the four-way friction shoulder design that allows full passive motion. The shoulder flexion and abduction unit is the most common and most functional.

Cosmetic Prosthesis

For some patients, cosmesis far outweighs the need or desire for a functional prosthesis. Some individuals are not able to operate a prosthesis. Often individuals whose upper extremity was amputated at a very proximal level prefer a cosmetic prosthesis and do not want a prosthesis with active components. Individuals with an FQ amputation or SD may do best with a simple shoulder cap to restore the profile of a normal shoulder (Fig. 31-16). The physician must know the patient and keep in mind that prescribing a prosthesis is typically a compromise between cosmesis and restored function. Hybrid systems of passive and active elements, with body-powered and externally powered components, are often the best choice.

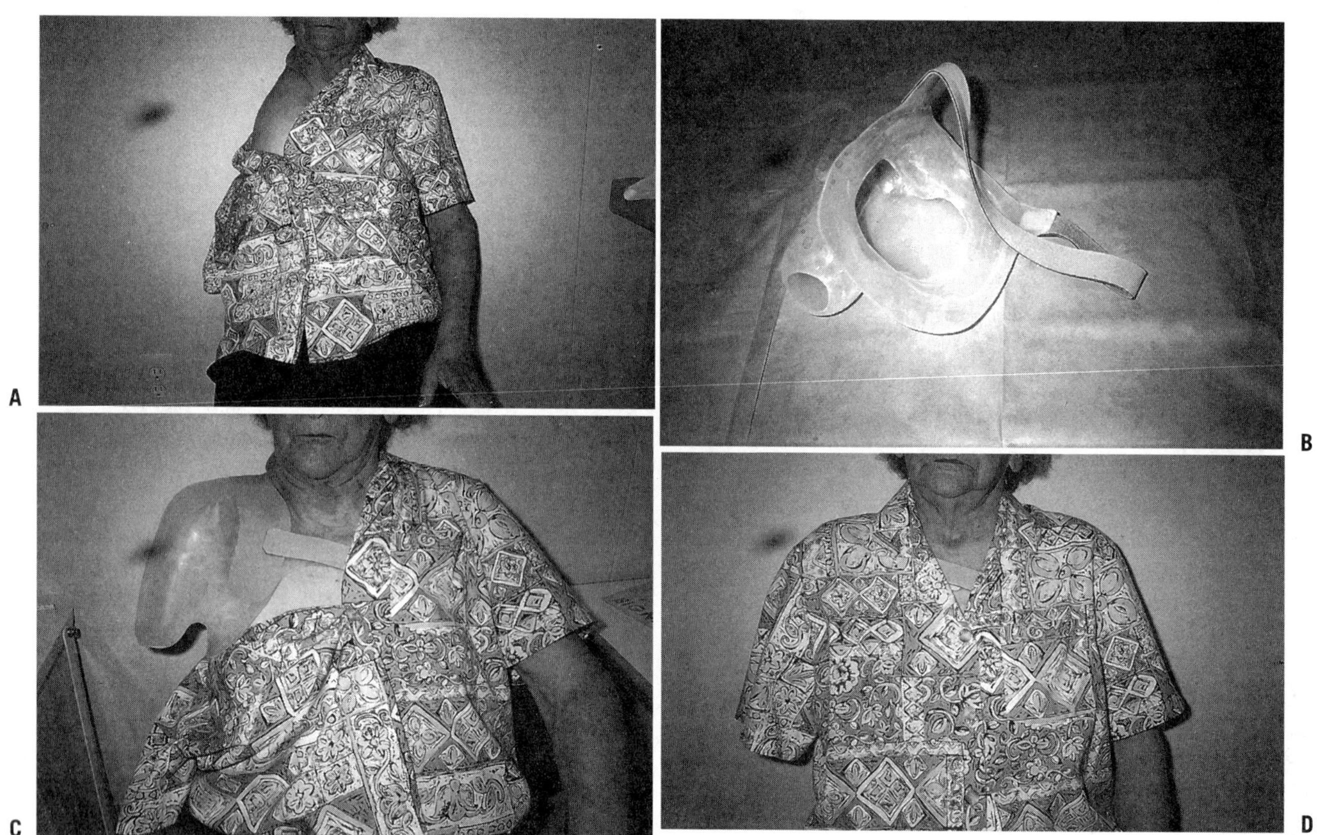

Figure 31-16. Forequarter amputation. Individuals who have had an amputation at this level often prefer a simple shoulder cap without other prosthetic components. This passive prosthesis restores the shoulder profile, improving the fit of clothing, but does not provide additional upper-extremity function.

PEDIATRIC PROSTHETICS

Upper-extremity limb loss in children is most often congenital. The etiology is highly variant, ranging from maternal infection, chemical or drug exposure, and amniotic band syndromes, to single gene mutations. Though some congenital limb deficiencies are associated with known syndromes, for example, craniofacial and thrombocytopenia absent radius (TAR) syndromes, or thalidomide exposure, the majority is of unknown etiology. The most common congenital limb loss is transverse deficiency of the proximal third of the left forearm (Fig. 31-17).

Acquired limb loss accounts for 40% of pediatric limb loss, typically involving a single limb; 60% involves the lower limb. Trauma is the most common cause; tumor and disease are next in frequency. With trauma, the limb loss is primarily due to power tool accidents, burns, and motor vehicle accidents. In the toddler and preschooler, power tools, such as lawn mowers, and household accidents are the primary causes. Regarding surgical amputations for disease, more than half are secondary to malignant tumors in preadolescents and adolescents.

Over the years, efforts have been made to classify and describe congenital limb deficiencies. Much of the terminology, being imprecise and ambiguous, generated confusion. The International Organization for Standardization (ISO), involving the work of the International Society for Prosthetics and Orthotics (ISPO), has developed a widely accepted classification system and standard terminology for congenital limb deficiency. There are two major classifications: transverse limb deficiencies and longitudinal limb deficiencies. The system is restricted to skeletal absence or reduction and does not consider the etiology or embryology. Since the classification is restricted to the absence or reduction of normal skeletal elements, radiography, or other methods to identify skeletal elements, is used. Lack of a skeletal element beyond a certain level is classified as a transverse deficiency. The limb has developed normally to a certain level, after which no further skeleton exists distally. In transverse limb deficiency, often limb bud remnants (often referred to as *nubbins*) are present. The transverse level is named by the terminal bone and the level at which no further skeletal elements exist. All other limb deficiencies are described as longitudinal deficiencies, that is, skeletal absence or reduction in the skeletal long axis of the arm or leg.

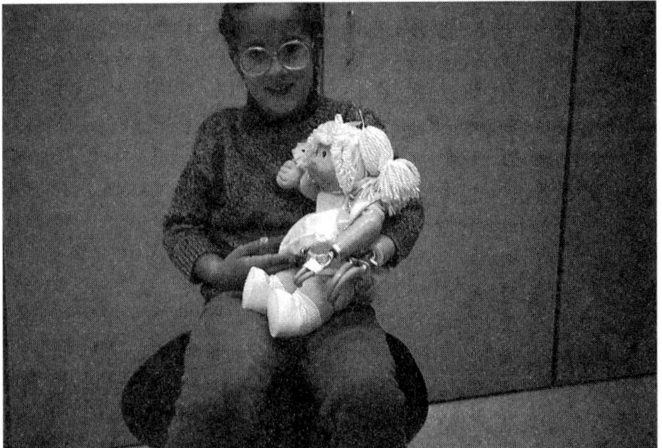

Figure 31-17. Transverse deficiency of the proximal part of the left forearm is the most common congenital limb deficiency.

The child with a congenital limb deficiency is fitted with a prosthesis in accord with the child's developmental stage. A child with an upper-extremity deficiency can be fitted with a passive hand prosthesis at 2 to 3 months old to facilitate the development of hand skills.

Children with partial hand amputations or congenitally absent digits are typically not fit with a prosthesis because of the sensory loss created by the device covering areas of sensation. Children are very adaptable and function very well without a prosthesis. Often, a prosthesis adds little function at this level. Like adults, opposition posts and pads can be used. Acceptance of these devices is variable and often are task specific. A child's acceptance is affected by the function provided by the device and by the attitude of parents or caregivers toward the prosthesis or orthosis.

Children with limb deficiency or loss at a more proximal level benefit from a prosthesis, and need to be fit at a young age before they develop compensatory techniques that preclude the use of a prosthesis. If a child has not been fitted and trained by the age of 2 years, the rejection rate is significantly higher than it is for those fitted before age 2. For the child with a congenital deficiency, a prosthesis must add function or the child will reject it. In the child with a traumatic or surgical amputation, the prosthesis provides both limb replacement and functional restoration. Children are very active and require prostheses that are durable and functional. Like adults, children who have had an amputation benefit from early prosthetic fitting.

Children require frequent refitting. A child may require socket modification or replacement to accommodate limb growth as often as every 3 to 6 months. Many of the previous prosthetic components can be reused in the replacement prosthesis. The use of multilayered sockets reduces the need for socket replacement as they can be easily modified to accommodate growth. Removable growth liners or flexible liners, which are composites of silicone and polyethylene, can reduce the frequency of socket replacement.

Cosmesis is important in pediatrics. Often the appearance of the prosthesis is more important to the parents than it is to the preschool child. Parents want the child to appear normal, as much for the child's sake as theirs. Once the child enters school, he or she becomes more concerned about appearance. Children, like adults, want to be accepted by peers and not perceived as "different" or odd.

Current technology produces smaller, simpler, and more durable myoelectric units. As a result, pediatric patients can be fitted at a very early age. Myoelectric systems are available for children who have undergone WD or a transhumeral amputation (50). The transradial myoelectric prosthesis is the most commonly prescribed for any age group.

The appropriate age to fit a child with a myoelectric prosthesis is debated. Some clinicians argue that a myoelectric prostheses can allow normal hand development earlier than body-powered systems do. Some rehabilitation centers fit children with myoelectric prostheses as early as 6 to 9 months old. Others wait until the child is of the preschool age and is proficient with a body-powered prosthesis. This approach maximizes the development of the residual limb and is less costly. These children become proficient with both body-powered and myoelectric systems.

Proponents of early fitting argue that children are developing pinch as early as age 3 to 4 months. These clinicians argue that these infants do not have the shoulder-arm coordination required for body-powered prostheses until the ages of 12 to 18 months. They propose that fitting the infant with a simple myoelectric prosthesis eliminates the problem of shoulder-arm incoordination and allows the child to learn pinch at an earlier age. Though prescribing myoelectric single-function TD for a child as young as 6 to 9 months is controversial, more clinicians are prescribing myoelectric prostheses at earlier ages (51,52). It is never appropriate for chronologic age to be the sole determinant of whether a child is or is not prescribed a myoelectric prosthesis. The child's needs, skills, and overall psychosocial situation determine which control system is most appropriate (50).

The young child who has undergone AE amputation is usually fitted with a static or friction elbow prosthesis. An active functional elbow, operated by cable or external power, is provided to older children. Often children with a long residual limb after transhumeral amputation function best with a body-powered system, rather than an externally powered one, since a body-powered system weighs less.

Like adults, children who have a very short residual limb after transhumeral, FQ amputation, or SD often reject prostheses. They must experience significant gains, particularly in terms of function, to tolerate the weight, the hassle, and other limitations of prostheses prescribed for this level.

Like adults, many older children do best owning both a body-powered prosthesis and a myoelectric one. They need a choice in TDs as well. Children with both a hook and hand TD, as well as a body-powered and a myoelectric prosthesis, can wear the prosthesis and TD appropriate for the situation. Overall, the best prosthetic choices are made when the rehabilitation team, the child, and the family work together to determine prosthetic options.

Children with more than one congenital limb deficiency are very challenging. The child with a unilateral upper-limb deficiency uses the prosthesis primarily as an assist device and uses the contralateral upper extremity as the dominant limb. The child with bilateral upper-extremity deficiency does not have this option. Ideally, the bilateral amputee needs to be independent with and without the prosthesis. Many children need to learn to use their feet for ADLs and other activities (e.g., writing). An experienced rehabilitation team is essential for the best outcome in these complex cases.

PRESCRIBING A PROSTHESIS

No two individuals are alike. No one prosthesis fits all patients. Prescribing an upper-extremity prosthesis requires the integration of a number of medical, rehabilitation, social, and economic factors. The rehabilitation team not only must assess the patient's needs, preferences, capabilities, and overall medical condition, but also must consider the anatomy of the residual limb, the functional status of the residual limb and proximal joints, the presence of any other impairments, and the individual's socioeconomic situation. If this information is synthesized and incorporated into the prosthetic restoration and rehabilitation program, the patient will receive the most appropriate prosthesis.

The essential components of a typical functional upper-extremity prosthesis are the socket, suspension system, control system, and TD. The suspension system includes cuffs and a harness. The control system is either body powered, externally powered, or a hybrid of both. The level of amputation determines whether a TD, wrist unit, elbow hinge or elbow unit, and shoulder component are needed. If the prosthesis is primarily cosmetic, few mechanic components, if any are needed (Fig. 31-18).

It is important to prescribe the most functional, comfortable, and cosmetic prosthesis for the individual. As an example, the most commonly prescribed "generic BE prosthesis" typically includes a VO split-hook TD, quick-disconnect wrist unit, flexible elbow hinge, double-wall laminated socket, single-control cable system, triceps cuff, and a figure-of-eight harness. For the "generic AE prosthesis," the same components are used but an elbow unit and a dual-control cable system are added.

PSYCHOSOCIAL IMPACT OF UPPER-EXTREMITY AMPUTATION

Each person who experiences an amputation grieves the loss of limb and function. Clinicians recognize that the grief process varies among individuals. However, many clinicians recognize that this process is very similar to the grief accompanying other major losses, such as divorce, terminal illness, and death of a loved one. The phases of grief, first described by Kubler-Ross in patients with

UNIVERSITY OF MICHIGAN HOSPITALS
ORTHOTICS & PROSTHETICS CENTER
UPPER EXTREMITY PROSTHETIC PRESCRIPTION

LIMB LOSS: Right/Left ________ DATE OF ONSET: ________

SPONSORING AGENCY: ________

Type of Prosthesis

______ Preparatory (provisional) ______ Definitive (final)

Control System

______ Endoskeletal (Manual): ________

______ Conventional (Body Powered):

______ Single Cable ______ Regular Cable

______ Dual Cable ______ Heavy Duty Cable

______ Cable (Replacement) ________

______ External Power:

______ Myoelectric: ________

______ Switch Control: ________

______ Hybrid: ________

Socket

______ Double Wall ______ Prep. Socket: ________

______ Liner ________ ______ Check Socket

Suspension System

______ Harness:

______ Figrue 8 ______ Chest Strap

______ Harness (Replacement) ______ Shoulder Saddle

____

______ Self-Suspending

Shoulder

______ Four-way Hinge ______ Shoulder Cap

Elbow

______ Internal Locking/Turntable ______ External Locking

______ Lift Assist ________

______ Powered: ________

______ BE Hinge:

______ Flexible ______ Cuff Attached to Socket

______ Rigid ______ Step-Up

Wrist

______ Friction ______ Powered Rotator

______ Quick Disconnect ______ Flexion Wrist

Terminal Device(s)

______ Mechanical Hand: ________ ______ Hook: ________

______ Powered Hand: ________ ______ Tool Kit

______ Glove ________ ________

Accessories

______ Compression Socks ______ Rubberbands ______ Electrodes

______ Limb Socks ______ Band-Applier ______ Batteries

________ ______ Battery Charger

Immediately after this prosthesis is provided to the patient, an Occupational Therapist will perform a prosthetic check-out, educate the patient about wear and care of the prosthesis and begin prosthetic controls and functional use training.

Prosthetist: ________ Physician: ________ Dr. # ________

ME2017349/DS Rev. 7/94	MEDICAL RECORD	University of Michigan Medical Center	**UPPER EXTREMITY PROSTHETIC PRESCRIPTION**

Figure 31-18. An upper-extremity prosthetic prescription form that accurately communicates the type of upper-extremity prosthesis prescribed. It also ensures that clinicians prescribe all the essential components and options specifically needed for each amputee.

terminal illness, are shock, denial, anger, depression, and acceptance (53–55).

Every individual feels a personal loss but the grief felt by the amputee is not directly proportional to the physical extent of limb loss. For example, the salesman who has lost his right hand may perceive the loss as deeply as the electrical lineman who has lost the entire upper extremity. The lineman may adjust more easily while the salesman experiences more grief because of the appearance of his hand for social greetings, whether at work or socializing. It is crucial for the rehabilitation team to be aware of the individual's response to amputation. Peer counselors can help the patient realize that "there is life after amputation." Referral to mental health professionals, ideally someone experienced working with individuals with limb loss, can assist individuals whose grieving exceeds the parameters of normal grief.

Every amputee eventually grieves, but not everyone does so at the same rate. Some reach acceptance quickly, while others are still grieving 10 years later. Clinicians report that the grief process lasts approximately 2 to 3 years. The individual's past experiences, cultural background, premorbid personality, coping skills, current interpersonal relationships, and support systems impact the individual's ability to achieve acceptance of the limb loss. Grieving is a dynamic process and may recur. Later events, such as a wedding, may remind the individual of the impact of the limb loss on personal appearance and life choices. Typically, the anger, irritability, and depression associated with the loss eventually resolve. Life resumes. The amputee works, socializes, and plays. The individual is different because of the amputation. The amputee does not like it, but it is okay. Life is different but not over. It is something the individual can live with. Unfortunately, some never reach this level of acceptance.

The amputee is not the only one who grieves. Family and loved ones also grieve, though less intensely. Children, who experience traumatic loss, tend to move through the grief process more quickly than adults. Parents of children with congenital limb deletions feel responsible and grieve deeply, while the infant is unaware of the deficiency. However, at a later age, when other children or adults react to the child's limb loss, the child learns that she or he is different. The child may grieve and wonder "Why do I have to be different?" The experiences of the various psychosocial and physical stages of maturation remind the amputee of the impact of limb loss on his or her life.

Limb loss is difficult at any age. Grief is painful. However, normal grief allows the person to adjust to the loss and to progress through rehabilitation to a full and productive life. The rehabilitation team must acknowledge the individual's loss and support the individual through the process. Direct discussions about limb loss, the personal and social impact, and prosthetic restoration and rehabilitation assist the amputee in accepting the loss. However, some patients need professional psychological assistance. Others thrive on their own.

PRE-PROSTHESIS MANAGEMENT

Ideally, one would like to begin prosthetic restoration and rehabilitation before amputation. However, most upper-extremity amputations are performed emergently. Generally, there is little time to prepare the individual for amputation or prosthetic restoration and rehabilitation.

If the surgery is elective, the patient, the physicians, and the rehabilitation team are able to collaborate and develop a treatment plan. There is also time to educate the patient about the level of amputation, preoperative and postoperative course, functional implications of the amputation, and available prosthetic and rehabilitation options. Additionally, the patient is counseled about phantom pain and sensation as well as psychosocial concerns.

Unfortunately, the patient and the members of the rehabilitation team typically do not meet until after surgery. However, patient assessment and education should begin as soon as possible. An initial assessment is performed. Information is collected about the individual's pre-amputation functional level, including vocational and recreational activities, upper-extremity dominance, and psychosocial situation. The initial assessment, or inventory, begins the process of determining the individual's prosthetic and rehabilitation needs. An individualized prosthetic rehabilitation program is initiated, integrating multiple factors including the status of the residual limb, the patient's overall functional status and general health, the person's financial resources, and the amputee's goals and expectations.

As a rule, ADL training does not begin until a person receives a prosthesis. If the individual becomes adept doing activities with one hand he or she is less likely to accept and use a prosthesis. Learning to be one-handed initially seems an acceptable option. However, after 20 or 30 years of performing activities with one hand, individuals who have not used an upper-extremity prosthesis frequently develop cumulative trauma syndromes of the back, neck, and the intact upper-extremity. Bilateral upper-extremity amputees are the exception to the rule. All efforts should be made to enable these individuals to begin feeding and performing ADLs as soon as possible, even before a prosthesis is available.

Other rehabilitation issues addressed early after amputation include wound management, edema and pain control, scar management, range of motion of the limb, and upper-extremity strength.

Wound Management

The surgical site requires close monitoring until healing is well established. The surgeon prescribes necessary postoperative limb care, including the type of dressing and incision care. Surgeons' opinions vary about when a surgical site can tolerate the fitting of a posthesis. Typically, the preparatory prostheses can be fit when small open wounds are present and healing is occurring uneventfully. In most cases, wounds tolerate prosthetic fitting within 2 to 3 weeks.

Edema Management and Early Limb Shaping

Edema control is important to enhance healing, reduce pain, and begin shaping the residual limb for prosthetic fitting. Initial compression of the residual limb is provided by a rigid dressing or elastic wrap or bandages. As mentioned earlier, a rigid dressing (cast) applied intraoperatively over the surgical dressing effectively limits postsurgical edema. However, compression is usually applied after the bulky surgical dressing is removed, which often occurs on postoperative day 1 if primary skin closure was performed. If skin grafting was performed, the application of compression is usually delayed 1 to 2 weeks.

The OT teaches the patient and family members how to apply appropriate compression. If the wound is draining, minimal dressing is applied over the incision before compression is applied. If the wound has no drainage, no dressing is required under the compression wrap. A figure-of-eight or herringbone elastic wrap technique is used to apply compression for transmetacarpal levels or shorter.

When the residual limb has healed, a custom-fitted compressive sock works well. A custom compressive garment very effectively stabilizes limb volume and is easy to don and doff. Clinical experience indicates that compression reduces phantom sensation and pain and controls scar formation. Usually, no more than two compression socks should be worn simultaneously. Some individuals find that they always need to wear a compressive garment to control limb volume and shape.

Range of Motion

After an uncomplicated amputation, the patient is instructed in active ROM exercises for all residual joints on the first postoperative day. If other injuries are involved, such as fractures, skin grafts, and tendon repairs, appropriate restrictions are observed. Full active ROM is expected for all joint motions with the exception of forearm or humeral rotation, which depends on the residual bone length. If full ROM has not been achieved after 1 week, passive ROM exercises are added.

Pain Management

Patients experience pain after an amputation. Postoperative incision pain can be controlled with appropriate postsurgical analgesia and resolves over a week or two. However, other types of pain may persist after the surgical recovery period. When managing pain, it is important to determine the etiology, for example, secondary to the pathomechanics of an arthritic joint or due to extrinsic factors such as an ill-fitting prosthesis. Phantom pain is a common but poorly understood problem.

Phantom Sensations and Phantom Pain

Phantom sensation and phantom pain are distinct syndromes. Phantom sensation, the perception a missing limb is still present, is a common postoperative experience. Typically, patients do not require treatment for these sensations. These "phantom feelings" are not painful but they can be annoying. The sensations change and fluctuate over time. The phenomena of telescoping and fading may also occur. With the phenomenon of telescoping, or regressive deformation, the phantom limb is perceived as shortening. Fading is the perception that the proximal part of the phantom limb is shortening and the most distal part of the phantom limb is regressing proximally; for example, the phantom hand feels as if it is at the stump site. These sensations (e.g., itching or tingling) occur more frequently after upper-extremity than lower-extremity amputation.

On the other hand, phantom pain is a painful sensation seemingly occurring in the missing limb or segment. The distribution of the perceived pain may or may not occur in a dermatomal pattern. Typically most prominent immediately postoperatively, the pain can range from mild to severe. Phantom pain is rare in children, especially before the age of 7 years. In general, phantom pain improves and resolves over time. However, a small percentage of patients experience persistent phantom pain that is debilitating.

Phantom sensation and phantom pain are puzzling experiences for the uneducated patient. Patients should be taught that these are not unusual experiences and that they are not "losing their mind" Teaching the patient about phantom sensation and pain reduces anxiety, which in itself heightens the perception of pain. Effective treatment is available for the pain.

Patients describe phantom pain in a number of ways: burning sensations, shooting pain, muscle cramping, as well as the sense that the limb is in a painful position. Typically, phantom pain is worse at night, after the extremity has been in a dependent position or after the prosthesis has been off for a period of time. Phantom pain is experienced mainly in the distal aspect of the phantom extremity. Sometimes, patients can identify specific points on their limb that trigger phantom pain. Examination of the residual limb can determine if these points correlate with neuromas, cysts, or sites of excessive weight bearing or pressure. In addition to an ill-fitting prosthesis or mechanical stimulation precipitating phantom pain, other precipitating factors occasionally reported include fatigue, micturition, defecation, and even yawning.

Strength and Endurance Training

Strength and endurance are required to operate a prosthesis successfully. Exercises are prescribed to improve the strength and endurance of muscles, particularly those muscles that will operate the prosthesis. This is particularly important in patients with known weakness around the glenohumeral joint and scapula.

PROSTHETIC CHECKOUT

When the patient receives any prosthesis, preparatory or definitive, the OT checks the prosthesis to make sure it is "just what the doctor ordered" (56). In addition to verifying that the prosthesis meets the specifications of the prosthetic prescription, the OT evaluates cosmesis, comfort, fit, control efficiency, stability of suspension, and the mechanical components of the prosthesis. Ideally, the prosthetist is present and makes the appropriate modifications before the amputee takes the prosthesis home (57).

The prosthesis should appear to be the same length, circumference, and shape as the sound extremity. The prosthesis should not have the same dimensions as the contralateral side or it would appear too large and bulky. Proper length is achieved when the end of the hook or the tip of the prosthetic thumb is level with the tip of the contralateral thumb with the arms extended at one's side (58–60). Length is important not only for appearance but also for the most effective use of the TD. For example, if the prosthesis is too long it will interfere with hand-to-mouth activities. The cosmetic glove covering the prosthetic hand needs to be similar in color to the sound hand. No glove will match the color of the intact hand exactly, but reasonably priced cosmetic gloves that provide a good match are available commercially.

Comfort is a major issue. The amputee will not wear a prosthesis that causes pain. The socket should provide even pressure on the residual limb. Pressure should be eliminated or reduced at bony prominences or neuroma sites. The socket should not leave red skin marks that last more than 15 to 20 minutes after removal of the prosthesis. Skin irritation, breakdown, or pain suggests an unsatisfactory fit. Modification of the socket fit or suspension system usually corrects these problems.

The prosthesis should permit maximal active ROM of the residual limb. Often this is not feasible with a very short residual forearm or Muenster-style sockets (41,61–63). Though harnessing systems may preclude full shoulder flexion or abduction, active shoulder flexion should be no less than 90 degrees (41).

The mechanical efficiency of the control system of a body-powered prosthesis is evaluated. Stable suspension of the prosthesis is also crucial. With a 25-kg axial load (i.e., 50 lb or one-third of the body weight of a child), the amount of socket displacement on the residual limb should not exceed more than approximately 2.5 cm (41,61–63). If the socket migrates more than 2.5 cm, the harness needs modification.

The checkout procedure is slightly different for the externally powered prosthesis. An experienced therapist listens to the electronics, monitors the speed of movement, and determines if the correct control muscle is utilized (e.g., wrist extensors for opening TD, not closing TD). In addition, the therapist checks the mechanical components of the prosthesis to determine that they are functioning properly.

PROSTHETIC TRAINING

Prosthetic training that focuses on the patient increases the likelihood that he or she will effectively use the prosthesis. Typically, patients learn to use the prosthesis by trial and error once they have been instructed in the specific control motions. Not all amputees approach activities using the same technique. Amputees who are experienced with tools tend to find training easier than those who are unfamiliar with tools. The OT acts as a facilitator, encouraging independent problem solving and providing guidance and assistance as needed. Only one therapist should do the training or the amputee will become confused by the different approaches. An experienced therapist who is a strong advocate of prosthetic use significantly increases the likelihood of successful prosthetic training (41). The amputee who is not fitted with a prosthesis during the 30-day golden period needs to relearn how to perform activities once the prosthesis is fitted. Having to abandon one-handed techniques and relearn prosthetic techniques reduces the likelihood that the individual will become a successful user of the prosthesis.

The individual must have realistic expectations regarding what the prosthesis can and cannot do. The amputee must consider the prosthesis as an assist. In a unilateral amputee, the prosthesis assumes the role of a nondominant upper extremity for activities. If the amputation involved the individual's dominant hand or arm, the contralateral limb assumes dominance. Typically, bilateral amputees use the longer residual limb as the dominant one.

Prosthetic training is divided into three distinct phases: orientation, controls training, and use training. During prosthetic orientation, the patient learns about prosthetic components. General instructions in the wear and care of the prosthesis are reviewed. During prosthetic controls training, the individual learns to operate all prosthetic components. The amputee must learn to operate the components smoothly and efficiently, avoiding strain or awkward movements. During prosthetic use training, the person learns to perform ADLs with the prosthesis. Bilateral tasks, such as cutting with scissors, cutting meat, and tying shoes, are emphasized.

Prosthetic Orientation

The patient first learns how to wear the prosthesis. Typically, the amputee learns to don and doff the prosthesis using either a pullover technique or a coat technique. The amputee initially wears the new prosthesis for periods of 30 to 60 minutes, and then gradually increases the wearing time. Within 1 or 2 weeks, the amputee should be comfortably wearing the prosthesis for an entire day. New amputees continue to wear shrinker socks or elasticized wraps when not wearing the prosthesis. This is required until the volume of the residual limb stabilizes, or indefinitely in patients with fluctuating limb volumes.

The wearer of a conventional, or body-powered, prosthesis is taught how many socks to wear and the indications for changing the number of socks. The amputee must learn how many rubber bands to put on the VO hook. Typically, the individual begins with about 1lb (0.5kg) of pressure, as measured by the pinchometer. The number of rubber bands is gradually increased until sufficient pressure is provided to meet the amputee's functional needs, that is, 3 to 15lb (1.35–6.75kg) of pressure. Generally, BE amputees need approximately 8lb (3.6kg) of pinch force, while AE amputees develop about 5lb (2.25kg) of pinch force with the VO hook.

The amputee is able to communicate effectively with the team once he or she learns to identify basic prosthetic components (64). Basic prosthetic concepts should be introduced as well. The prosthetic rehabilitation team, on the other hand, must learn to discuss aspects of prosthetic restoration and rehabilitation in lay terms.

Since many amputees require more that one TD, they must learn to switch from one TD to another and the indications for the various TDs. Users of conventional prostheses often learn to change cables and adjust the harness to improve control.

It is important for amputees to learn to care for limb socks, sockets, harnesses, cables, TDs, rubber bands, cosmetic gloves, and batteries. They are taught auditory and visual clues that indicate malfunction or deterioration. Amputees are to contact the prosthetist as soon as a malfunction is detected, to prevent further damage.

Conventional Prosthesis Controls Training

The patient learns the proper body mechanics and motions to operate all prosthetic components. Eventually, the amputee will perform the appropriate motions automatically. For most amputees, basic controls training is accomplished in 30 minutes.

Basic Controls Training

There are two parts to basic controls training: opening and closing the TD and learning to preposition it.

Opening and Closing the Terminal Device

The patient learns to open and close the TD and to activate the TD with the elbow and shoulder in different positions, including full flexion and full extension. For instance, the amputee learns to activate the TD using the control motions of humeral flexion, biscapular abduction, or shoulder depression.

Prepositioning the Terminal Device

The person learns to strategically place the TD in a position to grasp the object most easily. Using the sound hand, the unilateral amputee passively pronates or supinates the TD into the desired position. Next, the stationary finger of the hook or hand touches the object and the movable hook or fingers grasp the object. To position the TD, the bilateral amputee uses the other TDs or pushes the TD against the body or a stable object, such as the edge of a table. The friction wrist should be tight enough to maintain the hook or hand in position when the cable is activated. The bilateral amputee with a wrist flexion unit learns to position the unit and the TD close to the body, for activities such as toileting, eating, and shaving.

Above-Elbow Controls Training

In addition to the above-mentioned techniques, the AE amputee learns additional control techniques. Typically, an additional 30 minutes of training is necessary to learn these skills.

Elbow Flexion and Extension

The patient learns how to activate elbow flexion. With the elbow unlocked, the patient learns that humeral flexion causes the prosthetic elbow to flex. This is the same motion that operates the TD if the elbow unit is locked.

Elbow Locking Mechanism

The AE amputee learns to activate a second control cable for locking and unlocking the internally or externally hinged elbow. The amputee learns to use elbow nudging to lock and unlock the elbow hinges. Sometimes, this is a difficult motion to learn. This motion, often described as "down, back, and out," combines humeral extension and abduction with scapular downward rotation and depression to control the elbow hinges (48). There are other control motions for activating the elbow cable. Some prosthetists design the cable so it goes through a pulley on the shoulder saddle and then attaches to a belt loop. Shoulder elevation activates this system. The patient learns to listen for the clicking sounds made by the elbow locking cable as a cue to verify that the elbow lock is on or off. Elbow locking in various degrees of elbow flexion and extension is also learned.

Humeral Turntable

AE amputees who lack 5cm or more of humeral length benefit from a humeral turntable. The humeral turntable, located just proximal to the internal locking prosthetic elbow, requires passive prepositioning into the appropriate amount of internal or external rotation. The turntable must be tightened enough so that the selected position is maintained when the TD is activated.

Shoulder Disarticulation and Forequarter Controls Training

Control Motion

Typically, these individuals use chest expansion to activate the cable for TD use. This strap attaches both anteriorly and posteriorly to the prosthetic socket. Full cable excursion is often an unrealistic goal, and as a result, full voluntary TD opening is not achieved. Often the amputee is unable to provide sufficient strength to utilize a body-powered prosthesis and finds it is "more work than it is worth." For these individuals, externally powered components may be a good option.

Four-Way Friction Shoulder Hinge

If the patient chooses to have a shoulder unit, this type is a frequent choice. The patient is taught how to passively (manually) preposition the prosthetic arm in humeral flexion or extension, adduction or abduction, or any combination.

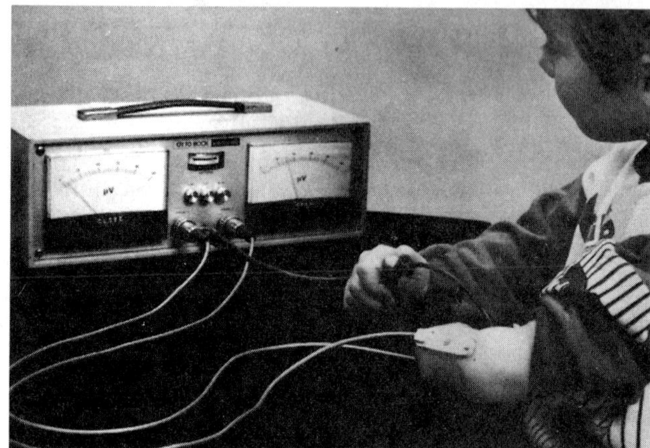

Figure 31-19. Electromyographic site selection and control evaluation are performed in preparation for fitting a myoelectric prosthesis.

Nudge Control

This button or lever mechanism is on the thoracic shell and enables the individual to engage or disengage the elbow lock. Typically, the amputee uses the chin to operate the nudge control. The individual passively positions the elbow into the position appropriate for the task and locks it. This option is selected when other motions are not available to control the prosthesis.

Externally Powered Controls Training

Myoelectric Site Selection and Training

Controls training for the myoelectric prosthesis is begun before the patient is fitted with the prosthesis. Selection and training of appropriate control sites is most important. An experienced therapist or prosthetist is essential to successful training (57).

The amputee must be able to generate sufficient muscle contraction to activate the myoelectric sensor contained in the prosthesis. Possible myoelectric control sites are tested using an electronic biofeedback system or a myoelectric tester that provides quantification of the electrical potential generated by the selected muscle site (Fig. 31-19). The most distal site with the strongest signal is chosen. As a rule, muscles that approximate normal motion are selected. For instance, wrist flexors and extensors are selected to close and open the TD of the BE prosthesis.

Control of muscle site signals is the basis of successful myoelectric prosthesis use. Dual-site control is preferred over the more difficult single-site control. With dual-site control, two muscles must be able to generate independently a sufficient electrical potential to operate the prosthesis without interfering with each other. Typically, the patient is taught to isolate antagonist muscles. For example, BE amputees learn to isolate the wrist flexors and extensors, while AE amputees learn to isolate the biceps and triceps. Some myoelectric systems are proportionally controlled; that is, the greater the muscle contraction, the faster the TD reacts or the greater the grip force produced. Amputees must learn to use proportional controls appropriately. Greater speed and more force do not translate into more control.

Amputees who are fit with the myoelectric AE prostheses often need to learn to perform quick co-contractions of the biceps and triceps to switch control between the elbow and hand. The prosthesis is in a hand mode except when co-contraction is used to switch it to the elbow mode. Like the TD, the elbow is controlled by the biceps and triceps. If the elbow is held in the same position for a brief period of time, the elbow automatically locks and the prosthesis automatically switches back to the hand mode.

Single-site electrodes are available for the individual who does not have two acceptable control sites or cannot isolate muscle contractions. In this case, the patient is taught to create a quick muscle contraction for one prosthetic action and a slow muscle contraction for another. This same control concept is used for activating powered wrist rotators.

Switch-Control Training

When myoelectric control sites are not available, other possible control motions (e.g., those that activate an on-off rocker, button, or pull switch) are considered. These control motions are usually proximal movements that are not used for normal ADLs, such as shoulder elevation. As mentioned earlier, chin nudge switches are occasionally used. Most of the controls training for this type of external power is conducted after the individual receives the prosthesis.

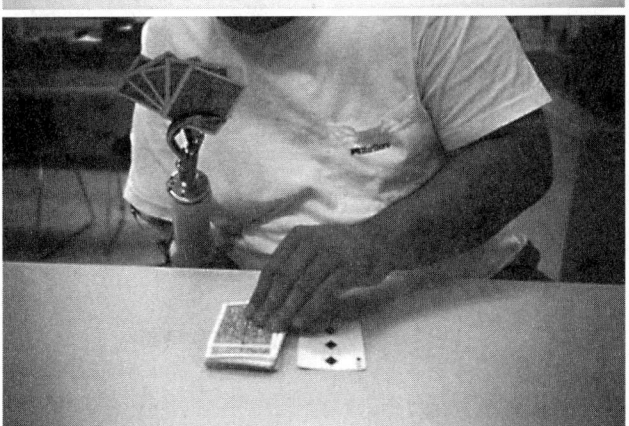

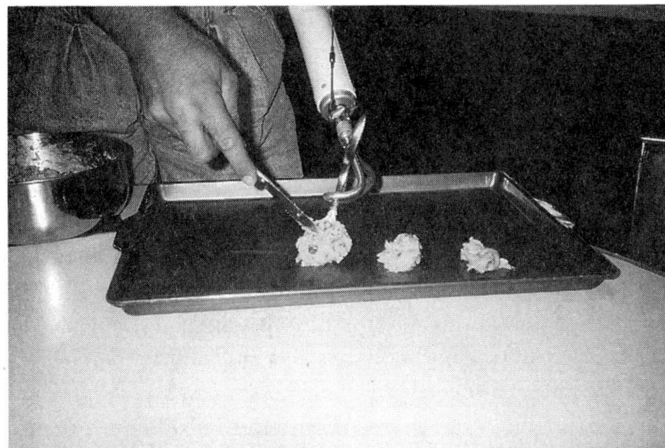

A

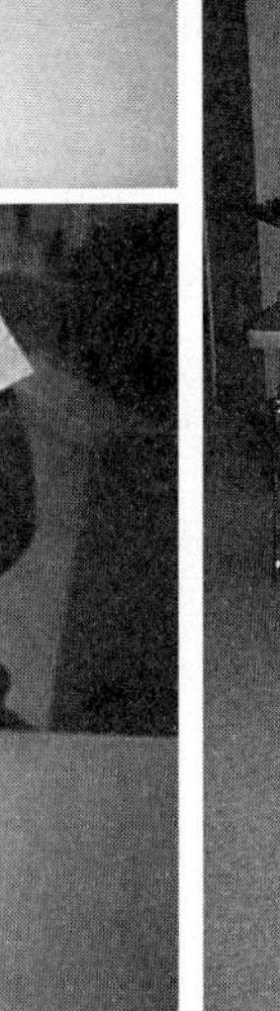

C

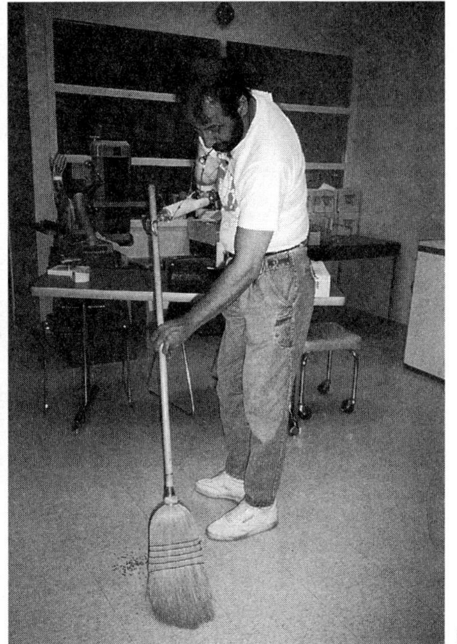

B

Figure 31-20. During prosthetic training, the amputee learns to perform a wide range of activities.

Use Training for Conventional or Externally Powered Prostheses

The study by Lake (65) demonstrated that amputees who receive prosthetic training show increased spontaneous use of the prosthesis as well as greater skill and efficiency. During this phase of training, the OT uses a variety of techniques. Initially, the therapist teaches the amputee to perform simple tasks with the prosthesis, and then introduces more difficult bilateral tasks (Fig. 31-20). The OT has the amputee grasp a variety of objects at different heights to improve control. Objects are graded in size and weight. To increase speed, the OT encourages minimal body movement, accurate TD prepositioning, and use of surroundings to facilitate task completion. The amputee learns both active and passive use of the TD. Whenever possible, the amputee is instructed to relax cable tension on the conventional prosthesis to avoid fatigue. Similarly, an amputee using a myoelectric prosthesis needs to relax the control-site muscles after activation of the myoelectric components.

During this stage of training, rubber bands are increasingly added to the VO hook, requiring the user to generate greater cable tension to operate the TD and secure an appropriate grip. Once the amputee is able to produce a pinch force of at least 3 lb (1.35 kg), functional tasks are taught, including tying shoes, cutting meat, and picking up objects. As available pinch force increases, the amputee also learns to grasp an object without squashing it. This is particularly important with a myoelectric TD that can generate high pinch forces.

While the unilateral amputee is typically trained as an outpatient, the bilateral amputee is best trained as an inpatient at a rehabilitation facility. Inpatient training allows more intensive instruction, training, and practice, effectively shortening the time from receipt of the prosthesis to active regular use. If both prostheses share a common harness, the patient learns to activate one TD without activating the other.

All ADL issues are addressed, including self-care, driving, home management, and vocational and leisure tasks (Fig. 31-21). Videotapes showing other amputees performing various ADL tasks are excellent training tools. Commercially made TDs are available for recreational activities such as baseball, gymnastics, weight lifting, and fishing.

The prosthesis is the primary adaptive device for the upper-extremity amputee. Other assistive devices should be kept at a minimum. Adaptive equipment is needed by some amputees, especially if they use a one-handed approach. Devices commonly used by the upper-extremity

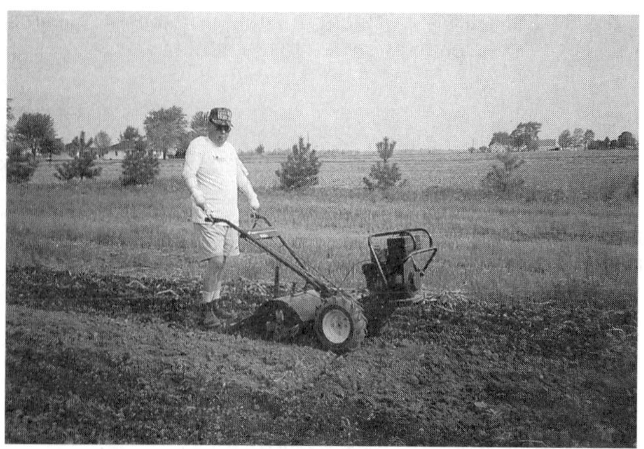

Figure 31-21. The individual with upper-extremity loss can learn to perform activities necessary for school or work.

amputee include rocker knives, cutting boards, or scrub brushes with suction cups to stabilize the object. Unilateral amputees may require turning knobs affixed to the steering wheel for turning when driving an automobile.

Bilateral Amputees

Persons with bilateral BE amputation can become completely independent in ADLs (Fig. 31-22). However, learning to do overhead activities is difficult. Individuals with bilateral amputations may require driving rings, button hooks, lever-type doorknobs, or ring pulls for zippers to achieve independence.

In addition to AE prosthetic training, children with congenital bilateral AE limb deficiencies should learn to use their feet as they would hands. These amputees frequently require a bidet for toileting. Telephones with a speaker phone work well for these individuals. Certain activities (e.g., dressing above the waist or cutting meat) are extremely challenging. Typically, these individuals, and amputees with more limb loss, require assistance from another person at various times during the day for certain activities such as bathing.

Amputees with bilateral SD or higher limb loss find it very difficult to don and doff prostheses independently

Figure 31-22. The occupational therapist trains an amputee to use the prosthesis to perform activities of daily living (ADLs).

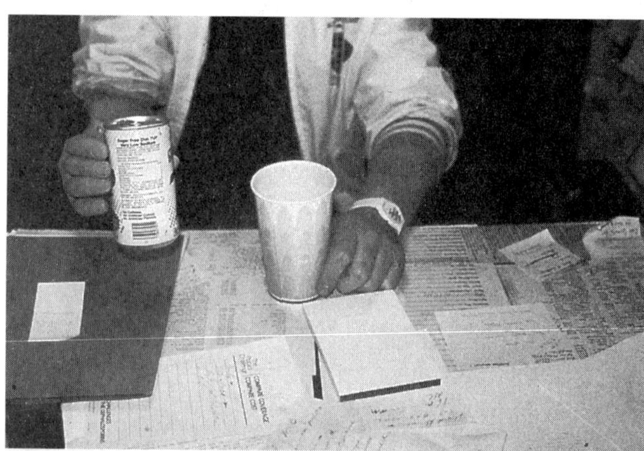

A

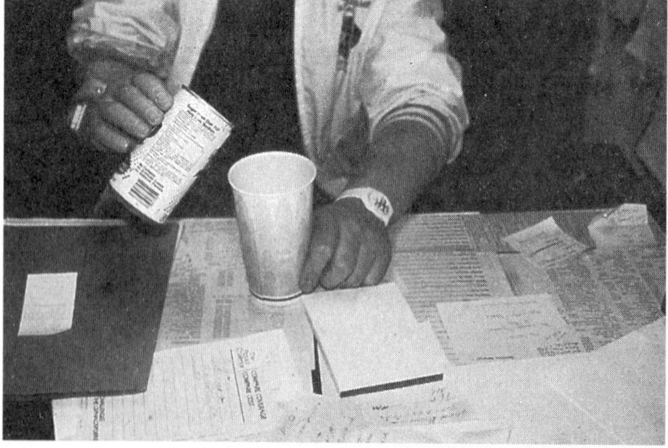

B

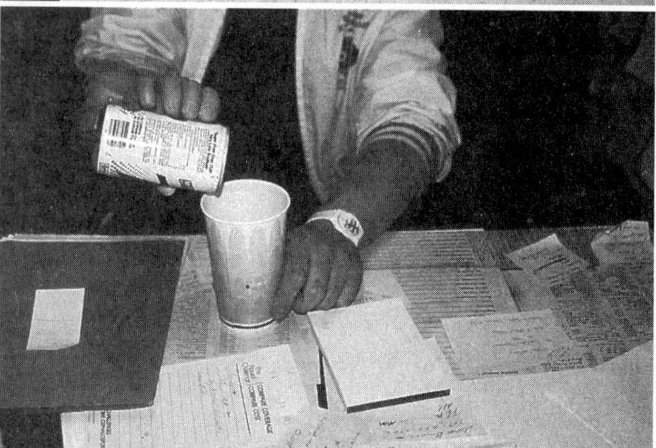

C

(48). They need an attendant at various times to assist them in performing specific tasks.

Prosthetic use training teaches the upper-extremity amputee realistic expectations for each prosthetic device. The length of time prosthetic training takes is extremely specific to each individual. Some will effectively self-train while others will require extensive occupational therapy training.

CONCLUSIONS

Prosthetic restoration and rehabilitation is a rapidly expanding field. A few basic points are important to remember. When upper-extremity amputation is necessary, the procedure needs to be viewed as part of a reconstructive and rehabilitation effort to restore upper-extremity function. When the surgical and rehabilitation decisions and interventions focus on the patient as an individual, he or she is able to achieve maximal function and independence in spite of limb loss.

APPENDIX I. AMPUTEE ASSOCIATIONS AND PUBLICATIONS

Ability (quarterly magazine)
P.O. Box 5311
Mission Hills, CA 91345

American Amputee Foundation
Tel: (501) 666-2523
Fax: (501) 666-8367
P.O. Box 250218
Hillcrest Station
Little Rock, AR 72225

AMP (quarterly magazine)
12-45 150th Street
Whitestone, NY 11357

Amputee Coalition of America (ACA)
Tel: (888) AMP-KNOW
Fax: (423) 525-7917
C/O Pam Trentham
900 E. Hill Ave, Suite 285
Knoxville, TN 37915-2568
(Annual spring conference and many other services)

National Amputation Foundation
Tel: (516) 887-3600
Fax: (516) 887-3667
73 Church Street
Malvern, NY 11565

National Amputee Fund
Tel: (800) 770-5090
6147 University Avenue
San Diego, CA 92115-5796
(Provide assistance with finding prostheses)

United Amputee Services Association, Inc.
Tel: (407) 395-1701
855 S. Federal Highway, Suite 212
Boca Raton, FL 33432
(Pamphlet: "A Survivor's Guide for the Recent Amputee")

APPENDIX II. UPPER-EXTREMITY PROSTHETIC MANUFACTURERS, DISTRIBUTORS, AND RESEARCH CENTERS

In United States

Fillauer, Inc.
Tel: (800) 251-6398 or (615) 624-0946
Fax: (615) 622-7836
P.O. Box 5189
2710 Amnicola Highway
Chattanooga, TN 37406
(Manufacturer/distributor prosthetic parts)

Health Related Products/Realastic
Tel: (800) 845-4566
Fax: (864) 229-1230
P.O. Box 3465
1704 Mathis Road
Greenwood, SC 29649
(Standard and custom polyvinyl chloride prosthetic gloves, silicone digits)

Hosmer Dorrance Corporation (Fillauer Subsidiary)
Tel: (800) 827-0070 or (408) 538-7748
Fax: (408) 379-5263
561 Division Street
PO Box 37
Campbell, CA 95008
(Myoelectric and conventional components;
NY Electric Elbow; NY Prehension Actuator,
NU-VA Synergistic Prehensor)

Liberty Technology
Tel: (508) 435-9061
Fax: (508) 435-8369
71 Frankland Road
Hopkinton, MA 01748
(Myoelectric components by developer
T. Wally Williams; Boston Elbow; distributor of all pediatric electronic components worldwide)

Life-Like Laboratories
2718 Hollendale Lane, Suite 400
Dallas, TX 75234
(Horst Bruckner, president; company makes custom silicone gloves, patented procedures, written articles)

Motion Control
(Fillauer Subsidiary)
Tel: (800) 621-3347
Fax: (801) 972-9072
3385 West 1820 South
Salt Lake City, UT 84104
(Harold Sears, PhD, vice-president and general manager; Utah Elbow, BE procontroller)

Otto Bock Orthopedic Industry
Tel: (800) 328-4058
Fax: (612) 519-6153
3000 Xenium Lane North
Minneapolis, MN 55441
(Originated in Germany, Otto Bock Hand, Greifer, Wrist Rotator, myoelectric components)

Pilot Hand Prostheses
Tel: (800) 441-HAND
Fax: (212) 489-7808
331 W. 57th Street, #109
New York, NY 10019
(Custom silicone gloves)

The Institute for Rehabilitation & Research
(TIRR) Amputee Center
Tel: (713) 797-5237
Fax: (713) 797-5904
1333 Moursund
Houston, TX 77030
(Diane Atkins-Jones, OTR, editor of *Comprehensive Management of Upper-Limb Amputee*, New York: Springer, 1989)

Therapeutic Recreation Systems (TRS)
Tel: (800) 279-1865
Fax: (303) 444-5372
2450 Central, Suite D
Boulder, CO 80301
(Bob Radocy, president; BE amputee developer of VC Adept and Grip hooks and numerous sports terminal devices, several videotapes for sale including one of sports)

United States Manufacturing Co.
Tel: (818) 796-0477
Fax: (818) 440-9533
P.O. Box 5030
180 N. San Gabriel Boulevard
Pasadena, CA 91107-0030
(Manufacturer quick disconnect wrist, mechanical elbows, books)

VA Rehabilitation Research and Development Service
Tel: (410) 962-1800
Fax: (410) 962-9670
E-mail: pubs@ballt-rehab.med.va.gov
103 South Gay Street
Baltimore, MD 21202-4051
(Myoelectric components: synergistic prehensor and elbow, puts out yearly research and development progress reports)

Outside United States

Centri Gummifabrik AB
Tel: 011-46-8580-31 165
Fax: 011-46-8580-81 128
Lidvagen 37S-17540
Järfälla, Sweden
(Powered hands, gloves, upper-extremity prosthetic components)

Hugh MacMillan Medical Centre
Tel: (416) 425-6220
Fax: (416) 425-6591
350 Rumsey Road
Toronto, ON, Canada M4G 1R8

Hugh Steeper (Roehampton) Ltd.
Tel: (01) 788-8165
237-239 Roehampton Lane
London SW15 4LB, England
(Steeper Hand, Systemteknik Hand,
Servo Hand, wrist units, Gripper powered hook)

Loth Fabenim
Tel: 011-31-3073-25 06
Fax: 011-31-3071-10 45
Netherlands

Orthopadie Brillinger
Tel: 011-49-7071-41 04 0
Fax: 011-49-7071-41 04 50
Germany

Otto Bock Orthopedic Industry
Tel: (800) 665-3327 or (905) 829-2080
Fax: (905) 829-1811
2897 Brighton Road
Oakville, ON, Canada L6H 5S3

Otto Bock Orthopadische Industrie KG
Tel: 011-49-055-27 8480
Fax: 011-49-055-27 72330
Postfach 1260
37105 Duderstadt, Germany

Systemteknik AB
Prosthetics and Orthotics Group
Tel: 011-46-876-70370
Vasavägen 76 S-18141
Lidingö, Sweden

David Trainer
Anaplastologist
Germany

University of New Brunswick
Prosthetics Research Centre Institute of Biomedical Engineering
Tel: (506) 453-4966 or 454-8283
Fax: (506) 452-1040
180 Woodbridge Street
Fredericton, NB, Canada E3B 4R3
(Annual myoelectric controls course and symposium on their system in August)

Variety Ability Systems (VASI)
Tel: (416) 698-1415 or (800) 891-4514
Fax: (416) 698-5860
3701 Danforth Avenue
Scarborough (Toronto), ON, Canada M1N 2G2
(Developer of "Cookie Crusher" children's myoelectric hand, hands, elbow, gloves)

APPENDIX III. UPPER-EXTREMITY AMPUTEE INFORMATION RESOURCES

American Academy of Orthotists and Prosthetics
Tel: (703) 836-7118
Fax: (703) 836-0838
1650 King Street, Suite 500
Alexandria, VA 22314
(*Journal of Prosthetics and Orthotics, Orthotics and Prosthetics Almanac*)

American Anaplastology Association
Tel: (415) 221-9775
493 Eighth Avenue
San Francisco, CA 94118
(cosmetic gloves, journal, annual conferences, international membership)

American Occupational Therapy Association (AOTA)
Tel: (301) 652-AOTA X288
Fax: (301) 652-7711
4720 Montgomery Lane
P.O. Box 31220
Bethesda, MD 20824-1220
(Video for sale/rent: "The Use of Upper Extremity Prostheses" by Art Heinze, OTR)

Area Child Amputee Center
Mary Free Bed Hospital and Rehabilitation Center
Tel: (616) 454-7988
Fax: (616) 454-3939
E-mail: amputee@mf brc.com
235 Wealthy Street, SE
Grand Rapids, MI 49503
(Pamphlets for sale: *Children With Limb Loss Handbooks* for families and teachers; *Children with Hand Differences: A Guide to Families*—also available in Spanish)

Association of Children's Prosthetic-Orthotic Clinics (ACPOC)
Tel: (847) 698-1637
Fax: (847) 823-0536
E-mail: king@aaos.org
6300 N. River Road, Suite 727
Rosemont, IL 60018-4226
(Annual spring conference and quarterly news bulletin)

Gillette Children's Hospital
Medical Media
Tel: (612) 229-3800
Fax: (612) 229-3833
200 East University Avenue
St. Paul, MN 55101
(Videos: "Upper Limb Options," "Did You Know. . . ," "The Team Approach," "Active Closing Terminal Device")

International Society for Prosthetics and Orthotics (ISPO)
Tel: 011-45-31 20 72 60
Fax: 011-45-31 20 75 01
ISPO Secretariat
Borgervaenget 5
2100 Copenhagen 0
Denmark
(International conferences every 3 years in different countries: 1998, 2001, 2004 also publishes *Prosthetics and Orthotics International*)

Northwestern University Medical School
Orthotic/Prosthetic Center
Tel: (312) 908-8006
Fax: (312) 503-6803
Prosthetic-Orthotics Education
345 East Superior Street
Chicago, IL 60611-4496
(Annual review courses)

Prosthetics and Orthotics Engineering
(monthly newsletter)
Lippincott-Raven Publishers
Tel: (800) 777-2295

Fax: (301) 824-7390
P.O. Box 1600
Hagerstown, MD 21741-9932

Rehabilitation Institute of Chicago Education and Training Material
Tel: (312) 908-2859
Fax: (312) 908-4451
345 East Superior, Room 1610
Chicago, IL 60611
(Video and guide for sale: "Upper-Limb Prosthetic Options for Kids: Below-Elbow")

University of Michigan Medical Center Occupational Therapy Division Department of Physical Medicine and Rehabilitation
Tel: (313) 936-7160
Fax: (313) 936-7016
University Hospital 1G225
1500 E. Medical Center Drive
Ann Arbor, MI 48109-0046
(Video for sale: "Tri-Membral Congenital Limb Deficiency—The Ultimate Challenge: Pregnancy and Child-Care")

VA Rehabilitation Research and Development Service
Tel: (410) 962-1800
Fax: (410) 962-9670
E-mail: pubs@ballt-rehab.med.va.gov
103 South Gay Street
Baltimore, MD 21202-4051
(*Journal of Rehabilitation Research and Development* and annual progress report)

REFERENCES

1. Hunter GA. Amputation surgery of the arm in adults. In: Murdoch G, Wilson AB Jr, ed. *Amputation: surgical practice and patient management.* London: Butterworth Heinemann, 1996: 305–312.
2. Beasley RW. General considerations in managing upper limb amputations. *Orthop Clin North Am* 1981;12:743–749.
3. Tooms RE. Amputation surgery in the upper extremity. *Orthop Clin North Am* 1972;3:383–395.
4. Baumgartner RF. The surgery of arm and forearm amputations. *Orthop Clin North Am* 1981;12: 805–817.
5. Wood MR, Hunter GA, Millstein SG. The value of stump split skin grafting following amputation for trauma in the adult upper and lower limb amputees. *Prosthet Orthot Int* 1987;11: 71–74.
6. Louis DS. Amputation. In: Green DP, ed. *Operative hand surgery.* 3rd ed. New York: Churchill Livingstone, 1993:53–98.
7. Kleinert H, Jablon M, Tsai T. An overview of replantation and results of 347 replants in 245 patients. *J Trauma* 1980;20:390–398.
8. Layton TR, Villella ER, Marrangoni AG. Traumatic forequarter amputation. *J Trauma* 1981;21: 411–412.
9. Goldner RD, Howson MP, Nunley JA, et al. One hundred eleven thumb amputations: replantation vs. revision. *Microsurgery* 1990;11:243–250.
10. Jaeger SH, Tsai T, Kleinert HE. Upper extremity replantation in children. *Orthop Clin North Am* 1981;12:897–907.
11. Wood MB, Cooney WP. Above elbow limb replantation: functional results. *J Hand Surg* 1986;11: 682–687.
12. Louis DS. To graft or not to graft—the finger tip. *J Hand Surg* 1985; 10A:439–440.
13. Murray JF, Carman W, MacKenzie JK. Transmetacarpal amputation of the index finger: a clinical assessment of hand strength and complications. *J Hand Surg* 1977;2: 471–481.
14. Wilson RL, Carter-Wilson MS. Rehabilitation after amputations in the hand. *Orthop Clin North Am* 1983;14:851–872.
15. Wood MB. Finger and hand replantation. *Hand Clin* 1992;8:397–408.
16. Brunelli GA, Brunelli GR. Reconstruction of traumatic absence of the thumb in the adult by pollicization. *Hand Clin* 1992;8:41–55.
17. Luchetti R. Wrist and forearm amputations. In: Peimer CA, ed. *Surgery of the hand and upper extremity.* Vol. 1. New York: McGraw-Hill, 1996:853–867.
18. Burkhalter WE, Hampton FL, Smeltzer JS. *Wrist disarticulation and below elbow amputation.* St. Louis: CV Mosby, 1981:174–182.
19. Akelman E, Weiss AC, Summerfield SL. Elbow arthrodesis, amputation and disarticulation. In: Peimer CA, ed. *Surgery of the hand and upper extremity.* Vol. 1. Peimer CA. New York: McGraw-Hill, 1996:573–582.
20. Ouellette EA. Wrist disarticulation and trans-radial amputation. In: Bowker JH, Michael JW, eds. *Atlas of limb prosthetics: surgical, prosthetic and rehabilitation principles.* 2nd ed. St. Louis: Mosby Year Book, 1992:231–241.
21. Marquardt E, Neff G. The angulation osteotomy of above elbow stumps. *Clin Orthop* 1974;104: 232–238.
22. Sim FH, Pritchard DJ, Ivins JC. Forequarter amputation.

Orthop Clin North Am 1977;8: 921–931.

23. Andersen-Ranberg F, Ebskov B. Major upper extremity amputation in Denmark. *Acta Orthop Scand* 1988;59:321–322.

24. Glynn MK, Galway HR, Hunter G, et al. Management of the upper limb deficient child with a powered prosthetic device. *Clin Orthop* 1986;209:202.

25. Heger H, Millstein S, Hunter GA. Electrically powered prostheses for the adult with an upper limb amputation. *J Bone Joint Surg [Br]* 1985;67:278.

26. Tooms RE. Acquired amputations in children. In: Bowker JH, Michael JW, eds. *Atlas of limb prosthetics: surgical, prosthetic and rehabilitation principles.* 2nd ed. St. Louis: Mosby Year Book, 1992:735–741.

27. Jain S. Rehabilitation in limb deficiency: the pediatric amputee. *Arch Phys Med Rehabil* 1996;77: S9–S13.

28. Kruger LM. Lower limb deficiencies, surgical management. In: Bowker JH, Michael JW, eds. *Atlas of limb prosthetics: surgical, prosthetic and rehabilitation principles.* 2nd ed. St. Louis: Mosby Year Book, 1992:795–834.

29. Aitken GT. The child with an acquired amputation. *Interclin Info Bull* 1968;7(8):1–15.

30. Pellicore RJ, Sciora J, Lambert CN, et al. Incidence of bone overgrowth in the juvenile amputee population. *Interclin Info Bull* 1974;18:1–8.

31. Lovett RJ. Osseous overgrowth in congenital limb deficient children. *J Assoc Child Prosthet Orthot Clin* 1987;22(2):26–28.

32. Helm PA. Burn rehabilitation: dimensions of the problem. *Clin Plast Surg* 1992;19:551–559.

33. Helm PA. Burn injury: rehabilitation management in 1982. *Arch Phys Med Rehabil* 1982;63:6–16.

34. Aitken GT. Surgical amputations in children. *J Bone Joint Surg [Am]* 1963;45:1735–1741.

35. Malone JM, Fleming LL, Roberson J, et al. Immediate, early, and late postsurgical management of upper limb amputation. *J Rehabil Res Dev* 1984;21:33–41.

36. Brenner CD. Prosthetic principles: wrist disarticulation and transradial amputation. In: Bowker JH, Michael JW, eds. *Atlas of limb prosthetics: surgical, prosthetic and rehabilitation principles.* 2nd ed. St. Louis: Mosby Year Book, 1992:241–249.

37. Malone JM, Childers SJ, Underwood J, et al. Immediate postsurgical management of upper extremity amputation: conventional, electric and myoelectric prosthesis. *Orthot Prosthet* 1981;35:1–9.

38. Burkhalter WE, Mayfield G, Carmona LS. The upper extremity amputee: early and immediate post-surgical prosthetic fitting. *J Bone Joint Surg [Am]* 1976;58:46–51.

39. Burrough S, Brook J. Patterns of acceptance and rejection of upper limb prostheses. *Orthot Prosthet* 1985;39:40–47.

40. Meier RH III. Evaluation of and planning for acquired upper limb amputee rehabilitation. In: Atkins DJ, Meier RH III, eds. *Comprehensive management of the upper limb amputee.* New York: Springer, 1989:16–21.

41. Atkins DJ. Adult upper limb prosthetic training. In: Atkins DJ, Meier RH, III, eds. *Comprehensive management of the upper limb amputee.* New York: Springer, 1989:39–59.

42. Muilenberg AL, LeBlanc MA. Body powered upper limb components. In: Atkins DJ, Meier RH III, eds. *Comprehensive management of the upper limb amputee.* New York: Springer, 1989:28–38.

43. Kitter AW. Current concepts review: myoelectric prostheses. *J Bone Joint Surg [Am]* 1985;67:654–657.

44. Millstein SG, Heger J, Hunter GA. Prosthetic use in adult upper limb amputees: a comparison of the body powered and electrically powered prostheses. *Prosthet Orthot Int* 1986;10:27–34.

45. Northmore-Ball MD, Heger H, Hunter GA. The below elbow myoelectric prosthesis with the hook and functional hand. *J Bone Joint Surg [Br]* 1980;62:363–367.

46. DeBear P. Functional use of myoelectric and cable driven prostheses. *J Assoc Child Prosthet Orthot Clin* 1988;23:60–61.

47. Radocy B. Upper-limb prosthetic adaptations for sports and recreation. In: Bowker JH, Michael JW, eds. *Atlas of limb prosthetics: surgical, prosthetic and rehabilitation principles.* 2nd ed. St. Louis: Mosby Year Book, 1992: 325–344.

48. Wilson AB. Upper-limb prosthetics, prosthetics training and stump care, and functional capacities of amputees and vocational rehabilitation. In: Wilson AB, ed. *Limb prosthetics.* New York: Demos, 1989:69–89.

49. McGrath BE. Humerus and shoulder region amputations. In: Peimer CA, ed. *Surgery of the hand and upper extremity.* Vol. 1. New York: McGraw-Hill, 1996: 403–424.

50. Trost FJ, Rowe D. Externally powered prostheses. In: Bowker JH, Michael JW, eds. *Atlas of limb prosthetics: surgical, prosthetic and rehabilitation principles.* 2nd ed. St. Louis: Mosby Year Book, 1992:767–778.

51. Scott RN, Porter PA. Myoelectric prosthesis: state of the art. *J Med Eng Technol* 1988;12:143–151.

52. Sorbye R. Myoelectric prosthetic fitting in young children. *Clin Orthop* 1980;148:343–340.

53. Novotky MP. Psychosocial issues affecting rehabilitation. *Phys Med Rehabil Clin N Am* 1991;2:373–393.

54. Romano MD. Psychosocial diagnosis and social work services. In: Kottke FJ, Lehman JF, eds. *Krusen's handbook of physical medicine and rehabilitation.* 2nd ed. Philadelphia: WB Saunders Company, 1990.

55. Kubler-Ross E. *On death and dying*. New York: Macmillan, 1969.

56. Fisher AG. Amputation and prosthetics. In: Trombley C, ed. *Occupational therapy for physical dysfunction*, 3rd ed. Baltimore, MD: Williams & Wilkins, 1989:604–624.

57. Hubbard S. Myoprosthetic management of the upper limb amputee. In: Hunter JM, Mackin EJ, Callahan AD, eds. *Rehabilitation of the hand: surgery and therapy*. 4th ed. St. Louis: CV Mosby, 1995:1241–1252.

58. Olivett BL. Conventional fitting of the adult amputee. In: Hunter JM, Mackin EJ, Callahan AD, eds. *Rehabilitation of the hand: surgery and therapy*. 4th ed. St. Louis: CV Mosby, 1995:1223–1240.

59. Carlyle L. Fitting the artificial arm. In: Klopsteg PE, Wilson PD, eds. *Human limbs and their substitutes*. New York: McGraw-Hill, 1954:637–652.

60. Carlyle L. *Using body measurements to determine proper lengths of artificial arms*. Pamphlet Series no. 2. Artificial Limbs Research Project, UCLA, 1951.

61. Wellerson TL. *A manual for occupational therapists on the rehabilitation of upper extremity amputees*. American Occupational Therapy Association. Dubuque: Kendall/Hunt, 1958.

62. *Upper-limb prosthetics, prosthetics and orthotics*. New York: New York University Postgraduate Medical School, 1986.

63. New York University. *Upper-extremity prosthetics and supplement*. New York: Prosthetics and Orthotics Publications, 1992:107.

64. Lehneis HR, Dickey R. Fitting and training the bilateral upper-limb amputee. In: Bowker JH, Michael JW, eds. *Atlas of limb prosthetics: surgical, prosthetic and rehabilitation principles*. St. Louis: Mosby Year Book, 1992:311–323.

65. Lake C. Effects of prosthetic training on upper-extremity prosthesis use. *J Prosthet Orthot* 1997;9: 3–9.

Chapter 32

Lower-Extremity Prosthetics and Rehabilitation

Miles O. Colwell
M. Catherine Spires
Leslie Wontorcik
Alicia J. Davis
Paul Cauley

Prosthetic restoration requires the integrated approach of a team of health care professionals to guide the amputee through the psychosocial and physical aspects of limb loss toward the goal of maximal personal and prosthetic rehabilitation. This approach involves a blending of the technical aspects of prosthetics with an understanding of the patient as a person, including perceived needs, physical capabilities, family expectations, and resources. An integrated team—including the orthopedic surgeon, general surgeon, vascular surgeon, nursing staff, physiatrist, physical therapist, prosthetist, occupational therapist, social worker, psychologist, vocational counselor, and recreational therapist—is often found in large prosthetic centers. Though not always in one building, many practitioners successfully coordinate these services in a comprehensive manner for their patients within the community. The goal is to preserve function. A comprehensive plan begins with the presurgical evaluation to determine salvageability of the limb versus level of amputation. Functional and quality-of-life outcomes should be factored into the surgical decision. Once the decision for amputation has been made, time permitting, pre-prosthetic evaluation and treatment should begin prior to surgery. The topic of pre-prosthetic management including wound care, edema control, pain relief, functional evaluation, and patient education followed by prosthetic prescription, construction, alignment, and gait training is expanded further in the sections that follow. An overview of additional issues relating to pediatric amputation and congenital limb deficiency is presented later in this chapter. The terms *team*, *prosthetic team*, and *rehabilitation team* refer to a team that includes each of the health care professionals just noted or, when not available, to the individuals who must coordinate all of these roles for the amputee.

HISTORICAL PERSPECTIVE

Prosthetic design and construction have run the gamut from simple crooked tree limbs, to the integration of sophisticated electronics with high-tech materials to provide sensory feedback and componentry that adjust the prosthesis's cadence and physical properties to meet the functional demands of the individual's varying activities. Bennett Wilson, Jr., in his book *Limb Prosthetics*, noted that the earliest known record of the use of a prosthesis is found in the writings of Herodotus's histories, written about 484 BC (1). The story is of a Persian soldier, Hegesistratus, who was imprisoned in stocks by the enemy and escaped by cutting off his foot, replacing it later with a wooden version. An artificial leg believed to be from 300 BC was unearthed from a tomb in Capua, Italy, in 1858 (1). The early prostheses were made by armorers from metal and wood, mostly for soldiers to conceal limb loss as they returned to their profession. The next evolution in design limited the use of metal in favor of lighter wood, with leather cuffs and straps attached to improve articulation of the joints. Early advances occurred mostly coincident with war and the need to rehabilitate larger numbers of young amputees.

Organized research in the United States began in 1945 as the result of limb loss during World War II. Programs in Europe were expanded. The patellar tendon–bearing (PTB) below-knee (BK) prosthesis, the quadrilateral socket, improved alignment techniques, and the integrated team approach to prosthetic management were developed. As instrumentation has improved, researchers have been able to record and understand the biomechanics of human function. The ongoing commercial development of synthetic rubber, silicones, plastics, high-strength lightweight metal alloys, graphite composites, resins, and microprocessors has increasingly improved the modeling of human function being provided by artificial limbs. Significant advancements in prosthetic componentry and rehabilitation are allowing more prosthetic users to improve their functional abilities at work and play. Fortunately the fundamental concepts and biomechanics remain the same as outlined in this chapter. Periodic updates, pictures, and supplements for this chapter via the CD-ROM will allow the busy practitioner to keep abreast of timely technological advances. Access to information via the Internet is expanding as well. The International Society for Prosthetics and Orthotics (Copenhagen, Denmark; Web site: http://www.i-s-p-o.org), other national organizations, and manufacturers are going on-line. Their home pages are a good source of specific product information and references.

ETIOLOGY AND INCIDENCE

The non-war-related causes for amputation fall into the following four main categories, in descending order of frequency: disease, trauma, tumor, and congenital maldevelopment. Exact figures are not available, but approximately 75% to 93% of all acquired lower-extremity loss is related to disease in individuals over the age of 60 years (United States). The majority of these amputations are performed secondary to peripheral vascular occlusive disease related to diabetic vessel disease, arteriosclerosis, immunologic vascular disease, or thromboembolism. Traumatic amputation accounts for 7% to 20% of lower-extremity amputations, mostly in the teenage through late-twenties age group. Tumor and malignancy result in 2.5 to 5.0% of all lower-extremity amputations. Tumors are the leading cause of childhood amputations. Congenital limb deficiencies are estimated to account for 1% to 3% (Table 32-1) (2–4). The ratio of distal amputation to proximal amputation may vary from region to region depending on the availability of health care. The National Center for Health Statistics reported approximately equal numbers of BK and above-knee (AK) amputations performed in acute care nonfederal hospitals (Table 32-2) (2).

The goal of the lower-extremity prosthesis is to preserve function. The phrase *preserve function* is an all-encompassing one and likely will have different meaning(s) depending on one's perspective. To the amputee it may mean anything from cosmesis, to being able to independently bear weight, transfer, and walk a few steps, to higher-level skills such as running a marathon, waterskiing, or mountain climbing. Preserving function is a process requiring the determination of realistic outcomes for the individual amputee. The team must assist the amputee in integrating the available medical, physical, technical, and appropriate psychosocial resources into a realistic "functional package" for that individual and his or her family. Psychological adjustment to amputation can be difficult. To assist the person adjusting to an amputation, the team needs to understand his or her value system. For the adult, this may be relatively constant, whereas for the child, this will likely change with progression to adulthood. The individual is affected by self-perception, internal expectations, and the expectations of the family and society. Cultural factors often need to be included in the rehabilitation plan. One individual may become an underachiever owing to depression, fear of injury, lack of knowledge, or overprotection by well-meaning family members. Another person,

Table 32-1: Estimated Incidence of Lower-Extremity Amputations, by Cause

Cause	Incidence
Disease	75%–93%
Trauma	7%–20%
Tumor	2.5%–5%
Congenital	<1%

Source: Data compiled from the U.S. National Center for Health Care Statistics.

Table 32-2: Estimated Number of Lower-Extremity Amputations, by Year and Type

Year	Total	Toe	Partial Foot	Below Knee	Above Knee
1984	129,000	41,000	—	32,000	33,000
1988	109,000	—	—	25,000	32,000
1994	135,000	56,000	11,000	33,000	32,000

Source: Data compiled from the U.S. National Center for Health Care Statistics.

in anger, denial, or a desire to overcome the impairment, may push the limits of overachievement, sometimes to the point of noncompliance, risking medical complications.

Physically, an amputee may still be quite capable of continuing to function at the preamputation level, though cultural factors may dictate drastic changes in his or her familial or societal role. Imagine the negative social stigma that a person with accidental limb loss might have to deal with living in a country where amputation is performed as punishment for criminal behavior. In another society, the head of the household may be perceived as unable to continue that role since he or she is no longer "whole." Physical and psychological adjustment can be difficult. The amputee may try to focus on "technology" to solve some of the adjustment issues. An example is the acquisition of a custom-sculpted, hand-painted, prosthetic cosmetic cover with real human hair to deal with an obsession with "looking normal," yet continuing to be quite unhappy with the prosthesis.

The amputee who is not satisfied with less than "normal" function often requests the latest high-tech componentry. There is a place for advanced prosthetics, but the team is cautioned to identify adjustment issues versus the true functional need for high-cost, high-tech prosthetic componentry before proceeding. "High tech" does not always equate with "high function"; the reverse can also be true. Using an expensive energy-storage foot may be appropriate for the strong, coordinated young runner. However, for the person with limited strength and poor balance, the same component may actually impede function and enhance the risk of falls. In this case, the relatively simple, solid-ankle cushioned-heel (SACH), prosthetic foot might improve the patient's function at a fraction of the cost.

Financial constraints may place limits on the amount of expensive technology that can be utilized in prosthetic restoration. When the individual has already had a significant physical loss, the team should try to balance the financial cost to the individual, the family, and society. A well-coordinated effort within the prosthetic team, including the patient, family, and payers, will ensure that the patient receives the best-overall outcome during the process of prosthetic restoration.

FUNCTION

Prosthetic restoration attempts to replace a lost limb and to restore function for the individual. Lower-extremity function is accomplished by a complex series of sensory feedback and motor-activating commands to produce controlled movement. The lack of sensory feedback and individual muscle control limits what function can be replaced with nonliving materials. Duplicating the natural function of a lower extremity involves understanding the determinates of gait, as well as the physics of ground force reaction lines and joint stability. The reader is referred to Chapter 12 on gait analysis for a detailed discussion of the function and kinesiology of the lower extremity and normal gait. Essentially normal balance, posture, upper-extremity strength, and trunk control are assumed for the initial discussion on using a lower-extremity prosthesis. Deficiencies in these areas are covered later as needed to deal with special situations.

Stability, ease of movement, energy efficiency, and the appearance of a natural gait are key elements to achieve with prosthetic use. To fully understand stability, one should review the ground force reaction vector during the phases of heel strike, foot flat, and toe off. This can be visualized as a line from the point of contact with the ground to the body's center of mass. The approximate center of mass is located 2 to 3 cm anterior to the S2 sacral segment. This center of mass varies during motion as well as with the change in body mass that occurs after amputation. To maintain balance and locomotion, the intact human leg utilizes an integrated muscle contraction-relaxation function to maintain joint stability, to control acceleration-deceleration forces, and to compensate for changes of alignment of the ground force reaction. Muscle action assists the transition from an extension to a flexion moment at the hip and knee. At toe off coordinated ankle plantarflexion, hip and knee flexion are achieved so swing through can be accomplished. The goal is to maintain stability at the prosthetic joint(s) by maintaining an appropriate corresponding extension moment as weight bearing is increased. Stability will be achieved when the ground force reaction line is in front of the axis of the knee joint and behind the axis of the hip joint in the sagittal plane, thus creating an extension moment. Since prostheses are made of nonliving materials, with a limited ability to change physical properties in the dynamic situation, a balance or trade-off is achieved between stability and mobility. The lower-extremity prosthesis can only partially mimic human motion and depending on the level of the amputation, the remaining muscles of the residual limb may have a difficult time compensating. This is particularly true for the AK amputation. Increased energy expenditure and gait deviation occur proportional to the amount of compensation needed. Proper alignment will minimize these problems. The reader is referred to references 5–10 for typical alignment problems, solutions, and gait analysis during prosthesis use.

AMPUTATION LEVEL

The basic surgical and rehabilitative principle used for choosing the level for lower-extremity amputation is to preserve as many functional joints, active muscles, and the longest lever arm (as determined by bone length) that will provide good postsurgical healing with full-thickness myocutaneous coverage. In the ischemic limb, noninvasive tests such as determination of ankle-brachial arterial blood pressure ratios combined with noninvasive Doppler waveform analysis or transcutaneous oxygen values may assist the surgeon in picking a level consistent with healing. Research for improved testing techniques and wound healing is ongoing, but there is no substitute for direct visualization of tissue blood flow during surgery to pick the final level of amputation. Major muscle groups should be surgically stabilized to each other (myoplasty) or to bone (myodesis). Less than optimum myocutaneous coverage may be considered when it means saving a potentially functional joint. The use of resilient, shock-absorbing silicone liners has greatly improved the success rate of fitting a prosthesis to a long, pointed residual limb with minimal myocutaneous coverage, scarred tissue, or skin grafts. The silicone liner and suspension systems also provide better containment and control for short residual limbs, owing to their intimate suction fit. Good healing and full-thickness myocutaneous coverage are still preferred over a longer but inadequately covered residual limb.

In the lower extremity, the preferred order for level of amputation is as follows: toe amputation, ray resection, transmetatarsal amputation, Syme amputation (disarticulation of the foot), BK amputation (at a level proximal to the junction of the middle and distal third of the leg), knee disarticulation, AK amputation (at a level 8 cm or more proximal to the knee joint so the femoral condyles are excised), hip disarticulation, and hemipelvectomy. Short AK amputations at or proximal to the greater trochanter are considered functionally as a hip disarticulation (11). The reader is referred to Chapter 93 for further details.

PRE-PROSTHETIC EVALUATION AND MANAGEMENT

Preoperative Management

One of the greatest preoperative benefits the team can provide is education of the patient about the process and probable outcomes. It is advised that the amputation team educate the person about the anticipated surgery, phantom sensations, the availability of pain relief, postoperative care of the residual limb, the timing of steps involved in prosthetic restoration, and what rehabilitative therapies will be needed. It is beneficial to the patient, the family, and the team to establish the anticipated postoperative functional goals with and without a prosthesis and the time required to achieve them. Critical pathways are recommended to coordinate the team and to improve the efficiency of patient care. Peer counseling by persons who have experienced the amputation process is of great benefit, particularly for the patient who is fearful of the surgery and doubts that there can be a good quality of life after amputation.

Past medical history, review of systems, social history, a detailed functional history, physical examination, and discussion with the patient about his or her expectations are needed to create a realistic patient profile (Table 32-3). Functionally there are three general outcomes. With prosthetic restoration, the amputee may be able to continue at his or her preamputation level of activity, improve function, or have an overall decline in functional level. The otherwise healthy patient who has had a traumatic lower-extremity amputation will often be able to return to the same basic daily activities—though dancing, running, and heavy work may require modifications and not be at the same high level. A person with deconditioning and a nonunion fracture, having undergone a year or more of treatment by attempted leg salvage, casts, crutches, surgery, and no weight bearing, would see his or her function greatly increase. A decrease in overall mobility after amputation is common in the person with other functional limitations such as dyspnea on exertion, claudication at a distance of one block, painful degenerative arthritis in the knee, poor balance, or aggravation of carpal tunnel syndrome when using a walker. Past medical history can be used to formulate specific questions for a focused review of systems and functional history to determine if the patient has any additional physical conditions that will impact therapies, prosthetic fitting, recommended prosthetic componentry, need for assistance, and anticipated goals. One should also incorporate in the plan any financial concerns, impact on employment, and changes in recreational activities.

The experienced clinician incorporates the information obtained from the medical history and review of systems into the evaluation of the patient and formulation of the treatment plan. The clinician will have learned whether the patient with peripheral vascular occlusive disease likely has limiting claudication in the nonamputated lower extremity. The location of bypass grafts may necessitate prosthetic socket or suspension modification to avoid compression of the graft. Limited blood flow in the residual limb may lead one to modify the use of postoperative compression from a rigid removable dressing or elastic wraps. In severe cases, suction suspension may be contraindicated because it can impede superficial blood flow. Diabetes often results in low vision, impaired balance, and loss of protective sensation, requiring the use of prosthetic components for maximum stability and pressure relief. Nerve damage, stroke, and prior injuries to other extremities may increase the need for restorative therapies to other body areas, for example, upper-extremity strengthening to facilitate transfers and the use of crutches or a walker. Modified hand grips and bracing may be needed to minimize aggravation of carpal tunnel syndrome, to hold an assistive device, or to protect areas of prior fractures, osteopenia, bone metastases, or joint deformities. The person who has had a BK amputation and has painful degenerative arthritis of the ipsilateral knee will likely need prosthetic modifications such as bimetal uprights and a

Table 32-3: Pre-prosthetic Evaluation—Medical and Functional History

Past medical history
- Anemia
- Arthritis/gout
- Bone cancer—metastases to bone
- Bursitis/tendinitis
- Cerebral vascular disease—stroke, weakness, impaired hand function, poor balance or ambulation
- Coronary artery disease—congestive heart failure, myocardial infarction, syncope, ejection fraction
- Deep vein thrombosis—fluctuating swelling
- Diabetes—retinopathy, peripheral neuropathy, foot ulcers
- Fractures—instability, internal hardware
- Malnutrition
- Nerve damage—weakness, loss of protective sensation, mononeuropathy (carpal tunnel syndrome)
- Osteopenia
- Peripheral vascular occlusive disease—vascular study results, bypass grafts and location
- Shoulder injury—rotator cuff injury, shoulder dislocation

Review of systems
- Balance and coordination—falls, difficulty ambulating in the dark or on uneven terrain
- Cardiac—angina, dyspnea, orthopnea, edema
- Gastrointestinal/urologic—osteotomy, incontinence, hernias
- Joint range of motion—of all extremities
- Mental status—difficulty following instructions, memory, compliance
- Musculoskeletal—joint pain or stiffness (any problems that will limit the use of an assistive device), backache, hand function
- Neurologic—fainting, dizziness, loss of balance, balance in the dark
- Pain—location, type, severity
- Peripheral vascular—claudication, venous stasis, swelling, pain
- Pulmonary—shortness of breath at rest, dyspnea on exertion, supplemental oxygen
- Sensation—numbness, burning pain, proprioception
- Strength—general weakness, focal weakness, endurance
- Usual weight and current weight
- Vision—sufficient to compensate for poor proprioception?

Social history
- Alcohol or pain medication use that may affect balance, pressure relief, or compliance
- Avocational pursuits—dancing, golf, hunting, martial arts, watersports, yoga
- Lives alone or has assistance
- Medical insurance—be aware of what direct costs might be charged to the patient
- Safety of physical environment—steps, throw rugs, multiple levels; location of bed, bath, and laundry
- Psychosocial—anger, fear, anxiety, depression
- Transportation—type, availability, independent or assisted
- Vocational history—type of work, hours, frequency of activities (sit, stand, kneel, bend, twist, lift, walk), category of work (light, medium, heavy), balance required (catwalks, ladders, stairs, uneven terrain), environment (dusty, wet)

Functional history
- Mobility—transfers, ambulation, distance, limitations, assistive device, wheelchair use
- Self-care—bathing, dressing, grooming, toileting
- Typical day—particularly activity level and interests (What was physical activity level prior to current medical condition? What would the person realistically want a typical day to be?)

thigh corset lacer to off-load and stabilize the knee. Osteomy bags, incontinence, and hernias frequently require creative modifications during prosthetic restoration for hemipelvectomy, hip disarticulation, or short AK amputations. Anemia, malnutrition, cardiac dysfunction, and pulmonary disease may need to be aggressively treated to promote wound healing, control edema, minimize orthostatic blood pressure changes, and enable the patient to tolerate rehabilitative therapies.

The patient's environment, finances, availability of personal assistance, and transportation will affect the rehabilitation plan. The healthy person with personal and financial resources may require some assistance in the short term but ultimately will be independent in most activities. After the initial postoperative hospitalization, outpatient rehabilitative therapies and prosthetic restoration are usually sufficient. There may be a need for a tub bench, crutches, or a wheelchair when the patient is having difficulties with the prosthetic fit, or for hand controls for safe operation of a vehicle. For the person with a borderline premorbid activity level, the additional impairment from an amputation may create enough disability that he or she cannot continue to live alone unless there are family, friends, or sufficient finances to hire help to go to the store, provide transportation, or assist with household chores. Inpatient rehabilitation, mobilization of community resources, home modifications, or alternative living arrangements may be necessary. The experienced team can identify many of these needs and begin to address them during pre-prosthetic education and therapy. The amputee, family, and employer often have questions about work and play. The team should be prepared to answer questions about future vocational and recreational abilities. If exact answers are not yet available, a plan and estimated time frame to determine the answers should be given.

Table 32-4 summarizes the goals of pre-prosthetic education and therapy.

Postoperative Management

Wound Care

The exact details of wound care are modified according to the patient's medical condition and preferences of the surgical team. A healthy person with good peripheral blood supply and primary closure of the wound may simply need the wound cleaned once a day, a gauze or nonstick bandage, and edema control with elastic wrapping or a rigid removable dressing (RRD). Another person with diabetes, malnutrition, borderline peripheral blood flow, and an open wound from a guillotine amputation because of infection will likely require meticulous wound care several times per day, antibiotics, nutritional supplements, edema control, skin traction, or eventual revision for surgical closure. Some facilities have hyperbaric oxygen therapy available, which may increase tissue oxygen concentrations and promote healing. In the medically compromised patient, there is a higher risk for suture abscess, sinus tracts, or osteomyelitis. The wound should be inspected on a regular basis for wound dehiscence, tracking, or an increase in redness, swelling, warmth, or drainage. Diagnostic ultrasound is useful to assess for fluid collections, while a bone scan or serial x-ray studies can be used to evaluate for osteomyelitis. Unless suture and staple removal is established by protocol, the surgeon will usually determine when this will occur and authorize progressive weight bearing on the residual limb. Some centers will use immediate postoperative casting and pylon attachment to begin progressive weight bearing on postoperative day 1 or 2, particularly for the otherwise healthy person. In this case, the total-contact casting remains in place up to 2 weeks before changing; thus, the wound is not inspected daily. The casting is removed early in the event of swelling, excessive pain, or drainage (12).

Residual Limb Care

Residual limb care should control edema, promote the formation of a cylindrical shape, prevent contractures, and provide strengthening as needed. The use of elastic wraps, elastic stockinette (Compresso-Grip), stump shrinker, or RRD is generally recommended to minimize the development of postoperative edema, and to shrink and assist in shaping the residual limb. Their use must be followed carefully in the residual limb with known moderate to severe ischemia. The compression may impair the blood supply by increasing the interstitial fluid pressure to the point of diminishing the ateriolar-venous pressure gradient and precipitate tissue anoxia. The RRD is a socket fabricated with plaster or fiberglass casting bandage over the distal end of the residual limb, typically in the operating room or recovery room as the person is coming out of anesthesia (13). The exact procedure may vary from center to center. The wound is covered with a small amount of fluffed gauze or 4 × 4 sheet gauze, then a single wrap of roll gauze, and a single-ply soft sock. Additional padding is recommended to prevent high pressure over bony prominences. Some centers use pressure-relief pads over a thin stump sock, then the casting material. Other practitioners prefer to use a five-ply stump sock and no pressure-relief pads. The five-ply sock technique is simpler and makes it easier to vary the thickness of the dressing over subsequent days, to accommodate volume changes and residual limb shape. The RRD also provides protection during transfers and in case of falls. It can be removed whenever the wound needs to be inspected and should be replaced immediately before edema develops

Table 32-4: Pre-prosthetic Education and Therapy—Summary Points
• Confirm the patient's understanding of why an amputation is necessary. Provide further education if needed. • Attempt to identify patient concerns or fears and address these. • Explain the totality of amputation, wound healing, residual limb care, rehabilitative therapies, prosthetic restoration, and gait training. • Inform the patient that he or she may experience phantom sensations or pain that is natural and usually manageable. • Provide general prosthetic knowledge. Show the patient a prosthesis and explain the basic functions, fabrication, and fit. • Explain the difference between the initial provisional (temporary) and definitive (permanent) prosthesis. Clarify that there will be periodic modifications to maintain fit and improve alignment. • Outline goals—anticipated functional outcome—and, as appropriate, deal with any unrealistic expectations. • Stress the importance of the patient's active participation and that the clinician's role is to provide knowledge, training, and equipment. • Provide an estimate of how much time will be involved for prosthetic restoration and rehabilitation.

and interferes with its fit. If it is left off for too long, using a thinner-ply sock or temporary elastic wrap should allow replacement of the RRD.

Elastic wraps are frequently used to control edema and assist with shaping the residual limb. Though inexpensive, they are labor-intensive and rely on use of proper technique. To ensure proper compression, they should be rewrapped four to six times a day with tension to create a distal to proximal pressure gradient. A herringbone pattern, pulling increased tension when going from posterior to anterior, is commonly used. If applied improperly, an elastic wrap may provide inadequate compression, or if applied too tightly proximally, can create a tourniquet effect resulting in more edema. Double-length 4-inch-wide elastic wraps may be used after BK amputation and 6-inch-wide wraps, after AK amputation. An elastic shrinker sock can provide uniform compression of the residual limb. The sock needs to be pulled on snugly against the distal end of the residual limb to prevent swelling into the toe of the sock. For the person who is not limited by pain or impaired hand function, the process of putting the sock on correctly is not labor-intensive and only requires a periodic resnugging. If the sock is not tolerated initially, one can try a larger size, less compression (such as using a Compresso-Grip stockinette), or transition to a stockinette after several weeks of wound healing. It is recommended that the patient wear a compressive device over the amputation site 24 hours a day except for during wound care and bathing. Rarely is a compression device worn at the same time as the prosthesis. It can be discontinued once the residual limb volume has stabilized. Some people are lifelong wearers of a compressive device, owing to mild residual limb swelling when they are not using their prosthesis. Others continue to wear one for protection, warmth, or pain control.

Time permitting, exercise instruction begins before surgery. The patient should be taught exercises to prevent contractures and facilitate strength. These should be resumed or taught as soon as possible postoperatively, barring any restrictions noted by the surgical team. Occasionally, increased wound tension or impaired wound healing requires modification of the exercise program. The patient should avoid early aggressive range of motion or muscle contractions across the region of the wound. Lying prone 10 to 15 minutes several times a day will minimize hip flexion contractures. The person should keep the knee extended when lying or sitting. Knee extension attachments are available for wheelchairs, or a padded board can be inserted between the chair frame and cushion. When compliance is difficult, one can consider using a knee immobilizer or cast, or crossing the knee joint when fabricating an RRD. The wound should be examined daily, more frequently in difficult situations, and modifications made as needed to prevent excessive pressure over bony prominences or the distal end of the residual limb.

PROSTHETIC PRESCRIPTION

The prosthetic prescription should include the diagnosis, patient's weight, activity level, and specifications regarding the suspension, socket type, socket-skin interface or liner if needed, joints, endoskeletal or exoskeletal system, and terminal device to be used. The functional goals established during the pre-prosthetic evaluation should be recorded and reviewed as they will influence the choice of componentry. It is essential that special considerations be noted, such as contractures, weakness, impaired sensation, poor balance, underlying bony deficits, and pressure-intolerant areas such as scars, skin grafts, burns, or bypass grafts. In a multidisciplinary amputee clinic, the prescription is generated by the consensus of the team with input from the physician, prosthetist, therapists, and in some countries, the case manager or coordinator who has financial approval. Technological advances in prosthetic componentry and health care are creating a demand for prostheses that allow a broader range of functional activities from basic mobility to track-and-field sports. New devices are available each year. The basics of prosthetic prescription will remain the same, but clinicians need to keep informed of the latest componentry, advances in functional restoration, and cost. Clinicians are advised to check with their local prosthetist, trade journals, and the prosthetic Internet pages concerning the detailed function, availability, and service of specific devices. A review of basic prosthetic componentry follows.

Components of a Lower-Extremity Prosthesis

The major components of a prosthesis are the socket, a skin-socket interface such as socks or a liner, a suspension system, articulating joints if needed, the pylon, and a foot. The terminal device is typically a foot but in some cases may be a nonslip rubber disk for water use or a custom-made device for a sporting activity. Prosthetic feet are broadly classified as energy storing or not energy storing and are made of a multitude of materials such as wood, foam, rubber, metal alloys, graphite, plastic polymers, and silicones. Ankle function is usually incorporated into the foot. In general, this reduces weight and results in fewer parts to service. A dedicated prosthetic ankle joint may be used in special situations, particularly during sports such as rowing, mountain climbing, or scuba diving. An AK prosthesis can be made without a knee joint but ambulation would appear choppy and labored as the person hikes the hip and circumducts the artificial leg to clear the ground and advance forward. To best compensate for the function lost from lower-extremity amputation, the AK prosthesis requires a knee joint and the hip disarticulation prosthesis should have a hip joint and knee joint. Joints have progressed from a simple hinge to complex multiaxis devices incorporating hydraulics, springs, friction devices, and electronics. The three broad categories of sockets are solid, solid with a liner, and solid windowed frame with a liner.

Liners vary from semirigid to flexible and are made from a large number of different materials, such as a dense foam, multidensity layered foam, multidurometer rubber, silicones, plastics, or a composite of several materials. Suspension systems to secure the prosthesis to the residual limb can be straps, wedges, sleeves, suction, or a combination.

Socket

The socket provides the weight-bearing interface between the patient's residual limb and the prosthesis. It must contain and protect the tissues of the residual limb while simultaneously controlling and transmitting the forces involved in standing and ambulation. A less than optimal fit can impair mobility, owing to loss of stability, increased energy consumption, and pain from excessively high pressure and tissue trauma. It is recommended that a skilled and knowledgeable prosthetist design and fit the socket because this is the critical link. The provisional (temporary or preparatory) socket will need to be modified to accommodate changes in volume and shape as postsurgical edema resolves, atrophy occurs, or the patient's weight fluctuates. The definitive (permanent) prosthetic socket is made when the shaping and shrinking process is complete and the residual limb volume has stabilized.

Aside from the immediate postoperative use of plaster or fiberglass bandage castings, there are two main approaches to socket fabrication. One is to create a positive plaster mold over which thermoplastics and resins can be vacuum formed, and the other is direct molding on the residual limb using low-temperature rapid-curing materials (resin-impregnated graphite braid) and uniform positive pressure (pneumatic cylinder). The positive plaster mold can be made by pouring plaster into a casting of the residual limb. Some centers have the equipment to laser scan the residual limb to create a mathematical contour map that can be electronically modified and used to direct an automated cutting machine to fabricate the custom mold. This process is referred to as "CAD-CAM," an acronym for "computer-aided design–computer-aided manufacture." Work is also being done on perfecting a computer-guided machine to directly cut the socket.

The socket is attached to joints or the foot via an endoskeletal or exoskeletal system. The exoskeletal system can be conceptualized as a hollow column. It consists of a shank made of a lightweight rigid foam that is shaped to match the patient's natural limb, then laminated with a hard resin or plastic shell. The laminated load-bearing shell is highly durable and transmits the patient's weight to the prosthetic foot. It is frequently used for active children and people engaged in activities such as construction or farming. Once laminated, the exoskeletal system is difficult to adjust, requiring sawing and relaminating the hard outer shell. Psychologically, some users, their family, and friends do not like the hard exoskeletal design since it is not soft to the touch like skin, muscle, or foam. This is sometimes overlooked by the cosmetic advantage of being able to laminate decorative designs. The endoskeletal system can be thought of as an internal weight-bearing pipe with a cosmetic non-load-bearing outer shell. It uses a lightweight metal or plastic pylon covered with soft, shaped foam for cosmesis. The endoskeletal systems are very modular in design, allowing easy interchangeability of components and alignment.

Hip Disarticulation/Hemipelvectomy (Transpelvic) Socket

A hip disarticulation prosthesis is used for true hip disarticulation and with a residual femur of less than 5 cm. The short residual femur is preferred because it can add to prosthetic stability. During hemipelvectomy, part or all of the ilium is removed. The prosthetic socket can be thought of as a bucket with a hole where the nonamputated leg fits through. This is accomplished by using a rigid frame to contain the tissues of the amputated side, buttocks, and contralateral ilium, as needed, with a flexible anterior shell that opens for donning of the prosthesis. In the case of hip disarticulation, most weight bearing occurs over the ipsilateral ischial tuberosity and gluteal tissues. The contralateral ischial tuberosity, sacrum, and ipsilateral remaining tissue are the weight-bearing areas for the hemipelvectomy socket. The proximal portion of the socket is contoured to fit into the space between the iliac crest and rib cage for control and to help suspend the prosthesis. If needed, the trim line can proceed to enclose the bottom few ribs of the rib cage and trunk to provide stability with additional control via trunk motion. Lightweight endoskeletal componentry is necessary. The prosthetic hip and knee joints have an extension assist for stability. The hip joint is mounted anteriorly for stability, with the goal of keeping it at or behind the ground force reaction vector. A single-axis or soft-heeled foot should be provided to quickly transition the ground force reaction vector in front of the knee and behind the hip units, creating a stabilizing extension moment across these joints. When needed, locking hip and knee joints can be added for further safety and stability during standing activities.

Above-Knee Socket (Transfemoral)

There are three main AK socket designs: the quadrilateral, the NSNA (normal shape, normal alignment) or CAT-CAM (contoured adducted trochanteric–controlled alignment method), and the flexible socket. The AK residual limb typically presents with anterior and posterior myofascial flaps sutured together (myoplasty) or anchored to bone (myodesis) with the femur in the center. The socket is designed to contain the soft tissues and effectively control the movement and force of the residual femur during standing and ambulation. Fluid dynamic studies have shown that a force placed on a fluid in a closed container generates a uniform, equally distributed opposing pressure. Typically the socket is a one-piece rigid container or "hard socket." The patient's weight is borne on the hydrostatic pressure generated when the soft tissue of the residual limb is contained and compressed in the socket. The residual limb is not a simple fluid; thus, modifications in socket design have transferred some weight bearing to pressure-tolerant areas such as the underlying ischial tuberosity.

The quadrilateral hard socket was the most commonly used AK socket from the 1940s into the 1980s. It is a relatively square socket with narrow anterior-posterior and wide medial-lateral dimensions. The posterior brim contains a broad flat posterior seat for weight bearing on the ischial tuberosity region. It does not cup or contain the ischial tuberosity. In the 1980s, observation and x-ray studies confirmed that the wide medial-lateral dimension allowed the proximal part of the residual femur to shift laterally, distally compressing the medial soft tissue of the residual limb and resulting in a lateral shift of the person's body relative to the socket during the stance phase. This led to the development of narrow medial-lateral sockets to minimize this movement.

The NSNA, CAT-CAM, and ischial-containment hard socket have wide anterior-posterior and narrow medial-lateral dimensions, providing medial-lateral compression of the soft tissues, which limits the lateral shift of the femur within the socket during the stance phase. This maintains a more anatomic alignment of the residual femur. The posterior-brim ischial seat includes a high posterior-medial wall that cups the ischial tuberosity, creating a bony lock of the socket to the ischium during the stance phase, further limiting lateral socket shift.

The flexible socket is a two-piece socket that has a hard, usually windowed, outer frame with a semiflexible plastic or silicon polymer socket inside it. The outer frame is a laminate of resin and a high-strength material such as graphite braid. The unit can be fabricated utilizing the same design contours of the quadrilateral or NSNA-type socket. The inner liner can be made of a relatively clear, low-temperature polymer that becomes more flexible as it warms from body heat. Depending on the properties of the chosen polymer, this can improve comfort, owing to the ability of the liner to change shape with the changes in weight-bearing forces or muscle activity, or to accommodate mild increased residual limb volume. Some prosthetists believe that the ability of the inner liner to expand and contract with muscle activity can improve proprioceptive feedback. Observing the residual limb–socket interface through the inner liner improves the accuracy and ease of identifying where to make adjustments.

Below-Knee Socket

In theory, total-contact and PTB are the two main categories of BK socket design. Most sockets fabricated are a hybrid of the two and the result is a total-contact PTB socket. The true total-contact socket distributes the pressure equally to all areas of the residual limb. The PTB socket is designed to put more force over pressure-tolerant areas. These typically are the patella tendon, the medial flare and shaft of the tibia, the soft tissues of the anterior compartment between the tibia and the fibula, the lateral shaft of the fibula, and the posterior compartment. This is accomplished by taking away material over these areas on the positive mold of the residual limb, resulting in a smaller dimension or tighter fit when the socket is casted. All other areas in the PTB socket receive partial contact but are not designed to transfer any significant force to the residual limb.

Syme Amputation Socket

The Syme amputation is a surgical disarticulation of the ankle, with shaving of the malleoli, slight trimming of the tibia, preservation of the weight-bearing distal tibial cartilage, and reattachment of the heel pad. Direct weight bearing on the residual limb is possible, allowing the amputee to stand and walk without a prosthesis. A prosthesis is recommended to normalize the speed, efficiency, and stability of ambulation. A Syme prosthetic socket is self-suspending by being narrow internally, just proximal to the bulbous flair of the malleoli. Early sockets used a posterior or medial door to open the narrow portion and allow the distal, bulbous end of the residual limb to pass through. Once closed, this door provided the suspension. The cutout for this door significantly weakens the socket. Expandable air bladders or compressible liners that allow the amputee to pull the bulbous portion of the residual limb past the narrow portion have allowed for the fabrication of solid sockets that are stronger and lighter. The foot for a Syme prosthesis has a low hindfoot profile, because there is limited space between the distal end of the socket and the ground.

Partial Foot Amputation Socket

Partial foot amputations are categorized as toe amputation, transmetatarsal amputation, disarticulation at the proximal metatarsal–midfoot level (Lisfranc), disarticulation at the midfoot-hindfoot level (Chopart), and removal of the foot except for preservation of the calcaneus and a large portion of the talus (Boyd). In the case of a simple toe amputation (i.e., one or more of the second through fifth toes), a simple piece of foam or wool can be placed in the shoe to take up the space and minimize movement within the shoe. The great toe aids in slowing down the transition from the foot-flat to the toe-off phase as well as imparting energy for forward propulsion. Without the great toe, there is the tendency to roll over the front of the foot too quickly, as well as having decreased push off. To normalize gait mechanics and provide some energy return during toe off, a great toe amputation is best dealt with by adding a spring steel shank to the sole of the shoe or inserting an orthotic foot plate with a foam toe filler. A rocker sole may be needed to create a smooth transition from foot flat to toe off. This technique also works well for transmetarsal amputations. Patients who have had a midfoot amputation, of the Chopart and Lisfranc types, can be fitted with a self-suspending split socket and a custom prosthetic foot. When ankle instability is not an issue, there are cosmetic advantages of a molded silicone partial foot with a zippered socket that goes over the ankle flair for suspension. When natural ankle stability is poor, a custom-fabricated prosthetic boot, a custom-molded posterior leaf, or bivalve ankle-foot orthosis (AFO) with partial foot filler can be used. Patients who have had a Boyd and Syme hindfoot amputation are fitted with a Syme prosthesis.

Suspension

Suspension of the prosthesis can be accomplished by contour of the residual limb, wedges, straps, belts, corsets, suction, or a combination of these (Table 32-5). There are two broad categories of suction suspension, which for the purposes of this chapter are called standard suction and silicon suction suspension (3S). Standard suction uses a form-fitting hard or semirigid socket into which the residual limb is pushed or pulled. The 3S system uses a formed, highly flexible interface material (silicon) shaped like a residual limb sock that is rolled onto the residual limb before it is fit into the rigid socket. This typically functions as a liner as well as the suspension system. The suspension is accomplished by providing an airtight seal between the material and the patient's residual limb. The vacuum created when the socket attempts to pull off the limb holds the prosthesis tightly. For standard suction suspension, the residual limb can be lubricated with lotion and pushed into the socket. Without lubrication, the residual limb is "pulled" into the socket by an elastic wrap or cotton sock

Table 32-5: Suspension

Suspension	Indications	Contra-indications	Actions	Advantages	Disadvantages
Suction Traditional Modified (gel suspension liners)	1. Smooth residual limb contour	1. Volume fluctuations	1. Precisely fitting socket with air expulsion valve 2. Socket seals directly against skin	1. Best proprioception 2. No pistoning 3. Lightweight 4. Easy to maintain	1. Need to maintain precise fit 2. May fall off if suction is lost 3. Need to maintain constant body weight
Anatomic/limb contour	1. Short BK residual limb 2. Knee disarticulation 3. Syme 4. Mild mediolateral knee instability	1. Obese or very muscular patient 2. Very long BK residual limb	1. The socket is contoured over some bony prominence, normally the femoral condyle or malleoli	1. Suspension is inherent part of socket 2. Less restrictive to circulation than a cuff strap in BK 3. Aids in knee stability for BK	1. Requires precise modification 2. High trim lines reduce cosmesis; more damage to clothing in BK 3. May require removable wedge or door.
Straps/belts	1. When other systems have failed 2. Past users 3. Anticipated volume changes	1. Must be careful not to compress blood vessels or bypass grafts	1. SC-cuff strap fits over femoral condyle 2. Waist belt 3. Suspenders	1. Adjustability 2. Ampillary suspension for at risk activities, e.g., sports 3. Unlikely that prosthesis could fall off	1. Chafing 2. Cumbersome 3. Bulky 1. Patient can overpower unit due to air compressing 2. Maintenance, weight, cost 1. Weight 2. Cost and maintenance

BK = below-knee; SC = supracondylar.

placed over the residual limb. The wrap or sock is threaded through and out the bottom of the socket and used to pull the residual limb into the socket. The person usually has to stand to load and off-load the residual limb in a pumping motion while simultaneously pulling on the sock to fit into the socket. This requires a moderate level of balance, upper-extremity strength, and hand function. The roll-on suction suspension component, being a separate piece, is fitted with a distal pin or strap to provide attachment to the prosthetic socket. This system can be put on while standing, sitting, or lying and can often be modified to accommodate limited hand function. Suction suspension is not recommended for use on residual limbs with poor blood flow.

Suction Suspension for the Above-Knee Prosthesis

Standard suction using a form-fitting hard socket, though not always the easiest for the user, is technologically the most simple. The next is to have a form-fitting semi-flexible liner inside a rigid frame. The rigid frame can be windowed to allow for some expansion and pressure relief in the system as well as to reduce weight. The patient must have a stable limb volume and the ability to stand to don a tight-fitting socket. In the United States, this has been a common system since the 1980s and well tolerated by younger patients with good strength and dexterity. The roll-on suction suspension system gained popularity in the mid to late 1990s in countries where cost and availability were not a limiting factor. Its advantages are increased absorption and dissipation of shear forces, the ability to accommodate volume changes by using a sock between it and the socket, and ease of application.

Suction Suspension for Above-Knee or Below-Knee Prosthesis

Standard suction sockets are rarely used for patients who have had a BK amputation, as the typical BK residual limb lacks the soft-tissue volume necessary to form an airtight seal. The roll-on suction suspension works well for AK and BK residual limbs. Its shear-absorbing properties minimize skin breakdown and improve comfort over bony prominences and scar tissue. Custom-molded, roll-on suction suspension systems can be used for irregularly shaped, excessively bony, or scarred residual limbs. Disadvantages of this system are cost and hygiene. The airtight seal traps moisture, creating an environment that favors the clogging of pores and the propagation of microorganisms such as bacteria and yeast. The suspension liner and residual limb must be washed daily with low-residue soap. Antibacterial soaps may be helpful. Soaps with deodorant and perfume additives should not be used. Some liner materials are not affected by rubbing alcohol. Cleaning the inner surface with rubbing alcohol at periodic intervals will assist in minimizing the colony count of microorganisms. It is recommended that the suspension liner be dried overnight before using. One should also check with the manufacturer for care and cleaning instructions specific to that product.

The Hypobaric sock is a standard prosthetic sock with a band of silicone added to provide an airtight seal between the patient's residual limb and the socket wall. The Hypobaric sock has been used for AK and BK residual limbs. The patient dons the sock, lubricates the silicone band, and slides the residual limb and sock into the prosthesis. The air is expelled through a one-way air valve. The patient can use multiple Hypobaric socks to accommodate volume changes in the residual limb.

The Flex-seal is a very flexible silicone diaphragm with a hole in the center that is positioned over the proximal part of the socket. The patient dons the prosthesis by inserting the residual limb through the hole against the diaphragm, which conforms to the residual limb shape and creates an airtight seal.

Suction Suspension for Below-Knee Prosthesis

A suspension sleeve can also become a type of suction suspension if the sleeve is made out of a material that is impermeable to air such as latex, neoprene, silicone, or polyurethane. The sleeve will fit over the proximal brim of the prosthesis and onto the patient's thigh, providing an airtight seal. Donning the prosthesis is accomplished by folding the sleeve onto the prosthetic socket, inserting the residual limb with stump socks and liner into the socket, and then pulling the sleeve onto the thigh.

Suspension Belts for Above-Knee Prosthesis

The total elastic suspension (TES) belt, Silesian band, and the combined hip joint with pelvic band and waist belt are the nonsuction suspension systems most frequently used for AK suspension. Occasionally a shoulder harness is used. The TES belt, made out of an elastic material such as neoprene, is fastened around the waist. It can be used as a primary suspension, but is mostly utilized as a secondary suspension in tandem with a suction system to help control rotation or provide a backup if suction is lost, to prevent the prosthesis from falling off.

The Silesian belt is the most often used belt system of suspension. Attachment starts near the brim of the posterolateral socket wall. The belt encircles the contralateral side of the patient's pelvis to fasten on the anterior wall of the prosthesis. It provides rotational control and minimizes lateral socket shift with less weight and bulk compared to the combined pelvic band and hip joint.

The combined hip joint with pelvic band and waist belt provides a strong, relatively rigid suspension system that can control rotational, anterior-posterior, medial-lateral, and superior-inferior movement. It consists of a single-axis hip joint fastened to the lateral socket wall with its center proximal and posterior to the greater trochanter. A rigid pelvic band is attached to the upright of the hip joint. The band, contoured to fit the patient's pelvis, is held in place by an attached waist belt. Due to the added bulk, weight, and decreased cosmesis, this system is mainly used where additional control and suspension are needed for the short AK residual limb, or the limb with hard-to-control redundant tissue, weakness, or the need for an exceptionally strong suspension.

The shoulder harness is a suspender-type strap attached to the anterior wall of the prosthesis at one end and the posterior wall of the prosthesis at the other and worn over the shoulder. It is generally used when proximal compression or suction is contraindicated over bypass grafts, when residual limb perfusion is poor, or as a last resort when other systems have failed.

Suspension Belts and Straps for Below-Knee Prosthesis

The supracondylar cuff strap fits just above the patient's femoral condyles and patella. Tabs attach it to the sides of the prosthesis. It secures the prosthesis during the swing phase and when it is unsupported during knee flexion such as when the patient is sitting on a high stool.

A fork strap attached to a waist belt can be used as an additional suspension, in situations where circumferential straps or sleeves are contraindicated or not tolerated. Extension assist is provided when a portion of the strap is elasticized and fastened under tension. It is forked to pass on either side of the patella, to minimize patellar compression when the person sits.

Limb Contour Suspension

Limb contour suspension of the prosthesis is achieved by narrowing the socket proximal to a wide area of the residual limb. Care must be taken not to impede venous return and create a choke syndrome. Traditionally this has been possible by using the femoral condyles at the knee or malleoli of the ankle. Careful casting and fitting are needed to closely follow the contours of the bony prominences. In the BK amputation patient, the supracondylar suspension system consists of high medial and lateral contoured walls that cover the femoral condyles. This is known as a supracondylar trim line. When the anterior brim of the socket is raised above the patella, it is known as a suprapatellar trim line. The narrowing needed for suspension can be achieved by a removable supracondylar wedge, a compressible nonremovable narrowing in the liner that the condyles can be pushed past during donning of the prosthesis, a removable medial wall, or a pneumatic device. This system provides good medial-lateral stability for patients with a short residual limb or unstable knee joint. It is also helpful for patients who have difficulty with straps or sleeves or who do not tolerate suction suspension. The patient who has had a Syme or partial foot amputation often uses supramalleolar suspension, as discussed previously in the corresponding sections an socket design.

Socket Inserts

Socket inserts or liners are used inside of a rigid solid or solid-framed socket to provide comfort by absorbing shock and distributing forces. A residual limb with limited tissue coverage, crevices, or sharp transitions traditionally requires a custom-molded liner. The advent of materials with some inherent flow and creep has resulted in the use of some pre-formed liners for these situations. The ultimate shape is controlled by the custom-formed outer socket. The polyurethane and silicon gel roll-on suction suspension systems (3S) are commonly used with the total-contact socket design, since the gel tends to act as a fluid and flows to equalize pressure within the socket. The expanded polyethylene foams are commonly used with the PTB-style socket. The polyethylene foams are resilient and perform well under the specific weight-bearing areas of the PTB socket design. The socket inserts can be layered in patients in whom day-to-day volume changes are expected to be beyond what can be accommodated by adjusting the ply of stump socks. This may be a person requiring dialysis or one who has moderate to severe congestive heart failure. Layers can be added and removed like an onion skin. The 3S systems are gaining in popularity as more hybrid sockets incorporate both total-contact and PTB features. The 3S system can also be used in patients with rapidly changing residual limb volume, by providing liners of several different thicknesses combined with residual limb socks. To maintain the liner-skin interface and suction, the socks are placed between the 3S liner and the socket.

Prosthetic Joints

Prosthetic joints are available to replace the loss of anatomic joints at the hip, knee, and ankle. Rotational units, derotational units, and quick-release units are available. Orthotic joints are often modified and incorporated into the prosthetic design to provide additional stability across the remaining joints. Instability may be due to ligamentous factors, weakness, or a short lever arm from a short residual limb. Supplemental orthotic knee joints are used most frequently, followed by hip joints. A dedicated prosthetic ankle unit is occasionally used for sporting activities such as scuba diving or rowing. Rotational units are used in the AK prosthesis when the prosthetic leg needs to be positioned, such as when the patient is sitting on the ground. Derotational units can be added if the tissues of the residual limb do not tolerate the torque developed from the repetitive twisting and turning activities, such as those required for assembly-line work or golf. Ankle and derotational units are not recommended as a first solution. The increased weight, often located at the distal end of the prosthesis, creates larger acceleration and deceleration forces, requiring more strength, energy expenditure, and socket suspension. For most activities, ankle function is successfully incorporated into the design of the prosthetic foot.

Prosthetic Knee Joints

The prosthetic knee has three functions: support during the stance phase, smooth control during the swing phase, and unrestricted flexion for sitting and kneeling. In the swing phase, the knee controls the speed and timing of knee flexion and extension. If flexion is too slow, the foot may not clear the ground or excessive hip flexion will be needed to compensate. If extension is too slow, the person's center of mass will fall behind the knee axis, causing it to buckle at heel strike. If acceleration is too fast, uneven heel rise and excessive terminal impact can occur. Control can be accomplished with a number of different systems: simple friction, pneumatics, hydraulic, and hybrid electronic systems.

There are two basic designs of prosthetic knees: the single axis and the polycentric axis. The single-axis system involves a simple hinge with a single pivot point. The polycentric-axis knee joint is designed to have continually changing instantaneous centers of rotation to mimic human knee function. The four-bar knee is a good example of how this is accomplished by the summation of rotations about multiple single-pivot points. The polycentric-axis knee joint is normally designed so that the initial instantaneous center of rotation is posterior to the patient's weight line. This allows the ground force reaction to be anterior to the center of rotation, creating a high degree of knee stability during the stance phase of gait. Other systems that enhance knee stability are weight-activated friction brakes (safety knee), manual locks, and hydraulic stance-phase control (Table 32-6). Advances will continue to be made to improve simulation of human knee function. "Stance flexion" mimics the normal knee flexion during the stance phase, thereby absorbing some of the shock of heel strike. Power-assisted joints are becoming feasible as miniature electric motors, batteries, sensors, and microprocessors are made smaller, lighter, longer lasting, and affordable. Pressure-sensitive sensors are being incorporated into artificial limbs to send electric signals to the skin of the residual limb. It is hoped that the brain will learn to interpret the sensory signals to the residual limb as feeling in the prosthetic limb (14).

Terminal Devices—Pylon, Ankle, and Foot

The human foot assists in providing deceleration from the heel-strike to the foot-flat phases, shock absorption, acceleration during toe off, and a stable base of support. It can be semipliable during the stance phase, adjusting to changes in terrain during ambulation, yet becomes a rigid lever arm for push off. Early terminal devices such as the peg leg provided support but none of the dynamic features of the human foot. The use of rubber bumpers and flexible mounts provided some dorsiflexion-plantarflexion, inversion-eversion, and transverse rotation. In the 1980s prototype designs of "dynamic-response feet" moved into production, providing energy-storage and -release features by successfully incorporating resilient resins, plastics, and graphite materials into prosthetic feet and pylons. The 1990s witnessed a large increase in the number and variety of dynamic-response feet and prototype designs of feet incorporating electronics for sensory feedback (14).

Pylon

Traditionally, the terminal device has been a prosthetic foot and a pylon, a simple structural tube or shell attaching the socket to the foot in a BK prosthesis, or the knee to the foot in an AK prosthesis. The majority of prostheses produced in the late 1980s used this simple technology. The sophistication of design and materials technology have progressed so the pylon can be designed to bend, store and release energy, absorb vertical shock, and provide or absorb axial rotation. The Air-Stance is a pylon designed to provide vertical shock absorption as well as axial rotation and can be used with most prosthetic feet. It uses an adjustable air chamber and piston that the user can vary to match changes in activities. The Re-Flex VSP is a shock-absorbing graphite leaf spring pylon that is integrated with a Flex-Foot to absorb vertical shock. The Flex-Foot is one of the earlier designs that extended the foot into the pylon. The carbon graphite shank enabled energy storage during the stance phase by "loading" the foot and pylon followed by releasing stored energy during toe off (Table 32-7).

Ankle

Ankle motion, except for sports or industrial-type work activities, is usually sufficiently incorporated into the properties of the prosthetic foot. There are several multiaxis ankle systems available that can be added to feet that have some limited capability for triplanar movement. One example is the Endolight Multi-Flex ankle. It is often added to the Seattle Light Foot to provide a multiaxis foot with some energy-storing characteristics. Rowing, swimming with fins, and mountain climbing are sports for which a prosthetic ankle joint is put to good use. Derotational units placed at ankle level have been helpful in managing excessive torque in sports such as golfing or when work duties require repetitive rotational movements. It is recommended that adding componentry at the ankle level be minimized. The extra weight at the distal end of the prosthesis (pendulum) produces more inertia and momentum, requiring more strength, energy expenditure, and suspension to control the acceleration and deceleration and the position in space of the prosthesis.

Prosthetic Feet

Prosthetic feet can be classified into four to six categories, achieving varying proportions of the five basic functions of a prosthetic foot: simulating anatomic joint function, absorbing shock, providing a stable weight-bearing base of support, replacing lost muscle function, and providing cosmesis. The main categories are the SACH, single-axis,

Table 32-6: Prosthetic Knees

Knee	Indications	Contra-indications	Action	Stability	Advantages	Disadvantages
Single-axis constant friction knee	1. Previous user 2. Good hip extensors 3. Long residual limb	1. Weak hip extensors 2. Hip flexion contracture 3. Patient with variable cadence	1. Constant friction 2. Extension aid (optional)	1. TKA alignment 2. Voluntary control (contraction of hip extensors)	1. Low cost 2. Simple design 3. Lightweight 4. Easy to maintain	1. Not cadence responsive (excessive heel rise and terminal impact with increased cadence)
Weight-activated stance-control knee (safety knee)	1. Short residual limb 2. Weak hip extensors 3. Hip flexion contracture 4. Insecure patient (poor balance)	1. Patient with variable cadence 2. Bilateral AK amputation	1. Constant friction in swing 2. Extension aid 3. Weight-activated brake in stance	1. Inherent in stance control 2. TKA alignment 3. Voluntary control (contraction of hip extensors)	1. Increased knee stability even with knee flexed up to 15 degrees	1. Maintenance and noise 2. Increased weight 3. Difficulty in jackknifing on stairs
Polycentric knee (most often 4-bar)	1. Knee disarticulation 2. Weak hip extensors 3. Short residual limb 4. Need for increased stance stability	—	1. Constant friction, pneumatic, and hydraulic models 2. Inherent shorting of shank in swing phase	1. Instantaneous knee center posterior to GFR line at full extension 2. TKA alignment	1. Shank swings under residual limb in knee disarticulation 2. Good stability	1. Weight (in some older models)
Pneumatic swing-phase control	1. Patient with variable cadence	1. Very active person 2. Inactive, limited ambulation	1. Piston travels in a cylinder forcing air through an adjustable valve, creating resistance 2. Air compressing can act as extension aid	1. TKA alignment 2. 4-bar knee models	1. Simpler, lighter, and less cost than hydraulic	1. Patient can overpower unit due to air compressing. 2. Weight, maintenance, cost
Hydraulic swing-phase control	1. Patient with variable cadence 2. Medium to long residual limb length 3. Very active patient	1. Inactive patient	1. Piston travels in a cylinder, forcing a fluid through a set of orifices and adjustable valves	1. TKA alignment 2. Voluntary control (contraction of hip extensors) 3. Hydraulic stance-phase control in SNS models	1. Excellent cadence response 2. Patient with SNS model can descend stairs step over step and downhills	1. Weight 2. Cost and maintenance

AK = above knee; TKA = trochanteric knee ankle line; SNS = swing and stance; GFR = ground force reaction.

multiaxis, solid-ankle flexible-keel, and dynamic-response (energy-storing) feet. An additional classification is hybrid electronic feet. Weight reduction, stability, and energy storage and release are key factors in decreasing the user's energy consumption and improving ambulation. When physically and financially available, the dynamic-response foot tends to be the prosthetic foot of choice since there are models that achieve all three of these factors (see Table 32-7).

The SACH foot features a solid wood keel extending

Table 32-7: Prosthetic Feet					
Feet	**Indications**	**Contraindications**	**Action**	**Advantages**	**Disadvantages**
SACH	1. Limited ambulation, such as transfer only 2. Patient with limited funding	1. Active patient	1. Plantarflexion simulated by compression of heel wedge	1. Moderate weight 2. Good durability 3. No moving parts 4. Minimal maintenance	1. Limited plantarflexion and dorsiflexion 2. Heel cushion deteriorates over time 3. Rigid forefoot provides poor shock absorption
Single axis	1. Short AK residual limb	1. Weight of foot 2. Plantarflexion can cause knee hyperextension at heel strike.	1. Plantarflexion simulated by compression of heel bumper and joint	1. Increased knee stability; plantar-flexion reduces knee flexion moment at heel strike 2. Plantarflexion resistance is adjustable	1. High maintenance 2. Increased weight 3. Noise from bumpers
Multiaxis	1. Uneven terrain 2. Residual limb with scars	1. Patient cannot tolerate added weight 2. Patient does not have access to maintenance	1. Provides motion in all three planes	1. Reduces torque on residual limb 2. Adjustability 3. Good shock absorption	1. Increased weight 2. Increased maintenance and noise
Dynamic response	1. Very active patient	1. Patient relies heavily on an ambulation aid	1. The keel of foot acts like a spring compressing in stance phase (storing energy) and rebounding at toe off (push off)	1. Reduces force at heel strike on contralateral side 2. Some designs are very lightweight	1. High cost

AK = above knee.

to the toe break with a soft cushion in the heel. The unit is covered with foam rubber shaped like a foot. The heel cushion provides some limited shock absorption at heel strike and simulates plantarflexion by shortening the time it takes to get the midfoot and forefoot in contact with the ground. The wooden keel provides an anterior lever arm for deceleration and stability during late stance. The SACH foot does not have dorsiflexion, inversion, eversion, or axial rotation. It is an economical, low-maintenance foot for the sedentary person who has had a BK or AK amputation.

The single-axis foot controls passive plantarflexion and dorsiflexion by the use of multidurometer rubber bumpers and a single-axis joint. Changing the bumpers determines how fast the forefoot contacts the ground. The faster the forefoot touches the ground, the sooner the ground force reaction line proceeds in front of the knee center of rotation to create a stabilizing extension moment. Stance-phase stability is excellent, making this a good choice for the sedentary person who has had an AK amputation.

The multiaxis foot is designed to incorporate ankle and foot motions to mimic plantarflexion, dorsiflexion, inversion, eversion, and rotation. Ball-and-socket joints, U-joints, steel tendons, and rubber and polymer bumpers have been utilized to create motion in all three planes. Statically, it may not feel as stable as the single-axis foot. Dynamically, it can reduce shear forces, absorb shock, and adjust to uneven terrain. It is a good choice for the active person who has had an AK or BK amputation and walks on uneven surfaces or needs to control torque and shear over scarred tissue or a bony prominence. The multiaxis foot is a good choice for the sedentary to moderately active person who has had an AK or BK amputation. Many of the dynamic-response feet provide the same features, as well as energy storage and release to create a more normal gait for the highly active person.

The dynamic-response foot has a flexible keel or a combination of a keel and pylon that compresses to store energy as the dorsiflexion moment "loads" the forefoot. Some push off occurs as energy is released during decompression at toe off. A broad range of performance characteristics is possible by varying the stiffness of the components. These are chosen according to height, weight, and activity level. The active amputee will tend to prefer the more aggressive dynamic-response foot (see Table 32-7).

PROSTHETIC EVALUATION

It is advisable that the amputee and the prosthesis be evaluated by the prosthetic team after fitting and alignment, but prior to major gait training, to ensure the overall fit and acceptability of the prosthesis. The ultimate outcome of the person's ability to use the prosthesis will not be known until he or she has gone through gait training. Having done a thorough pre-prosthetic evaluation, the team should have a good estimate of what to expect. A young, healthy person with no other medical problems likely will be able to proceed to sporting activities, whereas a person with significant cardiopulmonary disease may only be a household ambulator. Therapy orders should be updated to include additional physical limitations if re-evaluation confirms continued deficits and improvement is expected with further therapy. Before proceeding with therapy to achieve the desired goals, the team needs to assess the fit, comfort, fabrication, length, function, and appropriateness of the prosthetic componentry. The sedentary prosthetic user would not make full use of an expensive energy-storing foot. Likewise, the use of a multifunction knee unit would not be functionally or economically appropriate for the debilitated sedentary person with poor balance. A constant friction or safety knee would be a better choice. The patient should be observed with the prosthesis on while standing, sitting, and if possible, ambulating. The length of the prosthesis is checked once the person's residual limb is fully into the socket and there is equal weight bearing on both feet. Equal weight bearing can be approximated by suspending a plumb bob from the middle of the person's sacrum to just above the floor between the feet. The trunk and waist are shifted left or right as needed to center the plumb bob between the feet. (A clinic tape measure encased in a small round plastic casing can be used as a plumb bob.) Once the weight is centered, the examiner observes for equal heights of the iliac crests, posterior superior iliac spines, or anterior superior iliac spines. If these are unequal, shims of various thickness can be placed under the appropriate foot to level the pelvis. This thickness is then the amount that the prosthesis needs to be changed. Aside from asking the person if the socket fits comfortably, the examiner should check that there are no significant tissue rolls over the trim lines of the socket or suspension system, that there are no significant gaps between the socket and residual limb, and that the foot makes even contact with the floor. When the patient is sitting, the prosthesis should not pull off or rotate, the distance from the knee to the pelvis and height from the floor should be relatively equal for both limbs, and the prosthetic foot should touch the floor. During ambulation there should be no major medial or lateral shifts, excessive flexion or hyperextension of the knee, abnormally wide or narrow-based gait, pistoning of the prosthetic socket on the residual limb, or shifting of the person's body from side to side in compensation for improper fit. Excessive acceleration from heel strike to foot flat, trouble maintaining knee stability, and difficulties in proceeding from foot flat to toe off should be identified. If the prosthetist is present, minor adjustments should be made at this time. Pain over bony prominences should not occur if the fit is correct. The prosthetic socket should be removed and the residual limb closely inspected for signs of excessive pressure such as areas of deep sock marks or redness. The socket and liner should be modified and, if used, the ply of socks changed to correct this. At this stage, a prescription for physical therapy can be issued to begin gait training.

GAIT TRAINING

Therapy encompasses education in all areas of prosthetic use. This should include donning and doffing the prosthesis, adjusting the thickness or ply of residual limb socks, how to watch for areas of excessive pressure, implementation of a schedule for progressively increasing wearing time, residual limb care, and a home exercise program. If there is any concern regarding compliance or understanding safe prosthetic use, the prosthesis should remain at the therapy gym until the client can demonstrate safety in the following areas: donning and doffing the prosthesis, understanding of the need for progressively increasing wearing time, the ability to inspect the residual limb for areas of skin breakdown or increased pressure, safe transfers, and safe basic ambulation with or without an assistive device. Formal training with a therapist may last 1 week or several months, depending on the abilities of the amputee.

Therapy can be thought of as different phases in which the person achieves increasing functional levels. Initially the amputee is taught how to don and doff the prosthesis and transfer from sitting to standing. Weight shifting is then accomplished with the goal of even weight distribution on both lower extremities. Ambulation on level surfaces with an assistive device is next. The progression, as possible, is to learn to ascend and descend stairs, ambulate on uneven surfaces, and master ramps or inclines. The assistive device is weaned when strength, balance, and coordination are sufficient to do these safely. The therapist assists the amputee in learning how to perform a smooth, even reciprocal gait with appropriate balance on one leg, to tandem walk, to walk backwards, to hop, and to run. Transferring from the ground or floor should be accomplished. Ideally the prosthetic team will have a chance to periodically review the client's progress, evaluate the gait, check the fit of the socket, and make any needed adjustments for skin protection and improved gait.

COMMON PROBLEMS AND SOLUTIONS

Problems at the Residual Limb–Socket Interface

The lower-extremity amputee must bear the body weight on soft-tissue structures that were not designed for weight bearing. Total contact, when possible, provides a larger area over which to distribute the weight-bearing forces and increases sensory feedback. The socket is made to minimize forces over pressure-sensitive areas and provide loading over regions that are pressure tolerant. The pressure-tolerant areas of the transtibial residual limb include the patellar tendon, the pretibial muscles, the residual posterior muscles, the medial flare of the tibia, and the lateral fibula. Pressure-intolerant areas include the fibular head, tibial crest, hamstring tendons, and distal ends of the tibia and fibula. Failure to relieve pressure-sensitive areas causes skin breakdown, pain, and even abandonment of the prosthesis. A history of pain, skin redness or breakdown, change in the number of sock plies, or the inability to don or doff the prosthesis mandates evaluation of the fit of the socket. Direct external visualization, inspection of the fit through a transparent or translucent socket, observations of erythema or sock weave impressions on the skin of the residual limb, or the putty ball compression test can be used to assess the socket fit.

It is best to evaluate socket fit when the patient is standing and bearing weight on the prosthesis. For a transtibial amputee, the position of the patella relative to the location of the patellar tendon bar inside the socket can be determined by visual estimation, measurement, or examination of the skin over the patellar tendon for sock marks. For a transtibial socket with a standard trim line, the trim line typically falls at the midpatellar level. First, observe the position of the patella relative to the trim line. If the midpoint of the patella appears to be sinking below the brim of the socket ("setting sun"), the residual limb is sinking too far into the socket. This indicates that the socket system is too large, possibly due to weight loss, edema resolution, soft-tissue atrophy, or residual limb socks with an insufficient number of plies. Conversely, if the midpoint of the patella is above the socket brim ("rising sun"), the socket system is too small. Weight gain, edema, limb growth in the pediatric patient, or wearing socks with too many plies can cause this problem.

Proximal trim line sockets may not allow direct visualization of the patella. For prostheses with different trim lines, often a fixed point inside the socket corresponding to a known point on the residual limb can be identified. The distance from the point inside the socket to the proximal trim line can be measured. This same distance is marked where it can be visualized on the residual limb such as on the stump sock. The residual limb is placed back into the socket, and during weight bearing, the fit is assessed relative to the marked distance. A test socket made of clear acrylic or thermoplastic provides direct observation of the residual limb in the socket. Areas of excessive contact or lack of contact can be distinguished in these sockets. Frame sockets with clear or translucent flexible liners have become a frequent choice for the transfemoral-level amputee.

Sock marks, erythema, and compression of a putty ball can help assess the fit when direct visualization of the residual limb or limb-socket landmarks is not possible. When the prosthesis and limb socks first are removed, carefully inspect the residual limb for the presence of sock weave patterns on the skin of the residual limb. These impressions only last for a few moments. Heavier sock impressions correspond well to areas of greater contact with the socket. Less distinct impressions indicate less contact, whereas the absence of impressions suggests lack of contact. Erythema usually is not present on the residual limb when the socket and socks first are removed. It is normal to see erythema on the residual limb develop a few minutes after the socket is removed. If the prosthesis fits well, this erythema fades quickly, often within minutes, and should resolve in less than 20 minutes. If erythema in any area is excessive, persistent, painful, or tender on examination, there is a problem with the socket fit. Prolonged erythema on the AK residual limb at the proximal medial socket brim can occur if the adductor tissues roll over the socket brim (adductor roll) and not into the socket. This may occur from improper positioning of the adductor roll into the socket during donning, or from a socket that is too tight. Increased erythema in the region of the pubic symphysis may indicate a loose socket fit, allowing the residual limb to sink too deeply into the socket. Once adjustments are made in the socket–residual limb interface, re-evaluation of fit is imperative. Correction of socket fit problems can be verified by the absence of the undesirable erythema or sock impressions after prosthetic modification.

The putty ball compression test uses a small 1- to 2-cm ball of silicon or claylike material placed between the distal end of the residual limb and the socket interface. If residual limb socks and a liner are used, the ball is placed between the residual limb socks and the liner. It is recommended that the ball be wrapped in a thin piece of plastic to keep it from becoming enmeshed in the sock. Do not place it between the residual limb and the socks, as the socks may be pulled tightly up against the distal end of the residual limb, compressing the putty ball, but not really end bearing on the socket. The patient then is requested to walk for several minutes while wearing the prosthesis. The prosthesis is removed, and the putty ball examined. If the patient is achieving contact distally in the socket, the ball will be flattened. The degree of flattening is relative to the amount of contact or end bearing that is occurring in the socket. If the ball is not flattened or only slightly flattened, distal contact is insufficient.

Evaluation of distal contact inside a transfemoral socket can be accomplished by using a putty ball, just as in the case of the transtibial-level amputee. Direct palpation of the distal end of the residual limb inside the socket is possible if the transfemoral prosthesis has a traditional suction socket system that uses a distal valve. While the patients is standing in the prosthesis, the suction valve is removed. If the fit of the socket is correct, the soft tissues of the residual limb should fill the space of the removed valve and not permit the examiner's finger into the socket. If a space is visualized or the examiner's finger can enter the socket without obstruction, there is an obvious lack of contact. Complete contact in the area of the valve housing may be present, whereas total contact is inadequate elsewhere in the socket. If this is suspected, ask the patient to hike his or her pelvis on the amputated side. The residual limb will pull slightly out of the socket as suction is lost. This creates a small space for the clinician to insert his or her index finger into the distal socket. Caution: Be sure to position the finger with the palmer surface facing the distal end of the socket so the finger can flex as weight bearing occurs. The patient is asked to place weight on the prosthesis slowly while the examiner's finger monitors the degree of contact and pressure. Weight transfer must be done slowly, taking care not to pinch or even injure the examiner's index finger that is placed between the residual limb and the valve housing. If a void is noted, there is a lack of total contact. Lack of contact frequently is shown posteromedially or posterolaterally.

The transfemoral quadrilateral and ischial-containment sockets are designed to place significant weight bearing on the ischial tuberosity. If the ischial tuberosity contacts the ischial seat of the socket with no room for the examiner's finger between the socket and the residual limb, the prosthesis fits correctly with respect to proximal anatomic landmarks. The easiest way to evaluate this is to have the amputee flex the prosthetic knee while standing, and the examiner then locates the ischial tuberosity on the side of the amputation. With the examiner's index finger on the ischial tuberosity, the amputee is asked to extend the prosthetic knee and bear weight equally on both lower extremities. If the examiner's finger is pinched between the ischial tuberosity and the ischial seat of the prosthesis with little or no intervening space, the fit of the proximal socket is correct. If there is minimal contact with the examiner's finger, the residual limb is out of the socket and the socket is either too small or the liner-sock combination is too thick to properly fit into the socket. If the ischial tuberosity slides over and down into the socket and does not remain in contact with the ischial seat, the socket is too large. For the ischial-containment socket, the depression for containing the ischial tuberosity is located and the examiner's finger monitors the fit at this location. Caution: Be sure to position the finger with the palmer surface facing the distal end of the socket so the finger can flex as weight bearing occurs.

Phantom Pain and Sensation

Phantom sensation and phantom pain are not equivalent terms. Phantom sensation is the mental perception that a part of a missing limb still is present after amputation. It is a common postoperative experience. Phantom sensation is not painful and usually does not require treatment. Phantom pain, however, is the perception of painful sensation seemingly present in the missing limb or segment. The distribution of the perceived pain may or may not be in a dermatomal pattern. It is often most prominent immediately after amputation and ranges in severity from mild to severe. Phantom pain can be so severe that it interferes with all levels of functioning, including work and family life. Phantom pain rarely occurs in children, especially in those younger than 7 years (15). Phantom pain typically improves and eventually resolves with time. In a small group of patients, it may persist indefinitely. Phantom sensation and pain are puzzling to the uninformed patient. Patients need to know that these are usual experiences, they are not "losing their mind," and effective treatment is available for the pain. Anxiety, which can heighten the perception of pain, can be avoided with preoperative patient education.

The etiology for phantom pain is unknown. It has been compared to chronic pain, neuralgia, neural injury, and neuropathies. The pain generators and pathways can be peripheral, at the dorsal horn nerve root–spinal cord level, or central. As with any chronic pain, it is likely a mixture of all of these with variations from patient to patient. Please see Chapters 58 and 63 for further information.

Patients describe phantom pain many ways. They may experience burning, shooting, crushing, and cramping and the sense that the limb is positioned in a painful posture. Individuals typically report that phantom pain is worse at night, after the extremity has been in a dependent position or after the prosthesis has been off for a period. The pain tends to appear mainly in the distal aspect of the phantom extremity. At times, patients can identify specific points on the residual limb that trigger phantom pain. Careful examination of the residual limb can determine if these points correlate with neuromas, cysts, sites of excessive weight bearing, or pressure over specific nerves (e.g., the peroneal nerve at the fibular head). In addition to an ill-fitting prosthesis or mechanical stimulation precipitating phantom pain, other precipitating factors occasionally reported include fatigue, micturition, defecation, ejaculation, and even yawning.

Treatment of Phantom Pain

Phantom pain can be treated successfully. The treatment options include pharmacologic and nonpharmacologic physical and surgical interventions. Immediately after surgery, the analgesics used to treat surgical pain often control phantom pain; however, these medications eventually are ineffective because acute surgical pain and phantom pain are not the same neurophysiologically. If phantom pain occurs, low-dose tricyclic antidepressants (TCAs) such as nortriptyline or amitriptyline are the first drugs of choice. A "low dose" of 10 to 50 mg is frequently effective, though doses up to 150 mg are used in patients with more severe pain. With persistent phantom pain, periodic measurements of drug levels are helpful in determining whether the patient is taking the medication appropriately and the therapeutic serum levels are achieved. The anticholinergic side effects of these medications, especially in the elderly and patients with cardiac arrhythmia, can limit the their use. Antiseizure medications such as phenytoin, carbamazepine, and gabapentin can be used if the TCAs are ineffective or contraindicated. Full therapeutic anticonvulsant doses are most effective. For locally mediated pain, topical analgesics may work. Capsaicin, a derivative of capsicum oleoresin found in the common chili pepper plant, is a topical analgesic agent. It reduces the perception of pain by depleting the supply of the neurotransmitter substance P. The major advantages are the route of application and its nonsystemic effects. To be effective, capsaicin needs to be applied three to four times a day over the painful area. Capsaicin must be applied consistently for at least 2 to 3 weeks before its effectiveness can be determined. Testing over a small area of skin, not on the residual limb, is recommended. It should be discontinued if a rash forms. A burning sensation may occur locally when it is first used. This sensation resolves with repeated application. If it is not applied as prescribed, analgesia will not occur. Local irritation can occur if capsaicin comes into contact with eyes, mucous membranes, or open skin.

Nonpharmacologic treatment options often are overlooked. Transcutaneous electrical nerve stimulation (TENS) can provide sufficient neuromodulation of pain to reduce or eliminate the need for medication. TENS treatment can begin early in the postoperative period and has no significant side effects. Successful TENS therapy requires an experienced physical therapist to work with the patient to determine the most effective level of neurostimulation. Fitting with compression stockings or stump shrinkers early in the postsurgical period can reduce phantom pain and incision pain. Once the incision site has healed, physical modalities such as manipulation, vibration, or massage of the residual limb also can provide relief. Heat or cold applied to the residual limb after massage or manipulation is effective for some. Patients often report a significant reduction in phantom pain once weight bearing and prosthetic use begin. If anxiety or emotional stress is a significant factor in pain control, an experienced mental health professional can provide individual counseling or support-group therapy to teach patients effective methods of pain reduction and management (e.g., stress management, distraction, and hypnosis techniques).

In the refractory situation, as with other chronic pain syndromes, one may have to systematically work through treatments for peripheral, spinal cord level–, and brain level–mediated pain. Peripheral pain may respond to nonnarcotic analgesics, local anesthetics, anticonvulsants, and chemical sympathectomy. Physical interventions include feedback from the stump shrinker or socket, ultrasound, electrical stimulation, vibration, massage, thermal modalities, and acupuncture. Surgical intervention may be considered for neuroma excision, neurectomy, nerve fascicle ligation, rhizotomy, ganlionectomy, or sympathectomy. Treatment directed at spinal cord level–mediated pain includes narcotic analgesics, TCAs, neuroleptics, baclofen, and tizantidine. Epidural injections and spinal cord stimulators have been used to control phantom pain. Occasionally, dorsal column stimulation, chordotomy, and dorsal root entry zone (DREZ) sectioning have been utilized. Although extremely rare, there are reports of using brain stimulators and ablation brain surgery for the control of severe, refractory phantom pain (16).

Choke Syndrome

Choke syndrome is a swelling of the tissues that occurs when there is obstruction of venous outflow proximal to a potential space in the prosthetic socket into which the residual limb tissue can swell. Because arterial inflow is unimpeded and outflow is restricted, fluid accumulates in the area of inadequate contact. The obstruction to venous outflow is usually caused by tight proximal contact of the socket with the residual limb. Weight gain, edema from trauma or a medical condition, socks with too many plies, and do-it-yourself prosthetic modifications are the most frequent causes. The lack of total contact between the residual limb and the socket (potential space) distal to the proximal constriction may be secondary to distal tissue atrophy, compression of liner materials, removal or loss of a distal end–bearing pad, or socks with too many plies, preventing the residual limb from dropping all the way into the end of the socket. Swelling continues to occur in the soft tissues until contact with the socket wall occurs. Choke syndrome is the second most common dermatologic condition of the residual limb seen, after contact dermatitis to suspension sleeves.

Choke syndromes can be acute or chronic. The involved area has a sharply circumscribed round or oval margin, distinguishing it from cellulitis. When the residual limb is first examined after the prosthesis is removed, the skin may be cool to the touch and a dusky or purple color may appear after a few minutes. In approximately 5 minutes, the skin becomes red and warm to the touch as blood flow improves.

An acute choke syndrome is recognized by indurated red tissues that may have an orange-peel appearance, prominent skin pores, and skin changes that appear eczematous with open or weeping skin. Blisters may be present, especially on old scars. The skin eventually may macerate and leave an open, superficial ulcer if the constriction is allowed to continue. Pain may be the major complaint, especially after the prosthesis has been off for a brief time. The presence of choke syndrome does not exclude the possibility of a superimposed infection or carcinoma. Increased warmth, proximal advancement of the erythema, diffuse redness, foul odor, purulence, and constitutional symptoms suggest infection.

As the choke syndrome becomes chronic, the skin may take on a verrucose appearance with serous crusting. In the case of a chronic choke syndrome, the skin color may become brownish-orange from deposition of hemosiderin pigment in the skin. This latter change is a permanent condition. Venous stasis ulceration from the chronic venous hypertension can occur.

Except for the staining of the skin from hemosiderin deposition, all the changes associated with choke syndrome are reversible and resolve with correction of the prosthetic fit problem (i.e., restoration of total contact between the residual limb and the socket). Reducing the number of sock plies to improve distal contact, adding a proper-fitting distal end pad, and enlarging the proximal area of socket constriction are the most common modifications made to resolve a choke syndrome. The continuous use of a shrinker sock, even when wearing the prosthesis, may help prevent the occurrence of a choke syndrome in the individual with fluctuating edema.

The examiner is reminded of the importance of verifying residual limb contact with the socket by observation of sock weave impressions, performance of the putty ball compression test, or direct visualization. If the patient experiences pain from constriction at the distal end of the residual limb, this may be perceived as excessive weight bearing on the end of the residual limb. Additional sock plies may be added to reduce this excessiveness. However, the additional socks increase proximal constriction, prevent the residual limb from dropping into the socket, and create an even greater potential space distally into which swelling occurs. If the clinician does not recognize the choking phenomenon, he or she also can aggravate the problem by providing additional distal socket relief to relieve a misdiagnosed end-bearing problem.

Dermatologic Problems

The most frequently occurring dermatologic problems of the residual limb are contact dermatitis, folliculitis, sebaceous cysts, excessive sweating, and scar management. Contact dermatitis may present as an erythematous rash, edema, or if severe enough, oozing vesicles. Suspension sleeve, liner, and sock materials are common allergens. It is less common for someone to be allergic to the resins and plastics used for socket fabrication. Skin testing of materials is recommended when someone is highly allergic. Treatment is elimination of contact with the offending material by using a liner or switching to another material. The clinician should rule out the recent use of new laundry detergents, soaps, or skin lotions. Topical diphenhydramine (Benadryl), steroid, or skin creams are used depending on the severity. The clinician should observe for the development of superimposed infection. Prosthetic use may need to be stopped for several days.

Folliculitis and sebaceous cyst formation are found in areas of increased repeated shear or excessive weight-bearing contact. Excessive sweating and poor hygiene can exacerbate this. The medial tibial flare, popliteal fossa, and groin are common areas of involvement. One should ensure that the prosthetic socket, liner, and suspension fit well. Residual limb care should be changed, to keep pores open and minimize bacteria counts. More frequent washing and use of a wash cloth, antibacterial soaps without perfumes, warm soaks, or hot compresses should be instituted as needed. The residual limb socks should be cleaned and changed more frequently if sweat or hygiene is a problem. Liners and suspension systems that make direct contact with skin should be cleaned daily and allowed to dry overnight. Rubbing alcohol has been used to minimize bacterial counts on materials not adversely affected by it. Consult the prosthetist or manufacturer for verification. Excessive sweating may have to be dealt with by frequent sock changes or in the case of suction liners with which socks are not used, by a special antiperspirant such as Drysol.

Limbs with split-thickness grafts, extensive scarring, or skin adherence to underlying bone may develop blisters or tears from friction and repetitive traction. Scars with deep furrows may necessitate use of a shear-absorbing liner or pads custom fabricated to fill in the potential space, minimize local choke phenomena, prevent the rolling over of tissue at the margins, and control movement. Tissue mobilization to release adhesions, use of shear-absorbing liners (silicon gel or equivalent), and improvement of suspension comprise the first line of treatment. Repetitive movement–induced shear forces and weight bearing on the area can be decreased further with a thigh corset lacer, increased ischial weight bearing, or pelvic band and hip joint suspension.

In rare situations, there are residual limbs with little or no intervening subcutaneous soft tissue and only split-thickness skin graft coverage. The graft often is adherent to underlying bone. These tissues do not withstand the rigors of weight bearing in a prosthesis, and the result is skin breakdown. If prosthetic modifications are not successful, surgical intervention may be necessary. If surgical revision to a more proximal level would adversely affect the functional level of the amputee, the possibility of coverage with a vascularized muscle flap graft and meshed split-thickness skin graft should be considered in an effort to preserve function. The muscle flap provides subcutaneous padding and mobility for the overlying skin graft. The use of a meshed graft results in contraction of the skin graft with maturation that aids in providing an acceptable shape of the residual limb for prosthetic fitting.

PEDIATRIC LIMB LOSS AND PROSTHETICS

Children with congenital or acquired limb deficiency require not only the technical aspect of prosthetic restoration but also monitoring and intervention to assist them in reaching developmental, social, and psychological milestones. Acquired limb loss results from trauma, tumor, or disease. Most traumatic amputations involve accidents with power tools such as lawn mowers. Cancer is the most frequent disease leading to childhood amputation. Children with congenital limb deficiency may be seen in the clinic setting as soon as a few months after birth. The early visits are usually for counseling the parents. Education varies according to need but often includes care of the residual limb, precautions, acceptable activities, current and future therapy recommendations, criteria for revision surgery, expected functional goals, and cosmetic outcome. Short- and long-term financial planning may need to be discussed. Prosthetic restoration and counseling are ongoing processes as the child grows physically and emotionally into adulthood.

Approximately 60% of early childhood limb loss is a congenital limb deficiency and not acquired limb loss (17). The etiology is not always known. A few genetic syndromes, amniotic constriction bands, and teratogenic agents such as thalidomide and high-dose radiation have been identified. Technically these are "congenital skeletal deficiencies." Classification systems have been developed in an attempt to unify data collection. Patients with transverse deficiencies have a normal limb proximal to the level of termination, below which there is no limb. A total absence of the tibia, fibia, and all distal elements is considered a "transverse deficiency." The ISO/ISPO classification for this deficiency would be "leg transverse deficiency, total" (18). Longitudinal deficiencies refer to limbs with a reduction or absence of skeletal components while still having other components present below the affected part. If only the fibula is absent, the deficiency is a longitudinal type named "fibular longitudinal deficiency, total." This indicates that the femur is normal; the tibia, ankle, and foot are present; and the fibula is absent. The bones and tissues distal to the deficiency may not be normal. Previously this was named "fibular hemimelia," the definition of hemimelia being "longitudinal deficiency in which all or part of one long bone is missing." Common longitudinal deficiencies are fibular longitudinal deficiency, total/partial; proximal femoral focal deficiency (PFFD) or femoral longitudinal deficiency, partial; and tibial longitudinal deficiency, total/partial (Table 32-8).

The challenge for the team is to determine conservative management versus surgical revision and prosthetic restoration. Leg-length discrepancy may be minimized by shoe lifts, bracing, or surgery. If the foot is not functional, a Syme or Boyd amputation with prosthetic restoration may improve function. If there is hip or knee dysplasia and instability, orthotic bracing and surgical stabilization procedures are considered. In children with PFFD with a short femur, unstable knee, and preserved ankle-foot motion, knee fusion and a van Ness tibial rotationplasty allow the fitting of a transfemoral prosthesis modified to use the preserved ankle-foot motion as a knee joint.

The proper labeling tends to be disregarded as the child grows, especially if the congenital limb deficiency appears the same as an acquired limb loss or revision surgery has occurred to accommodate prosthetic restoration. "Surgical conversion has been estimated to be necessary in the management of 50% of lower extremity congenital deficiencies and only 8% of the upper extremity deficiencies" (3).

For children, the epiphysis (growth plate) should be saved whenever possible. A joint disarticulation amputation is preferred before a long-bone transverse amputation, whenever functional outcome will be similar. The benefits of saving the growth plate include a reduced leg-length discrepancy allowing the entire limb to grow, fewer fitting problems within the socket since the disarticulation surface tolerates direct weight bearing, and no bony overgrowth as occurs after cutting across a long bone. Approximately 12% of children with acquired limb loss will experience bony overgrowth (3). The result is a distal spike-like formation of bone that tends to grow faster than the overlying tissues and skin. A bursa may develop over the end of the sharp bone, or the end of the bone may protrude through the skin, resulting in the development of cellulitis or osteomyelitis. The shape of the limb may often be conical, come to a point, and create high focal pressure within a prosthesis. This also makes a suction fit difficult. If a roll-on suction suspension system is desired, an additional distal cup made of silicone can be used to minimize shear and increase the circumference of the distal end of the limb.

Prosthetic intervention should be considered at the time the child is beginning to pull up on the sound limb. This is usually around 9 to 15 months (19,20).

Alignment of the prosthesis should allow the patient optimum balance for standing and short steps. This alignment may need to be changed when the patient starts to walk. Formal physical therapy training sessions are used to teach the parents what to do with the child at home.

Table 32-8: Common Lower Extremity Longitudinal Deficiencies

Fibular longitudinal deficiency, total/partial (fibular hemimelia)
- Incidence: most common congenital deficiency, bilateral in 25% of cases
- Skeletal involvement
  - Hip: normal
  - Femur: usually normal, rare shortening
  - Knee: genu valgum
  - Fibula: absent total or partial, possible rudimentary piece
  - Tibia: often shortened, may have an anteromedial bow, possibly abnormal distal epiphysis
  - Ankle: possible joint surface abnormalities, instability, fusion of tarsals
  - Foot: equinovalgus deformity, absent lateral rays

Treatment
- Conservative: orthotic bracing for joint stability and minimize leg-length discrepancy, shoe lifts, hybrid orthotic incorporating prosthetic componentry
- Surgical: joint stabilization (fusion), leg-lengthening procedures, contralateral epiphysiodesis to stunt growth, tibial osteotomy, Syme or Boyd amputation if foot and ankle not functional or leg-length discrepancy no longer correctable with hybrid orthotic bracing

Femoral longitudinal deficiency, partial [proximal femoral focal deficiency (PFFD)]
- Incidence: 1:50,000 births, 10%–15% bilateral
- Skeletal involvement
  - Hip: coxa vara, possibly absent proximal femur, pseudarthrosis
  - Femur: total or partial absence, short
  - Knee: can be unstable
  - Fibula: often partial absence
  - Tibia: may be short
  - Ankle: variable bony abnormalities
  - Foot: frequent deformity
- Treatment
  - Conservative: orthotic bracing for joint stability and to minimize leg-length discrepancy, shoe lifts, hybrid orthotic incorporating prosthetic componentry
  - Surgical: joint stabilization (fusion), correction of coxa vara and pseudarthrosis, leg-lengthening procedures, knee disarticulation, Syme or Boyd amputation, van Ness tibial rotationplasty. Note: Prosthetic socket may need to have ischial containment to provide hip joint stability.

Tibial longitudinal deficiency, total/partial (tibial hemimelia)
- Incidence: 1:1,000,000 births
- Skeletal involvement
  - Hip: normal but can be associated with PFFD
  - Femur: normal but can be associated with PFFD
  - Knee: instability
  - Fibula: usually intact
  - Tibia: partial or total absence
  - Ankle: instability
  - Foot: varus deformity
- Treatment
  - Conservative: orthotic bracing for joint stability and to minimize leg-length discrepancy, shoe lifts, hybrid orthotic incorporating prosthetic componentry
  - Surgical: joint stabilization (fusion), leg-lengthening procedures, contralateral epiphysiodesis to stunt growth, knee disarticulation if quadriceps and knee motion not functional, Syme or Boyd amputation if foot and ankle not functional or leg-length discrepancy no longer correctable with hybrid orthotic bracing. Occasionally, centralization of fibula to create a tibia is attempted

Therapy is directed at incorporating the prosthesis into play activities of the young child. Much of this "therapy" is done at home. The physical therapist should perform periodic re-evaluation and instruction to advance the home program. Developmental milestones for the general pediatric population include the following: pulls self to standing at 6 to 10 months, stands alone well at 10 to 14 months, walks without support at 12 to 15 months, climbs up or down a few steps at 14 to 22 months, and walks heel to toe two of three attempts at 3½ to 5 years (20). Allowing for growth of the residual limb within the prosthesis is an important consideration in pediatric prosthetics. Children grow out of shoes and clothes fast enough, and a prosthesis is more costly and time-consuming to replace than clothing. One good way to allow for growth of the residual limb while still maintaining a proper fit is to incorporate growth liners within the socket. A growth liner may consist of two or more layers of material for the insert of the prosthesis. As the child grows and becomes too large for the insert, the inner layer can be removed, thus increasing the overall volume of the insert and allowing continued use of the prosthesis. While the child's limb may grow in length, it may have a reduction in overall volume due to loss of baby fat and pressures from the prosthesis. This can often be accommodated by increasing the number of sock plies worn by the patient. Often, the greater challenge for the prosthetic team is accommodating for the overall growth of the child in length, circumference, and foot size of the prosthesis. If permissible, endoskeletal components should be used to allow for greater ease in increasing the length of the prosthesis. This cannot be done with young pediatric patients or patients with long transtibial or transfemoral residual limbs. The overall length of the prosthesis is too short to accommodate the combined length of the endoskeletal fastening fittings. When an exoskeletal system is used, the increases in length can be accommodated by adding ankle spacer blocks below the foot attachment plate (easiest) or cutting the prosthesis and adding spacers below the socket and above the ankle area. The latter of these methods requires additional reinforcement. A fun cosmetic advantage of the exoskeletal prosthesis is the ability to laminate pictures or designs onto the surface. Fabric cloth may be chosen by the patient and incorporated on the socket in place of the standard skin pigmentation finishing. Children seem to enjoy this as it can make the prosthesis more of a conversation piece.

One of the pleasures of working with pediatric patients is their resilience and optimistic outlook. Often, their body image incorporates the prosthesis quickly and there are few emotional problems. On the other hand, the parents of the child, especially if one was somehow involved with the trauma leading to the amputation (i.e., lawn mower accidents), can increase the difficulty of the fitting process. Naturally, parents want their child to run and play as well as other children. Most parents adjust to their child's disability; however, a few will persist to push for a "better," "lifelike," or "natural" prosthetic fit, function, or cosmesis. These issues normally can be worked out by acknowledging the parents' concerns, discussing the limitations of man-made componentry, and explaining realistic options. Arranging peer counseling with another family is beneficial but not always initially accepted. When needed, one should encourage second opinions with other prosthetic teams.

Not all children adapt well. Some may have periods of difficulty at different stages of their physical and emotional development. Psychological conflict or crises can arise if they have low self-esteem or limited social support or perceive that their physical appearance is not acceptable to peers. Such issues should be explored during clinic visits. Counseling for the child and family members is recommended if the education and intervention provided in the clinic and prosthetic fitting sessions are not sufficient (22).

SPORTS

Sporting activities require advanced performance from the individual as well as from the prosthetic components. Each sport should be analyzed, particularly at the individual's anticipated activity level, to create a list of the desired functions to be performed by the prosthetic system. This will ultimately dictate the choice of components to be used with a properly fitting socket. A recreational runner will have different performance needs than a competitive runner. Prosthetic use requires increased energy output to achieve the same level of speed and power. Medical clearance, additional testing, or a controlled progressive exercise program may be needed to ensure that a person has sufficient cardiopulmonary reserve to safely engage in highly active sports.

When matching prosthetic components to an athlete's needs, it is important to review all available components. Rapid advances in new materials and applications make it impossible to list specific products. Table 32-9 lists many features and functions that are desired for various

Table 32-9: Prosthetic Features and Functions Desired for Sports

	Sports Activities							
Prosthetic functions	Biking	Hiking	Climbing	Golf	Watersports	Basketball	Football	Running
Secure suspension	×	×	×		×	×	×	×
Vertical shock absorption						×	×	×
Torque absorption		×		×		×	×	×
Knee stability		×				×	×	
Knee flexion >90 degrees	×		×					
Ankle dorsiflexion						×	×	×
Ankle plantarflexion						×	×	×
Ankle inversion		×	×	×		×	×	×
Ankle eversion		×	×	×		×	×	×
Energy-return plantarflexion						×	×	×
Waterproof					×			
Neutral buoyancy					×			
Grit and sand proof		×	×	×	×			
High strength		×				×	×	×

sporting activities. It is not an all-inclusive list but demonstrates the process of determining the features needed by the individual athlete. Once the features are determined, the team will need to review the currently available products and assemble the appropriate prosthetic system. A few specific examples are given. Depending on the user, further training by a physical therapist, peers, or specialized athletic clinics may be recommended. The International Society of Prosthetic and Orthotics home page (http://www.i-s-p-o.org/) has useful links to athletic events and associations throughout the world.

Although the athlete ultimately determines the final selection of the prosthetic component, it is essential that the selection process be based on a reasoned approach. The sport in question should be broken down into specific motions and forces to be achieved without benefit of muscular function. The following are some basic questions that should be included in all interviews of amputees as potential athletes:

1. What sport are you most interested in?
2. What are the requirements for your training (e.g., specific motions, running surfaces)?
3. What motions must the ankle achieve (active dorsiflexion, plantarflexion, inversion, eversion)?
4. Is transverse rotation at the ankle critical to the sport (e.g., golf, baseball)?
5. Will the prosthesis routinely be exposed to water (e.g., swimming, fishing)?
6. Will significant flexion or extension be required at the ankle and knee (e.g., bicycling, rowing, climbing)?
7. Does your sport involve high impact (e.g., motocross racing, long jump)?

Thorough analysis of the motions and forces involved in a particular sport will allow identification of the components best suited to achieve maximum performance. Table 32-9 will assist in the selection of components based on functional needs.

CONCLUSIONS

Improvements in neonatal care, trauma care, the management of multisystem failure, and surgical techniques for limb salvage, tumor resection, joint replacement, and amputation are resulting in more people living with limb deficiency. It is not uncommon to encounter a patient who has survived congenital problems, severe sepsis, electrocution, or cancer with resultant limb loss. Limb loss may not be the main functional limitation in some people with multisystem disease who previously would have been limited by comorbidities. Though not widely available in all countries, interventions such as retinal surgery, the opening of occluded coronary arteries, portable oxygen, or the control of renal failure are allowing people to remain active. These factors may affect prosthetic use and need to be considered during the pre-prosthetic evaluation. Frequently the team will need to provide education to assist a person in deciding between limb salvage procedures versus amputation. Early amputation and prosthetic use may return them to a higher activity level more quickly, minimizing the risks of medical complications as well as potentially lowering psychological and financial costs. Limb salvage may be the best option if the person has no significant medical comorbidities and can undergo multiple operations and rehabilitation. Once the decision for amputation has been reached, the level of amputation needs to be chosen. In general, the rule is to save as many natural joints and as much length as possible within the constraints of satisfactory healing and good tissue coverage. Restoring "function" is the key concept that needs to take into account not only the physical aspects of the person's residual limb but also the technical aspects of the anticipated prosthetic restoration. The availability of the prosthetic components, the skills of the prosthetist, and the overall capabilities of the amputee need to be considered. Individualized goals, therapy, and counseling are integral parts of the plan to assist the client to achieve maximal personal fulfillment and prosthetic restoration.

REFERENCES

1. Wilson AB. The history of limb prosthetics. In: *Limb prosthetics.* 6th ed. New York: Demos, 1989:1.
2. United States Department of Health and Human Services, Centers for Disease Control and Prevention. National Hospital Discharge Survey. Detailed diagnoses and procedures for patients discharged from short stay hospitals: annual summaries, 1984–1996. Series 13, Hyattsville, Maryland: National Center for Health Statistics.
3. Leonard JA, Meier RH. Prosthetics. In: De Lisa JA, ed. *Rehabilitation medicine: principles and practice.* Philadelphia: J.B. Lippincott, 1988:344.
4. McAnelly RD, Faulkner VW. Lower limb prostheses. In: Braddom RL, ed. *Physical medicine and rehabilitation.* Philadelphia: W.B. Saunders, 1996:289.
5. Sanders GT. Static and dynamic analysis. In: *Lower limb amputations: a guide to rehabilitation.* Philadelphia: F.A. Davis, 1986:415–475.
6. Hughes J. Biomechanics and prosthetics. In: Murdoch G, ed. *Amputation: surgical practice and patient management.* Oxford: Butterworth–Heinemann, 1996:13–22.
7. Picken RR. The below knee prosthesis and the above knee prosthe-

sis. In: Karacoloff LA, Hammersley CS, Schneider FJ, eds. *Lower extremity amputation: a guide to functional outcomes in physical therapy management.* Gaithersburg: Aspen Publishers, 1992:23–26, 31–36.

8. The amputee. In: Corel Medical Series, Comprehensives medical information on CD-ROM. Ontario: Corel Corporation, 1996.
9. Kapp S. Gait analysis of transtibial amputees. In: Bowker J, ed. *Atlas of limb prosthetics surgical, prosthetic, and rehabilitation principles.* 2nd edition. St. Louis: Mosby Year Book, 1992:471–476.
10. Mensch G. Prosthetics and prosthetic gait. In: *Physicial therapy management of lower extremity amputations.* Rockville: Aspen Publishers, 1986:232–335.
11. Chapter 1. The PRS management of amputations. Section II. General principles: level determination. In: Burgess EM, Romano RL, Zettl JH. *The management of lower extremity amputations.* Revised edition for World Wide Web. Seattle, 1996. URL: http://weber.u.washington.edu/~dboone/mlea/title.html.
12. Chapter 2. The below-knee amputation. Section IV. The below-knee immediate postsurgical prosthesis. In: Burgess EM, Romano RL, Zettl JH. The management of lower extremity amputations. Revised edition for World Wide Web. Seattle, 1996. URL:http://weber.u.washington.edu/~dbone/mlea/title.html.
13. Wu Y. Removeable rigid dressing for below-knee amputees. *Clin Prosthet Orthot* 1987;11:33–44.
14. Sabolich Sense of Feel System. Sabolich research and development department. Novacare, Oklahoma, 1999. Url:http://www.novacaresabolich.com/sof.html.
15. Vaida G, Friedmann LW. Postamputation phantoms—a review. In: Freidmann LW, ed. *Physical medicine and rehabilitation clinics of North America—prosthetics.* Philadelphia: W.B. Saunders, 1991:338.
16. Vaida G, Friedmann LW. Postamputation phantoms—a review. In: Freidmann LW, ed. *Physical medicine and rehabilitation clinics of North America—prosthetics.* Philadelphia: W.B. Saunders, 1991:339–345.
17. Tooms RE. Aquired amputations in children. In: Bowker JH, Michael JW, eds. *Atlas of limb prosthetics—surgical, prosthetic, and rehabilitation principles.* 2nd edition. St. Louis: Mosby Year Book, 1992:735.
18. Day HJB. *The ISO/ISPOI classification of congenital limb deficiency.* St. Louis: Mosby Year Book, 1992:743–748.
19. Hughes JH. *Pediatric limb deficiency.* Atlanta: Scottish Rite Children's Medical Center, 1994.
20. Cummings DR. Prosthetic considerations for the child with a limb deficiency (lower extremity). In: Herring JA, Birch JG, eds. *The child with a limb deficiency.* Rosemont, IL: American Academy of Orthopedic Surgeons, 1998:310.
21. Frankenburg WK, Dodds JB, Archer P, et al. *Denver II training manual.* 2nd edition. Denver: Denver Developmental Materials, Inc; 1992.
22. Varni JW, Setoguchi Y. Psychosocial factors in the management of children with limb deficiencies. In: Freidmann LW, ed. *Physical medicine and rehabilitation—clinics of North America—prosthetics.* Philadelphia: W.B. Saunders, 1991:395–404.

Chapter 33

Rehabilitative Optometric Interventions for the Adult with Acquired Brain Injury

Irwin Suchoff
Rosamond Gianutsos

One prerequisite for rehabilitation of any type is that appropriate diagnostic measures be undertaken first. Earlier in this volume (see Chapter 19), Seiller and Warren discussed issues concerning the screening, evaluation, and diagnosis of visual system dysfunction, including its high incidence following stroke, traumatic brain injury (TBI), and other forms of acquired brain injury (ABI). Nevertheless, even in spite of previous calls (1–8) for appropriate evaluation and diagnosis, in rehabilitation there is a huge service delivery problem in that evaluations of the visual system are minimized, deferred, or narrowly focused on eye health issues. All too often the patient with ABI has received an evaluation focused primarily on ocular and neurologic integrity and health. While these areas are of prime importance in the immediate posttrauma period, as the patient enters the rehabilitation arena, other functional aspects of the visual system become at least equally important. For example, cognitive rehabilitation can be seriously impeded if the patient is experiencing blurred or intermittent double vision that has not been diagnosed and managed.

It is important to understand the range of possibilities for intervention, to know how to implement a treatment plan, including which practitioners can be expected to play which roles, and to evaluate the outcome. It is often possible to bring about substantial improvement with basic "bread and butter" interventions, for example, a pair of +1 diopter lenses to give the accommodative-vergence system the boost it needs to provide binocular vision lost following ABI. Sometimes it is a matter of improving the fit of the lenses, especially bifocal or multifocal lenses. The high benefit-cost ratio of optometric intervention is yet another reason to pursue visual evaluation and rehabilitation.

There are times (e.g., when the patient is languishing in an ambiguous coma emergent state) when it is just as helpful to rule out visual problems as it is to identify them. Here again, the expertise of the rehabilitative optometrist is invaluable (9).

THE INVOLVED EYE CARE PROFESSIONS

Two professions, ophthalmology and optometry, are currently engaged in the ocular and visual care of the patient with ABI. Ophthalmology is a specialty of medicine, and is further divided into subspecialties: cataract, cornea, glaucoma, low vision, neuro-ophthalmology, pediatrics and strabismus, plastics and reconstructive, retina, and finally uveitis (10). In terms of the ABI patient, the neuro-ophthalmologist is most likely to be called on, particularly in the immediate posttrauma period. At this point, his or her expertise is essential in terms of patient management. At times, particularly in the case of accidents, the reconstructive or retinal ophthalmologist is needed. However, with the exception of the ophthalmologist specializing in low vision, in practice it is unusual for any of the other ophthalmologic specialists to play a significant role in rehabilitation. This is not meant to be a negative statement, for in general, ophthalmology is primarily a medical and surgical discipline. Indeed, the medical school graduate who is interested in rehabilitation is more likely to opt for a residency in physiatry.

Optometry specializes in primary eye care (11). The profession's scope of practice has been significantly extended with legislation authorizing the use of diagnostic and more recently, therapeutic pharmaceutical agents. For the present discussion, there has been and remains a distinct rehabilitative component in optometry. A prime example is optometric vision therapy, which has been defined as the art and science of developing visual abilities to achieve optimal visual performance and comfort (12). This is an integral part of optometry in that courses relating to the anatomy and physiology of the components of the accommodative and binocular systems, along with didactic and clinical components relating to the noninvasive therapeutic interventions for these systems, are included in the curricula of all the optometric educational institutions. The same case exists for the basic science and clinical applications of visual perception and low vision. Optometric students not only must show competence in these areas in school, but also are tested in this regard by the National Board of Examiners in Optometry. The profession's two major organizations, the American Optometric Association and the American Academy of Optometry, have particular subgroups representing the specialties of vision therapy and low vision. In addition, three other organizations, the Optometric Extension Program Foundation, the College of Optometrists in Vision Development, and the Neuro-optometric Rehabilitation Organization, are devoted to continuing education and representation of these areas. Consequently, while the neuro-ophthalmologist is most likely the eye care professional to be involved with the ABI patient during the hospitalization period, the optometrist with interest and expertise in vision therapy or low vision has been and is increasingly called on by members of the rehabilitation team, such as the physiatrist, occupational therapist, physical therapist, and neuropsychologist (5,13–15).

THE INTERFACE WITH COMPREHENSIVE REHABILITATION

Some larger rehabilitation centers have ongoing relationships with rehabilitative optometrists, who are essentially integrated into the team. When for a variety of practical reasons this has not occurred, the physiatrist (as coordinator) and occupational therapist (OT) are most likely to become involved with issues associated with vision. The OT's expertise in the practical, or as they would say functional, implications of interventions. The OT is the past master of activities of daily living (ADLs) and visual function is crucial to most ADLs. However, any member of the team should feel free to bring the issue to the attention of those who can do something and be prepared to support the treatment recommendations, even so simple as helping the patient to put on the correct pair of glasses. The neuropsychologist, speech-language pathologist, and vocational and educational therapists, who are likely to be working on reading and other near-point activities, should be well attuned to adjustments that have to be made for close vision.

Close working relationships have developed between OTs and eye care practitioners (1,4); however, at times the boundaries of professional responsibility are tested. What then is the role of the OT? In some respects, these practitioners have been the real pioneers who have reached out to eye care practitioners and encouraged them to become more involved in rehabilitation. In hospital and residential rehabilitation settings with no in-house eye care professional, OTs have frequently had to forge links with outside eye care professionals. In order to rationalize referrals, they have had to conduct fairly extensive screening procedures, for example, using stereoscopic vision screeners. This information has helped them formulate the referral issue and evaluate the response. When OTs have been able to accompany the patient to the eye care consultation, they have been able to assist in the communication of history, symptoms, and other observations, as well as to bring back the findings and recommendations to the family and the rest of the treatment team. However, the independent spirit that has made it possible for these therapists to bring these services to their patients has at times led to misunderstanding and the appearance, if not the fact, of overstepping the boundaries of their professional expertise. It is important for the physiatrist or case manager to recognize that it is imperative to have a close working relationship with eye care professionals and to understand the limitations of OTs and other therapists. Important as the OT's contribution is, it does not substitute for the active supervision of an eye care practitioner.

OPTOMETRIC REHABILITATION

A general rule for successful rehabilitation is that the caregiver fully discuss the diagnosed condition(s) with the patient and his or her family or significant others. Not only should the prognosis be addressed, but also, and perhaps even more important, is a thorough explanation of the behavioral and functional consequences of the condition(s). For example, in the patient with a left homonymous hemianopia (a loss of visual responsiveness on the left side of the field of view in each eye), one may anticipate frequent bumping into objects on the left, and ineffective scanning from the end of one line of text to the next. The individual may appear to "neglect" the left side, when in fact the problem should be identified as a product of the visual field cut. There should also be this type of communication with other members of the rehabilitation team, and other health care professionals. For example, the OT or neuropsychologist who is using computer programs for their aspects of rehabilitation should be fully cognizant that reading glasses, prescribed for a 20-year-old accident victim whose accommodative function has been compromised by oculomotor nerve (cranial nerve III) damage, should be used only for near-point activity, and that the patient's vision will be blurred when the glasses are used for distant vision.

Ocular Health

There is a relatively high incidence of blepharitis with or without an accompanying dry eye syndrome. Therapeutic measures for these conditions include patient education for lid hygiene, including lid scrubs and the use of ocular over-the-counter lubricants. Stroke patients often are diabetic or hypertensive and consequently are at risk for retinopathies and cataracts. These patients should be evaluated every 6 months, including with dilated funduscopic examination. The wearing of glasses with tinted lenses, as well as use of a hat with a visor, is a valuable intervention to reduce glare and soften bright environmental lighting conditions that are a common consequence of cataracts. Further, in the patient with new or worsening retinopathies, or cataracts that are compromising the patient's lifestyle, ophthalmologic consultation is frequently in order.

Refraction and the Prescribing of Glasses

Determining the degree of myopia, hyperopia, and astigmatism can be accomplished by objective means (i.e., static retinoscopy or automated refracting devices). However, determining the precise lens prescription is usually somewhat more time-consuming; the objective measures are not always in concordance with the patient's subjective experience. Some patients are unresponsive to lens changes over a relatively wide range, when based on Snellen chart criteria. It is productive to place lenses with the tentatively prescribed correction in a trial frame and engage the patient in real-life situations. Often, the increased clarity produced by the lenses will be appreciated when walking down a corridor, crossing the street, or looking for street signs.

It is essential to place the patient's refractive status in the context of the overall condition. Again, assume there is damage to cranial nerve III; for individuals with myopia of approximately 2.00 diopters, removing the glasses for most near-point visual activities is indicated, whereas hyperopes of any degree should be instructed to wear the glasses for all visual tasks. Indeed, for many hyperopes with cranial nerve III damage, a separate reading prescription is indicated. Diabetic patients should be forewarned that their refractive conditions are subject to change, depending on the degree to which the diabetes fluctuates (16).

Over the past several decades, great strides have been made in the options available for the most appropriate ophthalmic lens type for the particular patient. For the ABI patient, this can be particularly important because of the frequent use of prisms to compensate for a binocular dysfunction or a visual field defect. Prisms can cause chromatic aberrations that are sometimes more noticeable to the patient than the benefit of more comfortable clear and single binocular vision or the ability to perceive more of the compromised visual field. High index lenses afford the benefits of being thinner and lighter along with physically protecting the eyes. Lens materials such as polycarbonate and CR-39 have optical characteristics that can be optimal for the patient's refractive condition and for the incorporation of prism into the prescription. Further, antireflective coatings are a valuable option for the cataract or photophobic patient. Polycarbonate lenses are particularly effective in blocking harmful ultraviolet (UV) rays, which are etiologic factors in cataract formation and age-related macular degeneration.

Vertigo

As a result of head trauma or stroke, many patients have complaints of vertigo. Often, this is a result of a vestibular dysfunction. Substituting separate pairs of reading and distant glasses for bifocals helps some of these patients. Apparently, the head and eye movements involved in positioning the visual axes in the distant or near part of the multifocal lenses can often exacerbate the vestibular problem. Further, progressive addition bifocals are particularly disturbing to the dizzy patient; even many non-ABI patients need to adapt to the aberrations that are a consequence of the optical design of these "invisible" bifocal lenses. On the other hand, these progressive lenses can have particular advantages, including having only one pair of glasses to keep track of, being of variable strength for intermediate distances, and allowing for convenient adjustment to fluctuating needs.

Photophobia and Related Visual Phenomena

A not uncommon complaint of the ABI patient is an increased sensitivity to light, both outdoors and indoors. Further, some of these patients also remark on a perception of waviness or shimmering that is lessened in decreased lighting conditions. Lenses that absorb the shorter wavelengths of light (e.g., blue-tinted lenses) can relieve both the photophobia and the waviness or shimmering in a number of patients. While the type of tint may be determined by trial and error, recent research provided objective evidence to the patient's subjective reports of decreased symptoms with light-filtering lenses. Jackowski et al (17), in a controlled experiment, demonstrated that the use of Corning Photochromic Filtering lenses (CPF 450) increased contrast sensitivity and improved reading rates in TBI patients who became photophobic after trauma.

Optometric Vision Therapy (Visual Training)

This type of intervention is used to rehabilitate dysfunctions of the dynamic systems of vision, including eye movements (fixation, pursuit, and saccade), the accom-

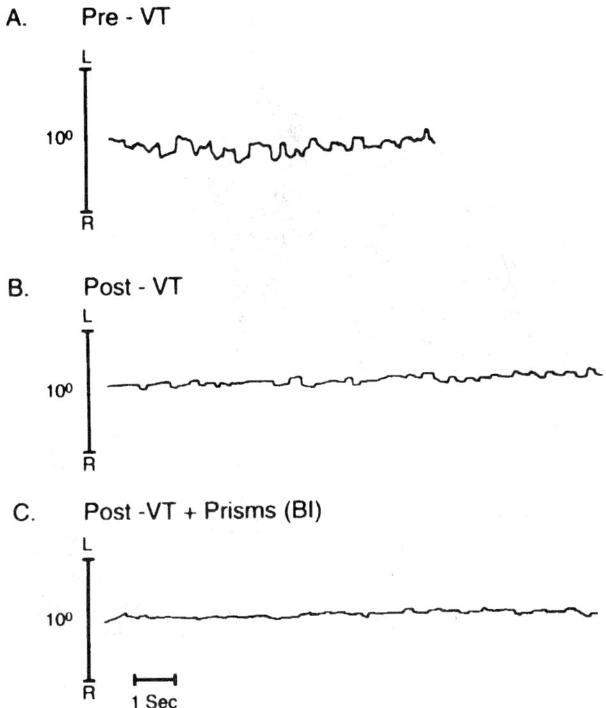

Figure 33-1. *A.* Pretherapy fixational movements of the right eye. Posttherapy fixational movements of the right eye without (*B*) and with (*C*) the 5.5–prism diopter base-in prism incorporated into the spectacle correction in each eye. Binocular viewing in all cases. (Reproduced by permission from Ciuffreda KJ, Suchoff IB, Marrone MA, Ahmann E. Oculomotor rehabilitation in traumatic brain-injured patients. *J Behav Optom* 1996;7:31–38.)

modative system, and the binocular system, ranging from constant strabismus, to intermittent strabismus, to the nonstrabismic anomalies of binocular vision and visual perception (2,18). There is also evidence that vision therapy is effective in controlling ABI-induced nystagmus (19).

Therapy to stabilize visual fixation ranges from using techniques that require sustained and accurate central fixation, such as filling in the circular portions of the letters "o," "b," and "d" contained on a newspaper page with a sharpened pencil, to using computer-based programs that require the patient to maintain fixation on a specific portion of the monitor screen, and respond by hitting the space bar or mouse when a predetermined number appears (20). The efficacy of such a regimen has been demonstrated by electronically based eye movement recordings (15) (Fig. 33-1).

Pursuit and saccadic eye movements are frequently impaired following ABI (21,22). When the latency and accuracy of these eye movements are compromised, the results can be devastating. Thus, the not infrequent observations of some ABI patients that they see the car while crossing the street, but cannot follow it . . . "I lose where it is" . . . can often be attributed to delayed or inaccurate visual pursuit. Saccadic eye movements are a prerequisite not only for accurate and effortless reading, but also for accurately sampling a new visual environment. Ron (23,24) conducted visual training with several TBI patients and gave objective evidence via infra-red eye movement recordings of enhanced pursuit and saccades. Further, he demonstrated that the improvements were beyond those attributed to the healing process.

Therapies to rehabilitate saccade and pursuit movements have long been an integral part of optometric vision therapy. In general, the goal is to equalize and maximize the performance of each eye as to latency, accuracy, and automaticity, in a purely visual fashion, that is, without active body, neck, or head movement. Then one proceeds to binocular techniques. Further, techniques to improve proprioceptive and kinesthetic awareness, or "feeling" of the extraocular muscles are used to enhance performance. Therapy proceeds from low to higher cognitive tasks as the individual gains increasing control over the saccade and pursuit movements. A popular technique for saccade therapy is the use of various electronically based devices that program random sequences of small light sources, which the patient is instructed to touch as each is lit. The speed and spatial complexity can be varied. Other advanced therapies for pursuits and saccades are available in computer programs that can be used for in-office and home procedures, some of which are listed in Table 33-1 (25). Others are described later in the section on interventions for visual field impairment.

Dysfunctions of the accommodative (focusing) mechanism are not uncommon in ABI patients (26). While the obvious immediate causes are trauma to cranial nerve III or the ciliary muscle, persistent accommodative dysfunctions (e.g., amplitude, flexibility, or sustenance) can be a consequence of anticholinergic or other medications that affect the parasympathetic nervous system. There is general agreement that the primary therapeutic measure is to prescribe the indicated convex lens power that enables the patient to attain clear near vision (8,27). Incorporating techniques that enhance all aspects of the accommodative response, such as decreasing latency and increasing flexibility, are often effective. These techniques challenge the ability of the patient first to quickly clear targets at near, then at far, and so on. The next step is to sustain clarity of the near target for increasing periods of time, and then instantly to clear the far target, and sustain its clarity for increasing periods of time, and so on. This type of "accommodative rock" can be carried out in free space, or with the aid of lenses, or lens and prism combinations (28) (Fig. 33-2). During the therapy, the patient's accommodative abilities should be closely monitored so that as improvement occurs, the convex lens prescription can be appropriately decreased in power.

Dysfunctions of the binocular system can be conceptualized on a continuum from constant strabismus, to intermittent strabismus, to nonstrabismic anomalies of

Table 33-1: Computer Resources for Optometric Rehabilitation

Name	Author(s)	Source
Computer Orthoptics	J. Cooper	American Vision Therapy[a]
Block Breaker	Y. Emura	http://www.emsoft.co.jp/block-e.htm
Functional Visual Fields	R. Gianutsos	Life Science Associates[b]
BISECT—Line Bisection	R. Gianutsos	Life Science Associates[b]
OPTOMEX—Optometric Scanning	R. Gianutsos	Life Science Associates[b]
VISMEM—Visual Memory	R. Gianutsos	Life Science Associates[b]
Jigsaws Galore	D. Gray	http://www.dgray.com/jigalo.htm
Visual Perception	S. Groffman	American Vision Therapy[a]
Vision 3D	M. Grossman & R. Cooper	http://www.vision3.com
Project Gutenberg	—	http://www.promo.net/pg/
VS	G. Kerkhoff and C. Marquardt	*J Neurosci Methods* 1995;63:75–84
Memory Jiggler	S. Moraff	http://www.moraffware.com
Morejongg	S. Moraff	http://www.moraffware.com
Computer Aided Vision Therapy	G. Vogel	Bernell Corporation[c]

[a] American Vision Therapy, PO Box 197, Cicero, IN 46034. Tel: 800-346-4925.

[b] Life Science Associates, 1 Fenimore Road, Bayport, NY 11705. Tel: 516-472-2111. Also, at Web site http://www.lifesciassoc.home.pipeline.com.

[c] Bernell Corporation, 750 Lincolnway East, PO Box 4637, South Bend, IN 46634-4637. Tel: 800-348-2225.

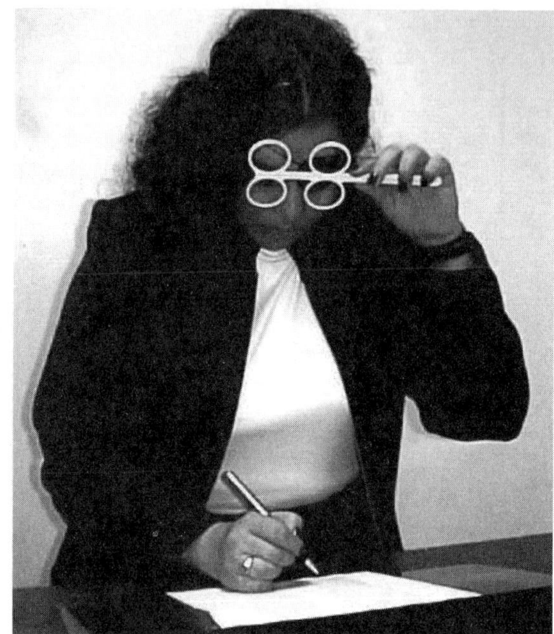

Figure 33-2. In the accommodative rock exercise, the patient holds "flipper" lenses that contain additional plus (magnification) lenses in one pair and additional minus lenses in the other. The task calls for attaining a clear image through one set of lenses and then flipping the lenses and using accommodation to attain a clear image as efficiently as possible. In the present illustration, an eye patch is worn and the exercise is monocular.

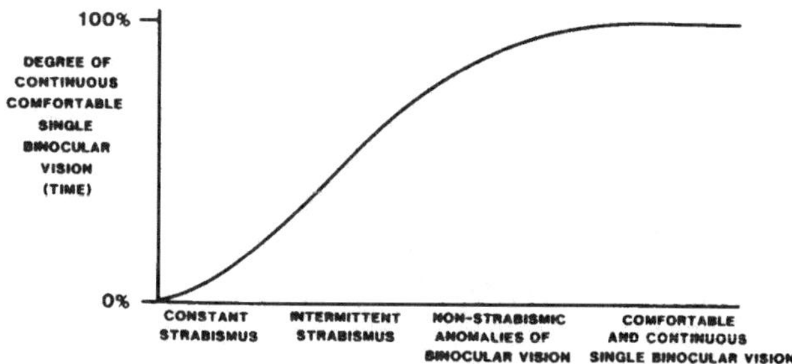

Figure 33-3. Continuum of dysfunctions of the binocular system. (Reproduced by permission from Suchoff IB, Petito GT. The efficacy of visual therapy: accommodative disorders and non-strabismic anomalies of binocular vision. *J Am Optom Assoc* 1986;57:119–125.)

binocular vision (Fig. 33-3). Patients with strabismus resulting from ABI most often do not make the adaptations that classically occur; there is little or no suppression-based amblyopia, or anomalous correspondence. Rather, even years after the accident or stroke, patients who are diplopic are told to either patch one eye or to "learn to live with it." One strategy has been to provide the patient with prism lenses that compensate for the eye turn, and then institute usual vision therapy to develop binocular vision (29). Basically, this is done by establishing single binocular vision with the eye in the primary position and the patient wearing the prism correction and then developing vergence binocular eye movements opposite to the direction of the turn (e.g., divergence in the case of esotropia, and convergence in exotropia). The primary method is to provide each eye with a discrete target that when combined with its counterpart, results in a meaningful visual percept. A number of devices have been developed for these purposes, so that it can be accomplished "in instrument" or in "free space" (Figs. 33-4 and 33-5). Targets that require various levels of binocular vision (i.e., superimposition, fusion, and stereopsis) are available. As the patient's ability in these tasks increases, it is usually possible to decrease the amount of prism in the patient's glasses. When it is believed that further progress cannot be made, active vision therapy is ceased, and the patient is monitored on a regular basis. In this manner, the patient is diplopia free without the use of a patch.

However, when further progress is possible, the same regimen is used for *nonstrabismic anomalies of binocular vision.*

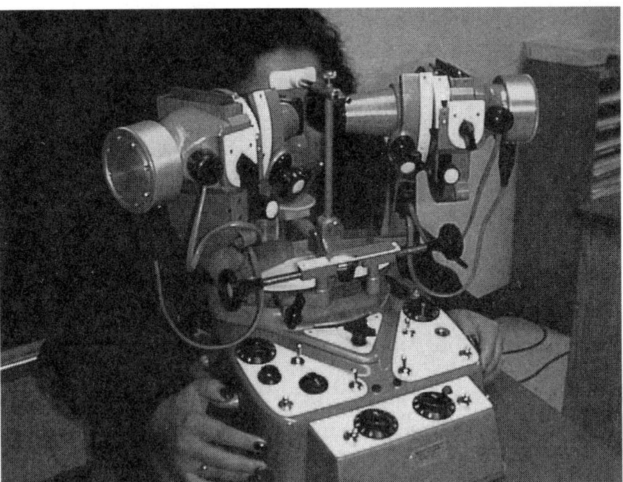

Figure 33-4. The troposcope is a device that allows one to present images to each eye and to determine precisely the separation of the two images. This separation corresponds to the deviation between the eyes in the absence of external stimuli that could promote fusion.

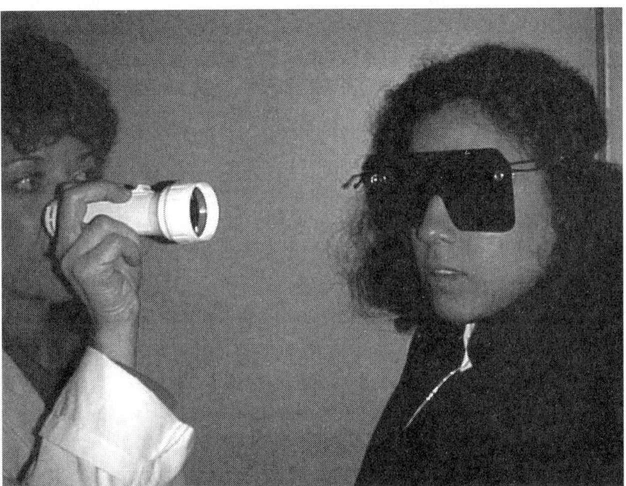

Figure 33-5. Worth 4 Dot test. The examiner shines a flashlight adapted so that it shines lights of red, white, and green. The examinee wears red/green anaglyphic glasses over the customary prescription. Under these circumstances, a person who uses both eyes will see all the lights.

This umbrella term classically encompasses the various vergence dysfunctions, for example, convergence and divergence insufficiency and excess, and vertical phorias for which the patient cannot compensate. However, an expanded classification has developed over the years (Table 33-2). Regimens and procedures to remediate these conditions have been fully described in the optometric literature (1,30–32). Further, once the patient has achieved sufficient binocular skills, exercises can be based on the stereograms available in popular books and computer programs (e.g., see Web page at http://www.vision3d.com). It is usually not difficult to motivate patients to use these attractive materials. The basis of these therapies is to maximally develop the quality, range, and sustenance of comfortable clear and single binocular vision by sequentially increasing the complexity of the cognitive and sensory-motor demands.

Table 33-2: An Expanded Classification of Vergence Dysfunctions
Fusional vergence dysfunction (skills case)
Convergence insufficiency
Pseudoconvergence insufficiency
Convergence excess
Divergence excess
Divergence insufficiency
Basic exophoria
Basic esophoria

While the synkinesis between accommodation and convergence is certainly a consideration in strabismic therapy, it takes on a key role in the rehabilitation of the nonstrabismic anomalies of binocular vision. Hence, the ultimate goal of therapy is to normalize this relationship, that is, to develop an appropriate or expected accommodative convergence to accommodation (AC/A) ratio. This is accomplished by developing a freedom between the two functions. In this instance, the patient is given techniques where, for example, convergence must be inhibited, in the interest of single vision, while accommodation is stimulated, or where accommodation is inhibited while convergence is stimulated. These techniques require the use of lenses or prisms that vary the accommodative and vergence demands, respectively.

In one of the best controlled efficacy studies, applying the single case experimental design, Kerkhoff and Stogerer (33,34) trained fusional convergence using three orthoptic devices (fusion trainer, prisms, and cheiroscope). Eleven of 12 ABI patients showed 1) no gains in baseline, 2) gains during treatment, and 3) maintenance of gains during a 10-month follow-up period. They also experienced gains in near-point acuity, stereopsis, and reading, together with a reduction in subjective symptoms associated with fusional deficiency (e.g., eyestrain and headache).

In general, there is increasing utilization of vision therapy for ABI patients. Morton (35), an ophthalmologist, proposed that this therapy uses repetition to retrain neural pathways that have been damaged, or to develop alternative pathways, and presented several case studies. Freed and Hellerstein (36) presented a more scientific demonstration of the efficacy of this type of optometric intervention. An experimental group of 18 patients with mild brain injury received a regimen of optometric rehabilitation, while 32 matched control subjects did not. At 12 to 18

Table 33-3: Functional Visual Field Assessment Procedures

Peripheral (to 20 Degrees)	Perifoveal (Central 4 Degrees)
REACT: Reaction Time Measure of Visual Field	INSPECT: Shape Inspection
SDSST: Single and Double Simultaneous Stimulation	FASTREAD: Tachistoscopic Reading
SOSH: Search for the Odd Shape	ERROR DETECT: Error Detection in Texts
SEARCH: Visual Search	

Source: Life Science Asssociates, 1 Fenimore Road, Bayport, NY 11705. Tel: 516-472-2111. Web site: lifesciassoc@pipeline.com.

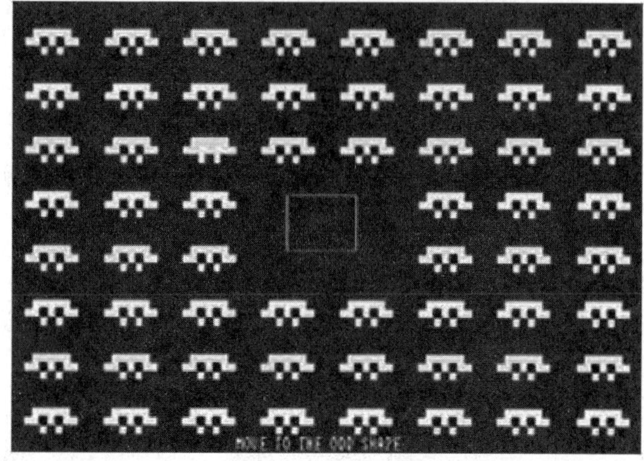

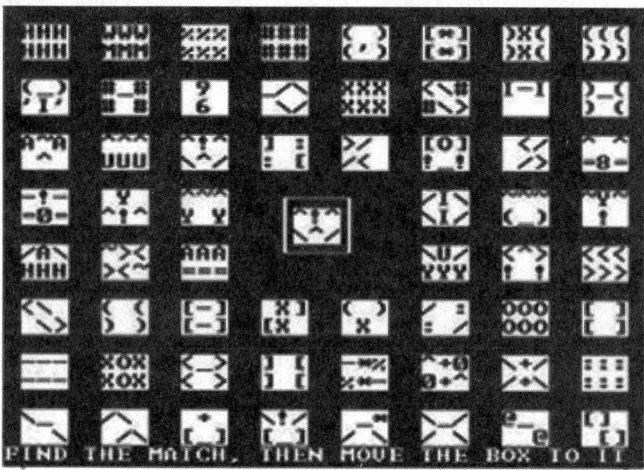

Figure 33-6. SOSH (*top panel*) and SEARCH (*bottom panel*) displays. With SOSH (Search for the Odd Shape) the task is to point to the shape ("Martian face") that is different ("sleeping"), in this case in the upper left of center. For SEARCH, one is to point to the shape in the peripheral array that matches the center shape exactly, again in the upper left. The examiner moves the center box with the arrow keys. Response time is the time from the stimulus onset to the beginning of a move that ultimately reaches the target.

months after therapy, the experimental group showed a significant decrease in pattern visually evoked cortical potential (VECP) abnormalities, as opposed to the control group.

Rehabilitation of Visual Field Impairments

Following brain injury, visual field impairment is fairly common, yet it is often undiagnosed or underdiagnosed. These problems are usually characterized by a lateralized differential pattern of response to visual stimuli. The loss may be relative or absolute, and the problem may involve the central (perifoveal) or the peripheral fields, or both.

Formal optometric diagnostic procedures, detailed elsewhere (5), include perimetry for the peripheral fields and testing using the Amsler grid for the central fields. Unfortunately, these assessment procedures present cognitive demands, which can limit their use with the ABI patient. Specifically the individual must sustain a focus of attention on a fixation point, while reporting on perceived events elsewhere in the field of view. In the case of threshold perimetry, in which the minimum light intensity seen at each point is mapped, these decisions may involve fine discriminations and rapid judgments. To help meet this diagnostic challenge, Gianutsos and Suchoff (5) recommend a modified two-person confrontation procedure and computerized functional visual field tests with norms (37).

Functional Visual Field Procedures

The functional visual field procedures, listed in Table 33-3, require responses to visual stimuli throughout a computer screen. In most instances, there is no fixation requirement and the speed of response to stimuli in different locations is measured. The functional visual field procedures have proved to be simple enough for most ABI patients to do and there are norms for both young and old adults (37). The procedures for the peripheral fields address responsiveness to the near periphery (about 30 degrees) and range from attentionally simple [e.g., Reaction Time Measure of Visual Field (REACT)] to complex [e.g., Search for the Odd Shape (SOSH) and Search for Shapes (SEARCH)], illustrated in Figure 33-6.

There are also functional visual field procedures for the perifoveal (central 4 degrees) fields: Shape Matching (INSPECT), Tachistoscopic Reading (FASTREAD), and two alternative forms of Error Detection in Texts (38). For assessment purposes, normative information is available (39). INSPECT (Fig. 33-7) requires a rapid same or different judgment and no verbal ability. In FASTREAD (Fig. 33-8), isolated words are flashed on the computer screen and the examinee says or types them. The procedure is adaptive in that following correct responses, the next item is presented faster and following incorrect ones, it is

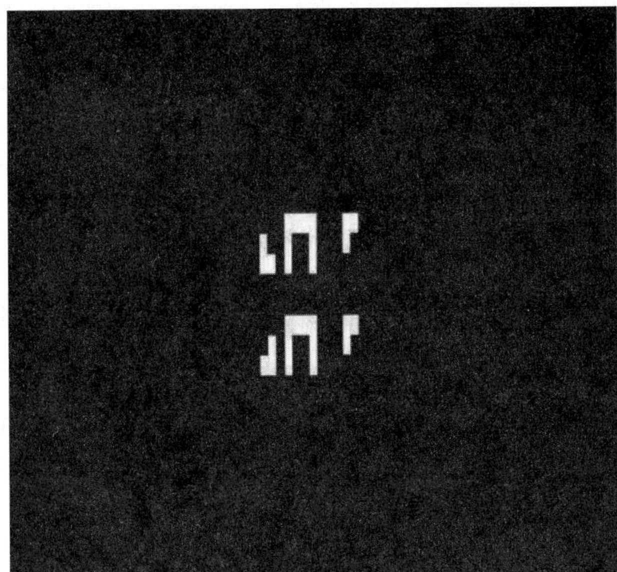

Figure 33-7. INSPECT display. The task is to press the left or right side button to indicate if the difference in the two shapes is on the left or right side. The computer reports decision times for stimuli that differ on the left and right.

presented more slowly. The nature and pattern of errors are analyzed. For example, POLICE may be changed to "POLICY," a right substitution, or to "LICE" a left truncation. Following brain injury, substitutional errors are more common than truncations and probably reflect macular sparing. Error Detection in Texts (Fig. 33-9) calls for proofreading of continuous text and affords a sensitive index of perifoveal hemi-imperception. Although errors are distributed equally on the left and right sides of the page, more often than not, the critical factor is whether the error occurs at the beginning or end of the word.

Optical Interventions for Visual Field Loss

Until fairly recently, rehabilitative interventions for visual hemifield impairment were limited to counseling and compensatory training. Fortunately, optical interventions are now being refined to complement, if not correct the problem. Optical interventions for visual field loss, reviewed by Cohen and Waiss (40), involve the use of displacing prisms or spectacle-mounted mirrors. Ground-in yoked prisms in the range of 6 to 12 diopters appear to be most useful. The base of each prism is placed in the same lateral direction in relation to the patient. In other words, the displacement is in the same direction in each eye. A pair of spectacles designed for a stroke survivor with an upper-right-quadrant field loss is illustrated in Figure 33-10. A different set of glasses with greater prismatic power than would be used for distance may be necessary for near-point work. The fit of the spectacle is important. Here we would especially recommend spring-loaded frames as they remain more consistently in place. Small oval lenses have less optical distortion and are lighter. Often the best response to these lenses is subjective, although the patient should be prepared not to expect a cure. Further, since the optical interventions do not fully correct the loss, it is essential to complement this intervention with awareness counseling, practice with feedback, and training in compensatory scanning.

Counseling

Typically, visual hemifield impairments caused by central nervous system injury are exacerbated by a loss of awareness. It is important to understand that this lack of awareness is inherent to some forms of sensory loss, as when the person with a hearing loss thinks others are not speaking clearly. Gianutsos (41) parallels this phenomenon with the unawareness all of us have for the rather substantial (the size of a fist at arm's length) visual field loss corresponding to our physiologic blind spot. She contrasts this with the heightened response to glare, which triggers immediate attempts to avoid or control. While this unawareness of neurologically produced visual field losses is sometimes profound, more often it is expressed as an underappreciation of the magnitude of the problem. Accordingly, there is much misinterpretation of the patient's behavior, and safety is compromised (42). It is therefore essential that rehabilitative interventions address the awareness issue. While a true subjective awareness of the lost vision often does not develop, as it would for a cataract or a retinal defect, it is possible for the patient to develop an intellectualized awareness of the problem. In other words, they can learn that if they cannot locate something, then it must be in the area covered by the visual field defect. Therefore, treatment must be directed toward increasing awareness of the visual field problem to the extent that it cannot be treated optically and by developing compensatory eye movements.

Practice with Feedback

Exercises that offer feedback organized by the location of the stimuli are useful for building both skill and awareness. Examples include cancellation (43,44), Error Detection in Texts, and common word-search and hidden-figure puzzles. These, especially error detection, tend to focus on central field impairments. Practice materials for error detection (38) can be created from texts downloaded from sources such as Project Gutenberg (see Web site http://www.promo.net/pg/), including famous speeches, short stories, and even whole books. These can be reformatted and edited with a word processor, as illustrated in Figure 33-9. Advanced computer spelling checkers, which highlight incorrectly spelled words, are particularly convenient for the creation of these materials, as one can see the errors and their distribution on the page.

Computerized tasks can have special value by offering immediate feedback to promote the development of

Figure 33-8. FASTREAD (Tachistoscopic Reading) printout. The display time (*horizontal bar*) decreases following correct reading, setting after a series of trials at an asymptotic level ("consistently best time," here approximately 0.04 second). The subject types the word seen and errors are printed for subsequent analysis. In this instance the individual has a profound macula invading homonymous right-upper-quadrant hemianopia (see Fig. 33-10), reflected in end of word substitutional ("CHAIR" → "CHAIN") and truncational ("BAND" → "BAN") errors.

```
                              FASTREAD

 DESIGNED BY:  ROSAMOND GIANUTSOS        PROGRAMMED BY:  AARON BEATTIE
  (C) 1995 LIFE SCIENCE ASSOCIATES       IBM COMPATIBLE VER #:  112295

        DISPLAY
  SEQ   TIME       STIMULUS  ->  RESPONSE

   1.    100        MOUSE
########################################
   2.     89        CRUISE
####################################
   3.     80        HAND
################################
   4.     71        GUIDE
############################
   5.     63        SOUR
#########################
   6.     56        LORE
######################
   7.     50        DELAY
####################
   8.     44        BANG
##################
   9.     39        PACK
################
  10.     35        MOUSE
##############
  11.     31        CRUSH
############
  12.     27        FIELDS  -> FIELD (R)

  13.     30        TRAIN
############
  14.     26        BONG
##########
  15.     23        MAID
#########
  16.     20        READ
########
  17.     17        NECK
#######
  18.     15        LORD
######
  19.     13        ASIDE  -> ASIA (R)
  20.     15        LOG  -> LORD (R)
  21.     17        SHOP
#######
  22.     15        RED
######

        DISPLAY
  SEQ   TIME       STIMULUS  ->  RESPONSE

  23.     13        ROOM
#####
  24.     11        FIELD
####
  25.      9        ZONE
####
  26.      8        READ
###
  27.      7        READ  -> READY (R)
  28.      8        WOOD
###
  29.      7        BOUND
###
  30.      6        DONE
##
  31.      5        RATS
##
  32.      4        BARK
##
  33.      3        NAIL  -> MAID (O)
  34.      4        JOIN  -> JOINT (R)
  35.      5        POOR  -> POUR (M)
  36.      6        ROPE
##
  37.      5        REEL
##
  38.      4        GUEST
##
  39.      3        IDEAL  -> IDEA (R)
  40.      4        BAND  -> BAN (R)
  41.      5        LORD
##
  42.      4        DONE
##
  43.      3        DELAY
#
  44.      2        CHAIR  -> CHAIN (R)
```

awareness. The computerized functional visual field tasks, described earlier, can be used for this purpose, as they offer different random versions on each administration. They also offer the individual opportunity to practice compensation and to determine the limits of compensation.

Training in Compensatory Scanning

Many tasks can be used as a tool for compensatory scanning. The classic task for nonaphasics is reading, both out loud and silently. Reading addresses the integrity of both the central fields (reading words accurately) and the peripheral fields (returning to the margin for left hemianopics reading languages that are printed from left to right and overall speed of reading for right hemianopics who have trouble scanning rapidly into their blind field). Weinberg et al (45) suggested the use of a colored line in the left margin to provide an anchor for left hemianopic readers. This technique can be very helpful for those who have peripheral field involvement.

Other visually complex tasks, such as completing mazes and jigsaw puzzles, are useful in building visual field scanning skills. Computerized versions of these tasks abound, and are becoming more and more visually rich with improved computers. A feature common to these tasks is the use of a computer mouse (or, often better for persons with limited motoric control, a trackball) to control the cursor on the screen. Developing the eye-hand coordination necessary for controlling the cursor in this fashion may be a special challenge for patients with visual field problems. Frequently it is a good idea to begin with a simple solitaire game on the computer—an insight that computer software manufacturers have long recognized, since solitaire is supplied with just about every computer that has a graphic user interface!

A dynamic scanning task, widely available under many names is Breakout. This task is like playing tennis off a backboard, except that the board is an array of bricks, which are removed by hitting them with the ball. The lateral movement of the paddle is typically under mouse (trackball) or joystick control. We use a "freeware" version (shown in Fig. 33-11) called BlockBreaker (see Web site http://www.emsoft.co.jp/block-e.htm) because it is very plain, has parameters affording a wide range of difficulty, and supplies meaningful scores.

A favorite among these computer exercises (or games) is Mahjongg, which goes under different names, such as Taipei, Shanghai, and Morejongg. This shape-matching exercise is visually appealing and presents constraints that challenge logic and sequencing. Morejongg (see Web site http://www.moraffware.com) is a multimedia

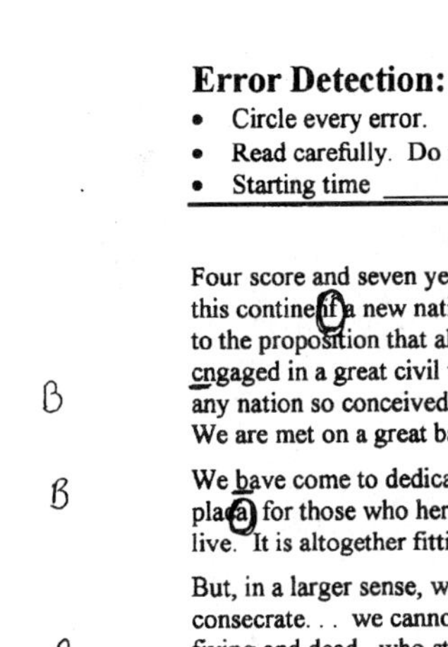

Error Detection:

- Circle every error.
- Read carefully. Do not go back over your work.
- Starting time _______ Ending time _______

Four score and seven years ago our fathers brought forth upon this continenf a new nation: conceived in libertg and dedicated to the proposition that all men are created equal. Now we are cngaged in a great civil war. . .testing whether that natiom or any nation so conceived and so dedicated. . . can long endure. We are met on a great battlefield of that war.

We bave come to dedicate a portion of that field as a tinal resting placa for those who here gave their lives that this nation might live. It is altogether fitting and proper that we ahould do this.

But, in a larger sense, we cannot dedicate. . .we cannot consecrate. . . we cannot hallow this ground. The hrave men, fiving and dead, who struggled here have consecrated it, fac above our poor power to add or detract. The world will little note, nor long remember, what we say here, but it can never forgef what they did here.

It is for us the living, rather, to be dedicated here to the vnfinished work which they who fought here have thus far so nobly advanced. It is rather for us to be here dedicated to the greaf task remaining before us. . .that from these bonored dead we take increased devotion to that cause for which they gave the last full measure of devotion. . . that we here highlv resolve that these dead shall not have died in vain. . . that this mation, under Cod, shall have a new birth of freedom. . . and that governmeni of the people. . .by the people. . .for the people. . . shall not perisb from this earth.

Lincoln's Gettysburg Address
given November 19, 1863
on the battlefield near Gettysburg, Pennsylvania, USA

	B	E
L	4	1
R	5	2

Figure 33-9. Error Detection in Texts. In the example there are 20 errors, half on the left and half on the right. Half of each of these is at the beginning of the word and half at the end. This famous text was downloaded from the Gutenberg Project Web site (http://www.promo.net/pg/), reformatted, and edited with a word processor.

version of this exercise that offers rich visual and auditory inducements to engage in the exercise (Fig. 33-12). Further, it yields scores (time and number of pieces remaining) that can be tabulated. The clinician enters this information on a spreadsheet that computes a rate of matching and a graph (Fig. 33-13) that reveals an overall trend, which can be very motivating for the patient (and the insurance company!).

Jigsaws Galore (see Web site http://www.dgray.com/jigalo.htm) is a program that preserves most of the features of the classic noncomputerized game and adds some useful ones. For instance, it keeps track of the time and number of pieces put together, information that can also be converted to a solution rate index and graphed. As illustrated in Figure 33-14, one can make jigsaws out of virtually any picture, including family photographs and scenes varying in complexity. Furthermore, the number, size, and orientation of pieces can be specified so that the difficulty can be controlled over a broad range. Like Mahjongg, the fun index for this exercise is high and patients engage in it eagerly on their home computers.

The value of the computer is that it is dynamic, it keeps track of performance automatically, and it is appealing. While the computer is not for everyone, it is a tool that can be invaluable. There is, however, no risk that the computer will replace therapists. While the computer may extend what is possible for therapists to do, the therapist is crucial in identifying appropriate tasks and parameters, introducing them and helping the patient to appreciate why the task is useful, advising on what methods should be used to improve performance, and counseling regarding the implications of the results.

Efficacy studies substantiating these techniques for promoting visual field awareness and compensation have been published by Kerkhoff and his colleagues (46,47), Scherzer (48), and researchers at the Rusk Institute in New York (43,45,49). Encouraging as these studies are, it is well to appreciate that visual field impairment remains one of the more challenging problems for optometric rehabilitation. The problem may persist and the individual lulled into thinking that the problem has been overcome. It is often useful to offer "booster doses"

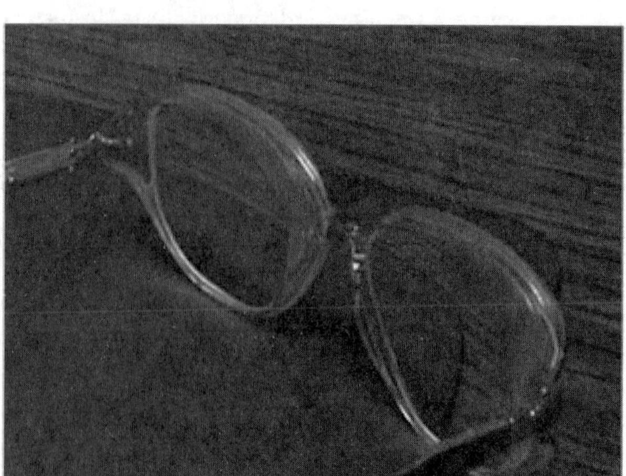

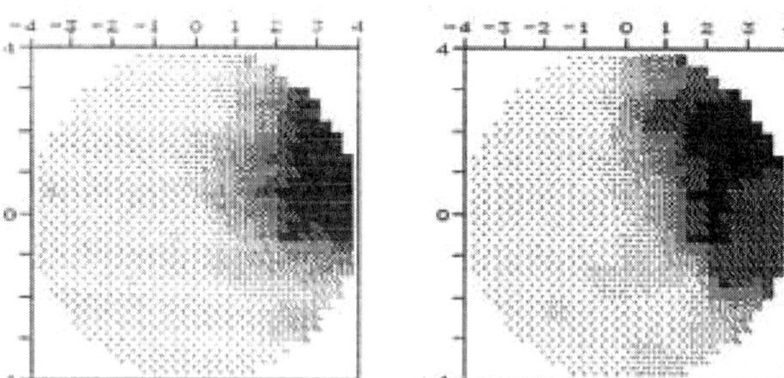

Figure 33-10. Spectacles (*upper panel*) with a yoked (bases up and right) prism used to assist an individual with an upper-right-quadrant (*lower panel*). The prisms displace the image down and to the left. In these reading glasses, the strength of the prism is greater than for distance viewing. Note that the visual fields shown are for the central 4 degrees and clearly show only a degree of macular sparing.

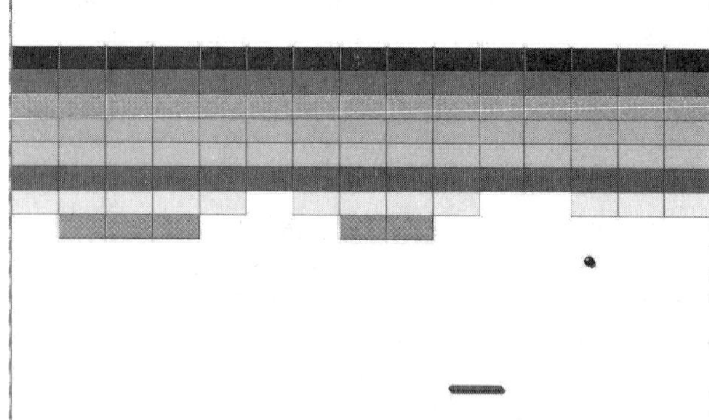

Figure 33-11. BLOCKBREAKER display. The bar at the bottom is the paddle that is controlled by rolling the trackball (or mouse) to the left and right. As the ball hits the bricks, they are removed. The ball bounces off the walls and the observer must engage in rapid visual pursuit, much as in the game of paddle tennis. The score is the number of bricks removed.

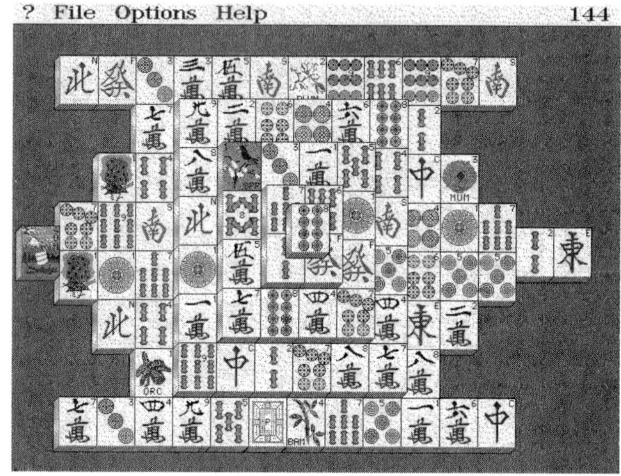

Figure 33-12. Mahjongg starting display from the program Shanghai: Dragon's Eye (Activision, Inc.). Visually, this stack of 144 attractively colored tiles is viewed slightly from the left. In computerized Mahjongg, the object is to match identical tiles, with the constraint that a piece cannot be covered by another piece and it must have a left or right edge exposed. Here the center (also the top of the stack) tile (eight balls) could be matched with one in the second row on the right, but not with the one in the third row from the bottom. As the exercise progresses, the computer reports the number of shapes remaining and elapsed time. From this, solution rate is the ratio of shapes matched per unit time.

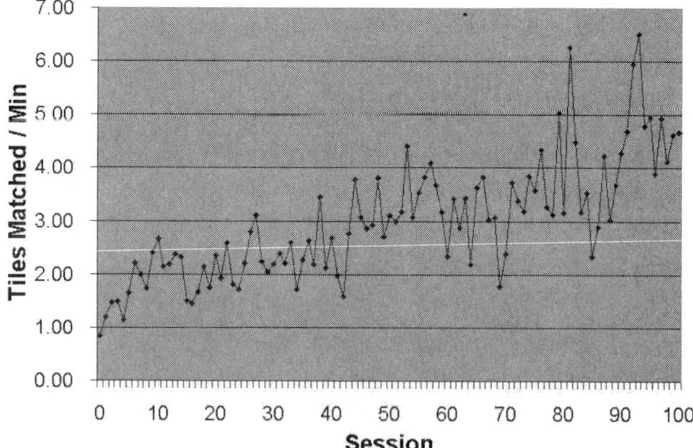

Figure 33-13. Progress on computerized Mahjongg of a patient after right-hemisphere cerebrovascular accident who has dense left homonymous hemianopia. For the most part, there was one session per week, although later on there were two sessions on 1 day. To minimize acuity issues, sessions 1 to 85 were conducted with tiles containing a large letter (disigned like a child's alphabet block). The dip at session 86 reflects the beginning of the more visually complex tiles shown in Fig. 33-12. The overall trend shows distinct progress; however, there was much session-to-session variation.

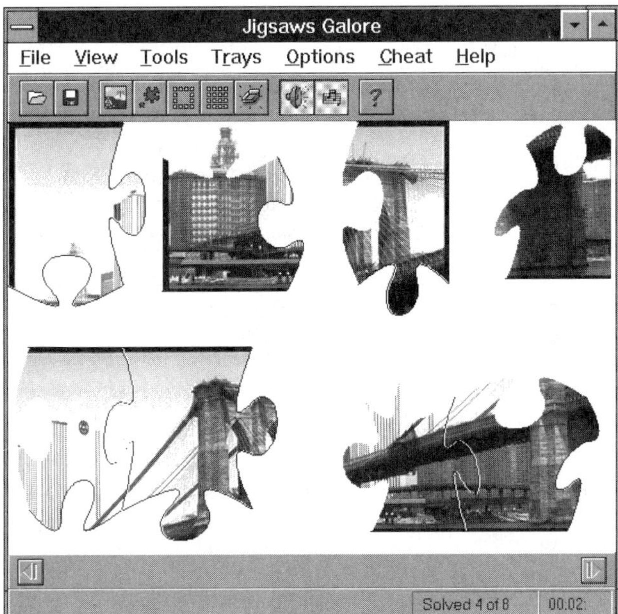

Figure 33-14. JIGSAWS GALORE, a computerized jigsaw puzzle. The pieces are moved by "dragging" them with the trackball or mouse, that is, pointing the cursor arrow to the desired piece, holding the button, moving the piece to the desired location, and releasing the piece. Correct juxtapositions are reinforced by an audible click and linking together. The computer reports the number of pieces solved and the solution time. One can create puzzles out of any computer image file and designate a wide range of difficulty (number of pieces). In the present instance, all pieces are shown in their correct orientation; however, one can allow rotation as an option. (Reproduced by permission from David Gray, http://www.dgray.com/jigalo.htm.)

of tasks with feedback to counter this tendency. Periodically, the individual with persistent visual spatial hemi-imperception needs to be reminded of the limits of compensation.

CONCLUSIONS

Importance of Comprehensive Evaluation

All too often following brain injury, visual problems remain undiagnosed. Diagnosis is a prerequisite for systematic rehabilitation to occur. Early, appropriate, and comprehensive evaluation is essential because of the primacy of vision in information processing and many visual problems do not reveal themselves subjectively.

Rehabilitative Optometry

Rehabilitative optometrists are the key service providers for such comprehensive diagnosis and functionally oriented treatment planning. They work most closely with OTs, physiatrists, neuropsychologists, and physical therapists, and are becoming an integral part of the treatment team. Consultation with ophthalmologists is appropriate when there is a need for ocular surgery or for the treatment of complicated ocular pathologies.

Visual Rehabilitative Interventions

Interventions include the treatment of ocular disease, prescription of lenses and prism, vision therapy, patient and family education and counseling, and environmental modifications. Computerized visual tasks have particular value as a therapy tool. Often conventional interventions (e.g., properly fit spectacles with correction) are overlooked or incorrectly applied following ABI. These all too common failures in the implementation of standard eye care occur, perhaps, because of the need for special clinical skill with this population.

Efficacy

Efficacy studies offer support for these approaches. The most difficult conditions to treat include visual field loss coupled with hemi-inattention, significant nystagmus, and optic nerve atrophy. In most instances, however, results range from at least helpful to, in some patients, a complete functional solution.

REFERENCES

1. Scheiman M, Wick B. *Clinical management of binocular vision heterophoric, accommodative and eye move-ment disorders.* Philadelphia: JB Lippincott, 1994.
2. Suchoff IB, Gianutsos R, Ciuffreda KJ, Groffman S. Vision impairment related to acquired brain injury. In: Silverstone B, Lang MA, Rosenthal B, Faye EE, eds. *The Lighthouse handbook on vision impairment and rehabilitation.* New York: Oxford University Press, in press.
3. Gianutsos R, Matheson P. The rehabilitation of visual perceptual disorders attributable to brain injury. In: Meier MJ, Benton AL, Diller L, eds. *Neuropsychological rehabilitation.* New York: Churchill Livingstone, 1987:202–241.
4. Anonymous. *Functional visual behavior: a therapist's guide to evaluation and treatment options.* Bethesda, MD: American Occupational Therapy Association, 1997.
5. Gianutsos R, Suchoff IB. Visual fields after brain injury: management issues for the occupational therapist. In: Scheiman M, ed. *Understanding and managing vision deficits: a guide for occupational therapists.* Thorofare, NJ: Slack, 1997:333–358.
6. Cohen AH. Acquired visual information-processing disorders: closed head trauma. In: Press LJ, ed. *Applied concepts in vision therapy.* St. Louis: CV Mosby, 1996:165–178.

7. Cohen AH. Optometry: the invisible member of the rehabilitation team. *J Am Optom Assoc* 1992;63:529. Editorial.

8. Cohen AH, Rein LD. The effect of head trauma on the visual system: the doctor of optometry as a member of the rehabilitation team. *J Am Optom Assoc* 1992;63:530–536.

9. Gianutsos R, Perlin R, Mazerolle KA, Trem N. Rehabilitative optometric services for persons emerging from coma. *J Head Trauma Rehabil* 1989;4(Special Issue): 17–25.

10. Lee PP, Jackson CA, Relles DA. Estimating eye care provider supply and workforce requirements. *Am Acad Ophthalmol* 1994;MR-516. Abstract.

11. Bowyer NK. Guest editorial: defining primary care. *J Am Optom Assoc* 1997;68:6–9.

12. Peachey GT. Principles of vision therapy. In: Press LJ, ed. *Applied concepts of vision therapy.* St. Louis: CV Mosby, 1997:9–20.

13. Gianutsos R. Working relationships between psychology and optometry. *J Behav Optom* 1991; 2:30–31.

14. Gianutsos R, Ramsey G. Enabling the survivors of brain injury to receive rehabilitative optometric services. *J Vis Rehabil* 1988;2: 37–58.

15. Ciuffreda KJ, Suchoff IB, Marrone MA, Ahmann E. Oculomotor rehabilitation in traumatic brain-injured patients. *J Behav Optom* 1996;7:31–38.

16. American Optometric Association. *Optometric clinical practice guideline; care of the patient with diabetes mullitus.* St. Louis: American Optometric Association, 1994.

17. Jackowski MM, Sturr JF, Taub HA, Turk MA: Photophobia in patients with traumatic brain injury: uses of light filtering lenses to enhance contrast sensitivity and reading rate. *Neurorehabilitation* 1996; 6:193–201.

18. Suchoff IB, Petito GT: The efficacy of visual therapy: accommodative disorders and non-strabismic anomalies of binocular vision. *J Am Optom Assoc* 1986;57:119–125.

19. Ciuffreda KJ, Tannen B. *Eye movement basics for the clinician.* St. Louis: Mosby Year Book, 1995.

20. Vogel G. Computer aided vision therapy. Cicero, In: American Vision Therapy, 1997. Abstract.

21. Hellerstein LF, Freed S, Maples WC. Vision profile of patients with mild brain injury. *J Am Optom Assoc* 1995;66:634–639.

22. Schlageter K, Gray B, Hall K, et al. Incidence and treatment of visual dysfunction in traumatic brain injury. *Brain Inj* 1993;7: 439–448.

23. Ron S. Plastic changes in eye movements in patients with traumatic brain injury. In: Fuchs AF, Becker W, eds. *Progress in oculomotor research.* New York: Elsevier North Holland, 1981:237–251.

24. Ron S. Can training be transferred from one oculomotor system to another? In: Roucoux A, Crommelinck M, eds. *Physiological and pathological aspects of eye movements.* London: Dr. W. Junk, 1982:83–88.

25. Groffman S. Treatment of visual perceptual disorders. *Pract Optom* 1993;4:76–83.

26. Falk NS, Aksionoff EB. The primary care optometric examination of the traumatic brain injury patient. *J Am Optom Assoc* 1992;63:547–553.

27. Manor RS, Heibronn YD, Sherf I, Ben-Sira I. Loss of accommodation produced by peristriate lesion in man? *J Clin Neuro-ophthalmol* 1988;8:19–23.

28. Miller KL, York RT, Goss D. Importance of proximity cues on the distance rock accommodative facility test. *J Behav Optom* 1996;7:93–96.

29. Coloruso EE, Rouse, MW. *Clinical management of strabismus.* Boston: Butterworth-Heinemann, 1993.

30. Press LJ. Accommodative and vergence therapy. In: Press LJ, ed. *Applied concepts in vision therapy.* St. Louis: CV Mosby, 1997:222–245.

31. Grisham JD. Treatment of binocular dysfunctions. In: Schor CM, Ciuffreda KJ, eds. *Vergence eye movements: basic and clinical aspects.* Woburn, MA: Butterworth, 1983:605–646.

32. Birnbaum MH. *Optometric management of nearpoint vision disorders.* Boston: Butterworth-Heinemann, 1993.

33. Kerkhoff G, Stogerer E. Treatment of fusional disorders in patients with brain damage [in German]. *Klin Monatsbl Augenheilk* 1994; 205:70–75.

34. Kerkhoff G, Stogerer E. Recovery of fusional convergence after systematic practice. *Brain Inj* 1994;8:15–22.

35. Morton RL. Visual dysfunction following traumatic brain injury. In: Ashley MJ, Krych DK, eds. *Traumatic brain injury rehabilitation.* Boca Raton, FL: CRC Press, 1995:171–186.

36. Freed S, Hellerstein LF. Visual electrodiagnostic findings in mild traumatic brain injury. *Brain Inj* 1997;11:25–36.

37. Hall C. Functional visual fields: norms for younger and older viewers. Master's thesis, Touro College, 1995.

38. Gianutsos R, Vroman GS, Matheson P, Glosser D. Computer programs for cognitive rehabilitation. Vol. 2. Further visual imperception procedures. Bayport, NY: Life Science Associates, 1983.

39. Medina-Constantino C. Norms for functional central visual field procedures. Bachelor's honor thesis, State University of New York at Purchase, 1997.

40. Cohen JM, Waiss B. An overview of enhancement techniques for peripheral field loss. *J Am Optom Assoc* 1993;64:60–70.

41. Gianutsos R. Vision rehabilitation after brain injury. In: Gentile M, ed. *Functional visual behavior: a*

therapist's guide to evaluation and treatment options. Bethesda, MD: American Occupational Therapy Association, 1997:321–342.

42. Diller L, Weinberg J. Evidence for accident-prone behavior in hemiplegic patients. *Arch Phys Med Rehabil* 1970;51:358–363.

43. Weinberg J, Diller L, Gordon WA. Training sensory awareness and spatial organization in people with right brain damage. *Arch Phys Med Rehabil* 1979;60:491–496.

44. Diller L, Weinberg J. Hemi-inattention and rehabilitation: the evolution of a rational treatment program. *Adv Neurol* 1977;18: 63–82.

45. Weinberg J, Diller L, Gordon WA, et al. Visual scanning training effect on reading-related tasks in acquired right brain damage. *Arch Phys Med Rehabil* 1977;58:479–486.

46. Kerkhoff G, Munssinger U, Meier EK. Neurovisual rehabilitation in cerebral blindness. *Arch Neurol* 1994;51:474–481.

47. Kerkhoff G, Munssinger U, Haaf E, et al. Rehabilitation of homonymous scotomata in patients with postgeniculate damage of the visual system: saccadic compensation training. *Restorative Neurol Neurosci* 1992;4:245–254.

48. Scherzer P. Rehabilitation following severe head trauma: results of the three-year rehabilitation program. *Arch Phys Med Rehabil* 1986;67:366–374.

49. Gordon WA, Hibbard MR, Egelko S. Perceptual remediation in patients with right brain damage: a comprehensive program. *Arch Phys Med Rehabil* 1985;66:353–359.

Chapter 34

Rehabilitation of the Patient Requiring Transplantation

Mark A. Young
Steven A. Stiens
Douglas McGill
Elizabeth Rittenberg
Douglas Slakey
Michael D. Freedman
Dilip S. Kittur

The role for the rehabilitation specialist in the preoperative conditioning and restorative aftercare of the transplantation patient has grown over the last decade. As transplantation surgery has gained wide acceptance as a therapeutic intervention for patients with hematologic and end-stage solid-organ pathology (See Table 34-1 for statistical analysis reflecting transplantation by organ donor and type, 1988–1996), the establishment of organ procurement protocols and an HLA registry for bone marrow transplantation has further facilitated "transplant matching" and survivorship (1). Besides restoring physiologic function, transplantation can enhance functional status, thereby improving the recipient's quality of life. Continuing refinements in surgical, antirejection, and infection-control strategies have optimized the treatment of transplantation patients, allowing quicker transition to rehabilitation centers and return to functional independence.

This chapter reviews the critical role rehabilitation plays in the functional and restorative care of the transplantation patient. It begins with a discussion of some general principles fundamental to proper rehabilitation management, followed by a more in-depth discussion of individual types of transplant surgeries and their implication for the rehabilitative and restorative process. The major transplant procedures addressed are cardiac, liver, pulmonary, kidney, bone marrow, intestinal, pancreas, and neural transplantations. Data citing the statistical prevalence of individual procedures is noted in Figure 34-1.

Due to the complexity of this broad, highly technical subject, the task of preparing and organizing this chapter has been divided among a national interdisciplinary panel of rehabilitation physicians and transplantation physicians—each with his or her own area of expertise. This chapter represents a pioneering effort as rehabilitation texts have not traditionally devoted entire chapters to this fledgling physiatric domain. The technologic breakthroughs in transplant sciences over the past decade have truly created a "new frontier" for physiatrists, necessitating comprehensive clinical literature devoted to the subject (2).

TRANSPLANTATION REHABILITATION

General Principles

As with most dimensions of rehabilitative care, optimal management of the transplantation patient requires a structured, multidisciplinary team effort. The essence of the rehabilitation process is that all its components are integrated (3,4). The "transplant rehabilitation team" ideally consists of a physiatrist, physical therapist, occupational therapist, transplant surgeon, internist, social worker, case manager, clinical pharmacologist, nutritionist, and nurse. Since functional deficits secondary to end-organ failure often predate the patient's transplant surgery, the physiatrist coordinates the rehabilitative aspects of the patient's treatment and should perform a baseline functional assessment *prior* to surgery.

The responsibility of physical medicine and rehabili-

Table 34-1: U.S. Organ Donors by Organ and Donor Type—1988 to 1996

Year	Organ/Donor Type								
	Kidney			Liver			Pancreas		
	Cadaveric	Living	Total	Cadaveric	Living	Total	Cadaveric	Living	Total
1988	3880	1812	5692	1835	0	1835	577	5	682
1989	3817	1902	5719	2377	2	2379	799	4	803
1990	4308	2095	6403	2871	14	2885	951	2	953
1991	4269	2393	6662	3167	22	3189	1066	1	1067
1992	4277	2533	6810	3335	33	3368	1004	3	1007
1993	4609	2851	7460	3764	36	3800	1243	2	1245
1994	4798	3008	7806	4095	60	4155	1360	2	1362
1995	4997	3289	8286	4324	45	4369	1286	7	1293
1996	5036	3489	8525	4452	52	4504	1295	12	1307

Year	Organ/Donor Type								
	Heart			Lung			Overall		
	Cadaveric	Living	Total	Cadaveric	Living	Total	Cadaveric	Living	Total
1988	1785	8	1793	130	0	130	4084	1825	5909
1989	1782	8	1790	191	0	191	4019	1916	5935
1990	2168	12	2180	275	1	276	4512	2124	6636
1991	2198	4	2202	395	4	399	4528	2424	6952
1992	2247	1	2248	527	0	527	4521	2570	7091
1993	2442	2	2444	790	12	802	4861	2903	7764
1994	2526	3	2529	918	31	949	5100*	3102	8202
1995	2503	0	2503	908	41	949	5357*	3375	8732
1996	2459	1	2460	750	12	762	5417*	3553	8970

* Of the total number of cadaveric donors for 1994–1996, the number of non-heart beating donors, by year: 1994, 48 non-heart beating donors (0.9% of cadaveric donors in 1994); 1995, 44 non-heart beating donors (0.8% of cadaveric donors in 1995); 1996, 70 non-heart beating donors (1.3% of cadaveric donors in 1996).

Source: UNOS OPTN data as of September 4, 1997.

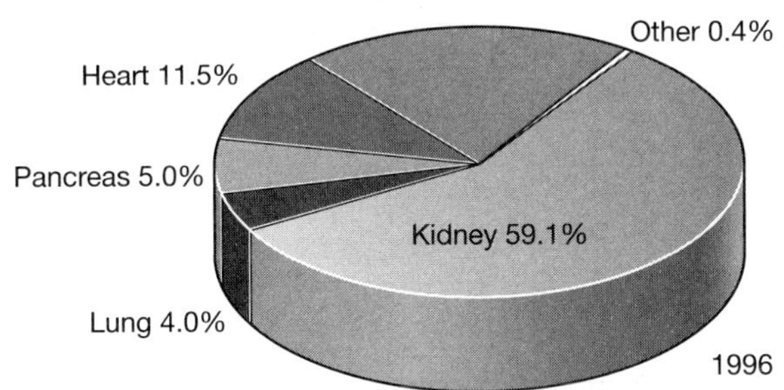

Figure 34-1. U.S. organ transplants (n = 20,354). Source: UNOS Scientific Registry data as of September 15, 1997.

tation specialists (as well as the entire therapy team) is to offer early evaluation, advise on acute preventive and maintenance strategies, and provide counseling and education to family members. The objectives include decubitus prophylaxis, bowel and bladder maintenance, contracture prevention, thromboembolic deterrence, and development of splinting and positioning protocols, where relevant. Since transplantation candidates are often deconditioned to the point of immobilization, the rehabilitation specialist must also focus on preventing the musculoskeletal and cardiovascular effects of a bed-bound state.

For transplantation patients, special attention must be paid to the unique psychosocial and emotional stresses associated with organ transplantation (5). The psychiatric aspects of transplantation include coping with disease chronicity, indefinite organ donor waiting periods, and other socioeconomic strains that can significantly alter the rehabilitation process. It is the role of the transplant team social worker and psychologist to address these issues, within the context of the *entire* team.

Upon screening for deficits in functional ability and medical status after transplantation, the physiatrist supervises the implementation of physical therapy and occupational therapy services. With the increase in numbers of posttransplantation patients requiring short-term mechanical ventilation, the rehabilitation team, under physiatric and pulmonary medicine direction, may play an instrumental role in promoting weaning from respiratory support. As with other disease processes, physiatry can also help to enhance swallowing and communication functions in the occasional posttransplantation patient with these complications (6–8).

Establishment of an efficacious transplantation-therapy prescription should be based on a comprehensive review of the medical record, with emphasis on the underlying medical, socioeconomic, and psychological needs of the patient (9). Individualization of the therapy plan is always imperative. Since transplantation patients frequently have many medical comorbidities, the inclusion of detailed precautions in every prescription is essential (10).

Review of General Physiatric Principles in Transplantation

A significant early challenge facing the physiatrist is the need to counter the ill effects of deconditioning and immobilization in the transplant patient. Virtually all organ systems can be adversely affected by the bed-bound state, impacting negatively on functional independence. Although many complications in the transplant patient can be avoided through early physiatric intervention, we have limited this background discussion to five major areas: skin, musculoskeletal, contractures, cardiovascular, and thromboembolic complications.

Skin

Skin breakdown (i.e., pressure ulcers) may be a serious complication of prolonged immobilization in transplant patients, just as it is a major potential hazard among all hospitalized patients. One study documented a 9.2% incidence of pressure ulceration among hospitalized patients (11). Decubitus and pressure ulcerations can develop when soft tissue overlying a major bony structure, such as the ischium, trochanter, or sacrum, becomes compressed against a supporting structure such as a wheelchair, operating table, or bed. Prolonged compression can lead to necrosis. Although superficial tissues are principally affected during the early stages of the process, damage to more deeply seated structures such as fat, muscle, and bone can ensue. Since transplant operations are often lengthy, not infrequently spanning 8 to 14 hours, the possibility of protracted immobilization leading to skin breakdown is great. During the postsurgical phase, patients may be especially susceptible to infection, owing to immunologic incompetence. Patients receiving steroids may be especially prone to skin fragility. Microbiologic intrusion of ulcers may occur. Urinary incontinence, a potential risk factor for ulcer development, may complicate transplantation recovery. Excess moisture can result in skin compromise and tissue necrosis by interfering with oxygen and nutrient delivery to the tissue (12).

Local, environmental, metabolic, and systemic factors in the transplant patient can predispose to skin ulceration. Skin maceration, edema, sheer forces, and thermal factors can contribute. Classic studies in the physiatry literature demonstrated that pressures ranging from 20 mm Hg and upward are necessary to produce skin breakdown (13). Metabolic and systemic issues heightening the risk of pressure ulceration in the transplant patient include malnutrition, anemia, and hormonal imbalance.

Anemia, frequently a pretransplantation characteristic of bone marrow and kidney transplant recipients, can be a significant contributing factor since it is associated with cell hypoxia and necrosis. Malnutrition, an almost universal attribute of liver transplant patients, can cause protein and albumin deficiencies, further preventing optimal healing of pressure ulcers. In addition, metabolic and hormonal deficiencies such as diabetes and adrenal cortical imbalance can impair metabolism, causing healing delays. The posttransplantation rehabilitation patient with reduced bed mobility is at risk for further worsening of integumentary status caused by sheer forces and stresses imposed during transfer activities. Since rehabilitation patients are often diabetic, vigilant insulin regulation is essential for the prevention of ischemic ulcers. Patients with toxic and metabolic neuropathies may have insensate skin with disordered sensory feedback systems, which further predisposes to skin denudation.

Management and Transplant Rehabilitation

The most economical and proactive technique to control ulcer formation is through *prevention.* The rehabilitation specialist rendering consultative input to the transplant team should emphasize optimization of nursing, medical, and nutritional care, as well as patient and family education. Institutional adoption of a pressure ulcer and wound documentation tracking form for transplant patients is imperative (Fig. 34-2).

Timely prescription of pressure-relief devices and a turning-positioning protocol will also help to avert the damaging consequences of skin ulcer formation. After transplantation (especially during the acute stage), the patients often experience difficulty with bed mobility and turning, due to the presence of multiple, life-sustaining intravenous and hyperalimentation lines, tubes, and catheters. Optimally, a turning program should include 2 hours with the patient on the side, 2 hours on the opposing side, and 2 hours in the supine position (14). For patients with sacral skin compromise, prone positioning when feasi ble can help to unload the area and promote skin healing (Fig. 34-3A). Anatomic areas most vulnerable to breakdown are the sacrum and heels. By avoiding elevation of the head of the bed, pressure reduction over the sacrum can be achieved. Optimal protection of the heels can be accomplished by placing a pillow under the calves to elevate the leg 15 degrees, thereby "unloading" the heels (Fig. 34-3B). Heel boots can also be worn, for added protection. Since transplant patients may be positioned on their sides for prolonged durations, the trochanteric skin must be protected. Patients can be positioned in a modified side-lying position in which the inferior leg is placed in 20 degrees of flexion at the hip and knee. The superior leg is extended at the hip and flexed 35 degrees at the knee to ensure that the foot is comfortably postured posteriorly (Fig. 34-3C).

Since transplant patients are often treated with a multitude of medications that can exert a potential effect on skin integrity and fragility, including steroids and

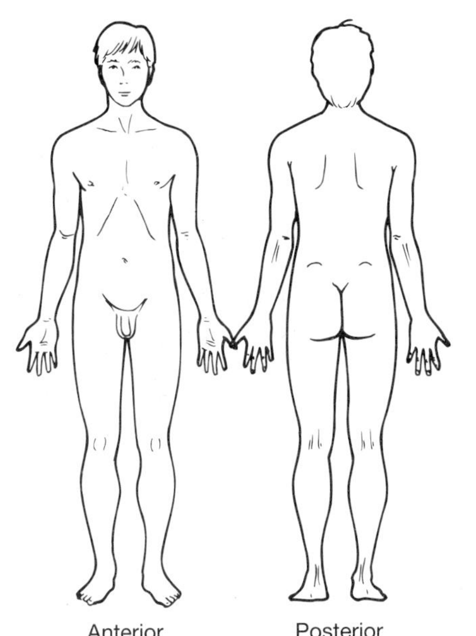

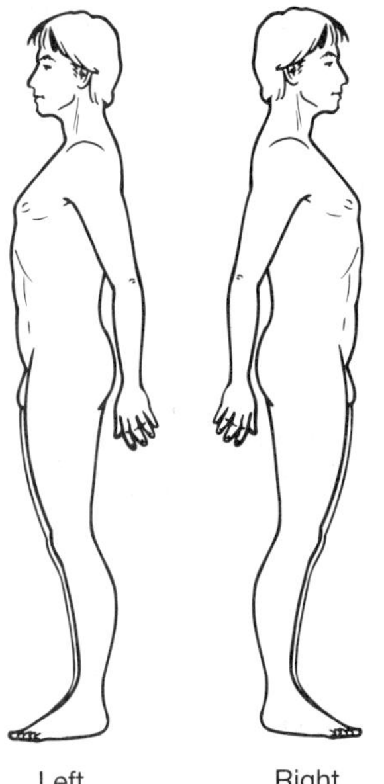

IDENTIFY ULCER BY CIRCLING AREA AND NUMBER AREA CIRCLED

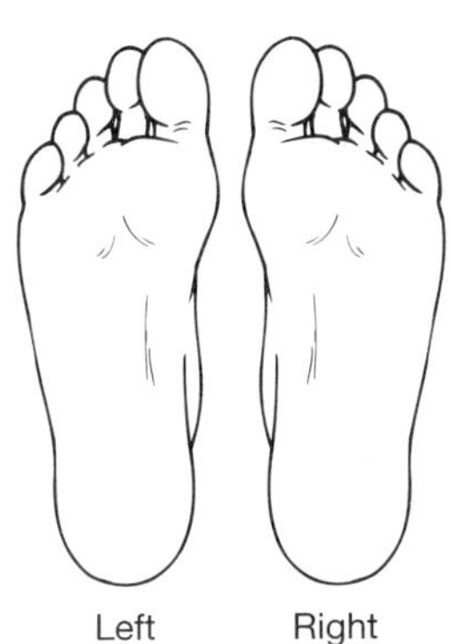

Key

Wound bed color	Tissue in wound bed & %	Type of exudate	Odor	Edema	Peri-wound skin condition
R- Red Y- Yellow M- Mixed (specify) B- Black	G- Granulation S- Slough E- Eschar M- Mixed N- Necrotic % 25/50/75/100	0- None S- Serous S/S- Serosang P- Purulent L- Light M- Moderate H- Heavy	0- None M- Mild F- Foul	0- None 1+ Mild 2+ Moderate 3+ Severe P- Pitting	I- Intact R- Reddened D- Denuded M- Macerated

Stage of Ulcer

Stage I	Stage II	Stage III	Stage IV
Reddened area does not fade in 30 minutes with relieving pressure	Partial thickness skin loss or blister	Full thickness skin loss with subcutaneous involvement	Full thickness skin loss with muscle and or bone involvement

Date & Initials	Location number	Stage	Size W x L cm	Depth	Under-mining	Wound bed color	Tissue in wound bed & %	Type of exudate	Odor	Edema	Peri-wound skin cond.	Comments

Figure 34-2. Sample pressure ulcer and wound documentation record.

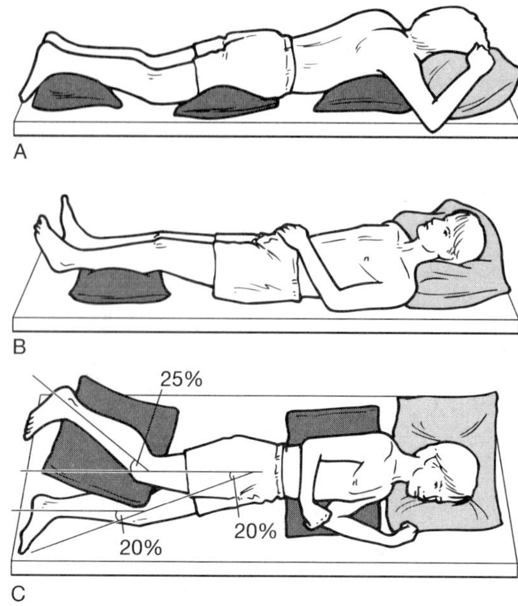

Figure 34-3. Turning-position protocol. *A.* Prone positioning. *B.* Elevation of calves. *C.* Side-lying position.

immunosuppressants, a careful review of inciting agents should be made. Maintenance of optimal skin hydration and water balance (avoiding excessive wetness or dryness) helps to sustain skin integrity. Maintaining proper nutrition is also essential in sustaining proper oxygenation to the skin. Since transplant patients often are "tethered" to a variety of catheters, enteral tubes, and drains, special attention must be made to ensure skin cleanliness and optimal mounting of these devices. New techniques for mounting tubes to maximally protect the skin have been described (15). The role of wound care products must be considered (Table 34-2).

Therapeutic mattresses and cushioned inserts that provide an additional measure of protection by reducing pressure should be considered for transplant patients. Options include the pressure air mattress, the air fluidized bed, and the kinetic bed.

Muscular System

Effort must be made to mobilize transplant patients as early as possible following surgery, since immobility can have a harmful effect on muscle size and strength. Bed-bound transplant patients may experience cardiovascular deconditioning, which can contribute to perceived muscle weakness. Early studies from the physical medicine and rehabilitation literature demonstrated that bed rest can lead to a 10% to 15% net strength loss per week (16). Muscle bulk may decrease to half of its original volume after a month. Transplant patients taking steroids may be at even greater risk for development of proximal muscle weakness. While all muscular structures of transplant patients are at risk for strength diminution, the earliest muscle groups to develop weakness are in the legs and trunk. Weakness in the antigravity musculature can have harmful functional consequences. Weakness of the quadriceps, gluteus maximus, and back extensors may lead to profound deficits in stair climbing and ambulation. Bone marrow transplant patients with chronic graft versus host disease may experience an added dimension of weakness resulting from soft tissue tightening, stiffness, and contractives (17).

Aerobic endurance can also be adversely affected in immobilized transplant patients who experience a significant decrement in metabolic activity related to reduced muscle activity. A decrease in oxidative capacity as well as a lowered tolerance to lactic acid and oxygen debt are responsible in part for poor endurance and reduced activity tolerance (18).

Although strength building and maintenance programs in transplant patients need to be individualized, it is generally recognized that strength can be maintained by daily contractions of 20% or more of maximal tension sustained for several seconds or a vigorous contraction of 50% of maximal tension performed for 1 second. Loss of strength or muscle bulk can be prevented further by electrical stimulation applied to isolated muscles. Two exercise programs that can help to maintain strength and decrease venous stasis include quadriceps sets and ankle pumps (Fig. 34-4). Cardiovascular fitness can be fostered by upright positioning on a tilt table, which enhances orthostatic tolerance and helps to strengthen antigravity muscles.

Skeletal System

Transplant patients often face formidable metabolic challenges that can add to the burden imposed by immobilization. Multiple risk factors for the development of osteoporosis in patients receiving transplantation are listed in Table 34-3. Since healthy bone structure and function depend on the forces that act on the bone (19), early ambulation is *critical.* Osteopenia and deterioration in bone structure are observed in animals and humans subjected to a weightless state or prolonged immobilization. Amplification of osteoclastic activity (bone loss) and inhibition of osteoblastic activity (bone growth) are thought to occur with immobilization. Several sequential stages of bone loss exist (19), and the rates of loss differ by patient demographics. In general, the rate of bone loss is linked to age, gender, and medical profile. Hormonal aberrations also have been linked to osteopenia (20). Osteoporosis caused by disuse can be forestalled through isometric and isotonic exercises (21). A number of important pharmacologic and physiatric therapies exist for osteoporosis (Table 34-4).

Contractures and Physiatric Intervention

Defined as a restriction in active or passive range of motion due to decreased stretchability of subcutaneous tissues, ligaments, muscles, joint capsules, or synovia, contractures in transplant patients can be attributable to either

Table 34-2: Properties and Common Uses of Five Major Classes of Wound-Care Products in Transplantation

	Properties	Uses
Transparent membranes	Moist healing principle Semipermeable Allows O_2 exchange Prevents bacterial entry Promotes epithelial migration	Prevents shear and friction Stage I, II, and shallow III ulcers Clean, granulating, nondraining Autolysis Secondary dressing Change when leaks or excess fluid
Hydrocolloids	Occlusive barrier Forms gel with wound exudate Creates moist wound environment Prevents bacterial contamination Available in wafers, paste, powder, or granules	Stage I, II, III, and some IV ulcers Minimal to moderate exudating wounds Prevents shear and friction Secondary dressing Aids in liquefaction, nonsurgical debridement Change when leaks (if <24 hr, try another dressing)
Hydrogels	Water, polyethylene oxide or other compound Primary wound covering Provides moist wound environment Various absorption abilities Good for patient comfort Nonadherent to wound bed	Stage II, III, and some IV ulcers Burns Autolysis—softens eschar Granulating or necrotic wounds
Alginate dressings	Hydrophilic, nonwoven fiber converts to gel Calcium and sodium exchange Creates moist environment Nonadherent to wound Available in packing or sheets	Light to heavily draining wounds Stage II, III, and IV ulcers Burns, vascular ulcers, graft sites May be used with infected wounds Can pack deep wounds to fill deadspace
Foam dressings	Semipermeable, absorptive, nonwoven, polyurethane dressing Combines moist healing and absorbancy No dressing residue in wound Nonadherent to wound Thermal insulation Comfortable, trauma-free removal Can be used with topicals	Minimal to moderate draining wounds Donor sites Burns (1st and 2nd degree) Pressure ulcers Wound dehiscence Skin tears

Adapted from Cuttino C. Dermal Wound Management in Long Term Care Settings Conference. Houston. Texas, February 1994. King of Prussia, PA: Health Management Publications, 1994.

intrinsic or extrinsic factors. Intrinsic factors include the shortening of collagen fibers in unstretched muscles, as might occur in transplant patients who have been bed bound without any therapy. As discussed later in this chapter, bone marrow transplant patients with chronic graft-versus-host disease (CGVHD) frequently develop "scleroderma-like" contractures, presumably ascribable to poorly defined intrinsic factors. Extrinsic factors that might predispose transplant rehabilitation patients to contracture development include an imbalance of agonists and antagonists as a result of paralytic, spastic, or biomechanical conditions. Muscles crossing 2 joints are first to shorten, when normal range is not preserved. Muscles commonly susceptible to contractures include the hamstrings, rectus femoris, tensor fasciae latae, erector spinae, and gastrocnemius muscles. In a study of 62 patients with bone marrow transplant–associated CGVHD, a significant percentage had range of motion abnormalities (unpublished data).

Prevention and Therapeutic Intervention

Unfortunately, the "position of comfort" (supine with pillows behind the head, flexed hips, flexed knees, and ankles plantarflexed) is a major culprit in the pathogenesis of contractures. Key elements of the contracture prevention and rehabilitation routine should include discontinuation of bed rest, use of proper positioning, and early joint mobilization. In the event that the transplant recipient requires more prolonged bed confinement, specific, bedside, targeted stretching and positioning techniques need to be enforced.

Mechanical appliances and specialized contracture-prevention medical equipment can be utilized. Use of a firm mattress can prevent excess hip flexion and other dysfunctional positions. Trochanteric rolls can be employed to maintain neutral position and to prevent hip external rotation and abduction. To prevent plantarflexion, a foot board or posterior ankle splints may be used. Since the arms are

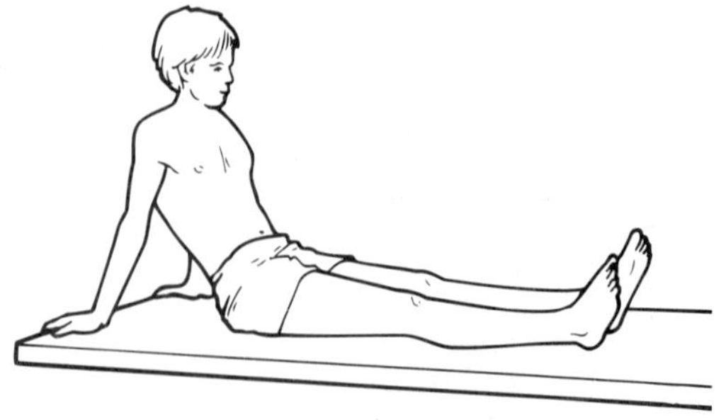

A **Quad Sets**

Tighten muscles on top thigh by pushing knee down into table.
Hold for .... seconds.
Perform .... repititions
.... times/day.

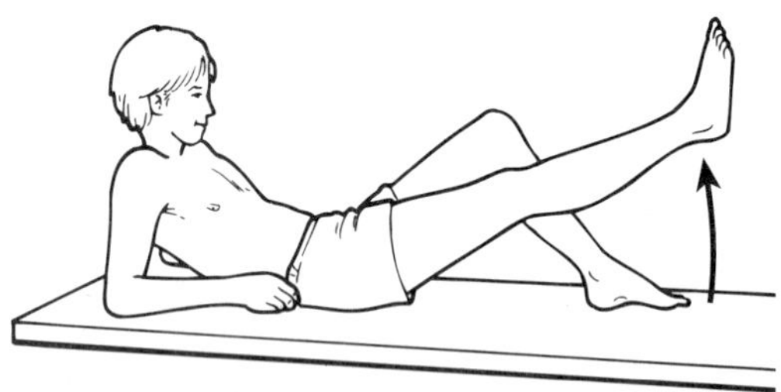

B **Straight Leg Raise**

Tighten muscles in front of thigh then lift leg 8-10 inches from surface, keeping knee locked.
Perform .... repititions
.... times/day.

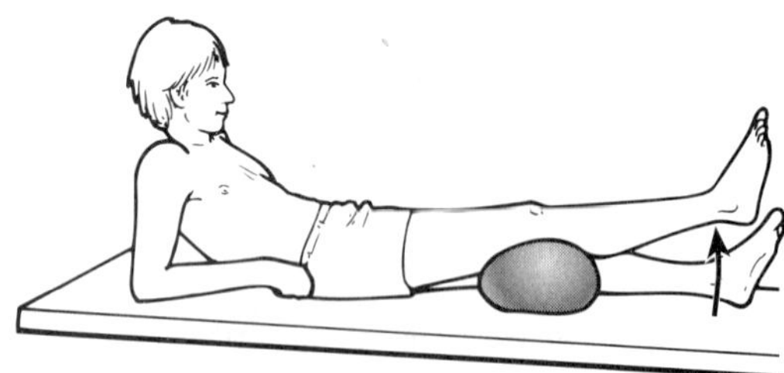

C **Terminal Knee Extension**

With knee bent over a bolster, straighten knee by tightening muscle on top of thigh. Keep bottom of knee on bolster. Perform .... repititions
.... times/day.

Figure 34-4. Muscle-strengthening exercises.

also prone to contracture, a properly placed pillow can maintain the arm in neutral rotation and abduction, thereby preventing tightness in the arm adductors and internal rotators. For patients with weakness in the upper extremity, a palmar roll or hand splint can be used to optimally position the hand, thumb, and finger joints.

If tightness exists in a joint, the primary means of treatment is active and passive range of motion exercises with a sustained terminal stretch. For mild contracture, a short sustained stretch lasting 20 to 30 minutes twice a day may be effective (22). Stretch can be enhanced by judiciously applying thermal modalities prior to movement (23,24).

Table 34-3: Risk Factors for Osteoporosis in Transplantation

Genetic
Female gender
Family history of osteoporosis
Small stature
Caucasian, Asian, or American Eskimo ethnicity
Homocystinuria, osteogenesis imperfecta
Dietary and Lifestyle
Malnutrition, anorexia nervosa
Low calcium intake/absorption
Vitamin C or D deficiency
? High-protein diet
Alcohol and tobacco
Sedentary lifestyle/immobilization
Secondary Causes of Osteoporosis
Endocrine disorders
Hyperprolactinemia
Hyperparathyroidism
Hyperthyroidism
Diabetes mellitus
Acromegaly
Glucocorticoid insufficiency or excess
Hypogonadism
Menopause
Surgery
Drugs
Congenital origin
Bone marrow expansion or replacement
Chronic illness
Cyanotic congenital heart disease
Renal insufficiency
Hepatic insufficiency
Chronic diarrhea or malabsorption
Rheumatoid arthritis
Metabolic acidosis
Drugs
Thyroid hormone over-replacement
Corticosteroids
Antiestrogens
Antiandrogens
Carbonic anhydrase inhibitors
Chronic lithium
Immunosuppressives
Anticonvulsants
Prolonged high-dose heparin

Adapted from Bellantoni M, Madoff DM. Osteoporosis and back pain: diagnosis, treatment, and prevention. [Young MA, Lavin R, eds.]. *Spinal Rehabil* 1995;9:641–656.

Cardiovascular System

A progressive rise in the resting heart rate by 0.5 beats/min occurs in bed-bound patients. The net effect of this phenomenon is "immobilization tachycardia" in which an abnormal pulse with submaximal exertion occurs. Follow-

Table 34-4: Therapies for Osteoporosis in Transplantation
Physiatric intervention
Heat and massage
Muscle strengthening and stretching
Gait stabilization and fall prevention
Bracing and assistive devices
Calcium supplementation
Antiresorptive agents
Established
Estrogen replacement therapy
Subcutaneous calcitonin
New
Bisphosphonates
Experimental
Tamoxifen
Nasal calcitonin
Sodium fluoride
Parathyroid hormone

Adapted from Bellantoni M, Madoff DM. Osteoporosis and back pain: diagnosis, treatment, and prevention. [Young MA, Lavin R, eds.]. *Spinal Rehabil* 1995;9:641–656.

ing 2 weeks of bed rest, a 15% reduction in stroke volume occurs, attributable to lower-extremity pooling of blood and blood volume reduction. With prolonged immobility, as might occur during the posttransplantation phase, oxygen consumption ($\dot{V}O_2$) or maximal oxygen consumption ($\dot{V}O_2max$) declines dramatically. Transplant patients may experience postural hypotension resulting from the circulatory system's inability to adjust to the upright position. Dizziness, light-headedness, vertigo, tachycardia, and decreased systolic pressure are symptoms. Measures that can be instituted to counteract orthostatic hypotension in transplant recipients include early mobilization and conditioning exercises, when approved by the transplant team. Other helpful interventions include increasing fluid and salt intake, tilt-table tolerance building, and use of reclining backs, elevating leg rests, abdominal binders, and compression stockings. Pharmacotherapy with sympathomimetic agents such as ephedrine and phenylephrine can be employed.

Venous Thromboembolism Prevention

Potential causes of mortality in hospitalized transplant rehabilitation patients are deep vein thrombosis and pulmonary embolism. Increased age and length of immobilization are highly correlated. Stasis, intimal injury, and hypercoagulability (Virchow's triad) are thought to be the significant factors underlying the high incidence of thromboembolic events.

Subcutaneous heparin and support stockings are two traditional interventions used to prevent thromboembolic complications in transplant rehabilitation patients. A regimen of 5000 units administered subcutaneously twice daily is customary, although the heparin-associated thrombocytopenia and thrombosis syndrome (HATT) can rarely occur (25). The risk of bleeding in posttransplantation patients must be carefully weighed against the benefits of anticoagulation. Since patients with generalized weakness, deconditioning, incoordination, and poor balance are often at risk for falls and other exercise-induced mishaps during therapy, treatment modalities that diminish the risk of bleeding may be advantageous. The recent introduction of low-molecular-weight heparin may hold promise because of the lower associated incidence of bleeding (26).

Transplant patients, like so many other surgical patients, often have underlying bleeding tendencies that contraindicate anticoagulation; therefore, nonpharmacologic treatment options are often needed (27). Intermittent pneumatic compression has also proved helpful, although its use is limited to patients without lower-extremity encumbrances or occlusive bandages. Since pulmonary embolism is a significant cause of mortality among asymptomatic rehabilitation patients and often results in thousands of preventable deaths annually, the impact of sudden alterations in intrathoracic and intra-abdominal pressures associated with the Valsalva maneuver as a cause for clot propagation should be further studied (28). Vena cava filter insertion should be carefully considered for patients with bleeding proclivities who are ineligible for other forms of prophylaxis.

Rehabilitation Before and After Cardiac Transplantation

Since the first successful cardiac transplant procedure was performed in 1967 by Dr. Christian Barnard in Capetown, South Africa (18-day posttransplantation survival span), survival rates have improved steadily. The growing success of cardiac transplantation is partially attributable to surgical refinements associated with greater numbers of procedures completed annually as well as improved rejection-prevention methodology. The emergence of cyclosporine in 1983 and other more recent potent antirejection pharmaceuticals, in addition to the use of endocardial biopsy to detect early rejection, has further improved outcomes.

Epidemiology

During the first decade following introduction of the procedure (1967–1977), the 90-day actuarial survival rate rose to 60% (29). By 1990, more than 2000 cardiac transplant procedures were performed internationally, with a perioperative mortality of 10% and 5-year survival rate of 69% (30). Projections for the year 2000 estimate that more than 40,000 people will survive heart transplantation (31). Currently up to 73% of heart transplant recipients live at least 4 years (31). Patient survival rates according to diagnosis are listed in Table 34-5.

The ultimate success of a cardiac transplant proce-

Table 34-5: Heart Transplants (Patient Survival Rates at 1 Month and at 1, 3, and 5 Years)

		1 Month Survival		1 Year Survival			3 Year Survival		5 Year Survival	
Primary Diagnosis	N_{94-95}	%	Std. Err.	%	Std. Err.	N	%	Std. Err.	%	Std. Err.
Coronary Artery Disease	1911	91.5	0.6	84.0	0.9	7387	76.0	0.5	68.4	0.6
Cardiomyopathy	1909	96.1	0.4	88.2	0.8	6816	78.0	0.5	70.1	0.7
Congenital Heart Disease	300	87.8	1.9	73.4	2.6	1178	66.3	1.5	63.7	1.6
Valvular Heart Disease	96	93.5	2.6	87.8	3.4	562	76.6	1.8	71.3	2.1
Other	46	83.8	5.6	75.7	6.8	194	76.2	3.2	67.1	4.1
Unknown	9	n.c.	n.c.	n.c.	n.c.	37	n.c.	n.c.	n.c.	n.c.
Overall	4271	93.3	0.4	85.1	0.6	16174	76.2	0.4	68.9	0.4

The survival rates were computed using the Kaplan-Meier method. N_{94-95} denotes the number of transplants in 1994–1995 for which a survival time could be determined. N denotes the number of transplants from October 1987 through December 1995 for which a survival time could be determined. n.c. denotes not calculated for the unknown categories.
Source: UNOS Scientific Registry data as of September 15, 1997.

dure is critically dependent on initial candidate selection. This often has important implications for the rehabilitative and restorative process, as many of the same factors used to determine "transplant suitability" can impact on patients' participation and performance in a structured post-transplantation exercise therapy program.

Indications for Cardiac Transplantation

The indications for cardiac transplantation must always be considered carefully. Although many patients currently enrolled in structured cardiac rehabilitation programs are potential candidates to receive transplants, those with documentable evidence of declining cardiac function and irreversible heart disease should be given priority. A review of patients' general health, anticipated changes in quality of life after transplantation, and risk for complications must be thorough. Tayler and Bergin (32) suggested that the procedure be considered in patients who 1) demonstrate severely reduced $\dot{V}O_2$max to less than 14/mL/kg/min or 40% of predicted with severe limitations in life activity, 2) have severe angina without successful revascularization, 3) have life-threatening recurrent arrhythmia uncontrolled by medicine or electrophysiologic means, or 4) have congestive heart failure (CHF) consistently uncontrollable by all medical therapy. It is notable that CHF is the most common indication for heart transplantation in major medical centers, internationally. Less common reasons for cardiac transplantation include idiopathic cardiomyopathy. Transplantation for postpartum cardiomyopathy, an extremely rare occurrence, has been reported in the rehabilitation literature (33).

Many of the guiding principles of traditional cardiac rehabilitation should be observed for the cardiac transplant patient. A systematic and structured exercise program should be administered as part of a comprehensive cardiac rehabilitation program (34). Since physiatric consultative input is often sought before transplantation, an effective pretransplantation program must be formulated. A cardiac rehabilitation program for patients with CHF must be individualized.

Congestive Heart Failure: Pathophysiology and Rehabilitation Intervention

Since pretransplantation patients with CHF often experience constant fatigue and breathlessness, these symptoms severely blunt their capacity to carry out many activities essential to their self-care and life roles. Although "old school" philosophy advocated rest and avoidance of vigorous exercise due to the concern that it could lead to decompensation of cardiocirculatory status, recent evidence supports a role for exercise. Studies of the aerobic exercise capacity of patients with left ventricular diastolic dysfunction did not demonstrate a consistent relationship between peak exercise performance, peak oxygen uptake, and left ventricular ejection fraction (35). Exercise training may impede skeletal muscle blood flow without a significant change in cerebral hemodynamics. Recently, investigators uncovered many peripheral circulatory effects in patients with CHF that in some studies were amenable to limited carefully dosed exercise.

The fatigue and decreased exercise experienced by CHF patients can be explained as follows: A person's capacity for oxygen utilization is correlated with exercise cardiac output. In CHF, exercise cardiac output is reduced and the proportion of blood flow to the legs and arms is proportionately reduced (36). Supportive of this explanation is evidence of atrophy (37) and impaired blood flow through skeletal muscles. A potential mechanism is the reduction in small-vessel vasodilative capacity. Histologic studies noted a predominance of type II (fast twitch) muscle fibers in patients with CHF (37).

The neurohumoral changes that have been observed include elevated levels of renin, catecholamines, atrial natriuretic factor, and arginine vasopressin. The sensitivity of both arterial and cardiopulmonary mechanoreceptors is diminished, contributing to excessive sympathetic excitation. Spirometric studies of heart transplant candidates show restrictive patterns attributed to cardiac enlargement infringing on lung fields. This effect is reversible with transplantation (38). The changes contribute to increased peripheral resistance and may shunt some circulation away from the muscles.

Exercise training, if properly dosed and administered on a regular schedule, can potentially reduce many of these effects. Studies demonstrated reduced resting catecholamine levels, enhanced heart rate variability, increased vagal tone, normalized resting heart rates, and modest increases in peak oxygen uptake after periods of training as long as 10 weeks (39). Introduction of low-level resistive exercise training into cardiac rehabilitation regimens has been achieved without complications. To date there is little information available about the effect of moderate- to high-resistance weight training on cardiovascular recovery.

The Cardiac Transplant Process

Should medical and rehabilitation management of CHF prove ineffective, patients come under consideration for cardiac transplantation. The most common transplant procedure is orthotopic, which includes an anastomosis of the donor heart to the recipient's atria and great vessels (Fig. 34-5) (32). An infrequently utilized and less successful procedure is heterotopic placement of the donor heart, by grafting it into place to pump in parallel with the recipient's failing heart.

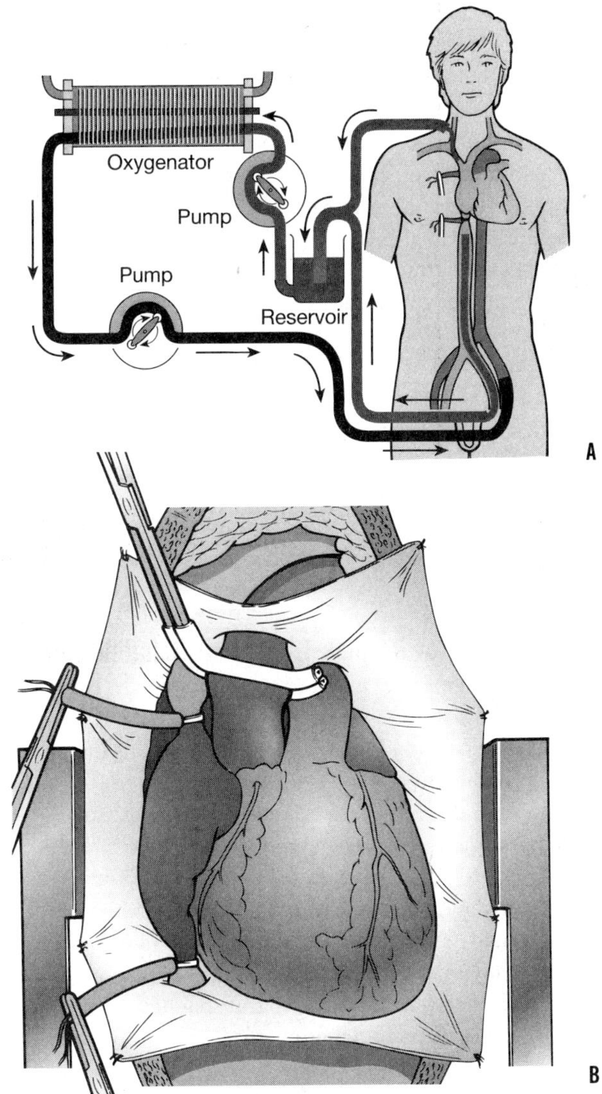

Figure 34-5. Heart transplantation. *A.* Diagram of extracorporeal circulation; superior and inferior venae cavae cannulated by catheters introduced, respectively, via internal jugular vein and saphenofemoral junction, thus leaving operative field free. *B.* Recipient's thorax opened by midline sternum—splitting incision; pericardium incised longitudinally and stitched to wound edges; tapes passed around venae cavae and tightened as patient is placed on extracorporeal circulation; aorta clamped. (Broken lines indicated levels for transection of aorta and pulmonary trunk.)

Physiology of the Transplanted Heart

In the normally innervated heart, the sympathetic nervous system exerts both a chronotropic effect and an ionotrophic effect. The sympathetic nervous system augments venous return, stroke volume, and cardiac output. Orthotopic cardiac transplantation results in complete denervation of the heart (40,41). Denervation of the transplanted heart results in loss of autonomic nervous system modulation and a reliance on circulating catecholamines for augmentation of heart rate during physical activity. The resting heart rate of the denervated heart is higher than normal and is not altered by carotid massage, Valsalva maneuver, or body position. The denervated heart reaches its maximum rate more slowly than the normal heart. The return of heart rate to baseline after exercise is more gradual in the denervated heart (40,41). Initially, this change in heart rate is mediated by a rise in circulating catecholamine levels. In a normally innervated heart, an increase in cardiac output occurs largely as a result of an increase in heart rate. The transplanted heart, despite its loss of autonomic nervous system modulation of heart rate, is able to increase its cardiac output in response to dynamic exercise (42). Early in exercise the increase in cardiac output results from the Frank-Starling mechanism and augmented preload. Despite this compensating mechanism, the cardiac output of the denervated transplanted heart may be lower than that of normal hearts both at rest and during exercise. The transplanted heart shows decreased exercise tolerance as well as lower oxygen uptake at submaximal exercise intensities (43,44).

During the immediate postoperative period, cardiac contractility is impaired. There is frequently an elevation of right and left atrial pressures, and a mild resting tachycardia, 10 to 15 beats/min higher than the expected rate at rest. This sinoatrial rate is released due to loss of vagal innervation. The rate is unaffected by carotid massage, position changes, or Valsalva maneuver. There is evidence of prolonged left ventricular relaxation with exercise (45).

The transplanted heart responds to meet the cardiovascular demands of exercise slowly through mechanical and humoral mechanisms. Ventricular preloading via the Frank-Starling effect increases stroke volume. As exercise proceeds, circulating catecholamine levels increase the heart rate and ejection fraction.

Over time there may be some sympathetic reinnervation of the heart. Sympathetic reinnervation is detectable as soon as 5 months after cardiac transplantation and may contribute to chronotropic effects and modulate vasomotor tone (46,47).

Cardiac perfusion is increased with exercise in spite of changes in sympathetic innervation (48). Coronary ischemia does not appear to explain the decreased exercise capacity of cardiac transplant patients.

The Philosophy of Cardiac Transplant Rehabilitation

Cardiac rehabilitation can continue immediately after surgery if the patient is hemodynamically stable in the perioperative period. The series of interventions for cardiac rehabilitation after transplantation is similar to those utilized after myocardial infarction (49). Cardiac rehabilitation is a person-centered participative interdisciplinary process that seeks to enhance the patient's personal effectiveness through cardiac disease prevention, cardiovascular and psychological functional improvement, and role reintegration (49).

Cardiac rehabilitation after transplantation emphasizes independence and achievement by the whole person (50,51). The process, like all rehabilitation interventions, starts with the interview of the patient as a person. The patient's personal goals and expectations in life roles drive the rehabilitation process. The medical history, physical examination, and review of the laboratory findings provide measures of cardiovascular and functional impairment (52–54). The first phase, phase I, of cardiac rehabilitation runs from the time of hospitalization to discharge and focuses primarily on overcoming impairments: weakness, decreased endurance, hypotension, and tachycardia. Very specific tasks help prepare the patient for his or her anticipated level of independence at the time of discharge: dressing, bathing, cooking, stair climbing, and so on. A program for modifying the risk factors for coronary artery disease is started before transplantation and continued beyond phase III as needed. Phase II is outpatient training with aerobic conditioning to achieve reacquisition of full activity and integration of diet and lifestyle changes. Phase III rehabilitation includes outpatient training in the home, community, or hospital. During this phase, the patient integrates successful medication use according to the prescribed schedule, exercise regimens, and diet to his or her lifestyle.

Phase III has been described as the maintenance phase because disability-appropriate behaviors have already been integrated into the patient's routines and lifestyle. During this period the patient monitors himself or herself as the individual cardiac rehabilitation program is carried out.

Preparation for exercise with a patient who has recently received a donor heart requires consideration of the physiologic effects of an orthotopic heart transplant on circulatory function. Before transplantation, the patient is either deconditioned with CHF or maximally conditioned based on protocols for exercise in the CHF patient (34). The goal of the cardiac rehabilitation team is to utilize the renewed capacity for increased cardiac output to overcome the peripheral effects of chronic CHF in the past.

Complications Associated with Cardiac Transplantation

The physiatrist caring for the cardiac transplant patient must be cognizant of the numerous complications associated with transplantation. A major complication is acute rejection and may be signaled by symptoms of CHF such as decreased exercise tolerance, development of peripheral edema, diastolic gallop, and premature atrial contractions. Another serious complication, chronic rejection, is an insidious process. The development of coronary atherosclerosis can manifest as sinoatrial node malfunction, myocardial ischemia, infarct, CHF, and sudden death in the cardiac transplant patient. It occurs without angina, owing to the denervated myocardium. Immunosuppressive drugs can prevent rejection but have numerous side effects and implications for the rehabilitation patient. Cyclosporine can cause interstitial edema, ankle edema, renal dysfunction, HTN, tremor, hirsutism, sexual dysfunction, liver damage, and death (55,56). Azathioprine may cause leukopenia and pancytopenia. Prednisone may result in HTN, cushingoidism, psychic derangement, myopathy, osteoporosis, and aseptic necrosis of bone (55).

Neurologic complications of cardiac transplantation are common and include seizures, central nervous system (CNS) infections, stroke, metabolic encephalopathy, acute psychosis, and neoplasm. CNS infections by opportunistic organisms, particularly fungi and viruses, are the most common neurologic complications. Infarcts can result from air emboli, particulate matter emboli, or inadequate cerebral perfusion during surgery (57). Vertebral compression fracture can result from osteoporosis. Neoplasm may appear de novo as a result of immunosuppression of the nervous system (14).

Psychosocial Adaptation to Heart Transplant

Since the emotional reaction to heart transplantation can be complex and intense, it is important that the rehabilitation psychologist be available to meet patients' emotional needs (59). Patients may go through psychological stages similar to those identified by Kubler-Ross in the dying patient. Denial, anger, bargaining, depression, and acceptance are typical reactions experienced by those facing death. The clinician should remember that all patients respond differently and prediction of their needs cannot be made without continuous reassessment. Each patient's spectrum of emotions has important implications for the rehabilitation team. Often heart transplant patients and their families are subjected to a great deal of stress, necessitating psychological support. The families are learning to cope with the chronicity of the disease state. Patients must extend their body image to incorporate a foreign organ sometimes from a donor of the opposite sex. Furthermore, episodes of organ rejection can result in depression.

Due to a prolonged period of disability secondary to the chronic nature of the illness, financial problems are common. The length of the pretransplant absence from work in combination with socioeconomic factors including education, prior employment status, and age seem to be the best predictor of return to work (60). During the postoperative period, patients quickly realize that they have traded an extended life for a new set of symptoms and complications. Christopherson et al noted that patients with specific goals are more likely to make an easier transition to the home setting (20). For people with young children, eager to see the growth and development of their offspring, the integration of child-care activities of daily living is a significant component of any physical medicine and rehabilitation program (33).

REHABILITATION OF PERSONS WITH RENAL IMPAIRMENT: RENAL FAILURE THROUGH TRANSPLANTATION

Epidemiology of Renal Failure and Rationale for Physiatric Intervention

Renal failure brings a high cost to society. Conservative estimates of the annual incidence of renal failure count 50 new terminal renal failure patients per million persons in the United States. Although recently the effect of the increased numbers of renal transplantations coupled with an increased survival rate for grafts has resulted in a shift away from a primarily dialysis population toward a group with functioning transplanted kidneys (61). Rehabilitation physicians frequently have the opportunity or the responsibility for surveillance of renal dysfunction or the maintenance of patients with early renal failure. Prevention of renal deterioration through regular screening of creatinine clearance, and imaging of the urinary tract in patients at risk for obstructive uropathy, is an important part of physiatric intervention. Patients with spinal cord dysfunction have been historically associated with renal deterioration (62). Inclusion of renal screening tests and partnership with the primary care physicians of patients undergoing rehabilitation ensure success in maintenance of function.

The constellation of treatment alternatives for renal impairment can be compared in various ways, for example, duration of patient survival, community reintegration, vocational achievement, cost-effectiveness, and quality of life. Dialysis can best be understood as a bridge from uncompensated renal failure to transplantation. Renal transplantation contributes to a better quality of life than does dialysis (63). Although as many as 50% to 60% of patients with end-stage renal disease (ESRD) could benefit from transplantation, only 10% of the ESRD population receives transplants annually. Encouragingly, over 90% of polled individuals would donate a kidney to a family member in need and at least 60% would accept some medical risks to do so (64). Over 92% of donors believe their health was not adversely affected and more than 96% reaffirmed their decision to donate regardless of the graft's success or financial sacrifices (65).

Physiatric Assessment

The physiatric assessment of persons with renal failure focuses on confirmation of the diagnosis and identification of associated impairments, disabilities, and handicaps. During the acute phase of renal failure, patients may complain of fatigue, weight gain, weakness, apathy, and intellectual decline (66). A history and review of the chart can reveal other associated diagnoses that frequently lead to or complicate renal failure. Diagnoses that are commonly associated with chronic renal failure include diabetes mellitus, hypertension, and atherosclerosis (66,67).

During the interview, the physiatrist should explore patients' past, to derive the best understanding of their activity and life goals. A review of life activity 6 months prior to the renal failure provides a baseline that can guide plans for reattainment of life roles. After dialysis, functional improvement can still be expected. In a longitudinal study of patients with ESRD, 50% were caring for themselves at initiation of dialysis, and improvements in the Karnofsky activity scales were noted at 6 months and after 2 years on dialysis (68). A review of patients' current function, role performance, and environment emphasizes recognition of situations that could tax endurance or present barriers for persons on dialysis. The examiner must attempt to discriminate between learned maladaptive dependency versus effective goal-directed energy conservation. Retrospective sociospatial-behavioral mapping systematically identifies the activities and the environments with which patients interact. Patients report where they went and who they are with for periods of a week at a time. These activities can become goals and the environment may be subject to adaptive manipulation to further enable patients (69,70).

The examination focuses on confirmation and quantification of impairments as well as assessments of potential capacity for compensatory capabilities. Resting pulse and blood pressure provide information on cardiovascular conditions and fluid status. The presence and distribution of edema should be noted. Examination of the chest should include auscultation to screen for pulmonary edema and percussion to detect pleural effusions. The effect of previously acquired impairments on success in rehabilitation after renal failure is significant; the examination must assess for visual loss, limb amputation (71), prior myocardial infarction, and evidence of previous stroke (67).

The physiatric history should include a review of systems that addresses potential complications of ESRD and associated conditions that could affect functional performance. In particular, diabetes and hypertension are often associated with ESRD. Visual deficits at night and with small print can occur. Dysesthesias as well as other sensory and motor deficits from neuropathy are common. Dysequilibrium and muscle cramping can develop owing to electrolyte imbalances before and after dialysis. Other symptoms that may be amenable to treatment include nausea, vomiting, fatigue, and intestinal disturbances (constipation, diarrhea, cramping). Review of bowel function is essential as ingested oral antacids, analgesics, and ion-exchange resins and hypomotility can cause constipation. Maintenance of regularity and prevention of fecal impaction (72) can be achieved by applying treatments used for neurogenic bowel management (73).

In addition to the general physical examination, the rehabilitative evaluation of ESRD patients should disclose and quantify the severity of impairments and disabilities. Weight should be related to the ideal body weight, the date of last dialysis, fluid intake, and urine production, if any. Visual acuity should be assessed. Strength can be quantified myometrically and endurance can be measured with timed ambulation over a standard course. Deficits in lower-extremity muscle and gait performance of renal transplant candidates have been successfully quantified using muscle dynamometer force measurements and the sit-to stand-to sit test (74). These data can be supplemented with psychomotor performance data such as reaction time and finger dexterity (75). Standardized tests can be used to demonstrate improvements in performance after dialysis and renal transplantation (66).

Rehabilitation Interventions

The initial interventions on behalf of persons with renal organ failure are primarily medical within the biomedical model. A diagnosis is made based on the specific pathophysiology. Evaluation then proceeds to quantification of organ impairment. Medical treatment includes metabolic manipulations to enhance kidney function or to minimize the physiologic demands of dysfunction (66). During the period an attempt is made to avoid transplantation and maintain maximal patient function. During palliative medical care, the role of rehabilitation includes person-centered management to achieve life goals in spite of the pathophysiologic process and secondary effects (76).

The sequence for rehabilitation of patients with renal dysfunction follows the same pattern as with other conditions (76). The initial assessment includes an interview focused on patients' immediate and ultimate life goals. Assessment of renal impairment and secondary effects requires some knowledge of nephrology and endocrinology. A review of symptoms provides a background for quantification of disability. Inquiry about patients' perceived challenges in life roles and vocational aspirations is a prerequisite for interventions that undermine handicapping barriers.

Reduction in disability begins with reachievement of essential life tasks such as basic activities of daily living, and then advancement to patients' goal-specific activities (77). Work simplification through planning a daily schedule and organizing tasks allows for greater endurance in life activities. Dialysis shunts can affect upper-extremity endurance for repetitive and strenuous activities. Assessment of upper-extremity work with a screen for focal fatigue allows for recognition of the steal syndrome, which causes pain due to a deficiency blood flow to working muscle (77).

Adapted persons must fundamentally perform their roles within their chosen environment (69,70). It is at the environmental interface that much of the quality of life (78) is experienced. Psychosocial adaptation is a process driven by multiple factors that contributes to and stems from compliance and full participation in chosen life activities. Full societal participation by the patient helps reconcile the socioeconomic costs of care (79).

Exercise Prescription for Patients with Renal Impairment

Chronic renal failure stresses cardiovascular function. Sodium and water retention increase preload at the right and left ventricles. Hypertension worsened by the increased circulatory volume increases afterload and contributes to ventricular hypotrophy, increased stiffness, and decreased compliance. Patients with moderate renal function may compromise renal perfusion with aerobic exercise. The diseased kidney is unable to maintain a glomerular filtration rate or conserve water under stress (80). Patients who produce urine should be well hydrated before and after exercise. Anemia results in an increased plasma volume and demands increased cardiac output. Electrolyte imbalances that can cause cardiac depression are only partially compensated by dialysis. Counting the pulse and assessment of regularity before and after exercise can detect arrhythmias.

The capacity for sustained exercise by persons receiving dialysis for ESRD is markedly impaired (81). The specific etiology of this deficit has not been fully elucidated. Exercise intolerance is likely affected by a variety of interacting factors. Some of the contributing factors include anemia, cardiovascular deconditioning, and skeletal muscle factors. The fatigue occurring with exercise has been attributed to low circulating red blood cell volumes. Increases in work capacity have been correlated with total

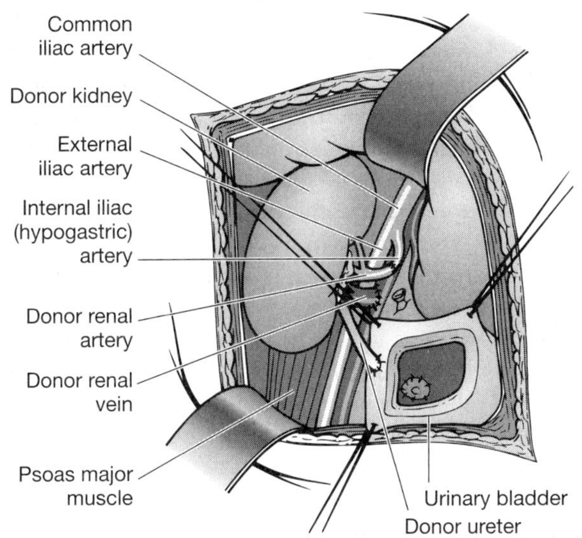

Figure 34-6. Donor kidney implanted in right iliac fossa; renal artery anastomosed end to end with internal iliac artery; renal vein end to side with external iliac vein; ureter implanted into bladder.

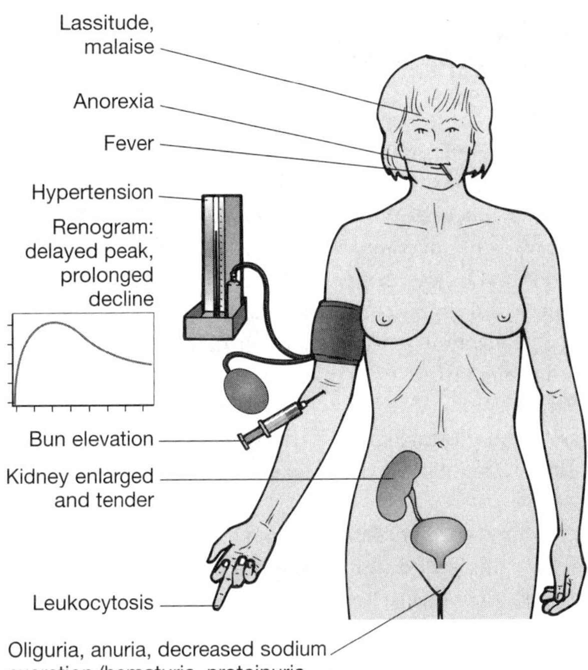

Figure 34-7. Clinical manifestations of rejection.

hemoglobin. Total hemoglobin is apparently a major determinant for adaptive increases in work capacity after renal failure (82). Peripheral circulatory factors have also been linked to the decrease in exercise tolerance of persons with ESRD (83). Grafts for hemodialysis contribute to arteriovenous shunting and increase cardiac work. At the muscle level, there is a preponderance of type II muscle fibers, with evidence for impaired glycolytic activity and defective excitation-contraction coupling (84). One study evaluated subjects with renal transplants within 6 to 152 months who completed a 6-month resistive and aerobic exercise program on a three-times-per-week schedule (85). Subjects successfully increased their exercise tolerance by 33%. $\dot{V}O_2$ increased but none of the subjects could exercise aerobically at an intensity to allow peak $\dot{V}O_2max$ to be estimated. Blood lactate levels remained low. As a result, exercise limitations were attributed to muscle weakness (85).

Rehabilitation Through Renal Transplantation

Transplantation offers a reasonable solution for all the primary impairments of renal failure and effectively mediates many of the secondary effects as well (68). It is important for the physiatrist to have a good understanding of the basic anatomy relevant to kidney transplantation (Fig. 34-6). Patients who develop sufficiently stable renal function after transplantation have demonstrated improvement in exercise capacity (82), although elderly patients are less apt to show improvement (86) and impaired exercise tolerance as compared with control levels persists after transplantation. The continued impaired tolerance for exercise is likely to be multifactorial (92); exercise malfunction could be related to anemia (82) and left ventricle dysfunction, as well as persistent intramuscular effects (83). The constellation of drugs used to prevent rejection can also contribute to weight gain. Rejection is still a common phenomenon and should be detected early (Fig. 34-7). Regular exercise is recommended to prevent excess weight (87).

Prolonged and intensive immune suppressive therapy utilized to prevent rejection after organ transplantation is complicated by an increased incidence of cancer. The overall cancer incidence in transplant recipients ranges from 4% to 18%. As many as 54% of these tumors are skin cancers, which occur with greater frequency in proportion to the duration of sunlight exposure. Tumors that are more common after organ transplantation include squamous cell carcinoma of the skin, non-Hodgkin lymphoma, Kaposi sarcoma, in situ carcinomas of the uterine cervix, carcinomas of the vulva and perineum, hepatobiliary carcinomas, and a variety of sarcomas (88). The incidence of carcinomas that commonly arise in the general population (lung, heart, prostate, colon, invasive uterine, cervical tumor) has not been observed to increase (88).

Patients who receive transplants are more likely to return to work than are those on dialysis. A study of patients utilizing dialysis identified 25% who work outside the home and 33% who work in the home (89). In a study published in the late 1970s with 132 subjects, 62% to 90% of the subjects who had received a transplant up to 12 years before were still productively active (90).

Patients requiring hemodialysis for renal failure due to diabetes frequently have other deficits preventing full vocational rehabilitation such as visual impairments, limb amputation, myocardial infarction, and stroke (67).

REHABILITATION BEFORE AND AFTER LUNG TRANSPLANTATION

Overview

The first single-lung transplantation was attempted in 1963 by Dr. James Hardy at the University of Mississippi (91), but the first successful lung transplantation with long-term survival was not accomplished until 1983, in Toronto, Ontario, by Dr. Joel Cooper (92). In 1986 in Toronto the first successful double-lung transplantation was accomplished. Since that time, the number of lung transplantations has increased dramatically from 130 in 1988 to 944 in 1995 (93). Two-year survival rates are now at 62% for single-lung transplantation and 72% for double-lung transplantation (94), with 5-year survival rates at only 45% (95).

Lung transplantation is performed for both congenital and acquired end-stage pulmonary diseases. Diseases such as chronic obstructive pulmonary disease (COPD), α_1-antitrypsin deficiency, cystic fibrosis, pulmonary hypertension, idiopathic pulmonary fibrosis, sarcoidosis, and lymphangioleiomyomatosis causing severe lung damage are all indications for lung transplantation (95). Contraindications for lung and heart-lung transplantations include history of carcinoma or sarcoma with possibility of recurrence, ongoing infection, multisystem disease, hepatic or renal dysfunction, poor medical compliance, and substance abuse (92). While single-lung transplantation allows the other lung to be transplanted into another recipient, double-lung transplantation is necessary in the setting of severe infection in both lungs or, as in the case of cystic fibrosis, when the remaining lung could affect the transplanted lung. A single case of a patient with cystic fibrosis undergoing bilateral below-knee amputation who develops postoperative hemiparesis has been described in the literature (96).

COPD and the less common variant, α_1-antitrypsin deficiency account for about 40% of lung transplantations performed, usually single-lung transplantation. Mal and Andreassian performed the first successful single-lung transplantation for COPD in 1988 (92). Patients undergoing transplantation for emphysema have the highest survival rate for any lung transplant population, about 80% at 1 year for both single-lung and bilateral transplantation and 65% for bilateral transplantation and 51% for single-lung transplantation at 4 years. The best predictor of survival is the postbronchodilator forced expiratory volume in 1 second (FEV_1). In COPD, bilateral lung transplantation, as opposed to single-lung transplantation, offers better improvement in FEV_1, but with only a slight improvement in the 6-minute walk test and aerobic exercise testing (95).

Cystic fibrosis patients are also candidates for lung transplantation. Double-lung transplantation is currently the operation of choice because of the risk of infection to the allograft from the native lung if only a single lung is transplanted. Negative predictive factors are a FEV_1 of less than 30% of predicted, a partial pressure of oxygen (pO_2) of less than 55 mm Hg, partial pressure of carbon dioxide (pCO_2) higher than 50 mm Hg, female gender, and age less than 18 (95). Lobes from living related donors have been used for bilateral lobar transplantation in about 54 patients (as of 1996). The donors have been parents with ABO compatibility and the results compare favorably with those of cadaveric lung transplantation. This remains a controversial technique because of the operative and postoperative risks posed to the healthy donors; however, it may be utilized as a salvage technique when there is no lung available for the patient who is decompensating rapidly (95,97).

Primary pulmonary hypertension and Eisenmenger syndrome (pulmonary hypertension with cardiac defects) account for about 10% of lung transplantations and 60% of heart-lung transplantations. Medical therapy such as calcium channel blockers or prostacyclin are tried before transplantation is considered. Both single-lung and bilateral transplantations are choices, with cardiopulmonary bypass generally required. The 1-year survival rate has been reported to be 62%, the lowest overall 1-year survival rate for major diagnoses (95).

In the early days of transplantation, idiopathic pulmonary fibrosis was the single indication for lung transplantation. Now, 15% of all lung transplantations are done for idiopathic pulmonary fibrosis, making this the second most indicated diagnosis for the procedure. Negative predictive factors for long-term survival prior to transplantation are male gender, a fibrotic rather than inflammatory lung histology, and failure of medical therapy. The 1-year survival rate is 64% (95). Ten percent of sarcoid patients progress to the point where lung transplantation is a necessity, accounting for 1.5% of transplantations. Sarcoid can reappear following the procedure; however, for patients so affected by sarcoid, lung transplantation is the only available option (95).

Lymphangioleiomyomatosis, a rare lung disease of unknown etiology that was first described in the medical literature in 1937, is a disease of smooth-muscle proliferation, affecting mostly women of childbearing age. The proliferation of muscle cells occludes the lungs, usually causing an obstructive lung pattern. The 1-year survival rate reportedly is 69%, and the 2-year survival rate, 58%. Single-lung transplantation is usually performed, but occasional bilateral transplantation and rarely heart-lung transplantation are done (98).

In a study of 17 pediatric patients younger than 25 months who underwent lung transplantation at two centers between July 1990 and February 1995, the survival rate was 71%, with one late death. At follow-up 22 months later, the survivors did not require supplemental oxygen and were small in stature but with a normal linear growth curve (99).

Complications and Medical Management

Medical management issues important to the physiatrist and rehabilitation specialists may affect therapy time and participation. It is of utmost importance to be able to understand the medical follow-up and complications after transplantation.

Most lung transplant patients are on a triple-drug regimen of cyclosporine, azathioprine, and prednisone to prevent acute and chronic rejections. Some new immunosuppressants being studied are tacrolimus (FK 506), sirolimus (rapamycin), mycophenolate mofetil, and leflunomide (100).

Bronchoscopy and lung biopsy are performed at regular intervals to assess the lung and ensure the patency of the airways. If acute rejection is suspected, then bronchoscopy will be performed. The procedure has been shown to diagnose rejection with a sensitivity of 72% to 94% and a specificity of 90% to 100%. Acute rejection may occur at any time, but in the first 4 to 6 weeks after transplantation, radiographic abnormalities may occur in conjunction with temperature elevation (even 0.5°C may be important) or a decrease in oxygenation or FEV_1 (10% is significant). After 6 weeks the radiographic study generally demonstrates no abnormalities in the setting of rejection. Most acute rejection episodes occur in the first 3 months after transplantation (97). Chronic rejection is manifested histologically as bronchiolitis obliterans and functionally as a deterioration in FEV_1, and is the single most important factor responsible for death after 1 year (101).

Infections, the most common cause of complications and early death, may manifest when the patient is on the rehabilitation unit. Cytomegalovirus infection is the most common viral infection and generally occurs 14 to 100 days postoperatively. Diagnosis is via bronchoscopy with lavage and biopsy and the infection is treated with gancyclovir. Fungal infections, such as with *Candida* species, *Aspergillus* organisms, and *Pneumocystis carinii*, although infrequent, appear most commonly between 10 and 60 days after transplantation. At one time, pneumocystis pneumonia occurred in 85% of patients; however, prophylactic treatment with trimethoprim-sulfa drugs has virtually eradicated this infection (97).

Immunosuppression is necessary after transplantation and includes azathioprine, cyclosporine, and prednisone for maintenance immunosuppression (97). Azathioprine may cause leukopenia, nausea, and vomiting, while cyclosporine may cause renal dysfunction, tremor, hypertension, and hirsutism. Prednisone has many side effects, one of which, steroid myopathy, may adversely affect rehabilitation progress. Posttransplantation lymphoproliferative disorder occurs in about 5% of lung transplant patients and generally occurs within 1 year after transplantation. The pathogenesis of the tumors involves the Epstein-Barr virus and effects of immunosuppression. Reduction in immunosuppression is the initial treatment and if necessary, chemotherapy may need to be initiated. Other types of cancer have been found in lung transplant patients. In areas of high sun exposure, the incidence of developing skin cancer is 21 times that of the normal population. Avoidance of excessive exposure to sunlight and use of sunscreens as well as regular dermatologic follow-up examinations should be emphasized (102).

Ineffective clearance of airway secretions may be difficult as there is no cough reflex below the anastomosis because of the denervation of the transplanted lung. There is also diminished mucociliary clearance. Chest physiotherapy, while an important part of postoperative care, must be monitored carefully as pulmonary hypertension may result. Postural drainage is recommended during the initial part of recovery (103).

Dorffner et al (104) found diaphragmatic dysfunction in 7.4% of patients in a series of 27 lung transplantations. This was diagnosed with ultrasound and found to correlate with a higher risk of pneumonia and intubation, suggesting that the phrenic nerve is mechanically damaged in lung transplant patients. This complication has been reported in patients after coronary bypass grafting, and is thought to be due to phrenic nerve injury secondary to cooling during surgery. However, since most lung transplant patients do not undergo bypass, the injury in lung transplant patients is believed to be mechanical.

Renal complications including nephrotoxicity can occur. Some renal impairment is found in most patients taking cyclosporine. This can present as acute or chronic. Chronic nephrotoxicity is often manifested by a rise in serum creatine level in the first 6 months.

Hypertension can be exacerbated by corticosteroids, but cyclosporine is thought to be the major factor. Hypertension is delayed in lung transplant patients, with onset occurring at a mean of 11 months. While difficult to control, calcium channel blockers have a protective effect against cyclosporine-induced nephrotoxicity and are the most frequently used (102).

Endocrine and metabolic abnormalities are noted in lung transplant patients. Heterotopic ossification can occur in lung and liver transplant recipients. In patients described in case reports, it developed at the elbows, causing a loss of function as well as pain. Two of the patients had ulnar and median neuropathies. Common factors noted were encephalopathy, use of wrist restraints, and possible perioperative positioning (105). Osteoporosis is found in 45% of patients before transplantation and in 73% after transplantation. Before transplantation, the loss is thought to be due to corticosteroids, immobility, and malnutrition. Posttransplantation osteoporosis has been correlated with total steroid dose. Prophylactic therapy such as calcium supplementation, vitamin D analogues, biphosphates, and calcitriol have all been used and should be started within 6 months after transplantation (102).

Hyperlipidemia with elevations in total cholesterol and triglyceride levels have been documented but Kesten et al (106) found no evidence of deteriorating left ventricular function in patients with hyperlipidemia 5 years after lung transplantation. Irregularities in menstruation can occur, but 19 of 20 patients in one review found that menses resumed within 1 year after surgery. Contraception should be addressed as pregnancy could possibly occur. Hyperglycemia secondary to corticosteroid use is commonly found. Cyclosporine has also been implicated in the development of diabetes after transplantation. Blood glucose levels and glycosylated hemoglobin should be checked periodically. Dietary modification, weight loss if applicable, and insulin treatment are all appropriate therapeutic measures. Oral hypoglycemics may cause prolonged hypoglycemia if hepatic dysfunction is present and cyclosporine has been noted to have adverse interactions with oral hypoglycemics (102).

Fenton and Cicale (107) described three patients in whom sigmoid colon diverticular perforation developed within 4 weeks of transplantation. It is believed to be related to intense immunosuppression, perioperative hypoperfusion, and increased intraluminal pressure secondary to narcotics and bowel stimulants. Gastroparesis and gastric and peptic ulcer disease can occur after lung transplantation. Metoclopramide for gastroparesis should be used with caution because of the CNS effects and interactions with other drugs. Cimetidine can raise cyclosporine levels, requiring more frequent monitoring of drug levels (102). Hypercoagulopathy resulted in left cerebrovascular accident and right hemiparesis with ischemic necrosis of both lower extremities in one patient; bilateral below-knee amputation was performed on postoperative day 20 (108).

Assessment and Rehabilitation Before and After Transplantation

Because of the deteriorating nature of end-stage pulmonary disease, patients come into surgery severely deconditioned. This, added to the stress of surgery, and immobilization contribute to the poor functional abilities of the patient. Rehabilitation includes a role for pulmonary reconditioning and remobilization, two cornerstone principles of rehabilitation. Lung transplantation involves pulmonary and cardiopulmonary rehabilitation both before and after surgery.

Exercise limitations both before and after transplantation may be due to several factors. Muscle disuse and atrophy limit the work rate and $\dot{V}O_2max$, along with a decreased maximal heart rate during exercise. Nutritional status may be poor and steroid use may lead to steroid myopathy, limiting aerobic performance. There is ventilation-perfusion mismatching after transplantation, but usually not so severe as to be the primary limitation to exercise performance. Cardiac abnormalities associated directly with the lung transplants are not common (109).

Before transplantation, the patient is evaluated with pulmonary function tests, exercise testing using the 6-minute walk test, exercise staging test, or a modified Bruce protocol (110). A sample protocol is provided in Table 34-6. Formal cardiopulmonary testing is usually not performed preoperatively. The 6-minute walk test is an objective test of physical fitness and can be performed in a short time without placing seriously ill patients at high medical risks. The test is done with the patient walking as quickly as possible over a standard course (111). Measurements taken include the distance walked, the number of rest breaks, pulse, and respiratory rate. If necessary, the patient is monitored with oximetry. Craven et al (110) found that 50% of patients accepted as transplant candidates were able to walk 300 to 400 m at the initial assessment. According to Howard et al (109), two centers found that none of the transplant candidates were able to complete stage 0 of a modified Bruce protocol and all demonstrated severe hypoxemia during testing. The rehabilitation management of lung transplant patients has been described (112).

After Transplantation

Williams et al (113) demonstrated that even in double-lung transplant recipients with near-normal spirometry and diffusion capacity and single-lung transplant recipients showing less, but substantial improvement, exercise capacity is reduced (Table 34-7). Forty-four percent of predicted work in single-lung transplant recipients was noted at 3 months after transplantation and 48% up to 2 years after transplantation, with double-lung transplant recipients showing about the same improvement in maximum work capacity (46% at 3 months and 51% two years postoperatively) (Fig. 34-8).

Exercise limitation in single-lung transplant patients is not thought to be due to abnormalities of gas exchange and ventilation-perfusion after surgery but rather to peripheral factors and an overall reduction in aerobic capacity (109). The decrease in exercise reserve may be caused by the amount of deconditioning and muscle atrophy present because of the severe limitations prior to surgery. Almost no patients who have exercise limitations are found to have problems with ventilation that could cause the limitations. Although exercise capacity is decreased in patients who received a single-lung transplant for COPD, it should be sufficient enough to perform the activities of daily living (114). To this end, aggressive rehabilitation programs, lasting longer than 3 months, including home programs may increase the maximum work capacity in lung transplant patients (113).

Lung transplant patients have psychosocial needs that are different from those of traditional pulmonary rehabilitation patients. A study at Duke University addressed these concerns. Crouch et al (115) found that pretransplantation patients are anxious about surgery and subsequent recovery. After the procedure they are con-

Table 34-6: Sample Protocol				
Phase	**Time**	**MET Level**	**Exercise**	**Pulmonary**
Assessment	When determined a candidate	Initial maximal MET level determined	6-min walk test, exercise treadmill test or modified Bruce treadmill test	Oximetry and supplemental O_2 to keep saturation at > 85%
Preoperative	Assessment time to transplantation	Determined by initial assessment, advance when RPE is < 5	Treadmill, light calisthenics, light weight training	Oximetry and supplemental O_2 to keep saturation at > 85%
Phase I-A	Extubated	2	ROM emphasizing upper and lower extremities transfers, bed mobility; begin postoperative patient education	Chest PT, incentive spirometer
Phase I-B	Extubation to transfer from ICU, two times a day	2	Begin ambulation twice a day, active ROM exercises	Wean off supplemental O_2 so that saturation > 95%
Phase II	Day 5 to discharge, two times a day	4	Ambulation up to 2000 ft/day, stair climbing (1 flight), flexibility and strengthening exercises, 6-min walk test prior to discharge	Monitor O_2 saturation, FEV_1, and FVC
Phase III	discharge to 3 mo, 3–5 days a week	Advanced when RPE < 5	Treadmill (> 80% maximum heart rate), bike ergometer, rowing machine, nautilus (3 wk postop)	
Phase IV	3 mo and beyond after transplantation	—	6-min walk and modified Bruce treadmill test every 3–6 mo for first year	

MET = metabolic equivalent; RPE = rating of perceived exertion from Borg scale; ROM = range of motion; PT = physiotherapy; FEV_1 = forced expiratory volume in 1 second; FVC = forced vital capacity.
Source: From PT, Craven, Howard.

cerned about not having their oxygen tank near as a safety measure. However, after transplantation, they have the possibility of participating in future life events such as attending college or family occasions. The goal of psychosocial rehabilitation is to provide appropriate support, and help establish short-term as well as long-term goals. Chaparro (101) looked at the status of lung transplant patients beyond 5 years and found that almost three-fourths were active and employed full-time, with no difference between the double-lung and single-lung transplant groups.

New Advances

An artificial lung is being tested that would provide a "bridge" between the time when a patient's lung has failed

Table 34-7: Pulmonary Function Testing Before and After Transplant

	FEV$_1$ Pretransplant	(% Pred) Posttransplant	FVC Pretransplant	(% Pred) Posttransplant
Single Lung Transplant				
OLD	19%	61%	52%	78%
PF	48%	69%	46%	68%
PPH	82%	95%	82%	97%
Bilateral lung transplant	20%	101%	57%	92%

OLD, obstructive lung disease; PF, pulmonary fibrosis; PPH, primary pulmonary hypertension.
Source: *Ann Surg* 1995;221:25.

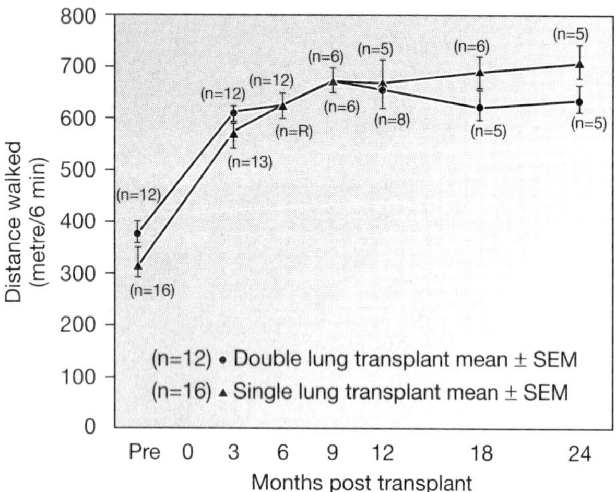

Figure 34-8. The 6-minute walk test: single and double lung transplant recipients. The total distance walked in 6 minutes is measured. Pretransplant, the test is performed with supplemental oxygen; posttransplant, without supplemental oxygen. (Reproduced by permission from Williams TJ, Grossman RF, Maurer JR. Long-term functional follow-up of lung transplant recipients. *Clin Chest Med* 1990;11:347–358.)

and when a donor lung is available. The device is planted in the chest cavity and is composed of tubes that exchange carbon dioxide for oxygen. The oxygen comes from an external source. Problems encountered are excessive thinning of the blood, which is necessary to make the device effective, and the force of the blood over the device, which can lead to inflammation by activating white blood cells.

LIVER TRANSPLANTATION

The growth and success of liver transplantation, as for other solid-organ transplantations, has changed dramatically during the past decade. The first human liver transplant trials were performed at the University of Colorado in 1963. Development of the procedure and its application did not progress significantly until the 1980s when cyclosporine became available. This revolutionized immunosuppression, making long-term survival after transplantation a reality. In 1996, 4058 liver transplantations were performed in the United States. Although this number has increased steadily, it has not kept pace with demand. In late 1997, there were almost 9000 patients awaiting liver transplantation within the United States. The current 1-year survival rates of 80% to 90% and the expected 5-year patient survival rates of 70% or higher highlight the importance of quality of life after liver transplantation. Nicholas et al (116) have surveyed quality of life parameters in a cohort of 346 patients who underwent orthotopic liver transplant. Critical to enhancing this quality of life is a concerted effort by the transplant team to ensure adequate rehabilitation of the transplant patient postoperatively.

Effects of Liver Disease Before Transplantation

When patients are referred for liver transplantation, their liver failure can be divided into two broad categories. Fulminant hepatic failure, such as occurring after ingestion of a toxin or due to viral hepatitis, typically occurs in patients who are previously healthy and with little warning. It is not unusual for these patients to require urgent transplantation within days or weeks of the first appearance of illness. Consequently, these patients tend to be well nourished, and generally in normal health prior to the onset of liver disease. Their rehabilitation needs are similar to those of any patient undergoing a major surgical procedure and their rehabilitation would be expected to be fairly rapid. The second broad category of liver disease, into which most of the patients receiving liver transplants fall, is that of chronic liver disease. Many diseases can lead to chronic liver failure, including chronic hepatitis C, alcoholic cirrhosis, autoimmune diseases, primary biliary cirrhosis, sclerosing cholangitis, inborn errors of metabolism such as α_1-antitrypsin deficiency, and a number of less common diseases. Consistent among all patients awaiting liver transplantation is significant hepatocellular dysfunction. This may be manifested by any of a combination of elevated prothrombin time, hypoalbuminemia, thrombocytopenia, and leukopenia secondary to splenomegaly; ascites; portal hypertension, which may be severe requiring frequent endoscopic procedures and blood transfusions; and neurologic dysfunction, which can vary from mild fatigue and forgetfulness to severe fatigue requiring absence from work or disability. In advanced disease, hepatic encephalopathy may necessitate hospitalization prior to transplantation. The loss of the ability to function is particularly important with respect to rehabilitation issues. This loss is related to both mental consequences of liver disease and physical loss of actual muscle mass and malnutrition. Patients who have full-time employment may be forced to reduce their workload to part-time or even stop completely. The ability to carry on activities of daily living, caring for children, or pursuing commonplace tasks may be significantly impaired. In fact, many patients report that they must sleep at midday to avoid succumbing to exhaustion, and frequently do not have the energy to leave the house. Compounding this may be forgetfulness and tremor such as asterixis, which further limit the patient's ability to perform activities of daily living.

Malnutrition in pre–liver transplantation patients is related to a variety of factors. Fatigue may impair the ability to cook and decrease the desire to eat. Blood chemistry abnormalities such as hyperbilirubinemia may make the patient nauseated and anorexic. Protein losses through ascites may exacerbate the patient's negative nitrogen balance. This culminates in loss of muscle mass and increased fragility of the skin. The combination of fatigue, chronic illness, and malnutrition decreases the patient's level of physical activity and endurance. Cardiopulmonary deconditioning frequently ensues.

Predictors of Outcome

Traditionally, the assessment of liver transplantation outcome has been divided into three time periods. The first is operative survival; the second, 30-day survival; and the third is long-term survival. The predictors of operative and 30-day survival relate primarily to patients' medical condition at the time that the transplant operation is undertaken. The Childs-Pugh classification, which reflects synthetic functional reserves of the liver, along with the patient's age, level of consciousness, and UNOS status are important predictors of operative survival. Thirty-day survival, which is primarily in-hospital survival after transplantation, relates largely to the function of the new liver after it is implanted and reperfused and complicating factors such as nonfunction of the graft, technical failures, rejection, and infection. The long-term survival of the transplant patient is more difficult to predict, but is an area of active research. Factors such as recurrence of viral hepatitis and refractory rejection may impact long-term survival.

Impact of Rehabilitation

Directed rehabilitation during the posttransplantation period primarily affects patients' time to functional recovery and improved quality of life. Aggressive physical therapy started early in the postoperative period is necessary to combat the effects of the chronic disease state. A comprehensive rehabilitation approach for the liver transplant patient is outlined in the literature (117). Efforts must be made to replete the patient nutritionally to aid in recovery of muscle mass, bone strength, and the overall feeling of well-being. Inpatient physical therapy is especially important to increase patients' mobility, which aids in recovery of pulmonary and cardiovascular status. Physical therapy should be directed not only at maximizing patients' mobility, but also at ensuring adequate strength and reserve for safety within the home after discharge. Attention also has to be directed toward neurologic status, as there may be residual effects of pretransplantation encephalopathy.

Psychosocial stresses are not unusual in the early posttransplantation period. Patients and their families may have had unrealistic expectations about the speed of recovery or be distressed by any complications that may have occurred. In addition, medications given to prevent rejection such as high-dose steroids may cause periods of sleeplessness or depression, which can delay patients' willingness and ability to participate in the rehabilitation program. If these issues are understood and addressed by the transplant team, directed physical therapy can continue. Rehabilitation also must include occupational therapies directed at re-establishing the ability to concentrate and perform detailed tasks. Some patients may have been out of the workforce for a considerable amount of time, lost their jobs, and be interested in vocational rehabilitation as part of the directed rehabilitation process.

Outpatient Postoperative Recovery

The fundamental goal of liver transplantation is to return patients to their predisease state, enabling them to be productive members of society. For most patients, this transition is marked by either a return to employment or a return to being able to carry on the duties of running a household and caring for their family. Quantifying patients' progress after they are discharged from the hospital is an important part of the rehabilitation process. By quantifying functional status, the physiatrist can provide the transplant team with progress updates and realistic expectations and goals over time. In addition, directed strategies regarding physical and occupational therapy can be established and altered as necessary in order to shorten the length of time to full recovery.

Using reproducible tests to monitor quality of life is an important aspect of posttransplantation rehabilitation. Several recent studies attempted to validate quality of life measurements in the liver transplant population. Lowe et al (118), using the Nottingham Health Profile, found that high levels of quality of life similar to those of the general population could be expected following transplantation. Pennington (119) showed a decreased quality of life, especially when transplant patients were denied job opportunities due to perceived physical limitations and concerns about long-term health. Although never studied, the hypothesis that directed rehabilitation as a regular part of the transplant protocol would produce an increase in the functional capacity of patients after transplantation is attractive.

Preemptive Rehabilitation

Another potential use of rehabilitation is in the pretransplantation period. It is not unusual for patients to wait 12 to 24 months for a donor liver to become available for transplantation. During this period, inactivity, fatigue, chronic illness, and malnutrition result in loss of cardiopulmonary reserve, muscle mass, ability to concentrate, and a sense of well-being. Depending on the degree of resultant disability, a significant delay in posttransplantation recovery may follow.

Therefore, the pretransplantation period potentially, provides an opportunity for intervention designed to minimize the loss of functional reserve. By participating in physical therapy, cardiovascular conditioning, nutritional counseling, and occupational therapy when indicated, the patient may be in a better physiologic state at the time of transplantation.

Conclusions

Liver transplantation offers patients with end-stage liver disease a real hope for functional recovery. However, severe liver disease results in significant losses of physical and mental capacity during the pretransplantation waiting period. The physiatrist and rehabilitation team can be an important part of the transplant team facilitating recovery. The potential for pretransplantation therapy in concert with postoperative inpatient and outpatient therapy can speed the recovery and improve patients' sense of well-being and quality of life.

TRANSPLANTATION IN THE NERVOUS SYSTEM

Transplantation of neural tissue is poised to play a significant role in the future of transplantation rehabilitation. The first evidence of nerve regeneration is found in studies of the peripheral nervous system. The earliest evidence dates to the 1960s and primarily involves plastic surgery studies of the return of sensation in skin grafts and repaired digits after amputation. The evolution of knowledge in this area has led to the use of nerve grafting as a widely accepted treatment for certain traumatic nerve injuries.

The current focus of research on neural regeneration is in the CNS. While current research activities primarily involve preclinical and clinical trials, some promising findings have been documented. Much of the foundation of these discoveries revolves around the grafting of fetal nerve tissue. This rapidly expanding dimension of transplantation research has documented successful function of graft tissue in the mammalian CNS.

The initiation of cerebral transplantation began in clinical trials in the 1980s in patients with Parkinson disease. The theory behind the transplantation approach in these patients was to replace the dopamine-deficient striatum of the patient with functional dopaminergic grafts. Prior animal studies had demonstrated the feasibility of the approach. In addition to the dopamine production by the grafts, findings in the animal model also suggested that transplant neurotrophic factors contributed to transplantation-related improvements (120). The two primary sources of graft tissue utilized in humans were the chromaffin cells of the adrenal medulla and the cells of the fetal ventral mesencephalon. While the induction of host-derived fiber sprouting was documented in the caudate nucleus following adrenal tissue grafting, fetal mesencephalon neurons demonstrated a more vibrant survival as well as extensive reinnervation of the parkinsonian striatum (121). In addition, the sequelae of perioperative psychosis and delirium following adrenal tissue transplantation appeared less common with fetal mesencephalon transplants (122).

The clinical trials reported primarily involved patients with severe parkinsonian traits or Parkinson disease symptoms refractory to pharmacologic interventions. Numerous studies demonstrated improvements in neurologic function. Clinical improvement as manifested by improved scores on the Hoehn-Yahr scale and the Unified Parkinson Disease Rating Scale has been documented (123), as has bilateral motor improvement for speed of movements. The quality of these movements improved most notably on the side contralateral to the graft (124). Long-term clinical benefits have been documented. Improvements in the verbal memory cluster index have been observed for up to 2 years postoperatively (125), and the persistence of clinical improvements in motor function, for up to 5 years (126). In addition to monitoring clinical improvements in the manifestations of Parkinson disease, care of transplantation patients may also require a controlled decrease of L-dopa intake due to transient post-operative heavy dyskinesias (124), as well as monitoring of immunosuppressive therapy (123).

Another challenging focus of CNS transplant therapy is in the treatment of spinal cord injury. The discovery of successful propagation of CNS tissue in vitro has led to attempts to reproduce the phenomenon in vivo. The theory behind successful transplantation involves the establishment of mechanical and chemical guidance for neural growth, the provision of cellular structures to repair damaged pathways, and the supplementation of modulating factors to improve neural circuit formation (127).

A variety of graft tissues have been used in attempts to restore the function of the injured adult mammalian spinal cord. These include fetal CNS tissue, neural support cells, and olfactory bulb neurons. Targets of repair techniques include both pathways within the CNS and connections between the CNS and the peripheral nerves.

In addition to the survival of grafted tissue and the establishment of new circuits, the restoration of functional synapses and regeneration along specific pathways to end-organ tissues have been demonstrated with the transplantation of neurons into the CNS. Experimental findings also reveal trophic effects of grafted tissue on native neurons as well as the prevention of retrograde cell death (128,129). There is evidence of functional synapses between avulsed dorsal root afferents and fetal spinal cord transplants, and experimental evidence that grafted embryonic motor neurons may facilitate the re-establishment of pathways to targeted musculature (130–132). Use of continually replaced cells, such as those of the olfactory bulb, also restored function of the injured spinal cord (133).

Other discoveries involve the use of neuronal support cells. The transplantation of oligodendrocyte-lineage cells was shown to lead to the restoration of myelin segments oriented parallel to nerve tracts (134). In addition, the integration of grafted Schwann cells into a host corticospinal tract was demonstrated, with preservation of linear orientation. An induction of astrocyte hypertrophy was also noted, preserving the astrocytic skeleton across the transplant region (135).

Future advances continue to expand the knowledge of nervous system pathophysiology and the reversal of abnormal function due to a disease process or injury. The implantation of serotonergic neurons into the spinal cord alleviates chronic neuropathic pain from peripheral nerve injuries. In addition, genetic engineering may lead to further methods of treatment by developing and implanting cell lines that could deliver inhibitory neurotransmitters in the case of chronic pain (136), or possibly neurotrophic factors in the case of spinal cord injury. The discovery of the gene responsible for Parkinson disease has opened the possibility of gene therapy for this patient population (137).

INTESTINAL TRANSPLANTATION

The experience related to transplantation of the small bowel is mainly from clinical trials and current preclinical trials. The majority of transplantations of the intestine have been utilized in the pediatric population to treat short-bowel syndrome. In addition, irreversible intestinal failure, esophageal bypass, and massive abdominal evisceration for aggressive tumor debulking are indications for intestinal transplantation (138). Survival rates are similar to those for lung transplant recipients. Intestinal transplants have included small bowel with or without colon as well as small bowel and liver (139). Outcome studies are more favorable for isolated bowel transplantation than for combined bowel-liver transplantation (140).

Patients who receive intestinal transplants are often dependent on total parenteral nutrition prior to surgery, and may be nutritionally compromised in addition to deconditioned. Further impairment of function may be acquired through complications of the procedure and the recovery period. Immunosuppression is required, and there is the risk of rejection and graft-versus-host disease. Cytomegalovirus infection, posttransplantation lymphoproliferative disorder, and obliterative arteriopathy have been reported (141).

Research continues in preclinical and clinical studies to minimize the risk of rejection and graft-versus-host disease, as well as advance the early detection of rejection. Laminin and hyaluronic acid have been suggested as markers of both initial transplant function and early detection of posttransplantation rejection, as has acetaminophen absorption tests (142,143). Mucosal biopsy has also been suggested as a useful method to detect rejection and differentiate rejection from other pathologies (141).

PANCREATIC TRANSPLANTATION

Transplantation of the pancreas, first performed in 1966, is being used to treat patients with severe complications of type I diabetes mellitis. The initial transplantations were performed with whole pancreas with a duodenal segment and enteric drainage. This procedure was refined using duct injection to obliterate exocrine tissue. Due to marginal success, further refinements were made to include a closed loop segment of duodenum for anastomosis to the bladder for exocrine drainage. The surgical modifications as well as immunosuppression have dramatically increased both patient and graft survival rates to the range of 80%.

Many of the patients considered for transplantation have advanced diabetic complications including peripheral neuropathy, retinopathy, and cardiovascular pathology. In addition, postoperative complications can further debilitate the patient. There is the risk of urologic complications, infection, and rejection (145). Prolonged ileus has been reported in the acute postoperative period.

More recent procedures include combining the pancreas graft with a renal transplant. The survival rates for patients under the age of 45 and without severe cardiovascular disease approach those of renal transplantation alone (146). Further evolution in pancreas transplantation research, in addition to advances in immunosuppression and improved detection of rejection, include transplantation of islet cells and genetic engineering. Adenovirus vectors have been used for genetic transfection of pancreatic epithelial cells for the treatment of pancreatic adenocarcinoma (147).

REHABILITATION AFTER BONE MARROW TRANSPLANTATION

With bone marrow transplantation's (BMT) growing utilization as a therapeutic alternative for patients with hematologic malignancies, aplastic anemia, and a variety of inherited disorders, an increasing number of rehabilitation, functional, and quality of life issues are emerging. The international availability of multiple donor registries has greatly enhanced "transplant matching" and survivorship, creating a major role for physiatrists and other rehabilitation professionals in the functional aftercare of these patients.

Since advances in the early detection and therapeutic management have allowed more people with cancer to live longer, functional issues are becoming more prevalent. Conservative estimates are that 4 million people have survived 5 years or longer with cancer as a diagnosis, leaving many of these survivors with physical deficits and psychosocial issues that impact on their quality of life. For those who have undergone BMT, there is an additional dimension of soft-tissue and musculoskeletal disability that must often be reckoned with. Utilizing early rehabilitation intervention, the disability imposed by cancer and cancer therapy can be profoundly reduced.

Many underlying factors independent of the bone marrow transplant are thought to contribute to the functional limitation imposed by cancer. Factors that contribute to disability include:

- Pain
- Fatigue
- Effects of chemotoxic agents
- Generalized deconditioning secondary to immobility
- Impaired nutrition
- Diminished immune function
- Psychological effects
- Neurologic and cardiac abnormalities.

Patients undergoing bone marrow transplant are often committed to several weeks of hospital confinement and months of close medical surveillance. This along with the underlying disease and its therapeutic management can lead to several major complications, including immobility, skin disruption, contractures, cognitive-perceptual deficits, peripheral nerve sequelae, myopathies, lymphedema, pain, and psychosocial alteration.

The Oncology Rehabilitation/Bone Marrow Transplant Team can serve the cancer patient's rehabilitation needs in the following ways:

- Formulation of customized rehabilitation team plan
- Maintenance of strength
- Improving endurance and conditioning
- Promoting flexibility
- Breathing exercises
- Reconditioning exercises
- Work simplification exercises
- Work simplification strategies
- Energy conservation techniques
- Education of patient and family

Table 34-8: Therapeutic Modalities and Techniques to Improve or Maintain ROM in Patients with GVHD

Type of Intervention	Joint	Therapy[a]
Preventive[b]	Hand	Resting hand splint
	Elbow	Air cast, molded splint made of aquaplast, fiberglass serial cast that can be bivalve and padded for skin protection
	Hip	Prone positioning
	Knee	Knee immobilizer
	Ankle	AFO, resting foot splint, high-top sneakers
Restorative[c]	Shoulders	Ultrasound and ROM, therapeutic exercise (AAROM), strengthening of antigravity muscles
	Elbow	Serial casting (bivalve and/or dynamic splints)
	Wrist/hand	Serial casting (bivalve and/or dynamic splints)
	Knee/ankle	Dynamic splint and/or serial cast

[a] Splints may be applied to restore and prevent complications with local changes and prevent further contractures. Application of splints is dependent on which joint is affected.

[b] Preventive therapy is joint focused, based on the location of sclerodermatous changes.

[c] Restorative therapy is applied if the loss of ROM is progressing and/or potentially limiting the patient functionally.

Source: Grant J, Young MA, Pidcock FS, Christenson JR. Physical medicine and rehabilitation management of chronic graft vs. host disease. Rehabil Oncol 1977;15:13–15.

- Nutritional counseling
- Psychological counseling
- Team conferencing/module discussion.

A Pretransplantation Approach

Prior to transplantation, prophylactic conditioning exercises and aerobic therapeutics should be emphasized. Getting the patient as "fit" as possible is a critical objective. This includes working on flexibility, bolstering strength via resistive training, enhancing aerobic endurance, and highlighting functional activity. Specific aerobic exercise protocols for bone marrow recipients have been described that can correct fatigue and loss of physical performance (148).

As with most areas of cancer rehabilitation, special emphasis must be placed in the following areas: skin integrity preservation, monitoring and maintenance of joint range of motion, and incentive spirometry and deep breathing.

Bone Marrow Transplant and Musculoskeletal Disability

Musculoskeletal disability associated with CGVHD is an increasingly recognized long-term complication of BMT. As an immune-mediated illness arising in 40% of patients who have survived 100 days following transplantation of HLA-identical sibling bone marrow, CGVHD is the leading complication of allogeneic BMT (148,149). The worldwide prevalence of CGVHD and its musculoskeletal and soft-tissue sequelae has grown significantly. While early CGVHD may adversely influence multiple organ systems, advanced disease often leads to a disabling array of musculoskeletal, dermal, and connective tissue pathologies that can adversely influence functional status. Sclerodermatous skin eruptions, skin ulcerations, soft-tissue induration, and muscle atrophy often stem from a massive immunologic assault. As the disease progresses, cumulative effects frequently include restriction in articular flexibility and limitations in ADls.

Physiatric Intervention in Graft vs. Host Disease

The essential multidisciplinary approach in the management of chronic graft vs. host disease has been described (150). Clinical features of GVHD often resemble systemic sclerosis including sclerodermatous skin eruptions, oral and ophthalmic lesions, and immunosuppression and neurologic involvement. In situations where GVHD is left untreated, patients develop contractures that can lead to immobility. Owing to the diffuse and progressive nature of sclerodermatous chronic GVHD, serial rehabilitation management within an interdisciplinary team setting is essential.

Range of Motion Abnormalities

Patients diagnosed with GVHD who do not exhibit signs of scleroderma can benefit from patient education to prevent generalized weakness and preserve strength. A home program is provided that emphasizes stretching of hip flexors, hamstrings and heel cords. Emphasis is also placed on aerobic conditioning to prevent fatigue and restore cardiopulmonary endurance.

For those patients who have been diagnosed with active sclerodermatous GVHD, with or without fascial involvement, emphasis is placed on therapeutic modalities and techniques to improve or maintain ROM through stretching and splinting. Splinting can play an important role (Table 34-8).

Table 34-9: Transplant Milestones in the United States and Canada

Year	Transplant
1954	First successful kidney transplant* Dr. Joseph E. Murray, Brigham & Women's Hospital, Boston, MA
1966	First successful pancreas transplant Drs. William Kelly and Richard Lillehei, University of Minnesota, Minneapolis, MN
1967	First successful liver transplant* Dr. Thomas Starzl, University of Colorado Health Sciences Center, Denver, CO
1968	First successful heart transplant Dr. Norman Shumway, Stanford University Hospital, Stanford, CA
1981	First successful heart-lung transplant Dr. Bruce Reitz, Stanford University Hospital, Stanford, CA
1983	First successful single lung transplant Dr. Joel Cooper, Toronto Lung Transplant Group, Toronto General Hospital, Canada
1986	First successful double lung transplant* Dr. Joel Cooper, Toronto Lung Transplant Group, Toronto General Hospital, Canada
1989	First successful living-related liver transplant Dr. Christoph Broelsch, University of Chicago Medical Center, Chicago, IL
1990	First successful living-related lung transplant Dr. Vaughn A. Starnes, Stanford University Medical Center, Stanford, CA

* This transplant was the first of its kind in the world.

THE FUTURE OF TRANSPLANTATION REHABILITATION: ROAD TO FUNCTIONAL INDEPENDENCE

With refinement in surgical technique and advancement of knowledge in the transplant sciences have come dramatic increases in the numbers and kinds of transplant operations performed each year. Many major milestones have been achieved in transplant science (Table 34-9). This phenomenon has created a major market demand for rehabilitative aftercare and restorative services. The specialist in physical medicine and rehabilitation plays a dynamic role in the care of this challenging population. Maximizing function and minimizing dependence through intensive physiatric intervention will enable patients to enjoy an enhanced quality of life in the wake of organ transplantation.

ACKNOWLEDGMENTS

The authors wish to acknowledge the editorial assistance and support provided by Dr. Leon Reinstein, Mr. Eric

Kwon, Terry Morris, PA, M. Malloy and Novartis Pharmaceutical. This chapter is dedicated to the remembrance of "Uncle Danny" Koningsberg, a valiant organ transplant recipient whose memory lives on.

REFERENCES

1. Grant J, Young MA, Vogelsang G, et al. Graft vs. host disease following bone marrow transplant: a physiatric challenge. *Arch Phys Med Rehabil* 1996;77:1996. Abstract.
2. Young MA. Review of *Physical medicine and rehabilitation*, edited by Randall L. Braddom: *JAMA* 1997.
3. Kutner NG. Rehabilitation revisited. *Transplant Proc* 1993;25:2506–2507.
4. Chyatte SB. In: Chyatte SB, ed. *Rehabilitation in chronic renal failure*. Baltimore: Williams & Wilkins, 1979:28.
5. Riether AM, Smith SL, Lewison BJ, et al. Quality of life changes and psychiatric and neurocognitive outcome after heart and liver transplantation. *Transplantation* 1992;54:444–450.
6. Tippett DC, Siebens AA. Using ventilators for speaking and swallowing. *Dysphagia* 1991;6920:94–99.
7. Young MA. Rehabilitation makes dysphagia easier to swallow. *J Clin Gastroenterol* 1993;17:179.
8. Tippett DC, Siebens AA, Lynch CQ, French JJ. Oral communication in tracheotomized and ventilator-dependent individuals. *Arch Phys Med Rehabil* 1990;71:789.
9. Marin E, Coladner A. Therapeutic prescriptions in PM&R. In: O'Young B, Young MA, Stiens SA, eds. PM&R secrets. Philadelphia: Hanley and Belfus, 1997:509–513.
10. Young MA, Young M. Rehabilitation of the transplantation patient: an international perspective. Second Mediterranean Congress on Physical Medicine and Rehabilitation, Valencia, Spain, May 20–23, 1998. Abstract.
11. Meehan M. Multisite pressure ulcer prevalence survey. *Decubiti* 1990;3(4):14–17.
12. Caly CH, Chimoskey JE, Holloway GA. The effects of pressure loading on blood flow in human skin. In: Kennedy RM, ed. *Bedsore biomechanics*. Baltimore: University Park Press, 1976:69–77.
13. Kosiak M. Etiology and pathology of ischemic ulcers. *Arch Phys Med Rehabil* 1959;40:62–69.
14. Dowling AS. Pressure sores: their cause, prevention and treatment. *Md State Med J* 1970;19(4): 131–134.
15. Young MA, Ehrenpreis E. Pressure sensitive dressings: a new technique for stabilizing NG tubes and Foley catheters in rehabilitation patients. *Arch Phys Med Rehabil* 1988;69:787.
16. Mueller EA. Influence of training and inactivity on muscle strength. *Arch Phys Med Rehabil* 1970;51:449–462.
17. Grant J, Young MA, Pidcock FS, Christenson JR. Physical medicine and rehabilitation management of chronic graft vs. host disease. *Rehab Oncol* 1997;15:13–15.
18. Henriksson R, Reitman JS. Time courses of change in human skeletal muscle succinate dehydrogenase and cytochrome oxidase activity and maximal uptake with physical activity and inactivity. *Acta Physiol Scand* 1977;99: 91–97.
19. Jaworski ZFG, ed. *Proceedings of the First Workshop on Bone Histomorphometry*. Ottawa: University of Ottawa Press, 1976:254–256.
20. Swartz CM, Young MA. Male hypogonadism and bone fracture. *N Engl J Med* 1988;318:996.
21. Bellantoni M, Madoff DM. Osteoporosis and back pain: diagnosis, treatment and prevention. [Young MA, Lavin R, eds.]. *Spinal Rehabil* 1995;9:641–656.
22. Kottke FJ, Pauley DL, Ptka RA. The rationale for prolonged stretching for correction for shortening of connective tissue. *Arch Phys Rehabil Med* 1966;47: 345–352.
23. Young MA, Kornhauser SH. Thermal electromedicine and the management of pain. *Phys Ther Forum* 1992:20–21.
24. Reitman CA, Esses SI. Modalities, manual therapy and education: a review of conservative measures. In: Young MA, Lavin R, eds. *Conservative care and spinal rehabilitation: state of the art.* Philadelphia: Hanley & Belfus, 1995.
25. Young MA. Ehrenpreis ED, Ehrenpreis M, Kirschblum S. Heparin-associated thrombocytopenia and thrombosis syndrome in a rehabilitation patient. *Arch Phys Med Rehabil* 1989;70: 468–470.
26. Ginsberg JS, Merli GJ, Young MA. New options for deep vein thrombosis. *Patient Care* 1998; Jan:91–100.
27. Young MA. Subcutaneous compared with intravenous heparin for deep vein thrombosis. *Ann Intern Med* 1992;117:265. Letter.
28. Berkin D, Young MA, Johnston JR. Valsalva maneuver: a risk factor for pulmonary embolism? *Arch Phys Med Rehabil* 1993;74:669. Abstract.
29. Solis E, Kaye MP. The registry of the International Society for Heart Transplant. *J Heart Transplant* 1986;5:2–5.
30. Kriett JM, Kaye MP. The registry of the International Society for Heart Transplant. *J Heart Transplant* 1991;10:491–498.
31. Mills R. Cardiac transplantation problems and opportunities. *Intensive Care Med* 1991;6:96–97.
32. Taylor A, Bergin J. Cardiac transplantation for the cardiologist not trained in transplantation. *Am Heart J* 1995;129:578–592.

33. Latlief G, Young MA. Cardiac transplantation rehabilitation in a post-partum female. *Arch Phys Med Rehabil* 1994;Sept. Abstract.

34. McKelvie R, Teo K, McCartney N, Humen D. Effects of exercise training in patients with congestive heart failure: a critical review. *J Am Coll Cardiol* 1995;25: 786–789.

35. Franciosa JA, Park M, Levine TB. Lack of correlation between exercise capacity and indexes of resting left ventricular performance in heart failure. *Am J Cardiol* 1981;47:33–39.

36. Muller A, Batin P, Evans S. Regional blood flow in CHF. *Postgrad Med* 1992;96:478–481.

37. Manicini D, Walter G, Reichek N, Lenkinski R. Contribution of skeletal muscle atrophy to exercise intolerance and altered muscle metabolism in heart failure. *Circulation* 1992;85:1364–1373.

38. Hosenpud J, Stibolt T, Atwal K, Shelley D. Abnormal pulmonary function specifically related to congestive heart failure: comparison of patients before and after cardiac transplantation. *Am J Med* 1990;88:493–502.

39. Coats A, Adamopoulos S, Radaelli A, et al. Controlled trial of physical training in chronic heart failure: exercise performance, hemodynamics, ventilation, and autonomic function. *Circulation* 1992;85:2119–2131.

40. Horak AR. Physiology and pharmacology of the transplanted heart. In: Cooper DKC, Lanza RP, eds. *Heart transplantation.* Lancaster: MTP Press, 1984:147–156.

41. Kavanagh T, Yacoub MH, Martins DT, et al. Cardiorespiratory responses to exercise training after orthotopic cardiac transplantation. *Circulation* 1988;77:162–171.

42. Squires RW. Exercise training after cardiac transplantation. *Med Sci Sports Exerc* 1991;23:686–694.

43. Pope SE, Stinson EB, Daughters GT, et al. Exercise response of the denervated heart in long-term cardiac transplant recipients. *Am J Cardiol* 1980;46:213–218.

44. Savin WM, Haskell WL, Schroeder JS, et al. Cardio-respiratory responses of cardiac transplant patients to graded symptom limited exercise. *Circulation* 1980;62:55–60.

45. Paulus W, Bronzwaer J, Felice H, Kishan N. Deficient acceleration of left ventricular relaxation during exercise after heart transplantation. *Circulation* 1992;86:1175–1185.

46. Wilson R, Christensen B, Olivari M, Simon A. Evidence for structural sympathetic reinnervation after orthotopic cardiac transplantation in humans. *Circulation* 1991;83:1210–1220.

47. Di Carli M, Tobes M, Mangner T, Levine A. Effects of cardiac sympathetic innervation on coronary blood flow. *N Engl J Med* 1997;336:1208–1215.

48. Krivokapich J, Stevenson L, Kobashigawa J, Huang S. Quantification of absolute myocardial perfusion at rest and during exercise with positron emission tomography after human cardiac transplantation. *J Am Coll Cardiol* 1991;18:512–517.

49. Lehman J, Stiens SA, Halar E. Cardiac rehabilitation: In: O'Young B, Young MA, Stiens SA, eds. *PM&R secrets.* Philadelphia: Hanley & Belfus, 1997:190–195.

50. Badenhop D. The therapeutic role of exercise in patients with orthotopic heart transplant. *Med Sci Sports Exerc* 1995;27(7): 975–985.

51. Block E, Montemayor J, Adler J, Alba A. Influence of exercise on a heart transplant patient. *Arch Phys Med Rehabil* 1990;71:153–155.

52. Joshi A, Kevorkian G. Rehabilitation after cardiac transplantation. *Am J Phys Med Rehabil* 1997;76:249–254.

53. Kappagoda C, Haennel R, Serrano-Fiz S, Davies D. The hemodynamic responses to upright exercise after orthotopic cardiac transplant. *Arch Phys Med Rehabil* 1993;74: 484–489.

54. Kavanagh T. Physical training in heart transplant recipients. *J Cardiovasc Risk* 1996;3:152–159.

55. Grant J. Corticosteroid side effects for PT. *Phys Ther* 1994;2:55–60.

56. Stovin PGI, English TAH. Effects of cyclosporin on the transplanted heart. *Heart Transplant* 1987; 6:180–185.

57. Hotson JR, Pedley TA. Neurologic complications of cardiac transplantation. *Brain* 1976;99:673–694.

58. Niset GC, Coustry-Degre, Degre S. Psychosocial and physical rehabilitation after heart transplantation: 1 year follow-up. *Cardiology* 1988;75:311–317.

59. Mai F. Psychiatric aspects of heart transplantation. *Br J Psychiatry* 1993;163:285–292.

60. Botsford 1995. Review of the literature on heart transplant and recipient return to work.

61. Novello A. Ethical, social, and financial aspects of end-stage renal disease. In: Saunders W, ed. *Management of the patient with renal failure.* Vol. 2. Philadelphia: WB Saunders, 1991:2424–2443.

62. Patrick G, Mahony J, Disney A. The prognosis for end-stage renal failure in spinal cord injury and spinal bifida—Australia and New Zealand, 1970–1991. *Aust N Z J Med* 1994;24:36–40.

63. Simmons R, Abress L. Quality of life and rehabilitation differences among alternate end-stage renal disease therapies. *Transplant Proc* 1988;20:379–380.

64. Spital A. Living kidney donation: still worth the risk? *Transplant Proc* 1988;20:1051–1058.

65. Smith M, Kappel D, Province M, et al. Living-related kidney donors: a multicenter study of donor education, socioeconomic adjustment and rehabilitation. *Am J Kidney Dis* 1986;8:223–233.

66. Chyatte S. Rehabilitation medicine in chronic renal failure. In: Chyatte S, ed. *Rehabilitation medicine in chronic renal failure.* Baltimore: Beverly Press, 1979: 28–45.

67. Lowder G, Perri N, Friedman E. Demographics, diabetes type, and degree of rehabilitation in diabetic

patients on maintenance hemodialysis in Brooklyn, *J Diabetes Complications* 1988;2:218–226.

68. Carlson D, Johnson W, Kjellstrand C. Functional status of patients with end-stage renal disease. *Mayo Clinic Proc* 1987;62:338–344.

69. Shamberg S, Stiens S, Shamberg A. Personal enablement through environmental modifications. In: O'Young B, Young MA, Stiens, S, eds. *PM&R Secrets.*: Hanley & Belfus, 1997:86–93.

70. Stiens S. Personhood, disablement, and mobility technology: personal control of development. In: DB G, Quatrano LA, ML L, eds. *Designing and using assistive technology: the human perspective.* Towson, MD: Paul Brookes, 1998:29–49.

71. Garrison S, Merritt B. Functional outcome of quadruple amputees with end-stage renal disease. *Am J Phys Med Rehabil* 1997;76:226–230.

72. Welch J, Schweizer R, Bartus S. Management of antacid impactions in hemodialysis and renal transplant patients. *Am J Surg* 1980;139:561–568.

73. Stiens S, Bierner-Bergman S, Goetz L. Neurogenic bowel dysfunction after spinal cord injury: clinical evaluation and rehabilitative management. *Arch Phys Med Rehabil* 1997;78:S86–S102.

74. Bohannon R, Smith J, Hull D, et al. Deficits in lower extremity muscle and gait performance among renal transplant candidates. *Arch Phys Med Rehabil* 1995;76:547–551.

75. Hester E, Taylor S. *Hester evaluation system users' manual*, 1976.

76. Stiens S, O'Young B, Young M. The person, disablement and the process of rehabilitation. In: O'Young B, Young MA, Stiens S, eds. *Physical medicine and rehabilitation secrets.* Philadelphia: Hanley & Belfus, Mosby, 1997:1–4.

77. Birnbaum A, Victor-Gittleman B. Occupational therapy for chronic renal disease patients. In: Kutner DC, ed. *Rehabilitation and the chronic renal disease patient.* Jamaica: Spectrum, 1985: 123–133.

78. Ahlmen I. Part B. Quality of life of the dialysis patient. In: Nissenson A, Fine R, Gentile D, eds. *Clinical dialysis.* 3rd ed. London: Prentice Hall, 1995:1466–1479.

79. de Aguiar JA. The socioeconomic problems of chronic renal failure: what can we do about them? *Contrib Nephrol* 1989;71: 164–168.

80. Taverner D, Craig K, Mackay I, Watson ML. Effects of exercise on renal function in patients with moderate impairment of renal function compared to normal men. *Nephron* 1991;57:288–292.

81. Painter P, Zimmerman S. Exercise in end-stage renal disease. *Am J Kidney Dis* 1986;7:386–394.

82. Clyne N, Jogestrand T, Lins LE, Pehrsson SK. Factors influencing physical working capacity in renal transplant patients. *Scand J Urol Nephrol* 1989;23:145–150.

83. Kempeneers G, Noakes TD, van Zyl-Smit R, et al. Skeletal muscle limits the exercise tolerance of renal transplant recipients: effects of a graded exercise training program. *Am J Kidney Dis* 1990;16:57–65.

84. Painter P. Exercise in end-stage renal disease. *Exercise Sports Sci Rev* 1988;16:305–309.

85. Kempeneers GLG, Myburgh KH, Wiggins T, et al. Skeletal muscle limiting exercise tolerance of renal transplant patients: effects of a graded exercise training program. *Am J Kidney Dis* 1990;14:57–66.

86. Nyberg G, Hallste G, Norden G, et al. Physical performance does not improve in elderly patients following successful kidney transplantation [see comments]. *Nephrol Dial Transplant* 1995;10:86–90.

87. Feber J, Dupuis JM, Chapuis F, et al. Body composition and physical performance in children after renal transplantation. *Nephron* 1997;75:13–19.

88. Penn I. Tumors after renal and cardiac transplantation. *Hematol Oncol Clin North Am* 1993;7:431–445.

89. Gutman R, Stead W, Robinson R. Physical activity and employment status of patients on maintenance dialysis. *N Engl J Med* 1981;304:309–313.

90. Mabee M, Tilney N, Vineyard G, Wilson R. Rehabilitation profile of kidney transplant patients. *Am J Surg* 1978;136:614–617.

91. Ross DJ, Water PF, Mohsenifar Z, et al. Hemodynamic responses to exercise after lung transplantation. *Chest* 1993;103: 46–53.

92. Grover FL, Fullerton DA, Zamora MR, et al. The past, present and future of lung transplantation. *Am J Surg* 1997;173:523–533.

93. UNOS OPTN/SR Annual Report. 1996.

94. Williams TJ, Patterson GA, Mcclean PA, et al. Maximal exercise testing in single and double lung transplant recipients. *Am Rev Respir Dis* 1992;145: 101–105.

95. Edelman JD, Kotloff RM. Lung transplantation. A disease-specific approach. *Clin Chest Med* 1997;18:627–644.

96. Powell HJ, Trovato M, Reinstein L, et al. Rehabilitation management of a lung transplantation patient with postoperative hemiparesis and bilateral below-knee amputation. *Arch Phys Med Rehabil* 1997;78:1054. Abstract.

97. Davis RD, Pasque MK. Pulmonary transplantation. *Ann Surg* 1995;221:14–28.

98. Boehler A, Speich R, Russi EW, Weder W. Lung transplantation for lymphangioleiomyomatosis. *N Engl J Med* 1996;335: 1275–1280.

99. Bridges ND, Mallory GB, Huddleston CB, et al. Lung transplantation in infancy and early childhood. *J Heart Lung Transplant* 1996;15:895–902.

100. Hausen B, Morris RE. Review of immunosuppression for lung transplantation: novel drugs, new uses for conventional immunosuppressants, and alternative strategies. *Clin Chest Med* 1997;18:353–366.

101. Chaparro C, Scavuzzo M, Winton T, et al. Status of lung transplant recipients surviving beyond five years. *J Heart Lung Transplant* 1997;16:511–516.

102. Maurer JR, Tewari S. Nonpulmonary medical complications in the intermediate and long-term survivor. *Clin Chest Med* 1997;18:367–382.

103. Meyer SB, Bass M, Ash R, et al. Postoperative care of the lung transplant recipient. *Crit Care Nurs Clin North Am* 1996;8:239–252.

104. Dorffner R, Eibenberger K, Youssefzadeh S, et al. Diaphragmatic dysfunction after heart or lung transplantation. *J Heart Lung Transplant* 1997;16:566–569.

105. Munin MC, Balu G, Sotereanos DG. Elbow complications after organ transplantation. Case reports. *Am J Phys Med Rehabil* 1995;74:67–72.

106. Kesten S, Mayne L, Scavuzzo M, Maurer J. Lack of left ventricular dysfunction associated with sustained exposure to hyperlipidemia following lung transplantation. *Chest* 1997;112:931–936.

107. Fenton JJ, Cicale MJ. Sigmoid diverticular perforation complicating lung transplantation. *J Heart Lung Transplant* 1997;16:681–685.

108. Powell HJ, Trovato M, Reinstein L, et al. Rehabilitation management of a lung transplantation patient with postoperative hemiparesis and bilateral below-knee amputations. *Arch Phys Med Rehabil* 1997;78:1054.

109. Howard DK, Iademarco EJ, Trulock EP. The role of cardiopulmonary exercise in lung and heart lung transplantation. *Clin Chest Med* 1994;15:405–420.

110. Craven JL, Bright J, Dear CL. Psychiatric, psychosocial, and rehabilitative aspects of lung transplantation. *Clin Chest Med* 1990;11:247–257.

111. Fitts SS, Guthrie MR. Six minute walk by people with chronic renal failure. *Am J Phys Med Rehabil* 1995;74:54–58.

112. Langlois LP, Crook R, Reinstein L, et al. Rehabilitation management of lung transplantation patients with neuromuscular complications. *Arch Phys Med Rehabil* 1995;76:1056. Abstract.

113. Williams TJ, Grossman RF, Maurer JR. Long-term functional follow-up of lung transplant recipients. *Clin Chest Med* 1990;11:347–358.

114. Gibbons WJ, Bryan CL, Calhoon JH, Jenkinson SG. Cardiopulmonary exercises responses after single lung transplantation for severe obstructive disease. *Chest* 1991;100:106–111.

115. Crouch RH, Schein RL. Integrating psychosocial services for lung volumes reduction and lung transplantation patients into a pulmonary rehabilitation program. *J Cardpulm Rehabil* 1997;17:16–18.

116. Nicholas JJ, Oleske D, Robinson LR, et al. The quality of life after orthotopic liver transplantation: an analysis of 166 cases. *Arch Phys Med Rehabil* 1995;75:431–435.

117. Tuel SM, Meythaler JM, Cross LL. Inpatient comprehensive rehabilitation after liver transplantation. *Am J Phys Med Rehabil* 1991;70(5):242–245.

118. Lowe D, O'Grady JG, McEwen J, Williams R. Quality of life following liver transplantation: a preliminary report. *J R Coll Phys Lond* 1990;24:43–46.

119. Pennington JC. Quality of life following liver transplantation. *Transplant Proc* 1989;21:3514–3516.

120. Ahlskog JE. Cerebral transplantation for Parkinson's disease: current progress and future prospects. *Mayo Clin Proc* 1993;68:578–591.

121. Kordower JH, Goetz CG, Freeman TB, Olanow CW. Dopaminergic transplants in patients with Parkinson's disease: neuroanatomical correlates of clinical recovery. *Exp Neurol* 1997;144:41–46.

122. Price LH, Spencer DD, Marek KL, et al. Psychiatric status after human fetal mesencephalic tissue transplantation in Parkinson's disease. *Biol Psychiatry* 1995;38:498–505.

123. Spencer DD, Robbins RJ, Naftolin F, et al. Unilateral transplantation of human fetal mesencephalic tissue into the caudate nucleus of patients with Parkinson's disease. *N Engl J Med* 1992;327:1549–1555.

124. Peschanski M, Defer G, N'Guyen JP, et al. Bilateral improvement and alteration of L-dopa effect in two patients with Parkinson's disease following intrastriatal transplantation of foetal ventral mesencephalon. *Brain* 1994;117(Pt3):487–499.

125. Sass KJ, Buchanan CP, Westerveld M, et al. General cognitive ability following unilateral and bilateral fetal ventral mesencephalic tissue transplantation for treatment of Parkinson's disease. *Arch Neurol* 1995;52:680–686.

126. Lopez-Lozano JJ, Bravo G, Brera B, et al. Long-term improvement in patients with severe Parkinson's disease after implantation of fetal ventral mesencephalic tissue in a cavity of the caudate nucleus: 5-year follow up in 10 patients. *J Neurosurg* 1997;86:931–942.

127. Zompa EA, Cain LD, Everhart AW, et al. Transplant therapy: recovery of function after spinal cord injury. *J Neurotrauma* 1997;14:479–506.

128. Miya D, Giszter S, Mori F, et al. Fetal transplants alter the development of function after spinal cord transection in newborn rats. *J Neurosci* 1997;17:4856–4872.

129. Mori F, Himes BT, Kowada M, et al. Fetal spinal cord transplants rescue some axotomized rubrospinal neurons from retrograde cell death in adult rats. *Exp Neurol* 1997;143: 45–60.

130. Itoh Y, Waldeck RF, Tessler A, Pinter MJ. Regenerated dorsal root fibers form functional synapses in embryonic spinal cord transplants. *J Neurophysiol* 1996;76:1236–1245.

131. Houle JD, Skinner RD, Garcia-Rill E, Turner KL. Synaptic evoked potentials from regenerating dorsal root axons within fetal spinal cord tissue transplants. *Exp Neurol* 1996;139:278–290.

132. Nogradi A, Vrbova G. Improved motor function of rat hindlimb muscles induced by embryonic spinal cord grafts. *Eur J Neurosci* 1996;8:2198–2203.

133. Li Y, Field PM, Raisman G. Repair of adult rat corticospinal tract by transplants of olfactory ensheating cells. *Science* 1997;277(5334):2000–2002.

134. Rosenbluth J, Schiff R, Liang WL, et al. Xenotransplantation of transgenic oligodendrocyte lineage cells into spinal cord-injured adult rats. *Exp Neurol* 1997;147:172–182.

135. Li Y, Raisman G. Integration of transplanted cultured Schwann cells into the long myelinated fiber tracts of the adult spinal cord. *Exp Neurol* 1997; 145(2Pt1): 397–411.

136. Eaton MJ, Santiago DI, Dancausse HA, Whittemore SR. Lumbar transplants of immortalized serotonergic neurons alleviate chronic neuropathic pain. *Pain* 1997;72:50–69.

137. Chase TN, A gene for Parkinson disease. *Arch Neurol* 1997;54: 1156–1157.

138. Raffensperger JG, Luck SR, Reynolds M, Schwarz D. Intestinal bypass of the esophagus. *J Pediatr Surg* 1996;31:38–46.

139. Grant D. Current results of intestinal transplantation. The International Intestinal Transplant Registry. *Lancet* 1996; 347(9018):1801–1803.

140. Beath SV, Needham SJ, Kelly DA, et al. Clinical features and prognosis of children assessed for isolated small bowel or combined small bowel and liver transplantation. *J Pediatr Surg* 1997;32: 459–461.

141. Lee RG, Nakamura K, Tsamandas AC, et al. Pathology of human intestinal transplantation. *Gastroenterology* 1996;110: 1820–1834.

142. Muller AR, Platz KP, Heckert C, et al. Laminin and hyaluronic acid as indicators for initial transplant function and acute rejection after small bowel transplantation. *Langensbecks Arch Chir Suppl Kongressbd* 1997; 114:201–204.

143. Miyauchi T, Ishikawa M, Tashiro S, et al. Acetaminophen absorption test as a marker of small bowel transplant rejection. *Transplantation* 1997;63:1179–1182.

144. Lee RG, Nakamura K, Tsamandas AC, et al. Pathology of human intestinal transplantation. *Gastroenterology* 1996;110(6): 1820–1834.

145. Hickey DP, Baktharatsalam R, Bannon CA, et al. Urological complications of pancreatic transplantations. *J Urol* 1997; 157:2042–2048.

146. Pirson Y, Squifflet JP. Combined kidney-pancreas transplantation: what are the costs and benefits, who are the recipients? *Presse Med* 1997;26:905–907.

147. Vickers SM, Sampson LS, Phillips JO, et al. Adenoviral vector infection of the human exocrine pancreas. *Arch Surg* 1997;132:1006–1009.

148. Vogelsang GB, Wagner JE. Graft-versus-host disease in bone marrow transplantation. *Hematol Oncol Clin North Am* 1990; 4(3):625–635.

149. Vogelsang GB, Farmer ER, Hess AD, et al. Thodidomide for the treatment of chronic graft vs. host disease. *N Engl J Med* 1992;324(14):1055–1058.

150. DeMeyer ES. Multidisciplinary team contributions in the management of chronic graft vs. host disease: a case study. *Oncol Nursing Forum* 1995;22:360. Abstract.

Chapter 35

Cognitive Rehabilitation

Brenda B. Adamovich

DEFINITIONS

Cognitive retraining is a systematic approach to improve cognitive functions, in order to improve overall functional skills, that have been impaired following damage to the central nervous system. Restorative approaches are used to restore specific cognitive functions, such as attention, memory, and problem solving. Compensatory approaches seek to bypass the deficit area and teach the patient how to use certain strategies to solve functional problems.

Ben-Yishay and Piasetsky (1) suggested that cognitive retraining activities were not effective for retraining lost functions. Instead, patients became more efficient at utilizing their residual cognitive and perceptual skills.

Cognition is inferred from behavior (2). Cognition includes the use of processes and knowledge to 1) make decisions as to the most appropriate and functional way to interact with the environment, 2) execute these decisions, 3) monitor responses to determine the appropriateness and accuracy of these decisions, and 4) adjust behavior if it is determined to be inappropriate or inaccurate (3). Specific cognitive processes include attention, perception, discrimination, organization, recall, reasoning, and executive functioning or metacognitive skills. These processes are impaired to varying degrees following widespread, diffuse brain damage due to closed head injury (4). Impaired cognitive processes can result in both disabilities and handicaps.

The International Classification of Impairments, Disabilities and Handicaps (ICIDH) developed by the World Health Organization (5) defines *impairment* as resultant losses of psychological or physical function. *Disability* is defined as the restricted ability to perform, or the functional consequences of an impairment manifested in integrated activities represented by tasks and skills. *Handicap* is defined as a social disadvantage resulting from the impairment or disability. Handicaps following traumatic brain injury (TBI) that prevent the fulfillment of a normal life can affect physical independence, vocational status or return to work, return to school, return to family roles, and establishment of a support network.

Cognitive impairments can cause disabilities in social interactions and interpersonal or pragmatic communication, which lead to problems with social adjustment and result in a handicap. A disability in pragmatic communication can include an inability to comprehend subtlety in language, as in metaphorical and figurative use, and a reduced ability to draw conclusions and to give coherence to narrative. Mildly impaired brain injury patients have diminished executive functioning (metacognitive) skills, making them appear unusual to others in the community. [*Metacognition* means "knowing about knowing" (6).] *Executive functioning* refers to the ability to formulate goals, develop plans, and effectively execute a plan (7). Executive skills include self-awareness in goal setting, planning, self-directing/initiating, self-inhibiting, self-monitoring, self-evaluating, and flexible problem solving (8). A person who lacks these skills appears to be egocentric, rude, impulsive, disinhibited, stubborn, denying, or incoherent.

Social disabilities following TBI, can be due to cognitive, personality, emotional, and behavioral impairments ranging from mild mood and personality changes to severe psychosis. Ylkvisaker et al (9) attributed reduced social skills to 1) poor awareness and perception of social and communication events; 2) inadequate retrieval of rules of social interactions; 3) reduced ability to take alternative perspectives; 4) disorganization at the level of introducing, maintaining, and terminating topics of conversation; and 5) disinhibition and weak self-monitoring of verbal and nonverbal behavior which may result in repetition of information, making inappropriate and offensive remarks, and demonstrating poor comprehension for spoken utterances.

Wehman et al (10) suggested that key barriers to employability relate to cognitive issues. Examples of such barriers are poor learning and memory abilities, impaired self-awareness, and preexisting and postinjury dysfunctional behavior including substance abuse and other psychological problems. People lose jobs because of poor social or interpersonal skills, not because of deficient task performance. Getting along with coworkers, accepting criticisms and supervision, following instructions, completing tasks, and being consistent in attendance and attitude are qualities desired by most employers (11). Haffey and Lewis (12) listed barriers to job placement and retention following TBI, including cognitive-communicative disorders, emotional and social behavior control problems, psychomotor and cognitive processing slowness, and inadequate interpersonal and social skills.

EFFICACY OF COGNITIVE REHABILITATION

To date, there is a lack of empirical evidence supporting the efficacy of cognitive rehabilitation for the restoration of overall cognitive functions, as well as the efficacy of direct cognitive retraining of specific functions such as memory (13–16). The prediction of outcomes is complicated by the uniqueness of every injury. One person with a serious injury may appear to make excellent recovery while another person with a mild injury may show long-lasting deficits. Outcome measurement is further complicated by the heterogeneity of the brain-injured population, with differing severities of neuropsychological and emotional deficits and differing premorbid factors such as age, educational level, family support, financial status, educational skills, and so forth. Recovery rates vary depending on variables such as age, severity of injury, site or location of injury, preinjury intellectual abilities, physical and mental status, time since injury, and postinjury social and medical support systems (17).

The arguments against cognitive rehabilitation have been weak evidence for its validity and efficacy, and an inadequate basis in theory (18). Butler and Namerow (19) criticized cognitive rehabilitation for lacking a basis in neuropsychological theory. Yet, Ben-Yishay and Diller (18) stressed that this criticism ignores the work of Luria (20) and more recent studies of neutral plasticity (21) which point toward a theoretical basis for brain injury rehabilitation. Ben-Yishay and Diller (18) noted that investigators operating within a psychological/learning framework based the application of cognitive rehabilitation interventions following brain injuries on clinical studies utilizing stroke, learning disabled, mentally retarded, and aged populations. Benedict (22) and Levin (23) reported that there was no evidence that cognitive remediation was efficacious; however, both investigators believed it was worth pursuing with multicenter clinical trials.

Cope et al (24) reported that cognitive rehabilitation can produce significant improvements in cognitive functioning that are not likely to be due to the results of spontaneous recovery alone. These authors suggested the need for future research to clarify the specific role of cognitive rehabilitation in the recovery process.

Studies designed to measure the effectiveness of cognitive retraining reported statistically significant improvements in scores on a number of tests of cognitive impairments which were the targets of the remedial training. Bond and Brooks (25) administered the Wechsler Adult Intelligence Scale (WAIS) to 40 patients following TBI at 3-month intervals for up to 2 years after injury. They reported that most of the recovery on the cognitive tasks assessed by the WAIS occurred during the first 6 months after TBI. Klonoff et al (26) reported that 76% of brain-injured children and adolescents made statistically significant improvements in the recovery of cognitive functions over 5 years. Thomsen (27) evaluated a 44-year-old man 2 years after TBI and reported marked cognitive impairments. Twelve years later, he had only mild cognitive impairments, suggesting continuous and gradual improvement in cognitive functioning for 14 years after the injury occurred. Sbordone et al (28) and Terayama et al (29) studied 20 patients and 42 patients following TBI, respectively, and reported that the majority of subjects showed cognitive improvements for as long as 10 years after injury. Yet, some investigators found that cognitive improvements did not generalize and did not result in large, clinically meaningful changes in the patients' overall capacity in the functional domains studied (1,30–35). These investigators concluded that cognitive remediation is meaningful only if it is embedded in, and systematically coordinated with, other rehabilitation interventions and if cognitive remedial exercises are done in such a way as to improve overall problem-solving abilities in a more holistic approach. Brain-damaged individuals are concrete thinkers and have difficulty transferring what they have been taught from one context to the next.

Kaplan and Corrigan (36) conducted a study to determine if measures of impairment reflected disturbances in functional outcome after brain injury. Ratings on the Orientation Group Monitoring System (OGMS) were compared to ratings on the Functional Independence

Measure (FIM). The OGMS is a scale developed to prospectively measure cognitive impairment after coma to the end of posttraumatic amnesia. The FIM is a measure of disability. Significant positive relationships were found between measures of cognition (OGMS) and measures of functional status (FIM). The authors suggested that cognition contributes to and can be used as a predictor of functional abilities.

On the other hand, Butler and Namerow (19) and Volpe and McDowell (37) found cognitive rehabilitation to be of no value. They criticized studies obtaining positive results as being due to poor experimental design. They pointed out that single-case-design studies were inadequate because they were not hypothesis driven, gave insufficient consideration to alternative explanations, and did not allow for generalization to other cases due to the absence of an adequate taxonomy of brain injury. Group designs were also criticized because of their inability to rule out natural recovery, invalid psychometric instruments, and the lack of a relationship between psychometric outcome measures and the cognitive rehabilitation treatments. These authors (19,37) suggested that cognitive rehabilitation lacks a sound rationale and that improvements noted following cognitive rehabilitation are practice effects rather than genuine gains in skill.

Cognitive rehabilitation is a relatively new field. The number of research studies in this area is on the increase, and hopefully, these studies will provide insight regarding specific treatment protocols that produce the most efficacious results. At this point, cognitive rehabilitation is a promising field.

COGNITIVE REHABILITATION MODELS

Benedict (22) referred to a classification of restorative versus compensatory approaches to cognitive rehabilitation. This distinction is analogous to treating an impairment (i.e., a disturbance in the structure of an organism due to underlying pathology) versus treating a disability (i.e., a difficulty in carrying out a functional act in a given situation) (38). These treatment theories also have been described as basic skill learning versus direct skill training (39). Restorative approaches designed to treat impairments have been highly criticized, particularly with regard to their impact on functional abilities. Compensatory approaches are more accepted than restorative approaches as they are generally used to improve functioning in real-life, daily activities.

Several investigators (18,39) found that basic skill learning or treatment of general cognitive processes can result in an improvement in functional skills. Other investigators (40) advocate for direct skill training of functional tasks following TBI. Gordon and Hibbard (41) and Adamovich (42) suggested that a combined treatment approach would result in the most efficacious training following TBI. Combined treatment would include training of cognitive processes in conjunction with the learning of actual functional skills during simulated and community-based activities; the cognitive processes provide a basic foundation that crosses over to many skills and behaviors, and they are necessary if generalization is to occur. It is impossible to train every skill that a person will need following TBI.

Ben-Yishay and Diller (18) advocated multimodal interventions consisting of both restorative and substitutive approaches. Restorative approaches dissect an impaired area of cognitive functioning and present tasks to restore competence. Theories of instruction and general learning such as "scaffolding" should be considered. Scaffolding is a restorative approach. Collins et al (43) wrote of "scaffolds of skill training in which previously trained abilities are used to train new abilities." This is similar to Bruner's notion (44) of a "spiral curriculum in education in which previously learned materials are repeated in increasing level of detail as the child advances through a school system."

Adamovich et al (4) proposed a similar treatment hierarchy in which cognitive tasks are presented, progressing from easy to difficult levels of cognition in a gradual, step-by-step fashion. Performance on a cognitive task can be analyzed in several ways. One way is to focus on questions involving competence levels, for example, the ability to process information (including the amount and complexity of the information), the speed with which information can be processed, the length of time information is retained, and the efficiency with which it can be applied. A second way is to focus on questions involving control processes.

Prigatano (30) and Ben-Yishay et al (1) described holistic or milieu-oriented neurologic rehabilitation, which includes cognitive retraining activities with psychotherapy activities within the context of a day treatment program. In order to progress, patients are made aware of their deficits and try methods of compensation using actual vocational or work trials.

Ben-Yishay and Prigatano (45) outlined six stages in their holistic approach: *engaging* patients in rehabilitation activities, progressive *awareness* of their problems, *mastery* of compensatory techniques for cognitive deficit, *control* of compensatory activities, *acceptance* of their deficits, and finally, the *emergence* of a new identity. According to Ben-Yishay and Diller (18), personal variables that interfere with cognitive rehabilitation include a lack of awareness of deficits, the extent of cognitive deficits, and impaired generalization.

COGNITIVE REHABILITATIVE METHODS

Treating Impairments

Cognitive retraining can be provided in both individual and group therapy sessions. Treatment ranges from a low-

Table 35-1: Hierarchy of Cognitive-Communicative Processes
Arousal/alerting
Perception, low-level selective attention
Discrimination
Organization
Recall
High-level thought processing
Convergent thinking
Deductive reasoning
Inductive reasoning
Divergent thinking
Multiprocess reasoning

level stimulation program to high-level treatment that focuses on reasoning and problem solving. Specific cognitive activities are presented according to the hierarchy of skills suggested by Adamovich and Henderson (46).

A diagnostic/treatment hierarchy of cognitive processes proposed by Adamovich et al (4,42,46) is presented in Table 35-1. The hierarchy was designed for two purposes: to establish a diagnostic battery that is directly applicable to treatment, and to establish an organized approach to the rehabilitation of attention, information processing, and cognition. Based on the diagnostic assessment, clinicians begin treatment at the level in the hierarchy where the patient began to have difficulty and progress in a step-by-step fashion through the hierarchy from easy to difficult levels of processing. It is important to know that a division between the levels is somewhat artificial in that the clinician may be working on the most difficult tasks at one level and the easiest activities at the next level. Attention is the focus of early treatment, yet it is essential that the attentional skills continue to improve as the patient moves through the treatment continuum. Memory skills must also continually improve as more complex processing places a greater load on memory. Information-processing considerations during all levels of treatment include the stimuli selected to accomplish each task, the mode of presentation of the stimuli (e.g., simultaneous versus sequential), the stimulus presentation rate, the response time, and the use of feedback to modify responses.

Prigatano (47) suggested various clinical guidelines for conducting cognitive retraining activities: 1) The therapist should know that even mild problems can cause significant deficits in day-to-day activities. 2) The therapist should be aware that most patients do not fully recognize the severity or impact of their cognitive deficits. 3) Differences in performance from training activities should be recorded to measure behavioral outcomes. 4) Training materials should be interesting and appropriate to the patient's background and interests. 5) Microcomputers cannot be used to retrain anything that can be used to provide interesting tasks.

Attention

Brain-injured patients have difficulty initiating, sustaining, shifting, and inhibiting the inappropriate shifting of attention. Attentional deficits include perseveration, distractibility, impulsivity, and disinhibition. Specific treatment techniques include varying concepts, rates, and sequences; varying length and intensity of work periods; utilizing techniques to focus attention and facilitate rehearsal; avoiding the presentation of repeating cues; and using instructions to increase self-monitoring. Techniques that focus attention include addressing the person by name before initiating a task, waiting for eye contact, touching the patient, or using start-up phrases such as "Are you ready?" Therapy should begin utilizing pertinent, meaningful stimuli and gradually move to less familiar stimuli. If a person is capable of attending for 5 minutes, changing tasks at the end of a 5-minute period might help increase attentional duration and allow for a longer treatment session.

Ben-Yishay et al (48) reported improved attention at 6 months after training utilizing their technique, the Orientation Remedial Module (ORM). The technique focused on more efficiently using the patient's residual cognitive and perceptual skills than on retraining functions. Wilson (40) reported that reality orientation sessions for groups of patients with TBI or stroke resulted in improved performance in attention and recall.

Perception

Visual and auditory perceptual tasks include tracking and scanning; perception of sounds, words, and objects; tracing or copying; following simple commands; and naming objects.

Discrimination

With discrimination tasks, the number and degree of similarity of stimuli that compete with the most pertinent or most salient stimulus or stimuli should be gradually increased. Activities begin with the visual discrimination of colors, shapes, and sizes, followed by the discrimination of pictures, words, sentences, and situations. The level of cognitive functioning must be considered for all functional tasks. For example, if a patient is able to discriminate between only two items at a time, only two foods should be placed on a food tray at a time, or only two articles of clothing should be given during a dressing activity.

Organization

Organizational activities include categorization, closure, and sequencing tasks. Categorization is the grouping of items by physical attributes, meaningful units, function, likenesses, and differences. Closure activities include the identification of missing elements of pictures, letters, words, sentences, stories, conversations, and situations. Sequencing activities include the sequencing of visual information from smallest to largest or lightest to darkest, with progression to the sequencing of letters, words, sentences, and steps to functional activities such as taking a shower, making coffee, and shopping.

Organizational skills are essential for all functional activities. An individual can be capable of completing the individual steps of an activity but be unable to sequence the entire activity. For example, a person might sit all day, intending to take a shower, get dressed, or make a sandwich, but not know what to do first, second, and so on. What might appear at first glance to be an initiation problem is actually an inability to deal with the sequencing of a task that is too complex for that person.

Treatment must focus on the gradual progression from the sequencing of two steps, such as taking the lid off the toothpaste and putting toothpaste on a toothbrush, to three steps, and so on. Patients will experience success and greater levels of independence if their level of cognitive functioning is considered during all activities.

Memory

Memory deficits are the result of ineffective encoding of information, inadequate storage of information, difficulty with retrieving information, and the inability to cope with interferences. Two general approaches to the treatment of memory disturbances after TBI include the development of internal retrieval strategies and the provision of external memory aids. Individuals with TBI usually have long-lasting memory deficits that require both types of memory treatments. Ponsford et al (49) reported the existence of memory problems, reduced speed of thinking, concentration difficulties, problems with planning and organization, impulsiveness, and decreased initiative in the majority of 175 TBI patients studied 2 years after injury. Memory remediation studies have been problematic because 1) the specific nature of memory impairments is not adequately isolated, and 2) there is little agreement about how to define a memory deficit (41). Ryan and Ruff (50) found that attention and memory training was effective for mildly or moderately impaired persons with TBI, but not for a severely impaired group. This suggests that individual differences can be an implied variable in treatment effectiveness.

Parenté and DiCesare (51) suggested that memory strategy training will not be effective with every person with brain injury. All memory strategies require an individual to attend initially. Varying degrees of working memory are also necessary. Parenté and DiCesare outlined strategies for memory retraining including domain-specific training, sensory-memory training, attention-concentration training, rehearsal, academic therapy, stimulation therapy, and memory strategy training. Reportedly, a literature review indicated that attention-concentration training and domain-specific training can be highly effective after brain injury. Brain-injured patients also benefit from rehearsal, imagery, translation of verbal text, verbal labeling, and number chunking.

Domain-specific training requires the simulation of what the person with brain injury will encounter when he or she enters the work world. The training conforms to an A-B: A^1-B^1 paradigm that predicts maximum transfer (15).

Attention-concentration training is a hierarchy of therapy tasks at each of five levels: focused attention, selective attention, sustained attention, alternating attention, and divided attention. This method has been shown to improve attention deficits (52).

Rehearsal training requires patients to rehearse information subvocally. Craine and Gudeman (53) demonstrated the effectiveness of this technique. Parenté and DiCesare (51) found that subvocal rehearsal of information yielded remarkable improvement in memory functioning because it sustains information in working memory and facilitates encoding.

Academic therapy involves relearning functional skills, often as a precursor to job training. Wilson (54) demonstrated that the preview, question, read, state, and test (PQRST) system improves the retention of text material. Glasgow et al (55) utilized the approach to improve the recall of written material in a 22-year-old woman with high-level memory deficits following a closed head injury that occurred 3½ years earlier. They reported a consistent improvement in memory over a 10-day period, with generalization of the strategy to everyday life activities. Schacter and Glisky (15) and Parenté et al (56) used an A-B:C-B intervention model such that the therapy and real-world materials differed. Persons with brain injury were taught to scan the iconic store in glimpses that are too fast to rely on eye muscle control for scanning. This training improved performance on tests of reading comprehension and word recognition.

In six brain-injured persons, Parenté and DiCesare (51) found improved recall of written materials using a training technique that required the patients to translate mentally into their own words what they read.

Other techniques found to improve attention and recall include reality-orientation group therapy (57), attention training (58), and prospective memory training (52).

Stimulation therapy is the oldest form of memory retraining; it requires repetitive drills. The generalization of learned skills to functional tasks has been questioned since tasks, stimuli, and required responses are often not relevant to real-life situations (35,51,59–61). However, several investigators (49,62–64) reported that this technique has resulted in improved performance on standardized tests.

Strategy training is another memory retraining technique. Recall strategies include verbal description in which an adequate explanation of items and concepts to be recalled is provided by the client or clinician; visual imagery in which objects, scenes of a story or situation, and maps or layouts in space are mentally pictured; chunking in which information is visually or aurally organized into segments that coincide with the patient's memory span; categorization of information to improve recall of that information (e.g., when required to remember items to be purchased at a grocery store, the patient should group the items into categories such as dairy products, frozen foods, meats, etc.); rehearsal, in which information to be recalled is drilled; associations based on semantic relationships (e.g., can-crutches and day-night), acoustic relationships (e.g., dew-shoe), or visual relationships (e.g., desk-dresser); temporal or spatial ordering in which events in episodic and semantic memory are recalled by remembering certain landmark events associated with the event to be recalled or those that occurred at a similar point in time; and mnemonic devices in which specific memory tricks are used to increase associative learning through paired association. For an example of a mnemonic device, during encoding, new words or bits of information are chained or paired to a pre-established set of keywords and phrases or a familiar sequence of known locations using several mnemonic systems. A peg system links or pegs new items to existing items, for example, a rhyming peg is *one* = *bun*, a phonetic peg is *two* = *n* (2 down strokes), and a loci peg involves items linked to familiar locations. The substitution-word system is based on linking a visual image with a word, for example, to remember the name *Cameron*, visualize a camera on his balding head (outstanding facial feature). The link system links lists of items together in generally a funny way to facilitate retrieval, for example, to remember bologna and milk, picture a cow eating bologna as the farmer milks her.

Parenté and DiCesare (51) suggested that memory strategy training will not be effective with every person with brain injury. All memory strategies require an individual to attend initially. Varying degrees of working memory are also necessary.

Wilson (54), Patten (65), Jones (66), and Crovitz (67) reported that imagery training is effective. However, Lorayne and Lucas (68) found only limited, short-term improvement with imagery training. Moffat (69), Schacter and Crovitz (70), and Schacter and Glisky (15) questioned the maintenance and generalization of imagery training to real-life situations.

Moffat (69) emphasized that the practical applications of imagery training are limited by encoding demands, which are often beyond the capacities of persons with brain injury. Parenté and DiCesare (51) found that imagery or embedded sentence training did not improve the short-term memory of 10 clients with TBI. However, improved performance resulted when number chunking and verbal labeling (a technique of associating something new with something already familiar) were used.

Patten (65) studied the benefit of associations for patients with dominant-hemisphere lesions. A peg system was used in which 10 peg words were learned and 10 random words were associated to constant images. This investigator suggested that the peg system technique results in improved memory for patients with TBI. Wilson and Moffat (57) suggested that mildly brain-injured patients benefit from this technique; however, they suggested that patients with pronounced unilateral damage in either hemisphere may not benefit as they may fail to recall the words or the peg words due to difficulty in forming verbal or visual associations.

Sohlberg et al (71) reported a significant and steady increase in the prospective memory ability of a 51-year-old brain-injured man with severe memory impairment who participated in their prospective memory training program.

Memory aids are similar to the type of memory aids that non-brain-injured individuals utilize, such as a calendar, appointment book, notepads, daily logs and diaries, memo books, lists, structured routines, alarms to remind a person to complete a task, tape recorders, and microcomputers. Prosthetic devices are used to help organize, recall, and utilize information for daily living activities. A variety of prosthetic memory aids, including checklists, electronic signaling devices, telememo devices, and personal directories, have been successfully used by brain injury persons to provide cues for daily activities (51,54,72,73). Sohlberg and Mateer (74) reported the successful training of a patient to use a memory notebook. However, prosthetic devices can be limiting because they can be misplaced or neglected by the patient (69,75). Patients with TBI can often be extremely effective in dealing with a faulty memory if they are willing to utilize memory aids faithfully to compensate for memory deficits. Probably the least conspicuous and most effective memory aid is the use of a watch alarm to remind a person to look at his or her appointment book. This strategy works quite well if the patient remembers to note all necessary appointments and information in the appointment book. Schacter and Glisky (15) concluded that memory is not like a muscle that becomes stronger with exercise. These investigators suggested that patients with memory disorders can be taught to use complex compensational devices to organize functional tasks. Wilson (54) is also a proponent of this theory.

Reasoning

Reasoning activities generally begin with practice in the clinic but must be extended to practice in real-life situations. Several types of reasoning should be addressed, beginning with the most concrete and extending to the most abstract forms. Convergent thinking involves the identification of main points or central themes. Deductive reasoning requires step-by-step problem solving. Inductive reasoning, more abstract, is a part of such diverse activities as cause-and-effect analysis, analogous thinking, and the formulation of antonyms and synonyms. Divergent thinking consists of unique abstract concepts such as homographs, absurdities, idioms, and proverbs.

Use of Computers

Computers can be helpful in the treatment of attention, concentration/persistence, visual localization, visual scanning, visual tracking, reaction time, memory, hand-eye coordination, and specific cognitive tasks. With computers, stimuli can be presented in a highly controlled manner and the client is required to compete only with himself or herself. This can provide a sense of control over therapy and progress, which leads to increased motivation and feelings of self-worth. Accurate, objective, and immediate feedback is received and patients tend to enjoy using computers.

According to Wilson (40), clinicians should consider the following when selecting computer programs: consistent, controlled levels of difficulty within a task; lesson- or file-generating capability; concise, easy-to-follow instructions; consistent response format; accurate and age-appropriate content; degree of supervision required; friendly, unambiguous, and informative feedback; control of variables or parameters (i.e., length of time that a stimulus is displayed, length of response delay time, task speed, number of trials per set, level of difficulty, type of prompts, size of stimuli, timing, and type of reinforcements); and method of keeping and reporting data.

All computer treatments designed to assist in the overall cognitive rehabilitation program should be under the direction and supervision of a professional rehabilitation specialist. Computers should never be used as a substitute for the clinician. Since aides often work with clients during computer sessions, clinicians also should know how to appropriately use support personnel. Cognitive remediation cannot occur using only a computer and an aide; computers, like workbooks, are merely tools.

Executive Functioning

Executive functioning, according to Lezak (7), is the ability to formulate goals, develop a plan, and effectively execute a plan. Treatment of higher-level patients following TBI should include the assessment and treatment of executive functioning. Impaired executive functioning can increase the difficulty of reintegrating the patient into the home, community, school, or workplace. As stated earlier, there are seven concepts specific to executive system problems (metacognitive dysfunction): self-awareness in goal setting, planning, self-directing/initiating, self-inhibiting, self-monitoring, self-evaluating, and flexible problem solving (8).

Executive functioning deficits are thought to be a consequence of frontal lobe damage (76). Levin and Kraus (21) also discussed pathophysiologic and neuroimaging evidence suggesting that the frontal lobes are involved in closed head injury. They suggested that even though damage to the brain is often diffuse with closed head injury, specific cognitive behavioral and mood disorders can be attributed to frontal lobe damage directly or indirectly. They indicated that treatment and rehabilitation require a multidisciplinary approach that includes education of the patient and family and modification of the patient's home and work environments. Executive functioning deficits probably become most evident when the patient leaves the rehabilitation center and attempts to function in his or her home and community. These deficits should be a focus of all outpatient community re-entry programs and probably can best be treated with individual and group therapy, along with specific activities in the community, home, and work designed to practice target behaviors. Individual and group therapy sessions should focus on the identification of individual strengths and weaknesses, insight, self-evaluation, self-monitoring, and utilization of feedback. According to Cicerone and Giacino (64), at some level the treatment of executive function deficits must attempt to re-establish psychological processes that link social and environmental demands and the deliberate response of the individual. The goal, in other words, is a remediation of behavior that is initially under external control. The behavior is gradually internalized and brought under the patient's own control to be applied spontaneously in varied situations.

Prigatano (30) proposed a four-step process to improve ineffective interpersonal skills resulting from the interaction between cognitive impairments and psychosocial behavioral impairments: 1) improvement of attentional skills to reduce generalized cognitive confusion, 2) awareness of strengths and deficits through group and individual counseling, 3) recognition of the need for compensation behaviors, and 4) understanding of the impact of cognitive deficits on interpersonal skills. Fryer and Fralish (77) and Ben-Yishay and Prigatano (45) stressed a cognitive rehabilitation approach that focuses on the elimination of impairments and the removal of barriers, to improve functional disabilities and increase competence in everyday life.

FUNCTIONAL OUTCOMES OF COGNITIVE RETRAINING

Cognitive remediation is a relatively new field and there is little research on the effectiveness of cognitive rehabilitation in the improvement of functional activities. Even though several studies have documented the efficacy of cognitive remediation, critics have cited the lack of generalization, the slow pace of learning, and the finding of improved test scores rather than improved functional behavioral outcomes (41,78–80). Meaningful functional gains that improve the level of independence in day-to-day activities are used to judge the benefit of rehabilitation. Yet, existing functional assessment tools lack reliability and validity. Adamovich (81) conducted a study to compare the functional communication ratings of registered nurses and speech-language pathologists on the FIM. Fourteen patients with left-hemisphere brain damage and 14 patients with right-hemisphere brain damage served as subjects. The nurses assigned significantly higher FIM scores than did speech-language pathologists when rating the communication of left-hemisphere–damaged patients. However, nurses and speech-language pathologists provided the same average rankings of patients from least to most impaired. Follow-up analysis revealed potential reasons for the discrepancies, including the fact that the nurses and speech-language pathologists were using different evaluation procedures.

Adamovich (82) conducted a retrospective review of admission and discharge FIM scores for 479 patients representing seven diagnostic groups: left cerebrovascular accident (CVA), right CVA, TBI, other neurologic disorders, and spinal cord injury. The TBI group improved significantly beyond the levels of the RCVA, LCVA, and other neurologic disorder groups. The greatest improvement for the TBI group was on the following items: upper-body dressing, memory, problem solving, social interaction, comprehension, and expression.

The most efficacious approach to the retraining of complex behavior is one that includes retraining of both cognitive processes and specific functional skills. Training of cognitive processes provides the necessary foundation for the more complex task of learning new skills and behaviors. Adamovich (83) conducted an investigation to compare communicative effectiveness in a traditional therapeutic clinical setting (a picture description task) versus a functional community-based setting using a standardized scoring system (84) to quantify the informativeness and efficiency of connected speech. Thirteen brain-injured subjects comprised three groups: LCVA (N = 5), RCVA (N = 4), and TBI (N = 4). A younger normal group (N = 4) and an older normal group (N = 5) served as controls. All groups, non-brain-injured and brain-injured, evidenced better performance during the functional community-based activity condition compared to the picture description task, based on an increase in the number and percentage of correct information units.

Schacter and Glisky (15) successfully utilized domain-specific training to improve the skills of brain-injured individuals in functional tasks. This technique requires the matching of task demands to those in the real world by simulating what the person will encounter in the real world. An A–B : A^1–B^1 paradigm that predicts maximum positive transfer using training materials similar to the evaluation world was used. The investigators reported the successful training of functions after the tasks were simulated and trained.

Gianutsos and Gianutsos (62) used an A–B : C–D stimulation therapy model in which the task elements and cognitive response sets are unlike anything the person will encounter after leaving therapy. They correlated improved performance on an information-processing task with improved performance on a test of verbal recall.

Substitute of compensatory approaches to cognitive remediation requires metacognitive abilities. These metacognitive skills are necessary to appropriately utilize compensatory strategies for impaired executive functions. Metacognitive skills are often a focus of group therapy sessions. Specific group therapy techniques for a variety of cognitive skills will be presented in Chapter 39, on community re-entry.

CONCLUSIONS

Cognitive processes include perception, discrimination, organization, recall, and problem solving. Cognitive rehabilitation is a relatively new field, with a paucity of research on the effectiveness of cognitive retraining in improving functional abilities. Functional gains that improve the level of independence in day-to-day activities are used to judge the benefit of rehabilitation. Yet, many existing functional assessment tools lack reliability and validity. There is need for a standardized protocol to assess functional outcomes after TBI—one that includes valid and reliable measures of functional abilities (including measures of both disability and handicap) in the home, community, school, and workplace. Functional assessment tools are essential to adequately evaluate the benefit of specific treatment techniques on functional outcomes.

Cognitive retraining programs should include the retraining of both cognitive processes and specific meaningful functional skills in real-life situations in each patient's home and community. Fortunately, the number of studies supporting the efficacy of cognitive rehabilitation programs have continued to increase over the past several years. Although the field of cognitive rehabilitation is relatively new and continually evolving, its future appears to be promising.

REFERENCES

1. Ben-Yishay Y, Piasetsky E. Rehabilitation of cognitive and perceptual deficits in persons with chronic brain damage. A comparative study. In: Diller L, et al, eds. *Annual progress report.* R.T. Center, NIHR grant no. G008300039, 4. 1985.
2. Mann L, Sabatino DA. *Foundations of cognitive process in remedial and special education* Rockville; MD: Aspen Systems, 1985.
3. "Cognitive Rehabilitation Guidelines," 1986.
4. Adamovich BB, Henderson JA, Auerbach S. *Cognitive rehabilitation of closed head injured patients.* San Diego: College-Hill, 1985.
5. World Health Organization (WHO). *The international classification of diseases.* 10th revision. Geneva: WHO, 1980:25–31.
6. Flavell J. Metacognition and cognitive monitoring. *Am Psychol* 1979;34:6–11.
7. Lezak MD. The problem of assessing executive functions.

Int J Psychol 1982;17:281–297.

8. Ylvisaker M. Cognitive and psychosocial outcome following head injury in children. In: Hoff JT, Anderson TE, Cole TM, eds. *Mild to moderate head injury.* Oxford: Blackwell Scientific, 1987:203–216.

9. Ylkvisaker M, Szekeres HK. Topics in cognitive rehabilitation therapy. In: Ylvisaker M, Gobble E, eds. *Community re-entry for head injured adults.* Boston: Little, Brown, 1987:174–175.

10. Wehman P, Kreutzer J, West M, et al. Employment outcomes of persons following traumatic brain injury: pre-injury, post-injury and supported employment. *Brain Inj* 1989;3:397–412.

11. Wilms W. Vocational education and job success: the employer's view. *Phi Delta Kappa* 1984;65:347–350.

12. Haffey WJ, Lewis FD. Programming for occupational outcome following traumatic brain injury. *Rehabil Psychol* 1989;34:147–159.

13. Miller JD, Pentland B, Berrol S. Early evaluation and management. In: Rosenthal M, Bond MR, Griffith ER, Miller JD, eds. *Rehabilitation of the adult and child with traumatic brain injury,* 2nd ed. Philadelphia: F.A. Davis, 1990: 21–49.

14. Grimm BH, Bleiberg J. Psychological rehabilitation in traumatic brain injury. In: Filskov S, Boll T, eds. *Handbook of clinical neuropsychology.* New York: John Wiley & Sons, 1986:495–527.

15. Schachter DL, Glisky EL. Memory remediation: restoration, alleviation and acquisition of domain specific knowledge. In: Uzzell B, Gross Y, eds. *Clinical neuropsychology of intervention.* Boston: Martinus Nijhoff, 1986:257–282.

16. Newcombe F. Rehabilitation in clinical neurology: neuropsychological aspects. In: Vinken P, Bruyn GW, Klawans HH, eds. *Handbook of clinical neurology.* Amsterdam: Elsevier Science, 1985:609.

17. Stratton MD, Gregory RJ. Review of subject after traumatic brain injury: a discussion of consequences. *Brain Inj* 1994;8:631–645.

18. Ben-Yishay Y, Diller L. Cognitive remediation in traumatic brain injury: update and issues. *Arch Phys Med Rehabil* 1993;74:204–213.

19. Butler RH, Namerow NW. Cognitive retraining in brain injury rehabilitation: a critical review. *J Neurol Rehabil* 1988;2:97–103.

20. Luria AR. *Restoration of function after brain injury.* New York: Macmillan, 1963.

21. Levin HS, Kraus MF. The frontal lobes and traumatic brain injury. *J Neuropsychiatry Clin Neurosci* 1994;6(4):443–454.

22. Benedict RR. The effectiveness of cognitive remediation strategies for victims of traumatic head injury: a review of the literature. *Clin Psychol Rev* 1989;9:608–626.

23. Levin HS. Cognitive rehabilitation, unproven but promising. *Arch Neuro* 1990;47:223–224.

24. Cope DN, Cole JR, Hall KM, Barkan H. Brain-injury: analysis of outcome in a post-acute rehabilitation system. Part 1: general analysis. *Brain Inj* 1991;5:111–126.

25. Bond MR, Brooks DN. Understanding the process of recovery as a basis for the investigation of rehabilitation for the brain injured. *Scand J Rehabil Med* 1976;8: 127–133.

26. Klonoff H, Low MD, Clark C. Head injuries in children: a perspective five year follow up. *J Neurol Neurosurg Psychiatry* 1977;40:1211–1219.

27. Thomsen IV. Neuropsychological treatment and long-term follow-up in an aphasic patient with very severe head trauma. *J Clin Neuropsychol* 1981;3:43–51.

28. Sbordone RJ, Liter JC, Pettler-Jennings P. Recovery of function following severe traumatic brain injury: a retrospective 10-year follow-up. *Brain Inj* 1995;9:285–299.

29. Terayama Y, Meyer JS, Kawamura J. Cognitive recovery with long-term increases of cerebral perfusion after head injury. *Surg Neurol* 1991;36:335–342.

30. Prigatano GP, et al. *Neuropsychological rehabilitation after brain injury.* Baltimore: Johns Hopkins University Press, 1986.

31. Scherzer BP. Rehabilitation following severe head trauma: results of a three year program. *Arch Phys Med Rehabil* 1986;67: 366–374.

32. Ben-Yishay Y, et al. Relationships between aspects of anterograde amnesia and vocational aptitude in traumatically brain damaged patients: preliminary findings. In: Ben-Yishay Y, ed. *NYU rehabilitation monograph,* no. 61. 1980:55.

33. Ben-Yishay Y, et al. Rehabilitation of cognitive and perceptual defects in people with traumatic brain damage: a five year clinical research study. In: Ben-Yishay Y, ed. *NYU rehabilitation monograph,* no. 64. 1982:127.

34. Ezrachi O, et al. Rehabilitation of cognitive and perceptual defects in people with traumatic brain damage: a five year clinical research study: results of the second phase. In: Ben-Yisha Y, ed. *NYU rehabilitation monograph,* no. 66. 1983:53.

35. Prigatano GP, Fordyce DJ, Zeiner HK, et al. Neuropsychological rehabilitation after closed head injury in young adults. *J Neurol Neurosurg Psychiatry* 1984;47: 505–513.

36. Kaplan CP, Corrigan JD. The relationship between cognition and functional independence in adults with traumatic brain injury. *Arch Phys Med Rehabil* 1994;75: 643–647.

37. Volpe BT, McDowell FH. The efficacy of cognitive rehabilitation in patient with traumatic brain injury. *Arch Neurol* 1990;47: 220–222.

38. Diller L. Neuropsychological rehabilitation. In: Meier MJ, Benton AL, Diller L, eds. *Neuropsychological rehabilitation.* London: Churchill Livingstone, 1987:1–17.

39. Levin HS, Eisenberg HM, Benton AL, eds. *Frontal lobe function and dysfunction.* New York: Oxford University Press, 1991.

40. Wilson B. Memory therapy in practice. In: Wilson B, Moffatt N, eds. *Clinical management of memory problems.* London: Croom Helm, 1984:89–112.

41. Gordon WA, Hibbard M. The theory and practice of cognitive remediation. In: Kreutzer J, Wehman PE, eds. *Cognitive rehabilitation for persons with traumatic brain injury: a functional approach.* Baltimore: Paul H. Brookes Publishing Co, 1991:13–22.

42. Adamovich BLB. Traumatic brain injury. In: LaPoint LL, ed. *Aphasia and related neurogenic language disorders.* 2nd ed. New York: Thieme Medical, 1997.

43. Collins A, Brown JS, Newman SE. Cognitive apprenticeship: teaching the crafts of reading, writing and mathematics. In: Resnick LB, ed. *Knowing, learning, and instruction: essays in honor of Robert Glaser.* Hillsdale, NJ: Erlbaum, 1989.

44. Bruner JS, ed. *Toward a theory of instruction.* New York: WW Norton & Company, Inc, 1996.

45. Ben-Yishay Y, Prigatano GP. Cognitive remediation. In: Rosenthal ER, Griffith M, Griffith ER, et al, eds. *Rehabilitation of the adult and child with traumatic brain injury.* 2nd ed. Philadelphia: Davis, 1990:393–400.

46. Adamovich BLB, Henderson J. *Scales of Cognitive Ability for Traumatic Brain Injury* (SCATBI). Chicago: Riverside Publishing, 1992.

47. Prigatano GP, Klonoff PS, Bailey I. Psychosocial adjustment associated with traumatic brain injury: statistics BNI neuro-rehabilitation must beat. *BNI Q* 1987;3:10–17.

48. Ben-Yishay Y, Silver S, Piasetsky E, Rattok J. Relationship between employability and vocational outcome after intensive holistic cognitive rehabilitation. *J Head Trauma Rehabil* 1987;2:35–49.

49. Ponsford JL, Olver JH. A profile of outcome: 2 years after traumatic brain injury. *Brain Inj* 1995;9: 1–10.

50. Ryan TV, Ruff RM. The efficacy of structured memory retraining in a group comparison of head injured patient. *Arch Clin Neuropsychol* 1988;3:165–179.

51. Parenté R, DiCesare A. Retraining memory: theory, evaluation and application. In: Kreutzer JS, Wehman PE, eds. *Cognitive rehabilitation for persons with traumatic brain injury: a functional approach.* Baltimore: Brookes, 1991.

52. Sohlberg MM, White O, Evans E, Mateer C. Background and initial case studies into the effects of prospective memory training. *Brain Inj* 1992;6:129–138.

53. Craine JF, Gudeman HE, eds. *Rehabilitation of brain function: principles, procedures, and techniques of neurotraining.* Springfield, IL: Charles C. Thomas, 1981.

54. Wilson BA. *Rehabilitation of memory.* New York: Guilford, 1987.

55. Glasgow RE, Zeiss RA, Barrera MD, Lewinsohn P. Case studies on remediating memory deficits in brain damaged individuals. *J Clin Psychol* 1977;33:1049–1054.

56. Parenté FJ, Anderson-Parenté JK, Shaw B. Retraining the mind's eye. *J Head Trauma Rehabil* 1989;4:53–62.

57. Wilson BA, Moffat N, eds. *Clinical management of memory problems.* Rockville, MD: Aspen Systems, 1984.

58. Sohlberg MM, Mateer CA. Effectiveness of an attention training program. *J Clin Exp Neuropsychol* 1987;9:117–130.

59. Godfrey H, Knight R. Cognitive rehabilitation of memory functioning in amnesic alcoholics. *J Consult Clin Psychol* 1985;43:555–557.

60. Schachter D, Rich SS, Stampp H. Remediation of memory disorders: experimental evaluation of the spaced-retrieval technique. *J Clin Exp Neuropsychol* 1985;7: 79–96.

61. Cermak LS. Imagery as an aid to retrieval for Korsakoff patients. *Cortex* 1975;11:163–169.

62. Gianutsos R, Gianutsos J. Rehabilitating the verbal recall of brain injured patients by mnemonic training: an experimental demonstration using single case methodology. *J Clin Neuropsychol* 1979; 1:117.

63. Ruff RM, Marshall LF, Crouch J, et al. Predictors of outcome following severe head trauma: follow-up data from the Traumatic Coma Data Bank. *Brain Inj* 1993;7:101–111.

64. Cicerone KD, Giacino JT. Remediation of executive function deficits after traumatic brain injury. *Neuropsychol Rehabil* 1992;2:12–22.

65. Patten BM. The ancient art of memory: usefulness in treatment. *Arch Neurol* 1972;26:28–31.

66. Jones MK. Imagery as a mnemonic aid after left temporal lobectomy: contrast between material specific and generalized memory disorders. *Neuropsychologia* 1974;12:21–30.

67. Crovitz LS. Memory retraining in brain-damaged patients: the airplane list. *Cortex* 1979;15:131–134.

68. Lorayne H, Lucas J. *The memory book.* New York: Ballantine Books, 1974.

69. Moffat N. Strategies of memory therapy In: Wilson BA, Moffat N, eds. *Clinical management of memory problems.* Rockville, MD: Aspen, 1984:63–88.

70. Schacter DL, Crovitz HF. Memory function after closed head injury: a review of quantitative research. *Cortex* 1977;13:150–176.

71. Sohlberg MM, Mateer CA, eds. *Introduction to cognitive rehabilitation: theory and practice.* New York: The Guilford Press, 1989.

72. Kreutzer JS, Wehman P, Morton MV, Stonnington HH. Supported employment and compensatory strategies for enhancing vocational outcome following traumatic brain injury. *Brain Inj* 1988;3: 205–223.

73. Fowler R, Hart J, Sheahan M. A prosthetic: an application of the prosthetic environment concept. *Rehabil Counsel Bull* 1972;15: 80–85.

74. Sohlberg MM, Mateer CA. Training use of compensatory memory books: a three-stage behavioral approach. *J Clin Exp Neuropsychol* 1989;11:871–891.

75. Harris J. External memory aids. In: Gruneberg M, Morris P, Sykes RN, eds. *Practical aspects of memory.* London: Academic, 1978:172–179.

76. Alexander MP, Benson DF, Stuss DT. Frontal lobes and language. *Brain Lang* 1989;37:656–691.

77. Fryer J, Fralish K. Cognitive rehabilitation. In: Deutsch PM, Fralish KB, eds. *Innovations in head injury rehabilitation.* Albany, NY: Matthew Bender, 1989:7-1–7-35.

78. Brooks N, McKinlay W, Symington D, et al. Return to work within the first seven years of severe head injury. *Brain Inj* 1987;1:5-29.

79. Gloag D. Rehabilitation after head injury: cognitive problems. *BMJ* 1985:290:834–837.

80. Hart T, Hayden MD. The ecological validity of neuropsychological assessment and remediation. In: Uzzell BP, Gross Y, eds. *Clinical neuropsychology of intervention.* Boston: Martinus Nijhoff, 1986:21–50.

81. Adamovich BLB. Pitfalls in functional assessment: a comparison of FIM ratings by speech-language pathologists and nurses. *Neurorehabilitation* 1992;2(4):42–51.

82. Adamovich BLB. Functional outcomes: assessment and intervention considerations. (in press).

83. Adamovich BLB. Comparisons of connected speech effectiveness using traditional therapeutic methods and functional community based activities with neurologically impaired adults. Presented at the Clinical Aphasiology Conference, Newport, RI, 1996.

84. Nicholas LE, Brookshire RH. A system for scoring main concepts in the discourse of non-brain-damaged and aphasic speakers. *Clin Aphasiol* 1993;21:87–99.

Chapter 36

Adaptive Systems: Adaptive Seating and Assistive Technology

Susan L. Garber
Thomas A. Krouskop
Kevin Magee
Mary Frances Baxter
Roger E. Levy

INTRODUCTION

Assistive technology has been defined as "any item, piece of equipment or product system, whether acquired commercially off the shelf, modified or customized, that is used to increase, maintain or improve the functional capabilities of individuals with disabilities" (1). Included within this definition are devices that run the gamut from simple durable medical equipment such as canes, walkers, adaptive utensils, and seating and mobility devices, to high-technology systems for augmentive communication, environmental control, and computer access. Historically, assistive technology had its beginnings in the early 1970s with the establishment of the federally funded Rehabilitation Engineering Centers (2). Each center focused on a particular problem faced by persons with physical impairments and integrated the skills of clinicians and engineers to solve these problems. Since that time, there has been a dramatic expansion of technology into practically every aspect of care for persons with severe physical impairments. Technology impacts on seating, positioning, and mobility; activities of daily living; employment and education; and even leisure activities. All of these technological systems and devices have one principal purpose: to assist the person with physical limitations to achieve his or her highest level of personal autonomy.

The Rehabilitation Act defines rehabilitation technology as "the systematic application of technologies, engineering methodologies, and scientific principles to meet the needs of and address the barriers confronted by individuals with disabilities in areas which include education, rehabilitation, employment, transportation, independent living, and recreation. The term encompasses rehabilitation engineering, assistive technology devices, and assistive technology services" (3). It is evident from this definition that the provision of rehabilitation technology services (adaptive systems) is more than a product. Rehabilitation technology is, in fact, a process.

The first step in the process of providing technology to a person with a physical impairment is to define the problem or the issues to be resolved. Although barriers to functional independence may appear obvious, and easily remedied by technology, environmental, social, and lifestyle considerations must not be overlooked. Therefore, a hierarchy of devices and systems has evolved from which the technology is selected (Table 36-1). Within this hierarchy of devices or systems to be provided, one should first consider compensatory strategies, which are solutions with no hardware associated with them. Such compensatory strategies might include task or work flow restructuring. Task restructuring may include taking nonessential tasks that are barriers to completing a job and trading with another employee for a task that the impaired individual can complete. For example, if an employee is unable to file, perhaps he or she can take additional phone duty. Changing work flow may be as simple as changing the position of equipment or reversing items on a desk that was set up for a right-handed individual for easy left-handed operation.

Table 36-1: Hierarchy of Technological Devices
1. Compensatory strategies, e.g., task restructuring, work flow restructuring
2. Off-the-shelf technologies
3. Customized devices

However, often it is not one single barrier that needs to be overcome, but multiple problems which cannot be solved by a single compensatory strategy.

Next in the hierarchy of devices or systems is off-the-shelf technology. There has been a veritable explosion in the numbers of products and assistive devices on the market today. Everything from therapist-constructed devices for activities of daily living to the most sophisticated systems for environmental control and augmentive communication have become more readily available. However, even off-the-shelf devices may require custom modification such as special mounting hardware or adaptation of the switching or control apparatus for better access. The major problem often encountered with off-the-shelf devices is that the consumer of these devices may see only a brochure or a picture of the device in a catalogue and does not have the opportunity to have a hands-on trial with the device. If the device is purchased, it may meet the individual's needs or it might be discarded soon after purchase for any one of a number of reasons. These include problems with fit, function, durability, and unrealistic expectations. Another major problem derived from the expansion in the number of systems and devices available for persons with physical impairments is that today, professionals in the field of rehabilitation in general, and specifically rehabilitation technology, are finding it increasingly difficult to keep pace with the newest developments. Therefore, clinicians who recommend devices and systems may not be able to provide the most current information to the clients they serve.

The last category in the hierarchy of technological devices is the individually customized device. This group may require expensive materials and fabrication methods as well as a great deal of time allocated to train the user in its proper operation and maintenance. For this reason, it is essential that a budget for materials, construction, and training be developed and explained. It is also important to identify strategies for the ongoing maintenance of the device or system. Who will pay for it? What will the individual use when the device is out for repair or upgrading? Will the system or device be upgraded as new technology is developed?

The next step in the process, and one that is often ignored or not adequately considered, is the setup and training with the equipment. It is essential that the individual knows exactly how the equipment should be set up and has time to learn the device so that mastery in its use can be achieved. It must be remembered that there is always a learning period when one is trying out a new device or new technology, and if the end user's perception is that it is not beneficial or worth the effort, then the device or technology will never be used.

The last step in the process of providing rehabilitation technology is the follow-up. To determine whether the technology has made a difference in a person's life, it will be necessary to develop a mechanism for communicating with the user over time. Such issues as device utilization, satisfaction, and maintenance must be addressed. At each step in the process of providing rehabilitation technology, it may be necessary to redefine and reassess the individual's abilities and the limitations or barriers to be overcome. In some cases, major physical, psychological, or social changes can impact on the original recommendations. Medical complications, family and financial problems, and living arrangements can alter dramatically the utilization of prescribed devices. One final factor that needs to be addressed is that evaluating for and providing rehabilitation technology must be a team effort, with the end user as the key member of the team.

Within the last decade, the technology applied specifically to rehabilitation of physically impaired persons has become more sophisticated and to a great extent, more expensive. Conversely, insurance providers are reluctant, if not outright refusing, to fund much of this equipment. Federal legislation, such as the Americans with Disabilities Act of 1990 (4) and the Technology-Related Assistance for Individuals with Disabilities Act of 1988 (5), has resulted in better access to the technological advances available (6–8). Nevertheless, studies have shown that often the equipment is not provided or once provided, has not lived up to its expectations (9). One of the frequently cited obstacles to obtaining technology is the lack of information about technological systems by both persons with impairments and the professionals with whom they work (7). However, information dissemination has improved with the publication of relevant material in the *Technology Special Interest Section Newsletter* of the American Occupational Therapy Association (AOTA), the *Assistive Technology Guide* published by AOTA, Rehabilitation Engineering Society of North America (RESNA) publications such as the journal *Assistive Technology*, and consumer publications such as *Accent on Living*, ABLEDATA, *Team Rehab*, *New Mobility*, *Paraplegia News*, and *Sports n' Spokes*.

CATEGORIES OF ADAPTIVE SYSTEMS

In this chapter, the following categories of adaptive systems are addressed: seating, positioning, and mobility devices; robotics; environmental control systems; augmentive communication systems; and computers. Although these categories may be more in the realm of high technology, it must be clear that equipment and devices described as low technology are no less important, since often they can provide the consumer with enhanced independence and quality of life.

SEATING, POSITIONING, AND MOBILITY

Seating and mobility comprise the foundation from which persons with severe physical impairments can achieve autonomy. This derives from the fact that the wheelchair and seating system are the first pieces of equipment that allow the individual to interact with his or her environment and to begin the process of regaining personal control over activities of daily living. For this reason, the wheelchair and seating system must provide comfort, stability, and balance while helping to prevent secondary complications such as contractures and pressure ulcers. Although wheeled vehicles can be traced back 5000 years, the idea that a wheelchair must be sized for the person using it and must fit the user's expected lifestyle has developed only since World War II. The philosophy of rehabilitation that encompasses independence, self-care, and vocational and avocational pursuits evolved at the conclusion of World War II when clinicians began to recognize the need to provide wheelchairs that met individual patient's requirements. The objective selection of wheelchair cushions was unheard of before the early 1970s (10). Today, therapists carry out comprehensive seating evaluations that not only include the wheelchair and seat cushion, but also address the back unit as well, hence, the seating conceptualization (11).

Prior to the 1980s, wheelchair seating was categorized as either seating for pressure relief or seating for positioning. Seating for pressure relief usually was reserved for individuals with spinal cord injury, whereas seating for positioning initially was developed specifically for children with cerebral palsy (12). Individuals in nursing homes and those who had strokes were largely ignored with regard to their seating needs, a fact that has not changed dramatically since that time.

The perfect seating surface would have the following characteristics:

- Minimizes the pressure under the bony prominences
- Controls the pressure gradient in the tissue
- Provides stability for performing functional activities
- Allows independent or assisted weight shifts
- Allows transfers
- Controls the temperature at the tissue interface
- Controls the moisture at the skin surface
- Is lightweight
- Is low cost
- Is durable
- Minimizes deformities

Unfortunately, a support system that incorporates all of these characteristics for every user does not yet exist and the rehabilitation professional must use judgment to create the best possible match between available products and the needs of the person being treated.

Table 36-2: Criteria for the Selection of Seating Systems
Intrinsic variables
Diagnosis—including attention to absent or diminished sensation
Tissue history—previous breakdowns, surgical repair, stress
Body build
Magnitude and distribution of interface pressures
Extrinsic variables
Number of hours spent on the seating surface each day
Types of activities performed while on the seating surface
Usage environment—temperature, humidity, continence
Living arrangements—level of personal autonomy
Type of wheelchair
Compatibility with wheelchair and other assistive devices
Ease of patient follow-up

Technology for Pressure Management

The prescription of appropriate and effective wheelchair seating, including cushions, is a complex process that involves therapists, physicians, and the patient and family. Therapists employ a number of strategies to select cushions, including objective assessments using mechanical, electrical, or computerized devices that quantitatively monitor the magnitude and location of pressure. The technology, however, must be applied in combination with issues of clinical judgment such as identifying lifestyle factors specific to each individual (13–15). Two groups of client-related variables must be considered when prescribing a seating system; the intrinsic factors and extrinsic factors are shown in Table 36-2. Technological advances in seating for persons vulnerable to pressure ulcers include 1) alarm systems, 2) support surfaces, 3) evaluation tools, and 4) computer-generated and interactive educational materials.

Alarm Systems

Alarm systems were developed to remind persons, especially those with impaired sensation, to shift their weight regularly to prevent pressure ulcers (16,17). At preset intervals, the alarm system "reminded" the person to shift his or her weight. Unfortunately, these alarm systems were not successful in reducing the occurrence of pressure ulcers, first because it was not possible to determine what sitting interval was "safe" for a specific person and second, because the alarms were intrusive and resulted in too much attention being drawn to the person. Finally, these

Table 36-3: Various Seating Systems and Their Advantages and Limitations

Product Class	Advantages	Limitations
Air-filled products	Lightweight Easy to clean Effective with many people Promotes even distribution of pressure Reduces shear	Subject to puncture Repair difficulty Must monitor inflation routinely May compromise user stability May exacerbate postural deformities
Fluid-filled products	Easy to clean Effective with a broad group of users Promotes even distribution of pressure Skin temperature control	Often heavy May compromise user stability May exacerbate postural deformities Subject to puncture Repair difficulty Weight
Gel-filled products	Effectively reduces shear Easy to clean Shock absorbency	Must be stored flat Puncture susceptibility Life expectancy Not washable
Foam products	Lightweight Cost Can be easily modified Many variations	Support properties change with time
Combination products	Easily modified Easily customized	Components may be lost Fitting Weight

systems were limited by timing parameters and data storage limitations. Many of the systems developed never left the hospital or laboratories in which they were developed; they simply were not applicable to the lifestyles of the persons for whom they were designed.

Support Surfaces

Wheelchair cushions are frequently prescribed for persons with absent or diminished sensation or mobility. Their primary purpose is to reduce the pressure between an individual and the seating surface, especially the wheelchair. Many cushions are on the market today and can be fit into convenient classes based on the type of materials used. These categories and their advantages and disadvantages are described in Table 36-3.

Effective wheelchair cushions reduce interface pressure, promote sitting balance and stability, and provide comfort. It is important to note, however, that the wheelchair cushion neither prevents nor heals pressure ulcers. Rather, the wheelchair cushion is one element within a comprehensive approach to pressure ulcer prevention and management. Other important factors include careful daily skin inspection, weight shifts, hygiene, and diet. One other factor that must not be overlooked is the wheelchair cushion's compatibility with the wheelchair itself and any accessory equipment attached to it, such as back cushions or custom-designed contoured or molded seat and back systems. Assessments for wheelchair cushions should be individualized for each person and should be repeated on a regular basis. Seating requirements change as people age. Therefore, seating must change also to accommodate anatomic and physiologic changes that occur as part of the normal aging process.

Methods to Evaluate the Effectiveness of Pressure Relief Systems

Unfortunately, we do not currently have a clinically measurable tissue viability factor that permits us to evaluate the status of the tissue and predict when the tissue is in danger of dying (18,19). A number of technologies have been developed to help assess the effectiveness of a support surface selected to reduce the risk of developing a pressure ulcer (20,21). The primary methods that have been used either clinically or experimentally include the following:

Blood flow measurements

Detection of reactive hyperemia

Surface thermography

Measurements of tissue deformations

Intratissue pressure measurements

Interface pressure measurements

Each of these modalities has limitations. These limitations should be considered when a technology is being used to document the efficacy of the support surface selected for a client.

Measurements of tissue deformations and intratissue pressures have been used only in experimental situations (18). To date, the only means to image directly the deformations that the tissues undergo when loaded is magnetic resonance imaging (MRI). The problem of placing the client and support surface in the imaging system and the time and cost associated with using the equipment have limited the use of tissue deformation imaging to small experimental situations. However, the concept of directly monitoring the tissue deformation so that it can be controlled and limit the disruption of transport phenomena in the tissue continues to be an area of research interest. Wick catheters have been used for a number of years to measure directly the pressures that exist in the extracellular fluid. Experimentally, they have been used successfully, but clinically they have limited value since they are invasive and require multiple insertion points to provide a useful description of the pressures in the loaded tissue.

Clinically, detection of reactive hyperemia has been used most universally to evaluate the effectiveness of the support surface. The problem with this modality is that it is not predictive and its use is time-consuming since the technique requires the client to use the support surface until the tissue reacts to it with an unblanchable reddened area that persists for more than 5 minutes. To measure blood flow to evaluate the performance of a support surface, Doppler flow transducers are often used (22). These devices often only detect flow in the tissue closest to the surface, the top 3 to 5 mm, and blood flow in this layer of tissue is mostly for thermal regulation: Only about 5% of the flow is needed to provide nourishment for the cells. Moreover, flow at the surface, due to the numerous shunts, is not a clear indicator of flow in the deeper tissues, the area where pressure ulcers first develop. Measurements of the temperatures of the skin surface also have been used clinically, but the equipment is expensive and the sensitivity of the technique has never been established clinically.

In the experience of many people (23–25), the most reliable, easily used method in the clinical environment is to measure interface pressure. Interface pressure, while not a perfect predictor, does permit the clinician to select the support surface that provides the lowest peak pressures as well as the best pressure distribution over the supported tissue. While interface pressures provide "snapshot" data, they can be used to compare the relative effectiveness of different products available at a particular institution.

When interface pressures are used as a screening tool for product selection, care must be taken to ensure that the data being used for the comparison are indeed comparable (26). Generally, interface pressure data collected using different instrumentation or by different investigations are not comparable. The instrumentation used to measure interface pressures affects the readings; the size, shape, and positioning of the pressure sensor affect the absolute value of the pressure being monitored. One method of making the data collected by different groups comparable is to have the data presented as percentages of the interface pressure measured on a standard surface rather than as absolute pressure readings. Making relative measurements involves collecting data when the subjects are supported on a standard surface like a new Staphcheck-covered hospital mattress or the unpadded sling seat of a wheelchair, and using these readings as the base for the relative readings. This technique greatly reduces the differences in the readings that are due to the operating characteristics of the instrumentation used to make the measurements.

Further complicating the issue of selecting a support surface is the continuing confusion about the importance of maintaining interface pressure below 32 mm Hg. It must be remembered that 32 mm Hg is an average value for the capillary pressure in the fingertips of young healthy male volunteers: In the literature, the range of capillary pressures is from less than 20 mm Hg to over 40 mm Hg. Capillary pressures as low as 12 mm Hg have been reported in geriatric patients. Moreover, interface pressure measurements do not necessarily reflect the actual pressures acting on the capillaries. Therefore, keeping interface pressures below 32 mm Hg may be a useful guideline but does not ensure that flow in the capillaries will be uninterrupted.

The absolute value of the interface pressure readings provides very little information that is useful to the clinician, and interface pressure readings should only be used to make relative judgments about the effectiveness of various products. By only considering the products that produce the lowest interface pressures, the care provider can eliminate products that are not effective for a particular user.

Technical Advances in Pressure Ulcer Education

Within the last decade, computer technology has been incorporated into the educational programs for health care professionals and their patients. Computer-assisted instruction (CAI) and interactive videodisc (IVD) are being used with increasing frequency to teach caregivers about a wide variety of topics, including pressure ulcer prevention and management. These technologies have been more widely accepted in recent years and have proved to be effective and cost-efficient (27).

Seating for Positioning

In the 1970s, a team of clinicians and engineers, working primarily with children with cerebral palsy, recognized that traditional wheelchairs and cushions were inadequate to meet the needs of these children (28). Seating systems for these children had to address such issues as head and neck verticality, lumbar spine support, hip flexion and abduction, and arm support so that mobility and function would be maximized. Off-the-shelf and readily available modular inserts provided therapists with relatively low-cost interchangeable components that addressed specific physical and functional needs of the child. These included headrests, side bolsters, pommels, lap trays, shoe holders, and seats that were available within a facility and individualized to each patient. These components often were attached to a reclining-back wheelchair in an effort to minimize abnormal reflexes and tone.

Custom Seating

In recent years, advances in materials and computer technology have expanded the seating industry. Contouring, position-in-space, and computer-aided design and manufacture (CAD/CAM) provide highly specialized seating, positioning, and mobility systems for individuals with severe skeletal abnormalities such as scoliosis, kyphosis, lordosis, joint contractures, dislocations, and other bony and soft-tissue deformities. Customization helps to reduce muscle tone and inhibit abnormal postural reflexes.

Although the seating system is designed to provide comfort and support and to enhance functional performance, it will not correct skeletal anomalies.

Contouring and position-in-space are two approaches for customizing a seating system. Each can be used independently or in combination with each other or with other seating techniques (29). For individuals with severe skeletal deformity or imbalanced muscle tone, contouring evenly distributes body contact over large surface areas. Among the techniques that constitute contouring are the sculpting of blocks of foam, adjustable modular linkage systems (Matrix), enclosed bead systems, foam-in-place, commercially fabricated systems, and computer shape sensing. Most of these methods are labor-intensive and expensive and often require modification even after construction appears complete (29).

Two methods of foam-in-place seating are used currently: direct and indirect. In the direct technique, foam-producing chemicals are poured into a bag that has been placed under and around the body. This method is fast, relatively inexpensive, and comfortable for the patient, and reduces pressure. However, it is difficult to use with individuals who have increased muscle tone or sensitivity to heat or whose position is difficult to maintain (29). The indirect foam-in-place method requires a custom molding frame as does the fabrication of commercially contoured seats and computer-generated shape sensing. The molding frame simulates the optimum seated position and produces a model of the person's body. The resulting castings of both the seat and the back can be used independently or as cojointed parts of the seating system. After the patient is removed from the molding frame, a plaster cast is made directly on the frame. The cast is then used as the mold for the foam and can be completed on-site or it can be sent to an outside vendor for commercial fabrication. If the seating system is completed on-site, it can be modified and adapted more efficiently.

Computer shape sensing is used to produce contoured seating. In this technology, evaluation data are entered into a machine that produces an exact copy. Two approaches are currently used. The first requires that the patient sit on sensors embedded in a foam cushion. The resulting digital printout is scanned by a machine which produces a finished cushion that corresponds to the contour information recorded on the printout. The second method requires the use of a bead-filled fitting chair. A stylus traces the contours of the imprint left by the person's body after he or she is removed from the chair. This produces digitized data which are then fed into a machine that produces a contoured cushion (29). In a recent study, the CAD/CAM method was found to be significantly better than the hand-sculpting methods in terms of on-site fabrication time, although there were no significant differences with regard to initial fitting time, final fitting time, clinician insert rating, and client satisfaction (30).

Table 36-4: Relationships Between Seating Purpose and Performance Criteria

Performance Criteria	Purpose		
	Comfort	Posture Control and Positioning	Pressure Management
Life expectancy	x	x	x
Moisture control	x		x
Temperature control			x
Pressure control	x		x
Service requirements	x	x	x
Fail safety	x	x	x
Infection control			x
Flammability	x	x	x
Friction control	x	x	x

Position-in-space systems such as the tilt-in-space models change the position of the person in the chair in space without changing the seat-to-back angle. This technology provides an individual who has severe physical impairments, abnormal tone and reflexes, and limited endurance with the ability to use multiple positions in space to maximize function and mobility. An individual can perform activities from an upright or anteriorly tilted position and return to neutral or posteriorly tilted positions as necessitated by the change in activity or the need to rest. These technologies have reduced the need for restraints such as straps, lap boards, and knee blocks and have enhanced the cosmetic acceptability of these devices. Furthermore, they allow the individual to use his or her upper extremities for functional activities rather than for stabilization (29).

When prescribing a seating system, it is important to remember the purpose that the seating system is to fulfill. For the seat to accomplish its purpose, the clinician must consider the relation between that purpose and the criteria that define the system's performance. These relations are summarized in Table 36-4.

ROBOTICS

Rehabilitation robotic systems that interact with humans consist almost universally of the following components: the robotic device, the computer that controls the robot, the human user, devices for communication between the human and the computer, and instruments for monitoring the surrounding environment (31–34). A major difference between rehabilitation robotics systems and many other robotics systems is that often the human must occupy portions of the robot's workspace, and even come in direct contact with the robot at times, such as when the robot is expected to assist in activities of daily living (35–37). This poses a safety hazard for the user that does not exist in industrial robot systems, since safety standards governing industrial systems are based on the principle that a human should never occupy a robot's workspace when the robot is activated (35,38). Thus, separate safety standards for rehabilitation robotics systems should be developed in order to optimize safety for the systems' users. Safety should be considered in the design and construction phases of a system as well as in the implementation phase (39–43).

The key to the user's safety is the realistic expectation he or she has of the system. The user should not only be aware of the robot's strength, range of motion, and achievable speeds, but also understand the expected failure rate on each of these parameters. There must be a comprehensive training period during which the user is acquainted with the new system's performance, advantages, and limitations (44).

There are few commercially successful examples of robot arms frequently used for "pick-and-place" tasks (36,45–47). In rehabilitation robotic systems the robot arm might be mounted to a workstation (31,37,41,47–53), wheelchair (47,48,53–58), or mobile base (46,48,50,59,60). Many robot arms are "anthropomorphic," that is, kinematically similar to human arms, because this design is fairly space efficient and not too difficult either to design or to control (61). Of the various types of end effectors—devices attached to the end of the arm for picking up objects—simple clamping grippers are the most common. While more sophisticated hands are being developed, they are still prohibitively large and expensive at this time (42,49,60,62).

Two entities share responsibility for the control of a rehabilitation robot: the user and the robot's computer. There is essentially a trade-off between control of the robot by the user and automatic control of the robot by the computer (63–65). If the user delegates control of the robot to the computer, then the user is free to devote attention to other things. However, because the robot's computer does not possess human reasoning and judgment, it may make decisions that are inappropriate or even dangerous. On the other hand, if the user does not delegate control to the computer, then operating the robot can require virtually all the user's attention to accomplish even the most simple tasks (63).

Programming a computer to be "intelligent" (66) can allow it to exercise more control over the robot but still make decisions that are safe and satisfying to the human user (36). Many approaches to artificial intelligence have been developed, including expert systems, fuzzy logic, genetic algorithms (GAs), and genetic programming (GP). An expert system is a set of information that has been encoded in the form of rules, usually "if-then" rules typically elicited from a human expert's knowledge of a situation (67–69). A major limitation of traditional expert systems is their inability to process imprecise information. Fuzzy logic provides a quantitative way of handling the ambiguity and imprecision inherent in linguistic communication (66,69,70). This hallmark of fuzzy logic is potentially of great value to any system in which a human is frequently interacting with a robot, since human users often provide imprecise information to the computer, yet expect it to control the robot precisely as they wish (60,66).

Another type of intelligent computer control, Artificial Neural Network (ANN), is based on function of a human brain in that a large number of simple "neurons" are connected together to perform complex computational tasks (71). In robotics, often there is no attempt to create an accurate model of the brain; rather, ANNs are used as a programming tool for representing information that is not easily represented by other methods, such as procedural (as opposed to declarative) knowledge (60,70,72).

GAs and GP are artificial intelligence methodologies based on the genetic variation, environmental fitness competition, and sexual reproduction found in living organisms (73). In GAs, character strings are reproduced; in GP, computer programs and functions are reproduced. In both GAs and GP, the "population" of individuals is generated randomly, and the members of the population that are most useful in solving the problem in question are bred together to produce new and hopefully more useful individuals (74). This process repeats until an acceptable solution is achieved. Examples of applications for GAs include automatic path determination for a mobile robot (75), and for GP include the processing of the myoelectric signals necessary to control a multifingered prosthetic hand (76).

Inasmuch as the user must be able to communicate to the robot's computer, the system must include input devices—devices for recoding a user-generated signal into one that the computer is able to interpret (57,61). Common input devices include "joystick" hand controllers (58,77); switches operated by mouth, chin (77,78), breath (35,77), or small movements of arms or hands (33,79); and head-movement transducers (37,42). Other input devices include speech recognition (41,42,50,78,80,81), myoelectric signal detection (42,82), and vision systems programmed to recognize facial features (81,83) or hand shapes (84), or to track eye gaze (85).

In addition to the need for the user to communicate to the computer, there often exists a need for the user to receive information from the computer (61). This information is presented on devices called *displays*. The point is not just to output or display the information, but rather to effectively communicate it to the user. Human factor engineering must be employed to design and construct effective displays (61,86). A special challenge is encountered when a user is lacking one or more of the five senses. In this case, alternative display types, called *sensory substitution systems*, are designed to present information to one of the senses that the user possesses (87–89).

Information about the status of the robot and the environment needs to be obtained and presented to both the user and the computer. Sensors do the work of gathering this information (42). The information is then transmitted to the computer in a form it can interpret, and is often presented to the user through a display. Ultrasonic (39,90–94), infrared (39,42,90), and visible light (such as machine vision) sensors (39,51,60,66,81,94) often are used for object and obstacle detection (95). Contact with the environment can be detected with simple switches, and contact intensity can be measured with "tactile sensors" such as force-sensitive resistors and force moment transducers (46). "Whisker"- and "antenna"-style sensors can actually detect shapes of obstacles and objects (96). Internal robot sensors collect robot status data such as the position, velocity, and acceleration of the robot arm, and the magnitude and direction of any forces or torques acting on the robot (48). Recently robots have even employed odor sensors for navigation tasks (97).

The entire system—the robot, its computer, the user, the input devices, the displays, and the sensors—must interact successfully with the surrounding environment. Because even the most "intelligent" computers do not approach the complexity of the human brain, robots cannot reliably function in an environment designed for humans. Thus, sometimes the environment must be adapted for the robot (48,98). For example, radio transmitters can be installed in a building enabling a mobile robot to triangulate its position much more accurately than it could calculate using internal robot sensors. Or, if a standard path is to be followed, a simple strip of magnetic tape on the floor can keep a robot on track. For manipulation tasks to which humans routinely apply a great deal of dexterity, special handles can be mounted on objects, rendering them much easier to manage for a robot arm with a simple gripper. Some of these adaptations are similar to those an occupational therapist would make for a person with a physical impairment, whether or not a robot would be involved; thus, occupational therapists or similar professionals are well suited for the work of designing such adaptations (44).

Robotic systems have been developed and evaluated within clinical facilities in which persons with severe physical limitations participate in dynamic rehabilitation programs (99). Most of these systems are voice activated and microprocessor based. Despite their technological glamour and mystique, robots have yet to live up to their potential for providing assistance to persons with physical impairments, primarily because the technology has not yet advanced to a usable form (31–34). Future acceptance of robotics will depend on cost-benefit analyses, reliability, and durability, as well as on knowledgeable professionals who must train in the use of these systems (100).

ENVIRONMENTAL CONTROL

The earliest environmental control units (ECUs), designed in England in the 1960s, were developed for persons with poliomyelitis and high-level quadriplegia (101). The primary purpose of this technology is to provide individuals with severe limitations in motor function with the opportunity to achieve greater levels of functional independence and quality of life in their home, work, school, and leisure environments (102–104). The ECU remotely controls electronic items in these environments. The primary methods by which ECUs transmit signals are by radio frequency, infrared, or ultrasound. In the radio frequency method, each item to be operated has its own module which is plugged into a wall socket. The appliances are then plugged into the modules (104). Several different electrical devices can be controlled with one ECU because each module is set to pick up different frequency signals. Radio frequency units are relatively inexpensive, readily available commercially in retail stores, and easy to install and do not have to be in the same room to operate. However, they only turn items off or on and each appliance requires separate modules (104).

Infrared units operate when a high-frequency light beam is sent directly from the ECU base unit to an infrared-compatible appliance such as a stereo, video recorder, or television. Some infrared modules also function similarly to the radio frequency units and can control on-off functions (104).

Ultrasound signals operate appliances in the same way as radio frequency in that only the modules pick up the ultrasonic transmission. They are easy to install and use existing house wiring. However, they are expensive, must be in the same room as the appliances to be operated, and work only with TASH ECUs (104).

The evaluation process for ECUs consists of three major elements: method of access, identifying ECU needs, and funding (104). Access to the ECU is accomplished by mouth stick, switch, or voice. Mouth stick access requires good head and neck control. This access method is simple, inexpensive, and easy to learn and can be used with switch access (104). However, it may be aesthetically unpleasant to some, requires a mounting system, can result in neck and jaw pain, and makes speaking difficult while in use (104). Switch access is recommended for individuals with limited neck mobility and head control. This access method is very versatile because the switches are controlled by the movements most easily and efficiently accomplished by the person. These include movements of the head, lips, tongue, jaw, eye, eyelid, and eyebrow. This method of ECU access requires that the switch scan through the entire menu (e.g., lights for a specific area, TV, telephone) until it reaches the desired item, at which time the person hits the switch. Pneumatic switches can be operated using a sipping or puffing movement which requires only that the individual be able to perform lip closure. Switches are readily available in a wide range of price categories. However, they break down easily and the user may experience physical fatigue from repetitive motions (104). In the voice access method of ECU activation, the ECU responds to voice commands through direct selection, eliminating scanning through the menu. Voice access is more aesthetically pleasing and faster to respond than switch access. However, it is the most expensive method of access and usually requires extensive training. Furthermore, reliability is decreased with fluctuation in voice quality and it is time-consuming for those who are ventilator dependent (104).

Defining the specific ECU needs of the individual user is the next phase in the process of providing an ECU to a person with a severe physical impairment. A number of issues must be discussed with the potential users if an ECU is to be maximally functional. Will someone be with them throughout the entire day and night? Will they be in their residence all day or will they be going out to attend work, school, or leisure activities? What are their interests? How will they get assistance in the event of an emergency? Is the ECU to be used from both the wheelchair and the bed (104)?

Funding the purchase of an ECU is a challenge in the current climate of controlling health care costs. Documented proof of medical necessity is required in most cases and even then, the request may be denied. The consumer and his or her family will need assistance and direction in seeking the funds for this equipment. Often it may come from fund-raisers within a community (e.g., churches, Kiwanis, Rotary) or from organizations such as Easter Seals. Outcome studies that demonstrate the benefits and cost savings derived from the use of ECUs by persons with severe physical impairments are virtually nonexistent (105). Third-party payers will continue to deny funding for this type of equipment if clinicians cannot provide data that clearly illustrate its utility and efficacy. Furthermore, the clinicians who prescribe ECUs and teach patients to use them need to be better educated about this technology.

AUGMENTATIVE COMMUNICATION AND COMPUTER ACCESS

Both verbal and written communication are vital to functional living in all stages of life. Persons communicate to make wants and needs known, to express ideas, and to discuss. In infancy and the early stages of life, methods of communication include facial expressions, gross gestures, and simple vocalizations. These are used to communicate innate needs. As we develop and mature, communication is continually refined and further enhanced with language skills, subtle facial expressions, and body language and gestures. Persons born with physical and cognitive disabilities may have difficulty developing these refinements in communication. They may not be able to effectively read and use the subtle facial expressions and complex language nuances that make communicating most effective. Conditions that may interfere with the development of communication skills include cerebral palsy, autism, and other congenital conditions. Other persons develop or acquire conditions that preclude them from communicating either temporarily or permanently. These conditions include spinal cord injuries, head injuries, and degenerative neuromuscular conditions such as muscular dystrophy and amyotrophic lateral sclerosis (ALS). Other persons with temporary or permanent laryngeal blockage will also be unable to verbalize. The conditions that can lead to temporary or permanent loss of voice include intubation, spinal cord injury, and cancers of the head and neck (Fig. 36-1).

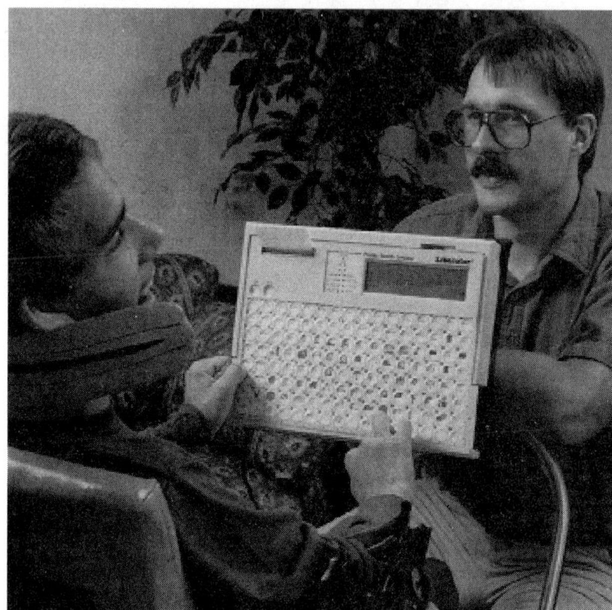

Figure 36-1. An augmentative communication device is used for a communication interaction. (Courtesy of the Prentke Romich Co., Inc.)

Historic Overview

The use of gestures and written word to convey messages has always been an alternative for lack of vocalization. There is evidence that prehistoric humans used gestures and vocalizations to express basic needs. Manual signing and gestures were also used by deaf individuals in early Rome, among monks who took vows of silence, and by explorers in eighteenth-century America to communicate with Native Americans (106). According to Zangari et al (106), augmentative and alternative communication (AAC), as it is known today, seems to have its beginnings in the 1950s. Advances in medicine and rehabilitation pioneered in the 1940s for veterans were being applied to individuals with mild and moderate cognitive impairments. In the 1960s social and political changes increased the awareness of the abilities of persons with disabilities and provided a foundation for the next three decades of AAC development. Links between the fields of technology and communication habilitation developed and from these links, advances in communication devices grew. In the 1970s AAC had significant growth in research, technology, and understanding of the linguistics of communication. Communication devices based on microprocessor technology were first available commercially in the 1970s. The first international symbol set was introduced by Charles Bliss in Canada (107). The Blissymbols is a combination of pictographic, ideographic, and arbitrary components and it is still used today. There was a tremendous expansion and dissemination of knowledge during the 1980s as well as an attempt to develop standards for the field of AAC. In 1981, the American Speech-Language Hearing Association (ASHA) formulated guidelines for the delivery of AAC services that included the determination of an AAC device versus continued oral training (106,108). Then in 1989, ASHA (109) defined the practice of AAC: "Augmentative and alternative communication is an area of clinical practice that attempts to compensate (either temporarily or permanently) for the impairment and disability patterns of individuals with severe expressive disorders (i.e., the severely speech-language and writing impaired)."

The technological advances continued through the 1980s, and a greater variety of communication devices and options became available. This trend has continued into the 1990s. Improvements in access options and voice synthesis offered greater flexibility and usability of communication aids. In addition to technological advances, there are major changes in the social/political arenas. Economic recession forced changes in the delivery of health care and some facilities that had provided evaluation and service delivery of AAC technology were forced to close. New service delivery options are still being explored. In the 1990s there are more options available in a wider range of prices and with greater functions. The consumers also have become more knowledgeable about what is available (110–113). The future can hold only increased availability and options for persons with disabilities.

Communication Systems

Communication is rarely done through a single mechanism. All persons use a combination of speech, tone of voice, gestures, body language, and written language in combination to communicate. These can be called *communication systems*. There are two commonly acknowledged categories of communication systems, unaided and aided systems. Unaided communication systems typically include vocalizations, gestures, facial expressions, and body language. Also included in unaided systems are the sign languages, including American Sign Language, signing exact English, and keyword signing.

The field of AAC usually encompasses aided communication systems. Aided communication systems involve mechanical, physical, and electronic devices that enhance the unaided abilities of the individual. A person who requires an aided system most typically does not have sufficient control of his or her voice and therefore needs augmentative or alternative ways of communicating. Aided communication systems have four components: the actual device or computer, the symbol set used to represent the language concepts, the communication techniques used including the access method and output options, and the communication strategies. Because the actual aids and devices change quickly with advances in technology, little mention of commercially available devices will be made. The rest of this section addresses the symbol set and the communication techniques currently used in AAC. Specific strategies for increasing the effectiveness of communication are beyond the scope of this text and the reader is referred to more in-depth texts on AAC (109,113,114).

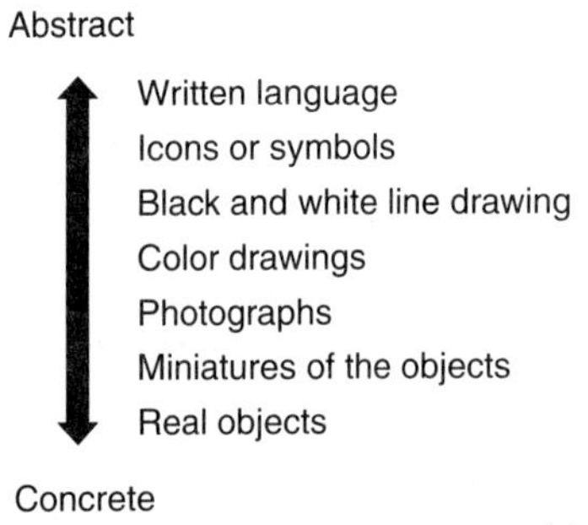

Abstract

- Written language
- Icons or symbols
- Black and white line drawing
- Color drawings
- Photographs
- Miniatures of the objects
- Real objects

Concrete

Figure 36-2. A hierarchy of symbol sets used in the representation of language. (Adapted from Church G, Glennen S. *The handbook of assistive technology.* San Diego: Singular Publishing, 1992.)

Symbol Sets

Most AAC aids and devices use symbol sets to represent language and provide a means for message formulation. Symbols range in hierarchy from very simple to complex and from concrete to abstract (Fig. 36-2) (110,111). At the simple end of the hierarchy are real objects where the actual object is used to communicate an idea. This is observed in very young children who point to a ball or cup to indicate that they want to play ball or want a drink. Persons with mental retardation need the concreteness of real objects. The communication level for these persons may be only choice making.

The hierarchy moves into miniature objects where smaller replicas of the objects are used. They may look like the object in shape and color. Photographs of the object are next in the hierarchy, with the color image being more recognizable and therefore more concrete than the black and white image. Photographs can be used to depict objects, persons, places, activities, and actions. Line drawings are the next symbols in the hierarchy. As with photographs, color line drawings are more recognizable than black and white drawings and the more the drawing looks like the object the more concrete it is. Picture Communication Symbols (PCS) (115) are examples of line drawings (Fig. 36-3). There are more than 1800 simple drawings in the PCS set representing objects, people, activities, and actions.

The next level in the hierarchy are the symbol sets. There are several symbol sets from which to choose and various rationales for the development of each. Only a few are described here.

Pic Syms (see Fig. 36-3) are line drawing symbol sets that combine predrawn and user-drawn symbols. Pic Syms were developed according to a defined set of principles (116) and the new symbols are generated using these same principles.

Blissymbolics (see Fig. 36-3) were first developed by Charles Bliss (107) and include approximately 100 basic symbols that are used singly or in combination with other symbols to form messages. This symbol set was first developed as an international language so people with varying languages would have a basis for communication.

Minspeak (Fig. 36-4) is defined as "minimum effort speech" (117) and is an iconic association coding system. The icons were developed to represent many ideas and the user assigns words or ideas to the symbols that are meaningful to the user. For example, one of the symbols or icons is a yellow sun with a smiling face. This icon could mean sun, sunny, yellow, happy, hot, or morning. Combine this symbol with the watch icon and the idea of morning becomes more obvious. This encoding allows for several concepts to be stored with a limited number of symbols.

At the abstract end of the hierarchy is orthography or written language (see Fig. 36-2). Orthographic symbols directly correspond to the spoken language and are the most arbitrary of the symbol sets because they do not resemble what they represent. Orthographic sets require higher cognitive skills because they are capable of generating unique expressions and novel messages. They are the most flexible of the symbol sets. Braille and Morse code are classified as orthographic symbol sets (110–112).

Access Modes

The access mode refers to the methods or ways in which the individual physically approaches and uses the AAC device or system. Persons who cannot effectively and efficiently use their hands to type on a keyboard must use alternative methods or body parts to access the computer, communication system, or other device. There are two general categories of access mode, direct selection and indirect or scanning selection.

Direct selection allows the user access to each item in the selection set at any time. Using a computer keyboard with the fingers is the most common example of direct selection. This is also the faster and most efficient method of access. Direct selection also can be accomplished by means of a head or mouth stick, an adaptive pointer, or other body part. Devices that respond to direct selection include a wide variety of keyboards such as large, expanded keyboards and small, minikeyboards. Touch-sensitive screens or membrane surfaces are considered to be accessed through direct selection. Keyboards that require depression of a key provide additional feedback to the user via the tactile and auditory systems and may be useful for individuals with visual impairments. The touch membranes and touch screens require very little pressure for activation and may be an advantage for individuals with diminished strength and endurance. The system of eye gaze is a method of direct selection that was used prior to the development of electronic and computerized systems. Eye gaze can be used to point to objects or pictures. The Etran system is a clear Plexiglas board with symbols, letters, and so on, on it (Fig. 36-5). The user gazes at the symbols while the "listener" follows the eye gaze to determine what is being communicated.

The newer generations of AAC systems include several devices that operate with a switch-activated direct selection mode. These devices use switches as substitutes for a keyboard. Figure 36-6 shows a variety of switches. Up to 12 digital (voice) messages can be stored depending on the device. Each message is accessed through switch activation. Obviously, very little information can be stored, but these are excellent for initiating AAC training, or for temporary use in the case of an intubated individual. Light and optical pointers are also included in the direct selection category (110–112). Through the use of laser light, light-emitting diodes (LEDs), or sonar or infrared technology, the individual accesses the selections on the communication device or computer.

When a person is unable to use direct selection because of motoric limitations, the method of indirect selection may be required (118,119). Indirect selection is an access method in which intermediate steps are involved in the selection process. Scanning provides systematic presentation of the symbol set choices. The individual then uses one or more switches (see Fig. 36-6) to "select" the desired symbol or keystroke. Examples of symbol or selection sets include graphic keyboard images such as alphabet, icons, or pictures. Other scanning access can be for textual keyboard characters, or a menu of computer commands.

Scanning arrays come in many forms. The simplest scanning arrays to understand and use are circular and linear. Both of these present the symbols one at a time in sequence. Circle scanning presents each symbol sequentially in a circular pattern. Linear scanning presents the symbols in a left-to-right pattern as in reading. Both of these are cognitively easy to learn since they only involve a one-step process. They are, however, very slow and the rate of communication is compromised.

Row-column scanning and group-item scanning are used to speed up the communication process. In row-column scanning, each entire row is presented at a time. When the desired row is selected, each symbol in the row

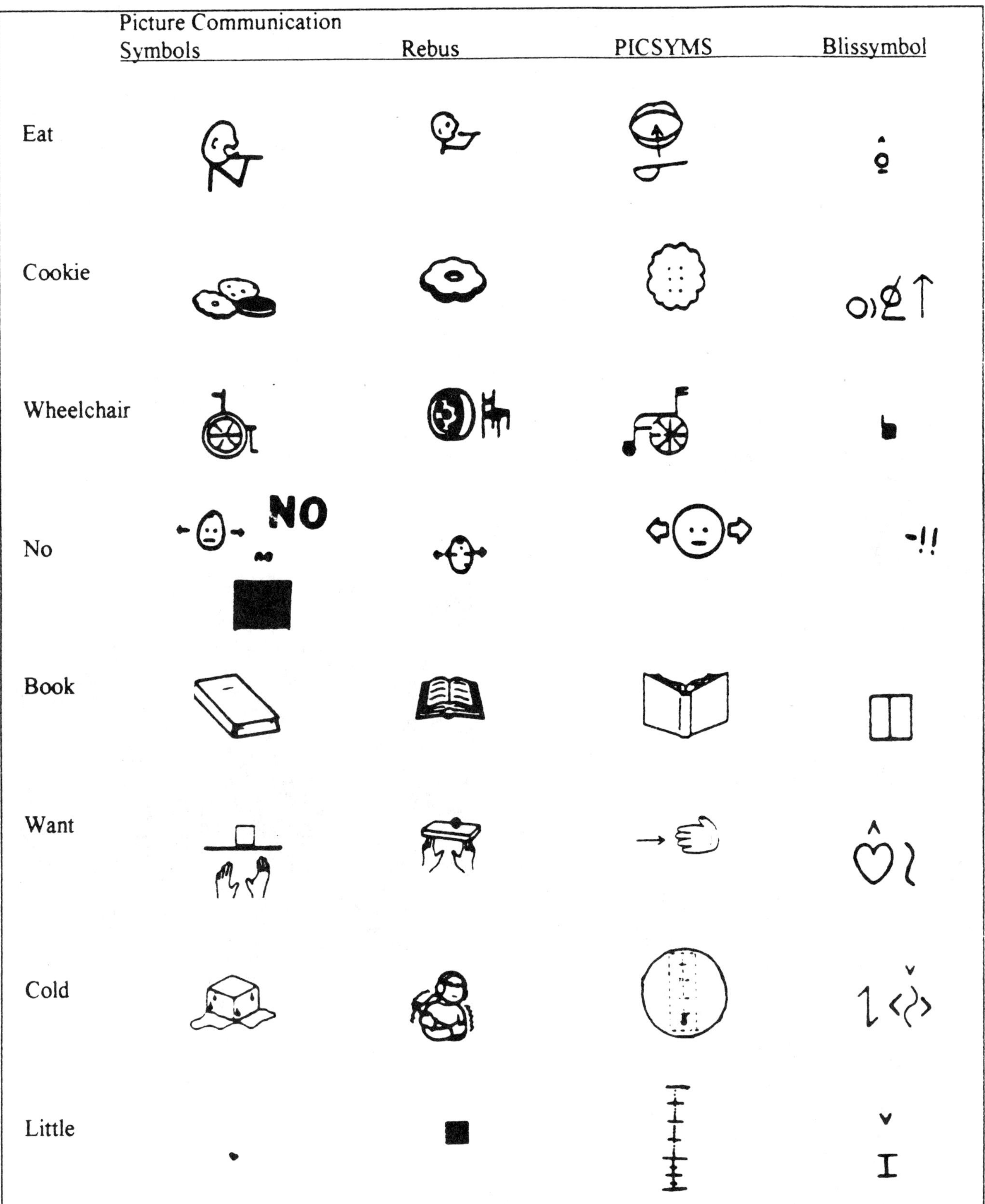

Figure 36-3. Examples of vocabulary symbols from four symbol sets. (Adapted from Brandenburg S, Vanderheiden G. Communication board design and vocabulary selection. In: Bernstein L, ed. *The vocally impaired: clinical practice and research.* Allyn & Bacon, 1988.)

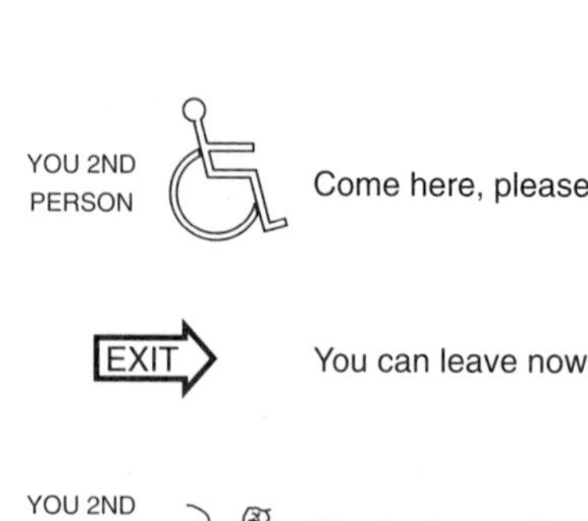

YOU 2ND PERSON — Come here, please.

You can leave now.

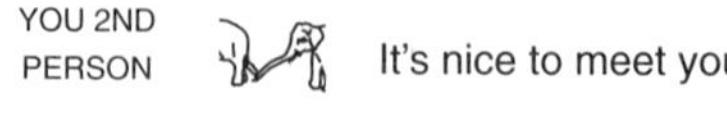

YOU 2ND PERSON — It's nice to meet you

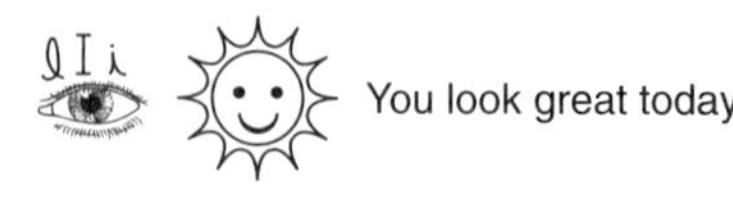

You look great today!

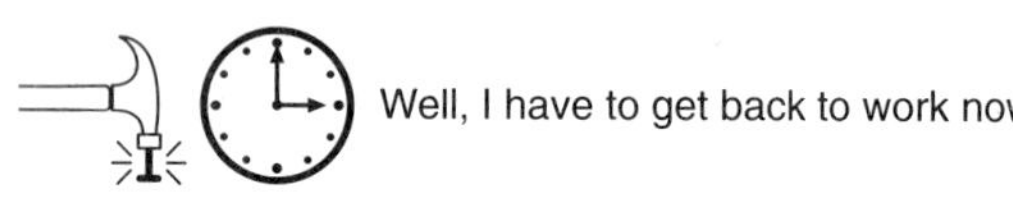

Well, I have to get back to work now.

What are the chances of that happening?

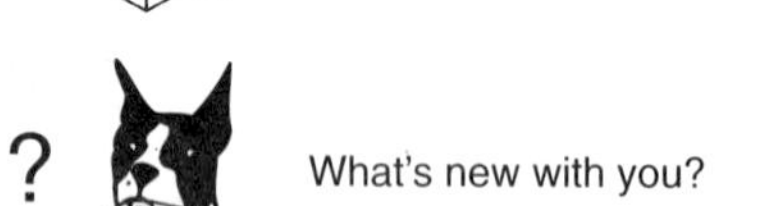

What's new with you?

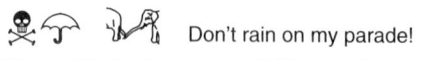

Knock knock joke.

Goodbye! Come back soon.

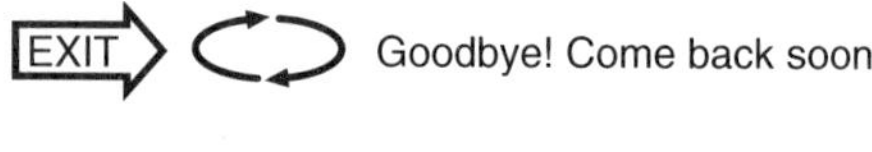

I am soooo happy!

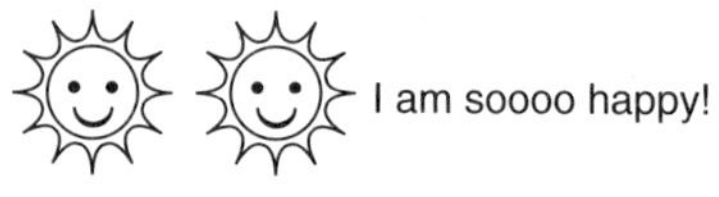

Don't rain on my parade!

Figure 36-4. Examples of Minspeak symbol sequences. (Reproduced by permission from Romich B. *Liberator manual.* Wooster, OH: Prentke Romich, 11.)

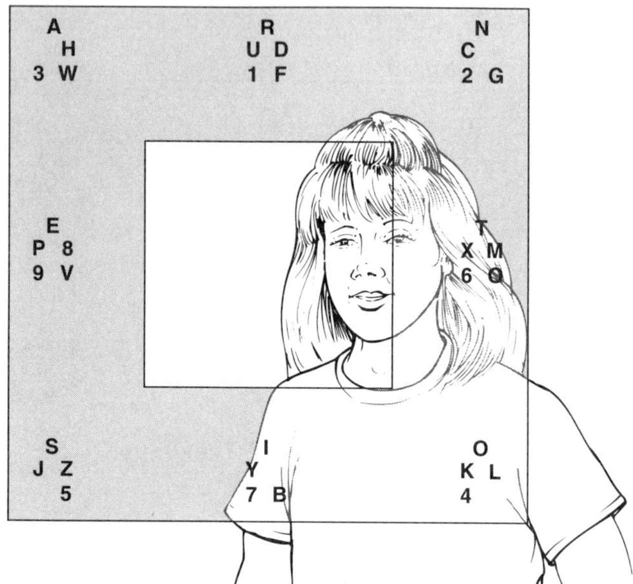

Figure 36-5. A child using a clear Plexiglas Etran communication board.

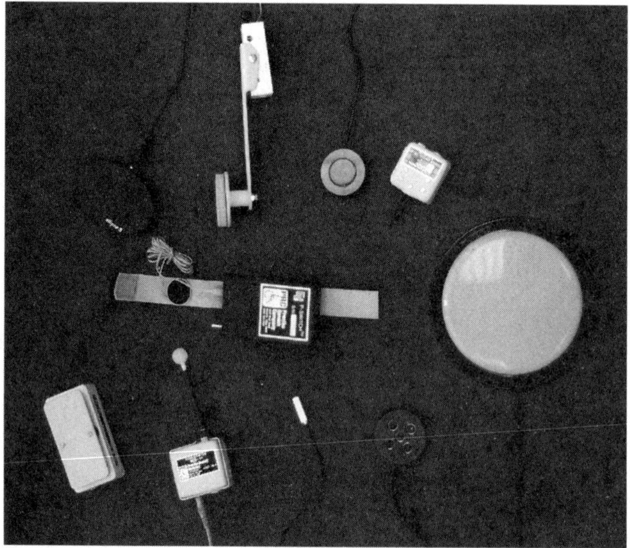

Figure 36-6. Examples of different switches. Clockwise from the upper-right corner: Don Johnston Bass Switch, TASH Buddy Switch, Zygo Leaf Switch, TASH Micro Light Switch, Toys For Special Children Ultimate Switch, and Able Net Big Red Switch.

is presented until the user selects the desired symbol. Group-item scanning has many variations, but basically the symbols are presented in groups, usually based on their location on the device such as the upper right quadrant or lower left quadrant. The groups are presented sequentially until a group is selected, then symbols in the group are presented one at a time until the desired symbol is selected. Figure 36-7 displays several scanning arrays. Each of these scanning arrays involves two or more steps and therefore, higher cognitive function.

It can be beneficial to consider scanning as an option even if the individual appears to be able to access via direct selection. Individuals who fatigue easily may benefit from scanning arrays that require less physical effort than direct access methods require. Sometimes, a person will be able to utilize direct selection methods, but will have very slow access times. They may be faster using a scanning access method. Another time scanning might be consid-

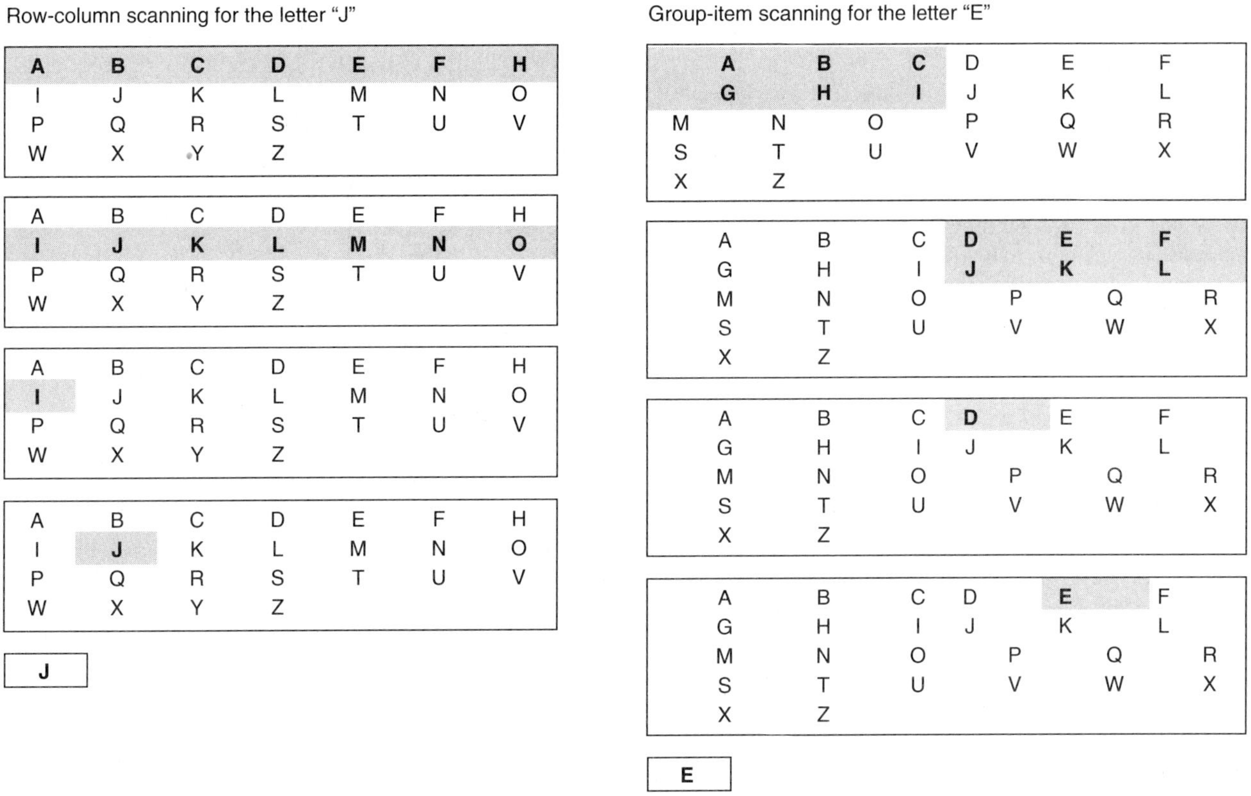

Row-column scanning for the letter "J"

A	**B**	**C**	**D**	**E**	**F**	**H**
I	J	K	L	M	N	O
P	Q	R	S	T	U	V
W	X	Y	Z			

A	B	C	D	E	F	H
I	**J**	**K**	**L**	**M**	**N**	**O**
P	Q	R	S	T	U	V
W	X	Y	Z			

A	B	C	D	E	F	H
I	J	K	L	M	N	O
P	Q	R	S	T	U	V
W	X	Y	Z			

A	B	C	D	E	F	H
I	**J**	K	L	M	N	O
P	Q	R	S	T	U	V
W	X	Y	Z			

J

Group-item scanning for the letter "E"

A	**B**	**C**	D	E	F
G	**H**	**I**	J	K	L
M	N	O	P	Q	R
S	T	U	V	W	X
X	Z				

A	B	C	**D**	**E**	**F**
G	H	I	**J**	**K**	**L**
M	N	O	P	Q	R
S	T	U	V	W	X
X	Z				

A	B	C	**D**	E	F
G	H	I	J	K	L
M	N	O	P	Q	R
S	T	U	V	W	X
X	Z				

A	B	C	D	**E**	F
G	H	I	J	K	L
M	N	O	P	Q	R
S	T	U	V	W	X
X	Z				

E

Figure 36-7. Examples of row-column scanning and group-item scanning.

ered is when the individual's selection process is very inaccurate as a result of tremors, ataxia, or other incoordination. Accuracy and speed can be enhanced in these situations with scanning requiring less finite control of movement (112,113,118,119).

Output

In order for communication to be effective, the output of the system must be considered. The output of the device or system must be an intelligible method of transmitting messages (110–112,120). Augmentative and alternative systems have printed, visual, voice, or combinations of output modes available to the user.

Visual displays include LED and liquid crystal display (LCD) screens, with LCD being more common than LED displays. The LCD or LED screens provide the user with a small printed display of what is being typed. This display is temporary and is replaced quickly as more is typed. These displays provide the user with visual feedback as keys are selected. The displays can also assist the user and listener in clarifying missed or misunderstood messages. The visual display can be read versus repeating the message. Visual displays can also be an advantage when the environment or situation requires quiet communication.

Communication is greatly enhanced with voice or speech output (110–112). Almost all of the current AAC devices have the capability of producing speech output. There are basically two forms of voice output: digitalized and synthesized speech. Digitalized speech produces a natural-sounding quality of speech. Very simplistically, digitalized speech works and sounds like a tape recording, although the technology is much more complicated than simple tape recording. The disadvantage of digitalized speech is that it requires a tremendous amount of memory. This has implications in the amount of information that can be stored in a single portable system. As the technology improves, the memory constraints will be less of an issue. Another disadvantage of this type of speech output is that the messages must be prerecorded for the individual. Although this may work for young children or individuals with cognitive impairments, individuals wishing to be autonomous may not want to depend on someone else to record their messages for them.

Synthesized speech is more frequently used in AAC devices. Early forms of synthesized speech, like the Echo synthesizer, were very robotic sounding and difficult to understand (106,110,113). Advances in speech output have increased the intelligibility and variability of the sound of speech output. DecTalk is currently the most widely used synthesizer in AAC devices. DecTalk provides 10 distinct voices in both male and female tones as well as the capability to create additional voices.

Text to speech is used when a person wants to

produce novel messages or a large amount of prestored information. Text to speech can be produced only on AAC devices that have synthesized speech. The process of text to speech involves converting the written text into corresponding phonemes plus adding pronunciation information such as stress, prosody, and segmentation. The English language has so many pronunciation variations that the software requires extensive knowledge of pronunciation exceptions. In addition, many AAC devices and systems are programmable for different pronunciations and even a variety of languages.

Printed output is provided in the form of paper printouts. AAC devices that have paper output usually have letter spelling capabilities. Messages printed on paper are useful when the message is lengthy or to aid in clarity. Paper output can be in the form of small ticker tape strips of paper or adding machine–type paper. Some AAC devices can be connected to computer printers to produce longer messages. The ability to produce longer messages such as questions and speeches ahead of time can greatly increase the rate of communication as well as increase the chance of getting the message across effectively.

At this point it is important to discuss written communication as a form of augmentative communication. In writing, the anticipated result is the "hard copy" or words printed on paper. Many of the more sophisticated AAC devices can be attached to a printer and used as a word processor. If the person still has vocalization, but has physical limitations that preclude traditional writing or typing, he or she may need assistance with written communication. At the low end of the technology spectrum, there are a variety of splints and writing aids that can assist a person in pencil and paper tasks. The occupational therapist usually has an array of these available. For computer access, there are also a wide array of options available. Keyboards can be adapted or alternative keyboards can be recommended to enhance access. Keyguards are usually plastic or metal covers for the keyboard with holes for each key. The holes isolate the keys so that a person with limited coordination, tremors, or excessive motions can isolate the keys and reduce typing errors. Also, keyguards may be used with a mouth stick, head wand, or handheld typing aid. These aids provide the person with the ability to use the regular keyboard when they have limited isolated finger movement. Each is a stick or wand that is attached or held by the respective body part and is used for typing.

There are a variety of keyboards available that provide alternative access such as the expanded keyboards and minikeyboards. Expanded keyboards are larger than normal and often can be programmed so that the keys are different sizes. These are typically used for children with excessive or inaccurate movements. Minikeyboards or small keyboards are much smaller than normal and are used when a person has limited motion, as is often observed in persons with neuromuscular diseases. Minikeyboards can also be useful for persons with decreased endurance or someone using a mouth stick or head wand.

In addition to the ACC access methods mentioned, some access methods are specific to computer access. Most of these are in the form of software programs. Virtual or on-screen keyboards can be used when access with the hands is not an option. Virtual keyboards can be accessed through scanning methods mentioned previously or alternative mouse access. Software has been designed and is available to provide for voice input (the computer types what is spoken), to change the configuration of the keyboard, to slow down the response and acceptance rate of the computer, or to provide for scanning or Morse code entry, to name a few. There are also programs that provide abbreviation expansion and word prediction. In abbreviation expansion, the individual types in an abbreviation, such as "OT," and the computer responds with the whole word or phrase, in this case *occupational therapy*. Word prediction speeds up typing by predicting which is the next letter and word being typed. This is based on statistics for letter combinations. For example, after the person types "t," the computer might then offer "h" or "e." As more is typed, the options are narrowed and the final word may be predicted or offered after three or four letters of the word are input. Both of these can be useful in reducing fatigue, increasing typing rate, and decreasing errors.

Evaluation

Prior to the evaluation, background information should be gathered and a needs analysis conducted (Fig. 36-8). Background information includes medical history, education, and communication history as well as current assessment reports (speech-language pathologists, occupational therapy, physical therapy). The needs analysis helps identify the deficits in the person's communication options and pinpoints the communication components that are needed, such as speech output and printer support. The needs analysis can also identify environments in which the communication process needs augmentation (111,112).

Evaluation of a person for AAC is a very time-consuming and information-intensive process. There are many factors to be considered that will affect the successful outcome of the evaluation (113,114,120). The evaluation should include the motoric, cognitive, language, and social skills of the person as well as the environments in which the person functions. For this reason, an effective evaluation of a person for AAC should always include a team of professionals, ideally led by a speech-language pathologist. An effective evaluation will predict a future match for the augmentative communication device (Fig. 36-9).

The evaluation should begin with effective positioning, which includes assessment of wheelchairs and seating systems. Proper positioning has been demonstrated to facilitate more effective movement in persons with physical disabilities (121,122). As part of the positioning assessment, consideration should be given to all the positions that the

Area of need:

1. What physical positions does the individual need to be in while using an augmentative or alternative communication (AAC) system?
   - Lying supine
   - Lying prone
   - Sitting in bed
   - In arm restraints
   - In a variety of positions

2. During what activities does the AAC system need to be available?
   - Moving from room to room
   - Carrying the device while walking
   - Independently positioning the device
   - Communicating within a manual/electric wheelchair
   - Simultaneously accessing the device & wheelchair controls
   - Accessing the device while using a lap tray
   - Accessing the device while the chair is tilted at _____%
   - Communicating while being transported

3. With what other equipment use will the AAC system be employed?
   - While orally intubated
   - While using a tracheostomy tube (a tube that goes into the airway below the larynx)
   - While using an oxygen mask
   - While using environmental control units

4. Within what environments will the AAC system be used?
   - Noisy or quiet room
   - Movie theater
   - Restaurant
   - Dimly lit room

5. With whom does the individual communicate?
   - Anyone visually or hearing impaired
   - More than one listener
   - An unfamiliar partner

6. What will the AAC system be used for?
   - To answer questions
   - To ask questions
   - To provide unique information
   - To convey basic medical needs

7. What output modes are important to the individual?
   - Produce a printed copy
   - Take notes
   - Use a telephone
   - Volley from writing to speaking

Figure 36-8. Needs assessment. (Reproduced by permission from Mann WC, Lane JP. *Assistive technology for persons with disabilities.* 2nd ed. Baltimore: American Occupational Therapy Association, 1995.)

person is in throughout the day and which positions have specific or different communication requirements. A child may spend part of the day in side-lying or prone positions and may not be able to use established methods of accessing the communication device. In this situation, other access options must be considered.

Motor Abilities

The evaluation of motor function is important to determine the most appropriate access method(s) or options. The intent of the evaluation of motor function is to determine five factors: speed, accuracy, control, reliability of the movement, and endurance (110,111). These factors will help determine the optimum position and access mode for the communication device so that the user is as fast as possible without jeopardizing accuracy or endurance. These five factors should be kept in mind throughout the evaluation and subsequent follow-up visits.

Observation of the client is the first step in the evaluation of motor function. Observations are done ini-

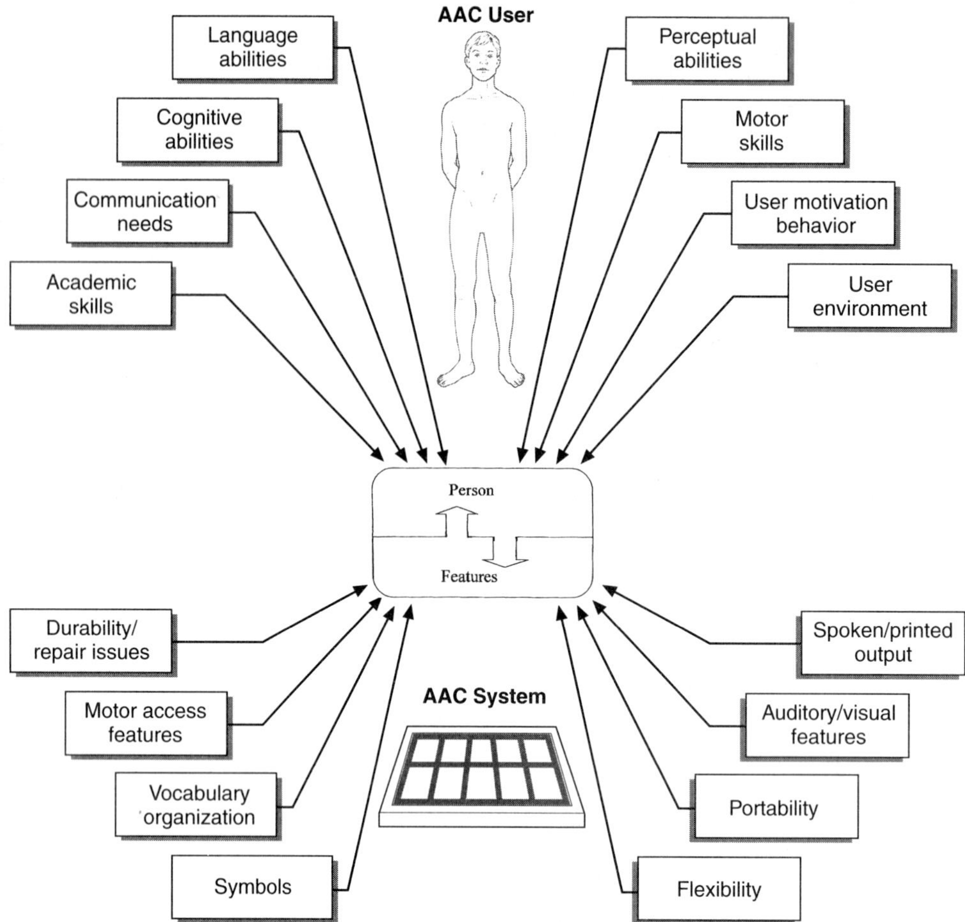

Figure 36-9. A model for assessing individuals to predict the optimum features of augmentative and alternative communication (AAC) devices. (Adapted from Glennen SL, DeCoste DC. *Handbook of augmentative and alternative communication.* San Diego: Singular Publishing, 1996.)

tially and throughout the evaluation process to determine the quantity and quality of the person's responses. For example, postural adjustments and repositioning switches or communication devices will affect the person's abilities in the five factors just mentioned. Readjustments may affect the person's comfort level, acceptance or rejection of devices, and so on (121,122). Facial expressions and body language will suggest much about the individual's response to the position, device, or interactions.

Since direct selection is considered the most efficient access, evaluation for direct access should be done first (119). The hands should always be considered as the first access method. A quick and effective observation in the initial meeting can help determine the feasibility of using the hands for access. If the hands are not an option for access, then the clinician systematically evaluates the person for consistent reliable motions. The sequence for evaluation usually begins with upper-body motions, specifically the upper extremities and head. In addition to gross head motions, motions of the mouth, eyes, and other facial muscles are assessed (110,112,122). The trunk, legs, and feet are evaluated for reliable motion if the upper-body motions are not effective and consistent (Fig. 36-10).

Cognitive and Language Abilities

In order to use an AAC system or device, certain cognitive skills are needed. These basic skills include the following abilities (110–112)

1. To remain alert and attend to the task
2. To visually or auditorily track events in the environment
3. To comprehend cause-and-effect relationships
4. To express preferences and make choices through current modes of communication
5. To remember objects, people, and events
6. To associate graphic symbols with objects, persons, or events

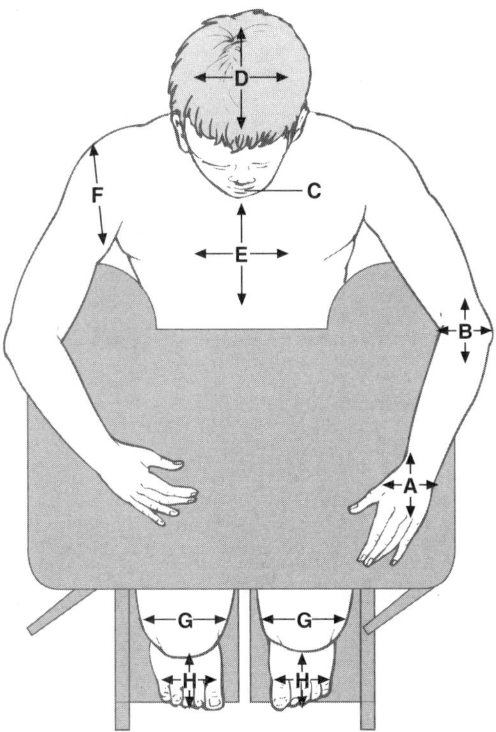

A Hand control – up/down and left/right hand movement

B Arm/elbow control – movement of the elbow outwards or sliding the arm forward and backward

C Mouth/tongue/lip or puff/sip control

D Head control – forward/backward and left/right movement of the head

E Chin control – forward/backward and left/right movement of the chin, as with a chin controlled joystick

F Shoulder control – elevation/depression or protraction/retraction of the shoulder

G Leg/knee control – inward/outward movement of the knee

H Foot control – left/right and up/down movement of the foot

Figure 36-10. Progression of evaluation of motor function for switch access.

These abilities are assessed through structured tasks and observations. The team will assess basic cognitive skills to determine how the individual's cognitive abilities will affect learning and use of an AAC device or system. Basic skill training will be required if there are deficiencies in cognitive abilities before effective use of a sophisticated system can be implemented. As an example, switch training with computer games and battery-operated toys can aid in the development of sustained attention and foster the understanding of cause-and-effect relationships.

Assessments in the areas of speech, language, and literacy are conducted by the speech-language pathologist, with input from family members and school or work personnel. This information is used to determine the appropriate communication devices, vocabulary, and symbol sets and whether the individual can use text-based communication systems.

Environments

In the evaluation process, the environments in which the person functions and the AAC system that will be utilized need to be considered. A person may have a variety of communication devices for different situations and environments (111). As an example, a dedicated device with text to speech would be the main communication device. This device can be attached to an external printer when needed in a school or office environment. The voice is turned off in situations when quiet is necessary, as when asking polite or private questions or at the library. If the person functions in environments that are not friendly to technological devices, some of the low-tech options will need to be considered for these environments. A person who goes to the pool or the beach should not be precluded from communicating in these environments. A low-tech communication board dedicated to messages related to the pool, beach, or other technologically challenged environments would supplement the person's high-tech device.

A child in school may have a variety of low-tech communication boards dedicated to different environments. A common example of this is a communication notebook. The notebook is composed of several pages and each page has a variety of pictures dedicated to a specific activity, task, or environment. There may be a page for requesting wants and needs such as a drink or to go to the bathroom. Other pages may be related to lunchtime, therapy time, activities done in a specific class, the community, or at home.

The Future

Future developments in AAC will be in two areas. First, the technological innovations are developing at a rapid pace and have a significant impact in this field. The AAC devices will continue to be easier to use and more intelligible. The technology, however, is limited in its application if the physical, sensory, cognitive, and psychosocial issues are not well understood. The second area of development and change needs to be in the process of evaluating, training, and integrating AAC in daily lives and fostering acceptance of AAC. Evaluation and therapeutic protocols will need to continue to be developed. As knowledge in these two areas grows, so will the successful integration of AAC into the lives of individuals.

CONCLUSIONS

Technology can contribute significantly to enhancing the personal autonomy and lifestyle of persons with physical disabilities. However, it must be emphasized that technology only provides tools and these tools must be used with judgment in order to achieve the desired results.

APPENDIX I. COMMUNICATION AID MANUFACTURERS

Ablenet
1081 Tenth Avenue S. E.
Minneapolis, MN 55414-1391
1-800-322-0956

Adaptivation
PO Box 626
Ames, IA 50010-0626
1-800-723-2783
http://users.aol.com/adaptaac

Communication Devices
2433 Government Way, Suite A
Coeur d'Alene, ID 83814-3630
1-800-60 HOLLY
E-mail: hollycom@rand.nidlink.com

Crestwood Company
6625 North Sidney Place
Milwaukee, WI 53206-3259
1-414-352-5678
E-mail: crestcomm@aol.com

Don Johnston Incorporated
PO Box 639
Wauconda, IL 60084-0639
1-800-999-4660
http://donjohnston.com

Innocomp
26210 Emery Road, Suite 302
Warrensville Heights, OH 44128-5771
1-800-382-8622
http://sayitall.com

Intellitools
55 Leveroni Court, Suite 9
Novato, CA 94949-5751
1-800-899-6687
E-mail: info@intellitools.com
http://www.intellitools.com

Mayer-Johnson Company
PO Box 1579
Solana Beach, CA 92075-7579
1-619-550-0084
E-mail: MayerJ@aol.com

Prentke Romich Company
1022 Heyl Road
Wooster, OH 44691-9744
1-800-262-1984
http://www.dialup.oar.net
/~Pprco/index.html

Sentient Systems Technology
2100 Wharton Street, Suite 630
Pittsburgh, PA 15203-1942
1-800-344-1778
E-mail: sstsales@sentient-sys.com
http://www.sentient-sys.com

Tash International
91 Station Street, Unit 1
Ajax, Ontario, L1S 3H2 Canada
1-800-463-5685
E-mail: tashcan@aol.com

Words+
40015 Sierra Highway, Building B#145
Palmdale, CA 93559-2101
1-800-869-8521
E-mail: wwwordspls@aol.com

Zygo Industries
PO Box 1008
Portland OR 97207-1008
1-800-234-6006

REFERENCES

1. O'Day BL, Corcoran RJ. Assistive technology: problems and policy alternatives. *Arch Phys Med Rehabil* 1994;75:1165–1169.
2. Hobson DA. RESNA: yesterday, today and tomorrow. *Assist Technol* 1996;8:131–143.
3. Rehabilitation Act of 1973 (Public Law 93-112) and its Amendments of 1986 (Public Law 99-506), 29 USC § 701.
4. Americans with Disabilities Act of 1990 (Public Law 101-336), 42 USC § 12101.
5. Technology-Related Assistance for Individuals with Disabilities Act of 1988 (Public Law 100-407), 20 USC § 2201.
6. Individuals with Disabilities Education Act of 1990 (Public Law 101-476), 20 USC § 1401.
7. Post KM. The promise of assistive technology. *Am J Occup Ther* 1993;47:965–967.
8. Hammel JM, Smith RO. The development of technology competencies and training guidelines for occupational therapists. *Am J Occup Ther* 1993;47:970–979.
9. Mann WC, Hurren D, Tomita M. Comparison of assistive device use and needs of home-based older

persons with different impairments. *Am J Occup Ther* 1993;47:980–987.

10. Garber SL, Krouskop TA, Carter RE. A system for clinically evaluating wheelchair pressure relief cushions. *Am J Occup Ther* 1978;32:565–570.

11. Trefler E, Tooms RE, Hobson DA. Seating services for the physically disabled: a twelve year experience. In: *Proceedings of the Third International Seating Symposium "Seating the Disabled."* Memphis, TN: 1987:37–43.

12. Garber SL. A classification of wheelchair seating. *Am J Occup Ther* 1979;10:652–654.

13. Cardi MD. Guidelines for selecting wheelchair cushions. In: *Physical disabilities special interest section newsletter.* Bethesda, MD: American Occupational Therapy Association, 1988;11:3–4.

14. Garber SL. Wheelchair cushions: a historical review. *Am J Occup Ther* 1985;39:453–459.

15. Henderson B (compiler). *Seating in review—current trends for the disabled.* Winnipeg, Canada: Otto Bock Orthopedic Industry of Canada, 1989.

16. Anathan PR, Srinivasan TM, Antia NH, Ghista DN. Pressure warning system for patients with insensitive feet to avoid ulceration. In: Kenedi RM, Cowden JM, Scales JT, eds. *Bedsore biomechanics.* Baltimore: University Park Press, 1975:207–210.

17. Fordyce WE, Simons BC. Automated training system for wheelchair pushups. *Public Health Rep* 1968;93:527–528.

18. Reddy N, Reswick J, Krouskop T. Predictors of soft tissue viability. In: *Care, treatment and prevention of pressure sores.* Washington, DC: Paralyzed Veterans of America, 1985.

19. Krouskop T. Tissue trauma management. In: *Care, treatment and prevention of pressure sores.* Washington, DC: Paralyzed Veterans of America, 1985.

20. Krouskop T, Noble P, Garber S, Spencer W. The effectiveness of preventive management in reducing the occurrence of pressure sores. *J Rehabil Res Dev* 1983;20:74–83.

21. Krouskop TA, Garber SL, Cullen BB. Factors to consider in selecting a support surface. In: Krasner D, ed. *Chronic wound care: a clinical source book for healthcare professionals.* King of Prussia, PA: Health Management Publications, Inc., 1990:142–151.

22. Gibson T, Barbenel J, Evans J. Biomechanical concepts and effects. In: Kenedi R, Cowden J, Scales J, eds. *Bedsore biomechanics.* Baltimore: University Park Press, 1975:25–30.

23. Reswick J, Rogers J. Experience at Rancho Los Amigos Hospital with devices and techniques to prevent pressure sores. In: Kenedi R, Cowden J, Scales J, eds. *Bedsore biomechanics.* Baltimore: University Park Press, 1975:301–310.

24. Reddy N, Palmieri V, Cochran G. Evaluation of transducers performance for buttock-cushion interface pressure measurements. *J Rehabil Res Dev* 1984;21:43–50.

25. Ferguson-Pell MB, Ball F, Evans J. Interface pressure sensors: existing devices, their suitability and limitations. In: Kenedi R, Cowden J, Scales J, eds. *Bedsore biomechanics.* Baltimore: University Park Press, 1975:189–197.

26. Krouskop TV, van Rijswijk L. Standardizing performance-based criteria for support surfaces. *Ostomy Wound Manage* 1985;41:33–47.

27. Bolwell C. Using computers as instructional technology in the pressure ulcer field. *Decubitus* 1993;6(4):20–25.

28. Trefler E, Tooms RE, Hobson DA. Seating for cerebral-palsied children. *Interclin Info Bull* 1978;17:1–8.

29. Currie DM, Hardwick K, Marburger RA, Britell CW. Wheelchair prescription and adaptive seating. In: DeLisa JA, ed. *Rehabilitation medicine principles and practices.* 2nd ed. Philadelphia: JB Lippincott, 1993:563–585.

30. Lemaire ED, Upton D, Paialunga J, et al. Clinical analysis of a CAD/CAM system for custom seating: a comparison with hand-sculpting methods. *J Rehabil Res Dev* 1996;33:311–320.

31. Dallaway JL, Jackson RD, Timmers PHA. Rehabilitation robotics in Europe. *IEEE Trans Rehabil Eng* 1995;3(1):35–45.

32. Hillman MR. A feasibility study of a robot manipulator for the disabled. *J Med Eng Technol* 1987;11(4):160–165.

33. Harwin WS, Rahman T, Foulds RA. A review of design issues in rehabilitation robotics with reference to North American research. *IEEE Trans Rehabil Eng* 1995;3(1):3–13.

34. Lees D, Lepage P. Will robots ever replace attendants? Exploring the current capabilities of rehabilitation robots. *Int J Rehabil Res* 1994;17:285–304.

35. Brich GE. Development and methodology for the formal evaluation of the Neil Squire Foundation Robotic Assistive Appliance. *Robotica* 1993;11:529–534.

36. Dallaway JL, Mahoney RM, Jackson RD, Gosine RG. An interactive robot control environment for rehabilitation applications. *Robotica* 1993;11:541–551.

37. Ishii S, Tanaka S, Hiramatsu F. Meal assistance robot for severely handicapped people. *Proc IEEE Conf Robot Autom* 1995;11:1308–1313.

38. New Robotics Safety Standards. *Occup Hazards* 1992;54(10):55.

39. Graham JH. Sensory-based safeguarding of robotic systems. *Int J Robot Autom* 1994;9(4):141–148.

40. Davies B, Hibberd R. A safe communication system for wheelchair mounted medical robots. *Comput Control Eng J* 1996;7:216–221.

41. Taylor B, Cupo ME, Sheredos SJ. Workstation robotics: a pilot study of a desktop vocational assistant robot. *J Occup Ther* 1993;47:1009–1013.

42. Napper SA, Seaman RL. Applications of robots in rehabilitation. *Robots Auton Syst* 1989;5:227–239.

43. Engelhardt KG. An overview of health and human services robotics. *Robots Auton Syst* 1989;5:205–226.

44. Cheatham JB, Magee KN. Rehabilitation robotics and environmental control systems. *Phys Med Rehabil State Art Rev* 1997;11(1):133–149.

45. Kassle M. Robotics for health care: a review of the literature. *Robotica* 1993;11:495–516.

46. Presiding B, Hsia TC, Mittelstadt B. A literature review: robotics in medicine. *IEEE Eng Med Biol* 1991;9:13–22.

47. Stanger CA, Anglin C, Harwin WS, Romilly DP. Devices for assisting manipulation: a summary of user task priorities. *IEEE Trans Rehabil Eng* 1994;2:256–265.

48. Kwee HH. Rehabilitation robotics—softening the hardware. *IEEE Eng Med Biol* 1995;14:330–335.

49. Gomsjo G, Neverdy H, Eftring H. Robotics in rehabilitation. *IEEE Trans Rehabil Eng* 1995;4:77–83.

50. Van der Loss HFM. VA/Stanford rehabilitation robotics research technology to the field of rehabilitation. *IEEE Trans Rehabil Eng* 1995;3:46–55.

51. Harwin WS, Ginige A, Jackson RD. A robot workstation for use in education of the physically handicapped. *IEEE Trans Biomed Eng* 1988;35:127–131.

52. Hillman MR, Pullin GM, Gammie AR, et al. Development of a robot arm and workstation for the disabled. *J Biomed Eng* 1990;12:199–204.

53. Pullin G, Gammie A. Current capabilities of rehabilitation robots. *J Biomed Eng* 1991;12:199–204.

54. Buhler C, Hoelper R, Hoyer H, Humann W. Autonomous robot technology for advanced wheelchair and robotics aids for people with disabilities. *Robot Auton Syst* 1995;14:213–222.

55. Wellman P, Krovi V, Kumar V. An adaptive mobility system for disabled. In: *Proceedings of the IEEE Conference on robotics and automation* 1994;10:2006–2011.

56. Wellman P, Krovi V, Harwin W. Design of a wheelchair with legs for people with motor disabilities. *IEEE Trans Rehabil Eng* 1995;3:343–454.

57. Schraft RD. Mechatronics and robotics for service applications. *IEEE Robot Automat* 1994;1:31–35.

58. Bach JR, Zeelenberg AP, Winter C. Wheelchair mounted robot manipulators. *Am J Phys Med Rehabil* 1990;69:53–59.

59. Regalbuto MA, Krouskop TA, Cheatham JB. Toward a practical mobile robot aid system for people with severe physical disabilities. *J Rehabil Res Dev* 1992;29:19–26.

60. Gruver WA. Intelligent robotics in manufacturing service, and rehabilitation: an overview. *IEEE Trans Ind Electr* 1994;41:4–11.

61. Van Vliet P, Wing AM. A new challenge—robotics in the rehabilitation of the neurologically motor impaired. *Phys Ther* 1991;71:50–58.

62. Gosine RG, Harwin WS, Furby LJ, Jackson RD. An intelligent end effector for a rehabilitation robot. *J Med Eng Technol* 1989;13:37–43.

63. Cammoun R, Detriche JM, Lauture F, Lesigne B. Clinical evaluation of the "Master" robot system and development of a new version. *Robotica* 1993;11:535–539.

64. Cooper RA. Intelligent control of powered wheelchairs. *IEEE Eng Med Biol* 1995;14:423–431.

65. Bourhis G, Pino R. Mobile robots and mobility assistance for people with motor impairment. *IEEE Trans Rehabil Eng* 1996;4:7–11.

66. Kawamura K, Peters RA, Bagchi S, Ishkarous M. Intelligent robotic systems in service of the disabled. *IEEE Trans Rehabil Eng* 1995;3:14–21.

67. Dojat M, Pachet F. An extendable knowledge-based system for the control of mechanical ventilators. *Proceedings of the Fourteenth Annual International Conference on the IEEE Engineering in Medicine and Biology Society.* 1992;14:920–921.

68. Callaghan SM, Voland G. Extracting knowledge for examples: induction of heuristic rules for wheelchair prescription. *J Intell Robot Syst* 1995;14:133–153.

69. Giarratano J, Riley R. *Expert systems: principles and programming.* Boston: RWS-Kent, 1994.

70. Kosko B. *Neural networks and fuzzy systems: a dynamical systems approach to machine intelligence.* Englewood Cliffs, NJ: Prentice Hall, 1992.

71. Wasserman PD. *Neural computing: theory and practice.* New York: Van Nostrand Reinhold, 1989.

72. Dubrawski A, Crowley JL. Self-supervised neural system for reactive navigation. *Proc IEEE Conf Robot Autom* 1994;2076–2082.

73. Goldberg DE. *Genetic algorithms in search, optimization and machine learning.* Reading. MA: Addison-Wesley, 1989.

74. Koza JR. *Genetic programming: on the programming of computers by means of natural selection.* Cambridge: MIT Press, 1992.

75. Zhao M, Ansari N, Hou ESH. Mobile manipulator path planning by a genetic algorithm. *J Robot Sys* 1004;11(3):143–153.

76. Fernandez JJ, Farry KA, Cheatham JB. Waveform recognition using genetic programming: the myoelectric signal recognition problem. In: Koza JR, Goldberg DE, Fogel DB, eds. *Genetic Programming: Proceedings of the First Annual Conference.* Cambridge: MIT Press, 1996:63–71.

77. Hillman MR, Pullin GM, Gammie AR, et al. Clinical experience in rehabilitation robotics. *J Biomed Eng* 1991;12:239.

78. Leung P. Robotics in rehabilitation. *J Rehabil* 1988;54:6–7.

79. Topping M. Early experience in the use of the "Handy 1" robotics aid

to eating. *Robotica* 1993;11: 525–527.

80. Brown MK, Buntschuh BM, Wilpon JG. SAM: a perceptive spoken language understanding robot. *IEEE Trans Syst Man Cyber* 1992;22:1390–1402.

81. Kara A, Kawamura K, Bagchi S. Reflex control of a robotic aid system to assist physically disabled. *IEEE Control Syst* 1992;2(3):71–77.

82. Farry K, Walker ID. Myoelectric teleoperation of a multifingered artificial had. *Seventh World Cong Int Soc Pros Ortho* 1992.

83. Goble JR, Suarez PF, Rogers SK, et al. A facial feature communications interface for the non-vocal. *IEEE Med Bio* 1993;12:46–48.

84. Ishibuchi K, Takamura H, Koshino F. Real time hand shape recognition using pipe-line image processor. *Proc IEEE Int Workshop Robot Human Comm* 1992:111–116.

85. Hu B, Qui MH. A new method for human-computer interaction using eye gaze. *Proc IEEE Int Conf Sys Man Cyber* 1994: 2723–2728.

86. Lees DS, Leifer LJ. A graphical programming language for robots opening in lightly structured environments. *Proceedings of the IEEE International Conference on Robotics and Automation* 1993;9: 648–653.

87. Damper RI. A multifunction domestic alert system for the deafblind. *IEEE Trans Rehabil Eng* 1995;3:354–359.

88. Tachi S, Tanie K, Komoriya K, Minoru A. Electrocutaneous communication in a guide dog robot (MELDOG). *IEEE Trans Biomed Eng* 1985;32: 461–469.

89. Kaczmarck KA. Sensory augmentation and substitution. In: Bronzion JD, ed. *The biomedical engineering handbook.* Boca Raton: CRC Press, 1994:2100–2082.

90. Engelberger JF. Health-care robotics goes commercial: the "HelpMate" experience. *Robotica* 1993;11:517–523.

91. Adnan S. Design, analysis, implementation, and control of a mobile robotics testbed for telepresence. PhD dissertation, Rice University, Houston, 1992.

92. Shoval S, Borenstein J, Koren Y. Mobile robot obstacle avoidance in a computerized travel aid for the blind. *Proc IEE Conf Rob Autom* 1994;10:2023–2038.

93. Bell DA, Borenstein J, Levine SP, et al. An assistive navigation system for wheelchair based upon mobile robot obstacle avoidance. *Proc IEEE Conf Rob & Automat* 1994;10:2019–2022.

94. Cincuin P, Bainville E, et al. Computer assisted medical interventions. *IEEE Eng Med Biol* 1995;14:254–263.

95. Bourhis B, Horn O, Agostini Y. Location and high-level planning for a powered wheelchair. *Proc IEEE Int Conf Syst Man Cyber* 1994:2629–2634.

96. Kaneko M, Kanayama N, Tsuji T. 3-D Active antenna for contact sensing. *Proc IEEE Conf Robotics Autom* 1995;12:1113–1119.

97. Russell A, Thiel D, Mackay-Sim A. Sensing odour trails for mobile robot navigation. *Proc IEEE Conf Robot Autom* 1994;11: 2627–2677.

98. Engelberger JF. *Robotics in service.* Cambridge: MIT Press, 1989.

99. Glass K, Hall K. Occupational therapists' views about the use of robotic aids for people with disabilities. *Am J Occup Ther* 1987;41:745–747.

100. Garber SL, Gregorio TL, Pumphrey N, Lathem P. Selfcare strategies for persons with spinal cord injuries. In: Christiansen C, ed. *Ways of living.* Rockville, MD: American Occupational Therapy Association, 1994:189–225.

101. Jenkins R: POSSOM: new communication aid. *Special Ed* 1967;56(1):9–11.

102. Garrison J. Emergency signaling for a person with quadriplegia and extraordinary respiratory risk. *Arch Phys Med Rehabil* 1989;63:180–181.

103. Vanderheiden G. Computers can play a dual role for disabled individuals. *BYTE* 1982;7(9): 136–162.

104. Graf M, Severe E, Holle A. Environmental control unit considerations for the person with high-level tetraplegia. *Top Spinal Cord Inj Rehabil* 1997; 2(3):30–40.

105. Holme SA, Kanny EM, Guthrie MR, Johnson KL. The use of environmental control units by occupational therapists in spinal cord injury and disease services. *Am J Occup Ther* 1997;51: 42–48.

106. Zangari C, Lloyd LL, Vicker B. Augmentative and alternative communication: an historical perspective. *Augment Altern Commun* 1994;10: 27–59.

107. Bliss C. *Semantography.* Sydney, Australia: Semantography Publications, 1965.

108. Browder JA, Anderson DE, Meek M. Augmentative communication, evolution, and progress for nonspeaking children. *Dev Behav Pediatr* 1986;7: 335–339.

109. American Speech-Language-Hearing Association. *Augmentative communication: an introduction.* Rockville, MD: ASHA, 1986.

110. Angelo J. *Assistive technology for rehabilitation therapists.* Philadelphia: FA Davis, 1997.

111. Church G, Glennen S. *The handbook of assistive technology.* San Diego: Singular Publishing, 1992.

112. Mann WC, Lane JP. *Assistive technology for persons with disabilities.* 2nd ed. Baltimore: American Occupational Therapy Association, 1995.

113. Glennen SL, DeCoste DC. *Handbook of augmentative and alternative communication.* San Diego: Singular Publishing, 1996.

114. Buekelman DR, Mirenda P. Augmentative and alternative communication, management of severe communication disorders in children and adults. Baltimore: Paul H. Brooks, 1992.

115. *Augmentative communication products.* Solana Beach, CA: Mayer-Johnson Company, 1994.

116. Carlson F. *Picsyms categorical dictionary.* Lawrence, KS: Baggeboda Press, 1985.

117. Baker B. Using images to generate speech. *Byte* 1986;3:160–168.

118. Angelo J. Comparison of three computer scanning modes as an interface method for persons with cerebral palsy. *Am J Occup Ther* 1992;46:217–222.

119. Higgenbotham DJ. Evaluation of keystroke savings across five assistive communication technologies. *Augment Altern Commun* 1992;8:258–272.

120. Light J, Beesly M, Collier B. Transition through multiple augmentative and alternative communication systems: a three-year case study of a head injured adolescent. *Augment Altern Commun* 1988;4:2–14.

121. McEwen IR, Karlan GR. Assessment of effects of positioning on communication board access by individuals with cerebral palsy. *Augment Altern Commun* 1989;5(4):235–242.

122. Reichle J, York J, Sigafoos J. *Implementing augmentative and alternative communication. Strategies for learners with severe disabilities.* Baltimore: Paul H. Brooks, 1991.

Chapter 37

Wheeled Mobility

Charles E. Levy
Michael L. Boninger
Marianne McDermott
and Theresa Frasca Berner

A core value of physiatry is dedication to the removal of barriers that limit people with disabilities from expressing their full human potential. Wheeled mobility, properly prescribed and fit, equals liberation to millions; unfortunately, millions more worldwide remain constrained for lack of financial resources, advocacy, and expertise. This chapter is designed to assist clinicians in prescribing wheeled mobility devices. Algorithmic flowcharts are provided to guide practitioners through the intricate maze of available componentry, and a glossary of terms is included (Appendix I). Of course, wheelchairs and scooters are only the foundation on which appropriate seating and assistive technology rest (see Chapter 36). It is the successful integration of these elements that truly enables our users. Another core value of physiatry discussed is reliance on the interdisciplinary team.

PATIENT HISTORY AND PHYSICAL EXAMINATION IN THE CONTEXT OF SEATING AND POSITIONING

The history taking and physical examination are directed at achieving three critical goals: determining or confirming the diagnosis; assessing the patient's functional abilities, limitations, and social support; and identifying the resources available to procure an appropriate device.

First, the physician must establish the diagnosis and understand the prognosis. Most patients will present with a known diagnosis, and it is usually not necessary to repeat the work-up. However, the clinician must scrutinize the medical history sufficiently to screen for alternative diagnoses and comorbidities that might change the patient's treatment plan or prognosis. A patient with Guillain-Barré syndrome may present with limitations in strength and endurance similiar to those of a patient with amyotrophic lateral sclerosis. The former would be expected to regain abilities while the latter's condition would most likely decline; therefore, their wheelchair prescriptions would be markedly different. Even when the diagnosis is uncertain, a complete work-up makes it possible to generate a reasonable prescription by extrapolation, based on the past course of the disease.

The next questions to be answered are, Will the patient be enabled by a wheeled mobility device? If so, what kind? These questions demand not only consideration of the patient's immediate motor and cognitive abilities, but also consideration of issues of transport and environment. A power chair that is too heavy to be transported or too wide to fit in the office or home will not be used, despite the fact that the patient may be able to sit with an improved posture and maneuver the device in the clinic.

The assessment should include how the device will be procured. The typical list price in the United States in 1997 for a new, lightweight, foldable wheelchair was $1100 to $2500 (1). Powered wheelchairs commonly cost between $4000 and $18,000. This does not include additional costs of adaptive seating, positioning, and assistive technology systems. Most patients are not prepared to pay out-of-pocket for a new wheelchair, and there are usually restrictions to the amount provided by public assistance and private insurance. Alternatives include buying used or floor models or trade-ins, or using community resources such as the Multiple Sclerosis Society. State bureaus dedicated to vocational rehabilitation will often help purchase equipment deemed necessary, as part of efforts to return a client to work. When any single source fails, a combination of resources may succeed. The American Medical Association publishes a book that describes the essential components of a letter of medical necessity and the sources of funding on a state-by-state basis (2).

Because most funding sources, both private and public, will provide only one chair every 5 years, it is paramount that the physician provide an accurate prescription the first time. The ideally prescribed chair maintains or improves the patient's best posture, is easy to operate, maximizes function, is appropriate to the intended environments, is aesthetically satisfying to the patient, is mechanically sound, and is backed by reliable and accessible sales and manufacturers' representatives. Unfortunately, for many patients, the ideal device does not exist. For these patients, the knowledgeable physician is indispensable in helping to guide them to an acceptable compromise.

To ensure that the optimal device is selected, kinesiologic, biomechanical, pathophysiologic, psychosocial, and technical parameters must be considered. A team approach where members of different disciplines and perspectives collaborate and solve problems with the patient is recommended. While no discipline has a franchise on any particular body of knowledge, certain tasks are typically assumed by different specialists.

Members of the wheeled mobility team include, but are not limited to the following:

1. Patient/family/caregivers (core members)
2. Physician (physiatrist) (core member)
3. Physical therapist (core member)
4. Occupational therapist (core member)
5. Local wheelchair vendors (core members)
6. Rehabilitation technology engineer (core member if the team is to address other issues of assistive technology such as augmented communication or environmental control units)
7. Speech pathologist (core member if the team is to address other issues of assistive technology such as augmented communication or environmental control units)
8. Wheelchair manufacturers
9. Social worker
10. Case manager
11. Education professional (teacher or administrator)
12. Vocational rehabilitation counselor
13. Nurse
14. Peer counselor

The most important members of the team are the *patient, family members*, and *caregivers*. From these individuals, the rest of the team learns of the patient's goals, aspirations, and functional capacity. As a patient tries different proposed solutions, his or her feedback guides the team to the final prescription.

The physician is responsible for assessing and communicating the pathophysiology and prognosis of the client's disease and identifying intrinsic limiting factors (e.g., spasticity, pain). This is accomplished by providing the other professionals with a thorough report of the history, physical findings, and psychosocial status of the client. The physician is also ultimately responsible for the written prescription and for medical justification of the wheelchair and seating system once input has been given by team members.

Physical therapists and *occupational therapists* evaluate the client's range of motion and strength to identify fixed deformities or structural abnormalities that will affect the wheelchair prescription. These therapists also provide valuable information about the client's functional level that may affect the appropriateness of certain components. Functional areas include capability to use power mobility or manual propulsion, ability to perform pressure relief maneuvers, ability to transfer to and from the wheelchair, and ability to ambulate. Often the therapist has already developed a trusting working relationship with the patient. In these cases, the therapist is in an ideal position to function as an advocate for the patient, ensuring that all questions and concerns have been addressed.

The *speech pathologist* is consulted to determine how seating and positioning affect swallowing and communication. The *rehabilitation technology engineer* provides information about current research and design of mechanics and electronics as related to the wheelchair and other assistive technology options.

Local wheelchair vendors (dealers) share their knowledge of currently available equipment. They also provide insight to the complex issues of funding policies for wheelchair purchases. The vendors are responsible for providing the wheelchair that is prescribed for the client. They may also be responsible for providing trial equipment prior to formulation of the final wheelchair prescription and loaner equipment prior to final delivery of the prescribed wheelchair. Upon delivery, the vendor should assemble the wheelchair and instruct the patient on its use and maintenance. The physician must maintain an independent view from the vendors, since the vendors may be tempted to provide equipment based on what they have in stock, or what will be most profitable, instead of what is best for the patient.

Manufacturers' representatives are informative about new and existing products. They are also a valuable source for loaner equipment. They may have the discretion to sell items at a reduced price in special circumstances. They may have discontinued stock that can be supplied to needy patients at a substantial discount.

The *social worker* or *case manager* communicates with the funding agency regarding the client's needs and the wheelchair prescription. In turn, he or she communicates to the team the stipulations and limitations of the client's funding source. Alternative funding is often researched and suggested by the social worker. The social worker can fill in detailed information regarding the psychological and social framework that surrounds the patient.

Nurses may be consulted for input to the wheelchair prescription if the patient has questionable skin integrity or a history of pressure ulcers. They may also be involved in solving problems associated with bowel and bladder management.

Educational professionals and *vocational counselors* provide input involving school and work accessibility. Educators are able to provide information about the client's performance and optimal positioning during the school day. Vocational counselors, in addition to adapting the work environment, often obtain funding for the mobility device or seating adaptations.

A mobility-impaired *peer counselor* can represent the patient's interests and perspectives, while guiding the patient through the selection process. Decisions endorsed by the peer gain credibility and thus are more likely to meet patient approval. This person must have the maturity and intelligence to avoid overgeneralizing from his or her personal experiences, conditions, and preferences, to be truly useful to the team.

Rational decision making for the wheeled mobility prescription can be accomplished by asking a series of questions as outlined in the flowcharts provided. In the following discussion, the general terms *wheelchair* and *powered wheelchair* will include scooters unless otherwise noted. Likewise, the term *chair* is used as shorthand for *wheelchair*.

It is obvious that those with bilateral lower-limb paralysis require a wheelchair while those with sufficient endurance and functional gait do not. On occasion, however, patients will present with limited ability to ambulate. For these patients, the key is to determine what limits their walking. A psychological or medical approach may be in order if fear, pain, or vertigo limits ambulation. Gait instability may be best treated with a directed course of physical therapy or bracing. Patients who can maintain ambulation will more easily access counters and navigate tight corners (i.e., bathrooms). They will retain the psychological benefit of engaging others face-to-face at a standing level. Upright weight bearing preserves certain physiologic advantages, such as better maintenance of bone density. Therefore, every option should be explored to preserve walking in those who are capable. However, the physician should not be reluctant to recommend a wheelchair or scooter for the marginally ambulatory individual. The proper device can enhance mobility and preserve energy, expanding participation in desired activities.

After it has been determined that a seated mobility device is necessary, then one must choose between manually propelled and power wheelchairs. Because manual chairs are lighter, are less prone to mechanical failure, are easier to transport, and provide continued cardiovascular challenge, they are preferred over power chairs. For those who lack the endurance or strength for self-propulsion and possess the requisite cognitive and perceptual skills, powered mobility is preferred. Of course, an option is for a separate person to push the patient in a manual chair. Disabilities commonly served by manual chairs include disease processes that spare either both arms at the C7 spinal cord level and below (such as spinal cord injuries or lower-limb amputation) or one side of the body (such as hemiplegia due to stroke). Power mobility often serves those with spinal cord injuries of C6 and above, neuromuscular diseases such as Duchenne muscular dystrophy, or neurologic diseases that sap strength and endurance such as multiple sclerosis or amyotrophic lateral sclerosis. Individuals with nonneurologic diseases of endurance and strength, such as rheumatologic, pulmonary, and cardiovascular diseases, may also benefit from power mobility (Algorithm 37-1).

MANUAL WHEELCHAIR PRESCRIPTION

To understand how wheelchairs are dispensed, one must understand the complex interrelationships among three parties who have different agendas: insurers, of which Medicare is the largest single payer in the United States; wheelchair vendors (for-profit private concerns); and the physician-patient team. Although insurers have the mission of paying for needed equipment, they have a conflicting interest to control cost. Vendors, the equipment providers, no matter how well intentioned, must look to the bottom line to remain in business. The patient generally wants what is best for himself or herself, but is usually not well informed about the various equipment options available, particularly immediately after a mobility-impairing injury or illness. The physician, in partnership with the patient, must mediate between these forces in the patient's interest. In the background is the fourth player, the manufacturer.

Medicare has classified manual wheelchairs from the heaviest to the lightest: standard (>36 lb), lightweight (≤36 lb), high-strength lightweight (<34 lb with a lifetime warranty on the side frames and cross-braces, and a sectional or adjustable back), and ultralightweight chair (<30 lb with an adjustable axle and a lifetime warranty on the side frames and cross-braces) (3). Almost all rigid-frame chairs are ultralightweight chairs. All major manufacturers warrant their wheelchairs for patients weighing up to 250 lb. A few manufacturers offer lightweight, high-

Algorithm 37-1. Is Wheeled Mobility Necessary?

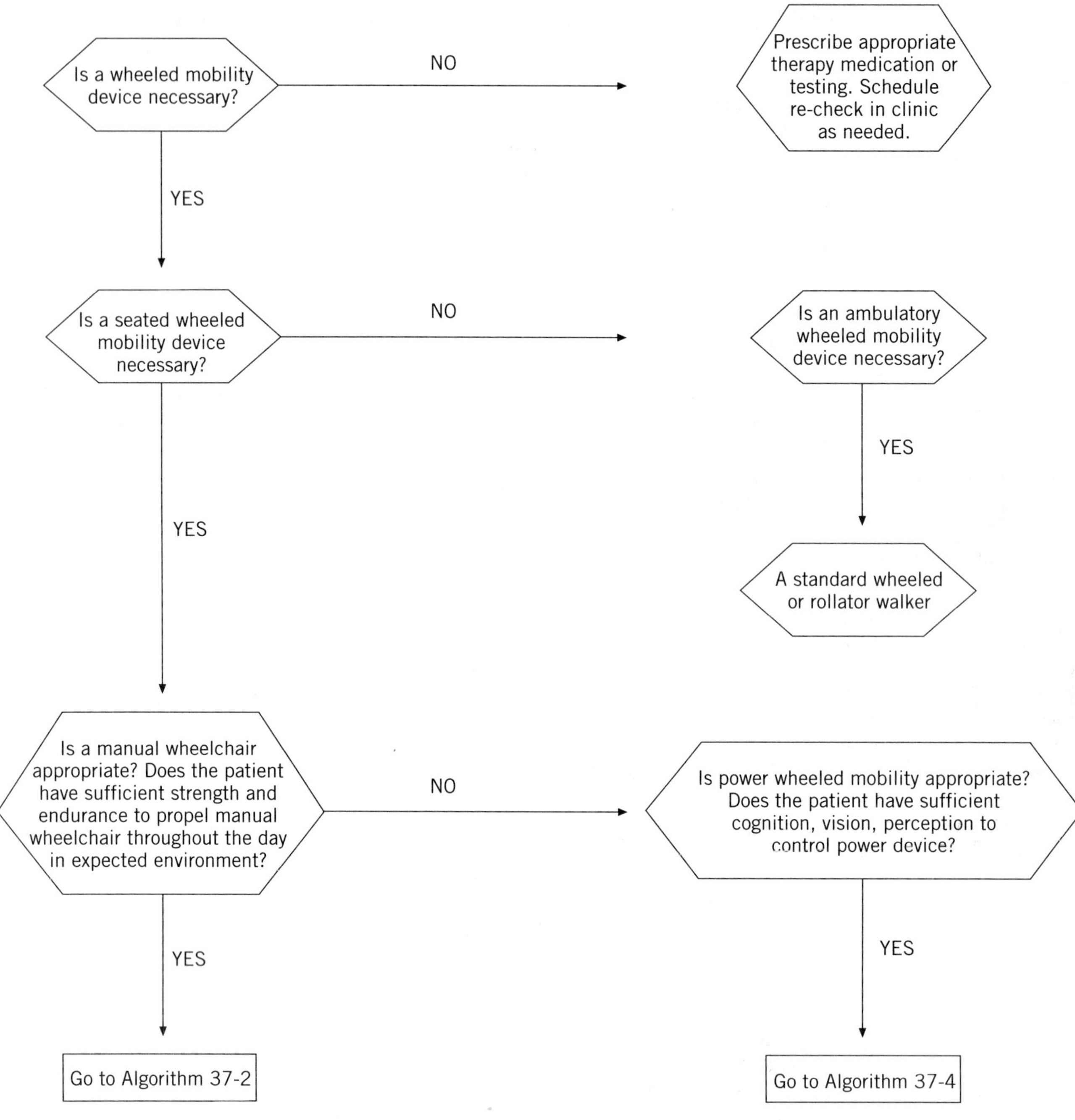

strength lightweight, and ultralightweight chairs warranted to 300 lbs. As would be expected, the lighter the chair, the more expensive it is.

Standard wheelchairs are more difficult to propel and transport; they offer little in terms of adjustability, and are often manufactured with fixed armrests and footplates, and less-expensive materials (Fig. 37-1). Thus, standard wheelchairs are nearly always the cheapest. They may be adequate for some patients who need a chair only temporarily, for example, following a hip replacement. *Lightweight* chairs also have fixed-height armrests, although they are detachable. To take advantage of the full spectrum of adjustability and options, one must look to *high-strength lightweight* and *ultralightweight* chairs. Cooper et al (4,5) investigated the life of various wheelchairs using the International Standards Organization standards, and concluded that in the long run, ultralightweight chairs may be the most economic investment for active users. They found that despite a higher initial cost, ultralightweight wheelchairs were on average 2.3 times less expensive than lightweight chairs

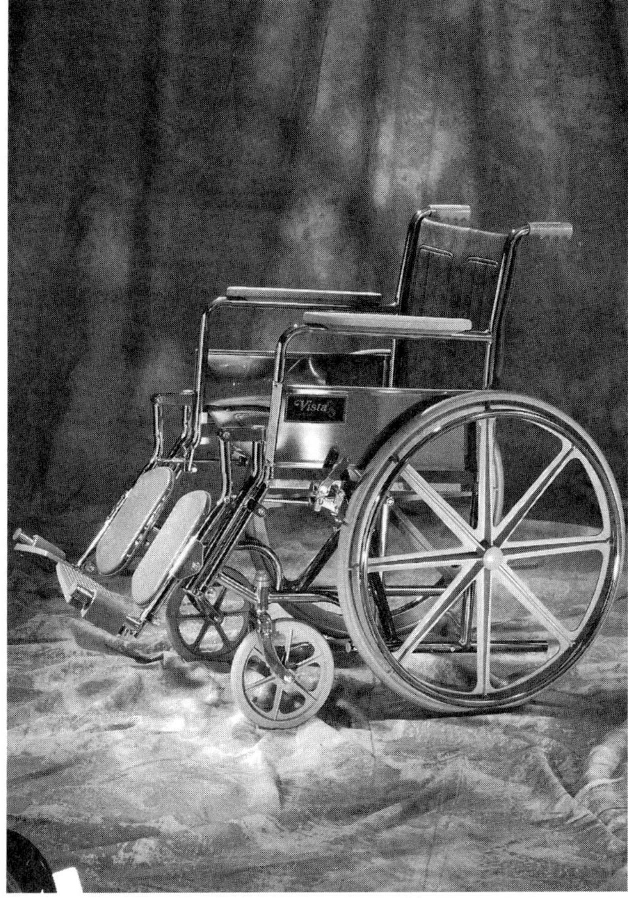

Figure 37-1. A standard weight wheelchair with a sling back, fixed full-length armrests, mag wheels, solid tires, and elevating leg rests.

and 3.4 times less expensive than standard chairs over time because they are so much more durable. This claim assumes that the user would keep the same chair until failure, that failure would necessitate purchase of a new wheelchair (as opposed to repair), and that the user would replace the lightweight or standard wheelchair with an identical model.

Medicare, in order to contain costs, requires that patients meet an escalating set of criteria to be eligible for a lighter, stronger chair. The patient's functional status must be verified on a form signed by a physician. As an example, a Medicare recipient is eligible to receive a standard wheelchair if the individual would be confined to a bed or chair without a wheelchair. In order to receive a lightweight chair, the user also must be unable to propel a standard chair, but be able to propel a lightweight chair. For a high-strength lightweight chair, the patient must self-propel "while engaging in frequent activities that cannot be performed in a standard or a lightweight wheelchair" or "require a seat width, depth, or height that cannot be accommodated in a standard, lightweight or hemi-wheelchair *and* spends at least 2 hours per day in the wheelchair" (3). A high-strength lightweight wheelchair will seldom be approved if the duration of need is expected to be less than 3 months. While ultralightweight chairs may be the most desirable because of their ease of wheeling, durability, and styling, they are generally also the most expensive. Medicare approves ultralightweight wheelchairs only on a case-by-case basis. There is no set formula that other insurers follow. Some third-party payers will allow a set fee, others will allow negotiation, while others provide no payment for durable medical equipment.

The patient's physician can play an important role in obtaining an appropriate wheelchair. The vendor is required to follow a physician's prescription and cannot legally substitute. If the physician specifies that the patient is to receive a rigid-frame wheelchair, the vendor cannot provide a folding-frame wheelchair. However, if the physician prescribes an item that is beyond the profit margin that the vendor will accept, the vendor can refuse to fill the prescription. Some vendors are more persistent than others at pursuing third-party funding, and are more willing to take financial risks for the patient's benefit. Knowledgeable physicians, particularly those who refer many patients, may influence the vendor to liberalize their policy. It is ultimately the physician's responsibility to prescribe the most appropriate wheelchair for the patient. Physicians are most likely to be successful in this when they are knowledgeable about the vendors, the manufacturers, and the available stock.

Patients are able to participate in this process to variable degrees. Many newly injured patients will be so burdened by the difficulties of recovery and adjustment to disability that they will have little ability to navigate the complexities of wheelchair prescription. The physician must be able to accurately assess the patient's needs, abilities, and ambitions, to guide him or her to the proper device. Five years later, after much personal experience and observation of others, the same patient may have formed strong opinions with regard to features and brand names he or she desires. At that time, the physician acts as an objective knowledgeable counselor to the patient to consult and a bridge to resources to help the patient procure the right equipment.

As already mentioned, standard, lightweight, high-strength lightweight, and ultralightweight wheelchairs are all warranted to 250 lb. However, active patients exceeding 225 lb may put such wear and tear on a lightweight frame that a heavy-duty frame is indicated. *Heavy-duty frames* are warranted up to 300 lb; beyond 300 lb, an *extra-heavy-duty wheelchair* is recommended. Physicians and vendors place themselves at risk for legal liability if they prescribe or provide a frame that does not meet the patient's weight requirements. Extra cross-braces and gussets (reinforcement) may be available from some manufacturers to upgrade the weight tolerance of a specific frame (Algorithm 37-2).

After the weight tolerance of the frame has been chosen (standard, lightweight, high-strength lightweight,

Algorithm 37-2. Deciding the Appropriate Frame Manual Wheelchair

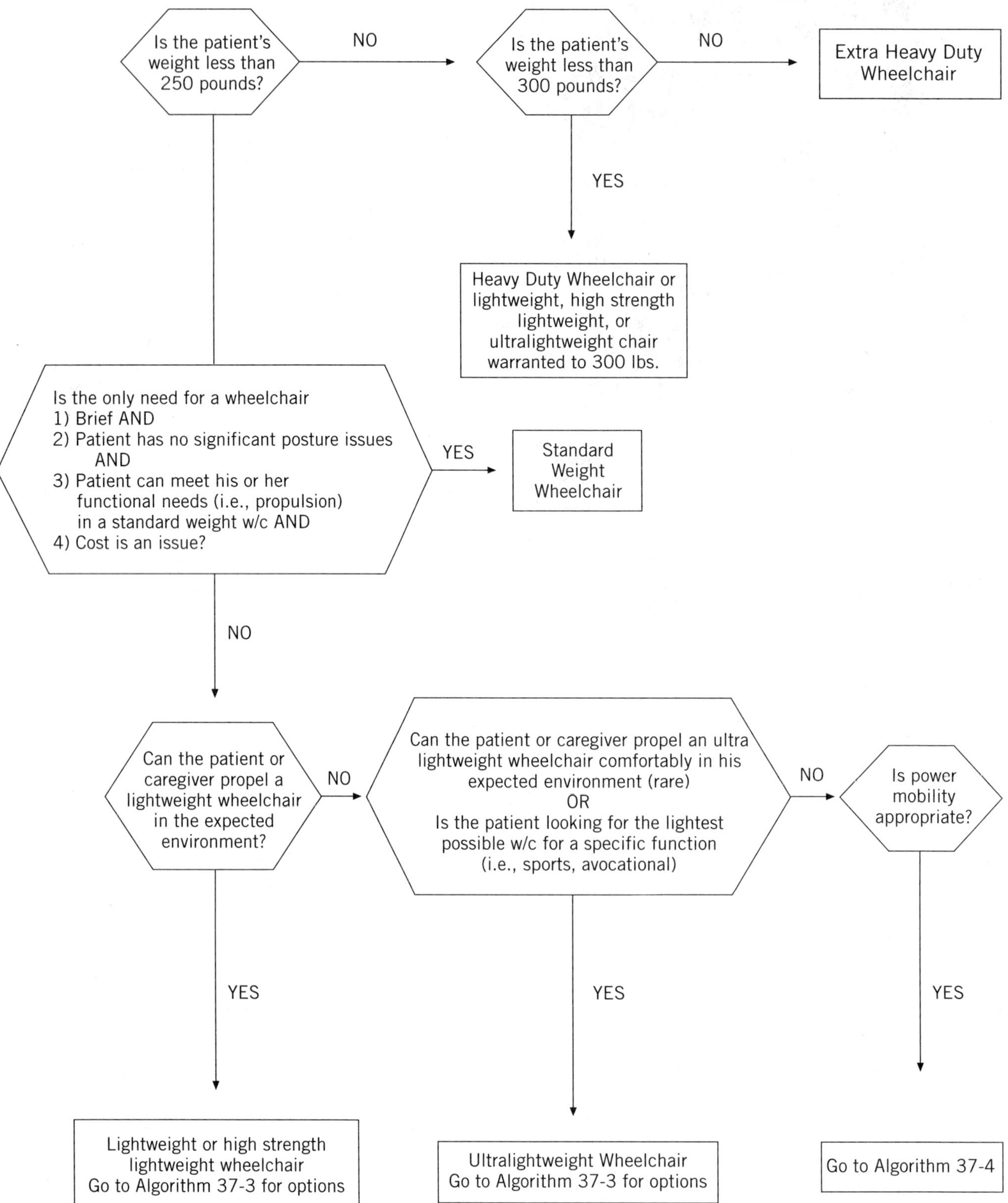

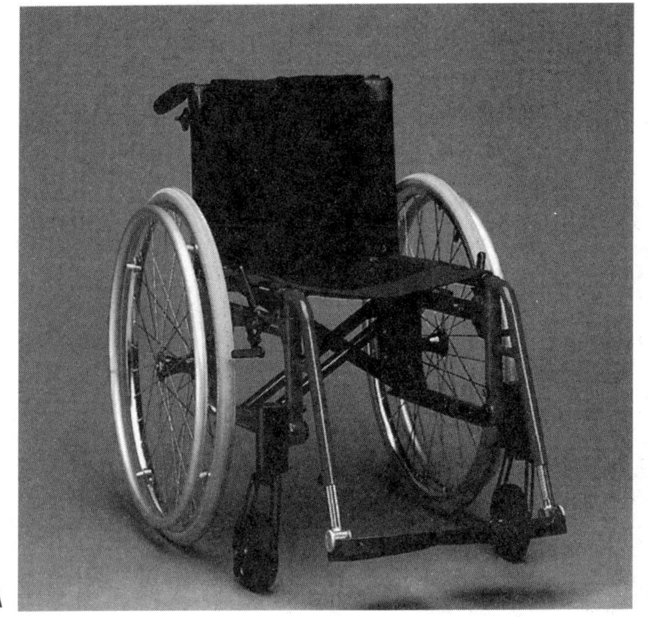

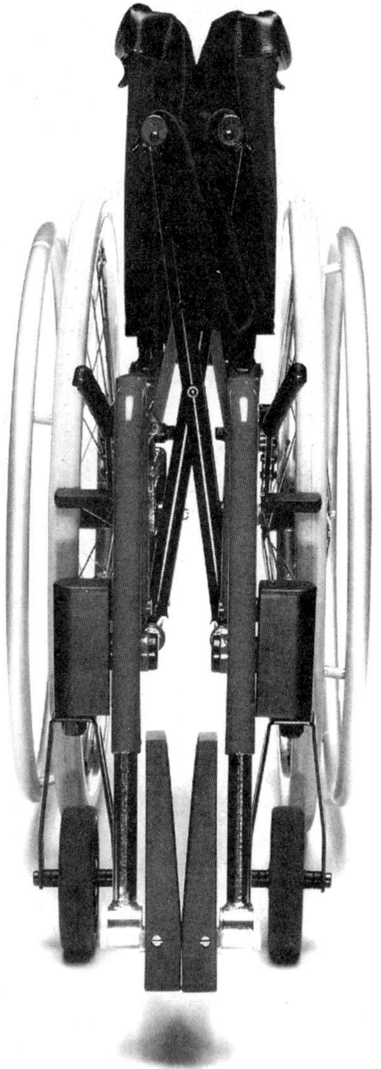

Figure 37-2. *A.* A folding frame wheelchair ready to wheel. *B.* A folding frame wheelchair in the folded position.

ultralightweight, heavy duty, or extra heavy duty), the next decision is "foldability" of the frame.

Frames come in two types of configuration, *foldable* and *rigid* (Figs. 37-2 and 37-3). These names are somewhat misleading since both types fold. Foldable frames have cross-braces underneath and fold like accordions. In most rigid-frame wheelchairs, the back folds forward and the wheels pop off. Most users describe the ride and the "feel" of a rigid chair as more responsive. This has been attributed to the fact that most folding-frame chairs "flex" to allow them to collapse. Rigid chairs are generally more durable and slightly lighter than the comparable foldable chair. More time, dexterity, and planning are needed to break down a rigid chair. Specifically, the back must be folded to the seat, and then the wheels are usually removed. This can constitute a significant obstacle to transporting a rigid-frame chair in a car. Although the vast majority of able-bodied caretakers will find it convenient to simply pull upward on the seat to collapse a folding chair, some people with disabilities may find the bulk of a folding chair more cumbersome to transport. Rigid chairs usually have quick-release axles (described in detail later), which are more prone to break and carry a small amount of risk of becoming disengaged while the user is wheeling. The typical user of a rigid-frame chair is a younger spinal cord–injured individual, while older individuals with hemiplegia secondary to stroke would typically be seated in a folding-frame chair. Another type of rigid-frame chair is a manual *tilt-in-space* chair (Fig. 37-4). These chairs allow a caregiver to reposition the patient while maintaining a constant seat-to-back angle. Manual tilt-in-space wheelchairs are large, heavy, and difficult to transport. A *hybrid* chair is foldable but does not use a cross-brace (Fig. 37-5). When assembled, the hybrid chair appears identical to a rigid-frame chair. It is a little heavier and more difficult to fold than the typical rigid chair, but when folded is very compact.

The prescription can now be organized sequentially

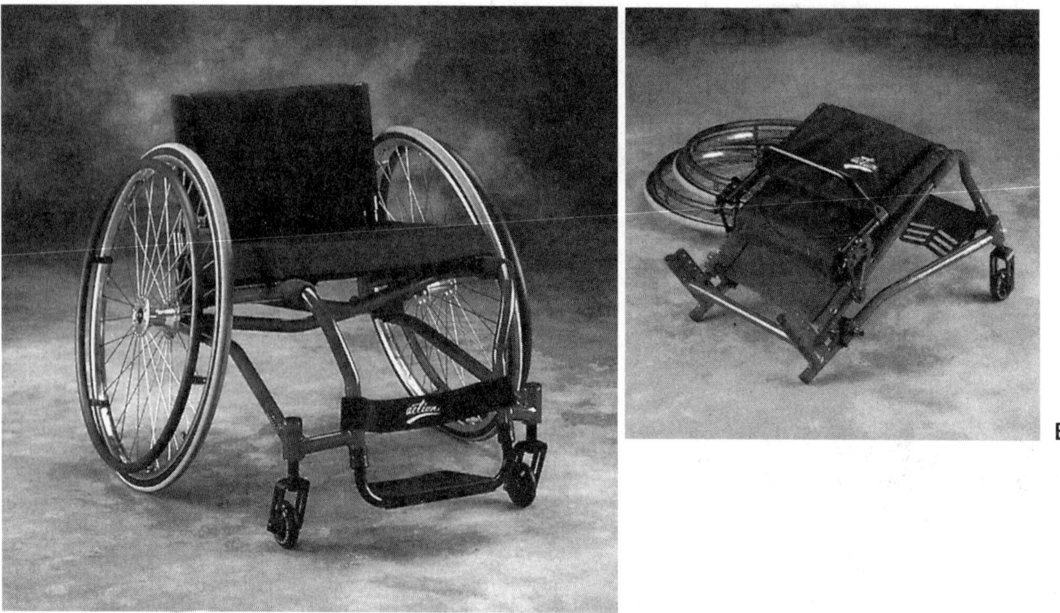

Figure 37-3. *A.* A rigid frame wheelchair ready to wheel. *B.* A rigid frame wheelchair in the folded position.

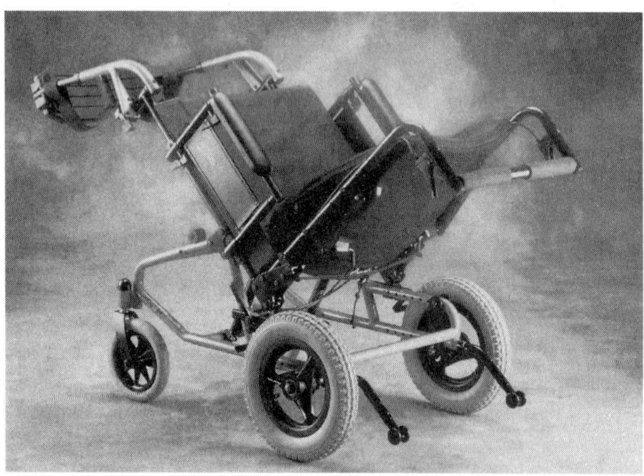

Figure 37-4. A manual tilt-in-space wheelchair in the tilted position.

from the push handles (the posterior-superior corner) to the front casters (the anterior-inferior corner). Decisions are guided by the goal of maximally enhancing a client's mobility and function, with the least amount and expense of equipment (Algorithm 37-3 and Appendix II).

Push handles, as their name suggests, can be used by a helper to push the chair. The helper can easily grasp push handles to negotiate stairs or curbs. Push handles also function as a fulcrum for those with poor trunk stability (i.e., individuals with tetraplegia) to wrap one arm around while reaching with the other. In a similar fashion, push handles can anchor maneuvers that aid the relief of pressure on the patient's buttocks and thighs. They also act as brackets from which backpacks can be suspended. Users with good arm strength and trunk balance (i.e., paraplegic individuals injured at a midthoracic level or lower) may perceive push handles as a sign of dependence and choose chairs without them. Sports wheelchairs often lack push handles.

The *sling back* is the most common wheelchair back. A fabric is simply suspended between the canes. In its most crude form, the material will be a nonbreathable synthetic that is bolted onto the chair. A better alternative is an easily removable, washable nylon. Sling backs are prone to fatigue over time. This can promote kyphosis and place the shoulders at a biomechanical disadvantage. An option available on many lightweight chairs is an *adjustable-tension* sling back that incorporates horizontal straps at preset intervals (Fig. 37-6). Besides combating material fatigue, these can be loosened or tightened to provide lumbar support and to increase trunk stability. When more support is needed, a *solid back* may be the solution. *Prefabricated solid backs* come in a variety of heights, depths, and contours. Most can be easily mounted and removed using special brackets. *Custom backs* can be individually fabricated for the hard-to-fit (i.e., individuals with fixed spinal deformities). *Lateral supports* can be attached to the canes in order to add further trunk stability.

A folding wheelchair requires a sling seat (it is hard to fold a solid seat); some rigid chairs come equipped or can be fitted with a *solid seat pan.* Like sling backs, sling seats fatigue over time. As they sag, the femurs of the seated person internally rotate and adduct, which can lead to contractures. To prevent this, a *solid seat insert* (often a wooden board) can be added beneath the cushion (often inside the cover). One manufacturer offers an adjustable-tension sling seat as a low-cost, low-technology positioning aid. Alternatively, cushions with a stiff, bowed undersurface

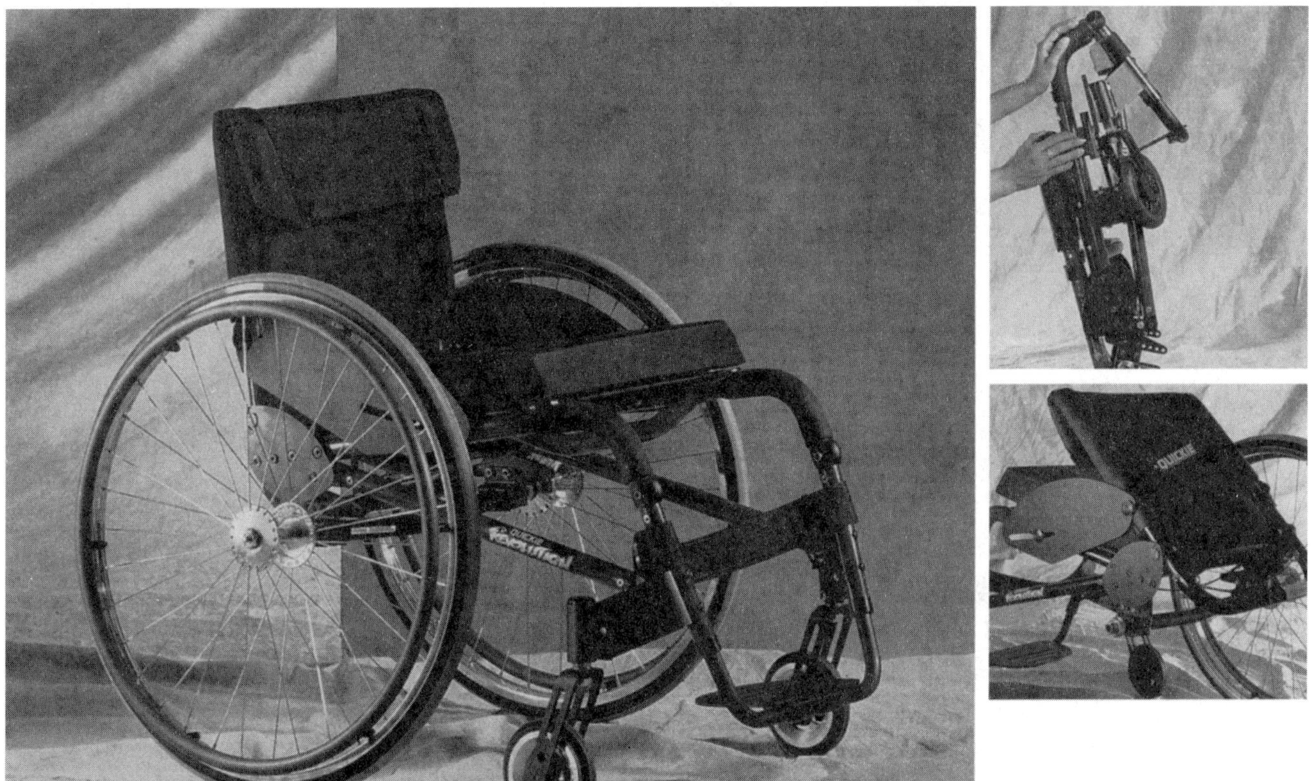

Figure 37-5. *A.* A hybrid wheelchair ready to wheel. *B.* A hybrid frame wheelchair in the folded position.

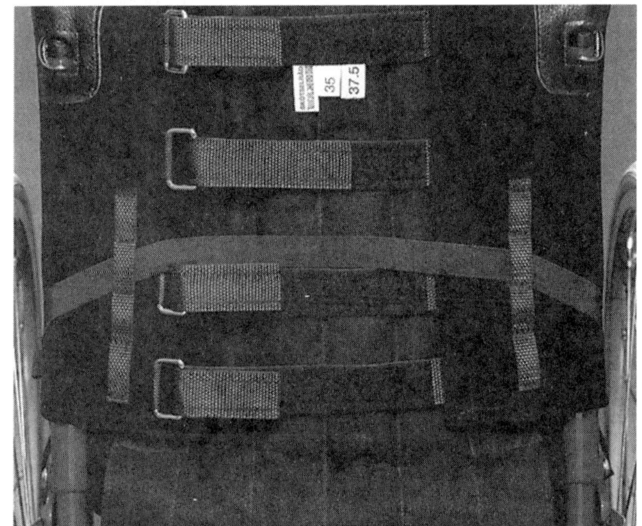

Figure 37-6. An adjustable-tension sling back.

can be selected to accommodate the sagging of the sling seat. See Chapter 36 for a full discussion of custom seating and cushion options.

Armrests can be divided into tubular and nontubular styles. The least amount of armrest is the *tubular armrest*, which is found almost exclusively on rigid chairs. Because tubular armrests tend to bend under pressure, they are most appropriate for those who can transfer without having to push off from the armrest, such as persons with spinal cord injuries at the lumbar or low thoracic level who have good trunk balance and some functional abdominal musculature. These detachable armrests provide a surface for the forearm to be stationed, and are easy to remove. They come in a shorter, desk length and a longer full length. An option with tubular (and other) armrests is a *clothing guard*, which fits between the user and the wheel to prevent the user's apparel from getting soiled.

Nontubular armrests provide a more stable surface for push-offs than do tubular armrests. Nontubular armrests vary in three dimensions: length (desk length versus full length), adjustability (height adjustable versus fixed height), and attachment to the frame versus detachability. *Desk-length* armrests are prescribed more commonly in our clinics. They allow a wheeler to approach a table almost as closely as an able-bodied person sitting on a static chair. A few patients will require *full-length* armrests for better leverage or forearm support; they can be detached for side-to-side transfers. The height-adjustable feature provides for elevation or depression of the arm pad depending on a given user's stature. To aid side-to-side transfers and to increase access to the user, a detachable armrest is recommended. A *flip-back armrest* is a kind of detachable armrest

Algorithm 37-3. Manual Wheelchair Options

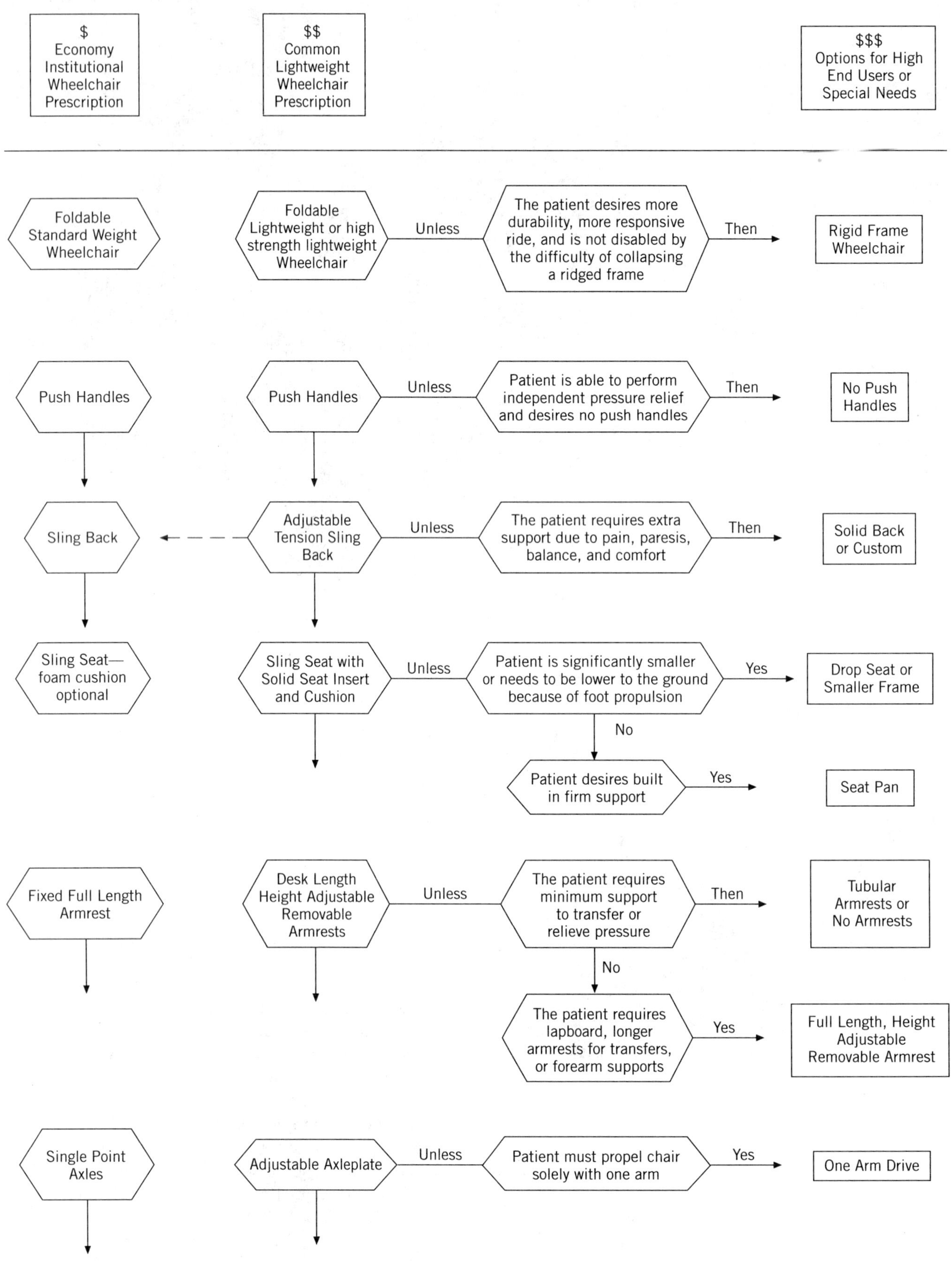

Algorithm 37-3. *Continued*

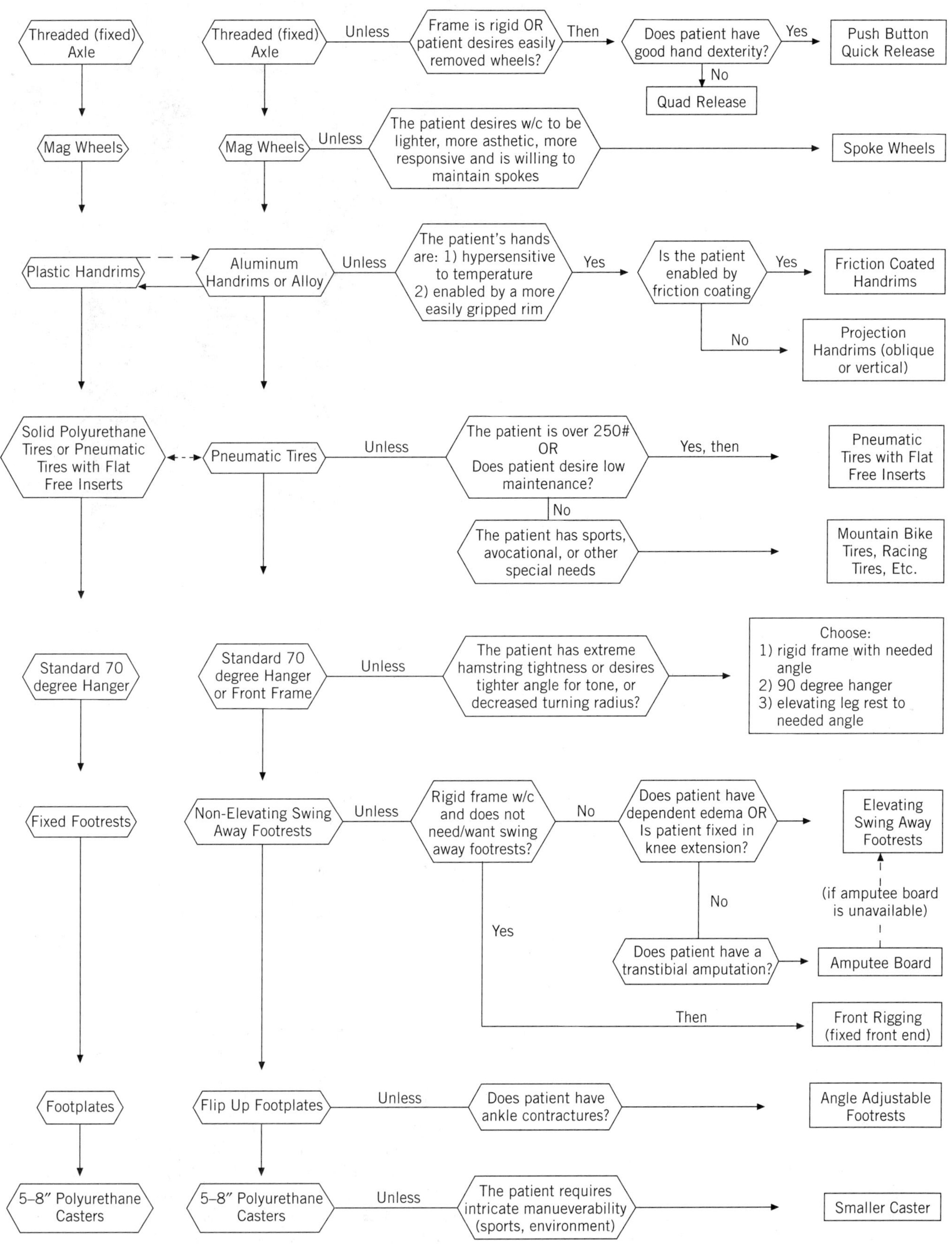

that pivots at the posterior post. It is often more convenient to pilot a flip-back armrest than to completely remove the standard removable armrest. *Height-adjustable, detachable, desk-length armrests* are standard equipment on most lightweight folding wheelchairs.

Fixed, full-length armrests are often standard equipment on standard frame wheelchairs. They cannot be adjusted to the individual user, and cannot be removed for side-to-side transfers.

A one-half *lap tray* is helpful in positioning the shoulder of the hemiplegic to decrease pain and the extent of subluxation. Arm troughs can also serve this purpose. A full lap tray gives a greater surface area on which can be placed environmental control units. The full lap tray can also function as a gentle restraint.

Axle plates allow for adjustment of axle position. Many less expensive chairs are manufactured with a single, fixed axle position. Other chairs with a fixed axle allow for the addition of an axle plate so that the chair can be modified to the patient's needs. More expensive, lightweight and ultralight chairs commonly come with the ability to adjust axle position either through an axle plate or by another mechanism. A curious terminology has been attached to the axle plate. An axle plate that allows repositioning of the axle anterior to or vertically from its original position has traditionally been called an *adjustable axle plate.* An axle plate that allows the wheel to be repositioned posterior to the posterior upright of the frame is called an *amputee axle plate.* Lower-limb amputees experience a posterior shift of their seated center of gravity (COG) when they lose any part of the lower limb. While many unilateral transtibial amputees will not require that the axle be repositioned, the great majority of transfemoral or bilateral transtibial amputees do require an axle adjustment. Vertical repositioning is valuable for clients of shorter or taller stature and those who require the wheelchair to be close to the ground for effective foot propulsion. Besides changing the COG, adjusting the axle will often change the seat angle.

For users who have control of one upper limb only, *one-arm drive* is available (Fig. 37-7). In the United States, the common configuration equips the wheel underneath the functioning arm with two push rims. The outer rim is connected to the ipsilateral wheel; the inner rim is connected via a shaft to the contralateral wheel. Another system more common in Europe uses a lever arm that is pumped to move both wheels. The handle can be turned to direct the chair by guiding the casters. These chairs are heavier than comparable manual chairs. Cognitively impaired individuals will be challenged by attempting to manage guidance and propulsion with the same limb.

Starting from the center of the wheel and working outward, the important considerations are type of axle (threaded or removable), type of strut (mag or spoked), type of push rim, and type of tire.

The *wheel axle* is the shaft on which the wheels rotate.

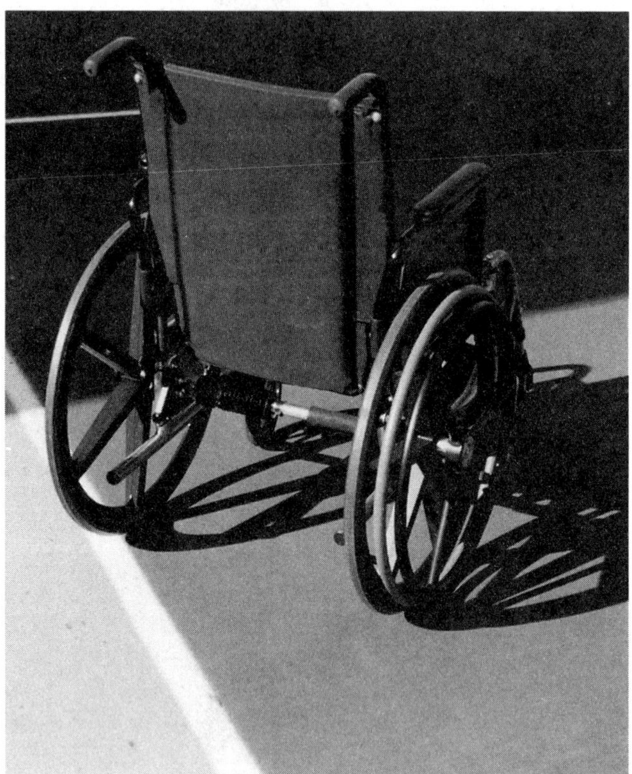

Figure 37-7. A one-arm drive wheelchair. Note the dual push rims at the right wheel and the axle connecting the outer rim to the left wheel.

Axles can be *threaded* (standard on foldable chairs) or *quick release* (standard on rigid chairs to permit easier transport in cars). As their name implies, quick-release axles allow the wheel to be detached with a push of a button. For those who have difficulty pushing a button, a larger lever release consisting of a looped nut that is attached to the axle (called *quad release*) may be enabling.

Wheels may be attached to the rim either with a metal spoke as seen on most bicycles (spoke wheel) or by several struts made of plastic or composite material (mag wheel). *Spoke wheel* rims are lighter than the comparable mag wheel, and may provide a smoother ride. However, spokes tend to loosen and break more easily than the struts of a mag wheel, and thus require more maintenance.

Mag wheels were so named because magnesium strips were used to connect the rim to the center of the wheel. Now, mag wheels are usually made of plastic. They are durable and require little or no maintenance and therefore are more commonly prescribed than their spoked counterparts. Another advantage of mag wheels is that the central hub may be narrower than a spoked hub. This is a consideration when trying to minimize the width of the chair.

Push rims are usually made of aluminum or a similar alloy, although plastic and other composites are available on some less expensive models. Smooth metal push rims can be coated with rubber or vinyl. This option offers the advantage of making the chair easier to push by increasing friction between the hand and the push rim. Unfortunately this same friction can lead to burns when attempting to slow down the chair. Therefore, gloves are especially recommended for those who choose coated push rims. Another disadvantage of the coated push rim is poor durability. These special push rims may have to be replaced as often as once a year. To increase grip further for users with impaired hand function, plastic tubing can be woven around the rim. When this fails, *projections* (quad knobs), which can be *vertically* or *obliquely* oriented, can be considered. These are typically used to improve the propulsive force in individuals with a C6 spinal cord injury. It is important to note that for the majority of individuals with a C6 injury, manual wheelchair use is not practical due to limitations in strength, balance, and endurance.

Conceivably, tires can come in all of the variety of sizes, diameters, and treads that are available for bicycles. Standard adult tire diameters are 20, 22, 24, and 26 inches; are 1¾ inches wide; are available as solid, smooth polyurethane, or treaded; and are filled with either air or a "flat-free" material. Racing- and mountain-bike tires may be indicated for particular sports or avocational uses; these are available on some models for an additional charge. The preferred tire is an air-filled *pneumatic* tire because it is the lightest, and gives the most cushioning. However, it demands periodic attention to maintain proper inflation. These tires are also prone to flats and are likely to fail for persons whose weight approaches or exceeds 250 lb. Therefore, some may prefer a *flat-free insert*. Although this is less shock absorbent, it is not subject to weight limitations on the user and requires very little upkeep. The *solid polyurethane* tire requires the least maintenance. It is suitable for predominantly indoor, noncarpeted (i.e., institutional) surfaces.

The standard *hanger* angle of 70 degrees from horizontal situates the knees in a relatively neutral position while avoiding collision with the casters when the chair is turned. A 60-degree hanger may be necessary to accommodate knee extension contractures, but increases the turning radius. A hanger angle of 90 degrees or greater accommodates hamstring contractures. The greater the hanger angle, the easier it is to turn the chair because the moment of inertia is decreased. Greater hanger angles also allow tighter turning radii. Bending the knees beyond 90 degrees often requires the ankles to accommodate by bending in dorsiflexion. Also the casters must be made smaller or be outset to avoid the footrest. While this posture may help inhibit tone, care must be taken to avoid knee flexion contractures. Chairs with hanger or frame angles of 90 degrees or more typically serve individuals with paraplegia who are committed to maintain a quadriceps stretching regimen.

The legs and feet are usually supported on either a swing-away *removable footrest* (the only option for most foldable chairs) or a *front rigging* (the only option for most rigid chairs). The swing-away removable footrest, as its name implies, can be rotated away from the frame of the chair or entirely removed. This allows the feet to touch the ground, which is required for stand and pivot transfers or foot propulsion. A common option is *flip-up footplates* to allow the user to reach the floor without having to move the hanger. *Heel loops* limit the posterior excursion of the foot; foot straps can help to position the foot on the plate, but must be released for transfers. Footplates may also be made with the angle of attachment adjustable to accommodate plantarflexion contractures.

Elevating leg rests usually come with a calf pad and can be helpful to control edema. Elevating leg rests are available with more proximally located calf pads for new transtibial amputees to aid in the prevention of knee flexion contractures. Another option is the amputee slot board that fits under the seat cushion and projects to support the residual limb.

Front rigging requires the user to lift his or her legs beyond the footplates when transferring. Front rigging can be adapted with a one-piece *swing-away footplate*, but this requires the user to be able to bend to reach and manipulate the footplate.

Unlike the main tires, solid *casters* are preferred to air-filled ones because the air-filled casters are large and bulky and deflate frequently. One great advantage of air-filled casters is that they reduce the impact transmitted to the frame, and thus may extend the frame's life (4). Standard caster sizes of 6 to 8 inches in diameter allow easy rolling over a variety of terrains, while still fitting with a standard 70-degree hanger. Smaller casters (available as small as 2-inch "Roller Blade" wheels) can accommodate more severe hanger angles and also turn more sharply. Although they function well in the gym, they are more easily caught in grates, tall carpets, and uneven or muddy terrains.

Standard safety features include a positioning belt, wheel locks, and antitip devices. The physician may be legally liable if these are not included in the prescription and the patient subsequently comes to harm that might have been prevented were these items prescribed. The *positioning belt* for most users will be a simple lap belt with a push button or air line buckle, although Velcro closures may be needed for those with insufficient finger dexterity. Whether these actually improve safety has not been determined. Patients with significant spasticity may require elaborate chest straps to control posture. *Wheel locks* hold the chair in position and prevent rolling. Locking requires more effort than releasing; for those with marginal strength, the locks can be set as either *push-to-lock* or *pull-to-lock*, depending on the user's preference. *Extensions* can increase leverage to ease locking and unlocking and to facilitate reaching to the opposite side for hemiplegics, but require a greater range of motion and can interfere with transfers. *Scissor locks* are located on the frame tubing that runs anterior-posterior, and have the advantage of being completely hidden when disengaged. This is useful for certain sports activities where otherwise the thumb has a proclivity to be caught during vigorous wheeling. However, scissor locks are harder to reach and more difficult to use. *Grade aids* are small cam mechanisms that attach to the wheel near the wheel lock and when engaged, prevent the wheel from slipping backward. This option can ease propulsion up longer inclines. When properly adjusted, *antitip devices* reduce the likelihood of a chair toppling backward. Unfortunately, they also block "wheelies," which may be required to jump curbs or to climb inclines.

ADJUSTING A MANUAL CHAIR FOR SPECIFIC PATIENT NEEDS

Wheelchairs should be adjusted to fit individual users. As stated before, high-strength lightweight and ultralightweight chairs generally offer the maximum in flexibility of adjustment (some chairs in these categories have less adjustability to decrease the weight, such as sports-specific chairs or custom-fabricated chairs). A number of studies have shown that adjusting the setup of a wheelchair affects the efficiency of propulsion, as well as the forces borne by the upper limbs (6–9). There is reason to believe that improved positioning and optimal propulsion technique reduce the risk of upper-limb injury (10). Features that can be modified include the seat angle, seat-to-back angle, axle position, camber, and footrest height. In general, a posture of 95 degrees between the spine and femur and 90 degrees between the femur and tibia is encouraged. These settings are impractical or unobtainable for many patients, thus influencing which wheelchair should be selected. Fixed deformities or poor abdominal tone (i.e., lower to middle thoracic spinal cord injuries and above) may necessitate that the seat-to-back angle be increased. Certain solid backs come with hooks that allow an extra 25 degrees in recline. Some chairs offer adjustable positioning for the canes. In other instances, bent canes can be obtained. The angle of the seat can be adjusted so that the sacrum sits even lower relative to the knees (*dump*). This can combat the tendency to slide out of a chair, and can prevent the pelvis from falling into a posterior tilt. As the pelvis tilts posteriorly, the lumbosacral region of the spine falls into kyphosis. With kyphosis, chest expansion is limited, leading to restricted inspiration, and the shoulders are put into a position of mechanical disadvantage, thereby confining reach.

Positioning the axle properly in relationship to the patient's seated COG is critical for safety and best propulsion (11,12). As the axle approaches the COG from the posterior, the chair will lose rear stability, and tend to tip backward. The shorter wheelbase provided by an anteriorly placed axle offers advantages, such as decreased rolling resistance, decreased downhill turning tendency, improved maneuverability, improved efficiency of propulsion, and usually improved portability. Conversely, placement of the axle posteriorly away from the COG will increase rear stability, but also will make popping wheelies more difficult (which are often necessary to negotiate curbs), and increase the turning radius. In general, the height of the axle should be adjusted so that the elbow is at a 90-degree angle when the hands are on the top of the push rims.

Camber is present when the distance between the top of the wheel is less than the distance at the bottom. Typically, the camber angle is 3 to 9 degrees from the vertical. Increasing the camber by moving the bottom of the wheel outward increases the ease of propulsion, as well as the lateral and rear stability of the wheelchair. However, the turning radius is increased. Because of improved responsiveness of wheelchairs with camber, larger camber angles are often used in sports. Although there are several advantages to increased camber, it does increase the overall width of the wheelchair, making it more difficult to get through standard door frames and to manipulate in tight areas. Increasing the camber angle can cause the wheels to toe out, lower the seat height, and decrease rear stability, requiring further adjustment of the chair.

A common problem is the wide patient who must navigate in a narrow environment. However, a few "tricks" can be used to decrease chair width. First, wraparound armrests can be employed. Wraparound armrests offer structural placement of the posterior upright of the armrest behind the canes of the chair, decreasing the overall width of the chair typically by 1.5 inches (standard armrests are seated alongside the canes). A more severe hanger angle will decrease the turning radius. Mag wheels tend to be narrower than spoke wheels. On many chairs the wheels can be placed closer to the center of a threaded axle. Some chairs are equipped with axle plates exterior to the posterior uprights. The axle plate can be relocated interiorly. Push rims can have their connecting brackets shortened or be removed entirely. Foldable chairs can come with a device that attaches to the armrest and to the seating tube underneath the fabric of a sling seat. By twisting a handle or turning a lever, the distance between the seating tube and the armrest is shortened, which has the effect of partially folding the chair, thus making the chair less wide. The beauty of this system is that it can be operated by the person occupying the chair. As soon as the operator has traversed the narrow doorway, the chair can be restored to its original width by turning the lever in the opposite direction.

POWER WHEELCHAIRS AND SCOOTERS

Problem solving for powered mobility is very similar to that for manual chairs, except there are generally fewer options from which to choose. The largest question is whether to prescribe a scooter, a power chair with easily detachable batteries, or a power-base power wheelchair. As always, the patient's participation and choice are essential to generating a successful prescription.

Powered mobility can be wonderfully liberating, but it is expensive, misapplication of this complex technology will only frustrate users. As the willingness of society to extend its resources to the people with disabilities diminishes, physicians must step forward to become forceful advocates for dispensation of truly useful equipment. Likewise, physicians should not shrink from withholding elaborate items that do not contribute to the patient's function. Four criteria should be met before powered mobility is authorized. First, the physician must be convinced that the patient's needs cannot be met with lesser equipment. Manual wheelchairs and walkers are lighter, easier to transport, and more mechanically reliable than powered mobility. Next, the patient must demonstrate sufficient vision and judgment to guide a powered chair safely. If this is questioned, vendors can often lend the patient an appropriate device in a controlled setting for a few days to see if the expected benefit is achieved. On rare occasions, a caregiver, instead of the patient, will be able to guide the chair. Third, patients must be enabled by the use of powered mobility in the intended environment. A scooter that works well in the clinic may be too long to fit in the office. Lack of proper ramps may make it impossible for the power chair to enter or leave the home. Finally, a plan for transporting the device to the intended environment should be established. Where public transportation is impractical or unavailable, the patient or family may have to invest in an adapted van. The services performed in a wheeled mobility device clinic include exploring and solving as many of these issues as possible (Algorithm 37-4).

Of the three power mobility options, *scooters* are the least expensive but also the least adaptable (Fig. 37-8). They are said to carry less of "the stigmata of disability." They come in three- and four-wheel designs; three-wheel designs are most common. Four-wheel designs may offer increased traction stability and power but at the cost of increased price, weight, and turning radius. The typical scooter seat is a swiveling bucket seat or captain's chair. Recently, some models have added seats that allow for limited customized posture control and seating protection. One common scooter option uncommonly found in power wheelchairs is the powered elevating seat (usually 2–7 inches), which can aid transfers and reach. Most scooters can be disassembled for transport in a car. The heaviest part, the transaxle, typically weighs 35 to 40 lb, which will present a challenge to some users. Appropriate larger cars may be equipped with *a trunk lift*, an assistive device to aid in the transfer of a scooter or wheelchair into the rear of a vehicle. Disadvantages of scooters (despite recent innovations) include that they do not allow much modification or customization of the seat, have longer wheelbases, and are slower and generate less torque than comparable power chairs; three-wheeled scooters have less lateral stability on

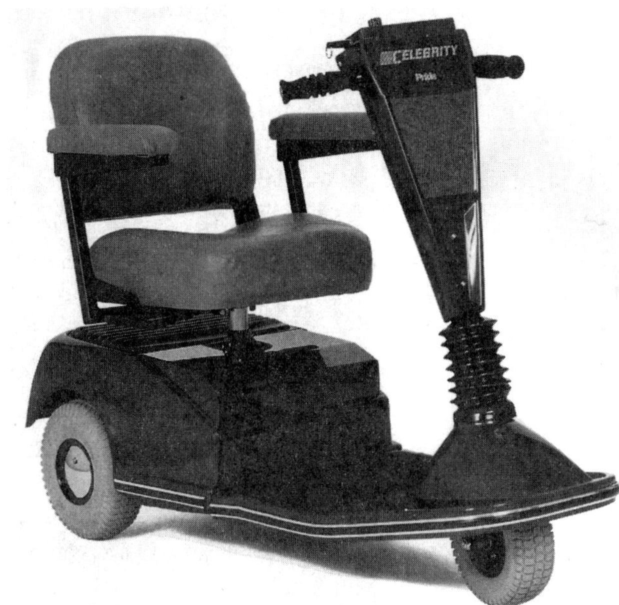

Figure 37-8. A three-wheeled scooter.

uneven terrain. Because of their length, scooters may not fit on some forms of public transportation (buses) that accept power chairs. The longer wheelbases translate to a longer turning radius. The tiller steering mechanism is mechanically similar to handlebars on a bicycle, demanding coordinated bimanual strength. Despite these negatives, for clients who are able to ambulate short distances, the scooter offers a well-accepted, cheaper alternative to the power chair. A typical scooter user is the patient with peripheral vascular disease, multiple sclerosis, arthritis, or pulmonary or cardiac disease whose ambulation is limited by endurance or ataxia. Very seldom are those with insufficient endurance to tolerate ambulation fit enough to propel a manual wheelchair.

Scooters are not practical for the nonambulatory. These individuals are most enabled by power wheelchairs (the term *electric chair* is already in use, referring to a device for capital punishment, and thus is discouraged in rehabilitation contexts). The choice of an easily transportable power wheelchair (*folding-frame power chairs* with detachable batteries or *rigid-frame power chairs* with detachable modular components) eliminates many options available in power-base power wheelchairs (Figs. 37-9 and 37-10). The options jettisoned include powered recline or tilt-in-space, a ventilation tray for oxygen, and environmental control units (Algorithm 37-5). These power chairs can only be directed by a joystick controller. As in manual chairs, folding frames are less durable. The main advantage of folding-frame power chairs is that they can be transported in many ordinary automobiles with simple disassembly. Further, they offer virtually all of the static seating options found in manual chairs. The rigid-frame chairs with the modular motors are probably more durable, but more difficult to transport in a car. One option available in some

Algorithm 37-4. Power Mobility Options

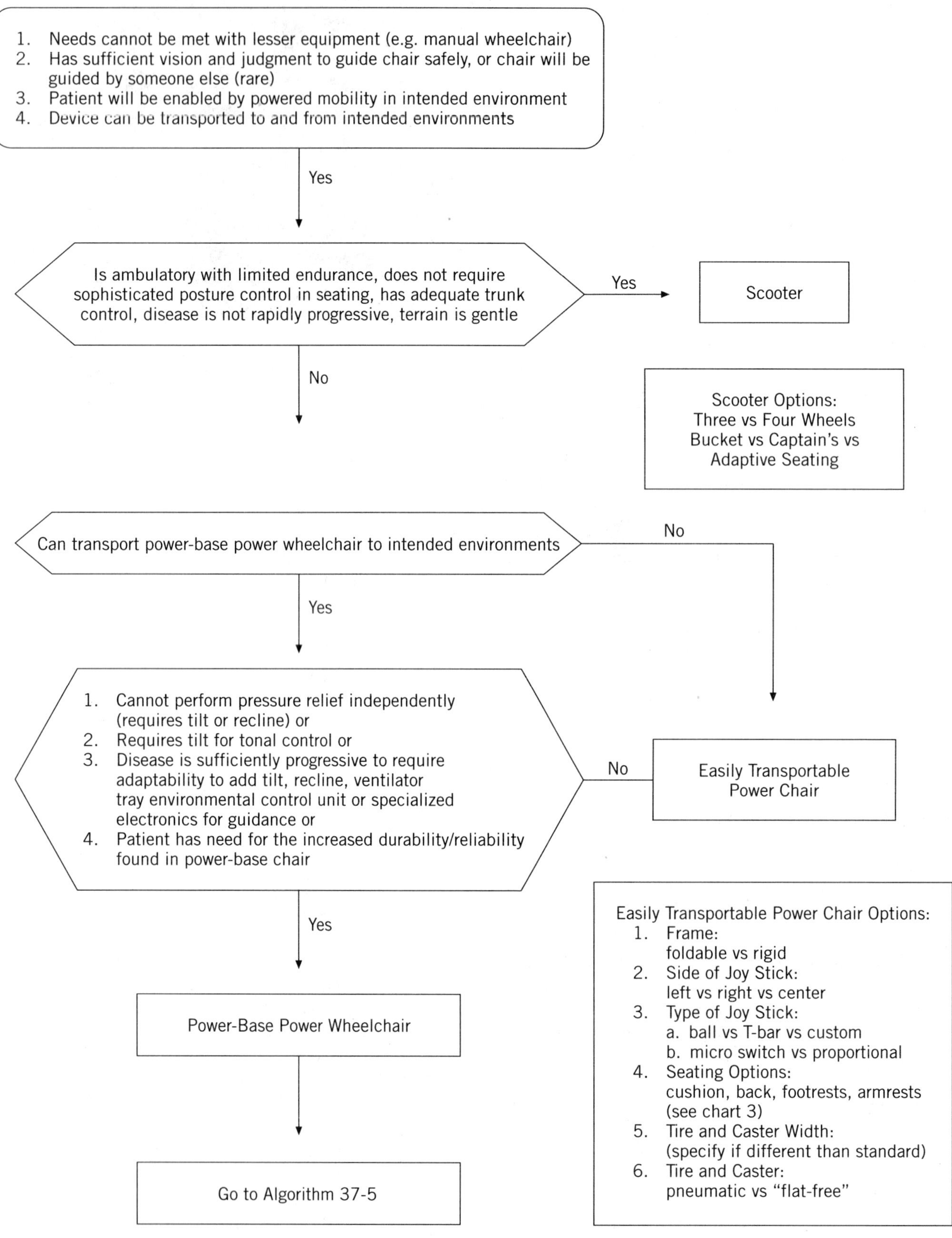

Prerequisites for Powered Mobility
1. Needs cannot be met with lesser equipment (e.g. manual wheelchair)
2. Has sufficient vision and judgment to guide chair safely, or chair will be guided by someone else (rare)
3. Patient will be enabled by powered mobility in intended environment
4. Device can be transported to and from intended environments
Yes
Is ambulatory with limited endurance, does not require sophisticated posture control in seating, has adequate trunk control, disease is not rapidly progressive, terrain is gentle
Yes
Scooter
Scooter Options:
Three vs Four Wheels
Bucket vs Captain's vs
Adaptive Seating
No
Can transport power-base power wheelchair to intended environments
No
Yes
1. Cannot perform pressure relief independently (requires tilt or recline) or
2. Requires tilt for tonal control or
3. Disease is sufficiently progressive to require adaptability to add tilt, recline, ventilator tray environmental control unit or specialized electronics for guidance or
4. Patient has need for the increased durability/reliability found in power-base chair
No
Easily Transportable Power Chair
Yes
Power-Base Power Wheelchair
Go to Algorithm 37-5
Easily Transportable Power Chair Options:
1. Frame:
foldable vs rigid
2. Side of Joy Stick:
left vs right vs center
3. Type of Joy Stick:
a. ball vs T-bar vs custom
b. micro switch vs proportional
4. Seating Options:
cushion, back, footrests, armrests
(see chart 3)
5. Tire and Caster Width:
(specify if different than standard)
6. Tire and Caster:
pneumatic vs "flat-free"

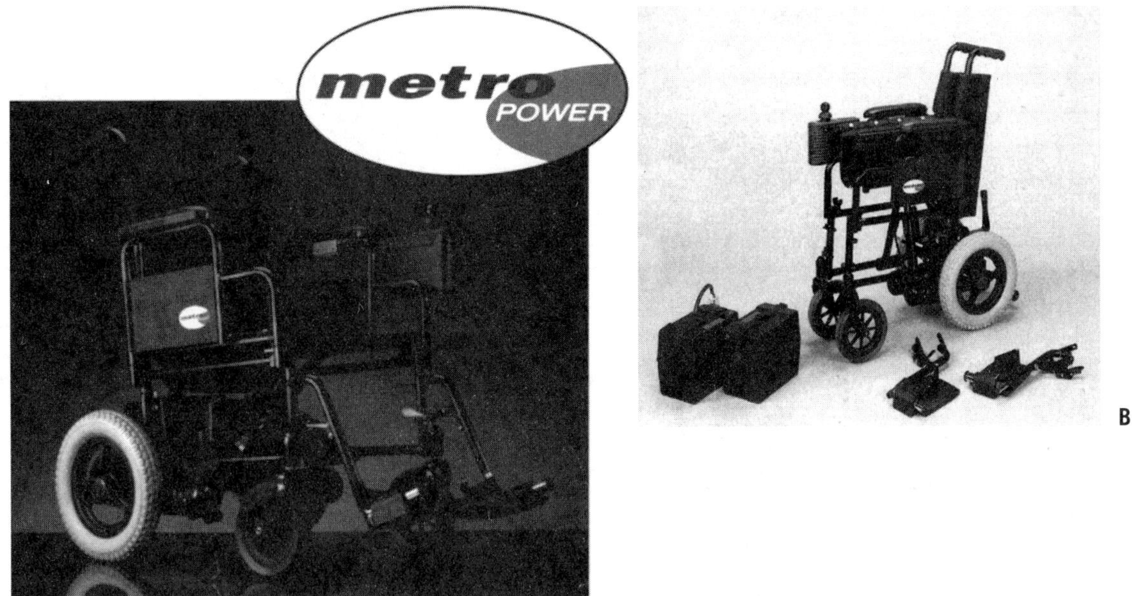

Figure 37-9. *A.* A folding frame power wheelchair ready to drive. *B.* A folding frame power wheelchair folded with all its component parts.

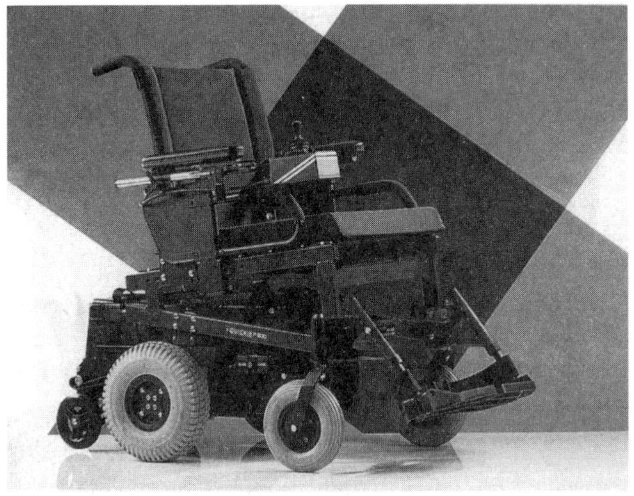

Figure 37-10. A rigid framed power wheelchair.

rigid-frame power chairs is a conversion kit with standard-size wheels (i.e., 24-inch diameter) to transform the chair into a manual wheelchair (albeit, a heavy one). The profile of a folding-frame power chair user overlaps that of the scooter user, except that he or she might require a smaller turning radius, more posture control, or improved accessibility to public transportation. Individuals with paraplegia who cannot transport a power-base power chair may find a solution in foldable power wheelchairs.

Two types of drive are available, *direct* and *belt driven.* In direct-drive chairs the axles are driven by a geared assembly connected directly to a drive shaft. Belt-driven chairs depend on a rubberized belt to translate rotation from the driveshaft to the wheel. Belt-driven chairs are less mechanically efficient and more prone to breakdown. Virtually all folding power chairs are directed by a *joystick.* Typically this is attached to the left or right armrest, to be guided by the least impaired or the dominant hand. A few patients will be best served by a drive placed in a central position on a lap tray. While a standard joystick topped with a *ball* can be easily manipulated by a normal hand, a *T-bar*, or a *custom-made hand piece*, may be necessary for those with reduced grip. Joysticks can be switch controlled or proportionally controlled. *Microswitch controlled* means that the patient can choose one of four directions to travel at a constant preset speed. Switch controls can be either latched (as found in sip-and-puff systems described below) or momentary. *Momentary* means that the wheelchair travels in a certain direction as long as the controller is pushed in that direction. When the controller is released, the chair stops. *Proportional controls* allow the user to choose any direction, and increase the speed in proportion to how far the joystick is deflected from neutral. Proportional control is generally easier to master and yields a smoother ride. Tires and casters may be true pneumatics or filled with a flat-free insert. If a user has a particular need for increased traction, a wider tire may be ordered with the caveat that wheelchair width will increase. Beyond this, the folding power wheelchair prescription should include the back angle if different from the standard angle, the type of back and cushion, specification of the armrest, specification of the footrest, and standard safety features such as a positioning belt and antitip devices (see Manual Wheelchair Prescription for a description of some of these options). Wheel locks should be specified only if there is a special need, since power chairs are always "in gear" unless the motor is manually disengaged.

Power-base power wheelchairs are made up of an

Algorithm 37-5. Power Wheelchair Options

SEATING

Patient is able to do own pressure relief, tone is normal or well controlled? — Yes → Static Seating

No

Unable to perform pressure relief and not limited by hypertonicity? — Yes → Recline System

No

Requires pressure relief but cannot tolerate recline (hypertonic or contracted)? — Yes → Tilt-in-Space

No

Requires tilt-in-space for positioning, and additionally requires recline for pressure relief? — Yes → Tilt-in-Space plus Recline

SPECIALS

Unable to rise from a seated position but capable of rising from an elevated and/or forward tilted position? — Yes → Elevated, Forward Tilt

Requires upright posture? — Yes → Standing Frame

NAVIGATIONAL CONTROL
(Choose momentary or latch switch, or proportional)

Able to manipulate a standard joystick? — Yes → Joystick with Ball

No

Able to operate a T-bar control? — Yes → Joystick with T-Bar

No

Able to manipulate custom handpiece? — Yes → Joystick with Custom Handpiece Laser Switch Control

No

Unable to direct chair with hands, but normal chin movement? — Yes → Chin Control (cup vs stick)

No

Able to direct chair with head? — Yes → Head Controls (rear mounted joystick vs magnetic vs laser switch)

No

Unable to direct chair with head? — Yes

MOUTH CONTROLS:

New user: (Most common system for experienced users) — Yes → Sip and Puff (proportional control not available)

No

Good tongue coordination, not disabled by the application of a retainer. Desire to run a computer or environmental control unit? — Yes → Tongue Touch Microswitch (proportional drive not available)

No

Possible alternatives to tongue touch microswitch or sip and puff — Yes → Voice control, EMG/EEG control

702 Part III Therapeutic Interventions

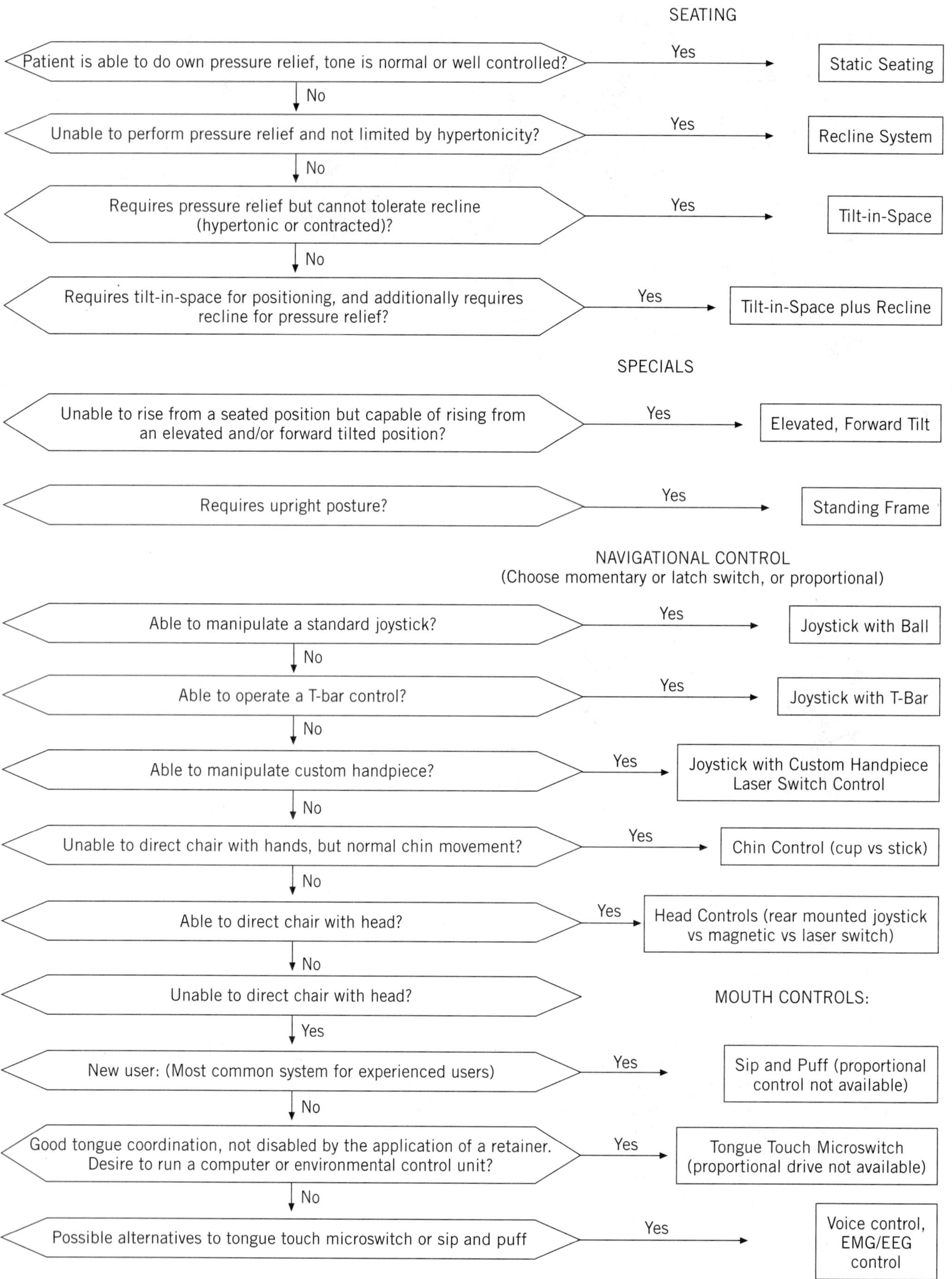

integrated power base consisting of the motor, frame, rear wheels, and front casters, to which a *seating system*—the seat, back, armrests, controller, and footrests—is then chosen and attached (Fig. 37-11). Power-base chairs cannot be easily broken down to component parts by users, and in the great majority of time are transported as a whole (i.e., they do not fit in automobiles). It is generally believed that power-base chairs are more rugged and durable than folding-frame chairs. Most power-base chairs feature a motorized rear wheel; a few offer front-wheel or mid-wheel drives. As their names suggest, the drive wheels are behind the front casters in a rear-wheel-drive chair and in front of the rear casters in a front-wheel-drive chair (Fig. 37-12) (13). Mid-wheel-drive (or center-wheel-drive) chairs employ three sets of wheels: one pair of rear casters, one pair of drive wheels in the center, and one pair of caster-size wheels anteriorly to prevent forward tipping. Front- and mid-drive chairs tend to position the drive wheels closer to the center of the chair, yielding a smaller turning radius. A smaller turning radius allows greater maneuverability, which can be of particular benefit to those who live or work in confined environments (Fig. 37-13). With more of the user's weight over the drive wheels, traction is improved. There is a tendency, however, to pitch forward

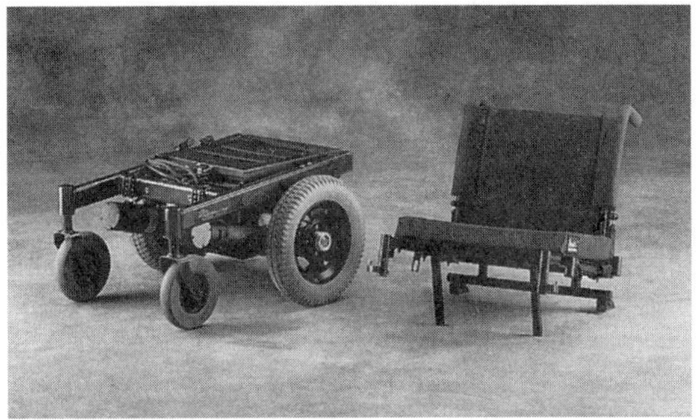

Figure 37-11. A power base and its detachable seating system.

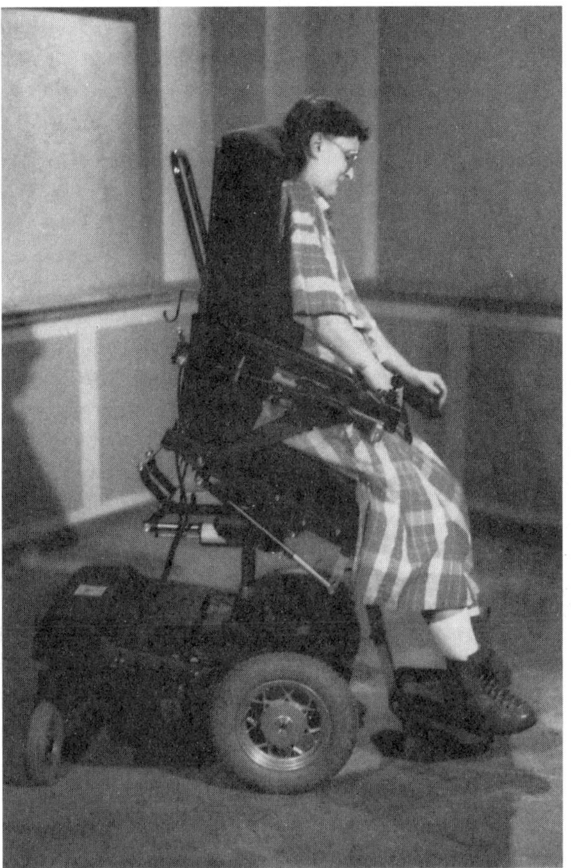

A

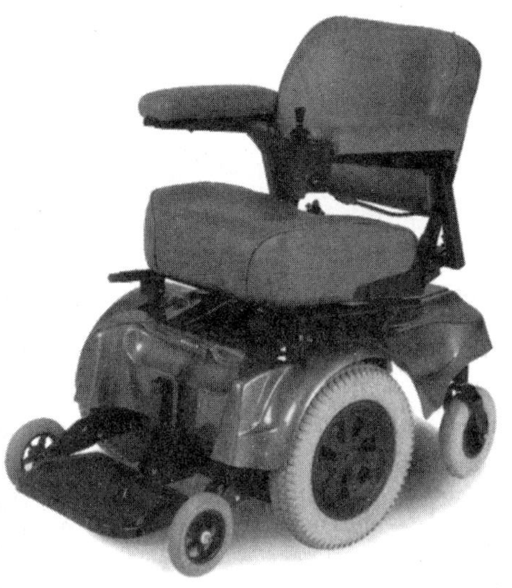

B

Figure 37-12. Front- and mid-wheel drive. *A.* Front-wheel-drive wheelchair. The user is a 30-year-old woman with fibrodysplasia ossificans progressiva, a slowly progressive disease of heterotopic ossification. Unregulated bone growth in the soft tissue has locked her spine, pelvis, femurs, and ankles in the position seen in the photograph. This power wheelchair includes a custom foam-in-place seating system. The chair itself features front-wheel drive that allows a smaller turning radius, a seat elevator, and a posterior power tilt of 30 degrees with a custom anterior tilt of an additional 30 degrees. The combination of these features allows the user to easily transfer into the chair, interact with others in an upright position, and achieve pressure relief at various degrees of tilt (13). *B.* Mid-wheel-drive wheelchair with a captain's chair.

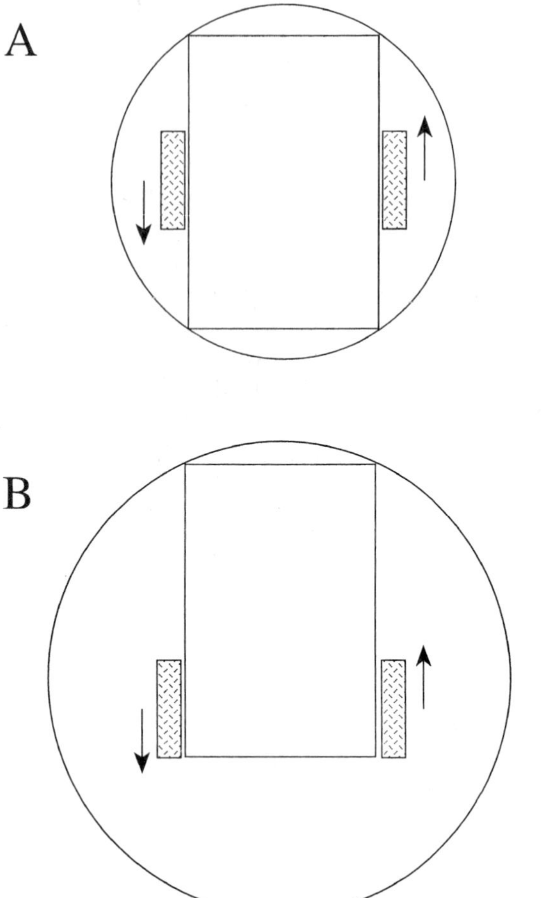

Figure 37-13. Schematic representations of the turning radii of front- or mid-wheel-drive versus a rear-wheel-drive wheelchair. The turning radius is determined by the distance between the driver's feet and the axle. The *smaller lateral rectangles* represent the drive wheels turning in opposite directions. The *larger rectangle* represents the wheelchair frame. The *circle* represents the turning radius. The *arrows* represent the wheels turning in opposite directions to allow the chair to turn. In *A*, the drive wheels are located at the center of the chair; the turning radius is smaller than in *B*.

while braking, which can be a disadvantage for those with poor trunk stability. Also, at higher speeds there is a greater tendency for instability. Therefore, the manufacturer may set the maximum speed available in a front- or mid-wheel-drive chair to less than that of an equivalent rear-wheel-drive chair (14).

Power-base wheelchairs offer an array of adjustability to accommodate those who are ventilator dependent with a vent tray; those who need power recline, tilt-in-space, or both; and those who need complex electronics to best operate environmental control units or to guide the chair without a hand-operated joystick. Patients with sufficiently progressive diseases (i.e., amyotrophic lateral sclerosis) are often better served with a power-base chair even if they do not need the above options at the time of evaluation.

Patients who cannot perform their own pressure relief are at risk for developing pressure ulcers. For these patients, *low-shear power recline* offers periodic repositioning to avoid skin breakdown. Power recline is also a means of postural realignment for those who are in their chairs for many hours or sleep in their chairs. Automatic power-elevating footrests or manual elevating footrests usually accompany power recline. Although it may seem counterintuitive, manual elevating leg rests operated by a helper may be preferred to automatic leg rests, which elevate every time the back is lowered. This automatic elevation can greatly increase the length of the chair, and users may prefer to choose when this is to occur. An option on some power chairs is power-elevating leg rests that can be activated separately from the recline system. The *tilt-in-space* feature can also accomplish pressure relief, and is particularly useful for those with contractures or hypertonicity who cannot tolerate power recline. The greatest disadvantage of a tilt-in-space system includes back flow of urine from the leg bags for those with Foley catheters. Occasionally a patient will have spasticity or risk of skin ulceration that can be best treated with a combination of power tilt and recline. Patients using either tilt-in-space or recline systems will almost certainly need a headrest added to the chair.

With modern technology, virtually any body movement that is under voluntary control can serve to operate a power chair. Possibilities have expanded with the application of laser switches. These switches project a set length of laser light and can be attached throughout the wheelchair frame. When the beam is interrupted (by toe movement as an example), a switch is activated. Still, the vast majority of those unable to operate a hand-controlled joystick are fitted with controls operated at the chin first, then by the head, and then by the mouth if the preceding option is not feasible. *Chin controls* can be either proportional or microswitch operated. Proportional control is generally easier to learn but requires more endurance than latched controls. A variety of devices can be attached at the end of the chin control joystick; cups are easy to operate, but experienced users may prefer a simple thin rod that extends horizontally to the chin and is less cosmetically obtrusive. Head controls can receive their input by a rear-mounted joystick, by sensors sensitive to motion as detected by perturbation of a magnetic field, or by laser light switches. An advantage of head control is a relatively unobstructed view of the face. For those who lack usable head movement, *mouth controls* can be utilized. The *sip-and-puff* system is the established standard. Pneumatic switches activated by small changes in mouth pressure control speed and direction. The switches can be operated by persons with little breath support and even those on ventilators. A newer system utilizes microswitches mounted in an oral retainer and activated by the tongue. Besides guiding the chair, patients can operate environmental control units and access desktop or laptop computers. Voice-activated controls have been explored, but are not currently available to the general public. Another potential source of guidance is the signal generated by electroencephalographic or electromyographic activity as detected by electrodes placed on the forehead.

WHAT ABOUT BRAND NAMES?

Within a category of chair, is there any objective guide to compare one manufacturer's chair to another? The International Standards Organization working with the Rehabilitation Engineering and Assistive Technology Society of North America (RESNA) has developed a set of standards for testing wheelchairs (15). The standards cover methods to test everything from durability to stability. Because the U.S. Department of Veterans Affairs requires this information for any chair that they purchase, many manufacturers have collected these data. However, it is not yet routinely available to the public. We encourage physicians, users, and other interested parties to demand this information, because we believe such action will lead to greater compliance among manufacturers. Independent research comparing wheelchairs is in its infancy.

Because objective information is lacking, physicians must guide patients by subjective measures, such as experience with particular chairs, a company's reputation, previous record of availability of parts, and price (when relevant). Sometimes specific desirable features are available only in one model. Often, however, several candidates may fit the user's needs, or no chair will fit perfectly. Ultimately, the decision is the patient's.

AESTHETICS

It may be impossible for the able-bodied person to truly understand the meaning of a chair to the user. Wheelchairs, so critical in everyday mobility, quickly become an extension of the user. Wheelers will be attracted to the image that they perceive the chair to project. Some will opt for an attention-grabbing style with bright colors and bold styling, while others will look for a chair that blends into the background in a business environment. As is true in so much of rehabilitation, a patient's happiness and compliance are proportional to the patient's sense of involvement and control over his or her recovery. Ideally, the patient would have an unlimited time to try out all available makes before deciding on a specific model. While this may not be feasible, the physician should insist on a trial period with as many chairs as available.

A FEW COMMENTS ON PEDIATRIC WHEELCHAIRS

Unfortunately, text limitations in this chapter preclude going into the detail necessary to fully cover pediatric wheelchairs and seating. General commonsense issues should be kept in mind. Seating for the child is a much more dynamic process. Even for nonprogressive conditions such as cerebral palsy, as the child grows, the wheelchair and seating system must also grow. Because of this constantly changing picture, power chairs more commonly utilize a power base, enabling seating components to be changed. Manual wheelchairs are also designed to accommodate growth. When working with children, it is crucial to realize how important mobility is to development. When appropriate, children should be placed in mobility devices that allow them to explore as soon as possible. Once again, an interdisciplinary approach that ensures involvement of the schools and their therapists is essential.

WHAT IF MONEY WERE NO OBJECT (OR, WHAT WOULD WE THINK WAS REASONABLE IF WE WERE MOBILITY IMPAIRED?)

This chapter has attempted to deal with the acquisition of wheelchairs in a logical and pragmatic fashion. It follows the assumption that any specific user must choose only one device. However, if cost were not a consideration, most users would be best served by having more than one chair. For those able to propel a manual chair, an ultralight model (folding or rigid . . . or both!) would be best for daily use. A power wheelchair for longer excursions might be desirable to conserve energy and reduce wear and tear on the rotator cuff and the rest of the upper limb. Standing chairs and standing frames come in a number of combinations, such as power drives and lift, manual lifts and drive, and manual drive with a power lift. In addition to providing the wheelchair user with the ability to interact with people at eye level, these chairs may slow the development of osteoporosis by restoring upright weight bearing, discourage contractures, and improve cardiac function. If financially feasible, many of our patients would appreciate one (or two . . .). Finally, our athletically inclined users would have at least as many sports-specific sports chairs as needed to be able to compete on the basketball court, the race track, the tennis court, or wherever. Of course, the manual wheelchair users, as well as all of our power wheelchair users, would have a lift in their vans with appropriate tie-down equipment so they would be as safe in their car as able-bodied drivers.

Our power wheelchair users would also be offered standing frame wheelchairs. Even those who are able to perform pressure relief independently would have alternate chairs with low-shear recline and tilt-in-space systems. This would allow them to change positions, perhaps just to relax or take a nap, a luxury the able-bodied take for granted. The input device for the power wheelchair would work with environmental control units and provide computer access.

The above is not meant to be taken whimsically. Although expensive in immediate dollars, many arguments can be mounted that a more liberal allocation of resources saves dollars in the long run. The ultralight wheelchairs last longer, possibly saving the expense and lost time of replacing a less expensive chair. In addition, manual wheelchair users are at great risk for carpal tunnel syndrome (16–19) and shoulder injuries (20–24). The part-time use of a power chair not only may increase the life of the manual chair, but also may prevent overuse injuries. Recline and tilt-in-space systems protect against pressure sores (as do appropriate cushions). Better interface between a power chair user and his or her environment may lessen the caregiver burden and improve productivity for both the patients and their caregivers. These pragmatic arguments do not begin to address the psychological, spiritual, and moral dimensions of a society's treatment of its members with disabilities as reflected in its commitment to the allocation of resources.

ACKNOWLEDGMENTS

We are extremely grateful for the generous help of the following individuals: Beth McCarty, OT, Lance McCartney, Matthew Misali, R. David Neal, Mike Mulesky, Gregory M. "Bear" Kiger, Dan Wagner, Ron Trager, Chuck Carlson, Dave Nebraska, Robert Spencer, Jr., and Rory A. Cooper, PhD. We give special appreciation to R. Lee Kirby, MD, for his thoughtful review of this manuscript.

APPENDIX I: GLOSSARY

Adjustable Axle Plate—Axle plate that allows for anterior-posterior adjustability or upward-downward adjustability or a combination of both. Adjusting the position of the wheel allows the chair to be fit to the user in the best position for propulsion and stability.

Adjustable Tension Back—An option on sling-back wheelchairs that uses a series of horizontal straps to provide better, more customized support and to battle the fatigability of the material as it ages.

Amputee Axle Plate—A particular kind of adjustable axle that allows the wheel to be repositioned posteriorly to accommodate for posterior shift in the center of gravity that accompanies lower-limb amputations.

Amputee Board—A board that can be inserted on the seat to keep the knee extended for transtibial amputees.

Antitip Device—An important safety feature that consists of small wheels placed on a post extended from the rear of the wheelchair to prevent it from tipping backward.

Armrest—Added to wheelchairs to provide balance and stability by allowing the user to rest his or her elbows. They also assist with push-off for pressure relief and aid in sitting-to-standing maneuvers.

Belt-Driven Power Wheelchair—A type of power wheelchair that has belts connecting the right and left motors to each of the rear wheels.

Brake Extensions—Tubes placed over the wheel locks that allow patients with upper-extremity weakness to easily lock the wheels of the chair by increasing the leverage and accessibility of the wheel locks.

Camber—The angle of the wheel in relation to vertical. As the camber angle increases, the distance between the bottom of the wheels is increased and the distance between the top of the wheels is decreased.

Casters—The small wheels found typically on the front of the wheelchair.

Chin Control—A drive mechanism that allows the user to operate the wheelchair using his or her chin to push a post. Chin controls are a type of joystick.

Clothing Guard—Fits between the user and the wheel to prevent the user's apparel from getting soiled.

Desk-Length Armrests—Armrests that are cut away to allow easy access to tables and desks.

Detachable Armrests—Armrests that can be easily removed from the chair to ease transfers.

Direct-Drive Power Wheelchair—A type of power wheelchair in which the rear wheels are connected directly to the motor and gear box.

Dump—An adjustment of the seat angle so that the sacrum sits even lower relative to the knees. This can combat the tendency to slide out of a chair, and can prevent the pelvis from falling into a posterior tilt. However, this can make transfers more difficult.

Elevating Leg Rests—Adjustable-height leg rests that can position the knee from 90 degrees of flexion to full extension. Common indications include to support a postsurgical knee at a specific angle, to decrease edema, and to support a limb after transtibial amputation. Elevating leg rests usually come with calf supports.

Fixed Armrests—Armrests that are not able to be removed from the wheelchair.

Flat-free Inserts—A gel-filled inner tube that replaces the air-filled tube in pneumatic tires to increase durability of the tire.

Flip-Back Armrest—A detachable armrest that pivots at the posterior post, which is more convenient than complete removal of the standard removable armrest.

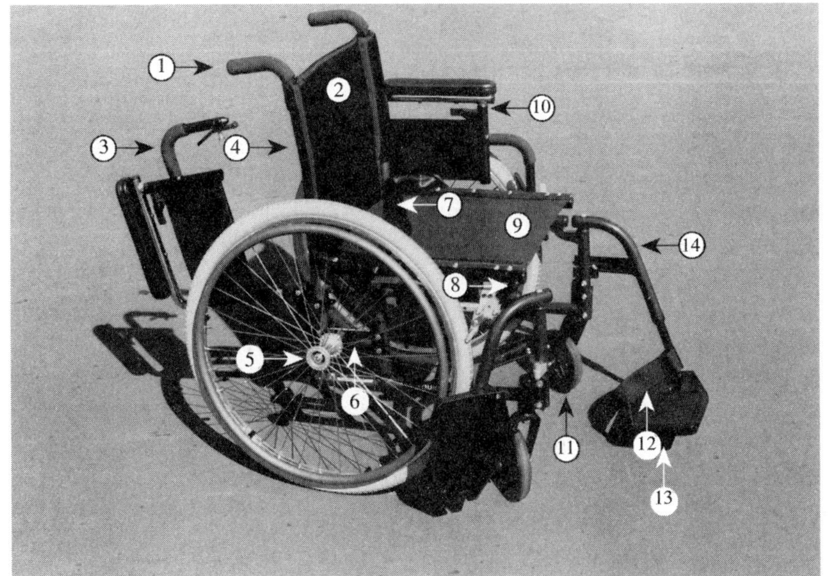

Figure 37-A1. Components of a foldable wheelchair. 1. Push handle. 2. Sling back. 3. Flip back armrest. 4. Cane. 5. Push button quick release axle. 6. Adjustable axle plate. 7. Positioning belt. 8. Push to lock wheel lock. 9. Sling seat. 10. Desk length adjustable height armrest. 11. Caster. 12. Heel loop. 13. Flip-up foot plate. 14. 70 degree swing-away detachable hanger.

Flip-Up Footplate—A hinged footplate that can be swung laterally to allow the feet to touch the ground. Being able to flip up allows easier transfers and safer sitting-to-standing.

Foldable Wheelchair—Wheelchair with at least one cross-brace underneath the seat that allows the wheelchair to fold. (Fig. 37-A1).

Folding-Frame Power Wheelchair—A portable power wheelchair that allows the battery packs to be removed so that the chair can be broken down to fit into a car. The frame is similar to that of a folding manual chair as it has a cross-bar and removable footrests. A disadvantage is that the wheelchair is heavy and difficult to lift into high trunks.

Footplates—A platform under the foot that provides stability and pressure distribution during sitting. Footplates can be made of composite, aluminum, or steel, with composite being standard.

Front Rigging—The fixed front end of a wheelchair, including a footplate, found on most manual rigid-frame chairs.

Full-Length Armrests—Armrests that extend from the back of the wheelchair to the front edge of the seat.

Grade Aid—A variation of a wheel lock that consists of spring-loaded teeth which prevent the wheelchair from rolling backward when on ramps or inclines.

Hanger—Attaches the footplate to the chair. Front hangers can be fixed, swing away, or rigid. Removable hangers may aid in transfers.

Head Control—A method to direct a power wheel chair. Input is transformed from a rear-mounted joystick, by sensors sensitive to motion as detected by perturbation of a magnetic field, or by laser light switches. An advantage of head control is a relatively unobstructed view of the face.

Height-Adjustable Armrests—Armrests that offer the ability to alter the height to several different levels.

Joystick—A power wheelchair guidance device that is usually operated by hand but can be activated by arm, elbow, chin, mouth, tongue, or head systems. The joystick can be a standard straight projection or can be either a T-bar or "stadium post" (a T-bar with side supports to assist with balancing the hand while driving). A joystick looks similar to its counterpart in video games.

Lap Tray—A surface (usually wood or clear Plexiglas) attached to the armrests. Lap trays are used to support one or both upper limbs for individuals who require extra support due to paralysis, edema, or upper-limb impairments. Plexiglas is generally preferred as it is aesthetically more appealing and allows the individual greater view of the lower body. The trays usually come in two sizes, full trays or half trays. Full trays are composed of one solid piece that rests on both armrests of the wheelchair and provides maximal support. Half trays are usually made for either the right or the left upper extremity and support one arm only. Half trays are often used by persons with hemiparesis.

Lateral Supports—Guides that can be attached to either cane to position the trunk more securely.

Low-Shear Power Recline—A method where either the back or the seat slides over a fixed surface in a compensatory fashion to reduce shear forces on the skin when the user reclines.

Mag Wheels—Wheels constructed of magnesium or a plastic material that connects the rim to the center of the wheelchair.

Microswitching System—A type of switch mechanism on a power wheelchair that produces an all-or-none response by activating switches in either an "on" or an "off" position.

Momentary Drive—A type of drive in which the power wheelchair travels in a certain direction as long as the controller is pushed in that direction.

Mouth Control—A power wheelchair drive mechanism used when an individual cannot utilize an extremity or chin for operation of a power chair. Examples include sip and puff, or tongue touch.

One-Arm Drive—A mechanism for wheelchair propulsion and steering with a single upper limb. In the United States, the common configuration equips the wheel underneath the functioning arm with two push rims. The outer rim is connected to the ipsilateral wheel; the inner rim is connected via a shaft to the contralateral wheel. Another system more common in Europe uses a lever arm that is pumped to move both wheels. The handle can be turned to direct the chair by guiding the casters. These chairs are heavier than comparable manual chairs.

Pneumatic Tires—Tires consisting of an air-filled inner tube covered with a rubber casing.

Polyurethane Tire—A type of hard tire best suited for indoor and institutional settings.

Positioning Belt—A lap harness that resembles an automobile safety belt. It can be used for positioning as well as a safely feature. It can be found with buckle or Velcro closures. For positioning, the belt should be placed anterior and inferior to the anterior superior iliac spine so that the pelvis is held in good alignment. This belt prevents the user from accidentally exiting the chair.

Power-Base Power Wheelchair—A modular power wheelchair design where the seating system is a completely separate system from the base. The base includes the frame, wheels, motor, battery, and drive.

Projections—See Quad Knobs.

Proportional Drive—A type of switch mechanism on a power wheelchair that responds proportionally to the amount of displacement of the joystick from neutral. Speed increases proportionally with the degree of displacement.

Pull-to-Lock Wheel Locks—Wheel locks that are engaged with a pulling movement (elbow flexion). This configuration places the lock handle in a vertical position when the lock is engaged. The disadvantage of this is an increased risk of scraping the buttock during a swing-through transfer. Greater clearance of the wheel as well as the lock must be ensured during the transfer. See Push-to-Lock Wheel Locks.

Push Handles—Handles projecting off the rear of the wheelchair back posts. These can be used by a caregiver to push the wheelchair.

Push Rims—Push rims are the smaller-diameter rims slightly lateral to the wheels. They are used for upper-limb propulsion of a manual wheelchair.

Push-to-Lock Wheel Locks—Wheel locks that are engaged with a pushing movement (elbow extension). This configuration is easy to lock. However, in the unlocked position the lock handle protrudes from the wheel, and may be more likely to catch the thumb. See Pull-to-Lock Wheel Locks.

Quad Knobs—Projections placed onto the hand rim of a wheelchair. They can be vertical or set at a 45-degree angle. They are used for individuals with very poor grip strength, such as those with tetraplegia.

Quad Release Axle—A type of removable axle that is attached to a looped nut, which allows for quick removal of the wheels by an individual with poor manual dexterity.

Quick-Release Axle—Axle that can be easily removed using a push-button mechanism.

Removable Footrests—Footrests that easily detach from the chair to increase portability and allow foot propulsion.

Rigid-Frame Manual Chair—Wheelchair frame that has a boxlike configuration beneath the seat. These frames are not foldable (Fig. 37-A2).

Rigid-Frame Power Wheelchair—A type of portable power wheelchair that allows the battery and power supply to be removed for transport in a car. The frame is not foldable. Although the rigid frame offers more stability, it is awkward to fit into most cars.

Scissor Locks—A type of wheel lock usually found on sports chairs. They are mounted under the seat, to the front right and left corners of the chair. They are positioned so that they cannot catch a thumb during self-propulsion. They are also out of visual field, which may be more aesthetically appealing. A disadvantage is that one must have good stability and sitting balance to reach the brakes.

Scooter—A three- or four-wheeled power mobility device with a swivel chair and directed with a mechanical tiller.

Sip and Puff—A power wheelchair steering mechanism allowing oral control of the chair. One hard puff usually facilitates drive forward while a soft puff translates driving to the right or left; a hard sip stops the chair.

Sling Back—The back of the wheelchair consisting of a piece of material suspended between the back rails (posts) of the chair.

Sling Seat—Seat consisting of a piece of material suspended between the seat rails of the wheelchair.

Solid Back—Back of a wheelchair consisting of rigid material covered with softer, supporting material.

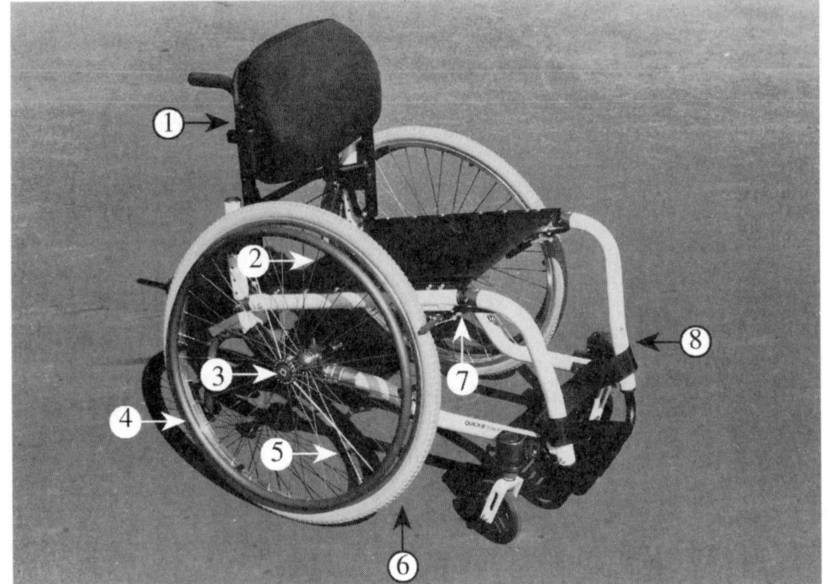

Figure 37-A2. Common components found on a rigid wheelchair. 1. Solid back (optional on either a foldable or a rigid wheelchair). 2. Seat is "dumped." 3. Large quick release button. 4. Pushrim. 5. Spoke wheels. 6. Pneumatic treaded tires. 7. Scissor brakes. 8. Fixed front rigging.

The solid back is placed between the posterior uprights (canes).

Solid Seat—Seat of a wheelchair consisting of a rigid material, usually metal or wood, placed between or soldered to the seat rails of the chair.

Solid Seat Insert—A board made of rigid material, often wood, that is placed between the sling seat and the wheelchair cushion to provide better support for the pelvis and femur.

Spoked Wheels—A standard type of wheel used for wheelchairs. Spokes are usually made of metal wires as commonly seen in bicycle wheels. Although these wheels are usually lighter than mag wheels, they tend to loosen and must be retightened periodically.

Swing-Away Footrests—Footrests that can be moved laterally from the front of the chair without detaching from the chair, to ease transfers and standing.

T-Bar—A T-shaped joystick used when the individual has poor arm strength or endurance, ataxia, or decreased coordination, or with a new user who is mastering the skill of driving a motorized wheelchair.

Threaded Axle—A nonremovable axle.

Tilt-in-Space-System—A seating system in which the entire seat and back can be tilted as a single unit, maintaining the back-to-seat angle. It is most often used for clients with muscle spasticity. A disadvantage is that it is not easily disassembled for transport.

Trunk Lift—A mechanism to aid in transferring scooters and power wheelchairs into vehicles. These are usually mounted to the rear of the vehicle and are often motorized.

Tubular Armrest—One-piece nonadjustable armrest that has a rounded or tubular configuration.

Wheel Axle—Shaft on which the wheels rotate.

Wheel Lock—Important safety feature that allows the wheels to be fixed so the chair does not move.

Wheel Lock Extensions—Extension placed on standard wheel locks to increase leverage and shorten the distance needed to reach the wheel lock.

Wraparound Armrest—Armrest that offers structural placement of the posterior upright of the armrest behind the posterior rails of the chair, decreasing the overall width of the chair by approximately 1.5 inches.

APPENDIX II: MANUAL WHEELCHAIR PRESCRIPTION FORM

<u>Manual Wheelchair Prescription Form</u>

Physician ________________ *Date of Rx* __________ *Measurements: Hips* __________ *Shoulders* __________

Pt. Name ______________________________________ *Seat to Mid Scapula* __________

Diagnosis ______________________________________ *Back to Knee* ____ *Knee to Heel* ________

1. **Construction** ❑ Standard ❑ Lightweight ❑ Lightweight high strength ❑ Ultralightweight
❑ Heavy duty ❑ Extra heavy duty ❑ Hemiheight ❑ Other ________________

2. **Frame** ❑ Folding ❑ Rigid ❑ Hybrid

3. **Push Handles** ❑ Yes ❑ No

4. **Back** ❑ Sling ❑ Adjustable tension ❑ Solid ❑ Brand___ Size___ ❑ Custom molded

5. **Seat** ❑ Sling ❑ Sling with solid seat insert ❑ Solid pan seat
❑ Adjustable tension sling Size ___________

6. **Cushion** ❑ Foam ❑ Contoured foam ❑ Fluid filled ❑ Air filled ❑ Honeycomb
❑ Other ❑ Brand_____ Size______

7. **Armrest** ❑ Tubular OR
a) ❑ Full length vs. ❑ Desk length
b) ❑ Fixed vs. ❑ Detachable ❑ Flip back
c) ❑ Fixed height vs. ❑ Adjustable height

8. **Chair Axle** ❑ Single point ❑ Adjustable ❑ Other

9. **Wheel Axle** ❑ Threaded ❑ Quick release ❑ Quad release

10. **Wheels** ❑ Mag ❑ Spoke

11. **Hand Rims** ❑ Plastic ❑ Aluminum/Alloy ❑ Friction coated ❑ Projections (oblique or vertical)
❑ None ❑ One-arm hand drive Right/Left

12. **Tires** ❑ Solid ❑ Pneumatic tires ❑ Pneumatic tires with flat-free inserts ❑ Mountain tire
❑ Racing tire ❑ Other ________________

13. **Hanger** ❑ 60 ❑ 70 ❑ 80 ❑ 90 ❑ Other _____________

14. **Calf Pad** ❑ Yes ❑ No

15. **Footrest** ❑ Fixed ❑ Swing away detachable ❑ Folding front rigging ❑ Elevating
❑ Amputee board ❑ Fixed front rigging (rigid chair)

16. **Footplates** ❑ Flip up ❑ Angle adjustable ❑ Rigid platform ❑ Detachable platform

17. **Casters** ❑ Solid ❑ Pneumatic ❑ 3 ❑ 5 ❑ 7 ❑ 8 ❑ 9 ❑ Other ________

18. **Safety Features** ❑ Positioning belt ❑ Antitips ❑ Wheel locks: Push-to-lock / Pull-to-lock / Scissor
❑ Grade Aids ❑ Lateral support(s) ❑ Location: _________________

19. **Accessories** ❑ Full lap tray ❑ Half lap tray (Right or Left) ❑ Lumbar support ❑ Brand:____________
❑ Manual recline ❑ Manual tilt-in-space

20. **Misc.** ____

REFERENCES

1. Anonymous It's the wheel thing, 14th annual survey of lightweight wheelchairs. *Sports Spokes* 1996;22:3–19.

2. Schwartzberg JG, Kakavas VK. Guidelines for the use of assistive technology: evaluation, referral, prescription. 1994; Abstract.

3. *Region B DMERC Supplier Manual.* Revision no. 12. Indianapolis: Admina Star Federal Inc., December 1997.

4. Cooper RA, Robertson RN, Lawrence B, et al. Life-cycle analysis of depot versus rehabilitation manual wheelchairs. *J Rehabil Res Dev* 1996;33:45–55.

5. Cooper RA, Gonzalez J, Lawrence B, et al. Performance of selected lightweight wheelchairs on ANSI/RESNA tests. *Arch Phys Med Rehabil* 1997:1138–1144.

6. Brauer RL, Hertig BA. Torque generation on wheelchair handrims. In: *Proceedings 1981 Biomechanics Symposium, ASME/ASCE Mechanics Conference*, Colorado. 1981:113–116.

7. Brubaker CE, Ross S, McLaurin CA. Effect of seat position on handrim force. *Proceedings 5th Annual Conference on Rehabilitation Engineering*, Houston, TX. 1982:111.

8. Ruggles DL, Cahalan T, An KN. Biomechanics of wheelchair propulsion by able-bodied subjects. *Arch Phys Med Rehabil* 1994;75:540–544.

9. Gaines RF, Zomlefer MR, Zhao W. Armstroke patterns of spinal cord injured wheelchair users. *Arch Phys Med Rehabil* 1984;65:618. Abstract.

10. Boninger ML, Robertson RN, Wolff M, Cooper RA. Upper limb nerve entrapments in elite wheelchair racers. *Am J Phys Med Rehabil* 1996;75:170–176.

11. Brubaker CE. Wheelchair prescription: an analysis of factors that affect mobility and performance. *J Rehabil Res Dev* 1986;23:19–26.

12. Cooper RA. *Rehabilitation engineering applied to mobility and manipulation.* London: Institute of Physics Publishing, 1995.

13. Levy CE, McCarty B, Berner TF. Mobility challenges and solutions in fibrodysplasia ossificans progressiva. *Arch Phys Med Rehabil* 1996;77:986.

14. Maddox S. Front- and mid-wheel drive: a new era arrives for power chairs. *New Mobility* 1988;9(52):29–33.

15. Axelson P, Minkel J, Chesney D. *A guide to wheelchair selection: how to use the ANSI/RESNA wheelchair standards to buy a wheelchair.* Washington, DC. Paralyzed Veterans of America, 1994.

16. Aljure J, Eltorai I, Bradley WE, et al. Carpal tunnel syndrome in paraplegic patients. *Paraplegia* 1985;23:182–186.

17. Gellman H, Chandler DR, Petrasek J, et al. Carpal tunnel syndrome in paraplegic patients. *J Bone Joint Surg [Am]* 1988;70:517–519.

18. Tun CG, Upton J. The paraplegic hand: electrodiagnostic studies and clinical findings. *J Hand Surg [Am]* 1988;13:716–719.

19. Davidoff G, Werner R, Waring W. Compressive mononeuropathies of the upper extremity in chronic paraplegia. *Paraplegia* 1991;29:17–24.

20. Pentland WE, Twomey LT. The weight-bearing upper extremity in women with long term paraplegia. *Paraplegia* 1991;29:521–530.

21. Gellman H, Sie I, Waters RL. Late complications of the weight-bearing upper extremity in the paraplegic patient. *Clin Orthop* 1988;233:132–135.

22. Bayley JC, Cochran TP, Sledge CB. The weight-bearing shoulder. The impingement syndrome in paraplegics. *J Bone Joint Surg [Am]* 1987;69:676–678.

23. Wylie EJ, Chakera TM. Degenerative joint abnormalities in patients with paraplegia of duration greater than 20 years. *Paraplegia* 1988;26:101–106.

24. Nichols PJ, Norman PA, Ennis JR. Wheelchair user's shoulder? Shoulder pain in patients with spinal cord lesions. *Scand J Rehabil Med* 1979;11:29–32.

Chapter 38

Therapeutic Recreation

Peggy Holmes-Layman

The value of recreation lies in its relation to one's quality of life. Quality of life is intermeshed with a person's social, emotional, physical, and mental spheres of behavior. Recreation significantly affects these same four areas of behavior. Recreational and leisure activities help a person to experience restoration, rejuvenation, relaxation, friendships, competence, skill development, improved physical conditioning, an uplift in spirit, and numerous other challenges and self-growth opportunities. All the benefits possible through recreation and leisure are also important to individuals with disabilities and individuals undergoing rehabilitation and change. The certified therapeutic recreation specialist is the professional whose expertise is to have an in-depth understanding of the role of leisure and recreation in one's life; to direct the utilization of leisure and recreation as an intervention for health change, adjustment, and improvement; to educate clients about leisure and recreation awareness, attitudes, and resources; and to facilitate recreational and leisure experiences. This chapter describes the profession of therapeutic recreation and its place in the physical medicine and rehabilitation process.

IMPORTANCE OF LEISURE AND RECREATION TO HEALTH AND THE QUALITY OF LIFE

Common knowledge supports the idea that there are numerous positive benefits to personal involvement in leisure and recreational activities. The leisure and recreational activities that we engage in have a holistic effect, interweaving with our emotional, physical, social, and cognitive aspects. Various empirical researchers have documented the effects that recreational activities have on physical and emotional well-being, as well as their social, economic, and environmental benefits (1,2). The physical benefits are numerous, as physical activity counteracts a sedentary lifestyle with its related health risks. The psychological benefits of recreational pursuits include reducing stress and positively impacting depression (1). Other concepts tied to participation in leisure and recreation are intrinsic rewards and self-determination (3).

Intrinsically motivated experiences are most often associated with leisure and recreational behaviors (3). In a 1984 article, Iso-Ahola and Weissinger provided empirical evidence supporting the idea that psychological, physical, and mental health is positively and significantly related to intrinsically motivated recreation and leisure. They also presented an argument that intrinsic motivation is a personality trait most often developed through recreational and leisure experiences (4). Also discussed have been results of involvement in leisure and recreation such as self-integration, a sense of freedom, and demonstration of mastery (5). Relaxation, creativity, building relationships, getting in touch with nature, testing oneself, companionship, trying something new, and just feeling good are all reasons people give as to why their leisure and recreational activities are important to them (5).

Leisure and recreation have also been discussed in

the literature in terms of their effect on health. Exactly what the word *health* means has had diffferent interpretations, from the absence of disease to a vigorous holistic state of being. The latter definition is the one adhered to by the World Health Organization. Its definition describes *health* as "a state of complete physical, mental, and social well-being, not merely the absence of disease or infirmity" (6). It puts an emphasis on looking at the individual from a holistic viewpoint; it considers contextual factors and recognizes the role of personal fulfillment (7).

An integrated and inclusive definition of *health* is a major component in the many changes experienced in the mid-1990s in the field of health care throughout the United States. A heightened awareness of illness prevention and patient education in the social, emotional, physical, and cognitive areas is being incorporated into what it means when an organization or entity is involved with providing "health" care (8).

The term *quality of life* and how its meaning interfaces with health are concerns of the health care industry (6,9). In reviewing research on recreational participation and quality of life, Iso-Ahola (10) summarized that a person's perceived quality of life and psychological well-being are positively influenced by active recreational participation.

There seems to be adequate evidence to indicate that leisure and recreation and their multifaceted benefits are integral to a broad, holistic definition of health. Therefore, services that consider the role of leisure and recreational activities can enhance the quality of life as it is tied to health.

HISTORICAL OVERVIEW OF LEISURE AND RECREATION AS AN ALLIED HEALTH SERVICE

Recreational activities such as dancing, music, and chanting were used in the earliest times, the prehistoric period, to affect disease and disability (11). Such use of recreation and leisure was greatly influenced by the health care orientations of societies as they evolved. Carter et al (6) discussed the purposeful recreational activity used by Phillippe Pinel, a French physician, in the late 1700s and early 1800s when activities such as physical exercise, chess, and gardening were prescribed for patients (11). By the 1930s the field of therapeutic recreation was beginning to be identified and its value as an intervention, as well as its diversionary aspect, was utilized (11). After World War II an expansion in the use of recreational services was evident in military and veterans hospitals.

Therapeutic recreation has traditionally drawn from both the recreation and health care professions. The first formal training of recreation personnel took place in 1926 and the first formal training in "hospital recreation" occurred in the 1950s (6). Attempts to create a professional organization for the field of therapeutic recreation can be traced to the American Recreation Society (and its hospital recreation section) in the 1940s. These early efforts at organization eventually developed in 1966 into the first fully representational national organization, the National Therapeutic Recreation Society (a branch of the National Recreation and Parks Association). As health care and human services experienced changes, another professional organization, the American Therapeutic Recreation Association, was created in 1984, independent of any larger public organization. Today these two professional organizations are the main ones representing therapeutic recreation specialists.

The important role that therapeutic recreation services has taken in allied health care was widely discussed by Paul Haun, a physician, in the 1960s. His notion of this service is elucidated in the following excerpt relating the roles of medicine and recreation (12):

> The medical case for play is straightforward enough. It is an essential aspect of healthy life and constitutes the natural rhythmic alternative to work. Having an established place in the community, its extension into the hospital environment acts as a potent normalizer that effectively dispels some of the inevitable threat of cultural isolation and social rejection. . . . It affords the patient a physiological escape from somatic pain and disruptive emotional experiences. It capitalizes upon and supports the nonpathological elements of his personality. It constitutes a path by which he may return from the malignant equilibrium of defensive withdrawal, first to the make-believe universe of the play world and then, after finding this tolerable, to the yet tighter discipline of prosaic day-to-day existence. It offers a gratifyingly wide opportunity for instinctual discharge in socially acceptable channels without the need for complicated sublimations. It gives the patient the safety of an *as if* relationship in the reestablishment of his emotional investment in the world of things and of people.
>
> Competently administered and skillfully presented, it encourages the timid, disarms the aggressive, motivates the lethargic, calms the restless and diverts the melancholic. As a necessary part of a hospital environment, genuinely attuned to the needs of the sick, it merits our serious attention. . . . The strength of the recreation movement is that it thinks about people and in so doing goes beyond the limitations of medicine. . . . While not curative in itself, it helps create the milieu for successful treatment. An apprehensive, resentful, or despondent patient is a chancy patient therapeutically. . . . I think of recreation as a way of taking the patient out of himself, of directing him to forget for the time being a weakness or handicap. I see in recreation a device for marshalling the hidden strengths upon which the patient has been unable to call; an interlude that leaves him a little happier, a little more confident, a little more refreshed. I believe that in recreation we have the high road to motivation; that as a reasonably predictable by-product of a reawakened interest in things that are fun to do, we find a hardening in the patient's determination to get well.

The value of therapeutic recreation services has the support of many allied health professionals and organizations. In 1988, the Council on the Accreditation of Rehabilitation Facilities (CARF), recognized the Certified Therapeutic Recreation Specialist (CTRS) credential for the first time. And in 1992, the Joint Commission of the Accreditation of Hospital Organizations (JCAHO) formally recognized therapeutic recreation within its standards as a rehabilitation treatment.

CURRENT RANGE OF SERVICES OFFERED THROUGH THERAPEUTIC RECREATION

Therapeutic recreation is a helping profession and has been involved in an allied health role in a wide variety of settings including those servicing the areas of gerontology, mental retardation, substance abuse, physical medicine and rehabilitation, psychiatry and mental health, pediatrics, and community services (13). There are several models of therapeutic recreation service delivery, and much discussion about its philosophical base.

A useful model for therapeutic recreation service delivery that integrates the various philosophical views has been proposed by Carter et al (6) and is presented in Figure 38-1.

Carter et al (6) described the four areas of service as diagnosis/needs assessment, treatment/rehabilitation, education, and prevention/health promotion. The nature of service will vary from that of intervention to that of facilitating leisure experience, depending on the setting and the client's needs. Therapeutic recreation services are unique

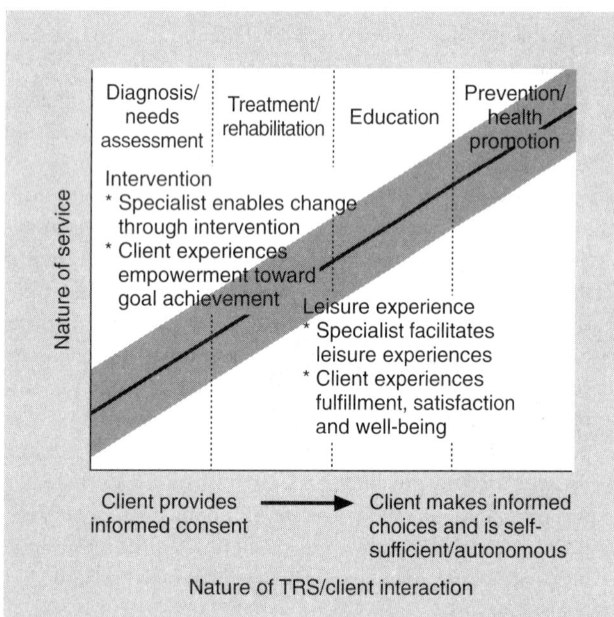

Figure 38-1. Therapeutic recreation (TR) service (TRS) model.

in that each individual situation directs the development of the intervention plan so that although protocols are used, they are always personally tailored. Diagnosis, treatment, education, and prevention can occur in the same therapeutic recreation program and all be used with the same client. For example, the therapist and a client with poor long-term memory may decide on a plan calling for the client to write in a journal, using it as a memory tool. That same patient may gain a sense of satisfaction and enjoyment during a community reintegration trip to a local restaurant. In the model shown in Figure 38-1, the line (and surrounding gray area) points to the dynamic relationship that occurs; one can be working on a treatment goal, and also experience enjoyment in the process. The line is intended to move up and down depending on the service philosophy that is prevalent in any one agency (6).

Recreational therapists go through a process of assessing the client; planning an intervention based on the needs identified by the assessment and, with the client's input, implementing that plan; and evaluating the progress the client has made toward the set goals. In the assessment process, a recreational therapist identifies a client's needs and functions in the physical, emotional, social, cognitive, and leisure areas of behavior and will utilize a variety of techniques to attain a full picture of the client's situation. The recreational therapist brings an emphasis on psychosocial concerns and their impact on rehabilitation and recovery (14). Interviews with the client and sometimes the family, observations of the client and the client's interactions with family, staff, and peers, and information from other disciplines found in the medical chart and provided in interdisciplinary team meetings are all potential sources of meaningful information. Also assessed are the leisure interests, needs, and desires of the client. A recreational therapist will also focus on abilities as well as *dis*abilities or problems that a client may be experiencing during the assessment and intervention process.

The uniqueness that therapeutic recreation brings to the effort of the treatment team is a traditionally based holistic approach and an in-depth understanding of leisure and recreation in relation to recovery, rehabilitation, health promotion, and quality of life.

When the therapist is drawing up the intervention plan, the client is as involved as is possible. This is especially important because what is defined as *leisure* will be different for each individual; therefore, the unique perspective of each client must be considered during the development of the therapeutic recreation intervention plan. The recreational therapist may work in groups or with individuals on a one-to-one basis, but it is always with the knowledge of the individual in his or her unique life context.

The certified therapeutic recreation specialist will evaluate the progress the client is making toward the outlined goals. How often this is done is influenced by the facility, the population it serves, and the way the facility operates. In many settings, the intervention plan and the client's progress are shared with a treatment team on a regular basis. When these goals are reviewed, they are then adjusted or revised as needed. When the client is discharged from an inpatient program, the therapist will write up a discharge summary and make recommendations for activities and involvements that will further recovery and ensure integration and involvement in meaningful personal and community pursuits.

In order to become eligible to take the national examination to qualify as a certified recreational therapist, a person can follow one of three paths: 1) an academic path where one must complete an undergraduate degree in therapeutic recreation, recreation or leisure with an option in therapeutic recreation, or a major in recreation or leisure (this must be done through an accredited college or university); or 2) two equivalency paths based on "specific academic preparation and full-time, paid work experience" (15).

Undergraduate college and university programs require the student to take several courses covering therapeutic recreation content, courses covering recreation content, and courses in supportive disciplines including anatomy and physiology, abnormal psychology and other social sciences, and health and human service courses. Students must complete an intensive internship as well. Upon graduation and with certification there are a wide variety of settings in which a therapeutic recreation specialist can work. An entry-level salary will range from approximately $18,000 to $31,000 per year, with a higher range available to those in administrative positions (16). There are approximately 15,000 certified therapeutic recreation specialists in the United States, and the number of positions is growing faster than the average for all occupations through the year 2006 (17).

RECREATIONAL THERAPISTS IN REHABILITATION SETTINGS

Across the various settings where therapeutic recreation is utilized, a diversity of outcomes is sought by therapeutic recreation specialists for their clients. In preliminary research done by Riley and Shank (14) the outcomes of concern for a recreational therapist were 1) functional limitation outcomes (defined as "outcomes associated with the ability of the individual to perform an action or accomplish a task using physical, cognitive, social or psychological abilities and adaptive devices or compensatory strategies; ability to perform these actions are within a range consistent with the purpose of an organ or organ system") (e.g., bowel and bladder, perceptual/sensory, motor coordination, etc.); 2) disability outcomes [defined as "outcomes associated with the ability to perform tasks, activities and roles to levels expected within physical and social contexts (school, work, family, leisure, community)"]; and 3) societal limitation outcomes (defined as "outcomes associated with social policy, services and opportunities that maintain or increase full participation in society"). These outcome categories were taken from a model of clinical outcome areas published by the National Center for Medical Rehabilitation Research (14).

Recreational therapists in rehabilitation settings are mainly engaged in treatment, leisure education, and community reintegration. In going through the process of assessment, planning, implementation, and evaluation, a variety of assessment tools are used. Some of the most common are the Ross Information Processing Assessment, the Ohio Functional Assessment (for assessing cognitive skills), and a variety of leisure interest surveys. The typical treatment interventions address endurance, balance, attention to task, cognition, motivation, problem solving, sequencing, gross motor coordination, and strength in the upper and lower extremities.

As in other settings, the recreational therapist in physical medicine and rehabilitation is concerned with problems in the various domains of behavior. These areas are discussed in the following paragraphs.

Social Outcomes

Typically in rehabilitation settings, the therapeutic recreation emphasis is in the area of social interaction as represented in the Functional Independence Measure (FIM) assessment tool (18). Social concerns, therefore, cover a wide variety of interaction and interpersonal problems as well as patient-staff relations and passive-aggressive behaviors (19). Typical patient problems that are dealt with under this behavioral domain include minimal, slow, or inappropriate responses to others; not initiating conversations; interrupting or dominating conversations with others; difficulty in getting along with others; not respecting personal boundaries; manipulating conversations for compliments or sympathy; inability to say "no" to others; avoiding staff contact; challenging group leader's authority; continually seeking staff approval or reassurance; and being unable to take direction from a male (or female) leader (19).

Emotional Outcomes

In the emotional domain, areas of concern include group performance and emotional expression problems. Recreational therapists are also concerned with making an impact on manipulative behaviors and flexibility.

Problems that are targeted include fear of failing in group situations; being easily distracted or upset by environmental milieu; frustration hindering participation; expressing no emotional response; explosive, unpredictable behavior; neglect of physical appearance due to depression; seeking attention through threats or action of self-injurious behavior; fearful of leaving the treatment center; and lack of insight into mental illness (19).

Cognitive Outcomes

Typical concerns and problem areas in the intellectual domain of behavior include inability to comply with verbal directions; inability to make decisions for self; being easily distracted or having a short attention span; being a poor judge of safety; having difficulty in following conversations; and having a poor short- or long-term memory, among other things (19). The FIM area of problem solving is covered when examining some of these issues with a client.

Physical Outcomes

Physical disability has a great impact on the affected person as well as the family. The ability to cope and adjust to disability varies according to the individual but most persons with physical disabilities have a variety of common experiences with the following: stress, social isolation, diminished self-concept, and depression (20).

Problems often encountered in the physical domain of behavior that are of concern to recreational therapists include low endurance; tiring easily; lethargy; difficulty hearing; poor hand-eye coordination; and being capable, but unwilling to propel one's own wheelchair (19).

Leisure Outcomes

In the leisure domain of behavior, areas of concern for recreational therapists include unawareness of the importance of leisure; lack of motivation for leisure involvement; having limited leisure skills; lack of transportation or companionship, or the presence of financial or other barriers to leisure; and use of alcohol as a barrier to leisure involvement (19).

CONCLUSIONS

Recreational therapists in the disability and rehabilitation fields have varied responsibilities. They play an integral role on the treatment team and have a unique niche in terms of the service they provide. The holistic orientation, the emphasis on ability and enjoyment, and the impetus therapeutic recreation gives to "hope" all contribute to a patient's adjustment and recovery. Where there is concern for quality of life, therapeutic recreation is a worthy component of the services hospital and health facilities provide.

REFERENCES

1. Sefton JM, Mummery WK. *Benefits of recreation research update.* State College, PA: Venture, 1995.
2. Driver BL, Brown PJ, Peterson GL, eds. *Benefits of leisure.* State College, PA: Venture, 1991.
3. Dattillo J, Kleiber DA. Psychological perspectives for therapeutic recreation research: the psychology of enjoyment. In: Malkin M, Howe CZ, eds. *Research in therapeutic recreation: concepts and methods.* State College, PA: Venture, 1993:57–66.
4. Iso-Ahola SE, Weissinger E. Leisure and well being: is there a connection? *Parks Recreation* 1984;18(6):40–44.
5. Kelly JR. *Leisure.* Englewood Cliffs, NJ: Prentice Hall, 1990.
6. Carter MJ, VanAndel GE, Robb GM. *Therapeutic recreation: a practical approach.* St. Louis: Times Mirror/Mosby, 1995.
7. Austin DR, Crawford ME. *Therapeutic recreation: an introduction.* Needham Heights, MA: Allyn & Bacon, 1996.
8. Clinical practice competencies: preparing for the 21st century. Presented at The American Therapeutic Recreation Association Annual Conference, San Francisco, CA. September 1996:18–22.
9. Bungay KM, Ware JE. Measuring and monitoring health-related quality of life. In: *Current concept series.* Kalamazoo, MI: The Upjohn Co., 1993.
10. Iso-Ahola SE. *The social psychology of leisure and recreation.* Dubuque, IA: Wm. C. Brown, 1980.
11. O'Morrow GS, Reynolds RP. *Therapeutic recreation: a helping profession.* Englewood Cliffs, NJ: Prentice Hall, 1989.
12. Haun P. Recreation: a medical viewpoint. A monograph compiled and edited by Avedan EM, Arje FB. Arlington, VA: National Park and Recreation Association, 1977.
13. *American Therapeutic Recreation Association Newsletter* 1997; 13:5.
14. Riley B, Shank J. Congruency of clincal outcomes among therapeutic recreation practitioners. Presented at the American Therapeutic Recreation Association's annual conference, San Francisco, CA, September 1996:18–22.
15. *National Council for Therapeutic Recreation Certification Newsletter* 1998;Spring:3.
16. Skalko T. Working as a recreational therapist in physical rehabilitation settings. In: Morgan BJ, Palmisano JM, eds. *Therapists' and allied health professionals care directory: a practical, one-step guide to getting a job as an allied health specialist.* Detroit, MI: Visible Ink Press, 1993.
17. *Bureau of Labor Statistics Occupational outlook handbook.* Washington, DC: U.S. Department of Labor, Jan 1998, Bulletin 2500.

18. *Guide for the uniform data set for medical rehabilitation (including the FIM instrument)*. A division of UB Foundation Activities Inc., Buffalo, NY, 1997.

19. Hogberg P, Johnson M. *Reference manual for writing rehabilitation therapy treatment plans.* State College, PA: Venture, 1994.

20. Berryman D, James A, Trader B. The benefits of therapeutic recreation in physical medicine. In: Coyle CP, Kinney WB, Riley B, Shank JW, eds. *Benefits of therapeutic recreation: a consensus view.* Ravensdale, WA: Idyll Arbor, 1991:235–287.

Chapter 39

Community Re-entry

Brenda B. Adamovich

Community re-entry programs focus on the training of functional skills necessary to successfully complete activities of daily living in real-life, natural situations in an individual's home, community, school, or workplace. These programs assist individuals in the integration of skills acquired during earlier phases of rehabilitation with actual, real-life situations. Community re-entry can take place in a variety of settings including traditional outpatient settings, day-treatment programs, transitional living centers, residential community programs, vocational and educational programs, and community colleges. The number of community re-entry programs has increased from two or three in the United States in 1979 to 200 in 1989, and even more today.

Kneipp (1) discussed the advantages of community-based treatment, which included 1) relevancy to the individual's life, which is inherently motivating; 2) provision of opportunities to integrate various approaches to cognitive rehabilitation to achieve objectives and outcomes that are meaningful for the individual; 3) opportunities to assess the individual's abilities to meet the unique demands of his or her own environment; 4) opportunities to observe, first-hand, the noninjury factors (e.g., family dynamics, peer culture) that affect the individual's ability to achieve his or her personal goals; 5) increased generalization; 6) higher level of success with meaningful activities; 7) greater awareness of the individual consequences of actions; and 8) promotion of empowerment and inclusion. It was suggested that even a naturalistic setting may not be sufficient because brain-injured individuals frequently have difficulty generalizing their skills across settings. It is often necessary to conduct therapy in the patient's own home and community. Cervelli (2) suggested that normalized daily living experiences are necessary to help the disabled individual address specific goals such as keeping appointments, handling money, using transportation, and performing other activities necessary for successful, day-to-day, independent functioning. Sohlberg and Mateer (3) stated "experience has shown that greater functional gains can be achieved when mechanisms to apply improved cognitive abilities to naturalistic settings are pursued."

Several disciplines generally participate in community re-entry programs. These include speech-language pathology, psychology, occupational therapy, physical therapy, recreational therapy, and vocational counseling.

TREATMENT MODELS

The New York University Head Trauma Program is a model developed by Ben-Yishay and Prigatano (4). It is a holistic program for outpatients with traumatic brain injury. Phase one is a 20-week cycle that includes assessment and intensive remedial treatment in a "therapeutic community" of 10 patients, plus their families, and the treatment team, which consists of five to six psychologists and two vocational counselors. Phase two is the individualized, "tailored-designed" phase of treatment geared to prepare the patient for productive work. Patients are then placed at actual work sites for guided occupational trials. The specific treatment sessions include the following:

1. One-half-hour sessions at the beginning of each day to foster orientation to the objectives and procedures of the program and the motivation to apply oneself; awareness and acceptance of deficiencies; habitual use of necessary compensatory mnemonic aids; and the capacity to objectively assess daily progress and set concrete goals in the presence of peers and staff.
2. Two hours of cognitive remedial training in the areas of attention; concentration and psychomotor speed of response; eye-hand coordination and fine-motor dexterity; visuoconstructional abilities; visual information processing (perceptual analysis, spatial organization, and visual problem solving); and logical reasoning.
3. A community meeting held each day to foster a sense of belonging; improve appropriateness of social behavior; foster sociability; enhance ability and willingness to comply with social rules of conduct; and increase self-esteem and realistic acceptance of the patient's own situation.
4. A weekly, 2-hour, multiple family group meeting to provide guidelines for managing the patient at home; in-depth understanding of the purpose, techniques, and results of the program; and mutual support.

Patient-family counseling is provided according to need. Patients are required to prepare two special parties for the significant others. Patients are also required to make presentations in front of the entire therapeutic community. These presentations are personal statements prepared with the assistance of staff. They are videotaped and are used clinically to further enhance each patient's self-esteem and reinforce the commitment to adopting a realistic attitude about the rehabilitation process. The last week of each cycle is devoted to reassessment. Phase two lasts from 3 to 6 months and is designed according to each individual's abilities. It involves intensive, individual, prevocational, remedial explorations and training, followed by in vivo guided work trials (usually within the setting of the medical center) and personal or small-group counseling (4).

Fryer and Haffey (5) described an outpatient program that included cognitive retraining, individual and group psychological counseling sessions, and role-playing problem-solving strategies. Patients who achieved 90% mastery of all four types of tasks achieved adequate community readaptation. Fryer and Haffey also developed a residential community re-entry model utilizing a cognitive restructuring approach in which specific cognitive barriers to the performance of residential and community survival skills and the results were used to develop strategies for organizing and retrieving information critical to task performance. The purpose was to alter the way an individual performed the task rather than trying to improve cognitive competence. Sixty-four percent of the patients in the study with traumatic brain injury achieved acceptable levels of community readaptation following participation in the program, and every patient demonstrated reductions in disability from admission to discharge. One group of patients benefited from the cognitive retraining method and another group benefited from the cognitive restructuring approach. A small number of patients did not benefit from either program.

Kneipp (1) described a model for cognitive remediation that is a community re-entry program. Her model contained the following elements: individualized, personalized program; variable scheduling; combination of individual and group interventions; transdisciplinary, extended one-on-one approach; systematic reduction of therapy and staff support; and ongoing functional observations.

Johnston and Lewis (6) described their residential community re-entry program for survivors of brain injury and strokes. It led to long-lasting improvements in independent living and productive activities, with a decrease in the requirement for supervision and an increase in paid employment, educational activities, and household management. The program required the development of client-centered goals. Clinical interventions were selected to attain outcomes such as return to paid work or to school or to other prevocational roles, behavioral control, ability to perform activities of daily living, and cognitive remediation.

Cook (7) advocated for behaviorally based training and education programs. These programs included an in-depth interdisciplinary vocational evaluation with consideration for premorbid job characteristics and interests; exploration of vocational choices, matching interests and skills; realistic appraisal of the magnitude of the discrepancy between the vocational goal, abilities, limitations, and effectiveness of compensatory strategies; ongoing counseling to confront problems, deal with stressors, and reinforce client's skills and assets; a prescriptive behaviorally based training plan that maximizes cognitive, physical, and behavioral abilities, and compensatory techniques and adaptations; work trials; and job placement.

GROUP TREATMENT

Group therapy is frequently used in community re-entry programs to focus on the interaction of cognitive functions and psychosocial behavior. Group treatment sessions can be an effective way to work on metacognitive/executive functioning skills. Groups can be designed to focus on interpersonal interactions, social skills, empathic abilities, social awareness, and recognition and acceptance of deficits. Group sessions provide an opportunity for peer support, peer review, and the practice of compensatory techniques that were established in individual therapy sessions in a more natural setting (8). Deaton (9) reviewed the following benefits of group therapy sessions: Subtle cognitive-behavioral deficits emerge in the more real-life situation in which there are multiple distractions, a degree of unpredictability, and numerous sources of input; social networks lessen social isolation and loneliness, and the focus on appropriate social interaction skills prepares the individuals for return to the community; groups are more cost-effective in a time when there are too few cognitive rehabilitation therapists and when some insurers do not reimburse for cognitive rehabilitation; improved motivation and insight occur with peer confrontation and motivation; and techniques can be practiced in a less-threatening environment.

Criteria for group membership should take into account verbal comprehension and verbal expression skills, intellectual functioning, ability to control aggressive and disruptive behavior, and homogeneity in that the area of weakness is shared by all group members (9–11). A few examples of group therapy activities are described in the following sections.

Interpersonal Interaction Group

The responsibility for doing a presentation on an assigned topic is rotated among group members. A video recording is made of each presentation. Utilizing the video recording, all group members evaluate the session using an objective form. Each person evaluates himself or herself as a speaker or listener during the group session. Specific areas of evaluation include presentation of organized, sequential information; conveyance of main point; ability to use abstract information; ability to use feedback; too little or excessive information; irrelevant information; redundant information; observation of rules; appropriate topic switching; obscurity or ambiguity; and style of communication. Pragmatic behaviors can also be evaluated; these include behavior appropriate to the situation, eye contact, turn taking, initiation of conversation, use of gestures, affect, speed of response, posture, rate, intonation, social distance, group support, ability to profit from cueing, and willingness and ability to modify behavior. Prutting and Kirchner (12) developed a pragmatic protocol to rate pragmatic skills during group interactions.

Listeners also can be evaluated for their use of appropriate questioning strategies and the abilities to interpret information abstractly, to request repetitions when needed, to identify missing information, to give feedback, and to identify the main point.

Several investigators reported functional improvements in social skills as a result of group treatment that addressed interpersonal interactions, verbal and nonverbal communication, and pragmatic skills (3,13–18).

Social Skills Group

The ability of each group member to cooperate and accept group decisions can be evaluated following participation in an assigned social activity such as planning special menus, birthday parties, outings, and family open houses. The ability of each group member to adjust behavior appropriately with regard to verbal output, dress, and gestures can also be evaluated following assigned role-playing activities. Specific activities include a party with friends versus a job interview, or a family dinner versus dinner with a new date.

Empathic Abilities Group

On a rotating basis, the conflict resolution skills of each group member can be evaluated following the role playing of a dispute between two friends according to a script prepared by the clinician or a subcommittee of group members. Specific abilities to be evaluated include the ability to determine reasons for the dispute (deductive reasoning), the ability to determine premises or assumptions of each person, the ability to establish compromise, the ability to test solutions, and the ability to negotiate a compromise (complementary reasoning).

Personal and Social Adjustment Group

In individual sessions, personal statements are established and rehearsed. For example, a client might be required to make a statement regarding two personal strengths, for example, "I am a person who . . ." (19). Video recordings are made of the individual session and are critiqued by the client and clinician. After the client has mastered the individual session, a presentation is made to the entire group. A self-evaluation and group evaluation are made of the video recording of the group session using a system to score awareness, understanding, assimilation, and acceptance.

Life Skills Group

A list of activities can be generated by the group members. Role playing in the group setting can be followed by actual community experiences. Activities include giving and following directions, shopping, using public transportation, using emergency skills, preparing meals, managing a household, using leisure and recreational time, managing time, managing personal care attendants, and writing letters.

Cognitive Skills Group

Groups can be used to teach and practice cognitive skills and strategies in the areas of organization, memory, and problem solving. Problem-solving groups provide opportunities to apply cognitive strategies, improve cognitive flexibility, and decrease impulsivity. Real-life problems are presented and steps are taught and rehearsed to solve the problems, such as locking keys in the car, locating a car in a parking garage, and arriving late to a scheduled appointment.

RETURN TO WORK OR SCHOOL

Handicaps following traumatic brain injury that prevent the fulfillment of a normal life role include physical independence, vocational status or return to work, return to school, return to family roles, and establishment of a support network. The ability to return to work or school is often used as an index of outcome following traumatic brain injury since survivors are often young adults of work or school age with an average life span. Webb et al (20) studied 116 subjects 2 years after traumatic brain injury occurred. Their findings suggested that employment was the strongest contributor of improved quality of life.

Vocational/educational outcome after injury is of crucial importance as it helps to reduce financial and emotional stress to the brain-injured individuals and their families as well as costs to society. A significant proportion of the costs of traumatic brain injury can be linked directly to discouraging rates of postinjury employment (21). Less than 30% of persons with traumatic brain injury will enter or re-enter the competitive work force (22). As a result of their research, Wehman et al (23) found that individuals with traumatic brain injury who return to work do so in less-demanding or menial positions, sheltered employment, or volunteer work. Many activities that were previously handled automatically and easily prior to the brain injury will require a great deal of concentration and effort, with some tasks beyond current capabilities after the brain injury.

Ponsford et al (24) stressed the need for ongoing community-based support and assistance in dealing with practical difficulties and psychological problems that individuals experience after return to the community. These investigators studied 175 patients with traumatic brain injury who had undergone intensive rehabilitation 2 years after injury. Two-thirds of these individuals reported cognitive, behavioral, and emotional deterioration even though the majority of the individuals were physically independent and competent in personal and domestic activities of daily living. A third of the group were still reliant on assistance with community skills and transport. More than half of those who previously had a job were not working 2 years after the injury. Cope et al (25) measured the outcomes of 192 subjects recovering from brain injury at 6, 12, and 24 months after discharge versus discharge from a community-based acute rehabilitation program. The community-based program focused on activities of daily living in as close to a real-world environment as possible. Posttreatment scores revealed an increase in the number of persons living at home, competitive employment, productive activities, and independence.

Klonoff et al (26) conducted an outcome study of subjects 2 to 4 years after brain injury occurred, and reported that behavioral difficulties tended to increase with time. The difficulties included being more belligerent, slowed motorically, socially withdrawn, negative, socially obstreperous, confused, and talkative. Johnson and Lewis (6) conducted an outcome study of 82 brain-injured subjects 1 year after discharge from a residential community re-entry program. Results suggested an increase in independent living activities such as self-care, mobility, and communication. Emotional distress and maladaptive social behaviors decreased in frequency. Stress decreased and social life improved.

Wehman et al (23) developed the use of supported employment as a method of vocational rehabilitation. Supported employment emphasizes placement into actual competitive employment sites with the necessary support to succeed. The support includes a job coach who works with the individual and the employer to educate coworkers and to make accommodations on the job (27).

Adolescents and young adults experience a disproportionately high incidence of brain injury compared to other age groups. Residual cognitive and behavioral deficits, even if subtle, can interfere with successful return to school. Brain-injured students who return to high school, adult education programs, trade schools, community colleges, and 4-year colleges and universities have unique needs. For example, they often need assistance in getting from class to class, organizing their notebook, planning their assignments, and recognizing problems when they arise; cognitive remediation classes; socialization groups; transportation tutors; adaptive equipment and assistance with note taking; and counseling and job placement. The key to success in educational endeavors often depends on the awareness of the institution to the unique learning needs of the brain injured and the willingness of the institution to accommodate resources to meet these needs. Return-to-work programs and work-hardening programs, which have been developed for injured workers who have not experienced brain injury, can be adapted quite effectively for patients with traumatic brain injury. They need to include vocational testing to determine specific job potentials, work hardening to train job-specific skills, job coaching and on-the-job training, and evaluation. Special considerations include determination of a program to meet each individual's needs; education of each individual regarding specific limitations; training of the necessary skills including filling out a job application and being interviewed, and job-related strengths and weaknesses; and supervised work trials provided through job simulation, sheltered workshops, and community work sites.

Dawson and Chipman (28) surveyed 454 individuals with traumatic brain injury 13 years, on average, after the injury occurred. The study was designed to investigate the determinants of three handicaps: physical independence, work, and social integration. The prevalence of long-term handicap was high, with 66% of the sample reporting the need for ongoing assistance with some activities of daily living, 75% not working, and 90% reporting some limitations or dissatisfaction with their social integration. The determinants of the handicaps included age (older), gender (female), level of education (primary school or less), living alone, physical environmental barriers, and specific motor and personal care disabilities. Limited data were collected on behavioral dysfunction or cognitive impairment in this study. The only behavioral dysfunction included was learning disability, and the only cognitive impairment included was memory difficulty.

Ip et al (29) studied factors predicting return to work or school following traumatic brain injury. Forty-five subjects were studied retrospectively with regard to sociodemographics, chronicity, indices of severity, physical impairment, and cognitive functioning. The generalizability of the predictive model was then tested on a sample of 20 subjects. The performance IQ score of the Wechsler Adult Intelligence Scale—Revised was found to be the most significant predictor of return to work or school. Other variables causing brain-injured individuals to be most at risk for not returning to work or school were age (older), a high percentage of reported alcohol abuse, and lower levels of performance on perceptual-motor tasks on psychometric tests. Brain injury severity as measured by the Glasgow Coma Scale and coma duration, time after injury, and physical impairment were not significantly related to return to work or school.

Crépeau and Scherzer (30) conducted a review of the literature and used a meta-analysis to combine and compare the results of available independent studies. Of 140 studies identified, 41 met inclusion criteria: limited exclusively to individuals with traumatic brain injury, at least one quantitative predictor or severity indicator measure, and one measure of return to work. Among the pretrauma predictors, age was only related to work status in studies that included subjects older than 60 years, while gender and number of years of education had a minimal relationship to employment outcome. Executive functioning and flexibility were highly correlated to employment outcome. Memory correlations with return to work were divergent among the 10 studies in the analysis. Pretrauma and early recovery predictors such as coma duration and posttraumatic amnesia were only marginally associated with vocational outcome. Better predictors were postcoma activity level, posttrauma neurological and motor sequelae, and duration of hospitalization.

Ruff et al (31) investigated outcome as a function of employment status or return to school in severely brain-injured patients. The three most potent predictors were intactness of verbal intellectual power, speed of information processing, and age. A higher return rate to school versus work was suggested to be a result of the educational system's adaptability. Ponsford and Olver (32) studied 254 patients 2 years after traumatic brain injury occurred. Their results revealed that the Disability Rating Scale score, Glasgow Coma Scale score, and age correlated significantly with employment status 2 years after traumatic brain injury.

Ben-Yishay and Prigatano (4,10) suggested a model for a rehabilitation program after acute brain injury that focused on return to work or school. The program focused on insight into disabilities and on emotional and behavioral problems that provide significant barriers to the rehabilitation of cognitive and physical disabilities. Their assumption was that a major cause of the inability to return to work was the lack of understanding and awareness of higher cerebral deficits. Prigatano et al (33) reported that 9 (50%) of 18 graduates were in age-appropriate activities (work, homemaking, or school) at 8 to 33 months after program completion. Ben-Yishay et al (34) reported that 53 (56%) of 94 graduates were competitively employed and an additional 20 (21%) were in sheltered or supported work at 12 months following program completion.

Malec et al (35) evaluated the outcomes of individuals with brain injuries following a group-oriented treatment program. A comprehensive, integrated, post–acute injury outpatient rehabilitation program, similar to those described by Ben-Yishay and Prigatano (4), was followed with these exceptions: Participants were admitted continuously, not as a group; there was no set length of treatment; and work trials were provided in actual community placements rather than as clinical work activities. From admission to program completion, the percentage of those living with no supervision increased from 59% to 93%, the percentage of those in transitional or competitive work placements increased from 7% to 59%, and the unemployment rate decreased from 76% to 31%. At 1-year follow-up, independent living and employment gains were maintained. Individuals entering treatment less than 1 year after injury showed greater gains than did individuals injured more than 1 year prior to admission. However, both the early and late intervention groups showed significant changes on the outcome measures. Other neuropsychological measures on admission did not significantly predict outcome. More extensive disabilities and reading ability had a negative impact on outcome. Cope et al (25) and Johnson and Lewis (6) also found that outcome was related to severity of disability and that early treatment (<6 months after injury) resulted in more improvement.

Wehman (36) and Sowers and Powers (37) found that supportive employment was an effective treatment approach to allow persons who have had traumatic brain injury to return to work. Wehman et al (21) completed a review of the literature and further analysis of 87 persons who secured competitive employment through a specialized, traumatic brain injury supported employment program. The authors concluded that supported employment with individual job coaches is a successful means of assisting individuals with severe traumatic brain injury to re-enter the workforce.

Fraser and Wehman (38) suggested that the literature on vocational rehabilitation for traumatic brain injury revealed variable outcomes due to methodologic differences, such as a lack of uniformity in severity of traumatic brain injury, in neuropsychological test batteries used, in operational definitions of successful employment outcome, in preinjury and postinjury emotional and behavioral functioning, in varying periods of follow-up, and in vocational interventions. These authors suggested the need for a standardized protocol for assessing functional vocational outcomes.

CONCLUSIONS

Community re-entry programs that focus on the treatment of daily living skills in real-life situations within each individual's home, community, school, and workplace result in the greatest improvement in functional outcomes. Group therapy is often used to improve interpersonal interactions, social skills, empathic abilities, social awareness, and recognition and acceptance of deficits. The ability to return to work or school is often used as an index of outcome. Further research is needed to continue the development and to assess the efficacy of these programs.

REFERENCES

1. Kneipp S. Cognitive remediation within the context of a community reentry program. In: Kreutzer JS, Wehman PH, eds. *Cognitive rehabilitation for persons with traumatic brain injury: a functional approach.* Baltimore: Paul H. Brookes, 1991:239–250.
2. Cervelli L. Re-entry into the community and systems of posthospital care. In: Bond MR, Griffith ER, Miller JD, Rosenthal M, eds. *Rehabilitation of the adult and child with traumatic brain injury.* 2nd ed. Philadelphia: FA Davis, 1990:463–475.
3. Sohlberg MM, Mateer CA. Training use of compensatory memory books: a three-stage behavioral approach. *J Clin Exp Neuropsychol* 1989;11:871–891.
4. Ben-Yishay Y, Prigatano GP. Cognitive remediation. In: Rosenthal ER, Griffith M, Griffith ER, Bond MR, Miller JD, eds. *Rehabilitation of the adult and child with traumatic brain injury.* 2nd ed. Philadelphia: FA Davis, 1990:393–400.
5. Fryer LJ, Haffey WJ. Cognitive rehabilitation and community readaptation: outcomes from two program models. *J Head Trauma Rehabil* 1987;2:51–63.
6. Johnston MV, Lewis FD. Outcomes of community re-entry programmes for brain injury survivors. Part 1: independent living and productive activities. *Brain Inj* 1991;5:141–154.
7. Cook JV. Returning to work after traumatic head injury. In: Bond MR, Griffith ER, Miller JD, Rosenthal M, eds. *Rehabilitation of the adult and child with traumatic brain injury.* 2nd ed. Philadelphia: FA Davis, 1990:493–505.
8. Adamovich BLB. Traumatic brain injury. In: LaPoint LL, ed. *Aphasia and related neurogenic language disorders.* 2nd ed. New York: Thieme Medical, 1997.
9. Deaton AV. Group interventions for cognitive rehabilitation, increasing the challenges. In: Kreutzer JS, Wehman PH, eds. *Cognitive rehabilitation for persons with traumatic brain injury.* Baltimore: Paul H. Brookes, 1991:191–199.
10. Prigatano GP. *Neuropsychological rehabilitation after brain injury.* Baltimore: Johns Hopkins University Press, 1986.
11. Wilson BA, Moffat N, eds. *Clinical management of memory problems.* Rockville, MD: Aspen Systems, 1984.
12. Prutting CA, Kirchner DM. Applied pragmatics. In: Gallagher TM, Prutting CA, eds. *Pragmatic assessment and intervention issues in language.* San Diego: College Hill, 1983:29–64.
13. Alexy WD, Foster M, Baker A. Audio-visual feedback: an exercise in self-awareness for the head injured patient. *Cogn Rehabil* 1983;1(6):8–10.
14. Helffenstein DA, Wechsler FS. The use of Interpersonal Process Recall (IPR) in the remediation of interpersonal and communication skill deficits in the newly brain-injured. *Clin Neuropsychol* 1982;4:139–143.
15. Brotherton FA, Thomas LL, Wisotzek IE, Milan MA. Social skills training in the rehabilitation of patients with traumatic closed head injury. *Arch Phys Med Rehabil* 1988;69:827–832.
16. Gajar A, Schloss PJ, Schloss CN, Thompson CK. Effects of feedback and self-monitoring on head trauma youths' conversation skills. *J Appl Behav Anal* 1984;17:353–358.
17. Schloss PJ, Thompson CK, Gajar AH, Schloss CN. Influence of self-monitoring on heterosexual conversational behaviours of head trauma youth. *Appl Res Ment Retard* 1985;6:269–282.
18. Hartley LL, Griffith A. A functional approach to the cognitive-communicative deficits of closed head injured clients. *Tex J Audiol Speech Pathol* 1989;14(2):37–42.
19. Ben-Yishay Y, Diller L. Cognitive remediation in traumatic brain injury: update and issues. *Arch Phys Med Rehabil* 1993;74:204–213.
20. Webb CR, Wrigley M, Yoels W, Fine P. Explaining quality of life for persons with traumatic brain injuries 2 years after injury. *Arch Phys Med Rehabil* 1995;76:1113–1119.
21. Wehman PH. Cognitive rehabilitation in the workplace. Cognitive rehabilitation for persons with traumatic brain injury, a functional approach. 1991;20:269–288.

22. Brooks N, McKinlay W, Symington D, et al. Return to work within the first seven years of severe head injury. *Brain Inj* 1987;1:5–19.

23. Wehman P, Kreutzer J, West M, et al. Employment outcomes of persons following traumatic brain injury: pre-injury, post-injury and supported employment. *Brain Inj* 1989;3:397–412.

24. Ponsford JL, Olver JH, Curran C, Ng K. Prediction of employment status 2 years after traumatic brain injury. *Brain Inj* 1994;9:11–20.

25. Cope DN, Cole JR, Hall KM, Barkan H. Brain-injury: analysis of outcome in a post-acute rehabilitation system. Part 1: general analysis. *Brain Inj* 1991;5:111–126.

26. Klonoff PS, Snow WG, Costa LD. Quality of life in patients 2 to 4 years after closed head injury. *Neurosurgery* 1986;19:735–743.

27. Willer B, Corrigan JD. New concepts Whatever It Takes: a model for community-based services. *Brain Inj* 1993;8:647–659.

28. Dawson DR, Chipman M. The disablement experienced by traumatically brain-injured adults living in the community. *Brain Inj* 1995; 9:339–353.

29. Ip RY, Dornan J, Schentag C. Traumatic brain injury: factors predicting return to work or school. *Brain Inj* 1995;9:517–532.

30. Crepéau F, Scherzer P. Predictors and indicators of work status after traumatic brain injury: a meta-analysis. *Neuropsychol Rehabil* 1993;3:5–35.

31. Ruff RM, Marshall LF, Crouch J, et al. Predictors of outcome following severe head trauma: follow-up data from the Traumatic Coma Data Bank. *Brain Inj* 1993; 7:101–111.

32. Ponsford JL, Olver JH. A profile of outcome: 2 years after traumatic brain injury. *Brain Inj* 1995;9:1–10.

33. Prigatano GP, Fordyce DJ, Zeiner HK, et al. Neuropsychological rehabilitation after closed head injury in young adults. *J Neurol Neurosurg Psychiatry* 1984;47:505–513.

34. Ben-Yishay Y, Silver S, Piasetsky E, Rattok J. Relationship between employability and vocational outcome after intensive holistic cognitive rehabilitation. *J Head Trauma Rehabil* 1987;2: 35–49.

35. Malec JF, Smigielski JS, DePompolo RW. Goal attainment scaling and outcome measurement in postacute brain injury rehabilitation. *Arch Phys Med Rehabil* 1991;72:138–143.

36. Wehman P. Supported employment: model implementation and evaluation. In: Kreutzer JS, Wehman P, eds. *Community integration following traumatic brain injury*. Baltimore: Paul H. Brookes, 1990:185–204.

37. Sowers J, Powers L. Job design strategies for persons with physical and multiple disabilities. In: Sowers J, Powers L, eds. *Vocational Preparation and Employment of Students with Physical and Multiple Disabilities.* Portland: Oregon Research Institute, 1989.

38. Fraser RT, Wehman P. Traumatic brain injury rehabilitation: issues in vocational outcome. *Neurorehabilitation* 1995;5:39–48.

Chapter 40

Competitive Employment for Persons with Disabilities: Overcoming the Obstacles

Paul Wehman
Valerie Brooke
Michael West
Pam Sherron Targett
Howard Green
Katherine Inge
John Kregel

The employment of persons with disabilities is a major goal that society must attend to much more seriously. It is a doable and solvable problem. For example, within the past 5 years, an enormous amount of attention has been directed to helping or encouraging persons on welfare to enter the workplace. These efforts seem, at least in the short term, to be paying off; yet a similar effort has not been made to help individuals with disabilities enter the workforce. The ability to be employed is important for many reasons, but there are at least four obvious ones. First, working in competitive employment provides an opportunity to receive wages and benefits that can lead to greater independence and mobility in the community at large. Second, being productive on a daily basis in a meaningful vocation is critically important to self-esteem and dignity. Third, establishing new friendships and networks of social support in the community is almost always facilitated by having a job within a career path. And finally, the extraordinary costs associated with maintaining persons with disabilities on Social Security disability rolls is a highly nonproductive and inefficient use of human potential in this country. It is now reaching the level of being politically unacceptable. This high level of entitlement leads to larger federal deficits and ultimately works against the perceptions that society has of people with disabilities.

Between 1985 and 1994 the number of people with disabilities who receive Disability Insurance (DI) and Supplemental Security Income (SSI) benefits from the Social Security Administration (SSA) has increased from 4.2 million to 7.2 million (1). These figures are dramatic indeed because of the enormous expenditures associated with long-term payment of Social Security cash benefits. For example, in 1994 the SSA reported that the DI program and SSI program provided $53 billion in cash benefits to the 7.2 million people. Yet the Louis Harris Poll (2) indicated that *the majority* of these people want to work. Since there have been substantive advances in assistive technology, rehabilitation technology, and medicine, it is reasonable to ask, why is there such a perplexing problem of extremely high unemployment for persons with disabilities?

The challenge to individuals working in the disability field is to try and more effectively understand *why* persons with disabilities have been unable to break into the competitive labor force. What are the specific reasons why this has not occurred to a greater extent? What are the specific barriers and what role do they play in blocking the vocational wishes and aspirations of persons with disabilities? Once these factors are well understood, careful advocacy and political action can begin to resolve some of the more challenging ones.

In this chapter, several specific reasons for this important societal dilemma are discussed. But first, it is important to understand that the issue of unemployment of persons with disability is seldom on the political agenda. *We cannot resolve these problems until politicians, policymakers, consumer groups, and professionals push this problem front and center onto the political agenda, in a similar way that welfare reform has occurred.* We must learn to speak with one voice regarding the importance of employment in the life of persons with disabilities and their respective families. The barriers that have blocked employment (and that are discussed in the balance of this chapter) are ultimately solvable, but none of them can be removed without key people in public policy positions being aware of the problems and understanding that people with disabilities want to work and can work.

HEALTH CARE BENEFITS AND SOCIAL SECURITY ADMINISTRATION POLICY

Perhaps the most imposing barrier to employment for persons with disabilities is potential loss of income assistance and health care benefits through programs administered by the SSA and the Health Care Financing Administration (HCFA). The two major SSA disability programs are SSI and DI. While the two have different eligibility criteria, under both programs individuals with disabilities must prove themselves to be *incapable* of engaging in substantial gainful activity (SGA), currently defined as earnings of over $500 per month, to be eligible for benefits.

For many individuals with disabilities, full-time employment with health benefits is not an option due to low levels of job skills, local labor market conditions, limitations in stamina or endurance, or the need to commit substantial amounts of time to personal care needs or treatments. Yet if they obtain part-time employment, they risk losing cash and other benefits, particularly medical coverage under Medicaid (in most states linked to eligibility for SSI) or Medicare (linked to eligibility for DI). This economic disincentive persuades most beneficiaries to limit their earnings to less than SGA or, more commonly, not to enter the labor market at all (3).

The impact of economic disincentives for SSA beneficiaries to return to work has become all too clear to the SSA, the Congress, and the American public. As stated already, from 1985 to 1994, the number of annual SSA disability benefit recipients grew from 4.2 million to 7.2 million, a 70% increase, and cash benefits grew from $23.1 billion to $52.6 billion, a 66% increase (4). The primary causes for this growth are 1) increasing numbers of applications, particularly from younger individuals and those with mental impairments, and 2) very low rates of return to the workforce for those who become beneficiaries (5).

The SSA has instituted corrective measures to reduce the disincentives of employment for beneficiaries, such as referral to state vocational rehabilitation services, trial work periods, continuing eligibility for Medicare, deduction of impairment-related work expenses from taxable earnings, and allowing beneficiaries to exclude income from the calculation of SGA using a Plan for Achieving Self-Sufficiency (PASS). However, according to a recent report by the General Accounting Office (4), few SSI or DI beneficiaries know about these incentives or understand how to access them, and thus these incentives have virtually no impact on return to work.

Medicaid and Medicare reforms at the federal and state levels may have significant impact on health benefits and employment for persons with disabilities. During the 1995 to 1996 legislative year, the 104th Congress and the president considered several reform proposals, including changing the nature of Medicaid from an entitlement to block grants to the states. All of the proposals placed caps on the anticipated growth of program expenditures and gave increased control to the states regarding eligibility and benefits. In addition, states are increasingly moving Medicaid and Medicare beneficiaries into managed care systems, through either reform of state programs or privatization (6). Managed care, a concept that has become the standard in employer-sponsored health insurance programs, is characterized by 1) cost containment through utilization management ("gatekeepers"), prior authorization of services, and a single-payer system; 2) shared risk between the beneficiary and the provider; and 3) use of management information systems to assess measurable outcomes and benefits.

There is little disagreement that Medicaid and Medicare reforms are needed for the programs to remain viable. However, the reforms that are eventually instituted could have dramatic effects on entitlements to health care, long-term care and services, and unemployment rates for persons with disabilities (7).

CHANGING ECONOMY

As important as health benefits are, the fact remains that the strength of the economy in a given area will greatly influence job marketability. Almost every day, newspapers and business news on television report that certain businesses are reorganizing or reducing their workforce. However, based on reports from the National Alliance of Business publication *Workforce Economics* (8), new jobs are being created and unemployment is stable. Even with the baby boomers joining the labor market in the 1970s and 1980s, employing millions of people, the labor market has yet to reach the saturation point. Given these figures, we must ask ourselves about the two-thirds of disabled Americans between the ages of 16 and 64 who are unemployed. Are people with disabilities being left behind in the American dream as our economic and labor market demands change?

Ask any job developer to name one of the biggest reasons given by business for not hiring, and they will tell you that it is due to the economy! *Cutbacks, downsizing, outsourcing, streamlining,* and *slow sales* are words we hear when trying to locate employers with job openings. Is the economy really in bad shape? What are the changes that have occurred over the past few years that hinder applicants with disabilities from securing suitable and productive employment in this country? Will this trend continue into the twenty-first century?

The Bureau of Labor Statistics, the Organization for Economic Cooperation and Development, and the McKinsey Global Institute recently provided new comparative data on economic performance (9). These data show the following:

- The U.S. economy has been creating jobs at a much faster rate than its international competitors.
- A larger percentage of the population is working in this country than in other countries.
- The job market is drawing into the economy even workers who have been idle.
- Employment growth is concentrated in sectors of the economy requiring more education and in jobs at the higher end of the occupational ladder.
- Unemployment in the United States is stable.
- U.S. productivity is growing.

In looking at these data it would appear things are going pretty well for most Americans. However, since statistics and recent studies show that people with disabilities are unemployed at such a high percentage rate as compared to other groups in this country, why is the changing economy keeping citizens with disabilities out of the workforce?

In the December 1995 issue of *Workforce Economics* (9) the Bureau of Labor Statistics reported that the jobs the U.S. economy is creating are concentrated in industries requiring more education. In addition, this issue reported that employment in the higher-ended occupations is growing rapidly in the United States. From 1980 to 1990, the United States created jobs in higher-ended occupations such as professional, technical, administrative, and managerial positions at a rate twice as high as that in Japan, Germany, and France. As all of us who work in the field of disability know, individuals with disabilities, especially people with the most severe disabilities, usually do not find employment in the higher-ended occupations. Individuals with disabilities are usually facing an uphill battle in securing the education, work experience, and technical skills that will allow them the opportunity to secure jobs with higher wages, good benefits, and the possibility for upward mobility. As we know, individuals with severe disabilities usually have to settle for entry-level jobs, low wages, and no promise of advancing in a career ladder. With the ever-changing economy, businesses are requiring more productivity from their current employees. Employers are requiring their current workers to cross-train so they may assume some of the job duties created by downsizing. In the past, it was common for businesses to look favorably on the idea of job restructuring or job carving to accommodate special needs; however, companies seem to be giving multiple duties to existing employees rather than hiring individuals to perform a specialized job.

The economy is always changing based on a number of different factors. Whether it be politics, government rules and regulations, employment and education programs, consumer demands, or world events, the economy will look vastly different each year. People and programs need to stay informed and be prepared for the changes. It may not be the fault of the economy that people with disabilities are grossly unemployed, but rather that the programs and services designed to enable these individuals to prepare for and enter employment need to keep up with the pace and the trends of the changing economy and employment opportunities in America.

IMPACT OF PREPARATION IN SCHOOLS

The lack of preparation and training in schools is also a major contributor to unemployment of persons with disabilities. While there have been major strides toward demonstrating the best practices that lead to successful transition from school to work, the majority of young people with disabilities continue to lag behind their peers without disabilities in postschool outcomes. A number of follow-up studies have been completed since the 1980s. They indicate that students with severe disabilities leave school only to join the ranks of those who are unemployed or underemployed (10–14).

Since 1985, SRI International of Menlo Park, California, has conducted a National Longitudinal Transition Study of Special Education Students (13). This project, conducted for the Office of Special Education Programs of the U.S. Department of Education, has been gathering information concerning how well students with disabilities are being served under the Individuals with Disabilities Education Act (IDEA). Included in the study are more than 8000 youths with disabilities. Some of the results include the following:

Employment Outcomes:

- Youths with disabilities do not achieve competitive employment at comparable levels to their able-bodied peers ($p < 0.001$).
- Some of the youth with multiple disabilities in the study were not employed when surveyed in 1987 or 1990. Of those employed, 10.2% lost their jobs during this time period.
- Some of the youth with mental retardation were not employed when surveyed in 1987 or 1990. Of those who were employed, 12.9% lost employment during this time period.
- Some of the youth with orthopedic impairments were not employed when surveyed in 1987 or 1990. Of those who were employed, 5.6% lost employment during this time period.

Independent Living Outcomes:

- Only 13.4% of the youth with multiple disabilities in the study were living independently 3 to 5 years after graduation.
- Only 23.7% of the youth with mental retardation in the study were living independently 3 to 5 years after graduation.
- Only 38% of the youth with orthopedic impairments were living independently 3 to 5 years after graduation.

These findings reveal the relatively poor transition outcomes for students with severe disabilities, indicating a need to provide services that facilitate successful postschool outcomes.

The newly funded systems change projects in supported employment were surveyed by the Rehabilitation Research and Training Center at Virginia Commonwealth University at the April 1996 meeting (15); it was indicated that the current availability of transition programs in these states is low and that the programs are of low quality. The states surveyed included Alabama, Hawaii, Massachusetts, Mississippi, Ohio, Rhode Island, South Dakota, Texas, and West Virginia. More specifically, 100% of the funded states identified the need to improve the existing transition programs as one of their top three priorities for supported employment systems change during the national meeting in April 1996. Some of the issues identified include the following:

- Large school districts often provide group work experiences but individual experiences are not as frequent, because coordinators do not have time to individualize arrangements/opportunities.
- There needs to be better coordination strategies between school-to-work professionals and supported employment professionals.
- Vocational rehabilitation is providing services for students with mild-to-moderate disabilities, but students with severe disabilities are not being served.
- *Information dissemination* to enhance awareness of supported employment options for students, along with training activities, is needed to provide more opportunities for community-based work experience and job outcomes for students. The target audience includes transition team members, counselors, special education teachers and coordinators, students and family networks, and service providers.

Students with disabilities who live in rural communities are confronted with additional barriers to successful transition outcomes. Sarkees and Veir (16) estimated that more than two-thirds of the schools in this country can be defined as residing in a rural area. Many of these school systems lack qualified school system personnel knowledgeable about transition service options available to students with disabilities. In addition, they often have not received training in the best-practices techniques that have been developed through model demonstration projects nationally.

Even teachers who reside in urban areas may have limited access to information. It has been suggested that school teachers work mainly in isolation from other professionals. They interact with their colleagues only for a few moments each day. Other related-services personnel also may be providing services in isolation from each other, even though "best practices" for transition calls for a collaborative approach to programming. For instance, Inge (17) surveyed occupational therapists in the public schools who worked with transition-age students with severe disabilities. She asked how many times a week the occupational therapists had at least 15 minutes to discuss each student in their caseload with other team members. Only 7.2% of the respondents indicated that they had 15 minutes more than once a week to discuss each student with other team members; 12.1% indicated once a week; 18.6% had about two to three times a month; 26.2% had about once a month; and 11.4% indicated that they never had time to discuss or review students in their caseload with other team members. Most other members of the nation's workforce collaborate, exchange information, and develop new skills on a daily basis (18).

Although parent participation in the decision-making process has been mandated, many parents continue to arrive at the Individualized Education Program (IEP) meeting to be presented with a completed plan. A lack of knowledge and information is an even greater problem for those parents who have low incomes or who are minorities. In addition, participants at the National Meeting for Supported Employment Systems Change (April 1996) indicated that parents do not have the needed information to assist their sons and daughters in making successful transition outcomes (15). Specifically, they often are not aware of the major strides that have been made in the area of community employment for individuals with severe disabilities. Training on how to obtain the needed support services once their sons and daughters leave the school system must be developed and provided to facilitate positive postschool outcomes.

TRANSPORTATION

The lack of available, affordable transportation is an employment barrier that cuts across virtually all disability groups (19). For many individuals with disabilities, such as those with epilepsy, visual impairments, mental retardation, or severe physical impairments, driving is restricted by law or by individual limitations. For members of other disability groups (such as psychosocial impairments) who are unemployed, financial constraints may prohibit ownership of an automobile. In either case, the result is that many individuals with disabilities must rely on either public transportation or alternative modes of transportation in order to enter the job market.

Community mobility is a necessary prerequisite not only for employment, but also for inclusion in social and recreational activities and use of community resources and facilities. A study of self-determined adults with disabilities conducted by West et al (20) found that transportation and independent mobility in the community were major factors in developing self-determination. Having means of accessing different environments increased the range of options in the areas of work, socialization, recreation, and housing. Being mobile also enabled individuals to exercise control, allowing them to decide where and how they lived, rather than relinquishing that control to service agencies, family members, or others.

The Americans with Disabilities Act of 1990 (ADA) mandated that public transportation facilities and vehicles, including buses, vans, rail cars, and so on, be accessible to persons with disabilities (21). While much progress has been made in improving access to transportation systems, many individuals with disabilities have not been affected because of 1) lack of voluntary compliance or overall cutbacks on routes in response to the ADA, or 2) absence of transportation systems in their communities (22–24).

In the absence of public transportation, creative solutions to transportation barriers must be employed, particularly in rural areas or in situations where individuals may be unable to move close to their jobs. Some of these options include the following:

1. Using a personal assistant, friend, or family member to assist with transportation
2. Ride sharing with a coworker, possibly with reimbursement for expenses
3. Arranging for transportation through paratransit services or other human service agencies
4. Locating jobs within companies (such as some hospitals and nursing facilities) that offer employee transportation for those in need
5. Assisting individuals with disabilities to locate work-at-home jobs, such as self-employment, on-line data entry, and child care

PROFESSIONAL ATTITUDES

The evolution of supported employment services has required rehabilitation professionals, families, customers of rehabilitation services, employers, service providers, and policy makers to examine their values. Before the availability of supported employment, the values related to sheltered employment programs can be traced back to a time when people with disabilities and their families wanted an alternative to staying home. The programmatic emphasis concerned providing a reliable routine and a safe, well-supervised environment. The philosophical foundation for community-based employment services for individuals with cognitive and other developmental disabilities shifted in the 1980s from sanctioning facility-based services to a preferred endorsement of integrated, supported employment (25). This shift has been reflected in federal policy. The Rehabilitation Act has continued to move away from segregated employment options toward integrated employment. The Rehabilitation Act Amendments of 1992 (26) contain major program changes that are intended to promote consumer choice, self-determination, and the ability for consumers to pick jobs and careers that they wish (27).

Supported employment has been about community-integrated jobs with commensurate wages and benefits (28–30). Supported employment's philosophical foundation and implementation strategies challenge the practice of providing services that remove people with disabilities from the mainstream of community activity. Supported employment, from its inception, has been based on the values listed in Table 40-1.

Rehabilitation professionals increasingly espouse a customer-driven, community-based employment philosophy. However, there has been no systematic attempt to assess integrated employment efforts against the

Table 40-1: Supported Employment Values
Commensurate wages and benefits—People with disabilities should earn wages and benefits equal to that of coworkers performing the same or similar jobs.
Community—People need to be connected to the formal and informal networks of a community for acceptance, growth, and development.
Everyone can work—Everyone, regardless of the level or the type of disability, has the capability and right to perform a job.
Focus on abilities—People with disabilities should be viewed in terms of their abilities, strengths, and interests rather than their disabilities.
Ongoing supports—Customers of supported employment services will receive assistance in assembling the supports necessary to achieve their ambitions as long as they need supports.
Real jobs—Employment occurs within the local labor market in regular community businesses.
Right to the opportunity—Regardless of their disability, everyone has the right to an opportunity to work in the employment of their choice.
Self-determination—Everyone has the right to make decisions for themselves.
Systems change—Traditional systems must be changed to ensure customer control, which is vital to the integrity of supported employment.

Source: Adapted from Brooke V, Inge K, Armstrong AJ, Wehman P. *Supported employment handbook: a consumer-driven approach for persons with significant disabilities.* Richmond, VA: Virginia Commonwealth University, Rehabilitation Research and Training Center, 1997.

customer-driven values base that drives the initiative. One way to obtain a "snapshot" of how professionals have operationalized supported employment philosophical values is to look at the known outcomes. National studies have documented the impressive rates of growth for integrated employment services since 1986. Nationally, supported employment has grown from only 9882 participants in fiscal year 1986 to approximately 140,000 participants in fiscal year 1995 (31). State mental retardation/developmental disabilities agencies reported that 32,471 persons received integrated employment services in 1993 (32). According to fiscal year 1995 Status 26 Closure Data reported by the Rehabilitation Services Administration, there were 8481 sheltered employment closures compared with 18,142 supported employment closures (33). Interest and demand for supported employment services has expanded.

However, implementation efforts are slowing and investment in supported employment seems to be dropping off (34). Some providers have experienced a significant drop in the numbers of referrals for supported employment services. Others have experienced an increase in the numbers of customers being turned down for authorization of funding for supported employment services. Providers are increasingly hearing "supported employment cost too much." It appears that costs are increasingly being used as a reason for denying services. Vocational rehabilitation providers can put cost controls on services, such as paying no more than a certain amount for a service, but they cannot say to an individual that the program is too expensive.

A closer look at the individuals who have had the opportunity to access supported employment services reveals that the majority have mild-to-moderate levels of disabilities. A study for fiscal year 1995 indicates that 87.5% of persons receiving supported employment have a primary disability classification of mental retardation or mental illness. Persons with a variety of other disabilities account for the remaining 12.5% (31). Thus, despite the espoused value and regulatory emphasis on supported employment being for persons who are considered to have the most severe disabilities, the data indicate that these individuals are not accessing supported employment services.

McGaughey, Kiernan, McNally, Gilmore, and Keith (35) recently conducted a survey to examine the service patterns across integrated and segregated employment sectors and to determine if the development of integrated employment has reduced the utilization of segregated services. They documented that integrated employment services have been added to the existing continuum, rather than replacing segregated services. Two-thirds of all participants entered facility-based programs in 1991. Also, 50% of the providers either plan to start facility-based services, maintain current capacity, or increase facility-based services, indicating that professionals have not operationalized service outcomes that are in line with the espoused customer-driven, community-based employment philosophy.

Supported employment implementation and the intended outcomes depend on the availability of quality staff to provide those services (36). A survey of personnel shortages and training needs in vocational rehabilitation (37) revealed that state directors of vocational rehabilitation have difficulty finding providers of supported employment services. Analysis of the data collected from providers indicates that a shortage of qualified supported employment personnel exists. Cohen and Pelavin (37) estimated that over 200 providers of supported employment services hired personnel who are educationally qualified but minimally skilled. Hanley-Maxwell et al (38) stated that academic training programs face difficulties in the preparation of supported employment personnel due to departmental lines, inflexible teaching load requirements, and threats of perceived duplication. Low salaries contribute to the difficulty with hiring qualified supported employment personnel and may influence the opinion that this position does not have professional status.

In addition, decisions related to supported employment services are frequently based on available funding streams, cost of services, the professional's best guess on what is appropriate for the customer, and her or his perception of the viability of a successful outcome (case closure) rather than on individual customer needs. In other situations, rehabilitation personnel simply do not believe that individuals with severe disabilities can work productively in the community labor force despite the customer's desire to do so. Continued mixed messages reflected in referral procedures, funding priorities, state regulations, and state licensure requirements only impede the expansion of integrated employment services.

Many individuals with disabilities have characterized their typical relationships with employment service providers as paternalistic or as "professionals know best" attitude (39). Complaints such as "he just doesn't appreciate the job that I got him," "supported employment costs too much," "she should be grateful for her slot in the workshop, several of my clients have no job," or "he has unrealistic expectations, he could never work in the banking industry" have commonly been made by professionals. When professionals view persons with disabilities as "dependent and in need of being sheltered from the community," employers, family members, and the general public accept this same attitude (40). The result is the continuation of negative attitudes and stereotypic images of persons with disabilities throughout the general public and a continued high rate of unemployment for individuals with disabilities.

It is clear that several professionals have a role to play in the implementation of supported employment. Vocational rehabilitation counselors, job coaches, special and vocational educators, case managers, rehabilitation facility staff, vocational evaluators, occupational therapists, physical therapists, and rehabilitation engineers all assume responsibilities. Despite the rapid growth and acceptance of supported employment, implementation has been delayed by a lack of belief in the employability of individuals with disabilities, an absence of innovative approaches to reducing service delivery costs, the unavailability of trained personnel, and the lack of wide-scale adoption of service intervention strategies by providers (37). Many of the individuals functioning in supported employment roles have not been trained to utilize the skills specific to their disciplines in a community environment, with customers having the most severe disabilities, or in a customer-driven environment. Service providers must adapt to service provision being in integrated settings and the changing expectations of their funding agencies, customers, family members, employers, and the community at large.

CONCLUSION

Employment holds the key to undoing the all-too-common segregated and dependency scenario among people with disabilities in our society. For most adults it is the employment arena where informal networks of supports are developed, goal setting is learned, decision making is fine tuned, and adult growth and self-esteem occur. Yet for years, people with disabilities have been denied equal access to the many benefits of employment because sheltered work was their primary rehabilitation option. However, sheltered work demonstrated low transition rates to competitive employment and lacked community integration. These factors have encouraged the national development and expansion of supported employment as an alternative service delivery model. In addition, growth in supported employment has also been encouraged by individuals with significant disabilities requiring a variety of new and innovative workplace supports to achieve their career goals.

Developing incentives and strong alliances with the business community are key to overcoming the obstacles that are reviewed in this chapter. The business community is looking for new sources of labor, and people with disabilities represent an untapped labor source. Programs and services designed to prepare or assist people with disabilities to access employment must keep pace with economic trends and our changing national workforce.

If large numbers of people with disabilities are going to access employment, disability benefit programs must begin to develop policies that are committed to this movement. Greater national attention must be paid to ensuring health care benefits, creating incentives, and expanding workplace supports for persons interested in transitioning to work or returning to work. To reach this goal disability benefit programs must stop segmenting employability programs and issues on the basis of gender, race, age, and most importantly, disability.

REFERENCES

1. Government Accounting Office. *People with disabilities: federal programs could work together more efficiently to promote employment.* Washington, DC: General Accounting Office, 1996.
2. *N.O.D./Harris Survey of Americans With Disabilities.* New York: Louis Harris & Associates, 1994.
3. Bowe FG. Statistics, politics, and employment of people with disabilities. *J Disability Policy Studies* 1993;4:83–91.
4. General Accounting Office. *SSA disability: program redesign necessary to encourage return to work.* Washington, DC: General Accounting Office, 1996.
5. Rupp K, Scott CG. *Determinants of duration on the disability rolls and program trends.* Presented at the SSA/ASPE conference on the Social Security Administration's disability programs, Washington, DC, July 20–21, 1995.
6. Bergman A. Keynote address at the Seminar on Managed Care Options for People with Developmental Disabilities, American Association on Mental Retardation, Chicago, IL, September 19, 1996.
7. Braddock D, Hemp R. Medicaid spending reductions and developmental disabilities. *J Disability Policy Studies* 1996;7:1–32.
8. National Alliance of Business. *Work America: To Prepare Workers, Employers and Educators on Skill Standards.* Vol. 12, Issue 11. Washington, DC: National Alliance of Business, 1996.
9. National Alliance of Business. *Work America: Workforce Economics, The Opportunity Economy.* Vol. 1, Issue 3. Washington, DC: National Alliance of Business, 1995.
10. Brodsky MM. A five year statewide follow-up of the graduates of school programs for trainable mentally retarded students in Oregon. Unpublished doctoral dissertation, University of Oregon, Eugene, OR, 1983.
11. Halpern A. A methodological review of follow-up and follow-along studies tracking school leavers from special education. *Career Dev Exceptional Individuals* 1990;13:13–27.
12. Haring K, Lovett D. A study of the social and vocational adjustment of young adults with mental retardation. *Educ Training Ment Retard* 1990;25:52–61.
13. Wagner M. *Trends in postschool outcomes of youth with disabilities: findings from the National Longitudinal Transition Study of Special Education Students.* Menlo Park, CA: SRI International, 1993.
14. Wehman P, Kregel J, Seyfarth J. Transition from school to work for individuals with severe handicaps: a follow-up study. *J Assoc Persons*

Severe Handicaps 1985;10: 132–136.

15. Virginia Commonwealth University, Rehabilitation Research and Training Center on Supported Employment. *Proceedings of the National Meeting for Supported Employment Systems Change, Leesburg, Virginia.* Richmond, VA: Virginia Commonwealth University, Rehabilitation Research and Training Center, 1996.

16. Sarkees MD, Veir C. Transition for special needs learners in rural areas: isolation creates unique problems. *Journal* 1988:23–26.

17. Inge KJ. A national survey of occupational therapists in the public schools: an assessment of current practice, attitudes, and training needs regarding the transition process for students with severe disabilities. Doctoral dissertation, Virginia Commonwealth University, Richmond, VA, 1995.

18. Lane C, Cassidy S. Technology and systematic educational reform. In: Portway PS, Lane C, eds. Guide to teleconferencing distance & learning. Livermore, CA: Applied Business teleCommunications, 1994:134–193.

19. President's Committee on Employment of People with Disabilities and Arkansas Research and Training Center in Vocational Rehabilitation. *Employment priorities for the '90s for people with disabilities.* Washington, DC: Government Printing Office, 1992. Publication No. 58:1611.

20. West M, Barcus M, Brooke V, Rayfield RG. An exploratory analysis of self-determination of persons with disabilities. *J Vocational Rehabil* 1995;5:357–364.

21. Architectural and Transportation Barriers Compliance Board. *Americans with Disabilities Act: accessibility guidelines for buildings and facilities, transportation facilities, and transportation vehicles.* Washington, DC: Architectural and Transportation Barriers Compliance Board, 1994.

22. National Council on Disability. *The Americans with Disabilities Act: ensuring equal access to the American dream.* Washington, DC: National Council on Disability, 1995.

23. National Council on Disability. *Voices of freedom: America speaks out on the ADA: a report to the president and Congress.* Washington, DC: National Council on Disability, 1995.

24. Weller B. Unmet needs for developmental disabilities services. *Popul Environ J Interdisciplinary Serv* 1994;15:279–302.

25. Kiernan WE, McGaughey MJ, Schalock RL. Employment environments and outcomes for adults with developmental disabilities. *Ment Retard* 1988;26: 279–288.

26. Rehabilitation Act Amendments of 1992, PL 102–569. (October 29, 1992). Title 29, U.S.C. 701 Section 101 (c).et seq: U.S. Statutes at Large, 100, 4344–4488.

27. Wehman P, Kregel J. At the crossroads: supported employment ten years later. In: Wehman P, John Kregel J, eds. *New directions in supported employment.* Richmond, VA: Virginia Commonwealth University, Rehabilitation Research and Training Center, 1994.

28. Wehman P, Moon MS, eds. *Vocational rehabilitation and supported employment.* Baltimore: Paul H. Brookes, 1988.

29. Wehman P. *Competitive employment; new horizons for severely disabled individuals.* Baltimore: Paul H. Brookes, 1981.

30. Mank DM, Rhodes LE, Bellamy GT. Four supported employment alternatives. In: Kiernan WE, Stark JA, eds. *Pathways to employment for adults with developmental disabilities.* Baltimore: Paul H. Brookes, 1986:139–153.

31. Wehman P, Revell G, Kregel J. Supported employment: a decade of rapid growth and impact. *Am Rehabil* 1998, in press.

32. Kiernan W, Gilmore D, Butterworth J. Integrated employment: evolution of national practices. In: Kiernan W, Schalock R, eds. *Integrated employment: current status and future directions.* Washington, DC: American Association of Mental Retardation, 1997:17–29.

33. Brooke V, Revell G, Green H. Long-term supports using an employee-directed approach to supported employment. *J Rehabil* 1998;64:38–45.

34. Virginia Commonwealth University, Rehabilitation Research and Training Center on Supported Employment. *National Marketing Initiative for Supported Employment: Executive Summary.* Richmond, VA: Virginia Commonwealth University, Rehabilitation and Training Center, 1994.

35. McGaughey MJ, Kiernan WE, McNally LC, et al. Beyond the workshop: national trends in integrated and segregated day and employment services. *J Assoc Persons Severe Handicaps* 1995;20:270–285.

36. Wehman P, Parent W. Critical issues in planning vocational services in the 1990's. In: Rowitz L, ed. *Mental retardation in the year 2000.* New York: Springer, 1992:251–267.

37. Cohen J, Pelavin D. *1992 Survey of personnel shortages and training needs in vocational rehabilitation.* Washington, DC: Pelavin and Associates, 1992.

38. Hanley-Maxwell C, Szymanski EM, Parent W, Shriner KF. Supported employment: revolution, passing fad, or a remake of an old song? *Rehabil Educ* 1990;4:233–246.

39. Brooke V, Barcus M, Inge K, eds. *Consumer advocacy and supported employment: a vision for the future.* Richmond, VA: Virginia Commonwealth University, Rehabilitation Research and Training Center, 1992.

40. Chumbley C, Collins M, Elliott J, et al. Supported employment service issues. In: Brooke V, Barcus M, Inge K, eds. *Consumer advocacy and supported employment: a vision for the future.* Richmond, VA: Virginia Commonwealth University, Rehabilitation Research and Training Center, 1992:14–32.

Chapter 41

Animal-Assisted Therapy

Denise H. Widmar
Katherine A. Feuillan

THE HUMAN-ANIMAL COMPANION BOND

Pets and animals have played an integral part in humans' lives throughout history. This is demonstrated in customs, legends, and religions. Domestication is a genetic process based on social interactions between humans and animals. It is viewed as evolutionary, occurring gradually and naturally where situations were predisposed for the domestication process, due to sharing of the environment. Humans used animals as hunting companions. They cared for wild herds as they protected their domestic stock against predators (1).

Records of dog domestication range back to the end of the Pleistocene period and Paleolithic age. Evidence of dog remains found in an Iraqi cave dates back approximately 12,000 years (1). Evidence of dogs in America dates back to at least 3500 BC, having come to this continent via the land bridges across the Bering Strait. They interbred with American wolves, moving throughout the hemisphere.

Cat domestication began when the dog had been fully domesticated for several thousand years. Egyptian artifacts date back to 2600 BC. A tomb dating back to 1900 BC contained skeletal remains of 17 cats with small milk pots. However, it was not until the first century AD that cats appeared in Europe (1). In the Middle Ages, horses and dogs provided companionship, travel, and hunting for their masters (2).

In the seventeenth century, domestic cats were brought to America for rodent control. In the nineteenth century, cats were viewed as a means of disease control and were viewed as clean animals because of their grooming skills (1).

In a survey of dog and cat owners, 99% of respondents considered their pets a family member, and 91% have photographs of their pets. Ninety-seven percent talk to their pets at least one time a day; 98% of dog owners and 91% of cat owners believe their pets are aware of their humans' needs (3).

Cats and dogs function in many ways for humans, from work to companionship. Humans have coexisted and interacted with animals throughout time. Today, 80% of American homes that have pets consider them very important family members (4).

A major distinction between animals for entertainment and animals for therapy is the human-animal companion bond. The bond is the interrelationship between humans and animals. The relationship that develops when the person has a strong attachment to the animals and that animal is responsive to the owner's needs is what defines the bond (5). True animal-assisted therapy (AAT) occurs when this bond is used therapeutically (2).

HISTORY OF ANIMAL-ASSISTED THERAPY

AAT is the use of animals to improve a person's physical, emotional, and social well-being. The healing power of animals dates back to 800 to 900 AD (4). Pets listen to our problems, give us devotion, make us feel secure, improve our self-esteem, and treat us, their owners, with unconditional love (6). Pets have become an important therapy tool in various settings and populations such as hospitals and nursing homes.

For several centuries, horseback riding has been used with the physically disabled (7). In seventeenth- and eighteenth-century England, pets were found to give the mentally retarded a "purposeful routine" (8). Written reports using animals in therapy date back to the 1790s in England at the York Retreat run by the Society of Friends. William Tuke, a Quaker merchant, believed animals could improve the outlook and personality of the emotionally disturbed. He perceived that patients could learn responsibility and control of their behaviors through working with farm animals roaming the grounds of the retreat (9).

Florence Nightingale believed that animals had an impact on the health of her patients. She believed that a small pet was a great companion for the sick. In 1860, she carried a pet owl in her pocket while doing rounds (10). In 1867, in Bielfeld, West Germany, the Bethal facility used animals in the treatment of epileptics. During the Crimean War and World War II, pet therapy was used for convalescing soldiers. The Army Air Force Convalescent Center in Pawling, New York, was the subject of one of the first documented reports on the use of animals in the United States. Dogs, horses, and farm animals were used in diversional treatment of airmen undergoing rehabilitation. Unfortunately, when the war ended, so did the collection of data (6,8).

The first acknowledgment of the human-animal bond is attributed to Boris Levinson, who in 1969, published "Pet Oriented Child Psychotherapy." Levinson cited the psychological and physiologic benefits of the human-animal bond, generating the acceptance in the academic and medical world of the use of animals in psychiatric treatment. He used his dog, Jingles, in psychotherapy sessions with children. He conceptualized it was easier to communicate with a "safe" animal before reaching out to a person. He believed pets created an environment that strengthened the family and facilitated normal childhood development (2,4).

In the 1970s, serious research into the advantages of animal companionship revealed a wide range of benefits to humans. Further investigation throughout the 1980s and 1990s regarding therapy animals demonstrated psychological and physiologic benefits for diverse conditions, including reduced blood pressure, increased survival rate of coronary care patients, and reduced cholesterol levels. Assist animals have been used in a variety of interventions. These include relaxation techniques, enhancing self-concept, expressing emotions, reaching withdrawn and alienated people, increasing rate of recovery, and boosting morale.

APPROACHES

The Delta Society established the Definitions Development Task Force of the Standards Committee in 1991 to provide a clear understanding of the terms used in programs: animal-assisted activities (AAAs), animal-assisted therapy (AAT), and human-animal support services (HASSs) (including pet fostering, pet loss counselors, veterinarians, trained volunteers, animal behaviorists, animal trainers, grief counselors, K-9 units, and self-help coordinators) (11). Many professionals who understand the medical model incorporate AAT and AAAs as an intervention. Each treatment team member is guided by the specific discipline delivery model. For example, the occupational therapist could have the patient stroke a dog to achieve the treatment goal of increasing active range of motion, utilizing assessments and evaluation processes. Thus, the entire process is one using an interdisciplinary approach (12).

AAT, using animals as a means of intervention for human problems, is viewed as therapeutic (2). It is goal directed, based on an assessment, individualized measurable goals, treatment, and follow-up evaluation. The Task Force defined AAT as a goal-directed intervention in which an animal meeting specific criteria is an integral part of the treatment process. AAT is delivered and directed by a health/human service provider working within the scope of the profession. AAT is designed to promote improvement in human physical, social, emotional, and cognitive functioning. It is provided in a variety of settings, may be administered in group or in individual settings, and is then documented and evaluated. AAT specialists demonstrate expertise in incorporating animals as a treatment modality and are knowledgeable about animals (11). Options utilized in AAT are listed in Table 41-1 (13). Goals are listed in Table 41-2 (2,13,14).

AAAs are defined by the Delta Society Task Force of the Standards Committee as "providing opportunities for motivational, educational, and/or recreational benefits to enhance quality of life. AAAs are delivered in a variety of environments by a trained professional, paraprofessional, or volunteer in association with animals that meet specific criteria . . . who possesses specialized knowledge of animals and the populations with which they interact" (11).

Table 41-1: Animal-Assisted Therapy Treatment Options
• Interactive—one-to-one basis; dogs used the most in this method; may follow commands. • Group—animals used in a group setting; may follow commands; dogs and other animals also used. • Passive—focus on groups of animals, such as small birds or fish, may or may not be handled by patients.

Source: *Handbook for animal-assisted activities and animal-assisted therapy.* Delta Society, 1992.

Table 41-2: Animal-Assisted Therapy Goals		
Endurance	Range of motion	Use of weaker side (upper extremity, lower extremity)
Visual tracking	Attention to neglected side	Cognitive tasks—memory
Following directions and attention	Giving command (verbal or gestures) to dogs	Balance
Ambulation	Wheelchair mobility	Coma stimulation

Sources: References 2, 13, 14.

Together, the AAA specialist and animal interact with people in schools, health care facilities, and other residential and treatment locations.

Persons leading AAA programs may have specialized training and can include paraprofessionals, animal shelter workers, technicians, and activity directors. AAA programs promote socialization, motivation, education, and recreation to enhance the quality of life (11). AAAs do not require measurable goals, charting, or individual assessment. Pets greet patients, promote socialization, and stimulate patients to reminisce about their own pets (4).

MODELS

Service Animals

Service animals are trained to assist people with various disabilities, including but not limited to visual or hearing deficits, spinal cord injury, acquired immunodeficiency syndrome (AIDS), and chronic pain, and those recovering from trauma or depression. Some of the tasks for which animals can be trained include guiding people with visual impairments, discriminating sounds for people with hearing impairments, assisting people with mobility and item retrieval, sensing and alerting owners to oncoming seizures, and providing general companionship and emotional support (15).

Dogs trained through Seeing Eye (Morristover, ND), an organization dedicated to training service dogs, have been used to assist the visually challenged since 1929. Only two people were enrolled in the first Seeing Eye dog training class. Today, Seeing Eye has increased their training to help up to 300 persons with visual impairments with independence and mobility skills each year (16). Guide dogs are trained to lead their blind masters in both rural and urban settings. They are taught to tolerate loud noises, as well as negotiate elevators, escalators, steps, revolving doors, and turnstiles (15).

Hearing or signal dogs are trained to alert persons with hearing impairments to important sounds or noises such as doorbells, sirens, or a baby's cry. These dogs can also help create a feeling of safety for the owner. Training with a hearing dog requires approximately 4 to 6 months (17). After the dogs are trained, additional training must occur simultaneously between the owner and dog.

According to the Delta Society, "consideration of a person as a (service animal) candidate should include not only the diagnosis of a chronic disability but also the person's ability to function on a daily basis" (15). Typical questions regarding the patient's ability to benefit from the use of a service animal might include the following (15):

- How difficult are the activities of daily living?
- Would the person have better stamina if the dog performs tasks for him or her?
- Would the service dog help the person exercise more or be more physically mobile?
- Would the dog provide the needed assistance to help the person stay employed?

Although service animals are predominantly dogs, other species have been used. An organization called Helping Hands trains Capuchin monkeys as "hands" for persons with tetraplegia. This organization began in 1979 to help many high-level tetraplegics regain a sense of independence, a more positive outlook, a life of companionship, and higher self-esteem. The monkeys are trained to respond to voice commands. Tasks they might perform on behalf of the patients include turning lights on and off; pushing buttons on the television, VCR, or microwave; combing the patient's hair; or even scratching an itch for the patient (18).

Programs

Programs may be carried out on an individual or group basis. Individual sessions are beneficial to patients with anxiety, limited pain tolerance, and hypertension. Group sessions are beneficial to patients who have common needs, promoting socialization and reality orientation (19).

Three primary types of methods are used in an AAA/AAT program: visitation, residential, and personal pet visitation. Visitation programs are conducted by volunteers who bring their own pets to facilities, such as Pet Partners of the Delta Society. Residential animals are pets who reside in the facility and are available on a regular basis for therapy or visitation. Personal pet visitation occurs when pets visit their "ill owners" in a health institution (10).

In visiting programs, animals are brought in, based on the facility's needs. The Delta Society, and regional organizations such as Caring Critters (Houston, TX), prepares volunteers and screens pets for visitation programs. Workshops are conducted by Delta Society trainers or other certified instructors to educate volunteers on the application of AAT and patient populations to promote safe programs, policies (infection control, hygiene, expectations prior to visiting, ability to control the animal, and suitability), and risk management (20,21). The temperament of the animals is tested. Trainers evaluate their reactions to strangers, loud noises, physical contact (ear, and fur tug), and objects such as walkers, intravenous poles, and wheelchairs. The testing is designed to evaluate the animal and handler as a team.

In Caring Critters, seasoned volunteers and "team leaders," under the guidance of a person in charge of temperament testing, evaluate the owner-animal team (20). The Pet Partners program registration process requires the owner to attend a workshop or home study course. The animal must pass a health examination and skills and aptitude evaluation (22).

A typical visit may consist of the following steps (20,21):

1. Patients who are appropriate to visit are identified by facility staff or a team leader of the AAT organization.
2. Patients or families give consent for visitation.
3. Volunteers are given data necessary for a successful visit.
4. The volunteer and the pet visit with patients. Visits may include petting, watching pet tricks, socializing, and reminiscing about one's own pets.
5. Visits range from a few minutes to approximately 15 minutes. The length of time depends on the stamina of the patient, pet and owner team, and facility/AAT organization policies. The owner needs to be aware of symptoms of stress in the animal.
6. After the visit, information is shared with facility staff and AAT organization team leaders. "Team leaders" or liaisons document observations, interactions, interventions, problems, and suggestions. Emergency situations and concerns need to be reported immediately.

The feedback from pet visitation programs usually is overwhelmingly positive. Patients who received visits from dogs interacted with them enthusiastically and reported that it was the most beneficial event occurring during their hospitalization (23). Resident pets, such as a dog, cat, fish, rabbit, hamster, or bird, have become common in nursing homes, rehabilitation centers, and hospitals. They help to decrease the unfamiliar and institutional atmosphere of the facility. They are readily available and can be utilized in therapy sessions or visitations. Caretaking responsibilities can be managed by high-level patients supervised by staff. AAT helps fill the loss of the caretaker role by providing the patient with the opportunity to nurture a living creature, thus giving a sense of purpose to what often seems like an empty existence (24).

The ultimate responsibility for care falls to the staff. A designated staff member needs to ensure the pet is cared for, with backup assistance available. Policies, veterinarian visits, food, financial responsibilities, and monitoring visits and interactions must be overseen (14).

Personal pet visitation programs promote bonds between humans and animals. Pets are viewed as family members and can be therapeutic for the patients, human family members, and also the pets. The pet needs to be clean and in good health. Written policies for this specialized program and approval must be obtained from the facility.

A study conducted at the Sepulveda VA hospital intermediate-care unit examined the therapeutic role of a cat mascot. The cat could sit on a patient's lap, allowing the patient to hug, pet, and talk to it. Some patients picked up the cat and carried it; others watched and talked to it from a distance. Conversations ranged from expressions of ownership or possessiveness to observations about the cat's activities. Overall, a significant increase in socialization was reported in patients who were exposed to animal mascots. The patients were more affectionate with the cat, creating a more pleasant environment. Patients' reality orientation was fostered by their realizations of the cat's needs for care and feeding (25).

Patients admitted to a cardiac care unit and cardiac observation unit at UCLA Medical Center were allowed 120 pet visits over a 6-month period. Participants completed a survey comprising five questions with eight positive and eight negative adjectives as possible responses. One hundred percent replied that the visits made them happier, calmer, and less lonely and recommended the service to others. One-half of the patients expressed a preference for hospitals that allow animal visits and recommended that the frequency of such visits be increased (26).

Depending on policies and procedures, animal visits may take place in a variety of locations, from the hospital grounds to the intensive care unit. Pets brought into the hospital need to be in a carrier or on a leash. Communication is essential among families and the staff for a successful visit. The greater attachment a person had to a pet signified the better one's mental and physical health (27).

Hippotherapy

The term *hippotherapy* derives from the Greek "hippos," meaning horse. Thus, hippotherapy literally means treatment with the help of a horse. Specially trained physical therapists and occupational therapists use this medical treatment for patients with movement dysfunction (28).

During hippotherapy, the horse influences the patient rather than the patient influencing the horse. The patient is positioned on and actively responds to the movement of the therapy horse. The therapist directs the movement of the horse, analyzes the patient's responses, and adjusts the treatment accordingly. The goals of hippotherapy are to improve the patient's posture, balance, mobility, and function (28).

Therapeutic riding, in the literal sense, has existed since 1951. Madame Liz Hartel of Denmark, who was diagnosed with poliomyelitis, brought recognition to the field by winning the silver medal for Grand Prix Dressage at the 1952 Helsinki Olympic Games after she had rehabilitated herself through riding. The Pony Riding for the Disabled Trust was formed in England in 1958, and the Community Association of Riding for the Disabled was formed in North America in 1960. Subsequently, the Cheff Center for the Handicapped was founded in Michigan in the late 1960s, and the North American Riding for the Handicapped Association (NARHA) was organized in 1970 (29).

Therapeutic riding consists of three approaches—medicine, sport, and education. While each area has its own goals and methods, the areas overlap, complement, and support each other.

The sport approach consists of adapting equine activities so people with physical, mental, and psychological impairments can participate in sport activities such as riding, vaulting, and driving. The education approach involves teaching the skills needed for sport riding. It is also a means to achieve educational and therapeutic goals. The medicine approach uses the horse to achieve physical, psychological, cognitive, and behavioral goals. This approach involves a team comprising medical professionals, the therapeutic riding instructor, and the rider (30).

There has been significant progress in research on therapeutic riding since 1986. Most of the research has been on the therapeutic or rehabilitative benefits, especially as applied to those with physical impairments. The research conducted since 1986 has concentrated primarily in the areas of balance, sensory-motor programming, strength, coordination, and posture (31).

Therapeutic riding consists of using a specially trained horse, a therapeutic riding instructor, and volunteers who lead the horse, walk alongside, and ride behind if necessary. Instructors should be trained through the NARHA or the Cheff Center to ensure the quality of the program. The value of therapeutic riding is contingent on the ability of the horse to interact well with the patient. The benefits of hippotherapy are listed in Table 41-3 (28,32).

Table 41-3: Benefits of Hippotherapy

Physical benefits (27)
- The horse's movement provides the sensory input of a precise, repetitive pattern of movement very similar to the movement of a person's pelvis during normal human gait—the three-dimensional movement of the horse's back simulates human gait.
- Mobilization of pelvis, lumbar region of spine, and hip joints
- Normalization of muscle tone
- Development of head and trunk postural control
- Improvement of endurance, symmetry, and body awareness

Cognitive, emotional, and social benefits (31)
- Improved self-esteem
- Improved confidence
- Improved group and didactic interaction
- Improved concentration and attention span

THERAPEUTIC BENEFITS

The benefits of AAT have been observed and studied for many years. Animals can serve as the ears, eyes, or arms for persons with disabilities (33). They can assist a patient's rehabilitative potential in enhancing or developing functional skills, often more quickly and less painfully than with traditional therapies. Overall, the benefits of AAT fall into four categories: social, physical, emotional, and cognitive.

Social Benefits

Research indicates that people benefit from AAT socially by increasing interaction with others and psychologically by promoting a sense of well-being. Animals seem to increase the initiation of socialization by facilitating patients to ask questions about the animals. Animals can also improve social skills by getting people to talk softly and slowly to the animals. On satisfaction surveys, patients report feelings of increased happiness, calmness, more feelings of love, and less loneliness while interacting with animals (26). Research studies demonstrated that AAT provides patients with companionship, affection, love, nurturance, and a sense of being needed (34). Corson noted that at Ohio State University patients who did not respond well to more traditional approaches demonstrated "improvement in terms of responsiveness, communication, apparent increased self-respect, and independence." The pet becomes a focus of attention—an accepting, receptive, willing listener (35).

Socially, dogs assist with a person's social interaction, including making eye contact and taking turns during an activity. It can be easier to promote initiation and interaction in a setting where people have come together because of an affinity for dogs (36). An animal is something that can be talked to as well as talked about. Animals are a safe, nonthreatening, neutral topic for discussion and one to which nearly everyone can relate. Animals are a natural topic for reminiscence, which is beneficial in facilities working with the elderly or patients who are confused. By having an animal present, people with language deficits feel more at ease, so they may talk more. A person's affect is also usually much brighter when an animal is present. Service dogs also have socializing benefits (37).

People with mobility challenges who rely on wheelchairs and utilize service dogs were studied before and after obtaining their dogs. The specific hypothesis tested was that the acquisition of a service dog would increase the number of friendly approaches by persons with whom the dog was unfamiliar. Subjects reported a significantly higher number of social greetings from adults and children on typical shopping trips with the dog, as compared to those received on trips before the subject had the dog or recent trips when the dog was not present. Subjects with service dogs reported more approaches than a control group without dogs. Subjects also increased their evening outings after obtaining dogs (37).

Physical Benefits

The relationships between humans and their companion animals have psychological and physiologic benefits. Simply stroking a cat or dog reduces blood pressure and heart rate, while survival after a heart attack is greater for those who have a pet. Pet owners are better able to overcome minor ailments. Dogs can sometimes predict when their owners are about to suffer seizures. Animals help patients to relax and sleep. They also have provided comfort at their owners' death beds (38).

Animals provide many physical benefits, including tactile, visual, auditory, and olfactory stimulation. This is especially useful for therapists working with patients with decreased levels of arousal, patients in a coma, or those emerging from a coma. "Touch is a vital necessity for human beings," says Aaron Katcher. "There's something very comforting [in using animals in therapy], especially to touch deprived people—the aged, people with AIDS, or the chronically sick" (39). A visual benefit is increased tracking toward a side of neglect for a brain-injured patient. Animals that can talk—bark, meow, or chirp—may elicit a verbal response. Animals also stimulate the sense of smell through their shampoo or their natural odor.

Additional physical benefits include increased range of motion, balance, strength, and fine- and gross-motor skills. A person with a spinal cord injury can work on upper-body control and balance to help reduce atrophy. The use of a therapy dog also can help someone walk again by increasing coordination and balance. Petting an animal can increase strength and movement on the weakened side of a stroke survivor (36). In brushing a dog, a patient can work on eye-hand coordination and fine-motor skills. Sitting balance, trunk rotation, and standing balance can be improved with the use of animals.

Emotional Benefits

Pets can provide companionship, something to care for, pleasurable activity, something pleasurable to watch, a source of constancy and security, and opportunities for play, laughter, and comfort. Pets clearly can help overcome loneliness (24). Therapy Dogs, Inc. suggests that dogs make the hospital less institutional and less frightening for young patients and visitors. The animals frequently take the patient's mind off pain to allow more productive therapy. Animals provide unconditional positive acceptance and can help increase self-esteem in depressed individuals (40). Animals make it easier for patients to express emotions. Animals may be a link to reality and may also provide an opening to discussions of fear and trust (41).

Children with severe emotional disturbances undergoing animal-oriented therapy improve their ability to control their impulses and understand others. Those undergoing similar therapies without animals saw no such improvement (42).

Animals also motivate people to participate in therapies. A study on the effects of companion animals on lonely people found that AAT can be an important source of stimulation and physical contact with the outside world for residents whose limitations prevent them from participating well or at all in other programs (43).

Unexpected benefits to staff morale have also been noted. "Watching a depressed patient's smiling face while having his chin licked by a black and tan mutt is enough to raise any caregiver's spirits" (19). One would be hard pressed to conduct an AAT session without physicians, therapists, and family members stopping by for "therapy."

Cognitive Benefits

Animals provide consistent reactions to patients. Particular breeds are consistent in appearance. Animals tend to make people more aware of their environment by drawing their gaze and engaging the mind. As patients anticipate AAT sessions, they become more oriented to day and time (19). Eye tracking and differences in heart rate while an animal is present can indicate progress for a patient emerging from a coma (41). Animals can also benefit people who have attention deficits, lengthening their attention spans and focusing their attention (19). Cognitive abilities can be improved by learning new skills or relearning previous ones. Animals may be used to assist patients in following commands, sequencing steps, and problem solving.

Another major cognitive area is memory. Patients may be asked to recall an animal's name or recall commands to use with an animal. For reality orientation, a patient may be asked to identify parts of the animal such as the ears or tail, or to identify the type of animal or color. Animals offer continuity in their relationships and focus patients' attention on the present.

RESEARCH

The majority of research in AAT has addressed outcomes with cardiac conditions. Friedman found that pet owners who had been hospitalized with coronary artery disease had significantly higher rates of survival after 1 year than did non-pet owners (44). Fifty-eight percent of survivors had one or more pets. Twenty-three percent of non-pet owners and 6% of pet owners died within 1 year of hospitalization (45).

Studies since 1980 have investigated further the variables of blood pressure, skin temperature, and stress level using animal interventions. In a study of stress management (46), heart rates of children during resting and reading aloud were monitored both with and without the presence of a friendly dog. The situations were randomly tested. The researcher controlled the variable that the children did not speak to or touch the dog. Blood pressures were consistently higher when the children were reading aloud in comparison to the resting period. When the dog was present at the beginning of the random situations, blood pressures were significantly lower, even during the stressful circumstances of reading aloud (7,46). No differences were noted in the children's responses to various dogs used. The results demonstrated that the presence of an unfamiliar dog in a mildly stressful situation leads to decreased blood pressure (46). Other studies reported similar results (5,9,47).

Katcher and others compared normotensive and hypertensive individuals observing fish swimming in an aquarium versus subjects looking at a poster or an identical empty aquarium. The individuals who looked at the fish had significantly lower blood pressure for a longer period than did those looking at an empty tank or poster (7). They also observed 42 dental patients watching fish in an aquarium prior to dental surgery. Positive results included increased patient compliance, decreased pain perceptions, and an increased hypnotic effect. Since watching fish is an effective means of relaxation, the activity can also be used to decrease anxiety in heart disease patients (7).

Seven hundred eighty-four pet owners and 4857 non-pet owners participated in a 3-year study investigating risk factors for cardiovascular disease. Participants completed a risk factor questionnaire addressing smoking habits, alcohol intake, exercise, dietary habits, diabetic history, and family history.

Blood pressure was measured and a blood sample obtained. After the cardiac assessment, participants were asked if they owned a pet. The results indicated that the pet owners had significantly lower systolic blood pressure and plasma triglyceride levels. Male pet owners between ages 30 and 60 and women over 40 years old had significantly lower systolic blood pressure, lower plasma triglyceride levels, and lower plasma cholesterol levels (48,49). Other lifestyle risk factors such as exercise, body mass, and eating habits did not influence the results (50). An ancillary study indicated that pet ownership lowers anxiety and increases the 1-year survival rate after a myocardial infarction (51).

Schuelke et al (45) conducted a study to determine if petting a companion dog with whom an attachment bond existed could promote a cue for relaxation in hypertensive patients. Blood pressure, heart rate, and peripheral skin temperature were determined at 1-minute intervals with a 3-minute rest period. No differences in systolic and diastolic blood pressures were observed between subjects petting a companion dog or a control dog. However, individuals exhibited an increased peripheral skin temperature while petting a companion dog, demonstrating that finger temperature is a more sensitive parameter to determine relaxation than is blood pressure. This study suggests that petting a companion dog is an excellent way to relax and train the individual to exert control over the autonomic nervous system, cuing the body to rest (45).

The 1992 study by Anderson et al (4) showed that pet owners had a reduced risk of cardiovascular disease, versus non-pet owners. Patronek and Gleckman (51) found that pet ownership increases the survival rate due to the influence of psychosocial factors that decrease the risk of coronary artery disease.

The effects of a residential poodle on terminally ill patients and nursing staff were researched in a hospice setting (52). A pretest, posttest, follow-up interviews, observations, and videotaping involved 14 patients and 15 staff. Attitudes, behaviors, and interaction changes were studied. The resident dog facilitated staff-patient interactions, eased patient-visitor relations, and improved staff-patient morale. Patients identified as loners did not bond with the dog, nor did they negatively affect the study's results. The most frequently observed behavior consisted of a relaxing or comforting effect on the patients and staff (52).

Serpell indicated that dog owners had fewer minor health problems and took recreational walks of increased number and length (51).

A final study of 938 Medicare patients in southern California reported that non-pet owners had 16% more doctor appointments per year than did pet owners and 20% more than dog owners (39).

Many studies have been conducted on the use or presence of an animal with chronically ill people. Raveis examined the effects of cat and dog ownership on the emotional well-being of cancer patients and their family members. The findings suggest that a companion animal in the household may lead to better psychological adjustment for the caregiver. Previous observations noted the integral role that pets play in the adjustment of children to illness or loss of a parent (24).

Albert (53) wrote about visiting people who have AIDS. These patients may exhibit opportunistic infections, psychiatric disorders, or nervous system disorders. Animals who act as companions for people with AIDS or human immunodeficiency virus (HIV) infection "reduce feelings of isolation and loneliness by their very presence, both physical and emotional. An animal by its very constancy remains present even if human relationships are lost due to fear" (34). The animals provide patients with affection, support, nurturance, and acceptance. Animals also help reduce stress; provide varying levels of communication, continuity, and support; and enable patients to feel valued and needed.

Carmack (34) noted the enhanced relationship between decreased stress levels and the immune system.

Table 41-4: Research Studies Supporting Benefits of Animal-Assisted Therapy (AAT)		
Author	**Sample**	**Results**
Social		
Brickel (1979)	19 nursing staff of a geriatric hospital surveyed	Responsiveness, pleasure, and reality therapy increased as a result of the presence of resident cats.
Friedman et al (1983)	36 hospitalized cardiovascular patients interviewed who owned dogs	Eighty percent of this population received information about their pets, opening up lines of communication with other people.
Madder (1989)	10 physically challenged school-aged children in wheelchairs with service dogs and without dogs	Children in wheelchairs with service dogs received significantly more smiles and conversation than did children without dogs.
Psychological		
Muggford (1975)	30 elderly home residents given birds to care for and compared with a control group of subjects without birds	Improvement of self-concept and attitude toward others was shown.
Sebkova (1977)	20 people tested in a laboratory setting and a home environment with or without a dog present	An overall decrease in anxiety was measured in both settings, with more attention given to the dog in the laboratory setting.
Fila (1991)	1 case study of a hospitalized patient who had become depressed, withdrawn, and expressed hopelessness	AAT visits from a guinea pig promoted laughter, talking, and feelings of relaxation.
Physiologic		
Anderson et al (1992)	5741 subjects seen at a free clinic for cardiovascular screening	Pet owners showed significantly lower systolic blood pressure and triglyceride levels than did non-pet owners.
Friedman et al (1980)	92 hospitalized patients with an admitting diagnosis of either myocardial infarction or angina pectoris	Pet ownership correlated with survival, regardless of type of pet.
Riddick (1985)	22 elderly apartment residents	The presence and care of fish in an aquarium correlated with positive changes in blood pressure and overall leisure activity.

Source: Cole KM, Gawlinski A. Animal-assisted therapy in the intensive care unit. *Nurs Clin North Am* 1995;30:529–537.

No special precautions are needed when visiting patients; the only real concern is to protect their delicate immune-suppressed systems. Moreover, visitors pose a greater risk of passing on infection to the patient than do animals. For 3½ years, the National Institutes of Health has documented health screening and visits to offer proof to other facilities concerned about zoonoses that healthy animals do not transmit diseases to patients (54).

Scientific research has begun to validate the role of service dogs for people with disabilities. In 1995, Karen Allen found that people with disabilities who had service dogs scored higher for psychological well-being, self-esteem, and community integration, and required 78% fewer personal assistant hours. This represents significant potential savings in health care costs.

A review of the literature indicates that further research studies should include larger population groups. More data are needed on grief and loss of companion animals, human-animal contact and diseases, and health benefits to animals involved in interactions, to give further evidence of animals' impact on humans (51).

Table 41-4 provides further examples and results of research (26).

ESTABLISHMENT OF A PROGRAM

Policies

Liability

When one is first starting an AAT program, it is important to review all existing liability policies for possible exclusions or restrictions that may apply in the facility (14). The review might be done by the legal counsel for the facility. When completed, each patient visit for AAT should be documented and reviewed regularly to ensure compliance with the established policies.

Volunteers must be informed of the ethics of confidentiality and instructed in protecting the dignity, privacy, and anonymity of the patients. Some facilities require the volunteer to sign an affidavit of confidentiality before engaging in any volunteer activities. Volunteers should be instructed not to discuss a patient in front of other patients or families and not to use the patient's name when describing a visit. Volunteers should always work under the supervision of a staff member or therapist to reduce the chances of negligence. Volunteers should never relate to clients in a "clinical" manner unless specifically instructed to do so by a physician, nurse, or therapist. Volunteers need to understand that the most innocent act—giving a drink of water or moving a limb, for example—could be detrimental to the patient's health or well-being. Any mishaps should be reported and documented immediately. Each facility should ensure the establishment of written guidelines for managing such incidents and responding immediately to animal and volunteer problems to preserve high morale among the volunteer team members.

Regulations will vary between facilities depending on the type of animal therapy program used. Regulations may include the type of identification the volunteer or animal wears during the visits, the duration and length of each visit, and infection control policies. Place of visitation and documentation of the program can also be written into the regulations. Volunteer guidelines could include parking information, where to enter the building, where animals may relieve themselves, and where volunteers should put scooped stools. If a facility utilizes a therapy group, the group might provide insurance coverage for certified volunteers.

Infection Control

Zoonoses are diseases or infections that are transmitted from animals to humans. Animals are the main reservoirs of these diseases. According to the latest veterinary medical resources, approximately 160 diseases can be transmitted from animals to humans. Fortunately, most of these diseases are extremely rare, and the chances of transmission from a healthy animal are minimal (55).

Western equine encephalitis and eastern equine encephalitis are two diseases that can be transmitted by horses to people. General precautions include insect control and up-to-date vaccination of horses. Awareness, education, precautions, and proper health care programs (e.g., good hand-washing practices) are the best preventive mechanisms.

The other leading health hazards to patients in therapy programs are allergies to animals and bites from animals. Allergies should be noted on the patient's chart, and volunteers must be informed about patients with allergies. Contact with animals must be avoided for these patients. If a volunteer is accompanied by an animal, even more than once a week, the animal should be bathed and groomed before each visit. Animals cannot be in rooms where patients are eating or where food preparation is taking place.

Animal bites can be minimized by effective temperament testing of each animal. Although animal behavior can be unpredictable, the chances of a good-tempered, calm animal biting a patient are generally minimal. However, in the unlikely event of an animal bite, the incident should be reported and documented immediately.

Though AAT programs have had relatively few reported problems with infections, it is important that the facility maintain detailed infection control policies. All animals used in a therapy program must have current veterinary forms on file with the facility. These forms must be updated annually for vaccinations and every 6 months for results of stool samples. In addition, facility policies must include guidelines for preventive health care for visiting animals. Before beginning a program, an animal should be observed for 14 days if it has not previously been owned by the volunteer (14). Patients at high risk for infection include pregnant women who can be at risk for toxoplasmosis if they are changing the litter for a cat, persons with immunosuppressed diseases (i.e., HIV infection), and children with poor hygiene habits (20). Common transmittable diseases include ringworm, toxoplasmosis, and salmonellosis. Most zoonoses can be prevented by good hygiene and healthy maintenance of the animal.

Temperament Testing

Animal temperament testing is of utmost importance in protecting the health and well-being of the patients. Temperament testing is an observation of an animal's reactions to unusual or stressful conditions in a controlled environment. This testing simulates conditions that can and do arise during AAT visits. Some programs require that dogs be trained in basic obedience. Other programs do not require formal training but stress that the animal must be easily controlled by the handler.

Unacceptable behavior consists of, but is not limited to, scratching, lifting leg, growling, snapping at or biting people or other animals, excessive or uncontrollable barking, and nervous or aggressive behavior states (20). Retesting of dogs may be required every 2 years and facility visits at least four times per year to retain certification (14). Team leaders or staff members may also request that an animal be retested at any time if a change in behavior is noted.

The temperament test should be conducted by a qualified animal handler or trainer through an established program. Any handler who displays unsportsmanlike conduct or who is seen to kick, strike, or otherwise roughly mishandle a dog at any time during a test shall be dismissed from the test (56). The basic components of the temperament test are listed in Table 41-5.

Generally, animals that fail temperament tests can be

Table 41-5: Basic Components of Animal Temperament Testing
• Obedience demonstration (if required) • The animal's reaction to a stranger approaching the owner • Reaction of the animal to a stranger approaching to talk to and pet the animal • The animal's reaction to unfamiliar objects it might encounter such as wheelchairs, walkers, etc • Reaction of the animal to physical contact and mild painful stimuli such as pulling an ear or touching paws, tail, etc • The animal's reaction to crowds • The animal's reaction to a different handler than the owner • Continual evaluation of the animal's ability to socialize with other animals in the facility

Sources: References 20, 56.

Table 41-6: Terms and Definitions from the Delta Society's Task Force Meeting of the Standards Documentation Committee
Assessment—a process to determine the needs of the client or population receiving services Objectives—a method to obtain goals, such as the patient will comb the dog three strokes with the left hand Documentation—a process for recording interactions and significant events, including participants, responses, and recommendations for the future Evaluation—a method to determine whether progress has been made toward previously stated goals

Source: Task Fosce of the Standards Committee, Definition Development Task Force, Delta Society, Tucson, AZ, 1991, February 1–3.

retested if the reasons for not passing have been remediated. Some programs require an interval of 2 months between tests, but other programs require up to 6 months.

Quality Management

Documentation is a vital part of AAT programs. It substantiates the work, justifies the program and reimbursement, protects liability, sets standards, provides animal protection protocols, and measures patients' progress. For AAA visitation programs, documentation is less extensive than for AAT programs. The date and time of the visit, the patient's, animal's, and volunteer's names, and basic interactions are recorded. Both functional and cognitive changes may be gradual, but records help indicate progress. Examples of a resident evaluation are shown in Appendix I.

Written protocols and policies give direction to the type of documentation required. AAT sessions are recorded so documents are available for physicians and other team members to review each patient's progress (57). Table 41-6 provides definitions of relevant terms.

The assessment of cognitive, physical, psychosocial, and behavioral strengths and deficits identifies the patient's diagnosis and the reason for referral to the AAT program, and assists in treatment planning. Assessment includes the number and type of pets owned, duration as a pet owner (since childhood or length of time with a particular pet), interactions and skills with the animal (dog shows, how pet was viewed in the patient's or family's life), and current animal interests (2,14).

Documentation of the interventions after the AAT session can be achieved by using a variety of techniques such as the Subjective/Objective/Assessment/Plan (SOAP) method progress note. Some facilities use a goal-directed format developed specifically for AAT. (See Appendix II for examples of AAT progress notes.) An evaluation is conducted to compare results and skill building, to identify progress toward goals, and to establish new short-term goals.

To provide a successful program, careful plans and protocols need to be established so that acceptance of AAT grows as a modality. A quality program must then address risk management and safety concerns. To keep abreast of current trends and practices, the handlers should belong to a reputable organization such as the Delta Society.

Pet Partners of the Delta Society has a national registration system and provides training and evaluation for volunteers and pets. To become registered, the volunteers complete a training program. The pet must pass a health and aptitude screening test. Volunteers receive training through certified instructors at many sites—humane and veterinary organizations, clubs, and health care facilities. In population centers without the benefit of certified instructors and workshops, the Delta Society has developed a Pet Partners home study course containing articles and a videotape covering information to prepare the volunteer.

The dog, cat, bird, and any animal that might be used for AAT must pass the health, skills, and temperament tests given by a veterinarian and certified Pet Partners animal evaluator. The Delta Society requires registration of the handler/animal team every 2 years (22).

The screening guarantees that the animals used are clean, free from disease, and of the right temperament. These documents are on file for use in case of any incident (bite, scratch). Caring Critters of Houston, Texas, has a similar program established to educate and train handler/animal teams.

A trained handler/animal team from an approved program ensures protection from financial liability. Organizations such as the Delta Society and Caring Critters

Table 41-7: Risks of Animal-Assisted Therapy (AAT) Program
Risk to humans: person tripped, bitten, scratched, infected by a zoonotic disease; human-animal companion bond broken if AAT program ends or animal dies
Risk to animals: abuse, neglect, not receiving veterinary check-ups, inadequate basic needs (food, water, shelter)
Risk to the field of AAT: administration hesitant to invest in AAT; insurer not providing necessary liability; administration needs to be informed, contact for insurance
Risk to the AAT Program: benefits not occurring from AAT intervention

Source: Westbrook GJ. Animal-assisted therapy: risks and risk-minimalization procedures. *Contin Care* 1988:26–27.

provide insurance and pay premiums through a group policy (20).

It is important for volunteers to follow policies to prevent a possible incident. Owners need to be attentive to their pets and recognize stress and changes. Volunteers need to be familiar with patients so that safety is adhered to. The facility needs to have protocols established for any emergency or incident that might occur. An incident needs to be reported immediately to the proper authorities.

Four main risks are involved in an AAT program: risk to humans, risk to animals, risk to the field of AAT, and risk of the AAT program not achieving the planned benefits (Table 41-7).

Volunteers should be instructed to remain calm when a potentially compromising situation occurs. This helps prevent the incident from being misunderstood. When such a situation occurs, it is important to stop the activity, seek first aid if necessary, and explain to the staff what actually transpired. Due to staff or animal stress, it may be best to terminate the visit. An incident report including all pertinent data needs to be completed as soon as possible. Participants in the Pet Partners program need to report the occurrence within 48 hours to the Delta Society. The Delta Society will make a decision regarding future visits with the pet, probation, or re-evaluation (58).

The program coordinator needs to be knowledgeable about animals, animal suitability to the facility, budgetary needs, volunteers, patient referrals to AAT, frequency of visits, length of program, training of the animal, and animal familiarity with hospital equipment (59).

Goals and Methods

Animals may be used by all members of the treatment team, providing a different focus according to their discipline. Nurses may focus on psychosocial issues; recreation therapists may focus on leisure skill development and community re-entry. Occupational therapists may focus on activities of daily living skills; physical therapists, on motor skills; and speech therapists, on communication skills.

The goals and methods for AAT are limited only by one's imagination. Unless there are medical or psychological contraindications, everyone can benefit from this intervention. Table 41-8 provides examples of goals and methods that can be used, and is not all inclusive but is meant to serve as a basis to start a program.

Volunteers

Volunteers are essential to the success of any AAT program. Volunteers may serve as animal handlers, program coordinators, fund raisers, and publicity coordinators for the program and facility. It is important to recognize the reasons why people volunteer for the program. Stavishinsky (61) studied nursing home volunteers' expectations and experiences in Upstate New York. The subjects of the study were community members and college students working in a pet therapy program. They brought companion animals to various institutions on a weekly basis. Visiting pets and people re-created an aura of domesticity for residents who had been cut off from homes and families by age or illness. The self-image that volunteers developed in their role was reflected by the domestic perceptions of the residents. Most came to see themselves as family and friends to patients, rather than visitors, strangers, or adjunct staff. The factors that influenced how volunteers felt about what they did and whether or not they continued with their work over a long period of time included personal motives, prior experience with this kind of work, career orientations, and preconception of the elderly and of nursing homes.

As the study suggested, people volunteer for a variety of reasons. Many are altruistic or have a general interest in sharing their loving animals with other animal lovers. The study further noted that volunteering is an emotionally demanding experience that some people manage more successfully than others. While certain individuals find the costs of this unexpected intimacy too high, others discover significant rewards in what one person called "selfish altruism" (61).

When one is developing a volunteer program, three primary areas must be considered: recruitment, training, and retention. Potential volunteers can be recruited from many sources. Bernard (14) suggested contacting obedience and breed clubs. These resources also may be helpful in recruiting a dog trainer to administer temperament testing. Another possible source is the local veterinarian's office. Beyond direct contacts, a facility might print small brochures or handouts for distribution in the waiting rooms of veterinary clinics. This also provides a way to advertise a facility's unique program in the community. Providing information at dog, cat, or horse show booths is a good recruiting strategy. Many facilities use a packet or brochure stating the goals of the program, steps to

Table 41-8: Animal-Assisted Therapy (AAT) Goals and Methods	
Goals	**Methods**
Social*	
Improve socialization, interaction and cooperation around others, and reality orientation, group participation and communication	Practice teaching an animal something new Learn about animal, then introduce animal to others Give animal verbal commands or hand signals Engage in play with an animal Develop a cooperative plan to accomplish something with an animal Remember and repeat specific information about the animal Ask questions about animals Play animal-related games such as animal charades Share favorite animal stories with group Introduce self or animal to others Reminisce about past experience with pets
Improve body awareness	Identify body parts on animal, then on self
Increase eye contact	After explaining activity, have person look at therapist, then repeat the instructions
Emotional*	
Reduce anxiety	Give appropriate affection to an animal
Increase self-esteem by stating positive affirmation of oneself	Reminisce about animals the person has known Generalize animal behavior to trust human behavior or circumstances
Address grieving/loss issues	Receive apparent acceptance from an animal
Improve ability to express feelings	Reminisce about past animal losses
Reduce isolation, boredom, loneliness	Observe and interpret animal behaviors
Brighten affect/mood	Receive affection from an animal
Provide opportunities to succeed	Identify one positive characteristic about the animal, then one positive characteristic about oneself
Decrease feelings of hopelessness	Provide opportunities for success when interacting with animal Engage in play with an animal Take animal for a walk Focus on animal or an aquarium during painful procedures or chemotherapy
Physical	
Increase trunk rotation	Place animal to side of patient to help patient rotate the body toward animal Place grooming tools in a position to facilitate trunk rotation when grooming a large animal such as a horse
Improve fine-motor skills	Manipulate buckles, clasp, on collars and leashes Feed animal small treats to utilize finger dexterity Open containers that hold treats for animal
Improve ambulation	Walk a dog Walk to get items for the animal Walk to animal placed at end of parallel bars
Improve wheelchair mobility	Place animal on lap and wheel to designated station or through obstacle course Have a large dog pull the wheelchair Have patient propel wheelchair to get items needed for the animal
Improve upper-extremity range of motion	Have patient groom or pet the animal Hold animal in front of patient and encourage patient to reach for animal
Improve supination	Have patient throw ball underhanded to animal Place animal so patient can stroke under belly with palm of hand of the affected side
Improve crawling/preambulation	Child will crawl to animal placed in visual field
Improve standing/balance	Stand while grooming animal Stand in standing frame while grooming animal
Improve trunk control	Patient to reach for grooming equipment and bringing self to sitting position Reach to pet/groom animal while handler holds animal away from patient When finished with activity, patient will hand animal to someone else

Table 41-8: (*Continued*)

Goals	Methods
Improve safe use of walker	Patient will put grooming supplies in walker basket and ambulate to animal
Increase endurance/strength	Remain and participate in therapy for entire session Use of weights during session
Increase bilateral use of extremities	Use both sides of body
Follow hip precautions	Use adaptive equipment to pick up items from floor such as a collar or toy
Use of affected side	Place animal on affected side for patient to cross mid-line and use weak side
Cognitive	
Improve sequencing	Have patient follow 1-, 2-, or 3-step commands Identify steps to giving animal a bath
Increase attention span	Demonstrate eye contact Follow through with task
Increase memory	Have patient recall animal's name, breed, age, etc. Vary recall delay time Have patient give command such as "sit" to dog, then remember to release dog from the command
Increase orientation	Have patient describe AAT session and why they are there Identify what kind of animal patient is working with, color, body parts, etc.
Sensory stimulation	Use animal for tactile stimulation Move animal from side to side to encourage visual tracking Have animal bark, meow, chirp, or jingle collar tags or bells for auditory stimulation
Word-finding tasks	Sentence completion tasks
Carry over skills to self	Use of brush or comb on animal Learn safety awareness when caring for animal at home
Leisure skills development	Provide resources for animal clubs in community
Community re-entry setting	Walk animal in community

* Please note that the methods do not correspond directly with the listed social and emotional goals, but overlap in their efficacy, while the physical and cognitive goals are organized to demonstrate a one-to-one relationship between the goal and the method.

Source: Fine AH, Fine NM. Broadening the impact of services and recreational therapies—section 2: animal assisted therapy. In: Fine AH, Fine NM, Zapf SA, et al, eds. *Therapeutic recreation for exceptional children: let me in, I want to play.* 2nd ed. Springfield, IL: Charles C. Thomas, 1996:270–288.

certification, and a contact number for more information. In addition, facilities may post flyers at pet stores that may also choose to help sponsor the program. The media is also an excellent source of publicity and recruitment. Often facilities invite the press or a local television crew to observe the program in progress. Overall, however, the best form of recruitment is word of mouth. As Bernard (14) stated, "Quality, not quantity is important; better to have five or six excellent owners and dogs and grow slowly, than to compromise the program's standards."

Once volunteers have been recruited, thorough training is essential to overcome their inexperience in working with persons with disabilities. They need to know what to expect from patients, staff, and facility. Training must include orientation to the special populations with whom they will be working and the policies and procedures of the facility. AAT training programs such as Pet Partners through the Delta Society or a similar local program are recommended.

Without proper training, many obstacles may arise. Volunteers discontinue service because their visits are not "working," or making a difference to the people they visit. Lack of communication can lead to disharmony or disillusionment.

Volunteers appreciate seeing patients' progress. Bernard (14) recommended rescheduling the same patient and animal team for several visits. When visits run smoothly, volunteers want to return. According to Davis (62), long-term, consistent programs provide the most benefits to patients and volunteers and are the most efficient.

Patient Referrals

A review of the literature indicates that programs approach referrals and protocols in various ways, through consent forms, physician's orders, evaluations performed by an AAT specialist, and referral forms. Assessments need to be completed prior to the initiation of interventions and should identify functional skills that can be addressed through AAT.

A treatment plan with long- and short-term goals needs to be developed to identify deficits and incorporate specific tasks with the animals. Evaluation of the patient's performance is documented and compared from session to session (11).

Indications include stroke patients, orthopedic patients, patients who have had general surgery, and AIDS patients. Therapy can benefit those who are self-conscious about their bodily appearance, since animals accept humans unconditionally. Other patients include those with impaired communication, impaired physical mobility, poor self-esteem, poor coping ability, or limited social skills. For patients in need of stress management, animals can be used for distraction and pain or anxiety reduction. Animals promote awareness of their environment and reality orientation (19).

Respect is given to patients who dislike, fear, or are allergic to animals or who wish to decline services (35). Patients who have had recent surgery (e.g., splenectomy) are more susceptible to infection (e.g., dog saliva bacteria) (10). Contraindications to AAT include patients with open wounds, delicate skin, or multiple intravenous lines. Patients who have a tendency to violence or unpredictable behavior may provoke or hurt the animals. Traditional modalities are used to meet these patients' goals (19,63).

The cardiac care unit and the cardiac observation unit at the UCLA Medical Center in Los Angeles established criteria for patient inclusion and exclusion in their AAT program (Table 41-9) (26).

The NARHA established contraindications and precautions for therapeutic riding for prospective patients diagnosed with any of the disabilities or behaviors listed in Table 41-10 (64).

Using animal-assisted therapy or therapeutic riding as a treatment modality is an excellent complement to human love and compassion.

Table 41-9: Inclusion and Exclusion Criteria

Inclusion Criteria	Exclusion Criteria
Post–myocardial infarction	Immunosuppressed
Angina	Splenectomy
Pretransplantation	Dog allergies
Cardiomyopathy	Tuberculosis
Congestive heart failure	Posttransplantation

Source: Cole KM, Gawlinski A. Animal-assisted therapy in the intensive care unit. *Nurs Clin North Am* 1995;30:529–537.

Table 41-10: North American Riding for the Handicapped Association Contraindications and Precautions for Therapeutic Riding

	Contraindications	
Moderate agitation with severe confusion, gross disruptive behavior	Unstable spine, including subluxation at cervical levels	Severe osteoporosis
Uncontrollable seizures	Pathologic fractures (e.g., osteogenesis imperfecta)	Acute stage of arthritis
Exacerbation of multiple sclerosis	Open pressure sores or wound	Drug dosages causing physical states inappropriate to riding settings
Hemophilia	Atlanto axial instability	Spondylolisthesis
Coxarthrosis	Detached retina	Acute herniated disk
Any spinal fusion, organic or operative	Anticoagulant medications	CVA 2 degrees to unclipped aneurysm or presence of other aneurysms
CVA 2 degrees to angioma that was not totally resected	Complete quadriplegia secondary to spinal cord injury	Structural scoliosis > 30 degrees; excessive kyphosis or lordosis; hemivertebrae
Any patient the therapist is not completely comfortable/confident treating		
	Additional Precautions and Possible Contraindications for Therapeutic Riding	
Prolonged use of phenytoin, can cause osteoporosis	Incontinence	Hydrocephalus, with presence of shunt(s)
Sensory deficits	Heterotrophic ossification	Significant allergies to horse hair, dust, hay, etc.
Recent surgery	Serious cardiac condition	Dislocation, subluxation, dysplasia of hip(s) with significant restriction or asymmetry
Craniotomy	Diabetes	Peripheral vascular disease
Obesity	Abnormal fatigue	Arnold-Chiari malformation
History of skin breakdown or grafting over weightbearing areas	Tethered cord	History of substance abuse resulting in fragile blood vessels

CVA = cerebrovascular accident.

Source: Contraindications for therapeutic riding: precautions and possible contraindications for therapeutic riding. In: *NARHA workshop notebook.* Denver, CO: North American Riding for the Handicapped Association, 1991:E7.

ACKNOWLEDGMENTS

We want to take this opportunity to thank the people and organizations who gave us the confidence and support to contribute to this work: Dr. Susan Jan Garrison, Medical Director, Rehabilitation Center at the Methodist Hospital and advocate of AAT; Brian Padjen, MA; Pam Cornell; Marilyn Trail, MOT, OTR, BCN; Edens Houston; Caring Critters; Sue Zapf, MOT, OTR, CTRS; Jack Mosgrove; Anne and Carl Grossman; Tomas Ramos, Zeiss Photographers, Houston, Texas; David Austin, PhD, CTRS; and Gerald J. Widmar, BSME.

DEDICATION

This chapter is dedicated to the significant animal "therapists" in our lives, T.C. (T.I.R.R. Cat), Tinka, Felix, and our companion animals, Tiger, Buddy, Chaos, and Serenity who gave us the inspiration to pursue this form of intervention with our patients. In memory of Maxine (1978–1996).

APPENDIX I: VISITATION REPORTS

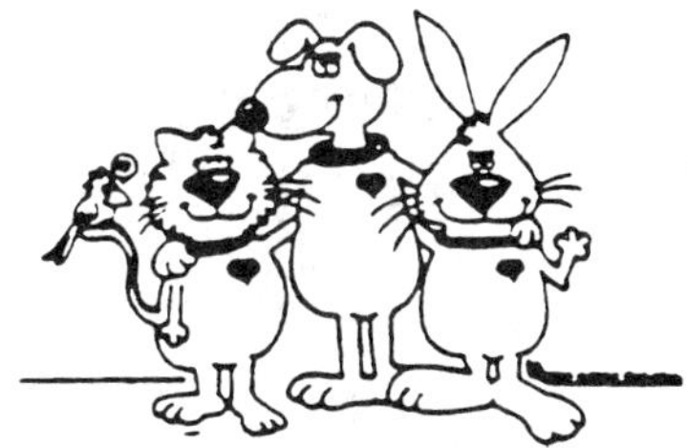

Caring Critters
Animal-Assisted Therapy
VISITATION EVALUATION

FACILITY VISITED: ______________________________

DATE: ______________________ **TIME OF DAY:** ______________

VOLUNTEER	PET'S NAME OR DESCRIPTION (Breed, Color, Size, Age)
1.	
2.	
3.	
4.	
5.	

❖ Problems Encountered: (Can be concerning animals, staff, facility, residents/patients, etc.)

❖ Good News and "Warm Fuzzies":

❖ How Did You Feel About Today's Visit?

❖ Suggestions: (Different animals, time in facility, variation in activity, etc.)

Reproduced with permission from *Caring Critters animal assisted therapy: volunteer handbook.* Houston, TX: Caring Critters, 1994.

APPENDIX I: (*Continued*)

CARING CRITTERS
ANIMAL-ASSISTED THERAPY
RESIDENT EVALUATION

NAME OR ROOM NO.	LOOKED AT ANIMAL	TALKED TO ANIMAL OR VOLUNTEER	TOUCHED ANIMAL	UNABLE TO VISIT (Resident Asleep or NI)	EMOTIONAL RESPONSE (Smiled, Excited, Angry, Cried, Etc.)

DATE: ____________________

Volunteer(s): ____________________ Pet(s): ____________________

Reproduced with permission from *Caring Critters animal assisted therapy: volunteer handbook.* Houston, TX: Caring Critters, 1994.

APPENDIX II: SAMPLE ANIMAL-ASSISTED THERAPY FORMS

ANIMAL ASSISTED THERAPY
Progress Note

______ Initial ______ Interim ______ Discharge Date of Initial TX: ______

Diagnosis: ______

Primary Occupational Therapist: ______

S: ______

______

______

O: Please refer to O.T. note for specific evaluation results.

A: Patient continues to benefit from ANIMAL ASSISTED THERAPY
secondary to: ______

______

Patient is limited by: ______

______

______

______

Gains have been noted in: ______

______

______

______

P: Goal areas which will be focused on for the next two weeks include:

______ Right UE Left UE Bilateral UE: PROM AAROM AROM
______ UE Strengthening: RUE ____ lbs. LUE ____ lbs.
______ Fine Motor Coordination
______ Endurance
______ Coma Stimulation
______ Cognitive Activities: Memory ____ Sequencing ____ Orientation ____
______ Perceptual Activities
______ Sitting Balance: Static ____ Dynamic ____
______ Standing Balance: Static ____ Dynamic ____
______ Wheelchair Mobility
______ Pet Care/Safety in Home
______ Other ______

Patient will be seen 2, 3, 5x's a week.

Date: ______ Therapist: ______

Reproduced with permission from Bernard S. *Animal assisted therapy: a guide for health care professionals and volunteers.* Whitehouse, TX: Therapet, 1995.

Rehabilitation Treatment Plan
Animal–Assisted Therapy

Patient: ______________________ Age: __________ Date: __/__/__

Diagnosis:

____

Therapist: ______________________ Physician: ______________________

Precautions: ____

Briefly describe patient's present level of functioning (Physical/Cognitive):

____

Work on:	___Right	___Left	___ Midline
Encourage use of:	___RUE*	___LUE*	
	___RLE*	___LLE*	
	SS Weights:	RUE ____lbs.	LUE ___ lbs.
Work with patient:	___Wheelchair	___ Mat	___ Bed
	___Other ______________________		
Transfers require:	___Maximum	___Moderate	___ Minimum
	___Supervision Assistant		

ACTIVITIES WHICH WOULD BE APPROPRIATE:

_____ Encourage visual tracking.
_____ Self-assisted over midline.
_____ Visually follow verbal command.
_____ Physically follow verbal command.
_____ Yes/No verbal response.
_____ Memory retention.
_____ Verbal repetition.
_____ Communication device.
_____ Facial and breathing exercises.
_____ Hand strength and coordination.
_____ Gross motor skills.
_____ Fine motor skills.
_____ Conversation/verbal communication skills.

* Definitions: RUE—Right Upper Extremity; RLE—Right Lower Extremity; LUE—Left Upper Extremity; LLE—Left Lower Extremity

Reproduced with permission from Bernard S. *Animal assisted therapy: a guide for health care professionals and volunteers.* Whitehouse, TX: Therapet, 1995.

APPENDIX II: (*Continued*)

Animal Assisted Therapy Referral

Patient: ______________________ Room: ________ Age: ____________
Therapist: ______________________ See Pt.: 2 3 5 x's week
Diagnosis: ______________________ Physician: ______________________
Precautions: ____
Briefly describe Pt.'s Physical/Cognitive Status: ______________________________
____

Work with Dog on: Right Left Midline

Encourage use of: Right Left BUE Add weights: RUE _____ LUE ____

Work with Patient: W/C Mat Bed Sidelying Other: ______________________

Transfers Require: Max Mod Min Supervision

Activities which would Be Appropriate Include:
________ Try to get patient to focus/track dog. Watch for any visual tracking.
________ Move patient's hand over the dog. Ask patient to look at his hand as they pet the dog. Ask patient to try and reach out for dog.
________ Have patient look on command to the dog's head, tail, or other body parts.
________ Have patient touch the body parts that the therapist names.
________ Have patient try to respond with head shakes, or "yes" "no" cards to simple questions about the dog.
________ Have the patient try to name the body parts that the therapist touches.
________ Have patient try to answer simple questions about the dog.
________ Have patient try to pucker and blow on dog's ear or fur, or blow bubbles for the dog to catch.
________ Have patient try to pet the dog using one hand, or both hands together.
________ Have patient brush dog.
________ Have patient throw a ball for the dog to retrieve.
________ Have patient play tug-of-war with the dog to increase BUE and trunk strength.
________ Have patient try to remember several facts about the dog and try to recall them to work on memory.
________ Other: ____

Animal Assisted Therapy
Feedback Form

Patient's Name: ______________________________

Diagnosis: ______________________________

Primary Therapist: Room: ____________ Date: ______________________________

________________ has been scheduled for Animal Assisted Therapy.

Patient will be seen 2 3 5 x's a week at __________ o'clock. Please add this to patient's daily schedule cards and alert him of his schedule change.

Goals which will be concentrated on include:

____ RUE LUE BUE: PROM AAROM AROM
____ UE Strengthening: RUE: ___ lbs. LUE: ___ lbs.
____ Fine Motor Coordination
____ Endurance
____ Coma Stimulation
____ Cognitive Activities: Memory Sequencing Orientation
____ Perceptual Activities
____ Sitting Balance: Static Dynamic
____ Standing Balance: Static Dynamic
____ Wheelchair Mobility
____ Other: ______________________________

If you have any questions or changes, please contact me at extension 2328.

____

Therapist's Name

Reproduced with permission from Bernard S. *Animal assisted therapy: a guide for health care professionals and volunteers.* Whitehouse, TX: Therapet, 1995.

ANIMAL-ASSISTED ACTIVITIES AND THERAPY EVALUATION SHEET

Date: ______________________________

Legend: ↑ Improvement
↓ Deterioration
Θ No Change

Patient Name	Socialization	Communication	Anxiety Level	Reality Orientation	Attention	Concentration	Engagement	Affect and Mood

Other Comments:

SOCIALIZATION
Interpersonal relationships; the level and appropriateness of an individual's interrelations within the group.

COMMUNICATION
The patient's ability to express him/herself within the context of the group and the activity.

ANXIETY LEVEL
How the individual responds to stimuli and modulates his/her responses.

REALITY ORIENTATION
The patient's ability to relate appropriately to the context of the group and the surroundings.

ATTENTION SPAN
How long the patient attends to the group and the activity, how long before becoming distracted by other stimuli.

CONCENTRATION
How well the patient focuses attention.

ENGAGEMENT
The relative level of the patient's involvement with the activity; how well s/he becomes an active participant.

AFFECT AND MOOD
How the patient feels about him/her self as expressed verbally, by body language, and by facial expressions.

APPENDIX II: (*Continued*)

Occupational & Recreational Therapy Animal Assisted Therapy Documentation Form

Patient Name: ______________________________ Date: __________ Unit: ________

Circle the number of those that apply:

DIAGNOSIS:

1. Schizophrenia
2. Major Depression
3. Manic Depressive
4. Personality Disorder
5. Conduct Disorder
6. ADHD
7. PDD or Autistic
8. Alcohol/Drug Addiction
9. Eating Disorder
10. PTSD
11. Learning Disabled
12. Mental Retardation
13. Head Injury
14. Other ____________

PRECAUTIONS:

1. Suicide
2. Elopement
3. Aggressive
4. 1:1 Supervision
5. Hallucinations, Delusions
6. Animal Abuse History
7. Seizures
8. Cardiac
9. Diabetes
10. Hearing Impairment
11. Speech Impairment
12. Vision Impairment
13. Cognitive Impairment
14. Allergies:
15. Other: ____________

GOAL REPORT:

Mark number of goal if circled on your patient, circle if goal *met* or *not met* then provide any comments pertinent to goal:

GOAL# MET/NOT MET COMMENTS: ______________________________

GOAL# MET/NOT MET COMMENTS: ______________________________

GOAL# MET/NOT MET COMMENTS: ______________________________

GOAL# MET/NOT MET COMMENTS: ______________________________

TEAM GOALS LIST CIRCLE NUMBER OF THOSE THAT APPLY:

1. To Increase Leisure Awareness and Participation: Pt. to participate in AAA/AAT activity when scheduled on unit in order to increase functional independence in leisure opportunities. To provide opportunities for the reinforcement and support of other treatment programs.

2. To Stimulate Cognitive Development and Affective Responses: Pt. resets appropriately to visitation, follows conversation, initiates conversation, and answers questions appropriately.

3. To Increase Memory: After cues, Pt. to remember pet's name, age, breed, and gender for either short term memory (remembers 10 minutes later) or long term memory (remembers the next day or next visit).

4. To Increase Verbalization: Pt. to participate at least 1 time in conversation during visit, pt. may have slow speech so give time to answer.

5. To Decrease Non-Productive Behavior: Pt. to stop non-productive behavior (rocking, biting nails, pacing etc.) with only_____ verbal cues while participating in AAA/AAT.

6. To Increase Expression of Feeling: Pt. to express feelings about visitation, animals, or how Pt. is feeling that day. To provide opportunities for Pt. to express feelings in a therapeutic environment.

7. To Increase Attention Span And Concentration: Pt. to have demonstrated good eye contact and follow through on task while participating in AAA/AAT.

Reproduced with permission from Fine AH, Fine NM. Broadening the impact of services and recreational therapies—section 2: animal assisted therapy. In: Fine AH, Fine NM, Zapf SA, et al, eds. *Therapeutic recreation for exceptional children: let me in, I want to play.* 2nd ed. Springfield, IL: Charles C. Thomas, 1996:270–288.

APPENDIX II: *(Continued)*

THERAPEUTIC RECREATION ANIMAL ASSISTED THERAPY REPORT FORM

PATIENT NAME: ________________________ DATE: ____________ ROOM#: ______________

CIRCLE ONE OF THE FOLLOWING:
UNIT: 2A/REHAB 2A/ORTHO 2B/SNF 1A/PSYCH OTHER ______________________________

CIRCLE NUMBER OF THOSE THAT APPLY:

DIAGNOSIS:

1. CVA STROKE LEFT SIDED WEAKNESS
2. CVA STROKE RIGHT SIDED WEAKNESS
3. CVA STROKE BILATERAL INVOLVEMENT
4. LEFT/RIGHT HIP FRACTURE
5. LEFT/RIGHT TOTAL HIP REPLACEMENT
6. LEFT/RIGHT TOTAL KNEE REPLACEMENT
7. FRACTURE/MULTIPLE FRACTURES
8. NEUROMUSCULAR DISEASE
9. DECONDITIONED
10. HEAD INJURY/TRAUMA
11. PARALYSIS
    A.) HEMI—ONE SIDE L OR R
    B.) PARA—LOWER EXTREMITY
    C.) QUAD—ALL EXTREMITY
12. SPINAL STENOSIS OR INJURY
13. CHRONIC PAIN
14. MULTIPLE TRAUMA
15. OTHER ______________________

PRECAUTIONS:

1. CARDIAC/BLOOD PRESSURE
2. SEIZURE PRECAUTIONS
3. SWALLOWING/DYSPHAGIA
4. HIP PRECAUTIONS
5. WEIGHT BEARING LIMITATIONS
6. BLEEDING PRECAUTIONS
7. IMPAIRED VISION
8. BLIND
9. LEFT OR RIGHT NEGLECT
10. SPEAKS FOREIGN LANGUAGE
11. SPEECH IMPAIRMENT
    A.) APHASIA—EXPRESSIVE/RECEPTIVE
    B.) DYSARTHRIA—SLURRED SPEECH
    C.) ANOMIA—WORD FINDING PROBLEMS
12. HARD OF HEARING/DEAF
13. DIETARY RESTRICTIONS—nothing by mouth no thin liquids, diabetic, pureed.
14. OTHER ______________________

GOAL REPORT:

MARK NUMBER OF GOAL IF CIRCLED ON YOUR PATIENT CIRCLE MET OR NOT MET THEN PROVIDE ANY COMMENTS PERTINENT TO GOAL

GOAL# MET/NOT MET COMMENTS: ______________________________

GOAL# MET/NOT MET COMMENTS: ______________________________

GOAL# MET/NOT MET COMMENTS: ______________________________

GOAL# MET/NOT MET COMMENTS: ______________________________

GOAL# MET/NOT MET COMMENTS: ______________________________

TEAM GOALS LIST CIRCLE NUMBER OF THOSE THAT APPLY:

1. PARTICIPATION GOAL—To facilitate self expression. To provide an environment for the integration of diverse physical, mental, social, and emotional skills. To provide opportunities for the reinforcement and support of other treatment programs. To provide opportunity for experiencing enjoyment or contentment, and provide normalcy to a rehab hospital environment.
2. TO STIMULATE COGNITIVE DEVELOPMENT AND AFFECTIVE RESPONSES—Patient reacts appropriately to visitation, follows conversation, initiates conversation, and seems to answer appropriately.
3. TO INCREASE VERBALIZATIONS—Encourage speech and communication; patient may have slowed responses so give ample time to answer.
4. TO ASSIST IN THE ADJUSTMENT OF CONDITION OR DISABILITY—Note if patient makes any depressive comments or fears related to their situation.
5. INCREASE ENDURANCE—sitting and participation.
6. INCREASE TRUNK CONTROL—sitting in bed or wheel chair in good position.
7. INCREASES VISUAL AND BODY AWARENESS—Are they aware of the affected side during visit do they attempt to use affected side.
8. IMPROVE BILATERAL USE OF EXTREMITIES UPPER/LOWER—Patient is able to use both sides of the body note if patient completes this task independently or with cuing verbal or visual.
9. IMPROVE SEQUENCING—Patient is able to complete a 2, 3, 4, step instruction or has difficulty with this task.
10. INCREASE STRENGTH AND RANGE OF MOTION—Patient made attempts to reach and hold the pets.
11. INCREASE BED MOBILITIES—Patient was able to roll and scoot maneuver in bed to get closer to the animals.
12. INCREASE WHEEL CHAIR MOBILITY—Patient propelled wheel chair to get closer to the animals.
13. INCREASE ATTENTION SPAN AND CONCENTRATION—Good eye contact able to follow the conversation.
14. INCREASE AMBULATION—Patient walked from bed to chair with assist/without assist to sit and play with animals.
15. INCREASE MEMORY—Cue patient to remember one pet's name, age, gender and breed for carryover the next day but do not tell them they may be quizzed.
16. DECREASE ANXIETY—Select one to two pets and give each one 15 strokes to calm patient preferably with eyes closed.
17. PROVIDE OPPORTUNITY FOR BONDING ESTABLISH FRIENDSHIP—Encourage patient to talk to the pet.
18. INCREASE ARTICULATION AND CLARITY OF COMMUNICATION—Ask patient to repeat slowly if not understood.
19. INCREASE ORIENTATION—Ask patient to tell you where they are and why, possibly a current event. (cue them if necessary).
20. INCREASE CONTACT WITH COMMUNITY/FAMILY—Note any comments about fear of re-entry into the community or home environment.

APPENDIX III: ORGANIZATIONS

The following is a list of organizations promoting AAT and the human-animal bond.

1. Alpha Affiliates, Inc.
   103 Washington Street, Suite 362,
   Morristown, NJ 07960-6813
   (973) 539-2770
   FAX (973) 644-0610

A nonprofit all-volunteer organization founded in 1987, dedicated to promoting the benefits on interactions between people and animals. Resource materials are available, such as:

   a. A video titled "Making a Difference," promoting "safety and effectiveness" in pet visitation/therapy. Cost $19.95 + $3.00 S/H.
   b. Certificates of recognition offered to volunteers meeting the criteria.
   c. A registry of volunteers available free to facilities. Requests need to be made on facility letterhead paper.
   d. "Pet Visitation/Therapy You and Your Dog Can Make a Difference," by Kathy Diamond Davis. Provides data on getting started after passing a certification program on AKC's Canine Good Citizen Test.
   e. Advance Directives for Pet Care, a kit on preparing for care of a pet when unforeseen circumstances occur. Cost $5.00.

2. Pet Information Bureau.
   1710 Rhode Island Avenue, N.W.
   Washington, DC 20036
   (202) 452-1515

3. The Latham Foundation
   Latham Plaza Building
   Clement and Schiller Streets
   Alameda, CA 94501
   Established in 1985, for "promoting respect for all life through education."

4. Canine Companions for Independence
   P.O. Box 446
   Santa Rosa, CA 95402-0446
   (707) 528-0830 or (800) 572-2275
   The first organization in 1975 that pioneered the idea of service dogs.

5. Handi-Dogs, Inc.
   P.O. Box 12563
   Tucson, AZ 85732
   (602) 326-3412
   Alamo Reaves, Executive Director

6. Delta Society
   Century Building
   289 Perimeter Road East
   Renton, WA 98055-1329
   (425) 226-7357
   FAX (425) 235-1076

The Delta Society, a nonprofit organization founded in 1977, is an international center undertaking research, service, and education in the field of human-animal interactions. Its mission is "to promote animals helping people improve their health, independence, and quality of life."

   a. Pet Partners Program/AAT is a service that trains volunteers and screens pets for programs in various facilities prior to visits. There are 200 pet partner teams, working in 45 states and four other countries, assisting over 35,000 people a year. The Delta Society also trains clinicians on how to train animals to work with people with disabilities. The Delta Society has established health regulations for animals to decrease the fears of animal transmitted infections and/or injury.
   b. National Services Dog Center, assists people with disabilities to achieve independence in their environment with service dogs.
   c. "People and Pets," teaches individuals and families with companion animals to promote health and well-being.
   d. Publications, newsletters, quarterly magazines, and journals addressing needs of volunteers, the general public, and professionals (22).

7. Hearing Dog Program
   The American Humane Association
   1500 West Tufts Avenue
   Englewood, CO 80110
   (303) 762-0342
   Kris Winship, Assistant Program Manager

8. Leader Dogs for the Blind
   P.O. Box 5000
   1039 South Rochester Road
   Rochester, MI 48307
   (313) 651-9011

9. Love on a Leash
   3809 Plaza Drive, #107-309
   Oceanside, CA 92056
   (619) 630-4824
   Liz Palika

10. PAWS—Pets Are Wonderful Support
    P.O. Box 460489
    San Francisco, CA 94146-0489
    (415) 824-4040

Support for pet owners with aids and assistance in care of companion

Other Locations:

PAWS, Los Angeles
8272 Sunset Boulevard
West Hollywood, CA 90046
(213) 466-1845

PAWS, San Diego
1278 University Avenue
P.O. Box 178
San Diego, CA 92103
(619) 234-PAWS

PAWS, St. Louis
4579 Lacleda
St. Louis, MO 63108
(314) 350-8047

11. The Institute of Animal Assisted Therapy (IAAT)
    823 Shader Street, Suite #1
    San Francisco, CA 94117
    (415) 750-7271

An organization based on the human-animal bond, recognizing the human need for comfort. Information on infection control guidelines is available.

12. Pet Assisted Therapy Facilitation Certificate Program
    Pearl Salotto, State University of New York
    (401) 463-5809

13. Pet Information Bureau
    1710 Rhode Island Avenue, N.W.
    Washington, DC 20036
    (202) 452-1525

14. The Eden Alternative
    RR #1, Box 31B4
    Sherburne, NY 13460
    (607) 674-5232
    Dr. William Thomas

15. Therapy Dogs, Inc.
    2416 E. Fox Farm Rd.
    Cheyenne, WY 82007
    (307) 638-3223
    Ann Butrick

Nonprofit organization, founded in 1990, bringing together therapy dogs and people in nursing homes, prisons, and hospitals countrywide.

16. Therapy Dogs International (TDI)
    91 Wiman Avenue
    Staten Island, NY 10308
    (908) 429-0607

Organization of qualified volunteers providing therapy dogs for visitation to various facilities. TDI is a part of a long-term study researching the bond of dogs and the geriatric population and Alzheimer disease. Contact the Delta Society for facilities in your area.

17. The Chenny Troupe
    1504 North Wells Street
    Chicago, IL 60610
    (312) 280-0266
    FAX (312) 642-2488
    Francie Glatt

The nonprofit organization began as a model based on a pediatric program utilizing MK Rainbow Therapy Dog Club, Inc., in Chicago. In 1991, the Junior League of Chicago, Inc. committed their support of the members to institute an AAT program. The executive director and volunteers visit a number of facilities in the Chicago area and serve many functions in the organization—marketing, fundraising, education, research, certification of dogs, and training.

18. The San Francisco Society for the Prevention of Cruelty to Animals
    2500 16th Street
    San Francisco, CA 94103-6589
    (415) 554-3000
    (415) 554-3060 (AAT program)
    Frank Burnett, Coordinator of San Francisco's program

The San Francisco SPCA has trained volunteers and visited facilities for 16 years. In 1995, 99 different facilities and 27,565 people were seen through the AAT program.

19. Paws with a Cause Headquarters
    1235 100th Street SE
    Bryon Center, MI 49315
    1-800-253-PAWS
    (616) 698-0688

20. Pets, Washington, DC
    1747 Connecticut Avenue, N.W.
    Washington, DC 20009
    (202) 234-PETS

Supports and provides resources for pet owners with AIDS.

21. Pet Owners with AIDS/ARC Resource Service, Inc. (POWARS)
    P.O. Box 1116
    Madison Square Station

New York, NY 10159
(212) 744-0842

Supports and provides resources for pet owners with AIDS.

22. Pets Support Network
1824 12th Avenue
Seattle, WA 98122
(206) 328-2780

Supports and provides resources for pet owners with AIDS.

23. Action AIDS
P.O. Box 1625
Philadelphia, PA 19105
(215) 981-0088

Supports and provides resources for pet owners with AIDS.

24. Marin Humane Society
171 Bel Marin Keys Boulevard
Novato, CA 94949
(415) 883-4621

Supports and provides resources for pet owners.

25. Companion Animal Support and Assistance Network (CASAN)
P.O. Box 4963
Louisville, KY 40204
(502) 451-2676

26. The Assistance Dog United Campaign (ADUC)
P.O. Box 2804
Rohnert, CA 94927
(707) 585-0300
(707) 537-1960

Established in 1991 for research, education, and development of the assistance dog. They promote training, placement, acceptance of assistance dogs, and breeding. They raise money to help the disabled obtain assistant dogs. The cost to train dogs ranges from $4000 to $10,000 and may take years to obtain the appropriate type of dog needed.

27. Therapy Pet Pals of Texas
Kathryn Lashmit
807 Brazos Street, Suite 312
Austin, TX 78701

28. North American Riding for the Handicapped Association, Inc. (NARHA)
P.O. Box 33150
Denver, CO 80233
(800) 369-RIDE
(303) 452-1212

The purpose is to promote equestrian activities for the disabled. It provides education, instructor's insurance coverage, guidelines for riding programs, and precautions for the disabled.

29. Local organizations also sponsor AAT/AAA programs. Contact the Delta Society for facilities in your area. Some SPCA agencies also have programs and may be a resource, i.e., SPCA, San Francisco. In the Houston area, three programs serve local facilities:

Caring Critters
P.O. Box 16279
Houston, TX 77222
Voice Mail: (713) 957-5319

Human-Animal Pet Partnership of Texas
5905 Heather Drive
League City, TX 77573
Sue Zaph, MOT, CTRS

Paws for Caring
740 Mulberry
Bellaire, TX 77401
(713) 667-8114
Jan Hassler

APPENDIX IV: PUBLICATIONS AND VIDEOS

The following is a list of publications available as resources for AAT programs.

1. *Alpha Bits*, official quarterly publication of Alpha Affiliates, Inc. Provides news and reviews of events and literature related to human-animal interactions. See Appendix III for address. Subscription rates $10/yr in U.S.; $12/yr outside U.S.
2. *Good For Your Animals, Good For You.* "How to Live and Work with Animals in Activity and Therapy Programs and Stay Healthy" by David Waltner-Toews and Andrea Ellis; illustrations by Doug Schaeffer. Published in 1994 by the University of Guelph, Guelph, Ontario, Canada N1G-2W1 for the PET TRUST with assistance from Effem Foods, Ltd. Distributed by the Delta Society.
3. *The Latham Letter*, published quarterly by the Latham Foundation. Latham Plaza Building, Clement and Schiller Streets, Alameda, CA 94501.
4. *How to Start a Pet Therapy Program: A Guidebook for Health Care Professionals*, by P. Arkow. Latham Plaza

Building, Clement and Schiller Streets, Alameda, CA 94501.

5. *Alert Newsletter*, sponsored by the Delta Society. Addresses issues faced by people with disabilities who have service dogs. Published six times a year. Cost $6.00.
6. *Anthrozoos*, sponsored by the Delta Society. Published quarterly. A multidisciplinary, referenced scientific journal that addresses interactions between humans and animals. Cost $40/yr.
7. *Animal Assisted Therapy—A Guide for Health Care Professionals and Volunteers*, by Shari Bernard, OTR. Addresses initiating an AAT program, selecting and testing animals, referrals, reimbursement, legal issues, documentation, volunteers, and treatment plans. Available from Therapet, L.L.C., P.O. Box 1696, Whitehouse, TX 75791. Costs $32 + $2 S/H.
8. *Therapy Dogs—Training Your Dog to Reach Others*, by Kathy Diamond Davis. Addresses training a dog to become a therapy dog and the owner's role and responsibilities. Published by Howell Book House, Macmillan Publishing Company, 866 Third Avenue, New York, NY 10022.
9. "Heart of a Hero"—Canine Companions for Independence. 1994. Thirteen-minute video. Closed captioned. P.O. Box 446, Santa Rosa, CA 95402. (707) 528-0830.
10. *INTERACTIONS*, sponsored by the Delta Society on a quarterly basis. Addresses issues about companion animals and ways the animals enrich human lives. Complimentary to Delta Society members; subscription rate $35.00/yr.
11. *Pet Partners Newsletter*, sponsored by the Delta Society for Pet Partners. Addresses practical tips and effective animal-assisted activities. Subscription: $6.00 a year (6 times a year).
12. The Delta Society has videotapes on a variety of topics: animals with children, patients with AIDS, seniors; for use in hospitals, classrooms, corrections housing; pet loss; service dogs; and therapeutic riding. A catalog is available for $3.00 with rental, descriptions, and purchase prices.

REFERENCES

1. Young M. The evolution of domestic pets and companion animals. *Vet Clin North Am Small Anim Pract* 1985;15:297–309.
2. Gammonley J, Yates J. Pet projects: animal assisted therapy in nursing homes. *J Gerontol Nurs* 1991;17:12–15.
3. Voith V. Attachment of people to companion animals. *Vet Clin North Am Small Anim Pract* 1985;15:289–295.
4. Niego M. Rx: animals. *ASPCA Animal Watch* 1992;12:9–13.
5. Baun M, Oetting K, Bergstrom N. Health benefits of companion animals in relation to the physiologic indices of relaxation. *Holist Nurs Pract* 1991;5:16–23.
6. Beck A, Katcher A. *Between pets and people: the importance of animal companionship.* New York: GP Putnam's Sons, 1983:159, 165.
7. Friedman E. The value of pets for health and recovery: Waltham Symposium 20: pets, benefits and practice. *J Small Anim Pract* 1990;31(12):8–17.
8. Mornhinweg G, Voignier R. Holistic nursing interventions. *Orthop Nurs* 1995;14(4):20–23.
9. Wolcott J. Hospitals going to dogs—willingly. *Puget Sound Business J* 1993;13: 24–25.
10. Haggar V. Good companions. *Nurs Times* 1992;88(44):54–55.
11. Task Force Meeting of the Standards Committee, Definition Development Task Force. Delta Society, Tucson, AZ, 1991, February 1–3.
12. Pfau H, Fila D, Howie A, Kirwin S. Practical application of AAT by health care professionals. Presented at the Delta Society tenth annual conference, Portland, OR, October 10–12, 1991.
13. *Animal assisted therapy options.* Delta Society handout 1992;4:20–22.
14. Bernard S. *Animal assisted therapy: a guide for health care professionals and volunteers.* Whitehouse: Therapet, 1995.
15. Duncan SL. *Health care options: service dogs for people who have disabilities.* Renton, WA: Delta Society, 1995.
16. The Seeing Eye expands. *Alpha Bits* 1993;4:5.
17. Texas Hearing & Service Dogs, Inc. brochure. Austin: Texas Hearing & Service Dogs, 1995.
18. Monkeys—companionship and independence. *Alpha Bits* 1996;7(2):2–3.
19. Barba BE. The positive influence of animals: animal-assisted therapy in acute care. *Clin Nurse Spec* 1995;9:199–202.
20. *Caring Critters animal assisted therapy: volunteer handbook.* Houston: Caring Critters, 1994.
21. *Handbook for AAA/AAT—Delta Society.* 2nd ed.
22. Delta Society. *Animals helping people–people helping animals. Animals in hospitals resource*

packet. Portland, OR: Delta Society, 1996.

23. Williams LA. Impact of a pet visitation program in an acute care facility. Presented at the Delta Society ninth annual conference, Portland, OR, October 11–13, 1990.

24. Duncan SL. Loneliness: a health hazard of modern times. *Interactions* 1995;13:5–9.

25. Brichel C. The therapeutic roles of cat mascots with a hospital-based geriatric population: a staff survey. *Gerontologist* 1979;19:368–372.

26. Cole KM, Gawlinski A. Animal-assisted therapy in the intensive care unit. *Nurs Clin North Am* 1995;30:529–537.

27. Martin S. Ask the experts. *Crit Care Nurs* 1993;13:74.

28. Sayler PJ. Selecting the hippotherapy horse. In: Engel BT, ed. *Therapeutic riding programs: instruction and rehabilitation.* Durango: Barbara Engel Therapy Services, 1992:86.

29. Potter T, Evans WJ, Nolt JR. Therapeutic horseback riding. *J Am Vet Med Assoc* 1994;204:1.

30. *NARHA instructor workshop notebook.* Denver, CO: North American Riding for the Handicapped Association, 1992:A1, B27.

31. DePauw DP. Review of research in therapeutic riding. In: Engel BT, ed. *Therapeutic riding programs: instruction and rehabilitation.* Durango: Barbara Engel Therapy Services, 1992:43–44.

32. Engel BT. Therapeutic riding: its benefits, professions, and divisions. In: Engel BT, ed. *Therapeutic riding programs: instruction and rehabilitation.* Durango: Barbara Engel Therapy Services, 1992:35–38.

33. McLaughlin C. Bow-wow: what a difference animal assistance can make. *Adv Phys Ther* 1996;7(4):10–11, 34.

34. Carmack BJ. The role of companion animals for persons with AIDS/HIV. *Holist Nurs Pract* 1991;5(2):24–31.

35. Rosenkoetter M. Health promotion: the influence of pets on life patterns in the home. *Holist Nurs Pract* 1991;5(2):42–51.

36. LaCosse GM. Pet therapy Chenny Troupe style. *Dog World* 1994;79(9):32–38.

37. Hart LA, Hart BL, Bergin B. Socializing effects of service dogs for people with disabilities. *Anthrozoos* 1987;1(1):41–44.

38. Howe C. The healing power of animals. *Nurs Stand* 1995;9(4):45.

39. Orey C. Dogs who comfort. *GOOD DOG!* 1995;2:4, 8.

40. *Therapy Dogs Incorporated: Member Handbook.* Cheyenne: Therapy Dogs Inc., 1994.

41. Voelker R. Puppy love can be therapeutic, too. *JAMA* 1995;274:1897–1899.

42. Bowker M. The pet prescription. *New Physician* 1991;40(7):13–17.

43. Ptak AL. Studies of loneliness: recent research into the effects of companion animals on lonely people. *Interactions* 1995;13(1):7–9.

44. Friedman E, Katcher A, Lynch J, Thomas S. Animal companions and one-year survival of patients after discharge from a coronary care unit. *Public Health Rep* 1980;95:307–312.

45. Schuelke S, Trask B, Wallace C, et al. Physiological effects of the use of a companion animal dog as a cue to relaxation in diagnosed hypertensives. *The Latham Letter* 1991/92; Winter.

46. Friedman E, Katcher A, Thomas S, et al. Social interaction and blood pressure: influence of animal companions. *J Nerv Ment Dis* 1983;171:461–465.

47. Fick K. The influence of an animal on social interactions of nursing home residents in a group setting. *Am J Occup Ther* 1993;46:529–534.

48. Good for the heart? *DVM* 1992;23:18–20.

49. Anderson W, Reid C, Jennings G. Pet ownership and risk factors for cardiovascular disease. *Med J Aust* 1992;157: 298–301.

50. Does pet ownership reduce your risk for heart disease? *Interactions* 1992;10(3):11–13.

51. Rowan A, Beck A. Editorial: the health benefits of human-animal interactions. *Anthrozoos* 1994;7(2):85–89.

52. Chinnar T, Dalziel F. An exploratory study on the viability and efficacy of a pet-facilitated therapy project within a hospice. *J Palliat Care* 1991;7(4):13–20.

53. Albert T. Visiting people who have AIDS. *Pet Partners* 1996;6(2):1–2.

54. Pet Partners offer comfort, delight children with AIDS. *Pet Partners* 1992;2:4.

55. Schantz PM. Preventing potential health hazards incidental to the use of pets in therapy. *Anthrozoos* 1990;4(1):14–23.

56. Chenny Troupe volunteer manual. Chicago: Rehabilitation Institute of Chicago, 1994:12.

57. Delta Society. Keeping track of visits. *Pet Partners* 1995;5:1.

58. Delta Society. How to handle a mishap. *Pet Partners* 1993;3: 2.

59. Westbrook GJ. Animal-assisted therapy: risks and risk-minimalization procedures. *Contin Care* 1988; Feb:26–27.

60. Fine AH, Fine NM. Broadening the impact of services and recreational therapies—section 2: animal assisted therapy. In: Fine AH, Fine NM, Zapf SA, et al. eds. *Therapeutic recreation for exceptional children: let me in, I want to play.* 2nd ed. Springfield, IL: Charles C. Thomas, 1996:270–288.

61. Stavishinsky JS. Intimacy, domesticity and pet therapy with the elderly: expectation and experi-

ence among nursing home volunteers. *Soc Sci Med [Med Psychol Med Sociol]* 1992;34:1325–1334.

62. Davis KD. Conserving your facility's animal-handling volunteers: people issues. *Alpha Bits* 1994;5(3):2.

63. Breske S. Animal-assisted therapy: anything but a pet peeve. *Adv Phys Ther* 1993;4:22–23.

64. Contraindications for therapeutic riding: precautions and possible contraindications for therapeutic riding. In: *NARHA workshop notebook.* 1991:E7.

Chapter 42

Speech, Language, and Hearing Intervention in Adults

Fabiane M. Hirsch
Pelagie M. Beeson

Speech-language pathologists and audiologists work with individuals across the life span to assess and remediate communication disorders due to congenital, developmental, and acquired impairments. The focus of this chapter is the management of communication disorders acquired after normal speech and language have developed, that is, problems typically addressed in the adult population. Acquired communication disorders may result from nervous system damage affecting the cognitive, linguistic, sensory, or motor abilities. Or, they may result from dysfunctional behaviors, such as vocal misuse, or significant changes in structural anatomy, such as following laryngectomy. The rehabilitation of patients with acquired communication disorders typically includes efforts to promote the restitution of normal structure and function, the relearning of lost or impaired functions, and the development of compensatory strategies to overcome persistent impairments. Treatment approaches are influenced by issues such as time after onset of the impairment (acute versus chronic), whether the disorder is progressive or static, as well as other factors such as motivation, medical status, and overall cognitive function.

The adult communication disorders reviewed in this chapter are often seen in medical settings across the spectrum of acute care, inpatient and outpatient rehabilitation centers, as well as speech, language, and hearing clinics. A sampling of current treatment approaches is reviewed across an array of communication disorders. Emphasis is given to behavioral treatment as the most common intervention approach; however, pharmacologic, surgical, and prosthetic interventions are discussed as well. Although this chapter focuses on the roles of speech-language pathologists and audiologists, their work frequently is accomplished in a dynamic, interdisciplinary context.

ACQUIRED IMPAIRMENTS OF LANGUAGE OR COGNITION

Aphasia

Aphasia is the most common acquired language impairment in adults, affecting approximately 1 million Americans (1). Aphasia results from brain damage to the language-dominant hemisphere, typically the left, and comprises disturbances of spoken language, auditory comprehension, reading, and writing. Treatment of aphasia is directed toward one or more language modalities (including verbal, written, and gestural) with the following goals: (1) to maximize the recovery of language skills, (2) to assist in the development of compensatory strategies, and (3) to assist aphasic individuals in their adjustment to the difference between their prior and residual language abilities (2).

The language profile of individuals with aphasia varies in accordance with lesion location, extent of brain damage, and premorbid brain organization for language. Most clinicians characterize the language profile by examination of verbal expression, auditory comprehension, and verbal repetition, as well as reading and writing abilities.

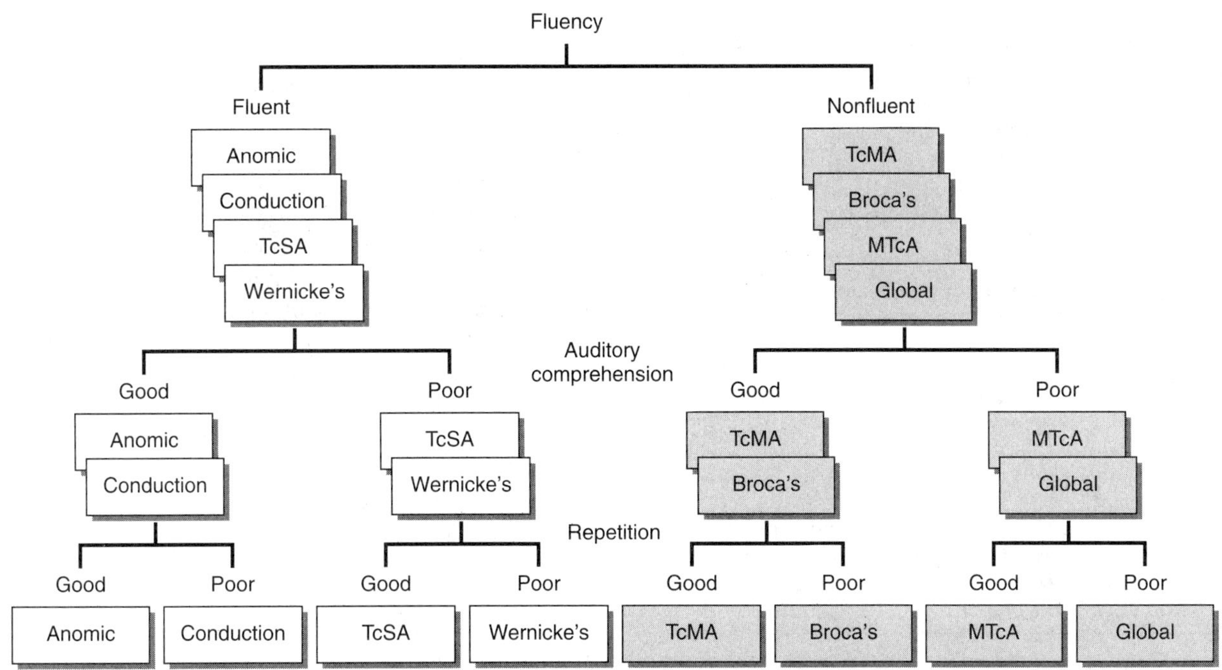

Figure 42-1. Decision tree for the classification of aphasia into eight classic types. Decisions are based on fluency, auditory comprehension, and repetition abilities. TcSA = transcortical sensory aphasia; TcMA = transcortical motor aphasia; MTcA = mixed transcortical aphasia. (Reproduced by permission from Beeson PM, Bayles KA. Aphasia. In: Nussbaum PD, ed. *Handbook of neuropsychology and aging.* New York: Plenum, 1997:300.)

Standardized tests are useful to sample language behaviors and profile the nature and severity of aphasia (3–5), thus providing a starting point for treatment planning and a basis for posttreatment comparison. Informal observation and nonstandardized assessment procedures that probe specific communication behaviors also provide information useful for guiding the treatment plan.

There are eight classic aphasia syndromes that have proved useful for characterizing language profiles (Fig. 42-1). Specification of aphasia type does not lead to the prescription of a particular treatment, but it does provide information regarding relative strengths and weaknesses, the likely evolution of the language profile, and the prognosis for recovery. Naming is impaired in all aphasia types, but aphasia syndromes vary with regard to speech fluency, auditory comprehension, and the ability to repeat (6,7). The decision tree shown in Figure 42-1 shows how aphasia types are generally classified. Four aphasia types are considered to be fluent: conduction, Wernicke's, transcortical sensory (TcSA), and anomic aphasias. They are characterized by plentiful verbal output consisting of well-articulated, easily produced utterances of relatively normal length and prosody (variations of pitch, loudness, rhythm). The nonfluent aphasias, which include Broca's, global, transcortical motor (TcMA), and mixed transcortical (MTcA) aphasias, are characterized by sparse, effortful utterances of short phrases and disrupted prosody. Auditory comprehension is a relative strength in Broca's, conduction, transcortical motor, and anomic aphasias, and a weakness in Wernicke's, global, transcortical sensory, and mixed transcortical aphasias. The ability to repeat sentences is relatively preserved for individuals with anomic aphasia and all three types of transcortical aphasia, but is impaired in the other aphasia types.

Treatment plans are tailored to the specific patient and take into consideration the nature of the impairment, overall cognitive abilities, and residual language processes, as well as the time after onset and functional needs of the individual. A sizable literature on treatment offers guidance for treatment planning. Some of the notable treatment approaches for aphasia include language stimulation techniques (8,9), programmed treatment approaches (7), psycholinguistic approaches (10), and treatments derived from cognitive processing models (11–13). Treatment also includes the development of strategies to maximize communication despite significant or persistent language impairment (14). Examples of treatment approaches are reviewed in the following sections relative to specific impairments.

Treating Aphasic Naming Impairment

Naming impairment is a feature of all aphasia types; consequently, treatment to enhance word finding is common in aphasia therapy. Naming failure can result from a breakdown at various stages of the lexical retrieval process, so a variety of treatment procedures may be appropriate. Treatment protocols may employ a cuing hierarchy that facilitates word retrieval (15–17). The goal of such therapy is to

Table 42-1: Example of Cuing Hierarchy for Naming

1. What is this? (Confrontation naming.)
2. Can you tell me something about it? What is it used for? What do you call it?
   (Semantic elaboration by the patient may result in lexical retrieval.)
3. It is used for writing. It is a _________.
   (Semantic elaboration by the clinician followed by sentence completion may serve to stimulate lexical retrieval.)
4. I write with a _________. (Completion of high-probability sentence or phrase may evoke the correct response.)
5. I write with a (placement for /p/) _________. (High-probability sentence followed by cue for articulatory placement.)
6. I write with a pe_________. (High-probability sentence followed by phonemic cuing may evoke the correct response.)
7. It's a pencil. Say pencil. _________ (Imitation.)

enhance lexical retrieval in a structured paradigm in order to increase the likelihood that such responses return to volitional control. Treatment may proceed from the easiest (i.e., most supported) to the hardest task, progressing as response stability is attained at each level. For example, tasks may progress from naming in imitation, then naming in response to an initial syllable cue, then naming in sentence completion, and finally spontaneous naming. Alternatively, responses may be elicited following a progression from the most difficult to the easiest task, as shown in Table 42-1. A semantic and phonemic cuing progression is provided until the target response is achieved, at which time the cues are incrementally reduced until independent naming is achieved, in essence, progressing again to the hardest task. In effect, this procedure serves to provide only the support that is necessary to elicit the response, and through reduction of support, allows patients to work toward the establishment and maintenance of independent, correct responses.

Treating Disorders of Verbal Expression in Connected Speech

Connected speech requires retrieval of content words embedded in the appropriate syntactic structure and with the appropriate morphologic markers (e.g., word endings to mark tense or number). Treatment approaches for verbal expression are tailored to the specific nature of the individual's verbal output. In particular, individuals who lack grammatical structure, for example, those with Broca's aphasia, may be treated with methods designed to expand the complexity and length of their utterances. The clinician typically implements a treatment progression that is consistent with the relative difficulty of syntactic constructions (2,7,18). For example, simple declarative constructions would be the focus of treatment before future tense.

In contrast to the reduced grammatical structure, or agrammatism, seen in nonfluent aphasia, individuals with fluent aphasia may produce confusing grammatical structures characterized by incorrect word order and morphologic endings, referred to as *paragrammatic speech.* Treatment for such individuals may be directed toward a reduction of excessive verbal output and an increase in self-monitoring of the content and quality of spoken output, with an emphasis on the efficient conveyance of meaning. Treatment may also include efforts to reduce perseverative responses that interfere with attempts to produce meaningful utterances (7), a problem that occurs with nonfluent as well as fluent aphasia.

When verbal expression deficits are severe, treatment includes the identification, development, and use of compensatory communication strategies, such as the use of gestures, drawing, and assistive devices (including *low-tech* communication books and *high-tech* computers). Systematic training of these techniques increases their effectiveness (7,19).

Treating Auditory Comprehension Deficits

Auditory comprehension is typically impaired to some extent in all patients with aphasia, but may range from a mild difficulty understanding syntactically complex utterances to a severe inability to understand single words. Treatment for auditory comprehension targets the level of breakdown and provides structured tasks that require processing of auditory input at progressively higher levels of difficulty. Some treatment protocols emphasize auditory input alone, whereas other procedures include visual (pictured or written) input along with the auditory stimuli (20). The task continuum may proceed from comprehension of single words to phrases (e.g., simple commands), to more complex sentences (e.g., yes/no questions, understanding descriptions, following directions), and ultimately to comprehension of spoken discourse. Other linguistic features that influence task difficulty are taken into consideration; examples include grammatical category (e.g., nouns are easier to process than prepositions) and syntactic structure (e.g., negatives and reflexive pronouns are easier to comprehend than tense, word order, and relative clauses) (21). Auditory comprehension can also be improved by tasks that do not specifically target auditory processing, yet require attention to auditory input (7).

Treating Acquired Reading and Writing Impairments

Acquired reading impairment (alexia) can occur in relative isolation, but more frequently coexists as part of an aphasia syndrome. Literate adults typically read by whole-word recognition, but can sound out words when necessary. Brain damage can disrupt either or both of these reading processes, resulting in various acquired alexia syndromes. Treatment procedures for acquired alexia are not as well established as treatments for auditory comprehension or verbal expression, but there is increasing attention to this clinical area. Individuals with pure alexia, who do not recognize whole words, often adopt a letter-by-letter reading strategy, whereby words are recognized only after their component letters are sequentially identified. This strategy is relatively successful but painfully slow, requiring treatment to increase reading rate (22,23). Individuals who fail to recognize words but can convert letters to their associated sounds can read by phonologic decoding. This syndrome, called *surface dyslexia*, results in reading errors for irregularly spelled words and confusion with homophones. Two other syndromes, deep dyslexia and phonological dyslexia, are characterized by word recognition deficits and an inability to "sound out" words. Treatment can be directed toward strengthening the link between the semantic concept and written words (24,25), or reestablishing letter and sound correspondences (26). Many individuals with acquired alexia have impairments at several stages of processing, so that treatment protocols are multifaceted.

Acquired writing problems (agraphia) often reflect language impairments including word-finding difficulties and problems with sentence construction, but writing can also be disturbed because of problems specific to retrieval of the written word form, letter selection, motor planning, and motor control. Treatment for agraphia associated with language impairment is directed toward facilitating recall of spelling or the use of a compensatory strategy that takes advantage of sound-to-letter correspondences, or both (27). Treatment of the direct spelling route aims to strengthen the link between word meanings and their written representation. The use of sound-to-letter correspondences can be exploited as a compensatory strategy whereby words are sounded out and each sound is converted to its corresponding letter. Some treatment approaches serve to rebuild writing skills in an item-specific manner (i.e., word by word), whereas other procedures target the remediation of processes that improve spelling for a broader corpus of words. In some patients, writing problems that arise from more peripheral deficits that interfere with letter formation can be compensated for by the use of typewriters or word processors; other patients require treatment directed at the written formation of letters and words.

Pragmatic Approaches to Language Intervention for Aphasia

Therapeutic intervention for aphasia includes the development of strategies that facilitate successful communication despite the language impairment. These approaches are not directed toward remediation of the language deficits, but rather focus on optimal use of residual communication abilities. This may include the use of nonverbal communication, such as intonation, facial expression, gesture, and drawing, but may also encompass verbal strategies. Conversational coaching, for example, is a treatment approach whereby individuals with aphasia are taught to develop and rehearse useful "scripts" that provide the necessary support for spoken communication (14). Training to maximize communication involves family members and other significant communicators because the shift from predominantly spoken communication to more holistic approaches is not always a natural one (28).

Communication Disorders Associated with Right Hemisphere Damage

Right hemisphere damage may result in language impairments similar to those experienced by individuals with aphasia, such as word retrieval problems and comprehension deficits, but more prominent effects are typically noted in extralinguistic and nonlinguistic behaviors that may themselves have an impact on communication (29). Extralinguistic features that may be impaired include thought organization, mental flexibility, and pragmatic skills. Because of impaired thought organization, patients with right hemisphere damage may be unable to recognize the gist, or main idea, of a conversation or event, even though they recognize the individual components. As a result, they often have difficulty accurately inferring meaning, both from conversation and from the environment in general, giving the appearance of confusion or disorientation. Impaired thought organization may also be revealed in the patient's verbal expression, which is characteristically rambling and tangential, often providing much detail but missing the main point. Reduced mental flexibility may be evident in a patient's inability to recognize all possible meanings of a word or phrase with resultant literal interpretation of figurative language, such as idioms, proverbs, and metaphors. For example, the phrase "he hit the roof" may be interpreted literally, rather than as implying anger. Processing of humor, irony, and sarcasm may be similarly impaired. Lack of mental flexibility may also result in difficulty appropriately revising an interpretation of a situation when new information necessitates a change, and in changing topics effectively in conversation. Finally, pragmatic skills necessary for good conversational interactions may be compromised by right hemisphere damage. The natural give-and-take of conversational exchange may be violated by inappropriate interruptions and failure to utilize eye contact to maintain a communicative interaction. Unresponsiveness to facial expressions, body language, and prosodic cues that convey meaning and emotion also can contribute to miscommunication and poor interpersonal interactions. The production of prosodic variation may also be disturbed, yielding monotone speech that may be misinterpreted in conversation, or may result in diagnostic errors for affective disorders, such as depression.

Nonlinguistic deficits associated with right hemisphere damage that may interfere with communication include left neglect and attention impairments. Despite intact sensory function, patients with left neglect fail to respond to information in the left visual field or on the left side of the body. Left neglect may result in inattention to communication partners situated in the left hemifield, errors in reading due to missed letters or words on the left side of the page, and written output limited to the right side of the paper, often with progressively larger left margins. Impaired attention, which may actually encompass left neglect, may limit the ability of a patient to attend to environmental cues, to sustain concentration during conversation and other tasks, and to selectively pay attention to important information.

Intervention for the cognitive-communication impairments associated with right hemisphere damage may be directed toward remediation of the underlying deficit or development of compensatory strategies. Sample tasks for treatment are provided in Table 42-2. Simulated functional activities incorporating several of the tasks in Table 42-2 allow the practice of necessary skills for real-world situations. For example, calling to make a dinner reservation requires looking up a phone number in a phone book, dialing the number correctly, interacting with the hostess, and recording the information for later reference. Recording these tasks on audiotape or videotape allows the clinician and patient to analyze the patient's performance together, in order to facilitate recognition of deficits, determine mutual goals, and demonstrate improvement over time. Much frustration may be avoided by explaining deficits associated with right-hemisphere damage to caregivers and family members and teaching them ways to compensate for possible difficulties in daily life.

Table 42-2: Treatment Tasks for Management of Right-Hemisphere Communication Disorders

Deficits	Treatment Tasks
Thought organization	Story retelling Responding to divergent questions on topics of interest Describing pictures, events, etc Organizing steps for completing multistep tasks Developing narratives Performing simulated functional activities (calling the doctor, making trip reservations, etc)
Mental flexibility	Generating multiple meanings of words Identifying inconsistencies in narratives Interpreting figurative language (idioms, proverbs, metaphors)
Pragmatic skills	Participating in spontaneous conversation (one-on-one or in group) on current events or topics of interest Recognizing indicators of emotion from photographs, intonation, etc Practicing production of varied intonation patterns
Attention/left neglect	Performing cancellation tasks Bisecting lines Drawing symmetric objects Reading words, sentences, and paragraphs Copying written information and writing spontaneously Implementing compensatory strategies, such as using a brightly colored marker to note the left margin of the page during functional reading and writing

Dementia

Dementia is an acquired impairment of intellectual functioning that may affect cognition, memory, language, and visuospatial skills, as well as emotion and personality (30). Assessment of cognitive and communication abilities contributes to the differential diagnosis process, serves to monitor the progression of the syndrome, and provides information necessary for the development of environmental intervention techniques, caregiver training, and family counseling.

The management plan for dementia should address issues affecting both language comprehension and production. To facilitate comprehension, caregivers may be trained to reduce the length and syntactic complexity of spoken utterances, increase the redundancy and availability of contextual cues, as well as use gestures, pictures, and written words to supplement spoken language. Reducing distractions can also markedly improve communicative interactions. The spoken output of individuals with dementia is often characterized by anomia, empty utterances, and perseveration in the early stages, and may be reduced to unintelligible jargon or mutism in the later stages. Listeners can employ strategies to reduce communication failure by structuring conversation, providing concrete choices, and redirecting attention.

Communication may be impaired further by reduced speech intelligibility, most notably in patients with a subcortical dementia, such as dementia associated with Parkinson disease or Huntington disease. Treatment for speech production disorders is discussed in the section on motor speech disorders. Memory books that contain biographical sketches, pictures of family and friends, and schedule information may act not only as external memory aids, but also as valuable resources to stimulate communicative interaction (31).

MOTOR SPEECH DISORDERS

The Dysarthrias

The dysarthrias are a collection of speech disorders characterized by paralysis, weakness, or incoordination of the speech musculature, with resultant deficits in oral communication (32). Dysarthria may result from a disruption of any of the processes critical for speech production, including respiration, phonation, articulation, resonance, or prosody.

Eight dysarthria types have been identified according to their underlying neuropathology and distinctive speech characteristics (33). *Flaccid dysarthria* results from lower motor neuron damage with resultant weakness and reduced tone of the speech musculature. The prominent speech characteristics include hypernasality, imprecise consonant production, breathy voice, and monopitch. The particular constellation of these deficits reflects the lesion location. Flaccid dysarthria may result from surgical or other traumatic injury, but it is also associated with diseases such as myasthenia gravis, botulism, poliomyelitis, Guillain-Barré syndrome, muscular dystrophy, progressive bulbar palsy, and acquired immunodeficiency syndrome (AIDS)–related complications such as cryptococcal meningitis. Flaccid dysarthria may also result from vascular disorders, such as brain stem stroke and Wallenberg's lateral medullary syndrome.

Spastic dysarthria arises from bilateral upper motor neuron damage that results in combined effects of excessive muscle tone and muscle weakness. Speech characteristics may include imprecise consonants, strained-strangled vocal quality, low pitch and pitch breaks, and slow speech rate. Patients with spastic dysarthria often complain of their speech being slow and effortful. Possible causes include brain stem strokes, bilateral hemisphere infarcts, multi-infarct dementia, leukoencephalitis, primary lateral sclerosis, and traumatic brain injury.

Damage to the cerebellum and its connections may result in *ataxic dysarthria*, which is characterized by reduced tone and incoordination of speech muscles. Speech often contains irregular articulatory breakdowns, excess and equal stress, imprecise consonants, and distorted vowel sounds. Patients may complain of the "drunken" quality of their speech. Degenerative diseases, such as Friedreich's ataxia, are the most common etiology; however, vascular lesions, cerebellar tumors, traumatic brain injury, severe hypothyroidism, and neurotoxic levels of anticonvulsant and antidepressant medications may also be associated with ataxic speech characteristics.

Hypokinetic dysarthria results from damage to the basal ganglia and their connections and is characterized by muscle rigidity and reduced force and range of movement. Patients may complain of having a weak voice and a rapid rate of speech. This is the only dysarthria type in which an increase of speech rate may be noted. Other deviant speech characteristics may include harsh or breathy vocal quality, monopitch, monoloudness, reduced stress, short phrases, and imprecise consonants. Parkinson's disease is the prototypic disease associated with hypokinetic dysarthria; however, patients with late-stage Alzheimer or Pick disease and those with a history of repeated head trauma may also demonstrate these features.

In contrast to hypokinetic dysarthria, basal ganglia damage may alternatively result in *hyperkinetic dysarthria*. This dysarthria type may be associated also with damage to the cerebellum or related extrapyramidal tracts. Hyperkinetic dysarthria is characterized by the presence of involuntary movements that disrupt normal speech prosody. Subtypes of hyperkinetic dysarthria can be identified according to the site of the lesion and the form of the speech disorder. For example, perceptual speech features of diseases with characteristic choreiform movements, such as Huntington disease, typically include variable speech rate, inappropriate silences, excess loudness variations, sudden forced inspiration or expiration, and voice stoppages. Other subtypes include those associated with dystonia, dyskinesia (such as tardive dyskinesia), myoclonus, tics (such as Tourette syndrome), spasm, and essential tremor.

When two or more dysarthria types are found in combination, a diagnosis of *mixed dysarthria* is accepted. Mixed dysarthrias may be found in patients with amyotrophic lateral sclerosis, which typically results in spastic-flaccid dysarthria; multiple sclerosis, which may result in spastic-ataxic dysarthria among other combinations; Friedreich's ataxia, which most often results in ataxic-spastic dysarthria; and progressive supranuclear palsy, which is typically associated with hypokinetic, spastic, and ataxic signs. Mixed dysarthrias may also be associated with Shy-Drager syndrome, toxic-metabolic conditions such as Wilson disease, brain stem or multiple strokes, and infectious diseases such as meningitis, encephalitis, and AIDS.

The final two dysarthria types are cited less frequently in clinical practice but appear to be gaining support as valid dysarthria diagnoses (33). *Unilateral upper motor neuron dysarthria* results from damage confined to one cerebral hemisphere, in contrast to spastic dysarthria which results from bilateral damage. Weakness and incoordination on the side of the face and tongue opposite the lesion location may result in disordered articulation, but are often mild and temporary. Patients may complain of slurred speech, a "heavy" lower face, or a "thick" tongue. Stroke is the most common cause of unilateral upper motor neuron dysarthria.

When a dysarthria profile reflects unusual or contradictory signs so that the above-described classifications are not appropriate, the label *motor speech disorder, type undetermined* may be most appropriate. It may well be that all distinct dysarthria types have not yet been recognized. This category allows clinicians and researchers to keep an open mind to the possibility of determining additional dysarthria types.

With such an assortment of neuropathologies and speech characteristics under the dysarthria umbrella, it is not surprising that there is no single treatment strategy for managing dysarthria. The vast array of treatment approaches may be generally classified as medical, prosthetic, and behavioral (33). Medical intervention encompasses pharmacologic and surgical management aimed directly or indirectly at improving speech intelligibility. Prosthetic intervention involves introduction of a prosthetic device to compensate for impaired speech function. Behavioral intervention typically forms the bulk of speech-language pathology services and includes clinician-directed activities designed to improve physiologic support for speech, implement facilitative speaking strategies, utilize alternative or augmentative communication (AAC) systems, and change the communication environment to best accommodate the needs of dysarthric individuals. Treatment is typically directed toward one or more of the speech production processes (respiration, phonation, articulation, resonance, and prosody) with the overall goal of maximizing the effectiveness, efficiency, and naturalness of communication (34).

Respiration

The respiratory system provides the primary aerodynamic force necessary for speech production. Reduced respiratory support can significantly affect speech intelligibility, particularly when there is inadequate air pressure to produce speech sounds. Prosthetic or behavioral management may be indicated to achieve adequate respiratory support to maintain consistent subglottal air pressure for speech.

Prosthetic assistance for respiratory function may include binding the abdomen in order to increase expiratory force during speech (34). Abdominal binding may be used with patients who have spinal cord injuries and requires careful medical supervision. For other patient populations, positioning devices may be used to make adjustments in the patient's position in a wheelchair or bed, to improve respiratory support for speech.

Behavioral techniques may be directed toward improving the physiologic function of respiration for speech or compensating for impaired function. Physiologic function may be strengthened by speech or nonspeech activities; however, speech activities are often preferred because of their closer association to the goal of functional communication. Nonspeech activities might include blowing exercises using air pressure transducers and on-line feedback to achieve increased respiratory drive for speech (34). An analogous speech activity would include vowel prolongation on a single breath with on-line feedback for loudness and duration. Pushing and pulling exercises that require the patient to generate physical force can be utilized to increase subglottal air pressure during phonation. Compensatory behavioral strategies include training the patient to inhale more deeply prior to speaking, initiate speech at the inspiratory peak rather than after partial exhalation, and use shorter phrases in conversation to ensure speech is loud enough to be heard throughout each phrase.

Phonation

Phonation is the production of voiced sound by vibration of the vocal folds. Vocal quality disturbances associated with dysarthria may be relatively trivial in some patients, but may significantly compromise intelligibility in others. Medical interventions may be indicated to improve phonatory quality (33). For example, patients with laryngeal hypofunction due to paralysis or weakness may benefit from laryngoplasty, a surgical procedure to improve vocal fold approximation. Teflon and collagen injections into the vocal folds share this goal. For vocal fold overadduction, as observed in adductor spasmodic dysphonia, medical treatment may include recurrent laryngeal nerve resection or injections of botulinum toxin (Botox) to reduce the hyperfunction. Prosthetic intervention for dysarthric phonation disorders may include a portable amplification system to increase loudness, or an artificial larynx to provide a stronger vibratory source for speech.

If laryngeal tension and hyperadduction are the presenting problems, relaxation techniques, such as yawn-sigh exercises and laryngeal massage, may be appropriate. Therapy may also include practice initiating speech with a breathy onset or sigh. For laryngeal hypofunction, behavioral management may include techniques to maximize vocal cord adduction, such as controlled coughing, pushing, and pulling. The Lee Silverman Voice Treatment (LSVT) is a well-documented program shown to improve loudness and overall speech intelligibility of individuals with Parkinson disease (35). The LSVT focuses on increased loudness as a means to achieve more effortful speech production that serves to overcome (or minimize) the hypofunction associated with Parkinson disease.

Articulation

Imprecise articulation is common with dysarthria and may result in significantly impaired speech intelligibility. Medical interventions such as injection of Botox to treat oral mandibular dystonia may be appropriate to improve movement of the articulators. Antispasticity and tremor-reducing medications also may improve articulatory precision. Prosthetic approaches to improve articulation are not common, but a bite block placed between the lateral upper and lower teeth may facilitate intelligible speech in patients with jaw-opening dystonia or Parkinson disease (33).

Behavioral approaches to improve articulation include some nonspeech activities, such as strengthening, relaxation, and stretching exercises; however, speech activities are the primary focus of articulation treatment. Treatment may include a combination or hierarchical ordering of tasks such as 1) imitation exercises following an articulatory model provided by the clinician; 2) phonetic placement activities in which articulators such as the lips and tongue are manually placed in the correct positions to provide tactile feedback for reinforcement of correct articulatory positions; 3) speech production using pictures and mirrors to facilitate accurate placement; 4) phonetic derivation in which intact nonspeech gestures are used to achieve a target, for example, using blowing to facilitate production of the /u/ sound; 5) exaggeration activities in which speech is slowed and individual articulations are exaggerated; 6) minimal contrast activities in which pairs of words with minimal contrasts, for example, "pie-bye," are practiced to solidify the articulatory differences required to make the distinction between similar sounds clear; and 7) intelligibility drills in which words and sentences are produced in drill-like fashion to secure precise articulatory placement (33). Tasks are selected and ordered so that correct articulation is facilitated and stabilized, and successful generalization outside the therapy environment is achieved. Recordings on audiotape and videotape are useful for providing feedback and documenting change over time.

Resonance

Normal speech production requires rapid elevation and relaxation of the soft palate, or velum, to affect changes in resonance features that distinguish oral and nasal sounds. Dysfunction of the velopharyngeal mechanism can result in abnormal resonance and inadequate oral pressure for consonant production. Velopharyngeal hypofunction is common with dysarthria and results in hypernasality and reduced intraoral pressure that may significantly reduce speech intelligibility. Velopharyngeal hyperfunction is less common, but can result in hyponasality, or denasality, which is recognizable as the speech that accompanies a "stuffy nose." Resonance may also be disturbed in patients with dysarthria where the timing of motor movements is disturbed.

Pharyngeal flap surgery, although popular for decreasing hypernasality in children with velopharyngeal insufficiency following adenoid removal or cleft palate repair, is not typically employed for the treatment of dysarthria. More commonly, a prosthesis that lifts the soft palate is fitted by a prosthodontist to manage hypernasality. This prosthesis consists of a plate that is fitted to the hard palate and typically anchored to the teeth. The posterior extension of the lift elevates the velum to approximate the posterior pharyngeal wall, thus reducing the strength and movement required to close the velopharyngeal opening.

Behavioral management approaches to improve velopharyngeal closure may include velar stimulation (e.g., pressure, icing, brushing) or strengthening techniques (blowing, sucking), but these are often ineffective (33). Postural management, such as use of a reclining wheelchair, may reduce hypernasality by using gravity to approximate the velum to the posterior pharyngeal wall. Unfortunately, important pragmatic aspects of communication, such as eye contact, can be compromised by implementing such postural changes. If velopharyngeal closure can be achieved, but is inconsistent, speech production tasks may be used to increase awareness and to monitor appropriate resonance for increasingly complex speech tasks.

Prosody

Rate of speech is a key prosodic feature and may constitute a primary focus of dysarthria therapy. Management can include implementation of devices, such as delayed auditory feedback (DAF) instruments, pacing boards, or metronomes. The goal is to decrease speech rate in an effort to increase intelligibility. An alphabet board can be used similarly; the combination of first-letter identification and decreased rate can significantly improve intelligibility of a severely dysarthric speaker. Treatment that does not rely on external devices can also be pursued. Simply pacing syllable production by tapping the hand or finger on the arm of a chair may be sufficient to adequately reduce speech rate. Rhythmic cuing in which the patient reads a passage as the clinician points to each word in a rhythmic fashion, can be useful practice for developing a slower speaking rate (33). The management approach depends on the patient's motivation and success during attempts at using the different techniques.

Attempts to improve the naturalness of speech, typically by normalizing stress patterns, may also be a focus of therapy. An approach that examines what a patient uses naturally to signal stress, whether it be pitch changes, loudness changes, syllable prolongation, or other strategies, is a good start. Subsequent speech activities can incorporate and build on these findings. Tasks may be highly structured initially, for example, utilizing pitch changes appropriately during recitation of a small set of sentences. A progression to scripted conversation and then spontaneous speech may follow. Recording on audiotape can be invaluable in providing feedback at all levels.

The treatment approaches mentioned thus far have all focused on improving the speech of the dysarthric speaker. Techniques aimed at improving actual communicative interactions, that is, techniques directed toward both the speaker and the listener in conversation, complement the more traditional deficit-oriented approaches. Dysarthric speaker strategies may include informing the communication partner about the nature of the speech problem, explaining any augmentative devices being used, providing the topic before initiating the details of a conversation, decreasing the length of utterances, and maintaining eye contact. The patient must act as his or her own advocate to ensure the communication of wants and needs. Listener strategies may include ensuring minimal background noise and adequate lighting, maintaining face-to-face contact, utilizing any needed hearing and vision aids, confirming understanding of the speaker's output, and asking for clarification as needed. Responsibility for many of the techniques falls on both members of the communication dyad, and agreement between partners on approaches to repair communication breakdowns is critical. Videotaping of interactions with subsequent critique of approaches can facilitate development of the most effective system.

Apraxia of Speech

Apraxia of speech (AOS), like dysarthria, is a motor speech disorder. Unlike dysarthria, however, neuromuscular function of the speech mechanism is considered to be intact in apraxia. AOS is a disturbance of motor programming for the positioning and movement of the articulators for speech production that can exist in the absence of muscle weakness. As such, a patient with AOS appears to be able to formulate the desired message and has the muscle function to perform the appropriate movements to produce the message, but has difficulty planning these movements. This describes AOS in its purest form. In clinical reality, however, AOS frequently co-occurs with aphasia or dysarthria, making it difficult to isolate the apraxic component.

The most common cause of apraxia of speech is stroke, with lesions usually found in the left posterior frontal or parietal lobe, the insula, or the basal ganglia. Tumor or trauma affecting these areas may also result in AOS. Less often, degenerative neurologic diseases such as multiple sclerosis, corticobasal degeneration, primary progressive aphasia, and Creutzfeldt-Jakob disease may be associated with AOS (33).

Apraxic speech is characterized as slow, labored, and effortful, and marred by inconsistent articulation errors, typically consonant and vowel distortions and substitutions. Speech initiation may be disturbed, and patients often appear to grope for correct articulatory positions. Syllable repetitions are also quite common. In addition, apraxic speech often has altered prosody and unusual stress patterns.

Treatment for AOS, as for dysarthria, aims to maximize the effectiveness, efficiency, and naturalness of communication. AOS management focuses, however, on reestablishing the motor programs or the ability to program speech movements, rather than on improving physiologic speech processes (33). Management for AOS relies predominantly on behavioral techniques but can include medical and prosthetic approaches. Pharmacologic interventions (e.g., anticoagulants to prevent stroke, antibiotics to prevent infection) and surgical interventions (e.g., endarterectomy, tumor removal, aneurysm repair) may indirectly affect the nature and severity of AOS, but no medications or surgical procedures are specifically designed to improve AOS. Prosthetic management may include implementation of AAC devices as simple as letter boards or as complex as electronic devices. Equipment for vibrotactile stimulation (36), electrolarynx for patients with phonatory difficulties (37), and electromyographic feedback to induce relaxation (38), have been used with reported success but are not common treatment practices for AOS.

Behavioral management for AOS typically focuses on articulation and prosody. Suitable goals and activities vary according to the nature and severity of the apraxia, but some common components pervade most treatments for AOS. These include careful selection and ordering of stimuli to achieve a continuum of task difficulty, utilization of imitation tasks incorporating both visual and auditory modalities, and intensive drill to re-establish automaticity of speech production (33).

For patients with severe AOS characterized by muteness or unreliable vocalization, activities may focus on eliciting any form of vocal or verbal response. Tasks may include attempts at producing automatic speech sequences (e.g., counting, saying days of the week, reciting prayers), completing predictable phrases (e.g., "salt and __"), singing familiar songs, and pairing words with automatic gestures (e.g., hand wave with verbal production of "hi"). If the patient is unable to perform any of these tasks, it may be necessary to regress to tasks aimed at improving oral motor control of nonspeech movements. For example, goals may include establishing voluntary control of jaw opening and closure, tongue protrusion and elevation, and lip pursing (39).

For patients with moderate to severe AOS characterized by articulatory errors or syllable repetitions, activities may include facilitation of correct articulatory placements through manual adjustment or use of nonspeech gestures (e.g., blowing to produce lip rounding for /u/ as in "who"). Once isolated sounds have been achieved, attempts can be made to shape these sounds into syllables, words, and phrases (e.g., hum "m," add a vowel to form "ma," add a following consonant to form "mom," and finally develop into a two-word phrase "my mom") (32). A number of formal intervention programs have been utilized in the treatment of patients with moderate to severe AOS (33). These include the eight-step continuum of Rosenbek et al (40), prompts for restructuring oral muscular phonetic targets (PROMPT) (41), melodic intonation therapy (MIT) (42), multiple input phoneme therapy (MIPT) (43), and voluntary control of involuntary utterances (VCIU) (44). Selection of an appropriate treatment protocol is dependent on the specific characteristics of the patient with AOS.

For patients progressing to multisyllable utterances, an appropriate activity may be a phonetic contrast task in which the patient produces word pairs with minimal differences in voicing, vowel sound, or manner or place of articulation (e.g., "to-do," "to-tie," "to-shoe," "to-boo"), to help gain control of articulation across syllables. Similarly, contrastive stress tasks in which varying stress patterns are elicited in sentence production may be appropriate to improve speech prosody. Rate control activities using finger tapping, a pacing board, or a metronome may also be beneficial. Patients with mild AOS also may be taught to self-monitor and self-correct errors in longer and more complex verbal outputs. Tasks may include making sentences with target words or generating narratives about newspaper articles, movies, and so forth (33). Group therapy for AOS may provide the ideal opportunity to practice learned skills in both structured and spontaneous conversation in a supportive environment. Strategies for improving interactions between communication partners, such as reducing background noise, maintaining eye contact, and clarifying the topic of conversation, complement the traditional techniques aimed directly at remediating the apraxia itself.

STRUCTURAL IMPAIRMENTS OF THE SPEECH MECHANISM

Altered Articulators

Impaired speech intelligibility can result not only from motor deficits, but also from alteration of the anatomic structures involved in speech production. Causes include facial trauma, abnormal growths, altered dentition, and surgical resections, such as glossectomy (removal of the tongue or a portion thereof). Intervention approaches vary according to the nature of the anomaly. Medical intervention such as surgical removal of a confounding growth or surgical restoration of altered facial structures may be indicated. Prosthetic intervention may include introduction of a maxillary obturator for patients with structural deficiencies of the hard palate (45) or proper fitting or relining of dentures for edentulous patients. Behavioral management for structural impairments often focuses on determination and implementation of compensatory oral gestures designed to achieve speech that is acoustically acceptable (45); that is, speech that *sounds right.* For example, a patient with a total glossectomy may learn to produce an approximation of a /d/ sound by touching the lower lip to the upper teeth, or a patient with a shortened upper lip may use similar labiodental (lip to teeth) approximations for bilabial consonants such as /b/ and /p/ (45).

Laryngectomy

When the vocal cords are removed, as in the case of laryngectomy, the sound source for speech is lost, often with devastating consequences for communication (46). Laryngectomees can benefit from utilization of one of a variety of available prosthetic sound sources. An electronic artificial larynx, often referred to as an *electrolarynx*, is a device that provides a vibratory source to replace that lost due to the removal of the vocal cords. Intraoral and neck-type devices are available: Intraoral devices transmit sound from a small transducer through a plastic tube into a patient's mouth, whereas neck-type devices, when held firmly against a patient's neck, transmit sound to the oral cavity through the neck tissues (47). Alternatively, a voice prosthesis may be surgically introduced via a tracheoesophageal puncture technique (48). This surgery involves insertion of a voice prosthesis known as a *duckbill* into a fistula created between the trachea and the esophagus. The duckbill is a one-way valve that permits air from the lungs to enter the esophagus when the patient exhales, setting into vibration a segment of the pharyngeal and esophageal muscles, which then act as a vibratory sound source for speech.

An alternative approach for laryngectomees includes teaching esophageal speech, a technique in which the patient learns to trap air in the esophagus and use esophageal-pharyngeal vibration as the sound source for speech (49).

Regardless of the sound source, patients may be taught to maximize intelligibility by exaggerating articulatory movements, slowing speech rate, and shortening phrase length.

Tracheostomies

Normal communication is significantly disrupted when pulmonary airflow is diverted to an opening in the neck before it reaches the vocal cords, as in the case of tracheostomies. Speech production is further complicated in patients who have lost normal respiratory function and must be mechanically ventilated. Patients undergo a tracheostomy or become ventilator dependent for a number of different reasons, including but not limited to respiratory conditions such as chronic obstructive pulmonary disease and acute upper-airway infections, vascular conditions such as stroke, degenerative diseases such as amyotrophic lateral sclerosis and AIDS, obstructive tumors, and trauma.

Management for the communication impairment may include oral and nonoral approaches (50). Oral approaches are typically preferred, as they most closely approximate normal conversation, but depend on the adequacy of the vocal mechanism. If vocal folds are intact and vibrate properly, attempts may be made to re-establish normal phonation. In order to do this, external devices or supplemental techniques are implemented. For example, a "talking" tracheostomy tube that uses an outside air source, such as an air tank, may be introduced. Alternatively, tracheal occlusion may be employed so that the tracheostomy tube is closed off either by simply placing a finger over the port during exhalation or by affixing a one-way speaking valve. The valve allows air to enter the tracheostomy tube during inhalation but does not allow air to exit during exhalation; thus, air is directed to the vocal cords. The appropriateness of each of the mentioned devices depends on the size and type of tracheostomy tube in place, the patient's respiratory status, the patient's anxiety level, and other factors. If phonation is not possible through implementation of the above-mentioned techniques, for example, if the vocal cords are damaged, an alternative vibratory sound source, such as the electrolarynx discussed earlier, may be introduced.

If oral communication is not possible or is unreliable, nonoral approaches must be considered (50). Most patients with new tracheostomies have a period of time during which oral communication is contraindicated. With no means of verbal communication, it is important that an alerting system, such as a specialized call light or independent alarm system, be established and some form of yes/no system, such as an eye blink or eye gaze system, be introduced so that the patient can alert family and staff to emergency situations and express basic needs. Family and staff must be trained in all techniques to maximize the safety and the quality of life of the patient. If short-term nonoral approaches are indicated, low-tech devices such as alphabet boards, patient-specific communication books, and dry-erase boards may be introduced. When long-term nonoral approaches are needed, a variety of nonelectronic and electronic devices are available. Some electronic devices are highly specialized and can include voice or visual output, word prediction, abbreviation expansion, memory for patient-specific vocabularies, and Internet access. Some systems also include options for environmental control, whereby the user can turn on the lights, turn off the television, answer the phone, and control other devices in his or her surroundings. Careful review of features of such systems and careful evaluation of cognitive skills, motor skills, and communication needs facilitate determination of the best choice for each individual patient.

VOICE DISORDERS

Voice disorders may result from neurologic impairment, as discussed in the context of motor speech disorders, and laryngeal malignancy, as addressed in the laryngectomy discussion; however, many acquired voice disorders are related to vocal hyperfunction, the hyperadduction of the vocal cords that may accompany behaviors such as yelling, prolonged or loud speaking, and chronic throat clearing and coughing (47,49,51). Vocal hyperfunction may result in vocal cord thickening, vocal nodules, polyps, or contact ulcers. Attempts to compensate for these structural changes may lead to further vocal hyperfunction, with a resultant reciprocal relationship between pathology and function. Vocal hyperfunction, however, may also be functional without pathology, as in psychological conversion disorders (47).

Intervention for acquired voice disorders begins with an evaluation by an otolaryngologist to determine if medical intervention such as surgical removal of a vocal nodule or prescription of appropriate medications is indicated (51). Following such intervention, or if medical attention is deemed unsuitable, behavioral approaches may be pursued. Behavioral intervention typically involves two paths: 1) identification of vocal abuse and misuse and reduction in the occurrence of these behaviors, and 2) determination of approaches that facilitate the patient's best voice and practice of these approaches in therapy (49). Many facilitating approaches have been identified for the treatment of vocal hyperfunction (47,49,51). Those appropriate for any given patient depend on their demonstrated success in achieving a better voice during trials in therapy. One commonly used approach to reduce vocal hyperfunction is a yawn-sigh technique in which a patient is instructed to yawn, thus opening wide the mouth and pharynx during inhalation, and to lightly phonate on exhalation. The relaxed phonation is extended to produce single-word and multiword productions while maintaining openness of the pharynx and light voicing. Another approach is differential relaxation in which particular muscles, typically around the face, neck, and shoulders, are deliberately relaxed and tensed. Changes to more optimal pitch and loudness may also be the focus of treatment. The speech-language pathologist can determine the optimal combination of approaches for helping the patient achieve the best voice possible. Treatment programs for vocal hyperfunction are typically followed by a vocal hygiene program designed to prevent further vocal abuse and misuse (49).

HEARING DISORDERS

According to the National Center for Health Statistics (52), about 20 million Americans report having some form of hearing problem. The majority of adult hearing loss is sensorineural in nature, reflecting dysfunction of the inner ear, the auditory nerve, or central auditory pathways. Sensorineural hearing loss in adults may be associated with noise exposure, ototoxic drugs, Meniere disease, or aging (presbycusis). A small percentage of hearing-impaired adults have impairment resulting from outer- or middle-ear problems that disrupt the transmission of acoustic energy to the inner ear. Such conductive hearing losses may result from the buildup of cerumen (wax) in the ear canal, eardrum perforation, middle-ear infection, or damage to the bones of the middle ear. In some patients, hearing loss can have mixed etiology with conductive and sensorineural components. Conductive hearing losses are often amenable to medical or surgical intervention; however, sensorineural losses typically are permanent.

Audiologists provide comprehensive hearing assessment that serves to determine 1) the nature and degree of hearing loss; 2) the need and appropriateness of amplification; and 3) the psychosocial, emotional, and educational impact of the hearing impairment. Audiologic assessment may prompt referral for medical intervention. It may also lead to subsequent fitting of a hearing aid, if appropriate, and will guide the aural rehabilitation program. The complexities of the audiologic examination and hearing aid selection are not covered in this chapter, but clearly these are areas of rapid change and technological advances [for a current review, see (53)]. The focus here is on aural rehabilitation activities that complement audiologic assessment and hearing aid selection. *Aural rehabilitation* refers to any attempts to maximize the communication skills of a hearing-impaired individual (54). An aural rehabilitation program is designed to meet the individual's needs and goals, and may include any appropriate combination of the following: 1) hearing aid orientation, 2) implementation of other assistive listening devices (ALDs), 3) counseling, 4) introduction and implementation of facilitative communication strategies, and 5) auditory and visual training.

Hearing Aid Orientation

After the audiologist and patient have determined that a hearing aid is appropriate, and suitable amplification has been selected, an orientation protocol is typically initiated. Such a protocol includes: 1) making physical adjustments to the new aid; 2) training the patient, family members, and caregivers on the use and care of hearing aids; and 3) implementing a program of graduated listening activities to familiarize the patient with hearing aid use. Physical adjustments may include refining the internal hearing aid settings or modifying the earmold as needed. Training includes instruction on the proper insertion and removal of the earmold, volume settings, and special functions, such as use of the telecoil for telephone use, as well as care and cleaning of the aid, battery use, and proper storage of the aid. Such training is provided not only to the wearer, but also to the caregivers. To facilitate adjustment to a new hearing aid, a graduated listening program may be implemented in which the patient begins using the hearing aid for only short periods of time each day within limited environments, and gradually progresses to longer periods of use and more complex listening situations that include unfamiliar persons, groups, and environs with increasing background noise.

Assistive Listening Devices

In some cases, a hearing aid may not be appropriate or adequate for a given individual in a given setting, and other assistive amplification devices may be considered (54). Some ALDs improve hearing by placing a microphone close to the sound source, thus reducing the effects of competing noise and reverberation. Frequency-modulated (FM) systems, for example, provide wireless transmission of radio waves from a microphone placed at the sound source. These radio waves are received and amplified by an instrument worn by the hearing-impaired individual. Such systems are increasingly common in movie theaters, classrooms, and auditoriums. FM systems can also be used for personal amplification in a one-on-one conversation through use of a small microphone by the speaker and an FM receiver by the listener. Alternatively, hardwire systems can be used that consist of a microphone worn or held by the speaker and attached directly to the listener's receiver by a wire. Similar hardwire devices are available for use with television or radio. Portable and built-in telephone amplifiers, as well as hearing aids equipped with telecoils, can be helpful to improve hearing for telephone use. For hearing-impaired persons unable to make auditory use of the phone, telecommunication devices for the deaf (TDDs), which use teletypewriters at both the callers' and receivers' ends, can afford these individuals the convenience of instantaneous distance communication. Finally, visual alerting devices may be established for fire or smoke alarms, the doorbell, telephone, or alarm clock.

Counseling

Critical to the success of any aural rehabilitation program is comprehensive patient and family counseling. Counseling includes provision of information about the function of the ear, causes of hearing loss, interpretation of the audiologic examination, description of the usefulness and limitations of hearing aids and other assistive devices, and instruction on self-advocacy in communicative interactions. For new users of hearing aids, counseling helps them develop realistic expectations and may help them deal with the common new-user complaints that hearing is not returned to normal (i.e., sound distortions persist) and background noise is amplified and distracting. Counseling also serves to give hearing-impaired individuals confidence to inform others of their communication needs (55).

Communication Strategies

Simply providing amplification is often not enough to restore receptive communication skills for hearing-impaired individuals. Instruction may be needed to develop specific strategies to minimize and repair communication breakdowns (54). Important strategies to minimize breakdowns include turning off the television or radio when a conversation is initiated, closing the door or window or moving to a quieter location to reduce background noise, and positioning oneself optimally to receive all possible visual cues from the speaker. Repair strategies include asking the speaker to provide the topic of conversation, to repeat or rephrase what was said, to spell a questionable word, and to speak more slowly and clearly. The other partner in the communication dyad also has a significant role to play in minimizing and repairing communication breakdowns. For example, written communication using a portable dry-erase board or simply a pen and paper can often facilitate repair of breakdowns. Table 42-3 lists additional strategies that the partner can employ in speaking with a hearing-impaired individual.

Auditory and Visual Training

Hearing-impaired individuals need to make the most of their residual hearing and visual input to maximize their communication. Auditory training may include tasks of discrimination and identification of speech sounds, words, and sentences with varying levels of background noise or other distractions (56). Auditory training is typically paired with training to improve speechreading, a technique that

Table 42-3: Speaker Strategies for Talking with a Hearing-Impaired Individual

Environmental considerations
Reduce background noise (turn off TV, close door, move to quieter room)
Get the listener's attention before beginning to speak
Face the hearing-impaired individual when speaking; do not speak while turned away
Ensure light is on your face, rather than behind you
Avoid chewing food or gum while speaking
Ensure your mouth and eyes are clearly visible; do not cover with hands
Speech considerations
Overtly introduce the topic of conversation and any topic changes
Slow speech rate as needed, but not so much as to be insulting
Avoid yelling, as this often gives the facial appearance of anger
Write names and other proper nouns
Speak clearly; avoid both mumbling and overexaggeration of mouth movements

encompasses comprehension of all avenues of visual communication, such as facial expressions and gestures, in addition to traditional lipreading, the recognition of speech sounds by the configuration of the speaker's mouth (56). Training for visual speech identification includes an analytic approach to improve recognition of speech sounds in isolation with subsequent progression to recognition of words and sentences, and a synthetic approach, in which patients learn to recognize the general meaning of a complete oral utterance rather than each individual sound (56). Because many speech sounds look the same (e.g., /p/, /b/, and /m/) and articulatory movements are often too fast to be readily distinguishable, speechreading is typically taught in conjunction with other approaches. Communication groups provide excellent opportunities for hearing-impaired individuals to practice the skills learned in auditory and visual training (57).

FUTURE DIRECTIONS

Some of the basic principles and treatment methods for acquired communication disorders in adults have long traditions in the fields of speech-language pathology and audiology, whereas other approaches reflect new theoretical and technological advances. Communication disorders and sciences intersect the knowledge base of many disciplines including cognitive science, psychology, linguistics, neurology, physiology, education, electronics, and computer technology, to name a few. The dynamic interaction of basic science, clinical research, and application leads to an ever-changing, ever-expanding fund of knowledge from which treatment decisions are made. A resultant trend is toward clinical specialization within the professions, and specialty recognition is rapidly developing. Through continued research efforts, the future promises exciting developments in treatment approaches for the generalist and specialist alike.

ACKNOWLEDGMENTS

This work was supported, in part, by National Multipurpose Research and Training Center grant DC-01409 from the National Institute on Deafness and Other Communication Disorders.

REFERENCES

1. American Heart Association. *Caring for a person with aphasia.* Dallas: American Heart Association, 1994.
2. Rosenbek JC, LaPointe LL, Wertz RT. *Aphasia: a clinical approach.* Austin, TX: Pro-Ed, 1989.
3. Goodglass H, Kaplan E. *Boston Diagnostic Aphasia Examination.* Philadelphia: Lea & Febiger, 1983.
4. Helm-Estabrooks N. *Aphasia Diagnostic Profiles.* Chicago: Riverside Publishing, 1992.
5. Kertesz A. *Western Aphasia Battery.* San Antonio: Psychological Corporation, 1982.
6. Goodglass H. *Understanding aphasia.* Boston: Academic, 1993.
7. Helm-Estabrooks N, Albert ML. *Manual of aphasia therapy.* Austin, TX: Pro-Ed, 1991.
8. Duffy JR. Schuell's stimulation approach to rehabilitation. In: Chapey R, ed. *Language intervention strategies in adult aphasia.* 3rd ed. Baltimore: Williams & Wilkins, 1994:146–174.
9. Jenkins JJ, Pabon-Jimenez E, Shaw RE, Sefer JW. *Schuell's aphasia in adults: diagnosis, prognosis, and treatment.* 2nd ed. Hagerstown: Harper & Row, 1975.
10. Shewan CM, Bandur DL. A psycholinguistic approach to aphasia. In: Chapey R, ed. *Language intervention strategies in adult aphasia.* 3rd ed. Baltimore: Williams & Wilkins, 1994:184–206.
11. Caramazza A, Hillis AE. Where do semantic errors come from? *Cortex* 1990;26:95–122.
12. Hillis AE. Contributions from cognitive analyses. In: Chapey R, ed. *Language intervention strategies in adult aphasia.* 3rd ed. Baltimore: Williams & Wilkins, 1994:207–219.
13. Mitchum CC. Traditional and contemporary views of aphasia: impli-

cations for clinical management. In: Roth EJ, Olson DA, eds. *Topics in stroke rehabilitation.* Frederick: Aspen, 1994:14–36.

14. Holland AL. Pragmatic aspects of intervention in aphasia. *J Neurolinguistics* 1991;6: 197–211.

15. Hillis AE. Efficacy and generalization of treatment for aphasic naming errors. *Arch Phys Med Rehabil* 1989;70:632–636.

16. Linebaugh CW, Lehner LH. Cueing hierarchies and word retrieval: a therapy program. In: Brookshire RH, ed. *Proceedings of the conference on clinical aphasiology.* Minneapolis: BRK Publishers, 1977:19–31.

17. Weidner WE, Jinks AF. The effects of single versus combined cue presentations on picture naming by aphasic adults. *J Commun Disord* 1983;16: 111–121.

18. Gleason JB, Goodglass H, Ackerman N, et al. Retrieval of syntax in Broca's aphasia. *Brain Lang* 1975;2:451–471.

19. Weinrich M, Steele RD, Carlson GS, et al. Processing of visual syntax in a globally aphasic patient. *Brain Lang* 1989;36:391–405.

20. Gardiner G, Brookshire RH. Effects of unisensory and multisensory presentation of stimuli upon naming by aphasic subjects. *Lang Speech* 1972;15:342–357.

21. Pierce RS, Patterson JP. Treatment of auditory comprehension impairment. In: Wallace GL, ed. *Adult aphasia rehabilitation.* Boston: Butterworth-Heinemann, 1996:175–192.

22. Beeson PM. Treatment for letter-by-letter reading: a case study. In: Helm-Estabrooks N, Holland AL, eds. *Approaches to the treatment of aphasia.* Singular clinical competence series. San Diego: Singular Publishing Group, 1998:153–177.

23. Moyer SB. Rehabilitation of alexia: a case study. *Cortex* 1979;15:139–144.

24. Behrmann M. The rites of righting writing: homophone remediation in acquired dysgraphia. *Cogn Neuropsychol* 1987;4:365–384.

25. DePartz M-P, Seron X, Van der Linden MV. Re-education of surface dysgraphia with a visual imagery strategy. *Cogn Neuropsychol* 1992;9:369–401.

26. DePartz M-P. Re-education of a deep dyslexic patient: rationale of the method and results. *Cogn Neuropsychol* 1986;3: 149–177.

27. Carlomagno S, Iavarone A, Colombo A. Cognitive approaches to writing rehabilitation: from single case to group studies. In: Riddoch MJ, Humphries GW, eds. *Cognitive neuropsychology and cognitive rehabilitation.* Hillsdale: Lawrence Erlbaum Associates, 1994:485–502.

28. Holland AL, Halper AS. Talking to individuals with aphasia: a challenge for the rehabilitation team. *Aphasiology* 1996;2:27–37.

29. Myers PS. Right hemisphere syndrome. In: LaPointe LL, ed. *Aphasia and related neurogenic language disorders.* 2nd ed. New York: Thieme, 1997:201–225.

30. Cummings JL, Benson DF. *Dementia: a clinical approach.* 2nd ed. Boston: Butterworth-Heinemann, 1992.

31. Bourgeois MS. *Conversing with memory impaired individuals using memory aids: a memory aid workbook.* Gaylord: Northern Speech Services, 1992.

32. Darley FL, Aronson AE, Brown JR. *Motor speech disorders.* Philadelphia: WB Saunders, 1975.

33. Duffy JR. *Motor speech disorders: substrates, differential diagnosis, and management.* St. Louis: Mosby, 1995.

34. Yorkston KM, Beukelman DR, Bell KR. *Clinical management of dysarthric speakers.* Boston: Little, Brown, 1988.

35. Ramig LO, Countryman S, Thompson L, Horii L. A comparison of two forms of intensive speech treatment for Parkinson disease. *J Speech Hear Res* 1995;39:1232–1251.

36. Rubow RT, Rosenbek J, Collins M, Longstreth D. Vibrotactile stimulation for intersystemic reorganization in the treatment of apraxia of speech. *Arch Phys Med Rehabil* 1982;63:150–153.

37. Simpson MB, Clark AR. Clinical management of apractic mutism. In: Square-Storer P, ed. *Acquired apraxia of speech in aphasic adults.* London: Taylor and Francis, 1989:241–266.

38. McNeil MR, Prescott TE, Lemme ML. An application of electromyographic feedback to aphasia/apraxia treatment. In: Brookshire RH, ed. *Clinical aphasiology conference proceedings.* Minneapolis: BRK Publishers, 1976:151–171.

39. Dworkin JP. *Motor speech disorders: a treatment guide.* St. Louis: Mosby–Year Book, 1991.

40. Rosenbek JC, Lemme ML, Ahern MB, et al. A treatment for apraxia of speech in adults. *J Speech Hear Disord* 1973;38:462–472.

41. Square P, Chumpelik D, Adams S. Efficacy of the PROMPT system of therapy for the treatment of acquired apraxia of speech. In: Brookshire R, ed. *Clinical aphasiology conference proceedings.* Minneapolis: BRK Publishers, 1985:319–320.

42. Sparks R, Helm N, Albert M. Aphasia rehabilitation resulting from melodic intonation therapy. *Cortex* 1974;10:303–316.

43. Stevens E, Glaser L. Multiple input phoneme therapy: an approach to severe apraxia and expressive aphasia. In: Brookshire RH, ed. *Clinical aphasiology conference proceedings.* Minneapolis: BRK Publishers, 1983:148–155.

44. Helm NA, Barresi B. Voluntary control of involuntary utterances: a treatment approach for severe aphasia. In: Brookshire R, ed. *Clinical aphasiology conference proceedings.* Minneapolis: BRK Publishers, 1980:308–315.

45. Bernthal JE, Bankson NW. *Articulation and phonological disorders.* 2nd ed. Englewood Cliffs: Prentice-Hall, 1988.

46. International Association of Laryngectomees. *First steps: helping words for the laryngectomee.* New York: American Cancer Society, 1992:40.

47. Stemple JC, Glaze LF, Gerdeman BK. *Clinical voice pathology: theory and management.* 2nd ed. San Diego: Singular Publishing Group, 1995.

48. Singer MI, Blom ED. An endoscopic technique for restoration of voice after laryngectomy. *Ann Otol Rhinol Laryngol* 1980;89:529–533.

49. Boone DR, McFarlane SC. *The voice and voice therapy.* 5th ed. Englewood Cliffs: Prentice-Hall, 1994.

50. Dikeman KJ, Kazandjian MS. *Communication and swallowing management of tracheostomized and ventilator-dependent adults.* San Diego: Singular Publishing Group, 1995.

51. Dworkin JP, Meleca RJ. *Vocal pathologies: diagnosis, treatment, and case studies.* San Diego: Singular Publishing Group, 1997.

52. Sándor G. Hearing a new market. *Am Demograph* 1994;16:48–55.

53. Tobin H. *Practical hearing aid selection and fitting.* Monograph 001. Baltimore: Department of Veterans Affairs, 1997.

54. Kaplan H. Communication problems in the hearing-impaired elderly: what can be done? *Pride Inst J Long Term Home Health Care* 1988;7:10–22.

55. Alpiner JG, Kaufman KJ, Hanavan PC. Overview of rehabilitative audiology. In: Alpiner JG, McCarthy PA, eds. *Rehabilitative audiology: children and adults.* 2nd ed. Baltimore: Williams & Wilkins, 1993:3–16.

56. Schow RL, Nerbonne MA. *Introduction to aural rehabilitation.* 2nd ed. Austin, TX: Pro-ed, 1989.

57. Montgomery AA. Management of the hearing-impaired adult. In: Alpiner JG, McCarthy PA, eds. *Rehabilitative audiology: children and adults.* 2nd ed. Baltimore: Williams & Wilkins, 1993:311–330.

Chapter 43

Driver Rehabilitation and Personal Transportation: The Vital Link to Independence

Carol Beatson
Rosamond Gianutsos

In technically advanced societies, driving has become an integral part of daily living for all aspects of adult life. For people with disabilities whose mobility has become severely curtailed, driving represents the ultimate freedom, the means by which to attain their highest level of independence and autonomy over their lives.

On the other hand, medical and health professionals have a responsibility toward society as a whole, as well as toward the person with a disability, to ensure that the best advice is given regarding safe control of an automobile. Weighing the issues involved is often a difficult task for medical and health professionals. It calls for sensitivity and diplomacy and an understanding of the disability and its progression. As well as medical and functional information, knowledge of the person's level of insight and the likelihood of the person displaying responsible behavior, as a direct result of the disability or originating from his or her actual personality traits, will have a bearing on the final recommendations regarding the advisability of driving. Despite extensive research, no firm conclusions have been drawn regarding which specific cognitive deficits may constitute a barrier to driving. However, the literature shows a consensus of the need for assessment to be carried out on several levels, including medical, psychological, and functional levels, including, if deemed safe to do so, an on-road driving assessment. The difficulty of separating individual skills as predictors of actual performance was recognized by Evans (1), who nonetheless commented that "perhaps a distinction should be made between perceptual-motor skills and total performance."

In comparison to the attention given to assessing brain-injured drivers, little emphasis has been found in the literature regarding the driving safety of those with physical disabilities but without brain injuries. The studies that did focus on physical disability demonstrated that given the correct vehicle adaptations, driving safety is not compromised (2–5).

This chapter provides an introduction to the issues involved in driver assessment for a wide range of disability types. It outlines several models of driving skill theory, examines the steps to be followed when assessing driving skill, and discusses aspects of behavior and environment that impinge on the person's ability to drive safely.

FRAMES OF REFERENCE

Before approaching comprehensive driver assessment, it is necessary to have a well-formed philosophy of what is to be evaluated, what relevance it has to the task of driving, and by what process the final decision will be made. Three frames of reference, developed between 1979 and 1992, are examined here. While it appears that the first two models have evolved independently of each other, similarities are present in their approach, in which the multiple factors that comprise the complex task of driving are described. Because each model adds a different dimension to the issues involved in driver assessment, they are all worthy of consideration. The development of theoretical models in driver assessment is now addressed through these three frames of reference.

Perceptual Information Processing Model of the Driving Task

Described by Simms (6), the focus of this model is on the internal processing methods of multiple, constantly changing, incoming visual stimuli by which the driver is bombarded during the driving task. The person's driving safety will depend on the rapid interpretation and accurate responses to this information. Comprehensive visual screening, especially in regard to restriction in visual fields, is an essential first step in the assessment process.

Environmental Information

The first stage of Simms's model includes the ability to perceive traffic engineering, advisory signs, and roadway design, as well as the presence and movement of other road users.

Attentional and Perceptual Mechanisms

The second stage of the model characterizes the person's ability to gather and form the complex environmental information into a meaningful picture within a compressed time frame. Simms commented that essential visual perceptual skills at this level include "scanning, tracking and figure-ground discrimination."

Logical Analysis and Decision Making

This stage describes the ability to interpret information gathered and combine it with already existing knowledge of the driving task, in order to make the most appropriate decisions. It involves the continuous, accurate assessment of risk in a wide variety of potentially hazardous situations, which are constantly changing.

Response

The final stage of Simms's model is the time frame in which the person makes a physical response. A prerequisite is to have accurate control of the vehicle, which may require vehicle modifications as well as, in our experience, full control over at least two out of four limbs.

Hierarchical Model of Task Performance in Car Driving

This model is hierarchical in that each level impacts on the other, thus affecting the way in which the driver performs. "Dealing with Danger," an unpublished summary report by Michon of a workshop in 1979, described a three-tier model of driving skill. Michon's report was outlined by van Zomeren et al in 1987 (7).

Strategic Level

The first level of Michon's model describes the skill of planning the drive in advance. It involves making decisions about the best route to take, what time of day is preferable, anticipated traffic density, expected weather, and the level of wellness or tiredness of the driver. As the person is not yet behind the wheel, the pressure caused by the time required to make decisions on the strategic level is low. It also involves more global decision making, for example, whether to spend the extra money for antilock brakes and dual air bags—even where to live and work. Clinical experience has shown the importance of understanding the driver's ability to address the strategic level, especially among those who lack insight about their actual abilities or who do not acknowledge their failing level of health.

Tactical Level

Skills in the tactical level involve the driver's actual behavior while driving and decisions on which these are based. Examples offered by van Zomeren et al (7) include "adapting one's speed when entering a residential district, switching on the headlights when rain reduces visibility, or deciding to pass another car." The time frame in which to respond at the tactical level is moderate. In psychological terms, the tactical level is a very broad description of function. Inasmuch as the tactical level calls for prospective thinking and action, there is an emphasis on the first three levels of Simms's model (environmental information, attentional and perceptual mechanisms, logical analysis and decision making). The outcomes of faulty cognitive mechanisms have been clarified by van Zomeren et al (7), thus adding another dimension to the approaches outlined in Simms's model. Impairments on the tactical level may include "impulsivity [which] is attributed to disinhibition or reduced cognitive control." "Poor judgement" is "derived from poor estimation of risks and inadequate adaptation of speed to traffic conditions."

Operational Level

The final level of Michon's model includes the automatic decisions and practiced responses of a driver. It involves the ability to position the vehicle and steer it accurately, to use the primary and secondary driving controls, and to monitor and avoid potential hazards both in the present and a few seconds ahead. Impairments in the operational level are listed by van Zomeren et al (7) as falling "into five general categories: 1) inadequate visual scanning of traffic and environment, 2) problems in spatial perception and orientation, 3) poor tracking, 4) slowness in acting and 5) confusion when more complex actions have to be carried out." The operational level encompasses the last two levels in Simms's model (logical analysis and decision making, and response). The time frame in which to respond at the operational level is limited and an ever-present factor.

The Michon/van Zomeren model is less about skills than about the driving task and, therefore, the skills identified by Simms will find expression at both the tactical and operational levels. Further, the Michon/van Zomeren model has interesting implications for on-road assessment. First, an explicit attempt should be made to address the tactical level. For instance, one might ask the person to find a way to reverse direction ("Oops, we should have gone the other way . . .") or to find a safe way to pull off the road. Second, the strategic level needs to be addressed, but, by definition, it cannot be while driving.

A Cybernetic Model of Driving

A study in 1991 by Galski et al (8) considered elements of the earlier frames of reference and further refined them. They went one step further than developing a hypothetical model and investigated its effectiveness in clinical practice. The researchers tested the cybernetic model for its use in evaluating fitness to drive after brain injury, and reported predictive validity of the model. The cybernetic model is complex, featuring layers of skills that continuously interact with each other.

General Driving Program

This level holds knowledge of the road rules as well as learning from repeated past experiences of driving. It is not a static body of knowledge but rather a changing database of information that is constantly updated by new experiences. "It initiates and directs all driving related activities" in routine and repeated situations (8). In this sense, the general driving program is an expansion of Michon's tactical and operational levels. Impairment of the general driving program may derive from loss of memory for past learning or reduced ability to use past learning in new situations.

Executive Component

The executive component is activated by the intention to drive. It guides the preparatory activities for driving and signals the calculation and construction coprocessor to become active.

Specific Driving Program

As a decision has now been made to drive, this level organizes the elements of destination, route, and so on, as described in Michon's strategic level. In addition, the specific driving program directs four additional systems to commence operation.

Sensory Input

This involves the scanning of global information being received from the body's visual, auditory, proprioceptive, and kinesthetic sensors. Whereas routine driving requires a low demand on this level, new situations demand more precisely directed sensory monitoring. Impairment may create delays in processing.

Calculation and Construction Coprocessor

In order to interpret the ever-changing three-dimensional environment, the driver makes use of this level to "calculate, integrate and coordinate the incoming sensory information" (8). This involves visual-perceptual skills including "distance, depth, spatial relationships, velocity and gradients" (8).

Motor Output

Similar to Michon's operational level, motor output includes the physical tasks of vehicle control, such as steering, braking, and accelerating. In addition, Galski et al (8) refined the concept by considering the need to perform a single action, or a combination of actions, as well as the degree of effort required to ensure safe passage of the vehicle.

Resident Diagnostic Program

The final level checks the entire system's function. It is a generic system covering "cognitive-perceptual-physical skills, executive processes (e.g., planning, goal setting, monitoring performance, regulating behavior) and psychological factors (e.g., personality, emotions, beliefs) in all activities" (8). Impairment in this area is likely to affect insight into one's own abilities and reduce safe driving behaviors.

DISABILITIES AND CASE EXAMPLES OF DRIVER REHABILITATION

A broad spectrum of disabilities or conditions is served by driver rehabilitation and if there is any subdivision, it has to be according to the presence of 1) physical disability and 2) cognitive impairment. These are summarized in Table 43-1, together with remarks and observations based on our clinical experience. The wide scope of disabling conditions and their impact on driving often present unique challenges to persons who would be driver rehabilitation specialists. We have chosen two of our more complicated cases to illustrate what can be involved and what can be accomplished. The first, whom we shall call Patient A, was treated in New Zealand, which will account for the steering wheel positioned on the right side of the vehicle. He had physical disability secondary to spinal cord injury. The second, Patient B, was treated for cognitive and behavioral sequelae of a severe traumatic brain injury. Parts of his case have been reported elsewhere (9). Together, they represent the two broad domains of disability, physical and cognitive, which are of concern for driver rehabilitation.

Patient A: Spinal Injury with Incomplete Paraplegia and Cauda Equina Syndrome

Once his condition had stabilized, Patient A was admitted to a spinal rehabilitation facility for rehabilitation. For driver assessment, this meant that his abilities did not remain static and gradual recovery occurred over several months, making it difficult to predict his final vehicle and equipment needs with any certainty. He was referred for driver or passenger assessment near the end of his inpatient stay at the spinal unit.

Functional Ability

Patient A initially presented with patchy cutaneous sensory loss and some return of movement in all limbs, but this

Table 43-1: Disability Diagnoses Served by Driver Rehabilitation

Disability	Diagnosis	Comments
PC	Acquired brain injury	TBI, CVA, post tumor. Check for associated physical weakness or impaired coordination. CVA: may need modifications and retraining.
PC	Parkinson disease	Caution for on-road if festinating gait is present. Later stage: medication effects may wear off quickly. Insight may be poor.
C	Dementia	Age associated and usually fit; HIV infection. Ensure support person is involved when discussing outcomes.
PC	Frail elderly	Unwell or slow recuperation following illness. Social issues weigh heavily.
P	Multiple sclerosis	Check vision, incoordination, muscle weakness. Monitor slow deterioration. May need hand controls and retraining.
P	Muscular dystrophy	Mild: driver, but keep open for review. Severe: passenger, often a child; may be disabled but growth is normal. Expect and monitor deterioration.
P	Motor neuron disease	Check driving at onset. Deterioration can be rapid. May quickly become a passenger.
PC	Cerebral palsy	Learner drivers will need extra lessons.
PC	Spina bifida—hydrocephalus	Learner drivers will need extra lessons.
C	Psychiatric (schizophrenia)	Often referred during discharge planning.
PC	Spinal injuries	"Occult" brain injury must be suspected.
	Complete/incomplete	Function is likely to improve dramatically. Prescribe modifications
	Paraplegia	with caution.
	Tetraplegia (Quadriplegia) C2–C3, C3–C4, C5–C6, C6–C7	Capable of transfers and independent wheelchair stowage. Need body support for travel as passengers. Need extensive modifications for driving.
P	Children with developmental delay	Travel as passengers. Check projected changes to mobility equipment and health of principal caregiver.
P	Amputees	May be hypersensitive to touch: check grip on wheel, key, hand
	Upper limbs	brake, gear select.
	Finger(s)	Modification to artificial limb for steering. Modify secondary driving
	Through wrist	controls.
	Above/below elbow	Check position of pedals. May need guides.
	Lower limbs	Check vision and cognitive function if secondary to diabetes.
	Through ankle	Using artificial limbs on pedals is unsafe because there is no sensory
	Above/below knee	feedback (i.e., proprioception, pressure, vibration). Add hinged left
	Bilateral/unilateral	accelerator or hand controls and retrain.
P	Ankylosing spondylitis	High seat for access. Check vision and add wide-angle mirrors. Check again for blind spots as results are not always safe.
P	Arthritis	May complicate other conditions.
	Osteoarthritis	High seat for transfers. Check grip strength.
	Rheumatoid arthritis	Systemic involvement causes fatigue. Pace daily activities. Check shoulder range of motion and strength for steering, use of pedals, seat height and positioning, modify key and small levers and switches.
P	Brachial plexus lesions	Modify car for one-arm driving.
P	Back injury	Check seating and ergonomics; may need substantial seat reupholstery and/or change of vehicle.
P	Chronic pain	Usually cannot be of help, especially if driving exacerbates. Pace daily activities.
P	Occupational overuse syndrome	Was repetitive strain injury. Usually in upper limb. Pace and modify as for rheumatoid arthritis.
P	Postpolio syndrome	Fatigue main new factor over existing weakness in arm or leg. May have scoliosis. Review ergonomics of driving; update modifications and/or car for ease of use. Pace driving to within fatigue levels.

P = physical disability, requiring a musculoskeletal approach; C = brain insult, requiring a cognitive approach; PC = requires both musculoskeletal and cognitive approaches; TBI = traumatic brain injury; CVA = cerebrovascular accident; HIV = human immunodeficiency virus infection.

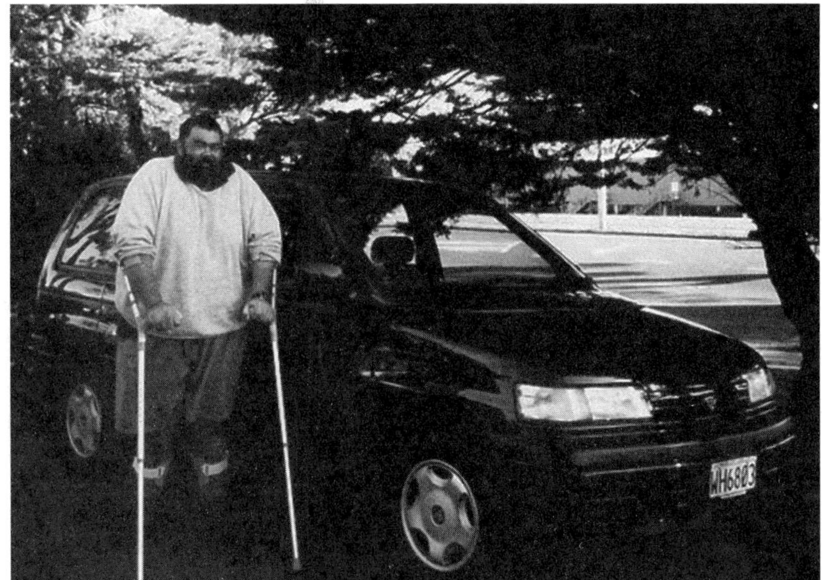

Figure 43-1. Patient A with incomplete tetraplegia uses elbow crutches for short distances and a fixed-frame wheelchair for longer journeys.

was not sufficiently functional for walking, driving, or independent transfers. He was confined to a wheelchair. At that time, it seemed his only option was to access a van via a wheelchair loader and to travel as a passenger. A further complicating factor was his large body size. This had major implications for driver assessment. It also meant that his occupational therapist and physiotherapist at the spinal unit gave special attention to equipment for daily living in all areas, especially wheelchair prescription and housing modifications. They also lobbied Patient A's funding agent to take into account not only his injury but also his ergonomic needs, a complication that hindered his rehabilitation and discharge planning.

Life Roles

Prior to his injury, Patient A was employed as an industrial chemist in a tertiary educational facility. He is married and the father of two 4-year-old boys (twins). In order to readjust their lives and to make the most of their earning capacities, Patient A and his wife decided to swap roles. His new role was to organize the care for his children during the day and to continue with distance learning by correspondence at the same time. This meant that he was determined, if possible, to drive. Traveling as a passenger simply did not fulfill his goals as a parent and a spouse.

Improvement in Function

The assessment and follow-up continued over a period of 3 months. During this time he steadily progressed to independent transfers and the use of elbow crutches. At this stage, we established that he had sufficient return of movement and upper-limb strength to enable him to use hand controls on a car with power steering. Therefore, the remaining obstacles to driving were a) how to stow an outsized fixed-frame wheelchair and b) what vehicle to choose (Fig. 43-1).

Vehicle Selection and Teamwork

With supervision from his occupational therapist at the spinal unit, Patient A quickly established that he was unable to stand up from a standard car seat. Furthermore, even with his tall height, he was unable to access the seat of four-wheel-drive vehicles, which were too high. Eventually, he discovered that the range of "people movers," a van-shaped car, seemed ideally suited to his needs. They cost more than twice the available car purchase grant. Static assessment of the first car was conducted with Patient A, his occupational therapist, the driver assessor specialist, and a vehicle modifications engineer. Although he could easily get into and out of the driver's seat, we found difficulties with seat positioning, and the potential creation of pressure areas on his thighs from the hand brake on one side and the contours of the driver's door on the other. It would require substantial modification. Another make of a similar vehicle had substantially more leg room and better seating support, and could be modified at less cost (Fig. 43-2).

Vehicle Modification and Teamwork

Patient A lives in the suburbs of a large city and would principally be driving short distances on sealed roads in relatively busy traffic. As a family, they would like to travel farther across the city on the freeway or out of town for vacations in rural areas. Both journeys require traveling at high speeds, which would affect the stability of an externally mounted, outsized fixed-frame wheelchair, which would essentially act as a large sail on top of the car. After discussions with the manufacturer of a car-top wheelchair carrier about safety risks, we decided against this modification. Instead, we agreed that although it was not ideal, Patient A should aim to stow the wheelchair in the level-access trunk, while seated safely at the opening to the trunk.

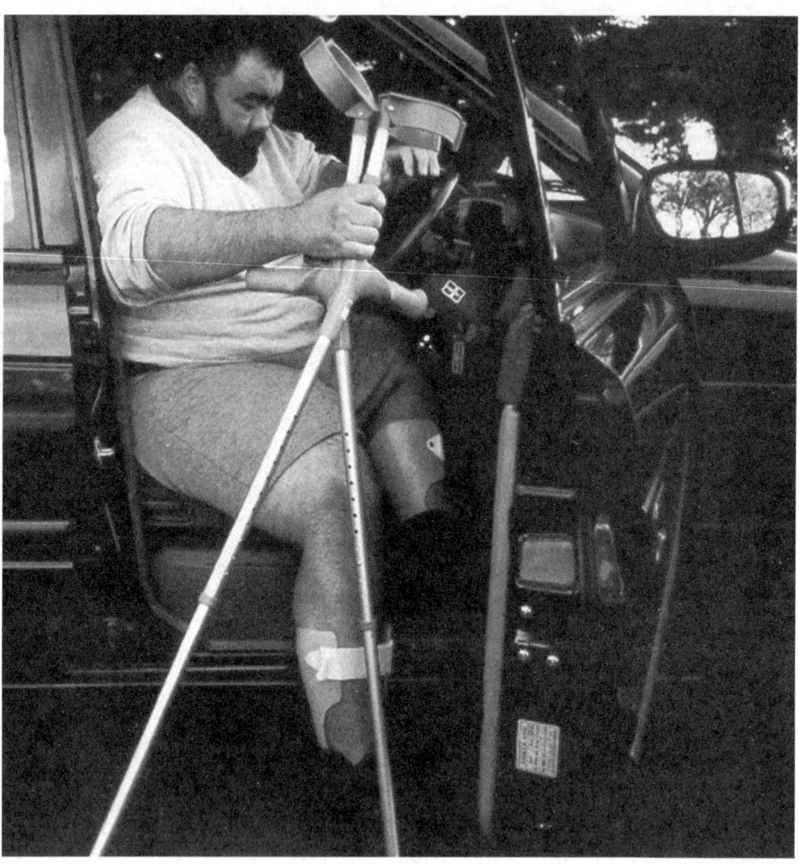

Figure 43-2. Patient A getting into the driver's seat. Weak muscles combined with heavy limbs make this a slow process.

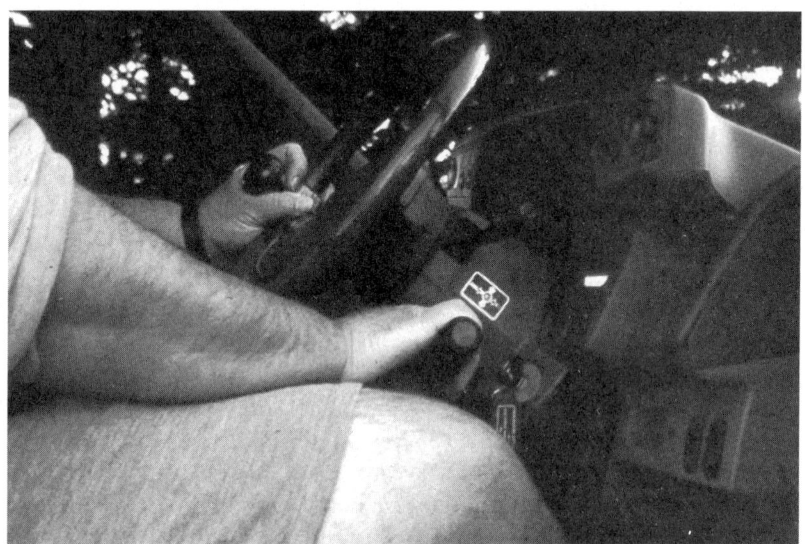

Figure 43-3. Patient A demonstrates hand controls and steering wheel spinner. Even in the most ideal vehicle, space for equipment was limited.

The following vehicle modifications were identified at a further follow-up assessment, with an additional team member, a vehicle upholsterer.

1. Add hand controls (Fig. 43-3).
2. Add steering wheel spinner (see Fig. 43-3).
3. Hinge accelerator pedal out of range of the right foot (Fig. 43-4).
4. Remove contours on driver's door and replace with flat panel.
5. Remove seat belt stalk from side of seat and replace on floor, to eliminate pressure areas and for ease of access.
6. Remove third row of seats in rear to make room for wheelchair.

7. Add central locking system to increase security and reduce walking.
8. Extend runners to the rear on the driver's seat by 75 mm to allow more leg room when seated (Fig. 43-5).
9. Install two hand grips on driver's door opening to aid in transferring.

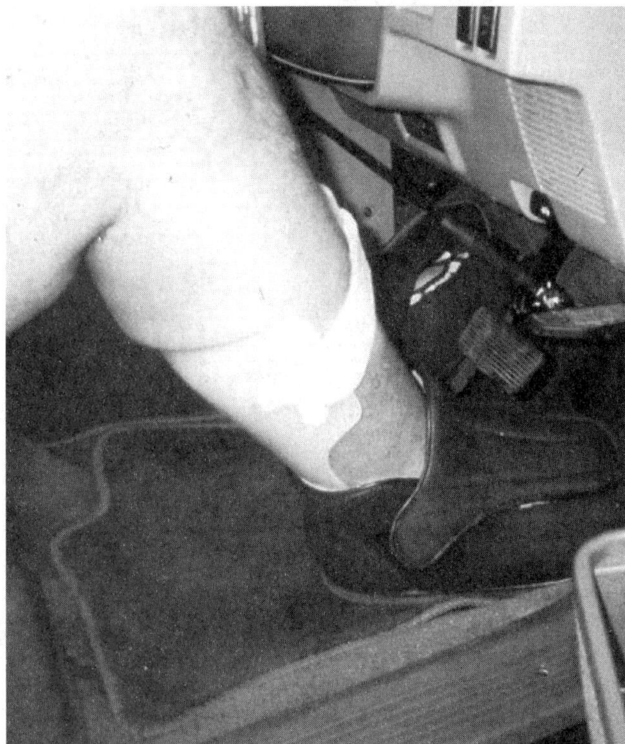

Figure 43-4. Foot positioning: Wearing an ankle-foot orthosis in a restricted space and weak thigh muscles make foot positioning difficult. This photograph shows the right accelerator pedal hinged out of the way for safety.

Due to his size and special needs, we had not been able to place Patient A in an adapted vehicle to test his practical driving abilities. Therefore, on collection of the vehicle, he was given driver education, concentrating on the safe use of hand controls. He quickly understood their use and within 40 minutes, was driving the vehicle as though he had had plenty of practice.

This project aided Patient A's return home and was integral in re-establishing a normal life following severe spinal injury. He regularly uses the vehicle to transport his sons to and from school and has enjoyed short weekend visits to the country. He is able to stow his wheelchair in the trunk, while maintaining his balance and has not found any difficulties achieving this on a variety of terrains. Patient A returned to the workshop on one occasion to add a further vehicle modification, which we had overlooked. On those days when he felt unwell, and needed to visit his doctor, it was difficult for him to access the front passenger seat. Therefore, the seat was also positioned 75 mm farther back to allow him sufficient leg room to travel as a passenger in addition to being a driver (see Fig. 47-5).

Patient B: Cognitive and Behavioral Sequelae of Traumatic Brain Injury

Patient B survived a head-on collision but had multiple trauma, including orbital and skull fractures and massive brain injury. He was evaluated and treated with an individualized technology-augmented cognitive rehabilitation program, in which driving was an important, but by no means the only component. By the time he was first seen a year after the accident, he was ambulatory and expressed (solo and a capella) great confidence in his ability to drive. His family did not trust his judgment to stay at home alone for anything other than short intervals and he was totally dependent on others to drive him where he needed to go. [It never ceases to amaze us how often people who are not safe in crossing the street on foot (or in a wheelchair) seek

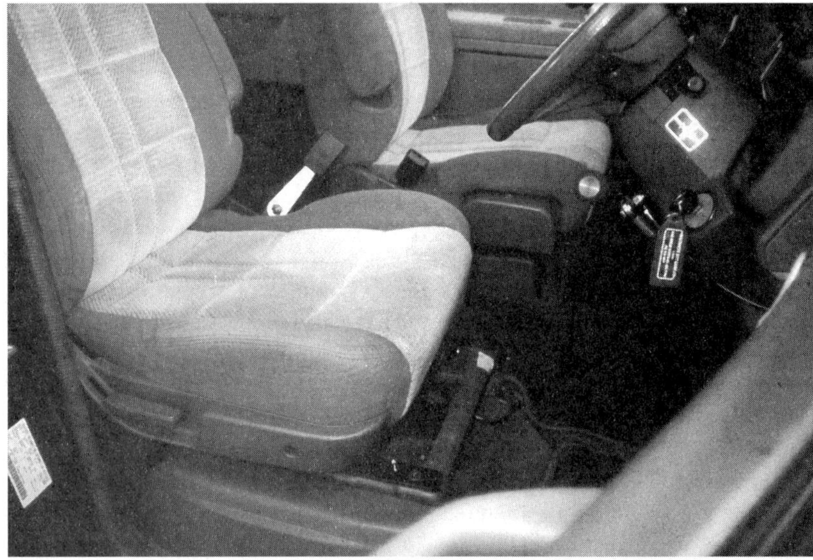

Figure 43-5. The driver's seat was substantially repositioned to the rear to enable Patient A to sit in it. A seat belt extension, which can be seen between both seats, enables him to locate and engage the seat belt.

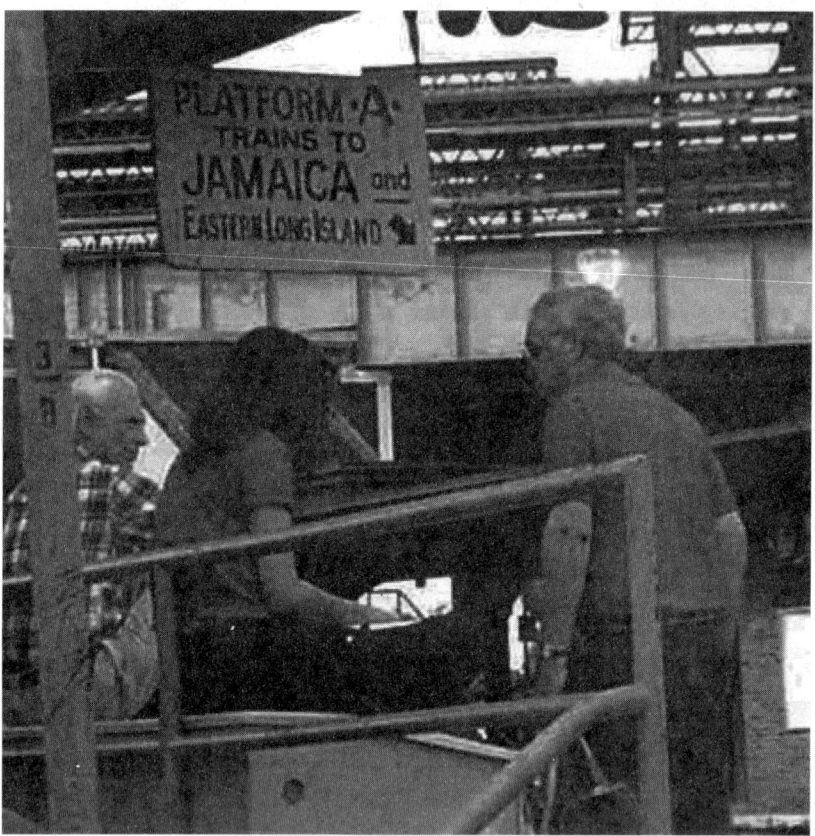

Figure 43-6. Patient B's use of the train was an important component of his driver rehabilitation and has continued to be part of his mobility plan.

to drive.] Initially, Patient B's obsession with driving was directed to mobility on foot and use of public transportation. With supervision and safety awareness training, he became independent on the train (Fig. 43-6). This achievement was psychologically uplifting and he has continued to use this mode of travel on longer trips, especially into urban areas.

Patient B would have angry outbursts and become easily frustrated. On each such occasion he would attest to having learned his lesson, that the problem would not occur again. He was persuaded that he had to earn the confidence and trust of others—that his own confidence was not sufficient, as his judgment was always to be "optimistic" rather than realistic. He agreed that he would have to remain outburst free for at least 3 months before he could expect others to find him sufficiently trustworthy to even consider assessment for resumption of driving. It took him 9 months to reach this goal.

Patient B had significant attentional problems (e.g., with simultaneous information processing and mental flexibility), binocular dysfunction (affecting depth and other forms of visual perception), impulsivity, and visual agnosia (failure to recognize some objects in his direct line of sight). These problems were addressed in his cognitive rehabilitation and optometric treatment programs. Some exercises were identified for their specific relevance to skills needed for safe driving, for example, visual closure. These exercises showed him concretely the standards that he needed to meet and demonstrated that others were taking his goal of driving seriously.

Throughout this time, the clinician's observations of Patient B's reasoning and behavior were complemented by information offered by family members and other professionals. It was clear that much improvement was needed before he would garner family support for his driving. Formal predriving assessment was initiated gradually and explicitly made contingent on achieving consistently acceptable behavior and judgment.

Since Patient B was under optometric care, formal vision screening was not needed; however, his binocularity problems were identified as potential issues for judgment of distances, for example, following and stopping. His visual perceptual agnosia was characterized as a "look no see" problem, regularly brought to his attention in whatever contexts it occurred, and explicitly related to driving, for example, "Gee, Officer, I didn't even see him. . . ."

Formal assessment of judgment and information-processing abilities related to driving was accomplished with the Elemental Driving Simulator (9), illustrated in Figure 43-7. On this rudimentary computer-based simulation, performance relative to a norm group of drivers is compared to self-appraisal. Patient B predicted that he would score average or better on all scales; however, it took him four attempts, separated by at least a month, to attain scores on all subscales within two standard deviations of

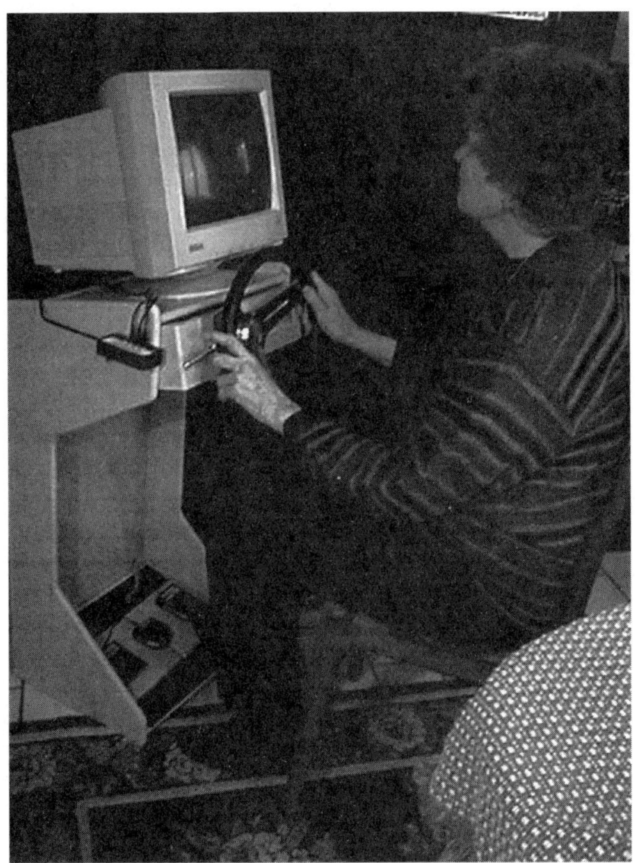

Figure 43-7. Elemental Driving Simulator (EDS) standard model. An IBM-compatible personal computer (not shown) controls a dynamic display of a schematic roadway and peripheral stimuli. The patient controls the lateral position of the "car" using the steering wheel and uses the turn signal to make responses. For hemiparetics, the foot pedals are used for responding.

the mean—a clinical cutoff corresponding to the second percentile.

An on-road behind-the-wheel assessment was then scheduled and as it happened Patient B was observed by two experienced driver rehabilitation specialists, one of whom recommended further cognitive rehabilitation and the other thought it was time to begin driving lessons. Although he had already made great progress, Patient B was still a marginal candidate for driving. Once authorized by his insurance carrier, he began lessons with a local commercial driving school instructor who was experienced with drivers with disabling conditions. The coordinating driver rehabilitation specialist observed the first lesson, which also served as an independent evaluation, and remained in close communication with the driving instructor. After 2 months of lessons, the instructor encouraged Patient B to begin practice driving. His family was not eager to work with him in this regard and Patient B was to obtain his own car and insurance and satisfy legal requirements (his license, by now, had expired and he had to notify the licensing authorities of his condition and obtain medical clearance to continue driving—see Appendix I, which details the applicable legal requirements). He obtained an oversized center-mounted rearview mirror (Fig. 43-8).

His practice and guidelines for driving now came into the direct oversight of the coordinating driver rehabilitation specialist. The following system remained in effect for approximately 1 year before Patient B achieved a modicum of meaningful independence in his driving:

1. Driving log: Patient B was to record each trip, including time, distance, objective, and observations.
2. Monthly observation drive: The itinerary for this 2-hour drive was proposed by Patient B based on where he wanted to go and felt was within his capa-

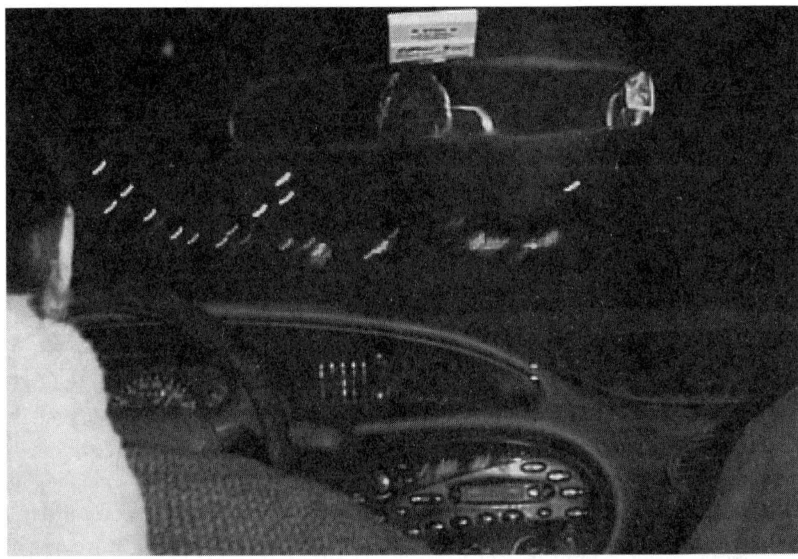

Figure 43-8. Oversized center-mounted rearview mirror.

bilities. Initially, over half the proposed routes were determined to be unsafe, usually because of traffic density and left turns. This method worked especially well as it gave the patient an opportunity to demonstrate his advancing appreciation of factors that impact on the safety of different routes. He learned how to use route planning to reduce risk. Computerized local street maps were helpful in this planning, both for Patient B and the driver rehabilitation specialist, who was not particularly familiar with Patient B's community. Over the months, the list of approved routes grew.

3. Patient B agreed to limit his driving strictly to daytime driving along approved routes. He adhered to these guidelines quite consistently, and there were no serious mishaps and only one lapse in which he drove some friends at the day center to lunch.

For a year Patient B's driving consisted of observed drives and limiting himself to approved routes. Because he showed excellent progress, he was given leeway to select his own routes within 10 miles from home. Since his depth perception continued to impact his judgments of gap and following distances at night, night driving was proscribed. A year later, a nighttime drive was scheduled and he demonstrated sufficiently improved skill that the driver rehabilitation specialist felt comfortable relaxing the night driving restriction. The patient's wife never clearly endorsed his driving, a fact that continues to frustrate him; however, she stopped objecting. He has now been driving for 3 years and has safely driven 25,000 miles locally. It has allowed him to resume part-time work and to pursue avocational and social activities.

LEVELS OF ASSESSMENT

With these examples in mind, we turn now to a systematic consideration of assessment of driving competencies and adaptive equipment needs. Specialist assessors can categorize the levels of assessment into three main sections:

1. Drivers with musculoskeletal impairment, which can be mild to severe. Mild impairment typically involves a range of adaptations to a car, or simply a change of vehicle to suit the ergonomics of the driver's disability in a more satisfactory way. These drivers can be readily evaluated using an adapted vehicle, which is essential equipment within a driver assessment program.

   Drivers with severe impairment who wish to drive from their wheelchair require a very detailed appraisal of their abilities, a precise understanding of the range of remote-controlled driving adaptations available on the market, and an understanding of which vehicles are suited to this type of adaptation. As these modifications are costly, careful prescription is needed, taking into account the person's activity tolerance, muscle strength, trunk balance, range of movement of all limbs, and potential safety while driving. In Britain and the United States, a number of companies specialize in the manufacture and installation of complex, computerized, "zero effort" driving controls into suitable vehicles.

2. Drivers with cognitive impairment, which can also range from mild to severe. The complexities of assessing the function of a driver with brain damage requires skilled attention when a return to driving is desired. Evaluation of aging drivers whose skills have deteriorated to a potentially unsafe level uncovers a whole range of social and emotional issues that they must begin to face. This aspect of driver assessment requires skilled evaluation and intervention and the support of a team to confirm and implement the assessor's findings.

3. Drivers with both musculoskeletal and cognitive impairment. This involves not only a comprehensive cognitive assessment approach but also specific evaluation for ergonomic fit of a vehicle and adaptive driving controls. It is well to be mindful of the potential for the multiplicative impact of disabilities. For example, hand controls may be easy for a cognitively intact person to learn. However, the person with mild cognitive impairments may exhibit excessive attentional constriction, hemi-inattention, or impulsivity when driving with hand controls. For drivers with variable and deteriorating conditions such as multiple sclerosis and Parkinson disease, complex issues arise involving the impact of musculoskeletal impairment on cognitive skills. Specialist assessors and close team work with the person's family or caregivers and the physician are needed to achieve an acceptable outcome. With a condition that is expected to progressively decline, the driver rehabilitation specialist should make it clear that the issue is not whether to stop driving, but when and how to do so. Along with the patient and treatment team, the driver rehabilitation specialist is to identify guidelines for making these decisions.

Although advances have been made in determining which skills affect driving safety, agreement has yet to be reached on the exact assessment battery to use. However, it is here that the multidisciplinary approach has particular value, with an on-road drive representing the final advancing vote. Essential team members include a physician, a psychologist, an occupational therapist, and a driving instructor, with other specialists such as an eye care specialist (optometrist or ophthalmologist) and vehicle modification engineer on call as needed.

While the literature focuses on providing comprehensive driver assessment services from within a large treatment facility, there is also a trend toward community-based assessment services. At this stage, the client's condition has generally stabilized and he or she has been, or is about to be, discharged from inpatient residential treatment.

Many drivers with musculoskeletal impairment who are medically stable already reside in the community and seek specialist assessment services as a further step toward independent living. A stable level of function enhances the assessment process. It enables the compilation of a realistic prescription for adaptive equipment that is suited to the individual's tested and observed abilities. Therefore, it is an advantage to see physically disabled drivers months or even years after hospital-based rehabilitation is complete.

In such a setting, the occupational therapist acts as coordinator and works closely with the client's general medical practitioner or rehabilitation team and family to obtain appropriate medical screening in preparation for driving. In community-based services, a team structure exists in different facilities, both commercial and service based, and members are called on at appropriate stages of the assessment and vehicle adaptation continuum. In New Zealand, for example, community-based, private occupational therapy services provide a focus of coordination for much of the driver assessment services. However, this may only work well in areas with a relatively low population density, such as New Zealand (population, approximately 3.5 million) (10). A significant advantage of community-based services is that they make it possible to evaluate the potential of persons with some cognitive limitations who may still be able to drive along familiar routes in their own communities.

In order to reduce the risk to the person with a disability, the assessing staff, and the public at large, efforts have concentrated on developing a screening battery prior to going on the road. The following section overviews the approaches to assessment that are commonly utilized in clinical practice and for which research has shown favorable outcomes.

Off-Road Screening Approaches

The exact range of off-road screening tools that are useful in assessing people with brain injury remain ill-defined. However, reliable results are reported in facilities where a multidisciplinary approach has been taken.

Medical Fitness

The first level of assessment is by the physician, to determine whether the person intending to drive is in a sufficiently stable condition to permit driving. If the recommended multidisciplinary driver assessment and rehabilitation services are available, the physician's emphasis should be on those medical conditions that are not apparent or intermittently produce symptoms incompatible with safe driving. These conditions include epilepsy, problems with cardiac function and circulatory efficiency, metabolic disorders including poorly controlled diabetes, and visual, neurologic, and psychiatric disorders. Essentially, the physician is being relied on to address those conditions that might not manifest themselves during clinical or behind-the-wheel assessment.

Medical screening guidelines have been developed by medical organizations and are recognized by licensing authorities. Several countries, for example, Australia (11), New Zealand, United Kingdom, Canada (12), and the United States, have manuals containing guidelines on medical fitness to drive, which usually can be obtained through the local licensing authorities or the local medical society. While these guidelines vary, in general they describe a range of medical conditions, with few guidelines on assessing cognitive function. As Gianutsos et al (13) commented, "The physician is thus placed in the difficult position of rendering an opinion both about complex cognitive functions . . . as well as driving, a domain of performance in which they have had no training or experience other than as drivers themselves." We would urge physicians in this position to seek input from other rehabilitation specialists, particularly occupational and physical therapists, and for those persons known or suspected to have cognitive/behavioral impairment, neuropsychologists. Increasing numbers of therapists are specializing in driver rehabilitation and in the United States there is a professional organization, the Association of Driver Educators for the Disabled, as well as Certified Driver Rehabilitation Specialist (CDRS) recognition (14,15). Also, in 1996, the New Zealand Association of Occupational Therapists inaugurated the first Special Interest Group in Driver and Passenger Assessment/Rehabilitation, with the aim of providing introductory and continuing education for occupational therapists in driver and passenger assessment.

Physical Skills

In the literature, no clear direction has been given in practical terms on where to place emphasis on assessing people with musculoskeletal versus cognitive impairments. In the practical setting, clinical reasoning must be used to determine the appropriateness of encompassing the whole assessment battery for people with spinal injuries and musculoskeletal impairments only. Comments on musculoskeletal impairment in this chapter are drawn from extensive clinical experience in assessing and training drivers with physical disability.

There is limited information detailing which physical skills should be measured in relation to driving and which test is to be used. In 1995 Sprigle et al (16) "surveyed 403 evaluators throughout the United States" to clarify the "methods, equipment and criteria used when assessing an individual's ability to drive." Although there was little agreement on the predictive ability of clinical evaluations, most people agreed that measurement of the following skills was important: "brake reaction time, steering reaction time, eye-hand coordination, brake force, steering force, gas force, range of motion, sensation, manual muscle strength, fine motor coordination, grip strength and pinch strength." However, not everyone used these assessments all the time. "Driving characteristics were determined most commonly by observing the task while in an evaluation vehicle, except brake reaction time . . . ," which was measured by one of three different types of equipment. Overall, simple, inexpensive techniques were used for evaluation and the majority of evaluators were satisfied with their evaluation equipment. Sprigle et al (16) concluded that "acceptable physical performance levels that could be used in driver assessment are typically unavailable to evaluators who measure driving characteristics." This was confirmed by the findings of Korner-Bitensky et al (17) who stated that "the development and testing of a standard assessment that accurately predicts driving performance will be an enormous challenge for the profession."

Throughout the assessment, the focus should be on the abilities that are relevant to the driving task from a functional perspective. In order to gauge which vehicle adaptations are most appropriate, the occupational therapist pays close attention to those actions that are difficult or impossible for the driver to perform. When considering the physical demands of driving a vehicle, in relation to any level of musculoskeletal impairment, it is useful to think of the driving compartment as a capsule, with all driving controls located on the frontal plane of the driver's body. If the capsule is divided into four segments, one for each limb, it is then easy to assign the car controls in each of the segments to each of the four limbs. This provides a convenient method of approaching functional assessment for the physical tasks involved in driving.

Upper Limbs

Physical assessment includes functional assessment of upper-limb range of movement, muscle strength, and coordination. Using the capsule concept just described, the right and left upper limbs need to be able to reach as high as the sun visor, as far laterally as the door and gear lever, and as far in front as the dashboard. These movements need to be rapid, accurate, and able to be carried out simultaneously with other tasks and without visual direction. In order to steer, one or both limbs need to be able to cross the midline in a resisted arc, which is important to be able to complete several full, resisted rotations of the steering wheel during maneuvers such as parking. Coordination and strength for steering are essential. But the exact amount of strength needed depends on the resistance from the steering wheel in the type of vehicle to be used. One older driver with Parkinson disease appeared to have adequate strength for steering the assessment vehicle: a late model car with power steering. However, his car was old and without power steering. When driving his own car, he struggled to steer the car smoothly around corners, due to his loss of muscle strength. Sharp turns at intersections were especially hazardous because of the wide arc needed to control the vehicle; he narrowly missed parked vehicles, pedestrians, and road engineering barriers.

The driver who is a "manual" wheelchair user will need sufficient arm strength and dexterity to dismantle and stow the wheelchair either inside or on top of the car. Trunk stability and upper-limb strength are also essential to enable access to the driver's seat.

Sufficient hand function and grip strength are needed to open the driver's door and to operate driving controls, which require a wide range of hand grips and dexterity. Drivers recovering from partial tetraplegia who have return of function to most of their body, but who have a completely flaccid hand, experience many problems, for instance, opening the driver's door. Unlocking can be achieved with an adapted key held between both wrists and the application of forearm movement. Alternatively a remote-controlled device eliminates this effort. However, because of the flaccid hand and absence of any muscle tone to achieve hook grip, the ability to lever up the door catch to open the car is absent. This is an important barrier. If they cannot gain access to the car, they simply will not be driving.

A range of adaptations exist for gaining control over the steering wheel when only one upper limb is functional or when arm strength is adequate but hand function is absent. Illustrated in Figure 43-9, these include a steering wheel spinner knob, tri-pin, and bi-pin. In New Zealand, a glove and pin attachment to the steering wheel results in appropriate contact with the steering wheel and a less bulky steering wheel modification. None of the devices described here cross the center of the steering wheel. In any vehicle with a driver's air bag, steering wheel adaptations that cross the center of the wheel are dangerous. On release of the air bag, the attachment will be forcibly removed and is likely to cause serious injury to the driver.

Lower Limbs

Based on the capsular driving compartment concept described earlier, there are few controls within the two segments occupied by the lower limbs: namely, the accelerator, brake, and clutch pedals and sometimes a foot-operated hand brake in the upper left segment of the lower limbs. Although relatively few in number, these controls are crucial to the safe operation of a motor vehicle and functional evaluation needs close attention.

Lower-limb range of movement is necessary to achieve a relaxed sitting position with at least 90 degrees of hip and knee flexion. Drivers who have had knee arthrodesis will need close evaluation of the suitability of their own vehicle. When they are seated in the vehicle, their foot is forced up underneath the dashboard area. The driver's seat will need to be pushed farther back, to relieve the situation. But this can result in the upper-limb controls being positioned out of reach. To relieve this situation, seating adaptations allow the affected leg to rest at a lower angle by scooping out a channel for the thigh.

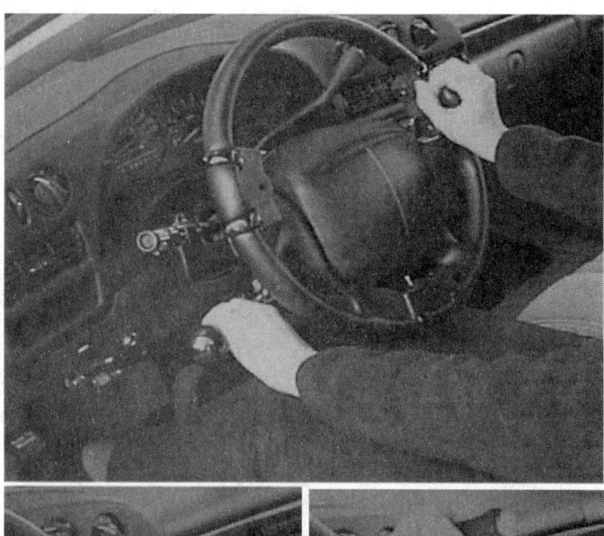

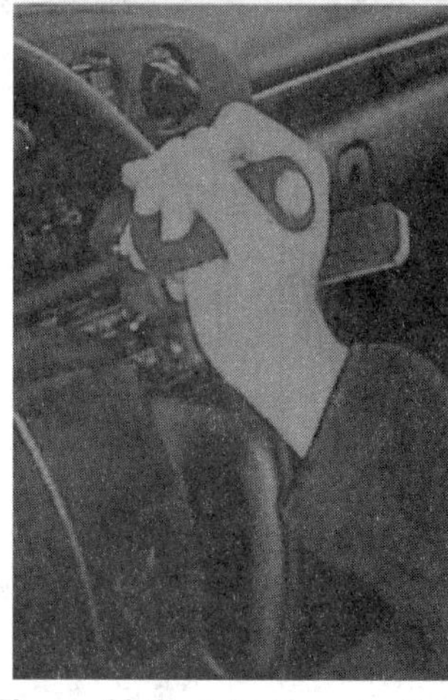

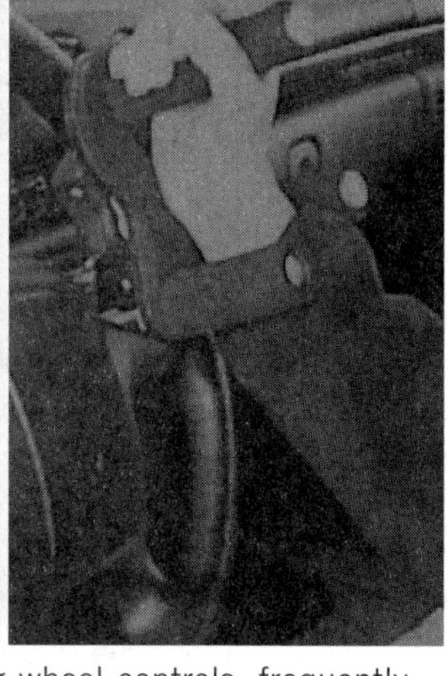

Figure 43-9. Adaptive steering wheel controls, frequently used with tetraplegic drivers, allow for a range of upper-limb abilities. *Top.* Steering wheel spinner in the right hand gives full control over the wheel, even on sharp turns. Hand controls operate the brake and accelerator pedals. *Lower left.* A bi-pin is used for those with active wrist extension. *Lower right.* Tri-pin firmly supports the wrist and stabilizes the hand of drivers with tetraplegia. Both bi-pins and tri-pins attach to the steering wheel through a pin that fits the steering wheel clamp.

Hip adduction and abduction movements are small but need to be performed with strength and accuracy. Knee extension is required for rapid, forceful braking in unexpected situations. Intact ankle plantarflexion and dorsiflexion are necessary to provide fine control over acceleration and braking. Because of the lack of ankle control, footdrop is not compatible with safe driving. Clients with footdrop who have attempted to drive report feeling puzzled that their car was constantly gathering speed. They did not relate this to their disability at the time.

Sensory feedback from proprioceptors is essential to safety. Proprioceptor impairment can result in missing the brake when stopping or confusion between the position in space of the clutch, brake, and accelerator. Causes of impaired proprioception most commonly seen in a driver assessment case load, and which can be overlooked, are trauma to nerves or joint surfaces in the lower limbs, incomplete spinal injury, mild cerebrovascular accident, multiple sclerosis, referred pain and patchy sensation from a back injury, lower-limb amputation with prosthesis, and knee-ankle-foot orthoses. Unsafe driving methods used by drivers with these disabilities may include using their hands to apply pressure to their knee for varying amounts of acceleration; achieving braking by using their hand to lift the leg from the accelerator to the brake pedal; only being able to locate the pedals in daylight as they rely on visual cues for foot movement; using their left foot on all pedals instead of using their right foot; and amputees driving with prostheses who report missing the foot pedals and accelerating instead of braking.

Lower-limb muscle endurance is another important factor in determining whether it is advisable to use the lower limbs for driving. Where there is any question of intermittent function, such as in multiple sclerosis, it is always advisable to perform the assessment during the days or activities that result in the lowest level of function. There is often a desire from drivers with intermittent leg function to use their legs on good days and hand controls on off days. Clinical experience from reports of a number of clients who have done so suggests that this can lead to involvement in crashes, probably because the person does not consistently use one driving technique.

Spinal Injury

The ability to raise the head to see the roadway ahead of the vehicle and maintain this position during driving is essential. Difficulty in head rotation will indicate the need for wide-angled mirrors and retraining to use them correctly. People with rheumatoid arthritis, ankylosing spondylitis, reflex sympathetic dystrophy, and cervical injuries such as severe whiplash are frequently affected. In order to bring the reduced vision to the clients' attention, it is useful to make a "map" of the blind spots, using cones or markers on the ground around them while they are seated. Translating this to the car can help convince people of the need to compensate for the gaps with the use of mirrors and to open them to acceptance of retraining.

Following a stroke, spinal rotation can be markedly restricted, probably due to the imbalance of the muscles in the trunk and spinal regions. This results in difficulty when turning to reverse the car and may require new learning with the use of mirrors in order to achieve safe maneuvers. An estimation of sitting balance is important for people with weak trunk musculature because upper-body stability is essential to maintain full control of the vehicle when cornering.

Visual Skills

The importance of visual skills for driving cannot be overemphasized. For instance, Wylie (18) estimated that

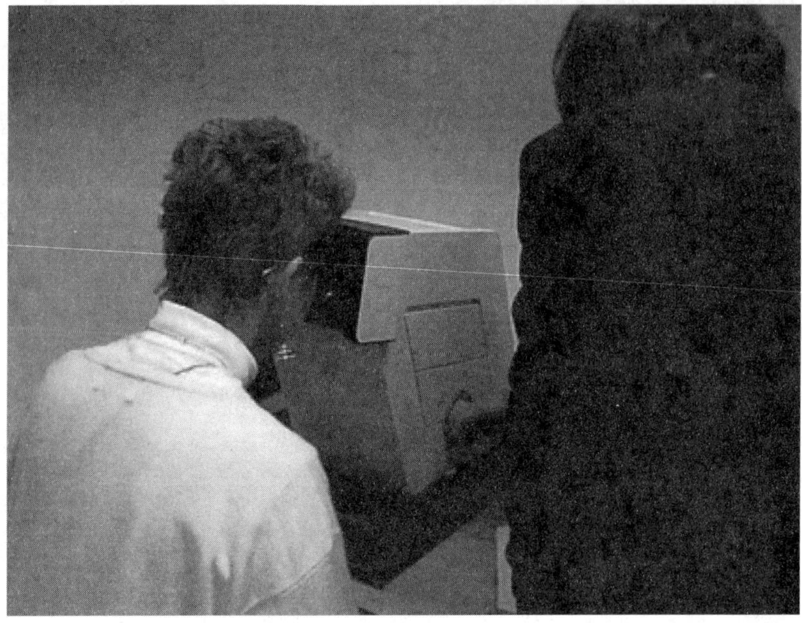

Figure 43-10. Stereoscopic vision screening testing device at the Easter Seals Mobility Center, Meriden, CT. This model is made by Stereoptical and other models are produced by Titmus and Keystone.

approximately 90% of the information processed while driving is taken in through the visual system. Nevertheless, some have raised questions, citing the importance of higher-order attentional processing (19) and instances where persons with significant visual impairments have been able to drive safely (20,21). In attempting to resolve this apparent contradiction, Gianutsos (22) cited the multiplicative effects of combinations of disabilities, whereby substantial isolated disability can be managed, but in combination with another disability (not necessarily substantial) the resulting effect is magnified outside safe limits. So an individual might be able to compensate for isolated visual field impairment or an oculomotor problem, but not both.

Strano (23) discussed the relationship of visual acuity to road engineering signage. In brief, when visual acuity is reduced, the time available to react to visual stimuli is equally reduced. Since visual fields are neither routinely nor periodically checked, and people with visual field losses may remain unaware (24), there are drivers with visual field loss. However, in most medical guidelines, homonymous hemianopia is deemed incompatible with safe driving. Quadrantanopia is a barrier to driving in at least one Australian state (11). Strano (23) discussed the difference in quadrants and their impact on driving. In her experience, upper-quadrant hemianopia will have more serious implications on driving than lower-quadrant defects. From an international perspective, relative seriousness of left- or right-quadrant hemianopia will depend on which side of the road the person should be driving. Visual fields are rarely seen to improve over time, even with retraining. Within optometry there are new optical interventions for visual field loss that may also enable otherwise intact persons with field loss to drive safely (24–28). Strano (23) also recommended that better compensatory field of vision can be obtained by "placing the [side rearview] mirror well forward on the front fender." Wide-angle mirrors can also be helpful, although the type and placement must be considered carefully so that confusion does not substitute for increased information.

Low lighting conditions, tiredness, ill health, and stress also negatively impact mild visual defects (23). Monocular vision produces a decrease in the available visual field and impaired depth perception (23). A wing mirror fitted to the side of the missing eye may be helpful. Careful evaluation and monitoring are essential under these circumstances.

Many driver rehabilitation specialists use a stereoscopic vision testing device, such as the one illustrated in Figure 43-10. In a few minutes these devices can be used to test acuity, binocular vision and stereopsis, and color vision and to screen for responsivity in the horizontal peripheral field. Some include measures of contrast sensitivity, which has been found to correlate with at-fault crashes (29). Computerized protocols for measuring the functional visual field (24,30) or the useful field of view (19,31) have particular value, as problems in these areas have obvious and demonstrated relationships to safe driving and are often poorly recognized by the individual with impairments.

Cognitive Skills

Driving is such a complex skill, requiring efficient, integrated functioning on all levels under pressure of time, that the relative importance of the skills involved is inherently difficult to define. Some facilities have used extensive neuropsychological testing (8,32) while others have reported success with specific computer assessment of a relatively small range of cognitive skills (9,13,33).

Cognitive skills that appear to be important for a positive outcome in driver assessment are visual discrimination, nonverbal reasoning, sequencing, spatial orientation, visual scanning, figure-ground discrimination, visual tracking, and right-left orientation (6). In 1992 Galski et al (8) found "visual perception . . . visual spatial analysis and synthesis, visuomotor coordination . . . planning, organising and executing test operations . . . scanning and attention, particularly selective sustained attention, . . . to be important in the prediction of actual performance." Galski et al (8) went on to warn that "many deficits in cognition did not adversely effect safe driving and were not equally important in predicting driving performance." Over the years, we have known, for example, people with profound recent memory impairment and aphasia who have sustained safe driving records. While these factors can serve as multipliers of other disabilities, they are not per se incompatible with safe driving. Carmella Strano was heard to observe at a conference that what counts is how the person deals with such problems; for example, does he impulsively cross several lanes of traffic to make a turn for which he had forgotten to prepare?

Others may bring loss of contact with reality to the clinician's attention, if not directly observed. While the implied lack of awareness has serious implications for driving safety, fortunately, there are usually others who recognize the need to intervene at this point to dissuade or prevent the person from driving. In these cases, it may not be productive to confront the individual, but rather to advise the family to assist with alternative mobility and to avoid the issue, if necessary, by removing or disabling the vehicle.

To the list of factors that need not be emphasized in the evaluation, we should add variables, such as glare sensitivity, of which most drivers are aware and experience as barriers to driving safely.

A validated screening assessment battery, The Stroke Drivers Screening Assessment, was developed by Nouri and Lincoln in Nottingham, England (34). This assesses concentration, nonverbal reasoning, and (British) road sign recognition. It takes approximately 1 hour to administer and is intended for use by a variety of health professionals as an initial screening tool to identify those who are definitely unfit to drive a car. In the United States, the Cognitive Behavioral Driver's Inventory (CBDI) (35) was developed psychometrically [normed (36) and validated (37)]; however, it lacks face validity (does not look to the client as if he or she has a relationship to driving) and its clinical utility is thereby reduced.

Complex, but noninteractive driving simulators, such as the Doron Driver Analyzer illustrated in Figure 43-11, originally intended for learner driver education, do have face validity, but have not been shown to predict the outcome of driving performance for people with disabilities (8,13). Simulation has much potential if it offers a dynamic interactive task that has a look and feel of driving (9,38–41). For instance, the authors of two computer programs developed specifically for the detection of impairment in brain-injured drivers in Christchurch, New Zealand (4), and New York, United States, (13), reported validity when computer results were compared to on-road driving skills (9) and driver self-reported limitations (42). In using computerized assessment and on-road evaluations with 261 drivers over 62 years old, McKnight and Lange (43) reported that "cognitive deficits evidenced the strongest association with unsafe (driving) performance."

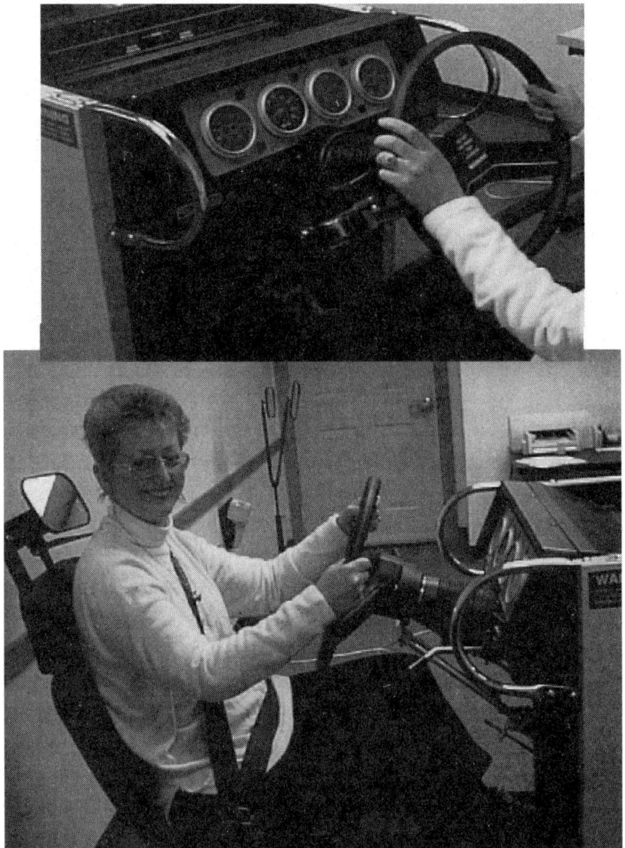

Figure 43-11. Doron Driver Analyzer at the Easter Seals Mobility Center. When performing the simulation, the patient would be viewing a video projected on a large screen directly ahead. The console is physically realistic; however, the task is not interactive (i.e., nothing that the patient does changes the display).

The success of computer-based programs is undoubtedly due to the unique ability of the computer to provide interactive, multiple information-processing tasks, at speeds similar to those of the human brain. They take less time to administer and can rapidly analyze and present results. The need to assess global skills at rapid speeds in real time may account for why pen and paper assessment processes have difficulty in predicting the outcome of driving safety. Experienced driver rehabilitation specialists, such as Amy Campbell of the Easter Seals Mobility Center (Meriden, CT), have dropped the paper and pencil procedures altogether, citing their lack of either face or empirical validity (personal communication, 1995).

Knowledge of Road Law

For people with brain impairment, additional tests examine knowledge of road law and decision making when presented with a variety of traffic situations, using road signs, slides, or videotapes (44).

Client and Family Interviews

Important information regarding premorbid driving habits, past driving experience, current license status, and general personality traits can be gained from the client and a close family member or friend. Although the information obtained is subjective, family and client interviews may add greater understanding of a wide range of lifestyle issues related to driving and place into context otherwise puzzling objective assessment findings.

It is important to remember that driving is not an end in itself, but merely a means to achieve a lifestyle goal as well as to carry out important life roles. Therefore, if one can understand the person's life roles in relation to driving, then final advice can be given in terms of which roles can be continued safely and which will need to be revised.

In-Car Static Assessment

This assessment takes place in the practical setting: in a vehicle. For people with minimal physical disabilities, it is preferable to view their needs in relation to the car that they would normally be driving. For people with cognitive impairment only and no physical disability, this stage will be carried out rapidly and with minimal detail, as part of the preparation for an on-road drive.

For most musculoskeletal driving assessments, a specially adapted vehicle with dual-control brake and accelerator will be required. The aim of this stage of assessment is to identify the actions that the person can easily perform and to develop a detailed prescription for driving adaptations. As this phase usually involves a large amount of detail, the use of a printed checklist is essential. A sample list is provided in Figure 43-12. One outcome of the static assessment may be that the current vehicle is clearly unsuited to the client's ergonomic needs and it should be replaced with another of more suitable design.

Mobility Aids

If the goal is for fully independent function, depending on the level of musculoskeletal impairment, the type of mobility aids and method of stowage inside the vehicle will need careful consideration. For instance, because of its awkward shape, a lightweight fixed-frame wheelchair, with wheels removed, is much more difficult to stow inside a car than a similar folding-frame wheelchair. This is most noticeable in a four-door vehicle, where the driver's door pillar and the steering wheel restrict the space available. Drivers with limited mobility may use a wheelchair for longer journeys outdoors (e.g., for shopping) and elbow crutches for short distances indoors. Therefore, consideration will need to be given as to how the wheelchair is to be stowed, who will accomplish this, and whether the car design allows for safe mobility when negotiating door openings.

Access

For some people, it is an accomplishment to achieve mobility as passengers. In this group are teenagers and adults with multiple handicaps, including physical and mental disabilities ranging from moderate to severe. It also includes former drivers who are no longer fit to do so. Whether in cars or vans, there are issues associated with method of access, stowage of mobility equipment, safety requirements, and caregivers.

The height of the driver's seat, width of the door opening, shape of the seat, and amount of leg room once inside may all impact on the functional ability and safety of the driver with a physical disability. The exact method of transfer into and out of the vehicle has a large impact on vehicle selection. If transfer from wheelchair to seat is not possible or contraindicated, then a van rather than a car will be required. If the driver is a permanent user of an electric wheelchair, a suitable vehicle must be selected to allow adequate head clearance when entering and exiting the vehicle, as well as when sitting in the driver's seat. As illustrated in Figure 43-13, floors of vans can be substantially lowered in order to achieve access. In addition to access to the van via a wheelchair hoist and specialist driving controls, appropriate wheelchair securing and safety belts will also be required. Assessment for people who intend to drive from their wheelchair is complex, involving specific decisions about the need for costly equipment, which this chapter does not aim to explore; detailed information should be sought from specialist driver assessors.

A variety of issues concerning access to the driver's seat of a car become a problem depending on the type of impairment. For instance, people with back injuries experience difficulty due to restricted or painful spinal flexion and rotation. This is magnified in a sports car that is low to the ground. Older people with arthritic conditions in their spine also experience this difficulty. In this respect, there is an ergonomic mismatch. On the one hand, drivers cannot reduce their body dimensions and have difficulty folding their body into a flexed position and on the other, car design has evolved to leaving a small hole in the car frame for the driver to squeeze through at the door opening.

STATIC ASSESSMENT:

DRIVER ACTIVITY ANALYSIS

Name: .... *Date:* ..../..../.... *Vehicle used:* ....

1. TRANSFERS

2. DOOR OPENING
   Key: lock & unlock

3. SEAT
   Adjust & tilt
   Seat belt

3. STEERING WHEEL
   Grip
   Turn
   Right/Left arm used to steer

4. BRAKE PEDAL Right/Left leg used for braking

5. ACCELERATOR PEDAL Right/Left leg used for accelerating

6. CLUTCH PEDAL

7. GEAR LEVER Engage through gears

8. HAND BRAKE

9. REAR VIEW MIRROR

10. SUN VISOR

11. WING MIRROR/S

12. IGNITION Insert key and start engine

13. HORN

14. WIPERS

15. TURN SIGNAL

16. LIGHTS

17. HEATER/DE-MISTER

18. TRUNK

Recommendations:

Figure 43-12. Form for static, in-car assessment.

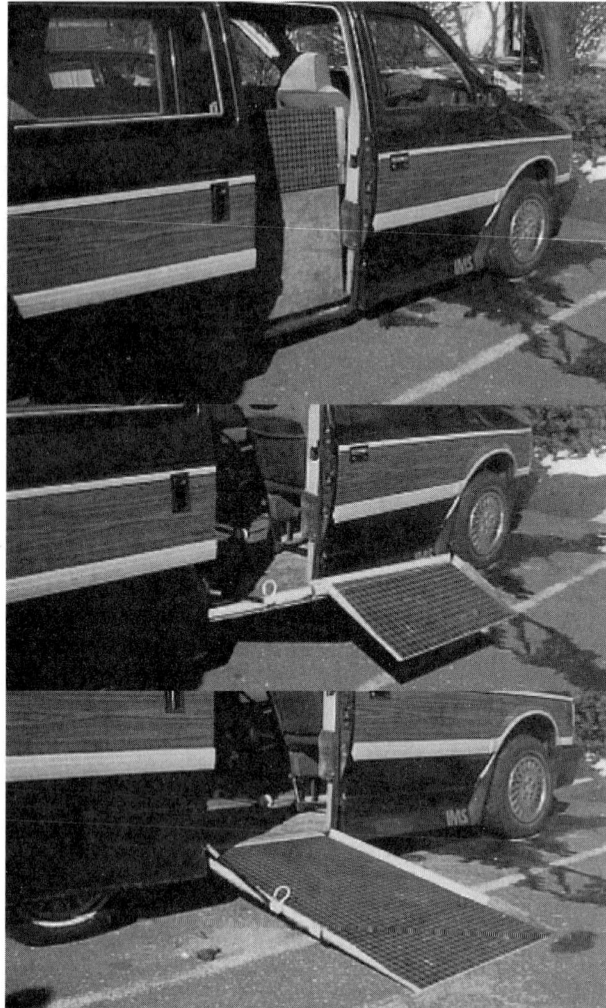

Figure 43-13. Adapted van at the Easter Seal Mobility Center. The floor has been lowered by 10 inches on this van. A side-mounted hoist installed in a van allows self-loading and driving from a wheelchair. *Top.* The door opens by remote-controlled switch. *Middle.* The hoist lowers automatically. *Bottom.* Hoist in wheelchair loading/unloading position.

Primary Driving Controls

For convenience of clinical reasoning, New Zealand occupational therapists distinguish primary and secondary driving controls. Primary controls are those essential to the driving task, that is, steering wheel, brake, accelerator, clutch, seat belt, and turn signal. They are used most frequently in optimum daylight driving conditions and therefore carry high priority in determining whether driving is possible. During in-car assessment, it is important to attend to these first.

Drivers with a spinal injury who use hand controls often need extra space to rest their legs, in order to avoid kinking the catheter tube and to maintain body balance. To enable this, the right-sided accelerator pedal can be hinged out of the way. This is also an important safety precaution when lower-limb extensor spasm is present, as a hinged accelerator ensures that unwanted acceleration is not applied during spasm. During driver training, one paraplegic client had a recurring problem of simultaneous extensor spasm in his right leg and flexor spasm in his left leg that interfered with the steering wheel. The spasms seemed to be triggered by anxiety and were noted during complex traffic situations. He was advised by the assessor to see his physician for a review of antispasmodic medication. There was a reduction in spasm sufficient to allow him to pass the practical driver's test without anxiety-produced lower-limb spasm.

In the absence of reliable function in the right leg, and when an automatic vehicle is used, a left-sided accelerator pedal can be added. Retraining is important so that the driver can use the same movement under all driving circumstances. In order for other people to also use the vehicle, it is standard practice to hinge the right accelerator so that it is out of the way but available for normal use. Reports of minor scrapes in driveways and garages caused by friends and family who attempt to drive the modified car illustrate the importance of ensuring the client is well educated in safety precautions.

Short drivers may require a range of driving adaptations including raising the height of the foot pedals. At the same time, it is necessary to reduce the length of the seat base to ensure that knee flexion is possible. A raised false floor gives the driver greater body stability when driving. Kleinberger and Summers (45) reported that severe or fatal air bag–induced injuries are more likely to occur in short female drivers (1.60 m) who do not wear a safety belt and who sit closer than 10 inches to the steering wheel. Therefore, it is imperative that satisfactory methods be found to enable the seat belt to be worn and the air bag mechanism to be turned off when it cannot be safely deployed.

Secondary Driving Controls

The remaining in-car controls represent the actions taken intermittently when driving, many of which can be adapted for easy use or operated by remote control. Frequently requested remote-control functions include adjusting headlights, controlling windshield wipers, and opening and closing windows. Special attention will need to be paid to drivers with marked hand impairment, such as that caused by rheumatoid arthritis, tetraplegia, severe hand trauma, and upper-limb amputation. In considering this list, the roles and lifestyle of the driver become important. For instance, daily use of fee-paying parking buildings means that it is essential for the driver to be able to operate the driver's window quickly; and the driver's desire for music while driving will influence what type of switches are appropriate on the radio or cassette or CD player.

On-Road Assessment

Issues

Many debates have arisen over the reliability and validity of using actual on-road driving for behavioral and cognitive assessment; nevertheless, it is an essential component of driver rehabilitation. Indeed a standard of care is evolving (46) to the effect that no one should be allowed to resume driving without an on-road assessment. This is not to say that everyone should be taken out on the road. Nor does it mean that performance on the road test overrides the outcome of the in-clinic assessment. Realistically, the aim is to determine whether persons with a disability are likely to be able to cope with driving in their locality, mostly on familiar routes, in order to pursue their goals and life roles. Whether drivers are likely to drive more than this or for extended periods outside familiar areas will have been discovered during client and family interviews. By this stage of assessment, hopefully anyone clearly unsuited for driving has been screened out of the program.

During the assessment of drivers with musculoskeletal impairment only, the on-road drive fulfills a slightly different role. Having established what range of adaptive driving equipment is likely to be suitable, the next step is to confirm in practice that drivers are actually able to use the equipment safely. There is a substantial learning curve when changing any type of driving technique, whether complex or simple. Sufficient time must be allowed for drivers to determine that they have full control over the vehicle before entering traffic flows. Essentially, they have become learner drivers again and will require competent instruction in order to feel safe in the new environment. The assessor needs to be aware of the emotional dynamics happening at this stage, and to stop and diffuse problems at any sign of unease. Drivers with low self-esteem may not feel confident in their abilities to drive; if they were injured in a motor vehicle crash, their first time back in the driver's seat may have heavy emotional significance; or they may simply have difficulty coordinating their limbs in a new way to achieve vehicle control. The use of an adapted vehicle with dual controls is essential to safety when assessing or retraining drivers who are new to driving with a disability.

Because occupational therapists (with their deep commitment to function) and most clients are impressed by the face validity of the on-road assessment, it is perhaps in order to introduce some considerations to modulate this enthusiasm, and to inspire improvements. First, "the" road test means many things to many people. Therefore, the tests actually used have no norms or established reliability and validity. In other words, the road test given to most clients does not even begin to meet the most basic standards for psychological tests and measurements (47). Interestingly enough, there have been attempts to develop a standardized road test (48,49) and substantial effort went into establishing its reliability. This "Michigan" test—unknown to most therapists in the United States—was adopted and adapted in New Zealand for evaluating advanced learner drivers (50). Implementation in each locality calls for extensive study of the level of skills accepted by the police for safe driving, establishment of a route containing a wide variety of driving conditions, and documentation during and after the 40-minute on-road drive. The documentation for each locale is several centimeters thick (about the size of a large urban telephone directory). Examiners receive 2 weeks of specialized training. Needless to say, the practical hurdles are significant, especially for community-based services. There is a major need to develop a practical on-road assessment protocol that can be implemented in different locations, with norms and acceptable levels of measurement reliability.

Then again, it would still be necessary to demonstrate that the test is a valid index of the individual's ability to drive safely. The appearance of validity, while clinically essential, is not sufficient. The vexing issue faced by all attempts to proving the validity of a given measure of driving, whether off-road or on-road, is the lack of an independent criterion. For older drivers free of overt neurologic diagnoses but with possible age-associated cognitive decline, one can attempt to use recent driving record—but even that is influenced by reporting and recording variables. A fundamental problem for measurement (but not for safety) is the fact that most older drivers limit themselves when their capabilities decline (42). Statistically, the validity coefficients shrink when poorly performing subjects maintain good driving records, because they drive very little.

Even if such a protocol were available, it would constitute a limited sample of performance, and being watched could cause the individual to be nervous, or at least, on their best behavior. Indeed, one insightful therapist looks for just this capability: Does the client recognize that the testing situation calls for one's "best behavior"? (51).

The face validity of the road test is a significant plus, but even if the psychometric limitations could be resolved, it would not be a complete assessment, its functionality notwithstanding. With off-road procedures aimed at assessing cognitive skills only, it is possible to simulate the types of crisis situations and to measure performance in precise quantitative ways. The most demanding aspects of driving can be safely condensed into a practical time frame. The more the off-road procedure simulates driving (i.e., has face validity), the more clinically effective it will be.

Many therapists have developed expertise to conduct on-road evaluations, through choosing quiet roads to minimize risk and then graduating the client to drive through increasingly busier areas. Some also become qualified driving instructors. Another approach recommended by trainers of occupational therapists as driver assessors in

Australia, and now accepted as standard practice, is for the therapist to collaborate with an experienced local driving school instructor with an interest in working with drivers with disabilities. The therapist observes and records findings from the back seat, free of the responsibility to ensure that the vehicle is operated safely. Under some circumstances, after observing the driving instructor, the therapist may feel comfortable enough to rely on the instructor's report. In uncomplicated cases where the individual has done very well on the in-clinic assessments, it may be sufficient to have a report from a local driving instructor.

If the coordinating therapist is not participating in the on-road evaluation, it is important to structure the process in such a way that the final recommendations remain in his or her hands so that all the findings and medical information are taken into account. While the on-road assessment may be the final step in the process, the results should not be the last word. For instance, off-road screening can show marked deficits in some areas of cognition that are not observed while on the road. At the least, the driver should be counseled by the therapist following the on-road drive and be made aware of what factors may constitute risky driving situations.

Finally, we must acknowledge that the state of the art in road testing is the "sweat index"—a global integration of the examiner's objective observations and subjective comfort level, signaled by his or her autonomic nervous system.

Routes

A review of published clinical practice (33,52) shows that occupational therapists, working with driving instructors, progress the client through a series of routes of increasing complexity. Fox et al (52), in Sydney, Australia, used four "standard assessment driving routes of increasing complexity . . . each requiring about 50 minutes to complete. The least complex drive is conducted within the Centre grounds, and the most complex in heavy density traffic incorporating freeway driving, road map navigation and multistorey car park manoeuvres where appropriate."

During this time, observations are recorded on a printed sheet that lists predetermined risk factors. van Zomeren et al (7) compiled an extensive list of commonly found driving faults. In New Zealand, driving instructors now use an Advanced Assessment and Training Report (53) as part of a three-tier licensing system. Occupational therapists in New Zealand are also using this same assessment approach. "The purpose of the assessment is to require drivers to demonstrate that they are skilled in the areas of Hazard Identification, Judgement, Manipulating Controls and Observing Traffic Regulations." The assessment is to last 40 minutes. The route "will, where practicable include suburban highway and motorway [freeway] conditions with at least 20 minutes of the time spent in busy city / town situations. (Medium to heavy traffic conditions should be sought)" (53).

An informal review of on-road assessment protocols in use in many driver rehabilitation programs indicates that the emphasis is on the operational level (i.e., mechanical skills). As suggested earlier, consideration should be given to incorporating the tactical level into the assessment. While examiner preparation and standardization call for a fixed route, this very fact removes the opportunity for tactical decision making regarding the route, unless the assessor specifically allows for it, for example, by asking the driver toward the end of the drive, "Can you find your way back now?"

COMMUNITY INTEGRATION

From the functional perspective of occupational therapy, besides formal assessment, it is helpful to examine the reality of the client's actual situation more fully.

Environmental Data

Terrain

Knowledge of the area in which the person with a disability intends to drive is an important aspect. Understanding the area and risks inherent for a particular disability will help to bring a practical focus for the client and family. Demonstrating a realistic understanding of the client's situation is likely to aid adherence to any recommendations made.

If the area is hilly with winding roads, then methods to maintain upper-body balance when cornering will be essential for people with weak trunk stabilizing muscles. Evaluation or prescription of the design of the driver's seat will also be necessary.

If a client with a back complaint is likely to be driving over rough ground, over poorly maintained or unsealed roads in rural areas, or over tram and railway tracks in the city, then no intervention is likely to be successful as it is the environment that is compounding the disability. If the vehicle is a light van or truck and the driver's seat is positioned over the front axle, the effect is to amplify every jolt on the road. In this instance, the vehicle and the terrain may become the prime focus of advice to the client. For instance, in the short term, the goal may be to avoid driving or to find alternative routes, and in the medium to long term to change the vehicle as well as the place of residence.

To illustrate, a client who recently had spinal surgery correctly identified the poorly maintained roads near his country home as a barrier to his return to work. However, he did not realize the importance of changing his vehicle from a four-wheel-drive vehicle with hard suspension to that of a sedan with highly absorbent suspension. He drove both vehicles over the same route. Whereas the four-wheel-drive seemed to magnify every small bump on the road, the sedan simply absorbed them.

For someone with cognitive or psychiatric impairment who is prone to concentration lapses, the monotony of driving on long, straight roads, such as on the freeway or in the Australian outback, is likely to contribute to a crash.

Climate

Weather factors specific to the driver's locality also need consideration. People with impaired contrast sensitivity may not be able to drive safely in mountainous areas where there is poor illumination during fog, drizzle, or snow. People with poor glare recovery may also be affected by oncoming headlights at night as well as environmental factors. For instance, during summer months in Auckland, New Zealand, commuters traveling west into the sun are at high risk of accidents due to what has become known as "sunstrike" (i.e., being dazzled by glare from the sun).

Behavioral

Galski et al (8) found that "behavioral measures . . . showed significant correlations to driving performance in traffic . . . it indicated that drivers who manifested specific [safety compromising] behaviors achieved poor outcomes in traffic." In his book, *Traffic Safety and the Driver*, Evans (1) devoted an entire chapter to driver behavior. Driver behavior is not what the driver can do but what the driver in fact does do. It is initially surprising to discover that in a study of the safety of racing car drivers and closely matched comparison drivers, "on a per year basis, the racing drivers had substantially more crashes and more violations, especially speeding violations." Evans provided a great deal of evidence that "we drive as we live." Evans (1) continued, "If his personal life is marked by caution, tolerance, foresight and consideration for others, then he would drive in the same way. If his personal life is devoid of these desirable characteristics then his driving will be characterized by aggressiveness. . . ." Therefore, when one is assessing drivers who lack insight, such as those with frontal lobe impairment and unresolved psychiatric conditions (the impulsiveness of hypermania, delusional thoughts or voices, unstable mood levels), assessment battery results must be interpreted with caution. During off-road assessment, additional emphasis therefore will need to be placed on safety-compromising behaviors.

Ethical and Legal Issues

Professional experience and even some data (54) reveal that many practitioners are unaware of their responsibilities to their patients regarding driving. Some useful articles are available on this subject (55,56). Gianutsos formulated a statement on "What happens to your New York State driver's license after a brain injury?" addressed to patients. She had the statement reviewed for accuracy by the New York State Department of Motor Vehicles. It is included as Appendix I and readers are encouraged to adapt it to their own jurisdictions. (They may adapt and distribute it if they acknowledge the source and send her a copy.)

Some rehabilitation specialists adopt a "don't ask, don't tell" posture regarding driving. It is safe to assume that all patients who were drivers are would-be drivers, no matter how severe their disabilities. Apprehensive about a negative decision, if there are no significant physical disabilities, they may not seek advice on the issue. However, as Antrim and Engum (57) emphasized, there is no legal safety in rehabilitation facilities' avoiding the issue of driving. Nor is ignorance of the applicable law an excuse.

In most jurisdictions there is an agency that controls licensure (e.g., the Department of Motor Vehicles in individual states in the United States, the Ministry of Transport in New Zealand, and the Roads and Traffic Authority in Australia). In some cases these agencies are national and in others, state or provincial. There is a legal code that governs this agency, as well as statutes that detail its practices. These rules include what medical and visual standards must be met for initial licensure and renewals. The most significant issue for rehabilitation professionals is whether and how the existence of a disability comes to the attention of the licensing agency. The range of possibilities includes mandatory reporting by health care providers, optional reporting with immunity (against claims of violation of confidentiality), reporting by the individual prior to resumption of driving, and reporting upon renewal of licensure. In the United States six to eight of the states have some form of mandatory reporting. British Columbia has an interesting variation with what could be called "mandatory reporting to the individual" (i.e., a mandate to raise the issue and make recommendations) followed by reporting to the licensing agency in those instances where noncompliance comes to the provider's attention. Because there is such a wide range of possibilities, it is essential for practitioners to find out from their local licensing agency what the law is.

Prior to initiation of the driving advisement process, it is important to have an explicit statement about what will be offered, individual responsibilities, and to whom the resulting information will be sent. Gianutsos uses a "Memo of Understanding" for this purpose, offered as Appendix II, which can be adapted and used to meet individual needs. It is recommended that the patient receive a written copy of the resulting report and recommendations. We have received a legal opinion that it is not sufficient to make an entry in the patient's medical record about recommendations given orally.

Helping patients return to safe independent mobility is part of our clinical mission. While the legal aspects may be daunting, we must give patients access to every resource and clinical insight we can marshal. If the outcome is not favorable, they need to know why: They may not be entitled to a license, but they are entitled to an explanation. Further, we need to offer constructive, and often creative, suggestions regarding mobility alternatives.

ACKNOWLEDGMENTS

Special appreciation is due to Michael Bannister, whose talents and contributions are many, for his assistance with graphics and to Amy Campbell, OTR/L, of the Easter Seals Mobility Center in Meriden, CT, for her collegial input, data collection, and allowing us to photograph.

APPENDIX I. WHAT HAPPENS TO YOUR NYS DRIVER'S LICENSE AFTER BRAIN INJURY?

Rosamond Gianutsos, Ph.D.

Neuropsychologist

Certified Driver Rehabilitation Specialist (Assoc. of Driver Educators for the Disabled)

Cognitive Rehabilitation Services, 38-25 52nd St. Sunnyside, NY 11104

Dr. Gianutsos was a member of the NYS DMV's Medical Advisory Board which met in 1988–89 to review policy. She chaired the Subcommittee for the Elderly and Disabled Driver. She is not currently associated with the DMV. The information below represents her own views and, while every effort has been made to assure accuracy, not official DMV policy.

Whether you can drive safely is NOT what this is about: **If you have survived a brain injury and you want to drive again, first take the matter up with your doctors and therapists.**

What follows IS information about the NYS Department of Motor Vehicles' (DMV) rules and procedures concerning your driver's license. For the moment, we assume that you hold a valid NYS operators license to drive an ordinary private car. For trucks, buses and other commercial vehicles the rules are much stricter if you drive interstate.

Your license remains valid until it expires or DMV takes action to suspend or revoke it. Suspension and revocation actions can be taken for many reasons, including too many points for moving violations or involvement in a crash in which someone was killed. DMV can review your qualifications for licensure if they receive a complaint from another person, including a health care professional who is treating you. However, health care professionals are not encouraged to make reports as you can file a lawsuit for violation of your privacy: The law does not afford them immunity.

So the answer to the question of what happens to your license is, simply, nothing.

Well . . . not quite.

An issue may come up when you renew your license depending on your answers to the questions which DMV asks all drivers on renewal (which are similar to the questions asked applicants for new licenses). **Your answers may trigger a request for medical information and a review.** The renewal form is the MV-2M. An older form (MV-2) dated 1/89 is still being distributed. A word to the wise: **interpret these questions literally and answer them honestly**. It is in your interests to inform the DMV about your status and to keep a copy of any records of your having done so. Should you have a serious accident, no one will be able to claim that you got, or kept, your license when you were not competent and should have known better.

What are the DMV license renewal questions?

- **Since you applied for a license, or since your last renewal was issued: Have you had, or are you being treated for, any of the following, or has a previous condition gotten worse?**

- **Convulsive disorder, epilepsy, fainting or dizzy spells, or any condition which causes unconsciousness**
- **Heart ailment**
- **Hearing impairment**
- **Lost use of leg, arm, foot, hand or eye**

A review occurs if you answer "yes" to any of the questions.

What kind of health care provider can fill out the DMV forms? The form will often be quite specific. Usually a medical doctor who has treated you in the last 3 months will do; however, in cases of seizure disorders (recurring periods of unconsciousness) a neurologist or neurosurgeon will be needed. The DMV may accept a report from a neuropsychologist or other qualified individual. Such a person should be prepared to explain why they are qualified, and this may add to the time it takes to resolve the matter.

The DMV has a Medical Review Unit (Medical Review Unit Driver Improvement Bureau, New York State Department of Motor Vehicles, Empire State Plaza, Albany, NY 12228 (518 474-0774) which has a medical consultant; however, there is no standing Medical Advisory Board.

If you require a medical report, the doctor will have to sign the following statement: "***The patient's medical condition would not interfere with his/her safe operation of a motor vehicle.***"

Specific Conditions

Vision

- If you can read at **20/40 or better** on an ordinary eye chart (with or without glasses), you meet DMV's requirements. If you are aphasic (have language problems), you can have an eye doctor certify on a DMV form which the doctor usually can supply.
- If you have **lost the use of one eye**, you can still qualify to drive a car, but can not drive commercially.
- If your **acuity is between 20/40 and 20/70**, you must submit a report by an eye doctor. These are the only circumstances in which you will have to meet the DMV's requirements for **visual field**: a span of what you can normally see with one eye (140 degrees, or almost 40% of the perimeter of a circle). If you have a "**homonymous hemianopia**" (don't see one half of the field of view in each eye), you will NOT meet this standard. Strictly speaking, if your acuity is good, you could have tunnel vision and still qualify for a NYS license. This is an obvious **loophole in the regulations**. In many states and most of the rest of the world, you would not even be considered for a license with such a loss of vision. If you have a visual field problem or "neglect," you will have a difficult time compensating, especially in busy, complex or new situations, or when you are tired or distracted. Most important, you are probably under-aware of your loss—you literally may not see any problem! . . . not because you deny or neglect it. The human nervous system normally fills in the gaps (which is only a problem when there are substantial gaps in the field of vision).

Any Condition Which Causes Unconsciousness

- This item used to be "loss of consciousness" and is the one which often leads to medical review for people who were unconscious for a period of time following a head injury. Unless you have a seizure condition (see below), you may have your primary care physician fill out form MV80-U based on an examination performed within the last 120 days.

Seizures

- Officially, you must be seizure free for a year. In practice, the DMV may accept 6 months. The MV80-U form must be filled out by a board certified/eligible neurologist or neurosurgeon based on an examination performed within the last 120 days.

Tips:

- **Renew early** if you anticipate Medical Review. You can renew as much as 6 months before your license expires. Do not wait for DMV to send you renewal forms. The Medical Review process takes time, up to 6 weeks they estimate. If you have to supply further information, it's another 6 weeks. Begin early and you won't be grounded while they review it.
- **Renew late** if you need time to recover. You have up to 2 years following your license expiration to renew using ordinary procedures. While, during that year, you can not drive, you will not necessarily have to take a written or road test and be treated like a new driver.

Comment

Some people think it is shocking that doctors are not required to report people with conditions which might affect driving to DMV. This "mandatory reporting" exists in a handful of states and is inconsistently applied, like the 55 mph speed limit. It forces your doctor to wear two hats: as your doctor and as an agent of the state. Some drivers would not seek treatment if they thought it might jeopardize their license. Given the right information, in an understandable form, the vast majority of drivers will, perhaps reluctantly, make the right decision.

APPENDIX II. *DRIVING ADVISEMENT: MEMO OF UNDERSTANDING*

between ________________ (examinee) and ______________________ (examiner)

The computerized driving advisement procedures (Functional Visual Fields and Elemental Driving Simulator) have been developed to help people find out if they have necessary cognitive skills for driving safely. Driving is a very serious matter, because, as many of us are painfully aware, grave injury can be caused by crashes. Not only do drivers risk their own safety, but also that of other drivers, passengers, pedestrians and cyclists as well. It is hoped that these services will give useful information to help would-be drivers to make informed decisions.

1. **Conclusions based on comparison with how safe drivers do**. What kinds of conclusions can be drawn from these procedures? First, we have tested safe drivers of varying ages on these procedures and will be able to compare how you do to how they did. If you fall within their range of scores, however, you are not guaranteed to be safe on the road. Or, if you fall outside the normal range, it may not mean that you would be unsafe. Hopefully, this information would give you something to consider in your decision making.
2. **Cognitive only**. These procedures are designed to address the cognitive skills that a content analysis of driving showed to be important. Other areas must also be checked, including: vision, motor function, and neurological status.
3. **Does not replace road test**. Whatever conclusions either of us draws based on how you do on these tasks should ordinarily be verified by a specialized in-vehicle, on-the-road test by a driving evaluator who has been fully informed of your background.
4. **Legal requirements are your responsibility**. It is up to you to see that you satisfy the requirements of the law, including having a valid driver's license or learner's permit and insurance. New York State law requires that you answer DMV's questions about disabilities when you renew your license.
5. **Report**. This evaluation is, therefore, strictly advisory. You will receive a summary and explanation of your performance, together with my conclusions and recommendations. I will send the report to a third party only with your written authorization. If an insurance company is paying for these services, your signature below permits me to send a copy of my report to the company.

Our signatures below signify that we have both read and acknowledge the above statement.

____________________________ (examinee signature)

____________________________ (examiner signature)

____________________________ (date)

____________________________ (date)

Address to which report should be sent:

REFERENCES

1. Evans L. *Traffic safety and the driver.* New York: Van Nostrand Reinhold, 1991.
2. Gurgold GD, Harden DH. Assessing the driving potential of the handicapped. *Am J Occup Ther* 1978;32:41–46.
3. Sivak M, Olson PL, Kewman DG, et al. Driving and perceptual/cognitive skills: behavioral consequences of brain damage. *Arch Phys Med Rehabil* 1981;62:476–483.
4. Jones JG, McCann J, Lassere MN. Driving and arthritis.

Br J Rheumatol 1991;30: 361–364.

5. Bardach JL. Psychological factors in handicapped drivers. *Arch Phys Med Rehabil* 1971;52:328–332.

6. Simms B. Perception and driving: theory and practice. *Br J Occup Ther* 1985;48:363–366.

7. van Zomeren AH, Brouwer WH, Minderhoud JM. Acquired brain damage and driving: a review. *Arch Phys Med Rehabil* 1987;68:697–705.

8. Galski T, Bruno RL, Ehle HT. Driving after cerebral damage: a model with implications for evaluation. *Am J Occup Ther* 1992;46:324–332.

9. Gianutsos R. Driving advisement with the Elemental Driving Simulator (EDS): when less suffices. *Behav Res Methods Instr Comp* 1994;26:183–186.

10. Beatson CJ. Transport technology: New Zealand perspectives. *Work J Prev Assess Rehabil* 1997;8:271–280.

11. *Drivers and riders: Guidelines for medical practitioners.* NSW, Australia: Roads and Traffic Authority, 1993:3.

12. *Physicians' guide to driver examination.* 5th ed. *Can Med Assoc J* 1991;(suppl):1–64.

13. Gianutsos R, Campbell A, Beattie A, Mandriota FJ. A computer-augmented quasi-simulation of the cognitive prerequisites for resumption of driving after brain injury. *Assist Technol* 1992;4:70–86.

14. Pierce S. A roadmap for driver rehabilitation. *Occup Ther Pract* 1996;(Oct):30–38.

15. Pierce SL. The team approach to transportation assessment. *Work J Prev Assess Rehabil* 1997;8: 239–252.

16. Sprigle S, Morris BO, Nowachek G, Karg PE. Assessment of the evaluation procedures of drivers with disabilities. *Occup J Res* 1995;15:147–164.

17. Korner-Bitensky N, Sofer S, Kaizer F, et al. Assessing ability to drive following an acute neurological event: are we on the right road? *Can J Occup Ther* 1994;61:141–148.

18. Wylie EJ. Vision and driving. *Can J Optom* 1978;40:70–74.

19. Owsley C. Vision and driving in the elderly. *Optom Vis Sci* 1994;71:727–735.

20. Ramsey WE. *Low vision and driving. Driving instruction course: focus on the handicapped.* College Park, MD: American Automobile Association, 1990.

21. Chapman BG. Driving with the bioptic. *J Vis Rehabil* 1995;9:19–22.

22. Gianutsos R. Driving and visual information processing in cognitively at risk and older individuals. In: Gentile M, ed. *Functional visual behavior: a therapist's guide to evaluation and treatment options.* Bethesda, MD: American Occupational Therapy Association, 1997:321–342.

23. Strano CM. Effects of visual deficits on ability to drive in traumatically brain-injured population. *J Head Trauma Rehabil* 1989;4(2):35–43.

24. Gianutsos R, Suchoff IB. Visual fields after brain injury: management issues for the occupational therapist. In: Scheiman M, ed. *Understanding and managing vision deficits: a guide for occupational therapists.* Thorofare, NJ: Slack, 1997: 333–358.

25. Gottlieb DD. *Enhancing awareness, increasing safety, and returning to driving for patients with visual field loss and neglect.* Washington, DC: Neuro-optometric Rehabilitation Association, International, 1993.

26. Gottlieb DD, Freeman P, Williams M. Clinical research and statistical analysis of a visual field awareness system. *J Am Optom Assoc* 1992;63:581–588.

27. Waiss B, Cohen J. The utilization of a temporal mirror coating on the back surface of the lens as a field enhancement device. *J Am Optom Assoc* 1991;63:576–580.

28. Cohen JM, Waiss B. An overview of enhancement techniques for peripheral field loss. *J Am Optom Assoc* 1993;64:60–70.

29. Brown J, Greaney K, Mitchel J, et al. *Predicting accidents and insurance claims among older drivers.* Southington, CT: ITT Hartford Insurance Group, 1993.

30. Suchoff IB, Gianutsos R, Ciuffreda KJ, et al. Vision impairment related to acquired brain injury. In: Silverstone B, Lang MA, Rosenthal B, Faye EE, eds. *The Lighthouse handbook on vision impairment and rehabilitation.* New York: Oxford University Press, 1999 (in press).

31. Ball K, Owsley C. The useful field of view test: a new technique for evaluating age-related declines in visual function. *J Am Optom Assoc* 1993;64:71–79.

32. Gouvier WD, Maxfield MW, Schweitzer JR, et al. Psychometric prediction of driving performance among the disabled. *Arch Phys Med Rehabil* 1989;70:745–750.

33. Jones R, Giddens H, Croft D. Assessment and training of brain-damaged drivers. *Am J Occup Ther* 1983;37:754–760.

34. Nouri FM, Tinson DJ, Lincoln NB. Cognitive ability and driving after stroke. *Int Disabil Stud* 1992; 9(3):110–115.

35. Engum ES, Cron L, Hulse CK, Pendergrass TM, Lambert W. Cognitive Behavioral Driver's Inventory. Cogn Rehabil 1988; 6(5):34–50.

36. Engum ES, Womac J, Lambert EW, Pendergrass T. Norms and decision making rules for the cognitive behavioral driver's inventory. *Cogn Rehabil* 1988;6(6):12–18.

37. Engum ES, Lambert EW, Scott K, et al. Criterion-related validity of the Cognitive Behavioral Driver's Index. *Cogn Rehabil* 1989;7(4):22–31.

38. Aaronson D, Eberhard J. An evaluation of computer-based driving systems for research, assessment, and advisement. *Behav Res Methods Instr Comp* 1994;26:195–197.

39. Schiff W, Arnone W, Cross S. Driving assessment with computer-video scenarios: more is sometimes better. *Behav Res Methods Instr Comp* 1994;26:192–194.

40. Blaauw GJ. Simulator and instrumented car: a validation study. *Hum Factors* 1982;24:473–485.

41. Rossi DG, Flint SJ. *An evaluation of mature driver performance.* New Mexico Highway and Transportation Department, Traffic Safety Bureau, Transportation Programs Division, 1988.

42. DeLibero V. *Self-appraisal and driving simulator performance in younger and older drivers.* Touro College, School of Health Sciences, Santa Fe, NM, Department of Occupational Therapy, 1995. MA thesis.

43. McKnight AJ, Lange JE. Automated screening techniques for drivers with age related ability deficits. In: *Conference presentations of the 41st annual meeting of the Association for the Advancement of Automotive Medicine.* Orlando, FL: Association for the Advancement of Automative Medicine, 1997:79–93.

44. Weaver JK. *Driver performance test II.* Palm Harbor, FL (4660 Brayton Terrace South, Palm Harbor, FL 34685): Advanced Driving Skills Institute, 1990.

45. Kleinberger M, Summers L. Mechanisms of injuries for adults and children resulting from airbag interaction. In: *Conference presentations of the 41st annual meeting of the Association for the Advancement of Automotive Medicine.* Orlando, FL: Association for the Advancement of Automotive Medicine, 1997:405–420.

46. Subcommmitee on Driver Evaluation and Training for Individuals with Disabilities. *Final report.* Albany, NY: New York State Vocational and Educational Services for Individuals with Disabilities (VESID), 1993.

47. Committee to Develop Standards for the Educational and Psychological Testing of The American Educational Research Association, The American Psychological Association, and The National Council on Measurement in Education. *Standards for educational and psychological testing.* Washington, DC: American Psychological Association, 1985.

48. Vanosdall F, Rudisill M, Alexander L, et al. *Michigan road test implementation project. Final report: pilot implementation of the Michigan driver performance test.* Vol. I. Ann Arbor, MI: Michigan State Police, Michigan Office of Highway Safety Planning, 1980.

49. Forbes TW, Nolan RO, Schmidt FL, Vanosdall FE. Driver performance measurement based on dynamic driver behavior patterns in rural, urban, suburban and freeway traffic. *Accid Anal Prev* 1975;7:257–280.

50. Wright PG, Perkins WA. *The implementation of a "Michigan" style driving test in New Zealand—a preliminary evaluation.* Wellington, New Zealand: Land Transport Division, Ministry of Transport, 1989:181.

51. Mitchell S. Brain injury and memory deficits in driver rehabilitation. Meeting of the Association of Driver Educators for the Disabled—Northeast, Albany, NY, October 1994.

52. Fox GK, Bashford GM, Caust SL. Identifying safe versus unsafe drivers following brain impairment: The Coorabel Programme. *Disabil Rehabil* 1992;14(3): 140–145.

53. Brown R, Eagle L, Swenson SC, et al. *Learning system for driving instructors.* Wellington, New Zealand: Land Transport Division, Ministry of Transport, 1992; 2. Road User Standards.

54. Pidikiti RD, Novack TA. The disabled driver: an unmet challenge. *Arch Phys Med Rehabil* 1991;72:109–111.

55. Bedway B. What's your responsibility for older patients who drive? *Med Econ* 1992;69:114–123.

56. O'Neill D. The doctor's dilemma: the aging driver and dementia. *Int J Geriatr Psychiatry* 1992; 7:1–5.

57. Antrim JM, Engum ES. The driving dilemma and the law: patients' striving for independence vs. public safety. *Cogn Rehabil* 1989;7:16–19.

Chapter 44

Music Therapy

Suzanne E. Jonas

"Music hath charms to soothe the savage breast; To soften rocks, or bend a knotted oak." William Congreave, in "The Mourning Bride"

Music therapy is increasingly being utilized in physical and cognitive rehabilitation programs. As health care organizations place more emphasis on functional independence in life activities, music therapy can address the functional needs of this population in the areas of cognition, communication, physical functioning, activities of daily living, and psychosocial functioning. According to the Joint Commission on Accreditation of Healthcare Organizations (1), the range of services offered in physical rehabilitation programs may include but is not limited to ". . . audiology, creative arts therapies, dental, dietetic, educational, occupational therapy, physical therapy, prosthetic and/or orthotic, psychological, recreational therapy, rehabilitation engineering, rehabilitation medicine, rehabilitation nursing, social work, speech-language pathology, and vocational rehabilitation services."

Although the number of music therapists working in rehabilitation programs is still relatively low, the use of music and sound for treating psychological and physical ills has been in existence since antiquity in all cultures and in many different forms. In ancient Greece, Apollo was the god of both music and medicine. And it was Pythagoras of Samos who is credited with being the father of music therapy in the sixth century BC. He taught his students that certain musical chords and melodies produced definite responses within the body. He demonstrated that the right sequence of sounds played on an instrument could cure bodily pain, soothe the pangs of bereavement, calm anger, and still desire. His philosophy encompassed music healing, science, mathematics, medicine, and nutrition based on the premise that the universe and all its creations are founded and governed by the laws of music and vibration. His philosophy dominated Mediterranean culture for 800 years.

In ancient Rome, music was considered as high an endeavor as science and a builder of one's character. Hippocrates, the "Father of Medicine," is said to have taken his patients suffering from mental illness to the Temple of Aesculapius to listen to the stirring music. And the physician Paracelsus practiced what he called a "musical medicine": Specific compositions were played for specific maladies: mental, moral, and physical. Although the ancient art of healing with music all but vanished in Europe after the fall of the Roman Empire and assisted by Cartesian science, its application as a specific means of therapeutic intervention is being rediscovered and researched in the twentieth century. Ironically, wars have been a major influence in bringing the use of music back as a healing agent in our century. The initial application of music therapy was in veteran's hospitals where it gradually evolved along two main lines: passive—listening to music; and active—singing, playing an instrument, and exercising. In the United States, the National Association for Music Therapy (NAMT) and the American Music Therapy Association (AMTA) were organized to support the ancient art.

DEFINITION OF MUSIC THERAPY

Music therapy involves the building of a relationship between a patient and a specially trained therapist, using music as the basis for communication. The current field is a broad one, encompassing psychotherapeutic, educational, instructional, behavioral, pastoral, supervisory, healing, recreational, and interrelated-arts applications of music and sound. Formally trained music therapists work in a variety of settings with a wide variety of patients. A newer branch is medical music therapy, which refers to the functional uses of music in medical specialties, to 1) affect health directly, 2) support or enhance medical treatment or procedures, 3) combine with therapist or medical treatment in equal importance, 4) become part of the therapeutic relationship, and 5) reduce distress related to specific illnesses (2). The use of music and sound in medicine is rapidly growing and being recognized once again as a viable treatment modality. The International Society for Music in Medicine conferences demonstrate the wide variety of applications and research in this field from analgesia to urology (3), as does the recent compilation of research in music therapy by both the NAMT (4) and CAIRSS. The latter is a bibliographic database of music research literature containing over 11,000 citations from articles published in more than 2000 different journals in 25 languages in 54 countries. It is maintained by the Institute for Music Research at the University of Texas at San Antonio (5).

The tremendous value of music is its ability to simultaneously influence mind, body, spirit, and emotions. Used regularly, like any prescribed medication, music is an effective outlet for feelings of stress; is an assistant in clarifying issues; and is effective for decreasing symptoms and increasing the body's own healing mechanisms. And music that touches our spirits can assist us in both transcending and transforming emotional and physical suffering. Table 44-1 is a current summary of all the proven ways that music affects our being. By its very nature it is a holistic treatment.

Table 44-1: Responses to Musical Experience

Mind	Body	Spirit	Emotions
Brain waves	Pulse rate	Socialization	Anxiety
Concentration	Blood pressure	Memories	Fear
Creativity	Circulation	Transpersonal realms	Apprehension
Aural development	Muscular energy	Imagery	Anger
Attention	Respiration	Ego	Loneliness
Synchronicity	GSR	Id	Happiness
Imagery	Pupil size	Superego	Excitement
	Autonomic nervous system	Patriotism	Expression
			Aura
	Pain		Depression
	Sleep		

Source: Reproduced by permission from Jonas SE. *Take two tapes and call me in the morning*. 2nd ed. Haydenville, MA: Music & Medicine, 1996.
GSR = Golvanic skin response.

HOW MUSIC WORKS

Physics has demonstrated that all matter is composed of one basic substance or energy, and each living and nonliving thing is a unique vibrating system determined by characteristic frequencies of vibration or rhythm. Or, as composer/researcher Randall McClellan (6) stated, "This whole universe is one great symphony and around us everything and every creature of this Earth continually resonates to that symphony, adding its own voice according to natural harmonic law." As human beings, we have a specific vibrational rate that makes us different from whales and trees. Each part of us—heart, eye, knee, and so on—also has its own frequency, as do the individual cells that make up these parts. One theory of disease propounds that when the normal frequency of a body part increases or decreases too dramatically, mutated or deformed cells are produced and disease occurs. The body part is "out of tune." Some of the influencers of change in frequency are emotions, chemicals, strong electromagnetic waves, and sound waves.

Music is organized sound; sound is vibration. The vibrations that constitute music differ from the random and irregular vibrations of noise. Musical tone creates a regular, evenly timed sine wave that repeats itself. So, even though we may criticize a piece of music as "noise," if the tones used in the music have regular sine waves, then it is indeed music.

While most of us intuitively know that "Music hath charms," exactly how music makes its way into our thinking and why it affects our bodies is still being researched. Results so far demonstrate the following:

1. As sound vibrations enter the outer ear, the eardrum vibrates at the same frequency as the sound source and transfers the vibrations to the inner ear where it is transformed into electrical impulses. The impulses go to the cochlear nuclei in the medulla oblongata in the brain stem. Continuing their journey, the impulses divide into two paths: to the neocortex through the pons and medial geniculate nucleus of the thalamus, and to the auditory cortical areas in the limbic system through the reticular formation. The impulses are then transferred throughout the entire body (6).
2. As the electrical impulses cross the corpus callosum, memory may be activated and synchronicity of the hemispheres may occur through entrainment principles (7).

3. Music may be able to stimulate the production of endorphins to produce feelings akin to love, and to decrease pain (7).
4. Musically naive persons have higher α brain waves in the right hemisphere, and respond to music almost equally in both hemispheres during listening. Musicians have higher α waves in the left hemisphere, and perceive melody and chords with the left hemisphere (8).
5. Music is the only outside stimulus that automatically stimulates the two hemispheres: Lyrics, beat, rhythm, and notation, stimulate the left one; harmony, intonation, creativity, and overall flow stimulate the right one (9).
6. Harvard professor Howard Gardner demonstrated that it is the music/sound portion of the brain that develops first.

USE OF SOUND IN MUSIC THERAPY

Returning to the above discussion of physics and vibrations, each object has its own vibratory rate (i.e., resonance). One way in which the resonance can be altered is through entrainment. The ancient Egyptian and Greek civilizations used these principles and techniques for healing in their temples. In this process, the powerful rhythmic vibrations of one object cause the less powerful vibrations of another object to lock in step and oscillate with the more powerful object. This is demonstrated in a field of fireflies, which if allowed to remain in close proximity to one another for a period of time, will synchronize their blinking.

Another way of changing frequency is to match the resonant frequency of an object to implode it, to break it up. An example of this would be the opera singer who sings a note that has the same resonant frequency as a crystal wine glass, with the result that the wine glass shatters.

The most widely recognized and accepted use of frequency application is the field of ultrasonics, where in medicine high frequencies are used to generate heat that can penetrate to the deep tissues of the body.

Hemi-Sync

In the 1830s the German experimenter H. W. Dove discovered the phenomenon of binaural beats. These are beats that are generated in the human brain as a result of hearing different externally generated frequencies in each ear. For instance, if a tone of 200 beats/min was played in the right ear and a tone of 210 beats/min in the left, the brain would "hear" the difference in the beats and generate its own frequency of 10 beats/min. No one ever "hears" the binaural beats. The late Robert Monroe, formerly a composer in the communications industry, used this theory to develop an auditory guidance system to heighten selected awareness and performance while establishing a relaxed state. Based on entrainment principles, the system involves sending specific frequencies to each ear to assist in entraining the separate areas of the hemispheres to equal electromagnetic environments, to enhance the free-flowing exchange of information between hemispheres (10). The resulting synchronicity of the hemispheres greatly increases learning, healing, and meditative abilities. The Monroe Institute in Faber, Virginia, has produced dozens of tapes to assist in synchronizing the hemispheres and achieving optimal brain wave states. The frequencies are embedded in ocean surf sounds, "pink noise," or nonrhythmic music. Several tapes are just music, but the majority are guided relaxation exercises to assist in decreasing a variety of symptoms or increasing certain skills. The results from regular usage of the tapes can be dramatic, as the brain is trained to operate at an optimal level.

MUSIC IN MEDICINE

The physiologic effects of music are in direct correlation to the specific characteristics of each musical selection. For example, a stirring Sousa march will affect bodily processes differently than a Brahms waltz. To understand the prescriptive aspect of music, it is necessary to explore the components of music, as they are the determiners in deciding which music is appropriate under specific circumstances.

Beat/pulse is the strongest component of music, the "toe-tapping" aspect. It is a primitive, automatic response.

Rhythm is the regular division of time into long and short patterns. Think of the dance, the cha-cha. The basic rhythm is one-two-cha-cha-cha. The beat falls on one, two, then the first and last cha. In the widest sense, beat and rhythm are the organizing principles of our world and our lives. Rhythmic sound creates a resonance with the natural clocks of the brain that control physiologic function and behavior (i.e., brain waves, heart rate, respiration, and ultradian cycles or alertness, sleepiness, urination, and hunger). People who have upset their rhythmic cycles can be greatly assisted in re-establishing these rhythms with the use of music with a consistent beat and rhythm.

Melody is a succession of tones used in a meaningful way added to rhythm. Usually it is the first thing people in Western society listen for in a piece of music, unless the rhythm is overpowering. It is the "tune" we whistle or hum or add words to. Melody is theorized as corresponding to our thoughts—both are linear, have a beginning, a middle, and an end, and exist singularly. Researchers have found music with simple rhythm and melody to be very successful in assisting cognitive functioning.

Harmony is the sounding together of two or more tones, with the effect of adding depth and richness. It is a relatively recent phenomenon, having been added in

Western music in the tenth century. The addition of notes under or over the melody give music its character of being consonant (pleasant, peaceful, stable) or dissonant (unpleasant, difficult to listen to, disconcerting). Harmony corresponds with our various emotions. Music contains emotion that can assist our releasing of stored emotions to bring harmony back to our physiology.

Tempo is the overall speed of performance. This is correlated to a system of beats per minute much like our own energy system. If we want to raise or lower our pulses by listening to music, all we need to do is use a piece of music that is higher or lower in tempo than our own pulse, and our body will attempt to match the tempo, especially if we have ingested certain drugs.

Timbre is the characteristic quality of the sound produced by a voice or instrument. A cello has a timbre very different from a trombone, though both can play the identical notes.

Volume is how loud or soft the music is.

Pitch is the frequency of a sound. Piccolos and violins are high-pitched instruments, while string basses and tubas are low pitched.

BASIC MUSIC MEDICINE INTERVENTIONS

Basic music medicine can be implemented by conscientious nurses and therapists with success by adhering to the following considerations and recommendations. First, decide on the purpose of the application of music/sound: What does one want the music/sound to do for the patient? Then consider the variables in success: the presentation; assessment of the patient's mental, physical, and listening states; appropriate recommendation; and *consistency*. A music therapy checklist is included to assist in this process (Table 44-2).

Variables Affecting Success

The ability of music/sound to enter one's system and be therapeutic depends on a number of variables: a person's physiologic state, mental state, and willingness to identify with the music; a therapist's appropriate prescriptive recommendation based on knowing the components of music and their effect; and the presentation of the modality to the patient.

Physiologic State

Stated simply, how bad a person feels physically determines how willing he or she is to listen to music. For instance, most people in extreme pain will not even try music as an analgesic, but will usually choose a pain shot or pill, preferring the instant effect.

Mental State

Just as with the physical state, a person experiencing extreme emotions such as depression, grief, or anger may not be wholly receptive to music's charms. However, playing music that matches the patient's mood can assist the patient in discharging the emotion, which will decrease emotional and physical suffering. The practitioner must be willing to assist the patient with this process by being supportive rather than directive. Once catharsis has occurred, the patient is usually more open to listening to other music.

Willingness to Listen

A person needs not only to be willing to identify with the music, but also to become involved in it for it to be healing. Factors to consider are preference for instrumental or vocal music, sociocultural background, age, and musical preferences.

Table 44-2: Music Therapy Checklist

Date ________ Time ________ Patient ________________ Room ________

Patient Diagnosis ________________ Sex ________ Age ________

Medications ________________

Physical Disabilities ________________

Music Therapy Objectives

1. Symptom Change

________Decrease Anxiety	________Stabilize Heart Rate
________Increase Energy	________Raise/Lower Blood Pressure
________Decrease Pain	________Change Mood
________Decrease Light-headedness	________Decrease Respiratory Distress
________Bladder Control	________Decrease Insomnia/Wakefulness

2. Physical Therapy

________Gait Control	________Muscle Strengthening/Mobility

3. Occupational Therapy

________During AM Routine to Increase Energy	________Muscle Strengthening/Mobility

4. Speech Therapy

________Increase Concentration/Focus

5. Emotional Adjustment

________Relieve Boredom	________Increase Socialization

Presentation of Music as Medicine

For successful intervention, music tapes must be presented as an important part of the patient's treatment and given the same weight as medications. Therefore, the implementor must present the therapy in a convincing and structured way. For example, "I recommend (or Dr. so and so recommends) the use of an audiotape to assist in decreasing your pain so you don't have to rely on medications. This is a successful intervention and promoted by our unit. You will be listening to this tape three times a day. We will help you and try to keep you from being disturbed while you listen. I think now is a good time to start." There are several points to keep in mind: 1) Be positive. 2) Show firm belief in the modality. 3) Be direct—do not ask what they think about it. (Remember, to be effective, music should be thought of as a medication.) 4) Promote the positive outcome of self-control and decreasing reliance on chemicals. 5) Help the patient in carrying out the schedule, that is, assist with the tape player, and *do not interrupt* when the patient is listening.

BODY

The Relaxation Response

We are endowed with two gross, innate, biobehavioral responses—the stress response and the relaxation response—which are in direct contrast to one another. "The stress response is characterized physiologically by increased heart rate and blood pressure and by the narrowing of blood vessels, and catecholamine releases; emotionally, by the subjective experiences of discomfort, fear, and rage; and bio-socially, by the flight-fight response" (11). As defined by Herbert Benson (12), the leading researcher on this effect, the relaxation response "is a reduction in the activity of the sympathetic nervous system . . . that brings on bodily changes that decrease heart rate, lower metabolism, decrease the rate of breathing, and bring the body back into a health[y] balance," "emotionally, by subjective experiences of comfort and trust along with receptivity to new information; and biosocially, by an increased capacity for social interaction and bonding." The relaxation response is one of the key variables in a person's ability to heal. As shown in Tables 44-1 and 44-3, certain music can achieve this effect, thereby assisting the patient's healing process.

Symptom Reduction

Symptom reduction addresses some of the same psychological and physiologic symptoms so readily treated with medications. As a result of modern technology and decades of research determining music's effect on symptomatology, several conclusions and recommendations can be made (see Table 44-3). The tapes recommended in the table are a result of my work in rehabilitation and have been found to be highly successful. The importance of listening according to an established schedule cannot be stressed too often. This assists in establishing new patterns in the body. As an example, an anti-anxiety music program should include listening to tapes at least three times per day, whether or not the patient is feeling increased anxiety; anti-insomnia tapes *must* be listened to every night. When the programs are faithfully followed, not only are patients able to learn some control over their own functioning, but also the need for medications is decreased, other therapies are performed more easily and successfully, and the patient's own sense of hopefulness and control increases.

Pain Reduction

There are currently three theories as to music's effectiveness in relieving suffering (7).

Gate Control Theory

This theory proposes that pain can be influenced by cognitive activities such as anxiety, attention, and suggestion, acting at the earliest levels of sensory transmission. Distraction elicits responses that are incompatible with pain responses, and for this reason, is an effective maneuver for reducing anxiety and, thereby, pain. In other words, one cannot think about two things at once; one focuses either on the pain or on something else. Music can be an effective method of pain relief through its ability to distract.

In this respect, it is important to use music to which the patient will listen. Patients in truly terrible pain are often unable to respond to very soft music. In patients with extreme pain, the music must match the level of tension and anxiety to be an effective relaxant and distraction. In working with leukemic children undergoing a short but extremely painful procedure, researchers found "the children, with few exceptions, clamored for Michael Jackson, and, headphones in place, sailed through the ordeal!" I found similar results with chronic pain patients. If the pain level was low, pleasant music and guided relaxation tapes worked well to decrease the pain, but when the pain was rated by patients to be above 6.5 on a scale of 1 to 10, where 10 is the most painful, then something else was needed to decrease the pain.

Pleasure Theory

The second theory holds that pain reduction occurs when the patient is distracted enough to listen to certain music perceived as uplifting or relaxing. This music and resulting perception stimulate the brain to release endorphins, which relieve pain by acting on certain receptors in the brain and body. In other words, if the patient in a lower level of pain can be distracted by music perceived as relaxing and pleasant, then the body will release its own pain medication, and both mind and body will find peace.

Vibrational Theory

A new theory of pain reduction has recently been postulated to relate to vibrational theory. When a part of the

Table 44-3: Symptom Reduction			
Symptom	**Music Components**	**Suggested Tape***	**Listening Routine**
Anxiety/hypertension	Soft, calm, consonant,	Patient's choice	Daily + PRN
	Simple melodies	Ison: "Balance"	Daily + PRN
	Low-pitched instruments	Jonas: "Color Relax/The Beach"	Daily + PRN
		Surf sounds	Daily + PRN
	Guided relaxation	Hemi-Sync: "Deep Relaxation"	3×/day
		"H + Relax"	3×/day
		"Cloudscapes"	Daily
Bladder function	Any music with strong, flowing water sounds	Dexter and Gordon: "Secret Fountain"	PRN
Cardiac distress	Calm, even rhythms	Strauss waltzes	PRN
		Chopin waltzes	
	Guided imagery	Jonas: "Cardiac Healing"	4×/day
	Music with added heart beat	"Sweet Baby Dreams"	Intermittent + PRN
Depression	Lively, fun, recognizable	Patient's choice	PRN
		Hymns, big band music	PRN
	Imagery producing	Jonas: "Music for Imaging"	1×/day + PRN
Insomnia	Slow, quiet, imagery producing	Rachmaninoff: *Vespers*	Nightly
		Weber: *Lullaby*	Nightly
	Guided relaxation	Hemi-Sync: "Sound Sleeper"	Nightly
		"Sleepy Locust"	Nightly
		"Flying Free"	Nightly
		"Deep Relaxation"	Daily
Pain	Attention grabbing	Patient's choice	PRN
		Jonas: "Chakra Meditation"	Daily
	Guided relaxation	Jonas: "Color Relax/The Beach"	Daily
		Jonas: "Pain Control"	Daily
		Hemi-Sync: "Deep Relaxation"	2×/day
		"Energy Walk"	2×/day
Respiratory distress	Calm	Ison: "Balance"	Daily
	Guided relaxation	Hemi-Sync: "Deep Relaxation"	3×/day
		"H + Lung Repairs"	3×/day

PRN = as required.
* Most tapes are available through Music & Medicine, Walland, TN. www.musicandmedicine.com.

body is "out of tune" and relaying strong pain signals, the vibrational rate of that part is strong, unstable, and chaotic. Gentle, slow vibrations of music will not be strong enough to influence it. However, if the vibrations applied are stable and their rate close to that of the pain, they will create a resonance that entrains, and the pain will decrease. Music therapist Mark Rider (13) found that listening to a formulated music tape that exhibited a definite mood shift from unpleasant to pleasant, and from an unstable meter to a comfortable meter, significantly reduced pain and muscle tension levels, and stimulated more imagery than other types of music tested.

Using the theory of entrainment, I compiled a tape, "Pain Control" (available from Music & Medicine, 5A Meadow Oak Lane, South Deerfield, MA 01379), for intense pain that contains a short relaxation exercise (distraction principle) followed by highly rhythmic minimalist music to entrain, ending with ocean surf (pleasure/release of endorphins). Patients are instructed to continue listening to side 2, which contains soothing, pleasant classical music. Though the patients stated they did not like the minimalist music, they all reported significant and lasting pain reduction, particularly if they listened to both sides of the tape. Rider (14) also found in his research that the imagery stimulated by the music contributes to the reduction of pain, as a further pleasant distraction that deepens the listening experience.

Pain Prescriptives

In summary, for effective use of music to mediate pain, the following must be kept in mind:

1. Have the patient assess the level of pain on a scale of 1 to 10.
2. If pain is rated 6 or lower, the music to use should be of a soothing, pleasant nature. The patient's preference can be considered. Guided relaxation tapes are highly recommended as they teach the patient how to decrease pain in the future. Highly recommended are "Deep Relaxation," "Color Relax/The Beach," "Chakra Meditation," and "H+ Relax" (all available from Music & Medicine, Walland, TN. www.musicandmedicine.com.).

3. Music that stimulates pleasant images has greater pain reduction qualities than does "new age," rock, or jazz, which usually increases tension in the body.
4. Children in high levels of pain do well with their own choice of music.
5. If pain is rated above 6, entrainment tapes appear to have the greatest effect; "Pain Control" is most successful.

Physical Therapy

An increasing number of studies have demonstrated the effect of music on one's motor system (15). Music serves to increase the general mobility, muscular strength and coordination, gait and balance, and social interaction of patients. They are able not only to increase their range of motion while listening to music, but also to increase their tolerance for repetition. It is the rhythmic element of music that has been noted to override poorly established motor patterns. A recent experiment conducted at Colorado State University studied rhythmic auditory stimulation with stroke patients (16). Metronome pulses were embedded in music that was listened to through headphones. Patients showed improved cadence, stride, and foot placement with lasting effects. It appears that the beat excites and shapes activity in the motor system of the brain, which helps organize and integrate complex movement. In this therapy, it is not music's emotional or motivational value but the entrainment effect on movement frequencies.

There are several factors to consider when implementing music in physical therapy (15,17):

1. Given the complexity of neuromuscular and skeletal disorders, a therapist needs to operationally define with care the areas to be changed and then select the appropriate activities and music.
2. Patients respond best to familiar tunes with which they can identify.
3. Simple music, with a clear and distinctive beat and rhythmic pattern, is essential.
4. The tempo of the music is crucial: It must match the activity; for example, for side-to-side weight shifting in a sitting position, use music of 58 to 63 beats/min. Patients need to be able to comfortably keep up with the tempo, which decreased straining.
5. Music should suit the desired movement; for example, stretch movements require flowing melodies, while foot tapping requires a heavier, more punctuated orchestration.
6. Each new pattern of movement should be rehearsed prior to its performance with music; some verbal cuing is necessary from the therapist throughout the session.
7. Group sessions demonstrate the greatest gains in both physical and social interaction between participants. Familiar music stimulates spontaneous singing, whistling, or humming and decreases anxiety. Opportunities to reach and touch another appear to be very beneficial; that is, patients sit in a circle close enough for them to touch one another and perform goal-oriented movements of reaching to touch a neighbor's shoulder, knee, hand, or foot.

Dance in a group format has also been used for patients with a variety of physical disabilities, including leg amputation, stroke, or rheumatoid arthritis. The patients significantly increased their enjoyment of exercise and rest, as well as bettered their scores in range of motion.

The Stroke Recovery Series of Hemi-Sync tapes contains several tapes to accompany exercise. The tapes are listened to through headphones, while the listener is lying down. The focus is on both sides of the body and imagining movements. I used these with several patients who had hemiparesis resulting from stroke. The treatments were administered in sessions scheduled between physical therapy and occupational therapy sessions. Although difficult to assess, the patients believed that the exercises contributed to their recovery. These patients were noticeably less anxious during subsequent physical therapy sessions and had more positive attitudes. The Monroe Institute has collected many case studies demonstrating the effectiveness of Hemi-Sync tapes for patients who have had a cerebrovascular accident (18). Common themes of improvement were increased feelings of relaxation, continued improvement even after 2 years, increased ability to image, and decreased pain.

Occupational Therapy

Although there has been little research on music applied in this area, I find music to be useful as background in the morning while patients are bathing and getting dressed. Lively, familiar music assisted in raising spirits and decreasing the time needed to perform these tasks. Individual music making is also very useful in this therapy. Patients who had played an instrument prior to their impairment are encouraged to bring their instrument to the occupational therapy session to assist in increasing range of motion and flexibility. Playing rhythm instruments like maracas to music also increases range of motion, once again demonstrating the importance of rhythmic stimulation on motor functioning.

MIND

Speech Therapy

Several studies have demonstrated music's effectiveness in assisting organized, recognizable speech in traumatic brain-injured (TBI) patients (19). Aphasic patients with left-hemisphere damage who are unable to produce normal speech are often able to sing their thoughts to familiar music (20). Melodic intonation therapy is a treatment approach that utilizes the client's unimpaired ability to sing to facilitate spontaneous and voluntary speech. Starting with the singing of short phrases to known melodies, the patient progresses to chanting sentences in more normal inflection patterns of speech (21).

Singing also increased verbal intelligibility and improved rate of speech in TBI patients in a study comparing the effects of singing and rhythmic interventions (19). The use of melody was a key variable.

Background music during speech therapy sessions can also facilitate a decrease in anxiety and an increase in focusing ability. Several suggestions are Mozart's symphonies no. 1 to 17 and flute sonatas, and Superlearning tapes (available from Superlearning, 450 Seventh Avenue, New York, NY 10123; telephone: (212) 279-8450). Superlearning is a program that uses the research of Soviet-bloc scientists on the use of music in learning. Their results show that Baroque music (classical music from the seventeenth and early eighteenth centuries) creates a relaxed state that lowers blood pressure; synchronizes heart beat and brain waves to slower, more efficient rhythms; and promotes hemisphericity, the synchronization of the right and left hemispheres. In this country, Sheila Ostrander and Lynn Schroeder (22) incorporated these findings into tapes that use rhythm, breathing, and music of 60 beats/min.

Several speech therapists with whom I have worked, have tried the Hemi-Sync tape "Concentration," with notable results over a period of time. Played softly through headphones, the Hemi-Sync signals assisted in increasing attentiveness, organization, and short-term memory. Patients remarked how much easier it was to accomplish the tasks presented. The Stroke Recovery Series also contains some speech exercise tapes.

Music Therapy According to Rancho Los Amigos Levels of Brain Injury

In addition to the above, the use of music and sound with brain-injured patients includes coordinating the Rancho Los Amigos levels of cognitive function with interventions (23). Many former level I coma patients are able to recall activities and people who were around them at various times in the hospital. Coma patients who were read to from their favorite books or were played their favorite music often remember, and thank the people who did so. The general goal of assessment for the level II or III coma client is to determine what kind of musical stimulus produces alerting or orienting responses. The stimulus is played for 10 to 15 seconds, followed by 30 seconds of silence. A verbal cue may be given to prepare the client. The stimuli should include as wide a variety of instrumental sounds as possible. Careful observations and recordings should be made to compare the data. In one study (24) a music therapist improvised wordless singing based on the tempo of the patient's pulse and breathing pattern. When any reaction on the part of the patient was observed, the phrase was repeated. When the therapist first began to sing, there was a slowing down of the heart rate. Then the heart rate rose rapidly and sustained an elevated level until the end of contact, a period of approximately 10 minutes. The patient's encephalogram showed a desynchronization from τ rhythm to α or β rhythm; there were grabbing movements of the hand and turning of the head and then the eyes opened to the return of consciousness.

Music therapy can also assist to increase client awareness of the environment. One technique involves giving feedback about the client's behavior in song (e.g., improvise songs about clothing, random movements, weather, date, and time). Familiar songs about the season or day can also be sung. Music and Hemi-Sync music can be used with inpatients to calm them and to assist in impulse control.

Clients functioning at Rancho Los Amigos levels IV to VI are given the opportunity to use strengths in addressing goals ranging from active responsiveness to following simple functional directives. A patient may respond with more accuracy to directives and questions that are sung rather than spoken (25). For instance, Gervin (26) sang one- and two-stage commands to TBI patients during dressing, to promote independence. Using music familiar to the patients, they would sing in response, learning the sequential steps for dressing. This is much like the songs we sang as children to learn activities. This song technique is very successful with patients who have left frontal lobe damage or bilateral damage.

Playing soothing, instrumental music with an even beat and tempo in the background gives the patient an alternative focus and quiet environment. Several Hemi-Sync tapes have been useful: "Cloudscapes," "Midsummer Night," and "Remembrance" (all available from Music & Medicine, Walland, TN. www.musicandmedicine.com.).

Outpatients who sustained concussions have benefited from Hemi-Sync tapes to decrease headaches, irritability, fatigue, sleeplessness and anxiety, as well as to improve concentration. I recommend "H + Brain Repairs and Maintenance" and "Deep Relaxation" (both available from Music & Medicine). The Monroe Institute also has a collection of case studies documenting improvement related to the listening of their tapes (27). Common themes from these cases include increased energy, concentration, and verbal and written communication; decreased anxiety; and improvements even after 6 years.

EMOTIONS

Shamans, medicine men and women, and psychiatric personnel have utilized music, chanting, or drumming to create an atmosphere of heightened emotion in which to heal. In these situations, the music helps to center one's attention on the ritual and intent, and to intensify the feelings of the participants. Many studies have demonstrated music's ability to evoke memories, increase or decrease emotional states, and change moods (7). As the medical establishment refocuses on the importance of emotions in the healing process, the use of music is a natural adjunct to assist in decreasing anxiety and depression. A perfect example is the 75-year-old widower who had a mild cerebrovascular accident on the left side, with resulting right hemiparesis. He was angry, belligerent, and uncooperative. He refused to listen to any audiotapes until the therapist made a deal to delay psychological testing with him if he would take a music tape for the evening. He would not choose a tape so he was given a tape of love songs sung by Linda Rondstadt. The next morning his nurses immediately wanted to know what was said to him and what was on the tape. Apparently he had listened to the music several times, wept, and slept peacefully, all without communicating with the staff. When he awoke, he was a new man, cooperative, cheerful, and ready to fully participate in his rehabilitation program. When he returned to the therapist to complete the battery of psychological tests, he only would say that the tape was beautiful and how good it made him feel. He would disclose no more. When people find themselves suddenly incapacitated *and* hospitalized, they experience a loss of control and a sense of helplessness that can quickly change to hopelessness and depression. In these situations music can be a constant companion and friend. It is important to allow patients to listen to their favorite music, be it opera, big band music, hymns, or show tunes; whatever they will willingly listen to will help. Patients begin to smile, relax, and in general feel better from listening to familiar music. They also begin to talk about the music with each other, trade tapes, and improve socially.

The addition of a live performer is also a bonus. Patients will sing, move, tap, clap, smile, hum, laugh, cry, and feel happier from the experience.

SPIRIT

When medical professionals and the public talk about mind-body health, the suggestion is that it is about gaining mental control of physical functions. However, patients who do not consciously put their mind to healing often appear to recover from their physical afflictions. A part of us transcends our humanness, a part that is wise—the spirit. Our mentally identified culture has a tendency to deny mystery, to deny the spiritual. The Institute of Noetic Sciences has compiled a collection of thousands of well-documented cases of people who have recovered from an illness when all mental, medical, and chemical means have been exhausted. The cases are from various medical journals throughout the world and we can safely assume there are thousands more from medical practitioners that have not made it into the journals. I have personally encountered many of them, one of whom illustrates this point. When I first met "Mary," she was 27 and admitted with multiple infarcts of unknown cause that left her entire body weak with some right-side paresis. She related her medical history, which included the following: At 16 years old, she was diagnosed with cervical cancer and her physician initiated a 6-week course of chemotherapy. At the end of the 6 weeks, she felt worse, and the condition of the cancer had not changed; her physician recommended further chemotherapy. She felt hopeless and sick and elected not to continue the treatment. Her physician told her to prepare to die and gave her no more than 6 months to live. She adopted an "I don't care attitude," got married, and set off on a trip across the United States with her husband to explore the country. They did what they pleased, when they pleased, and had fun. Two years later, still alive, she returned to the same obstetric/gynecology office to have a pregnancy test. Not only were they surprised to see her, but also they found only scar tissue in her cervix. As for her later hospital stay, no treatment or diagnosis was useful, so she discharged herself and disappeared into the world.

What then is the spiritual? Rachel Naomi Remen (28) found it easier to say what it is than what it is not. She stated it is not morals, ethics, the psychic, or religion. The spirit is something that is an essential part of human nature; something in all of us seeks to connect with it. Certain pieces of music, largely classical, have the ability to connect with this inner self. The music is many sided and able to touch all parts of ourselves: mind, body, emotions. It is healing music; it transcends our current condition. Several recommended pieces are Jonas's "Soul Music" (available from Music & Medicine), Handel's *Messiah*, Rachmaninoff's *Vespers*, Mozart's *Vesperae Solemnas*, and the second movement of Beethoven's Symphony no. 6.

Imagery

Many researchers are studying the effects of visualization on healing. Psychologist and researcher Jeanne Achterberg, while studying a group of terminally ill cancer patients, found that the most reliable way of predicting how they would fare against their disease was their mental imagery—more accurate even than immune component levels in the blood. The study results were corroborated by Robert Trestman (29). In the arena of music therapy, an important psychological treatment is guided imagery and music developed by Helen Bonny, a music therapist (30). One of the most noticeable reactions to listening to music is the images that are evoked. They can be useful in understanding one's process, disease, emotions, and relationships.

One dramatic case comes to mind. A cardiac patient was given a tape of classical music ("Music for Imaging," by Jonas, available from Music & Medicine). After 10 minutes of listening, he was sobbing and took off the headphones. As he eventually calmed enough to talk, he said the music had evoked buried memories of many years ago when as an alcoholic he beat his wife and son, the latter nearly to death. It had been decades since he had seen them. The attending nurse listened empathetically and allowed him to go through complete catharsis, with the result that his physical condition stabilized and he could participate in therapies.

Listening to image-producing music can assist in transporting oneself out of the present, resulting in decreases in anxiety, fear, pain, and boredom.

CONCLUSIONS

Music has tremendous value in medicine. It has the ability to simultaneously influence the mind, physiology, emotions, and spirit. Used regularly, like medications, music and sound are effective change agents to assist in healing. The basic recommendations given in this chapter can be administered by staff. However, just like the nursing profession, professionally trained music therapists are the best ones to perform music therapy. The NAMT and AMTA are working very hard to have music therapy be included in third-party reimbursements. Physicians who have found music useful in the medical setting should inform insurance companies. This holistic, powerful medium needs to be included in everyone's life.

REFERENCES

1. Joint Commission on Accreditation of Healthcare Organizations. *Accreditation manual for hospitals.* Oakbrook Terrace, IL: 1992.
2. Maranto C. A comprehensive definition of music therapy with an integrative model for music medicine. In: Spintge R, Droh R, eds. *MusicMedicine.* St. Louis: MMB Music, 1992:23–24.
3. Spintge R, Droh R, eds. *MusicMedicine.* St. Louis: MMB Music, 1992.
4. Furman C, ed. *Effectiveness of music therapy procedures: documentation of research and clinical practice.* 2nd ed. Silver Spring, MD: National Association for Music Therapy, 1996.
5. Eagle C. An introductory perspective on music psychology. In: Hodges D, ed. *Handbook of music psychology.* San Antonio, TX: University of Texas at San Antonio, 1996:1–29.
6. McClellan R. *The healing forces of music.* Rockport, MA: Element, 1991.
7. Jonas SE. *Take two tapes and call me in the morning.* 2nd ed. South Walland, TN: Music & Medicine, 1996.
8. McElwain JJ. The effect of spontaneous and anylized listening on the evoked cortical action in the left and right hemispheres of musicians and non-musicians. *J Music Ther* 1979;16:180–189.
9. Maduale P. *When listening comes alive.* Norval, Ontario, Canada: Moulin Publishers, 1993.
10. Atwater FH. *The Monroe Institute's Hemi-Sync process.* Faber, VA: Monroe Institute, 1988.
11. Dafter R. Why "negative" emotions can sometimes be positive: the spectrum model of emotions and their role in mind-body healing. *Advances J Mind/Body Health* 1996;12(2):8.
12. Benson H. *The relaxation response.* New York: Avon Books, 1975:26.
13. Rider MS. Entrainment mechanisms are involved in pain reduction, muscle relaxation and music-mediated imagery. *J Music Ther* 1985;22:183–192.
14. Rider MS. Treating chronic disease and pain with music mediated imagery. *Arts Psychother* 1987;14:113–120.
15. Staum MJ. Music for physical rehabilitation: an analysis of literature from 1950–1993 and applications for rehabilitation setting. In: Furman CE, ed. *Effectiveness of music therapy procedures: documentation of research and clinical practice.* Washington, DC: National Association for Music Therapy, 1988:65–104.
16. Marwick C. Leaving the concert hall for clinic, therapists now test music's "charms." *JAMA* 1996;275:267–268.
17. Cross P, et al. Observations on the use of music in rehabilitation of stroke patients. *Physiother Can* 1984;36:197–201.
18. The Monroe Institute. *Stroke recovery: case study reports.* Faber, VA: The Monroe Institute, 1996.
19. Adamek M, Shiraishi I. Music therapy with traumatic brain-injured patients: speech rehabilitation, intervention models, and assessment procedures (1970–1995). In: Furman C, ed. *Effectiveness of music therapy procedures: documentation of research and clinical practice.* 2nd ed. Silver Spring, MD: National Association for Music Therapy, 1996:267–279.
20. Greschwind N. Specializations of the human brain. In: *The brain.* New York: Freeman, 1979:114.
21. Sandness M. The role of music therapy in physical rehabilitation programs. *Music Ther Perspect* 1995;13:75.
22. Ostrander S, Schroeder L. Superlearning. 1979.
23. Claeys S. The role of music and music therapy in the rehabilitation of traumatically brain-injured clients. In: Harvey A, ed. *Music and health.* Louisville, KY: Music for Health Services Foundation, Eastern Kentucky University, 1988:118–139.
24. Adridge D. Where am I—music therapy applied to coma patients. *J R Soc Med* 1990;83:345–346.

25. Claeys MS, Miller AC, Dalloul-Pampersad R, Kollar M. The role of music and music therapy in the rehabilitation of traumatically brain injured clients. *Music Ther Perspect* 1989;6:71–77.

26. Gervin AP. Music therapy compensatory technique utilizing song lyrics during dressing to promote independence in the patient with a brain injury. *Music Ther Perspect* 1991;9:87–90.

27. The Monroe Institute. *Brain injury: case study reports.* Faber, VA: The Monroe Institute, 1996.

28. Remen RN. *Spirit: resource for healing. Ins Noetic Sci J* 1988;Autumn:5–9.

29. Barasch MI. *The healing path.* New York: Penguin Books, 1994:154–155.

30. Bonny H, Savory L. *Music and your mind.* New York: Harper & Row, 1973.

Chapter 45

Adjunctive Treatment Approaches for Injured Musicians

Jan Dommerholt
Richard N. Norris
Michèle Masset

During the past two decades, there has been growing interest in music medicine in the United States as well as abroad (1–6). In 1983, the first "Medical Problems of Musicians" conference was conducted in conjunction with the Aspen, Colorado Music Festival, quickly followed by multiple other arts medicine conferences throughout the world. Numerous studies investigating the prevalence, incidence, and nature of musicians' injuries were presented and published (7–14). Roach et al (15) demonstrated that instrumentalists have a higher prevalence of musculoskeletal complaints than do noninstrumentalists. While often musicians' ailments are thought to be performance related, non-musical-related upper-extremity trauma is very common and can be a major source of disability (16,17). Irrespective of the cause, the result is a limitation in musical performance and physical function. In response to the increased awareness and knowledge base, several arts medicine associations were started, including the International Arts Medicine Association (IAMA) (18) and the Performing Arts Medicine Association (PAMA), as well as special interest groups or sections within the American Occupational Therapy Association, the American Physical Therapy Association, and the American Congress of Physical Medicine and Rehabilitation. This chapter reviews several aspects of the physiatric examination and treatment of musicians. Particular attention is paid to those areas that differ considerably from the examination and treatment of more common patient populations. The physiatrist must consider multiple factors in the treatment of musicians. As musicians tend to be more demanding, many of the treatment interventions are considered "adjunctive" approaches.

MEDICAL EXAMINATION

Although pain is the most common complaint of musicians seeking medical attention (7), physicians interested in the field of music medicine must be aware of the broader context in which the medical problems of musicians exist. Physical complaints may be the result of playing the musical instrument or be attributed to the particular work environment of musicians. Physicians and other health care providers must be sensitive to musicians' relationships to their musical instruments, their peers, teachers, and relatives (19,20). Serious musicians will spend many hours every day studying, rehearsing, and performing, and music has become the main focus of their lives, or as Rachmaninoff stated, "I am 85% musician and only 15% of me is human" (21). While it is not necessary for physicians to be musicians themselves, familiarity with the demands of musical performance, the design and postural demands of musical instruments, the musician's work environment, and the psychosocial aspects of musicians' lives is an essential element of the treatment approach (22). In addition, to be recognized as an expert in music medicine by both musicians and medical colleagues, knowledge of neuromusculoskeletal anatomy, kinesiology, physiology, and pathophysiology is required. The physician must be prepared to study literature related to music pedagogy, technical aspects of musical instruments, cumulative trauma disorders, spinal disorders, ergonomics and biomechanics, occupational therapy, physical therapy, and alternative treatment approaches (23).

Musicians tend to be reluctant to consult medical practitioners. Most work-related musculoskeletal injuries are not associated with a distinct trauma, and compared to other occupational groups, musicians may be even more reluctant to report injuries or recurrent complaints of pain. Many musicians started playing at a very young age on instruments that may have been too large. They may have learned that assuming strained postures is required for playing the instrument. For professional musicians, the competition is often so severe that "playing through pain" may seem the only option out of fear of loss of employment, income, or career advancement. Past experiences with health care providers may have been unsatisfactory, since few medical professionals have specialized in music-related injuries. Health care providers may not fully appreciate the complex work environment of many musicians. Musicians' beliefs about illness may be quite different from those of physicians (24). Occasionally, musicians may blame themselves as responsible for the injury and choose consciously or subconsciously to ignore it (25). There may be financial reasons or lack of adequate health insurance to cover medical expenses (7). Within the context of a managed health care environment, musicians, as well as other patients, may not have direct access to medical specialists, although their medical care requirements may not be easily managed by primary care practitioners (26).

The examination of musicians follows the general principles that apply to all musculoskeletal or physiatric medicine (27). The keys to eliminating pain problems and returning injured musicians to playing the instrument are a proper diagnosis, the formulation of the initial hypothesis, the development and implementation of the treatment plan, and interventions in the most suitable sequence. In addition to the standard comprehensive neuromusculoskeletal evaluation, the initial examination must include an extensive music-specific history, and an analysis of the musician's playing posture and technique. Bogduk (28) outlined the complexity of the differential diagnosis and the determination of the primary causal factor or combination of factors. Only through a thorough review of the causes and contributing factors of disease and dysfunction can the physiatrist establish an accurate diagnosis and develop a functional treatment plan. Pain may be primarily nociceptive, or peripheral neurogenic or may have central or autonomic features. There may be a significant affective contribution to the pain presentation (29,30). In addition to possible medical causes of pain, the physiatrist must consider the possible contributions of joint dysfunction (31,32), neurogenic (33) or myogenic causes (34,35), posture dysfunction (36), and muscle imbalances (37).

Physically, musicians tend to be deconditioned and exhibit poor posture and poor muscular endurance. Musical instruments are not ergonomically designed and force the performer to assume and maintain asymmetric postures for sustained periods of time. As a result, most injuries of musicians are musculoskeletal disorders (38), including entrapment neuropathies (39,40), disk herniations (41), tendinitis (42), thoracic outlet syndrome (43), and overuse injuries (44). Upper-body and back musculoskeletal injuries are most common. Psychologically, performance anxiety is one of the most common complaints of musicians (45,46). In addition, musicians have to cope with the stress of perfection in artistic performance and interpretation (47). Since the physical and psychological demands on musicians vary for each instrument and each individual, each musician must be assessed on the basis of professional and personal demands (48). Specific protocols for treatment are appropriate only when they consider the musician's individual status and perspective in the clinical decision-making process (38).

TREATMENT CONSIDERATIONS

There are two distinct, although overlapping, treatment phases: the acute phase and the "return-to-play" phase (38,49). During the acute phase, common sports medicine principles apply to promote healing, including the regimen of rest, ice, compression, and elevation (RICE) (50). Dennett and Fry (51) recommended total rest of the affected extremity for prolonged periods of time, based on biopsy findings of nonspecific fiber ratio changes in their study of the first dorsal interosseous muscle. Total rest is also advocated by Taubman, who is quoted as having said, "Take three or four months of rest, then call me if the pain has not disappeared or if, when playing is resumed, the pain returns" (52). Since most music-related injuries are repetitive motion disorders associated with prolonged abnormal postures, muscle imbalances, and movement disorders, prolonged rest, as recommended by Dennett, Fry, and Taubman, will most likely result in further development of muscle imbalances and increased complaints of pain and other symptoms (38,53). A modification of playing activity is always indicated; however, this can be achieved by reducing the intensity or duration of playing. Choosing an easier repertoire, or taking more frequent breaks may be sufficient (38,54). With severe inflammation, complete rest is indicated for as long as 1 week (50).

During the return-to-play phase, musicians are encouraged to learn new practice techniques, perform specific conditioning exercises, and improve static and dynamic postures. Emphasis is placed on movement re-education, increasing work tolerances, and gradually returning to full musical and daily activities. Injured musicians usually miss playing so much, and often have so much anxiety about being away from their instruments, that as soon as they start to feel somewhat recovered, they attempt to leap prematurely back to their usual routine. When the musician is ready to return to the instrument, the physiatrist may develop a detailed written return-to-play schedule that includes periods of playing and frequent breaks. To avoid disrupting the flow of practice, during the breaks the musician can listen to a recording of what he or she has just practiced. It is inadequate and inappropriate for a physician merely to advise the player who is ready to return to playing to "go back little by little." This is too vague and open to misinterpretation. The value of a written schedule is that it minimizes the risk of further excessive muscle overloading (55). Players must be advised to adhere to the schedule even if they feel that they can do more. The use of a clock or timer is helpful. It may be advisable to start with only 5 minutes once or twice a day. A brief physical warmup should precede playing and a cooldown period should follow playing, and if there is still some pain or discomfort, the involved muscles may be iced down for about 10 minutes after the playing session. The return-to-play schedule can and should be modified to suit the individual player. In addition to the warmup and cooldown, musicians are encouraged to begin with moderately easy pieces or études. A metronome may be beneficial. The musician should gradually work in different tempi to facilitate full recovery of neuromuscular control mechanisms. As the condition improves, the player may resume technically more difficult materials for prolonged periods of time. Therefore, the progression involves modifications in tempi, duration, and technical difficulty of the material (38,49). Further scientific studies are needed to evaluate current rehabilitation strategies and to determine the most appropriate and effective approach.

EDUCATION

The primary focus of any medical intervention should be to return the musician to the prior level of performance. The crucial role of the physiatrist and other members of the rehabilitation team in educating musicians cannot be overemphasized. Education in the etiology, biomechanics, neurophysiology, and prevention of musculoskeletal injuries is an essential component of the return-to-play process. Musicians should become familiar with those factors that predispose them to injury (38,56). Few musicians have received formal training in injury mechanisms and prevention of injuries. In general, music schools do not include courses in anatomy, kinesiology, pathology, and injury prevention (57), although Spaulding (58) demonstrated that a comprehensive teaching curriculum can reduce the incidence and prevalence of music-related injuries. Often, musicians have deeply rooted beliefs, theories, and convictions about their instruments, their past and current teachers, their practice and performance habits, and their health status. To be an effective educator, the musician-patient must have the opportunity to develop a therapeutic relationship with the physician. Physicians must realize that such a therapeutic relationship is established especially during the first contact between the musician and the physician (59). During the first visit, the physician develops a diagnosis and communicates with the musician regarding the diagnosis, the treatment plan, and the prognosis. Several studies demonstrated that the more confident the physician is in the diagnosis, the better the outcome is (60,61). For example, the treatment team may recommend certain instrument modifications to avoid excessive stretching of the fingers. In general, musicians will only agree to such modifications on the basis of a solid and trusting therapeutic relationship. Providing the musician with written information regarding the diagnosis, exercises, posture, and other treatment components further facilitate patient satisfaction and less health care utilization; however, a brochure cannot replace the health care provider (62). Treatment approaches combining education with exercises, stress management, and other modalities are superior to education only (63). A critical analysis of teaching behaviors of health care providers is needed. Gahimer and Domholdt (64) demonstrated that teaching behaviors of physical therapists did not correspond well to the therapists' perceptions of their teachings, or to the patients' or supervisors' perceptions.

From an ergonomic perspective, the development of localized muscle fatigue in musicians with overuse injuries is more important than lack of muscle strength (65). Clinicians must realize that a simple measurement of grip strength is a poor indicator of muscular endurance and does not assess the functional ability to play the musical instrument (66). In some situations musicians suddenly increase the amount of playing time; for example, when they attend summer camps or start music school, the daily playing time may immediately increase from less than 3 hours to as much as 8 hours. Considering that localized muscle fatigue and subsequent complaints of muscle pain and decreased motor control can arise from sustained muscular work (67), musicians must understand that a more gradual increase in playing time may prevent the onset of musculoskeletal problems. Prolonged playing without regular interruptions is another etiologic factor for localized muscle fatigue. The postures and movements required to play instruments challenge the musculoskeletal system. Prolonged static contractions, as in the left supraspinatus when playing the viola, are common. There are few scientific studies of static muscle loading specifically in musicians (68); however, studies of other occupations may be applicable. In a study of newspaper employees, Burt et al (69) found an 11% prevalence of shoulder symptoms. The symptoms were related to performing static work tasks with unsupported arms. The biomechanical demands of musicians are still in need of further research; however, from a biomechanical perspective, there are many similarities between musicians and computer operators (70). Most musical tasks require prolonged static postures with unsupported arms (i.e., when playing the violin, trombone, or drums). Localized muscular fatigue is characterized by increased intramuscular pressure, decreased blood flow to the muscles, and accumulation of metabolites (71,72). According to Lindström et al (73), vascular compromise occurs when the relative force exceeds 15% to 20% maximum voluntary contraction (MVC). Bystrom and Fransson-Hall (74) demonstrated that 10% MVC was unacceptable for repeated 5-second handgrip contractions. Although music making is considered "light" work, musicians perform highly skilled and coordinated repetitive motions at very high speeds requiring precision and dexterity (47). Patterns of repetitive muscular activity are important in the development of muscular pain (75). Magnusson and Pope (76) recommended that static muscle load should not exceed 2% to 5% MVC, while Johnson (77) advocated limiting constrained muscular loading to less than an hour. Poor or sustained postures contribute significantly to the musculoskeletal problems of musicians. Even minimal abduction can cause significant increases in intramuscular pressure (78,79). The anterior and middle deltoid, the upper trapezius, the supraspinatus, and the infraspinatus muscles are more susceptible to muscle fatigue when the arm is held at or above shoulder level (80). Therefore, playing musical instruments like the flute, violin, or viola may lead to impaired circulation and chronic muscle damage (81). It is noteworthy that music pedagogist Dorothy Taubman believed that muscular fatigue is always the result of incorrect technique and "incoordination" and not of overuse (52,82).

The health care provider should explain common injury mechanisms and recommend that practice sessions be limited to a maximum of 45 minutes, with a break of no less than 10 minutes. Musicians may not be able to eliminate the highly repetitive nature of musical performance, and frequent breaks are therefore the only option to prevent overuse injuries (83). Short sessions and regular breaks allow the musculoskeletal system to relax, and one may continue to practice for several hours in this fashion. Difficult passages or those that require awkward fingering should be practiced in short segments of not more than 5 minutes each (38). The musician may go through the actual physical motions of playing without the instrument (49), what Menuhin referred to as "shadow playing" (84); engage in sight-reading the music; and review the fingering and dynamics mentally rather than physically. When a musician changes teachers, he or she should consider reducing the normal practice schedule and slowly increase it to previous levels, since different teachers may promote different techniques with significantly different biomechanical demands (85). When a musician is switching to another instrument (i.e., from violin to viola, from guitar to piano, or from one piano to another one with stiffer action), similar modifications must be made (86).

When addressing postural disorders in musicians, it is important to realize that instrument-specific patterns of postural dysfunction may exist due to instrument-specific biomechanical loading (38). Arm and hand positions vary for different instruments. An individual's anthropometric dimensions may not match the size of the instrument, forcing the player to use excessive reach, trunk rotation, or forward head posture (87,88). Different instruments require different techniques and place unique biomechanical demands on the player (85,89).

The physician and rehabilitation team members must consider both playing postures and nonplaying postures. Common postural and muscle imbalances seen with musicians are forward head posture with posterior cervical rotation, pronated shoulders, increased thoracic kyphosis and loss of lumbar lordosis with posterior pelvic rotation, scoliosis, external rotation and valgus deformity of the left shoulder and arm in violinists, and ulnar deviation of the wrists (38,50). In the forward head posture, the C7–T1 motion segment carries most of the load (65), predisposing the musician to neck, shoulder, and upper-limb pain (90,91). Forward head posture alters the embouchure of wind instrumentalists, the free way space, and the airflow. Posture and respiratory function are closely related not only for wind instrumentalists but also for other musicians. Optimum control of posture and breathing patterns is essential for the musical performance (92,93). Musicians should be instructed in abdominal breathing patterns. Abdominal breathing allows the thoracic region of the spine to maintain its dynamic stability, and it decreases the load on the auxiliary respiratory muscles, including the scalenes (94). Eventually, abdominal breathing should be incorporated into the musical performance. Even when a musician is aware of postural demands, certain musical tasks may contribute to temporary postural adjustments, as seen in trumpeters playing high notes (95). These changes may be dependent on the individual's anthropometric dimensions and breathing physiology (96).

Musicians should be made aware of potential errors in technique, as they can contribute to overuse problems. Some educators believe that all musicians' ailments are the result of poor technique rather than overuse (52,97); however, their opinions are contradicted by the results of biomechanical studies (75–80). While there is much confusion and disagreement among music teachers (98,99), physiatrists and other health care providers can play an important role in further defining the biomechanical and physiologic parameters of music making. Common errors include playing with excessive muscle tension, as often seen when playing with inadequate or improperly fitted chin rests and shoulder rests (68), when playing a poorly maintained instrument, or when playing forte (100). Several authors (98,99,101–103) suggested that musicians may play louder and with greater force than necessary, and with body and finger positions that result in unnecessarily high tendon and joint forces. In general, musicians should play as much as possible with their joints in the neutral position.

Excessive wrist flexion or extension may also predispose the musician to entrapment syndromes, including carpal tunnel syndrome (104). The combination of repetitive finger movements, wrist flexion and extension, and gripping force can result in overuse problems and affect the pressure in the carpal tunnel (105).

Other factors to review with the musician include nonmusical activities, including sports participation, knitting, computer work, gardening, mechanical work, and sleeping, as the positions and motions required of each of these activities can cumulate into overuse injuries and tendinitis. The repertoire is another potential contributor. Certain musical pieces require excessive hand span or very rapid finger movements, possibly beyond the anatomic-physiologic limits of the performer (22,88). Playing primarily modern music may be more stressful than playing a more classical repertoire (106).

THERAPEUTIC INTERVENTIONS

Physical Therapy

Physical therapists play a key role in the treatment and prevention of acute and chronic musculoskeletal pain and postural disorders in musicians. During the acute stage, standard physical therapy modalities including ice, heat, electrotherapy, and ultrasound can be applied (107,108). Almost all injured musicians will benefit from hands-on physical therapy including soft-tissue (35,109), joint (110,111), or neurodynamic mobilizations (112–114). Mobilizations are indicated for both subacute and chronic conditions. Musicians tend to exhibit significant muscle imbalances in the upper quadrant, described as "the upper crossed syndrome" (115); therefore, soft-tissue therapies are very useful to restore function, normalize tissue tone and extensibility, and reduce pain. The performing arts physical therapist should consider myofascial pain syndrome as a possible cause of pain in musicians, since it is a common diagnosis and because the treatment is specific and effective (116–118).

Many of the problems could be prevented by a regular conditioning program; however, physical conditioning is not usually part of the standard repertoire of the average musician. Musicians tend to be sedentary and deconditioned. As many musicians have never exercised, the concept of a regular conditioning program must be introduced carefully. The performing arts physical therapist should develop an appropriate and individualized exercise program for each musician, with appreciation of the characteristic patterns of postural and phasic muscles (37,119). A comprehensive exercise program for musicians should include exercises to restore dynamic pelvic and vertebral stabilization, motor control, flexibility, muscle balances, strength, endurance, and breathing patterns with and without the musical instrument. The individual components must be integrated into total motor patterns (120). Flexibility training is probably the most important component of the program (121). Considering the different postural and biomechanical demands of various musical instruments, the therapist may consider instrument-specific stretches (38). Postural exercises must address the alignment of all kinetic chain properties of the whole body, with the pelvis as the center (121). Since several musical instruments are large and heavy (i.e., the cello, bass, harp, and various percussion instruments), particular attention should be paid to lifting and carrying techniques. Real-time video feedback is particularly useful in reinforcing postural corrections.

Video Feedback

Video analysis and feedback can provide additional adjunctive modalities in the treatment of musicians. Locating the video monitor in front of the musician and the camera to the side or rear allows musicians to see their postures from various angles while playing the instrument. Video recordings of the musician's hands may give insight in the complex movement patterns of playing the instrument both clinically and for research purposes (122). Many hand and finger movements are performed beyond the human capacity to register and analyze (123,124). After the session is recorded, the physician, therapist, musician, and teacher will be able to closely review and analyze in slow motion the movements and playing technique, and make suggestions to minimize unnecessary stressors accordingly.

Biofeedback

Surface electromyography (EMG) is a noninvasive, reliable, and quantitative method to analyze and visualize muscle contractions, muscle fatigue, posture imbalances, and movement patterns (125,126). In addition, surface EMG can be applied therapeutically for purposes of muscle retraining, posture awareness, relaxation, and pain management (127). Within the context of physical therapy, there is a significant lack of normative data on the application of surface EMG to define the biomechanical and kinesiologic parameters of musical performance (128). Using synchronized surface EMG and sound recordings, Bejjani et al (85,129) evaluated the functional performance of pianists and violinists. Naill and McNitt-Gray (130) recorded the EMG activity of various muscles associated with different playing techniques on the cello, while Moore (131) studied the bowing and vibrato techniques of cellists. Philipson et al (132) established that musicians playing with pain use significantly more muscle force than do those without complaints of pain. Heuser and McNitt-Gray (133,134) used surface EMG to study the embouchure parameters of trumpet players. Levy et al (68) evaluated the effect of the presence of a shoulder rest on the muscular loading of different shoulder and arm muscles in violinists. Over 30 years ago, Polnauer and Marks (135) recorded muscle activity during violin playing using indwelling electrodes and in 1971, Szende and Nemessuri (136) published a comprehensive review of the physiology of violin playing.

Only a few case studies in the literature described using surface EMG for clinical and pedagogic purposes. LeVine and Irvine (137) used EMG to alter the tension patterns in the left hand during violin and viola playing, while Levee et al (138) applied biofeedback to achieve relaxation of facial muscles in a woodwind player. By recording muscle activity at rest or during musical performance, one can document localized increases in muscle tension and provide a baseline for biofeedback training. Using multiple-channel biofeedback training in addition to correcting posture and technique, musicians can learn how to actively engage the muscles required to maintain the posture and to play the instrument, while relaxing those muscles that are irrelevant for musical performance. Small portable biofeedback units with auditory feedback are sufficient to increase the musician's awareness of muscle tension during an at-home program; however, in the clinical setting computerized visual feedback is preferred, as it is difficult for a performer to concentrate simultaneously on the sound of the instrument and the sound of an audiosignal biofeedback machine. The computer's monitor can be placed in front of the musician (i.e., on top of the piano). The screen can display the EMG signals of various muscles, providing the musician with instant feedback. For further analysis, the raw EMG signal must be processed to receive adequate information about the state of muscle tension. Most commonly the root mean square integrated EMG is used (125,126,139).

Acupuncture

Several authors have promoted the use of acupuncture in the treatment of instrumental musicians and singers (140–143). In a population of string, wind, and keyboard musicians, acupuncture was determined to be successful in 95.5% of those with musculoskeletal problems, and 77.7% of those with neurologic disorders (144). Such highly successful outcomes allowed the majority of the musicians to continue with their musical careers. The upper-body musculoskeletal problems for which acupuncture has been successful include osteoarthritic pain of the hand or shoulder, tennis elbow, acute or chronic myogenic headache or neck pain, and acute or chronic back pain (145,146). Patients with myogenic headaches experienced the same degree of relief when undergoing treatment with either acupuncture or physical therapy (147). Moreover, the combination of acupuncture and standard drug therapy was five times superior to that of drug therapy alone (148). Lehman et al (149) examined the long-term improvement of pain reduction in patients who had chronic low-back pain by comparing electroacupuncture therapy and transcutaneous electrical nerve stimulation (TENS), and found that acupuncture was significantly more effective. Acupuncture also was more effective than nonsteroid antirheumatoid drugs in patients with osteoarthritis of the humeroscapular joint, after 2 weeks of treatment (150).

Acupuncture is based on an ancient, 5000-year-old practice, whose earliest historical account may be traced to the emperor Huan Di (2697–2597 BC), the legendary author of *Nei Jing*, a book often considered the first medical text, that comprises the foundation of acupuncture as it is known today. Over the course of centuries and various Chinese dynasties, this medical technique was continually refined and perfected in terms of its diagnostic treatment (151). Taoism, the basis of Chinese philosophy, assumes that a given phenomenon can only be understood in relation to the whole, while at the same time, everything in nature exhibits perpetual motion and is undergoing a continuous process of change (152). The dual concepts of Yin and Yang comprise the reunion of two opposite aspects that exist in all phenomena and objects. This kinetic duality exists in relation to each other as well as to the external environment and explains the process of natural changes (153). From the traditional Chinese perspective, human physiology and pathology are based on the five metaphysical elements—wood, fire, earth, metal, and water. Each of these five elements incorporates a physical, physiologic, emotional, and environmental component. Each element manifests itself on the surface of the body in the form of a discrete meridian, which acts as a pathway to the flow of the life force known as *Qi* (154). According to traditional acupuncture, Qi is the fundamental substance that regulates the normal activities of the human body. Qi includes a material aspect, which allows life to manifest itself, as well as an energy aspect, responsible for various physiologic activities and emotional states of the organism. Like a river traversing the earth, the smooth and regular flow of Qi and blood nourishes all aspects of the body and mind (155).

The occurrence of disease results from a relative imbalance between the Qi (Yang) and blood (Yin), which may lead to either an excess or a deficiency in a specific area of the body. Each meridian allows the practitioner to first determine the nature and localization of the problem, and then to treat it. One such problem is referred to by the term *Bi syndrome*, characterized by obstruction or blockage, and generally designating conditions characterized by pain, including the sensation of heaviness in the joints or muscles, and often accompanied by swelling and a reduction in the range of motion. Bi syndrome is caused by two factors: the invasion of an external pathogenic factor, such as wind, cold, heat, or dampness, and a weakened body that allows the pathogen to invade the organism and thereby disturb the free flow of Qi and blood to the meridians (156). Another category of problem, primarily emotional and physiologic in nature, is manifested by anxiety, stress, depression, or dysfunction of the internal organs, and is due to the overexertion of the body, along with poor nutritional and other lifestyle habits. Such problems ultimately weaken the mental and physiologic functions of the body by affecting the internal organs and their respective meridians on the surface. Finally, the traumatic overuse of specific parts of the body, including repetitive motion disorders or poor posture, may impair the flow of Qi and blood into the meridians, muscles, joints, and skin. This may give rise to a local problem or a generalized problem relating to the meridian that crosses the traumatized part of the body.

The main problems experienced by musicians relate to repetitive movements and stress and anxiety. Repetitive motion disorders place stress on the same tendons, connective tissues, or joints, and primarily involve the upper part of the body and the back, thereby creating acute inflammatory or chronic degenerative musculoskeletal conditions. Stress and anxiety disorders are often related to the nature of performance (46). Acupuncture has demonstrated its analgesic effects on the body by increasing pain thresholds, while also positively affecting the autonomic nervous system, thereby improving metabolic functions (157). Because of the holistic approach of Chinese medicine, both physical and emotional components are continuously related. The liver meridian controls muscular tension and stress, while the kidney meridian controls bones and anxiety. The treatment of one aspect will necessarily influence the other.

Within traditional Chinese medicine, different modalities can be applied to treat musculoskeletal conditions and to regulate the meridians (140):

- Acupuncture: the insertion of needles into the body with the intent of reaching the Qi and blood of a given meridian. Relative to the nature of the specific problem, different manipulation is applied to stimulate or reduce the circulation of Qi.
- Heat (Moxa): a compressed herb called *Artemesia vulgaris*, which can be used in different forms, burned either directly on the skin, on top of a needle, or on a stick.
- Tuina: a Chinese therapeutic massage agent that increases the pain threshold, increases the range of motion, and reduces the physical side effects of stress.
- Chinese herbs: able to accelerate bodily repair by reducing swelling and regulating the metabolism. Herbs can be applied either as a topical agent or may be ingested for more general affect on the body as a whole.
- Tai chi chuan: a slow-motion exercise that was created as a marshal art and that affects the body and mind, reduces stress, lubricates the joints, and improves coordination.
- Serica therapy: combines traditional Chinese medicine principles with anthroposophical medicine, and utilizes colored silk swatches. Serica therapy is a newly developed approach based on the German-Dutch "Meridian therapy" (158,159).

During recent years, many researchers and clinicians have adopted a more neurophysiologic approach to acupuncture, especially in the field of pain management (157,160,161). Traditional acupuncture points appear to correspond to superficial peripheral nerve endings (162). The analgesic effects of acupuncture are modulated through activation of sensory receptors in the skin, muscle, or other innervated structures, and by a complex system of neural loops in the central nervous system (157). Several endogenous opioid substances, including dynorphin, endorphin, and enkephalin, facilitate acupuncture analgesia (157,163). Electroacupuncture at 4 Hz can increase endorphin levels and at 100 Hz, dynorphin levels (164). Other applications of needling for analgesia were developed by Gunn (165,166), Baldry (167), and Waumsley (168).

Clearly, acupuncture has a place among other forms of therapy in providing relief to the common physical afflictions specific to musicians; its timely application as a form of preventive therapy can also provide health improvements to musicians by exploiting the well-documented physical and mental benefits inherent in this ancient form of traditional Chinese medicine (169).

ALTERNATIVE MOVEMENT THERAPIES

The treating physician may consider the use of alternative or adjunctive movement therapies in the treatment of musicians. Many musicians may already have consulted other disciplines prior to seeking medical advice: the Alexander technique, the Feldenkrais method, the Mensendieck system, the Pilates method, or approaches initiated by musicians, such as Lister-Sink's "Freeing the Caged Bird" approach (16,170,171). The performing arts physician is encouraged to study these approaches, philosophies, concepts, and treatment techniques and incorporate them into the overall treatment program where appropriate, even though there is a limited body of research supporting them (172,173).

The Alexander Technique

Developed by the Australian Shakespearean actor Frederick M. Alexander (1869–1955) after episodes of recurrent loss of his voice, the Alexander technique considers the correct relationships between the head, neck, and back as essential for proper movement and functioning (174,175). This relationship is referred to as *the primary control.* The Alexander technique is very popular with musicians and singers. The approach is very gentle, however, goal oriented. The goal is not to alleviate or treat symptoms, but to improve kinesthetic awareness, posture, and movement and to inhibit unnecessary effort. The Alexander technique can inhibit habitual and learned responses that may interfere with normal functioning (176). A typical lesson includes verbal instructions with tactile and kinesthetic feedback. The student will experience which muscles are tense, and how that tension can be relieved. Through specific relaxation training, the student will learn consciously and subconsciously new, more efficient movement patterns. During more advanced lessons, the musician-student will learn new movement patterns while playing the instrument. Typically, 25 to 30 lessons are required to accomplish the basic goals of the Alexander technique (16). Physicians considering the Alexander technique for their patients should make sure that the teacher is certified through the Alexander Guild.

The Feldenkrais Method

Following a knee injury, the Israeli physicist Moshe Feldenkrais (1904–1984) developed what is now known as the *Feldenkrais method*. By applying his knowledge of physiology, anatomy, neurology, psychology, and the martial arts, Feldenkrais believed that previous experiences determine current functioning. By interrupting negative habitual patterns of movement, the body will develop improved self-awareness and sensory-motor integration. The Feldenkrais method emphasizes self-exploration and encourages each person to find the optimal style of movement without imposing rigid rules or standard of "correct posture." The Feldenkrais method is thought to reprogram the neuromotor and central nervous system. The notion of "self-image" is central to the Feldenkrais theory. As in the Alexander technique, Feldenkrais practitioners have received several years of training leading to certification. Feldenkrais developed two interrelated approaches: group lesson called *Awareness through Movement* and individual hands-on approach called *Functional Integration*. With Awareness through Movement, participants are guided through gentle active movement sequences to develop new patterns of movement and self-image. With Functional Integration, the practitioner's touch directs the person's body through movements (177,178). The Feldenkrais method may be less threatening for musicians than a more common physical conditioning program.

The Mensendieck System

The Dutch Mensendieck therapist Ans Samama has promoted the Mensendieck system and its applications for musicians (179). Bess Mensendieck (1862–1957) developed her approach to correct body and movement awareness of women. Samama and colleagues further developed the Mensendieck system into an elaborate posture correction system based on the conscious recognition of faulty and corrected movement patterns. Although not commonly used in the United States, many European musicians consult with Mensendieck therapists. Through cognitive training, musicians become aware of their movement patterns and are taught how to assume and maintain correct posture with and without the musical instrument. A distinction is made between posture/balancing muscles and playing muscles, and the musician learns which muscles to contract when. *Correct posture* is defined as a biomechanical alignment of body parts maintained by conscious contractions of specific muscle groups. Several components of the Mensendieck system are appropriate for musicians.

The Pilates Method

Although there is no research documenting the use of the Pilates method for musicians, anecdotal evidence suggests that musicians can certainly benefit from working out on Pilates equipment. The Pilates method became popular among dancers, after Joseph Pilates opened an exercise studio in New York in 1923. The most significant difference from the other approaches is the use of various exercise equipment, developed by Pilates while imprisoned during World War I. The equipment includes the Pilates Universal Reformer, the Pilates Cadillac, and several other pieces (The Pilates Studio, 2121 Broadway, Suite 201, New York City, NY 10023). The Pilates method aims to repattern the neuromusculoskeletal system and has similarities with the Alexander technique, the Feldenkrais method, and proprioceptive neuromuscular facilitation (180). The Pilates method is appropriate for beginners as well as advanced students and can easily be used in the rehabilitation of injured musicians. The Pilates method can be used to improve muscle strength, muscle endurance, cardiovascular endurance, and postural awareness (181,182). As with the Alexander technique and the Feldenkrais Method, physicians should consider a practitioner's educational program. Training programs are available through the Pilates Studio and through Current Concepts' "Balanced Body" Program (Current Concepts Corp., 7500 14th Avenue, Suite 23, Sacramento, CA 95820 USA).

"Freeing the Caged Bird"

Barbara Lister-Sink, an accomplished piano soloist, developed the "Freeing the Caged Bird" approach together with physical therapist Glenna Batson. According to Lister-Sink, a pianist's musicality is comparable to "a songbird caged inside a body," when the pianist's technique is restricted by poor posture and skeletal misalignment, accumulated muscle tension, and a misunderstanding of basic biomechanical principles (102,103). The "Freeing the Caged Bird" approach has seven steps that emphasize education, posture and movement awareness, and stress-free piano technique and performance. Lister-Sink produced an excellent educational video outlining her approach (WingSound, P.O. Box 10912, Winston-Salem, NC 27108; Tel/fax (910) 945-2304). The video is appropriate for both health care providers and musicians. Physicians are encouraged to consider Lister-Sink's program for their injured pianists, especially when comprehensive treatment options are not available locally. Most serious pianists will consider traveling to North Carolina, if recommended by their treating physician.

DOCUMENTATION

Considering the increasing demands of the health care system and managed care organizations, it is important to document treatment outcomes (183,184). Bengtson and Schutt (44) recommended using a functional index when treating musicians. The index defines outcome as the musicians' self-reported amount of time currently played on their instrument(s) in hours per week divided by the amount of time they had played their instrument(s) prior to experiencing medical problems:

$$\frac{\text{Time currently played (hr/wk)}}{\text{Time played (hr/wk) before problems}} \times 100\%$$
$$= \%\ \text{Return to play}$$

Since the functional index is a self-report scale, and does not consider that musicians may have symptoms and "play through pain" prior to consulting a medical practitioner, the "Functional Grading of Severity of Injury" for musicians may be more accurate (185):

- Grade 1: pain limited to one site and brought on by playing the instrument.
- Grade 2: pain in two or more sites with a high work load, and possibly some loss of coordination. Physical signs may be present; however, there is no interference with other uses of the hand.
- Grade 3: pain persisting while away from the instrument. There is early involvement of other uses of the hand with a possible loss of coordination, or strength. Physical findings include persistent tenderness of the upper-limb structures. The musician has difficulty maintaining a high work load.
- Grade 4: pain persisting at rest, at night, or both. The musician has pain with most uses of the hand, including activities of daily living. A normal work load is challenging.
- Grade 5: the musician has no functional use of the hand. The musical career stops or is seriously threatened.

Most overuse injuries are grade 1 (29.6%), 2 (28.8%), or 3 (21.9%). It is fairly common for musicians to experience stiffness rather than pain during the early stages of dysfunction.

CONCLUSIONS

Working with musicians can be very challenging, owing to the complex nature of musical performance, but also very rewarding. Musicians tend to be very motivated patients, who often are desperate trying to find answers. Physiatrists interested in performing arts medicine should consider multiple factors in the examination and treatment of musicians. While many aspects of musicians' care are similar to those of other patient populations having overuse syndromes, musicians require sensitivity to their particular needs, the artistic nature of their profession, and the specific neuromusculoskeletal demands. Physiatrists are encouraged to consider the outlined adjunctive therapy approaches as part of the overall management strategy.

REFERENCES

1. Fry HJH. Occupational maladies of musicians: their cause and prevention. *Int J Music Educ* 1984;4:59–63.
2. *The seventh annual symposium on medical problems of musicians and dancers.* Snowmass, CO: Cleveland Clinic Foundation, 1989.
3. Lederman RJ, Brandfonbrenner AG. Medical problems of musicians: introduction and overview. *Cleve Clin Q* 1986;53(1):1–2.
4. Kersing W. *Medici voor Musici, conference proceedings.* Hilversum, Netherlands: Kersing, 1985.
5. Mischakoff A. *Sforzando! Music medicine for string players.* Urbana, TX: American String Teachers Association, 1985.
6. Roehmann FL, Wilson FR. *The biology of music making: proceedings of the 1984 Denver conference.* St. Louis, MO: MMB Music, 1988.
7. Amadio PC, Russoti GM. Evaluation and treatment of hand and wrist disorders in musicians. *Hand Clin* 1990;6:405–416.
8. Fry HJH. Incidence of overuse syndrome in the symphony orchestra. *Med Probl Perform Art* 1986;2:51–55.
9. Fry HJH. Prevalence of overuse in Australian music schools. *Br J Ind Med* 1987;44:35–40.
10. Larsson L, Baum J, Mudholkar GS, et al. Nature and impact of musculoskeletal problems in a population of musicians. *Med Probl Perform Art* 1993;8:73–76.
11. Lederman RJ. Peripheral nerve disorders in instrumentalists. *Ann Neurol* 1989;16:640–646.
12. Lockwood AH. Medical problems in secondary school-aged musicians. *Med Probl Perform Art* 1988;3:129–132.
13. Manchester RA, Flieder D. Further observations on the epidemiology of hand injuries in music students. *Med Probl Perform Art* 1991;6:11–14.
14. Sakai N. Hand pain related to keyboard techniques in pianists. *Med Probl Perform Art* 1992;7:63–65.
15. Roach KE, Martinez MA, Anderson N. Musculoskeletal pain in student instrumentalists: a comparison with the general student population. *Med Probl Perform Art* 1994;9:125–130.

16. Blum J, Ahlers J. Verletzungen und Rehabilitation. In: Blum J, ed. *Medizische Probleme bei Musikern.* Stuttgart: Georg Thieme Verlag, 1995:163–175.

17. Dawson WJ. Upper extremity injuries in high level instrumentalists: an end-result study. *Med Probl Perform Art* 1990;5:109–112.

18. Lippin RA. Arts medicine: a call for a new medical specialty. *Phila Med* 1985;81:14–15.

19. Ostwald PF. Psychodynamics of musicians; the relationship of performers to their musical instruments. *Med Probl Perform Art* 1992;7:110–113.

20. Johnson C. Evaluation of the injured musician: role of the instrument. In: Bejjani FJ, ed. *Current research in arts medicine.* Chicago: a capella books, 1993:363–364.

21. Neuhaus H. *Die Kunst des Klavierspiels.* Köln: Gerig, 1967.

22. Wagner C. Physiologische und pathophysiologische Grundlagen des Musizierens. In: Blum J, ed. *Medizinische Probleme bei Musikern.* Stuttgart: Georg Thieme Verlag, 1995:2–29.

23. Materson RS, Dommerholt J. Industrial, spine, and related rehabilitation. *Phys Med Rehabil Clin N Am* 1996;7:107–123.

24. Cherkin D, Deyo RA, Berg AO. Evaluation of a physician education intervention to improve primary care for low back pain. 1: Impact on patients. *Spine* 1991;16:1173–1178.

25. Quarrier NF. Performing arts medicine; an evolving specialty. *J Orthop Sports Phys Ther* 1993;17:90–95.

26. Melvin JL. The health care environment and physiatric practice. *Phys Med Rehabil Clin N Am* 1996;7:5–12.

27. Cole A, Herring SA. Role of the physiatrist in management of musculoskeletal pain. In: Tollison CD, Satterthwaite JR, Tollison JW, eds. *Handbook of pain management.* Baltimore: Williams & Wilkins, 1994:85–95.

28. Bogduk N. The sources of low back pain. In: Jayson M, ed. *The lumbar spine and back pain.* Edinburgh: Churchill Livingstone, 1992:61–88.

29. Butler D. Moving in on pain. In: Shacklock MO, ed. *Moving in on pain.* Chatswood: Butterworth-Heinemann, 1995:8–12.

30. Butler DS, Shacklock MO, Slater H. Treatment of altered nervous system mechanics. In: Boyling JD, Palastanga N, eds. *Grieve's modern manual therapy.* Edinburgh: Churchill Livingstone, 1994:693–703.

31. Dvorák J, Dvorák V. *Manual medicine; diagnostics.* Stuttgart: Georg Thieme Verlag, 1990.

32. Langley JC. Spinal manipulation and physical rehabilitation. In: Tollison CD, Satterthwaite JR, Tollison JW, eds. *Handbook of pain management.* Baltimore: Williams & Wilkins, 1994:96–107.

33. Butler DS. *Mobilisation of the nervous system.* Melbourne: Churchill Livingstone, 1991.

34. Gerwin R. Myofascial back and neck pain. In: Young MA, Lavin RA, eds. *Physical medicine and rehabilitation state of the art reviews.* Vol. 9. Philadelphia: Hanley & Belfus, 1995:657–671.

35. Gerwin RD, Dommerholt J. Treatment of myofascial pain syndromes. In: Weiner R, ed. *Pain management: a practical guide for clinicians.* Vol. 1. Boca Raton, FL: St. Lucie Press, 1997:217–229.

36. Mannheimer JS. Prevention and restoration of abnormal upper quarter posture. In: Gelb H, ed. *New concepts in craniomandibular and chronic pain management.* London: Mosby-Wolfe, 1994:93–161.

37. Janda V. Muscles and motor control in cervicogenic disorders; assessment and management. In: Grant R, ed. *Physical therapy of the cervical and thoracic spine.* New York: Churchill Livingstone, 1994:195–216.

38. Norris RN, Dommerholt J. Orthopädische Probleme und Rehabilitation bei muskuloskeletalen Störungen. In: Blum J, ed. *Medizische Probleme bei Musikern.* Stuttgart: Georg Thieme Verlag, 1995:116–159.

39. Lederman RJ. Neurological problems of performing artists. In: Sataloff RT, Brandfonbrenner AG, Lederman RJ, eds. *Textbook of performing arts medicine.* New York: Raven, 1991:171–204.

40. Lederman RJ. Entrapment neuropathies in instrumental musicians. *Med Probl Perform Art* 1993;8:35–40.

41. Newmark J, Rybock JD. Post-traumatic cervical disc herniation in a professional bass player. *Med Probl Perform Art* 1990;5:89–90.

42. Markison RE. Tendinitis and related inflammatory conditions seen in musicians. *J Hand Ther* 1992;5:80–83.

43. Roos DB. Thoracic outlet syndrome in musicians. *J Hand Ther* 1992;5:65–72.

44. Bengtson KA, Schutt AH. Upper extremity musculoskeletal problems in musicians; a follow-up survey. *Med Probl Perform Art* 1992;7:44–47.

45. Fishbein M, Middlestadt SE, Ottatic V, et al. Medical problems among ICSOM musicians: overview of a national survey. *Med Probl Perform Art* 1988;3:1–8.

46. Sternbach DJ. Stress in the lives of musicians—on stage and off. In: Bejjani FJ, ed. *Current research in arts medicine.* Chicago: a capella books, 1993:475–478.

47. Byl NN, Arriaga R. Treating the injured musician. *PT Mag Phys Ther* 1993;1:62–68.

48. Novak CB. Physical therapy management of thoracic outlet syndrome in the musician. *J Hand Ther* 1992;5:73–79.

49. Norris RN. Return to play after injury: strategies to support a musician's recovery. *Work* 1996;7:89–93.

50. Lowe C. Treatment of tendinitis, tenosynovitis, and other cumulative trauma disorders of musicians' forearms, wrists, and hands . . . restoring function with hand therapy. *J Hand Ther* 1992;5:84–90.

51. Dennett X, Fry HJH. Overuse syndrome: a muscle biopsy study. *Lancet* 1988;1:905–908.

52. Pratt RR. An interview with Dorothy Taubman. *JIAMH* 1989;4(2):15–39.

53. Higgs PE, Mackinnon SE. Repetitive motion disorders. *Annu Rev Med* 1995;46:1–16.

54. Teitz CC. Overuse injuries. In: Teitz CC, ed. *Scientific foundations of sports medicine*. Toronto: Decker, 1989:299–328.

55. Kibler WB. Concepts in exercise rehabilitation. In: Leadbetter W, Buckwalter JA, Gordon SL, eds. *Sports induced inflammation*. Chicago: American Academy of Orthopaedic Surgeons, 1990:759–769.

56. Mastroianni T. Technique born free. *Piano Q* 1986;134:56–59.

57. Blum J, Mastroianni T, Norris R. Musikschulen und -hochschulen und ihre präventiven Aufgaben bezüglich zukünftiger Erkrankungen bei Musikern. In: Blum J, ed. *Medizische Probleme bei Musikern*. Stuttgart: Georg Thieme Verlag, 1995:40–44.

58. Spaulding C. Before pathology: prevention for performing artists. *Med Probl Perform Art* 1988;3:135–139.

59. Deyo RA, Diehl AK. Patient satisfaction with medical care for low back pain. *Spine* 1986;11:28–30.

60. Bass MJ. The physician's action on the outcome of illness in family practice. *J Fam Pract* 1986;23(1):43–47.

61. Bush T, Cherkin D, Barlow W. The impact of physician attitudes on patient satisfaction with care for low back pain. *Arch Fam Med* 1993;2:301–305.

62. Friedrich M, Cermak T, Maderbacher P. The effect of brochure use versus therapist teaching on patients performing therapeutic exercise and on changes in impairment status. *Phys Ther* 1996;76:1082–1088.

63. Nordin M. Education and training. In: Nordin M, Andersson GBJ, Pope MH, eds. *Musculoskeletal disorders in the workplace; principles and practice*. St. Louis: Mosby, 1997:234–241.

64. Gahimer JE, Domholdt E. Amount of patient education in physical therapy practice and perceived effects. *Phys Ther* 1996;76:1089–1096.

65. Magnusson M. Posture. In: Nordin M, Andersson GBJ, Pope MH, eds. *Musculoskeletal disorders in the workplace: principles and practice*. St. Louis: Mosby, 1997:74–84.

66. Nordin M. The skeletal muscle. In: Nordin M, Andersson GBJ, Pope MH, eds. *Musculoskeletal disorders in the workplace: principles and practice*. St. Louis: Mosby, 1997:33–44.

67. Chaffin DB. Localized muscle fatigue: definition and measurement. *J Occup Med* 1973;15:346–354.

68. Levy CE, Lee WA, Brandfonbrenner AG. Electromyographic analysis of muscular activity in the upper extremity generated by supporting a violin with and without a shoulder rest. *Med Probl Perform Art* 1992;7:103–109.

69. Burt S, Hornung R, Fine LJ. *NIOSH health hazard evaluation report HETA 89-250-2046*. Cincinnati: National Institute for Occupational Health and Safety, 1990.

70. Grant A. Homo-Quintadus, computers and rooms (repetitive ocular orthopedic motion stress). *Optom Vis Sci* 1990;67: 297–305.

71. Edwards RTH, Hill DK, McDonell M. Myothermal and intramuscular pressure measurements during isometric contractions of the human quadriceps muscle. *J Physiol* 1973;224:58–59.

72. Edwards RTH. Human muscle function and fatigue. *Ciba Found Symp* 1981;82:1–18.

73. Lindström L, Kadefors R, Petersen I. An electromyographic index for localized muscle fatigue. *J Appl Physiol* 1977;43:750–754.

74. Bystrom S, Fransson-Hall C. Acceptability of intermittent handgrip contractions based on physiological response. *Hum Factors* 1994;36:158–171.

75. Veiersted KB, Westgaard RH, Andersen P. Pattern of muscle activity during stereotyped work and its relation to muscle pain. *Int Arch Occup Environ Health* 1990;62:31–41.

76. Magnusson M, Pope M. Epidemiology of the neck and upper extremity. In: Nordin M, Andersson GBJ, Pope MH, eds. *Musculoskeletal disorders in the workplace: principles and practice*. St. Louis: Mosby, 1997:328–335.

77. Johnson B. Measurement and evaluation of local muscle strain in the shoulder during constrained work. *J Hum Ergol (Tokyo)* 1982;11:73–88.

78. Järvholm U, Palmerud G, Karlsson D, et al. Intramuscular pressure and electromyography in four shoulder muscles. *J Orthop Res* 1990;9:609–619.

79. Järvholm U, Palmerud G, Styf J, et al. Intramuscular pressure in the supraspinatus muscle. *J Orthop Res* 1988;6:230–238.

80. Herberts P, Kadefors R, Broman H. Arm positioning in manual tasks. An electromyographic study of localized muscle fatigue. *Ergonomics* 1980;23:655–665.

81. Larsson SE, Bengtsson A, Bodegård L, et al. Muscle changes in work related chronic myalgia. *Acta Orthop Scand* 1988;59:552–556.

82. Wilson F. Dorothy Taubman and Fernando Laires. *Piano Q* 1987;139:56–59.

83. Armstrong TJ, Martin BJ. Adverse effects of repetitive loading and

segmental vibration. In: Nordin M, Andersson GBJ, Pope MH, eds. *Musculoskeletal disorders in the workplace: principles and practice*. St. Louis: Mosby, 1997:134–151.

84. Menuhin Y. *The complete violinist*. New York: Summit Books, 1986.

85. Bejjani FJ, Ferrara L, Xu N, et al. Comparison of three piano techniques as an implementation of a proposed experimental design. *Med Probl Perform Art* 1989;4:109–113.

86. Cameron DMA, McCutcheon J. Experiences of guitar students who begin to study piano as a second instrument. *Med Probl Perform Art* 1992;7:75–82.

87. Kopfstein-Penk A. *The healthy guitar*. Arlington, VA: Kopfstein-Penk, 1994.

88. Wagner C. Success and failure in musical performance; biomechanics of the hand. In: Roehmann FL, Wilson FR, eds. *The biology of music making. Proceedings of the 1984 Denver Conference*. St. Louis: MMB Music, 1988:154–179.

89. Brockman R, Tubiana R, Chamagne P. Anatomic and kinesiologic considerations of posture for instrumental musicians. *J Hand Ther* 1992;5:61–64.

90. Aprill C, Dwyer A, Bogduk N. Cervical zygopophyseal joint pain patterns. II. A clinical evaluation. *Spine* 1990;15:458–461.

91. Fukui S, Ohseto K, Shiotani M, et al. Referred pain distribution of the cervical zygopophyseal joints and cervical dorsal rami. *Pain* 1996;68:79–83.

92. Brouw NAB. *Stem en lichaam*. Alphen a/d Rijn: Stafleu, 1983.

93. Balfoort B. *Houding, adem en keel; Fundamenten voor zangers, blazers en sprekers*. Baarn: Bosch & Keuning, 1985.

94. Carriere B. Therapeutic exercise and self-correction programs. In: Flynn TW, ed. *The thoracic spine and rib cage; musculoskeletal evaluation and treatment*. Boston: Butterworth-Heinemann, 1996:287–307.

95. Bejjani FJ, Halpern N, Lewis E. Standing postures of trumpeters. In: Oborne DJ, ed. *Contemporary ergonomics*. London: Taylor & Francis, 1986:217–221.

96. Halpern N, Bejjani FJ. Postural kinematics of trumpet playing. In: *Proceedings of the North American Congress on Biomechanics*. Montreal: NACB, 1986:57–58.

97. Lehrer S, Weiss J, Kark P. Misuse syndrome in musicians: combined medical and musical approach. In: Bejjani FJ, ed. *Current research in arts medicine*. Chicago: a capella books, 1993:365–367.

98. Taubman D. A teacher's perspective on musicians' injuries. In: Roehman FL, Wilson FR, eds. *The biology of music making. Proceedings of the 1984 Denver conference*. St. Louis: MMB Music, 1988: 144–153.

99. Wilson F. Fernando Laires and Dorothy Taubman part one. *Piano Q* 1987;138:36–39.

100. Havas K. *Stage fright, its causes and cures with special reference to violin playing*. London: Bosworth, 1989.

101. Wolf FG, Kenae MS, Brandt KD, et al. An investigation of finger joint and tendon forces in experienced pianists. *Med Probl Perform Art* 1993;8: 84–95.

102. Lister-Sink B. Rethinking technique. *Clavier* 1994:29–33.

103. Lister-Sink B. An holistic, hands-on approach to teaching injury-preventive technique. *South Med J* 1993;85(2).

104. Gelberman RH, Herginroeder PT, Hargens AR, et al. The carpal tunnel syndrome: a study of carpal tunnel pressures. *J Bone Joint Surg [Am]* 1981;63:380–383.

105. Szabo RM, Chidgey LK. Stress carpal tunnel pressures in patients with carpal tunnel syndrome and normal patients. *J Hand Surg [Am]* 1989;14: 624–627.

106. Furhmeister ML, Wiesenhütter E. *Metamusik; Psychosomatik der Ausübung zeitgenössischer Musik*. München: JF Lehmanns Verlag, 1973.

107. Michlovitz SL. *Thermal agents in rehabilitation*. Philadelphia: FA Davis, 1996.

108. Prentice WE. *Therapeutic modalities in sports medicine*. St. Louis: Times Mirror/Mosby, 1990.

109. Cantu RI, Grodin AJ. *Myofascial manipulation; theory and clinical application*. Gaithersburg: Aspen, 1992.

110. Schneider W, Dvorák J, Dvorák V, et al. *Manual medicine; therapy*. Stuttgart: Georg Thieme Verlag, 1988.

111. Maitland GD. *Vertebral manipulation*. Oxford: Butterworth-Heinemann, 1986.

112. Elvey RL. Peripheral neuropathic disorders and neuromusculoskeletal pain. In: Shacklock MO, ed. *Moving in on pain*. Chatswood: Butterworth-Heinemann, 1995:115–122.

113. Slater H, Butler DS, Shacklock MO. The dynamic central nervous system: examination and assessment using tension tests. In: Boyling JD, Palastanga N, eds. *Grieve's modern manual therapy*. Edinburgh: Churchill Livingstone, 1994:21–38.

114. Shacklock MO. Clinical application of neurodynamics. In: Shacklock MO, ed. *Moving in on pain*. Chatswood: Butterworth-Heinemann, 1995:123–131.

115. Janda V. Muscle strength in relation to muscle length, pain, and muscle imbalance. In: Harms-Rindahl K, ed. *Muscle strength*. Edinburgh: Churchill Livingstone, 1993:83–91.

116. Moran CA. Using myofascial techniques to treat musicians. *J Hand Ther* 1992;5:97–101.

117. Fricton JR. Myofascial pain syndrome: characteristics and epi-

demiology. *Adv Pain Res* 1990;17:107–127.

118. Skootsky SA, Jaeger B, Oye RK. Prevalence of myofascial pain in general internal medicine practice. *West J Med* 1989; 151:157–160.

119. Janda V. *Muscle function testing.* London: Butterworths, 1983.

120. Walpin LA. Posture: the process of body use; principles and determinants. In: Gelb H, ed. *New concepts in craniomandibular and chronic pain management.* London: Mosby-Wolfe, 1994:13–76.

121. Sahrmann SA. Adult posturing. In: Kraus S, ed. *TMJ disorders; management of the craniomandibular complex.* New York: Churchill Livingstone, 1988:295–309.

122. Winold H. High speed photography of cello playing. In: Roehman FL, Wilson FR, eds. *The biology of music making. Proceedings of the 1984 Denver conference.* St. Louis: MMB Music, 1988:180–182.

123. Lippmann HI. A fresh look at the overuse syndrome in musical performers: is "overuse" overused? *Med Probl Perform Art* 1991;6:57–60.

124. Wilson FR. *Tone deaf & all thumbs; an invitation to music-making.* New York: Vintage Books, 1987.

125. Sella GE. *Muscles in motion.* Martins Ferry: Sella, 1993.

126. Sella GE. *Neuro-muscular testing with surface EMG.* Martins Ferry: Sella, 1995.

127. Arena JG, Blanchard EB. Biofeedback and relaxation therapy for chronic pain disorders. In: Gatchel RJ, Turk DC, eds. *Psychological approaches to pain management.* New York: Guilford, 1996:179–230.

128. Kai-Nan A, Bejjani FJ. Analysis of upper-extremity performance in athletes and musicians. *Hand Clin* 1990;6:393–403.

129. Bejjani FJ, Ferrara L, Pavlidis L. A comparative electromyographic and acoustic analysis of violin vibrato in healthy professional violinists. *Med Probl Perform Art* 1989;4:168–175.

130. Naill R, McNitt-Gray J. Surface EMG as a method for observing the muscle activation patterns associated with strategies of string depression used by cellist. *Med Probl Perform Art* 1993;8:7–13.

131. Moore GP. The study of skilled performance in musicians. In: Roehman FL, Wilson FR, eds. *The biology of music making. Proceedings of the 1984 Denver conference.* St. Louis: MMB Music, 1988:169–190.

132. Philipson L, Sörbye R, Larsson P, et al. Muscular load levels in performing musicans as monitored by quantitative electromyography. *Med Probl Perform Art* 1990;5:79–82.

133. Heuser F, McNitt-Gray JL. EMG potentials prior to tone commencement in trumpet players. *Med Probl Perform Art* 1991;6:51–56.

134. Heuser F, McNitt-Gray JL. EMG patterns in embouchure muscles of trumpet players with asymmetrical mouthpiece placement. *Med Probl Perform Art* 1992;8: 96–102.

135. Polnauer F, Marks M. *Sensomotor study and its application to violin playing.* Urbana, TX: American String Teachers Association, 1964.

136. Szende O, Nemessuri M. *The physiology of violin playing.* London: Collet's Ltd., 1971.

137. LeVine WR, Irvine JK. In vivo EMG biofeedback in violin and viola pedagogy. *Biofeedback Self Regul* 1984;9:161–168.

138. Levee JR, Cohen MJ, Rickles WH. Electromyographic biofeedback for relief of tension in the facial and throat muscles of a woodwind musician. *Biofeedback Self Regul* 1976;1:113–120.

139. Flor H, Miltner W, Birbaumer N. Psychophysiological recording methods. In: Turk DC, Melzack R, eds. *Handbook of pain assessment.* New York: Guilford, 1992:169–190.

140. Dai K, Hou X, Shen X. Acupuncture-moxibustion and related techniques for artists. In: Bejjani FJ, ed. *Current research in arts medicine.* Chicago: a capella books, 1993:323–325.

141. Li Y. Treating voice disorders with acupuncture of acupoint "Li." In: Bejjani FJ, ed. *Current research in arts medicine.* Chicago: a capella books, 1993: 523–525.

142. Pi J, Zhang Y. Acupuncture treatment of vocal fold hypertrophy. In: Bejjani FJ, ed. *Current research in arts medicine.* Chicago: a capella books, 1993:527–529.

143. Molsberger A. Akupunktur bei Musikerkrankungen. In: Blum J, ed. *Medizische Probleme bei Musikern.* Stuttgart: Thieme Verlag, 1995:160–162.

144. Schnorrenberger CC. Die Behandlung von Bewegungsstörungen und andere Berufskrankheiten bei Musikern mittels Akupunktur. *Das Orchester* 1984;32: 1047–1061.

145. Chaitow L. *The acupuncture treatment of pain.* Rochester: Healing Arts Press, 1990.

146. Molsberger AE, Hille E, Molsberger F, Schulitz KP. Der Künstler als orthopädischer Patient. *Dtsch Arzteblatt* 1989;33: A2292–A2295.

147. Ahonen E. Acupuncture and physiotherapy in the treatment of myogenic headache patients: pain relief and EMG activity. In: Bonica JJ, ed. *Advances in pain research and therapy.* New York: Raven, 1983.

148. Loh L, Nathan PW, Schott GD, Zilkha KJ. Acupuncture vs medical treatment for migraine and muscle tension headaches. *J Neurol Neurosurg Psychiatry* 1984;47:333–337.

149. Lehman TR, Russell DW, Spratt KF, et al. Efficacy of electro-acupuncture and TENS in the

rehabilitation of chronic low back pain patients. *Pain* 1986;26:277–290.

150. Junnila SYT. Acupuncture superior to piroxicam in the treatment of osteoarthrosis. *Am J Acupunct* 1982;10:341–346.

151. Larre C. *La voie du ciel.* Paris: Desclee de Brouwer, 1987.

152. Grenier J. *L'esprit du Tao.* Paris: Flammarion, 1973.

153. Bichen Z. *Traite de'alchimie et de physiologie Taoiste.* Paris: Les Deux Oceans, 1979.

154. Auteroche B, Navailh P. *Le diagnostic en medecine Chinoise.* Paris: Maloine, 1983.

155. Xinnong C. *Chinese acupuncture and moxibustion.* Beijing: Foreign Languages Press, 1987.

156. Maciocia G. *The foundations of Chinese medicine.* New York: Churchill Livingstone, 1989.

157. Liao SJ, Lee MHM, Ng LKY. *Principles and practice of contemporary acupuncture.* New York: Marcel Dekker, 1994.

158. Dommerholt J. Meridian therapy—a new European concept. *Phys Ther Forum* 1990;3(5):8–11.

159. Heidemann C. *Meridiantherapie.* Freiburg: Heidemann, 1986.

160. Evans D. Acupuncture. In: Raj PP, ed. *Practical management of pain.* St. Louis: Mosby–Year Book, 1992:934–944.

161. Gaupp LA, Flinn DE, Weddige RL. Adjunctive treatment techniques. In: Tollison CD, Satterthwaite JR, Tollison JW, eds. *Handbook of pain management.* Baltimore: Williams & Wilkins, 1994:108–135.

162. Liu YK, Varela M, Oswald R. The correspondence between some motor points and acupuncture. *Am J Chin Med* 1975;3:347–358.

163. Han JS, Xie GX, Zhou ZF. Acupuncture mechanism in rabbits studied with microinjection of antibodies against β-endorphins, enkephalin, and substance P. *Neuropharmacology* 1984;23:1–5.

164. Han JS, Xie GX, Ding XZ, Fan SG. High and low frequency electro-acupuncture analgesia are mediated by different opioids. *Pain* 1984;2(suppl):543.

165. Gunn CC. *Treating myofascial pain: intramuscular stimulation for myofascial pain syndromes of neuropathic origin.* Seattle: University of Washington, 1989.

166. Gunn CC. *The Gunn approach to the treatment of chronic pain.* Edinburgh: Churchill Livingstone, 1996.

167. Baldry PE. *Acupuncture, trigger points and musculoskeletal pain.* Edinburgh: Churchill Livingstone, 1993.

168. Waumsley C. *Practical needling for physiotherapists.* Schaffhausen: Myopain Kurse, 1996.

169. Thomas M, Lundeberg T. Does acupuncture work? *Pain Clin Updates* 1997;4(3):1–4.

170. Rosenthal E. The Alexander technique and how it works: work with three musicians. *Med Probl Perform Art* 1987;2:53–57.

171. Spire N. The Feldenkrais method: an interview with Anat Baniel. *Med Probl Perform Art* 1989;4:59–62.

172. Miller B. Alternative somatic therapies. In: White AH, Anderson R, eds. *Conservative care of low back pain.* Baltimore: Williams & Wilkins, 1991:120–133.

173. Strohecker J, ed. *Alternative medicine: the definitive guide.* Puyallup: Future Medicine Publishing, 1994.

174. Barlow W. *The Alexander technique.* New York: Alfred A. Knopf, 1973.

175. Knebelman S, Ralson Dressler P, Mathews Brion M, et al. The essentials of the Alexander technique. In: Gelb H, ed. *New concepts in craniomandibular and chronic pain management.* London: Mosby-Wolfe, 1994:177–185.

176. Murphy M. *The future of the body; explorations into the further evolution of human nature.* Los Angeles: Jeremy P. Tarcher, 1993.

177. Feldenkrais M. *Awareness through movement.* New York: Harper & Row, 1977.

178. Rywerant Y. *The Feldenkrais method; teaching by handling.* New Canaan: Keats Publishing, 1983.

179. Samama A. *Muscle control for musicians.* Utrecht: Bohn, Scheltema & Holkema, 1981.

180. Knott M, Voss DE. *Proprioceptive neuromuscular facilitation.* Philadelphia: Harper & Row, 1968.

181. Friedman P, Eisen G. *The Pilates method of physical and mental conditioning.* New York: Warner Books, 1980.

182. Swaim K. An alternative therapy: Pilates® method. *PT Mag Phys Ther* 1993;1(10):55–58.

183. Stewart DL, Abeln SH. *Documenting functional outcomes in physical therapy.* St. Louis: Mosby, 1993.

184. Scott RW. *Legal aspects of documenting patient care.* Gaithersburg: Aspen, 1994.

185. Fry JHH. Overuse syndrome of the upper limb in musicians. *Med J Aust* 1986;144:182–185.

Part IV.

Specific Concerns

Chapter 46

Deconditioning and Bed Rest

Kamala Shankar
Sanjiv Jain

The natural state of the human body is one of motion. Humans have evolved, as has all animal life, with the ability to move through space in order to obtain the necessities of life including food, water, and shelter. A high level of activity and physical conditioning was needed in order to survive. With the development of more socialized forms of living and certainly with the advent of a modern industrialized society, the direct connection between survival and the physical ability to "hunt and gather" was severed. Vast numbers of individuals now live sedentary lives and are deconditioned compared with the level of conditioning at which humans evolved to function. Whereas primitive man's activities of daily living (ADLs) resulted in a high level of conditioning, we must now add "exercise" to our ADLs to achieve this same level. To explore the effects of this change in activity, large epidemiologic studies have been performed. They have provided evidence relating a lack of "exercise" with several pervasive, life-threatening diseases including coronary heart disease, hypertension, diabetes mellitus, and osteoporosis (1).

The importance of physical activity to maintain health is not new to the medical literature, with references found in the writings of Hippocrates, Maimonides, and Mendez and in the ancient Indian medical text, the Ayurveda, to mention a few (2,3). Nonetheless, either in the treatment of disease or as a consequence of disease, extended periods of inactivity and bed rest occur. For example, in the late 1800s and early 1990s it was common practice to prescribe 6 to 8 weeks of complete bed rest after a myocardial infarction (MI) occurred. In many diseases, inactivity and bed rest comprised a treatment modality that allowed the body to heal with few sequelae. With further experience and research, as well as with the drive to bring health care costs down, the periods of hospitalized bed rest are being dramatically reduced. Revisiting the example of the patient with an MI, depending on the extent of damage, mobilization typically begins by day 2, without an increase in morbidity and mortality and thereby avoiding the many complications of prolonged bed rest. Despite many advances, patients, especially those with a typical rehabilitation diagnosis, undergo periods of bed rest and immobility that result in deconditioning. Table 46-1 provides examples of causes of immobility.

Deconditioning per se means loss or decrease of a prior state of physical conditioning. Hypothetically this can be divided into mild, moderate, and severe deconditioning. In general, considering the relatively sedentary life of most individuals in Western society, many of us are functioning at a level of mild deconditioning where we have difficulty with maximal activity (e.g., running, swimming, "exercising"). A level of moderate deconditioning is measured by difficulty with normal (submaximal) activity such as walking down the street, shopping, and cutting the lawn. Severe deconditioning is evidenced by difficulty with minimal activity and self-care such as that seen in patients after a prolonged stay in an acute hospital unit who are too deconditioned to get out of bed, secondary to medical complications. The functional limitations of a severely

Table 46-1: Examples of Causes of Immobility*
Multiple trauma/orthopedic injuries
Spinal cord injuries
Cerebrovascular accidents
Prolonged hospitalizations
Multiple medical problems/multiple organ failure
Severe cardiovascular/pulmonary disease
Myocardial infarction
Complications of pregnancy
Back pain
Severe deconditioning

* A significant element of the period of immobility is iatrogenic "physician-prescribed" bed rest.

deconditioned individual with resultant complications can be examined in relation to each organ system. In the musculoskeletal system, there may be a loss of antigravity muscle strength with an inability to transfer and an inability to stand, secondary to hip and knee flexion contractures. Functional limitations of the cardiopulmonary system may include an inability to stand secondary to orthostatic hypotension and a severely reduced pulmonary reserve (oxygenation), resulting in shortness of breath during minimal exertion. This limits the patient's ability to perform ADLs and is only exacerbated rather than improved with further inactivity, regardless of the primary disease process. This "cycle" of inactivity and bed rest leading to further deconditioning in turn, makes it more difficult for the patient to get out of bed and thus results in further deconditioning. The effects of deconditioning involve a spectrum of change that can be seen at all levels of activity, from the highly trained athlete who does not work out during the off season, to the sedentary general population, to the hospitalized rehabilitation patient. In any person at any level of deconditioning, with a concerted effort it is possible to improve the level of conditioning to achieve a higher level of functioning and improve quality of life.

To evaluate the specific pathophysiologic changes that occur with bed rest, many studies have been performed over the past 50 years. A typical study design (from which much of the knowledge on the subject is derived) is as follows: A group of healthy, young (early 20s) men are admitted to the hospital and restricted to "bed rest." The level of inactivity imposed varies, with the most restrictive (4) requiring subjects to wear a lower-body cast and to use a bed pan. More typical, and less restrictive studies simply ask volunteers to remain horizontal in bed, and allow them to transfer with assistance to the wheelchair and to use the commode for self-care. Difficulties with this study design arise from the fact that volunteers who are young and healthy are more mobile in bed and physiologically different from the typical hospitalized rehabilitation patient. Monitoring compliance and closely limiting time in the wheelchair for hygiene and toileting were important factors in the better studies. These data provide a foundation for basic changes that occur under conditions of bed rest, though the magnitude of changes found often varied in studies, likely because of differing study designs. In the ill, deconditioned elderly patient, many of the effects of bed rest are magnified. Many of the studies on bed rest have sprung from the space program and the use of bed rest as a model for weightlessness. As such, the emphasis of some of these studies and their treatment interventions are not directly relevant. However, as often occurs as a by-product of the space program, considerable important and useful information has been generated and is referenced as appropriate.

As indicated, prolonged bed rest and inactivity are unnatural states of the human body. As such, numerous physiologic adaptations occur (in all organ systems), with often negative consequences. Furthermore, the physiologic effects of bed rest and deconditioning are superimposed on whatever the primary disease process may be. The salient pathophysiologic adaptations of bed rest on relevant organ systems are discussed, with every effort made to reference classic, clinically relevant, and recent studies.

CENTRAL AND PERIPHERAL NERVOUS SYSTEMS

Much of the psychological sequelae of bed rest stems from the secondary factors of sensory deprivation and loss of independence. Several factors contribute to the relative sensory deprivation of the bed-rested patient. These include the isolation of a private, unfamiliar hospital room; the inability to effectively manipulate one's environment (secondary to neurologic sequelae from the primary disease, e.g., stroke, traumatic brain injury, and spinal cord injury or severe deconditioning); the relatively common findings of decreased visual or hearing acuity in the elderly (compounded by a lack of convenient access to glasses and hearing aids); the lack of social stimulation (secondary to the patient's being removed from the circle of friends and family by being hospitalized); and the frequent loss of sensation secondary to the patient's primary disease (5).

A prospective study by Ishizaki et al (6) of nine, young, healthy subjects confined to bed for 20 days found a tendency for the development of depression and neurosis, using Zung's Self Rating Depression Scale and the General Health Questionnaire. In other studies with imposed sensory deprivation and bed rest, subjects experienced alterations in affect, perception, and cognition (5,7). Changes in affect included anxiety, fear, depression, and rapid mood changes (7). Changes in perception included disorientation to time and the perception that time was passing slowly (8), the appearance of hallucinations, a lowered pain threshold, and an increased auditory threshold (9,10). Changes in cognition that have been found include decreased concentration (5) and impairments in judgment and problem solving (11). A prospective study with 18 healthy subjects after 30 days of bed rest (both with and without exercise training) (12) found no alterations in mood or performance test results, further supporting the idea that secondary factors such as sensory deprivation rather than primary effects, are leading to these alterations in hospitalized rehabilitation patients. Increased environmental stress in the form of poor caretaker-patient relationships has been suggested to increase psychotic manifestations in bedfast elderly in Japan (13). Apathy, withdrawal, irritability, and uncooperative behavior often occur as well, and significantly impair the patient's motivation and ability to participate in a rehabilitation program. Table 46-2 lists major psychosocial complications of immobility.

Every attempt should be made to keep the patient stimulated, oriented, and socially integrated into the milieu of the unit. Examples of environmental interventions include using semiprivate or four-person rooms (i.e., avoid private rooms), encouraging family and friends to visit, arranging visits from clergy and volunteers, arranging group activities, and taking the patient outside (even if in bed). Adapting the patient's room by making the phone accessible and using adaptations such as headphones, keeping hearing aids and glasses easily available (while taking extra care that they are not lost in the laundry or on food trays), encouraging the family to bring in the patient's favorite music, books on tape, and photographs, and instituting other such commonsense measures provide a more user-friendly environment and keep the patient involved and stimulated.

Peripheral nerve compression is one potential direct complication of immobility. Common sites for compression neuropathies include the peroneal nerve at the fibular head and the ulnar nerve at the retrocondylar groove. Although footdrop can occur secondary to peroneal compression, severe weakness and subsequent contracture of the gastrocnemius muscle and Achilles tendon are the more common etiologic factors in the bed-rested patient.

Table 46-2: Major Psychosocial Complications of Immobility
Depression
Loss of control
Loss of motivation
Feeling of helplessness
Loss of independent activities of daily living
Loss of avocational and social pursuits
Loss of vocation

CARDIOVASCULAR SYSTEM

Many of the changes that occur in the cardiovascular system become more intuitive by understanding the fluid shifts that accompany bed rest and the body's responses to them (Fig. 46-1). In a normal healthy individual, moving from the supine to the erect position shifts 500 to 700 mL of fluid from the thorax into the legs, secondary to the force of gravity. The body adapts to this shift of fluid (which has been described as a *functional hemorrhage*) by several compensatory mechanisms, including the carotid and aortic mechanoreceptors (baroreceptors) and the cardiopulmonary mechanoreceptors (14). In the erect position, with less blood volume in the thorax, there is a decreased "stretch" in the mechanoreceptors, which produces pressor responses such as increased heart rate and contractility, vasoconstriction, venoconstriction, and antidiuresis. These responses combine to maintain adequate systolic blood pressure and cerebral perfusion.

In the supine position, the reverse occurs. There is a shift of 500 to 700 mL of blood volume from the lower body to the central thorax. This *central fluid shift* has the immediate effect of increasing venous return to the heart

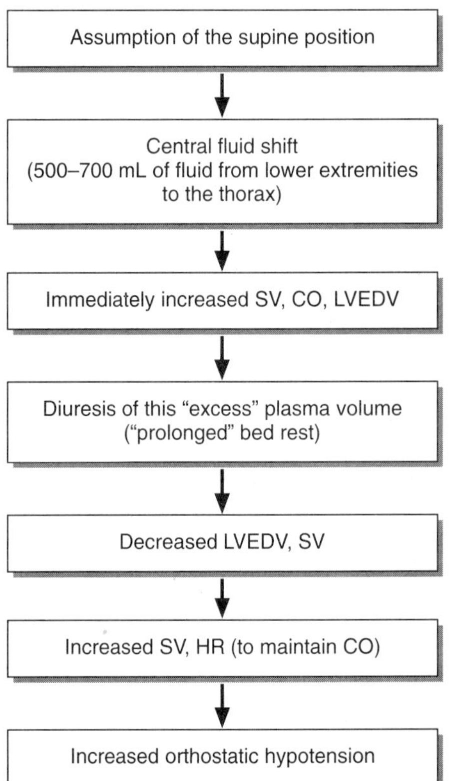

Figure 46-1. Fluid shifts and cardiovascular adaptations to bed rest. SV = stroke volume; CO = cardiac output; LVEDV = left ventricular end-diastolic volume; HR = heart rate.

Table 46-3: Major Cardiac Complications of Immobility
Increased heart rate
Decreased stroke volume
Atrophy of cardiac muscle
Decreased VO_2max (with exercise)
Central fluid shift
Orthostatic hypotension

VO_2max = maximum oxygen consumption.

and thus increasing ventricular and diastolic volume and consequently stroke volume. Compensatory adaptations are quickly mediated by increased stretch of the afore mentioned mechanoreceptors, with resultant depressor responses.

With prolonged bed rest, the relatively increased central blood volume is adapted to by depressed levels of aldosterone and antidiuretic hormone, with a resultant diuresis. Thus, the net effect is a decreased blood and plasma volume. From this decrease, it follows that the stroke volume is lower, the resting heart rate is higher (to maintain resting cardiac output), and the maximum oxygen consumption (VO_2max), which is a function of maximum cardiac output, is decreased. In addition, there is increased orthostatic intolerance (or postural hypotension) as there is less blood volume. Table 46-3 lists the major cardiac complications of immobility. Although fluid shifts do not account for all of these changes independently, and some conflicting research findings exist, understanding this conceptual model will allow one to understand and reason out the major cardiovascular changes that occur with bed rest.

Cardiovascular Changes at Rest

After the acute changes develop in response to taking the supine position, as soon as within 24 hours of bed rest, the prolonged changes with bed rest begin to occur (see Fig. 46-1) (15,16).

According to the majority of studies on prolonged bed rest, the generally accepted finding is that the resting heart rate increases by ½ beat/min each day for the first 3 to 4 weeks and then plateaus (4,17–20). Depending on the duration of bed rest, the heart rate increases by around 4 to 15 beats/min (14). For example, in one study, resting heart rate increased from 69 to 79 beats/min after 20 days of bed rest (21). The etiology for this rise in pulse has not been shown, although theories include compensation for the decrease in blood volume or an imbalance in the autonomic nervous system (22–24). Quantification of this blood volume loss revealed that plasma volume losses occur early with bed rest, with a 5% decrease in 24 hours, 10% in 6 days, and 20% decrease in 14 days (25), with a range of 6% to 20% total plasma volume loss noted in different studies (26,27). Incidentally, plasma volume decreases more in men than in women (28). The autonomic imbalance can take the form of decreased vagal tone or decreased sensitivity to vagal stimulation (29) or opposite sympathetic-mediated effects (22,30). Other studies demonstrated no change in resting heart rate with prolonged bed rest (30,31). These studies postulated that any slight motion of the subjects prior to measuring the heart rate can lead to erroneously elevated "resting" heart rate levels.

As noted previously, stroke volume is decreased, left ventricular end-diastolic volume is decreased, and cardiac output is relatively unchanged or decreased (17,21,31–36). A decrease in left ventricular size occurs with bed rest (17,21,32) or as a result of decreased activity (37), and atrophy of cardiac muscle develops with chronic disuse (38). In addition, Doppler ultrasound studies showed that cerebral blood flow is maintained at the expense of blood flow to the lower body (21).

Cardiovascular System Response to Exercise after Bed Rest

As would be expected, the ability of the cardiovascular system to respond to exercise after a prolonged period of disuse is diminished. Remembering that plasma volume is decreased with prolonged bed rest partially explains many of these changes. At any level of submaximal exercise (in either the supine or the erect position) there is an abnormally large increase in heart rate in individuals after a period of bed rest compared with control subjects who have not been placed on bed rest (2,4,17,32,39,40). Although many of the previously noted adaptations (such as decreased stroke volume, cardiac output, and an altered autonomic system) may contribute, orthostatic stress has been proposed as the most important factor in limiting exercise tolerance after bed rest (in otherwise healthy, middle-aged men) (34). Classic studies by Taylor et al (32) and Saltin et al (17) demonstrated an increase in heart rate by about 30 beats during submaximal exercise performed after 3 weeks of bed rest, compared with the heart rate while performing the same activity prior to bed rest. Stroke volume and cardiac output are reduced by about 25% and 15%, respectively, with submaximal exercise and by about 30% and 26% at maximal exercise (17,41). The finding by Hung et al (36) of decreased left ventricular end-diastolic volume in the supine position after bed rest supports the concept that decreased ventricular filling rather than depressed myocardial function are responsible for these lower values. Similarly, VO_2max, which is a measure of cardiovascular fitness and reserve, is reduced (by 15%–46%) after exercise in the upright position (16,17,34).

Recovery from Bed Rest

There is no consensus on the rate of recovery following bed rest, but as a rule of thumb, it generally takes at least as long as the period of bed rest to return to baseline levels for heart rate, VO_2max, and other parameters. One 20-day bed rest study involving five women and nine men found that despite exercise training, women had a persistent decrease in VO_2max after 8 to 9 weeks of recovery following bed rest (42).

Orthostatic Intolerance

Prolonged bed rest produces a profound orthostatic intolerance. During sitting or standing after a period of bed rest, an otherwise healthy individual commonly experiences symptoms of orthostatic hypotension including dizziness, light-headedness, sweating, tachycardia, and even fainting. This dramatic effect is often exacerbated in the elderly or ill and requires careful monitoring and care in hospitalized patients. Much of the literature on this topic stems from the need to understand and prevent orthostatic hypotension from occurring to astronauts during the critical reentry and landing phase of their mission when their period of "bed rest" (weightlessness) ends and they are again subjected to the forces of gravity.

Alterations of the normal orthostatic response include a markedly elevated heart rate, decrease in pulse pressure, decrease in systolic blood pressure, and diminished stroke volume. In a study by Chobanian et al (41), heart rate upon standing increased by 32% after 3 days of bed rest, by 62% after 1 week of bed rest, and by 89% after 3 weeks of bed rest.

There is incomplete understanding of the mechanism for this intolerance. The effect can be explained partially by a decreased circulating plasma volume and increased venous pooling with inadequate venous return upon standing. However, this intolerance cannot be explained completely by decreased plasma volume, as replacement of the volume (by oral saline solution and mineralocorticoids) improves but does not resolve the orthostatic intolerance (43,44). Other effects that possibly contribute as well include altered autonomic nervous functioning (45) such as reduced cardiac vagal activity, without a change in cardiac sympathetic activity (23), or impaired cardiac baroreceptor reflex responses (46), though this is still in dispute (24,47–49).

Thrombogenesis

Bed rest increases the risk of clot formation, leading to deep vein thrombosis and thereby pulmonary embolism. Bed rest reduces the muscular action pumping blood through the calves and thereby increases the stasis of blood. Many rehabilitation patients have paralysis of a lower extremity, further contributing to the relative stasis of blood in that extremity. In addition, the red blood cell mass initially remains constant with bed rest, then begins to decrease, though not at the same rate, as plasma losses increase, leading to an increased hematocrit and blood viscosity (2). This increased blood viscosity, as well as increased platelet aggregation and blood fibrinogen levels (2,50,51), also creates a more thrombogenic environment (52,53). Table 46-4 lists the major vascular complications of immobility. The risk of deep vein thrombosis in nonambulatory cerebrovascular accident patients is five times greater than that for ambulatory patients, with the affected extremity involved 10 times more than the uninvolved extremity (54).

Table 46-4: Major Vascular Complications of Immobility
Decreased blood flow
Increased platelet adhesiveness
Increased fibrinogen level
Increased risk for deep vein thrombosis and pulmonary embolism

A rheologic study of two patients with sickle cell disease and leg ulcerations demonstrated an improvement in erythrocyte deformability with bed rest, which in turn may have aided in healing their ulcers by improving the blood supply (55).

Prevention and Treatment of Cardiovascular Complications

Avoidance of prolonged bed rest is the most important intervention to prevent cardiovascular deconditioning from occurring. The reduction in the duration of bed rest prescribed after MI from 2 to 3 months at the turn of the century to 1 or 2 days today dramatically illustrates such an adjustment (56). Redistributing the blood volume back into the lower extremities to avoid the central fluid shift and resultant diuresis is of primary importance in reducing some of the effects of cardiac deconditioning (20). Using mechanisms such as sitting or quiet standing during the bed rest period (14) may decrease orthostatic intolerance. Also effective, though more relevant for space travel, is the use of lower-body negative-pressure devices or reverse-gradient garments to induce venous pooling, as well as oral saline loading to prevent or minimize plasma volume losses and thereby prevent orthostatic intolerance and changes in heart rate and VO_2max (35,43,44,57). No significant improvement in orthostatic intolerance was noted with isometric or isotonic bed exercises (16,19,39). Furthermore, light exercise bicycling in a supine position does not prevent a decline in VO_2max (16,42,58).

RESPIRATORY SYSTEM

Bed rest predisposes the patient to atelectasis, decreased oxygenation, and the development of pneumonia. Upon assumption of the supine position there are several immediate effects on the respiratory system. The diaphragm moves to a more cephalad position, with a resultant decrease in thoracic size (59,60). In addition, the central fluid shift results in increased blood in the thorax, further

Table 46-5: Major Respiratory System Complications of Immobility
Increased respiratory rate
Increased forced vital capacity
Increased ventilation-perfusion mismatch
Increased atelectasis*
Decreased ciliary action*
Decreased cough*
Diaphragm elevation
Increased risk for pulmonary embolism
Increased risk for pneumonia

* Postulated.

reducing the available space for lung expansion and aeration. Thus, upon taking the supine position, there is an immediate decrease in lung volumes, most markedly in the residual volume (61). In addition, whereas in the upright position quiet tidal breathing is mainly caused by rib expansion, in the supine position the abdominal muscles predominate (62). Rib cage motion accounts for 68% of tidal volume during sitting while in the supine position abdominal motion accounts for 68% of tidal volume (63). With prolonged bed rest it is generally accepted (although not scientifically proved) that several physiologic changes occur due to gravity. While supine, it is thought that there is pooling of mucus in the dependent (posterior) portion of the bronchial tree, whereas the upper (ventral) bronchial wall dries out. Coupled with impaired ciliary function in the affected airway and a less effective cough (secondary to weakened abdominal musculature), the patient has more difficulty clearing secretions and is predisposed to mucous plugging, atelectasis, and upper and lower respiratory tract infections. Beckett et al (61) found, after 11 to 12 days of bed rest in normal subjects, a small increase in forced vital capacity and total lung capacity and no change in functional residual capacity and residual volume. Other studies did not find significant changes in pulmonary function values with bed rest (16,26). Table 46-5 lists the major respiratory system complications with bed rest.

Because of alterations in blood supply and aeration that occur in the supine position, a mismatch in lung ventilation and perfusion occurs and leads to decreased arterial oxygenation (60,64–67). Prolonged immobility and bed rest may lead to intercostal muscle and joint contractures, more shallow breathing, and an increased respiratory rate. These changes further impair the patient's oxygenation and thereby limit endurance and the ability to make functional gains. Furthermore, the development of a pneumonia in such a deconditioned patient can quickly become life-threatening (68).

Interventions to minimize the effects of bed rest include early mobilization, frequent changes in position, deep breathing and incentive spirometry, adequate hydration, and adequate coughing. Aggressive pulmonary toilet with chest percussion, postural drainage, oropharyngeal suctioning, and in some patients, intermittent positive-pressure breathing treatments with normal saline solution, acetylcysteine (Mucomyst), or bronchial dilators may be needed. A prospective study of elderly bed-bound patients that utilized povidine-iodine to clean patients' mouths and had patients sit up for 2 hours after meals to avoid aspiration demonstrated a reduced number of febrile days compared to a control group, presumably by minimizing respiratory tract infections (69). Another important intervention is adequate prophylaxis against the development of deep vein thrombosis as well as prompt evaluation and treatment to avoid a potentially fatal pulmonary embolism.

MUSCLES

At bed rest there is a decrease in muscle strength (or torque around a joint) of approximately 1% per day (depending on the study, 0.7%–1.5%/day). The amount of strength that is lost plateaus at 20% to 50%. Many variables in different studies, including length and relative restrictiveness of the bed rest, the force measurement techniques employed, and the type of muscle testing (isometric versus isotonic) used, partially explain this variability. Loss of strength is consistently greatest in the postural muscles (such as the low-back muscles) and weight-bearing lower-extremity muscles (such as the quadriceps and gastrocnemius-soleus muscle groups). For example, in a classic study by Dietrick et al (4), cast immobilization for 6 to 7 weeks resulted in a 6.6% loss in elbow flexor, 8.7% loss in shoulder flexor, 13.7% loss in dorsiflexor, and 20.8% loss in the plantarflexor strength. Many studies since found a similar pattern for loss of muscle strength (70–72). Upper-extremity muscles are significantly less involved, as the finding of preserved handgrip strength in patients on bed rest illustrates (73). Paralleling this loss in strength of postural and lower-extremity muscles is loss of muscle mass and increased muscle atrophy. A 17-week bed rest study by LeBlanc et al (74) demonstrated a 30% loss of volume in ankle extensors, a 16% to 18% loss in the quadriceps, a 9% loss in the intrinsic lower-back muscles, and no volume loss in the upper-extremity muscles. These results are consistent with those of other studies (75,76). Furthermore, it appears likely that loss of strength and muscle volume occurs relatively rapidly during the early part of bed rest (75,76), with one study demonstrating a 3% volume loss in the thigh muscles within 7 days of bed rest, as quantified by magnetic resonance imaging (77,78). It should be noted that bed rest alone does not completely unweight the bones, and healthy young individuals on bed rest use their back and leg muscles a significant amount in moving about in the bed, compared with elderly, deconditioned, rehabilitation patients without the ability to reposition themselves

Table 46-6: Major Musculoskeletal Complications of Immobility
Muscles
Loss of muscle strength (weight bearing)
Decreased muscle mass
Decreased tendon and ligament strength
Contractures
Decreased number of sarcomeres in series
Decreased ATP and glycogen stores
Increased fatigability of muscle
Bones
Osteoporosis (weight bearing primarily)
Heterotopic ossification
Cortical thinning at ligament insertion sites
Joints
Flexion contractures
Cartilage degeneration
Fibrofatty connective tissue infiltration
Synovial atrophy
Fusion
Osteoarthritis*

* Controversial.

freely. Table 46-6 lists the major musculoskeletal complications of immobility.

On the anatomic and histologic level, many changes occur to the muscles, though many of these findings have been derived from animal studies. Animal studies (particularly rat studies) found that type I slow-twitch fiber muscles were predominantly affected by bed rest, compared with type II fast-twitch fibers (79–82). This finding is consistent with the relatively high cross-sectional area of type I fibers in the antigravity muscles most affected with disuse, and in humans it may be anatomic position and function rather than fiber type that is more important (3,83). In addition, the postural role of physiologic extensors explains their greater atrophy with immobility compared with flexors (84). In a 30-day bed rest study, Dudley et al (83,85) noted little difference in the magnitude of atrophy of type I compared with type II fibers.

Additional changes with immobilization include a decrease in protein synthesis (86,87) and an increase in relative collagen content and cross-linkage (88). The number of sarcomeres in the series decreases with muscles kept in a shortened position (89–91). A decrease in the strength of the myotendinous junction (92) and changes in muscle electrical activity (93) have been found. Furthermore, fatigability of the muscles increases, possibly because of decreased levels of adenosine triphosphate and glycogen stores, more rapid accumulation of lactic acid, and a decreased ability of muscles to utilize fatty acids after a period of immobility (94–96). The extent of atrophy is significantly increased if the muscle is kept in its contracted position, while stretching the muscle slows or prevents atrophy (87,89,90,97–100).

Interventions to minimize changes in the muscles during bed rest, as expected, involve early mobilization and activity. Studies have demonstrated that relatively intense exercises in bed (isokinetic or isotonic) can be used to maintain muscle strength (40,72,101), especially for the anterior thigh muscles compared with the hamstrings (102). Early weight-bearing activities should modify the decline in muscle strength as well (103). Performing daily exercises can help maintain muscle function. Techniques such as electrical stimulation (used more frequently by athletes trying to minimize loss of muscle bulk while wearing a cast secondary to a fracture) can decrease atrophy due to inactivity (104,105).

JOINTS

Immobility and bed rest often result in joints not regularly moving through their full range of motion and no longer being subjected to normal weight-bearing forces. This condition leads to the development of joint contractures. Immobilization leads to changes in the collagen, ligaments, and muscles surrounding the joint, resulting in reduced range of motion and a decreased ability to withstand stress (59,106). There is fibrofatty proliferation of connective tissue within the joint cavity, with the development of atrophic synovium and deterioration of the subchondral bone (107,108). The articular cartilage can become necrotic in areas of contact and develop fissures in other areas (106,109). Typical contractures that develop with prolonged bed rest include the hips or knees in a flexed position and the ankles plantarflexed. Less common upper-body contractures with bed rest include the fingers flexed, the elbows flexed, the shoulders internally rotated, and the thorax flexed. Interventions to minimize the development of contractures involve early mobilization and maintenance of full range of motion through active or passive range-of-motion exercises. There is no consensus on the frequency of exercises required, although performing them twice daily appears to be effective. The patient and family should become actively involved in this aspect of care early in the rehabilitation course. Proper positioning and the use of a foot board to prevent ankle plantarflexion are important considerations in the deconditioned bed-rested patient.

BONES

The primary factor in stimulating bone formation is the stress of weight bearing, which is largely eliminated in the supine position. Thus, bed rest and immobilization lead to disuse osteoporosis documented by both increased calcium excretion and decreased bone density. Bone loss occurs primarily in weight-bearing bones such as the vertebral bodies, the long bones of the legs, the calcaneus, and the metacarpals. Bone mineral density of the vertebral bones decreases by about 1% per week of bed rest (110,111), which is nearly 50 times the predicted involutional bone loss (112). Another study demonstrated a 25% to 40% loss in calcaneous bone mass after 30 to 36 weeks of bed rest (113). About 25% of U.S. women over the age of 50 will develop a fracture of one or more vertebral bones related to osteoporosis (114). Non-weight-bearing bones such as the radius and ulna lose significantly less bone, and the skull in some studies actually showed an increase in bone mineral density (perhaps owing to new weight bearing in the supine position) (110,115). Nishimura et al (110) concluded that early in bed rest, initially increased bone matrix resorption without activation of osteoclasts resulted in rapid decalcification without any discernible change in anatomic structure.

A separate 17-week bed rest study (116) demonstrated a small increase in intervertebral disk height of only about 1 mm. With 5 weeks of bed rest, disk height returned to baseline after a few days of ambulation, but after 17 weeks of bed rest, the disk area remained increased even after 6 weeks of ambulation.

Although lack of muscle activity and therefore decreased tension imposed on the bone may contribute to bone loss, supine isometric or isotonic exercise during bed rest only minimally affects bone loss. Interventions to minimize bone loss with bed rest involve early weight bearing and mobilization (117). Quiet standing for several hours per day significantly reduces bone loss and hypercalciuria (118,119). In a study looking at the biochemical parameters of bone turnover during bed rest, the use of intranasal salmon calcitonin was suggested as being effective in counteracting the early increase in bone resorption induced by immobilization (120). During a 30-day bed rest study, there was no loss in knee proprioception, although daily isokinetic exercise training improved proprioceptive tracking above baseline levels (121).

Fetal immobility secondary to neuromuscular disease results in thin, hypomineralized, elongated bones and joint contractures in the newborn infants and is believed to be secondary to the reduction in intrauterine motion of the fetus (122).

Immobilization Hypercalcemia

High serum calcium levels occur more often in adolescent males after trauma, particularly spinal cord injury, and is not typically seen with immobilization alone. Symptoms include nausea, vomiting, weakness, change in mental status, and hypotonia. There may finally be a progression to coma. Symptomatic hypercalcemia may occur a couple of weeks to a few months after immobilization (123). Treatment includes intravenous hydration, diuretics, and calcitonin or etidronate or both.

Heterotopic Ossification

Abnormal bone growth around a joint (heterotopic ossification) or in muscle (myositis ossificans) is not usually seen secondary to immobility alone. It occurs more often after neurologic trauma (such as spinal cord injury and traumatic brain injury) or after direct trauma (such as muscle contusions or bone fractures) with superimposed immobility. Effective treatment is not available but involves maintenance of range of motion and a functional position, and though controversial, the use of nonsteroidal anti-inflammatory medications such as indomethacin (Indocin) or diphosphonates such as etidronate.

Table 46-6 lists the major musculoskeletal complications of immobility.

METABOLIC AND ENDOCRINE SYSTEMS

It appears that there is a decrease in the basal metabolic rate with bed rest (4,32), with one study demonstrating a 13% drop in males and a 21% drop in females after 10 days of bed rest (124). Other studies, however, demonstrated no change in the basal metabolic rate (3,16). Total body weight remains unchanged with bed rest (125,126); however, lean body mass is decreased while body fat is increased (127–129). Body temperature remains normal during bed rest, but is minimally higher than expected during submaximal exercise after bed rest (130,131).

Beginning by the third day of bed rest (126), peripheral muscle develops a decreased sensitivity to insulin, resulting in a decrease in glucose tolerance (132). Serum glucose levels remain normal; however, there is a progressive delay in the peak insulin concentration and an increase in the total insulin response after a glucose tolerance test, depending on the duration of the bed rest (78,126). Evidence also suggests increased secretion of insulin in response to glucose by beta cells of the pancreas (133). A decrease in norepinephrine excretion by 35% was found after 14 days of bed rest, without a change in renal dopamine production. This sympathetic inhibition despite a decreased plasma volume (caused by the central fluid shift and subsequent diuresis with prolonged bed rest) may partially explain the orthostatic intolerance experienced after prolonged bed rest (134).

It has been postulated that physically conditioned individuals (individuals with a higher VO_2max) have greater changes in serum carbohydrate and electrolyte levels, and orthostatic intolerance, compared with unconditioned individuals after a period of bed rest. A study by Zorbas et al (135) demonstrated a significant decrease in serum glucose, cortisol, aldosterone, testosterone, and triiodothyronine levels and an increase in serum thyroxine, potassium, sodium, and chloride levels after 30 days of bed rest in physically conditioned subjects (VO_2max = 69 mL/kg/min), compared with physically unconditioned subjects (VO_2max = 44 mL/kg/min). Chronic hyperhydration (subjects who consumed an additional 26 mL of water per kilogram of body weight and 0.10 mg of sodium per kilogram of body weight daily) of the physically conditioned subjects during the period of bed rest normalized all of these biochemical changes. Similarly, chronic hyperhydration improved VO_2max and orthostatic intolerance in the conditioned subjects compared with controls. These improvements are thought to be mediated by increasing circulating blood volume to counteract the hypohydration caused by bed rest (135).

Serum erythropoietin titers are not depressed during bed rest, but total red blood cell volume is decreased and hematocrit is elevated secondary to the reduction in plasma volume (136).

Nitrogen

There is a daily net nitrogen loss with bed rest. The loss of nitrogen with bed rest in the young healthy individual is about 2 g/day via urinary excretion, and begins by day 5 or 6 of bed rest and persists throughout the period of inactivity. A reduction in muscle activity, muscle atrophy, and decreased protein synthesis leads to hypoproteinemia (129,137). Initially during recovery after bed rest, nitrogen continues to be lost, then undergoes a period of decreased excretion (excretion below normal baseline level) in order to recover losses, and eventually returns to normal levels (4).

Other Losses

There is increased excretion of electrolytes including potassium, sodium, and chloride during bed rest, although serum levels remain normal (27,41,138,139). The losses in sodium and potassium occur early during bed rest, paralleling the losses in plasma volume. There are losses in phosphorus that parallel calcium losses (140) and in sulfur that follow nitrogen losses (4). There is also a loss of zinc during bed rest, likely secondary to bone loss and muscle atrophy (141). Copper levels do not decrease during bed rest but copper does accumulate with zinc during the recovery period after bed rest (141).

Calcium

Calcium is lost during bed rest via fecal and urinary routes, paralleling losses in bone mass. In a 17-week bed rest study, calcium absorption decreased by 22%, urinary excretion increased, but serum calcium levels remained unchanged (142). Total body calcium is lost by about 0.5% per month (143,144). Absorption of 1,25-dihydroxyvitamin D is also decreased (by 17% in the same study) during bed rest (142). Parathyroid hormone levels are relatively unchanged (or minimally decreased) during bed rest, with no change in serum calcitonin or prolactin levels (142). Disuse osteoporosis caused primarily by increased bone resorption is consistent with these findings.

INTEGUMENTARY SYSTEM

The occurrence of pressure sores is a very common problem in patients with limited mobility or at bed rest (see Chapter 50). Considering their common occurrence, the potentially devastating medical consequences, the high cost of care, and the pain and disability they cause, prevention is of paramount importance. Pressure ulcers occur when there is extrinsic pressure that is greater than the capillary perfusion pressure (30 mm Hg) for a prolonged time, resulting in ischemia to the affected tissues. Typical locations for ulcer development are over bony prominences including 1) the sacrum (in the supine position), 2) the ischial tuberosities (in the sitting position), 3) the heels (in the supine position), 4) the greater trochanters (in the side-lying position) and 5) the occiput, especially in children owing to their relatively enlarged heads (in the supine position).

Essential for ulcer development is pressure (145), with sheer forces, friction, and moisture traditionally believed to be the primary factors contributing to ulcer formation (145–147). A recent prospective study on pressure sore development in a general hospital population found an incidence of 12.9% for grade 2 ulcer development, with nonblanchable erythema, lymphopenia, immobility, dry skin, and decreased body weight as independent significant risk factors (148). In the rehabilitation patient population, contractures, spasticity, impaired sensation, altered mental status, and incontinence often exist and significantly increase the risk for ulcer development. Dependent edema also occurs with immobility and further impairs circulation in at-risk tissue. Complications of pressure sores include excessive metabolic needs and protein loss, cellulitis, osteomyelitis, sepsis, and ultimately death.

Prevention of pressure sores is an achievable and highly desired goal. This involves, among other interventions, identification of at-risk patients; education of patient, family, and staff; selection of proper bedding; proper positioning; frequent turning; adequate nutrition; maintenance of continence; and proper skin care.

If a pressure sore develops, treatment involves prompt identification of the etiology and complete pressure relief without causing excessive pressure in other areas. Usually conservative management is appropriate, with dressing changes, enzymatic or sharp debridement, and the use of a special bed if the ulcer is large or if it is otherwise difficult to achieve pressure relief (149,150). Adequate nutrition including protein, vitamin C, and zinc supplements, if needed, should be provided (145). Systemic antibiotics are indicated for sepsis, cellulitis, or osteomyelitis or to prevent bacterial endocarditis in susceptible individuals. Rarely, surgical flap closure is needed, and in the most severe cases, amputation may be necessary. An ongoing review of established protocols and how effectively they are being followed is an important factor in reducing the development of pressure sores (151).

GENITOURINARY SYSTEM

There are several effects of prolonged bed rest on the genitourinary system. These include increased diuresis, hypercalciuria, increased renal stone formation, urinary

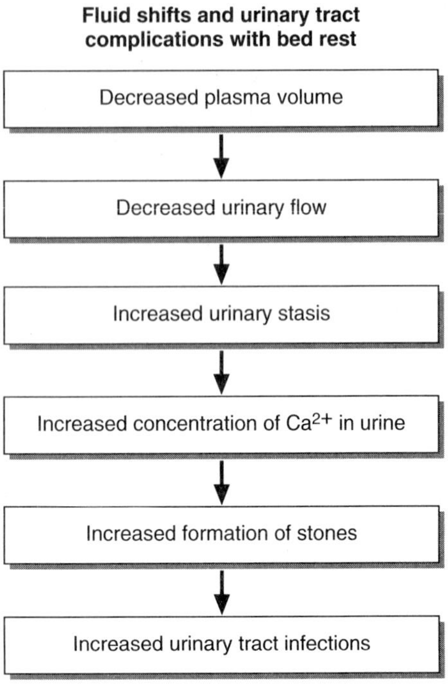

Fluid shifts and urinary tract complications with bed rest

Decreased plasma volume
↓
Decreased urinary flow
↓
Increased urinary stasis
↓
Increased concentration of Ca^{2+} in urine
↓
Increased formation of stones
↓
Increased urinary tract infections

Figure 46-2. Fluid shifts and urinary tract complications with bed rest.

retention, bladder distention, urinary stasis, and increased urinary tract infections (Fig. 46-2). With prolonged bed rest, hypercalciuria and hyperphosphaturia increase the propensity to form calcium-containing renal stones (152). Renal stones in turn increase the risk for, and make it more difficult to eradicate, urinary tract infections, by providing a nidus for bacterial growth. Difficulty in emptying the bladder in the supine position without the assistance of gravity, and weakened abdominal musculature may lead to increased urinary retention and incomplete emptying of the bladder, with increased postvoid residual volumes. The resultant urinary stagnation further increases the risk for both urinary tract infection and stone formation. Limited animal studies suggest that with immobilization there may be a decrease in spermatogenesis and changes in androgen secretion (153,154).

Bed rest functionally leads to an increase in urinary incontinence. In community-dwelling elderly, the rate of urinary incontinence is 5% to 15%. This rate increases to 40% to 50% in these patients after 1 day of hospitalization (155). Factors likely related to this marked increase include immobility, environmental barriers such as placement of urinals and bedpans, intravenous lines, inability for staff to respond quickly enough, direct medication effects, and medications that alter sensorium. Incontinence in turn leads to significant psychological stress for patients as well as increases the risk for skin breakdown. Urinary incontinence also significantly increases the cost and labor intensiveness of care that must be provided for the patient. In a study of caregivers of elderly confined to a bed at home, depressive symptoms in caregivers and perceived level of burden of care were associated with the amount of urinary incontinence of the person for whom they were caring (156).

Interventions to improve management of the genitourinary system include providing adequate fluid intake, instituting a timed void program, having the patient void on the commode or upright whenever possible, and avoiding the use of instrumentation. If indicated, however, intermittent catheterization to ensure adequate drainage of the bladder may be needed. Appropriate evaluation of urinary incontinence should be undertaken if it is not identified as a physiologic consequence of bed rest. In a study of elderly patients at a long-term-care facility, urologic causes commonly found included unstable detrusor function, sphincter weakness, and overflow incontinence, and typical nonurologic causes included behavioral problems, immobility, and medications (157). In addition, there should be prompt treatment of urinary tract infections based on culture results, and evaluation and treatment of renal stones if they are found in patients with persistent urinary tract infections. Not infrequently, in the elderly immobilized patient, work-up of a change in mental status may reveal a urinary tract infection. A high index of suspicion and prompt intervention are necessary to avoid the potentially life-threatening complications of pyelonephritis and sepsis.

GASTROINTESTINAL SYSTEM

Several common problems related to prolonged bed rest and inactivity involve the gastrointestinal system. Constipation is associated with bed rest at any age, though it is more frequently seen in the elderly (158). The prevalence of constipation in one study of the elderly (158) was 12% in the community, 41% in acute geriatric wards, and 78% in long-stay geriatric wards, with similar findings in other studies (159,160). Decreased peristaltic activity (64) including increased bolus transit time through the esophagus (161) and stomach (162,163) and decreased small-bowel motility (64) while in the supine position have been noted. Dehydration (secondary to decreased fluid intake and reduced plasma volume) and lack of physical activity also tend to increase constipation.

Not uncommonly after a patient's acute medical problems have resolved and upon transfer to the rehabilitation ward, it becomes apparent that several days have passed since the patient's last bowel movement. Constipation often results in fecal impaction. The size of the rectal vault is increased in patients with fecal impaction (>500 mL compared with the normal volume of 200 mL). These physiological data may suggest that some elderly patients develop fecal impaction secondary to blunted rectal sensation and subsequent failure to detect the fecal mass until it becomes too large to expel (158). Difficulty in defecating in the supine position and using a bedpan further increases the risk of constipation. Overflow

Table 46-7: Example of a Bowel Training Program (BTP) for Immobilized Patients

1. Institute a daily BTP at the same time each day.
2. Perform the program up on the commode (if possible).
3. Preferred time is 1/2 hr after a meal (to take advantage of the gastrocolic reflex).
4. Use a suppository [i.e., glycerin or bisacodyl (Dulcolax)] and/or anal stretch (digital stimulation) if the patient does not have a bowel movement on his or her own.
5. Use daily an oral stool softener [docusate sodium (Colace 250 mg)] if stools are hard.
6. Use daily dose of senna (i.e., Senokot 1 tablet) 8 hr before BTP.
7. Add fiber or supplementary fiber (Metamucil 1 tbsp) to diet.

incontinence related to fecal impaction is the most common cause of diarrhea in the elderly (164). According to a cost-analysis study in Canada in 1992, immobility is the strongest predictor of the amount of nursing time spent dealing with incontinence. Incontinence (urinary and fecal) added nearly $10,000 to the cost of care annually per patient in a long-term-care facility (9).

Although bed rest subjects typically note a decreased appetite, they normally were given only standard hospital trays for the length of the bedrest. A separate 20-day bed rest study allowed patients to eat their favorite foods when they showed lack of appetite for hospital food, and found that patients maintained or increased their appetite during the period of bed rest (124). Increased gastric acidity secondary to decreased bicarbonate secretion has been noted during bed rest (165).

Early mobilization, toileting on the commode, and adequate fluid intake are important interventions to prevent or decrease constipation. A daily bowel program can include using dietary fiber (166), using stool softeners, having the patient get up on the commode at the same time every day, ensuring adequate fluid intake, using suppositories, and judiciously using laxatives. Table 46-7 provides an example of a bowel training program. If the patient initially has fecal impaction, manual evacuation and enemas may be required. Patient medications should also be reviewed to avoid ones with constipating side effects.

CONCLUSIONS

Physical, psychological, environmental, cultural, and social factors influence the total outcome of immobility and deconditioning. Immobility can be focal such as immobilization of the knee after a femoral fracture, or it can be generalized such as bed rest after acute illness such as an MI. Deconditioning is more a compilation of pathophysiologic changes to different organ systems resulting in impairments that can lead to functional limitations causing psychological and physical disabilities and handicaps. Prolonged immobility and deconditioning may lead to a decrease in functional capacity including, in moderate cases, impairing an individual's ability to perform ADLs such as cooking, shopping, and driving. In the elderly population, a fear of falling, poor motivation, and depression can diminish the ability to perform basic functional skills such as ambulation and predisposes them to further deconditioning. In extreme cases, even self-care skills like hygiene, eating, and toileting may be affected, and may result in the necessity for long-term-care placement. In a long-term-care setting, often there is inadequate support to regularly mobilize the patients. The use of restraints and medications, unfortunately, may also severely impair mobility and must be guarded against. It is important to note that the same level of immobility may produce different levels of impairment, disability, and handicap in different people.

Bed rest and immobility are far from benign states without sequelae. They result in deconditioning and negatively affect every major organ system. The effects are superimposed on the patient's primary disease process, and soon become more significant a problem than the primary disease. Minimizing the period of inactivity and proactively preventing or minimizing complications during this period are essential management strategies for treating bed-rested, immobilized, and deconditioned patients.

DEDICATION

We dedicate this chapter in memory of Mani Shankar, who passed away suddenly in April of 1998.

REFERENCES

1. Siscovick DS, LaPorte RE, Newman JM. The disease-specific benefits of physical activity and exercise. *Public Health Rep* 1985;100:180–188.
2. Greenleaf JE. Physiological responses to prolonged bed rest and fluid immersion in humans. *J Appl Physiol* 1984;57:619–633.
3. Buschbacher RM. Deconditioning, conditioning and the benefits of exercise. In: Braddom RL, ed. *Physical medicine and rehabilitation.* 1st ed. Philadelphia: WB Saunders, 1996:687–708.
4. Dietrick JE, Whedon GD, Shorr E. Effects of immobilization upon various metabolic and physiologic functions of normal men. *Am J Med* 1948:3–36.

5. Downs FS. Bed rest and sensory disturbances. *Am J Nurs* 1974;74:434–438.

6. Ishizaki Y, Fukuoka H, Katsura T, et al. Psychological effects of bed rest in young healthy subjects. *Acta Physiol Scand Suppl* 1994;616:83–87.

7. Ryback RS, Lewis OF, Lessard CS. Psychobiologic effects of prolonged bed rest (weightless) in young, volunteers (study II). *Aerosp Med* 1971;42: 529–535.

8. Smith MJ. Changes in judgment of duration with different patterns of auditory information for individuals confined to bed. *Nurs Res* 1975;24:93–98.

9. Borrie MJ. Davidson HA. Incontinence in institutions: costs and contributing factors. *Can Med Assoc J* 1992;147:322–328.

10. Zubek JP, Bayer L, Milstein S, Shephard JM, Behavioral and physiological changes during immobilization plus perceptual deprivation. *J Abnorm Psychol* 1969;74:230–236.

11. Halar EM, Bell KR. Rehabilitation's relationship to inactivity. In: Kottke FJ, Lehmann JF, eds. *Krusen's handbook of physical medicine and rehabilitation.* 4th ed. Philadelphia: WB Saunders, 1990:1113–1133.

12. DeRoshia CW, Greenleaf JE. Performance and mood-state parameters during 30-day 6 degrees head-down rest with exercise training. *Aviat Space Environ Med* 1993;64: 522–527.

13. Ohi G, Kai I, Ichikawa S, Miyama T, Naka K. Psychotic manifestations in the bed-fast elderly—a preliminary communication. *J Hum Ergol (Tokyo)* 1989;18:237–240.

14. Winslow EH. Cardiovascular consequences of bed rest. *Heart Lung* 1985;14:236–246.

15. Lathers CM, Charles JB. Comparison of cardiovascular function during the early hours of bed rest and space flight. *J Clin Pharmacol* 1994;34:489–499.

16. Stremel RW, Convertino VA, Bernauer EM, Greenleaf JE. Cardiorespiratory deconditioning with static and dynamic leg exercise during bed rest. *J Appl Physiol* 1976;41:905–909.

17. Saltin B, Blomqvist G, Mitchell JH, et al. Response to exercise after bed rest and after training. *Circulation* 1968;38(5 suppl): VII1–78.

18. Taylor ML. The effects of rest in bed and of exercise on cardiovascular function. *Circulation* 1968;38:1016–1017.

19. Miller PB, Johnson RL, Lamb LE. Effects of moderate physical exercise during four weeks of bed rest on circulatory functions in man. *Aerosp Med* 1965;36: 1077–1082.

20. Convertino VA, Sandler H, Webb P, Annis JF. Induced venous pooling and cardiorespiratory responses to exercise after bed rest. *J Appl Physiol* 1982;52:1343–1348.

21. Takenaka K, Suzuki Y, Kawakubo K, et al. Cardiovascular effects of 20 days bed rest in healthy young subjects. *Acta Physiol Scand Suppl* 1994; 616:59–63.

22. Crandall CG, Engelke KA, Convertino VA, Raven PB. Aortic baroreflex control of heart rate after 15 days of simulated microgravity exposure. *J Appl Physiol* 1994;77:2134–2139.

23. Crandall CG, Engelke KA, Pawelczyk JA, et al. Power spectral and time based analysis of heart rate variability following 15 days head-down bed rest. *Aviat Space Environ Med* 1994;65: 1105–1109.

24. Haruna Y, Suzuki Y, Kawakubo K, Gunji A. Orthostatic tolerance and autonomous nervous functions before and after 20-days bed rest. *Acta Physiol Scand Suppl* 1994; 616:71–81.

25. Johnson PC, Driscoll TB, Carpentier WR. Vascular and extravascular fluid changes during six days of bedrest. *Aerosp Med* 1971;42:875–878.

26. Greenleaf JE, Bernauer EM, Young HL, et al. Fluid and electrolyte shifts during bed rest with isometric and isotonic exercise. *J Appl Physiol* 1977;42:59–66.

27. Greenleaf JE. Physiology of fluid and electrolyte responses during inactivity: water immersion and bed rest. *Med Sci Sports Exerc* 1984;16:20–25.

28. Fortney SM, Turner C, Steinmann L, et al. Blood volume responses of men and women to bed rest. *J Clin Pharmacol* 1994;34:434–439.

29. Goldberger AL, Goldwater D, Bhargava V. Atropine unmasks bed-rest effect: a spectral analysis of cardiac interbeat intervals. *J Appl Physiol* 1986;61: 1843–1848.

30. Lathers CM, Charles JB. Use of lower body negative pressure to counter symptoms of orthostatic intolerance in patients, bed rest subjects, and astronauts. *J Clin Pharmacol* 1993;33: 1071–1085.

31. Beck L, Baisch F, Gaffney FA, et al. Cardiovascular response to lower body negative pressure before, during, after ten days head-down tilt bedrest. *Acta Physiol Scand Suppl* 1992;604:43–52.

32. Taylor HL, Henschel A, Brozuek J, Keys A. Effects of bedrest on cardiovascular function and work performance. *J Appl Physiol* 1949:223–239.

33. Melada GA, Goldman RH, Luetscher JA, Zager PG. Hemodynamics, renal function, plasma renin, and aldosterone in man after 5 to 14 days of bed rest. *Aviat Space Environ Med* 1975;46:1049–1055.

34. Convertino V, Hung J, Goldwater D, DeBusk RF. Cardiovascular responses to exercise in middle-aged men after 10 days of bedrest. *Circulation* 1982;65:134–140.

35. Lathers CM, Charles JB, Schneider VS, et al. Use of lower body negative pressure to assess changes in heart rate response to orthostatic-like stress during 17

weeks of bed rest. *J Clin Pharmacol* 1994;34:563–570.

36. Hung J, Goldwater D, Convertino VA, et al. Mechanisms for decreased exercise capacity after bed rest in normal middle-aged men. *Am J Cardiol* 1983;51:344–348.

37. Maron BJ, Pelliccia A, Spataro A, Granata M. Reduction in left ventricular wall thickness after deconditioning in highly trained Olympic athletes. *Br Heart J* 1993;69:125–128.

38. Katsume H, Furukawa K, Azuma A, et al. Disuse atrophy of the left ventricle in chronically bedridden elderly people. *Jpn Circ J* 1992;56:201–206.

39. Greenleaf JE, Wade CE, Leftheriotis G. Orthostatic responses following 30-day bed rest deconditioning with isotonic and isokinetic exercise training. *Aviat Space Environ Med* 1989;60:537–542.

40. Greenleaf JE, Bernauer EM, Ertl AC, et al. Isokinetic strength and endurance during 30-day 6 degrees head-down bed rest with isotonic and isokinetic exercise training. *Aviat Space Environ Med* 1994;65:45–50.

41. Chobanian AV, Lille RD, Tercyak A, Blevins P. The metabolic and hemodynamic effects of prolonged bed rest in normal subjects. *Circulation* 1974;49:551–559.

42. Kashihara H, Haruna Y, Suzuki Y, et al. Effects of mild supine exercise during 20 days bed rest on maximal oxygen uptake rate in young humans. *Acta Physiol Scand Suppl* 1994;616: 19–26.

43. Lathers CM, Charles JB. Orthostatic hypotension in patients, bed rest subjects, and astronauts. *J Clin Pharmacol* 1994;34:403–417.

44. Bungo MW, Charles JB, Johnson PC Jr. Cardiovascular deconditioning during space flight and the use of saline as a countermeasure to orthostatic intolerance. *Aviat Space Environ Med* 1985;56:985–990.

45. Hughson RL, Yamamoto Y, Maillet A, et al. Altered autonomic regulation of cardiac function during head-up tilt after 28-day head-down bed-rest with counter-measures. *Clin Physiol* 1994;14:291–304.

46. Eckberg DL, Fritsch JM. Influence of ten-day head-down bedrest on human carotid baroreceptor-cardiac reflex function. *Acta Physiol Scand Suppl* 1992;604:69–76.

47. Pannier B, Lacolley P, Laurent S, et al. Effects of twenty-four hours of bed rest with head-down tilt on cardiopulmonary baroreflex control: preliminary study. *J Hypertens Suppl* 1989;7:S38–S39.

48. Melchior FM, Fortney SM. Orthostatic intolerance during a 13-day bed rest does not result from increased leg compliance. *J Appl Physiol* 1993;74:286–292.

49. Convertino VA, Doerr DF, Guell A, Marini JF. Effects of acute exercise on attenuated vagal baroreflex function during bed rest. *Aviat Space Environ Med* 1992;63:999–1003.

50. Buczynski A, Kedziora J, Wachowicz B, Zolynski K. Effect of bed rest on the adenine nucleotides concentration in human blood platelets. *J Physiol Pharmacol* 1991;42:389–395.

51. Wang JS, Jen CJ, Chen HI. Effects of exercise training and deconditioning on platelet function in men. *Arterioscler Thromb Vasc Biol* 1995;15:1668–1674.

52. Kaperonis AA, Michelsen CB, Askanazi J, et al. Effects of total hip replacement and bed rest on blood rheology and red cell metabolism. *J Trauma* 1988;28:453–457.

53. Ernst E, Schmidt-Pauly E, Muhlig P, Matrai A. Blood viscosity in patients with bone fractures and long term bedrest. *Br J Surg* 1987;74:301–302.

54. Miyamoto AT, Miller L. Pulmonary embolism in stroke: prevention by early heparinization of venous thrombosis detected by iodine-125 fibrinogen leg scans. *Arch Phys Med Rehabil* 1980;61: 584–587.

55. Keidan AJ, Stuart J. Rheological effects of bed rest in sickle cell disease. *J Clin Pathol* 1987;40:1187–1188.

56. Pashkow FJ. Issues in contemporary cardiac rehabilitation: a historical perspective. *J Am Coll Cardiol* 1993;21:822–834.

57. Hargens AR. Recent bed rest results and countermeasure development at NASA. *Acta Physiol Scand Suppl* 1994;616:103–114.

58. Chase GA, Grave C, Rowell LB. Independence of changes in functional and performance capacities prolonged bed rest. *Aerosp Med* 1966;37:1232–1238.

59. Harper CM, Lyles YM. Physiology and complications of bed rest. *J Am Geriatr Soc* 1988;36:1047–1054.

60. Marini JJ, Tyler ML, Hudson LD, et al. Influence of head-dependent positions on lung volume and oxygen saturation in chronic airflow obstruction. *AM Rev Respir Dis* 1984;129: 101–105.

61. Beckett WS, Vroman NB, Nigro D, et al. Effect of prolonged bed rest on lung volume in normal individuals. *J Appl Physiol* 1986;61:919–925.

62. Sharp JT, Goldberg NB, Druz WS, Danon J. Relative contributions of rib cage and abdomen to breathing in normal subjects. *J Appl Physiol* 1975;39: 608–618.

63. Druz WS, Sharp JT. Activity of respiratory muscles in upright and recumbent humans. *J Appl Physiol* 1981;51:1552–1561.

64. Downey RJ. The physiology of bedrest. In: Downey JA, Myers SJ, Gonzalez EG, Lieberman JS, eds. *The physiological basis of rehabilitation medicine*. 2nd ed. Boston: Butterworth-Heinemann, 1994:447–479.

65. Cardus D. O_2 alveolar-arterial tension difference after 10 days

recumbency in man. *J Appl Physiol* 1967;23:934–937.

66. Nikolaenko EM, Katkov VE, Gvozdev SV, et al. Pulmonary blood flow and arterial blood oxygenation in healthy men after seven days of hypokinesia. *Hum Physiol* 1984;10:204–208.

67. Trimble C, Smith DE, Cook TI, Trummer MJ. The effect of supine bedrest upon alveolar-arterial oxygen gradients and intrapulmonary shunting in normal man. *J Thorac Cardiovasc Surg* 1972;63:873–879.

68. Beck-Sague C, Banerjee S, Jarvis WR. Infectious diseases and mortality among US nursing home residents. *Am J Public Health* 1993;83:1739–1742.

69. Meguro K, Yamagauchi S, Doi C, et al. Prevention of respiratory infections in elderly bed-bound nursing home patients. *Tohoku J Exp Med* 1992;167:135–142.

70. Gogia P, Schneider VS, LeBlanc AD, et al. Bed rest effect on extremity muscle torque in healthy men. *Arch Phys Med Rehabil* 1988;69:1030–1032.

71. Dudley GA, Duvoisin MR, Convertino VA, Buchanan P. Alterations of the in vivo torque-velocity relationship of human skeletal muscle following 30 days exposure to simulated microgravity. *Aviat Space Environ Med* 1989;60:659–663.

72. Germain P, Guell A, Marini JF. Muscle strength during bedrest with and without muscle exercise as a countermeasure. *Eur J Appl Physiol* 1995;71: 342–348.

73. Greenleaf JE, Van Beaumont W, Convertino VA, Starr JC. Handgrip and general muscular strength and endurance during prolonged bedrest with isometric and isotonic leg exercise training. *Aviat Space Environ Med* 1983;54:696–700.

74. LeBlanc AD, Schneider VS, Evans HJ, et al. Regional changes in muscle mass following 17 weeks of bed rest. *J Appl Physiol* 1992;73: 2172–2178.

75. LeBlanc A, Gogia P, Schneider V, et al. Calf muscle area and strength changes after five weeks of horizontal bed rest. *Am J Sports Med* 1988;166:624–629.

76. Berry P, Berry I, Manelfe C. Magnetic resonance imaging evaluation of lower limb muscles during bed rest—a microgravity simulation model. *Aviat Space Environ Med* 1993;64: 212–218.

77. Ferrando AA, Stuart CA, Brunder DG, Hillman GR. Magnetic resonance imaging quantitation of changes in muscle volume 7 days of strict bed rest. *Aviat Space Environ Med* 1995;66:976–981.

78. Shangraw RE, Stuart CA, Prince MJ. et al. Insulin responsiveness of protein metabolism in vivo following bedrest in humans. *Am J Physiol* 1988;255: E548–E558.

79. Appell HJ. Muscular atrophy following immobilization. Review. *Sports Med* 1990;10:42–58.

80. Asmussen G, Miersch H, Soukup T. The influence of suspension hypokinesia on contractile properties of slow and fast twitch muscles of young growing and adult rats. *Biomed Biochim Acta* 1989;48(5–6):S426–S431.

81. Desplanches D, Mayet MH, Sempore B, Flandrois R. Structural and functional responses to prolonged hindlimb suspension in rat muscle. *J Appl Physiol* 1987;63:558–563.

82. Kasper CE, McNulty AL, Otto AJ, Thomas DP. Alterations in skeletal muscle related to impaired physical mobility: an empirical model. *Res Nurs Health* 1993;16:265–273.

83. Dudley GA, Gollnick PD, Convertino VA, Buchanan P. Changes of muscle function and size with bedrest. *Physiologist* 1989;32(1 suppl):S65–S66.

84. Kilmer DD. Functional anatomy of skeletal muscle. In: Shankar K, ed. *Physical medicine and rehabilitation: state of the art reviews.* Vol. 10. Philadelphia: Hanley & Belfus, 1996:1–14.

85. Hikida RS, Gollnick PD, Dudley GA, et al. Structural and metabolic characteristics of human skeletal muscle 30 days of simulated microgravity. *Aviat Space Environ Med* 1989;60:664–670.

86. Booth FW, Seider MJ, Early change in skeletal muscle protein synthesis after limb immobilization of rats. *J Appl Physiol* 1979;47:974–977.

87. Goldspink DF, Morton AJ, Loughna P, Goldspink G. The effect of hypokinesia and hypodynamia on protein turnover and the growth of four skeletal muscles of the rat. *Pflugers Arch* 1986;407:333–340.

88. Savolainen J, Vaananen K, Vihko V, et al. Effect of immobilization on collagen synthesis in rat skeletal muscles. *Am J Physiol* 1987;252:R883–R888.

89. Herbert RD, Balnave RJ. The effect of position of immobilisation on resting length, resting stiffness, and weight of the soleus muscle of the rabbit. *J Orthop Res* 1993;11:358–366.

90. Spector SA, Simard CP, Fournier M, et al. Architectural alterations of rat hind-limb skeletal muscles immobilized at different lengths. *Exp Neurol* 1982;76:94–110.

91. Williams PE. Use of intermittent stretch in the prevention of serial sarcomere loss in immobilised muscle. *Ann Rheum Dis* 1990;49:316–317.

92. Kannus P, Jozsa L, Kvist M, et al. The effect of immobilization on myotendinous junction: an ultrastructural, histochemical and immunohistochemical study. *Acta Physiol Scand* 1992;144:387–394.

93. Duchateau J, Hainaut K. Effects of immobilization on contractile properties, recruitment and firing rates of human units. *J Physiol (Lond)* 1990;422:55–65.

94. Booth FW. Physiologic and biochemical effects of immobilization on muscle. *Clin Orthop* 1987;219:15–20.

95. Booth FW, Seider MJ. Recovery of skeletal muscle after 3 mo of

hindlimb immobilization in rats. *J Appl Physiol* 1979;47: 435–439.

96. Rifenberick DH, Max SR. Substrate utilization by disused rat skeletal muscles. *Am J Physiol* 1974;226:295–297.

97. Baker JH, Matsumoto DE. Adaptation of skeletal muscle to immobilization in a shortened position. *Muscle Nerve* 1988:11:231–244.

98. Jarvinen MJ, Einola SA, Virtanen EO. Effect of the position of immobilization upon tensile properties of the rat gastrocnemius muscle. *Arch Phys Med Rehabil* 1992;73:253–257.

99. Loughna P, Goldspink G, Goldspink DF. Effect of inactivity and passive stretch on protein turnover in phasic and postural rat muscles. *J Appl Physiol* 1986;61:173–179.

100. Loughna PT, Goldspink DF, Goldspink G. Effects of hypokinesia and hypodynamia upon protein turnover in hindlimb muscles of the rat. *Aviat Space Environ Med* 1987;58:A133–A138.

101. Greenleaf JE, Bernauer EM, Ertl AC, et al. Work capacity during 30 days of bed rest with isotonic and isokinetic exercise training. *J Appl Physiol* 1989;67: 1820–1826.

102. Ellis S, Kirby LC, Greenleaf JE. Lower extremity muscle thickness during 30-day 6 degrees head-down bed rest with isotonic and isokinetic exercise training. *Aviat Space Environ Med* 1993;64:1011–1015.

103. Brown M, Hasser EM. Weight-bearing effects on skeletal muscle during and after simulated bed rest. *Arch Phys Med Rehabil* 1995;76:541–546.

104. Buckley D, Kudsk KA, Rose B, et al. Transcutaneous muscle stimulation promotes muscle growth in immobilized patients. *J Parenter Enter Nutr* 1987;11: 547–551.

105. Gould N, Donnermeyer D, Ashikaga T. Transcutaneous muscle stimulation as a method to retard muscle disuse atrophy. *Clin Orthop* 1982;164:215–220.

106. Langenskiold A, Michelsson JE, Videman T. Osteoarthritis of the knee in the rabbit produced by immobilization. Attempts to achieve a reproducible model for studies on pathogenesis and therapy. *Acta Orthop Scand* 1979;50:1–14.

107. Enneking WF, Horwitz M. The intra-articular effects of immobilization on the human knee. *J Bone Joint Surg [Am]* 1972;54:973–985.

108. Smith RL, Thomas KD, Schurman DJ, et al. Rabbit knee immobilization: bone remodeling precedes cartilage degradation. *J Orthop Res* 1992; 10:88–95.

109. Akeson WH, Amiel D, Abel MF, et al. Effects of immobilization on joints. *Clin Orthop* 1987;219:28–37.

110. Nishimura Y, Fukuoka H, Kiriyama M, et al. Bone turnover and calcium metabolism during 20 days bed rest in young healthy males and females. *Acta Physiol Scand Suppl* 1994;616:27–35.

111. Krolner B, Toft B. Vertebral bone loss: an unheeded side effect of therapeutic bed rest. *Clin Sci* 1983;64:537–540.

112. Riggs BL, Wahner HW, Dunn WL, et al. Differential changes in bone mineral density of the appendicular and axial skeleton with aging: relationship to spinal osteoporosis. *J Clin Invest* 1981;67:328–335.

113. Donaldson CL, Hulley SB, Vogel JM, et al. Effect of prolonged bed rest on bone mineral. *Metabolism* 1970;19: 1071–1084.

114. Lukert BP. Vertebral compression fractures: how to manage pain, avoid disability [see comments]. *Geriatrics* 1994;49:22–26.

115. LeBlanc AD, Schneider VS, Evans HJ, et al. Bone mineral loss and recovery after 17 weeks of bed rest. *J Bone Miner Res* 1990;5:843–850.

116. LeBlanc AD, Evans HJ, Schneider VS, et al. Changes in intervertebral disc cross-sectional area with bed rest and space flight. *Spine* 1994;19:812–817.

117. Buckwalter JA. Activity vs. rest in the treatment of bone, soft tissue and joint injuries. *Iowa Orthop J* 1995;15:29–42.

118. Issekutz B Jr, Blizzard JJ, Birkhead NC, Rodahl K. Effect of prolonged bed rest on urinary calcium output. *J Appl Physiol* 1966;21:1013–1020.

119. Saltzstein RJ, Hardin S, Hastings J. Osteoporosis in spinal cord injury: using an index of mobility and its relationship to bone density. *J Am Paraplegia Soc* 1992;15:232–234.

120. van der Wiel HE, Lips P, Nauta J, et al. Intranasal calcitonin suppresses increased bone resorption during short-term immobilization: a double-blind study of the effects of intranasal calcitonin on biochemical parameters of bone turnover. *J Bone Miner Res* 1993;8:1459–1465.

121. Bernauer EM, Walby WF, Ertl AC, et al. Knee-Joint proprioception during 30-day 6 degrees head-down bed rest with isotonic and isokinetic exercise training. *Aviat Space Environ Med* 1994;65:1110–1115.

122. Rodriguez JI, Garcia-Alix A, Palacios J, Paniagua R. Changes in the long bones due to fetal immobility caused by neuromuscular disease. A radiographic and histological study. *J Bone Joint Surg [Am]* 1988;70:1052–1060.

123. Meythaler JM, Tuel SM, Leland LC. Successful treatment of immobilization hypercalcemia using calcitonin and etidronate. *Arch Phys Med Rehabil* 1993;74:316–319.

124. Haruna Y, Suzuki Y, Kawakubo K, et al. Decremental reset in basal metabolism during 20 days bed rest. *Acta Physiol Scand Suppl* 1994;616:43–49.

125. Suzuki Y, Murakami T, Haruna Y, et al. Effects of 10 and 20 days bed rest on leg muscle mass and strength in young subjects. *Acta*

Physiol Scand Suppl 1994; 616:5–18.

126. Yanagibori R, Suzuki Y, Kawakubo K, et al. Carbohydrate and lipid metabolism after 20 days of bed rest. *Acta Physiol Scand Suppl* 1994;616: 51–57.

127. Fuller JH, Bernauer EM, Adams WC. Renal function, water and electrolyte exchange during bed rest with daily exercise. *Aerosp Med* 1970;41:60–72.

128. Greenleaf JE, Bernauer EM, Juhos LT, et al. Effects of exercise on fluid exchange and body composition in man during 14-day bed rest. *J Appl Physiol* 1977;43:126–132.

129. Krebs JM, Schneider VS, Evans H, et al. Energy absorption, lean body mass, and total body fat changes during 5 weeks of continuous bed rest. *Aviat Space Environ Med* 1990;61: 314–318.

130. Greenleaf JE, Reese RD. Exercise thermoregulation after 14 days of bed rest. *J Appl Physiol* 1980;48:72–78.

131. Greenleaf JE. Energy and thermal regulation during bed rest and spaceflight. *J Appl Physiol* 1989;67:507–516.

132. Stuart CA, Shangraw RE, Prince MJ, et al. Bed-rest-induced insulin resistance occurs primarily in muscle. *Metabolism* 1988;37:802–806.

133. Mikines KJ, Dela F, Tronier B, Galbo H. Effect of 7 days of bed rest on dose-response relation between plasma glucose and insulin secretion. *Am J Physiol* 1989;257:E43–E48.

134. Goldstein DS, Vernikos J, Holmes C, Convertino VA. Catecholaminergic effects of prolonged head-down bed rest. *J Appl Physiol* 1995;78:1023–1029.

135. Zorbas YG, Naexu KA, Federenko YF. Blood serum biochemical changes in physically conditioned and subjects during bed rest and chronic hyperhydration. *Clin Exp Pharmacol Physiol* 1992;19:137–145.

136. Dunn CD, Lange RD, Kimzey SL, et al. Serum erythropoietin titers during prolonged bedrest; relevance to the "anaemia" of space flight. *Eur J Appl Physiol* 1984;52:178–182.

137. Stuart CA, Shangraw RE, Peters EJ, Wolfe RR. Effect of dietary protein on bed-rest-related changes in whole-body-protein synthesis. *Am J Clin Nutr* 1990;52:509–514.

138. Giannetta CL, Castleberry HB. Influence of bedrest and hypercapnia upon urinary mineral excretion. *Aerosp Med* 1974;45:750–754.

139. Greenleaf JE, Stinnett HO, Davis GL, et al. Fluid and electrolyte shifts in women during +Gz acceleration after 15 days' bed rest. *J Appl Physiol* 1977;42:67–73.

140. Hulley SB, Vogel JM, Donaldson CL, et al. The effect of supplemental oral phosphate on the bone mineral changes during prolonged bed rest. *J Clin Invest* 1971;50:2506–2518.

141. Krebs JM, Schneider VS, LeBlanc AD, et al. Zinc and copper balances in healthy adult males during and after 17 wk of bed rest. *Am J Clin Nutr* 1993;58:897–901.

142. LeBlanc A, Schneider V, Spector E, et al. Calcium absorption, endogenous excretion, and endocrine changes during and after long-term bed rest. *Bone* 1995;16(4 suppl):301S–304S.

143. Schneider VS, McDonald J. Skeletal calcium homeostasis and countermeasures to prevent disuse osteoporosis. *Calcif Tissue Int* 1984;36(suppl 1):S151–S144.

144. Whedon GD. Disuse osteoporosis: physiological aspects. *Calcif Tissue Int* 1984;36(suppl 1):S146–S150.

145. Goode PS, Allman RM. The prevention and management of pressure ulcers. *Med Clin North Am* 1989;73:1511–1524.

146. Evans JM, Andrews KL, Chutka DS, et al. Pressure ulcers: prevention and management. *Mayo Clin Proc* 1995;70:789–799.

147. Perez ED. Pressure ulcers: updated guidelines for treatment and prevention. *Geriatrics* 1993;48:39–44.

148. Allman RM, Goode PS, Patrick MM, et al. Pressure ulcer risk factors among hospitalized patients with activity limitation. *JAMA* 1995;273:865–870.

149. Charles MA, Oldenbrook J, Catton C. Evaluation of a low-air-loss mattress system in the treatment of patients with pressure ulcers. *Ostomy Wound Manage* 1995;41:46–48, 50, 52.

150. Young JB, Dobrzanski S. Pressure sores. Epidemiology and current management concepts. *Drugs Aging* 1992;2:42–57.

151. Kresevic DM, Naylor M. Preventing pressure ulcers through use of protocols in a mentored nursing model. *Geriatr Nurs* 1995;16:225–229.

152. Hwang TI, Hill K, Schneider V, Pak CY. Effect of prolonged bedrest on the propensity for renal stone formation. *J Clin Endocrinol Metab* 1988;66:109–112.

153. Vernikos J, Dallman MF, Keil LC, et al. Gender differences in endocrine responses to posture and 7 days of -6 degrees head-down bed rest. *Am J Physiol* 1993;265:E153–E161.

154. Cockett AT, Elbadawl A, Zemjanis R, Adey WR. The effects of immobilization on spermatogenesis in subhuman primates. *Fertil Steril* 1970;21:610–614.

155. Creditor MC. Hazards of hospitalization of the elderly. *Ann Intern Med* 1993;118:219–223.

156. Flaherty JH, Miller DK, Coe RM. Impact on caregivers of supporting urinary function in noninstitutionalized, chronically ill seniors. *Gerontologist* 1992;32:541–545.

157. Pannill FCD, Williams TF, Davis R. Evaluation and treatment of urinary incontinence in long term care. *J Am Geriatr Soc* 1988;36:902–910.

158. Read NW, Celik AF, Katsinelos P. Constipation and incontinence in the elderly. *J Clin Gastroenterol* 1995;20:61–70.

159. Donald IP, Smith RG, Cruikshank JG, et al. A study of constipation in the elderly living at home. *Gerontology* 1985;31:112–118.

160. Everhart JE, Go VLW, Johannes RS, et al. A longitudinal survey of self-reported bowel habits in the United States. *Dig Dis Sci* 1989;34:1153–1162.

161. Dooley CP, Schlossmacher B, Valenzuela JE. Modulation of esophageal peristalsis by alterations of body position. Effect of bolus viscosity. *Dig Dis Sci* 1989;34:1662–1667.

162. Moore JG, Datz FL, Christian PE, et al. Effect of body posture on radionuclide measurements of gastric emptying. *Dig Dis Sci* 1988;33:1592–1595.

163. Mojaverian P, Vlasses PH, Kellner PE, Rocci MLJ. Effects of gender, posture, and age on gastric residence time of an indigestible solid: pharmaceutical considerations. *Pharm Res* 1988;5:639–644.

164. Kinnunen O, Jauhonen P, Salokannel J, Kivela SL. Diarrhea and fecal impaction in elderly long-stay patients. *Z Gerontol* 1989;22:321–323.

165. Sjovall H, Forssell H, Haggendal J, Olbe L. Reflex sympathetic activation in humans is accompanied by inhibition of gastric HCO_3^- secretion. *Am J Physiol* 1988;255:G752–G758.

166. Grant LP, Wanger LI, Neill KM. Fiber-fortified feedings in immobile patients. *Clin Nurs Res* 1994;3:166–172.

Chapter 47

Spasticity and Abnormalities of Muscle Tone

Ross D. Zafonte
Elie Elovic

The clinical dilemma associated with the constellation of symptoms known as *spasticity* has left clinicians caring for such patients perplexed over the last century. No clear practice of treatment had been established, and indeed definitions were somewhat unclear. The functional consequences of spasticity were rarely considered and are still not appreciated in many acute care settings. Thus, the need for rather standard nomenclature, evaluation, and paradigms of treatment is established. This chapter provides a review of the terminology, pathophysiology, and treatment of this symptom complex.

DEFINITIONS

Spasticity is a clinical syndrome that results in an increase in a voluntary reflex to stretch. Clinically one appears to see hyperactive reflexes, spread of reflex phenomena, and increased tone. The increased "tone" is associated with a reduction of the threshold angle at which the stretch reflex is elicited (1). Thus, there exists the concept of hypertonia, whereas decreased response to stretch represents hypotonia. This concept is discussed in further detail when the neurophysiology of this syndrome is approached. *Rigidity* represents an increase in passive stretch that exists throughout the passive range of motion, unlike spasticity which is angle or rate dependent (2).

THE UPPER MOTOR NEURON SYNDROME

This syndrome is caused by a lesion above the level of the α motor neuron and the peripheral neuronal system. It is characterized by a constellation of symptoms that include weakness, exaggerated reflexes, decreased motor control, and extensor-plantar responses. This syndrome exists in contradistinction to the lower motor neuron syndrome in which weakness, hyporeflexia, and atrophy predominate (2). While believed to be a negative phenomenon, the upper motor neuron syndrome, specifically its component of spasticity, can sometimes be used in a functional manner.

MECHANISMS OF SPASTICITY

First described by Little in 1843 (3), spasticity is found in various conditions affecting the central nervous system (CNS). However, we are still not able to describe in detail the pathophysiology associated with this symptom complex. This problem is probably due in part to the differences in spasticity seen in various neurologic populations, as well as the fact that no single pathway alone can be identified as its source. Denny-Brown's statement in 1980 (4) may best relay this point: "Spasticity is a complex disability not identifiable with any single reflex or neurotransmitter." In fact, the data seem to reveal the involvement of many pathways and neurotransmitter systems in this condition.

Motor Control

The motor control system is responsible for sensory feedback, reflex activity, coordination of movement, and actual volitional control. It involves numerous cortical, subcortical, brain stem, and spinal neurons and pathways. The final common pathway for the entire system is the motor unit in the peripheral nervous system. Afferent and efferent nerve fibers are involved in this densely connected system, and muscle excitation and inhibition are the results.

Motor Unit

The motor unit described by Sherrington (5) consists of an α motor neuron and all muscle fibers under its control. These units have different fiber types with different firing rates and threshold recruitment patterns based on the demands and purpose of the individual unit. The two major fiber types are type I and type II. Type I fiber–containing units are small, red, oxidative, and slow to fatigue. These type I units are responsible for the baseline "tonic" activity of muscles. Type II fibers are large, white, anaerobic, fatigable, powerful units that are mobilized normally when increased speed or power is required of the contracting muscle. While these types represent two extremes, there are numerous hybrids in the middle of these extremes (6,7). In the normal functioning motor system, the units have normal angles of motion activity, in addition to coordination of agonist and antagonist firing. Katz et al (8) discussed the disturbance created by co-contraction of agonist and antagonist muscles in addition to muscles firing at angles different from their normal peak areas of activity. The loss of the normal recruitment and decruitment pattern may play a key role in spasticity.

Motor Unit Regulation

To control motor activity, there needs to be a feedback system that integrates information about the motor unit, agonists, and antagonists. There also must be a means of regulation and coordination of stimulation to all muscles around the joint that is to be moved. The information required includes muscle length, speed of movement, position of joint, and muscle tension. Integration of an immediate response occurs via monosynaptic reflexes, while higher-level processing is involved at spinal and supraspinal levels. Each unit responds to inhibitory and excitatory influences; thus, when excitatory influences exceed inhibitory input, the motor unit fires.

Muscle Spindle and Golgi Tendon Organs

The muscle spindle is attached in parallel to the main muscle mass, which contains afferent (type Ia and II) fibers that provide information about the rate of change and position of the muscle to the spinal column. As a muscle contracts, the spindle would be placed at less tension, much like a volleyball net becomes lax as the poles are brought closer together. This lessening of tension would make feedback information through the entire range of motion difficult to obtain. To alleviate this problem, the spindle has its own motor fibers controlled by efferent γ motor neurons that fire in concert with the α motor neuron to maintain tension of the spindle, thus allowing the spindle to be on stretch (7). Monosynaptic reflexes, such as the knee jerk reflex, are created quite simply by placing the muscle at stretch with the Ia afferents, causing the α motor neuron to fire. The Golgi tendon organs found in the muscle tendons are via the Ib fibers and their related interneurons, and place the brakes on muscle contraction by facilitating antagonist and inhibiting agonists. Thus, they serve to impose a ceiling effect on muscle contraction and prevent musculotendinous injury (9).

Spinal Interneurons

Spinal interneurons are critical to the discussion of motor control and spasticity in specific type Ia and Ib interneurons, Renshaw cells, and propriospinal interneurons. The type Ib interneurons are connected to the type Ib afferents from the Golgi tendon organs (9). As mentioned earlier, their purpose is to place a ceiling on the maximum tension generated by the muscle. These interneurons receive input from supraspinal and propriospinal sources. Type Ia interneurons receive input from the type Ia neurons from the muscle spindle. They facilitate agonist activity of the Ia spindle firing, and more importantly, reciprocally inhibit antagonist muscles. This action prevents the futility of agonist and antagonist muscles co-contracting. Type Ia interneurons are influenced by the supraspinal input, and the loss of Ia interneuronal reciprocal inhibition allows for co-contraction (10).

The Renshaw cell receives input from the α motor neuron, and through the process of recurrent inhibition shuts off the α motor neuron and its agonists. In addition, it sends off input to the antagonist Ia interneuron, inhibiting the so-called inhibition and thus, promoting antagonist function (11). The loss of Renshaw cell function makes it difficult to perform motor movements that require tight control of reciprocal inhibition (12). Renshaw cells are under the influence of spinal and supraspinal input. Shefner et al (13) demonstrated that in spinal cord injury, Renshaw cell recurrent inhibition is increased.

The propriospinal interneurons are a complex set of neurons that traverse both the white matter and the gray matter of the spinal cord. They are important in controlling many patterns of movement. In animals, walking behavior can be elicited by stimulating these neurons (7).

Supraspinal Influences

Rothwell et al (14) demonstrated the presence of corticomotorneuronal pathways that are task specific for truncal balance and initiation of fine patterns of hand movements. These connections are from the primary motor cortex, and injury there typically leads to loss of function rather than spasticity (14). The extrapyramidal cells from the prefrontal region, supplementary motor region, and the cingulate gyrus as well as the postcentral gyrus of the parietal lobe are just some of the sources of fibers for the corticospinal pathways (15). The main extensor pathways are the pontine medial reticulospinal and lateral vestibulospinal tracts. The pontine system is facilitatory to the α and γ motor neurons of the extensors. This system receives some input from the sensory motor cortex. The lateral vestibular tract arising from the vestibular nucleus of Dieters found in the ventromedial portion of the cord terminates at the motor neuron in the spinal cord. Stimulation results in inhibition of flexors and facilitation of extensor α and γ motor neurons. The nucleus of the cerebellum also has an excitatory influence on extensor pathways (7,11,16).

The medullary lateral reticular formation works to inhibit extensor pathways. It is subject to excitation from the cortex and therefore is less active with cortical injury. The pathway forms inhibitory influences on the α and γ neurons by synapsing on the motor neurons, type Ia interneurons, and type Ib system (17).

The corticospinal, corticoreticulospinal, and corticorubrospinal tracts in the cat all show significant flexor facilitation. Through interneurons the corticorubrospinal tract excites flexor motor neurons and inhibits extensors. In addition, the medullary reticulospinal tract is a predominant part of a largely flexor-oriented system (7,17).

PATHOPHYSIOLOGY OF THE UPPER MOTOR NEURON SYNDROME

There exist multiple explanations of the clinical symptoms seen in the upper motor neuron syndrome, yet all remain with some question marks.

Prior theory had introduced the concept that intrinsic properties of the muscle were responsible for the changes seen in the patient with spasticity (18). This theory is based on tensile changes in the muscle that occur without concomitant changes in motor unit firing; however, this theory does not account for reflex changes and is generally not accepted.

Studies with cat models led to the belief that "gamma rigidity" with resultant hyperexcitability explained the hyperreflexia and velocity-dependent resistance to movement. This hypothesis is based on an increased reactivity of the muscle spindle to stretch, thus, resulting in a hyperactive response (19). Work by Hagbarth (20) employing microneurography failed to confirm such activity.

Delwaide (21) suggested an alternative theory that spasticity is a result of a loss of descending facilitatory influences on Ia interneuron inhibition. The inability for the antagonist muscle to shut off results in increased velocity-dependent resistance to movement mediated by the muscle spindle.

More recently introduced is the concept that in spasticity the motor neuron pool is continuously in a higher state of readiness to fire. In other words, it remains more depolarized; thus, little excitation would be needed to reach the threshold. This condition may occur because of the loss of tonic inhibitory influences from the supraspinal level. Some have expressed the belief that the ionic properties of the membrane itself are changed as well.

Theories that also may serve to complement the prior explanations of the upper motor neuron syndrome include central collateral sprouting (22), presynaptic dysinhibition (21), and denervation hypersensitivity (23). Of additional interest is the potential role neurotransmitters may have in the clinical upper motor neuron syndrome. Serotonin and substance P appear to have significant roles in neuronal responses. Animal work demonstrated a significant prolongation of responses when serotonin is liberated. Serotonin also facilitated extensor responses in animals (24).

NEUROPHYSIOLOGIC TESTING IN SPASTICITY

Quantification of spasticity is a difficult and challenging endeavor. Various methods have been developed and many are under investigation. Some of the most commonly employed methods are discussed here.

Electromyographic Analysis

Electromyographic (EMG) analysis of patients with upper motor neuron dysfunction reveals that the rate of firing is slower than that seen in patients with lower motor neuron weakness. Surface-EMG burst activity is often seen in the antagonist muscle when the agonist has undergone reflex activation (25).

H-reflex

In 1918, in a set of fascinating experiments, Hoffman described a compound muscle action potential associated with ankle and knee jerk reflexes, the so-called H-reflex. The short-latency compound muscle action potential is designated as the *M response*. Subsequent work by Magladery and McDougal (26) further clarified issues by describing centrifugal discharges from motor neurons, designated as the *F response*. Comparison of the maximum amplitude of the H-reflex to that of the M response has been employed to assess spasticity. When excitability of the motor neuron pool is increased, as in spasticity, the ratio of the maximum amplitude of the H-reflex to that of the M response (H max/M max ratio) is increased (27). Thus, the H-reflex amplitude is larger because of the increased excitability of the motor neuron pool (28). However, there has been disappointing correlation between the H max/M max ratio and the clinical severity of spasticity (29). H-reflex excitability curves are determined by double stimulation of the tibial nerve at the popliteal fossa. These H-reflexes demonstrate various phases of hypo-excitability or hyperexcitability. They appear to demonstrate alteration in patients with CNS disturbance (30,31). These responses, however, are not considered stable and may well be affected by peripheral nerve phenomena (32). The reproducibility of these responses is less than desired, and their true relationship to clinical spasticity is in question. H-reflexes may be used to assess type Ib fibers from the Golgi tendon organs. There may be impairment of type Ib inhibition in patients with significant spasticity. Paired H-reflex studies employing a collision technique have been used to assess recurrent inhibition (33) but the results have been less than consistent.

Tonic Vibration Reflex

Vibratory stimulation in normal subjects will generally result in inhibition of reflex responses. Thus, the utility of the tonic vibration reflex may be in the assessment of presynaptic inhibition. This vibrator reflex is diminished in patients with the clinical spastic syndrome (34). The ratio of the maximum amplitude of the H-reflex with vibration to that without vibration is increased in the patient with spasticity. Again, however, there is less than optimal correlation with the clinical severity of spasticity. In addition, prolonged vibration may lead to a suppression of the response.

F-wave Response

F-waves provide a window to measure the general excitability of the motor neuron pool. While H-reflexes are recorded with submaximal stimulus, the F-wave is best elicited by supramaximal stimuli. The F-wave is not a reflex and reflects a "bounce back" traveling via the motor neuron pool antidromically and orthodromically. In patients with significant chronic spasticity, the persistence and amplitude of the F-wave may be increased (35). The ratio of the maximal F-wave amplitude to the maximal M response is also increased (36).

Flexor Reflex Responses

The flexor responses are recorded by assessing EMG activity over the tibialis anterior after stimulation of the flexor reflex or the sole of the foot. Typically a twofold response is produced. A first component appears at 50 to 60 msec and a later response is noted at between 110 and 400 msec. The role of the first response appears to be withdrawal of the foot, while the second response is responsible for maintaining the slower withdrawal of a limb from a noxious stimulus (37). In patients with CNS disturbance, a stimulus may elicit continuous EMG activity at a longer latency. The utility of these responses also remains in question (25).

Lumbosacral Evoked Potential

The lumbosacral response is elicited by stimulation of the tibial nerve and the response is measured by detection over the T12 spinous process. The response elicited produces three deflections: a positive 1 (P1), a positive 2 (P2), and a negative deflection (S). The P2 deflection may be reflective of presynaptic inhibition. Work with spinal cord patients showed a decrease in P2 responses in patients receiving baclofen (38).

Central Conduction

In 1876 Ferrier was able to stimulate the motor cortex of monkeys using faradic stimulation. Today transcranial electrical stimulation and now more importantly, transcranial magnetic stimulation have been employed to evaluate spasticity and motor control. Protocols have been developed to produce maps of the motor cortex in humans. Abnormal central motor conduction times have been demonstrated in several spastic conditions. Transcranial magnetic stimulation has been found to be useful in finding incomplete lesions in the spinal cord injury population. This modality holds some significant promise for the assessment of motor dysfunction in the CNS-injured population.

Pendulum Testing

There exists a model for evaluating spastic muscle groups, most classically the quadriceps and hamstring muscles. The subject is placed in a supine position with the knees bent over the edge of a table, and the lower limb is allowed to fall from a fully extended position. Measurements of the angular motion of the knee joint are obtained. Sinusoidal patterns of angular motion are typical in normal subjects; however, this is not the case in patients with upper motor neuron syndrome. The torque measurement at a constant velocity may be the best measure. EMG activity can also be recorded.

CLINICAL ASSESSMENT AND QUANTIFICATION

The clear goal of spasticity assessment and quantification is to provide information on movement dysfunction and its impact on functional status.

Spasticity Not Always Dysfunctional

Spasticity is a symptom complex that may be influenced or induced by external stimuli. It is notable that spasticity may be worsened by a number of neuromedical conditions. Assessment for and treatment of these underlying conditions should be considered a primary point of spasticity evaluation and management.

Spasticity produces some positive consequences that must be detailed as well. Spastic patients often utilize their spasticity to facilitate transfers or ambulation. Therapeutic procedures do not always improve voluntary motor control and functional status, and in some patients, may have a negative impact on real-life concerns. Spasticity may also help to maintain muscle tone. While controversial, spasticity may have a role in the prevention of osteoporosis, deep venous thrombosis, and general venous return.

Many patients, however, have experienced the numerous negative consequences of spasticity. Spasticity has been associated with pain, decreased range of motion, contractures, poor perineal hygiene, skin lesions, fractures, and an increased risk for heterotopic ossification. Motor dysfunction and impairment of functional status are hallmarks of the spastic syndrome (39).

Clinical Evaluation

The clinical evaluation requires an assessment of the limitations in either passive or voluntary movement. Manual testing for stretch-induced spastic response, hyperactive tendon jerks, and postural dysfunction is imperative. Observation for patterned synergies is also necessary (40).

Measurement Scales

Since its original development, the Ashworth scale has been used widely. It is a five-point scale used to rate the severity of muscle tone. Modifications of the Ashworth scale have added additional intermediate grades and have a reasonable interrater reliability. Yet, there exists significant criticism of this scale. Critics have been concerned about the grouping of patients in the middle to lower categories. In addition, this scale does not distinguish spasticity from other disorders that increase tone.

Functional scales such as Fugl-Meyer are helpful in designating capacity to perform activities but do not directly measure the severity of spasticity. Traditional measures such as the Barthel and the Functional Independence Measure (FIM) assess the amount of assistance a person may need. While these tasks may be impeded by spasticity, the focus of these scales is not assessment of spasticity severity. The Tufts Assessment of Motor Performance (TAMP) is a 32-item scale for the assessment of motor performance (41). The TAMP has measures to assess efficiency of movement, and work is being done to further assess the role of this measure in the evaluation of the patient with spasticity.

Work remains to be done to better classify and quantify spasticity. Measures that capture meaningful clinical information that can be transferred to numerical values are sought after.

TREATMENT MODALITIES

Clinical Paradigms

The goal of any evaluation process is to determine the extent and success of any treatment. Spasticity treatment needs to be approached in a logical manner.

Positioning

It has been well observed that altering body position may change overall tone in patients with the upper motor neuron syndrome. The presence of spasticity can impair normal range of motion. Positioning of the patient, especially in the acute care setting, is important to reducing overall patterns of spasticity. Positioning goals must include improved alignment and symmetry of body position. Proper positioning can cause relaxation of muscle tone and may be needed to take advantage of various reflex responses. Placing the patient in a position of mechanical advantage in order to retain maximal possible function is the key. Positions such as scissored posture (bilateral hip extension, adduction, internal rotation), windswept position (hip flexion, abduction, external rotation on one side and relative hip extension, adduction, and internal rotation on the other), and frog-leg position reinforce negative reflex patterns. Postural alignment may well need to be combined with additional methods to improve overall tone. Proper position in a wheelchair is, of course, essential to any antispasticity program. The general rule of hips at 90 degrees, knees at 90 degrees, and good overall posture will often lead to a profound reduction in overall tone. The reader is referred to Chapter 36 on wheelchair seating for details.

Physical Modalities

Often physical modalities are employed to assist in an overall or regional reduction in tone. They include agents such as cold, heat, electrical stimulation, and mechanical vibration. These methods are often short-lived, yet have limited side effects when applied appropriately. These modalities may work via pain relief, thus decreasing spasticity either regionally or overall.

Cold

Cold application is not a new method, yet it remains relatively effective. Cold may inhibit monosynaptic stretch reflexes. In addition, a decrease in receptor sensitivity occurs after removal of the cold (42). Cold is generally applied for 10 to 20 minutes. Active exercises should begin shortly after application of the cold since the spasticity-inhibiting effects of cold last only 30 minutes. Care must be taken to protect the skin from burning, especially in those patients who are insensate. In addition, there have been reports of cold hypersensitivity. Vapocoolant spray has also been recommended as a method to apply cold to a local region. Vapocoolant spray such as flurומethane or ethyl chloride is applied to the spastic muscle. The patient's face should be protected during application (43). Vapocoolant spray may act by decreasing skin receptor activity.

Heat

Heat may be applied using a variety of methods. Ultrasound, paraffin, superficial heat, and whirlpool are the most useful modalities in the patient with spasticity. The effect of heat is of a rather short duration (44). Superficial heat may be administered for 10 to 20 minutes. The immersion method for paraffin treatment is often difficult to perform in the spastic patient with significant tone or contracture. Heat may have a calming effect on patients; however, in the agitated brain-injured patient, application, especially via whirlpool, may increase the agitation and behavioral dysfunction. Ultrasound increases elasticity secondary to its heating effects. One should avoid heat application in individuals with insensate regions or vascular flow dysfunction and in pregnant patients, and over the carotid sinus or ocular cavity. In general, application of heat should be followed by stretching for maximal effect.

Electrical Stimulation and Vibration

Electrical stimulation has been advocated to decrease spasticity; however, it again is a relatively short-acting modality. The stimulation can be applied to inhibit or fatigue a spastic muscle. In addition, stimulation of the antagonist of the spastic muscle will lead to relaxation and reciprocal inhibition. Electrical stimulation can be accomplished by functional electrical stimulation, neuromuscular electrical stimulation, or high- and low-voltage stimulation of the spinal cord.

Vibration can be employed to facilitate muscle contraction. High-frequency vibration applied to the antagonist can cause reciprocal inhibition of the spastic muscle (45). Low-frequency vibration may have general relaxation effects.

Massage

Massage may produce a sense of general well-being and relaxation. There is no distinct evidence for an increase in endogenous opiates after massage. The utility of massage in the patient with significant spasticity is not yet clear.

Casting and Splinting

Most useful in individuals where treatment is focused on a particular extremity, casting or splinting, or both, can be remarkably effective. Splinting appears useful in both the acute and postacute stages of treatment. However, splinting does not reduce EMG activity in the spastic muscles. In the upper extremity, some controversy still exists as to whether dorsal or volar splints reduce spasticity to a greater degree. No strong data exist to draw conclusions as to whether static or dynamic splints are clearly superior. Casting can be a very effective method of approaching spasticity treatment. Care must be taken to observe for skin changes and circulation dysfunction. Casts may be bivalved and function as a static splint. Potential mechanisms of action include elongation of the muscle fibers' elastic structure. Elbow dropout casts for elbow flexor spasticity allow for elbow extension and prevent elbow flexion. Otis et al (46) demonstrated the benefit of long-term casting for spasticity.

Pharmacotherapy

A significant part of the arsenal employed to treat generalized spasticity is the use of pharmacologic agents. Numerous agents have been tested in the past and have shown benefit in certain populations. It is important to realize that such treatments as casting, splinting, and nerve blocking are all local, while the effects of pharmacologic agents are more global. When many of the patient's muscles demonstrate evidence of the upper motor neuron syndrome, medications may be the methodology of choice.

Benzodiazepines

The most commonly used member of this class is diazepam. It is the oldest medication that is still in use to treat spasticity. Its site of action in the CNS is the brain stem reticular formation and spinal polysynaptic pathways (47). It potentiates presynaptic inhibitory effects of γ-aminobutyric acid (GABA) at GABA-A receptor sites.

Diazepam decreases resistance to passive range of motion, deep tendon reflexes, and painful spasms. Dosing begins at 2 mg twice a day, increasing to 2 mg/week to a maximum of 60 mg/day. Diazepam is most commonly employed in patients with spinal cord injury, but is also used for multiple sclerosis and cerebral palsy. The value of diazepam in patients with acquired brain injury is still in question. Side effects include sedation, decreased memory, weakness, ataxia, decreased coordination, and depression (48). There also remains the real possibility of developing drug dependence with the use of any benzodiazepines.

Baclofen

Baclofen is a GABA-B analogue that is also centrally acting on polysynaptic inhibitory pathways (8). The parameters affected by baclofen include reduction in spasms and clonus, decrease in resistance to stretch, and reduction in deep tendon reflexes. Baclofen is used to treat complete and incomplete spinal cord lesions, painful spasms, and multiple sclerosis (49–53). The utility of baclofen for disorders of a cerebral origin is not clear. Baclofen begins at 5 mg twice to three times a day and can be titrated up 5 to 10 mg day/week. A maximum dose of 80 mg is often discussed; however, doses as high as 300 mg have been used (8). The side effects of baclofen include sedation, fatigue, weakness, nausea, dizziness, paresthesias, hallucinations, and reduction of seizure threshold. Rapid withdrawal may produce hallucinations or seizures (48).

Dantrolene Sodium

Unlike the other agents discussed, dantrolene works in the periphery at the sarcoplasmic reticulum by inhibiting the release of calcium. This inhibition effectively uncouples muscle contraction from excitation (8). This action occurs in both extrafusal and intrafusal fibers. The changes in the intrafusal fibers may change spindle sensitivity. Dantrolene's effect is primarily on fast-twitch fibers. Its effect on maximal voluntary capacity is limited. Dantrolene decreases resistance to range of motion as well as reduces clonus, spasm, and tone. It is recommended for spasticity of cerebral origin, including cerebral palsy and stroke. Its role in spasticity of spinal origin is not clear. Dantrolene is best known for its potential liver toxicity; therefore, prior to initiating therapy, one must check liver enzyme levels. The starting dose is 25 mg twice a day. It can be increased 25 to 50 mg/week to a maximum dose of 400 mg/day (54). The side effects of dantrolene include weakness, paresthesias, nausea, and diarrhea. Utili et al (55) reviewed the rate and occurrence of liver damage with the use of dantrolene. It occurs rarely, at a rate of 1.8% when treatment is longer than 60 days, and is usually reversible. Women over 30 years old receiving long-term treatment at doses higher than 400 mg are at highest risk (55).

Clonidine

Clonidine is an α_2-adrenergic agonist that has been utilized to treat spasticity due to spinal cord injury. Many patients have experienced improvement with doses of 0.1 mg twice a day or less. Recent evidence indicates favorable results with transdermal clonidine as well (56). Adverse effects of clonidine include hypotension, syncope, nausea, vomiting, and cognitive concerns in patients with spasticity of cerebral origin. However, a recent report showed beneficial effects of clonidine in the treatment of patients with acquired brain injury (57).

Tizanidine

While not yet available in the United States, tizanidine has been shown by numerous studies to have many benefits (54,58–61). It is an imidazoline derivative as well as having α_2-agonist effects. It also possesses antinociceptive and anticonvulsant effects. However, its relevance to spasticity treatment is not known. The α_2 agonist manifests activity, thus decreasing the release of excitatory amino acids at the spinal cord level and cerulospinal pathways. This results in reduced clonus, resistance to passive stretch, tone, and muscle spasms (62).

Tizanidine appears to have fewer side effects than many of the other antispasticity medications. Weakness, sedation, nausea and vomiting, dry mouth, and dizziness have been noted. Dosing begins at 2 mg two to three times a day, which can be increased 4 mg every 4 to 7 days to a maximum of 36 mg/day (48).

Other Medications

Numerous other medications have been tried to treat spasticity. The results have been mixed, and a discussion of all the different medications that have been attempted to treat spasticity is beyond the scope of this chapter.

Efforts to demonstrate the efficacy of cyclobenzaprine in the treatment of spasticity demonstrated no effect (63). However, tetrahydrocannabinol (THC), the active agent in marijuana, has been reported to decrease spasticity (64). Progabide is an active GABA agonist at both the A and B receptor sites (65). Its utility appears to be limited by the side effects of weakness, fever, and liver dysfunction. Glycine is a neurotransmitter that has decreased spasticity in animal models; further trials are needed to evaluate its efficacy in humans. One small study of seven patients demonstrated a subjective improvement in symptoms (66). Vigabatrin is an anticonvulsant not yet avaliable in the United States. It increases levels of GABA by inhibiting the breakdown of GABA (67). An interesting newer class of medications is being derived from drugs with NMDA antagonist activity.

Intrathecal Medications

Intrathecal delivery of baclofen was first described by Penn et al (68). Recent studies demonstrated efficacy in the treatment of spasticity due to spinal cord injury and cerebral palsy. A recent initial investigation showed promise in patients with acquired brain injury (69). A pump is implanted surgically and medication is delivered to the subarachnoid space in an attempt to obtain higher efficacy and avoid many of the CNS side effects (70). The costs are relatively high, and complications can include rare infection, baclofen overdosage, pump dysfunction, and tube kinking. Clonidine has also been advocated as an intrathecal medication and may serve as an adjuvant to intrathecal baclofen (71). Intrathecal baclofen does hold reasonable promise, especially for the patient with severe or intractable spasticity. Further investigation of treatment efficacy is underway.

Nerve Blocks, Motor Points, and Chemical Neurolysis

In essence, the performance of nerve blocks consists of creating a lower motor neuron lesion to treat an upper motor neuron problem process. The key to all decision making is maximizing functional status of the patient with the least amount of side effects.

Glenn (72) defined *nerve block* as the application of chemical agents to the nerve to impair function, either temporally or permanently. He further defined *chemical neurolysis* as a nerve block that impairs conduction by means of destruction of a portion of the nerve. Motor point blocks are performed lower down the nerve terminal trunk, where only fibers that control activity to the injected area will sustain an effect (72).

Purpose of Nerve Blocks

Nerve blocks can serve as either a diagnostic or a therapeutic procedure, depending on the agent used. As a diagnostic procedure, the use of an anesthetic nerve block can differentiate between a dynamic or static deformity of a contracted joint. It also allows the patient to test-drive the results of the block to evaluate functional changes. This may well be an important item prior to attempting chemical neurolysis or orthopedic intervention. Temporary blocks may also be helpful when used in combination with serial casting. One must be careful not to cast the extremity in the maximal obtainable range of motion after a temporary block has been induced, for tone may well return once the block wears off.

Nerve blocks with neurolytic agents are used to treat functional issues, improve quality of life, reduce pain, increase range of motion, break synergy patterns, improve position, and improve hygiene (72,73).

Performance of Nerve Blocks

The actual act of performing a nerve block is relatively similar regardless of the agent used. The nerve is localized electronically, if possible, first at the skin and then below the skin, using an insulated needle with only the electrically active tip exposed. A stimulator that is capable of delivering a pulse wave at 1 Hz is connected to the needle. The stimulator must be capable of delivering varying amounts of current, and the clinician should have the needle tip close enough to the nerve that a current less than 1.0 mA is required to activate the target spastic muscles.

Motor nerve or motor point blockade occurs at a point distal to the main branch. With this method, sensory fibers in mixed nerves can be spared the effects of neurolytic agents. Motor point blockade is somewhat more time-consuming than mixed nerve blockade and requires a more cooperative patient (72,73). Books such as that by Warfel (74) may be helpful in acquainting the clinician with finding motor points; however, these books are aids only and do not replace electrical localization.

Agents for Nerve and Motor Blockade

Agents employed for nerve blocks can be broken down into two categories: anesthetic and neurolytic. Lidocaine has the advantage of a quick onset of action; bupivacaine has a longer duration of effect.

Phenol and ethanol are the most common neurolytic agents. Phenol has a direct anesthetic effect and a subsequent neurolytic effect. Typical concentrations of phenol are 5% to 7%, with some believing that the higher concentration produces a more effective blockade. Typical neurolytic effects of a motor point block last from 3 to 9 months, while nerve blocks may last as long as 12 to 18 months (72,73).

Side Effects and Complications of Nerve Block

It is critical for the treatment team to identify functional goals prior to any procedure. Even if performed successfully, nerve blocks can cause excessive weakness, change in kinesiologic pattern, and loss of beneficial spasticity. Bleeding, swelling, pain, and deep venous thrombosis are rare possible complications. Dysesthesias occurring after blockade have been reported in 3% to as many as 32% of patients. This percentage seems quite high as we have experienced a much lower incidence of this complication. The concentration of the agent employed as well as the experience of the individual performing the block may play a significant role. Injection of sensory-rich nerves like the median may predispose one to dysesthesias, while nerves such as the obturator and the musculocutaneous are much less likely to cause this condition. Dysesthesia can be treated with modalities and membrane-stabilizing anticonvulsants or antidepressants. If it is resistant to initial treatment, reblockade will usually relieve the symptoms (72,73).

Botulinum Toxin

Botulinum toxin, as available in the United States, is the lyophilized form of purified botulinum toxin A, produced by *Clostridium botulinum*. Of the seven toxin serotypes available, A is the most biologically active. Its clinical efficacy is mediated by its binding to receptor sites at the neuromuscular junction and inhibiting the release of acetylcholine. In contrast to nerve and motor point blocks, which require electrical localization, botulinum toxin, once injected, will actually be transported to the nerve terminal, simplifying its use (75,76).

Adverse reactions to botulinum toxin A have been very rare. There is some systemic absorption of the product and concern exists regarding the formation of antibodies (77,78). Yablon (79) reported on a low incidence of side effects (<2%) with no long-term sequelae. Simpson (80) showed the efficacy of this agent in upper-extremity spasticity for stroke survivors.

Therapeutic doses are normally in the 100- to 400-unit range. There is a wide window for therapeutic versus fatal doses. For the primate, a lethal dose is 40 units/kg, or roughly 3000 units for the 70-kg man (81).

Clear concerns do exist, however. Botulinum toxin A has a duration of action of 3 to 6 months (75), which may be sufficient in some patients yet rather short in others. As yet, botulism toxin A is approved for blepharospasm and dystonia but its use for spasticity is an off-label use. A final concern is economic—the cost of a single vial of botulinum toxin is over $300. One must consider the functional needs of the patient and the cost of less expensive and more expensive interventions when deciding upon a treatment regimen. Further work is necessary to clarify the role of all these medications.

Neurosurgical Approaches

Rhizotomies have been advocated as treatment for the patient with severe spasticity. Anterior rhizotomies have been associated with significant anterior denervation atrophy and their practical utility has been thought to be limited. Posterior rhizotomy was first performed in 1913, as a treatment for spasticity (82). Percutaneous radiofrequency rhizotomy was first reported in 1974. Kasdon and Lathi (83) noted a significant improvement in spastic hypertonia in the patients they evaluated. Selective dorsal rhizotomies have been used most frequently in the cerebral palsy population. Roots are selected secondary to functional needs and the particular patterns they produce. It is generally advisable to avoid complete sections of all rootlets at one level, since this produces anesthesia.

Dorsal route entry-zone lesions produce lesions in the posterior substantia gelatinosa and typically these lesions are used to treat pain. By extending the lesions, abnormal motor responses can be decreased (84).

Myelotomy or cordotomy was reported by Bischoff to be of value in spasticity and has been advocated as a treatment for severely spastic patients (85). The Bischoff T-shaped myelotomy may result in the loss of bladder and bowel function. In addition, this procedure is rather complex. Placement of a stimulator in the spinal cord has been reported by some to have excellent results (86). Barolat et al (86) reported a percutaneous method to stimulator placement. Long-term results have been modest and it is clear that any blinding of the patient is not possible.

Orthopedic Procedures

Orthopedic surgical procedures have played an important role in the management of the spastic patient. The goals of surgical intervention are to improve function, increase mobility, and correct or prevent severe deformity. Clearly a cooperative patient is essential, and often an aggressive therapy program is required postoperatively.

The split anterior tibial transfer procedure is performed to reduce excessive supination of the foot. In this procedure the tendon of the tibialis anterior is split and a portion of the tendon is driven into the cuneiform and cuboid bones to generate an eversion force (87). Significant pes cavus can be defined as a decrease in the angle below 140 degrees. This condition can be treated early with a plantar fasciotomy, and in later stages, a lateral wedge osteotomy of the calcaneus may be needed (88).

A shortening of the Achilles tendon may require a Z-lengthening procedure. Care must be taken to determine preoperatively that this procedure will not result in kinematic changes that will further impair ambulation.

Knee flexion contractures may require hamstring-lengthening procedures and postoperative casting. Hip flexion remains a difficult concern and may require iliopsoas tenotomy if the patient remains with a flexion contracture of more than 20 degrees after more conservative treatment (89). Patients with severe spasticity may develop hip subluxation. This can be treated with adductor myotomies, or if not successful, femoral osteotomy. Successful upper-extremity procedures focus on the restoration of hand hygiene, improved grasp, and key pinch.

REFERENCES

1. Lee W, Boughton A. Absence of stretch reflex gain enhancement in voluntarily activated spastic muscle. *Exp Neurol* 1987;98:317–335.
2. Gans BM, Glenn MB. Introduction. In: Glenn MB, Whyte J, eds. *The practical management of spasticity in children and adults.* Philadelphia: Lea & Febiger, 1990:1–7.
3. Little WJ. Course of lectures on the deformities of the human frame. Lecture 9. *Lancet* 1843;1:350–354.
4. Denny-Brown D. Historical aspects of the relation of spasticity to movement. In: Feldmann RG, Young RR, Koella WP, eds. *Spasticity: disordered motor control.* Chicago: Year Book Medical, 1980:1–16.
5. Sherrington CS. On plastic tonus and proprioceptive reflexes. *Q J Exp Neurol* 1909;2:109–156.
6. Henneman E. Skeletal muscle: the servant of the nervous system. In: Mountcastle VB, eds. *Medical physiology.* 14th ed. St Louis: CV Mosby, 1980:674–702.
7. Whitlock JA. Neurophysiology of spasticity. In: Glenn MB, Whyte J, eds. *The practical management of spasticity in children and adults.* Philadelphia: Lea & Febiger, 1990:8–33.
8. Katz RT, Elovic EP, Glenn MB, Meythaler JM. Spasticity management in the patient with brain injury. American Academy of PM&R; Orlando. 1995:715–735.
9. Moore JC. The Golgi tendon organ: a review and update. *Am J Occup Ther* 1984;38:227–236.
10. Hultborn H, Illert M, Santini I. Convergence on interneurons mediating the reciprocal Ia inhibition of motorneurones. *Acta Physiol Scand* 1976;96:193–201.
11. Brooks VB, ed. *The neural basis of motor control.* New York: Oxford University Press, 1986.
12. Katz RT, Pierrot-Deseilligny E. Recurrent inhibition of motorneurons in patients with upper motor neuron lesions. *Brain* 1982;105:103–124.
13. Shefner JM, Berman SA, Sarkarati M, et al. Recurrent inhibition is increased in patients with spinal cord injury. *Neurology* 1992;42:2162–2168.
14. Rothwell JC, Thompson PD, Day BL, et al. Stimulation of the human motor cortex through the scalp. *Exp Physiol* 1991;76:159–200.
15. Turton A, Fraser C, Flament W, et al. Organization of cortico-motorneuronal projections from the primary motor cortex; evidence for task related function in monkey and in man. In: Thrilmann AF, Burke DJ, Rymer WZ, eds. *Spasticity: mechanisms and management.* Berlin: Springer, 1993:8–24.
16. Brodal A, ed. *Neurological anatomy in relationship to clinical medicine.* New York: Oxford University Press, 1981.
17. Magoun HW, Rhines R. An inhibitory mechanism in the bulbar reticular formation. *J Neurophysiol* 1946;9:165–171.
18. Dietz V, Berber W. Normal and impaired regulation of muscle stiffness in gait: a new hypothesis about muscle hypertonia. *Exp Neurol* 1983;79:680–687.
19. Granit J. The gamma loop in the mediation of muscle tone. *Clin Pharmacol Ther* 1964;5:837–847.
20. Hagbarth KE. Exteroceptive, proprioceptive and sympathetic activity recorded with microelectrodes from human peripheral nerves. *Mayo Clin Proc* 1979;54(6):353–364.

21. Delwaide PJ. Human monosynaptic reflexes and presynaptic inhibition. In: Esmedt JE, eds. *New developments in electromyography and clinical neurophysiology*. Basel: Karger, 1973:508–522.
22. McCouch GP. Sprouting as a cause of spasticity. *J Neurophysiol* 1958;21:205–216.
23. Cannon WB, Haimovici H. The sensitization of motorneurons by partial denervation. *Am J Physiol* 1939;126:731–740.
24. Willis WD. The raphe-spinal system. In: Barnes CD, eds. *Brainstem control of spinal cord function*. New York: Academic, 1984:141–214.
25. Delwaide PJ. Contribution of human reflexes studies to the understanding and management of the pyramidal syndrome. In: Shahani BT, ed. *Central EMG*. Boston: Butterworth, 1984:77–109.
26. Magladery J, McDougal D. Electrophysiologic studies of nerve and reflex activity in man. *Bull Johns Hopkins Hosp* 1950;86:265–282.
27. Mathews W. Ratio of the maximum H reflex to maximum M response as a measure of spasticity. *J Neurol Neurosurg Psychiatry* 1966;29:201–204.
28. Shanhani B, Cros D. Neurophysiologic testing in spasticity. In: Glenn M, Whyte J, eds. *The practical management of spasticity in the adult and child*. Philadelphia: Lea & Febiger, 1990:34–43.
29. Katz R, Rovai G, Brait C, et al. Objective quantification of spastic hypertonia: correlation with clinical findings. *Arch Phys Med Rehabil* 1992;79:339–347.
30. Taborikova H, Sax D. Conditioning of H reflexes by a preceding subthreshold H reflex stimulus. *Brain* 1969;92:203–207.
31. Little J, Halar E. H-reflex changes following spinal cord injury. *Arch Phys Med Rehabil* 1985;66:19–22.
32. Pannizza M, Nilsson J, Hallett M. Optimal stimulus duration for the H-reflex. *Muscle Nerve* 1989;12:576–579.
33. Pierrot-Deseilligny E. Electrophysiological assessment of the spinal mechanisms underlying spasticity. *Electroencephalogr Clin Neurophysiol Suppl* 1990;41:264–273.
34. Lance J, DeGail T, Neilson P. Tonic and phasic spinal cord mechanisms in man. *J Neurol Neurosurg Psychiatry* 1966;29:535–544.
35. Eisen A, Odusote K. Amplitude of the F wave; a potential means of documenting spasticity. *Neurology* 1979;29:1306–1309.
36. Fisher M. F/M ratios in polyneuropathy and spastic hyperreflexia. *Muscle Nerve* 1988;11:217–222.
37. Hallet M, Shanhani B, Young R. EMG analysis of stereotyped voluntary movements in man. *J Neurol Neurosurg Psychiatry* 1975;38:1154–1162.
38. Kofler M, Donoan W, Loubser P, et al. Effects of intrathecal baclofen on lumbosacral and cortical somatosensory evoked potentials. *Neurology* 1992;42:864–868.
39. Esquenazi A, Hirai B. Assessment of gait dysfunction in patients with spastic stroke or brain injury. In: Katz R, eds. *Spasticity: state of the art reviews*. Philadelphia: Hanley & Belfus, 1994:523–533.
40. Mayer N, Esquenazi A, Keenan M. Analysis and management of spasticity, contracture and impaired motor control. In: Horn L, Zasler N, eds. *Medical rehabilitation in traumatic brain injury*. Philadelphia: Hanley & Belfus, 1996:411–458.
41. Gans B, Mann N, et al. Description and interobserver reliability of the Tufts Assessment of Motor Performance. *Am J Phys Med Rehabil* 1988;67:202.
42. Knutson E. Topical cryotherapy in spasticity. *Scand J Rehabil Med* 1970;2:159–163.
43. Travell J. Ethyl chloride spray for painful spasm. *Arch Phys Med Rehabil* 1952;33:291–298.
44. Lehmann J, De Lateur B. Diathermy and superficial heat and cold therapy. In: Krusen F, eds. *Handbook of physical medicine and rehabilitation*. 1996.
45. Hagbarth K, Eklund G. The effect of muscle vibration in spasticity, rigidity and cerebellar disorders. *J Neurol Neurosurg Psychiatry* 1968;31:207–213.
46. Otis J, Root L, Kroll M. Measure of plantar flexor spasticity during treatment with tone reducing casts. *J Pediatr Orthop* 1985;5:682–686.
47. Tseng T, Wang S. Locus of action of centrally acting muscle relaxants diazepam and tybamate. *J Pharmacol Exp Ther* 1971;178:350–360.
48. Whyte J, Robinson KM. Pharmacologic management. In: Glenn M, Whyte J, eds. *The practical management of spasticity in the adult and child*. Philadelphia: Lea & Febiger, 1990:201–226.
49. Basmajian JV. Lioresal (baclofen) treatment of spasticity in multiple sclerosis. *Am J Phys Med Rehabil* 1975;54:175–177.
50. Basmajian JV, Yucel V. Effects of a GABA-derivative on spasticity. *Am J Phys Med Rehabil* 1974;53:223–228.
51. Duncan GW, Shanhani B, Young RR. An evaluation of baclofen treatment for certain symptoms in patients with spinal cord lesions. *Neurology* 1976;26:441–446.
52. Feldman RG, Kelly-Hayes M, Conomy JP, et al. Baclofen for spasticity in multiple sclerosis. *Neurology* 1978;28:1094–1098.
53. Hudgson P, Weightman D. Baclofen in the treatment of spasticity. *BMJ* 1971;4:15–17.
54. Katz RT, Campagnolo DI. Pharmacologic management of spasticity. In: Katz RT, eds. *Spasticity: state of the arts review*. Philadelphia: Hanley & Belfus, 1994:473–480.
55. Utili R, Boitnott JK, Zimmerman HJ. Dantrolene associated hepatic injury: incidence and character. *Gastroenterology* 1977;72:610.
56. Weingarden S, Belen J. Clonidine transdermal system for treatment of spasticity in spinal cord injury. *Arch Phys Med Rehabil* 1992;73:876–877.

57. Dall J, Harmon R, Quinn C. Use of clonidine for treatment of spasticity arising from various forms of brain injury: a case series. *Brain Inj* 1996;10:453–458.

58. United Kingdom Tizanidine Trial Group. A double blind placebo controlled trial of tizanidine in the treatment of spasticity caused by multiple sclerosis. *Neurology* 1994;44:S70–S78.

59. Wallace JD. Summary of combined clinical analysis of controlled clinical trials with tizanidine. *Neurology* 1994;44:S60–S68.

60. Nance PW, Bugaresti J, Shellenberger K, et al. Efficacy and safety of tizanidine in the treatment of spasticity in patients with spinal cord injury: North American Study Group. *Neurology* 1994;44:S44–S51.

61. Smith C, Birnbaum G, Carter JL, et al. Tizanidine treatment of spasticity caused by multiple sclerosis: results of a double blind placebo controlled trial. US Tizanidine Study Group. *Neurology* 1994;44:S34–S43.

62. Coward DM. Tizanidine: neuropharmacology and mechanism of action. *Neurology* 1994;44:S6–S11.

63. Ashby P, Burke D, Rao S, et al. Assessment of cyclobenzaprine in the treatment of spasticity. *J Neurol Neurosurg Psychiatry* 1972;35:599–605.

64. Petro DJ, Ellenberger C. Treatment of human spasticity with delta-9-tetrahydrocannabinol. *J Clin Pharmacol* 1981;21:S413–S416.

65. Mondrup K, Pedersen E. The clinical effect of the GABA-agonist, progabride, on spasticity. *Acta Neurol Scand* 1984;69:200–206.

66. Stern P, Bokonjic R. Glycine therapy in 7 cases of spasticity. *Pharmacology* 1974;12:117–119.

67. Grant S, Heel R. Vigabatrin: a review of its pharmacodynamic and pharmacokinetic properties and therapeutic potential in epilepsy and disorders of motor control. *Drugs* 1991;41:899–926.

68. Penn R, Savoy S, Corcos D, et al. Intrathecal baclofen for severe spinal spasticity. *N Engl J Med* 1989;320:1517–1521.

69. Methyaler J, Devivo M, Hadley M. Prospective study on the use of bolus intrathecal baclofen for spastic hypertonia due to acquired brain injury. *Arch Phys Med Rehabil* 1996;77:461–465.

70. Bucholz RD. Management of intractable spasticity with intrathecal baclofen. In: Katz RT, eds. *Spasticity: state of the arts review.* Philadelphia: Hanley & Belfus, 1994:565–578.

71. Middelton J, Walker S, Molloy A, et al. Intrathecal clonidine and baclofen in the management of spasticity and neuropathic pain following spinal cord injury. *Arch Phys Med Rehabil* 1966;77:824–829.

72. Glenn MB. Nerve blocks. In: Glenn M, Whyte J, eds. *The practical management of spasticity in the adult and child.* Philadelphia: Lea & Febiger, 1990:227–258.

73. Glenn MB. Nerve blocks for the treatment of spasticity. In: Katz RT, ed. *Spasticity: state of the arts review.* Philadelphia: Hanley & Belfus, 1994:481–505.

74. Warfel JH, ed. *The extremities, muscles and motor points.* 6th ed. Philadelphia: Lea & Febiger, 1993.

75. O'Brien C. Clinical pharmacology of botulinum toxin. In: O'Brien C, Yablon S, eds. *Management of spasticity with botulinum toxin.* Littleton: Postgraduate Institute for Medicine, 1995:3–6.

76. Jankovic J, Brin MF, Comelia CL. Botulinum toxin; chemistry, pharmacology, toxicity and immunology. In: Jankovic J, Brin MF, Comelia CL, eds. *Botulinum toxin treatment of cervical dystonia.* New York: Churchill Livingstone, 1994:6–19.

77. Green P, Fahn S, Diamond B. Development of resistance to botulinum toxin type A in patients with torticollis. *Mov Disord* 1994;9: 213–217.

78. Zuber M, Sebald M, Bathien N, et al. Botulinum antibodies in dystonic patients treated with type A botulinum toxin: frequency and significance. *Neurology* 1993;43:1715–1718.

79. Yablon SA, Agana BT, Ivanhoe CB, Boake C. Botulinum toxin in severe upper extremity spasticity among patients with traumatic brain injury: an open-labeled trial. *Neurology* 1996;47(4):939–944.

80. O'Brien CF, Simpson DM, Alexander DN, et al. A randomized, double-blind, placebo-controlled study to evaluate the use of botulinum toxin type A in the treatment of spasticity [Abstract]. Neurology 1995;45(suppl 4): A329.

81. Scott BA, Suzuki D. Systemic toxicity of botulinum toxin by intramuscular injection in the monkey. *Mov Disord* 1988;3:333–335.

82. Foerster O. On the indications and results of the excision of posterior spinal nerve roots in men. *Surg Gynecol Obstet* 1913;26:463–475.

83. Kasdon D, Lathi E. A prospective study of radiofrequency rhizotomy in the treatment of posttraumatic spasticity. *Neurosurgery* 1984;15:526–529.

84. Sindou M, Jeanmonod D. Microsurgical procedures in the peripheral nerves and the dorsal root entry zone for the treatment of spasticity and pain in the lower limbs. *Neurosurgery* 1989;24:655–670.

85. Kasdon D. Controversies in the surgical management of spasticity. *Clin Neurosurg* 1986;33:523–529.

86. Barolat G, Mylebust J, Hemmy D, et al. Immediate effects of spinal cord stimulation in spinal spasticity. *J Neurosurg* 1985;62(4): 558–562.

87. Keenan M. Surgical decision making for residual limb deformities following traumatic brain injury. *Orthop Rev* 1988;27:102–109.

88. Keenan M, Perry J, Jordan C. Factors affecting balance and ambulation following stroke. *Clin Orthop* 1988;182:165–171.

89. Keenan M. Hamstring release for knee flexion contractures in spastic adults. *Clin Orthop* 1988;236:221–226.

Chapter 48

Rehabilitation of Joint Contractures

Kevin M. Means

Contractures are well-known adversaries of the physiatrist and rehabilitation team. They can be either a consequence of or a contributor to immobility. Perry (1) presented a good historical perspective on contractures as they relate to the relative merits and consequences of immobility. Other adverse effects of immobility and bed rest are discussed in detail elsewhere in this section of the textbook. Contractures can affect persons of any age or gender. However, aged, neurologically impaired, and chronically disabled persons, including many patients cared for by the physiatrist, are at increased risk for contracture development because they are more likely to be at least partially immobilized.

Rehabilitation of a patient with a contracture may be extremely challenging, especially when the contracture is of long duration or involves multiple joints or limbs. Fortunately, many contractures are preventable if appropriate measures are initiated. The wise physiatrist will learn to recognize the underlying pathologic conditions, contributing factors, and secondary changes associated with the development of contractures so that rehabilitation measures can be employed, and whenever possible, the contractures can be avoided.

DEFINITION AND CLASSIFICATION

A *contracture* is defined as a persistent or chronic loss of the range of motion (ROM) of a body part or joint due to a pathologic shortening or "contraction" of the soft connective tissue structures in or around the body part or joint. Contractures may limit motion virtually anywhere. This chapter focuses on joint contractures in which soft tissue overlying a joint is contracted to limit joint ROM. Trauma, infection, inflammatory or degenerative processes, pain, structural or mechanical alterations, and immobilization are factors that commonly precipitate the development of contractures. The loss of motion of the joint is often accompanied by functional limitations and deformity. Halar and Bell (2) reported an anatomically based system for classifying contractures (Table 48-1).

Arthrogenic contractures are associated with pathologic or structural changes *within* the joint, such as the degeneration and inflammation seen with various arthritic disorders, joint infection, prolonged joint immobilization, or trauma to the articular synovium, cartilage, or joint capsule. Arthrogenic contractures are typified by intra-articular synovial proliferation and fibrosis associated with the edema and pain seen with rheumatoid arthritis. Involvement of the joint capsule can occur when inflammation is present, resulting in capsular fibrosis, or when collagen fiber shortening occurs in the capsule, because of inadequate positioning of the joint. In capsular fibrosis, the ROM limitation is multidirectional or multiaxial.

Soft-tissue joint contractures are limitations in the joint ROM caused by pathologic changes *outside* the joint and joint capsule. The collagen fiber proliferation and shortening seen in the soft tissues surrounding the joint are similar to the changes seen with arthrogenic contractures. Common precipitants are inflammation, trauma, infection,

Table 48-1: Anatomic Classification of Contractures	
Arthrogenic contracture	
Etiology	Intra-articular pathology or structural incongruency (e.g., degeneration, inflammation, infection, immobilization, or trauma to synovium, cartilage, or joint capsule)
Key features	Intra-articular synovial proliferation, fibrosis, edema, pain; capsular fibrosis with multidirectional, multiaxial ROM limitation
Extra-articular soft-tissue contracture	
Etiology	Collagen fiber proliferation and shortening of soft tissues surrounding the joint precipitated by inflammation, trauma, infection, or immobilization
Key features	Periarticular soft tissue: pathologic fibrosis and hyperplasia with ROM limitation in one plane or axis only (e.g., infrapatellar contracture syndrome) Skin and subcutaneous tissue: pathologic inflammatory or proliferative infiltration (e.g., scleroderma, burns, infection, trauma) Tendons and ligaments: inflammatory infiltration, shortening with alteration of mechanical load characteristics (e.g., tendonitis, bursitis, ligament injury)
Myogenic contracture	
Etiology	Shortening of muscles crossing a joint due to intrinsic causes, such as trauma (bleeding, immobilization, edema), inflammation (myositis), degenerative changes (muscular dystrophy), ischemia (diabetes, peripheral vascular disease, immobilization); or extrinsic causes (spasticity, paralysis/paresis, malpositioning or immobilization in a shortened position)
Key features	Restructuring of muscle tissue components; muscle fiber loss; collagen, fibrofatty, and connective tissue infiltration of muscle fibers; fibrosis; necrosis; muscle imbalance; and change in mechanical properties

ROM = range of motion.
Source: Adapted from Halar EM, Bell KR. Contractures and other deleterious effects of immobility. In: DeLisa JA, ed. *Rehabilitation medicine principles and practice.* Philadelphia, JB Lippincott, 1988:448–462.

and immobilization. In contrast to the ROM limitations when seen there is joint capsule involvement, the ROM limitation due to soft-tissue contractures is usually in one plane or axis only. Various types and layers of soft tissues, including the skin and subcutaneous tissue, tendons, and ligaments, may be involved. Pathologic changes from numerous conditions commonly lead to inflammatory infiltration, tissue shortening, and alteration of the physical properties of soft tissue.

Myogenic joint contractures are ROM limitations that occur because of changes (usually shortening) of *muscle* crossing a joint. Myogenic contractures may be due to intrinsic (structural) or extrinsic (secondary) causes or a combination of both. Examples of intrinsic causes include trauma with intramuscular hemorrhage, immobilization, intramuscular edema, inflammatory conditions such as myositis, degenerative conditions like muscular dystrophy, and ischemia of diabetes or peripheral vascular disease. Examples of extrinsic causes of myogenic contracture include disorders of muscle tone, weakness and paralysis, inadequate limb positioning, and prolonged immobilization of muscles in a shortened position.

Depending on the underlying etiology, myogenic contractures have various pathologic features. Inflammation, trauma, ischemia, and hemorrhage result in rearrangement of cellular and extracellular muscle tissue components. Degenerative conditions tend to cause muscle fiber loss; necrosis; muscle fiber infiltration by collagen, fat, and connective tissue; fibrosis; or necrosis. Extrinsic conditions, such as paralysis, disorders of muscle tone (spasticity, rigidity), and mechanical malpositioning, directly or indirectly result in muscle shortening. Prolonged shortening of muscle results in gradual replacement of normal loose connective tissue in muscle with dense connective tissue composed primarily of type I collagen.

ETIOLOGY AND PATHOPHYSIOLOGY OF CONTRACTURES

Many clinical conditions precipitate contracture formation, either in isolation or when superimposed with underlying immobilization. These conditions include congenital absence; deformity or imbalance of muscles or muscle groups; neurogenic weakness or spasticity, which often causes an imbalance of opposing agonist and antagonist muscle groups acting across a joint; and degenerative, septic, traumatic, and inflammatory arthritides, which are usually associated with joint pain. All these conditions restrict joint ROM, albeit through different mechanisms. This suggests that joint movement is required in order to preserve normal ROM in a limb.

Normal Joint Physiology

Normal synovial joints contain articular cartilage at the ends of the adjoining bones; a joint cavity that is outlined by the synovium and the articular cartilage; synovial fluid within the joint cavity; the joint capsule that envelops the joint cavity; ligaments that cross the junction of the adjoin-

Table 48-2: Studies Describing Pathophysiologic Changes in Joints Associated with Contracture Development

Author(s)	Model Used	Major Findings
Ely and Mensor (1933) (6)	Dogs	Dogs immobilized in casts for 1–10 mo developed changes in articular cartilage, including reduced thickness, decreased number of matrix cells, changes in staining properties.
Hall (1963) (7)	Rats	Rats immobilized for 1–4 mo developed articular cartilage changes similar to those found by Ely and Mensor.
Evans et al (1960) (8)	Rats	An immobilized rat knee, allowed to bear weight, developed proliferation of fibrofatty connective tissue and muscle atrophy within 2 wk; within 60 days, fibrous adhesions developed between the fibrofatty connective tissue and underlying cartilage surfaces.
Thaxter et al (1965) (9)	Rats	Immobilized rat knees with and without weight bearing developed fibrofatty connective tissue proliferation and adhesions at 45 days; changes were slightly worse in the immobilized weight-bearing rats.
Hall (1963) (7)	Rats	In immobilized mature rats, early degeneration of apposed joint surfaces occurred, in contrast to immature rats who developed thickening of apposed areas and no degeneration until 53 days.
Enneking and Horowitz (1972) (10)	Humans	Amputation and autopsy knee specimens from patients immobilized for 12 mo had fibrofatty proliferation and fibrosis of the joint space.

ing bones to support and reinforce the capsule; muscles that act across the junction to produce movement of the adjoining bones relative to each other; and tendons that extend from muscles to form their bony attachments. Joint capsules, tendons, and ligaments are types of connective tissues that are composed of collagen fibers and fibroblast cells in a parallel arrangement and an extracellular matrix composed of proteoglycans and water. Also contained in the matrix are polysaccharide complexes called *glycosaminoglycans*. Among the glycosaminoglycans commonly found in joint capsules and ligaments are chondroitin 4- and chondroitin 6-sulfate, hyaluronic acid, dermatan sulfate, and keratin sulfate (3).

The Effect of Immobilization on Joints

Numerous investigators have studied the pathophysiologic changes in the joint and surrounding soft connective tissues that accompany contracture formation. Akeson et al (4), and more recently, Nicholas (5) reviewed literature on this topic. Most of the studies reviewed [summarized in Table 48-2 (6–10)] used animal models and immobilization as the sole precipitating etiologic condition for contracture formation.

Ely and Mensor (6) described articular cartilage changes in the joints of dogs immobilized from 1 to 10 months. After immobilization, the staining properties of the articular cartilage changed. The thickness of the cartilage and the number of matrix cells were decreased. Hall (7) reported similar findings using immobilized adult rats. Evans et al (8) also studied the immobilized knee joints of adult rats. The rat limbs were immobilized but were allowed to bear weight. Proliferation of fibrofatty connective tissue was seen within 2 weeks, and became more extensive at 30 days. From 30 to 60 days, adhesions developed between the fibrofatty connective tissue and the underlying cartilage surface. Beyond 60 days, ulcerations were found in areas of the cartilage subject to compression, and erosive fibrovascular proliferation extended beneath the cartilage to subchondral bone. Thaxter et al (9) found similar connective tissue changes in immobilized rat knee joints with and without weight bearing.

Akeson et al (11) also reviewed the work of himself, his colleagues, and others on the biochemical changes seen in the fibrous connective tissue of immobilized joints. These changes include a mild (3%–6%) decrease in the water content of the connective tissue matrix and periarticular structures, and a moderate (20%–40%) decrease in the glycosaminoglycans hyaluronic acid, chondroitin 4- and 6-sulfate, and dermatan sulfate. A decrease in glycosaminoglycans results in reduced buffering of the matrix between collagen fibers, which increases the tendency for cross-linkage between adjacent fibers at crossover points. There is also increased collagen turnover and a slight (5%) reduction in collagen mass, due to a slightly higher rate of degradation of old collagen compared to the rate of new collagen synthesis. The new immature collagen is more disorganized, owing to the increased metabolic turnover. In ligaments, a similar increase in the turnover of fibrils occurs. In an immobilized joint, without the normal physical stimulation of motion, ligaments around the joint undergoing increased collagen turnover have new fibrils that appear disorganized. These fibrils lack the ordered parallel array of normal fibrillar matrix. Accordingly, the ligaments will have a reduced ability to resist tensile forces (12,13).

Ennecking and Horowitz (10) used amputation and autopsy specimens of persons who had been immobilized for at least 12 months. Synovial fibrofatty proliferation was found within the joint space, and fibrous ankylosis of the joint space was observed. These changes are similar to those found in the immobilized-animal studies. Together, these biochemical changes produce a fibrous, more tightly bound mesh of connective tissue matrix in and around a joint, with less lubrication and extensibility than normal.

Effect of Immobilization on Skeletal Muscle

Clinically, some contractures are associated with or are produced, at least in part, by changes in skeletal muscles that act across immobilized joints. Several investigators using animal and human experimental models have studied muscle responses to immobilization. Many of these studies are summarized in Table 48-3 (8,14–20).

Perhaps the most obvious change in muscles around an immobilized joint is atrophy. Evans et al (8), in their work with immobilized knee joints of rats, noted muscle atrophy within 2 weeks of immobilization. Booth (19) also reported skeletal muscle atrophy in the hind limbs of immobilized rats; however, in his study, the atrophy was noted within 1 to 3 days of immobilization. Peak atrophy occurred between 3 to 8 days. Lindboe and Platou (20) also studied rats with the knee immobilized in 15 degrees of flexion, and reported a 14% to 17% decrease in muscle fiber size after only 72 hours of immobilization. MacDougall et al (14) immobilized the elbow joints of healthy persons in casts for 5 weeks. After cast removal, the volunteers had a 5% decrease in arm circumference and a 35% decrease in elbow extension strength. In a later study among healthy persons, MacDougall et al (15) also found a decreased mean cross-sectional area of type II muscle fibers and decreased strength of the elbow extensors after 5 to 6 weeks of immobilization of elbows in casts. Using ankle and knee joints of cats immobilized at 90 degrees for 17 to 29 weeks, Mayer et al (16) found reduced motor unit tetanic force output, loss of maximal twitch, and decrease in type I and IIA fiber size.

Skeletal muscle in an immobilized limb has lower levels of adenosine triphosphate and glycogen and higher levels of lactic acid concentration. Witzmann et al (17) found decreased tetanic tension in three different hind-limb muscles at 1 to 3 days of immobilization. In rat experiments, using intermittent pulses of electrical stimulation of the soleus muscle, Witzmann et al (18) found that peak tension declined more rapidly after 6 weeks of hind-limb immobilization compared with nonimmobilized

Table 48-3: Studies Describing Pathophysiologic Changes in Muscle Associated with Contracture Development

Author(s)	Model Used	Major Findings
Evans et al (1960) (8)	Rats	Rat knees developed muscle atrophy within 2 wk of immobilization, in addition to the connective tissue changes noted in Table 48-2.
MacDougall et al (1977) (14)	Humans	Healthy persons immobilized in elbow casts for 5 wk had a 5% decrease in arm circumference and a 35% decrease in elbow extension strength.
MacDougall et al (1980) (15)	Humans	Healthy persons with an elbow immobilized in a cast after 5–6 wk had a decrease in the mean cross-sectional area of type II muscle fibers and a decrease in elbow extension strength.
Mayer et al (1981) (16)	Cats	Ankle and knee joints of cats immobilized at 90 degrees for 17–29 wk resulted in reduced motor unit tetanic force output, loss of maximal twitch, and decrease in type I and IIA fiber size.
Witzmann et al (1982) (17)	Rats	Decreased tetanic tension found in 3 different hind-limb muscles at 1–3 days of immobilization.
Witzmann et al (1983) (18)	Rats	Peak tension from intermittent pulses of electrical stimulation of the soleus muscle declined more rapidly after 6 wk of hind-limb immobilization compared to controls, suggesting increased fatigability. Lower levels of ATP and glycogen and higher levels of lactic acid concentration were also found in the immobilized soleus muscles.
Booth (1987) (19)	Rats	Skeletal muscle atrophy in the hind limbs of immobilized rats starts within 1–3 days, with peak loss occurring during the subsequent 5 days.
Lindboe and Platou (1984) (20)	Humans	Lower limbs immobilized in a hip-to-ankle cast with the knee in 15 degrees of flexion had a 14%–17% decrease in muscle fiber size after 72 hr of immobilization.

control limbs. This indicates that muscles of immobilized limbs have increased fatigability. Collectively, these animal and human studies demonstrated a consistent reduction of muscle size (atrophy) and strength and an increase in fatigability in response to immobilization ranging from a few days to a few weeks.

CONTRACTURE BIOMECHANICS

Data from studies using animal models and humans with immobilized joints indicate that contractures are associated with biomechanical changes. In a contracture, the soft-tissue length is shortened and the viscoelastic properties of the soft tissue are changed. The ROM of the joint decreases and movement, accomplished within the available range, is more difficult because of increased stiffness of the joint. This increased stiffness, or increase in the effort or torque required to move a joint with a contracture, is the result of the periarticular soft-tissue viscoelastic changes (13,21). Muscles acting across a joint with a contracture shorten and become atrophied. Normally, the strength of muscle contraction is a function of its physiologic resting length and cross-sectional area. Accordingly, muscles around a joint contracture become weaker, as their contractile length and area are reduced.

Clinically, depending on location, the limb or body part with a joint contracture is less likely to participate in or perform functional tasks. Ankle, knee, or hip contractures commonly interfere with normal ambulation and mobility patterns and result in high energy costs when the patient adapts by using postural substitutions to compensate. An ankle plantarflexion contracture of at least 15 degrees, for example, prevents normal progression of loading over the supporting foot during the stance phase. This results in premature heel-off during the mid-stance phase and excessive weight bearing by the metatarsal heads. To compensate, the patient will often attempt to lean the trunk forward during the stance phase or hyperextend the knee, which can result in genu recurvatum. This compensatory motion results in increased energy expenditure by the trunk muscles to maintain trunk control (1).

Perry et al (22) found that knee flexion contractures between 15 and 30 degrees will increase demand on the quadriceps to support the body weight during the stance phase by increasing tension from 22% to 51% of normal strength. The work by Potter and Kirby (23) supported the findings of increased quadriceps activity. They demonstrated a linear increase in electromyographic activity of the vastus lateralis during standing with simulated knee flexion contractures of increasing magnitude (0–40 degrees). This increased muscle activity greatly increases energy cost and reduces endurance during standing and walking. Knee flexion contractures also impair standing balance by altering the center of pressure (24). The nonambulating, supine patient with knee flexion contractures may be prone to developing pressure sores on the heels or sacrum.

A hip flexion contracture of 30 degrees reduces hip extension and is accommodated by increasing the lumbar lordosis, by walking in increased plantarflexion with excessive weight bearing on the metatarsal heads, and by standing with the unaffected knee in flexion to equalize limb height. These substitutions also increase energy cost during standing and walking. Because the hamstring muscles cross both the hip and the knee joints, patients with a hip flexion contracture shorten their hamstring muscles and may also develop a secondary knee flexion contracture. A hip adduction contracture may occur in isolation or in association with a hip flexion contracture. If the abnormal adduction is unilateral, scissoring during the swing phase of gait may impair ambulation. Bilateral hip adduction contractures will have a more pronounced effect on ambulation and may compromise perineal hygiene in the nonambulating patient. Patients with several joints affected by contractures or other limitations have markedly increased energy costs and limited ability to compensate posturally.

Activities of daily living other than ambulation, such as feeding, grooming, dressing, and reaching and grasping objects, are typically affected by impaired ROM associated with upper-limb joint contractures. However, in wheelchair or crutch users, lower-limb amputees, persons with spinal cord injury, and other persons who routinely depend on use of the upper limbs for locomotion and mobility tasks, the presence of upper-limb joint contractures may profoundly affect these important functions.

SPASTICITY AND CONTRACTURE FORMATION

Young and Wiegner (25) suggested that joint contracture formation in the presence of spasticity may differ from that in joints that are merely immobilized. Spasticity is a pathologic increase in the tone and stretch reflexes of a muscle, due to a loss of the normal inhibitory control by upper motor neuron pathways. Spasticity is often associated with other clinical signs, such as muscle rigidity, weakness, and clonus. A detailed discussion of spasticity is provided in Chapter 47. Although the contribution to contracture formation from spasticity is a well-known clinical phenomenon, relatively sparse objective reports exist on the development of spasticity-related contractures.

Descending upper motor neuron pathways in the cerebral cortex, brain stem, or spinal cord directly or indirectly influence the excitatory or inhibitory activity of α motor neurons, γ motor neurons, Golgi tendon organs, Renshaw cells, and muscle spindles. Pathologic lesions or conditions affecting upper motor neuron pathways, such as stroke, spinal cord injury, cerebral palsy, traumatic brain injury, and multiple sclerosis, result in diminished regulatory influence and loss of voluntary motor control. Spontaneous, uncontrolled, primitive-type hyperactive reflexes and pathologically increased muscle tone ensue (Fig. 48-5) (26). It is this increase in muscle tone and accompanying paralysis or weakness, not just the immobility, that favors posturing of an affected limb in a position that can lead to contracture formation. In addition to the biochemical changes in joint synovium, ligaments, cartilage, and surrounding muscle described earlier, gross changes in muscle, including increased rigidity in the relative absence of voluntary contraction and muscle shortening in the absence of voluntary contraction, add a muscle stiffness factor to joint contractures. This additional factor may cause molecular and gross changes that differ from the changes caused by immobilization alone.

PHYSIATRIC ASSESSMENT

Appropriate physiatric management of a contracture begins with a careful clinical assessment of the patient. This assessment should include a review of the medical history for predisposing or associated factors, a determination of the joint or joints involved, and a classification of the contracture type. Neurologic evaluation is also warranted to assess the integrity of this system. A functional neuromuscular examination will identify the functional impact of the contracture. An accurate determination of the ROM of the involved joint(s) is critical to determine the severity of involvement and to provide a baseline for subsequent measurements if intervention is planned.

CONSERVATIVE TREATMENT

Range of Motion and Stretching

Despite the best prevention efforts of patients, caregivers, and health care personnel, contractures do occur. Treatment options for an established contracture include a combination of 1) active and active-assisted ROM exercises, 2) inhibition of shortened agonist muscles, and 3) sustained passive stretching (Table 48-4). Active ROM exercises attempt to reduce the contracture through activation of (antagonist) muscles that oppose the muscle shortened by the contracture (e.g., extensor muscles in the case of a flexion contracture). This activation may not be possible in the presence of neurologic disease. In active-assisted ROM exercises, active movement by the patient in the direction opposing the contracture is assisted by a helper.

Table 48-4: Principles of Conservative Treatment and Prevention of Contractures
Active range of motion (opposing muscles shortened by the contracture)
Active-assisted range of motion to weak agonist muscles (muscles opposing those shortened by the contracture)
Selective inhibition of shortened muscle(s)
Passive stretching (with or without therapeutic heating)
Manual stretch
Orthoses
Serial casting
Traction/pulley devices
Functional positioning

Passive stretching differs from passive ROM exercises. The former implies an attempt to take the range of an involved joint beyond its present limit. The duration of the stretch will usually vary with the severity of the contracture. Other practical limiting factors in stretching are the endurance of the therapist applying the stretch and the tolerance level of the patient who might be uncomfortable during the stretch. Manually applied stretching typically continues for 30 to 120 seconds. Stretching of longer duration is usually applied with the use of mechanical devices.

The duration of mechanical stretching will usually vary depending on the severity of the contracture and the tolerance of the patient. Although there is no consensus on rating the severity of a contracture, estimation of contracture severity may take factors into account other than ROM. These factors could include chronicity, degree of functional impairment, or presence of associated spasticity.

For contractures that are relatively mild (limited to approximately 80%–95% of functional ROM), sustained stretching for 20 to 30 minutes twice a day has been suggested (27,28). For more severe contractures (<80% of the functional ROM), stretching for a duration of 30 to 45 minutes or longer may be necessary. Several methods for applying prolonged stretch, using a variety of limb-weighting and mechanical pulley systems, have been described (29–33). These techniques are used most often on large joints, such as the hip, knee, and shoulder. Although literature support for these techniques is scant and has methodologic limitations, low-load, prolonged stretching can reduce contractures and may be superior to manual stretching techniques.

For severe contractures, application of therapeutic heat to the affected joint capsule or musculotendinous junction can enhance the effectiveness of stretching—the elasticity of connective tissue increases when heated in the therapeutic range (40°–43°C) (34,35). Ultrasound is established as a popular method of heating contractures of large joints or joints covered by abundant layers of tissue (36,37). However, depending on the size and location of the involved joint, other heating modalities may accomplish similar objectives. For example, contractures of small, relatively superficial joints, such as metacarpophalangeal or interphalangeal joints, may be more easily heated with a paraffin bath immersion.

Therapeutic stretching with or without heat takes advantage of the elastic properties of contractile tissue and the viscous or plastic properties of contractile and noncontractile tissue. Elastic properties represent spring-like behavior in response to a stretch where the elongation is temporary or recoverable. Viscous properties refer to permanent linear deformation that remains after the stretching force is removed. High-force, short-duration stretching favors elastic tissue deformation, whereas low-force, long-duration stretching favors permanent viscous deformation desirable to reduce contractures (29,38). Serial addition of new sarcomeres accounts for increased length in muscle. This lengthening occurs in response to prolonged stretching of tissue over a several-week period (33,39–41). In noncontractile connective tissue, length increases when the force of stretching elongates the tissue.

Regardless of method, all stretching must be applied with caution. Tendon rupture, joint dislocation, and bone fracture are possible complications from overly aggressive stretching. High-force stretching is more likely to result in structural weakening of connective tissues than is low-force stretching, especially at lower tissue temperatures (35,38). Also, increasing the distance from the joint axis to the point on a limb where the stretching force is applied will greatly increase the magnitude of the force and the risk of injury.

Dynamic Splinting, Pulley Systems, and Serial Casting

Dynamic Splints

Dynamic splints, also called *low-load prolonged stretch* (LLPS) orthoses, are used to reduce contractures by applying prolonged, low-intensity stretching across the joint. Dynamic splints employ a static-base orthosis, usually on the dorsal or ventral aspect of a limb. The static supporting part of the orthosis extends just proximal to the joint with the contracture. The joint itself is usually left unencumbered to allow movement in the direction of contracture reduction. A separate part of the dynamic splint supports part of the limb or digit immediately distal to the involved joint. Tension is applied to this distal part of the limb or digit and across the involved joint, through the use of an elastic band, wire, or spring device, opposing the direction of the contracture shortening. For example, extension is applied for a flexion contracture. This allows persistent tension that is adjustable during the course of treatment. Some dynamic splints are "homemade" out of thermoplastic materials. Commercial prefabricated dynamic splints are available and have been used for reduction of contractures at hand, wrist, knee, and ankle joints.

Mixed results have been reported using dynamic splints for the treatment of flexion contractures of the knee, elbow, and proximal interphalangeal joints of the hand (42–48). Important factors to consider in the use of dynamic splinting for contracture reduction include capacity for patient compliance, the type and chronicity of the pathologic process contributing to the contracture (e.g., progressive systemic sclerosis versus central nervous system disease), the amount of time the splint is applied, and the duration of treatment. Dynamic splints are commonly worn for 8 to 10 hours; however, longer and shorter durations have been reported (45).

Passive Weight and Pulley Systems

An alternative approach to applying low-intensity stretch to reduce joint contractures is the use of a passive weighted traction or pulley system (29,30,32,33). These techniques have been used primarily for flexion contractures of the large joints (hips and knees) of the lower limb. The patient is positioned on a table or bed for stabilization. A stretch force (against the direction of the contracture shortening) is applied across the joint by pulling the free part of the limb (leg or thigh) into extension with a weighted traction apparatus. Similar forces can be generated either by having the patient lie supine with the hip joint supported (and padded) but most of the thigh and leg extending off the table unsupported, or by lying prone with the knee joint supported but the leg partially extending past the table. The weight of the unsupported limb and added weight to the distal limb (thigh or ankle) from a weighted traction and pulley apparatus produce extension force to help reduce the contracture. Weights of 2 to 5 kg or 5% to 10% of body weight have been used. Authors have suggested a treatment time of 20 to 30 minutes or more for 3 to 5 days, depending on patient tolerance. This method of contracture reduction reportedly is better tolerated than high-intensity, brief-duration, manually applied stretching (32). Contracture reductions in the 20- to 70-degree range and greater have been reported (30,32,33).

Serial Casting

Another method of contracture reduction that is popular and well established is the application of serial casting. In serial casting, the joint contracture is measured and cast padding is applied to protect nerves and bony prominences on the part of the limb to be enclosed in the cast. The affected joint is then manually stretched to reduce the contracture, and held in a position of maximally tolerated stretch while a plaster or fiberglass cast is applied.

After the initial cast is worn for several days, the process is repeated as a series of casts are applied at weekly intervals. Between cast changes, the limb is inspected for pressure areas (subsequent cast modifications or padding adjustments are made as necessary). The joint ROM is remeasured, and the limb is taken through its maximum possible range prior to reapplication of the cast. Some protocols call for cutting and removing half of the cast (bivalving). This leaves half of the cast to maintain the joint in stretch and converts the cast into a splint, which can be removed to facilitate better hygiene and allow the skin to be checked for pressure areas. This type of cast is called a *drop-out cast.*

Serial casting has been used to reduce adult and pediatric contractures in a variety of upper- and lower-limb joints, including elbow flexion, wrist extension, knee flexion, and ankle plantarflexion contractures. Favorable results have been reported using serial casting alone or in combination with other methods to reduce contractures. These reports included contractures associated with burns and congenital and acquired neuromuscular disorders (49–55).

ENHANCEMENT OF TREATMENT

An important way to enhance the effect of other methods of contracture treatment is to encourage use of the affected limb in functional activities between or during (as possible) treatment. These activities could include bed mobility, transfers, self-care, and other activities of daily living, as well as standing and in some cases ambulation. Use of the limb for functional activities can aid the objectives of contracture reduction and may even assist in preserving or enhancing function of uninvolved joints and limbs.

When a contracture is associated with increased abnormal muscle tone, an attempt to reduce the abnormal tone with available therapeutic modalities or pharmacologic intervention may enhance the rate and outcome of contracture reduction. For contractures associated with an intact nerve supply, strengthening exercises, relaxation techniques, and biofeedback may also enhance the effect of contracture reduction treatments. There is also evidence that electrical stimulation, with constant direct current, may be a useful adjunct therapy for contracture reduction in the future (56,57).

PREVENTION

Contractures may develop in a few days to weeks under the right conditions. Conversely, contracture treatments may require several weeks to months, even under ideal circumstances. The time and effort (expense) required to successfully reduce a contracture add to the already increasing costs of rehabilitation and other segments of our health care system. The human cost of contractures, in terms of disability, is difficult to quantify but can be devastating. These factors make it imperative that the physiatrist and other rehabilitation team members aggressively initiate measures to prevent contractures from developing.

Contracture prevention should be integrated into the nursing care plan or home care plan (58). The patient who is temporarily or permanently immobilized should be progressively remobilized as early as possible. Passive, active-assisted, or active ROM exercises should be employed routinely. Placing paretic patients in appropriate positions of function, rather than positions of perceived comfort, can help them to gain or maintain mobility. Finally, education of the patient and family about the effects of immobility and the preventive aspects of mobility is an essential part of the rehabilitation process.

For the surgical patient after hip and knee operative procedures, continuous passive motion (CPM) machines have been used widely to both prevent and reduce contractures by obtaining functional ROM (59,60). A CPM machine is an electrically powered mechanical device on which the patient places his or her thigh and leg, usually while lying supine (59). The CPM machine passively flexes the hip and knee simultaneously at variable rates of speed before returning to extension. ROM settings and speed of the flexion-extension cycles are varied according to patient comfort and the condition being treated. Usually, CPM is prescribed for intermittent use. Slow and gradually increasing passive motion is well tolerated. Although CPM machines have been used most commonly for hip and knee mobilization, more recently, CPM machines have been manufactured for use with shoulder, elbow, wrist, and hand joints (61).

SURGICAL TREATMENT

Despite the best preventive efforts of the rehabilitation team, some contractures do not respond to conservative measures and may require surgical intervention. The risks, benefits, and goals of surgical contracture release should be carefully considered. Whenever possible, corrective surgery for contractures should be performed by a surgeon experienced in the evaluation, surgical technique, and postoperative management of contractures. Several authors have described surgical procedures for the correction of contractures of upper-limb joints due to various pathologic etiologies. Instead of presenting an exhaustive review, some representative reports of some of these procedures are summarized here.

Surgical Correction of Upper-Limb Contractures

Surgical correction is indicated for upper-limb contractures after failure of conservative treatment, in order to restore lost functional use. Mih and Wolf (62) reported on surgical procedures for a series of pediatric patients with elbow capsular contractures. The contractures in most of their nine patients were of a traumatic etiology. All had had unsuccessful conservative therapy prior to surgical referral. A lateral approach was used to release the anterior and posterior capsules. The authors reported an average improvement in elbow extension from 47 to 15 degrees and in mean angle of flexion from 102 to 124 degrees, and a total arc of motion increase from 55 to 108 degrees, by an average of 17 months after surgery. Their patients were treated postoperatively with ROM exercises and splinting.

Husband and Hastings (63) reported similar favorable results in a series of seven patients with elbow contractures. Their study included preoperative and postoperative assessments of functional activities on a 12-point scale. The scores improved from a mean of 5.1 points to a postoperative mean of 10.4 points.

In a series of 12 patients with elbow flexion contractures, Jones and Savoie (64) reported a mean postoperative improvement of 35 degrees. They described the use of an arthroscopic technique for release of the elbow joint capsule. Their study did not include functional assessment.

Abbiati et al (65) described a new surgical procedure for releasing chronic flexion contractures of the proximal interphalangeal joint of the fingers. Their midlateral approach, surgical incision of the accessory collateral ligament and flexor sheath, and excision of the volar plate and check-rein ligaments, is combined with postoperative use of a dynamic splint and active and passive ROM exercises. In their series of 19 patients with a preoperative extension deficit that ranged from 70 to 90 degrees, 11 patients (57.9%) achieved full extension of the proximal interphalangeal joint and 8 patients achieved a decrease in extension deficit range from 10 to 15 degrees. No functional assessment was included in their study.

Surgical Correction of Lower-Limb Contractures

Lower-limb contractures commonly interfere with important functional activities including transfers, standing, and ambulation. Contractures can alter the joint biomechanics and energy requirements involved in these activities, which can make them difficult to impossible to perform. Many surgical procedures for the correction of lower-limb contractures have been reported in the literature. Surgical lengthening of the associated muscle tendons, with or without muscle transfer, has been the mainstay of corrective procedures.

Frawley et al (66) reviewed the results of anterior surgical release of hip flexion contracture in a series of 38 children (57 hips) with spina bifida. All patients had a preoperative flexion contracture greater than 30 degrees. A good postoperative outcome, defined as flexion deformity less than 30 degrees, was achieved in 43 hips (75%). Surgical results were unrelated to age or neurologic level, but correlated well with ambulation ability at the time of evaluation.

Szalay et al (67) reported on a series of 29 pediatric patients with extension-abduction contractures of the hip because of cerebral palsy. These patients were unable to sit adequately. The mean age of patients in this series was 10.5 years and several had associated spasticity, athetosis, or rigidity. Most (17) of the patients in the series were successfully treated with conservative measures (stretching, active ROM, wheelchair modification). However, 12 patients required surgical correction, which included proximal hamstring release with or without section of the gluteus maximus insertion into the iliotibial band and femur. Ten patients also required release of either the joint capsule or the external rotators of the hip. All patients had a good outcome and regained the ability to sit in a wheelchair.

Surgical Correction of Burn Wound Contractures

Various types of surgical procedures are available to treat burn wound contractures, depending on the amount of scarring of the skin adjacent to the contracture, the anatomic area involved, the size and extent of the contracture, and the patient's functional needs. Kraemer et al (68) reviewed 53 patients seen for surgical correction of burn contractures. In their series, the incidence of contractures requiring surgical release was almost four times as high (7.8%) in children treated acutely for burns, compared to adults (2%). The most common anatomic areas involved were the hand (35%), the head and neck (30%), and the axilla (21%). Surgical release of the contracture followed by closure of the skin defect with either a skin graft, Z-plasty, or a rotational flap was the most common procedure. Successful functional outcome after surgery depended primarily on anatomic site of the contracture, with better results obtained for hand contractures and the worst results obtained for head, neck, and axilla contractures. Patient demographics, type of operation, and timing of surgery did not affect surgical outcome.

Keenan et al (69) described a procedure for surgical release of the hamstring tendons for correction of knee flexion contractures in 30 patients (46 limbs). The patients in their series had spasticity from central nervous system disorders (stroke, brain injury, spinal cord injury, multiple sclerosis) and 26 (87%) were nonambulatory. Following hamstring release, the average knee position improved from 61.4 degrees of flexion preoperatively to 6 degrees of flexion postoperatively. Thirteen (43%) of the patients regained the ability to ambulate. The authors noted that 5 patients (16.7%) had postoperative complications, including 2 patients who eventually required amputation.

Marshall et al (70) described a similar hamstring release procedure that they used in a prospective series of 28 patients with myelomeningocele who had knee flexion contractures. The mean knee flexion contracture, which was 39 degrees prior to surgery, improved to 5 degrees postoperatively. Ten patients in this series were nonambulators, with involvement at a thoracic neurosegmental level, and remained nonambulatory. Surgery in nonambulators was performed to improve transfers and sitting. Patients with involvement at a L3–L4 neurosegmental level and to a lesser extent, those with a L5–S1 involvement had the most marked improvement in walking ability. Of these patients, 4 preoperative nonambulators became nonfunctional ambulators, 3 nonfunctional ambulators became household ambulators, 4 household ambulators became community ambulators, and 3 community ambulators remained so postoperatively. Although the indications for surgery were reported in this study, no mention of attempted conservative management of the contractures was included.

Damron et al (71) retrospectively reviewed the results of surgical lengthening of the Achilles tendon for gastrocnemius-soleus (ankle plantarflexion) contracture in patients with cerebral palsy. Surgical correction resulted in highly significant initial improvement in dorsiflexion of 25 degrees, from a 17-degree lack of dorsiflexion to 8 degrees of positive dorsiflexion. Improvements were maintained for 7 years postoperatively. Curiously, the average arc of motion was not significantly different postoperatively. The initial level of ambulation was improved in 55% of the patients and maintained in 45%. The authors also reviewed the records of 68 additional cerebral palsy patients with ankle plantarflexion contractures who were not treated surgically. Among this nonsurgical group, no significant spontaneous improvement in ankle dorsiflexion was noted and in only 12 (18%) did the ambulation level improve. Seven (11%) in this group showed a decrease in ambulation level. It should be noted that no conservative alternative to surgical treatment in the nonsurgical group was described.

Mulier et al (72) reviewed several surgical procedures for ankle plantarflexion contracture associated with varus deformity of the hindfoot (equinovarus deformity). They described results of a modified procedure (split posterior tibial tendon transfer combined with Achilles tendon lengthening) to correct equinovarus deformity in 17 children with spasticity. Tendon lengthening combined with tendon transfer procedures for spastic or paralytic contracture attempts to restore equilibrium around the joint. Excellent or good results with marked improvement in the ankle and foot deformity and qualitative gait improvements were reported. Outcome was poor in 2 patients in whom the procedure failed due to technical errors.

CONCLUSIONS

Many time-honored nonsurgical treatments for contractures are available to the physiatrist and rehabilitation team. Surgical procedures have improved. Recent reports in the expanding body of literature on contracture treatment include more information about functional assessment and outcomes. New adjunct therapies for the treatment of contracture and its contributing factors appear to be on the horizon. This therapeutic progress suggests that the incidence of contractures, especially in the rehabilitation setting, should decrease in the future. Despite the advancement of therapeutic techniques, the best treatment of contractures continues to be prevention, through vigilance and early intervention by an experienced rehabilitation team.

REFERENCES

1. Perry J. Contractures: a historical perspective. *Clin Orthop* 1987;219:8–14.
2. Halar EM, Bell KR. Contractures and other deleterious effects of immobility. In: DeLisa JA, ed. *Rehabilitation medicine principles and practice*. Philadelphia: JB Lippincott, 1988:448–462.
3. Stolov WC. Musculoskeletal problems: mobility problems of the muscle-joint unit. In: Basmajian JV, Kirby RL, eds. *Medical rehabilitation*. Baltimore: Williams & Wilkins, 1984.
4. Akeson WH, Woo SLY, Amiel D, et al. The connective tissue response to immobility: biochemical changes in periarticular connective tissue of the immobilized rabbit knee. *Clin Orthop* 1973;93:356–362.
5. Nicholas JJ. Joint contractures. *Phys Med Rehabil Clin N Am* 1994;5:803–813.
6. Ely LW, Mensor MC. Studies on the immobilization of the normal joint. *Surg Gynecol Obstet* 1933;57:212–215.
7. Hall MC. Cartilage changes after experimental immobilization of the knee joint of the young rat. *J Bone Joint Surg [Am]* 1963;45:36–44.
8. Evans EB, Eggers GWN, Butler JK, Blumel J. Experimental immobilization and remobilization of rat knee joints. *J Bone Joint Surg [Am]* 1960;42:737–758.
9. Thaxter TH, Mann RA, Anderson CE. Degeneration of immobilized knee joints in rats. *J Bone Joint Surg [Am]* 1965;47:567–572.
10. Enneking WF, Horowitz M. The intra-articular effects of immobilization on the human knee. *J Bone Joint Surg [Am]* 1972;54:973–985.
11. Akeson WH, Amiel D, Abel MF, et al. *Clin Orthop* 1987;219: 28–37.
12. Woo SLY, Matthews JV, Akeson WH, et al. Connective tissue response to immobility: correlative study of biomechanical measurements of normal and immobilized rabbit knees. *Arthritis Rheum* 1975;18:257–263.
13. Woo SL-Y, Gomez MA, Seguchi Y, et al. Measurement of mechanical properties of ligament substance from a bone-ligament-bone preparation. *J Orthop Res* 1983;1:22–29.
14. MacDougall JD, Ward GR, Sale DG, Sutton JR. Biochemical adaptation of human skeletal muscle to heavy resistance training and immobilization. *J Appl Physiol* 1977;43:700–703.
15. MacDougall JD, Elder GCB, Sale DG, et al. Effects of strength training and immobilization on human muscle fibres. *Eur J Appl Physiol* 1980;43:25–34.
16. Mayer RF, Burke RE, Toop J, et al. The effect of long-term immobi-

lization on the motor unit population of the cat medial gastrocnemius muscle. *Neuroscience* 1981;6:725–733.

17. Witzmann FA, Kim DH, Fitts RH. Hindlimb immobilization: length-tension and contractile properties of skeletal muscle. *J Appl Physiol* 1982;53:335–345.

18. Witzmann FA, Kim DH, Fitts RH. Effect of hindlimb immobilization on the fatigability of skeletal muscle. *J Appl Physiol* 1983;54:1242–1247.

19. Booth FW. Physiologic and biochemical effects of immobilization on muscle. *Clin Orthop* 1987;219:15–20.

20. Lindboe CF, Platou CS. Effect of immobilization of short duration on the muscle fiber size. *Clin Physiol* 1984;4:183–189.

21. Woo SL-Y, Gomez MA, Young-Kyun W, Akeson WH. Mechanical properties of tendons and ligaments. II. The relationships of immobilization and exercise on tissue remodeling. *Biorheology* 1982;19:397–408.

22. Perry J, Antonelli D, Ford W. Analysis of knee joint forces during flexed knee stance. *J Bone Joint Surg [Am]* 1975;57:961–967.

23. Potter PJ, Kirby RL. Relationship between electromyographic activity of the vastus lateralis while standing and the extent of bilateral simulated knee-flexion contractures. *Am J Phys Med Rehabil* 1991;70:301–305.

24. Potter PJ, Kirby RL, MacLeod DA. The effects of simulated knee-flexion contractures on standing balance. *Am J Phys Med Rehabil* 1990;69:144–147.

25. Young RR, Wiegner AW. Spasticity. *Clin Orthop* 1987;219:50–62.

26. Botte MJ, Nickel VL, Akeson WH. Spasticity and contracture. *Clin Orthop* 1988;233:7–18.

27. Bohannon RW. Effect of repeated eight minute muscle loading on the angle of straight leg raising. *Phys Ther* 1984;64: 491–497.

28. Bohannon RW, Larkin PA. Passive ankle dorsiflexion increases after a regimen of tilt table: wedge board standing. *Phys Ther* 1985;65:1676–1678.

29. Sapega AA, Quedenfeld TC, Moyer RA, Butler RA. Biophysical factors in range of motion exercise. *Physician Sports Med* 1981;9:57–65.

30. Kottke FJ, Pauley DL, Ptak RA. The rationale for prolonged stretching for correction of shortening of connective tissue. *Arch Phys Med Rehabil* 1966;47:345–352.

31. Rizk TE, Christopher RP, Pinnels RS, et al. Adhesive capsulitis (frozen shoulder): a new approach to its management. *Arch Phys Med Rehabil* 1983;64:29–32.

32. Light KE, Nuzik S, Personius W, Barstrom A. Low-load prolonged stretch vs. high-load brief stretch in treating knee contractures. *Phys Ther* 1984;64:330–333.

33. Bohannon RW, Chavis D, Larkin P, et al. Effectiveness of repeated prolonged loading for increasing flexion in knees demonstrating postoperative stiffness. *Phys Ther* 1985;65:494–496.

34. Lehmann JF, Masock AJ, Warren CG, Koblanski JN. Effect of therapeutic temperatures on tendon extensibility. *Arch Phys Med Rehabil* 1970;51:481–487.

35. Warren CG, Lehmann JF, Koblanski JN. Elongation of rat tail tendon: effect of load and temperature. *Arch Phys Med Rehabil* 1971;52:465–474.

36. Lehmann JF, deLateur BJ, Warren CG, Stonebridge JB. Heating of joint structures by ultrasound. *Arch Phys Med Rehabil* 1968; 49:28–30.

37. Lehmann JF, Fordyce WE, Rathbun LA, et al. Clinical evaluation of a new approach in the treatment of contracture associated with hip fracture after internal fixation. *Arch Phys Med Rehabil* 1961;42:95.

38. Taylor DC, Dalton JD, Seaber AV, Garrett WE. Viscoelastic properties of muscle-tendon units; the biomechanical effects of stretching. *Am J Sports Med* 1990;18: 300–309.

39. Tabary JC, Tabary C, Tardieu C, Tardieu G. Physiological and structural changes in the cat soleus muscle due to immobilization at different lengths by plaster casts. *J Physiol* 1972;224: 231–244.

40. Tardieu C, Tabary JC, Tabary C, Tardieu G. Adaptation of connective tissue length to immobilization in the lengthened and shortened position in cat soleus muscle. *J Physiol (Paris)* 1982;78:214–220.

41. Williams PE, Goldspink G. Changes in sarcomere length and physiological properties in immobilized muscle. *J Anat* 1978;127:459–468.

42. Hepburn G, Crivelli K. Use of elbow Dynasplint for reduction of elbow flexion contracture: a case study. *J Orthop Sports Phys Ther* 1984;5:269–272.

43. Seeger MW, Furst DE. Effects of splinting in the treatment of hand contractures in progressive systemic sclerosis. *Am J Occup Ther* 1987;41:118–121.

44. Jansen CM, Windau JE, Bonutti PM, Brillhart MV. Treatment of a knee contracture using a knee orthosis incorporating stress-relaxation techniques. *Phys Ther* 1996;76:182–186.

45. Nuismer BA, Ekes AM, Holm MB. The use of low-load prolonged stretch devices in rehabilitation programs in the Pacific Northwest. *Am J Occup Ther* 1997;51:538–543.

46. Callahan AD, McEntee P. Splinting proximal interphalangeal joint flexion contractures: a new design. *Am J Occup Ther* 1986;40:408–413.

47. Prosser R. Splinting in the management of proximal interphalangeal joint flexion contracture. *J Hand Ther* 1996;9: 378–386.

48. Steffen TM, Mollinger LA. Low-load, prolonged stretch in the treatment of knee flexion contractures in nursing home residents. *Phys Ther* 1995;75:886–897.

49. Moseley AM. The effect of casting combined with stretching on passive ankle dorsiflexion in adults with traumatic head injuries. *Phys Ther* 1997;77:240–247.

50. Booth BJ, Doyle M, Montgomery J. Serial casting for the management of spasticity in the head-injured adult. *Phys Ther* 1983;63:1960–1966.

51. Cherry DB, Weigand GM. Plaster drop-out casts as a dynamic means to reduce muscle contracture. A case report. *Phys Ther* 1981;61:1601–1603.

52. Zander CL, Healy NL. Elbow flexion contractures treated with serial casts and conservative therapy. *J Hand Surg [Am]* 1992;17:694–697.

53. Johnson J, Silverberg R. Serial casting of the lower extremity to correct contractures during the acute phase of burn care. *Phys Ther* 1994;75:262–266.

54. Cusick BD. Splints and casts. Managing foot deformity in children with neuromotor disorders. *Phys Ther* 1988;12:1903–1912.

55. Ridgway CL, Daugherty MB, Warden GD. Serial casting as a technique to correct burn scar contractures. A case report. *J Burn Care Rehabil* 1991;12:67–72.

56. Akai M, Shirasaki Y, Tateishi T. Electrical stimulation on joint contracture: an experiment in rat model with direct current.

57. Tart RP, Dahners LE. Effects of electrical stimulation on joint contracture in a rat model. *J Orthop Res* 1989;7:538–542.

58. Getz PA, Blossom BM. Preventing contractures: the little extras that help so much. *RN* 1982;December:45–48.

59. Richardson WJ, Garrett WE. Clinical uses of continuous passive motion. *Contemp Orthop* 1985;10:75–79.

60. Frank C, Akeson WH, Woo SL-Y, et al. Physiology and therapeutic value of passive joint motion. *Clin Orthop* 1984;185:113–125.

61. Bentham S, Brereton WDS, Cochrane IW, Lyttle D. Continuous passive motion device for hand rehabilitation. *Arch Phys Med Rehabil* 1987;68:248–250.

62. Mih MD, Wolf FG. Surgical release of elbow-capsular contracture in pediatric patients. *J Pediatr Orthop* 1994;14:458–461.

63. Husband JB, Hastings H. The lateral approach for operative release of post-traumatic contracture of the elbow. *J Bone Joint Surg [Am]* 1990;72: 1353–1358.

64. Jones GS, Savoie FH III. Arthroscopic capsular release of flexion contractures (arthrofibrosis) of the elbow. *J Arthroscopic Surg* 1993;9:277–283.

65. Abbiati G, Delaria G, Saporiti E, et al. The treatment of chronic flexion contractures of the proximal interphalangeal joint. *J Hand Surg [Br]* 1995;20: 3:385–389.

66. Frawley PA, Broughton NS, Menelaus MB. Anterior release for fixed flexion deformity of the hip in spina bifida. *J Bone Joint Surg [Br]* 1996;78:299–302.

67. Szalay EA, Roach JW, Houkom JA, et al. Extension-abduction contracture of the spastic hip. *J Pediatr Orthop* 1986;6:1–6.

68. Kraemer MD, Jones T, Deitch EA. Burn contractures: incidence, predisposing factors, and results of surgical therapy. *J Burn Care Rehabil* 1988;9:261–265.

69. Keenan MA, Ure K, Smith CW, Jordan C. Hamstring release for knee flexion contracture in spastic adults. *Clin Orthop* 1988;236:221–226.

70. Marshall PD, Broughton NS, Menelaus MB, Graham HK. Surgical release of knee flexion contractures in myelomeningocele. *J Bone Joint Surg [Br]* 1996;78:912–916.

71. Damron TA, Greenwald TA, Breed AL. Chronologic outcome of surgical tendoachilles lengthening and natural history of gastroc-soleus contracture in cerebral palsy. *Clin Orthop* 1994;301:249–255.

72. Mulier T, Moens P, Molenaers G, et al. Split posterior tibial tendon transfer through the interosseus membrane in spastic equinovarus deformity. *Foot Ankle Int* 1995;16:754–759.

Chapter 49

Movement Disorders, Including Tremors

Kathleen D. Francis
Allen J. Rubin

Movement disorders are characterized by intrusions of involuntary movements or impairment or loss of extrapyramidal modulation of movements. Ataxia, which arises from cerebellar dysfunction, and paresis, which arises from pyramidal tract dysfunction, are typically considered separate from movement disorders and are not discussed here. Such disorders generally either are structural diseases of the basal ganglia or its related nuclei, or result from neurochemical dysfunction in neuronal projections to or from the basal ganglia. Clinically, abnormalities in movement, posture, and tone predominate. Disorders of perception, cognition, and emotion are often present as concomitant features (1).

Traditionally, these disorders have been referred to as *extrapyramidal*, since the basal ganglia were thought to project to the spinal cord via pathways distinct from the pyramidal tract. More recently it has become apparent that the basal ganglia project through multiple feedback loops to the cerebral cortex and thence to the spinal cord through the pyramidal tract, but the term *extrapyramidal* has persisted.

Essentially, patients with movement disorders can have only two types of defects: a positive defect, referring to the presence of an unwanted involuntary movement (e.g., chorea, tremor, dystonia), or a negative defect, that is, the inability to perform a desired movement (e.g., akinesia, bradykinesia). When positive signs predominate, the disease is classified as *hyperkinetic*, while preponderance of negative defects leads to classification as *hypokinetic* (Table 49-1). Parkinson disease is the classic example of a hypokinetic disorder, while dystonia and essential tremor are examples of hyperkinetic disorders. The classification remains a useful one, although these distinctions become blurred in many conditions, such as in Huntington disease (HD), which is characterized as largely hyperkinetic in the early and mid stages, with hypokinetic features often becoming prominent late in the course.

Extrapyramidal movement disorders tend to share certain characteristics, such as abolishment of the abnormal movements during sleep and exacerbation with anxiety or excitement. Some, such as tics and certain dystonias, may be transiently suppressed voluntarily or elicited by particular stimuli, while others cannot be inhibited by any volitional action.

ANATOMY AND NEUROPHYSIOLOGY

There are five major subdivisions of the movement control system: 1) cerebral cortex, including motor, premotor, and somatosensory cortices; 2) basal ganglia and related nuclei; 3) cerebellum; 4) brain stem; and 5) spinal cord.

The motor system functions both in a hierarchical fashion, with each higher group of neurons controlling a lower group, and in parallel circuits, which permit each area to act independently on the final common pathway, allowing commands from higher levels to modify or supersede lower-order reflex behavior. With regard to central motor control, both the basal ganglia and the cerebellum

Table 49-1: Partial List of Movement Disorders, Classified as Hypokinetic or Hyperkinetic

HYPOKINETIC	HYPERKINETIC
Idiopathic Parkinson disease	Akathisia
Secondary/acquired parkinsonism	Ataxia
Drug or toxin induced	Athetosis
Multi-infarct/frontal lesions	Dentatorubropallidoluysian atrophy (DRPLA)
Postencephalitic	Dystonia
Traumatic	
Parkinson plus	Huntington disease
Shy-Drager syndrome	Myoclonus
Progressive supranuclear palsy	Neuroacanthocytosis
	Restless legs syndrome
Olivopontocerebellar atrophy	Sydenham chorea
	Secondary chorea
Parkinson–amyotrophic lateral sclerosis-dementia complex of Guam	Tardive dyskinesia
	Tics
	Tremor
	Wilson disease
Multisystem atrophy	

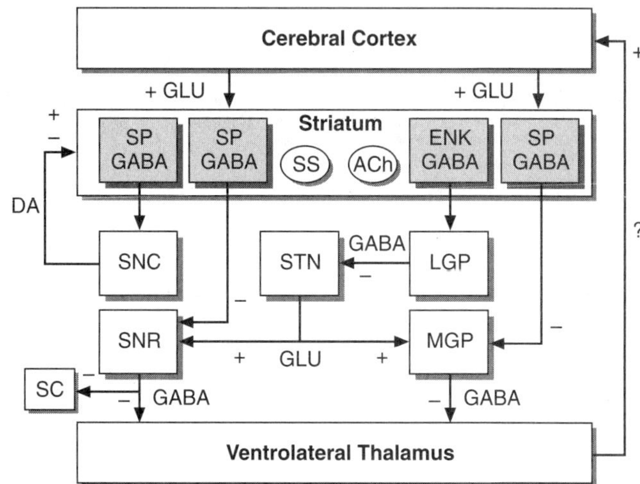

Figure 49-1. Schematic of the basal ganglia circuits involved in motor control. Terms in larger letters indicate the nuclei; those in smaller letters indicate neuromodulators and neurotransmitters utilized in the pathways. The *arrowheads* indicate the direction of transmission, with the *plus* and *minus signs* used to denote excitatory or inhibitory action, respectively, of the neurotransmitter involved. ACh = acetylcholine; DA = dopamine; ENK = enkephalin; GABA = γ-aminobutyric acid; GLU = glutamate; LGP = lateral globus pallidus; MGP = medial globus pallidus; SC = superior colliculus; SNC = substantia nigra pars compacta; SNR = substantia nigra pars reticulata; SP = substance P; SS = somatostatin; STN = subthalamus nucleus. (Repoduced by permission from Young AB, Penney JB. Biochemical and functional organization of the basal ganglia. In: Jancovic J, Tolosa E, eds. *Parkinson's disease and movement disorders.* 2nd ed. Baltimore: Williams & Wilkins, 1993:2.)

send outputs to the cortical precentral motor and premotor areas via separate pathways through the thalamus, which integrates these dual influences on movement and posture and channels them through thalamocortical fibers to the corticospinal and other descending spinal pathways from the cortex. Movement disorders as described in this chapter relate primarily to abnormalities in the basal ganglia–thalamocortical circuits rather than those directly involving the cerebellum. There are several such circuits (Fig. 49-1) originating in distinct cortical areas, interacting with separate regions of the striatum, and returning to their respective cortical areas, which appear to play important roles in skeletomotor, oculomotor, cognitive, and limbic functions.

Anatomy of the Basal Ganglia

The basal ganglia is composed of the caudate, putamen, and globus pallidus (Fig. 49-2). The caudate and putamen together are known as the *striatum* or *neostriatum*, the two structures being composed of identical cell types and fused anteriorly. The globus pallidus has two segments, the internal and the external, also known respectively as the *medial* and *lateral globus pallidus*. The basal ganglia are functionally related to the thalamus, subthalamic nucleus, and substantia nigra; because of the intimate functional relationship, the latter two structures are often regarded as part of the basal ganglia.

The neostriatum comprises the main *input* area for the basal ganglia, receiving glutamatergic, somatotopically organized afferents from the motor, sensory, and association cortices; dopaminergic input from the substantia nigra; and excitatory projections from the thalamus.

The *output* stages of the system are composed chiefly of the medial globus pallidus (MGP) and the substantia nigra pars reticulata (SNR). These two structures form one somatotopically organized nucleus separated by the internal capsule. The output of the SNR and MGP is inhibitory and projects in part to the thalamus, which in turn projects to the cortical supplementary motor area, frontal eye fields, pons, and superior colliculus. MGP neurons exert a tonic inhibitory effect on the thalamus. It appears that phasic increases and decreases of MGP/SNR output result in inhibition or facilitation, respectively, of movements initiated at the cortical level.

The basal ganglia seem to function through a balance of inhibition and disinhibition via two circuits called the *direct* and *indirect motor pathways* (2). Striatal outputs are projected over a direct pathway, from the striatum to the MGP/SNR, and an indirect pathway, from the

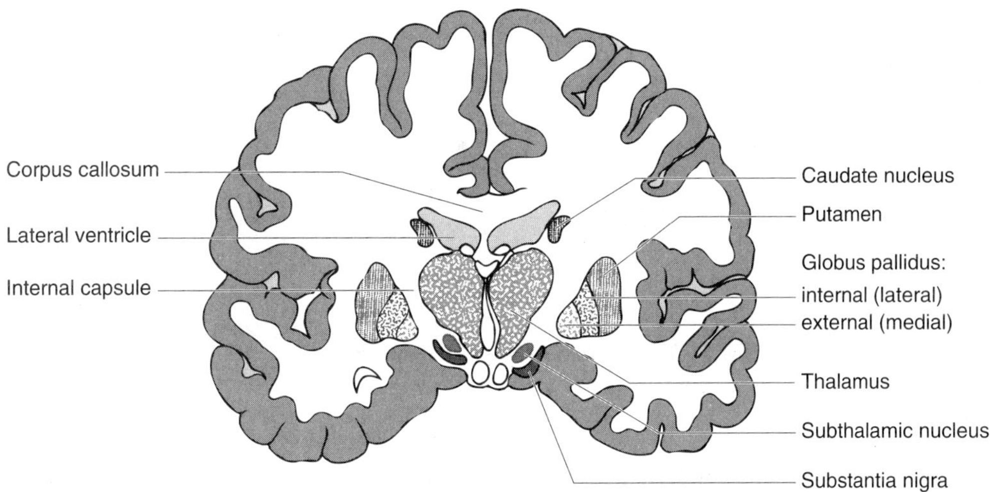

Figure 49-2. Simplified coronal section of the brain, depicting the basal ganglia and related structures.

striatum via a parallel circuit through the lateral globus pallidus and subthalamic nucleus to the MGP/SNR. The direct and indirect pathways function together to control movement. The direct and indirect pathways function together to control movement, acting as parallel systems to initiate and sustain movement while suppressing unwanted movements (Fig. 49-3).

More specifically, a defect in the direct pathway leads to disinhibition and overactivity of the MGP, resulting in augmented inhibition of the thalamus, such as occurs in Parkinson disease. The effect of a defect in the indirect pathway is disinhibition of the thalamus, such as occurs in chorea and hemiballism. The localization of dystonia has not been fully elucidated but may involve decreased activity of both pathways. Effects of this balance of inhibition and disinhibition are expressed through the thalamocortical completion of the "loop" (Fig. 49-4).

The diseases expressing involuntary alteration of movement control also frequently involve disturbances of perception, cognition, and emotion, and may be complicated by dysautonomia. These features arise from three factors: 1) more widespread selective neuronal degeneration not confined to the basal ganglia; 2) involvement of associated parallel loops interconnected with cortical (particularly frontal) and subcortical regions subserving these other cerebral functions; and 3) involvement of neurotransmitter systems other than the dopamine system, particularly serotonergic and noradrenergic systems.

Problems arising outside the central nervous system often reflect altered central and peripheral autonomic regulation, or as in the case of the altered energy needs in HD, reflect intrinsic defects in energy metabolism. The "movement disorders" and "extrapyramidal" designations are somewhat misleading, driven by the most obvious visible aspect of the diseases. In contrast, clinical management problems often arise because of the associated features of these disease-affecting, *nonmotor* aspects of function. Moreover, the rehabilitation of these diseases must necessarily address comprehensively all components of dysfunction, as well as the effects of chronic or progressive disease.

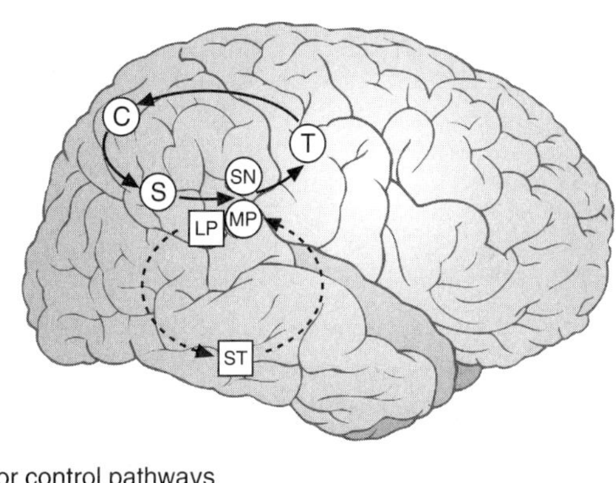

Motor control pathways

a) Direct system ————

b) Indirect system - - - - - - - -

Key:

C Cortex
S Striatum
MP Medial pallidum
LP Lateral pallidum
SN Substantia nigra
T Thalamus
ST Subthalamic nucleus

Figure 49-3. Direct and indirect pathways through the basal ganglia. The direct pathway (*solid line*) appears to be important in sustaining appropriate movements. The indirect pathway (*dotted line*) seems to suppress unwanted movements. C = cortex; S = striatum; MP = medial pallidus; LP = lateral pallidus; SN = substantia nigra; T = thalamus.

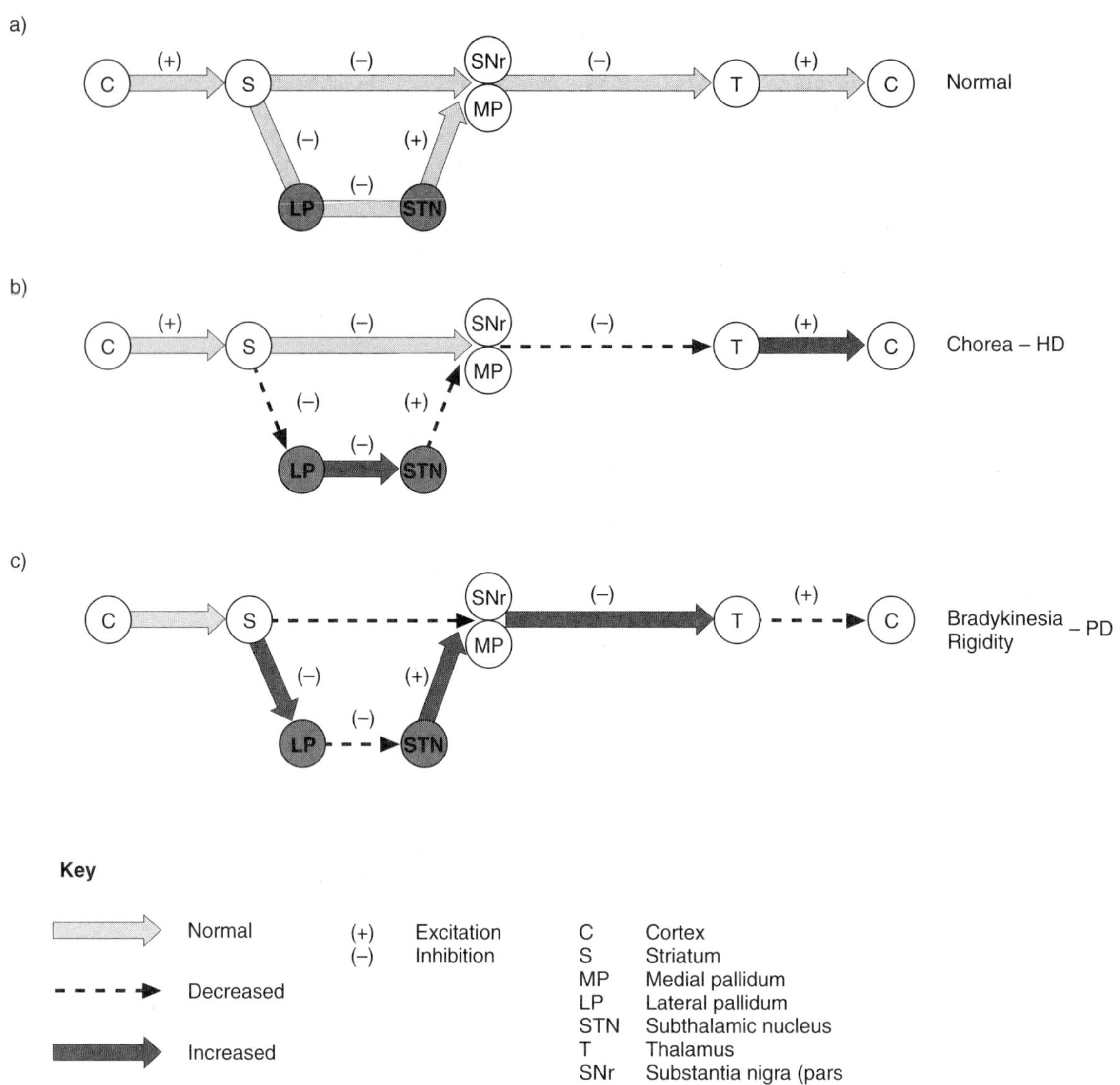

Figure 49-4. Simplified schematic depicting direct and indirect basal ganglia circuits in normal and disordered states. *A.* Normal balance of inhibition and disinhibition through direct and indirect pathways resulting in normal thalamic output to the cortex, and thus normal movement patterns. *B.* Underactivity of the indirect pathway resulting in the chorea typical of Huntington disease (HD). *C.* Underactivity of the direct pathway and overactivity of the indirect pathway resulting in the bradykinesia and rigidity seen in Parkinson disease (PD). (+) = excitation; (–) = inhibition; C = cortex; S = striatum; LP = lateral pallidus; STN = subthalamic nuclei; MP = medial pallidus; T = thalamus; SNR = substantia nigra pars reticulata.

SPECIFIC MOVEMENT DISORDERS

Movement disorders may be most conveniently classified as hypokinetic or hyperkinetic and are discussed in this context here. However, it is important to realize that these distinctions are somewhat artificial, and that various combinations of hypokinetic and hyperkinetic movements may be found in a single patient or within a single diagnosis. Therefore, diagnostic considerations and management strategies must be individualized and often readjusted as manifestations of the specific disease process evolve.

Hypokinetic Movement Disorders

Parkinson Disease

Parkinson disease encompasses a spectrum of related disorders that includes the idiopathic form and secondary or acquired forms, including drug- or toxin-induced, postencephalitic, and vascular parkinsonism. *Parkinson plus* is a term that refers to a group of multisystem, neurodegenerative disorders displaying parkinsonian signs along with other neurologic deficits. Included in this designation are Shy-Drager syndrome, progressive supranuclear palsy, olivopontocerebellar atrophy, Parkinson–amyotrophic lateral sclerosis–dementia complex of Guam, and multisystem atrophy. Idiopathic Parkinson disease is the most common form, and accounts for 75% of all cases of neurodegenerative Parkinson disease. Diffuse Lewy body disease is a recently characterized, pathologically distinct disease combining features of parkinsonism, dementia, and neuropsychiatric disturbance.

In addition to the neurodegenerative form of Parkinson disease, a number of conditions with "parkinsonian" features may present in rehabilitation practice. These include hydrocephalus, frontal ablative or mass lesions, neuroleptic intoxication or the effects of pharmacologic dopamine receptor blockade, lacunar state or multiple cerebral infarctions, traumatic or pugilistic parkinsonism, and hypoparathyroidism.

Clinical Presentation

Classically, Parkinson disease is characterized by bradykinesia associated with asymmetric rigidity, resting tremor, and postural instability. A multitude of other signs and symptoms are variably present, reflecting impairment of motor, autonomic, cognitive, emotional, cranial nerve, and musculoskeletal systems.

Tremor occurring at rest is the presenting complaint in over half of patients with idiopathic neurodegenerative Parkinson disease and generally consists of a typical "pill-rolling" motion at a frequency of 3 to 5 Hz that is suppressed by activity and sleep and intensified by fatigue and stress. It does not usually result in significant disability except in those individuals with associated action tremor. Rest tremor in Parkinson disease typically is lateralized asymmetrically.

Rigidity in Parkinson disease may be of the lead-pipe or cogwheeling type. Lead-pipe rigidity is characterized by relatively smooth resistance to passive movement throughout the available range (similar to bending a lead pipe); it is independent of velocity and occurs more or less equally in flexors and extensors. Cogwheel rigidity has a ratchety pattern, and may reflect a superimposition of tremor on rigidity.

Although patients may complain of paresthesias and sometimes pain, objective deficits in sensation are not characteristic. Cognitive deficits occur in approximately 25%, and depression, in approximately one-third.

The leading cause of death in patients with Parkinson disease, either idiopathic or other forms, is pneumonia. In one study, the second leading cause of death in advanced parkinsonism was pulmonary embolism secondary to deep venous thrombosis associated with prolonged immobility (4). This warrants careful monitoring and possibly low-dose anticoagulation, weighing the risk of hemorrhage in patients with postural instability.

For a complete discussion of Parkinson disease and its variants, please refer to Chapter 75.

Hyperkinetic Movement Disorders

Tremor

There are two basic categories of tremor: physiologic (normal) and pathologic (abnormal). Physiologic tremor is a normal phenomenon occurring in all muscle groups during the waking state; most often it is barely apparent to the naked eye. The frequency ranges from 8 to 12 Hz, with slightly slower frequencies noted during childhood and old age (5). In certain states, such as anxiety or fatigue, the physiologic tremor may be exaggerated and become more pronounced. Many cases of tremor presenting clinically are attributable to accentuated physiologic tremors, particularly due to inadvertent adverse side effects of medications or metabolic conditions. These include thyrotoxicosis, hypoglycemia, and hyperadrenergic states. Common drugs that augment physiologic tremor include steroids, lithium, calcium channel blockers, valproic acid, β-adrenergic agonists, theophylline, and caffeine.

Tremor can be classified by frequency, appearance, or cause (Table 49-2). Pathologic tremors are generally classified according to the principal conditions in which they occur and are of four basic types: rest tremor, postural tremor, kinetic tremor, and intention tremor. *Action tremor* is a term that refers to both postural and kinetic tremors. Rest tremor, as the name implies, is present when the affected body part is at rest. Postural tremor occurs when a static posture, such as outstretched arms, is maintained. Kinetic tremor is provoked by voluntary activities such as writing or pouring liquids, while intention tremor is most pronounced in the terminal iterative adjustment required with targeted maneuvers.

Tremor of a particular type is often characteristic of a certain clinical or anatomic diagnosis, such as rest tremor in parkinsonism, postural or action tremors in essential

Table 49-2: Classification of Tremor by Mode of Occurrence and Frequency

		Appearance		
Frequency (Hz)	Cause	Rest Tremor	Action Tremor	Intention Tremor
8–12	Physiologic	–	+	±
	Enhanced physiologic	–	++	+
4–12	Benign essential	–	+++	+
	Severe essential	++	++++	++
3–5	Parkinson—rest	++++	++	+
	Parkinson—postural	+	+++	+
4–5	Rubral	++	+++	++++
	Cerebellar	–	+	+++

– = absent; + = present; ++ = common feature; +++ = prominent feature; ++++ = very prominent feature; ± = may be present.

tremor, and intention tremor in cerebellar disease. Tremors of different types or pathologic origins may occur independently or be concurrent and superimposed. Pathologic tremors are discussed here as they occur in clinical and diagnostic settings.

Parkinsonian (Rest) Tremor

Parkinsonian tremor occurs at a frequency of 3 to 5 Hz, most characteristically in the distal aspects of the upper extremities, although it may be seen in the feet and buccal-oral-lingual muscles, albeit less often. Electromyographically, it has been shown to consist of alternating bursts of activity in opposing muscle groups while the limb is in a relaxed attitude. Mild rest tremor is suppressed or diminished during volitional activity, and for this reason rarely results in significant functional disability; however, severe rest tremor can be very disabling. Like most movement disorders, rest tremor disappears during sleep. Although the frequency of the tremor is relatively constant, the amplitude may increase with emotional stress or anxiety. Anticholinergic and dopaminergic medications may ameliorate the tremor, and a dramatic response has also been obtained with stereotactic thalamotomy or pallidotomy in selected patients.

Parkinsonian tremor is discussed more fully in Chapter 75.

Intention and Action (Postural and Kinetic) Tremors

Intention tremor occurs in conjunction with cerebellar disease, and is present only during fairly precise, exacting movements. The tremor is absent at rest and during the first part of a movement, but intensifies as fine adjustments are required, producing an irregular side-to-side oscillation at 2 to 3 Hz as the target is approached (e.g., during finger-to-nose testing).

Action tremor occurs either during active maintenance of a static posture (postural tremor) or throughout the range of a particular movement (kinetic tremor). Although action tremor is accentuated when greater precision is required, the degree of augmentation is less than that seen with intention tremor. It is characterized electromyographically by synchronous bursts of activity in agonist and antagonist muscles simultaneously, in contrast to parkinsonian tremor (5). Postural tremor should be distinguished from asterixis, which consists of irregular lapses of sustained posture characterized by electromyographically silent periods of 35 to 200 msec, evoked best during active dorsiflexion of the outstretched hands.

There are several types of action tremors, the most frequently observed being essential or familial tremor.

Essential Tremor

Essential tremor (ET) is a monosymptomatic, heritable movement disorder that is often minimally disabling and thus often fails to come to the attention of medical professionals. It is generally considered to be the most common movement disorder, although the prevalence rates reported in the literature vary widely, from 0.0005% to 5.5%, depending on the population studied and the diagnostic criteria used (6). ET appears to be inherited in an autosomal dominant pattern, with a family history reported in about 50% of cases. There is great variability in age at onset and clinical expression. Some authors reported 100% penetrance after age 70 (7); onset most frequently occurs after age 40, and prevalence increases with age.

Clinical Presentation

Tremor is the sole clinical manifestation of this disorder, with mild associated abnormalities in gait and tone only occasionally reported. The tremor is a typical rhythmic oscillating movement produced by alternating or simultaneous contractions of reciprocally innervated antagonistic muscles. It is usually postural, that is, accentuated or provoked by maintenance of a fixed posture (8), although it may also be seen at rest or with action. The tremor most frequently affects the hands, is often unilateral at onset with progression to bilaterality, and affects the lower extremities only in later stages, if at all. Tongue, head, or voice may be affected, generally in association with hand tremor, although any of these regions may be involved in isolation. Primary writing tremor is precipitated by pronation of the forearm and results in a pronation-supination tremor that may make handwriting impossible. This must be distinguished from writer's cramp, a segmental dystonia.

The frequency of ET varies from 4 to 12 Hz, and classification schemes based on frequency have been proposed, along with other classifications based on response to medication and electromyographic (EMG) activity. None has been universally accepted.

Progression of the disease is characterized by an increase in the amplitude of the tremor with advancing years or by extension of the tremor to previously unaffected body parts. Tremor may also be accentuated in the short term by various factors, including fatigue, emotional stress, sexual arousal, extremes of temperature, and central nervous system stimulants (8,9). A unique feature of ET is its sometimes remarkable attenuation with alcohol, often even in small amounts. Like most movement disorders, it generally remits during sleep. The diagnosis of ET is not associated with increased mortality.

Diagnosis

The diagnosis of ET is made on a clinical basis (Table 49-3). A positive family history and reduction of tremor with alcohol are supportive of but not required for diagnosis. It is sometimes misdiagnosed, most frequently as early Parkinson disease; the confusion is compounded by the fact that parkinsonian signs such as cogwheeling and rest tremor may be found in patients with ET, and postural tremor is not uncommon with Parkinson disease. The differential diagnosis includes other neurologic diseases that may have tremor as a clinical manifestation, including mul-

Table 49-3: Diagnostic Criteria for Essential Tremor
1. Intermittent or constant tremor of the hands, head, or voice.
2. Tremor is of the postural and/or kinetic variety.
3. No other neurologic abnormalities related to systemic or other neurologic disease.
4. No other medical explanation for tremor, e.g., not taking drugs known to cause tremor.
5. Positive family history of tremor supports the diagnosis.
6. Reduction of tremor with alcoholic beverages supports the diagnosis.

Source: Reproduced by permission from Hubble JP, Busenbark KL, Koller WC. Essential tremor. *Clin Neuropharmacol* 1989;12:462.

tiple sclerosis, HD, Wilson disease, and degenerative cerebellar disorders. Many studies have described the occurrence of postural tremor in patients with focal or generalized dystonias, and tremor may also occur with hereditary and acquired peripheral neuropathies. Drug- and toxin-induced tremor, such as that seen with the administration of valproic acid or lithium, must also be excluded. Systemic illness (e.g., thyrotoxicosis) may precipitate tremor resembling ET.

Treatment

Disability in ET results mainly from an impairment of fine motor skills and embarrassment with attendant social withdrawal. Many patients can be effectively treated now, although the responses to different therapeutic interventions vary depending on the type and location of the tremor.

Most patients respond to alcohol with a transient but dramatic decrease in tremor, and small amounts of alcoholic beverages prior to meals or other events may be acceptable. At one time, the incidence of alcoholism among patients with ET was thought to be excessive, but more recent studies have not supported this belief (10). The results of studies on the efficacy of propranolol for ET have been conflicting, but success has been sufficient to make this the drug of choice in the treatment of most patients with ET, using 240 to 320 mg/day in divided doses or in a single dose of a long-acting preparation (11–13). Symptomatic relief is obtained in an estimated 50% to 70% of patients, with responses varying from dramatic to nonexistent (6). Responses consist of a reduction in tremor amplitude, with no significant effect on frequency. Relative contraindications to the use of propranolol are mainly associated with its β-blocking action, and include heart failure, second- or third-degree atrioventricular block, bronchospastic disease, and insulin-dependent diabetes mellitus in which adrenergic manifestations of hypoglycemia may be blocked (6).

Other β-blockers may also be effective for ET. Metoprolol, a relatively selective β_1 antagonist, may be better tolerated in bronchospastic patients, although caution must still be exercised (14). Nadolol may be effective in patients who respond to propranolol, and its long half-life allows a more convenient once-daily dosing schedule (15).

The antiepileptic primidone has been shown to significantly reduce tremor. In one study primidone reduced hand tremor an average of 60%, and was more effective than propranolol (16). Primidone has been used in doses of 50 to 1000 mg/day, but doses of 250 mg/day were found to be as effective as higher doses (17). Tolerance is sometimes limited by nausea and dizziness, especially with initial doses, but the side effects tend to abate after several days.

Phenobarbital has occasionally been used with success for ET, but is generally thought to be ineffective. Benzodiazepines have limited efficacy for ET, and the benefits reported may be due to their anxiolytic effect; however, clonazepam does appear to be effective for intention tremor and orthostatic truncal tremor (18,19).

Many other agents including antiparkinsonian drugs have been tried as treatment for ET, without consistent responses. Propranolol and primidone remain the drugs of choice, with the side effect profile often dictating which one is most appropriate for a given patient. In some patients, therapy with both these agents is required for optimal control. Hubble et al (6) suggested one useful model for approaching drug therapy in ET (Fig. 49-5). Surgical therapy represents a useful alternative for patients with severe disabling unilateral tremor that is not adequately controlled by medication. Stereotactic thalamotomy, lesioning the ventral intermediate or ventral anterior nucleus of the thalamus, has resulted in improvement in up to 90% of patients (20). The mortality rate for thalamotomy is less than 0.3%. The morbidity associated with unilateral thalamotomy is usually transient, and most frequently consists of transitory hemiparesis, dysarthria, or cognitive deficit. With bilateral thalamotomy, the deficits may be more severe and persistent, and such surgery must be approached with caution.

Rehabilitation Considerations

Behavioral therapies including biofeedback, relaxation therapy, hypnosis, and psychotherapy have been used with limited success in the treatment of various tremors including ET. Improvements that do occur may be related to a decrease in muscle tension. Weighted cuffs have been used to dampen the tremor amplitude during activities, but may augment postural tremor.

Chorea, Ballism, and Dyskinesia

Chorea is a term derived from the Greek word for "dance" and refers to rapid, irregular, involuntary jerking or twitching movements with a random pattern of occurrence. Choreiform hyperkinetic movement disorders share a final common pathway of disinhibition of the thalamus from

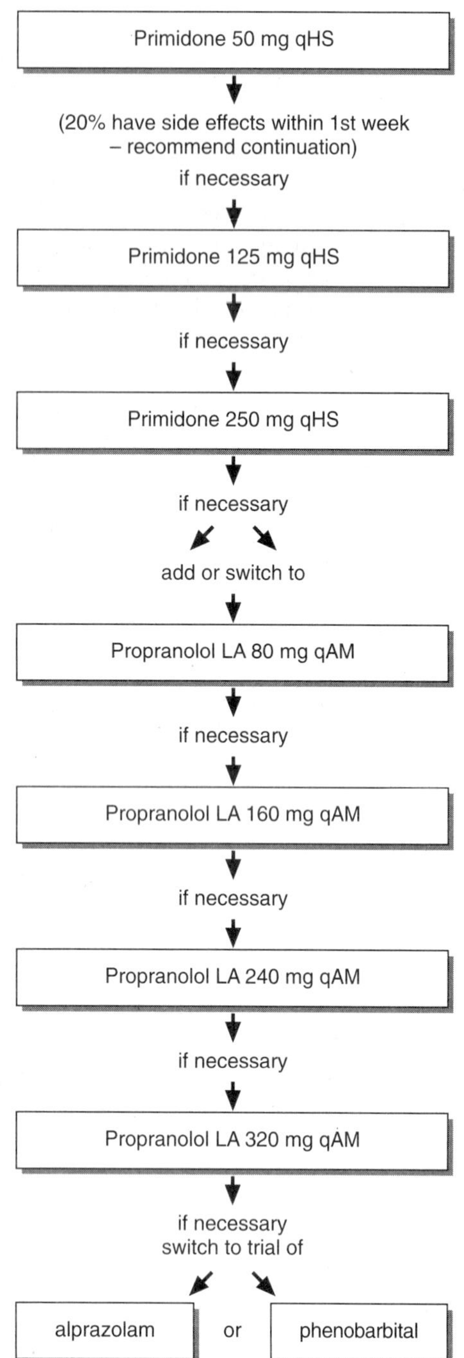

Figure 49-5. A suggested algorithm in the treatment of essential tremor. (Adapted with permission from Hubble JP, Busenbark KL, Koller WC. Essential tremor. *Clin Neuropharmacol* 1989;12:475.)

deficient subthalamic inputs. Chorea may be associated with other hyperkinetic movements including athetosis, which describes a writhing quality of the movements, and dystonia and ballism, which are described below.

A lesion (typically infarction) of the subthalamus or its projections classically causes large-amplitude, flinging-writhing movements called *ballism* in contralateral limbs. The course of ballism is variable. In the extreme, it can result in exhaustion and persist until death, but more often the involuntary movements wane over months and may merge into a choreiform disorder.

Dyskinesia is a general term implying a movement indistinguishable from chorea. The term is employed in settings where the movement is induced by a drug or toxin, for example, in response to excessive treatment with dopaminergic medicines. Tardive dyskinesia is one of the late-emerging movement disorders that follow use of dopamine receptor blockade agents, occurring especially after prolonged use of neuroleptics.

Treatment of these movement disorders varies with the cause. When the disorder is related to drug use, elimination of the *offending* medications will be helpful. In patients with tardive dyskinesia, cumulated exposure to neuroleptics should be minimized, or eliminated if possible. In patients with psychoses, consideration should be given to the use of atypical antipsychotics such as clozapine, as the effects of tardive dyskinesia can be disfiguring, impairing, prolonged, and in some patients, permanent. Vitamin E has demonstrated modest effects in some patients.

Huntington Disease

HD is a hereditary degenerative neuropsychiatric disorder affecting mainly the basal ganglia, but involving widespread areas of the central nervous system. It is characterized by progressive motor, cognitive, and psychiatric abnormalities usually presenting in adult life.

Genetics

The disorder is inherited in an autosomal dominant pattern, so that each offspring of an affected parent has a 50% chance of inheriting the gene. The genetic defect responsible for HD has been localized to the short arm of chromosome 4, and consists of an abnormally long trinucleotide sequence of DNA base pairs (cytosine-adenine-guanine: CAG) (21). Elucidation of the gene product and its relationship to the pathogenesis and manifestations of HD remains incomplete. Testing individuals for the abnormal gene involves amplification and counting of the repetitive length of the CAG trinucleotides within the HD gene region. Currently a repeat length of 40 or longer is believed to signify a high probability of HD (22), and is considered a positive result. Repeat lengths of 36 to 40 may be predictive of HD, but are associated with reduced penetrance. Repeat lengths of 35 and shorter are thought not to be predictive of HD, but only lengths of 28 and less are thought to be predictably stable in intergenerational transmission.

Neuropathology

Histologically, prominent loss of medium spiny neurons in the striatum is noted, with severe atrophy of the caudate and putamen on a macroscopic level. There is also loss of cortical neurons, along with marked changes in other areas such as the thalamus and brain stem. The movement disorder is attributed to striatal atrophy, while dementia is believed to relate to both cortical and subcortical pathology.

Onset of the disease is insidious and most commonly occurs between the ages of 35 and 50; however, onset has been observed at any time from childhood to old age. The duration of disease after diagnosis is variable, but death occurs an average of 15 to 20 years after onset. Some patients die earlier from falls or suicide, and in some a slowly progressive course over more than two decades is seen. The most common causes of death are attributed to bulbar dysfunction and are related to aspiration, including aspiration pneumonia and acute suffocation. The second leading cause of death is cardiovascular disease (23). In long-term-care settings, a disproportionate number of deaths due to the use of restraints have occurred among HD patients.

Clinical Presentation

The three cardinal manifestations of the disease are abnormal movements, cognitive deficits, and psychiatric disturbance. Initial signs and symptoms may consist of subtle decreases in mental speed and flexibility, along with irritability, depression, or loss of interest in activities. Early motor signs include fidgetiness, clumsiness, and abnormal ocular motility.

Motor disease consists of involuntary movements such as chorea, dystonia, and motor restlessness, as well as impaired voluntary movements including bradykinesia, rigidity, dyscoordination, motor impersistence, and deficient postural reflexes. Although the chorea is the most prominent motor sign, the voluntary motor disturbances are actually more disabling, and ultimately result in rigidity and an inability to initiate any voluntary movements.

Abnormal movements may involve the facial, axial, and limb muscles, with grimacing, shrugging of the shoulders, and jerking movements of the limbs seen early in the course. Ambulation often intensifies the movements, resulting in a characteristic "Huntington ataxia," a weaving, dancing, stuttering gait that is not seen in any other disorder. During the course of the disease, postural instability, dystonia, and parkinsonian features increase, becoming predominant in late disease, while chorea tends to increase in early and mid stages but wanes in advanced disease.

Loss of motor control also affects the muscles of deglutition and articulation, and dysphagia and speech impairments are inevitable complications of HD. Swallowing deficits are seen in all HD patients, but vary somewhat depending on whether hypokinetic or hyperkinetic characteristics of the disease predominate. All phases of the swallowing mechanism are affected. Speech is impaired, affected by a combination of poor respiratory support, inadequate control of the laryngeal mechanism, and impaired articulation, along with cognitive and language difficulties (24,25). In advanced HD, caloric needs are frequently increased, while a concomitant progression of bulbar dysfunction occurs. Consequently, cachectic states result as the need and the difficulty in providing nutrition increase together.

Cognitive deficits affect 100% of patients and are often noticed first as deterioration in performance in the workplace as the patient experiences difficulties organizing and sequencing tasks and information. Increasing impairments in memory, calculations, verbal fluency, visuospatial abilities, and judgment occur with disease progression.

Psychiatric disturbances occur commonly in HD patients, and often present several years before the onset of other symptoms. Initial symptoms commonly include depression (approximately 20%–40%), bipolar disorder, and apathy. Frank psychosis occurs in about 5%. Frontal syndromes, including disinhibited and rarely, inappropriate sexual behavior, are seen. The rate of suicide in HD is higher than that of the general population (26). Unlike other populations, suicide in these patients can occur in the absence of depression, deriving instead from the convergence of impulsivity, cognitive impairment, pessimism, and a loss of sustaining relationships and hedonic resources. As the disease progresses, psychiatric symptoms often worsen, especially irritability, which sometimes leads to aggressive or antisocial behavior, and apathy. Depressive symptoms tend to lessen late in the course, although in some patients depression persists until death.

Juvenile-onset HD (Westphal variant) occurs with greater frequency in paternal transmission and with increased numbers of trinucleotide repeats in the abnormal gene. It is characterized by bradykinesia, rigidity, and dystonia, rather than chorea, and may be associated with tremors and seizures. In general, the course is more rapidly progressive than that of adult-onset disease.

Staging

A rating scale for staging HD has been developed based on the patient's functional capacity in vocational, domestic, financial, and self-care domains (27), and has been incorporated into a more comprehensive clinical rating instrument, The Unified Huntington's Disease Rating Scale (UHDRS) (28). The latter has proved valuable for assessment and monitoring in both clinical management and research and includes evaluations of neurologic, cognitive, behavioral, and functional status.

In a general sense, however, HD can be divided into early, middle, and late stages. Early-stage HD is characterized by subtle deficits in coordination, minor involuntary movements, difficulty thinking through problems, and persistent episodes of depressed or irritable mood. In middle-stage HD, chorea and problems with voluntary movement become more prominent and disabling, and are accompanied by increasing gait ataxia, and progressive dysarthria and dysphagia. Cognitive decline continues, and renders the patient unable to maintain employment or carry out household responsibilities. Greater supervision for safety and assistance with activities of daily living (ADLs) become necessary. Late-stage HD generally requires nursing home care. Although severe chorea may persist in some patients, rigidity and bradykinesia generally predominate, and the patient becomes bedridden and nonverbal. Dementia becomes more global, but with relative preservation of recognition and comprehension.

Therapeutic Strategies

Medical management to date has been symptomatic and palliative, but recent advances in research elucidating the genetic basis and possible pathophysiologic mechanisms of HD have raised hopes for future preventive and even curative therapies. In the meantime, medical strategies focus on the four main areas of concern: movement disorders, cognition, emotional disturbance, and functional adaptation. Because HD is a complex convergence of these areas, is highly variable from individual to individual, and encompasses most aspects of other movement disorders as components of dysfunction, it represents a model for the approach to the neurorehabilitative treatment of degenerative movement disorders in general.

Identified components of dysfunction in HD may be addressed using the usual class of medications for that symptom (clonazepam for myoclonus, baclofen for spasticity, benzodiazepines for anxiety, etc). Many components of HD may be refractory to pharmacologic treatment, particularly the cognitive decline, or limited in effectiveness, for example, in the treatment of spasticity and dystonia. Treatments for the psychiatric and emotional aspects of HD are relatively more successful, and lead to a profound benefit in overall functioning.

Symptomatic pharmacologic treatments target each individual component, with priority given to the most functionally impairing components so as to avoid polypharmacy. In particular, it is noted that neuroleptics (commonly, haloperidol) may be very much overused for HD. Haloperidol suppresses chorea or psychosis, where its use is well indicated, but at the same time may lead to more impairing problems of depression, apathy, failure of initiative, increased dysphagia, and increased parkinsonism. Importantly, typical neuroleptics have only limited effectiveness for temperamental lability and irritability (for which they are commonly used), where selective serotonin reuptake inhibitor (SSRI) antidepressants (fluoxetine and others), anticonvulsants (carbamazepine), and atypical antipsychotics (risperidone) in low dose may have greater benefit. For a symptom-by-symptom guideline for the treatment of HD, the reader is referred to *A Physician's Guide to the Management of Huntington's Disease* (29).

Because language comprehension and features of personality are generally well preserved in HD, pharmacologic approaches to problems should not displace an attempt to understand the unique experience and resources of the affected individual, where this is available through communication.

Rehabilitation Considerations

General rehabilitation goals in HD, as in most other neurodegenerative diseases, include optimizing functional independence for as long as possible while promoting safety and prevention of injuries, and avoiding complications such as contractures, loss of muscle mass, deconditioning, respiratory compromise, musculoskeletal pain syndromes, and social withdrawal. In today's medical insurance environment, in the setting of a prolonged degenerative disease process, rehabilitation interventions must be relatively brief, individualized, and goal directed, with the focus on creative solutions to specific problems and documentation of the goals achieved.

Movement and Cognitive Strategies

As a complement or an alternative to the medical strategies just described, chorea can also be treated with nonpharmacologic interventions such as trunk weights, comfortable positioning in a semireclining chair with adequate padding to prevent injury from high-amplitude chorea, and alleviation of hunger and anxiety whenever possible, as these may exacerbate choreic movements. One must keep in mind that suppression of chorea frequently does not result in functional improvement, and treatment specifically directed at chorea often need not be initiated unless the chorea is disabling or very distressing to the patient.

Dystonia, rigidity, and spasticity are more disabling than chorea, causing gait impairment, recurrent falls, ADL deficits, and eventual loss of mobility sufficient to necessitate wheelchair use. Contractures and scoliosis can also result from prolonged hypertonia and abnormal postures. Appropriate physical and occupational therapy, along with judicious use of medications, can aid in reducing spasticity and parkinsonian symptoms, and these measures should be employed aggressively to preserve functional mobility. Loss of ambulation signifies a profound loss of control and independence to these patients, and the use of rolling walkers, medial or lateral flanges added to footwear to improve stability, personal safety equipment such as helmets, and home adaptations such as railings, grab bars, padding on hard or sharp surfaces, and appropriate floor textures can aid in preserving ambulation safely for as long as possible.

Workplace adaptations may also prolong the patient's ability to remain employed. As endurance declines, adaptations such as moving a desk closer to a frequently used copy machine may permit better function. Tasks should be divided into subcomponents to decrease their complexity, schedules organized to provide more structure, and frequent alternation of tasks eliminated. Noise and distraction in the environment should be minimized, and situations avoided in which impaired balance or coordination may have disastrous results (e.g., climbing ladders or catwalks, or operating dangerous equipment).

Cardiovascular exercise is important for maintaining and improving endurance, strength, coordination, and a sense of well-being. Swimming is an excellent activity for HD individuals, as is the use of a stationary bicycle. Aerobic equipment, adapted for use by persons with impaired balance and coordination, is often available in community gyms.

Communication

In patients with HD, a combination of dysarthria, dysphonia, impaired language skills, and cognitive deficits results in progressive deterioration of communication abilities. Speech pathologists can play a vital role in helping the patient and caregivers maintain communication for as long as possible, with early interventions designed to reduce the rate of speech, improve self-monitoring, and enhance respiratory control and phonation (25). In later stages, priority is given to establishing a functional communicative system with family and caregivers, encouraging greater use of forced-choice formats such as yes/no questions or multiple choice, as well as use of communication boards or computerized augmentative communication systems in selected patients. Training of caregivers in effective listening strategies is important, including use of cuing, feedback, gestures, and allowance of increased response time for the patient.

Swallowing and Nutrition

The person with HD typically develops significant dysphagia in the middle and late stages, and in fact "dysphagia is the most common cause of death in HD, either directly from suffocation or aspiration, or indirectly from starvation" (24). With the use of a videofluoroscopic swallowing study, the speech-language pathologist and physician can accurately diagnose the nature of the swallowing impairment and design appropriate interventions. These may involve changes in food consistency, optimal positioning during feeding, and employment of compensatory techniques for safe and efficient swallowing. Such interventions are doubly important in these patients, for whom caloric needs are considerably greater than in normal persons. It is not unusual for patients to require as many as 5000 cal/day to maintain good general health and average body weight.

Fluid requirements seem to be increased as well, and dehydration is a risk, particularly in the warm weather or in patients in a late stage who cannot communicate requests for fluids. Use of thickeners, straws, weighted cups, nonskid plates with built-up rims, baby spoons to minimize bolus size, and large-handled utensils may prolong independent eating and drinking. However, when self-feeding begins to require excessive energy, time, and concentration, or significant weight loss occurs, progressive assistance with feeding should be instituted.

Seating and Positioning

Most HD patients, even those still able to ambulate independently, have difficulty sitting comfortably. They tend to slide down in chairs, bearing weight on the lumbosacral region of the spine rather than the ischial tuberosities. Risk of aspiration is increased by failure to maintain an upright position, and choreic movements lead to injuries from chairs without proper padding. Appropriate positioning is also important in enabling the individual with HD to interact optimally with his or her environment.

Important considerations in providing proper seating and positioning for HD patients include solid, sturdy foot support; minimal use of restraints; adequate padding of sharp or hard surfaces; appropriate design for use at tables or with a lap tray; and provision for maximal ease of transfers. In many patients, chorea is reduced or exacerbated in certain positions, and this information should be incorporated into seating and positioning techniques. In patients with large-amplitude trunk movements, chest straps may be necessary to enhance safety.

Sydenham Chorea

Sydenham chorea is an acute choreic disorder often accompanied by irritability, cognitive dysfunction, and emotional disturbance; it generally occurs in childhood in association with rheumatic fever. The onset may be gradual or sudden, and over 80% of cases occur between the ages of 5 and 15, with girls affected twice as often as boys. Symptoms of rheumatic fever may take the form of arthritis, pericarditis, endocarditis, or myocarditis, and are seen in at least 75% of patients at some point before, during, or after the onset of choreic manifestations (30). The disorder is self-limited, usually resolving completely within 2 years. Fatalities are unusual and nearly always result from cardiac complications, which occur in about 20% of patients.

The disorder is characterized by rapid irregular movements of the limbs, trunk, and face; weakness and incoordination; hypotonia; and psychological manifestations. Symptoms vary considerably in severity, from mild restlessness and incoordination to disabling chorea and weakness, and are often exacerbated by emotional or physical stress. In about 35% of patients, motor symptoms are worse on one side of the body and in a small percentage, are entirely confined to one side.

On examination, motor impersistence (inability to sustain voluntary muscle contractions) and incoordination related to involuntary movements in antagonist muscles during volitional activities are seen. On extension of the arms, a characteristic hand posture (Warner hand) is often noted in which the wrist is sharply flexed and the fingers hyperextended at the proximal and terminal phalanges Except for involuntary movements of facial and oropharyngeal muscles, cranial nerves are unaffected, and there are no sensory deficits. Muscle stretch reflexes may be increased, decreased, or absent, and extensor plantar responses are unusual. The results of routine laboratory and cerebrospinal fluid studies are usually normal, and diagnosis is made clinically. The differential diagnosis includes tardive dyskinesia related to neuroleptics or phenytoin, familial benign chorea, and systemic lupus erythematosus in which chorea may be a rare early sign.

Treatment is symptomatic, and should include rest and reduction of environmental stimuli. In patients with severe or disabling movements, neuroleptics initiated at low doses and titrated carefully may be utilized. Valproic acid and steroids have been reported as helpful.

Dystonias

Dystonia refers to a syndrome of involuntary sustained or spasmodic muscle contractions involving the same group of muscles in a repetitive and patterned manner, frequently leading to twisting and other abnormal movements and postures (31).

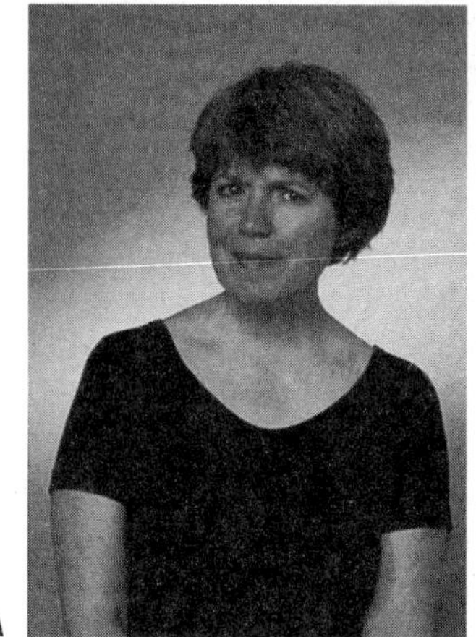

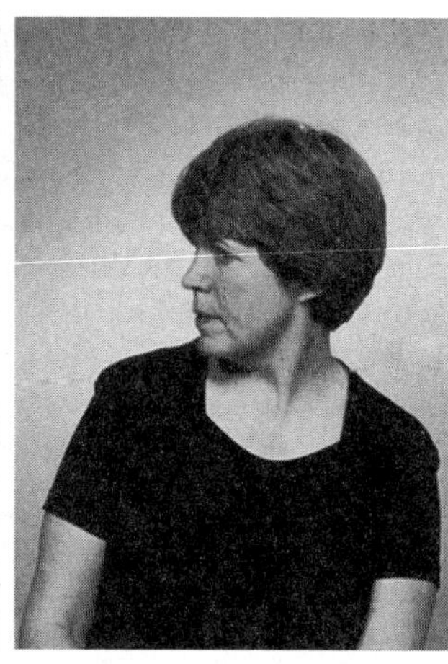

A B

Figure 49-6. *A.* Patient with cervical dystonia characterized by left lateral rotational torticollis. Note the prominence of the right sternocleidomastoid. *B.* Nearly complete resolution following treatment with botulinum toxin. [Photo courtesy of WE MOVE (Worldwide Education and Awareness for Movement Disorders).]

Clinical Presentation

Although dystonic movements are usually continual, variations are seen in which the dystonia fluctuates depending on the time of day (diurnal dystonia) or occurs in abrupt episodes (paroxysmal dystonia) (31). As with most movement disorders, dystonia may be influenced by fatigue, anxiety, relaxation, or sleep (32). Dystonic movements may be slow or rapid and are nearly always enhanced by voluntary movement ("overflow"); some can be transiently suppressed by a contactual stimulus such as a hand placed on the ipsilateral or contralateral side of the face or neck in the patient with spasmodic torticollis. It is often associated with either dystonic or essential-type tremor, the former being most evident when the individual attempts to move in a direction opposing the dystonic contraction, and the latter persisting regardless of direction.

Dystonic movements may vary in duration from less than a second (myoclonic dystonia) to seconds, minutes, hours, weeks, or longer. When dystonic movements are sustained for weeks or longer, they may lead to permanent fixed contractures. The functional impact of dystonia varies from barely noticeable to severely disabling, with some patients unable to ambulate or participate effectively in ADLs; occasionally, muscle contractions are severe enough to cause muscle breakdown and myoglobinuria (33).

Etiology and Classification

Dystonia may be symptomatic (i.e., secondary to a wide variety of neurologic diseases, drug intoxication, metabolic disease, or hypoxic brain damage) or may be idiopathic. It may also be classified by distribution (focal, segmental, multifocal, generalized, or hemidystonia), or age at onset (childhood or adult onset). Idiopathic dystonia may be either sporadic or inherited, with heritable childhood-onset dystonia particularly common among Ashkenazi Jews. Secondary dystonia may result from virtually any metabolic or structural lesion affecting the brain, especially lesions involving the basal ganglia or rostral brain stem structures. Dopamine antagonists including neuroleptics and gastrointestinal drugs such as metoclopramide are an important cause of both acute and tardive drug-induced dystonias

Focal dystonia involves a single body part, with cervical dystonia or torticollis being the most common idiopathic focal dystonia. *Torticollis* refers to spasmodic rotation of the head (Fig. 49-6A), which is seen most frequently, while anterocollis, retrocollis, and laterocollis describe positions of flexion, extension, and lateral bending. Often the clinical picture involves a combination of these abnormal postures. Other craniocervical dystonias include blepharospasm, oromandibular dystonia, and laryngeal dystonia. Focal limb dystonias most frequently begin as action- or task-specific dystonia, with writers' cramp the most commonly observed example; similar dystonias occur during typing, feeding, or playing musical instruments. In 20% to 30% of patients, focal dystonias progress to involve adjacent or other parts of the body; that is, they become segmental or multifocal.

Treatment and Rehabilitation

The options in the management of dystonias (Table 49-4) have traditionally been threefold, consisting of medications, surgery, and physical therapy. These approaches have been limited in efficacy, and in the case of the first two, often associated with an unacceptable spectrum of side effects.

During the past decade, however, botulinum toxin has become a powerful therapeutic tool in improving the symptomatic treatment of focal dystonias, and appears to be the treatment of choice for blepharospasm, cervical dys-

Table 49-4: Guidelines for Symptomatic Treatment of Dystonia

Generic Name	Trade Name	Daily Dosage (mg)	Mechanism of Action
Trihexyphenidyl	Artane	6–40	Anticholinergic
Benztropine	Cogentin	4–15	Anticholinergic
Orphenadrine	Norflex	200–800	Anticholinergic
Clonazepam	Klonipin	1–12	Serotonergic; relaxant
Lorazepam	Ativan	1–16	Relaxant
Diazepam	Valium	10–100	Relaxant
Cyclobenzaprine	Flexeril	20–60	Relaxant
Chlordiazepoxide	Librium	10–100	Relaxant
Baclofen	Lioresal	40–120	Antispastic; GABA agonist; substance P antagonist
Primidone	Mysoline	50–800	Antiepileptic; antitremor
Valproate	Depakote	500–1500	Antiepileptic; GABA-T inhibitor
Carbamazepine	Tegretol	600–1600	Antiepileptic
Levodopa/carbidopa	Sinemet (CR)	75/300–200/2000	Dopamine precursor
Bromocriptine	Parlodel	10–60	Dopamine agonist
Lisuride	—	1–10	Dopamine agonist
Pergolide	Permax	0.5–5.0	Dopamine agonist
Pimozide	Orap	2–10	Dopamine agonist
Lithium	Lithobid	600–1800	Antidopaminergic
Tetrabenazine	Nitoman	50–300	Monoamine depleter and blocker
Combination:			
Tetrabenazine		75 mg/day	—
Pimozide		6–25 mg/day	—
Trihexyphenidyl		6–30 mg/day	—
Botulinum A toxin	Botox	5–400 units	Blocks acetylcholine release at neuromuscular junction
Surgery—thalamotomy or peripheral denervation			—

Source: Reproduced by permission from Jancovic J, Fahn S. Dystonic syndromes. In: Jancovic J, Tolosa A, eds. *Parkinson's disease and movement disorders.* 2nd ed. Baltimore: Williams & Wilkins, 1993:363.

tonia (see Fig. 49-6B), and hemifacial spasm (34,35). The neurotoxin is produced by the gram-negative bacterium *Clostridium botulinum*, and acts by irreversibly inhibiting the presynaptic release of acetylcholine at the neuromuscular junction. Of the seven immunologically distinct serotypes, only type A is approved for clinical use. The doses vary depending on the target muscle bulk and desired clinical effect, from 50 units for small muscles to a maximum recommended dose of 400 units in large muscles, and the number of injection sites per muscle varies similarly, generally from two to six.

Selection of appropriate muscles should be based on careful clinical assessment of the maximally involved muscles and clear delineation of the goals (e.g., improved function, hygiene, or pain relief). Initial needle placement in the chosen muscle is based on anatomic landmarks, with EMG localization of muscle twitch at 2 to 3 mA often utilized for more precise placement near the motor end-plate. The onset of clinical effect is seen within 1 to 3 days, and the peak physiologic effect at 2 to 6 weeks after the time of injection. The duration of effect varies from 4 weeks to 6 months; repeated injections are required to maintain a therapeutic effect in most patients.

The side effects of botulinum toxin injections are generally transient and related to local weakness or pain, or in occasional patients, the development of antibodies that lead to resistance. The other major limitation at this point is the high cost of ongoing botulinum toxin therapy.

Systemic pharmacologic therapy benefits about a third of patients and consists of a wide variety of medications including anticholinergics, benzodiazepines, antiparkinsonian drugs, anticonvulsants, baclofen, tetrabenazine, and lithium (31). Successful drug therapy often requires combinations of these medications, with choices generally guided by empirical trials and side effect profiles. Dosages should be increased slowly over the course of weeks or months until therapeutic benefit is optimized or side effects occur. In most patients, discontinuation of the drugs requires tapering to prevent withdrawal symptoms.

Surgical options for intractable dystonias include peripheral denervation procedures such as ramusectomy/rhizotomy, and transection of the spinal accessory nerve for cervical dystonia, stereotactic thalamotomy for generalized dystonia, and muscle excision or section in the treatment of blepharospasm or torticollis. Because of the risk of significant comorbidity, these approaches are reserved for patients with disabling dystonia in whom other treatment modalities have been exhausted.

Various physiatric therapies and modalities have been employed with limited success in the symptomatic treatment of dystonias. These include relaxation training, sensory stimulation, biofeedback, transcutaneous electrical nerve stimulation (36), and percutaneous dorsal column stimulation. Stretching and bracing may aid in preventing or reducing the contractures associated with prolonged abnormal positions, especially when utilized in conjunction with the medical treatments previously described.

Occupational therapy is important for ADL training, proper positioning and seating for patients whose mobility is impaired, and provision of adaptive equipment to enhance function. Speech therapists can offer training and communication aids for patients with oromandibular or laryngeal dystonia, and help prevent complications in patients with transient dysphagia resulting from botulinum toxin injections. Vocational rehabilitation may aid individuals in job retraining or adaptation of the workplace where appropriate.

Finally, because dystonias may be significantly disabling and have a profound effect on the patient's personal, vocational, and emotional life, psychological counseling and support groups are a vital adjunct to medical and physical approaches in the multidisciplinary management of this disorder.

Neuroacanthocytosis

Neuroacanthocytosis refers to a condition in which various neurologic deficits, including chorea, dystonia, seizures, and dementia, are associated with the presence of abnormal erythrocytes (acanthocytes). In some patients, tics, parkinsonism, and neurogenic muscular atrophy are seen (37). The most consistent neuropathologic changes consist of atrophy and neuronal loss in the basal ganglia, most notably in the caudate nucleus (38). Peripheral muscle weakness and wasting have been noted, often reflecting neuronal loss in the anterior horns of the spinal cord.

The most difficult clinical and neuropathologic distinction is between neuroacanthocytosis and HD, but with discovery of the expanded trinucleotide repeat in the HD gene, genetic testing can now reliably distinguish the two.

Hepatolenticular Degeneration (Wilson Disease)

Wilson disease is an autosomal recessive disorder of copper metabolism, associated with cirrhosis of the liver and degeneration of the basal ganglia. The gene defect has been localized to the long arm of chromosome 13. The disease affects all races, with a worldwide prevalence of about 30 per million (39).

The abnormal copper metabolism results in deposition of the metal in the liver, brain, kidneys, and corneal tissue primarily. Signs and symptoms, mainly relating to liver and brain damage, generally appear between the ages of 11 and 25, although cases of earlier and later onset have been observed. Patients may display signs of liver damage, including jaundice or ascites, at any point in the disease; in some, cirrhosis is asymptomatic. Intracorneal ring-shaped pigmentations called Kayser-Fleischer rings are seen in virtually all patients with cerebral symptoms, and may require slit-lamp examination for detection.

Various brain structures are affected in Wilson disease, but the most striking changes are seen in the basal ganglia. Neurologic manifestations reflect primarily motor dysfunction, and include tremor (commonly a ballistic, large-amplitude proximal "wing-beating" tremor of the arms), rigidity, dystonic movements, dysarthria, contractures, and muscle spasticity. Behavioral abnormalities occur in about 25% of patients, while seizures are relatively rare. The neurologic picture may be so variable from patient to patient that no "typical" presentation emerges.

Characteristic findings on imaging studies include ventricular dilatation, generalized atrophy, and abnormal MRI signals in the caudate, putamen, subcortical white matter, mid brain, and pons (40).

Treatment is directed toward initiating a negative copper balance, both by restricting dietary intake or absorption of copper and by chelation therapy with penicillamine or other "decoppering" agents. Precipitous deterioration has occurred when chelation therapy is initiated too vigorously. Potassium sulfate or zinc taken with meals helps to minimize copper absorption. In some patients, addition of levodopa to the treatment regimen improves dystonia. Careful management can lead to a significant remission of symptoms and improvement in long-term survival.

Akathisia

Akathisia refers to an internal sense of motor or cognitive restlessness and an inability to maintain a fixed position or posture. Individuals affected will often march or rise frequently, and may mistake their symptoms for anxiety. Akathisia may be a side effect of many drugs, particularly neuroleptics, but also SSRIs [paroxetine (Paxil), fluoxetine (Prozac), sertraline (Zoloft)]. Treatment consists of removing the provocative medication, if possible. As a secondary strategy, symptomatic benefit has been reported with propranolol or propoxyphene.

Myoclonus

Myoclonus refers to rapid shock-like contractions of muscle groups in an asymmetric distribution, resulting in irregular movements resembling twitches or jerks. These may occur singly, may be repeated several times in a group of muscles (sometimes referred to as *segmental myoclonus*), or may be more widespread and irregularly repetitive (*polymyoclonus*).

Myoclonus can occur with many neurodegenerative diseases, both familial and sporadic. It can be seen in association with seizure disorders of various types; with progressive dementias; in certain slow virus syndromes such as Creutzfeld-Jakob disease; in metabolic disorders including a variant of Gaucher disease; and in lithium, strychnine, and tetanus intoxications. Viral encephalitis and suppurative meningitis, uremia, advanced Alzheimer disease, and anoxic encephalopathy have all been associated with myoclonus (5). In the latter, a phenomenon called *intention myoclonus* has been described in which ballistic movements, especially when directed at a target, elicit a series of irregular myoclonic jerks (41).

CONCLUSIONS

Movement disorders encompass a complex and heterogeneous group of diseases, many of them neurodegenerative and progressive in nature, leading to profound disability in many patients of all ages. Regrettably, many such patients have been diagnosed and then left to cope with their functional deficits, with little or no input from rehabilitation professionals. This generally occurs because of a misguided feeling on the part of many health providers that in disorders for which there may be no cure, "nothing can be done."

In fact, as one can see from the preceding discussion, the quality of life for many persons with movement disorders can be significantly enhanced with optimal rehabilitation management. Physiatric interventions should be relatively brief and goal directed for these often chronic and progressive conditions, with concomitant attention to medical management, patient and family education, and provision of an appropriate long-term home exercise program.

The key to effective rehabilitation services for persons with movement disorders is a flexible and holistic approach, emphasizing innovative and individualized solutions to specific problems, with attention to all aspects of the patient's life, including medical, functional, psychological, and social. No other health professional is better suited to such an approach than the rehabilitation specialist, and it is hoped that as awareness of the potential benefits of rehabilitation interventions increases in both the medical and lay communities, more individuals with movement disorders will have access to these crucial services.

REFERENCES

1. Saint-Cyr JA, Taylor AE, Nicholson K. Behavior and the basal ganglia. *Adv Neurol* 1995;65:1–28.
2. Albin RL, Young AB, Penney JB. The functional anatomy of basal ganglia disorders. *Trends Neurosci* 1989;12:366–375.
3. Strange PG. Dopamine receptors in the basal ganglia: relevance to Parkinson's disease. *Mov Disord* 1993;8:263–270.
4. Mosewich RK, Rajput AH, Shuaib A, et al. Pulmonary embolism: an underrecognized yet frequent cause of death in parkinsonism. *Mov Disord* 1994;9:350–352.
5. Adams RD, Victor M. *Principles of neurology.* 5th ed. New York: McGraw-Hill, 1993:83–85.
6. Hubble JP, Busenbark KL, Koller WC. Essential tremor. *Clin Neuropharmacol* 1989;12: 453–482.
7. Larsson T, Sjogren T. Essential tremor. A clinical and genetic population study. *Acta Psychiatr Neurol Scand* 1960;36(suppl): 1–176.
8. Larsen TA, Calne DB. Essential tremor. *Clin Neuropharmacol* 1983;6:185–206.
9. Cleeves L, Findley LJ. Variability in amplitude of untreated essential tremor. *J Neurol Neurosurg Psychiatry* 1987;50:704–708.
10. Koller WC. Alcoholism in essential tremor. *Neurology* 1983;33: 1074–1076.
11. Winkler GF, Young RR. Efficacy of chronic propranolol therapy in action tremors of the familial, senile or essential varieties. *N Engl J Med* 1974;290: 984–988.
12. Koller WC. Dose-response relationship of propranolol in essential tremor. *Arch Neurol* 1986;35:42–43.
13. Koller WC. Long-acting propranolol in essential tremor. *Neurology* 1985;36:106–108.
14. Koller WC, Biary N. Metoprolol compared to propranolol in the treatment of essential tremor. *Arch Neurol* 1984;41:171–172.
15. Koller WC. Nadolol in the treatment of essential tremor. *Neurology* 1983;33:1074–1075.
16. Findley LJ, Cleeves L, Calzetti S. Primidone in essential tremor of the hands and head: a double-blind controlled clinical study. *J Neurol Neurosurg Psychiatry* 1985;481:911–915.
17. Koller WC, Royse V. Efficacy of primidone in essential tremor. *Neurology* 1986;36:121–124.
18. Biary N, Koller WC. Kinetic-predominant tremor: effect of clonazepam. *Neurology* 1987;37:471–474.
19. Heilman KM. Orthostatic tremor. *Arch Neurol* 1984;4:880–881.
20. Bertrand C. Stereotactic and peripheral surgery for the control of movement disorders. In: Barbeau A, ed. *Disorders of movement.* Lancaster: MTP Press, 1981:191–208.
21. Huntington's Disease Collaborative Research Group. A novel gene containing a trinucleotide repeat that is expanded and unstable on

Huntington's disease chromosomes. *Cell* 1993;72:971–983.

22. Albin R, Tagle D. Genetics and molecular biology of Huntington's disease. *Trends Neurosci* 1995;18:11–14.

23. Haines JL, Conneally PM. Causes of death in Huntington's disease as reported on death certificates. *Genet Epidemiol* 1986;3: 417–423.

24. Klasner ER. Managing swallowing difficulties associated with Huntington's disease. Cambridge, ON: Huntington Society of Canada, 1990.

25. Klasner ER. Managing the communication and speech difficulties associated with Huntington's disease. Huntington Society of Canada, 1990.

26. Morris M. Psychiatric aspects of Huntington's disease. In: Harper PS, ed. *Huntington's disease.* London: WB Saunders, 1991:81–126.

27. Shoulson I, Kurlan R, Rubin AJ, et al. Assessment of functional capacity in neurodegenerative movement disorders: Huntington's disease as a prototype. In: Munsat T, ed. *Quantification of neurologic deficit.* Stoneham, MA: Butterworths, 1989:271–284.

28. Huntington Study Group. Unified Huntington's disease rating scale: reliability and consistency. *Mov Disord* 1996;11:136–142.

29. Ranen NG, Peyser CE, Folstein SE. *A physician's guide to the management of Huntington's disease.* New York: Huntington's Disease Society of America, 1993.

30. Carter S. Sydenham chorea. In: Rowland LP, ed. *Merritt's textbook of neurology.* 8th ed. Philadelphia: Lea & Febiger, 1989:645–647.

31. Jancovic J, Fahn S. Dystonic disorders. In: Jancovic J, Tolosa A, eds. *Parkinson's disease and movement disorders.* 2nd ed. Baltimore: Williams & Wilkins, 1993: 337–397.

32. Fish DR, Sawyers D, Allen PJ, et al. The effect of sleep on the dyskinetic movements of Parkinson's disease, Gilles de la Tourette syndrome, Huntington's disease and torsion dystonia. *Arch Neurol* 1991;48:210–214.

33. Jancovic J, Penn AS. Severe dystonia and myoglobinuria. *Neurology* 1982;32:1195–1197.

34. Jancovic J, Schwartz PA. Botulinum toxin injections for cervical dystonia. *Neurology* 1990;40: 277–281.

35. Williams A. Consensus statement for the management of focal dystonias. *Br J Hosp Med* 1993;50: 655–660.

36. Foley-Nolan D, Kinirons M, Coughlan RJ, O'Connor P. Post-whiplash dystonia well-controlled by transcutaneous electrical nervous stimulation (TENS): case report. *J Trauma* 1990;30:909–910.

37. Rinne JO, Daniel SE, Scaravilli F, et al. Neuropathological features of neuroacanthocytosis. *Mov Disord* 1994;9:297–304.

38. Bird TD, Cederbaum S, Valpey RW, Stahl WL. Familial degeneration of the basal ganglia with acanthocytosis: a clinical, pathological and neurochemical study. *Ann Neurol* 1978;3:253–258.

39. Menkes JH. Disorders of mental metabolism. In: Rowland LP, ed. *Merritt's textbook of neurology.* 8th ed. Philadelphia: Lea & Febiger, 1989:538–544.

40. Starosta-Rubinstein S, Young AB, Kluin K, et al. Clinical assessment of 31 patients with Wilson's disease: correlations with structural changes on magnetic resonance imaging. *Arch Newol* 1987;44:365–370

41. Lance JW, Adams RD. The syndrome of intention of action myoclonus as a sequel to hypoxic encephalopathy. *Brain* 1963;87:111.

Chapter 50

Prevention and Management of Pressure Ulcers

Gary M. Yarkony

Although considered an "old subject" by some, pressure ulcers have not been neglected in the literature. Acute care facilities, hospitals, nursing homes, and homes have increasing numbers of aged persons. Although people today are living longer and healthier than in past generations, there are also more people with chronic illness and longer periods of immobility and disability. Hospitalized patients are more often the severely ill. Thus, a thorough consideration of pressure ulcers, their etiology, structure, prevalence, and amelioration is mandated.

Pressure ulcers are frequently referred to as *decubitus ulcers*, *bed sores*, *ischemic ulcers*, and *pressure sores*. The principal etiologic factors are pressure and shear, resulting in the sloughing of necrotic tissue. The incidence and location vary according to patient age, underlying medical conditions, type of institution, and other factors. Prevalence in acute care hospitals has been reported as ranging from 9.2% to 4.7% (1,2). Nursing homes have demonstrated a 17.4% prevalence at the time of admission, with an incidence of pressure ulcer development during a 1-year period ranging from 9.5% at year 1 to 21.6% by year 2 (3).

Estimates of pressure ulcer prevalence range from 3% to 14% among patients in acute care hospitals and from 15% to 25% on admission to skilled nursing facilities (2,4). The most common sites of development are the sacrum, the ischium, the trochanters, and the ankles and heels (1,5).

This chapter reviews the relevant literature on pressure ulcers from the late 1950s to the present. It includes some earlier references and recent areas of research, such as growth factors and new technologies for pressure relief in beds.

SKIN ANATOMY AND PHYSIOLOGY

The largest organ of the body, the skin, accounts for approximately 15% of body weight, about 10 kg, and has a surface area of 1.5 to 2.0 m^2 (6,7). It is an active dynamic organ with numerous functions (8). It serves as a barrier to microorganisms and protects against injuries from mechanical, chemical, thermal, and osmotic forces. The skin is involved in thermoregulation and maintenance of fluid balance. It is involved in the synthesis of vitamin D and has the capacities of both absorption and excretion. The skin is an extensive sensory organ and it can display emotion through expressions and vascular reflexes.

Skin is composed of two layers, the epidermis and the dermis. The avascular epidermis, or outer layer, is composed of stratified squamous keratinizing epithelium derived from the ectoderm. The dermis, derived from mesenchyme, is composed of vascularized, irregularly arranged fibroelastic tissue that provides nourishment to the epidermis (9). Thick skin with a thick epidermis covers the palms of the hands and soles of the feet while thin skin covers the remainder of the body. Beneath the skin is the subcutaneous tissue, often called the *hypodermis* or *superficial fascia*, which is composed of loose connective tissue and adipose tissue. The dermis is anchored by fibrous bands containing collagen that attaches to the underlying fascia or periosteum, resulting in limited skin movement. Beneath the fatty hypodermis is the fascial tissue and the muscle tissue that cover the bone.

The epidermis protects against environmental influences and against harmful fluid loss. This proactive function is provided by the outermost stratum corneum, which contains keratin (a protein complex) and a mixture of complex lipids. The epidermis is renewed every 3 to 4 weeks, forming the horny layer (stratum corneum) as cells reproduce and die while moving in an orderly fashion to the surface. The keratinization process occurs in 85% of the cells of the epidermis known as *keratinocytes*. Keratinization is not equivalent to formation of the stratum corneum, as cells in the vagina and oral mucosa keratinize without forming a stratum corneum. The remaining cells, the *melanocytes*, produce the pigment melanin, which is responsible for skin color and ultraviolet light protection. Langerhans cells in the epidermis are involved in the immune reactions of the epidermis. The stratus germinativum, the inner layer, grows mitotically to regenerate the epidermis and produce vitamin D.

The dermis (7,9) is the thick layer of connective tissue beneath the epidermis. It is composed of two layers, the papillary layer (the thin outer layer of the dermis of loose connective tissue) and an inner reticular layer of dense, irregularly arranged connective tissue. The papillary layer is a highly vascular area that provides nourishment for the epidermis. The connective tissue of the dermis provides support and strength, and the elastin and reticulum fibers provide elasticity. The vasculature, in addition to nourishing the epidermis and removing waste, assists in the regulation of body temperature and skin color (8).

Thin skin contains many appendages—the hair, sebaceous glands, apocrine sweat glands, and nails—that serve many functions (9). Sebaceous glands produce sebum, which keeps skin and hair supple, controls skin pH, and has antibacterial and antifungal effects. Sweat glands are less numerous in thin skin than in thick skin and assist in cooling. Thick skin has more eccrine sweat glands, but some are present throughout the body. Apocrine sweat glands are present in the axilla, the areolae of the breasts, and the pubic and perineal regions and do not secrete until puberty (9). There are many kinds of sensory receptors in skin, grouped into two categories: free nerve endings and encapsulated nerve ends. These sensory receptors can be described functionally as mechanoreceptors, which respond to touch and pressure; stretch thermoreceptors for temperature changes; and nociceptors that respond to skin irritants (9). Lymph vessels in the dermis remove excess fluids and store protein (8).

ETIOLOGY

Although numerous factors are involved in any individual with a pressure ulcer, it is clear that pressure over bony prominences is the key etiologic factor. Trumble (10) described the relationship between pressure intensity and duration in 1930. Kosiak's (11–13) classic studies were the first to define the relationship between pressure and time. He described a parabolic relationship between pressure and time, indicating that higher pressures cause ulceration in a shorter time period than do lower pressures. This relationship was determined by using dogs, which as animal models are not as relevant to humans as are pigs, whose skin more closely resembles human skin.

The studies in pigs by Daniel et al (14) showed a curve similar to the one described by Kosiak. The curve for paraplegic animals was similar in shape, but the orders for time and magnitude were reduced (14). This change was attributed to impaired mobility and sensation, incontinence leading to skin maceration, and atrophy of soft tissues leading to increased interface pressure at bony prominences. Pressure that exceeds the mean blood pressure on the back leads to a cessation of skin blood flow (15). Pressure is more concentrated in the area of the muscle and fat adjacent to the bone (16). In contrast to Kosiak, Daniel et al (17) determined that these tissues are more susceptible to pressure and may show signs of damage prior to evidence of damage to the skin (18). Tissue that is atrophied, scarred, or secondarily infected has an increased susceptibility or pressure (14–19). Skin can be damaged by intermittent pressures in excess of mean capillary pressures, resulting in endothelial damage and platelet thrombosis (20). Moderate stresses, although within physiologic limits, can result in damage to the skin if repeated frequently (21).

Shearing force is the second key factor in the development of "presshear ulcers." (The word *presshear* indicates the two major factors in the development of skin ulceration: pressure and shear. The term *presshear ulcers* is proposed as more accurate than *pressure ulcers* to describe these lesions.) Shear is an applied force that causes an opposite parallel sliding motion in the planes of an object (22). It has been described as "more disastrous than the more vertical pressure," as it cuts off large areas of vascular supply. For one example, shearing forces affect the sacrum when the head of the bed is elevated for an immobilized person who is supine (23). Shear can significantly decrease the amount of pressure needed to occlude blood flow (24). Elderly persons tend to develop higher shearing forces while sitting, further predisposing them to pressure ulcers (25). Friction applies mechanical forces to the epidermis, resulting in increased susceptibility to ulceration (26).

Moisture secondary to incontinence or perspiration can result in skin maceration and predispose patients to pressure ulceration (26). Anaerobic waste products that accumulate due to occlusion of lymphatic vessels have been hypothesized to contribute to tissue necrosis (27), and this development is hypothesized to be mediated by emotional stress (28). The results of a small, poorly controlled study suggested that smoking cigarettes, which contain nicotine, a peripheral vasoconstrictive agent, increases the risk of pressure ulceration (29).

Although pressure and shear are still considered the major causes of pressure ulcers, many factors must be considered in the treatment plan for persons considered to be at risk.

PERSONS AT RISK

Any person who is immobilized or has an immobilized body part in a cast is at risk for pressure ulcer development (30). Hospitalized patients who are bed or chair bound are at increased risk of developing pressure ulcers if they have hypoalbuminemia, fecal incontinence, or fractures (2). Malnourished or vitamin-deficient patients are at increased risk of pressure development (6,31–38). Norton and Braden (34) and the Dutch Consensus Conference (35) developed scales that assess physical and mental activity, continence, sensation, and other factors to identify persons at risk (Table 50-1). Elderly persons, particularly those in hospitals or nursing homes, are at particular risk of pressure ulcer development for several reasons. Ischemia can be induced more easily in elderly persons than younger persons, and they may develop more shear while sitting (25). The mean pressure and the calculated total pressure per hour of bed occupation (referred to as *impulse pressure* in the study) on the sacrums of elderly persons are increased in elderly as compared to younger subjects who are in bed (36). Aging skin, with its associated physical, structural, physiologic, and immunologic changes, may have a major impact on pressure ulcer development (6,37). Aged skin has a diminished barrier function, increased susceptibility to shearing forces, and decreased vascularity. Body build may impact on an individual's susceptibility to pressure ulcer development. Thinner persons may develop higher pressures over bony prominences than the average-weight or obese patients (38,39).

Table 50-1: The Dutch Consensus Meeting for the Prevention of Pressure Sores Risk Score*

	Score			
Variable	0	1	2	3
Mental status	Normal	Listless, depressed, frightened	Severely depressed, psychotic, apathetic	(Semi) comatose
Neurology	Normal	Minor disorders, minor loss of strength	Loss of sensation, partial hemiparesis (points × 2)	Hemiparesis (points × 2), paraparesis below TH5 (× 3), above TH6 (× 4)
Mobility	Normal	Limited, walks with help	Almost bedridden	Totally bedridden
Nutritional status	Good	Moderate, no food for several days	Bad, no food for a week	Emaciated
Nutritional intake	Normal, good appetite	Parenteral	No appetite, insufficient feeding	None
Incontinence	None	Occasionally urinary	No control but catheter in place	Total for urine and excrement
Age (yr)	< 50	50–59	60–69	> 70
Temperature (°C)..	> 35.5 < 37.5	> 37.4 < 38.5	> 38.4 < 39.0	< 35.6 > 38.9
Medication	None	Corticosteroids, sedatives, anticoagulants	Tranquilizers, chemotherapy, oral antibiotics	Parenteral antibiotics
Diabetes	None	Diet only	Diet and oral medication	Diet and insulin

TH = thoracic sensory segment.

* A score > 8 indicates a patient is at risk.

Source: Reproduced by permission from Hofman A, Geelkerken RH, Wille J, et al. Pressure sores and pressure-decreasing mattresses: controlled clinical trial. *Lancet* 1994;343:458–571.

Psychological adjustment affects a person's ability to follow through on prescribed skin care regimens. Depressed persons and those prone to self-neglect may develop pressure ulcers due to a lack of follow-through on self-care needs (40,41). Poor home care, poor advice from caregivers, and inadequate care in general hospitals by persons not familiar with skin care principles in paralyzed persons may contribute to pressure ulcer development (42). Persons with spinal cord injury are well known to be at high risk for pressure ulcer development (43,44). A spinal cord–injured person's risk may be enhanced immediately after injury by prolonged immobilization on spine boards, and his or her risk is inversely related to systolic blood pressures (45).

PRESSURE ULCER ASSESSMENT

Assessment of pressure ulcers requires 1) a description of the wound and surrounding tissue, 2) assignment of a grade, and 3) measurement of its size. Adequate description is essential for staff communication as well as for research purposes. Wounds covered with necrotic tissue or eschar should be debrided to determine the grade of the wound.

Ulcers are generally graded or staged based on erythema of the skin or depth of the ulcer (Table 50-2) (4,46,47). The most commonly used system was developed by Shea (47) and uses four grades and the description "closed pressure sore" to record the presence of large cavities accessible through a small sinus on the skin surface. The Yarkony-Kirk scale (46) is considered more useful than Shea's despite having more grades. One study comparing the Yarkony-Kirk scale to Shea's indicated a higher inter-rater reliability for the Yarkony-Kirk scale (46). This scale includes a distinct classification of a red area and a healed area to allow for recognition of sites of future breakdown, and describes the depth of a wound by the tissue observed at the base of the wound. The National Pressure Ulcer Advisory Panel (4) developed a different scale as a step toward developing a universally accepted classification. This scale is described as combining several of the most commonly used staging systems. However, it has not been verified or accepted as a standard (49). The International Association for Enterostomal Therapy has developed a separate classification (48). To date, no study has compared the use of these numerous systems to each other or their relative utility in the evaluation and treatment of pressure ulcers. Future research is needed in this area.

Other systems, not specific to any type of wound, include the use of color to describe wounds (49,50). Yellow indicates soft necrotic tissue, black indicates adherent

Table 50-2: Comparison of Three Pressure Ulcer Classifications

Yarkony-Kirk Classification (46)	Shea Classification (47)	National Pressure Ulcer Advisory Panel (4)	
1. Red area A. Present > 30 min but < 24 h B. Present > 24 h	1. Limited to epidermis, exposing dermis; includes a red area	Stage I:	nonblanchable erythema of intact skin: the heralding lesion of skin ulceration
2. Epidermis and/or dermis ulcerated with no subcutaneous fat observed	2. Full thickness of dermis in the junction of subcutaneous fat	Stage II:	partial-thickness skin loss involving epidermis and/or dermis; superficial ulcer presenting clinically as an abrasion, blister, or shallow crater
3. Subcutaneous fat observed, no muscle observed	3. Fat obliterated, limited by the deep fascia undermining of skin	Stage III:	full-thickness skin loss involving damage or necrosis of subcutaneous tissue that may extend down to, but not through, underlying fascia; ulcer presents clinically as a deep crater with or without undermining of adjacent tissue
4. Muscle/fascia observed but no bone observed	4. Bone at base of ulceration	Stage IV:	full-thickness skin loss with extensive destruction, tissue necrosis, or damage to muscle, bone, or supporting structure (e.g., tendon, joint, capsule)
5. Bone observed, but no involvement of joint space	5. Closed large cavity through a small sinus		
6. Involvement in the joint space; pressure sore healed			

necrotic tissue, and red indicates a wound ready to heal with granulation tissue.

Numerous techniques have been described to measure the size and depth of a pressure ulcer. Generally the ulcer is measured at its maximum dimensions and depth is indicated. It is then diagrammed, traced, or photographed (51). One recent study compared acetate tracings, the Kundin device (a six-pronged measuring device), and photography with digital analysis. Acetate tracings can provide the most accurate description of the wound area (52) but require manual or computer planimetry once the tracings are completed. Photography requires special equipment and an image analysis system. The Kundin measuring device consistently underestimates the area (53). Other more complex techniques not generally applicable in the clinical setting include use of dental impression materials (54,55) and analysis of photographs with a computer taken over a polyester grid (56). Sinography may be used when clinical assessment of a tunneling ulcer is not adequate (57–59). A radiopaque dye is instilled into the wound and plain x-ray films made to determine the depth and extent of the lesion. These wounds are described by Shea as "closed" (47).

Bates-Jensen et al (60) developed a Pressure Sore Status Tool as a means of clinically describing a pressure ulcer, including the location, shape, and 13 items, including size, depth, edges, undermining necrotic tissue, exudate, surrounding skin, and evidence of healing. They proposed future research areas to study use of this tool. The need for training and complexity make the use of this technique in care settings questionable.

PATHOLOGY

Kosiak (12), in studies of dogs, proposed that with pressure, degeneration occurs equally in tissue at all levels, as opposed to only from bone outward. He later described edema, loss of cross-striation and myofibrils, hyalinization, and phagocytosis by neutrophils and macrophages in normal and paraplegic rats. He determined that there were no differences in paraplegic and normal rats in studies that were done less than 24 hours after section of the spinal cord (13).

Dinsdale (61) described changes in the skin of swine due to friction. Friction initially removes the stratum corneum. The superficial cells at the epidermis separate from the basal cells because their bridges are brittle. With pressure and friction, superficial dermis becomes hyperemic, then eosinophilic, and with increasing pressure, there is hemorrhage and leukocyte infiltration in the capillaries of the dermis. The superficial dermis then becomes necrotic (61). Since friction can be affected by the amount of moisture on the skin, with low rates of sweating, friction increases, yet with maximal sweating there is a decrease as compared to dry skin (62). The studies in swine by Daniel et al (17) showed that initial damage occurs in deep muscle with progression toward the skin. As discussed earlier, his animal model in swine is more appropriate than Kosiak's dog model. At high pressures of short duration (500 mm Hg for 9 hours) or low pressures of long duration (100 mm Hg for 10 hours), skin is intact, but deep muscle damage occurs. At high pressures of long duration (800 mm Hg for 10 hours) or low pressures of prolonged duration (200 mm Hg for 15 hours), there is damage from muscle to the subcutaneous tissue and lower dermis, but superficial skin and hair growth are intact. With long-duration pressure (600 mm Hg for 11 hours, 200 mm Hg for 16 hours), a visible skin lesion is present at 1 week and full-thickness destruction occurs (17). With septicemia, bacteria can localize at the sites of pressure application and encourage breakdown at lower pressures (14). Given confirmation of this early muscle damage, turning patients at least every 2 hours to prevent pressure ulcerations is a sound practice (12,13,30).

Witkowski and Parish (63) described a sequence of capillary and venule dilatation followed by edema of the papillary dermis and a perivascular infiltrate in human skin, followed by platelet aggregates, red blood cell engorgement, and perivascular hemorrhage. As these vascular changes occur, the sweat glands and subcutaneous fat show signs of necrosis with eventual epidermal necrosis. This study demonstrated no correlation with pressure amount and duration and no indication if shearing had occurred. Tissues were taken from various sites, but deep tissues were not studied (63).

COMPLICATIONS

Pressure ulcers that become infected can lead to local abscess formation and cause septicemia or osteomyelitis. Infection of an ulcer is recognized by extensive surrounding inflammation and induration, purulent drainage, and fever (64). A foul odor is generally associated with the presence of anaerobes (65). Swab culture results and deep tissue culture results do not always concur, and deep tissue culture results vary depending on the site of the lesion (65). A technique known as *irrigation-aspiration* has a 97.6% concordance for aerobes and a 91.8% concordance for anaerobes when compared with biopsy (66). As pressure ulcers heal and granulation tissue appears, the bacterial counts drop. Aerobic organisms (*Staphylococcus aureus*, *Streptococcus*, *Pseudomonas*, *Proteus*) and anaerobic organisms (*Clostridia*, *Bacteroides*) may be involved. Use of antibiotics is generally limited to systemic infection and lesions with surrounding cellulitis; there has been debate about their use (30,67). Foul-smelling necrotic tissue can be removed by debridement, wound cleansing, and saline wet-to-dry dressing. Topical or oral administration of metronidazole may be beneficial in treating infected ulcers not responsive to local care (68,69).

Soft-tissue and pelvic abscesses can develop secondary to pressure ulcers. The soft-tissue abscess may present as spontaneous rupture or may be aspirated. Computed tomography is of value in identifying these abscesses (70,71).

Osteomyelitis in bone beneath a pressure ulcer can impair healing of an ulcer, result in repeated breakdown, impair healing of surgically repaired wounds, and result in spread of infection. Although a variety of methods have been suggested to obtain this diagnosis (72,73), bone biopsy still is the definitive diagnostic procedure. The results of nuclear medicine scans are often positive because of local bone disease and soft-tissue infection (74), and the appearance on plain x-ray films alone does not always correlate directly with osteomyelitis (73). A positive finding on a plain x-ray film, a white blood cell count of 15,000/μL, and an erythrocyte sedimentation rate of 120 mm/hr or greater is presumptive evidence of osteomyelitis. A recent study indicated that plain x-ray films can identify osteomyelitis with greater accuracy than computed tomography (75).

Bacteremia, a potentially life-threatening complication of pressure ulcers, resulted in a mortality rate of over 50% in one series (76). Surgical debridement of the ulcer, along with administration of appropriate antibiotics, is essential (77,78).

Marjolin ulcer, a malignant degeneration of a chronic pressure ulcer that is usually present for more than 20 years, is a rare (< 0.5%) complication (79–83). Clinical signs include pain, increasing discharge, foul odor and bleeding, and verrucous hyperplasia (84–88). Biopsy remains the definitive diagnostic method. Metastasis to inguinal nodes is common (89,90).

MEDICAL MANAGEMENT

When treating a pressure ulcer, it is important to treat the entire person and not focus solely on the ulcer. Since pressure ulcers are attached to people, a person's general medical condition, nutrition, and social situation must be considered. These factors are critical in healing the ulcer and preventing recurrence.

Wound healing occurs in a continuum that has been described in three stages (8). The inflammatory phase lasts up to 3 days. A fibrin clot is formed as platelets aggregate to prevent bleeding. To cause further platelet aggregation, platelets release the following substances: factors chemotactic for leukocytes, proteolytic enzymes that initiate couplement activation, and growth factors. Thrombocytopenia may diminish the rate of wound healing. Leukocytes remove foreign material, and macrophages remove bacteria and debris. Macrophages are essential cells and release angiogenic substances and stimulate fibroblasts (91), whose growth is enhanced by low oxygen and high lactate levels. Fibroblasts, which appear at 48 to 72 hours, synthesize collagen elastin and proteoglycans. The proliferation phase occurs next until the wound is healed. Granulation tissue develops and contracts. Collagen synthesis and angiogenesis occur as new epithelium, with its silvery appearance, and covers the wound. A maturation process occurs after the wound is healed and continues for years as the scar is observed to shrink and thin out from reorganization. Fading of the scar is due to regression of capillaries.

Ensuring adequate nutrition should be a routine part of all medical management irrespective of the patient's risk for pressure ulcers. When a pressure ulcer develops, nutritional status must be reassessed. Mulholland et al (31) were the first to demonstrate diminished plasma protein levels in persons with pressure ulcers. Malnutrition may occur in hospitalized patients in general, medical, and surgical wards (92). Nursing home patients with pressure ulcers may have low cholesterol, albumin, and zinc levels and may be anemic in spite of a high-protein calorie diet administered via feeding tubes (93). A nursing home study using serum albumin, total lymphocyte count, and somatic protein as markers determined that patients with pressure sores were more severely malnourished (33). Adequate protein intake correlates with potential for ulcer healing (94).

Maintaining adequate protein, calories, and fluid intake to prevent negative nitrogen balance and dehydration is essential (95,96). Water is needed in excess of 1 L/day, and 1.5 to 2.0 g of protein is needed per kilogram of body weight (95). The major source of calories should be from carbohydrates (95). Protein balance can be assessed by serum albumin and transferrin levels and nitrogen balance studies may also be helpful. Numerous studies have been done on zinc and its impact on pressure ulcers (32), particularly since zinc is required for protein synthesis and repair (97). Since elevated zinc levels (> 400 mg/dL) can interfere with macrophage function, zinc supplements are recommended only for persons who are zinc deficient (95,98,99). Iron should be supplemented only in iron-deficient individuals. Vitamin C, which is required for collagen synthesis and needed in levels above the basic requirement, has been the subject of several studies (100,101). In a double-blind, placebo-controlled study on 20 patients with pressure ulcers, vitamin C supplementation of 1 g/day in divided doses improved the rate of pressure ulcer healing. Excess ascorbic acid is metabolized to oxalic acid and may increase the risk of kidney stones (95). This risk has not been studied in pressure ulcer patients. Persons with pressure ulcers should receive the basic requirements of all vitamins and trace elements and appropriate treatment should be given if they are anemic.

TREATMENT OF THE ULCER

There is no definitive study of the most effective way to treat pressure ulcers. The outline here is based on the results of both animal and human studies. Many studies have explained what is dangerous to use. Other studies have found one treatment better than another. There are no clear guidelines as to possible controls when studying the use of a new dressing, for instance. No study has systematically compared various treatments with a standard nontoxic control. Individual patients may vary in their clinical responses, perhaps responding better to one dressing despite a finding that it may result in slower healing. For instance, when patients are switched from wet-to-dry dressings to an occlusive dressing as the wound improves, healing may stop until a saline dressing is reapplied. The generally accepted principles of pressure ulcer management are described. Further study is needed to determine the ideal moist-wound healing environment as products continue to proliferate without adequate study.

The first step in the treatment of a pressure ulcer after removing pressure is the elimination of necrotic tissue. Debridement may be surgical, mechanical, osmotic, chemical, enzymatic, autolytic, or ingestive by the use of maggots (102,103). Necrotic tissue is a barrier to wound contraction and epithelialization and a nidus for infection. Surgical debridement, generally done with a scalpel, is the most efficient method of debridement. A newer method of surgical debridement is vaporization with a carbon dioxide laser. The laser can debride bone as well as soft tissue. Wet-to-dry dressing can remove small amounts of necrotic tissue and is useful to remove residual necrotic tissue after a partial surgical debridement. Since these dressings will remove healthy tissue as well, they should be discontinued when the wound is clean. Hydrotherapy requires the time of staff members and is generally not necessary. Autolytic debridement can occur under an occlusive dressing but is quite slow; thus, it is more efficient to debride the wound before using an occlusive dressing. Enzymatic debridement agents contain either fibrinolysin-deoxyribonuclease trypsin, papain, collagenase, or sutilains. These materials require several treatments and are more expensive than simple debridement or wet-to-dry dressing changes.

The general principles that should be used in healing ulcers, as well as some commonly used toxic substances that should be avoided, are reviewed here, but it is not possible to review the risks and benefits of all dressings, potions, salves, liniments, and concoctions that have been proposed to treat pressure ulcers. Unfortunately, much research in pressure ulcer treatment includes numerous uncontrolled studies, and some discussions of potentially useful dressings compare them with "control" dressings containing toxic substances (104, 105). Thus, the reported findings on any particular product should be viewed with caution. Also, in any particular study, staff interest will focus on new devices, as demonstrated by one study using a placebo device that supposedly emitted electromagnetic waves. This device was judged to be effective by the hospital staff (106). Since staff awareness increases with any study of pressure ulcer, all the patients may show improvement no matter what treatment is being used.

Much of the interest in wound healing in a moist environment began with Winters study in domestic pigs (107). A moist-wound environment resulted in enhanced epithelialization that stimulated growth of underlying connective tissues (107). Hinman and Maibach (108) confirmed these benefits in humans and described how eschar in an air-exposed wound inhibits migration of epithelium. Knighton et al (109) studied the hypoxic wound environment under occlusive dressings and concluded that local wound hypoxia encourages angiogenesis and capillary growth. In comparisons of hydrocolloid dressings, wet-to-dry dressings, polyurethane film, and air exposure in an animal model, Alvarez et al (110) confirmed improved wound healing in a moist environment and described damage to the new epithelium when the polyurethane films and gauze were removed. Several studies concerned with infection under occlusive dressings (111–114) demonstrated lower rates of infection with these dressings and indicated that they may protect wounds from invasion by bacteria. Occlusive dressings should not be applied to grossly infected wounds. Falanga (115) reviewed the question of which occlusive dressing to use. Premature removal can cause epithelial damage, and granulating wounds that do not epithelialize while covered with an occlusive dressing should be switched to a nonadherent dressing. Occlusive dressings should not be placed over severe dermatitis surrounding a wound. Hydrocolloid dressings may have a modest cost benefit in treating pressure ulcers when compared to saline-soaked gauze (116), but may not be as effective as gauze in lesions that expose muscle (117). Calcium alginate dressings, made of a polysaccharide from brown seaweed, were recently introduced in the United States (118,119). They have been devised to handle wounds with large amounts of exudate, but scientific documentation of their benefit is lacking. The studies on occlusive dressings and other moist dressings did not uniformly control for nutritional status or allow for determining which patients would benefit most from a particular dressing.

Careful consideration must be given to the application of topical agents to pressure ulcers. Povidone-iodine (Betadine), a topical antiseptic, contains iodine, which can be absorbed through the skin and mucosal surfaces, resulting in increased serum iodine concentrations (120–122). Iodine absorption can result in metabolic acidosis, hypernatremia, hyperosmolarity, and renal failure and has been associated with hypothyroidism and hyperthyroidism. Povidone-iodine (1%) is also toxic to fibroblasts, as are 3% hydrogen peroxide, 0.5% sodium hypochlorite, and 0.25% acetic acid (123). These substances are not recommended.

Topical antibiotics such as bacitracin, silver sulfadiazine, and combinations of neomycin, bacitracin, and polymyxin B may enhance epidermal healing (102,115, 123). This effect may not be explained by their antimicrobial activity (124). Topical antibiotics may be effective in wounds that are not healing after several weeks or those that are continuing to produce exudate. Agents such as silver sulfadiazine and triple antibiotic ointment that have a broad spectrum of action may be used (125,126). Our clinical experience indicates that they are beneficial when used with a nonadherent gauze on superficial ulcerations. These agents are particularly helpful on superficial open areas that cannot hold an occlusive dressing or are not responsive to one.

Electrical stimulation as a treatment for pressure ulcers has been the subject of numerous studies (127–131), which were recently reviewed (132). Many of these studies had a poor sample size or were poorly controlled. The clinical effectiveness of electrical stimulation techniques has not been established. Further study is needed to determine the benefits and cost-effectiveness of electrical stimulation; this is particularly important because a therapist's time may be required to apply electrical stimulation.

GROWTH FACTORS

Growth factors are naturally occurring proteins that are secreted from platelets and macrophages and are believed to direct the migration of cells into wounds and orchestrate the process of repair (8,133).

Epidermal growth factor increases mitosis in epidermal cell cultures and granulation tissue, and may enhance epithelialization. It increases glycosaminoglycan synthesis in dermal fibroblast cultures, and increases glycolysis, fibronectin, and nucleic acid synthesis. In animal studies, the recombinant epidermal growth factor enhanced epithelialization in partial-thickness wounds (134,135).

The fibroblast growth factor, which occurs in acid and basic forms stimulates endothelial cell growth and blood vessel growth in vivo (8,135). Transforming growth factor β (TGFB1) (135,136) is released from platelets and has a direct effect on collagen synthesis, causing it to mature more rapidly. It inhibits the differentiation of fibroblasts in myofibroblasts, possibly because its presence reduces the need for wound contraction as increased cellular matrix is synthesized.

Platelet-derived growth factor (PDGF) is chemotactic for fibroblasts, smooth muscle cells, neutrophils, and mononuclear cells (137,138). It induces an inflammatory response and a provisional matrix synthesis in wounds that is greater compared with normal wounds. The differentiation of fibroblasts is affected by PDGF in the same manner as by TGFB1, as described earlier. PDGF derived from recombinant DNA is currently being studied in humans. Autologous platelet–derived wound-healing factors are also being used in nonhealing wounds (139, 140). These factors are prepared by using an individual's platelet-rich plasma, extracting the platelets, and suspending them in a buffer solution that is activated with thrombin and made into a salve. Robson et al (141) reported that persons treated with high doses (100 μg/mL) of recombinant PDGF BB showed improved healing of the pressure ulcers. Lower doses tested were not effective. This study is not believed to be conclusive because of the small sample size and statistical significance level ($p = 0.12$) (133). Studies by Knighton et al (139) and Atri et al (140) using platelet extracts may contain a more natural combination of factors needed to stimulate wound healing, as opposed to a single growth factor. However, in these studies the types of patients and the content of the extracts were not controlled, the sample size was small, and the content of the growth factors in each extract was not known. Further studies using defined preparations in large well-controlled studies are needed (133). Although PDGF and its preparations have been studied the most extensively, compared to other growth factors, it is too early to recommend their usage.

Growth factors or extracts of autologous human platelets may play a major role in the treatment of pressure ulcers in the future. Further study is needed to determine the indications, the cost-effectiveness, the type of ulcers that will benefit optimally from growth factors, and the incorporation of their use in overall patient management.

SURGICAL REPAIR

Davis (142) is credited with the first report of using a skin flap in treatment of a pressure ulcer. He undercut and shifted flaps of skin and subcutaneous tissue. A large series of repairs reported by Conway and Griffith (143) in 1956 described several principles of surgical treatment: excision of the ulcer, surrounding scar tissue and underlying bursas, and removal of underlying bone. Surgical management included careful hemostasis and a muscle flap to fill in deep holes and provide a well-vascularized pad. They used split-thickness skin grafts and advancement or rotation flaps, as well as large flaps with skin and fat, and avoided scars over the site of the ulcer (143). Myocutaneous flaps are now the primary means of surgical management (18,19).

Muscle is more metabolically active than skin and more sensitive to pressure (18,19), and its effectiveness as a cover for pressure ulcers has been called into question. Anatomic dissections reveal that myocutaneous flaps are being placed over bony prominences not normally covered by muscle. The muscle in these flaps will atrophy (18,19). A recent series for which myocutaneous flaps were used indicated that in 69% of patients and 61% of sores, ulceration recurred as early as 9.3 months (144). Clearly, this treatment is not a definitive cure for pressure ulcers.

New flaps that rotate innervated, vascularized tissue, to allow for sensory input and hopefully decrease recurrence, are being studied (145–147). Placement of these flaps may require multiple surgical stages. Further study is needed to determine the indications and effectiveness of the innervated flaps. The current literature is based on case reports.

Repair of a pressure ulcer should be accompanied by an educational program in the rehabilitation setting to teach methods to prevent recurrence and to reassess equipment and attendant care needs. Specific surgical techniques have been described and illustrated by Agris and Spira (5). Pressure sores not responding to medical management and not amenable to surgical repair have resulted in amputation of the lower extremities. This condition generally occurs in the patient with multiple ulcerations and severe osteomyelitis (148). Although in the past amputation has been considered an appropriate surgical technique to aid rehabilitation, it is now used as a last resort when standard medical and surgical repair are not possible (149).

PREVENTION

The methods and the technologies used to prevent pressure ulcers depend on the setting. In a hospital setting, the basis for prevention is adequate nursing care (150). Most persons can be treated with proper bed positioning and turning every 2 hours. Bony prominences should be checked every 2 hours and hyperemia of the skin should resolve in 30 minutes. Turning techniques should avoid shearing the soft tissues. Patients should be alternated between their backs and sides and placed prone if medically indicated. Care should be taken to avoid pressure over bony prominences. The prone position has larger low-pressure areas and smaller high-pressure areas (151). Difficulties develop in the acute care setting when turning is limited or not possible because of the medical condition or because pressure ulcers prohibit various positions. This problem led to the development of numerous beds and bed overlays to prevent pressure ulcers.

It is not possible to review in detail the large number of products available. The literature is insufficient to make recommendations as to cost-effectiveness and appropriate patient characteristics for specific mattresses. Further study is needed in this area. The majority of studies are case reports or uncontrolled studies. Recent controlled studies of low-air-loss beds and pressure-decreasing mattresses indicated their effectiveness in preventing and treating pressure ulcers.

Mattress overlays can be static pads or alternating-pressure pads and are designed to reduce pressures during recumbency (151,152). Alternating-pressure pads have periods of high and low pressure and there is great variability in their effectiveness. At least 4 inches of convoluted foam is needed, as 2 inches provide no protection for the trochanters (152). Although these pads may reduce pressures below those of a standard bed, pressures can be raised by spasms, posture changes, and muscle contractions. Alternating-pressure air mattresses are costly in that they require a constant supply of electricity, are noisy, and are subject to puncture and breakdown (153). Water beds are bulky, making turns and lifting difficult, and the patient cannot sit up (153). Pressures over the shoulder area are high on water beds (154).

Numerous models of pressure-reducing mattresses are available. Through the use of special surface coverings and foam or other internal padding, they attempt to reduce peak interface pressures of the person. These mattresses appear to reduce the risk of pressure ulcer development when their use is incorporated into a program of risk assessment and standard prevention techniques (35,155). The inability to blind the staff to the nature of the mattress being studied is a problem with all the studies performed.

Low-air-loss beds (air flotation), which support the patient on an air-permeable fabric through which air is continuously pumped, produce consistently fewer pressures than do standard beds or water beds (156). Pressures in the areas of bony prominences are consistently less than capillary pressures (156). Pressures on low-air-loss are equivalent to those on air-fluidized beds if these beds are adjusted properly. If not, they can be less effective than static beds (157).

Air-fluidized beds use a process that makes granules behave like a liquid by forcing warm air through beads covered by a woven polyester sheet (94,158). Adverse effects include fluid loss, dehydration, dry skin, scaly skin, and epistaxis from the flow of dry air. With these beds, confusion and disorientation due to the sensation of floating may develop, thick pulmonary secretions can occur, turning and repositioning may be difficult, and pressure ulcers can develop. The size and weight of the bed can be a problem and the microspheres can leak. The therapy is expensive (159). These beds have a bactericidal effect because of the sequestration and desiccation of microorganisms by the ceramic beads (160,161).

One large controlled study comparing alternating-air mattress overlays and water beds with standard mattresses demonstrated a decrease in pressure ulcer development with the air or water mattress. The study was done over a 10-day period in an acute care hospital (153). Low-air-loss beds, compared to foam mattresses, allowed improvement in the healing of pressure ulcers in a nursing home study (162). A recent study in an intensive care unit setting showed that low-air-loss beds are associated with a decrease in the development of pressure ulcers. They are also believed to be cost-effective in this setting (163).

The majority of studies testing the effectiveness of air-fluidized beds was uncontrolled (164–166). Allman et al (94) compared air-fluidized beds to standard therapy in a large general hospital population. Air-fluidized beds appeared to improve pressure ulcer healing, although they did not eliminate the development of new ulcers. Further study is needed to determine the cost-effectiveness of these beds and the optimal treatment periods. These beds may be particularly useful in the intensive care unit (158) or for postoperative pressure ulcer patients, although controlled studies in these areas are needed (167).

Rotating beds are used in trauma units for conditions such as acute spinal cord injury. These beds are not practical in rehabilitation or home settings because they interfere with transfers and therapy. They are useful to prevent pressure ulcers in persons who must be immobilized in the supine position.

In the rehabilitation setting, minimal-air-loss and air-fluidized beds are generally used for short periods because they are impractical and too expensive for home use. Turning tolerance is determined on a mattress and overlay suitable for home use. Patient and family education in prevention and early intervention at home becomes the key to preventive measures.

Wheelchair cushions are available in several forms to help prevent pressure ulcers. They are generally filled with gel, foam, air, or water. They do not eliminate the need for pressure relief maneuvers in the wheelchair and do not decrease pressures at the ischium below the capillary pressure (168). Their benefits vary and there is no ideal cushion. Gel cushions will maintain skin temperature but cooling of the cushion after 3 hours is necessary to maintain this effect. Foam cushions will increase the temperature of the seating surface, while water-filled cushions will cause a decrease. An air-filled cushion with multiple cells causes an increase in the humidity and temperature of the seating surface as well, but this increase is less than that resulting from foam cushions (169,170). Air-filled cushions require the user to monitor air pressure, which can be a problem if the person is not responsible (171). Foam cushions have a life span of 6 months (172). Contoured foam cushions, compared to standard foam, gel, and multiple-cell air-filled cushions, reduced pressure and improved posture and balance in studies involving less than 10 patients (173,174).

Pressure relief maneuvers should be encouraged to prevent ulceration. Numerous devices have been developed to measure their frequency and encourage follow-through (151,175). Many spinal cord–injured persons are able to sit for prolonged periods and not develop pressure ulcers, but clinical experience indicates that this is not a universal finding.

There are numerous supports designed to decrease or totally eliminate pressure on the heel while in bed. The most effective ones are designed to elevate the heel from the bed completely, to eliminate pressure (176). Doughnut-shape devices decrease blood flow to the area in the center and should not be used (30).

Electrical stimulation is currently being studied as a means to prevent pressure ulcers. Electrical stimulation of the gluteus maximus muscles increases local blood flow and produces a change in the contour of these muscles. The utility and cost-effectiveness of this technique require further study (177,178).

AGING SKIN

Multiple factors result in the aging of skin: intrinsic factors, biologic aging, and extrinsic photoaging. The effects of genetics, hormonal influence, and diet have not been quantified and should be studied. It is believed that 90% of the cosmetic problems associated with aging are due to ultraviolet radiation, and the American Academy of Dermatology has concluded that the majority of undesirable clinical features associated with skin aging are due to photoaging (179).

Skinfold thickness measurements, an anthropometric analysis used to calculate indirectly the body's adipose mass, follow a triphasic pattern with aging (180). Skinfold thickness is measured with a caliper. The skinfold thickness of infants falls until age 20. There is a plateau from age 20 to 60, and then a massive loss occurs. Youthful change is believed to occur secondary to dehydration, followed by a reduction in the synthesis of collagen and then degradation of collagen. One study of skin biopsy specimens (181) revealed epidermal thickness decreases of 7.2% per decade in men and 5.7% per decade in women. In men and women, dermal thickness decreased 6% per decade. The thickness of the superficial dermis decreased until age 50, after which there was an increase in thickness, while the overall thickness of the dermis decreased.

Skin surface changes occur with aging and are more marked and accelerated with photoaging (182). Aged skin is scaly and dry as a result of changes in the stratum corneum and the hydrolipid emulsion. The microrelief changes and the surface area in contact with the environment increases. Reduced functioning of the sebaceous glands and sweat glands results in a decrease in the hydrolipid emulsion, which in turn leads to a decreased number of normal skin flora (saprophytic bacteria). Saprophytic bacteria inhibit the growth of parasitic microorganisms. With intrinsic aging the skin appears smooth with visible angiomas. The surface is dry, itchy, and wrinkled and the epidermis is acanthotic and parakeratotic with atypical cells. Elderly individuals have difficulty neutralizing alkaline substances so alkaline soaps and cleansing measures that remove the hydrolipid emulsions should be avoided (182).

The aged stratum corneum undergoes many changes. The cells change and are larger due to a slow turnover, with keratinocytes displaying parakeratosis. Intercellular spaces are widened and filled with a hard cementing substance. Transepidermal water loss is increased and penetration of some substances is less inhibited. The stratum corneum's ability to retain water is decreased, resulting in increased stiffness and cleft formation. The epidermis flattens because of loss of papillae and will peel off more readily from a shearing force (133).

Pigmentary changes also occur with aging skin (183). After age 30 the number of melanocytes decreases by 10% to 20% per decade. Exposed skin will have twice as many pigment cells as unexposed skin, as sunlight stimulates the epidermal melanocyte system. The tanning response is impaired. Sun-exposed skin will have irregular pigmentation or hyperpigmentation. Pigmented lesions such as ephelides (freckles), actinic lentigines, pigmented solar keratoses, and seborrheic keratoses develop. The hair grays due to loss of melanocytes from hair follicles. Melanocytic nevi (moles) actually decrease with age. Hypopigmented moles may occur as well; therefore, sunbathing and the use of sunlamps are discouraged. There are fewer Langerhans cells in the aged epidermis, resulting in an altered immunologic state (184).

Atrophy and changes in the architectural organization of the aging dermis are the predominant cause for the appearance of old skin (185). The production of macromolecules decreases with age, resulting in decreased hydration. Collagen is lost from the dermis. Aged collagen is thicker and structural changes result in an exaggerated tensile strength that predisposes to tearing injuries (186). Structural changes in elastic fibers result in a loss of resiliency after stretching, predisposing individuals to injury of the underlying tissue. There is a decrease in vascularity of the dermis, particularly the papillary dermis. This decrease may be due to the decreased number of mast cells that stimulate capillary migration. These changes predispose individuals to contact dermatitis as the clearance of foreign substances is diminished.

The skin appendages are affected by aging as are other skin structures (184). The number of hair follicles diminishes, although this is more prominent on the scalp of some men than others. Beard growth in men peaks at 40 years and declines after 70. Hair follicle structure is unchanged with age, except for a loss of melanocytes. Sebaceous glands remain constant in number, may increase in size, and produce less sebum (184,186). The staining characteristics of eccrine sweat glands changes, and function and density are diminished (6). Decreased apocrine sweating occurs with aging, especially in females (6). The elderly have less body odor and less need for deodorants. Kligman et al (6) described this as "an unsung benefit of growing old."

There is a diminution of the physiologic functioning of aging skin (187,188). Because of the thinning of the epidermis and flattening of the dermal-epidermal junction, the skin of the elderly is more subject to detachment and blister formation. Epidermal tissue repair declines with age, and there is a general slowing of wound healing. The barrier function of the stratum corneum is impaired, but this impairment is not uniform for all substances. Clearance of foreign substances by the dermis is decreased due to changes in the vascularity. Changes in the vascularity of the skin, decreased sweating, and decreased subcutaneous tissue may predispose the elderly to heat stroke. Decreased sensory perception occurs in the elderly, and they have an increased threshold for pain. Free nerve endings are not modified but pacinian and Messner corpuscles undergo disorganization and degeneration. The conversion of vitamin D in the skin is decreased, as there is a 75% decrease in 7-dehydrocholesterol content; thus, vitamin D must be supplemented in the diet. A deficiency of vitamin D in adults can result in osteomalacia and disturbances of mineral ion metabolism and parathyroid hormone secretion.

A decline of cell-mediated immunity occurs with aging (189). Langerhans cells are diminished by 20% to 50% in areas of the skin protected from the sun and are further diminished in sun-exposed areas. The absolute number of T cells is also reduced. B-cell numbers are not affected by age, but increased autoantibody production occurs. Elderly skin produces less epidermal cell thermocyte-activating factor. This factor increases the response of T cells in the skin. These changes result in a decrease in the intensity of the skin's delayed hypersensitivity reactions and an increased risk of photocarcinogenesis. The increased susceptibility of the elderly to skin infections is a result of the immune changes, decreased tissue perfusion, and delayed wound healing.

A recent study compared sacral pressures in the elderly with those in young subjects on mattresses. Pressure measurements were described in two ways. Mean pressure over time was measured and a pressure impulse was calculated. Impulse pressure is the measured pressure recorded at 2-second intervals expressed as the total pressure that would be applied per hour of bed occupation. Both mean pressures and pressure impulses were increased in the elderly as compared with younger subjects (190). This may partially explain the susceptibility of certain elderly individuals to the development of pressure ulcerations.

Pharmacologic Agents and Skin Aging

As skin aging increases the risk of pressure ulcers, it is important to be aware of methods to prevent skin aging or decrease its impact since the sun has a major impact on aging of skin, the most reliable means of reducing the effects of ultraviolet radiation would be to limit exposure (191). In individuals who are not willing to limit sun exposure, sunscreens are recommended. Sunscreens generally are ultraviolet B (280–315 nm)–absorbing molecules. The ability of sunscreens to prevent skin cancer is not well documented. Sunscreens may encourage prolonged exposure to the sun and increase the risk of skin cancer, as they may not protect against the immunosuppression that allows tumors to occur. In sun-sensitive skin types, a tan may not protect against DNA damage, and therefore may not protect against skin cancer. Sunscreens that do not encourage overexposure to the sun may be protective against skin cancer. Sunscreens with a sun protection factor (SPF) around 2 may be useful as they inhibit changes in the dermis associated with photoaging, but they do not prevent erythema. When sunscreens are used as part of a personal care regimen without increasing sun exposure, they may be beneficial in preventing sun-induced cancer. An example of this would be protecting exposed areas during non-sunbathing activities.

Tretinoin (all-*trans*-retinoic acid), used topically for the treatment of acne (192,193), reversed the effects of photoaging when applied daily for 4 months (192). It is an inhibitor of human skin collagenase, an enzyme in the papillary dermis that is capable of degrading collagen. Its use increases epidermal-dermal anchoring fibrils. Clinically it reduces wrinkling of the skin and improves skin color. There is an increased number of saprophytes and more uniform pigmentation; shine and gloss are restored to the skin (182,192). Tretinoin can cause increased keratinocyte proliferation, increased keratohyalin granule formation, decreased keratinocyte cohesion, decreased melanocyte activity, altered composition of keratin, and production of mucin. The changes not only will improve the skin's appearance but also may decrease skin infection and other complications of aging skin. Tretinoin is currently being investigated as a treatment for premalignant and malignant skin conditions (192).

AGING SKIN AND PRESSURE ULCERS

Although the studies on aging skin have not specifically studied people with disabilities, it is likely that their immobility will cause these individuals to be subject to the same, if not greater, consequences from these changes. The surface changes, drying of the skin, decreased barrier function, and decreased number of saprophytic bacteria will increase the risk of cellulitis. The diminished ability of skin to clear foreign substances, the decreased barrier function, and the altered immune response will lead to an increased risk of contact dermatitis. Both of these risks will be further enhanced in individuals with disabilities who are incontinent. Efforts to maintain proper skin hygiene, using nonirritating, nonalkaline soaps and maintaining the proper balance for good hygiene without removing the protective coatings of the epidermis, must be encouraged. Sun exposure in people with disabilities must be limited and the use of sunscreens in chronically exposed areas encouraged.

The structural age-related changes in the skin that may lead to the development of pressure ulcers are of particular concern. Aged skin has an increased susceptibility to shearing forces, which can lead to a peeling off of the epidermis. The changes in the collagen structure also increase the risk of a tearing injury to the dermis and the onset of pressure ulceration from combined pressure and shear. The decreased vascularity of the dermis will further predispose the skin to the development of ischemia from pressure.

The changes in skin that occur with aging have several implications for individuals with disabilities. Sitting and turning tolerance may diminish, and individuals may develop pressure ulcers at previously acceptable levels of tolerance. These ulcers may be developing as family members, who themselves are aging, are diminished in their ability to assist with care needs. The individual with spinal cord injury may require hospital admission to repair ulcers and to upgrade their sitting tolerance postoperatively. One study determined that in older people with spinal cord injuries, the risk of developing pressure ulcers increases with age but the length of time after injury is equally important (194). Other factors included poor care at home or poor advice from caregivers. Inadequate equipment may play a part in the development of pressure ulcers, as poor seating systems and improper wheelchair cushions or mattresses can lead to pressure ulceration.

Based on the changes in aging skin, it is necessary to increase the number of follow-up visits for older people. Skin should be monitored for infection and for areas of early breakdown. Personal hygiene needs of the individuals should be assessed to ascertain proper skin care with proper cleansing agents. Individuals should be educated to be aware of potential changes in their sitting and turning tolerance. Fortunately, the skin is readily amenable to physical examination and does not require regularly scheduled diagnostic or laboratory procedures. Nutritional assessment is necessary to ensure an adequate nutritional status to prevent and heal skin ulceration.

REFERENCES

1. Meehan M. Multisite pressure ulcer prevalence survey. *Decubitus* 1990;3:14–17.
2. Allman RM, Larade CA, Noel LB, et al. Pressure sores among hospitalized patients. *Ann Intern Med* 1986;105:337–342.
3. Brandeis AH, Morris JN, Nash DJ, Lipsitz VA. The epidemiology and natural history of pressure ulcers in elderly nursing home residents. *JAMA* 1990;264:2905–2909.
4. National Pressure Ulcer Advisory Panel. *Pressure ulcers. Incidence, economics, risk assessment. Consensus development conference statement.* Rockville, MD: National Pressure Ulcer Advisory Panel, 1989:5–6.
5. Agris J, Spiro M. Pressure ulcers: prevention and treatment. In: *CIBA clinical symposia.* Vol. 3. CIBA Pharmaceutical Company, 1979.
6. Kligman AM, Grove GI, Balin AK. Aging of human skin. In: Finch CE, Schneider EL, eds. *Handbook of the biology of aging.* New York: Van Nostrand Reinhold, 1985:820–842.

7. Geneser F. *Textbook of histology.* Philadelphia: Lea & Febiger, 1987.

8. Rudolph R, Shannon MI. The normal healing process. In: Englstein WH, ed. *New directions in wound healing.* Princeton, NJ: ER Squibb & Sons, 1990:7–24.

9. Cormack DG. *Ham's histology.* Philadelphia: JB Lippincott, 1987.

10. Trumble HC. The skin tolerance for pressure and pressure sores. *Med J Aust* 1930;2:724–726.

11. Kosiak M, Kubicek WG, Olson M, et al. Evaluation of pressure as factor in production of ischial ulcer. *Arch Phys Med Rehabil* 1958;39:623–629.

12. Kosiak M. Etiology and pathology of ischemic ulcer. *Arch Phys Med Rehabil* 1959;42:62–68.

13. Kosiak M. Etiology of decubitus ulcers. *Arch Phys Med Rehabil* 1961;42:19–29.

14. Daniel RK, Wheatley D, Priest D. Pressure sores and paraplegics: an experimental model. *Ann Plast Surg* 1985;15:41–49.

15. Larsen BK, Holstein P, Lassen NA. On the pathogenesis of bedsores. *Scand J Plast Reconstr Surg* 1979;13:347–350.

16. Rueler JB, Cooney TG. The pressure sore: pathophysiology and principles of management. *Ann Intern Med* 1981;94:661–666.

17. Daniel RK, Priest DL, Whestley DC. Etiologic factors in pressure sores: an experimental model. *Arch Phys Med Rehabil* 1981;62:492–498.

18. Nola GT, Vistnes LM. Differential response of skin and muscle in the experimental production of pressure sores. *Plast Reconstr Surg* 1980;66:728–733.

19. Daniel RK, Faibusoff B. Muscle coverage of pressure points: the role of myocutaneous flaps. *Ann Plast Surg* 1982;8:446–452.

20. Barton AA. The pathogenesis of skin wounds due to pressure. In: Kenedi RM, Couden JM, Scales JT, eds. *Bedsore biomechanics.* Baltimore: University Park, 1916:55–62.

21. Brand PW. Pressure sores the problem. In: Kenedi RM, Couden JM, Scales JT, eds. *Bedsore biomechanics.* Baltimore: University Park, 1916:19–23.

22. *Dorland's illustrated medical dictionary.* 27th ed. Philadelphia: WB Saunders, 1988:1514.

23. Reichel SM. Shearing force as a factor in decubitus ulcer in paraplegics. *JAMA* 1958;166: 762–763.

24. Bennett L, Kavner D, Lee BY, Trainer FA. Shear vs pressure as causative factors in skin blood flow occlusion. *Arch Phys Med Rehabil* 1979;60:309–314.

25. Bennett L, Kavner D, Lee BY, et al. Skin blood flow in seated geriatric patients. *Arch Phys Med Rehabil* 1981;52:392–398.

26. Dinsdale SM. Decubitus ulcers: role of pressure and friction in causation. *Arch Phys Med Rehabil* 1974;55:147–152.

27. Krouskop TA, Reddy NP, Spencer WA, Secor JW. Mechanisms of decubitus ulcer formation: a hypotheses. *Med Hypotheses* 1978;4:37–39.

28. Krouskop TA. A synthesis of the factors that contribute to pressure sore formation. *Med Hypotheses* 1983;11:255–267.

29. Lamid S, El Ghatit AZ. Smoking, spasticity and pressure sores in spinal cord injured patients. *Am J Phys Med* 1983;62: 300–306.

30. Allman RM. Pressure ulcer among the elderly. *N Engl J Med* 1989;320:850–853.

31. Mulholland JH, Tui C, Wright AM, et al. Protein metabolism and bed sores. *Ann Surg* 1948;118:1015–1023.

32. Breslow R. Nutritional status and dietary intake of patients with pressure ulcers: review of research literature 1943–1989. *Decubitus* 1991;4: 16–21.

33. Pinchcofsky-Devis GD, Kaminski MU Jr. Correlation of pressure sores and nutritional status. *J Am Geriatr Soc* 1986;34:435–440.

34. Agency for Health Care Policy and Research. *Pressure ulcers in adults: prediction and prevention.* Agency for Health Care Policy and Research publication no. 92-0047. Rockville, MD: US Department of Health and Human Services, 1992:13–17.

35. Hofman A, Geelkerken RH, Wille J, et al. Pressure sores and pressure-decreasing mattresses controlled clinical trial. *Lancet* 1994;343:458–571.

36. Clark M, Rowland LB. Comparison of contact pressures measured at the sacrum of young and elderly subjects. *J Biomed Eng* 1989;11:197–199.

37. Yarkony GM. Aging skin, pressure ulcerations, and spinal cord injury. In: Whiteneck GG, ed. *Aging with spinal cord injury.* New York: Demos, 1993:39–52.

38. Garber SL, Krouskop TA. Body build and its relationship to pressure distribution in the seated wheelchair patient. *Arch Phys Med Rehabil* 1982;63:17–20.

39. Garber SL, Campion LJ, Krouskop TA. Trochanteric pressure in spinal cord injury. *Arch Phys Med Rehabil* 1982;63:549–552.

40. Anderson TP, Andberg MM. Psychosocial factors associated with pressure sores. *Arch Phys Med Rehabil* 1979;60:341–346.

41. Gordon WA, Harasymiw S, Bellile S, et al. The relationship between pressure sores and psychosocial adjustment in persons with spinal cord injury. *Rehabil Psychol* 1982;27:185–191.

42. Thiyagorajan C, Silver JR. Aetiology of pressure sores in patients with spinal cord injury. *BMJ* 1984;289:1487–1490.

43. Young JR, Burns PE, Bowen AM, McCutchen R. *Spinal cord injury statistics.* Phoenix: Good Samaritan Medical Center, 1982.

44. Stover SL, Fine PR, eds. *Spinal cord injury: the facts and figures.*

Birmingham: The University of Alabama at Birmingham, 1986.

45. Mawson AR, Biundo PR Jr, Neville P, et al. Risk factors for early occurring pressure ulcers following spinal cord injury. *Am J Phys Med Rehabil* 1988;67: 123–127.

46. Yarkony GM, Kirk PM, Carlson C, et al. Classification of pressure ulcers. *Arch Dermatol* 1990:126;1218–1219.

47. Shea JD. Pressure sores: classification and management. *Clin Orthop* 1975;112:89–100.

48. Mash N. *Standards of care dermal wounds: pressure sores.* Irving, CA: International Association of Enterostomal Therapy, 1987.

49. Cuzzell JZ. The new RYB color code. *Am J Nurs* 1988;88: 1342–1346.

50. Moriorty MB. How color can clarify wound care. *RN* 1951;51:49–54.

51. Dealy C. Measuring a wound. *Nursing* 1991;4:29.

52. Thomas AC, Wysocki AB. The healing wound: a comparison of three clinical useful methods of measurement. *Decubitus* 1990;3:18–25.

53. Kundin JI. A new way to size up a wound. *Am J Nurs* 1989;89:206–207.

54. Covington JS, Griffin JW, Mendiw RK, et al. Measurement of pressure ulcer volume using dental impression materials: suggestion from the field. *Phys Ther* 1989;69:690–694.

55. Resch CS, Kerner E, Robson MC, et al. Pressure sore volume measurement: a technique to document and record wound healing. *J Am Geriatr Soc* 1988;36:444–446.

56. Anthony D, Barnes E. Measuring pressure sore accurately. *Nursing Times* 1984;80:33–35.

57. Putnam T, Calenoff L, Betts HB, Rosen JS. Sinography in management of decubitus ulcers. *Arch Phys Med Rehabil* 1978;59: 243–246.

58. Borgstrom PS, Ekberg O, Lasson A. Radiography of pressure ulcers. *Acta Radiol* 1988;29: 581–584.

59. Hooker EZ, Sibley P, Nemchausky B, Lopez E. A method for quantifying the area of closed pressure sores by sinography and digitometry. *J Neurosci Nurs* 1988;20:118–127.

60. Bates-Jensen BM, Uredevoe DL, Brecht ML. Validity and reliability of the pressure sore status tool. *Decubitus* 1992;5: 20–28.

61. Dinsdale SM. Decubitus ulcers in swine: light and electron microscopy study of pathogenesis. *Arch Phys Med Rehabil* 1973;54:51–56.

62. Sulzberger MB, Cortese TA Jr, Fishman L, Wiley HS. Studies on blisters produced by friction. I. Results of linear rubbing and twisting technics. *J Invest Dermatol* 1966;47:456–465.

63. Witkowski JA, Parish LC. Histopathology of the decubitus ulcer. *J Am Acad Dermatol* 1982;6:1014–1021.

64. Sugarman B. Infection and pressure sores. *Arch Phys Med Rehabil* 1985;66:177–179.

65. Sapico FL, Ginunas VJ, Thornhill-Joyner M, et al. Quantitative microbiology of pressure sores in different stages of healing. *Diagn Microbiol Infect Dis* 1986;5:31–38.

66. Ehrenkranz NJ, Alfonso B, Nerenberg D. Irrigation-aspiration for culturing draining decubitus ulcers: correlation of bacteriological findings with a clinical inflammatory scoring index. *J Clin Microbiol* 1990;28: 2389–2393.

67. Daltrey DC, Rhodes B, Chattwood JG. Investigation into microbial flora of healing and non-healing decubitus ulcers. *J Clin Pathol* 1981;34:701–705.

68. Baker PG, Haig G. Metronidazole in the treatment of chronic pressure sores and ulcers. *Practitioner* 1981;225:561–573.

69. Gomulin IH, Brandt JL. Topical metronidazole therapy for pressure ulcer of geriatric patients. *J Am Geriatr Soc* 1983;31: 710–712.

70. Firooznia H, Rafii M, Golimbu C, et al. Computerized tomography of pressure sores, pelvic abscess, and osteomyelitis in patients with spinal cord injury. *Arch Phys Med Rehabil* 1982;63:545–548.

71. Firooznia H, Rafaii M, Golimbu C, Sokolow J. Computerized tomography in diagnosis of pelvic abscess in spinal-cord-injured patients. *Comput Radiol* 1983;7:355–341.

72. Sugarman B. Pressure sores and underlying bone infection. *Arch Intern Med* 1987;147:553–555.

73. Thornhill-Joynes M, Gonzales F, Stewart CA, et al. Osteomyelitis associated with pressure ulcers. *Arch Phys Med Rehabil* 1986;67:314–318.

74. Sugarman B. Osteomyelitis in spinal cord injury. *Arch Phys Med Rehabil* 1984;65:132–134.

75. Lewis VL Jr, Bailey MH, Pulawski G, et al. The diagnosis of osteomyelitis in patients with pressure sores. *Plast Reconstr Surg* 1988;81:229–232.

76. Bryan CS, Dew CE, Reynolds KL. Bacteremia associated with decubitus ulcers. *Arch Intern Med* 1983;143:2093–2095.

77. Galpin JE, Chow AW, Bayer AS, Guze LB. Sepsis associated with decubitus ulcers. *Am J Med* 1976;61:346–350.

78. Rissing JP, Crowder JG, Dunfee T, White A. Bacteroides bacteremia from decubitus ulcers. *Am J Med* 1976;61:346–350.

79. Berkwits L, Yarkony GM, Lewis V. Marjolin's ulcer complicating a pressure ulcer: case report and literature review. *Arch Phys Med Rehabil* 1986;67:381–383.

80. Dumurgier C, Pujol G, Chevallery J, et al. Pressure sore carcinoma: a late but fulminant complication

of pressure sores in spinal cord injury patients: case report. *Paraplegia* 1991;29:390–395.

81. Treves N, Pack GT. Development of cancer in burn scars: analysis and report of thirty-four cases. *Surg Gynecol Obstet* 1930;51:749–782.

82. Schlosser RJ, Kanar EA, Harkins HN. Surgical significance of Marjolin's ulcer with report of three cases. *Surgery* 1956; 39:645–653.

83. Giblin T, Pickrell K, Pitts W, Armstrong D. Malignant degeneration in burn scars. Marjolin's ulcer. *Ann Surg* 1965;162:291–297.

84. Bereston ES, Ney C. Squamous cell carcinoma arising in chronic osteomyelitic sinus tract with metastasis. *Arch Surg* 1941;43:257–268.

85. Dunn JE Jr, Levin EA, Linden G, Harzfeld L. Skin cancer as cause of death. *Calif Med* 1965;102:361–363.

86. Fitzgerald RH, Brewer NS, Dahlin DC. Squamous-cell carcinoma complicating chronic osteomyelitis. *J Bone Joint Surg [Am]* 1976;58:1146–1148.

87. Johnson LL, Kempson RK. Epidermoid carcinoma in chronic osteomyelitis diagnostic problems and management: report of ten cases. *J Bone Joint Surg [Am]* 1965;47:133–145.

88. McAnally AK, Dockerty MB. Carcinoma developing in chronic draining cutaneous sinuses and fistulas. *Surg Gynecol Obstet* 1949;88:87–96.

89. Taylor GW, Nathanson IT, Shaw DT. Epidermoid carcinoma of extremities with reference to lymph node involvement. *Ann Surg* 1941;113:268–275.

90. Glass RL, Spratt JS Jr, Perez-Mesa C. Fate of inadequately excised epidermoid carcinoma of skin. *Surg Gynecol Obstet* 1966;122:245–248.

91. Nathan CF, Murray HW, Cohn ZA. Current concepts: the macrophage as an effector cell. *N Engl J Med* 1980;303: 622–662.

92. Bristian BR, Blackburn GL, Vitale J, et al. Prevalence of malnutrition in general medical patients. *JAMA* 1976;235:1567–1570.

93. Bruslow RA, Hallfrish J, Goldberg AP. Malnutrition in tube fed nursing home patients with pressure sores. *J Parenter Enter Nutr* 1911;15:663–668.

94. Allman RM, Walker JM, Hart MK, et al. Air-fluidized beds or conventional therapy for pressure sores: a randomized trial. *Ann Intern Med* 1987;107:641–648.

95. Silane M, Oot-gironmini B. Systemic and other factors that affect wound healing. In: Eaglstein WH, ed. *New directions in wound healing.* Princeton: ER Squibb & Sons, 1990:39–54.

96. Constantian MB, Jackson HS. Biology and care of the pressure ulcer wound. In: Constantian M, ed. *Pressure ulcers: principles and techniques of management.* Boston: Little, Brown, 1980:69–100.

97. Hallbook J, Lanner E. Serum-zinc and healing of venous leg ulcers. *Lancet* 1972;2:780–782.

98. Williams CM, Lines CM, McKay EC. Iron and zinc status in multiple sclerosis patients with pressure sores. *Eur J Clin Nutr* 1988;42:321–328.

99. Norris JR, Reynolds RE. The effect of oral zinc sulfate on decubitus ulcers. *J Am Geriatr Soc* 1971;8:211–216.

100. Hunter T, Rajai KT. The role of ascorbic acid in the pathogenesis and treatment of pressure sores. *Paraplegia* 1971;8:211–216.

101. Taylor TV, Rimmer S, Day B, et al. Ascorbic acid supplementation in treatment of pressure-sores. *Lancet* 1974;11:544–546.

102. Witkowski JA, Parish LC. Debridement of cutaneous ulcers: medical and surgical aspects. *Clin Dermatol* 1992;9:585–591.

103. Baxter CR, Rodeheaver GT. Interventions: hemostasis, cleansing, topical, antibiotics, debridement and closure. In: Eaglstein WH, ed. *New directions in wound healing.* Princeton: ER Squibb and Sons, 1990:71–82.

104. Yarkony GM, Kramer E, King R, et al. Pressure sore management: efficacy of a moisture reactive occlusive dressing. *Arch Phys Med Rehabil* 1984;65:597–600.

105. Gorse GT, Messner RL. Improved pressure sore healing with hydrocolloid dressings. *Arch Dermatol* 1987;123:766–771.

106. Fernie GR, Dornan J. The problems of clinical trials with new systems for preventing or healing decubiti. In: Kenedi RM, Couden JM, Scales JT, eds. *Bedsore biomechanics.* Baltimore: University Park, 1916:315–320.

107. Winter GD. Formation of scab and rate of epithelialization of superficial wounds in skin of young domestic pig. *Nature* 1962;193:293–294.

108. Hinman CD, Maibach H. Effect of air exposure and occlusion on experimental human skin wounds. *Nature* 1963;200:377–378.

109. Knighton DR, Silver IA, Hunt TK. Regulation of wound-healing angiogenesis—effect of oxygen gradients and inspired oxygen concentration. *Surgery* 1981;90:262–270.

110. Alvarez OM, Mertz PM, Eaglstein WH. Effect of occlusive dressings on collagen synthesis and re-epithelialization in superficial wounds. *J Surg Res* 1983;35:142–148.

111. Varghese ML, Balin AK, Carter M, Caldwell D. Local environment of chronic wounds under synthetic dressings. *Arch Dermatol* 1986;122:52–57.

112. Katz S, McGinley K, Leyden JT. Semipermeable occlusive dressing. *Arch Dermatol* 1986;40:58–62.

113. Mertz PM, Marshall DA, Eaglstein WH. Occlusive wound dressings to prevent bacterial invasion and wound infection. *J Am Acad Dermatol* 1985;12:662–668.

114. Hutchinson JT, McGuckin M. Occlusive dressings: a microbiologic and clinical review. *Am J Infect Control* 1990;18:257–268.

115. Falanga V. Occlusive wound dressing: why when which? *Arch Dermatol* 1988;124:872–877.

116. Xakellis GC, Chrischilles EA. Hydrocolloid vs saline-gauze dressing in treating pressure ulcers: a cost-effectiveness analysis. *Arch Phys Med Rehabil* 1992;73:463–469.

117. Seburn MD. Pressure under management in home health care: efficacy and cost effectiveness of moisture vapor permeable dressing. *Arch Phys Med Rehabil* 1986;67:726–729.

118. Fowler E, Papen JC. Evaluation of an alginate dressing for pressure ulcers. *Decubitus* 1991;4:47–52.

119. Chapius A, Dollfus P. The use of calcium alginate dressings in the management of decubitus ulcers in patients with spinal cord lesions. *Paraplegia* 1990;28:269–271.

120. Dela Drux F, Brown DH, Leikin JB, et al. Iodine absorption after topical administration. *West J Med* 1987;146:43–45.

121. Sherry KR, Duthie EH Jr. Thyrotoxicosis induced by topical iodine application. *Arch Intern Med* 1990;150:2400–2401.

122. Aronon GR, Friedman SJ, Doedeus DJ, Lavell KJ. Increased serum iodide concentration from iodine absorption through wounds treated topically with povidone-iodine. *Am J Med Sci* 1980;279:173–176.

123. Lineaweaver W, Howard R, Soucy D, et al. Topical antimicrobial toxicity. *Arch Surg* 1985;120:267–270.

124. Geronemus RG, Mertz PM, Eaglstein WH. Wound healing: the effects of topical antimicrobial agents. *Arch Dermatol* 1979;115:1311–1314.

125. Bendy RH Jr, Nuccio PA, Wolfe E, et al. Relationship of quantitative wound bacterial counts to healing of ducubiti: effect of topical gentamicin. *Antimicrob Agents Chemother* 1964;4:147–155.

126. Kacan TO, Robson MC, Heggers TP, Ko F. Comparison of silver sulfadiazine, povidone-iodine and physiologic saline in the treatment of chronic pressure ulcers. *J Am Geriatr Soc* 1981;29: 232–235.

127. Kloth LC, Feedar JA. Acceleration of wound healing with high voltage, monophasic, pulsed current. *Phys Ther* 1988;68:503–508.

128. Wolcott LE, Wheeler PC, Hardwicke HM, Rowley BA. Accelerated healing of skin ulcers by electrotherapy: preliminary clinical results. *South Med J* 1969;62:795–801.

129. Carley PJ, Wainapel SF. Electrotherapy for acceleration of wound healing: low intensity direct current. *Arch Phys Med Rehabil* 1985;66:443–446.

130. Alvrez OM, Mertz PM, Smerbeck RV, Eaglstein WH. The healing of superficial skin wounds is stimulated by external electrical current. *J Invest Dermatol* 1983;81:144–148.

131. Alkers TK, Gabrielson AL. The effect of high voltage galvanic stimulation on the rate of healing of decubitus ulcers. *Biomed Sci Instrum* 1984;20:99–100.

132. Yarkony GM, Roth EJ, Cybulski GR, Jaeger RJ. Neuromuscular stimulation in spinal cord injury. II: prevention of secondary complications. *Arch Phys Med Rehabil* 1992;73:195–200.

133. Hotta SS, Holohan TV. *Procuren: a platelet-derived wound healing formula.* Health technology review no. 2. Agency for Health Care Policy and Research, publication no. 92-0065. Rockville, MD: U.S. Department of Health and Human Services, 1992.

134. Mertz PM, Davis SC, Arakawa Y, Cohen A. Pulsed rh EGF treatment increased epithelialization of partial thickness wounds. *J Invest Dermatol* 1988;90:558. Abstract.

135. Falanga V, Zitelli JA, Eaglstein WH. Wound healing. *J Am Acad Dermatol* 1988;191:559–563.

136. Pierce GF, Vande Berg T, Rudolph R, et al. Platelet-derived growth factor and transforming growth factor beta selectively modulate glycosaminoglycans, collagen and myofibroblasts in excisional wounds. *Am J Pathol* 1991;138:629–646.

137. Antoniades HN, Scher CD, Stiles CD. Purification of human platelet-derived growth factor. *Proc Natl Acad Sci USA* 1979;76:1809–1813.

138. Pierce GF, Brown D, Mustoe TA. Quantitative analysis of inflammatory cell influx, procollagen type I synthesis and collagen cross linking in incisional wounds: influence of PDGF-BB and TGF B therapy. *J Lab Clin Med* 1991;117:373–382.

139. Knighton DR, Ciresi KF, Fiegel VD, et al. Stimulation of repair in chronic, nonhealing, cutaneous ulcers using platelet-derived wound healing formula. *Surg Gynecol Obstet* 1990;170:56–60.

140. Atri SC, Misra J, Bisht D, Misra K. Use of homologous platelet factors in achieving total healing of recalcitrant skin ulcers. *Surgery* 1990;108:508–512.

141. Robson MC, Phillips LG, Thomason A, et al. Platelet-derived growth factor BB for the treatment of chronic pressure ulcers. *Lancet* 1992;339:23–25.

142. Davis JS. The operative treatment of scars following bedsores. *Surgery* 1938;3:1–7.

143. Conway H, Griffith BH. Plastic surgery for closure of decubitus ulcers in patients. *Am J Surg* 1956;91:946–975.

144. Disa JJ, Carlton JM, Goldberg NH. Efficacy of operative care in pressure sore patients. *Plast Reconstr Surg* 1992;89: 272–278.

145. Spear SI, Kroll SS, Little JW III. Bilateral upper-quadrant (inter-

costal) flaps: the value of protective sensation in preventing pressure sore recurrence. *Plast Reconstr Surg* 1987;80: 734–736.

146. Daniel RK, Terzis JK, Cunningham DM. Sensory skin flaps for coverage of pressure sores in paraplegic patients: a preliminary report. *Plast Reconstr Surg* 1976;58:317–328.

147. Dibbell DG. Use of a Long Island flap to bring sensation to the sacral area in young paraplegics. *Plast Reconstr Surg* 1974;54:220–223.

148. Lawton RL, DePinto V. Bilateral hip disarticulation in paraplegics with decubitus ulcers. *Arch Surg* 1987;122:1040–1043.

149. Chase RA, White WL. Bilateral amputation and rehabilitation of paraplegics. *Plast Reconstr Surg* 1959;24:445–455.

150. Rehabilitation Institute of Chicago. *Division of Nursing Rehabilitation nursing procedures manual.* Rockville, MD: Aspen, 1990:179–203.

151. Lindan O, Greenway RM, Piozza JM. Pressure distribution on the surface of the human body. 1. Evaluation in lying and sitting positions using a "bed of springs and nails." *Arch Phys Med Rehabil* 1965;46:378–385.

152. Krouskop TA, Williams R, Krubs M, et al. Effectiveness of mattress overlays in reducing interface pressures during recumbency. *J Rehabil Res Dev* 1985;22:7–10.

153. Andersen KE, Jensen O, Kuarning SA, Bach E. Decubitus prophylaxis: a prospective trial on the efficiency of alternating-pressure air mattresses and water-mattresses. *Acta Derm Venereol* 1982;63:227–270.

154. Redfern SJ, Jeneid PA, Gillingham ME, Lunn HF. Local pressures with ten types of patient support systems. *Lancet* 1973;2:277–280.

155. Bell JC, Mathews SD. Results of a clinical investigation of four pressure reduction replacement mattresses. *J ET Nurs* 1993;20: 204–210.

156. Dean LS, Krall S, Wharton GW. A comparison study of the pressure relief characteristics of two air flotation beds. In: San Francisco, CA: American Spinal Injury Association, 1986:274. Abstract.

157. Krouskop TA. The role of mattresses and beds in preventing pressure sores. In: Lee BY, Ostrander LE, Cochran GVB, Shaw WW, eds. *The spinal cord injured patient: comprehensive management.* Philadelphia: WB Saunders, 1991:244–250.

158. Thomson CW, Ryan DW, Dunkin LJ, et al. Fluidized-bead bed on the intensive therapy unit. *Lancet* 1980;1:568–570.

159. Nimit K. *Public Health Service assessment guidelines for home air-fluidized bed therapy.* Washington, DC: US Government Printing Office, 1989.

160. Sharbaugh RJ, Hargest TS. Bactericidal effect of the air-fluidized bed. *Am Surg* 1971;37:583–586.

161. Sharbaugh RJ, Hargest TS, Wright FA. Further studies on the bactericidal effect of the air fluidized bed. *Am Surg* 1971;37:583–586.

162. Ferrell BA, Osterwell D, Christenson P. A randomized trial of low-air-loss beds for treatment of pressure ulcers. *JAMA* 1993;269:494–497.

163. Inman KJ, Sibbald WJ, Rutledge FS, Clark BJ. Clinical utility and cost-effectiveness of an air suspension bed in the prevention of pressure ulcers. *JAMA* 1993;269:1139–1143.

164. Greer DM, Morris EJ, Walsh NE, et al. Cost-effectiveness and efficacy of air-fluidized therapy in the treatment of pressure ulcers. *J Enterostomal Ther* 1988;15:247–251.

165. Parish LC, Witkowski JA. Clinitron therapy and the decubitus ulcer. *Int J Dermatol* 1980;19:517–518.

166. Bennett RG, Bellantoni MF, Ouslander JG. Air fluidized bed treatment of nursing home patients with pressure sores. *J Am Geriatr Soc* 1989;37:235–242.

167. Dolezal R, Cohen M, Schultz RC. The use of clinitron therapy unit in the immediate postoperative care of pressure ulcers. *Ann Plastic Surg* 1985;14: 33–36.

168. Souther SG, Carr SD, Vistnes LM. Wheelchair cushions to reduce pressure under bony prominences. *Arch Phys Med Rehabil* 1974;55:460–464.

169. Seymour RJ, Lacefield WE. Wheelchair cushion effect on pressure and skin temperature. *Arch Phys Med Rehabil* 1985;66:103–108.

170. Stewart SFC, Palmieri V, Cochran GVB. Wheelchair cushion effect on skin temperature, heat flex, and relative humidity. *Arch Phys Med Rehabil* 1980;61: 229–233.

171. Krouskop TA, Williams R, Noble P, Brown J. Inflation pressure effect on performance of air-filled wheelchair cushions. *Arch Phys Med Rehabil* 1990;71:655–658.

172. Ferguson-Pell M, Cochran GVB, Palmieri V, Branski JB. Development of a modular wheelchair cushion for spinal cord injured persons. *J Rehabil Res Dev* 1986;23:63–76.

173. Sprigle SH, Faisant JE, Chung KC. Clinical evaluation of custom-contoured cushions for the spinal cord injured. *Arch Phys Med Rehabil* 1990;71:655–658.

174. Sprigle S, Chung KC, Brubaker CE. Reduction of sitting pressures with custom contoured cushions. *J Rehabil Res Dev* 1990;27:135–140.

175. Patterson RP, Fisher SV. Sitting pressure-time patterns in patients with quadriplegia. *Arch Phys Med Rehabil* 1986;67:812–814.

176. Pinzur MS, Schumacher D, Reddy N, et al. Preventing heel ulcers: a comparison of prophylactic body support systems. *Arch Phys Med Rehabil* 1991;72: 508–510.

177. Levine SP, Ken RL, Gross MD, et al. Blood flow in the gluteus maximus of seated individuals during electrical muscle stimulation. *Arch Phys Med Rehabil* 1990;71:682–686.

178. Levine SP, Kett RL, Cederna PS, Brooks SV. Electrical muscle stimulation for pressure sore prevention: tissue shape variation. *Arch Phys Med Rehabil* 1990;71:210–215.

179. Leyden JJ. Clinical features of ageing skin. *Br J Dermatol* 1990;122(suppl 3):S1–S3.

180. Hall DA, Blackett AD, Zajac AR, et al. Changes in skin fold thickness with increasing age. *Age Ageing* 1981;10:19–23.

181. Branchet MC, Boisnic S, Frances C, Robert AN. Skin thickness changes in normal aging skin. *Gerontology* 1990;36:28–35.

182. Raab JP. The skin surface and stratum corneum. *Br J Dermatol* 1990;122(suppl 3):S37–S41.

183. Ortonne JP. Pigmentary changes of the aging skin. *Br J Dermatol* 1990;122(suppl 3):S21–S28.

184. Montagna W, Carlisle K. Structural changes in ageing skin. *Br J Dermatol* 1990;122(suppl 3S):61–70.

185. Lapier CM. The aging dermis: the main cause for the appearance of old skin. *Br J Dermatol* 1990; 122(suppl 3):S5–S11.

186. Fenske NA, Lober CW. Structural and functional changes of normal aging skin. *J Am Acad Dermatol* 1986;15:571–585.

187. Cerimele D, Celleno L, Serri F. Physiological changes in ageing skin. *Br J Dermatol* 1990;122(suppl 3):S13–S20.

188. Stuttgen G, Ott A. Senescence in the skin. *Br J Dermatol* 1990;122(suppl 3):S43–S48.

189. Thivolet J, Nicolas JT. Skin aging and immune competence. *Br J Dermatol* 1990;122(suppl 3):S77–S81.

190. Clark M, Rowland LB. Comparison of contact pressures measured at the sacrum of young and elderly subjects. *J Biomed Eng* 1989;11:197–199.

191. Young AT. Senescence and sunscreens. *Br J Dermatol* 1990; 122(suppl 3):S111–S114.

192. Goldfarb MT, Ellis CN, Voorhees JJ. Topical tretinoin: its use in daily practice to reverse photoageing. *Br J Dermatol* 1990; 122(suppl 3):S78–S91.

193. Woodley DT, Zelickson AS, Briggaman TA, et al. Treatment of photoaged skin with topical tretinoin increases epidermal-dermal anchoring fibrils: a preliminary report. *JAMA* 1990;263:3057–3059.

194. Thiyagoarjan C, Silver JR. Aetiology of pressure sores in patients with spinal cord injury. *BMJ* 1984;289:1487–1490.

Chapter 51

Neurogenic Bladder

David Chen
Yeong-Chi Wu

Bladder function is frequently impaired in patients with neurologic disorders and other medical conditions. Recognition of the problem and effective treatment and management are essential in the setting of rehabilitation, to allow patients to achieve their functional potential and prevent medical complications.

A detailed description of normal renal and bladder anatomy, neuroanatomy, and physiology is beyond the scope of this chapter; numerous other textbooks cover these areas in greater depth. Following a brief overview of normal anatomy, neuroanatomy, and physiology, the focus in this chapter turns to methods of evaluation and assessment, types of bladder dysfunction, and management and treatment options for the neurogenic bladder. Finally, the potential complications of the neurogenic bladder are described.

RENAL AND BLADDER ANATOMY AND PHYSIOLOGY

Anatomy

Upper Urinary Tract

The kidneys are a pair of bean-shaped organs that lie posterior to the peritoneum against the psoas major muscles. They lie alongside the vertebral column from T12 to L3, with the right kidney slightly lower than the left. Each kidney has a renal cortex (composed of glomeruli and convoluted tubules) and a collecting system (composed of pyramids, papillae, minor and major calyces, and renal pelvis).

The ureters are expansile, thick-walled muscular tubes, approximately 25 cm in length, that originate from the renal pelvis. Peristaltic waves in the walls of the ureters propel the urine from the kidney to the bladder.

Lower Urinary Tract

The urinary bladder is a muscular sac that functions as a reservoir for temporarily storing urine prior to its elimination from the body. The wall of the bladder is composed primarily of smooth muscle, called the *detrusor urinae.* This muscle consists of three layers: external and internal layers of longitudinal fibers, and a middle layer of circular fibers. Near the bladder neck, these muscle fibers form the involuntary internal sphincter.

The bladder trigone is located at the base and is demarcated by the openings of the ureters and urethra. The ureters pass obliquely through the bladder wall in an inferomedial direction into the bladder. An increase in bladder pressure presses the walls of the ureter together and prevents urine from backing up into the ureter from the bladder.

The urethra, functioning as the final channel through which urine is eliminated, begins in the bladder neck and ends at the external urethral orifice. The male urethra is approximately 15 cm in length and is divided into prostatic, membranous, and penile parts. A voluntary external sphincter, composed of a band of striated muscular fibers, is located in the male in the area of the membranous part. The female urethra is only about 4 cm in length and is surrounded by the sphincter urethra muscle along almost its entire length. This muscle functions as the external sphincter in the female.

Neurologic Innervation

Carrying out the storage and elimination functions of the bladder system requires not only the proper functioning of the various components of the upper and lower urinary tracts, but also the coordinated influence of the complex central and peripheral neural control mechanisms.

Functions of the lower urinary tract are influenced by parasympathetic, sympathetic, and somatic innervations (Fig. 51-1). Parasympathetic innervation originates in the inferomediolateral gray matter at the S2–S4 region of the spinal cord. These efferent fibers travel through the pelvic nerves and subsequently end at smooth muscle cholinergic receptors in the detrusor muscle of the bladder. Stimulation of these receptors results in contraction of the bladder.

Sympathetic innervation originates in the intermediolateral gray matter at the T11–L2 region. The sympathetic efferent fibers travel through the lumbar paravertebral ganglia and then travel to the lower urinary tract via the hypogastric nerves. These nerves ultimately synapse at α- and β-adrenergic receptors within the bladder and urethra. β-Adrenergic receptors are found primarily in the body of the bladder and stimulation of these receptors results in smooth muscle relaxation. α-Adrenergic receptors are found predominantly near the base of the bladder and in the prostatic part of the urethra, and stimulation results in smooth muscle contraction in both areas.

Somatic innervation, which is primarily to the external urethral sphincter, originates in the pudendal nerve nucleus at the S2–S4 region and travels via the pudendal nerve to the striated muscle of the external sphincter.

Afferent innervation from the lower urinary tract, which carries exteroceptive and proprioceptive sensory stimuli from the bladder and urethra, also is carried via the pelvic, hypogastric, and pudendal nerves.

Central nervous system influence over bladder function is believed to occur via several micturition centers located at various points in the cerebral cortex, basal ganglion, cerebellum, pons and sacral region of the spinal cord. The act of micturition itself is predominantly due to reflex activity that occurs in the sacral micturition center. Descending signals to the sacral micturition center from the higher suprasacral centers (especially the cerebral cortex and basal ganglion) are primarily inhibitory in nature. The pontine micturition center appears to have a significant role in coordinating detrusor and sphincter activity (1).

Normal Physiology and Function

The kidneys function to remove excess water, electrolytes, and products of protein metabolism from the blood. The by-product of this effort is urine, which is further concentrated and ultimately excreted into the collecting system of the kidneys.

In each kidney, the collecting system is made up of multiple minor and major calyces that converge into the renal pelvis. From each renal pelvis originates a ureter, which is a muscular duct that carries the urine to the bladder via peristaltic waves.

The bladder serves as a storage vesicle for urine until it can be properly eliminated from the body. Normally, the bladder is a very compliant system, which serves its storage function. During normal bladder filling, intravesical pressure rises very slowly (accommodation) despite a large increase in volume. In addition, there is a gradual increase in proximal urethral resistance, and in activity in the pelvic floor and external urethral sphincter. All of this activity serves to promote the urine storage function of the bladder

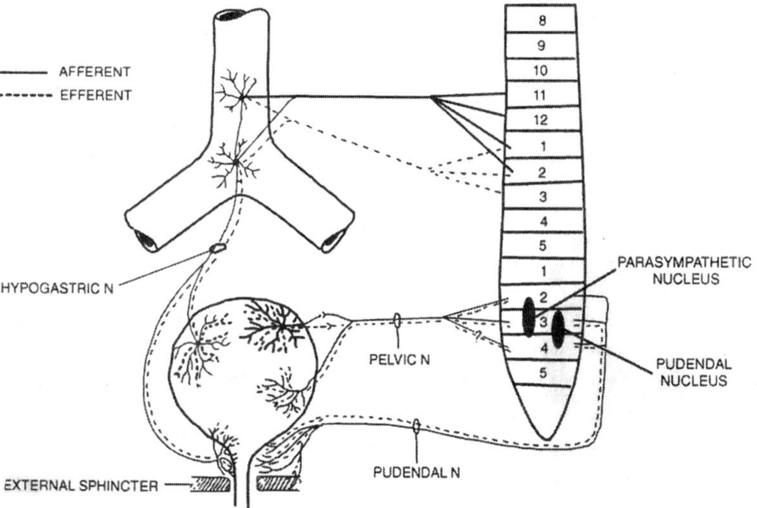

Figure 51-1. Neurologic innervation of the kidneys and bladder.

and maintain continence. When a specific intravesical pressure is reached, the sensation of bladder distention is perceived, but the individual is able to voluntarily suppress the need to void. As bladder volume and pressure continue to increase further, a threshold is reached when the need to void can no longer be suppressed. Normal voiding occurs voluntarily with the coordinated relaxation of the external urethral sphincter and pelvic floor, and contraction of the bladder detrusor muscle, which forces urine out of the bladder and also reshapes the proximal urethra, resulting in a decrease in bladder outlet resistance.

EVALUATION AND ASSESSMENT OF BLADDER DYSFUNCTION

History and Physical Examination

A thorough history obtained from the patient or a family member is necessary to ascertain the status of the patient's voiding pattern and the symptoms for which the patient seeks treatment. It is valuable to know whether any symptoms were present prior to the recent events or illness. A diary of voiding activity is often helpful in gaining an understanding of the patient's daily fluid intake, output, frequency of incontinent episodes and voiding pattern. Knowledge of any coexisting medical condition (i.e., diabetes or congestive heart failure), current usage of medications, and the primary neurologic diagnosis is necessary to determine the type of bladder dysfunction responsible for the patient's symptoms, and options for treatment. With the information and findings from physical examination and results of appropriate diagnostic tests, one can develop an appropriate and effective treatment plan.

A complete and thorough physical examination should focus on specific areas to gain further information to help improve the treatment and management of the person with bladder dysfunction. Specific attention should be made to the perineal region, including the assessment of skin integrity and sensation and the status of pelvic floor support. When appropriate, establishing a neurologic level (both motor and sensory levels), the presence of cutaneous reflexes, and the presence of significant spasticity is important in understanding the patterns of voiding disorders and prescribing effective bladder management regimens.

In men, it is important to make an assessment of the prostate gland during rectal examination; however, the overall size does not necessarily reflect the degree of urethral obstruction (2).

In women, a vaginal examination should focus on the degree of pelvic and vaginal support and atrophic changes of the vaginal mucosa.

The neurologic examination should also include an assessment of the patient's mental and cognitive status. Alterations in level of consciousness, orientation, communication ability, and memory may contribute to voiding dysfunctions and dictate options for bladder management.

Diagnostic Tests

A number of diagnostic and evaluative tests are available to assess the integrity and function of the upper and lower urinary tracts. The decision of which test to perform on an individual depends on the primary or underlying disease process or neurologic condition, the status of bladder function, and information gained from the history and physical examination. The timing and frequency for any of these tests are based in part on the chronology of the voiding dysfunction and the likelihood of involvement of the upper or lower urinary tract, or both. For example, diagnostic measures focused on the upper urinary tract should be considered when there are signs or symptoms, such as fevers, chills and hematuria, suggestive of pyelonephritis or other upper tract disorders. On the other hand, for progressive urinary incontinence in an elderly woman, attention most likely would be directed to the lower urinary tract.

In a number of chronic conditions such as multiple sclerosis and spinal cord injury, the ongoing potential for changes in bladder function and development of upper and lower urinary tract complications necessitates regular, periodic scheduling of tests as a surveillance measure (3). The long-term use of particular bladder management techniques, such as indwelling catheters, which have been associated with an increased risk of squamous cell carcinoma, also may dictate the regular scheduling of surveillance tests (3).

A number of diagnostic and evaluative tests are available to assess the structure and function of the upper and lower urinary tracts. Several of the most commonly used tests are briefly described including indications for use, limitations, advantages, and disadvantages.

Intravenous Pyelogram

The intravenous pyelogram (IVP) or excretory urogram is a radiologic procedure that involves the intravenous administration of a contrast dye, followed by serial plain film imaging of the kidneys and ureters over a period of time (Fig. 51-2). Structural abnormalities of the kidneys, collecting systems, and ureters may be found with this test. The addition of tomograms with an IVP often is valuable when evaluating for kidney tumors and ureteral tumors or stones. The disadvantages of this procedure include the inconvenience of a need for preparation prior to the test, the potential for allergic reaction to the contrast dye, and the radiation exposure (4).

Renal Ultrasound

Renal ultrasound is a noninvasive diagnostic modality that has largely replaced the IVP, especially when focusing on the kidneys for evidence of chronic obstruction, hydronephrosis, or renal stones. (Fig. 51-3). This procedure has limited value for visualizing the ureters, but with the bladder partially filled, it may be used to assess bladder wall thickness and the presence of stones. The advantages

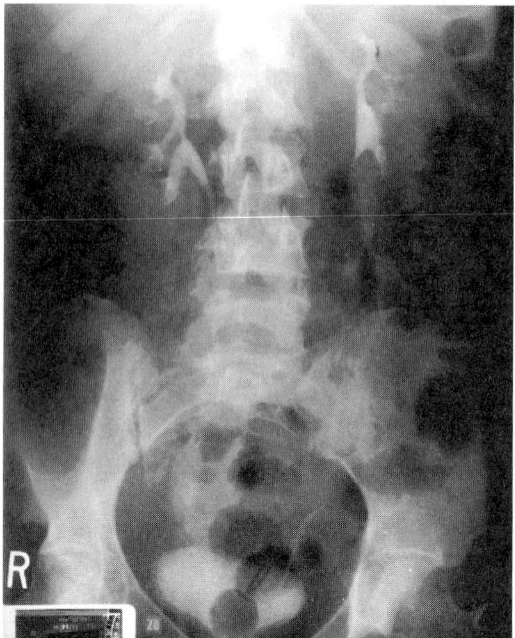

Figure 51-2. Image from an intravenous pyelogram study showing normal structure of the kidney, collecting systems, and ureters.

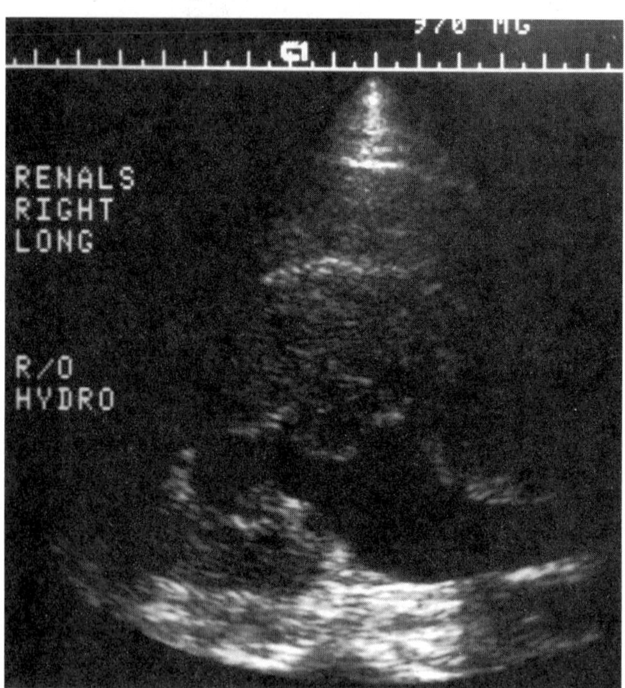

Figure 51-3. Ultrasound image showing evidence of marked hydronephrosis.

of renal ultrasound are that the disadvantages with IVP are avoided, the procedure is generally well tolerated, and if needed, if can be done at the bedside. The major disadvantage is the limited ability to visualize the ureters unless there is significant dilatation (5).

Renal Scan

Periodic evaluation and follow-up of actual renal function may be accomplished with a radioisotope renal scan. A determination of the glomerular filtration rate, creatinine clearance, and differential renal function can also be made with this test. The primary advantage of this study is that the results are a reflection of actual function rather than anatomic changes. Conversely, limitations of the renal scan stem from its decreased anatomic resolution so that kidney stones and minor dilatation of the collecting system may not be detected (6).

Cystogram

The cystogram is similar to the IVP in that the result of the procedure is a visual assessment of anatomic detail and any abnormalities, in this case, of the bladder. In addition, this test may also reveal the presence of ureteral reflux. The procedure is performed by instilling the contrast dye into the bladder via a urethral catheter, followed by taking a series of plain film images of the bladder and lower ureters.

Urodynamic Study

The purpose of the urodynamic study is to record the neurophysiologic function of the detrusor and external urethral sphincter. The study is of value in patients with impairment of storage or discharge of urine. The urinary bladder functions as a container, a system that involves pressure generated in the bladder and resistance at the urethral outlet level. The difference between the orthodromic pressure and antidromic resistance determines whether urine is stored in or discharged from the bladder. Therefore, monitoring the change of the intravesical pressure as well as the external urethral sphincter activity simultaneously is necessary. During urodynamic study, information regarding the following areas is collected:

1. Bladder-filling sensation
2. Electromyographic (EMG) findings of the external urethral sphincter, especially the presence of voluntary control
3. Cystometrogram (pressure change in the bladder) and sphincter EMG (outlet resistance) relationship during
    a. Gradual bladder filling
    b. Crede or Valsalva maneuver, or abdominal tapping
    c. Anal stretch
4. Urethral pressure profile
5. Sacral reflex latency

Documenting Bladder-Filling Sensation

Since micturition is a part of an individual's daily activities, the sensation of bladder fullness is important for the

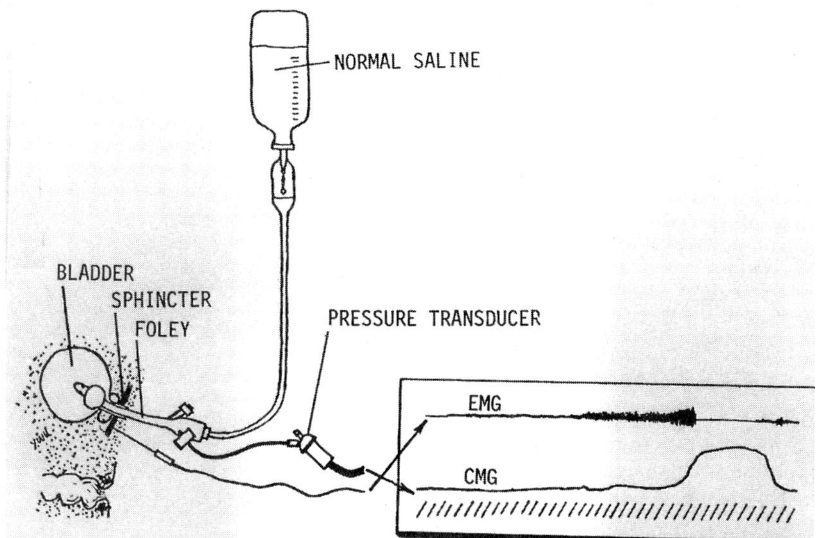

Figure 51-4. Setup for cystometrogram/sphincter electromyographic (EMG) study.

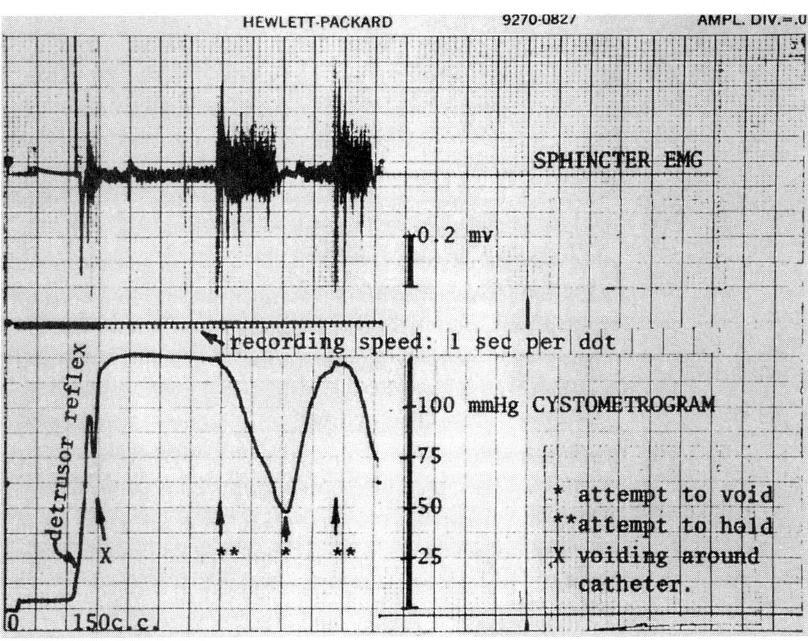

Figure 51-5. Cystometrogram/sphincter EMG recording from a patient with C5–C6 incomplete spinal cord injury. The patient had voluntary control of the toes in both feet and the urethral sphincter. He was also able to void (*asterisk*) or hold (*double asterisk*) the urine upon command.

individual to prepare for bladder emptying. During the urodynamic study, it is necessary to document the presence of the bladder-filling sensation, and at what capacity the patient experiences urgency.

Electromyographic Study of the External Urethral Sphincter

Once the EMG electrode is placed in the external urethral sphincter, look for the patient's ability to "voluntarily" contract and relax the urethral sphincter upon command. The presence of volitional contraction or relaxation of the external urethral sphincter indicates an intact connection between the cerebral cortex and the urethral sphincter and is a very favorable sign for regaining normal bladder function. It is often seen in patients with incomplete spinal cord injury (e.g., central cord syndrome, Brown-Séquard syndrome) and in patients with hemiplegia.

Cystometrogram/Sphincter Electromyographic Study

This procedure documents the time relationship between intravesical pressure and sphincter EMG activity. It shows whether the detrusor muscle and external sphincter muscle are acting coordinately (synergia) or against each other (dyssynergia). While the bladder is filled with normal saline solution to a maximal amount of 500 mL, the pressure change in the bladder and the EMG activity of the external urethral sphincter are simultaneously recorded (Figs. 51-4 and 51-5). During the study, several responses are observed (7):

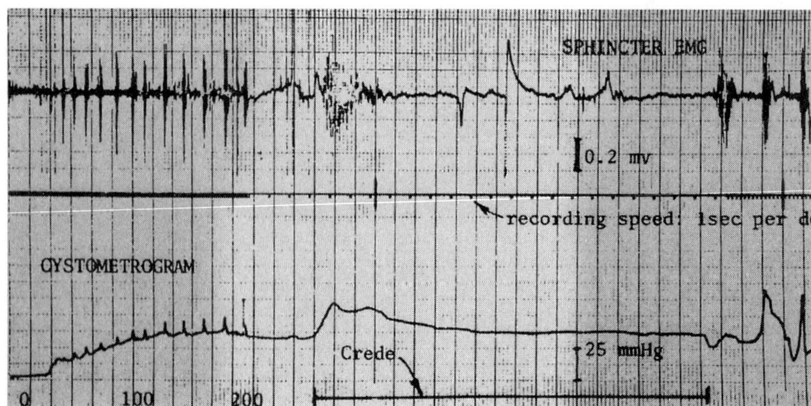

Figure 51-6. Cystometrogram/sphincter EMG recording from a patient with T4–T5 complete spinal cord injury. Note the gradual buildup of intravesical pressure with intermittent bursts of sphincter activity. The Crede maneuver induced a transient increase, followed by a prolonged (18-second) silent period of sphincter activity, suggesting detrusor-sphincter synergia. This phenomenon is rarely seen in patients with complete spinal cord injury.

Detrusor Contraction During Gradual Bladder Filling

Detrusor contraction is indicated by a sudden rise of the intravesical pressure. It occurs voluntarily in normal individuals during voiding as well as involuntarily in patients following noxious stimulation. It occurs at 300- to 400-mL capacity in normal conditions and at 50- to 200-mL capacity in the spastic bladder (Fig. 51-6), and is absent in patients during spinal shock or with lower motor neuron lesions. Three factors are important in analyzing the detrusor reflex:

1. Bladder capacity at the time when detrusor reflex occurs. This capacity indicates the amount of urine that can be held in the bladder before involuntary voiding (incontinence) occurs.
2. Maximal pressure in the bladder during detrusor contraction. The maximal orthodromic pressure produced in the bladder is compared with the antidromic resistance at the external urethral sphincter (measured from urethral pressure profile, discussed later). The difference between the intravesical pressure and the urethral resistance determines the direction of urine flow.
3. Sphincter EMG activity during detrusor contraction. This activity determines the pattern of detrusor-sphincter synergia or dyssynergia. In the presence of increased sphincter activity in patients with detrusor-sphincter dyssynergia, voiding will be incomplete and potentially harmful to the upper urinary tract due to back pressure from high outlet resistance (8).

Crede or Valsalva Maneuver or Abdominal Tapping

Since these techniques are often used by patients for bladder evacuation, it is important to document whether these techniques are achieving a favorable condition: relaxation of the external urethral sphincter muscle and increased pressure in the bladder (see Fig. 51-6). In most spinal cord injury patients with complete upper motor neuron lesions, these maneuvers tend to induce both increased intravesical pressure and increased sphincter activity.

Anal Stretch Response

Anal stretch, rather than anal stimulation, inhibits both the detrusor and urethral sphincter contraction in many patients with complete spinal cord injury. If this condition is present, the patient with normal hand function can be taught to perform the anal stretch and apply the Valsalva maneuver simultaneously to achieve bladder emptying (Fig. 51-7). Anal stretch can effectively inhibit the bulbocavernosus reflex and relax the urethral sphincter. It can be a simple solution when encountering difficulty in catheterizing a patient who has a spastic sphincter (9–11).

Urethral Pressure Profile

The change of pressure (outlet resistance) in the urethra is recorded during slow withdrawal of a water-filled catheter (Fig. 51-8). Comparison of the peak pressure in the urethra with the intravesical pressure recorded on the cystometrogram provides information about the possibility of bladder emptying (Fig. 51-9).

Sacral Reflex Latency

The bulbocavernosus reflex is routinely checked as part of the clinical evaluation. Its presence, however, only suggests an intact reflex arc. More precisely, it can be tested by the sacral reflex latency study. Abnormally prolonged or absent latency of the sacral reflex is suggestive of involvement somewhat along the reflex arc. Sacral latency study is done by stimulating the glans penis and recording the response from the external urethral sphincter.

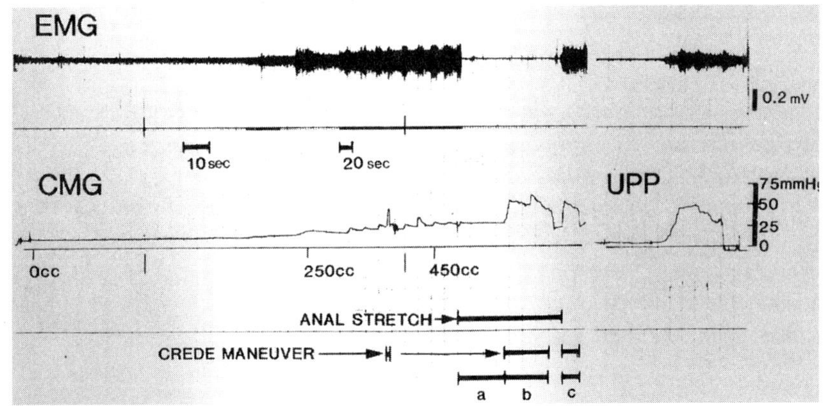

Figure 51-7. Cystometrogram/sphincter EMG recording from a patient with C8 complete spinal cord injury revealing detrusor-sphincter dyssynergia. The Crede maneuver alone (*C*) increased the sphincter activity and intravesical pressure, while anal stretch alone (*A*) significantly reduced the sphincter activity. The combination of anal stretch and Crede maneuver resulted in a favorable condition for bladder emptying: relaxation of urethral sphincter and increase of intravesical pressure (*B*).

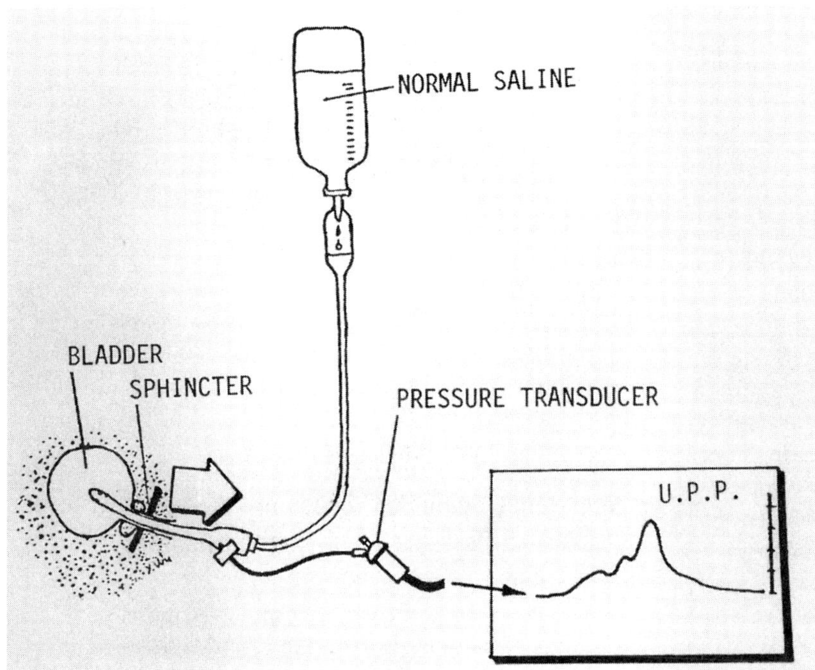

Figure 51-8. Setup for urethral pressure profile study.

Cystoscopy

Cystoscopy permits direct visualization of the interior of the bladder. Indications for cystoscopy include hematuria that cannot be attributed to urinary tract infection, renal or bladder stones, or trauma, as from intermittent catheterization or an indwelling catheter; recurrent urinary tract infections, especially when the bacteria is a stone-forming organism (e.g., *Proteus mirabilis*); and significant calculus formation, which may result in frequent obstruction of indwelling catheters. Because of the increased risk for bladder carcinoma in individuals with indwelling catheters, it has been suggested that cystoscopy be performed on a regular basis for early detection of this complication, especially in persons who have had indwelling catheters for longer than 10 years (3,12).

PATTERNS OF BLADDER DYSFUNCTION

Management of the neurogenic bladder has evolved from advances in the understanding of the pathophysiology of micturition and care techniques during the past decades. The following sections provide a different perspective for care of bladder dysfunction using a theoretical "care model." After all, the physiologic phenomena of the urinary bladder follow simple physical principles: To store urine, the outlet resistance is higher than the bladder pres-

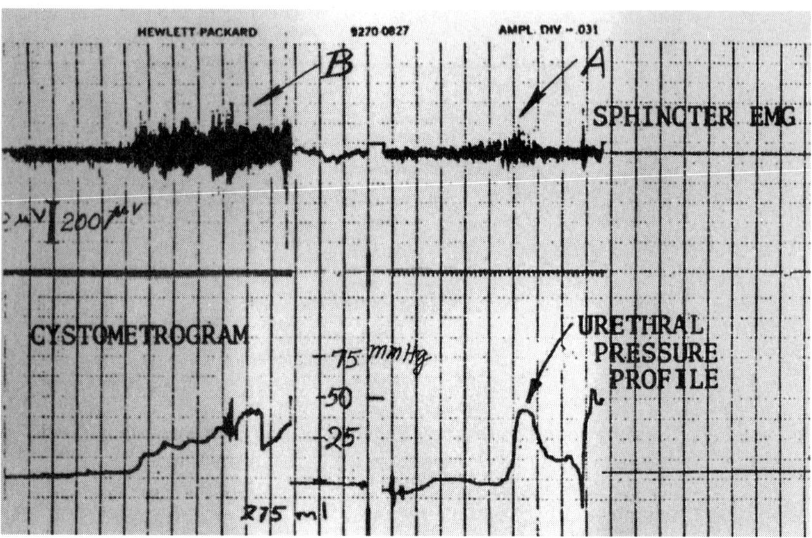

Figure 51-9. Cystometrogram/sphincter EMG and urethral pressure profile study on a patient with C5–C6 motor complete quadriplegia. The patient exhibited a typical detrusor-sphincter dyssynergia. The higher urethral resistance compared to the intravesical pressure caused persistent incomplete bladder emptying. If the sphincter were more active at point A than at point B, the peak pressure in the urethra would be much higher.

sure; to discharge urine, the bladder pressure must be higher than the outlet resistance. Although the following care model is quite different from what has been traditionally stressed in the past, one might find this approach useful and practical in managing bladder dysfunction due to various causes.

Neurogenic "Sphincter" Rather Than "Neurogenic Bladder" as the Cause for Bladder Dysfunction

Under normal conditions, the bladder functions as a reservoir to store and to expel urine at will. Once there is any involvement of the neurocontrol of the bladder and urethral sphincter, both retention and expulsion of urine may be affected; that is, there is an inability to hold urine until preparation is made for urination, or to urinate completely when ready. An inability to retain urine results in incontinence and an inability to expel urine results in urinary retention. Urinary incontinence is a "psychosocial problem" and can be managed by a collecting device, frequently timed voiding, or use of anticholinergic agents. On the other hand, urinary retention causes "medical complications," such as urinary infection or renal dysfunction, and therefore requires careful management. With this in mind, it would be feasible to focus the discussion on dysfunction of micturition first and the problem of urinary storage later.

There are three steps involved in normal micturition: 1) Sensory feedback informs the individual whether or not the bladder is full. 2) When the bladder is full and voiding is desired and preparations made, the detrusor muscle contracts. 3) While the detrusor contracts, the external urethral sphincter relaxes. At that moment, the increased pressure in the bladder pushes urine out through the relaxed outlet.

In dealing with the neurogenic bladder, one needs to understand which of the three steps is compromised. For example, in a spinal cord–injured person, awareness of bladder fullness may be impaired but could be compensated for by suprapubic palpation. The necessary bladder pressure from detrusor contraction might be produced by the Crede maneuver. Unfortunately in the person with severe spinal cord injuries, a substitute for relaxing the external urethral sphincter to achieve an opening of the outlet structure often is absent.

For stroke patients, sensation may be intact while the detrusor and urethral sphincter are unable to function for urine storage, but act coordinately for micturition. Thus, the common problem in stroke after the acute phase, if there is no structural outlet obstruction, is urinary incontinence rather than urinary retention.

"Neurogenic Sphincter" Leads to "Increased Intravesical Pressure" and "High Residual Urine Volume"

An inability to relax the external sphincter muscle during micturition leads to an increased outlet resistance, which in turn produces increased intravesical pressure and high residual urine volumes. Once increased intravesical pressure persists for a prolonged period, dilatation of the upper urinary tracts becomes inevitable. Meanwhile the high volume of residual urine breaks down the bladder defense mechanism and causes bacteriuria (8).

The primary problem in neurogenic bladder, therefore, is not due to impaired detrusor function but mainly from altered external urethral sphincter function. Practically, the impaired urethral sphincter rather than the detrusor should be blamed for bladder dysfunction. Therefore, in managing the neurogenic bladder, efforts should be aimed at solving two problems: high intravesical pressure and high residual urine because of impairment of the external urethral sphincter.

CLASSIFICATIONS

Many classifications have been used to describe bladder dysfunction. Each has its merit and clinical values. Based on the level of motor neuron involvement, the neurogenic bladder can be classified as follows:

1. Upper motor neuron–type bladder, complete or incomplete
2. Lower motor neuron–type bladder, complete or incomplete

Another classification is based somewhat on the function of the urinary bladder:

1. Spinal shock bladder
2. Uninhibited bladder
3. Reflex bladder, coordinated or uncoordinated
4. Autonomous bladder
5. Motor paralytic bladder
6. Sensory paralytic bladder
7. Mixed upper and lower motor neuron bladder

From a patient care viewpoint, bladder dysfunction is analogous to motor impairment of the limbs. The patient's potential to ambulate is determined by the presence of residual motor control in key gait muscles, rather than by the level of spinal cord injury or the presence of spasticity. Similarly, whether the bladder is to function again depends not on involuntary detrusor contraction, but the residual function of the external urethral sphincter. Therefore, classification of the neurogenic bladder is more practical if it is based on the patient's ability to achieve external urethral sphincter opening during the event of voiding, as follows:

1. The ability to voluntarily control the external urethral sphincter through the residual intact cerebrospinal pathway
2. The ability to induce synergic reflexic opening of the external urethral sphincter using cutaneous or other stimulation
3. The ability to perform intermittent self-catheterization with normal hand function

Based on this concept, the neurogenic bladder can be classified into four groups:

1. Group C: Patients with voluntary cortical control to relax the external urethral sphincter during micturition belong in this group (see Fig. 51-6). They are patients with very incomplete spinal cord injury, such as Brown-Séquard syndrome or central cord syndrome; patients with early multiple sclerosis; and patients with hemiplegia. Voluntary contraction and relaxation of the external urethral sphincter can be observed during the EMG study. Clinically, almost all patients with voluntary contraction and relaxation of the anal sphincter during rectal examination and voluntary movement of toes on one or two sides will have coordinated detrusor-sphincter function and would be expected to regain normal bladder function.
2. Group S: About 10% to 15% of patients with complete spinal cord injury and loss of cortical control of the external urethral sphincter may achieve synergic reflexic sphincter relaxation using the Crede, Valsalva, or tapping maneuver (see Fig. 51-7). A coordinated detrusor-sphincter pattern can be observed during the urodynamic study.
3. Group T: Patients with complete tetraplegia or bilateral hemiplegia do not have cortical control or spinal synergic relaxation of the external urethral sphincter. In addition, they do not have normal hand function for self-catheterization (see Fig. 51-10). Bladder emptying cannot be achieved by voluntary means, or by perineal stimulation. Urethral catheterization can only be done by the caregiver.
4. Group P: Patients with loss of both cortical control and spinal synergic control of the external urethral sphincter, but have normal hand function to perform intermittent self-catheterization or anal stretch for bladder emptying belong in this group. Most complete paraplegic patients have this type of neurogenic bladder. Patients with severe peripheral neuropathy with low intravesical pressure are considered to have this type of bladder dysfunction.

TREATMENT AND MANAGEMENT OF BLADDER DYSFUNCTION

Since no single management method can be used indiscriminately for all types of bladder dysfunction, it would be logical to apply one of the most suitable methods to the particular type of bladder disorder after taking into consideration the medical, social, and economic factors (Fig. 51-10). For example, for a patient with incomplete spinal cord injury and partial voluntary control of the toes and anal sphincter, an external catheter can be provided initially until normal bladder function returns. For any patient with no volitional control of the urethral sphincter but with detrusor-sphincter synergia, cutaneous stimulation may be used to induce voiding while the external catheter may be needed to prevent incontinence. With complete tetraplegia and dyssynergic sphincter function, one of three approaches may be considered: indwelling catheterization, external sphincterotomy, and suprapubic cystostomy. Completely paraplegic patients may use intermittent catheterization, anal stretch, or external sphincterotomy.

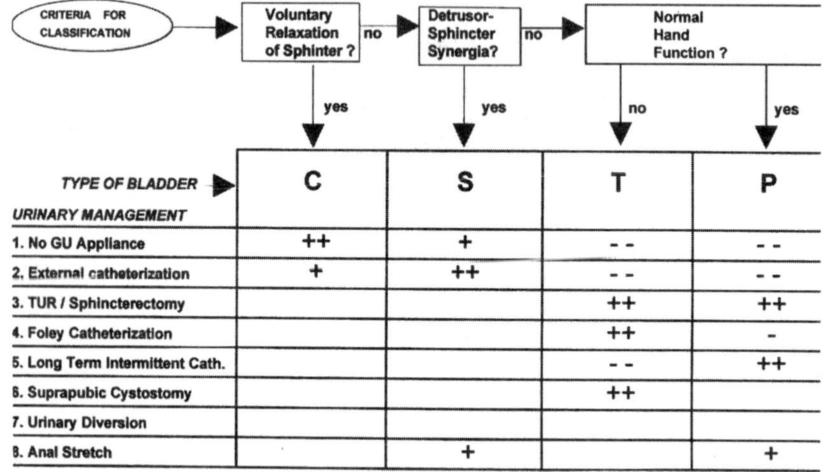

TYPE OF BLADDER	C	S	T	P
URINARY MANAGEMENT				
1. No GU Appliance	++	+	- -	- -
2. External catheterization	+	++	- -	- -
3. TUR / Sphincterectomy			++	++
4. Foley Catheterization			++	-
5. Long Term Intermittent Cath.			- -	++
6. Suprapubic Cystostomy			++	
7. Urinary Diversion				
8. Anal Stretch		+		+

Figure 51-10. Total bladder algorithm. The " + " and " ++ " signs indicate recommended care methods. The " – – " sign indicates nonrecommended methods.

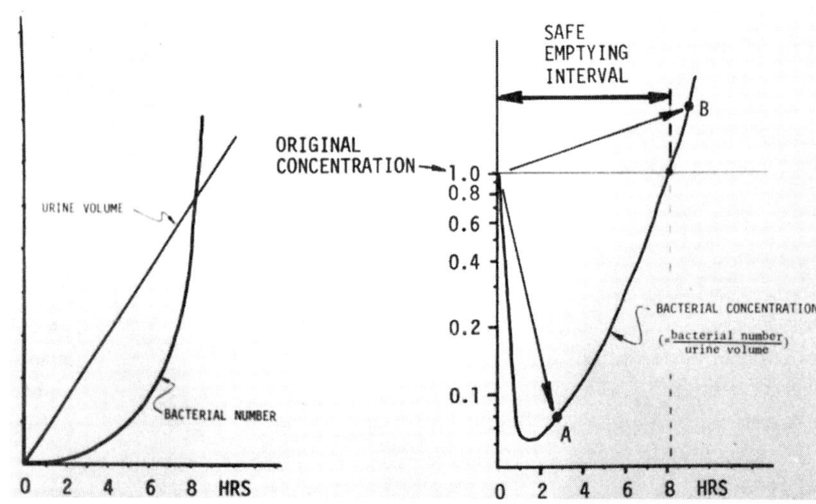

Figure 51-11. Changes of bladder urine volume, total bacterial number, and bacterial concentration in the bladder after voiding. The safe emptying interval (SEI) is the interval from the time of previous emptying to the time when the bacterial concentration returns to the original level.

Theory of Safe Emptying Interval

The higher incidence of urinary tract infection in persons with impaired bladder function, such as in those with spinal cord injury, is in part due to the breakdown of the natural defense mechanism. Dilution of the residual urine and periodic evacuation of urine from the bladder protect it from urinary infection. When one has a high volume of infected residual urine, there is a high starting total bacterial population that leads to rapid overgrowth of the bacteria. Delaying bladder emptying allows the residual bacteria more time to multiply in the bladder.

This basic model for understanding the natural defense mechanism of the bladder against infection has been explained with a mathematical model. (13–17). For more than a decade we have conceptually and mathematically re-examined the dynamic defense mechanism of bladder against infection in a manner similar to that of Hinman and Cox (14) and used a concept of "safe emptying interval" (SEI) for clinical management of urinary tract infection.

With the assumption that the urinary bladder without an indwelling catheter works as a container and the presence of bacteria is limited to the bladder, the bacterial concentration changes constantly and predictably due to the growth of the bacterial population on one hand and the addition of sterile urine from the kidneys on the other. After voiding, urine from the kidney is added to the residual urine in the bladder at a linear rate (14,17), while the remaining bacteria increase in number at an exponential rate (left curve, Fig. 51-11). This results in an initial reduction of the bacterial concentration, which is then followed by a rapid return to and surpassing of the original concentration (right curve, Fig. 51-11). The interval from the time of previous emptying to the time when the bacterial concentration returns to the original level is clinically important and is defined as the SEI (17). Within this SEI, the bacterial concentration is lower than its level at the time of previous emptying. Once passing the SEI, the bacterial concentration becomes higher than its original level. It is apparent that a "decrease" or "increase" of the bacte-

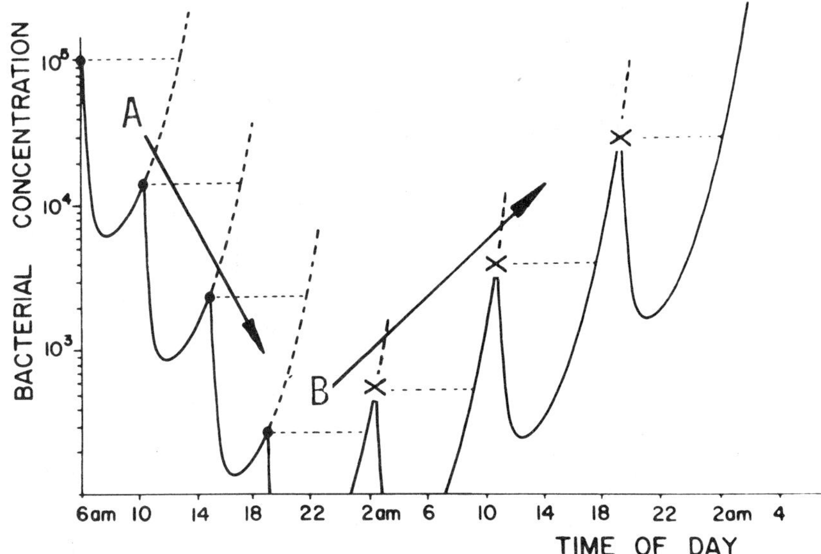

Figure 51-12. Bladder emptying within (*dots*) or after (*crossmarks*) the safe emptying interval results in a decrease (*A*) or an increase (*B*) in bacterial concentration.

rial concentration in the urine is determined by whether the bladder is emptied "within" or "after" the SEI (Fig. 51-12). Since the SEI is a result of several variables, the same voiding interval may result in an increased bacterial concentration in one patient but a decreased concentration in another.

The Wu bladder graph (Fig. 51-13), a slide rule–like graph evolved from a mathematical equation discussed by previous researchers, can be used easily to determine the SEI. This is done by tracing from the residual urine amount (Ro), to the estimated urine volume (Vt) in the bladder at the next voiding, then to the bacterial doubling time (D), and finally to the SEI (see Fig. 51-13). For example, if patient A has a residual urine amount of 50 mL, bladder capacity (or urine volume at the time of the next voiding) of 300 mL, and an infection with bacterial doubling time of 60 minutes, the SEI will be about 2.5 hours. This is obtained by tracing on the Wu bladder graph from point A (Ro = 50), to A′ (Vt = 300), to A″ (D = 60), and finally to A‴ (SEI = 2.5 hours).

Significance of the Wu Bladder Graph

The only way one can maintain sterile urine or eliminate bacteriuria is to have the bladder emptied within the SEI. This is done 1) by voiding more frequently so that the actual bladder emptying interval is shorter than the SEI, or 2) by increasing the SEI so that it is longer than the actual bladder emptying interval. To empty the bladder more frequently is a matter of willingness by the individual. Increasing the SEI, however, can be achieved reducing the residual urine volume, increasing the bladder urine

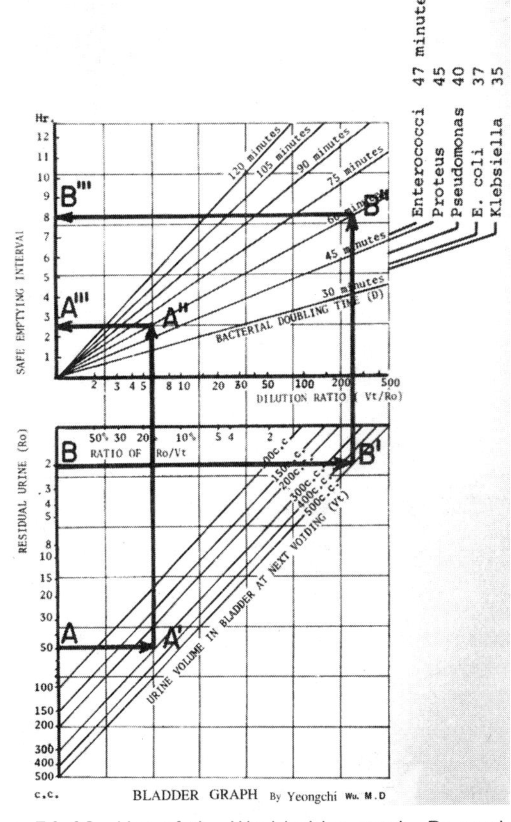

Figure 51-13. Use of the Wu bladder graph. By applying known variables of residual urine volume (Ro), bladder urine volume (Vt), and bacterial doubling time (D), the safe emptying interval can be obtained in a few seconds. The in vivo bacterial doubling times of common organisms are listed at the side of the graph.

volume, and prolonging the bacterial doubling time (Fig. 51-14).

Each of the variables affects the SEI differently. Assuming the bladder urine volume and bacterial doubling time remain constant, there will be an inverse parabolic relationship between the residual urine and the SEI. In other words, a patient with low residual urine volume can void less frequently whereas another patient with high residual urine volume must void more frequently to avoid bladder infection. Consequently, it is incorrect to assume any certain volume as the acceptable residual urine amount without, at the same time, taking into account the frequency of actual bladder emptying (Fig. 51-15).

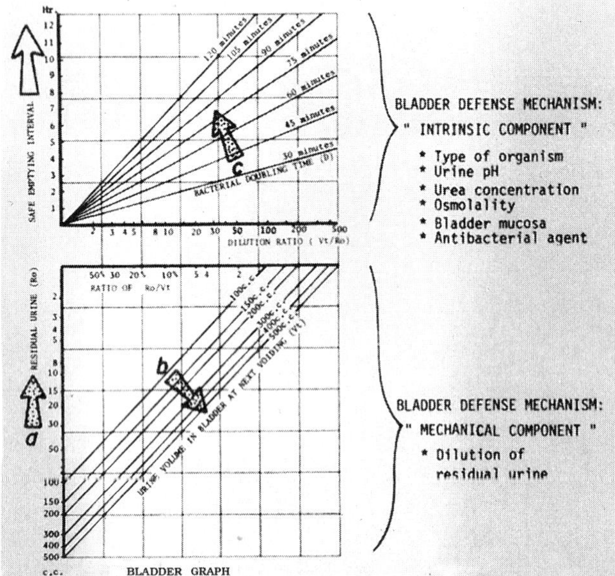

Figure 51-14. The safe emptying interval can be prolonged by one or a combination of the following: (*A*) reduction of residual urine volume (*Ro*), (*B*) larger bladder capacity (Vt) for larger mechanical dilution of residual urine, and (*C*) prolongation of the bacterial doubling time (*D*).

Components of the Bladder Defense Mechanism Against Infection

The bladder graph (see Fig. 51-14) shows two distinct components of the bladder defense mechanism: The upper portion is the "intrinsic component," and the lower portion is the "mechanical component." The intrinsic component consists of factors that affect the bacterial doubling time, such as the type of organism, urine pH, urea concentration, osmolality, antibacterial effect of the bladder mucosa, and the use of antibacterial agents. The mechanical component is the ratio of residual urine to the bladder urine volume at the next voiding. From this bladder graph, one can appreciate that a reduction of residual urine, an increase in the bladder volume, and a prolongation of the bacterial doubling time result in an extension of the SEI.

Since the change of bacterial concentration is related to the time relationship between actual bladder emptying and the SEI, any clinical study to determine the effectiveness of a given antibacterial agent (that affects only the bacterial doubling time) for bladder infection would be theoretically inadequate if residual urine and the bladder urine volume (both are mechanical components) as well as the "frequency" of voiding were not controlled.

Nonsurgical Bladder Management

Bladder Training

Bladder training is a commonly used term even though it is not clearly defined. To some extent, bladder training using the intermittent catheterization technique may be considered as a "range of motion" exercise of the bladder. Just like "range of motion" exercise to the paralyzed legs, intermittent catheterization alone may not be expected to change the uncoordinated detrusor-sphincter to a coordi-

Figure 51-15. Relationship between the residual urine volume (Ro) and the safe emptying interval when the bladder urine volume (Vt) and bacterial doubling time (D) remain unchanged. Ct = bacterial concentration t minutes after previous bladder emptying; Co = the original bacterial concentration immediately after voiding.

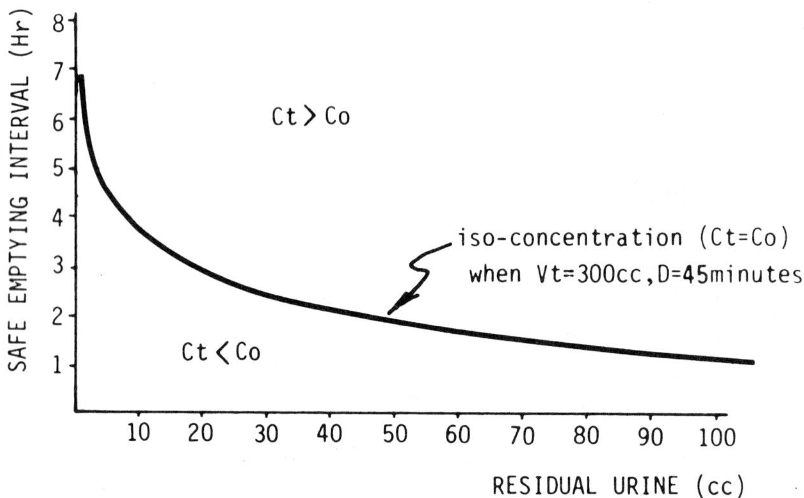

nated pattern. However, if there is a chance of eventual return of bladder function, avoiding bladder contracture by intermittent catheterization is desirable.

Anal Stretching

In patients, mostly those with complete spinal cord injury and detrusor-sphincter dyssynergia, anal stretch (not anal stimulation) will inhibit the activity of the external sphincter and allow a reduced outlet resistance. During the time when the anal sphincter is stretched, performing a Valsalva or Crede maneuver to increase abdominal pressure may allow the urine in the bladder to be drained through the relaxed outlet (see Fig. 51-7).

Anal stretch is a very important technique for patients with complete spinal cord injury for both periodic evacuation of urine and insertion of an indwelling catheter. This phenomenon was reported initially in 1961 and more than a decade later (9–11).

When practical, anal stretch can replace intermittent catheterization so that the number of daily urethral catheterizations is reduced and the chance of contamination often associated with instrumentation can be reduced.

Urine Collection Devices

A number of methods are available for the collection and storage of urine, depending on the status of bladder function and the ability of the patient to manage the specific bladder-emptying technique. The ideal urine collection device is one that effectively empties and collects urine from the bladder, minimizes the potential for skin breakdown and other complications in the perineal region, minimizes the potential for urinary infection and other renal complications, and is compatible with the patient's lifestyle and daily routine.

Protective Undergarment

Individuals who have the ability to adequately empty their bladder, but experience occasional incontinence due to control problems may be adequately managed with a protective undergarment to prevent soiling of their clothing. There are a variety of disposable, commercially available undergarments and protective liners available to serve this purpose. Problems with these undergarments trapping moisture and causing skin breakdown have been decreased with the use of highly absorbent materials that maintain a dry lining against the covered skin. Some patients resist the use of the undergarments because of the perceived social stigma.

External Condom Catheters

In men with adequate detrusor contractions, reflexic or voluntary, and without external sphincter dyssynergy so that fairly complete bladder emptying is occurring, the use of external condom catheters is an option. Individuals utilizing intermittent catheterization who also have spontaneous voids between catheterizations also may utilize this method of urine collection. Unfortunately, this is not a viable option for women because no reliable system has been developed that is clinically effective. Attention has to be paid to placement of and tolerance for the condom, as there is the potential for penile skin breakdown and allergic reaction to the condom material and adhesive. Use of newer materials and adhesives has reduced the number of these complications. Although the incidence of urinary tract infection is lower than the incidence associated with indwelling catheters or intermittent catheterization, it remains a risk, owing to the potential to collect bacteria in the condom; therefore, attention to hygiene is essential (18). Men with a smaller or a retractile penis may encounter difficulties applying and keeping the condom catheter on, thereby limiting its use and effectiveness.

Indwelling Catheters

An indwelling urethral catheter is commonly used in the early period of an acute medical process, such as a spinal cord injury, when there is associated bladder dysfunction and a need to accurately monitor fluid intake and output. In most cases, attempts to remove the catheter and use an alternative method of bladder management and urine collection should be made. In instances where no other method is effective or the patient does not have the ability or assistance to carry out an alternative regimen, use of an indwelling catheter may be the only option. Chronic indwelling catheters are associated with an increased risk of urinary tract infections, bladder stones, urethral injury, penile-scrotal fistula, squamous metaplasia, and squamous cell carcinoma (19,20). Proper care of the catheter and adherence to certain measures are essential to minimize the risk of these potential complications. These measures include changing the catheter monthly, maintaining adequate fluid intake and urine output to ensure free urine flow and reduce sediment in the catheter, frequent emptying of the leg bag to prevent overdistention of and back pressure on the bladder, and proper placement of the catheter and tubing to minimize traction to the urethra. Interestingly, there has been a recent suggestion that the complication rates associated with indwelling catheters are no higher than those of other management methods (19,20). This may be due in part to a greater awareness of these potential complications and stricter adherence to suggested periodic surveillance studies such as renal ultrasound and cystoscopy. An alternative method using an indwelling device is the suprapubic tube cystostomy, which is described in greater detail later. This method is also associated with many of the complications found with urethral catheters.

Intermittent Catheterization

In persons who are unable to spontaneously and completely empty their bladder and who have functional use of their hands or the consistent availability of a caregiver, intermittent catheterization is probably the preferred method of bladder management. The sterile technique for intermittent catheterization was originally proposed for the management of patients with acute spinal cord injury in the mid-1960s, and continues to be a common practice today in many acute care settings to minimize the risk of nosocomial infection (21). The clean technique, which is easier and less expensive to perform than the sterile technique, was proposed a decade later and has become a generally accepted and widely utilized method of intermittent catheterization in the outpatient setting (22).

An effective intermittent catheterization program requires attention to a balanced fluid intake throughout the day so that the output volume with each catheterization is not greater than 400 mL. To minimize the potential for upper urinary tract complication and to prevent incontinence between catheterizations, a low-pressure bladder is desired and may necessitate the use of anticholinergic agents. The time interval between catheterizations will vary in different individuals, depending in part on the volume of fluid intake and output, and may range from every 4 to 8 hours. In general, the interval should be within the SEI for the prevention of urinary infection, or catheterization should occur when the bladder is full, to avoid incontinence or reflux.

While in most patients, intermittent catheterization is generally the preferred method of bladder management, in some, such as obese individuals, women with significant hip adduction spasticity, noncompliant patients, or persons with inconsistent availability of assistance, it may not be feasible. Although the risks are less than those associated with indwelling catheters, bladder stones and urinary tract infections remain potential complications (23,24). In those who experience repeated urinary tract infections, changing to the sterile technique and the use of various touchless disposable catheter kits are available options.

Pharmacologic Agents

Depending on the type of bladder dysfunction, the use of medications may be a useful adjunctive treatment in the overall management of the neurogenic bladder. The various classes of pharmacologic agents and specific medications, and situations in which their use may be beneficial, are described.

Anticholinergic Agents

Anticholinergic agents are probably the most commonly used class of medications for the treatment of bladder dysfunction, most specifically to suppress uninhibited detrusor contractions. The use of an agent with these properties would theoretically suppress reflex detrusor activity, allowing an individual to avoid incontinence between catheterizations and to maintain a high-compliance, low-pressure bladder. Three commonly used drugs with anticholinergic effects include propantheline bromide, oxybutynin chloride, and hyoscyamine sulfate. Propantheline bromide is the most frequently used agent and is generally administered in doses of 7.5 to 30.0 mg three or four times a day. Oxybutynin chloride is administered in a dose of 5 to 10 mg three or four times a day and is unique in that it also has a direct relaxing effect on smooth muscle in addition to its anticholinergic properties. Because of this additional effect, oxybutynin in solution directly instilled in the bladder may be effective in reducing reflex detrusor activity in persons who are not able to tolerate the medication orally (25,26). At the present time, however, there is no commercial preparation of oxybutynin in a liquid form. Hyoscyamine sulfate, a commonly used agent for spastic and irritable bowel disorders, has recently gained popularity for use for bladder dysfunction. It is available as a rapidly acting sublingual tablet and a sustained-release capsule. One additional agent, imipramine, is known to have anticholinergic activity at low dosages and may have a synergistic effect when used with oxybutynin.

Cholinergic Agents

In persons with decreased bladder contractility and incomplete emptying, the use of an agent with agonist activity on cholinergic muscarinic receptors in the detrusor would appear to be ideal. Bethanechol is a cholinergeric agonist that has been commonly used to improve bladder contractility. Unfortunately, this agent has not been widely effective, and has met with little success in individuals with detrusor areflexia (27,28). Because of the potential for increasing intravesical pressure, this agent should not be used in persons with detrusor-sphincter dyssynergia or other bladder outlet obstructions.

Adrenergic Antagonist Agents

Adrenergic antagonist agents with specific activity for α_1 receptors are commonly used to decrease bladder outlet resistance and improve bladder emptying. In addition, patients who experience sweating and other symptoms of autonomic dysreflexia during reflex voiding benefit from the use of these agents for symptom relief. Phenoxybenzamine, which has both α_1- and α_2-adrenergic activity, and agents with more specific α_1 activity, such as prazosin and terazosin, have been used. Although effectiveness and benefits have been seen in men with bladder outlet obstruction, such as in those with benign prostate hypertrophy, the same results have not been consistently reported in persons with neurogenic bladder dysfunction such as detrusor-sphincter dyssynergy (29). This difference may be attributable to the fact that there is a greater concentration of α_1 receptors in the bladder neck, proximal part of the urethra, and prostate smooth muscle than in the external urinary sphincter (30).

Adrenergic Agonist Agents

There are limited reports of the beneficial effects of α-adrenergic agonist agents for the treatment of urinary incontinence due to inadequate urinary sphincter tone (31). Ephedrine and phenylpropanolamine are the two most commonly used agents. It is important to emphasize that these agents be used cautiously in individuals with potentially high-pressure bladders (i.e., bladder with low compliance or with hyperreflexic detrusor activity) so as not to increase further the intravesical pressure and increase the risk of ureteral reflux and upper urinary tract complications.

Miscellaneous Agents

Various other medications have been used in the treatment of specific voiding disorders, or have been noted to have effects on bladder function, but are not being used clinically on a routine basis.

A course of estrogen supplementation is often effective in postmenopausal women who experience urinary stress incontinence due to atrophy of the urethral epithelium (32).

Two agents that appear to depress detrusor activity are intrathecal baclofen and terodiline. When administered intrathecally for the treatment of spinal spasticity, baclofen suppresses detrusor reflex activity, which may result in a higher-compliance bladder (33). Any potential for its use in the management of bladder dysfunction has yet to be determined. Terodiline is a calcium channel blocker reported to have the ability to suppress detrusor instability and hyperreflexia (34,35). Additional clinical studies will determine whether any benefit can be obtained from its use.

Surgical Management

A number of surgical options are commonly considered in particular situations of bladder dysfunction when more conservative measures are not effective. The more frequently performed procedures are designed either to enhance effective bladder drainage, to reduce resistance to bladder emptying, or to increase the storage capacity of the bladder.

Suprapubic Catheterization

Suprapubic catheterization is essentially a variant on use of the indwelling urethral catheter except that the catheter is placed in the bladder by cystostomy, bypassing the urethra. The greatest benefit of this procedure is that the urethra is free of the catheter, which avoids the accompanying risks of urethral injury. In addition, a larger-diameter catheter may be used suprapubically to enhance bladder drainage and decrease the problem of catheter occlusion from urinary sediment. Similar to an indwelling urethral catheter though, use of a suprapubic catheter is associated with an increased risk of urinary tract infection and bladder stones (36,37). The long-term use of this method may also lead to a contracted, small-capacity bladder, and urine leakage through the urethra and around the suprapubic tube (36).

Sphincterotomy

Transurethral sphincterotomy has been used frequently in men with detrusor-sphincter dyssynergy, to reduce resistance to bladder emptying and maintain low intravesical pressures. In persons unable to perform intermittent catheterization and preferring to avoid use of an indwelling catheter, sphincterotomy is an option, provided they have adequate reflex voiding and are able to use an external condom catheter (which unfortunately excludes women). The procedure is usually performed by incising the striated external sphincter through the full thickness of the muscle. An anteromedial location is preferred to avoid possible nerve injury and resultant impotence (38). Although the procedure is effective in appropriate patients, the long-term potential for recurrent obstruction is an issue (39). A potential solution to this problem, and an alternative to sphincterotomy, that has recently completed clinical trials is the use of an implantable stainless-steel mesh stent (40). This potentially reversible device expands and holds the sphincter open, and has the advantages over sphincterotomy of decreased risks of bleeding with the procedure itself, erectile and ejaculatory dysfunction, and recurrent obstruction. Additional long-term studies will determine whether stent migration is a potential issue and the effect of the presence of an implanted foreign material.

Bladder Augmentation and Continent Diversion

In individuals with significant detrusor hyperreflexia or low-compliance, small-capacity bladders that fail to respond to anticholinergeric medications and who experience difficulty maintaining continence with various bladder-emptying methods, bladder augmentation is often an effective procedure (37). In many of these individuals, an additional procedure, the creation of a continent catheterizable stoma, may further improve bladder management (37). Bladder augmentation is performed to achieve a larger bladder capacity while maintaining low intravesical pressure. In this procedure, a segment of colon or ileum is excised with its mesentery intact and detubularized. It is then anastomosed to the bladder, which has been previously bivalved, creating an enlarged reservoir with a capacity of 500 to 600 mL. The patient may still be required to perform intermittent catheterization to empty the bladder, so patient motivation and compliance are important factors to consider prior to surgery. Potential long-term complications of this procedure include chronic bacteriuria, increased mucus in the urine, stone formation, and neoplastic changes in the bladder (37,41,42).

A continent diversion may be performed in a number of different situations. In individuals who have sustained traumatic injuries to the bladder or the urethra that make the use of indwelling catheters or intermittent catheterization difficult, construction of an ileal or colon conduit is an alternative option for urinary drainage.

Similar to colostomies, the proper application and use of an external collection appliance are essential to minimize the risk of potential complications such as stomal stenosis and skin irritation and breakdown. In persons who have difficulty performing intermittent catheterization, such as women or persons with significant spasticity, creating a catheterizable stoma or opening in the abdomen in conjunction with bladder augmentation is also a viable option. This procedure has allowed many individuals to be more independent in effectively managing their bladder (37).

Electrical Stimulation

A number of techniques utilizing electrical stimulation in some form have been proposed to improve bladder function, but the clinical applications remain limited (43). Despite differences in these various techniques, they share the common objectives of regaining the storage function of the bladder, achieving complete bladder emptying, and in patients with voiding disorders such as urge incontinence or detrusor-sphincter dyssynergia, decreasing and stabilizing bladder overactivity. Electrical stimulation has been used to strengthen specific pelvic floor muscles in order to improve urinary continence (44). Direct means of utilizing electrical stimulation to alter bladder function that have been proposed include percutaneous pelvic floor stimulation, anal sphincter stimulation, dorsal penile nerve stimulation, and transurethral stimulation (45–48). Recently, there have been several promising reports of an implanted neurostimulation system that involves the stimulation of the sacral anterior roots to produce voiding in persons with inadequate emptying due to impaired detrusor function (Fig. 51-16). Division of the posterior sacral roots is also recommended to increase bladder capacity and restore bladder compliance (49). Clinical studies on a developed neurostimulation system are currently underway in the United States.

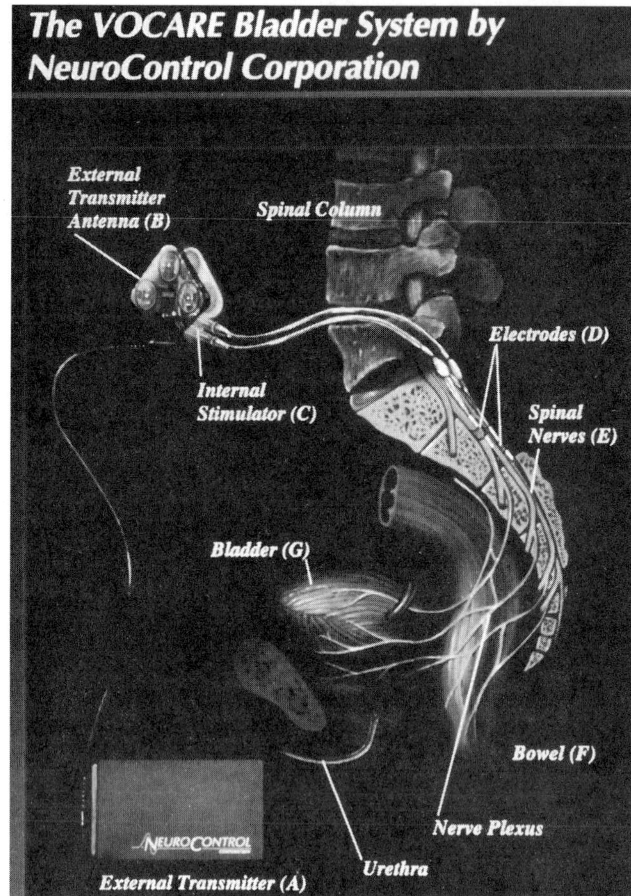

Figure 51-16. VOCARE bladder system. An implanted neurostimulation system that involves the stimulation of the sacral anterior roots, producing detrusor contraction and enhanced bladder emptying.

POTENTIAL COMPLICATIONS

Urinary Tract Infection and Bacteriuria

For decades, the terms *bacteriuria* and *urinary tract infection* have been used interchangeably. At a consensus validation conference, organized by the National Institute on Disability and Rehabilitation Research, on the prevention and management of urinary tract infections among persons with spinal cord injuries, *urinary tract infection* was defined as "bacteriuria (>10^5 bacteria per ml of urine) with tissue invasion and resultant tissue response with signs and/or symptoms" (50). On the other hand, presence of bacteria in the urine without associated signs or symptoms is referred to as *bacteriuria* (50).

Urinary infection in patients with neurogenic bladder, especially those with spinal cord injury, is a very important problem because of the high morbidity and mortality rates related to urinary complications. Frequent infection, reinfection, and relapse infection as well as the development of antibiotic-resistant organisms led to the difficulty of deciding whether or not to treat urinary tract infection in spinal cord injury patients. Questions are often raised regarding urinary infection versus bacterial colonization, localization of urinary infection, and short-term versus long-term antibacterial therapy.

With the presence of an indwelling catheter, the patient inevitably will acquire bacteriuria no matter what kind of preventive measures are taken. Since a "catheterized" urine specimen rather than a spontaneous "midstream" specimen is often obtained from spinal cord injury patients, the conventional criteria for "significant bacteriuria" in neurologically intact individuals as originally defined are not applicable to those with neurogenic bladder (51,52). With impaired sensation, the classic symptoms of dysuria, frequency, urgency, and suprapubic pain are not reliable in the spinal cord injury population, whereas gross pyuria indicates an increased risk of morbidity for untreated urinary infection (53).

Localization of Urinary Tract Infection

Once bacteriuria is confirmed, distinction between upper and lower urinary tract infection is clinically important because of the potential for renal damage in patients with upper tract infections. Patients with renal infection given conventional short courses of antibacterial therapy for 1 or 2 weeks have an inordinate frequency of relapse. Repetitive and insufficient antibiotic therapies also cause selection of highly resistant organisms, which is another potential problem in the hospital setting.

The Fairley bladder washout procedure for localizing the site of urinary infection (54), and the modified Fairley test (55) are too complicated for routine clinical application. The antibody-coated bacteria screening was not accepted as a useful procedure for the spinal cord injury population (56). A simplified method with some diagnostic and therapeutic value using modified bladder irrigation and dip-slide semiquantitative bacterial counting was tested at the Rehabilitation Institute of Chicago (57,58). In our modified washout test, the bladder is irrigated with 50 mL of normal saline solution for 20 times with or without the initial instillation of diluted povidone-iodine (Betadine) solution (1 : 1 dilution with normal saline solution). Three urine specimens, obtained before irrigation, after irrigation, and 90 minutes after irrigation, are collected for semiquantitative bacterial counting using dip-Slide procedure. In addition to the change of bacterial concentration, the change of total bacterial population is also compared with the postirrigation bacterial concentration and population. Since the bladder irrigation is expected to suppress the growth of residual bacteria during its lag phase of growth for at least 2 hours, any dramatic increase in the total bacterial population would indicate migration of the bacteria from either the upper urinary tract or the prostate. Further clinical data are being collected to define the usefulness of this procedure.

Monitoring Bacteriuria

Because of the high incidence of recurrent urinary tract infection, there should be frequent monitoring to reduce the morbidity rate from untreated urinary infection. Home monitoring of bacteriuria and pyuria will be important for the prevention of secondary complications following spinal cord injury. Possible methods for such home monitoring are use of the dip-Slide for semiquantitative bacterial counting and dip-Stick for detection of nitrite and leukocyte esterase (58). The dip-Slide culture and dip-Stick method are simple procedures and can be taught to most patients and families. Long-term use could be part of a self-care program to monitor and to adjust the bladder care program, such as the need to increase the frequency of micturition or intermittent catheterization when bacteriuria is detected.

Management of Asymptomatic Bacteriuria

It is current practice not to treat asymptomatic bacteriuria with antibiotics, because of the concern of selection of highly resistant organisms. If one refers to the basic bladder defense mechanism as described with the Wu bladder graph, it is clear that to prevent or eliminate bacteriuria, the bladder must be emptied constantly with the SEI. This was clearly demonstrated by the experiment by Hinman and Cox (14). When volunteer medical students were inoculated with *Escherichia coli* and asked to void every 3 hours, bacteriuria was completely eliminated in less than 72 hours without the use of any antibacterial agents. Frequent bladder emptying also explains the low risk of urinary tract infection in patients with spinal cord injury or multiple sclerosis using clean intermittent catheterization for bladder care (22).

In managing asymptomatic bacteriuria in the setting of an indwelling catheter, one should attempt to follow this approach:

1. Make sure the indwelling catheter is free of any blockage due to sediment or kink or an overfilled urinary bag.
2. Increase fluid intake to ensure adequate urinary output.

When there is no indwelling catheter present, one should follow this approach:

1. Void or perform intermittent catheterization frequently within the SEI, usually 4 to 6 hours, or whenever the bladder is full.
2. Attempt to reduce the residual urine volume by intermittent catheterization rather than spontaneous voiding.

Renal Calculi

Persons with bladder dysfunction appear to be at increased risk for the development of renal and bladder calculi (Fig. 51-17). Renal and ureteral stones have been found in approximately 1.1% of persons with spinal cord injury during the first year following injury. Overall, renal calculi develop in approximately 8% of all spinal cord–injured persons (59).

The cause for the development of many of these renal stones is believed to be upper urinary tract infections. In addition to infections, other risk factors for stone formation include complete cervical neurologic injuries, presence of vesicoureteral reflux, previous history of bladder calculi, hypercalcemia due to immobilization, and infections in which the organism is of the *Klebsiella*, *Serratia*, or *Proteus* species (59–61). Persons with indwelling urethral catheters also appear to be at greater risk for stone formation,

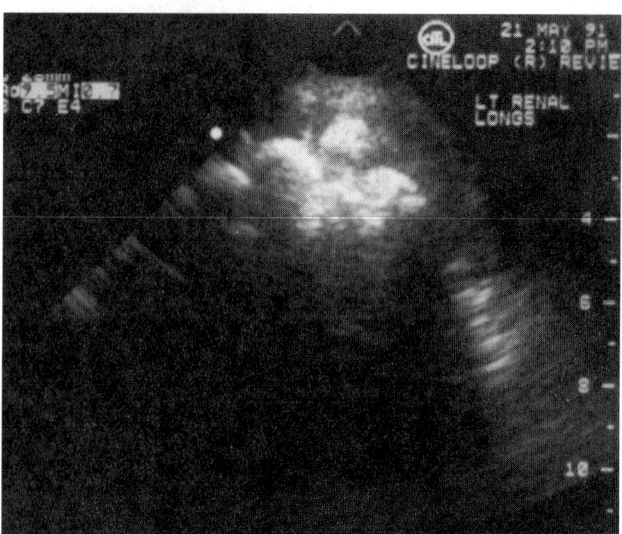

Figure 51-17. Nephrolithiasis. Renal ultrasound image showing extensive nephrolithiasis that obstructs all normal features of the kidney.

although individuals on intermittent catheterization also can develop bladder stones.

Bladder calculi are easily managed with electrohydraulic lithotripsy. The electrical probe is passed into the bladder through a cystoscope. A series of electrical shocks are then delivered to break up the stones, and the fragments are washed out through the cystoscope. Renal stones can also be treated with extracorporeal shock wave lithotripsy (ESWL) or percutaneous ultrasonic lithotripsy. On occasion, a ureteral stent may be temporarily inserted to facilitate passage of the fragments following ESWL. Ureteral calculi can be managed by several methods. With the use of a ureteroscope, smaller stones can be directly visualized, grasped, and removed. For larger stones, an ultrasonic probe may be used to break up the stone.

Ureteral Reflux and Hydronephrosis

Elevated intravesical pressure may result in the development of vesicoureteral reflux and hydronephrosis in persons with neurogenic bladder dysfunction. Increased bladder pressure may be secondary to hyperreflexic detrusor activity, low bladder compliance due to fibrotic changes from recurrent bladder infections, or increased outlet resistance as is found with detrusor-sphincter dyssynergy. Persistent vesicoureteral reflux has been frequently associated with renal damage and deterioration of function in persons with spinal cord injury (62,63). In addition, the presence of bacteriuria with ureteral reflux greatly increases the risk for the development of pyelonephritis, renal and ureteric stone formation, hydronephrosis, and deterioration of renal function.

Decreasing intravesical pressure and preventing and treating urinary tract infections are the goals for preventing and managing ureteral reflux and hydronephrosis. Frequently an intermittent catheterization program and the use of anticholinergic medications are effective. In individuals who do not respond to these conservative measures, bladder augmentation to increase bladder compliance, or in men, a sphincterotomy can prevent further renal damage.

Bladder Cancer

Persons with chronic indwelling catheters appear to have an increased risk for developing carcinoma of the bladder. Kaufman et al (64) reported that 13% of persons with spinal cord injury who had long-term indwelling catheters developed bladder cancer. Locke et al (65) reported an 8% incidence of squamous cell carcinomas in spinal cord–injured individuals with indwelling catheters for at least 10 years. In spinal cord–injured persons who develop persistent hematuria or recurrent urinary tract infections, evaluation of the upper urinary tracts, urine cytology, and cystoscopy should be performed to rule out a malignant process. In individuals who have had an indwelling urethral or suprapubic catheter for longer than 10 years, urine cytology studies should be performed on an annual basis to screen for bladder cancer. In addition, some authors (3) recommend that cystoscopy be performed as part of a routine, annual urologic evaluation.

REFERENCES

1. Arsdalin KV, Wein AJ. Physiology of micturition and continence. In: Krane RJ, Siroky MB, eds. *Clinical neuro-urology.* 2nd ed. Boston: Little, Brown, 1991:25–82.
2. Girman CJ, Jacobsen SJ, Guess HA, et al. Natural history of prostatism: relationship among symptoms, prostate volume and peak urinary flow rate. *J Urol* 1995;153:1510–1515.
3. Chancellor MB, Rivas DA. Voiding dysfunction due to spinal cord injury. *AUA Update Series* 1995;14:282–287.
4. Kellet MJ, Fry IK. Methods of investigation. In: Grainger RG, Allison DJ, eds. *Diagnostic radiology: an Anglo-American textbook of imaging.* New York: Churchill Livingstone, 1986: 1045–1049.
5. Rao KG, Hackler RH, Woodlief RM, et al. Real time renal sonography in spinal cord injury patients: prospective comparison with excretory urography. *J Urol* 1986;135:72–77.
6. Maisey M. Nuclear medicine. In: Grainger RG, Alison DS, eds. *Diagnostic radiology: an Anglo-American textbook of imaging.* New York: Churchill Livingstone, 1986:1051–1058.
7. Diokno AS, Koff SA, Bender LF. Periurethral striated muscles activity in neurogenic bladder dysfunction. *J Urol* 1974; 112:743–749.

8. Hinman F. Obstruction: back pressure or residual volume and laminar flow. *J Urol* 1971;105:702–708.

9. Gans BM, Zimmerman T, Stolov WC. Urinary catheterization in severe sphincter spasticity: report of two cases. *Arch Phys Med Rehabil* 1975;56:498.

10. Donovan WH, Clowers MD, Macri D. Anal sphincter stretch: a technique to overcome detrusor-sphincter dys-synergia. *Arch Phys Med Rehabil* 1977;58: 320–324.

11. Wu Y, Nanninga JB, Hamilton BB. Inhibition of the external urethral sphincter and sacral reflex by anal stretch in spinal cord injured patients. *Arch Phys Med Rehabil* 1986;67: 135–136.

12. Kaufman JM, Fam B, Jacobs SC, et al. Bladder cancer and squamous metaplasia in spinal cord injury patients. *J Urol* 1977;118:967–971.

13. Cox CE, Hinman F. Experiments with induced bacteriuria, vesical emptying and bacterial growth on the mechanism of bladder defense to infection. *J Urol* 1961;86:739–748.

14. Hinman F, Cox CE. The voiding vesical defense mechanism: the mathematical effect of residual urine, voiding interval and volume on bacteriuria. *J Urol* 1966;96:491–498.

15. Boen JR, Sylwester DL. The mathematical relationship among urinary frequency, residual urine and bacterial growth in bladder infection. *Invest Urol* 1965;2:468–473.

16. O'Grady F, Cattell WR. Kinetics of urinary tract infection. II. The bladder. *Br J Urol* 1966;38:156–162.

17. Wu Y. Total bladder care for the spinal cord injured patient. *Ann Acad Med Singapore* 1983;12:387–399.

18. Giroux J, Perkash I. In vitro evaluation of current disinfectants for leg bags. *J Am Paraplegia Soc* 1985;8:13–15.

19. Dewire DM, Owens RS, Anderson GA, et al. Comparison of urological complications associated with long-term management of quadriplegics with and without chronic indwelling urinary catheters. *J Urol* 1992;147:1069–1072.

20. Chao R, Clowers D, Mayo ME. Fate of upper urinary tracts in patients with indwelling catheters after spinal cord injury. *Urology* 1993;42:259–262.

21. Guttmann L, Frankel H. The value of intermittent catheterization in the early management of traumatic paraplegia and tetraplegia. *Paraplegia* 1966;4:63–84.

22. Lapides J, Diokno AC, Silber SJ, Lowe BS. Clean, intermittent self-catheterization in the treatment of urinary tract disease. *J Urol* 1972;107:458–462.

23. Chai T, Chung AK, Belville WD, Faerber GJ. Compliance and complications of clean intermittent catheterization in the spinal cord injured patient. *Paraplegia* 1995;33:161–163.

24. Bakke A, Vollset SE, Hoisaeter PA, Irgens LM. Physical complications in patients treated with clean intermittent catheterization. *Scand J Urol Nephrol* 1993;27:55–61.

25. Madersbacher H, Jilg G. Control of detrusor hyperreflexia by the intravesicle instillation of oxybutynin hydrochloride. *Paraplegia* 1991;29:84–90.

26. Mizunga M, Miyata M, Kaneko S, et al. Intravesical instillation of oxybutynin hydrochloride therapy for patients with a neuropathic bladder. *Paraplegia* 1994;32:25–29.

27. Finkbeiner AE. Is bethanechol chloride clinically effective in promoting bladder emptying? A literature review. *J Urol* 1985;134: 443–449.

28. Light JK, Scott FB. Bethanechol chloride and the traumatic cord bladder. *J Urol* 1982;128: 85–87.

29. Chancellor MB, Erhard MJ, Rivas DA. Clinical effect of alpha-1 antagonist terazosin on external and internal urinary sphincter. *J Am Paraplegia Soc* 1993;16: 207–214.

30. Awad SA, Downie JW, Lywood DW, et al. Sympathetic activity in the proximal urethra in patients with urinary obstruction. *J Urol* 1976;115:545–547.

31. Wyndaele JJ. Pharmacotherapy for urinary bladder dysfunction in spinal cord injury patients. *Paraplegia* 1990;28:146–150.

32. Fantl JA, Cardozo L, McClish DK. The Hormones and Urogenital Therapy Committee. Estrogen therapy in the management of urinary incontinence in post-menopausal women: a meta-analysis. First report of The Hormones and Urogenital Therapy Committee. *Obstet Gynecol* 1994;83:12–18.

33. Steers WD, Meythaler JM, Haworth C, et al. Effects of acute bolus and chronic continuous intrathecal baclofen on genitourinary dysfunction due to spinal cord pathology. *J Urol* 1992;148:1849–1855.

34. Tapp A, Fall M, Norgaard J, et al. Terodiline: a dose titrated multicenter study of the treatment of etiopathic detrusor instability in women. *J Urol* 1989;142:1027–1031.

35. Ekstrom B, Andersson K-E, Mattiasson A. Urodynamic effects of intravesical instillation of terodiline in healthy volunteers and in patients with detrusor hyperactivity. *J Urol* 1992;148:1840–1844.

36. Barnes DG, Shaw PJR, Timoney AG, Tsokos N. Management of the neuropathic bladder by suprapubic catheterisation. *Br J Urol* 1993;72:169–172.

37. Hollander JB, Diokno AC. Urinary diversion and reconstruction in the patient with spinal cord injury. *Urol Clin North Am* 1993;20:465–474.

38. Yalla SV, Fam BA, Gabilondo FB, et al. Anteromedian external urethral sphincterotomy: technique, rationale and complications. *J Urol* 1977;117:489–493.

39. Vapnek JM, Couillard DR, Stone AR. Is sphincterotomy the best management of the spinal cord

injured bladder? *J Urol* 1994;151:961–964.

40. Chancellor MB, Rivas DA, Linsenmeyer T, et al. Multicenter trial in North America of Urolume urinary sphincter prostheses. *J Urol* 1994;152:924–930.

41. Dykes EH, Ransley PG. Gastrocystoplasty in children. *Br J Urol* 1992;69:91–95.

42. Nurse DE, McInerney PD, Thomas PJ, Mundy AR. Stones in enterocystoplasties. *Br J Urol* 1996;77:684–687.

43. Schmidt RA. Advances in genitourinary neurostimulation. *Neurosurgery* 1986;19:1041–1044.

44. Domoulin C, Seaborne DE, Quiriou-DeGiardi C, Sullivan SJ. Pelvic-floor rehabilitation, part 2: pelvic-floor reeducation with interferential currents and exercise in the treatment of genuine stress incontinence in post-partum women—a cohort study. *Phys Ther* 1995;75:1075–1081.

45. Wheeler JS, Walter JS, Zaszczurynski PJ. Bladder inhibition by penile nerve stimulation in spinal cord injury patients. *J Urol* 1992;147:100–103.

46. Lyne CJ, Bellinger MF. Early experience with transurethral electrical bladder stimulation. *J Urol* 1993;150:697–699.

47. Ishigooka M, Hashimoto T, Sasagawa I, et al. Electrical pelvic floor stimulation by percutaneous implantable electrode. *Br J Urol* 1994;74:191–194.

48. Petersen T, Just-Christensen JE, Kousgaard P, et al. Anal sphincter maximum functional electrical stimulation in detrusor hyperreflexia. *J Urol* 1994;152: 1460–1462.

49. Creasey GH. Electrical stimulation of sacral roots for micturition after spinal cord injury. *Urol Clin North Am* 1993;20:505–515.

50. National Institute on Disability and Rehabilitation Research. The prevention and management of urinary tract infections among people with spinal cord injuries. *J Am Paraplegia Soc* 1992;15:194–207.

51. Kass EH. Asymptomatic infection of urinary tract. *Trans Assoc Am Physicians* 1956;69:56.

52. Kass EH. The meaning of significant bacteriuria. *JAMA* 1963;184:727–729.

53. Peterson JR, Roth EJ. Fever, bacteriuria and pyuria in spinal cord injured patients with indwelling urethral catheters. *Arch Phys Med Rehabil* 1989;70: 839–842.

54. Fairley K, Bond A, Brown R, Habersberger P. Simple test to determine the site of urinary tract infection. *Lancet* 1967;2:427–428.

55. Giroux J, Perkash I. Limited value of the Fairley test in urological infections in patients with neuropathic bladders. *J Am Paraplegia Soc* 1985;8:10–12.

56. Merritt JL, Keys TF. Limitation of the antibody-coated bacteria test in patients with neurogenic bladder. *JAMA* 1982;247: 1723–1725.

57. Guttmann D, Naylor GRE. Dipslide aid to quantitative urine culture in general practice. *Br Med J* 1967;3:343–345.

58. Cohen SN, Kass EH. A simple method for quantitative urine culture. *N Engl J Med* 1967;277:176–180.

59. DeVivo MJ, Fine PR. Predicting renal calculus occurrence in spinal cord injury patients. *Arch Phys Med Rehabil* 1986;67: 722–725.

60. Hall MK, Hackler RH, Zampieri TA, Zampieri JB. Renal calculi in spinal cord injured patients: association with reflux, bladder stones, and Foley catheter drainage. *Urology* 1989;34: 126–128.

61. Kohli A, Lamid S. Risk factors for renal stone formation in patients with spinal cord injury. *Br J Urol* 1986;158:588–591.

62. McGuire EJ, Woodside JR, Borden TA, Weiss RM. Prognostic value of urodynamic testing in the myelodysplastic patient. *J Urol* 1981;126:205–209.

63. Gerridzen RG, Thijssen AM, Dehoux E. Risk factors for upper tract deterioration in chronic spinal cord injury patients. *J Urol* 1992;147:416–418.

64. Kaufman JM, Fam B, Jacobs SC, et al. Bladder cancer and squamous metaplasia in spinal cord injury patients. *J Urol* 1977;118: 967–971.

65. Locke JR, Hill DE, Walzer Y. Incidence of squamous cell carcinoma in patients with long-term catheter drainage. *J Urol* 1985;133: 1034–1035.

Chapter 52

Neurogenic Bowel

Kamala Shankar
Elaine Date
Inder Perkash

The term *neurogenic* is applied to functions originating in the nervous tissue or induced, controlled, or modified by nervous factors. In this chapter, the term denotes neurologic deficit caused by abnormally altered neural tissue. The term *bowel* means gut. The gastrointestinal (GI) system is composed of the oropharynx, esophagus, stomach, intestines, and associated glands (liver, pancreas, etc). The complex process of ingestion, digestion, subsequent absorption of nutrients, and ultimate elimination of fecal material is under the control of both neural and hormonal factors. Neurologic diseases can affect the bowel functions at several levels of innervation, by altering the electrical activity that controls the smooth muscles, the enteric nervous system, or the extrinsic neural pathways to the gut from the brain to the postganglionic fibers. In a rehabilitation setting, one is usually faced with neurogenic bowel secondary to extrinsic neural pathway lesions (e.g., strokes, spinal cord injury, diabetic neuropathy); hence, these are the focus here. This chapter begins with a review of the innervation and motility of the GI system, followed by discussion of neurogenic bowel disorders, their evaluation, and management.

INNERVATION OF THE BOWEL

The nerves, intrinsic and extrinsic nerves, play an important role in the motility of the GI tract. The central nervous system modifies the intrinsic nerves through the extrinsic nerves (1). The afferent supply consists of the sensory nerves in the GI tract, though the primary afferents, the vagal and splanchnic afferents, come from the central nervous system. The efferent supply from the central nervous system comes from the cranial nerves, somatic nerves, and autonomic nerves.

Afferent Nerve Supply

Sensory Receptors in the Gut

Sensory receptors are located in the mucosa, muscle, and serosal layers (2). The types of mucosal receptors are as follows:

1. Mechanoreceptors for touch, pressure, and stretch
2. Chemoreceptors for alkali, acid, glucose, and amino acids
3. Osmoreceptors
4. Thermoreceptors (cooling, warming, or both)
5. Nociceptors

The *mechanoreceptors* that respond selectively to mucosal pinching or stroking are present throughout the GI tract. Mechanoreceptors that respond to light touch are present in the pharynx and the anal canal. *Chemoreceptors* are generally small-diameter unmyelinated fibers. They do not fire spontaneously and are activated only by certain chemical substances. *Osmoreceptors* are generally present in the liver. They discharge at a rate proportional to the osmotic pressure of the solutions. Single-fiber recordings show that receptors that are activated by osmotic activity are multimodal, and are stimulated by mechanical, thermal, and other chemical stimuli (3). Thermoreceptors are sensitive to visceral cooling or warming and in some instances both. They are located in the esophagus, stomach, and small intestine. Thermoreceptors located in esophageal mucosa and submucosa are connected to unmyelinated afferent fibers in the vagus, while those in the parietal peritoneum are connected to splanchnic unmyelinated fibers (3). Sensory receptors in the anal canal (mucosal mechanoreceptors, thermoreceptors, and nociceptors) have free nerve endings and are connected to unmyelinated or thin myelinated fibers. *Tension receptors* are located throughout the GI tract in the muscle layer. These receptors are spontaneously active and have a low threshold for stretch or contractive stimulation (2). Muscle nociceptors may be represented by free nerve endings and are connected to unmyelinated fibers. Serosal and mesenteric sensory receptors are pressure sensitive (pacinian corpuscles). These receptors are located around the blood vessels and are sensitive to pressure and may monitor local changes in blood flow. They are rapidly adapting and are connected to myelinated fibers that are carried by splanchnic afferents (4).

Afferent Neurons

Vagal primary afferent neurons are bipolar or pseudobipolar and their cell bodies are located in the inferior ganglion (nodose) of the vagus (3). The peripheral processes of these neurons are predominantly distributed to a large variety of mucosal and muscle sensory receptors throughout the gut, including the esophagus, stomach, small intestine, gallbladder, liver, pancreas, and large bowel as far as the mid-transverse colon. The fibers from the nodose ganglion ascend rostrally through the jugular foramen into the medulla oblongata as the tractus solitarius.

Splanchnic primary afferents are T-shaped unipolar cells whose cell bodies are located in the dorsal root ganglion of the spinal cord from the T2 through the L3 level. The splanchnic afferents carry pain sensation as well as a wide variety of sensory information from various portions of the gut. The splanchnic nerve carries 20% afferents, whereas the vagus carries 80% afferents (3).

Enteric sensory neurons, whose cell bodies are located in the enteric plexuses, send processes that exit the gut wall and travel along the blood vessels to the prevertebral ganglia, where they make synaptic contact with postganglionic sympathetic neurons. Some enteric neurons carry information from one enteric ganglia to another (2).

Efferent Nerve Supply

This supply is shown in Figure 52-1. It involves both somatic and autonomic innervation.

Somatic control is limited to the entry of solid and liquid food into the oral cavity and esophagus and elimination of waste from the rectum. The striated muscles located at the proximal and distal ends of the alimentary canal are innervated by α motor neurons with myelinated axons. Acetylcholine is the neurotransmitter for these neurons. The axons carried in the ninth, tenth, and eleventh cranial nerves innervate the striated muscle of the pharynx. The muscles of mastication are supplied by the fifth cranial nerve, and the tongue muscle by the twelfth cranial nerve. The pudendal nerve, which has S2–S4 sacral roots, supplies the external anal sphincter, and the nerve at S4 also supplies the pelvic floor muscles (Fig. 52-2).

Autonomic control of the GI tract is mediated through sympathetic and parasympathetic nerves. The preganglionic sympathetic neurons to the gut are located in the intermediolateral columns of the spinal cord, at thoracolumbar segments. Preganglionic fibers are thin myelinated fibers approximately 3 μm in diameter. These fibers pass as ventral roots from peripheral nerve via white rami (myelinated) fibers and enter the paravertebral ganglia of the sympathetic chain. As they enter, they synapse with postganglionic fibers at that level or a level above and below (5).

Some of the preganglionic fibers synapse in more peripherally located prevertebral ganglia such as celiac, superior mesenteric, and inferior mesenteric ganglia (Fig. 52-3). Paravertebral sympathetic ganglia include 22 pairs of ganglia on both sides of the vertebral bodies that are interconnected by ascending and descending fibers in two nodular cords which extend from the base of the skull to the ventral coccyx. The specific ganglia involved in GI functions include the superior cervical ganglion (glands and smooth muscles of the head and neck), middle cervical and stellate ganglia (esophagus), 10 to 12 pairs of thoracic ganglia (stomach, small and large intestines), and 4 pairs of lumbar ganglia (colon).

Prevertebral sympathetic ganglia occur near major arteries. Celiac and superior mesenteric ganglia provide sympathetic supply to the stomach, small intestine, gallbladder, liver, kidneys, and spleen. The inferior mesenteric ganglion provides sympathetic supply to the colon.

Parasympathetic efferent projections consist of cranial (vagus) and sacral (pelvic splanchnic) nerves (Fig. 52-4). The dorsal motor nucleus where vagus nerve originates is located in the floor of the fourth ventricle in the medulla oblongata. The vagus provides parasympathetic innervation to practically all thoracic and abdominal viscera (up to the middle half of the transverse colon) except in the pelvic region. Sacral parasympathetic preganglionic neurons are located along the lateral aspect of the anterior gray horn in spinal cord segments S2–S4. These nerve roots join to form the nervi erigentes. These nerves join the superior hypogastric plexus to form the pelvic plexus. They supply the bladder, colon, and rectum. The preganglionic neurons of the parasympathetic pathway are generally believed to be cholinergic; however, some vagal parasympathetic neurons contain catecholamines and enkephalins.

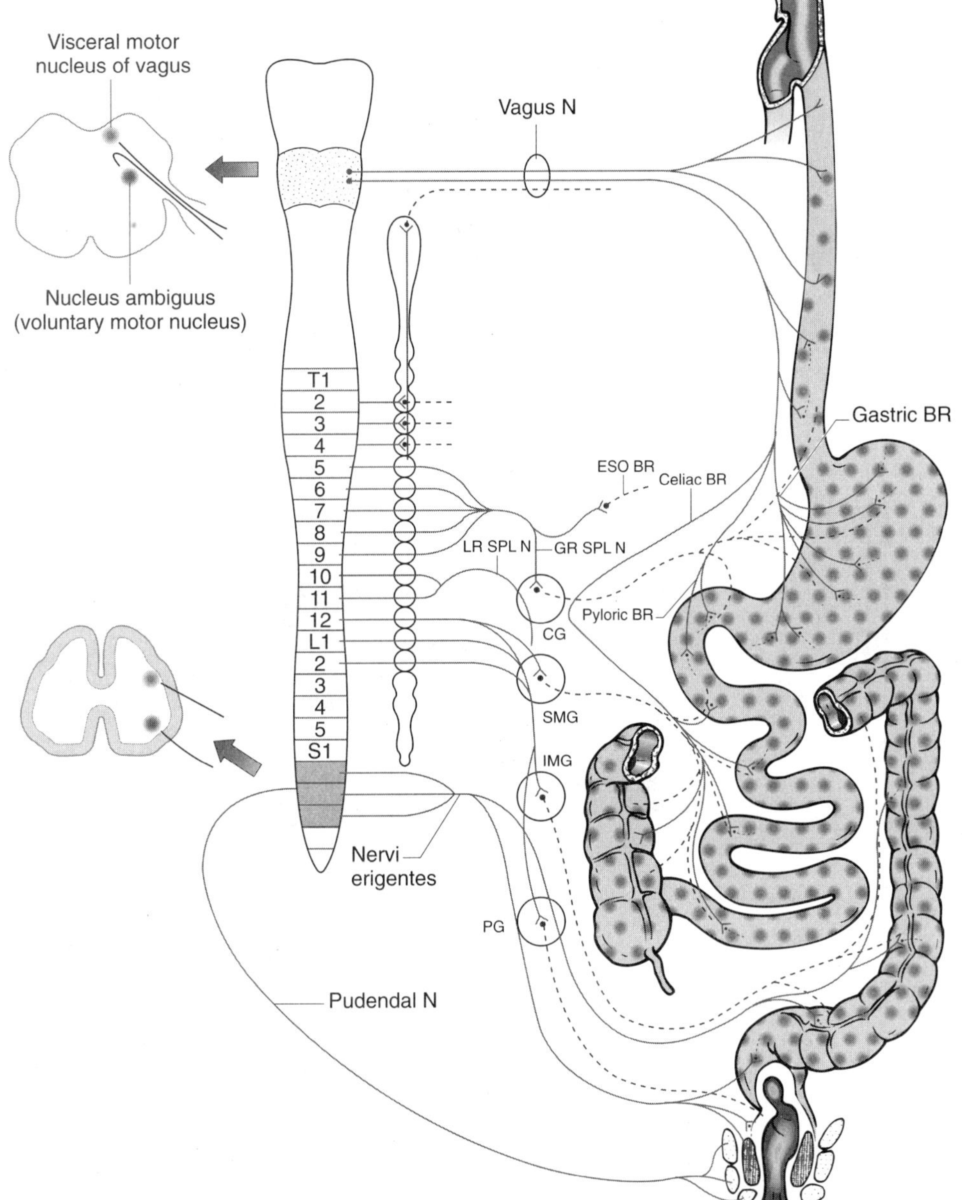

Figure 52-1. Efferent innervation of the gastrointestinal tract. The α motor neurons are depicted. They innervate skeletal muscle at either end of the gut. The α motor neurons to the pharynx and upper esophagus are present in the nucleus ambiguus and their axons are carried in the vagus nerve. The α motor neurons to the external anal sphincter are present in the Onuf nucleus and their axons are carried in the pudendal nerve. The sympathetic pathway consists of cell bodies of preganglionic neurons located in spinal cord segments T2 through L2. The preganglionic fibers are carried in the greater splanchnic nerve (GR SPL N), Lesser splanchnic nerve (LR SPL N), and smallest splanchnic nerve (not labeled) to terminate in the celiac ganglion (CG), superior mesenteric ganglion (SMG), inferior mesenteric ganglion (IMG), and pelvic ganglion (PG). The postganglionic sympathetic neurons are distributed in a segmental fashion to the gastrointestinal tract. The parasympathetic pathway consists of vagal and sacral outflows. The vagal pathway consists of preganglionic parasympathetic axons whose cell bodies are present in the dorsal motor nucleus of vagus. The vagal parasympathetics supply the gastrointestinal tract up to the right half of the colon. Sacral preganglionic parasympathetic fibers arising from neurons in spinal cord segments S2 to S4 (nervi erigentes) supply the left half of the colon, including the rectum and the internal anal sphincter. The postganglionic parasympathetic nerves and fibers are present intramurally in the gut wall. Sympathetic and parasympathetic nerves make extensive contacts with neurons in the enteric nervous system. (Redrawn with permission from Goyal RK, Crist JR. Neurology of gut. In: Sleisenger MH, Fordtran JS, eds. *Gastrointestinal disease.* 4th ed. Vol. 1. Philadelphia: WB Saunders, 1989:21–52.)

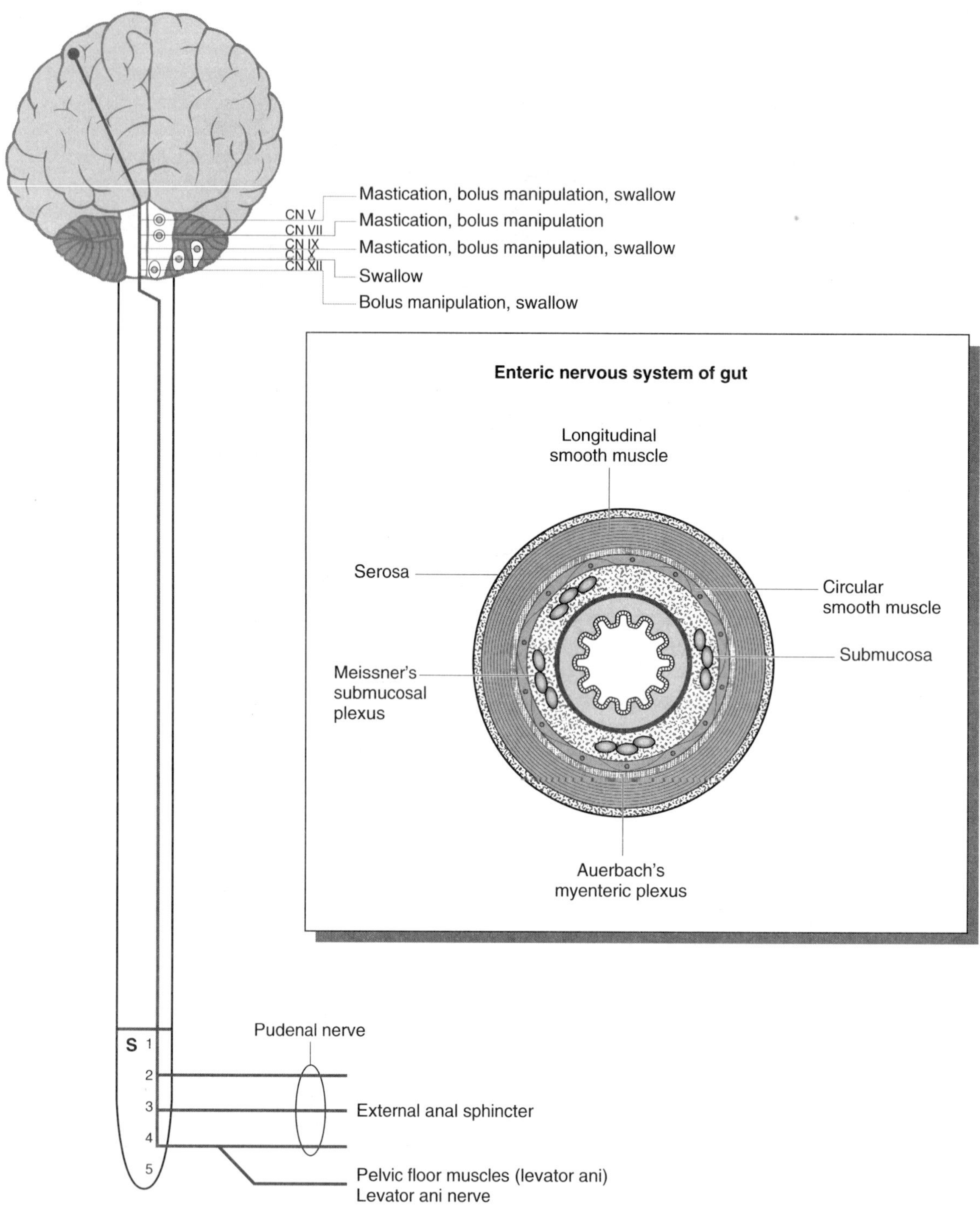

Figure 52-2. Somatic (voluntary) control of GI tract plus enteric nervous system. (Redrawn with permission from Ugalde V, Litwiller SE, Gater RD. Bladder and bowel anatomy for the physiatrist. In: Shankar K, ed. *Physiatric anatomic principles, state of the art reviews in physical medicine and rehabilitation.* Vol. 10. Philadelphia: Hanley & Belfus, 1996:547–569.)

Central Nervous System Connections

The central projections of the sensory cells in the nodose ganglia extend to the dorsal motor nucleus of the vagus. Neurons from the dorsal motor nucleus make extensive synaptic connections with the brain stem and hypothalamic nuclei.

The motor efferents to the GI tract (α motor neurons, vagal and sacral parasympathetic neurons, and thoracolumbar sympathetic neurons) receive projections from neurons in cortical and subcortical areas, including the limbic system, the hypothalamus, and various brain stem centers, and also directly from GI afferent neurons.

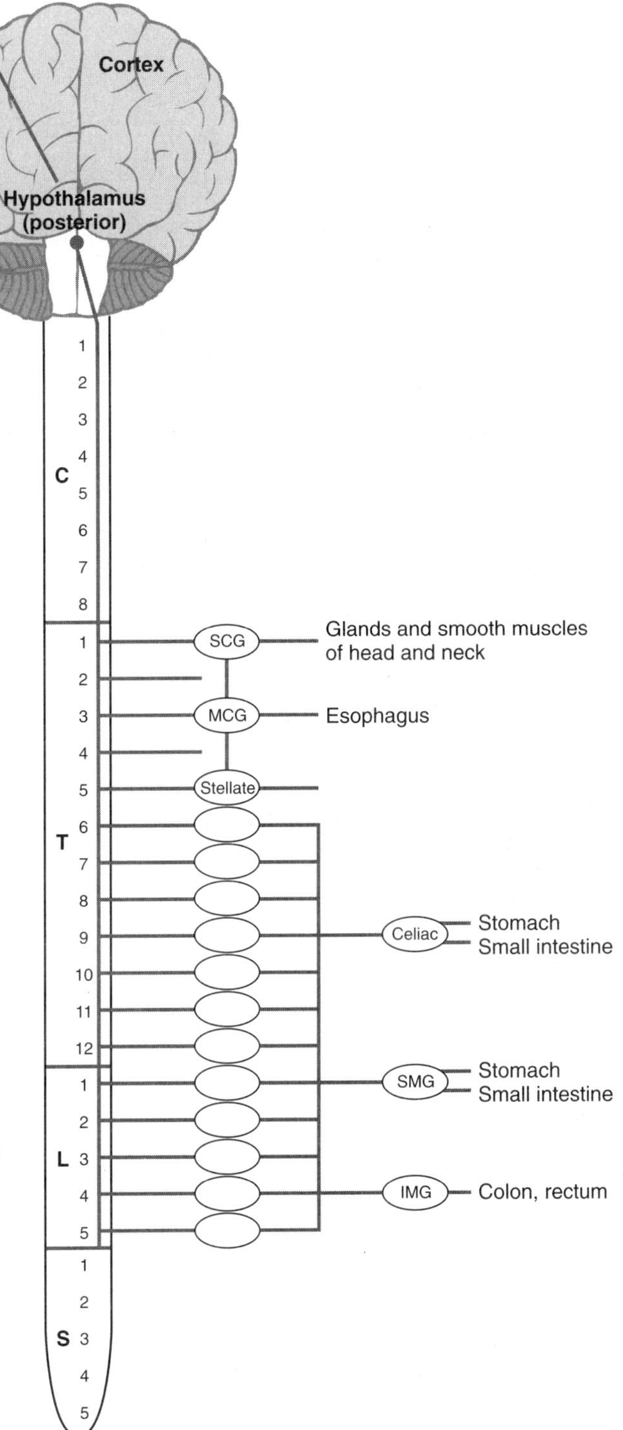

Figure 52-3. Sympathetic "innervation" to the GI tract. SCG = superior cervical ganglion; MCG = medial cervical ganglion; SMG = superior mesenteric ganglion; IMG = inferior mesenteric ganglion. (Redrawn with permission from Ugalde V, Litwiller SE, Gater RD. Bladder and bowel anatomy for the physiatrist. In: Shankar K, ed. *Physiatric anatomic principles, state of the art reviews in physical medicine and rehabilitation.* Vol. 10. Philadelphia: Hanley & Belfus, 1996:547–569.)

Enteric Nervous System

The intrinsic nervous system consists of two major and three minor networks of plexuses of neurons and their processes. The myenteric (Auerbach) plexus is located in between the outer (longitudinal) and inner (circular) smooth muscle layers. The Meissner plexus is found within the submucosal layer of the esophagus, the stomach, and the intestines and innervates both mucosal glands and smooth muscles to stimulate glandular secretion and motility of substances through the GI tract.

In the esophagus the myenteric plexus is an irregular network with sparse small ganglia. The myenteric plexus is more prominent in the stomach than in the esophagus. In the small bowel the myenteric plexus is very highly developed and consists of a regular network of interconnecting nerve bundles with ganglia. In the ascending and trans-

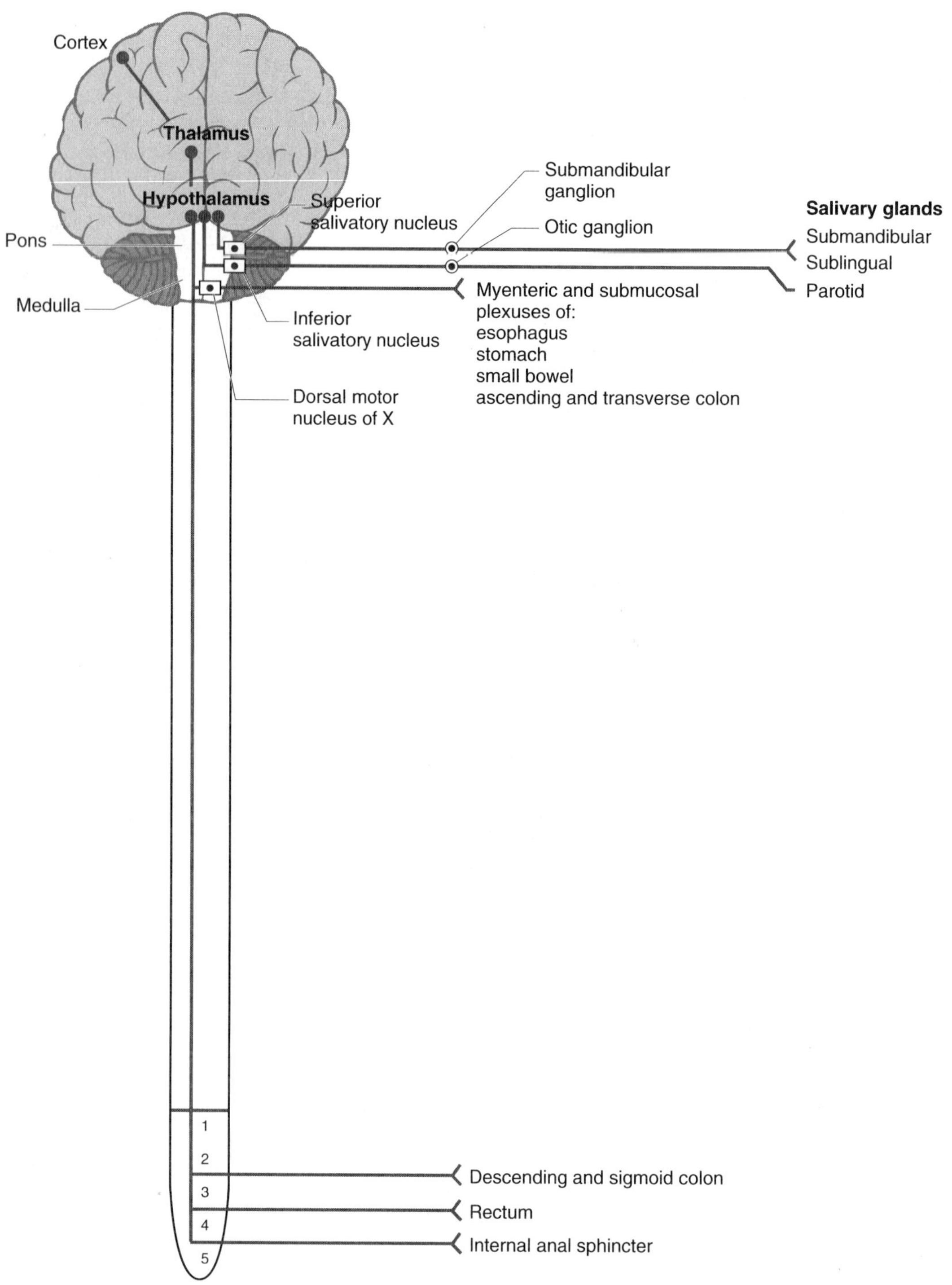

Figure 52-4. GI Innervation by the parasympathetic nervous system. (Redrawn with permission from Ugalde V, Litwiller SE, Gater RD. Bladder and bowel anatomy for the physiatrist. In: Shankar K, ed. *Physiatric anatomic principles, state of the art reviews in physical medicine and rehabilitation.* Vol. 10. Philadelphia: Hanley & Belfus, 1996:547–569.)

verse colon, the myenteric plexus is abundant and located mainly under taeniae coli (2). The myenteric ganglia are irregular and found less frequently along the colon. In the lower part of the anal canal, there are almost no myenteric ganglia. The Meissner plexus, like the myenteric plexus, varies in meshwork density and nerve cell content along the length of the gut.

In addition to the two major plexuses, three others are known: a subserous plexus, a deep muscular plexus, and a mucosal plexus. Enteric neurons are either sensory neurons, motor neurons, or interneurons. Enteric neurons utilize many neurotransmitter substances like acetylcholine, 5-hydroxytryptamine, peptide, substance P, enkephalin, and somatostatin.

FUNCTIONAL ASPECTS OF NERVOUS CONTROL

Somatic control of the external anal sphincter is important in maintaining fecal continence. The act of defecation occurs in response to distention of the mechanoreceptors within the rectal mucosa, which stimulates afferent responses to be conveyed to the spinal cord and cerebral cortex. At the cerebral cortex, awareness of rectal fullness and urge results in efferent impulses being conveyed through the pontine and sacral "defecation centers" with subsequent contraction of the levator ani and external sphincter. When conditions prevail, inhibitory influence from the cortex ceases and the intra-abdominal pressure rises. Reflex rectal contraction and relaxation of the internal anal sphincter occur with rectal distention. Voluntary relaxation of the external sphincter and levator ani allows subsequent expulsion of fecal matter from the rectal vault (5).

Sympathetic stimulation slows digestion by reducing motility and secretion of the GI tract. Sympathetic effects are more prominent in the stomach, small bowel, and large bowel than in the esophagus and rectum. Clinically, sympathetic stimulation generally leads to gastric stasis or adynamic or paralytic ileus (6). Surgical sympathectomy or visceral neuropathy involving sympathetic nerves (e.g., diabetic mellitus) usually results in diarrhea due to a loss of tonic inhibitory effects of sympathetic nerves on small-intestine motility and intestinal secretions (7).

The parasympathetic nervous system has the main function of promoting digestion and bolus motility. Vagal effects are prominent in the proximal part of the GI tract. Cervical vagotomy causes a loss of the primary esophageal peristalsis associated with swallowing. Bilateral truncal vagotomy leads to a decrease in gastric acid secretion, which is clinically used in the treatment of peptic ulcers. The sacral parasympathetic nerves exert important effects on colorectal motility and the internal anal sphincter. Sacral parasympathetic damage leads to an impaired defecation reflex and constipation.

Pacemaker cells within the enteric plexuses are responsible for the basal electrical rhythm within the GI tract, which results in peristalsis. Gastric contractions occur at a frequency of 3 to 5 per minute, the duodenum contracts at a rate 10 to 12 per minute, and the transition occurs at the level of the pylorus (5).

As gastric motility occurs, chyme moves through the small bowel under control of the *enteric nervous system*. The small intestine is also under the influence of several hormones and neurotransmitters—neuropeptides, serotonin, opioid peptides, and histamine (8). The motility of the colon is more irregular and reliant on extrinsic innervation. Many neuropeptides including substance P, gastrin, enkephalin, and cholecystokinin stimulate colonic motility whereas vasoactive inhibitory peptide slows colonic motility.

Clinical syndromes like achalasia (in the esophagus) and Hirschsprung disease (in the colon) are examples of complete loss of the enteric neurons.

PATHOPHYSIOLOGY

Uninhibited Bowel

Dysfunction is caused by neurologic lesions interfering with the cortical interrelationships with the pontine defecation center. Patients with stroke, brain injury, or other supraconal lesions, when stimulated by anorectal filling, can maintain fecal continence owing to the intact pontine defecation center (9).

Upper Motor Neuron Bowel Dysfunction

When neurologic lesions interrupt the pontine defecation center, such as in spinal cord injury above the conus medullaris, there is evidence that with rectal filling, not only the internal but also the external anal sphincter relax (10). Defecation occurs by mass contraction mediated through the myenteric plexus of the colon. By mechanical and chemical stimulation of the rectal mucosa, similar results are seen, probably by stimulating the myenteric plexus and spinal reflex. UMN colon has been described as spastic.

Lower Motor Neuron Bowel Dysfunction

When lesions of the conus destroy either the sacral defecation center or the related nerve supply to the rectum and anus, there is denervation of the external sphincter, which results in a patulous external anal sphincter, and with rectal filling, the internal sphincter relaxes (11). With distention of the colon and rectum, stimulation of the myenteric plexus of the colon does occur, which leads to mass action peristalsis and internal sphincter relaxation. Lower motor neuron lesions result in both rectal stasis, drier stool because of the prolonged transit time, and at times incontinence of feces.

SITE OF LESIONS IN THE NERVOUS SYSTEM

A practical anatomic approach to the classification of neuromuscular disorders affecting gut motility is shown in Table 52-1. This table provides a useful approach for clinical evaluation of neurogenic bowel. The interrelationships among the three areas of control make it difficult to determine the exact focus of pathology, and in many instances both extrinsic and intrinsic neural functions are affected. This section focuses on the extrinsic nervous system pathology leading to GI disorders. Figure 52-5 shows the site of neural lesions and their effects.

Table 52-1: Neuromuscular Disorders Affecting Gastrointestinal Motility

Enteric nervous system
- Idiopathic, degenerative, or inflammatory disorders of the myenteric plexus
- Some disorders of the enteric nervous system may be associated with diseases that affect extrinsic neural control

Extrinsic nervous system
- Peripheral nerves
  - Acute (e.g., Guillain-Barré syndrome)
  - Chronic (e.g., diabetes mellitus, amyloidosis)
  - Autonomic nervous system degenerations (e.g., idiopathic orthostatic hypotension, pandysautonomia)
  - Spinal cord (e.g., injury, multiple sclerosis)
  - Brain stem (e.g., tumor)
  - Higher centers (e.g., parkinsonism)

Smooth muscle
- Infiltration of muscle by generalized disease (e.g., amyloidosis, scleroderma)
- Generalized muscle disease affecting the gut (e.g., dermatomyositis, dystrophia myotonica, other muscular dystrophies)

Source: Modified with permission from Camilleri M. Disorders of gastrointestinal motility in neurological disease. *Mayo Clin Proc* 1990;65:825–846.

Brain

Cortical and hypothalamic lesions usually produce uninhibited-type bowel. The cerebral cortex is responsible for somatic (voluntary) function and to some extent can influence autonomic functions (5). Impairments in cognition following cortical lesions may negatively impact several components of normal GI functions, including mastication, swallowing, and defecation. Lesions of the anterior hypothalamus may impair parasympathetic functions, resulting in adynamic ileus, whereas posterior hypothalamic lesions can alter sympathetic control over the gut, leading to GI hypermotility (5). Constipation is common in patients with parkinsonism, which can be influenced by gut hypomotility, generalized hypokinesia, and the effects of anticholinergics and dopamine antagonists (12).

Brain Stem

Brain stem strokes and lesions are known to be associated with abnormal esophageal and gastric motility (5), intestinal and colonic pseudo-obstruction (13), and an inability to perceive rectal distention and impaired anorectal inhibitory reflex (10). Cranial nerves V, VII, IX, X, XI, and XIII may be involved in pons and medullary lesions, leading to impairments in mastication and swallowing.

Spinal Cord

During the acute phase following spinal cord injury, there is adynamic ileus, but subsequently this condition improves (14). Following recovery from the spinal shock, gastric and small-intestine functions return to normal, partly because of the prevertebral parasympathetic influence of the vagus nerve, which supplies the esophagus, stomach, small intestine, and proximal portions of the colon (5). Some possible effects on the GI tract are shown in Table 52-2 according to the level of spinal cord lesions. Injury at a single level of the spinal cord leaves the majority of autonomic functions intact at a spinal cord reflex level, whereas input from the brain is lost.

Table 52-2: Spinal Cord Injury, Impairments as Related to the Level of Lesions

Level of Lesion	Effect	Impairments
Cervical, upper thoracic	Impaired sympathetic control in the lower esophagus, stomach, and small bowel	Increase in gastric and small-intestine motility
Midthoracic level	Unopposed parasympathetic-mediated gastric acid release Sparing of lumbar and sacral control centers	Increased risk for gastric ulcer Effects on small bowel less pronounced Motility in left colon remains preserved
Lumbar	Removal of inhibitory influence to large bowel if lesion is at L2–L4 Relative preservation of parasympathetic influence from sacral cord control centers (S2–S4)	Increased colonic tone Preservation of the defecation reflex arc
Sacral level of cord or cauda equine	Loss of parasympathetic influence to the left bowel, unopposed sympathetic action Lesions involving S2–S4 α motor neurons	Impaired colonic motility and atonic internal anal sphincter Flaccid, areflexic external anal sphincter Loss of defecation reflex

Effects on Various Parts of the Gastrointestinal Tract

Esophagus and Stomach

No clinical data indicate esophageal dysfunction. The high incidence of pneumonitis, in both acute and chronic quadriplegics, raises the question of whether aspiration is due to gastroesophageal reflex or abnormalities in upper

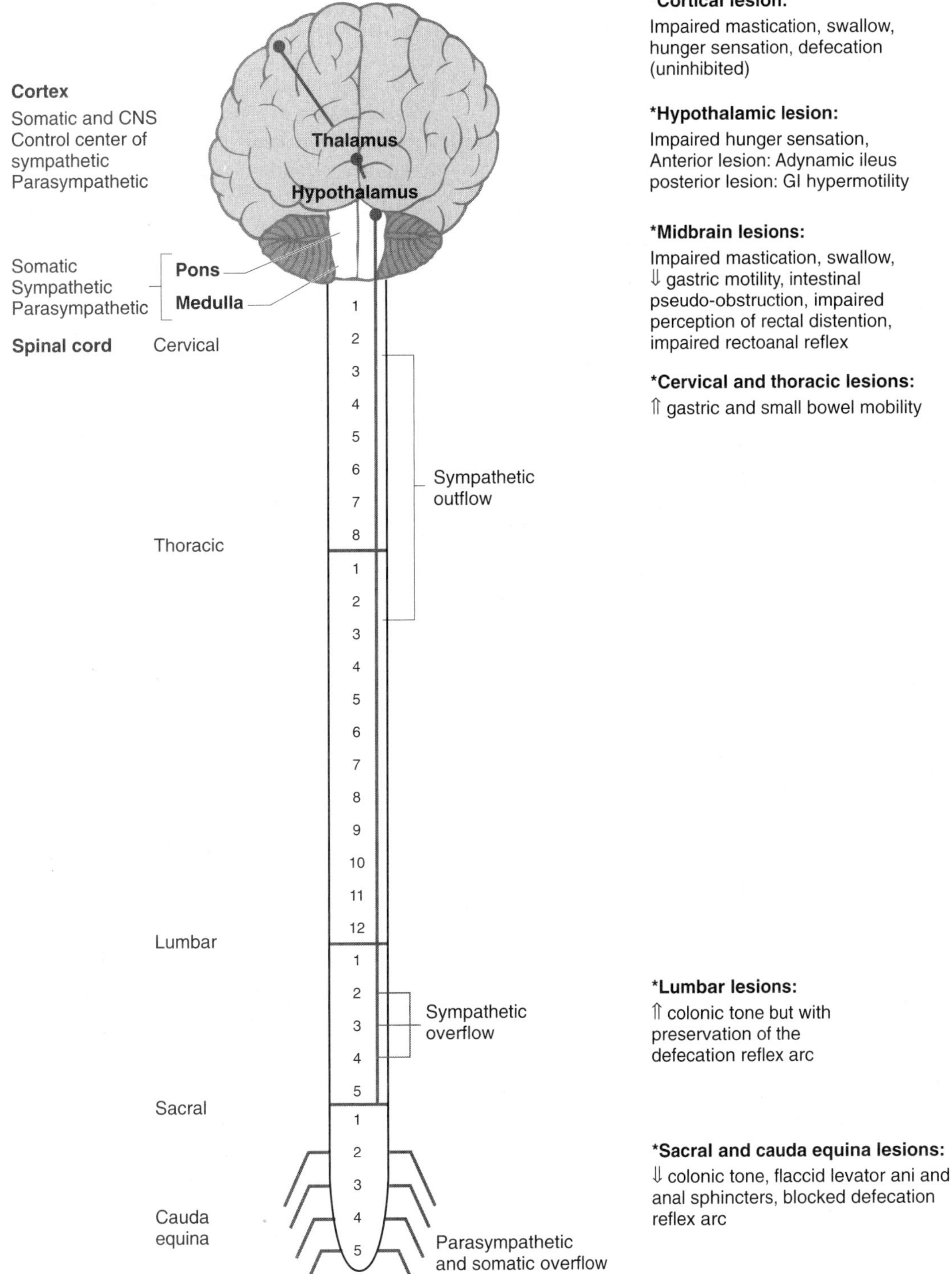

Figure 52-5. Effect of neural lesions in GI function. CNS = central nervous system. (Redrawn with permission from Ugalde V, Litwiller SE, Gater RD. Bladder and bowel anatomy for the physiatrist. In: Shankar K, ed. *Physiatric anatomic principles, state of the art reviews in physical medicine and rehabilitation.* Vol. 10. Philadelphia: Hanley & Belfus, 1996:547–569.)

esophageal sphincter function. Gastric motility and emptying effects are not well documented yet, but in quadriplegics they are abnormal (15). Delayed postprandial gastric emptying has been documented. Aerophagy (swallowing of the air) is fairly common in quadriplegic patients. Acute gastric dilatation is not rare. Gastric dilatation has been noted on x-ray studies of many long-term quadriplegic patients with chronic abdominal distention (15).

Small Bowel

No specific abnormalities are seen in spinal cord injury patients. Small-bowel obstruction is rare. Small-bowel gas distention is attributable to the same problems as in the stomach, such as aerophagia and failure of eructation, with passage of air down the small bowel (15).

Gallbladder

Risk of chololithiasis appears to have increased 29% compared with 4% in an autopsy series of 38 patients with spinal cord injuy and matched control (16). Resting volume and ejection fraction of gallbladder were reduced, whereas emptying time and residual volume remained normal in an ultrasound study. No specific abnormalities were noted (15).

Colon and Rectum

Most GI problems in patients with chronic spinal cord injury are noted in the colon. Abnormalities in transport, storage, and evacuation have been identified. Approximately one-fourth of spinal cord injury patients develop chronic complaints related to the lower GI tract (17). Most of these problems are noticed about 4 to 5 years after the injury occurred. The most common GI problems in spinal cord injury patients are fecal impaction, colonic distention, abdominal bloating, constipation, and nonfunctional or prolonged evacuation.

Anus

In spinal cord injury patients the anal resting tone appears normal, but reflex relaxation with rectal distention is observed. Because of loss of central control, there is a high incidence of incontinence. In essence, spinal cord injury patients have more devastating effects in the lower GI tract than in the upper GI tract.

Anorectal Reflex

As feces pass from the colon to the rectum, the rectum stretches, which leads to reflex relaxation of the internal sphincter, which then allows the feces to enter the anal canal. In normal people, the urge to defecate is controlled by accommodating feces in the rectum. In spinal cord injury patients in whom this reflex is still present, any distention of the rectum leads to the relaxation of the internal sphincter. However, the external anal sphincter, which normally is under voluntary control, does not relax in spinal cord injury patients. Therefore, evacuation is facilitated by anal stretch prior to a bowel management program. Also, introduction of a suppository helps to cause rectal wall stretch, and this mass action of the colon results in easy evacuation. Anal digital stretch also seems to create a reverse reflex in which anal sphincter relaxation causes rectal wall contraction and expulsion of the feces. Anorectal manometric examination can help define this reflex.

BOWEL DISORDERS FROM PERIPHERAL NEUROPATHIES

Acute peripheral neuropathies such as Guillain-Barré syndrome are known to cause GI disturbances like gastric dilatation and adynamic ileus. Acute viral infections may result in nausea, vomiting, abdominal cramps, constipation, or pseudo-obstruction. In chronic peripheral neuropathy such as seen with diabetes mellitus or amyloidosis, the extrinsic system is affected. GI symptoms, nausea, and constipation are exceedingly common in patients with diabetes. Gastric emptying is slow and contractions of the antrum are reduced. There is decreased post-prandial duodenojejunal phasic pressure activity (Fig. 52-6) and nonpropagated uncoordinated bursts of contractions in the proximal portion of the small bowel compared with normal finding (see Fig. 52-6). Some patients have diarrhea or fecal soiling. This may result from dysfunction of the anorectal sphincter or abnormal rectal sensation. Also, osmotic diarrhea from bacterial overgrowth due to small-bowel stasis or rapid transit from uncoordinated small-bowel activity may occur. Histologic studies of the vagus nerve revealed a severe reduction in the density of unmyelinated axons and thinning of the surviving axons (18).

In diabetic patients with diarrhea, histologic studies showed in sympathetic neurons, dendritic swelling of the postganglionic neurons in the prevertebral and paravertebral ganglia (19) and reduced fiber density in the splanchnic nerves.

Amyloid neuropathy can lead to diarrhea and steatorrhea. Patients with amyloid neuropathy demonstrate uncoordinated, nonpropagated phasic pressure bursts in the small bowel (20). Severe reduction in the number or degeneration of ganglion cells has been noted, without extensive deposition of amyloid in the enteric plexus, in familial amyloid neuropathy (21). Manometric studies can help differentiate neuropathic and myopathic types of amyloid gastroenteropathy (20).

EVALUATION

GI symptoms may develop in the setting of lesions in any part of the nervous system. One way of analysis is to follow Table 52-3. All systems should be evaluated by obtaining a detailed history, including of medication use. Abdomen should be checked for bowel sounds, tenderness, and rigidity. Rectal exam should be given to check sphincter tone, consistency of stool, presence of hemorrhoids, and prostate size in males.

Screening of a patient with visceral autonomic neuropathy must include tests that identify occult causes of peripheral neuropathy such as lung tumors or amyloidosis (22). Neurological exam helps identify the level of injury and verify whether it is an upper motor neuron or lower motor neuron lesion.

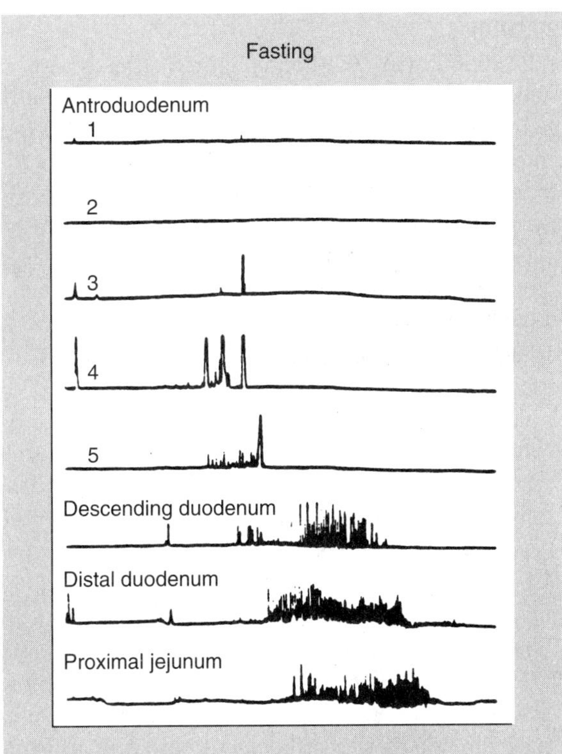

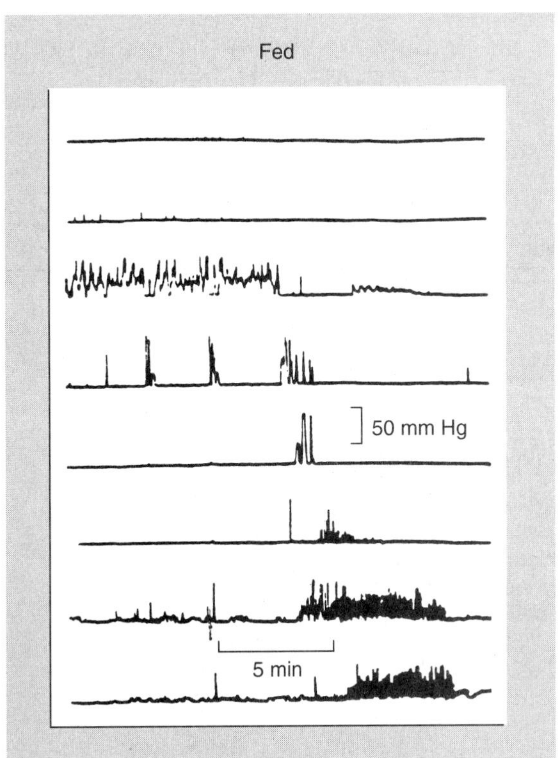

Figure 52-6. Classic abnormalities in manometric profile of diabetic gut dysmotility. Note the absence (leads 1 through 5) of the antral component of the fasting interdigestive motor complex and the abnormal propagation of activity front (phase III) through the proximal part of the small bowel (retrograde propagation between leads 6 and 7). In the postprandial period, the frequency of antral contractions is reduced, phasic and tonic pressure activity is prominent at the level of the pylorus, and the meal fails to inhibit the interdigestive motor complex (Redrawn with permission from Colemont LJ, Camilleri M. Chronic intestinal pseudo-obstruction: diagnosis and treatment. *Mayo Clin Proc* 1989;64:60–70.)

Assessment of GI motility and transit time is helpful to identify motor functions of the gut and to distinguish between neuropathic and myopathic disorders (23). Neuropathic conditions show a picture of uncoordinated but normal-amplitude phasic peak pressures, whereas myopathic conditions show contractions of considerably reduced amplitude in the affected regions on manometry (22). Such studies do not distinguish between intrinsic and extrinsic neuropathies.

After spinal cord injury the ascending colon is most affected because vagal innervation ends at the middle of the transverse colon. The left halves of the colon and rectum are supplied by sacral parasympathetic fibers. Therefore, any lesion above the conus would result in a loss of central control. One of the major bowel problems in spinal cord injury patients is a dysfunction of the colon and rectum. The colonic transit time is prolonged. The mean total colonic transit time in patients with spinal cord injuries is 81 ± 11 hours; in normal persons it is 39 ± 5 hours (24) Most patients spend ½ to 1 hour on bowel programs. At times patients may spend more than 1 hour, which usually is associated with very prolonged colonic transit time. If the transit time is longer than 120 hours, patients may need transverse colostomy to alleviate the constant abdominal sympatry.

MANAGEMENT

Dietary Management and Supplements

Since there is loss of the gastrocolic reflex as well as a slowed transit time through the bowel (25) in the patient with an upper or lower motor neuron injury, the stool consistency and evacuation from the rectum must be controlled. Ensuring a high dietary fiber intake can increase the bulk and soften the stool (26). Fiber can be obtained in the everyday diet, such as in fruits, vegetables, and cereal products, or it can be purchased as a supplement such as wheat bran. The dietary fiber is a bulking agent that increases the retention of water in stool.

- Polycarbophil is a dietary fiber available in tablet form.
- Psyllium can be purchased as a supplement in products such as Metamucil; the undigested fiber has water-holding capacity, and there is also bulking due to the increased bacterial mass following partial fiber

Table 52-3: Components in the Evaluation for Extrinsic Neurologic Disease in Patients with Gastrointestinal Motor Dysfunction

Component	Specific Features
History	Postural dizziness, control of blood pressure Disturbances of vision Sweating Urinary disturbances or infections Sensory or motor deficits
Medications	Calcium channel blockers, anticholinergic agents, antiarrhythmic drugs, antipsychotic agents, antihypertensive agents
Past history	Diabetes mellitus, spinal cord injury
Family history	Amyloidosis, other neuropathy
Examination	Blood pressure and pulse (with patient supine and standing) Pupils (size, reaction to light) Cranial nerves Sensation Motor function
Studies	Gastrointestinal manometry RR-interval (electrocardiographic) responses to Valsalva maneuver and pulse rate variation (oscillation) with deep breathing Pupillary responses to 0.1% epinephrine, 0.125% pilocarpine, 5% cocaine drops Thermoregulatory sweat test Quantitative sudomotor axon reflex test (to iontophoresed acetylcholine) Blood pressure and plasma norepinephrine (with patient supine and standing) Screen for peripheral neuropathy Magnetic resonace imaging of the brain/brain stem

Source: Modified with permission from Camilleri M. Disorders of gastrointestinal motility in neurological disease. *Mayo Clin Proc* 1990;65:825–846.

digestion (27). Psyllium is now available in flavored powders as well as wafers, to make it more palatable.

- Dioctyl sodium sulfosuccinate or docusate sodium is a stool softener that probably has a detergent effect on the stool. It may also increase fluid accumulation in the gut.
- Senna concentrate tablets are available in tablet form alone or in combination with docusate sodium in one tablet. Senna is a vegetable or fruit derivative that is a neuroperistaltic stimulant. It is also available in suppository form.

Suppositories

Rectal suppositories are often used on a chronic basis in patients with neurogenic bowel. They are inserted into the rectum against the rectal wall and can take from 15 to 60 minutes to take effect. The tip can be coated with petroleum jelly before insertion in patients with hemorrhoids or irritation in the rectal region. Orthotics for the insertion of suppositories are available for patients with low-cervical or incomplete quadriplegia so that they can perform their own bowel program independently.

- Bisacodyl is available as a suppository (e.g., Dulcolax) and as medication to be taken orally. It works to stimulate sensory nerve endings to produce parasympathetic reflexes, which then create increased peristaltic colonic contractions (27). In one study, polyethylene glycol-based bisacodyl suppositories reduced bowel program time by half compared with vegetable oil-based bisacodyl suppositories (28).
- Glycerin suppositories are also available; these tend to be somewhat less irritating to the patient with residual GI sensation. The precise action of glycerin is not well known, but it has been suggested that it causes dehydration of exposed tissues to produce an irritant effect.

Bowel Training Program for Patients with Upper Motor Neuron Bowel Dysfunction

The bowel training progran (BTP) is essential to begin as early as possible, as soon as the acute ileus stage has resolved. Patients should ideally start on an everyday program, in the evening or in the morning. It is useful to perform the BTP shortly after a meal (breakfast or dinner) so that the natural peristalsis may assist somewhat in the program. The regular BTP, at least initially, should consist of a suppository and digital stimulation with a gloved finger. If there is stool in the vault, this should be cleaned out, then the suppository inserted with a gloved, lubricated finger. Digital stimulation refers to a circular movement and gentle stretching of the anus to stimulate the defecation reflex. After 10 minutes, the digital stimulation can be repeated. It normally takes 20 to 30 minutes for evacuation from the suppository. If at all possible, the patient should be transferred to a commode during the program to allow gravity to assist. Eventually, the BTP can be changed to an every-other-day program; some patients need to maintain an everyday program to avoid accidents during daily activities.

Bowel Training Program for Patients with Lower Motor Neuron Bowel Dysfunction

Since lower motor neuron lesions result in atonic bowels, manual evacuation is frequently necessary. Firmer stools often help with manual evacuation so fluid restriction and avoidance of too many stool softeners are necessary. As with the upper-motor-neuron program, rectal suppositories, digital stimulation, and upright posture are useful. Maintenance of a regular schedule (e.g., every day between 8 and 9 AM) for the BTP helps promote success in avoiding accidents. Patients should be taught to avoid Valsalva forces during transfers to prevent expulsion of stool (29). During bowel case procedure for LMN patients, bowel care should be started with patients in the seated position and digital stimulation initiated. Intermittent Valsalva force and abdominal wall contraction along with transabdominal massage of the colon in a clockwise manner helps advance the stool (29). Digital removal is repeated with digital stimulation until there is no further palpable stool.

COMPLICATIONS

Complications related to neurogenic bowel include hemorrhoids, impaction, colonic diverticuli, rectal prolapse, perirectal abscess, megacolon, and colonic cancer. Some helpful strategies are a high-fiber diet to maintain a soft stool, supporting pelvic flow with a gel or air cushion, and following a regular schedule of bowel programs (29).

CONCLUSION

Management of neurogenic bowel involves comprehensive bowel programs to prevent incontinence and produce adequate evacuation, keeping in mind diet and oral and rectal medications, physical activity and a regular bowel case regimen.

ACKNOWLEDGMENT

We thank Ron J. McLeod for typing this chapter.

REFERENCES

1. Rattan S. Neural regulation of gastrointestinal motility: nature of neurotransmission. Med Clin North Am 1981;65:1129–1145.
2. Goyal RK, Crist JR. Neurology of the gut. In: Sleisenger MM, Fordtran JS, eds.: *Gastrointestinal disease.* 4th ed. Vol. 1. Philadelphia: WB Saunders, 1989;21–52.
3. Mei N. Intestinal chemosensitivity. *Physiol Rev* 1985;65:211.
4. Floyd K, Hick VE, Morrision JF. Mechanosensitive afferent units in the hypogastric nerve of the cat. *J Physiol* 1976;259:457–471.
5. Ugalde V, Litwiller SE, Gater RD. Bladder and bowel anatomy for the physiatrist. In: Shanker K, ed. *Physiatric anatomic principles, state of the art reviews in physical medicine and rehabilitation.* Vol. 10. Philadelphia: Hanley & Belfus, 1996:547–569.
6. Grabella G. Structure of muscle and nerves in the gastrointestinal tract. In: Johnson LR, ed. *Physiology of the gastrointestinal tract.* New York: Raven, 1987: 335–381.
7. Graffer H, Ekelund M, Hakanson R, et al. Effects of upper abdominal sympathectomy on gastric acid, serum gastrin and catecholamines in the rat gut. *Scand J Gastroentrol* 1984;19: 711–716.
8. Costa M, Brookes SJH. The enteric nervous system. *Am J Gastroenterol* 1994;89:S129–S137.
9. Opitz JI, Thorsteinsson G, Schutt AM, et al. Neurogenic bladder and bowel. In: Delisa JA, ed. *Rehabilitation medicine—principles and practice.* Philadelphia: JB Lippincott, 1988:492–515.
10. Weber J, Denis P, Mihout B, et al. Effect of brainstem lesion on colonic and anorectal activity: study of three patients. *Dig Dis* 1985;30:419–425.
11. Stass WE Jr, Formal CS, Gershkoff AM, et al. Rehabilitation of the spinal cord injured patient. In: Delisa JA, ed. *Rehabilitation medicine—principles and practice.* Philadelphia: JB Lippincott, 1988:635–659.
12. Kupsky WJ, Grimes MM, Sweeting J, et al. Parkinson's disease and megacolon: concentric hyaline inclusions (Lewy bodies) in enteric ganglion cells. *Neurology* 1987;37:1253–1255.
13. Reynolds BJ, Eliassion G. Colonic pseudo-obstruction in patients with stroke. *Am Neurol* 1977;1:305.
14. Fealey RD, Szurszewski JH, Merritt JL, DiMango EP. Effect of traumatic spinal cord transection on human upper gastrointestinal motility and gastric emptying. *Gastroenterology* 1984; 87:69–75.
15. Cosom BC, Stone JM, Perkash I. Gastrointestinal complications of chronic spinal cord injury. *J Am Paraplegia Soc* 1991;14: 175–181.
16. Apstein MD, Dalecki-Chipperfield K. Spinal cord injury is a risk factor for gallstone disease. *Gastroenterology* 1992;87: 966–968.
17. Stone JM, Nino-Murcia M, Wolfe A, Perkash I. Chronic gastrointestinal problems in spinal Cord injury VA patients: a prospective analysis. *Am J Gastroenterol* 1990;85: 1114–1119.
18. Guy RJC, Dawson JL, Garrett JR, et al. Diabetic gastroparesis from autonomic neuropathy: surgical considerations and changes in vagus nerve morphology. *J Neurol Neurosurg Psychiatry* 1984;47: 686–691.
19. Hensley GP, Soergel KH. Neuropathologic findings in diabetic diarrhea. *Arch Pathol* 1968;85: 587–597.
20. Camilleri M, Malagelanda J-R, Stanghellini V, et al. Gastrointestinal motility disturbances in patients with orthostatic hypotension. *Gastroenterology* 1985;88: 1852–1859.

21. Ikeda S-I, Makishita H, Oguchi K, et al. Gastrointestinal amyloid deposition in familial amyloid polyneuropathy. *Neurology* 1982;32:1364–1368.

22. Camilleri M. Disorders of gastrointestinal motility in neurological disease. *Mayo Clin Proc* 1990;65:825–846.

23. Malagelada J-R, Camilleri M, Stanghellini V. *Manometric diagnosis of gastrointestinal motility disorders.* New York: Thieme, 1986.

24. Niro-Murcia M, Stone JM, Chang PJ, Perkash I. Colonic transit in spinal cord–injured patients. *Invest Radiol* 1990;25:109–112.

25. Banwell JG, Creasey GM, Aggarwal AM, Mortimer JT. Management of the neurogenic bowel in patients with spinal cord injury. *Urol Clin North Am* 1993;20:517–526.

26. Weingarden SI. The gastrointestinal system and spinal cord injury. *Phys Med Rehabil Clin N Am* 1992;3:765–781.

27. *Physician's desk reference.* New York: Three Rivers Press, 1995.

28. Stiens SA. Reduction in bowel program duration with polyethylene glycol based bisacodyl suppositories. *Arch Phys Med Rehabil* 1995;76:674–677.

29. Stiens SA, Bergman SB, Goetz LL. Neurogenic bowel dysfunction after spinal cord injury: clinical evaluation and rehabilitative management. *Arch Phys Med Tehabil* 1997;78:S86–S102.

30. Cervero F, Connell LA, Lawson SN. Somatic and visceral primary afferents in the lower thoracic dorsal root ganglia of the cat. J Comp Neurol 1984;228:422–431.

Chapter 53

Heterotopic Ossification: Diagnosis and Management

Jay V. Subbarao

HISTORY AND NOMENCLATURE

Ossification of soft tissues is a pathologic process and can be of a hereditary progressive variety or idiopathic form. Riedel (1) in 1883 first described the relationship between soft-tissue ossification and neurologic disorders. Unlike the calcification of soft tissues seen in the setting of chronic granulomatous infections, heterotopic ossification (HO) is a true bone formation. DeJerine and Ceillier (2) observed that the ossification was juxtamuscular and interfascicular.

Previously this ossifying process was described by different names based on presumed etiopathology (Table 53-1). Soft-tissue ossification can be classified into three forms: 1) ossification seen in patients with neurologic disorders such as spinal cord injury (SCI), brain injury, burns, and other medical conditions; 2) traumatic myositis ossificans that is always associated with evidence of direct trauma; and 3) congenital myositis ossificans progressiva or fibrodysplasia ossificans progressiva (FOP), which is inherited in an autosomal dominant manner with full penetrance and variable expression. FOP is associated with skeletal malformations in addition to the soft-tissue ossification (3,4). Detailed discussion of traumatic myositis ossificans and FOP is beyond the scope of this chapter.

In 1918 DeJerine and Ceillier (2), in a classic review of HO, labeled it as "Paraosteo Arthropathies (POA) of paraplegic people." They noted that POA is characterized by the presence of more or less abundant osseous malformations near joints and bones but without morphologic alterations to the bones. The designation *POA* is misleading because there is no true arthropathy seen in these patients. The term *myositis ossificans* is misleading because there is no evidence of an inflammatory process in the muscle fibers, the ossification occurs in the interfascicular plane, and quite often the muscle necrosis is due to extrinsic pressure. The muscle necrosis, edema, and hypersensitivity reaction in the tissues surrounding the HO and osteoporosis are only consequences of HO, not causes (5).

Incidence

The incidence of HO reported in the literature varies from 16% to 53% (6,7). The incidence reported largely depends on the patient population studied, the interval from the onset of the condition to the time of the study, the investigations utilized, whether data collection was prospective or retrospective, and the duration of follow-up (8). The majority of the studies reported a 20% to 30% incidence in SCI patients (3,7–18) and in patients with traumatic brain injury (TBI) (19–22). A prospective study of 111 pediatric patients with TBI reported a 22.5% incidence (22). The peak incidence of HO is noted from 4 to 12 weeks (8,14) but frequently may occur between 2 and 5 months after onset of the deficit. However, late-onset HO in SCI patients is not uncommon, hence the need for long-term follow-up (8). HO is a frequent complication following total hip arthroplasty (THA); however, the reported incidence varies widely from 15% to 90%, with significant

Table 53-1: Old Terminology
Neurogenic ossifying fibromyopathy
Osteosis neuratica
Paraosteoarthropathy
Myositis ossificans
Ectopic ossification

amounts of HO found in 1% to 27% of patients (23–27). A 1% to 3% incidence of HO was found in patients with burns, but a tertiary rehabilitation center reported a 35.3% incidence (28–32). Joint ankylosis, with severe functional limitations, occurs only in 8% to 10% of patients with HO (18,33).

Risk Factors

The level of lesion, age, sex, and race has no significant correlation with HO formation (34). Lal et al (35) and Bravo-Payno et al (36) reported a higher incidence of medical complications including pressure ulcers and increased spasticity in patients with HO. However, it appears that those conditions are merely associated with HO and are not causative factors. Similarly, Hurvitz et al (37) and Ritter and Vaughan (26) described the risk factors for TBI patients and patients undergoing THA, respectively. Male patients with osteoarthritis and proliferative osteophytes are at risk for HO following hip arthroplasty. Patients with neurologic lesions that are complete and are of traumatic origin tend to have a higher incidence of HO. Hurvitz et al (37) reported that children older than 11 years who were in a coma had a greater risk for extensive HO formation. The incidence of HO in pediatric and geriatric patients with SCI and TBI is generally lower than that in adult patients.

Researchers suggested an association of human leukocyte antigens such as HLA-B18, HLA-B27, and HLA-DW7 (38–42). However, such a relationship has not been conclusively established (43).

LOCATION

The most common joints where HO occurs are the hips and knees in the lower extremity and shoulders and elbows in the upper extremity (12,16) (Fig. 53-1). However, HO has been found in other locations (44) including the spinal column (see Fig. 53-1). It may be unilateral or bilateral, but not all joints in a paralyzed extremity develop HO. In patients with neurologic disorders, HO always occurs below the neurologically impaired segments.

ETIOLOGY

The etiology of HO remains unknown. HO is a true ossification. Histologic studies demonstrate a demarcated zone of fibroblastic proliferation, leading to chondroblasts and finally resulting in osteoblastic change, with blood vessels and haversian canal formation (Fig. 53-2). Histologically HO cannot be distinguished from the callus seen in fracture healing. The initial step in this ossification process is the metaplasia of fibroblasts. Many local and systemic factors have been considered as triggering mechanisms for the metaplasia (5,45–50). However, to date there is no known mechanism. Michelsson et al (46,47) found that repeated forcible mobilization of an immobilized knee joint caused ossification in the quadriceps muscle in rabbits. Changing the position of the knee joint during mobilization changed the location of ossification (46,47). Interestingly, the amount of HO did not increase with denervation of the extremities (46). However, these findings are not collaborated by clinical experiences. Injection of autologous blood did not result in bone formation (47), but HO did develop after a suspension of bone marrow cells was implanted in the muscle. These osteoprogenitor cells did not require any additional stimulus for bone formation (51). Cells in the extraskeletal sites, called *inducible osteoprogenitor cells* (IOPCs), can be induced to form new bone. A number of bone growth factors and bone morphogenetic proteins, and manipulation of local environmental factors have been extensively researched in animals (48,50,51), but thus far the factors leading to HO formation in humans are not known. Ekelund et al (52) and Renfree et al (53) studied the effect of injecting sera into the muscle of the experimented animals from patients with SCI or head injuries on the proliferation of osteoblasts, without con-

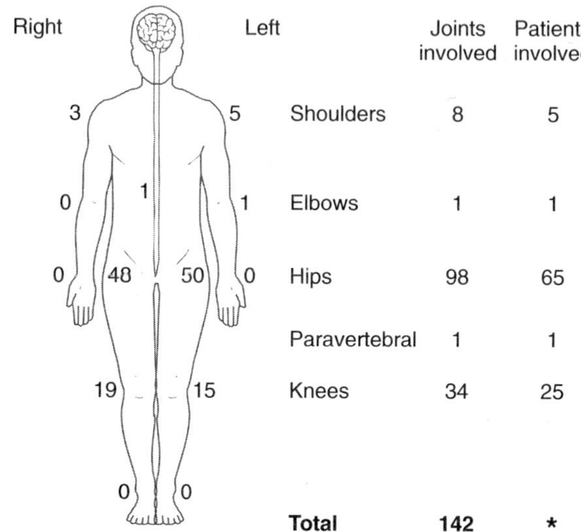

	Joints involved	Patients involved
Shoulders	8	5
Elbows	1	1
Hips	98	65
Paravertebral	1	1
Knees	34	25
Total	**142**	*

Figure 53-1. Location and incidence of heterotopic ossification in 77 patients, as determined by prospective x-ray survey of 250 spinal cord injury patients. The total (*asterisk*) for the number of patients involved is more than 77 because some patients had multiple joint involvement. (Reproduced by permission from Stover S. Heterotopic ossification after spinal cord injury. Baltimore: Williams & Wilkins, 1986.)

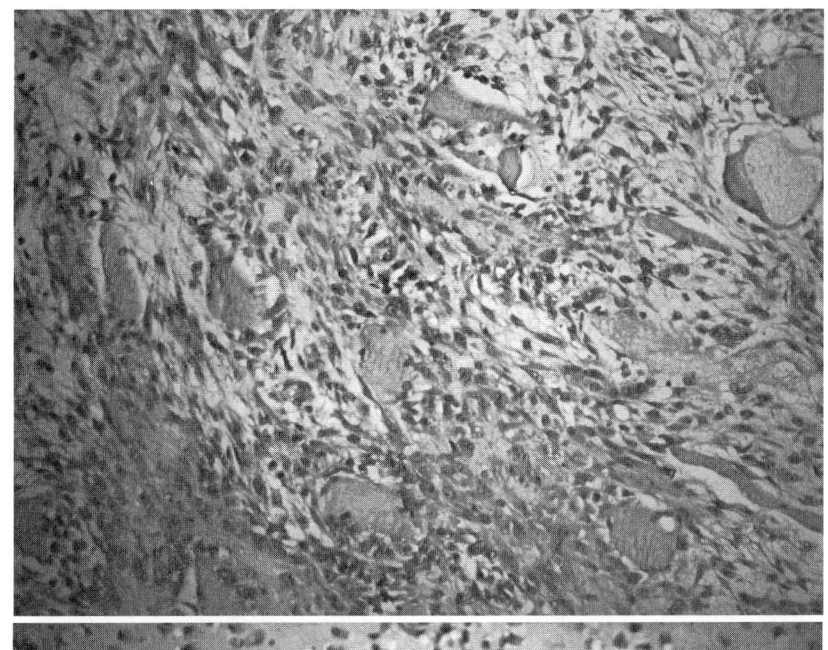

A

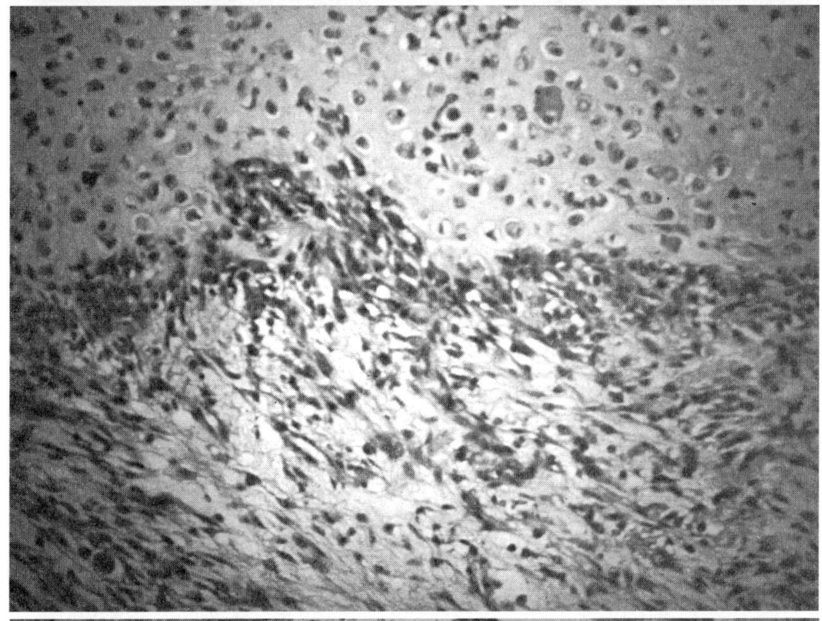

B

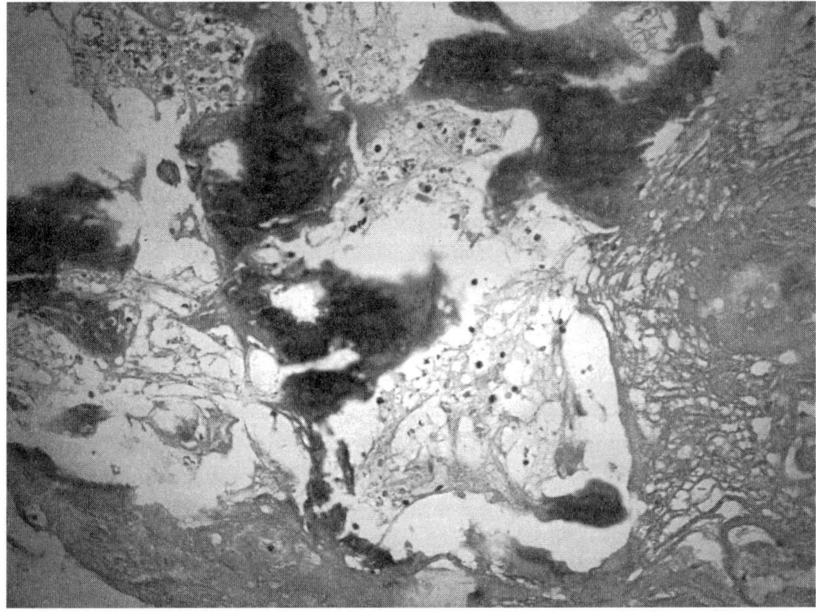

C

Figure 53-2. *A*. Fibroblasts with hyperchromatic and pleomorphic nuclei infiltrating the muscles. *B*. Cartilage with fibroblastic proliferation. *C*. Bone formation with osteoblastic activity.

vincing conclusions. Traumatic myositis ossificans is the only clinical condition that can mimic the experimental studies (54,55).

DIAGNOSIS

HO may present with a sudden onset of redness and swelling near a large joint in the impaired extremity (15). Initially the swelling is fairly localized but after 7 to 10 days the edema will be indurated and a palpable mass may be noted. At a later stage, edema may be noted distal to the lesion, secondary to compression from HO. Systemic features such as fever and chills are rare. In patients with incomplete lesions and those with nonneurologic lesions, pain is a common presenting symptom.

The pathognomic feature of HO, in addition to the above-described inflammatory signs, is the decreasing range of motion (ROM) of the joint involved. Minimal joint effusion may also be seen. In patients presenting with the above clinical picture, other medical complications such as deep vein thrombosis, septic arthritis, impending pressure ulcer, and cellulitis should be eliminated. Unfortunately, venous thrombosis and pressure ulcer may coexist with HO, thus complicating the diagnosis and management (14,56–58). The loss of ROM in the joint remains a clear distinguishing feature between HO and the venous thrombosis and pressure ulcers except septic arthritis. Aspiration of the joint will reveal findings of "infected synovial fluid" and a positive culture in the setting of septic arthritis; fever and leukocytosis are also common. Other clinical conditions that mimic HO include local trauma with hematoma, fracture, and osteomyelitis (5,14). A combination of an unexplained increase in spasticity in the extremity, loss of ROM in the joint, and inflammatory signs should alert the clinician to the possibility of HO in patients with neurologic deficits. HO is quite often detected as an incidental finding in patients who undergo radiologic studies of the extremity or urologic assessments. Some of these patients may not be able to recall any previous episode of acute symptoms.

INVESTIGATIONS

There is no single laboratory or imaging study that can accurately predict patients at high risk of developing HO. Roentgenologic studies may reveal only diffuse swelling in the first 7 to 10 days, and calcification should occur prior to noting significant changes on the x-ray film. Thus, routine x-ray studies are of no value in the early stages of HO. Elevated serum alkaline phosphatase (SAP) levels are often detected in patients with clinically significant HO (5,59–61). The SAP level may be elevated in patients with fractures and other skeletal or hepatic abnormalities. Thus, elevation of SAP from a normal value or previously abnormal level in a patient, with the above-described clinical presentation is strongly indicative of HO. The SAP elevation may coincide with the clinical presentation but does not correlate with the severity of the lesion or the number of lesions. Nicholas (62) reported that SAP elevations always precede the x-ray findings. Elevated levels of creatinine phosphokinases and total urinary hydroxyproline have been observed in SCI patients with HO (63–65).

The three-phase bone scan using technetium 99m–methylane diphosphonate is very commonly utilized for diagnosing HO, monitoring progress, and establishing inactivity of HO (56,66–72). Images are obtained during 1) dynamic blood flow, 2) a static phase after completion of injection, and 3) 2 to 3 hours after the injection (Fig. 53-3). The first two phases of the scan indicate hyperemia and blood pooling, which are precursors of the ossification process and thus are of greater value. For patients with inflammatory signs, elevated SAP levels, and positive findings on images taken during the first or second phase of the three-phase bone scan, treatment should be instituted as soon as possible.

The activity noted on the radionuclide bone images may subside in 12 to 18 months, thus indicating a "burnout" of the HO. Some clinicians observe signs of increased radionuclide uptake for prolonged periods and thus continue management (3,73). However, the scan will be positive if there is reactivation (74). Performing surgical resection, when the bone scan demonstrates no activity, this is considered to minimize the risk of recurrence. Routine x-ray films of long-standing lesions may reveal a trabeculated pattern with "bridging lesions" across the joint, resulting in ankylosis. The lack of flocculation and "fluffy appearance" is also indicative of mature bone formation. Osteoporosis may be seen adjacent to the lesion (5).

Finerman and Stover (75) categorized HO occurring around the hip into six grades: grade 0—no heterotopic ossification; grade 1—a small amount of bone on the lateral aspect; grade 2—a small amount of bone medially and laterally; grade 3—a greater amount of bone, particularly on the lateral aspect; grade 4—a greater amount of bone both medially and laterally; and grade 5—apparent ankylosis. Though the investigators utilized this as a grading scale, there is considerable subjectivity. More importantly, the grading system does not take into consideration the functional implications of HO. For example, as shown in Figure 53-4, a small amount of HO at the shoulder and the hip forming a "bridge across the joint" can result in severe functional loss similar to that in a patient with extensive HO (Fig. 53-4C). Thus, the grading system is of very little clinical significance.

Computed tomography (76) and magnetic resonance imaging can be utilized to demarcate the relationship of blood vessels, nerves, and muscles to the HO prior to planning surgical resection. The role of these advanced studies in the diagnosis of HO has not been well established. Rossier et al (77) noted "circulatory changes to be more frequent when there is POA in the segment examined and

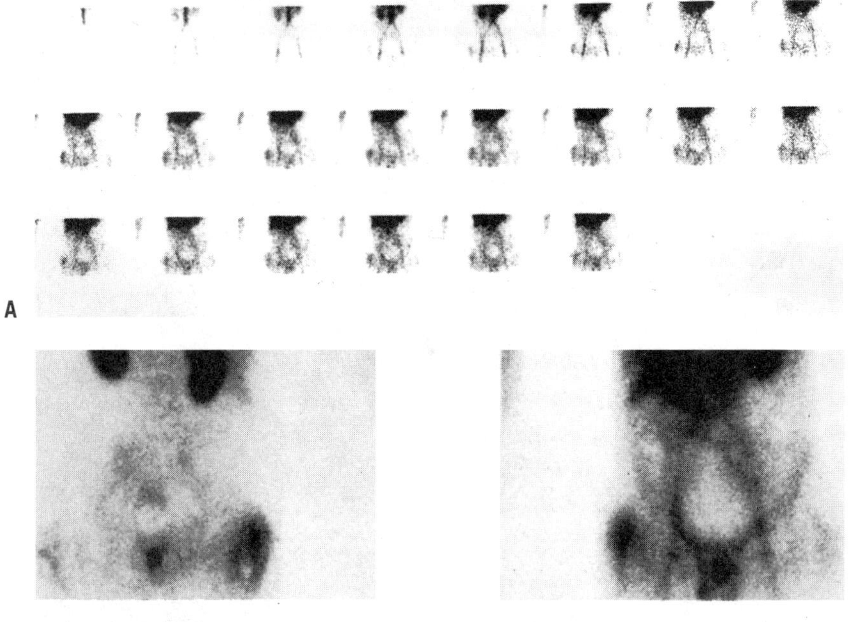

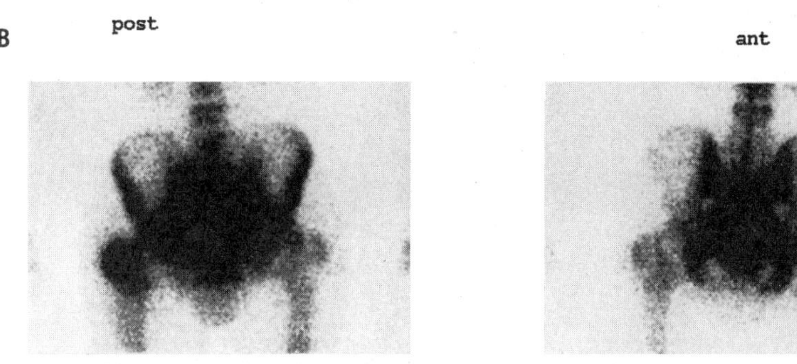

Figure 53-3. Three-phase radionuclide bone imaging using Tc99M MDP. *A*. Blood-flow study showing moderate hyperemia in the area of right greater trochanter. *B*. Blood-pool study showing moderate hyperemia in the same areas. *C*. Delayed static image showing a well-circumscribed area of markedly increased radio tracer intake in the intertrochanter area.

it consists of an opening of the arterio-venous shunts, easily determined by angiography." Angiography is rarely used to diagnose HO but may help delineate the relationship of major vessels in patients with extensive HO.

MANAGEMENT

Garland (3) reviewed the natural history of HO and emphasized the need for understanding the normal clinical course and minor variations between the different etiologic factors within similar patient populations. "This variation only occurs in a small percentage of a given population, but this variation, because of etiology or the inherent trait within the patient or both, causes continuing confusion for physicians" (8). He observed that the SAP elevations and findings on radionuclide and roentgenographic studies were closely correlated in the majority of patients. The activity was noted to have subsided in 6 months in a majority of the patients, and in patients who required surgical resection, the abnormalities in SAP and imaging continued for longer durations. Garland (8) also noted that TBI patients with severe cognitive deficits and spasticity tended to have extensive bone formation, required surgical resection, and demonstrated recurrence after surgery. Van der Linden (78) reported spontaneous regression of HO. A thorough understanding of the natural history and early diagnosis are essential for planning appropriate management strategies.

Table 53-2 enumerates the modalities utilized in the treatment of HO. Cryotherapy and ultrasound were tried in the earlier days but are rarely considered now.

Prophylaxis

The prophylactic use of medications for the prevention of HO has been studied mostly in SCI (16,79–84) and THA patients (84). The results of these studies are variable. Stover et al (81) conducted a double-blind, multi-institutional study of 166 SCI patients. Eighty-two patients

Figure 53-4. *A.* X-ray of shoulder showing heterotopic ossification bridging between the scapula and humerus. *B.* X-ray of hip showing ossification bridging between the greater trochanter and the iliac region. *C.* AP view of pelvis showing massive ossification across both hip joints with sparing of the articular surfaces.

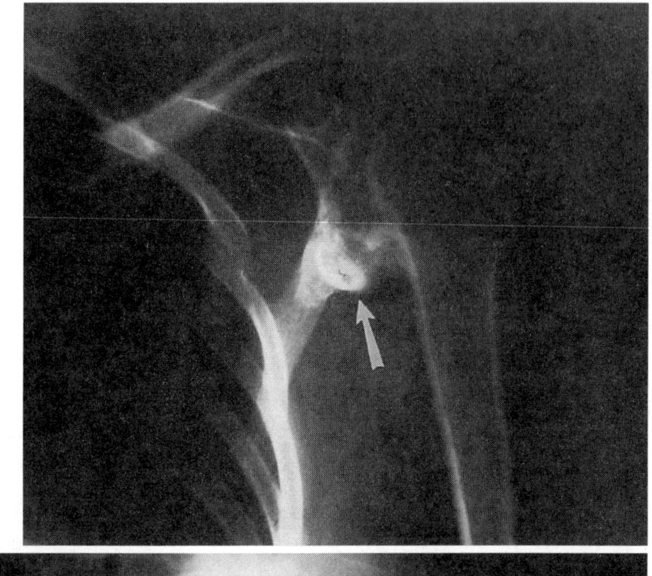

A

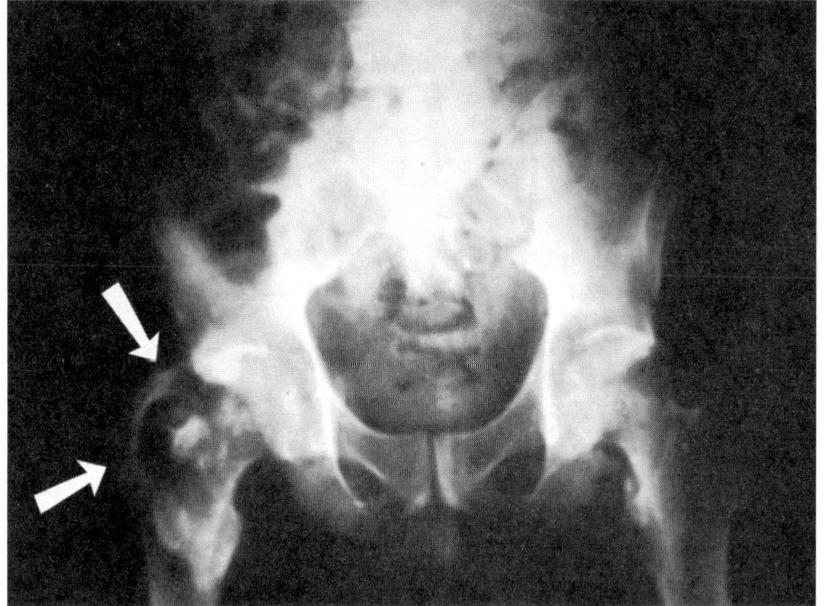

B

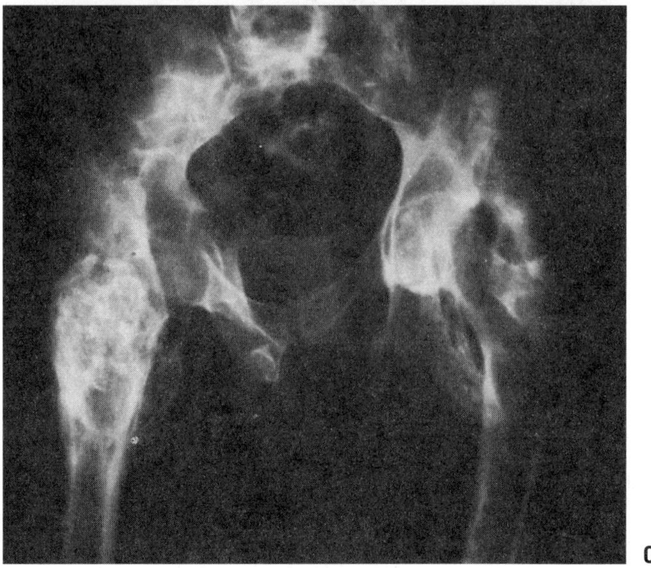

C

Table 53-2: Treatments Available
1. Passive and active range of motion exercises 2. Medications to arrest progression (e.g., EHDP, anti-inflammatories) 3. Radiation to the involved joint 4. Immobilizing the joint in the optimal functional position 5. Manipulation of the involved joint 6. Surgical resection 7. Ultrasound 8. Cryotherapy

were treated with etidronate disodium, 20 mg/kg for 2 weeks and 10 mg/kg for another 10 weeks, and 84 were included in the placebo group. However, the treatment was started 20 to 121 days after injury. The x-ray findings were graded from 0 to 4, with grade 4 revealing extensive ossification and invariably leading to ankylosis.

The authors noted that up to the time when the treatment was discontinued, the HO in the etidronate disodium–treated group was significantly less ($p < 0.05$) compared with the placebo-treated patients. They observed that some ossification may still occur after the drug is discontinued and that the final incidence of HO in the treated and placebo group was about the same, but the amounts of HO and functional limitations in the treated group were considerably less. The drawbacks of this study are 1) that only x-ray films were used to monitor the HO, and thus early stages of HO formation may not have been diagnosed; and 2) that the treatment was not started until 20 to 121 days after injury, and thus, true "prevention" was not possible because the pathologic processes leading to HO may have been established prior to initiating therapy. Routine prophylaxis with etidronate disodium for all SCI or TBI patients may not be justifiable, as only 20% to 30% of patients develop clinically significant HO and only 8% to 10% of patients develop severe functional limitations. Prophylactic use of medications to prevent recurrence after surgical resection (3,8,73,85) and forceful mobilization is well established (86). Use of anti-inflammatory medications and other pharmacologic agents such as warfarin, tenoxicam, ketorolac, calcitonin, and vitamin K, and use of radiation for the prevention of recurrence following surgical excision or THA have been extensively studied (10,83,85,87–101). The timing, duration, and dosage of such treatments are still not uniform. Administration of indomethacin, 25 mg three times a day for at least 3 weeks starting from the first postoperative day, is a common practice. Using smaller doses and delaying the start of therapy for 5 days do not appear to result in a poor outcome. Gebuhr et al (95) observed that 500 mg of naproxen given twice daily for 8 days reduced the incidence of HO in patients who underwent cemented THA compared to the control group.

Role of Medications and Mechanism of Action

The anti-inflammatory medications inhibit the formation of prostaglandins and related substances (102,103). Indomethacin is known to inhibit the differentiation of mesenchymal cells into osteogenic cells, thus reducing the formative and resorptive phases of bone remodeling (5,102).

Ethane-1-hydroxy-1,1-diphosphonate (EHDP) has been extensively studied in experimental animals, and was found to inhibit the precipitation of calcium phosphate from clear solutions (104–106). EHDP absorbs calcium hydroxyapatite crystals and thus blocks crystal growth and mineralization and delays the dissolution of crystals (6,18,80,104,105). EHDP blocks the amorphous calcium phosphate transformation into crystalline hydroxyapatite without inhibiting the nucleation phase (99,105,106). Garland (3) recommended a 20-mg/kg dose for up to 6 months because the research showed that the "activity" continues up to 6 months in the majority of the patients. However, the duration and dosage should be individualized, because a small percentage of patients may have evidence of continued elevation of SAP levels or increased uptake on bone scans. Subbarao et al (73) observed no deleterious effects in two patients who required EDHP for longer than 2 years. Unfortunately there are no published reports of a large patient series demonstrating the efficacy or deleterious effects of larger doses and long-term therapy (107,108). The elevation of serum phosphorus levels in patients taking EHDP was dose related and did not have any other clinical implications. Fracture healing in the spine and extremities and healing of the osteotomized trochanter were not delayed by use of EHDP (81,108). There are very few side effects reported with the use of this medication. Gastrointestinal disturbances such as nausea and vomiting were noted in 10% to 20% of patients. The symptoms were eliminated with divided doses given ½ hour before meals (16,82). Banovac et al (109) studied 27 consecutive patients with acute-onset HO and treated them with 300 mg of intravenous disodium etidronate daily for 3 days. After 3 days, the medication was continued orally at 20 mg/kg/day for 6 months. They noted rapid decrease in the soft-tissue swelling in 20 of 27 patients.

Radiation

Ayers et al (110) reviewed the role of radiation therapy in the prevention of HO in high-risk patients. Patients with diffuse idiopathic skeletal hyperostosis (DISH syndrome) or hypertrophic osteoarthritis and patients with evidence of ipsilateral or contralateral HO are considered to be the "high-risk group" to develop HO following THA (26, 27,111). The implications of radiation therapy in patients with a cementless prosthesis have been studied and techniques to avoid a delay in bone ingrowth into the prosthesis have been developed (25). Single versus multiple doses and timing of the radiation have been extensively researched (92,112–114). Ionizing radiation exerts its greatest influence on rapidly dividing cells by altering nuclear DNA. Some researchers postulated that radiation prevents the differentiation of mesenchymal cells into osteoblasts. Prospective studies on the effect of preoperative versus postoperative radiotherapy for the prevention of HO showed that preoperative radiation at the operative site 4 hours prior to elective surgery was as effective as postoperative radiation after 72 hours (113,114). Radiation therapy is rarely utilized for the management of HO in SCI patients because of the effect of radiation on the skin, leading to chronic indolent decubiti (73). Chantraine and Minaire (63) reported favorable results after radiation of HO sites in SCI patients. Schaeffer and Sosner (115) treated established bone with radiation therapy; however, this is not a common clinical practice.

Role of Exercise and Physical Therapy

Experimental studies in animals by Michelsson et al (46,47) and others (45) showed new bone formation following ROM exercises and forcible manipulation. The hematoma is considered to be a precursor to the development of HO. The investigators postulated that forcible stretching, joint mobilization, and manipulation will lead to soft-tissue bleeding, thus an increased incidence of HO. A majority of the patients with SCI or TBI undergo rehabilitative therapies that consist of ROM exercises and stretching; however, only 20% to 30% of patients develop HO and it may involve only one joint even though the other extremities are managed similarly. There is no comparable research in patients with SCI or TBI to substantiate the above findings in animal experiments. Not having these patients perform such ROM exercises will result in a very poor functional outcome and predispose them to secondary complications such as pressure ulcers and contractures. The benefits outweigh the possible risks, thus, ROM exercises and stretching should be performed by these patients. However, the timing of physical therapy in patients who develop acute symptoms of HO is controversial. Forcible stretching and mobilization should not be prescribed to these patients until the acute inflammatory signs, increased uptake on the radionuclide scans, and elevated SAP levels have stabilized (44,47). The joint, however, should be rested in a functional position, and a gentle active assisted ROM exercise should be initiated as soon as possible. The role of continuous passive ROM machines has not been evaluated in these cases. The exercise program should aim at achieving painless, full range of movement, by starting with gentle stretching and splinting as needed (10,16,73). The joint should not be totally immobilized unless ankylosis is an expected end result. In such patients, the joint is immobilized in an optimal functional position. Subbarao (116) reported the spontaneous development of pseudoarthrosis in two SCI patients with extensive HO. These patients were able to retain functional ROM in the involved joints. Similarly, An et al (117) found pseudoarthrosis in the shoulder of a patient with encephalitis. ROM exercises performed before HO has matured will mold the HO, and thus help to retain function in the extremity despite radiologic evidence of HO.

Manipulation and Joint Mobilization

Manipulation of a joint, with functional limitations secondary to HO, is done with a goal to improve the ROM of the joint and thus minimize residual functional loss (86). While theoretically this approach appears to be rational, it is controversial because manipulation leads to fresh hematoma and thus to an increased risk of additional new bone formation. In addition, there is an increased risk of fractures of the long bones because of the secondary osteoporosis seen in these patients. Thus, manipulation should not be prescribed for patients who are prone to these complications (73). Garland et al (86) reported good results following manipulation of joints in patients with TBI and recommended a manipulation every 1 to 2 months, but cautioned against manipulating more than a total of three times.

Surgical Resection

Surgery is recommended to increase joint mobility and minimize functional limitations or to prevent secondary complications such as pressure ulcers and compression of neurovascular structures due to ankylosis (8,10,18,31, 32,73,82,83,118–121). The success of surgery depends on patient selection and timing. The HO should be quiescent, as evidenced by normal SAP levels, lack of activity on radionuclide scans, and x-ray films revealing maturity (3,16,17,73). Most researchers agree that surgical intervention should be delayed for 12 to 18 months; however, the above-mentioned parameters can be utilized as criteria to determine the timing of surgery. Persistent severe spasticity generally leads to a poor functional outcome and recurrence after surgical resection of HO in SCI and TBI patients. Patient selection with well-defined goals and infection-free status is essential for good outcome. Delayed wound healing, excessive bleeding, superficial and deep infection, fractures, and recurrence of HO are commonly reported complications (6,16,73,120,121). Preoperatively, infection in skin and urinary tract should be eliminated, and appropriate antibiotic coverage should be prescribed for the immediate postoperative period. In SCI and other severely impaired individuals, secondary complications of bed rest should be avoided by instituting a good reconditioning and restorative rehabilitation program.

Postoperatively, anti-inflammatory drugs, EDHP, or radiation (in THA patients) are frequently prescribed. As already stated, radiation is not recommended for SCI patients. Indomethacin, 25 mg three times a day, or EHDP, 20 mg/kg of body weight, for 3 months is frequently recommended. At the end of 3 months, if there is an indication of increased activity on radionuclide bone scans, the

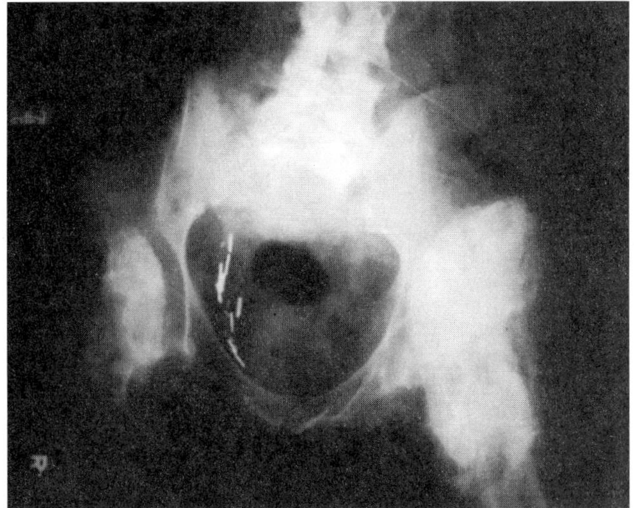

A

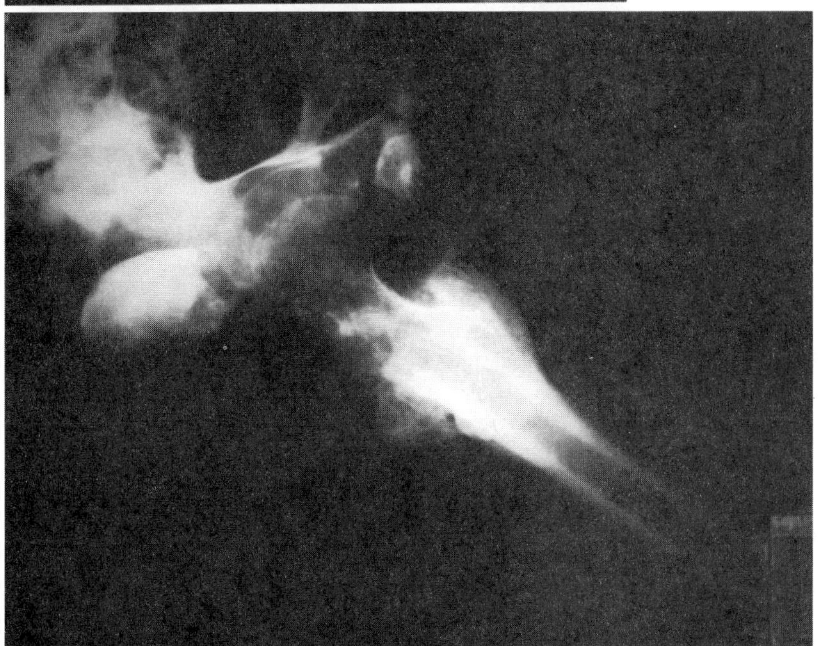

B

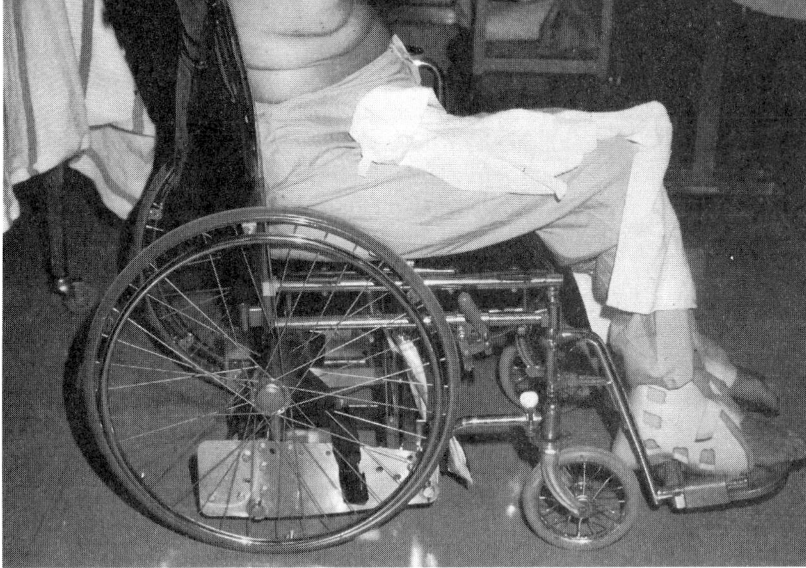

C

Figure 53-5. *A*. X-ray of pelvis (AP view) showing massive ossification across the joint. *B*. X-ray of hip after wide excision. *C*. Patient sitting in a wheelchair after the resection of HO.

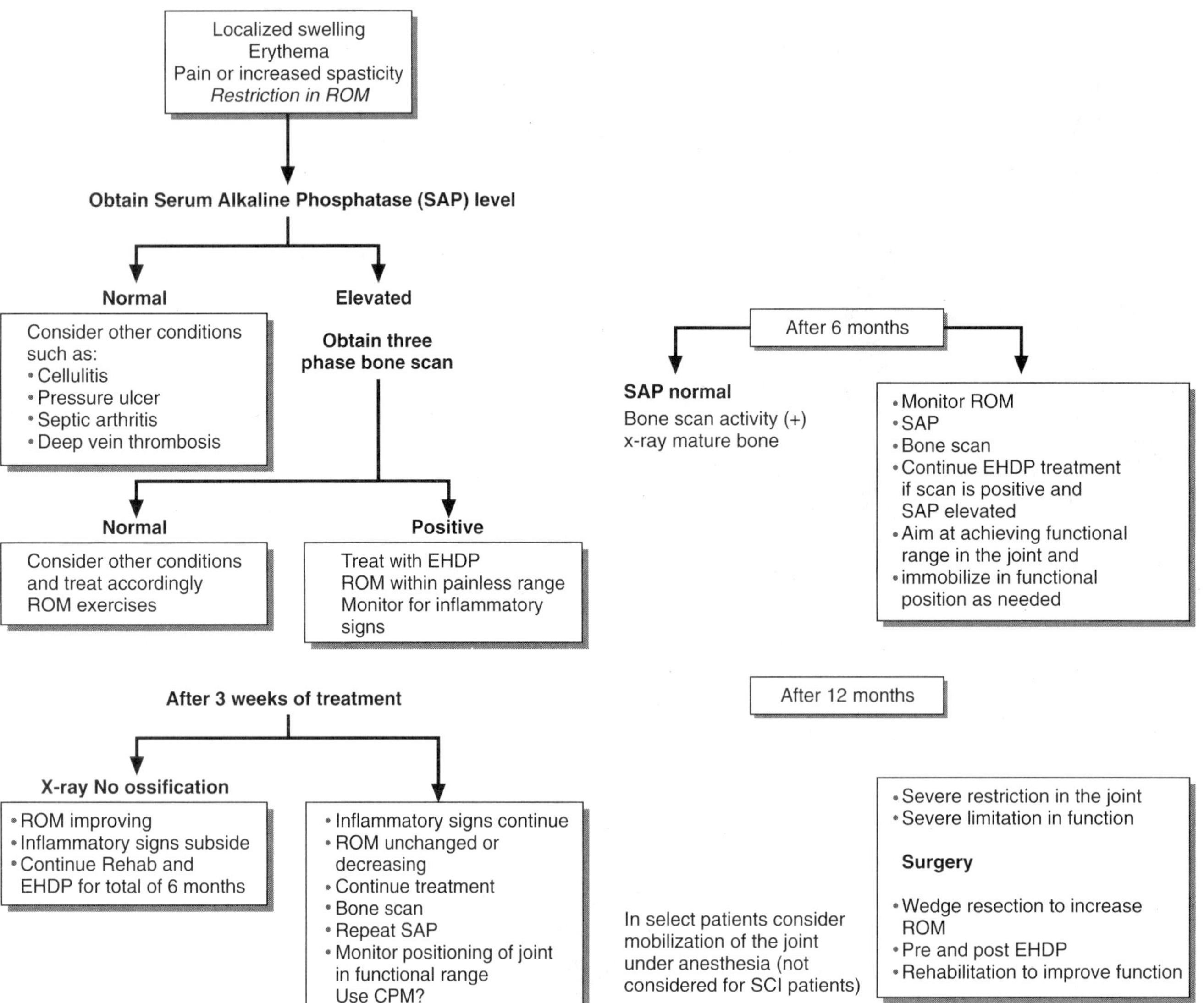

Figure 53-6. Suggested algorithm for the management of heterotopic ossification in patients with spinal cord injury (SCI) or traumatic brain injury. This algorithm is only a proposed scheme and guide; each patient should be evaluated individually and treated accordingly. EHDP = ethane-1-hydroxy-1,1-diphosphonate; ROM = range of motion; CPM = continuous passive motion.

medication is continued. There is no agreement on how long such therapy should be continued.

Garland et al (8) summarized the various approaches utilized to resect HO in patients with TBI. It is noted that the large joints such as the hips, knees, shoulders, and elbows are the ones most frequently submitted for surgery (3,121–124). To increase the ROM, wedge resection is done more frequently than wide excision of HO (33, 122,123). Contrary to the common clinical practice, Frischhut et al (124) reported good results following early removal of HO without waiting for "maturation" of the bone.

Postoperatively the joint is properly positioned using foam wedges so that the correction obtained by surgery can be maintained and stretch on the incision and pressure ulceration can be prevented. Gentle ROM exercises of the joint are initiated 72 hours after surgery, mainly to promote drainage of the hematoma (73). The intensity of therapy is gradually increased to incorporate retraining in functional activities such as sitting in the wheelchair and utilizing the upper extremity. ROM and strengthening exercises of the uninvolved extremities should be prescribed to prevent deconditioning (73). Fracture of the femoral neck and shaft fractures in osteoporotic bones have been reported (16). Peterson et al (31) reviewed the surgical management in postburn patients and emphasized a similar postoperative treatment plan.

Radiologic evidence of recurrence of HO is quite common (6,16,33) but results of surgical resection should be evaluated by the long-term functional gains. Subbarao et al (73) followed five SCI patients who underwent resection of HO to regain their ability to sit in the wheelchair. They followed the patients for an average of 2 years and 3 months and reported good results (Fig. 53-5). Good results from surgical management have also been reported for TBI and THA patients (8,17,27). Subbarao et al (73) emphasized that patient selection, identification of a distinct functional goal, education of the patient regarding potential complications, prolonged rehabilitation, and a good team approach contribute to an optimal functional outcome. An appropriate wheelchair seating system should be prescribed to maximize the long-term result's of surgery.

CONCLUSIONS

HO is a pathologic process in which soft tissues undergo ossification. The etiology is unknown. Patients with neurologic deficits develop HO in the proximal joints. An incidence of 20% to 30% is commonly reported and 8% to 10% of those patients develop severe functional limitations. The risk factors are better understood for patients undergoing arthroplasty; hence, prophylactic management with medications or radiation is commonly utilized for these patients. Routine prophylaxis in patients with SCI, TBI, or burns cannot be justified. Early diagnosis and treatment with EHDP or other anti-inflammatories will result in good functional outcomes. Elevated SAP levels, activity on radionuclide bone scans, and restriction in ROM are indicative of HO. A small percentage of patients require surgery to improve function. Joint manipulation to produce pseudoarthrosis has been utilized in TBI patients. An algorithm (Fig. 53-6) is proposed for the diagnosis and management of HO in patients with SCI or TBI.

ACKNOWLEDGMENTS

The author thanks Ms. Vaunda Bray from the Hines Comprehensive Rehabilitative Services for her assistance in preparation of this chapter.

REFERENCES

1. Riedel B. Demonstration line durch ach Hagiges Umhergehen total destruirten kniegelnkes von einem pantienten mit stichverletzing des ruckans. *Verh Dtsch Ges Chirurg* 1883;12:93.

2. Dejerine Mme, Cecillier A. Para-osteo-arthropathies des paraplegiques par lesion medullaire: (etude clinique et radiographique). *Ann Med* 1918;5:497–535.

3. Garland DE. A clinical perspective on common forms of acquired heterotopic ossification. *Clin Orthop* 1991;263:13–29.

4. Rosenfeld SR, Kaplan FS. Progressive osseous heteroplasia in male patients: two new case reports. *Clin Orthop* 1995;317:243–245.

5. Kewalrammani LS. Ectopic ossification. *Am J Phys Med* 1977;56:99–121.

6. Garland DE. Clinical observations on fractures and heterotopic ossification in the spinal cord and traumatic brain injured populations. *Clin Orthop* 1988;233:86–101.

7. Stover SL, Hataway CJ, Zeiger HE. Heterotopic ossification in spinal cord-injured patients. *Arch Phys Med Rehabil* 1975;56:199–204.

8. Garland DE, Hanscom DA, Keenan MA, et al. Resection of heterotopic ossification in the adult with head trauma. *J Bone Joint Surg* [*Am*] 1985;67: 1261–1269.

9. Damanski M. Heterotopic ossification in paraplegia: a clinical study. *J Bone Joint Surg* [*Br*] 1961;43:286–299.

10. Garland DE, Shimoyama ST, Lugo C, et al. Spinal cord insults and heterotopic ossification in the pediatric population. *Clin Orthop* 1989;245:303–310.

11. Hardy AG, Dickson JW. Pathological ossification in traumatic paraplegia. *J Bone Joint Surg* [*Br*] 1963;45:76–87.

12. Hernandez AM, Forner JV, Fuente T, et al. The particular ossifications in our paraplegics and tetraplegics: a survey of 704 patients. *Paraplegia* 1978–1979;16:272–275.

13. Hossack DW, King A. Neurogenic heterotopic ossification. *Med J Aust* 1967;1:326–328.

14. Hsu JD, Sakimura I, Stauffer ES. Heterotopic ossification around the hip joint in spinal cord injured patients. *Clin Orthop* 1975;112:165–169.

15. Freehaer AA, Urick R, Mast WA. Particular ossification in spinal cord injury. *Med Serv J Can* 1966;22:471–477.

16. Stover SL. Heterotopic ossification after spinal cord injury. In: Bloch RF, Basbaum M, eds. *Management of spinal cord injuries*. Baltimore: Williams & Wilkins, 1986:284–301.

17. Tibone J, Sakimur I, Nickel V, Hsu JD. Heterotopic ossification around the hip in spinal cord-injured patients: a long term follow-up study. *J Bone Joint Surg* [*Am*] 1978;60: 769–775.

18. Wharton GW, Morgan TH. Ankylosis in the paralyzed patient. *J Bone Joint Surg* [*Am*] 1970;52:105–112.

19. Garland DE, Blum CE, Waters RL. Periarticular heterotopic ossification in head injured adults: incidence and location. *J Bone Joint Surg* [*Am*] 1980;62: 1143–1146.

20. Mendelson L, Grosswasser Z, Najenson T, et al. Periarticular new bone formation in patients suffering from severe head injuries. *Scand J Rehabil Med* 1975;7:141–145.

21. Mital MA, Garber JE, Stinson JT. Ectopic bone formation in children and adolescents with head injuries: its management. *J Pediatr Orthop* 1987;7:83–90.

22. Citta-Pietrolungo TJ, Alexander MA, Steg NL. Early detection of heterotopic ossification in young patients with traumatic brain injury. *Arch Phys Med Rehabil* 1992;73:258–262.

23. Ahrengart L. Periarticular heterotopic ossification after total hip arthroplasty, risk factors and consequences. *Clin Orthop* 1991;263:50–58.

24. Lewallen DG. Heterotopic ossification following total hip arthroplasty. *Instr Course lect* 1995; 44:287–292.

25. Purtill JJ, Eng K, Rothman RH, Hozack WJ. Heterotopic ossification: incidence in cemented versus cementless total hip arthroplasty. *J Arthroplasty* 1996;11:58–63.

26. Ritter MA, Vaughan RB. Ectopic ossification after total hip arthroplasty: predisposing factors, frequency, and effects on results. *J Bone Joint Surg* [*AM*] 1977; 59:345–351.

27. Ahrengart L, Lindgren U. Functional significance of heterotopic bone formation after total hip arthroplasty. *J Arthroplasty* 1989; 4:125–131.

28. Tepperman PS, Hilbert L, Peters WJ, Pritzker KPH. Heterotopic ossification in burns. *J Burn Care Rehabil* 1984;5:283.

29. Holguin PH, Rico AA, Garcia JP, Del Rio JL. Elbow ankylosis due to postburn heterotopic ossification. *J Burn Care Rehabil* 1996;17:150–154.

30. Koch BM, Wu CM, Randolph J, Eng GD. Heterotopic ossification in children with burns: two case reports. *Arch Phys Med Rehabil* 1992;73:1104–1106.

31. Peterson SL, Mani MM, Crawford CM, et al. Postburn heterotopic ossification: insights for management decision. *J Trauma* 1989; 29:365–369.

32. Varghese G, Williams K, Desmet A, Redford JB. Nonarticular complication of heterotopic ossification: a clinical review. *Arch Phys Med Rehabil* 1991;72: 1009–1013.

33. Wharton GW. Heterotopic ossification. *Clin Orthop* 1975; 112:142–149.

34. Scher AT. The incidence of ectopic bone formation in post-traumatic paraplegic patients of different racial groups. *Paraplegia* 1976;14:202–206.

35. Lal S, Hamilton B, Heinemann A, Betts HB. Risk factors for heterotopic ossification in spinal cord injury. *Arch Phys Med Rehabil* 1989;70:387–390.

36. Bravo-Payno P, Esclarin A, Arzoz T, et al. Incidence and risk factors in the appearance of heterotopic ossification in spinal cord injury. *Paraplegia* 1992;30:740–745.

37. Hurvitz EA, Mandac BR, Davidoff G, et al. Risk factors for heterotopic ossification in children and adolescents with severe traumatic brain injury. *Arch Phys Med Rehabil* 1992;73:459–462.

38. Larson JM, Michalski JP, Collacott EA, et al. Increased prevalence of HLA-B27 in patients with ectopic ossification following traumatic spinal cord injury. *Rheumatol Rehabil* 1981;20:193–197.

39. Minnaire P, Betuel H, Girard R, Pilochery G. Neurologic injuries, paraosteoarthropathies, and human leukocyte antigens. *Arch Phys Med Rehabil* 1980;61:214–215.

40. Weis S, Grosswasser A, Ohri A, et al. Histocompatibility (HLA) antigens in heterotopic ossification associated with neurological injury. *J Rheumatol* 1979;6:88–91.

41. Hunter T, Dubo HIC, Hildahl CR, et al. Histocompatibility antigens in patients with spinal cord injury or cerebral damage complicated by heterotopic ossification. *Rheumatol Rehabil* 1980;19:97–99.

42. Seignalet J, Boulin M, Pelissier J, et al. HLA and neurogenic paraosteoarthropathies. *Tissue Antigens* 1983;21:268–269.

43. Garland DE, Alday B, Venos KG. Heterotopic ossification and HLA antigens. *Arch Phys Med Rehabil* 1984;65:531–532.

44. Meythaler JM, Tuel SM, Cross LL, Mathew MM. Heterotopic ossification of the extensor tendons in the hand associated with traumatic spinal cord injury. *J Am Paraplegia Soc* 1992;15:229–231.

45. Crawford CM, Varghese G, Mani MM, Neff JR. Heterotopic ossification: are range of motion exercises contraindicated? *J Burn Care Rehabil* 1986;7:323–327.

46. Michelsson JR, Rauschning W. Pathogenesis of experimental heterotopic bone formation following temporary forcible exercising of immobilized limbs. *Clin Orthop* 1983;176:265–272.

47. Michelsson JR, Franroth G, Andersson LC. Myositis ossificans following forcible manipulation of the leg: a rabbit model for the study of heterotopic bone formation. *J Bone Joint Surg* [*Am*] 1980;62:811–814.

48. Wlodarski KH. Bone histogenesis mediated by nonosteogenic cells. *Clin Orthop* 1991;272:8–15.

49. Ostrowski K, Wlodarski K. Induction of the heterotopic bone formation. In: Bourne GH, ed. *The biochemistry and physiology of* bone. Vol. 3, New York: Academic, 1971:299.

50. Urist MR, Nakagawa M, Nakata N, Nogami H. Experimental myositis ossificans. Cartilage and bone formation in muscle in response to a diffusible bone matrix-derived morphogen. *Arch Pathol Lab Med* 1978;102:312–316.

51. Friedenstein AJ, Piatezky-Shapiro J, Petrakova KV. Osteogenesis in

transplants of bone marrow cells. *J Embryol Exp Morphol* 1966;16:381–390.

52. Ekelund A, Brosjo O, Nilsson O. Experimental induction of heterotopic bone. *Clin Orthop* 1991;263:102–112.

53. Renfree KJ, Banovac K, Hornicek FJ, et al. Evaluation of serum osteoblast mitogenic activity in spinal cord and head injury patients with acute heterotopic ossification. *Spine* 1994;19:740–746.

54. Silver JR. Heterotopic ossification: a clinical study of its possible relationship to trauma. *Paraplegia* 1969–1970;7: 220–230.

55. Snoecx M, DeMuynck M, Van Laere M. Association between muscle trauma and heterotopic ossification in spinal cord injured patients: reflections on their causal relationship and the diagnostic value of ultrasonography. *Paraplegia* 1995;33:464–468.

56. Haselkorn JK, Britell CW, Cardenas DD. Diagnostic imaging of heterotopic ossification with coexistent deep-venous thrombosis in flaccid paraplegia. *Arch Phys Med Rehabil* 1991; 72:227–229.

57. Perkash A, Sullivan G, Toth L, et al. Persistent hypercoagulation associated with heterotopic ossification in patients with spinal cord injury long after injury has occurred. *Paraplegia* 1993;31:653–659.

58. Yarkony GM, Lee MY, Green D, Roth EJ. Heterotopic ossification pseudophlebitis. *Am J Med* 1989;87:342–344.

59. Furman R, Nicholas JJ, Jivoff L. Elevation of serum alkaline phosphatase coincident with ectopic bone formation in paraplegic patients. *J Bone Joint Surg* [*Am*] 1970;52:1131–1137.

60. Kjaersgaard-Andersen P, Pedersen P, Kristensen SS, et al. Serum alkaline phosphatase as an indicator of heterotopic bone formation following total hip arthroplasty. *Clin Orthop Related Res* 1988;234:102–109.

61. Mollan RAB. Serum alkaline phosphatase in heterotopic para-articular ossification after total hip replacement. *J Bone Joint Surg* [*Br*] 1979;61:432–434.

62. Nicholas JJ. Ectopic bone formation in patients with spinal cord injury. *Arch Phys Med Rehabil* 1973;54:354–359.

63. Chantraine A, Minaire P. Para-osteo-arthropathies, *Scand J Rehabil Med* 1981;13:31–37.

64. Klein L, Van Den Noort S, DeJack JJ. Sequential studies of urinary hydroxyproline and serum alkaline phosphatase in acute paraplegia. *Med Serv J Can* 1966;22:524–533.

65. Mysiw WJ, Tan J, Jackson RD. Heterotopic ossification: the utility of osteocalcin in diagnosis and management. *Am J Phys Med Rehabil* 1993;72:184–187.

66. Drane W. Myositis ossificans and the three-phase bone scan. *AJR Am J Roentgenol* 1984;142: 179–180.

67. Freed JH, Hahn H, Menter R, Dillon T. The use of the three-phase bone scan in the early diagnosis of heterotopic ossification (HO) and in the evaluation of Didronel therapy. *Paraplegia* 1982;20:208–216.

68. Mulheim G, Donath A, Rossier AB. Serial scintigrams in the course of ectopic bone formation in paraplegia patients. *AJR Am J Roentgenol* 1973;118:865–869.

69. Orzel JA, Rudd TG. Heterotopic bone formation: clinical, laboratory, and imaging correlation. *J Nucl Med* 1985;26:125–132.

70. Prakash V, Lin MS, Perkash I. Detection of heterotopic calcification with (99mTc pyrophosphate) in spinal cord injury patients. *Clin Nucl Med* 1978;3:167–169.

71. Suzuki Y, Hisada K, Takeda M. Demonstration of myositis ossificans by (99mTc pyrophosphate) bone scanning. *Radiology,* 1974;3:663–664.

72. Tanaka T, Rossier AB, Hussey RW, et al. Quantitative assessment of para-osteo-arthropathy and its maturation of senal radionuclide bone images. *Radiology* 1977;123:217–221.

73. Subbarao JV, Nemchausky BA, Gratzer M. Resection of heterotopic ossification and Didronel therapy—regaining wheelchair independence in the spinal cord injured patient. *J Am Paraplegia Soc* 1987;10:3–7.

74. Vento JA, Sziklas JJ, Spencer RP, Rosenberg RJ. "Reactivation" of (Tc 99m MDP) uptake in heterotopic bone. *Clin Nucl Med* 1985;10:206–207.

75. Finerman GAM, Stover SL. Heterotopic ossification following hip replacement or spinal cord injury. Two clinical studies with EHDP. *Metab Bone Dis Rel Res* 1981;4,5:337–342.

76. Bressler E, Marn C, Gore R, Hendrix R. Evaluation of ectopic bone by CT. *AJR Am J Roentgenol* 1987;148:931–935.

77. Rossier AB, Bussat P, Infante F, et al. Current facts on para-osteo-arthropathy (POA). *Paraplegia* 1978;11:36–78.

78. Van der Linden AJ. Spontaneous regression of neurogenic heterotopic ossification. *Int Orthop* 1984;8:25–27.

79. Garland DE, Betzabe A, Venos KG, Vogt JC. Diphosphonate treatment for heterotopic ossification in spinal cord injury patients. *Clin Orthop* 1983;176:197–200.

80. Meade S, Cain HD, Kelly RE, Liebgold H. Periarticular calcification in paraplegics: attempted treatment with disodium edetate. *Paraplegia* 1963;1:62–68.

81. Stover SL, Hahan HR, Miller JM III. Disodium etidronate in the prevention of heterotopic ossification following spinal cord injury (preliminary report). *Paraplegia* 1976;14:146–156.

82. Stover SL, Niemann KMW, Miller JM III. Disodium etidronate in the prevention of postoperative recurrence of heterotopic ossification in spinal cord injury

patients. *J Bone Joint Surg [Am]* 1976;58:683–688.

83. Spielman G, Gennarelli TA, Rogers CR. Disodium etidronate: its role in preventing heterotopic ossification in severe head injury. *Arch Phys Med Rehabil* 1983; 64:539–542.

84. Thomas BJ. Heterotopic bone formation after total hip arthoplasty. *Orthop Clin North Am* 1992; 23:347–358.

85. Ritter MA. Indomethacin: in adjunct to surgical excision of immature heterotopic bone formation in a patient with a severe head injury. *Orthopedics* 1987; 10:1379–1381.

86. Garland DE, Razza BE, Waters RL. Forceful joint manipulation in head-injured adults with heterotopic ossification. *Clin Orthop* 1982;169:133–138.

87. Biering-Sorenson F, Tondevold E. Indomethacin and disodium etidronate for the prevention of recurrence of heterotopic ossification after surgical resection: two case reports. *Paraplegia* 1993;31:513–515.

88. Gebuhr P, Sletgard J, Dalsgard J, et al. Heterotopic ossification after hip arthroplasty: a randomized double-blind multicenter study tenoxicam in 147 hips. *Acta Orthop Scand* 1996;67:29–32.

89. Burssens A, Thiery J, Kohl P, et al. Prevention of heterotopic ossification with tenoxicam following total hip arthroplasty: a double-blind, placebo-controlled dose-finding study. *Acta Orthop Belg* 1995;61:205–211.

90. Buschbacher R, McKinley W, Buschbacher L, et al. Warfarin in prevention of heterotopic ossification. *Am J Phys Med Rehabil* 1992;71:86–91.

91. Elmstedt E, Lindholm TS, Nilsson OS, Tornkvist H. Effect of ibuprofen on heterotopic ossification after total hip replacement. *Acta Orthop Scand* 1985;56:25–27.

92. Ahrengart L, Lindgren U, Reinholt FP. Comparative study of the effects of radiation, indomethacin, prednisolone, and ethane-1-hydroxy-1,1-diphosphonate (EHDP) in the prevention of ectopic bone formation. *Clin Orthop* 1988; 229–265.

93. Fingerroth RJ, Ahmed AQ. Single dose 6GY prophylaxis for heterotopic ossification after total hip arthroplasty. *Clin Orthop* 1995;317:131–140.

94. Pritchett JW. Ketorolac prophylaxis against heterotopic ossification after hip replacement. *Clin Orthop* 1995;314:162–165.

95. Gebuhr P, Wilbek H, Soelberg M. Naproxen for 8 days can prevent heterotopic ossification after hip arthroplasty. *Clin Orthop* 1995;314:166–169.

96. Guillemin F, Maindard D, Rolland H, Delagoutte JP. Antivitamin K prevents heterotopic ossification after hip arthroplasty in diffuse idiopathic skeletal hyperostosis: a retrospective study in 67 patients. *Acta Orthop Scand* 1995;66:123–126.

97. Kjaersgaard-Andersen P, Nafei A, Teichert G, et al. Indomethacin for prevention of heterotopic ossification: a randomized controlled study in 41 hip arthroplasties. *Acta Orthop Scand* 1993;64:639–642.

98. Kjaersgaard-Andersen P, Schmidt SA. Indomethacin for prevention of ectopic ossification after hip arthroplasty. *Acta Orthop Scand* 1986;57:12–14.

99. Kjaersgaard-Andersen P, Schmidt SA. Total hip arthoplasty: the role of anti-inflammatory medications in the prevention of heterotopic ossification. *Clin Orthop* 1991;263:78–86.

100. Russell RG, Smith R, Diphosphonates—experimental and clinical aspects. *J Bone Joint Surg [Br]* 1973;55:66–86.

101. MacLennan L, Keys HM, Evarts CM, Rubin P. Usefulness of post-operative hip irradiation in the prevention of heterotopic bone formation in a high risk group of patients. *Int J Radiat Oncol Biol Phys* 1984;10:49–53.

102. Nilsson OS, Bauer HCF, Brosjo O, Tornkvist H. Influence of indomethacin on induced heterotopic bone formation in rats: importance of length of treatment and of age. *Clin Orthop Related Res* 1986;207:239–245.

103. Vane JR. Inhibition of prostaglandin synthesis as a mechanism of action for aspirin-like drugs. *Nature* 1971;231:232–235.

104. Spielman G, Gennarelli TA, Rogers CR. Disodium etidronate: its role in preventing heterotopic ossification in severe head injury. *Arch Phys Med Rehabil* 1983;64:539–542.

105. Fleisch H. Diphosphonates: history and mechanisms of action. *Metab Bone Dis Related Res* 1981;3:279–287.

106. Nollen AJG. Effect of ethylhydroxydiphosphonate (EHDP) on heterotopic ossification. *Acta Orthop Scand* 1986;57:358–361.

107. Lindholm TS, Bauer FC, Rindell K. High doses of the diphosphonate EHDP for the prevention of heterotopic ossification: an experimental and clinical study. *Scand J Rheumatol* 1987;16:33–39.

108. Flora L, Hassing GS, Cloyd GG, et al. The long-term skeletal effects of EHDP in dogs. *J Bone Joint Surg* 1981;3:289.

109. Banovac K, Gonzalez F, Wade N, Bowker JJ. Intravenous disodium etidronate therapy in spinal cord injury patients with heterotopic ossification. *Paraplegia* 1993;31:660–666.

110. Ayers D, Pellegrini VD, McCollister EC. Prevention of HO in high risk patients by radiation. *Clin Orthop* 1991;263:87–93.

111. Spry NA, Dally MJ, Benjamin B, et al. Heterotopic bone formation affecting the hip joint is preventable in high risk patients by post-operative radiation. *Australas Radiol* 1995;39:379–383.

112. Healy WL, Lo TC, DeSimone AA, et al. Single-dose irradiation for the prevention of heterotopic ossification after total hip arthro-

plasty. A comparison of doses of five hundred and fifty and seven hundred centigray. *J Bone Joint Surg* [*Am*] 1995;77:590–595.

113. Pellegrini VD Jr, Gregoritch SJ. Preoperative irradiation for prevention of heterotopic ossification following total hip arthroplasty. *J Bone Joint Surg* [*Br*] 1996;78:870–881.

114. Seegenschmiedt MH, Martus P, Goldmann AR, et al. Preoperative versus postoperative radiotherapy for prevention of heterotopic ossification (HO): first results of a randomized trial in high-risk patients. *Int J Radiat Oncol Biol Phys* 1994;30:63–73.

115. Schaeffer MA, Sosner J. Heterotopic ossification: treatment of established bone with radiation therapy. *Arch Phys Med Rehabil* 1995;76:284–286.

116. Subbarao JV. Pseudoarthrosis in heterotopic ossification in spinal cord-injured patients. *J Phys Med Rehabil* 1990;69:88–90.

117. An HS, Ebraheim N, Kim K, et al. Heterotopic ossification and pseudoarthrosis in the shoulder following encephalitis. *Clin Orthop* 1987;219:291–298.

118. Hastings H II, Graham TJ. The classification and treatment of heterotopic ossification about the elbow and forearm. *Hand Clin* 1994;10:417–437.

119. Wainapel SF, Rao PU, Schepsis AA. Ulnar nerve compression by heterotopic ossification in a head injured patient. *Arch Phys Med Rehabil* 1985;66: 512–514.

120. Armstrong-Ressy CT, Weiss AA, Ebel A. Results of surgical treatment of extraosseous ossifications in spinal cord injuries. *Proc Annu Clin Paraplegia Conf* 1957;6:22.

121. Stover SL, Niemann KMW, Tulloss JR. Experience with surgical resection of heterotopic bone in spinal cord injury patients. *Clin Orthop* 1991; 263:71–77.

122. Moore TJ. Functional outcome following surgical excision of heterotopic ossification in patients with traumatic brain injury. *J Orthop Trauma* 1993;7: 11–14.

123. Roberts JB, Pankratz DG. The surgical treatment of heterotopic ossification at the elbow following long-term coma. *J Bone Joint Surg* [*Am*] 1979;61: 760–763.

124. Frischhut B, Stockhammer G, Saltuari L, et al. Early removal of periarticular ossification in patients with head injury. *Acta Neurol* 1993;15:114–122.

Chapter 54

Vision Impairment and Blindness

Stanley F. Wainapel

A PHYSIATRIC PERSPECTIVE ON VISION IMPAIRMENT

In 1991 more than 3 million Americans had survived a cerebrovascular accident (CVA) and were living with varying degrees of residual neurologic or functional deficits (1). At about the same time, another survey found that almost 4.3 million Americans were experiencing visual impairment sufficiently severe to prevent them from reading ordinary newspaper print despite the use of corrective lenses (2). Given the high prevalence of disabilities due to CVA, it is not surprising to find that stroke rehabilitation occupies its own chapter in this book, as it has in all previously published general rehabilitation medicine texts. What is surprising is that visual impairment and blindness—even more prevalent disorders—have been almost totally overlooked in these texts (3) as well as in the rehabilitation medicine literature (4,5).

There is considerable irony in the relative neglect of vision rehabilitation by physiatrists, for history confirms the close links between rehabilitation medicine and vision rehabilitation: The first civilian vision rehabilitation program was established at the Veterans Administration Hospital in Hines, Illinois, within its Rehabilitation Medicine Department (6). Such a close association is understandable given the simultaneous impetus to vision and medical rehabilitation provided by the injuries sustained by the soldiers during World War II. The blind veteran, the amputee veteran, and the paraplegic veteran all posed formidable challenges to the postwar medical and social service systems. The shared roots of vision rehabilitation and rehabilitation medicine are manifested in their structural similarities:

1. A focus on function rather than disease
2. Attention to psychosocial and vocational dimensions
3. An interdisciplinary approach to treatment using a team of specially trained professionals

The analogies go even deeper, however: The orientation and mobility instructor is comparable to the physical therapist; the rehabilitation teacher is comparable to the occupational therapist; low-vision enhancement techniques correspond to orthotics; and substitutes for lost vision (e.g., Braille, guide dog) correspond to prosthetics.

There are several compelling reasons for physiatrists to become increasingly familiar with the special problems associated with vision impairment and blindness. On the most basic level, this loss of vision is a commonly encountered cause of disability and handicap in its own right. Isolated vision impairment results in significant deficits in basic and instrumental activities of daily living (ADLs) as well as declines in social function (Table 54-1) (7–10). Moreover, loss of vision is a significant risk factor for falls (11,12). Felson et al (13) demonstrated this dramatically using data from the Framingham Eye Study, finding a markedly increased prevalence of hip fractures among visually impaired older persons (Table 54-2). Since vision loss is more common with advancing age, the physiatrist is

Table 54-1: Effects of Vision and/or Hearing Loss on Self-Care

	VA-HA (*n* = 948) (%)	VA-HI (*n* = 106) (%)	VI-HA (*n* = 118) (%)	VI-HI (*n* = 20) (%)	x^2
Sex					
Men	308 (32.4)	44 (41.5)	24 (20.4)	9 (45.0)	13.3**
Women	640 (67.6)	62 (58.5)	94 (79.6)	11 (55.0)	
Years of schooling					
<3	601 (63.4)	72 (67.9)	85 (72.0)	16 (80.0)	6.0
>3	347 (36.6)	34 (32.1)	33 (28.0)	4 (20.0)	
Financial status					
Good	198 (20.8)	19 (18.0)	17 (14.4)	1 (5.0)	6.6
Sufficient	424 (44.7)	46 (43.3)	54 (45.7)	11 (55.0)	
Insufficient	326 (34.5)	41 (38.7)	47 (39.8)	8 (40.0)	
Mood (mBDI)					
Normal (<22)	677 (71.4)	60 (56.7)	57 (48.3)	9 (45.0)	
Low (23–44)	224 (23.7)	37 (34.9)	49 (41.5)	6 (30.0)	45.7***
Very low (45–66)	47 (4.9)	9 (8.4)	12 (10.2)	5 (25.0)	
Self-sufficiency (IADL):					
Dependent (>1)	87 (9.2)	22 (20.8)	21 (17.1)	6 (30.0)	
Indep. (0–1)	861 (90.8)	84 (79.2)	97 (82.9)	14 (70.0)	25.4***
Cognition (MSQ)					
Impaired (>2)	28 (3.0)	5 (4.7)	6 (5.1)	3 (15.0)	
Not imp. (0–2)	920 (97.0)	101 (95.3)	112 (94.9)	17 (85.0)	9.9*
Social relationships (self)					
Low (<12)	237 (25.0)	36 (34.0)	57 (48.4)	10 (50.0)	
Middle (13–24)	464 (48.9)	54 (50.9)	44 (37.2)	7 (35.0)	38.9***
High (25–36)	247 (26.1)	16 (15.1)	17 (14.4)	3 (15.0)	
Physical health status					
Good (5)	648 (68.3)	69 (65.1)	83 (70.3)	11 (55.0)	
Border (6–10)	263 (27.7)	32 (30.2)	25 (21.2)	8 (40.0)	8.8
Poor (11–20)	37 (4.0)	5 (4.7)	10 (8.5)	1 (5.0)	
Sick days in bed					
None	821 (86.6)	89 (84.0)	96 (81.4)	15 (75.0)	
1–7	73 (7.7)	11 (10.4)	11 (9.3)	4 (20.0)	8.4
8–14	24 (2.5)	3 (2.8)	4 (3.3)	0 (0.0)	
>15	30 (3.2)	3 (2.8)	7 (6.0)	1 (5.0)	

VA = Adequate visual function; HA = Adequate hearing function; VI = Visual impairment; HI = Hearing impairment. Financial status and housing conditions are self-rated. Numbers in brackets are percentage for each group. *P < 0.05; **P < 0.01; ***P < 0.001.
Source: Carabellese C, Appollonio I, Rozzini R, et al. Sensory impairment and quality of life in community elderly population. *J Am Geriatr Soc* 1993;41:401–407. Reprinted by permission of the American Geriatrics Society.

particularly likely to encounter patients with combined visual and neuromusculoskeletal disabilities such as the blind stroke patient (14) or the blind amputee (15). The frequency of such combinations is confirmed by a 1989 retrospective survey of 191 consecutive admissions to a rehabilitation medicine unit, 7.0% of which involved patients with severe visual impairments in addition to other nonvisual disabilities (16). Finally, the advent of managed care makes it more necessary for physiatrists to conceptualize their specialty as a component of primary care for persons with disabilities, and it would be difficult to support such a concept unless its practitioners are aware of vision rehabilitation services and at least able to give their patients access to them. This chapter does not emulate the comprehensive overview of vision rehabilitation found in full-length volumes such as those by Faye (17) or Walsh and Blasch (18), but it should provide a conceptual and practical framework for those unfamiliar with this subject.

CLASSIFICATIONS, CAUSES, AND CONSEQUENCES OF VISION IMPAIRMENT

It is a widely held misconception that vision loss is synonymous with total blindness. The reality is that most visually impaired individuals have at least some degree of useful residual sight, even if limited to perception of light, shadows, or movement. Classification of the degree of vision loss requires a formal assessment of visual acuity (using a standardized Snellen-type eye chart) and visual fields (using manual or computerized perimetry). Based on these test results, two critical levels of vision impairment can be identified:

Table 54-2: Association of Vision Impairment and Risk of Hip Fracture

Visual Acuity	Cumulative Incidence Rate of Hip Fracture (%)	Unadjusted RR (95% CI)*	Multivariate Adjusted RR (95% CI)*
Good vision both eyes	63/2131 (3.0%)	1.00	1.00
Any impaired vision in either eye	47/502 (9.4%)	3.28 (2.25–4.79)	1.73 (1.13–2.65)
Moderately impaired vision in at least one eye	29/342 (8.5%)	2.95 (1.90–4.58)	1.54 (0.95–2.49)
Good eye—Moderate eye	19/215 (8.8%)	3.08 (1.84–5.15)	1.94 (1.13–3.22)
Moderate eye—Moderate eye	10/127 (7.9%)	2.73 (1.40–5.32)	1.11 (0.55–2.24)
Poor vision in at least one eye	18/160 (11.3%)	4.01† (1.61–6.78)	2.17† (1.24–3.80)
Good eye—Poor eye	5/89 (5.6%)	1.92 (0.77–4.78)	1.50 (0.60–3.75)
Moderate eye—Poor eye	9/44 (20.5%)	7.78 (3.87–15.64)	2.82 (1.33–5.96)
Poor eye—Poor eye	4/27 (14.8%)	5.49 (2.00–15.07)	2.46 (0.87–6.99)

* Results of Cox models with unadjusted model testing vision as sole predictor of hip fracture and multivariate model adjusted for age, sex, Metropolitan Relative Weight, alcohol use, and, in women, estrogen use.

† Test for linear trend (good—good; moderate impairment in at least one eye; poor vision in at least one eye), $P < 0.01$.

Source: Felson D, Anderson JJ, Hannan MT, et al. Impaired vision and hip fracture: the Framingham study. *J Am Geriatr Soc* 1989; 37:495–500. Reprinted with permission of the American Geriatrics Society.

1. *Legal blindness*: corrected visual acuity of less than 20/200 in the better eye, or visual field of 20 degrees or less in the better eye
2. *Low vision*: corrected visual acuity between 20/70 and 20/200, or visual field of over 20 degrees in the better eye

Although these definitions are to some extent arbitrary and exclude a considerable variety of significant eye problems such as monocular blindness, diplopia, and loss of color vision, they are important for the physiatrist in terms of entitlement for services as well as functional implications. Legal blindness was defined by the Social Security Act of 1935 and is widely utilized as the benchmark for entitling a person to receive formal vision rehabilitation services from specialized state agencies for the blind or visually impaired. Low-vision acuity deficits correspond to the inability to read ordinary-size newsprint, which translates functionally into a significant reading disability. Greater degrees of visual loss are usually described in terms other than acuity or field measurements, for example, finger counting, hand movement, and light perception.

Visual deficits can be more clearly classified into those that affect acuity and those that affect visual fields. Acuity deficits may be discrete, in which case they are labeled *scotomas*, or they may be diffuse, as would be produced by cataracts. Visual field deficits are either central or peripheral in type; the former is characteristic of macular degeneration while the latter is characteristic of glaucoma or retinitis pigmentosa. These distinctions are illustrated in Figures 54-1, 54-2, and 54-3, which present a simulation of the visual losses associated with diabetic retinopathy (multiple scotomas), retinitis pigmentosa (tunnel vision), and age-related macular degeneration (loss of central vision), respectively. These photographs explain the different functional consequences of such disorders: Tunnel vision impacts on mobility without undue restriction of reading or facial recognition, while central vision loss produces precisely the opposite effects.

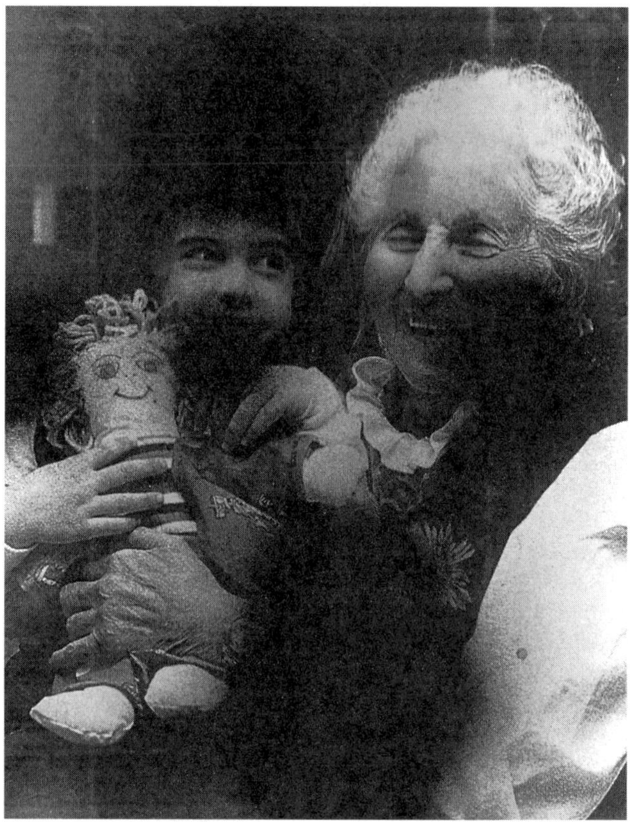

Figure 54-1. Visual consequences of diabetic retinopathy. (Photograph Courtesy of the Jewish Guild for the Blind.)

The most frequently encountered etiologies for vision impairment or blindness vary with age. Among children

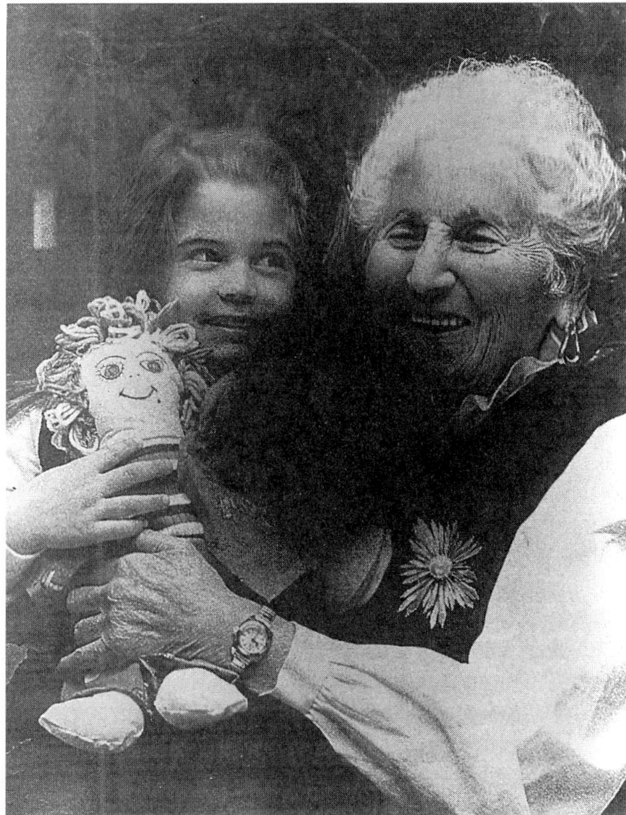

Figure 54-2. Visual consequences of macular degeneration. (Photograph Courtesy of the Jewish Guild for the Blind.)

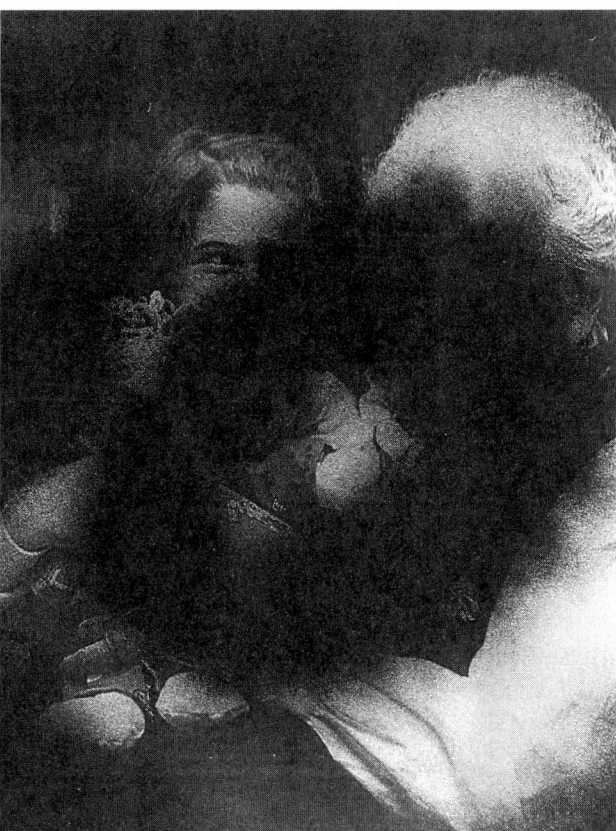

Figure 54-3. Visual consequences of glaucoma. (Photograph Courtesy of the Jewish Guild for the Blind.)

and young adults, retinopathy of prematurity, congenital cataract, and retinitis pigmentosa are frequent causes, although they remain relatively uncommon causes of disability overall. In middle-aged adults, diabetic retinopathy is the most common cause of blindness, and it remains a significant cause of vision impairment in the older adult as well. Vision impairment progressively increases in proportion to age, and by the age of 85 or older its prevalence has reached 27% (19). Geriatric patients comprise about two-thirds of the total population with vision impairment (2), and in the great majority of them, the cause is one of the following: cataracts, age-related macular degeneration, glaucoma, or diabetic retinopathy (20). Additional etiologic factors that should be of significance in physiatric practice are the optic neuritis associated with multiple sclerosis and the visual deficits associated with CVAs or traumatic brain injury.

PHYSIATRIC ASSESSMENT AND REFERRAL TO VISION REHABILITATION SERVICES

Until vision loss is severe or total, it can often be difficult to detect unless it is specifically sought out by history and physical examination. A particularly high index of suspicion should be maintained by the physiatrist when evaluating elderly patients who may be presenting other more visible disabilities. It is not sufficient to inquire whether the patient has any eye diseases; the more significant question to ask is whether there is difficulty of function associated with vision problems, such as difficulty in reading, identifying faces, ambulating, or performing normal daily activities. The physical examination should include a screening for visual acuity and gross visual field testing. It should also be remembered that along with vestibular function and proprioception, vision is one of the major factors required for normal upright stance (21), and thus must be considered whenever a patient has problems of balance or falling. Extraocular movements should be assessed with particular care in patients with suspected multiple sclerosis or brain stem strokes, both of which can produce disabling diplopia.

More detailed evaluation of visually impaired patients involves the participation of an ophthalmologist or optometrist, either of whom can clarify the degree of visual loss and treatment options. Additionally, these professionals can provide written certification of the patient's eligibility for formal vision rehabilitation services if he or she meets the criteria for legal blindness. In such cases, the state agency serving this population assigns a social worker or rehabilitation counselor to coordinate rehabilitation services. These services can include any of the following:

1. Orientation and mobility instructor: assists in teaching special ambulation techniques such as the use of the long white cane, guide dog, electronic vision devices, and sighted guide technique
2. Rehabilitation teacher: instructs the patient in special techniques required for daily activities and recommends special devices to assist in these tasks
3. Low-vision assessment: specialized evaluation by a trained optometrist who will prescribe low-vision devices that enhance or substitute for lost vision
4. Social worker: assists the patient in coping with vision loss, its associated emotional stresses, and the social changes it produces
5. Rehabilitation counselor: provides evaluation and assistance in educational and vocational activities

The similarity between the medical and the vision rehabilitation systems was already emphasized at the outset of this chapter, but the disparities between these systems need to be highlighted as well. Vision rehabilitation is much less medically oriented and is performed at facilities separate from the hospitals, clinics, or offices that provide medical rehabilitation. Funding sources are similarly distinct, with vision rehabilitation being paid mainly from budgets controlled by the specific state agency for the blind and visually impaired. Such funds have traditionally favored young vocational or educational candidates at the expense of older individuals, who form the majority of the visually impaired population. However, Massof et al (22) have begun to bridge the fiscal gap between medical and vision rehabilitation by proposing a service model in which vision care services would be reimbursed by Medicare as part of a medical rehabilitative paradigm. This proposed fusion of systems highlights the need for greater knowledge by physiatrists about the principles of vision rehabilitation.

BASIC PRINCIPLES OF VISION REHABILITATION

Vision rehabilitation techniques can be divided into two basic components. *Vision enhancement* involves devices or strategies that maximize residual visual function. *Vision substitution* goes a step farther by providing an alternative to total or near-total vision loss. Table 54-3 outlines the 10 primary components of vision rehabilitation; note that the five vision enhancement techniques start with the consecutive letters E through I, and the five vision substitution techniques start with the consecutive letters S through W.

Table 54-3: Ten Basic Strategies for Vision Rehabilitation

Enhancement of residual vision
*E*nlargement of image
*F*ield expansion
*G*lare reduction
*H*eightened contrast
*I*llumination
Substitution for lost vision
*S*elf-care activities
*T*actile substitution
*U*ltrasonic mobility devices
*V*ocal substitution
*W*alking devices

Vision Enhancement

Enlargement

There are numerous methods to provide varying degrees of image enlargement for visually impaired individuals. By far the most ubiquitous are prescription spectacles or contact lenses, which may be all that is required to normalize sight. When greater amounts of magnification are required, however, these are supplemented by a variety of low-vision aids whose appropriate prescription is usually provided by optometrists. Magnifiers come in a sometimes bewildering number of shapes and sizes. Figure 54-4 illustrates several of these: the plastic reading bar, the traditional magnifying glass, and the more recently developed halogen illuminated stand magnifier. The latter has the advantage of leaving the hands free, avoiding problems associated with arthritis or movement disorders such as Parkinson disease, and allowing for a fixed focal length. As will be mentioned later, the addition of illumination gives even greater enhancement to impaired vision. Monocular (Fig. 54-5) or binocular spectacle-mounted telescopic magnifiers are less frequently prescribed and used. They may be helpful as hand-held devices to read street names when a visually impaired person is walking in an unfamiliar environment.

The magnifiers and telescopes discussed have the advantage of relatively low cost and a high degree of portability, but they also have the disadvantage of relatively limited magnification capacity and of producing rapid visual fatigue in the user. The closed-circuit television (CCTV) videomagnifier (Fig. 54-6) eliminates much of this fatigue by heightening contrast through image reversal, and it has the capacity to enlarge images anywhere between 3 and 60 times the normal size, making it valuable for individuals with very poor central acuity. On the other hand, it is relatively large and rather expensive. Smaller portable models have been developed in recent years. It is worth noting that some CCTV devices have been reimbursed under Medicare, albeit after considerable efforts and written appeals.

A much simpler approach to magnification is the use of enlarged print for books, periodicals, and computer screens. The *New York Times* and *Readers Digest*, among others, have large-print editions, and large-print books have become increasingly popular, particularly with older readers. Many computer programs have the capacity for print enlargement, and several specialized software packages are available.

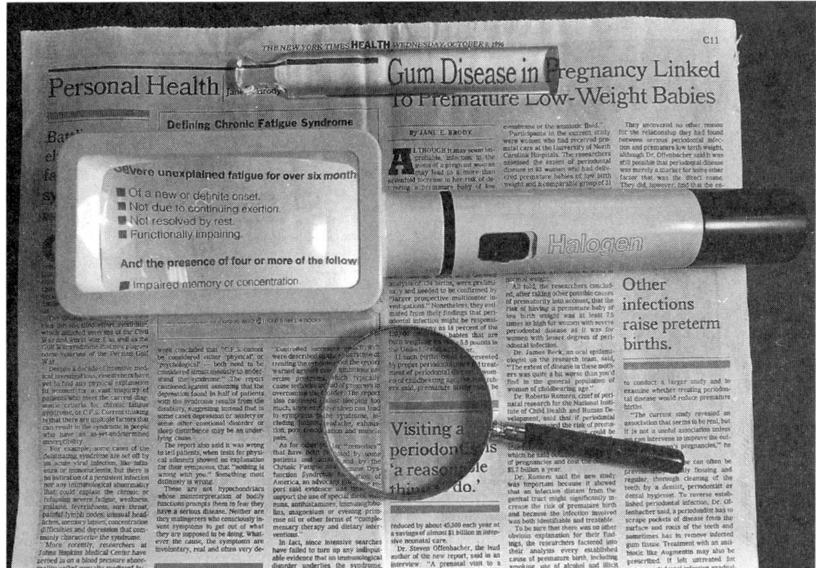

Figure 54-4. Hand-held and stand magnifiers.

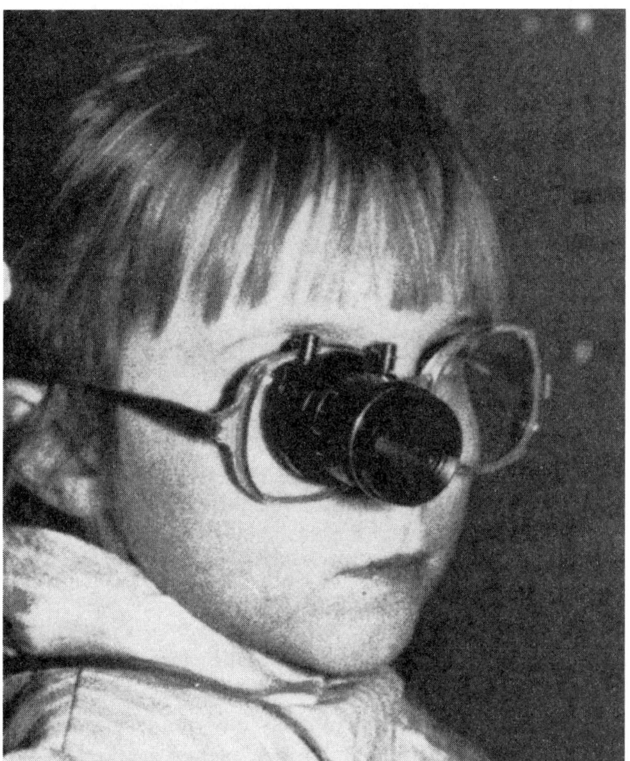

Figure 54-5. Monocular telescope mounted on glasses for reading. (Photograph Courtesy of Resources for Rehabilitation, Lexington, MA.)

Field Expansion

Visual field deficits such as hemianopsia and tunnel vision resulting from glaucoma or retinitis pigmentosa can produce significant problems with mobility. Mirrors or Fresnel prisms have been used to shift vision from the affected to the unaffected visual field in brain-injured individuals with associated homonymous hemianopsia. These devices presume a sufficient degree of cognitive and perceptual ability to allow for the integration of these transferred images into a coherent environmental gestalt. Similar techniques have been applied to the central visual loss associated with age-related macular degeneration. The contracted visual fields associated with glaucoma or retinitis pigmentosa can be expanded by the relatively simple and inexpensive expedient of reversing a pair of binoculars or opera glasses, although this can also be accomplished with spectacle-mounted prisms. The major disadvantage of this approach is that it makes the image appear much smaller and farther away from the patient, which requires a significant readjustment by the user (23).

An often-overlooked intrinsic form of field expansion is the technique of eccentric fixation and viewing, which can be learned and used effectively by patients with macular degeneration or other conditions that impair central vision. This method requires considerable practice and must be done under the close supervision of a trained optometrist (24).

Glare Reduction, Heightened Contrast, and Illumination

Magnification and field expansion form the twin pillars of low-vision rehabilitation, but they are primarily directed toward the remediation of deficits due to intrinsic eye disease. They are supplemented by a triad of factors that are externally generated by the environment rather than the eyes. Eliminating these factors or reducing them to a more tolerable level greatly improves visual function. The physiologic changes that accompany the aging process, such as nuclear sclerosis, pupillary constriction, and reduced color sensitivity (25) make these factors particularly problematic among older adults with cataract or macular degeneration.

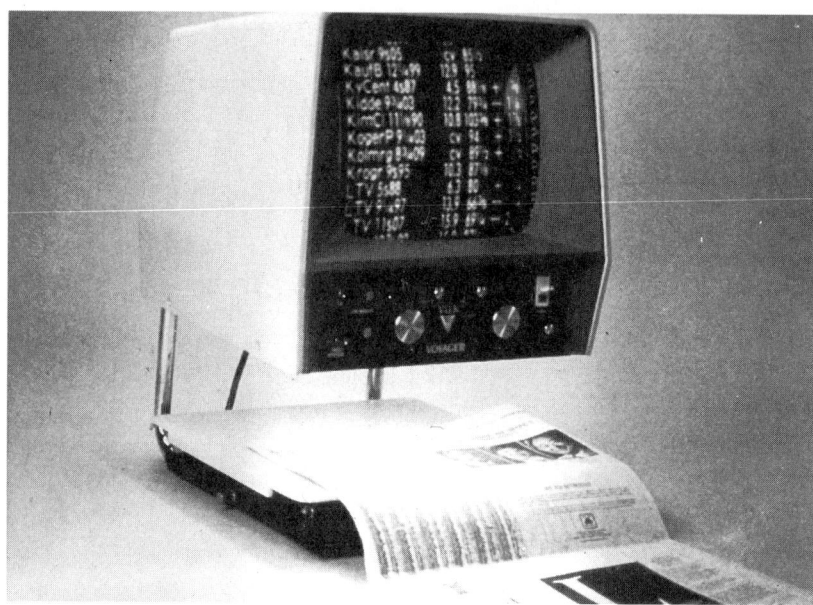

Figure 54-6. Closed-circuit television (CCTV) videomagnifier with reversal image. (Photograph Courtesy of Resources for Rehabilitation, Lexington, MA.)

Heightened glare sensitivity is exacerbated by sunlight or poorly located artificial illumination. Sunglasses, especially those that selectively block the blue part of the visible spectrum, are useful, but the precise shade or color to be used must be carefully chosen so that adequate light reaches the retina. A hat with a broad brim or a visor will reduce glare from light sources above the patient without interfering with color perception and can markedly reduce visual fatigue. Magazines or books with high-gloss pages will produce glare problems for the reader; a clear photocopy of the desired pages can eliminate this problem but is impractical when dealing with multiple pages. The image-reversal feature found with the CCTV is useful in this respect but entails considerable additional expense.

Contrast and glare problems frequently coexist, as in the glossy white magazine page with relatively thin black print, but they also occur in the environment by virtue of poorly chosen colors in public spaces. An unfortunately all-too common example is the typical hospital or nursing home corridor that presents a shiny floor whose color is almost identical with that of the walls. A greater awareness by architects and developers of health care facilities is necessary to avoid such faulty environmental planning (26).

Simple devices and techniques can greatly heighten contrast and therefore improve impaired visual function. Bold writing pens or felt-tipped ones make writing easier to decipher, and paper with thicker lines is also helpful. A common and inexpensive assistive device is the typoscope (Fig. 54-7), a piece of black material with apertures cut into it that direct the visually impaired user to the correct place for writing checks, addressing envelopes, or writing letters (27). Every physician who has attended a lecture can appreciate the contrast enhancement obtained by using 35-mm slides with white writing on a black background, as well as the users of computers who change the color display on their monitors for maximal contrast.

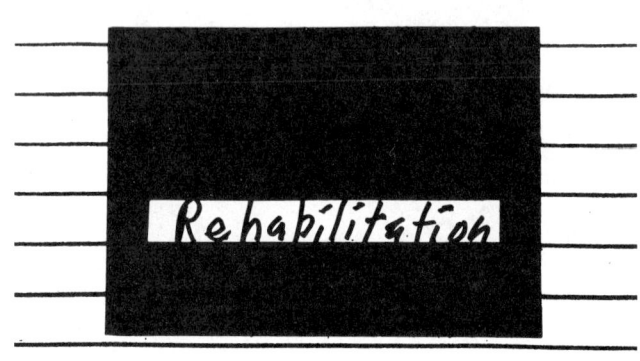

Figure 54-7. Typoscope, heavy line paper, and bold writing pen for heightened contrast.

Adequacy of illumination is the sine qua non of vision enhancement. Unfortunately it is often overlooked by physicians, patients, and planners of health care facilities, not to mention restauranteurs or hoteliers. A simple incandescent light that can be adjusted in distance and direction is probably the most important low-vision aid. Halogen and fluorescent lighting have their advantages, but the former can seem too harsh and the latter may produce glare or visual fatigue. Full-spectrum halogen and fluorescent bulbs that simulate natural sunlight are currently available.

Vision Substitution

When all the above-mentioned vision enhancement techniques do not suffice for the visually impaired patient, substitutes for vision loss must be considered. It should not be construed that these are only applicable to the totally blind person, however, for many are used by individuals with some residual sight.

Self-Care Techniques

The rehabilitation teacher in the vision rehabilitation system corresponds to the occupational therapist, focusing on the performance of ADLs. Vision loss interferes with many of these ADLs, including kitchen activities, shopping, grooming, and dressing. Labeling kitchen appliances with raised-dot markings can allow safer use of the stove, oven, and toaster. Braille (see below) can be used to label cans or packages for easier retrieval. Dollar-bill denominations can be identified if they are folded in different patterns prior to placing them in a wallet or pocketbook. Clothing identification is facilitated by Braille labels or other tactile cues (e.g., embossed letters for specific colors, geometric shape hung on a shirt with stripes). The rehabilitation teacher will frequently do a home visit as part of the evaluation process and recommend environmental modifications that will enhance safety or independence.

Tactile Substitution

It is a common misconception that blind people have extraordinary tactile sensitivity. The truth is that they have to become increasingly dependent on touch and therefore attend to tactile stimuli more thoroughly than the normally sighted individual. A number of important techniques and devices make use of this fact. Braille is a tactile language that utilizes raised dots in patterns based on a six-dot "cell" that can be perceived by the fingers after a period of study. Grade I Braille includes symbols for all letters and numbers as well as punctuation marks. It is generally used for labeling and is easier to master than the more complex grade II Braille, which has more than 250 symbols for letter combinations as well as individual letters, and is the main format for books or computer output. Older persons and those with sensory or coordination problems in the hands (e.g., neuropathy, cerebellar disease, multiple sclerosis) may find it difficult or impossible to use or even learn Braille, but younger persons may become extremely fluent with it. Another tactile technique is the Optacon, a device that converts written material or diagrams into vibrations that are felt with the fingers. With the Optacon, it is possible for a blind physician to "read" electrocardiograms, for instance (28). A less complex use of tactile ability involves placing raised dots at key locations on kitchen dials, permitting a blind person to set the oven or toaster to appropriate levels.

Ultrasonic Travel Aids

Sonic devices have been employed by blind individuals to improve their mobility and as adjuncts to the more commonly used white cane or guide dog (18,29). The Pathsounder is hung around the neck and is especially helpful for blind persons in wheelchairs. Its stationary position limits its use to providing warnings about upcoming objects directly ahead of the user. The Mowat Sensor is held in the hand and thus can be moved to face different directions; it has been mounted on a walkerette for patients with combinations of neuromusculoskeletal and visual deficits (29). The Sonic Guide is the most sophisticated of these devices; it is mounted on a pair of glasses and provides lateralized cues about upcoming objects by producing sounds in the appropriate ear.

Vocal Substitution

One of the most ubiquitous and valuable vision substitution options involves the use of verbal output via recorded material or synthetic speech. Recorded books and magazines are widely available through the Talking Books program of the Library of Congress, giving the print-disabled individual (dyslexia also qualifies for inclusion in the program) access to an enormous quantity of superbly read literature in a convenient four-track cassette format that is mailed to the user free of charge. Recordings for the Blind and Dyslexic (Princeton, NJ) has more than 75,000 recorded books that complement the Talking Books program by including many textbooks that should be invaluable for visually impaired students. Commercial recorded books have become increasingly popular in recent years and are found in bookstores as well as libraries. The American Printing House for the Blind (Lexington, KY) distributes cassette recordings of *Readers Digest* and *Newsweek* magazines at no charge. A specially adapted recorder is required to accommodate the extra-slow playing speed ($^{15}/_{16}$ inches/sec) of the cassettes; a large but portable one is given to Talking Books recipients at no charge, and smaller models can be purchased for $150 to $250.

"Talking" technology has been greatly improved with newer types of synthetic speech output. It is now possible to purchase talking watches, thermometers, weight scales, sphygmomanometers, glucometers (for visually impaired diabetics), and calculators. On a more sophisticated level, computers can be modified using synthetic speech software to provide excellent voice output that facilitates computer use by blind individuals who are unable or unwilling to use Braille output. When this technology is combined with a scanner and optical-character recognition (OCR) software, it enables totally blind individuals to read typed or printed matter such as books, magazines, and letters.

Walking Techniques

Ambulation training is supervised by the orientation and mobility instructor, who corresponds to the physical therapist. Ambulation aids and techniques taught by the orientation and mobility instructor include the following:

1. Sighted guide. This refers to the correct manner in which a visually impaired person walks in the company of a sighted person. The former holds

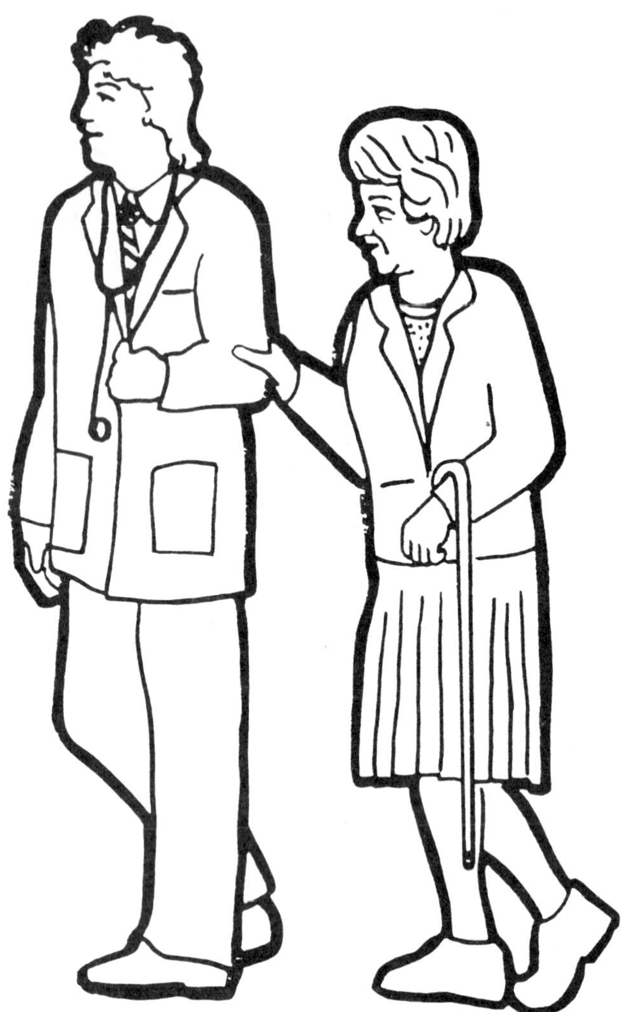

Figure 54-8. Sighted guide technique. (Courtesy of The Lighthouse, Inc., New York, NY.)

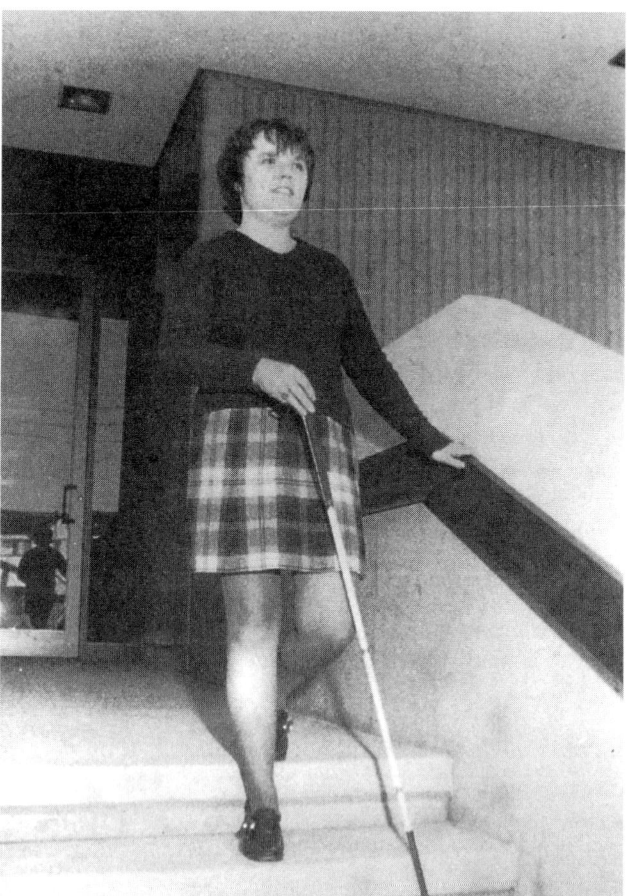

Figure 54-9. Descending stairs using a long white cane. (Reproduced by permission from Cole RG, Rosenthal BP. *Remediation and management of low vision.* St. Louis: Mosby, 1996.)

onto the sighted person's arm just above the elbow and walks a step behind in order to get advance feedback about upcoming changes in terrain or direction. A series of maneuvers and signals have been devised to facilitate walking using this technique, which should be learned by every physician and health care worker who is likely to encounter visually impaired or blind patients (Fig. 54-8).

2. Long white cane. Unlike its shorter counterpart, the long cane is not a support device. It acts as an extension to the visually impaired person's sense of touch and also identifies the user as having a visual impairment. The cane is tapped or swept from left to right in front of the user in a pattern that mimics the alternate two-point crutch gait pattern. With correct training, totally blind persons can be enabled by the long cane to negotiate everyday environmental hazards such as stairs (Fig. 54-9). One of the less desirable aspects of cane use is its function as a stigma symbol (30), causing others to assume that the cane user is totally blind; this can be partly remedied with telescoping or folding canes that can be kept in a less conspicuous place until they are needed for ambulation. The more sophisticated laser cane provides extra information on obstacles at head level and warns of drop-offs up to 12 feet ahead by emitting three laser beams in varying directions and giving audible feedback when obstacles are detected. However, it is more expensive and requires special training, so it has not replaced the standard long white cane as the most common ambulation aid for the blind.

3. Guide dog. The advantages of a guide dog for the blind are many, including security, companionship, and a potentially greater freedom of movement once the dog and the master have established a trusting and efficient working relationship. Accomplishing this involves extensive training of both participants separately and together. Disadvantages must also be considered when determining whether a blind person is an appropriate candidate for a guide dog. The dog needs to be cared for by its owner, including grooming and regular walking as

exercise for the dog. Also, the energy and speed of the dog may make it unsuitable for older or less vigorous patients.

SPECIAL ISSUES FOR THE PHYSIATRIST

The overlap of vision rehabilitation and physiatry creates a number of challenging situations in which the physiatrist's expertise is particularly crucial for successful outcome. These cases clearly highlight the need for a closer integration between the two systems and their practitioners.

Human aging produces multiple system impairments that often link visual and neuromuscular problems. In some cases the link is even causal in type, as with the visually impaired person who falls and sustains a hip fracture (13). More frequently the association is indirect and reflective of simultaneous aging changes in multiple organ systems. A study of 220 consecutive stroke admissions found that 7 patients were also blind or visually impaired, often having their visual loss for years preceding the stroke. Despite their double disability, 4 of these patients returned to their homes, and all but one showed significant benefits in function during their rehabilitation (14). Similarly, in the study by Altner et al (15), 8 of 12 blind amputees became prosthetic users; Fisher (31) reported on two other blind amputees with equally positive results. These data attest to the potential for success in rehabilitating these doubly disabled individuals and should be considered as an antidote to any possible therapeutic nihilism by practitioners who have not encountered such patients.

Prescribing wheelchairs for visually and neuromuscularly impaired individuals is a real challenge to the physiatrist. Visual loss need not be a contraindication to wheelchair use but requires careful consideration and evaluation. One-arm drive chairs allow the concomitant use of a long white cane in the contralateral hand. An ultrasonic mobility device can also be hung over the neck of a wheelchair user who propels the chair with both hands. Motorized wheelchairs for visually impaired patients should have their maximal speed set lower than usual, for greater safety (29,32).

The diabetic patient deserves separate mention since the visual and neuromuscular problems have the same etiology. Additionally, diabetes produces autonomic neuropathy that can have a negative impact on exercise tolerance during rehabilitation. Bernbaum et al (33) evaluated 29 visually impaired diabetic patients in terms of their pulse changes with respiration, blood pressure responses to position changes, and the occurrence of postural hypotension. Twenty-eight subjects had abnormal respiratory pulse variation (parasympathetic neuropathy), 23 had abnormal postural blood pressure responses (sympathetic neuropathy), and 9 developed orthostatic hypotension. The use of seated or recumbent bicycle exercise was recommended. These results are important to keep in mind when one is

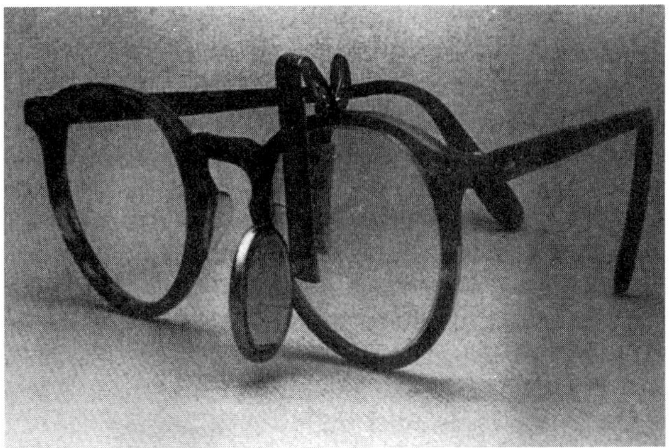

Figure 54-10. Spectacle-mounted mirror for homonymous hemianopsia. (Reproduced by permission from Cole RG, Rosenthal BP. *Remediation and management of low vision.* St. Louis: Mosby, 1996.)

prescribing exercise for diabetic patients, many of whom have rehabilitation problems such as amputations, peripheral neuropathy, or cardiac disease.

Vision problems resulting from acquired brain injury such as CVA and traumatic brain injury are associated with visual sequelae that may adversely affect functional outcome. Although both of these conditions are dealt with in detail elsewhere in this book, it is worth reiterating some of the major aspects of the vision problems likely to be part of the rehabilitation of these patients.

The most frequent visual deficits associated with CVA are homonymous hemianopsia and visual neglect, both of which are most frequently seen after right-sided cerebral damage. Compensatory strategies are taught but these may not be successful in all patients, particularly when there is severe perceptual-motor dysfunction or anosognosia. A mirror mounted on a pair of spectacles (Fig. 54-10) may help to transfer images to the intact portion of the visual field. A recent study (34) suggested that monocular (right eye only) patching plus computer-generated stimulation of the affected visual field may be beneficial.

The visual consequences of traumatic brain injury may be more difficult to document because of the degree of associated cognitive deficits, but they are nonetheless more common than would be recognized unless they are specifically sought out by detailed and often time-consuming optometric evaluation. Gianutsos et al (35) found that 36 of 55 severely head-injured patients had visual problems and that the great majority of these were remediable, and resulting in favorable effects on overall rehabilitation performance.

FUTURE TRENDS IN VISION REHABILITATION

The association between the vision rehabilitation and medical rehabilitation systems, which has strong historical precedents, seems to be experiencing a renaissance in recent years. The optometric literature has increasingly argued in favor of a physiatrically oriented model, with members of the vision rehabilitation team assuming the roles of physical and occupational therapists for visually impaired patients (22). It has also been suggested that Medicare funding sources be tapped through this model, using profound vision loss as a disability diagnosis. Such activities argue strongly for the increased involvement of physiatrists in vision rehabilitation programs. There is a large market and patient source to be found here, and fruitful associations can be forged with optometric and ophthalmologic professionals. There are many research areas to be explored in which the physiatrist's expertise can be invaluable; functional assessment is perhaps the most urgently needed one.

Technology continues to advance at a dizzying pace and vision rehabilitation is no exception. Computer systems have grown increasingly sophisticated and accessible to trained visually impaired individuals. Voice-activated programs promise to extend computer access even to the patient without useful vision or arm function. New challenges are created by the visually oriented format of graphical-user interface, but it is likely that future techniques will overcome even this hurdle. In many ways the greatest obstacle may be the relatively high cost of this technology; however, the Kurzweil Reading Machine, which cost almost $30,000 in the early 1980s, is now available at about one-sixth of the original price. Computer-generated vision enhancement is one of the most exciting prospects for the future, as is the use of computer and satellite tracking for a new level of electronic navigation. These are not science fiction fantasies but are actually in the development stage at this time.

REFERENCES

1. American Heart Association. *Heart and stroke facts: 1994 statistical supplement.* Dallas: American Heart Association, 1993.
2. Nelson KA, Dimitrova E. Severe visual impairment in the United States and in each state, 1990. *J Vis Impairment Blind* 1993;87:80–86.
3. Goodpasture RC. Rehabilitation of the blind. In: Krusen FH, Kottke FJ, Ellwood PM, eds. *Handbook of physical medicine and rehabilitation.* 2nd ed. Philadelphia: WB Saunders, 1971.
4. Lupinacci M. Physiatric management of the visually impaired disabled patient. *Curr Concepts Rehabil Med* 1990;5:6–13.
5. Wainapel SF. Vision rehabilitation: an overlooked subject in physiatric training and practice. *Am J Phys Med Rehabil* 1995;74:313–314.
6. Koestler FA. *The unseen minority: a history of the blind in America.* New York: American Foundation for the Blind, 1976.
7. Carabellese C, Appollonio I, Rozzini R, et al. Sensory impairment and quality of life in community elderly population. *J Am Geriatr Soc* 1993;41:401–407.
8. Branch LG, Horowitz A, Carr C. The implications for everyday life of incident self-reported visual decline among people over age 65 living in the community. *Gerontologist* 1989;29:359–365.
9. Rudberg M, Furner SE, Dunn JE, Cassel CK. The relationship of visual and hearing impairments to disability: an analysis using the Longitudinal Study of Aging. *J Gerontol* 1993;48:M261–M265.
10. Marx MS, Werner P, Cohen-Mansfield J, Feldman R. The relationship between low vision and performance of activities of daily living on nursing home residents. *J Am Geriatr Soc* 1992;40:1018–1020.
11. Tinetti M, Inouye S, Gill T, Doucette J. Shared risk factors for falls, incontinence, and functional dependence. *JAMA* 1995;273:1348–1353.
12. Tobis JS, Block M, Steinhaus-Donham C, et al. Falling among the sensorially impaired elderly. *Arch Phys Med Rehabil* 1990;71:144–147.
13. Felson D, Anderson JJ, Hannan MT, et al. Impaired vision and hip fracture: the Framingham study. *J Am Geriatr Soc* 1989;37:495–500.
14. Wainapel SF. Rehabilitation of the blind stroke patient. *Arch Phys Med Rehabil* 1984;65:487–489.
15. Altner PE, Rusin JJ, DeBoer A. Rehabilitation of blind patients with lower extremity amputations. *Arch Phys Med Rehabil* 1980;61:82–85.
16. Wainapel SF, Kwon YS, Fazzari PJ. Severe visual impairment on a rehabilitation unit: incidence and implications. *Arch Phys Med Rehabil* 1989;70: 439–441.
17. Faye EE. *Clinical low vision.* Boston: Little, Brown, 1984.
18. Walsh R, Blasch BB. *Foundations of orientation and mobility.* New York: American Foundation for the Blind, 1983.
19. Havlik RJ. *Aging in the eighties. Impaired senses for sound and light in persons aged 65 years and over. Preliminary data from the Supplement on Aging to the National Health Interview Survey; United States, Jan-June, 1984. Advanced Data from Vital and Health Statistics.* DHHS publication no. (PHS) 86-1250. Hyattsville, MD: U.S. Department of Health and Human Services, 1986.
20. Kahn HA, Liebowitz HM, Ganley JP. The Framingham Eye Study: outline and major prevalence findings. *Am J Epidemiol* 1977;106:17–32.

21. Stones MJ, Kozma A. Balance and age in the sighted and blind. *Arch Phys Med Rehabil* 1987;68:85–89.

22. Massof RW, Dagnelie G, Deremeik JT, et al. Low vision rehabilitation in the U.S. health care system. *J Vis Rehabil* 1995; 9:3–31.

23. DiStefano AF, Aston SJ. Rehabilitation for the blind and visually impaired elderly. In: Brody SL, Ruff DL, eds. *Aging and rehabilitation: advances in the state of the art.* New York: Springer, 1986:203–217.

24. Cole RG, Rosenthal BP. *Remediation and management of low vision.* St. Louis: Mosby, 1996.

25. Kenney RA. *Physiology of aging.* 2nd ed. Medical, Chicago: Year Book Medical, 1989.

26. Welch P, ed. *Strategies for teaching universal design.* Boston: Adaptive Environments, 1995.

27. Rosenthal BP, Cole RG. *Functional assessment of low vision.* St. Louis: Mosby, 1996.

28. Hartman D, Hartman CW. Disabled students and medical school admission. *Arch Phys Med Rehabil* 1981;62:90–91.

29. Coleman CL, Weinstock RF. Physically handicapped blind people: adaptive mobility techniques. *J Vis Impairment Blind* 1984;78:113–117.

30. Goffmann E. *Stigman: notes on the management of spoiled identity.* New York: Simon and Schuster, 1963.

31. Fisher R. Rehabilitation of the blind amputee: a rewarding experience. *Arch Phys Med Rehabil* 1987;68:382–383.

32. Williams S. Teaching visually impaired adults with a neuromuscular disorder. *J Vis Impairment Blind* 1983;77:382–385.

33. Bernbaum M, Albert S, Cohen JD. Exercise training in individuals with diabetic retinopathy and blindness. *Arch Phys Med Rehabil* 1989;70:605–611.

34. Butter C, Kirsch N. Combined and separate effects of eye patching and visual stimulation on unilateral neglect following stroke. *Arch Phys Med Rehabil* 1992;73:1133–1139.

35. Gianutsos R, Ramsey G, Perlin R. Rehabilitative optometric services for survivors of acquired brain injury. *Arch Phys Med Rehabil* 1988;69:573–578.

Chapter 55

Sexual Aspects of Physical Disability

Stanley H. Ducharme

Medical interest in sexuality and sex therapy has its roots in the pioneering work of Masters and Johnson, which was originally published in the 1960s (1). Their work in human sexual response marked a new era in which sexuality became a legitimate area of clinical work and scientific investigation. Clinical observations from their laboratory were widely reported in the media of that era and ultimately served as an important component of the sexual revolution of the 1960s. In addition, the treatment techniques developed by Masters and Johnson served as a foundation for clinical sex therapy and have been extensively utilized in the treatment of male and female sexual dysfunctions. Since that time, the field of sex therapy has undergone tremendous growth as new advances in medicine and psychology have expanded our understanding of human sexuality and behavior (2). Moreover, interest in sexuality and sex therapy has become an interdisciplinary activity that spans a broad scope of theoretical approaches and medical treatments.

For people with disabilities, the acceptance of sexuality as a justifiable and sanctioned area of rehabilitation has been much more controversial (3). Historically, people with disabilities received little information on sexuality and were often regarded as nonsexual and incapable of an intimate relationship. This misperception not only has persisted in the general population but has been equally prevalent in the medical community as well. In spite of the similarities in sexual functioning for people with and those without disabilities, the tendency has been to emphasize the differences between the two groups and to view people with disablility as being sexually impaired (4). Obviously, this tendency goes much deeper than issues of sexuality and is a reflection of society's general discomfort of people with disabilities. In reality, the sexual rights and responsibilities of people with disabilities are identical to those of all other people. Everyone, regardless of disability, has the right to sexual information and expression and the right to develop the fullest potential in all aspects of life.

The history of addressing sexual issues during the rehabilitation process dates back only to the 1970s when Theodore and Sandra Cole developed the "Sexual Attitude Reassessment" (SAR) program to train rehabilitation professionals (5). These early workshops quickly gained in popularity throughout the rehabilitation community and for many years were offered at major medical facilities in the United States and Canada. The focus of these programs was on values clarification and communication. Their purpose was to increase the practitioner's level of comfort with and awareness of sexual issues among people with disabilities. In these ways, the SAR programs were very successful, but they tended not to provide the counseling skills necessary to assist individuals in their sexual adjustments after disability. To some extent during the 1970s, the idea of sexual education for people with disabilities was academic. People in rehabilitation were beginning to recognize the need for sexuality services, but there was little agreement as to how and when these services should be provided. There was also little agreement as to who should provide sexual education services, and often patients left rehabilitation with no information because various members of the rehabilitation team assumed that other disciplines had addressed sexual concerns (6). Such lack of coordination for sexuality services and the failure to address these concerns in various team meetings simply perpetuated the notion that information on sexuality was of little importance to people with disabilities. Ultimately, people with disabilities themselves began to demand further information regarding their sexual functioning and their capacity to have children.

To clarify issues discussed in this chapter, it is important first to define *sexuality*. *Sexuality* is the integration of the physical, emotional, intellectual, and social aspects of an individual's personality that express maleness or femaleness. Sexuality is an expression of the total personality evident in everything done by a person (7). Interactions with others, personal hygiene, speech, dress, and expressions of affection are all an important part of sexuality. Given this broad definition, sexuality may be regarded as an avenue toward intimacy and may be directly or indirectly affected by the presence of a disability. Disabilities such as blindness, burns, and cancer, for example, may not directly impair genital functioning but can affect communication, body image, and self-esteem. Ultimately, disruptions in these areas may compound physical and psychological well-being and result in various secondary conditions requiring medical treatment (8).

ANATOMY AND PHYSIOLOGY OF HUMAN SEXUALITY

Throughout the health care professions, it is recognized that an understanding of sexual anatomy and physiology is a prerequisite to further consideration of sexual diagnostic and treatment issues. Although the interaction of psychological and physical factors is nowhere more obvious than in sexual behaviors, a basic review of physiologic factors provides a framework for further discussion.

Male Sexual Anatomy

The sexual organs of the male consist of a complex combination of tubes, glands, valves, and muscles that work together to produce sperm, store it, and deliver it outside of the body (Fig. 55-1). The penis consists of three cylindrical bodies of erectile tissue. The paired corpora cavernosa lie parallel to each other and just above the corpus spongiosum, which contains the urethra. The male urethra, which acts as the conduit for both urinary and genital systems, extends from the internal meatus in the urinary bladder to the external meatus at the tip of the penis. It is divided into three regional segments: prostatic, membranous, and penile. The penile segment of the urethra is the longest and extends about 15 cm in the adult male. It has a ventral concave curve in its proximal segment, which is continuous with the membranous urethra until it reaches the lowest level of the symphysis pubis, where it continues into the free part of the penis as the pendulous urethra (9).

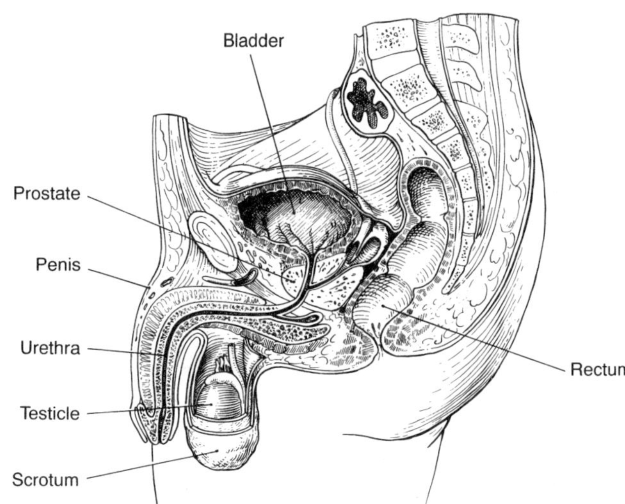

Figure 55-1. Male sexual anatomy.

The erectile tissues of the penis consist of irregular sponge-like networks of vascular spaces interspersed with arteries and veins. The distal portion of the corpus spongiosum expands to form the glans penis. Each cylindrical body is covered by a fibrous coat of tissue, the tunica albuginea, and all three corpora are enclosed in a covering of dense fascia. At the base of the penis, the corpora cavernosa diverge to form the crura, which attach firmly to the pubis and ischium. The blood supply to the penis derives from terminal branches of the internal pudendal arteries.

Erection occurs as a result of vasocongestion within the spongy tissue of the penis. When the penis is flaccid, the vascular spaces in the erectile tissue are relatively empty; with arteriolar dilation, blood flows into the network of sinuses in the spongy tissue, and increased hydraulic pressure results in enlargement and hardening of the penis. When the rate of arterial inflow of blood is matched by the rate of venous return, a state of equilibrium is reached and the erection is maintained. The role of venous blockade in the process of erection is uncertain, but detumescence occurs as a result of venous outflow exceeding arterial input.

The scrotum is a thin sac of skin containing the testes. Involuntary muscle fibers are an integral part of the scrotal skin; these muscle fibers contract as a result of exercise or exposure to cold, causing the testes to be drawn upward against the perineum. These alterations in the scrotum are important thermoregulators for this reason: Since spermatogenesis is temperature sensitive, elevation of the testes in response to cold provides a warmer environment by virtue of body heat, whereas loosening of the scrotum permits the testes to move away from the body and provides a larger skin surface area for the dissipation of intrascrotal heat (10). The scrotum is divided into two compartments by a septum.

The testes are the male reproductive organs and function as the site of spermatogenesis and also play an important role in the production of sex steroid hormones. The testes lie within the scrotal sac, suspended by the spermatic cords. Spermatozoa are produced in the seminiferous tubules of the testes while steroid hormone production occurs in the Leydig cells located in the interstitial tissue. Although architecturally these tissues are admixed within the testes, the two functions are under separate control from the pituitary gland (11). The glandular structure of the testes is about 4 to 5 cm long and 2 to 3 cm thick. The blood supply to the testes is closely associated with that to the kidney because of their common embryologic origin.

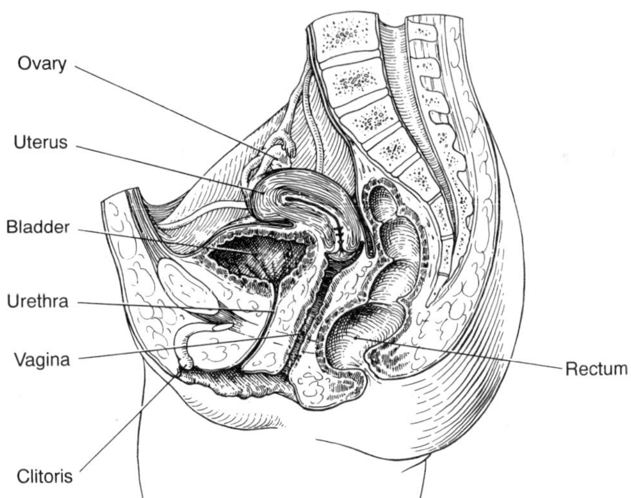

Figure 55-2. Female sexual anatomy.

Female Sexual Anatomy

The external genitalia of a woman are called the *vulva* and consist of the labia majora, the labia minora, the clitoris, and the perineum. Bartholin glands, which open on the inner surfaces of the labia minora, may be considered functionally within the context of the external genitals, although their anatomic position is not in fact external. The appearance of the female genitalia varies considerably from one woman to another, including variations in size, pigmentations, shape of the labia, location of the clitoris, and location of the urethral meatus and the vaginal outlet.

The female urethra is about 4 cm long and about 6 mm in diameter. It begins at the internal meatus and runs anteroinferiorly behind the symphysis with a gentle ventral curvature firmly adherent to the anterior wall of the vagina. Except during the passage of urine, the urethral lumen is stellate in shape and completely occluded. The entire urethra is rich in elastic and collagen fibers. The female urethra is much more readily dilatable than the male urethra (11).

The clitoris itself contains very sensitive nerves that react when stimulated by either psychological or physiologic factors. It is located at the point where the labia majora meet anteriorly and is made up of two small erectile cavernous bodies enclosed in a fibrous membrane surface and ending in a glans or head. The clitoris is richly endowed with free nerve endings, which are extremely sparse within the vagina. The clitoris is not known to have any function other than serving as a receptor and transducer for erotic sensation. The tip of the clitoris is covered by a small area of tissue usually referred to as the *clitoral hood*. This hood tends to protect the sensitive nerves located in the clitoris. The size and shape of this hood varies among women and is not related to the amount of sexual pleasure that a woman can receive when she is sexually stimulated (10).

The internal genitalia of the female include the vagina, cervix, uterus, fallopian tubes, and ovaries (Fig. 55-2). These structures may show considerable variation in size, spatial relationship, and appearance as a result of individual differences as well as reproductive history, age, and presence or absence of disease.

The mouth of the cervix provides a point of entry for spermatozoa into the upper female genital tract and also serves as an exiting point for menstrual flow. The endocervical canal contains numerous secretory crypts that produce mucus. The consistency of cervical secretions varies during various phases of hormonal stimulation throughout the menstrual cycle. At the time of ovulation, for example, cervical secretions become thin and watery; at other times of the cycle, these secretions are thick and viscous, forming a mucous plug that blocks the cervical os (12).

The vagina is a soft tube that is several inches long and can extend during sexual intercourse. It exists more as a potential space than as a balloon-like opening. In the unstimulated state, the walls of the vagina are collapsed together. The walls of the vagina are completely lined with a mucosal surface that is now known to be a major source of vaginal lubrication; there are no secretory glands within the vaginal walls, although there is a rich vascular bed.

The uterus is a muscular organ that is situated in close proximity to the vagina. The lining of the uterus and the muscular component of the uterus function quite separately. The myometrium is important in the onset and completion of labor and delivery, with hormonal factors thought to be the primary regulatory mechanism. The endometrium changes in structure and function depending on the hormonal environment. Under increasing estrogenic activity, the endometrium thickens and becomes more vascular in preparation for the possible implantation of a fertilized egg.

The fallopian tubes or oviducts originate at the uterus and open near the ovaries, terminating in finger-like extensions called *fimbriae*. The fallopian tube is the usual site of fertilization; the motion of cilia within the tube combined with peristalsis in the muscular wall results in the transport of the fertilized ovum to the uterine cavity.

The Sexual Response Cycle

The sexual response cycle, originally proposed by Masters and Johnson, is regarded as the most accepted description of the physiologic and behavioral aspects of sexuality (13). These phases have been defined as excitement, plateau, orgasm, and resolution and were originally determined by extensive laboratory studies. The phases are observed in both men and women, although the demarcation between stages is somewhat arbitrary for both sexes and is dependent on such factors as age and general health.

Excitement Phase

Excitement occurs in response to sexual stimulation because of either touch (i.e., reflexogenic) or imagination (i.e., psychogenic) in both men and women. This stage is governed mainly by the parasympathetic nervous system through the S2, S3, and S4 levels via the cauda equina. The sympathetic nervous system (T11–L1) is also involved, but to a lesser extent (14). Psychogenic stimuli can be both facilitatory and inhibitory, and the degree of stimulation necessary to achieve physiologic arousal is affected by psychological stimulation. Libido is also affected by general health, neurotransmitters, serotonin, dopamine, depression, anxiety, relationship issues, and medication. Both men and women show increases in muscle tension, breathing rate, heart rate, and blood pressure.

In men, the excitement stage is characterized by penile erection as a result of vasocongestion in the spongy tissue. The scrotum contracts and the testes are brought close to the body. In some men, nipple erection occurs as well.

In women, the excitement stage is characterized by vaginal lubrication, with vasocongestion leading to a transudate of fluid (10). Other changes include expansion of the inner two-thirds of the vagina and elevation of the uterine body, cervix, and labia majora. The clitoris enlarges as well. The nipples become erect, and the breasts may swell.

Plateau Phase

The plateau stage consists of the high level of sexual arousal that precedes the threshold levels required to trigger orgasm. The duration of the plateau phase varies considerably, depending on the length of time necessary to reach orgasm. If stimulation is ineffective during this phase, the body will show a gradual reduction of the physiologic phenomena that are characteristic of this phase.

In men, vasocongestion continues in the following way: The penis enlarges further and can deepen in color. The testes elevate and rotate anteriorly, coming to rest against the perineum.

In women, the process of vaginal expansion, clitoral engorgement, and nipple erection continues. A redness known as a *sex flush* may spread over parts of the abdomen, breasts, and chest wall.

Extragenital features of this stage seen in men and women include further changes in tachypnea, tachycardia, elevated blood pressure, and generalized myotonia. With continued stimulation, the individual will enter the third phase of sexual response.

Orgasm Phase

Masters and Johnson (1) theorized that orgasm is triggered by a neural reflex arc once the orgasmic threshold is reached. For both men and women, this stage is under control of the sympathetic nervous system. If no major psychological issues emerge, the individual will progress through one or more orgasms. Intensity and duration of the orgasm vary from individual to individual and depend on arousal, psychological, and physiologic features.

In the male, accessory sex organ contraction concentrates seminal fluid, which consists of live sperm and prostatic seminal vesicle and vas deferens secretions. The man first experiences a felling of ejaculatory inevitability. The internal sphincter of the bladder closes to ensure the forward propulsion of seminal fluid. Orgasm is experienced as rhythmic contractions of the pelvic muscles, prostate, and penile shaft.

In the female, orgasm is also experienced as rhythmic muscular contractions of the uterus, anal sphincter, and the outer one-third of the vagina. In many women, more diffuse experiences are noted as well, including peripheral muscular contractions and changes in electroencephalographic (EEG) activity (15).

Resolution Phase

Males undergo a refractory period immediately after ejaculation. Further ejaculation cannot occur although an erection is possible. The length of this refractory period varies and tends to be affected by factors such as arousal, age, and general physical health. The refractory period for young men may be as short as 10 minutes compared to over 1 hour for an elderly man. Women do not experience a refractory period after the initial orgasm and have the potential to experience several successive orgasms if stimulation continues. During the resolution stage, vasocongestion and the changes that have occurred during the previous phases tend to reverse. The process is generally more rapid for men than for women.

PHYSICAL AND PSYCHOLOGICAL ASSESSMENT

A comprehensive physical assessment is an important part of the patient's work-up. The assessment of the patient's sexual functioning has several objectives: 1) to legitimize the patient's concerns about sexuality and to provide an opportunity for discussion of this topic; 2) to involve the patient (and couple) fully in the decision and treatment process; and 3) to identify the physical, psychological, and social correlates of the sexual functioning (16). An understanding and empathic evaluation can serve as both a challenge and a reward for the patient and the health care provider. Specifying the details of specific sexual functioning—how it occurs—is necessary but not sufficient. Fundamental to long-term positive outcome is assessing (and treating if indicated) the relevant physical features, psychological issues, and relationship concerns brought about by the person's sexual functioning. Developing a solid therapeutic alliance and enlisting the patient's participation comprise the bedrock on which a positive assessment can be completed (17).

Attitude of the Examiner

A gentle, organized, and empathetic approach is the most useful. In order to be successful, the physician or rehabilitation professional must form an alliance with the patient and the couple. It is crucial that the atmosphere be safe, open, and nonjudgmental. The professional must speak in a language that is understandable to the patient and be flexible to the patient's needs, without having a rigid agenda. The clinician must be able to follow subtle leads so that difficult and sensitive material can be expressed. A sensitivity to nonverbal expressions of anxiety and conflict is highly valued and will lead to a more positive outcome (18). Comfort with the topic and one's own sexuality is essential to conveying acceptance and safety to the patient (19). The absence of self-understanding about sexuality may lead the physician to do harm to the patient and a disservice to the medical profession. Regardless of personal style on the part of the professional, validating the patient's experience, supporting any feelings of loss, and being empathetic to the degree of difficulty involved in the disclosure are "basic skills" for clinical inquiry (20).

The examiner must realize that the person with a disability may require more time in pre-examination preparation because of issues such as transfers to the examination table, emptying of the urinary bag, undressing or dressing, history taking, and speech and cognitive impairments. Professional and ancillary staff that may be assisting should be knowledgeable in both attitude and skills most helpful to the patient. The examiner should be clear as to the goals of the assessment and the problems that may occur, such as bladder and bowel accidents.

The examiner should use the opportunity of the examination to discuss issues of sexually transmitted diseases (STDs), especially if the patient is sexually active in nonexclusive relationships (21). Open-ended questions can often be extremely valuable and provide additional information that may be especially sensitive for the patient to discuss. An example of one such question is, "Is there anything else that I have not asked that would be helpful for us to discuss?" This is also the time in which education about symptoms, condom use, and safe sex techniques should be provided to the patient. Most patients, female and male, are not aware of the signs or symptoms of STDs, nor are they aware of the fact that a significant portion of the infected population is without symptoms. Depending on the sexual history, some patients should be screened for infection.

Physical Examination

Female Patient

The female patient should be positioned on the examining table to ensure a sense of stability. This may require safety belts, extra pillows, as well as ancillary staff members to assist the patient and the examiner. Having an ancillary person on each side and the examiner at the foot of the table during the genital-rectal examination allows the examiner to conduct the examination with good control over safety and to maximize this opportunity for evaluation. As a matter of practice, bladder and bowel care should be completed before the examination. Just prior to the examination, the bladder should be emptied. Necessary steps should also be taken to empty the lower bowel, as assessment can be inaccurate if the lower bowel is distended because of a stool. For example, a determination of diaphragm size, for the female, can be incorrect if the stool distends the vagina and alters the examiner's perception of distance from the symphysis to the posterior fornix (22).

Breast examination is essential. Breast self-examination should be taught, or arrangements should be made for the patient to have her breast examined every 3 months. If the patient is at high risk for breast cancer, the examination should be completed on a monthly basis. If the patient is unable to conduct the examination, a relative, visiting nurse, or personal care attendant should perform the examination. Breast palpation should include the neck, supraclavicular and ancillary nodes, and the nipples to check for discharge.

Women with disabilities can have special concerns about their breasts. Concerns from women with congenital disability may reflect feelings of inadequacy and lack of sexuality. For a woman with a traumatic injury, the sense of loss may include the breast. This may reflect a sense of loss of one's femininity and the ability for childbearing. Other women have reported that their breasts, along with their neck and shoulders, were the most arousable (23). The patient must be given ample time to discuss these concerns if the examiner believes that issues such as these are a concern for the woman.

Before the pelvic examination, placement of a pad on the examining table may be helpful in case of a bladder accident. Flaccid buttocks may need extra cushioning on the examining table as well. This provision is especially important if there are any signs of redness indicating skin breakdown. Feet can be secured in stirrups with elastic wraps or other bandages. It is important to note that the labia minora and majora of women who use wheelchairs may appear more atrophic than age would suggest. This appearance is usually due to muscular atrophy from injury (24). Speculum insertion must be conducted gently and carefully. Care should be taken to test the temperature of the instrument prior to insertion, as it is possible to trigger autonomic dysreflexia with a speculum that is too cold.

Several more points should be noted. A mirror should be available to demonstrate findings to the patient. This form of education to the patient should be an ongoing part of the entire physical examination. Observation and inspection of the skin of the lower back, the buttocks, and the genitals should be conducted at the time of the examination. Inspection of the clitoris, by retraction of the clitoral hood, should be performed by employing gentle contact. Bimanual examination of the vagina and rectum, including occult blood testing, should be performed on each patient. Finally, in obtaining Papanicolaou smears, samples from the endocervix and the exocervix should be gathered before any STD samples are obtained. This ensures that any abnormal cells are retrieved for cytologic evaluation and not lost to the microbiology laboratory analysis.

Male Patient

The classic male genital examination should be conducted. Special care and attention should be paid to the skin of the penis and foreskin. As with all patients, concerns about body image will be important and merit special attention. Routine blood chemistry tests, hormonal assays, determination of the sensory threshold of the genital area, vascular assessment, neurologic evaluation of male sexual dysfunction, and nocturnal penile tumescence monitoring with sleep EEG should be included in a comprehensive work-up (25). In addition to the sexual history taking, obtaining knowledge of all medications used, prescription and nonprescription, should be part of the assessment.

When the examination has been completed, skin around the genital and rectal areas should be gently washed. Plain tap water will dissolve water-soluble jelly. Cornstarch or talc should be used to avoid moisture and all fabric edges should be checked to avoid skin breakdown. Assistance with dressing and transfers should be provided as needed.

Psychological Assessment

A number of authors have emphasized physicians' increasing awareness of the importance of including a sexual history as part of the standard database (25–27). One reason the sexual history is relevant is the high incidence of sexual dysfunction in a medical patient population, including people with physical disabilities. Another reason is the high incidence of STDs that often go undiagnosed. Regardless, the sexual history provides the physician with a valuable perspective in understanding the patient's values, relationships, overall adjustment, and health-maintaining behaviors. The sexual history also provides the patient with the opportunity to ask questions about sexual adjustment as well as his or her own unique physical abilities.

A simplified sexual history often includes such areas as the patient's past and current sexual functioning, partner satisfaction, relationship history, medications used, behavioral repertoire, traumatic events such as abuse, and specific difficulties brought on by the illness or disability (28). A nonjudgmental stance that respects the values and preferences of the patient is necessary to maintain rapport, to foster the patient's autonomy, and to promote candor. Most training programs include specific opportunities for the practitioner to understand and evaluate his or her own values so that he or she does not impose them on the patient (29). Open-ended questions tend to promote this nonevaluative atmosphere. Naturally, this nonjudgmental attitude must stop short of sanctioning attitudes or practices that are psychologically or physically harmful to the patient and his or her sexual partner.

The language of the interview should be neither too casual nor too technical. In reality, many patients have some anxiety about sexual topics and the language of the interviewer will set the tone for the patient to discuss the topic and to ask questions of a sensitive nature. The interviewer models a sensitive and matter-of-fact attitude while listening carefully to the attitudes expressed by the patient's verbal and nonverbal behavior. More difficult topics are generally reserved for later in the interview, when greater rapport and trust have already been established. As a general rule, it is a good idea to ask if the patient or partner would find it helpful to speak with someone knowledgeable about sexuality and disability in order to gain more information or to discuss the topic in more depth. Referral may then be made to physicians such as urologists and physiatrists or other professionals such as nurses, psychologists, or social workers.

SEXUALITY AS A DEVELOPMENTAL ISSUE

The theory of developmental tasks was originally discussed by the psychologist Eric Erikson (30). These stages represent the critical periods of development from birth to death. The first three stages of development represent infancy and childhood. They reflect the achievement of trust, autonomy through mobility, and the ability to explore the environment. Even at these early stages in life, sexual behaviors and curiosity are quite typical and expected. This is true for children with and without disabilities.

As individuals move through life, they encounter a number of tasks set by their cultural milieu and by themselves as biologic entities. These developmental tasks are particularly critical as they must be mastered if children are to develop more mature social and interpersonal skills. When disability occurs, not only are the current developmental tasks threatened, but the persons, at least temporarily, regress to an earlier stage of development. This regression has broad implications for an individual's psychological and sexual adjustment. Because the person's sense of masculinity or femininity is an integral part of these developmental milestones, disability can create confusion and conflict in both gender identity and gender role, identity and role being different aspects of the same process. For people with disabilities, confusion regarding both gender identity and gender role can make the adjustment process more difficult, especially without adequate role models and sources of emotional support.

Gender identity is the inner experience of one's self as male or female; *role* is the outward expression of that identity (31). Without resolution of these conflicts, more complex tasks such as the formation of relationships and the achievement of a positive self-esteem may never occur. Thus, for a person with a disability, a healthy sexual adjustment and the ability to achieve intimacy depend on successful resolution of the developmental tasks at the time of injury or onset of illness.

The developmental process can be further complicated for young people with gay and lesbian orientations. More than simply a matter of having a same-sex partner, gay and lesbian identity is similar in scope to ethnic or racial identity, involving identification with the values of a discrete subculture (32). The process of forming a gay or lesbian identity evolves in stages from confusion and conflict around the emerging awareness of the same-sex urges to acceptance. For the person with a disability, the presence of homosexual issues can further complicate an already difficult sexual adjustment.

Congenital disabilities often prevent the child from gaining essential information about the body. Overprotection by parents, discouragement of sexual exploration, and a lack of adequate socialization often add confusion to male and female roles. Since identity is formulated before the age of 3 years, confusion regarding sexuality lends itself to later feelings of inferiority and difficulty relating to members of the opposite sex. Children with a disability are often isolated from peers and may regard themselves as "not equal" to their playmates (33). These deficits in the early sexual education of a child can easily become more difficult to manage later in life.

During puberty and adolescence, the achievement of sexual identity and acceptance in peer group relationships are the goals to be accomplished. As the adolescent grows and enters young adulthood, one of the primary developmental tasks is the development of intimacy and the concurrent strivings toward independence. Traumatic injury at this time threatens these important peer relationships and fosters dependency on the family unit. Adolescents with a disability often feel unattractive and ashamed of their bodies. Subsequently, they feel unwanted by the opposite sex and incapable of establishing a meaningful relationship. Without a sense of sexual identity, even late adolescents can lack the ability to make vocational and educational decisions or to assume responsibility for their own behavior. Thus, future emotional growth is threatened.

Aging is also an often overlooked developmental stage (34,35). Although the reality is that elders can continue to be sexually active throughout the life span, internalized negative attitudes can inhibit sexual expression in later years. The stigma against aging is even greater in the disabled community than in the culture at large and is experienced with fear at earlier ages than for individuals without disability.

SEXUAL ADJUSTMENT

Adjustment to a physical disability or illness is a gradual process that occurs over an extended period of time. The individual must mourn the losses and ultimately develop coping strategies that will validate the meaningfulness of the new postinjury life. Successful adjustment depends on the recognition that choice is still available and is influenced by many factors such as age at onset, quality of social supports, physical health, gender, and type of illness or injury.

Successful sexual adjustment also requires the same gradual, and sometimes painful, emotional process. Losses need to be grieved so that the remaining strengths can be developed and nurtured. Because of different personality styles, however, not everyone completes this difficult adjustment. Some individuals, for example, may have experienced more profound earlier periods of grief and trauma because of early emotional, physical, or sexual abuse (36). Perhaps there were few emotional supports during childhood, and the grieving may have extended for prolonged periods of time. The resolution of predisability psychological issues may be necessary for the individual to master the demands and responsibilities of living with a disability.

After onset of a traumatic disability, individuals frequently go through a period of reduced sexual drive or performance. Others go through a period of sexual acting out, presumably to validate their survival and sexual identity. However, substantial numbers of people fail to resume an active sex life after injury because of misinformation, problems of adjustment, or shame regarding body image and function (7). Those who do assume an active sex life after injury are often advised by rehabilitation staff members to keep separate the roles of sexual partner and care provider (37,38). Having one's sexual partner provide intimate medical care can be destructive to the relationship. Mixing these roles often places one member in a needy, helpless position while the other member is perceived as powerful and giving. Such an unequal balance of power in a relationship tends to dilute feelings of intimacy and to be the source of feelings of resentment and anger.

To the extent that a person with a disability can learn to value his or her new sexual abilities, as opposed to trying to regain the same sexual expressions that existed before the injury, and to establish a positive level of communication, the person will achieve a satisfying sexual adjustment. These adjustments, however, often come slowly after a period of intense grieving and sadness. Many individuals find that emotional relationships and physical intimacy do not occur for many months following discharge from the rehabilitation center. Even then, the process can be slow and painful. Sexual experimentation may or may not be a part of this adjustment process, depending on the individual's ability to take risks and tolerate feelings of vulnerability.

People with disabilities who achieve success in their sexual functioning often do so because of increased communication and a willingness to experiment with developing romance and intimacy as well as technique. They are secure enough to realize that not every experiment will work and they value nongenital erogenous zones. They are typically more comfortable with their own bodies and continue to feel a sense of self-worth and self-respect (39,40). As a result, partners also feel validated and perceive the sexual relationship to be warm, caring, and mutually enjoyable.

The importance of communication cannot be overstated. The development of skills in communication about sexual topics and of methods of pleasure is the single most critical aspect of successful sexual adjustment. Specific and immediate communication between partners can relieve intense feelings of anxiety, fears of rejection, and concerns about physical safety. For this reason, psychological counseling and education about sexuality while the patient is in rehabilitation must emphasize these areas and provide the individual with the opportunity to develop and strengthen these skills.

Although psychological considerations need to be addressed in all discussions regarding sexuality, physical functioning is equally important. Often in rehabilitation, it can be extremely supportive and helpful to the patient if a sensitive discussion regarding physical capabilities is provided as soon as the individual is ready. Usually, the patient will indicate his or her readiness by asking questions regarding attractiveness, dating, relationships, and intimacy. Even if the individual does not raise these concerns during hospitalization, it is usually appropriate for staff members to offer information if the patient seems interested and curious. Such topics as libido, erections, orgasms, lubrication, fertility, mobility, sensation, and bladder functioning are all relevant to the sexual functioning of people with disabilities (29,41).

SEXUAL DESIRE

Inhibited sexual desire is a highly prevalent dysfunction, affecting possibly up to 50% of sex cases seen in clinical settings (42–44). Although no data currently exist, this figure is probably higher for people with disabilities. Now known as hypoactive sexual desire disorder, it is characterized by persistently low or absent sexual fantasies and desire for sexual activity not caused by substance abuse or a primary psychiatric disorder. It is not uncommon for individuals with desire disorders to present themselves to the rehabilitation clinic with a variety of other sexual difficulties in addition to the primary problem of low desire. Couples may also present without a desire disorder but with desire discrepancy (where the partner's levels of desire are at variance with one another). Attempts are underway to clarify the diagnosis and the concept of normal desire and to standardize treatment. In patients with a psychiatric disturbance or severe reactive depression, the treatment is generally longer and outcomes less certain. Considerable research is still needed in this area of sexual dysfunction.

The sudden onset of disability or the more chronic issues of malaise, pain, fatigue, or stress can contribute to decreased libido (45). Low desire after onset of a traumatic disability is, for the most part, of limited duration. As adjustment proceeds, sexual desire often returns slowly and on a steady basis. The level of depression after disability occurs may in fact be the single greatest factor in determining the level of desire for sexual activities. If depression is more severe, or if there are substantial relationship issues that emerge after the onset of disability (or that were present before the onset of disability), the return of sexual desire may be more protracted and may require counseling or medications for it to resolve. Depressions associated with disability are complex medical problems that require an in-depth evaluation and treatment plan. Often a psychiatric or psychological consultation may be warranted. In other instances, the precipitating factors responsible for the loss of sexual desire may be less apparent. Additional effort will be required to unravel the chain of events responsible for diminishing the libido. Changes in sexual desire may also be somewhat variable over time, depending on the emotional well-being of the person with the disability and his or her partner.

In addition to traumatic disability, many chronic illnesses and medications can result in inhibited sexual desire, either temporarily or permanently (42,46). Neuroendocrine disorders, cancer, heart disease, renal failure, liver disease, chronic lung disease, drug or alcohol addiction, and multiple sclerosis are among the conditions that can have a physical effect on sexual desire. Also, numerous medications may inhibit desire. Included are antihypertensives (propranolol, methyldopa), neuroleptics and sedatives (diazepam, phenobarbital), mood active drugs (phenelzine sulfate, alprazolam), cancer chemotherapy, glaucoma medications, and anticonvulsives (44,47). Even serotonin reuptake inhibitors, which are used to treat depression, which itself reduces desire, can result in loss of desire and other sexual dysfunctions.

MALE SEXUAL FUNCTIONING

The capacity to achieve erections is often altered in most men who sustain damage to the central nervous system. This typically includes injuries such as spinal cord injury and stroke as well as progressive disabilities such as multiple sclerosis and diabetes. Men with congenital disabilities such as cerebral palsy and muscular dystrophy typically retain the ability to achieve erections but more often report difficulties in mobility, positioning, and communication. If erections are altered, such as with spinal cord injury, the man may still be capable of reflexogenic erections. This is especially true with men who have sustained upper motor neuron lesions. Although these erections may not be suitable for penetration, they can usually be achieved and sustained by ongoing manual stimulation of the genital area. Some authors suggested that techniques such as stuffing can be mutually satisfying to the couple, while others discussed the importance of medical interventions to improve erection quality (37,48,49).

Sensory disturbances are also a prominent symptom in many of the patients with disabilities that affect central nervous system functioning. Many individuals report a complete loss of sensation below the level of the lesion. Other men who have partial sensation may experience some sparing of sensation in the genital area, although these areas may not be as sensitive as prior to the onset of disability. For example, the man may be able to differentiate hard touch but be unable to experience soft touch or stroking. Areas of intact sensation, usually above the level of injury, are often considered hypersensitive and can be another source of erotic pleasure. For other men, these areas can be a source of pain and are to be avoided during times of sexual behavior. Intensely erotic areas that are often used in sexual activity may be at the nipple line or in the vicinity of the ears, scalp, and neck. Because of the wide variations among different individuals, it is important to encourage patients and their partners to experiment with sexual functioning in order to gain a better understanding of their own unique situations.

In recent years, procedures such as penile injections, implants, vacuum constrictive devices (that fit over the penis), as well as various surgical procedures have gained increased popularity for men with neurogenic erectile difficulties (Figs. 55-3 and 55-4). Despite problems associated

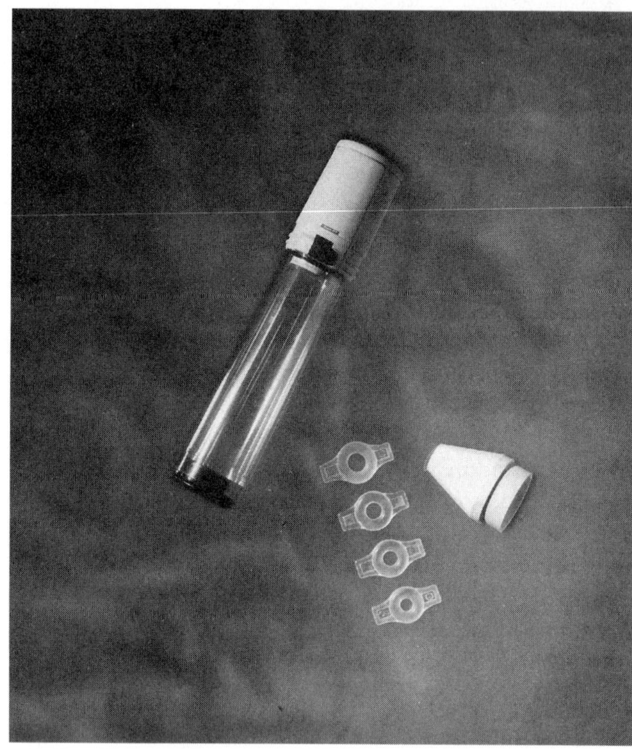

Figure 55-3. Response battery-powered vacuum erection system. (Courtesy of Mentor Urology.)

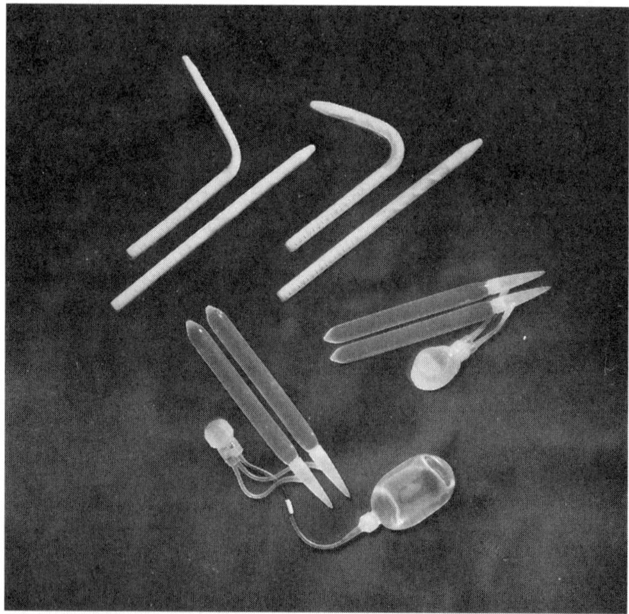

Figure 55-4. Inflatable and bendable penile implants. (Courtesy of Mentor Urology.)

with these various devices such as corporal scarring, infection, and mechanical failure, patient satisfaction has generally been positive (50). Dissatisfaction has usually been caused by size of the penis, firmness of the erection, temperature of the penis, or difficulty in manipulating the device. Other couples have reported a loss of spontaneity with love making and a feeling that use of a mechanical device seems unnatural and a deterrent to their sexual expression.

Alternative methods of delivering drugs to the erectile bodies have also been widely discussed and evaluated. Originally, it appeared that one of the most promising forms of treatment was the application of nitroglycerin plasters directly to the penile shaft (51). In pilot studies, however, transdermal nitroglycerin, minoxidil, and prostaglandin E failed to induce rigid erections, apparently because of insufficient transfer of the drug through the skin (52).

Recently, the use of injections of alprostadil (Caverjet) has resulted in a major breakthrough in the treatment of erection problems for men with and without disabilities. Developed by the UpJohn Company, alprostadil was the first drug approved by the FDA for the treatment of erection problems. The drug received clearance by the FDA in July 1996, and was quickly made available in over 30 countries including the United States, France, Spain, Italy, and the United Kingdom.

As with other injection therapies, alprostadil is administered by a small needle into the corpus cavernosum. It relaxes the smooth muscle, which in turn enhances blood flow into the penis, creating an erection. Men receive the initial treatments by a medically trained professional, in order to determine the dosage and to learn the injection technique. For men with limited hand functioning, the injections are performed by their sexual partners. After these initial injections, the man and his partner take the medication home and use it whenever they desire. Usually injection therapies can be used once a day and up to three times per week.

Pain in using various injection medications does seem to be a common feature, although to date no data on this side effect exist for men with or without disabilities. Naturally, the amount of pain perceived depends on the amount of intact sensation after the onset of disability. Other side effects from the various injection therapies may include scarring, bleeding, and prolonged erections, known as *priapism* (53,54). Other medications commonly used for injections include papaverine and phentolamine as well as prostaglandin E. These medications, although experimental in nature, have been used for several years and the side effects may be less pronounced, especially with good training as to the technique. Because their erection problems are usually not vascular in nature, men with disabilities often find that small doses of these medications have a very significant positive impact on erection quality.

Other methods of drug delivery to the erectile bodies are currently under investigation. For example, the administration of alprostadil to the urethra mucosa for transfer to the erectile bodies has recently gained attention and is now available with prescription. Transurethral alprostadil appears to be effective with men of various age groups who demonstrate erectile dysfunction from a variety of organic causes. Side effects from this method of administration seem to be minor and were limited to penile pain in a minority of men in the initial studies (55).

Oral medications to improve erections are clearly the cutting edge in erection research around the world. There will be a tremendous market for oral medications once FDA approval has been obtained. Currently medications such as Viagra (Sildenafil) from Pfizer Pharmaceutical Company have great potential for men with erection problems. Other centers are doing clinical testing on various hormone therapies to improve male sexual functioning. The results of these studies seem very promising and breakthroughs are happening on a regular basis.

The ability to diagnose and treat infertility in men is another area that continues to improve. For men with disabilities of the central nervous system, fertility rates have generally ranged anywhere from 1% to 10% (56). Reports of pregnancies initiated were typically undocumented and anecdotal. Problems were due to either difficulties of sperm retrieval or poor sperm quality. Newer methods of retrieving sperm through electroejaculation and vibratory stimulation are demonstrating very positive results (57). In other cases, surgical sperm aspiration coupled with in vitro fertilization is offering new hope for couples wishing to have children. In other men, techniques to reduce testicular temperatures are having positive results on spermatogenesis and sperm production.

Of the advanced procedures, intracytoplasmic sperm injection (ICSI) has offered hope to many couples for whom poor sperm quality has been an issue (58). With ICSI, sperm is collected from the man through an assisted ejaculatory procedure if necessary. A single sperm is then injected directly into the egg, which was retrieved through a surgical procedure. Once the egg has been fertilized, it is then placed back in the uterus. Because of the effectiveness of the ICSI procedure, a growing number of reproductive clinics are adopting the procedure and using it for men with poor sperm motility and quantity.

As a result of these new procedures, the possibility of parenthood for people with disabilities has changed greatly. Ten years ago, men were often told that fatherhood was not possible after onset of a disability and were discouraged in their hopes of having a child. Currently, if the man with a disability has sperm, there is the potential for fatherhood. Rehabilitation professionals who provide education to their patients need to realize that these new procedures are available and that parenthood is possible.

FEMALE SEXUAL FUNCTIONING

The literature on sexuality for women with disabilities has historically lagged behind the research being conducted for men with disabilities. One author suggested that age-old myths regarding female sexuality, cultural stereotypes, and the low incidence of traumatic disability in women are to blame (59). This situation seems to be changing, however, as women's sexuality and wellness have become an increasing priority for funding sources such as the National Institute on Disability and Rehabilitation Research and the National Institutes for Health. In spite of the growing attention to this area, there are still many unanswered questions that have far-reaching implications for the woman with a disability.

For the most part, changes in the female genital tract are most common after neurologic trauma or disease. These changes include vaginal lubrication, labial swelling, clitoral swelling and regression, and changes in the perception of orgasm. Most of the reports on female sexual changes following disability, however, tend to be anecdotal with little scientific basis. Since many of the findings tend to be self-reports, some researchers (59) suggested that the existing data are inaccurate and that this method is insufficient to obtain objective, quantifiable data on sexual arousal (Table 55-1).

One of the few scientific studies that examined sexual relationships following spinal cord injury was conducted by Sipski and Alexander (66). They questioned 25 female spinal cord–injured patients about sexual activities and frequency of sex before and after spinal cord injury. Ten subjects (40%) resumed sexual activities within 6 months of injury and an additional 6 (24%) resumed sexual activity within 2 years after injury. Frequency of activity also decreased after the onset of disability. Whereas 16 (64%) of the women had engaged in sexual activity at least weekly before the injury, only 12 (48%) were as active after the injury. The number of sexual partners was also evaluated and no significant difference was noted for the number of partners before injury versus after injury for the group as a whole or based on neurologic injury. Finally, whereas sexual intercourse was the woman's favorite sexual activity before the injury occurred, kissing, hugging, and touching were preferred after the injury.

Many aspects of a woman's sexuality, including libido or desire, arousal, response, and specific sexual behaviors, may be altered after a traumatic injury. Complications encountered by women with traumatic disabilities include management of autonomic hyperreflexia (drastic changes in blood pressure), management of bowel and bladder continence, and management of spasticity. In some women with multiple sclerosis or spinal injury, lubrication may become reflexogenic, facilitating penetration of the vagina. Changes in desire and arousal may result from the impact of changes in her physical status on her perception of herself, from role changes that may occur as a result of injury, or from the anger and depression that often accompany the onset of a disability (22).

Current research on female sexuality now appears to be exploring issues related to vaginal contractions, intensifying perception of the orgasm, and stimulating vasodilation of the pelvic region. All require further investigation but seem to indicate a renewed interest in the field and a commitment to understanding female sexuality and disability. Most importantly, newer research is providing a renewed sense of hope for women with

Table 55-1: Sexual Response in Women with Complete Spinal Cord Lesions

Level of Injury	Sexual Response
C1–C3	Reflex lubrication. Altered sexual sensations during excitement and plateau phases. Severe respiratory difficulties may impair sexual activity. No change in sexual desire. Fertility remains unchanged.
C4–C5	Reflex lubrication likely. Psychogenic lubrication unlikely. Oral sex possible. Erotic zones above clavicle likely.
C6	Most common level of injury. Sensation same as for injury at C4–C5. Holding and caressing possible.
C7–C8	Increased potential for use of hands.
T1	Same as for injury at C7–C8 but with increased manual dexterity.
T2–T5	Sensation from level of diaphragm. Reflex clitoral erection and lubrication. Possible orgasm from nipple and breast stimulation.
T6–T10	Reflex erection of clitoris, labial swelling, and reflex lubrication with stimulation. Vaginal tone generally intact. No genital sensation at rest. Genital sensation altered during excitement phase.
T10–T12	Water-soluble lubricant needed for intercourse due to absence of reflex and psychogenic lubrication. No genital sensation during excitement and plateau phases.
Below T12–S1	Response to direct stimulation present but much less than lesions above T11. Lubrication is psychogenic. At rest, internal genitals sensate, external genitals insensate.
L1–L2	Psychogenic erection of clitoris, lubrication, labial swelling, and skin flush possible but unlikely.
L3–L4	Psychogenic reactions unlikely.
L5–S1	Clitoral erection and lubrication unlikely.
S2–S4	No reflex clitoral erection. No genital sensation at rest. Vagina remains well lubricated.

Source: Data from Weinberg (60), Zasler (61), Berard (62), Glass (63), Sipski and Alexander (64), and Whipple (65).

disabilities, offering important applications for clinical practice (65).

Of special note in the current research on women are new data regarding orgasms in women with spinal cord injury. Sipski and Alexander (67) demonstrated that a large percentage of women with spinal cord injury achieved orgasm regardless of the pattern or degree of neurologic injury. Furthermore, they ascertained that no consistent characteristics have been identified to predict which women with spinal cord injury would be able to achieve orgasm. These new data seem to indicate that education of women regarding their sexuality plays an important role in their overall sexual adjustment and is a determining factor in their general sexual satisfaction. These studies have had vast implications on previous assumptions regarding women with disabilities and have sparked renewed interest in the physiologic sexual responses in women following the onset of disability.

An area that has been particularly neglected is the issue of menstruation in women who have sustained traumatic injury. Yet, the role of motherhood and the emotional issues connected with this cannot be overestimated. Menses is important to a woman; it reinforces her belief in herself as a woman, which in turn affects her self-esteem (68).

Cessation in the menstrual cycle may occur for a number of reasons other than menopause or pregnancy. These reasons may include changes in hormone secretion, severe psychological disturbances, or significant trauma such as spinal cord injury. Concerns about menstruation are typical early in the rehabilitation program.

Menstrual periods generally continue after onset of a traumatic disability, with a temporary post injury interruption of menses occurring for at least 6 months. In women with spinal cord injury, rates of temporary amenorrhea range from 44% to 58% in research samples (64,68,69). The nature of the disability tends not to be associated with an interruption of menses. In some studies, there were changes in cycle length, duration of flow, amount of flow, and changes in amount of menstrual pain after the onset of disability. Ovulation in most disabilities tends to be unaffected because the location of the ovaries makes them less susceptible to changes in body temperature (70). Menstrual self-care should include frequent changing of tampons and absorbent pads to guard against the risk of infection, toxic shock, and pressure sores. Concerns about reduced fertility, with most disabilities, are unfounded, and conception should not be a problem for most disabled women (71).

The issue of birth control is somewhat problematic for women with disabilities. However, Zasler (61) suggested that in the age of acquired immunodeficiency syndrome (AIDS), the choice is no longer so controversial: Unless the relationship is monogamous and long-standing, the safest method is a thick latex condom with a spermicidal foam or jelly containing nonoxynol-9. This method is believed to protect against AIDS and other STDs. Limiting the number of sexual partners is also recommended for AIDS prevention. The combination of a diaphragm and foam is also thought to reduce risk, but the limited dexterity of many women with disabilities makes it difficult to insert and remove; reduced sensation also prevents detection of an incorrectly placed diaphragm, which might cause irritation and subsequent bladder infection. The partner or personal care attendant might assist in placing the device (72).

Birth control pills are known to increase the risk of blood clots, signified by leg pain, in the general population. Women with mobility impairments are already at higher risk for developing blood clots because of reduced circulation in the lower extremities and may not be able to sense the warning pain. For this reason, some health experts consider their use contraindicated; however, no empirical studies have been conducted to document the increased risk (64). Those people who do recommend the pill for women with reduced mobility argue that the new low-dose pill minimizes the risk. Blood clots are more common in the first 6 months following traumatic injury, so delay in prescribing birth control pills until that time and provision of frequent follow-up checks—usually twice per year—should minimize the risk (72).

Patients who have a disability and become pregnant often face a wide variety of medical issues that are not as common among the general population. These include an increased risk of urinary tract infection, anemia, sepsis, pressure sores, unattended births, and autonomic hyperreflexia, and difficulty with transfers toward the end of pregnancy. Therefore, proper follow-up by an obstetrician knowledgeable about disability is essential. In reality, however, finding such a medical professional may be difficult and the obstetrician may need ongoing consultation with the physiatrist in order to address disability specific issues.

It follows that to improve the sexual satisfaction of women with disabilities, new treatments must be developed and documented. New data on reproduction and wellness must be communicated to women who have disabilities. These may include medical treatments such as the use of biofeedback and vibratory stimulation or psychological approaches such as patient education or new forms of sexual counseling (23). Only then will women begin to have the information that they deserve regarding their bodily processes and sexuality.

STAFF TRAINING AND INSTITUTIONAL ISSUES

Staff training in sexuality is a critical feature of any comprehensive rehabilitation program. This training must include programs aimed at values clarification as well as those that provide specific information on disability and sexuality. In addition to the training curriculum, administrative support of the sexuality program must be evident to staff members, families, and patients alike. This administrative approval establishes a positive therapeutic environment where openness, empowerment, and caring are the foundations of the rehabilitation process.

Although not all staff members need be sex counselors, all should feel comfortable with the topic of sexuality and communicate a sense of openness about the topic. This necessitates an awareness of one's own values and reactions to sexually related issues. Generally, anxiety, shame, and discomfort about sexuality are common (29,73). Putting this anxiety aside and becoming aware of our personal reactions to sexual issues is a long process that requires sensitization, education, and practice. Often a first step in reducing this tension is acknowledging one's feelings to another person. In a work setting, a peer support group or discussion with a colleague can be especially helpful in overcoming personal barriers about sexuality.

In addition to processing personal feelings about sexuality, specific information on sexuality and disability must also be taught to staff members. Without correct up-to-date information about sexuality, staff members will only add confusion to an already difficult topic. Even worse, the patient and partner could be given incorrect information that will have a negative effect on their overall adjustment and relationship. An ongoing lecture series is often helpful in this regard. Typical issues addressed in such a program include sexual anatomy and physiology, effects of medications, physical functioning, treatment options such as penile injections and implants, counseling techniques, professional roles, and gay and lesbian issues.

Staff members should be able to facilitate positive sexual identity for all rehabilitation patients, including exposure to healthy role models. Patients require specific information on medications, sexual techniques, communication styles, as well as complications such as dysreflexia that may be experienced when using a vibrator or during childbearing.

The development of a sexuality committee within a facility is often the method of choice in addressing ongoing sexual issues and problems (73). Ideally, a member of the administration should serve on the committee. His or her presence validates the committee's function and provides a sense of security, safety, and recognition to its members. The development of institutional guidelines and procedures is usually the first task of the committee and often its most important function. It is essential that the committee establish guidelines on some of the most sensitive interactions that occur in the day-to-day functioning of the institution. Typically issues to be addressed include such matters as whether to establish a privacy room, public versus private masturbation, sexual activity with a partner, dissemination of birth control information and supplies, prevention of sexual assault, prevention of STDs, and policies concerning the relationships between patients and staff members.

Most often in-service education programs will raise concerns about staff-patient interactions. This interaction is usually the primary area of staff anxiety, and sensitive discussion is most often welcomed and appreciated. In addition, an overview of behavior modification techniques can be helpful. This overview should be especially geared to sexual issues and should be combined with theoretical discussions of reinforcement schedules and behavioral contingencies. Finally, the importance of limit setting and professional boundaries should be discussed and emphasized.

CONCLUSIONS

For people with disabilities, there are multiple restrictions on the expression of sexuality. These stem from cultural biases, social ignorance, and unfounded fears regarding the person with a disability. For homosexual men and women, these fears and biases are significantly intensified, and there is a serious lack of information and resources available in the area of sexual health. The responsibility of medical professionals is to achieve a balance between protecting the rights and privacy of hospitalized patients and providing a safe and enriching environment. As staff attitudes are retrained away from control and from imposing restrictive values, a therapeutic environment that fosters self-esteem and sexual growth will unfold in the rehabilitation setting.

In the last decade, we have witnessed tremendous progress in the areas of sexuality and disability. However, there is much left to be done so that men and women from all sexual orientations are included in this revolution. What once began as a passing fad outside of mainstream rehabilitation has now become an accepted standard of practice for the rehabilitation team. Education about sexuality is a critical component of the rehabilitation process. More importantly, people with disabilities are now recognized as having the same rights, needs, and desires as all people.

REFERENCES

1. Masters WH, Johnson VE. *Human sexual response.* Boston: Little, Brown, 1966.
2. Krane RJ. Surgical implants for impotence: implications and procedures. In: Santen R, Swerdloff R, eds. *Male reproductive dysfunction; diagnosis and management of hypogonadism, infertility and impotence.* Baltimore: Marcel Dekker, 1986:227–243.
3. Cole TM, Glass DD. Sexuality and physical disability. *Arch Phys Med Rehabil* 1977;58:585–586.
4. Ducharme S. Sexuality and disability. In: DellOrto AE, Marinelli

RP, eds. *Encyclopedia of disability and rehabilitation.* New York: Macmillan, 1995:668–673.

5. Cole TM, Chilgren R, Rosenberg P. A new program of sex education and counseling for spinal cord injured adults and health care professionals. *Int J Paraplegia* 1973;8:111–124.

6. Ducharme S. Innovations in sexual health for men with spinal cord injury. *Sex Update* 1991;4(1):8–12.

7. Ducharme SH, Gill KM, Biener-Bergman S, Fertitta LC. Sexual functioning: medical and psychological aspects. In: DeLisa JA, ed. *Rehabilitation medicine: principles and practice.* Philadelphia: JB Lippincott, 1993:763–782.

8. Cole SS, Cole TM. The handicapped and sexual health. In: Comfort A, ed. *Sexual consequences of disability.* Philadelphia: George Stickley, 1978:37–45.

9. Steers WD. Neuroanatomy and neurophysiology of erection. *Sex Disability* 1994;12:17–29.

10. Kolodney RC, Masters WH, Johnson VE, Biggs MA. *Textbook of human sexuality for nurses.* Boston: Little, Brown, 1979:9–30.

11. Walsh R, Retik A, Stamey T, Vaughan P. Diagnosis and management of male sexual dysfunction. In: William R, ed. *Campbell's urology.* 6th ed. Philadelphia: WB Saunders, 1992:50–67.

12. Victor JS. *Human sexuality.* Englewood Cliffs, NJ: Prentice Hall, 1980:13–25.

13. Spark R. *Male sexual health: a couple's guide.* Mount Vernon, NY: Consumer Union, 1991: 28–35.

14. Freed MM. Traumatic and congenital lesions of the spinal cord. In: Kottke FJ, Stillwell KG, Lehmann JF, eds. *Krusen's handbook of physical medicine and rehabilitation.* 3rd ed. Philadelphia: WB Saunders, 1982:645–671.

15. Fisher S. *The female orgasm: psychology, physiology and fantasy.* New York: Basic Books, 1972.

16. Kaplan HS. *The evaluation of sexual disorders: psychological and medical aspects.* New York: Brunner/Mazel, 1983.

17. Leiblum R, Rosen RC. *The principles and practice of sex therapy: update for the 1990's.* New York: Guilford, 1989.

18. Smith AD. Psychologic factors in the multidisciplinary evaluation and treatment of erectile dysfunction. *Urol Clin North Am* 1988;15:41–51.

19. Kaplan HS. *The new sex therapy.* New York: Random House, 1974.

20. Levine SB, Althof SE. Psychological evaluation and sex therapy. In: Mulcahy JJ, ed. *Diagnosis and management of male sexual dysfunction: topics in clinical urology.* New York: Igaku-Shoin Medical, 1997:74–88.

21. Derogatis LR. Psychological assessment of psychosexual functioning. *Psychiatr Clin North Am* 1980;3:113–131.

22. Gill KM, Ducharme SH. Female sexual functioning. In: Frankel HL, ed. *Handbook of clinical neurology.* Amsterdam: Elsevier Science, 1992:331–345.

23. Sipski ML, Alexander CJ. Female sexuality after spinal cord injury: current knowledge and future directions. *Top Spinal Cord Inj Rehabil* 1995;1(2):1–11.

24. Zwerner J. Yes, we have troubles but nobody's listening; sexual issues of women with spinal cord injury. *Sex Disability* 1982;5:158–171.

25. Ende J, Rockwell S, Glasgow M. The sexual history in general medical practice. *Arch Intern Med* 1984;144:358–361.

26. LoPiccolo L, Heiman J. Sexual assessment and history interview. In: LoPiccolo J, LoPiccolo L, eds. *Handbook of sex therapy.* New York: Plenum, 1978:103–113.

27. Wincze JP, Carey MP. *Sexual dysfunction: a guide for assessment and treatment.* New York: Guilford, 1991.

28. Schumacher S, Lloyd C. Assessment of sexual dysfunction. In: Gregoire H, ed. *Behavioral assessment: a practical handbook.* Elmsford, NY: Pergamon, 1976:76–102.

29. Medlar T, Medlar J. Nursing managment of sexual issues. *J Head Trauma Rehabil* 1990;5:46–51.

30. Erikson E. *Childhood and society.* New York: WW Norton, 1953.

31. Kauth MR, Kalichman SC. Sexual orientation and development: an interactive approach. In: Diamantt L, McAnulty RD, eds. *The psychology of sexual orientation, behavior and identity.* Westport, CT: Greenwood, 1995:81–104.

32. Nichols M. Low sexual desire in lesbian couples. In: Leiblum S, Rosen R, eds. *Sexual desire disorders.* New York: Guilford, 1988:387–412.

33. Rousso H. Special considerations in counseling clients with cerebral palsy. *Sex Disability* 1993;11:99–109.

34. Glover BH. Sex counseling. In: Reichel W, ed. *The geriatric patient.* New York: HP Publishing, 1978.

35. O'Connor CE, Stilwell EM. Sexuality, intimacy and touch in older adults. In: Reichel W, ed. *Clinical aspects of aging.* Baltimore: Williams & Wilkins, 1989:258–281.

36. Lew M. *Victims no longer: men recovering from incest and other sexual child abuse.* New York: HarperCollins, 1995:11–20.

37. Ducharme S, Gill K. *Sexuality after spinal cord injury: answers to your questions.* Baltimore: Paul Brookes, 1997:17–31.

38. Vermote R, Peuskens J. Sexual and micturition problems in multiple sclerosis patients. *Sex Disability* 1996;14:73–83.

39. Kroll K, Levy Klein E. *Enabling romance: a guide to love, sex and relationships for the disabled.* Bethesda, MD: Woodbine House, 1995:51–61.

40. Dunn M, Lloyd E, Phelps GH. Sexual assertiveness in spinal cord injury. In: Bullard DG, Knight SE,

eds. *Sexuality and physical disability.* St. Louis: CV Mosby, 1981:249–257.

41. Zasler N. Sexuality and neurologic disability; an overview. *Sex Disability* 1991;9:11–29.

42. Bullard DG. The treatment of desire disorders in the medically ill and physically disabled. In: Leiblum SR, Rosen RC, eds. *Sexual desire disorders.* New York: Guilford, 1988:348–384.

43. Zilbergeld B, Ellison CR. Desire discrepancies and arousal problems in sex therapy. In: Leiblum SR, Pervin LA, eds. *Principles and practice of sex therapy.* New York: Guilford, 1980:223–247.

44. Beck JG. Hypoactive sexual desire: an overview. *J Consult Clin Psychol* 1995;63:919–927.

45. Gilbert DM. Sexuality issues in persons with disabilities. In: Braddom RL, ed. *Physical medicine and rehabilitation.* Philadelphia: WB Saunders, 1996:605–629.

46. Kaplan HS. *The sexual desire disorders: dysfunctional regulation of sex motivation.* New York: Brunner/Mazel, 1995:266–309.

47. Wilson GD. The psychology of male sexual arousal. In: Gregoire A, Pryor JP, eds. *Impotence: an integrated approach to clinical practice.* London: Churchill Livingstone, 1993:16–27.

48. Basile G, Goldstein I. Medical treatment of neurogenic impotence. *Sex Disability* 1994;12:81–95.

49. Ami Sidi A. Vasoactive intracavernous pharmacotherapy. *Urol Clin North Am* 1988;15:99–100.

50. Mulcahy JJ. Update on penile prostheses. *Curr Opin Urol* 1991;1:152–155.

51. Sonksen J, Biering-Sorenson F. Transcutaneous nitroglycerin in the treatment of erectile dysfunction in the spinal cord injured. *Paraplegia* 1992;30:554–557.

52. Kim ED, McVary KT. Topical prostaglandin E for the treatment of erectile dysfunction. *J Urol* 1995;153:1828–1830.

53. Kerfoot WW, Carson CC. Pharmacologically induced erections among geriatric men. *J Urol* 1991;146:1022–1024.

54. Levine SB, Althof SE, Turner LA, et al. Side effects of self-administration of intracavernous papaverine and phentolamine for the treatment of impotence. *J Urol* 1989;141:54–57.

55. Padma-Nathan H, Hellestrom WJ, Kaiser FE, et al. Treatment of men with erectile dysfunction with transurethral alprostadil. *N Engl J Med* 1997;336:1–7.

56. Seftel AD, Oates RD, Krane JJ. Disturbed sexual function in patients with spinal cord disease. *Neurol Clin* 1991;9:757–777.

57. Bennett CJ. Sexual dysfunction and electroejaculation in men with spinal cord injuries: a review. *J Urol* 1988;139:453–470.

58. Brackett N, Nash M, Lynne C. Male fertility following spinal cord injury: facts and fiction. *Phys Ther* 1996;11:1224–1241.

59. Mccluer S. Reproductive aspects of spinal cord injury in females. In: Leyson JFJ, ed. *Sexual rehabilitation of the spinal cord injured patient.* Clifton, NJ: Humana, 1991:181–196.

60. Weinberg JS. Human sexuality and spinal cord injury. *Nurs Clin North Am* 1982;17:407–419.

61. Zasler ND. Sexuality issues after spinal cord injury. *Spinal Cord Inj Connector* 1988;4:22–28.

62. Berard EJ. The sexuality of spinal cord injured women: physiology and pathophysiology. *Paraplegia* 1989;27:99–112.

63. Glass DD. Diagnosis of sexual dysfunction in spinal cord injured women. In: Lyson JF, ed. *Sexual rehabilitation of the spinal cord injured patient.* Clifton, NJ: Humana, 1991:131–147.

64. Sipski ML, Alexander CJ. Female sexuality following spinal cord injury. *Spinal Cord Inj Psychosoc Proc* 1991;4(2):49–52.

65. Whipple B. Female sexuality. In: Lyson JF, ed. *Sexual rehabilitation of the spinal cord injured patient.* Clifton, NJ: Humana, 1991:19–38.

66. Sipski ML, Alexander CJ. Sexual activities, response and satisfaction in women pre and post spinal cord injury. *Arch Phys Med Rehabil* 1993;74:1025–1029.

67. Sipski ML, Alexander CJ, Rosen R. Physiological parameters associated with psychogenic sexual arousal in women with complete spinal cord injuries. *Arch Phys Med Rehabil* 1995;76:811–819.

68. Axel SJ. Spinal cord injured women's concerns: menstruation and pregnancy. *Rehabil Nurs* 1982;9:10–15.

69. Comarr AE. Observations of menstruation and pregnancy among female spinal cord injured patients. *Paraplegia* 1966;3: 263–272.

70. Sandowski CL. *Sexual concerns when disability strikes.* Springfield, IL: Charles C Thomas, 1989.

71. Nygaard I, Bartscht KD, Cole S. Sexuality and reproduction in spinal cord injured women. *Obstet Gynecol Surv* 1990;45:727–732.

72. Mccarren M. Birth control for spinal cord injured women. *Spinal Network* 1989;8:41–43.

73. Ducharme S, Gill K. Sexual values, training and professional roles. *J Head Trauma Rehabil* 1990;5:38–45.

Chapter 56

Substance Abuse and Disability

John W. Cassidy

Since the dawn of self-awareness, mankind has attempted to find ways to alter consciousness, first mystically and then chemically. Today the available licit and illicit choices number in the hundreds. The lifetime prevalence of alcoholism and drug addiction is as high as the prevalence of all other psychiatric disorders combined (1). Thus, early in his or her career, every rehabilitation clinician will be confronted with these problems. Therefore, in this chapter I focus on the common disorders seen in clinical settings and provide a framework for diagnosis and management. Furthermore, I attempt to avoid the confusing and ever-changing psychiatric nosology found in many texts on the general subject of "substance use." To that end, I use the term *addiction* to describe the general rubric subsuming both abuse and dependence, and I substitute *drug* for *substance* for reasons enumerated below. Furthermore, alcohol addiction, or alcoholism, is not considered separately from other drug addictions, unless there is a clinical rationale for doing so.

DEFINITIONS

The *Diagnostic and Statistical Manual of Mental Disorders*, fourth edition (DSM-IV) of the American Psychiatric Association remains the standard by psychiatrists for diagnosing substance-related disorders (2). Like any specialty, a unique lexicon has evolved to define and classify these conditions. (See Appendix I.) In many circumstances, however, this language has become a barrier to communication. In its attempt to be all-inclusive and avoid terms with pejorative connotations, the DSM-IV criteria for diagnosing these disorders are confusing. Although the words *substance* and *abuse* or *use* have become inextricably linked in the psychiatric literature to describe drug addiction, their use is not helpful in extending an understanding of these disorders to nonpsychiatrically trained professionals. The term *substance* refers to a drug of abuse (including alcohol), a medication, or a toxin. As such, the substance-related disorders refer to a number of conditions caused by the taking of a drug of abuse, to the side effects of a medication, and to toxin exposure (2). In most clinical settings, however, alcohol and other drug addictions are the problems that cause and increase morbidity in physiatric patients. Medication side effects are managed by the clinician responsible for overseeing or prescribing the drug in question, and toxin exposure, although a cause precipitating rehabilitation, rarely continues once a patient enters treatment. Thus for all practical purposes, drug addiction is the comorbid issue requiring a rehabilitation treatment team's attention.

Abuse was a term substituted for *addiction* during the evolution of the *Diagnostic and Statistical Manual* (3) in an attempt to find a less pejorative term than *addiction*. Historically, it is a behavioral term and has been characterized as improper use or misuse of a drug (substance) outside of the boundaries established by "a society" (2). *Abuse* connotes use that is voluntary, unethical, and immoral—hardly less judgmental than the discarded *addiction*. To move away from this connotation, the DSM-IV replaces *abuse* with *use* in the general categorization of these disorders.

Also from the historic perspective, *dependence* emphasized the physiologic consequences of alcoholism or other drug addiction, focusing on pharmacologic tolerance and symptomatic withdrawal. Given the fact that cocaine, one of the most irresistible drugs known to man, produces virtually no physiologic withdrawal syndrome, it becomes clear why pharmacologic dependence does not capture the construct of addiction.

So what, then, is addiction? It is what we generally consider it to be: uncontrollable preoccupation with and compulsive use of a drug despite the problems associated with such use, be they physical or psychosocial or both. The individual loses control over the use of the drug, denies it, tries to stop using it, and fails. The drug assumes a central position in the individual's life, and as the condition worsens, other aspects of existence pale in comparison. Eventually both social and occupational functioning are compromised. Denial and subterfuge are always associated with addiction, and thus cloud an external observer's ability to identify the problem early in its course. However, Miller (3) correctly asserted that "relapse is the *sine qua non* of diagnosing addictive behavior." Physiologic and pharmacologic markers of addiction, such as tolerance and withdrawal, may or may not accompany the disorder. *Tolerance* occurs when an individual develops a need for increasing amounts of the drug to produce the same effect he or she felt when first exposed to it (2). It is also seen when, with continued use, the same dose of the drug has diminished effectiveness. The development of tolerance has more to do with the drug chosen for abuse rather than the extent of its use, per se. For example, patients prescribed narcotic analgesics for pain control very quickly find that the doses initially ordered are inadequate to provide sustained relief. Classically, *withdrawal* is a physical syndrome that occurs with a reduction in or cessation of use of a drug (2). The response seen also depends on the drug used, but is usually stereotypic for each pharmacologic class. These physiologic markers may occur with legitimate use of a medication. The benzodiazepine class of anxiolytics is known to generate tolerance and with abrupt discontinuation of high doses, a recognizable withdrawal syndrome, which may include major motor seizures. Yet many patients benefit from their use and few develop the other behavioral concomitants of addiction listed earlier.

Drug intoxication is a common experience and is characterized by reversible psychological, behavioral, and physiologic reactions that are caused by use of a psychoactive drug. For example, alcohol, a central nervous system (CNS) depressant, produces intoxication by impairing the function of the frontal systems, leading to impaired attention, disinhibition, and reduced arousal. These deficits can produce transient disability in driving and judgment. The intoxication syndrome is again dependent on the drug under consideration, but can vary from individual to individual and depend on environmental circumstances. Some individuals become jovial when drunk, others belligerent. In social situations alcohol may lead to increased public interaction; however, when the individual drinks alone, sedation may be the prominent effect. Evidence of intoxication can be obtained from the patient's history, physical examination, or laboratory studies of urine or blood. However, intoxication is not a reliable indicator of addiction. This is particularly true with classes of drugs that produce rapid tolerance, such as narcotic analgesics, anxiolytics, and alcohol. With these drugs, a patient may be quite addicted and yet not evidence signs of intoxication during an evaluation. Under these circumstances, laboratory analysis may be the only evidence substantiating heavy use.

Many addicts use a number of drugs in sequence or simultaneously and are therefore described as poly-addicts or multiple-drug users. As an example, the stimulant addict finds the soporific effects of alcohol helpful at night when sleep has been difficult to attain and under these circumstances becomes an alcoholic as well. Although most addicts have a preferred drug of abuse, multiple-drug use has become increasingly common, especially in younger age groups. Fully 80% of alcoholics under age 30 abuse another drug in addition to alcohol (4). Thus, it behooves the clinician to broaden the discussion of drug use beyond a single agent.

Another area of concern is *comorbidity*. Historically drug addiction has been conceptualized as being secondary to another primary psychiatric disorder. This view was particularly common during the "drug as self-medication" phase of understanding addiction. The alcoholic was seen as medicating his or her depression with alcohol in an attempt to reclaim a more normal mood. Contemporary thinking suggests that the reverse is actually true (3). Alcohol itself produces the depression, and the alcoholic continues to drink despite inducing depression he or she finds so intolerable. Thus, alcoholism is the primary disorder. Treat the alcoholism, and the depression may remit spontaneously; an attempt to treat the depression without recognizing the alcoholism and in most cases, the mood disorder remains refractory to intervention. Certainly, psychiatric disorders and addiction can occur together, but identification of the psychiatric condition as primary is fraught with danger.

CLASSIFICATION

The common classes of drugs of abuse from the DSM-IV (2) are listed in Table 56-1. Street names for many of these drugs are listed in Table 56-2.

From the pharmacologic perspective, many of the drugs listed cluster into categories that help a clinician anticipate the issues expected to surface as an addictive cycle evolves. *Alcohol*, sedatives, hypnotics, and many anxiolytics are *CNS depressants* and as such are grouped together. The lifetime prevalence of alcoholism is 29% for

Table 56-1: Common Classes of Drugs of Abuse
Alcohol
Ethanol
Amphetamine
Dextroamphetamine
Methamphetamine
Phenmetrazine
Methylphenidate
Diethylpropion
Caffeine
Cannabis
Marijuana
Cocaine
Hallucinogens
Lysergic acid (LSD)
Methylenedioxymethamphetamine (MDMA) and
Congeners
Atropine
Psilocybine
Mescaline
Inhalants
Toluene
Gasoline
Carbon tetrachloride
Amyl nitrate
Nitrous oxide
Nicotine
Opioids
Opium
Morphine
Methadone
Heroin
Oxycodone
Phencyclidine (PCP)
Sedative, hypnotics, and anxiolytics

men and 7% for women (5). *Benzodiazepines* are the principal nonalcohol CNS depressants used today, both licitly and illicitly. They are among the most widely prescribed medications in the world. Fortunately, however, abuse of these drugs occurs infrequently. Interestingly, the elderly are at increased risk with these medications, which are given to treat anxiety and insomnia, two common problems of maturity. *Barbiturates* comprise another class of CNS depressants; however, in recent years the use and abuse of these drugs have been supplanted by the benzodiazepines. While tolerance is well recognized as a problem associated with alcohol consumption and barbiturate use, it is a somewhat more controversial phenomenon in those who abuse benzodiazepines. Nonetheless, all produce a withdrawal syndrome. Table 56-3 outlines the alcohol withdrawal syndrome.

Delirium tremens, or the "DTs" as they are colloquially known, is a potentially life-threatening withdrawal syndrome seen with heavy alcohol abuse and must be managed expediently by experienced physicians. The symptoms of delirium tremens are listed in Table 56-4.

Alcohol and barbiturates impair working memory and exacerbate frontal system deficits, making either a poor mix with brain injury. Alcohol is also a toxin to many human organ systems, notably the liver, and many alcoholics die from hepatic failure (cirrhosis) and its complications. It also crosses the placenta into the fetus and can produce the fetal alcohol syndrome, a major cause of mental retardation.

The benzodiazepine withdrawal syndrome is outlined in Table 56-5. It can be difficult to differentiate this syndrome from the underlying condition that the benzodi-

Table 56-2: "What's in a Name?"

Common Name	Street Name
Amphetamine	Bennies, speed, black and white, black bombers, brain ticklers, brownies, cartwheels, dexies, hearts, jolly bean
Methamphetamine	Speed, Chris, crystal meth, crink, double bubble
MDMA	ADAM, ecstasy, booty juice (in liquid), chocolate chips, clarity, doctor, E, essence
Cocaine	Coke, snow, flake, gold dust, blow, jam, toot, nose candy, Angie, Bernie, big rush, California cornflakes, dream, lady
Alkaloidal cocaine	Crack, rock, free-basing, baseball, beemers, baby T, Bill Blass, caps
LSD	Acid, window panes, sunshine, purple haze, white lightning, blotter acid, barrels, Bart Simpsons, battery acid, brown dots
Cannabinoids	Marijuana, Acapulco gold, airplane, grass, bale, bar, pot, weed, Black Bart, Mary Jane, puff, hashish, ganja, bhang, hemp
Heroin	Smack, TNT, horse, snow, white junk, Mexican brown, H, stuff, big Harry, bozo, Carga, Chinese red, dirt, dyno, Estuffa
Morphine	Dreamer, hard stuff, Ms Emma, morf, first line, God's drug, hows, Mister blue
Fentanyl and derivatives	China white, Persian white, Apache, friend, Goodfellas, great bear, king ivory
PCP	Angel dust, aurora borealis, black whack, busy bee, CJ, crazy Eddie, cyclones, crystal joint, energizer, elephant

Table 56-3: Alcohol Withdrawal Syndrome
Alcohol craving
Tremor, irritability
Nausea
Sleep disturbance
Tachycardia
Hypertension
Sweating
Perceptual distortion
Seizures (12–48 hr after last drink)

Source: O'Brien CP. Drug addiction and drug abuse. In: Hardman JG, Limbird LE, eds. *Goodman & Gilman's, the pharmacologic basis of therapeutics.* 9th ed. New York: McGraw-Hill, 1996:563.

Table 56-4: Symptoms of Delirium Tremens
Severe agitation
Confusion
Visual hallucinations
Fever, profuse sweating
Tachycardia
Nausea, diarrhea
Dilated pupils

Source: O'Brien CP. Drug addiction and drug abuse. In: Hardman JG, Limbird LE, eds. *Goodman & Gilman's, the pharmacologic basis of therapeutics.* 9th ed. New York: McGraw-Hill, 1996:563.

Table 56-5: Benzodiazepine Withdrawal Symptoms
Following moderate drug usage:
Anxiety, agitation
Increased sensitivity to light and sound
Paresthesias, strange sensations
Muscle cramps
Myoclonic jerks
Sleep disturbance
Dizziness
Following high-dose usage:
Seizures
Delirium

Sources: O'Brien CP. Drug addiction and drug abuse. In: Hardman JG, Limbird LE, eds. *Goodman & Gilman's, the pharmacologic basis of therapeutics.* 9th ed. New York: McGraw-Hill, 1996:564.

azepine was originally prescribed to treat. Many patients, therefore, confuse withdrawal with a return of anxiety and insomnia and become reluctant to discontinue use of the benzodiazepine despite requests to do so.

Psychostimulants are the broad classification subsuming amphetamine and its related congeners, caffeine, and cocaine. Stimulants increase CNS levels of excitatory neu-

Table 56-6: Symptoms of Stimulant Withdrawal
Dysphoria, depression
Sleepiness, fatigue
Cocaine craving
Bradycardia

Source: O'Brien CP. Drug addiction and drug abuse. In: Hardman JG, Limbird LE, eds. *Goodman & Gilman's, the pharmacologic basis of therapeutics.* 9th ed. New York: McGraw-Hill, 1996:571.

Table 56-7: Marijuana Withdrawal Syndrome
Restlessness
Irritability
Mild agitation
Insomnia
Sleep EEG disturbance
Nausea, cramping

Source: O'Brien CP. Drug addiction and drug abuse. In: Hardman JG, Limbird LE, eds. *Goodman & Gilman's, the pharmacologic basis of therapeutics.* 9th ed. New York: McGraw-Hill, 1996:573.

rotransmitters such as dopamine, norepinephrine, and epinephrine, often producing euphoria. These drugs are frequently used and highly addictive. Caffeine is the most widely utilized psychotropic drug in the world, and it has been estimated that 23 million Americans have experimented with cocaine and that 640,000 people use the drug weekly (6). Binge use of these agents is common and ceases only when the user's current supply is exhausted. Tolerance develops to each, but the associated withdrawal syndrome is mild and rarely requires acute medical intervention. Table 56-6 lists the signs and symptoms associated with stimulant withdrawal.

Cardiovascular system toxicity is occasionally seen and must cross the placental barrier to potentially affect the fetus. High doses can produce paranoia and other symptoms mimicking psychosis.

At one time *cannabinoids* were classified with the hallucinogens; however, during recent years they have been segregated from "psychedelics," as "hallucinations" are not prominently associated with their use. Rather they produce complex behavioral reactions that are highly dependent on the environment in which they are used and the expectations of the user. Most report positive feelings, such as "giddiness," anxiolysis, and disinhibition as well as increased hunger during social use. Tolerance occurs rapidly, but the withdrawal syndrome is mild or nonexistent. Table 56-7 lists the reported symptoms of withdrawal.

There is no evidence to suggest that uncomplicated marijuana use irreparably damages the CNS, although working memory may be impaired up to several weeks after cessation of heavy use. However, there have been recent reports (7,8) that it does serve as a "gateway drug" and increases the risk of abuse of other drugs, especially narcotic analgesics.

Although DSM-IV classifies drugs that alter perception and produce abnormalities in thought content as "hallucinogens," this is a misnomer since not all agents produce these phenomena. A more accurate descriptor is "psychedelic agents." Toxic doses can produce paranoia (an abnormality in thought content) in the absence of hallucinations. The most popular of these drugs in the United States are lysergic acid (LSD), phencyclidine (PCP), and methylenedioxymethamphetamine (MDMA). Although the prevalence of use tends to be cyclic, current estimates are that nearly 12% of young adults have experimented with them at some point in their lives (9). Pharmacologically their hallucinogenic effects appear to be associated with affinity for the serotonin 5-hydroxytryptamine type 2 (5-HT_2) receptor, although most agents have complex interactions with a number of receptor subtypes. PCP binds to the *N*-methyl-D-aspartic (NMDA)–type glutamate receptor, blocking the effects of this excitatory amino acid neurotransmitter. There is evidence to suggest that uncontrolled release of this neurotransmitter during traumatic brain injury (TBI) is associated with delayed (8–24 hours) neuronal death. MDMA has produced degeneration of serotonergic neurons in animal models, but this effect has not been demonstrated in humans.

Repeated and frequent use of psychedelics is uncommon; therefore, tolerance, although theoretically possible, is rarely seen clinically, and frank withdrawal syndromes are equally rare. High-dose PCP abuse has been associated with hallucinations and assaultive behavior, with some patients progressing to coma, associated with hypertension, and fixed and dilated pupils.

Inhalants form a heterogeneous class of abusable drugs, ranging from toluene (from model airplane glue) to amyl nitrate ("poppers"). Solvents produce significant systemic toxicity in addition to intoxication. Cerebral degeneration, peripheral neuropathy, cardiac arrest, bone marrow suppression, and hepatic and renal failure have all been reported with prolonged abuse. Amyl nitrate produces rapid dilation of smooth muscle and therefore vasodilation. Nitrous oxide produces euphoria, analgesia, and finally loss of consciousness. Binge use of amyl nitrate and nitrous oxide is common and therefore few cases of tolerance, withdrawal, and frank systemic toxicity have been reported.

As a class, *opioids* are known as *narcotic analgesics*. They also influence mood, often producing euphoria, along with pain relief. Naturally occurring agents, derived from the opium poppy, and synthetically manufactured drugs bind with CNS "opium receptors" to produce their characteristic clinical effects. Tolerance rapidly develops to these agents and a characteristic withdrawal syndrome is seen 6 to 12 hours after ingestion of a short-acting agent (e.g., heroin) and at 72 to 84 hours with long-acting ones (e.g., methadone) (Table 56-8).

Table 56-8: Opioid Withdrawal

Symptoms	**Signs**
Regular withdrawal	
Craving for opioids	Pupillary dilation
Restlessness, irritability	Sweating
Increased sensitivity to pain	Piloerection ("gooseflesh")
Nausea, cramps	Tachycardia
Muscle aches	Vomiting, diarrhea
Dysphoric mood	Increased blood pressure
Insomnia, anxiety	Yawning
	Fever
Protracted withdrawal	
Anxiety	Cyclic changes in weight, pupil size
Insomnia	Respiratory center sensitivity
Drug craving	

Source: O'Brien CP. Drug addiction and drug abuse. In: Hardman JG, Limbird LE, eds. *Goodman & Gilman's, the pharmacologic basis of therapeutics*. 9th ed. New York: McGraw-Hill, 1996:568.

Heroin is the prototype drug of abuse from this class of medications. Impure and dilute forms are administered intravenously, but purer forms, with higher concentrations of the drug, can be successfully administered by inhalation, vitiating the need for injection. It is estimated that there are over 1 million "heroin addicts" living in the United States. Overdose, leading to respiratory arrest, usually results from widely varying purities of the available street drug. Toxic systemic effects from the drug itself appear to be minimal.

PREVALENCE

As might be imagined, the prevalence of addiction depends on the drug in question, the population studied, and the method of case finding used. The facts of addiction—the use of illicit drugs is a felony in many legal jurisdictions, denial and duplicity are hallmarks of these disorders, and intoxication is an unreliable marker of dependence—lead to epidemiologic studies that generally underestimate the extent of drug abuse in the general population. The often-cited Epidemiologic Catchment Area Study (1) completed in 1988 reported the lifetime prevalence of alcoholism as 15% and that of "drug abuse and dependence" ranged from 9% to 20%. As noted in the introduction, the merged rate of these conditions is equivalent to the prevalence of all other primary psychiatric disorders combined.

Thus, with a base rate of nearly 35% in the general population, comorbidity with rehabilitation diagnoses is inevitable, particularly in younger patients (10). Drubach et al (11) examined over 300 patients admitted to a TBI rehabilitation hospital between 1988 and 1991. They reported that 30% of these patients admitted to a history of alcoholism, 29% to alcohol and other drug addiction, and 8% to other drug addiction alone. Age was a significant factor in drug choice, as older patients more often abused alcohol while younger ones used other drugs alone or in combination with alcohol. Drug use was highly correlated with sustaining a brain injury as a result of violence, such as that caused by gunshot wound or blunt cranial trauma. Of additional interest in this study was the finding that 30% of those admitting to drug abuse had a prior history of head injury as well. Lindenbaum et al (12) reviewed the toxicology screens of 169 patients admitted to an urban trauma center and found that nearly 50% of those sustaining trauma as a result of violent crimes tested positively for illicit drugs, more than 30% for drugs and alcohol, and more than 6% for ethanol alone.

The Substance Abuse Task Force of the National Brain Injury Foundation (13) noted that more than 30% of brain injury survivors had an identifiable problem with chemical dependence before trauma. In a very recent study, Soderstrom and colleagues (14) found even higher rates of psychoactive substance abuse in seriously injured, trauma center patients. Due to cognitive impairment, severely brain injured patients were excluded from the study. Of the over 1100 patients enrolled in this project, nearly 55% had a diagnosis of psychoactive substance use disorders during their lifetimes. At the time of the study, nearly 25% were alcohol dependent and another 20% were dependent on other drugs.

Data on the prevalence of addiction in other common rehabilitation populations such as those with spinal cord injury, stroke, orthopedic injuries, or burns are not readily available. Hospital-based spinal cord injury and stroke services request few consultations for help with these disorders. Stroke can be caused by drug abuse in younger populations. In these circumstances, the comorbid issue must be confronted actively but it is generally apparent. Orthopedic programs that deal with chronic pain are frequent referral sources, especially if patients with "back pain" are highly represented in the group. Often these individuals were prescribed narcotic analgesics early in their treatment, developed tolerance to the analgesic effects, increased the dose of the medication on their own, and ultimately found their use of the drug escalating out of control.

In elderly populations, abuse of prescribed sedative and hypnotic agents generally presents with hospitalization and unexpected withdrawal when the patient is not prescribed the offending agent(s). On occasion, a urinary drug screening test at the time of admission will reveal the presence of potentially habit-forming compounds in concentrations high enough to suggest regular and heavy use.

UNDERSTANDING ADDICTION

As late as 50 years ago, alcoholism and other drug addictions were considered defects of character and a sign of moral turpitude. This assessment prevailed despite the fact that the construct of alcoholism as a "disease" process was first proposed by Benjamin Rush in 1870. He wrote that in this diseased state, alcohol was the causal agent; loss of control over drinking, its characteristic symptom; and abstinence, its only cure. However, it was E. M. Jellinek's *The Disease Concept of Alcoholism* (15), published in 1960, that popularized this notion among the general population. The growth of self-help groups, beginning with Alcoholics Anonymous (AA), has had both positive and negative effects in this evolution. On the one hand, they have advanced acceptance of addiction and its treatment, but on the other, they have obfuscated some components of the disease model, particularly by resisting psychopharmacologic treatment of these disorders and by reincorporating spirituality into its conceptual matrix.

Awareness of predisposing risk factors aids the detection of these disorders. Early longitudinal studies of alcoholics by Valliant (16) focused primarily on cultural factors that increased individual risk. One striking factor in the United States was ethnic background; those of Irish extraction were seven times more likely to manifest alcohol dependence than were those of "Mediterranean" heritage. Increasing northern latitude also heightened the risk. The cultural forces adduced to explain these findings centered on enforced childhood and adolescent abstinence coupled with tolerance of public, adult male drunkenness. Potential psychiatric comorbidity was also implicated, but subsequent work revealed that only those diagnosed with schizophrenia and antisocial personality disorder were at a higher risk than the general population.

Heritable influences have also been studied. Discerning the individual contributions of nature and nurture in the production of any clinical condition is always fraught with difficulty; however, studies evaluating the etiology of the addictive disorders have found a greater influence of genetic factors than environmental ones. Merikangas (17) reviewed a number of family studies and convincingly concluded that the risk of alcoholism was sevenfold higher among first-degree family members of alcoholics than in the general population. Narcotic analgesic dependence followed a similar pattern, with nearly a 14-fold increase in risk of addiction among first-degree relatives of opiate abusers. Adoption studies (18–20), where one of the probands is adopted into a nonalcoholic family, also support the conclusion that heritable, nonenvironmental factors have substantial influence on the development of this disorder. However, the influence does not follow any currently identifiable pattern of inheritance and no identifiable genetic marker has yet been found. A twin study (21) looking at drug addiction found that monozygotic concordance was significantly higher than dizygotic concordance.

This study suggests that the expression of these traits is a complex interaction of constitutional diatheses, upbringing, and personal experiences.

Premorbid personality characteristics have not been particularly helpful in identifying this patient population. Early beliefs about the alcoholic personality appear to have been constructed based on the effects of alcohol rather than the converse. However, antisocial personality disorder (2) conveys the highest risk of any psychiatric disorder for the development of alcoholism or drug addiction. Adoption studies (18–20) found that antisocial personality disorder is also heritable and that these two disorders may have a common, but still unidentified, genetic precursor. However, depression, anxiety, and passivity did not predict the development of these disorders.

Finally, contemporary research suggests that there are common neurochemical substrates that produce a vulnerability to drug addiction. Such research primarily points to limbic system dysfunction, specifically in the ventral tegmentum, nucleus accumbens, locus ceruleus, dorsal raphe nucleus, and periaqueductal gray area. These regions contain the somas of the neurons that are the major producers of dopamine, norepinephrine, serotonin, and the endogenous opioids. Alcohol and other drugs of abuse influence the production, release, and degradation of these important classes of neurotransmitters that ultimately impact mood, drive states, and instinctual behavior (22).

DIAGNOSIS AND EVALUATION

The single most important factor in diagnosing addiction for the rehabilitation professional is considering its possibility in the midst of a myriad of other problems. Acute care records are often sketchy in areas involving "social history" unless the trauma patient reeks of alcohol on presentation to the emergency department. However, most level I neurotrauma centers routinely order measurement of blood alcohol concentrations (BAC) and urinary drug screens on all patients. Requesting these records is vital in establishing whether the neurotrauma patient was under the influence of drugs at the time of the accident. However, as noted already, there is not a one-to-one correspondence between intoxication and addiction. When one is searching for problems with drug addiction, these screening laboratory studies produce both false-positive and false-negative results. False-positive results generally occur in the context of having received a licit drug of potential abuse from the medical team before or upon admission to the emergency department for the relief of pain, to facilitate intubation, and so on. False-negative results occur when the addicted patient has not used the drug of abuse within the period of detection by common laboratory tests. Cannabinoids can be detected for up to 14 days after repeated use, but evidence of cocaine, opiates, amphetamines, and barbiturates is present for only 2 to 4 days after use. In the Soderstrom study noted earlier (14), the rates for false-negative results on BAC and urinary drug screen tests were approximately 12% and 4%, respectively.

Table 56-9: CAGE Questionnaire

1. Have you ever felt you should *C*ut down on your drinking?
2. Have people *A*nnoyed you by criticizing your drinking?
3. Have you ever felt bad or *G*uilty about your drinking?
4. Have you ever taken a drink first thing in the morning to steady your nerves or get rid of a hangover? (*E*ye opener).

Scoring

Two or more positive answers suggest that the existence of alcohol-related problems is very probable.

Source: Seppa K, Makela R, Sillanaukee P. Effectiveness of the alcohol use disorders identification test in occupational health screenings. *Alcohol Clin Exp Res* 1995;19:999–1003.

For better or worse, the "gold standard of diagnosis" remains the clinical history, supplemented by appropriate screening tools and instruments. These screening tools include the so-called CAGE questionnaire, CAGE being an acronym created by using the first letters of the words cut, annoyed, guilty, and *eye opener*. Table 56-9 lists the full questionnaire. The CAGE questionnaire can be modified for drug abuse screening by replacing the words "drink" and "drinking" with "drug" and "drug use." A shortened version of the Michigan Alcoholism Screening Test, known as the S-MAST, can also be used to screen for alcoholism but has less use in other drug-addicted populations. Table 56-10 provides this screening tool. The CAGE questionnaire has been shown to be a credible screening tool for alcoholism in primary care settings (sensitivity, 74%–89%; specificity, 79%–95%) and by extension, should be of equal benefit in rehabilitation patients, barring significant cognitive impairment or speech and language disorders.

However, the final diagnosis of these disorders rests with fulfilling the criteria of the DSM-IV, generally evaluated by using the psychoactive substance use section of the Structured Clinical Interview for the *Diagnostic and Statistical Manual* (SCID) (23). This is considered a "criterion standard" against which screening instrument results can be assessed. However, one must be trained in its use and therefore, such an evaluation is best deferred to an appropriate consulting clinician.

Thus, the approach to the diagnosis of alcoholism and drug addiction in most acute rehabilitation settings should include the following:

1. Review initial medical records for historical or laboratory evidence of use at the time of presentation to acute care.

Table 56-10: S-MAST Questionnaire
1. Do you feel you are a normal drinker?
2. Do your relatives and friends think of you as a normal drinker?
3. Have you already attended a meeting of Alcoholics Anonymous?
4. Have you already lost friends or companions because of drink?
5. Have you already had problems at work because of drink?
6. Have you neglected your responsibilities, your family, or your work for 2 days running or more because you drink too much?
7. After you have had a lot to drink, have you ever had an attack of *delirium tremens*, felt severe shaking, heard voices, or had any visual hallucinations?
8. Have you ever sought help from anyone because of your drinking habits?
9. Have you ever been in a hospital because of drink?
10. Have you ever been arrested for drunk driving or for driving after having a drink?

Source: Pokorny AD, Miller BA, Kaplan HB. The brief MAST: a shortened version of the Michigan Alcoholism Screening Test. *Am J Psychiatry* 1972;129:342–345.

2. If not already done, consider ordering a urinary drug screen test if the patient presents to rehabilitation within the time period needed to detect most drugs of abuse.
3. Obtain a social history and ask "probe questions" about any use of alcohol, licit, or illicit "recreational drugs."
4. If the answer to any probe question is "yes," administer the CAGE questionnaire for addiction, modified for drug addiction, or the S-MAST.
5. In patients with compromised cognition or aphasia, laboratory studies may be supplemented by interviewing a family member or "significant other." However, such outside sources are less reliable than the history given by the patient.
6. If screening evaluations suggest addiction, refer the patient for formal psychiatric, psychological, or social service consultation.
7. Suggest use of the SCID by consultants.
8. If addiction is confirmed, further medical evaluation is indicated to survey for potential end-organ damage and systemic illness. For example, alcoholism can produce direct toxic effects to the liver, leading to hepatic disease and cirrhosis. Intravenous heroin use can lead to the acquired immunodeficiency syndrome (AIDS) when materials contaminated with human immunodeficiency virus are used to inject the drug.

TREATMENT

Alcohol

Because of its life-threatening nature and delayed presentation, one condition that every physician must be able to recognize and treat is delirium tremens caused by withdrawal from alcohol. This syndrome generally presents within 48 to 96 hours after the last ingestion of alcohol and manifests itself by producing profound confusion, visual hallucinations, and severe autonomic dysregulation (see Table 56-4). General treatment involves close observation, hydration, nutritional support, and the judicious use of intravenous benzodiazepines.

Vigilant nursing care is vital as the onset of delirium tremens is often heralded by a major motor seizure. Intravenous access must be immediately established and hydration initiated with normal saline solution. Preparations with glucose are avoided until thiamine is administered intravenously to avoid the risk of Wernicke-Korsakoff syndrome. In most circumstances, 200 mg of thiamine administered intravenously is adequate to prevent this complication, and should be routinely given. To mitigate bleeding diathesis, any patient with a prolonged prothrombin time is also parenterally administered 5 to 10 mg of vitamin K. In any patient with a past history of alcohol-related withdrawal seizures, 1 g of magnesium sulfate is given intramuscularly every 6 hours for 2 days. Indices of malnutrition, such as lowered total protein and albumin levels, necessitate dietary consultation, supplemental folic acid (1 g/day), and increased caloric support.

If seizures continue, the patient, by definition, has developed status epilepticus. This is a major neurologic emergency and necessitates transfer to an intensive care setting. However, its emergent management centers on administering diazepam, 10 mg, by slow intravenous push. If intravenous access is unavailable or becomes compromised, intramuscular lorazepam, 2 mg, is preferable to diazepam because it is more reliably absorbed following injection. Rectal administration of 10 mg of diazepam or suppository-compounded diazepam is also acceptable. Repeated doses are given every 2 to 5 minutes until the seizures abate. The vast majority of patients respond to such interventions; those who do not respond require intravenous administration of phenytoin. The intravenous administration of this drug is fraught with hazards, especially due to cardiovascular complications, and is best done with continuous blood pressure and electrocardiographic monitoring. If no alternative exists, very, very slow intravenous loading to 1 g (up to 50 mg/min, but preferably in unmonitored situations no faster than 25 mg/min *by the clock*) in normal saline solution may be lifesaving.

When experiencing marked agitation and hallucinosis, the patient may require restraints. Vest restraints are best supplemented by bilateral wrist and ankle reatraints, as these patients frequently compromise their intravenous access, strike out at the staff, and disrupt any orthopedic appliances. Hallucinations are best managed by short-term administration of low-dose, high-potency antipsychotic medications, such as haloperidol. Although some theoretical objections have been raised to the use of this class of medications in the brain injured, clinically significant complications are not seen with low doses given for brief periods. Haloperidol, 2 to 5 mg, is given intravenously. Rarely do patients require more than 15 mg/day administered for 48 to 96 hours.

Less severe withdrawal is managed with oral medications. Thiamine and folate, 100 mg and 1 mg four times per day, respectively, are given with a once-daily multivitamin supplement. In patients with a past history of withdrawal seizures, magnesium sulfate, 1 g every 6 hours for 2 days, is given and then discontinued. Although chlordiazepoxide was historically the benzodiazepine of choice under these circumstances, there is little pharmacologic reason to choose it over diazepam. Thus, I prefer to administer 10 mg of diazepam orally to the patient who manifests objective signs of withdrawal such as tremulousness, tachycardia, and hypertension. Appropriate objective guidelines are contained within Table 56-11. If the patient is not sedated within an hour of administration, another 10 mg is given every hour until sedation is achieved. Most patients respond to 10 mg and this dose is continued every 6 hours for the next 24 hours. Recurring symptoms are managed by additional doses of 10 mg given as needed every 2 hours. After 24 hours, the dose is tapered to extinction by approximately 10% to 15% of the total first-day dose each day. For example, if the patient requires a total of 40 mg of diazepam on day 1, he would be given 35 mg in divided doses on day 2, 30 mg on day 3, and so on, until he is completely off this medication.

If the patient's withdrawal from alcohol does not interfere with the ability to participate in rehabilitation, referral to a specific outpatient substance abuse treatment program can be deferred until discharge. Recent studies, although somewhat controversial, suggested that there are at least three effective nonpharmacologic treatment approaches to alcoholism. In a large multicenter study (24), "Project MATCH," more than 1700 patients were studied after completing one of three 12-week treatment programs. Researchers randomly assigned a third of the participants to a "cognitive-behavioral coping skills program" that taught techniques to enable patients to achieve and maintain sobriety. These skills included coping with potential drinking situations, managing thoughts and feelings about alcohol, and learning effective ways to decline offered alcoholic beverages. Another third were enrolled in "motivational enhancement therapy" that mobilized the patients' own resources to effect behavioral change by fostering motivation to initiate or maintain change, consolidating commitment to change, and monitoring and encouraging progress with sobriety. The final third attended "12-step facilitation" designed to prepare and encourage participation in AA.

All three therapies produced equally encouraging results at 1 year after treatment. Using three consecutive drinking days as an indicator of relapse, the investigators found that all patients were abstinent for 80% of the post-treatment period. According to this criterion, less than 40% of the patients had a relapse during the 12 months following their participation in the study.

Random outpatient urinary tests for alcohol provide one mechanism of evaluating compliance with the request for abstinence during rehabilitative treatment. The specimens must be obtained under observation to avoid adulteration or substitution of the specimen. Although most laboratories have developed measures to detect sample dilution or adulteration, they are at best rudimentary and become a source of never-ending contention with patients who "test negative" but fail laboratory "integrity checks."

A number of medications have been adjunctively used in the treatment of alcoholism. Disulfiram (Antabuse) blocks the metabolism of alcohol, resulting in the accumulation of acetaldehyde. Acetaldehyde produces flushing, nausea, and vomiting following the ingestion of alcohol. With regular use of this medication, impulsive consumption of alcohol may be mitigated by a patient's wish to avoid such noxious reactions. However, this inhibitory effect is short-lived if the medication is discontinued. Thus, compliance is a major issue for patients whose commitment to sobriety is not firmly established.

Naltrexone, and opiate antagonist, was recently approved by the U.S. Food and Drug Administration (FDA) for use in the treatment of alcoholism. For some patients, alcohol appears to elevate CNS levels of endogenous opioids such as endorphins and enkephalins, thereby producing a sense of euphoria along with frontally mediated disinhibition. Based on this theory and on research with animal models, two double-blind, placebo-controlled patient trials were undertaken recently to evaluate its efficacy in humans. Both studies demonstrated drug efficacy; however, this result was obtained in the context of supportive outpatient counseling (25,26). Recent European experience (27) with another drug, acamprosate, has also been positive. Acamprosate appears to be a γ-aminobutyric acid (GABA) antagonist that blocks the CNS brain reward systems mediated by this inhibitory neurotransmitter, thereby reducing the drive to consume alcohol.

Other Central Nervous System Depressants

With the advent of benzodiazepine sedative-hypnotics, the use of barbiturates and other nonbenzodiazepine sedatives has greatly declined. However, an occasional geriatric patient will present with secobarbital addiction, following years of use for insomnia. Its abrupt discontinuation following stroke will precipitate the withdrawal syndrome outlined in Table 56-5. If the type and dose of the barbiturate are known, it may be gradually tapered by 10% to 15% each day until extinction. Even under these

Table 56-11: Withdrawal Assessment Scale

Name.. **Hospital number..**

Temperature (per axilla) 1 37.0–37.5°C 2 37.5–38.0°C 3 Greater than 38.0°C			
Pulse (beats per minute) 1 90–95 3 100–105 5 110–120 2 95–100 4 105–110 6 Greater than 120			
Respiration rate (inspirations per minute) 1 20–24 2 Greater than 24			
Blood pressure (diastolic) 1 95–100 mmHg 3 103–106 mmHg 5 109–112 mmHg 2 100–103 mmHg 4 106–109 mmHg 6 Greater than 112 mmHg			
Nausea and vomiting (Do you feel sick? Have you vomited?) 0 None 4 Intermittent nausea with dry heaves 2 Nausea with no vomiting 6 Nausea, dry heaves, vomiting			
Tremor (arms extended, fingers spread) 0 No tremor 4 Moderate with arms extended 2 Not visible—can be felt fingertip to fingertip 6 Severe even with arms not extended			
Sweating (observation) 0 No sweat visible 4 Beads of sweat visible 2 Barely perceptible, palms moist 6 Drenching sweats			
Tactile disturbances 0 None 2 Mild itching or pins and needles or numbness 4 Intermittent tactile hallucinations (for example, bugs crawling) 6 Continuous tactile hallucinations			
Auditory disturbances (loud noises, hearing voices) 0 Not present 2 Mild harshness or ability to frighten (increased sensitivity) 4 Intermittent auditory hallucinations (appears to hear things you cannot) 6 Continuous auditory hallucinations (shouting, talking to unseen persons)			
Visual disturbances (photophobia, seeing things) 0 Not present 2 Mild sensitivity (bothered by the lights) 4 Intermittent visual hallucinations (occasionally sees things you cannot) 6 Continuous visual hallucinations (seeing things constantly)			
Hallucinations 0 None 2 Non-fused auditory or visual 1 Auditory, tactile or visual only 3 Fused auditory and visual			
Clouding of sensorium (What day is this? What is this place?) 0 Oriented 2 Disoriented for date by no more than two days 3 Disoriented for date 4 Disoriented for place (re-oriente if necessary)			
Quality of contact 0 In contact with examiner 2 Seems in contact, but is oblivious to environment 4 Periodically becomes detached 6 Makes no contact with examiner			
Anxiety (Do you feel nervous?) (observation) 0 No anxiety; at ease 4 Moderately anxious, or guarded 2 Appears anxious 6 Overt anxiety (equal to panic)			
Agitation (observation) 0 Normal activity 4 Moderately fidgety and restless 2 Somewhat more than normal activity 6 Pacing, or thrashing about constantly			

Table 56-11: (*Continued*)

Name.. Hospital number..			
Thought disturbances (flight of ideas) 0 No disturbance 2 Does not have much control over nature of thoughts 4 Plagued by unpleasant thoughts constantly 6 Thoughts come quickly and in a disconnected fashion			
Convulsions (seizures or fits of any kind) 0 No 6 Yes			
Headache (Does it feel like a band around your head?) 0 Not present 4 Moderately severe 2 Mild 6 Severe			
Flushing of face 0 None 1 Mild 2 Severe			
Total			
Date			
Time			

Source: Foy A, March S, Drinkwater V. Use of an objective clinical scale in the assessment and management of alcohol withdrawal in a large general hospital. *Alcohol Clin Exp Res* 1988;12:360–364.

Table 56-12: Pentobarbital Challenge Test

Clinical manifestations
Mild—agitation, anxiety, nausea, vomiting, tachycardia, postural hypotension, hyperreflexia, tremor
Severe—seizures, delirium, hypothermia, cardiovascular collapse

Management
There is significant morbidity and mortality, making hospitalization mandatory in most cases. Pentobarbital tolerance test and detoxification as follows:

Day 1
When the patient is no longer intoxicated, give pentobarbital 200 mg PO.
If intoxication results (nystagmus, ataxia, or dysarthria), patient's 6-hour pentobarbital requirement is 100–200 mg. If patient *falls asleep*, he or she was already probably not addicted.
If no intoxication, give an additional 100 mg PO q2h until intoxication develops.
Total dose required to produce intoxication is the patient's 6-hour requirement.
Multiply by 4 to calculate 24-hour pentobarbital requirement.
Phenobarbital substitution. After 24-hour pentobarbital requirement is calculated, substitute phenobarbital 30 mg or each 100 mg of pentobarbital. Give this amount of phenobarbital in three divided doses for 48 hours.

Day 2
Give 24-hour phenobarbital requirement as given on day 1.

Day 3 and thereafter
Subtract 30 mg/day of phenobarbital (beginning with the AM dose) from the total dose given on day 1 until the patient is detoxified. If signs of intoxication develop, eliminate a single dose and resume treatment 6–8 hours later. If signs of withdrawal develop, give 60–120 mg of phenobarbital PO or IM immediately.

Mixed opiate-sedative dependence. Maintain temporarily on methadone and withdraw patient from sedatives first, then from methadone.

Source: Weiss RD, Mirin SM. Alcohol-related emergencies. In: Hyman SE, ed. *Manual of psychiatric emergencies*. 2nd ed. Boston: Little, Brown, 1988:236.

circumstances, rebound insomnia is likely and may require short-term management with a benzodiazepine. However, this rebound does not mean that an underlying sleep disorder remains. Therefore, the benzodiazepine should be discontinued within a few weeks.

If the type and dose of the barbiturate are not known, a pentobarbital challenge test is performed according to the guidelines in Table 56-12. Owing to its long half-life and cross-reactivity, phenobarbitol is substituted for the pentobarbital and the patient is gradually tapered from this agent.

Withdrawal from benzodiazepines can be accomplished similarly, but most often the patient is tapered from the drug itself using the guidelines just suggested. Substitution of diazepam or clorazepate for shorter-acting agents such as oxazepam (Serax) or lorazepam (Ativan) may smooth the tapering process and mitigate the need for barbiturate substitution. It is essential, however, that the treating clinician be familiar with the dosage equivalents of the substituted agent because of the wide variation in potency among drugs in this class of medications. This familiarization is particularly important with alprazolam (Xanax). After detoxification, the prevention of relapse generally requires referral to an outpatient treatment program similar to what was described for alcoholism.

For the unwitting, iatrogenically addicted patient, more specific diagnosis of the underlying psychiatric condition that first led to the prescription of the drug may lead to the recommendation of non-habit-forming alternatives. For example, many patients with insomnia experience this problem as a symptom of depression. Prescription of a sedating antidepressant may ameliorate both the depression and the insomnia, without the potential for addiction. I also described the use of trazodone (Desyrel), a non-habit-forming heterocyclic antidepressant, for the management of primary insomnia in the brain-injured patient (28). Of particular importance, trazodone induces sleep that closely mimics that achieved without medications. This mitigates suppression of rapid eye movement (REM) sleep and lengthens stage IV sleep, which promotes restful, restorative sleep. Hypotension is a well-described side effect of this agent, especially at higher doses. The risk of hypotension may be lessened if the agent is taken following a light snack and right before the patient wishes to retire for the night.

Psychostimulants

Most psychostimulants facilitate the presynaptic release of dopamine and norepinephrine (amphetamine, dextroamphetamine, methamphetamine, and diethylpropion) or block their reuptake (cocaine). The withdrawal syndrome seen with such agents (see Table 56-5) rarely requires medical intervention. However, many addicts report depression as a component of the so-called psychostimulant "crash" that occurs following abstinence. Most studies report a gradual diminution of this syndrome within 1 to 3 weeks after drug discontinuation (29). However, a significant minority of patients will continue to evidence signs and symptoms of melancholia (2) and should be treated with antidepressant medications. Some studies suggested the preferential use of desipramine, a tricyclic antidepressant that inhibits monoamine reuptake (30). However, unlike the majority of the abused drugs, desipramine preferentially inhibits the reuptake of norepinephrine and not dopamine.

Preliminary studies using bupropion (Wellbutrin) also suggested its use in similar circumstances. Fluoxetine (Prozac) reportedly reduces cocaine craving in some patients, while ameliorating underlying depression or a depressive diathesis (31). Psychosocial treatments center on referral to Cocaine Anonymous (CA) or similar groups.

Cannabinoids and Psychedelic Agents

The withdrawal syndrome from marijuana is mild and does not require medical attention. An occasional patient may report persistent depression following abstinence that can be treated with the antidepressant medications. However, there is now relatively convincing evidence that marijuana serves as a "gateway" drug. Therefore, multiple-drug addiction should be assessed in all patients found to have cannabinoids in their urine following routine testing.

LSD is the most potent of the commonly abused psychedelic drugs. Although there is no known withdrawal syndrome, some patients present with severe agitation following use. Accompanying disorders of thought content, such as paranoia and hallucinations, generally respond to antipsychotic agents. If intravenous administration is required, haloperidol remains the drug of choice. However, when oral administration is possible, two newer agents are available to mitigate the extrapyramidal movement disorder seen with older agents. Risperidone (Risperdal) and olanzapine (Zyprexa) recently were approved by the FDA for use in idiopathic psychotic disorders and by extension have been used in combating the hallucinogenic effects of LSD. Doses of risperidone range from 2 to 6 mg, while 5 to 20 mg is the standard for olanzapine. "Flashbacks" are occasionally seen with this drug as well. These experiences occur in a small percentage of former LSD users and are characterized by false, fleeting perceptions in the peripheral visual fields, flashes of color, geometric pseudohallucinations, and positive afterimages. Fatigue, stress, entry into a dark environment, and cannabinoid use apparently precipitate them. The visual component of the disorder is stable in approximately 50% of these patients and represents a permanent alteration of the visual systems (32).

PCP abuse can also cause hallucinosis accompanied by extreme agitation. Rarely, patients present with persistent psychotic states that require treatment with antipsychotics. Psychosocial interventions generally require referral to Narcotics Anonymous (NA) and long-term outpatient psychiatric therapy.

Opioids

Given their use for the management of acute pain, opioids or narcotic analgesics are frequently abused both during and after rehabilitation for both orthopedic injuries and "back pain." Because tolerance to the analgesic effect of these agents develops so rapidly, patients become rapidly addicted and uncontrollable and escalate their use. Drug-seeking behavior manifests itself in multiple office calls requesting additional medication due to "lost prescriptions" and other semiplausible excuses; use of multiple pharmacies; weekend calls to the service when the primary

Table 56-13: Diagnosis and Treatment of Opioid Withdrawal
Objective signs of opiate withdrawal
Pulse is 10 beats/min over baseline* or >90 in the absence of a history of tachycardia if baseline is unknown.
Systolic blood pressure is 10mm Hg over baseline or >160/95 in the absence of known hypertension.
Dilated pupils.
Sweating, gooseflesh, rhinorrhea, or lacrimation.
Treatment
Administer methadone, 10mg PO q4h prn, when two of the four criteria above are met; decrease by 5mg/day to zero.

* Baseline refers to the patient's vital signs 1 hour after receiving 10mg of methadone. For a patient who has received no methadone, these baseline vital signs should be estimated according to what one would expect from the patient's age, sex, and general health.

Source: Weiss RD, Mirin SM. Alcohol-related emergencies. In: Hyman SE, ed. *Manual of psychiatric emergencies.* 2nd ed. Boston: Little, Brown, 1988:234.

physician is "off call"; emergency room visits for "migraine" headaches; and so on. Ultimately, "doctor-shopping" begins as the patient becomes increasingly desperate for the medication in high-enough doses to overcome substantial tolerance and is embarrassed by his or her own behavior or when it is finally confronted by the treating physician. Finally, some patients will go to the streets to illegally obtain the drug, often graduating to a more potent, illicit agent.

Detoxification may require admission to an inpatient "pain program." A full description of a such a program is beyond the scope of this chapter, but is covered in greater detail in Chapter 58. In general, however, most programs compound the patient's medication of abuse and gradually taper it on a pre-prescribed schedule that does not permit use as needed. A critical guiding principle in treating opiate withdrawal is to respond to the patient's objective clinical signs rather than subjective symptoms. When signs of withdrawal occur, oral administration of methadone, 10mg, is often enough to eliminate them. Methadone should be administered when two of the four objective criteria listed in Table 56-13 are met.

Another, less complicated approach involves the use of clonidine, an α_2-adrenergic receptor agonist prescribed primarily as an antihypertensive agent. Clonidine ameliorates many of the adrenergically mediated symptoms of withdrawal, such as nausea, vomiting, sweating, tachycardia, and hypertension, by reducing the presynaptic release of norepinephrine from the locus ceruleus. It is available orally and as a transdermal patch (Catapres-TTS) in doses ranging from 0.1mg/day/week to 0.3mg/day/week. Most young patients require the 0.3-mg application, but higher doses can be achieved by using additional patches or administering the medication orally. Doses up to 0.6mg/day have been routinely used in this patient population as long as the blood pressure is closely monitored to avoid symptomatic postural hypotension. Treatment is usually continued for 2 weeks, and then the medication is tapered and discontinued. However, clonidine does not treat muscular cramping or the "opioid craving" that accompanies full-blown withdrawal.

Long-term management is best accomplished psychiatrically. This assertion is especially true if agonist maintenance with methadone is contemplated. Occasionally patients are treated with naltrexone for reasons similar to those outlined for alcoholism.

INTEGRATED TREATMENT

Much has been made of integrating the treatment of drug addiction into most, if not all, rehabilitation programs. Paradoxically, however, this development has occurred as the average length of stay in most acute rehabilitation settings has been reduced to a historic nadir. Such pressure for discharge makes treatment impractical if not impossible. Therefore, identification, detoxification (if necessary), and referral are the only viable options available to most clinicians.

In postacute, day-treatment settings, where the length of stay ranges from 6 to 24 weeks, integrated treatment becomes more feasible. Rehabilitation centers that focus on chronic pain must integrate the treatment for addiction into their programs. Unfortunately, the handicaps that devolve from addiction are often more debilitating than the underlying physical condition itself. As noted already, a full discussion of these constructs exceeds the reach of this chapter and the interested reader is referred to Chapter 58.

The premorbid risk factors associated with TBI are intimately related to problems with drugs and alcohol. These include youthfulness, male gender, impulsivity coupled with risk taking, learning disabilities, and primary psychopathology. Of course, the best predictor of the future is the past, and not surprisingly patients at greatest risk for drug addiction after an injury has occurred are those who were addicted prior to their injuries. The frontal system dysfunction that accompanies most, if not all, severe TBI untethers the tenuous self-control of these individuals and often exacerbates their premorbid problems. Furthermore, TBI leads to an inevitable downward drift in both socioeconomic status and the "quality" of the individuals who choose to associate with the "survivor." This combination of impaired self-control and association with "the wrong crowd" is fertile soil for the growth and maintenance of addiction.

Reversal of such a cycle is extremely difficult. No program or therapist has a behavioral reinforcer stronger

Table 56-14: Modified 12-Step Program for Traumatic Brain Injury (TBI) Patients

1. Admit that if you drink and/or use drugs, your life will be out of control. Admit that the use of substances after having had a TBI will make your life unmanageable.
2. You start to believe that someone can help you put your life in order. This someone could be God, an AA group, counselor, sponsor, etc.
3. You decide to get help from others or from God. You open yourself up.
4. You will make a complete list of the negative behaviors in your past and current behavior problems. You will also make a list of your positive behaviors.
5. Meet with someone you trust and discuss what you wrote in step 4.
6. Become ready to sincerely try to change your negative behaviors.
7. Ask God for the strength to be a responsible person with responsible behaviors.

Reprinted courtesy of Alcoholics Anonymous.

than a direct-acting CNS drug of abuse. It is well known that laboratory animals will forsake even food and water for solubilized cocaine. Environmental prosthesis is often the only remedy. However, this is an expensive proposition that requires residential placement.

In such settings the staff is required to substitute its intact executive functioning for that of the patient. Access to drugs and alcohol is restricted and random screening is implemented to detect any unsuspected breakdown of primary defenses. With time, cravings tend to wane, and some patients will be able to incorporate the externally imposed structure into themselves. A shift in the individual's position on drug abuse is generally heralded by movement away from viewing treatment as imprisonment toward a sense that "working with the program" is consistent with a more "normalized" life. As this occurs, the patient is gradually exposed to a broader range of environments, including some that will invariably offer access to drugs and alcohol.

Furthermore, both education and a "12-step" program can then be started. Suggested modifications to the standard AA 12-step program for the brain injured are included in Table 56-14. Once the patient leaves treatment, medications as well as random drug screening are continued.

I have found that the combination of the duplicity of the addict and the anosognosia of the brain injured precludes successful individual counseling. Group and family therapies are somewhat more successful because relapse can be actively confronted by those not constrained by therapeutic neutrality.

Attendance at community-based AA, CA, or NA meetings must be continued. It is best to pair a non-brain-injured "sponsor" with a participating brain injury survivor. When necessary, sponsors should "rotate" to avoid the burnout associated with supervision of the cognitively and behaviorally impaired. Backup access to a therapist should be provided to permit support should the patient's sponsor be unavailable or the patient feel that relapse is imminent. Sadly, such supports are often needed for the remainder of the individual's life.

CONCLUSIONS

Given that very often the only good outcome from rehabilitation is associated with not needing it in the first place, it behooves all of us to work toward the prevention of the problems caused by drug abuse and alcoholism. These problems range from falls leading to broken hips, to motor vehicle accidents producing severe brain injury. Thus, we know that the diagnosis and treatment of preinjury substance abuse will reduce both the incidence and the severity of many rehabilitation-related diagnoses. Furthermore, of the many pitfalls a rehabilitation patient faces, drug abuse can prove to be the most handicapping. These disorders have a way of consuming an individual's life and leave few footholds for treatment or for community reintegration. It is therefore necessary for rehabilitation professionals to have a basic understanding of the diagnosis and management of these life-threatening disorders.

APPENDIX I. DSM-IV CRITERIA FOR SUBSTANCE USE DISORDERS

Criteria for Substance Dependence

A maladaptive pattern of substance use leading to clinically significant impairment or distress, as manifested by three or more of the following, occurring at any time in the same 12-month period:

1. Tolerance, as defined by either of the following:
   a. A need for markedly increased amounts of the substance to achieve intoxication or desired effect.
   b. Markedly diminished effect with continued use of the same amount of the substance.
2. Withdrawal, as manifested by either of the following:
   a. The characteristic withdrawal syndrome for the substance.
   b. The same or a closely related substance is taken to relieve or avoid withdrawal symptoms.
3. The substance is often taken in larger amounts or over a longer period than was intended.
4. There is a persistent desire or unsuccessful efforts to cut down or control substance use.
5. A great deal of time is spent in activities necessary to obtain the substance or recover from its effects.

6. Important social, occupational, or recreational activities are given up or reduced because of substance use.
7. The substance use is continued despite knowledge of having a persistent or recurrent physical or psychological problem that is likely to have been caused or exacerbated by the substance.

Criteria for Substance Abuse

Maladaptive pattern of substance use leading to clinically significant impairment or distress, as manifested by one or more of the following, occurring within a 12-month period:

1. Recurrent substance use resulting in a failure to fulfill major role obligations at work, school, or home.
2. Recurrent substance use in situations in which it is physically hazardous.
3. Recurrent substance-related legal problems.
4. Continued substance use despite having persistent or recurrent social or interpersonal problems caused or exacerbated by the effects of the substance.

The symptoms have never met the criteria for substance dependence for this class of substance.

Criteria Substance Intoxication

1. The development of a reversible substance-specific syndrome due to recent ingestion of or exposure to a substance.
2. Clinically significant maladaptive behavioral or psychological changes that are due to the effect of the substance on the central nervous system (e.g., belligerence, mood lability, impaired judgment, etc) and develop during or shortly after use of the substance.
3. The symptoms are not due to a general medical condition and are not better accounted for by another mental disorder.

Criteria for Substance Withdrawal

1. The development of a substance-specific syndrome due to the cessation of or reduction in substance use that has been heavy and prolonged.
2. The substance-specific syndrome causes clinically significant distress or impairment in social, occupational or other important areas of functioning.
3. The symptoms are not due to a general medical condition and are not better accounted for by another mental disorder.

REFERENCES

1. Robbins LN, Helzer JE, Przybeck TR, et al. Alcohol disorders in the community: a report from the epidemiologic catchment area. In: Rose RM, Barrett J, eds. *Alcoholism: origins and outcomes.* New York: Raven Press, 1988: 219–224.
2. *Diagnostic and statistical manual of mental disorders.* 4th ed. Washington, DC: American Psychiatric Press, 1994.
3. Miller NS. *Addiction psychiatry.* New York: Wiley-Liss, 1995.
4. Galizio M, Maish SA. *Determinants of substance abuse.* New York: Plenum, 1985:383–424.
5. Grant BF, Harford TC, Dawson D, et al. Prevalence of DSM-IV alcohol abuse and dependence: United States 1992. *Alcohol Health Res World* 1994;18: 243–248.
6. O'Brien CP. Drug addiction and drug abuse. In: Hardman JG, Limbird LE, eds. *Goodman & Gilman's, the pharmacological basis of therapeutics.* 9th ed. New York: McGraw-Hill, 1996:557–577.
7. Labouvie E, Bates ME, Pandina RJ. Age of first use: its reliability and predictive utility. *J Stud Alcohol* 1997;58:638.
8. Golub A, Johnson BD. The shifting importance of alcohol and marijuana as gateway substances among serious drug abusers. *J Stud Alcohol* 1994;55: 607–614.
9. Substance Abuse and Mental Health Services Administration. *Preliminary estimates from the Drug Abuse Warning Network: 1993 preliminary estimates of drug-related emergency department episodes.* Advance report No. 8. Rockville, MD: US Department of Health and Human Services, Substance Abuse and Mental Health Services Administration, 1994.
10. Sparadeo FR, Gill D. Effects of prior alcohol use on head injury recovery. *J Head Trauma Rehabil* 1989;4:75–82.
11. Drubach DA, Kelly MP, Winslow BA, Flynn JPG. Substance abuse as a factor in the causality, severity, and recurrence rate of traumatic brain injury. *Md Med J* 1993;40:989–993.
12. Lindenbaum GA, Carrol SF, Daskal I, Kapusnick R. Patterns of alcohol and drug abuse in an urban trauma center: the increasing role of cocaine abuse. *J Trauma* 1989;29:1654–1658.
13. *Substance Abuse Task Force: White Paper.* Washington, DC: National Head Injury Foundation, 1988.
14. Soderstrom CA, Gordon GS, Dischinger PC, et al. Psychoactive substance use disorders among seriously injured trauma center patients. *JAMA* 1997;277: 1769–1774.
15. Jellinek EM. *The disease concept of alcoholism.* New Brunswick, NJ: New Haven College and University Press (in association with Hillhouse Press), 1960.

16. Valliant GE. *The natural history of alcoholism: causes, patterns and paths to recovery.* Cambridge, MA: Harvard University Press, 1983.

17. Merikangas KR. The genetic epidemiology of alcoholism. *Psychol Med* 1990;20:11–22.

18. Goodwin DW, Schulsinger F, Lermansen L, et al. Alcohol problems in the adoptees raised apart from alcoholic biological parents. *Arch Gen Psych* 1973;28:238–243.

19. Cadoret RJ, Cain CA, Grove WM. Development of alcoholism in adoptees raised apart from alcoholic relatives. *Arch Gen Psych* 1980;37:561–563.

20. Pickens RW, Svikis DS, McGue M, et al. Heterogeneity in the inheritance of alcoholism. *Arch Gen Psych* 1991;48:19–28.

21. Goodwin DW. Alcoholism and genetics. *Arch Gen Psychiatry* 1985;42:171–174.

22. Miller NS, Gold MA. A hypothesis for a common neurochemical basis for alcohol and drug disorders. *Psychiatr Clin North Am* 1993;16:115–116.

23. Spitzer RL, Williams JB, Gibbon M, First MB. *Structured Clinical Interview for DSM III-R.* Washington, DC: American Psychiatric Press, 1990.

24. Project MATCH Research Group. Matching alcoholism treatments to client heterogeneity: Project MATCH postdrinking outcomes. *J Stud Alcohol* 1997;58:7–29.

25. Volpicelli JR, Alterman AI, Hayashida M, O'Brien CP. Naltrexone in the treatment of alcohol dependence. *Arch Gen Psychiatry* 1992;49:876–880.

26. O'Malley SS, Jaffe AJ, Chang G, et al. Naltrexone and coping skills therapy for alcohol dependence. *Arch Gen Psychiatry* 1992;49:881–887.

27. Sass H, Soyka M, Mann K, Zieglgasberger W. Relapse prevention by acamprosate: results from a placebo-controlled study on alcohol dependence. *Arch Gen Psychiatry* 1996;53:673–680.

28. Cassidy J. Insomnia. *J Head Trauma Rehabil* 1991;6(4):81–83.

29. Satel SL, Price LH, Palumbo JM, et al. Clinical phenomenology and neurobiology of cocaine abstinence: a prospective inpatient study. *Am J Psychiatry* 1991;148:1712–1716.

30. Gawin FH, Kleber HD, Byck R, et al. Desipramine facilitation of initial cocaine abstinence. *Arch Gen Psychiatry* 1989;46: 117–121.

31. Batki SI, Manfredi LB, Jacob P, Jones RT. Fluoxetine for cocaine dependence in methadone maintenance: quantitative plasma and urine cocaine/benzoylecgonine concentrations. *J Clin Psychopharmacol* 1993;13:243–250.

32. Abraham HD. Visual phenomenology of the LSD flash. *Arch Gen Psychiatry* 1983;40:884–889.

Part V.

Medical Rehabilitation for Diagnostic Groups

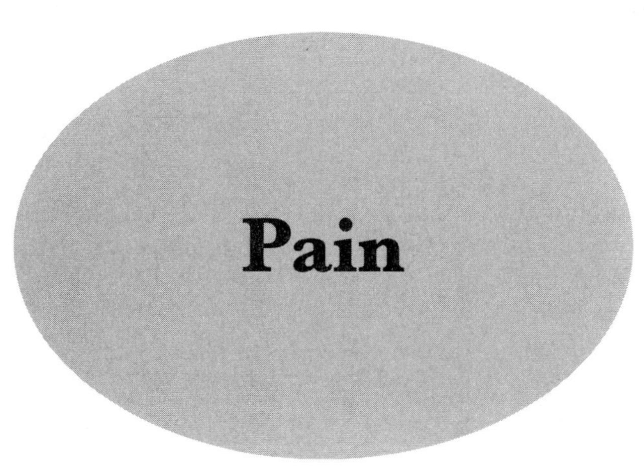

Pain

Chapter 57

Acute Pain

Steve M. Gnatz
Martin Childers

It is only great pain, that slow protracted pain which takes its time and in which we are as it were burned with green wood, that compels us philosophers to descend into our ultimate depths and to put from us all trust, all that is good-hearted, palliated, gentle, average, wherein perhaps our humanity previously reposed. I doubt whether such pain "improves"—but I do know it deepens us. Friedrich Nietzsche

Evil being the root of mystery, pain is the root of knowledge. Simone Weil

Almost everyone has experienced pain at one time or another. Pain is the most common reason why patients seek treatment by a physician. The "hard-wired" pain signal warns us of danger and potential tissue damage. However, pain is a complex interplay of peripheral and central nervous system (CNS) processes that are incompletely understood. Our external and internal environments have become recognized as a significant factor in the interpretation of the pain signal. If pain continues despite the removal of the stimulus, the pain may lose its adaptive value and result in significant physical and psychosocial disability.

The goal of this chapter is to provide on overview of how the physiatrist can use his or her special talents and training to provide the best possible functional outcome for the patient with pain. An overview of the mechanisms of acute pain and a framework for diagnosis and treatment of the patient who presents with an acutely painful condition is presented. Subsequent chapters delve more deeply into individual syndromes of pain.

The emergent treatment of acutely painful conditions may not be seen as cause for referral to the physiatrist. In fact, most acute pain can be eliminated by discontinuing the source of tissue damage, resting the damaged part, and the use of simple analgesia. Nonetheless, early effective treatment of acute pain was been theorized to decrease the likelihood of the development of chronic pain (1). Also, the physical restoration of many painful conditions can be enhanced by physical medicine techniques (2,3). Usually a referral is received when simple interventions by primary care physicians have not eliminated the pain or if significant loss of function has occurred. However, it is also becoming common practice in some areas for the physiatrist to act as the primary physician for persons who are injured on the job or have musculoskeletal complaints. An acute exacerbation of a chronic pain condition may also prompt a renewal of evaluation and treatment. Therefore, a good working knowledge of the diagnosis and treatment of acute pain problems is required of the physiatrist.

NEUROANATOMY AND NEUROPHYSIOLOGY OF THE PAIN PATHWAYS

Physiology and Pathophysiology of Pain

In the past, it was believed that pain and nociception were one and the same (4). However, while pain processes are still poorly understood, recent studies have begun to shed some light on the complex neural interactions by which pain is experienced. No longer is it acceptable to believe that pain is simply a hard-wired, stimulus-response phenomenon. According to Chapman (5), "pain is not the consequence of a passive brain registering tissue trauma, but rather the product of an active brain forming subjective experience in response to sensory signaling."

Acute Pain Pathway

From the skin, the myelinated A-delta fibers rapidly carry to the CNS the "first pain" or the sharp, sticking pain associated with an acute injury that can be readily localized (6). The smaller, slower, unmyelinated C fibers carry more noxious, burning "second pain" that lingers long after the inciting stimulus has gone. These first-order neurons synapse in the dorsal horn of the spinal cord on second-order nociceptive-specific and wide dynamic range neurons. At the level of the CNS, a significant filtering of the information supplied by these peripheral nerve fibers occurs (7). In the spinal cord this filtering may consist of facilitation or inhibition of the transmission of impulses. Facilitation or hyperexcitability of the dorsal horn neurons, the so-called windup, may occur when there is temporal summation of the nociceptive afferent barrage. It has been suggested that this process is caused by the release of amino acids and neuropeptides and *N*-methyl-D-aspartate (NMDA) receptor stimulation, with resulting hyperalgesia and allodynia (8). Several other chemical mediators are purportedly involved in the central sensitization process; the interested reader is referred to recent reviews (9,10). Substance P, an 11–amino acid peptide, has been identified as a peripheral neurotransmitter in the dorsal horn of the spinal cord. Endogenous opioids, such as β-endorphin and enkephalins in the CNS and periphery, modulate pain in an inhibitory manner. The CNS has a rich system of facilitatory neuroendocrine and genetic mechanisms for the perpetuation of nociceptive input. Awareness and management of the central sensitization processes are important in the discussion of "preemptive analgesia" and the treatment of subacute and chronic pain problems.

On the inhibitory side, the stimulation of large-diameter, sensory fibers associated with afferent vibratory and proprioceptive sensation causes central inhibition of nociceptive input at the dorsal horn level by "closing the gate" (7). The gate theory of pain is the principle on which many common treatments for pain control such as transcutaneous electrical nerve stimulation (TENS) rely.

Pain impulses ascend the spinothalamic and spinoreticular tracts to project on the lateral and medial thalamic nuclei and the brain stem, respectively. Projection of these impulses to the sensory cortical areas brings the pain to consciousness and allows localization to the body parts of origin. At the level of the brain, complex neural networks, termed a *neuromatrix* by Melzack (7), maintain the image of our body and may "remember" and perpetuate pain, for example, phantom limb pain. The finding of a correlation between pain and pathologic abnormalities prior to amputation and subsequent phantom limb pain seems to support this concept (11).

There is also evidence of higher CNS inhibition of afferent nociceptive input by descending pathways from the brain. This phenomenon has been observed particularly in war-time, when wounded soldiers would not even consciously recognize that they had been injured until after the battle and they finally paid attention to their injuries. This form of higher CNS inhibition of pain may explain some of the cultural differences in pain perception or at least expressed pain behavior (12).

Referred Pain and Convergence Projection Theory

The discussion so far has focused on the pain pathways from the skin to the CNS. It is important to note that another, possibly more important, mechanism comes into play when considering pain arising from deeper anatomic structures such as the muscles, ligaments, tendons, bones, joints, and visceral organs. This mechanism is called *referred pain* (13).

Our skin is the only organ that has the luxury of precise pain localization. The afferent neurons that supply the skin outnumber those to the viscera and deep somatic structures by 10 to 1 (14). Relatively large areas of somatosensory cortical representation make discrimination of pain and other sensations especially sensitive on the face and hands. The deep somatic and visceral organs do not enjoy this kind of cortical representation and must find other ways of representing sensation at a cortical level.

The neuroanatomic and physiologic bases for referred pain have been a matter of controversy in the medical literature over the past 50 years. It was theorized that referred pain was produced locally at the peripheral nerve level due to the release of chemical substances (15). That idea has been disregarded (16). The main evidence against this mechanism is that an injection of an anesthetic agent at the source of referred pain will abolish both the local and the referred pain. This finding has important bearing on the discussion of the generation and treatment of myofascial trigger points. Another argument against the peripheral generation of referred pain is the time delay noted between the injection of saline solution in the proximal muscles and the experience of the referred pain afterward (17).

Once a peripheral mechanism was ruled out, the next logical place for referred pain generation was at the dorsal root ganglia or dorsal root entry zone of the spinal cord. Most of the experimental work in the last 30 years has focused on referred pain mechanisms at the spinal cord level. An excellent review of much of this basic science work is available (18).

Microelectrodes have been used to stimulate various individual axons involved in the somatosensory process, both peripherally and centrally. These microelectrode studies have led to the conclusion that there is come specificity of the cutaneous nociceptive fibers peripherally. As discussed earlier, stimulation of the A-delta fibers of the skin produces a sensation of a sharp pricking or stinging nature, whereas stimulation of the C fibers produces a dull, aching, or burning pain. To date, no such fibers have been conclusively found to produce specific deep somatic or visceral sensations. The sensation produced by the stimulation of deep somatic and visceral afferent fibers instead is a poorly localized, diffuse aching pain that may be referred to the skin.

While it is theorized that cutaneous sensory afferents have specific second-order neurons that carry their impulses to the higher levels of the CNS, the deep somatic and visceral fibers must synapse on "convergent" or multisensory neurons, losing some of their specificity (19,20). Since all three groups (cutaneous, deep somatic, and visceral) synapse on these second-order multisensory neurons, it is clear that afferent input from a deep somatic structure such as a muscle would require a significant amount of interpretation by the CNS and such input may not be able to be perceived as arising from that deep somatic structure alone.

Confirmatory evidence for the convergence theory has come from animal studies. Retrograde labeling of a cutaneous nerve to the shoulder with simultaneous labeling of a motor branch to the diaphragm with a different color dye showed that the two dyes could be found in some of the same dorsal root ganglion cells (21). Therefore, a retrograde motor signal generated at the diaphragm may converge with a sensory afferent fiber from the shoulder. The brain might interpret this input as arising from the skin of the shoulder, either in addition to or instead of the muscle where it really originated. Because of this need for CNS discrimination and filtering of this incoming afferent information, several theories, discussions of which are beyond the scope of this chapter, have evolved (19,22,23).

Convergence projection theory and referred pain have an important role in many acute, subacute, and chronic pain syndromes. Referred pain may arise from any deep somatic or visceral structure that is supplied with afferent fibers. Most vascularized and metabolically active structures of the body receive some sensory fibers. A few notable non-pain-producing structures are hyaline cartilage, some ligamentous structures, and the nucleus pulposus. It should be noted that the attachments of many structures such as synovium and periosteum are richly supplied with pain fibers, so that a cartilage tear produces pain by inflammation and disruption of the surrounding tissues, even though the cartilage itself does not contain nociceptors.

Referred pain from viscera includes such examples as myocardial infarction with pain referred to the chest wall, back, left arm, or jaw, and gallbladder disease or diaphragmatic irritation with referred pain to the shoulder. Visceral referred pain is not discussed further in this chapter but can be an important consideration in pelvic and abdominal pain problems.

Bone and joint structures can be the originating points of referred pain. Examples include degenerative hip arthropathy with referred pain to the knee and temporomandibular joint pain referred to the ear, sinuses, or muscles of the head and neck (see Chap. 62).

Deep somatic structures that may be the origin of referred pain include the periosteum, joints, some ligaments, tendons, annulus fibrosus, fascia, and muscles. Certainly one of the most common, if still poorly understood, deep somatic referred pain syndromes is myofascial pain (24). Pain originates in the myofascial "trigger point" and is referred in a pattern that is not dermatomal, myotomal, or sclerotomal but instead follows a pattern that is recognizable and reproducible (25). Studies with normal subjects showed that local tenderness to palpation of muscle is common, yet true trigger points with pain referred to another area are present in only 5% to 12% of normal subjects (26). Any muscle can be involved in this process. The referred pain usually projects distally in the limbs and caudally in the neck. It may be associated with autonomic phenomena such as piloerection, flushing, sweating, and skin temperature changes. Additionally, visceral symptoms such as nausea and even vomiting may result from stimulation of the trigger area. Reflex weakness of the affected muscle can occur.

It may be helpful clinically to distinguish between myofascial pain syndromes and the more generalized fibromyalgia, although these two diagnoses may be two ends of the same scale (27) (see Chap. 61).

Major mixed nerves are not included in this scheme as they usually contain cutaneous afferents and when damaged, would elicit a radiating or projected pain. Still the distinction is not entirely clear, since the deep somatic afferents may travel through the major nerves. There has been controversy as to whether myofascial trigger points are a form of neural referred pain (28). Moreover, there is some evidence that local compression or irritation of nerve fibers in the region of trigger points may be partly responsible for their hyperirritable properties (29).

While sometimes difficult to do clinically, it may be helpful to consider the physiologic distinction between radiating (or projected) pain, where the pain originates at a point (e.g., the cervical nerve root) and follows a dermatomal pattern distally, and true referred pain, where this continuity may or may not be present (30). These two forms of pain are generally readily differentiated from localized pain (Table 57-1). With radiating pain, the brain interprets the pain as arising in the entire dermatome, although the damage is localized. This type of pain is usually neuropathic in quality. Occasionally, late neuroma formation may play a role in the perpetuation of symptoms when nerve injury has occurred (31). Referred pain has a dull aching and burning character, whereas radiating pain is generally sharp and searing. The distinction between these two types of pain is not clear-cut, since referred pain may take on some characteristics of radiating pain and vice versa. Often patients with referred pain complain of negative symptoms such as numbness, "deadness" or "woodenness" in the referred pain zone of the limb.

Table 57-1: Characteristics of Three Types of Pain

Referred Pain	Radiating Pain	Local Pain
Deep somatic*	Nerve	Tendonitis
Myofascial	Radiculopathy	Laceration
Dull, aching	Sharp, searing	Sharp
Poorly localized	Moderately well localized	Well localized
Paresthesias	Paresthesias	None
Rare dysesthesia	Dysesthesia	None
Subjective swelling	No swelling	Real swelling
Autonomic symptoms	Autonomic, sympathetic	Rare autonomic
Unique reference pattern for trigger points	Reference pattern Dermatomal pattern	No reference
Nondermatomal loss of sensation	Dermatomal loss of sensation	With or without loss of sensation
Diffuse tenderness in reference zone	Tenderness, local or diffuse	Localized tenderness
Muscle weakness on a reflex basis	Muscle weakness on a neurogenic basis	No muscle weakness except antalgic

* Deep somatic, originating from skeletal, joint, ligament, deep tendon, muscle, or fascial tissues.

Source: Reproduced by permission from Gnatz SM. Referred pain syndromes of the head and neck. *Phys Med Rehabil State Art Rev* 1991;5:585–596.

They may complain of a subjective feeling of swelling, despite no observable edema.

ETIOLOGY

Acute pain can usually be linked to a precipitating event, most often involving a specific trauma or injury. The acute injury may damage tissue directly, for example, tearing a ligament or muscle. In this case, the pain provides an incentive for the person to rest and allow regenerative and repair processes to occur. Other possible pain etiologies include overuse syndromes and improper posture or body mechanics. These processes may lead to pain through "microtrauma" or fatigue. Systemic or localized degenerative, inflammatory, infectious, or malignant processes can be causes or contributors to acute pain syndromes. Table 57-2 lists the causes of acute pain. In the majority of patients, the history will reveal the cause of the pain, with the physical examination and diagnostic studies providing confirmation and documentation of clinical impressions.

To understand the patient with pain, it must be assumed that all pain is real; however, the way in which it is perceived varies widely. Pain that is incapacitating to one person may be taken in stride by another, or the same person under different conditions. There is no objective measure of pain. The quantitation of function and subjective perception of pain must be used as an approximate measure of the effects of pain on the host.

Transition from Acute to Chronic Pain

Generally, acute pain is defined as lasting up to 2 weeks; subacute, between 2 weeks and 6 months; and chronic pain, longer than 6 months. These definitions are entirely artificial, however. The longer pain persists, the less likely complete resolution becomes. This statement assumes that an adequate search for etiologic and contributing factors has been performed, and that any etiologic or perpetuating factors have been controlled to the extent possible. Significant psychosocial overlay, lack of insight, or secondary gain motives bode poorly for recovery (see Chap. 58). Patients who are adaptable and educable and who show a willingness to take responsibility for aspects of the treatment within their control generally have a better outcome to their pain problem (32).

ASSESSMENT

Observation

First, and often neglected, is a thorough observation of the patient who complains of pain. How does the patient walk down the hall, sit in the waiting room, or act during the examination? Pain has many complex psychosocial aspects, and observation of the patient's pain behavior when alone versus when being examined may provide significant insight and information to the physician. This is not to say that any patient who exhibits pain behavior in public but not while alone is malingering. However, the physician will want to know what, if any, emotional overlay is present, in order to completely evaluate the patient.

History

The history taking should be directed at obtaining pain descriptors that help identify a specific syndrome or category into which the patient falls. Identifying a pain syndrome will assist in organizing the proper work-up needed to provide an accurate diagnosis, and once established, develop a rational treatment plan. Patients will not always fit into a specific known syndrome or category and it is better to keep an open mind, leaving patients undiagnosed rather than "pigeonholed" into an erroneous diagnosis.

Pain can be characterized using the mnemonic PQRST: *p*rovocative and palliative factors, *q*uality, *r*egion-radiation, *s*everity, and *t*emporal characteristics. Many types of pain are diffuse and difficult for the patient to

Table 57-2: Classification of Causes of Musculoskeletal and Neuropathic Pain

I. Intrinsic causes of musculoskeletal and neuropathic pain
  A. Skeletal abnormalities
    1. Fracture
    2. Neoplasm, primary or metastatic
    3. Infection, osteomyelitis
    4. Paget disease
    5. Osteoporosis
    6. Endocrinologic, hyperparathyroidism
    7. Arteriovenous malformations, aneurysms
    8. Hematologic, sickle cell, multiple myeloma
  B. Joint abnormalities
    1. Synovitis, capsulitis, diskitis
    2. Joint effusion, hemarthrosis
    3. Osteoarthritis
    4. Rheumatic disease, rheumatoid arthritis, etc
    5. Disk derangements
    6. Joint instability, ligamentous laxity
    7. Biomechanical abnormalities
    8. Neoplasms, primary or metastatic
    9. Vasculitides
  C. Ligaments
    1. Trauma, sprains, rupture
    2. Chronic laxity
    3. Contracture
    4. Neoplasms
    5. Infection
  D. Muscles, tendons, fascia
    1. Myofascial pain, fibromyalgia
    2. Trauma, strains, tears, ruptures
    3. Inflammatory conditions, polymyositis
    4. Infectious conditions, trichinosis, etc
    5. Polymyalgia rheumatica
    6. Vasculitides
    7. Metabolic, exercise induced, cramps
    8. Ischemic, claudication, compartment syndrome
    9. Neoplasms
    10. Contracture, biomechanical abnormalities
    11. Overuse syndromes
    12. Nutritional, avitaminosis
    13. Toxins, venom, etc
  E. Nerve structures
    1. Entrapment, compression
    2. Trauma, stretch, laceration
    3. Deafferentation, neuromas
    4. Reflex sympathetic dystrophy, causalgia
    5. Neuritis, neuralgia, tics
    6. Peripheral neuropathy, diabetes, toxins
    7. Ischemia, vasculitis
    8. Infection, herpes, AIDS
    9. Neoplasms
II. Extrinsic cause of musculoskeletal pain
  A. Other organs referring pain to the musculoskeletal system
    1. Heart: myocardial infection, angina
    2. Lungs: pleuritis, tumors (especially pancoast)
    3. Eyes: infection, strain
    4. Ears: infection, tumors
    5. Nose and sinus: infection, abscess, tumors
    6. Throat and teeth: infection, tumors
    7. Central nervous system: tumors, neuromas, neurofibromas, infections, vascular abnormalities and accidents, supratentorial factors

describe. Often a diagram and pain-rating scale will be helpful. Identification of an acute traumatic event should be sought. A complete medication and treatment history is essential if one is not to repeat previous unsuccessful attempts at treatment. Occasionally, pain patients will have been to many physicians in their quest to cure the pain. The quickest way to lose their confidence is to prescribe something that was tried unsuccessfully in the past.

A history of prior diagnostic testing will prevent duplication. Records of these diagnostic tests, operative reports, therapists' notes, consultants' notes, and psychosocial information, if available, may provide additional background.

A history of the job site conditions and job description is critically important if the pain is related to an on-the-job injury.

A history of prior painful conditions and the approximate time for recovery may give a clue about individual variability in healing and the patient's expectations about time away from work because of the injury.

A history of the current and past social situation including vocational, family, and interpersonal stresses should be sought. The ability to cope with these types of stressors has been correlated with outcome in patients with fibromyalgia and probably can be generalized to most patients with pain (33). The current functional limitations in activities of daily living, endurance for exercise, and dependence on adaptive equipment will help characterize the extent of disability. A person who is already significantly functionally limited may have little "reserve" to avoid the effects of a painful problem. The existence of litigation and other aspects of secondary gain may be strong motivators against improvement and should be noted (34).

Physical Examination

The physical examination of the pain patient is a directed neuromuscular and joint examination with the purposes of identifying the painful structures and documenting variations from the norm that may interfere with function. While details of the examination will depend on what is found in the history, certain elements will be constant. Alterations in muscle strength, sensation, and deep tendon reflexes are sought. Often patients in pain cannot participate in manual muscle testing because of the increase in pain the examination produces. It should be noted that "give-way" weakness is not always an indication of poor cooperation on the patient's part, but rather may be a manifestation of reflex muscle weakness on the basis of pain.

The search for dermatomal or root level dysfunction of sensory and reflex systems should be systematic. If dysfunction is found, sensory dysfunction and reflex changes are hard neurologic signs which are difficult to voluntarily produce. However, muscle atrophy on the basis of immobility or disuse may contribute to decreased muscle stretch reflexes.

Examination of any involved (and sometimes uninvolved) joint structures for effusion, erythema, warmth, decreased range of motion, deformity, and palpation of tendons and ligamentous structures may lead to a particular diagnostic entity.

Palpation of muscle is important to evaluate for trigger points or tight bands of muscle that when pressed, cause referred pain in a characteristic pattern. These are the hallmark of myofascial pain. Palpation of muscle may also point the examiner in the direction of specific painful muscle disorders such as polymyositis, polymyalgia rheumatica, and exercise-induced muscle pain. Observation for dystonic movements and cramps in the muscles of writers, performing artists, and athletes may be informative.

Specific maneuvers such as the straight-leg raising test, Tinel sign, Hoffman sign, or Finkelstein test may be required to add weight to the suspected diagnosis.

Pain Measures

Subjective rating scales of pain are a useful adjunct to the history and physical examination data. Several of the scales have a good track record and are reliable (35). For the visual analogue scale, the patient is asked to place a mark on a line representing a scale from 1 to 10, indicating the amount of pain that he or she is experiencing at that time. At repeated testing the patient's progress can be monitored. The McGill pain questionnaire goes into more detail about the aspects of pain that the patient is experiencing. The algometer has been shown to be a reliable device for quantitation of muscular tender points (36).

Quantitation of Function

As part of the diagnostic work-up, it may be helpful to obtain quantitative measures of certain physical parameters, using, for example, dynamometer or functional capacity testing. It should be noted, however, that similar to muscle strength testing, quantitative physical capacity testing is less reliable in the presence of pain. However, if valid, the data may be useful as a baseline for monitoring progression in the patient's therapy program.

Other Tests

Laboratory examination will help when the tests ordered are directed by the specific diagnosis suspected. Testing for rheumatoid factor, antinuclear antibody (ANA), creatine phosphokinase (CPK), sedimentation rate, and others may point the evaluation in a particular direction, usually toward a rheumatologic or autoimmune etiology for the pain. Radiographic findings may also aid in the diagnosis by identifying fractures, dislocations, or other bone and joint pathology as a cause of pain. Magnetic resonance imaging can be utilized to identify abnormalities of the muscle, tendons, and ligaments, providing better resolution than x-ray studies.

Electromyography (EMG) may be performed by the physiatrist to evaluate the continuity of the neuromuscular system. It should be used as an extension of the physical examination. EMG may provide confirmatory data for diagnoses such as radiculopathy, neuropathy, myopathy, and disorders of the myoneural junction.

TREATMENT

Preemptive Analgesia

It has been suggested that early effective analgesia for acute pain problems may decrease the incidence of chronic pain (1), although this theory has been challenged on both an experimental (9) and a clinical basis (37).

Physiatric Modalities in the Treatment of Acute Pain

Physical modalities may be useful in the patient with acute pain. The modalities are discussed in Chapter 24. For acute pain management, rest of the damaged structure is essential for recovery. Passive modalities are appropriate initially for a short period of time, to allow the tissues to repair themselves. This philosophy is in contrast to the management of chronic pain, where the patient usually needs mobilization due to underuse and passive modalities alone are not indicated (38). It is important to consider that contracture of collagenous structures including tendon, ligament, and joint capsules occurs rapidly in patients with painful range of motion (ROM), especially if edema is present (39). These patients require gentle passive ROM exercises to avoid the vicious cycle of pain leading to immobility, followed by tissue contracture, which when challenged to move, leads to increased pain. Similarly, atrophy of immobilized and painful muscle should be avoided, if possible, through the use of isometric exercise.

The physical modalities of heat, cold, electricity, sound, and water are used to accomplish the goals of increased function while minimizing pain (3). Both heat and cold provide analgesic effects. Heat is useful for both acute and chronic pain, for inducing analgesia and muscle relaxation and because of its effect on the stretchability of collagen. (40). Cold may be more beneficial for acute pain for its ability to control edema. Heat may exacerbate edema if present. The general guidelines of applying cold for the first 24 to 48 hours after an acute injury has occurred and heat thereafter are time tested (41).

Conventional TENS (high-frequency, low-intensity electrical stimulation) may be more effective for acute pain than chronic pain (42). Electroacupuncture decreased nociception in an animal model through an endogenous opioid pathway (43,44).

Medications

Medications provide a useful tool in the management of acute pain. The mechanism of action of the medication will provide a theoretical framework for determining which drug should be initiated for any given acute pain problem (45) (Table 57-3).

Patients may be given numerous medications by other health professionals if they have had pain for any length of time. It is important to know which medications were tried, which were effective, and how they were taken, in order to rationally prescribe pharmacologic adjunct therapy for the rehabilitation program.

Nonsteroidal anti-inflammatory drugs (NSAIDs) such as ibuprofen (Motrin), diclofenac (Voltaren, Cataflam), and naproxen (Naprosyn, Anaprox) have both analgesic and anti-inflammatory properties (46). While there is significant variability between agents, usually the anti-inflammatory effect is obtained at two to four times the analgesic dosage. Generally, the NSAIDs with a longer half-life [e.g., piroxicam (Feldene), nabumetone (Relafen), and etodolac (Lodine)] may yield better compliance for patients who must be on NSAIDs for longer periods of time, but do not afford as quick an analgesic effect after a dose is taken. While significantly less expensive, plain aspirin has more gastrointestinal intolerance and less anti-inflammatory effect than do the other NSAIDs. NSAIDs may produce gastrointestinal complications slowly and insidiously after prolonged use. Other side effects of NSAIDs include fluid retention and rarely, renal problems. Nonetheless, kidney and liver function should be monitored in the elderly or any patient with a history of renal or liver dysfunction.

A new class of cyclooxygenase 2 inhibitors (47) may offer an enhanced anti-inflammatory effect with less chance of gastrointestinal intolerance. However, none of these agents were commercially available at the time of this writing.

Muscle relaxants such as cyclobenzaprine (Flexeril), methocarbamol (Robaxin), and carisoprodol (Soma) may be indicated for the short-term treatment of muscle spasm if present. Carisoprodol has some potential for abuse (48). Cyclobenzaprine may also be useful in the long term, or intermittently, in low doses at bedtime for patients with fibromyalgia or myofascial pain who have a disturbed sleep pattern (49). Drowsiness is associated with these agents, which makes them potentially dangerous for certain patients (e.g., machine operators) and for when mental alertness is required for safety. They should not be taken with alcohol.

Amitriptyline (Elavil, Endep) is a tricyclic antidepressant with excellent analgesic properties, probably based on the blockade of serotonin and norepinephrine reuptake (50). It is used as a first-line agent for fibromyalgia and neuropathic pain syndromes (51–53). It can be effective for pain relief in doses much lower than those used for depression (54). Usually 25 to 100 mg at bedtime is sufficient for sleep and pain control, versus 300 to 450 mg/day for depression. The side effects include drowsiness, which is limited by giving the drug at bedtime, and anticholinergic effects (dry mouth, urinary retention, etc). Fatal cardiac arrhythmias from tricyclic overdose can occur at low doses, especially in the elderly (55). It is important to prescribe small amounts, without refills, or use an alternative drug for anyone suspected of suicidal potential. Other tricyclic antidepressant drugs, including doxepin and nortriptyline, have been used in the same manner as amitriptyline (56,57). They may have less anticholinergic effect, but otherwise the side effect profiles are similar.

Newer antidepressants, such as fluoxetine (Prozac), venlafaxine (Effexor), and paroxetine (Paxil) that tend to have more CNS stimulant action do not seem to work as well clinically for sleep and pain control as do the older, more sedating antidepressants (50). This finding further reinforces the theory that it is not the antidepressant effect of the tricyclic compounds, but some other quality (such as the restoration of a normal sleep cycle) that results in pain control.

Other drugs that may occasionally be useful in some pain patients are phenytoin (Dilantin) and carbamazepine (Tegretol) (58,59). These anticonvulsant medications probably control pain through their membrane-stabilizing effects

Table 57-3: A Framework for Medication Management in Patients with Acute Pain

Type of Pain	NSAIDS	MR	TCA	MSA	CLO	CCB	NARC
Acute fractures	—	—	—	—	—	1	—
Sprain/strain	1	2	—	—	—	—	—
Joint inflammation	1	—	—	—	—	—	—
Neuropathic	2	—	1	3	4	5	—
Osteoarthritic	1	—	2	—	—	—	3
Fibromyalgia/ Myofascial pain	2	1	1	—	—	—	—
Reflex sympathetic dystrophy	—	—	1	2	3	4	—

NSAIDS = nonsteroidal anti-inflammatory drugs; MR = muscle relaxants; TCA = tricyclic antidepressants; MSA = membrane-stabilizing agents; CLO = clonidine; CCB = calcium channel blockers; NARC = narcotics. 1 = drug of first choice; 2 = second choice; etc.

on nerve fibers. Along with mexiletine, they fall into a class of sodium channel–blocking agents that have been particularly useful in neuropathic pain states (60). However, any lancinating or burning pain may respond to these agents. Both phenytoin and carbamazepine have significant hepatic and hematologic side effects that require careful monitoring. They should not be considered first-line agents for acute pain problems. The anticonvulsant gabapentin (Neurontin) has been useful in a variety of painful conditions (61) (Childers M, unpublished data, 1996). Gabapentin has a better side effect profile and may be as effective as the other anticonvulsants, making its consideration a better choice for an early intervention.

Clonidine is a centrally acting α-adrenergic agonist with antinociceptive properties (62–65). It may have the added benefit of diminishing the adverse effects of narcotic withdrawal (66). Clonidine may be useful for pain control when administered epidurally or orally. Its main side effect is hypotension when given orally. Clonidine may be initiated orally at a low dose (0.05–0.10 mg/day) and gradually titrated to a higher dose. It has the added advantage of being available in a transdermal form so that patients who have adapted well to the oral regimen can be switched to a patch, which offers better compliance.

Dextromethorphan is a cough suppressant and expectorant that is also a NMDA receptor antagonist (67). The results of using this medication clinically have been disappointing, despite the fact that there is good basic science research offering a mode of action in pain control (68,69).

Mexiletine (Mexitil) is an oral analogue of lidocaine that may offer some analgesic properties, particularly for neuropathic pain (70,71). However, it was ineffective for dysesthetic pain in spinal cord–injured patients (72). The side effects are rare cardiac arrhythmias.

Calcium channel blockers may have a role when it is difficult to control pain, particularly neuropathic pain, that of reflex sympathetic dystrophy, and bone pain (73–75). The mechanism of action is not known, but may be related to vasodilation, anti-inflammatory effects, or modulation of calcium channels of the C fibers involved in nociception (76,77). The main side effect is hypotension.

Despite recent calls for more liberalization of the use of narcotic analgesics for benign pain syndromes (78), rarely are narcotics indicated for the treatment of any acute or subacute pain other than for anesthesia, emergency, or very acute situations. The main problem clinically with the use of narcotics in any setting other than the very acute setting is tolerance. The patient quickly needs increasing doses of narcotics because of this tolerance. There is experimental evidence that narcotics are not effective for chronic (nonnociceptive) pain (79). Eventually, the narcotic is not helping the pain at all but has become a problem in and of itself. Additionally, more recent data show that increased opioid receptor sensitivity may occur in the nervous system when the "trough" level of narcotics is reached (80). While currently there is no experimental evidence of this, it makes intuitive sense that the ongoing administration of exogenous opioids may interfere with endogenous opioid pathways, making nonpharmacologic interventions that use this final common pathway (e.g., electroacupuncture, strenuous exercise, etc) less effective.

Benzodiazepines such as diazepam (Valium) and lorazepam (Ativan) are generally contraindicated for any acute pain problems that do not involve a significant component of anxiety. All benzodiazepines, while initiating the onset of sleep, will interfere with deeper stages of sleep (81) and may be counterproductive in the treatment of subacute to chronic muscle pain syndromes such as fibromyalgia.

Zolpidem tartrate (Ambien) is a nonbenzodiazepine hypnotic that is proposed to work through the α-subunit of the γ-aminobutyric acid (GABA) receptor to produce sleep and muscle relaxation. It reportedly does not have the side effect of interference with stages 3 and 4 sleep that benzodiazepines have (82). Nonetheless, the results in patients with fibromyalgia and subacute muscle pain have not been impressive, although long-term, controlled trials are lacking at this time.

Other Methods of Treatment

Interventional pain management may fall within the realm of the physiatrist who is familiar with spinal injections, indications, and potential complications. Some patients may benefit from procedures that need to be performed by other pain specialists with appropriate training. Table 57-4 lists a number of interventions that may benefit patients with acute or chronic pain.

Physiatrists skilled in peripheral injection techniques and competent in the management of potential complications may perform a number of interventional pain procedures in an outpatient setting. Such procedures may further provide a synergistic benefit with physical modalities and pharmacologic treatments of pain. Practitioners skilled in the diagnosis and treatment of low-back pain may safely perform a number of procedures including lumbar facet blocks, lumbar epidural injections, sacroiliac injections, and piriformis trigger point injections.

Facet-induced back pain may be considered a diagnosis of exclusion, since there is no clear pathognomonic clinical presentation (83). The diagnosis is supported by reproduction of pain during arthrography and abolition of pain following injection of anesthetic agents. Patients with facet pain may have localized tenderness over the facet joints and, local muscular spasm and lack neurologic deficits. Facet pain syndrome has been reported in patients with restricted motion in extension and rotation (84). Signs of nerve root irritation, such as with the straight-leg raising test, are usually negative. Contraindications to facet block include coagulopathy and systemic or local infection at the injection site.

Table 57-4: Interventions That May Benefit Patients with Acute or Chronic Pain	
Physiatric Procedure	**Indication**
I. Neural blockade	
A. Atlanto-occipital/atlantoaxial injections	Cervical headache syndromes
B. Sphenopalatine ganglion block	Facial pain
C. Occipital nerve block	Headache, occipital neuralgia
D. Stellate ganglion block	Sympathetic-mediated pain syndromes
E. Cervical epidural injection	Radiculopathy, spondylosis
F. Facet block	Facet syndrome
G. Thoracic epidural injection	Postherpetic pain, radiculopathy
H. Intercostal nerve block	Rib fracture, postoperative pain
I. Lumbar epidural block	Radiculopathy, spinal stenosis
J. Lumbar sympathetic nerve block	Sympathetic-mediated pain syndrome
K. Caudal epidural block	Same as for lumbar epidural block
L. Sacroiliac joint block	Sacroiliac joint syndrome
II. Neurolysis (phenol or radiofrequency ablation)	
A. Facet neurolysis	Facet pain
B. Lumbar sympathetic neurolysis	Sympathetic-mediated pain
C. Medial branch block	Facet pain
III. Neuroaugmentation	
A. Spinal cord stimulation	Radiculopathy, sympathetic-mediated pain
B. Peripheral nerve stimulation	Same as above
IV. Spinal opioids (epidural)	Same as for lumbar epidural injections
V. Image-guided deep trigger point injections (fluoroscopy, computed tomography, ultrasound)	
A. Psoas	Psoas syndrome
B. Piriformis	Piriformis syndrome
C. Quadratus lumborum	Myofascial back pain syndrome

Facet joint injections are performed under fluoroscopic imaging, from a 45-degree angle, with the patient in the prone position. Small amounts of contrast dye are injected to verify penetration of the zygapophyseal joint prior to injection of 1.0 to 1.5 mL of a local anesthetic or steroid preparation.

A medial branch block can anesthetize the facet by anesthesia of the posterior rami that innervate the joint. Arthrography is not needed for medial branch blockade. For lumbar facets, the medial branch block is performed by introducing a spinal needle approximately 5 cm lateral from the midline and directed obliquely toward the medial edge of the transverse process. Since one medial branch of the posterior ramus arises from the nerve at the same level as the joint, and the other from the segmental level above, two injections are necessary to effectively block a single facet joint (85).

A diagnostic sacroiliac joint block (86–88) may be indicated for individuals suspected of sacroiliac joint dysfunction who have not responded to less invasive treatment after 3 to 4 weeks and continue to have symptoms that interfere with daily activity. Fluoroscopic-guided injections are performed, owing to the configuration of the joint (89) and the difficulty of localization without the use of imaging guidance (86,90,91). A technique has been described (86) in which the sacroiliac joint is visualized radiographically in the prone patient with the contralateral hip raised 10 to 30 degrees from the table. A small-bore spinal needle may be precisely advanced in small increments until the tip of the needle can be visualized as a dot superimposed on the sacroiliac joint. As the needle enters the joint, an arthrogram confirms the position prior to the introduction of diagnostic or therapeutic agents.

Recent studies examined the ability to diagnose sacroiliac joint syndrome by history and physical examination alone (88,90–94). Diagnostic sacroiliac joint blocks may confirm a suspected diagnosis of sacroiliac joint syndrome. Therapeutic treatment with local injection of a corticosteroid and anesthetic may facilitate a rehabilitation program for acute pain due to sacroiliac joint dysfunction.

Lumbar epidural nerve block using local anesthetics may be indicated as a diagnostic tool in the evaluation of back, groin, pelvic, abdominal, genital, rectal, and lower-extremity pain (95). Local anesthetics or steroids may be administered via the lumbar approach to the epidural space for a variety of pain syndromes including lumbar radiculopathy, low-back pain syndromes, spinal stenosis, phantom limb pain, vertebral compression fractures, diabetic polyneuropathy, chemotherapy-related neuropathic pain syndromes, postherpetic neuralgia, and sympathetic-mediated pain syndrome (96–99).

Identification of the epidural space may be accomplished by a variety of techniques, including imaging under fluoroscopy. The patient may be placed in a prone, seated, or lateral decubitus position. Based on the “loss of resistance” technique, bony landmarks or imaging studies are used to identify midline structures to determine the vertebral level appropriate for needle insertion. Under sterile conditions, a 3.5-inch, 18-gauge Tuohy or Hustead needle (used to enhance proprioceptive feedback of the needle in the practitioner's hands) is inserted in the midline after a small amount of local anesthetic is infiltrated into the skin and supraspinous and interspinous ligaments. The needle stylet is removed, and a saline- or air-filled glass syringe is attached. While continuous pressure is applied to the plunger of the syringe, the needle is advanced until a loss of resistance is encountered upon penetration of the epidural space. With fluoroscopy, the depth of the ligamentum flavum can be determined by advancing the needle tip off the lamina and into the ligamentum flavum. Local anesthetics or steroids are administered directly into the epidural space following confirmation of the needle position.

Transforaminal epidural injections of corticosteroids or anesthetics (also known as selective epidural or selective nerve root block) may place medications more reliably in the anterior epidural space where the most pain-sensitive structures are located (100). A needle angled at the inferior aspect of the pedicle superior to the exiting nerve root (the 6-o'clock position of the round pedicle) is guided by fluoroscopic imaging. Transforaminal epidural injections may identify or confirm a specific nerve root as a pain generator when the diagnosis is not clear based on clinical examination.

Contraindications to epidural steroid injection include infection, anticoagulation, coagulopathy, and hypovolemia. Risks associated with this procedure include inadvertent dural puncture, epidural hematoma and subsequent neurologic deficit, epidural abscess, and systemic infection (101). Application of local anesthetics and opioids to lumbar or sacral nerve roots may lead to urinary retention.

Piriformis muscle syndrome is characterized by signs and symptoms of sciatic nerve compression by a contracted, hypertrophic piriformis muscle as the nerve passes through the pelvis (102–104). The patient often presents with a history of trauma to the buttocks, and physical examination reveals buttock tenderness from the sacrum to the greater trochanter with referred pain in a sciatic distribution (105). Intramuscular injections of anesthetic agents or botulinum toxin (106,107) in the piriformis muscle may be accomplished most accurately using imaging techniques, such as fluoroscopy, to avoid neurovascular structures and precisely localize the muscle. A 22-gauge spinal needle directed toward the piriformis muscle, but lateral to the sciatic nerve, will usually elicit a twitch response from the muscle. A small amount of radiocontrast agent injected through the needle should verify needle placement by outlining the muscle fiber orientation in relation to the bony anatomy. Following needle placement verification, syringes are changed, and the agent of choice is injected into the muscle.

Trigger point injections of muscles can be helpful if an isolated painful point in the muscle with referral of the pain (a trigger point) can be identified (108). One milliliter to 2 mL of 0.5% procaine or 1% lidocaine without epinephrine (which causes vasoconstriction) is used. Injection into and needling of the trigger point spreads out the muscle fibers and can provide relief of pain. The addition of a corticosteroid to the local anesthetic has not been shown to provide any additional effect and may add significant side effects (109). In fact, a similar quantity of normal saline solution may be as effective in dispersing the trigger point but does not provide the immediate pain relief of the anesthetic agent (110). Application of ultrasound to the injected area may provide longer lasting relief than injection alone. Patients should be instructed to apply heat and perform stretching exercises after trigger point injections, to prolong the relief. However, trigger points tend to recur unless a coordinated effort is made to eliminate the causative factors.

The spray and stretch technique using fluoromethane or a vapocoolant spray can also be effective if muscle tension of large muscles is a problem (111). This modality works by the counterirritant effect, similar to TENS and topical agents such as liniments or Ben-Gay.

Capsaicin cream is occasionally useful, particularly in patients with painful neuropathies, postherpetic neuralgia, or osteoarthritis (112,113). Its active ingredient is the extract of hot pepper. It has an analgesic effect due to blocking of C-fiber conduction and the inactivation of pain-related neuropeptides, including substance P, from the nerve terminals in the skin (114). Patients should be warned not to touch their eyes or oral or genitorectal areas until they have thoroughly washed their hands after applying capsaicin cream. Sometimes they will have to apply the cream several times a day for several weeks before significant results are noted (115). These considerations often limit the effectiveness of capsaicin clinically.

Therapeutic massage may be useful for short-term, acute muscle tension (116). Massage is labor-intensive, however, and unless the patient has funds available to hire a masseur, it is less likely to be useful in the long term than are other modalities. There are many ways patients can utilize self-massage, including using devices on the market that help to reach muscular areas not generally accessible to the individual for self-massage.

The use of manipulation in the treatment of musculoskeletal disorders remains controversial. There is some evidence that properly applied manipulative techniques may be useful for facet joint arthropathy of the cervical spine and acute low-back pain (117,118). Nonetheless, unsubstantiated claims to remove all pain and questionably trained providers continue to make manipulation a risky modality for many patients with pain. Many chiropractors also use traditional physical therapy modalities, further muddying the question of the effectiveness of manipulation as an independent intervention. The prescription of intermittent and never-ending "adjustments," without development of a home program of exercise, fosters dependence on the part of the patient and may serve to increase the cost to the health care system in general.

Phonophoresis and iontophoresis are specialized modalities that cause the passage of drugs, particularly steroids, through the skin by the use of ultrasound and electrical current, respectively. Phonophoresis has been recommended for several acute pain states (119–121). Similarly, iontophoresis may have beneficial effects in acute pain syndromes (122–126). There is some controversy as to whether phonophoresis is any more effective than ultrasound alone (127,128). Both of these treatments may be less effective than direct injection of a corticosteroid for inflammatory conditions, but have the advantage of being noninvasive (129).

Functional electrical stimulation (FES) of the muscle involves using electrical current to cause a muscle contraction (3). It may be helpful in some cases of peripheral nerve injury to inhibit atrophy. In partially innervated muscle, FES used in conjunction with surface EMG biofeedback may help retrain and strengthen affected muscle. Occasionally, for pain of longer duration, FES may be helpful to rebuild muscles that have weakened with disuse.

Exercise is an important adjunctive therapy for patients with pain. The ideal combination of rest and exercise is a difficult concept for patients and practitioners alike. When acute inflammation of the muscle or joint is present, rest is necessary to allow healing to occur. However, muscle weakness and joint contracture can take place very rapidly when there is complete immobility. The key to proper management of the inflamed tissue is passive ROM up to, but not past, the point of pain. The power required to move the joint may be provided by a therapist or by the patient after proper training. Causing pain during ROM exercises of the joint will only restart the vicious cycle of pain, immobility, contracture, and increased pain.

Isometric exercise may be initiated even in the setting of acute joint inflammation. When combined with surface EMG biofeedback techniques, isometric contraction and relaxation of the muscle can easily be coordinated (130).

Therapeutic exercise of a painful joint in the subacute period begins with gentle passive ROM exercises up to, but not past, the point of pain following application of a suitable heating modality (usually hot pack or ultrasound). This will maximize the ROM and minimize the pain. As inflammation subsides, the therapist allows the patient to become more active in the isotonic use of muscles around the joint, ultimately concentrating more on strengthening through resistive exercise. The timing of this program is highly variable depending on the tolerance of the patient, and requires close follow-up by both the therapist and the prescribing physiatrist.

It is a common misconception that patients with acute or subacute pain need strengthening exercise. It is difficult, if not impossible, to strengthen painful muscles. Developing a muscle training response requires forces applied to the muscle and other tissues that will not be tolerated by the patient in pain, and no progress will be made. General aerobic conditioning may be beneficial in the treatment of diffuse muscle pain syndromes such as fibromyalgia (131).

The three-stage treatment protocol of pain relief—modalities, ROM and flexibility exercises to regain the normal resting length of the muscles and other tissues, and then gradual strengthening to protect from further injury—will help ensure a safe and successful recovery.

EMOTIONAL SUPPORT

Supportive counseling by either a professional or a layperson, as well as other lifestyle adjustments, may provide added effectiveness in the treatment of pain. Most often, acute pain patients have anxiety about the presence of pain and the prognosis for recovery. Emotional support may be as simple as reassurance from the physician about the expectations for recovery. Occasionally patients will require more formal emotional or psychological support. Patients may be sensitive about the psychological overlay associated with their pain. It is generally accepted that if pain proceeds from acute to chronic, the "typical" pain psychological profile emerges, as opposed to a predisposition to pain behavior based on some intrinsic psychological weakness (132). Nonetheless, one's first meeting with the patient is usually not a good time to suggest seeing a psychologist. Instead, the patient should be allowed to gain some confidence in the clinician's ability to control the pain acutely using the techniques advocated here, and then to educate them about the usefulness of long-term lifestyle adjustments in the management of pain if necessary.

Secondary gain, both monetary and emotional, can be a persuasive and often a totally subconscious motivating factor to continue pain behavior. The ways that patients use their pain and the reasons why they need to keep their pain must be addressed before patients can hope for recovery.

CONCLUSIONS

The diagnosis and treatment of pain is an endeavor as old as medicine itself, yet pain mechanisms remain incompletely understood. Careful history taking, a thorough physical examination, and judiciously applied diagnostic studies will help the physiatrist arrive at a satisfactory approach to the treatment of the pain patient. Many treatment alternatives are available. The physical medicine modalities can be highly efficacious for acute musculoskeletal pain, yielding a good outcome in the vast majority of patients. However, the spectrum of acute to chronic pain should be borne in mind since all chronic pain patients at one time had acute pain. It may be helpful to recognize any psychosocial or behavioral issues early, as this will allow for the planning of comprehensive pain treatment.

REFERENCES

1. Suzuki H. Recent topics in the management of pain: development of the concept of preemptive analgesia. *Cell Transplant* 1995;4(suppl 1):S3–S6.
2. Minor MA, Sanford ML. Physical interventions in the management of pain in arthritis: an overview of research and practice. *Arthritis Care Res* 1993;6:197–206.
3. Sawyer M, Zbieranek CK. The treatment of soft tissue after spinal injury. *Clin Sports Med* 1986;5:387–405.
4. Loeser JD, Cousins MJ. Contemporary pain management. *Med J Aust* 1990;153:208–213.
5. Chapman CR. Neuromatrix theory: do we need it? *Pain Forum* 1996;5:139–142.
6. Cross SA. Pathophysiology of pain. *Mayo Clin Proc* 1994;69:375–383.
7. Melzack R. Gate control theory: on the evolution of pain concepts. *Pain Forum* 1996;5: 128–138.
8. Arendt-Nielsen L, Peterson-Felix S. Wind-up and neuroplasticity: is there a correlation to clinical pain? *Eur J Anesthesiol* 1995;12(suppl 10):1–7.
9. Dickenson AH. Central acute pain mechanisms. *Ann Med* 1995;27:223–227.
10. Woolf CL. A new strategy for the treatment of inflammatory pain: prevention or elimination of central sensitization. *Drugs* 1994;47(suppl 5):1–9.
11. Weiss SA, Lindell B. Phantom limb pain and etiology of amputation in unilateral lower-extremity amputees. *J Pain Symptom Manage* 1996;11:3–17.
12. McGrath PA. Psychological aspects of pain perception. *Arch Oral Biol* 1994;39(suppl): 55S–62S.
13. Gnatz SM. Referred pain syndromes of the head and neck. *Phys Med Rehabil State Art Rev* 1991;5:585–596.
14. Janig W. Neuronal mechanisms of pain with special emphasis on visceral and deep somatic pain. *Acta Neurochir Suppl (Wien)* 1987;38:16–32.
15. Lewis T. *Pain.* New York: Macmillan, 1942.
16. Anonymous. Annotations, referred pain. *Lancet* 1967;2:1245.
17. Torebjork HE, Ochoa JL, Schady W. Referred pain from intraneural stimulation of muscle fascicles in the median nerve. *Pain* 1984;18:145–156.
18. Sessle BJ, Hu JW, Amano N, et al. Convergence of cutaneous, tooth pulp, visceral, neck and muscle afferents onto nocioceptive and non-nocioceptive neurones in the trigeminal subnucleus caudalis (medullary dorsal horn) and its implications for referred pain. *Pain* 1986;27:219–235.
19. Ruch TC. Pathophysiology of pain. In: Ruch T, Patton HC, eds. *Physiology and biophysics.* Philadelphia: WB Saunders, 1979:272–342.
20. Cervero F, Tattersall JEH. Somatic and visceral integration in the thoracic spinal cord. *Prog Brain Res* 1986;67:189–203.
21. Laurberg S, Sorensen KE. Cervical dorsal root ganglion cells with collaterals to both shoulder skin and the diaphragm. A fluorescent double labelling study in the rat. A model for referred pain? *Brain Res* 1985;331:160–163.
22. Wall PD. The gate control theory of pain mechanisms. A reexamination and re-statement. *Brain* 1978;101:1–18.
23. Fields HL, Busbaum AI. Brain stem control of spinal pain-transmission neurons. *Annu Rev Physiol* 1978;40:217–248.
24. Travell JG, Simons DG. *Myofascial pain and dysfunction.* Baltimore: Williams & Wilkins, 1983.
25. Travell J. Myofascial trigger points: clinical view. In: Bonica JJ, Albe-Fessard, eds. *Advances in pain research and therapy.* Vol. 1. New York: Raven, 1976:919–926.
26. Sola AE, Rodenberger ML, Gettys BB. Incidence of hypersensitive areas in the posterior shoulder muscles. A survey of two hundred young adults. *Am J Phys Med* 1956;34:585–590.
27. Simons DG. Myofascial pain syndromes: where are we? Where are we going? *Arch Phys Med Rehabil* 1988;69:207–212.
28. Quintner JL, Cohen ML. Referred pain of peripheral nerve origin: an alternative to the "myofascial pain" construct. *Clin J Pain* 1994;10:243–251.
29. Arroyo P. Electromyography in the evaluation of reflex muscle spasm. *J Fla Med Assoc* 1966;53:29–31.
30. Travell J, Bigelow NH. Referred somatic pain does not follow a simple "segmental" pattern. *Fed Proc* 1946;5:106.
31. Buxbaum JD, Myslinski NR, Myers DE. Dental management of orofacial pain. In: Tolleson CD, ed. *Handbook of chronic pain management.* Baltimore: Williams & Wilkins, 1989:303–304.
32. Pilowski I, Chapman CR, Bonica JJ. Pain, depression and illness behavior in a pain clinic population. *Pain* 1977;4:183–192.

33. Buckelew SP, Murray SE, Hewett JE, et al. Self-efficacy, pain and physical activity among fibromyalgia subjects. *Arthritis Care Res* 1995;8:43–50.

34. Weintraub MI. Chronic pain in litigation. What is the relationship? *Neurol Clin* 1995;13: 341–349.

35. Ekblom A, Hansson P. Pain intensity measurements in patients with acute pain receiving afferent stimulation. *J Neurol Neurosurg Psychiatry* 1988;51:481–486.

36. Reeves JL, Jaeger B, Graff-Radford SB. Reliability of the pressure algometer as a measure of myofascial trigger point sensitivity. *Pain* 1986;24:313–321.

37. Woolf CJ, Chong MS. Preemptive analgesia—treating post-operative pain by preventing the establishment of central sensitization. *Anesth Analg* 1993;77:362–379.

38. Sternbach RA. Acute vs chronic pain. In: Wall PD, Melzack R, eds. *Textbook of pain.* Edinburgh: Churchill Livingstone, 1984:173–177.

39. Lehmann JF, ed. *Therapeutic heat and cold.* 3rd ed. Baltimore: Williams & Wilkins, 1982.

40. Lehmann JF, Masock AJ, Warren CG, et al. Effects of therapeutic temperatures on tendon extensibility. *Arch Phys Med Rehabil* 1970;51:481–487.

41. Schmidt KL, Oh VR, Rocher G, et al. Heat, cold and inflammation. *Rheumatology* 1979;38:391–404.

42. Shafer N, Kitay G. Transcutaneous electrical nerve stimulation and pain relief: an overview. *Am J Electromed* 1987;2:9–13.

43. Pomeranz B, Cheng H. Supression of noxious responses in single neurons of the cat spinal cord by electroacupuncture and its reversal by opiate antagonist naloxone. *Exp Neurol* 1979;64:307.

44. Sjolund BH, Terenius L, Erickson MBE. Increased cerebrospinal fluid levels of endorphin after electro-acupuncture. *Acta Physiol Scand* 1977;100:382–384.

45. Ananth J. Psychopharmacological agents in physical disorders. *Psychother Psychosomati* 1992;58:13–31.

46. Bellamy N. Treating musculoskeletal disease with NSAIDs. Practitioner's guide. *Can Fam Physician* 1996;42:482–492.

47. Vane JR, Botting RM. Mechanism of action of anti-inflammatory drugs. *Scand J Rheumatol Suppl* 1996;102:9–21.

48. Rust GS, Hatch R, Gums JG. Carisoprodol as a drug of abuse. *Arch Fam Med* 1993;2:429–432.

49. Campbell SM, Gatter RA, Clark S, et al. A double blind study of cyclobenzaprine in patients with primary fibrositis. *Arthritis Rheum* 1985;28:S40.

50. Max MB, Lynch SA, Muir J, et al. Effects of desipramine, amitriptyline and fluoxetine on pain in diabetic neuropathy. *N Engl J Med* 1992;326:1250–1256.

51. Goldenberg DL, Felson DT, Dinerman H. A randomized controlled trial of amitriptyline and naproxen in the treatment of patients with fibromyalgia. *Arthritis Rheum* 1986;29:1371–1377.

52. Carette S, McCain GA, Bell DA, et al. Evaluation of amitriptyline in primary fibrositis. *Arthritis Rheum* 1986;29:655–659.

53. Watson CPN, Evans RJ, Reed K, et al. Amitriptyline versus placebo in post-herpetic neuralgia. *Neurology* 1982;32:671–673.

54. McQuay HJ, Carroll D, Glynn CJ. Dose response for analgesic effect in chronic pain. *Anaesthesia* 1993;48:281–285.

55. Glassman AH, Roose SP. Risks of antidepressants in the elderly: tricyclic antidepressants and arrhythmia—revising risks. *Gerontology* 1994;40(suppl 1):15–20.

56. Max MB. Antidepressants as analgesics. In: Fields HL, Liebeskind JC, eds. *Pharmacological approaches to the treatment of chronic pain: new concepts and critical issues. Prog Pain Res Manage* Vol. 1. Seattle: IASP Press, 1994:229–246.

57. Clifford DB. Treatment of pain with antidepressants. *Fam Physician* 1985;31:181–185.

58. Swerdlow M. Anticonvulsant drugs and chronic pain. *Clin Neuropharmacol* 1984;7: 51–82.

59. Swerdlow M, Cundhill JG. Anticonvulsant drugs used in the treatment of lancinating pain: a comparison. *Anaesthesia* 1981;36:1129–1132.

60. Tanelian DL, Victory RA. Sodium channel-blocking agents: their use in neuropathic pain conditions. *Pain Forum* 1995;4: 75–80.

61. Mellick GA, Mellick LB. Gabapentin in the management of reflex sympathetic dystrophy. *J Pain Symptom Manage* 1995;10:265–266.

62. Eisenach JC, Dewan DM, Rose JC, Angelo JM. Epidural clonidine produces antinociception, but not hypotension, in sheep. *Anesthesiology* 1987;66:496–501.

63. O'Neill TP, Haigler HJ. Effects of clonidine on neuronal firing evoked by a noxious stimulus. *Brain Res* 1985;327:97–103.

64. Shafar J, Tallett ER, Knowlson PA. Evaluation of clonidine in prophylaxis of migraine. *Lancet* 1972;1:403–407.

65. Tan YM, Croese J. Clonidine and diabetic patients with leg pains. *Ann Intern Med* 1986; 105:633.

66. Washton AM, Resnick RB. Clonidine in opiate withdrawal: review and appraisal of clinical findings. *Pharmacotherapy* 1981;1: 140–146.

67. Elliott KJ, Brodsky M, Hyanansky A, et al. Dextromethorphan shows efficacy in experimental pain (nociception) and opioid tolerance. *Neurology* 1995;45(12 suppl 8):S66–S68.

68. Price DD, Mao J, Frenk H, Mayer DJ. The *N*-methyl-D-aspartate receptor antagonist dextromethorphan selectively reduces temporal summation of second pain in man. *Pain* 1994;59:165–174.

69. McQuay HJ, Carroll D, Jadad AR, et al. Dextromethorphan for the treatment of neuropathic pain: a double blind randomised controlled crossover trial with integral N-of-1 design. *Pain* 1994;59:127–133.

70. Chabal C, Jacobsen L, Mariano A, et al. The use of oral mexiletine for the treatment of pain after peripheral nerve injury. *Anesthesiology* 1992;76: 513–517.

71. Stracke H, Meyer U, Schumaker H, Federlin K. Mexiletine in the treatment of diabetic neuropathy. *Diabetes Care* 1992;15: 1550–1555.

72. Chiou-Tan F, Tuel SM, Johnson JC, et al. Effect of mexiletine on spinal cord injury dysesthetic pain. *Am J Phys Med Rehabil* 1996;75:84–87.

73. Wright JM. Review of the symptomatic treatment of diabetic neuropathy. *Pharmacotherapy* 1994;14:689–697.

74. Prough DS, McLeskey CH, Poehling GG, et al. Efficacy of oral nifedipine in the treatment of reflex sympathetic dystrophy. *Anesthesiology* 1985;62: 796–799.

75. Barbosa LM, Gauthier VJ, Davis CL. Bone pain that responds to calcium channel blockers. A retrospective and prospective study of transplant recipients. *Transplantation* 1995;59: 541–544.

76. Gurdal H, Sara Y, Tulunay FC. Effects of calcium channel blockers on formalin induced nociception and inflammation in rats. *Pharmacology* 1992;44: 290–296.

77. Chapman SR, Pogrel JW, Yaksh TL. Role of voltage-dependent calcium channel subtypes in experimental tactile allodynia. *J Pharmacol Exp Ther* 1994;269:1117–1123.

78. Hegarty A, Portenoy RK. Pharmacotherapy of neuropathic pain. *Semin Neurol* 1994;14:213–224.

79. Arner S, Meyerson BA. Lack of analgesic effect of opioids on neuropathic and idiopathic forms of pain. *Pain* 1988;33:11–23.

80. Kanjhan R. Opioids and pain. *Clin Exp Pharmacol Physiol* 1995;22:397–403.

81. Borbely AA, Acherman P. Ultradian dynamics of sleep after a single dose of benzodiazepine hypnotics. *Eur J Pharmacol* 1991;195:11–18.

82. Blois R, Gaillard JM, Attali P, Coquelin JP. Effect of zolpidem on sleep in healthy subjects: a placebo-controlled trial with polysomnographic recordings. *Clin Ther* 1993;15:797–809.

83. TePoorten BA. The piriformis muscle. *J Am Osteopath Assoc* 1969;69:150–160.

84. Jackson RP. The facet syndrome. Myth or reality? *Clin Orthop* 1992;279:110–121.

85. Dupuis PR. The anatomy of the lumbar spine. In: Kirkalky-Willis WH, ed. *Managing low back pain.* New York: Churchill Livingstone, 1988:42.

86. Hendrix RW, Lin PJ, Kane WJ. Simplified aspiration or injection technique for the sacro-iliac joint. *J Bone Joint Surg [Am]* 1982;64:1249–1252.

87. Maugars Y, Mathis C, Vilon P, Prost A. Corticosteroid injection of the sacroiliac joint in patients with seronegative spondylarthropathy. *Arthritis Rheumat* 1992;35:564–568.

88. Schwarzer AC, Aprill CN, Bogduk N. The sacroiliac joint in chronic low back pain. *Spine* 1995;20:31–37.

89. Lavignolle B, Vital JM, Senegas J, et al. An approach to the functional anatomy of the sacroiliac joints in vivo. *Anat Clin* 1983;5:169–176.

90. Fortin JD, Aprill CN, Ponthieux B, Pier J. Sacroiliac joint: pain referral maps upon applying a new injection/arthrography technique. Part II: clinical evaluation. *Spine* 1994;19:1483–1489.

91. Fortin JD, Dwyer AP, West S, Pier J. Sacroiliac joint: pain referral maps upon applying a new injection/arthrography technique. Part I: asymptomatic volunteers. *Spine* 1994;19: 1475–1482.

92. Osterbauer PJ, De Boer KF, Widmaier R, et al. Treatment and biomechanical assessment of patients with chronic sacroiliac joint syndrome *J Manipulative Physiol Ther* 1993;16:82–90.

93. Potter NA, Rothstein JM. Intertester reliability for selected clinical tests of the sacroiliac joint. *Phys Ther* 1985;65: 1671–1675.

94. Dreyfuss P, Dryer S, Griffin J, et al. Positive sacroiliac screening tests in asymptomatic adults. *Spine* 1994;19:1138–1143.

95. Waldman SD. Lumbar epidural nerve block. In: Waldman SD, ed. *Interventional pain management.* Philadelphia: WB Saunders, 1996:325–332.

96. Waldman SD, Waldman KA. Reflex sympathetic dystrophy of the knee following arthroscopic surgery: successful treatment with neural blockade utilizing local anesthetics. *J Pain Symptom Manage* 1992;7:243–245.

97. White AH, Derby R, Wynne G. Epidural injections for the diagnosis and treatment of low-back pain. *Spine* 1980;5:78–86.

98. Waldman SD. Acute herpes zoster and postherpetic neuralgia. *Intern Med* 1990;11:33–38.

99. Woodward JL, Herring SA, Windsor RE, et al. Epidural procedures in spine pain management. In: Lennard TA, ed. *Physiatric procedures in clinical practice.* Philadelphia: Hanley & Belfus, 1995:260–291.

100. Derby R, Bogduk N, Kine G. Precision percutaneous blocking procedures for localizing spinal pain. Part 2. The lumbar neuroaxial

compartment. *Pain Dig* 1993;3:175–188.

101. Bromage PR. Complications and contraindications. In: Bromage PR, ed. *Epidural analgesia.* Philadelphia: WB Saunders, 1978:654–711.

102. Retzlaff EW, Berry AH, Haight AS, et al. The piriformis muscle syndrome. *J Am Osteopath Assoc* 1974;73:799–807.

103. Parziale JR, Hudgins TH, Fishman LM. The piriformis syndrome. *Am J Orthop* 1996;25: 819–823.

104. Barton PM. Piriformis syndrome: a rational approach to management. *Pain* 1991;47:345–352.

105. Beatty RA. The piriformis muscle syndrome: a simple diagnostic maneuver [see comments]. *Neurosurgery* 1994;34:512–514.

106 Jankovic J, Brin MF. Therapeutic uses of botulinum toxin. *N Engl J Med* 1991;324:1186–1194.

107 Coffield JA, Considine RB, Simpson LL. The site and mechanism of action of botulinum neurotoxin. In: Jankovic J, Hallett M, eds. *Therapy with botulinum toxin.* New York: Marcel Dekker, 1994:3–14.

108. Travell JG, Simons DG. *Myofascial pain and dysfunction.* Baltimore: Williams & Wilkins, 1983.

109. Gottlieb NL, Riskin WG. Complications of local corticosteroid injections. *JAMA* 1980;243: 1547–1548.

110. Frost FA, Jessen B, Siggard-Andersen J. A controlled, double blind comparison of mepivacaine injection versus saline injection for myofascial pain. *Lancet* 1980;1:499–500.

111. Travell J. Myofascial trigger points: clinical view. In: Bonica JJ, Albe-Fessard D, eds. *Advances in pain research and therapy.* Vol. 1. New York: Raven, 1976:919–926.

112. Winter J, Bevan S, Campbell EA. Capsaicin and pain mechanisms. *Br J Anaesth* 1995;75:157–168.

113. Rains C, Bryson HM. Topical capsaicin. A review of its pharmacological properties and therapeutic potential in post-herpetic neuralgia, diabetic neuropathy and osteoarthritis. *Drugs Aging* 1995;7:317–328.

114. Dray A. Mechanism of action of capsaicin-like molecules on sensory neurons. *Life Sci* 1992;51:1759–1765.

115. Craft RM, Porreca F. Treatment parameters of desensitization to capsaicin. *Life Sci* 1992;51:1767–1775.

116. Goats GC. Massage—the scientific basis of an ancient art: part 2. Physiological and therapeutic effects. *Br J Sports Med* 1994;28:153–156.

117. Maigne R. Manipulation of the spine. In: Basmajian JV, ed. *Manipulation, traction and massage.* 3rd ed. Baltimore: Williams & Wilkins, 1985:77–78.

118. Twomey LT. A rationale for the treatment of back pain and joint pain by manual therapy. *Phys Ther* 1992;72:885–892.

119. Griffin JE, Echternach JL, Price RE, et al. Patients treated with ultrasonic driven hydrocortisone and with ultrasound alone. *Phys Ther* 1967;47:594–601.

120. Wing M. Phonophoresis of hydrocortisone in the treatment of temporomandibular joint syndrome. *Phys Ther* 1982;62: 32–33.

121. Pottenger FJ, Ranalfa BL. Utilization of hydrocortisone phonophoresis in US Army physical therapy clinics. *Milit Med* 1989;154:355–358.

122. Delacerda FG. A comparative study of three methods of treatment for shoulder girdle myofascial syndrome. *J Orthop Sports Phys Ther* 1982;4:51–54.

123. Bertolucci LE. Introduction of antiinflammatory drugs by iontophoresis: double blind study. *J Orthop Sports Phys Ther* 1982;4:103–108.

124. Swezey RL. Rheumatoid arthritis: the role of the kinder and gentler therapies. *J Rheumatol* 1990;17(suppl 25):8–13.

125. Garagiola U, Dacatra U, Braconaro F, et al. Iontophoretic administration of pirprofen or lysine soluble aspirin in the treatment of rheumatic diseases. *Clin Ther* 1988;10:553–558.

126. Lark MR, Gargarosa LP. Iontophoresis: an effective modality for the treatment of inflammatory disorders of the temporomandibular joint and myofascial pain. *Cranio* 1990;8:108–119.

127. Muir WS, Magee FP, Longo JA, et al. Comparison of ultrasonically applied vs. intra-articular injected hydrocortisone levels in canine knees. *Orthop Rev* 1990;19:351–356.

128. Oziomek RS, Perrin DH, Herold DA, Denegar CR. Effect of phonophoresis on serum salicylate levels. *Med Sci Sports Exerc* 1991;23:397–401.

129. Theib U, Kuhn I, Lucker PW. Iontophoresis—is there a future for clinical application? *Methods Find Exp Clin Pharmacol* 1991;13:353–359.

130. Ferraccioli G, Ghirelli L, Scita F, et al. EMG biofeedback training in fibromyalgia syndrome. *J Rheumatol* 1987;14:820–825.

131. McCain GA. Role of physical fitness training in fibrositis/fibromyalgia syndrome. *Am J Med* 1986;81(suppl 3A): 73–77.

132. Gamsa A. Is emotional disturbance a precipitator or a consequence of chronic pain? *Pain* 1990;42:183–195.

Chapter 58

Chronic Pain

John C. King

What is different about chronic pain that it deserves a chapter distinct from acute pain? How does duration influence the pathophysiology, management, and understanding of pain? These questions may initially seem difficult to answer. The effects of time in the pain experience, however, do make a difference in clinical presentation and treatment. The human being is a dynamic organism and responds to its ongoing experiences. When these experiences include pain, adaptations occur, many of which contribute to the difficulty in successfully treating the underlying painful conditions.

Pain is defined by the International Association for the Study of Pain as "an unpleasant sensory and emotional experience associated with actual or potential tissue damage or described in terms of such damage" (1,2). This intrinsically subjective experience is essential for protection and warning about potential harm. When pain becomes chronic, it sometimes loses its protective effects and no longer provides any sensory experience of value. If this occurs, the subjective pain experience ceases to be an important biologic symptom, and can become the disabling problem itself. Chronic pain, at that point, only serves to add emotional suffering, physical disability, and potential social handicap to the individual.

Chronic pain can be subdivided into two major classifications according to the presence or absence of progressive ongoing tissue destruction. The former is often a cause of pain associated with malignancies. Cancer pain can often be successfully managed through both acute pain management techniques and special techniques peculiar to cancer management, described more fully in Chapter 91. In this subcategory of chronic pain, the experience of pain does signal ongoing tissue destruction and continues to be an important biologic symptom. The pain experience is also self-limited in duration by the often terminal nature of the disease process. However, the more common situation in chronic pain is that of no ongoing tissue destruction, despite the ongoing unpleasant experience of pain. Because of the lack of progressive tissue damage, the experience has been referred to as the *chronic benign pain syndrome*, *chronic intractable benign pain syndrome*, or simply the *chronic pain syndrome* (3). In this syndrome, the pain signals no longer serve to warn of ongoing harm. The continuous aversive affective experience leads to physical, emotional, and social adaptations that are often found to be harmful and countertherapeutic. Recognizing these maladaptations will allow more successful interventions toward diminishing the suffering associated with chronic pain.

Chronic pain is variously defined. Most research has considered ongoing pain of longer than 6 months as the minimum criterion. Others have used 3 months, and still others define *chronic pain* in terms of any pain that persists longer than the expected healing time for the involved tissues (3,4). This latter definition presupposes recognizing all tissues that were injured. It also sometimes flows from the misconception that upon healing, all tissue nociception will cease, and thus seeks alternative sources for the pain experience.

Acute pain is emotionally unpleasant, by the definition of pain. However, the emotional involvement of acute pain patients does not seem to interfere with effective treatment and indeed tends to reinforce compliance. However, the emotional involvement seen in chronic pain patients is aversive to many providers as it seems to thwart effective interventions instead of reinforce them. This element is sometimes viewed as a lock closing the door to effective intervention. This perception is incomplete and faulty as it does not recognize the complete human experience of pain. Providers who maintain only this perspective will continue to be frustrated and defeated in their management of the physically impaired, chronic pain patient. A more effective conceptualization and comprehensive approach to the chronic pain sufferer that will enhance goal-directed care is described further in this chapter.

EPIDEMIOLOGY

Whereas acute pain is a ubiquitous and protective transient experience, chronic pain is not an expected experience. Those rare individuals born congenitally insensate have shortened life spans and rarely reach adulthood with intact appendages (5). Therefore, acute pain is biologically desirable as a protective and thereby beneficial experience. The most common sites of acute pain are the head, including the throat, and the lower extremities, followed by the abdomen, upper extremities, and chest (6,7). Chronic pain has a different pattern of distribution and is rarely felt to be a beneficial experience.

Chronic pain has reached epidemic proportions in the United States. Pain resulting from cancer affects 1 million (and perhaps 20 million worldwide). There are more than 36 million people with chronically painful arthritis, 70 million with episodic or ongoing back pain, 29 million with chronic headaches, and 23 million others with chronically painful conditions such as myofascial pain syndromes, cardiac and visceral pain syndromes, deafferentation pain states such as phantom limb pain, and sympathetically mediated pain conditions (8,9). The back is the most common site of chronic pain (6). Back pain accounts for half of all workers' compensation cases and accounts for 19 million of the 40 million annual visits to physicians due to chronically painful conditions (9,10). Ten million Americans are disabled by low-back pain, which is the most common cause of disability before the age of 45 years (11), and the third most common cause behind heart disease and "arthritis and rheumatism" among 45 to 64 year olds (12). Despite its frequency, the cause of low-back pain remains unclear for 85% of episodes (13). For patients without an obvious cause of the pain found at their initial presentation, only 2% of those with persistent back pain may require surgery (14), an additional 1.5% are subsequently found to have systemic disease causing the back pain (15,16), and even fewer have cancer as the cause (16), yet two-thirds of patients are concerned that they may have a serious underlying illness (17). Headaches have a higher prevalence, with 29 million people suffering from recurrent moderate to severe head pain, and cause slightly more lost workdays per year, but low-back pain results in higher medical costs as well as 250 million workdays lost each year (8,10). Over 30 million Americans have osteoarthritis, including 24 million with moderate to severe pain and 100,000 who cannot ambulate to the bathroom owing to its severity. The prevalence of osteoarthritis is 20% for those over age 35 years, affecting 2% of those under 45 years old, 30% of those 45 to 64 years old, 68% of those between 65 and 69 years old, and almost all individuals over 80 years old. Though low-back pain is the most common cause of chronic work disability in industrialized nations, in underdeveloped countries knee osteoarthritis is the most common chronic pain cause for work impairment (18,19).

COST

The cost of chronic pain can be measured most easily in terms of its economic impact. The cost of emotional suffering is staggering and often this suffering leads to significant and profound disability and handicap. Disruptions in the labor force and the retraining of new workers and injured workers also add to the costs associated with chronic disabling pain. In 1986 in the United States, approximately $79 billion was spent on medical care, disability compensation, and litigation due to chronic pain (8). Medical care for low-back pain alone costs over $14 billion per year (10). Only ten percent of the patients, the ones with the more chronic pain, accounted for 78% of the cost (20). A cost of more than $11 billion per year can be extrapolated from the prevalence of and additional medical expenses encountered by osteoarthritis sufferers (8,21).

ETIOLOGIES

Pain is the most common complaint that leads patients to seek medical care (7). Chronic pain begins with acute pain. Up to 80% of all chronic pain sufferers have an identifiable initiating physical traumatic event, and the musculoskeletal system is most commonly involved. A recent text listed over 2000 diagnoses to consider, categorized according to the region of the body affected (7). Excluding a few time-limited causes such as acute infections or catastrophic ones such as ruptured aneurysms, the same differential diagnoses apply to chronic pain. Even among the exception of acute infections, granulomatous disease processes and osteomyelitis can contribute to chronic pain etiologies. Table 58-1 presents a more condensed list of the common differential diagnoses to be considered.

Some of the most common painful conditions encountered by the physiatrist are the following: myofascial

Table 58-1: Etiologies of Chronic or Recurrent Pain

- Psychological pain factors
  - Psychological factors contributing to chronic pain, includes depression +/– anxiety
  - Malingering / factitious pain
  - Conversion disorder / psychogenic pain
  - Somatic preoccupation / symptom magnification / hypochondriasis
  - Delusions from psychosis
  - Secondary gain
- Nerve pain
  - Polyneuropathy, most commonly due to diabetes, alcohol, toxins, AIDS sensory neuropathy
  - Nerve trauma, scar pain
  - Amputation, neuroma
  - Sympathetic-mediated pain
  - Focal nerve entrapments
  - Chronic inflammatory demyelinating polyradiculoneuropathy
  - Porphyric polyneuropathy
  - Cryoglobulin neuropathy
  - Mononeuritis multiplex
- Deafferentation syndromes
  - Focal and mononeuropathies
  - Polyneuropathies
  - Polyradiculoneuropathies
  - Nerve root avulsions
  - Postherpetic neuralgia
  - Neurolytic sensory procedures
  - Nerve laceration and stretch injuries
  - Postfrostbite neuropathy
  - Phantom pain
  - Central pain (thalamic) syndromes
- Head Pain
  - Muscle tension headaches
  - Vascular (migraine) headaches
  - Temporomandibular dysfunction
  - Temporalis tendonitis
  - Sinusitis
- Facial pain
  - Trigeminal neuralgia
  - Glossopharyngeal neuralgia
  - Nervus intermedius neuralgia (Ramsay Hunt syndrome)
  - Sphenopalatine neuralgia
  - Carotiditis
  - Referred dental/TMJ pain
- Neck pain
  - Whiplash strain
  - Myofascial
  - Degenerative disk disease
  - Osteoarthritis/spondylosis
  - Cervical radiculopathy
  - Myelopathy
  - Rheumatoid joint inflammation (especially atlantoaxial)
  - Spondyloarthropathics (such as ankylosing spondylitis)
- Thoracic pain
  - Myofascial
  - Recurrent vertebral fractures secondary to osteoporosis +/– associated biomechanical strain
  - Rib fractures
  - Pleuritis
  - Referred pain such as chronic pancreatitis, gallstones, renal disease, angina
- Low-back pain
  - Muscle/ligamentous strain/sprain
  - Myofascial
  - Facet osteoarthropathy
  - Degenerative disk disease
  - Spinal stenosis
  - Arachnoiditis
  - Inflammatory arthritides such as ankylosing spondylitis,
  - Reiter syndrome, rheumatoid arthritis
  - Spondyloarthropathy
  - Disk disruption +/– herniation +/– radiculopathy
  - Vertebral tuberculosis (Pott disease)
  - Vertebral osteomyelitis
- Visceral pain
  - Cardiovascular disease (angina)
  - Peripheral vascular disease includes claudication, phlebitis, and chronic lymphedema
  - Gastroesophageal reflux
  - Peptic ulcer disease
  - Pancreatitis
  - Gallstones
  - Bowel obstructions
  - Diverticulitis
  - Inflammatory bowel disease
  - Irritable bowel syndrome
- Genitourinary
  - Urinary retention
  - Referred renal/urethral disease
  - Herpes simplex retroperitoneal mass
- Male
  - Prostatitis
  - Urethral stricture
  - Testicular torsion
  - Peyronie disease
  - Myofascial pelvic pain
- Female
  - Uterine diseases
  - Endometriosis
  - Myofascial pelvic pain
  - Idiopathic pelvic pain
  - Mittelschmerz
  - Dysmenorrhea
  - Premenstrual syndrome
  - Ectopic pregnancy
- Joints
  - Trauma +/– internal derangement
  - Osteoarthritis
  - Postinfectious or postbleed arthropathy
  - Rheumatoid arthritis
  - Lyme disease
  - Reiter syndrome
  - Other inflammatory arthritides
  - HIV-associated arthritis
  - Sarcoid arthritis
  - Gout/pseudogout
- Bone
  - Pathologic fractures due to osteoporosis, osteomalacia, metabolic disease, and tumor
  - Metastasis and primary bone tumors
  - Nonhealing stress fractures
  - Paget disease
- Muscle/Tendon/Bursa
  - Myofascial
  - Chronic overuse syndromes
  - Tendonitis
  - Bursitis
  - Fibromyalgia
  - Metabolic deficiency myalgias
  - Polymyositis
  - Polymyalgia rheumatica
  - Trichinosis
  - Eosinophilia-myalgia syndrome
  - Eosinophilic fasciitis
  - Polyarteritis nodosa
  - Sarcoidosis
- Cancer
  - Visceral distention/erosion
  - Neural compression/invasion
  - Bony erosion
  - Chemotherapeutic, radiation, and surgical complications

AIDS = acquired immuno-deficiency syndrome; TMJ = temporomandibular joint; HIV = human immuno-deficiency virus.

pain syndromes including fibromyalgia; cumulative trauma disorders—a new name for presumed overuse microinjuries that accumulate to cause muscle, tendon, or bursae injuries with possible secondary nerve compromises including carpal tunnel syndrome and possibly idiopathic low-back pain; deafferentation pain from many conditions including polyneuropathy, phantom pain from amputations, spinal cord injury, multiple sclerosis, or stroke causes for central pain; reflex sympathetic dystrophy, a type of sympathetically mediated pain syndrome; and neuroma hypersensitivity pains. Many specific interventions exist for these particular syndromes but most are relatively ineffective, and thus these conditions frequently present to the physiatrist as chronic pain complaints (1,9,11).

The diagnoses in Table 58-1 are only a starting point for understanding chronic pain. These diagnoses represent the initiating or precipitating acute pain processes. They must be appreciated and appropriately managed by medical interventions, though typically fewer than 5% of chronic pain patients will have a curable medical etiology (22). Once pain becomes chronic, simple medical management alone may be insufficient to ameliorate the physical disability and suffering that can result from a chronic pain problem.

Etiology of the Chronic Pain Syndrome

Chronic pain is not uncommon and most often is not disabling. Many professional athletes report pain throughout their season yet continue to perform at physically demanding, strenuously high levels. Surveys of industrial work settings yield a cross-sectional prevalence of between 15% and 30% of active productive workers reporting pain on that day (23–27). Up to 80% of Americans will experience low-back pain sufficient to seek medical attention at some point in their life (28,29). Most will have recurrences, yet by 4 weeks the pain in 90% will have resolved, but at 6 months as many as 3% continue to have persistent pain that interferes with their desired activities (30). Even this 3% yields millions of chronic low-back pain sufferers. One measure of disability is the loss of ability to perform productive employment. Return to work rates among patients with chronic pain do not correlate with either the type of pain or the self-reported severity of pain (31). This very nonintuitive result suggests that more than just a response to nociception is occurring in the disability due to chronic pain.

Patients who experience a new pain for the first time have no track record to know empirically how to deal with the unpleasant experience. This coupled with their anxiety over the cause often leads to physician visits. Patients' initial reactions to a new pain are called *respondent* because these reactions are, in a sense, reflexive and are not guided by any past learning experiences. After many days, patients will find different methods for dealing with their pain according to what seems helpful, not just what seems helpful to the pain but what is helpful to the person overall. An example is a person dropping a brick on the foot. The initial reaction may be hopping around while holding that foot in the air. However, as days pass, the patient will not continue this behavior but will adopt different strategies according to what seems to help. This may include propping the foot up during the day. However, this behavior may be avoided if the patient's income depends on sales activities that preclude such a posture. Here a social issue, generating income, may interfere with what otherwise was physically helpful. When behavior changes from a purely reflexive to a more educated learned response, it is called *operant* behavior (32,33). The helpful factors operate to alter the behavior from what one might otherwise expect to spontaneously arise.

While this is part of learning theory, learning in this context does not mean education or even a conscious accumulation of facts. It only means the individual is being influenced. Unfortunately pain is only one of many factors that influence behavior. Intrapersonal desires and goals, interpersonal relationships, and psychological, spiritual, vocational, avocational, family, legal, and social factors all influence how humans are likely to act.

Behavior is important because of the subjective nature of the pain experience. The only means clinicians have to measure pain, especially chronic pain, is by what patients say and how they act, i.e., by their behavior. Physicians can measure some physiologic correlates to pain, such as increased sympathetic tone in the setting of acute pain, but these correlates do not indicate what the *subjective* level of discomfort is. Anxiety and other stressors contribute to this subjective experience such that the dysphoria does not necessarily result from only pain. However, with chronic pain, little in the way of increased sympathetic tone occurs. This does not invalidate the existence of pain; it merely means that sympathetic responses accommodate over time. Other correlates exist but none have the precision to indicate the degree of nociception the patient may be experiencing. (*Nociception* means the neurologic and tissue-level biochemical changes that from past experience are interpreted to signal actual or potential harm.) The patients' behavior, what they say and how they act, is all clinicians can observe to evaluate the degree of pain experienced, especially in the clinical setting. Clinicians cannot feel or measure the pain directly; they can only subjectively observe and report patients' demonstrated behaviors, which are correlated to the suspected pathology.

A major problem in the assessment of the chronic pain patient is correctly interpreting what factors are affecting the presenting behavior. In the acute pain situation, insufficient time has elapsed for other factors to obscure the respondent's behavior, and a pretty good estimate of a patient's level of nociception can be obtained by the behavior, both verbal report and activity. For the chronic pain patient, much time has passed. Innumerable factors may be contributing. Figure 58-1 illustrates how

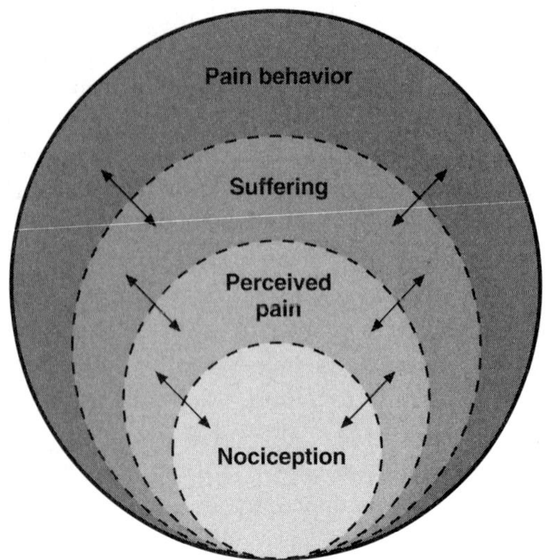

Figure 58-1. Interactive model of the pain experience. Only the outer layer, behavior, can be observed. Several layers of processing intervene and interact before nociception is expressed. (Redrawn by permission from King JC, Dumitru D, Walsh NE. Rehabilitation of the pain patient: a U.S. perspective. *Pain Dig* 1992;2:106–126.)

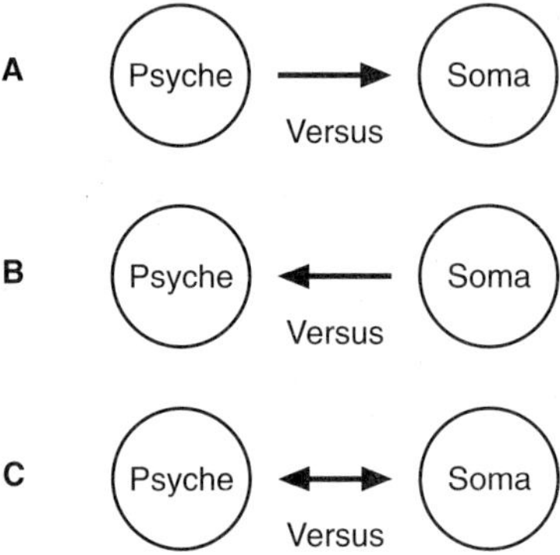

Figure 58-2. Dichotomous views of the interactions of mind and body. *A.* Mental factors affect the body. Physical problems such as pain are due to influences from the mind, such as a manifestation of depression. *B.* Mental problems are caused by physical problems. Physical pain leads to mental problems such as depression. *C.* A two-way street exists, with mental problems affecting physical conditions and physical problems affecting the mental condition. All three views do not fully capture the human experience. These two aspects (mind and body) of personhood cannot be effectively separated or treated in isolation.

some of the experiences associated with pain interact to influence the final product and the only part that can be directly observed, the patient's behavior. The patient's behavior is what the patient says or does. This conceptualization does not try to separate the physical experience from the emotional experience of pain. They occur together and are inseparably linked by the definition of what pain is. Theories that try to separate and then approach only one portion of the problem are likely to fail, since the complete experience is neither understood nor fully managed. A great deal of the frustration experienced by many clinicians in the care of the chronic pain sufferer can result from such faulty conceptualizations, illustrated in Figure 58-2, and the incomplete approaches they engender.

When the usual time for a tissue to heal has past, yet pain persists, often clinicians are aware that additional factors, psychological or social factors, are contributing. A referral to a psychologist or psychiatrist at that point forms an attempt to treat these factors. If the referral is made without concurrent coordinated physical interventions, then the psychologist or psychiatrist will also fail, as they may only address one portion or aspect of the problem. To be successful in the rehabilitation of the chronic pain patient, physiatrists must recognize all the issues interplaying with the pain experience so that all issues affecting disability and rehabilitation can be addressed in a coordinated and comprehensive manner. Physical medicine training often ideally prepares clinicians to effectively treat the more common causes for chronic pain, which are musculoskeletal syndromes. Psychological skills must be equally honed to help one both to interact with these challenging patients in a therapeutic manner, and to appreciate more fully the approaches necessary to help these patients become extricated from their suffering experiences. Coordination of their rehabilitation requires expertise in both arenas.

Chronic Pain Syndrome Evaluation Flowsheet

Figure 58-1 helps one to recognize how the pain experience can psychologically evolve. Any aspect of life that contributes to suffering, such as loss of employment or avocational activities, will influence the perception of suffering caused by the pain. Overattentiveness to the nociception will enhance pain perception and thereby also increase suffering. *Suffering*, defined here as an experience that is perceived to decrease the quality of one's life, is a key factor in determining what patients will be difficult to manage. Figure 58-3 illustrates the sequence of steps encountered by the pain patient that can lead to the untoward effects called the *chronic pain syndrome*, and itemizes how the less complicated chronic pain patient avoids this pitfall (3,34,35).

All patients bring a preexisting set of cultural, psychological, and adaptation skills, strengths, and weaknesses to the pain experience. No one "naturally" knows how to best manage a pain problem, but reacts according to what seems to help. Each step in Figure 58-3 is affected by these factors, and the response at any step interacts with the others. The first step is to experience nociception. A purely conversion disorder without any physical basis can occur but is a rare cause (only a few percent) (36) for chronic

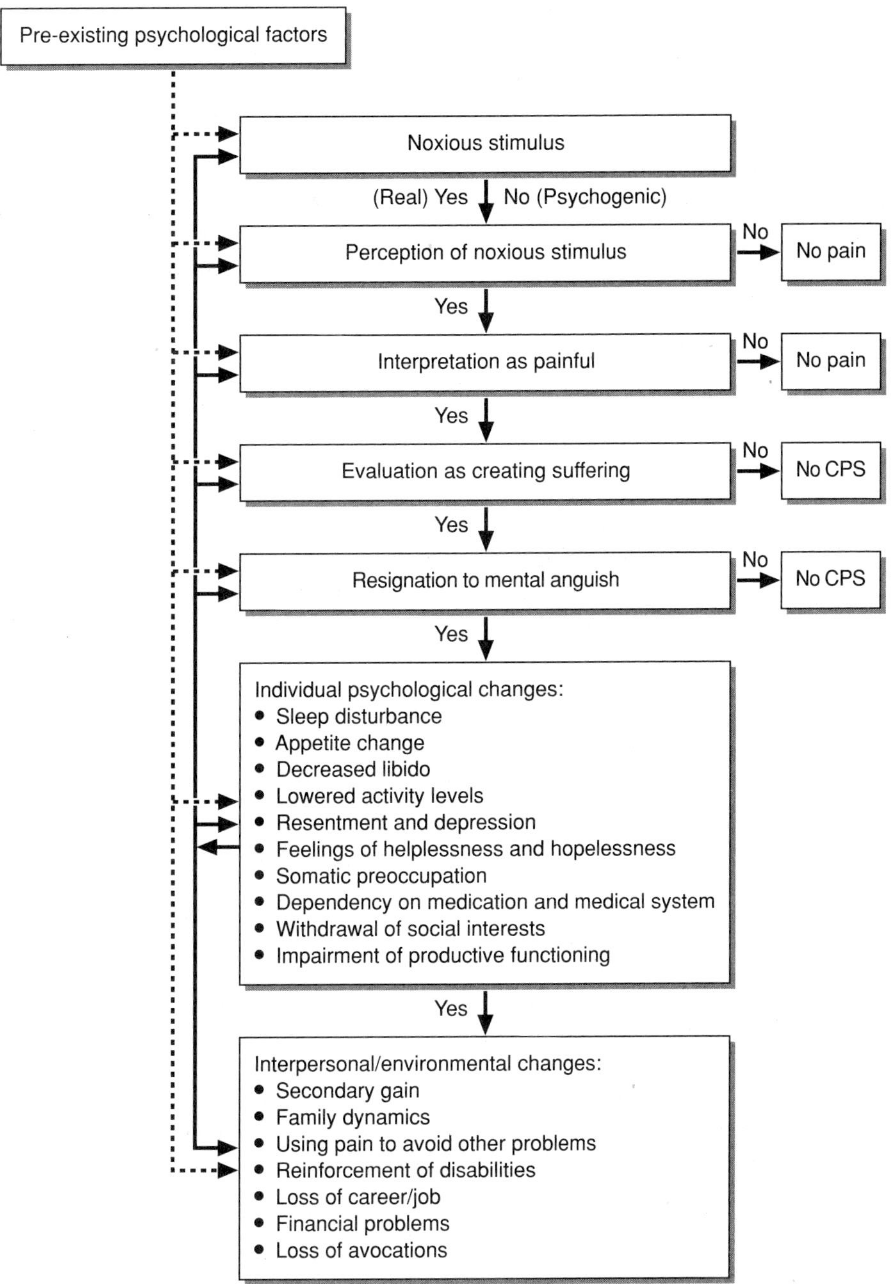

Figure 58-3. Evolution of the chronic pain syndrome (CPS). (Redrawn by permission from King JC, Kelleher WJ. The chronic pain syndrome: the inpatient interdisciplinary rehabilitative behavioral modification approach. In: Walsh NE, ed. *Rehabilitation of chronic pain: physical medicine and rehabilitation state of the art reviews.* Philadelphia: Hanley & Belfus, 1991:167.)

pain. Most patients with pain have had an identifiable precipitating traumatic physical event. Sometimes when a cure is not readily achieved and there are clearly psychological factors at work, one can be tempted to shift to the paradigm in Figure 58-2 of the problem being all psychological. However, before such a judgment can be justified, more than simply normal physical findings and normal results on laboratory or imaging studies must exist. The findings on a physical examination may be normal because it was inadequately or incompletely performed. I rarely perform all possible examinations, and the depth of the examination usually does not exceed the differential diagnosis. So if I have not thought of all the possibilities, I may well fail to appropriately examine for the actual cause of the pain. Laboratory studies cannot as yet demonstrate, in a cost-effective manner, such common problems as muscle strains, tendonitis, or chronic bursitis. Many of the etiologies listed in Table 58-1 may go undiagnosed by routine laboratory and imaging studies. In addition to a thorough physical examination showing normal findings, and normal laboratory results, the patient should show a nonphysiologic pain pattern before the clinician suspects purely psychogenic causes. An example of a nonphysiologic pain pattern is a patient who cannot ride elevators because the acceleration and deceleration induce severe sacral pain, yet tolerates jumping into the air and landing heels first. This pattern is not consistent with physics or physiology. So this rare patient is considered to have purely psychogenic pain, or a type of conversion disorder.

The next step in Figure 58-3, after having some form of nociception, is to perceive that nociception. This also is not a universal process. Most of us have had the experience of removing our clothing at night and discovering a bruise that we had not perceived previously. Tissue damage occurred and we can be reasonably certain nociception occurred, but it was not perceived. Athletes also know that they perceive their injuries much more intensely after the competition than during it, even though the time since their onset is longer. Just as having nociception does not guarantee perception, perceiving nociception does not necessarily indicate ongoing tissue damage. Many have experienced pain upon striking their ulnar nerve at the elbow. This "funny bone" experience is often described as painful, yet it is not evidence of ongoing tissue damage. It occurs from midaxonal excitation of the ulnar nerve, and this nerve volley has lingering effects for several seconds. Peripheral nerves are not normally very excitable in their midaxonal regions but can become so after trauma, such as striking of the very superficially exposed ulnar nerve at the elbow when it is prone. This is one reason why fusion surgeries are sometimes considered for low-back pain. It is believed that normal movements are provoking pain in abnormal tissues even though they are not causing additional damage. There is no necessary link between the perception of pain and ongoing tissue injury. Indeed, one of the most important roles physiatrists have in their comprehensive assessment of the chronic pain patient is to determine whether the patient's ongoing pain signals have physiologic value. Does the pain indicate a static process or ongoing progressive destruction, such as occurs in the minority of chronic pain patients, for example, those who have a progressive malignancy?

The next process in Figure 58-3 is to evaluate that perception as pain. If a patient describes a sensation in terms other than pain, it is not pain. A pressure sensation, itch, or irritation is not pain unless the patient states it is painful. Similar nociceptive events, such as childbirth, have wide ranges of perceived pain and its expression.

The next consideration is the most crucial for determining who will progress into the multitude of complications commonly seen in chronic pain patients. Does the patient evaluate the experience of pain as creating suffering or a decrement in his or her quality of life? Most patients do not consider pain as adding to the quality of life, though it is biologically beneficial for protection. The negative emotional experience is evaluated by most patients as lessening the quality of their lives. This seemingly reasonable step leads to incredible psychosocial problems. Patients can have nociception that they perceive as pain for longer than 6 months and have few or none of the problems listed at the bottom of Figure 58-3. However, these patients, such as burned-out rheumatoid arthritis patients, do not evaluate their pain in terms of decreasing the quality of their life. They make statements such as, "I don't let it get the best of me," "I haven't stopped yet," or "I don't let it get in my way" (37). Such patients meet the technical definition of chronic pain, yet rarely report to physicians, and have so few of the common problems associated with patients whose lives are devastated by chronic "benign" pain. Because of these differences, a term—*chronic pain syndrome*—was chosen to describe the associated set of factors that commonly complicate the management of the latter chronic pain sufferer (3,34,35). This syndrome is *not* a primary diagnosis; it represents a set of complications that arise directly from the ongoing experience of nociception from a primary etiology. Patients who do not evaluate their pain as creating suffering are unlikely to progress to the complications of the chronic pain syndrome listed in the boxes at the bottom of Figure 58-3, though they do technically have chronic pain. In these patients, more typical medical management approaches are usually sufficient, including for a small subset perhaps even chronic opioid dosing (38). These chronic pain patients do not require the extensive resources needed to successfully manage the behavioral and emotional disturbances of the devastated, chronic pain syndrome patient.

Subsequently in the psychological evolution of the chronic pain syndrome, illustrated in Figure 58-3, patients can develop a woeful resignation to suffering. This can be one of the more aggravating features of such patients. It is a learned helplessness response from the passive role typically required of patients in acute medical care, as well as a response developing from the many ineffective measures already tried by the time the pain process has become chronic. It is a psychologically self-defeating cognitive approach that sends the negative self-message, "Woe is me, no one can do anything to help me." Leriche (39), describing this reaction to the chronic pain experience, stated, "In a very short time it will convert the brightest spirit into a being haunted, driven upon himself, thinking only of his disease, selfishly indifferent to everything and everybody, and constantly obsessed by the dread of recurrent spasms of pain." These patients present as passive inactive victims who assume no responsibility for their behaviors. Their approach is often, "Doctor, what are you going to do for me?" and suggestions for purposeful or responsible activity on their part are met with resistance.

The Physician's Approach to the Chronic Pain Syndrome Patient

The physician's approach at this point is critical. With chronic pain syndrome being a learned response over many months, it cannot be reversed by simply insisting that the patient "shape up" and perform. This helpless-hopeless attitude can also be terribly reinforced by taking a posture of pitying the patient and allowing for incapacity that is not structurally necessary. It is natural to become empathetic with the suffering of the patient, and from that subjective experience one may be tempted to make harmful underestimates of the patient's physical abilities to perform. This often results in the patient becoming handicapped iatrogenically by an arbitrary pessimistic prognostication, defeating rehabilitation before it ever begins. A more helpful approach is to respect the patient, treat the patient as a competent adult, and express the expectation of the high levels of functional return possible with physical rehabilitation.

The attitude of being a victim, continually suffering from pain, leads to many individual psychological changes, which can be better understood from this context. Depression leads to sleep disturbance (if not already present owing to the pain disorder), appetite changes and weight changes, decreased sexual interest and function (to which the primary pain problem may also be contributing), withdrawal of social interests, and withdrawal from avocational activities (to which the pain disorder may also be contributing). Lowered activity levels are common and may be iatrogenic. The concept of kinisophobia, or the fear of moving, is a common problem, even for patients who do not report increased pain with activities (40).

Resentment and anger can result from the many medical failures these patients have endured. Often a patient appears angry with the examiner upon first introduction, possibly because that clinician represents the medical field that thus far has failed the patient's expectations. One must be careful to recognize and to not react to this anger, so that it does not interfere with developing the necessary therapeutic relationship of trust.

Somatic preoccupation is both common and countertherapeutic. Many patients, and unfortunately health care providers as well, conceptualize themselves mechanically, for example, as an automobile. They assume if there is a problem, it can be fixed, and if the fix does not work, then one must have had a bad mechanic. Because of this, many patients hope that if they can just give their physicians enough details, the physicians will be able to solve the problem. Others pay close attention because their pain is alarming to them and they are anxious about what might occur next. Unfortunately, concentrating on a painful area of the body tends to increase the perception of signals from that area and actually intensifies the pain experience. Despite noble intentions, such concentration on the body, or somatic preoccupation, is countertherapeutic.

Dependency on medication and the medical system is another common characteristic of the chronic pain syndrome patient that must be diminished if rehabilitation toward optimal function and independence is a goal. One beneficial outcome commonly measured in chronic pain programs is the number of health care provider visits in the subsequent year compared to the previous year. The number of visits is often effectively reduced 20% or more from the number of pretreatment visits for the same period of time. Muscle relaxants and narcotics when used chronically create physical dependence. Narcotics especially tie patients to the medical system by usually requiring monthly refills, which often requires physician's visit as well. Some physicians will repetitively use noncurative procedures to ameliorate the pain, thus also maintaining dependency of the patient on the medical care system.

Impairment of productive functioning is the most expensive aspect of chronic pain problems, and the aspect physiatrists are most adept at considering and rehabilitating. From a purely acute medical model, productive functioning is irrelevant and even relatively contraindicated if it is believed to contribute to the ongoing pain. This is one reason why many chronic pain patients are iatrogenically made inactive, which after deconditioning, results in iatrogenic impairment independent of the impairments caused by the presenting problem (41–43).

These problems add to and are affected by interpersonal and social problems. Pain can be used for secondary gain. The fact that an employee remains off work because the disability pay after taxes is greater than the working pay after taxes does not mean that the employee has no pain. It just means that pain, and especially pain behavior such as not working, are reinforced by factors that tend to help more if the employee remains unemployed. Likewise, pain behaviors can be reinforced by family dynamics. In America, single-parent homes are becoming more common. A disabling pain problem is more likely to persist if it allows the parent to devote more desired time to child rearing, but would not persist if the parent would rather be away from the children. A pain behavior such as rubbing one's hip will become more common if it results in benefit. For example, if a patient's spouse were to offer to take out the garbage after seeing the patient rub the hip, and the patient does not really like to take out the garbage, the likelihood of that behavior (rubbing the hip) just increased, whether done consciously or not. Remember, pain is common in the workplace among active workers. What I am talking about here are pain behaviors or responses to that pain experience, not intrinsic capabilities.

Most often, loss of a career or job leads to depression and to financial problems, not gains (44). These patients do not just quit productive functioning but also quit fun activities, leaving more time for the individual psychological changes of Figure 58-3 such as depression and somatic preoccupation to develop. These losses then add to the perception of pain and its associated suffering, creating the miserable individual identified as the chronic pain syndrome patient. A physician's approach must recognize this complication and broaden his/her intervention to also address this common set of disability maladaptations that add to the patient's pain problem.

TREATMENT

Treatment most often was initiated in the acute phase. Ideally, if the pain problem persists into a subacute phase [approximately 1-month duration (45)], a more comprehensive assessment occurs, with factors affecting recovery of function addressed and acute intervention adjusted, recognizing the risk of emerging chronic pain and its possible complication of chronic pain syndrome. Modalities and other short-term interventions such as administration of narcotic and muscle relaxant medications are gradually replaced by more active physical interventions and use of potentially long-term effective medications such as tricyclic antidepressants, anticonvulsants, and nonsteroidal anti-inflammatory drugs (NSAIDs). Unfortunately many patients continue to be managed as though their problem has only persisted a few days, and chronic pain patients may become physically deconditioned, dependent on narcotics and tranquilizers, and no closer to a resolution or return to work than during their first days off from work.

Physical inactivity is only helpful during the acute inflammatory phase of an injury, and activities should be rapidly resumed unless an obvious risk of structural damage is present (i.e., recent fracture or severe ligamentous injury). Bed rest used to treat low-back pain, for example, was shown to be just as beneficial when restricted to 3 days as for longer periods (46). When prolonged restrictions to activities are imposed, muscle and eventually connective tissue strength diminishes, eventually to the point of disabling patients from their former duties (42,43). Thus, despite an ongoing pain problem that otherwise does not prevent work, work abilities can become impaired simply by allowing passive deconditioning to occur.

One must distinguish between patients already developing chronic pain syndrome and those with chronic pain who do not manifest such life disruptions. The latter should continue to be treated according to the medical model, recognizing the importance of adding physical rehabilitation measures to their regimens. The former require additional interventions from care providers by an interdisciplinary team coordinating care to reverse the maladaptive learned behaviors while proceeding with physical rehabilitation. Both groups warrant additional, initial medical investigation to ensure that all reasonable curative procedures or interventions have been exhausted and that there are no dangerous underlying medical conditions that intrinsically limit the amount or type of physical restoration pursued. Despite frequent, dubious physician-imposed restrictions, such intrinsic physical limitations do not commonly exist (47).

Medications

Narcotics are typically underutilized in the acute pain situation (48). Though widely discrepant findings exist, it is generally believed that less than 0.1% of patients treated with narcotics for acute pain become addicted (38,49,50). In patients with chronic pain, tolerance limits the effectiveness of opioids. Even data on chronic opioid use for nonmalignant pain demonstrate the need for escalating doses over time [approximately 5-mg increase of an intramuscular morphine equivalent/day/year in a closely monitored group (51)]. The most compelling demonstration is the multitude of patients tapered off such medications, as is common in a multidisciplinary rehabilitation approach, whose pain is no more than it was when they were on high chronic doses of opioids (37,47). Such patients also report subjective benefits of "feeling more alive," which may have to do with the emotional and motivational blunting effects of narcotics (37). Narcotic tolerance does not develop as rapidly in animal models, when each dosing is preceded by tissue injury (50,52). This underrecognized fact may account for the more effective narcotic use observed in cancer patients, as compared to those with chronic pain due to benign diseases. When narcotics are used chronically in patients with benign disease, improvements in function or return to work do not occur consistently, despite self-reporting subjective benefit (50,51). Narcotic pain medications appear to have only a very limited place in the rehabilitation of the patient with chronic pain due to benign disease, perhaps best reserved to transiently treat a new or emerging pain problem that is different from the original chronic pain complaint. Some advocate using opioids as any other chronic pain medication, with limited trials to see if sustained benefits can be obtained. Recognizing the known hazards of dependence and possible addiction, strict guidelines (Table 58-2) are offered and preclude use in most patients with chronic pain syndrome (item 2 in Table 58-2, which was expanded by the author to include "a chaotic home environment"). The very fact that chronic opioid dosing requires dependence on medical prescribers leads opioids to be a lower-priority choice in the spectrum of medications used to rehabilitate a dependent chronic pain patient.

All muscle relaxants are centrally acting tranquilizers (53). The approach to certain intermittent pain problems, such as incapacitating migraine headaches, has frequently been to sedate the patients so they sleep through the experience. Physiologic pain is not experienced during sleep. However, this is not a reasonable long-term solution to chronic nonremitting pain. Many muscle relaxants are from the benzodiazepine family and have been shown to increase hostility and depression after 8 weeks of routine use (53). These effects clearly are not desirable in the chronic pain syndrome patient. None of the muscle relaxants have proved to be effective in chronically decreasing muscle tone (53–56). Thus, little rationale exists for their use, except to blunt life's experiences,

Table 58-2: Proposed Guidelines in the Management of Opioid Maintenance Therapy for Nonmalignant Pain

1. Should be considered only after all other reasonable attempts at analgesia have failed.
2. A history of substance abuse, severe character pathology, and chaotic home environment should be viewed as relative contraindications.
3. A single practitioner should take primary responsibility for treatment.
4. Patients should give informed consent before the start of therapy; points to be covered include recognition of the low risk of true addiction as an outcome, potential for cognitive impairment from the drug alone or from coadministration of sedative/hypnotics, likelihood that physical dependence will occur (abstinence possible with acute discontinuation), and understanding by female patients that children born when the mother is receiving opioid drugs will likely be physically dependent at birth.
5. After drug selection, doses should be given on an around-the-clock basis; several weeks should be agreed upon as the period of initial dose titration, and although improvement in function should be continually stressed, all should agree to at least partial analgesia as the appropriate goal of therapy.
6. Failure to achieve at least partial analgesia at relatively low initial doses in the nontolerant patient raises questions about the potential treatability of the pain syndrome with opioids.
7. Emphasis should be given to attempts to capitalize on improved analgesia by gains in physical and social function; opioid therapy should be considered complementary to other analgesic and rehabilitative approaches.
8. In addition to the daily dose determined initially, patients should be permitted to escalate dose transiently on days of increased pain; two methods are aceptable: a) prescription of an additional 4–6 "rescue doses" to be taken as needed during the month; b) instruction that one or two extra doses may be taken on any day, but must be followed by an equal reduction of dose on subsequent days.
9. Initially, patients must be seen and drugs prescribed at least monthly. When stable, less frequent visits may be acceptable.
10. Exacerbations of pain not effectively treated by transient, small increases in dose are best managed in the hospital, where dose escalation, if appropriate, can be observed closely and return to baseline doses can be accomplished in a controlled environment.
11. Evidence of drug hoarding, acquisition of drugs from other physicians, uncontrolled dose escalation, or other aberrant behaviors must be carefully assessed. In some cases, tapering and discontinuation of opioid therapy will be necessary. Other patients may appropriately continue therapy within rigid guidelines. Consideration should be given to consultation with an addiction medicine specialist.
12. At each visit, assessment should specifically address:
    a. Comfort (degree of analgesia).
    b. Opioid-related side effects.
    c. Functional status (physical and psychosocial).
    d. Existence of aberrant drug-related behaviors.
13. Use of self-report instruments may be helpful but should not be required.
14. Documentation is essential and the medical record should specifically address comfort, function, side effects, and the occurrence of aberrant behaviors repeatedly during the course of therapy.

Source: Reproduced by permission from Fields HL, Liebeskind JC, eds. *Pharmacological approaches to the treatment of chronic pain. Pain research and management.* Vol. 1. Seattle: IASP Press, 1994.

and significant contraindications exist for chronic dosing (35,56).

Long-term effective medications include neuropathic pain agents, such as tricyclic antidepressants; anticonvulsants; and other medications not associated with tolerance and dependency such as NSAIDs and acetaminophen. One must recall that NSAIDs possess both analgesic and anti-inflammatory properties. Typically their analgesic effect is obtained at lower doses than what is required for anti-inflammation, and NSAIDs have a ceiling effect for analgesia. This means that higher doses do not necessarily result in greater analgesia, but can result in greater side effects. Since it is often unclear whether inflammation is a component of a chronic pain problem, an empiric trial at an anti-inflammatory dose seems reasonable, but should be tested by periodic withdrawal. If pain increases the first day off the NSAID but then becomes relatively stable over the next 10 days, it is likely that only analgesic effects are occurring. In this scenario, consideration should be given to using the lowest dose of the NSAID that continues to provide analgesia, or changing to acetaminophen, to minimize the risks of side effect. On the other hand, a progressive crescendo pattern of pain beginning about 3 days after discontinuation and accelerating over the next 2 weeks suggests an inflammatory response that was being controlled adequately by the NSAID, and the higher dose should be continued. If no change in perceived pain occurs, the NSAID can be discontinued as it is ineffective. Though anticonvulsants and tricyclic antidepressants require 1- to 2-month trials before efficacy can be determined, the efficacy of NSAIDs can usually be determined within 1 to 2 weeks (57).

Often few or no medications seem to benefit the patient, or the side effects preclude the use of many of them. Frequently, medications are not necessary to optimally manage a chronic pain patient and one should not feel compelled to use them if not found to be effective. This point will not be reached quickly in the therapeutic process, but a conscious effort should be made to eliminate necessary medications. Physiatrists more than others should feel comfortable in managing disease processes without medications. However, only one physician should manage all medications for the chronic pain patient and an agreement as to who this individual will be must be established early among all treating physicians.

REHABILITATION

The first step in the rehabilitation of a pain patient is the identification and listing of the patient's problems. Medical, psychosocial, and disability issues should be considered, recognizing that treatments can be specifically targeted to each. A set of time-limited, specific, measurable, desired goals should be established with the patient. The comprehensive treatment plan should include goal-directed interventions to address each problem. The development of this list of problems requires a comprehensive evaluation, possibly by professionals from a multitude of disciplines.

A simple office visit that approaches a chronic pain problem as an acute pain problem will only contribute to the long list of ineffectual interventions tried, and further contribute to the hopelessness and helplessness engendered by such an approach to the chronic pain syndrome patient. Table 58-3 points out some of the significant differences between acute and chronic pain management (58). Because by definition chronic pain has existed so long, and has typically defied diagnosis and cure by multiple providers, it cannot be managed as efficiently as simple acute pain. One of the greatest challenges the physiatrist has is establishing a trusting relationship that will allow the patient to physically participate in therapeutic exercises safely, despite ongoing chronic pain. This level of trust cannot be established during a quick interview and cursory physical examination. Additional time must be allotted to perform a complete and comprehensive assessment. This additional time helps the clinician to understand the pain problem as well as it can be understood, and to establish baselines from which to monitor the patient's progress, as well as to judge safety for participation in physical rehabilitation.

Table 58-3: Acute Versus Chronic Pain

Acute	Chronic
Physicians trained in evaluation and diagnosis	Physicians typically less interested and less trained
Short evaluation and treatment course	Long evaluation and treatment course
Pain a biologic symptom	Pain a disease
Pain plus anxiety	Pain plus depression
Medications as needed	Nonnarcotic analgesics, antidepressants preferred
Little addiction concern	Polyaddiction concern
Diagnosis straightforward	Diagnosis complex
Cure likely	Cure usually not achieved

Source: Reproduced by permission from Grabois M. Chronic pain: evaluation and treatment. In: Goodgold J, ed. *Rehabilitation medicine*. St. Louis: Mosby-Year Book, 1988:663–674.

Pain Centers

A multitude of different types of pain centers have proliferated over the last two decades. There are four primary classifications (59): major comprehensive pain center, comprehensive pain center, syndrome-oriented pain center, and modality-oriented pain center (45). The first two types are interdisciplinary as are many of the syndrome-oriented (headache center, low-back center, etc) programs. The organization of such pain centers has been addressed (60,61). The degree of rehabilitation emphasis, however, is quite variable, and such emphasis may not be present in even the largest of centers. In 1985, physiatrists in the United States directed 35 of 217 such programs identified. Anesthesiologists were the most common, directing 96 programs (62).

Anesthesiology pain experts are frequently adept at pain-alleviating procedures and medication approaches. Many such experts direct comprehensive interdisciplinary programs that address a multitude of the psychosocial as well as the physical problems of chronic pain syndrome (63). The field of pain management is a shared discipline, with pain center directors commonly representing at least one of seven specialties and with professionals of almost all medical disciplines called on as consultants (62). Comprehensive texts describe in detail the pathophysiology, treatment rationale, treatment approaches, and outcome statistics for the many different pain syndromes listed in Table 58-1 (63–68). The unique contribution brought to chronic pain management by the physiatrist is the expertise to focus musculoskeletal and psychosocial knowledge to the comprehensive rehabilitation of these complex and very involved patients.

Interdisciplinary Pain Rehabilitation Team

Rehabilitation of the chronic pain syndrome patient often requires an interdisciplinary team. Typically, physical therapists, occupational therapists, recreational therapists, specially trained behaviorally oriented nurses, and psychologists with behavioral orientation, plus the patient and a rehabilitation-oriented physician with expertise in the interaction of physical exercise and pathology are required. The input based on assessments by these professionals is combined to coordinate a comprehensive approach that addresses all the needs of the patient and will allow the patient to reintegrate fully and actively into life with as few restrictions as possible.

Physical therapy provides baseline measures of capabilities and ongoing monitoring during progressive reconditioning exercise, eventually translating into "work hardening," which is more job-specific therapy. A safe rate of progression is determined physiologically. Patients start well within their initial capabilities, at perhaps half their baseline ability. They are given specific daily quotas to meet during each exercise session. Patients are required to perform their quota, regardless of the chronic pain level, and to do no more and no less. New problems are reported and evaluated, but not the initially comprehensively evaluated chronic pain.

Occupational therapy helps reinforce proper body posture and positioning during various activities of daily living, and assists with ergonomic assessments and job modifications. Pacing skills are reinforced. Many chronic pain patients are hard-driving, intense individuals who develop a pattern of excessive bed rest and inactivity interspersed with outbursts of activity beyond their conditioning. An example is the patient who after several days in bed decides to clean out the entire garage since he is feeling better. This overuse results in pain exacerbation and another prolonged period of inactivity, which over time leads to progressive deconditioning and re-exacerbations. This pattern is difficult to break. Occupational therapy can provide one medium for monitoring and modifying this countertherapeutic behavior.

Recreational therapy is essential for reversing the maladaptive loss of avocational skills and providing outlets that help maintain physical conditioning. Compliance can be enhanced by incorporating increased activity into pleasurable pursuits instead of simply prescribing a rote set of home exercises. Avocational activities are also distracting and thus therapeutic for minimizing the pain experience. Community re-entry skills can also be pursued with professional supervision by therapeutic recreation specialists.

Inpatient Chronic Pain Rehabilitation

Should inpatient treatment be necessary, then specially trained behaviorally oriented nursing staff is required. The routine approach of inquiring about comfort and pain, which is quite appropriate for the acute pain patient, only focuses the chronic pain patient on the pain, which will intensify the pain experience and is thus countertherapeutic. Instead, praise must be given for increased activity, socialization, and self-care. Inpatient care is required when insufficient motivation or excessive anxiety would preclude successful narcotic tapering and termination as an outpatient. If the home environment provides so many reinforcers for illness behavior that success on an outpatient basis is unlikely, then inpatient admission should be considered.

If inpatient management is needed for behavior modification, then all appropriate acute medical interventions and evaluations, including diagnostic studies, should be completed prior to considering such an admission. It may be appropriate to admit a patient for certain diagnostic and therapeutic procedures and even physical rehabilitation measures during that admission, but behavior modification is severely compromised during such an admission and likely should not be attempted in that setting. The pursuit of diagnostic studies or procedures, which are more easily approved by third-party payers when they are performed during inpatient admissions, continues to place the patient in a passive dependent position, hoping for the elusive cure. This focus is not compatible with the desired shift in emphasis toward optimal self-management. It would be inappropriate for nursing staff and others to not inquire regarding the patient's levels of pain if the patient has just undergone a procedure, thus impairing an ideal behavioral approach. Once an admission is required for the purpose of refocusing the patient's behavior toward a more active, healthy, and productive approach, then all factors need to be in place to reward increased activity and diminish the patient's responses toward the physiologically unhelpful pain. Using such pain-relieving medical procedures to reward performance again results in confusion of the focus from independent self-management, a goal of rehabilitation, to dependence on the medical care provider, though improvements in performance have been obtained by this behavioral approach (68). Some authors have described behavioral approaches as "learning to live with the pain," but it involves far more. It involves being safely rehabilitated back to capable levels, which usually results in less pain, not more, by the end of the programs, despite increased activity levels and increased ability to safely lift weights (39,47,69–82).

The family and significant others must be trained during this inpatient time in methods to reinforce healthy behaviors and maintain gains in the home environment. They must be taught why and how to avoid reinforcing illness behaviors, which is often done inadvertently with the best of intentions. Training of family and significant others is essential to maintain the strength, endurance, and flexibility gains made in therapy. The patient became deconditioned and incapacitated in the environment from which he or she came. If no training occurs, the same reinforcers will be there, and regression can be anticipated.

Psychological Interventions

The psychologist's role is to help identify the factors that may be reinforcing or complicating the pain experience. Despite many useful tools such as the Minnesota Multiphasic Personality Inventory (MMPI) (83,84), the less often used MMPI-2 (85), Symptom Checklist-90 (SCL-90) (86,87) or revised SCL-90-R (88), Million Behavioral Health Inventory (89), Oswestry Scale (90), Beck Depression Inventory (91), Illness Behavior Questionnaire (92), Schedule of Recent Experiences (93), and Medical Outcome Study (94), and measures of the pain experience such as the McGill Pain Questionnaire (95), Million Visual Analog Scale (96), Quantified Pain Drawing (97), and Pain

Diaries (32), the most important psychological assessment is the structured behaviorally oriented interview (39,45), such as the Illness Behavior Assessment Schedule (98). A search for purely psychogenic conversion factors may help in excluding certain patients from unnecessary surgical and medical interventions, but is seldom helpful in planning comprehensive effective treatment. "Faking" the profile of a disabling painful condition by naive subjects was not found to be possible on the SCL-90-R (99). The MMPI has validity scales to check for internal consistencies. Typical responses of chronic pain patients tend to differ from those attempting malingering, and such instruments may be helpful in identifying the patients with unusual motivations. The structured behavioral interview helps to identify more specifically the contributing psychological factors so that plans can be made to modify these factors. The MMPI is ubiquitous in chronic pain centers, and offers some helpful information. However, contrary to helping predict success in surgical interventions (75,100), the MMPI has not been of any predictive value in determining successful outcomes for behaviorally oriented, physical rehabilitation participants (101–103). Elevated MMPI scores do return to more normal levels after a physical reconditioning, behavioral, and work rehabilitation program, suggesting that such changes may be the result of and not the cause of the patient's pain problem (42).

The psychologist must help coordinate the team's interventions, which are done in concert to avoid sending mixed messages to the patient. A patient "contract," a written document signed by the patient, significant others, and all team members, can also help in establishing the basic ground rules for what is expected from each participant (39). These patients will sometimes try to split the team and play one member off another. To avoid this, frequent staff meetings, sometimes several per week, must be held to analyze and unify by consensus the approaches taken.

Individual and group therapy with the psychologist is often necessary to deal with stress management, relaxation training, and the typical catastrophic self-talk common to these patients (104). Such thoughts as "My head is going to explode" are clearly alarming and will worsen a tension headache. Patients can be taught to monitor themselves for such irrational talk (i.e., they do not really believe their head is going to explode) and to provide more reassuring and rationale messages such as "I've had headaches like this before. It will pass." This form of therapy is called *rationale emotive therapy*, which with cognitive behavioral therapy can be significantly helpful in decreasing the suffering of the chronic pain syndrome patient (37,105).

The physician must be aware that every activity has an underlying meaning to the patient. Thus any tests or alterations in therapy should be discussed and coordinated with the team, once a comprehensive interdisciplinary team approach has been initiated. The reason to work with such a team is that one provider cannot possibly tackle all the psychosocial, cognitive, and rehabilitation issues presented by the complicated chronic pain syndrome patient. The psychologist also provides behavioral guidance, which is not intuitive to most health care providers. Examples of helpful behavioral approaches for physicians to use with chronic pain patients are listed in Table 58-4 (104).

Table 58-4: Ten Steps to Help Chronic Pain Patients

1. Accept patients' pain as real. Find out *why* they hurt, not whether they hurt.
2. Protect patients from unnecessary invasive procedures.
3. Set realistic goals. Expect to manage rather than cure.
4. Evaluate chronic pain in terms of what patients do, not what they say.
5. Let patients know that *you* are the expert on medications and procedures.
6. Shift patients to oral, time-contingent medications (not prn).
7. Prescribe exercises to start at easily achieved levels, but increase at a preset rate.
8. Educate patients' families to encourage increased activity.
9. Focus your attention on patient activity rather than on pain.
10. Help patients get involved in pleasurable activities. Remember, people who have something better to do don't hurt as much.

Source: Reproduced by permission from Fordyce WE, Fowler RS, Lehmann JF, DeLateur BJ. Ten steps to help patients with chronic pain. *Patient Care* 1978;12:263.

The Physiatrist's Role

The physician's primary role is to verify that no ongoing destructive disease process is occurring and to monitor the patient for ongoing safe participation in physical rehabilitation, while optimizing medical management, by modifying and minimizing drug therapy and protecting the patient from unnecessary and potentially harmful invasive procedures. The initial assessment should be comprehensive enough to determine whether any invasive procedures or surgical interventions could reasonably, not just potentially, benefit the patient. Any interventions that could reasonably benefit the patient should be pursued prior to initiating comprehensive rehabilitation. Simple physical rehabilitation may not have even been tried and likewise should be exhausted prior to considering comprehensive rehabilitation. However, the more components of the chronic pain syndrome the patient exhibits, the less likely simple outpatient therapy will be of benefit, and this too may become an unreasonable pursuit in the absence of a comprehensive approach.

If no ongoing progressive destruction is occurring, then the chronic pain is not providing helpful information.

The chronic pain experience must be discerned from any new-onset pains or changes in the previous chronic pain. Patients must be instructed that the physician is responsible for their safety and they must report any new changes to the physician and not to other team members. It is not therapeutic for patients to spend their hours in therapy discussing their same old pain and how it is affecting their exercise. If any new changes occur or patients are concerned about the safety of proceeding, they must discuss this with their monitoring physician. The physiatrist is the expert on pathology and its interactions with exercise. Any concerns by the therapists likewise should be discussed with the physician, ideally during each team staff meeting, unless urgency requires earlier consultation. These concerns should not be discussed in isolation with the patient, except to offer referral back to the treating physician, to help avoid further team-splitting strategies.

Very seldom do intrinsic lesions preclude eventual rehabilitation (47). Most of the impairments of chronic pain patients are due to disuse and not neurologic or intrinsic structural loss. Especially for patients who have had low-back fusions, postoperative restrictions are given not only acutely but indefinitely, despite there being little to no justification in the literature. Thus, the treatment itself "created" the impairment, which is consistent with the rating procedures of the American Medical Association's *Guides to the Evaluation of Permanent Impairment* (106). Such restrictions, in the absence of clinical evidence, should be evaluated on the basis of physiologic rationale, and not simply surgical opinion, which may rest on a vested interest in protecting placed hardware (68). The patient and his or her desires should take precedence. If the pain continues as incapacitating, functionally it cannot get worse, and only in the highly unlikely event of relevant structural failure occurring many months postoperatively does the patient need to be considered for rehabilitation.

OUTCOMES

The character and intensity of pain do not determine who remains on the job or who returns to work (27,31). Many factors do predict return to work (31). These are listed in Table 58-5 (107–109). Some cannot be controlled, others can. It is important to consider all these factors when planning a patient's comprehensive rehabilitation. Clearly there are many social and intrapersonal issues that more effectively predict return to work than does the intrinsic pathology.

Initiating rehabilitation can often be facilitated by baseline measures of capabilities. These measures can be as simple as establishing capabilities for each of the initial exercises to be pursued, or as sophisticated as an initial functional capacity evaluation. The latter is more costly and can be misused to legally establish the patients' level of abilities. It can be helpful to target the deficits and to

Table 58-5: Twelve Factors That Enhance Return to Work for Chronic Pain Patients

Noncontrollable
1. Younger patient
2. Good work history

Partially controllable
3. Satisfying job
4. Better educated patient
5. No substance abuse or self-destructive behaviors
6. Time-limited, lesser, or no compensation benefits
7. No pending litigation

Controllable factors
8. Fewer psychotropic medications
9. Fewer surgeries
10. Shorter time off work before rehabilitation
11. A more "return to work" directive approach in therapy
12. Primary, secondary, and tertiary gain factors not continuing operative in perpetuating pain

Sources: References 107–109.

measure overall progress, and was used effectively in one outpatient 56-hour/week program with an almost 80% rate of return to work (110). Functional capacity evaluations are of great use to psychologically reassure both the employer and the patient, who may still have pain, that the patient can safely return to his or her former job once physical rehabilitation and work-hardening programs are complete.

The physical rehabilitation component often consists of an initial phase of general reconditioning and restoration of activities of daily living. Depending on the severity of involvement, narcotic dependence, and the home environment, this component may require inpatient admission. This phase is usually followed by more intense aerobic conditioning combined with more occupation-specific strengthening and endurance training. An improved level of conditioning is predictive of fewer future episodes of low-back pain, and is an effective intervention for diffuse myofascial pain syndromes and fibromyalgia (111). These somewhat generalized programs are followed by work-hardening programs where actual on-the-job skills are performed and work endurance is developed. Once the patient safely performs 8 hours/day, transition back to the workplace occurs. The job reintegration is often accompanied by an on-site ergonomic assessment, both to make suggestions to the employer and to verify that all aspects of the employee's job tasks have been addressed in rehabilitation. Return to work should be seen as part of the process of rehabilitation, not just an end point (31,112).

Outcome measures are essential to document success. Most comprehensive, behaviorally oriented, physical rehabilitative programs have objective success rates of approximately 50% to 70% for return to work and function (39,45,72,74,78,79,81,82,110,113–120). This range is similar to the percentages reported for subjective benefits after a second lumbar surgery, which has no guarantee that return to work will result. The costs are also similar (121,122). Recidivism rates are reasonably low, at around 10% of those who were initially successful after 1 to 2 years (39,45,47,72,74,78,79,81,82,113–119,123). Inpatient programs are more successful than outpatient programs and longer inpatient programs also correlate with better outcomes (37,124). Owing to the high initial costs, however, most managed care programs insist on additional outpatient care, even when this may be a repetition of care previously shown to be ineffective. This approach represents false economy, since the overall lifetime savings, considering the cost of drugs, future medical expenses, and disability payments, in 1981 was up to $200,000 for each successfully rehabilitated patient. For fewer than 14% of these chronic pain patients, treatment in comprehensive behavioral rehabilitation programs costs more than no intervention (113). Unfortunately many pain centers and pain experts do not have a rehabilitation focus, and continue passive interventions, seeking patients' subjective benefits only. These interventions are costly, but more importantly are ineffective in restoring abilities. In some measure, because of this, many third-party payers are quite skeptical of any pain program. Documenting objective success rates by establishing baseline measures of function and reporting return-to-work rates as one "gold standard" to document functional restoration can be essential in marketing the efficacy and cost-effectiveness of such a program to third-party payers.

CONCLUSIONS

Pain does not preclude active work. Neither the type nor the severity of pain predict who returns to work. Other factors have a major impact. Rehabilitation reverses many of these factors, and may allow a return to full function, including return to work. As in many areas of rehabilitation medicine, a cure of the underlying disorder is not required for rehabilitation to be successful (125). The costs of incapacitating pain are enormous. If universally employed, rehabilitation can significantly reduce these costs. Management of the full set of complications that can result from the human experience of chronic pain, called the chronic pain syndrome, will allow successful reintegration of affected patients into active life and society. The dramatic increase in quality of life possible for these individuals through comprehensive rehabilitation lessens their suffering and perceived levels of pain (39). Success in chronic pain management depends on a focus toward active rehabilitation and comprehensive management of the full set of complications that comprise the chronic pain syndrome.

REFERENCES

1. Wall PD, Melzack R. *Textbook of pain.* 2nd ed. New York: Churchill Livingstone, 1989:1–3.
2. International Association for the Study of Pain Subcommittee on Taxonomy. Classification of chronic pain: descriptions of chronic pain syndromes and definitions of pain terms. *Pain Suppl* 1986;3:S1–S225.
3. Bonica JJ. Definitions and taxonomy of pain. In: Bonica JJ, ed. *The management of pain.* Vol. 1. 2nd ed. Philadelphia: Lea & Febiger, 1990:18–27.
4. Bonica JJ. Evolution of multidisciplinary/interdisciplinary pain programs. In: Aronoff GM, ed. *Pain centers: a revolution in health care.* New York: Raven, 1988:9–32.
5. Scadding JW. Peripheral neuropathies. In: Wall PD, Melzack R., eds. *Textbook of pain.* 3rd ed. New York: Churchill Livingstone 1994:669.
6. Crook J. The prevalence of pain complaints in a general population. *Pain* 1984;18:299–314.
7. Wiener SL. *Differential diagnosis of acute pain by body region.* New York: McGraw-Hill, 1993.
8. Bonica JJ. General considerations of chronic pain. In: Bonica JJ, ed. *The management of pain.* Vol. 1. 2nd ed. Philadelphia: Lea & Febiger, 1990:180–196.
9. Walsh NE, Dumitru D, Ramamurthy S, Schoenfeld LS. Treatment of the patient with chronic pain. In: DeLisa JA, ed. *Rehabilitation medicine: principles and practice.* Philadelphia: JB Lippincott, 1993:973–995.
10. Kriegler JS, Ashenberg ZS. Management of chronic low back pain. A comprehensive approach. *Semin Neurol* 1987;7:303–312.
11. Tollison CD, Satterthwaite JR, Tollison JW. *Handbook of pain management.* Baltimore: Williams & Wilkins, 1994.
12. Wildes CS. National Center for Health Statistics. *Limitation of activity due to chronic conditions, United States, 1969–1970.* Rockville, MD: U.S. Department of Health, Education and Welfare Publication. Series 10, No. 80. 1973.
13. White AA, Gordon SL. Synopsis: workshop on idiopathic low-back pain. *Spine* 1982;7:141–149.
14. Currey HL, Greenwood RM, Lloyd GG, Murray RS. A prospective study of low back pain. *Rheumatol Rehabil* 1979;18:94–104.
15. Liang M, Komaroff AL. Roentgenograms in primary care

patients with acute low back pain: a cost-effective analysis. *Arch Intern Med* 1982;142:1108–1112.

16. Deyo RA, Diehl AK. Cancer as a cause of back pain: frequency and diagnostic strategies. *Clin Res* 1987;35:738A.

17. Deyo RA, Diehl AK. Patient satisfaction with medical care for low back pain. *Spine* 1986;11:28–30.

18. Brandt KD. Osteoarthritis. In: Isselbacher KJ, Braunwald E, Wilson JD, eds. *Harrison's principles of internal medicine.* 13th ed. New York: McGraw-Hill, 1992:1692–1701.

19. Hicks JE, Gerber LH. Rehabilitation of the patient with arthritis and connective tissue disease. In: DeLisa JA, ed. *Rehabilitation medicine: principles and practice.* 2nd ed. Philadelphia: JB Lippincott, 1993:1047–1081.

20. Snook SH. The costs of back pain in industry. In: Deyo RA, ed. *Back pain in workers: state of the art reviews in occupational medicine.* Philadelphia: Hanley & Belfus, 1988:1–6.

21. Gabriel JNA, Crowson CS, O'Fallon WM. Costs of osteoarthritis: estimates from a geographically defined population. *J Rhematol* 1995;22:23–25.

22. Swanson DW, Swenson WM, Floreen AC. Program for managing chronic pain. I. Program description and characteristics of patients. *Mayo Clin Proc* 1976;51:401–408.

23. Crook J, Weir R, Tunks E. An epidemiological follow-up survey of persistent pain sufferers in a group family practice and specialty pain clinic. *Pain* 1989;36:49–61.

24. Bigos SJ, Battie MC, Spengler DM, et al. A prospective study of work perceptions and psychosocial factors affecting the report of back injury. *Spine* 1991;16:1–6.

25. Biering-Soreensen F. A prospective study of low-back pain in a general population. 1. occurrence, recurrence, and etiology. *Scand J Rehabil Med* 1983;15:71–79.

26. Valkenburg HA, Haaven HC. The epidemiology of low back pain. In: White AA, Bordon SL, eds. *AAOS symposium on idiopathic low back pain.* St. Louis: CV Mosby, 1982:9–22.

27. Jefferson JR, McGrath PJ. Back pain and peripheral joint pain in an industrial setting. *Arch Phys Med Rehabil* 1996;77:385–390.

28. Kelsey JL, White AA. Epidemiology and impact of low back pain. *Spine* 1980;5:133–142.

29. Frymoyer JW. Back pain and sciatica. *N Engl J Med* 1988;318:291–300.

30. Nachemson AL. The natural course of low back pain. In: White AA, Gordon SL, eds. *AAOS symposium on idiopathic low back pain.* St. Louis: CV Mosby, 1982:46–51.

31. Aronoff GM, McAlary PW, Witkower A, Berdell MS. Pain treatment programs: do they return workers to the workplace? In: Deyo RA, ed. *Back pain in workers: state of the art reviews in occupational medicine.* Philadelphia: Hanley & Belfus, 1988:123–136.

32. Fordyce WE. *Behavioral methods for chronic pain and illness.* St. Louis: CV Mosby, 1976.

33. Fordyce WE, Fowler RJ, Lehmann JF, et al. Operant conditioning in the treatment of chronic pain. *Arch Phys Med Rehabil* 1973;54:399–408.

34. Berdell MS. The development, implementation, and evolution of a biopsychology program within a multidisciplinary inpatient chronic pain center: an operational manual. In: Aronoff GM, ed. *Pain centers: a revolution in health care.* New York: Raven, 1988:115–129.

35. King JC, Goddard MJ. Pain rehabilitation. 2. Chronic pain syndrome and myofascial pain. *Arch Phys Med Rehabil* 1994;75:S9–S14.

36. Walters A. Psychogenic regional pain alias hysterical pain. *Brain* 1961;84:1–128.

37. King JC, Kelleher WJ. The chronic pain syndrome: the interdisciplinary rehabilitative behavioral modification approach. In: Walsh NE, ed. *Rehabilitation of chronic pain: state of the art reviews in physical medicine and rehabilitation.* Vol. 5. Philadelphia: Hanley & Belfus, 1991:165–186.

38. Portenoy RK. Opioid therapy for chronic nonmalignant pain: current status. In: Fields HL, Liebeskind JC, eds. *Pharmacologic approaches to the treatment of chronic pain: new concepts and critical issues. Progress in pain research and management.* Vol. 1. Seattle: IASP Press, 1994.

39. Leriche R, Young A, transl, ed. *Surgery of pain.* Baltimore: Williams & Wilkins, 1939.

40. Kori SH, Miller RP, Todd DD. Kinisophobia: a new view of chronic pain behavior. *Pain Management* 1990;Jan/Feb: 35–43.

41. Bigos S, Bower O, Braen G, et al. Acute low back problems in adults. Clinical practice guideline, quick reference guide number 14. AHCPR publication no. 95-0643. Rockville, MD: U.S. Department of Health and Human Services, Public Health Service, Agency for Health Care Policy and Research, December 1994.

42. Mayer TG, Gatchel RJ. *Functional restoration for spinal disorders: the sports medicine approach.* Philadelphia: Lea & Febiger, 1988.

43. Buschbacher RM. Deconditioning, conditioning, and the benefits of exercise. In: Braddom RL, ed. *Physical medicine and rehabilitation.* Philadelphia: WB Saunders, 1996: 687–708.

44. Averill PM, Novy DM, Nelson DV, Berry LA. Correlates of depression in chronic pain patients: a comprehensive examination. *Pain* 1996;65:93–100.

45. King JC, Dumitru D, Walsh NE. Rehabilitation of the pain patient: a U.S. perspective. *Pain Dig* 1992;2:106–126.

46. Deyo RA, Diehl AM, Rosenthal M. How many days of bedrest for acute low back pain? A randomized clinical trial. *N Engl J Med* 1986;315: 1064–1070.

47. King JC, Stedwill JE. Can active duty chronic pain patients be rehabilitated to full active duty? *Am J Phys Med Rehabil* 1994;73:331–337.

48. Bonica JJ. History of pain concepts and therapies. In: Bonica JJ, ed. *The management of pain.* Vol. 1. 2nd ed. Philadelphia: Lea & Febiger, 1990:2–17.

49. Porter J, Jick H. Addiction rare in patients treated with narcotics. *N Engl J Med Letter.* 1980; 302:123.

50. Schug SA, Merry AF, Acland RH. Treatment principles for the use of opioids in pain of nonmalignant origin. *Drugs* 1991;42:228–239.

51. Portenoy RK. Chronic opioid therapy in non-malignant pain. *J Pain Symptom Manage* 1990;5:S46–S62.

52. Colpaert FC, Niemegeers CJE, Janssen PAJ, Maroli AN. The effects of prior fentanyl administration and of pain on fentanyl analgesia: tolerance to and enhancement of narcotic analgesia. *J Pharmacol Exp Ther* 1980;213:418–426.

53. Lipman RS. Pharmacotherapy of anxiety and depression. *Psychopharmacol Bull* 1981;171:91–103.

54. Basmajian JV. Cyclobenzaprine hydrochloride effects on skeletal muscle spasm in the lumbar spine region and neck: two double-blind controlled clinical and laboratory studies. *Arch Phys Med Rehabil* 1978;59: 58–63.

55. Greenblatt DJ, Shader RI, Abernathy DR. Current status of benzodiazepines. *N Engl J Med* 1983;309:410–416.

56. Dellemijn PLI, Fields HL. Clinical review: do benzodiazepines have a role in chronic pain management? *Pain* 1994; 57:137–152.

57. Brooks PM. Nonsteroidal antiinflammatory drugs. In: Klippel JH, Dieppe PA, eds. *Rheumatology.* St. Louis: CV Mosby, 1994:10.1–10.6.

58. Grabois M. Chronic pain: evaluation and treatment. In: Goodgold J, ed. *Rehabilitation medicine.* St. Louis: Mosby-Year Book, 1988:663–674.

59. Carron H. *International directory of pain centers/clinics.* Oak Ridge, IL: American Society of Anesthesiologists, 1979.

60. Grabois M, McCann MT, Schramm D, et al. Chronic pain syndromes: evaluation and treatment. In: Braddom RL, ed. *Physical medicine and rehabilitation.* Philadelphia: WB Saunders, 1996:876–891.

61. Aronoff GM, McAlary PW. Organization and function of the multidisciplinary pain center. In: Aronoff GM, ed. *Evaluation and treatment of chronic pain.* Baltimore: Williams & Wilkins, 1992:55–74.

62. Brena SF. Pain control facilities: patterns of operation and problems of organization in the U.S.A. *Clin Anesth* 1985;3:183–195.

63. Bonica JJ, ed. *The management of pain.* Vols. 1 and 2. 2nd ed. Philadelphia: Lea & Febiger, 1990.

64. Wall PD, Melzack R, eds. *Textbook of pain.* 3rd. ed. New York: Churchill Livingstone, 1994.

65. Aronoff GM, ed. *Pain centers: a revolution in health care.* New York: Raven, 1998.

66. Raj PP, ed. *Practical management of pain.* 2nd ed. St. Louis: Mosby-Year Book, 1992.

67. Ramamurthy S, Rogers JN, eds. *Decision making in pain management.* St. Louis: Mosby-Year Book, 1993.

68. Tollison CD, ed. *Handbook of chronic pain management.* Baltimore: Williams & Wilkins, 1989.

69. Fordyce WE, McMahen R, Rainwater G, et al. Pain complaint-exercise performance relationship in chronic pain. *Pain* 1981;10:311–321.

70. Aronoff GM, Evans WO. A review of follow up studies of multidisciplinary pain units. *Pain* 1983;16:1–11.

71. Cassisi JE, Sypert GW, Salamon A, Kapel L. Independent evaluation of a multidisciplinary rehabilitation program for chronic low back pain. *Neurosurgery* 1989;25:877–883.

72. Chapman SL, Brena SF, Bradford LA. Treatment outcome in a chronic pain rehabilitation program. *Pain* 1981;11: 255–268.

73. Cinciripini PM, Floreen A. An evaluation of a behavioral program for chronic pain. *J Behav Med* 1982;5:375–389.

74. Guck TP, Skultety FM, Meilman PW, Dowd ET. Multidisciplinary pain center follow-up study: evaluation with a no treatment control group. *Pain* 1985;21:295–306.

75. Hammonds W, Brena SF, Unikel ID. Compensation for work-related injuries and rehabilitation of patients with chronic pain. *South Med J* 1978;71:664–666.

76. Linton SJ. Behavioral remediation of chronic pain: a status report. *Pain* 1986;24:125–141.

77. McArthur DL, Cohen MJ, Gottlieb HJ, et al. Treating chronic low back pain. I. Admissions to initial follow-up. *Pain* 1987;29:1–22.

78. McArthur DL, Cohen MJ, Gottlieb JH, et al. Treating chronic low back pain. II. Long-term follow-up. *Pain* 1987;29:23–38.

79. Roberts AH, Reinhardt L. The behavioral management of chronic pain: long-term follow-up with comparison groups. *Pain* 1980;8:151–162.

80. Sturgis ET, Schaefer CA, Sikora TL. Pain center follow-up study of treated and untreated patients. *Arch Phys Med Rehabil* 1984;65:301–303.

81. Tollison CD, Kriegel ML, Downie GR. Chronic low back pain: results of treatment at the pain therapy center. *South Med J* 1985;78:1291–1295.

82. Tyre TE, Anderson DL. Inpatient management of the chronic pain patient: a one-year follow-up study. *J Fam Pract* 1981;12:819–827.

83. Graham JR. *The MMPI. A practical guide.* 2nd ed. New York: Oxford University Press, 1987.

84. Hathaway SR, McKinley JC. *Minnesota Multiphasic Personality Inventory Manual.* New York: Psychological Corporation, 1976.

85. Graham JR. *MMPI-2. Assessing personality and psychopathology.* 2nd ed. New York: Oxford University Press, 1993.

86. Deragotis LR, Lipman RS, Covi L. The SCL-90: an outpatient psychiatric rating scale. *Psychopharmacol Bull* 1973;9:13–28.

87. Derogatis LR, Rickels K, Rock AF. The SCL-90 and the MMPI: a step in the validation of a new self-report scale. *Br J Psychiatry* 1976;128:280–289.

88. Derogatis LR, Cleary PA. Confirmation of the dimensional structure of the SCL-90-R: a study in construct validation. *J Clin Psychol* 1977;33:981–989.

89. Million T, Green CJ, Meagher RB: *Million Behavioral Health Inventory.* 3rd ed. Minneapolis: Interpretive Scoring System, 1982.

90. Fairbank JC, Davies JD, Couper J, et al. The Oswestry low back pain disability questionnaire. *Physiotherapy* 1980;66:271–273.

91. Beck A. *Depression: clinical experimental and theoretical aspects.* New York: Harper & Row, 1967.

92. Pilowsky I, Spence ND. *Manual for the Illness Behavior Questionnaire.* 2nd ed. Adelaide: University of Adelaide, 1984.

93. Holms IH, Rahe RH. The social readjustment rating scales. *J Psychosom Res* 1967;11:213–218.

94. Stewart AL, Hays RD, Ware JE. The MOS short-form general health survey: reliability and validity in a patient population. *Med Care* 1988;26:724–735.

95. Melzak R. The McGill Pain Questionnaire: major properties and scoring methods. *Pain* 1975;1:277–299.

96. Million R, Nilsen KH, Jayson MI, Baker RD. Evaluation of low back pain and assessment of lumbar corsets with and without back supports. *Ann Rheumat Dis* 1981;40:449–454.

97. Mooney V, Cairns D, Robertson J. A system for evaluating and treatment of chronic back disability. *West J Med* 1976;124:370–376.

98. Pilowsky I, Bassett D, Barrett R, et al. The illness behavior assessment schedule: reliability and validity. *Int J Psychiatr Med* 1983–1984;13:11–28.

99. Wallis BJ, Bogduk N. Faking a profile: can naive subjects simulate whiplash responses? *Pain* 1996;66:223–227.

100. Gentry WD. Chronic back pain: does elective surgery benefit patients with evidence of psychological disturbance? *South Med J* 1982;75:1169–1170.

101. Herron LD, Pheasant HC. Changes in MMPI profile after low back surgery. *Spine* 1982;7:591–597.

102. Love AW, Peck CL. The MMPI and psychological factors in chronic low back pain: a review. *Pain* 1987;28:1–12.

103. Maruta T, Swanson DW, Swenson WM. Chronic pain: which patients may a pain-management program help? *Pain* 1979;7:321–329.

104. Fordyce WE, Fowler RS, Lehmann JF, DeLateur BJ. Ten steps to help patients with chronic pain. *Patient Care* 1978; 12:263.

105. Turk DC, Meichenbaum D, Genest M. *Pain and behavioral medicine: a cognitive behavioral perspective.* New York: Guilford, 1983.

106. Doege TC, ed. *Guides to the evaluation of permanent impairment.* 4th ed. Chicago: American Medical Association, 1993.

107. Kelsey JL, Golde AL. Occupational and workplace factors associated with low back pain. In: Deyo RA, ed. *Back pain in workers: state of the art reviews in occupational medicine.* Philadelphia: Hanley & Belfus, 1988:7–16.

108. Deyo RA. The role of the primary care physician in reducing work absenteeism and costs due to back pain. In: Deyo RA, ed. *Back pain in workers: state of the art reviews in occupational medicine.* Philadelphia: Hanley & Belfus, 1988:17–30.

109. Aronoff GM, McAlary PW, Witkower A, Berdell MS. Pain treatment programs: do they return workers to the workplace? In: Deyo RA, ed. *Back pain in workers: state of the art reviews in occupational medicine.* Philadelphia: Hanley & Belfus, 1988:123–136.

110. Mayer TG, Gatchel RJ, Kishino N, et al. A prospective short-term study of chronic low back pain patients utilizing novel objective functional measurement. *Pain* 1986;25:53–68.

111. McCain GA. Role of physical fitness training in the fibrositis/fibromyalgia syndrome. *Am J Med* 1988;81(suppl 3A):73–77.

112. Catchlove R, Cohen K. Effects of a directive return to work approach in the treatment of workman's compensation patients with chronic pain. *Pain* 1982;14:181–191.

113. Steig RL, Williams RC, Gallagher LA. Multidisciplinary pain treatment centers. *J Occup Med* 1981;23:94–102.

114. Anderson TP, Cole TM, Gullickson G, et al. Behavioral modification of chronic pain: a treatment program by a multidisciplinary team. *Clin Orthop* 1977;129:96–100.

115. Finlayson RE, Maruta T, Morse RM, Martin MA. Substance dependence and chronic pain: experience with treatment and follow-up results. *Pain* 1986;27:175–180.

116. Gottlieb HJ, Koller R. Low back pain comprehensive rehabilitation program: a follow-up study. Arch Phys Med Rehabil 1982;63:458–461.

117. Malec J, Cayner J, Harvey RF, Timming RC. Pain management: long-term follow-up of an inpatient program. *Arch Phys Med Rehabil* 1981;62:369–372.

118. Mayer TG, Gatchel RJ, Mayer H, et al. A prospective two-year study of functional restoration in industrial low back injury. *JAMA* 1987;258:1763–1767.

119. McCann VJ, Redford JB, Jacobs RR. Long-term effectiveness of a multidimensional treatment program for persons with low back pain. *Pain Suppl* 1981;1:S225. Abstract.

120. Vasudevan SV, Lynch NT, Abram S. Effectiveness of an ambulatory chronic pain management program. *Pain Suppl* 1981;1:S272. Abstract.

121. Aronoff GM, Crue BL, Seres JL. Pain centers: help for the chronic pain patient. a dialogue. In: Aronoff GM, ed. *Pain centers: a revolution in health care.* New York: Raven, 1988:1–8.

122. Lipson M. Evolution of pain center. Hospital issues. In: Aronoff GM, ed. *Pain centers: a revolution in health care.* New York: Raven, 1988:157–166.

123. Newman RI, Seres JL, Yospe LP, Garlington B. Multidisciplinary treatment of chronic pain: long-term follow-up of low-back pain patients. *Pain* 1978;4:283–292.

124. Williams ADdeC, Richardson PH, Nicholas MK, et al. Inpatient vs. outpatient pain management: results of a randomised controlled trial. *Pain* 1996;66:13–22.

125. Stolov WC, Hays RM. Evaluation of the patient. In: Kottke FJ, Lehmann JF, eds. *Krusen's handbook of physical medicine and rehabilitation.* 4th ed. Philadelphia: WB Saunders, 1990:1–9.

Chapter 59

Low-Back Pain

Andrew J. Haig

PAIN, PATHOLOGY, AND PERFORMANCE

Low-back pain implies a complaint of pain anywhere between the rib cage and the gluteal folds. The simple definition defies our collective experience with this complex disorder. Indeed the physiatrist must continuously keep in mind the relationships and lack of relationships between pain, pathology, and performance—the "three P's." The vast differences in strategies for prevention, acute management, rehabilitation, and chronic management make this disorder a challenge. The whole paradigm changes for the pediatric population, athletes, and the elderly, as compared to the injured worker. And the physiatrist's role is seldom only that of a clinician. Often the physiatrist's greatest impact is that of a team leader and administrator.

Since long before industrial society, before physiatrists, lawyers, and insurance companies, humans have always had low-back problems. Ancient medical texts described a variety of traction methods, herbal potions, and physical modalities to treat the problem (1). But the disease and the culture were different then. In the decades after World War II, progress in medical science allowed physicians the ability to deal with dangerous spinal pathology such as tuberculosis, fracture, and tumor in a more direct fashion, with more success. But at the same time, and in a process not completely unrelated, society became cursed with pathology that is less easily quantified and less treatable. One representative study showed that the incidence of low-back pain in America is 70% (2). The number of people with disability from back pain has grown exponentially. Meanwhile, in an isolated native Australian "aborigine" village, the inhabitants showed no evidence of back pain behavior or disability, even though they admitted to its presence (3).

Given the risk factors for acquiring back pain (4) and for becoming disabled from the pain (Table 59-1) (5), one may draw conclusions as to why the problem has increased in modern society. Repetitive, unchanging physical activity on the job, vibration and velocity from motor vehicles, and work environments designed for the product, not the producer, are twentieth-century phenomena. Legal rewards for documenting causation, a health care system that rewards productivity in terms of number of treatments rather than patient outcomes, and an increasingly technical and anonymous workplace dismotivate modern workers and their allies. Finally, as Robert Addison, MD, former chief of staff at the Rehabilitation Institute of Chicago taught, "Chronic back pain transforms socially unacceptable disabilities into socially acceptable disabilities." It is possible that some of the problems seen in the spine clinic have always been disabling, but appeared in other forms in earlier societies. Patients who have chronic back disability may also have problems with substance abuse, physical abuse, learning disability, mild traumatic brain injury, depression, anxiety, and even occasionally Sigmund Freud's nemesis, hysteria. A challenge for the holistically oriented physiatrist is to effectively eliminate both the ancient

Table 59-1: Risk Factors for Low-Back Pain

Category of Factor	Known Risk Factors	Factors Not Associated
Constitutional	Age Physical fitness Abdominal muscle strength Flexor/extensor balance Muscular insufficiency	Sex Weight Height Davenport index
Postural/ structural	Severe scoliosis Some congenital anomalies Narrowed spinal canal Spondylolisthesis Fractures Multilevel degenerative disk disease Spondyloarthropathies	Lordosis Disk space narrowing Schmorl nodes Spina bifida Osteophytes
Environmental Occupational	Smoking Heavy lifting Twisting Bending Stooping Floor surface conditions Prolonged sitting Vibration (vehicular and nonvehicular)	
Psychosocial	Anxiety Depression Hypochondriasis Somatization Work dissatisfaction Stress Hysteria	Psychoses Most neuroses
Recreational	Golf Tennis Football Gymnastics Jogging Cross-country skiing	Snowmobiling Downhill skiing Ice hockey Baseball Other sports
Other	Multiple births Possible genetic clustering	

Source: Frymoyer JW, Cats-Beril W. Predictors of low back pain disability. *Clin Orthop* 1987;221:89–98.

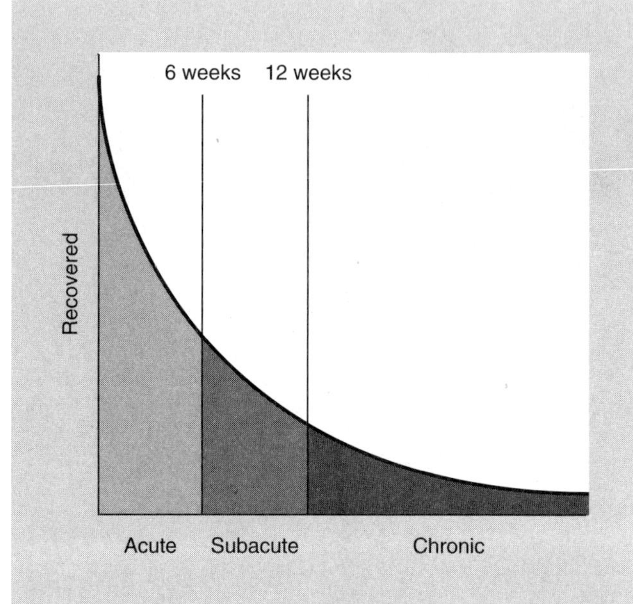

Figure 59-1. Acute, subacute, and chronic low-back pain are defined by the time after onset, but have vastly different prognoses if left untreated.

problem of back pain and the modern problem of back pain disability.

The treating physician cannot easily assess his or her own effectiveness. Both the natural history of low-back pain and the subjectivity of patient outcomes interfere with assessment. Numerous studies showed that most patients get better regardless of treatment (6–8). But they do not get better in a gradual, predictable way. Patients with a first episode of back pain have a 60% chance of recurrence within the year (9). The placebo effect in pain patients has been demonstrated to be 60% (10). Patient reports of pain relief to the physician are colored by the lopsided nature of the physician-patient relationship. As we have learned through the stormy and controversial scientific history of another well-known relapsing-remitting disease, multiple sclerosis, clinical intuition cannot predict effectiveness of treatment. Only carefully designed clinical research can lead the physician away from quackery toward effective treatment.

The research-based protocols for the management of acute low-back pain are abundant and controversial (11). The *Guidelines for Management of Acute Low Back Problems in Adults* from the U.S. Agency for Health Care Policy Research (AHCPR) probably describe a simple approach to the problem (12).

Using the vertical line at the 12-week point in Figure 59-1 (13) as a divider, one can see that low-back pain is really two diseases: the acute one with expected spontaneous resolution, and the chronic one. Evidence suggests that persons disabled from low-back pain for more than 6 months have a 40% chance of ever returning to meaningful work. Those who remain out of work for more than 1 year have a 20% chance, while 2 years of disability almost ensures permanent unemployment (14). Fortunately, modern comprehensive rehabilitation can radically change these percentages. But for a given person, the point at which acute pain becomes chronic is often only seen in retrospect. Given this complex, but basic understanding of low-back pain, the discussion now continues along the lines of the "three P's."

PAIN

As an entity, pain is dealt with elsewhere in this text. It is discussed here primarily to differentiate it from performance. Almost all structures in the low back, with the exception of the deepest parts of the intervertebral disk, carry pain fibers (15). Stimulation of pain fibers in most of these areas (the facet joints, posterior ligaments, muscles, periosteum) can result in local or radiating pain. When previously damaged nerve roots in the lumbar region are stimulated, signals that had traveled up other spinal pathways travel instead through the pain pathways (16). Repetitive painful stimulation results in central amplification and spread of the pain sensitivity. Thus, an injury that has completely repaired, and biomechanically is normal, may still generate pain signals not unlike those from a previous state in which pain warned the patient of a significantly dangerous lesion. Pain may not correlate with performance.

While perception of a stimulus as painful is similar for most persons, pain tolerance may be vastly different, depending on past experience, culture, and current consequences of pain behavior. Pain behavior may also differ substantially among individuals and interpretation of that pain behavior by clinicians may also vary (17,18). While clinicians can measure changes in pain, they cannot yet prove its existence in a given patient. The score a patient reports on a 10-point visual analogue pain scale can reflect anything from a noxious stimulus in the annulus fibrosus to bad advice from an unscrupulous attorney.

Many treatments for pain are independent of the presumed pathology. Given a placebo effect in pain patients of about 60% (10), it is not surprising that confusion exists regarding the multitude of treatments that have not been subjected to adequate randomized controlled trials. Bed rest is probably not effective after the first 2 days, and has side effects (19,20). Traction, electrical stimulation, heat, cold, ultrasound, phonophoresis, iontophoresis, acupuncture, and other treatments have not been shown to be effective. Applied by a clinician, these can become quite expensive (12,21). On the other hand, evidence for the effectiveness of nontreatment and resumption of usual activity is rather compelling (6,19).

Medications have not been proved to improve function in persons with back problems, but a number of randomized controlled trials have validated the use of certain drugs to relieve the pain itself (22,23). A number of nonsteroidal anti-inflammatory drugs (NSAIDs) have been demonstrated to be effective in the management of low-back pain. One may presume that any of them would be effective. Table 59-2 lists a number of these medicines, including their cost and side effect profiles (22,24–26). No research has compared NSAIDs to acetaminophen, which is very inexpensive and has a much more favorable side effect profile and similar analgesic properties in other situations.

Back muscle "spasm" has been treated with drugs used to treat hyperreflexia and spasticity, including dantroline sodium, diazepam, and baclofen (Lioresal). Other "antispasm" drugs have unknown effects, but work better than placebo. These include carisoprodol and cyclobenzaprine. Tricyclic antidepressants work for pain syndromes in general, and probably for low-back pain (27). In patients with depression and chronic pain, these antidepressants are probably the drugs of first choice over more modern antidepressants. The use of other drugs for chronic pain is dealt with elsewhere in this text.

Narcotic analgesics have a place in the management of severe acute pain not controlled by NSAIDs or acetaminophen, but their effectiveness in the management of chronic pain is controversial at best. Given the high incidence of addictive disorders in the population and the side effects of sleep disruption, constipation, concentration problems, and depression, many chronic back pain rehabilitation programs require patients to stop these medications before participation.

In extreme cases, pain is sometimes treated with operative measures. Pumps with morphine or baclofen, or electrical stimulators may be implanted into the spinal canal, with varying effects. Dorsal column ablation and thalamotomy are heroic procedures that await an appropriate population.

PATHOLOGY

As already pointed out, most patients get better whether the diagnosis is right or wrong. Most patients will also leave the physician's office without an exclusive diagnosis (14). Quickly one realizes that the day-to-day rewards to the clinician in looking for a diagnosis are not great. But some back problems can kill. And the most dangerous disorders often present with only a few subtle differences from the benign ones. Physicians training in our spine program learn the habit of answering two questions for each patient they see: "What is the likely diagnosis?" and "If I'm wrong, what other dangerous diagnosis could there be?"

Stedman's Medical Dictionary (28) defines disease as "an interruption, cessation or disorder of body functions, systems, or organs . . . characterized by at least two of these criteria: A recognizable etiologic agent or agents; an identifiable group of signs and symptoms; consistent anatomical alterations."

Over the years, back pain management has been haunted by misunderstanding of this basic principle. The medical history of sciatica is illustrative. Early in this century Yeoman (29) reported on thousands of "successful" operations for "piriformis syndrome." Now his patients' complaints would likely be explained as related to disk herniation. In the 1930s, Mixter and Barr first performed a diskectomy for relief of sciatica. Their predecessors thought disk herniations were chondromas, since they were found so often at autopsy in persons without obvious disease. Mixter and Barr's patient recovered (as did most of Yeoman's patients) and an epidemic of spine surgery swept the industrialized world. (Folklore has it that Mixter and Barr's famous patient came from Vermont, where the

Table 59-2: Medications for Low-back Pain (Non-Radiating and Radiating)

Class	NSAID	Brand Name	Typical Oral Dose (mg)	Cost/Month ($) Brand	Generic	Side Effects
Carbolic Acids	Aspirin	Multiple	975 TID	—	4	Tinnitus
	Salsalate	Disalcid	1500 BID	36	17	Lower GI effect/renal risk
	Choline magnesium trisalicylate	Trilisate, Tricosal	1500 BID	51	27	Lower GI effect/renal risk
	Diflunisal	Dolobid	500 BID	//	59	Lower GI effect/renal risk
Acetic Acids	Diclofenac	Cataflam, Voltaren	75 BID	80	65	Worse risk for liver disease
	Etodolac	Lodine	300 BID	83	75	Low GI effect
	Indomethacin	Indocin	50 TID	85	29	Risk of headaches Avoid in renal disease
	Sulindac	Clinoril	200 BID	77	63	Better for renal disease
	Tolmetin	Tolectin	400 TID	98	69	
	Ketorolac	Toradol Acular	10 QID	155	—	
Propionic Acids	Ibuprofen	Advil, Motrin, Nuprin	600 QID or 800 TID	34	21	Aseptic meningitis
	Fenoprofen	Nalfon	600 TID	70	43	
	Flurbiprofen	Ansaid	100 TID	123	101	
	Ketoprofen	Orudis	75 TID	104	91	
	Naproxen	Naprosyn	500 BID	78	67	Avoid in renal disease
	Oxaprozin	Daypro	1200 QAM	71	—	
Enolic Acids	Phenylbutazone	N.A.	100 TID	—	16	Liver disease
	Piroxicam	Feldene	20 QD	82	62	
Fenamic Acids	Meclofenamate	Meclofenamate	50 QID	—	48	
Naphthylalkanones	Nabumetone	Relafen	1000 QD	66	—	Low gastric irritation (comparable to using Etodolac)
"Muscle Relaxants"	Cyclobenzaprine	Flexeril	10 TID	93	77	Anticholinergic
	Carisoprodol	Soma	350 QID	242	14	Drowsiness
	Baclofen	Lioresal	10 QID	—	43	Drowsiness
	Diazepam	Valium	10 QHS	33	6	Drowsiness, depression, addiction

"local MD," an orthopedic surgeon, had figured out that the disk was pushing on a nerve. He reassured his patient, to no avail, that the problem would resolve on its own) (30). Now there is evidence that this "disease" indeed is prevalent on computed tomography (CT) scans (31) and magnetic resonance images (MRIs) in 30% to 60% of asymptomatic persons (32,33). Disk herniation is considered one step in a degenerative cascade that may or may not result in symptoms (34). Inflammation, rather than actual compression, is implicated as a cause for pain (35). For patients who have symptoms, conservative management, not surgery, is the treatment of choice (36).

Systemic Disorders

Nonmechanical causes for back pain include abdominal processes such as aortic aneurysm, renal infection or calculi, peritonitis, and tumor, and systemic illnesses such as sickle cell anemia and acute intermittent porphyria (Table 59-3). The routine history taking, therefore, includes questions about the family history and the patient's general health, including fevers, night sweats, weight loss, hematuria or melena, breast or testicular masses, diabetes, recent infection, surgery, sinus or bladder symptoms, smoking, alcohol use, intravenous drug use, immune disorders including human immunodeficiency virus (HIV) disease, and peripheral musculoskeletal complaints.

Confirmation of the diagnosis may be difficult. Determinations of the complete blood cell count and sedimentation rate are appropriate screening tests for suspicious cases, but the results may be negative at times in the course of an infection. Serum protein electrophoresis and bone scanning may demonstrate myelomas or other tumors. MRIs will detect many tumors or infections.

The relationship between polyarthritis and low-back pain is complex. Spondylotic arthropathies such as ankylosing spondylitis, Reiter syndrome, psoriatic arthropathy, and intestinal arthropathy can cause pain (37). A history of dry eyes, urethritis, diarrhea, psoriatic skin lesions, enthisopathy (frequent tenderness at the bone-tendon interface) remissions and relapses, or a dramatic response to NSAIDs may be obtained. Sacroiliitis as demonstrated on x-ray films is the sine qua non of spondylitic arthropathies,

Table 59-3: The Differential Diagnosis of Low-Back Pain

- Systemic causes of back pain
  - Aortic aneurysm
  - Renal infection
  - Renal calculi
  - Peritonitis
  - Tumors
  - Metabolic disorders
    - Porphyria
    - Sickle cell disease
    - Renal osteodystrophy
  - Seronegative spondylitic arthritis
    - Ankylosing spondylitis
    - Reiter syndrome
    - Arthritis of ulcerative colitis
    - Psoriatic arthritis
  - Other arthritis
    - Diffuse idiopathic skeletal hyperostosis (DISH)
    - Scheuermann epiphysitis
    - Rheumatoid arthritis—uncommon
    - Gout
  - Connective tissue disorders
    - Marfan syndrome
    - Ehlers-Danlos syndrome
  - Myopathy
  - Inflammatory radiculopathy
- Dangerous local causes of back pain
  - Tumor
  - Disk space infection
  - Epidural abscess
  - Fractures
  - Osteoporosis with fracture
  - Disk herniation
  - Spinal stenosis
  - Spondylolisthesis
    - Congenital
    - Isthmic
    - Degenerative
    - Traumatic
    - Tumor related
  - Failed back surgery syndrome
  - Arachnoiditis
  - Not fully proven entities
    - Sacroiliac joint dysfunction
    - Facet joint syndrome
    - Internal disk disruption
    - "Manipulable" lesions
- Local pathology that mimics radiating low-back pain
  - Osteoarthritis of the hip
  - Aseptic necrosis of the femoral head
  - Sciatic nerve injury due to pressure, stretch, or piriformis muscle entrapment
  - Cyclic sciatica—endometriosis on the sciatic nerve
  - Intrapelvic masses—benign or malignant
  - Peroneal (fibular) nerve entrapment at the fibular head

but is a late finding and is often missed on plain x-ray studies of the spine. Angled sacroiliac views are and bone scans may be helpful, but serologic studies such as for HLA-B27 and correlated clinical history and examination findings may be more appropriate on initial presentation. There is a wide variety of expression of these disorders, so an acute pain episode cannot be automatically attributed to them.

Diffuse idiopathic skeletal hyperostosis (DISH) is seen not infrequently on x-ray films as flowing calcification and ossification along the anterolateral aspect of at least four contiguous vertebral bodies, relative preservation of disk height, and absence of intra-articular bony ankylosis of the sacroiliac and apophyseal joints (37). Middle-aged and elderly men are affected most commonly. It may be asymptomatic or present as stiffness and pain.

Connective tissue disorders such as Marfan syndrome and Ehlers-Danlos syndrome are sometimes first detected in the spine clinic. Affected patients may present with multiple disk herniations, mechanical pain related to hypermobility, or rarely, aortic aneurysm (38). The possibility of dangerous cardiac arrhythmia and aortic aneurysm needs to be considered when prescribing rehabilitation exercises or drugs such as tricyclic antidepressants for these patients. It is possible that a familial predisposition to multiple disk herniations is a less serious form of connective tissue disorder. In my experience, patients with scleroderma, another connective tissue disorder associated with tight skin, commonly have chronic low-back pain; the precise etiology of this is not certain.

Fibromyalgia is recognized as a syndrome, although the pathophysiology is not yet established. Based on history and physical examination findings, patients with this syndrome may respond to a number of treatments, including appropriate sleep, exercise, and tricyclic antidepressants (39).

Osteoarthritis perhaps presents the most confusing relationship between arthritis and low-back pain. The pathophysiology and epidemiology of this disorder in the spine are complex. Population-based radiologic studies demonstrated that osteoarthritis of the spine, "degenerative joint disease," is not a disease at all, but correlates primarily with age, physical activity history, and heredity. With a few exceptions, x-ray findings of osteoarthritis in the spine do not relate to the presence or absence of pain (40,41).

Prospective evidence suggests that psychiatric disease is most commonly a consequence, or a relatively unrelated coexisting condition, but not often a direct cause of chronic low-back disability (5). Depression (42) and anxiety (43) are often concomitants. The small number of frustrating cases in which hysteria, Munchausen syndrome, or malingering is the cause of chronic complaints occupy a disproportionately large part of the cerebral cortex of the spine physician.

Waddel et al (44) showed that the presence of nonanatomic pain symptoms, regardless of cause, result in a poor outcome after surgery, even if local anatomic pathology is present. Waddel's signs include nonanatomic sensory loss, less than a full effort on strength testing, pain during presumably painless maneuvers such as superficial skin palpation or axial compression, and a positive "distracted" straight-leg raise test (done while seated—perhaps while pretending to look at the sole of the foot or performing a Babinski reflex).

Primary neurologic disorders may predispose for, directly cause, or complicate the diagnosis of low-back pain. Severe neurologic disorders ranging from stroke to hereditary neuropathies may change mobility so that pain occurs from awkward motion or poor positioning.

Myopathies such as polymyositis may present as low-back and hip pain (45). Generalized peripheral nerve diseases, especially polyradiculopathies and mononeuritis multiplex, can present with focal nerve root disorders, which in the presence of minor back complaints may be mistaken as evidence for disk herniation or another anatomic lesion (46).

Local Pathology

The discussion of local pathology begins with dangerous causes, both because they are important to detect and because the entities are more clearly provable. Then disorders that seem to fit more clearly into the category of "diagnosis" are described. As the discussion progresses to the entities with less disastrous consequences, it becomes more challenging to define entities as specific "diseases," and the word *syndrome* seems more appropriate. Finally, it is important to recognize entities that appear unusual, or atypical, but have not been correlated with any "recognizable etiologic agent or agents; identifiable group of signs and symptoms; or consistent anatomical alterations" (28).

Dangerous Local Pathology

Infection, tumor, fracture, and cauda equina syndrome are the most significant and dangerous local disorders (see Table 59-3). Diskitis (47) and osteomyelitis (48) are uncommon, but difficult to detect. Classically, patients with tumor present with night pain, or pain not relieved while lying down, but this is neither a sensitive nor a specific indicator (49).

An unstable fracture with a risk for paraplegia needs to be detected immediately. Unless the patient has had substantial trauma or is over the age of 60, the yield of x-ray films is very low. In a person at risk the diagnosis should be pursued while spinal cord precautions are maintained. CT (as opposed to MRI) is a second test of choice, and bone scan has a high yield after the first few days. Compression fractures are usually stable and without neurologic deficit. They can be treated conservatively with bracing and pain relief measures. Predisposing factors including osteoporosis, tumor, and balance disorders should be considered.

Cauda equina syndrome—*progressive* paralysis of the lumbar and sacral nerve roots, usually caused by a large central disk herniation—is an uncommon surgical emergency. It may present as radiating low-back pain, but also may be more insidious, with a complaint of central, nonradiating low-back pain and bowel or bladder dysfunction. There is substantial literature to document that affected patients do better with emergent surgical treatment compared to conservative treatment (50). In patients with a moderate suspicion for cauda equina syndrome, rectal tone and perianal sensation should be evaluated. In most patients, MRI will document the pathology. It is most often a large central disk herniation at L4–L5. Other causes may be spondylolisthesis or rarely, benign cysts or other space-occupying lesions. For the physiatrist, the acute presentation of cauda equina syndrome is less problematic than is rehabilitating patients who are perceived to be at risk for it. It is useful to know that cauda equina syndrome occurs in only 2.5% of patients with disk herniations (51). The literature otherwise provides no data on which to base exercise precautions.

Common Local Pathology

Disk herniation is suggested when a patient presents with new radiating pain to below the knee. Physical examination findings may include a radicular pain pattern, neurologic deficit, and a positive finding on the straight-leg raising test. High lumbar disk herniations present a diagnostic challenge, since the pain usually does not radiate below the knee and the neurologic deficit is different from that of the more common L4–S1 herniations (52). Most persons with symptomatic disk herniations recover within a few months (53,54). Imaging studies are probably not helpful in most patients whose pain slowly resolves. In those who continue to have disabling pain after 6 weeks, the odds of other factors being causative increase, and the presence or absence of a definitive diagnosis may guide treatment and activity restrictions, and validate symptomatology.

Treatment of disk herniation varies more with the practitioner than with the presentation. Surgical treatment works in the short term, but has no advantages in the long term (53,54). The morbidity and expense are criticized. Surgical outcomes are worse in persons who have abnormal results on psychological tests (e.g., Minnesota Multiphasic Personality Inventory), in patients involved in litigation, and in patients who exhibit two or more of Waddel's "nonorganic pain" signs (44,55,56). On the other hand, the decision to seek surgical relief may be driven by other social factors, especially short-term financial hardship (57). Medical factors including the presence of diabetes or polyneuropathy may adversely affect surgical outcomes (58).

Epidural cortisone injections have gained popularity, and evidence supports their efficacy (59). The dosage of steroid, the number and timing of injections, and the route of injection (caudal, paralumbar, or via a nerve root sleeve) are debated. No studies have compared epidural to oral steroids. Numerous other treatments thought to be specific to disk disease have been proposed, but not validated.

Kirkaldy-Willis's degenerative cascade model suggests that disk degeneration may lead to two disorders other than disk herniation (34). Tears of the annulus fibrosis can presumably cause pain, but there is currently no way to demonstrate that a specific episode of pain was caused by an annular tear, and no specific treatments for this disorder are proven. With degeneration, the disk space narrows and the facet joints settle on each other, causing degeneration of these joints. Again, no specific clinical picture has been described, although pain relief induced by injection of these joints is thought to indicate "facet joint syndrome" (60). The use of such injections either to relieve pain in the long term or to guide treatment is still unproved.

Spinal stenosis occurs when the spinal canal is small relative to its contents either centrally or at the lateral recess where the nerve root exits (61). Congenital stenosis can occur in otherwise normal persons and in persons with growth disorders such as achondroplastic dwarfism. Acquired stenosis, the most common type, is found primarily in persons over the age of 50. It is usually the result of degenerative changes in the facet joints and the vertebra-disk margin, perhaps accompanied by hypertrophy of the posterior longitudinal ligament or the facet joint capsular ligaments. Symptoms include "neurogenic claudication"—leg pain during walking. Peculiar symptoms including tolerance for bicycling despite difficulty walking, pain walking downhill greater than that walking uphill, and lack of pain relief unless bent forward help to differentiate this from vasogenic claudication, which also occurs in older persons.

The size and shape of the spinal canal as seen on CT scans or MRIs correlate, but not perfectly, with the presence of symptoms and neurologic damage. In general, a canal with an anterior-posterior dimension less than 1.5 cm may be symptomatic, and one with a diameter less than 1.0 cm is quite likely to be symptomatic. "Trefoil"-shaped spinal canals are more likely to be symptomatic than are more rounded ones. Medication and lifestyle modification, perhaps exercises to increase the spinal and hip range of motion, and epidural cortisone injections are appropriate conservative forms of treatment. Surgical treatment has reasonable success when conservative treatment fails (62).

There are five types of spondylolisthesis: the most common, isthmic spondylolisthesis; congenital spondylolisthesis, caused by mismatch of the size of the posterior elements; traumatic spondylolisthesis, caused by severe trauma in adults or children; degenerative spondylolisthesis, caused by laxity of ligaments with age; and the very rare tumor-related spondylolisthesis (63).

Isthmic spondylolisthesis is usually a childhood-onset disorder, but it may also require treatment in adulthood. Microfractures of the pars interarticularis occur related to repeated minor trauma, classically in participants of sports such as gymnastics, football, or swimming using the butterfly stroke. These microfractures, termed *spondylolysis*, can sometimes be seen as the classic "Scottie dog with a broken neck" on oblique x-ray films. If they stretch to lengthen the distance between the vertebral body and the posterior elements, the lower vertebra shifts posteriorly in relation to the upper one. This type of childhood process is called *isthmic spondylolisthesis*. Grade I, II, III, IV, or V slippage correlates with less than 25%, 25% to 50%, 50% to 75%, 75% to 100%, or more than 100% slippage of one vertebra on another. In childhood and young adulthood, this active process can be painful, and continued trauma may worsen the slippage. On the other hand, a slippage of less than grade I does not increase the incidence of pain in adults (64).

Detection of spondylolisthesis is usually by plain anteroposterior and lateral spine x-ray films. Occasionally oblique x-ray studies are necessary to detect the lesion, but routine oblique films are overused. Bone scanning, preferably with single-photon emission CT images, are sensitive to active repair. Treatment is symptomatic. It is thought that physical exercise should be limited in athletes until the bone scan demonstrates less activity. Occasionally, bracing is used in the symptomatic population.

Disruption of the sacroiliac joint has been debated as a cause of low-back pain for decades. Recent evidence seems to support this etiology. Sacroiliac joint injections and manipulation may offer local treatment for these lesions (65).

Scoliosis might be termed a local back disorder, but recent evidence suggests that "idiopathic" scoliosis is actually a subtle muscle disease (66). The diagnosis of idiopathic scoliosis requires elimination of other neuromuscular disorders and focal deformities of the spine. While a discussion of the diagnosis and treatment of juvenile idiopathic scoliosis is beyond the scope of this chapter, it is important to note that minor scoliosis in adults is not an explanation for back pain. In fact, the risk for back pain increased over the normal risk only when the angle of deformity was over 60 degrees in one epidemiologic study (14).

Other pathologic processes seem to make common sense, but are quite difficult to prove. There are no criteria for the diagnoses of muscle strain or ligament sprain, for instance. Clinicians skilled in manual medicine often find, on detailed examination of the spine, a number of abnormalities at multiple levels that are correctable by manipulation: "manipulable lesions." While interobserver reliability for such lesions has not been demonstrated, most reviews concluded that manipulation is successful in relieving acute pain (12,21). There is insufficient support to claim that manipulation improves function (e.g., return to work), that more than a few treatment episodes are needed, or that there is any effect on chronic pain. One suspects that "manipulable lesions" may well become a more standard part of the diagnostic terminology as more practitioners, many of whom are physiatrists, quantify their findings.

Failed back surgery syndrome is an all too common disorder. The removal of paraspinal muscle mass results in pain in the long term (67). Violation of the thecal sack may cause arachnoiditis. Fusions may fail. Regardless of the cause, rehabilitation often includes dealing with either frustration and anger at the health care system, or paradoxically an illogical sense that another operation will solve the problem. Only in patients with clear-cut recurrent disk herniation or pathology such as severe instability or stenosis is reoperation a consideration.

Arachnoiditis, or clumping and scarring of the lumbar nerve roots, is essentially unknown in the nonoperated spine (68). The chronic unrelenting pain of arachnoiditis may occasionally be accompanied by progressive neurologic deficit. To date, no treatments specific to the pathology in the back are effective, but nonspecific pain management techniques may be helpful.

Uncommon Disorders and Nonspinal Musculoskeletal Disorders

Rare hypothesized causes for local pain include a compartment syndrome, reported in one patient (69), and entrapment of the posterior primary ramus of the nerve root in a small ligament that crosses the pedicle (70).

Other musculoskeletal problems can present as back pain, or in combination with benign back syndromes, take on the appearance of more significant disorders. Arthritis of the hip (including avascular necrosis of the femoral head in younger persons) can present as back pain. Distal entrapment neuropathies, such as fibular nerve injury at the femoral head and sciatic nerve injury in the gluteal region, can be mistaken for radiating spinal pain. This "pseudo-radicular syndrome" is seen in a small percentage of patients referred for spinal electromyography (EMG) (71). Coccyx pain, or coccydynia is seen occasionally (72).

Diagnostic Tests

The history and physical examination are key to diagnosing even the most advanced or complex back pain. They are all that is required to diagnose more simple acute pain (73). At the end of a successful history taking, a positive physician-patient relationship has been established, possible dangerous pathology has been suspected, the probable diagnosis has been established, patient goals are understood, and any barriers to recovery or compliance have been unearthed. The physical examination rules out neurologic deficits, assesses for gross orthopedic deformities, and assesses pain behavior.

From a diagnostic standpoint, the history should contain medical facts regarding history of previous back problems and the results of any previous diagnostic tests and treatment. Past medical history should include any personal history of cancer, arthritis, infection, or systemic diseases that might predispose to infection. The review of systems should include fever, incontinence, symptoms suggesting metastatic or metabolic disorders, and psychiatric issues including depression and drug use. The findings that suggest serious disease have been termed *red flags* in the AHCPR's guidelines for management of acute low-back problems (12). The review and history must screen for other processes that might interfere with treatment choices. For example, the presence of gastrointestinal ulcers, renal disease, or cardiac disease may interfere with medication prescription. Unrelated orthopedic disorders, cardiac disease, or diabetes may interfere with exercise prescription. The social history must include current work status, any legal or financial issues pertaining to the injury, and other stressors that might interfere with recovery. Given the misinformation about back pain that is prevalent in both society and the medical professions, it is useful to understand the patient's perceptions about the diagnosis, treatment options, restrictions, and prognosis.

The history of the back problem itself focuses on the physical examination and subsequent diagnostic tests. History taking is greatly augmented by the use of pain drawings which have value both as psychological and as musculoskeletal diagnostic tools (74,75). Insidious onset, pain worse while recumbent or at night, pain not relieved or worsened by positions of movement, and pain associated with illness are worrisome. A history of minor trauma is not helpful except perhaps in persons at risk for osteoporosis. More significant trauma such as a motor vehicle accident requires treatment of the problem as a presumed unstable fracture until proved otherwise. Pain that is getting better will probably continue to do so, while worsening pain suggests the need for a definitive diagnosis, if one can be obtained. The location of the pain provides hints. Nonradiating pain can occasionally be the result of a central disk herniation. Pain that radiates to below the knee suggests a low lumbar root lesion, while anterior thigh pain suggests an upper root lesion. Either can occur, however, with lesions of bones, joints, or muscles. Leg pain worsened with ambulation suggests stenosis.

The physical examination includes a neurologic screen that tests two muscles and a reflex representing each of the lumbar roots. This overlap, demonstrated in Table 59-4, allows one to more accurately differentiate root syndromes from focal neuropathies, other neurologic syndromes, and inconsistent effort, which may occur for a number of reasons. Nerve tension signs including the straight-leg raise test for the lower roots and the prone leg raise test for the upper roots can add support to the diag-

Table 59-4: Neurologic Examination for Lumbar Root Lesions*

Root	Primary Muscle	Secondary Muscle	Reflex
S2, 3, 4	Anal sphincter	?	Bulbocavernosus?
S1	Ankle plantarflexors	Hip extensors	Achilles
L5	Great toe extensor	Hip internal rotators	Medial hamstring
L4	Knee extensors	Hip adductors	Patellar
L2, 3	Hip flexors	?	?
L1	?	?	?

* Note that the three most commonly involved roots are tested via muscles from two different nerves and a reflex.

nosis, although they reflect subjective interpretation. The mechanical examination at its most basic (which is usually sufficient) includes reproduction of the pain by palpation of the entire spine and the sacroiliac joints, and examination of pain and limitations with the spine in flexion and extension.

This routine examination is quite good at assessing most provable causes of back pain. At its conclusion, the examiner should pause to consider other parts of the neurologic, musculoskeletal, or general medical examination that might assist in making more uncommon diagnoses; other lesions that may mimic back pain; or problems that may interfere with subsequent rehabilitation. A high index of suspicion may lead to an examination of the lower sacral nerve roots including perianal sensation and rectal sphincter control. A more advanced manual examination may become quite sophisticated in assessing subtle abnormalities that may respond to manipulative or manual therapy. Discussion of the scope of such an examination is beyond this text.

Other diagnostic tests should be used judiciously. Without evidence for a dangerous cause of low-back pain, plain x-ray films yield little, increase cost, and increase exposure to radiation (76). If a patient is not progressing after a few weeks and if the pain is not radiating, x-ray studies may be a first choice, more because they are inexpensive than because they are either sensitive or specific (76). Oblique films are of little use unless a spondylolysis is suspected and not detected on the two routine (anteroposterior and lateral) films (77).

"Red flags" or unresolved radiating pain usually lead to a more advanced imaging test. MRI is quickly superseding CT as the test of choice because of its ability to provide soft-tissue detail and multiplanar images. These tests are not perfect, with substantial false-positive rates and less common false-negative findings (31–33,78,79).

In the setting of negative MRI findings and a high index of suspicion, or positive MRI findings that do not make clinical sense, the next question to ask is whether the problem suggests a bone or nerve lesion. In the case of a nonradiating, mechanical-type pain, especially that relieved by anti-inflammatory medications, a bone scan may be the test with the next best yield. At any hint of radiation, numbness, or tingling, EMG is more likely helpful.

While EMG is discussed elsewhere in this text, the physiatrist's role in performing EMG for low-back problems deserves special comment here. The indications for EMG have changed drastically from the time when it was the only noninvasive test for disk herniation (80). EMG is only indicated when the results of the test will substantially change treatment. Table 59-5 lists common circumstances where this may be true. EMG of the paraspinal muscles has proved sensitive to clinical syndromes and is somewhat specific to root levels, but only when the test is done in a carefully quantified fashion (81,82). Although H-reflex, F-waves, somatosensory evoked potentials, and other neurodiagnostic parameters have value in certain circumstances, the venerable needle examination is usually the most sensitive and specific electrodiagnostic test.

Table 59-5: Indications for Electrodiagnostic Testing in Patients with Low-Back Problems

Absolute
1. Patients with symptoms suggestive of cauda equina syndrome and nondiagnostic imaging tests results.

Relative

When added information will alter treatment plans and:
1. Imaging studies show an abnormality that does not correlate with symptoms.
2. Imaging findings are normal despite clinical suspicion.
3. There is a suspicion of polyneuropathy, myopathy, or entrapment neuropathy.
4. It is clinically important to determine the age of the lesion.
5. It is clinically important to demonstrate which of numerous anatomic lesions in the spine is causing radicular symptoms.
6. Severe paralysis requires a determination of prognosis in order to decide on bracing options.

Uncertain
1. For medicolegal purposes to document the presence or absence of a lesion in light of unclear imaging studies.
2. To provide a prognosis for incomplete nerve damage.

Usually not indicated
1. As a first-line test in the diagnosis of radiating low-back pain.
2. To corroborate with clearly abnormal or clearly normal imaging findings and consistent clinical findings on examination.

A number of invasive radiologic diagnostic tests exist. The oldest, myelography, is quickly becoming obsolete, although it still holds an advantage in the rare patient in whom nerve impingement occurs with standing or with movement. Diskography, often in combination with CT, is commonly used to diagnose disk disruption (83). Pain reproduction is as important as an actual demonstration of disk disruption on film, when interpreting diskography results (84). The benefit of making such a diagnosis is debated, however. Facet joint injection with an anesthetic and possible steroids may not be as specific as once thought, though it may lead to relief of pain for an unknown period of time and might lead to consideration of more permanent treatments such as radiofrequency ablation of the posterior primary ramus of the nerve root that innervates the joint. Similarly, sacroiliac joint injection may confirm pathology there (85,86). Pain relief from selective nerve root blocks may be useful for both diagnosis and treatment (87).

Finally, a number of laboratory tests may be appropriate. Most notable are the complete blood cell count and sedimentation rate, which can detect uncommon but disastrous infections. With a high index of suspicion, one should not hesitate to repeat these tests, as the results may be negative for disk infections for some time. Work-up for cancer, a topic beyond the scope of this discussion, may include measurements of alkaline phosphatase and serum protein electrophoresis. Suspected rheumatologic disorders may be diagnosed by tests for antinuclear antibodies, rheumatoid factor, or uric acid or blood typing for HLA-B27.

PERFORMANCE

Treatment of performance problems in persons with low-back pain (otherwise known as rehabilitation!) is often not separated from treatment of the pain or pathology. Indeed, exercise programs such as the McKenzie approach (88), dynamic lumbar stabilization (89), and others (90) may both decrease pain and improve strength and flexibility performance.

It is worthwhile, however, to separate the "three P's." First of all, a lot of the disability and handicap that result from an episode of back pain are not directly related to the pathology or pain. Chronic pain patients are often profoundly deconditioned in terms of strength, endurance, and flexibility. Reconditioning can be accomplished. They often develop psychiatric problems, including depression and anxiety, that are readily treated with psychotherapy and drugs. Finally, the handicap, or disadvantage in society, often is confounded by premorbid conditions including poor education, learning disabilities, and poor understanding of an employers expectations, and can be improved by patient education and mediation between the patient, family, and employer.

Successful treatments of performance deficits early after injury have included reassurance (91), directed return to work (92), facilitated communication between employers and injured employees (93), back school education (94), and limitation of bed rest (20).

As problems become more chronic, approaches such as work hardening and work conditioning may help (95). Work hardening includes simulated job activity and reconditioning, while work conditioning is primarily exercise. Although work hardening is popular and probably effective, it is supported by surprisingly little research (96). Work conditioning with graduated return to actual work costs less and is gaining in popularity, despite a lack of convincing outcome research.

Very chronic pain syndromes, including work disability lasting longer than 3 months, have been effectively treated with an approach termed *functional restoration.* This complex and challenging type of program is based on the premise that patients must be responsible for their own destiny. Separate studies by Mayer et al (97) and Hazzard et al (98) demonstrated an 80% rate for return to work by program completers and only a 40% success rate for "insurance denial" control subjects. The research support for functional restoration has been challenged, but a more effective alternative has not been presented (99).

"Diagnostic tests" of performance may be helpful in a number of clinical circumstances: Tests that detect deficits in strength, coordination, endurance, flexibility, or emotional stability are helpful in guiding treatment choices. Rissanen et al (100) showed that very simple tests actually outperform complex and expensive ones in predicting response to rehabilitation. Unfortunately, based on only the most crude evidence (101,102), "functional capacity tests" have also been used to predict future ability or inability to perform work activities. Clinical judgment regarding reversibility of deficits, similarity of the test to actual long-term life activity, and the effect of the specific pathology must be used in addition to test scores when the tests have no known predictive value.

The law often requires "proof" of disability and handicap. Again, there is no objective system to provide such proof. Measures of spinal range of motion, as required by the American Medical Association's *Guides to the Evaluation of Permanent Impairment* (103) are quite inconsistent (104) and correlate minimally with actual disability. The physician simply is left either to report results as required in the jurisdiction that asks the question, or in the absence of specific rules, to use clinical judgment.

SPECIAL CIRCUMSTANCES

Primary Prevention

The physiatrist's role in primary prevention is expanding as rehabilitation and occupational medicine share roles. Common strategies have included screening for risk factors, ergonomic redesign of the home or worksite, preventative exercise, and wearing of devices such as corsets. Of all of these, only environmental redesign has received substantial support as a successful strategy. At the job site, "nonspecific" health measures including smoking cessation and mental health support may have an effect on back pain disability, if not the back pain itself. A thoughtful assessment of the problem must take into consideration both effectiveness and cost-effectiveness. One must consciously avoid strategies that make technical sense but support a societal trend to equate pain with disability.

Children with Back Pain

Back pain is unusual before the teen years. Although most children have benign causes for pain, prominent concerns include the possibility of important congenital malformation, neural axis tumors, and psychiatric disorders. Adolescents, especially girls, may require treatment of idiopathic scoliosis (66) (a diagnosis made only after neurologic and orthopedic disorders are ruled out). Scheuermann epiphysitis, a disorder of the vertebral growth plate causing thoracic kyphosis and back pain, is not uncommon (105).

Athletes

Athletes with back pain are susceptible to the usual causes, including "idiopathic" factors. Special concerns include spondylolysis and spondylolisthesis in contact sports such as football and sports that require hyperextension of the spine including gymnastics and butterfly-stroke swimming. Isolated trauma may fracture a posterior element of the vertebra including a spinous process or transverse process. Imbalance in training efforts, such as in rowing, may predispose athletes to back pain. Treatments need to focus on improving training or competition strategies, and providing adequate warm-up. Even when competition is precluded during recovery, the athlete can almost always participate in noncontact conditioning and skill building.

Older Persons

There are many concerns regarding the diagnosis and treatment of low-back pain in older persons. After the age of 55, the risks of cancer and osteoporosis are increased. The incidence of both spinal stenosis and its differential diagnosis, vascular claudication, is increased. Exercise treatment may not be well understood by a generation (especially women) who were never exposed to the pleasures of athletic exercise. Exercise in general is often difficult for patients with cardiac disease, emphysema, or osteoarthritis. Flexion exercises should be avoided in persons with osteoporosis. Medications are riskier, with an increased risk of gastrointestinal bleeding with NSAIDs and an increased risk of falls with narcotics and tricyclic antidepressants. On the other hand, this population is often not pushed by the need to work or physically care for a young family.

Persons with Other Disabilities

Persons with preexisting neurologic or orthopedic disabilities may present with back pain related to their immobility, their increased seated posture, or asymmetric or uncoordinated movements in gait. The usual diagnostic and treatment considerations of able-bodied persons cannot be ignored, but oftentimes modification of the primary disorder (through bracing, spasticity drugs, correction of contracture) or of an assistive device (such as wheelchair modification, transfer improvement, etc) results in success.

PUTTING IT ALL TOGETHER—THE PHYSIATRIST'S ROLE IN TRIAGE

The physiatrist is ideally trained to manage the diverse disorder called low-back pain (see Appendix I). Acutely, training in physical medicine, kinesiology, exercise physiology, psychology, and sometimes manual medicine, injection technology, and electrodiagnosis, allows the physiatrist to identify and treat almost all back problems. While an influential study suggesting the only difference between different care providers was cost did not include physiatrists (106), there is evidence to indicate that a physiatric approach is more effective than a primary care approach to acute back injury (93) and that spine specialists are more able to identify patients who are at risk for chronicity than are primary care specialists (5). When patients do become chronic, there is a consensus that a multidisciplinary team is required (12,21). The physiatrist's roots in inpatient rehabilitation are not wasted.

The physiatrist is often called on to take a leadership role in rehabilitation teams, or in multispecialty diagnostic and treatment teams. This is a unique opportunity to improve care for persons with back pain. An efficient triage system has a direct impact on the extent of back pain disability, by eliminating delays in return to work. Responsive paperwork and other communications with employers, insurers, and the referring physician have the same effect. It is often a major challenge to develop a mutual team treatment philosophy that focuses on enabling rather than disabling. A prospective outcome measurement system not only is important in the modern business-like environment of health care, but also is an effective way to help the team improve through a continuous quality improvement process.

CONCLUSIONS

This chapter discussed in depth a number of specific aspects of low-back pain. Of necessity, the new physician will simplify by dealing with only a few dimensions of this problem in a given patient. Unfortunately, since up to 90% of patients with low-back pain will leave without a valid diagnosis, and 90% will be cured regardless of a physician's efforts, it is especially easy to become older without becoming wiser. The physician who truly becomes an expert will do so by struggling to deal with pain, pathology, and performance—all of the complexity inherent in this disorder. Over time he or she will learn to see not so much the dimensions themselves as the exceptions to the rules. This is the true definition of expertise.

APPENDIX. TRIAGE: A SIMPLISTIC APPROACH TO DIFFICULT LOW-BACK DISABILITY PROBLEMS

Acute (0–6 weeks): How concerned are you about the pain?

Trivial pain? Physician institutes directed return to activity, prescribes nonnarcotic pain medicine, and teaches "first aid" strategies.

Activity-limiting pain? Patient and physician develop activity limitations together. Nonnarcotics and specific physical therapy follow frequently until patient is fully active.

Neurologic deficit or "red flags"? Physician limits activity, performs diagnostic tests if "red flags" present, prescribes pain medication, and performs frequent follow-up until patient is fully active.

Subacute (6–12 weeks): To make a diagnosis or not?

Getting better? Perform no diagnostics.

Not getting better? Most likely obtain MRI. Possibly request bone scan or EMG. Occasionally order x-ray studies or other tests.

Chronic (>12 weeks): What's left to offer?

No clear diagnosis? Order any reasonable tests.

Deconditioned? Recommend exercise program.

Psychosocial barriers to recovery? Prescribe drugs and refer to counselor.

Deconditioned and psychosocial barriers? Institute multidisciplinary rehabilitation (e.g., functional restoration).

Stable emotionally and physically, but still suffering? Use medications, surgical treatments, or experimental treatments.

None of the above: Help the patient to exit the health care system.

REFERENCES

1. Richardson JG, Ford WH, Vanderbeck CC. *Medicology.* New York: University Medical Society, 1905:1393.

2. Frymoyer JW, Pope MH, Rosen J, Goggin J. Epidemiologic studies of low back pain. *Spine* 1980;5:419–423.

3. Honeyman PT, Jacobs EA. Effects of culture on back pain in Australian aboriginals. *Spine* 1996;21:841–843.

4. Frymoyer JW. Helping your patients avoid low back pain. *J Musculoskeletal Med* 1984:65–74.

5. Frymoyer JW, Cats-Beril W. Predictors of low back pain disability. *Clin Orthop* 1987;221: 89–98.

6. Indahl A, Velund L, Reikeraas O. Good prognosis for low back pain when left untampered: a randomized clinical trial. *Spine* 1995; 20:473–477.

7. Roland M, Morris R. 1982 Volvo award in clinical science: a study of the natural history of back pain—part I: development of a reliable and sensitive measure of disability in low-back pain. *Spine* 1983;8:141–144.

8. Roland M, Morris R. 1982 Volvo award in clinical science: a study of the natural history of low-back pain—part II: development of guidelines for trials of treatment in primart care. *Spine* 1983;8: 145–150.

9. Berquist-Ullman M, Larsson U. Acute low back pain in industry: a controlled prospective study with special reference to therapy and confounding factors. *Acta Orthop Scand Suppl* 1977;170:1–117.

10. Turner JA, Deyo RA, Loeser JD, et al. The importance of placebo effects in pain treatment and research. *JAMA* 1994;271: 1609–1614.

11. Steven ID, Fraser RD. Spine update: clinical practice guidelines. Particular reference to the management of pain in the lumbosacral spine. *Spine* 1996;21: 1593–1596.

12. Bigos A, Bowyer O, Braeng G, et al. Acute low back problems in adults. Clinical practice guideline no. 14. AHCPR publication no. 95-0642. Rockville, MD: Agency for Health Care Policy and Research, Public Health Service, U.S. Department of Health and Human Services, December 1994.

13. Andersson GBJ, Svensson HO, Oden A. The intensity of work recovery in low back pain. *Spine* 1983;8:880.

14. Frymoyer JW. Back pain and sciatica. *N Engl J Med* 1988; 318:291–300.

15. Bogduk N, Tynan W, Wilson AS. The nerve supply of the human lumbar intervertebral disk. *J Anat* 1981;132:39–56.

16. Bonica JJ. General considerations of chronic pain. In: Bonica JJ, ed. *The management of pain.* 2nd ed. Philadelphia: Lea & Febiger, 1990:180–196.

17. Bate MS, Rankin-Hill L. Control, culture, and chronic pain. *Soc Sci Med* 1994;39:629–645.

18. Cherkin DC, Deyo RA, Wheeler K, Cilo MA. Physicians' views about treating low back pain: the result of a national survey. *Spine* 1995;20:101–109.

19. Malmivaara A, Hakkinen U, Aro T, et al. The treatment of acute low back pain—bed rest, exercises, or ordinary activity? *N Engl J Med* 1995;332: 351–355.

20. Deyo RA, Kiehl AK, Rosenthal M. How many days of bed rest for acute low back pain? A randomized clinical trial. *N Engl J Med* 1986;315:1064–1092.

21. Quebec Task Force on Spinal Disorders: scientific approach to the assessment and management of activity-related spinal disorders: a monograph for clinicians. *Spine* 1987(suppl);12:S22–S30.

22. Saag KG, Cowdery JS. Spine update—nonsteroidal anti-inflammatory drugs: balancing

benefits and risks. *Spine* 1994;19:1530–1534.

23. Porter RW, Ralston SH. Pharmacological management of back syndromes. *Drugs* 1994;48: 189–198.

24. Haig AJ. Back to school: N.S.A.I.D.'s in muscle and tendon injuries. Presented at the American Academy of Physical Medicine and Rehabilitation annual assembly, Orlando, FL, November 18, 1995.

25. Schnitzer TJ. NSAID's in orthopedic practice: management guidelines for arthritis patients. *Contemp Orthop* 1995;30: 383–389.

26. Medical Economics Data Production Company. *Physician's desk reference.* 49th ed. Montvale, NJ: Medical Economics, 1994.

27. Alcoff J. Controlled trial of imipramine for chronic low back pain. *J Fam Pract* 1982;14: 841–846.

28. Stedman TL. *Stedman's medical dictionary.* 23rd ed. Baltimore: Williams & Wilkins, 1976.

29. Yeoman W. The relation of arthritis of the sacro-iliac joint to sciatica. *Lancet* 1928;2: 1119–1122.

30. Frymoyer JW, Donaghy RM. The ruptured intervertebral disc. Follow-up report on the first case fifty years after recognition of the syndrome and its surgical significance. *J Bone Joint Surg Am* 1985;67:1113–1116.

31. Wiesel SW, Tsourmas N, Feffer HL. 1984 Volvo award in clinical sciences: a study of computer-assisted tomography: I. The incidence of positive CAT scans in an asymptomatic group of patients. *Spine* 1984;9:549–551.

32. Jensen MC, Brant-Zawadzki MN, Obuchowski N, et al. Magnetic resonance imaging of the lumbar spine in people without back pain. *N Engl J Med* 1994; 331:69–73.

33. Deyo RA. Magnetic resonance imaging of the lumbar spine: terrific test or tar baby? *N Engl J Med* 1994;331:115–116.

34. Kirkaldy-Willis WH, Wedge JH, Yong Hing K, Reilly J. Pathology and pathogenesis of lumbar spondylosis and stenosis. *Spine* 1978;4:319–328.

35. Franson RC, Sall JS, Saal JA. Human disk phospholipase A_2 is inflammatory. *Spine* 1992;17(6 suppl):5129–5132.

36. Saal JA, Saal JS, Herzog RJ. The natural history of lumbar intervertebral disc extrusions treated nonoperatively. *Spine* 1990;15: 683–686.

37. Rodman GP, Schumacher HR, Zvaifler NJ, eds. *Primer on the rheumatic diseases.* 8th ed. Atlanta: Arthritis Foundation, 1983:85–88, 151–152.

38. Tallroth K, Malmivaara A, Laitinen ML, et al. Lumbar spine in Marfan's syndrome. *Skel Radiol* 1995;24:337–340.

39. Yunus MB, Kalyan-Raman UP, Kaylan-Raman K. Primary fibromyalgia syndrome and myofascial pain syndrome: clinical features and muscle pathology. *Arch Phys Med Rehabil* 1988;69:451–454.

40. Witt I, Vestergaard A, Rosenklint A. A comparative analysis of x-ray findings of the lumbar spine in patients with and without lumbar pain. *Spine* 1984;9: 298–300.

41. Frymoyer JW, Newberg A, Pope MH, et al. Spine radiographs in patients with low-back pain. *J Bone Joint Surg [Am]* 1984; 66:1048–1055.

42. Krishnan K, France RD, Pelton S, et al. Chronic pain and depression. I: classification of depression in chronic low back pain patients. *Pain* 1985;22: 279–287.

43. Krishnan K, France RD, Pelton S, et al. Chronic pain and depression. II: symptoms of anxiety in chronic low back pain patients and their relationship to subtypes of depression. *Pain* 1985;22: 289–294.

44. Waddel G, McCulloch JA, Kummel E, Venner RM. Nonorganic physical signs in low-back pain. *Spine* 1980;5:117–125.

45. Mitz M, Chang GL, Albers J, et al. Electromyographic and histological paraspinal abnormalities in polymyositis/dermatomyositis. *Arch Phys Med Rehabil* 1981; 62:118–121.

46. Bastron JA, Thomas JE. Diabetic polyradiculopathy: clinical and electromyographic findings in 105 patients. *Mayo Clin Proc* 1981;56:725–732.

47. Honan M, White GW, Eisenberg GM. Spontaneous infectious diskitis in adults. *Am J Med* 1996;100:85–89.

48. Stefanovski N, Van Voris LP. Pyogenic vertebral osteomyelitis: report of a series of 23 patients. *Contemp Orthop* 1995;31: 159–164.

49. Delamarter RB, Sachs BL, Thompson GH, et al. Section II—general orthopaedics: primary neoplasms of the thoracic and lumbar spine—an analysis of consecutive cases. *Clin Orthop* 1990;256:87–100.

50. Kostui J, Harrington I, Alexander D, et al. Cauda equina syndrome and lumbar disk herniation. *J Bone Joint Surg [Am]* 1986; 68:386–391.

51. Spangfort EV. The lumbar disk herniation: a computer aided analysis of 2504 operations. *Acta Orthop Scand Suppl* 1972;142: 61–77.

52. Albert TJ, Balderston RA, Heller JG, et al. Upper lumbar disk herniations. *J Spinal Disord* 1993; 6:351–359.

53. Hakelius A. Prognosis in sciatica: a clinical follow-up of surgical and nonsurgical treatment. *Acta Orthop Scand Suppl* 1970; 129:1.

54. Weber H. Lumbar disc herniation: a controlled prospective study with ten years of observations. *Spine* 1983;8:131–140.

55. Spengler DM, Freeman C, Westbrook R, Miller JW. Low

back pain following multiple lumbar spine procedures: failure of initial selection? *Spine* 1980; 5:356–360.

56. Wiltse LL, Rocchio PD. Preoperative psychological tests as predictors of success of chemonucleolysis in the treatment of the low back pain syndrome. *J Bone Joint Surg [Am]* 1975;57:478–483.

57. Shartzman L, Weingarten E, Sherry H, et al. Cost-effectiveness analysis of exteended conservative therapy versus surgical intervention in the management of herniated lumbar intervertebral disc. *Spine* 1992; 17:176–182.

58. Simpson JM, Silver CP, Balderston RA, et al. The results of operations on the spine in patients who have diabetes mellitus. *J Bone Joint Surg [Am]* 1993;75:1823–1829.

59. Bowman SJ, Wedderburn L, Whaley A, et al. Outcome assessment after epidural corticosteroid injection for low back pain and sciatica. *Spine* 1993;18: 1345–1350.

60. Dreyer SJ, Dreyfuss PH. Low back pain and the zygoapophyseal (facet) joints. *Arch Phys Med Rehabil* 1996;77:290–300.

61. Ciricillo SF, Weinstein PR. Lumbar spinal stenosis. *West J Med* 1993;158:171–177.

62. Turner JA, Ersek M, Herron L, et al. Patient outcomes after lumbar spinal fusions. *JAMA* 1992;268: 907–911.

63. Lawhon SM, Ballard WT. Spondylolisthesis: a review of the literature. *Contemp Orthop* 1990; 21:27–35.

64. Saraste H. Long term clinical and radiological follow up of spondylosis and spondylolisthesis. *J Pediatr Orthop* 1987;7: 631–638.

65. Oh TH, Brander VA, Hindere SR, Alpinen N. Rehabilitation in joint and connective tissue diseases. 2. Inflammatory and degenerative spine diseases. *Arch Phys Med Rehabil* 1995;76:S41–S46.

66. Gunnoe BA. Adolescent idiopathic scoliosis. *Orthop Rev* 1990;19:35–43.

67. Sihvonen T, Herno A, Paljarvi L, et al. Local denervation atrophy of paraspinal muscle in postoperative failed back syndrome. *Spine* 1993;18:575–581.

68. Dolan RA. Spinal adhesive arachnoiditis. *Surg Neurol* 1993;39: 479–484.

69. Styf J, Lysell E. Chronic compartment syndrome in the erector spinae muscle. *Spine* 1987; 12:680–682.

70. Fisher MA, Kaur D, Houchin J. Electrodiagnostic examination, back pain, and entrapment of posterior rami. *Electromyogr Clin Neurophysiol* 1985;25: 183–189.

71. Saal JA, Dillingham MF, Gamburd RS, Fanton GS. The pseudo radicular syndrome: lower extremity peripheral nerve entrapment masquerading as lumbar radiculopathy. *Spine* 1988;13: 926–930.

72. Maigne JY, Guedj S, Straus C. Idiopathic coccygodynia—lateral roentgenograms in the sitting position and coccygeal discography. *Spine* 1994;19: 930–944.

73. Deyo RA, Rainville J, Kent DL. The rational clinical examination: what can the history and physical examination tell us about low back pain? *JAMA* 1992;268: 760–765.

74. Parker H, Wood PLR, Main CJ. The use of the pain drawing as a screening measure to predict psychological distress in chronic low back pain. *Spine* 1994;20: 236–243.

75. Mann NH, Brown MD, Enger I. Expert performance in low-back disorder recognition using patient pain drawings. *J Spinal Disord* 1992;5:254–259.

76. Liang M, Komaroff AL. Roentgenograms in primary care patients with acute low back pain: a cost effective analysis. *Arch Intern Med* 1982;142: 1108–1112.

77. Scavone JG, Latshaw RF, Widener WA. Anteroposterior and lateral radiographs: an adequate lumbar spine examination. *Am J Radiol* 1991;136:715–717.

78. Janssen ME, Bertrand SL, Joe C, Levine MI. Original research: lumbar herniated disk disease: comparison of MRI, myelography, and post-myelographic CT scan with surgical findings. *Orthopedics* 1994;17:121–127.

79. Modic MT, Masaryk T, Boumphrey F, et al. Lumbar herniated disk disease and canal stenosis: prospective evaluation by surface coil MR, CT and myelography. *AJR Am J Roentgenogr* 1986; 147:757–765.

80. Knuttson B. Comparative value of electromyographic, myelography, and clinical neurological examination in the diagnosis of lumbar root compression syndrome. *Acta Orthop Scand Suppl* 1961;49: 1–133.

81. Haig AJ, LeBreck DB, Powley SG. Paraspinal mapping: quantified needle electromyography in persons without low back pain. *Spine* 1995;20:715–721.

82. Haig AJ. Clinical experience with paraspinal mapping II: a simplified technique that eliminates three fourths of needle insertions. *Arch Phys Med Rehabil* 1997; 78:1185–1190.

83. Antti-Poika I, Soini J, Tallroth K, et al. Clinical relevance of discography combined with CT scanning: a study of 100 patients. *J Bone Joint Surg* [Br] 1990;72:480–484.

84. Weinstein J. The pain of discography. *Spine* 1988;13: 1344–1348.

85. Fortin JD, Dwyer AP, West S, Pier J. Sacroiliac joint pain referral maps upon applying a new injection/arthrography technique: part I: asymptomatic volunteers. *Spine* 1994;19:1475–1482.

86. Fortin JD, Aprill CN, Ponthieux B, Pier J. Sacroiliac joint: pain referral maps upon applying a new injection/arthrography technique: part II: clinical evaluation. *Spine* 1994;19:1483–1489.

87. Haveisen DC, Smith BS, Myers SR, Pryce MC. The diagnostic accuracy of spinal nerve injection studies: their role in the evaluation of recurrent sciatica. *Clin Orthop* 1985;198:179–183.

88. Donelson R. The McKenzie approach to evaluating and treating low back pain. *Orthop Rev* 1990;19:681–686.

89. Saal JA. Dynamic muscular stabilization in the nonoperative treatment of lumbar pain syndromes. *Orthop Rev* 1990;19:691–700.

90. Koes BW, Bouter LM, Beckerman H, et al. Physiotherapy exercises and back pain: a blinded review. *BMJ* 1991;302:1572–1576.

91. Thomas KB. General practice consultations: is there any point in being positive? *BMJ* 1987; 294:1200–1202.

92. Catchlove R, Cohen K. Effects of a directive return to work approach in the treatment of workman's compensation patients with chronic pain. *Pain* 1982; 14:181–191.

93. Haig AJ, Linton P, McIntosh M, et al. Aggressive early medical management by a specialist in physical medicine and rehabilitation: effect on lost time due to injuries in hospital employees. *J Occup Med* 1990;32:241–244.

94. Linton SJ, Kamwendo K. Low back schools: a critical review. *Phy Ther* 1987;67:1375–1383.

95. Thomas LK, Hislop HJ, Waters RL. Physiological work performance in chronic low back disability: effects of a progressive activity program. *Phy Ther* 1980;60:407–411.

96. Sachs BL, David JF, Olimpio D, et al. Spinal rehabilitation by work tolerance based on objective physical capacity assessment of dysfunction: a prospective study with control subjects and twelve month review. *Spine* 1990; 15:1325–1332.

97. Mayer TG, Gatchel RJ, Mayer H, et al. A prospective two-year study of functional restoration in industrial low back injury: an objective assessment procedure. *JAMA* 1987;258:1763–1782.

98. Hazard RG, Fenwick JW, Kalisch SM, et al. Functional restoration with behavioral support: a one-year prospective study of patients with chronic low-back pain. *Spine* 1989;14:157–161.

99. Teasell RN, Harth M. Functional restoration: returning patients with chronic low back pain to work: revolution or fad? *Spine* 1996;21:844–847.

100. Rissanen A, Alaranta H, Sainio P, Harkonen H. Isokinetic and non-dynamometric tests in low back pain patients related to pain and disability index. *Spine* 1994; 19:1963–1967.

101. Pedersen DM, Clark JA, Johns RE, et al. Quantitative muscle strength testing: a comparison of job strength requirements and actual worker strength among military technicians. *Mil Med* 1989;154:14–18.

102. Cady LD, Bischoff DP, O'Connell ER, et al. Strength and fitness and subsequent back injuries in fire fighters. *J Occup Med* 1979;21:169–172.

103. American Medical Association. *Guides to the evaluation of permanent impairment.* 3rd ed, revised. Chicago: American Medical Association, 1990.

104. Gill K, Drag MH, Johnson GB, et al. Repeatability of four clinical methods for assessment of lumbar spinal motion. *Spine* 1988;13:50–53.

105. Lowe TG. Scheuermann's disease. *J Bone Joint Surg [Am]* 1990;72:940–945.

106. Carey TS, Garrett J, Jackman A, et al. The outcomes and costs of care for acute low back pain among patients seen by primary care practitioners, chiropractors, and orthopedic surgeons. *N Engl J Med* 1995;333:913–917.

Chapter 60

Cervical Pain

Susan J. Dreyer
Andrew J. Cole

Neck pain is a common and often misunderstood complaint among both the able-bodied and the disabled populations. There are many causes of neck pain and practitioners must be able to use their knowledge of cervical anatomic structures and innervation to discern the precise cause of a patient's neck pain. Visceral causes of neck pain rarely result in neck pain alone and are usually accompanied by other characteristic features. Differentiating visceral from musculoskeletal neck pain is usually straightforward. Potentially painful musculoskeletal structures include the bones, muscles, ligaments, facet (zygapophyseal) joints, and intervertebral disks. Neural structures including the dorsal root ganglia and nerve roots can also mediate pain. Cervical muscles may be sprained or torn, resulting in both neck and referred pain (1). The occipitoatlantal (OA), atlantoaxial (AA), and cervical facet joints can also cause both axial and referred pain (2–6). In addition, the cervical disks have been implicated as cervical pain generators (7–10). Despite these various (and often overlapping) pain patterns, neck pain complaints are often attributed to "cervical spondylosis." However, neck pain can occur in the absence of cervical spondylosis (11) and cervical spondylosis can occur in the absence of neck pain (12). Furthermore, the radiographic changes of spondylosis occur almost equally among individuals with neck pain symptoms and asymptomatic persons (13). Understanding potential diagnoses is critical to optimizing intervention and outcomes.

The exact prevalence of neck pain is unknown, as it is often included along with back pain in studies of spinal pain or with shoulder pain because of their shared referral zones. Studies of Swedish forest and industrial workers 15 to 49 years old found a prevalence of 35% to 71% (14,15). Other authors surveying the general adult population (ages 18–65) found 18% suffered from neck and/or shoulder pain (16). A similar 1-year prevalence of 16% to 18% was noted in a Finnish study (17). The frequency of neck problems increases with age (16–18). Degenerative changes of the spine have been noted in 30 year olds and are ubiquitous by age 70 (19). Physically demanding jobs are also associated with an increase in neck complaints (16).

This chapter focuses on the anatomy and biomechanics of the cervical spine in the context of common cervical conditions including muscular strains, ligamentous sprains, facet joint injuries, cervical disk injuries, and cervical spondylosis. The neck is designed to allow maximal flexibility while still providing stability and protection of the vital neural and vascular structures passing between the body and the head. It is imperative that clinicians understand the structure of the neck and cervical spine in order to fully understand the diseases, injuries, and degenerative conditions that affect it.

A thorough discussion of all cervical diagnoses and treatment is beyond the scope of this chapter. For more detailed reviews, the reader is referred to Chapter 61 for myofascial pain, Chapter 64 for neck pain in sports and performing arts, Chapters 23 and 24 for physical agents and modalities, Chapter 25 for injection techniques, and Chapter 26 for therapeutic exercise.

FUNCTIONAL ANATOMY AND BIOMECHANICS

The seven cervical vertebrae and their supporting elements provide the stability and flexibility needed to control motion and distribute forces applied to the spine while allowing safe passage of delicate neural and vascular structures. The cervical vertebrae increase in size with caudal progression, to help support increasing loads but remain smaller than their thoracic and lumbar counterparts (20,21). Although the vertebral bodies are relatively small in the cervical region, the spinal canal is more capacious at the cervical vertebral level than at any other part of the spine. Within the cervical spine the transverse diameter generally decreases with caudal progression; the sagittal diameter generally decreases slightly from C1 to C3 and then remains relatively constant. Lateral radiographs allow for an estimation of canal diameter and the diagnosis of congenital spinal stenosis (22,23).

The First Cervical Vertebra

The first and second cervical vertebrae are unique in both appearance and function, whereas the third, fourth, fifth, sixth, and seventh cervical vertebrae are similar (24–27). The first cervical vertebrae, the *atlas*, is a ring of bone composed primarily of an anterior arch, lateral masses, posterior arch, and bilateral inward projections of bone called *tubercles* that give rise to the transverse ligament. The atlas lacks a vertebral body, its ring-like structure functions as a "washer" between the occiput and C2 (26). Weight bearing occurs through the right and left lateral masses (24,26,28,29). A compressive force to the head while the cervical spine is straight may lead to a burst fracture of C1, a *Jefferson fracture*, or to a burst fracture of the lower cervical spine. If the neck is flexed and compressed at the time of injury, disruption of the posterior ligament occurs and may lead to an unstable segment. Hyperflexion injuries may cause either unstable "teardrop" fractures of the anterior inferior corner of the vertebral body or typically stable wedge compression fractures. If rotational forces are added to the flexion force, "jumped" or locked facet(s) may result. Hyperextension may result in fracture of the posterior arch of C1.

The superior kidney-shaped concave facet surfaces of C1 face upward and inward to support and articulate with the paired convex occipital condyles, which face downward and outward (24–26,30). Active flexion around the transverse axis of the OA joint has a 15-degree range, whereas active extension has a range of 20 degrees. This OA flexion and extension represent approximately 50% of all flexion and extension occurring in the cervical spine (31) and can be pictured as the nodding that occurs around an imaginary axis through the ears. Impingement of the anterior margin of the foramen magnum on the dens creates a bony limit to further flexion. Side bending of approximately 5 degrees occurs around a sagittal axis. Minor amounts of active rotation may also occur and have been reported to be up to 8 degrees (26,27,32–36). The OA joint configuration, its capsule, the ligamentum nuchae, the tectorial membrane, the alar, and possibly apical ligaments all provide stability for the OA joint (27). In general, the ligaments of the cervical spine provide both stability and significant proprioceptive feedback during physiologic motion; they also help absorb energy during trauma (37,38).

The Second Cervical Vertebra

The second cervical vertebra, the *axis*, has a large body that projects cephalad as the odontoid process, also called the *dens*. The dens is the phylogenetically displaced body of the atlas and serves as a pivot around which the atlas rotates. The transverse ligament confines the odontoid process to the anterior third of the atlantal ring, permitting free rotation of the atlas on the dens and axis as well as ensuring stability during flexion, extension, and lateral bending (39). Rupture of the transverse ligament results in an unstable cervical spine and possibly death if the dens moves posteriorly and impinges on the spinal cord. The C1–C2 joint is further stabilized by the right and left alar ligaments, which connect the lateral aspect of the apex of the dens to the ipsilateral medial aspect of the occipital condyle and anchor the skull to the axis. They help control excessive lateral and rotational motions, but not flexion or extension. The alar ligaments provide the next line of support against any further anterior translation of the atlas on the axis after rupture of the transverse ligament. If the alar ligaments fail, there remains no other significant barrier to prevent spinal cord compression (24,40–42). Rupture of the transverse ligament should be suspected if the transverse diameter of the atlas is 7 mm or greater than the transverse diameter of the axis on an anteroposterior open-mouth projection of C1–C2. (27,43). A severe cervical flexion injury may cause an AA dislocation and rupture of the transverse and alar ligaments. Without ligamentous restraints, the atlas may translate anteriorly, resulting in impingement of the spinal cord between the odontoid process and the posterior rim of the atlas. Normally the alar ligaments also function to limit rotation between C1 and C2 (44). "Hangman's fracture" involves fracturing the pedicles of C2, often with anterior displacement of the body of C2 in relation to C3. Other extension injuries include the unstable hyperextension sprain often accompanied by extensive spinal cord damage with little change on radiographs other than prevertebral soft-tissue swelling.

The AA joint allows for 40% to 50% of bilateral rotation, nearly half of the rotation provided in the cervical spine. The OA and AA joints provide roughly 60% of the axial rotation of the entire cervical spine (45,46). The mobility of the AA joint is the greatest of any joint in the spine (24–26). The large amount of rotation that occurs at the AA joint can result in traction or kinking of a vertebral artery.

The transverse processes of C1 through C6, and usually C7 have transverse foramina that house and protect the vertebral arteries. With rotation to or beyond 30 degrees, kinking of the contralateral vertebral artery may occur, and with rotation to 45 degrees, the ipsilateral vertebral artery may also kink, resulting in reduced circulation to the brain stem and upper spinal cord (29,45,47,48). Kinking and consequent reduced circulation may develop because of trauma (49), inappropriate cervical manipulation (20,47,50), cervical traction (12), cervical degenerative joint disease, or a therapeutic exercise that creates a rotational subluxation or dislocation of the atlas on the axis (47,49).

The Lower Cervical Vertebrae

The third through seventh cervical vertebrae are similar in appearance and function. Table 60-1 summarizes the available range of motion for the middle and lower cervical segments. The vertebral bodies are ovoid and are wider than they are tall. The bilateral raised uncinate processes (or hooks) that are located posterolaterally correspond to similar beveled surfaces, located on the inferior aspect of the superior vertebral body. These "uncovertebral joints," also known as *joints of Luschka*, are not present in the embryologic development of the cervical spine but arise as a consequence of the degenerative and adaptive changes of anular tissue to loads and stresses (24–26). Hypertrophy may result in foraminal stenosis and radicular symptoms.

Cervical Intervertebral Disks

The cervical vertebrae are connected anteriorly by an intervertebral disk between adjacent levels. These disks, made of an outer annulus fibrosus and an inner nucleus pulposus, are biconvex and conform to the concavity of the vertebral bodies. Cervical disk height is greater anteriorly and thus contributes to normal cervical lordosis. The thickest disk is located at C6–C7. Only the outer one-third to one-half of the annular fibers in adults have a vascular supply. The remainder of the annulus and the entire nucleus pulposus are avascular. Nutrition of the inner annular fibers and the nucleus pulposus occurs by diffusion (39,51). The annular fibers that contain the disk are made up of 10 to 20 circumferential collagenous lamellae. Although the direction of inclination alternates with each lamella, the fibers within each lamella are oriented 35 degrees from the horizontal. Therefore, rotation and translation are more likely to injure the annulus because resistance can be offered only by half of the available lamellae—those with their fibers oriented in the direction of motion (51).

The annulus, particularly the middle third, is innervated by both nocioceptors and mechanoreceptors (52,53). Painful stimulation of the receptors is generated by structural disruption of the intervertebral disk or the chemically mediated inflammatory effect of phospholipase A_2. Proprioceptive information is thought to be transmitted by the pacinian corpuscles and Golgi tendon organs, which are particularly numerous in the posterolateral region of the outer third of the annulus (23,39,51,53–56). The intervertebral disk transmits compressive loads throughout a range of motion, but it prevents excessive stress concentrations by slowing the rate at which an applied force is transmitted

Table 60-1: Active Range of Motion of the Cervical Spine

	Combined Flexion/Extension (± x-axis rotation)		One-Side Lateral Bending (z-axis rotation)		One-Side Axial Rotation (y-axis rotation)	
Interspace	Limits of Ranges (degrees)	Representative Angle (degrees)	Limits of Ranges (degrees)	Representative Angle (degrees)	Limits of Ranges (degrees)	Representative Angle (degrees)
Middle						
C2–C3	5–16	10	11–20	10	0–10	3
C3–C4	7–26	15	9–15	11	3–10	7
C4–C5	13–29	20	0–16	11	1–12	7
Lower						
C5–C6	13–29	20	0–16	8	2–12	7
C6–C7	6–26	17	0–17	7	2–10	6
C7–T1	4–7	9	0–17	4	0–7	2

Sources: Reproduced by permission from Stratton SA, Bryan JM. Dysfunction, evaluation, and treatment of the cervical spine and thoracic inlet. In: Donatelli B, Wooden M, eds. *Orthopaedic physical therapy.* 2nd ed. New York: Churchill Livingstone, 1983:77–102.

through the cervical spine. The disk diverts some of the force by temporarily stretching annular fibers and thus protects each of the underlying vertebrae from receiving the entire force at one time. Stress concentrations are also minimized by a posterior nuclear shift during flexion and an anterior nuclear shift during extension (21,30,39,51).

Facet Joints

Posterolaterally the cervical segments are connected by facet or zygapophyseal joints. Their fibrous capsules are lined with synovium and their articular surfaces covered with hyaline cartilage. The facet capsule is richly innervated by both nocioceptors and mechanoreceptors. There are even more mechanoreceptors in the cervical facet capsules than in their lumbar counterparts, thus enhancing cervical proprioception (39,51,57). The orientation of the cervical facet joints provides resistance to anterior translation and assists in weight bearing (39,58,59). From C2–C3, the facet joints' articular planes are oriented at approximately 45 degrees from the horizontal, and with caudal progression this inclination increases slightly. The articular planes of the facet joints are oriented 70 to 85 degrees to the sagittal plane. The C2–C3 facet is considered transitional anatomically and biomechanically, because it joins the upper cervical spine, allowing primarily rotation, and flexion and extension of the lower cervical spine (21,26,60). The limits and ranges of rotation of the middle and lower cervical regions of the spine are presented in Table 60-1. Cervical facet menisci are thought to help transmit load by increasing the surface area of contact when articular facets come together (51,61,62). With age the meniscus narrows and retracts between childhood and the fourth decade (63).

Ligaments

The principal ligaments supporting the middle and lower portions of the cervical spine include the posterior and anterior longitudinal ligaments (PLL and ALL), the interspinous ligament, the ligamentum nuchae, and the ligamentum flavum. The ALL runs along the anterior surface of the vertebral column from the sacrum to the axis, where it then merges with the anterior AO membrane. The PLL is located along the posterior surface of the vertebral bodies and also runs the length of the spine. The PLL is widest in the cervical spine and becomes the tectorial membrane proximal to the atlas. The tectoral membrane attaches to the clivus and basilar portion of the occipital bone. The anterior and posterior longitudinal ligaments provide significant stability to the intervertebral joints. The PLL limits flexion and distraction (21,25,46). The articulations between the vertebral arches are maintained by the supraspinous ligaments; the interspinous ligaments, which are poorly developed in the cervical spine; and the segmental ligamentum flavum. The supraspinous ligament evolves into the ligamentum nuchae. Both the ligamentum nuchae and interspinous ligaments limit flexion and anterior horizontal displacement. Because it has a great deal of elastic tissue, the ligamentum flavum also helps limit flexion of the cervical spine (21,29,46,64,65). The anterior and posterior longitudinal ligaments and the interspinous ligaments have a nerve supply that may be similar to their lumbar counterparts (66–68). The ligamentum flavum does not have a nerve supply (44).

Cervical Spinal Cord and Nerves

The cervical spinal cord is somatotopically arranged. This arrangement facilitates the diagnosis of upper motor neuron injury. A regular series of dorsal rootlets, or fila, arises from the dorsolateral sulcus of the spinal cord, and a less regular series of ventral rootlets arises from the ventrolateral aspect of the spinal cord. These rootlets form the dorsal and ventral spinal nerve roots, respectively. To help stabilize the spinal cord, the denticulate ligaments anchor lateral expansions of the pia mater surrounding the spinal cord to the internal aspect of the dural sac. The dorsal and ventral roots are also invested with pia mater and are surrounded by an arachnoid sleeve, which is inside the overlying dural sleeve. These two roots are enclosed within a funnel-shaped dural sac that tapers toward the intervertebral foramen. The dorsal and ventral nerve roots become separately enclosed in arachnoid and dural sleeves at the entrance to the foramen. At the level of the dorsal root ganglion, which is located near the outer orifice or just lateral to the foramen, the arachnoid layer ends and thus allows spinal fluid within the subarachnoid space to surround the nerve slightly past the interforaminal level (24,44,69). The mixed spinal nerve has only a dural sheath that then blends imperceptibly into the epineurium. The epineurium gives rise to the perineurium and endoneurium. These tissues invest the spinal nerve and provide it with structural integrity. The dorsal and ventral roots within the dural sheath are supported only by the pia mater that surrounds them. The spinal nerves divide into anterior and posterior rami.

The cervical posterior rami supply the intrinsic spinal musculature and the overlying skin. The fifth through eighth cervical anterior primary rami and first thoracic anterior primary rami form the brachial plexus. The epineurium of the fourth, fifth, and sixth cervical anterior primary rami is anchored to the periosteum of the transverse processes at the same level, and one level above, the fascial prolongation of the PLL, the scalene muscle group, and the adventitial coating of the vertebral artery fix the spinal nerve against the transverse process (24,44,70–72).

Burners and *stingers* describe the most common athletic neurologic injury and are most frequently caused by traction forces that increase the acromion to head distance, resulting in traction to the cervical roots or the brachial plexus. Although less common, burners and stingers may also be caused by compression created by dynamic narrowing of the neural foramen with cervical extension, lateral bending, or rotation and axial loading (20,70). Normal cervical anatomy affords two distinct mechanisms that protect nerves from moderate traction injury. With lateral traction, the funnel-shaped dural sac impacts into the inner aspect of the intervertebral foramen, providing resistance to further lateral displacement of the nerve (24,44,70,72). Another way the nerve is protected is by the anchoring of the epineurium to the transverse processes, PLL, and the scalene muscle groups. This anchoring also provides resistance to lateral traction forces (24,44,70,72). Because it lacks a perineurium, the weakest portion of the peripheral nerve is located at the junction of the spinal cord with the dorsal and ventral rootlets. If traction forces are excessive, nerve rootlet avulsion, a preganglionic lesion, can occur. Unlike postganglionic lesions, which are amenable to surgical repair, preganglionic lesions have no significant possibility of successful surgical repair (42).

Cervical Muscles

The muscles that create cervical spine movement can be divided into three functional groups: 1) capital movers, which flex and extend the head; 2) cervical movers, which flex and extend the cervical spine; and 3) the rotators and lateral flexors (44,73). Table 60-2 lists these muscle groups. The *capital flexors* flex the head on the neck. The *capital extensors* attach to the skull and move the head on the neck (25,44,74). The *cervical flexors*, flex the cervical spine. The *cervical extensors* originate on the cervical spine and attach to the cervical spine and upper thoracic vertebrae and ribs (24–26). They can extend the cervical spine and alter its curvature (44,74,75).

The main mass of the extensor groups overlie the AA area as well as the C6–T1 levels, and the bulk of flexor muscle groups are at the C4–C5 level; these muscle groups are thought to be at sites of major stress (76). The muscles that rotate and laterally flex the cervical spine are listed in Table 60-2 (25,74).

Motion of the lower cervical spine occurs in conjunction with that of the upper thoracic spine. Cervical spine motion mediated by the splenius, longissimus, semispinalis cervicis, and semispinalis capitis creates stress and motion of the upper thoracic spine from T1 to T6 because of their distal attachment to these vertebrae (26,74). This may be one reason why cervical spine dysfunction, particularly postural abnormalities, can create thoracic spine dysfunction and pain, and vice versa.

Table 60-2: Muscles Controlling and Neck Head Motion

Capital extensors
- Rectus capitis posterior minor
- Rectus capitis posterior major
- Obliquus capitis superior
- Obliquus capitis inferior
- Longissimus capitis
- Semispinalis capitis
- Splenius capitis

Cervical extensors
- Splenius cervicis
- Longissimus cervicis
- Semispinalis cervicis

Capitol flexors
- Longus capitis
- Rectus capitis anterior and lateralis
- Hyoid
- Suprahyoid

Cervical flexors
- Sternocleidomastoid
- Scalenus anterior and medius

Cervical rotators and lateral flexors
- Sternocleidomastoid
- Scalenus (anterior, medius, and posterior)
- Splenus capitis
- Splenus cervicis
- Longissimus capitis
- Levator scapulae
- Longus colli
- Iliocostalis cervicis
- Multifidi
- Intertransversarii
- Obliquus capitis inferior and lateralis

Degenerative Changes and Biomechanics

The primary biomechanical function of the neck is to support the head and provide the ability to position the head in space. Trauma and the normal degenerative process can compromise a cervical motion segment's biomechanical properties that handle applied forces. Cervical spondylosis is found most often at the C5–C6 level, followed by the C6–C7 and C4–C5 levels (12). Spondylosis may result in central or foraminal stenosis, progressive thinning of the facet joint articular cartilage, sclerosis, and reactive bone formation of the facet joints. In spondylosis the annulus may become stiff and break down with changes in the annular collagen type. Annular fissures and herniated nucleus pulposus may then occur (77,78). Herniated disks are most often found posterolaterally where the rate of curvature of the annulus is greatest. Recall that the annulus is thicker anteriorly. Anterior vertebral body traction spurs, posterior vertebral body osteophytes and bony bar formation, osteophytosis of the uncovertebral joints, thickening of the ligamentum flavum, and calcification of the PLL are other degenerative changes that may compromise normal cervical biomechanics (13,42,59,79–82). Exercise may promote improved diskal nutrition and collagen alignment, strength, and flexibility. Exercise may also improve muscular strength and flexibility. All of these factors can protect the motion segment from applied forces (83,84).

DIAGNOSIS

The spectrum of cervical spine injuries ranges from simple muscle strains and ligamentous sprains to potentially fatal bone and neurovascular injuries. The most common presenting complaint in cervical injuries is neck pain; however, some cervical problems present as referred pain such as interscapular pain or with neurologic changes such as numbness and weakness. A careful history and detailed physical examination along with judicious use of ancillary tests such as magnetic resonance imaging (MRI) and electrodiagnostic studies are the keys to accurate diagnosis of cervical disorders. A precise diagnosis facilitates an effective treatment plan.

History

The diagnosis of musculoskeletal neck pain begins with triaging the presenting signs and symptoms to quickly identify any life-threatening injuries (e.g., an unstable cervical spine fracture). Once the patient has been determined to be safe from immediate harm, additional historical information should be gathered to help narrow the diagnostic possibilities (Table 60-3). Duration of symptoms, mechanism of onset (traumatic, atraumatic), exact location and quality of pain, history of similar pain in the past, constitutional symptoms, past medical history, age, social history, and family history will guide the diagnostic thought process. With likely diagnoses in mind, one proceeds to the clinical examination. The physical examination focuses on three areas: the patient's presentation (abnormal postures, guarding, pain behavior, etc), a detailed neurologic examination, and a careful segmental examination of the neck.

Shoulder complex pain syndromes may easily be confused with pain emanating from the cervical spine. Acromioclavicular joint synovitis may recreate C5 pain. Subacromial bursitis may mimic C5 or C6 pain patterns. A rotator cuff tear may mimic neurologic loss associated with C5 or C6 root lesions. Glenohumeral joint synovitis associated with osteoarthritis or adhesive capsulitis may be felt in any radicular pattern. Abnormal neural tissue tension also may be a source of pain and can mimic almost any cervical pain pattern, particularly a radiculopathy (85). These lesions can usually be differentiated from cervical sources of pain given a careful history, physical examination, response to physical therapy, and possibly differential contrast-enhanced fluoroscopically guided injections. The subacromial bursa, acromioclavicular joint, glenohumeral joint, cervical facet, cervical nerve root, or cervical epidural space may be targeted in varying combinations, depending on the physician's working diagnosis (40,86,87).

Table 60-3: Historical Red Flags

Finding	Possible Implication
Fever and weight loss	Infection, tumor
Night pain with recumbency	Spinal cord tumor
Morning stiffness >1 hr	Spondyloarthropathy, rheumatoid arthritis
Acute localized bone pain	Fracture, bone tumor

Vascular injuries in the cervical spine may result iatrogenically (27,29,45,47,48,88,89,90), from cervical athletic trauma (90a), or from cervical spondylosis (62). An acute hyperextension injury, occurring in football (90a), soccer, rugby, and equestrian sports, for example, may produce vertebral artery ischemia or thrombosis. Momentary feelings of paralysis or tingling of the limbs may occur. Compression and spasm of the spinal arteries may produce acute paralysis, numbness, and tingling in the lower limbs and then in the upper limbs. The athlete may recover even before being transported from the field (90a). The vertebral arteries are most vulnerable at the OA area by hyperextension and compression injuries (91–93). Brief neurologic brain stem signs and symptoms secondary to vasospasm as well as cervicomedullary infarction and death due to thrombosis have been reported (83,91). A transient ischemic attack or stroke in the internal carotid–middle cerebral artery region may develop if these arterial systems are injured by extreme cervical lateral flexion, or extension or by a direct blow to the anterolateral part of the neck (91). A automobile's shoulder harness restraint that is improperly positioned (allowed to ride over the neck rather than shoulder region) may also cause direct trauma to the internal carotid artery.

Although burners and stingers have already been discussed, one further point deserves mention. If avulsion of the first thoracic nerve rootlets from the spinal cord occurs, interruption of the preganglionic *sympathetic fibers* that supply the eye can occur. The ocular portion of Horner syndrome may result (24). Other problems that can mimic cervical pain or refer pain to the cervical region include *thoracic outlet syndrome*, *thoracic facet* or *costovertebral joint synovitis*, *spinal cord tumors*, *lung pathology*, and *upper-extremity peripheral nerve entrapments* (40,79,94,95).

Physical Examination

Inspection of the patient's habitus and behavior provides valuable clues to potential etiologies of the neck pain. Postural abnormalities such as a forward-thrust head and rounded shoulders place strain on the posterior muscles and ligaments. Acute torticollis is often visible upon first entering the room. Inconsistency between functional activities such as turning to address the physician who has just moved across the room and range of motion testing during the physical examination point toward symptom amplification or malingering. Inspection for symmetry may identify atrophy and possibly fasciculations. Atrophy may result from either disuse due to pain or from denervation. Thus, even before touching the patient for the physical examination, the astute clinician is able to gather important information regarding the patient's condition.

Range of Motion

Accurate assessment of cervical range of motion requires radiographic evaluation (96). Clinically accepted estimates of range of motion utilize a single or double inclinometer method (97). Normal cervical active range of motion includes 60 degrees of flexion, 75 degrees of extension, 45 degrees of side bending or lateral flexion bilaterally, and 80 degrees of rotation bilaterally. Essentially if a patient is able to touch his or her chin to the chest with the mouth closed, gaze upward positioning the face almost horizontal to the ground, touch the ears to the neutral shoulder, and turn the head so the chin contacts each shoulder, the cervical range of motion is normal (98).

Palpation

Palpation of the neck is best achieved with the patient supine and the examiner standing behind the patient's head. The examiner cups his or her hands to support the neck while allowing the fingertips to meet in the midline. It is important to elicit the patient's cooperation and relaxation. Starting in the midline just below the ridge of the skull, C2 is the first spinous process encountered. The spinous process of C1 is typically not palpable owing to its small size and position deep in the soft tissues. The spinous processes of C3–C6 are examined by palpating the successive boney projections caudal to C2. Each is approximately a fingerbreadth below the more superior level. The vertebra prominens or the C7 spinous process is the largest and most prominent of the cervical spinous processes. The vertebra prominens moves with flexion and extension of the neck whereas the large T1 spinous process does not. A shift in the alignment of the cervical spinous processes may indicate fracture or dislocated facet joints. Significant, focal tenderness over one spinous process may indicate fracture or other boney lesion. Tenderness between the spinous process may reflect injury to the superior nuchal ligament, which runs from the inion of the skull to the C7 spinous process. At the base of the skull, the greater occipital nerves exit on each side of the inion. The greater occipital nerves may become inflamed and painful after trauma to the posterior part of the skull. Moving the fingers laterally, the cervical paraspinal muscles are encountered and any tenderness or local tissue texture changes are noted. Active and latent trigger points are sought. The fingers then move laterally where the facet joints may be palpated, approximately 1.5 cm off the midline between the semispinalis medially and the longissimus muscle laterally. Localized tenderness may be further assessed by gently gliding each segment below C2, assessing for restriction in lateral translation. The facets may also be palpated laterally. Lateral palpation is especially useful as there is less soft-tissue mass than on posterolateral palpation of the facet joints.

While the patient is still supine, the anterior neck structures may be assessed. Anterior palpation should be performed one side at a time to avoid bilateral interruption of cerebral flow in the setting of an occluded carotid artery. Any tenderness in the sternocleidomastoid and scalene muscles is noted. The anterior strap muscles (sternohyoid, sternothyroid, and omohyoid) are also examined. Deep behind the trachea and esophagus and anterior to the vertebral bodies lie the longus colli and longus capitis muscles. During deep anterior palpation, the cervical disks may be felt. Anterior landmarks include the horseshoe-shaped hyoid bone at the level of C3; the thyroid cartilage, commonly known as Adam's apple, at C4; and the first cricoid ring, which lies beneath the thyroid cartilage and is at the level of C6. Lateral to C6 is Chassaignac tubercle, an important landmark for stellate ganglion blocks and anterior surgery. While examining the anterior neck structures, one should note any unusual swelling such as lymphadenopathy, soft-tissue edema, or thyroid gland goiter.

Scapular and glenohumeral motion should also be tested to determine if any potential shoulder pathology is contributing to the patient's complaints. As previously discussed, it is not uncommon for neck pathology to present with pain radiating to the shoulder. At times, shoulder pathology also refers pain to the neck.

Neurologic Examination

All neck injuries require a detailed neurologic examination. Special attention is given to the synthesis of the potential injury level based on the physical findings. In addition to distinguishing normal from abnormal, the physician must determine how the abnormal findings are related: Has there been an injury to a single nerve root? Is there evidence of spinal cord damage? Table 60-4 lists the corresponding reflex, key muscle groups, and key sensory areas for each neurologic level. Pathologic reflexes such as the Hoffmann, Babinski, and inverted radial reflexes suggest an upper motor neuron injury. A positive jaw jerk implies that the injury is systemic or above the level of the spinal cord. The Spurling maneuver reproduces radicular symptoms into the upper extremity by applying a light compressive force (<10 lb) to a rotated and extended spine. This combination of rotation, extension, and compression narrows the intervertebral foramen and will intensify any symptoms due to compression of the spinal nerve root in the foramen. Spurling maneuvers are often positive in the setting of spinal stenosis and acute herniated disks.

Table 60-4: Neurologic Level

Neurologic Level	Reflex	Key Muscles/Motions	Key Sensory Zones
C5	Biceps	Deltoideus, biceps	Lateral brachium
C6	Brachioradialis	Wrist extension, biceps	Lateral antebrachium, thumb
C7	Triceps	Wrist flexion, grip	Middle finger
C8	None	Finger flexors, hand intrinsics	Medial antebrachium
T1	None	Interossei	Medial brachium

CERVICAL STRAINS AND SPRAINS

Muscular strain and *ligamentous sprains*, common noncatastrophic injuries, are often associated with a restriction of vertebral motion. A cervical strain is produced by an overload injury to the muscle-tendon unit due to excessive forces on the cervical spine.

Almost 85% of neck pain results from acute or repetitive neck injuries or chronic stresses and strain (99). Neck strain is really more of a clinical syndrome describing nonradiating neck pain associated with acute or static stresses. The etiology is believed to be elongation and tearing of muscles or ligaments. Secondary edema, hemorrhage, and inflammation may occur. Many cervical muscles do not terminate in tendons but instead attach directly to bone by myofascial tissue that blends into the periosteum (38). The response of the muscles to injury is contraction, with recruitment of surrounding muscles in an attempt to splint the injured muscle.

A forward head posture often causes cervical pain. Poor postural habits are usually acquired at a young age when the patient learns that slumping the thoracic spine requires no energy expenditure. With the thoracic spine flexed, the spinal balance is disrupted. The resulting forward-placed head creates chronic cervical pain and often drives a patient to attempt to compensate by thrusting the head farther forward, exacerbating the condition. This posture can be summarized as increased kyphosis of the thoracic spine, secondary increased lordosis of the cervical spine initially, and increased capital extension. This forward head posture results in muscle length adaptations that alter normal spinal biomechanics. Later, a decrease in midcervical lordosis results along with adaptive soft-tissue changes as capital extension is maintained. Over time, the body attempts to keep the eyes horizontal using greater capital extension (26,100–102). Normal motion undertaken in this poor postural environment produces abnormal muscular strain, particularly of the levator scapulae, upper trapezius, sternocleidomastoid, scalene, and suboccipital muscles. Other adaptations associated with this posture include a retruded mandible, rounded shoulders, and protracted scapulae with tight anterior muscles and stretched posterior muscles (26,90,103). Patients with these postural abnormalities may develop secondary *myofascial pain* that can cause referral zone pain (94).

A strain typically involves stretching or tearing of muscle fiber. With greater injury forces, a *somatic dysfunction* may result in vertebral motion restriction. The levels of restriction can be isolated with great accuracy by a skilled examiner (104,105). The pathomechanics of these restrictions are not known. Possible explanations include entrapment of synovial material or a meniscoid (61), hypertonic contracted musculature (9), changes in nervous reflex activity such as sympathicotonia (106) or gamma bias (107), and abnormal stresses on an unguarded spine (108). With extreme forces, fracture, dislocation, and neurologic injury may occur.

Patients with cervical strains present with complaints of neck pain, headache, and occasional extremity or chest pain. Typically the pain has a dull and aching quality and is aggravated by any motion. There may be guarding and limitation of motion due to the pain. Palpation nearly always reveals tenderness but no true spasm. The most commonly involved muscles are the upper trapezius and sternocleidomastoid muscles. Neurologic findings are normal. Radiographs typically appear normal or reveal only nonspecific straightening of the spine due to muscle contraction.

Treatment of neck sprain varies with the degree of pain. Physical modalities may be used to relax the muscles. Acetaminophen and nonsteroidal anti-inflammatory medications aid in controlling the pain. Muscle relaxants have a sedative effect, which can be useful in inducing sleep. Light cervical traction may reduce pain and diminish spasm. A cervical collar, worn especially at night when the patient is most at risk at placing the neck in a position of further strain, is often beneficial. Graduated return to activities should begin 2 to 4 weeks after the injury and the patient's exercise program should include strengthening. Physical therapy can be beneficial in reducing neck pain and improving mobility (109). Judicious use of trigger point injections of local anesthetic may be helpful in breaking reflex spasm and relieving pain. Treatment of cervical sprain and strains is nonsurgical. Most patients improve within 8 weeks. Whiplash injuries may require longer to heal and are discussed under facet injuries. If significant pain persists past 4 to 8 weeks, flexion and extension radiographs may be useful to exclude late instability. Occasionally a cervical sprain-strain can persist for months or years. A type of posttraumatic myofascial pain may result from an acute cervical sprain-strain.

MYOFASCIAL PAIN

Myofascial pain syndrome involves pain and autonomic responses referred from active myofascial *trigger points* (110) in the muscle. Myofascial trigger points are hyperirritable areas within a taut band of skeletal muscle or in the muscle's fascia that are painful on compression. Typically palpation of these trigger points causes pain in a predictable referral pattern. Normal muscle tissue does not exhibit these characteristics. Pressure over a trigger point may produce a pathognomonic twitch response, a visible contraction of the muscle. Myofascial trigger points are thought to begin after a muscular strain, with the affected area becoming a site of sensitized nerves with altered metabolism. Active trigger points cause pain, whereas latent trigger points restrict range of motion and produce weakness of the affected muscle without the patient being aware of the tender area until the examination. Latent trigger points may persist for years after a patient recovers from an injury and may become active and create acute pain in response to minor overstretching, overuse, or chilling of the muscle (26,111). For further discussion of myofascial pain and its treatment, the reader is referred to Chapter 61.

CERVICAL DISK INJURIES

Repetitive microtrauma or an excessive single load may injure a cervical disk via an *annular fissure* or *herniated nucleus pulposus* (HNP) (105). Depending on the size and location of the lesion, pain from the disk injury may result from inflammation (54,56) or compression of local nervous or vascular tissue (86). The pain may be radicular or axial, or both. Patients with an HNP without radiculopathy usually complain of neck and interscapular pain aggravated by cervical flexion or extension and relieved with traction (26,112–114). Lateral disk herniation may compress a cervical nerve root, resulting in radiculopathy. Radiculopathy may include pain radiating down the arm, paresthesias in a dermatomal pattern, weakness in the appropriate myotome, as well as associated changes of the reflexes. Radicular pain becomes worse with positional foraminal compression maneuvers and with cervical extension and rotation (i.e., Spurling maneuver). The pain of radiculopathy is often relieved with cervical traction (26,112–114). The annual incidence of cervical HNP with radiculopathy is 5.5 per 100,000 in Rochester, Minnesota (80). The peak incidence for cervical HNP is at the ages of 45 to 54 years; HNP is only slightly less common in the 35 to 44-year-old group. C5–C6 is the most commonly affected level, followed by C6–C7 and C4–C5. The combined prevalence of C5–C6 and C6–C7 HNPs accounts for 75% of cervical disk herniations (79,115). Of these disk herniations, 23% were attributed to a motor vehicle accident. Cigarette smoking and frequent lifting are associated with a higher risk of HNP (115).

Cervical radiculopathy must be differentiated from peripheral nerve entrapments: C6 radiculopathy must be differentiated from high median neuropathy; C8 radiculopathy, from ulnar neuropathy; C5 radiculopathy, from shoulder and hand tendinitis; and C6 or C7 radiculopathy, from DeQuervain and extensor tendinitis of the wrist (94). Carpal tunnel syndrome may mimic a cervical radiculopathy or may occur concomitantly as a "double crush" injury.

Patients with cervical disk herniations often report a history of neck pain for days to weeks prior to the onset of arm pain. As time passes, radicular complaints overshadow axial ones. Physical examination typically reveals a loss of range of motion and occasional torticollis with the head tilted toward the side of the disk herniation. If the disk herniation is causing radiculopathy, appropriate changes in reflex, strength, and sensory examinations may be noted (see Table 60-4). Manual muscle testing has greater specificity than reflex or sensory abnormalities (116). Radicular pain is often exacerbated by compression of the neural foramen (Spurling maneuver) and relieved by abduction of the affected arm (117).

Electromyography (EMG) may be useful in assessing for radiculopathy in patients with deficits of questionable neurologic origin. The accuracy of EMG is 80% to 90% and improves with the more classic presentation and findings on physical examination. False-negative EMG findings may occur if there is selective involvement of only the sensory fibers of the root, if the electromyographer fails to study the cervical paraspinal muscles and an adequate sampling of the peripheral muscles, or if the test is performed within the first 3 weeks after presentation.

Imaging of the cervical spine can confirm the clinical diagnosis. Plain radiographs may appear normal or show evidence of spondylosis. Cervical MRI allows for the best assessment of disk herniations. However, 19% of asymptomatic individuals may have abnormalities including disk protrusion (118).

Treatment of cervical disk herniation is primarily nonoperative. Rest and immobilization are important, usually requiring a few days of bed rest with bathroom privileges.

Typically the pain will begin to ease within 2 weeks of restricted activities. At that point it is important to taper use of the cervical orthotic and begin gentle reactivation. Most patients will be able to return to restricted-duty work. Medication includes nonsteroidal anti-inflammatory drugs, and muscle relaxants for their soporific effects. Occasionally a short course of oral narcotics is required. The need for narcotics can be minimized by adequate rest and patient education. Cervical traction can provide dramatic relief and consideration should be given to training the patient in the use of a home unit. With a unit at home, patients can use it two or three times a day for 15-minute sessions. The efficacy of traction has not been scientifically proved with a randomized controlled trial, but it is commonly used and thought to be of benefit (119). Therapeutic modalities may also provide temporary analgesia but should only be used acutely. Exercises begin with isometrics to prevent atrophy and progress to gentle stretching and finally strengthening. The use of a cervical pillow, a soft pillow tied in the middle with a ribbon to allow cradling of the neck, or a cervical collar at night often improves sleep. A patient's posture should be corrected and the patient should be taught to avoid prolonged static postures, especially those involving cervical extension.

Despite appropriate conservative care, approximately a small percentage of patients presenting with acute cervical radiculopathy will continue to have significant and debilitating arm pain and possibly persistent neurologic deficits. These patients should be referred for surgical consultation after a minimum of 6 weeks to 3 months of conservative care. Patients without neurologic deficit or significant arm pain do not benefit from surgical intervention over the long run (120).

CERVICAL MYELOPATHY

Posterior disk herniations often in combination with degenerative osteophytes may lead to compression of the spinal cord and result in cervical myelopathy. Patients with cervical myelopathy frequently have difficulties with balance and a stooped, wide-based, jerky gait. Spasticity is nearly uniformly present while radicular pain is present in about one-third of patients (121). Patients may experience loss of dexterity, nonspecific weakness, numbness, and paresthesias of the upper extremities. Bladder incontinence is uncommon. The Lhermitte sign may be present. Lower motor neuron deficits at the level of the cervical lesion and upper motor neuron signs below the lesion may be found on physical examination.

Lower-extremity symptoms may occur before upper-extremity difficulties. Patients often have trouble describing their symptoms but frequently report difficulty walking, peculiar sensations, spontaneous leg movement, shuffling of their feet, and fear of falling. The clinical presentation is often variable, depending on the number and location of levels involved (122,123). There are five cervical spondylotic myelopathic clinical syndromes: 1) lateral, causing radicular arm pain, often unilateral; 2) medial, presenting with bilateral lower-extremity involvement but no pain; 3) combined medial and lateral syndromes, upper-extremity radicular pain with lower-extremity clumsiness; 4) anterior, causing painless unilateral upper-extremity weakness; and 5) vascular, the least common. Symptoms generally begin insidiously in patients over 55 years old.

Cervical spinal cord neurapraxia may occur, particularly given certain predisposing factors that may cause the anteroposterior diameter of the spinal canal to narrow. These factors include developmental spinal stenosis, instability, HNP, and spondylosis. Hyperflexion or hyperextension injuries of the cervical spine may further decrease the size of an already stenotic central canal. These forced injuries may result in brief but abrupt mechanical compression of the spinal cord, causing transient interruption of motor or sensory function distal to the lesion. Both arms, both legs, or all four extremities may be involved. These bilateral findings help differentiate spinal cord neurapraxia from radiculopathy or from brachial plexus injury, both of which are almost always unilateral. By definition, the neurologic deficit associated with cervical spinal cord neurapraxia is transient and completely reversible (22,123,124).

Physical examination typically reveals hyperreflexia including positive Babinski and Hoffmann signs, and gait abnormalities of a stooped, wide-based shuffling pattern. Sensory changes usually involve the spinothalamic tract (pain temperature) or posterior columns (vibration and proprioception).

Radiographs often demonstrate advanced degenerative changes. Congenital stenosis should be assessed. The Pavlov ratio is the anteroposterior diameter of the canal divided by the anteroposterior diameter of the corresponding vertebral body. Values less than 0.8 suggest stenosis. If the Pavlov ratio is less than 0.8, stenosis should be excluded using more advanced imaging techniques such as computed tomograpy (CT) myelography or MRI. EMG and nerve conduction studies may be helpful to rule out myopathies and neuropathies. Somatosensory evoked potentials (SEPs) are typically abnormal.

Cervical myelopathy should be treated conservatively at first unless there has been rapid onset of symptoms or clear progression. However, only 50% of patients or fewer improve. Surgical decompression aims to halt the progression of the disease; recovery of neural function is variable (125,126).

Conservative therapy for cervical myelopathy includes immobilization in a rigid orthosis, rest, nonsteroidal anti-inflammatory medication, physical therapy avoiding aggressive stretching or manipulation, and occasionally epidural steroid injections (see Chap. 25).

Surgical intervention achieves better outcomes in the early stages of the disease as it aims to halt progression rather than restore neurologic function. Anterior cervical diskectomies, anterior corpectomies, and arthrodesis and posterior laminoplasty are all methods of decompressing the cervical spine. Cervical myelopathy is generally a slowly progressive disease with episodes of increased symptoms. Occasionally (approximately 20%) slow progression without remission is encountered. Only 5% to 15% of patients improve and the myelopathy does not progress (127–129).

CERVICAL FACET JOINT INJURIES

The cervical facet (zygapophyseal) joints are responsible for a significant portion of chronic neck pain. The first report on the prevalence of cervical facet pain in patients with chronic neck pain documented that 26% of the sample population achieved relief with zygapophyseal joint blocks, and estimated that up to 63% of the population whose joints had been investigated experienced painful cervical facet joints (130). A more recent study found the prevalence of chronic cervical facet pain after whiplash injuries to be 54% (131). Over 1 million whiplash injuries occur each year in the United States (132). Twenty percent to 40% of these patients with whiplash injuries experience symptoms that persist for years. It quickly becomes apparent that the cervical facet joint is a significant source of chronic neck pain. Established referral zones for the cervical facet joint (2,6) overlap both myofascial and diskogenic pain patterns (Fig. 60-1).

Cervical facet pain typically presents as unilateral, dull, aching neck pain with occasional referral into the occiput or interscapular regions, depending on the cervical facet joint injured. Neurologic findings should be normal. Palpation often reveals regional soft-tissue changes in

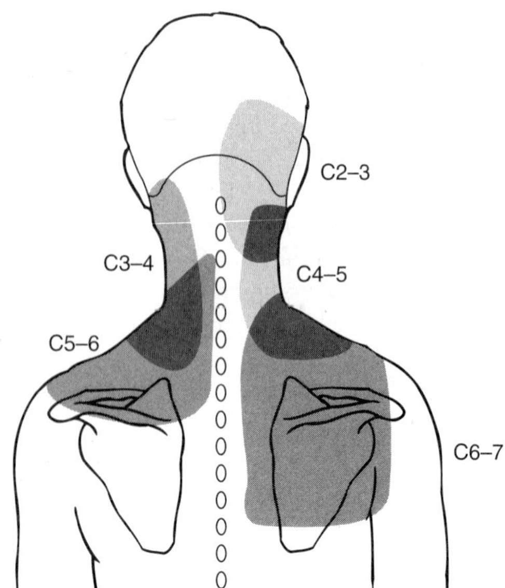

Figure 60-1. Composite map of the distribution of pain from cervical zygapophyseal joint injections. (Reproduced by permission from Dwyer A, Aprill C, Bogduk N. Cervical zygapophyseal joint pain patterns. 1: a study in normal volunteers. *Spine* 1990;15:453.)

response to the underlying injury. Palpation laterally along the facet joints will often reveal an area of focal tenderness and altered mechanics corresponding to the injured facet (133). Findings on traditional imaging studies (x-ray, MRI, CT scans) are typically unremarkable although incidental disk pathology may be noted. Presently clinical suspicion of facet injuries is best confirmed by diagnostic intra-articular facet injections or blockade of the facet nerve supply, that is, medial branch blocks (see Chap. 25) (131,134).

Treatment of cervical facet joint injuries remains controversial. Intra-articular corticosteroid injections for the treatment of whiplash facet pain are ineffective (104). Their potential use for more degenerative/inflammatory conditions of the spine needs to be determined by well-designed studies on carefully selected patient populations. Typical conservative care of cervical facet joint injuries without dislocation includes nonsteroidal anti-inflammatory drugs, postural exercises and education, use of a cervical pillow, active and passive stretching, positional releases and manual therapy, specific strengthening, and short-term judicious use of modalities to facilitate the above interventions. Unfortunately as in other cervical injuries, no studies on documented, isolated cervical facet pain exist to guide the practitioner through the most cost-effective and efficacious algorithm.

In patients with recalcitrant, disabling neck pain due to documented facet nociception, radiofrequency neurotomies of the medial branches may be an effective long-term pain control measure (135). Radiofrequency heat can be used to interrupt the innervation of the facet joint and thereby halt the noxious stimuli.

CERVICAL SPONDYLOSIS

Cervical spondylosis occurs gradually and as a result of aging. The C5–C6 segment is most commonly and severely involved. Over time the cervical intervertebral disk degenerates owing to loss of water content of the nucleus pulposus and loss of annulus fibrosus elasticity. These changes result in loss of the disk space height and narrowing of the foramen. If degeneration of the disk is accompanied by posterior disk protrusion, further compromise of the canal and roots may occur. The vascular supply also diminishes. Over time these changes result in irregular transmission of forces though that segment and secondary injury to the ligaments and facet joint complex. Instability of the segment stimulates osteophyte growth as the body tries to fuse or stabilize the injured area.

Cervical spondylosis typically presents in patients over 40 years old with neck or referred pain without known antecedent trauma. Headaches are common, especially if the upper cervical segments are involved. Approximately 15% of subjects may present with tinnitus or vertigo and 5% may give a history of syncope due to vertebrobasilar insufficiency (121).

Physical findings are typically fairly normal. At times a restriction in cervical range of motion is noted. Palpation usually reveals midline tenderness. Radiographs are positive for cervical spondylosis in 70% of persons over 70 years old (136), but there is no correlation between radiographic abnormalities and symptoms (137–139). MRI is usually not indicated, partially because of its high false-positive rates. One study found degenerative cervical disks in 62% of asymptomatic persons over 40 years. However, no degenerative disks were noted in persons younger than 30 years (140). The diagnosis of cervical spondylosis is one of exclusion.

Treatment for cervical spondylosis includes use of a cervical orthosis for a few days, activity modifications, oral nonsteroidal anti-inflammatory drugs, ergonomic evaluation of daily activities and work, isometric exercise, moist heat applied at home, and possibly facet joint injections in combination with an exercise program. Surgery is generally not indicated.

CONCLUSIONS

Neck pain is a complex, subjective experience with a variety of musculoskeletal causes that generally can be treated nonoperatively. Accurate diagnosis rests heavily on a careful history and physical examination. Imaging studies are important tools used to support or refute a suspected diagnosis. Treatment of musculoskeletal neck pain generally follows rehabilitative principles: Functional deficits are identified, realistic goals set, and a multifaceted treatment program is initiated to control pain and to restore range of motion, strength, and function.

REFERENCES

1. Feinstein B, Langton JNK, Jameson RM, et al. Experiments on pain referred from deep somatic tissues. *J Bone Joint Surg [Am]* 1954;36:981–997.
2. Aprill C, Dwyer A, Bogduk N. Cervical zygapophyseal joint pain patterns. II: a clinical evaluation. *Spine* 1990;15:458.
3. Busch E, Wilson PR. Atlanto-occipital and atlanto-axial injections in the treatment of headache and neck pain. *Reg Anesth* 1989;14(S2):45.
4. Dreyfus P, Stratton S. The use of the low energy laser, electroacuscope, and neuroprobe in sports medicine: a current review. *Physician Sportsmed* 1993;21:47–56.
5. Dreyfuss P, Rogers J, Dreyer S, et al. Atlanto-occipital joint pain: a report of three cases and description of an intraarticular block technique. *Reg Anesth* 1994;19:344–351.
6. Dwyer A, Aprill C, Bogduk N. Cervical zygapophyseal joint pain patterns. I: a study in normal volunteers. *Spine* 1990; 15:453.
7. Cloward RB. Cervical diskography: a contribution to the etiology and mechanism of neck, shoulder and arm pain. *Ann Surg* 1959;150:1052–1064.
8. Hodgkinson A. Neck pain localisation by cervical disc stimulation and treatment by anterior interbody fusion. *J Bone Joint Surg [Br]* 1979;52:789.
9. Janda V. Muscles, central nervous regulation and back problems. In: Korr IM, ed. *Neurobiologic mechanisms in manipulative therapy.* New York: Plenum, 1978.
10. Kikuchi S, MacNab I. Localisation of the level of symptomatic cervical disc degeneration. *J Bone Joint Surg [Br]* 1981;63:272–277.
11. Heller CA, Stanley P. Lewis-Jones B, et al. Value of x-ray examinations of the cervical spine. *BMJ* 1983;287:1276–1279.
12. Gore DR, Sepic SB, Gardner GM. Roentgenographic findings of the cervical spine in asymptomatic people. *Spine* 1986;11: 521–524.
13. Friedenberg Z, Miller W. Degenerative disc disease of the cervical spine. *J Bone Joint Surg [Am]* 1963;45:1171–1178.
14. Hult L. The Munkfors investigation. *Acta Orthop Scand Suppl* 1954;17:1–38.
15. Hult L. Cervical, dorsal, and lumbar spinal syndromes. *Acta Orthop Scand Suppl* 1954;17:39–102.
16. Westerling D, Jonsson BG. Pain from the neck-shoulder region and sick leave. *Scand J Soc Med* 1980;8:131–136.
17. Takala J, Sievers K, Klaukka T. Rheumatic symptoms in the middle-aged population in southwestern Finland. *Scand J Rheumatol Suppl* 1982;47:15–29.
18. Anderson GBJ. The epidemiology of spinal disorders. In: Frymoyer JW, ed. *The adult spine: principles and practice.* New York: Raven, 1991:137.
19. Heine J. Uber die arthritis deformans. *Virchows Arch Pathol Anat* 1926;260:521–663.
20. Panjabi M, Duranceau J, Goel V, et al. Cervical human vertebrae quantitative three-dimensional anatomy of the middle and lower regions. *Spine* 1991;16: 861–869.
21. Panjabi M, Vasavada A, White A. Cervical spine biomechanics. *Semin Spine Surg* 1993;5: 10–16.
22. Herzog RJ, Wiens JJ, Dillingham MF, et al. Normal cervical spine morphometry and cervical spinal stenosis in asymptomatic professional football players: plain film radiography, multiplanar computed tomography, and magnetic resonance imaging. *Spine* 1991;16:S178–S188.
23. Hickey D, Hukins S. X-ray diffraction studies of the arrangement of collagen fibers in human fetal intervertebral disc. *J Anat* 1980;131:81–90.
24. Johnson R. Anatomy of the cervical spine and its related structures. In: Torg JS, ed. *Athletic injuries to the head, neck, and face.* 2nd ed. St. Louis: Mosby–Year Book, 1991.
25. Parke WW, Sherk HH. Normal adult anatomy. In: Sherk HH, Dunn EJ, Eismon FJ, et al. *The cervical spine.* 2nd ed. Philadelphia: JB Lippincott, 1989: 11–32.
26. Stratton SA, Bryan JM. Dysfunction, evaluation, and treatment of the cervical spine and thoracic inlet. In: Donatelli B, Wooden M, eds. *Orthopaedic physical therapy.* 2nd ed. New York: Churchill Livingstone, 1993: 77–122.
27. White AA, Panjabi MM. *Clinical biomechanics of the spine.* 2nd ed. Philadelphia: JB Lippincott, 1990.
28. Dvorak J, Dvorak V. *Manual medicine diagnostics.* New York: Thieme-Stratton, 1984.
29. Selecki B. The effects of rotation of the atlas on the axis: experimental work. *Med J Aust* 1969; 1:1012.
30. Kapandji I. Physiology of the joints. In: *The trunk and vertebral column.* Vol. 3. Edinburgh: Churchill Livingstone, 1974: 170–250.
31. Lehmkuhl LD, Smith LK. Head, neck, and trunk. In: Lehmkuhl LD, Smith LK, eds. *Brunnstrom's clinical kinesiology.* 2nd ed. Philadelphia: FA Davis, 1983: 337–359.
32. Clark C, Goel V, Galles K, et al. Kinematics of the occipito-atlanto-axial complex. *Trans Cervical Spine Res Soc* 1986;8: 24–27.
33. Depreux R, Mestdagh H. Anatomic functionelle de l'articulation sousoccipitale. *Lille Med* 1974;19:122.

34. Dvorak J, Panjabi M, Gerber D, et al. Functional diagnostics of the rotary instability of the upper cervical spine: an experimental study in cadavers. *Spine* 1987;12:197.

35. Field J, Hawkins R, Hensinger R, et al. Deformities. *Orthop Clin North Am* 1978;9:955.

36. White A, Panjabi M. The basic kinematics of the human spine. *Spine* 1978;3:13.

37. Brand RA. Knee ligaments: a new view. *J Biomech Eng* 1986;108:106–110.

38. Press JM, Herring SA, Kibler WB. Rehabilitation of musculoskeletal disorders. In: *The textbook of military medicine.* Borden Institute: Office of the Surgeon General, 1996.

39. Dreyfus P. The cervical spine: non-surgical care. Presented at Tom Landry Sports Medicine and Research Center, Dallas, TX, April 8, 1993.

40. Cole AJ, Reid M. Clinical assessment of the shoulder. *J Back Musculoskel Rehabil* 1992;2(2): 7–15.

41. Dvorak J, Panjabi M, Novotny J, et al. In vivo flexion/extension of the normal cervical spine. *J Orthop Res* 1991;9:828–834.

42. Saal JS. Brachial plexus injuries. Presented at the Cervical Spine and Upper Extremity in Sports and Industry. San Fancisco, San Francisco Spine Institute, April 1, 1990.

43. Glasgow S. Upper cervical spine injuries (C1 and C2). In: Torg JS, ed. *Athletic injuries to the head, neck, and face.* 2nd ed. St. Louis: Mosby–Year Book, 1991:457–468.

44. Calliet R. Functional anatomy. In: Calliet R, ed. *Neck and arm pain.* Philadelphia: FA Davis, 1981:1–41.

45. Fielding J. Cineroentgenography of the normal cervical spine. *J Bone Joint Surg [Am]* 1957;39: 1280–1284.

46. White AA, Panjabi MM. The problem of clinical instability in the human spine: a systematic approach. In: *Clinical biomechanics of the spine.* 2nd ed. Philadelphia: JB Lippincott, 1990:277–378.

47. Barton J, Margolis M. Rotational obstruction of the vertebral artery at the atlantoaxial joint. *Neuroradiology* 1975;9:117.

48. Marks MR, Bell GR, Boumphrey FR. Cervical spine injuries and their neurologic implications. *Clin Sport Med* 1990;9: 263–278.

49. Weinstein S, Cantu R. Cerebral stroke in a semi-pro football player: a case report. *Med Sci Sports Exerc* 1991;23: 1119–1121.

50. Schellas K, Latchaw R, Wendling L, et al. Vertebrobasilar injuries following cervical manipulation. *JAMA* 1980;244:1450.

51. Bogduk N, Twomey LT. *Clinical anatomy of the lumbar spine.* 2nd ed. New York: Churchill Livingstone, 1991.

52. Bogduk N, Windsor H, Inglis A. The innervation of the cervical intervertebral discs. *Spine* 1988;13:2–8.

53. Mendel T, Wink CS, Zimny M. Neural elements in human cervical intervertibral discs. *Spine* 1992;17:132–135.

54. Franson R, Saal J. Human disc phospholipase A_2 in inflammatory. *Spine* 1992;17(suppl 6): S129–S132.

55. Hickey D, Hukins D. Relation between the structure of the annulus fibrosus and the function and failure of the intervertebral disc. *Spine* 1980;5:100–116.

56. Saal J, Franson R, Dobrow R, et al. High levels of inflammatory Phospholipase A_2 activity in lumbar disc herniations. *Spine* 1990;15:674–678.

57. Benzon HT. Epidural steroids for lumbosacral radiculopathy. *Adv Pain Res Ther* 1990; 13:231.

58. Bland JH. *Disorders of the cervical spine: diagnosis and medical management.* Philadelphia: Saunders, 1987.

59. Parke W. Correlative anatomy of cervical spondylotic myelopathy. *Spine* 1988;13:831.

60. Lysell E. Motion in the cervical spine. An experimental study on autopsy specimens. *Acta Orthop Scand Suppl* 1969;123:1.

61. Bogduk N, Engle R. The menisci of the lumbar zygapophyseal joints: a review of their anatomy and clinical significance. *Spine* 1984;9:454–460.

62. Lewin T, Moffet B, Viidik A. The morphology of the lumbar synovial intervertebral joins. *Acta Morphol Neerl Scand* 1962;4:299–319.

63. Yu S, Sether L, Haughton V. Facet joint menisci of the cervical spine: correlative MR imaging and cryomicrotomy study. *Radiology* 1987;164:79–82.

64. Dvorak J, Panjabi M. Functional anatomy of the alar ligaments. *Spine* 1987;12:183–189.

65. Jia L, Shen Q, Chen D, et al. Dynamic changes of the cervical ligamental flavum in hyperextension-hyperflexion movement and their measurement. *Chin Med J* 1990;103:66–70.

66. Jackson H, Winklemann R, Bickel W. Nerve endings in the human lumbar spine and related structures. *J Bone Joint Surg [Am]* 1966;48:1272–1281.

67. Roofe P. Innervation of annulus fibrosus and posterior longitudinal ligaments. *Arch Neurol Psychiatry* 1940;44:100.

68. Wyke B. The neurological basis of thoracic spinal pain. *Rheum Phys Med* 1970;10:356–367.

69. Dyson M. Therapeutic applications of ultrasound. In: Nyberg WL, Ziskin MC, eds. *Biological effects of ultrasound: clinics in diagnostic ultrasound.* New York: Churchill Livingstone, 1985:121–133.

70. Frykholm R. Cervical nerve root compression resulting from disc

degeneration and root-sleeve fibrosis: a clinical investigation. *Acta Chir Scand Suppl* 1951; 160.

71. Herring SA, Weinstein SM. Electrodiagnosis in sports medicine. *Phys Med Rehabil* 1989;3: 809–822.

72. Sunderland S. Meningeal-neural relations in the intervertebral foramen. *J Neurosurg* 1974;40:756.

73. Perry J, Nickel V. Total cervical-spine fusion for neck paralysis. *J Bone Joint Surg [Am]* 1959;41:37–60.

74. Warwick R, Williams PL. *Gray's anatomy.* 35th ed. Philadelphia: WB Saunders, 1973.

75. Mennel J. *Back pain.* Boston: Little, Brown, 1960.

76. Torg J, Vegso M, O'Neill M, et al. The epidemiologic, pathologic, biomechanical, and cinematographic analysis of football-induced cervical spine trauma. *Am J Sports Med* 1990;18: 50–57.

77. Krag M. Biomechanics of the cervical spine: including bracing, surgical constructs, and orthoses. In: Frymoyer JW, ed. *The adult spine: principles and practice.* New York: Raven, 1991: 929–965.

78. Wilder D, Porter JM, Frymoyer J. The biomechanics of lumbar disc herniation and the effect of overload and instability. *J Spinal Disord* 1988;1:16–32.

79. Kelsey J, Githens P, Walter S, et al. An epidemiological study of acute prolapsed cervical intervertebral disc. *J Bone Joint Surg [Am]* 1984;66:907–914.

80. Kondo K, Molgaard C, Kurland L, et al. Protruded intervertebral cervical disc. *Minn Med* 1981;64:751–753.

81. Lester JP, Windsor RE, Dreyer SJ. *Medical management of the cervical spine.* New York: Churchill Livingstone, 1996.

82. Lestini W, Wiesel S. The pathogenesis of cervical spondylosis. *Clin Orthop* 1989;239:69.

83. Saal J. Flexibility training. In: Saal JA, ed. *Physical medicine and rehabilitation: rehabilitation of sports injuries.* Philadelphia: Hanley & Belfus, 1987: 537–554.

84. Smith W. Exercise and the intervertebral disc. In: Hochschuler SH, ed. *The spine in sports.* Philadelphia: Hanley & Belfus, 1990:3–10.

85. Butler D. Adverse neural tension disorders based on the spinal canal. In: *Mobilization of the nervous system.* Melbourne: Churchill Livingstone, 1991:231–246.

86. Derby R. Cervical injection procedures. Presented at Cervical and Lumbar Spine: State of the Art '91. San Francisco, San Francisco Spine Institute, March 24, 1991.

87. Dvorak J, Dvorak V. Differential diagnosis and definition of the radicular and spondylogenic (nonradicular) pain syndromes. In: *Manual medicine diagnostics.* 2nd ed. New York: Thieme-Stratton, 1990:63–64.

88. Ferrel W, Nade S, Newbold P. Inter-relation of neural discharge; intraarticular pressure, and joint angle in the knee of the dog. *J Physiol* 1986;373: 353–365.

89. Haldeman S. Spinal manipulative therapy in sports medicine. *Clin Sports Med* 1986;5:277–293.

90. Kulund D. Athletic injuries to the head, face, and neck. In: *The injured athlete.* 2nd ed. Philadelphia: JB Lippincott, 1988:267–299.

90a. Saunders H. *Evaluation, treatment and prevention of musculoskeletal disorders.* 2nd ed. Minneapolis: Viking Press, 1985.

91. Cantu R. Head and neck injuries. In: Mueller FO, Ryan AJ, eds. *Prevention of athletic injuries: the role of the sports medicine team.* Philadelphia: FA Davis, 1981:201–213.

92. Schneider R, Reifel E, Crisler HO, Oosterbaum BG. Serious and fatal football injuries involving the head and spinal cord. *JAMA* 1961;177:362.

93. Schneider R, Gosch H, Norrell H. Vascular insufficiency and differential distortion of brain and cord caused by cervicomedullary football injuries. *J Neurosurg* 1970;33:363.

94. Saal J. Diagnostic decision making: where do all the pieces fit? Presented at Cervical and Lumbar Spine: State of the Art '91. San Francisco, San Francisco Spine Institute, March 24, 1991.

95. Wilbourn AJ, Porter JM. Thoracic outlet syndromes. *Spine State Art Rev* 1988;2:597–625.

96. Kottke FJ, Mundale MO. Range of mobility of the cervical spine. *Arch Phys Med Rehabil* 1959;40:379.

97. *AMA guides to the evaluation of permanent impairment.* 4th ed. Chicago: American Medical Association, 1995.

98. Braddon RL. Management of common cervical pain syndromes. In: Delisa JA, ed. *Rehabilitation medicine: principles and practice.* 2nd ed. Philadelphia: JB Lippincott, 1993:1037.

99. Jackson R. Cervical trauma: not just another pain in the neck. *Geriatrics* 1982;37:123.

100. Grieve G. Common patterns of clinical presentation. In: Grieve GP, ed. *Common vertebral joint problems.* 2nd ed. London: Churchill Livingstone, 1988:164.

101. Kendall FP, Kendall-McCreary E. *Muscles: testing and function.* 3rd ed. Baltimore: William & Wilkins, 1983.

102. Rocabado M. *Diagnosis and treatment of abnormal craniocervical and craniomandibular mechanics.* Knoxville, TN: Rocabado Institute, 1981.

103. Janda V. *Muscle function testing.* London: Butterworths, 1983.

104. Lord SM, Barnsley L, Bogduk N. The utility of comparative local anesthetic blocks versus placebo-

controlled blocks for the diagnosis of cervical zygapophysial joint pain. *Clin J Pain* 1995;11: 208–213.

105. Saal JA, Herzog RJ, Saal JS. The natural history of lumbar intervertebral disk extrusions treated nonoperatively. *Spine* 1990;15:683–686.

106. Korr I. Sustained sympathicotonia as a factor in disease. In: Korr IM, ed. *Neurobiologic mechanisms in manipulative therapy.* New York: Plenum, 1978.

107. Korr I. Proprioceptors and somatic dysfunction. *J Am Osteopath Assoc* 1975;74:638.

108. Clarke K. An epidemiologic view. In: Torg JS, ed. *Athletic injuries to the head, neck, and face.* St. Louis: Mosby–Year Book, 1991:15–27.

109. Koes BW, Bouter LM, van Mameren H, et al. The effectiveness of manual therapy, physiotherapy and treatment by the general practitioner for nonspecific back and neck complaints: a randomized clinical trial. *Spine* 1992;17:28.

110. Hubbard DR, Berkhoff GM. Myofascial trigger points show spontaneous needle EMG activity. *Spine* 1993;18: 1803–1807.

111. Travell HH, Simons DG. *Myofascial pain and dysfunction: trigger point manual.* Baltimore: Williams & Wilkins, 1983.

112. Colachis S, Strohm B. Cervical traction: relationship of traction time to varied tractive force with constant angle of pull. *Arch Phys Med Rehabil* 1965;46:815.

113. Colachis S, Strohm B. A study of tractive forces and angle of pull on vertebral interspaces in the cervical spine. *Arch Phys Med Rehabil* 1965;46:820.

114. Valtonen E, Kiurn E. Cervical traction as a therapeutic tool: a clinical analysis based on 212 patients. *Scand J Rehabil Med* 1970;2:29.

115. Kelsey JL, Githens PB, O'Connor T, et al. Acute prolapsed lumbar intervertebral disc. An epidemiologic study with special reference to driving automobiles and cigarette smoking. *Spine* 1984;9:608–613.

116. Yoss RE, Corbin KB, McCarthy CS, et al. Significance of symptoms and signs of localization of involved root in cervical disc protrusion. *Neurology* 1957; 7:673.

117. Beatty RM, Fowler FD, Hanson EJ Jr. The abducted arm as a sign of ruptured cervical disc. *Neurosurgery* 1987;21:731.

118. Boden SD, McCowin PR, Davis DO, et al. Abnormal magnetic-resonance scans of the cervical spine in asymptomatic subjects: a prospective investigation. *J Bone Joint Surg [Am]* 1990;72:1178–1184.

119. Ellenberg MR, Honet JC, Treanor WJ. Cervical radiculopathy. *Arch Phys Med Rehabil* 1994;75:342.

120. Dillin W, Booth R, Cuckeler J, et al. Cervical radiculopathy: a review. *Spine* 1986;11:988–991.

121. Crandall PH, Batzdorf U. Cervical spondylotic myelopathy. *J Neurosurg* 1966;25:57.

122. Bernhardt M, Hynes R, Blume H, et al. Cervical spondylotic myelopathy. *J Bone Joint Surg [Am]* 1993;75:119–128.

123. Gamburd RC. Sports related cervical injuries. Presented at Cervical and Lumbar Spine: State of the Art '91. San Francisco, San Francisco Spine Institute, March 24, 1991.

124. Torg JS, Fay CM. Cervical spinal stenosis with cord neurapraxia and transient quadriplegia. In: Torg JS, ed. *Athletic injuries to the head, neck, and face.* St. Louis: Mosby–Year Book, 1991:533–552.

125. LaRocca H. Cervical spondylotic myelopathy: natural history. *Spine* 1988;13:854.

126. Phillips DG. Surgical treatment of myelopathy with cervical spondylosis. *J Neurol Neurosurg Psychiatry* 1973;36:879.

127. Clarke E, Robinson PK. Cervical myelopathy: a complication of cervical spondylosis. *Brain* 1956;79:483.

128. Lees F, Turner JWA. Natural history and prognosis of cervical spondylosis. *BMJ* 1963; 2:1607.

129. Symon L, Lavender P. The surgical treatment of cervical spondylotic myelopathy. *Neurology* 1967;17:117.

130. Aprill C, Bogduk N. The prevalence of cervical zygapophyseal joint pain: a first approximation. *Spine* 1992;17:744–747.

131. Barnsley L, Lord SM, Wallis BJ, et al. The prevalence of chronic cervical zygapophysial joint pain after whiplash. *Spine* 1995;20:20–25.

132. Evans RW. Some observations on whiplash injuries. *Neurol Clin* 1992;10:975–997.

133. Jull G, Bogduk N, Marsland A. The accuracy of manual diagnosis for cervical zygapophyseal joint pain syndromes. *Med J Aust* 1988;148:233–236.

134. Barnsley L, Bogduk N. Medial branch blocks are specific for the diagnosis of cervical zygapophyseal joint pain. *Reg Anesth* 1993;18:343–350.

135. Lord SM, Barnsley L, Wallis BJ, et al. Percutaneous radiofrequency neurotomy for chronic cervical zygapophyseal-joint pain. *N Engl J Med* 1996;335: 1721–1726.

136. Heller JG. The syndromes of degenerative cervical disease. *Orthop Clin North Am* 1992;23:381.

137. Clark CR. Cervical spondylotic myelopathy: history and physical findings. *Spine* 1988; 13:847.

138. Epstein NE, Epstein JA, Carras R, et al. Coexisting cervical and lumbar spinal stenosis: diagnosis and management. *Neurosurgery* 1984;15:489.

139. Yiannikas C, Shahani BT, Young RR. Short-latency somatosensory-evoked potentials from radial, median, ulnar, and peroneal nerve stimulation in the assessment of cervical spondylosis: comparison with conventional electromyography. *Arch Neurol* 1986;43:1264.

140. Pavlov H, Torg JS, Robie B, et al. Cervical spinal stenosis: determination with vertebral body ratio method. *Radiology* 1987;164:177.

Chapter 61

Myofascial Pain

Robert D. Gerwin

Chronic pain is a major cause of personal distress and is of social concern, resulting in a significant loss of productivity and costing literally billions of dollars yearly in medical care. Myofascial pain syndromes (MPSs) account for a substantial portion of the chronic pain spectrum, standing alone as primary causes of disability and complicating other problems as secondary causes of pain and suffering. Myofascial pain is pain of muscular origin, although the term implies, and certainly includes, pain originating in the fascial covering of muscle. It is muscle pain of a very specific type, and is not to be confused with the pain of inflammatory myopathies or fibromyalgia. MPS is a common occurrence after injury, resulting in so-called soft-tissue pain. The pain can be intermittent and mild, causing little discomfort, or excruciating, debilitating, and totally disabling. MPS commonly occurs in association with other musculoskeletal disorders like zygapophyseal or facet joint injuries and disk herniations, or as a complication of other conditions like ureteral lithiasis, myocardial infarction, and osteoarthritis. It can be acute, or it can persist for many years, and still be treatable. MPS can complicate recovery from cervical and lumbar laminectomy, as part of a postlaminectomy pain syndrome. It is seen with repetitive movement or "overuse" syndromes that occur in many diverse occupations. It mimics other conditions like radiculopathy, anginal pain, and migraine, and is therefore to be considered in the differential diagnosis. In short, MPS is a common and important cause of treatable pain that is underrecognized, and therefore undertreated, although it is readily diagnosable by physical examination.

This chapter describes the clinical features of MPS and of the myofascial trigger point (MTrP). As the trigger point (TrP) is the clinical sign that is necessary for the diagnosis of MPS, the physiology underlying each of the features of the TrP, such as referred pain and tenderness, is reviewed insofar as it is known. Current evidence about the nature of the TrP itself is reviewed and studies supporting the reliability of the identification of the TrP are analyzed.

The pain syndromes that have been associated with individual muscle TrPs are well described in the two-volume text on myofascial pain written by Travell and Simons (1,2), and are not repeated here. However, the interactions of individual muscles affected by MTrPs and their interaction as functional units, especially in chronic cases, causing widespread pain, are discussed, as these are the most common presentations seen in the clinic. Finally, the current state of the treatment of MPS is reviewed.

HISTORICAL BACKGROUND

Interest in pain originating in muscles and ligaments developed in the 1930s, about the time that interest in herniated vertebral disks and radiculopathies developed following their identification in 1934, which ultimately directed attention away from muscle and toward nerve root compression as a cause of pain. Edeiken and Wolferth (3) in 1936 reported that muscle injury resulted in referred pain. Kellgren, in a series of papers in 1938 to 1939, reported that injection of hypertonic saline solution into muscle produced patterns of referred pain, and that palpation of tender areas in muscle in symptomatic individuals also produced referred pain. Injection of procaine into the tender areas relieved local tenderness, diminished referred pain symptoms, and restored normal movement to the affected limb (4–7). Travell extended the clinical observations and theoretical concepts about pain of muscular origin in a body of work that spans four decades, and culminated in the two-volume text entitled *Myofascial Pain and Dysfunction: The Trigger Point Manual* written with Simons (1,2). For a listing of Travell's publications, see her contribution to the proceedings of the First International Conference on Myofascial Pain and Fibromyalgia (8). Travell and her colleagues defined single-muscle MPSs through meticulous observations of literally thousands of patients. These observations formed the basis for the more recent work on the nature of myofascial pain and its associated phenomena, most notably referred pain, and on the nature of the TrP itself. A detailed historical review of the literature on muscle pain was written by Simons in 1975 (9).

The cardinal feature of MPS is the MTrP. It distinguishes MPS from all other causes of muscle pain and is characterized by the features shown in Table 61-1 (p. 1073) (1). The diagnosis of MPS reflects the practitioner's skill in identifying these characteristic features by physical examination. Treatment involves inactivation of the MTrP for immediate relief, and identification and correction of the factors that led to the establishment of the MPS in the first place, or that impede the recovery process. Thus, the practitioner must assess the patient for postural dysfunction, impaired spinal joint function, pelvic rotations, leg-length inequalities, and work- and recreation-related physical and mental stresses. Systemic factors like nutritional or hormonal deficiencies or insufficiency states are often seen in persons with chronic (>6 months) MTrP pain (1,10,11).

EPIDEMIOLOGY

The prevalence of MPS in a general internal medicine clinic (12) was 9%, and MPS accounted for 30% of patients who listed pain as a complaint. A study of 200 young men and women (13) selected from an Air Force basic training program who were examined by trained physical therapists for hypersensitive areas in the muscles of the shoulder region and for referred pain patterns found that 49.5% had hypersensitive areas in at least one of the muscles examined, and 62.5% had hypersensitivity in more than one muscle. Referred pain was found in 25% of those with hypersensitivity. This study did not look for the presence of taut bands or local twitch responses. Nonetheless, hypersensitivity or tenderness was found in half the subjects, and referred pain, a more precise marker for MTrPs, was found in 12.5% of the entire group. Eighty-five percent of patients with benign pain seen in a chronic pain clinic had MPS that contributed to the cause of their pain (14). Sixty-five percent of postpolio survivors had MTrPs with tender, taut bands, plus the variable presence of local twitch responses and referred pain (Gerwin RD, unpublished data, 1993). Among 250 consecutive patients with chronic low-back pain (15), 94 (38%) had MPS as a cause of their low-back pain, as opposed to 57 (23%) who had herniated disk syndrome.

Among 296 patients with chronic head and neck pain evaluated in a university dental clinic, 55.4% had pain primarily due to MPS (16). Sixty subjects with fibromyalgia syndrome (FMS) and an equal number of subjects with regional pain syndrome and of control subjects were examined for tender points (TePs) and MTrPs (17). Forty-one percent of FMS subjects had one or more TrPs, most commonly in the trapezius muscles. In 58.5% of the FMS subjects with TrPs, stimulation of the TrP reproduced the subject's pain, and constituted an active TrP. A comprehensive examination for MTrPs in 96 subjects with musculoskeletal pain identified 25 subjects who fulfilled the criteria for FMS, the remainder having MPS (11). In this longitudinal study with an average observation period of 7.8 months (range, 1–36 months), 18 (72%) of those with FMS had MTrPs that were clinically significant causes of pain. In a study of interrater reliability (18), nearly all subjects had tenderness and taut bands in the sternocleidomastoid and extensor digitorum muscles, and MTrPs, active or latent. Latent TrPs with tenderness in a taut band, and either localized twitch responses to stimulation or referred pain, are common phenomena, and not restricted to persons with symptomatic musculoskeletal pain. Nonetheless, one can conclude from studies on the prevalence of MPS in different clinical settings that MPS is an important cause of pain. Moreover, if one looks carefully, latent MTrPs can be found in persons without pain. These considerations raise the additional issues of 1) what is required in order to make a diagnosis of MPS, and 2) what is the significance of the TrP if it can be found in persons without pain. The first question is addressed in the section on interrater reliability of MTrP examination. As to the second issue, the TrP is similar to the arthritic joint of osteoarthritis. It may have anatomic changes, but may not be symptomatic at all times. Pain may occur only when the joint is physically stressed, such as after walking a long distance. Symptomatic treatment may be all that is required in such cases. Similarly, muscle may respond to physical stress by developing taut bands that are tender to palpation, but may not be spontaneously painful until subjected to an unusual load. The study by Sola et al (13) is of interest in this regard, as it showed that a substantial number of young persons in basic training have muscle tenderness, and some have referred pain from muscle. The study of polio survivors, moreover, demonstrated that over half of those with MTrPs had latent or nonpainful TrPs at the time of the examination. Thus, TrPs can be present in physically active persons and in persons with physical disabilities, and yet not necessarily cause pain or require treatment. When the MTrP is symptomatic, producing pain, restricting motion, or otherwise causing dysfunction, it should be specifically treated.

CLINICAL MYOFASCIAL PAIN SYNDROMES

A particular pain problem is identified as MPS when one or more MTrPs can reproduce all or part of the individual's pain picture. This can be seen graphically when the patient indicates the sites of pain on a body diagram, and demonstrated on the physical examination when TrPs in certain muscles reproduce the pain. TrP pain is both local at the TrP and distant, at the referred pain zone that is usually distal to the TrP. When individual muscles are examined for TrPs, single muscle syndromes are identified. The pain that is experienced from a MTrP is a combination of the local pain that may be more or less appreciated, and the pain that is felt in the zone of referred pain, which may be the predominant pain sensation. The person suffering from an MPS may complain only of the pain felt in the referred pain zone. This can be very confusing, as treatment directed toward the perceived pain, but not toward the primary TrP, may be unsuccessful for no obvious reason.

MTrPs may refer pain to contiguous or nearby sites. Thus, upper trapezius muscle TrPs refer pain into the ipsilateral posterior part of the neck. Pain from MTrPs may also be felt in remote sites, such as upper trapezius muscle TrPs that refer pain to the ipsilateral side of the jaw and temple (Fig. 61-1). Once recognized, the referred pain patterns can be used to identify the muscle harboring the MTrP. A pain distribution involving the shoulder, arm, and hand may be the manifestation of a TrP in the infraspinous muscle, the biceps or scalene muscles, the triceps, the coracobrachial muscle, the pectoralis major and minor muscles, or the serratus posterior superior. However, the nuances of pain are different for the TrPs in each of these muscles, and activation of the TrP is different, so that localization of pain to the anterior or posterior region of the shoulder helps identify the offending muscle. Examination of specific muscles for TrPs can then identify the actual TrPs that reproduce the patient's pain. This process is actually not difficult, and can be quite rewarding when the patient informs the examiner that this indeed is the cause of the problem. Review articles well describe single-muscle TrP pain syndromes (19–22).

MPS is more often the result of MTrPs in many muscles, affecting a region or even appearing as widespread pain involving three or four regions of the body

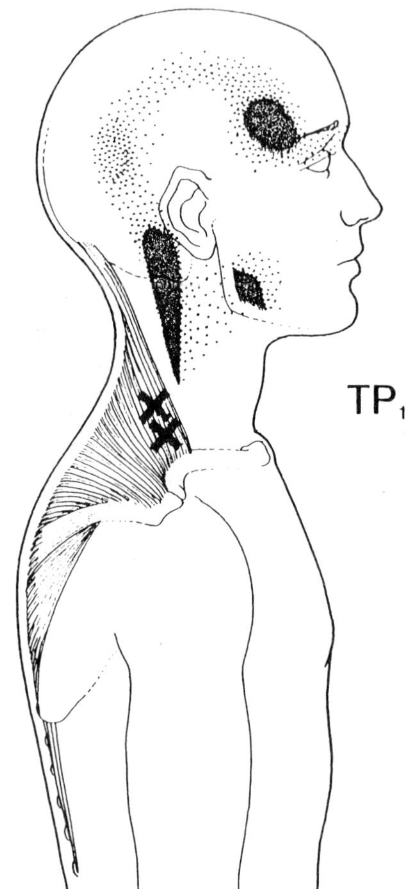

Figure 61-1. Referred pain patterns from the trapezius muscle. The primary referred pain zone is denoted by *solid markings*, and the spill-over zone is noted by *stippling*. The common areas of trigger points are noted by *X*'s. Mechanical stimulation of the trigger zone gives rise to pain in the referral zones. (Reproduced by permission from Travell JG, Simons DG. *Myofascial pain and dysfunction: the trigger point manual*. Vol. 1. Baltimore: Williams & Wilkins, 1983.)

(11). The spread of MTrPs and therefore of myofascial pain occurs as a result of the development of TrPs in dysfunctional muscle units and in the muscles in the referred pain zone.

FUNCTIONAL MUSCLE UNITS

Muscles work together in functional units that extend force or stabilize a body part when they act as agonists, or in opposition as antagonists, sometimes to limit or restrain movement, as the sternocleidomastoid muscles do in relation to the extensor muscles of the neck. When one muscle in a functional unit is impaired, as when it is weakened or shortened because of TrPs, other muscles in that unit must take up the load, or will be affected by an abnormal balance between agonist and antagonist. A good example is one of the paired bilateral muscles in the trunk, the quadratus lumborum. Together, the paired muscles act to extend the back and to limit flexion produced by the iliopsoas muscles. If one quadratus lumborum muscle is injured, its extensor function is assumed by the contralateral quadratus lumborum and by the deep and superficial paraspinal muscles. These muscles can become overloaded and develop TrPs. Pelvic tilt caused by shortening of the quadratus can result in a functional scoliosis, with resultant stress on trunk, shoulder, and neck muscles. The quadratus lumborum muscles also stabilize the trunk and pelvis, the extensor group of gluteal and hamstring muscles, and anteriorly the flexor group of iliopsoas, abdominal, and quadriceps muscles. Weakness and shortening of any one of these muscles produce an imbalance that overloads the other muscles in the group, and can result in the development of MTrPs in them. Similarly, when there is weakness of the serratus anterior muscle, it may fall onto the latissimus dorsi and the pectoral muscles to stabilize the scapula, thereby overloading these muscles and causing TrPs to form in them. In this way, there can be a regional spread of MTrPs.

The spread of MTrPs from one region to another becomes understandable, when one considers that muscles have multiple actions. For example, the iliopsoas acts as a trunk flexor, synergistic with the abdominal muscles when the thoracolumbar region of the spine is flexed, and acts as a hip flexor, synergistic with the rectus femoris head of the quadriceps muscle. Dysfunction of the iliopsoas can affect either of its agonist muscles. The rectus femoris muscle also acts at two joints, distally acting on the knee as an extensor and stabilizer in conjunction with the vastus medialis and lateralis. Hence, dysfunction of the iliopsoas can affect the function of the vastus medialis and lateralis muscles and lead to the development of TrPs in them, causing the MPS to spread through the muscular chain. Rosen (23) coined the term *gateway muscles* to indicate that certain muscles are key to the spread of the MPS across regional groups. The latissimus dorsi is another such muscle, one that links the shoulder and the hip, as it inserts superiorly in the humerus, medially from the seventh thoracic vertebral spinous process downward through the entire lumbar vertebrae, and inferiorly to the iliac crest and the sacrum. Its major action is adduction of the arm at the shoulder, but it also assists in hyperextension of the trunk and in lateral tilting of the pelvis (24). Dysfunction secondary to TrP-induced weakness and restricted range of motion can affect the functioning of both the shoulder and the pelvis. In this manner, MPS can spread from one region to another as the condition becomes chronic. Side-to-side spread of TrP pain is easily understood as many axial muscles are paired and both sides share functions as agonists and oppose functions as antagonists. This is readily seen in the quadratus lumborum where the two muscles are agonists in extension of the trunk, and antagonists in lateral flexion. Vertical spread of MTrPs occurs through the involvement of muscles like the paraspinal muscles and the latissimus dorsi that act as bridging muscles.

Another mechanism facilitates the spread of MPS through the body, and that is the involvement of postural muscles. Surface electromyography (EMG) can monitor simultaneous muscle function at different sites in the body. Dysfunction of postural muscles in the leg, in the gastrocnemius-soleus complex, for example, alters activity in the muscles that control head and neck posture, including the sternocleidomastoid muscle.

Individuals suffering from an injury may complain only about the most prominent pain, but if examined comprehensively, can be found to have widespread active MTrPs. This does not mean that they have a disease like fibromyalgia, but that the MPS is not restricted to a single region. Such a finding has significant implications for treatment, as correction of postural dysfunction becomes an important element of the physical therapy program. Treatment must include distant areas of the body that have a far-reaching effect, as the example of the gastrocnemius-soleus complex effect of the sternocleidomastoid muscle shows.

NEUROPHYSIOLOGY OF THE MYOFASCIAL TRIGGER POINT

The MTrP poses some very serious questions that have perplexed clinicians. What is the physical representation of the MTrP? No pathologic change in muscle has been associated with the MTrP. What is the nature of the tenderness that occurs in muscle in the absence of any inflammation and only nonspecific signs of degeneration (25)? No specific or consistent biochemical changes have been found in the MTrP. High-energy phosphates were found to be reduced in the TeP of the trapezius muscles in fibromyalgia patients, indicating a metabolically stressed area (26), but there has been no further characterization of a metabolic aberration in the TrP. How does a MTrP in one area of a muscle produce pain that is felt at a distance (referred pain)? Patients often complain of pain in the zone of referred pain (e.g., above the eye or in the parietal region in muscular headache), without being aware of the muscle origin of the pain (e.g., in the sternocleidomastoid muscle). There are no direct sclerotomal, dermatomal, nerve, or vascular connections between most of the referred pain zones and their primary trigger area. How does an MTrP become chronic and lead to persistent MPS? How is it that the pain of even chronic MPS is rapidly eliminated once the MTrP is inactivated? Are there electrodiagnostic abnormalities that are unique to the TrP zone? The neurophysiologic models of pain perception must address these questions. The known plasticity of the nervous system as it responds to noxious stimulation can explain much of the clinical phenomena that clinicians see. Some of the answers to these questions come as the result of studies of pain physiology in tissues other than muscle, and some are derived from the study of muscle specifically. These topics are now considered with reference to the existing neurophysiologic literature.

The nature of the MTrP itself has not been understood until quite recently when Hubbard and Berkoff (27) reported that the MTrP sustained spontaneous EMG activity not seen in adjacent nontender muscle. They postulated that the activity was generated in the intrafusal muscle spindle fibers. Travell (28) in 1959 reported a high-frequency repetitive EMG discharge from the trigger area with the muscle at rest, while a neighboring area in the same muscle was electrically silent. In a series of studies, Simons et al (29–32) elaborated on the finding of spontaneous electrical activity of the MTrP, which they called *SEA*. These authors identified a zone in the taut band in which SEA was found. Such abnormal activity is considered to come from the motor end-plate because of its electrical characteristics, although Hubbard (33) thinks that it emanates from the muscle spindle because of its response to pharmacologic manipulation. Normal and abnormal sites of activity indicate that the trigger zone contains both functionally abnormal and normal loci that they consider to be myoneural junctions or motor end-plates.

Simons (34) proposed that an energy crisis within the muscle forms the basis of the taut band found in muscle. In this model, injury to the sarcoplasmic reticulum leads to a release of ionized calcium, which activates the contraction of local sarcomeres. Contraction of sarcomeres is an energy-consuming action, but the contraction compromises local capillary blood flow, limiting the supply of glucose and oxygen to the muscle. The subsequent shortage of oxygen within the MTrP could limit the production of ATP, impair the function of the calcium pump, and result in sustained muscle contraction of the taut band.

The Physiologic Basis of Tenderness and Referred Pain

The hallmark of MPS is the MTrP that has as its foremost characteristic an exquisitely tender point in a taut band. The other features of the MTrP would not occur without this characteristic change in muscle. The TeP in the taut band is both a physical structure and a psychophysiologic response. The taut band is palpable in accessible muscles and can be visualized by ultrasound (35). It has both hyperalgesia and allodynia.

Muscle pain is like other visceral pain in that it is dull and poorly localized, in contrast to cutaneous pain that is sharp and well localized. The sharp, well-defined pain of cutaneous tissues is mediated by thinly myelinated group III A-delta fibers that conduct at a rate of about 20 m/sec, whereas muscle pain is mediated by slowly conducting group IV C fibers (see Chap. 57) (36). Free nociceptive nerve endings are not found in muscle fibrils, but instead are located in close relation to arterioles and capillaries. The central terminations of the dorsal root ganglion (DRG) neurons of group III A-delta and group IV nociceptive C fibers are in laminae I and V of the dorsal horn (37). Both A-delta and C fibers in muscle are sensitive to naturally occurring pain-producing substances like bradykinin, 5-hydroxytryptamine, and histamine (38,39). The receptive fields of these nociceptor afferent nerves tend to be small and restricted (40). Many of the dorsal horn neurons receive input from many receptive fields, however. Furthermore, they receive input from cutaneous noxious stimuli and from visceral stimuli (41). Thus, muscle is supplied with afferent nociceptor nerve endings that are sensitive to pressure and to chemical stimulation, and that activate dorsal horn neurons that receive input from multiple muscle sites (receptive fields) and from deep tissues. Furthermore, sensitization occurs in muscle nociceptors as it does in other skin and other tissues (42).

Substance P (SP) is a neuropeptide that modulates nociception by activating nociceptor neurons. It can induce a long-lasting depolarization of the dorsal horn neuron cell membrane (43), which in turn can lead to opening of the *N*-methyl-D-aspartate (NMDA) ion channel. Entrance of calcium ions through the NMDA channel leads to a cascade of events that activates the neuron and releases substances that spread activation to other cells. Thus, release of SP by activation of nociceptive afferents can enhance the activation of dorsal horn nociceptors, contributing to the sensitization of dorsal horn neurons. The effect of SP is enhanced by the presence of calcitonin gene–related peptide (CGRP).

Hyperexcitability of dorsal horn neurons in response to experimental myositis is due to activation of neurokinin 1 (NK-1) and NMDA receptors. In addition, superfusion of the spinal cord with SP causes dorsal horn cells to establish new connections with C-fiber nociceptors, accounting in part for the appearance of new receptive fields and the referred pain phenomena seen in MPSs (44).

Thus, two key features of the MTrP, tenderness and the presence of referred pain, have their origin in the ability of the nervous system to modulate afferent nociceptive activity, as noted. Tenderness is an expression of sensitization. Referred pain is an expression of activation of afferent input from remote sites.

Sensitization is the increase of nociceptive responsiveness of the afferent receptor or its dorsal horn cell. High-threshold mechanoreceptor neurons or wide-dynamic-range (WDR) neurons respond to nociceptive stimulation by becoming like low-threshold mechanoreceptor neurons. Bradykinin injected into muscle produces an acute myositis that lowers the threshold to other peripheral nociceptive stimuli like pinch. These neuroplastic changes are most effectively produced by slowly conducting unmyelinated C fibers or thinly myelinated A fibers (45).

The dorsal horn neuronal receptive field enlarges and the mechanical threshold to stimulation is lowered, in response to sensitization. Similar to referred pain in MPS, distant islands of pain-sensitive receptive fields occur that are not contiguous with the primary area of pain.

Pain referral, both to contiguous receptive fields and to distant remote receptive fields, is an essential feature of the TrP that distinguishes it from a fibromyalgia TeP. Some of the frequently occurring myofascial referred pain patterns involve pain of headache in the temple, forehead, or scalp associated with sternocleidomastoid muscle TrPs; posterior neck pain associated with trapezius muscle TrPs; and sacroiliac and hip pain associated with quadratus lumborum TrPs.

Referred pain is not a phenomenon unique to the MTrP, but is well known throughout clinical medical practice, for example, in cases of esophageal pain referred to the lower chest wall; anginal pain referred to the arm, the neck, and the throat; ureteral pain referred to the torso flank; and prostate pain referred to the leg (46). Referred pain originating in muscle TePs was described in 1938 by Kellgren (4). The phenomenon of referred pain was further studied by Travell, who with Simons published the pain referral patterns of single-muscle myofascial syndromes (1,2).

The mechanism of referred pain has been elucidated by neurophysiologic studies performed in the last two decades. This subject is discussed in Chapter 57. The mechanisms that underlie convergence of input from several different receptive fields onto a single neuron are illustrative of a phenomenon that occurs in muscle as well as in skin and viscera (41). Studies by Yu and Mense (47) showed that a sizable percentage of dorsal horn neurons have convergent input from deep somatic tissues (muscle) and cutaneous and visceral receptors. In fact, no dorsal horn nociceptive-responsive neuron was exclusively responsive to muscle stimulation only. Every neuron responsive to deep muscle pain was responsive to mechanical stimulation of the skin as well (41). Thus, referred pain to dissociated areas of muscle and skin, and to or from viscera, is characteristic of muscle pain as well as the pain of other tissues, and is consistent with the referred pain patterns that are seen in persons with MPS (48). Facilitation of nociceptive brain stem neuronal activity, with increased sensitivity and with enlargement of neuronal receptive fields, is also seen when a muscle irritant like mustard oil is injected into the masseter muscle (49). This area is relevant to the myofascial pain dysfunction syndrome associated with MTrPs in the masticatory muscles and muscles of facial expression.

Acute myositis produced by injecting carrageenan into the gastrocnemius-soleus muscle of the rat acutely increased the number of neurons responding to A- and C-fiber input, increased the number of neurons receiving input from more than one nerve, and increased the number of receptive fields. These changes are consistent with findings from previous studies in which bradykinin was injected into muscle to induce nociception. Sensitization occurred peripherally and centrally, and there was an increase in the size and number of receptive fields (50).

The majority of referred pain zones from MTrPs are located distal to the TrP. This was also the situation in over 70% of the neurons with convergent input from deep muscle receptors and skin (49).

Referred pain can also result from the branching of peripheral afferent nerve fibers distal to the DRG, innervating muscle in two or more zones or viscera, or both. Input from one branch can activate other branches antidromically, producing an axon reflex, for example, or signal by means of chemical transmitters that another area was activated. Two branches may run in the same peripheral nerve to two separate sites in muscle. Different conduction velocities in single fibers excited distally indicate that the nerve in question has two distal branches (51).

Finally, descending supraspinal influences alter the responsiveness of the dorsal horn. Descending tonic inhibition modulates dorsal horn nociceptive neuron activity. Cold block of the spinal cord abolishes or decreases the inhibitory influence, resulting in sensitization of nociceptive neurons and an increase in their receptive fields (52). Cold block of the spinal cord selectively disinhibits activity of dorsal horn cells receiving input from deep (muscle) nociceptors compared to cutaneous nociceptors, suggesting that muscle pain is selectively controlled (50). Modulation of descending tonic inhibition of muscle and visceral nociceptive activity is partly mediated by opioid receptor–related synapses (53). Mense (54) summarized the data relating to referral of muscle pain, discussing the mechanisms cited here. The convergence-projection mechanism best explains the clinical and experimental data, taking into account two modifications that Mense suggested: the activation of previously ineffective connections to the dorsal horn, possibly related to the release of SP, and the appearance of new receptive fields due to central sensitization spread to adjacent spinal segments.

The persistence of tenderness in the MTrP can result from an increase in the sensitivity of nociceptor afferents or from an increase in the excitability of dorsal horn neurons. Low-frequency repetitive activation of these afferents results in summation of the action potential. Postsynaptic depolarization progressively increases, producing a larger action potential with repeated stimulation ("wind-up"). Activation of membrane NMDA receptors is involved in the maintenance of central sensitization, and may promote prolonged hyperalgesia in chronic MPSs (55).

Temporal and spatial summation of experimental noxious muscle stimulation increases pain intensity and referred pain, similar to the clinical condition of MPS, though the inciting stimuli are different (56).

The neurophysiologic studies cited earlier and reviewed recently (46,57–59) established the basis for sensitization and for referred pain mechanisms. However, all of these studies were short-term ones based on tissue injury. Application of these findings to the clinical condition of acute or chronic myofascial pain is an extrapolation to a situation in which there is no identifiable inflammatory or other injury to muscle. However, these mechanisms are so universal in different experimental models that study different tissues that it seems only reasonable they would apply to the pain generated by the MTrP. Moreover, a quantitative study of muscle tenderness in headache (60) showed that the pain stimuli-response function for pressure versus pain was qualitatively different in myofascial pain subjects than in control subjects, suggesting that there is nociceptive reception by low-threshold mechanosensitive afferent fibers (or sensitized high-threshold mechanosensitive receptors) and sensitized dorsal horn neurons, a finding consistent with the results of the short-term animal experiments cited earlier in which a peripheral nociceptive stimulus caused sensitization of peripheral and central receptors and neurons.

These considerations have definite practical implications for MPS, as they indicate the possibilities for modulation of pain from TrPs by a number of treatment approaches. Inhibition and facilitation of pain transmission and of changing receptive fields can alter TrP pain perception and perhaps TrP activity itself. Postural effects on TrP point activity were not addressed in these experiments, but are clinically important. Inactivation of MTrPs in one muscle, by injection of a local anesthetic, alters the activity in TrPs in another muscle, emphasizing the importance of these modulating factors (61,62).

Sinaki et al (63) proposed that the cause of muscle pain in MPS and FMS was prolonged sustained load or tension on a muscle. However, they did not discuss the mechanism of sustained pain in their model in the same kind of physiologic terms that are being discussed here.

An alternative view of the nature of MTrPs is that the pain of MPS is not caused by MTrPs in skeletal muscle at all, but rather is the expression of secondary hyperalgesia related to peripheral nerve injury like cervical or lumbar radiculopathy, or more likely, to central sensitization (64). Referred pain is considered the result of the expansion of receptive fields of dorsal horn neurons, as described earlier in this chapter. The MTrP is not considered to be a primary muscular disorder. Current thinking holds that central sensitization is an integral part of TrP phenomena. The mechanism of the development of the TrP is unknown, but is likely to be related to dysfunction of the motor end-plate.

Local Twitch Response

The local twitch response elicited by mechanical stimulation of the taut band is an unequivocal sign of an MTrP, whether active or latent. Only the taut band in which the TeP is found contracts, not the entire muscle. A burst of high-amplitude electrical activity accompanies the contraction (Fig. 61-2) (65). It can be elicited by needling a TrP, and sometimes is produced only by needling when it is not elicited by strumming or snapping palpation. The local twitch response is a confirmatory sign that a TrP is present when it occurs during therapeutic needling in a TrP identified by the presence of a taut band and tenderness. There is no EMG difference between a local twitch response produced by strumming or snapping palpation and that produced by needling (66), so they are considered to have the same diagnostic meaning. EMG studies have shown a latency suggestive of a spinal reflex (67). Interruption of the proximal nerve greatly diminishes, but does not abolish the local twitch response (68). In animal models of MTrPs (69–71), there is no difference between the EMG characteristics of the local twitch response elicited from the taut band of a mammal (canines and rabbits) and that elicited from a human MTrP. In these studies, as in the human studies, blocking the proximal nerve (afferent sensory, efferent motor) mechanically by transection, chemically, or by rendering the nerve ischemic markedly reduces or eliminates the local twitch response. Transection of the spinal cord in the experimental animal model caudal to the level of the nerve to the muscle stimulated produced only a transient loss of the ability to elicit the local twitch response, while transection of the peripheral nerve permanently abolished it. Thus, the local twitch response is a spinal cord reflex requiring an intact peripheral nerve. The mechanism of activation of the response and its relation to inactivation of the TrP are not known.

DIAGNOSIS

Diagnosis of MPS is made by physical examination. As always, the history provides the context of the pain problem: the events at onset; the progression or course of the problem; modifying activities that make the pain better or worse; the distribution of the pain; the effects of prior treatment; and any social disruption at work, in family relations, and in self-esteem. However, the history in MPS can only be suggestive. The diagnosis is based on the identification of the MTrP. The TrP is distinguished from simple muscle tenderness first by the presence of a taut band, and second by the presence of referred pain, and a local twitch response when the TrP is mechanically stimulated. The TrP exists in a latent form that is asymptomatic (13), although even TrPs can restrict motion and cause intermittent discomfort. An active TrP is defined as one that is spontaneously painful at rest or with activity (1). Mechanical stimulation of an active TrP, by palpation or by needling, reproduces the patient's usual pain, which is an important diagnostic observation. The diagnostic process involves an overall evaluation of possible factors that could explain the patient's symptoms. The diagnosis of MPS is not one of exclusion, but is based on positive findings. Thus, pain in the shoulder must include the usual differential diagnostic considerations of local shoulder dysfunction, including rotator cuff syndrome, impingement syndrome, bursitis, cervical disk disease, and intrinsic bone disorders such as enchondromas. MTrPs can occur

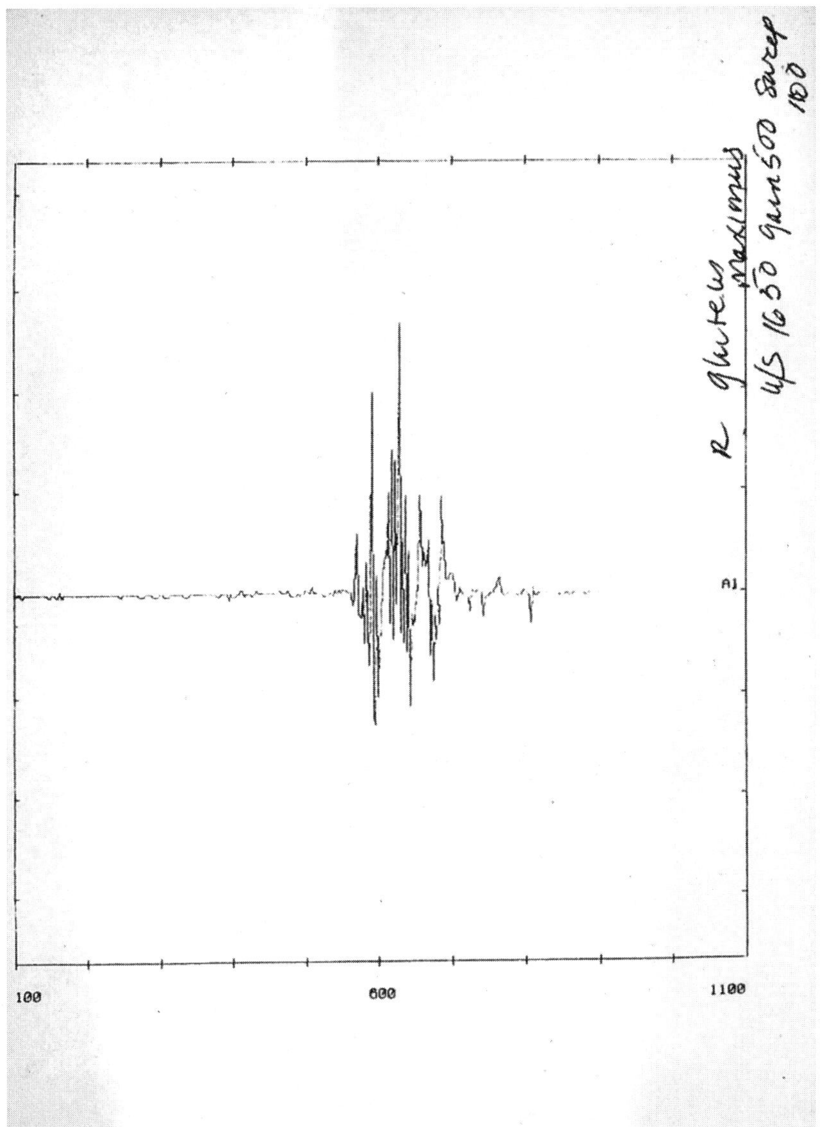

Figure 61-2. The polyphasic compound motor unit discharge of the taut band when stimulated by an electromyographic needle. The gain is 500 µV. The sweep is 100 msec.

with any of these conditions, and the presence of active TrPs should not be construed to mean that MPS is the sole cause of the pain. Anterior shoulder pain can be caused by any of the conditions just mentioned, and also can be caused by TrPs in the infraspinous, biceps, anterior scalene, anterior deltoid, and coracobrachial muscles. A comprehensive examination for TrPs will include all of these muscles. When TrPs that reproduce the pain are identified, MPS can be invoked either as a primary cause of pain or as part of a secondary pain syndrome.

The examiner must be able to identify the physical features of the TrP with confidence in order to make a diagnosis of MPS. The key physical features associated with a MTrP are listed in Table 61-1. The reliability of the examination of these physical signs has been subjected to study within the past decade.

Table 61-1: The Physical Features Associated with a Myofascial Trigger Point
1. Exquisite tenderness in a taut muscle band
2. Referred pain elicited by mechanical stimulation of the trigger point
3. Local twitch or contraction of the taut band when the trigger point is mechanically stimulated
4. Reproduction of the patient's spontaneous pain pattern when the trigger point is mechanically stimulated
5. Weakness without muscle atrophy
6. Restricted range of motion of the affected muscle
7. Autonomic dysfunction associated with the trigger point, such as changes in skin or limb temperature and piloerection

Tenderness is the most universal of the palpatory findings. It has indeed been the most studied physical sign of the TrP. A palpatory index (PI) of muscle and joint tenderness was developed as part of a craniomandibular index in the evaluation of patients who had myofascial pain dysfunction syndrome affecting the muscles of the temporomandibular joint (TMJ) or who had pain referred to the facial structures from head or neck MTrPs (72). Palpation of extraoral muscles for tenderness was found to be reproducible over time and among examiners, and was considered to be a reliable examination technique. The indices were shown to be valid in that they did represent the severity of craniomandibular pain and dysfunction. The PI correlated better with myofascial pain dysfunction than with internal derangements of the TMJ, indicating a better correlation with muscle tenderness than with joint dysfunction (73).

Attempts to quantify the measurement of tenderness have led to the use of a pressure threshold meter or algometer (74). This technique was found to be valid and reliable as a measure of TrP sensitivity (75,76) and as a way to assess the effectiveness of treatment (77,78). Pressure pain threshold was found to be reliable as a measurement of muscle tenderness, but did not correlate with the presence of referred versus local pain associated with muscle tenderness (79). The technique has been used to differentiate FMS from regional musculoskeletal pain syndromes and an absence of pain (80). Pressure algometry by itself, or combined with tissue compliance measurement to identify taut bands, fibrotic tissues, or muscle spasm, has been recommended for wider clinical use in the diagnosis and assessment of patients with musculoskeletal pain (81–83). One study comparing pressure dolorimetry and digital palpation for tenderness performed by examiners blinded to the diagnoses showed that both techniques separated FMS and MPS patients from control subjects, that both techniques showed high intrarater and interrater reliability, but that neither technique could discriminate between FMS and MPS, nor did either method correlate well with the location of the pain complaint (84). This study is important for establishing the reliability of the examination techniques of pressure dolorimetry and of digital palpation in the identification of tenderness. The inability to distinguish FMS from MPS is not surprising, however, since both have tenderness as a necessary finding and the study did not look at the unique features of the TrP that distinguish it from a TeP. Moreover, since referred pain is common from TrPs in MPS patients, and since many FMS patients also have MTrPs in addition to TePs (11), one would expect that at least some of the subjects' pain sites would be referred pain zones distant from the TeP. Hong et al (85) studied the pressure threshold for referred pain arising from TrPs and found that the force of compression needed to elicit referred pain was less (lower pressure threshold) in active TrPs and served to discriminate active from inactive TrPs.

Another device that quantitates the force of palpation when assessing muscle tenderness is the palpometer, a pressure-sensitive plastic film attached to the palpating finger. It has intrarater and interrater reliability both for the technique and for the evaluation of tenderness in subjects (86). The palpometer has been used to quantitate pain pressure thresholds in clinical research and its use has contributed to an understanding of the nature of muscle pain, as noted previously (64,87).

A study establishing the reliability of six of the major physical features of the MTrP, extending beyond the limited assessment of tenderness only, was recently performed (18). The absence of such a study had led to the criticism that the examination of the TrP was unreliable and invalid (88). Prior to this study (19), three attempts had been made to study interrater reliability for examination of two or more physical features of the MTrP. A preliminary study (89) did not demonstrate interrater reliability among four different examiners. A subsequent study among physical therapists (90) reported poor agreement among examiners evaluating tenderness and referred pain and reproduction of pain, the latter two features combined into one assessment, in persons with low-back pain. Despite methodologic shortcomings, they achieved 76% to 79% agreement for the features evaluated. However, there was low statistical significance, and reliability of the examination was not established. A third study (91) actually found tenderness, taut bands, and reproduction of pain in persons with low-back pain to be reliable signs among different examiners, but could not evaluate the features of local twitch responses or referred pain because of lack of sufficient numbers of positive responses. In the study by Gerwin et al (18), agreement among examiners was evaluated for identification of the physical features of the MTrP itself, but not with any relation to a particular diagnosis, since the study focused on the reliability of identifying physical features. Five features of the TrP were evaluated—tenderness, taut bands, local twitch responses, referred pain, and Rep P—as well as a global assessment of the TrP (present active, present latent, and absent). Interrater reliability was high for all of the features studied in most, but not all instances, and varied with both the muscle being examined and the feature being sought. The feature that was least reliable, and therefore the most difficult to identify, was the local twitch response. Agreement was highly reliable for the global assessment of TrP presence (active or latent) or absence.

The minimum features required to distinguish an MTrP from a TeP of FMS are tenderness and taut bands, that is, a TeP in a taut band. The presence of referred pain or a local twitch response is confirmatory, and makes the identification of an MTrP more certain. Each of these two features may be elicited when needling a TrP even when neither is elicited by manual examination. Reproduction of the patient's usual pain is considered necessary to call a TrP "active," since an active TrP is spontaneously painful. Nevertheless, some TrPs may change from latent to active and back again depending on the state of physical activity, rest, or stress. Based on the results of this study, one should not expect to identify all features of an MTrP by manual examination in each and every muscle. Some muscles are more difficult to examine than others, and some features of the TrP are more difficult to elicit than others. Moreover, the study showed that some training is necessary in order to attain the manual skill necessary to examine muscle well for TrPs. However, training should not be lightly undertaken, lest it be inadequate. The preliminary study by Wolfe et al (89) showed that 2 hours of training was not sufficient for rheumatologists skilled in the identification of fibromyalgia TePs to gain the required skill to identify MTrPs. Nice et al (90) could not achieve the desired level of competence among a group of physical therapists who practiced palpation of two target muscles "until they felt capable of using the technique on patients." A 5-hour training program was not sufficient to train eight examiners (six of them dentists) to achieve high agreement on examination of the head and neck for temporomandibular disorders (92). However, a general practitioner was able to teach medical students over a 3-month period to examine for TrPs well enough to achieve significant interrater reliability for the features of tenderness, jump sign (an involuntary sudden withdrawal or jump), and recognition of their usual pain (91). Workshops that offer 15 to 20 hours of instruction enable practitioners to identify TrP features in most commonly affected muscles, but there has been no formal study showing that training novices in a weekend workshop is effective.

Thermography

Attempts to diagnose MPS objectively have led to the use of algometry, discussed already, and to thermography. Thermographic findings are suggestive of or compatible with MTrPs, but not sensitive to their presence and not specific. Typical findings are "hot spots" that occur eccentrically over TrPs, creating a mottled, asymmetric pattern (93,94). The usefulness of the technique in the diagnosis of MPS has been debated (95,96). Variability in the findings possibly relates to differences in examination techniques, lack of discrimination between active and latent TrPs, and a disregard for the skin temperature changes that can occur in the referred pain zones of MTrPs. A decrease in temperature emitted over the referred pain zone occurs following compression of the TrP (95), demonstrating both the physiologic changes associated with TrP treatment and the autonomic nervous system alterations in association with the TrP. Infrared thermography is preferred because it is more sensitive than liquid crystal thermography and avoids potential changes in the TrP that might result from contact of the liquid crystal film against the skin. Identification of a taut band, the minimal discriminatory finding that distinguishes the MTrP, requires manual examination. Hence, there seems to be little need to employ thermography in the clinical diagnostic protocol at this time.

Other Laboratory Studies

The MTrP taut band is visible with high-resolution B-mode ultrasound. This technique allows visualization of the localized twitch in the taut band of the MTrP when stimulated by insertion of a hypodermic needle (35). Thus, the physical response of the TrP to treatment can be documented, and a permanent record can be made.

No other laboratory studies have shown positive results or abnormalities in MPSs. This includes all other imaging studies (x-rays, computed tomography, and magnetic resonance imaging). Magnetic resonance spectroscopy is still being studied, but no significant results have been described in association with MPS. The results of blood tests, both hematologic profiles and chemistries, are normal. Tests of autoimmune disorders, nutritional and metabolic disorders, and hormone function also show normal results. The routine EMG is normal unless the needle is put directly into the TrP, eliciting the SER activity described by Hubbard and Berkhof (27). Any abnormality seen in any of these studies, except for the finding of SEA, it not directly related to the TrP, but represents a coexisting disease or dysfunction. Coexisting disorders can be important causes of the MTrP and can be related to their maintenance. Thus, nerve root irritation or radiculopathy can initiate MPS with TrPs in muscles innervated by the affected root. Iron insufficiency is quite common in women with MPS, but is not a known cause of the TrP itself. The same is true of low levels of vitamin B_{12}. They are seen in some patients with chronic MPS (see below), but are not thought to be directly related to the development of the TrP. General laboratory studies do need to be done, however, in order to identify the important coexisting disorders that can complicate MPS and that may interfere with recovery. The history and physical examination determine which studies are appropriate for each patient. Certainly, the person with low-back pain and radiating pain and weakness in a leg deserves an evaluation for disk disease and lumbosacral radiculopathy. Degenerative disease of the hip can cause MTrPs to occur in the psoas, tensor fasciae latae, gluteal, piriform, and adductor muscles of the thigh, and may well need to be treated directly by physical therapy and perhaps by hip replacement.

Surface EMG is being used to evaluate muscle function in persons with MPS (97). It shows asymmetries in the activity of affected paired muscles. It can identify specific muscles that contribute to postural dysfunction and functional muscle unit imbalance, and objectively demonstrates dysfunction in a muscle containing TrPs.

CLINICAL SYNDROMES

The single-muscle syndromes that characterize MTrPs have been well described by Travell and Simons in the two-volume text they coauthored (1,2). However, a number of clinical syndromes are the result of regional MPS or the result of involvement of a number of muscles in a functional muscle unit. These syndromes are worthy of specific mention.

Myogenic Headache

Headache is a common complaint, and the attempt to place headaches into a heuristic classification has led to a detailed and somewhat complicated description of the varieties of headache by the International Headache Society (98). This headache classification emphasizes *descriptive* characteristics like pulsating, throbbing, band-like, and laterality; *duration* divided into hours, or days; *frequency* as less than or greater than 15 days per month; and associated autonomic and brain stem symptoms like nausea, vomiting, and photophobia. However, the occurrence of both migraine and tension headache in the same individual is common (99). One-third of patients with chronic tension-type headaches have migraine headaches, and both photophobia and phonophobia occur during tension headaches (100). The location of the ache and clinical characteristics are often the same in the two types of headaches. The term *benign recurring headache* has been used to describe these overlapping headache syndromes (99). Many of these headaches have a myofascial basis that explains their similarity. Rogers and Rogers (101) similarly proposed that MTrPs may cause at least chronic or episodic tension-type headache. Muscle tenderness, pressure pain threshold, and EMG have been studied extensively in association with headache (102–105). Pericranial muscles are more tender in headache patients than non-headache subjects, even between headaches. Tenderness increases during the headache phase, however. It is not clear whether any MTrP characteristics other than tenderness or pressure pain thresholds (e.g., taut bands or referred pain) were measured in these studies. EMG activity in the headache subjects was normal; there was no pain-induced increase in muscle activity. These findings suggest that the increase in tenderness of pericranial muscles represents a reversible sensitization of central nociceptors as occurred in the experimental studies of Mense (59) and Sessel (49) and their colleagues cited previously. This issue has also been studied in posttraumatic headaches characterized as chronic, frequent, tension-type headache, with some subjects having additional intermittent migraine-like headaches (106). Myofascial "irritability" was evaluated by muscle palpation over seven preselected sites in a fixed palpation protocol of using 4-kg/cm^2 pressure for 1 second. Muscle tenderness was related to the presence and severity of headache. In a more recent study using the palpometer described earlier, Jensen (105) found that rolling palpation of the finger over the muscle at different pressure intensities identified not only tenderness, but also a pressure-related response that suggested a stimulus-response relation in tension-type headache. This suggested that the qualitatively altered response to painful stimulation represents a change in the processing of sensory information from myofascial tissues. In all of these studies, tenderness was the main criterion for the definition of myofascial pain. The other physical features of the MTrP were not evaluated.

Muscle involvement in headache goes beyond mere tenderness, however. MTrPs play three distinct roles in headache. First, TrPs act as a local source of pain. Second, they act as a source of referred pain to the neck and head. Third, the pain from the TrP could activate the trigeminal-vascular system.

In addition to producing local pain in the neck and especially in the shoulder, and the discomfort often preceding or accompanying headache, TrPs in these areas refer pain to the occiput, the vertex, the temple, the forehead, and the periorbital region (1). TrPs in the trapezius muscle, for example, refer pain to the neck and suboccipital regions, the temple, the parietal area, and the mastoid area. Sternocleidomastoid TrPs refer pain to the periorbital region, in a distribution like that of cluster headache. The sternocleidomastoid muscle TrPs also refer pain to the occiput, the forehead, and sometimes the vertex of the head. Temporal muscle TrPs cause a local tenderness as well as supraorbital pain. Orbicularis oculi and zygomaticus muscle TrPs produce a headache pain pattern along the nose and medial canthus to the supraorbital region, resembling what many patients describe as a "sinus headache." Occipitofrontal muscle TrPs cause a local supraorbital and parietal headache. Splenius capitis and cervicis TrPs are important causes of vertex and "behind the eye" or periorbital headaches that can often be readily relieved by TrP compression (see Treatment). Semispinalis cervicis and capitis TrPs produce occipital and temple headaches, respectively. Thus, all of the unilateral or band-like headaches; occipital, parietal, or temporal headaches; and all of the frontal, sinus, or behind- or around-the-eye headaches can be caused by TrPs in one or more of the cranial or pericranial muscles, and can be diagnosed by careful manual examination.

The diagnosis of headache as a manifestation of MPS of the head, neck, and shoulder muscles can lead to a specific local treatment of the acute headache, and to prophylactic therapy to prevent future headache. This concept extends Olesen's construct of a vascular-supraspinal-myogenic model of headache (107) by giving more weight to the myogenic factor in all headache varieties. Therefore, MTrPs should be sought for by physical examination as one of the direct and treatable causes of headache.

There are other mechanisms of headache production in which MTrPs may play a role, in addition to the direct referral of pain to the cranium. Moskowitz (108) proposed that vascular (migrainous) headache results from the disturbance between the trigeminal nerve and the cerebral blood vessels that are one of its target organs. Neural activation releases vasoactive neurotransmitters that produce sterile inflammation or neurogenic edema. The release of substance P (SP) from perivascular nerves produces vasodilation and increased vascular permeability. These changes are thought to be related to the development of the migraine attack. Trigeminal sensory nerve fibers become sensitized to nonnociceptive stimuli such as mechanical pressure or vascular pulsations. One type of sensory input that could activate the trigeminal complex and initiate the chain of events that lead to headache is the MTrP that occurs in cervical or cranial muscle. Input of nociceptive stimuli from the cervical muscles innervated by nerve roots at the C5 or higher levels reaches the descending subnucleus caudalis of the trigeminal nerve. These stimuli could activate the trigeminal-vascular system and could also refer pain to the forehead, because trigeminal fibers from the ophthalmic division descend the farthest down this sensory nucleus.

Temporomandibular Joint Dysfunction

This pain syndrome often primarily involves the muscles of mastication and facial expression rather than the joint itself, and is commonly referred to as the *myofascial pain dysfunction syndrome* (See Chap. 62) (109). Pain is felt in the side of the head and at the TMJ itself, and is referred from the masseter muscles to the face. The postural muscles of the neck (sternocleidomastoid and the posterior cervical muscles) frequently contain TrPs that also refer pain to the head. The pain is more likely to be a constant, unilateral side-of-head pain rather than a more typical muscular tension headache. Patients complain of unilateral pain, although it may change sides, of a more or less constant nature that may last for days or weeks, thereby distinguishing the headache from a true paroxysmal migraine that has a beginning and an end. They point to the side of their head, from the jaw joint up to the temple, as the primary site of pain, although they may also have forehead and neck pain. A comprehensive history and physical examination, including examination of the jaw and neck muscles, jaw motion, and TMJ capsule tenderness, is a reliable and valid tool in establishing the diagnosis (73). Key diagnostic features are tenderness of the intraoral, extraoral, and neck muscles, impaired jaw mobility, and TMJ capsular noise and tenderness. The masseter muscles, both superficial and deep, are tender and taut bands are readily identified in the superficial masseter. The pterygoid muscles are also tender and shortened, and may pull the joint meniscus or disk into an anterior position that interferes with movement of the condyle. The neck muscles are frequently tender, especially the sternocleidomastoid muscle, which helps to adjust the position of the head and to stabilize it while chewing and talking. Taut bands are readily palpated in these muscles, eliciting referred pain from the MTrPs in these muscles. Since head position during talking and chewing is modified by jaw movement, the position of the mandible and the state of the muscles that control its movement are part of the same functional muscle unit as the neck and shoulder muscles that control head and neck posture (e.g., the sternocleidomastoid, the scalenes, the splenii, and the levator scapulae). A screening diagnostic test based on the clinical examination for specific signs of jaw dysfunction, tenderness of the TMJ itself, and pain with passive jaw opening and lateral jaw movement has a high specificity and sensitivity for identification of myofascial pain dysfunction syndromes (110). Understanding the relationship between the TMJ-related muscles and the muscles of the neck and shoulder facilitates the resolution of cranial muscle pain perpetuated by MTrPs outside of the jaw, and of head and neck muscle pain perpetuated by MrTPs in the muscles of mastication.

Cervical Vertigo

Individuals with whiplash and those with myofascial pain dysfunction syndrome frequently complain of dizziness, usually indicating imbalance rather than vertigo. Two causes of imbalance from whiplash include vestibular concussion and perilymphatic fistula of the round or oval window. In addition, two MPSs can lead to dizziness. In one myofascial syndrome, TrPs in the clavicular head of the sternocleidomastoid muscle cause a sense of displacement of the head with respect to the body, resulting in postural imbalance that can be seen during the Romberg test or tandem walking with the eyes closed (1). True vertigo can occur, especially with a sudden change in position like turning over in bed. Inactivating the TrPs manually or by injection with a local anesthetic can immediately resolve the sense of disequilibrium. In the second MPS causing dizziness, postural reflexes that involve cervical muscle afferent input are impaired (111,112). The inactivation of posterior cervical MTrPs, alone or with inactivation of sternocleidomastoid TrPs, reduces or eliminates the disequilibrium, difficulty focusing, and dizziness. Functional postural impairment has been noted in persons with mechanical neck pain, all of whom had tender neck muscles and all of whom showed a decrease in dizziness and pain and an improvement in postural performance following physiotherapy to the neck (113).

Cervical Whiplash

Whiplash occurs when the head and neck move forcefully or abruptly in extension or flexion (more often in extension) or in some form of rotational or torsional motion. The consequences of cervical whiplash include neck pain, headache, visual disturbance, dizziness, weakness, paresthesias, cognitive disorders, and psychological disturbance (114,115). Many patients with cervical whiplash have MTrP pain (MPS) as part of the clinical constellation. The muscles most often involved are those of the neck and shoulder region, most notably the sternocleidomastoid, the splenii and the semispinalis capitis, the trapezius, the levator scapulae, and the pectoral muscles. Few studies have examined the role of the MTrP in cervical whiplash.

Nonetheless, MTrPs are clinically significant causes of pain or other symptoms (116–118). The MTrPs can be identified in the usual manner by palpation and reproduction of the symptoms of headache, neck ache, or dizziness. Effective treatment of the MTrPs reduces the pain, increases the range of motion, and corrects the imbalance. Disequilibrium, tinnitus, blurred vision, and headache can result from whiplash-induced sternocleidomastoid MTrPs, and can be eliminated or reduced by inactivating the cervical MTrPs.

A form of thoracic outlet syndrome caused by MTrPs can occur after cervical whiplash. Thirty-seven patients who had tingling of the symptomatic hand during hyperabduction maneuvers and upper-limb hyperesthesia and weakness improved after appropriate physical therapy and TrP injections in the pectoralis minor muscle (117). A second mechanism of thoracic outlet syndrome occurs when MTrPs are present in the scalene muscles (119). The brachial plexus passes between the anterior and medial scalene muscles (the scalene compartment) and can be compressed by hypertrophied or contracted scalene muscles. When the scalene muscles have MTrPs with taut bands, they are shortened. Shortened scalene muscles pull the first rib upward, narrowing the space between the first rib and the clavicle through which the neurovascular bundle passes, and compressing the lower cervical roots comprising the brachial plexus. Treatment of this form of thoracic outlet syndrome requires inactivation of the scalene muscle MTrPs. In addition, the breathing pattern should be examined, as chest breathing utilizes the scalene muscles as accessory respiratory muscles. Chest breathers must learn diaphragmatic breathing to prevent overloading and shortening of the scalene muscles. A final important cause of thoracic outlet syndrome symptoms that can occur following cervical whiplash and other injuries to the upper back and neck are MTrPs originating in the anterior scalene or infraspinous muscles. Referred pain from firm palpation of these MTRPs can reproduce the pain in the shoulder and arm that is typical of thoracic outlet syndrome.

Postlaminectomy Pelvic Pain Syndrome

This syndrome is an all too frequent cause of persistent pain after surgery for lumbar radiculopathy. The pain is commonly related to MTrPs in the quadratus lumborum, iliocostal, deep paraspinal, gluteal, piriform, psoas, adductor, and hamstring muscles. Referred pain from the gluteus minimus, entrapment of the sciatic nerve by the piriform, and TrPs in the hamstrings mimic signs of radiculopathy.

Pelvic Pain Syndromes

Among the causes of pelvic pain are MTrPs in the adductor magnus muscle and in the levator ani, which produce poorly localized deep pelvic pain. The two parts of the levator ani, the pubococcygeal muscle and the iliococcygeal muscle, attach to the anococcygeal body; the latter muscle also attaches to the coccyx. Coccydynia can be caused by levator ani MTrPs, the levator ani being exquisitely tender to manual palpation by rectal examination. Pain may be referred to the coccyx or elsewhere in the pelvis. The palpating finger sweeps around the circumference of the anus, identifying local regions of increased muscle tautness and tenderness. These areas are manually stretched by the examining finger. A mixture of lubricant and lidocaine (e.g., viscous lidocaine) makes the examination more tolerable. This condition is seen in persons who have been in motor vehicle accidents where there has been considerable force from the seat back against the pelvis, in persons who have fallen onto their buttocks and sacrum, and in those who have had genitourinary tract infections, including men with prostatitis. Disorders of bladder function commonly occur in women with this kind of pain syndrome. TrPs in the urethral sphincter cause a sense of constant bladder irritation and of a need to void. TrPs seldom occur in these muscles alone, and are usually accompanied by TrPs in the adductor magnus muscle, which refers pain deep into the pelvis, and to other muscles in the area, including the abdominal, iliopsoas, piriform, and gluteal muscles. In addition to the MTrPs, spinal-pelvic dysfunctions (lumbar rigidity, ilial rotations, and sacroiliac joint hypomobility) cause pain or perpetuate the MPS.

Phantom Pain

Stump pain and phantom limb pain cause persistent discomfort and disability after amputation. Central pain mechanisms and local nerve injury, including the development of neuromas, are thought to be responsible for many of these pain syndromes. However, MTrPs in the stump muscles can be a source of readily treatable pain. The leg muscles that tend to shorten and develop MTrPs in patients with above-knee amputations are the psoas and adductor muscles. Passive movement can be greatly restricted because of these MTrPs. TrP injections and stretching the muscles can produce rapid, almost immediate relief. One gentleman with a traumatic amputation of the thumb had clinically important MTrPs in the remnant of the first dorsal interosseous muscle, and also in the infraspinous muscle, both of which caused pain in the hand. Injection of these TrPs altered his phantom pain, first increasing it and subsequently eliminating it. This case was an illuminating example of the interaction between the dysfunctional muscle associated with the amputation and the plasticity of central nervous system nociception.

TREATMENT

Treatment is intended to relieve pain and to restore normal function both of the postural muscle patterns and of the whole individual. Central to this purpose is the inactivation or elimination of the MTrP. Therefore, the treatment must be directed toward the MTrP itself, and to those mechanical, general medical, and psychological factors that sustain and aggravate the MPS. Correction of work-related or recreational postural stresses and encouragement to resume normal activity are also part of the treatment. Inactivation of the MTrP is done through one or a combination of manual and invasive techniques.

Intermittent Cold and Stretch

Travell (120) expanded the use of a cold stimulus in her work with acute sprains, referred viscerosomatic pains like those associated with cardiac ischemia, and MPS, using a vapocoolant that she thought produced a local block. The action of the vapocoolant spray can now be understood as an activation of myelinated, low-threshold, mechanothermal-sensitive nonnociceptive cutaneous receptors that inhibit nociceptive C-fiber input according to gate control theory (121) and thereby allow stretching of the painful muscle. In a detailed discussion of the stretch and spray technique, Travell and Simons (1) described its use in the treatment of MPS, and emphasized the importance of the stretch in the inactivation of the MTrP. The spray is directed in an oblique angle onto the skin at a slow rate of about 10 cm/sec, taking care not to frost the skin. The spray is first directed toward the TrP in the affected muscle, and is then swept in a few parallel lines over the muscle toward the referred pain zone. While the vapocoolant is applied, the muscle is gradually stretched until the maximum stretch is achieved or a barrier is reached. Stretch for each muscle is always opposite its direction of action. Heat is applied after stretching in order to reduce poststretching discomfort.

The goal of treatment is the inactivation of the MTrP through the lengthening of the affected muscle. Use of the tactile and thermal vapocoolant stimulus is one way of facilitating stretch and achieving this goal, but other techniques are also effective.

Manual Therapy

A technique that can be as effective as intermittent cold and stretch, and as easy to use, is postisometric relaxation. Lewit (122) described this method well, along with the technique of respiratory facilitation that enhances postisometric relaxation. The muscle to be stretched is brought to its barrier, the point at which resistance prevents further stretching without force. The subject then exerts a gentle force against the operator's hand, in the direction of the action of the muscle, opposite the stretch. Lewit (122) reported that activation of as little as 10% to 15% of the muscle fibers is sufficient to produce the desired effect. The operator holds the part stationary, preventing loss of the stretch already gained; thus, the contraction is isometric. Following 5 to 15 seconds of isometric contraction, the subject "lets go" and the stretch is repeated. A considerable increase in the stretch is usually achieved by this method. This technique is more effective for increasing the range of motion in the passive straight-leg raising test than is myofascial release leg pull (manual traction of the leg) (123).

Lewit also used the known effect of respiration on muscle contraction and relaxation to further enhance the stretch produced by postisometric relaxation. Exhalation enhances muscle contraction and inhalation facilitates relaxation, except for the respiratory muscles, which act in just the opposite way. The technique can be taught readily to patients for their own use in self-directed stretching.

TrP compression, sometimes called *ischemic compression*, is effective in relaxing the taut band and relieving pain. Firm pressure is exerted directly over the TrP zone. After an initial tenderness, there is a decrease in pain within 15 to 20 seconds. Within 60 to 90 seconds of continued pressure, the tenderness is gone and the taut band can be felt to relax. The TrP is then stretched locally, and the muscle stretched to its full length.

Repeated rhythmic tapping (percussion) of the TrP results in a decrease in pain and relaxation of the taut band after 8 to 12 taps, similar to the effect of TrP compression. Stretching of the muscle is important in maintaining the improvement. Patients can perform this technique themselves in accessible muscles.

Other manual techniques including Rolfing, deep friction massage, myofascial release, muscle stripping massage, and reciprocal inhibition are methods of relaxing and stretching muscle that are well described in standard texts of physical medicine and physical therapy, and are not discussed here except to note that they, too, are effective in the inactivation of MTrPs. Intermittent cold and stretch, moist heat, ultrasound, and deep pressure massage each are more effective than no treatment or placebo in the reduction of pain from active MTrPs (124).

Trigger Point Injection

Inactivation of the MTrP can be accomplished by insertion of a needle into the trigger zone of the MTrP. Lewit (125) used dry needling in the management of myofascial pain, a technique termed *intramuscular stimulation* by Gunn et al (126). Lewit's motor point localization of soreness in muscle identifies tenderness and taut bands that are similar to or identical with MTrPs. Dry needling of MTrPs in paraspinal muscles is effective in the treatment of pain associated with lumbosacral radiculopathy (127). Hong (128) compared dry needling to injection of local anesthetic (lidocaine). He found that both techniques produced an immediate reduction in the pain intensity and in the pain threshold and improvement in the range of motion, provided that a local twitch response was elicited by the procedure. This shows that the essential action producing inactivation of the TrP is the mechanical effect of the needle, although the mechanism by which needle stimulation produces a local twitch response, relaxation of the taut band, and an almost immediate reduction in pain is not known. Hong (128) found that dry needling, though effective in relieving pain, caused more postinjection soreness than did injection of lidocaine, which he attributed to the need to do more needle insertions into the muscle in order to elicit and eliminate local twitch responses with dry needling. As a consequence, he speculated, there is more intramuscular hemorrhage associated with dry needling, accounting for the pain.

TrP injections with local anesthetics are more commonly performed than dry needling without anesthetics. Kellgren (4) infiltrated tender areas in muscle with a local anesthetic and eliminated muscle pain in his subjects. Hendler et al (129) found that muscle tension measured by surface EMG over the TrP decreased significantly with injection of a local anesthetic. One injection technique is described in detail by Hong (130), although many variations of holding the syringe and stabilizing the trigger zone exist. Travell and Simons (1) recommended use of procaine diluted to 0.5%, because procaine is metabolized locally by procaine esterase, and the effective half-life is as short as 10 to 15 minutes. If a local nerve block is inadvertently produced, numbness and weakness resolve shortly. Patients can become very upset if they leave the clinic with a numb or weak limb, which can happen when a local anesthetic with a longer half-life is used.

The local twitch response is a reliable objective sign that the taut band has been entered. The patient's report that the usual pain is reproduced ("that's my pain!") or that referred pain accompanies an injection is also a reliable sign that the trigger zone has been entered.

Injection into the trigger zone is continued until there is no further response, indicating that all TrPs in that zone are inactivated. The taut bands should be palpably relaxed when the TrP zone is inactivated. The needle is repeatedly pulled back to the skin and reangled slightly to enter an adjacent area in the trigger zone, until the area is cleared of active TrPs. When that occurs, the needle is withdrawn and firm pressure is applied for hemostasis. Vitamin C, one 500-mg timed-release tablet taken daily, is recommended during the time of TrP injections, to reduce bleeding in the muscle.

All TrPs in a functional muscle unit should be addressed, the key TrPs that seem to be clinically responsible for the pain syndrome injected until they are inactivated, and the remainder treated manually. TrP injections are performed to effectively stretch the muscle, which is an essential part of the treatment. Moist heat applied afterward decreases posttreatment muscle soreness. Anesthetic-medicated patches relieve any local skin discomfort caused by the injections.

Baldry (131) described one variation of the TrP injection technique, called *superficial dry needling.* A fine needle like an acupuncture needle is placed over the tender ("ouch") spot. This technique has been reported to be effective, though no controlled study has been done to confirm this.

Injection of materials other than local anesthetics has been advocated. Most commonly, corticosteroids have been injected, although no well-designed study has demonstrated the superiority of this technique over dry needling or the use of local anesthetics. Injection of ketorolac may also be useful, though the study results are preliminary. Botulinum toxin currently is perhaps the most actively studied agent used as an alternative to local anesthetic (132,133). The rationale is that long-lasting inactivation of motor end-plate activity produced by blocking the release of acetylcholine from the cholinergic presynaptic terminal will allow the muscle to recover function without a recurrence of TrP activity.

TrP injection therapy can fail for a variety of reasons (Table 61-2). Most commonly, inadequate injection into the primary or important TrPs leads to failure. Inadequate hemostasis leads to muscle pain and spasm. Inadequate stretching, either just after the injection or in follow-up programs at home, leads to recurrence of the TrP. Nontechnical factors associated with a lack of efficacy of TrP injection therapy combined with physical therapy are unemployment, constant rather than intermittent pain, and failure to achieve relief with analgesic medications (134). Fibromyalgia as a coexisting condition is also associated with decreased pain relief as measured by pain threshold assessment. In one study, postinjection soreness was greater and lasted longer in subjects with fibromyalgia. The soreness was improved by 2 weeks following TrP injection therapy, but the fibromyalgia group never did as well as those without fibromyalgia (135).

Table 61-2: Reasons for Failure of Trigger Point Injections to Relieve Pain

1. Missing the trigger point (injecting the taut band, but not the trigger point)
2. Injection into an inactive, rather than active, trigger point
3. Inadequate hemostasis
4. Inadequate stretching
5. Treating only part of the functional muscle unit, or treating only the secondary or satellite trigger point
6. Inadequate follow-up treatment (home program) by the patient
7. Unemployment
8. Constant pain (in contrast to intermittent pain)
9. Lack of pain relief with analgesics

The complications of TrP injections (Table 61-3) serve to warn that muscle injection is a potentially dangerous, invasive technique. Care must be taken to avoid injecting into internal organs. Pneumothorax is the most common consequence of organ puncture. Nerve injury from the penetrating needle is heralded by sudden, severe, electric shock–like pain traveling in the distribution of the nerve. These complications are best avoided by careful attention to anatomic landmarks and knowledge of underlying structural relationships. Attention to hemostasis will

Table 61-3: Complications of Trigger Point Injections
1. Local hemorrhage into a muscle
2. Vasodepressive syncope
3. Allergic reactions, including anaphylaxis
4. Local muscle edema (myoedema)
5. Infection
6. Penetration of a viscus or solid organ
7. Pneumothorax
8. Local nerve block
9. Nerve injury
10. Muscle spasm
11. Anesthetic toxicity

avoid the common problem of bleeding into the muscle and the accompanying muscle pain. Vasodepressive syncope is avoided by having the patient recumbent while receiving injections into the TrP.

Pharmacologic Therapy

There is a paucity of studies on drug treatment for MPS, perhaps because there is no biochemical or metabolic disturbance thought to be related to the development or maintenance of the MTrP that is seen as being amenable to drug therapy. Therefore, the same principles that apply to treatment of nonmalignant pain of any source are applied to the treatment of MPS.

Nonprescription analgesics are preferred initially. Prescription analgesics may be used during the introduction of TrP therapy. Sleep disturbance caused by pain is treated, usually by relieving the pain at night. This can be done through the use of analgesics at bedtime, or the use of an antidepressant drug that increases serotonin and norepinephrine blood levels and combines a sedative effect and a pain modulation effect. Nonsteroidal anti-inflammatory drugs (NSAIDs) and muscle relaxants are commonly used, but there is no proof that they offer any particular advantage. The combination of a mild narcotic and an NSAID produces a synergistic effect. One study evaluated sumatriptan as a treatment of temporal muscle myofascial pain–related headache, and found that it was not effective (136). All drug therapy should be regarded as temporary, and should be used for pain relief while the underlying condition of the MPS is treated specifically.

PERPETUATING FACTORS

The problem of chronic MPS has been touched on in the previous discussion of MTrP spread. Although the majority of persons with acute MPS improve within a short time, some continue to suffer from the condition for many months or even years. TrPs that develop as a result of an injury or other cause may seem to develop a life of their own and persist long after the original trauma has passed. Mechanical factors that constantly or recurrently overload muscle are potential causes of persistent TrPs and continued pain (1). The role of repetitive strain or cumulative trauma as a cause of painful syndromes such as carpal tunnel syndrome is controversial (137). The issue is relevant to MPS, where attention to ergonomic factors has a positive effect on recovery. Particular attention is directed toward correction of stressful postures. The head-forward, rolled-shoulder posture is associated with MTrPs in the posterior cervical muscles, the pectoral muscles, and the trapezius and levator scapulae muscles. In the low back, sacral and pelvic dysfunctions associated with leg-length discrepancies, hypomobility of the sacroiliac junction, and ilial rotations and upslip are associated with persistent TrPs in the quadratus lumborum, longissimus, psoas, and piriform muscles; the adductor muscles of the thigh; and the gluteal muscles. Examination of the low back and pelvis is done with the patient standing, walking, and bending. Any asymmetry of pelvic motion is rechecked with the patient seated on the examination table, which stabilizes the ilium and focuses attention on hypomobility of the sacroiliac joint. Lumbar motion is assessed during flexion and lateral bending, and mobility of the sacroiliac joint is evaluated. When necessary, correction of asymmetries can be accomplished using gentle mobilization techniques and muscle energy techniques. These corrections, and lengthening of the quadratus lumborum muscle, should always be done before recommending use of a lift to raise the heel of an apparently short leg, because the mechanical factors that produce the same effect can be corrected directly when found. Torsions of the cervical and thoracic regions of the spine, associated with scoliosis, also overload muscle, and lead to recurrent TrPs when there has been an acute MPS.

GENERAL MEDICAL PERPETUATING FACTORS

Though long suspected as being important (1), there has been little documentation of an association between inadequate concentrations of essential nutritional elements such as vitamins, which act as enzyme cofactors, or low levels of hormones such as thyroid hormone, and chronic MPS. Preliminary studies showed that inadequacies of iron as indicated by serum ferritin, vitamin B_{12}, folic acid, and thyroid hormone levels are likely to be associated with chronic MPS (11,100). Many patients complain of being cold, and have either insufficient serum ferritin, insufficient thyroid hormone, or insufficient folic acid. The difference between deficient and insufficient levels is that deficiency states produce well-defined clinical disorders, such as pellagra from vitamin C deficiency, or anemia from iron deficiency. Insufficiency states produce more subtle changes, but when a careful history is taken, clearly abnormal function is reported. For example, many with both MPS and borderline results on thyroid function tests are cold; do not tolerate wet, cold weather; are constipated; have dry skin, thinning hair, and mild pretibial edema; and fatigue easily. Ferritin at a level of 15 to 20 ng/mL is sufficient to prevent iron deficiency anemia, but is low enough to be associated with depletion of nonessential iron stores in muscle, liver, and bone marrow and to produce coldness and fatigability. Correction of these states is associated with symptomatic improvement, and probably better responses to both TrP injection therapy and physical therapy.

Vitamin C has the value of improving vascular integrity and decreasing intramuscular bleeding when treating MPS with TrP injections, and in reducing muscle cramps one to several days after strenuous exercise.

In addition, other medical conditions seem to be associated with diffuse, widespread MTrPs, in a manner similar to that seen in persons with hypothyroidism. Women with recurrent vaginal yeast infections seem to be particularly prone to this, and to have a virulent form of MPS. A history of frequent bladder infections or respiratory infections treated with antibiotics is often associated with recurrent "yeast" infections in these women and suggests that they may be harboring *Candida albicans* in the bowel or vagina. Empiric treatment can result in notable diminution in their muscle pain, but the numbers are so small as to preclude any real study of this association. There is no evidence to support a candidiasis hypersensitivity syndrome, however (138). Elevated uric acid levels in men and in postmenopausal women also seem to be a risk factor for persistent MTrPs. Parasitic infections, especially amoebic infestation, appear to be a risk factor, and a history of possible exposure should lead to examination of the stool.

Identification of ergonomic risk factors, particularly those in the workplace, is important in order to correct poor body mechanics. Photographs of the individual at work can help identify poor layout of work tools and equipment. Back, neck, and shoulder stressors can be identified and corrected by this means (139). Postures that promote chronic shortening of the hip flexors can be treated by specific stretching techniques of the psoas muscle, and correction of sitting or lying postures. Alternative ways of lifting or carrying can relieve shoulder loading.

A perpetuating factor that must be considered in the chronic patient, and in the subject who does not respond as expected, is psychological stress. The TrP in the trapezius muscle specifically responds to a psychological stressor, while the adjacent nontender muscle does not (140). Psychological stress or distress does not inevitably lead to MPS, nor does it always accompany it. Nevertheless, persons with chronic MPS, like other persons with chronic pain of any sort, are subject to disruptions in their lives because of pain. They may be unable to work, or their jobs may have to be modified, affecting their income or the possibilities of advancement. Their role as caregiver or breadwinner may be impaired, or the relationships in their lives may be inverted, so that the support they once could give they must now receive. Their ability to participate in family or social relationships, including sexual relations, may be greatly altered. These stresses can be associated with a worsening or persistence of MPS (141). Somatization was more prevalent in persons with chronic low-back MPS than in those with herniated disk syndromes (15). Depression is a likely comorbid factor in chronic or widespread myofascial pain, and has an adverse impact on the pain (142–144).

CONCLUSIONS

MPS is a common cause of pain, particularly of chronic pain, and is a complicating factor of many other conditions like disk disease and stroke. Its defining feature, the MTrP, is also the target of treatment, which involves inactivation of the TrP by manual or invasive means, and correction of the biomechanical factors that may have initiated the condition or that perpetuate it. A search for and correction of the medical and psychological factors associated with the condition and related to its persistence must be undertaken. Once these are identified and properly treated, the pain can usually be reduced or eliminated, with a consequent return to normal or useful activity.

REFERENCES

1. Travell JG, Simons DG. *Myofascial pain and dysfunction: the trigger point manual.* Vol. 1. Baltimore: Williams & Wilkins, 1983.
2. Travell JG, Simons DG. *Myofascial pain and dysfunction: the trigger point manual.* Vol. 2. Baltimore: Williams & Wilkins, 1992.
3. Edeiken J, Wolferth CC. Persistent pain in the shoulder region following myocardial infarction. *Am J Med Sci* 1936;191: 201–210.
4. Kellgren JH. A preliminary account of referred pains arising from muscle. *BMJ* 1938;1: 325–327.
5. Kellgren JH. Observations on referred pain arising from muscle. *Clin Sci* 1938;3: 175–190.
6. Kellgren JH. On the distribution of pain arising from deep somatic structures with charts of segmental pain areas. *Clin Sci* 1939;4:35–46.
7. Lewis T, Kellgren JH. Observations relating to referred pain, visceromotor reflexes and other associated phenomena. *Clin Sci* 1939;4:47–71.
8. Travell JG. Chronic myofascial pain syndromes. In: Fricton JR,

Awad EA, eds. *Advances in pain research and therapy*. Vol. 17. New York: Raven, 1990:129–137.

9. Simons DG. Muscle pain syndromes. *Am J Phys Med* 1975;54:289–311; 1976;55:15–42.

10. Gerwin RD, Gervitz R. Chronic myofascial pain: iron insufficiency and coldness as risk factors. *J Musculoskel Pain* 1995;3(suppl 1):120. Abstract.

11. Gerwin RD. A study of 96 subjects examined both for fibromyalgia and myofascial pain. *J Musculoskel Pain* 1995;3(suppl 1):121. Abstract.

12. Skootsky SA, Jaeger B, Oye RK. Prevalence of myofascial pain in general internal medicine practice. *West J Med* 1989;151: 157–160.

13. Sola AE, Rodenberger ML, Gettys BB. Incidence of hypersensitive areas in posterior shoulder muscles. A survey of two hundred young adults. *Am J Phys Med* 1955;34:585–590.

14. Fishbain DA, Goldberg M, Meagher BR, et al. Male and female chronic pain patients categorized by DSM-III psychiatric diagnostic criteria. *Pain* 1986; 26:181–197.

15. Cassisi JE, Sypert GW, Lagana L, et al. Pain, disability, and psychological functioning in chronic low back pain subgroups: myofascial versus herniated disc syndrome. *Neurosurgery* 1993;33:379–385.

16. Fricton JR, Kroening R, Haley D, Siegert R. Myofascial pain syndrome of the head and neck: a review of clinical characteristics of 164 patients. *Oral Surg* 1985;60:615–623.

17. Granges G, Littlejohn G. Prevalence of myofascial pain syndrome in fibromyalgia syndrome and regional pain syndrome: a comparative study. *J Musculoskel Pain* 1993;1(2):19–35.

18. Gerwin RD, Shannon SR, Hong C-Z, et al. Interrater reliability in myofascial trigger point examination. *Pain* 1997;69:65–73.

19. Simons DG, Travell JG. Myofascial pain syndromes. In: Wall PD, Melzack R, eds. *Textbook of pain*. Edinburgh: Churchill Livingstone, 1984:263–276.

20. Simons DG, Travell JG. Myofascial origins of low back pain. *Postgrad Med* 1983;73:66–108.

21. Simons DG. Myofascial pain syndromes. In: Basmajian JV, Kirby RL, eds. *Medical rehabilitation*. Baltimore: Williams & Wilkins, 1984:209–215, 313–320.

22. Simons DG. Myofascial pain syndromes due to trigger points. In: Goodgold J, ed. *Rehabilitation medicine*. St. Louis: CV Mosby, 1988:686–723.

23. Rosen NB. Physical medicine and rehabilitation approaches to the management of myofascial pain and fibromyalgia syndromes. *Baillieres Clin Rheumatol* 1994;8:887–889.

24. Basmajian JV, De Luca CJ. *Muscles alive*. 5th ed. Baltimore: Williams & Wilkins, 1985:270–271.

25. Drewes AM, Andreason A, Schroder HD, et al. Pathology of skeletal muscle in fibromyalgia: a histo-immuno-chemical and ultrastructure study. *Br J Rheumatol* 1993;32:79–83.

26. Bengtsson A, Henricksson KG, Larsson J. Reduced high-energy phosphate levels in the painful muscles in fibromyalgia. *Arthritis Rheum* 1986;29: 817–821.

27. Hubbard DR, Berkoff GM. Myofascial trigger points show spontaneous needle EMG activity. *Spine* 1993;18:1803–1807.

28. Travell J. Symposium on mechanism and management of pain syndromes. *Proc Rudolf Virchow Med Soc* 1959;16:128–135.

29. Simons DG, Hong C-Z, Simons LS. Nature of myofascial trigger points, active loci. *J Musculoskel Pain* 1995;3(suppl 1):62. Abstract.

30. Simons DG, Hong C-Z, Simons LS. Spontaneous electrical activity of trigger points. *J Musculoskel Pain* 1995;3(suppl 1): 124. Abstract.

31. Simons DG, Hong C-Z, Simons LS. Spike activity in trigger points. *J Musculoskel Pain* 1995;3(suppl 1):125. Abstract.

32. Simons DG, Hong C-Z, Simons LS. Prevalence of spontaneous electrical activity at trigger spots and at control sites in rabbit skeletal muscle. *J Musculoskel Pain* 1995;3:35–48.

33. Hubbard DR. Chronic and recurrent muscle pain: pathophysiology and treatment, and a review of pharmacologic studies. *J Musculoskel Pain* 1996;4: 123–143.

34. Simons DG. Referred phenomena of myofascial trigger points. In: Vecchiet L, Albe-Fessard D, Lindbloom U, Giamberadino MA, eds. *New trends in referred pain and hyperalgesia*. Amsterdam: Elsevier Science, 1993:341–357.

35. Gerwin RD, Duranleau D. The identification of the myofascial taut band by ultrasound. *Muscle Nerve* 1997;20:767–768. Letter.

36. Cross SA. Pathophysiology of pain. *Mayo Clin Proc* 1994;69:375–383.

37. Mense S, Craig AD. Spinal and supraspinal terminations of primary afferent fibers from the gastrocnemius-soleus muscle in the cat. *Neuroscience* 1988;26:1023–1035.

38. Mense S, Schmidt RF. Activation of group IV afferent units from muscle by algesic agents. *Brain Res* 1974;72:305–310.

39. Mense S. Nervous outflow from skeletal muscle following chemical noxious stimulation. *J Physiol* 1977;267:75–88.

40. Mense S, Meyer H. Different types of slowly conducting afferent units in cat skeletal muscle and tendon. *J Physiol* 1985;363:403–417.

41. Hoheisel U, Mense S. Response behavior of cat dorsal horn neu-

rones receiving input from skeletal muscle and other deep somatic tissues. *J Physiol* 1990;426:265–280.

42. Mense S, Meyer H. Bradykinin-induced modulation of the response behavior of different types of feline group III and IV muscle receptors. *J Physiol* 1988;398:49–63.

43. Zieglgansberger W, Tulloch IF. Effects of substance P on neurones in the dorsal horn of the spinal cord of the cat. *Brain Res* 1979;166:273–282.

44. Mense S. Biochemical pathogenesis of myofascial pain. *J Musculoskel Pain* 1996;4: 145–162.

45. Wall PD, Woolf CJ. Muscle but not cutaneous C-afferent input produces prolonged increases in the excitability of the flexion reflex in the rat. *J Physiol* 1984;356:443–458.

46. Fields HL. *Pain.* New York: McGraw-Hill, 1987:82–95.

47. Yu X-M, Mense S. Response properties and descending control of rat dorsal horn neurons with deep receptive fields. *Neuroscience* 1990;39:823–831.

48. Hoheisel U, Mense S, Simons DG, Yu X-M. Appearance of new receptive fields in rat dorsal horn neurons following noxious stimulation of skeletal muscle: a model for referred muscle pain? *Neurosci Lett* 1993; 153:9–12.

49. Hu JW, Sessle BJ, Raboisson P, et al. Stimulation of craniofascial muscle afferents induces prolonged facilitatory effects in trigeminal nociceptive brainstem neurons. *Pain* 1992; 48:53–60.

50. Hoheisel U, Koch K, Mense S. Functional reorganization in the rat dorsal horn during an experiment myositis. *Pain* 1994;59:111–118.

51. McMahon SB, Wall PD. Physiological evidence for branching of peripheral unmyelinated sensory afferent fibers in the rat. *J Comp Neurol* 1987;261:130–136.

52. Wall PD. The laminar organization of dorsal horn and effects of descending impulses. *J Physiol* 1967;188:403–424.

53. Yu X-M, Hua M, Mense S. The effects of intracerebroventricular injection of naloxone, phentolamine and methysergide on the transmission of nociceptive signals in rat dorsal horn neurons with convergent cutaneous-deep input. *Neuroscience* 1991;44:715–723.

54. Mense S. Referral of muscle pain: new aspects. *Am Pain Soc J* 1994;3:1–9.

55. Woolf CJ, Thompson WN. The induction and maintenance of central sensitization is dependent on *N*-methyl-D-aspartic acid receptor activation; implications for the treatment of post-injury pain hypersensitivity states. *Pain* 1991;44:293–299.

56. Graven-Nielsen T, Arendt-Nielsen L, Svensson P, Jensen TS. Quantification of local and referred muscle pain in humans after sequential i.m. injections of hypertonic saline. *Pain* 1997;69:111–117.

57. Gerwin R. Neurobiology of the myofascial trigger point. *Baillieres Clin Rheumatol* 1994;8:747–762.

58. Hong C-Z. Pathophysiology of myofascial trigger point. *J Formos Med Assoc* 1996;95:93–104.

59. Mense S. Nociception from skeletal muscle in relation to clinical muscle pain. *Pain* 1993;54:241–289.

60. Bendtsen L, Jensen R, Olesen J. Qualitatively altered nociception in chronic myofascial pain. *Pain* 1996;65:259–264.

61. Carlson CR, Okeson JP, Falace DA, et al. Reduction of pain and EMG activity in the masseter region by trapezius trigger point injection. *Pain* 1993;55:397–400.

62. Knapp L, Atchison JW, Shapiro R, et al. Electromyographic and kinematic analysis of the painful hemiplegic shoulder before and after subscapularis motor point block. *Arch Phys Med Rehabil* 1996;77:925–926. Abstract.

63. Sinaki M, Merritt JL, Stillwell GK. Tension myalgia of the pelvic floor. *Mayo Clin Proc* 1977;52:717–722.

64. Quintner JL, Cohen ML. Referred pain of peripheral nerve origin: an alternative to the myofascial pain construct. *Clin J Pain* 1995;11:243–251.

65. Fricton JR, Auvinen BA, Dykstra D, Schiffman E. Myofascial pain syndrome: electromyographic changes associated with the local twitch response. *Arch Phys Med Rehabil* 1985;66:314–317.

66. Simons DG, Dexter JR. Comparison of local twitch responses elicited by palpation and needling of myofascial trigger points. *J Musculoskel Pain* 1995;3:49–61.

67. Dexter JR, Simons DG. Local twitch response in human muscle evoked by palpation and needle penetration of a trigger point. *Arch Phys Med Rehabil* 1981;65:521–522.

68. Hong C-Z. Persistence of local twitch response with loss of conduction to and from the spinal cord. *Arch Phys Med Rehabil* 1994;75:12–16.

69. Simons DG, Stolov WC. Microscopic features and transient contraction of palpable bands in canine muscle. *Am J Phys Med* 1976;55:65–88.

70. Hong C-Z, Torigoe Y. Electrophysiologic characteristics of localized twitch responses in responsive taut bands of rabbit skeletal muscle fibers. *J Musculoskel Pain* 1994;2:17–43.

71. Hong C-Z, Torigoe Y, Yu J. The localized twitch responses in responsive taut bands of rabbit skeletal muscle fibers are related to the reflexes at spinal cord level. *J Musculoskel Pain* 1995;3:15–33.

72. Fricton JR, Schiffman EL. Reliability of a craniomandibular index. *J Dent Res* 1986;65:1359–1364.

73. Fricton JR, Schiffman EL. The craniomandibular index: validity. *J Prosthet Dent* 1987;58: 222–228.

74. Fischer AA. Pressure threshold measurement for diagnosis of myofascial pain and evaluation of treatment results. *Clin J Pain* 1987;2:207–214.

75. Reeves JL, Jaeger B, Graff-Radford SB. Reliability of the pressure algometer as a measure of trigger point sensitivity. *Pain* 1986;24:313–321.

76. Delaney GA, McKee AC. Inter- and intra-rater reliability of the pressure threshold meter in measurement of myofascial trigger point sensitivity. *Am J Phys Med Rehabil* 1993;72: 136–139.

77. Jaeger B, Reeves JL. Quantification of changes in myofascial trigger point sensitivity with the pressure algometer following passive stretch. *Pain* 1986;27:203–210.

78. Cote P, Mior SA, Vernon H. The short-term effect of a spinal manipulation on pain/pressure threshold in patients with chronic mechanical low back pain. *J Manipulative Physiol Ther* 1994;17:364–368.

79. Ohrbach R, Gale EN. Pressure pain thresholds, clinical assessment, and differential diagnosis: reliability and validity in patients with myogenic pain. *Pain* 1989;39:157–169.

80. Granges G, Littlejohn G. Pressure pain threshold in pain-free subjects, in patients with chronic regional pain syndromes, and in patients with fibromyalgia. *Arthritis Rheum* 1993;36: 642–646.

81. Fischer AA. Documentation of myofascial trigger points. *Arch Phys Med Rehabil* 1988;69:286–291.

82. Fischer AA. Pressure algometry (dolorimetry) in the differential diagnosis of muscle pain. In: Rachlin E, ed. *Myofascial pain and fibromyalgia: trigger point management.* St. Louis: Mosby, 1994:121–142.

83. Magora A, Vatine JJ, Magora F. Quantification of musculoskeletal pain by pressure algometry. *Pain Clin* 1992;5:101–104.

84. Tunks E, McCain GA, Hart LE, et al. The reliability of examination for tenderness in patients with myofascial pain, chronic fibromyalgia, and controls. *J Rheumatol* 1995;22:944–952.

85. Hong C-Z, Chen Y-N, Twehous D, Hong D. Pressure threshold for referred pain by compression on the trigger point and adjacent areas. *J Musculoskel Pain* 1996;4:61–79.

86. Bendtsen L, Jensen R, Jensen NK, Olesen J. Muscle palpation with controlled finger pressure: new equipment for the study of tender myofascial tissues. *Pain* 1994;59:235–239.

87. Bendtsen L, Jensen R, Jensen NK, Olesen J. Pressure-controlled palpation: a new technique which increases the reliability of manual palpation. *Cephalalgia* 1995;15:205–210.

88. Bohr TW. Fibromyalgia syndrome and myofascial pain syndrome: do they exist? *Neurol Clin North Am* 1995;13:365–384.

89. Wolfe F, Simon DG, Fricton J, et al. The fibromyalgia and myofascial pain syndromes: a preliminary study of tender points and trigger points in persons with fibromyalgia, myofascial pain syndrome and no disease. *J Rheumatol* 1992;19:944–951.

90. Nice DA, Riddle DL, Lamb RL, et al. Interrater reliability of judgements of the presence of trigger points in patients with low back pain. *Arch Phys Med Rehabil* 1992;73:893–898.

91. Njoo KH, Van der Does E. The occurrence and inter-rater reliability of myofascial trigger points in the quadratus lumborum and gluteus medius: a prospective study in non-specific low back pain patients and controls in general practice. *Pain* 1994;58:317–323.

92. Dahlstrom L, Keeling SD, Fricton JR, et al. Evaluation of a training program intended to calibrate examiners of temporomandibular disorders. *Acta Odontol Scand* 1994;52:250–254.

93. Diakow PRP. Thermographic imaging of myofascial trigger points. *J Manipulative Physiol Ther* 1988;11:114–117.

94. Fischer AA. Diagnosis and management of chronic pain in physical medicine and rehabilitation. In: Ruskin AP, ed. *Current therapy in physiatry.* Philadelphia: WB Saunders, 1984: 123–154.

95. Kruse RA Jr, Christiansen JA. Thermographic imaging of myofascial trigger points: a follow-up study. *Arch Phys Med Rehabil* 1992;73:819–823.

96. Swerdlow B, Dieter JN. An evaluation of the sensitivity and specificity of medical thermography for the documentation of myofascial trigger points. *Pain* 1992;48: 205–213.

97. Donaldson CCS, Skubick DL, Clasby RG, Cram JR. The evaluation of trigger-point activity using dynamic EMG techniques. *Am J Pain Manage* 1994;4: 118–122.

98. Headache Classification Committee of the International Headache Society. Classification and diagnostic criteria for headache disorders, cranial neuralgias and facial pain. *Cephalalgia* 1988;8(suppl 7):1–96.

99. Marcus D. Differentiating migraine from tension headaches: a real or artificial distinction? *Am Pain Soc Bull* 1991;1(6):1–9.

100. Langemark M, Olesen J, Jensen TS, et al. Clinical characterization of patients with chronic tension headache. *Headache* 1988;28:590–596.

101. Rogers EJ, Rogers RJ. Tension type headaches, fibromyalgia, or myofacial pain. *Headache Q* 1991;2:273–277.

102. Jensen K, Tuxen C, Olesen J. Pericranial muscle tenderness and pressure-pain threshold in the temporal region during common migraine. *Pain* 1988;35:65–70.

103. Jensen R, Rasmussen BK, Pedersen B, Olesen J. Muscle tenderness and pressure thresholds in headache. A population study. *Pain* 1993;52:193–199.

104. Bovim G. Cervicogenic headache, migraine, and tension-type headache. Pressure-pain threshold measurements. *Pain* 1992;51:169–173.

105. Jensen R. Mechanisms of spontaneous tension-type headaches: an analysis of tenderness, pain thresholds and EMG. *Pain* 1995;64:251–256.

106. Duckro PN, Chibnall JT, Greenberg MS. Myofascial involvement in chronic post-traumatic headache. *Headache Q* 1995;6:34–38.

107. Olesen J. Clinical and pathological observations in migraine and tension-type headache explained by integration of vascular, supraspinal and myofascial inputs. *Pain* 1991;46:125–132.

108. Moskowitz MA. The trigeminovascular system. In: Olesen J, Tfelt-Hansen P, Welch KMA, eds. *The headaches*. New York: Raven, 1993:97–104.

109. Sharav Y, Benoliel R. Temporomandibular pain. In: Vaeroy H, Merskey H, eds. *Progress in fibromyalgia and myofascial pain*. Amsterdam: Elsevier Science, 1993:237–252.

110. Schiffman E, Haley D, Baker C, Lindgren B. Diagnostic criteria for screening headache patients for temporomandibular disorders. *Headache* 1995;35:121–124.

111. Biemond A, De Jong JMBV. On cervical nystagmus and related disorders. *Brain* 1969;92:437–458.

112. Bogduk N. Cervical causes of headache and dizziness. In: Grieve G, ed. *Modern manual therapy of the vertebral column*. Edinburgh: Churchill Livingstone, 1986:289–302.

113. Karlberg M, Magnusson M, Malmstrom E-M, et al. Postural and symptomatic improvement after physiotherapy in patients with dizziness of suspected origin. *Arch Phys Med Rehabil* 1996;77:874–882.

114. Barnsley L, Lord S, Bogduk N. Whiplash injury. *Pain* 1994;58:283–307.

115. Bogdan PR, Sturzenegger M. The effect of accident mechanisms and initial findings on the long-term outcome of whiplash injury. In: Allen ME, ed. *Musculoskeletal pain emanating from the head and neck: a proceedings issue*. New York: Haworth, 1996:47–60.

116. Baker BA. The muscle trigger: evidence of overload injury. *J Neurol Orthop Med Surg* 1986;7:35–43.

117. Hong C-Z, Simons DG. Response to treatment for pectoralis minor myofascial pain syndrome after whiplash. *J Musculoskel Pain* 1993;1:89–131.

118. Hohl M. Soft-tissue injuries of the cervical spine. *Clin Orthop* 1975;109:42–49.

119. Sucher BM. Thoracic outlet syndrome—a myofascial variant: part I. Pathology and diagnosis. *J Am Osteopath Assoc* 1990;90:686–704.

120. Travell JG. Basis for the multiple uses of local block of somatic trigger areas (procaine infiltration and ethyl chloride spray). *Miss Valley Med J* 1949;71:13–21.

121. Melzack R, Wall PD. Pain mechanisms: a new theory. *Science* 1965;150:971–978.

122. Lewit K. *Manipulative therapy in rehabilitation of the locomotor system*. 2nd ed. Oxford: Butterworth-Heinemann, 1991:26–28, 190–192.

123. Hanten WP, Chandler SD. Effects of myofascial release leg pull and sagittal plane isometric contract-relax techniques on passive straight-leg raise angle. *J Orthop Sports Phys Ther* 1994;20:138–144.

124. Hong C-Z, Chen Y-C, Pon CH, Yu J. Immediate effects of various physical medicine modalities on pain threshold of an active myofascial trigger point. *J Musculoskel Pain* 1993;1(2):37–53.

125. Lewit K. The needle effect in relief of myofascial pain. *Pain* 1979;6:83–90.

126. Gunn CC, Milbrandt WE, Little AS, Mason KE. Dry needling of muscle motor points for chronic low-back pain. *Spine* 1980;5:279–291.

127. Chu J. Dry needling (intramuscular stimulation) in myofascial pain related to lumbosacral radiculopathy. *Eur J Phys Med Rehabil* 1995;5:106–121.

128. Hong C-Z. Lidocaine versus dry needling to myofascial trigger point. *Am J Phys Med Rehabil* 1994;73:256–263.

129. Hendler N, Fink H, Long D. Myofascial syndrome: response to trigger-point injections. *Psychosomatics* 1983;24:990–999.

130. Hong CZ. Myofascial trigger point injection. *Crit Rev Phys Rehabil Med* 1993;5:203–217.

131. Baldry PE. *Acupuncture, trigger points, and musculoskeletal pain*. Edinburgh: Churchill Livingstone, 1993:91–110.

132. Cheshire WP, Abashian SW, Mann JD. Botulinum toxin in the treatment of myofascial pain syndrome. *Pain* 1994;59:65–69.

133. Yue SK. Initial experience in the use of botulinum toxin A for the treatment of myofascial related muscle dysfunctions. *J Musculoskel Pain* 1995;3(suppl 1):22. Abstract.

134. Hopwood MB, Abram SE. Factors associated with failure of trigger point injections. *Clin J Pain* 1994;10:227–234.

135. Hong C-Z, Hsueh T-C. Difference in pain relief after trigger point injections in myofascial pain patients with and without fibromyalgia. *Arch Phys Med Rehabil* 1996;77:1161–1166.

136. Dao TTT, Lund JP, Remillard G, Lavigne GJ. Is myofascial pain of the temporal muscles relieved by oral sumatriptan? *Pain* 1995;62:241–244.

137. Hadler NM. *Occupational musculoskeletal disorders.* New York: Raven, 1993:190–223.

138. Dismukes WE, Wade JS, Lee JY. A randomized, double-blind trial of nystatin therapy for the candidiasis hypersensitivity syndrome. *N Engl J Med* 1990;323:1717–1723.

139. De Wall M, van Riel MPJM, Snijders CJ. The effect on sitting posture of a desk with a 10° inclination for reading and writing. *Ergonomics* 1991;34:575–584.

140. McNulty WH, Gevirtz RN, Hubbard DR, Berkoff GM. Needle electromyographic evaluation of trigger point response to a psychological stressor. *Psychophysiology* 1994;31:313–316.

141. Zautra AJ, Marbach JJ, Raphael KG, et al. The examination of myofascial face pain and its relationship to psychological distress among women. *Health Psychol* 1995;14:223–231.

142. Cassisi JE, Sypert GW, Friedman EM, Robinson ME. Pain, disability, and psychological functioning in chronic low back pain subgroups: myofascial versus herniated disc syndrome. *Neurosurgery* 1993;33:379–385.

143. Faucett JA. Depression in painful chronic disorders: the role of pain and conflict about pain. *J Pain Symptom Manage* 1994;9:520–526.

144. Kuch K, Cox B, Evans RJ, et al. To what extent do anxiety and depression interact with chronic pain? *Can J Psychiatry* 1993;38:36–38.

Chapter 62

Temporomandibular Joint Disorders

Steve M. Gnatz

The first modern description of the constellation of symptoms that we call temporomandibular joint (TMJ) syndrome is usually ascribed to Costen in 1934 (1). He described pain in the area of the jaw joint that occurred in many people after removal of their teeth. Costen theorized that changes in dental occlusion or the way that the teeth are aligned could lead to a biomechanical dysfunction of the TMJ and subsequent pain. However, changes in dental occlusion are just one of the many causes of pain in the area of the TMJ and may not be as important in the development and maintenance of this syndrome as once thought (2,3). Pain or dysfunction of the TMJ or surrounding tissues affects up to 80% of the population at some time in their life (4). Between 6% and 12% of those who develop TMJ symptoms will develop a chronic or relapsing and remitting course with pain that may necessitate therapeutic intervention (5–7). This syndrome is a major contributor to painful conditions of the head and neck and can cause significant disability in terms of eating and communicating (8). The symptoms may be related to the jaw joint itself or referred to other head and neck structures (9).

TMJ syndrome is somewhat of a misnomer and abandonment of the term has been suggested because it is nonspecific (10). The addition of the term *temporomandibular myofascial pain dysfunction syndrome* (TMPDS) may be more descriptive of the true scope of the problem. Current concepts of the differentiation between TMJ syndrome, or internal derangements of the craniomandibular apparatus, and myofascial pain dysfunction (MPD) syndrome are discussed in this chapter. Further complicating the issue of terminology are the differences in training between dentists, who are involved in the evaluation of dental pain syndromes but may not be well acquainted with muscle or joint disorders, and physicians who are unfamiliar with the craniomandibular apparatus and causes of orofacial pain in general.

It is helpful for the clinician to ascertain the extent of true joint versus myofascial pathology and their respective contributions to the symptoms, both for diagnostic and for therapeutic decision making. Figure 62-1 shows how the clinical entities of myofascial pain, fibromyalgia, and temporomandibular pain and dysfunction syndromes might interact and overlap. With proper diagnosis and treatment, the patient with TMPDS can do well and a significant disability can be avoided. However, when the symptoms are chronic, patients should be aware that a "cure" comes more from adaptation and lifestyle adjustment than from elimination of pain.

DIFFERENTIAL DIAGNOSIS

A complete differential diagnosis of pain involving the TMJ and associated structures contains at least 70 items (Table 62-1). For the purposes of this chapter, the following pain problems are delineated: MPD; internal derangement of the TMJ; combinations of TMJ and myofascial problems (the "true" TMPDS); and inflammatory, autoimmune, and other "nonbenign" conditions.

While most patients with temporomandibular dysfunction present with pain that can be localized to the jaw joint, there is a significant component of referred pain that may mask the true origin of the symptoms (11). All patients who complain of headache should be screened for temporomandibular dysfunction (12). There is a high incidence of temporomandibular dysfunction found in "post-traumatic headache" patients (13). In one study, 11% of patients who had a chief complaint of neck pain were ultimately diagnosed as having temporomandibular dysfunction (13). It may be helpful to think of TMJ and MPD syndromes as a spectrum, as shown in Figure 62-2. In this scheme, the most severe symptoms occur in category 4, a combination of joint dysfunction and myofascial pain.

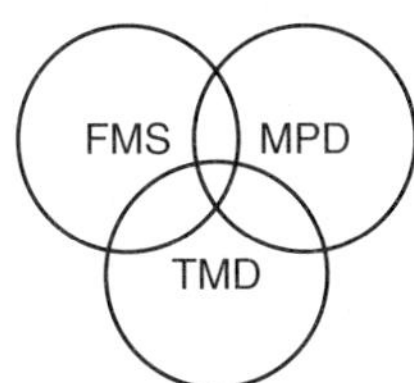

Figure 62-1. Overlap of the clinical entities of fibromyalgia syndrome (FMS), myofascial pain dysfunction (MPD), and temporomandibular dysfunction (TMD).

Internal derangements of the TMJ are more likely to be acute and ascribed to a known incident of trauma. In one study, 79% of patients who demonstrated a TMJ disk dislocation gave a history of a traumatic incident (14). However, even those with myalgia alone had a 54% history of trauma related to the TMJ. Essentially, internal derangements represent problems with the disk and the ligaments that tether the disk in place. If these ligaments are torn or stretched, the disk is free to be displaced within the joint and locking may occur. The disk itself may be torn or damaged. In less severe conditions, only a pop or click and deviation of the jaw with opening will be noted. Internal derangement may or may not be painful by itself, depending on chronicity. An internal derangement is almost always acutely painful, but if the nonbony structures can compensate, the patient may become relatively pain free later. An internal derangement of the TMJ is usually a subluxation or dislocation of the disk. This most often

Table 62-1: Classification of Causes for Head and Neck Pain

Intrinsic causes of craniomandibular pain

1. Skeletal abnormalities
   - A. Fracture
   - B. Neoplasm, primary or metastatic
   - C. Infection, osteomyelitis
   - D. Paget disease
   - E. Osteoporosis
   - F. Endocrinologic, hyperparathyroidism
   - G. Arteriovenous malformations, aneurysms
   - H. Hematologic, sickle cell, multiple myeloma
2. Joint abnormalities
   - A. Synovitis, capsulitis, diskitis
   - B. Joint effusion, hemarthrosis
   - C. Osteoarthritis
   - D. Rheumatic disease, rheumatoid arthritis, etc
   - E. Disk derangements
   - F. Joint instability, ligamentous laxity
   - G. Biomechanical abnormalities
   - H. Neoplasms, primary or metastatic
   - I. Vasculitides
3. Ligaments
   - A. Trauma, sprains, rupture
   - B. Chronic laxity
   - C. Contracture
   - D. Neoplasms
   - E. Infection
4. Muscles, tendons, fascia
   - A. Myofascial pain, fibromyalgia
   - B. Trauma, strains, tears, ruptures
   - C. Inflammatory conditions, polymyositis
   - D. Infectious conditions, trichinosis, etc
   - E. Polymyalgia rheumatica
   - F. Vasculitides
   - G. Metabolic, exercise induced, cramps
   - H. Ischemic, claudication, compartment syndrome
   - I. Neoplasms
   - J. Contracture, biomechanical abnormalities
   - K. Overuse syndromes
   - L. Nutritional, avitaminosis
   - M. Toxins, venom, etc
5. Nerve structures
   - A. Entrapment, compression
   - B. Trauma, stretch, laceration
   - C. Deafferentation, neuromas
   - D. Reflex sympathetic dystrophy, causalgia
   - E. Neuritis, neuralgia, tics
   - F. Peripheral neuropathy, diabetes, toxins
   - G. Ischemia, vasculitis
   - H. Infection, herpes, AIDS
   - I. Neoplasms

Extrinsic causes of craniomandibular pain

1. Other organs referring pain to the craniomandibular apparatus
   - A. Heart: myocardial infarction, angina
   - B. Lungs: pleuritis, tumors (especially Pancoast)
   - C. Eyes: infection, strain
   - D. Ears: infection, tumors
   - E. Nose and sinus: infection, abscess, tumors
   - F. Throat and teeth: infection, tumors
   - G. Central nervous system: Syringomyelia, Arnold-Chiari, spasmodic torticollis, tumors (especially acoustic neuromas, neurofibromas, and other slow growing), infections, vascular abnormalities and accidents, and supratentorial factors

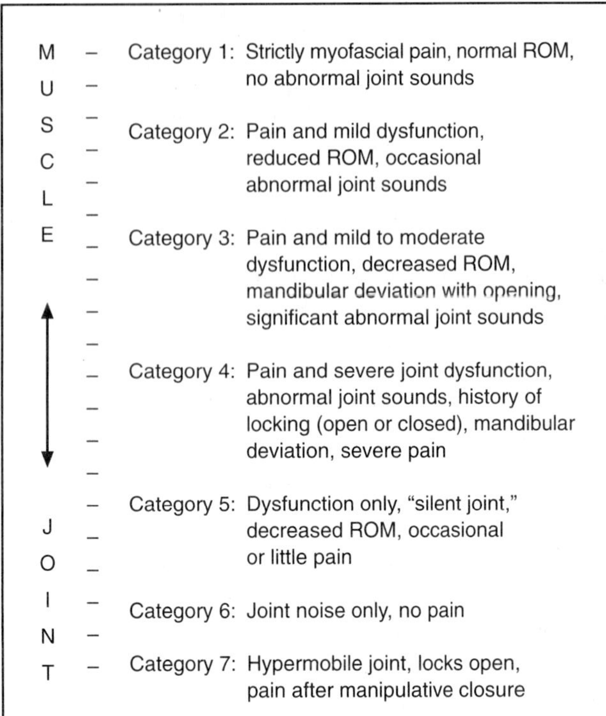

Figure 62-2. Categories of patients with temporomandibular or myofascial pain dysfunction. ROM = range of motion. (Adapted from Murphy GJ. American Association of Newomuscular Studies Seminar 1988.)

occurs in an anterolateral direction but other abnormal movements are possible (15). The capsule of the joint may become stretched or torn. The coronoid of the mandible may contact the cranial fossa without the cushioning effect of the disk, leading to pain and dysfunction. Ultimately disk and joint degeneration may occur. Fibrosis and scarring may limit range of motion. Bony ankylosis may occur. Chronic biomechanical and musculoligamentous stresses may cause the disk and ligaments to become damaged as well. Long-standing internal derangement may lead to degenerative changes in the joint such as obliteration of the joint space and osteophytes.

MPD involves painful muscular or musculoligamentous structures as the primary problem. While the etiology of MPD syndrome is unknown, it is thought to be multifactorial (see Chap. 61). A combination of genetic predisposition, biomechanical abnormalities, stress, and trauma lead to a vicious cycle of muscular pain, immobility, contracture, and more pain. There is some evidence now of a lack of high-energy phosphates (ATP, etc) in myofascially involved muscles, but whether this is cause or effect remains to be seen (16).

Myofascially involved muscle is essentially normal muscle. The pathology is thought to be primarily a physiologic abnormality of the muscle that causes it to remain in spasm. The symptoms vary with time and other factors (e.g., weather) (17). The pain may decrease with age as the muscles thin and lifestyles become more sedentary. However, the judicious use of nontraumatic aerobic exercise may play a role in altering the pathophysiology of the muscle. Females are affected at least three times more than males for reasons unknown.

Trigger points and referred pain patterns are the rule in the muscles of the head and neck. Usually this is a regional myofascial pain syndrome, but if more generalized, the symptoms may be part of fibromyalgia. In a pure MPD syndrome, the TMJ is only secondarily involved and is anatomically normal. However, with long-standing myofascial abnormalities, some joint dysfunction may develop and the patient may need to be reclassified.

A combination of TMJ dysfunction and myofascial pain is, by far, the most common scenario seen in clinical practice. Determination of the individual contributions of the joint versus muscle abnormalities will be helpful in planning the work-up and treatment. Affected patients will have various levels of muscle and joint involvement. Usually there is a multifactorial etiology, and while many patients have a history of joint trauma, the relationship of trauma as a cause is not as clear-cut as with internal derangement alone. A combination of stress, trauma, occlusal abnormalities, and genetic predisposition (among other factors) conspires to produce the resulting symptoms.

Inflammatory, autoimmune, carcinomatous, and other nonbenign reasons for pain around the head and neck are significantly less common than the causes just listed. Nonetheless, they are important to consider and rule out, if possible, since they may be potentially curable or at least treated in ways significantly different from the other causes. Most often these patients present with symptoms that will distinguish them from the patient with "benign" TMPDS, such as diffuse joint pain, swelling, Raynaud phenomenon, or cranial nerve findings that may be the clue to a less benign etiology. There is rarely a history of trauma. They may fall into the wrong age or sex group for myofascial problems (i.e., older men) (18). Their symptoms are more likely to be progressive and unrelenting instead of the typical waxing and waning pattern of TMPDS. The TMJ is usually involved late in the course of rheumatoid arthritis, so that there is rarely diagnostic uncertainty with this disease (19). However, the TMJ has been noted to be involved earlier in patients with systemic lupus erythematosus (20). The diagnostician should be aware that other, more rare causes of TMJ symptoms may occasionally be present, particularly in elderly individuals, and should proceed with the diagnostic work-up accordingly (18,21).

ANATOMY

The human TMJ is a remarkable structure (22). It is the only joint in the body that is really two joints linked together by a bony bridge (the mandible). Therefore, processes that affect one joint ultimately will affect both. Both joints must be treated simultaneously, despite the fact that the biomechanical stresses may be quite different on the individual joints. It is impossible to rest (or exercise) only one TMJ. The joint itself is relatively unconstrained; that is, it relies primarily on surrounding muscles and ligaments for stability. In this respect, the TMJ is more like the shoulder than the hip, where inherent stability is provided by the bony coupling of the femur and acetabulum. The unconstrained nature of the TMJ gives it remarkable freedom of movement (and in humans, a remarkable adaptability in food sources), but at the cost of biomechanical stress on the nonbony structures of the temporomandibular apparatus (23).

The articulation of the condyle of the mandible in the temporal bone fossa is a biomechanically complex arrangement likened to a "saddle" joint (24). There is a fibrocartilaginous disk between the bony structures. This disk is tethered in place by ligaments, which also contain the disk's blood supply. The disk is capable of regeneration and remodeling due to the presence of a blood supply and the qualities of fibrocartilage (cf. the lack of these restorative abilities in the hyaline cartilage of the knee) (25). However the disk's ability to repair itself is limited, particularly in the relatively less vascular anterior portion. Also, inflammatory chemical mediators such as prostaglandin E_2 and leukotriene B_4 may contribute to the "degenerative spiral" associated with long-standing TMJ dysfunction (26). During opening and closing, the joint goes through a process of rotation and translation to effect jaw movement. Initially, the condyle of the mandible rotates in the craniomandibular fossa and then "slides" or translates down the fossa to maximize jaw opening. The process is reversed in closing the jaw. The muscles of mastication provide the power for this process. The muscles that act to close the jaw are more numerous and stronger than those that open the jaw since gravity aids in jaw opening. Lateral deviation of the jaw is also an important movement and in fact, the jaw is capable of circumduction as required for grinding.

The anatomic relationships of the TMJ contribute to the pain referral patterns noted clinically. The proximity of the TMJ to the trigeminal ganglion and fifth cranial nerve pathways may help explain the common facial and neck symptoms. Occipital and temporal structures are also common recipients of referred pain (9). The presence of hearing loss, tinnitus, or disequilibrium may be explained by the proximity of the TMJ to otic structures and spasm of the tensor tympani muscle (27,28). Dysphagia or a subjective sensation of choking may occur with voluntary throat musculature spasms (13).

The manner in which the teeth contact, called *occlusion*, is another important anatomic consideration in TMJ function (and dysfunction) (2,29). The loss of posterior support (e.g., when posterior molars are removed) was one of the first occlusal problems to be associated with TMPDS and is still called *Costen syndrome*. However, there is not a direct relationship between occlusion and temporomandibular dysfunction (3). Poor occlusion is not a sure indicator that a given person will develop TMPDS, nor can it be said that someone with "perfect" occlusion will not develop the syndrome (30). More germane is the ability of the muscular and ligamentous structures to adapt and compensate for bony and structural abnormalities and asymmetries. When these nonbony elements are able to compensate, they will function normally and without pain. Tight, stressed, myofascially involved muscles and fibrotic, scarred ligaments have difficulty compensating for the changes in structural conditions. There is some evidence that the muscular dysfunction of TMDPS is similar to the cranial dystonias (31).

One of the most common malocclusions seen is called *overclosure*. This occurs when patients clench or "brux" (grind) their teeth. Over long periods of time, the surfaces of the teeth are worn away, changing the biomechanical relationship of the TMJ. Most often this change is compensated for by the nonbony elements, the temporomandibular apparatus remains balanced, and the person remains asymptomatic. However, when the nonbony elements cannot compensate, the patient becomes symptomatic. The process of bruxism and subsequent overclosure is one of the most amenable to treatment, since a splint placed between the upper and lower teeth will replace the lost height and rebalance the biomechanics of the joint (32). Many other malocclusions are correctable by splinting or other dental treatments, but the clinician should be aware of the lack of a direct correlation between occlusion and response to splint therapy (33).

HISTORY TAKING IN PATIENTS WITH PAIN IN THE TEMPOROMANDIBULAR JOINT AREA

The patient with MPD will complain of pain in the muscular areas of the head and neck. Generally the pain is described as tightness, soreness, or stiffness but occasionally may be sharp or even hyperesthetic. Muscle contraction–type headaches involving the temporal or occipital areas are most common, but pain may be generalized or unilateral. Painful or limited jaw motion may be reported, but joint locking or noise suggests internal derangement. The patient may complain of ear symptoms such as tinnitus, fullness in the ears, or hearing loss. Also vestibular symptoms such as vertigo, dizziness, or nausea may be noted. Pain behind the eyes, blurring of vision, and occasionally photophobia may be reported. Many patients interpret their problems as originating in the sinus area, as this is a common referred pain zone for pterygoid muscle spasm. Tooth and gum complaints, swallowing difficulty, and autonomic phenomena such as sweating or lacrimation are occasionally reported.

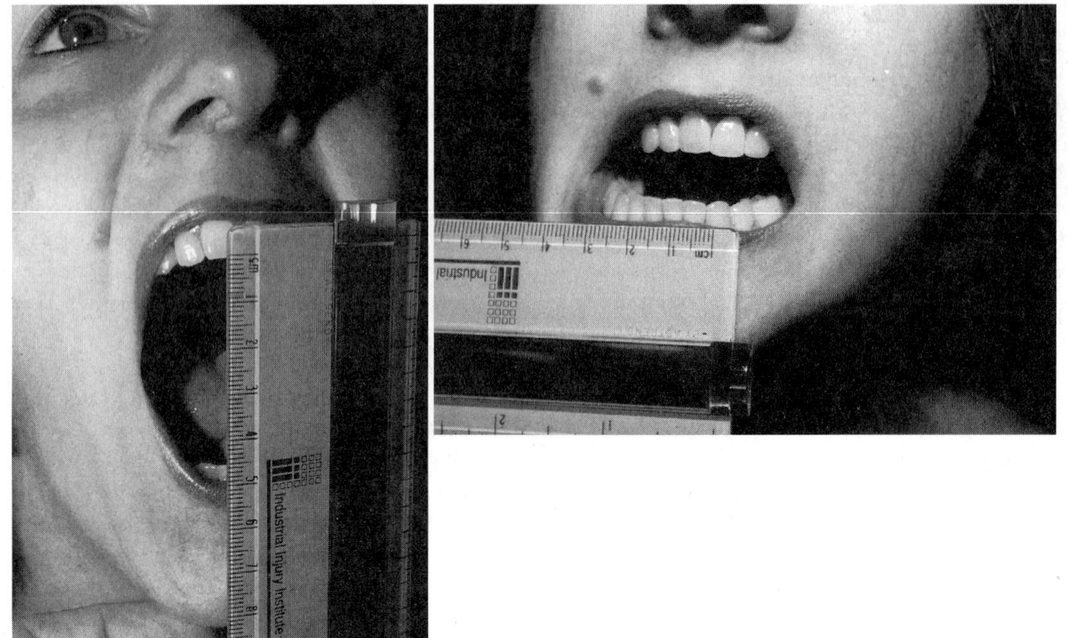

Figure 62-3. *A, B.* Interincisal distance measurement and lateral deviation measurement.

A thorough history of the pain pattern should include the characteristics, onset, and location of pain (a pain diagram may be helpful); the duration and severity of pain; exacerbating and remitting factors; and any neurologic symptoms. Any cervical trauma or whiplash-type injury including that caused by a deployment of air bags should be documented (14,34). A history of bruxism, excessive chewing, smoking, nail biting, or other dysfunctional oral habits should be sought. While both the patient with internal derangement and MPD may complain of painful or limited movement of the jaw, with an internal derangement there is more likely to be significant joint noise such as a clicking, popping, or grinding associated with motion of the jaw. The jaw may lock open or closed and require the patient to manipulate the jaw back into alignment. The patient may complain that the jaw deviates to one side during opening of the mouth or of a difficulty with enunciation.

A review of systems for contributing medical problems such as anemia and thyroid abnormalities may be revealing. Also the sleep pattern should be noted. Information on current and past medication usage and the presence of psychosocial stressors will round out the history.

The history of orthodontic procedures may be obtained, but the relationship between these and the subsequent development of TMPDS is unclear. This question of whether prior orthodontic treatment may be a precipitating factor in TMJ problems has been evaluated. No increase in TMJ symptomatology or signs at 10 years in patients treated orthodontically was seen when compared to age- and sex-matched control subjects (35). Similarly, a large prospective study in the United States found no correlation between orthotic treatment and onset of TMJ symptoms (36). In fact, the association of TMJ dysfunction with "natural" occlusal problems (such as severe overbites or crossbites) left untreated seems to be higher than that of TMJ dysfunction with orthodontic treatment (37).

PHYSICAL EXAMINATION

Examination of the TMJ should begin with observation for any facial asymmetry or swelling. The presence of erythema or warmth, or both, around the joint may indicate inflammation. The interincisal distance (Fig. 62-3) should be measured as an indicator of range of motion of the TMJ (normal > 40 mm). Lateral deviation should be measured and limitation noted (normal > 8 mm, in each direction). Protrusive movement of the mandible should also be evaluated (normal > 8 mm) (29). Any lateral deviation with opening should be noted. In the event of anterolateral disk dislocation (the most common type), the jaw will laterally deviate toward the dislocated side. The joint should be palpated and any tenderness noted. This can be done by placing the fingers over the joint, just in front of the ear, or by inserting the small finger in the external ear canal. During opening and closing, the presence of a click, pop, or crepitation may be appreciated with the fingers or a stethoscope. These sounds may be associated with various abnormalities of joint and disk pathology, but can also be appreciated occasionally in painless joints. Occlusion should be checked and the measurement of overclosure measured (normal = 18 mm, gumline to gumline as shown in Fig. 62-4).

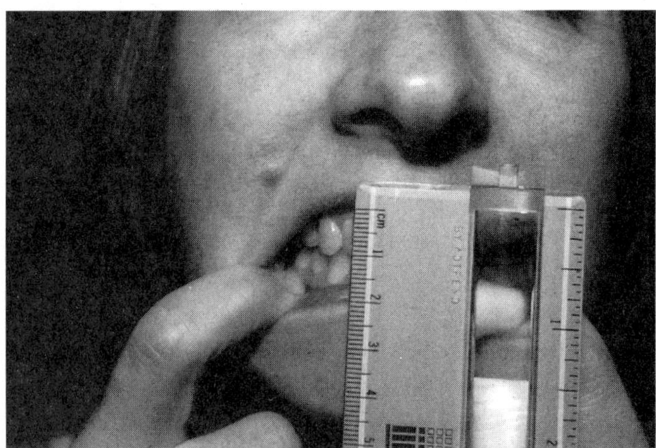

Figure 62-4. Gumline-to-gumline measurement to evaluate for overclosure.

A thorough examination of the muscles of the head and neck should be performed by palpation, to identify local tenderness, spasm, tightness, or true trigger points. The muscles, including the masseter, pterygoid, temporal, sternocleidomastoid, occipital, cervical, hyoid, trapezius, levator scapulae, and pectoral muscles at a minimum, should be examined both intraorally and extraorally. The range of motion of the cervical spine should be examined. Range of motion of the peripheral joints may be important as there is a correlation between peripheral joint hypermobility and TMJ dysfunction (38–41). A neurologic examination of the cranial nerves and peripheral nerves should be performed. The joints of the limbs should be examined for signs of systemic arthropathy. Generalized muscle tenderness may be a sign of myositis or fibromyalgia, if present. The posture should be evaluated. Most commonly, a forward-head posture is noted but the entire skeletal axis should be examined for contributing postural abnormalities such as scoliosis, pelvic obliquity, or leg-length discrepancy (42).

When evaluating a patient with cervical extension-flexion injury (whiplash), one must be aware that the symptoms related to the TMJ are often delayed by several weeks (43). The reason for this delay is unclear, but may relate to a slow inflammatory response in the joint or surrounding tissue. The signs and symptoms may show primarily myofascial or joint (internal derangement) characteristics (44,45).

Patients who have undergone surgical procedures on the TMJ represent a distinct problem for the diagnostician. There is a growing body of literature that indicates that TMJ implants may be associated with significant problems (46–50). Specifically, a significant foreign body reaction including granulomas that may erode into the cranial fossa can occur. There has been a call to remove certain TMJ implants, and patients require close monitoring for signs of an aggressive foreign body reaction even after the removal of the implants (47).

IMAGING AND OTHER DIAGNOSTIC TESTING

Radiologic imaging will aid in the identification of internal derangement of the TMJ. Plain radiographs taken in a transcranial view give gross information about the joint space, which if lost, suggests dislocation of the disk. Degenerative changes and osteophytes may be noted on plain films of both the TMJ and the cervical region. There is little role for tomography (plain or computed) unless a bony abnormality is suspected. The gold standard for evaluating the nonbony elements of the TMJ space is magnetic resonance imaging (MRI) (51,52). MRI can show disk subluxation or dislocation (53). The limitation of routine MRI is that it only shows static abnormalities and fails to evaluate the motions of the joint dynamically. This will hopefully become less of a limitation as dynamic MRI develops (54). This dynamic information may currently be gathered by such means as the mandibular kinesiograph; however, this technology requires significant skill in interpretation (55,56). Arthrography should be reserved for preoperative diagnostic use as it is invasive and can precipitate joint capsule tears. While arthrography is believed to be useful and more sensitive than MRI in some centers, it has been replaced by MRI in other centers (57,58). Bone scanning may be helpful to determine the cellular activity of bone related to the level of inflammation present (59).

MPD remains a clinical diagnosis in that there is no specific laboratory or radiologic test for this disorder. Surface electromyography (EMG) may be useful in the monitoring of patient progress (60) and in biofeedback training, but is of limited usefulness in the diagnosis of myofascial problems because of the wide range of normal values. Thermography may be helpful in the documentation of trigger points and joint inflammation but its specificity remains to be documented (61,62). Medical problems that can lead or contribute to muscle pain should be ruled out by appropriate laboratory testing (63). Anemia and thyroid abnormalities (either hypothyroidism or hyperthyroidism) are the most common contributing medical problems and can be ruled out by a complete blood cell count (CBC) and thyroid function tests (triiodothyronine resin uptake, thyroxine, thyroid-stimulating hormone). Occasionally, hypocalcemia or other endocrinologic problems may contribute to muscular pain. Rarely, hypovitaminosis is identified as a contributing factor.

Psychological tests such as the Minnesota Multiphasic Personality Inventory (MMPI) or other batteries may be helpful in quantifying psychosocial makeup and coping ability, yet these studies are limited in the prediction of good results from a therapy plan (64,65).

SPLINTING

Splinting (intraoral device or orthotic) may be helpful in the treatment of many types of temporomandibular disorders (66,67). The splint should be specifically designed to counteract forces and compensate for postural abnormalities that are found. Generally, the design and fabrication of the splint is best left to a qualified dental professional. There are several schools of thought on the design of these devices, and a significant amount of conflict exists in the dental literature at this point regarding the efficacy of the various philosophies. It is generally advisable to consider the fabrication and use of a splint before "nonreversible" forms of occlusion adjustment such as grinding or building up of the tooth structure (68).

The use of a splint is ideally combined with other interventions (such as medications or physical therapy) to maximize the effectiveness of treatment (69). Splinting decreases the EMG activity of the muscles of mastication (70,71). Splints may be used 24 hours a day, only during activities such as chewing or talking that aggravate symptoms, or at night to discourage bruxism, depending on the situation. Many patients can ultimately be weaned from the splint as their symptoms improve, or more permanent correction of their bite may be advisable if they are not weanable.

Splinting can result in reduction of the disk and other soft-tissue structures of the TMJ and should be attempted as a first-line therapy prior to any consideration of joint surgery (72).

TREATMENT

First, the patient with temporomandibular dysfunction should be reassured of the benign nature of most causes of symptoms (73,74). It should be stressed that acute symptoms will most likely respond well to a brief period of rest, mild analgesics, and gradual remobilization of the tissues. If the syndrome has become chronic, patients may be informed that it generally has a waxing and waning course and that long-term strategies of pain management are required (75). Lifestyle adjustment may be needed.

An algorithm for treatment may be followed (76). A well-coordinated program of general aerobic conditioning may be warranted if the person has aspects of fibromyalgia or diffuse muscle pain (77). Short courses of physical therapy during times of exacerbations of symptoms may be very helpful to break the "vicious cycle," but these should be discontinued as soon as the patient is able to take over the management of the muscular problems with a home program. The physical therapy program is aimed at relieving pain through the modalities of heat, ultrasound, cold, and electrical stimulation, followed by relaxation and range of motion exercises for the contracted musculoligamentous structures (63,78). The spray and stretch technique may be helpful and local injection of a local anesthetic into true trigger points may also help to break the pain cycle (79). Only when significant pain reduction has been achieved and all structures are at or near their normal resting lengths should any strengthening be attempted. These patients generally do not require major strengthening programs but more generalized aerobic fitness to counteract the abnormal muscle physiology. They should be placed on a program that emphasizes stretching and flexibility, attention to posture, muscle relaxation, and self-massage techniques (80).

All clinical studies that evaluated treatments in the medical and dental literature up until 1989 have been reviewed (81). These studies usually compared one treatment regimen to another and rarely involved control groups or randomization, limiting their utility. A study comparing four treatment modalities (short-wave diathermy, electrical stimulation, ultrasound, and laser) to placebo for temporomandibular dysfunction found all four treatments to be better than placebo but not significantly different from each other (82).

Medications of the tricyclic antidepressant class, such as amitriptyline, in low doses may help to restore a normal sleep pattern and provide some analgesia (83). Nonsteroidal anti-inflammatory drugs (NSAIDS) are generally not as useful for MPD as for TMJ derangements and osteoarthritis. Similarly, oral steroids offer no benefit in MPD. Muscle relaxants, especially cyclobenzaprine, which is chemically related to amitriptyline, may be of benefit. Occasionally, drugs such as carbamazepine and gabapentin may be helpful, particularly if there is an element of neuropathic pain (84). All potentially habit-forming medications (such as narcotics and benzodiazepines) should be avoided in the management of any long-term pain problem (85).

Internal derangement is one of the few indications for surgical intervention in patients with TMPDS. Even so, surgery should not be required in the vast majority of these patients (86). Arthroscopic procedures may be less traumatic to the joint than an open procedure, but selection for which patient can be operated arthroscopically is a decision to be discussed with the surgeon. Generally, ligamentous injuries and disk derangements that do not require diskectomy may be amenable to an arthroscopic approach. Nonetheless, diskectomy may have some effectiveness in pain relief, but should be considered a "salvage procedure" (87). When disk dislocation or subluxation is the result of abnormal muscle biomechanics and spasm, these factors must be corrected or the surgery is doomed to failure (88). Splinting allows for effective management of certain internal derangements, and since the disk is capable of remodeling and repair, this avenue should be explored prior to the consideration of surgical intervention (89).

The physical therapy modalities may be applied to the patient with internal derangement. For an acute derangement, more rest than exercise is needed. As inflammation subsides, a program of active and passive range of motion exercises and gradual strengthening will be required. Cold may be more useful than heat in an inflamed TMJ. Iontophoresis with steroid may be helpful to reduce inflammation as well. Ultrasound should be avoided if acute joint inflammation is present, but can be used over an osteoarthritic or chronically deranged joint if needed. All postoperative patients (including those who had arthroscopic surgery) should be given a thorough rehabilitation program in physical therapy as soon as possible (90,91).

Anti-inflammatory medications play a more important role in the management of internal derangement than of MPD. NSAIDs or even a short course of oral steroids may be effective in reducing inflammation after an acute dislocation or in the patient with long-standing degenerative joint disease. Steroid may be injected directly into the TMJ, but this is rarely indicated (92,93).

Heating muscle and joint tissues produces several beneficial effects. Analgesia and relaxation of muscle tension can be obtained. Heat increases the blood supply to the affected area by vasodilation and increases enzymatic activity. By the same token, heat can increase the inflammatory response and may increase the rate of destruction in rheumatoid joints. Heating allows collagenous structures to be stretched more effectively in the setting of joint or tendon contractures (94,95).

Despite general agreement on the efficacy and usefulness of heat in treating the TMJ patient, studies that isolate and document an independent therapeutic effect are lacking.

Many different forms of heating are available. The most common are hot pack (hydrocollator pack), diathermy, and ultrasound. Hydrocollator packs come in a size specifically designed to cover the posterior cervical muscles and the TMJ region. Diathermy is rarely used, primarily because of the contraindication to use around the eyes. Ultrasound may be effective, especially if a smaller head is used in the area of the joint. The effect of ultrasound and other heating modalities on the intra-articular temperature of the relatively superficial TMJ has not been studied.

Because of its analgesic and relaxant properties, heat is usually a first-line agent in the treatment of TMJ symptoms, barring any contraindication. Which heating modality to choose and the placement will be directed by the location of the pain-producing structures. The patient can continue to utilize superficial heat in a home program with one of the "moist heat" pads available.

When it comes to prescription of an exercise regimen, the ideal combination of rest and exercise is a difficult concept for patients and practitioners alike. When acute inflammation of the muscle or joint is present, rest is necessary to allow healing to occur. However, muscle weakness and joint contracture can take place very rapidly when there is complete immobility. Due to its masticatory function, the jaw is difficult to immobilize. Rest of the joint can be aided by adherence to a liquid diet. However, patient compliance for such a diet is limited. The key to proper management of the inflamed TMJ is passive range of motion up to, but not past, the point of pain. The power required to exercise the joint may be provided by a therapist or by the patient after proper training. Causing pain during range of motion exercises of the joint will only restart the vicious cycle of pain—immobility, contracture, more pain.

Isometric muscle contraction may be initiated even in the presence of acute joint inflammation. When combined with surface EMG biofeedback techniques, isometric contraction and relaxation of the masseter or temporal muscles can easily be coordinated. Therapeutic exercise of the TMJ at this stage should be limited to gentle passive range of motion up to, but not past, the point of pain after application of a suitable heating modality and isometrics. As inflammation subsides, the patient should be encouraged to become more active in the isotonic use of muscles around the TMJ, ultimately concentrating more on strengthening through resistive exercise. The timing of this program is highly variable, depending on the tolerance of the patient, and requires close follow-up by the prescribing physiatrist.

Rocabado (96) described a program of exercise that is composed of six instructions to be performed six times a day with six repetitions of each. The sequence is easily taught to the patient for use at home. It encompasses the normal movements of the TMJ as well as posturing of the head and neck. Position names and their potential therapeutic benefits (in parentheses) include rest position of the tongue (vertical rest position), controlled TMJ rotation (range of motion), rhythmic stabilization technique (isometric contraction of the jaw in all directions), cervical joint liberation (range of motion), axial extension of the cervical spine (posture), and shoulder girdle retraction (range of motion). Other TMJ exercise programs have been described (63,97).

While there is no objective evidence that any particular exercise program is more effective than simple range of motion and posture exercises in the control and prophylaxis against TMJ symptomatology, the Rocabado program encompasses many of the known therapeutic movements into an easy-to-learn and memorable sequence.

Transcutaneous electrical nerve stimulation (TENS) is one of the few modalities that has been submitted to controlled testing for efficacy in TMJ dysfunction (98–100). The results have been equivocal and, to date, have failed to demonstrate an independent therapeutic effect of this modality. Of the two basic types of TENS—conventional high-frequency, low-intensity TENS and low-frequency, high-intensity TENS—only conventional TENS has been evaluated in controlled studies. Low-frequency, high-intensity forms of electrical stimulation such as functional electrical stimulation (FES) and high-voltage galvanic stimulation (HVGS) may reduce muscle pain and increase muscle circulation and strength (101). The tetanic muscle contraction produced by these forms of therapy may be painful, and less well tolerated in the area of the face than other modalities.

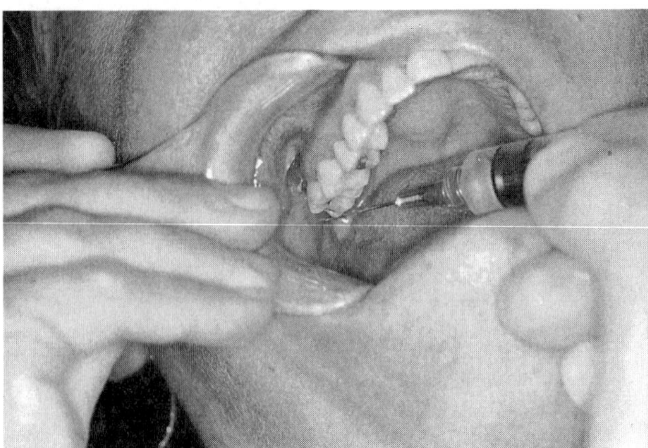

Figure 62-5. Injection into a pterygoid trigger point.

Interferential electrical stimulation may be more well tolerated than FES if the equipment is available, but its usefulness in TMPDS has not been established (102).

Using surface EMG activity, the patient can be taught to monitor the contraction and relaxation of muscles. The electrical muscle activity is picked up by electrodes over the belly of the muscle (usually the masseter) and is amplified and displayed to the patient in a quantitative manner. The patient then gets visual or auditory feedback of the muscle activity level that is present. With practice the patient can learn to relax these muscles, first with, then without the biofeedback machine.

Clinical studies showed EMG biofeedback to be effective in the treatment of TMPDS (103–105).

Trigger point injections may be helpful if the patient has "true" trigger points that can be identified by palpation. These trigger points may be in muscles that are difficult to access, such as the pterygoids (Fig. 62-5). Injection into the trigger point with 0.5 to 1.0 mL of 1% lidocaine without epinephrine may provide relief for a week or longer and allow the patient to progress in therapy (106). The addition of corticosteroids to the injectate does not provide any additional effectiveness (106). The use of heat after trigger point injection may increase its effectiveness (106). Based on a case report, botulinum toxin has been advocated for the spasm associated with TMPDS (107).

Cryotherapy utilizing ice packs and fluoromethane spray also may be helpful in the treatment of MPD (106,108).

Iontophoresis may have beneficial effects under circumstances involving significant TMJ inflammation, but its effectiveness remains to be documented by well-controlled studies (109). Phonophoresis has been reported to be helpful for temporomandibular disorders; however, the effects are more likely based on the effects of heat rather than the introduction of steroid into the joint (110). One study found no statistically significant differences in intra-articular hydrocortisone levels between the phonophoresis and external application treatments, in the knee or shoulder joints of dogs (111).

Patients with chronic TMJ pain (like chronic pain of any origin) often have complex psychosocial and stress-related influences interplaying on the disease process (63,112). Nonetheless, patients with TMPDS are less likely to be disabled from work than are patients with low-back pain (113). They often have been treated by many health professionals and may become disillusioned, feel isolated, and be depressed. It is often difficult to separate somatization accompanying depression from physiologic pain. Such patients are easy marks for pseudoscientific quacks who may make wild promises and use unproved and sometimes dangerous methods in their treatment of these patients (114). More often, however, well-meaning health care professionals recommend irreversible forms of therapy (such as surgery or changes in tooth structure) that add iatrogenic injury to the list of causes of their symptoms. Education of these patients will keep the temptation to undergo "miracle cures" to a minimum.

Physical therapy modalities can provide only temporary relief of pain and muscle tension. Long-term gains will be made through lifestyle adjustment using relaxation techniques, stress management, and ongoing home programs of exercise (115). The ultimate goal is to make the patient responsible for the day-to-day maintenance and preventive treatment of the disorder. Prolonged treatment with physical modalities without a specific goal or end point is fiscally irresponsible and generates dependency of the patient on the health care system.

CONCLUSIONS

Because TMPDS is the result of a complex interrelation of musculoskeletal, psychological, and anatomic abnormalities of which we have limited knowledge, a coordinated team effort is required if the patient is to improve. This should include a thorough history, physical examination, and careful diagnostic testing to rule out surgical pathology and identify the painful structures. Treatment with medications, correction of occlusal problems, and rest should be followed by an intensive, planned rehabilitation program utilizing physical modalities, patient education, and adequate psychological support to provide the patient with the best chance of a good functional recovery.

REFERENCES

1. Costen JB. A syndrome of ear and sinus symptoms dependent upon disturbed function of the temporomandibular joint. *Ann Otol Rhinol Laryngol* 1934;43:1–15.

2. Lipp MJ. Temporomandibular symptoms and occlusion: a review of the literature & the concept. *J Colo Dent Assoc* 1991;69: 18–21.

3. Perry HT. Temporomandibular joint dysfunction: from Costen to the present. *Ann Acad Med Singapore* 1995;24:163–167.

4. Klausner JJ. Epidemiology of chronic facial pain. *J Am Dent Assoc* 1994;125:1604–1611.

5. Lipton JA, Ship JA, Larach-Robinson D. Estimated prevalence and distribution of orofacial pain in the United States. *J Am Dent Assoc* 1993;124:115–121.

6. Schiffman EL, Fricton JR, Haley DP, Shapiro BL. The prevalence and treatment needs of subjects with temporomandibular disorders. *J Am Dent Assoc* 1990; 120:295–303.

7. Dworkin SF, Huggins KH, LeResche L, et al. Epidemiology of signs and symptoms in temporomandibular disorders: clinical signs in cases and controls. *J Am Dent Assoc* 1990;120: 273–281.

8. Foreman PA. Temporomandibular joint and myofascial pain dysfunction—some current concepts, part 1: diagnosis. *NZ Dent J* 1985;81:47–52.

9. Gnatz SM. Referred pain syndromes of the head and neck. *Phys Med Rehabil State Art Rev* 1991;5:585–596.

10. Kirk WS. The TMJ syndrome: is it a reasonable diagnostic term? *N C Med J* 1988;49:574–578.

11. Campbell CD, Loft GH, Davis H, Hart DL. TMJ symptoms and referred pain patterns. *J Prosthet Dent* 1982;47:430–433.

12. Schiffman E, Haley D, Baker C, Lindgren B. Diagnostic criteria for screening headache patients for temporomandibular disorders. *Headache* 1995;35: 121–124.

13. Gelb H, Bernstein I. Clinical evaluation of two hundred patients with temporomandibular joint syndrome. *J Prosthet Dent* 1983;49:234–243.

14. Pullinger AG, Seligman DA. Trauma history in diagnostic groups of temporomandibular disorders. *Oral Surg Oral Med Oral Pathol* 1991;71:529–534.

15. Ryan DE. Temporomandibular disorders. *Curr Opin Rheumatol* 1993;5:209–218.

16. Bengtsson A, Henriksson KG, Larsson J. Reduced high-energy phosphate levels in painful muscle in patients with primary fibromyalgia. *Arthritis Rheum* 1986;29:817–819.

17. Raphael KG, Marbach JJ. A year of chronic TMPDS: relating patient symptoms and pain intensity. *J Am Dent Assoc* 1992;123:49–55.

18. MacRae DL. Head and neck pain in the elderly. *J Otolaryngol* 1986;15:224–227.

19. Larheim TA, Storhaug K, Tveito L. Temporomandibular joint involvement and dental occlusion in a group of adults with rheumatoid arthritis. *Acta Odontol Scand* 1983;41:301–309.

20. Bade DM, Lovasko JH, Montana J, Waide FL. Acute closed lock in a patient with lupus erythematosus: case review. *J Craniomandib Disord Facil Oral Pain* 1992;6:208–212.

21. Ficarra B, Nassif J. Temporomandibular joint syndrome: diagnostician's dilemma—a review. *J Med* 1991;22:97–121.

22. Piette E. Anatomy of the human temporomandibular joint. An updated comprehensive review. *Acta Stomatol Belg* 1993;90:103–127.

23. Baragar FA, Osborn JW. A model relating patterns of human jaw movement to biomechanical constraints. *J Biomech* 1984;17:757–767.

24. Bermejo-Fenoll A, Puchades-Orts A, Sanchez del Campo F, et al. Morphology of the meniscotemporal part of the temporomandibular joint and its biomechanical implications. *Acta Anat* 1987;129:220–226.

25. Mongini F. Influence of function on TMJ remodeling and degenerative disease. *Dent Clin North Am* 1983;27:479–493.

26. Quinn JH, Bazan NG. Identification of prostaglandin E_2 and leukotriene B_4 in the synovial fluid of painful dysfunctional temporomandibular joints. *J Oral Maxillofac Surg* 1990;48:968–972.

27. Esposito V, Leisman G, Frankenthal Y. Neuromuscular effects of temporomandibular joint dysfunction. *Int J Neurosci* 1993;68:205–207.

28. Chan SWY, Reade PC. Tinnitus and temporomandibular pain-dysfunction syndrome. *Clin Otolaryngol* 1994;19:370–380.

29. Nowlin TP, Nowlin JH. Examination and occlusal analysis of the masticatory system. *Dent Clin North Am* 1995;39:379–401.

30. Baker RW, Catania JA, Baker RW. Occlusion as it relates to the TMJ: a study of the literature. *NY State Dent J* 1991;57:36–39.

31. Raudino F. Is temporomandibular dysfunction a cranial dystonia? An electrophysiological study. *Headache* 1994;34:471–475.

32. Nelson SJ. Principles of stabilization bite splint therapy. *Dent Clin North Am* 1995;39:403–421.

33. Gray RJM, Davies SJ, Quayle AA, Wastell DG. A comparison of two splints in the treatment of TMJ pain dysfunction syndrome. Can occlusal analysis be used to predict success of splint therapy? *Br Dent J* 1991;170:55–58.

34. Garcia R. Air bag implicated in temporomandibular joint injury. *Cranio* 1994;12:125–127.

35. Dibbets JM, van der Weele LT. Orthodontic treatment in relation to symptoms of the temporomandibular joint. A 10 year study report of the University of Groningen study. *Am J Orthod Dentofacial Orthop* 1987;91:193–199.

36. Rendell JK, Norton LA, Gay T. Orthodontic treatment and temporomandibular disorders. *Am J Orthod Dentofacial Orthop* 1992;101:84–87.

37. Mohlin B, Pilley JR, Shaw WC. A survey of craniomandibular disorders in 1000 12-year-olds. Study design and baseline data in a follow-up study. *Eur J Orthod* 1991;13:111–123.

38. Westling L, Mattiasson A. General joint hypermobility and temporomandibular joint derangement in adolescents. *Ann Rheum Dis* 1992;51:87–90.

39. Bates RE, Stewart DM, Atkinson WB. The relationship between internal derangements of the temporomandibular joint and systemic joint laxity. *J Am Dent Assoc* 1984;109:446–447.

40. Westling L, Carlsson GE, Helkimo M. Background factors in craniomandibular disorders: with special reference to general joint hypermobility, parafunction and trauma. *J Craniomandib Disord Facial Oral Pain* 1990;4:89–98.

41. Buckingham R, Braun T, Harinstein D, et al. Temporomandibular joint dysfunction syndrome: a close association with systemic joint laxity (the hypermobile joint syndrome). *Oral Surg Oral Med Oral Pathol* 1991;72:514–519.

42. Braun BL. Postural differences between asymptomatic men and women and craniofacial pain patients. *Arch Phys Med Rehabil* 1991;72:653–656.

43. Benoliel R, Eliav E, Elishoov H, Sharav Y. Diagnosis and treatment of persistent pain after trauma to the head and neck. *J Oral Maxillofac Surg* 1994;52:1138–1147.

44. Weinberg S, LaPointe H. Cervical extension-flexion injury (whiplash) and internal derangement of the temporomandibular joint. *J Oral Maxillofac Surg* 1987;45:653–666.

45. Ernest EA. The orthopedic influence of the TMJ apparatus in whiplash: report of a case. *Gen Dent* 1979;27:62–64.

46. Kulber DA, Davos I, Aronowitz JA. Severe cutaneous foreign body giant cell reaction after temporomandibular joint reconstruction with Proplast-Teflon. *J Oral Maxillofac Surg* 1995;53:722–723.

47. Estabrooks LN, Fairbanks CE, Collett RJ, Moyer DJ. Letter to the editor: appropriateness of recommendations for management of temporomandibular joint implants. *J Oral Maxillofac Surg* 1994;52:656–657.

48. Anonymous. Recommendations for management of patients with temporomandibular joint implants. *J Oral Maxillofac Surg* 1993;51:1164–1172.

49. Trumpy IG, Lyberg T. In vivo deterioration of Proplast-Teflon temporomandibular joint interpositional implants: a scanning electron microscope and energy-dispersive x-ray analysis. *J Oral Maxillofac Surg* 1993;51: 624–629.

50. Gundaker WE. Serious problems with Proplast-coated TMJ implant. Rockville, MD: U.S. Food and Drug Administration, *FDA Safety Alert* Dec. 28, 1990.

51. Mafee MF, Heffez L, Campos M, et al. Temporomandibular joint: role of direct sagittal CT air-contrast arthrogram and MRI. *Otolaryngol Clin North Am* 1988;21:575–588.

52. Krasnow AZ, Collier BD, Kneeland JB, et al. Comparison of high-resolution MRI and SPECT bone scintigraphy for noninvasive imaging of the temporomandibular joint. *J Nucl Med* 1987;28:1268–1273.

53. Katzberg RW, Westesson P, Tallents RH, et al. Temporomandibular joint: MR assessment of rotational and sideways disk displacements. *Radiology* 1988;169:741–748.

54. Bell KA, Miller KD, Jones JP. Cine magnetic resonance imaging of the temporomandibular joint. *J Craniomandib Pract* 1992;10:313–317.

55. Cooper BC, Alleva M, Cooper DL, Lucente FE. Myofascial pain dysfunction: analysis of 476 patients. *Laryngoscope* 1986; 96:1099–1106.

56. Kerstein RB, Wright NR. Electromyographic and computer analysis of patients suffering from chronic myofascial pain-dysfunction syndrome: before and after treatment with immediate complete anterior guidance development. *J Prosthet Dent* 1991;66:677–686.

57. Westesson P, Rohlin M. Diagnostic accuracy of double-contrast arthrotomography of the temporomandibular joint: correlation with postmortem. *AJR* 1984;143: 655–660.

58. Hermans R, Termote JL, Marchal G, Baert AL. Temporomandibular joint imaging. *Curr Opin Radiol* 1992;4:141–147.

59. Keller DC. Ready for phase II—quantitative radionuclide bone scanning. *J Gen Orthodont* 1992;3:5–10.

60. Cooper BC, Cooper DL, Lucente FE. Electromyography of masticatory muscles in craniomandibular disorders. *Laryngoscope* 1991;101:150–157.

61. Gratt BM, Sickles EA. Thermographic characterization of the asymptomatic temporomandibular joint. *J Orofacial Pain* 1993;7:7–14.

62. Weinstein SA, Weinstein G. A protocol for the identification of temporomandibular disorders by standardized computerized electronic thermography. *Clin J Pain* 1987;3:107–112.

63. Travell JG, Simons DG. *Myofascial pain and dysfunction.* Baltimore: Williams & Wilkins, 1983.

64. Schwartz RA, Green CD, Laskin DM. Personality characteristics of patients with myofascial pain-dysfunction (MPD) system unresponsive to conventional therapy. *J Dent Res* 1979;58: 1435–1439.

65. Schnurr RF, Rollman GB, Brooke RI. Are there psychologic predictors of treatment outcome in temporomandibular joint pain

and dysfunction? *Oral Surg Oral Med Oral Pathol* 1991;72:550–558.

66. Okeson JP, Hayes DK. Long-term results of treatment for temporomandibular disorders: an evaluation by patients. *J Am Dent Assoc* 1986;112:473–476.

67. Vallon D, Ekberg EC, Nilner M, Kopp S. Short-term effect of occlusal adjustment on craniomandibular disorders including headaches. *Acta Odontol Scand* 1991;49:89–96.

68. Harkins S. Letter to the editor. *J Prosthet Dent* 1991;65:153.

69. deFelicio CM, Rodrigues da Silva MAM, Mazzetto MO, Centola ALB. Myofunctional therapy combined with occlusal splint in the treatment of temporomandibular joint dysfunction-pain syndrome. *Braz Dent J* 1991;2:27–33.

70. Shan SC, Yun WH. Influence of an occlusal splint on the integrated electromyography of the masseter muscles. *J Oral Rehabil* 1991;18:253–256.

71. Kotani H, Abekura H, Hamada T. Objective evaluation of bite plate therapy in patients with myofascial pain dysfunction syndrome. *J Oral Rehabil* 1994;21:241–245.

72. Chen CW, Boulton JL, Gage JP. Effects of splint therapy in TMJ dysfunction: a study using magnetic resonance imaging. *Aust Dent J* 1995;40:71–78.

73. Yunus MB. Diagnosis, etiology, and management of fibromyalgia syndrome: an update. *Compr Ther* 1988;14:8–20.

74. Semble EL, Wise CM. Fibrositis. *Am Fam Physician* 1988;38:129–139.

75. Grzesiak RC. Psychologic considerations in temporomandibular dysfunction: a biopsychosocial view of symptom formation. *Dent Clin North Am* 1991;35:209–226.

76. Gray RJM, Davies SJ, Quayle AA. A clinical approach to temporomandibular disorders: 7 treatment planning, general guidelines and case histories. *Br Dent J* 1994;177:171–178.

77. McCain GA, Bell DA, Mai FM, Halliday PD. A controlled study of the effects of a supervised cardiovascular fitness training program on the manifestations of primary fibromyalgia. *Arthritis Rheum* 1988;31:1135–1141.

78. dos Santos J. Supportive conservative therapies for temporomandibular disorders. *Dent Clin North Am* 1995;39:459–477.

79. Travell J. Identification of myofascial trigger point syndromes: a case of atypical facial neuralgia. *Arch Phys Med Rehabil* 1981;62:100–106.

80. Heinrich S. The role of physical therapy in craniofacial disorders: an adjunct to dental pain management. *J Craniomandib Pract* 1991;9:71–75.

81. Gnatz SM. Temporomandibular joint syndrome: a critical review. *CRC Crit Rev Rehabil* 1990;2:1–10.

82. Gray RJM, Quayle AA, Hall CA, Scholfield MA. Physiotherapy in the treatment of temporomandibular disorders: a comparative study of four treatment methods. *Br Dent J* 1994;176:257–261.

83. Clifford DB. Treatment of pain with antidepressants. *Am Fam Physician* 1985;31:181–185.

84. Swerdlow M. Anticonvulsant drugs and chronic pain. *Clin Neuropharmacol* 1984;7:51–82.

85. Arner S, Meyerson BA. Lack of analgesic effect of opioids on neuropathic and idiopathic forms of pain. *Pain* 1988;33:11–23.

86. Dolwick MF, Dimitroulis G. Is there a role for temporomandibular joint surgery? *Br J Oral Maxillofac Surg* 1994;32:307–313.

87. Takaku S, Toyoda T. Long-term evaluation of discectomy of the temporomandibular joint. *J Oral Maxillofac Surg* 1994;52:722–726.

88. Israel HA. Current concepts in the surgical management of temporomandibular joint disorders. *J Oral Maxillofac Surg* 1994;52:289–294.

89. Moses JJ, Topper DC. A functional approach to the treatment of temporomandibular joint internal derangement. *J Craniomandib Disord Facil Oral Pain* 1991;5:19–27.

90. Bertolucci LE. Postoperative physical therapy in temporomandibular joint arthroplasty. *J Craniomandib Pract* 1992;10:211–220.

91. Wilk BR, McCain JP. Rehabilitation of the temporomandibular joint after arthroscopic surgery. *Oral Surg Oral Med Oral Pathol* 1992;73:531–536.

92. Murtagh J. Musculoskeletal medicine tip: injection into temporomandibular joint. *Aus Fam Physician* 1992;21:688.

93. Ahlqvist J, Legrell PE. A technique for the accurate administration of corticosteroids in the temporomandibular joint. *Dentomaxillofac Radiol* 1993;22:211–213.

94. Lehmann JF. *Therapeutic heat and cold.* 3rd ed. Baltimore: Williams & Wilkins, 1982.

95. Lehmann JF, Masock AJ, Warren CG, et al. Effects of therapeutic temperatures on tendon extensibility. *Arch Phys Med Rehabil* 1970;51:481–487.

96. Rocabado M. Arthrokinematics of the temporomandibular joint. *Dent Clin North Am* 1983;27:573–594.

97. Gelb H. Effective management and clinical treatment of the craniomandibular syndrome. In: Gelb H, ed. *Clinical management of head, neck and TMJ pain and dysfunction.* Philadelphia: WB Saunders, 1977:338–343.

98. Block SL, Laskin DM. The effectiveness of transcutaneous nerve stimulation (TNS) in the treatment of unilateral MPD syndrome. *J Dent Res* 1980;59:519.

99. Wessberg GA, Caroll WL, Dinham R, Wolford LM. Transcutaneous electrical stimulation as an adjunct in the management of myofascial pain-dysfunction syndrome. *J Prosthet Dent* 1981;45:307–314.

100. Gold N, Greene CS, Laskin DM. TENS therapy for treatment of MPD syndrome. *J Dent Res* 1983;62:244.

101. Eisen RG, Kaufman A, Green CS. Evaluation of physical therapy for MPD syndrome patients. *J Dent Res* 1984;63 (special issue):344.

102. Taylor K, Newton RA, Personius WJ, Bush FM. Effects of interferential current stimulation for treatment of subjects with recurrent jaw pain. *Phys Ther* 1987; 67:346–350.

103. Dohrmann RJ, Laskin DM. An evaluation of electromyographic biofeedback in the treatment of myofascial pain-dysfunction syndrome. *J Am Dent Soc* 1978;96: 656–662.

104. Trott PH Goss AN. Physiotherapy in diagnosis and treatment of the myofascial pain dysfunction syndrome. *Int J Oral Surg* 1978;7: 360–365.

105. Flor H, Birbaumer N. Comparison of the efficacy of electromyographic biofeedback, cognitive-behavioral therapy, and conservative medical interventions in the treatment of chronic musculoskeletal pain. *J Consult Clin Psychol* 1993;61: 653–658.

106. Travell J, Simons DG. *Myofascial pain and dysfunction: the trigger-point manual.* Baltimore: Williams & Wilkins, 1983:85, 86, 228, 254.

107. Girdler NM. The use of botulinum toxin to alleviate facial pain. *Br J Hosp Med* 1994;52: 363.

108. Hargreaves AS, Wardle JJM. The use of physiotherapy in the treatment of temporomandibular disorders. *Br Dent J* 1983;155:121–124.

109. Lark MR, Gangarosa LP. Iontophoresis: an effective modality for the treatment of inflammatory disorders of the temporomandibular joint and myofascial pain. *Cranio* 1990;8:108–119.

110. Wing M. Phonophoresis with hydrocortisone in the treatment of temporomandibular joint dysfunction. *Phys Ther* 1982;62: 32–33.

111. Muir WS, Magee FP, Longo JA, et al. Comparison of ultrasonically applied vs. intra-articular injected hydrocortisone levels in canine knees. *Orthop Rev* 1990;19: 351–356.

112. Garro LC. Narrative representations of chronic illness experience: cultural models of illness, mind, and body in stories concerning the temporomandibular joint (TMJ). *Soc Sci Med* 1994; 38:775–788.

113. Keefe FJ, Dolan E. Pain behavior and pain coping strategies in low back pain and myofascial pain dysfunction syndrome patients. *Pain* 1986;24:49–56.

114. Dodes JE, Schissel MJ. The role of physicians in dental quackery. *N Y State J Med* 1993;93: 116–117.

115. Greene CS, Laskin DM. Long-term evaluation of conservative treatment of myofascial pain-dysfunction syndrome. *J Am Dent Assoc* 1974;89: 1365–1368.

Chapter 63

Complex Regional Pain Syndrome

Wade S. Kingery

Reflex sympathetic dystrophy syndrome (RSDS) is a term coined by Evans in 1946 to describe a syndrome of pain, vasomotor instability, and dystrophy in the extremity (1). The RSDS terminology has enjoyed widespread usage (525 MEDLINE references from 1990 to 1995), but its definition is ambiguous and its acceptance hardly universal, with over 40 different names for this syndrome appearing in the medical literature.

The International Association for the Study of Pain (IASP) has recognized several problems with the RSDS terminology, which is often applied to patients without clinical evidence of sympathetic abnormality or dystrophy. The IASP (2) advocates using the terms *complex regional pain syndromes (CRPS) type I* and *type II.*

CRPS type I (RSDS) is defined as a syndrome that usually starts after a noxious event, is not limited to the distribution of a single peripheral nerve, and is disproportionate to the inciting event. The diagnosis requires 1) pain, allodynia, or hyperalgesia disproportionate to injury; 2) evidence at some time of edema, changes in skin blood flow, or abnormal sudomotor activity in the region of pain; and 3) no other conditions that would otherwise account for the degree of pain and dysfunction.

CRPS type II (causalgia) is defined as a syndrome that starts after a nerve injury, and is not necessarily limited to the distribution of the injured nerve. The diagnostic criteria are the same as those for CRPS type I. The exclusion diagnoses include unrecognized local pathology (e.g., fracture, strain, sprain), traumatic vasospasm, cellulitis, Raynaud disease, thromboangiitis obliterans, and thrombosis.

PATHOPHYSIOLOGY

Allodynia and Aβ Low-Threshold Mechanoreceptors

There is considerable experimental evidence that the mechanical allodynia observed in some patients with CRPS and neuralgia is mediated by Aβ low-threshold mechanoreceptors, which normally have no nociceptive function (3). Ischemic compression block of the limb selectively eliminates allodynia to light touch before it causes loss of warmth and heat pain sensation (4), while differential local anesthetic block of the involved nerve causes loss of temperature sensation before loss of allodynia and light touch (5). Patients have nearly the same stimulus intensity thresholds for both the detection of and a pain response to transcutaneous electrical nerve stimulation (TENS) over the allodynic skin (6). Such low-current strengths should only activate the Aβ fibers, which normally cannot mediate pain. Latencies for the detection of pain in the allodynic limb are the same as those for touch in the contralateral limb, which is further evidence for myelinated fiber mediation of allodynia (5).

The low-threshold mechanoreceptor mediation of allodynia is attributed to altered or sensitized central nervous system processing of normal Aβ primary afferent impulses. The allodynia seen in CRPS and neuralgia patients closely resembles the allodynia created in soft-tissue injury experiments in normal volunteers (7). Both the CRPS and soft-tissue injury allodynia are mediated by Aβ primary afferents (8), while the mechanical hyperalgesia often seen in CRPS and soft-tissue injury experiments appears to be mediated by unmyelinated fibers (4,9,10). Both neuropathic and soft-tissue injury–induced allodynia are probably dynamically maintained by ongoing nociceptive afferent activity (11,12).

There are extensive clinical and experimental data regarding dynamic central nervous system adaptations to pain, but the neural process leading to allodynia has yet to be identified (13). One of the mysteries of CRPS is that both soft-tissue trauma and nerve injuries can develop into clinically identical chronic pain syndromes. The similar features of the allodynia seen with experimental soft-tissue injury, CRPS, and neuralgic pain indicate a possible common pathophysiology that may respond to a single pharmacologic approach.

Sympathetic Hyperactivity

Despite clinical evidence of sympathetic hyperactivity in some CRPS patients (hyperhidrosis, vasoconstriction), the experimental evidence for increased sympathetic efferent activity is equivocal. Microneurographic recordings of sympathetic fibers in the involved limb are normal (14,15). The cold pressor test can be ineffective in CRPS limbs, indicating a loss of the normal sympathetic efferent reflex (16–18). After a peripheral nerve block there is a greater increase in subcutaneous blood flow on the asymptomatic side, indicating a lower resting sympathetic vasomotor tone in the affected hand (19).

Plasma levels of norepinephrine and its intracellular metabolite 3,4-dihydroxyphenylethyleneglycol (DHPG) can be reduced in the affected limb compared to the contralateral side (20,21). Neuropeptide Y is also released from the sympathetic vasomotor neurons and its plasma concentration is reduced in CRPS limbs if allodynia is present (22). Deafferentation adrenergic supersensitivity may occur, with an increased venous responsiveness to norepinephrine observed in some CRPS patients, in both the affected and the unaffected extremity (23).

There may be a loss of cholinergic sensitivity in CRPS patients, with a reduction in the cholinergic sudomotor response. The sympathetic skin potential amplitudes can be reduced (24), and iontophoresed acetylcholine usually causes a diminished hidrotic response in the CRPS limb (25). End-organ supersensitivity is a possible explanation for some symptoms of adrenergic hyperactivity, but there is no scientific consensus on the pathophysiology of the sympathetic abnormalities in CRPS (26).

Sympathetically Maintained Pain

The limited success of controlled trials with regional and systemic adrenergic blockade in CRPS is surprising in light of the frequent analgesia reported with local anesthetic sympathetic ganglion blocks (SGBs) and the long-term pain relief observed with surgical sympathectomy. Except for three sympathetic block studies, all the SGB and surgical sympathectomy studies are outcome series without controls. One study found local anesthetic SGBs to be superior to morphine SGBs, but this was a small study without a randomized, double-blinded protocol, no placebo effect, no quantitative outcomes, and no statistical analysis (27). Two SGB trials found no difference between SGB and "active" control agents (28,29), but there is considerable evidence that the "active" controls used in these studies (guanethidine and phentolamine) are ineffective analgesics for CRPS.

There is also evidence that the pain relief from SGB is not related to the adequacy of the sympathetic block as determined by skin temperature change (30,31). Classic clinical findings of CRPS (generalized pain, allodynia, edema, vasomotor instability) were not predictive of a positive SGB response in a large series of SGB-treated patients with chronic pain and heterogeneous symptoms and signs (25). SGB has been advocated as a diagnostic tool to identify CRPS patients with sympathetically maintained pain (SMP) and as a therapeutic procedure that could cure CRPS in some patients (32). Placebo-controlled trials with quantitative sensory testing are necessary to determine if SGB in CRPS patients provides short-term analgesia without afferent fiber blockade of the plexus.

If guanethidine intravenous regional blocks (IVRBs) and intravenous phentolamine do not provide analgesia in CRPS, what clinical evidence supports the concept of SMP? Electrical stimulation of the decentralized thoracic sympathetic ganglia in CRPS patients elicited tingling and burning pain in uncontrolled investigations (33,34). About 20% of neuralgia patients reported increased spontaneous and evoked pain after norepinephrine was subcutaneously injected or iontophoresed into the hyperalgesic skin, but there were no saline-treated control subjects in this study to evaluate for possible negative placebo effects (35). Intradermal injection of phenylephrine (an α-adrenergic agonist) caused increased pain and hyperalgesia in a CRPS patient (36), but intravenous phenylephrine administered in a randomized, double-blind trial did not cause an exacerbation of spontaneous or evoked pain in CRPS patients (37).

The hypothesis that some CRPS patients have pain that is partially or completely maintained by the sympathetic nervous system (26,38) has not been supported by controlled trials and appears to have lost ground in recent years (37,39–42). Randomized controlled clinical trials are required to establish the presence of a significant component of SMP in CRPS.

Inflammation

The edema, redness, and warmth frequently seen in CRPS patients can resemble autoimmune diseases or infection. Several controlled trials have indicated that CRPS can be successfully treated with anti-inflammatory corticosteroids

(43,44). A scintigraphy study using indium 111–labeled immunoglobulin G demonstrated increased vascular permeability for macromolecules in early CRPS, which was not related to limb blood flow (45). Despite this evidence for an inflammatory process in CRPS, sedimentation rates, antigen titers, autoimmune antibody levels, and blood cell counts are normal, and histologic studies demonstrate little or no inflammatory cell infiltrate (46,47). It has been proposed that a peripheral release of the neuropeptide substance P from the unmyelinated nociceptive afferents could cause the vasodilatation and plasma extravasation seen in CRPS (40,41). Inflammation and hyperalgesia due to peripheral cytokines or neuropeptide release after soft-tissue or nerve injury comprise another possible etiology for CRPS and neuropathic pain (48,49).

Psychological Aspects

It has been theorized that certain personality traits or psychiatric illnesses predispose a person to the development of CRPS following an injury (50). Patients without objective clinical findings to explain their symptom amplification may represent a conversion reaction or a psychogenic pain phenomenon. Munchausen syndrome or malingering may also present with symptoms and signs mimicking CRPS (51). Functional recovery in CRPS can be hindered by volitional or inadvertent behaviors, such as immobilization and disuse of the limb, that may persist even after the pain has resolved (52). CRPS patients may also have the same psychological issues as any chronic pain patient, including operant conditioning, cognitive issues, coping skills, chemical dependency, depression, anxiety, and fear. There is no consensus regarding any of the psychological issues in CRPS and the efficacy of psychophysiologic interventions is unknown (41,51,53–56).

CLINICAL FEATURES

Epidemiology

Most large civilian CRPS series include more women than men (47,57). The female preponderance in the older patient population (57) probably reflects the higher incidence of fractures in elderly women (58,59). Sex is not a predisposing factor for the development of CRPS after a fracture has occurred (58). There is no predilection for the dominant side, but approximately 5% of patients have bilateral symptoms (47). The upper extremity is affected almost twice as often as the lower extremity (47,57). The shoulder is painful with limited range in 21% to 53% of cases involving the hand (58,60). The median age of 829 CRPS patients referred to one clinic was 42 years, and the condition was rarely seen in patients younger than 10 or older than 70 (47). When this syndrome occurs in children and adolescents, it has a clinical presentation and therapeutic response similar to those observed in adults. Children are more likely to have lower-extremity involvement (61,62).

Incidence

The incidence of CRPS is dependent on the diagnostic criteria, type of injury, care of the injury, time elapsed between the injury and initial assessment, and the sex and age of the subjects. The annual incidence of CRPS for the community of Freidburg, Germany, was estimated at roughly 1 per 5000 persons per year (57).

Many diseases, injuries, and drugs have been associated with CRPS (Table 63-1). The incidence of CRPS ranges from 1% to 28% following peripheral nerve injury (32,63,64), 5% to 20% after myocardial infarction (65,66), and 23% to 26% after stroke (43,67). Prospective studies of Colles or tibial shaft fractures found a 28% to 37% incidence of mild CRPS at 8 to 17 weeks following injury (58,59,68). The severity of the fracture is a predisposing factor for the development of CRPS (58). A literature review of the conditions frequently associated with CRPS found that 27% of all CRPS patients had soft-tissue trauma, 27% had idiopathic or miscellaneous etiologic factors, 25% had a fracture, 6% had a myocardial infarction, 6% had central nervous system disease, 5% had spinal cord or diskogenic disease, and 4% had peripheral nerve injuries (46).

Progression

The clinical course of CRPS has been divided into three overlapping stages (69,70). The first "acute" stage lasts 3 to 6 months, characterized by pain, tenderness, swelling, and vasomotor disturbances. The second "dystrophic" stage,

Table 63-1: Causes of Complex Regional Pain Syndrome
Antituberculous drug administration
Barbiturate and other anticonvulsive drug administration
Cardiac surgery
Cerebrovascular disease with hemiplegia
Cervical spine disease, such as arthritis and diskogenic disorders
Convulsive disorders (?)
Fractures, especially Colles fracture
Hemiplegia of other causes
Herpes zoster with postherpetic neuralgia
Hysterical personality (?)
Idiopathic
Ischemic heart disease
Nerve injuries (including entrapment mononeuropathies, radiculopathies, plexopathies, needle injection injuries)
Painful lesions of the rotator cuff
Peripheral neuropathy
Primary central nervous system disorders
Pulmonary tuberculosis
Spinal cord lesions
Surgical trauma (including amputation, scars, manipulation, tight casts, adhesions)
Trauma, major or minor (including crush, lacerations, ischemia, sprain, tendonitis, repetitive motion injuries)
Tumors

lasting another 3 to 6 months, presents a partial reduction in these symptoms, with trophic changes appearing in the skin and bone. The third "atrophic" stage evolves into marked skin and bone atrophy, with severe contractures. The third stage is chronic, and the patient is left with a shiny, cool, contracted, and usually painless extremity.

These three stages of CRPS are difficult to distinguish in a specific individual, with considerable fluctuation of symptoms over time (46). A prospective study of 829 CRPS patients failed to identify a three-stage evolution of symptoms and signs (47). There were no significant differences in the incidence of skin atrophy and contractures in the acutely and chronically affected patients, but the incidence of edema does gradually decrease over time and the incidence of trophic bone changes increases after several months. There is no correlation between symptom duration and resting skin blood flow (71). An IASP workshop concluded that neither the staging nor the grading of the different CRPS clinical presentations offered any utility from a descriptive, diagnostic, or therapeutic viewpoint (38).

Prognosis

The prognosis for CRPS is variable and may be adversely affected by the duration and severity of the symptoms. Prospective studies demonstrated a 28% to 31% incidence of mild CRPS type I symptoms soon after tibial (68) or Colles (58) fractures, with 86% to 93% of these CRPS patients having spontaneous resolution of their pain within a year. A prospective study of guanethidine regional blocks in early CRPS type I patients found that only 35% of the subjects had resolution or near resolution of their pain during the 6-month study (42). The difference between these outcomes probably reflects the severity of the CRPS in the respective patient populations, with the fracture studies including all patients with persistent pain and joint tenderness, and the guanethidine study including only patients referred to pain clinics with allodynia, hyperalgesia, or hyperesthesia.

CRPS type II patients from World War II also had a gradual improvement of symptoms, with a dramatic reduction of pain in 57% to 68% of patients at 6 months and in 90% to 91% by 12 to 17 months (63,72). These CRPS type II outcomes were not based entirely on the natural resolution of the disease since surgical sympathectomies were performed in 20% of the patients in one series (72) and 3% in the other series (63), and many patients had surgical explorations of their nerves.

The prognosis for the chronic CRPS patient is poor, with less than 10% reporting resolution 4 to 18 years after onset (35,73). CRPS may also recur in the same or a different limb after it has resolved, with a 1.8% annual incidence of recurrence (74).

Symptoms

Symptoms start within a day of the triggering event in about 75% of patients, but may develop weeks or months later (47). The symptoms can appear in the hand, foot, a single digit, the knee, hip, shoulder, trunk, or face. Spontaneous pain is common, with a deep, diffuse distribution variously described as burning, throbbing, pressing, shooting, or aching. There may be an orthostatic aspect, with increased spontaneous pain with the limb dependent, decreasing with limb elevation. The area of pain usually exceeds the distribution of a single peripheral nerve or myotome (57).

Evoked pain or abnormal sensation is also a common feature. Pain is usually elicited by passive or active range of motion in the involved limb. Allodynia is observed in 8% to 41% of CRPS patients (37,57), with pain to light touch, moving stimuli, vibration, mild thermal stimulation, or low-intensity electrical stimulation such as produced with a TENS unit. Hyperpathia can be seen with exaggerated responses to painful stimuli, which are delayed in onset, persist after the stimulus, and spread beyond the stimulus site.

Usually the patient notes differences in skin temperature between the affected and unaffected limbs, and frequently notes edema or skin color changes in the affected extremity (47).

Signs

Hyperalgesia and hypoalgesia to heat, cold, and mechanical stimuli can be observed. Mechanical hyperalgesia is almost always observed with dolorimetry, which is instrumented nociceptive pressure threshold testing over the distal articular surfaces (58,59,68,75). Heat and cold hyperalgesia in the affected extremity is identified in less than half of CRPS patients evaluated with instrumented nociceptive threshold testing (37).

Skin blood flow is usually abnormal at some point during the disease, with a red, blue, or white skin tint. Side-to-side skin temperature differences are usually greater than 2.5°C, with the affected extremity either warmer or cooler (76). There is often an abnormal sweat response, with either hypohidrosis or hyperhidrosis. Edema is present in most patients at some point in the development of the syndrome. There can be tight, shiny skin; loss of skinfolds over digits; pitting or nonpitting edema; and increased circumference, skin thickness, or volumetric measures compared to the contralateral side (Fig. 63-1). Motor function is usually impaired, with weakness, atrophy, and loss of active range of motion (47,57). A fine postural or action tremor can be seen (77). Rarely, in chronic cases of CRPS, a dystonia may develop (78).

Trophic skin changes, including abnormal nail growth, increased or decreased hair growth, palmar or plantar fibrosis, thin glossy skin, and hyperkeratosis, are seen in 30% to 40% of patients (47,76). Patchy bone demineralization is observed in 50% of chronically affected patients, especially in a periarticular distribution. All these clinical features of CRPS may also be observed in patients with no history of pain (47,59).

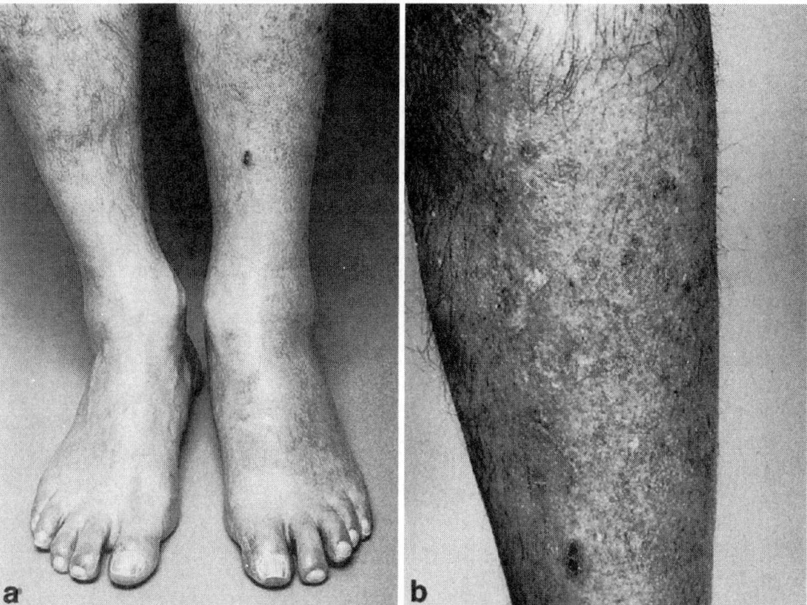

Figure 63-1. *a.* Edema and erythema in the left foot of a man who developed severe allodynia and spontaneous pain after a total knee arthroplasty with a subsequent severe axonotmetic peroneal mononeuropathy. *b.* Dry, scaly skin and hair loss over the anterolateral surface of the lower part of the leg.

Histology

Histologic changes are seen in the synovial tissues of the hand in CRPS patients, with subsynovial fibrosis, edema, and proliferation of the synovial lining cells and capillaries (46). Minimal inflammatory cell infiltrate with a few perivascular lymphocytes was observed. Histologic evidence of iron deposition in the shoulder periarticular tissues of hemiplegic patients with shoulder and hand pain suggested a history of microtrauma and bleeding (43). The shoulder synovium in these patients also had signs of granulation tissue and perivascular leukocytic infiltration.

DIAGNOSTIC TESTING

Clinical Examination

Although the clinical examination is the gold standard of diagnosis, there is no definitive clinical diagnostic criteria for CRPS. There are a minimum of three IASP diagnostic criteria for CRPS type I, all of which can be established from the clinical examination and history (2): 1) The patient must have persistent pain disproportionate to injury, allodynia, or hyperalgesia. 2) At some point in the disease there must be a clinical sign or symptom of sympathetic abnormality. This sign or symptom can be an objective or subjective cold or warm limb, red or cyanotic skin, hyperhidrosis or hypohidrosis, or edema. 3) There cannot be any other diagnosis that would otherwise account for the symptoms.

The clinical diagnostic criteria for CRPS type II are the same as for CRPS type I, except there must be evidence of nerve injury, and the pain, allodynia, or hyperalgesia can be limited to the distribution of the injured nerve, or in a generalized area including the territory of the injured nerve. Careful clinical examination of CRPS type I patients can often identify occult nerve injuries. One series utilizing von Frey monofilament, vibration, and two-point discrimination tests, provocative clinical tests, and nerve conduction studies found an 86% prevalence of mononeuropathies in 35 patients with CRPS in the hand (79). A thorough neurologic examination, including quantitative sensory testing and electrodiagnosis, has been advocated for the evaluation of the CRPS patient (51,80).

Numerous methods or algorithms have been developed for the clinical diagnosis and grading of CRPS, often subdividing subjects into categories such as definite, probable, possible, and unlikely CRPS (81,82). No single clinical diagnostic or grading methodology has been widely utilized in treatment trials or in the evaluation of new diagnostic tests for CRPS, making it difficult to compare outcome data.

Dolorimetry

Tenderness to palpation over the distal articular surfaces is a common finding in CRPS and the degree of joint tenderness has been correlated to the patient's pain (59,68,83). Joint tenderness has also been associated with loss of range of motion, edema, and vasomotor instability (59). The joint tenderness can be quantitated by a pressure measurement device called a *dolorimeter* or *algometer.* Several scoring methods have been employed in CRPS trials to measure mechanical hyperalgesia. Values derived from this technique have been used as diagnostic criteria for CRPS (68,75,84). The specificity is 95% in asymptomatic subjects and the sensitivity for CRPS in recent fracture patients is 100% in the hand and 92% in the foot (85–87). Dolorimetry can give quantitative data on the natural progression of the hyperalgesia (68,87) and its response to treatment (75,88,89).

Sympathetic Ganglion Blocks with Local Anesthetics

Local anesthetic is injected into the lumbar or stellate (Fig. 63-2) paravertebral sympathetic ganglia (90). A successful SGB is confirmed when the finger or toe skin temperature significantly increases (see Fig. 63-2b). Temporary relief of pain (usually a 50% reduction) indicates SMP. False-positive findings may result from a placebo effect, which should be controlled for with randomized, blinded saline injections, but this has not been reported in the literature. False-positive findings can also result from blocking adjacent afferents in the brachial or lumbar plexus, and must be excluded by careful sensory function testing after the block (31).

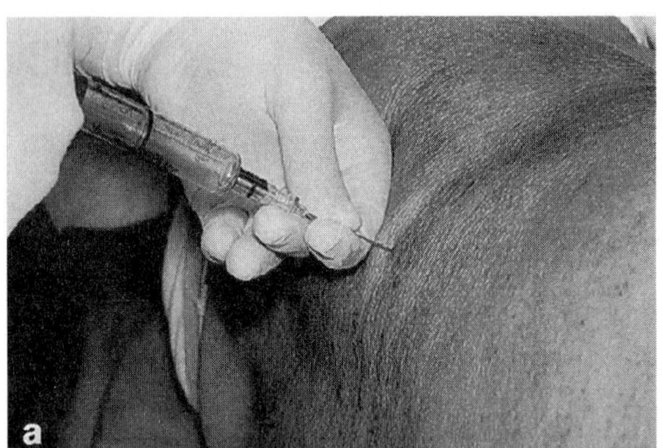

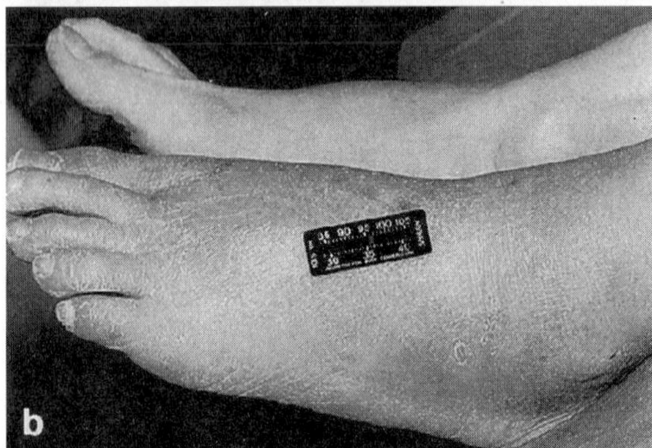

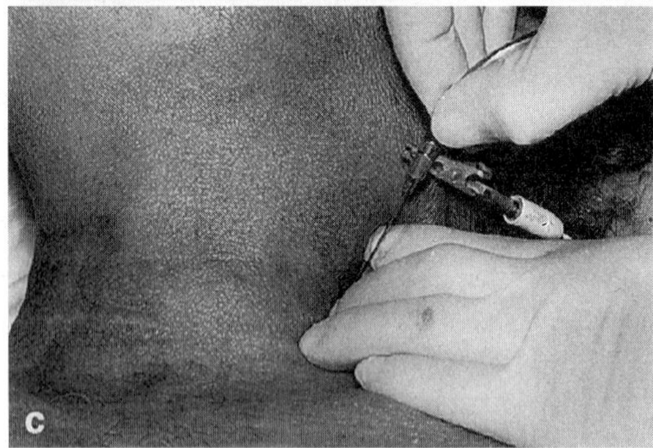

Figure 63-2. *a.* A posterior, paravertebral, L2–L4 approach for a lumbar sympathetic block. *b.* A successful lumbar sympathetic block, indicated by a rise in foot temperature to over 35°C. *c.* An anterior, paratracheal C6 approach for a stellate ganglion block, using a needle-sterile tubing-syringe technique, which allows optimal needle control.

Guanethidine Intravenous Regional Blocks

Intravenous injection of guanethidine into an extremity distal to a suprasystolic cuff can deplete norepinephrine from postganglionic axons, which can initially cause a brief pain, followed by days of symptom relief (91). Pain relief after the guanethidine treatment would indicate SMP.

Phentolamine Test

Phentolamine, an α_1, α_2-adrenergic antagonist, is continuously infused intravenously after an initial blinded placebo saline infusion. Frequent monitoring of visual analog pain scales may demonstrate a 50% reduction of spontaneous pain, indicating SMP (29).

Quantitative Autonomic Testing

Skin temperature asymmetry between the affected and contralateral side has frequently been noted in CRPS. Early CRPS is associated with warmer limbs and late CRPS, with cooler limbs (25). Quantitation of skin temperatures with infrared telethermography and video thermography has been advocated for the diagnosis and for tracking the progression of CRPS. The problem with this approach for diagnosis and staging is that the sensitivity and specificity are low, there is great variability in the progression of the disease with regards to temperature, and the skin temperature patterns are unstable over multiple recordings (92).

The cold stressor test has been used in CRPS patients to evaluate the duration of skin temperature drop in the asymptomatic contralateral limb after it is immersed in 15°C to 20°C water for 1 minute. There is a prolonged reduction in skin temperature in the noninvolved limb before returning to baseline (93), but this is not a specific finding for CRPS and similar results are observed in other chronic pain patients (94).

Doppler flowmetry has been used to measure skin blood flow in CRPS patients. Patients with a sensation of limb warmth are more likely to have increased skin blood flow, and patients with a sensation of limb coolness tend to have decreased skin blood flow, but there is no relation between skin blood flow and the duration of symptoms (71).

The sympathetic skin response is an electrical measurement of glabrous skin depolarization caused by sudomotor activation following noxious electrical stimulation. This test has been used in CRPS patients with simultaneous bilateral recordings over the palms or soles while stimulating the middle of the forehead. An abnormal skin response is a delayed latency, a diminished amplitude, or a different waveform morphology compared to the contralateral side. The sympathetic skin response test has a 63% sensitivity for clinically diagnosed CRPS (24).

A combined sudomotor and skin temperature evaluation has also been proposed (95). Sudomotor evaluation is performed by recording resting sweat output and a quantitative sudomotor axon reflex test (QSART), with bilateral recording capsules attached bilaterally to the forearm and hand, or foot and distal part of the leg. This is recorded for 5 minutes over the four sites simultaneously, using sudometers. The QSART measures an evoked sweat response to iontophoretically applied 10% acetylcholine and a depressed QSART has the highest specificity (58%) of any single autonomic test (25). Skin temperature is recorded with infrared telethermography at 14 different sites bilaterally and 0.5°C unidirectional asymmetries at three or more sites are considered abnormal. Skin temperature asymmetry had the highest sensitivity (62%) for clinical CRPS. Combinations of these three laboratory tests reportedly give a 100% sensitivity and 77% specificity for the diagnosis of CRPS, compared to clinical diagnostic criteria (95).

Radionuclide Bone Scans

A three-phase bone scan is performed after injection of 20 mCi of technetium 99m–labeled radioisotope, with images obtained immediately, 10 minutes, and 2 hours after injection. A diffuse asymmetric uptake in the affected limb can be seen in the early scan, and an asymmetric periarticular accumulation of tracer can be seen later (Fig. 63-3). Kozin et al (75) reported an 86% sensitivity, but only a 60% specificity for bone scanning, compared to clinical diagnosis. A recent review found a wide range in the reported sensitivity of the three-phase bone scan (50%–100%), and concluded that bone scanning is probably more sensitive in early and in clinically obvious CRPS (96). The specificity of the three-phase bone scan in asymptomatic limbs is 77% (97).

After sympathectomy, CRPS patients with normal bone scans will develop the classic CRPS bone scan pattern, even when the sympathectomy has no effect on the symptoms (98). The increased bone blood flow and periarticular bone turnover seen on the positive bone scan may reflect diminished sympathetic activity in the CRPS patient. Another variant of abnormal bone scan in CRPS is decreased periarticular activity on blood pool and delayed images (Fig. 63-4), which is presumed to be caused by vasoconstriction (99,100).

X-ray Studies

Patchy demineralization at the periarticular surfaces may appear within 3 weeks after injury (101). Later in the disease there may be subperiosteal bone reabsorption with a ground-glass appearance and tunneling of the cortices and endosteal surface of the bone (Fig. 63-5). Approximately half of CRPS patients will develop these dystrophic bone changes (47), but these changes are nonspecific and may be seen with any disuse syndrome.

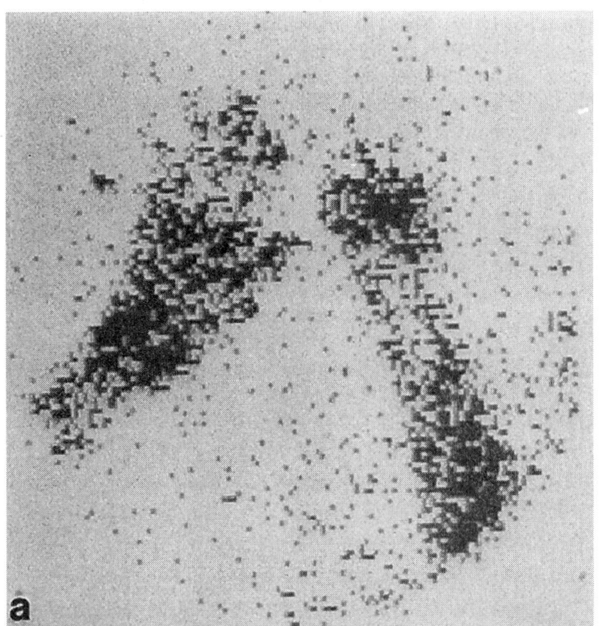

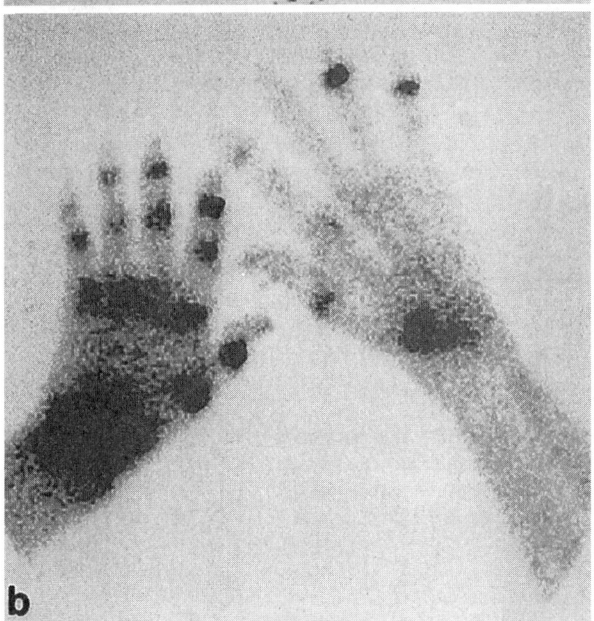

Figure 63-3. A typical triple-phase bone scan in a patient with complex regional pain syndrome involving the right hand. *a.* The first-phase spot view demonstrates increased perfusion in the right hand within a minute after intravenous administration of 20 mCi of technetium 99 m–labeled diphosphonate. *b.* The third-phase delayed scan 3 hours after injection demonstrates diffusely increased periarticular uptake.

Magnetic Resonance Imaging

Magnetic resonance (MR) imaging with contrast enhancement has been advocated as a diagnostic test of CRPS. At least one abnormal finding was seen on MR images in 88% of CRPS patients in one series (102). The abnormal

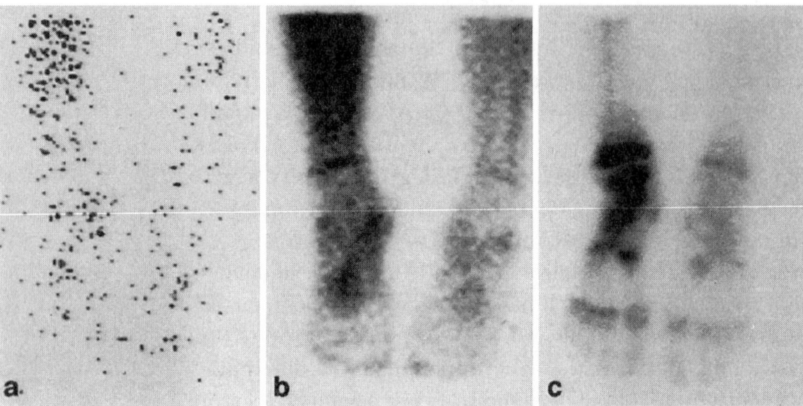

Figure 63-4. An atypical triple-phase bone scan in a patient with complex regional pain syndrome involving the left foot. *a.* The first-phase spot view demonstrates decreased perfusion in the left foot within a minute after injection. *b.* The second-phase blood pool scan taken 5 minutes after injection also shows decreased perfusion. *c.* A decreased periarticular uptake is seen in the third-phase delayed scan.

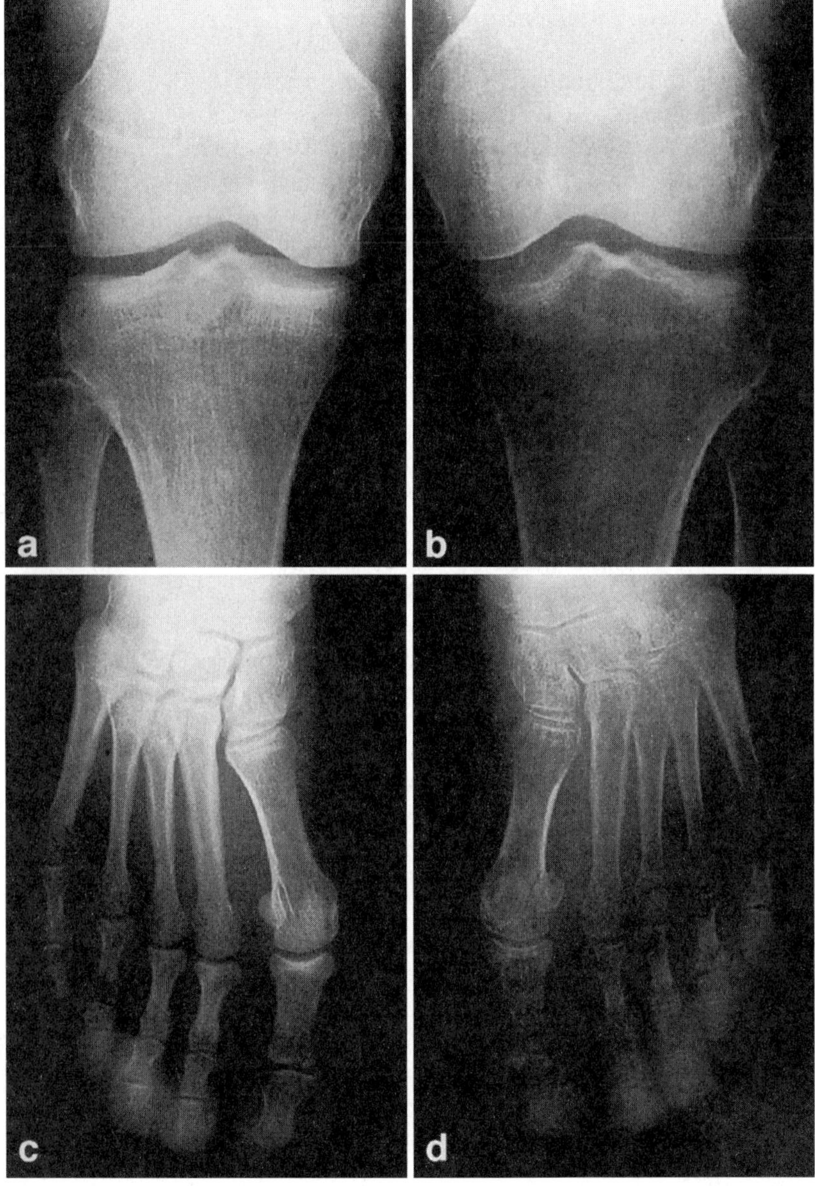

Figure 63-5. Radiographs of the feet and knees of a patient who developed complex regional pain syndrome in the left foot after an ankle sprain. A generalized loss of density and patchy translucencies are clearly visible in the left knee (*b*), compared to the uninvolved side (*a*). The left foot (*d*) has subchondral bone resorption with cortical translucencies and a severe osteopenia with a ground-glass appearance, while the uninvolved side (*c*) appears normal.

findings in this study included thickening or thinning of skin, muscle atrophy, edema, or soft-tissue enhancement. No control subjects were evaluated with this method and the MR findings usually did not add to the clinical findings of edema and dystrophy. MR imaging of bone marrow changes has not proved useful in the diagnosis of CRPS (103).

Ischemia Test

Supersystolic tourniquet application to the CRPS limb can reduce pain within 1 to 2 minutes (57). Ischemic pain relief was reported to predict a positive response to SGB and was proposed as a diagnostic test for CRPS.

TREATMENT

Physical Therapy

Physical therapy is widely recommended as a first-line treatment for CRPS and is usually used in conjunction with sympathetic blocks and pharmacotherapy (46), but its efficacy is unknown. A 1984 CRPS review stated "the role of physical therapy . . . remains an area of controversy replete with anecdotal comments" (104). Since that review, there have been no controlled trials for modalities, edema control, stretching, strengthening, splinting, desensitization, TENS, friction massage, or stress loading as treatment for CRPS. Early physical therapy has been advocated for CRPS, since earlier treatment correlates with better outcome (105,106).

The control groups in two large calcitonin trials used early CRPS patients (8 weeks after trauma), and these control groups had a similar reduction in pain during the 8-week trial period. One trial gave its control patients an eight-week course of active and passive physical therapy within the pain-free range of movement, positive pressure treatments for edema, lymphatic drainage or whirlpool, TENS, and cooling (107), while the other trial gave its control subjects no treatment of any kind (89). Placebo intranasal saline treatments were given for 3 to 4 weeks to both control groups, and after 8 weeks the reduction in pain was virtually identical (55% to 57%) for both the physical therapy group and the no-treatment control groups. This comparison illustrates the need for randomized trials to distinguish between the spontaneous resolution of pain in early CRPS and possible effects of physical therapy.

The primary goal of physical therapy is to mobilize the involved extremity. Patients tend to guard the involved limb, avoiding movement and functional use, sometimes even after their pain resolves. Continued immobilization aggravates the edema and weakness, and can eventually lead to an atrophic, severely contracted limb. When the edema has converted into scar tissue and the ligaments have shortened, the prognosis for functional use is poor (108).

Some authors have advocated passive range of motion and stretching as tolerated (109,110), while others have recommended avoiding any painful activities that may result in exacerbation of the disease (43,104). Increasing use of the hand for dressing, eating, and oral-facial hygiene is encouraged, and progressive resistive exercises have also been used for CRPS (111).

Prolonged heating of the involved limb has also been recommended (106,109,112), which when combined with active or passive range of motion exercises can help mobilize joint contractures. Static and dynamic splinting has been used to prevent and treat contractures (108). Forceful mobilization of the limb after induction of a local anesthetic IVRB has also been used for CRPS contractures (106,113). Intra-articular injection of high volumes of anesthetic and contrast material into the frozen shoulder ruptures the shoulder capsule, which can cause immediate pain relief and recovery of shoulder mobility (114).

Edema control is also a primary objective in CRPS, initially using elevation of the extremity, compression garments, and friction massage for treatment. If edema persists, a pneumatic pressure pump with pressures up to 40 to 60 mm Hg can be used. Following the pump treatment, compression is continued with an elastic bandage wrap or compression garment and the limb is elevated again. The patient is advised to avoid holding the limb in a dependent position, and to frequently mobilize it to reduce edema (107,115–117).

Various modalities have also been used to reduce pain and sensitivity in the CRPS limb. Local heat or cold can be applied with paraffin baths, contrast baths, or icing. Fluidotherapy or whirlpool hydrotherapy can provide heat while the patient is mobilizing the limb. TENS has been frequently used for analgesia in CRPS patients (118–121). Some patients may be unable to tolerate TENS directly over sensitive skin or an involved nerve, with an allodynic response to mild electrical stimulation (6). Desensitization of the allodynic limb has been advocated, with initial gentle stroking with cotton, progressing to materials with increasing friction and coarseness to touch (115).

A novel modality for the treatment of CRPS is ultrasound over the sympathetic ganglia (122) or peripheral nerves (123). Goodman (122) and Portwood et al (123) proposed that low-dose ultrasound (0.5–1.5 watt/cm^2) can block nerve impulses. There are several questions regarding the safety and efficacy of ultrasound treatments for CRPS. High-dose ultrasound can cause cavitation of neural tissue and irreversible paralysis in animals (124). Low-dose ultrasound (1–3 W/cm^2) applied over human lumbar sympathetic ganglia does not raise the temperature of the foot more than 1 to 2°C, which does not indicate a successful SGB (125,126).

Most patients have a transient aggravation of symptoms after physical therapy (47), and analgesics or TENS with therapy can increase pain tolerance in therapy and help patients overcome excessive protectiveness o the involved limb (127). It has been recommended that exercise should be increased as tolerated, but if the patient has increased pain persisting for more than an hour after a treatment session, the exercise routine should be reduced to a more comfortable level (110).

Sympathetic Ganglion Blocks with Local Anesthetics

Serial SGBs have been advocated as a treatment for CRPS, with complete and lasting relief reported in 18% to 59% of patients (32). There are no randomized placebo-controlled trials for serial SGBs in CRPS, but one randomized parallel trial found no outcome differences between a series of eight SGBs and a series of four guanethidine IVRBs (28). One large study retrospectively compared selected unmatched control subjects with patients who had four or more lumbar SGBs (128). There was no statistical analysis, but at a 3-year follow-up 11% of control subjects and 12% of patients were pain free, and 41% of control subjects and 65% of patients had some improvement. Some studies used indwelling catheters for continuous anesthetic infusion into the sympathetic ganglion for 2 to 26 days (129,130). A long-term block can be achieved by injection of phenol into the sympathetic ganglia (131), with extended relief reported in 38% of CRPS patients (98).

Intravenous Regional Blocks

IVRBs for CRPS originally used guanethidine (91). An intravenous line was placed distally in the painful limb and a pneumatic tourniquet was placed around the proximal limb. The limb was exsanguinated and the tourniquet inflated to 50 to 100 mm Hg above systolic pressure. Guanethidine was then infused with a local anesthetic or saline solution, and 15 to 30 minutes later the cuff was released. Numerous other intravenously administered regional block drugs have since been tried in CRPS. The drugs include reserpine (132), lidocaine and corticosteroid (106), ketorolac (133), bretylium (134), ketanserin (135), atropine (136), and droperidol (137). The outcomes of controlled IVRB studies are discussed later in the controlled trials section.

Peripheral Nerve Block with Local Anesthetics

Local anesthetic blocks of peripheral nerves reduced spontaneous and evoked pain in CRPS patients in a distribution outside of the blocked nerve, or proximal to the block site (12). Bupivacaine blocks of peripheral nerves in patients with neuralgia provided pain relief of variable duration, with 66% of patients noting a prolonged reduction in pain lasting from 12 hours to 6 days (138). A series of local anesthetic blocks of the suprascapular nerve have been advocated as a treatment for the frozen shoulder component of CRPS (139). No controlled trials have examined serial nerve block treatments for CRPS.

Epidural Anesthetic Block

A long-term sympathetic and somatic blockade can be achieved with an indwelling epidural catheter continuously infusing local anesthetic or opioid. This treatment has been used for CRPS of the knee (140). The infusion can be continued for as long as 7 days, with manipulation and continuous passive motion of the knee if the anesthetic is titrated so the patient is pain free. Opiates can also be infused epidurally, providing pain relief without a complete motor block, which allows ambulation.

Surgery

Sympathectomy

Surgical sympathectomy for CRPS was first performed by Spurling in 1930 (141). Numerous war-time sympathectomy series claimed complete relief of burning pain in 50% to 100% of CRPS type II patients, but there were no controlled trials and CRPS in the majority of these patients would have spontaneously resolved without treatment (32,64). Recent civilian studies claimed 61% to 74% success rates (full use of extremity) after sympathectomy for CRPS, but these retrospective studies did not include controls, standard diagnostic criteria, or objective outcome measures (142–144). The study with the longest follow-up found that sympathectomy outcome was highly correlated with symptom duration, and no patient with symptoms for more than 12 months had complete relief from surgery (142). The response to SGB was predictive of the long-term surgical outcome in this study.

A less invasive alternative to surgical sympathectomy is radiofrequency sympatholysis, a technique that involves insertion of an insulated needle percutaneously into the sympathetic ganglia and then heating of the tip of the needle to 70°C for 120 seconds (131). This technique was reported effective in 25% of CRPS patients (145). Another alternative to open surgical sympathectomy is endoscopic sympathectomy (146).

The most common postoperative complication of sympathectomy is a transient sympathetic neuralgia seen in 25% to 46% of patients (142,144,147). While postsympathectomy neuralgia has been considered a self-limited problem, some cases of persistent symptom exacerbation after sympathectomy have been reported (98). Repeat sympathectomies have been performed, with a more extensive surgical sympathectomy relieving pain in some patients (144). Some patients have contralateral sympathetic crossover innervation, requiring bilateral sympathectomy for relief (144,148,149).

Amputation

Amputation of the painful extremity provides long-term pain relief in only 7% to 30% of CRPS patients, but in carefully selected patients it may improve mobility or self-care (52,150). Frequently after amputation the CRPS recurs in the stump, and sometimes develops in another extremity (150).

Decompression of Nerve Entrapments

Occult nerve entrapments are a surgically treatable cause of CRPS and should be evaluated for by clinical examination and electrodiagnostic studies. One series of 22 early CRPS patients who failed to respond to corticosteroids and exercise had good pain relief following surgical decompression of the carpal tunnel, with 91% returning to work (151). Another series of 20 CRPS patients had good results from surgical decompression of various nerve entrapments, including carpal and cubital tunnel syndrome and entrapment involving the Guyon canal, posterior interosseous nerve, and the superficial radial nerve (79).

Reanastomosis or Grafting of Severed Nerves

Successful nerve regeneration after reanastomosis or grafting of severed nerves is associated with a reduction in pain, allodynia, and hyperalgesia (152–155). Not all axons successfully reinnervate their original target end-organs after reanastomosis or grafting, and this may explain why some patients do not develop significant pain relief after these procedures (156,157).

Neuroablative Procedures

Neuroablative procedures ranging from neurolysis, neurectomy, rhizotomy, cordotomy, mesencephalic tractotomy, thalamotomy, cingulotomy, and resection of the frontal and parietal cortex have been tried in the management of CRPS. All have had disappointing long-term outcomes (64).

Implantable Nerve Stimulators

Implantable nerve stimulators may provide long-term relief in 25% of CRPS patients (158). Implantable stimulators have been used on the peripheral nerve (159) and in the epidural space over the spinal cord (121,160,161). Epidural stimulation can provide a mild analgesia to heat-evoked pain (1°C) compared to placebo stimulation, but the effectiveness of epidural stimulation reportedly wanes over time (162).

Controlled Drug Trials

Tables 63-2 to 63-5 summarize 27 controlled trials that investigated 15 different treatments for CRPS. Table 63-2 illustrates that guanethidine IVRBs in CRPS patients are ineffective analgesics compared to placebo or no treatment (42,88,132,163,164). One study found a decrease in spontaneous pain relative to baseline levels at 1 hour after a guanethidine IVRB, but a later study by the same investigators failed to demonstrate any guanethidine effect (39,165). One trial demonstrated a better recovery in early CRPS after 3 weeks of topical dimethylsulfoxide (DMSO) than after six guanethidine blocks (166).

Numerous other drugs have been used in controlled IVRB trials (see Table 63-3). Bretylium (which depletes norepinephrine in the postganglionic axon) was used in a single small trial that demonstrated a significant difference between the duration of the analgesia following bretylium and lidocaine IVRBs (20 ± 18 days vs 2.7 ± 4 days) (134). Effective analgesia was also observed for more than 3 weeks following several ketanserin blocks (a serotonin type 2 receptor antagonist) in another small trial (135). The results of these two trials, with a combined total of 16 patients, need to be confirmed in larger-scale investigations before any conclusions can be drawn. Two trials with reserpine (which depletes norepinephrine in the postganglionic axon) did not demonstrate any short- or long-term benefits over placebo (132,163). Atropine (a muscarinic cholinergic antagonist) and droperidol (an α-adrenergic antagonist) had no analgesic effects following IVRBs for chronic CRPS (136,137).

Table 63-4 lists eight more controlled drug trials for CRPS. Corticosteroids were effective analgesics in several trials with early CRPS patients (43,44). Braus et al (43) claimed a long-term, or curative effect 20 weeks after a short course of oral corticosteroids, but the placebo-controlled phase of this trial only lasted 4 weeks. Calcitonin administered subcutaneously or by intranasal spray over 3 to 4 weeks in early CRPS patients had mixed results, with two studies finding no difference between the calcitonin-treated and control groups (89,167), and one study showing a benefit after 3 weeks of calcitonin treatments (107). Epidural clonidine (an α-adrenergic agonist) had a short-term analgesic effect in chronic CRPS, but there were significant sedation and hypotension issues and the continuous epidural infusion resulted in frequent infections (168). Intravenous ketanserin had no short-term analgesic effects in a small crossover trial (169).

Intravenous systemic phentolamine studies have had conflicting results (see Table 63-5). Two studies examined the phentolamine response in CRPS after an initial saline placebo infusion. One study (29) found 45% of patients had significant short-term relief with phentolamine, but a much larger study (37) found only 9% of patients had significant relief. Verdugo and Ochoa (37) found that after starting the intravenous saline solution, some patients developed a progressive placebo analgesia. They attributed the phentolamine analgesia observed in 9% of their patients, and in 45% of the patients in Raja et al's study (29), to the problem of starting the phentolamine infusion during the progressive development of the placebo analgesia, which could be confused with a phentolamine effect.

An additional randomized crossover study by Verdugo and Ochoa (37) using intravenous phentolamine and phenylephrine (an α-adrenergic agonist) demonstrated that 17% of subjects had significant relief of ongoing pain with phenylephrine and 9% had significant relief with phentolamine. These data indicate there is probably either no phentolamine analgesia, or possibly a short-term effect in a small subset of CRPS patients (170).

There are no SGB trials with placebo controls, but

Table 63-2: Controlled Trials of Intravenous Regional Guanethidine Blocks in Complex Regional Pain Syndrome (CRPS)

Trial	Subjects and Design	Diagnosis (Duration of Symptoms)	Treatment (Guanethidine)	Control Treatment (Tourniquet Time)	Outcome Measure and (Follow-up)	Results: Guanethidine vs Control	Results: Control
Glynn et al, 1981 (165)	n = 28 C, SB	+SGB, 4/7 symptoms and signs of CRPS (?)	G: 10 mg in 10 mL saline, 1 block	Saline: 10 mL, 1 block, (10 min)	VAS(I) (1 hr)	S at 1 hr (NS at 1 wk from baseline)	NS at 1 hr
Bonelli et al, 1983 (28)	n = 9 P, O, R	4/6 signs of CRPS G—(18) and SGB —(28 wk)	G: 20 mg in 25 mL saline, 4 blocks	SGB: B 15 mL, 0.5%, 8 blocks	VAS(I) (16 days)	NS at all times	S at 1 hr, persists to 16 days
Rocco et al, 1989 (132)	n = 12 C, DB, R	+SGB, allodynia, pain, vasomotor	G: 20 mg in 50 mL 0.5% L, 1 block	L: 50 mL, 0.5% (20 min)	VAS(I) (90 min) NPS (1 wk)	NS at all times	avg VAS ↓ 72% at 90 min
Blanchard et al, 1990 (163)	n = 12 C, DB, R	+SGB, signs and symptoms (2.9 yr)	G: 20 mg UE, 30 mg LE, in 30–50 mL saline, 1 block	Saline: 30–50 mL (20 min)	↓VAS(I) > 50% = relief (until no relief)	NS at all times	83% with relief at 30 min
Field and Atkins, 1993 (88)	n = 10 P, O	Colles Fx, ↓ range vasomotor, edema dolorimetry (12 wk)	G: ? mg ? mL 2–4 blocks, and physical therapy	Physical therapy	5 physical measures (24 wk)	NS except for dolorimetry at 20 and 24 wk	?
McGlone et al, 1993 (164)	n = 20 C, DB	Signs and symptom (?)	G: 15 mg, 30 mL 0.3% L, 1 block	L: 30 mL, 0.3%	VAS(I) and (1 wk)	S at 1 hr (NS at 1 wk from baseline)	S at 1 hr, NS at 7 days
Geertzen et al, 1994 (166)	n = 13 P, O, R	3/6 symptoms and signs of CRPS (3–12 wk)	G: ? mg, ? mL, 6 blocks	DMSO (50% in water) topical 4 × day for 3 wk	VAS(I), 3 clinical scales, ADLs (9 wk)	S worse than DMSO at 7 and 9 wk	S, combined score was better than G at 7 and 9 wk
Jadad et al, 1995 (39)	n = 8 C, DB, R	+G block, 4/7 symptoms and signs of CRPS (?)	G: 10 and 30 mg UE, 20 and 30 mg LE in 25–50 mL saline, 1 block	Saline: 25 mL UE, 50 mL LE, (15 min)	VAS(I) (R) (1 wk, then until pain at baseline)	NS at all times	Avg VAS ↓ 37% over 1 hr, 14% over 1 wk
Ramamurthy et al, 1995 (42)	n = 20 P, DB, R	allodynia, hyperalgesia (6 wk)	G: 20 mg UE, 40 mg LE, 30–75 mL 0.5% L, 1, 2, or 4 blocks	L: 30–50 mL UE 40–75 mL LE, 0.5%, 0–3 block (20 min)	MPQ and Global Evaluation (4 days to 26 wk)	NS at 4 days (no dose response for G to 26 wk)	Avg MPQ ↓ 27% after 4 days

n = number of subjects in smallest group after randomization; P = parallel; C = crossover; DB = double-blind; SB = single-blind; R = randomized; O = open; S = significant; NS = not significant; UE = upper extremity; LE = lower extremity; G = guanethidine; L = lidocaine; B = bupivacaine; DMSO = dimethylsulfoxide; SGB = sympathetic ganglion block; VAS = visual analog scale for pain; (I) = intensity; (R) = relief; ADLs = activities of daily living; MPQ = McGill pain questionnaire; NPS = numeric pain scale; q = each; Fx = fracture; avg = average.

three SGB trials did use "active" controls. A six-patient crossover study (27) found that SGB with bupivacaine gave short-term pain relief compared to a morphine ganglion block, but the morphine control subjects had no placebo effect and there were no quantitative outcome measures (see Table 63-4). Another short-term crossover study compared an SGB to low doses of intravenous phentolamine in 20 patients, and found no difference between these treatments (29). Both the SGB and the systemic phentolamine reduced (>50% drop in visual analog scale) ongoing pain in half of the patients, with a high correlation of positive responses between the two treatments (see Table 63-5). A parallel study compared eight SGBs to four guanethidine IVRBs, both administered over 16 days (28). There was no difference in analgesia between the treatments over the ensuing 12 weeks, with the mean pain intensity scores dropping 50% (see Table 63-2).

Several important points emerge from the literature on CRPS controlled trials. There is no evidence of analgesia with guanethidine or reserpine IVRBs in CRPS. Oral corticosteroids may offer analgesia in early CRPS, but a curative effect has not been established. The other drugs

Table 63-3: Controlled Trials of Intravenous Regional Drug Blocks in Complex Regional Pain Syndrome (CRPS)

Trial	Subjects and Design	Diagnosis (Duration of Symptoms)	Treatment Drug	Control Treatment (Tourniquet Time)	Outcome Measure (Follow-up)	Results: Drug vs Control	Results: Control
Hord et al, 1992 (134)	n = 12 C, DB, R	+SGB, +cold stress test, hx of CRPS (?)	Bretylium 1.5 mg/kg in 40–60 mg 0.5% L, 2 blocks	Lidocaine 0.5% 40 mL UE, 60 mL LE, 2 blocks (20 min)	VAS(R) > 30% = relief (until no relief)	S difference avg duration of relief with bretylium 20 days vs L 3 days	Duration avg relief with L 3 days
Hanna and Peat, 1989 (135)	n = 9 C, DB, R	Pain, vasospasm edema, atrophic, duration (2.1 yr)	Ketanserin 10 mg UE, 20 mg LE, 30 mL saline, 2 blocks	Saline 30 mL, 2 blocks (15 min)	VAS(I) (2 wk)	S at 1 wk, 2 wk, from baseline	NS at 1 wk
Rocco et al, 1989 (132)	n = 12 C, DB, R	+SGB, allodynia, pain, vasomotor (?)	Reserpine 1.5 mg in 50 mL 0.5% L, 1 block	Lidocaine 0.5% 50 mL, 20 min	VAS(I) 90 min and NPS (1 wk)	NS at all times avg AVS ↓ 72% at 90 min	Avg VAS ↓ 72% at 90 min
Blanchard et al, 1990 (163)	n = 12 C, DB, R	+SGB, signs and symptoms (2.9 yr)	Reserpine 0.5 mg UE, 1 mg LE, 30–50 mL saline, 1 block	Saline 30–50 mL (20 min)	↓VAS(I) > 50% = relief (until no relief)	NS at all times	83% with relief at 30 min
Glynn et al, 1993 (136)	n = 33 C, DB, R	+Guanethidine IVRB (7 yr)	Atropine 0.6 mg in 10 mL saline, 2 blocks	Saline 10 mL (10 min)	VAS(I) (R) 1 hr, CS (q hr/1 wk)	NS at all times	Avg VAS ↓ 29% at 60 min
Kettler and Abram, 1988 (137)	n = 6 C, DB, R	+SGB, clinical signs CRPS (3.1 yr)	Droperidol 2.5 mg in 30–50 mL saline, 1 block	Saline 30 mL UE, 50 mL LE (15 min)	VAS(I) (q day/2 wk)	1/5 with ↓VAS > 40%	3/4 with ↓ VAS > 40%

n = number of subjects in smallest group after randomization; C = crossover; DB = double-blind; R = randomized; S = significant; NS = not significant; UE = upper extremity; LE = lower extremity; L = lidocaine; Res = reserpine; SGB = sympathetic ganglion block; NRB = intravenous regional block; VAS = visual analog scale for pain; (I) = intensity; (R) = relief; CS = categorical scale; q = each; avg = average; hx = history; NPS = numeric pain scale.

that are reportedly effective for CRPS [bretylium IVRB (134), ketanserin IVRB (135), intranasal calcitonin (107), epidural clonidine (168), and intravenous phentolamine (29)] need further study to resolve conflicting results, to improve the methodology, and to confirm single reports.

Seven CRPS studies followed patients for 3 months (or longer). Only prednisone provided effective analgesia for 3 months when compared to placebo (44). Three studies found no outcome differences between guanethidine IVRBs compared to placebo (163), SGBs (28), or multiple guanethidine IVRB treatments (42). One study found no analgesic effect for repeated guanethidine IVRBs compared to physical therapy, except for a reduction of dolorimetry scores developing 5 months after the completion of guanethidine treatments (88). Reserpine IVRBs (163) and intranasal calcitonin (89) were also ineffective long-term analgesics in CRPS.

A total of 48 controlled pharmacotherapy trials for peripheral neuropathic pain (PNP), excluding central nervous system injury and trigeminal neuralgia, were identified. Neuropathic pain includes neuralgia and painful polyneuropathy. Neuralgia is spontaneous or evoked pain in the distribution of a single nerve. Painful polyneuropathies are usually symmetric and distal, affecting the feet and sometimes the hands. These conditions may present with or without paresthesia, hypoesthesia, hyperalgesia, and allodynia. Table 63-6 summarizes the controlled treatment trials for PNP. The patients in these trials were not usually evaluated for symptoms or signs of abnormal sympathetic function associated with the pain, which if present would also classify the patients as having CRPS type II.

Tricyclic antidepressants provide moderate analgesia for thermal-, mechanical-, and electrical-evoked pain in normal subjects (171–173). Antidepressants also can produce partial pain relief in diabetic (174–182), postherpetic (183–187), and peripheral nerve injury (188) patients with PNP. Both spontaneous and evoked PNP is relieved (187), but the long-term analgesic efficacy has not been established. The plasma concentration probably correlates with the analgesic effect (177,179,184) and the pain relief appears to be independent of the antidepressant effect of these drugs (174,176,179,185). Most successful trials used tricyclic antidepressants, but some serotonin receptor reuptake inhibitors may also provide analgesia (179,181), although probably not as effectively as the tricyclics.

The tricyclics are initiated with a low bedtime dose (10 or 25 mg) and gradually increased on a weekly basis up

Table 63-4: Controlled Drug Trials in Complex Regional Pain Syndrome (CRPS)

Trial	Subjects and Design	Diagnosis (Duration of Symptoms)	Treatment Drug	Control Treatment	Outcome Measure (Follow-up)	Results: Drug vs Control	Results: Control
Christensen et al, 1982 (44)	n = 10 P, SB, R	4/7 signs and symptoms (13 wk)	Prednisone 30 mg/day for 12 wk	Placebo 3 × day up to 12 wk	Clinical scale (12 wk)	S at 12 wk	Clinical scale ↓28% at 12 wk
Braus et al, 1994 (43)	n = 17 P, SB, R	CVA, Kozin's criteria for definite CRPS (6–8 wk)	Methylprednisolone, 32 mg/day for 2 wk, then taper over 2 wk	Placebo 4 × d for 4 wk	Clinical scale (4 wk)	Avg clinical scale ↓65% at wk 4	No change in clinical scale at 4 wk
Gobelet et al, 1986 (167)	n = 10 P, O, R	Symptoms and signs of CRPS (7 wk)	Calcitonin, s.c. 100 U/day for 3 wk, physical therapy	Physical therapy	Clinical scales (8 wk)	NS at all times	S at 3 wk for pain, edema, ROM
Gobelet et al, 1992 (107)	n = 33 P, DB, R	Kozin's criteria for definite CRPS (9 wk)	Calcitonin intranasal 300 U/day for 3 wk, physical therapy	Saline intranasal 3 × day for 3 wk, physical therapy	Clinical scales (8 wk)	S at wk 8 for pain and ROM	S at wk 1 for pain and ROM
Bickerstaff and Kanis, 1991 (89)	n = 20 P, DB, R	Colles Fx, ↓ROM, edema, vasomotor, dolorimetry (8 wk)	Calcitonin intranasal 400 U/day for 4 wk	Saline intranasal 2 × day for 4 wk	Pain% and 3 physical measures (12 wk)	NS at all times	Pain% all 3 measures improved over 12 wk
Rauck et al, 1993 (168)	n = 26 C, DB, R	+SGB, pain, edema, hyperalgesia (3.8 yr)	Clonidine 300 µg and 700 µg epidural in 10 mL saline	Saline 10 mL epidural	VAS(I) and MPQ (6 hr)	S on VAS, MPQ from baseline for both doses	NS from baseline
Glynn and Casale, 1993 (27)	n = 6 C	+G block, upper-limb pain (2.1 yr)	Bupivacaine 0.5% 10 mL SGB × 1	Morphine 5 mg in 10 mL saline SGB	Patient report of relief (1 hr)	4/6 complete pain relief after SGB	No relief in any patient
Bounameaux et al, 1984 (169)	n = 9 C, DB, R	Signs and symptom (?)	Ketanserin i.v. bolus 10 mg	Placebo i.v. bolus	Clinical scale (25 min)	No change at 25 min	No change at 25 min

n = number of subjects in smallest group after randomization; P = parallel; C = crossover; DB = double-blind; SB = single-blind; R = randomized; O = open; S = significant; NS = not significant; ROM = range of motion; G = guanethidine; SGB = sympathetic ganglion block; VAS = visual analog scale for pain; (I) intensity; MPQ = McGill pain questionnaire; Pain% = the % of patients with residual pain; Fx = fracture; CVA = cerebrovascular accident; s.c. = subcutaneous; avg = average; i.v. = intravenous.

to 150 mg/day if analgesia is inadequate. Serum concentrations may help guide the clinician in adjusting dosages in patients with a poor response (189), but in many patients (7%–58%) tricyclic antidepressants either do not provide good analgesia or have side effects that limit the effective dosage (190). The mechanism of the tricyclic analgesia is unknown, but these drugs block norepinephrine and serotonin reuptake, block α_1-adrenergic receptors, reduce sympathetic efferent activity, and block the hyperalgesia induced by intrathecal *N*-methyl-*D*-aspartate (190,191).

Intravenous lidocaine infusion has no analgesic effect on ischemic and thermal-evoked pain in normal subjects at serum levels below 4 µg/mL (192–194), but higher serum levels of lidocaine are probably analgesic. Controlled studies in diabetic (195), postherpetic (196), and peripheral nerve injury (197) patients with PNP demonstrated short-term analgesia with intravenous lidocaine. Allodynia can be relieved (197) and analgesia is achieved at mean serum levels below 4 µg/mL (192,196). Topical lidocaine applied over postherpetic neuropathic painful skin provides a modest short-term analgesia when compared to placebo or lidocaine application over a contralateral site (198).

Mexiletine is an orally administered lidocaine analogue that has been tested in several PNP trials at doses between 450 and 750 mg/day. The higher doses provided effective analgesia in small controlled studies of diabetic (199) and peripheral nerve injury (200) patients with PNP. One large multicenter controlled trial just failed to obtain a significant analgesic effect with 225 to 675 mg/day in diabetic PNP patients (201). Retrospective analysis indicated that a subset of the patients in this study with symptoms of stabbing or burning pain did have an analgesic response, but this needs confirmation in a prospective study.

Anticonvulsant analgesia in diabetic patients with PNP was examined in four randomized, crossover-design,

Table 63-5: Controlled Phentolamine Trials in Complex Regional Pain Syndrome (CRPS)

Trial	Subjects and Design	Diagnosis (Duration of Symptoms)	Treatment: Phentolamine	Control Treatment	Outcome Measure (Follow-up)	Results: Phentolamine vs Control	Results: Control
Raja et al, 1991 (29)	n = 20 C, DB	Pain and Hyperalgesia (3.1 yr)	Phentolamine 25–35 mg i.v. over 15–40 min (after saline)	Saline i.v. for 1st 8–36 min (avg 21 min) before drug	↓VAS > 50% = pain relief (1 hr)	9/18 with relief	2/20 patients had >80% ↓ VAS(I)
Raja et al, 1991 (29)	n = 20 C, O, R	Pain and hyperalgesia (3.1 yr)	Phentolamine 25–35 mg i.v. over 15–40 min (after saline)	SBG with 0.25% bupivacaine 10 mL UE, 20 mL LE	↓VAS > 50% = pain relief (1 hr)	NS	9/18 with relief after SGB
Verdugo and Ochoa, 1994 (37)	n = 76 C, SB	IASP 1986 criteria for CRPS, with ongoing pain (?)	Phentolamine 35 mg i.v. over 30 min (after saline)	Saline i.v. for 1st 30 min before drug and 30 min after drug	NPS ongoing and evoked (allodynia and pressure) NPS > 50% = pain relief (1 hr)	NS, 9% relief of ongoing pain, 3% relief of allodynia, and 6% relief of deep pressure pain	29% relief of ongoing pain, 28% relief of allodynia, 18% relief of pressure pain
Verdugo and Ochoa, 1994 (37)	n = 23 C, DB, R	IASP 1986 criteria for CRPS, with ongoing pain (?)	Phentolamine 35 mg i.v. over 20 min, saline i.v. 20 min at start and end of protocol	Phenylephrine 500 µg i.v. over 20 min, either before or after phentolamine	NPS ongoing and evoked (allodynia and pressure) ↓NPS > 50% = pain relief (1 hr)	NS, 9% relief of ongoing pain, 11% relief of allodynia, and 15% relief of deep pressure pain	17% relief of ongoing pain, 0% relief of allodynia, 8% relief of pressure pain

n = number of subjects in smallest group after randomization; C = crossover; DB = double-blind; SB = single-blind; R = randomized; O = open; IASP = International Association for the Study of Pain; NS = not significant; avg = average; i.v. = intravenous; UE = upper extremity; LE = lower extremity; SGB = sympathetic ganglion block; VAS = visual analog scale for pain; (I) = intensity; NPS = numeric pain scale; Tx = treatments.

double-blinded trials. None of the studies adjusted the anticonvulsant dosage to maintain target serum levels. The phenytoin (300 mg/day) results are mixed, with one trial reporting effective analgesia after 2 weeks (202) and another investigation finding no analgesic effect at 23 weeks (203). Carbamazepine (600 mg/day) had an analgesic effect in one arm and not in the other arm of a crossover study at 7 days, but there was no combined data analysis for all subjects (204). Another study found greater than 50% relief on the investigator global evaluation scale in 66% of carbamazepine (600 mg/day)-treated patients and 20% of placebo-treated patients after 2 weeks of treatment, but no statistical analysis was performed (205).

The analgesic properties of 0.075% capsaicin applied topically four times a day over painful skin were investigated in four polyneuropathy (206–209) and two postherpetic (210,211) PNP studies. The investigator global evaluation for symptom relief at the end of the treatment (4–8 weeks) indicated capsaicin was better than placebo in three trials (206,209,211), with two other trials showing a trend for greater improvement in the capsaicin groups (207,210). Patients frequently noted burning, erythema, or both after topical application of capsaicin, which may prevent continued use and makes true patient blinding in these trials problematic. It is interesting to note that only one capsaicin study used an active topical placebo (methyl nicotinate), which caused erythema and stinging in some patients. This trial also had the largest placebo effect (67%) and was the only trial that did not demonstrate a trend in favor of capsaicin (208).

Two trials tested transdermal clonidine patches (0.3 mg/day) applied over painful skin in diabetic neuropathy patients. Both studies found no clonidine analgesia over 3 to 6 weeks of continuous treatment, but a subset of the total patient population, identified by retrospective (212) and prospective (213) criteria, did have analgesia. Another trial found that a single oral dose of clonidine (0.2 mg) provided significant analgesia in postherpetic neuralgia patients (214). Continuous infusion of epidural clonidine (30 µg/hr) for 14 days had no effect on patient-controlled morphine analgesia requirements, but did significantly reduce the reported pain intensity in a study of cancer patients with neuropathic pain (215).

Nonsteroidal anti-inflammatory drugs had mixed results in several neuropathic pain trials. A small single-blinded, crossover study found ibuprofen (2400 mg/day) or sulindac (400 mg/day) to be effective analgesics for diabetic PNP (216). This trial demonstrated a gradual decline in patient global symptom scores over the 8-week course of nonsteroidal anti-inflammatory treatment. A 4-week course of piroxicam (20 mg/day) was ineffective in a large double-blind, parallel, randomized trial of lumbosacral radiculopathy patients (217). A single dose of ibuprofen (800 mg) had no analgesic effect in a large crossover trial of postherpetic neuralgia patients (214). A single dose of a topical aspirin–diethyl ether mixture provided analgesia for a

Table 63-6: Controlled Drug Trials on Peripheral Neuropathic Pain				
Drug	**Route**	**Neuropathy**	**Analgesia**	**References**
Antidepressants	Oral	Diabetic	Yes	174–182
		Postherpetic	Yes	183–187
		Nerve injuries	Yes	188
Lidocaine	Intravenous	Diabetic	Yes	195
		Postherpetic	Yes	196
		Nerve injuries	Yes	197
	Topical	Postherpetic	Yes	198
Mexiletine	Oral	Diabetic	Yes	199
			No*	201
		Nerve injuries	Yes	200
Phenytoin	Oral	Diabetic	Yes	202
			No	203
Carbamazepine	Oral	Diabetic	Yes	204
			Yes	205
Capsaicin	Topical	Diabetic	Yes	209
				206
			No	207
		Polyneuropathy	No	208
		Postherpetic	Yes	211
			No*	210
Clonidine	Transdermal	Diabetic	No*	212, 213
	Oral	Postherpetic	Yes	214
	Epidural	Cancer-neuropathic	Yes	215
Nonsteroidal anti-inflammatory	Oral	Diabetic	Yes	216
		Radiculopathy	No	217
		Postherpetic	No	214
	Topical	Postherpetic	Yes	218
Morphine	Intravenous	Nerve injuries	Yes	224
			No	223
		Postherpetic	Yes	196
Codeine	Oral	Postherpetic	No	214
Propranolol	Oral	Nerve injuries	No	219
Lorazepam	Oral	Postherpetic	No	214
Phentolamine	Intravenous	Polyneuropathy	No	220

* Subset of patients had analgesia.

mean duration of 4.6 hours in a small crossover study of acute and postherpetic neuralgia patients (218).

Several other drugs were ineffective in PNP patients. A 2-week course of propranolol (a β-adrenergic antagonist, 240 mg/day) did not provide relief in peripheral nerve injury patients (219). Lorazepam (a benzodiazepine, 0.5–6.0 mg/day) for 6 weeks had no analgesic properties in postherpetic neuralgia patients (214). Intravenous systemic phentolamine was ineffective analgesia for polyneuropathy patients with spontaneous and evoked PNP (220).

Intravenous morphine produces analgesia for evoked pain in normal subjects, in both a dose- and a plasma concentration–dependent manner (221,222). Several controlled trials examined the analgesic efficacy of opioids in chronic PNP patients. No significant analgesic effect was seen in 40 postherpetic neuralgia patients following a single 120-mg dose of codeine (214). Another study used eight neuropathic pain patients who had failed prior opioid therapy and were scheduled for intracerebral or dorsal column stimulators. Intravenous morphine (15 mg) provided partial relief in only one of these patients (223).

Two other placebo-controlled trials (196,224) used high doses (0.3 mg/kg) of intravenous morphine and demonstrated short-term analgesic effects in neuropathic pain patients. Opioid analgesia has been correlated to dose and serum drug levels in neuropathic patients (196,225). Evoked pain can also be transiently relieved with morphine in most patients with postherpetic neuralgia (196). There is a wide range of analgesic responses to opioids in both neuropathic and nociceptive pain patients, and some data suggest that neuropathic pain is less opioid responsive than nociceptive pain (225). The only study to look at serum morphine levels and analgesia in PNP demonstrated significant analgesia with a mean peak serum level of 68 ng/mL (196), which is less than the median effective concentration for analgesia seen in normal subjects for electrically evoked dental pain (222).

Watson (226) recommended guidelines for the use of opioids in postherpetic neuralgia. The use of opioids in PNP should be a last resort. Administration of oxycodone, 5 to 10 mg every 4 hours, is a practical therapeutic approach. Patients with a history of chemical dependency should be excluded and there should be one prescriber and one dispenser. Patients need to be seen regularly to monitor pain and record drug utilization.

The PNP trial literature indicates that tricyclic antidepressants are effective in approximately half of the patients, and these drugs have been recommended as first-line agents for all PNP except trigeminal neuralgia (227,228). Mexiletine can provide analgesia for some PNP patients, especially those with stabbing or burning pain. The capsaicin trials indicated a modest analgesic effect, but the trial data may be biased by inadequate patient blinding. Anticonvulsants may also have analgesic effects in neuropathic pain, but the data are contradictory. The clonidine and nonsteroidal anti-inflammatory trials also had mixed results, and further testing is required to confirm an analgesic role in PNP. Potent opioids can provide effective analgesia for PNP, but because of the inherent risks should be used as a last resort. Propranolol, lorazepam, and intravenous phentolamine have been ineffective as analgesics in various neuropathic PNP states.

Long-term clinical trials are needed to establish whether these agents are effective for chronic treatment of PNP. The two PNP trials that examined analgesic efficacy for 3 months (or longer) demonstrated no relief with phenytoin (203) or capsaicin (208). Side effects limit the clinical utility of the PNP treatments, and none of these treatments are advocated as curative. Anecdotal evidence suggests that analgesics that are effective for neuropathic pain may also help some CRPS patients, but there is almost no overlap in the controlled trial literature between PNP and CRPS treatments. The only therapies used in both conditions were intravenous phentolamine and epidural clonidine. Intravenous phentolamine was found ineffective in PNP (220) and in CRPS (37), while epidural clonidine provided analgesia in PNP (215) and CRPS (168) patients.

Despite the clinical trial data demonstrating successful pain relief with several drug regimens, pharmacotherapy for PNP is frequently ineffective. A survey of 188 specialist physicians experienced in treating neuropathic pain (229) revealed that only a minority would rate their analgesia results as good or excellent with antidepressants (40%), anticonvulsants (35%), opioids (30%), and simple analgesics (18%). This lack of success may reflect an inadequate dosage of medication, the development of drug tolerance, adverse side effects terminating the treatment, or modest analgesic effects that do not relieve a major component of the patient's pain.

CONCLUSIONS

To quote the late Dr. Bonica "notwithstanding the vast amount of neurophysiological and neuropathological evidence acquired since Weir Mitchell and Letievant, we are not much nearer to the understanding of the mechanism of causalgia" (32). Understanding the pathogenesis of CRPS does not appear to be in our grasp, but randomized controlled trials can help lay a foundation for the effective treatment of CRPS.

APPENDIX: IASP DEFINITIONS OF PAIN TERMS (2)

Allodynia: pain due to a stimulus that does not normally provoke pain.

Hyperalgesia: an increased response to a stimulus that is normally painful.

Hyperesthesia: increased sensitivity to stimulation, includes allodynia and hyperalgesia.

Hypoalgesia: diminished pain in response to a normally painful stimulus.

Hypoesthesia: decreased sensitivity to stimulation, excluding the special senses.

Paresthesia: an abnormal sensation, whether spontaneous or evoked.

REFERENCES

1. Evans JA. Sympathectomy for reflex sympathetic dystrophy: report of 29 cases. *JAMA* 1946;132:620–623.
2. Merskey H, Bogduk N. *Classification of chronic pain: descriptions of chronic pain syndromes and definitions of pain terms.* 2nd ed. Seattle: IASP Press, 1994.
3. Gracely RH, Price DD, Roberts WJ, Bennett GJ. Quantitative sensory testing in patients with complex regional pain syndrome (CRPS) I and II. In: Janig W, Stanton-Hicks M, eds. *Reflex sympathetic dystrophy: a reappraisal. Progress in pain research and management.* Vol. 6. Seattle: IASP Press, 1996:151–172.
4. Ochoa JL, Yarnitsky D. Mechanical hyperalgesias in neuropathic pain patients: dynamic and static subtypes. *Ann Neurol* 1993b;33:465–472.
5. Campbell JN, Raja SN, Meyer RA, Mackinnon SE. Myelinated afferents signal the hyperalgesia associated with nerve injury. *Pain* 1998b;32:89–94.
6. Price DD, Long S, Huitt C. Sensory testing of pathophysiological mechanisms of pain in patients with reflex sympathetic dystrophy. *Pain* 1992;49:163–173.
7. Koltzenburg M, Torebjork HE, Wahren LK. Nociceptor modulated central sensitization causes mechanical hyperalgesia in acute

chemogenic and chronic neuropathic pain. *Brain* 1994;117: 579–591.

8. Torebjork HE, Lundberg LER, LaMotte RH. Central changes in processing of mechanoreceptive input in capsaicin-induced secondary hyperalgesia in humans. *J Physiol* 1992;448:765–780.

9. Kilo S, Schmelz M, Koltzenburg M, Handwerker HO. Different patterns of hyperalgesia induced by experimental inflammation in human skin. *Brain* 1994;117: 385–396.

10. Koltzenburg M, Lundberg LER, Torebjork HE. Dynamic and static components of mechanical hyperalgesia in human hairy skin. *Pain* 1992;51:207–219.

11. LaMotte RH, Shain CN, Simone DA, Tsai EP. Neurogenic hyperalgesia: psychophysical studies of underlying mechanisms. *J Neurophysiol* 1991;66:190–211.

12. Gracely RH, Lynch SA, Bennett GJ. Painful neuropathy: altered central processing maintained dynamically by peripheral input. *Pain* 1992;51:175–194.

13. Coderre TJ, Katz J, Vaccarino AL, Melzack R. Contribution of central neuroplasticity to pathological pain: review of clinical and experimental evidence. *Pain* 1993;52:259–285.

14. Casale R, Elam M. Normal sympathetic nerve activity in a reflex sympathetic dystrophy with marked skin vasoconstriction. *J Auton Nerv Syst* 1992;41: 215–219.

15. Wallin G, Torebjork E, Hallin R. Preliminary observations on the pathophysiology of hyperalgesia in the causalgic pain syndrome. In: Zotterman Y, ed. *Sensory functions of the skin in primates with special reference to man.* Oxford: Pergamon, 1976: 489–502.

16. Bej MD, Schwartzman RJ. Abnormalities of cutaneous blood flow regulation in patients with reflex sympathetic dystrophy as measured by laser Doppler fluxmetry. *Arch Neurol* 1991;48:912–915.

17. Rosen L, Ostergren J, Fagrell B. Skin microvascular circulation in the sympathetic dystrophies evaluated by videophotometric capillaroscopy and laser Doppler fluxmetry. *Eur J Clin Invest* 1988;18:305–308.

18. Rosen L, Ostergren J, Roald OK, Fagrell B. Bilateral involvement and the effect of sympathetic blockade on skin microcirculation in the sympathetic dystrophies. *Microvasc Res* 1989;15: 309–318.

19. Christensen K, Henridsen O. The reflex sympathetic dystrophy syndrome. *Scand J Rheumatol* 1983;12:263–267.

20. Drummond PD, Finch PM, Smythe GA. Reflex sympathetic dystrophy: the significance of differing plasma catecholamine concentrations in affected and unaffected limbs. *Brain* 1991;114:2025–2036.

21. Harden RN, Duc TA, Williams TR, et al. Norepinephrine and epinephrine levels in affected versus unaffected limbs in sympathetically maintained pain. *Clin J Pain* 1994;10:324–330.

22. Drummond PD, Finch PM, Edvinsson L, Goadsby PJ. Plasma neuropeptide Y in the symptomatic limb of patients with causalgic pain. *Clin Auton Res* 1994;4:113–116.

23. Arnold JMO, Teasell RW, MacLeod AP, et al. Increased venous alpha-adrenoceptor responsiveness in patients with reflex sympathetic dystrophy. *Ann Intern Med* 1993;118:619–621.

24. Rommel O, Tegenthoff M, Pern U, et al. Sympathetic skin response in patients with reflex sympathetic dystrophy. *Clin Auton Res* 1995;5:205–210.

25. Chelimsky TC, Low PA, Naessens JM, et al. Value of autonomic testing in reflex sympathetic dystrophy. *Mayo Clin Proc* 1995; 70:1029–1040.

26. Janig W. The puzzle of "reflex sympathetic dystrophy": mechanisms, hypotheses, open questions. In: Janig W, Stanton-Hicks M, eds. *Reflex sympathetic dystrophy: a reappraisal. Progress in pain research and management.* Vol. 6. Seattle: IASP Press, 1996:1–24.

27. Glynn CJ, Casale R. Morphine injected around the stellate ganglion does not modulate the sympathetic nervous systems nor does it provide pain relief. *Pain* 1993;53:33–37.

28. Bonelli S, Conoscente F, Movilia PG, et al. Regional intravenous guanethidine vs. stellate ganglion block in reflex sympathetic dystrophies: a randomized trial. *Pain* 1983;16:297–307.

29. Raja AN, Treed RD, Davis KD, Campbell JN. Systemic alpha-adrenergic blockade with phentolamine: a diagnostic test for sympathetically maintained pain. *Anesthesiology* 1991;74: 691–698.

30. Treede RD, Davis KD, Campbell JN, Raja SN. The plasticity of cutaneous hyperalgesia during sympathetic ganglion blockade in patients with neuropathic pain. *Brain* 1992;115:607–621.

31. Dellemijm PLI, Fields HL, Allen RR, et al. The interpretation of pain relief and sensory changes following sympathetic blockade. *Brain* 1994;117: 1475–1487.

32. Bonica JJ. Causalgia and other reflex sympathetic dystrophies. In: Bonica JJ, ed. *Advances in pain research and therapy.* Vol. 3. New York: Raven, 1979: 141–166.

33. Walker AE, Nulsen F. Electrical stimulation of the upper thoracic portion of the sympathetic chain in man. *Arch Neurol Psychiatry* 1948;59:559–560.

34. White JC, Sweet WH. *Pain and the neurosurgeon.* Springfield: Charles C Thomas, 1969.

35. Torebjork E, Wahren LK, Wallin G, et al. Noradrenaline-evoked pain in neuralgia. *Pain* 1995;63:11–20.

36. Davis KD, Treede RD, Raja SN, et al. Topical application of clonidine relieves hyperalgesia in patients with sympathetically

maintained pain. *Pain* 1991;47: 309–317.

37. Verdugo R. Ochoa JL. Sympathetically maintained pain. I. Phentolamine block questions to concept. *Neurology* 1994;44: 1003–1010.

38. Boas RA. Complex regional pain syndromes: symptoms, signs, and differential diagnosis. In: Janig W, Stanton-Hicks M, eds. *Reflex sympathetic dystrophy: a reappraisal. Progress in pain research management.* Vol. 6. Seattle: IASP Press, 1996: 79–92.

39. Jadad AR, Carroll D, Glynn CJ, McQuay HJ. Intravenous regional sympathetic blockade for pain relief in reflex sympathetic dystrophy: a systemic review and a randomized double-blind crossover study. *J Pain Symptom Manage* 1995;10:13–20.

40. Dotson RM. *Causalgia-reflex sympathetic dystrophy-sympathetically maintained pain: myth and reality. AAEM international symposium on neuropathic pain.* Charleston: Johnson Printing Company, 1992:33–38.

41. Schott GD. An unsympathetic view of pain. *Lancet* 1995;345:634–635.

42. Ramamurthy S. Hoffman J, Group GS. Intravenous regional guanethidine in the treatment of reflex sympathetic dystrophy/causalgia: a randomized, double-blind study. *Anesth Analg* 1995; 81:718–723.

43. Braus DF, Krauss JK, Strobel J. The shoulder-hand syndrome after stroke: a prospective clinical trial. *Ann Neurol* 1994; 36:728–733.

44. Christensen K, Jensen EM, Noer I. The reflex sympathetic dystrophy syndrome response to treatment with systemic corticosteroids. *Acta Chir Scand* 1982;148:653–655.

45. Oyen WJG, Arntz IE, Claessens RAMJ, et al. Reflex sympathetic dystrophy of the hand: an excessive inflammatory response? *Pain* 1993;55:151–157.

46. Kozin F. Painful shoulder and the reflex sympathetic dystrophy syndrome. In: McCarty DJ, Koopman WJ, eds. *Arthritis and allied conditions.* Vol. 2. 12th ed. Philadelphia: Lea & Febiger, 1993: 1643–1676.

47. Veldman PHJM, Reynen HM, Arntz IE, Goris RJA. Signs and symptoms of reflex sympathetic dystrophy: prospective study of 829 patients. *Lancet* 1993;342: 1012–1016.

48. Watkins LR, Maier SF, Goelhler LE. Immune activation: the role of pro-inflammatory cytokines in inflammation, illness responses and pathological pain states. *Pain* 1995;63: 289–302.

49. Levine JD, Fields HL, Basbaum AI. Peptides and the primary afferent nociceptor. *J Neurosci* 1993;13:2273–2286.

50. Lankford LL. Reflex sympathetic dystrophy. In: Flynn JE, ed. *Hand surgery.* 3rd ed. Baltimore: Williams & Wilkins, 1982: 656–670.

51. Ochoa JL. Guest editorial: essence, investigation, and management of "neuropathic" pains: hopes from acknowledgment of chaos. *Muscle Nerve* 1993; 16:997–1008.

52. Szeinberg-Arazi D, Heim M, Nadvorna H, et al. A functional and psychosocial assessment of patients with post-Sudeck atrophy amputation. *Arch Phys Med Rehabil* 1993;74: 416–419.

53. Van Houdenhove B, Vasquez G, Onghena P, et al. Etiopathogenesis of reflex sympathetic dystrophy: a review and biopsychosocial hypothesis. *Clin J Pain* 1992;8:300–306.

54. Lynch ME. Psychological aspects of reflex sympathetic dystrophy: a review of the adult and paediatric literature. *Pain* 1992;49: 337–347.

55. Bruehl S, Carlson CR. Predisposing psychological factors in the development of reflex sympathetic dystrophy. *Clin J Pain* 1992;8:287–299.

56. Covington EC. Psychological issues in reflex sympathetic dystrophy. In: Janig W, Stanton-Hicks M, eds. *Reflex sympathetic dystrophy: a reappraisal. Progress in pain research and management.* Vol. 6. Seattle: IASP Press, 1996:191–215.

57. Blumberg H, Janig W. Clinical manifestations of reflex sympathetic dystrophy and sympathetically maintained pain. In: Wall PD, Melzack R, eds. *Textbook of pain.* 3rd ed. Edinburgh: Churchill Livingstone, 1994:685–697.

58. Bickerstaff DR, Kanis JA. Algodystrophy: an under-recognized complication of minor trauma. *Br J Rheumatol* 1994; 33:240–248.

59. Atkins RM, Duckworth T, Kanis JA. Features of algodystrophy after Colles' fracture. *J Bone Joint Surg [Br]* 1990;72: 105–110.

60. Veldman PHJM, Goris JA. Shoulder complaints in patients with reflex sympathetic dystrophy of the upper extremity. *Arch Phys Med Rehabil* 1995;76: 239–242.

61. Wilder RT. Reflex sympathetic dystrophy in children and adolescents: differences from adults. In: Janig W, Stanton-Hicks M, eds. *Reflex sympathetic dystrophy: a reappraisal. Progress in pain research and management.* Vol. 6. Seattle: IASP Press, 1996:67–77.

62. Stanton RP. Malcom JR, Wesdock KA, Singsen BH. Reflex sympathetic dystrophy in children: an orthopedic perspective. *Orthopedics* 1993;16:773–779.

63. Echlin F, Owens RM, Wells WL. Observations on major and minor causalgia. *Arch Neurol Psychiatry* 1948;62:183–203.

64. Sunderland S. *Nerves and nerve injuries.* 2nd ed. Edinburgh: Churchill Livingstone, 1978.

65. Johnson AC. Disabling changes in the hands resembling sclerodactylia following myocardial infarction. *Ann Intern Med* 1943;19:321–331.

66. Russek HI. Shoulder-hand syndrome following myocardial infarction. *Med Clin North Am* 1958;42:1555–1566.

67. Ouwenaller CV, Laplace PM, Chantraine A. Painful shoulder in hemiplegia. *Arch Phys Med Rehabil* 1986;67:23–26.

68. Sarangi PP, Ward AJ, Staddon GE, Atkins RM. Algodystrophy and osteoporosis after tibial fractures. *J Bone Joint Surg [Br]* 1993;75:450–452.

69. Steinbrocker O, Argyros TG. The shoulder-hand syndrome: present status as a diagnostic and therapeutic entity. *Med Clin North Am* 1958;42:1533–1553.

70. Miller DS, deTakats G. Post-traumatic dystrophy of the extremities. *Surg Gynecol Obstet* 1941;125:558–582.

71. Kurvers HAJM, Jacobs MJHM, Beuk RJ, et al. The influence of local skin heating and reactive hyperaemia on skin blood flow abnormalities in patient with reflex sympathetic dystrophy (RSD). *Eur J Clin Invest* 1995;25:346–352.

72. Sunderland S, Kelly M. The painful sequelae of injuries to peripheral nerves. *Aust N Z J Surg* 1948;18:75–118.

73. Griepp ME. Thomas AF. New thoughts on reflex sympathetic dystrophy syndrome. *J Neurosci Nurs* 1990;22:313–316.

74. Veldman PHJM, Goris RJA. Multiple reflex sympathetic dystrophy. Which patients are at risk for developing a recurrence of reflex sympathetic dystrophy in the same or another limb. *Pain* 1996;64:463–466.

75. Kozin F, Ryan LM, Carerra GF, Soin JS. The reflex sympathetic dystrophy syndrome (RSDS). III. Scintigraphic studies, further evidence for the therapeutic efficacy of systemic corticosteroids, and proposed diagnostic criteria. *Am J Med* 1981;70:23–30.

76. Baron R, Blumberg H, Janig W. Clinical characteristics of patients with complex regional pain syndrome in Germany with special emphasis on vasomotor function. In: Janig W, Stanton-Hicks M, eds. *Reflex sympathetic dystrophy: a reappraisal. Progress in pain research and management.* Vol. 6. Seattle: IASP Press, 1996:25–48.

77. Deuschl G, Blumberg H, Lucking CH. Tremor in reflex sympathetic dystrophy. *Arch Neurol* 1991;48:1247–1252.

78. Bhatia KP, Bhatt MH, Marsden CD. The causalgia-dystonia syndrome. *Brain* 1993;116: 843–851.

79. Monsivais JJ, Baker J, Monsivais D. The association of peripheral nerve compression and reflex sympathetic dystrophy. *J Hand Surg [Br]* 1991;16:337–338.

80. Verdugo R, Ochoa JL. Use and misuse of conventional electrodiagnosis, quantitative sensory testing, thermography, and nerve blocks in the evaluation of painful neuropathic syndromes. *Muscle Nerve* 1993;16: 1056–1062.

81. Wilson PR, Low PA, Bedder MD, et al. Diagnostic algorithm for complex regional pain syndromes. In: Janig W, Stanton-Hicks M, eds. *Reflex sympathetic dystrophy: a reappraisal. Progress in pain research and management.* Vol. 6. Seattle: IASP Press, 1996:93–106.

82. Mevorach DL. Measurement and differential diagnosis of sympathetic pain syndromes. In: Tollison CD, Satterthwaite JR, eds. *Sympathetic pain syndromes: reflex sympathetic dystrophy and causalgia. Physical medicine and rehabilitation: state of the art reviews.* Vol. 10. Philadelphia: Hanley & Belfus, 1996:229–235.

83. Davidoff G, Morey K, Amann M, Stamps J. Pain measurement in reflex sympathetic dystrophy syndrome. *Pain* 1988; 32:27–34.

84. Field J, Protheroe DL, Atkins RM. Algodystrophy after Colles fractures is associated with secondary tightness of casts. *J Bone Joint Surg [Br]* 1994;76:901–905.

85. Sarangi PP, Ward AJ, Smith EJ, Atkins RM. The use of dolorimetry in the assessment of post-traumatic algodystrophy of the foot. *Foot* 1991;1:157–163.

86. Atkins RM, Kanis JA. The use of dolorimetry in the assessment of post-traumatic algodystrophy of the hand. *Br J Rheumatol* 1989;28:404–409.

87. Bryan AS, Klenerman L, Bowsher D. The diagnosis of reflex sympathetic dystrophy using an algometer. *J Bone Joint Surg [Br]* 1991;73:644–646.

88. Field J, Atkins RM. Effect of guanethidine on the natural history of post-traumatic algodystrophy. *Ann Rheum Dis* 1993;52:467–469.

89. Bickerstaff DR, Kanis JA. The use of nasal calcitonin in the treatment of post-traumatic algodystrophy. *Br J Rheumatol* 1991;30:291–294.

90. Stanton-Hicks M, Raj PP, Racz GB. Use of regional anesthetics for diagnosis of reflex sympathetic dystrophy and sympathetically maintained pain: a critical evaluation. In: Janig W, Stanton-Hicks M, eds. *Reflex sympathetic dystrophy: a reappraisal. Progress in pain research and management.* Vol. 6. Seattle: IASP Press, 1996:217–237.

91. Hannington-Kiff JG. Relief of Sudeck's atrophy by regional intravenous guanethidine. *Lancet* 1977;1:1132–1133.

92. Sherman RA, Karstetter KW, Damiano M, Evans CB. Stability of temperature asymmetries in reflex sympathetic dystrophy over time and changes in pain. *Clin J Pain* 1994;10:71–77.

93. Herrick A, El-Hadidy K, Marsh D, Jayson M. Abnormal thermoregulatory responses in patients with reflex sympathetic dystrophy syndrome. *J Rheumatol* 1994; 21:1319–1324.

94. Cooke ED, Glick EN, Bowcock SA, et al. Reflex sympathetic dystrophy (algoneurodystrophy): temperature studies in the upper limb. *Br J Rheumatol* 1989;28:399–403.

95. Low PA, Wilson PR, Sandroni P, et al. Clinical characteristics of patients with reflex sympathetic dystrophy (sympathetically maintained pain) in the USA. In: Janig W, Stanton-Hicks M, eds. *Reflex sympathetic dystrophy: a reappraisal. Progress in pain research and management.* Vol. 6. Seattle: IASP Press, 1996:49–66.

96. Lee GW, Weeks PM. The role of bone scintigraphy in diagnosing reflex sympathetic dystrophy. *J Hand Surg [Am]* 1995;20:458–463.

97. O'Donoghue JP, Powe JE, Mattar AG, et al. Three-phase bone scintigraphy asymmetric patterns in the upper extremities of asymptomatic normals and reflex sympathetic dystrophy patients. *Clin Nucl Med* 1993;18:829–836.

98. Mailis A, Meindok H, Papagapiou M, Pham D. Alterations of the three-phase bone scan after sympathectomy. *Clin J Pain* 1994;10:146–155.

99. Heck LL. Recognition of atypical reflex sympathetic dystrophy. *Clin Nucl Med* 1987;12:925–928.

100. Intenzo C, Sung K, Millin J, Park C. Scintigraphic patterns of the reflex sympathetic dystrophy syndrome of the lower extremities. *Clin Nucl Med* 1989;14:657–661.

101. Bickerstaff DR, Charlesworth D, Kanis JA. Changes in cortical and trabecular bone in algodystrophy. *Br J Rheumatol* 1993;32:46–51.

102. Schweitzer ME, Mandel S, Schwartzman RJ, et al. Reflex sympathetic dystrophy revisited: MR imaging findings before and after infusion of contrast material. *Radiology* 1995;195: 211–214.

103. Koch E, Hofer HO, Sialer G, et al. Failure of MR imaging to detect reflex sympathetic dystrophy of the extremities. *AJR* 1991;156:113–115.

104. Schutzer SF, Gossling HR. The treatment of reflex sympathetic dystrophy syndrome. *J Bone Joint Surg [Am]* 1984;66:625–629.

105. Rosen PS, Graham W. The shoulder-hand syndrome: historical review with observations on seventy-three patients. *Can Med Assoc J* 1957;77:86–91.

106. Poplawski ZJ, Wiley AM, Murray JF. Post-traumatic dystrophy of the extremities. *J Bone Joint Surg [Am]* 1983;65:642–655.

107. Gobelet C, Waldburger M, Meir JL. The effect of adding calcitonin to physical treatment on reflex sympathetic dystrophy. *Pain* 1992;48:171–175.

108. Moberg E. The shoulder-hand-finger syndrome as a whole. *Acta Chir Scand* 1955;109:284–292.

109. Johnson EW, Pannozzo AN. Management of shoulder-hand syndrome. *JAMA* 1966;195:152–154.

110. Steinbrocker O. The shoulder-hand syndrome: present perspective. *Arch Phys Med Rehabil* 1968;49:388–395.

111. Watson HK, Carlson L. Treatment of reflex sympathetic dystrophy of the hand with an active "stress loading" program. *J Hand Surg [Am]* 1987;12:779–785.

112. Plewes LW. Sudek's atrophy in the hand. *J Bone Joint Surg [Br]* 1956;38:195–203.

113. Duncan KH, Lewis RC, Racz G, Nordyke MD. Treatment of upper extremity reflex sympathetic dystrophy with joint stiffness using sympatholytic Bier blocks and manipulation. *Orthopedics* 1988;11:883–886.

114. Rizk TE, Gavant ML, Pinnals RS. Treatment of adhesive capsulitis (frozen shoulder) with arthrographic capsular distension and rupture. *Arch Phys Med Rehabil* 1994;75:803–807.

115. Subbarao JV, Blair SJ. Reflex sympathetic dystrophy syndrome. In: Mehta AJ, ed. *Rehabilitation of fractures. Physical medicine and rehabilitation: state of the art reviews.* Vol. 9. Philadelphia: Hanley & Belfus, 1995: 31–50.

116. Priebe MM, Holmes SA. Reflex sympathetic dystrophy syndrome: physical medicine strategies. In: Tollison CD, Satterthwaite JR, eds. *Sympathetic pain syndromes: reflex sympathetic dystrophy and causalgia. Physical medicine and rehabilitation: state of the art reviews.* Vol. 10. Philadelphia: Hanley & Belfus 1996:289–296.

117. Frazer FW. Persistent post-sympathetic pain treated by connective tissue massage. *Physiotherapy* 1978;6:211–212.

118. Kesler RW, Saulsbury FT, Miller LT, Rowlingson JC. Reflex sympathetic dystrophy in children: treatment with transcutaneous electric nerve stimulation. *Pediatrics* 1988;82:728–732.

119. Meyer GA, Fields HL. Causalgia treated by selective large fibre stimulation of peripheral nerve. *Brain* 1972;95:163–168.

120. Richlin DM, Carron H, Rowlingson JC, et al. Reflex sympathetic dystrophy: successful treatment by transcutaneous nerve stimulation. *J Pediatrics* 1978;93: 84–86.

121. Robaina F, Rodriguez JL, Vera JA, Martin MA. Transcutaneous electrical nerve stimulation and spinal cord stimulation for pain relief in reflex sympathetic dystrophy. *Stereotact Funct Neurosurg* 1989;52:53–62.

122. Goodman CR. Treatment of shoulder-hand syndrome. *N Y State J Med* 1971;71:559–562.

123. Portwood MM, Liebermann JS, Taylor RG. Ultrasound treatment of reflex sympathetic dystrophy. *Arch Phys Med Rehabil* 1987; 68:116–118.

124. Anderson TP, Wakim KG, Herrick JF, et al. Experimental study of effects of ultrasonic energy on lower part of spinal cord and peripheral nerves. *Arch Phys Med* 1951;32:71–83.

125. Lota MJ. Electronic plethysmographic and tissue temperature studies of effect of ultrasound on blood flow. *Arch Phys Med Rehabil* 1965;46:315–322.

126. Schroeder KP. Effect of ultrasound on the lumbar sympathetic

nerves. *Arch Phys Med Rehabil* 1962;43:182–185.

127. Rizk TE, Christopher RP, Pinals RS, et al. Adhesive capsulitis (frozen shoulder): a new approach to its management. *Arch Phys Med Rehabil* 1983;65:29–33.

128. Wang JK, Johnson KA, Iistrup DM. Sympathetic blocks for reflex sympathetic dystrophy. *Pain* 1985;23:13–17.

129. Betcher AM, Bean G, Casten DF. Continuous procaine block of paravertebral sympathetic ganglions. *JAMA* 1953;151:288–292.

130. Linson MA, Leffert R, Todd DP. The treatment of upper extremity reflex sympathetic dystrophy with prolonged continuous stellate ganglion blockade. *J Hand Surg [Am]* 1983;8:153–159.

131. Haynsworth RF, Noe CE. Percutaneous lumbar sympathectomy: a comparison of radiofrequency denervation versus phenol neurolysis. *Anesthesiology* 1991; 74:459–463.

132. Rocco AG, Kaul AF, Reisman RM, et al. A comparison of regional intravenous guanethidine and reserpine in reflex sympathetic dystrophy: a controlled, randomized, double-blind crossover study. *Clin J Pain* 1989; 5:205–209.

133. Vanos DN, Ramamurthy S, Hoffman J. Intravenous regional block using ketorolac: preliminary results in the treatment of reflex sympathetic dystrophy. *Anesth Analg* 1992;74:139–141.

134. Hord AH, Rooks MD, Stephens BO, et al. Intravenous regional bretylium and lidocaine for treatment of reflex sympathetic dystrophy; a randomized double-blind study. *Anesth Analg* 1992;74:818–821.

135. Hanna MH, Peat SJ. Ketanserin in reflex sympathetic dystrophy. A double-blind placebo controlled cross-over trial. *Pain* 1989;38: 145–150.

136. Glynn CJ, Stannard C, Collins PA, Casale R. The role of peripheral sudomotor blockade in the treatment of patients with sympathetically maintained pain. *Pain* 1993;53:39–42.

137. Kettler RE, Abram SE. Intravenous regional droperidol in the management of reflex sympathetic dystrophy: a double-blind, placebo-controlled, crossover study. *Anesthesiology* 1988;69: 933–936.

138. Arner S, Lindblom U, Meyerson BA, Molander C. Prolonged relief of neuralgia after regional anesthetic blocks. A call for further experimental and systematic clinical studies. *Pain* 1990;43: 287–297.

139. Wassef MR. Suprascapular nerve block. *Anaesthesia* 1992;47:120–124.

140. Cooper DE, DeLee JC. Reflex sympathetic dystrophy of the knee. *J Am Acad Orthop Surg* 1994;2:79–86.

141. Spurling RG. Causalgia of the upper extremity: treatment by dorsal sympathetic ganglionectomy. *Arch Neurol Psychiatry* 1930;23:784–788.

142. AbuRahma AF, Robinson PA, Powell M, et al. Sympathectomy for reflex sympathetic dystrophy: factors affecting outcome. *Ann Vasc Surg* 1994;8: 372–379.

143. Herz DA, Looman JE, Ford RD, et al. Second thoracic sympathetic ganglionectomy in sympathetically maintained pain. *J Pain Symptom Manage* 1993;8: 483–491.

144. Olcott C, Eltherington LG, Wilcosky BR, et al. Reflex sympathetic dystrophy—the surgeon's role in management. *J Vasc Surg* 1991;14:488–495.

145. Rocco AG. Radiofrequency lumbar sympatholysis. *Reg Anesth* 1995;20:3–12.

146. Ahn SS, Machleder HI, Concepcion B, Moore WS. Thoracoscopic cervicodorsal sympathectomy: preliminary results. *J Vasc Surg* 1994;20:511–517.

147. Mockus MB, Rutherford RB, Rosales C, Pearce WH. Sympathectomy for causalgia. *Arch Surg* 1987;122:668–672.

148. Munn JS, Baker WH. Recurrent sympathetic dystrophy: successful treatment by contralateral sympathectomy. *Surgery* 1987;102:102–105.

149. Allen G, Samson B. Contralateral Horner's syndrome following stellate ganglion block. *Can Anesth Soc J* 1986;33:112–113.

150. Dielissen PW, Classen ATPM, Veldman PHJM, Goris RJA. Amputation for reflex sympathetic dystrophy. *J Bone Joint Surg [Br]* 1995;77:270–273.

151. Grundberg AB, Reagan DS. Compression syndrome in reflex sympathetic dystrophy. *J Hand Surg [Am]* 1991;16:731–736.

152. Braune S, Schady W. Changes in sensation after nerve injury or amputation: the role of central factors. *J Neurol Neurosurg Psychiatry* 1993;56:393–399.

153. Bruxelle J, Travers V, Thiebaut JB. Occurrence and treatment of pain after brachial plexus injury. *Clin Orthor* 1988;237:87–95.

154. Campbell JN, Raja SN, Meyer RA. Painful sequelae of nerve injury. In: Dubner R, Gebhart GF, Bonds MR, eds. *Proceedings of the 5th World Congress on Pain.* Amsterdam: Elsevier, 1988: 135–143.

155. Ochs G, Schenk M, Stuppler A. Painful dysesthesias following peripheral nerve injury: a clinical and electrophysiological study. *Brain Res* 1989;496:228–240.

156. Noordenbos W, Wall PD. Implications of the failure of nerve resection and graft to cure chronic pain produced by nerve lesions. *J Neurol Neurosurg Psychiatry* 1981;44:1068–1073.

157. Wynn-Parry CB, Withrington R. The management of painful peripheral nerve disorders. In: Wall PD, Melzack R, eds. *Textbook of pain.* 1st ed. New York: Churchill Livingstone, 1984;395–401.

158. Burchiel KJ, Taha JM. Surgical intervention for reflex sympa-

thetic dystrophy and causalgia. In: Tollison CD, Satterthwaite JR, eds. *Sympathetic pain syndromes: reflex sympathetic dystrophy and causalgia. Physical medicine and rehabilitation: state of the art reviews.* Vol. 10. Philadelphia: Hanley & Belfus, 1996:311–326.

159. Nashold BS, Goldner JL, Mullen JB, Bright DS. Long-term pain control by direct peripheral-nerve stimulation. *J Bone Joint Surg [Am]* 1982;64:1–10.

160. Barolat G, Schwartzman RJ, Woo R. Epidural spinal cord stimulation in the management of reflex sympathetic dystrophy. *Stereotact Funct Neurosurg* 1989;53: 29–39.

161. Robaina RJ, Dominguez M, Diaz M, et al. Spinal cord stimulation for relief of chronic pain in vasospastic disorders of the upper limbs. *Neurosurgery* 1989;24:63–67.

162. Marchand S, Bushnell MC, Molina-Negro P, et al. The effects of dorsal column stimulation on measures of clinical and experimental pain in man. *Pain* 1991;45:249–257.

163. Blanchard J, Ramamurthy S, Walsh N, et al. Intravenous regional sympatholysis: a double-blind comparison of guanethidine, reserpine and normal saline. *J Pain Symptom Manage* 1990;5:357–361.

164. McGlone F, Dean J, Dhar S. *A sympathetic response to sympathetic block in RSD. Proceeding of 7th World Congress on Pain.* Seattle: IASP Press, 1993:350.

165. Glynn CJ, Basedow RW, Walsh JA. Pain relief following post-ganglionic sympathetic blockade with iv guanethidine. *Br J Anaesth* 1981;53:1297–1301.

166. Geertzen JHB, deBruijn H, deBruijn-Kofman AT, Arendzen JH. Reflex sympathetic dystrophy: early treatment and psychological aspects. *Arch Phys Med Rehabil* 1994;75:442–446.

167. Gobelet C, Meier JL, Schaffner W, et al. Calcitonin and reflex sympathetic dystrophy syndrome. *Clin Rheumatol* 1986;5: 382–388.

168. Rauck RL, Eisenach JC, Jackson K, et al. Epidural clonidine treatment for refractory reflex sympathetic dystrophy. *Anesthesiology* 1993;81:1163–1169.

169. Bounameaux HM, Hellemans H, Verhaeghe R. Ketanserin in chronic sympathetic dystrophy. An acute controlled trial. *Clin Rheumatol* 1984;3:556–557.

170. Campbell JN, Raja SN. Reflex sympathetic dystrophy. *Neurology* 1995;45:1235–1236.

171. Poulsen L, Arendt-Nielsen L, Brosen K, et al. The hypoalgesic effect of imipramine in different human experimental pain models. *Pain* 1995;60:287–293.

172. Coquoz D, Porchet HC, Dayer P. Central analgesic effects of antidepressant drugs with various mechanisms of action: desipramine, fluvoxamine and moclobemide. *Schweiz Med Wochenschr* 1991;121: 1843–1845.

173. Bromm B, Meier W, Scharein E. Imipramine reduces experimental pain. *Pain* 1986;25:245–257.

174. Max MB, Culnane M, Schafer SC, et al. Amitriptyline relieves diabetic neuropathy pain in patients with normal or depressed mood. *Neurology* 1987;37:589–596.

175. Max MB, Kishore-Kumar R, Schafer SC, et al. Efficacy of desipramine in painful diabetic neuropathy: a placebo-controlled trial. *Pain* 1991;45:3–9.

176. Max MB, Lynch SA, Muir J, et al. Effects of desipramine, amitriptyline, and fluoxetine on pain in diabetic neuropathy. *N Engl J Med* 1992;326:1250–1256.

177. Kvinesdal B, Molin J, Froland A, Gram LF. Imipramine treatment of painful diabetic neuropathy. A double-blind crossover study. *JAMA* 1984;25:1727–1730.

178. Sindrup SH, Ejlertsen B, Froland A, et al. Imipramine treatment in diabetic neuropathy: relief of subjective symptoms without changes in peripheral and autonomic nerve function. *Eur J Clin Pharmacol* 1989;37:151–153.

179. Sindrup SH, Gram LF, Skjold T, et al. Clomipramine vs desipramine vs placebo in the treatment of diabetic neuropathy symptoms. A double-blind cross-over study. *Br J Clin Pharmacol* 1990;30:683–691.

180. Sindrup SH, Gram LF, Brosen K, et al. The selective serotonin reuptake inhibitor paroxetine is effective in the treatment of diabetic neuropathy symptoms. *Pain* 1990;42:135–144.

181. Sindrup SH, Bjerre U, Dejgaarde A, et al. The selective serotonin reuptake inhibitor citalopram relieves the symptoms of diabetic neuropathy. *Clin Pharmacol Ther* 1992;52:547–552.

182. Sindrup SH, Tuxen C, Gram LF, et al. The effect of mainserin on the symptoms of diabetic neuropathy. *Eur J Clin Pharmacol* 1992;43:251–255.

183. Kishore-Kumar R, Max MB, Schafer SC, et al. Desipramine relieves postherpetic neuralgia. *Clin Pharmacol Ther* 1990;47: 305–312.

184. Max MB, Schafer SC, Culnane M, et al. Association of pain relief with drug side effects in postherpetic neuralgia: a single-dose study of clonidine, codeine, ibuprofen, and placebo. *Clin Pharmacol Ther* 1988;43: 363–371.

185. Watson CPN, Evans RJ, Reed K, et al. Amitriptyline versus placebo in postherpetic neuralgia. *Neurology* 1982;32: 671–673.

186. Watson CPN, Evans RJ. A comparative trial of amitriptyline and zimelidine in postherpetic neuralgia. *Pain* 1985;23:387–394.

187. Watson CPN, Chipman M, Reed K, et al. Amitriptyline versus maprotiline in postherpetic neuralgia: a randomized, double-blind, cross over trial. *Pain* 1992;48:29–36.

188. Langhor HD, Stohr M, Petruch F. An open and double-blind cross-over study on the efficacy of

clomipramine (Anafranil) in patients with painful mono- and polyneuropathies. *Eur Neurol* 1982;21:309–317.

189. Sindrup SH, Gram LF, Skjold T, et al. Concentration-response relationship in imipramine treatment of diabetic neuropathy symptoms. *Clin Pharmacol Ther* 1990;47:509–515.

190. Max MB. Antidepressants as analgesics. In: Fields HL, Liebeskind JC, eds. *Progress in pain research and management.* Vol. 1. Seattle: IASP Press, 1994:229–246.

191. Eisenach JC, Gebhart GF. Intrathecal amitriptyline acts as an *N*-methyl-D-aspartate receptor antagonist in the presence of inflammatory hyperalgesia in rats. *Anesthesiology* 1995;83: 1046–1054.

192. Boas RA, Covino BG, Shahnarian A. Analgesic responses to i.v. lignocaine. *Br J Anaesth* 1982;54: 501–505.

193. Nielsen JC, Arendt-Nielsen L, Bjerring P, Carlsson P. Analgesic efficacy of low doses of intravenously administered lidocaine on experimental laser-induced pain: a placebo controlled study. *Reg Anesth* 1991;16:28–33.

194. Rowlingson JC, DiFazio CA, Foster J, Carron H. Lidocaine as an analgesic for experimental pain. *Anesthesiology* 1980;52:20–22.

195. Kastrup J, Petersen P, Dejgard A, et al. Intravenous lidocaine infusion—a new treatment of chronic painful diabetic neuropathy. *Pain* 1987;28:69–75.

196. Rowbotham MC, Reisner-Keller LA, Fields HL. Both intravenous lidocaine and morphine reduce the pain of postherpetic neuralgia. *Neurology* 1991;41: 1024–1028.

197. Marchettini P, Lacerenza M, Marangoni C, et al. Lidocaine test in neuralgia. *Pain* 1992;48:377–382.

198. Rowbotham MC, Davies PS, Fields HL. Topical lidocaine gel relieves postherpetic neuralgia. *Ann Neurol* 1995;37:246–253.

199. Dejgard A, Petersen P, Kastrup J. Mexiletine for treatment of chronic painful diabetic neuropathy. *Lancet* 1988;2:9–11.

200. Chabal C, Jacobson L, Mariano A, et al. The use of oral mexiletine for the treatment of pain after peripheral nerve injury. *Anesthesiology* 1992;76: 513–517.

201. Stracke H, Meyer U, Schumacher HE, Federlin K. Mexiletine in the treatment of diabetic neuropathy. *Diabetes Care* 1992;15: 1550–1555.

202. Chadda VS, Mathur MS. Double blind study of the effects of diphenylhydantoin sodium on diabetic neuropathy. *J Assoc Physicians India* 1978;26: 403–406.

203. Saudek CD, Werns S, Reidenberg MM. Phenytoin in the treatment of diabetic symmetrical polyneuropathy. *Clin Pharmacol Ther* 1977;22:196–199.

204. Wilton TD. Tegretol in the treatment of diabetic neuropathy. *S Afr Med J* 1974;48:869–872.

205. Rull JA, Quibrera R, Gonzalez-Millan M, Castaneda OL. Symptomatic treatment of peripheral diabetic neuropathy with carbamazepine (Tegretol): double blind crossover trial. *Diabetologia* 1969;5:215–218.

206. Capsaicin Study Group. Treatment of painful diabetic neuropathy with topical capsaicin, a multicenter, double-blind, vehicle-controlled study. *Arch Intern Med* 1991;151: 2225–2229.

207. Chad DA, Aronin N, Lundstrom R, et al. Does capsaicin relieve the pain of diabetic neuropathy? *Pain* 1990;42:387–388.

208. Low PA, Opfer-Gehrking TL, Dyck PJ, et al. Double-blind, placebo-controlled study of the application of capsaicin cream in chronic distal painful polyneuropathy. *Pain* 1995;62:163–168.

209. Scheffler NM, Sheitel PL, Lipton MN. Treatment of painful diabetic neuropathy with capsaicin 0.075%. *J Am Podiatr Med Assoc* 1991;14:288–293.

210. Watson CPN, Tyler KL, Bickers DR, et al. A randomized vehicle-controlled trial of topical capsaicin in the treatment of postherpetic neuralgia. *Clin Ther* 1993;15:510–526.

211. Bernstein JE, Korman NE, Bicker DR, et al. Topical capsaicin treatment of chronic postherpetic neuralgia. *J Am Acad Dermatol* 1989;21:265–270.

212. Zeigler D, Lynch SA, Muir J, et al. Transdermal clonidine versus placebo in painful diabetic neuropathy. *Pain* 1992;48:403–408.

213. Byas-Smith MG, Max MB, Muir J, Kingman A. Transdermal clonidine compared to placebo in painful diabetic neuropathy using a two-stage "enriched enrollment" design. *Pain* 1995; 60:267–274.

214. Max MB, Schafer SC, Culnane M, et al. Amitriptyline, but not lorazepam, relieves postherpetic neuralgia. *Neurology* 1988;38: 1427–1432.

215. Eisenach JC, Dupen S, Dubois M, et al. Epidural clonidine analgesia for intractable cancer pain. *Pain* 1995;61:391–399.

216. Cohen KL, Harris S. Efficacy and safety of nonsteroidal anti-inflammatory drugs in the therapy of diabetic neuropathy. *Arch Intern Med* 1987;147: 1442–1444.

217. Weber H, Holme I, Amlie E. The natural course of acute sciatica with nerve root symptoms in a double-blind placebo-controlled trial evaluating the effect of piroxicam. *Spine* 1993;11: 1433–1438.

218. Benedittis GD, Besana F, Lorenzetti A. A new topical treatment for acute herpetic neuralgia and post-herpetic neuralgia: the aspirin/diethyl ether mixture. An open-label study plus a double-blind controlled clinical trial. *Pain* 1992;48:383–390.

219. Scadding JW, Wall PD, Parry W, Brooks DM. Clinical trial of pro-

pranolol in post-traumatic neuralgia. *Pain* 1982;14:283–292.

220. Verdugo R, Campero M, Ochoa JL. Phentolamine sympathetic block in painful polyneuropathies. II. Further questioning of the concept of "sympathetically maintained pain." *Neurology* 1994;44:1010–1014.

221. Price DD, Von der Gruen A, Miller J, et al. A psychophysical analysis of morphine analgesia. *Pain* 1985;22:261–269.

222. Hill HF, Chapman CR, Saeger LS, et al. Steady-state infusions of opioids in human. II. Concentration-effect relationships and therapeutic margins. *Pain* 1990; 43:69–79.

223. Arner S, Meyerson BA. Lack of analgesic effect of opioids on neuropathic and idiopathic forms of pain. *Pain* 1988;33: 11–23.

224. Kupers RC, Konings H, Adriaensen H, Gybels JM. Morphine differentially affects the sensory and affective pain ratings in neurogenic and idiopathic forms of pain. *Pain* 1991;47:5–12.

225. Cherny NI, Thaler HT, Friedlander-Klar H, et al. Opioid responsiveness of cancer pain syndromes caused by neuropathic or nociceptive mechanisms: a combined analysis of controlled, single-dose studies. *Neurology* 1994;44:857–861.

226. Watson CPN. The treatment of postherpetic neuralgia. *Neurology* 1995;45(suppl 8):S58–S60.

227. Galer BS. Neuropathic pain of peripheral origin: advances in pharmacologic treatment. *Neurology* 1995;45(suppl 9): S17–S25.

228. Fields HL. Peripheral neuropathic pain: an approach to management. In: Wall PD. Melzack R, eds. *Textbook of pain.* 3rd ed. Edinburgh: Churchill Livingstone, 1994:919–995.

229. Davies HTO, Crombie IK, Lonsdale M, Macrae WA. Consensus and contention in the treatment of chronic nerve-damage pain. *Pain* 1991;47:191–196.

Sports and Performing Arts Medicine

Chapter 64

Head and Neck Injuries

Lori B. Wasserburger
Robert E. Windsor
Andrew J. Cole
Krystal Chambers

The most common sports injuries are due to overuse. Traumatic sprains and strains are the second most common sports injuries. Injuries to the cervical region of the spine are no exception, as the majority are a result of soft-tissue and mechanical dysfunction of the spine and its supporting structures (1). While these types of injuries may have long-term consequences, catastrophic injuries to the head and neck have the potential for significant morbidity and mortality. Fortunately, catastrophic injuries are rare. The risk of a catastrophic injury is more common in collision or contact sports and certain noncontact sports. Athletes who return to play too soon may suffer a new injury whose effects may be cumulative. Unlike musculoskeletal structures, which can regenerate, injured cell bodies of the brain or spinal cord may not completely regenerate. Therefore, brain injuries can result in long-term cognitive dysfunction and brain and spinal cord injury can cause sensory, motor, bowel, and bladder dysfunction.

EPIDEMIOLOGY

Injuries to the head and cervical region of the spine in athletes are not common (2), although they are the most frequent catastrophic injuries (3). The biomechanics of certain sports may predispose athletes to head and cervical spinal injuries. Such injuries are common in boxing, football, hockey, rugby, and other contact sports. Head injuries in boxing are caused by direct blows, resulting in rotational acceleration of the brain. The most common mechanism of cervical injury in both football and hockey is a blow to the top of the head with the neck slightly flexed and deceleration injuries due to a tackle, check into the boards, or throw to the mat (3–10).

A variety of different injury patterns occur in recreational athletes. As a whole, catastrophic neck injuries have a prevalence of 2 per 100,000 neck injuries (11). The majority of cervical spinal injuries occur during unsupervised recreational sports, such as diving, skiing, surfing, and trampolining. Diving injuries are the primary cause of cervical spinal injury in this group, accounting for 10% of all spinal injuries, with most resulting in neurologic injury (12). They are typically caused by an axial loading mechanism with hyperflexion.

Of the supervised sports, the majority of cervical injuries occur during collision or contact sports including football, rugby, wrestling, and hockey and noncontact sports such as gymnastics. Football and hockey neck injuries are typically produced by axial loading and hyperflexion or hyperextension forces. The incidence of nonfatal cervical spinal injuries in football players is high (13). In a series of adolescent athletes with cervical and brain trauma, 66% of the injuries were related to football (11). The incidence of fatal cervical spinal injuries in football remains low (13). However, 75% to 90% of fatalities in football are related to head and neck injuries (6,7,11,14).

The majority of cervical spinal injuries in athletics result in soft-tissue and mechanical dysfunction of the

Research, epidemiologic studies, and applied medicine have led to a reduction in the number and erity of sports-related injuries (10). A great number of head and neck injuries were noted in the 1950s and 1960s after introduction of the original models of the football helmet with a face mask. In the late 1970s the helmets were improved, resulting in a decline in the number of head injuries. There was, however, a concurrent increase in cervical spinal injuries and permanent quadriplegia. Similar trends were seen in hockey. It has been theorized that improved head protection encouraged athletes to use their head and neck to block, tackle, and check (13,15). Modern helmets allow players to think of their head as weapons, utilizing them to "spear" block and check or tackle their opponents, placing their cervical spines at increased risk for serious injury (1). After the introduction of uniform helmet standards, rule changes, and educational programs against spearing techniques, there was a decrease in the number of fatalities due to head injury, although spearing continued to account for the majority of cervical spinal injuries resulting in quadriplegia (6). Fortunately, the return to shoulder tackling techniques did not result in an increase in brachial plexus or shoulder injuries (6).

PATHOMECHANICS AND DIFFERENTIAL DIAGNOSIS OF HEAD INJURIES

The two major classifications of head injury are focal and diffuse (16). Focal brain injuries are posttraumatic intracranial mass lesions that include epidural hematomas (EDHs), subdural hematomas (SDHs), cerebral contusions, and intracerebral hematomas (ICHs). Diffuse brain injuries are posttraumatic injuries that do not demonstrate focal lesions. Diffuse brain injuries may occur without gross structural damage, or be associated with anatomic distortion (17). The nonstructural injuries are typically less serious and encompass the concussion syndromes. They are generally due to a transient physiologic "short circuit." Axonal disruption is considered diffuse axonal injury (DAI). The extent of injury is proportional to the degree the brain is accelerated (5). Additional factors favoring DAI are 1) impacts over large areas of the head, 2) more rotational than translational forces, and 3) greater lateral than sagittal forces (18). DAI is generally more severe than a concussion due to actual anatomic injury (19). Diffuse brain swelling is an anatomic change that may also occur on an acute or delayed basis with any of the diffuse or focal brain injuries. The ultimate morbidity and mortality from brain injury are proportional to the sum of the various pathophysiologic processes (i.e., focal brain syndromes and brain swelling) (5,16).

Brain injury may occur through a variety of mechanisms (5). Applied forces to the brain may be compressive, tensile, or shear, the latter occurring when forces are applied in a parallel direction. Shearing stresses are not well tolerated by neural tissue (18). A coup injury is caused by an injury to the resting head (i.e., direct trauma) and produces maximal injury beneath the site of impact (Fig. 64-1A). A contrecoup injury occurs when the moving head strikes an immobile object, producing maximal injury to the part of the brain opposite the side of impact (Fig. 64-1B). If the head is accelerating prior to impact, the brain lags behind, squeezing away the cerebrospinal fluid (CSF) and decreasing the cushioning effect provided by the CSF (5). These lesions are most common at the undersurface and tips of the temporal lobes. Football and hockey helmets have decreased the number of injuries secondary to direct trauma, and the acceleration and deceleration forces of the brain within the cranium.

Diffuse Brain Injury

Concussion

Cerebral concussion is often a vague term to describe many forms of nonfocal brain injury. It is generally caused by sudden acceleration or deceleration forces to the brain. Concussions are due to immediate temporary global disruption or "short circuiting" of neurologic function, which may include a loss of consciousness. The duration of unconsciousness directly correlates with the severity of concussion (20). When associated with a loss of consciousness, concussions do not last longer than 6 hours (20). When loss of consciousness lasts more than 6 hours, it should be assumed that there is axonal damage and the injury should be classified as DAI (19,20).

There are several published guidelines for the grading and management of concussions (1,21–23). When one is evaluating what initially appears to be a concussion, it is imperative to rule out other more significant intracranial pathology, as the latter will affect management and treatment decisions. The most recognized guidelines are those proposed by Cantu (21), the Colorado Medical Society (22), and Nelson et al (23) (Tables 64-1, 64-2, and 64-3). There are differences in each of these guidelines with regards to grading and return to play. It would appear that Cantu's guidelines are the most widely utilized by team physicians (24) (see Tables 64-1 and 64-2). By Cantu's guidelines, a grade I concussion is defined as *mild*. There is no loss of consciousness, although posttraumatic amnesia or a period of confusion may persist for less than 30 minutes. It has been estimated that grade I concussions constitute about 50% of concussions (25). Due to their minor symptoms, they often elude medical care. A grade II concussion is a *moderate* concussion. There may be loss of consciousness, although it lasts less than 5 minutes. Posttraumatic amnesia typically lasts no longer than 30 minutes. A grade III concussion is a *severe* concussion. There will be loss of consciousness for longer than 5 minutes or a period of posttraumatic amnesia for longer than 24 hours, or both. The Cantu grading system is more

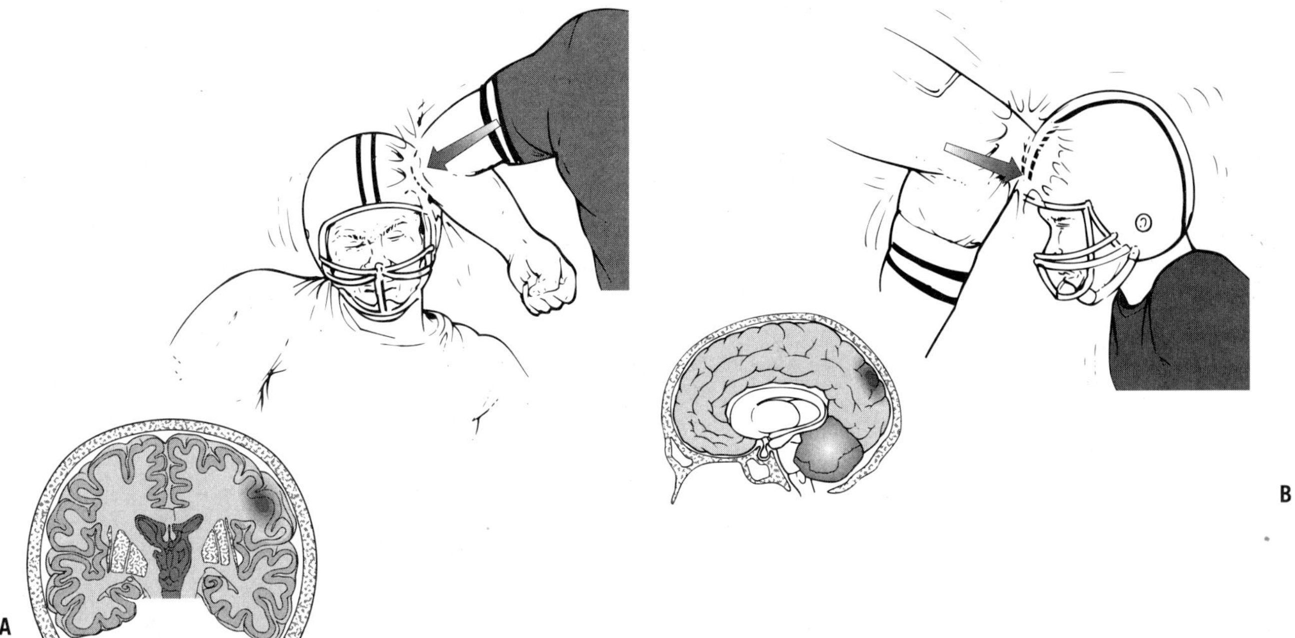

Figure 64-1. *A.* A coup injury. These injuries are produced by a blow to a stationary head and produce maximal effect at the side of impact. *B.* A contracoup injury. This injury occurs when the moving head strikes a stationary object, producing maximal injury to the side opposite the impact. (Adapted by permission from Berquist TH. *Imaging of sports injuries*. Gaithersburg, MD: Aspen, 1992.)

Table 64-1: Classification of Concussions

	Grade I, Mild	Grade II, Moderate	Grade III, Severe
Loss of consciousness	None	<5 min	>5 min
Posttraumatic amnesia	<30 min	<30 min	>24 hr

Source: Cantu RC. Guidelines for return to contact sports after cerebral concussion. *Phys Sports Med* 1988;13(10): 75–83.

concerned with the presence of posttraumatic amnesia or persistent postconcussive symptoms rather than loss of consciousness.

The Colorado guidelines (22) also delineate three grades of concussion (see Table 64-3). A grade I (*mild*) concussion is defined as confusion without amnesia and a grade II (*moderate*) concussion is defined as confusion with amnesia. All concussions with loss of consciousness are considered grade III (*severe*).

Nelson et al (23) define five classifications of concussion. Grades 0 to 2 are associated with neurologic symptoms but no loss of consciousness. A grade 3 concussion involves loss of consciousness for less than 1 minute and a grade 4 concussion, loss of consciousness for longer than 1 minute. The primary advantage of this system is that it allows classification of concussions without loss of consciousness, as grades 0 to 2.

Diffuse Axonal Injury

DAI is manifested by loss of consciousness at the time of impact. The loss of consciousness may persist beyond 6 hours, but is not caused by a focal mass lesion or ischemia due to diffuse brain swelling (26). The axonal injury results in microscopic hemorrhage and retraction balls of axoplasm; therefore, no neurodiagnostic study can determine definitively the degree of injury (27). Occasionally, the areas of axonal damage may coalesce and become visible on diagnostic images (28). Macroscopic changes detected by magnetic resonance imaging (MRI) will underestimate the degree of axonal injury verified by histopathologic studies (29,30). DAI usually is caused by shearing forces from acceleration or deceleration (17,30). This occurs maximally at sites where rotational gliding and shear forces develop owing to differential movement of one portion of the brain relative to another. These forces are concentrated at the junction of tissues of different density, such as the gray-white matter junction (17,28). Therefore, lesions are most severe in the lobar white matter, corpus callosum, and brain stem. The involvement becomes sequentially deeper in the brain with increasing severity of trauma (28,31). Athletes with DAI may have greater disturbances of consciousness than those with focal brain syndromes (29). DAI may result in permanent residual psychological or neurologic sequelae (32).

Diffuse Brain Swelling

Diffuse brain swelling can occur or coexist with any form of brain injury, from concussion to focal brain syndromes.

Table 64-2: Guidelines for Return to Contact After Concussion

	First Concussion	Second Concussion	Third Concussion
Grade 1 (mild)	May return to play if asymptomatic for 1 wk	May return to play in 2 wk, if asymptomatic at 1 wk	Terminate season, although athlete may return to play next season, if asymptomatic
Grade 2 (moderate)	May return to play after asymptomatic for 1 wk	Minimum of 1 mo out of competition, may return to play then if asymptomatic for 1 wk and consider termination of season, dependent on symptoms	Terminate season, although the athlete may return to play next season, if asymptomatic
Grade 3 (severe)	Minimum of 1 mo, may then return to play if asymptomatic for 1 wk	Terminate season, although may return to play next season if asymptomatic	

Source: Cantu RC. Guidelines for return to contact sports after cerebral concussion. *Phys Sports Med* 1988;13(10):75–83.

Table 64-3: Guidelines of the Colorado Medical Society

	Return to Play Recommendations		
Severity	First Concussion	Second Concussion	Third Concussion
Grade 1 (mild): confusion without amnesia; no loss of consciousness	May return to play if asymptomatic for at least 20 min	Terminate contest or practice for the day	Terminate season: may return in 3 mo if asymptomatic
Grade 2 (moderate): confusion with amnesia; no loss of consciousness	Terminate contest/practice; may return if asymptomatic for at least 1 wk	Consider terminating season, but may return if asymptomatic for 1 mo	Terminate season; may return to play next season if asymptomatic
Grade 3 (severe): loss of consciousness	May return after 1 mo if asymptomatic for 2 wk at that time; may resume conditioning sooner if asymptomatic for 2 wk	Terminate season; discourage any return to contact sports	

Source: Adapted with permission from the Colorado Medical Society Sports Medicine Committee. *Guidelines for the management of concussion in sports.* Denver: Colorado Medical Society, 1991.

It is not synonymous with cerebral edema, as this is an increase in brain water. Brain swelling is caused by a vascular reaction to head trauma. The extent of swelling does not always relate to the severity of the injury. The trauma leads to vasodilatation, with increased cerebral blood volume and increased intracranial pressure, with eventual cytotoxic brain edema and ischemia. This is a type of secondary lesion, as it develops consequent to the impact rather than by a direct effect. Secondary lesions are potentially preventable, as long as the initial injury is recognized and appropriate treatment provided. The effects of brain swelling are additive to the effects of focal brain injuries and may be more severe than the focal injury itself (16).

Brain swelling can occur acutely or on a delayed basis. More severe delayed brain swelling can cause a coma, after a mild concussion from which the athlete appears to initially recover (16). Minutes to hours after the injury occurs, the athlete becomes more lethargic before lapsing into deeper levels of consciousness. These athletes differ from those with DAI alone, as there is an interval between the initial disturbance of consciousness and the subsequent deeper level. Additionally (unless the swelling is associated with other focal brain lesions), there is no structural damage, so the swelling and its damaging results are potentially reversible.

Focal Brain Syndromes

Focal brain syndromes are caused by some form of intracranial hemorrhage, the leading cause of death from athletic injuries (33,34). Focal brain syndromes are subdivided into cerebral contusions and hemorrhagic lesions such as EDHs, SDHs, and ICHs. Traumatic hemorrhage results from injury to the cerebral vessels. The type of vessel damaged will determine the site and pattern of the hemorrhage.

Epidural Hematoma

An EDH results when there is bleeding into the epidural space, which is between the dura and the inner table of the periosteum (35). The hematoma is usually due to injury to an arterial vessel after a severe focal blow to the head (16). A skull fracture crossing the middle meningeal groove severing the middle meningeal artery occurs in 85% to 90% of subjects with EDHs (36). Approximately one-third of patients with EDH have a lucid interval immediately after the injury, which can lead to complacency regarding postinjury evaluation and management (33). With or without this lucid interval, there may be a progressive and potentially rapid decrease in consciousness, usually presenting within 1 to 2 hours of the injury (5). The athlete will often complain of a severe headache, then develop dilatation of the ipsilateral pupil and posturing on the side contralateral to the lesion (due to a shift of cerebral tissue across the midline) within 30 minutes to an hour. If missed, EDHs are universally fatal; therefore, prudence dictates that any athlete with a significant head injury be monitored frequently during the first 24 hours (5).

Subdural Hematoma

An SDH is usually caused by bleeding from the bridging veins between the brain and the cavernous sinus (35). The blood collects between the dura and the brain, and has a crescent-shaped appearance on MRI (31). SDHs are usually caused by rotational acceleration or deceleration injuries or contrecoup injuries (29). Most SDHs are located along the supratentorial convexity. Since bleeding is from the low-pressure venous system, the hematoma generally forms slowly. An athlete with an SDH may be asymptomatic or only have a headache. Signs or symptoms of increasing intracranial pressure may not be evident for hours, days, or weeks after the injury, depending on whether the SDH is acute or chronic. Most patients develop anisocoria or hemiparesis (34). Loss of consciousness is less likely to occur with SDH than with DAI, unless there is mass effect or another associated lesion (26). SDHs can be serious, as the series by Schneider (37) indicates. In this series, 24 of 69 patients underwent surgery or died within 6 hours of the injury. At times, SDHs may be associated with intracerebral bleeding as well.

Intracerebral Hematoma

ICHs occur when there is bleeding into the brain parenchyma and most often result from rotational shear to intraparenchymal arteries or veins. ICHs are most often located in the frontotemporal white matter or basal ganglia (31). Symptoms are determined by the location of the brain injury and may include paresis, sensory loss, and changes in language, cognition, or sensorium. Even athletes with significant intracerebral pathology may not have had a loss of consciousness or a focal neurologic deficit (16,33).

Cerebral Contusions

Cerebral contusions are bruises of the gray matter or cerebral cortex. They usually appear at the crests of the brain gyri at the undersurface of the frontal and temporal lobes (27). They are the second most common type of focal brain lesion (28). Due to their location, approximately 50% of cerebral contusions will have areas of hemorrhage within them (28,38). Athletes with isolated cerebral contusions usually recover well with only mild impairment, unless there is additional brain swelling or secondary brain stem injury. By themselves, contusions are usually not responsible for loss of consciousness (27).

Postconcussion Syndrome and Long-Term Sequelae

Postconcussion syndrome (PCS) is a constellation of symptoms such as headache, dizziness, fatigue, irritability, and impaired memory and ability to concentrate. PCS tends to occur in athletes after a minor head injury. While the neurologic findings are normal, neuropsychological testing may reveal subtle cognitive impairments. The duration of PCS depends on the extent and location of axonal injury, and psychological makeup. It has been proposed that PCS occurs infrequently in athletes, as they have more positive reinforcement for minimizing symptoms (39).

Dementia pugilistica or punchdrunk represents the cumulative effects of repeated brain trauma (32,40), described as a constellation of symptoms including dysarthria, impaired memory, slowed thought processes, personality disturbances, and cerebellar and parkinsonian-type symptoms (ataxia, tremors, rigidity, spasticity). Chronic brain damage is believed to be the most common detrimental effect of boxing trauma. Ryan (41) attempted to determine the rate of chronic brain injury from boxing, a sport in which the goal is to achieve a "knockout." Much of the data he collected were retrospective and as a result, often incomplete; however, a number of the studies on the brains of boxers demonstrated chronic encephalopathy with radiographic and postmortem examinations. There was an association between the number of fights and the severity of findings (41,42). Relatively few studies have documented chronic neuropsychological dysfunction in athletes with repeated head trauma (16). Ross et al (43) found that 90% of boxers had abnormal scores on visual and verbal memory portions of neuropsychological tests. When neuropsychological testing indicates subtle deficits, it may be difficult to distinguish whether they are due to a preexisting abnormality or are the earliest signs of brain injury due to trauma. The constellation of abnormalities on testing in visual and verbal memory, visual motor abilities, psychomotor coordination, attention, concentration, and ability for new learning usually indicates brain injury (42).

Posttraumatic Epilepsy

Posttraumatic epilepsy may occur immediately or as a late complication of head injury. There is a correlation with prolonged posttraumatic amnesia, depressed skull fractures, and ICH. Focal seizures occur most commonly with focal brain lesions. With acute epilepsy, the first seizure occurs within the first 24 hours of the injury and 50% of these occur within the first hour (20). Late epilepsy is defined as seizures that occur following the first week after the injury. The presence of electrophysiologic seizure activity immediately after injury does not have long-term predictive value regarding the persistence of seizure activity (44). In the absence of depressed skull fractures, ICH, or early epilepsy, the risk of late epilepsy is 1% (44). Prophylactic anticonvulsant therapy is usually recommended for 1 year after the occurrence of focal intracranial hemorrhage. The chance for seizure activity is less than 10% in athletes with concussions or cerebral contusions; therefore, anticonvulsant therapy is reserved for those who develop late epilepsy (45).

Second Impact Syndrome

Second impact syndrome was first described in 1973 (17,46). Saunders and Harbaugh (46) coined the phrase *second impact syndrome*. They postulated that catastrophic consequences may occur when an athlete who has sustained a concussion or other head injury sustains a second concussion or head injury before the symptoms associated with the first injury have fully abated. Second impact syndrome has occurred during football, hockey, and boxing. However, it could potentially occur in any sport in which the head is susceptible to impact (47).

With second impact syndrome, the second blow is often fairly minor and may not be a direct blow but one that causes acceleration forces to the brain (47). It may be of such minor consequence that the athlete may not lose consciousness. While the athlete may present with symptoms similar to a grade I concussion in the first seconds to minutes, the initially conscious athlete then often abruptly collapses into unconsciousness. The neurologic state rapidly deteriorates, with dilatation of the pupils, loss of eye movements, and eventual respiratory failure. Disruption of the blood autoregulatory system in an already compliant compromised brain is thought to be the causative factor of second impact syndrome (37,46–50). The dysfunctional autoregulatory system causes massive vascular engorgement within the cranium. As the cranial volume is restricted, expansion of the contents causes increased intracranial pressure. This increased pressure can lead to herniation of the uncal portion of the temporal lobes or of the cerebellar tonsils through the foramen magnum. Unfortunately, once brain herniation occurs, there is secondary involvement of the brain stem with coma, ocular involvement, and respiratory failure. These precipitous changes occur much more rapidly than do those associated with EDH.

Second impact syndrome is catastrophic, resulting in death in all reported cases. Cantu and Voy (47), reporting six cases of second impact syndrome, outlined the potential development of this syndrome in any athlete returning to contact sports before concussive symptoms from the initial injury have abated. Most important in the "treatment" of this particular syndrome is actual prevention. A thorough precompetition examination for any athlete attempting to return to a contact sport after a concussion or head injury is necessary. Unfortunately, many of the symptoms that persist after a concussion are subjective in nature. As a result, it is occasionally difficult to determine accurately whether all concussive symptoms have cleared if the athlete is anxious to return to play. There must be strict enforcement of the guidelines regarding return to play after the first, second, and third concussions (see Return to Play Criteria, later in this chapter).

Associated Head Injuries

Concussion and head injuries may be associated with other injuries to the head and face such as contusions and lacerations. Even when mild, facial lacerations may cause profuse bleeding. The presence of facial trauma may indicate that ocular or oromaxillofacial injuries are also present. The immediate management of these injuries is to stop the bleeding. If the bleeding has been adequately stopped and there is no evidence of associated brain, ocular, or maxillofacial injury, then the athlete may return to play.

Skull fractures may also occur with or without head injuries. Skull fractures should be suspected if there is an obvious deformity or palpable ridge. A basilar skull fracture should be suspected if there appears to be blood or CSF leakage from the external auditory canal, blood or CSF behind the tympanic membrane, retroauricular bruising, periorbital bruising, or CSF leaks from the nose (20). Skull fractures obviously require further evaluation prior to return to play, especially if there are depressed fragments.

PATHOMECHANICS AND DIFFERENTIAL DIAGNOSIS OF CERVICAL INJURIES

The anatomy of the cervical region of the spine allows maximum mobility while sacrificing the stability that the thoracic or lumbar regions have. The cervical spine is relatively stable in all planes of motion, unless rotational forces are applied (51). The severity and type of cervical injury produced are determined by the mechanism (magnitude and direction of the applied forces). Applied forces may flex, extend, compress, or rotate the spine. Anatomic factors make the cervical spine slightly more resistant to flexion than extension. Therefore, equivalent amounts of force may produce a more serious injury with extension than flexion (5). The mechanism of most cervical spinal injuries resulting in fracture or dislocation usually entails more than one force variable (52). Flexion injuries occur most commonly during football, hockey, rugby, or other collision sports (53). Flexion without axial loading may result in distraction and potential injury to the supraspinous and interspinous ligaments as well as facet capsules. Flexion with rotation is likely to cause facet subluxation (5).

Axial loading is the most common cause of athletic injuries to the cervical spine with or without a neural defect (5,10,54). Examples include a football player performing a spear tackle, a hockey player being checked into the boards head first, or a swimmer diving into a shallow body of water and striking his or her head on the bottom. During axial loading, the cervical spine is compressed between the decelerating head and the significant momentum and mass of the body. The energy-absorbing capabilities of the cervical musculature, as well as the diskogenic and ligamentous structures, help dissipate collision energy. In the anatomic position, the cervical spine has a lordotic posture. Flexing the neck to 30 degrees straightens the cervical spine and limits the energy-absorbing effects of the disks and muscles. This converts the spine into a straight segmented column, transmitting forces along its longitudinal axis, potentially injuring bones, disks, and ligamentous structures (Fig. 64-2) (10,54,55). Axial loading of the segmented column first results in compressive deformation. As the force increases, further angular deformation can occur. If the compressive force is not dissipated by controlled motion in the spinal segments, buckling occurs and fracture or dislocation, or both, result. Axial loading injuries can cause quadriplegia even at low-impact velocities (10,56).

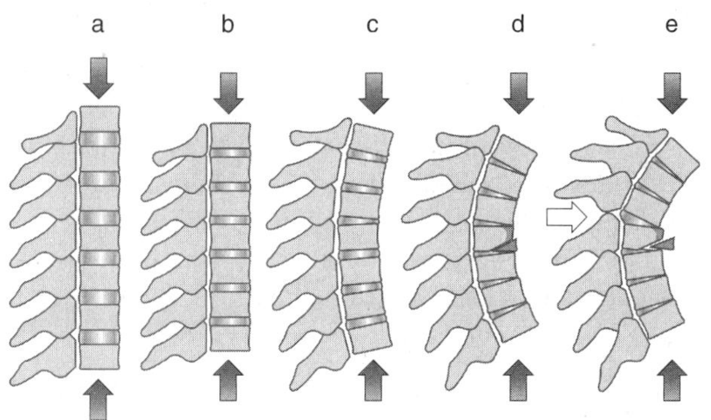

Figure 64-2. The axial loading mechanism causes the highest percentage of football-induced cervical injuries with or without quadriplegia (3,10,105). Axial loading straightens the segmented column of the cervical spine. Initial compressive deformation occurs at the intervertebral disks (*a*, *b*). The spine begins to buckle as compressive deformation peaks (*c*). Subsequent angular deformation along the segmented column results in potential fracture, ligamentous rupture, and dislocation. (Reproduced by permission from Anderson C. Neck injuries: backboard, bench or return to play? *Phys Sports Med* 1993;21(8):23–34.)

Soft-tissue Ligamentous Injury

Cervical sprains and strains result from the chronic overloading or acute injury of musculoligamentous structures in the cervical region. They are the most common noncatastrophic cervical injuries (15). Sprains and strains can cause local or referred pain and tenderness and limit cervical mobility. They can coexist with any other head, cervical, or shoulder girdle injury. Athletes may develop myofascial pain syndromes in the cervical, thoracic, and shoulder girdle muscles. Active myofascial trigger points can cause local or referred pain and tenderness (57). Latent myofascial trigger points can act to restrict motion, but later become active after overuse (57,58). Referred pain from a trigger point may mimic a cervical radiculopathy (58). Trigger points may be associated with a subjective alteration in sensation but no objective clinical findings.

Thoracic outlet syndrome (TOS) was first described by Rob and Sandoven in 1958 (59). The thoracic outlet is the space between the inferior part of the clavicle and the upper border of the first rib. The symptoms of TOS are caused by compression of the neurovascular bundle as it passes from the neck into the arm. TOS may result from dynamic or static factors. The athlete with chronic cervical disk or facet pain may develop compensatory soft-tissue and postural adaptations in the cervical or thoracic spinal region and shoulder girdle. Forward-head position with protracted shoulders, elevated scapulae, and tight anterior cervical and thoracic muscles can cause narrowing of the thoracic outlet dynamically (58). Fixed structural abnormalities such as a cervical rib, bifid rib, or excessive callus formation from an old clavicular fracture may also play a role in the development of TOS (60).

Compression of the neurovascular bundle may create a variety of symptoms including altered sensation, paresthesia, or weakness in C8 or T1 distribution (60,61). Pain, decreased temperature, weakness, and easy fatigability may be associated with arterial compression, whereas edema, aching pain, and distention of collateral vessels about the shoulder may occur with venous compression. This may be accentuated with arm elevation or rotation or extension head positions. Therefore, athletes in sports that require these positions may develop TOS on a dynamic basis.

Shoulder girdle complex pain may emanate from a number of different sources about the shoulder girdle. Owing to muscle attachments of cervical muscles to the scapula, pathology in the glenohumeral and acromioclavicular joint may produce neck pain. The "weakness" associated with rotator cuff tears may be confused with neurologic loss associated with C5 or C6 root lesions, injury to the upper trunk of the brachial plexus, or isolated suprascapular nerve injuries (62). The majority of cervical degenerative changes occur at the C5–C6 and C6–C7 levels, potentially affecting the C6 and C7 nerve roots; thus, older athletes may present with referred shoulder girdle pain. Diagnostic selective injections into the shoulder and cervical spinal joints may help distinguish between cervical and shoulder girdle pathology so a precise diagnosis can be made (15).

Intervertebral Disk Injuries

Cervical disk injuries may include the spectrum of annular tears, end-plate disruption, protrusions, extrusions, and degenerative disks. The natural history of the degenerative process due to repetitive microtrauma has been described and expanded upon as the degenerative cascade. Intervertebral disk herniations have been generally classified into four different categories, including a bulge, protrusion, extrusion, and sequestration. This is discussed in other sections of this text.

Repetitive compressive loading can cause vertebral end-plate fractures with extrusion of the nucleus into the vertebral body (51). Histologic studies from in vitro as well as surgical specimens reveal that annular material and end-plate fragments, along with nuclear material, may be present in the herniated portion of the disk. Athletes may demonstrate early degenerative disk changes or disk space narrowing due to repetitive cervical loading (13).

Athletes with symptomatic cervical intervertebral disk changes but without radiculopathy typically present with segmental neck pain, spasm, loss of motion, and referred pain in a nonradicular pattern. Symptoms may increase with lifting, vibration, and Valsalva maneuvers; lying supine or traction may provide relief. Generalized or advanced degenerative disk changes (without herniation) may be seen in the younger athletic population (63). A degenerative disk may result from cumulative trauma to the end-plate of the vertebral body and may or may not be symptomatic. Additionally, not all athletes with disk herniations present with axial or cervical pain. Some athletes may not demonstrate significant symptoms until they begin to develop radiculopathy. In Kumano and Yumeyama's series (64), athletes with cervical disk injuries that were able to be treated nonoperatively returned to full sporting activity. Those with myelopathy or instability did not return to preinjury sport levels.

Cervical Facet Pain

Facet pain may occur in isolation or in conjunction with signs and symptoms of diskogenic pain (65,66). Pain produced by cervical facets may be confused with cervical disk and shoulder girdle complex problems. Facet joint syndrome is characterized by dull, aching neck pain that may be associated with headache and scapular pain. Cervical motion may be limited segmentally by joint restrictions or diffusely by accompanying soft-tissue spasm. There may be local pain over the facet or secondary trigger points due to the spondylogenic reflex (67). A detailed history and a good manual examination will often help differentiate facet from diskogenic pain. Diagnostic selective spinal injections may help identify the pain generator in difficult cases (65).

Cervical Fractures, Dislocations, and Subluxations

There are several distinct cervical spinal fracture patterns. The type of fracture depends on the force and the relative position of the head, neck, and thorax at the time of injury (10,52,54) (Fig. 64-3). Burst fractures require a nearly neutral spinal position with an applied axial load. Axial loading with the load less than 1 cm anterior to neutral vertebral axis typically results in an anterior wedge fracture. The same axial load applied at a distance of more than 1 cm anterior to this vertebral axis causes buckling of the cervical spine with failure of the end-plate and disk. With either increasing forward application of the force or increasing force, additional structures including the interspinous ligaments may fail, potentially leading to facet dislocation.

The major consideration in the evaluation of fractures or subluxations is the presence of an unstable injury. Unstable injuries are those where there is enough damage to the anterior and posterior column that movement could cause damage to the cord or nerve roots (68). According to the National Center for Sports Injury Research (NCSIR), all cases of quadriplegia in the absence of spinal stenosis resulted from fracture or dislocation at the cervical spine (5).

Cervical subluxation injuries occur when the articulation between two vertebral levels is disturbed but the articular surfaces remain in contact. Cervical dislocations create separation of the two opposed vertebral articular surfaces and require injury to the intervertebral disk and ligamentous structures. Dislocations may occur at the level of the cervical facets. Unilateral facet dislocations are typically created by flexion forces combined with rotation under an axial load (69,70). They may be due to ligament injury only, without fracture. These dislocations are generally stable but are usually associated with neurologic involvement. Generally, bilateral facet dislocations are the result of significant ligamentous disruption and require surgical stabilization. The degree of instability is directly proportional to the ease of reduction (69). Bilateral facet dislocations are defined as more than 50% anterior displacement of the superior vertebral body on the inferior vertebral body on lateral radiographs (71). With either unilateral or bilateral facet dislocations, there may be complete or partial spinal cord injury.

Fractures, subluxations, and dislocations can occur alone or in combination at individual or multiple cervical vertebral levels. The lower cervical region of the spine (C4–C7) is the most common site for fracture and dislocation in athletics (52,72). Most athletic cervical spinal injuries are fractures of the vertebral body, with varying degrees of comminution or compression. A less severe injury includes a small chip fracture or anterior wedge compression fracture without involvement of the posterior elements or neurologic injury. Anterior-superior chip fractures are usually due to hyperflexion and may be unstable if there is tearing of the posterior longitudinal ligament.

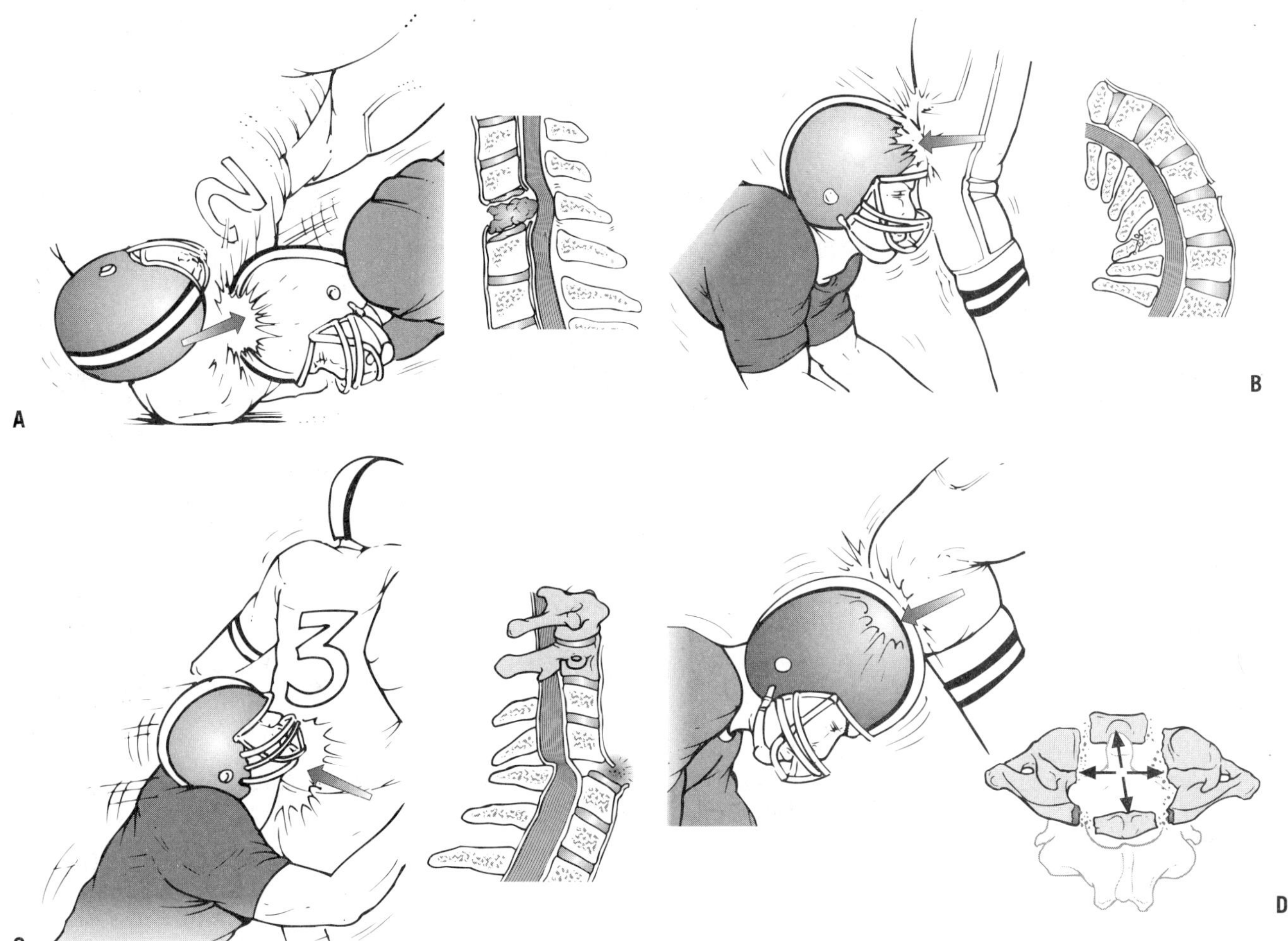

Figure 64-3. *A.* A burst fracture is a type of vertical compression injury. *B.* Hyperextension injury of the cervical spine with force applied to the facial region may result in tearing of the anterior disk or anterior longitudinal ligament in addition to posterior element fracture. *C.* Hyperextension injury of the cervical spine with force applied to the anterior cranium. *D.* Vertical compression injury resulting in a burst fracture of C2. (Adapted by permission from Berquist TH. *Imaging of sports injuries.* Gaithersburg, MD: Aspen, 1992.)

Anterior-inferior chip fractures are usually due to hyperextension and are generally stable unless there is injury of the posterior arch (52). When the forces applied to the spine are great enough to cause a burst fracture, both the anterior and the posterior column are damaged and therefore are unstable. Additionally, there may be propulsion of fracture fragments posteriorly into the central canal, potentially causing spinal cord injury (see Fig. 64-3A) (71). A teardrop fracture is named for the large triangular anterior fracture fragment of the vertebral body and is associated with neurologic involvement in 80% patients (52).

Fractures of the posterior elements of the lower cervical region of the spine are generally due to hyperextension forces. Dependent on head position and with hyperextension, posterior arch fractures may be associated with anterior disk or anterior longitudinal ligament injury (see Fig. 64-3B). These are generally unstable. The benign Clay Shoveler fracture is an avulsion fracture of the tip of the spinous process of C6, C7, or T1 (52). These fractures may occur with contact or excessive muscular contraction. If the fracture is at the tip of the spinous process and does not involve the lamina, it is a stable injury (73). Isolated fractures of the lamina are rare and usually due to compression with hyperextension, rotation, or lateral bending (52,56). Fractures of the lamina may extend into the base of the spinous process, creating an unstable injury (see Fig. 64-3C) (52). Isolated fracture of the facet or articular pillars of the lower cervical spine may be associated with radicular symptoms (52). Although fractures of the pedicle are most common at C2, they are seen in the lower cervical spine with hyperextension mechanisms. Up to 60% of articular pillar fractures and 80% of pedicle fractures missed on plain radiographs can be detected by computed tomography (CT) (52,75).

Injuries at the middle cervical level (C3–C4) are rare (76). The response to loading is different at C3–C4 than at the upper and lower cervical regions of the spine. Injuries at that level are generally not associated with fractures and are more likely to involve disk injury, subluxation, or facet dislocation (70,77). The National Football Head and Neck

Registry documented 885 injuries over 14 years. Only 2.8% involved C3–C4 and only 0.3% involved fractures at C3 (76). It is often more difficult to maintain reduction with subluxations or dislocations, but there may be a favorable response with improvement in neurologic deficits with early aggressive treatment (76).

Upper cervical (C1–C2) injuries are rare in athletics (2). When fractures occur, they are usually due to contact sports or accidents while riding motorcycles, race cars, snowmobiles, or similar vehicles. A Jefferson fracture is usually caused by a pure vertical axial load and results in disruption of the ring of the first cervical vertebra (see Fig. 64-3D) (69,70,78). As it can be caused by hyperextension forces, it is imperative to exclude associated lower cervical spinal fractures (79). When the posterior arch alone is fractured, union usually occurs uneventfully after immobilization. When fracture involves both the anterior and the posterior arch, it may be called a *burst fracture* even though it is stable (2). Burst fractures may be identified on a CT scan or open-mouth radiographs (52). Fielding and Hawkins (80) described rotatory fixation of the atlas on the axis, which may demonstrate no neurologic involvement or be associated with cord or vertebral artery injury.

Fractures of the odontoid process or pedicles of the axis (C2) comprise approximately 80% of the injuries (81). Fracture of the neural arch of C2 has been termed a *hangman fracture* (69), reflecting the hyperflexion-distraction forces that classically cause this injury. They may also be caused by flexion combined with compression or distraction and are considered traumatic spondylolisthesis of C2 (82). They are generally unstable injuries, although they will generally heal without surgical intervention (70).

Fractures of the odontoid process of C2 have been classified into three types, each differing in their relative stability and treatment (83). A type I odontoid fracture is a fracture of the odontoid tip, where the alar ligament attaches. It is considered to be stable (70,71). A fracture through the base of the odontoid is classified as a type II fracture and a fracture through the body of the axis is a type III injury. Type II fractures are unstable. Nonunion can be a sequela of type II fractures after bracing or casting (84). Odontoid fractures that appear unstable on extension radiographs or those with nonunion generally require surgical fusion (70).

Dislocations at the atlas and axis may be caused by fractures of the odontoid process of C2 or rupture of the transverse ligament of C1 (85). These dislocations are generally caused by axial loading (70). When either of these anatomic changes occur, anterior translation of C1 on C2 may develop. The spinal cord may become compressed between the posterior rim of C1 and the posterior aspect of the odontoid. As the spinal canal is quite large in this region, there is a relative safety factor for displacement before impingement or damage occurs to the cord (69). There may be no neurologic impairment or a complete spinal cord injury may occur. At this level, when neurologic injury occurs, it usually results in death due to loss of innervation to the diaphragm.

Transient Quadriplegia

Transient quadriplegia (TQ) was described first by Maroon (86) in 1977 as "burning hand syndrome" and later by Wilberger et al in 1987 (87). This was believed to be a variant of a central cord syndrome, with selective trauma of the central fibers of the spinothalamic tract. Credibility was given to the mechanism of neuropraxia of the spinal cord for TQ by a case reported by Wilberger et al (87). In this case, somatosensory evoked potentials demonstrated a reversible insult to sensory pathway conduction in the spinal cord (87). The athletes they identified did not have permanent neurologic loss. The etiology was believed to be a result of edema or vascular insufficiency in the cord. This phenomenon was later described by Torg and Pavlov (88,89) as *transient quadriplegia* and was considered a neuropraxic injury to the spinal cord. As a variant of a central cord syndrome, TQ is potentially very serious. The same mechanism of injury that can cause TQ can cause fractures and dislocations or complete versus incomplete spinal cord injury. TQ most commonly occurs during football, ice hockey, and boxing (89).

The typical symptoms of TQ are burning paresthesias and weakness in both arms, or three or four extremities. The symptoms usually resolve in 10 to 15 minutes, though resolution may take up to 36 to 48 hours (89). By definition, for the injury to be termed *transient* quadriplegia, there must be complete return of sensory and motor function and full pain-free cervical range of motion. Anything less than complete resolution of neurologic symptoms should be considered an incomplete spinal cord injury. Athletes with symptoms of TQ should be treated as having a significant spinal cord injury until proved otherwise.

The primary factor that appears to predispose an athlete to TQ is a decrease in the sagittal diameter of the spinal canal (89). This can occur in isolation or in combination with congenital anomalies, posttraumatic instability, intervertebral disk herniations, or developmental degenerative changes. The mechanism for TQ (as well as some forms of spinal cord injury) has been proposed to be a pincher mechanism at extremes of flexion or extension (90). When an athlete has a congenitally small spinal canal or has a moderately small spinal canal with superimposed developmental stenosis of any cause and the neck is subsequently hyperextended or hyperflexed, the spinal cord may be momentarily compressed between the lower edge of the upper vertebra and the upper edge of the vertebra below. This mechanism may cause a transient neuropraxia, a contusion in the cord, or potentially even more permanent neurologic sequelae. Another mechanism in which TQ may occur is through axial loading with the neck slightly flexed with straightening of the normal lordotic curve (10). However, this mechanism also usually requires some amount of congenital or developmental stenosis to be present. TQ may be associated with bony or ligamentous abnormalities in about 50% of athletes affected (89).

Spinal Cord Injury Syndromes

Trauma to the cervical spine can result in a wide variety of clinical spinal cord injuries depending on the severity or type of impact (12). Similar to brain injuries, there may be primary insults to the cord, such as contusion and hemorrhage, as well as secondary insults created by edema and ischemia (5). Intraspinal hematomas are the most common and subdural spinal hematomas are the second most common according to the (NCSIR) (5). Spinal cord injuries can be either complete or incomplete. In complete injuries, there is a total loss of sensory and motor spinal function below the level of the lesion. Complete spinal cord injuries are typically considered permanent, although improvement may eventually be noted at the involved spinal level due to a decrease in spinal cord swelling and neuropraxia.

There are a number of different incomplete spinal cord injury patterns, including the central, Brown-Séquard, and anterior and posterior spinal cord syndromes. There is great variability in the persistence of symptoms in these incomplete spinal cord injuries. Described by Schneider (68), *central cord syndrome* results in incomplete loss of motor function, with greater involvement of the upper extremities compared to the lower extremities, based on the topographic arrangement of the corticospinal tracts. The spinothalamic tracts are also involved, resulting in sensory dysfunction in the form of pain and burning paresthesias. The initial insult may be due to either hemorrhage or ischemia of the central portion of the cord. Depending on the severity of the lesion, there may be either complete or incomplete recovery.

Posterior spinal cord syndrome is seen infrequently. It is usually secondary to selective ischemia in the distribution of the posterior spinal artery. It results in loss of dorsal column function with preservation of the corticospinal and spinothalamic tracts. In contrast, the *anterior spinal cord syndrome* occurs when there is involvement of the anterior spinal artery. It supplies the anterior two-thirds of the spinal cord. As opposed to the central cord syndrome, this can involve the corticospinal motor tracts of the lower extremities. There is usually weakness or paresis of the lower extremities as well as impairment of sphincter and sexual function. Involvement of the spinothalamic tracts may result in pain and paresthesias in primarily the lower extremities. The *Brown-Séquard syndrome* typically involves one-half of the spinal cord. Therefore, there is loss of motor function ipsilaterally and pain and temperature on the contralateral side.

Cervical Radiculopathy

Radiculopathy may be due to nerve irritation or compression caused by degenerative changes in the disk or facet joint complex, in isolation or combination. A *radiculopathy* is any sensory, motor, or reflex abnormality secondary to nerve root injury (91). Radicular pain is experienced in a dermatomal, myotomal, or sclerotomal pattern of the involved nerve root. The athlete may experience pain that is deep, dull, and achy, or sharp, burning, or electric in quality, depending on whether there is primarily motor or sensory root involvement (92,93). The pain associated with radiculopathy follows a radicular pattern and numbness follows a dermatomal pattern (73,94). Weakness can be present when there is motor root compromise but must be differentiated from weakness due to pain or neuromuscular inhibition. The athlete with radiculopathy may present clinically with decreased cervical range of motion and signs of nerve root tension.

Radiculopathy tends to be more common in older athletes, though it may occur at any age. In 60% of athletes with traumatic cervical disk herniations without fracture or dislocation but sustaining neurologic deficits, either the C5 or C6 nerve roots are involved (64). Radiculopathy may be secondary to mechanical compression, inflammatory exudate, or both (95). Various types of injury may occur. Neuropraxia is typically caused by a reversible insult to the myelin sheath (96). A neuropraxic injury results in conduction failure across the injury site. The nerve distal to the lesion does not undergo wallerian degeneration and generally maintains normal physiologic properties. Axonal loss can occur with an insult great enough to damage the axons alone (axonotmesis) or the axons and their connective tissue support (neurotmesis) (96). The initial clinical findings may be no different in athletes with conduction block and axonal loss; however, 2 to 3 weeks after the injury, the athletes with axonal loss may begin to demonstrate characteristic electrophysiologic changes of fibrillation potentials and positive sharp waves in muscles supplied by the affected nerve(s) (96–98). Wallerian degeneration distal to the site of injury results in denervation of muscles supplied by the affected nerve root or trunk.

Brachial Plexus Lesions (Stinger, Burner)

Brachial plexus injuries are the most common "spine" injuries to athletes. It has been estimated that 50% to 70% of collegiate football players have at least one stinger or burner injury in their athletic careers and 57% suffer more than one (99–101). One series estimated the incidence to be 70% in football players (101). This may be underestimated because many athletes continue to play without reporting their injury. Brachial plexus injuries are most frequently encountered in players of contact or limited-contact sports such as football, hockey, and wrestling (97,102,103).

Typical symptoms of a stinger are sudden, unilateral upper-extremity burning, aching pain, or weakness for 2 to 15 minutes after the traumatic incident. Lower-intensity aching, weakness, and paresthesias may persist for hours to months. The C5–C6 roots or the upper trunk of the plexus are at greatest risk for these injuries. For at least one potential mechanism of injury, the C5–C6 roots are placed on the greatest stretch.

There is no clear consensus regarding the pathomechanics of stingers. The first mechanism requires simultaneous lateral flexion of the cervical spine contralateral to the symptomatic upper extremity and forceful shoulder depression ipsilateral to the symptomatic upper extremity, creating a traction injury to the brachial plexus (69,99,104–111) or nerve root (105,108,112,113) (Fig. 64-4A). The second suggested mechanism may occur with forceful cervical extension combined with rotation ipsilateral to the symptomatic arm, creating compression to the nerve root in the neuroforamen (63,100,104,105,114) (see Fig. 64-4B). This position is similar to that used in the Spurling maneuver. It has been suggested that the traction mechanism is more likely to occur in high school players who sustain stingers, whereas cervical nerve root injury secondary to the extension-rotation-compression mechanism is more likely to occur in professional players (97,104). This difference may be due to improved muscle strength and tackling and blocking techniques in the higher-level athletes (97). A grading system for stingers is provided by Clancy et al (99).

ON-FIELD AND IMMEDIATE MANAGEMENT

Evaluation of the athlete after potential concussion or head injury includes 1) determination of the athlete's orientation to person, place, and time; 2) assessment for post-traumatic and retrograde amnesia; 3) observation of facial expression; 4) evaluation of gait; 5) neurologic examination including cranial nerves; and 6) direct questioning (16,115). The Glasgow Coma Scale (GCS) is a simple and universal method for assessing an athlete's level of consciousness (116). The GCS evaluates verbal response, motor response, and eye opening and the scores range between 3 and 15. Most patients with minor brain injury score between 13 and 15 on the GCS and those with severe head injuries are comatose and score between 3 and 8.

After the athlete suffers trauma to the head, the physician may be uncertain of the diagnosis until the symptoms either evolve or resolve. An injured athlete may initially present with symptoms similar to a grade I concussion, but within minutes develop symptoms consistent with an EDH. Intermittent reassessment should occur and precautions given to the athlete, trainer, and parent when applicable. Immediate management of a concussion depends on its severity, and hinges on appropriate evaluation at the time of injury, as well as appropriate re-evaluation within the first 24 hours and ensuing weeks. As discussed previously, several classification scales have been recognized for the grading of concussion (21–23). Physiatrists must decide which system is most applicable and enforceable in the athletic population they cover.

The signs and symptoms that require emergency medical attention in athletes that have had head trauma are progressive or sudden impairment of consciousness, increasing headache, nausea, vomiting, unequal pupils, gradual rise in blood pressure, or diminution of pulse rate (115,117). The development of these symptoms alone or in combination may be signs of increasing intracranial pressure, necessitating immediate transport to a medical facility. Additionally, any focal neurologic deficit, skull fracture, or focal or generalized seizure is suggestive of a focal brain lesion and mandates transport to a medical facility (20). Management of brain injuries in the hospital setting is beyond the scope of this chapter.

It must be assumed that a "downed" athlete with impaired consciousness has both a head injury and a cervical spinal injury until proved otherwise

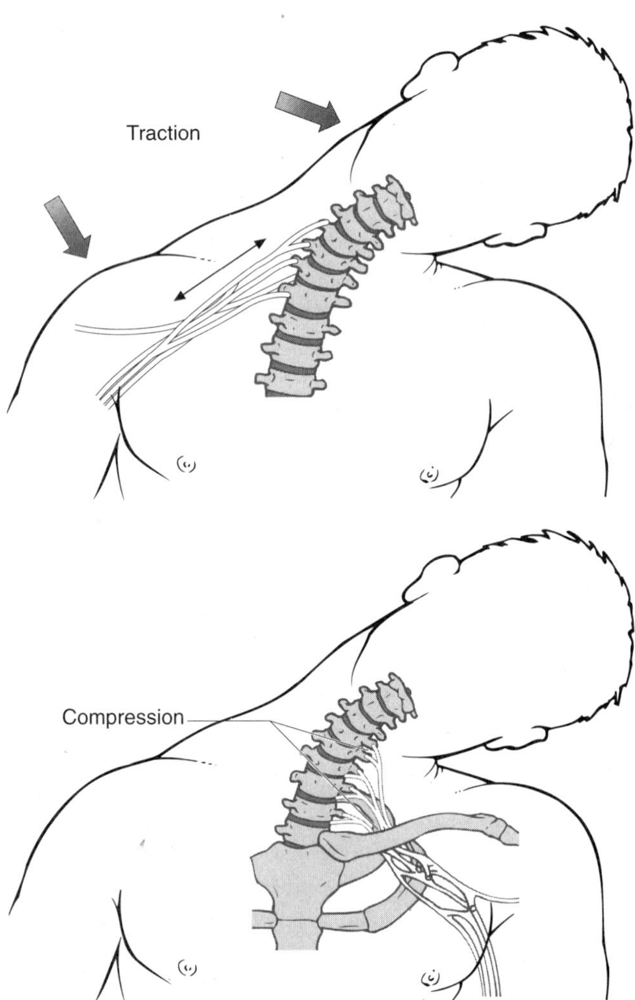

Figure 64-4. *A.* Traction to the brachial plexus may occur through lateral flexion of the head and neck away from the injured side and ipsilateral shoulder depression. *B.* Compression, often combined with extension and ipsilateral rotation, may injure the nerve roots. (Reproduced by permission from Sallis RE, Jones K, Knopp W. Burners: offensive strategy for an underreported injury. *Phys Sports Med* 1992;20(11):47–55.)

(1,5,16,73,104,115,117). The conscious athlete who is "down" yet complains of severe neck pain or symptoms consistent with TQ or a stinger must be treated initially as though he or she has a spinal cord injury (73). If the athlete is down on the playing surface at the time he or she is reporting the symptoms, the spine should be immobilized until the athlete has been evaluated more thoroughly. It is important to question the patient completely about the mechanism of injury and the presence or absence of cervical pain and sensory changes, weakness, and paresthesias in the arms and lower extremities. Additionally, the athlete should be questioned regarding prior cervical spinal, brachial plexus, and shoulder injuries (73). If the patient has persistent pain, stiffness, or increasing pain on gentle active range of motion, neurologic symptoms, or a self-perception that "something is wrong," the spine should remain immobilized until a definitive radiographic evaluation is performed. Algorithms can be used to guide the "on-field" assessment and management of head and neck injuries (Fig. 64-5).

It is important to know when and how to immobilize a patient with a potential cervical spinal or head injury (70,73). The main objective of immobilization is to prevent further injury. Approximately 50% of neurologic deficits are created after the initial traumatic event (2,55). Spinal cord injury occurs in the postinjury period in 5% to 10% of those injured (118). The athlete's level of consciousness should be assessed, as well as their response to pain and the presence of any unusual posturing, rigidity, flaccidity, pupillary response, or sensorimotor changes. The athlete should be immobilized until consciousness returns, there is no further evidence of cervical spinal injury, or a definitive evaluation is performed. In general, the head and neck should be immobilized in the neutral position or the position in which they are found (104,115).

After temporary immobilization, the physician should assess the athlete's airway, breathing, and circulation (ABC). If the athlete is breathing, the mouth guard is removed and the airway is maintained. If the athlete is not breathing or if breathing stops, an airway must be established. While the athlete is on the field or playing surface, the airway is secured by removing only the face mask. After the face mask has been removed, the oropharynx should be swept to clear the tongue or other obstructions. A jaw thrust may be performed, and basic cardiopulmonary resuscitation (CPR) should be instituted until emergency support arrives. If the initial maneuvers to restore an airway are unsuccessful and airway obstruction is suspected owing to malalignment of the neck, then gentle two-handed traction with slow turning to alignment may be attempted (69). Hyperextension or flexion movement of the neck should be avoided.

No attempt should be made to turn or move the athlete on to a spine board without proper assistance (70,104,115). A minimum of four people in addition to the team leader is required. The team leader controls the head, neck, and shoulders. When the athlete is face down, the team leader starts with the arms rotated and a second person assists in stabilizing the athlete's head and neck between the leader's forearms. Other members of the team position themselves at the knees, hips, trunk, and shoulders, and log roll the athlete upright or slide the athlete on to the spine board if already upright. The assistants ensure that the torso remains in alignment with the head and neck. Once the athlete is positioned safely on the spine board, additional support of the head and neck may be provided by placing a small roll under the neck, positioning sandbags on either side of the head, and strapping the head down to the board.

If the athlete is wearing a helmet, optimally it is removed only at an appropriate treatment facility, once neurologic examination and x-ray evaluation have been completed (70,104,105). The helmet is removed by detaching the chin strap, spreading the ear flaps, and gently pulling it off parallel to the cervical spine. The cervical spine is immobilized during this process while the head is supported by another person who reaches under the head and neck from below.

When the athlete walks off the playing field on his or her own power and complains of neck pain or gives symptoms consistent with a stinger or TQ, it is still important to obtain a complete history on the sidelines. This includes questions regarding the presence of neck pain, stiffness, and apprehension as well as the presence of neurologic symptoms in the extremities. The comprehensive sideline physical examination assesses postural alignment, deformity, soft-tissue spasm, and neurologic integrity. Manual muscle testing should evaluate strength of isolated muscle groups. When athletes have neck and shoulder pain, it is often difficult to perform a reliable manual muscle test. A practical method is to start with the arm at the side, with the elbow flexed to 90 degrees and in the neutral position of supination and pronation. The examiner may support and hold the elbow and humerus at the side, using the examiner's opposite arm to the one he or she is testing in the athlete, attempting to eliminate contraction of the proximal shoulder girdle muscles. (For example, if the athlete's right arm is being tested, the right arm is supported or immobilized at the athete's side with the examiner's left arm as he or she faces the athlete.) The athlete should be cautioned not to use substitution maneuvers such as shoulder shrugging or abducting the arm, unless that is being tested. From that position, 1) internal rotation tests the pectoral muscle (medial and lateral pectoral—C5–C8, T1), 2) external rotation tests the infraspinatus (suprascapular nerve—C), 3) elbow flexion preferentially tests the brachioradial and brachial muscles (musculocutaneous and radial nerves—C5, C6), 4) elbow extension tests the triceps muscle (radial nerve—C6–C8), 5) elbow flexion with supination tests the biceps (musculocutaneous nerves—C5, C6), and 6) isometric abduction from this position tests the deltoid muscle (axillary nerve—C5, C6).

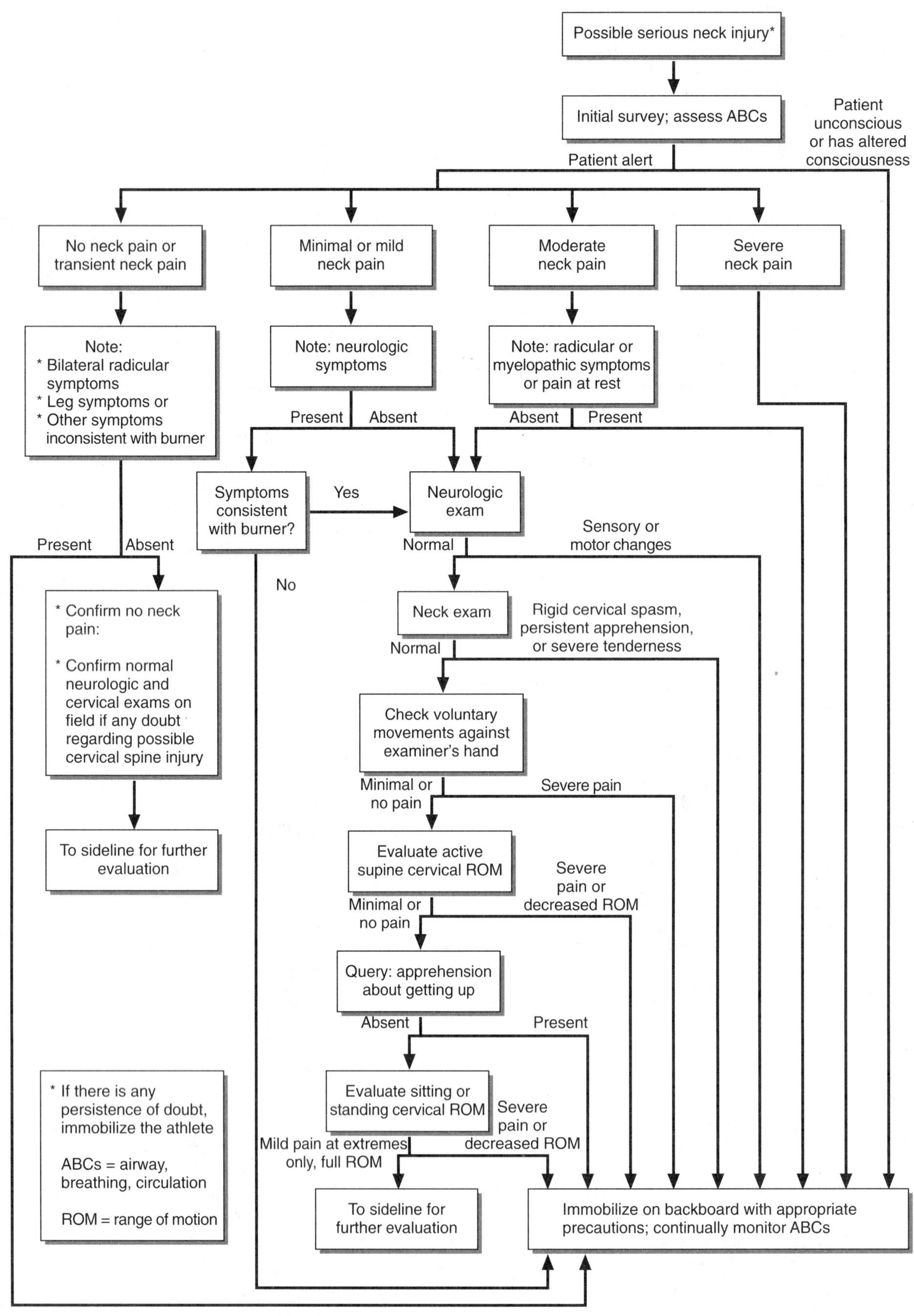

Possible serious neck injury*
Initial survey; assess ABCs
Patient unconscious or has altered consciousness
Patient alert
No neck pain or transient neck pain
Minimal or mild neck pain
Moderate neck pain
Severe neck pain
Note:
* Bilateral radicular symptoms
* Leg symptoms or
* Other symptoms inconsistent with burner
Note: neurologic symptoms
Note: radicular or myelopathic symptoms or pain at rest
Present
Absent
Absent
Present
Symptoms consistent with burner?
Yes
Neurologic exam
Sensory or motor changes
Present
Absent
Normal
No
* Confirm no neck pain:
* Confirm normal neurologic and cervical exams on field if any doubt regarding possible cervical spine injury
Neck exam
Rigid cervical spasm, persistent apprehension, or severe tenderness
Normal
Check voluntary movements against examiner's hand
Minimal or no pain
Severe pain
To sideline for further evaluation
Evaluate active supine cervical ROM
Severe pain or decreased ROM
Minimal or no pain
Query: apprehension about getting up
Absent
Present
* If there is any persistence of doubt, immobilize the athlete
ABCs = airway, breathing, circulation
ROM = range of motion
Evaluate sitting or standing cervical ROM
Severe pain or decreased ROM
Mild pain at extremes only, full ROM
To sideline for further evaluation
Immobilize on backboard with appropriate precautions; continually monitor ABCs
A

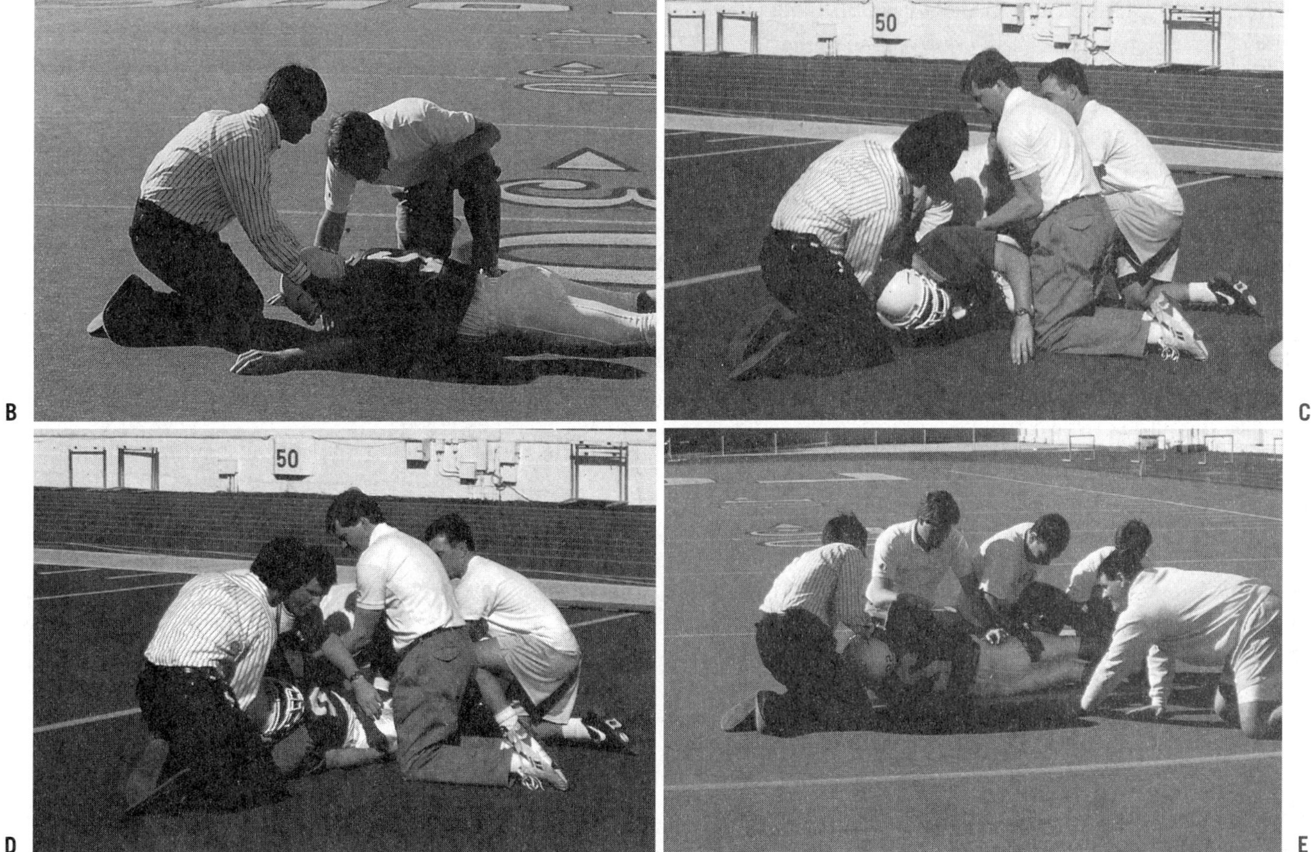

Figure 64-5. *A.* Algorithm for on-field assessment of head and neck injuries. (Reproduced by permission from Anderson C. Neck injuries: backboard, bench or play? *Phys Sports Med* 1993;21(8):23–34.) *B.* A face-down injured player is assessed for level of consciousness, presence of neck pain, or neurologic symptoms. *C.* If immobilization is required, the team leader grasps the trapezius area and inner shoulder pad while holding the head between the shoulder pads. When there are enough assistants available, a second person may assist in immobilizing the head and neck region. *D–E.* The team leader calls the signal to roll the athlete to the upright position or to the spine board.

Testing by this method is a quick screen and is tolerated by athletes with almost any neck or shoulder injury. If these tests are well tolerated, supraspinatus (suprascapular nerve), serratus anterior (long thoracic nerve), and trapezius (spinal accessory nerve) muscle strength may then be evaluated. A brief sensory examination seeks deficits in light touch, pinprick and proprioception. Evaluating the symmetry of reflexes on the right and left, comparing upper extremities to lower extremities, and examining for pathologic reflexes (Hoffman and Babinski) and clonus are important. The presence of Horner syndrome (miosis, anhydrosis, enophthalmos, and ptosis) or vasomotor changes in the extremity suggests injury to the sympathetic chain.

DIAGNOSTIC EVALUATION

Whether or not diagnostic imaging is performed after head trauma depends on the grade of concussion or brain injury and the presenting or developing symptoms. MRI is used increasingly over CT, owing to its sensitivity in evaluating anatomic pathology in athletes with moderate or severe concussions (31). It is more sensitive for visualizing DAI and focal brain syndromes such as inferior frontal and temporal lobe contusions (31,33). MRI is also more sensitive in detecting the edema of nonhemorrhagic contusions and contusions in the brain stem and posterior fossa (119). It also distinguished between intra-axial and extra-axial fluid collections. CT is superior for imaging and assessing bony detail in suspected fractures (5).

Evaluation by electroencephalography (EEG) has not proved to be a sensitive indicator of minor brain dysfunction (43). Some health care practitioners recommend neuropsychological testing as a sensitive means to monitor cumulative problems following a head injury, especially when making decisions with regards to allowing athletes to return to play (42). Unfortunately this is not always practical or cost-effective.

Radiographic Examination of the Cervical Spine

If there is suspicion of a severe cervical spinal injury, cervical x-ray studies should be performed immediately; otherwise, they can be performed within 24 hours after the injury (63). Bony or ligamentous injuries may be evident radiographically, by changes either in the configuration of the anatomic elements or in their alignment. Prior to "clearing" an athlete's cervical spine, plain radiographs should be obtained to rule out dislocation or instability, as well as potential congenital anomalies such as fused vertebrae, Klippel-Feil syndrome, or odontoid abnormalities, which may complicate return to play. This requires an adequate cross-table lateral radiograph taken while the athlete is still immobilized. All cervical vertebrae and the cervicothoracic junction must be well visualized. Boger straps (straps applied to the athlete's arms to create downward traction) may be utilized in the conscious athlete to acquire full visualization of the cervical spine at the cervicothoracic junction (71,104). A swimmer's view, with the arm closest to the cassette extended overhead, may be beneficial. If these attempts to fully visualize the cervical spine and the cervicothoracic junction are unsuccessful, CT may be necessary (71).

Lateral radiographs will allow evaluation of a number of critical elements (Fig. 64-6). It is one of the most important views for cervical spine trauma, as 90% of significant pathology is detected (52). However, when cross-table lateral views *alone* are utilized to screen for cervical injury, up to 20% of unstable fractures are missed (120). The height of the disk spaces should be equal at each level and uniform throughout a given disk space. The presence of significant prevertebral swelling is suggestive of a serious spinal injury. The prevertebral soft tissues anterior to C3 should not exceed 4 mm and at C5, it should be equal to or less than the sagittal dimension of the C5 vertebral body (72,121). The anterior and posterior margin of the vertebral bodies and spinolaminar line should demonstrate a continuous concave curve. Deviation of this arch could indicate ligamentous instability or muscle spasm. Unilateral facet dislocations can be visualized on lateral radiographs as an abrupt change in orientation of the vertebral bodies. The cervical spine will appear lateral in one region and more oblique in another (122).

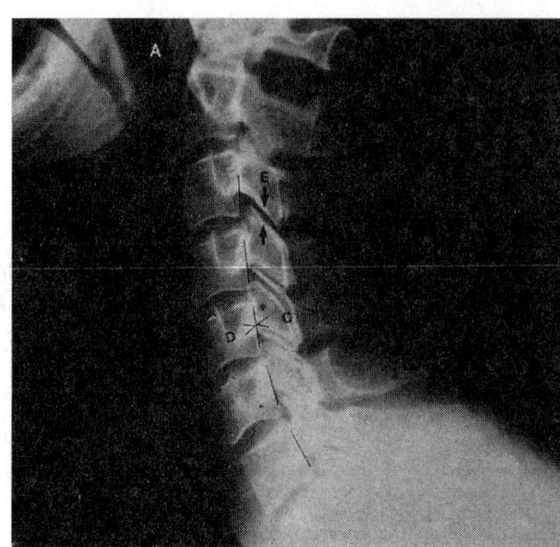

Figure 64-6. A normal lateral cervical spine radiograph. *A* = the atlanto-dens interval (ADI) (the distance between the anterior arc of C1 and the anterior aspect of the odontoid); C = the canal diameter (measured from the midpoint of the posterior aspect of the vertebral body to the nearest point of the spinal laminar line); D = the vertebral body diameter; E = superior and inferior facet joints. The *solid lines* represent the posterior aspects of the vertebral bodies. The Torg-Pavlov ratio is determined by dividing the canal diameter by the vertebral body diameter. (Reproduced by permission from Torg JS, Pavlov H, Geneuaro SE, et al. Neuropraxia of the cervical spinal cord with transient quadriplegia. *J Bone Joint Surg [Am]* 1986;68:1354–1370.)

Lateral radiographs also allow assessment of the atlanto-dens interval (ADI) (see Fig. 64-6). The ADI is the distance between the anterior arch of C1 and the anterior aspect of the odontoid and is normally less than 3 mm (123). An increase in the ADI between 3 to 5 mm on flexion and extension views generally indicates injury to the transverse ligament, and an increase of more than 5 mm indicates potential injury to the transverse, alar, and accessory ligaments (72,85).

An anterior-posterior view permits visualization of the alignment of the uncovertebral joints and the spinous processes. Deviation of these elements may be indicative of ligamentous instability (72). The tracheal air shadow should be midline. The disk spaces should be of equal height and uniform in the anterior to posterior dimension. An increase in the interpedicular distance at a given level compared to others is indicative of a burst fracture (71). Oblique views should be taken to better visualize the pedicles, lateral masses, intervertebral foramina, and facet joints (72). Standard plain film views should also include an open-mouth odontoid view. There should be no significant lateral overhang of the lateral masses of C1 on C2. A lateral overhang of over 7 mm on open-mouth odontoid views may indicate a ruptured transverse ligament or a Jefferson fracture (85,124). An open-mouth odontoid view will help determine the presence and location of a fracture. The latter is important for determining stability of the fracture (2). At times the posterior arch of C1 may project over the base of the odontoid, creating a horizontal radiolucent line, simulating a fracture (71).

Flexion of the cervical spine will normally produce narrowing of the anterior disk space with fanning or a gradual increase in the interspinous distance. The latter is more pronounced in the upper cervical region of the spine. Any increase in the degree of angulation and translation on flexion and extension lateral views of the vertebrae must be noted. Horizontal translation of more than 3.5 mm between adjacent vertebrae of the lower cervical region is considered to be significant (125). In adolescents it may be normal to have slight ligamentous laxity at C2–C3 and C3–C4, resulting in mild subluxation (1–2 mm) (5,52,125). The angle formed between lines drawn parallel to the inferior end-plates of adjacent vertebral bodies from C3 to C7 should not be more than 11 degrees (125). White and Panjabi (125) developed additional criteria for determination of clinical instability of the lower cervical spine (Table 64-4) (see Return to Play Criteria). If the athlete has residual neck stiffness and adequate flexion and extension films have not been obtained, the athlete should not be returned to competition (126). It is important to remember that radiographic features alone do not always correlate with the severity of injury or potential neurologic damage. An x-ray film taken after the injury does not consider the amount of energy that was dissipated through the spinal column at the time of the injury (73).

Congenital or developmental cervical stenosis in the sagittal plane may predispose an athlete to spinal cord injury. Congenital stenosis may be associated with other forms of congenital malformations such as hemivertebrae, congenital fusion, or spina bifida. These abnormalities may be more important criteria for exclusion from contact sports than a small degree of stenosis, as they may result in abnormal segmental motion. Developmental spinal stenosis may be a result of generalized local or segmental narrowing of the central or foraminal canal due to degenerative changes. Either soft-tissue or bony elements may cause encroachment on neural structures. The degenerative changes that can cause developmental stenosis are hypertrophy of the ligamentum flavum, osteophytic spurring of the vertebral body end-plates and uncinate processes, hyperostotic spurring of the ligamentum flavum, and hypertrophy of the anterior facet capsules.

Table 64-4: Checklist for the Diagnosis of Clinical Instability in the Lower Cervical Spine

Elements	**Point Value***
Anterior elements destroyed or unable to function	2
Posterior elements destroyed or unable to function	2
Relative sagittal plane transition 3.5 mm (measured on lateral flexion/extension films)	2
Relative sagittal plane rotation 11 degrees (measured on lateral films)	2
Positive stretch test	2
Nerve root damage	1
Abnormal disk narrowing	1
Dangerous loading anticipated	1

* Total of 5 or more indicates an unstable spine.
Source: Adapted with permission from White AA III, Punjabi M. *Clinical biomechanics of the spine.* 2nd ed. Philadelphia: JB Lippincott, 1990:38–79.

The most commonly utilized method for determining sagittal spinal canal diameter is to measure the distance between the middle of the posterior surface of the vertebral body and the nearest point on the spinal laminar line (71,126) (see Fig. 64-6). The normal sagittal diameter of the cervical canal below C3 is approximately 17 mm when measured on a lateral plain radiograph (127). According to Wolf et al (128), the normal spinal cord diameter is 15 mm or more. Kesler (129) and Countee and Vijayanathant (130) observed that a cervical sagittal canal diameter of less than 14 mm (at a target distance of 6 feet) fell below two standard deviations from the mean in any cervical segment. Despite standardized techniques, variable distances used in radiographic technique have altered interpretation.

Pavlov et al (126) attempted to resolve the problem of varying distances based on the x-ray technique by calculating the ratio of the spinal canal diameter to the sagittal width of the vertebral body. The ratio technique compensates for variations in radiographic technique, as both the sagittal diameter of the canal and that of the vertebral body would be affected in a similar manner by any magnification factors. In a study by Torg and Pavlov (88), many of the young athletes who had documented episodes of cervical cord neuropraxia had a Torg-Pavlov ratio of 0.8 or less in at least one or more levels.

In 1989, Herzog et al (131) calculated the Torg-Pavlov ratio of 80 professional football players with the San Francisco 49ers during training camp. Of the 464 cervical vertebral levels studied, there were 100 (approximately 25%) abnormal ratios. However, stenosis could be confirmed with multiplanar CT at only 12 of the 100 levels. Therefore, the sensitivity of the ratio was high (92%) but the specificity low (12%).

Penning (90) measured the sagittal diameter of the cervical spine during flexion and extension. The diameter was measured from the inferior portion of the superior vertebral body to the closest portion of the spinal laminar line of the inferior vertebra. The *pincher mechanism* occurs when the spinal cord is pinched between the aforementioned opposing bony processes of the spinal canal. If the sagittal diameter is less than 11 mm in extension, the potential for spinal cord compression exists (90). Hyperextension injuries may also cause infolding of the ligamentum flavum, which narrowed the central spinal canal by up to an additional 30% in one study or by 2 to 3 mm in another (128,132).

Cantu (133) proposed that bone measurements alone could not define spinal stenosis. MRI or CT myelography demonstrates the relative size of the spinal canal to the nerve tissue with the amount of functional reserve between the cord and the bony canal. Functional spinal stenosis is present when a spinal canal is so small that it obliterates the CSF around the cord or deforms the cord itself. In a small percentage of professional football players with spinal stenosis (defined as canal size measured by MRI two standard deviations below the mean), none experienced spinal cord symptoms or had functional cervical spinal stenosis (131). Yu et al (134) contended that a sagittal diameter of less than 15.5 mm and a cross-sectional diameter of less than 55 mm^2 places an athlete at risk for neurologic injury during extension. Some practitioners advocate that functional spinal stenosis is the greater concern, and if it coexists in an athlete who incurs spinal cord symptoms (even TQ), no further participation in contact or collision sports should be allowed (133,135). Cantu and Mueller (3) reported five athletes who became quadriplegic after TQ episodes, with two having clear evidence and three having equivocal evidence of functional spinal stenosis.

When one is evaluating stenosis by MRI or CT myelography, it is important to define the relative contributions of each degenerative component. CT without contrast enhancement will usually not adequately demonstrate neural impingement (136). CT myelography works well to differentiate between spondylitic spurs and disk herniations (137). MRI is superior to CT myelography or myelography alone for the anatomic evaluation of radiculopathy and myelopathy (138). It evaluates the effect of degenerative changes or developmental narrowing on neural structures (137), as well as the degree of dural and spinal cord compression (102). Due to MRI's superior soft-tissue imaging, it can also exclude a number of different pathologic processes that can mimic symptoms of cervical myelopathy, including demyelinating or metastatic disease and intradural or extradural spinal cord tumors.

Overall, MRI is superior to CT, except in demonstrating cervical spine fractures. If there is suspicion of an occult fracture, CT is the preferred imaging course. CT is useful for detecting fracture fragments in the spinal canal or neuroforamina. Coronal and sagittal reconstruction or three-dimensional processing enhances the information obtained. This requires 1.5-mm contiguous slices or 3-mm slices at 2-mm intervals for good images (52). Conventional tomography is often preferred for the evaluation of odontoid fractures, facet or posterior element fractures, or when the fracture planes may be parallel to the CT image plane (52).

TREATMENT AND REHABILITATION

Rehabilitation of head injuries depends on the specific diagnosis and any associated cranial or cervical injuries. The head-injured athlete may be able to perform aerobic and low-level progressive resistance exercises, depending on the intensity and type of postconcussion symptoms present. Clinical judgment must be utilized during the recovery phase when determining what types of conditioning the patient is capable of performing. The athletes with persistent cognitive dysfunction may require cognitive rehabilitation. Persistent lack of judgment and reaction time may preclude resumption of contact sports.

Rehabilitation of cervical spinal injuries must be diagnosis specific. This process was described by Kibler et al (139) and applied to cervical spine rehabilitation by Cole et al (15). It should address not only the primary source of pain, but also any secondary and tertiary sources. Subclinical adaptations that may not be painful or part of the active clinical symptom complex must also be treated to ensure complete rehabilitation.

From a tissue injury standpoint, cervical injuries may be classified as mild (class 1), moderate (class 2), severe (class 3), very severe (class 4), and catastrophic (class 5) (140). Most injuries that fall within the mild category are stable cervical sprains and strains and neuropraxic brachial plexus injuries. Most athletes with mild injuries do not require immobilization or surgery and may immediately begin a rehabilitation program. The injured region is loaded in a protected fashion to promote healing yet prevent the deleterious effects of immobilization. The moderate cervical injuries include anterior compression fractures and facet joint or intervertebral disk injuries. Management of athletes in this category may require a short period of immobilization followed by an appropriate rehabilitation program. Immobilization should be discontinued at the earliest opportunity. Cervical spinal injuries included in the severe category are fractures and unstable injuries with subluxation or dislocation without neurologic involvement. Very severe injuries include fractures or dislocations of the cervical spine that occur with partial or complete quadriplegia. Management of severe and very severe injuries always requires either immobilization or surgical stabilization prior to rehabilitation.

Injuries that can be treated with nonsurgical methods are 1) a stable isolated laminar or spinous process fracture and avulsions of the tip of the odontoid without neurologic impairment; 2) stable compression fracture of the vertebal body without neurologic deficit; 3) nondisplaced fractures of the lateral masses, without neurologic deficit; 4) soft-tissue or ligamentous injuries without detectable neurologic deficit; 5) some unstable cervical spine fractures or fracture dislocations without neurologic deficit; and 6) stable reduced facet dislocations without neurologic deficit (70,73). The latter are usually treated with a Minerva jacket/brace until lateral flexion-extension radiographs do not demonstrate instability. Fractures of the body of C2, the base of the odontoid, or Jefferson fractures are usually treated with a halo brace for 3 months (124). A C1 to C2 fusion usually follows if there is evidence of instability. Fusion incorporates the occiput when a posterior arch fracture associated with ligament rupture has not healed. Fractured odontoid bases have a high nonunion rate following immobilization and may later require a C1 to C2 fusion (124). Hangman fractures are usually treated with traction and reduction with subsequent application of a halo brace for 3 months. Residual instability is typically treated with a C2 to C3 anterior fusion. Unilateral facet dislocations without facet fracture reduce readily and may be treated with a halo brace. Postimmobilization instability may also require surgical stabilization.

Surgery is generally the recommended treatment for the following injuries: 1) most unstable fractures with or without neurologic deficit; 2) unstable ligamentous injuries without neurologic deficit with anterior subluxation of more than 20%, or unstable ligamentous injuries with neurologic deficit with less than 20% anterior subluxation; 3) type II and III atlantoaxial fractures and dislocations with nonunion or instability; and 4) unreduced comminuted cervical compression injuries (73). Bilateral facet dislocations may be treated with a halo brace or posterior interspinous wiring and fusion. The latter is typically preferred to expedite the rehabilitation process. Severe burst fractures with quadriplegia generally require anterior and posterior fusion with decompression of the canal.

After a cervical injury, it may be difficult to predict which injuries will lead to instability or a neurologic deficit. The guidelines established by White and Panjabi (125) were created to diagnose clinically significant instability. They were developed after a series of cadaver studies in which the various supporting structures were systematically sacrificed and the resulting instabilities in the spine noted. The systematic basis for determining instability utilizes a point value for elements present on clinical or radiographic examination. If the points total 5 or more, then the lower cervical spine should be considered clinically unstable (see Table 64-4). This checklist is applied after appropriate clinical examination and radiographic studies. Instability may require surgical stabilization.

Whether the athlete begins rehabilitation immediately or begins after a period of immobilization or surgery, progression through appropriate phases of rehabilitation is critical. The rehabilitation of any musculoskeletal injury is typically divided into three phases: 1) acute phase, 2) restoration phase, and 3) maintenance phase (139). When immobilization is not required for fracture or ligamentous healing, early motion is initiated in the acute phase of rehabilitation. The deleterious effects of immobilization and decreased joint motion on soft tissues and bone are well known (141–144). There is an increase in soft-tissue shortening and collagen fiber cross-linkages, resulting in increased stiffness and joint contracture. Muscle atrophy occurs very quickly following injury and immobilization. Estimates of decreases in muscular strength range between 1% and 5% per day (142). The injury itself may inhibit muscular action through neural or chemical mechanisms (145). While this initially helps to protect the injured region from further injury, it may accentuate abnormal biomechanics later on and thus must be controlled. Chemical mediators may cause inhibition of the agonistic muscle and spasm in the antagonistic muscle. Strengthening should proceed within a reasonably pain-free range of motion, as excessive pain during rehabilitation only reinitiates chemical and neural mechanisms that inhibit muscle contraction and initiate muscle spasm (63).

During the acute phase of rehabilitation, the signs and symptoms of tissue injury are treated (15). First, pain and inflammation are reduced. Restoration of pain-free range of motion and of normal resting muscle length and improved neuromuscular postural control must be addressed as rapidly as possible. When rigid immobilization is not required, passive bracing with a soft cervical collar may be beneficial for a short period of time. The collar should be weaned within the first 1 to 2 weeks. Education involves instructing the patient to develop an awareness of the aggravating activities, and solutions for relieving pain through positioning, stretching, and passive modalities. Joint protection and body mechanics should be taught so that the athlete does not reinjure the area during activities of daily living (ADLs).

Muscle atrophy and strength losses are minimized by isometric exercises or exercises in the pain-free range of motion. Low-impact conditioning of unaffected areas should continue if clinically appropriate to prevent a protracted reconditioning period. An active form of joint protection involves instruction in cervicothoracic stabilization training (CTST) (145). "Stabilization training optimizes the capacity of the cervicothoracic spine to absorb loads in all directions while it minimizes direct stress and strain on individual cervical tissues" (145). The goals of cervicothoracic stabilization are to 1) gain dynamic control of external spinal forces; 2) minimize repetitive injury to disks, facet joints, and other soft tissues; 3) promote healing of injured areas; and 4) attempt to alter the degenerative process (15,145).

Protective bracing, patient education, pharmacologic management, physical therapy modalities, manual therapy approaches, and diagnosis-dependent stretching and strengthening exercises may assist the athlete in progressing through the first phase of rehabilitation. At times, trigger point injections or fluoroscopically guided selective injections may be necessary to control an athlete's pain (146). Pharmacologic management and physical therapy modalities are covered in other sections of this textbook.

As mastery of preliminary exercises is achieved during the stabilization program, progressive activities are added to gain further dynamic control of cervicothoracic forces. Strengthening should address the cervical spinal, scapulothoracic, and thoracolumbar musculature. Isometric exercises are usually initiated with the patient in the supine position and then progression to the upright position. When isometric strengthening is tolerated, additional challenges are presented by increasing the range of motion and resistance. Neutral spine strengthening of the thoracic region and the interscapular musculature helps to counteract scapular elevation, protraction, and kyphosis, and emphasizes scapular retraction, depression, and thoracic extension. This is important, as overutilization of scapular stabilizers and abnormal scapulothoracic mechanics can also lead to an overload of cervical spinal structures (145,147). If the athlete moves too rapidly into progressive resistive exercises, he or she may not learn to isolate appropriate muscle groups and thus develop compensatory movement patterns. As kinesthetic awareness is developed, the program may be advanced. If the athlete begins to fatigue and precise repetitions cannot be performed, the exercise should be discontinued.

Significant adaptive soft-tissue shortening may occur after acute injury and must be addressed. Appropriate flexibility in the posterior cervical, anterior chest wall, interscapular, and rotator cuff musculature is critical. Efforts to achieve appropriate flexibility may include active or passive stretching and neuromuscular facilitation (103). In the acute phase of rehabilitation, tissues should be stretched in the second half of the tolerable range of motion with the patient in a neutral spinal posture. Superficial or deep soft-tissue mobilization, manual traction, and passive joint mobilization may be useful. Massage may help increase flexibility and improve circulation to expedite healing and removal of inflammatory by-products (148). Soft-tissue techniques help to decrease pain in the setting of shortened shoulder girdle musculature, expediting joint mobilization and restoration of normal joint mechanics. Passive joint motion through mobilization or manipulation stretches joint capsules, lubricates tissues, and induces metabolic changes in soft tissue, cartilage, and bone (149). Mobilization is the application of a force along the rotational or translational plane of motion of a joint. At times, high-velocity manipulation performed by a skilled clinician may be of benefit (149). Mechanical therapy based on the McKenzie method of assessment may also be useful in determining a directional preference of motion, so the athlete can be taught repetitive motions that may decrease pain from postural syndromes, soft-tissue dysfunction problems, or structural derangements (150).

When pain inhibits rehabilitation and aggressive conservative care, injection therapy may be beneficial. Trigger point injections at primary points of myofascial pain or at the end points of referred pain may decrease muscular tone and improve muscular flexibility (57). Diagnostic and fluoroscopically guided, contrast-enhanced, facet, selective nerve root, or epidural steroid injections provide therapeutic benefit by decreasing pain so that rehabilitation can progress (146).

The restorative phase of rehabilitation addresses both tissue overload and mechanical dysfunction. Decreased pain, improved cervical range of motion, soft-tissue length, and biomechanics are prerequisites to entering this phase. The goals of this phase of rehabilitation are to 1) eliminate the majority of the athlete's pain, 2) normalize spinal and shoulder girdle mechanics, and 3) improve neuromuscular control of the injured areas (15). Muscular re-education may be necessary during preliminary strength training to ensure that appropriate motor engrams are reinforced. Once motor coordination has been reinforced, the speed and duration of resistance may be increased. The final component of this phase includes functional conditioning and sports-specific training.

The last phase of rehabilitation is the maintenance phase. This phase is often omitted in many rehabilitation programs. It requires that there is functional, nonpainful spinal and shoulder girdle mechanics. In addition, appropriate flexibility, strength, and sports-specific skills are necessary (15). It is at this phase that the athlete usually returns to play; thus, essentially normal clinical findings on examination are required. In collision sports, contact techniques should be reviewed to ensure appropriateness. Dangerous axial loading and other at-risk techniques must be corrected prior to return to play.

RETURN TO PLAY CRITERIA

Return to Play After Concussion

Concussion management depends on its grade and the guidelines utilized (see Tables 64-1, 64-2, and 64-3). Available protocols require repeat assessments of the athlete at specific intervals. Strich (30) demonstrated that an athlete's chance of a repeat concussion may be four times greater than that of an athlete who has never had a concussion. However, Cantu (39) indicated that if the athlete has fully recovered from a concussion, the risk of subsequent concussion is not increased.

The lack of consensus on return to play between the guidelines by Cantu and Micheli (21), Nelson et al (23), and the Colorado Medical Society (22) has been described. All agree that return to play is not allowed as long as there are postconcussive symptoms. These guidelines differ in how long to wait to return to play after the symptoms clear. Time frames are empiric, since there is a paucity of influential scientific data. Additionally there is no simple, objective test to evaluate the severity of an injury or recovery from it. Return to play is often determined by the presence or absence of subjective symptoms. Although the guidelines differ on their timetable for return to play, each physician must adopt guidelines that are enforceable with athletes, coaches, and parents when applicable. The physician must remember that these are "guidelines" and that sound clinical judgment must be utilized on an individual basis.

The Colorado guidelines are stringent. As an example, even the briefest loss of consciousness is considered "severe" and hospital evaluation is recommended (22). There is no return to play until 1 month after the athlete is asymptomatic for 2 weeks. According to Cantu (21,39), a mild concussion mandates removal from competition with observation on the sidelines for a minimum of 30 minutes. The athlete may not return to play if there was loss of consciousness or persistent postconcussive symptoms such as headache, dizziness, disorientation, or concentration or memory problems during rest or exertion. Other postconcussive symptoms that may be demonstrated include diplopia, behavioral problems, generalized fatigue, and sleeping and eating disturbances. These symptoms may not be volunteered as concussion related and may only be revealed upon asking friends, relatives, and coaches. Cantu (39,151) recommends examination by the team physician prior to return to play. All symptoms must be resolved at rest and during exertion, prior to return to play.

After a second mild concussion, Cantu (39) recommends removal from competition for at least 2 weeks and evaluation with CT to ensure that there are no intracranial abnormalities prior to return to play. After being out of play for 2 weeks, return to play is allowed only if the symptoms have resolved for at least 1 week during rest and exertion. Current recommendations by the American College of Sports Medicine are that three grade I concussions terminate that athlete's season and that the athlete may not engage in a contact sport for a minimum of 3 months (21). At that time, the athlete may return to contact activity if he or she has been asymptomatic at rest and during exertion for that 3-month period.

A moderate concussion as defined by Cantu requires removal of the athlete from competition and immediate evaluation by the team physician. The athlete should have an emergency neurosurgical evaluation if there is a prolonged disturbance in consciousness. This grade concussion may necessitate CT or MRI within the first 24 hours. The athlete should be examined often for signs of potential intracranial pathology (151). After the first moderate concussion, the patient may return to competition as soon as 1 week after the resolution of symptoms during rest and exertion. After a second moderate concussion, return to contact should be suspended for at least 1 month. Termination of the season should be considered following a third moderate concussion. If there is any evidence of intracranial pathology on CT or MRI scans after the first or second grade II concussion, the season should be terminated.

A severe concussion by Cantu's definition mandates immediate transport from competition to an emergency room facility with advanced imaging capabilities and a neurosurgeon on call (39,151). Upon discharge from the medical facility, ongoing assessment will determine whether that athlete may return to play. If the brain scan is normal, the athlete may return to play 1 month after the injury if there have been no postconcussive symptoms for at least 1 week during rest and exertion. Noncontact conditioning drills may be resumed prior to that 1-month period, if the patient is totally asymptomatic. If the athlete should have a second severe concussion within the same season, the season is terminated.

Certain conditions will contraindicate return to contact or collision sports after concussion or other forms of brain injury. These include 1) the presence of persistent postconcussion symptoms; 2) spontaneous subarachnoid hemorrhage; 3) permanent central neurologic sequelae such as the presence of a homonymous hemianopsia, paresis, or organic dementia; or 4) posttraumatic seizure disorder (20). Clinical judgment must be utilized when determining whether to return an athlete to play when there are mild persistent abnormalities on neuropsychological tests, without other subjective or objective signs or symptoms.

Return to Play After a Cervical Injury

Torg (140) developed criteria for classifying cervical injuries as well as criteria for return to play for each class of injury. More recent recommendations for absolute, relative, and no contraindications for return to collision sports after cervical injuries are summarized in Table 64-5 (152).

After a mild cervical spine injury as defined by Torg (140), athletes who formally have been given a clinical diagnosis and who are asymptomatic and have full cervical range of motion, full muscle strength, and stability of the cervical spine on flexion and extension films may return to play (127). These injuries include cervical sprains, intervertebral disk injuries without neurologic involvement, and stable wedge compression fractures that are at least 3 months old.

The moderate group of cervical injuries include compression fractures and facet joint or intervertebral disk changes without neurologic involvement (140). Athletes within the moderate class of injuries who have a stable spine with subsequent full pain-free range of motion may participate with precautions. Either the underage athlete and parents, or the adult athlete need to be fully informed of the potential for further degenerative changes and problems associated with the injury, if there is a return to contact or collision sports. Clinical judgment must be used when considering return to play issues and the classification of the sport (contact/collision, limited contact/impact, strenuous noncontact) in an athlete with a herniated disk without neurologic involvement but with continued symptoms.

Cervical spinal injuries included in the severe category are 1) fractures with neurologic involvement, 2) unstable injuries with subluxation or dislocation, and 3) acute herniated intervertebral disks with neurologic involvement (140). Most athletes in the severe injury category will not return to contact or collision sports but may be able to return to less rigorous sports depending on residual symptoms. Decisions should be made on a case-by-case basis.

Neurologic abnormalities due to injuries around the foramen magnum and first two cervical segments preclude return to contact or collision sports. Return to contact sports may be considered after appropriate rehabilitation in athletes with successful one-level anterior interbody decompression and fusion for herniated nucleus pulposus or anterior instability, if they have full range of motion and strength (141). Congenitally or surgically fused segments may result in long-term sequelae to adjacent motion segments. The athlete should be thoroughly counseled regarding the possibility of intervertebral disk changes or

Table 64-5: Guidelines for Return to Contact After Cervical Injury
Absolute contraindications
Occipital or atlantoaxial instability
Atlantoaxial rotatory fixation
Healed upper cervical fractures except those that are relative contraindications
C1–C2 fusion
Lower cervical spine instability
Lower vertebral fractures: 1) vertebral body fracture with sagittal component; 2) vertebral body fracture with posterior column damage; 3) comminuted vertebral body fractures with displaced fragments into the spinal canal; 4) healed anterior or posterior element fracture with pain, limitation of motion, or associated neurologic findings; 5) healed displaced fractures of the lateral masses with facet incongruity
Acute disk herniation
Chronic disk herniation with associated pain, limitation of motion, or associated neurologic findings
Three-level anterior or posterior fusion
Relative contraindications
Healed nondisplaced Jefferson fractures
Healed type I and II odontoid fractures
Healed lateral mass fractures of C2
Healed fractures without pain, limitation of motion, or associated neurologic findings: 1) vertebral body compression fractures without sagittal component; 2) elements of the posterior ring
Conservatively or surgically treated disk disease with facet instability
Stable two-level fusion without pain, limitation of motion, or associated neurologic findings
No contraindication
Healed disk herniation, conservatively or surgically treated (diskectomy or fusion) without pain, limitation of motion, or associated neurologic findings
Healed stable compression or end-plate fractures without sagittal or posterior element component
Healed Clay Shoveler fracture
Spina bifida occulta without other segmentation anomalies

Source: Torg JS, Ramsey-Emrhein JA. Management guidelines for participation in collision activities with congenital, developmental or post-injury lesions involving the cervical spine. *Clin Sports Med* 1997;16:501–530.

herniation at an adjacent level (104,140). The level of the fused segment is taken into consideration. With each increasing cephalad level, the cervical spine is less able to absorb axial loading stresses and dissipate forces (104). Anterior or posterior fusion at more than a one-level prohibits return to contact sports (104,140). There is a significantly increased risk of injury above and below this longer lever-arm fusion mass. These athletes are considered on an individual basis for return to noncontact sports.

Very severe injuries include fractures or dislocations of the cervical spine that occur with partial or complete quadriplegia (140). Quadriplegia athletes may return to limited-contact or noncontact sports depending on the level of the lesion and availability of adaptive equipment. Many paraplegics and incomplete quadriplegics may return to limited-contact sports. Almost any sport is permissible as long as the risks of increased neurologic damage with falls are minimal, discussed, and accepted.

Return to Play After an Episode of Transient Quadriplegia

There continues to be controversy regarding return to play criteria following an episode of TQ (55,89,133,135). In making these decisions, the physician must consider spinal stability, functional reserve, spinal cord integrity, MRI results, electrophysiologic findings, and the athlete's expectations and goals regarding future sports participation. If instability has been ruled out and stenosis continues to be suspected, then MRI or CT is necessary.

If the athlete with TQ has normal findings on radiographic and neurologic examinations with full pain-free range of motion of the neck, then he or she may be permitted to play. Torg et al (70,89) believe that there is no evidence that an episode of TQ predisposes an athlete to permanent neurologic injury. Their retrospective interviews of athletes with spinal cord injury revealed no preceding incidents of TQ (88). More recently, Torg and Ramsey-Emrhein (152) proposed more stringent guidelines for return to contact or collision sports in athletes with an episode of TQ. A *relative contraindication* is one episode of cord neuropraxia and a ratio of 0.8 or less or intervertebral disk degenerative changes. A *relative/absolute contraindication* is one episode of cord neuropraxia associated with cord edema by MRI. An *absolute contraindication* is an episode of cord neuropraxia with associated instability, neurologic deficits persisting beyond 36 hours, or multiple episodes. The player (and parents) should be warned that there may be a greater risk for TQ, but not necessarily permanent neurologic damage.

The medical literature suggests that functional spinal stenosis predisposes to spinal cord injury and thus should prevent an athlete with an episode of TQ from returning to contact sports (55,133,135). The presence of a second episode mandates another complete work-up (153). Although normal imaging findings and neurologic work-up results allow return to competition, some practitioners think there should be serious discussion regarding termination of contact sports.

Return to Play After a Stinger

Decisions regarding return to play after a stinger should not be taken lightly and can pose diagnostic and prognostic challenges. Excluding other potential injuries besides a nerve root or plexus injury is important in making the appropriate decisions regarding return to play. All too often, athletes, trainers, and coaches assume the athlete has a stinger and do not consider a more serious injury.

Clancy et al (99) presented a grading scale for brachial plexus injuries in sports. Studies by Robertson et al (110) demonstrated that electromyography (EMG) was more sensitive than clinical examination in detecting neurologic changes; however, they were not included in return to play criteria. Most clinicians utilize lack of clinical weakness as the sole criterion for return to play. Complete electrophysiologic assessment would help to establish a specific diagnosis and prognosis when assessing athletes with prolonged neurologic deficits. Early electrodiagnostic examination is the best means of differentiating an incomplete, recovering brachial plexus lesion from a pure peripheral nerve lesion (97). Needle EMG is the most sensitive test for determining the presence of even mild axonal loss (97,154–156). Lack of paraspinal findings when spontaneous potentials can be found in a single root distribution does not rule out a more proximal radiculopathy. The detection of moderate spontaneous potentials at rest by needle EMG usually seen in the deltoid, biceps, supraspinous, and infrequently the brachioradial muscles in the context of clinical weakness is the most important electrodiagnostic factor in influencing return to play decisions in athletes with brachial plexus lesions (97,155). The presence of polyphasic potentials during motor unit recruitment without spontaneous potentials is not enough to withhold an athlete from play (97). Currently, use of serial EMG studies in influencing return to play decisions is not widespread (97).

An athlete with a resolving stinger should not be permitted to return to contact sports until he or she is asymptomatic. Specifically, this implies an absence of neck tenderness, muscle spasm or arm pain, numbness, or paresthesias. There must be adequate rehabilitation of any residual muscular weakness and the athlete must demonstrate normal biomechanics at the neck and shoulder girdle (111,157). The athlete's sports-specific biomechanics should be evaluated. It is important to note that athletes with brachial plexus lesions are not necessarily at risk for a spinal cord injury. However, the presence of associated neck injuries, TQ, peripheral nerve injuries, or shoulder injuries may occur alone or in combination with a brachial plexus lesion. Two or three stingers within one season preclude return to contact sports, owing to an increased risk of permanent nerve damage.

CONCLUSIONS

The increased size, speed, and strength of athletes has resulted in increased forces applied to their head and neck. Controlled spinal motion through adequate strength, flexibility, and endurance of the spinal segments will assist in buffering the forces that are applied to the cervical region of the spine. Emphasis should continue to be placed on appropriate preseason screening evaluations to identify those at risk for injury. Instruction to athletes, coaches, and trainers concerning appropriate sport technique and other preventative measures should continue.

When sports-related head and neck injuries do occur, appropriate evaluation and treatment require that the physiatrist have a thorough understanding of sports biomechanics and associated injury patterns. Appropriate on-field assessment will help to minimize catastrophic outcomes. A high index of suspicion is critical. A precise diagnosis is necessary to initiate appropriate management and subsequent rehabilitation of the injured athlete.

REFERENCES

1. Cantu RC. Head and neck injuries. In: Mueller FO, Ryan AJ, eds. *Prevention of athletic injuries: the role of the sports medicine team.* Philadelphia: FA Davis, 1991:201–203.
2. Torg JS. Anecdotal observations. In: Torg JS, ed. *Athletic injuries to the head, neck, and face.* 2nd ed. St. Louis: Mosby Year Book, 1991:3–14.
3. Cantu RC, Mueller FO. Catastrophic spine injuries in football, 1977–1989. *J Spinal Disord* 1990;(3):227–231.
4. Bishop PJ, Wells RP. Cervical spine fractures; mechanisms, neck loads, and methods of prevention. In: Castaldi CR, Hoerner EF, eds. *Safety in ice hockey.* Philadelphia: American Society for Testing and Materials, 1989:971–983.
5. Cantu RC. Head and spine injuries in youth sports. *Clin Sports Med* 1995;14:517.
6. Clark K. An epidemiologic view. In: Torg JS, ed. *Athletic injuries to the head, neck and face.* 2nd ed. St. Louis: Mosby Year Book, 1991:15–27.
7. Mueller FO, Blyth CS, Cantu RC. Catastrophic spine injuries in football. *Phys Sports Med* 1989;17(10):51–53.

8. Tator CH, Edmonds VE. National survey of spinal injuries in hockey players. *Can Med Assoc J* 1984;130:875.

9. Tator CH, Edmonds VE, Lapeczak L, et al. Spinal injuries in ice hockey players, 1966–1987. *Can J Surg* 1991;34:63–69.

10. Torg JS, Vegso JJ, O'Neil M, et al. The epidemiologic, pathologic, biomechanical, and cinematographic analysis of football induced cervical spine trauma. *Am J Sports Med* 1990;18:50–57.

11. Bruce PA, Schut L, Sutton LN. Brain and cervical spine injuries occurring during organized sports activities in children and adolescents. *Clin Sports Med* 1982;1:496.

12. Shields CL, Stauffer ES. Cervical cord injuries in sports. *Phys Sports Med* 1978;6:71.

13. Albright JP, Moses JM, Feldnick HG. Nonfatal cervical spine injuries in interscholastic football. *JAMA* 1976;236:1243.

14. Mueller FO, Blyth CS. Fatalities from head and cervical spine injuries occurring in tackle football: 40 years experience. *Clin Sports Med* 1977;6:185–196.

15. Cole AJ, Farrell JP, Stratton SA. Cervical spine athletic injuries: a pain in the neck. *Phys Med Rehabil Clin N Am* 1994;5(1):37–68.

16. Bruno LA, Gennarelli TA, Torg JS. Management guidelines for head injuries in athletics. *Clin Sports Med* 1987;6:17–29.

17. Hollborn AHS. The mechanics of brain injuries. *Br Med Bull* 1945:147–149.

18. Ommaya AK. Biomechanical aspects of head injuries in sports. In: Jordan BD, Tsairis P, Warren RF, eds. *Sports neurology.* Rockville, MD: Aspen, 1989.

19. Gennarelli TA. Cerebral concussion and diffuse brain injuries. In: Cooper PR, ed. *Head injury.* Baltimore: Williams & Wilkins, 1987:108–124.

20. Jordan BD. Head injury in sports. In: Jordan BD, Tsairis P, Warren RF, eds. *Sports neurology.* Rockville, MD: Aspen, 1989.

21. Cantu RC, Micheli LJ. *ACSM's guidelines for the team physician.* Philadelphia: Lea & Febiger, 1991:205–208.

22. Colorado Medical Society Sports Medicine Committee. *Guidelines for the management of concussion in sports.* Denver: Colorado Medical Society, 1991.

23. Nelson WE, Jane JA, Gieck JH. Minor head injury in sports: a new system of classification and management. *Phys Sports Med* 1984;12(3):103–107.

24. Swenson EJ Jr, McKeag DB. Minor head injury evaluation: current state of the art: results of survey completed by the AMSSM membership in 1994. Presented at the annual meeting of the American Medical Society for Sports Medicine, Orlando, Florida, June 1996.

25. Yarnell PR, Lynch S. The "ding" amnestic state in football trauma. *Neurology* 1983;23:196.

26. Gennarelli TA, Thibault LE, Adams JH, et al. Diffuse axonal injury and traumatic coma in the primate. In: Dacey RG, Winn HR, Rimel RW, Jane JA, eds. *Trauma of the central nervous system.* New York: Raven, 1985:169–193.

27. Mendelow AD, Teasdale GM. Pathophysiology of head injuries. *Br J Surg* 1983;70:641–650.

28. Gentry LR, Godersky JC, Thompson B, Dunn V. MR imaging of head trauma: review of distribution and radiopathologic features of traumatic lesions. *AJNR* 1988;9:101–110.

29. Adams JH. Head injury. In: Adams JH, Corsellis JN, Duchen LW, eds. *Greenfield's neuropathology.* 4th ed. New York: John Wiley, 1984:85–124.

30. Strich SJ. Shearing of nerve fibres as a cause of brain damage due to head injury: a pathological study of twenty cases. *Lancet* 1961;2:443–448.

31. Gentry LR. Head trauma. In: *Magnetic resonance imaging of the brain and spine.* New York: Raven, 1991:439–466.

32. Lavaca G. Boxer's encephalopathy. *J Sports Med Phys Fitness* 1963;3:87–92.

33. Bruno LA. Focal intracranial hematoma. In: Torg JS, ed. *Athletic injuries to the head, neck and face.* Philadelphia: Lea & Febiger, 1982:105–121.

34. Cooper PR. Post traumatic intracranial mass lesions. In: Cooper PR, ed. *Head injury.* Baltimore: Williams & Wilkins, 1997:238–284.

35. Moore KL. *Clinically oriented anatomy.* Baltimore: Williams & Wilkins, 1980:855–932.

36. Zimmerman RA, Bilaniuk LT. Computed tomography staging of traumatic epidural bleeding. *Radiology* 1982;144:809–812.

37. Schneider RC. *Head and neck injuries in football: mechanisms, treatment and prevention.* Baltimore: Williams & Wilkins, 1973.

38. Gentry LR, Godersky JC, Thompson B, Dunn V. Prospective comparative study of intermediate field MR and CT in the evaluation of closed head trauma. *AJNR* 1988;9:91–100.

39. Cantu RC. Guidelines for return to contact sport after cerebral concussion. *Phys Sports Med* 1986;14(10):75–83.

40. Casson IR, Siegel O, Sharm R, et al. Brain damage in modern boxers. *JAMA* 1984;251: 2663–2667.

41. Ryan AJ. Intracranial injuries resulting from boxing: a review (1918–1985). *Clin Sports Med* 1987;6:31–40.

42. Ross RJ, Casson IR, Siegel O, Cole M. Boxing injuries: neurologic, radiologic and neuropsychologic evaluation. *Clin Sports Med* 1987;6:41–51.

43. Ross RJ, Cole M, Thompson JS, Kim KH. Boxers: computed

tomography, EEG and neurological evaluation. *JAMA* 1983;249:211–213.

44. Jennet B. *Epilepsy after non-missile head injury.* Chicago: Year Book Medical, 1975.

45. Gruber R, Bubl R, Fruttinger V. Anticonvulsant therapy after juvenile craniocerebral injuries: a retrospective evaluation. *Z Kinderchir* 1985;40:199–202.

46. Saunders RL, Harbaugh RE. The second impact in catastrophic contact sports head trauma. *JAMA* 1984;252:538–539.

47. Cantu RC, Voy R. Second impact syndrome: a risk in any contact sport. *Phys Sports Med* 1995;23(6):27–34.

48. Bruce DA, Alive A, Bilaniuk K, et al. Diffuse cerebral swelling following head injuries in children: the syndrome of "malignant brain edema." *J Neuro Surg* 1981;54(2): 10–178.

49. Cantu RC. Second impact syndrome: immediate management. *Phys Sports Med* 1992;20(90): 55–66.

50. Kelly JP, Nichols JS, Philley CM, et al. Concussion in sports: guidelines for the prevention of catastrophic outcome. *JAMA* 1991;266:2867–2869.

51. Roaf R. A study of the mechanics of spinal injuries. *J Bone Joint Surg [Br]* 1984;42:810–823.

52. Berquist TH. *Imaging of sports injuries.* Gaithersburg, MD: Aspen, 1992.

53. Schneider R. The treatment of the athlete with neck, cervical spine and spinal cord trauma. In: Schneider RC, ed. *Sports injuries: mechanism, prevention and treatment.* Baltimore: Williams & Wilkins, 1985.

54. Burstein AH, Otis JC, Torg JS. Mechanics and pathomechanics of athletic injuries to the cervical spine. In: Torg JS, ed. *Athletic injuries to the head, neck, and face.* Philadelphia: Lea & Febiger, 1982:139–142.

55. Anderson C. Neck injuries: backboard, bench or return play? *Phys Sports Med* 1993;21(8):23–34.

56. Babcock JL. Cervical spine injuries. Diagnosis and classification. *Arch Surg* 1976;3:646.

57. Travell JH, Simmons DG. *Myofascial pain and dysfunction: trigger point manual.* Baltimore: Williams & Wilkins, 1983.

58. Stratton SA, Bryan JM. Dysfunction, evaluation and treatment of the cervical spine and thoracic inlet. In: *Orthopedic physical therapy.* 2nd ed. New York: Churchill Livingstone, 1993: 77–122.

59. Rob CG, Standoven A. Arterial occlusion complicating—thoracic outlet compression syndrome. *BMJ* 1958;2:709–712.

60. Roos DB. Congenital anomalies associated with the thoracic outlet syndrome of anatomy, symptoms, diagnosis and treatment. *Am J Surg* 1976;123: 771–778.

61. Kelly TR. Thoracic outlet syndrome: current concepts of treatment. *Ann Surg* 1979;190: 657–662.

62. Calliet R. *Shoulder pain.* Philadelphia: FA Davis, 1981.

63. Wiens JJ, Saal JA. Rehabilitation of the cervical spine and brachial plexus. *Phys Med Rehab State Art Rev* 1987;1:583–595.

64. Kumano K, Yumeyama T. Cervical disc injuries in athletes. *Arch Orthop Trauma Surg* 1986;105:223–226.

65. Barnsley L, Lord S, Bogduk N. Comparative local anaesthetic blocks in the diagnosis of cervical zygapophyseal joint pain. *Pain* 1993;55:99–106.

66. Dwyer A, Aprill C, Bogduk N. Cervical zygapophyseal joint pain patterns. I: a study in normal volunteers. *Spine* 1990;15:453.

67. Dreyfus P, Calodnex A. Cervical facet pain. *Pain Dig* 1993;3: 197–201.

68. Schneider RC, Cherry GR, Pantek H. Syndrome of acute central cervical spinal cord injury with special reference to mechanisms involved in hyperextension injuries of the cervical spine. *J Neurol Surg* 1954;11:546.

69. Jackson DW, Lohr FT. Cervical spine injuries. *Clin Sports Med* 1986;5:373–386.

70. Torg JS. Athletic injuries to the cervical spine. In: Jordan BD, Tsairis P, Warren RF, eds. *Sports neurology.* Rockville, MD: Aspen, 1989.

71. Pavlov H, Torg JS. Roentgen examination of cervical spine injuries in the athlete. *Clin Sports Med* 1987;6:751–766.

72. Thomas JC. Plain roentgenograms of the spine in the injured athlete. *Clin Sports Med* 1986;5:353–371.

73. Torg JS. Management guidelines for athletic injuries to the cervical spine. *Clin Sports Med* 1987;6:53–60.

74. Daffner RH. *Imaging of vertebral trauma.* Gaithersburg, MD: Aspen, 1988.

75. Acheson MB, Livingston RR, Stimade GK. High resolution CT scanning in the evaluation of cervical spine fractures: comparison with plain film examination. *AJR* 1987;148:1179–1185.

76. Torg JS, Vegso JJ, Sennett B. The National Football Head and Neck Registry; 14 year report on cervical quadriplegia (1971–1984). *Clin Sports Med* 1987;6:61–72.

77. Torg JS, Sennett B, Vegso JJ. Spinal injury at the level of third and fourth cervical vertebrae resulting from the axial loading mechanism: an analysis and classification. *Clin Sports Med* 1987;6:159–183.

78. Jefferson G. Fracture of the atlas vertebrae. *Br J Surg* 1920;7: 407.

79. Jevitch V. Horizontal fractures of the anterior arch of the atlas. *J Bone Joint Surg [Am]* 1986;68: 1094–1095.

80. Fielding JE, Hawkins RJ. Atlantoaxial rotatory fixation. *J Bone J Surg [Am]* 1977;59:39–44.

81. Burke JJ, Harris JH. Acute injuries of the axis vertebrae. *Skel Radiol* 1989;18:335–345.

82. Gehweiler JH, Osborne RL, Becker RF. *The radiology of vertebral trauma.* Philadelphia: Saunders, 1980.

83. Anderson LD, D'Alonzo RT. Fracture of the odontoid process of the axis. *J Bone Joint Surg* 1974;56:1663.

84. Cloward RB. Acute cervical spinal injuries. *Ciba Clin Symp* 1980;32:2.

85. Fielding JW, Cochran GV, Lawsing JF III, et al. Tears of the transverse ligament of the atlas. *J Bone Joint Surg [Am]* 1974;56: 1683–1691.

86. Maroon JC. "Burning hands" in football and spinal cord injuries. *JAMA* 1977;238:2049.

87. Wilberger JE, Abla A, Maroon JC. Burning hand syndrome revisited. *Neurosurgery* 1986;19:1038.

88. Torg JS, Pavlov H. Cervical spinal stenosis with cord neuropraxia and transient quadriplegia. *Clin Sports Med* 1987;6:115–133.

89. Torg JS, Pavlov H, Geneuaro SE, et al. Neuropraxia of the cervical spinal cord with transient quadriplegia. *J Bone Joint Surg [Am]* 1986;68:1354–1370.

90. Penning L. Some aspects of plain radiography of the cervical spine in chronic myelopathy. *Neurology* 1962;12:513–519.

91. Kirklady-Willis WH. Managing low back pain. 2nd ed. Edinburgh: Churchill Livingstone, 1988.

92. Feinstein B. Referred pain from paravertebral structures. In: Buerger AA, Tobis JS, eds. *Approaches to the validation of manipulative therapy.* Springfield, IL: Charles C Thomas, 1977: 139–174.

93. Feinstein B, Langton JNK, Jameson RM, et al. Experiments on pain referred from deep somatic tissues. *J Bone Joint Surg [Am]* 1954;36:981–997.

94. Rydevik B, Brown M, Lundborg G. Pathoanatomy and pathophysiology of nerve root compression. *Spine* 1984;9:7–15.

95. Saal J, Franson R, Dobrow R, et al. High levels of phospholipase A_2 activity in lumbar disc herniations. *Spine* 1990;15:683–686.

96. Dumitru D. *Electrodiagnostic medicine.* Philadelphia: Hanley & Belfus, 1995:585–642.

97. Herring SA, Weinstein SM. Electrodiagnosis in sports medicine. *Phys Med Rehabil State Arts Rev* 1989.

98. Wilbourne AJ, Aminoff MJ. Electrophysiologic examination in patients with radiculopathy. AAEE minimonograph #32. *Muscle Nerve* 1988;11:1099–1114.

99. Clancy WG, Brand RL, Bergfield JA. Upper trunk brachial plexus injuries in contact sports. *J Sports Med* 1977;5:209–215.

100. Poindexter DP, Johnson EW. Football, shoulder, and neck injury: a study of the "stinger." *Arch Phys Med Rehabil* 1984;65:601–602.

101. Sallis RE, Jones K, Knopp W. Burners: offensive strategy for an underreported injury. *Phys Sports Med* 1992;20(11):47–55.

102. Kulkarni MV, McArdle CB, Copanicky D, et al. Acute spinal cord injury: MR imaging at 1.5T. *Radiology* 1987;164:837–843.

103. Knott M, Voss DE. *Proprioceptive neuromuscular facilitation.* New York: Harper & Row, 1968.

104. Watkins RG. Neck injuries in football players. *Clin Sports Med* 1986;5:215–246.

105. Wroble RR, Albright JP. Neck and low back injuries in wrestling. *Clin Sports Med* 1986;5: 295–325.

106. Archambault JL. Brachial plexus stretch injury. *J Am Coll Health* 1983;31:256–260.

107. Bateman JE. Nerve injuries about the shoulder in sports. *J Bone Joint Surg [Am]* 1967;49: 785–792.

108. Funk FJ, Wells RE. Injuries of the cervical spine in football. *Clin Orthop* 1975;109:50–58.

109. Hunter C. Injuries to the brachial plexus: experience of a private sports medicine clinic. *J M Osteopath Assoc* 1982;91: 757–760.

110. Robertson WC, Eichman PL, Clancy WG. Upper trunk brachial plexopathy in football players. *JAMA* 1979;241:1480–1482.

111. Vegso JJ, Torg E, Torg JS. Rehabilitation of the cervical spine, brachial plexus, and peripheral nerve injuries. *Clin Sports Med* 1987;6:135–158.

112. Chrisman OD, Snook GA, Stanitis JM, et al. Lateral flexion neck injuries in athletic competition. *JAMA* 1965;192: 613–615.

113. Marshall TM. Nerve pinch injuries in football. *J K Med Assoc* 1970;68:648–649.

114. Rockett FX. Observations on the "Burner." Traumatic cervical radiculopathy. *Clin Orthop* 1982;164:18–19.

115. Vegso JJ, Lehman RC. Field evaluation and management of head and neck injuries. *Clin Sports Med* 1987;6:1–15.

116. Teasdale G, Jennet B. Assessment of coma and impaired consciousness: a practical scale. *Lancet* 1974;1:81–84.

117. Coady C, Stanish WD. Emergencies in sports: the young athlete. *Clin Sports Med* 1988;7: 625–640.

118. Rogers FA. Fractures and dislocations of the cervical spine: an end result study. *J Bone Joint Surg* 1957;39:341.

119. Cacayorin ED, Petro GR, Hochhauser L. Headache in the athlete and radiologic evaluation. *Clin Sports Med* 1987;6: 739–749.

120. Blahd WH Jr, Iserson KV, Bjelland JC. Efficiency of the posttraumatic cross table lateral view of the cervical spine. *J Emerg Med* 1985;2:243–249.

121. Weir DC. Roentgenographic signs of cervical injury. *Clin Orthop North Am* 1975;109:9.

122. Beatson TR. Fractures and dislocations in the cervical spine. *J Bone J Surg [Br]* 1963;45:21.

123. Hinck VC, Hopkins CE. Measurement of the atlanto dental interval in the adult. *AJR* 1965;84: 945–951.

124. Marks MR, Bell GR, Boumphrey FRS. Cervical spine fractures in athletes. *Clin Sports Med* 1990;9:13–29.

125. White AA III, Panjabi M. *Clinical biomechanics of the spine.* 2nd ed. Philadelphia: JB Lippincott, 1990:38–79.

126. Pavlov H, Torg JS, Robie B, et al. Cervical spinal stenosis: determination of vertebral body ratio method. *Radiology* 1987;164: 771–775.

127. Edwards WC, LaRocca H. The developmental segmental diameter of the cervical canal in patients with cervical spondylosis. *Spine* 1983;8:20–27.

128. Wolf BS, Khilanai M, Malis L. Sagittal diameter of the bony cervical canal and its significance in cervical spondylosis. *J M Sinai Hosp* 1956;23:283–292.

129. Kesler JT. Congenital narrowing of the cervical spinal canal. *J Neurol Neurosurg Psychiatry* 1975;38:1218–1224.

130. Countee RW, Vijayanathant. Congenital stenosis of the cervical spine: diagnosis and management. *J Natl Med Assoc* 1979;71:57–264.

131. Herzog RJ, Wiens JJ, Dillingham MF, et al. Normal cervical spine morphometry and cervical spinal stenosis in asymptomatic professional football players: plain film radiography, multiplanar computed tomography, and magnetic resonance imaging. *Spine* 1991;16:178–186.

132. Epstein VA, Epstein JA, Jones MD. Cervical spinal stenosis. *Radiol Clin North Am* 1977;15:215–281.

133. Cantu RC. Functional cervical spinal stenosis: a contraindication to participation in contact sports. *Med Sci Sports Exerc,* 1993;25:316–317.

134. Yu YL, Stevens JM, Kendall B, et al. Cord shape and measurements in cervical spondylitic myelopathy and radiculopathy. *AJNR* 1983;4:839–842.

135. Munnings F. Should athletes return to play after transient quadriparesis? *Phys Sports Med* 1991;19(10):127–134.

136. Daniel DL, Grogan JP, Johansen JG, et al. Cervical radiculopathy: computed tomography and myelography compared. *Radiology* 1984;151:109–113.

137. Herzog RJ. Selection and utilization of imaging studies for disorders of the lumbar spine. *Phys Med Rehabil Clin N Am* 1991;2:7–59.

138. Modic MT, Masaryk TJ, Mulopulos GP, et al. Cervical radiculopathy: prospective evaluation with surface coil MR imaging, CT with metrizamide and metrizamide myelography. *Radiology* 1986;161:753–759.

139. Kibler WB, Chandler TJ, Pace BK. Principles of rehabilitation after chronic tendon injuries. *Clin Sports Med* 1992;11:661–672.

140. Torg JS. *Athletic injuries to the head, neck, and face.* Philadelphia: Lea & Febiger, 1982.

141. Akeson WH, Woo SY, Amil D, et al. The connective tissue response to immobility. *Clin Orthop* 1973;93:356–362.

142. Mueller EA. Influence of training and inactivity on muscle strength. *Arch Phys Rehabil Med* 1970;51:449–462.

143. Noyes F, et al. Biomechanics of ligament failure: II. Analysis of immobilization, exercise and reconditioning effects in primates. *J Bone Joint Surg [Am]* 1963;56:154–162.

144. Salter RB, et al. Comparison of the affects of immobilization and continuous passive motion on surgical wound healing in rabbits. *Plast Reconstr Surg* 1986;78: 360–368.

145. Sweeny T, Prentice C, Saal JA, Saal JS. Cervicothoracic muscular stabilization techniques. *Phys Med Rehabil State Art Rev* 1990;4:335–359.

146. Windsor R, Washington K. Clinical review of specific selective spinal injections. In: Windsor R, Lox D, eds. *Soft tissue injury—diagnosis and treatment.* Philadelphia: Hanley & Belfus, 1977.

147. Saal JA. Rehabilitation of throwing in tennis related shoulder injuries. *Phys Med Rehabil State Art Rev* 1987;1:597–612.

148. Greenman F. Principles of soft tissue and articulatory (mobilization without impulse) technique. In: *Principles of manual medicine.* Baltimore: Williams & Wilkins, 1989.

149. Farrell JP. Cervical passive mobilization techniques: the Australian approach. *Phys Med Rehabil State Art Rev* 1990;4: 309–334.

150. McKenzie RA. *The cervical and thoracic spine: mechanical diagnosis and therapy.* New Zealand: Spinal Publications, 1990.

151. Cantu RC. Athletic head injuries. *Clin Sports Med* 1997;16: 531–542.

152. Torg JS, Ramsey-Emrhein JA. Management guidelines for participation in collision activities with congenital, developmental or post-injury lesions involving the cervical spine. *Clin Sports Med* 1997;16:501–530.

153. Wilberger JE, Maroon JC. Cervical spine injuries in athletes. *Phys Sports Med* 1990;18(3):57–70.

154. Wilbourne AJ. Electrodiagnostic diagnosis of plexopathies. *Neural Clin* 1985;3:511–529.

155. DiBenedetto M, Markey K. Electrodiagnostic localization of trau-

matic upper trunk brachial plexopathy. *Arch Phys Med Rehabil* 1984;65:15–17.

156. Trojaborge W. Electrophysiologic findings and pressure palsy of the brachial plexus. *J Neurol Neurosurg Psychiatry* 1977;40: 1160–1167.

157. Nissen SJ, Laskowski ER, Rizzo TD. Burner syndrome: recognition and rehabilitation. *Phys Sports Med* 1996;24(6):57–64.

Chapter 65

Shoulder Assessment and Management

W. Ben Kibler
Stuart E. Willick
Andrew J. Cole
Joel M. Press
Stanley A. Herring

In recent years, the incidence of injuries to the shoulder has increased owing to a heightened interest in physical fitness and a concomitant escalation in the level of participation in sports by the public (1). The athlete's shoulder is at high risk for injury because the shoulder girdle sacrifices stability for mobility in order to perform a wide array of movements demanded by sporting activities. A detailed knowledge of the anatomy and functional biomechanics, coupled with the appropriate history, physical examination, and ancillary testing, ensures an accurate diagnosis of shoulder injuries. The physiatrist specializing in sports medicine can then employ biomechanical principles to formulate optimal treatment plans that ensure successful outcomes. This chapter discusses the basic pathoanatomy of the shoulder and describes the pertinent history, physical examination, diagnostic testing, and rehabilitation programs for shoulder dysfunction in the athlete.

ANATOMY AND FUNCTIONAL BIOMECHANICS

The shoulder's extensive range of motion comes at the expense of anatomic and functional stability. Its motion is due to the simultaneous participation of the glenohumeral, sternoclavicular, acromioclavicular, and scapulothoracic articulations. Any injury to these structures or those that support them may cause pain or a loss of functional ability such as range of motion and strength. This creates a cycle of further pain, anatomic changes, and decreased athletic performance. A clear understanding of the anatomy and functional biomechanics of the shoulder and their relation to its stability is therefore essential.

The glenohumeral joint, an incongruous joint, is relatively unstable. The glenoid has a relatively shallow concave surface that articulates with the convex humeral head. These dissimilar articulating surfaces necessitate a gliding motion about a constantly changing axis of rotation (2). The shallow glenoid forces the glenohumeral joint to rely on the static stability provided by the glenoid labrum, joint capsule, and glenohumeral, coracohumeral, coracoacromial, and coracoclavicular ligaments. The static stabilizers are reinforced by the muscular dynamic stabilizers, in particular the rotator cuff and scapular stabilizing muscles (3).

The fibrocartilaginous glenoid labrum on the outer perimeter of the glenoid fossa enhances the stability of the glenohumeral joint by increasing the coverage of the humeral head from 25% to 75%, thereby restraining excessive movement of the head (4). The glenohumeral ligaments further enhance the static stability of the glenohumeral joint. The inferior glenohumeral ligament, the most significant static anterior and inferior stabilizer of the humeral head, is the major restraint preventing anterior

---

Portions of this chapter were adapted from
Cole AJ, Reid MD. Clinical assessment of the shoulder. *J Back Musculoskel Rehabil* 1992;2(2)7–15; and Press JM, Herring SA, Kibler WB. Rehabilitation of musculoskeletal injuries. In: *The textbook of military medicine*. Borden Institute, Office of the Surgeon General, (in press).

n of the humeral head during external rotation duction (4–10). The middle glenohumeral ligament rains external rotation of the joint between 60 and 90 degrees of abduction (5). The superior glenohumeral ligament provides antigravity support for the dependent arm.

The coracohumeral ligament assists the superior glenohumeral ligament in providing support for the dependent arm and restraint against external rotation of the joint below 60 degrees of abduction (5). The coracoacromial and coracoclavicular ligament complexes reinforce the acromioclavicular articulation, thereby helping stabilize the glenohumeral joint complex. The subscapularis tendon provides anterior static stability up to 90 degrees of abduction but thereafter shifts superior to the humeral head and no longer provides stability (11). The capsule arises from the glenoid fossa and inserts around the anatomic neck of the humerus. Arm position selectively tightens the capsule. At rest, the superior portion of the capsule is taut and the inferior portion lies in lax folds. Overhead elevation of the arm reverses these characteristics (2,6).

Scapular positioning plays a critical role in enhancing glenohumeral stability. The scapula sits at approximately 40 to 50 degrees from the coronal plane, placing the posterior half of the glenoid behind the glenohumeral joint and thus increasing posterior stability (12). Further stability is afforded by normal scapulothoracic motion, which serves to 1) optimally seat the humeral head in the glenoid during full range of motion (13,14); 2) elevate the inferiorly oriented glenoid fossa, helping to prevent excessive inferior movement of the humeral head (7); 3) minimize tensile stress on capsular ligaments and other supporting soft tissues that could otherwise be damaged (14); and 4) allow for the normal glenohumeral to scapulothoracic ratio range of 2 : 1 to 5 : 4 to be maintained (8,15,16).

Normal glenohumeral joint motion and stability also depend on proper functioning of the acromioclavicular and sternoclavicular joints. The acromioclavicular joint is a plane synovial joint that depends primarily on the acromioclavicular and coracoclavicular ligaments for its integrity (17). Because 50 degrees of clavicular rotation is required to allow a full 180 degrees of abduction, the acromioclavicular joint is subjected to continuous stress during arm motion (6,7). The sternoclavicular joint is a saddle-shaped synovial joint with an interposed disk separating its articular surfaces. Joint strength is provided by both ligamentous and diskal attachments (17). Motion at the sternoclavicular joint occurs almost exclusively during the first 90 degrees of arm elevation, during which every 10 degrees of elevation is accompanied by 4 degrees of clavicular elevation (15).

Dynamic stability of the glenohumeral joint is primarily ensured by the coordinated action of the rotator cuff and scapulothoracic muscle groups with the assistance of other muscles. The subscapularis, supraspinatus, teres minor, and infraspinatus muscles make up the rotator cuff. The confluence of their tendons surrounds the anterior, superior, and posterior portions of the joint.

The rotator cuff prevents any untoward glenohumeral motion through muscular "force couples" that assist the static stabilizers to maintain the instantaneous center of rotation of the glenohumeral joint within a 1-mm locus (13,14). *Internal rotation* by the subscapularis is assisted by the latissimus dorsi, pectoralis major, teres major, and anterior part of the deltoideus. The antagonists providing *external rotatory forces* include the teres minor, infraspinatus, and posterior part of the deltoideus. *Abduction* occurs by the action of middle portion of the deltoideus and supraspinatus. The rotator cuff muscles fire synergistically to create compressive force couples that counterbalance the vertical force vector of the middle part of the deltoideus and keep the humeral head securely seated in the glenoid fossa (15,18–20). The pectoralis major, latissimus dorsi, and teres major are the chief *adductors*. They gain some assistance from the coracobrachialis, long head of the triceps, teres minor, and posterior portion of the deltoideus. *Forward flexion* results from the action of the clavicular head of the pectoralis major, anterior part of the deltoideus, coracobrachialis, and biceps brachii. *Extension* results primarily from the action of the posterior fibers of the deltoideus, latissimus dorsi, and sternocostal fibers of the pectoralis major, and secondarily from the teres major and long head of the triceps (7–18).

The scapulothoracic articulation is also controlled by a series of counterbalanced dynamic muscular forces. The resulting coordinated motion reinforces the effect of the static stabilizers and ensures the stability of the glenohumeral joint by maintaining the proper relationship between the scapula and the humerus (Fig. 65-1) (7). *Elevation* of the scapula by the upper trapezius and levator scapulae with assistance from the rhomboideus major and minor is balanced by scapular *depression* due to contraction of the lower trapezius, lower fibers of the latissimus dorsi, serratus anterior, pectoralis major, pectoralis minor, and subclavius. *Upward rotation* is controlled by the upper and lower trapezius and serratus anterior, and is countered by the forces of the pectoralis minor, latissimus dorsi, lower pectoralis major, rhomboideus major and minor, and levator scapulae, which control *downward rotation*. *Protraction* by the pectoralis minor and major and serratus anterior is opposed by the *retractive forces* governed by the rhomboideus minor and major, middle trapezius, and latissimus dorsi (7,15,18).

Two additional anatomic observations deserve mention. Approximately eight bursae are distributed throughout the shoulder joint. These bursae allow motion of contiguous structures while minimizing frictional forces and potential secondary inflammation with its resultant pain (6,7,11,21). Altered shoulder biomechanics and excessive forces can cause inflammation and injury to the bursae. The final observation is that the biceps tendon arises from the superior glenoid rim and travels through

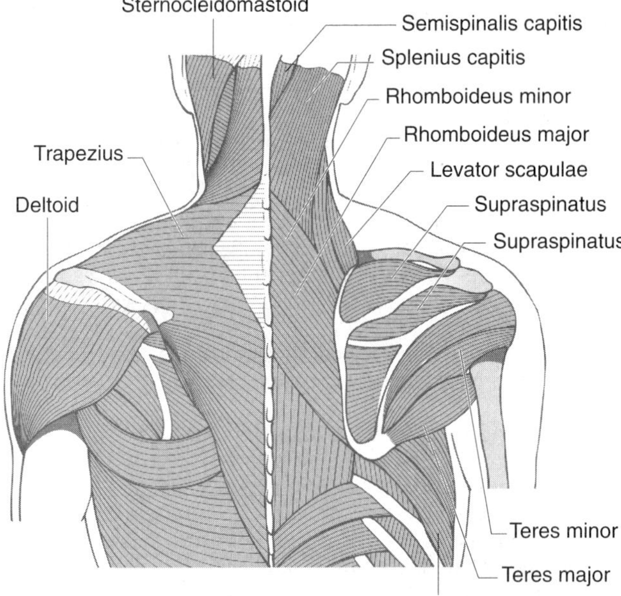

Figure 65-1. Dynamic stabilizers of the scapulothoracic articulation. (Reproduced by permission from Warwick R, Williams PL, eds. Gray's anatomy 35th British ed. Philadelphia: WB Saunders, 1973.)

the intertubercular groove. It is surrounded by its own synovial sheath. Because the tendon remains angulated around the medial wall of the groove except during external rotation, it is at risk for injury from traction, impaction, and shear forces (11,15,22).

HISTORY

By taking a detailed and accurate history, the physiatrist is able to form an initial differential diagnostic impression that could explain the athlete's degree of pain and disability. Then, a well-planned and focused physical examination is performed. A working diagnosis, based on the history and physical examination, is a further refinement of the differential diagnosis and will determine what further testing may be required to arrive at the correct final diagnosis. The key elements of the shoulder history are summarized in Table 65-1.

The athlete's age, hand dominance, sporting activities, mechanism of injury, and functional limitations provide initial diagnostic clues. Certain shoulder problems tend to be related to age; examples are calcific tendinitis, which generally occurs between the ages of 20 to 40, and rotator cuff degeneration, which is more often seen in older athletes. Important information can also be gleaned from the type of sport in which the athlete participates. Bicipital tendinitis and impingement should be considered in a water polo athlete engaged in repetitive overhead activity. The patient's tasks off the playing field may also contribute to a sports-related injury. For example, an assembly line worker who plays weekend softball may develop acute pain from a quiescent calcific tendinitis. If not due to repetitive microtrauma, the injury may be a result of direct trauma, such as a fall on an outstretched hand causing a glenohumeral joint dislocation. In addition, careful note should also be taken of all functional limitations. Finally, an occupational history will help determine how aggressive the patient's rehabilitation program needs to be. Clearly, a professional football player who must play within 3 days may require a more aggressive treatment program than someone who plays weekend games of touch football.

The location, quality, intensity, frequency, and course of the pain should be determined. Anterior pain suggests

Table 65-1: Key Elements of the Shoulder History
Demographics
Age
Hand dominance
Sporting activities
Occupation
Mechanism of injury
Acute traumatic
Overuse/repetitive
Position of shoulder at time of injury
Functional limitations
During sporting activities
During vocational activities
During activities of daily living
Symptoms
Pain
Location
Quality
Intensity
Frequency
Duration
Course
Exacerbating or alleviating positions and activities
Other
Sensory changes
Motor changes
Changes in skin color, texture, and temperature
Muscle spasms
Crepitus
Catching
Recurrent dislocations or sense of instability
Prior shoulder dysfunction
Previous symptoms and diagnosis
Previous work-up and imaging
Previous interventions and their effect
Kinetic chain history
Upper-limb symptoms
Neck and back symptoms
Hip and pelvis symptoms
Other musculoskeletal injuries

Source: Adapted from Cole AJ, Reid MD. Clinical assessment of the shoulder. *J Back Musculoskel Rehabil* 1992;2(2):7–15.

bicipital tendinitis, posterior pain might be due to a posterior labral tear, superior pain occurs with acromioclavicular joint injury, and global pain can occur with glenohumeral joint synovitis.

It is also important to note the quality of pain. Radicular pain tends to be sharp, burning, and radiating. Bone pain is deep, boring, and localized. Muscle pain can be dull, aching, and hard to localize. Vascular pain can be diffuse, aching, and poorly localized and may be referred to other areas of the body. Tendon pain such as that with calcific tendinitis tends to be hot and burning. The intensity of pain may wax and wane with particular motions associated with specific activities. Acromioclavicular pain tends to occur with arm motion above 90 degrees of abduction, as seen in basketball players. However, the initial pain associated with an idiopathic frozen shoulder tends to be constant but is particularly bad at night, and frequently awakens the athlete. Additionally, positions that help to relieve pain are important. For example, athletes whose symptoms diminish when their arms are held in a dependent position may be suffering from thoracic outlet syndrome. Finally, the course of symptoms over time can provide clues regarding the type and stage of the injury as in the progression of an adhesive capsulitis.

The possibility of nerve injury should be thoroughly investigated. In addition to questioning the patient about the quality of pain, the physician should note skin color and texture changes, wasting, paresthesia, numbness, and muscle spasm.

The initial evaluation should also include any history of prior shoulder pain, its work-up, diagnosis, and treatment. Special attention should be paid to the results of any testing procedures, including imaging and electrodiagnostic studies. Response to oral medications including nonsteroidal and steroid preparations and any side effects from them should be noted. The results of any selective injections (subacromial bursae, glenohumeral joint, bicipital tendon sheath, or acromioclavicular joint) should also be noted, and whether the injections were performed with fluoroscopic guidance. Finally, the details and results of prior rehabilitation or surgical procedures should be recorded (16,17,23,24).

PHYSICAL EXAMINATION

The physical examination should be focused and thorough, using the clinical impression gleaned from the history as a guide. The pertinent parts of the shoulder examination are summarized in Table 65-2. Athletes should be observed as they walk into a room. An upper extremity should swing in tandem with its opposite lower extremity, and the movements while patients disrobe should appear smooth and natural. Dividing the anatomy into anterior, lateral, posterior, and superior aspects permits an ordered inspection. The general contour of the shoulder (bony landmarks) should be observed. Any asymmetry, swelling, discoloration, muscle wasting, or significant change in posture should be noted. For example, a hollowed infraspinatus fossa may indicate a rotator cuff tear or suprascapular nerve lesion. Anterior prominence of the humeral head or a high-riding outer clavicle suggests glenohumeral dislocation or acromioclavicular separation, respectively.

Table 65-2: Key Elements of the Shoulder Examination

Observation
Walking, arm swing, disrobing, reaching, asymmetry, discoloration, atrophy, posture
Palpation
Sternum, sternoclavicular joint, clavicle, acromioclavicular joint, acromion, coracoid process, ribs, costal cartilage, greater tuberosity, muscles and tendons, axilla, cervical spine, elbow, wrist
Range of motion
Active, passive, total shoulder girdle vs isolated glenohumeral, spine, elbow, wrist
Vascular
Pulses, Adson test, Roos test, skin changes
Neurologic
Strength, sensation, reflexes, neural tension
Special tests
Yergason test, Speed test, drop arm, instability and apprehension tests, impingement tests, scapular slide
Ancillary tests
Plain radiographs, computed tomography (CT), CT arthrography, magnetic resonance imaging, electrodiagnosis, diagnostic injections

Source: Adapted from Cole AJ, Reid MD. Clinical assessment of the shoulder. *J Back Musculoskel Rehabil* 1992;2(2):7–15.

Palpation should include an evaluation of the sternum, sternoclavicular joint, clavicle, acromioclavicular joint, acromion, coracoid process, ribs and costal cartilages, humerus, greater tuberosity, bicipital tendon and groove, superficial rotator cuff muscles, and the axilla.

The degree and location of tenderness is often a reliable physical sign leading to an accurate diagnosis. For example, impingement is suggested by pain over the anterior part of the acromion and greater tuberosity. Tenderness over the posterior joint line could indicate joint pathology such as glenohumeral arthritis or a torn posterior labrum. Tenderness over the biceps tendon in the bicipital groove is a reliable sign of bicipital tendinitis.

Active and passive range of motion should be assessed. One important sign is pain with end-range stress. Crepitus can be soft or harsh with rotator cuff pathology or glenohumeral arthritis, respectively. When one is assessing true glenohumeral motion, it is important to eliminate substitution patterns by fixing the scapula at its inferior border. Routinely evaluated ranges of motion include active and passive measurements of total elevation, and external and internal rotation. Maximal elevation of the shoulder occurs in a plane somewhere between the coronal and sagittal planes, usually 15 to 20 degrees from the sagittal plane. The testing of external rotation begins with the arm resting comfortably at the side, elbow flexed 90 degrees, and the forearm in the sagittal plane. There is considerable variability among normal patients but one shoulder should not vary from the other in the same individual unless pathology is present. End-range internal rotation can be assessed by noting where the extended thumb touches an obvious anatomic landmark on the back. Abduction should be assessed to gain a more reliable impression regarding the presence of a painful arc commonly seen with impingement.

Several special tests are useful in the diagnosis of shoulder disorders: 1) the Yergason test and Speed test for bicipital tendinitis (Fig. 65-2); 2) the drop-arm test for a rotator cuff tear; 3) apprehension tests for shoulder instability (Fig. 65-3); 4) impingement tests for the impingement syndrome (Fig. 65-4); and 5) scapular slide test for abnormal scapulothoracic motion.

A vascular examination should include an assessment of distal pulses, general skin texture, color, temperature, hair growth, and alteration of sensation about and distal to the shoulder. The autonomic system should be assessed to help rule out reflex sympathetic dystrophy. Neurovascular compression or thoracic outlet syndrome tests include the Adson maneuver and hyperabduction test.

A focused neurologic evaluation will help rule out neurologic causes of shoulder symptoms. A motor evaluation should specifically test the anterior part of the deltoideus in the process of flexion and the middle part of the deltoideus and supraspinatus in the process of abduction. Additionally, it should test the external rotation generated by the posterior part of the deltoideus, infraspinatus, and teres minor, and the internal rotation generated by the subscapularis, latissimus dorsi, and pectoralis major. Strength testing is not complete without a full assessment of the scapular stabilizers.

The joints above and below the shoulder should be assessed during an evaluation. Cervical diskogenic or facet pain can result in altered cervical and shoulder motion. Furthermore, a cervical radiculopathy can cause strength deficits that may affect shoulder function and cause pain. Pain that radiates distal to the elbow generally arises from a cervical source. Examination of the elbow and wrist for median and ulnar nerve entrapment should also be performed (7,12,14,16,17,21,23–31).

ANCILLARY TESTS

Athletes with shoulder pathology often present with a decrease in athletic performance or nonspecific pain. While a properly performed history and physical examination should narrow the differential diagnosis, further testing is often required for confirmation of the working diagnosis, and to better delineate the severity of anatomic disruption. Ancillary tests commonly used to evaluate shoulder problems in athletes include radiologic examinations, diagnostic injection techniques, and electrodiagnostic studies. The indications and limitations of each should be appreciated.

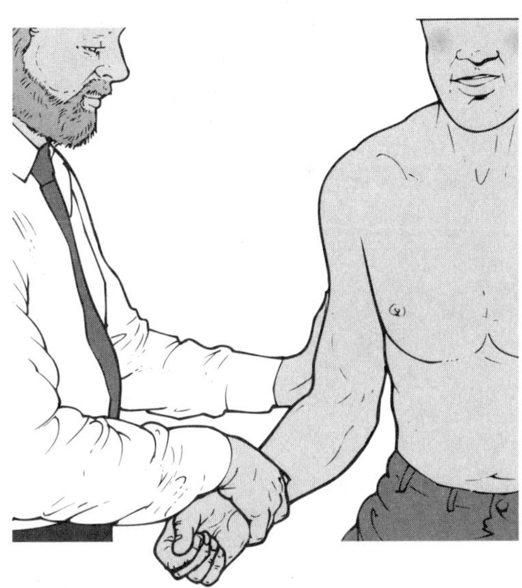

(a)

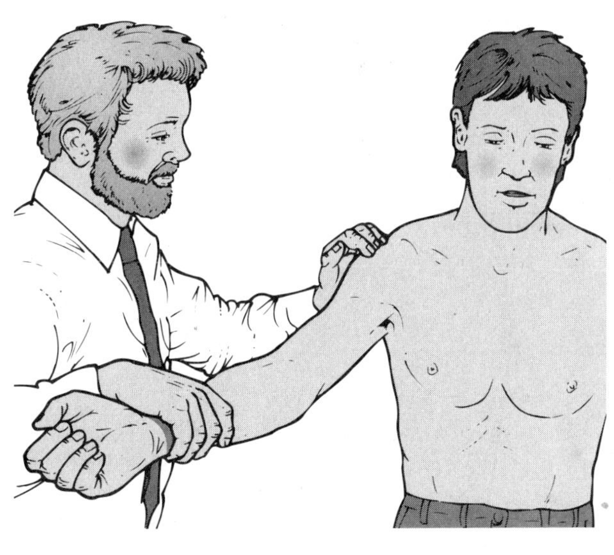

(b)

Figure 65-2. Yergason test (*a*) and Speed test (*b*) for bicipital tendinitis. (Reproduced by permission from Magee D, ed. *Orthopedic physical assessment.* Philadelphia: WB Saunders, 1992:117.)

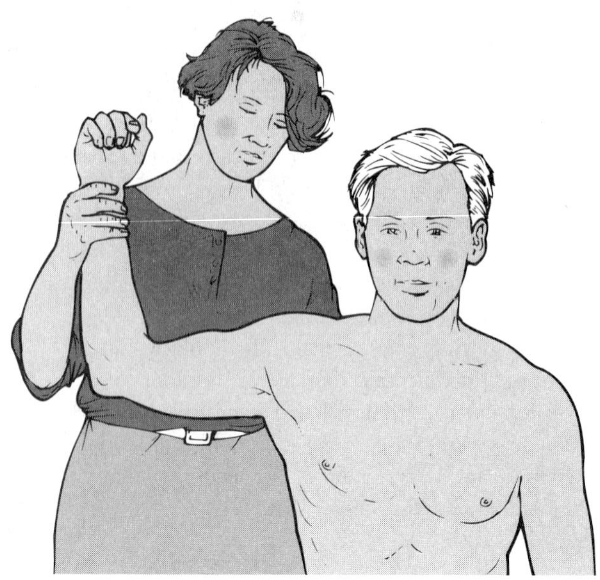

Figure 65-3. Rockwood test for anterior instability. If the athlete experiences apprehension or fear with passive abduction, external rotation, and extension, the test is positive for anterior glenohumeral instability. (Reproduced by permission from Magee D, ed. *Orthopedic physical assessment.* Philadelphia: WB Saunders, 1992:109.)

Imaging the Athlete's Shoulder

Conventional radiography is a good screening technique for osseous lesions such as degenerative changes of the glenohumeral and acromioclavicular joints, fractures, dislocations, erosions, or the unsuspected bony tumor. In many instances, however, shoulder pathology involves soft-tissue derangements for which plain radiographs will yield limited information. More sophisticated imaging studies may then be needed.

Imaging of Fractures and Dislocations

In acute bony trauma, plain radiographs may be used to assess fracture size, displacement, and rotation of major fragments. Frontal films with the humerus in internal and external rotation are invaluable for this assessment. Gross dislocation and associated impaction fractures of the humeral head, such as Hill-Sachs lesions (32) of the posterolateral part of the humeral head, and Bankart fractures of the anterior inferior aspect of the glenoid rim may be evaluated with these internal and external rotation views. The less common reverse Hill-Sachs and reverse Bankart fractures may also be seen. More precise delineation of fracture size and orientation, or subtle avulsion fragments, may be obtained by computed tomography

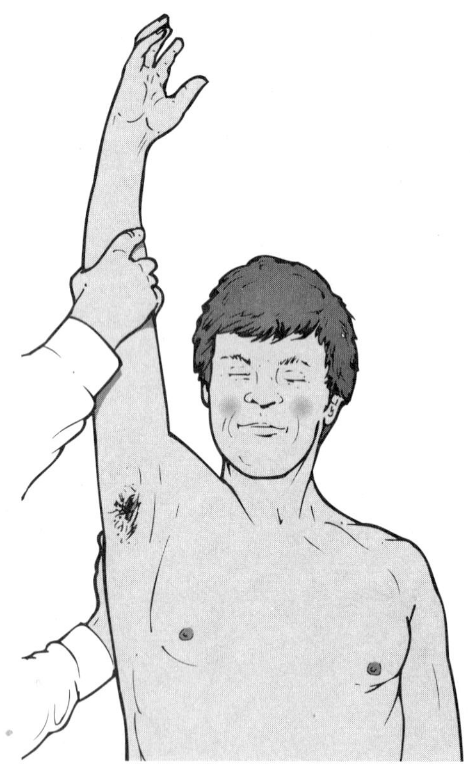

(a)

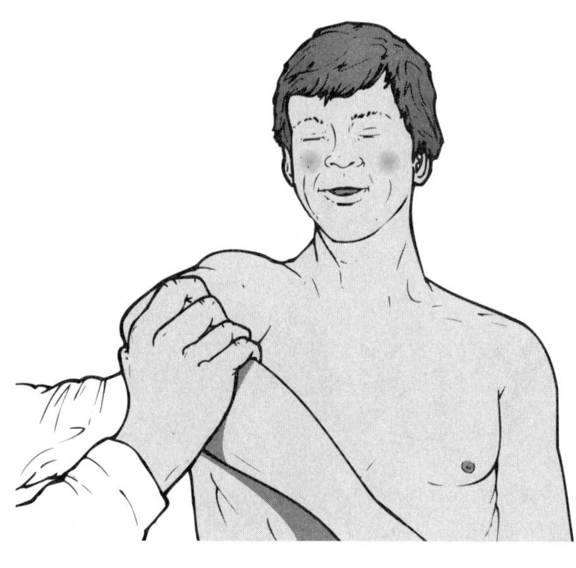

(b)

Figure 65-4. Rotator cuff impingement tests. *a, b.* The examiner attempts to reproduce the athlete's symptoms by bringing the greater tuberosity in closer opposition with the coracoacromial arch, thus narrowing the allowable space for the rotator cuff tendons. (Reproduced by permission from Magee D, ed. *Orthopedic physical assessment.* Philadelphia: WB Saunders, 1992:119.)

(CT). Bone scans, although less specific, may be more sensitive for equivocal or occult fractures. Magnetic resonance imaging (MRI) is also sensitive for occult fractures, as well as bone contusions and osteonecrosis.

Imaging of Rotator Cuff Derangement and Impingement Syndrome

Conventional radiographs may show gross osseous changes such as prominent hypertrophic degenerative changes of the acromioclavicular joint with inferior osteophyte formation, subacromial spur or enthesophyte formation, and the high-riding humeral head coming in close apposition to the inferior margin of the acromion. Gross narrowing of the subacromial space to less than about 5 to 7 mm on plain radiographs supports a clinical diagnosis of impingement syndrome (33,34) and possible associated rotator cuff derangement. Unfortunately, these plain film findings occur late in the evolution of impingement syndrome and are therefore of limited use when acute or subacute rotator cuff derangement is present. Furthermore, these radiographic findings are indirect as they do not demonstrate the rotator cuff itself. The other components of the coracoacromial arch that may contribute to clinical impingement are also not well delineated on plain radiographs. For example, the shape of the acromial undersurface (35,36) has been implicated in the natural history of rotator cuff tears and possibly also in clinical impingement. Yet conventional radiographs, including scapular Y views or outlet views, have not been found to be a reliable indicator of acromial shape. MRI, by its multiplanar tomographic capability, accurately evaluates acromial shape and orientation.

As with the acromion, the shape and orientation of the coracoid process is difficult to determine by conventional radiographs. When prominent, broad, and elongated, the coracoid may come in close apposition to the lesser tuberosity and impinge the subscapularis tendon with forward flexion and horizontal adduction of the humerus. This less common form of anterior or coracoid impingement syndrome may require CT or MRI to obtain adequate information about coracoid process morphology. In addition, coracoid fractures may be inadequately visualized by radiographs; CT may be needed to detect the fracture and assess fracture fragment displacement and orientation. MRI may be needed for full evaluation of all the soft-tissue structures that may encroach on the rotator cuff and contribute to clinical impingement, including a thickened coracoacromial ligament or extrinsic masses.

More direct imaging and visualization of the cuff is needed for earlier detection and clinical intervention in the natural history of rotator cuff derangement. Arthrography is very sensitive for the detection of full-thickness cuff tears, but somewhat less sensitive for partial-thickness tears of the inferior, or articular margin of the cuff. Partial tears of the superior, or bursal margin of the cuff cannot be seen by glenohumeral joint injection, and require a separate subacromial or subdeltoid bursal injection of contrast material. Assessment of the precise size and location of rotator cuff tears in both medial-lateral and anterior-posterior dimensions is important when planning operative strategies. Arthrography may be inadequate when such fine resolution is required.

Ultrasound has been used in the assessment of rotator cuff tears. In experienced hands sonography may be accurate for the evaluation of lateral tears close to the greater and lesser tuberosities. More medial tears under the acromion may be more difficult to evaluate because of penetration limits or artifact formation due to the intervening sound reflecting osseous structures.

MRI has become the gold standard imaging procedure for direct visualization and full evaluation of the rotator cuff (37–43). Morphologic and signal change in acute tendinitis or tendon or muscle strain or contusion may be seen. More chronic tendinosis with atrophy and degeneration may also be delineated. The size and location of full-thickness or partial-thickness tears (including both superior or bursal and inferior or articular margin partial tears) may be accurately determined. The relatively late findings of muscle atrophy and fatty infiltration, difficult to detect by other imaging modalities, may also be determined by MRI and may have prognostic significance.

Imaging of Glenohumeral Instability

Clinical instability is another major category of shoulder pain and dysfunction. Acute traumatic dislocations or more chronic recurrent dislocations may present with the humeral head still displaced, which may be apparent clinically. Plain radiographs serve to confirm the degree and direction of dislocation. Once the humeral head is reduced, plain radiographs may reveal associated Hill-Sachs or Bankart fractures. More subtle impaction fractures or bony fragments may require CT for adequate visualization. Plain radiographs will not reveal soft-tissue injury such as labral tears or detachments (44) or capsular tears. Conventional arthrography in acute injuries may show gross extravasation of contrast material through large capsular or labral defects. In more chronic instances, CT arthrography with its tomographic capability and high resolution may be needed for the detection of labral tears or attenuation. MRI is very promising as an accurate and sensitive means of visualizing the labral and capsular surfaces and substance (45) for degeneration, fraying, and tears. MRI is particularly useful in the more acute setting when large joint effusions may be present. These effusions serve as a native intra-articular contrast agent by outlining the labral and capsular surfaces. In more chronic settings, MRI arthrography with intra-articular injection of saline or diluted gadolinium-saline solutions may be needed to delineate more subtle labral tears.

Imaging of Other Causes of Shoulder Pain

Many of the other causes of shoulder pain involve soft-tissue derangements not well detected or evaluated by plain radiographs, bone scan, or CT. Biceps tendon tears may occasionally be seen by arthrography or CT arthrography. The more superficial or lateral tears may also be seen by ultrasound. Tendinitis or tendinosis, or degeneration, as well as tendon dislocation (46), may be better demonstrated by MRI. Extra-articular soft-tissue lesions such as para-articular ganglion cysts, which are associated with labral or capsular defects, may entrap the suprascapular nerve within the suprascapular notch or spinoglenoid notch (47), producing nonspecific deep shoulder pain that may be associated with atrophy and weakness of the supraspinatus and infraspinatus muscles. Such cysts are difficult to detect by physical examination because of their location and are not reliably demonstrated by most imaging modalities because they are located deep in the soft tissue. Again, MRI is the optimal imaging modality for accurate evaluation of ganglion cysts or other soft-tissue lesions along the course of the suprascapular nerve.

Other Ancillary Tests

Two other evaluations also deserve mention. Electrodiagnostic testing including nerve conduction studies and electromyography can help determine, for example, whether a cervical radiculopathy, brachial plexus injury, or axillary nerve injury may be present. Selective fluoroscopically guided injection of anesthetic or steroid into the subacromial bursae, glenohumeral joint, bicipital tendon sheath, or acromioclavicular joint can provide powerful evidence that a particular structure is the pain generator (7). Such injections may yield both diagnostic and therapeutic benefit.

DIFFERENTIAL DIAGNOSIS AND REHABILITATION

Differential Diagnosis

The rehabilitation plan relies on accurate diagnosis for success. Nonspecific diagnoses lead to nonspecific treatments and suboptimal outcomes.

There are many ways to categorize the differential diagnosis of shoulder dysfunction. A comprehensive differential diagnosis is presented in Table 65-3. The first step in narrowing the differential diagnosis is to rule out the most serious conditions. In the athlete who has suffered acute trauma, look first for vascular or neurologic injury or septic arthritis, as these can be catastrophic and may require emergent intervention. In the office setting, it is important to remember that athletes are patients first, and may suffer from the same ailments as nonathletes. Therefore, physiatrists must always keep in mind non-sports-related conditions that may present as shoulder pain, such as the rare tumor, metabolic and inflammatory disorders, and referred visceral pain.

Table 65-3: Differential Diagnosis of Shoulder Pathology

- Bone
  - Fractures
  - Avascular necrosis
  - Tumor
    - Primary
    - Metastatic
  - Paget disease
  - Osteomalacia
  - Hyperparathyroidism
- Ligament/labrum
  - Subluxation or dislocation
    - Glenohumeral joint
      - Bankart lesion of anterior capsule and ligaments
    - Acromioclavicular joint
    - Sternoclavicular joint
  - Coracohumeral ligament
  - Coracoacromial ligament
  - Coracoclavicular ligament
  - Glenohumeral ligaments
  - Instability possibly due to acute macrotrauma, chronic microtrauma, or inherent hyperelasticity
- Muscle/tendon
  - Rotator cuff tendinitis or tendinosis
    - Subscapularis tendon
    - Supraspinatus tendon
  - Biceps tendinitis or tendinosis
  - Biceps tendon rupture
  - Scapular stabilizer weakness
- Neurologic
  - Radiculopathy
  - Brachial plexopathy
    - Traumatic
    - Idiopathic (neuralgic amyotrophy or Parsonage-Turner syndrome)
  - Peripheral nerve lesion
    - Axillary nerve
    - Suprascapular nerve
    - Musculocutaneous nerve
- Vascular
  - Axillary vein thrombosis
  - Axillary artery aneurysm or intimal tear
- Inflammatory
  - Subacromial bursitis
  - Rheumatoid arthritis
  - Polymyalgia rheumatica
- Neoplastic
  - Bony tumors
  - Soft-tissue tumors
  - Primary vs metastatic
- Noninflammatory arthritis
  - Septic arthritis
  - Hemophilic arthritis
  - Osteochondromatosis
  - Posttraumatic or degenerative arthritis
- Referred visceral pain
  - Cardiac pain
  - Gastric ulcer
  - Cholecystitis/cholelithiasis

Nerve Injuries Affecting the Athlete's Shoulder

Sports medicine physiatrists are particularly well trained to diagnose neuropathies affecting the shoulder, because they are educated in the interaction between the nervous and musculoskeletal systems and trained in electromyography.

Nerve injury as a cause of shoulder dysfunction may be easily overlooked. Nerve injuries may be the result of a direct blow, compression, fracture, or traction. Lesions span the range of severity from neuropraxia to axonotmesis and neurotmesis. Neuropathies affecting the shoulder are often incomplete lesions and may be quite subtle. Although weakness, sensory loss, and pain are classic indicators of nerve injury, the first clue to the presence of a nerve injury in an athlete may be altered biomechanics and a drop in performance. Nerve injuries that can affect the athlete's shoulder have been described at the spinal cord, root, plexus, and peripheral nerve levels.

Cervical spinal cord injuries may be catastrophic or very mild. They are most commonly seen in sports involving high-speed impacts such as football, horseback riding, hang gliding, motorcycle and car racing, skiing, mountain climbing, and boxing (48–50).

The majority of shoulder girdle musculature, including the deltoideus, rotator cuff, and scapular stabilizers, are innervated by the C5 and C6 cervical roots. However, C7 and C8 contribute to the innervation of other muscles that act on the shoulder girdle, including lower fibers of the pectoralis major and latissimus dorsi and triceps. Cervical radiculopathy is a cause of shoulder weakness or altered biomechanics. The C5 and C6 roots and upper trunk of the brachial plexus are at particular risk during a collision that increases the angle between the neck and shoulder, which is the usual mechanism for the "stinger" seen in football players (51–53). Neurogenic thoracic outlet syndrome sometimes results from compression of the brachial plexus as it passes through the scalene muscles of athletes with particularly well-developed neck muscles, such as weight lifters and football linemen (54,55).

The axillary nerve, which innervates the deltoideus and teres minor, may suffer traction injury from inferior glenohumeral dislocation. It is also at risk as it courses through the quadrilateral space, either due to a proximal humerus fracture or possibly secondary to scar formation following rupture of the inferior glenohumeral ligament (the so-called quadrilateral space syndrome) (56,57). Long thoracic nerve injury presents as winging of the scapula, and may be seen in climbers who carry heavy backpacks. It has also been observed in backstroke swimmers (58), weight lifters, wrestlers, gymnasts, bowlers, golfers, and soccer, hockey, and football players (54,55,59).

A blow to the supraclavicular area, as might be delivered by a lacrosse or hockey stick, may injure the spinal accessory nerve as it passes under the upper trapezius. The athlete may complain of a shoulder ache, and will demonstrate a weak shoulder shrug on the affected side (60). The suprascapular nerve, which innervates the supraspinatus and infraspinatus, may also be injured by this mechanism. Difficulty with abduction and external rotation will result. Injury to the suprascapular nerve can also occur with anterior shoulder dislocations during bicycling (61), football (62), weight training (62), and archery (63). Entrapment of the suprascapular nerve may occur along its course through the suprascapular notch, and may result in pain with scapular movement, weakness, and altered biomechanics.

A Framework for Rehabilitation

There are five primary goals of the rehabilitation plan for an athlete's shoulder. First, the sports medicine physiatrist must establish an accurate diagnosis. A nonspecific diagnosis leads to nonspecific treatment and thus suboptimal outcome. Second, it is crucial to minimize the deleterious local effects of the acute injury. Third, the rehabilitation plan must not interfere with the normal healing process. Fourth, other components of general fitness must be maintained while the injured body part is healing. Finally, the athlete must be readied for return to normal athletic activity.

Complete and accurate diagnosis goes beyond identifying the primary site of anatomic disruption. In each injury, there are five separate elements comprising the musculoskeletal injury complex that may be identified as contributing to the production or continuation of symptoms (64). These elements include 1) the tissue injury complex—the actual area of anatomic disruption; 2) the clinical symptom complex—the group of symptoms the athlete experiences, such as pain, stiffness, and impaired performance; 3) the functional biomechanical deficit—the set of muscle inflexibilities, weakness, and imbalance that cause inefficient mechanics; 4) the functional adaptation complex—the set of functional substitutions that the athlete employs in an attempt to reduce pain and maintain performance; and 5) the tissue overload complex—the group of muscles and other soft-tissue structures that are subject to overload injury, thus causing or prolonging symptoms. These five elements are often interactive and additive, setting up a "vicious cycle" of continuing musculoskeletal problems.

During the acute stage of injury the initial goal is minimization of the deleterious local effects of the insult. Cryotherapy is very beneficial for acute control of pain and swelling. Cryotherapy lessens edema and reduces pain by decreasing arteriolar and capillary blood flow and decreasing muscle spasm (65–74). Cryotherapy can be applied in various manners, including crushed ice in a plastic bag, in an iced immersion tub, or as ice massage (68,69,71,75–77). Recovery proceeds faster if the initial swelling is limited (78). Compression with a shoulder wrap also aids in minimizing swelling. Nonsteroidal anti-inflammatory drugs (NSAIDs) serve the dual purpose of lessening inflammation and relieving pain. Acetaminophen may be used alone or with NSAIDs for relief of mild to moderate pain. More severe injuries, such as acute dislocations or fractures, usually require short-term narcotic analgesia. Other therapeutic modalities, such as transcutaneous electrical stimulation (TENS) and electric galvanic stimulation (EGS), can be very useful for the management of acute pain and swelling (79).

As the athlete progresses through the early stages of rehabilitation, it is important that therapies do not interfere with the normal healing process of the injured tissues. Brief immobilization may be required following glenohumeral subluxation or acromioclavicular sprain to allow the initial healing of disrupted ligamentous and capsular fibers. The time period of immobilization is individualized to the athlete and injury. In general, however, as pain and swelling diminish, gentle range of motion begins within 24 hours and progresses gradually in order to limit the formation of adhesions (80) and to promote proprioception retraining (81).

In the case of acute glenohumeral anterior dislocation, the initial brief period of immobilization should be followed by an extended 4- to 6-week period of relative protection. Abduction with external rotation, which causes anterior translation of the humeral head, is avoided. Early isometric strengthening of the rotator cuff and scapular stabilizing muscles stimulates collagen fiber growth and realignment in muscles, tendons, and ligaments (82–85) while minimizing the risk of further injury to these structures. The effects of immobilization on muscle are well documented (86–88) and emphasize the need for early therapies. Loss of muscle strength proceeds at a rate as high as 20% per week of immobilization (89), and atrophy may occur even faster if the muscle is braced in a shortened position (90). Immobilization has an adverse affect primarily on type I muscle fibers, which are crucial for shoulder maneuvers involving rapid acceleration, such as in pitching or volleyball (91–93). Significant changes also occur in the joint capsule, cartilage, and subchondral bone with prolonged immobilization (94). If prolonged shoulder immobilization is necessary, exercising the uninvolved shoulder helps by way of "cross-education" of the neuromuscular system. Such "cross-education" exercise can increase strength on the immobilized side by as much as 30% (95). Progressing therapies is a fine balance between protecting the tissue injury complex and restoring normal muscular balance and normal athletic function at the earliest possible time (82–96).

Maintaining other components of fitness during recovery from shoulder injuries is, in general, easier than during recovery from lower-limb injuries. Usually, the athlete can participate in aerobic exercises such as running or cycling, although high-impact activities may be too jarring. Strengthening and range of motion exercises of the lower limbs and contralateral upper limb should proceed. Strength and stretching work can also proceed in the involved upper limb, as long as the injured body part is protected. For example, a rotator cuff injury does not necessarily preclude (and may in fact require) early strengthening of scapular stabilizing muscles, biceps, triceps, and forearm muscles. Similarly, an athlete with a mild to moderate anterior labral injury will benefit from continuing cardiovascular training, strength and flexibility training in uninvolved limbs, and gentle internal rotation strengthening of the injured shoulder, while avoiding abduction and external rotation. As therapies progress, it is essential to identify and correct other problems along the kinetic chain and substitution patterns that either predated the injury or developed subsequently.

Strengthening exercises are usually done only in pain-free ranges. Therefore, pain-free range of motion exercises must progress in order to allow for progression of strengthening exercises. Once range of motion and light weight work is pain free in the full range of motions at the cervical, scapulothoracic, and glenohumeral articulations, the athlete is ready for sport-specific exercise, which is the last step prior to returning to play. Constant repetition with focus on perfecting the athletic movements required is necessary for the neurophysiologic learning process that helps develop coordinated skill patterns and smooth athletic engrams (97–99). Criteria for return to play should include resolution of the tissue injury and clinical symptom complex. Functional range of motion, adequate muscle strength, and ability to perform sport-specific activities are also necessary prior to return to play. The comprehensive rehabilitation plan does not end at this point, however. Rehabilitation of the athlete's shoulder must extend well beyond resolution of symptoms. If the functional biomechanical deficits and resultant adaptive substitution patterns are not addressed, the athlete remains at risk for recurrent injury or inability to attain the highest level of performance possible.

Principles of Rehabilitation of Specific Shoulder Injuries

Unfortunately, space does not permit discussion of all possible shoulder injuries encountered in athletics. We therefore focus on the most common injuries seen in a typical sports physiatry practice. The reader is referred elsewhere for a comprehensive review of other shoulder injury rehabilitation protocols (100–102).

Rehabilitation of Rotator Cuff Injuries

One of the most common upper-limb injuries seen in the athletic population is rotator cuff pathology and associated lesions such as labrum tears, bicipital tendinitis, and subacromial bursitis. Repetitive overhead activity is implicated in the pathomechanics of the injury. The musculoskeletal differential diagnosis includes acromioclavicular or glenohumeral arthritis, acute soft-tissue or bone contusion following trauma, and occult fracture of the greater tuberosity. The neuromuscular differential diagnosis includes cervical radiculopathy, brachial neuritis, axillary nerve entrapment in the quadrilateral space, suprascapular nerve entrapment, and musculocutaneous nerve entrapment in the biceps muscle. The visceral differential diagnosis includes referred pain from cardiac or gastrointestinal disorders.

Accurately identifying the five elements of the musculoskeletal injury complex precedes the formation of the rehabilitation plan. The tissue injury complex may be acute or subacute rotator cuff tendinitis, chronic rotator cuff tendinosis, or a frank rotator cuff tear. The clinical symptom complex includes the impingement sign with abduction and internal rotation, pain with isolated resistance of the supraspinatus, and a painful arc from 60 to 120 degrees of abduction. The functional biomechanical deficits include internal rotation inflexibility, external rotation weakness, and "lateral scapular slide" (64). The functional adaptation complex includes substitution patterns with alteration of the arm position during overhead activities such as throwing or lifting, "short arming" the throwing motion, and muscle recruitment from the anterior shoulder, forearm, or trunk. The tissue overload complex involves eccentric overload in the posterior shoulder capsule, posterior shoulder muscles, and scapular stabilizing muscles.

Nonsteroidal anti-inflammatory medication is appropriate in the acute phase for both its analgesic and anti-inflammatory effects. Corticosteroid injection into an inflamed subacromial bursa provides rapid relief of inflammation. The injectate must be correctly placed, however, because corticosteroid injected into musculotendinous structures can weaken these structures and increase the risk of rupture (103). Cryotherapy, TENS, and ultrasound have all been used to expedite resolution of inflammation of the bursa and rotator cuff tendons (104).

Gentle passive and active assisted range of motion may begin immediately. Particular attention should be paid to tightness of the external rotators with resultant limitation of internal rotation. Manual mobilization and cross-friction massage also help restore flexibility (105). Strengthening exercises begin isometrically. Isometric exercises should be done in all planes and various angles that do not produce pain. During recovery, new connective tissue is laid down along lines of stress (80,81). Isometric exercises provide the appropriate physical environment in which fibroblasts can make healthy, organized connective tissue, yet avoid untoward force and movement on the healing tendon. Once full, pain-free range of motion is achieved, the athlete progresses to isokinetic and isotonic strengthening exercises in all planes. External rotation should be strengthened preferentially over internal rotation to correct muscle imbalance. In addition to focusing on the rotator cuff itself, special emphasis is placed on fortifying the scapular stabilizers, which help to properly position the rotator cuff. Finally, once flexibility and strength have been regained, the athlete must complete sport-specific shoulder exercises prior to being allowed to return to play.

Rehabilitation of Glenohumeral Instability

Glenohumeral instability is also commonly seen in the athletic population. Instability may span the range from subclinical instability, to occasional, mild subluxation, to recurrent, gross dislocation. With acute dislocation, fractures of the glenoid and humerus must be considered in the differential diagnosis. Depending on the mechanism of injury, the nerve lesions mentioned in the preceding section may also occur.

As with any sports injury, identification of the five elements of the musculoskeletal injury complex aids in developing comprehensive rehabilitation strategies that address primary and secondary sites of pathology. The tissue injury complex is the anterior capsule, including the anterior labrum and glenohumeral ligaments. The clinical symptom complex may include anterior pain, a subjective sense of instability, loss of normal mobility, and deformity in the case of gross subluxation or dislocation. The functional biomechanical deficit is weakness of the anterior dynamic stabilizers, pectoralis major, and subscapularis. The functional adaptation complex varies with injury severity, but may include guarding the shoulder and avoiding abduction and external rotation. The tissue overload complex consists primarily of the anterior static stabilizers, especially the labrum and inferior glenohumeral ligament. The rotator cuff may also become overloaded as increased demand is placed on it to try and maintain normal glenohumeral alignment.

Acute traumatic dislocation in the competitive athlete will frequently require surgical repair. Acute dislocation or chronic laxity in the recreational athlete can often be successfully treated conservatively. Chronic glenohumeral subluxation or dislocation most commonly occurs in the anterior direction. If an acute dislocation has occurred, a period of immobilization aids initial healing of the capsuloligamentous lesion. Application of ice decreases tissue edema and pain. The time period for immobilization must be brief, however, to avoid disuse atrophy, shoulder stiffness, and maladaptive histologic changes in soft tissue and bone (94). Three to 6 weeks is adequate (106,107).

Gentle isometric strengthening can begin during the period of immobilization. Early motion is important for minimizing adhesions and preserving proprioceptive skills (80,81). The caveat is to avoid the combination of abduction, external rotation, and extension, which stresses the already damaged anterior capsule. Strengthening exercises should begin at less than 90 degrees of abduction and anterior to the coronal plane, so as to avoid anterior translation of the humerus (108). Strengthening exercises should target the dynamic anterior stabilizers, including the subscapularis, pectoralis major, and latissimus dorsi. Later, strengthening of the remaining shoulder muscles is initiated. Once range of motion and strengthening have progressed to the point that the athlete can assume a position of 90 degrees of abduction and external rotation without apprehension, sport-specific exercises may commence. The total period of rehabilitation may vary from 6 weeks to 6 months.

Rehabilitation of Acromioclavicular Injuries

Its superficial location and relatively large degree of clavicular rotation put the acromioclavicular joint at relative risk for traumatic injury. The usual mechanism of injury for acute acromioclavicular sprain or dislocation is a fall or blow onto the point of the shoulder, such that acromion is forced caudally relative to the clavicle (109). A grade II sprain consists of mild injury to the acromioclavicular and coracoclavicular ligaments with no frank anatomic disruption (110). A grade II sprain represents sufficient ligamentous injury to the acromioclavicular static stabilizers so as to allow for displacement of the acromioclavicular joint less than the width of the clavicle. A grade III sprain indicates complete loss of the integrity of the acromioclavicular and coracoclavicular ligaments (110).

Once again, the most complete rehabilitation plan can be outlined if all aspects of the musculoskeletal injury complex are appreciated. The tissue injury complex is the acromioclavicular joint and supporting ligaments. The clinical symptom complex includes tenderness with acromioclavicular joint palpation, pain with horizontal adduction, and gross deformity with "tenting up" of the top of the shoulder. Functional biomechanical deficits that may develop if the injury is left untreated include weakness of abduction and posterior capsule tightness. The functional adaptation complex includes alteration in normal scapulothoracic and glenohumeral motion. The tissue overload complex consists of the acromioclavicular and coracoclavicular ligaments.

To a large extent, the rehabilitation of acromioclavicular joint injuries depends on the degree of the sprain and the goals of the athlete. Obviously, a tennis player is more reliant on normal acromioclavicular motion than is a football lineman. Acutely, ice and compression are used to diminish pain and edema. Injection of anesthetic into the joint may serve both diagnostic and therapeutic purposes. Local padding serves to protect the area from additional insult.

Grade I joint sprains respond well to ice and NSAIDs, and return to usual sporting activities in 2 days to 2 weeks is common. Grade II sprains may benefit from the use of a sling to diminish strain on the joint until it is asymptomatic, a time period that may range from 1 to 4 weeks. As symptoms abate, gentle passive and active assisted range of motion exercises begin. Strengthening of the trapezius and other shoulder girdle musculature begins isometrically in pain-free positions, and progresses to light isotonic or isokinetic exercises as pain-free range of motion improves. Repetitive shoulder elevation should be kept to a minimum for the first 4 weeks of rehabilitation (111). The deformity present at the superior aspect of the shoulder, however, will likely persist (110).

The rehabilitation of grade III injuries follows a similar protocol as outlined above, but with a longer time frame. Grade III acromioclavicular separations tend to result in greater limitation of motion and have a higher potential for prolonged disability. In most cases, however, nonsurgical treatment is still the preferred course (110–112). A 5% to 10% incidence of significant problems with grade III acromioclavicular separations has been reported, regardless of whether or not surgical repair was performed (110). Conservative care includes use of a sling for comfort and to lessen the chance of further injury in the early postinjury stage. Ice and NSAIDs are used to reduce edema and pain. Narcotic analgesia may also be required for a few days. The sling is allowed to be removed for progressively longer periods to perform gentle range of motion exercises. If pain free, isometric exercises may begin early while the limb is in the sling. The sling is discontinued as symptoms allow (110). If progression to dynamic or sport-specific exercises is hampered by continued symptoms or if the cosmetic deformity is unacceptable to the athlete, then surgical referral for open repair is indicated. Surgical referral may also be indicated if the acromioclavicular separation causes a major shift in the position of the scapula owing to loss of support by the clavicle, in which case more pain symptoms may be expected, or if there is pressure to return the athlete to play rapidly.

One long-term complication of acromioclavicular separation is continued pain at the acromioclavicular joint due to posttraumatic degenerative changes in the joint. A simple procedure consisting of distal osteolysis of the clavicle usually provides good relief (113).

INDICATIONS FOR SURGERY

The need for surgical repair of an anatomic lesion varies with the nature of the injury, the athletic demands placed on the individual, and the philosophy of the physician and the athlete. In general, displaced fractures require surgical reduction. Many nondisplaced and minimally displaced fractures can be treated with brief immobilization followed by relative rest. Large rotator cuff tears and severe ligamentous injuries with instability in the competitive athlete are often best treated with surgical repair. Cervical radiculopathy with progressive neurologic deficit or intractable pain is also an indication for surgical intervention. Although acromioclavicular separations can be successfully treated conservatively, surgical repair is indicated in the competitive throwing athlete to speed return to competition and optimize mechanics. Surgical débridement of troublesome osteophytes can improve quality of motion and decrease pain. One example is resection of the distal 1 cm of the clavicle for the treatment of acromioclavicular arthritis. Regardless of the surgical procedure performed, the athlete will still require a presurgery and postsurgery rehabilitation program that maximizes range of motion, strength, muscle balance, endurance, and neuromuscular control.

CONCLUSIONS

The glenohumeral joint is relatively unstable and requires both static and dynamic stabilizing forces in order to function most efficiently. Any injury to the structures that directly or indirectly support it results in pain and loss of function. A thorough history, accurate physical examination, and appropriate ancillary testing will guide the astute clinician to the correct diagnosis. An appropriate treatment plan can then be developed to meet specific patient needs.

REFERENCES

1. Kelsey J, Pastides H, Bisbee G. *Musculoskeletal disorders: their frequency of occurrence and their impact on the population of the United States.* New York: Prodist, 1978.
2. Calliet R. *Shoulder pain.* Philadelphia: FA Davis, 1981.
3. Jobe F, Kvitne R. Shoulder pain in the overhead or throwing athlete and the relationship of anterior instability and rotator cuff impingement. *Orthop Rev* 1989;28l:963–975.
4. Saha A. Anterior recurrent dislocation of the shoulder. *Acta Orthop Scand* 1967;68:479–493.
5. Ferrari D. Capsular ligaments of the shoulder. *Am J Sports Med* 1990;18:20–24.
6. Perry J. Anatomy and biomechanics of the shoulder in throwing, swimming, gymnastics and tennis. *Clin Sports Med* 1983;2:247–270.
7. Saal J. Rehabilitation of throwing and tennis related shoulder injuries. *Phys Med Rehabil State Art Rev.* 1987:597–612.
8. Poppen N, Walker P. Normal and abnormal motion of the shoulder. *J Bone Joint Surg [Am]* 1976;58:185–201.
9. Saha A. Mechanics of elevation of glenohumeral joint: its application in rehabilitation of flail shoulder in upper brachial plexus injuries and poliomyelitis and in replacement of the upper humerus by prosthesis. *Acta Orthop Scand* 1973;44:668–678.
10. Slivka J, Resnik D. An improved radiographic view of the glenohumeral joint. *J Can Assoc Radiol* 1979;30:83–85.
11. Kent B. Functional anatomy of the shoulder complex. *Phys Ther* 1971;51:867–887.
12. Rockwood C, Matsen F, eds. *The shoulder.* Philadelphia: WB Saunders, 1990.
13. deLuca C, Forrest W. Force analysis of individual muscles acting simultaneously in the shoulder joint during isometric abduction. *J Biomech* 1973;6:385–393.
14. Kibler W. Role of the scapula in the overhead throwing motion. *Contemp Orthop* 1991;22:525–532.
15. Inman V, Saunders J, Abbott L. Observations of the functions of the shoulder joint. *J Bone Joint Surg [Am]* 1944;26:1–30.
16. Hawkins R. Physical examination of the shoulder. *Orthopedics* 1983;6:1270–1278.
17. Magee D, ed. *Orthopedic physical assessment.* Philadelphia: WB Saunders, 1992:90–142.
18. Hollingshead W, Jenkins D, eds. *Functional anatomy of the limbs and back.* Philadelphia: WB Saunders, 1981:72–111.
19. Weiner D, Macnab I. Superior migration of the humeral head. *J Bone Joint Surg [Br]* 1970;52:524–527.
20. Cole A, Kadaba M, McCann P, et al. Electromyographic study of the subscapularis. 52nd Annual Meeting of the American Academy of Physical Medicine and Rehabilitation, Phoenix, AZ. 1990;71:790.
21. Rowe C. *The shoulder.* New York: Churchill Livingstone, 1988:673.
22. Lucas D. Biomechanics of the shoulder joint. *Arch Surg* 1973;107:425–432.
23. Hoppenfeld S. *Physical examination of the spine and extremities.* New York: Appleton-Century-Crofts, 1976:1–35.
24. Kulund D. *The injured athlete.* Philadelphia: JB Lippincott, 1988:301–356.
25. Yergason R. Supination sign. *J Bone Joint Surg* 1931;13:160.
26. Neer CS. Anterior acromioplasty for the chronic impingement syndrome in the shoulder: a preliminary report. *J Bone Joint Surg [Am]* 1972;54:41–50.
27. Schwartz E, Warren R, O'Brien S, Fronek J. Posterior shoulder instability. *Orthop Clin North Am* 1987;8:409–419.
28. O'Brien S, Warren R, Schwartz E. Anterior shoulder instability. *Orthop Clin North Am* 1987;18:395–408.
29. Pappas A, Goss T, Kleinman P. Symptomatic shoulder instability due to lesions of the glenoid labrum. *Am J Sports Med* 1983;11:279–288.
30. Gerber C, Ganz R. Clinical assessment of instability of the shoulder. *J Bone Joint Surg [Br]* 1984;66:551–556.
31. Hawkins R, Kennedy J. Impingement syndrome in athletes. *Am J Sports Med* 1980;8:151–158.
32. Workman TL, Burkhard TK, Resnick D, et al. Hill-Sachs lesion: comparison of detection with MR imaging, radiography, and arthroscopy. *Radiology* 1992;185:847–852.
33. Fu FJ, Harner CD, Klein AH. Shoulder impingement syndrome: a critical review. *Clin Orthop* 1991;269:162–173.
34. Neer CS. Impingement lesions. *Clin Orthop* 1983;173:70–77.

35. Bigliani LU, Morrison DS, April EW. The morphology of the acromion and its relationship to rotator cuff tears. *Orthop Trans* 1986;10:126.

36. Morrison DS, Bigliani LU. The clinical significance of variations in acromial morphology. Presented at the Third Open Meeting of the American Shoulder and Elbow Surgeons, San Francisco, 1987.

37. Chandnani V, Ho C, Gerharter J, et al. MR findings in asymptomatic shoulders: a blind analysis using symptomatic shoulders as controls. *Clin Imaging* 1992;16:25–30.

38. Clark JM, Harryman DT II. Tendons, ligaments, and capsule of the rotator cuff. *J Bone Joint Surg [Am]* 1992;74:713–725.

39. Farley TE, Neumann CH, Steinbach LS, et al. Full thickness tears of the rotator cuff of the shoulder: diagnosis with MR imaging. *Am J Radiol* 1992;158:347–351.

40. Ho CP. Applied MRI anatomy of the shoulder. *J Orthop Sports Phys Ther* 1993;18:351–359.

41. Iannotti JP, Zlatkin MB, Esterhai JL, et al. Magnetic resonance imaging of the shoulder. Sensitivity, specificity and predictive value. *J Bone Joint Surg [Am]* 1991;73:17–29.

42. Kjellin I, Ho CP, Cervilla V, et al. Alterations in the supraspinatus tendon at MR imaging: correlation with histopathologic findings in cadavers. *Radiology* 1991;181:837–841.

43. Traughber PD, Goodwin TE. Shoulder MRI: arthroscopic correlation with emphasis on partial tears. *J Comput Assist Tomogr* 1992;16:129–133.

44. Snyder SJ, Karzel RP, Del Pizzo W, et al. SLAP lesions of the shoulder. *Arthoscopy* 1990;6:274–279.

45. Neumann CH, Petersen SA, Jahnke AH. MR imaging of the labral-capsular complex: normal variation. *Am J Radiol* 1991;157:1015–1021.

46. Cervilla V, Schweitzer ME, Ho C, et al. Medial dislocation of the biceps brachii tendon: appearance at MR imaging. *Radiology* 1991;180:523.

47. Fritz RC, Helms CA, Steinbach LS, Genant HK. Suprascapular nerve entrapment: evaluation with MR imaging. *Radiology* 1992;182:437–444.

48. Kewalramani LS, Krauss JF. Cervical spine injuries resulting from collision sports. *Int Med Soc Paraplegia* 1981;19:303–312.

49. Brooks WH, Bixby-Hammett DM. Prevention of neurologic injury in equestrian sports. *Phys Sports Med* 1988;16:84–95.

50. Harris JB. Neurologic injuries in winter sports. *Phys Sports Med* 1983;11:111–112.

51. Poindexter DP, Johnson EW. Football shoulder and neck injury: a study of the "stinger." *Arch Phys Med Rehabil* 1984;65:601–602.

52. Clancy WG Jr, Brand RL, Bergfeld JA. Upper trunk brachial plexus injuries in contact sports. *Am J Sports Med* 1977;5:209.

53. Herring SA, Weinstein SM. Electrodiagnosis in sports medicine. *Phys Med Rehabil State Art Rev* 1989;3:809–822.

54. Gregg JR, Labosky D, Harty M, et al. Serratus anterior paralysis in the young athlete. *J Bone Joint Surg [Am]* 1979;63:825–832.

55. Johnson TH, Kendall HO. Isolated paralysis of the serratus anterior muscle. *J Bone Joint Surg [Am]* 1955;37:567–574.

56. Cahill BR, Palmer RE. Quadrilateral space syndrome. *J Hand Surg* 1983;8:65–69.

57. Petrucci FS, Morelli A, Raimondi PL. Axillary nerve injury: 21 cases treated by nerve graft and neurolysis. *J Hand Surg* 1982;7:271–278.

58. Bateman JE. Nerve injuries about the shoulder in sports. *J Bone Joint Surg [Am]* 1967;49:785–792.

59. Goodman CE, Kenrick MM, Blum MV. Long thoracic nerve palsy: a follow-up study. *Arch Phys Med Rehabil* 1975;56:352–355.

60. Jordan BD, Tsairis P, Warren RF, eds. *Sports neurology.* Rockville, MD: Aspen, 1989.

61. Zoltan JD. Injury to the suprascapular nerve associated with anterior dislocation of the shoulder: case report and review of the literature. *J Trauma* 1979;19:103–106.

62. Goodman CE. Unusual nerve injuries in recreational sports. *Am J Sports Med* 1983;2:224–227.

63. Hashimoto K, Oda K, Kuroda Y, Shibasaki H. Case of suprascapular nerve palsy manifesting as selected atrophy of the infraspinatus muscle. *Rinsho Shinkeigaku* 1983;23:970–973.

64. Kibler WB. Clinical aspects of muscle injury. *Med Sci Sports Exerc* 1990;22:450–452.

65. Chambers R. Clinical uses of cryotherapy. *Phys Ther* 1969;49:245–249.

66. Drez D, Faust DC, Evans JP. Cryotherapy and nerve palsy. *Am J Sports Med* 1981;9:256–257.

67. Grana WA, Curl WL, Reider B. Cold modalities. In: Drez D, ed. *Therapeutic modalities for sports injuries.* Chicago: Year Book Medical, 1986:25–31.

68. Halvorson GA. Principles or rehabilitating sports injuries. In: Teitz CC, ed. *Scientific foundations of sports medicine.* Toronto: BC Decker, 1989:345–371.

69. Lehmann JF, DeLateur BJ. Cryotherapy. In: Lehmann JF, ed. *Therapeutic heat and cold.* Baltimore: Williams & Wilkins, 1982:563–602.

70. McMaster WC. Cryotherapy. *Phys Sports Med* 1982;10:112–119.

71. McMaster WC, Liddle S, Waugh TR. Laboratory evaluations of various cold therapy modalities. *Am J Sports Med* 1978;6:291–294.

72. Ork H. Uses of cold. In: Kuprian W, ed. *Physical therapy for sports.* Philadelphia: WB Saunders, 1982:62–68.

73. Quillen WS, Rouiller LH. Initial management of acute ankle sprains with rapid pulsed pneumatic compression and cold. *J Orthop Sports Phys Ther* 1982;4:39–43.

74. Sloan JP, Giddings P, Hain R. Effects of cold and compression on edema. *Phys Sports Med* 1988;16:116–120.

75. Grant AE. Massage with ice (cyokinetics) in the treatment of painful conditions of the musculoskeletal system. *Arch Phys Med Rehabil* 1964;45:233–238.

76. Lehmann JF, DeLateur BJ. Diathermy and superficial heat and cold therapy. In: Kottke FJ, Stillwell GK, Lehmann JF, eds. *Krusen's handbook of physical medicine and rehabilitation.* Philadelphia: WB Saunders, 1982:275–350.

77. Roy S, Irvin R, eds. *Sports medicine: prevention, evaluation, management, and rehabilitation.* Englewood Cliffs, NJ: Prentice-Hall, 1983.

78. Akeson WH. An experimental study of joint stiffness. *J Bone Joint Surg [Am]* 1961;43:1022–1034.

79. Marino M. Principles of therapeutic modalities: implications for sports injuries. In: Nicholas JA, Hershman EB, eds. *The upper extremity in sports medicine.* St. Louis: CV Mosby, 1990:195–244.

80. Frank G, Woo S, Amiel D, et al. Medial collateral ligament healing. A multidisciplinary assessment in rabbits. *Am J Sports Med* 1983;11:379.

81. Leach R. The prevention and rehabilitation of soft tissue injuries. *Int J Sports Med* 1982;3(1):18.

82. Dehn E, Torp RR. Treatment of joint injuries by immediate rehabilitation. *Clin Orthop* 1971;77:218–231.

83. Jarvinen M. Healing of crush injury in rat striated muscle. 2. A histological study of the effect of early mobilization and immobilization on the repair process. *Acta Pathol Microbiol Scand* 1975;A83:269–282.

84. Jarvinen M. Healing of crush injury in rat striated muscle. 3. A micro angiographical study of the effect of early mobilization and immobilization on capillary ingrowth. *Acta Pathol Microbiol Scand* 1976;A84:85–94.

85. Jarvinen M. Healing of crush injury in rat striated muscle. 4. Effect of early mobilization and immobilization on the tensile properties of gastrocnemius muscle. *Acta Chir Scand* 1976;142:47–56.

86. Muller EA. Influence of training and of inactivity on muscle strength. *Arch Phys Med Rehabil* 1970;51:449–462.

87. Booth FW. Time course of muscular atrophy during immobilization of hind limbs in rats. *J Appl Physiol* 1977;43:656–661.

88. Booth FW, Seider MJ. Effects of disuse by limb immobilization on different muscle fiber types. In: Pette D, ed. *Plasticity of muscle.* New York: de Gruyter, 1980.

89. Hettinger T, Mueller EA. Muskelleistung and muskeltraining. *Arbeitsphysiologie* 1953;15:111.

90. Paulos LE, Payne FC, Rosenberg TD. Rehabilitation after anterior cruciate ligament surgery. In: Jackson D, Drew D, eds. *The anterior cruciate deficient knee.* St. Louis: CV Mosby, 1987:291–314.

91. Eriksson E. Sports injuries of the knee ligaments: their diagnosis, treatment, rehabilitation and prevention. *Med Sci Sports Exerc* 1976;8:133.

92. Eriksson E, Haggmark T. Comparison of isometric muscle training and electrical stimulation supplementing isometric muscle training in the recovery after major knee ligament surgery. *Am J Sports Med* 1979;7:169.

93. Haggmark T, Eriksson E. Cylinder or mobile cast brace after knee ligament surgery: a clinical analysis and morphologic and enzymatic studies of changes in the quadriceps muscle. *Am J Sports Med* 1979;7:48.

94. Akeson V, Woo S, Amiel D. The connective tissue response to immobility: biomechanical changes in periarticular connective tissue of the immobilized rabbit knee. *Clin Orthop* 1973;93:356.

95. Saltin B, Nagar K, Costill DL, et al. The nature of the training response: peripheral and central adaptations to one-legged exercise. *Acta Physiol Scand* 1976;96:289–305.

96. Knight KL. Guidelines for rehabilitation of sports injuries. *Clin Sports Med* 1985;4:405.

97. Saal JS. Flexibility training. *Phys Med Rehabil State Art Rev* 1987;1:537–554.

98. Fahey TD. Physiologic adaptation to conditioning. In: Basmajian JV, ed. *Therapeutic exercise.* Baltimore: Williams & Wilkins, 1984.

99. Hams FA. Facilitation techniques and technological adjuncts in therapeutic exercise. In: Basmajian JV, ed. *Therapeutic exercise.* Baltimore: Williams & Wilkins, 1984.

100. Matsen FA, Lippitt SB, Siddles JA, Harryman DT, eds. *Practical evaluation and management of the shoulder.* Philadelphia: WB Saunders, 1994:65.

101. Brotzman SB, ed. *Clinical orthopedic rehabilitation.* New York: Mosby, 1996:91–142.

102. Andrews JR, Wilk KE, eds. *The athlete's shoulder.* New York: Churchill Livingstone, 1994.

103. Kennedy JL, Baxter-Willis R. The effects of local steroid injections on tendons: a biomechanical and microscopic correlative study. *Am J Sports Med* 1976;4:11–18.

104. Hawkins RJ, Kennedy JC. Impingement syndrome in athletics. *Am J Sports Med* 1980;8:151–163.

105. Sarfran MR, Garrett WE, Seaber AV. The role of warm-up in muscle injury prevention. *Am J Sports Med* 1988;16:123–129.

106. Simonet WT, Colfield RH. Prognosis in anterior shoulder dislocation. *Am J Sports Med* 1984;12:19.

107. Yoneda B, Welsh RP, MacIntosh DL. Conservative treatment of shoulder dislocation. *J Bone Joint Surg [Br]* 1982;64:254.

108. Turkel SJ, Panio MW, Marshall JL, Girgis FG. Stabilizing mechanisms preventing anterior dislocation of the glenohumeral joint. *J Bone Joint Surg [Am]* 1981;63:1208–1217.

109. Allman FL Jr. Fracture and ligamentous injuries of the clavicle and its articulation. *J Bone Joint Surg [Am]* 1967;9:774.

110. Bergfeld JA. Acromioclavicular complex. In: Nicholas JA, Hershman EB, eds. *The upper extremity in sports medicine*. St. Louis: CV Mosby, 1990;169–180.

111. Brems JJ. Degenerative joint disease in the shoulder. In: Nicholas JA, Hershman EB, eds. *The upper extremity in sports medicine* St. Louis: CV Mosby, 1990:235–250.

112. Cox JS. The fate of the acromioclavicular joint in athletic injuries. *Am J Sports Med* 1977;5:264.

113. Eskola A, Santavirta S, Viljakka HT, et al. The results of operative resection of the lateral end of the clavicle. *J Bone Joint Surg [Am]* 1996;78:584–587.

Chapter 66

Rehabilitation of Elbow Injuries

Steven L. Wiesner

An athlete's elbow joint and its associated neurovascular and soft-tissue structures may be injured as a result of repetitive upper-extremity forces or an acute, single traumatic event. An accurate diagnosis and appropriate rehabilitation must be based on an understanding of the relevant anatomy and functional biomechanics. Rehabilitation beyond symptom control involves controlling the inflammatory process and improving joint flexibility, muscular strength, endurance, and aerobic conditioning. To provide for timely healing, safe return to sport, and decreased risk of reinjury, the sport physiatrist must also address upper-extremity kinetic chain functioning, sporting techniques, training regimens, and proper equipment use.

RELEVANT ANATOMY AND BIOMECHANICS

Distal End of the Humerus

The distal end of the humerus consists of two condyles that form the articular surfaces of the trochlea and capitellum. The laterally situated capitellum serves as a buttress for lateral compression and rotational forces commonly encountered during throwing motions (1). The lateral epicondyle is located proximal to the capitellum and serves as an attachment site for the supinator-extensor muscle groups as well as the lateral collateral ligament. The radial fossa is located proximal to the capitellum and accommodates the radial head during flexion.

Owing to its oblique orientation, the spool-shaped trochlea, situated between the medial and lateral columns of the distal part of the humerus, contributes to the carrying angle. This angle is formed by the long axis of the humerus and the long axis of the ulna, while the arm is extended and supinated. In males, the normal angle is 5 to 10 degrees; in females, 10 to 15 degrees (2). The medial epicondyle is situated proximal to the trochlea and serves as the attachment site for the medial collateral ligament as well as the flexor-pronator muscles. Anterior and superior to the trochlea lies the coronoid fossa, while the olecranon fossa is situated posteriorly. The plane of flexion and extension is defined by the articulation of the trochlea and olecranon process (3).

Ulna and Radius

Inherent stability of the elbow is enhanced by the ulnohumeral joint. This joint is formed by the articulation of the greater sigmoid notch of the ulna and the trochlea. The opening of the sigmoid notch is angled 30 degrees posteriorly, allowing for maximum range of motion while maintaining articular conformity (4). The coronoid process forms the distal and anterior aspect of the notch, with the olecranon forming the proximal and posterior aspect. The medial aspect of the coronoid process provides the attachment site for the anterior portion of the medial collateral ligament and the ulnar portion of the pronator teres. The radial notch, also known as the lateral or lesser sigmoid notch, is located along the lateral aspect of the coronoid

. The cylindrically shaped radial head articulates the radial notch and is stabilized by the annular ligament. In forming the radiohumeral joint, the radial head also articulates with the capitellum. The radial neck is distal to the head, with the radial tuberosity forming the most distal aspect of the neck (4,5).

Ligamentous and Capsular Stability

Medial Collateral Ligament

The collateral ligaments are specialized thickenings of the medial and lateral capsule. The medial collateral ligament is composed of three bundles, a major anterior bundle, a thin posterior bundle, and a nonfunctional transverse ligament. The proximal attachment of the medial collateral ligament is at the inferior surface of the medial epicondyle in a somewhat medial position, with the anterior bundle being positioned posterior to the axis of rotation. The ligamentous fibers of the anterior portion insert along the medial aspect of the coronoid process and the posterior bundle inserts on the medial aspect of the posterior olecranon. The anterior bundle is the prime stabilizer of the joint, as it remains taut throughout the range of elbow motion (6,7). Sectioning of the posterior band, which is lax until approximately 60 degrees of flexion, causes minimal change in elbow stability (8). As the transverse ligament arises and inserts onto the ulna, it does not contribute to elbow stability (9).

Lateral Collateral Ligament and Annular Ligament

Compared to the medial ligamentous complex, the lateral ligamentous complex is less clearly defined and has greater anatomic variability. According to Morrey (5), the complex is composed of the radial collateral ligament, the lateral ulnar collateral ligament, the accessory lateral collateral ligament, and the annular ligament. The radial collateral ligament is a thickening of the lateral capsule. This ligament originates from the lateral epicondyle and has a diffuse attachment distally onto the annular ligament. The radial collateral ligament is taut throughout the normal range of flexion and extension, consistent with the origin being near the axis of rotation. Fibers from the lateral ulnar collateral ligament and posterior fibers from the radial collateral ligament merge as they attach to the ulna. The accessory lateral collateral ligament and the lateral ulnar collateral ligament insert on the ulna, without receiving any contribution from the posterior portion of the radial collateral ligament. Proximal fibers of the accessory lateral collateral ligament blend with fibers from the annular ligament. This band appears to further stabilize the annular ligament during varus stress.

The annular ligament originates and inserts onto the anterior and posterior margins of the radial notch. This ligament maintains contact of the radius with the ulna and limits distal migration of the radius. The annular ligament is funnel shaped and constitutes about four-fifths of the fibro-osseous ring. The remainder of the ring is formed by the radial notch. The anterior insertion becomes taut during supination and the posterior aspect tightens during pronation. Disruption of the annular ligament may cause a loss of articular congruity and deficits in forearm rotation. This may occur when the radial head is fractured (5,10).

Joint Capsule

The joint capsule surrounds the elbow joint. The anterior capsule is taut in extension and lax in flexion. The posterior capsule is redundant and allows for full range of motion at the elbow. The posterior capsule's redundancy also allows fluid to accumulate, which may result from certain inflammatory conditions (5,11).

Muscles

Wrist Extensors

The extensor muscles of the wrist and fingers originate from a common tendinous origin at the lateral distal region of the humerus and the epicondyle. The extensor muscle group consists of the extensor carpi radialis brevis (ECRB), extensor carpi radialis longus (ECRL), extensor carpi ulnaris (ECU), and extensor digitorum communis (EDC). The brachioradialis is discussed based on its functional role rather than its anatomic position (Fig. 66-1).

Elbow Flexors

The primary muscles that allow for elbow flexion include the brachioradialis, biceps brachii, and brachialis. The pronator teres and flexor carpi ulnaris are considered

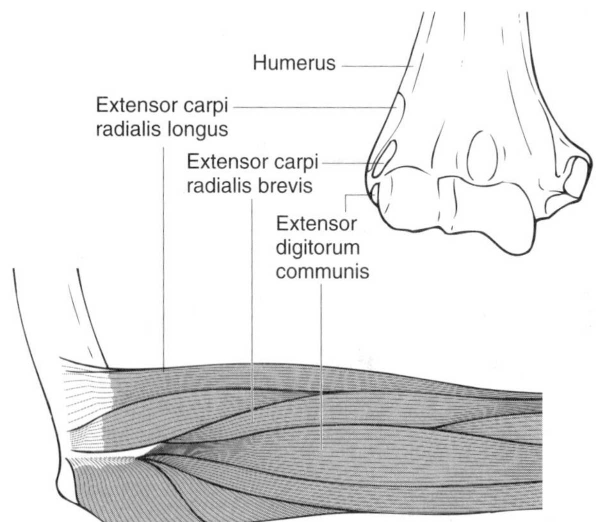

Figure 66-1. Anatomy of the musculotendinous structures arising from the lateral epicondyle. (Redrawn with permission from Plancher KD, Halbrecht J, Lourie GM. Medial and lateral epicondylitis in the athlete. *Clin Sports Med* 1996;15:283–305.

secondary contributors to elbow flexion (12). The brachioradialis originates from the lateral border of the humerus and the lateral intermuscular septum and inserts on the lateral side of the distal end of the radius. It provides the greatest mechanical advantage of the elbow flexors, adding speed and power. The biceps brachii is a major flexor of the elbow, with the two heads joining into a common tendon that passes anterior to the elbow before inserting on the radial tuberosity. Contraction of the biceps muscle produces elbow flexion and supination, owing to the bicep's insertion onto the radial tuberosity. Thus, in the pronated position the biceps functions more as a supinator than as an elbow flexor. The brachialis, although having the largest cross-sectional area of the flexors, suffers from a poor mechanical advantage as it crosses close to the axis of rotation. Unlike the biceps, however, the brachialis attaches to the ulnar tuberosity and does not contribute to pronation or supination, thereby being equally effective in flexing the forearm regardless of the position of forearm rotation (13).

Elbow Extensors

The primary elbow extensor is the triceps brachii. It is composed of three heads: the lateral and medial heads originating from the posterior aspect of the humerus and the long head originating from the infraglenoid tuberosity of the scapula. The three heads combine to insert onto the olecranon, with the attachment being separated by the olecranon bursa. Although various bursae about the elbow have been described, the most commonly involved bursal structure is the superficial olecranon bursa, which is frequently injured as a result of direct trauma and repetitive pressure or inflammatory conditions.

The anconeus originates from the lateral epicondyle, with insertion along the lateral side of the olecranon and ulna. It appears to assist in stabilization of the elbow joint against flexion or pronation-supination as well as serve as a secondary elbow extensor (13).

Flexor-Pronator Group

The flexor-pronator muscle group includes the pronator teres, flexor carpi radialis, flexor carpi ulnaris, and the palmaris longus. The muscles originate from the medial epicondyle via a common flexor tendon. The pronator teres is the most proximal and superficial of this group. The two heads arise from the medial epicondyle and the coronoid process of the ulna. The pronator teres inserts at the junction of the proximal and middle portions of the lateral aspect of the radius through a common musculotendinous unit. The muscle serves as a primary pronator of the forearm as well as a weak elbow flexor. The flexor carpi radialis and palmaris longus, when present, function as wrist flexors and may also assist with forearm pronation. The flexor carpi ulnaris is the most posterior of the flexor-pronator muscle group and functions as a wrist flexor and ulnar deviator, owing to its insertion into the pisiform (13).

Supinators

The supinator originates from the lateral aspect of the lateral epicondyle, the lateral collateral ligament, and the posterolateral surface of the ulna just below the radial notch (crista supinatoris). It courses inferiorly and laterally to insert diffusely onto the radius. As the name implies, the muscle serves as a supinator of the forearm and unlike the supination action of the bicep, the supinator muscle's effectiveness is not altered by the position of the elbow. The supinator is, however, believed to be a weaker supinator in comparison to the biceps (13).

Neurovascular Structures

Anatomy, Clinical Presentation of Injury States, and Treatment Principles

Peripheral nerve injuries may be caused by traction and friction forces from repetitive activities or as a result of acute compression. Electrodiagnostic evaluation in concert with a thorough history and physical examination is essential to assess the presence of nerve damage, localize the site of injury, delineate the severity of the dysfunction, and assist in proper patient management. The absence of conduction delays, amplitude reduction, or electromyographic abnormalities is not uncommon and does not exclude underlying neuropathic compromise (14).

Nonsurgical management may include the use of splinting techniques, anti-inflammatory medication and modalities for pain and inflammatory control, myofascial release techniques, flexibility and strengthening exercises, and when necessary, injections for both diagnostic and therapeutic purposes. Attention must also be given to proper sport and activity biomechanics (14).

Ulnar Nerve

The most common nerve injury at the elbow region involves the ulnar nerve. At the elbow, the ulnar nerve courses posterior to the medial epicondyle in the posterior condylar groove. The nerve then travels under an arch-like structure that bridges the origin of the two heads of the flexor carpi ulnaris, thereby creating a potential site for ulnar nerve compression. Branches of the ulnar nerve that innervate the flexor carpi ulnaris arise proximal to the arch, with branches to the ulnar portion of the flexor digitorum profundus being provided within the cubital tunnel (15).

According to Nirschl (16), the epicondylar groove can be divided into three zones: zone 1, proximal to the medial epicondyle; zone 2, at the medial epicondyle; and zone 3, distal to the medial epicondyle. The majority of ulnar nerve dysfunction is due to compression forces in zone 3, as the ulnar nerve passes through the two heads of the flexor carpi ulnaris (16). Osteophytic spurs, loose bodies, and rheumatoid synovitis more commonly cause damage in zone 2, whereas a tight medial intermuscular septum can cause compression of the ulnar nerve in zone 1 (17,18).

Increased tensile and traction forces on the ulnar nerve can develop as a result of a valgus instability, especially when accompanied by medial collateral ligament disruption (19–21). During full flexion, the ulnar nerve undergoes approximately 5 mm of stretch, with associated narrowing of the cubital tunnel as the overlying retinaculum becomes taut (22–25). Shoulder external rotation and abduction further increase the traction force on the ulnar nerve, with a sixfold increase in intraneural pressure noted during the cocked position of the throwing motion (26). Scar tissue formation due to previous injury or surgery, hypertrophy of the flexor-pronator group, hypermobility, and subluxation-dislocation of the nerve from its groove can cause abnormal compressive forces to the nerve (17,20,27). More proximal lesions that can lead to ulnar distribution symptoms include cervical dysfunction with C8 or T1 nerve root involvement, thoracic outlet syndrome, and entrapment at the arcade of Struthers.

Clinically, the athlete may report dysesthesias in an ulnar nerve distribution, pain from the medial aspect of the elbow to the hand, and a clumsy sensation in the hand. Weakness, atrophy, and deformity usually occur later with ongoing nerve injury. As the symptoms may not be present at rest, additional maneuvers can assist in the diagnosis. These provocative tests include sustained elbow flexion (to reproduce symptoms), repetitive flexion-extension motions (to observe for snapping sensation), and the Tinel test at the cubital tunnel. Electrodiagnostic evaluation may help to further localize the site of nerve damage and determine its severity (4,14,21,28).

Conservative treatment includes avoiding aggravating activities and padding the elbow to protect against further trauma (29). A rigid thermoplastic orthosis with the elbow in less than 45 degrees of flexion can be used to further limit elbow flexion. Initially, the splint is worn at all times, and as the symptoms improve, the orthosis should be worn only at night (30). The patient should maintain elbow strength through isometric and isotonic exercises within a 0- to 45-degree range of motion, thereby minimizing stretch to the ulnar nerve. When conservative care fails or significant motor denervation is identified, surgery is pursued. Ulnar nerve transposition is performed when subluxation-dislocation or valgus instability is present (16,21).

Harrelson (31) described a postoperative rehabilitation protocol following ulnar nerve decompression. A posterior splint set at 90 degrees of flexion is used for 7 days. Early grip and wrist exercises are initiated. At 7 days, the splint is removed for exercise and bathing, but extension for the last 15 degrees is avoided when out of the splint. By 3 weeks following surgery, the athlete has been weaned off of the splint and begins working on regaining end-range extension. Therapeutic exercise is progressed, with most individuals beginning a sport-specific interval training program by 8 weeks postoperatively.

Median Nerve

The median nerve and brachial artery travel beneath the bicep muscle and lie adjacent to the brachialis. The median nerve then passes under the bicipital aponeurosis and between the two heads of the pronator teres. At this level, it innervates the pronator teres, flexor carpi radialis, and palmaris longus. The anterior interosseous nerve arises approximately 5 to 8 cm distal to the lateral epicondyle, at the distal aspect of the pronator teres. The remainder of the median nerve travels beneath a fibrous arch formed by the proximal border of the flexor digitorum superficialis, ultimately passing through the carpal tunnel and into the hand (15).

In 1% of limbs an anomalous spur is found 3 to 5 cm above the medial epicondyle. The ligament of Struthers connects this spur to the medial epicondyle, creating a fibro-osseous tunnel through which the median nerve and brachial artery pass, thereby forming a site for potential compression. More commonly, compression of the median nerve occurs as it passes through the pronator teres (pronator teres syndrome). The pronator teres is usually spared as innervation to the muscle originates proximally.

Median nerve compression has been associated with repetitive, strenuous motion and muscle hypertrophy as seen in weight lifting, racquet sports, and underarm fastball pitching. Clinically, the patient will present with an insidious onset of poorly localized aching in the proximal, volar aspect of the forearm (32,33). When compression occurs at the pronator teres, pain is noted in the proximal part of the forearm, with symptoms increased on resistance to pronation and wrist flexion. Compression at the lacertus fibrosus causes pain in the proximal part of the forearm that increases during resisted supination and at 120 to 130 degrees of elbow flexion. Compression at the flexor digitorum superficialis arch causes pain on resisted long finger flexion (28). Unlike carpal tunnel syndrome, nocturnal dysesthesias are uncommon. Tenderness over the pronator teres and a positive Tinel sign may be found. When symptoms and functional deficits persist despite conservative treatment, especially with documented axonal loss, surgical intervention is indicated (28).

Injury to the anterior interosseous nerve (AIN) can result from aggressive forearm exercise and structural anomalies and may also be associated with acute brachial neuritis (34,35). Clinically, patients may report vague, activity-related pain in the proximal region of the forearm. Motor examination reveals an inability to maintain tip-to-tip contact of the thumb and index finger due to weakness of the flexor pollicis longus and flexor digitorum profundus, respectively. The pronator quadratus may also be weak. Electrodiagnostic testing noting denervation of the flexor digitorum profundus in the index finger, flexor pollicis longus, and pronator quadratus is diagnostic of AIN injury. Surgical intervention is considered if there is a limited response to conservative treatment after 8 weeks or if symptoms progress. Operative management involves exploration and decompression of the median nerve from the proximal part of the forearm to all of the branches of the AIN (35).

Radial Nerve

The radial nerve descends along the lateral aspect of the humerus and innervates the triceps and anconeus muscles before it courses anterior to the lateral epicondyle, where it innervates the brachioradialis and the ECRL muscles. The radial nerve then bifurcates and gives off a superficial branch that innervates the skin over the dorsal radial aspect of the wrist and hand. The deep motor branch courses around the posterior lateral aspect of the radius and through an arch in the supinator muscle (arcade of Frohse), providing innervation to the ECRB and supinator, before emerging posteriorly in the forearm as the posterior interosseous nerve (PIN). The PIN courses distally to innervate the remaining wrist and finger extensor musculature. Radial tunnel syndrome refers to injury of the PIN as it courses along the fibrous border between the laminae of the supinator muscle (28,36–39) (Table 66-1).

Patients with injury to the PIN may report an aching, burning-type pain at the anterior radial head and extensor wad region as well as paresthesias in the hand and lateral part of the forearm. Tenderness to deep palpation is noted at the border of the supinator, approximately 4 cm distal to the lateral epicondyle, and pain may be increased with resisted supination (4). Weakness can ultimately develop and can be identified by having the patient extend the wrist. The wrist will dorsiflex radially, indicating functioning of the extensor carpi radialis muscle groups but weakness of the ECU. Due to the anatomic and dynamic relationship between the ECRB and the PIN, posterior interosseous neuropathy can mimic and coexist in up to 10% of patients with chronic lateral epicondylitis (38). Diagnostic anesthetic injections can help identify the source of lateral elbow pain. If the symptoms are due to PIN involvement at the arcade of Frohse, then an injection 4 fingerbreadths (6 to 7 cm) distal to the lateral epicondyle may result in symptom improvement, whereas pain relief following an injection at the origin of the ECRB would be more consistent with lateral epicondylitis (40).

Table 66-1: Potential Sites of Compression in the Radial Tunnel Syndrome
1. Arcade of Frohse
2. Fibrous bands that tether the posterior interosseous nerve to the anterior radial head at the entrance to the tunnel
3. Medially situated tendinous margin of the extensor carpi radialis brevis muscle
4. Recurrent vascular arcade including the recurrent radial artery and vein which cross the nerve

Various provocative maneuvers may be used to increase compressive forces and tension on the nerve as it passes through the radial tunnel (37,39,41,42). Elbow flexion and forceful, resisted forearm supination may provoke pain as the nerve becomes compressed within the fibrous arcade. Symptoms created by compression of the radial nerve at the ECRB may be reproduced with the forearm fully pronated and the wrist flexed. A characteristic finding of pain on resistive extension of the long finger with the elbow extended has been associated with compression of the PIN, but symptoms related to lateral epicondylitis can also be worsened by this test. Therefore, resisted middle finger extension is not pathognomonic for PIN entrapment.

Electrodiagnostic evaluation can be useful in delineating the level of the lesion. The brachioradialis and ECRL are innervated proximal to the bifurcation of the main trunk of the radial nerve. Prior to entering the supinator muscle, the deep branch of the radial nerve innervates the supinator muscle itself and the ECRB. Therefore, these muscles are typically spared in the radial tunnel syndrome, whereas the distal muscles innervated by the PIN, including the EDC, the extensor digiti minimi, and the ECU, may demonstrate neuropathic changes (36).

Conservative treatment includes splinting to control supination and pronation motion. Surgical treatment is indicated when motor deficits persist for 8 to 12 weeks or when conservative management has been ineffective after 6 to 12 months. Surgical intervention involves decompression of the radial nerve within the radial tunnel and release of the ECRB (28,41,42).

Musculocutaneous Nerve and Lateral Antebrachial Cutaneous Nerve

The musculocutaneous nerve innervates the coracobrachialis, biceps, and brachialis muscles and terminates as the lateral antebrachial cutaneous nerve (LACN). The LACN travels laterally at the elbow and supplies sensation to the skin over the radial half of the forearm. Although compression neuropathies involving the LACN are rare in sports, they have been noted in pitchers, swimmers, and players of racquet sports (28,43,44). Injury is created by sudden supination to pronation motions with the elbow fully extended, as seen during the follow-through phase of the pitch. The site of compression is at the lateral margin of the bicipital aponeurosis (lacertus fibrosus) where the nerve is compressed between the biceps tendon and the brachial fascia. The injured athlete may note lateral elbow pain, dysesthesias, or sensory deficit consistent with the LACN distribution in the forearm and a positive Tinel sign at the elbow.

Nonsurgical treatment includes orthotic management with an elbow extension lag of 20 to 40 degrees, activity modification, and modalities. When symptoms persist, surgical intervention includes nerve release and possibly decompresson of the biceps tendon overlying the compression site (28).

FUNCTIONAL AND SPORT-SPECIFIC BIOMECHANICS

The elbow joint does not act in isolation but rather as an integral component of the upper-extremity kinetic chain. The joint serves as the anatomic link between the shoulder and the hand, thereby allowing for hand placement as well as transmission and absorption of upper-extremity force (45). Most activities of daily living require between 30 and 130 degrees of flexion and between 50 degrees of pronation and 50 degrees of supination. The articular orientation of the joint, however, allows for approximately 150 degrees of flexion, 75 degrees of pronation, and 85 degrees of supination, creating an arc of forearm rotation averaging 160 to 170 degrees (2,46).

Joint Motion, Stability, and Power Generation

The elbow joint is commonly described as a hinge joint, but complex motions are allowed through the combined movements of both flexion-extension and pronation-supination. Specifically, the ulnohumeral (trochlear) articulation is considered a uniaxial hinge joint allowing for one degree of freedom (i.e., flexion and extension). The radiohumeral and proximal radioulnar articulations allow for axial rotation, and can be considered a pivot-type joint (5). The axis of elbow flexion-extension is through the center of the trochlea and capitellum, with the axis of supination-pronation situated within the center of the radial head and the capitellum and along a line through the base of the ulnar styloid (8,47).

According to Morrey and An (9), 50% of elbow stability is a result of joint characteristics, namely, the ulnohumeral articulation, and 50% is capsuloligamentous, a function of the collateral ligaments and anterior capsule. Bony articulations restrict valgus stresses when the elbow is flexed less than 20 degrees or more than 120 degrees, with the medial collateral ligament, especially the anterior band, providing the stabilizing component during the remainder of the range of motion (4). The radiocapitellar joint serves as a secondary restraint to valgus stress when the anterior band of the medial collateral ligament is intact (48).

The lateral collateral ligament complex provides stability to varus stress, with the radial collateral ligament being taut throughout flexion and extension while the accessory collateral ligament is taut only with varus stress, and unrelated to flexion and extension positions. The lateral ulnar collateral ligament provides the primary restraint to varus posterolateral rotatory instability (4). Additional constraints to varus and valgus stress are provided by the olecranon and the anterior capsule when the elbow is extended (9,49).

Elbow extension is limited by the anterior capsule, the anterior bundle of the medial collateral ligament, and possibly the olecranon fossa fat pad (8). At end-range extension, the tip of the olecranon "locks" into the olecranon fossa, providing additional stability (11,13).

Force transmission depends on joint position, with maximum flexion force production generated between the range of 80 and 110 degrees of flexion (50). Extension strength is approximately 70% of flexion strength with a 3% to 8% difference between dominant and nondominant sides (8,51).

Selected Sport Biomechanics

Throwing

The overhand throwing motion is used for the football pass, javelin throw, tennis serve, and volleyball spike. The baseball pitch has been the most extensively analyzed (52–54). Regardless of activity, injury prevention depends on the efficient functioning of the kinetic chain. Energy transfer and upper-extremity acceleration are primarily generated by the lower extremities, pelvis, and trunk. The acceleration phase begins at the end of maximal external rotation of the shoulder (late cocking phase) and continues until ball release. The forearm and hand lag behind as the trunk and shoulder are brought forward, thereby imparting a valgus stress to the elbow. The acceleration phase ends and the follow-through phase begins at ball release. Vertical and horizontal control is maintained during the release phase by forearm pronation and wrist flexion.

Significant medial valgus-distraction forces and lateral compressive forces at the radiocapitellar joint are created by the rapid movement requirements at the elbow, especially during the late-cocking, acceleration, and follow-through phases. Medial distraction forces may lead to injuries of the medial collateral ligament, medial epicondyle, flexor-pronator group, and ulnar nerve. Lateral compressive forces and sheer stress at the radiocapitellar joint may result in capitellum and radial head pathology, and osteochondritis dissecans in the adolescent athlete (3,21) (Fig. 66-2). The high extension forces placed on the elbow during the acceleration phase and after ball release demand that the elbow flexors decelerate the rapidly moving forearm (54). If elbow extension is decelerated too rapidly, biceps tendon injury may occur owing to significant flexion forces (55). If extension is not adequately decelerated, injuries can occur as the olecranon is repetitively driven into the olecranon fossa (56). In the throwing athlete, selective muscular hypertrophy of the forearm flexors and bony hypertrophic changes of the humerus can develop. As a result, elbow flexion contractures have been noted in as many as 50% of professional pitchers, often with associated valgus deformities (33).

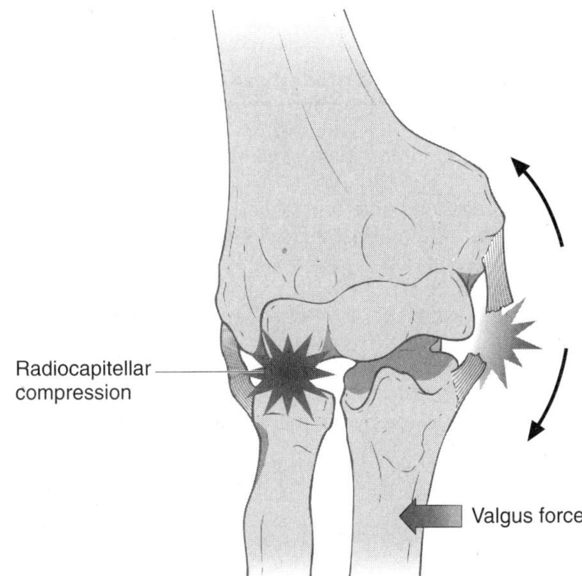

Figure 66-2. Sites of injury to the medial and lateral structures with valgus forces. (Redrawn with permission from Nirschl RP, Kraushaar BS. Assessment and treatment guidelines for elbow injuries. *Phys Sports Med* 1996;24:43–60.

Tennis

Elbow pain in tennis players is not uncommon. Up to 40% of players between the ages of 35 of 50 years develop elbow pain and dysfunction, with tennis elbow occurring four times more frequently in individuals over the age of 40 (21,57). Nirschl (58) noted that half of club players over the age of 30 had experienced symptoms related to tennis elbow, with lateral epicondylitis occurring five times more frequently than medial epicondylitis (58). Skill level can also be a determining factor for medial versus lateral epicondylar involvement. Recreational and novice players have a lateral to medial distribution of 90% to 10%, respectively, whereas highly skilled players have a distribution of 25% to 75%, respectively (59). Because of inconsistent muscle activity, which occurs in the less skilled tennis player, poorly coordinated body movements occur, thereby increasing the athlete's risk for upper-extremity pain and dysfunction (60).

Biomechanically, the elbow acts as a fixed component of the arm-racquet lever system and allows for energy transmission from the lower extremities, trunk, and shoulder to the ball. Proper stroke mechanics require that the force generated by body weight shift and trunk rotation be transferred efficiently to the racquet-ball interface, while maintaining the elbow and wrist in a relatively fixed position throughout ball contact (61). The four stages of the tennis serve include windup, cocking, acceleration, and follow-through. The forehand and backhand strokes can be broken down into three stages: stage I—racquet preparation; stage II—acceleration; and stage III—ball-strike and follow-through (62).

The wrist extensors and lateral epicondyle are especially susceptible to stress during the backhand stroke as the extensor muscle group concentrically contracts to stabilize the wrist and support the racquet (63). The highest electromyographic activity occurs in the ECRB during the acceleration and follow-through phases (61,64). The one-handed backhand requires greater strength since only one upper extremity is available to generate force. The two-handed backhand, on the other hand, allows for trunk rotation to generate force in the forward swing phase of the stroke, with the arms of both limbs moving with the trunk. Increased stability at the elbow occurs with the two-handed backhand, since forces at ball impact are transmitted through, rather than absorbed, by the elbow (61).

Increased stress at the medial epicondyle and flexor-pronator group may occur during powerful overhead serves, the late phase of the forehand stroke, and service strokes, owing to forceful forearm pronation and associated valgus forces, especially when accompanied by wrist snap (17,65,66). During the acceleration phase of the serve, which begins at maximal external rotation and ends at ball impact, the predominant forearm muscular activity occurs at the pronator teres and flexor carpi radialis (64). The biceps muscle helps decelerate forceful elbow extension, thereby preventing hyperextension in the late acceleration phase, prior to racquet-ball impact (67). Lateral epicondylar injury, due to subsequent eccentric load on the supinators, may also develop (60). Because increased forearm pronation creates a greater eccentric load on the posterior rotator cuff to decelerate the internally rotating humerus, rehabilitation not only must correct abnormal stroke mechanics, but also must address proper functioning of the entire upper-extremity kinetic chain (60).

INJURIES AND REHABILITATION MANAGEMENT

General Principles

Implementation of the proper treatment program requires that the sport physiatrist understand tissue injury, anatomic and functional deficits, and specific sport demands. The treating physician, therapist, and athletic trainer must be aware of the injured athlete's goals and expectations. The patient's history should include the mechanism of injury (acute, repetitive overload–chronic, or acute-on-chronic); previous injuries to the same or other parts of the kinetic chain; the nature and response to previous treatments; change in type, rate, frequency, duration, or intensity of the sport activity; and how the injury has affected the patient's athletic and non-sport-related functional activities. Acute injuries more commonly have a localized pain presentation, whereas chronic injuries present with more generalized symptoms. Patients with acute-on-chronic injuries may present with both localized and generalized complaints (3).

The physical examination includes inspection for anatomic malalignment. Malalignment may result from fracture, dislocation, prior injury with malunion, edema formation, musculotendinous disruption, or atrophy. Palpation can be helpful in localizing the source of pain. With range of motion evaluation, loss of mobility due to pain inhibition often has a soft "end feel" and associated muscle guarding, whereas mechanical loss of motion due to adhesive capsulitis or bony involvement has a firm end point. Varus and valgus stability is evaluated with the elbow flexed 20 to 30 degrees. On stress testing, laxity greater than that of the uninjured elbow or joint opening of more than 1 cm with a soft end point suggests collateral disruption (3). Posterolateral subluxation as a result of lateral collateral ligament disruption occurs with forced elbow extension, axial loading, and forearm supination. Neurovascular evaluation is mandatory, especially with acute trauma. A complete evaluation of upper-extremity kinetic chain function, including the cervical and scapular stabilizing musculature, completes the physical examination.

If fracture or dislocation is suspected, routine anteroposterior and lateral radiographs must be obtained. Axial and oblique views as well as comparison views of the noninjured extremity, especially in the pediatric or adolescent patient, may also be necessary. Radiographs may also be helpful to evaluate chronic degenerative or systemic disease processes. When loose bodies are suspected, arthrography or tomograms may be useful. Stress views, computed tomography (CT) arthrograms, and magnetic resonance imaging (MRI) may be considered to further delineate collateral ligament injury. When the diagnosis remains unclear despite the routine evaluation, bone scanning and serologic laboratory work-up may be helpful, especially to identify a stress fracture or a previously undiagnosed systemic process (3). Electrodiagnostic evaluation may be useful to determine if a nerve injury is present and may provide additional prognostic information.

The focus of treatment is on an active, patient participation model, minimizing the use of a prolonged passive treatment approach. Ongoing communication between the patient, therapist, coach, and the sports physiatrist ensures safe progression through the rehabilitation program.

Lateral Injuries

The most common injury to the lateral elbow complex is lateral epicondylitis. A few other problems, however, can also cause lateral elbow pain. Entrapment neuropathies such as posterior interosseous involvement may mimic lateral epicondylitis or coexist with it. Lateral compression injuries primarily involving the bony structures may occur secondary to abnormal compression forces at the radiocapitellar region. Referred pain may also create elbow pain (68) (Table 66-2).

Table 66-2: Differential Diagnosis of Lateral Elbow Pain

Lateral epicondylitis
Radial tunnel syndrome/posterior interosseous nerve entrapment
Musculocutaneous nerve entrapment
Posterolateral rotatory instability/lateral collateral ligament disruption
Osteochondritis dissecans
Radiocapitellar degenerative changes/loose body formation
Fractures–radial head, capitellum/distal end of humerus, lateral epicondyle
Chronic compartment syndrome of the anconeus muscle (1)
Cervical radiculopathy/referred pain processes

Lateral Epicondylitis

Lateral epicondylitis most commonly occurs in participants in racquet sports but is also seen in athletes participating in baseball, golf, fencing, and swimming (17,21,65,69,70). Factors that increase the likelihood of developing lateral epicondylitis in the tennis player include older age, lower skill level, increased frequency of play, force and flexibility deficiencies of the forearm extensor muscles, and lack of coordinated upper-extremity kinetic chain function.

The tennis player with lateral epicondylitis most commonly has developed altered backhand mechanics, whereby the elbow "leads" into the backhand swing. Additionally, excessive spin and repetitive peripheral rather than central ball-racquet contact create excessive rotational racquet torque, with increased demand on the extensor muscles of the wrist and elbow to help control these abnormal forces (59,71,72). Grabiner et al (73) noted that the grip on the racquet should be sufficiently firm to avoid excessive racquet rotation in off-center shots, but not so firm as to cause increased muscle fatigue and subsequent injury. When altered sport mechanics develop, the biomechanically inefficient position transfers forces to the extensor muscles of the forearm, rather than to the larger shoulder and trunk muscles. Kinetic chain dysfunction, therefore, may include strength and flexibility deficits of the wrist and finger extensors as well as weakness of the posterior shoulder musculature (50).

Clinically, the patient may present with pain and tenderness localized at the lateral epicondyle and over the origin of the ECRB, approximately 1 cm medial and distal to the lateral epicondyle (3,18). The pain is commonly increased during resisted wrist extension, especially with the elbow extended and the forearm pronated. Gripping and end-range passive wrist flexion can also precipitate the patient's complaints. Wrist extension weakness and a 10- to 15-degree loss of passive wrist flexion may ultimately develop (63).

To differentiate lateral epicondylitis from degenerative changes at the radiocapitellar joint, pain reproduction with axial pressure to the forearm, combined with gentle passive supination and pronation while maintaining the wrist in a neutral position, is suggestive for joint degeneration. Complaints of catching, locking, and crepitus are also consistent with intra-articular involvement (62). Anterior-posterior and lateral elbow radiographs can be helpful to assess for calcific deposits, degenerative changes, and loose body formation at the radiocapitellar joint (62). When radiocapitellar joint involvement is confirmed and conservative treatment fails, surgical intervention is often necessary for joint débridement and removal of marginal osteophytes and loose bodies (74).

The pathophysiology of lateral epicondylitis involves the forearm extensors, most commonly the ECRB and less commonly the ECRL and the anterior portion of the extensor communis tendon (59). Owing to repetitive microtrauma, the muscle-tendon unit is unable to meet the demands of the applied forces, thereby leading to microscopic rupture with the formation of subsequent mucinoid degeneration and reactive granulation tissue (63). Nirschl (16,17) described the pathologic process involving the tendon origin as *angiofibroblastic tendinosis*, which results from tensile overuse, fatigue, and possibly avascular changes secondary to anoxia and vascular thrombosis, as the changes appear consistent with a degenerative process, rather than primary inflammation. Inflammatory cells found within the tendon likely result from the repair process involving organization of granulation tissue and scar formation, rather than the direct pathologic process (75). If progressive insult occurs, partial, and more rarely, complete tears in the ECRB may develop.

Treatment Principles

Control of Pain and Inflammation

A period of relative rest during which the athlete avoids the activities leading to increased symptoms is strongly advised. Total immobilization should be used judiciously to minimize additional loss of motion and strength (59). In the highly acute phase, the use of a wrist orthosis with the wrist positioned in approximately 15 degrees of extension may help to rest the inflamed extensor musculature (76). Icing and nonsteroidal anti-inflammatory medication are most effective during the initial 2- to 4-week period. Additional modalities including high-voltage galvanic stimulation, iontophoresis, and whirlpool may help control pain and inflammation. As the acute inflammatory phase is controlled, the incorporation of heating techniques including ultrasound and phonophoresis, use of a large-head vibrator, and friction massage may improve tissue extensibility and muscle function (77,78). Modalities should not be considered the sole rehabilitative tool. Rather, they should be used to prepare the patient for a more aggressive and comprehensive therapy approach.

Proper Anatomic Healing and Restoration of Normal Tissue Functioning

Therapeutic exercise is initiated as the acute symptoms diminish. Restoration of full and pain-free range of motion of the joint and improvement of muscle flexibility and strength are the goals, with specific attention directed to the wrist and finger extensors. A comprehensive muscle reconditioning program includes multiplane and multijoint exercises that simulate normal functional activities (Table 66-3).

Wrist flexion mobility is increased by placing the wrist extensors on passive stretch while the elbow is extended. This sustained, pain-free stretch is held for 10 seconds and repeated for 5 to 10 repetitions, two or three times a day (14,79,80) (Fig. 66-3A). Myofascial release techniques are used to improve soft-tissue flexibility, with pressure applied along the borders of the dorsal forearm (81). End-range extension stretching, joint mobilization, and distraction maneuvers are used to improve the range of motion of elbow extension, especially in the presence of elbow flexion contractures (82).

Strength training is initiated as pain-free range of motion improves. Multiple-angle isometric exercises and manual resistance techniques within the patient's pain-free range are begun, initially targeting the wrist extensors. A progressive isotonic strengthening program is incorporated, and may include free weights (Fig. 66-4A) and a wrist roll (14) (Fig. 66-5A). Pronation-supination and radial-ulnar motions can be strengthened through the use of a weighted rod (14,31) (Fig. 66-6). During the early phase of rehabilitation, low resistance and high repetitions (25–40 repetitions) help improve muscle endurance and resistance to repetitive stress (59,60). Weight is then increased in 1- to 2-lb increments, up to a maximum of 5 to 7 lb, when the patient can comfortably perform two consecutive sets of 30 repetitions (3).

Once a functional range of motion at the wrist and elbow is achieved, isokinetic devices may help in detecting strength imbalances, as well as improving high-velocity strength and endurance (59,66). A submaximal treatment trial of wrist extension-flexion with the elbow flexed to 90 degrees is initiated. Following this trial, isokinetic speeds of 180 to 300 degrees per second are used to improve local muscular endurance. Positional progression occurs from wrist extension-flexion to forearm pronation-supination and finally to elbow extension-flexion (60).

Complex concentric-eccentric routines using resistive tubing are initiated, as guided by the patient's symptoms

Table 66-3: Flexibility and Strengthening of the Relevant Muscle Groups in Elbow Dysfunction
Elbow flexion-extension
Forearm pronation-supination
Wrist flexion-extension
Wrist radial-ulnar deviation
Hand intrinsics

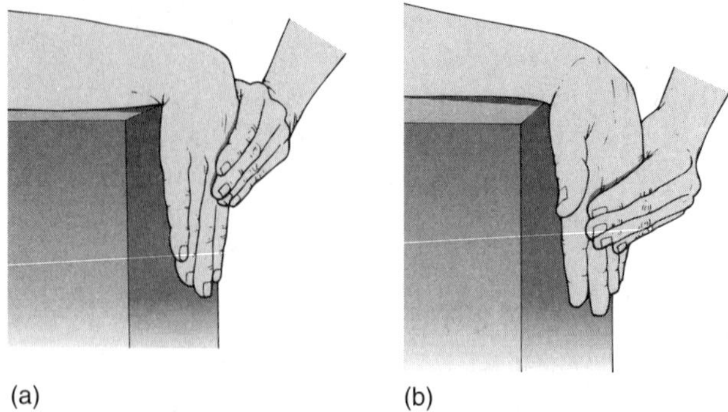

(a) (b)

Figure 66-3. Stretching of (*a*) the extensor muscle group and (*b*) the flexor muscle group.

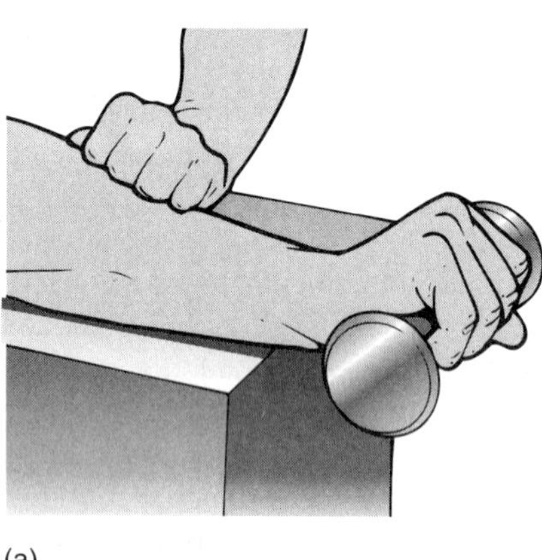

(a)

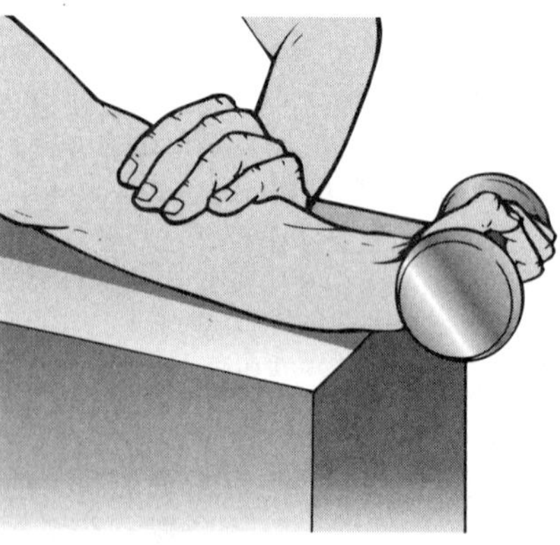

(b)

Figure 66-4. The use of hand-held free weights for strengthening (*a*) the extensor muscle group and (*b*) the flexor muscle group.

(14) (Fig. 66-7). Proprioceptive neuromuscular facilitation techniques are used to improve control of the elbow musculature and to upgrade functional patterns (83). Wall pulleys can provide further resistance during simulation of various sport activities, including the forehand, backhand, and overhead motions (63).

Kinetic Chain Performance and Cardiovascular Endurance

Anatomic and functional deficits of the cervical and thoracic regions of the spine and upper-extremity kinetic chain need to be evaluated, as the force and power provided by the trunk and lower extremities must be efficiently transferred through the shoulder complex to the elbow, forearm, wrist, and hand. Cervical dysfunction may inhibit efficient kinetic chain motion, since the cervical region serves as a fulcrum for the shoulders as the body rotates in relation to the ball. Deficits proximally may have a carryover effect at the elbow owing to the neck and shoulder's role in maintaining proximal stability and base of support for proper elbow placement. Specifically, an imbalance of tight internal shoulder rotators and weak external rotators transfers into abnormal overload patterns at the elbow (84,85). Epidemiologic studies in tennis players identified a high prevalence of shoulder and elbow injuries, highlighting the need for a comprehensive rehabilitation program. Priest and Nagel (86) reported that 74% of male and 60% of female tennis players had a history of shoulder or elbow injuries on the dominant side, with both the shoulder and the elbow of the dominant side being involved in 21% of men and 23% of women. Priest et al (87) studied 2633 recreational tennis players and noted a 31% incidence of tennis elbow. There was a 63% higher incidence of shoulder injury among players with tennis elbow than players without tennis elbow. Flexibility, strength, and muscular endurance of the uninvolved extremities as well as maintenance of overall body conditioning must not be overlooked at any stage of the rehabilitation process.

Specific Skill Retraining and Safe Return to Sport Activity

The focus of the rehabilitation program is directed at proper technique, equipment modification, and sport-specific skill reacquisition. Interval training involves increasing the frequency, intensity, and duration of a particular activity as guided by the athlete's symptoms (31,60,63,88,89). Thomas et al (80) recommend beginning sport-specific skill retraining when the patient has regained 80% of strength of the injured extremity. The activity is performed at a level low enough to prevent symptom recurrence, increasing the work volume and intensity by no more than 5% per day.

For the tennis player, controlling abnormal force transmission to the elbow is necessary to ensure proper tissue healing and prevent reinjury. Various interventions have been described to diminish abnormal energy absorption at the ball-racquet interface (16,59,63) (Table 66-4). Correcting improper backhand stroke and using the two-handed backhand allow the uninvolved extremity to absorb additional energy and thereby decrease lateral epicondylar stress. By evaluating and correcting altered stroke mechanics, Ilfeld (90) noted a 90% good to excellent

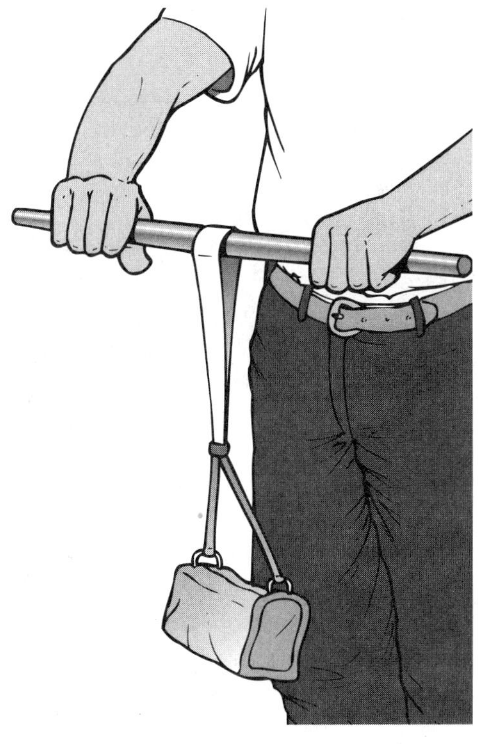

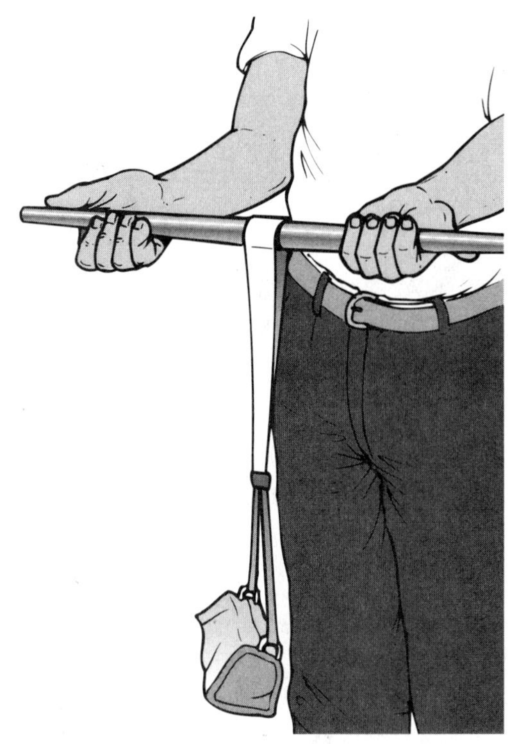

(a) (b)

Figure 66-5. The use of a wrist roll to strengthen (*a*) the extensor muscle group and (*b*) the flexor muscle group.

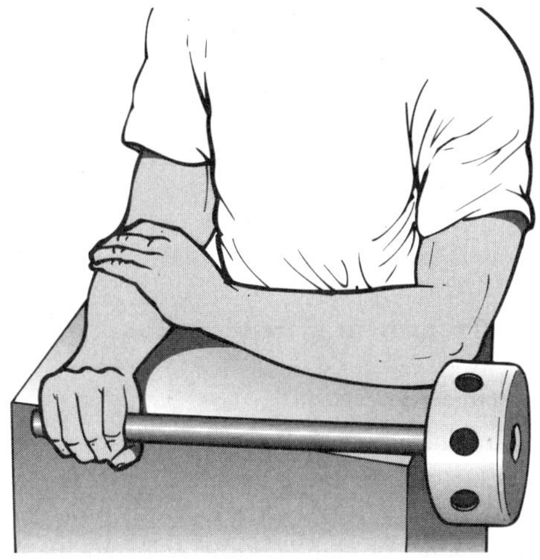

Figure 66-6. The use of a weighted rod to strengthen the muscles of pronation-supination.

Table 66-4: Methods to Decrease Abnormal Force Transmission to the Elbow Complex in the Tennis Player
Proper backhand mechanics including a two-handed stroke
Racquet characteristics
Low-range string tension: 50–55 lb
Midsize racquet heads
Proper grip size/grip padding
Lightweight graphite composite construction
Playing surface
Slower clay surface
Newer ball
Counterforce bracing

outcome in patients with a less-than-6-month history of epicondylitis and an 82% good to excellent outcome in patients with a more-than-6-month history of medial and lateral epicondylitis.

Lowering string tension by 3 to 5 lb, using racquets with midsized heads made of lightweight graphite composite, and playing with fresh balls can be helpful in minimizing stress at the elbow (59,91). The larger head and newer balls decrease arm vibration, while a lighter racquet shifts the effective moment arm closer to the elbow, thereby decreasing elbow torque (62,71). Proper grip size, as measured from the tip of the ring finger along the radial border to the proximal palmar crease, allows for use of the largest handle that the athlete's hand can comfortably control (92,93). The duration of maximal grip pressure also affects stress at the elbow. The skilled player grips the racquet submaximally through most of the stroke cycle, increasing grip pressure immediately prior to ball impact,

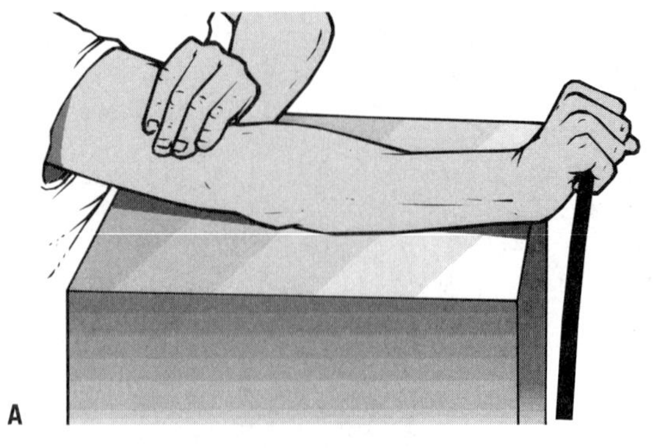

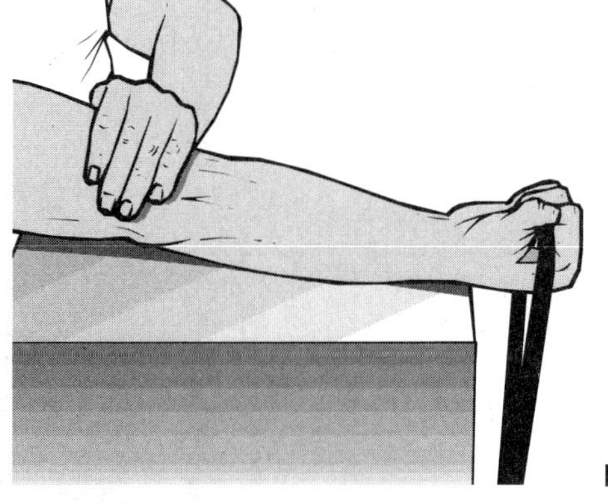

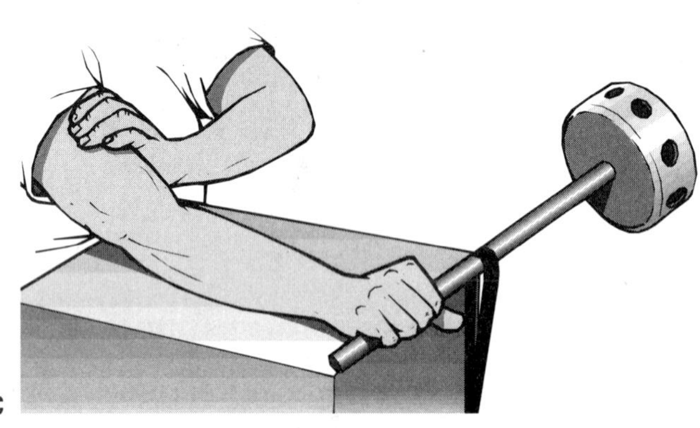

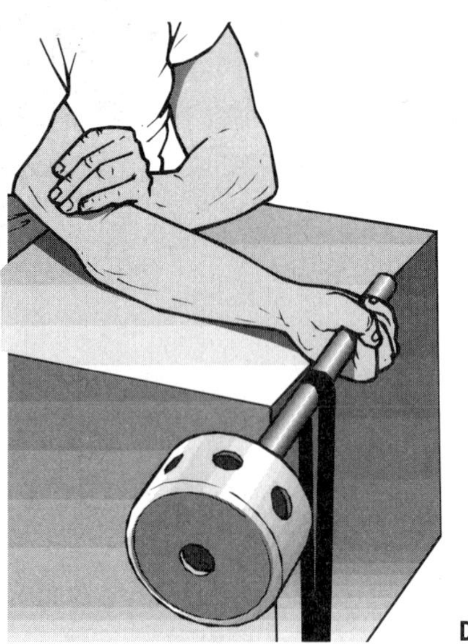

Figure 66-7. The use of resistive tubing for strengthening (*A*) the extensor muscle group, (*B*) the flexor muscle group, (*C*) the muscles of pronation, and (*D*) the muscles of supination.

thereby increasing efficiency and decreasing stress to the forearm musculature. The novice tennis player, on the other hand, has a longer duration of maximal gripping force (60,94). Hatze (95) noted that cushioned grip bands may further reduce vibration transfer to the forearm.

Counterforce bracing has been advocated for decreasing epicondylar load. The orthosis may prevent full muscular expansion, decrease the force of muscular contraction, create a new functional origin, and broaden the area of applied stress. Additionally, force may be transferred partially to the brace itself, bypassing the injured muscle, which is now situated above the orthosis (59,66,96,97). The orthosis can also be used during the acute phase to diminish force production on the injured muscle-tendon unit, thereby decreasing pain and inflammation and assisting with improved healing.

Finally, the physician and therapist must also evaluate what non-sport-related daily activities may be aggravating or limiting anticipated recovery.

Additional Treatment Considerations

Corticosteroid Injections

Local steroid injections may be considered for the athlete who has marked inflammation or who has lacked the anticipated response after 8 to 12 weeks of rehabilitation.

An injection, combining corticosteroid with a local anesthetic, at the point of maximal tenderness within the subaponeurotic space can provide diagnostic information and therapeutic results. Most commonly, the injection site is below the ECRB origin in the triangular recess formed by the medial slope of the lateral condyle and the ECRB tendon (59,62). The lack of resistance during the injection indicates that the injectant has not been deposited within the tendon. Following the injection, the patient is advised to avoid strenuous activities with the forearm for 2 weeks (63).

Since steroids depress fibroblastic and chondroblastic protein synthesis, with the increased risk for further weakening of connective tissues and poor tendon healing, their judicious use is recommended (3,98). A second injection may be beneficial if the initial injection provided some relief but with the subsequent return of symptoms and functional limitations. Injections should be only one component of a comprehensive rehabilitation program and should be spaced at least 1 month apart, with no more than three injections being applied to the same region within 1 year (21,69,99).

Surgical Intervention and Postoperative Rehabilitation

Various authors (41,59) have reported good to excellent outcomes with nonoperative management in 80% to 90% of their patients. When symptoms persist for more than 6 to 12 months, despite appropriate rehabilitation, surgical release and débridement of focal degeneration within the ECRB tendon origin may be necessary (16,21,100). MRI may help to confirm the diagnosis and stage the extent of local pathology (62). Potter et al (101) used MRI to help assess lateral epicondylitis and aid in surgical planning. They found 95% accuracy in the ability of MRI to document focal areas of scarring and collagen fibril disruption when compared with histologic findings.

Following surgery, the elbow is protected for 1 to 2 weeks in a posterior splint at 90 degrees, thereby allowing for active use of the wrist, hand, and shoulder. Flexibility exercises are started by postoperative day 3, with strength and endurance training beginning at 3 weeks. Modified sport patterns may begin at 6 weeks postoperatively. The tennis player may begin light hitting on a soft, clay surface for 20 to 25 minutes. The duration is increased every other day, so long as no pain occurs the following day. The athlete may return to competition when strength is normalized, and abnormal substitution patterns are resolved. Following surgery, full strength commonly returns by $4\frac{1}{2}$ months for lateral epicondylitis and $5\frac{1}{2}$ months for medial dysfunction (63,65).

Radial Head Fractures

Radial head fractures are the most common elbow fracture in adults and usually arise as a result of a fall onto the outstretched hand. Type I radial head fractures are undisplaced, whereas type II fractures are displaced with possible impaction, depression, and angulation. Type III fractures are comminuted and involve the entire radial head (Fig. 66-8). Type IV fractures include a concomitant dislocation (102,103).

Clinically, patients will report tenderness at the radial head region, with decreased mobility and pain during forearm rotation. Nonspecific elbow pain with an associated effusion can also be seen. The evaluation must also consider injuries to the capitellum and the distal radioulnar joint. Since most radial head fractures are nondisplaced or minimally displaced, radiographic findings may be subtle. In addition to the standard anteroposterior and lateral views, radiocapitellar oblique radiographs and views in varying degrees of radial rotation can also be useful when routine views are indeterminant (103).

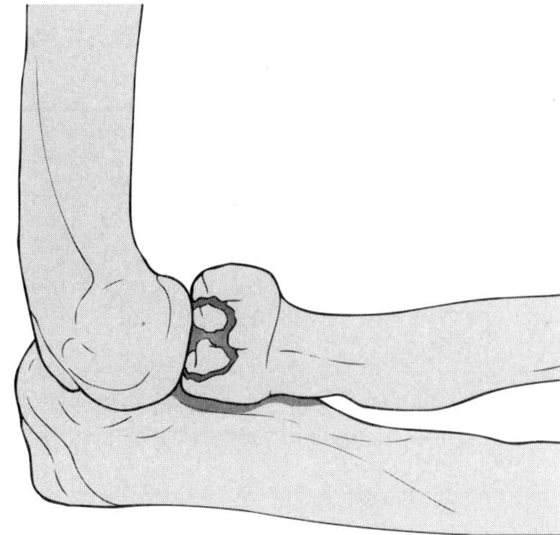

Figure 66-8. Type III radial head fracture with comminution.

Treatment is dependent on the type of radial head fracture, the amount of displacement, and the size of the fracture fragment. For type I nondisplaced fractures, a short period (3–5 days) of immobilization with the elbow flexed and the forearm in a neutral position is pursued. As pain decreases, active range of motion and conditioning of the elbow, wrist, and shoulder muscles are implemented. Repeat radiographs are obtained at 10 days and 3 weeks to evaluate for displacement. Most individuals are able to return to full activity within 4 weeks (79,104).

Types II and III fractures usually require open reduction and internal fixation (82). At 10 days to 2 weeks following surgery, active controlled motion in a hinged orthosis is initiated (105). Type IV fractures have a guarded prognosis for return to preinjury sporting activities. The risk for heterotopic ossification is increased, with sequelae including painful and restricted range of motion with associated functional limitations (79,103).

Medial Injuries

The differential diagnosis for injuries to the medial region of the elbow is provided in Table 66-5.

Medial Collateral Ligament Sprain, Flexor-Pronator Strain, and Medial Epicondylitis

Medial capsuloligamentous and flexor-pronator injuries most commonly occur as a result of repetitive elbow valgus stress. Since tension at the medial aspect of the elbow is initially resisted by the flexor-pronator group, muscle disruption, fibrosis, and elbow flexion contracture can occur (16,69). Bennett fascial compression syndrome is caused by hypertrophy of the flexor-pronator muscle group within the fascial compartment, usually seen with repetitive throwing activities. The hypertrophy leads to medial elbow

Table 66-5: Differential Diagnosis of Medial Elbow Pain
Medial epicondylitis
Flexor-pronator group strain or tear
Bennett fascial compression syndrome
Medial collateral ligament disruption (sprain or tear)
Medial epicondylar avulsion fracture
Valgus extension overload complex
Ulnar neuropathy or cubital tunnel syndrome
Osteophytic spurring
Loose bodies
Cervical radiculopathy—C8 or T1
Brachial trunk, plexus injury, thoracic outlet syndrome
Referred pain process

complex pain, usually noted after a few innings. Treatment includes proper warm-up exercises and waiting 3 to 5 days between pitching starts. Fasciotomies are rarely required (106). Medial epicondylitis results from microtears of the flexor-pronator muscle group at its attachment to the epicondyle. Associated ulnar neuropathy can be seen in up to 40% of individuals with medial epicondylitis, with symptoms usually occurring after prolonged activity (4,58,93).

Clinically, patients with flexor-pronator muscle strains present with pain, tenderness, and swelling radial to the medial epicondyle, while patients with medial epicondylitis will have pain more localized to the medial epicondyle. Symptoms may be increased with resisted wrist flexion and forearm pronation with the elbow extended as well as with passive wrist extension (63,69). Medial epicondylar pain may occur during the tennis forehand, serve, and overhead shots as a result of repetitive valgus elbow stress, wrist flexion, and pronation (64). Players who commonly apply a top spin to their stroke also increase their risk for medial epicondylitis due to the repetitive forced pronation motion (62). In the golfer, stress to the flexor-pronator complex occurs when the right-handed individual forces the head of the club down at the ball with the right arm rather than pulling the club through with the left arm and trunk. (79).

Repetitive valgus stress may also cause capsular and medial collateral ligamentous disruption (microtearing or complete rupture), osteophytes, and ulnar neuropathy. In addition to ulnar nerve compromise, the differential diagnosis of medial elbow pain also includes cervical radiculopathy, especially C8 lesions, lower trunk brachial plexus injuries, and thoracic outlet syndrome. In the throwing athlete, symptoms localized to the medial collateral ligament complex most commonly occur during the acceleration phase, with medial elbow pain also noted at ball release and ball impact (4,52,107).

When the medial collateral ligament has been injured, tenderness will be noted approximately 2 cm distal to the medial epicondyle (4). Valgus stress testing is performed to assess ligamentous integrity. The shoulder is externally rotated and the forearm supinated. The elbow is flexed 20 to 30 degrees, thereby eliminating the articular stability provided by the olecranon. The examiner stabilizes the humerus either by grasping the humerus above the condyles or by placing the patient's hand between the examiner's chest wall and arm. Once the humerus is stabilized, a valgus force is applied to the elbow. When the result is positive, medial opening with a less distinct end point is noted (27,107,108). Pain may also be precipitated by palpating the medial joint line beneath the medial collateral ligament while performing the stress test.

To assist in differentiating ulnar ligamentous injury from medial epicondylitis and pronator-flexor strains, resistance against wrist flexion and forearm pronation commonly will not lead to pain with pure collateral compromise. Additionally, laxity will not be noted on stress testing when only the flexor-pronator muscle group is involved (1). Radiographic changes in the athlete with medial collateral ligament disruption include medial osteophytosis of the proximal part of the ulna, with the potential development of heterotopic calcification following an avulsion fracture (1). Additional diagnostic evaluation may include MRI and CT arthrography. MRI can demonstrate irregularity of the medial collateral ligament and increased signal intensity within and adjacent to the medial collateral ligament due to hemorrhage and edema (109). Timmerman et al (110) noted that both CT arthrography and MRI are accurate in diagnosing a complete tear of the medial collateral ligament, but CT arthrography is superior in evaluating partial undersurface tears of the ligament.

Conservative Treatment

Treatment concepts for medial epicondylitis and flexor-pronator group strains are similar to those described for lateral epicondylitis. When symptoms are acute, the wrist may be immobilized in 10 degrees of palmar flexion to decrease tension on the flexor mass. In more severe cases where the pronator teres is involved, a splint that blocks forearm rotation can also be used (30). As pain and inflammation diminish, a therapeutic flexibility and strengthening program is initiated. Specific attention is directed to the flexor-pronator group, ensuring proper muscle balance with the wrist extensors (14,52) (see Fig. 66-3B, 66-4B, 66-5B, 66-7B). As in lateral epicondylitis, counterforce bracing with compression applied over the medial muscle mass may be helpful. The use of corticosteroid injections can be considered for more medial epicondylitis, but should be avoided with medial collateral ligament injuries, as the injections may lead to further attenuation of the ligament (4). Surgical intervention is indicated for recalcitrant injuries for which conservative treatment did not provide adequate pain relief or functional improvement.

Surgical Considerations Following Medial Collateral Ligament Injury

Chronic medial collateral ligamentous sprains may be associated with calcium deposits, loose bodies, or traction spurs arising from the coronoid process or medial epicondyle (69,105). Surgical intervention may be required for significant collateral ligament disruption or ulnar neuropathy associated with spurs. Surgical options for the medial collateral ligament include reconstruction or repair, with reconstruction of the ligament with the palmaris longus or short toe extensor tendons being the operation of choice (27,89). Conway et al (107) recommended that concomitant dissection and ulnar nerve transposition occur only when symptoms of ulnar neuropathy are present preoperatively or when pathology within the posterior compartment requires exposure through the cubital tunnel.

Rehabilitation protocols following medial collateral ligament reconstruction are well described (27,89,111). Postoperatively, the elbow is immobilized in a posterior splint set at 90 degrees of elbow flexion. During the second week, a range of motion brace preset at 30 to 90 degrees is provided, with motion being increased by 5 degrees of extension and 10 degrees of flexion in the subsequent weeks. Full motion is usually restored by 6 to 7 weeks. Positions that increase valgus force to the elbow are avoided during the first 4 to 6 months of the program. Strengthening exercises of the wrist and forearm may be started at 4 to 6 weeks, with elbow strengthening at 6 weeks. Initiation of an interval throwing program can begin at 3 to 5 months postoperatively, but windup motions are avoided until 6 months, owing to the added valgus force at the elbow. Shoulder and total body reconditioning, as well as monitoring to assess for complications related to inflammation or abnormal stress on the ligament substitute, must occur throughout the rehabilitation program. The postoperative rehabilitation program may last up to 12 months to allow the tendon graft to revascularize and assume the properties needed to withstand the forces generated at the elbow and for the adjacent tissues to develop the strength and endurance for safe sport return (21,89). Competitive pitching may be considered at 12 months postoperatively, if there is no pain while throwing and full shoulder, elbow, and forearm range of motion and strength have been achieved. Three innings are initially allowed, with at least 6 days of rest between outings. Usually by 18 months following surgery, the pitcher may return to the regular rotation (27). In the racquet player, serves and overhead smashes are usually avoided until 6 months postoperatively, with many tennis players requiring 1 full year before they are able to return to their preinjury level (62).

Posterior Injuries

Extensor Musculotendinous and Bursal Compromise

Tricep tendinitis mostly commonly arises from repetitive overload of the extensor musculature due to hyperextension forces as seen in throwers, weight lifters, shot-putters, and gymnasts (Table 66-6). In the gymnast, the elbow is exposed to further stress as it repetitively "locks" into hyperextension during upper-extremity weight-bearing activities, such as vaulting, balance beam, uneven parallel bar, and floor events. Management for tricep dysfunction includes inflammatory control and biceps strengthening, so that the elbow need not assume a hyperextended position(4,112,113).

Olecranon bursitis most commonly develops from repetitive pressure applied to the posterior elbow region or secondary to an acute impact. The athlete with olecranon bursitis presents with swelling in the posterior aspect of the elbow. Pain is more commonly associated with an acute event or infection. The patient may report discomfort with flexion past 90 degrees but range of motion is usually within functional limits. Radiographs may identify soft-tissue calcification, and in acute trauma, an olecranon or trochlear fracture may occur. Aspiration and bursal fluid analysis are indicated for the swollen bursa when septic arthritis is suspected. In the noninfectious situation, however, aspiration alone will not prevent fluid reaccumulation. Treatment includes the anti-inflammatory principles of rest through splinting, compression, cryotherapy and/or hourly warm soaks, and nonsteroidal anti-inflammatory medication. A pad with a relief over the bursa may decrease recurrences. Surgical excision of the bursa may be necessary in the chronic situation (4,74,114).

Stress fractures of the olecranon have occurred in javelin throwers and baseball players, with the presenting symptoms being posterior pain and limitation in performance and overall function. Posterior impingement secondary to repeated hyperextension and "lock-out" is commonly seen when the upper extremity is performing weight-bearing activities, such as in gymnastics. When the gymnast who performs repetitive axial loading and high-intensity training presents with elbow pain and loss of motion, stress fractures of the distal end of the humerus should be considered (115,116). Radiographs are usually unremarkable and further evaluation by bone scanning can lead to a definitive diagnosis. The treatment of choice remains operative management due to the high incidence of delayed union with immobilization (117–119).

Table 66-6: Differential Diagnosis of Posterior Elbow Pain
Triceps tendinitis or rupture
Olecranon bursitis
Olecranon fractures
Olecranon apophysitis
Valgus extension overload syndrome
Osteophytes
Loose body formation
Dislocation

Triceps rupture with associated avulsion fractures may occur owing to forceful, uncoordinated triceps contraction as seen during a fall or direct impact to the elbow. Triceps disruption also occurs in weight lifters and has been associated with anabolic steroid use and local steroid injections. Most tears occur at the tendon insertion, with fewer cases being noted at the musculotendinous junction. Clinical presentation includes pain and ecchymosis at the triceps insertion. There may also be a palpable defect. Elbow extension is limited and painful. Radiographs may demonstrate a small fleck of bone avulsed from the olecranon. Surgical intervention is the treatment of choice (4,120–122).

Valgus Extension Overload Syndrome

In the throwing athlete, most injuries to the posterior compartment occur from repetitive valgus forces generated at the posterior medial aspect of the elbow during the acceleration phase. As the triceps acts on the olecranon at follow-through, extension sheer stress is created, leading to further olecranon compression and fossal impingement (11,123). Repetitive articular compression during the tennis forehand and service strokes may also cause valgus overload to the posteromedial elbow complex. Loss of proper articulate congruity due to the hypertrophy of the distal end of the humerus and osteophyte formation at the posteromedial aspect of the olecranon tip may occur, leading to bony block and flexion contractures (21,124). Abnormal compression at the radiocapitellar joint may also develop, especially with medial collateral ligament disruption (62,125).

Clinically, pain and tenderness are noted at the posteromedial aspect of the elbow, often with swelling. The symptoms can be increased with extension and valgus stress testing. Patients may also report crepitus, catching, and frank locking when free fragments are present within the joint (11,123). Pitchers will often describe pain that increases early in the game, associated with a loss of control and leading to early ball release and highly thrown pitches. Tennis players will report similar symptoms with overhead serves as they reach full extension (27).

The valgus extension overload test helps to determine whether the pain is the result of posteromedial osteophytes abutting against the medial margin of the olecranon fossa. The test is performed by forcing the elbow into extension while exerting a valgus stress, thereby simulating the position of the upper extremity during the acceleration phase of the throw. At the same time, the examiner is palpating over the posteromedial area of the olecranon tip to elicit tenderness as well as crepitus. A positive test result occurs with reproduction of pain over the posterior and posteromedial region of the olecranon process (123,126). To assess for degenerative changes at the radiohumeral joint, gentle supination and pronation in varying degrees of elbow flexion are performed, while the examiner palpates the head of the radius, feeling for crepitus, popping, or reproduction of pain (126). Radiographic evaluation includes standard anteroposterior and lateral views, and an axial projection to more clearly identify posteromedial osteophytes (55). While radiographs can detect osteophytes and loose bodies, CT may assist in determining the three-dimensional anatomy (56).

Management includes controlling inflammation, therapeutic exercise, and proper throwing mechanics. Attention is directed to balanced bicep and tricep muscle functioning. With the use of resistive tubing to achieve both slow and fast contractions, the elbow is flexed with the shoulder positioned in 60 degrees of flexion. This isometric position is then released, leading to an eccentric phase. As the elbow reaches full extension, the individual concentrically flexes the elbow. Plyometric exercises with a weighted ball can be used to train the athlete to more efficiently transfer energy and stabilize the involved joints through eccentric and concentric control. (79,83). Strengthening of the wrist flexors and forearm pronators provides medial stabilization of the elbow during throwing and serving motions. Rotator cuff and scapular stabilizer flexibility, strength, and coordination training is indicated to ensure proper functioning of the more proximal musculature.

When bony sequelae develop, surgical intervention is usually required (16,69). Harrelson (31) described a postoperative protocol following arthroscopic removal of loose bodies and osteophytic excision. The initial phase includes gentle elbow motion in the surgical dressing on the day of surgery, upgrading to hand and wrist exercises on postoperative days 1 and 2. From days 3 to 7, passive elbow flexion-extension range of motion exercises as well as a 1-lb resistive strengthening component incorporating wrist curls and pronation-supination exercises are initiated. The intermediate phase begins at postoperative weeks 1 and 2 with the continuation of the progressive resistive exercises upgrading to five sets of 10 repetitions with 5- to 7-lb weights. The final advanced stage begins at postoperative weeks 4 to 6 and focuses on eccentric tubing exercises with the gradual return to athletic involvement through an interval throwing program. As a general guideline, elbow mobility should be at least 15 to 90 degrees 10 days after arthroscopy, upgrading to 10 to 100 degrees by 2 weeks. Full range of motion is usually obtained by 20 to 25 days postoperatively (79).

Elbow Instability and Dislocations

Elbow subluxations and dislocations most commonly occur from falls onto an outstretched hand. The flexing elbow undergoes an axial compressive force as the body approaches the ground, with an associated supination and valgus moment as the body rotates internally on the elbow. Most elbow dislocations occur posteriorly, based on the final resting position of the olecranon relative to the distal end of the humerus, with anterior dislocations occurring in only 1% to 2% of patients (79). Posterior elbow instability can be thought of as a continuum, consisting of three stages. In stage 1, as the lateral ulnar collateral ligament is disrupted, the elbow subluxates in a posterolateral direction. Clinically, patients describe vague elbow pain, recurrent locking, snapping, and instability. Instability with associated pain occurs when the elbow is extended and the forearm supinated (lateral pivot-shift). When this maneuver leads to apprehension, further evaluation under anesthesia is often recommended (49,127–129). Although conservative management can incorporate an elbow orthosis to maintain the forearm in pronation, treatment for symptomatic instability is usually surgical. Operative intervention involves reattachment of the avulsed lateral ulnar collateral ligament or reconstruction with a free tendon. Postoperatively, the extremity is immobilized for 4 weeks with the elbow flexed 90 degrees and the forearm fully pronated. A hinged orthosis is provided for the following 6 weeks, with a 30-degree extension block. Full activity is usually resumed within 6 months postoperatively (27,130).

In stage 2, there is further injury to both the anterior and posterior elbow complex, so that the medial edge of the ulna rests on the trochlea, giving the appearance that the coronoid is perched on the trochlea. In stage 3, the elbow dislocates fully (Fig. 66-9). Stage 3 is further classified. Stage 3A is when the anterior band of the medial collateral ligament is intact and the elbow is stable to valgus forces following reduction. In stage 3B, the entire medial collateral complex is disrupted, causing the elbow to be unstable in all directions (131).

With a complete posterior dislocation, the limb is held in 45 degrees of flexion and the olecranon is situated posteriorly. Differentiation between a posterior dislocation and a supracondylar fracture can initially be difficult, owing to associated swelling and olecranon positioning. With a supracondylar fracture, the normal alignment of the olecranon relative to the epicondyles is maintained.

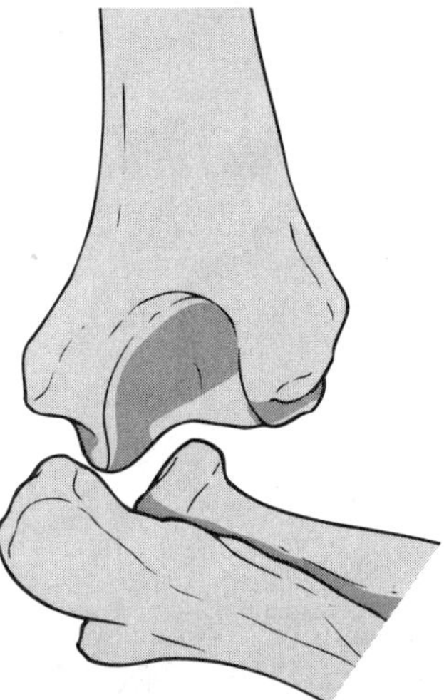

Figure 66-9. Stage 3 posterior dislocation. Stages 3A and 3B cannot usually be distinguished on radiographs.

With a posterior dislocation, however, the olecranon is displaced from the plane of the epicondyles.

Reduction, ongoing assessment of the neurovascular status, with particular attention to the brachial artery and median and ulnar nerves, and early protected range of motion to minimize the risk of flexion ankylosis are the basis of proper treatment (132,133). A postreduction rehabilitation program described by Harrelson (31) utilizes posterior splint immobilization at 90 degrees of flexion for 3 to 4 days. Rarely should immobilization exceed 2 weeks, as prolonged positioning leads to flexion contracture development and associated pain. The splint can be removed for active elbow flexion-extension and supination-pronation range of motion exercises after 3 to 4 days, avoiding valgus stress. By 10 days to 2 weeks the splint should be discontinued and a full elbow flexibility and strengthening program initiated. A hinged orthosis may also be used for up to 4 weeks postoperatively, allowing for 15 to 90 degrees of motion, if stability is a concern (79). Upon return to play, the elbow may be braced or taped to limit elbow hyperextension and provide for protection from valgus forces. Unstable dislocations require repair of the medial collateral ligament, with a longer period of joint protection.

Fractures occur in association with complete elbow dislocations in up to 50% of patients, with avulsions of the medial and lateral epicondyles and the radial head being seen most commonly (132).

Supracondylar Fractures

As with dislocations, supracondylar fractures occur most commonly from a fall onto an outstretched hand. Following forearm fractures, they are the second most common fracture in the skeletally immature population (134). Supracondylar fractures are classified based on the position of the distal humeral fragment. Extension fractures (type I), which are more common, have the distal humeral fragment displaced posteriorly, with potential damage to the brachial artery and associated nerves. The less common flexion fractures (type II) occur as a result of a direct blow to the posterior aspect of the flexed elbow, with the distal humeral fragment being displaced anteriorly (133). Radiographic assessment includes anteroposterior and lateral views (135) (Fig. 66-10). Oblique views with the elbow extended may help identify associated fractures of the radial head, coronoid, and condylar regions.

Due to the risk for neurovascular compromise, emergent orthopedic surgical referral is recommended. Casts should not be applied in the acute setting of a supracondylar fracture due to the potential for delayed swelling and subsequent vascular insult (compartment syndrome). When displacement is noted, which is the usual presentation, the most common treatment approach is open reduction and internal fixation. Following a stable reduction, active and active assisted pronation and supination exercises can be started within 2 to 3 days, with flexion-extension exercise initiated at 2 to 3 weeks (104,136,137).

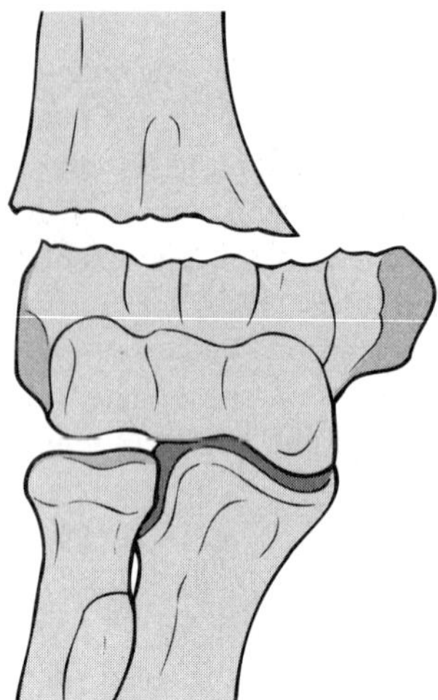

Figure 66-10. Anteroposterior view of a displaced supracondylar fracture in a 9-year-old child.

Anterior Injuries

The differential diagnosis for anterior elbow injuries is provided in Table 66-7.

Elbow hyperextension injuries can lead to anterior capsular disruption with damage to the median nerve, brachial artery, and the elbow flexor muscles. Clinically, patients present with swelling anteriorly and the inability to fully extend the elbow because of pain. Distal biceps tendinitis may develop as a result of repetitive flexion and supination motions, leading to tenderness at the distal insertion site, and pain and weakness on resisted supination and flexion. Conservative management for capsular strains and bicipital tendinitis involves a brief period of immobilization, usually lasting less than 5 days, followed by a comprehensive rehabilitation program. The therapy approach helps restore full range of motion and flexion and supination strength at the elbow (83,138).

Flexion Contractures

Morrey (139,140) classifed the cause of elbow stiffness into three categories:

1. Extrinsic causes that include contractures of the joint capsule, surrounding musculature, collateral ligaments, or ectopic bone formation
2. Intrinsic causes that include intra-articular adhesions, disruption of articular congruity, or loss of articular cartilage
3. Combined causes, such as seen with immobilization (extrinsic component) following an intra-articular fracture (intrinsic component)

The stiffness that develops following a fracture is related to the location of the fracture and is proportional to the length of time the joint is immobilized (141).

Since joint motion improves cartilage nutrition and bone remodeling, early range of motion exercises minimize the risk of contracture formation (142). When there is relatively minimal loss of mobility, rehabilitation can include joint mobilizations, contract-relax muscle energy techniques, flexibility and joint range of motion exercises, and ultrasound to improve collagen extensibility. Passive overpressure stretch can also be provided by having the patient hold a 2- to 4-lb weight or a resistive band while resting the upper extremity on a point proximal to the elbow joint. The stretch is then held for 10 to 12 minutes to provide for a sustained-duration, low-intensity force. Stretching must be performed so that the healing tissues are not overstretched and the patient's pain response is not increased. To determine the aggressiveness of stretching, the pain-resistance sequence is assessed in conjunction with the range of motion end-feel. With the proper degree of sustained stretch, collagen fiber elongation occurs, since pain and protective muscle guarding are minimized (83) (Table 66-8). To diminish the risk of myositis ossificans, aggressive high-force stretching is avoided (31,88). In the more chronic situation, with greater loss of elbow motion and absent intra-articular pathology, low-load sustained passive stretching techniques using dynamic orthotics,

Table 66-7: Differential Diagnosis of Anterior Elbow Pain
Anterior capsular strain or tear
Brachialis tendinitis
Biceps tendinitis
Distal biceps rupture
Ectopic bone formation
Annular ligament disruption
Loose body formation
Adhesions or synovitis
Distal physeal humeral fracture

Table 66-8: The Pain-Resistance Sequence to Assist in Determining the Degree of Passive Stretching
Pain before resistance
Acute lesion with an active inflammatory component.
Treatment focus is on diminishing pain and incorporating a *mild* stretch.
Pain with resistance
Subacute lesion with a mild inflammatory component.
Treatment incorporates a *moderate* stretch.
Resistance before pain
Chronic lesion without an active inflammatory component.
Treatment incorporates *aggressive* stretching.

Source: Adapted with permission from Wilk KE, Arrigo C, Andrews JR. Rehabilitation of the elbow in the throwing athlete. *JOSPT* 1993;17:305–317.

static adjustable splints with a turnbuckle screw, and serial casting have been recommended. These techniques allow for a gradual increase in range of elbow motion through the use of low-intensity, prolonged, controlled force generation (30,143–145). In the most recalcitrant cases of elbow arthrofibrosis, surgical intervention is pursued and can include interpositional and distraction arthroplasty, arthroscopic débridement, and total elbow replacement (146).

PEDIATRIC AND ADOLESCENT CONCERNS

The pathologic processes that occur in this age group develop often as a result of traction, compression, and shear forces applied to an immature skeleton whereby the epiphyseal growth plate serves as the weak link in the young athlete's musculoskeletal system. In addition to the growing epiphysis, joint laxity, underdeveloped musculature, articular surface softness, and bone immaturity must be considered in evaluating upper-extremity injuries in the skeletally immature athlete (147). The most common disorders in the young athlete include Little Leaguer's elbow and osteochondritis dissecans.

Little Leaguer's Elbow

Little Leaguer's elbow is an overuse injury resulting from repetitive valgus traction forces (traction apophysitis) at the origins of the medial collateral ligament and flexor-pronator musculature. This valgus stress, combined with compressive lateral forces, leads to partial or complete avulsion of the medial epicondyle ossification center (4,148). Osteochondral injuries to the capitellum and premature closure of the proximal radial epiphysis with increased risk for long-term growth deformity can also develop (33,69,149,150). Trabecular and cortical thickening as well as enlargement of the medial epicondyle epiphysis with fragmentation can be seen radiographically. As these findings may be present in both symptomatic and asymptomatic individuals, they are most likely stress reaction responses rather than true pathologic changes (21,134) (Fig. 66-11).

Various authors have investigated the prevalence of elbow dysfunction in the Little League population. The studies show that the incidence of elbow pain, anatomic impairment, and potential long-term functional limitations increase with age and exposure to pitching tasks (149,151–155).

Clinical Presentation and Management Options

The adolescent commonly complains of medial elbow pain that is increased with pitching and diminished with rest. There may also be a catching or locking sensation when a free fragment exists within the joint. In the pitcher, the number of pitches thrown per week and any recent change in technique, frequency, intensity, or duration should be noted (134). Point tenderness at the medial region with loss of full elbow extension may be noted. Radiographic evaluation includes anteroposterior and lateral views. Comparison views of the noninjured elbow can be helpful in determining if the medial epicondyle has separated from the adjacent humerus (134,156–158). Additional diagnostic studies, including gravity stress views, arthrography, CT arthrography, and MRI, can be considered in the more difficult situations (134).

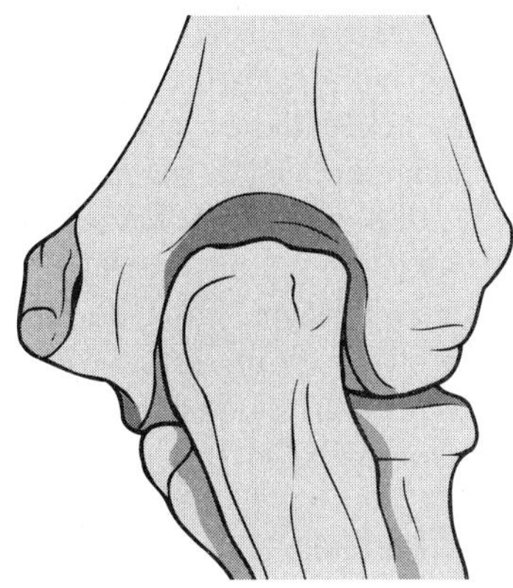

Figure 66-11. Medial humeral epicondylar overgrowth in a Little League pitcher. The epicondyle is larger and the epiphyseal plate lucency is increased.

In the patient without an avulsion fracture or disruption of the medial collateral ligament, treatment involves a brief period of immobilization, rest from aggravating activities, avoidance of throwing for 6 to 12 weeks, and inflammatory control. As the acute symptoms are controlled, anterior capsular stretching and upper-extremity kinetic chain reconditioning is incorporated. Complete cessation from throwing activities for the remainder of the season may be necessary if symptoms recur as the athlete attempts a return to pitching (31,74,159).

In the adolescent throwing athlete with an avulsion of the medial epicondyle, treatment is guided by fracture displacement and elbow stability. For minimal displacement of less than 5 mm and adequate stability, treatment is conservative, with immobilization for 3 weeks followed by joint range of motion and strengthening exercises. When the fragment is displaced more than 5 mm, or when instability exists, then open reduction with internal fixation and repair of the medial collateral ligament is pursued (134,135,148,152,160). The cornerstone of conservative management, however, is the prevention of elbow injuries in the young throwing athlete. Attention should be on a comprehensive conditioning program and instruction in proper pitching and delivery techniques. Curveball and other breaking pitches should be avoided in the skeletally immature athlete (i.e., athletes younger than 15 years), as the medial epicondyle epiphyseal center has yet to close (134,148,161). These pitches create greater tensile loads at the medial epicondyle as the forearm is "snapped" into supination. Vertical ball delivery is preferable to side-arm delivery to minimze the risk for developing elbow injuries (162). Additional prevention measures include limiting the number of innings pitched and the number of pitches thrown (163). Although limiting formal pitching to six innings per week with 3 days of rest between pitching turns is recommended, the informal practice sessions outside of the structured league setting and the amount of pitching during the off-season must not be overlooked (31). A useful guideline for progression of throwing is at a rate no more than 10% per week (164).

Osteochondritis Dissecans

Osteochondritis dissecans is a lesion of bone and articular cartilage, occurring between the ages of 13 and 17, that develops as a result of repetitive, traumatic lateral compression forces as seen in pitching and upper-extremity weight-bearing activities of gymnasts. This repetitive loading leads to compression of the radial head against the capitellum, with subsequent disruption of the tenuous vascular supply. Loose body formation, bony overgrowth of the radial head, arthritic changes, and permanent joint deformity with elbow dysfunction can ultimately occur. Early recognition and management are crucial to prevent long-term disability (21,69,161,165).

As described by Pappas (166), treatment and prognosis are guided by the stage of the disease. Group I is considered osteochondrosis (Panner disease) with fragmentation of the capitellum ossific nucleus but without loose body formation. The diagnosis is made as a result of an incidental finding on radiographs, with symptoms being minimal or nonexistent. The athlete is usually under the age of 12, and the prognosis is favorable. Treatment is activity restriction with the occasional need for immobilization, followed by restoration of full range of motion. Return to sporting activities is gradual and is permitted as long as the athlete remains asymptomatic (4).

Group II commonly occurs in the individual 13 years or older. The common presentation is an insidious onset of pain with activity. Radiographs may identify localized rarefaction in the capitellum and possible crater formation with a sclerotic rim. Loose body identification may require CT arthrography, and MRI can also be used to assess the status of the fragment and continuity of the overlying cartilage (167). Treatment is similar to that for group I, but arthroscopy may be required to delineate damage to the articular cartilage. To diminish cartilage incongruity and joint erosion in a lesion that has not completely fragmented, drilling or bone grafting or both may be required (21).

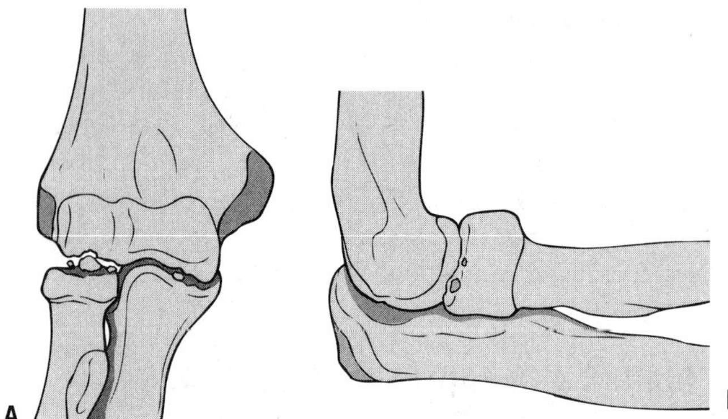

Figure 66-12. *A.* Oblique view of an elbow of a 16-year-old, who had been a baseball pitcher between the ages of 11 and 13, showing osteochondritis dissecans of the capitellum. *B.* Lateral view documenting a loose body within the joint.

Group III occurs in the older individual with loose body formation, associated locking or catching, flexion contractures, joint incongruity, and degenerative changes extending beyond the radiocapitellar joint. There can also be premature physeal closure and radial head enlargement (135,168) (Fig. 66-12). Treatment often involves arthrotomy, with the prognois being limited as a result of difficulty in reconstructing a congruous articulation (21).

CONCLUSIONS

Based on an accurate diagnosis, a comprehensive rehabilitation program for the athlete with an elbow-related disorder can be implemented in a timely and cost-effective manner. By addressing the anatomic and biomechanical functioning of the upper-extremity kinetic chain and understanding the sport-specific demands of the athlete, the physiatrist can appropriately advance the treatment program, thereby enhancing a favorable outcome with a safe return to sport and decreased risk of reinjury.

REFERENCES

1. Yocum LA. The diagnosis and nonoperative treatment of elbow problems in the athlete. *Clin Sports Med* 1989;8:439–451.
2. Magee DJ. Elbow joints. In: Magee DJ, ed. *Orthopedic physical assessment,* 2nd ed. Philadelphia: WB Saunders, 1992:143–167.
3. Nirschl RP, Kraushaar BS. Assessment and treatment guidelines for elbow injuries. *Phys Sports Med* 1996;24:43–60.
4. Caldwell GL, Safran MR. Elbow problems in the athlete. *Clin Sports Med* 1995;26:465–485.
5. Morrey BF. Applied anatomy and biomechanics of the elbow joint. *Instr Course Lect* 1986;35:59–68.

6. Regan WD, Korinek SL, Morrey BF, An KN. Biomechanical study of ligaments around the elbow joint. *Clin Orthop* 1991;271: 170–179.

7. Schwab GH, Bennet JB, Woods GW, Tullos HS. Biomechanics of elbow instability: the role of the medial collateral ligament. *Clin Orthop* 1980;146:42–52.

8. Morrey BF. Anatomy of the elbow joint. In: Morrey BF, ed. *The elbow and its disorders*, 2nd ed. Philadelphia: WB Saunders, 1993:16–51.

9. Morrey BF, An KN. Articular and ligamentous contributions to the stability of the elbow joint. *Am J Sports Med* 1983;11:315–319.

10. Anderson TE. Anatomy and physical examination of the elbow. In: Nicholas JA, Hershman EB, eds. *The upper extremity in sports medicine*. St. Louis: CV Mosby, 1990:273–288.

11. Andrews JR, Craven WM. Lesions of the posterior compartment of the elbow. *Clin Sports Med* 1991;10:637–651.

12. Fox GM, Jebson PJL, Orwin JF. Overuse injuries of the elbow. *Phys Sports Med* 1995;23: 58–66.

13. Hollinshead WH, Jenkins DB, eds. *Functional anatomy of the limbs and back*. 5th ed. Philadelphia: WB Saunders, 1981: 118–126, 137–147, 148–157.

14. Wiesner SL. Rehabilitation of elbow injuries in sports. *Phys Med Rehabil Clin N Am* 1994; 5:81–113.

15. Spinner M, ed. *Injuries to the major branches of the peripheral nerves of the forearm*. 2nd ed. Philadelphia: WB Saunders, 1978:80–157, 160–227, 230–266.

16. Nirschl RP. Elbow tendinosis-tennis elbow. *Clin Sports Med* 1992;11:851–870.

17. Nirschl RP. Prevention and treatment of elbow and shoulder injuries in the tennis player. *Clin Sports Med* 1988;4:289–308.

18. Plancher KD, Halbrecht J, Lourie GM. Medial and lateral epicondylitis in the athlete. *Clin Sports Med* 1996;15:283–305.

19. Childress HM. Recurrent ulnar nerve dislocation at the elbow. *Clin Orthop* 1975;108:168–173.

20. Glousman RE. Ulnar nerve problems in the athlete's elbow. *Clin Sports Med* 1990;9:365–377.

21. Jobe FW, Nuber G. Throwing injuries of the elbow. *Clin Sports Med* 1986;5:621–636.

22. Apfelberg FG, Larson SJ. Dynamic anatomy of the ulnar nerve at the elbow. *Plast Reconstr Surg* 1973;51:76–81.

23. Buehler MJ, Thayer DT. The elbow flexion test: a clinical test for the cubital tunnel syndrome. *Clin Orthop* 1988;233:213–218.

24. O'Drsicoll SW, Horil E, Carmichael SW, et al. The cubital tunnel and ulnar neuropathy. *J Bone Joint Surg [Br]* 1991;73:613–617.

25. Wadsworth TG. The external compression syndrome of the ulnar nerve at the cubital tunnel. *Clin Orthop* 1977;124:189–204.

26. Pechan J, Julius I. The pressure measurement in the ulnar nerve. A contribution to the pathophysiology of the cubital tunnel syndrome. *J Biomech* 1975;8: 75–84.

27. Johnston JJ, Plancher KD, Hawkins RJ. Elbow injuries to the throwing athlete. *Clin Sports Med* 1996;15:307–329.

28. Weinstein SM, Herring SA. Nerve problems and compartment syndromes in the hand, wrist, and forearm. *Clin Sports Med* 1992;11:161–188.

29. Jobe FW, Fanton GS, Elattrache NS. Ulnar nerve injury. In: Morrey BP, ed. *The elbow and its disorders*. 2nd ed. Philadelphia: WB Saunders, 1993:560–565.

30. Sailer SM, Lewis SB. Rehabilitation and splinting of common upper extremity injuries in athletes. *Clin Sports Med* 1995;14:411–446.

31. Harrelson GL. Elbow rehabilitation. In: Andrews JR, Harrelson GL, eds. *Physical rehabilitation of the injured athlete*. Philadelphia: WB Saunders, 1991:443–472.

32. Goodgold J, Eberstein A. Motor and sensory nerve conduction measurements. In: *Electrodiagnosis of neuromuscular diseases*. 3rd ed. Baltimore: Williams & Wilkins, 1983:104–153.

33. Spinner M, Spencer PS. Nerve compression lesions of the upper extremity. *Clin Orthop* 1974;104:46–67.

34. Eversmann WW Jr. Entrapment and compressive neuropathies. In: Green DP, ed. *Operative hand surgery*. 3rd ed. New York: Churchill Livingstone, 1993:1341–1385.

35. Plancer KD, Peterson RK, Steichen JB. Compressive neuropathies and tendinopathies in the athletic elbow and wrist. *Clin Sports Med* 1996;15:331–369.

36. Chu-Andrews J, Johnson RJ, Bruyninckx FL. Common injuries and entrapment syndromes involving the peripheral nerves. In: Chu-Andrews J, Johnson RJ, eds. *Electrodiagnosis. An anatomical and clinical approach*. Philadelphia: JB Lippincott, 1986:308–310.

37. Lutz FR. Radial tunnel syndrome: an etiology of chronic lateral elbow pain. *J Orthop Sports Phys Ther* 1991;14:14–17.

38. Roles N, Maudsley R. Radial tunnel syndrome: resistant tennis elbow as nerve entrapment. *J Bone Joint Surg [Br]* 1972;54: 499–508.

39. Spinner M. The arcade of Frohse and its relationship to posterior interosseous nerve paralysis. *J Bone Joint Surg [Br]* 1968;50: 809–812.

40. Werner CO. Lateral elbow pain and posterior interosseous nerve entrapment. *Acta Orthop Scand Suppl* 1979;174:1–62.

41. Crawford GP. The radial tunnel syndrome. *J Hand Surg [Am]* 1984;9:451–452.

42. Lister GD, Belsole RB, Kleinert HE. The radial tunnel syndrome. *J Hand Surg* 1979;4:52–59.

43. Bassett FH, Nunley JA. Compression of the musculocutaneous nerve at the elbow. *J Bone Joint Surg [Am]* 1982;64: 1050–1052.

44. Felsenthal G, Mondell DL, Reischer MA, Mark RH. Forearm pain secondary to compression syndrome of the lateral cutaneous nerve of the forearm. *Arch Phys Med Rehabil* 1984; 65:139–141.

45. Steinberg BD, Plancher KD. Clinical anatomy of the wrist and elbow. *Clin Sports Med* 1995;14: 299–313.

46. Boone DC, Azen SP. Normal range of motion of joints in male subjects. *J Bone Joint Surg [Am]* 1979;61:756–759.

47. London JT. Kinematics of the elbow. *J Bone Joint Surg [Am]* 1981;63:529–535.

48. Hotchkiss RN, Weiland AJ. Valgus stability of the elbow. *J Orthop Res* 1987;5:372–377.

49. An K-N, Morrey BF, Chao EYS. The effect of partial removal of the proximal ulna on elbow constraint. *Clin Orthop* 1986;209: 270–279.

50. Kapandji AI. *The physiology of the joints: upper limb.* Vol. 1. 5th ed. Edinburgh: Churchill Livingstone, 1982:88.

51. Askew LJ, An KN, Morrey BF, et al. Functional evaluation of the elbow: normal motion requirements and strength determinations. *Trans Orthop Res Soc* 1981;6:183.

52. Glousman RE, Barron J, Jobe FW, et al. An electromyographic analysis of the elbow in normal and injured pitchers with medial collateral ligament insufficiency. *Am J Sports Med* 1992;20: 311–317.

53. Jobe FW, Moynes DR, Tibone JE, et al. An EMG analysis of the shoulder in pitching. A special report. *Am J Sports Med* 1984;12:218–220.

54. McLeod WD. The pitching mechanism. In: Zarin B, Andrews JR, Carson WG, eds. *Injuries to the throwing arm.* Philadelphia: WB Saunders, 1985:22–29.

55. Andrews JR. Bony injuries about the elbow in the throwing athlete. *Instr Course Lect* 1985;36: 323–331.

56. Plancer KD, Minnich JM. Sports-specific injuries. *Clin Sports Med* 1986;15:207–218.

57. Ilfeld FE, Field SM. Treatment of tennis elbow. *JAMA* 1986;195: 67–70.

58. Nirschl RP. Lateral and medial epicondylitis. In: Morrey BF, ed. *Master techniques in orthopaedic surgery, the elbow.* New York: Raven, 1994:129–148.

59. Nirschl RP, Sobel J. Conservative treatment of tennis elbow. *Phys Sports Med* 1981;9:43–54.

60. Ellenbecker TS. Rehabilitation of shoulder and elbow injuries in tennis players. *Clin Sports Med* 1995;4:87–107.

61. Giangarra CE, Conroy B, Jobe FW, et al. Electromyographic and cinematographic analysis of elbow function in tennis players using single- and double-handed backhand strokes. *Am J Sports Med* 1993;21: 394–399.

62. Field LD, Altchek DW. Elbow injuries. *Clin Sports Med* 1995; 14:59–78.

63. Leach RE, Miller JK. Lateral and medial epicondylitis of the elbow. *Clin Sports Med* 1987;6:259–272.

64. Morris M, Jobe FW, Perry J, et al. Electromyographic analysis of elbow function in tennis players. *Am J Sports Med* 1989;17:241–247.

65. Nicola TL. Elbow injuries in athletes. *Prim Care* 1992;19:283–302.

66. Sobel J, Pettrone F, Nirschl R. Prevention and rehabilitation of racquet sports injuries. In: Nicholas JA, Hershman EB, eds. *The upper extremity in sports medicine.* St. Louis: CV Mosby, 1990:843–860.

67. Rhu KN, McCormick J, Jobe FW, et al. An electromyographic analysis of shoulder function in tennis players. *Am J Sports Med* 1988;16:481–485.

68. Gunn CC, Milbrandt WE. Tennis elbow and the cervical spine. *Can Med Assoc J* 1976;114: 803–809.

69. Cabrera JM, McCue FC. Nonosseous athletic injuries of the elbow, forearm, and hand. *Clin Sports Med* 1986;5: 681–700.

70. Coonrad RW: Tennis elbow. *Instr Course Lect* 1986;35:94–101.

71. Henning EM, Rosenbaum D, Milani TL. Transfer of tennis racket vibrations onto the human forearm. *Med Sci Sports Exerc* 1992;24:1134–1140.

72. Roetert EP, Dillman CJ, Groppel JL, Schultheis JM. The biomechanics of tennis elbow. An integrated approach. *Clin Sports Med* 1995;14:47–57.

73. Grabiner MD, Groppel JL, Campbell KR. Resultant tennis ball velocity as a function of off-center impact and grip firmness. *Med Sci Sports Exerc* 1983;15: 542–544.

74. Mehlhoff TL, Bennett JB. Elbow injuries. In: Mellion MB, Walsh WM, Shelton GL, eds. *The team physician's handbook.* Philadelphia: Hanley & Belfus, 1990: 334–345.

75. Regan WD, Word LE, Coonrad R, et al. Microscopic histopathology of chronic refractory lateral epicondylitis. *Am J Sports Med* 1992;20:746.

76. Brown M. The older athlete with tennis elbow. Rehabilitation concerns. *Clin Sports Med* 1995; 14:267–275.

77. Fillion PL. Treatment of lateral epicondylitis. *Am J Occup Ther* 1991;45:340–343.

78. LaFreniere JG. Tennis elbow: evaluation, treatment and prevention. *Phys Ther* 1979;59:742–746.

79. Andrews JR, Wilk KE, Groh D. Elbow rehabilitation. In: Brotzman SB, ed. *Clinical orthopaedic rehabilitation.* St. Louis: Mosby–Year Book, 1996:67–89.

80. Thomas DR, Plancher KD, Hawkins RJ. Prevention and rehabilitation of overuse injuries of the elbow. *Clin Sports Med* 1996;14:459–477.

81. Lee DG. Tennis elbow: a manual therapist's perspective. *J Orthop Sports Phys Ther* 1986;8: 134–141.

82. Chinn CJ, Priest JD, Kent BE. Upper extremity range of motion, grip strength, and girth in highly skilled tennis players. *Phys Ther* 1974;54:474–482.

83. Wilk KE, Arrigo C, Andrews JR. Rehabilitation of the elbow in the throwing athlete. *J Orthop Sports Phys Ther* 1993;17:305–317.

84. Dilorenzo CE, Parkes JC, Chmelar RD. The importance of shoulder and cervical injuries. *J Orthop Sports Phys Ther* 1990;11: 402–409.

85. Wells P. Cervical dysfunction and shoulder problems. *Physiotherapy* 1983;68:66–71.

86. Priest JD, Nagel DA. Tennis shoulder. *Am J Sports Med* 1976;4:28–42.

87. Priest JD, Braden J, Gerbierich JG. The elbow and tennis. Part I: an analysis of players with and without pain. *Phys Sports Med* 1980;8:80–87.

88. Anderson TE, Ciolek J. Specific rehabilitation programs for the throwing athlete. *Instr Course Lect* 1989;38:487–491.

89. Seto JL, Brewster CE, Randall CC, et al. Rehabilitation following ulnar collateral ligament reconstruction of athletes. *J Orthop Sports Phys Ther* 1991;14: 100–105.

90. Ilfeld FW. Can stroke modification relieve tennis elbow? *Clin Orthop* 1992;276:182–186.

91. Lehman RC. Surface and equipment variables in tennis injuries. *Clin Sports Med* 1988;7:229.

92. Adelsberg S. The tennis stroke: an EMG analysis of selected muscles with rackets of increasing grip size. *Am J Sports Med* 1986;14:139–142.

93. Nirschl RP. Muscle and tendon trauma: tennis elbow. In: Morrey BF, ed. *The elbow and its disorders.* 2nd ed. Philadelphia: WB Saunders, 1993:537–552.

94. Nirschl RP. Tennis elbow: joint resolution by conservative treatment and improved technique. *Phys Sports Med* 1984;12:168–182.

95. Hatze H. The effectiveness of grip bands in reducing racquet vibration transfer and slipping. *Med Sci Sports Exerc* 1992;24:226–230.

96. Harding WG. Use and misuse of the tennis elbow strap. *Phys Sports Med* 1992;20:65–74.

97. Nirschl RP. Tennis elbow. *Orthop Clin North Am* 1973;4:787–791.

98. Buckwalter JA. Pharmacologic treatment of soft tissue injuries. *J Bone Joint Surg [Am]* 1995;77:1902–1914.

99. Gorga PP, Brown M, Al-Obaidi S. Hydrocortisone and exercise effects on articular cartilage in rats. *Arch Phys Med Rehabil* 1993;74:463–467.

100. Nirschl RP, Pettrone FA. Tennis elbow. The surgical treatment of lateral epicondylitis. *J Bone Joint Surg [Am]* 1979;61:832–839.

101. Potter HG, Hannafin JA, Morwessel RM, et al. Lateral epicondylitis: correlation of MR imaging, surgical and histopathology findings. *Radiology* 1995;196: 43–46.

102. Mason ML. Some observations on fractures of the head of the radius with a review of one hundred cases. *Br J Surg* 1954;42:123–132.

103. Morrey BF. Radial head fracture. In: Morrey BF, ed. *The elbow and its disorders.* 2nd ed. Philadelphia: WB Saunders, 1993:383–404.

104. Ogle AA. Rehabilitation of upper extremity fractures. *Phys Med Rehabil State Art Rev* 1995;9:141–159.

105. DeHaven KE, Evarts CM. Throwing injuries of the elbow in athletes. *Orthop Clin North Am* 1973;4:801–808.

106. Bennett JB, Green MS, Tullos HS. Surgical management of chronic medial elbow instability. *Clin Orthop* 1992;278:62–68.

107. Conway JE, Jobe FW, Glousman RE, et al. Medial instability of the elbow in throwing athletes. *J Bone Joint Surg [Am]* 1992;74:67–83.

108. Jobe FW, Elattrache NS. Diagnosis and treatment of ulnar collateral ligament injuries in athletes. In: Morrey BF, ed. *The elbow and its disorders.* 2nd ed. Philadelphia: WB Saunders, 1993:566–572.

109. Mirowitz SA, London SL. Ulnar collateral ligament injury in baseball pitchers: MR imaging evaluation. *Radiology* 1992;185: 573–576.

110. Timmerman LA, Schwartz ML, Andrews JR. Preoperative evaluation of the ulnar collateral ligament by magnetic resonance imaging and computed tomography arthrography. Evaluation in 25 baseball players with surgical confirmation. *Am J Sports Med* 1994;22:26–31.

111. Jobe FW, Stark H, Lombardo SJ. Reconstruction of the ulnar collateral ligament in athletes. *J Bone Joint Surg [Am]* 1986;68: 1158–1163.

112. Kirby RL, Simms FC, Symington VJ, et al. Flexibility and musculoskeletal symptomatology in female gymnasts and age-matched controls. *Am J Sports Med* 1981;9:160–164.

113. Snook GA. Injuries in women's gymnastics. A 5-year study. *Am J Sports Med* 1979;7: 242–244.

114. Reilly JP, Nicholas JA. The chronically inflamed bursa. *Clin Sports Med* 1987;6:345–370.

115. Aronen JG. Problems of the upper extremity in gymnastics. *Clin Sports Med* 1985;4:61–71.

116. Feretti A, Papandrea P. Stress fracture of the trochlea in an adolescent gymnast. *J Shoulder Elbow Surg* 1994;3:399–405.

117. Hulko A, Orava S, Nikula P. Stress fractures of the olecranon in javelin throwers. *Int J Sports Med* 1986;7:210–214.

118. Nuber GW, Diment MT. Olecranon stress fractures in throwers. *Clin Orthop* 1992;278: 58–61.

119. Orava S, Hulko A. Delayed unions and nonunions of stress fractures in athletes. *Am J Sports Med* 1988;16:378–382.

120. Bach BR, Earren RF, Wickiewicz TL. Triceps rupture: a case report and literature review. *Am J Sports Med* 1987;15:285–289.

121. Sherman DH, Snyder SJ, Fos JM. Triceps tendon avulsion in a professional body builder: a case report. *Am J Sports Med* 1976; 12:328–331.

122. Tarsney FF. Rupture and avulsion of the triceps. *Clin Orthop* 1972; 83:177–184.

123. Wilson FD, Andrews JR, Blackburn TA, et al. Valgus extension overload in the pitching elbow. *Am J Sports Med* 1982; 11:83–88.

124. Andrews JR, Wilson FD. Valgus extension overload in the pitching elbow. In: Zarins B, Andrews JR, Carson WG, eds. *Injuries in the throwing athlete.* Philadelphia: WB Saunders, 1985:250–257.

125. Morrey BF, Tanaka S, An KN. Valgus stability of the elbow: a definition of primary and secondary constraints. *Clin Orthop* 1991;265:187–191.

126. Andrews JR, Wilk KE, Satterwhite YE, Tedder JL. Physical examination of the thrower's elbow. *J Orthop Sports Phys Ther* 1993; 17:296–304.

127. Morrey BF, O'Driscoll SW. Lateral collateral ligament injury. In: Morrey BF, ed. *The elbow and its disorders.* 2nd ed. Philadelphia: WB Saunders, 1993: 573–580.

128. Nestor BJ, O'Driscoll SW, Morrey BF. Ligamentous reconstruction for posterolateral rotatory instability of the elbow. *J Bone Joint Surg [Am]* 1992;74:1235–1241.

129. O'Driscoll SW, Bell DF, Morrey BF. Posterolateral rotatory instability of the elbow. *J Bone Joint Surg [Am]* 1991;73:440–446.

130. O'Driscoll SW, Morrey BF. Surgical reconstruction of the lateral collateral ligament. In: Morrey BF, ed. *Master techniques in orthopaedic surgery: the elbow.* New York: Raven. 1994: 169–181.

131. O'Driscoll SW. Classification and spectrum of elbow instability: recurrent instability. In: Morrey BF, ed. *The elbow and its disorders.* 2nd ed. Philadelphia: WB Saunders, 1993:453–463.

132. Hotchkiss RN, Green DP. Fractures and dislocations of the elbow. In: Rockwood CA, Green DP, eds. *Fractures in adults.* Vol. 1. 3rd ed. Philadelphia: JB Lippincott, 1991:739–841.

133. Hurley JA. Complicated elbow fractures in adults. *Clin Sports Med* 1990;9:39–57.

134. Ireland ML, Hutchinson MR. Upper extremity injuries in young athletes. *Clin Sports Med* 1995;14:533–569.

135. Gill TJ, Micheli LJ. The immature athlete. Common injuries and overuse syndromes of the elbow and wrist. *Clin Sports Med* 1996;15:401–423.

136. Millis MB, Singer I, Hall JE. Supracondylar fractures of the humerus in children: further experience with a study in orthopaedic decision making. *Clin Orthop* 1988;188:90–97.

137. Waddell JP, Hatch J, Richards RR. Supracondylar fractures of the humerus—results of surgical treatment. *J Trauma* 1988;28: 1615–1621.

138. Hotchkiss RN. Common disorders of the elbow in athletes and musicians. *Hand Clin* 1990;6: 507–515.

139. Morrey BF. Post-traumatic contracture of the elbow. Operative treatment, including distraction arthroplasty. *J Bone Joint Surg [Am]* 1990;72:601–618.

140. Morrey BF. Post-traumatic stiffness: distraction arthroplasty. In: Morrey BF, ed. *The elbow and its disorders.* 2nd ed. Philadelphia: WB Saunders, 1993: 476–491.

141. Knapp ME. Aftercare of fractures. In: Kottke FJ, Lehmann, JF, eds. *Krusen's handbook of physical medicine and rehabilitation.* 4th ed. Philadelphia. WB Saunders, 1990:749–753.

142. Salter RB, Simmonds DF, Malcolm BW, et al. The biological effect of continuous passive motion on the healing of full thickness defects in articular cartilage. *J Bone Joint Surg [Am]* 1980;62:1232–1251.

143. Middleton K. Range of motion and flexibility. In: Andrews JR, Harrelson GL, eds. *Physical rehabilitation of the injured athlete.* Philadelphia: WB Saunders, 1991:141–164.

144. Green DP, McCoy H. Turnbuckle orthotic correction of elbow-flexion contractures after acute injuries. *J Bone Joint Surg [Am]* 1979;61:1092–1095.

145. Zander CL, Healy NL. Elbow flexion contractures treated with serial casts and conservative therapy. *J Hand Surg [Am]* 1992;17:694–697.

146. Timmerman LA, Andrews JR. Arthroscopic treatment of post-traumatic elbow pain and stiffness. *Am J Sports Med* 1994;22: 230–235.

147. Ireland ML, Andrews JR. Shoulder and elbow injuries in the young athlete. Clin *Sports Med* 1988;7:473–493.

148. Pappas AM. Elbow problems associated with baseball during childhood and adolescence. *Clin Orthop* 1982;164:30–41.

149. Adams JE. Injuries to the throwing arm: a study of traumatic changes in the elbow joints of boy baseball players. *Cal Med* 1965;102:127–132.

150. Micheli LJ. Overuse injuries in children's sports: the growth factor. *Orthop Clin North Am* 1983;14:337–360.

151. Grana WA, Rashkin A. Pitcher's elbow in adolescents. *Am J Sports Med* 1980;8:333–336.

152. Gugenheim JJ, Stanley RF, Woods GW, et al. Little League survey: the Houston study. *Am J Sports Med* 1976;4:189–200.

153. Larson RL, Singer KM, Bergstrom R, et al. Little League survey: the Eugene study. *Am J Sports Med* 1976;4:201–209.

154. Pappas AM. Overuse syndromes of the shoulder and arm. *Adolesc Med State Art Rev* 1991;2: 181–212.

155. Takenoabu I, Ikata T. Baseball elbow of young players. *Tokushima J Exp Med* 1985; 32:57.

156. Ballinger PW. *Merrill's atlas of radiographic positions and radiologic procedures.* 6th ed. St. Louis: CV Mosby, 1986:82–93.

157. Belhobek GH. Roentgenographic evaluation of the elbow. In: Nicholas JA, Hershman EB, eds. *The upper extremity in sports medicine.* St. Louis: CV Mosby, 1990:289–292.

158. Bontrager KL, Anthony BT. *Textbook of radiographic positioning and related anatomy.* 2nd ed. St. Louis: CV Mosby, 1987:112–115.

159. Outerbridge AR, Micheli LJ. Overuse injuries in the young athlete. *Clin Sports Med* 1995;14:503–516.

160. Woods GW, Tullos HS. Elbow instability and medial epicondylar fractures. *Am J Sports Med* 1977;5:23–30.

161. Meyers JF. Injuries to the shoulder girdle and elbow. In: Sullivan JA, Grana WA, eds. *The pediatric athlete.* Park Ridge, IL: American Academy of Orthopaedic Surgeons, 1990: 145–153.

162. Albright JA, Jokl P, Shaw R, et al. Clinical study of baseball pitchers: correlation of injury to the throwing arm with method of delivery. *Am J Sports Med* 1978;6:15–21.

163. Torg JS, Pllack H, Sweterlisch P. The effect of competitive pitching on the shoulders and elbows of preadolescent baseball players. *Pediatrics* 1972;49:267–272.

164. Micheli LJ. Elbow pain in a Little League pitcher. In: Smith NJ, ed. *Common problems in pediatric sports medicine.* Chicago: Year Book Medical, 1989:233–241.

165. Singer KM, Roy SP. Osteochondrosis of the humeral capitellum. *Am J Sports Med* 1984;12: 351–360.

166. Pappas AM. Osteochondritis dissecans. *Clin Orthop* 1981;158: 59–69.

167. McManama GB Jr, Micheli LJ, Berry MV, et al. The surgical treatment of osteochondritis of the capitellum. *Am J Sports Med* 1985;13:11–21.

168. Bauer M, Jonsson K, Josefsson PO. Osteochondritis dissecans of the elbow: a long-term follow-up study. *Clin Orthop* 1992;284:156–160.

Chapter 67

Hand and Wrist Injuries

Richard N. Norris
William J. Dawson

THE ATHLETE

The hand and wrist are employed in virtually all types of sports activities by people of all ages and with varying degrees of physical expertise. Demands made of the athlete's hand are in many ways similar to those made of the instrumental musician's hand; effective performance by both groups requires multiple, rapid, precise, and complex repetitive motions of the fingers, hands, and wrists. Even small degrees of inaccuracy can profoundly affect the success of both musical and sports endeavors. However, athletes usually demand a greater degree of strength to properly perform their activities.

It is not surprising that the hand is one of the structures most commonly injured during sports participation (1,2). These injuries may occur during practice or competition as isolated, acute problems. Injuries to the hand frequently do not recur when the person returns to sports, following proper treatment. They also may arise from repetitive, forceful activities that have been traditionally labeled "overuse" conditions. In contrast to acute trauma, these injuries are more likely to recur, especially if the underlying conditions or practices are not modified as part of the rehabilitation process. The epidemiology of these conditions in athletes differs from that of instrumental musicians, for whom music-related trauma is unusual (3). Problems caused by overuse activities while making music are much more common, and the potential for recurrences is much greater in instrumentalists.

A third group of athletic injuries often seen by the treating physician may represent the greatest challenge to treatment skills and rehabilitative efforts. Many high-level sports participants sustain injuries that are either ignored or treated in a temporizing fashion, to allow the performer (often a professional or collegiate varsity player) to continue or finish the season (4). When these conditions are finally seen, late in their natural history, definitive treatment may not be possible and secondary or reconstructive methods may need to be employed. Results, despite often heroic rehabilitation efforts, are rarely as good as those obtained with timely primary treatment.

Many individuals, both young and old, participate in both music and sports or conditioning activities during any given period in their lives. Injuries and other difficulties occurring in this group demand that both areas of special hand needs be considered for acute care and rehabilitation (Tables 67-1 and 67-2).

Basic Principles

Optimal hand and wrist function requires full and comfortable ranges of joint motion, flexibility of periarticular structures and muscle-tendon units, full strength in both agonist and antagonist groups, stable bony architecture, and neuromuscular coordination of all parts sufficient to perform the necessary tasks. The philosophies and techniques of rehabilitation in the hand and upper extremity are essentially no different for the athlete or the instrumentalist. Whenever possible, the rehabilitation process should

Table 67-1: Upper-Extremity Sports Injury in Instrumentalists, 1984–1996

Type of Sport	No. of Patients
Ball sports	149
Basketball	(49)
Baseball, softball	(46)
Football (American)	(22)
Volleyball	(21)
Soccer	(8)
Snow sports	23
Skating	30
On land	(16)
On ice	(14)
Aquatic sports	6
Cycling	13
Racquet sports	5
Gymnastics	10
Track and field sports	2
Miscellaneous	24
Total	262

Table 67-2: Diagnoses of Upper-Extremity Sports Injury in 259 Instrumentalists, 1984–1996

Diagnosis Group	No. of Patients
Fractures	165
Fracture-dislocations	8
Dislocations	9
Ligament sprains	65
Muscle strains	16
Tendon injuries, closed	6
Lacerations	5
Crush injuries, contusions	10
Late effects of trauma	25
Total	309

begin sometime during the acute treatment phase of the injury or condition. It should involve use of both the injured part and the entire body, thus encouraging the athlete to maintain effective levels of conditioning and skills in the uninjured parts. Ideally, this overlap of treatment and rehabilitation will minimize the competitive athlete's frequent tendency to develop anxiety and depression when injury prevents participation, as well as shorten the total amount of time spent "on the sideline."

In general, rehabilitation of an injured part will follow a consistent pattern. Swelling and edema about the injury must be controlled or minimized before other gains can be made (5). Early, vigorous treatment actually can prevent swelling and its resultant joint stiffness (6). Following this, normal movement of joints and flexibility of muscle-tendon units must be regained. Next, muscle strength about the injured area must be redeveloped, and distant and uninvolved muscles also must be maintained in, or returned to, proper condition. When these goals have been met, the individual's needs for improved coordination may be dealt with; regaining proprioceptive control of the involved limb is an integral part of the process and plays a major role in prevention of further injury. The final element that must be regained prior to sports return is endurance, or the ability to use one's strength and motions in a repetitive manner without fatigue, pain, loss of coordination, or resultant new injury. In many cases, some degree of overlap of these elements may be possible during the rehabilitative period, further minimizing the duration of disability and time spent away from sports.

Techniques employed by the physician, therapist, and trainer should not be confined to those traditionally used in the office, gym, or training room. Sport-specific skills need to be redeveloped also, and this usually can be accomplished during the same time interval. Involvement of the athletic coach in regaining these skills is essential, to complete the entire rehabilitation process and to assist in preventing new or repeated injuries when the athlete returns to practice.

Mobilization

Nowhere else in the human body is there such a complex organization of joints and muscles as in the hand and wrist. This arrangement permits a wide spectrum of motions and forces in the limb, and allows the performance of both powerful and precision activities in a rapid and repetitious fashion. Restoration of these myriad functions requires not only a full range of joint motion but also supple muscle-tendon units and smooth tendon gliding.

Joint mobility may be regained through a series of concentric or translational exercises, stretching the tight ligaments and capsular tissues and facilitating the smooth gliding of articular cartilage surfaces. Active range of motion (ROM) exercises can be performed by the athlete after appropriate instruction, but translational movements (especially useful for stiff finger and wrist joints) must be performed by a therapist. It is necessary for the patient to regain a range of joint motion greater than that required to perform a given task. The additional range or "cushion" obviates the need for the joint to function consistently at the extremes of its range. Many athletes (gymnasts and divers, for example) require ranges of joint motion that would be considered excessive in a "normal" population; this degree of hyperextensibility must be regained in these individuals.

Active ROM exercises should begin as soon as possible after the injury, consistent with proper healing. Uninjured areas should be exercised from the beginning of treatment to prevent additional stiffness, which might result in more prolonged rehabilitation later.

A regimen of stretching and flexibility exercises for the muscles also should begin early in the treatment program. Not only will active muscle contraction assist in mobilizing edema in the injured limb, but also it prevents stiffness and facilitates normal tendon gliding. It is necessary to stretch both agonists and antagonists, and best results are achieved when the program is carried out at least three times a day (7). Stretching of tight intrinsic muscles must be included in this program when appropriate (Fig. 67-1), as should stretching of the retinacular system in the distal two phalanges of the fingers (Fig. 67-2).

A variety of mobilization techniques may be utilized, depending on the structures involved, the nature of the injury, and the athlete's needs. Active-assistive techniques may be employed in the early healing stages when pain would prohibit active methods alone. Passive stretching may be performed by the patient or therapist, and is one of the methods essential in facilitating the early ranges of tendon gliding after surgical repair. A variety of manual techniques also may be helpful, when performed by a therapist trained in their use. These would include myofascial release in the wrist and forearm, deep tissue or scar massage, and tendon and nerve gliding techniques (8).

Strengthening and Endurance

Although some improvement in muscle tone and power will occur during mobilization exercises, a more specialized program of strengthening is essential for resumption of full

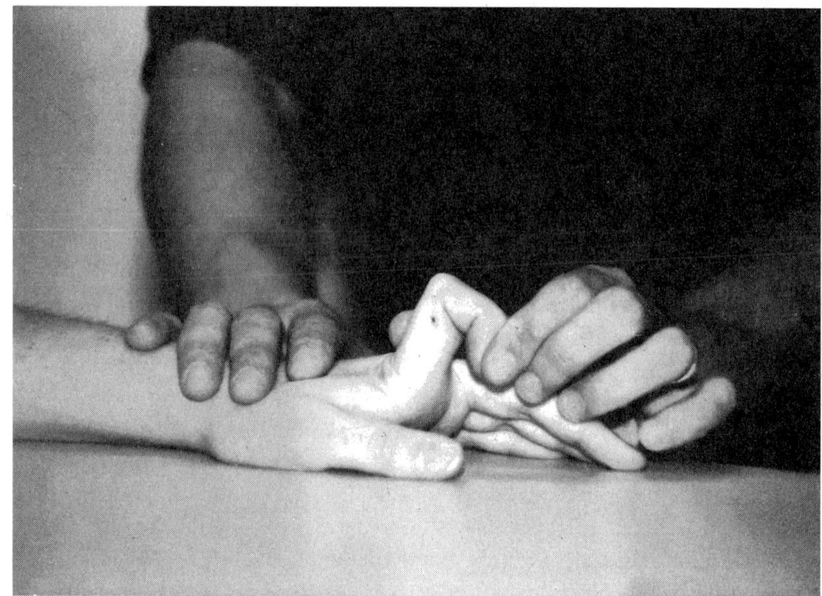

Figure 67-1. Technique of intrinsic muscle stretch. The metacarpophalangeal joint must be held in full passive extension while the two interphalangeal joints are passively stretched into maximum comfortable flexion, and held in that position for 5 seconds.

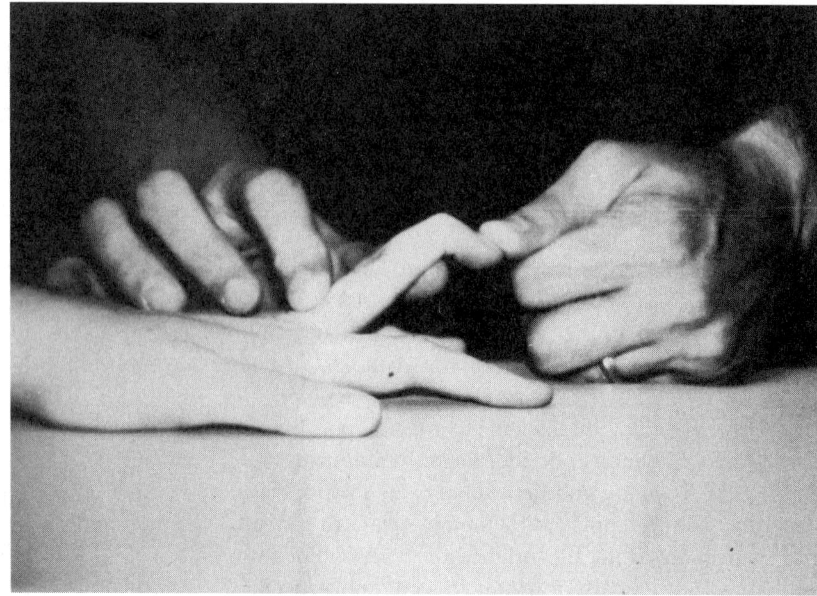

Figure 67-2. Technique of retinacular ligament stretch. The proximal interphalangeal joint must be held in full passive extension while the distal interphalangeal joint is passively flexed to its maximum comfortable extent, and held in that position for 5 seconds.

sports activities. This program also should include the uninjured muscle groups, since they have not usually maintained full conditioning levels during the period of acute treatment. As with mobility, function of uninjured areas should be maintained, with exercises for both agonist and antagonist groups instituted during the acute treatment phase.

The injured area may benefit by initiating early exercises. Isometric methods are frequently employed in this phase, since their use affords protection of injured joints from additional stress or injury caused by premature or improper motion. Later, progressive resistance programs can be employed effectively. Often strengthening is begun in the central range of available muscle and joint motion, and progressed toward the extremes as additional flexibility and mobility are regained. Isotonic techniques are usually added as joint ranges approach normal. Biofeedback may prove useful in those instances where co-contractions interfere with the efficiency of a specific exercise program.

Isokinetic exercises are usually initiated after isotonic routines have achieved their maximum benefit. The ultimate goal of such a program is active contraction of a muscle (group) against maximum resistance through a full arc of motion (9). Machines such as the Orthotron or Cybex help achieve this goal by permitting exercise in variables of range, speed, duration, and intensity of effort (Fig. 67-3). Slow training routines are effective for correction of residual strength deficits, while fast training is better for redeveloping power and endurance (10).

Coordination

Organized and repetitive patterns of musculoskeletal activity depend not only on adequate motion and strength, but also on proprioceptive skills and neuromuscular control. A variety of rehabilitative techniques may be employed to regain or improve this necessary element. Reciprocal stabilization routines and proprioceptive neuromuscular facilitation (PNF) are useful in restoring awareness and control in the injured or disused limb (11). Task-specific exercises that duplicate the physical requirements for a particular sports activity may be utilized "off the field" as well as during formal practice.

Modalities

Heat is one of the most useful adjuncts to both mobilization and strengthening. When used correctly, it increases local circulation and gently distends tissues, as well as assists in their desensitization; exercise efforts are enhanced under these favorable conditions. Heat may be applied in a variety of ways: heating pads or Hydrocollator packs, paraffin baths, fluidotherapy, direct immersion of the limb in a whirlpool bath, and ultrasound. The choice of application should be determined by the nature of the injury, the part involved, the training of the therapist, the availability of the apparatus, and any associated patient conditions or contraindications.

Cold is somewhat less commonly used during this stage of rehabilitation, but may be useful after an exercise session to minimize secondary swelling and discomfort. Ice or gel packs can be applied locally to specific areas as needed.

Massage of the hand, wrist, and forearm is a useful adjunct to the above-mentioned modalities, especially in the treatment of chronic edema. Mobilization of accumulated fluid by proximal to distal massage, with a lubricant used to protect the skin from undue friction, can speed the return of joint and tendon motions and minimize discomfort during exercise sessions.

High-voltage pulsed galvanic stimulation has proved quite effective in the treatment of extremity edema,

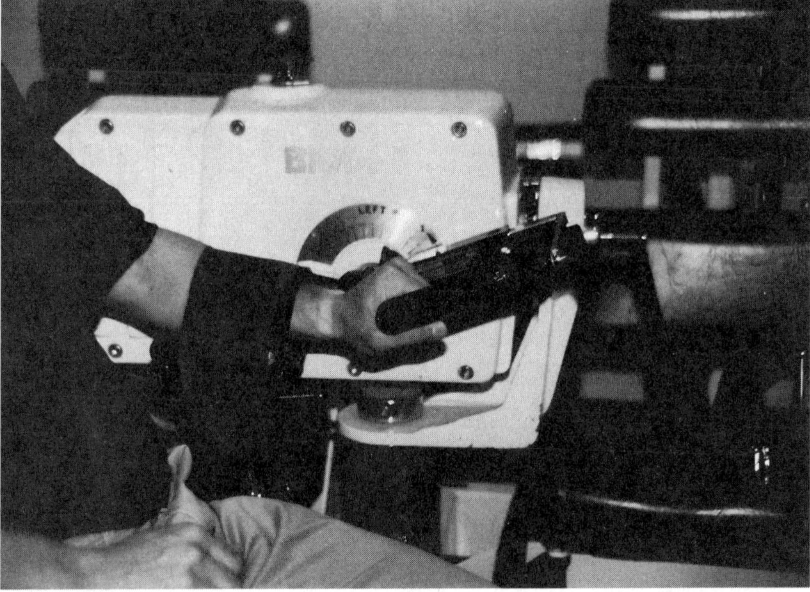

Figure 67-3. Biodex machine used for wrist motion and strength rehabilitation. All wrist ranges of motion (flexion/extension, pronation/supination, and radial/ulnar deviation) can be rehabilitated effectively in an isokinetic manner by this apparatus. Computerized printouts of each session can be used to document improvement in parameters such as motion, strength, and force over varying ranges of motion.

especially the chronic form that commonly occurs in a hand and forearm during cast treatment of wrist fractures. It also is indicated in patients with organized hematomas or chronic fibrous edema (12). This type of stimulation creates a muscle-pump action to facilitate blood flow, and usually is employed in conjunction with an active exercise program.

Orthoses

An orthosis can be defined as an appliance or apparatus used to support, align, prevent, or correct deformities, or to improve the function of movable parts of the body (13). Splints or other immobilization techniques are frequently employed during the treatment and healing stages of many hand and wrist injuries, and often may allow an earlier removal of casts or other forms of postoperative immobilization (9). As motion and strength of the injured area improve, continued protection by splinting or strapping is often necessary to facilitate the return of sport-specific skills and prevent new injury during this phase.

Some of the goals and ideals of splinting include 1) protecting the injured area from additional trauma during rehabilitation and sports return; 2) limiting excessive motion of the injured area; 3) regaining or improving motion in a stiff joint (14); 4) allowing the player to participate comfortably, effectively, and safely; and 5) being lightweight, compact, and unlikely to injure the patient or opposing players.

Splinting may be accomplished by wrapping an area with adhesive tape, or by using one of a variety of metallic, elastic, plaster, fiberglass, plastic, or cushioning devices, whether ready-made or custom fabricated. Each material has its own advantages, disadvantages, and indications for use, and many factors will govern the precise choice of material, type of splint construction, and duration of use. Details of various methods are discussed later under Rehabilitation of Specific Conditions.

Return to Sports Activity

Many factors enter into deciding when to allow an athlete to return to play following an injury (4). The decision should be made jointly by the treating physician, therapist(s), and the athlete's coach or trainer. Certain prerequisites seem obvious: The injured hand or wrist must be healed sufficiently to permit return without risking further trauma; joints should possess more than enough motion to accommodate the demands of the sport (13); muscles should be at preinjury strength and trained to handle the loads required for each individual sports activity (15); the athlete's entire body must be in proper condition as well (16), including restoration of cardiovascular fitness (13). Protective splinting may facilitate an earlier return to sports while protecting the affected area from further trauma (17,18). It may also serve a preventive function, especially if worn regularly thereafter for practice and competition.

Rehabilitation of Specific Conditions

Distal Phalanx and Distal Interphalangeal Joint Injuries

These injuries are usually caused by sports involving a ball (4). The so-called mallet finger injury to the extensor tendon insertion may also include an avulsion fracture of the dorsal lip of the distal phalanx, but the basic treatment is the same for both types. Static splinting of the distal interphalangeal joint in full extension is needed until the fracture is healed or the tendon can support the joint against gravity (at least 4–6 weeks). Gentle flexion is allowed thereafter (19), but full power of the flexor digitorum profundus should not be encouraged for several more weeks. Extension splinting is required at night and during sports for at least 1 month after it has been discontinued for gentle daily activities, and complete function may not be achieved for at least 3 months (20).

Avulsion of the flexor digitorum profundus tendon insertion on the distal phalanx is seen frequently in American football players, and usually in the ring finger when the digits are caught while grasping an opponent's jersey and then forcibly extended (21). The avulsion may or may not be accompanied by a small bony fragment from the distal phalanx (22). Surgical reattachment of the tendon is followed by 4 weeks of immobilization; the resulting tendon scarring and joint stiffness require a prolonged period of mobilization exercises, during which protective splinting of the hand and finger in flexion will allow the football player an earlier return to the field.

Proximal Interphalangeal Joint Fractures, Sprains, and Dislocations

These are the most common injuries seen in ball sports, especially baseball and softball (23). The majority do not require prolonged immobilization or surgical treatment, but nonetheless may result in persistent swelling and stiffness of the joint and require months of mobilization exercises and long-term protective splinting. Avulsion or tear of the central extensor tendon slip at the base of the middle phalanx requires continuous splinting of the joint in full extension for a minimum of 4 to 6 weeks, with the distal interphalangeal joint usually kept free to allow active flexion and prevent retinacular ligament contractures (19). Despite this program, a boutonnière deformity may develop, although this condition is seen more often in the untreated or incompletely treated injury. Rehabilitation of such a deformity must include a prolonged period of splinting, at least 6 to 9 months (24).

Fracture-subluxation of the proximal interphalangeal joint is sometimes underdiagnosed, or dismissed as a rather innocuous injury. However, the long-term disability from its inadequate treatment can seriously affect an athletic career (professional or otherwise). Early concentric reduction of the joint is mandatory and often requires internal fixation or open surgical methods. Prevention of full joint extension is necessary after any type of reduction for this injury, and extension block splinting (25) often is utilized to achieve this goal. Active flexion and extension exercises must be performed for many weeks after injury, and treatment of long-term losses of full extension may require dynamic extension splinting (14).

Thumb Metacarpophalangeal Joint

Tears of the ulnar collateral ligament are the most common sport-related injury to this joint, and are the most common hand injury incurred from skiing. Grade I and II sprains have incomplete tears of the ligament, without damage to the adductor tendon aponeurosis; these usually are treated with a thumb spica cast for a minimum of 4 weeks. Grade III injuries are associated with a complete tear of the ligament, which often is displaced superficially to the adductor aponeurosis (the so-called Stener lesion). Although the literature reflects some difference of opinion regarding the treatment of grade III tears, most authors advocate open surgical repair of the ligament (2,26). Regardless of the degree of collateral ligament sprain, prolonged splinting can protect the healing ligament during resumption of sports activity. Many athletes, especially those who have recurrent injuries, prefer preventive taping of this joint to using rigid splints (18). High-level competitive skiers and other athletes may require concomitant splinting of the interphalangeal joint for adequate protection during sports activity.

Wrist and Carpal Fractures and Dislocations

Details of classification, diagnosis, and treatment options for this group of injuries have been covered in many recent articles and texts (27–33) and are not discussed here. Rehabilitation principles relate primarily to treatment of the joint and periarticular stiffness that commonly follow most open or closed methods of treatment. Indeed, open reduction and rigid internal fixation of scaphoid and some distal radial fractures may actually permit a more rapid recovery of joint motion and strength, and afford the athlete an early return to participation while wearing a protective playing cast or brace (27,34). Treatment of distal radial fractures with external fixation devices may actually result in greater stiffness than with cast or open treatment (9), and may require prolonged exercise programs to restore mobility.

Secondary difficulties with more distal uninvolved structures are not uncommon with these types of trauma. Significant swelling of the hand and fingers following wrist fractures and dislocations may result in intrinsic muscle contractures in the hand (9), with the interosseous and lumbrical muscles being involved more than the thenar and hypothenar groups. This complication may be minimized by early, active ROM exercises of all joints that do not require immobilization. In established cases, however, correction often requires months of dynamic splinting and tedious active exercise.

Tendinitis

When one considers the multiplicity of tendons in the hand and wrist, and the wide variety of motions they produce, it is not surprising that repetitive, forceful activity during sports practice and competition frequently results in inflammatory problems (17). de Quervain tenosynovitis is common in participants in racquet sports and fishing, while strain and inflammation of the radial and ulnar wrist flexor tendons are seen in those who play golf, volleyball, or some racquet sports. Splinting is commonly employed during the acute phase of inflammation, but should be discontinued gradually and as soon as possible (8). Thereafter, exercises to improve tendon gliding should begin, thus decreasing the tendency for adhesions to develop from immobility and inflammation. Return of mobility should be followed by strengthening exercises, progressing from isometric through isotonic to isokinetic programs. Prevention of recurrences must also be stressed, since prophylatic splinting may interfere with the mobility required for certain sports.

THE MUSICIAN: OVERUSE INJURIES

Most of the rehabilitation concepts already discussed hold true for instrumental musicians as well as athletes. One of the main differences in types of injuries is the low incidence of macrotrauma and high incidence of repetitive microtrauma (overuse) in musicians as compared to athletes (3). Overuse injuries of the hand and wrist are common among instrumentalists (35–37). Fortunately, such injuries are largely preventable and can often be treated through a combination of proper care and a change in the habits or activities that caused them (38). The term *overuse injury* has been defined as a condition that occurs when any biologic tissue (muscle, bone, tendon, ligament, etc) is stressed beyond its physical or physiologic limits (39). Some histologic studies have revealed pathologic but nonspecific changes (40). Overuse injuries can be classified as acute or chronic. An acute overuse injury occurs following a specific incident of stressing the tissue beyond its limits. An example would be a musician who learns a new phrase or trill and is determined to master it before going to bed that evening. He or she practices it for 3 or 4 hours, and then wakes up the next day with a stiff and painful hand or arm. Chronic overuse injury takes place more insidiously over a longer period of time, starting out as a mild discomfort that becomes progressively severe over the course of weeks or months.

Symptoms

The most common indicator is pain or discomfort. Overuse injuries are commonly graded into five categories (41):

Grade 1—pain at one site only, and only while playing.

Grade 2—pain at multiple sites.

Grade 3—pain that persists well beyond the time when the musician stops playing.

Grade 4—all of the above; in addition, many activities of daily living (ADLs) begin to cause pain.

Grade 5—all of the above, but all daily activities that engage the affected body part cause pain.

Most overuse injuries fall into grade 1, 2, or 3. The earlier the symptoms are recognized and treated, the sooner and more completely recovery is likely to occur. In the earliest stages, overuse injuries may be experienced as stiffness without significant amounts of pain. Research in progress suggests that subtle loss of motor control or technique may be one of the earliest signs of overuse (42).

Principles of Rehabilitation

The injury that plagues the student or professional musician can usually be treated nonoperatively with success, especially in its early stages. However, it should be kept in mind that nonsurgical treatment is not always the conservative path and there are many conditions that respond quickly and reliably to surgical procedures. In situations of prolonged pain and disability, nonsurgical procedures should not be pursued indefinitely when surgery would correct the situation and allow the performer a rapid return to playing.

(Relative) Rest

Perhaps the most important treatment of all is rest. It is usually difficult for professional musicians to take time off to rest, so we must utilize the concept of "relative rest" from sports medicine (43). Depending on the severity of the injury, this may mean cutting back, rather than completely stopping practice and performances. It may be possible to modify or change the repertoire, such as avoiding piano pieces with large chord spans or broken or serial octaves or triple forte playing. Sometimes technique can be modified, such as having a violinist with a left finger sprain or arthritis minimize the use of vibrato in an orchestral setting, where it is less likely to be noticed. Acoustic steel-string guitar players can be advised to switch to lighter-gauge strings. For students, there is less justification for not markedly cutting back or stopping for a brief period of time when necessary. It is better to postpone an examination or an audition than to allow an injury to worsen. Relative rest basically means avoiding pain-producing activities.

Performance Resumption Following an Injury

The rehabilitation of upper-extremity injuries in musicians has two distinct, although overlapping, phases. Reducing pain or symptoms represents only the first stage. If the player has had to stop or significantly reduce playing during the healing phase, a graduated, methodical plan for returning to full musical and daily activities is essential to avoid emotionally and physically distressing relapses (44). Traditionally, the musician performs his or her specific tasks, but starts out at a greatly reduced level of duration and intensity. The process of gradually building up to normal activity is usually guided or supervised by the physician or therapist.

Historical Perspective

Injured musicians usually miss playing so much, and often have so much anxiety about being away from their instruments, that as soon as they start to feel somewhat recovered, they attempt to leap prematurely back to their usual routine, often with disastrous consequences. Fry (45) quotes Poore (1887) on this:

> Treatment: The most important point in treatment is rest. The excessive use of the hand must be discontinued, and it is often necessary to insist on this rather forcibly. Piano playing, if not prohibited altogether, must only be practiced to a degree short of that which causes pain or annoyance. It is often difficult to restrain the ardor of these patients in the matter of playing. Directly they feel in a small degree better, they fly to the piano; and I have known the progress of more than one case very seriously retarded by the undoing, as it were, of the good effect of rest by an hour's injudicious and prohibited practising.

Counseling the Patient

It is critical that the treating clinical team be fully educated in both the psychological and practical aspects of guiding patients through the difficult and often treacherous stages of resuming full musical activities so as to avoid the despair that can accompany setbacks, treatment failure, and career abandonment. Ideally, the treating physician or therapist will devote ample time to counsel the patient to avoid this common error and to exercise patience, restraint, and good judgment while recovering. It is a wise patient who is able to learn by the mistakes of others. Musicians should be reassured that they are not going to lose their technique during the course of a few weeks' rest, and that they can put their "downtime" to good use by working on music theory, harmony, sight-reading or solfège, critically listening to recordings, or learning something about the business aspects of music and career promotion.

Initial Stages

It is not always necessary to stop playing entirely. Often, reducing the intensity or time of playing, or both, choosing an easier repertoire, or taking more frequent breaks may suffice. It may be necessary to cancel or postpone performance commitments, examinations ("juries"), or auditions. If one hand is injured, the unaffected side may be able to continue playing. It is not necessary for the injured musician to be completely asymptomatic before beginning the reconditioning program. A person who is not yet ready or able to deal with the physical instrument can go through the motions of playing without the instrument, what Menuhin (46) referred to as "shadow" playing. It is advisable that the recovering player have the endurance to shadow play comfortably for 10 minutes or so prior to beginning a return to play schedule on the actual instrument.

The Return to Play Schedule

When the musician is ready to return to the instrument, a detailed return to play schedule is developed and reviewed (Table 67-3). It is inadequate and inappropriate for a clinician merely to advise the player who is ready to return to playing to "go back little by little." This is too vague and open to misinterpretation. The value of a written schedule is that it helps minimize the risk of overdoing things. Players must be advised to adhere to the schedule even if they feel that they can do more. The use of a clock or timer is helpful. The problem is that the effects of overuse are often not perceived at the time of activity; the pain may evolve over several hours or more.

It may be advisable to start with only 5 minutes once or twice a day, but if the injury was severe or the person has had to stop playing for a long time, he or she might begin cautiously with a single 2- or 3-minute period or even less and see how the injury feels later on or the next day. Fry (41) recommended an even more gradual approach, starting with 5 seconds twice a day. A brief physical warm-up should precede and a cooldown follow playing, and if there is still some pain or discomfort, the sore part may be iced down for 10 minutes or so after the playing session.

The return to play schedule can and should be modified to suit the individual player. In addition to the warm-up and cooldown, slow, easy pieces or études should be practiced initially. A metronome may be used initially at a medium setting and gradually increased to faster tempos by clicking up a notch or two every few days. Gradually progressing to slower tempos should also be practiced, as the control required to play very slowly can also be demanding. With time the player gradually resumes more technically difficult material. In summary, the progression encompasses three gradually increasing parameters: duration, tempo, and technical difficulty.

Review During Breaks

To avoid disrupting the flow of practice, Markison (47) recommended using a tape recorder during the break periods to critically review what has just been practiced. This suggestion is useful as it is difficult to critically listen to oneself while playing, due to the concentration required in reading, fingering, phrasing, and so on. More importantly, compliance with prescribed rest breaks is enhanced as the

Table 67-3: Returning to Play

Levels (3–7 Days at Each)	Play	*Rest*	Play	*Rest*	Play	*Rest*	Play	*Rest*	Play
1	**5**	*60*	**5**						
2	**10**	*50*	**10**						
3	**15**	*40*	**15**	*60*	**5**				
4	**20**	*30*	**20**	*50*	**10**				
5	**30**	*20*	**25**	*40*	**15**	*45*	**5**		
6	**35**	*15*	**35**	*30*	**20**	*35*	**10**		
7	**40**	*10*	**40**	*20*	**25**	*25*	**15**	*50*	**10**
8	**50**	*10*	**45**	*15*	**30**	*15*	**25**	*40*	**15**
9	**50**	*10*	**50**	*10*	**40**	*10*	**35**	*30*	**20**
10	**50**	*10*	**50**	*10*	**50**	*10*	**45**	*20*	**30**
Etc.									

- Start with slow and easy activity or pieces. Gradually progress to faster, more difficult tasks or pieces.
- In general, perform a maximum of 50 minutes' continuous work or play with a minimum of 10 minutes' rest.
- *Warm up* before working or playing!
- If pain occurs at any level, drop back to a level of comfort until able to progress without pain.

Source: Reproduced by permission from Norris RN. *The musicians' survival manual.* St. Louis: MMB Music, 1993.

musician has something musically "useful" to do during the breaks.

Instrument-Specific Rehabilitation Strategies

To provide care on a sophisticated level, it is necessary to modify the concept of a musician's return to play to address specific injuries and specific instruments. String players with de Quervain tendonitis of the right wrist should avoid using the proximal 4 to 6 inches of the bow, as the wrist often assumes the provocative position of flexion/ulnar deviation as the hand approaches the strings on the upbow. A pianist recovering from the same problem might avoid using the thumb on the black keys to avoid ulnar deviation. It may be easier for the pianist with a painful hand or forearm overuse condition to resume playing on a synthesizer or electronic keyboard, as the action requires less force. A guitarist may switch to lighter-gauge strings. Guitarists with problems in the left hand could place the capo (a type of clamp with a rubberized bar) on the third fret and detune the strings one and one-half steps to bring them back into pitch, thus decreasing the stress of wrist supination and shoulder external rotation required when playing on the first three frets. Since the distance between the frets decreases as one goes higher up the guitar's neck, the finger and hand stretch required for chords or intervals is also lessened.

Addressing Painful Daily Activities

During the acute phase of an overuse injury, daily activities often are a significant aggravating factor. Overlooking this factor can result in treatment failure. Intervention by an occupational therapist (OT) is critical at this point. The OT is skilled in counseling the patient regarding modifications of daily activities and in recommending the numerous devices available that have been developed for people with limited hand function or painful hands. These serve the purpose of joint protection and minimizing the stress of daily activities. Examples are jar "wrenches" to increase leverage, telephone holders or headsets to avoid sustained grasp, key holders to improve leverage and avoid pinch grip, and cylindrical foam sleeves for writing or eating utensils. Eaton (48) recommended using these devices primarily during the acute phase of injury to minimize physical stress on the tissues and weaning the patient as soon as possible from them in order to prevent tissue fragility secondary to overprotection.

Orthotics

An orthotic is a medical device, such as a splint or strap, applied to or around a bodily segment to help manage physical impairment or disability. Orthotics may be used in a number of different ways to help manage upper-extremity disorders. Orthotics can be applied to the upper extremity in the form of a splint or they can be applied to an instrument to help stabilize it or to lessen the amount of force required to control it (49–52).

Splints

Splints must be chosen according to the diagnosis and situation (53). If the chief complaint is night pain from clenching the fists during sleep, then a full-length resting splint is indicated. The full-length splint may also be necessary to prevent use of the injured hand when the chief complaint is pain during all daily activities. This would be particularly true if the dominant extremity is injured, since the dominant limb tends to be used automatically. Care must be taken not to provoke injury in the opposite arm by the unaccustomed, increased use of that side. Removing the splint hourly to perform gentle active movements and muscle contractions will minimize stiffness and soreness of the splinted part. Splints that are custom-molded by an OT can provide maximum comfort and optimal fit. Slings should be avoided, if possible, as there may be some risk of ulnar nerve compression from prolonged elbow flexion (54) and of shoulder stiffness.

For disorders affecting the thumb region, such as de Quervain tendonitis or carpometacarpal arthritis, a thumb spica splint is indicated. However, the practitioner must keep in mind that the spica still allows use of the hand and the patient may still continue to aggravate the injury through isometric contraction of the affected muscles. If a splint is not tolerated or complied with, a padded fiberglass cast may be used for a week or two, but will cause more stiffness than a removable splint. Both the splint and the cast should be "bubbled out" or relieved directly over the radial styloid to avoid direct, mechanical irritation of the tendons (55). In addition, the thumb must be aligned with the edge of the forearm, in slight ulnar deviation, so that the thumb extensor tendons are placed in the position of least tension (48).

Reduction of Static Loading

The static loading that occurs when the weight of a tool is sustained and supported by the hand has long been recognized as an etiologic factor in workers' injuries (56). Industry has addressed this by developing ways to suspend tools in order to remove the weight from the hand. This approach has also worked for musical instruments. For example, several devices on the market relieve the right thumb strain common to playing the clarinet. Freeing the right hand allows alternative fingerings that may be more efficacious. The support developed by Adam and Fry (57) has the advantage of working while the performer is in the seated or standing position. The thumb rest, however, has to be replaced by a small knob and thus the instrument can no longer be used without the support unless the thumb rest is replaced. The Weightlifter (Bob James, PO Box 2514, San Marcos, CA 92079) is a tripod support on which the bell of the instrument rests (Fig. 67-4). It can be used during sitting and standing. It is relatively heavy, making it somewhat impractical for travel. The FHRED (Quodlibet, 8278 E. Hinsdale Avenue, Englewood, CO 80112) is a lightweight, adjustable-height post that attaches to the thumb rest and rests on the seat between the player's legs. It can only be used while sitting. There are "end pins" that attach to the bell of the English horn in order to unload the weight from the right thumb. A flute post can be fabricated to transfer the weight of the flute from the hands to the left trapezius. This is particularly useful for the very young player or the musician playing with a right shoulder, arm, or hand injury. The soprano saxophone, usually a straight instrument, has to be held away from the frontal plane of the body. This angle renders a neck strap relatively ineffective in taking the load of the instrument off the right thumb. However, the soprano sax is now available with an angled neck. The resulting increased verticality allows the neck strap to take the majority of the weight of the instrument off the thumb.

Key Modifications

Woodwind instruments are especially amenable to key modification. The location of the flute keys may be customized to fit the player's hand, and the cluster of keys worked by the right little finger can be angled in toward the finger (John Lunn, 23 Fletcher Road, Newport, NH 03773), thus reducing strain (Fig. 67-5). The keys operated by the left fourth and fifth fingers can be lengthened in order to achieve a more neutral position for the left wrist.

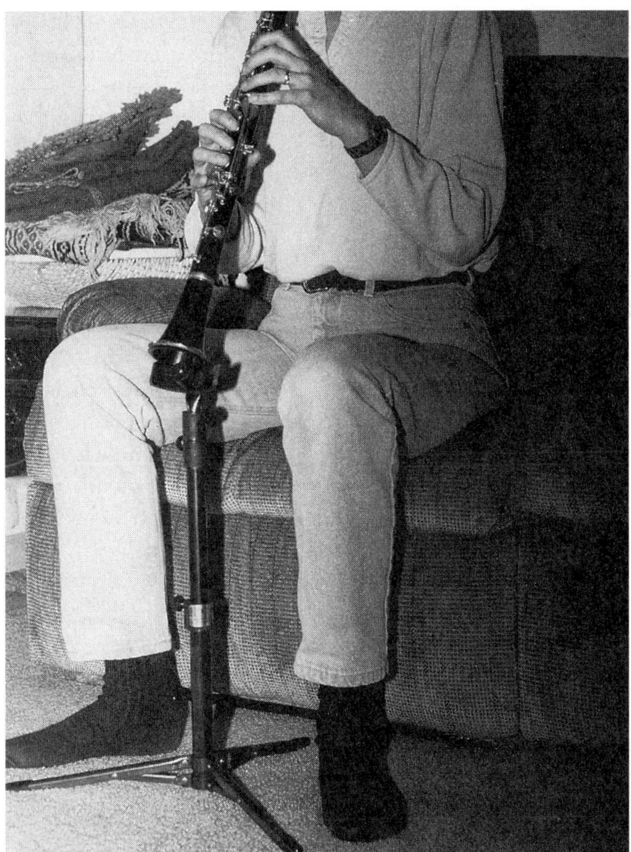

Figure 67-4. A support post takes the 2-lb weight of the clarinet off the right thumb, hand, and arm.

For children, in addition to these modifications, disks should be soldered to the keys for the right index, middle, and ring fingers, in such a way as to reduce the interkey distance, thus reducing hand strain. The levers that operate the valves on the French horn can be lengthened to provide greater leverage and widened to provide increased contact area. This is accomplished by soldering dimes onto the end of the levers. A hook-like device can be soldered onto the upright post of the trombone, significantly decreasing the stretch required for the left index finger to support the mouthpiece.

Nerve Compression

The common sites of nerve compression in the instrumentalist are the median nerve at the wrist (carpal tunnel syndrome) and the ulnar nerve at the elbow (cubital tunnel syndrome) (58). Less common sites are the digital nerve, entrapments of which are found mainly in those playing the flute (59), percussion, and bowed instruments, and the ulnar nerve at Guyon canal, compression of which is found in flutists (60).

Digital neuropathies are addressed by appropriate padding or orthoses. Carpal tunnel syndrome should be treated with splinting in 0 to 5 degrees of extension (although the splint is usually removed for practice or performance), medications (nonsteroidal anti-inflammatory or tricyclic agents), steroid injection (especially if flexor tenosynovitis is also present), and the nerve and tendon gliding exercises previously described. Biomechanical correction is key, as the carpal canal pressure increases dramatically with deviation in any direction from the neutral position (61,62). It is imperative to try to minimize wrist deviation if the musician is to keep playing during rehabilitation.

Anatomic Variations

Anatomic variations of the hands may be a significant factor in injury. Small hands can be a large problem, depending on the instrument and repertoire selected (63). The clarinet keys can and should be modified when the player lacks independent flexor digitorum sublimis (FDS) function. This condition, characterized by interconnections between the fourth and fifth FDS tendons (64), tends to restrict certain fingering motions on the clarinet. This problem is remediated by modifying the location of the keys. The lack of FDS independence may also create problems in guitarists (65), violinists, and violists (66). The Linberg anomaly (conjoined flexor digitorum profundus and flexor pollicis longus) (67) may cause problems in pianists or classical guitarists, as thumb adduction (as in arpeggios) or flexion (as when plucking) causes involuntary index flexion. Tenodesis of digital extensors may cause problems in violists (68). Variations in connective tissue extensibility—"hypermobility syndrome" (HMS)—is believed by some authors (69,70) to be a significant contributing factor to musical injuries and may explain the

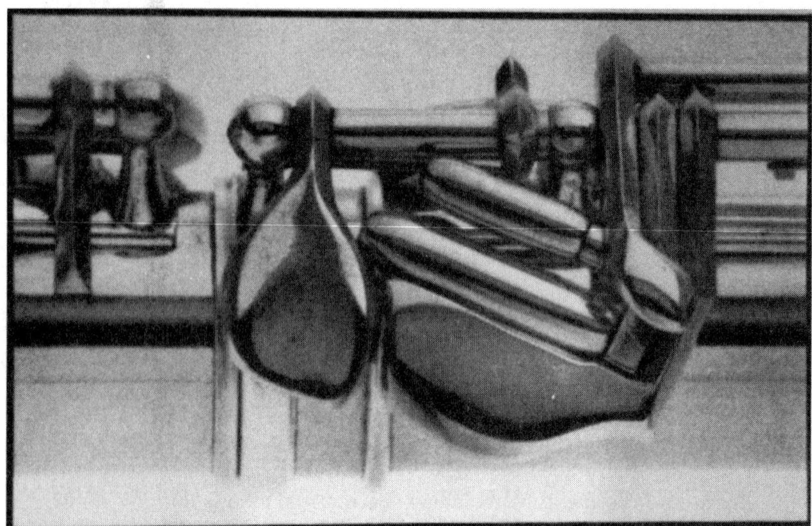

Figure 67-5. Modification of the foot-joint of the flute by angling the keys 45 degrees aligns the keys with the angle of approach of the right fifth finger, reducing strain.

statistically significant prevalence of hand injuries in professional female musicians when compared to their male counterparts (71).

Focal Dystonia, or Occupational "Cramp"

This condition, characterized by painless (and often progressive) loss of motor control, has been reported in the medical literature for centuries (72). It is associated with specific occupations such as writing, arts and crafts work, and music making. The common factor seems to be years of repetitive motion, although precipitating events, such as trauma or overuse (73), and biomechanical predisposition (74) have been proposed. The hand is usually the site of presentation. Stereotypical, unintentional movements of curling, extension, abduction, or adduction of the digits commonly occur. The condition can occur, however, in the oral musculature in woodwind or brass players, or in the vocal muscles in singers (spastic dysphonia). The dystonic pattern is usually highly task specific, at least in the early stages. The site of "lesion," if there is one, is not known. Diagnostic tests (electromyography, nerve conduction studies, imaging studies, blood tests, etc.) usually demonstrate findings within normal limits.

The incidence of the condition among musicians is low but the effect is devastating as there is no consistently effective treatment. Prolonged rest, psychotherapy, steroids, tricyclics, bromocryptine, biofeedback, botulinum toxin (75), and surgery have all been tried without success (76). Since the prognosis is so poor, the patient must be gently counseled and given a realistic appraisal of the situation. Depression following the diagnosis and prognosis is common and may require psychotherapy and career counseling. It is important not to mistake focal dystonia for potentially treatable conditions. A number of patients with this presentation turn out to have stenosing tenosynovitis of the flexor tendons, interphalangeal joint osteoarthritis, or overuse muscle spasms. For this reason, the diagnosis of focal dystonia should only be made when it is reasonably certain. A meticulous, detailed history and physical examination are critically important. Slow-motion video analysis is often helpful.

CONCLUSIONS

The treatment and rehabilitation of hand and wrist injuries in athletes and musicians are complex and challenging, owing to the extraordinary demands these highly competitive people place on these structures. The extra work and effort required of the treating team is made well worthwhile by the rewards of helping these patients back to the playing field and concert stage.

REFERENCES

1. Amadio PC. Epidemiology of hand and wrist injuries in sports. *Hand Clin* 1990;6:379–381.
2. Hankin FM, Peel SM. Sport-related fractures and dislocations in the hand. *Hand Clin* 1990;6: 429–453.
3. Dawson WJ. Experience with hand and upper extremity problems in 1000 instrumentalists. *Med Prob Perform Art* 1995;10: 128–133.
4. Dawson WJ. The spectrum of sports-related interphalangeal joint injuries. *Hand Clin* 1994;10: 315–326.
5. McEntee PM. Therapist's management of the stiff hand. In: Hunter JM, Schneider LH, Mackin EJ, Callahan AD, eds. *Rehabilitation of the hand.* 3rd

ed. St. Louis: CV Mosby, 1990: 328–341.

6. Curtis RM. Management of the stiff hand. In: Hunter JM, Schneider LH, Mackin EJ, Callahan AD, eds. *Rehabilitation of the hand.* 3rd ed. St. Louis: CV Mosby, 1990:321–327.

7. Hageman CE, Lehman RC. Stretching, strengthening and conditioning for the competitive athlete. *Clin Sports Med* 1988;7: 211–228.

8. Sailer SM, Lewis SB. Rehabilitation and splinting of common upper extremity injuries in athletes. *Clin Sports Med* 1995;14; 411–446.

9. Frykman GK, Nelson EF. Fractures and traumatic conditions of the wrist. In: Hunter JM, Schneider LH, Mackin EJ, Callahan AD, eds. *Rehabilitation of the hand.* 3rd ed. St. Louis: CV Mosby, 1990: 267–283.

10. Nicholas JA, Hershman EB, Posner MA. *The upper extremity in sports medicine.* St. Louis: CV Mosby, 1990.

11. Prokop LL. Upper-extremity rehabilitation: conditioning and orthotics for the athlete and performing artist. *Hand Clin* 1990;6:517–524.

12. Mullins PAT. Use of therapeutic modalities in upper extremity rehabilitation. In: Hunter JM, Schneider LH, Mackin EJ, Callahan AD, eds. *Rehabilitation of the hand.* 3rd ed. St. Louis: CV Mosby, 1990:195–220.

13. Press JM, Wiesner SL. Prevention: conditioning and orthotics. *Hand Clin* 1990;6:383–392.

14. Colditz JC. Dynamic splinting of the stiff hand. In: Hunter JM, Schneider LH, Mackin EJ, Callahan AD, eds. *Rehabilitation of the hand.* 3rd ed. St. Louis: CV Mosby, 1990: 342–352.

15. Kiefhaber TR, Stern PJ. Upper extremity tendinitis and overuse syndromes in the athlete. *Clin Sports Med* 1992;11:39–55.

16. Mayer V, Gieck JH. Rehabilitation of hand injuries in athletes. *Clin Sports Med* 1986;5:783–794.

17. Rettig AC, Patel DV. Epidemiology of elbow, forearm and wrist injuries in the athlete. *Clin Sports Med* 1995;14:289–297.

18. Gieck JH, Mayer V. Protective splinting for the hand and wrist. *Clin Sports Med* 1986;5:795–806.

19. Evans RB. Therapeutic management of extensor tendon injuries. In: Hunter JM, Schneider LH, Mackin EJ, Callahan AD, eds. *Rehabilitation of the hand.* 3rd ed. St. Louis: CV Mosby, 1990: 492–511.

20. Tubiana R. Injuries to the digital extensors. *Hand Clin* 1986;2:149–156.

21. Leddy JP, Packer JW. Avulsion of the profundus tendon in athletes. *J Hand Surg* 1977;2:66–69.

22. Schneider LH. Fractures of the distal interphalangeal joint. *Hand Clin* 1994;10:277–285.

23. Dawson WJ, Pullos N. Baseball injuries to the hand. *Ann Emerg Med* 1981;10:302–306.

24. Rosenthal EA. The extensor tendons. In: Hunter JM, Schneider LH, Mackin EJ, Callahan AD, eds. *Rehabilitation of the hand.* 3rd ed. St. Louis: CV Mosby, 1990:458–491.

25. Dobyns JH, McElfresh EC. Extension block splinting. *Hand Clin* 1994;10:229–237.

26. Dray GJ, Eaton RG. Dislocations and ligament injuries in the digit. In: Green DP, ed. *Operative hand surgery.* 3rd ed. New York: Churchill Livingstone, 1993:767–798.

27. Koman LA, Mooney JF III, Poehling GG. Fractures and ligamentous injuries of the wrist. *Hand Clin* 1990;6:477–491.

28. Amadio PC, Taleisnik J. Fractures of the carpal bones. In: Green DP, ed. *Operative hand surgery.* 3rd ed. New York: Churchill Livingstone, 1993:799–859.

29. Green DP. Carpal dislocations and instabilities. In: Green DP, ed. *Operative hand surgery.* 3rd ed. New York: Churchill Livingstone, 1993:861–927.

30. Milford L. Fractures of the hand. In: Crenshaw AH, ed. *Campbell's operative orthopaedics.* 7th ed. St. Louis; CV Mosby, 1987:183–228.

31. Putnam MD. Fractures and dislocations of the carpus including the distal radius. In: Gustilo RB, Kyle RF, Templeman D, eds. *Fractures and dislocations.* St. Louis: CV Mosby, 1993: 553–644.

32. Dobyns JH, Linscheid RL. Fractures and dislocations of the wrist. In: Rockwood CA, Green DP, eds. *Fractures in adults.* 2nd ed. Philadelphia: JB Lippincott, 1984: 411–509.

33. Palmer AK. Fractures of the distal radius. In: Green DP, ed. *Operative hand surgery.* 3rd ed. New York: Churchill Livingstone, 1993: 929–972.

34. Riester JN, Baker BE. Mosher JF, et al. A review of scaphoid fracture healing in competitive athletes. *Am J Sports Med* 1985;13: 159–161.

35. Fishbein M, Middlestadt SE, et al. Medical problems among ICSOM musicians: overview of a national survey. *Med Probl Perform Art* 1988;3:1–8.

36. Fry HJH. Incidence of overuse syndrome in the symphony orchestra. *Med Probl Perform Art* 1986;1:51–55.

37. Manchester RA. Further observations on the epidemiology of hand injuries in music students. *Med Probl Perform Art* 1991;6: 11–14.

38. Norris R. Overuse injuries: how string players can recognize, prevent and treat them. *Strings* 1989;(Nov/Dec)45–47.

39. Lederman RJ, Calabrese LH. Overuse syndrome in instrumentalists. *Med Probl Perform Art* 1986;1:7–11.

40. Fry HJH. Overuse syndrome: a muscle biopsy study. *Lancet* 1988;1:905–908.

41. Fry HJH. The treatment of overuse injury syndrome. *M Med J* 1993;42:277–282.

42. Fry HJH. Instrumental musicians showing technique impairment with painful overuse. *M Med J* 1992;41:899–903.

43. Gieck JH, Saliba EN. Application of modalities in overuse syndromes. *Clin Sports Med* 1987; 6:427–465.

44. Norris RN. Return to play after injury. In: Torch D, ed. *The musicians' survival manual.* St. Louis: International Conference of Symphony and Opera Musicians 1993:103.

45. Fry HJH. Overuse syndrome in musicians—100 years ago: an historical review. *Med J Aust* 1986;145:620–625.

46. Menuhin Y. *The compleat violinist.* New York: Summit Books, 1986:75.

47. Markison RE. Treatment of musical hands: redesign of the interface. *Hand Clin* 1990;6:525–544.

48. Eaton RG. Entrapment syndromes in musicians. *J Hand Ther* 1992; 5:91–97.

49. Smutz WP, Bishop A, Niblock H, et al. Load on the right thumb of the oboist. *Med Probl Perform Art* 1995;10:94–99.

50. Marion JD, Sheppard JE. An orthotic device to prevent thumb joint hyperextension following carpometacarpal arthritis surgery: a case study. *Med Probl Perform Art* 1991;10:90–92.

51. Anderson JI. Orthotic device for flutist's digital compression neuropathy. *Med Probl Perform Art* 1990;5:91–93.

52. Norris RN. Design for a right thumb rest for the flute based on physical analysis. *Med Probl Perform Art* 1990;10: 161–162.

53. Johnson CD. Splinting the injured musician. *J Hand Ther* 1992; 5:107–111.

54. Per Ohlin CO, Elmqvist D. Pressures recorded in ulnar neuropathy. *Acta Orthop Scand* 1985;56:404–406.

55. Norris RN, Dommerholt J. Orthopadische probleme und rehabilitation bei muskulo-skeletalen storungen. In: Blum J, ed. *Medizinische probleme bei musikern.* Stuttgart: Thieme Verlag 1995:129.

56. Armstrong TJ. Ergonomics and cumulative trauma disorders: symposium on occupational injuries. *Hand Clin* 1986;2: 553–565.

57. Fry HJH. Overuse syndrome in clarinetists. *Clarinet* 1987;14:48–51.

58. Lederman RJ. Entrapment neuropathies in instrumental musicians. *Med Probl Perform Art* 1993;8:35–40.

59. Norris RN. Clinical observations on the results of the 1991 NFA survey. *Flutist Q* 1996;21:77–80.

60. Wainapel SF, Cole JL. The not-so-magic flute: two cases of distal ulnar nerve entrapment. *Med Probl Perform Art* 1988;3:63–65.

61. Gelberman R. The carpal tunnel syndrome: a study of carpal canal pressures. *J Bone Joint Surg [Am]* 1981;63:380–383.

62. Rempel D. Musculoskeletal loading and carpal tunnel pressure. In: Gordon SL, Blair SJ, Fine LJ, eds. *Repetitive motion disorders of the upper extremity.* Rosemont, IL: American Academy of Orthopaedic Surgeons, 1995:123–132.

63. Kopfstein-Penk A. *The healthy guitar.* Bethesda: Kopfstein-Penk, 1994.

64. Austin GJ, Leslie BM, Ruby LK. Variations of the flexor digitorum superficialis of the small finger. *J Hand Surg [Am]* 1989;14: 262–267.

65. Watson HK. Achieving independent finger flexion: the guitarist's advantage. *Med Probl Perform Art* 1987; 2:58–60.

66. Norris RN. The "lazy finger" syndrome. In: Torch D, ed. *The musician's survival manual.* St. Louis: International Conference of Symphony and Opera Musicians, 1991:87–90.

67. Linberg RM, Comstock BE. Anomalous tendon slips from the flexor pollicis longus to the flexor digitorum profundus. *J Hand Surg* 1989;4:79–83.

68. Feinberg J, Brandt KD, Steichen JB. Tenodesis of the digital extensors in a violist. *Met Probl Perform Art* 1988;3:109–112.

69. Brandfonbrener AG. Joint laxity in instrumental musicians. *Med Probl Perform Art* 1990;5: 117–119.

70. Bejjani FJ, Stutchin S, Winchester R. Effect of joint laxity on musicians' occupational disorder. *Clin Res* 1984;32:660A. Abstract.

71. Middlestadt SE, Fishbein M. The prevalence of severe musculoskeletal problems among male and female symphony orchestra string players. *Med Probl Perform Art* 1989;4:41–48.

72. Hochberg FH. Occupational hand cramps; professional disorders of motor control. *Hand Clin* 1990;6:417–428.

73. Lederman RJ. Focal dystonia in instrumentalists. *Med Probl Perform Art* 1991;6:132–136.

74. Wagner C. Success and failure in musical performance: biomechanics of the hand. In: Roehman and Wilson, eds. *The biology of music making: proceedings of the 1984 Denver conference.* St. Louis: MMB Music, 1988:154–179.

75. Cole RA, Cohen LG, Hallett M. Treatment of musician's cramp with botulinum toxin. *Med Probl Perform Art* 1991;6: 137–143.

76. Bejjani FB, Kaye GM, Benham M. Musculoskeletal and neuromuscular conditions of instrumental musicians. *Arch Phys Med Rehabil* 1996;77:406–413.

Chapter 68

Overuse Injuries of the Hip and Pelvis

Robert P. Wilder
Michael C. Geraci, Jr.
Andrew J. Cole

Thirty percent to 50% of all sports injuries are caused by overuse (1–3). In the primary care setting, overuse injuries account for the majority of athletic injuries seen by physicians (4). For example, overuse accounted for more than 80% of hip and pelvis injuries presenting to a general sports medicine clinic (5). The etiology and management of pelvis and hip disorders, however, have not been documented as well as those for the more common injuries to the knee, lower leg, and foot. Understanding the basic anatomy and the etiology and treatment of overuse injuries in general, with additional attention paid to common injuries of the hip and pelvis, assists the physiatrist in treating patients who have sport-related musculoskeletal injuries.

ANATOMY

The bony pelvis is formed by the two paired innominate bones, the sacrum, and the coccyx. Each innominate bone consists of the fused ilium superiorly and the ischium and pubis inferiorly. The upper edge of the ilium, the iliac crest, ends anteriorly in the anterior superior iliac spine (ASIS) and posteriorly in the posterior superior iliac spine (PSIS). Other important ilial landmarks include the anterior inferior iliac spine (AIIS) anteriorly and the posterior inferior iliac spine (PIIS) posteriorly. The ASIS and PSIS are located at the ends of the iliac crest and can be easily palpated. The PIIS sits just above the sciatic notch (6–12).

The inferior aspect of the innominate bone is formed by the ischium posteriorly and the pubis anteriorly. The two innominate bones are firmly attached posteriorly to the sacrum through the sacroiliac joints (SIJs). The SIJs are classified as synovial joints surrounded by a fibrous capsule that is well formed anteriorly, but posteriorly may have tears and rents (6–8). Primary ligamentous support is provided by the relatively weak anterior sacroiliac ligament, the stronger posterior iliosacral ligament, and the interosseous ligaments. Accessory ligaments provide additional support and include the iliolumbar, sacrotuberous, and sacrospinous ligaments (6,9). The SIJ receives innervation from the L3–S3 nerves, with S1 providing the primary contribution (6,10). Shear, compressive, and other moment loads are created in the SIJ by a number of muscles including the erector spinae, quadratus lumborum, psoas major and minor, piriformis, latissimus dorsi, obliquus internus and externus abdominis, and gluteus maximus, medius, and minimus. The pelvis is attached anteriorly at the pubic symphysis.

The hip joint is a ball and socket formed between the pelvic acetabulum and the femoral head. The superior, anterior, and posterior margins of the acetabulum form its articular surface. The inferior margin, known as the *acetabular notch,* is a non-weight-bearing surface. A fibrocartilaginous labrum surrounds the acetabulum, encasing the femoral head and thus contributing to the joint stability (11,12).

The femoral neck bridges the femoral head to the shaft, angled medially approximately 125 degrees. Coxa vara exists when the angle of the neck to the shaft is decreased, and may contribute to increased shearing and torsional forces. Coxa valga exists when the angle is increased. Increased compressive forces may contribute to accelerated degeneration (11). The femur is also angled in the anteroposterior plane in approximately 15 degrees of anteversion (medial femoral torsion).

The capsule of the hip joint is reinforced along the anterior and posterior surfaces by the iliofemoral, pubofemoral, and ischiofemoral ligaments. The iliofemoral ligament (Y ligament of Bigelow) resembles an inverted Y arising from the AIIS, subsequently dividing and inserting into the femur at the greater trochanter and on the anterior aspect of the femur inferior to the intertrochanteric line. The iliofemoral ligament restrains hyperextension at the hip. The pubofemoral ligament primarily limits abduction and extension; the ischiofemoral ligament primarily limits extension. With the ligaments functioning as a group, the greatest stability is provided in extension, abduction, and external rotation. Therefore, the hip joint is least stable in flexion, adduction, and internal rotation, the most frequent position of hip dislocation (12).

Dual vascular supply is provided to the hip by a small artery to the femoral head in the ligamentum teres and by the medial and lateral circumflex arteries which pierce the capsule. Muscular action at the hip is summarized in Table 68-1 (11,13).

Table 68-1: Muscular Action at the Hip

Hip Action	Muscles Prime Movers	Muscles Assistant Movers
Flexors	Psoas Iliacus Pectineus Rectus femoris	Sartorius Tensor fasciae latae Gracilis Adductor brevis Adductor longus
Extensors	Gluteus maximus Semitendinosus Semimembranosus Biceps femoris (long head)	
Abductors	Gluteus medius	Gluteus minimus Tensor fasciae latae Sartorius Rectus femoris
Adductors	Adductor magnus Adductor longus Adductor brevis Gracilis Pectineus	
External rotators	Gluteus maximus Gemellus inferior Gemellus superior Obturator externus Obturator internus Quadratus femoris Piriformis	Adductor longus Adductor brevis Biceps femoris (long head) Sartorius Pectineus
Internal rotators	Tensor fasciae latae Gluteus minimus	Semitendinosus Semimembranosus Gracilis

CONCEPTS OF OVERUSE INJURY

Overuse injuries result from repetitive microtrauma that leads to inflammation and local tissue damage in the form of cellular and extracellular degeneration (14). This tissue damage can be cumulative, resulting in myositis, bursitis, ligament sprains, joint synovitis, cartilaginous degeneration, stress fractures, neuropraxic or axonal nerve injury, and tendinitis or tendinosis (1,14). The musculotendinous unit appears to be particularly susceptible to injury resulting from microtrauma caused by excessive eccentric loading (4,15). Acute injury results in the development of an inflammatory response. As inflammation becomes chronic, tissue changes occur, characterized by the development of young vascular elements with fibroblastic proliferation (angiofibroblastic hyperplasia), ultimately leading to tendon degeneration (4,16). The common etiology of overuse injuries is repetitive trauma that overwhelms the tissue's ability to repair itself (Fig. 68-1).

Both intrinsic and extrinsic factors contribute to overuse injuries (Table 68-2) (1,14,15). Intrinsic factors are biomechanical and physiologic abnormalities unique to a particular athlete; extrinsic factors primarily are related to training errors. In addition to injury-specific management, the management of overuse injuries addresses these risk factors. The interaction of such intrinsic and extrinsic factors with repetitive overuse leading to tissue injury and kinetic chain adaptations is also depicted by the viscious

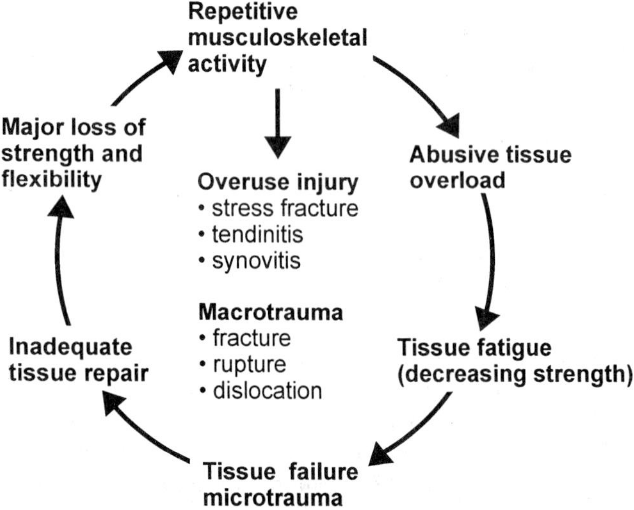

Figure 68-1. Cycle of repetitive overload, abuse, and activity leading to overuse injury. (Reproduced by permission from Virginia Sportsmedicine Institute, Arlington, VA.)

Table 68-2: Risk Factors That Contribute to Overuse Injuries

INTRINSIC	EXTRINSIC
Malalignment	Training errors
Muscle imbalance	Equipment
Inflexibility	Environment
Muscle weakness	Technique
Instability	Sport-imposed deficiencies

Source: Reproduced by permission from the Virginia Sportsmedicine Institute, Arlington, VA.

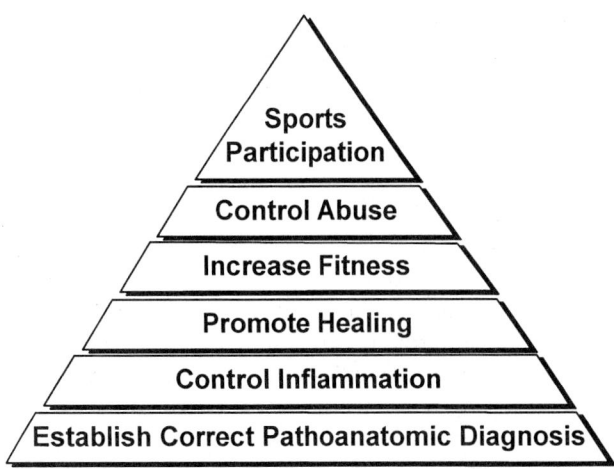

Figure 68-2. Overuse injury management pyramid (Reproduced by permission from Virginia Sportsmedicine Institute, Arlington, VA.)

overload cycle. According to Kibler et al (17), there are five complexes associated with the viscious cycle. The *tissue injury complex* describes the group of anatomic structures that have sustained damage. The *clinical symptom complex* comprises those symptoms and signs that manifest themselves due to the injury. The *tissue overload complex* encompasses the group of tissues subject to tensile overload. The *functional biomechanical deficit complex* includes the constellations of inflexibilities and muscle strength imbalances that can then alter normal biomechanics. Finally, the *subclinical adaptation complex* describes all of the substitute activities that are used to compensate for the altered biomechanics. Kibler's cycle underscores the necessity to address deficits throughout the kinetic chain in addition to injury-specific management in order to produce the most successful treatment.

REHABILITATIVE MANAGEMENT OF OVERUSE INJURIES

The diagnosis and management of overuse injuries requires a multidisciplinary approach. The clinician's principal responsibilities are to establish a correct pathoanatomic diagnosis and direct rehabilitation, which often involves enlisting the help of physical therapists, orthotists, athletic trainers, and coaches.

A comprehensive rehabilitation program following overuse injuries of the hip and pelvis emphasizes a series of stages leading to a return to participation in sports (Fig. 68-2). The steps build on one another yet overlap considerably. In addition, these basic management principles can be applied to the management of overuse injuries in general, although different tissues have unique characteristics and vary somewhat in response to treatment.

Establish Correct Pathoanatomic Diagnosis

Successfully treating an injured athlete requires correct identification of the injury. Vague diagnoses, such as groin strain or hip pointer, fail to clearly define the disorder. On the other hand, diagnoses such as adductor longus tendinosis or iliac crest apophysitis clearly define the injury.

Most overuse injuries can be diagnosed through a good history, physical examination, and selected radiographs.

The history is most important in establishing the diagnosis. In addition to injury-specific details, risk factors for athletic injury are identified: When did the injury first occur? Did the athlete recently purchase new equipment? Has the athlete changed training locations or training regimen? Does the pain occur only with sport activity or also with daily activities? Any history of previous injury also is significant.

A thorough physical examination will identify focal injury of the hip and pelvis as well as associated intrinsic alignment abnormalities and soft-tissue (musculotendinous or ligamentous) insufficiencies of the lumbar region of the spine, SIJ, knee, lower leg, foot, and ankle. Failure to identify muscle imbalance patterns and structural malalignment throughout the kinetic chain often sabotages an otherwise well-planned rehabilitation program. Radiographs, advanced imaging techniques, and electrodiagnostic studies can assist evaluation when clinically warranted (14).

Control of Inflammation

Though inflammation is required for proper healing of overuse injuries, an excessive or prolonged inflammatory response can become self-perpetuating and self-destructive (1). A prolonged inflammatory phase also invites disuse atrophy and generalized deconditioning. Therefore, controlling or suppressing inflammation is one of the primary goals of overuse treatment.

Relief of pain and inflammation is achieved through the principles of "PRICEMM"—*p*rotection, *r*est, *i*ce, *c*ompression, *e*levation, *m*edication, and *m*odalities. It is important to note that rest does not mean immobilization but rather elimination of the specific activities that cause pain. Preservation of fitness is of utmost importance; therefore, it is important to emphasize the activities an athlete *can* do in addition to those that should be avoided. Nonsteroidal anti-inflammatory drugs (NSAIDs) are helpful, as can be oral steroids (if symptoms are acute or particularly intense). Cortisone injections are used sparingly, as intratendinous injections can result in tendon atrophy or dissolution. Injections generally are reserved for patients for whom pain interferes with rehabilitative progress. Modalities that are most helpful include high-voltage electrical stimulation, ultrasound, ice, and heat. For tendinitis and tendinosis, electrical stimulation helps to reduce pain, inflammation, and spasm as well as enhance circulation. A continuous sensory stimulus at submotor intensity with a high pulse rate (>100 pulses/sec) for 20 to 30 minutes is recommended. Four to six sessions during 2 to 3 weeks usually are sufficient. Ultrasound is effective in facilitating tissue extensibility and enhancing blood flow in the deeper tissues (14).

Promotion of Healing

Failure to properly rehabilitate an athlete's initial injury can be an important risk factor for recurrent injury (14,18). Too often, efforts to control inflammation successfully relieve an athlete's pain, and then the athlete prematurely returns to sport activity. Athletes and health care professionals may fail to appreciate that rest and anti-inflammatory medications alone do not heal. Clinicians can ensure a successful return to sports only when inflammation control is combined with aggressive efforts to promote healing (14,16,19).

The goal of rehabilitative exercise is to restore injured tissue to normal or near-normal function. Early exercises enhance tissue oxygenation and nutrition, minimize unnecessary atrophy, and align collagen fibers to meet sport-induced stresses. Ultimately, exercise helps restore normal flexibility, strength, balance, endurance, and coordination. At the hip, it is essential to identify motion restrictions and begin flexibility exercises early for those areas that are restricted. Flexibility deficits are common at the hip, particularly the external rotators, flexors, hamstrings, and iliotibial band, and may create the basis for an injurious environment. Joint mobility and flexibility exercises also ensure proper orientation of collagenous tissue. Soft-tissue mobilization and myofascial techniques are useful adjuncts in restoring normal motion. Low-intensity, submaximal resistance exercises are advanced based on pain, inflammatory response to exercise, and healing time of specific tissues.

First, multiangle isometric exercises are performed submaximally in the pain-free range of motion, progressing to full effort. Isotonic exercises are initiated without weights in pain-free arcs and then advanced to full range of motion with weights as tolerated. Isokinetic exercises often are emphasized for athletes, since most sporting motions are performed at high speeds. Patients progress from short bouts of midspeed, limited range, submaximal effort to full-motion endurance bouts of varying speeds. Isotonic and isokinetic exercises are performed both concentrically and eccentrically. Proprioceptive neuromuscular facilitation (PNF) techniques, based on reciprocal muscle inhibition, are applied to enhance flexibility, strength, and muscular coordination. Rehabilitative exercise programs ultimately incorporate full-motion strengthening and balance antagonistic forces to allow the athlete to meet the demands of his or her own sport. Once normal strength and flexibility are restored, plyometrics can be incorporated to train the neuromuscular system to react quickly and forcefully, as is needed in sports. Coordination exercises and sport-specific drills are completed before returning to competition (14).

In addition to rehabilitative exercises, general body conditioning is important in promoting healing. General body conditioning enhances rehabilitation of a specific injury by 1) increasing regional perfusion through central and peripheral aerobics, 2) providing neurologic stimulus to the injured tissue through neurophysiologic synergy and overflow, 3) minimizing weakness of adjacent uninjured tissue, 4) minimizing negative psychological effects, and 5) controlling unwanted fat and accumulated weight.

It is also important to correct deficits in each link of the kinetic chain. Thus, the management of hip and pelvis disorders also should include evaluation and correction of weaknesses, functional imbalances, and malalignments in the spine, knee, foot, and ankle. Exercise of the contralateral uninjured limb is also useful due to the "cross-education" of the neuromuscular system (20).

Increase Fitness

People who have tissue that has above-normal (supranormal) strength, endurance, and power are optimally suited for the demands of sports. To elevate patients' repaired more-normal tissue to such above-normal levels, fitness exercises are introduced. These exercises involve sport-specific rehabilitative exercises and further general body conditioning (14).

A patient can begin sport-specific exercises once pain-free range of motion is achieved, and strength and endurance tests indicate a return to preinjury state. Sport-specific activities work the athlete's target tissues, providing neurophysiologic stimulus and redeveloping proprioceptive skills. Sport-specific agility, speed, and skill drills (including plyometrics, interactive eccentric/concentric muscle loading, anaerobic sprints, and interval training) coordinate interaction of the athlete's antagonistic and supporting muscles (14).

Athletes should continue sport-specific activities while increasing general body conditioning. Maintaining or enhancing preinjury fitness levels and correcting potentially injurious deficits are essential. Sport-specific activities increase regional perfusion as well as oxygen extraction for enhanced skeletal muscle activity. Athletes should continue to develop the central aerobic system to meet the demands of the skeletal muscle as a target organ and to facilitate a return to sports (14).

Control Abuse

The final step of overuse injury management is to control force loads to the previously injured rehabilitated tissue. Controlling abusive overload requires modifying the intrinsic and extrinsic risk factors that were identified through the history and physical examination. Control of abusive force loads is best accomplished by 1) improving training and sport technique, 2) bracing and wrapping the injured part, 3) controlling the intensity and duration of activity, and 4) appropriately modifying equipment (14).

Because abnormal biomechanics quickly promote reinjury, modification of improper sport technique is critical before the patient is allowed to return to the sport. Bracing and wrapping are used to control abuse during rehabilitation and when the athlete first resumes sport activity. Elastic wrapping or compressive shorts are particularly useful as an adjunct to rehabilitative exercise of muscle strains about the hip. Excessive intensity and duration most often lead to overuse injury; therefore, athletes should follow the basic training principles of progression and periodization. Appropriate equipment and sizing will help eliminate unnecessary abusive force loads (14).

Sport Participation

Traditionally, athletes have been allowed to return to activity when 1) pain has ceased, 2) they demonstrate full range of motion, and 3) the injured extremity demonstrates 80% to 90% of the strength (objectively measured through isokinetic or isotonic testing) of the uninjured extremity. These criteria, however, represent only the minimum required for athletic return. Athletes also must demonstrate adequate sport-specific function and be psychologically ready to return. When the athlete, coach, and physician are satisfied that these criteria have been met, the athlete can return safely to full activity (14,21).

DIAGNOSIS AND TREATMENT OF SPECIFIC DISORDERS

Overuse injuries of the hip and pelvis in sports are classified according to their anatomic location (i.e., anterior, posterior, or lateral) (Table 68-3). Treatment discussions detail rehabilitative exercises directed specifically at the hip and pelvis. However, it must be emphasized again that imbalances and abnormalities at each level of the kinetic chain (i.e., lumbar spine, knee, foot, and ankle) must also be identified and corrected.

Anterior Overuse Injuries

Quadriceps Strain

Strains of the quadriceps most commonly involve the rectus femoris and occur during sports involving sprinting, jumping, or kicking. Strains are graded as mild (grade I), moderate (grade II), or severe (grade III) (22–28) (Table 68-4). Factors that can increase the risk of quadriceps strain include tightness (especially the rectus femoris) or weakness (especially the vasti) of the quadriceps musculature, hamstring tightness, lack of sufficient warm-up or stretching prior to exercise, previous injury without rehabilitation, and overtraining (12).

The *functional adaptations* that persist when the return to activity is too early include greater reliance on the unaffected leg for upward propulsion in jumping activities, shortened running stride with reduced hip flexion, and reduced running velocity. Occasionally the athlete tries to maintain an externally rotated femur so the adductor group can be used to advance the thigh (12). Quadriceps strains must be distinguished from quadriceps contusions that result from impact trauma with secondary hematoma formation.

Table 68-3: Common Overuse Injuries of the Hip and Pelvis in Sports

Anterior	Posterior	Lateral
Quadricep strain /contusion	Hamstring strain	Greater trochanter bursitis
Adductor strain	Piriformis syndrome	Gluteus medius bursitis
Femoral stress fracture	Ischial bursitis	External snapping hip
Osteitis pubis	Sacroiliac joint dysfunction	Lateral hip pointer
Anterior hip pointer		Tensor fasciae latae syndrome
Internal snapping hip		Meralgia paresthetica

Table 68-4: Quadricep Strains

Grade	Severity	Description
I	Mild	Overstretch with minimal disruption of musculotendinous unit integrity. There is probably less than 5% fiber disruption. Patient experiences soreness with motion, but only minimal strength loss.
II	Moderate	Incomplete muscle tear. There is intramuscular bleeding with hematoma formation. Muscle strength is clearly compromised.
III	Severe	Complete rupture. Muscle function is essentially lost. Avulsion injuries are included in this category.

Diagnosis

The athlete complains of local pain and tenderness in the anterior aspect of the thigh. Pain may be gradual in onset or may be experienced suddenly during an explosive muscle contraction. Grade I strains result in pain with resisted active contraction and with passive stretching. Local spasm may be present. Athletes with grade I strains generally are able to continue sport activity. Grade II strains cause significant pain with passive and unopposed active stretching. Athletes with grade II strains generally are unable to continue sport activity. Complete tears of the rectus femoris are rare and are associated with a sudden violent contraction; a defect is palpable when the muscle is contracted. Radiographic studies rule out associated avulsion of the AIIS, especially in children. Myositis ossificans can be a complication of quadriceps strain and contusion and is identified by swelling, erythema, and a palpable hard mass. Confirmation is made by plain films or bone scans.

Treatment

Ice and NSAIDs are useful in limiting pain and inflammation. Pain-free stretching is instituted early to preserve range of motion. Associated tightness in the hamstrings and hip flexors and inhibition of the gluteus maximus must be corrected. Soft-tissue mobilization may assist with motion. Special emphasis is placed on strengthening exercises, because loss of strength may be marked and is actually considered to be a major predisposing factor to injury. Straight-leg raises are initiated with the patient in the supine position and progress to long sitting (i.e., sitting on a floor or mat with the knees extended). Short-arc quadriceps sets in pain-free ranges are expanded to full range as tolerated. Both concentric and eccentric exercises are performed. Attention is given to hip flexor and hamstring strength and flexibility to ensure muscular balance. Closed kinetic chain exercises at submaximal weight (i.e., leg press, partial squats) are initiated in short arcs and progress to full range. The stair-climber and bicycle are very effective, but isolated restrengthening of the injured leg is essential. Sport-specific functional retraining is completed before a return to sport.

Following a quadriceps contusion, loss of motion can be significant; therefore, special emphasis is placed on early maintenance of range of motion, particularly in flexion (29,30). Ryan et al (29) advocated maintenance of the hip and knee in pain-free flexion with the use of elastic wrap for 24 to 48 hours to minimize hematoma formation and preserve flexion range. Ice is applied several times daily. Active stretching is then performed in pain-free ranges only during the next 7 to 10 days. Soft-tissue therapy and electrical stimulation also are useful but are avoided during the first few days. Ultrasound is avoided as it has been implicated in the development of myositis ossificans (12). Multiangle isometric quadriceps contractions and isotonic exercises without weights in pain-free ranges are expanded to full range with weights as tolerated. Biking is used for strengthening and general fitness. When flexion of more than 120 degrees and strength of more than 85% of that on the uninjured side are attained, functional retraining should begin. Myositis ossificans, if present, is treated by the principles of PRICEMM. Prophylactic use of diphosphonates does not seem warranted. The use of NSAIDs such as indomethacin is common among clinicians, but has not been conclusively shown to halt the progression of the lesion (12). Follow-up radiographs and "cold" bone scans are useful in determining whether the lesion has become "mature" (12). Physical activity is gradually increased after maturity has been determined. On rare occasions, surgical excision of a mature lesion is necessary. This should generally be reserved for patients with pain and loss of range of motion persisting for 6 to 12 months after the lesion has matured (12).

Adductor Strain

Adductor or groin strain can result from an acute strain or from chronic angiofibroblastic tendinosis of the hip adductor group, particularly the adductor longus at the proximal musculotendinous junction, tendo-osseous insertion to the inferior pubic rami, or the muscle belly itself (31–35). Eccentric overload, such as that experienced during quick changes in direction from a stretched-out lunge position, is thought to be especially contributive (32–35). Ballistic stretching, which is advised in many exercise tapes and aerobics classes, often leads to groin strain.

Diagnosis

The *clinical symptom complex* presents as pain in the groin region worsened with passive abduction or active adduction and flexion against resistance. Primary muscle involvement can be established by reproducing the symptoms during resisted adduction in three positions of hip rotation: external rotation (adductor magnus), neutral (adductor longus), and internal rotation (pectineus) (22). Acute cases may be accompanied by swelling and ecchymosis. A palpable defect may be present, representing a tear. Also commonly seen is ipsilateral pelvic and hip pain, worse with walking or running. The *functional biomechanical deficits* center around tightness of the ipsilateral adductors and contralateral tensor fasciae latae. The ipsilateral gluteus medius and gluteus minimus will then become inhibited or weak, as well as the lower abdominal muscles. The *functional adaptation complex* includes an increase in lateral tilt of the pelvis where the contralateral side of the pelvis drops in the swing phase of gait. An ipsilateral inferior pubic rami dysfunction is often associated. The *tissue overload complex* is exhibited by excessive strain and inflammation of the lateral pelvic and hip structures, including the gluteus medius and gluteus minimus, as well as the trochanteric bursa. Along the kinetic chain, the tensor fasciae latae and iliotibial band as well as lateral knee structures and lumbar region of the spine have increased overload. The knee and, in particular, the patellofemoral joint are overloaded, as well as distal structures such as the shoulder, owing to altered pelvic stability. The abdominals are considered overloaded due to the position of the pubic rami inferiorly, which puts the abdominals on stretch, placing them at risk for tears. Finally, the adductors inhibit the contraction of the glutei after the propulsion phase of running (31).

Treatment

In acute cases, ice and NSAIDs are used to limit pain and inflammation. Elastic spica wrapping or compressive shorts helps control swelling and minimize pain during ambulation and sport activity. Rehabilitative exercise emphasizes full motion strengthening of the hip adductor group and flexibility. Functional deficits in the glutei, tensor fasciae latae, and pelvis are corrected. Strengthening involves both concentric and eccentric loading. PNF diagonal motions effectively exercise the muscles to promote balanced strength and flexibility around the joint. Soft-tissue mobilization and electrical stimulation are useful adjunctive treatments. In more chronic adductor strains, ultrasound is a useful modality to precede mobilization. Five or six treatments of deep friction massage to break up scar tissue before stretching may also be necessary. Flexibility and strength of the abductor group ensure muscular balance. Sport-specific activities should include the slide board (for side-to-side gliding) and lateral sprints.

Femoral Stress Fractures

Stress fractures of the hip or pelvis are uncommon, the incidence ranging from 0.05% to 0.22% of all running injuries and 3.2% to 4.0% of all stress fractures in athletes (5,36,37). Femoral stress fractures are more common, accounting for up to 10% of all stress fractures in runners (38). The majority of femoral stress fractures occur at the femoral neck. Femoral shaft stress fractures are less common and generally occur in the subtrochanteric region but can occur in the midshaft and distal regions as well (39,40).

Stress fractures result from accelerated bone remodeling in response to repeated stress (36,38,40,41). Several factors contribute to this excessive stress: repetitive microloads from pounding (which does not allow the bone time to heal with its normal reparative process) (38,42,43), the transmission of excessive force loads to bone secondary to surrounding muscle fatigue (38,44), and the repetitive action of muscular traction on bone (38,45,46). Butler et al (39) specifically speculated that subtrochanteric fractures are caused by excessive traction at the origin of the vastus medialis or adductor brevis, producing tension on bone. Femoral stress fractures should be included in the differential diagnosis of hip pain in all athletes, particularly in those with persistent pain, because of the risk of displacement or avascular necrosis of the femoral head.

Diagnosis

The athlete generally complains of nonspecific deep thigh or groin pain that is aggravated by activity and relieved by rest (36,38,39,40,47,48). Onset often is associated with a recent change in training (particularly an increase in distance or intensity) or a change in training surface. Physical examination may reveal normal hip motion and strength. Advanced cases will be associated with decreased strength and motion with pain on end rotation. Direct palpation over the involved bony area may elicit pain in patients with femoral shaft fractures, as will stressing the femur over the edge of the examining table, distal to the site of pain. Hopping on one leg may reproduce pain.

Initial x-ray findings often are negative, and as many as one-third of femoral stress fractures never show radiologic changes on plain films. Thus, bone scans should be ordered if suspicion is high, particularly if pain has persisted for more than 2 weeks (12).

With femoral neck fractures, the type of fracture must be differentiated. Compression-type injuries occur at the lower border of the femoral neck, and displacement is rare. Distraction-type fractures occur in the superior part of the neck; displacement is more common, thus necessitating internal fixation (40,49).

Treatment

Patients with nondisplaced femoral neck fractures are placed on crutches with partial weight-bearing status until pain is absent and radiologic follow-up indicates sufficient callus formation (3–8 weeks). During this time, the athlete should continue conditioning with non-weight-bearing activity (deep-water running, swimming, biking) as well as upper-extremity strengthening. Rehabilitative exercise restores muscle flexibility, strength, and balance. The stair-climber and stationary cross-country skiing machines are then useful for further conditioning. A gradual walking, jogging, and running program is followed before a return to sport activity. Correction of foot and leg malalignments and running gait pattern may help limit intrinsic stress. Displaced fractures require internal fixation. Femoral shaft fractures typically respond to a protracted period of weight-bearing rest (2–4 months).

Osteitis Pubis

Osteitis pubis represents a chronic inflammatory and overuse condition of the pubic symphysis and adjacent ischial rami (50–61). Most commonly associated with urologic procedures, prostatectomy, and childbirth, osteitis pubis also can occur in athletes and appears to be related to repetitive shear forces transmitted to the pubic symphysis during running and repetitive adductor contractions during kicking sports.

Diagnosis

The athlete typically complains of the gradual onset of discomfort in the lower abdomen or groin area that is worsened by sport activity and relieved by rest. Physical examination reveals point tenderness at the pubic tubercles, rectus abdominis insertion, adductor origin, and inferior pubic rami. Pain is intensified with sit-ups and resisted hip adduction. Range of motion is maintained. Radiographic studies may reveal a fraying or roughening of the periosteum of the pubic symphysis. However, x-ray signs may be delayed for as long as 4 weeks after the onset of symptoms; therefore, a bone scan may assist diagnosis in early stages.

Treatment

Almost all patients with osteitis pubis will respond to a period of relative rest (up to 1½–2 months) and anti-inflammatory medications, with a gradual return to sport activity. Soft-tissue flexibility and strength deficits and pelvic and SIJ dysfunction are corrected. Nonpainful fitness exercises such as swimming and deep-water running are undertaken as tolerated during this phase. Leg-length discrepancies and excessive pronation can be corrected with orthotic devices. Abdominal and adductor strengthening and adductor stretching should be performed in moderation. A corticosteroid injection into the pubic symphysis can be useful in refractory cases.

Anterior Hip Pointer

Anterior hip pointer refers to pain localized to the ASIS that may result from a direct blow in contact sports or from repetitive overuse strain of the sartorius (commonly in runners and gymnasts) (62,63).

Diagnosis

Pain and tenderness are localized at the ASIS. Passive hip extension increases symptoms, as do resisted hip flexion, external rotation, and abduction. Radiographic studies should be performed to rule out an avulsion of the ASIS.

Treatment

Early treatment emphasizes ice, NSAIDs, relative rest, ultrasound, and electrical stimulation. Subsequent management includes flexibility training and strengthening, most specifically of the hip flexors, abductors, and external rotators. Especially effective exercises include long-sitting, straight-leg raises with the hip externally rotated, as well as the PNF leg-diagonal flexion adduction, external rotation to extension, abduction, and internal rotation.

Internal Snapping Hip Syndrome

Internal snapping hip syndrome is most often caused by friction of the iliopsoas tendon over an osseous ridge on the lesser trochanter or the iliopectineal eminence (50,64). Less commonly, loose bodies, labral tears, and osteochondritis dissecans can be intra-articular sources of the snap (12).

Diagnosis

Patients complain of diffuse, aching pain in the anteromedial hip or groin region. A discrete area of tenderness to palpation generally is not present. An audible snap typically occurs with extension of the flexed, abducted, and externally rotated hip.

Treatment

Ice, NSAIDs, and electrical stimulation are used in acute cases. Superficial heating is followed by prolonged stretching of the hip flexors. Re-education of the antagonistic gluteus maximus helps restore proper balance. Soft-tissue mobilization assists flexibility and motion. Strengthening of the hamstrings promotes muscular balance. All hip motions should be evaluated for flexibility and strength deficits and appropriately exercised (31).

Refractory Groin Pain

In athletes with persistent groin pain for whom conservative measures fail, a broader differential diagnosis should be entertained (Table 68-5). Athletes with bursitis, nerve syndromes, and enthesopathy may respond to steroid injections in addition to physical therapy (32,33,35,65–69).

A small subset of athletes will experience long-standing groin pain despite aggressive conservative measures (medications, rest, physical therapy, massage, flexibility, strengthening). The athlete with athletic pubalgia presents with chronic exertional lower abdominal/inguinal pain near the pubic insertion, which is not explainable by a demonstrable hernia or other medical diagnosis. The pain progresses to involve the adductor longus tendon as well as the contralateral inguinal and adductor regions. The location of pain suggests injury to both the rectus abdominis and adductor longus muscles. Paramount to the diagnosis of athletic pubalgia is the exclusion of other

Table 68-5: Differential Diagnosis of Groin Pain in Athletes
Tendonitis (adductor, flexor, abdominal)
Pelvic/femoral stress fracture
Osteitis pubis
Snapping hip syndrome
Bursitis (iliopsoas)
Nerve entrapment (iliopectineal, obdurator)
Enthesopathy (inguinal ligament)
Pubalgia
Degenerative joint disease
Avascular necrosis of the hip
Lumbar referred pain
Genitourinary disease
Inguinal hernia
Systemic disease (rheumatologic, other)

causes of groin pain. Athletes who fail to respond to conservative management, including flexibility and strengthening of the abdominal and hip musculature, may benefit from surgical remediation, which includes attachment of the abdominal muscle firmly to the anterior pelvis and, in those cases with adductor pain, a partial adductor release also (70–73).

Posterior Overuse Injuries

Hamstring Strain

Hamstring strains are a common cause of posterior thigh pain in athletes and may present as acute, subacute, or chronic injury. These strains commonly occur in sprinters, hurdlers, jumpers, and athletes in other sports involving sudden sprinting such as soccer, football, tennis, and hockey. Excessive eccentric muscle force appears related to hamstring injury—many hamstring strains occur during the last part of the swing phase or at foot strike, during which time the hamstrings work maximally eccentrically to decelerate the leg. Factors related to hamstring injury include poor hamstring flexibility, strength, and endurance; muscular imbalance (such as a hamstring to quadriceps strength ratio <0.6 or compared with the uninjured hamstring group); lumbar degenerative joint disease; lumbar and SIJ dysfunction; increased neural tension; biomechanical inadequacies (i.e., excessive anterior pelvic tilt); and inadequate warm-up (22,74–77). The *tissue injury complex* can include all hamstring muscles, most commonly the short head of the biceps femoris.

Diagnosis

The *clinical symptom complex* includes pain in the posterior region of the thigh. The athlete with an acute strain may report a "pop" or a tearing sensation. Tenderness to palpation can be located throughout the muscle, including the origin at the ischial tuberosity, as well as the muscle belly and distal insertions. Pain is intensified with resisted knee flexion. Functional biomechanical deficits are identified. Flexibility often is decreased, and weakness of the involved hamstring group may be identified with manual muscle testing or more formal isokinetic testing. Tightness in the hip flexors and inhibition of the glutei may be identified; anterior pelvic tilting is not uncommon. Examination of the lumbar region of the spine is important, because muscle injury may be related to referred pain with subsequent muscle inhibition and weakness (22,35). Radiographic studies may be performed to rule out avulsion of the ischial tuberosity if suspected, particularly in younger athletes. Lumbar referred pain should also be considered in the athlete with posterior thigh pain, especially when a clear injury history is not present.

Treatment

Treatment of acute or subacute injuries follows the principles of PRICEMM, emphasizing ice, electrical stimulation, and pulsed ultrasound to minimize the extent of tissue damage. A neoprene thigh sleeve provides comfort and a possible counterforce effect. Active exercises within pain-free ranges of motion are begun soon after injury, as is stretching, ensuring proper orientation with collagen deposition. Strengthening of the hamstrings is advanced as tolerated and incorporates isometric, isotonic, and isokinetic exercise. Special emphasis ultimately is placed on eccentric loading. Isokinetic testing at 60 degrees/sec should demonstrate hamstring strength of at least 60% of quadriceps strength and no more than 10% deficit when compared with the uninjured leg. Soft-tissue therapy (transverse friction, transverse gliding, and myofascial release) is useful for increasing mobility and decreasing pain in the patient with chronic injury but is often unnecessary for acute injury if strengthening and flexibility are initiated early. Flexibility of the rectus femoris and hip flexors, and facilitation and strengthening of the vasti and glutei are important to provide muscular balance. Biomechanical factors, particularly excessive anterior tilt of the pelvis and leg-length discrepancies, should be corrected. Hypomobility and dysfunction of the lumbar region of the spine and SIJ must be corrected if present (22,35,75). Neuromobilization to mobilize the connective tissue of the sciatic nerve may also be effective. This on-off stretching technique helps stretch supporting neural and muscle connective tissue. Running is resumed at low speeds on flat terrain, with an emphasis on adequate warm-up and stretching before running and stretching and icing afterward. Trampoline and bounding drills are useful transition exercises. Athletes must demonstrate adequate sport-specific function before returning to competition.

Piriformis Syndrome

The piriformis muscle originates on the anterolateral aspect of the sacrum and passes posterolaterally through the sciatic notch, inserting into the upper border of the greater trochanter. The sciatic nerve typically exits the pelvis through the sciatic notch anterior to the piriformis muscle. In approximately 15% of the population, however, the sciatic nerve passes through the piriformis muscle itself. Pain may result from a strain or overload of the piriformis muscle or from pressure on the sciatic nerve, most commonly in patients in whom the sciatic nerve courses through the piriformis muscle (*tissue injury complex*) (22,50,78,79). A common cause of piriformis overload is a tight hip adductor with hip abductor inhibition. This leads to the piriformis substituting as an abductor (31).

Diagnosis

The *clinical symptom complex* consists of buttock and hip pain that may radiate down the posterior aspect of the leg. Passive internal rotation of the affected hip is limited and may increase pain (Freiberg sign) (80). Pain and weakness are present with resisted abduction or external rotation of the hip. Rectal examination will reveal distinct tenderness on the lateral pelvic wall that reproduces symptoms. Examination of the lumbar spine is important to rule out lumbar dysfunction. The structures within the *tissue overload complex* are the piriformis, gluteal muscles, gemelli, quadratus lumborum, and sacroiliac ligaments and the sciatic nerve. The *functional biomechanical deficits* include tight piriformis, external rotators, and adductors; hip abductor weakness; SIJ hypermobility; and lower lumbar spine dysfunction. *Functional adaptations* consist of ambulating with an externally rotated thigh, shortened stride length, and functional limb-length shortening (12). Any runner who develops buttock and varying lower-extremity paresthesias without evidence of radiculopathy should be considered to have piriformis syndrome (31).

Treatment

Treatment includes correcting dysfunction of the SIJ and pelvis. Prior to stretching of the piriformis or iliopsoas muscles, the hip joint capsule in its anterior and posterior portion should be mobilized, which will allow for more effective stretching of these muscles. Prolonged stretching includes hip flexion, adduction, and internal rotation in supine and standing positions. Soft-tissue therapy of the piriformis muscle, including longitudinal gliding combined with passive internal hip rotation as well as transverse gliding and sustained longitudinal release with the patient lying on one side, may be useful (22). Effective exercises include the knee-to-chest stretch in adduction, internal rotation in which the knee of the involved lower extremity is brought toward the opposite shoulder, and the adduction/external rotation stretches. Ultrasound or phonophoresis may be useful modalities. Local trigger point or corticosteroid injections may be useful for more recalcitrant cases (78,79). Correction of lumbar spine and SIJ dysfunction and hypomobility is important, particularly in patients in whom piriformis irritability and pain are related to lumbar disorders. Any strength or flexibility deficit at the hip is corrected with appropriate exercise.

Ischial Bursitis

Ischial bursitis, an inflammation of the ischial bursa, is often associated with proximal hamstring strains. It is not uncommon in cyclists (probably caused by prolonged sitting). It can also be seen in adolescent runners, often in conjunction with traction apophysitis.

Diagnosis

Tenderness is localized to the ischium. Isolated ischial bursitis can be differentiated from hamstring strains, because patients with isolated ischial bursitis generally will not complain of pain in the posterior thigh or demonstrate hamstring flexibility and strength inadequacies.

Treatment

Most patients with ischial bursitis respond to ice, NSAIDs, soft-tissue massage, relative rest, and avoidance of prolonged sitting. Hamstring strength and flexibility deficits are corrected as needed. When the cause is prolonged sitting, the patient's workstation should be modified to allow for activities to be conducted in a standing position and a cushion should be used during sitting. Corticosteroid injections can be helpful for persistent bursitis (12).

Sacroiliac Joint Dysfunction

The SIJ has been reported to be responsible for approximately 20% of low-back pain and referred pain (6,81). Pain at the SIJ can result from primary pain at the joint and the overlying soft tissues (sacral hilum and iliofibrocartilage, supporting ligaments, and joint capsule), or may be the result of referred pain (6). SIJ dysfunction, resulting from a biomechanical imbalance at the SIJ, is by far the most common painful condition affecting the SIJ. Up to 14 different patterns of imbalance have been reported, the most common being right anterior innominate rotation, followed in frequency by left posterior innominate rotation (31). Differential diagnoses include fracture, infections, inflammatory conditions (ankylosing spondylitis, psoriatic arthritis, Reiter disease), degenerative joint disease, metabolic disease (gout, calcium pyrophosphate disease), tumor, osteitis condensans ilia, reactive sacroiliitis as a late sequela of pelvic inflammatory disease, and referred pain (from lumbar disk or facet disease, radiculopathy, hip disease, or gluteal/multifidi trigger points). Pregnancy also results in relative hypermobility of the SIJ, which may predispose to ligamentous sprain (6).

Diagnosis

Patients with SIJ pain can complain of pain that is sharp, aching, or dull and generally localize the pain to the involved SIJ or PSIS (6,82) (Fortin JD. Personal observations, 1993). Due to a wide range of segmental innervation of the SIJ, pain can also be referred to the buttocks, groin, posterior thigh, or distally beyond the knee and even into the foot (6,81). Patients may give a history of trauma. Symptoms generally increase with joint motion, especially when changing from a sitting to standing position or during rotational movements. Pain is usually unilateral and tends to have a right-sided bias, with 45% right, 35% left, and 20% bilateral (6,7). Tenderness to palpation may be localized over the sacral sulcus and just medial to the PSIS (7). Asymmetry and pelvic rotation may be appreciated by palpation of the iliac crest and iliac spines. A variety of additional physical examination test categories have been recommended by various authors to clinically predict SIJ dysfunction, as follows: 1) soft-tissue examination for zones of hyperirritability; 2) evaluation of fascial and musculotendinous restrictions; 3) determination of length-strength muscle relationships; 4) postural analysis; 5) true leg-length determination; 6) functional leg-length determination (83–85); 7) osteopathic evaluation, including static and dynamic osseous landmark evaluation (structural testing) (63,65,66); 8) dynamic osteopathic screening tests

(84,86–89); 9) evaluation of regional tissue texture changes; 10) provocative testing, including traditional orthopedic tests such as the Gaenslen or Patrick test; 11) motion demand (articular spring) tests (90); 12) ligament tension tests (84); and 13) hip rotation testing (7). No test or combination of tests has been found to be pathognomonic of SIJ pain and dysfunction (6).

The absence of neurologic findings helps differentiate SIJ pain from lumbar referred pain (22). Radiographic testing is generally unrevealing in isolated SIJ dysfunction, but may be useful in ruling out fracture, infection, and inflammatory conditions, as well as associated lumbar disease. In recalcitrant cases or confusing presentations, a fluoroscopically guided, contrast-enhanced, intra-articular SIJ injection can be used for diagnostic as well as therapeutic purposes (6).

Treatment

Treatment of SIJ dysfunction must include the entire lumbopelvic complex and lower-extremity kinetic chain. A number of treatment techniques from various philosophies, including osteopathic, manual, and chiropractic, have evolved to help rehabilitate SIJ dysfunction. At this point, no research has recognized one treatment protocol as superior and the most successful rehabilitation programs may integrate aspects of each of these schools of thought (6).

The acute phase of rehabilitation addresses the *tissue injury complex* and *clinical symptom complex*. In SIJ dysfunction, the *tissue injury complex* involves the SIJ, including the sacral hyaline cartilage and iliofibrocartilage, supporting ligaments, and joint capsule. The *clinical symptom complex* involves the patient's primary complaint of local sacroiliac, buttock, and posterior thigh pain as well as referred pain to the groin, hip, and lower extremity. Pain and inflammation are controlled with NSAIDs and modalities including therapeutic cold and electrical stimulation. SIJ belts may help proprioception and decrease motion and pain (83,91). Patient education and a home exercise program are initiated early and built on throughout rehabilitation. Subsequent phases continue to address tissue overload complex, as well as functional biomechanical deficits and subclinical adaptation complex. *Functional biomechanical deficits* include associated soft-tissue dysfunction. In right anterior dysfunction, these include tightness in the ipsilateral adductors, rectus femoris, iliopsoas, quadratus lumborum, latissimus dorsi, and tensor fasciae latae. Weaknesses or inhibitions are identified in the ipsilateral glutei, lumbosacral paraspinal, and abdominal muscles (31). The *subclinical adaptation complex* includes pelvic rotation and subsequent lumbar dysfunctions. Various manual approaches include inhibitive techniques including positional release, functional techniques, general muscle stretching, and mobilization including muscle energy and direct oscillation. Manipulation using a high-velocity, low-amplitude, short-level arm thrust technique can be employed if needed. Following mobilization or manipulation, a maintenance exercise program is imperative to prevent recurrences (6,92,93). Leg-length discrepancies greater than ½ inch should be corrected (94). Manual therapy techniques also eliminate associated restriction in lumbar and pelvic motion. Flexibility and strength of soft tissues about the lumbar-pelvic-hip complex are enhanced. Aerobic conditioning is important throughout the rehabilitation program as tolerated. A home exercise program to maintain flexibility and strength is continued after rehabilitation is completed. In refractory cases, a fluoroscopically guided, contrast-enhanced injection may assist in decreasing pain as well as assisting subsequent mobilization and rehabilitation. Injections may also be directed toward the overlying muscles or ligaments (6).

Other, more invasive techniques have also been proposed for the treatment of SIJ pain. Prolotherapy or sclerotherapy has been employed to treat SIJ pain due to presumed laxity of the SIJ ligamentous complex. If followed with proper stretching, it is theorized that collagen will be laid down in an orderly fashion to help stabilize the joint. No controlled clinical study has proved the efficacy of this technique for SIJ pain, however, and therefore it should be considered only in refractory cases of hypermobility and performed only by clinicians with extensive experience in this technique (6). Fusion techniques exist for the SIJ, and should be considered only in patients with proven SIJ pain by diagnostic anesthetic blocks who have severe disabling symptoms and have failed to respond to all attempts at aggressive conservative care techniques (6). Any SIJ fusion should be bilateral, as unilateral fusion could cause significant biomechanical dysfunctions.

Lateral Overuse Injuries

Trochanteric Bursitis

Trochanteric bursitis represents an inflammation of the greater trochanteric bursa, often related to friction of the iliotibial tract as it crosses the greater trochanter.

Diagnosis

The *clinical symptom complex* includes pain and tenderness localized to the greater trochanter. Pain is reproduced with flexion of the hip from an extended position and resisted hip abduction as well as by stretching of the iliotibial tract. *Functional biomechanical deficits* consist of shortening of the tensor fasciae latae, rectus femoris, and hamstrings and weakness of the abductors. *Functional adaptations* include increased hip external rotation with an altered gait or running pattern (12,20).

Treatment

Early treatment includes relative rest, ice, NSAIDs, electrical stimulation, phonophoresis, and soft-tissue massage. A steroid injection at the area of tenderness over the greater trochanter may be useful for particularly intense or recalcitrant bursitis. Stretching of the iliotibial tract is emphasized, as well as flexibility of the external rotators, quadriceps, and hip flexors. Strengthening of the hip abductors and establishment of muscular balance between the adductors and abductors is also important. All motions at the hip are evaluated for strength and flexibility, and exercises are prescribed to establish balanced motion.

Gluteus Medius Bursitis

Gluteus medius bursitis results from inflammation of the gluteus medius bursa and often occurs in conjunction with gluteus medius tendinitis or tendinosis. This condition often is associated with excessive lateral tilt of the pelvis (22).

Diagnosis

Tenderness is localized immediately above the greater trochanter and is intensified by stretching the gluteus medius. *Functional biomechanical deficits* may include tight adductors and inhibited gluteus medius and minimus (31).

Treatment

Treatment includes relative rest, ice, NSAIDs, electrical stimulation, soft-tissue massage, re-education of the inhibited gluteus medius and minimus, and stretching of the adductors and abductors. If the pain is particularly severe, a steroid injection may be placed into the area of maximal tenderness above and behind the greater trochanter. Pelvic stability exercises are important in patients with bursitis associated with excessive lateral tilt.

External Snapping Hip Syndrome

The external snapping hip syndrome is caused by friction of the iliotibial band or the anterior border of the gluteus maximus on the greater trochanter.

Diagnosis

Pain is localized to the lateral part of the hip over the greater trochanter. An audible snap is heard during repetitive hip motion.

Treatment

Patients generally are markedly relieved by reassurance that this is not an intra-articular condition. Early treatment follows the principles of PRICEMM. Stretching of the iliotibial band and gluteus maximus is emphasized. Flexibility of the external rotators, hip flexors, and quadriceps is also addressed. Flexibility is enhanced by soft-tissue mobilization. Any deficit in strength or flexibility at the hip is addressed to provide balanced motions.

Lateral Hip Pointer

A lateral hip pointer consists of pain localized to the lateral iliac crest that usually represents a contusion resulting from a direct blow to the iliac crest in contact sports such as football and rugby. A lateral hip pointer also may result from acute strain or chronic overuse of the abductors (gluteus medius and minimus) and external oblique abdominal muscles.

Diagnosis

Pain and tenderness are localized to the lateral iliac crest. Swelling and ecchymosis may accompany traumatic injuries. Truncal side bending away from the affected hip increases pain, as does resisted abduction of the affected hip. Radiographic studies should be performed to rule out an iliac crest fracture (95–97).

Treatment

Initial treatment emphasizes ice, NSAIDs, electrical stimulation, and relative rest. Compression can be used for traumatic hip pointers; if a hematoma is present, aspiration may be useful. Management of overuse injuries emphasizes flexibility and strength of the hip abductors and external oblique muscles followed by balanced hip flexibility and strengthening. Soft-tissue mobilization is useful in regaining motion but should be avoided in the first 2 to 3 days following traumatic injury. Adequate hip padding is mandatory in contact sports.

Tensor Fasciae Latae Strain

Inflammation and ultimately angiofibroblastic changes can occur in the tensor fasciae latae, particularly where it passes over the greater trochanter. This overuse injury is common in runners and cyclists (50). Overload of the tensor fasciae latae is often seen with inhibition of the gluteus medius and minimus. This may be from tight hip adductors reciprocally inhibiting these abductors or simply as a response to painful stimuli.

Diagnosis

The onset of lateral hip pain generally is gradual and localized to the greater trochanter and distally along the tensor fasciae latae. There is often a history of a recent change in training regimen. The Ober test result is positive, revealing a tight iliotibial band. A snapping of the tensor fasciae latae as it passes over the greater trochanter and greater trochanteric bursitis also may be associated. Radiographic studies and bone scanning are performed if a femoral neck stress fracture is suspected.

Treatment

Initial treatment follows the principles of PRICEMM. Rehabilitative management is similar to that described for the external snapping hip syndrome and emphasizes flexibility of the iliotibial band, external rotators, hip flexors, and quadriceps followed by balanced flexibility and strengthening throughout the hip. Soft-tissue mobilization is a useful adjunctive treatment. Re-education of the inhibited hip abductors is also important.

Meralgia Paresthetica

This syndrome consists of pain and paresthesia in the lateral region of the thigh caused by irritation of the lateral femoral cutaneous nerve. Injury may occur by violent hip extension or by compression, most commonly at the inguinal ligament. Compression may be caused by a tight belt or clothing, obesity, or pregnancy.

Diagnosis

Decreased sensation is limited to the distribution of the lateral femoral cutaneous nerve. As this is a purely sensory nerve, motor deficits are not observed.

Treatment

Treatment includes correction of contributing factors such as weight loss or eliminating tight clothing and restrictive equipment. Neuroleptic medicines such as amitriptyline or carbamazepine may be useful. Refractory cases may respond to corticosteroid injections.

SPECIAL CONCERNS IN THE PEDIATRIC ATHLETE

Apophysitis and Apophyseal Avulsions

In younger athletes, the apophyseal attachment of tendons may be more likely injured than the myotendinous junction, as in adults. Common apophysites about the hip and pelvis involve the hamstring insertion at the ischial tuberosity, the sartorius insertion at the ASIS, the rectus femoris insertion at the AIIS, and the abdominal insertions at the iliac crest. Mild displacements are treated as per their respective soft-tissue injuries, although they may require a longer period of activity modification. More severe displacement may require orthopedic surgical intervention (22).

Legg-Calvé-Perthes Disease

Legg-Calvé-Perthes disease is an idiopathic avascular necrosis of the proximal femoral epiphysis. It occurs in children between the ages of 3 and 12 years, most commonly between 5 and 7 years. Boys are affected three to five times more frequently than girls and both hips are involved in 10% to 20% of patients (98–100).

Diagnosis

The affected athlete presents with a limp and vague pain in the groin, hip, thigh, or knee (any child with a vague knee pain should have a hip evaluation). Physical examination reveals variable shortening of the involved leg, which may accentuate a limp. Almost all affected children will have limited hip abduction and internal rotation when tested in both hip flexion and extension, even in early stages of the disease. Anteroposterior and frog-leg radiographs should be carefully scrutinized in suspected cases. Early disease is characterized by a dense epiphysis that is patchy, more distal, and uneven at the margins. A bone scan may be useful if x-ray findings are negative and clinical suspicion is high. Later stages show more involvement of the femoral head with cystic changes and fragmentation (98).

Treatment

Initial treatment is directed toward regaining range of motion and may include traction, range of motion exercises, and limited weight bearing.

Containment of the femoral head within the acetabulum is usually accomplished with an abduction orthosis; however, osteotomy may be necessary. If the physiatrist has not had experience treating this condition, orthopedic referral is mandated. In general, children diagnosed before the age of 5 years have a more favorable prognosis while those diagnosed after the age of 8 years have a less favorable outcome (98–101).

Slipped Capital Femoral Epiphysis

Both acute and chronic slips result in displacement of the capital femoral epiphysis through the growth plate relative to the femoral neck. Posterior medial slips are the most common and they are bilateral in approximately 60% of patients (98,102). The high-risk period for developing a slipped epiphysis is during periods of peak height velocity (10–13-years old for girls and 12–15-years old for boys) (98,103). Children large for their age or maturity are at higher risk (98).

Diagnosis

Children with a chronic slipped epiphysis may have a mild limp and complain of vague groin, hip, or knee pain. Medial knee pain, referred from the hip via the obturator nerve, may be the only complaint. As the slip develops, the affected child develops progressive out-toeing and a worsening limp. Acute slipped epiphyses result in severe pain and are more likely to be identified early. Physical examination reveals a decreased range of motion, especially in flexion, internal rotation, and abduction. The classic finding is a hip that externally rotates as it is passively flexed (98).

In normal hips, a line drawn through the center of the femoral neck should bisect the epiphysis on both the anteroposterior and frog-leg lateral radiographs (98,102). Comparison views are of questionable help as most slips are bilateral.

Treatment

Slipped epiphyses are considered a relative orthopedic emergency once the diagnosis is made. Even minimally displaced chronic slips are prone to sudden progression with a misstep or twist of the leg. Patients should be placed on non-weight-bearing crutches or bed rest pending orthopedic management (98).

CONCLUSIONS

The majority of athletic injuries of the hip and pelvis are caused by overuse. Most of these injuries will respond to adequate rehabilitative management, including correction of intrinsic and extrinsic risk factors and control of the abusive force loads that may have contributed to injury. In addition to injury-specific rehabilitation, imbalances and abnormalities at each level of the kinetic chain must be corrected to ensure optimal healing.

REFERENCES

1. Herring SA, Nilson KL. Introduction to overuse injuries. *Clin Sports Med* 1987;6:225–239.
2. Orava S. Exertion injuries due to sports and physical exercise: a clinical and statistical study of nontraumatic overuse injuries of the musculoskeletal system of athletes and keep-fit athletes. Thesis. University of Ouler, Finland, 1980.
3. Renstrom P, Johnson RJ. Overuse injuries in sports: a review. *Sports Med* 1985;2:316–333.
4. Puffer JC, Zachazewski JE. Management of overuse injuries. *Am Fam Phys* 1988;38:225–232.
5. Lloyd-Smith R, Clement DB, McKenzie DC, et al. A survey of overuse and traumatic hip and pelvis injuries in athletes. *Phys Sportsmed* 1985;13:131–141.
6. Cole AJ, Dreyfuss P, Stratton SA. The sacroiliac joint: a functional approach. *Crit Rev Phys Med Rehabil Med* 1996;8:125–152.
7. Bernard TN, Cassidy JD. The sacroiliac joint syndrome: pathophysiology, diagnosis, and management. In: Frymoyer JW, ed. *The adult spine: principles and practice.* New York: Raven 1991:2107–2130.
8. Lavignolle B, Vital JM, Senegas J, et al. An approach to the functional anatomy of the sacroiliac joints in vivo. *Anat Clin* 1983;5:169–176.
9. Weisl H. Ligaments of sacro-iliac joint examined with particular reference to their function. *Acta Anat* 1954;20:201–213.
10. Bradley KC. The anatomy of the backache. *Aust N Z J Surg* 1974;44:227–232.
11. Anderson LC, Blake DJ. The anatomy and biomechanics of the hip joint. *J Back Musculoskel Rehabil* 1994;4:145–153.
12. Young JL, Olsen NK, Press JM. Musculoskeletal disorders of the lower limbs. In: Braddom RL, ed. *Physical medicine and rehabilitation.* Philadephia: WB Saunders, 1996:783–812.
13. Rasch PJ, Burke RK. *Kinesiology and applied anatomy.* 4th ed. Philadelphia: Lea & Febiger, 1971.
14. O'Connor FG, Sobel JR, Nirschl RP. Five-step treatment for overuse injuries. *Phys Sportsmed* 1992;20:128–142.
15. Hess GP, Cappiello WL, Poole RM. Prevention and treatment of overuse tendon injuries. *Sports Med* 1989;8:371–384.
16. Nirschl RP. The etiology and treatment of tennis elbow. *J Sports Med* 1974;2:308–323.
17. Kibler BW, Chandler TJ, Pace BK. Principles of rehabilitation after chronic tendon injuries. *Clin Sports Med* 1992;11:661–671.
18. Ekstrand J, Gillquist J. Soccer injuries and their mechanisms: a prospective study. *Med Sci Sports Exerc* 1983;15:267–270.
19. Kibler WB, McQueen C, Uhl T. Fitness evaluations and fitness findings in competitive junior tennis players. *Clin Sports Med* 1988;7:403–416.
20. Press JM, Herring SA, Kibler WB. Rehabilitation of the combatant with musculoskeletal disorders. In: Zajtchuk R, ed. *Textbook of military medicine.* Washington, DC: Office of the Surgeon General, 1998:353–415.
21. McKeag DB. Criteria for return to competition after musculoskeletal injury. In: Cantu RC, Micheli LJ, eds. *ACSM's guidelines for the team physician.* Philadelphia: Lea & Febiger, 1991:196–204.
22. Brukner P, Khan K. *Clinical sports medicine.* Sydney, Australia: McGraw-Hill, 1993.
23. Jarvinen M. Muscle injuries. In: Renstrom PAFH, ed. *Clinical practice of sports injury prevention and care.* London: Blackwell, 1994:115–124.
24. Young JL, Laskowski ER, Rock M. Thigh injuries in athletes. *Mayo Clin Proc* 1993;68:1099–1106.
25. Zarins B, Ciullo JV. Acute muscle and tendon injuries in athletes. *Clin Sports Med* 1983;3:167–182.
26. Loosli AR, Quick J. Thigh strains in competitive breaststroke swimmers. *J Sport Rehabil* 1992;1:49–55.
27. Parker MG. Characteristics of skeletal muscle during rehabilitation: quadriceps femoris. *Athletic Training* 1981;18:122–124.
28. Ryan AJ. Quadriceps strain, rupture and charley horse. *Med Sci Sports* 1969;1:106–111.
29. Ryan JB, Wheeler JH, Hopkinson WJ, et al. Quadriceps contusions. *Am J Sports Med* 1991;19:299–304.
30. Aronen JG, Chromister RD. Quadricep contusions—hastening the return to play. *Phys Sportsmed* 1992;20:130–136.
31. Geraci MC. Overuse injuries of the hip and pelvis. *J Back Musculoskel Rehabil* 1996;6:5–19.

32. Estwanik JJ, Sloane B, Rosenberg MA. Groin strain and other possible causes of groin pain. *Phys Sportsmed* 1990;18: 54–65.

33. Smodlaka VN. Groin pain in soccer players. *Phys Sportsmed* 1980;8:57–61.

34. Martens MA, Hansen L, Mulier JC. Adductor tendinitis and muscular rectus abdominis tendopathy. *Am J Sports Med* 1987;15:353–356.

35. Muckle DS. Associated factors in recurrent groin and hamstring injuries. *Br J Sports Med* 1982;16:37–39.

36. Taunton JE, Clement DB, Webber D. Lower extremity stress fractures in athletes. *Phys Sportsmed* 1981;9:77–86.

37. Orava S. Stress fractures. *Br J Sports Med* 1980;14:40–44.

38. Jackson DL. Stress fracture of the femur. *Phys Sportsmed* 1991;19:39–43.

39. Butler JE, Brown SL, McConnell BG. Subtrochanteric stress fractures in runners. *Am J Sports Med* 1982;10: 228–232.

40. Lombardo SJ, Douglas WB. Stress fractures of the femur in runners. *Phys Sportsmed* 1982;10:219–227.

41. McBryde AM. Stress fracture in athletes. *J Sports Med* 1975; 3:212–217.

42. Branch HE. March fractures of the femur. *J Bone Joint Surg* 1944;26:387–391.

43. Walter NE, Wolf MD. Stress fractures in young athletes. *Am J Sports Med* 1977;5: 165–170.

44. Blat DJ. Bilateral femoral and tibial stress fractures in a runner. *Am J Sports Med* 1981; 9:322–325.

45. Stanitski CL, McMaster JH, Scranton PE. On the nature of stress fractures. *Am J Sports Med* 1978;6:391 –396.

46. Devas MB. Stress fractures in athletes. *J Sports Med* 1973; 1:49–51.

47. Belkin SC. Stress fractures in athletes. *Orthop Clin North Am* 1980;11:735 741.

48. Hershman EB, Mailly T. Stress fractures. *Clin Sports Med* 1990;9:183–214.

49. Devas MB. Stress fractures of the femoral neck. *J Bone Joint Surg [Br]* 1965;47:728–738.

50. Flynn TW. Pelvis and thigh injuries. In: Lillegard WA, Rucker KS, eds. *Handbook of sports medicine.* Boston: Andover Medical, 1993:123–134.

51. Hanson PG, Angevine M, Juhl JH. Osteitis pubis in sports activities. *Phys Sportsmed* 1978;4:111–114.

52. Pearson RL. Osteitis pubis in a basketball player. *Phys Sportsmed* 1988;16:69–72.

53. Koch RA, Jackson DW. Pubis symphysitis in runners. *Am J Sports Med* 1981;9:62–63.

54. Harris NH, Murray RO. Lesions of the symphysis in athletes. *BMJ* 1974;4:211–214.

55. Cochrane GM. Osteitis pubis in athletes. *Br J Sport Med* 1971; 5:233–235.

56. Fricker PA, Taunton JE, Ammann W. Osteitis pubis in athletes: infection, inflammation or injury? *Sports Med* 1991;12:266–279.

57. Howse AJG. Osteitis pubis in an Olympic road walker. *Proc R Soc Med* 1964;57:88–90.

58. McMurtry CT, Avioli LV. Osteitis pubis in an athlete. *Calcif Tissue Int* 1986;38:76–77.

59. Pyle LA. Osteitis pubis in an athlete. *J Am Coll Health Assoc* 1975;23:238–239.

60. Wiley JJ. Traumatic osteitis pubis: the gracilis syndrome. *Am J Sports Med* 1983;11: 360–363.

61. Williams JG. Limitation of hip-joint movement as a factor in traumatic osteitis pubis. *Br J Sports Med* 1978;12:129–133.

62. Reider B, Belniak R, Miller DW. Football. In: Reider B, ed. *Sports medicine: the school-age athlete.* Philadelphia: WB Saunders 1991:559–589.

63. Clancy WG. Running. In: Reider B, ed. *Sports medicine: the school-age athlete.* Philadelphia: WB Saunders, 1991:632–650.

64. Schaberg JE, Harper MC, Allen WC. The snapping hip syndrome. *Am J Sports Med* 1984;12: 361–365.

65. Ashby EC. Chronic obscure groin pain is commonly caused by enthesopathy: tennis elbow of the groin. *Br J Surg* 1994;81: 1632–1634.

66. Ekberg O, Persson NH, Abrahamsson P, et al. Longstanding groin pain in athletes. A multidisciplinary approach. *Sports Med* 1988;6:56–61.

67. Lovell G. The diagnosis of chronic groin pain in athletes: a review of 189 cases. *Aust J Sport* 1995;27:76–79.

68. Merrifield HH, Cowan RFJ. Groin strain injuries in ice hockey. *J Sports Med* 1973; 1:41–42.

69. Renstrom P, Peterson L. Groin injuries in athletes. *Br J Sports Med* 1980;14:30–36.

70. Malycha P, Lovell G. Inguinal surgery in athletes: the "sportsman's" hernia. *Aust N Z J Surg* 1992;62:123–125.

71. Polglase AL, Frydman GM, Farmer KC. Inguinal surgery for debilitating chronic groin pain in athletes. *Med J Aust* 1993;155:674–677.

72. Taylor DC, Meyers C, Moylan JA, et al. Abdominal musculature abnormalities as a cause of groin pain in athletes. *Am J Sports Med* 1991;13:239–242.

73. Thomas JM. Groin strain versus occult hernia: uncomfortable alternatives or incompatible rivals? *Lancet* 1995;345: 1522–1523.

74. Agre JC. Hamstring injuries: proposed etiological factors, prevention and treatment. *Sports Med* 1985;2:28.

75. Heiser TM, Weber J, Sullivan G, et al. Prophylaxis and management of hamstring muscle injuries in intercollegiate football players. *Am J Sports Med* 1984:12:368–370.

76. Liemohn W. Factors related to hamstring strains. *J Sports Med* 1978;18:71–76.

77. Paranen J, Orara S. The hamstring syndrome: a new diagnosis of gluteal sciatic pain. *Am J Sports Med* 1988;16:517–521.

78. Pace JB, Nagle D. Piriformis syndrome. *West J Med* 1976: 124:435–439.

79. Barton PM. Piriformis syndrome: a rational approach to management. *Pain* 1991;47:345–352.

80. Freiberg AH. Sciatica pain and its relief by operation on muscle and fascia. *Arch Surg* 1937; 34:377.

81. Schwarzer AC, Aprill CN, Bogduk N. The sacroiliac joint in chronic low back pain. *Spine* 1995; 20:31–37.

82. Fortin JD. Sacroiliac joint dysfunction—a new perspective. *J Back Musculoskel Rehabil* 1993;3:31–43.

83. Vleeming A, Stoeckart R, Snijders CJ. General introduction. In: Vleeming A, Mooney V, Dorman T, Snijders CJ, eds. *The integrated function of the lumbar spine and sacroiliac joint.* Rotterdam: Eco, 1992:3–64.

84. Beal MC. The sacroiliac problem: review of anatomy, mechanics, and diagnosis. *J Am Osteopath Assoc* 1982;81:667–679.

85. Lee D. The relationship between the lumbar spine, pelvic girdle, and hip. In: Vleeming A, Mooney V, Dorman T, Snijders CJ, eds. *The integrated function of the lumbar spine and sacroiliac joint.* Rotterdam: Eco, 1992: 464–478.

86. Bourdillon JF *Spinal manipulation.* 3rd ed. London: William Heinemann Medical Books, 1982.

87. Mitchell FL, Jr, Moran PS, Pruzzo NA. *An evaluation and treatment manual of osteopathic muscle energy techniques.* Valley Park, MO: Mitchell, Moran, and Pruzzo Associates, 1979:49–62, 109–155.

88. Bernard TN Jr, Kirkaldy-Willis WH. Recognizing specific characteristics of non-specific low back pain. *Clin Orthop* 1987;217: 266–280.

89. Dreyfuss P, Dreyer S, Griffin J, et al. Positive sacroiliac joint screening tests in asymptomatic adults. *Spine* 1994; 19:1138–1143.

90. Hesch J, Aisenbray JA, Guerino J. Manual therapy evaluation of the pelvic joints using palpatory and articular spring tests. In: Vleeming A, Mooney V, Dorman T, Snijders CJ, eds. *The integrated function of the lumbar spine and sacroiliac joint.* Rotterdam: Eco, 1992:435–459.

91. Vlemming A, Buyruk HM, Stoekart R, et al. Towards an integrated therapy for peripartum pelvic instability: a study based on the biomechanical effects of pelvic belts. *Am J Obstet Gynecol* 1992;166:1243–1247.

92. Cassidy JD, Kirkaldy-Willis WH, McGregor M. Spinal manipulation for the treatment of chronic low back and leg pain: an observational study. In: Buerger AA, Greenman PE, eds. *Empirical approaches to the validation of spinal manipulation.* Springfield, IL: Charles Thamas, 1985: 119–148.

93. Kirkaldy-Willis WH, Cassidy JD. Spinal manipulation in the treatment of low back pain. *Can Fam Phys* 1985;31:535–539.

94. Cibulka MT, Koldehoff RM. Leg length disparity and its effect on sacroiliac joint dysfunction. *Clin Manage* 1986; 6:10–11.

95. Butler JE, Eggert AW. Fracture of the iliac crest apophysis: an unusual hip pointer. *Sports Med* 1975;3:192–193.

96. Godshall RW, Hansen CA. Incomplete avulsion of a portion of the iliac crest epiphysis: an injury of young athletes. *J Bone Joint Surg [Am]* 1973;6: 1301–1302.

97. Clancy WG, Foltz AS. Iliac apophysitis and stress fractures in adolescent runners. *Am J Sports Med* 1976;4: 214–218.

98. Zukowski CW, Lillegard WA. Special considerations for the pediatric running population. *J Back Musculoskel Rehabil* 1996;6:21–35.

99. The prevention of sports injuries of children and adolescents. *Sidelines* 1993;3(2):3–4.

100. Wenger DR, Ward WT, Herring JA. Current concepts review: Legg-Calve-Perthes disease. *J Bone Joint Surg [Am]* 1991; 73:778–788.

101. Gross ML, Nasser S, Finerman GA. Hip and pelvis. In: De Lee JC, Drez D, eds. *Orthopedic sports medicine.* Philadelphia: WB Saunders, 1994: 1063–1085.

102. Hagglund G, Hansson LI, Ordeberg G, Sandstrom S. Bilaterality in slipped upper femoral epiphysis. *J Bone Joint Surg [Br]* 1988;70:179–191.

103. Kendig RJ, Field L, Fischer LC. Slipped capital femoral epiphysis, a problem of diagnosis. *J Miss State Med Assoc* 1993; 34(5):147–151.

Chapter 69

Rehabilitation of Knee Disorders

Joel M. Press
Jeffrey L. Young

The overwhelming majority of musculoskeletal problems of the knee can be solved nonsurgically. However, if aggressive conservative treatment is to be successful, the physiatrist coordinating patient care must have the skills to make an accurate diagnosis, generate a logical differential diagnosis, and formulate a precise rehabilitation program. The physiatrist should also be able to recognize when surgery is the best way to restore function and allow the patient to safely return to activity. Acquiring a working knowledge of all the musculoskeletal ailments involving the knee is a formidable task, and cannot be achieved by reading a single text. The purpose of this chapter is not to be encyclopedic, but rather to provide the foundation for establishing appropriate rehabilitation programs for knee injuries.

INJURY ANALYSIS AND REHABILITATION

Proper rehabilitation requires a thorough understanding of applied anatomy, biomechanics, and the "kinetic chain." The effects of a musculoskeletal injury are rarely, if ever, confined to a single joint, and rehabilitation programs must consider the alterations in anatomy and biomechanics that have occurred proximal, distal, and contralateral to the site of acute injury. The physiatrist must also be able to recognize the adaptations that have occurred in response to errors of training, particularly those induced by chronic musculotendinous overload. This section details a "template" for rehabilitation of musculotendinous overload injuries. Application of the template to specific knee problems follows.

Step 1. Establish an Accurate Diagnosis

Inherent to this task is recognizing how muscle overload injuries and tendon injuries may present. The vicious overload cycle model for analysis of musculotendinous injury induced by repetitive overload is presented in Figure 69-1. To aid those unfamiliar with this model, some clarification of the terminology is provided:

Tissue injury complex—the area of actual tissue disruption (1–5).

Clinical symptom complex—the symptoms associated with the dysfunction and injury (1–5)

Tissue overload complex—the tissue group being subjected to tensile overload (1–5)

Functional biomechanical deficit—inflexibilities and muscle strength imbalances that create altered mechanics (1–5)

Functional adaptation complex—functional substitutions used by the patient to try to maintain activity (1–5)

When the musculotendinous unit is subjected to tensile overload, damage occurs at a cellular level. This typically produces symptoms of pain, dysfunction, and instability, and also impairs athletic performance (1–3). If the extent of that overload is small (microtear) and nutri-

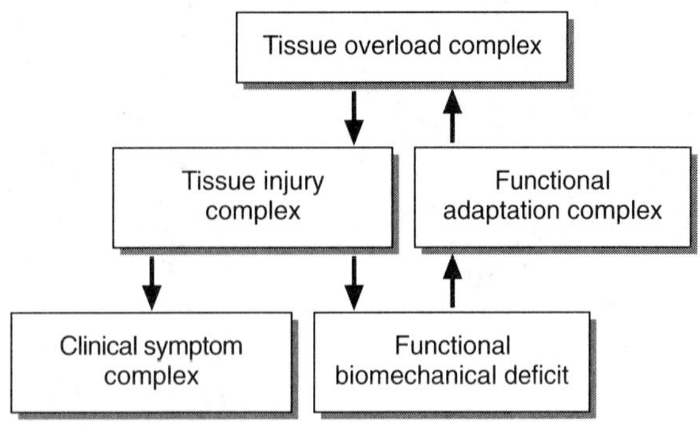

Figure 69-1. Vicious overload cycle model for musculotendinous injury.

tion and healing time are adequate, activities may be safely resumed. However, if the injury is not adequately treated and is allowed to progress (macrotear), healing is accompanied by the development of scar tissue and the development of subclinical adaptations such as loss of flexibility and loss of strength, or strength imbalances (1–3). This leads to further decrements in performance and biomechanical substitutions that perpetuate this "negative feedback vicious cycle" (Fig. 69-2), creating the chance for more overload and injury (1–3). Therefore, muscle injury may present as acute or chronic injury, as exacerbation of a chronic injury, or as a subclinical injury (3). Muscle "strain"-type injuries typically manifest themselves microscopically as a zone of myonecrosis confined to within 500 μm of the myotendinous junction (6). Tendon injuries present either as an acute inflammatory process superimposed on acute or chronic injury (tendinitis) or as a product of maladaptation and intratendinous degeneration unaccompanied by mediators of inflammation (tendinosis) (3,7). In tendinitis, the immediate treatment goal is relief of symptoms while in tendinosis, the immediate goal is restoration of function (3). Identification of the components of musculotendinous injury using the vicious cycle format facilitates understanding the functional consequences of the injury that require rehabilitation.

Step 2. Acute Management

Efforts are directed toward minimizing the effects of inflammation and controlling pain. The PRICE (*p*rotection, *r*elative rest, *i*ce, *c*ompression, and *e*levation) principle is followed. This is usually a period for judicious use of anti-inflammatory medications and pain-relieving modalities (3,5,8–10).

Step 3. Initial Rehabilitation

This phase continues to focus on the promotion of proper healing. Restoration of motion helps to reduce the effects of immobilization, with controlled tensile loading promoting ordered collagen growth and alignment. Identification of correctable biomechanical imbalances is initiated. Many rehabilitation programs fail because they do not progress beyond this step.

Step 4. Correction of Imbalances

The goals are to develop symmetric motion and symmetric strength. When motion is pain free, and when nearly full concentric strength is achieved, it is essential that an eccentric strengthening program be initiated. This is a critical step in developing a musculotendinous unit that is less likely to fail in the setting of future tensile stresses. Understanding the difference between closed kinetic chain (CKC) and open kinetic chain (OKC) exercises is also important. If, for instance, during knee flexion or extension, the foot is allowed to move freely through space, the system is called *open*. In an OKC system, the hamstrings cause flexion while the quadriceps cause extension. During CKC exercise for the lower limbs, the foot is kept immobile or maintains contact with a ground reactive force, and there is the creation of a multiarticular "closed chain." Rather than the near isolation of the large muscle groups seen during OKC exercises, performance of CKC knee flexion and extension results in "coactivation" of the hamstrings and quadriceps groups (11,12). Examples of CKC exercises are leg presses or partial squats (Fig. 69-3). These types of exercises strengthen agonist and antagonist muscles simultaneously via co-contraction and are more physiologic for lower-limb sporting activities (i.e., running). An OKC exercise, knee extension, is shown in Figure 69-4. Flaws in exercise technique are identified and training practices initiated if the patient is capable of full weight bearing under controlled conditions. Alternative aerobic conditioning exercises are encouraged. Beyond local icing, modalities are hardly ever indicated during this phase.

Step 5. Return to Normal Function

Cross training, aqua training, and the use of alternative conditioning formats give way to a gradual increase in activity-specific training and eventual resumption of full activity. Endurance, performance, power, and agility should also be restored.

APPLIED ANATOMY AND BIOMECHANICS

The knee should not be viewed as a simple "hinged joint." The knee proper actually consists of three joints: the tibiofemoral, patellofemoral, and tibiofibular. Actions at these joints are determined by local forces and by events occurring proximally at the hip, pelvis, and thigh and distally at the leg, ankle, and foot. Knee joint structures are frequently injured owing to muscular imbalances and mechanical dysfunctions occurring at other sites in the kinetic chain.

Integrity of the knee is maintained via a complex system of static and dynamic restraints. The knee joint is enveloped by an extensive synovial capsule. The capsule is an important secondary restraint to joint destruction. The joint capsule may be injured in combination with high-grade damage to the primary ligamentous structures. The

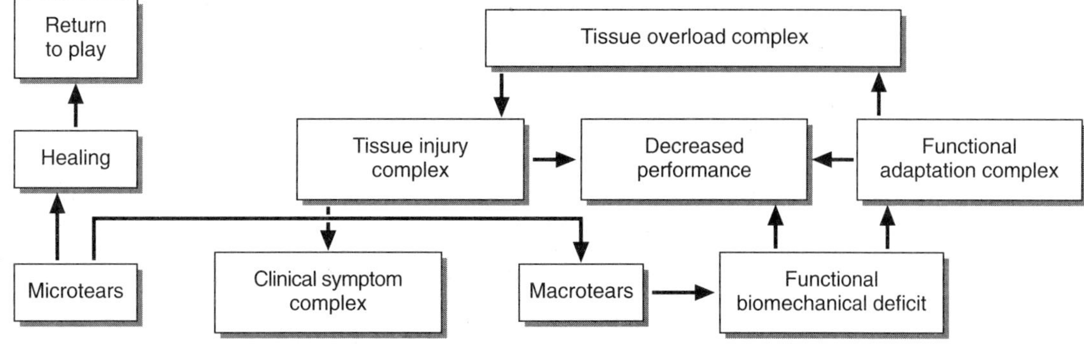

Figure 69-2. Negative feedback vicious overload cycle.

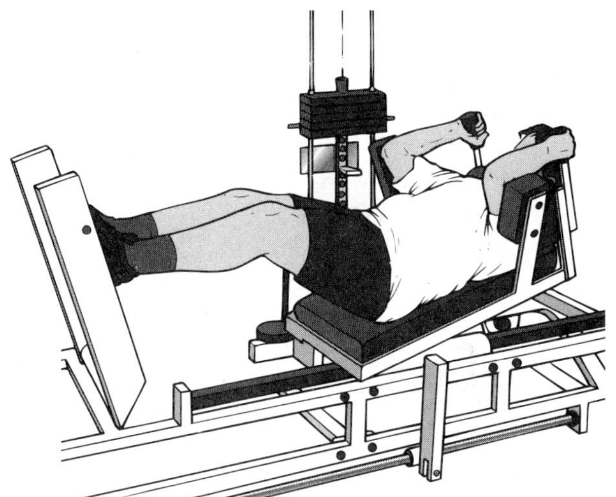

Figure 69-3. The leg press is an example of a closed kinetic chain exercise.

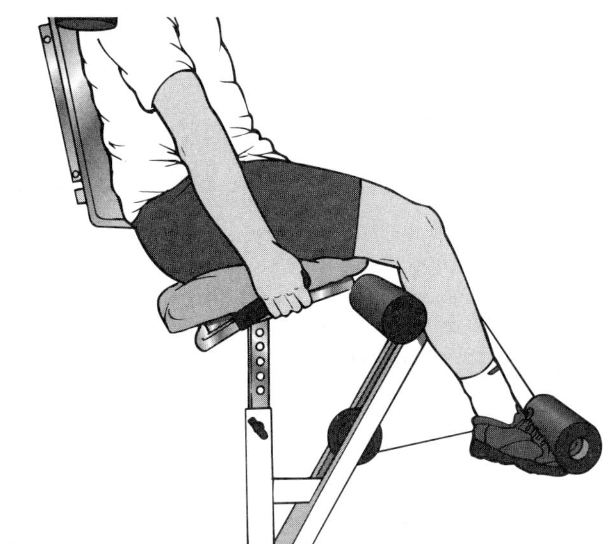

Figure 69-4. The knee extension is an example of an open kinetic chain exercise.

capsule blends into expansions of the patellar tendon anteriorly, the iliotibial band (ITB) laterally, and the semimembranosus tendon and the deep fibers of the tibial collateral ligament medially. Laterally, the fibular collateral ligament supports the capsule although it remains separate from the synovium. On the posteromedial corner, the capsule blends with the semimembranosus and the oblique popliteal ligament. At the head of the fibula, the posterior region of the capsule forms the arcuate ligament, below which the popliteus tendon enters the knee.

The primary static restraints to tibiofemoral translatory motion are the cruciate ligaments. Each cruciate ligament is described by its attachment to the tibial plateau. The anterior cruciate ligament (ACL) arises lateral and anterior to the tibial spine, and its fascicles fan out to form a broad-based attachment to the posteromedial aspect of the lateral femoral condyle. There are two primary groups of fascicles—the anteromedial bundle that tightens during knee flexion, and the larger posterolateral band that tightens during knee extension (13). Functionally, the ACL prevents anterior translation of the tibial plateau relative to the femur and aids in rotational control.

The posterior cruciate ligament (PCL) arises between the posterior junction of the tibial condyles and attaches to the inner aspect of the medial femoral condyle. The PCL is composed of an anterior band and a smaller posterior bundle (13). The PCL prevents posterior translation of the tibial plateau relative to the femur and provides secondary rotational stability. Both cruciate ligaments are intra-articular but extrasynovial structures.

The menisci are cartilaginous structures that assist the motion of the femoral condyles at the tibiofemoral joint. They deepen the articular surfaces, provide a thin layer of lubrication, and assist in shock absorption. In addition, the menisci guide the femur through a rolling and gliding motion combined with rotation. The menisci also limit extremes of flexion and extension. They have been shown to transmit approximately 50% of weight-bearing moments in extension and 85% in flexion (14,15). Viewed from above (Fig. 69-5), the menisci approximate incomplete circles, open at their central borders. The

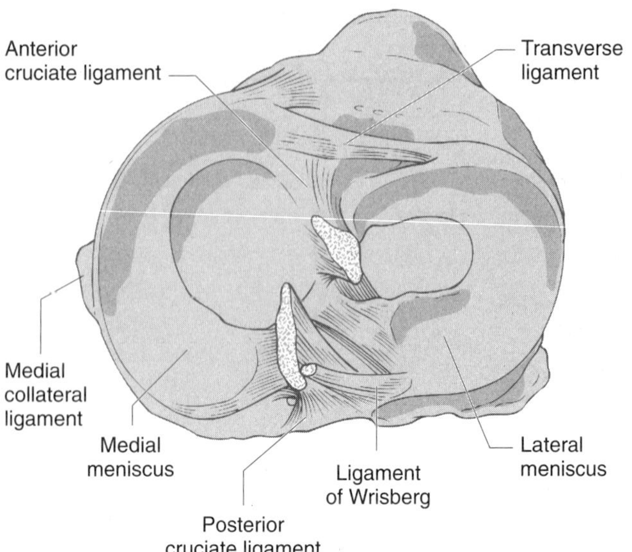

Figure 69-5. The menisci of the knee, viewed from above.

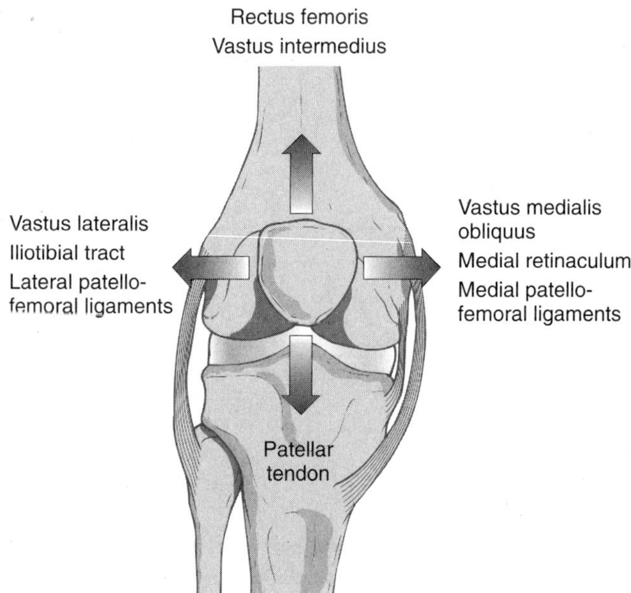

Figure 69-6. The patella is the centerpiece of all static and dynamic stabilizing forces on the patellofemoral joint.

medial meniscus is firmly attached to the medial collateral ligament (MCL) and the synovial capsule, while the lateral meniscus has a less significant bond to the capsule and is separate from the collateral ligament. This strong medial anchor restricts the mobility of the medial meniscus and might account for the high number of injuries of the posterior horn. Meniscal vascular support consists of a capillary plexus located in the thicker, peripheral one-third (16). Centrally, the meniscus is thinner and relies on the synovial fluid for diffusion of nutrients.

The two collateral ligaments control valgus and varus moments acting at the knee and help limit rotation of the tibia (17). The MCL consists of superficial and deep layers separated by a bursa. Superiorly, the ligament arises from the medial epicondyle and is anchored in the medial, proximal region of the tibia, with its deep layer attaching to the meniscal periphery. The lateral collateral ligament (LCL) courses from the lateral femoral condyle to the fibula, free of the meniscus and the synovial capsule.

The patellofemoral joint is essentially a soft-tissue joint under the control of numerous muscular and fascial structures. The patella is the centerpiece of all the static and dynamic stabilizing forces affecting the patellofemoral joint (Fig. 69-6). The extensor mechanism consists of the quadriceps muscle group, the patella, and the quadriceps and patellar tendons. The hamstrings act as antagonists to the anterior group. The iliotibial tract, lateral retinaculum, and patellofemoral ligaments provide a laterally directed pull, while the vastus medialis obliquus (VMO), medial retinaculum, and medial patellofemoral ligaments pull medially. These stabilizing forces, by compressing the patella against the femur, create a patellofemoral joint reaction force (PFJRF). The PFJRF becomes greater with increases in quadriceps tension and with increased knee

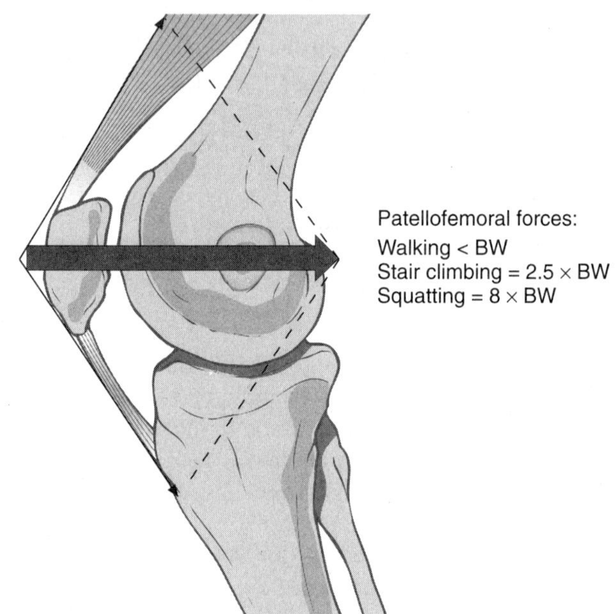

Figure 69-7. Force vector of patellofemoral joint reaction force.

flexion (Fig. 69-7). The approximate PFJRFs for walking, ascending stairs, and squatting approximate 0.5, 3.3, and 6 to 7 times body weight, respectively (18). The patellofemoral joint reaction stress (PFJRS) refers to the PFJRF per unit of contact area. A large PFJRF distributed over a large contact area produces a relatively lower degree of articular stress. A large PFJRF over a smaller area yields high articular stresses and heightens the chances of subchondral degenerative changes. The amount of patellofemoral contact area changes with knee flexion, as demonstrated in Figure 69-8. From full extension through the first 10 to 20 degrees of flexion, little contact occurs. Trochlear engagement then begins, with the inferior margin of both medial and lateral facets sharing the load (19). Between 20 and 90 degrees of flexion, there is increased proximal patellar and lateral edge contact, and at flexion over 90 degrees the odd facet makes contact (19). The patellofemoral contact areas are the greatest in the mid range (30–90 degrees).

SPECIFIC PROBLEMS OF THE KNEE

Although numerous musculoskeletal problems can affect the knee, this chapter focuses on the most common. Patellofemoral pain syndrome (PFPS) is a primary overload injury and the rehabilitation principles used to treat it are applicable to other overload injuries of the knee as well as some traumatic knee injuries.

Patellofemoral Pain Syndrome

PFPS is the most common knee problem encountered in an outpatient physical medicine and rehabilitation practice. It is the most common knee problem in runners (20). The differential diagnosis of anterior knee pain includes but is not restricted to infrapatellar bursitis, synovial plica, patellar tendinitis, quadriceps tendinitis, Osgood-Schlatter disease, osteochondritis dissecans, patellofemoral tracking disorder, and meniscal pathology. Factors that predispose individuals to patellofemoral pain include the presence of patella alta, increased Q angle, femoral anteversion, and excessive pronation (21–23). Clinicians should look for all of these factors as well as attempt to mobilize the patella superiorly, inferiorly, medially, and laterally to determine if any soft-tissue restrictions exist.

Complete and Accurate Diagnosis—Patellofemoral Pain

Tissue Injury Complex

Most often this complex includes the patellar cartilage, the synovium, and the tendon insertion into the patella (18).

Functional Biomechanical Deficit Complex

The deficits include insufficiency of medial quadriceps musculature; inflexibility of the ITB, lateral retinaculum, hamstrings, and gastrocnemius muscles (all of which either increase knee flexion or cause lateral tracking of the patella); hamstring muscle weakness; hip abductor and external rotator weakness (which causes increased medial rotation of the femur and further stress on the patellofemoral joint); imbalance of hip internal and external rotators (leading to increased torque at the knee); and excessive pronation. The functional biomechanical deficit may be the cause of the problem, the result of the problem, or both. Again, it is important to look for these deficits at the knee as well as proximally and distally.

Functional Adaptation Complex

In PFPS, this complex includes knee flexion contracture (loss of terminal knee extension), lateral patellar tracking, increased pain with running (often associated with a decreased stride length) and axial loading of the knee, and jumping off the opposite leg to avoid full loading of the involved knee. All of these adaptations will lead to inefficiencies in sporting performance and to tissue overload of other structures in the kinetic chain.

Tissue Overload Complex

Tissue overload occurs locally and distally along the kinetic chain. Locally, the lateral retinaculum and patellar tendon are overloaded. These structures are also part of the tissue injury complex. The hip external rotators may also suffer from overload. Because the hip external rotators may not

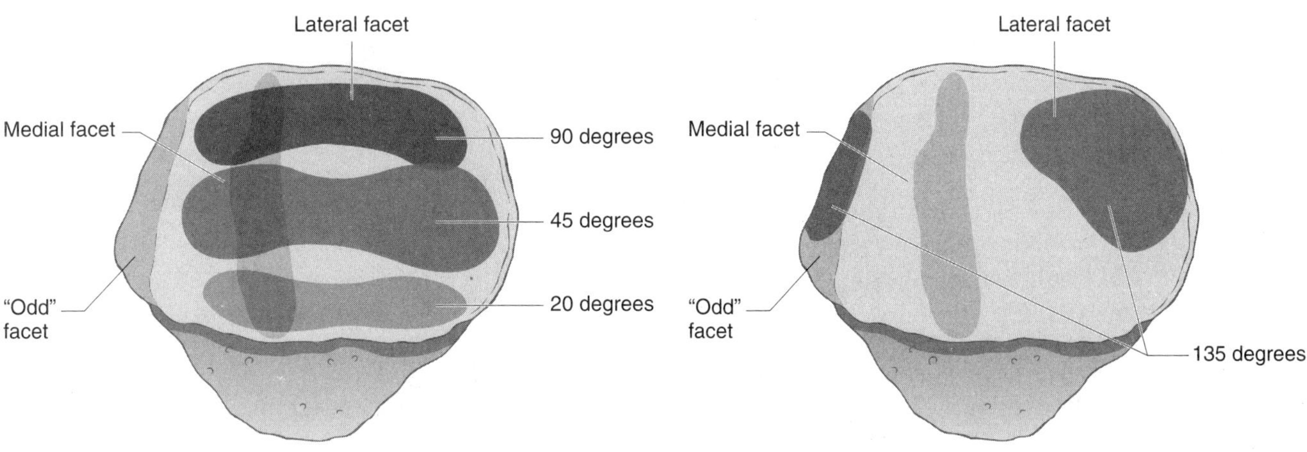

Figure 69-8. Patellofemoral contact areas at different degrees of knee flexion.

be strong enough to balance the internal hip rotators, increased medial femoral rotation occurs and increased patellofemoral shear results.

Rehabilitation of Patellofemoral Disorder

Acute phase (0–7 Days with Emphasis on the First 48 Hours)

The acute phase of rehabilitation of patellofemoral disorders focuses on treating the tissue injury complex and the clinical symptom complex. In most PFPSs, the actual symptoms are not the result of an acute inflammatory reaction or tendinitis but rather the result of a chronic repetitive overload creating cellular damage and degeneration with scar formation of the patellar tendon and lateral retinaculum. Acute painful presentation may also occur if inflammation is present. Under these conditions it is unlikely that acute treatment is necessary for more than 24 to 48 hours. If there has been true subluxation or dislocation of the patella, a much longer period of time may be necessary to control swelling and inflammation. Symptomatic treatment may start with judicious use of anti-inflammatory and pain medications and modalities. Intra-articular corticosteroid injection is rarely, if ever, indicated for patellofemoral symptoms. Therapeutic activities include relative rest (i.e., avoiding abusive or stressful activity to the knee but maintaining some motion of the injured part) and conditioning of other parts of the kinetic chain (i.e., riding a stationary bike using arms and uninvolved leg, arm ergometers, hip musculature strengthening). Cryotherapy is useful to decrease a joint effusion. This is particularly important because joint effusions can inhibit quadriceps function (24,25). Protected range of motion helps to avoid soft-tissue contracture. Initial muscle activity includes isometric exercise, often at multiple pain-free angles (26). Criteria for advancement to the recovery phase include resolution of edema, improved range of motion, and decreased pain.

Recovery Phase (5–7 Days to 5–7 Weeks)

The complexes involved in this phase are the tissue overload complex and the functional biomechanical deficit complex. Therapeutic activities include regaining lost flexibility, appropriate loading, resistive exercises, and kinetic chain and functional exercises aimed at improving patellar tracking.

Flexibility exercises focus on lower-extremity muscles, especially the ITB, rectus femoris, gastrocnemius, and hamstrings (26–28). The ITB is important because of the laterally deviating forces created by its insertion into the lateral aspect of the patella (29–31). It is critical to stabilize the patella while stretching the ITB and lateral retinaculum. A medially directed force applied to the patella by the therapist prevents stressing of the medial retinaculum and the patellofemoral joint. The ITB and lateral retinaculum then receive the intended stretch instead of only the ITB (Fig. 69-9). Manual medial glide and tilt of the patella may be employed to stretch specifically the tight lateral retinaculum (32) (Fig. 69-10). The hamstrings and gastrocnemius must be stretched properly because of their propensity to shorten and increase the PFJRFs with increasing flexion of the knee (Figs. 69-11 and 69-12). Gastrocnemius-soleus inflexibility causes compensatory pronation of the foot, resulting in increased tibial internal rotation and additional patellofemoral stress (22). The rectus femoris, if tight, affects patellar movement during knee flexion (22). A tight rectus femoris creates a patella alta. This is most prominent during hip flexion where the rectus femoris also functions as a hip flexor as well as a knee extensor. Patellar

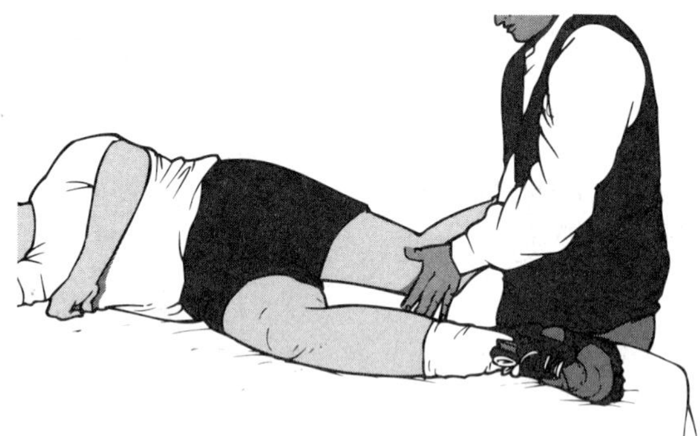

Figure 69-9. Iliotibial band stretch with the clinician applying medial pressure to the patella.

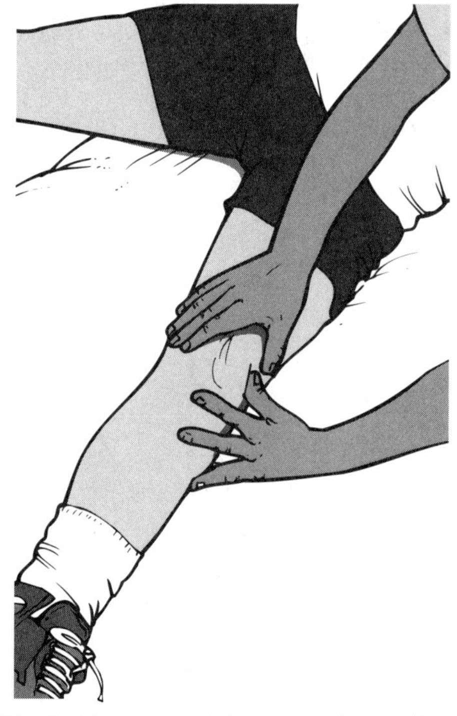

Figure 69-10. Manual medial glide of the patella performed by the patient.

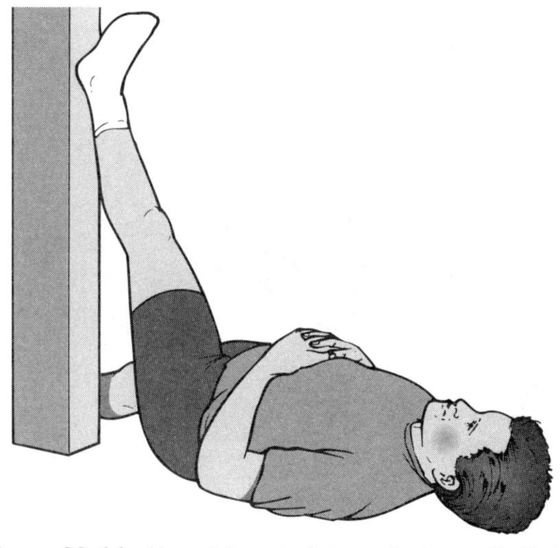

Figure 69-11. Hamstring stretch against a wall. Note the low back is flat and supported against the floor.

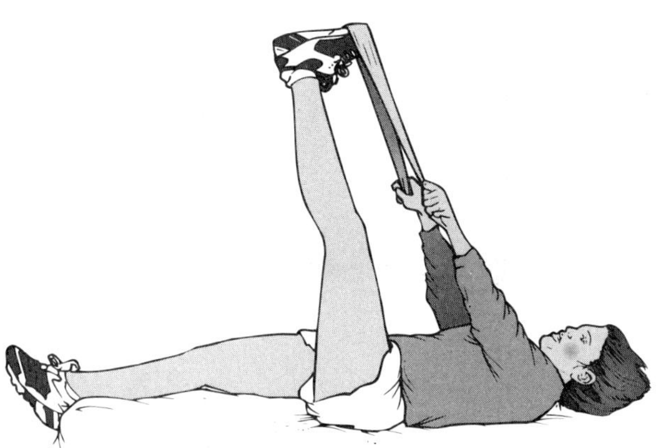

Figure 69-12. Hamstring stretch using a towel or theraband.

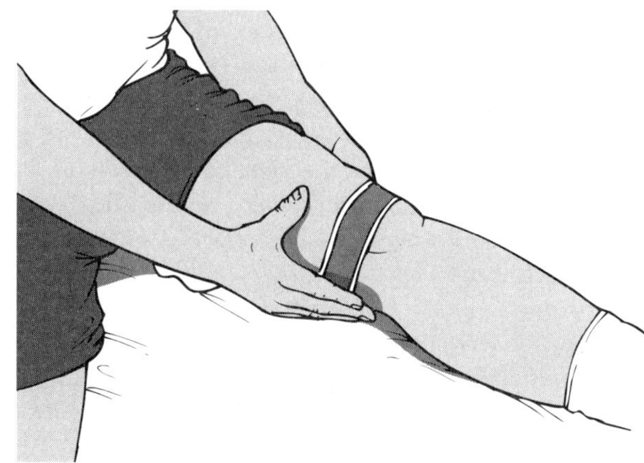

Figure 69-13. McConnell taping of the knee.

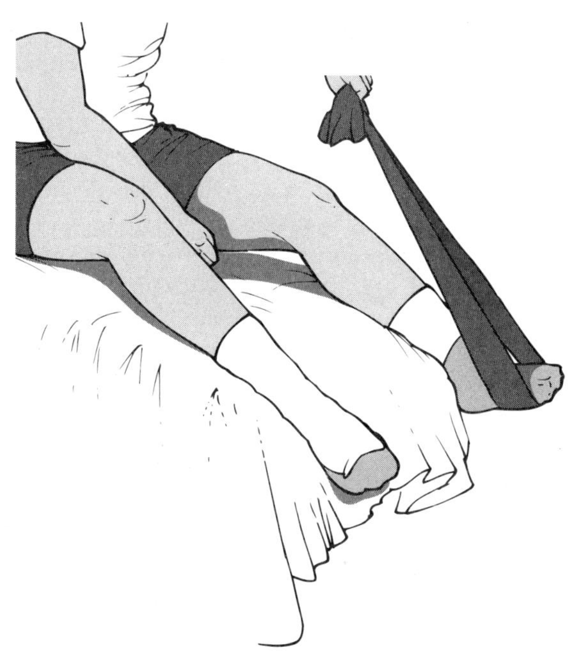

Figure 69-14. Strengthening of the foot supinators to decrease pronation using a theraband.

taping as described by McConnell may be used to correct patellar glide, tilt, and rotation (21,22) (Fig. 69-13).

Lower-extremity malalignment problems (i.e., genu varum, tibia vara, hindfoot varus, and forefoot pronation) can cause a compensatory subtalar joint pronation and obligatory internal tibial rotation, and must be corrected. Strengthening exercises of the supinators of the foot (i.e., posterior tibialis, invertors of the ankle) may also be instituted to decrease pronation (Fig. 69-14). Strengthening of the hip external rotators, to correct hip internal rotation–external rotation imbalance and a tendency toward an internally rotated femur, is also essential. Often, resolution of the tight ITB alone through aggressive stretching will not alleviate symptoms because the external rotators of the hip are still relatively weak. Orthotics may occasionally be necessary, although they should not be seen as an immediate solution to any weaknesses or imbalances.

All strengthening programs for patellofemoral pain must consider not only quadriceps strength but also what effect knee flexion angle and the type of exercise (OKC versus CKC) have on PFJFR. The goals of patellofemoral rehabilitation are maximizing quadriceps strength while minimizing PFJRF and PFJRS. Strengthening of the quadriceps and hip flexors is typically done via short-arc (−30 degrees of extension to 0 degrees) quadriceps exercises, although the selectivity of strengthening only the VMO is debatable (33–36). Selective VMO strengthening may possibly be enhanced by hip adduction exercises (37). Besides strengthening the VMO, hip adductor strengthening may also serve to give the VMO a stable origin from which to contract. Hanten and Schulthies (37) showed that during hip adduction, the electrical activity of the VMO is significantly greater than that of the vastus lateralis. Therefore, the use of hip adductor contraction in conjunction with quadriceps sets and straight-leg raises is recommended to facilitate VMO strengthening.

Often isometric contractions may strengthen the quadriceps muscles without the significant increase in PFJRFs that may occur with isotonic exercises. It is also important to know that articular cartilage is adversely affected by shear forces. Shear forces are theoretically reduced during isometric exercises. Articular cartilage may actually derive its nutrition through diffusion created by intermittently applied compression (33). Specifically, isometric contraction at 90 degrees of knee flexion maximizes compression forces and minimizes shear forces. At 90 degrees of knee flexion compared to 15 degrees of knee flexion, VMO activity is increased relative to vastus lateralis activity (33,38). Kannus and Niittymaki (39) showed that 70% of patients with patellofemoral pain symptoms of more than 2 months' duration had complete resolution of symptoms with only intense isometric quadriceps strengthening exercises with the knee in full extension. Wild et al (40) emphasized the importance of doing isometric contractions with the knee in full extension because 10 degrees of flexion of the knee reduces the effective muscle effort in the vasti group to an average of one-fourth of the muscle effort demonstrated in full extension.

Emphasis should be placed on strengthening lower-extremity muscles in the ranges where the PFJRF and PFJRS are lowest. During CKC exercises (leg presses), consistently less patellofemoral joint stress is generated in lower knee flexion ranges (<45 degrees of flexion) than during OKC (leg extension) exercises. As discussed earlier, when increased knee flexion angles are used (>50 degrees of flexion), OKC activities (leg extension) show less PFJRF and PFJRS than do CKC activities (leg presses) (41). Therefore, a biomechanically sound rehabilitation program, at least in terms of isometric strengthenging, should consist of CKC exercises near terminal extension (Fig. 69-15) and OKC exercises between 60 and 90 degrees of flexion (Fig. 69-16).

Strengthening in weight-bearing activities also needs to be done as soon as possible, as these are more physiologic. CKC exercises, with co-contraction of quadriceps and hamstring muscles, are important to reduce excessive forces across the patella (18,19,42). The same degree of force generation to maintain any degree of knee flexion is shared by these two major muscle groups. Shared forces help to reduce the amount of quadriceps tension needed to create a given position of knee flexion. Less PFJRF is generated. Partial squats (one-fourth of a full squat) also eccentrically load the knee and provide a more physiologic training technique. Most overload injuries are caused by eccentric overload. Therefore, it is essential for proper patellofemoral rehabilitation. Progression of strengthening exercises, especially those for the VMO muscle, continues, with an emphasis on developing sports-specific strengthening.

The position of the femur during knee extensor strengthening is also important. When the femur is internally rotated, knee extension is assisted by the tensor fasciae latae (TFL) muscle through its attachment into the ITB (43). This increases the lateral pull on the patella and thus decreases the effectiveness of the VMO (22,31). Therefore, an attempt should be made to position the femur in neutral or slight external rotation to avoid increased pull from the TFL.

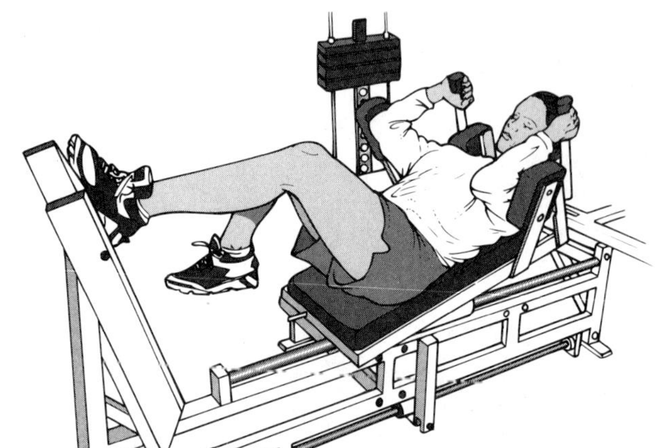

Figure 69-15. Closed kinetic chain strengthening of the lower extremity using a leg press.

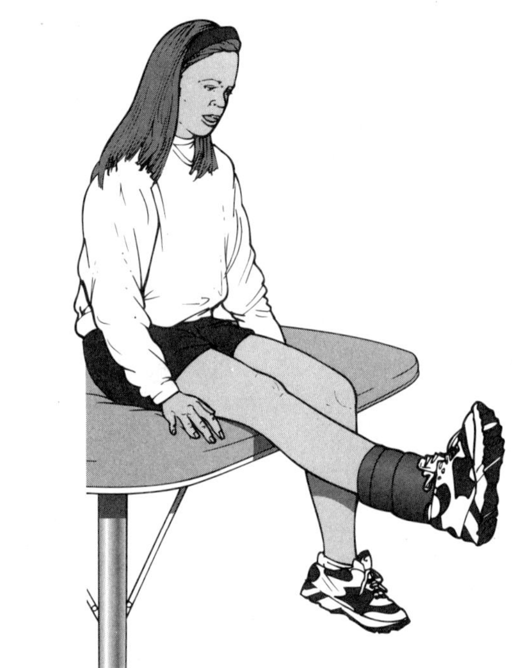

Figure 69-16. Open kinetic chain strengthening of the lower extremity using a free weight on the ankle.

Muscular imbalances between the medial and lateral rotators and adductors and abductors of the hip need to be addressed because increased medial femoral rotation and adduction cause excessive medial rotation and adduction of the hip during the stance phase of gait, with an associated increased valgus vector at the patellofemoral joint (22,32). Strengthening the external rotators with the leg slightly extended and adducted can accomplish appropriate strengthening of the external rotators at the same time the ITB is stretched (Fig. 69-17). Distally, a weak tibialis anterior muscle decreases foot control at heel strike and causes increased stress at the knee (44). Strengthening the anterior tibialis, as well as addressing footwear problems or other factors that increase stress at the ankle, must be part of a PFPS rehabilitation program.

Some controversy exists regarding the effects of patellofemoral taping and selective VMO training to improve patellofemoral tracking. McConnell claimed excellent outcomes in more than 90% of patients with patellofemoral pain using taping and a neuromuscular reeducation program (21,22). Selective training of the vastus medialis muscle using electromyographic (EMG) biofeedback or combining biofeedback with a graded exercise program can also be beneficial (45–47). Using EMG biofeedback to facilitate VMO control of the patella has also been described and may be of benefit in patellofemoral rehabilitation (22,48). The clinical benefits of taping, however, have not been proved. Bockrath et al (49) reported that patellofemoral taping caused no change in patellofemoral congruency or rotational angles as measured by Merchant views on x-ray films. These measurements were done statically at one specific flexion angle and no measures of dynamic motion were addressed. Nevertheless, a 50% reduction in reported pain on visual analogue scales was found when patellofemoral taping was used. Grabiner et al (34), in their extensive review of patellar neuromechanics, were unable to conclude that selective VMO strengthening is possible. Rather, they suggested that a generalized quadriceps strengthening effect is the outcome of these rehabilitation programs and that perhaps it is the achievement of a "threshold" for absolute VMO strength that leads to reacquisition of normal tracking. Under any circumstance, the problem with all of these studies is that full kinetic chain assessment was not performed. Dynamically, patients may be improving by these techniques because control at the level of the hip, the knee, or the ankle may be stabilizing the entire kinetic chain system. Examination of one joint in isolation is inadequate.

Criteria for advancement to the maintenance phase include absence of pain and inflammation, range of motion equal to that of the opposite side, strength at more than 75% of the normal side, and smooth kinetic motion.

Maintenance Phase

The complexes involved in the maintenance phase of a patellofemoral rehabilitation program include the functional biomechanical deficit complex and subclinical adaptation complex. Therapeutic activities are geared toward optimizing strength and flexibility, proprioception retraining, balance, plyometrics, and sport-specific activities. Agility drills, running, jumping, and kicking are stressed. A study by Powers et al (50) suggests that initial running activities may be started by running backward, as the peak patellofemoral joint compressive forces are less in backward compared with forward running at self-selected speeds. Use of a balance board to provide a basic proprioceptive stimulus to the knee could also ease the transition into more functional activities and could serve to improve kinesthetic sense of the knee (27).

In most cases, athletes are able to resume activity without knee bracing. However, the use of a knee sleeve with fenestration for the patella can occasionally be helpful (51). Knee sleeves may work by enhancing proprioception to the knee or warming the soft tissues of the knee. Greenwald et al (52) showed that patients who wear a patellofemoral brace have significantly improved levels of perceived knee stability and decreased levels of pain during activities of daily living and athletics. However, objective parameters showed no effect on knee flexion

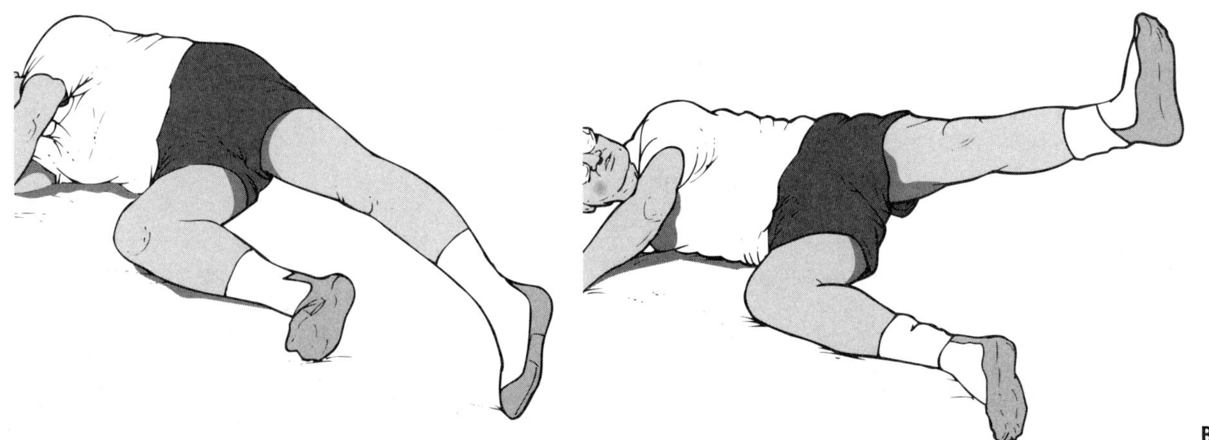

Figure 69-17. A. ITB stretch with the leg extended and adducted. B. Hip extend rotator strengthening with leg extended and actively abducted and externally rotated.

angle during gait or level walking, stair ascent, or stair descent. Use of knee braces should be restricted to competitive or high-demand situations. The more "supportive" a brace is, the more likely it is to promote muscular atrophy, particularly if it is worn constantly. Finestone et al (53) showed that a simple elastic knee sleeve was more effective than the more elaborate patellar braces for decreasing symptoms. Infrapatellar straps may also help decrease patellofemoral symptoms by increasing the area for force dissipation of the patellar tendon.

During the maintenance phase of rehabilitation, a thorough evaluation of sport-specific demands on the knee must occur. The athlete must demonstrate the ability to assume proper limb placement and coordinated patterns of muscle firing to prevent further patellofemoral overload. It is during this phase that more definitive equipment modifications are made. For example, the runner who continues to pronate excessively may be encouraged to purchase shoes with greater rear-foot control and a straight last. Analysis of a cyclist often reveals the need to adjust the bicycle seat height slightly higher or alter the cam type (54). A beginning power lifter may need reminders to maintain a position with the "toes-out" and hips externally rotated when performing squats.

Criteria for return to play include full range of motion, normal strength and balance, normal techniques, absence of pain, and evidence that a sport-specific progression has occurred.

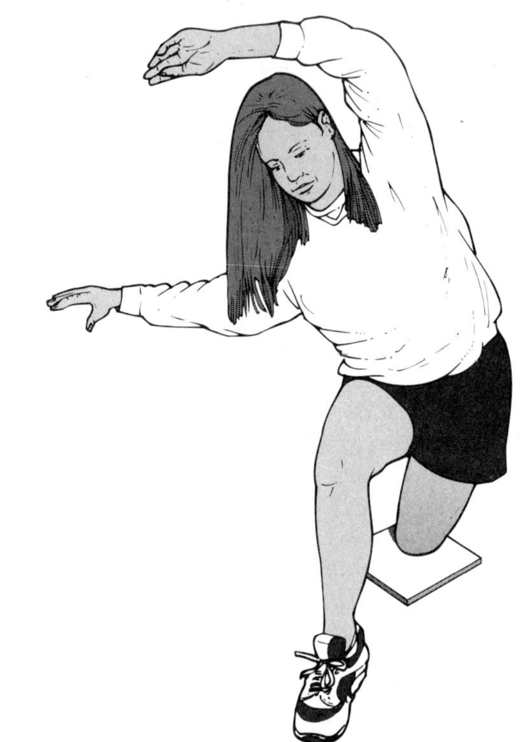

Figure 69-18. ITB stretching in a kneeling position.

Iliotibial Band Syndrome

The ITB is the extension of the TFL that extends down the lateral part of the leg to insert into the Gerdy tubercle along the lateral tibia. ITB syndrome is associated with painful sensation as the ITB slides back and forth over the lateral femoral condyle as the knee flexes and extends (55–57). Running on beveled surfaces, limb-length discrepancies, tibia vara, hyperpronation, and ITB contracture are all associated risk factors (55,57). The Noble compression test is a useful examination maneuver when an ITB friction syndrome is suspected. With the patient supine, and the knee positioned in 90 degrees of flexion, the examiner presses on or just proximal to the lateral epicondyle. The knee is then gradually extended. Pain occurring at about 30 degrees (as the ITB crosses the bony prominence) is a positive finding (56).

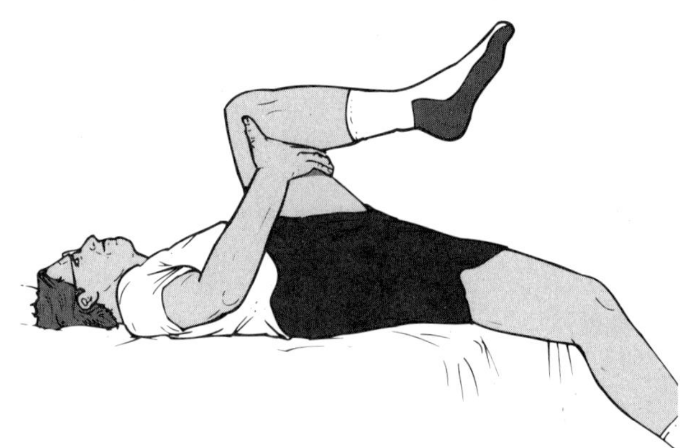

Figure 69-19. Hip flexor stretching with the ipsilateral leg hanging over the edge of the table.

The *tissue injury complex* is typically the ITB over the femoral condyle or at the Gerdy tubercle. The *clinical symptom complex* consists of localized pain over the lateral femoral condyle, worsened with running. The *functional biomechanical deficit* is the inflexible ITB, while the *functional adaptation complex* consists of functional pronation of the foot, external rotation at the hip, internal rotation of the lower leg, and lateral patellar tracking (5).

Rehabilitation of ITB syndrome consists of attempts to stretch the ITB, hip flexors, and gluteus maximus (Figs. 69-18 to 69-20). Correction of foot pronation is needed

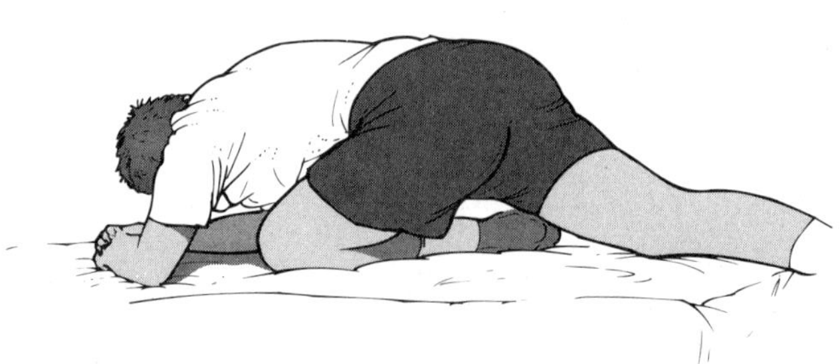

Figure 69-20. Gluteus maximus stretch in a prone position.

and the runner should run only on level surfaces, if at all. Swimming and stationary ski machines can help maintain fitness. Strengthening of the hip adductors, gluteus maximus, and TFL is emphasized. The adductors counter the pull of the tight ITB and the other muscles that give rise to the ITB (gluteus maximus and TFL) and must be strengthened to avoid overuse (5). Symptoms can take as long as 2 to 6 months to resolve (57). Occasionally, local injection of a combination of an anesthetic agent and a corticosteroid placed in the region of the lateral femoral condyle is helpful (5).

Bursitis

The anserine bursa separates the three conjoined tendons of the pes anserinus (semitendinosus, sartorius, and gracilis muscles) from the MCL and the tibia. Pes anserine bursitis is commonly seen in women with heavy thighs and osteoarthritis of the knees. The bursa also can become inflamed after direct trauma in athletes, especially soccer players. Patients complain of pain inferior to the anteromedial border of the knee near or below the joint line with ascension of stairs. The examiner can reproduce the symptoms by moving the knee in flexion and extension while internally rotating the leg. Palpation localizes the pain to the anserine bursa. Steroid injection is typically quite effective in reducing the inflammatory symptoms. The athlete at risk for direct trauma can benefit from padded protection around the knee. The rehabilitation program should emphasize stretching of the medial hamstrings and adductor muscles.

Prepatellar bursitis, colloquially referred to as housemaid's knee, is often the result of frequent kneeling, producing an effusion of the subcutaneous bursa at the anterior surface of the patella. The patient rarely complains of pain unless direct pressure is applied to the bursa. Occupational modifications should include patient education, avoidance of kneeling, and the use of knee pads when pressure must be applied to the patella. Rehabilitation should correct flexibility deficits in the quadriceps, hamstrings, and the triceps surae, while the swelling is reduced with the application of ice (58).

Acute Ligamentous Injuries

Primary and secondary restraints of the knee are frequently injured in occupational and recreational activities. It is beyond the scope of this chapter to provide a detailed description of all the surgical and nonsurgical management schemes for collateral and cruciate ligament injuries. However, regardless of surgical or nonsurgical routes of treatment, the patient will benefit from a rehabilitation program that emphasizes maximizing function at the lowest cost. Once an acceptable level of function has been achieved, the patient should be directed to continue a maintenance program to prevent reinjury. There are no single best "cookbook" recipes for success.

Anterior Cruciate Ligament

Partial or complete disruption of the ACL can be a disabling event for the athlete or worker. Frequently the patient describes an audible "snap" or "pop" while the lower limb undergoes hyperextension or rotational strain. The injury is painful and an acute hemarthrosis usually develops in the first hours following the insult. It is common to damage additional restraints of the knee at the same time. If the patient complains of "locking" or "clicking" and there is an associated restriction of range of motion, the clinician should be suspicious of an associated meniscal tear. An accurate diagnosis should be established to include each structure damaged, so an appropriate treatment plan is initiated.

Examination should begin with the uninvolved lower limb and progress to include all the joints in the kinetic chain on the involved extremity. Functional limitations should be observed during standing, ambulation, and squatting. Palpation should localize tenderness and note any effusion present. Careful examination for range of motion deficits is needed, using the uninvolved limb for comparison. Limitation of full extension can be seen with capsular distention but this also raises the possibility of a meniscal tear. Loss of ACL integrity can be demonstrated with a *Lachman maneuver* (Fig. 69-21) (59). The examiner

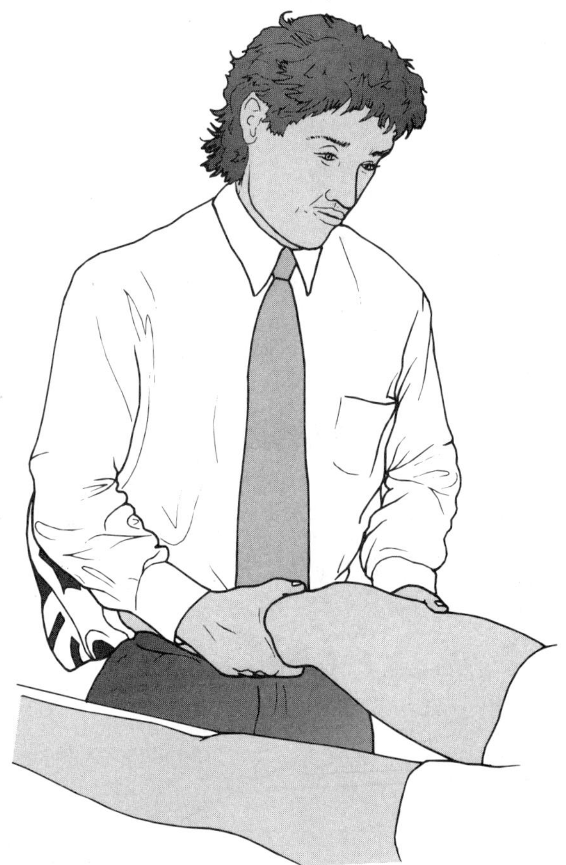

Figure 69-21. The Lachman maneuver.

attempts to introduce anterior tibial translation while the limb is kept in 15 to 20 degrees of knee flexion. With complete tears of the ACL, there is significant anterior tibial translation and a loss of a distinctive end feel. A partial tear will maintain a "soft" end feel, but tibial translation will be greater than that on the uninvolved side. Quantification of the tibial translation can be done with the use of an arthrometer. The *anterior drawer test* (Fig. 69-22), although technically easier for many clinicians to perform than the Lachman test, has significant limitations. In this position, with the knee flexed to 90 degrees, the hamstrings are at a mechanical advantage, and tibial translation will not be appreciated if there is any degree of hamstring activity. An associated meniscal tear can act like a "door jam" and provide a block to tibial motion in this position. If there is a PCL tear, a false-positive finding on the drawer test may ensue as the tibia is actually being brought back to its proper position from a position of tibial "sag" rather than truly being translated forward. The *pivot-shift test* further indicates anterolateral rotatory instability, and represents an increased risk for cartilaginous injury acutely or at a later date (17,60,61). The reader is referred to Losee's work for a detailed explanation of this test (61). Magnetic resonance imaging (MRI) is excellent for visualizing the disrupted ACL, as well as for assessing the presence of other coexisting injuries.

Acute treatment includes aggressive reduction of joint swelling, either via Cryocuff compression or aspiration of the hemarthrosis. Even if surgical reconstruction is planned, there is evidence to suggest that early (within the first 3 weeks) repair is not advisable due to an increased chance of graft arthrofibrosis developing (62). An appropriate "prehabilitation" should be initiated after the injury and continued until surgery or entry into an aggressive nonsurgical rehabilitation program. Isometric co-contractions of the quadriceps and hamstrings with protected weight bearing as tolerated are encouraged early on. Hyperextension of the knee should be avoided.

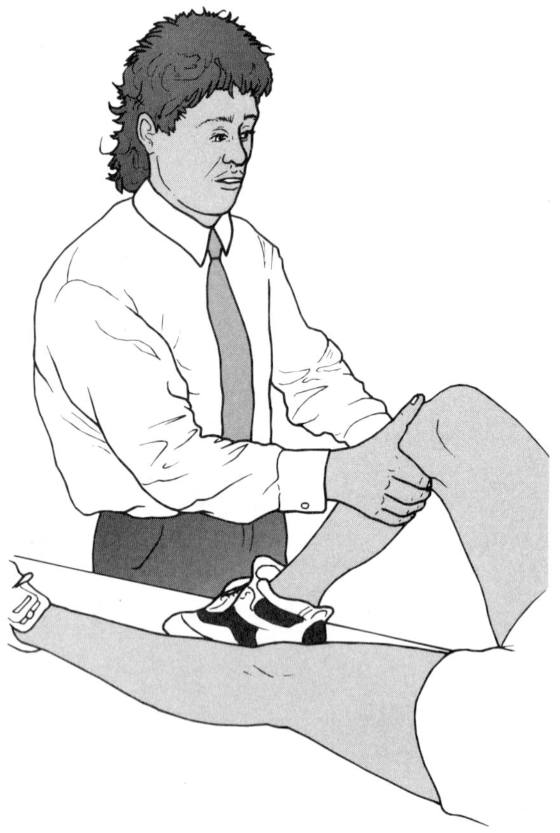

Figure 69-22. The anterior drawer test.

When reconstruction is performed, a number of materials and techniques can be used. The most common is the patellar tendon autograft using the middle one-third of the patellar tendon. The bone-patellar-bone graft offers excellent fixation and has been shown to be stronger than the original ACL (17,63). Following reconstruction, safe restoration of motion and weight bearing is emphasized. During the immediate postoperative period, continuous passive motion (CPM) can be utilized, even at home (with the patient instructed on the correct use of the device prior to hospital discharge). To maximize a patient's compliance, it is necessary to provide adequate pain relief in the immediate postoperative period. Controlling the effusion with compression, ice, and elevation is the first step. Electrical stimulation of the quadriceps to help prevent atrophy may be considered. Soft-tissue mobilization about the patella should be employed to restore patellar mobility and lessen the chance of adhesion formation.

It is important to gain full extension at the tibiofemoral joint during the first week to avoid a persistent extension block. Weight bearing with the knee in extension while wearing an immobilizer is required. If swelling and other soft-tissue restrictions preclude immediate extension, it may help to have the patient lie prone with a towel placed beneath the knee while an ankle weight is worn to provide a passive stretch. The patient can cycle on a stationary bike without resistance to facilitate motion. Once the swelling is controlled and extension is achieved, the next goal is re-establishment of a normal gait pattern. Crutch walking progresses from two crutches with partial weight bearing to one crutch and then none by the end of the first month. By this time most patients no longer need the immobilizer. CKC exercises to promote strengthening of the lower extremity are initiated. CKC exercises are theoretically preferable over the OKC type, owing to their reported lessening of tibiofemoral shear forces (12). However, even with CKC exercises, hyperextension and dynamic pivot shifting must be avoided. Leg presses, bicycles, and stair climbers may be used safely. Arm ergometry and trilimbed exercises are useful to maintain cardiovascular fitness during this period. By the end of the first month, the bony plugs from the graft should be healed and fixed into the surrounding tibial and femoral tunnels constructed at the time of surgery (17).

During subsequent weeks, further increases in range

of motion, restoration of baseline strength in both hamstring and quadriceps groups, and progression to functional activities occur (12,17). Exercises to develop appropriate strength and flexibility of hip abduction, adduction, extension, and flexion are essential for maintaining control of the affected limb. Cardiovascular efforts are continued on a stationary bike, and the position of the seat should be adjusted to avoid knee hyperextension. As the patient gains proprioceptive and muscular control of the lower extremity, progression to a cross-country ski machine, stair-climber, or slide board is encouraged. Hyperextension at the knee should be avoided, and the entire kinetic chain should show the proper synergistic pattern for each exercise to avoid unnecessarily stressing the reconstructed knee. Reviewing proprioceptive neurofacilitation patterning may be helpful in restoring proper mechanics during these functional skills. During the second to third months, the rehabilitation program should include unidirectional jogging. Once thigh circumference approximates that of the uninvolved limb (typically by the fourth to sixth months), functional bracing with a derotation brace may be considered. The brace provides some mechanical restraint and also probably enhances proprioceptive feedback (64).

Agility drills including jumping rope, lateral shuffling around cones, figure-eight drills, and carioca are included in the rehabilitation program. When the quadriceps, hamstrings, and primary movers of the hip show strength that is 90% or better in comparison to the uninvolved limb, and there is no evidence of a clinical pivot shift, the patient may return to full sporting and occupational activities. Although isokinetic testing provides some level of objectivity, functional ability is our preferred method to measure the effectiveness of a successful rehabilitation program and safe return to full activity.

Some patients elect to pursue a nonoperative course. The exercise program is virtually identical to that following surgery, but the use of a functional brace is instituted earlier to protect the tibiofemoral joint and the menisci from potential damage. Patients who are candidates for nonoperative management include those not motivated for postsurgical rehabilitation, those who wish to modify their lifestyle in order accommodate the ligamentous injury, those who do not have any other associated ligamentous or meniscal injuries, and those whose lifestyle is already sedentary. Some individuals, through aggressive exercise, can often return to high levels of athletic competition without surgery. Unfortunately, it is difficult to predict which patients will achieve this successful outcome at the time of injury. Under any circumstance, the success of nonoperative treatment requires both hard work and extensive patient education (63).

Posterior Cruciate Ligament

Acute tears of the PCL are not as common as ACL injuries. Isolated PCL injury occurs with direct trauma forcing the tibia posteriorly (such as when the knee hits a car dashboard during an automobile accident), with a fall on a flexed knee, or from knee hyperflexion (65). Unlike ACL injuries, the patient's symptoms can be vague. There is less pain, less restriction of motion, and generally, less hemarthrosis (65). Visual inspection will demonstrate posterior tibial translation with a positive "sag" sign. The result of the *reverse Lachman test* (directing the tibia posteriorly while the knee is in approximately 15–20 degrees of flexion) is positive. Roentgenographic examination should be completed to exclude a bony avulsion from the tibial insertion of the PCL. Presence of an avulsed bony fragment requires immediate surgical fixation. MRI can clearly demonstrate PCL injury.

Treatment of isolated injury to the PCL remains controversial. Most studies showed good functional outcomes with nonoperative treatment and aggressive rehabilitation (66–69). Since there are relatively few reports with long-term follow-up, patients treated conservatively should be monitored for premature tibiofemoral joint degeneration due to instability. Frequently, PCL insufficiency is accompanied by other ligamentous, meniscal, or capsular damage and might necessitate surgical reconstruction to manage joint instability (70). The MCL and the oblique popliteal ligament are commonly injured in conjunction with the PCL.

The treatment plan should be congruent with the patient's preinjury lifestyle, functional goals, and motivation for postoperative rehabilitation. Whether treated nonoperatively or with surgery, it is essential to reduce the effusion and regain full range of motion to re-establish neuromuscular control and normalize gait. Exercises should initially focus on CKC strengthening of the quadriceps and then progress to include the musculature of the hip and the hamstrings. As strength returns and atrophy is reduced, the patient should begin sport-specific agility drills and be able to return to full activity approximately 2 months after injury.

Medial Collateral Ligament

MCL injuries are quite common and are caused by direct trauma or overuse. Swimmers who use the breaststroke undergo repeated valgus strain and can develop irritation of the MCL. There are three degrees of damage and the first two, mild to moderate injuries, have good functional results with a nonsurgical approach and appropriate rehabilitation.

Grade I (mild) MCL strains demonstrate pain with palpation, but there is no evidence of valgus instability. Treatment is based on the type of injury and the demands of the patient's activity. In the case of a traumatic injury, pain and inflammation should be controlled with cryotherapy and possibly a limited course of nonsteroidal anti-inflammatory drugs (NSAIDs). The knee should be placed in a locked brace for the first few days and then progressed to a hinge brace. A strengthening and flexibility program should be employed to stabilize the knee and limit further injury. Athletes attempting a return to sports can wear the hinged brace for 1 to 2 months following injury.

Grade II (second-degree, moderate) injuries to the MCL are characterized by the inability to fully extend the knee due to pain and inflammation. The extracapsular fibers of the MCL are ruptured. There is mild to moderate instability with a valgus stress applied in knee flexion and there is swelling and hemorrhage. When one is implementing a treatment plan, it is important to recall that the ligament tightens in extension and is most relaxed in flexion. Therefore, a knee orthosis should restrict the last 20 to 30 degrees of extension for the first week while the effusion is reduced with the application of ice and compression. After the first week, a limited arc of motion (i.e., 20–75 degrees) is permitted. Early mobilization is encouraged within pain-free limits, and range of motion should be regained over a 3- to 4-week period. Full weight bearing in a brace that allows full flexion and extension begins near the end of the first month. Strengthening of the hip girdle and knee stabilizers is integrated into the rehabilitation program as the effusion is reduced and there is no exacerbation of pain. After 4 to 5 weeks, rehabilitation should include agility drills and sport-specific activities including lateral movements. Return to play criteria include 90% strength or better, minimal or no thigh atrophy, and no inhibition during agility drills (17).

Grade III (third-degree, severe) MCL tears demonstrate instability to valgus stress in both knee flexion and extension. Hemarthrosis usually develops within a few hours due to rupture of both the deep and superficial fibers. The treatment for grade III insufficiency remains controversial. It is essential that the knee is examined to rule out associated meniscal or cruciate ligament damage, which increases the chance that surgical repair is needed. It has been reported that isolated rupture of the MCL can undergo nonoperative treatment similar to that for a grade II tear (71–73). Conversely, Kannus and Niittymaki (39) reported deterioration of the knee after long-term follow-up of nonoperative treatment. However, closer review of this work reveals that one-third of their population with insufficiency of the MCL also had a Lachman maneuver of at least grade II, which could account for some of the unsatisfactory results with nonoperative care. Although the decision for surgical care remains controversial, the development of an appropriate treatment plan should focus on the patient's preinjury demands and motivation to return to biomechanically stressful activities. In the case of young, aggressive individuals wishing to return to their previous activities, surgical reconstruction with appropriate postoperative rehabilitation might be warranted. For patients who are able to modify their lifestyle, a nonoperative approach can achieve satisfactory functional results.

Lateral Collateral Ligament

The treatment program for isolated LCL injuries is similar to the nonoperative approach described for the MCL. However, the vulnerability of the peroneal nerve at the level of the fibular head must be kept in mind. The peroneal nerve may be injured during the initial trauma or may be subjected to pressure with improper taping or bracing, or frozen during cryotherapy. Grade III injuries are often associated with capsular or cruciate ligament insufficiency, giving rise to a rotational instability as well. These combination injuries require surgical reconstruction to avoid later degeneration of the joint and to allow return to more demanding activities (65).

Meniscal Lesions

Meniscal lesions are common in both sport and industry. Tears in the semilunar cartilages are most common in the posterior horn of the medial meniscus. Injury usually follows forceful rotation of the lower extremity while the foot is firmly placed on the ground. An effusion usually develops within 24 to 48 hours, in contrast to the rapid development of hemarthrosis seen with an acute ligament rupture. Damage may range from a small peripheral tear to a larger bucket-handle tear presenting with intense pain. The patient may describe a sensation of giving way or mechanical locking. Clinical examination will often reveal tenderness upon palpation of the joint line. The *McMurray test* (Fig. 69-23) is performed with varying degrees of tibial internal and external rotation combined with valgus or varus movement, while the limb is moved from full flexion to extension. The test result is positive if a "click" is produced or if pain is reproduced. Care must be taken not to be fooled by clicking from within the patellofemoral joint or the pseudomeniscal clicking produced by a plica. The posterior meniscus can be further loaded by having the patient attempt to squat or by the examiner taking the knee into deep flexion and introducing rotation. Intermittent locking can be a subtle sign or be more obvious in the setting of a large bucket-handle tear. MRI can be used to demonstrate a meniscal tear, but if mechanical symptoms exist, arthroscopy is probably the diagnostic test of choice. Arthroscopic evaluation is required when range of motion is severely limited, or if the knee joint is locked. Locking may be observed with osteochondral lesions, cruciate ligament rupture, bony avulsions, or meniscal impingement.

Treatment of meniscal lesions is dependent on the severity of the injury to the meniscus and the possibility of combined damage. In the absence of a locked knee, a period of observation to allow for pain control and reduction of the effusion can help delineate the most appropriate treatment. The presence of associated ligamentous tears or an inability to bear weight after 2 to 3 days suggests the need for arthroscopic evaluation. If the patient is able to regain full joint motion, reduction of swelling, and full strength (and high-intensity athletic competition is not planned), a nonoperative approach may be successful.

The surgical approach to meniscal tear management has changed significantly in the last 15 to 20 years. Total meniscectomy is no longer an acceptable treatment, and

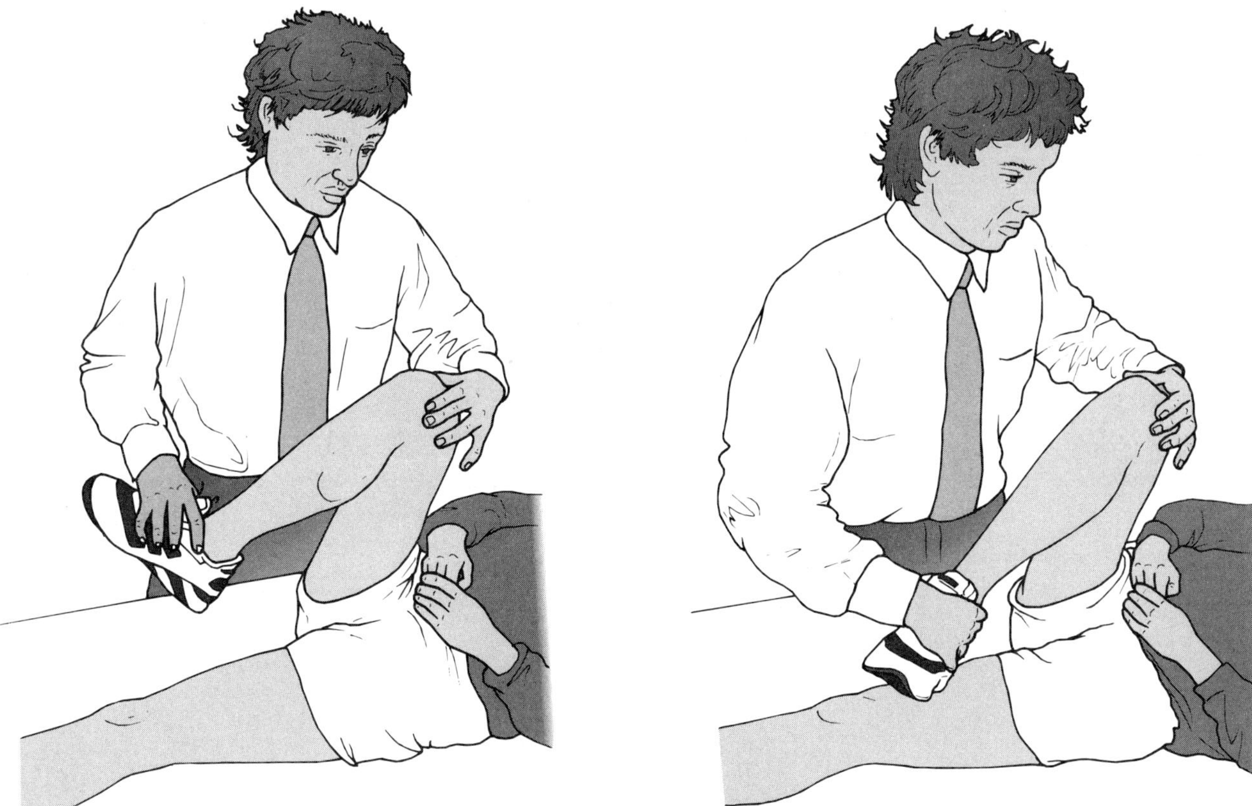

Figure 69-23. McMurray's test. The knee is brought in and out of flexion with internal and external rotatory loading. The examiner's fingers are on the joint line.

efforts are geared toward preserving as much of the cartilage as possible. The degenerative effects of meniscectomy described by Fairbanks (74) include joint space narrowing, ridging, and squaring of the condyles. Preservation of the meniscus reduces the development of such degenerative changes (75–77). Currently, efforts are made to repair the meniscus when possible and to remove as little of the meniscus as possible (78).

For the nonsurgically treated patient, early rehabilitation consists of reducing pain and swelling with institution of hamstring and ITB stretching and short-arc CKC activities. Pool-based exercise can facilitate recovery and allow the patient to maintain endurance. Use of a cane or crutches to unload the affected side is strongly recommended. Once symptoms are reduced, the intensity of the program is increased, but activities involving loading with rotation are avoided.

For the surgically treated patient, postoperative rehabilitation depends on the complexity of the repair. Once pain-free range of motion has been established and there is no joint line tenderness, the patient should return to full weight bearing. Return to weight-bearing activities too early or overly aggressive strengthening may induce effusion and an exacerbation of pain. If this occurs, the program should be modified and the patient returned to a partial weight-bearing status. Deep squatting should be avoided during the first 6 months (15). Progressive strengthening should focus on the quadriceps and hamstrings, and include the entire lower extremity.

Osteochondritis Dissecans

Osteochondritis dissecans is a lesion of subchondral bone with or without articular cartilage involvement (79). In the knee, the most common site for a subchondral lesion is at the interior portion of the medial femoral condyle. Lesions in the lateral condyle and in the patellar articular cartilage occur with less frequency. Chondral flaps and chondral loose bodies may also be present (80,81). Patients experience intermittent mechanical symptoms with or without pain. An effusion may be present. X-ray films should include a tunnel view to evaluate the intracondylar notch. Computed tomography is helpful in evaluating the bony lesions, while MRI can provide a more accurate view of the articular cartilage. Treatment is based on the staging of the lesion, and the patient's symptoms (79). Arthroscopic evaluation is indicated when there is separation of the lesion from the femur, mechanical locking, or chronic pain and effusion.

CONCLUSIONS

Rehabilitation of disorders of the knee requires an understanding of the relevant anatomy and biomechanics, combined with appropriate exercise physiology and training principles. With this knowledge, many knee injuries can be adequately rehabilitated nonoperatively and postoperatively and patients returned to full preinjury levels of activity.

REFERENCES

1. Kibler WB. Clinical aspects of muscle injury. *Med Sci Sports Exerc* 1990;22:450–452.
2. Kibler WB, Chandler TJ, Pace BK. Principles of rehabilitation after chronic tendon injuries. *Clin Sports Med* 1992;11: 661–671.
3. Kibler WB, Chandler TJ, Stracener ES. Musculoskeletal adaptations and injuries due to overtraining. *Exerc Sports Sci Rev* 1992;20: 99–126.
4. Kibler WB, Goldberg C, Chandler TJ. Functional biomechanical deficits in running athletes with plantar fasciitis. *Am J Sports Med* 1991;19:66–71.
5. Press JM, Herring SA, Kilber WB. Rehabilitation of the combatant with musculoskeletal disorders. In: Dillingham TR, Belandres PV, eds. *Rehabilitation of the injured combatant.* Vol 1. Washington, DC: Walter Reed Medical Center, 1998; 353–415.
6. Reddy AS, Reedy MK, Seaber AV, et al. Restriction of the injury response following an acute muscle strain. *Med Sci Sports Exerc* 1993;25:321–327.
7. Leadbetter WB. Cell-matrix response in tendon injury. *Clin Sports Med* 1992;11:533–578.
8. Herring SA, Kibler WB. Rehabilitation. In: Cantu RC, Micheli LJ, eds. *ACSM's guidelines for the team physician.* Philadelphia: Lea & Febiger, 1991:191–195.
9. Roy S, Irvin R. *Sports medicine: prevention, evaluation, management and rehabilitation.* Englewood Cliffs, NJ: Prentice-Hall, 1983:299–305.
10. Young JL, Laskowski ER, Rock M. Thigh injuries in athletes. *Mayo Clin Proc* 1993;68:1099–1106.
11. Draganich LF, Jaeger RJ, Kralj AR. Coactivation of the hamstrings and quadriceps during extension of the knee. *J Bone Joint Surg [Am]* 1989;71:1075–1081.
12. Shelbourne KD, Wilckens JH, Mollabashy A, et al. Accelerated rehabilitation after acute anterior cruciate ligament reconstruction. *Am J Sports Med* 1990;18: 292–299.
13. Main WK, Scott NW. Knee anatomy. In: Scott NW, ed. *Ligament and extensor mechanism injuries of the knee: diagnosis and treatment.* St. Louis: CV Mosby, 1991:17–18.
14. Ahmed AM, Burke DL. In vitro measurement of static pressure distribution in synovial joints in the tibial surface of the knee. *J Biomech Eng* 1983;105: 216–225.
15. Fu FH, Baratz M. Meniscal injuries. In: DeLee JC, Drez D Jr, eds. *Orthopaedic sports medicine.* Philadelphia: WB Saunders, 1994:1146–1248.
16. Arnoczky SP, Warren RF. Microvasculature of the human meniscus. *Am J Sports Med* 1982;10:90–95.
17. Dillingham MF, King WD, Gamburd RS. Rehabilitation of the knee following anterior cruciate ligament and medial collateral ligament injuries. *Phys Med Rehabil Clin N Am* 1994;5:175–194.
18. Ficat RP, Hungerford DS. *Disorders of the patellofemoral joint.* Baltimore: Williams & Wilkins, 1997.
19. Hungerford DS, Barry M. Biomechanics of the patellofemoral joint. *Clin Orthop* 1979;144:9–15.
20. Putnam CA, Kozey JW. Substantive issues in running. In: Vaughn CL, ed. *Biomechanics of sport.* Boca Raton, FL: CRC Press, 1989:2–33.
21. Hilyard A. Recent developments in the management of patellofemoral pain: the McConnell programme. *Physiotherapy* 1990;76: 559–565.
22. McConnell J. The management of chondromalacia patellae: a long term solution. *Aust J Phys* 1986;32:215–219.
23. Fulkerson JP, Kalenak A, Rosenberg TD, Cox JS. Patellofemoral pain. *Instr Course Lect* 1992;41:57–71.
24. Spencer J, Hayesk, Alexander I. Knee joint effusion and quadriceps inhibition in man. *Arch Phys Med Rehabil* 1984;65:171–177.
25. Fahrer H, Rentsch HU, Gerber NJ, et al. Knee effusion and reflex inhibition of the quadriceps. *J Bone Joint Surg [Br]* 1988;70:635–638.
26. O'Neill DB, Micheli LJ, Warner JP. Patellofemoral stress: a prospective analysis of exercise treatment in adolescents and adults. *Am J Sports Med* 1992;20:151–156.
27. Shelton GL, Thigpen LK. Rehabilitation of patellofemoral dysfunction: a review of literature. *J Orthop Sports Phys Ther* 1991;14:243–248.
28. Winslow J, Yoder E. Patellofemoral pain in female ballet dancers: correlation with iliotibial band tightness and tibial external rotation. *J Orthop Sports Phys Ther* 1995;22:18–21.
29. Punicello MS. Iliotibial band tightness and medial patellar glide in patients with patellofemoral dysfunction. *J Orthop Sports Phys Ther* 1993;17:144–148.
30. McNichol K. Iliotibial tract friction syndrome in athletes. *Can J Appl Sports Sci* 1981;6(2): 176–80.

31. Noble C. Iliotibial band friction syndrome in runners. *Am J Sports Med* 1980;8:232–234.

32. Beckman M, Craig R, Lehman RC. Rehabilitation of patellofemoral dysfunction in the athlete. *Clin Sports Med* 1989;8:841.

33. Boucher JP, King MA, Lefebvre R, Pepin A. Quadriceps femoris activity in patellofemoral pain syndrome. *Am J Sports Med* 1992;20:527–532.

34. Grabiner MD, Koh TJ, Draganich LF. Neuromechanics of the patellofemoral joint. *Med Sci Sports Exerc* 1994;261:10–21.

35. Doucette SA, Goble EM. The effect of exercise on patellar tracking in lateral patellar compression syndrome. *Am J Sports Med* 1992;20:434–440.

36. Cerney K. Vastus medialis oblique/vastus lateralis muscle activity ratios for selected exercises in persons with and without patellofemoral pain syndrome. *Phys Ther* 1995;75: 672–683.

37. Hanten WP, Schulthies SS. Exercise effect on electromyographic activity of the vastus medialis oblique and vastus lateralis muscles. *Phys Ther* 1990;70:561–565.

38. Stoles M, Young A. Investigations of quadriceps inhibition: implications for clinical practice. *Physiotherapy* 1984;70:425–428.

39. Kannus P, Niittymaki S. Which factors predict outcome in the non-operative treatment of patellofemoral pain syndrome? A prospective follow up study. *Med Sci Sports Exerc* 1994;26:289–296.

40. Wild JJ, Franklin TD, Woods GW. Patellar pain and quadriceps rehabilitation: an EMG study. *Am J Sports Med* 1982;10:12–15.

41. Steinkamp LA, Dillingham MF, Markel MD, et al. Biomechanical considerations in patellofemoral joint rehabilitation. *Am J Sports Med* 1993;21:438–444.

42. Reilly DJ, Martens M. Experimental analysis of quadriceps muscle force and patellofemoral joint reaction force for various activities. *Acta Orthop Scand* 1972;43:126–137.

43. Kaplan ED. The iliotibial tract. *J Bone Joint Surg [Am]* 1958;40:817–832.

44. Black JE, Alten SR. How I manage infrapatellar tendinitis. *Phys Sport Med* 1984;12:86–92.

45. LeVeau BF, Rogers C. Selective training of the vastus medialis muscle using EMG biofeedback. *Phys Ther* 1980;60:1410–1415.

46. Ingersoll CD, Knight KL. Patellar location changes following EMG biofeedback or progressive resistive exercise. *Med Sci Sports Exerc* 1991;23:1122–1127.

47. Wise HH, Fiebert IM, Kates JL. EMG biofeedback as treatment for patellofemoral pain syndrome. *J Orthop Sports Phys Ther* 1984;6: 95–103.

48. Felder CR, Leeson MA. *The use of electromyographic biofeedback for training the vastus medialis obliquus in patients with patellofemoral pain. Clinical protocol.* Montreal, Canada: Though Technology, 1990.

49. Bockrath K, Wooden C, Worrell T, et al. Effects of patella taping on patella position and perceived pain. *Med Sci Sports Exerc* 1993;25:989–992.

50. Powers CM, Maffucci R, Hampton S. Rearfoot posture in subjects with patellofemoral pain. *J Orthop Sports Phys Ther* 1995;22: 155–160.

51. Stanitski CL. Rehabilitation following knee injury. *Clin Sports Med* 1985;4:495.

52. Greenwald WE, Bagley AM, France EP, Paulos LE. A biomechanical and clinical evaluation of a patellofemoral knee brace. *Clin Orthop* 1996;324: 187–195.

53. Finestone A, Radin EL, Lev B, et al. Treatment of overuse patellofemoral pain. Prospective randomized controlled clinical trial in a military setting. *Clin Orthop* 1993;293:208–210.

54. Ericson MO, Nisell R. Patellofemoral joint forces during ergometric cycling. *Phys Ther* 1987;67:1365–1369.

55. Messier SP, Pittala KA. Etiologic factors associated with selected running injuries. *Med Sci Sports Exerc* 1988;20:501–505.

56. Noble CA. Iliotibial band friction syndrome in runners. *Am J Sports Med* 1980;8:232–234.

57. Sutker AN, Barber FA, Jackson DW, Pagliano JW. Iliotibial band syndrome in distance runners. *Sports Med* 1984;5:447–451.

58. Olsen NK, Press JM, Young JL. Bursal injections. In: Lennard TA, ed. *Physiatric procedures in clinical practice.* Philadelphia: Henley & Belfus, 1995.

59. Gurtler RA, Stine R, Torg JS. Lachman test revisited. *Contemp Orthop* 1990;20:145–154.

60. Galway RD, Beaupre A, MacIntosh DL. Pivot shift: a clinical sign of symptomatic anterior cruciate ligament insufficiency. *J Bone Joint Surg [Br]* 1972;54:763.

61. Losee RE, Johnson TR, Southwick WO. Anterior subluxation of the lateral tibial plateau: a diagnostic test and operative repair. *J Bone Joint Surg [Am]* 1978;60:1015.

62. Shelbourne KD, Nitz P. Arthrofibrosis in acute anterior cruciate ligament reconstruction: the effect of timing of reconstruction and rehabilitation. *Am J Sports Med* 1991;19:332–335.

63. Noyes FR, Butler DL, Paulos LE, et al. Inter-articular cruciate reconstruction. Perspectives on graft strength, vascularization, and immediate motion after replacement. *Clin Orthop* 1983;172: 710–717.

64. Barrack RL, Skinner HB, Buckley SL. Proprioception in the anterior cruciate deficient knee. *Am J Sports Med* 1989;17:1–6.

65. DeLee JC, Bergfeld JA, Drez D Jr, et al. The posterior cruciate ligament. In: DeLee JC, Drez D Jr, eds. *Orthopaedic sports medicine.* Philadelphia: WB Saunders, 1994:1374–1400.

66. Cross MJ, Powell JF. Long-term follow up of posterior cruciate ligament rupture: a study of 116 cases. *Am J Sports Med* 1984;12:292–297.

67. Fowler PJ, Messieh SS. Isolated posterior cruciate ligament injuries in athletes. *Am J Sports Med* 1987;15:553–557.

68. Paroli JM, Bergfeld JA. Long term results of nonoperative treatment of isolated posterior cruciate ligament injuries in the athlete. *Am J Sports Med* 1986;15:35–38.

69. Tietjens BB. Posterior cruciate ligament injuries. *J Bone Joint Surg [Br]* 1985;59:15–19.

70. Rubinstein RA Jr, Shelbourne DK. Diagnosis of posterior cruciate ligament injuries and indications for nonoperative and operative treatment. *Operative Techn Sports Med* 1993;1:99–103.

71. Hastings DE. The non-operative management of collateral ligament injuries of the knee joint. *Clin Orthop* 1980;147:22–28.

72. Indelicato PA. Non-operative treatment of complete tears of the medial collateral ligament of the knee. *J Bone Joint Surg [Am]* 1983;65:323–329.

73. Sandberg R, Balkfors B, Nilsson B, et al. Operative vs. non-operative treatment of recent injuries to the ligaments of the knee. *J Bone Joint Surg [Am]* 1987;69:1120–1126.

74. Fairbanks TM. Knee joint changes after meniscectomy. *J Bone Joint Surg [Br]* 1948;30:64–67.

75. Cox JS, Nye CE, Schaeffer WW, et al. The degenerative effects of partial and total resection of the medial meniscus in dogs' knees. *Clin Orthop* 1965;109: 178–183.

76. Levy M, Torzilli PA, Warren RF. The effect of medial menisectomy on anterior-posterior motion of the knee. *J Bone Joint Surg [Am]* 1982;64:883–888.

77. Lynch MA, Henning CE, Glick KR. Knee joint surface changes: long term follow-up of meniscus tear treatment in stable anterior cruciate ligament reconstructions. *Clin Orthrop* 1983;172: 148–153.

78. Miller MD, Ritchie JR, Harner CD. Meniscus surgery: indications for repair. *Operative Techn Sports Med* 1994;2:164–171.

79. Green W, Banks H. Osteochondritis in children. *J Bone Joint Surg [Am]* 1958;14:26.

80. Bradley J, Dandy DJ. Osteochondritis dissecans and other lesions of the femoral condyles. *J Bone Joint Surg [Am]* 1983;65:193.

81. Clanton TO, Delee JC. Osteochondritis dissecans: history, pathophysiology and current treatment concepts. *Clin Orthop* 1982; 167:50.

Chapter 70

Foot and Ankle Injuries

Christina Yun Lee

As humans evolved from quadrupedal to bipedal locomotion, a high degree of specialized foot and ankle mechanics was required. The structures in the foot and ankle are particularly vulnerable to injury when subjected to the high-impact forces of unaided bipedal weight bearing, such as those that occur during athletic activity and dancing. Numerous other extrinsic factors, including athletic shoe construction and dance and sports demands on the foot and ankle, place these structures at risk of injury. As a result, conditions of the foot and ankle are a common reason why athletes, dancers, and the general population alike visit their physician.

Physiatrists must have a clear understanding of foot and ankle biomechanics to provide accurate diagnoses and treatment protocols for lower-limb sports injuries. Running is an essential part of many athletic endeavors for the professional as well as for the leisure sport enthusiast. Studying the biomechanics of running will aid discussion of injuries of the foot and ankle. This chapter begins with a description of the anatomy of the foot, followed by a detailed description of the complexities of the running mechanism and how it affects the foot. Specific injuries of the foot, ankle, and leg are then reviewed as they are related to faulty foot biomechanics. Progression is then toward study of the anatomy, physical examination, diagnosis, and treatment of conditions of the ankle.

The portions of this chapter on foot anatomy and biomechanics were adapted from Geiringer SR. Functional biomechanics of running. *Phys Med Rehabil State Art Rev* 1997;11:569–582. The author is grateful to Dr. Geiringer for his assistance with this chapter.

THE FOOT

Anatomy

The foot is a unique structure in that it is composed primarily of bones, tendons, and ligaments. The muscular control of the foot is accomplished predominantly through the distal tendons of muscle masses originating in the leg or distal end of the thigh. The intrinsic muscles of the foot contribute supplementary roles in the overall biomechanical function of the foot. Given that the foot is meant to withstand repetitive weight-bearing forces, this design of the foot is not unexpected.

Hindfoot

The bones of the hindfoot are the talus and calcaneus (1) (Fig. 70-1). The trochlea, the superior portion of the talus, articulates with the distal end of the tibia. The posterior aspect of the trochlea narrows, thereby rendering the ankle joint minimally stable in plantarflexion. The distal, convex aspect of the talus comes into contact with the navicular bone. The smooth articular surfaces on either side of the talus accommodate the malleoli, while the calcaneus abuts much of the inferior portion of the talus. The calcaneus is the largest bone in the foot, with a rough and expansive

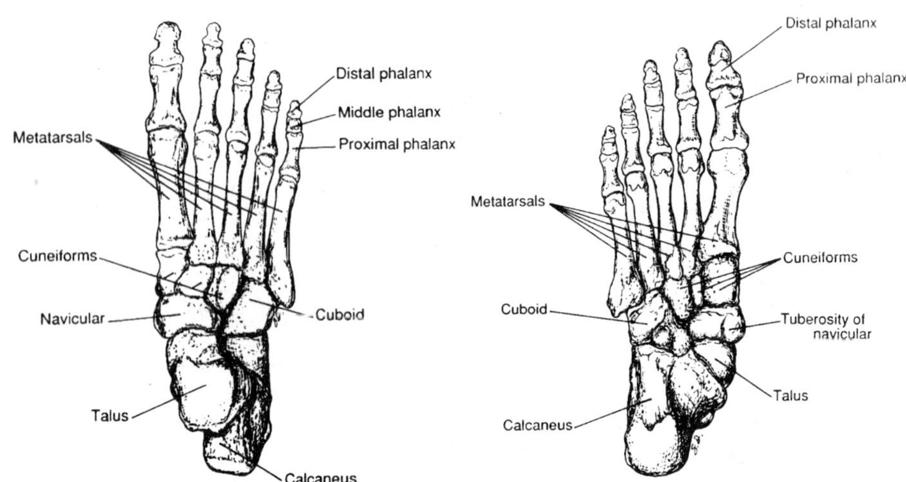

Figure 70-1. Bony anatomy of the foot. *Left.* Dorsal view. *Right.* Ventral (plantar) view. (Reprinted from *J Back Musculoskel Rehabil,* Vol. 5, Geiringer SR, The biomechanics of running, page 274, 1995, with kind permission from Elsevier Science Ireland Ltd., Bay 15K, Shannon Industrial Estate, Co. Clare, Ireland.)

posterior surface and three smooth surfaces at the anterior, superior portion where it contacts the talus. Its inferior aspect serves as the weight-bearing surface. The sustentaculum tali is a horizontal prominence off the superior, medial aspect of the calcaneus. One articular facet of the talus rests on this shelf and the plantar calcaneonavicular ("spring") ligament arises from it, providing important support for the arch. The plantar fascia originates from the bony tuberosity on the medial plantar surface of the calcaneus.

Midfoot

The midfoot is composed of the navicular, cuboid, and cuneiform bones. The navicular bone lies on the medial aspect of the foot and has an easily palpable medial tuberosity (1). The cuboid is placed lateral to the navicular, and the three cuneiform bones (medial, intermediate, and lateral) are distal to the navicular (1) (see Fig. 70-1). The bones of the midfoot are arranged as a compact unit, with a dorsal arch and with the plantar surface forming the transverse arch of the foot.

Forefoot

The individual phalanges and the metatarsals together make up the forefoot (1) (see Fig. 70-1). In the first digit of the foot, two phalanges with one interphalangeal joint exist. In the other digits of the foot, three phalanges comprise each toe, as in the hand. The metatarsals become increasingly short and thick as they progress from the lateral to the medial aspect of the foot, with the first metatarsal being the shortest and thickest. The medial and lateral cuneiform bones of the midfoot protrude more distally than the intermediate bone, resulting in the relative immobilization of the second metatarsal within the grip of the cuneiform bones.

Soft Tissues

The clinically significant foot ligaments can be found on the plantar surface (1). The long plantar ligament links the middle metatarsal, cuboid, and calcaneus bones, while the powerful, short plantar ligament attaches to the plantar surfaces of the cuboid and calcaneus bones. These ligaments, along with the plantar fascia, provide support to the longitudinal arch of the foot. The plantar fascia is a fibroaponeurotic structure that originates at the medial tubercle of the calcaneus. At its origin, the fascia is thickened and then broadens as it courses anteriorly. Transverse and oblique fibers join the fascial fibers at the midfoot and beyond.

The foot intrinsic muscles, except for the extensor digitorum brevis, are situated on the plantar aspect, (1). The muscles are arranged in four layers, and do not play a primary role in providing structural integrity for the foot. Except for the popliteus, all muscles originating in the leg cross the ankle and thereby act on the intervening joints (1,2). The muscles of the anterior compartment serve as dorsiflexors and invertors, whereas the lateral compartment muscles act as plantarflexors and evertors. The Achilles muscles also contribute as powerful plantarflexors with an added valgus force on the calcaneus. Further discussion of muscle function during the gait cycle can be found elsewhere in this textbook and in other sources (3).

Running and the Biomechanics of the Foot

Most sports activities involve running. Running itself is an extremely popular method of aerobic exercise for the young and old alike. While running or jogging is easily accomplished by most of us, it is actually a result of the synthesis of remarkably complex component parts into a fluid chain of linked events. Examination of the foot, with its unique but manifold biomechanical qualities and adaptations, can shed light on the essential role of running in the evolution and survival of our species. In everyday activities as well as in the awesome feats of elite athletes, our feet endure widely diverse surfaces, varied movements ranging from slow walks to sprints, and untold miles through the years. For some fortunate athletes, the feet survive these insults with little injury. For others, a running-related injury may occur. The sports physiatrist must have a detailed understanding of lower-limb mechanics, especially of the foot, so an accurate diagnosis can be made and an individualized treatment program developed. Treatment of primary injury, rehabilitation to prevent recurrences, and training to enhance athletic performance are the goals of rehabilitation.

During running, the foot comes into contact with the ground and ideally serves two purposes. First, the foot should absorb all of the energy on impact. Second, it should be rigid enough to prevent the limb from buckling above it. A balance between these two conflicting goals must be achieved in order for efficient biomechanical running to be attained. With isolation of each phase of the running cycle, analysis of the foot reveals a well-adapted biomechanical structure. Rigidity is first dominant at heel strike, preventing collapse of the leg. During the stance phase, flexibility of the foot is more crucial. Rigidity is once again most beneficial at toe off.

The subtalar joint, between the talus and calcaneus in the hindfoot, provides the important key to understanding foot motion. Movement in this joint occurs about an axis inclined 40 degrees up from horizontal and adducted 20 degrees from the midline (4), resulting in the familiar "mitered hinge" configuration of the joint (4). This arrangement allows several paired actions: plantarflexion-dorsiflexion, adduction-abduction, and inversion-eversion. These movements are linked at the subtalar joint, thereby allowing the combined motions of plantarflexion-adduction-inversion, and dorsiflexion-abduction-eversion. These movements correlate functionally with supination and pronation, respectively (4).

Motion at the calcaneocuboid and talonavicular joints in the midfoot is also linked to the subtalar joint. With eversion (or pronation) of the hindfoot and fixation of the forefoot in a weight-bearing position, the axes of the midfoot joints are aligned, allowing free, "unlocked" motion. With inversion (supination) of the hindfoot, alignment of the midfoot joint axes is not achieved. The joints are relatively "locked," resulting in decreased movement but more stability in the foot (4,5).

At the end of the stance phase, just before toe off, the metatarsophalangeal joints are in a fully dorsiflexed position. Internal rotation occurs around the head of the first metatarsal bone, planted to the ground. This motion can be represented as a clockwise pivoting of the left foot around the great toe. Simultaneously, the hindfoot externally rotates, with resultant tautness of the plantar fascia. This tightening of the fascia leads to elevation and rigidity of the arch of the foot, known as the *windlass mechanism* (6) (Fig. 70-2).

Most clinicians regard the beginning of the gait (or running) cycle to occur at heel strike, although some argue that toe off is more logical (7). The stance phase occurs as long as any portion of the foot or shoe is in contact with the ground, and the swing phase lasts until the heel contacts the ground again (8). Running is differentiated from walking by the introduction of a float phase, when both feet are off the ground at the same time, implying that stance occurs less than 50% of the time during the running cycle for each foot (3). With increasing running speed, the time spent in the float phase is prolonged relative to the duration of stance. Most long-distance runners land heel first. Others land foot flat, and sprinters land on the ball of the foot. Consequently, sprinters must modify their traditional concept of the running cycle. These athletes are also involved in high acceleration rates and speeds, leading them prone to a high incidence of hamstring and gluteal strains. Hamstring ruptures also occur commonly.

The biomechanics of the foot allow for the proper orientation of the foot during heel strike so as to avoid collapse of the leg. In preparation for landing, the foot is inverted at the end of the swing phase. Inversion at the subtalar joint is linked to the midfoot, and the joints there are locked. The foot contacts the floor in its rigid, supinated position (2), leading to the typical wear pattern at the lateral part of the heel of the running shoe.

Distribution of the weight-bearing forces becomes most important during the stance phase. Immediately after heel strike, the subtalar joint rapidly moves into eversion. In the midfoot, this transition is evident in the alignment of the joint axes and in the unlocking of the bony structure of the foot. By inference, some extent of pronation while running is normal as well as advantageous. The weight-bearing foot is in a flattened position, thus achieving greater surface area distribution (2,3) and reducing the risk of injury.

The windlass mechanism occurs at the end of the stance phase with toe off (see Fig. 70-2). Complete reversal of midfoot and hindfoot movement does not occur, but the arch is converted into a somewhat rigid structure by the taut plantar fascia. The foot can leave the ground in a relatively locked position (2). The swing phase then marks the interval when the foot cycles from eversion to inversion in preparation for the following heel strike.

The biomechanics of the lower limb in relation to the foot is also important to know when evaluating foot and ankle problems. At heel strike, external rotation of the femur and tibia results from the supinated and rigid posture of the foot. During the foot's transition to pronation-eversion, the thigh and leg move simultaneously into internal rotation (Fig. 70-3). In mid-stance, a valgus moment occurs at the knee with a resultant increased Q angle. When toe off is reached, the tibia, knee, and femur

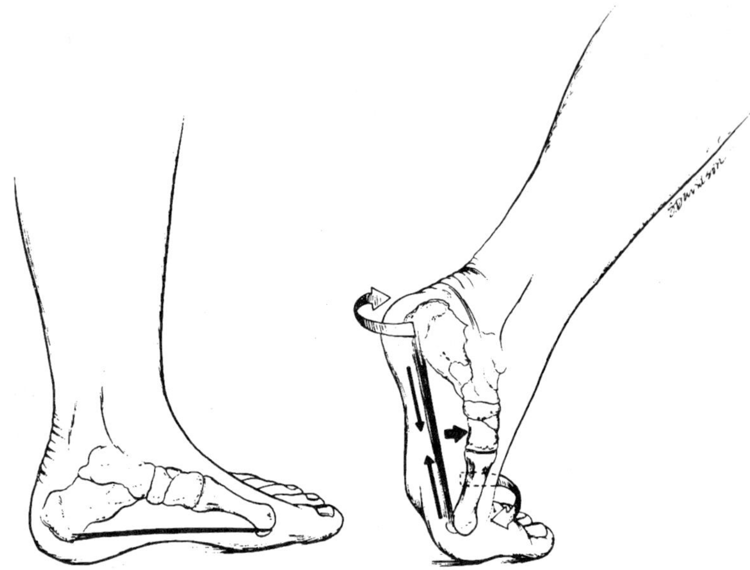

Figure 70-2. The windlass mechanism. At end-stance phase, the forefoot internally rotates around the first metatarsal head while the hindfoot externally rotates. This puts tension on the plantar fascia, increasing the height of the longitudinal arch and creating relative stability for push off. (Reprinted from *J Back Musculoskel Rehabil,* Vol. 5, Geiringer SR, The biomechanics of running, page 276, 1995, with kind permission from Elsevier Science Ireland Ltd., Bay 15K, Shannon Industrial Estate, Co. Clare, Ireland.)

have mostly regained neutral orientations as the windlass mechanism is activated. Similar to the foot during the swing phase, the lower limb cycles through internal rotation and then to external rotation in preparation for the next heel-strike phase (7). During the moments just after heel strike until mid-stance, the pelvic girdle and lumbar structures rotate inward toward the anterior midline and return to a nearly neutral position for much of the remainder of the running cycle (7).

Of paramount importance during running is the reduction and distribution of impact forces. Measurements of peak forces during running have been performed and scaled to multiples of body weight. These measurements have revealed forces up to 8 times body weight occurring at the Achilles tendon, 3 times body weight at the plantar fascia, up to 14 times body weight at the ankle joint, almost 7 times body weight at the patellar tendon, and 11 times body weight at the patellofemoral joint (9). During running simulations, the heel pad demonstrated an average absorption of 79% of impact energy, an amount that does not change even after a 10-km run. The peak ground reaction force is achieved 25 msec after heel strike (10). Both the ankle and the knee are effective at absorbing the transmitted energy (11). Rotation at the knee is minimized by movement at the subtalar joint (12). Following heel strike, the large two-joint muscles, including the gastrocnemius and rectus femoris, contribute to the transfer of energy in a proximal direction from the distal end of the limb (13). A reciprocal transfer of energy from the proximal to the distal end of the limb occurs at end-stance and toe off via these same muscles.

The more experienced runners do prove to be more economic in their energy expenditure (14). The beginner tends to use greater forces for propulsion and deceleration with increased variability in these forces. Physical attributes and metabolic composition have been linked to the optimal distance chosen by a runner for competition (15). Thus, natural selection does play a role in identifying sprinters and long-distance runners.

Intrinsic Factors and Their Relationship to Biomechanics

In addition to the fundamental principles of the biomechanics of running, several other important variables, including intrinsic and extrinsic factors, must be considered when clinically assessing the runner. Intrinsic factors (16) are those based within the neuromusculoskeletal system, including overpronation of the foot, patella alta, and distribution of shock absorption. These factors can contribute to poor biomechanics and can lead to potential injury.

Leg-length discrepancy (LLD) is one example of an intrinsic factor that may lead to injury in the athlete. One can expect to find some leg-length differences in the general population, but clinical experience suggests that LLD of more than 1 cm could result in injury. Other conditions such as stress fractures, vertebral disk injuries, and hip and back pain have been associated with LLD in runners (17). Other intrinsic or extrinsic causes need to be considered before prescribing heel lifts, particularly if the LLD has been present since bone maturation. Flexibility and strength problems in the leg and foot have been linked to plantar fasciitis (PF) (18), but whether these effects are causative or secondary is uncertain. Patellofemoral pain is associated with increased Q angle and diminished endurance of the quadriceps. These factors are likely causative in this particular condition (19).

Extrinsic Factors and Their Relationship to Biomechanics

Extrinsic factors are those that arise external from the neuromusculoskeletal system of the athlete (16). An extrinsic factor itself might pose a problem, or it may be the solu-

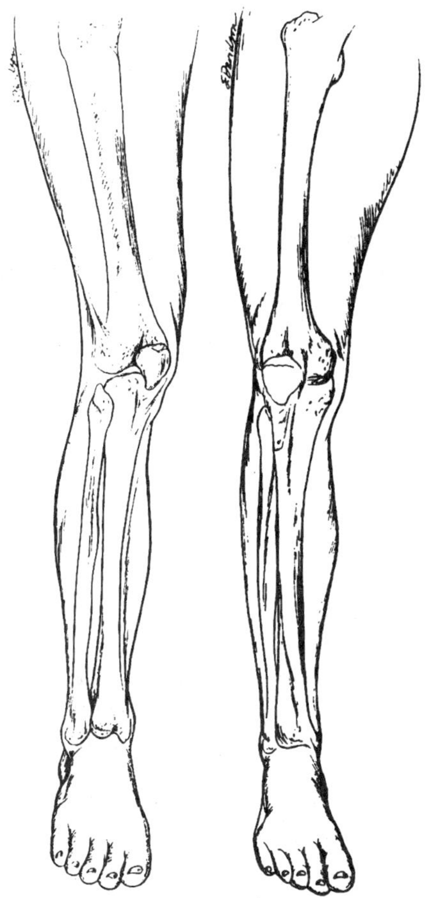

Figure 70-3. The linking of foot motion with lower-extremity mechanics. *Left.* Foot pronation is accompanied by tibial, femoral, and hip joint internal rotation, and a valgus posture at the knee with an increased Q angle. *Right.* Foot supination is accompanied by tibial, femoral, and hip joint internal rotation, with a neutral or varus posture at the knee. (Reprinted from *J Back Musculoskel Rehabil,* Vol. 5, Geiringer SR, The biomechanics of running, page 277, 1995, with kind permission from Elsevier Science Ireland Ltd., Bay 15K, Shannon Industrial Estate, Co. Clare, Ireland.)

tion used to correct an intrinsic factor. Orthoses, training errors, inadequate shoes, and a concrete running surface are examples of extrinsic deficits. Overuse injuries can result from many of these factors, particularly training errors (16).

The orthotic shoe insert is the most popular aid used by runners to correct biomechanical dysfunction. Runners use these inserts for many conditions, including overpronation and underpronation of the foot, patellofemoral pain, LLD, Achilles tendinitis, shin splints, and PF (20). In a study of 500 long-distance runners by Gross et al (20), 378 (75.6%) found their inserts beneficial and 450 (90%) continued to use them even after becoming asymptomatic. Orthoses are most useful when they are prescribed for the correction of clear mechanical problems such as overpronation or LLD. Prescriptions of custom or off-the-shelf orthoses should not be made if there is no obvious association beween the symptoms and the biomechanical problem. This also holds true for runners who may incidentally have an underlying deficit, but who are otherwise asymptomatic (21). Orthotic shoe inserts are most successful for the overpronated foot rather than for the rigid, supinated foot (22). Subtalar overpronation is controlled only minimally by rearfoot posting alone (23).

The engineering and design of the running shoe have advanced rapidly with the improvements in materials science technology. Countless innovative "energy-return" systems have been designed for the midsoles of shoes. These new shoes have been shown to have a beneficial but small influence on performance (24). The firm heel counter in current running shoes aids in controlling hindfoot movement, especially inversion and eversion. Jorgensen (25) showed that runners consume 2.4% less oxygen on average and reduce stresses on the musculoskeletal aspects of the leg when using these shoes. The improper running shoe can be an extrinsic cause of injury also. For joggers and less-experienced runners, overly worn outsoles may lead to decreased shock absorption and remote but severe outcomes, including stress fracture of the femoral neck (26).

Foot Injuries and Their Relationship to Biomechanics

Plantar Fasciitis

The plantar fascia is a strong fibroaponeurotic structure, akin to a ligament, that originates at the inferior medial calcaneal tuberosity (1). It aids in maintaining the integrity of the longitudinal arch of the foot, although the plantar fascia will relax some in the normal state with weight bearing. During the mid-stance of walking or the foot-flat phase of running, until toe off, the fascia flattens and stretches to the greatest degree. At the toe-off stage, the fascia tightens, pulling on its insertional points. The distal portion of the plantar fascia is divided into interdigitating fibers to ensure that no isolated "weak point in the chain" exists in the forefoot. The repetitive strain on the isolated, fixed attachment at the fascia's origin at the medial calcaneus can lead to the microtrauma of overuse, and the clinical syndrome of PF. With overpronation (Fig. 70-3), increased stress is placed on the calcaneal origin of the plantar fascia, rendering runners with pes planus more susceptible to the condition. Tightness of the gastrocnemius-soleus complex may also be a contributing factor, considering the valgus moment on the calcaneus from the soleus (27). Inadequate distribution of forces of impact with each step can lead to the presentation of a rigid, supinated foot in patients with PF (27). Finally, some investigators isolated nerve entrapment as the cause of heel pain (28–31), although this is less widely accepted.

PF is characterized by the predominant symptom of pain at the plantar surface of the heel, initially worse with running and with weight bearing immediately after arising from sleep. If the pain is left untreated, it can return with activity or persist throughout the day. When continued heel pain is coexistent with low-back or other joint pain, the practitioner must consider a seronegative spondyloarthropathy (28,32). The physical examination reveals a primary area of tenderness directly over the medial calcaneal tubercle, in addition to the possibility of overpronation and muscle tightness. Excessive wear of the outsole and weakening of the supporting structures of the midsole should be assessed by inspection of the running shoes. A horizontally oriented bone spur on the calcaneus might be present on radiographic studies (28,32). This is a common radiographic finding and must be thought of as a result of the fasciitis, *not* a cause. Bone forms new bone, such as the bony tuberosities at muscle attachments, in response to repeated traction. At the heel, the bone spur is oriented along the axis of the plantar fascia and develops at the fascia's calcaneal origin. Although on x-ray films it appears to be capable of generating pain, the spur does not need to be removed surgically (28,33–39). Occasionally, relief of the pain does occur with surgery because the fascia itself is also sectioned. It is more prudent to avoid disrupting the natural anatomy and to leave it intact if possible. Up to 15% of the general population has such spurs (35,37).

Acute management includes relative rest (16), icing, and anti-inflammatory medication taken for 7 to 10 days. It is rarely necessary to treat with corticosteroid injection around the affected heel region, and there is a distant chance of atrophy of the specialized fat pads within the weight-bearing heel pad. In addition to treating the acute condition, the practitioner must search for the biomechanical factors that can be rectified. Overpronation is a common intrinsic factor that can be corrected, perhaps with an in-shoe orthosis, especially if proper low-dye taping is consistently helpful (40). If valgus of the hindfoot is evident, a heel cup alone or an arch support with an integrated heel cup may be prescribed. Important extrinsic factors such as a worn-out shoe or always running against traffic flow should be considered. When running facing traffic on a banked road, the right (uphill) foot is persistently overpronated compared to the supinated left (downhill) foot. After the acute PF pain has resolved and the biomechanical deficits have been corrected, the athlete may follow a graduated program to increase running mileage or other activity.

Metatarsalgia

Running places a tremendous amount of force on the plantar surfaces of the metatarsal heads. The medial two or three metatarsal heads in particular are subjected to much of the high-impact force of running at mid-stance. As stated previously, some degree of pronation is normal and actually aids in dispersing the force of impact over a larger surface area of the sole. However, overpronation can lead to increased pressure on the metatarsal bones, pain with running, and ultimately pain even with walking. Physical examination reveals tenderness over the involved metatarsal heads as well as evidence of overpronation.

Pain relief is achieved by the treatment measures followed for PF, including acute intervention and use of orthotics to compensate for faulty biomechanics. Use of a longitudinal arch support may provide good relief. A metatarsal pad, appropriately placed just proximal to the metatarsal heads, might also be prescribed. The pad will transfer some of the load from the metatarsal heads to the fleshy part of the sole where the pad is located, providing rapid pain relief for many. Surgical removal of the metatarsal heads is rarely necessary.

Stress Fractures

Stress fractures of the foot and lower extremity are thought to occur as a result of an underpronating foot with a supinated posture. The theory is that a foot in this position cannot absorb shock effectively. The forces are focused on the metatarsal and calcaneus bones instead of over a larger area as occurs with the natural pronation in mid-stance (27). More recent arguments support abnormal muscular stress to a normal bone as the underlying causative factor leading to the stress fracture (41). However, this theory does not explain sufficiently the relationship of the supinated foot. Nevertheless, a dramatic increase in exercise activity is often an underlying factor. The second and third metatarsal shafts are particularly vulnerable to stress fractures (42–45). Physical examination reveals extreme point tenderness with palpation directly over the stress fracture, dropping off to no tenderness within 1 to 2 cm (46). The fracture may not be evident on plain x-ray films initially, but a bone scan is sensitive for revealing the remodeling bone even in the early stages (47).

The mainstay of treatment of a stress fracture is an alteration of the exercise routine. Relative rest (16) to achieve a nearly pain-free level, followed by a gradual increase in activity, usually constitutes successful treatment. Orthotic devices can also be useful. A cushioning longitudinal arch support can provide a filler for the midfoot space on impact if a high arch is an underlying cause. This corrective measure disperses the shock over a larger surface area. Since a large proportion of the general population does not have supinated feet, shoe manufacturers do not design their shoes for this group, and the proper amount of arch support should be added to the shoe. The athlete should also select a shoe with excellent cushioning features, and avoid running surfaces composed of asphalt or concrete.

Leg Injuries and Their Relationship to Biomechanics

Medial Tibial Stress Syndrome

The term *shin splint* has been used for years for a condition that is now known as *medial tibial stress syndrome* (MTSS)

(48). As more has been elucidated about the cause of this condition, MTSS has replaced *shin splint* as the accepted term. Increased third-phase scintigraphic uptake in the tibia at the attachment of the medial portion of the soleus reveals the site of the enthesitis resulting in MTSS (49).

MTSS is frequently diagnosed in runners and dancers and is the most common leg injury in these groups. Although there are numerous contributing biomechanical factors, the most common is excessive pronation of the foot and consequent increased internal tibial rotation during the stance phase of running (49–52), with additional stress on the soleus. A high velocity of midfoot pronation just after heel strike has also been implicated as a causative factor (27).

Clinically, the patient presents with a well-localized area of pain at the medial, distal aspect of the tibia, frequently after an increase in the intensity or duration of the exercise regimen. Initially, the symptoms are relieved rapidly with rest, but with continued running, pain can occur even at rest (52). The physical examination is remarkable for tenderness along a portion of the distal tibial shaft with possible minimal swelling (52). Excessive pronation of the midfoot, with or without valgus of the heel, can be observed. Abnormal mechanics are notable with rapid walking or running; therefore, it is important for the practitioner to observe the patient running.

Bone scan studies of MTSS will reveal diffuse, patchy areas of increased tracer uptake along the medial aspect of the tibia (53). Radiographs usually appear normal, and other diagnostic studies are not useful. Treatment for MTSS includes relative rest, anti-inflammatory medications, ice, and prevention with identification of any underlying biomechanical causative factors. The search for these problems should include distinguishing whether hindfoot valgus or midfoot pronation is the ultimate cause.

Other diagnoses to consider include tibial stress fracture and anterior compartment syndrome. A stress fracture can also occur after an abrupt increase in the exercise routine, but examination reveals a much more localized site of exquisite tenderness, with a 1- to 2-cm region affected and no pain immediately adjacent (46). Bone scanning can help in distinguishing a stress fracture from MTSS. With a stress fracture, intense uptake will appear in one area only, unlike the segmental uptake seen in the setting of MTSS (unless there are numerous stress fractures, which can be extremely difficult to differentiate from a stress syndrome). The anterior compartment syndrome is the most prevalent compartment syndrome. It often appears with the first sessions of running after a break of many months. Pain and tenderness are notably located in the muscle itself and not along the tibia. Walking will also elicit the pain and the athlete will ambulate with great care. The syndrome is usually self-limited, with the treatment consisting only of allowing the patient to run when the symptoms allow. The practitioner must identify acute compartment syndrome, as this is severe and requires emergent operative treatment.

Patellofemoral Syndrome

Much of the recent literature addressing this condition has focused on the proper accepted name. *Chondromalacia patella* should not be used as the name of a clinical condition, but rather should be used to describe the initial histopathologic changes seen in cartilage in some patients with patellofemoral syndrome (PS) (52). The classic presentation of PS is aching, anterior knee pain, precipitated by overuse, stair climbing, squatting, or prolonged sitting. These causative factors involve positions of knee flexion or loading of the flexed knee (54,55). Clicking of the joint is a common finding, while swelling is not.

Typical physical examination findings include pain with compression of the patella against the femoral condyles, pain with displacement from side to side, and pain with squatting. Numerous biomechanical factors can directly influence PS (56–60). Specifically, excessive pronation of the foot is often the culprit (61–63). In those cases, if pain relief is not achieved with the wearing of proper shoes, a change in running surface, and so on, treatment with orthotics may be necessary.

THE ANKLE

Anatomy

The ankle is primarily a hinge-type joint, with the malleoli gripping the trochlea tali much like a mortise and tenon configuration. The ankle joint allows for normal passive range of motion of 20 degrees of dorsiflexion and 50 degrees of plantarflexion (64). Due to the slightly wider trochlea anteriorly, the ankle joint is relatively unstable in plantarflexion and maximally stable in dorsiflexion.

Sports physiatrists need to consider three important ligament regions in the distal end of the limb when evaluating sports-related injuries of the foot and ankle (Figs. 70-4 and 70-5). On the medial aspect of the ankle joint is the thick deltoid ligament, a four-part structure that flares out from the medial malleolus of the tibia. It is composed of the anterior and posterior tibiotalar ligaments, the tibionavicular ligament, and the tibiocalcaneal ligament. The deltoid ligament protects against eversion injuries of the ankle. The plantar calcaneonavicular (or "spring") and medial talocalcaneal ligaments are also situated on the medial side of the foot. The spring ligament prevents downward displacement of the head of the talus, thereby helping to support the highest portion of the arch. Because some of the elasticity of the arch is attributed to it, it has been called the *spring ligament.* Three lateral ankle ligaments aid in minimizing inversion and in limiting posterior talar movement. The lateral ligaments include the posterior talofibular (PTFL), the anterior talofibular (ATFL), and the calcaneofibular (CFL) ligaments. Inversion sprains are much more common because of the relatively weak nature

Figure 70-4. The right ankle joint and its ligaments as viewed from (*A*) the medial aspect and (*B*) the lateral aspect. (Reproduced by permission from Snell RS. *Clinical anatomy for medical students.* 5th ed. Boston: Little, Brown, 1995:584.)

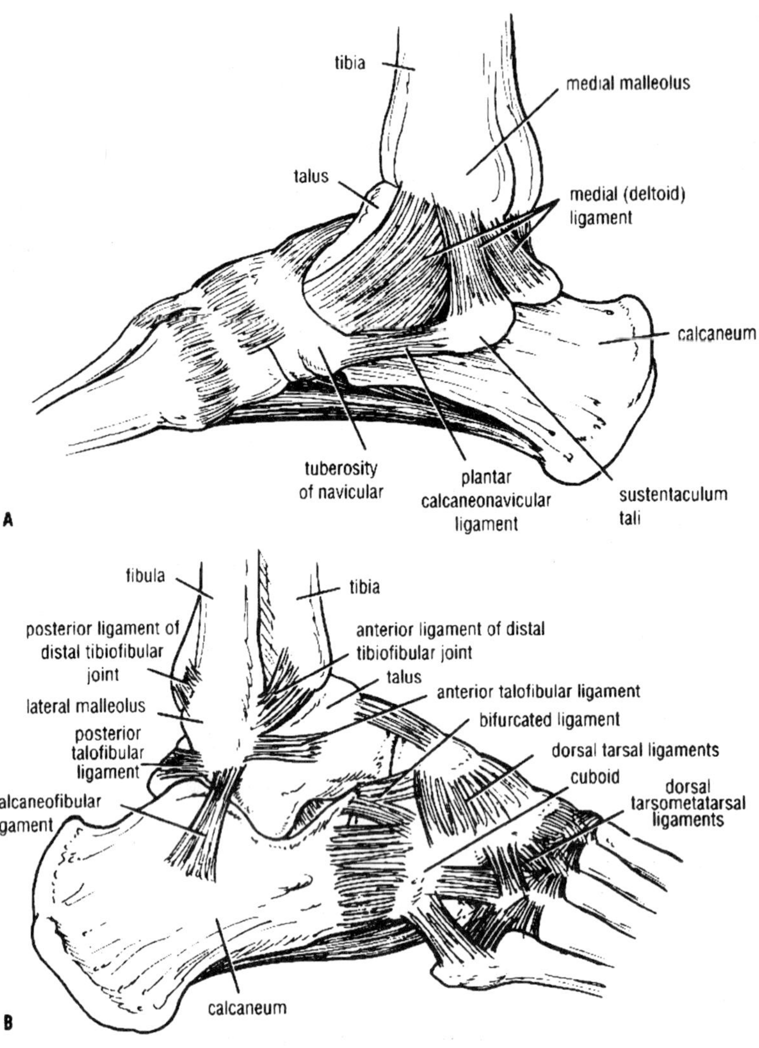

of the three lateral ligaments. In the plantarflexed and inverted position, the ATFL is particularly at risk for injury because of its relative increased tension and nearly vertical orientation. Most injuries of the ankle occur in this position. Finally, the tibiofibular syndesmosis joins the tibia and fibula anterolaterally. The syndesmosis consists of the anterior and posterior inferior tibiofibular ligaments, the interosseous ligament, and the interosseous membrane.

Numerous lower-limb muscles add protection and strength to the ankle region. These include the gastrocnemius, soleus, anterior tibialis, posterior tibialis, peroneus longus, peroneus brevis, flexor digitorum longus, and flexor hallucis longus muscles. The peroneus longus and brevis are the major dynamic stabilizers of the ankle.

The most important factor to consider regarding the lower-limb functional anatomy above the ankle is the "Q angle" at the knee (65). The Q angle is defined by the long axes of the femur and tibia (with the tibial line passing through the tuberosity and the midpoint of the patella), typically measuring 5 to 15 degrees in the valgus direction in normal knees. An increased Q angle may not itself cause running injuries, but it may reveal underlying abnormal biomechanics of the foot, knee, or hip. An example of such a case would be the patellofemoral joint, a frequent site of running injuries. The patella is lined posteriorly with cartilage and normally tracks smoothly over the femoral condyles. Clinically significant pathology may arise in conditions that cause altered patellar tracking, especially in a lateral direction. Q angles of 15 to 20 degrees or more may signal the underlying biomechanical cause.

Physical Examination of the Ankle

Examination of the ankle begins with careful assessment of the structures for localizing areas of swelling and maximal tenderness. A thorough examination must include palpation of the key ligaments, tendons, and bones in the foot, ankle, and distal region of the lower limb, including the lateral ankle ligaments, the syndesmosis, the posterior tibial and peroneal tendons, the Achilles tendon, the fifth metatarsal base and shaft, and the tibia and fibula. The bony structures must be scrutinized for possible fracture.

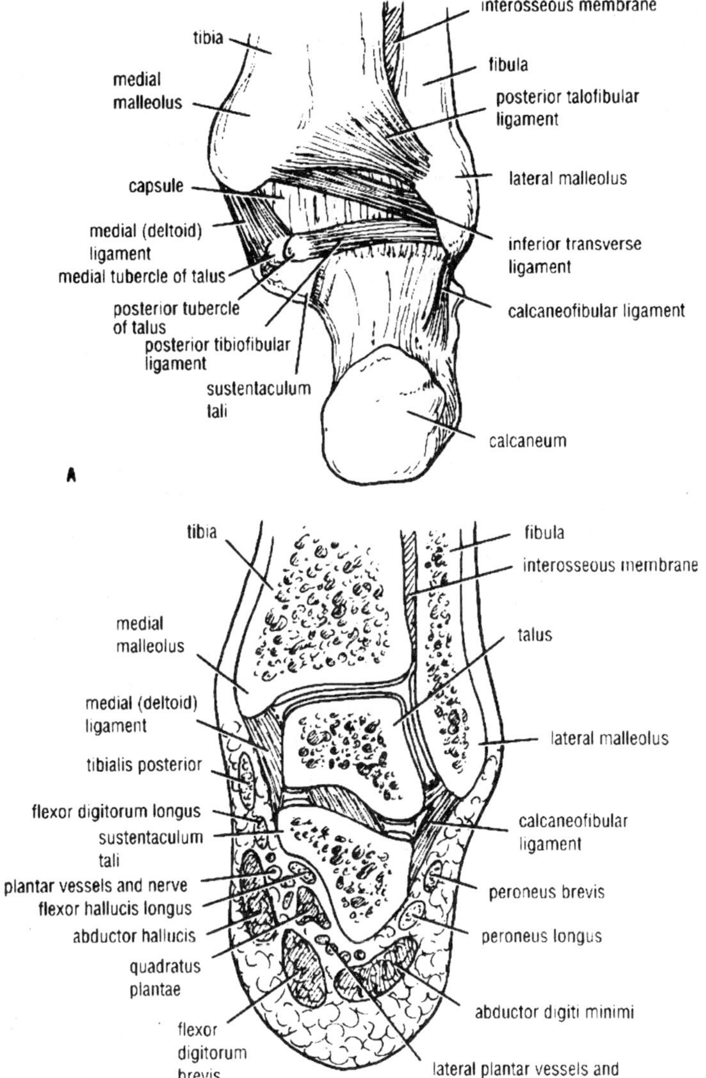

Figure 70-5. The right ankle joint as viewed from (*A*) the posterior aspect and (*B*) the coronal section. (Reproduced by permission from Snell RS. *Clinical anatomy for medical students.* 5th ed. Boston: Little, Brown, 1995:585.)

Several special stress tests should be included in the routine examination of an injured ankle. The reliability of these tests is highly dependent on the clinician's technique and on the patient's success in relaxing and cooperating.

The *anterior drawer sign* is elicited when ankle instability exists. It is an important manual stress test to evaluate the competence of the ATFL. The test is performed with the patient sitting with the knee flexed at 90 degrees and the foot in a few degrees of plantarflexion. While the heel is grasped and pulled forward, a posterior force is applied to the tibia. An ATFL stretch or tear is indicated if more than 5 mm of translation of the talus is achieved (52).

The *inversion (talar tilt) test* stresses the CFL. The medial part of the tibia is grasped in one hand and the lateral aspect of the talus and calcaneus is held in the other. With the ankle joint in neutral position, the examiner inverts the heel with force. Displacement of the talus is normally limited with a solid end point. A positive test result is indicated by an increase in the talar tilt with separation of the talus from the tibia (66).

The *eversion test* can be performed to demonstrate incompetence of the infrequently injured medial ligaments of the ankle. One hand grips the heel while the other holds the distal part of the lower limb. A positive test result is elicited if eversion stress results in increased prominence of the medial tibiotalar joint.

Injury to the inferior tibiofibular ligaments can be evaluated by the *transverse (side-to-side) stress test.* While holding the calcaneus in one hand and the tibia and fibula in the other, the examiner stresses the talus forcibly from side to side. A "clunk" may be detected with injury of the ligament as the talus contacts the tibia or fibula.

Syndesmosis injuries can be identified by the presence of tenderness over the syndesmosis as well as a positive *squeeze test* result. The fibula and tibia are squeezed together midway between the knee and ankle. A syndesmosis sprain is diagnosed if pain is reproduced at the distal syndesmosis. Syndesmosis sprains occur with 1% to 11% of sprained ankles and increase the risk of developing diastasis at the ankle joint (67).

Mechanism of Ankle Injury

Ankle injuries in the athlete and in the general population are common. In sport-related activities alone, injuries of the ankle comprise a large percentage of the total injuries: basketball, 45%; volleyball, 25%; and soccer, 31% (68). Eighty-five percent of ankle injuries are sprains (68). Of these, 85% are inversion sprains of the lateral ligaments (69,70). Deltoid or medial ligament eversion sprains make up 5% to 6% of ankle sprains, and syndesmosis injuries constitute 10% (69). With medial ligament injuries, there is a higher association of a lateral malleolar fracture or compromise of the interosseous membrane.

Ankle sprains are most common when the foot is plantarflexed. The injury occurs typically when the body weight is forced down on a plantarflexed and internally rotated ankle. The ATFL is often the first ligament injured when an inversion-plantarflexion stress is applied. The CFL is subsequently involved, and is frequently torn in association with the ATFL. With severe inversion sprains, the PTFL can be injured with possible concomitant posterior displacement of the talus. In sprained ankles that underwent surgery, 40% to 99% had a CFL tear in association with the ATFL (71,72). The deltoid ligament can be damaged in eversion injuries. Syndesmosis injuries can occur with inversion and dorsiflexion injuries or with rotational stress. Pain located anteriorly along with the inability to bear weight may signify injury to the syndesmosis.

Ankle ligament disruption can be described by a three-grade classification system (52,66). The classification scheme is based on pathology, function, and instability. *Grade I* injuries involve mild stretching of the ligament without a macroscopic tear. Minimal or no swelling is present and the joint is stable on testing. Point tenderness over the ligament may be evident, and range of motion may be mildly restricted. Functional ability is not impaired or only minimally so. After appropriate treatment, the athlete can return to sports within 7 to 10 days (72,73).

Grade II, or moderate, injuries represent a partial macroscopic tear with mild to moderate instability. Moderate swelling, tenderness, ecchymosis, or hemorrhage may be apparent. Range of motion may be restricted. The functional ability is compromised, demonstrated by a limp during walking and an inability to toe raise and to hop on the affected foot.

A *grade III* injury is severe with complete rupture of the ligament. Marked swelling with ecchymosis is present, along with pronounced instability with positive results on anterior drawer and varus laxity tests. Significant functional loss with an inability to bear weight fully and a limited range of motion accompanies this injury grade.

Radiographic Assessment

Plain radiographs of the ankle (including anteroposterior, lateral, and mortise views) are required if a moderate to severe injury is diagnosed. Fracture or diastasis of the ankle joint must be ruled out. Widening of the tibiofibular gap can be assessed by the mortise view to evaluate for a syndesmosis tear with diastasis. This view can also evaluate the distal ends of the tibia and fibula as well as the talus. Diastasis of the ankle can be further assessed on an external rotation stress radiograph. A tibiofibular gap on anteroposterior and mortise views of more than 6 mm signifies diastasis (66). Other common fractures seen on routine x-ray films could include osteochondral fractures of the talus, lateral process fractures of the talus, fracture of the anterior process of the calcaneus, and fractures of the medial or lateral malleolus (66). If fracture of a metatarsal is suspected, anteroposterior and oblique views of the foot should be obtained. Ankle arthrography is rarely performed to evaluate for ligament injury because of the availability of magnetic resonance imaging (MRI) and the current treatment protocols.

MRI can identify acute lateral ankle ligament injury accurately if periarticular hemorrhage, edema, loss of continuity of the ligaments, and an irregular or wavy contour is present (74). Other soft-tissue injuries such as deltoid ligament and peroneal tendon disruptions can be demonstrated with MRI (66). MRI also can be valuable in evaluating elongated or redundant ligaments, which can occur with chronic sprains. Because of the high costs involved, MRI is usually reserved for the assessment of chronic pain after inversion sprains.

Rehabilitation of the Ankle Sprain

The goal of rehabilitation is to prevent functional instability of the ankle. Severe injuries are more prone to develop residual instability than are mild injuries. Chronic functional instability is associated with mechanical instability and peroneal weakness.

Functional treatment of grade I or II lateral ligament injuries is the current treatment of choice with early controlled mobilization (71,75,76). Patients are able to return to normal activities more quickly with conservative treatment than with surgery. The potential complications of surgery are also avoided. Most importantly, prognosis is good to excellent: disability with grade I injury averages 8 days; that with grade II injury averages 15 days.

Treatment of the grade III ligament injury is controversial. Both operative and nonoperative treatments have been successful (72). Most studies comparing the surgical and nonsurgical treatment of acute lateral ankle ligament injuries have concluded that the nonsurgical approach is the most successful treatment for complete tears (72,73,77–80).

In the acute phase of treatment of the ankle sprain, the PRICE (*p*rotection, *r*est, *i*ce, *c*ompression, and *e*levation) principle is followed. Ice is diligently applied three times per day, with compression and elevation. Ankle support and protection should be provided with air cast splints, lace-up braces, or taping. Crutches are used until full weight bearing can be accomplished without pain. The patient can progress to the next phase of treatment when full weight bearing is comfortable and swelling and tenderness have decreased dramatically. For grade I or II injuries, a splint or brace is applied for 1 to 2 days. Grade III injuries receive a splint with subsequent functional treatment when the ankle is able to support weight while protected by a brace. The alternative treatment may be casting for at least 3 weeks.

Strengthening of the peroneal and ankle dorsiflexor muscles is achieved in the next phase with isometric, concentric, and eccentric exercises. Plantarflexion exercises are not emphasized, as increased plantarflexion may lead to increased ankle instability. Achilles tendon stretching is also performed to increase the range of motion in dorsifixion and decrease the incidence of the ankle sprain (81). Progression to the next phase is accomplished when normal range of motion in dorsiflexion is possible and no pain or swelling occurs after exercise.

In the final phase of rehabilitation, motor coordination with proprioception and conditioning exercises, as well as endurance training, are optimized. Finally, in preparation for the return of the athlete to full activity, sport-specific function is emphasized. Running routines with sudden acceleration and deceleration, along with jumping, landing, and turning, are included.

The use of postrehabilitation bracing with lace-up braces or taping is not required, but some patients with grade I and most with grade II or III injuries should have functional bracing, especially in high-risk sports. All patients with grade III sprains need to have protective bracing for at least 3 to 6 months after returning to full sports participation (75).

The mainstay of treatment for the ankle sprain is the nonoperative approach. Given the expense and potential morbidity of surgery, it is not recommended for routine use. Exceptions to this recommendation include the young athlete with complete tears of the ATFL and CFL who may require surgery acutely (82,83); a patient with chronic symptoms of lateral ligament instability and recurrent severe ankle sprains; a patient with a displaced osteochondral fracture of the talus; and an athlete with large avulsion fractures of the fibula that may indicate injury of the CFL.

CONCLUSIONS

Foot and ankle injuries in sports are a frequent occurrence. Understanding the fundamental biomechanical concepts of the distal aspect of the lower limb is a key component in the proper diagnosis and treatment of these injuries. Based on this knowledge as well as a careful clinical examination, sports physiatrists can design a proper rehabilitation program for the injured athlete. Rapid, but appropriate, return of the anxious athlete to the playing court, running track, or athletic field is the ultimate goal of the physician and the patient. With the information covered within this chapter, the clinician may be able to achieve this objective in a most timely and effective manner.

REFERENCES

1. Williams PL, Warwick R, Dyson M, et al, eds. *Gray's anatomy.* 37th ed. Edinburgh: Churchill Livingstone, 1989.
2. Geiringer SR. Foot injuries. In: Press J, Kibler W, eds. *Functional rehabilitation of sports injuries.* Gaithersburg, MD: Aspen, 1998: 284–293.
3. Ounpuu S. The biomechanics of walking and running. *Clin Sports Med* 1994;13:843–863.
4. Mann RA. Biomechanics of running. In: D'Ambrosia R, Drez D, eds. *Prevention and treatment of running injuries.* Thorofare, NJ: Slack, 1982:4–13.
5. Rose J, Gamble JG, eds. *Human walking.* 2nd ed. Baltimore: Williams & Wilkins, 1994.
6. Nuber GW. Biomechanics of the foot and ankle during gait. *Clin Sports Med* 1988;7:1–13.
7. DeVita P. The selection of a standard convention for analyzing gait data based on the analysis of relevant biomechanical factors. *J Biomech* 1994;27: 501–508.
8. Hreljac A. Preferred and energetically optimal gait transition speeds in human locomotion. *Med Sci Sports Exerc* 1994;25: 1158–1162.
9. Scott SH, Winter DA. Internal forces of chronic running injury sites. *Med Sci Sports Exerc* 1990;22:357–369.
10. Bobbert MF, Yeadon MR, Nigg BM. Mechanical analysis of the landing phase in heel-toe running. *J Biomech* 1992;25: 223–234.
11. Ounpuu S. The biomechanics of running: a kinematic and kinetic analysis. *Instr Course Lect* 1990;39:305–318.
12. Engsberg JR, Allinger TL. A function of the talocalcaneal joint during running support. *Foot Ankle* 1990;11:93–96.

13. Prilutsky BI, Zatsiorsky VM. Tendon action of two-joint muscles: transfer of mechanical energy between joints during jumping, landing, and running. *J Biomech* 1994;27:25–34.

14. Lees A, Bouracier J. The longitudinal variability of ground reaction forces in experienced and inexperienced runners. *Ergonomics* 1994; 37:197–206.

15. Brandon LJ, Boileau RA. Influence of metabolic, mechanical and physique variables on middle distance running. *J Sports Med Phys Fitness* 1992;32: 1–9.

16. Geiringer SR, Bowyer BL, Press JM. Sports medicine: the physiatric approach. *Arch Phys Med Rehabil* 1993;74: S428–S432.

17. McCaw ST. Leg length inequality. Implications for running injury prevention. *Sports Med* 1992;14: 422–429.

18. Kibler WB, Goldberg C, Chandler TJ. Functional biomechanical deficits in running athletes with plantar fasciitis. *Am J Sports Med* 1991;19:66–71.

19. Messier SP, Davis SE, Curl WW, et al. Etiologic factors associated with patellofemoral pain in runners. *Med Sci Sports Exerc* 1991;23:1008–1015.

20. Gross ML, Davlin LB, Evanski PM. Effectiveness of orthotic shoe inserts in the long-distance runner. *Am J Sports Med* 1991;19: 409–412.

21. Kannus VP. Evaluation of abnormal biomechanics of the foot and ankle in athletes. *Br J Sports Med* 1992;26:83–89.

22. Gross ML, Napoli RC. Treatment of lower extremity injuries with orthotic shoe inserts. *Sports Med* 1993;15:66–70.

23. Blake RL, Ferguson HJ. Effect of extrinsic rearfoot posts on rearfoot position. *J Am Podiatr Med Assoc* 1993;83:447–456.

24. Shorten MR. The energetics of running and running shoes. *J Biomech* 1993;26S:41–53.

25. Jorgensen U. Body load in heel-strike running: the effect of a firm heel counter. *Am J Sports Med* 1990;18:177–181.

26. Kupke MJ, Kahler DM, Lorenzoni MH, et al. Stress fracture of the femoral neck in a long distance runner: biomechanical aspects. *J Emerg Med* 1993;11: 587–591.

27. DeLee JC, Drez D, eds. *Orthopaedic sports medicine.* Philadelphia: WB Saunders, 1994.

28. Baxter DE, Thigpen CM. Heel pain-operative results. *Foot Ankle* 1984;5:16–25.

29. Bordelon RL. Subcalcaneal pain—a method of evaluation and plan for treatment. *Clin Orthop* 1983; 177:49–53.

30. Freeman C. Heel pain. In: Gould JS, ed. *The foot book.* Baltimore: Williams & Wilkins, 1988: 228–238.

31. Savastano AA. Surgical neurectomy for the treatment of resistant painful heel. *Rhode Island Med J* 1985;68:371–372.

32. DuVries HL. Heel spur (calcaneal spur). *Arch Surg* 1957;74: 536–542.

33. Ali E. Calcaneal spur in Guyana. *West Indian Med J* 1980;29:175–183.

34. Mann RA. *Surgery of the foot.* St. Louis: Mosby, 1986: 244–247.

35. Shmokler RL, Bravo AA, Lynch FR, Newman LM. A new use of instrumentation in fluoroscopically controlled heel spur surgery. *J Am Podiatr Med Assoc* 1988;78: 194–197.

36. Snook GA, Christman OD. The management of subcalcaneal pain. *Clin Orthop* 1972;82:163–168.

37. Tanz SS. Heel pain. *Clin Orthop* 1963;28:169–178.

38. Warren BL. Anatomical factors associated with predicting plantar fasciitis in long-distance runners. *Med Sci Sports Exerc* 1984;16: 60–63.

39. Warren BL, Jones CJ. Predicting plantar fasciitis in runners. *Med Sci Sports Exerc* 1987;19: 71–73.

40. Windsor RE, Deryer SJ, Lester JP. Overuse injuries of the leg, foot, and ankle. *Phys Med Rehabil Clin N Am* 1994;5: 195–213.

41. Berquist TH, Cooper KL, Pritchard DJ. Stress fractures. In: Berquist TH, ed. *Imaging of orthopedic trauma.* 2nd ed. New York: Raven, 1992:881–894.

42. Childers RL, Meyers DH, Turner PU. Lesser metatarsal stress fractures: a study of 37 cases. *Clin Podiatr Med Surg* 1990;7: 633–644.

43. Greaney RB, Gerber FH, Laughlan RL. Distribution and natural history of stress fractures in US Marine recruits. *Radiology* 1983;146:339–346.

44. Orava S, Puranen J, Ala-Ketola L. Stress fractures caused by physical exercise. *Acta Orthop Scand* 1978;49:19–27.

45. Pester S, Smith PC. Stress fractures in the lower extremities of soldiers in basic training. *Orthop Rev* 1992;21:297–303.

46. Geiringer SR. Rehabilitation of stress fractures. *Phys Med Rehabil State Art Rev* 1995;9: 93–103.

47. Keats TE. *Radiology of musculoskeletal stress injury.* Chicago: Year Book Medical, 1990:4–9.

48. Mubarak SJ, Gould RN, Lee YF, et al. The medial tibial stress syndrome. A cause of shin splints. *Am J Sports Med* 1982;10: 201–205.

49. Michael RH, Holder LE. The soleus syndrome: a cause of medial tibial stress (shin splints). *Am J Sports Med* 1985; 13:87.

50. McKenzie DC, Clement DB, Taunton JE. Running shoes, orthotics, and injuries. *Sports Med* 1985;2:334–347.

51. Messier SP, Pittala KA. Etiologic factors associated with

selected running injuries. *Med Sci Sports Exerc* 1988;20: 501–505.

52. Reid DC, ed. *Sports injury assessment and rehabilitation.* New York: Chuchill Livingstone, 1992.

53. Rupani H, Holder L, Espinola D, Engin S. Three-phase radionuclide bone imaging in sports medicine. *Radiology* 1985;156: 187–196.

54. Ficat RP, Hungerford DS. *Disorders of the patellofemoral joint.* Baltimore: Williams & Wilkins, 1977.

55. McConnell J. The management of chondromalacia patellae: a long term solution. *Aust J Phys Ther* 1986;32:215.

56. Dandy DJ, Poirier H. Chondromalacia and the unstable patella. *Acta Orthop Scand* 1975;46: 695–699.

57. Fox T. Dysplasia of the quadriceps mechanism. *Surg Clin North Am* 1975;55:199–226.

58. Sikorski J, Peters J, Watt J. The importance of femoral rotation in chondromalacia patella as shown by serial radiography. *J Bone Joint Surg* [*Br*] 1979;61:435–442.

59. Townsend PR, Rose RM, Radin EL, Raux P. The biomechanics of the human patella and its implication for chondromalacia. *J Biomech* 1977;10:403–407.

60. Turner MS, Smillie IS. The effect of tibial torsion on the pathology of the knee. *J Bone Joint Surg* [*Br*] 1981;63:296–298.

61. Buchbinder RM, Nappora NJ, Biggs EN. The relationship of abnormal pronation to chondromalacia of the patella in distance runners. *Pod Sports Med* 1979;69:159–162.

62. Clement DB, Taunton SE, Smart GW, McNicol KL. A survey of overuse running injuries. *Phys Sportsmed* 1981;9:47–58.

63. Pritchett JW. A statistical study of knee injuries due to football in high school athletes. *J Bone Joint Surg* [*Am*] 1982;64: 240–241.

64. Hoppenfeld S. *Physical examination of the spine and extremities.* Norwalk, CT: Appleton & Lange, 1976.

65. Gooch JL, Geiringer SR, Akau CK. Sports medicine: lower extremity injuries. *Arch Phys Med Rehabil* 1993;74:S438–S442.

66. Trevino SG, Davis P, Hecht PJ. Management of acute and chronic lateral ligament injuries of the ankle. *Orthop Clin North Am* 1994;25:1–16.

67. Hopkinson WJ, St. Pierre P, Ryan JB, et al. Syndesmosis sprains of the ankle. *Foot Ankle* 1990;10: 325–330.

68. Garrick JM. The frequency of injury, mechanism of injury, and epidemiology of ankle sprains. *Am J Sports Med* 1977;5: 241–242.

69. Balduini FC, Tetzlaff J. Historical perspectives on injuries of the ligaments of the ankle. *Clin Sports Med* 1982;1:3–12.

70. Garrick JG. Epidemiologic perspective. *Clin Sports Med* 1982;1:13–18.

71. Cass JR, Morrey BF, Katoh Y, Chao EY. Ankle instability: comparison of primary repair and delayed reconstruction after long-term follow-up study. *Clin Orthop* 1985;198:110–117.

72. Liu SH, Jason WJ. Lateral ankle sprains and instability problems. *Clin Sports Med* 1994;13: 793–809.

73. Lassiter TE, Malone TR, Garrett WE. Injury to the lateral ligaments of the ankle. *Orthop Clin North Am* 1989;20:629–640.

74. Schneck CD, Mesgarzedeh M, Bonakdarpour A. MR imaging of the most commonly injured ankle ligaments. *Radiology* 1992;184: 507–512.

75. Drez D, Young JC, Waldman D, et al. Nonoperative treatment of double lateral ligament tear of the ankle. *Am J Sports Med* 1982;10:197–200.

76. Kannus P, Renstrom P. Current concepts review: treatment for acute tears of the lateral ligaments of the ankle. *J Bone Joint Surg* [*Am*] 1991;73:305–312.

77. Freeman MAR. Instability of ruptures of the foot after injuries to the lateral ligament of the ankle. *J Bone Joint Surg* [*Br*] 1965;47:669–677.

78. Freeman MAR. Treatment of ruptures of the lateral ligament of the ankle. *J Bone Joint Surg* [*Br*] 1965;47:661–668.

79. Niedermann B, Andersen A, Bryde Andersen S, et al. Rupture of the lateral ligaments of the ankle: operation or plaster cast? A prospective study. *Acta Orthop Scand* 1981;52:579–587.

80. Kaikkonen A, Kannus P, Jarvinen M. Surgery versus functional treatment in ankle ligament tears. *Clin Orthop* 1996;326: 194–202.

81. McCluskey GM, Blackburn TA, Lewis T. Prevention of ankle sprains. *Am J Sports Med* 1976;4:151–157.

82. Clanton TO, Schon LC. Athletic injuries to the soft tissues of the foot and ankle. In: Mann RA, Couglin MJ, eds. *Surgery of the foot and ankle.* 6th ed. St. Louis: CV Mosby, 1993:1128–1130.

83. Clark BL, Derby AC, Power GRI. Injuries of the lateral ligament of the ankle. Conservative vs. operative repair. *Can J Surg* 1965;8:358–363.

84. Eastmond CJ, Rajah SM, Tovey D, Wright V. Seronegative pauciarticular arthritis and HLA-B27. *Ann Rheum Dis* 1980;39: 231–234.

85. Gerster JC. Plantar fasciitis and Achilles tendinitis among 150 cases of seronegative spondarthritis. *Rheumatol Rehabil* 1980;19:218–222.

86. Insall J, Falvoka K, Wise DW. Chondromalacia patella. *J Bone Joint Surg* [*Am*] 1976;58:1–8.

87. Minetti AE, Ardigo LP, Saibene F. The transition between walking and running in humans: metabolic and mechanical aspects at different gradients. *Acta*

Physiol Scand 1994;150: 315–323.

88. Rehrer NJ, Meijer GA. Biomechanical vibration of the abdominal region during running and bicycling. *J Sports Med Phys Fitness* 1991;31:231–234.

89. Viita Sala JT, Kuist M. Some biomechanical aspects of the foot and ankle in athletes with and without shin splints. *Am J Sports Med* 1983;11:125–130.

Chapter 71

Lumbar Spine Disorders

Frank J. E. Falco
Robert E. Windsor
Lori B. Wasserburger

The spine is subjected to rapid, constant repetitive loading during athletic activities. This can result in acute, chronic, or relapsing injuries. Despite relative hypertrophy of the vertebral bodies and increased muscular and ligamentous strength in the lumbar region of the spine compared to the remainder of the spine, acute or cumulative injuries can occur. Injuries are due to the magnitude, duration, or frequency of the imposed loads to the spine. The lumbar section of the spine has the greatest weight bearing demands and is more resistant to serious injury than is the cervical region.

ANATOMY AND PATHOMECHANICS

The lumbar region of the spine connects the thorax to the pelvis. It is typically composed of five lumbar vertebrae, although there may be as few as four and as many as six vertebrae. In addition, a number of normal anatomic variants may occur at the lumbosacral region. These include facet tropism, spina bifida occulta, unilateral fusion of the lowest lumbar vertebra to the sacral ala, a partially or completely lumbralized first sacral vertebra, and a partially or completely sacralized fifth lumbar vertebra. Facet tropism may be associated with an increased incidence of low-back dysfunction (1).

The spine with its specialized anatomy supports loading and guides movement while protecting the spinal cord and nerve roots. The lumbar vertebrae are well suited to bear heavy loads over long periods of time. They are larger than either the cervical or thoracic vertebrae. The vertebrae can be divided into anterior and posterior structures. The anterior portion is composed of large cylindrical vertebral bodies that have an external cortex, an inner medullary portion, and end-plates that abut the disk on either end of the body (Fig. 71-1). The cortex is innervated by the sinuvertebral nerves and gray ramus communicans and functions to provide tensile strength to resist vertical and torsional forces. The medullary tissue has a vascular plexus supported by a bony matrix, probably is not innervated, and functions to help nourish spinal structures such as the intervertebral disk and to make blood and lymphatic products. The end-plate is a fibrocartilaginous structure that is an interface between the disk and the vertebral body. Some investigators consider it a part of the disk while others consider it a part of the body. It is innervated by the sinuvertebral nerve and may be a source of chronic segmental pain following injury (1).

The posterior portion of the vertebrae is composed of the pedicle, lamina, spinous process, transverse process, and superior and inferior articular processes (see Fig. 71-1). The pedicle and the lamina together comprise the neural arch that helps house and protect the lumbar portion of the neuroaxis. The portion of bone connecting the superior articular processes to the lamina is known as the *pars interarticularis* (1,2). This region is occasionally damaged during activities that provide strong axial loads. The pars may also be congenitally incomplete. If it is incomplete for any reason, the condition is known as a *spondylolysis*. If

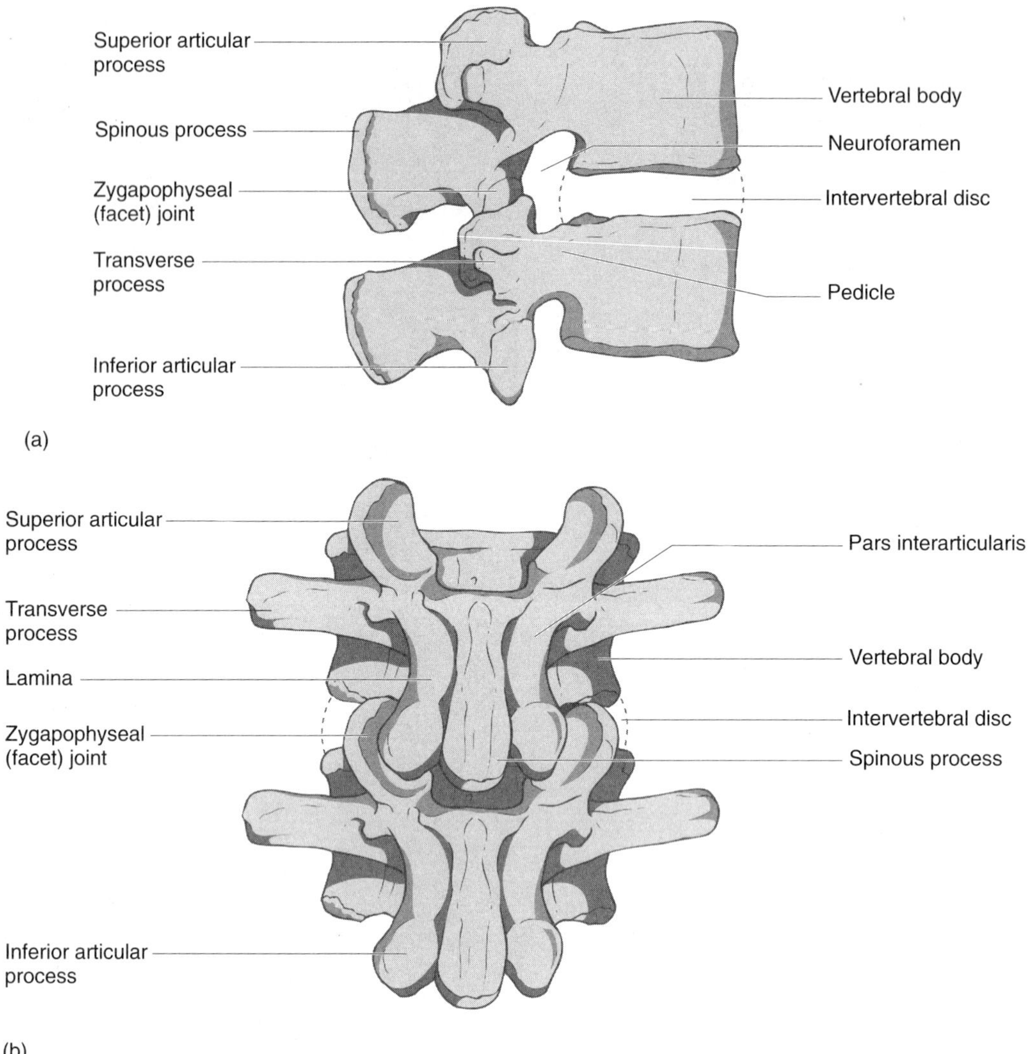

Figure 71-1. Lumbar vertebral segment. *a.* Lateral view. *b.* Posterior view. (Reproduced by permission from Bogduk N, Twomey LT. *Clinical anatomy of the lumbar spine.* 2nd ed. London: Churchill Livingstone, 1991.)

bilateral spondylolysis is present, then a slip of the superior vertebra on the inferior vertebra may occur. This is known as a *spondylolisthesis.* The spinous process provides a site for ligamentous and muscular attachment to the sagittal plane of the body. It helps to restrain hyperextension and may occasionally become injured with rapid hyperextension. The transverse processes also provide a broad site for both muscular and ligamentous attachment and may become injured following direct blunt trauma. Each articular process articulates with the complementary articular process from the adjacent vertebra to form the zygapophyseal (facet) joint. As an example, the right L4 superior articular process articulates with the right L3 inferior articular process to form the right L3–L4 facet joint.

The paired facet joints are diarthrodial synovial joints. The upper lumbar facet joints are oriented 45 degrees to the sagittal plane and the lower lumbar facet joints approach the coronal plane. The capsule attaches approximately 2 mm from the articular margin, resulting in a capsular capacity of 1 to 2 mm (3,4). The capsule contains a fibrocartilaginous meniscus that is thought to protect the articular surfaces of the facet joints during movement (1). The capsule helps resist flexion and torsion stresses to assist in protecting the posterior intervertebral disks (1). The capsule also resists backward sliding and excessive bending forces (3). The capsule is innervated by the medial branch of the dorsal primary ramus.

The facet joints help to guide rotation of one vertebra on another and to resist hyperextension and hyperrotation. They allow approximately 3 degrees of rotation and side bending of one vertebra on another. The upper lumbar facet joints primarily allow flexion and extension and resist side bending and rotation most, while the lower lumbar facet joints allow side bending and rotation and resist flexion (2).

A given facet joint bears 7% to 10% of the total

body weight. Increased weight bearing occurs with hyperlordotic postures, and maximal pressure occurs within the facet joint during hyperextension (5). Hyperextension allows the inferior articular process to slip past the superior articular process to impact on the laminae (6). Overloading the facet joint can result in injury to the articular cartilage or damage to the facet joint capsule (6).

The intervertebral disk has a fibrous outer structure known as the *annulus fibrosus* and a semifluid center known as the *nucleus pulposus* (Fig. 71-2). The outer structure is composed of 12 to 20 circumferential layers of collagenous ligamentous-like tissue oriented at 30 degrees from the horizontal in a clockwise or counterclockwise direction, with each layer alternating in direction. The outer layers are firmly attached to the osseous vertebral body while the inner layers are secured to the cartilaginous end-plate (7). The intervertebral disk is avascular at skeletal maturation. The outer one-third to one-half of the annulus has a nerve supply and thus may result in pain if injured (1). The anteriormost fibers are innervated primarily by the gray ramus communicans, the lateral fibers are innervated by the sinuvertebral nerve and direct branches from the anterior ramus, and the posterior portion is primarily innervated by the sinuvertebral nerve (Fig. 71-3). The inner annulus and nucleus have no innervation (1).

With its strong, flexible outer covering, semifluid center, and fibrocartilaginous end-plates, the disk works as a hydraulic mechanism. As axial loads are applied to the lumbar region of the spine, the nucleus expands radially and is reduced in height. The increased pressure generated by the nucleus is transmitted to the annular fibers and end-plate. The annulus develops tension and absorbs the load, and then undergoes elastic recoil after the load is removed. If the load is excessive, it can result in tearing of the annular fibers or fracturing of the end-plate (8). The disk also absorbs loads during flexion, extension, and lateral bending. Disk compression occurs in the direction of motion, with tensile forces applied to the contralateral annular fibers. This reduces the tensile strength of the disk by 50% during flexion. Tensile forces often create greater injury than compressive forces. Rotation stretches the annular fibers oriented in the direction of motion, while the remaining fibers are in a relaxed position. Therefore, flexion (or other directional movement) combined with twisting often causes annular injury and herniation (2,9). Injury of the outer, innervated portion of the annulus may be perceived as mild to severe local pain with or without radiation into the lower extremity depending on the extent of the injury. Multiple circumferential annular fissures may coalesce to form a radial fissure. A radial fissure predisposes to a protrusion and may later lead to disk extrusion. These fissures commonly occur at the posterolateral corner of the disk (10). This may be due to increased curvature and stress concentration in this region.

The anterior and posterior longitudinal ligaments (ALL and PLL, respectively) run longitudinally along the anterior and posterior aspects of the vertebral bodies (Fig. 71-4). The ALL is innervated by the gray ramus communicans and primarily resists hyperextension. The PLL resists hyperflexion and is innervated by the sinuvertebral nerves. The PLL does not extend to the posterolateral corner of the lumbar disk, which may contribute to the higher frequency of disk herniations at this location (1).

In general, the cervical and lumbar lordoses are mobile zone while the thoracic and sacral curves are less

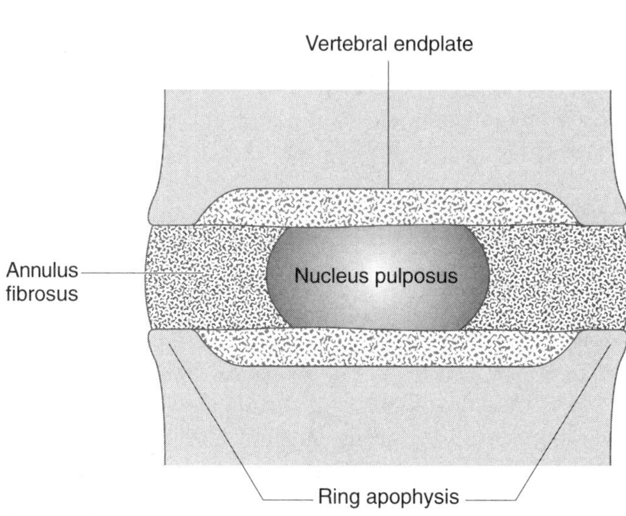

Figure 71-2. Intervertebral disk components. The annulus fibrosus encompasses the centrally located the nucleus pulposus. (Reproduced by permission from Bogduk N, Twomey LT. *Clinical anatomy of the lumbar spine.* 2nd ed. London: Churchill Livingstone, 1991.)

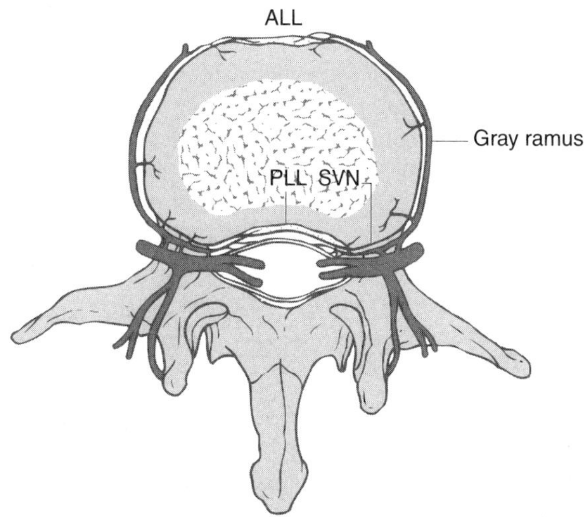

Figure 71-3. Innervation of the lumbar intervertebral disk. All = anterior longitudinal ligament; PLL = posterior longitudinal ligament; SVN = sinuvertebral nerve. (Reproduced by permission from Bogduk N, Twomey LT. *Clinical anatomy of the lumbar spine.* 2nd ed. London: Churchill Livingstone, 1991.)

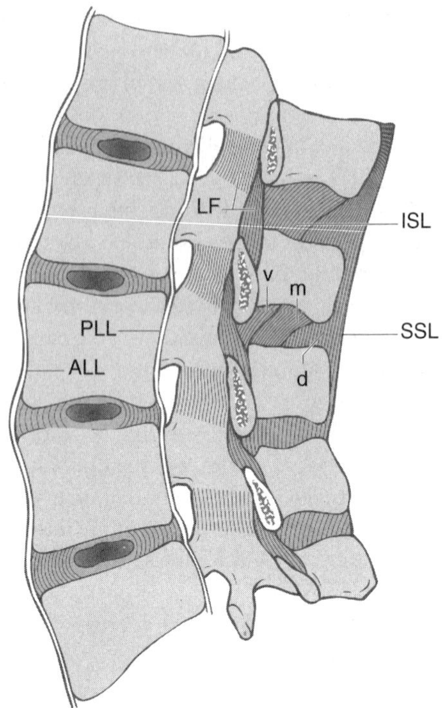

Figure 71-4. Lumbar spine ligaments. ALL = anterior longitudinal ligament; PLL = posterior longitudinal ligament; LF = ligamentum flavum; SSL = supraspinous ligament; ISL = interspinous ligament; v = ventral part; m = middle part; d = dorsal part. (Reproduced by permission from Bogduk N, Twomey LT. *Clinical anatomy of the lumbar spine.* 2nd ed. London: Churchill Livingstone, 1991.)

flexible. The curvilinear arrangement of the spine seen in the sagittal plane actually gives it increasing load-absorbing capabilities, allowing the spine to act like a spring (11,12). As the mobile areas of the spine alternate with relatively immobile zones, areas of increased stress are created at the cervicothoracic, thoracolumbar, and lumbosacral junction (13). The relative hypomobility at these transition points results in an increased incidence of injury to the osseous, soft-tissue, and neural elements. Fortunately, because the spinal cord ends proximal to the lumbosacral junction, injuries at that level do not produce the degree of catastrophic neural injuries seen at the cervicothoracic or thoracolumbar region (1,2,14).

The same biomechanical and physiologic forces that act on the sedentary spine act on the athlete's spine. Depending on the biomechanics of each individual sport, excessive forces may occur to a greater extent in the athlete's spine. Any factor that creates excessive demand can lead to injury. Mechanical loading may occur by repetitive fatigue overload, supramaximal overload, or unexpected overload (15). Each sport varies in this regard. An improper blocking or tackling technique or other sport technique, poor body mechanics, or improper training can lead to overload on both the mature and the skeletally immature spine. While the center of gravity normally passes anterior to the spine, subtle movements of the pelvis move the center of gravity's vector to pass through either the vertebrae or the posterior elements. This change in loading occurs only during active movement such as in a sport and can cause increased compressive loading of the anterior or posterior elements. Sports like gymnastics often cause fatigue overload, resulting in pars interarticularis stress reactions. Competitive weight lifters are predisposed to supramaximal overloads. Unexpected overloads result from falls or collisions and improper technique. The latter two types of overload can occur during nearly every sport and are difficult to prevent. Good coaching, proper technique, and safety measures may help to minimize fatigue overload and limit otherwise hazardous situations.

The ultimate result of the forces acting on the lumbar spine in athletes is determined by a given athlete's posture, muscular and ligamentous support system, and level of conditioning. Athletes have additional risk for injury based on their unique psychology. They are often encouraged to push through pain in their training and during competition, resulting in repetitive overload of spinal structures.

EPIDEMIOLOGY

Thoracolumbar spinal abnormalities are more common in athletes than nonathletes in the general population (16). The majority of lumbar spinal injuries occur during sports in which there is chronic repetitive loading of the spine. These loads may be axial, flexion-extension, or rotational. The region of the lumbar spine that is susceptible to injury in each sport is based on the biomechanics of that sport (15,17–34). In addition, impact to the lumbar spine from falls can result in more serious or acute trauma. This would include falls off gymnastic equipment; falls off the horse in equestrian sports and rodeo events; and falls during snow skiing, water-skiing, and all board sports. Tackles in football and rugby and checks into the boards during hockey can result in acute trauma as well. Almost any injury pattern can be seen with acute trauma.

Many of the epidemiologic studies are based on retrospective reviews. They often report low-back pain as a symptom, but do not indicate a specific diagnosis. The studies most often only report injury when the symptoms are severe enough to limit participation in sports. Many athletes continue to practice and compete despite chronic low-back pain. Additionally, due to the self-limited nature of many episodes of low-back pain, much of it goes unreported. Many prospective studies observe athletes for a short period of time and very few look at the long-term sequelae of sport-related lumbar injuries.

Any sport can create injuries or degenerative changes based on repetitive loading. Athletes are susceptible to degenerative disk changes at an early age (35). In the series from Horne et al (19) of competitive water ski jumpers, 45% demonstrated changes consistent with posttraumatic sequelae of the spine. Damage to the spine was associated with the age the subject began the sport and the length of participation in the sport. In general, 37% demonstrated evidence of vertebral wedging and 26 percent revealed evidence of Scheuermann disease. However, 100% of the skiers who began skiing before age 15 and continued jumping more than 9 years had radiographic evidence of damage. These degenerative changes were the result of repetitive axial loading microtrauma during landing and macrotrauma from falls. In comparing the sports of wrestling, gymnastics, tennis, and soccer, Sward et al (29,30,31) found that male gymnasts had the highest frequency of low-back pain. Additionally, 55% of male wrestlers demonstrated radiographic changes and the number of radiographic changes correlated with the severity of back pain (34).

Approximately 10% to 27% of collegiate football players experience lumbar spinal complaints (27,36). Nearly 50% of football linemen experience low-back pain in one season, and spondylolytic defects may occur in up to 33% (37). McCarrol et al (36) found that 13% of collegiate-level football players followed over a 5-year period have spondylolysis or spondylolisthesis. Semon and Spengler (27) noted a 21% incidence of spondylolisthesis in football players, but there was no apparent difference in lost playing time in this group compared to the group without spondylolisthesis.

A study of weight lifters and wrestlers found a five times increased incidence of spondylolysis and spondylolisthesis compared to the general population (34). There is a 10% incidence of spondylolysis defects in female gymnasts (21), four times the incidence in the general population. The rate of lumbar spinal injury in gymnasts was directly related to the level of competition (20). Similarly, magnetic resonance imaging (MRI) evidence of spinal abnormalities was noted in 9% of pre-elite, 43% of elite, and 63% of Olympic-level gymnasts (38). Hockey and basketball have not been associated with a high incidence of low-back injuries (39,40). As an example, injuries at the lumbosacral level during the 1990 to 1991 National Basketball Association season accounted for only 8.7% of the total number of injuries (41).

A number of noncontact sports are associated with low-back pain, with the majority of injuries due to repetitive forces or chronic postures. Injuries to golfers are usually of an overuse nature and are due to the large lateral bending, shear, compression, and torsional forces the spine is subjected to during the golfer's drive stroke (24). Low-back injuries are the most common injuries among amateur golfers (34.5%) and are fairly equal in incidence to left wrist injuries (23.7%) in professional golfers (24). In regard to professional golfers, 25% of men and 22.4% of women experience symptoms related to the lumbar spine. Up to 15% of nationally ranked swimmers have MRI evidence of spinal abnormalities (18). Nontraumatic lumbar injuries in bicyclists have an incidence of between 2.7% and 10% (33,42). These injuries are apparently due to chronic flexion postures.

DIFFERENTIAL DIAGNOSIS

Most episodes of low-back pain in an athlete resolve spontaneously or respond to conservative care within 1 to 2 weeks. Back pain that does not resolve fairly promptly or repeated recurrences of back pain may herald a more serious problem. Persistent pain in an athlete is rarely accompanied by secondary gain issues. The differential diagnosis of low-back pain in the athlete will depend on the sport, the level of competition, and age.

Younger athletes (<12 years) are more likely to have an inflammatory, infectious, neoplastic, or nonspinal cause of low-back pain (43). The adolescent athlete's skeletally immature spine reacts to abnormal or repetitive biomechanical forces differently than does the mature spine after the degenerative cascade has begun (14,44). The anterior structures such as the intervertebral disk in the mature athlete or the vertebral end-plates in the skeletally immature athlete are most susceptible to excessive or repetitive flexion, compression, or torsion forces. These forces can cause a herniated disk in a skeletally mature spine or damage to the ring apophysis and vertebral end-plate in the immature skeleton (43–45). The repetitive loads to which athletes' spines are subjected cause degenerative disk changes at an early age (16,19,46). Similarly, hyperlordotic postures or excessive and repetitive extension forces that would cause failure at the pars interarticularis in the adolescent might result in a facet or sacroiliac syndrome in the more mature athlete.

Intervertebral Disk Herniations

Luschka (39) was the first to describe the herniated disk, in 1858. Mixter and Barr, as early as 1934 (47), called attention to the pathoanatomy of the herniated disk and its relationship to radicular dysfunction from neural compression. Over the years, much attention has been directed at the lumbar disk as a source of back and lower-extremity pain. The pathogenesis and natural history of disk herniations have been investigated primarily with cadaveric specimens and advanced radiologic imaging techniques.

The disk bulge is considered to be a normal finding and is described as a symmetric extension of the posterior part of the disk beyond the end-plate. Intervertebral disk herniations that are anatomically abnormal have been generally classified into three different categories (48) (Fig. 71-5). The *protruding disk* is described as nuclear material that penetrates through the annular fibers without escaping the outside margin of the annulus. This is also known as a *contained disk herniation.* Nuclear material that extends outside the periphery of the annulus is called an *extruded disk.* A

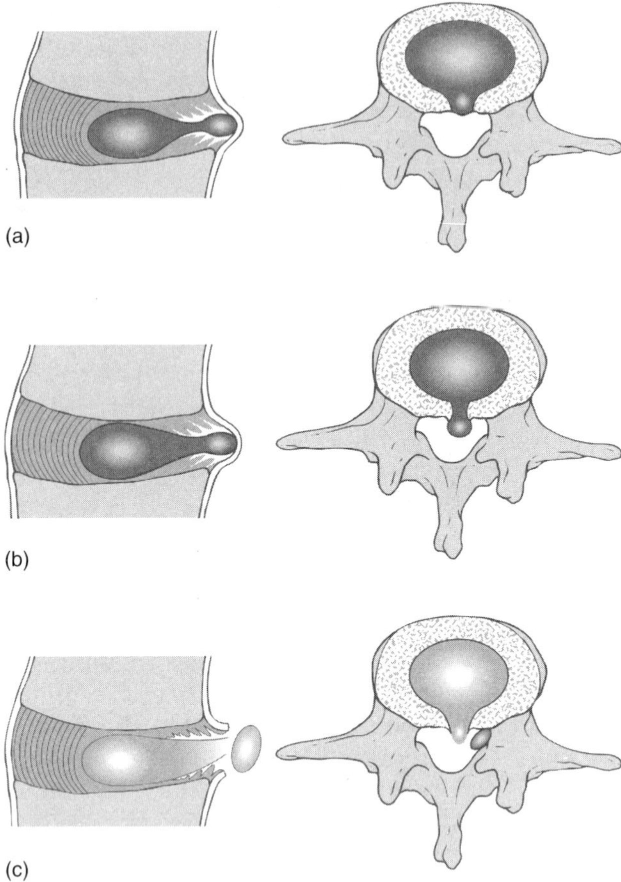

Figure 71-5. Intervertebral disk herniation classification. *a.* Disk protrusion. *b.* Disk extrusion. *c.* Disk sequestration. (Reproduced by permission from Modic MT, Masaryk TJ, Ross JS. *Magnetic resonance imaging of the spine.* 2nd ed. Chicago: Year Book Medical, 1994.)

sequestered disk is extruded disk material that has separated from the main body of the nucleus. The protruding disk is considered an *incomplete herniation* whereas the extruded or sequestered disk is referred to as a *complete herniation.* Histologic studies from in vitro as well as surgical specimens reveal that annular material and end-plate fragments are present along with nuclear material in the herniated portion of the disk (49).

Lumbar disk herniations are rarely the result of an isolated compressive or flexion insult. Instead, repetitive flexion, rotation, and compression forces produce mechanical failure at the posterior corners of the annulus, culminating in posterolateral disk herniations (50). Questioning typically reveals prior episodes of intermittent low-back pain. When diskogenic pain occurs at an early age, it is frequently associated with congenital variants or anomalies that subject the disk to abnormal forces (9). Although injury of the anterior segment in the adolescent spine is more likely to cause injury to the vertebral end-plate and ring apophysis, up to 10% of low-back pain in the 21-and-under age group is due to disk protrusion or herniation (49).

The athlete with diskogenic pain usually experiences increased pain with sitting, flexion, coughing, sneezing, or activities that increase intradiskal pressure (51). Not all patients with disk herniations present with lumbar pain (14). The size of the spinal canal and the time over which the herniation occurs play a role in whether significant axial pain is felt. Repetitive annular tears may produce more pain because the intradiskal pressure is maintained. Once the disk herniates and the annular pressure has been reduced, back pain may be reduced. Some athletes may not demonstrate significant symptoms until they begin to develop radiculopathy.

A radiculopathy is any sensory, motor, or reflex abnormality secondary to nerve root injury that typically occurs from mechanical compression or intense inflammation (38). Acute demyelination or axonal loss may occur as a result of sustained compression or inflammation. Neurologic deficits secondary to demyelination may be reversible whereas those secondary to axonal loss may not. Recovery from neurologic deficits is not usually completely reversible and may take up to 18 months to occur (52). The term *Radiculitis* in used to describe symptoms that occur in a radicular distribution but are not associated with neurologic signs.

Radicular pain is deep, dull, and achy or sharp, burning, and electric in quality, depending on whether there is primarily ventral motor or dorsal sensory root involvement (53,54). The pain associated with radiculopathy generally follows a radicular pattern in the hip, leg, and foot (55). While back pain may not be associated with radiculopathy, the athlete may demonstrate a lumbar list. Athletes with radiculopathy may have lower-limb numbness or weakness with or without pain. Lower-limb weakness can be present when there is significant motor root compromise but must be differentiated from weakness due to pain. The athlete with radiculopathy typically displays decreased lumbar range of motion and dural tension signs.

Most patients are treated with nonsteroidal anti-inflammatory drugs (NSAIDs) during the acute phase for control of pain and inflammation. An oral steroid taper provides a powerful anti-inflammatory effect and can be used in treating a radiculopathy that does not initially respond to NSAIDs. Steroids should not be given concomitantly with NSAIDs or aspirin products, to avoid potential side effects. Muscle relaxants can be used as adjuncts to analgesics on a short-term basis. Narcotics may be used sparingly for short periods of time.

Physical modalities are used initially for acute pain control and later on an as-needed basis only. Traction can be beneficial in reducing radicular symptoms. Centralizing pain and restoring normal posture and range of motion are important initial goals. Strengthening and stabilization comprise the next part of the rehabilitation process. The patient should go through a back school and be independent in following through with a home program at the time of discharge from rehabilitation to minimize recurrent episodes.

Individuals who progress slowly sometimes require the use of selective spinal injection procedures. Fluoroscopically guided and contrast enhanced lumbar epidural and selective nerve root blocks provide both diagnostic and therapeutic benefits. An epidural can provide enough relief to radiculopathy patients to expedite a rehabilitation program. Patients with mechanical low-back pain typically do not respond well to epidural procedures.

Internal Disk Disruption

The term *internal disk disruption* (IDD) was first used by H. V. Crock in 1970 (56) to describe pathologic changes in the internal structure of the disk. IDD is considered a chemically mediated abnormality of the nucleus pulposus or annulus fibrosus without a disk contour defect. This disorder is believed to result from trauma such as an end-plate fracture allowing direct contact between the nucleus and systemic blood supply (57–59). Exposure of normally cloistered nuclear material is theorized to result in a localized autoimmune process causing degradation of the nucleus and at times the peripheral annulus (60–63) (Fig. 71-6). Annular fiber deterioration may present as radial fissuring, which can extend into the innervated outer disk margins, potentially causing pain from mechanical or chemical irritation.

Annular tears are also believed to result from axial rotation injuries. The zygapophyseal joints limit rotation and serve to protect the annulus from twisting injuries. If further axial rotation occurs after zygapophyseal impaction, tearing of annular fibers may result (9,58,59). This may cause a concentric annular fissure. Further rotation may cause facet fracture (1). The risk for annular tearing is increased during rotation because only half of the annular fibers are able to resist this movement (1).

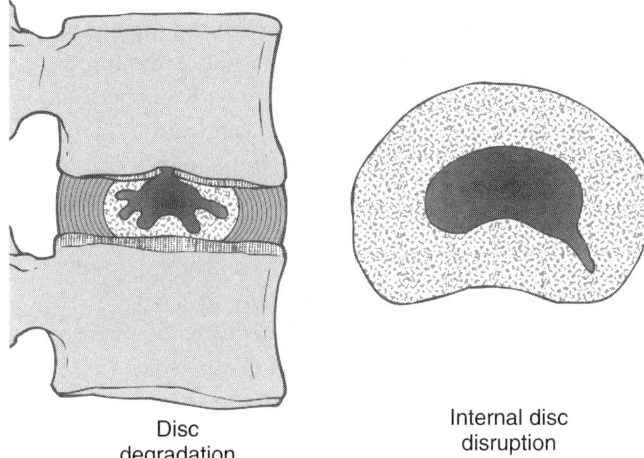

Figure 71-6. Disk degradation from autoimmune response initiated by an end-plate fracture, leading to internal disk disruption. (Reproduced by permission from Bogduk N, Twomey LT. *Clinical anatomy of the lumbar spine*. 2nd ed. London: Churchill Livingstone, 1991.)

Diskogenic pain is typically vague and diffuse in an axial distribution. Pain referred from the disk to the leg is usually in a nondermatomal pattern. Symptoms may vary according to changes in intradiskal pressure. Activities such as sitting, lifting, and Valsalva maneuvers may intensify symptoms, whereas lying supine may provide relief by decreasing intradiskal pressure. Vibration also has a tendency to exacerbate diskogenic pain (14).

Diskogenic pain is treated in a similar manner as lumbar radiculopathy. NSAIDs can be used initially to reduce inflammation and in conjunction with other medications to decrease pain and spasm. Rehabilitation efforts emphasize posturing and dynamic lumbar stabilization to reduce forces across the symptomatic disk level.

Lumbar Scheuermann Disease

Classic Scheuermann disease is diagnosed when end-plate irregularities are present and three consecutive vertebrae are wedged by 5 degrees or more (64,65). Lumbar Scheuermann disease is present when one or two vertebral bodies between T10 and L4 demonstrate end-plate irregularities. Patients with lumbar Scheuermann disease typically demonstrate anterior Schmorl nodes, as opposed to the central Schmorl nodes seen in the classic form (64). Anterior Schmorl nodes are often found in athletes (29,64,66). Central Schmorl nodes are due to herniation of nuclear material through the end-plate, whereas an anterior Schmorl node develops by rupture of the disk material through the anterior annulus (66). With an anterior or marginal Schmorl node, the disk material then continues through the cartilaginous layer between the ring apophysis and the vertebral body, as has been demonstrated by MRI (31). Disk degeneration then follows in all patients with Scheuermann disease of the lumbar spine, and they have an increased rate of degenerative disk changes compared to normal control subjects (67). Lumbar Scheuermann disease may be caused by a single traumatic flexion compression force or chronic repetitive loading (29,64,68). The former is typically the result of an end-plate fracture and therefore more likely to be symptomatic (29). A thoracolumbar spinal orthosis in extension is often required for symptom relief.

Vertebral Body Fractures

A number of different mechanisms of injury can cause fractures of the anterior spinal column. Mechanisms of injury may include hyperflexion, flexion with rotation, and axial loading with or without flexion.

Hyperflexion injuries are the most common mechanism of injury resulting in vertebral body fracture (69). A fracture most often results in compression of the anterior portion of the vertebral body. Uncomplicated compression fractures, by definition, involve only the anterior vertebral body and are inherently stable. The point of force in hyperflexion forces is focused at the middle of the intervertebral disk (7,69). Because the disks in the upper thoracic region of the spine are thinner, the resultant fracture is more of a true compression fracture. The disk in the lower thoracic and lumbar regions of the spine are larger and better shock absorbers. Rather than a compression fracture, herniation into the cartilaginous end-plate is more probable (70). Compression fractures are graded by quarters. Fifty percent compression or more of the anterior margin with associated disk space narrowing is more likely to have long-term sequelae, such as delayed instability (7,71). This may also be seen when there are several contiguous compression fractures (69).

Burst fractures involve two or three of the columns of the three-column spinal model. They are generally due to longitudinal compression without flexion, although they may occur with severe hyperflexion injuries without longitudinal compression. Herniation into the end-plate may occur, but disk or fracture fragments usually retropulse into the spinal canal. Therefore, they may be associated with neurologic injury (2,69). Burst fractures account only for 1.5% of all spinal injuries and are generally located at the T12 to L2 level, where the spinal cord or bulk of the cauda equina is present (72,73).

Flexion-rotation injuries are relatively rare, but are some of the most unstable of spinal injuries (70,74). Most injuries by this mechanism occur at the thoracolumbar junction, owing to the rapid transition of facet joint orientation. This injury is associated with a high incidence of neurologic injury (7,69). The extent of osseous injury determines treatment. Anterior compression fractures are treated in a Jewett extension brace or similar brace. Immobilization is continued for 1 to 3 months depending on the degree of injury and pain. Immobilization in extension is generally acceptable for the neurologically intact burst fracture (7). Burst fractures with neurologic compromise or fractures involving all three spinal columns require surgical stabilization.

Posterior Element Fractures

Posterior element fractures are more likely to present after a single traumatic incident, usually involving extension and rotation (70). Either fatigue fractures or facet syndrome can also occur with sports that involve repetitive loading in extension or rotation such as gymnastics, diving, and golfing. Athletes with either entity generally will experience pain on extension, will be neurologically intact, but may have referred proximal lower-extremity pain. Their clinical symptoms will often overlap with those of athletes with an acute fracture of the pars interarticularis without spondylolisthesis or radiculopathy (7,75,76).

Fractures of the posterior arch can occur at multiple locations, including the articular processes, and may result from forceful twisting injuries or direct trauma (26,77). Spinous process fractures are relatively rare but may occur as a result of flexion, extension, or muscle contraction. Transverse process fractures can occur in the lumbar region owing to forceful muscle contractions or direct trauma. If caused by the latter, they may be associated with renal or splenic injury or retroperitoneal hemorrhage (7). A high index of suspicion must be maintained, as the nonosseous injury is potentially more serious. Many athletes with a fracture of the posterior arch will present clinically similar to athletes with facet injury or pain. Radiographs should demonstrate the fracture, although the findings may be subtle. Further diagnostic study through computed tomography (CT) and bone scanning is beneficial in evaluating questionable fractures, as treatment will often differ.

Facet Syndrome

The term *facet syndrome* was coined by Ghormley in 1933 (78). Facet syndrome has been described as nonspecific low-back pain with a deep and achy quality. The syndrome is considered in a patient with low-back pain that radiates into the back and posterior part of the thigh. The patient can complain of symptoms that increase with twisting or backward bending of the lumbar spine. Physical examination findings typically reveal local paravertebral muscle tenderness to palpation. Radicular findings are commonly absent. Often the pain can be increased with hyperextension and rotation of the lumbar spine. Although these findings might be somewhat helpful in evaluating for lumbar facet syndrome, there are no history or examination findings unique for facet syndrome (79–81).

The facet joints are diarthrodial, with articular cartilage, a synovial membrane, and a richly innervated capsule. The lumbar facet joint is formed by the inferior articular process of the vertebra above with the superior articular process of the vertebra below. The joints are innervated by the posterior rami via the medial branch nerves.

Mooney and Robertson (82) evaluated the lumbar facet joint in a group of subjects with and without low-back pain using x-ray–controlled provocative hypertonic facet joint injections. The pain produced from the injections was described by the subjects and pain referral maps were constructed for both groups (Fig. 71-7). The pain mapping is often utilized in clinical practice to assist the physician in the evaluation for facet syndrome and other lumbar disorders such as radiculopathy.

Treatment for facet syndrome consists of medications, joint mobilization, rehabilitation, and injections. Lumbar facet joint blocks are effective in providing diagnostic information with regard to whether or not the facet joint is responsible for low-back pain symptoms (83,84). The long-term therapeutic benefit from intra-articular facet joint injections has been controversial (84,85). No studies have evaluated facet blocks with a comprehensive rehabilitation program and long-term outcome. Although further research is warranted, a subset of patient with facet joint pain may also benefit in the long term from denervation of the symptomatic joints (86).

Sacroiliac Joint Syndrome

The sacroiliac joint (SIJ) is formed by a fibrous capsule anteriorly and the interosseous ligament posteriorly; the posterior part of the capsule is often incomplete (87,88). The lateral branches of the posterior primary rami of potentially L3 to S3 innervate the posterior ligaments and rudimentary capsule. The anterior aspect of the SIJ is innervated primarily by L4 to S1 (89). Because of the potential for differing innervation of the SIJ, there may be different pain referral patterns (89).

SIJ dysfunction has been described to occur after a direct insult to the joint such as falling on the buttocks or from repetitive overuse such as twisting or lifting. Ipsilateral groin and posterior superior iliac spine pain correlate with SIJ dysfunction. The pain is often nonspecific and described as deep, vague, achy, and at times sharp. In an asymptomatic group, provocative fluoroscopic SIJ injections produced pain in the ipsilateral buttock extending into the posterolateral aspect of the thigh and occasionally into the leg (90) (Fig. 71-8).

The treatment is similar to that of facet syndrome, incorporating a combination of medication, joint mobilization, rehabilitation, and injection. Heel lifts for leg-length discrepancies and SIJ belts have also been used to treat this condition. No controlled studies have evaluated the effectiveness of SIJ injections in treating SIJ dysfunction with or without rehabilitation.

Maigne Syndrome

This syndrome was first characterized by Maigne as a lesion at the posterior column of the T12–L1 level (14). Injuries at the thoracolumbar junction are often overlooked when evaluating the athlete complaining of back pain. Sports that require repetitive loading of the spine with associated hip flexion and neck extension focus forces at the thoracolumbar junction. This would include sports such as weight lifting, hockey, and football. The thoracolumbar segment is vulnerable to injury when athletes are positioned with hips flexed and the neck in extension, as this region bears the load of further extension.

The athlete with Maigne syndrome may describe nonspecific thoracolumbar pain. They often present with symptoms similar to athletes with facet syndromes at other levels. Physical examination reveals tenderness to palpation of the involved thoracolumbar segment. The posterior rami of T12 or L1 spinal nerves pass caudally and laterally

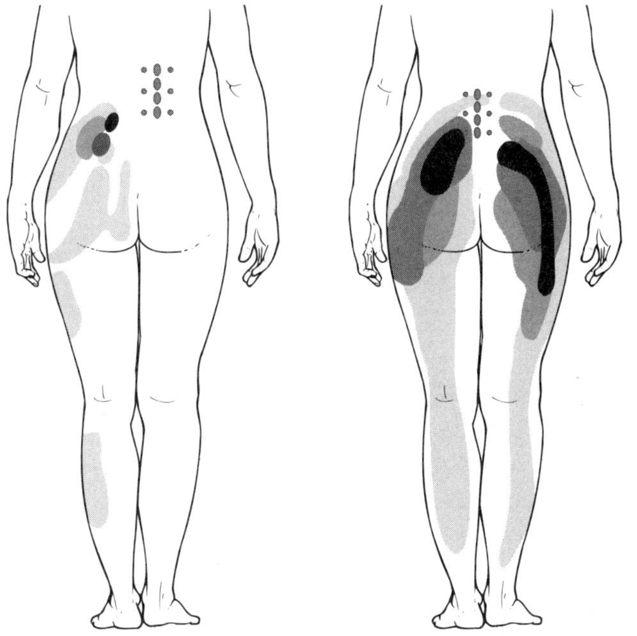

Normal Abnormal

Figure 71-7. Pain topography in individuals with (abnormal) and without (normal) low-back pain after provocative facet joint injections. (Reproduced by permission from Mooney V, Robertson J. The facet syndrome. *Clin Orthop* 1976;115:149.)

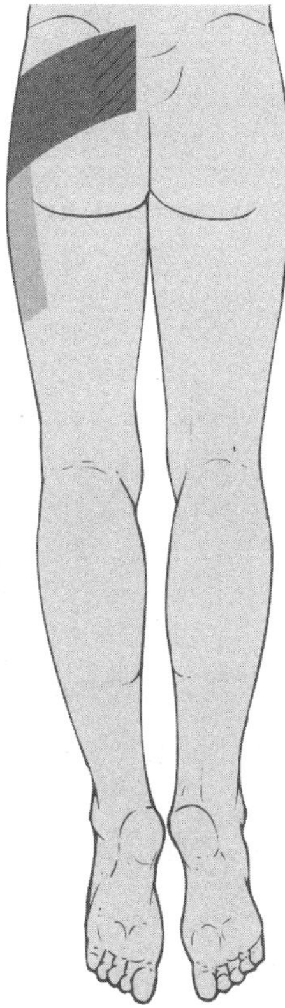

Figure 71-8. Pain topography in asymptomatic individuals after provocative sacroiliac joint injections. (Reproduced by permission from Fortin JD, Dwyer AP, West S, et al. Sacroiliac joint: pain referral maps upon applying a new injection/arthrography technique. Part I: asymptomatic volunteers. *Spine* 1994;19:1475–1482.)

to supply the cutaneous region at the iliac crest; therefore, associated findings may include pain in response to pinching or rolling the skin over the iliac crest or greater trochanter (14).

Lumbar Spondylolysis and Spondylolisthesis

The spectrum of injuries of the pars interarticularis region includes 1) pars stress reaction, 2) spondylolysis, and 3) spondylolisthesis. A pars stress reaction is actually a "pre-spondylolytic" lesion (Fig. 71-9). In the pars stress reaction there is increased bony reaction or bone turnover, evident on a bone scan or single-photon emission CT (SPECT) scan, but no lytic lesion has been identified either on plain films or CT scans (75). Spondylolytic defects may be either congenital or acquired (91–94). Five different types of spondylolysis have been described and classified: 1) dysplastic, 2) isthmic, 3) degenerative, 4) traumatic, and 5) pathologic (95,96). The isthmic variant tends to be the most important in the athletic population. Even this classification is further subdivided into the subtypes of acute fracture, pars elongation, and lytic lesion. In lytic isthmic lesions there is actual cleavage or separation of the pars interarticularis. This gap may be filled with fibrous scar or fibrocartilage. Spondylolysis may or may not be associated with spondylolisthesis. *Spondylolisthesis* is the term to indicate radiographic evidence of forward displacement of an upper vertebra over a lower vertebra. Most often, this is caused by bilateral pars defects, but may also occur with a unilateral spondylolytic lesion, an elongated pars interarticularis, or a severe, degenerative disk with segmental instability (97).

While biomechanical forces are definitely factors in the development of spondylolysis, it is generally believed that there is a genetic predisposition (91,98). A high familial incidence of spondylolysis has been reported, with Alaskan natives having an incidence of 50% to 60% (28,98). Approximately 4% to 6% of white adults have a pars defect on radiography, which is twice the incidence observed in blacks. The incidence of this defect may be increased by stresses created by excessive lumbar lordosis and dynamic loading (11). Genetic predisposition is supported by an absence of neural arch defects in other primates and nonbipedal mammals or in nonambulatory adult cerebral palsy patients (99). The incidence of spondylolysis is three times higher in males than females (100). This difference may be secondary to past differences in participation in sporting activities between males and females. However, more recently there has been a fourfold increase in the occurrence rate in female gymnasts (21,25).

Unilateral spondylolysis has been described, although it occurs less frequently than bilateral defects (101). The pars on the side opposite the defect is often thickened and sclerotic, possibly representing healing of a prior pars fracture or compensatory hypertrophy (102). At times, more than one level may be involved (92,103).

Trauma has a role in the development of spondylolysis which is supported by the 90% incidence of spondylolytic lesions occurring at the L5 level. This is the site of maximal shear and loading in the lumbar spine (11,17,104). Biomechanical properties at the transition zones lead to the L5 segment being the most commonly involved, with the L4 level the next most common. Additionally, a higher incidence of spondylolytic defects is seen in athletes who participate in sports that require repetitive or excessive flexion and extension of the spine, such as football, gymnastics, ballet, weight lifting, pole vaulting, diving, and baseball (18,36,76,105).

Analogies have been drawn between stress fractures and spondylolysis (106). The similarities are that they both can present with bony pain secondary to repetitive trauma.

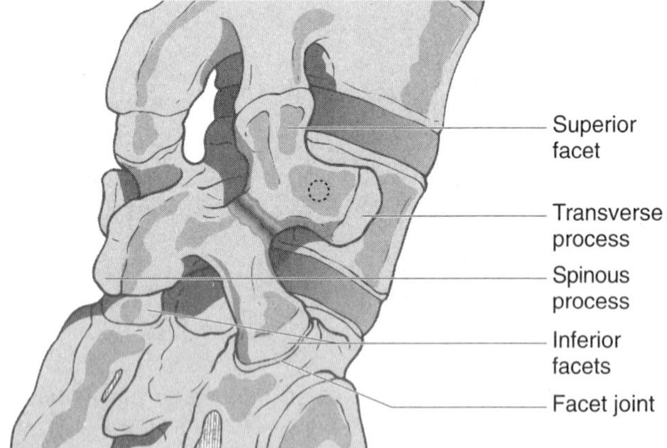

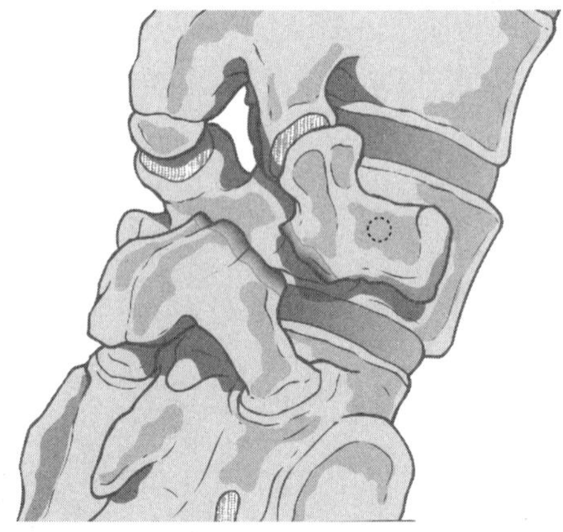

Figure 71-9. Spondylolysis and spondylolisthesis. The left figure reveals a spondylolysis with a defect at the pars interarticularis (collar on the Scottie dog). The right figure depicts spondylolisthesis with slippage of the vertebral body and subsequent widening of the collar or "decapitation" of the Scottie dog head. (Reproduced by permission from Reid DC, ed. *Sports injury assessment and rehabilitation.* London: Churchill Livingstone, 1992.)

They are dissimilar in that 1) spondylolytic lesions tend to develop at an earlier age than do stress fractures in most athletes, 2) there appears to be a genetic predisposition to spondylolysis, and 3) it may actually appear on radiography as a complete defect prior to the patient's complaints of pain (76,84,90,107). In addition, athletically acquired spondylolysis is unique in that it produces symptoms and usually presents later than the silent pars defects "picked up" on screening radiographs.

During the evaluation of the athlete with low-back pain and spondylolysis, one must determine whether the pars defect is of recent or long-standing onset. The examiner must also determine whether there is segmental instability in the patient with an actual defect. The history, physical examination, and radiographic imaging techniques will help to determine appropriate management. If the spondylolysis appears old on radiographs, a bone scan does not demonstrate increased uptake, and there is no instability pattern on flexion-extension radiographs, then relative rest and modification of activities may be all that is necessary to control pain and inflammation in the acute phase.

If the bone scan indicates ongoing bony turnover and a traumatic spondylolytic defect, then an antilordotic brace may be indicated (108). The use of antilordotic-type bracing remains controversial in this population. Some believe that avoidance of inciting activities, as well as a progressive lumbar stabilization program, is sufficient to allow healing (25). The presence of actual pars defects on radiographs tends to decrease the chance of healing even with adequate immobilization (44). Athletes with pars stress reactions (normal radiographs with an abnormal SPECT scan) and persistent symptoms benefit from use of an orthosis (108). This allows them to rest the injured area without requiring them to become totally sedentary and deconditioned. These athletes are more likely to heal completely. If the spondylolytic defect is believed to be a fracture caused by a single traumatic insult, cast immobilization (preferably with thigh spica) and a short period of recumbency is recommended prior to transitioning into the brace (108).

Once an athlete with a pars stress reaction has become asymptomatic or the bracing period is complete, rehabilitation may progress. This involves retraining the spine to perform sport-specific skills with a gradual progression from simple to increasingly demanding skills. These skills are performed while appropriate neutral spinal posture and good technique are maintained. The length of time spent in this phase of rehabilitation is highly variable and depends on the patient's level of conditioning and recurrence of symptoms.

In athletes with spondylolisthesis, the two factors that determine treatment and return to play criteria are the degree of slippage and the skeletal maturity of the athlete. The skeletally immature patient is at greater risk for progressive displacement and the greatest risk appears to be between ages 9 and 14 (46). Many of the criteria for return to activity for a grade 1 spondylolisthesis are the same as those for acute spondylolysis. If the displacement approaches the high end of a grade 2 lesion or greater and the athlete is asymptomatic after rehabilitation, he or she may return to athletic activities but should refrain from activities such as football, gymnastics, wrestling, or sports that entail axial loading (46,76). In addition, if the patient is skeletally immature, antilordotic bracing and careful observation may be required to prevent progression of slippage. Once skeletal maturity is reached, unless the degree of slippage is 50% or more, there is little likelihood of further displacement (76). The potential for nerve injury is present in patients with spondylolisthesis. The cauda equina may be compressed over the sacral dome, or traction may occur at the segmental level of instability, in athletes with more than a 25% slip (46,76).

Progression to grade 3 or 4 with intractable pain and dysfunction despite conservative care indicates surgery (97,104,109). Other indications for surgery are persistent deformity or abnormal gait, neurologic deficit, a more than 50-degree slip angle, and refractory pain (97,104,109). If the skeletally mature athlete with less than grade 3 slippage has had persistent pain for longer than 6 months despite excellent conservative care, and diagnostic studies have excluded other potential causes for the presence of pain, surgery may be indicated (91,110).

ON-FIELD ASSESSMENT

Most injuries of the lumbar spine are of a cumulative nature rather than secondary to major trauma. The injured athlete generally walks off the field and presents to the trainer or physician after a game. When the athlete is "down," he or she is treated similar to the athlete with a cervical spinal injury, in that immobilization is instituted until an initial assessment can be performed. Location of pain, presence of neurologic signs or symptoms, and increased pain with attempts at movement may require continued immobilization until a definitive evaluation or imaging studies are performed.

The initial clinical evaluation is used to create a working diagnosis on which treatment and rehabilitation are based. Nonspecific diagnoses often lead to nonspecific treatment and a protracted rehabilitation course (111). If the biomechanics of the injury are not evaluated and the factors that led to the injury are not corrected, then the athlete may have recurrent spinal problems. Important information to obtain from the patient is whether there was a gradual or acute onset after a particular play. The character and the intensity of the pain, and especially the relation of that pain to specific activities, are important to ascertain. Coughing, sneezing, lifting, bending forward, sitting, and at times lying supine can increase anterior segment loading, and therefore increase symptoms in a patient with an injury to the vertebral body or intervertebral disk (1,14). Alternately, extension, standing, walking, running, and lying on the stomach may increase posterior element loading, and therefore increase symptoms in a patient with facet or pars interarticularis pain (1,14). Any history of neurologic symptoms such as weakness, numbness, burning, tingling, or bowel or bladder dysfunction and other associated symptoms should also be elicited to exclude or confirm the presence of a concomitant neurologic lesion. Swelling, decreased range of motion, or nonaxial sites of pain as well as constitutional symptoms such as fever, weight change, loss of appetite, and skin rashes may indicate the presence of a connective tissue disorder or another medical or systemic process. This information can help avoid treatment for a "sports medicine injury" when there is actually a problem that will require more intensive evaluation and treatment.

Initial evaluation of low-back complaints requires a general inspection of the spine and peripheral joints, posture, and range of motion limitations. Pain generators suspected by the clinical history are further evaluated by palpation, neurologic examination, and provocative maneuvers.

The general skeletal examination includes assessment for anatomic dysfunction that may cause abnormal loads on the lumbar spine. Those that are correctable may facilitate recovery from the injury. Anatomic problems might include a leg-length discrepancy, pelvic obliquity, tight hamstrings, or other inflexibilities in the lower extremities. The presence of scoliosis, kyphosis, excessive lordosis, and compensatory lumbar shifts may also be present. Range of motion assessment evaluates for any segmental restrictions (either secondary to bony or soft-tissue abnormalities). It is often useful to test an athlete during and after repetitive motion, noting increasing or decreasing pain and centralization or peripheralization of pain distribution. Repetitive loading may be necessary to elicit pain that may not be present on a single range of motion. Pain secondary to muscular tightness or articular stiffness may actually improve with repetitive motion. Diskogenic pain usually increases or becomes more peripheral with repetitive forward flexion. Posterior element pain usually increases with repetitive extension.

Careful palpation may help identify a source of pain. Focal tenderness in a muscular region does not necessarily indicate that it is the primary pain generator. An area of secondary spasm or pain may actually be caused by an underlying primary pain generator. Areas of soft-tissue pain may also be due to overload or compensation for regions in the kinetic chain that are weak or painful.

Muscle weakness, alteration of sensation, or nerve root tension signs indicate the presence of radiculopathy. Subtle side-to-side strength asymmetry may be significant, as highly conditioned athletes often have "supernormal" strength compared to the average population. Repetitive strength testing through calf raises, heel walking, or squats may also bring out subtle weaknesses. Evaluation of the patient during functional activities such as forward and backward ambulation, squatting, and heel and toe walking may reveal compensatory postures or movements that give clues to the underlying pathology.

The athlete with an acute symptomatic disk lesion will tend to have pain on flexion activities, although extension during weight bearing will often cause pain as well in the presence of a large central or lateral herniation. The athlete may demonstrate nerve root tension signs or potentially neurologic changes in a nerve root distribution.

The patient with a symptomatic pars interarticularis lesion typically has segmental lumbar pain. There may be no restrictions of flexion and this may actually relieve the symptoms, while extension may be limited or cause pain. The patient may have diffuse tenderness in the paraspinal muscles or focal posterior element tenderness in the setting of spondylolysis. With a true spondylolytic lesion with spondylolisthesis there may be a palpable step-off of the spinous process (91,97). Symptomatic patients with spondylolisthesis will often demonstrate a hyperlordotic posture with associated tight hip flexors and hamstrings and weak abdominal musculature. Neurologic signs are typically not seen in the spondylolytic patient, but may be seen in those who have progressed to spondylolisthesis. The patient with acute posterior element pain such as fractures and facet syndrome may present in a similar fashion.

RADIOLOGIC IMAGING

Radiologic imaging is often necessary to evaluate back pain that is persistent beyond the initial few weeks of conservative treatment. Imaging studies may be ordered sooner in an athlete than a nonathlete, owing to the increased demands on their spines compared to the average population (112). Imaging studies may also help physiatrists make return to play decisions.

While plain anteroposterior and lateral films often appear normal, the presence of congenital variations such as sacralization or lumbarization of vertebra, hemivertebra, or spina bifida should be noted. The role of many of these congenital variations in the development of lumbar spinal problems is questioned, but spina bifida occulta is associated with a slightly higher incidence of spondylolysis compared to the incidence in the normal population. Other important observations include the shape of the vertebral bodies, loss of disk space height, and facet joint alignment or sclerosis.

Plain radiography is invaluable for demonstrating the presence of spondylolysis or the degree of "listhesis." Posterior oblique x-ray views are the most sensitive for revealing the classic spondylolytic lesion. This has the appearance of a "Scottie dog" with a collar (see Fig. 71-9). Occasionally, the pars interarticularis will appear elongated, but without interruption.

For spondylolytic defects with spondylolisthesis, standing lateral views are utilized for staging and monitoring. A number of other measurements can be performed on a standard lateral radiograph and include the lumbosacral joint angle, sacral inclination, and slip angle. The sacral inclination defines the angle created by the posterior aspect of the sacrum to the plumbline. The slip angle is the angle formed by a line drawn perpendicular to the superior end-plate of S1 and the inferior end-plate of L5. The sacro-horizontal angle is the angle between a line drawn parallel to the upper end-plate of the sacrum and the horizontal plane on a standing lateral radiograph. Sward et al (113) found no evidence of spondylolysis in athletes with a sacro-horizontal angle below 35 degrees but did find evidence in 50% with a sacro-horizontal angle above 60 degrees. The measurement with the greatest clinical application in a series of patients with isthmic spondylolysis/spondylolisthesis was the percentage of slip or degree of listhesis (114). The Meyerding method grades the amount of spondylolisthesis in quarters (94) (Fig. 71-10): grade 1 lesion, zero to 25% slippage of the upper vertebra on the lower vertebra; grade 2 lesion, 26% to 50% slippage; grade 3, 51% to 75% slippage; and grade 4, 76% to 100% slippage. Some investigators also include a grade 5 that implies more than 100% slip with inferior subluxation (91,97,115).

Hyperextension injuries of the lumbar spine may demonstrate widening of the disk spaces anteriorly or fracture of posterior elements on lateral films. At times it may be difficult to differentiate isolated posterior arch fractures from congenital defects or spondylolysis. Acute fractures will typically demonstrate irregular nonsclerotic margins. There are no plain film findings associated with athletes with facet joint pain. While there is an association between age and osteoarthritic changes, the incidence is equal in symptomatic and asymptomatic individuals with facet joint pain (116). Additionally, there are no radiographic findings diagnostic of SIJ pain problems. Only selective facet or SIJ injections under fluoroscopic and contrast-enhanced guidance diagnose the facet or SIJ as a source of the athlete's pain (117,118).

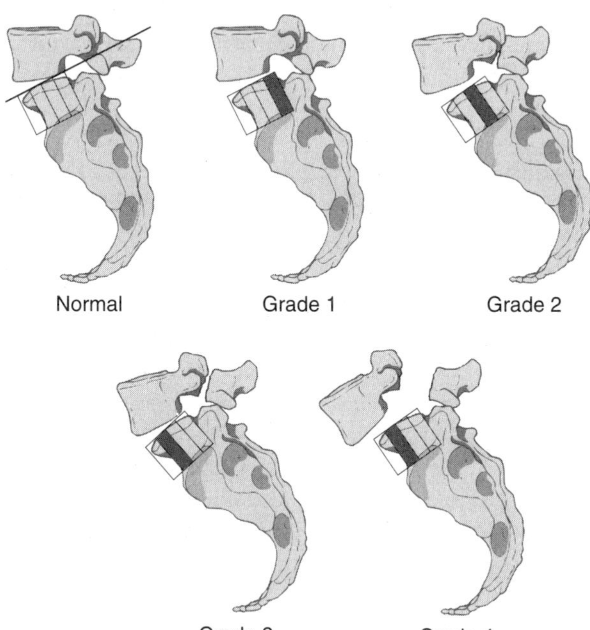

Figure 71-10. Spondylolisthesis grading system. (Reproduced by permission from Reid DC, ed. *Sports injury assessment and rehabilitation.* London: Churchill Livingstone, 1992.)

Flexion and extension x-ray studies are of value in the athlete who has had acute trauma or demonstrated spondylolisthesis because these x-ray films determine whether instability is present. Instability at the thoracolumbar junction may be seen in patients with Maigne syndrome (16,30,70). Films made with the patient in a side bending position may also demonstrate areas of focal segmental dysfunction (14). Burst fractures may be found by an increased interpedicular distance on the anteroposterior radiographic view or abnormalities in the posterior vertebral line on lateral radiographs (70,71). Interpedicular distance normally widens with caudal progression from L1 to L5. The height of the vertebral body posteriorly is usually 1.0 to 1.5 mm higher than the anterior margin; therefore, this finding should not be misinterpreted as an anterior vertebral body compression fracture. However, a posterior edge of the vertebral body that is not concave or at least straight may be a subtle indicator of buckling of the posterior cortex (70). Approximately 20% of unstable burst fractures are missed by using plain radiographs alone (71). CT more sensitively evaluates the true extent of injury. CT also will detect associated dural tears and epidural hematomas.

Athletes with a suspected pars interarticularis stress reaction or with a spondylolytic lesion of questionable duration should have a bone scan. Only 17% of chronic pars interarticularis lesions are associated with increased uptake on radionuclide imaging (119). Bone scan findings are nonspecific, but identify focal areas of active bone turnover seen in a stress reaction, fracture, apophysitis, tumor, or infection. SPECT has increased sensitivity and specificity compared to planar bone scanning; SPECT provides a better three-dimensional representation than does planar bone scanning (107,120). It can often distinguish whether increased uptake is in the ring apophysis, the pars interarticularis, or the facet joint. Serial SPECT scans may assist in monitoring the healing activity of a bony injury. A bone scan that shows a less hot or "warm" area after an initial scan early in the treatment course showed the same area to be "hot" may indicate healing of the pars defect.

MRI provides excellent resolution of soft-tissue abnormalities and demonstrates abnormalities of the intervertebral disk, the presence of nerve root or cord compression, and intradural or extradural tumors (121). MRI is often the study of choice in young athletes since significant bony degenerative changes are usually absent. MRI findings may be either normal or abnormal in the presence of IDD (122,123). Often, T2-weighted MRI may demonstrate decreased nuclear signal intensity. This reflects water loss from nuclear degradation (124). The presence of high-intensity zones within the posterior part of the annulus typifies radial annular fissures associated with IDD (125). Although MRI can demonstrate architectural abnormalities within the disk, it does not predict whether these changes are symptomatic (122,123). Provocative lumbar diskography can reveal whether or not internal disk findings such as annular disruption or disk degeneration are actually responsible for low-back pain symptoms (122,123,126–131).

MRI is excellent for visualizing the extent of disk degeneration in athletes with spondylolysis of the affected segment. Degenerative disk changes are more prevalent with this lesion at both the level of the lesion and the adjacent levels (121). When spondylolysis with spondylolisthesis is present at L5–S1, MRI can evaluate the extent of cephalocaudal stenosis of the intervertebral canal (132). MRI also visualizes hypertrophic fibrous tissue adjacent to the lysis, but will often miss ossified fragments contiguous to the defect (133).

CT offers a more detailed look at bony structures; therefore, it is often used for evaluating the anatomy of patients with pars interarticularis defects, fractures, or congenital abnormalities (hemivertebrae, other neural arch defects). Axial views of a lytic lesion through the pars interarticularis will demonstrate cleavage through the neural arch just above the plane of the articular facets (70,73). Dependent on its location in the pars, the defect can present an appearance similar to two facet joints. The zygapophyseal joint is distinguished from the lytic defect in that the former has a linear sclerotic articular margin. In addition to the lytic defect, CT may reveal arthritic changes in the facet joints or the "pseudobulging disk" of spondylolisthesis (89). Sagittal re-formation will demonstrate the association of the fracture line to the articular processes. This view is also optimal for visualizing stenosis of the central or intervertebral canals, which can be caused by fragmentation or hypertrophy of the pars defect, as demonstrated by thin-section CT. Different patterns of a healing pars fracture can be seen. There may be actual bridging with dense cortical bone or fibrocartilaginous material (121).

REHABILITATION

Rehabilitation of sport-related lumbar spinal injuries should be diagnosis specific and relevant to the athlete's clinical symptoms. The rehabilitation program must take into consideration the structures involved, the degree of tissue injury, and the optimum time frame for tissue healing. Kibler et al (134) described an elegant model for the treatment of musculoskeletal injuries. This model dictates treatment of not only the primary site of pain and dysfunction, but also all areas of dysfunction in the kinetic chain. The *tissue overload complex* includes tissues that are exposed to tensile overload. *Functional biomechanical deficits* are the various muscle imbalances of strength and flexibility that cause altered biomechanics. Subclinical adaptations often follow and are the substitute compensations for the tissue overload and the biomechanical deficit. The *tissue injury complex* is the point at which the tissue becomes injured and there is anatomic change. The *clinical symptom complex* comprises the signs and symptoms that result from the injury. In general, rehabilitation of lumbar spinal injuries is divided into three phases: 1) acute phase, 2) restorative phase, and 3) maintenance phase.

Acute Phase

Regardless of the diagnosis, the goals of the acute phase of rehabilitation are to reduce pain and inflammation. This phase includes restoration of nonpainful range of motion of the lumbar spine and normal resting muscle length. Therapeutic interventions may allow speedy progression through this phase. These interventions include but are not limited to patient education and body mechanics training, pharmacologic management, physical therapy modalities, manual therapy approaches, protective bracing, and diagnosis-dependent stretching and strengthening exercises. At times, trigger point injections or selective injections under fluoroscopically guided contrast-enhanced may expedite a reduction in pain and inflammation. Pharmacologic management and physical therapy modalities are covered in other sections of this textbook.

Patient Education

Patient education begins in this phase. The initial principles of back school and postural education involve instructing the athlete to develop awareness of any aggravating factors of the pain, develop solutions for relieving that pain, and find relieving positions. The therapist should teach active joint protection so that the athlete does not continually reinjure the area during simple activities of daily living (ADLs). Instruction in proper body mechanics during typical activities decreases the possibility of further reinjury. This assists in shortening the overall rehabilitation time.

Flexibility Training and Mobilization

Flexibility training is an essential component of the rehabilitation program. Appropriate flexibility through the lumbopelvic region and the lower extremities is critical to achieving balanced posture and decreasing strain on the injured tissues. Efforts to achieve appropriate flexibility may include manual soft-tissue techniques, passive stretching, static stretching, and neuromuscular facilitation. In the first phase of rehabilitation, flexibility should be initiated with static stretching in the middle or end of the tolerable range of motion. Significant adaptive soft-tissue shortening may occur after acute injury and must be addressed when present. Superficial or deep soft-tissue massage, manual traction, assisted stretching, and passive joint mobilization may be effective. Superficial massage may help increase flexibility and improve circulation to expedite healing and to remove inflammatory by-products (135). Pain may cause patterns of neuromuscular inhibition that promote abnormal lumbar postures. Soft-tissue techniques help decrease pain in shortened tissues, expediting joint mobilization and restoration of normal joint mechanics. Passive joint motion through mobilization stretches the joint capsules, lubricates the joint surfaces, and induces metabolic changes in soft tissue, cartilage, and bone. Mobilization is the application of a force along the rotational or translational plane of motion of a joint. At times, high-velocity low-amplitude manipulation may be of benefit in treating a dysfunctional segment (40).

McKenzie Treatment

Mechanical therapy based on the McKenzie principles of assessment and treatment may also be useful in determining a directional preference of motion, soft-tissue dysfunction problems, or structural derangements (136). The McKenzie method utilizes a simple categorization of examination findings into three syndromes: posture, dysfunction, and derangement. Exercises are primarily performed by repeated movements that are determined by the directional preference of motion and according to the syndrome classification.

Lumbar Stabilization

An active form of joint protection is a lumbar stabilization program (14,40,52,111). The stabilization concept revolves around the elimination of repetitive microtrauma, attempting to limit injury and thus allow healing. Stabilization training involves the coordinated co-contraction of abdominal and extensor muscles in a lumbar neutral position (40,52,111). The goal of this portion of therapy is to eliminate repetitive injury and encourage healing of the injured segment. Lumbar neutral is a position of optimum function in which the least amount of mechanical stress is applied to the lumbar spine. The neutral position is initially assisted by a therapist, since patients often are not aware of poor postural patterns. To be able to achieve this neutral spinal position, the athlete needs adequate flexibility of torso and lower-extremity musculature.

Selective Injections

Selective spinal injection procedures can be of benefit when pain continues to inhibit progress during the acute phase of rehabilitation. Trigger point injections at primary points of myofascial pain or at the end points of referred pain may decrease muscular tone and improve muscular flexibility (137). Depending on the diagnosis, fluoroscopically guided and contrast-enhanced facet, selective nerve root, or epidural steroid injections may be used to decrease pain and aid progress through the rehabilitation program (138).

Restorative Phase

The restorative phase of rehabilitation addresses both tissue overload and functional biomechanical deficits. Improved lumbar range of motion, soft-tissue length, and biomechanics are a prerequisite for initiating this phase of rehabilitation. Occasionally, manipulative or soft-tissue techniques may still be required. Strengthening is begun in simple planes of motion and progressed to more complex patterns. Muscular re-education may be necessary during preliminary strength training to ensure that proper muscle engrams are reinforced. Once motor coordination has been developed, the speed of repetition and amount of resistance may be increased. After appropriate static and dynamic stabilization has been achieved, the athlete may begin functional activities and conditioning.

Maintenance Phase

The final phase of rehabilitation is the maintenance phase. This requires full, nonpainful active and passive lumbar range of motion and an appropriate neutral posture during both static and dynamic activities. It is usually in this phase that the athlete returns to play. Thus, normal clinical findings including normal responses to provocative-type maneuvers are necessary. In collision sports, tackling or checking techniques should be reviewed to ensure appropriateness. It is important to understand the biomechanics of each sport such that the physiatrist can emphasize sport-specific training. Subclinical adaptations may be inherent to the athlete's sport and strategies to minimize them must be incorporated into the maintenance treatment program.

Sport-Specific Rehabilitation and Return to Play

In order to plan the appropriate rehabilitation program for the injured athlete, the physiatrist needs to understand the biomechanics involved for the sport involved as it relates to the injured body part. An in-depth analysis of lumbar spinal biomechanics as they apply to the athlete for different sports is beyond the scope of this chapter.

Football

Low-back pain is a common complaint for football players, especially linemen (139). The majority of lumbar spinal injuries are related to soft tissues and respond to treatment in a short period of time without long-term consequences. Persistent low-back pain complaints can be secondary to facet joint or intervertebral disk injury (140). There is a higher incidence of lumbar spondylolysis in football players than in the general adult population, presumably owing to repetitive hyperextension loads (139). Weight training has also been linked to lumbar spinal injuries in football players (141).

After recovery during the acute phase of the injury, the football player with a lumbar spinal injury undergoes an aggressive stabilization program. Increasing strength and flexibility is also emphasized during the restorative phase. Playing technique is analyzed and corrected to incorporate proper stabilization. The three-point stance for linemen and running backs is adjusted for balance and neutral spine posture. Upright defensive players and receivers are instructed on proper foot work to avoid movements that twist the spine. Return to play is contingent on pain-free movement and proper technique with spine stabilization (142).

Baseball

The treatment of lumbar spinal injuries in baseball players can be classified by position: pitcher, fielder, and hitter. The pitching motion places tremendous demands on the lumbar spine. It depends in large part on the coordinated muscular activities of the abdominal, lumbar, and gluteal muscles (143). Strengthening, flexibility, and conditioning of these muscles are imperative to achieve maximal pitching performance and to prevent lumbar spinal injuries.

A lack of flexibility can lead to torsional strain of the nondominant lumbar facet joints or SIJ. This is most commonly seen during spring training in pitchers who have not maintained an off-season fitness program. Weakness or fatigue in the abdominal, lumbar, or gluteal muscles can lead to poor pitching performance or injury to other body structures. These muscle groups provide stabilization of the spine and trunk and allow for the power and control generated during the pitching motion. If these muscles are weakened or deconditioned, the throwing arm works harder in an attempt to maintain pitching performance, which can lead to upper-extremity injuries (143).

Any painful disorder of the lumbar spine will have an impact on pitching performance by altering the intricate coordination of trunk muscles needed to stabilize the pelvis and spine. Rehabilitation efforts during the restorative and maintenance phases focus on strengthening and trunk stabilization. The pitcher must be able to achieve an adequate level of conditioning and stabilization, and demonstrate the ability to throw pain free before returning to play.

The same emphasis on trunk conditioning and stabilization applies in the treatment of the hitter as well as the pitcher. After the player progresses through the acute phase of treatment, the emphasis during the restorative phase centers on balance, flexibility, and strength. The hitter is trained without a bat. It is important to wait until the end of the restorative phase of treatment before allowing the hitter to swing the bat again. This allows for the correction of bad habits. The batting stance is evaluated for balance and base of support. Treatment includes stabilization and strengthening of the torso. The batter is taught to maintain muscle contraction through a full swing rotation. Strengthening is accomplished with resistance from the therapist during full range of motion and in the opposite direction. The hitter is allowed to start training with the therapist and coach on batting mechanics after successful completion of the restorative phase. The hitter returns to play after demonstrating the ability to swing the bat with proper mechanics and without pain.

The infielder and catcher are treated for lumbar spinal injuries in the same manner as someone who performs a lifting job at work. Proper spine stabilization technique in the squat position is emphasized during treatment. The player must be able to maintain proper spine mechanics during fielding as well as in the transition to and during throwing. As in pitching and hitting, the player is returned to play after demonstrating proper pain-free technique and mechanics.

Basketball

Ankle and knee injuries are more common in basketball than are lumbar spinal injuries. Most back injuries in basketball are sprain or strain disorders that occur from repetitive twisting and bending during a game. Off-balance jumping and landing can lead to intervertebral disk and facet joint injuries from asymmetric axial loading. The frequency of axial loading during a basketball game will exacerbate diskogenic and radicular symptoms, which can lead to further injury as well as suboptimal play. Treatment after the acute phase stresses lumbar stabilization. This is important since basketball players assume a crouched position to protect the basketball while dribbling and playing defense. It is important that the player slide and move the feet when in the defensive position and not rotate the spine. Return to play criteria include resolution of pain and demonstration of proper body mechanics.

CONCLUSIONS

The successful treatment of an athlete with a lumbar spinal injury begins by making the correct diagnosis. If the injury occurs on the playing field, the initial assessment must exclude a catastrophic spinal injury. Imaging studies are performed when appropriate to evaluate for fracture, disk herniation, spondylolysis, and spondylolisthesis. Aggressive acute treatment incorporates pharmacologic management, physical therapy techniques, bracing when necessary, and patient education. Lumbar stabilization, flexibility, and strength training are emphasized during the restorative phase of treatment. Playing technique is analyzed during the latter part of the restoration phase and modifications are made with instruction on proper body biomechanics. A return to play depends on the athlete's demonstration of proper playing technique incorporating a neutral spine posture and full pain-free lumbar range of motion.

REFERENCES

1. Bogduk N, Twomey LT. *Clinical anatomy of the lumbar spine.* 2nd ed. London: Churchill Livingstone, 1991.

2. White AA III, Panjabi M. *Clinical biomechanics of the spine.* 2nd ed. Philadelphia: JB Lippincottt, 1990.

3. Cyron BM, Hutton WC. The tensile strength of the capsular ligaments of the apophyseal ligaments. *J Anat* 1981;132: 145–150.

4. Glover JR. Arthrography of the joints of the lumbar vertebral arches. *Orthop Clin North Am* 1997;8:37–42.

5. Adams MA, Hutton WC. The mechanical function of the lumbar apophyseal joints. *Spine* 1983;8:327–330.

6. Yang KH, King AI. Mechanism of facet load transmission as a hypothesis for low back pain. *Spine* 1984;9:557–565.

7. Weinstein J, Weisel S. *The lumbar spine.* Philadelphia: WB Saunders, 1990.

8. Hochsculer S. *The spine in sports.* Philadelphia: Hanley & Belfus, 1990.

9. Aggrawal ND, Ravinder K, Kumar S, Mathur D. A study of changes in the spine in weightlifters and other athletes. *Br J Sports Med* 1979;13:58–61.

10. Adams MA, Hutton WC. The relevance of torsion to the mechanical derangement of the lumbar spine. *Spine* 1981;6:241–248.

11. Dietrich M, Kurrowskip. The importance of mechanical fractures and the etiology of spondylolysis: a model analysis of loads and stresses in human lumbar spine. *Spine* 1985;6:532.

12. Franco V, Nordin M. *Basic biomechanics of the skeletal system.* Philadelphia: Lea & Febiger, 1980:255–290.

13. Markolf K. Deformation of the thoracolumbar intervertebral joints in response to external loads. *J Bone Joint Surg [Am]* 1972;54:511–533.

14. Kirkklady-Willis WH. *Managing low back pain.* 2nd ed. New York: Churchill Livingstone, 1988.

15. Spencer CW, Jackson DW. Back injuries in athletes. In: Jordan BD, Tsairis, Warren RF, eds. *Sports neurology.* 159–179.

16. Hellstrom M, Jacobsson B, Sward L, et al. Radiologic abnormalities of the thoracolumbar spine in athletes. *Acta Radiol* 1990;31:127.

17. Cyrone BM, Hutton WC. Fatigue strength of the lumbar neural arch and spondylolysis. *J Bone Joint Surg [Br]* 1978;68:234.

18. Goldstein JD, Berger PE, Windler GE, et al. Spine injuries in gymnasts and swimmers: an epidemiologic investigation. *Am J Sports Med* 1991;19:463.

19. Horne J, Cockshott WP, Shannon HS. Spinal column damages from water ski jumping. *Skel Radiol* 1987;16:612.

20. Jackson D, Forman W, Benson B. Patterns of injuries in intercollegiate athletes: a retrospective study of injuries sustained in intercollegiate athletics in two colleges in a two year period. *Mt Sinai J Med* 1980;47:423.

21. Jackson DW, Wiltsee LL, Cirincinone RJ. Spondylolysis in the female athlete. *Clin Orthop* 1976;117:68–73.

22. Kernahan M, Kirkpatrick J, Stanish WD. An investigation into the incidence of low back pain in horseback riders. *Nova Scotia Med Bull* 1979:167–169.

23. Mahlamaki S, Soimakallio S, Michelsson JE. Radiologic finding in the lumbar spine of 39 young cross-country skiers with low back pain. *Int J Sports Med* 1988;9:196–197.

24. McCarrol JR, Gioe TJ. Professional golfers and the price they pay. *Phys Sports Med* 1982; 10:64.

25. Micheli LJ. Back injuries in gymnastics. *Cl* 1985;4:85–9

26. Omar MM, Levinsoh unusual fracture of the articular process in a skie *Trauma* 1979;19:212.

27. Semon RL, Spengler D. Significance of lumbar spondylosis in college football players. *Spine* 1981;6:172.

28. Stewart T. The age incidence of neural arch defects in Alaskan natives. *J Bone Joint Surg [Am]* 1953;3:937.

29. Sward L, Hellstrom M, Jacobsen B, et al. Acute injury of the vertebral ring apophysis and intervertebral disc in adolescent gymnasts. *Spine* 1990;15:144.

30. Sward L, Hellstrom M, Jacobsen B, et al. Back pain and the radiologic changes in the thoracolumbar spine of athletes. *Spine* 1989;15:124–129.

31. Sward L, Hellstrom M, Jacobsen B, et al. Disc degeneration and associated abnormalities of the lumbar spine in elite gymnasts: a magnetic resonance imaging study. *Spine* 1991;16:437.

32. Tator CH, Edmonds VE. National survey of spinal injuries in hockey players. *Can Med Assoc J* 1984;130:875.

33. Weiss BD. Nontraumatic injuries in amateur long distance bicyclists. *Am J Sports Med* 1985;13:187.

34. Wroble RR, Albright JP. Neck and low back injuries in wrestling. *Clin Sports Med* 1986;5:295–325.

35. Schneiderman G, Flannigan B, Kingston S, et al. MRI in the diagnosis of disc degeneration: correlation with discography. *Spine* 1987;12:276–281.

36. McCarrol JR, Miller JM, Ritter MA. Lumbar spondylolysis and spondylolisthesis in college football players. A prospective study. *Am J Sports Med* 1986;14: 404–406.

37. Ferguson RJ, McMaster JH, Stan-

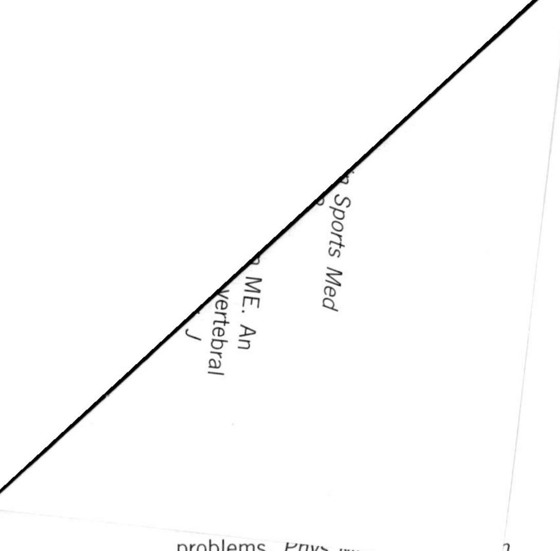

problems. *Phys Med* ... *N Am* 1991;2:187–203.

41. National Basketball Trainers Association. *NBTA injury reporting system, 1990–1991 season.* New York: National Basketball Association, 1991:1–6.

42. Bohlman JT. Injuries in competitive cycling. *Phys Sports Med* 1981;9:1117.

43. Anderson SJ. The pediatric and adolescent athlete with low back pain. *Phys Med Rehabil Clin N Am* 1991;2:157–185.

44. Letts M, McDonald P. Sports injuries to the pediatric spine. *Spine State Art Rev* 1990;4:49–83.

45. Epstein JA, Epstein NE, Marc J, et al. Lumbar intervertebral disk herniation in teenage children: recognition and management of associated anomalies. *Spine* 1982;9:427–432.

46. Spencer CW, Jackson DW. Back injuries in the athlete. *Clin Sports Med* 1981;2:191.

47. Mixter WJ, Barr JS. Rupture of the intervertebral disc with involvement of the spinal canal. *N Engl J Med* 1934;211:210–215.

48. Modic MT, Masaryk TJ, Ross JS. *Magnetic resonance imaging of the spine.* 2nd ed. Chicago: Year Book Medical, 1994.

49. Gordon SJ, Yang KH, Mayer PJ, et al. Mechanism of disc rupture. A preliminary report. *Spine* 1991;16:450–456.

50. Wilder DG, Pope MH, Frymoyer JW. The biomechanics of the lumbar disc herniation and the effect of overload and instability. *J Spinal Disord* 1988;1:1–32.

51. Jackson DW. Low back pain in young athletes: evaluation of stress reactions and discogenic problems. *Am J Sports Med* 1979;7:364.

52. Saal JA, Saal JS. Later stage management of lumbar spine problems. *Phys Med Rehabil Clin N Am* 1991;2:205–222.

53. Feinstein B. Referred pain from paravertebral structures. In: Buerger AA, Tobis JS, eds. *Approaches to the validation of manipulative therapy.* Springfield, IL: Charles C Thomas, 1977: 139–174.

54. Feinstein B, Langton JNK, Jameson RM, et al. Experiments on pain referred from deep somatic tissues. *J Bone Joint Surg [Am]* 1954;36:981–997.

55. Rydevik B, Brown M, Lundborg G. Pathoanatomy and pathophysiology of nerve root compression. *Spine* 1984;9:7–15.

56. Crock HV. A reappraisal of intervertebral disc lesions. *Med J Aust* 1970;1:983–989.

57. Farfan HF. A reorientation in the surgical approach to degenerative lumbar intervertebral joint disease. *Orthop Clin North Am* 1977;8:9–21.

58. Farfan HF, Cossette JW, Robertson GH, et al. The effects of torsion on the lumbar intervertebral joints: the role of torsion in the production of disc degeneration. *J Bone Joint Surg [Am]* 1970;52:497–568.

59. Farfan HF, Huberdeau RM, Dubow HI. Lumbar intervertebral disc degeneration. The influence of geometrical features on the pattern of disc degeneration—a post mortem study. *J Bone Joint Surg [Am]* 1972;54:492–510.

60. Bobechko WT, Hirsch C. Autoimmune response to nucleus pulposus in the rabbit. *J Bone Joint Surg [Br]* 1965;47:574–580.

61. Gertzbein SD. Degenerative disk disease of the lumbar spine: immunologic implications. *Clin Orthop* 1977;129:68–71.

62. Gertzbein SD, Tait JH, Devlin SR. The stimulation of lymphocytes by nucleus pulposus in patients with degenerative disk disease of the lumbar spine. *Clin Orthop* 1977;123:149–154.

63. Gertzbein SD, Tile M, Gross A, et al. Autoimmunity in degenerative disc disease of the lumbar spine. *Orthop Clin North Am* 1975; 6:67–73.

64. Blumenthal SL, Roach J, Herring JA. Lumbar Scheuermann's. A clinical series and classification. *Spine* 1987;12:930.

65. Wilcox PG, Spencer CW. Dorsolumbar kyphosis or Scheuermann's disease. *Clin Sports Med* 1986;5:343–351.

66. Alexander CJ. Scheuermann's disease: a traumatic spondylodystrophy? *Skel Radiol* 1977;1: 209.

67. Panjanen H, Alanen A, Erkintalo M, et al. Disc degeneration in Scheuermann's disease. *Skel Radiol* 1989;18:523.

68. McCall IW, Park WM, O'Brien JP, et al. Acute traumatic intraosseous disc herniation. *Spine* 1985;10:134–137.

69. Denis F. The three column spine and its significance on classification of acute thoracolumbar spine injuries. *Spine* 1983;8:817–831.

70. Berquist TH, Gehweiler, JA, Osborne RL, Becker RF. *The radiology of vertebral trauma.* Philadelphia: WB Saunders, 1980.

71. Ballock TR, Mackersie R, Abitbol JJ, et al. Can burst fractures be diagnosed with plain radiographs alone? *J Bone Joint Surg [Br]* 1992;74:147–150.

72. Berquist TH. *Imaging of orthopedic trauma.* 2nd ed. New York: Raven, 1991.

73. Gehweiler JA, Osborne RL, Becker RF. *The radiology of vertebral trauma.* Philadelphia: WB Saunders, 1980.

74. Kramer KM, Levine AM. Unilateral facet dislocation of the lumbosacral junction. *J Bone Joint Surg [Am]* 1989;69:140–142.

75. Jackson DW, Wiltse LL, Dingeman RD. Stress reactions involving the pars interarticularis in young athletes. *Am J Sports Med* 1981;9:304–312.

76. Cirillo JV, Jackson DW. Pars interarticularis stress reaction, spondylolysis and spondylolisthesis in gymnasts. *Clin Sports Med* 1982;4:991–996.

77. Mann DC, Keene JS, Drummond DS. Unusual causes of low back pain in athletes. *J Spinal Disord* 1991;4:337–343.

78. Ghormley RK. Low back pain with special reference to the articular facets, with presentation of an operative procedure. *JAMA* 1933;101:1733–1777.

79. Jackson RP, Jacobs RR, Montesano PX. Facet joint injection in low back pain: a prospective statistical study. *Spine* 1988;13:996–971.

80. Revel ME, Listrat VM, Chevalier XJ, et al. Facet joint block for low back pain: identifying predictors of a good response. *Arch Phys Med Rehabil* 1992;73:824–828.

81. Schwarzer AC, Aprill CN, Derby R, et al. The false positive rate of single lumbar zygapophysial joint blocks. *Pain* 1994;58:195–200.

82. Mooney V, Robertson J. The facet syndrome. *Clin Orthop* 1976; 115:149.

83. Schwarzer AC, Derby R, Aprill CN, et al. The value of the provocation response in lumbar zygapophyseal joint injections. *Clin J Pain* 1994;10:309–313.

84. Carette S, Marcoux S, Truchon R, et al. A controlled trial of corticosteroid injections into the facet joints for chronic low back pain. *N Engl J Med* 1991;325: 1002–1007.

85. Lilius G, Laasonen EM, Myllynen P, et al. Lumbar facet joint syndrome: a randomized clinical trial. *J Bone J Surg [Br]* 1989; 71:681–684.

86. Bogduk N, Long D. Percutaneous lumbar medial branch neurotomy. *Spine* 1980;5:193–200.

87. Schunke GB. Anatomy and development of the sacroiliac joint in man. *Anat Rec* 1938;72:313–331.

88. Bernard TN Jr, Cassidy JD. The sacroiliac joint syndrome—pathophysiology, diagnosis and management. In: Frymoyer JW, ed. *The adult spine: principles and practice.* New York: Raven, 1991:2107–2130.

89. Solonen KA. The sacroiliac joint in light of anatomical, roentgenological and clinical studies. *Acta Scand Suppl* 1957;27:1–127.

90. Fortin JD, Dwyer AP, West S, et al. Sacroiliac joint: pain referral maps upon applying a new injection/arthrography technique. Part I: asymptomatic volunteers. *Spine* 1994;19:1475–1482.

91. Fredrickson BE, Baker D, Holich NJ, et al. The natural history of spondylolysis and spondylolisthesis. *J Bone Joint Surg [Am]* 1984;66:699.

92. Wiltse LL. Spondylolysis in children. *Clin Orthop* 1961;21:156–163.

93. Wiltse LL, Widdelle EH Jr, Jackson DW. Fatigue fracture: the basic lesion in spondylolisthesis. *J Bone Joint Surg [Am]* 1975; 57:17.

94. Wiltse LL, Winter RB. Terminology and measurement of spondylolisthesis. *J Bone Joint Surg [Am]* 1983;65:768.

95. Newman P, Stone K. The etiology of spondylolisthesis with special investigation. *J Bone Joint Surg [Br]* 1963;45:39.

96. Teplick JG, Laffey PA, Berman A, et al. Diagnosis and evaluation of spondylolisthesis and/or spondylolisthesis on axial CT. *AJNR* 1986;7:479.

97. Bradford D. Spondylolysis and spondylolisthesis in children and adolescents. In: Bradford D, Hensinger R, eds. *Pediatric spine.* New York: Thieme & Stratton, 1985.

98. Win[illegible] tance i[illegible] *Joint Surg* [illegible]

99. Rosenberg N, Ba[illegible] Freidman B. Incide[illegible] spondylolysis in non-a[illegible] patients. *Spine* 1981;6:3[illegible]

100. Roche MB, Rowe GC. Incidence of separate neural arch in coincident bone variations. *J Bone Joint Surg [Am]* 1952;34:491.

101. Porter R, Park W. Unilateral spondylolysis. *J Bone Joint Surg [Br]* 1982;64:345.

102. Rothman SL. Computed tomography of the spine in older children and teenagers. *Clin Sports Med* 1986;5:247–270.

103. Ravichandran G. Multiple lumbar spondylolyses. *Spine* 1980;5: 552.

104. Boxall D, Bradford D, Winter R, et al. Management of severe spondylolisthesis in children and in adolescence. *J Bone Joint Surg [Am]* 6:479.

105. Ireland ML, Michaeli GJ. Bilateral stress fracture of the lumbar pedicles in a ballet dancer. *J Bone Joint Surg [Am]* 1989; 1987;69:140–142.

106. Hutton WC, Stott RJ, Cyrone BM. Spondylolysis a fatigue fracture? *Spine* 1977;2:202.

107. Collier BD, Johnson RP, Carrera GF, et al. Painful spondylolysis or spondylolisthesis studied by radiography and single photon emission computed tomography. *Radiology* 1985;154:207.

108. Bell DF, Ehrlich MG, Zaleske DJ. Brace treatment for symptomatic spondylolysis. *Clin Orthop* 1988; 236:192–198.

109. Hensinger RR, Lang J, MacEweng. Surgical management of spondylolisthesis in children and adolescents. *Spine* 1976;1:207.

110. Peck R, Wiltsee LL, et al. In situ arthrodesis without decompression for grade III or IV isthmic spondylolisthesis in adults who have severe Sciatica. *J Bone Joint Surg* 1989;71:62.

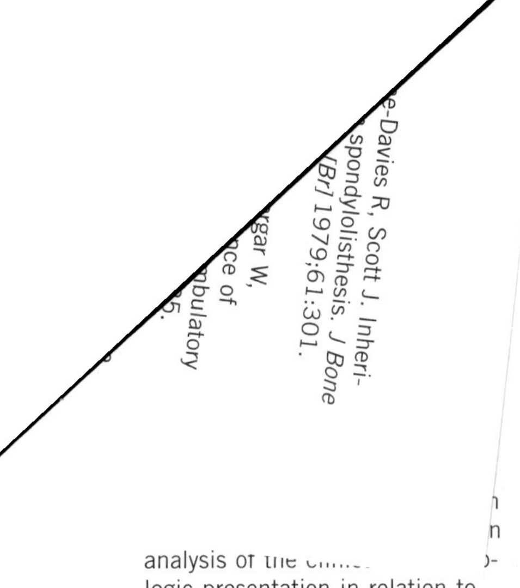

analysis of the ... logic presentation in relation to intraoperative findings and surgical results in 72 consecutive cases. *Acta Neurochir* 1992;110:154.

115. Wiltse LL, Newman P, MacNab I. Classifications of spondylolysis and spondylolisthesis. *Clin Orthop* 1976;117:23.

116. Magora A, Schwartz T. Relation between low back pain syndrome and X-ray findings. *Scand J Rehabil Med* 1976;8:115–125.

117. Schwarzer AC, Derby R, April CA, et al. The role of bone scintigraphy in chronic low back pain: comparison of SPECT and planar images and zygapophyseal joint injections. *Aust N Z J Med* 1982;22:185.

118. Cole AJ, Dreyfuss P, Stratton SA. The sacroiliac joint: Principles of treatment. In: Windsor R, Lox D, eds. *Soft tissue injuries—diagnosis and treatment*. Philadelphia: Hanley & Belfus, 1988:65–84.

119. Pennell RG, Maurer AH, Bonakdarpour A. Stress injuries of the pars interarticularis: radiographic classification and indications for scintigraphy. *AJR* 1985;145:763.

120. Bella HR, Summerville D, Trevess, et al. Low back pain in adolescent athletes: detection of stress injury to the pars interarticularis with SPECT. *Radiology* 1991;180:5 09–512.

121. Herzog RJ. Selection and utilization of imaging studies for disorders of the lumbar spine. *Phys Med Rehabil Clin N Am* 1991;2:7–59.

122. Gibson MJ, Buckley J, Mawhinney R. Magnetic resonance imaging and discography in the diagnosis of disc degeneration. A comparative study of 50 discs. *J Bone Joint Surg [Br]* 1986;68: 369–373.

123. Horton WC, Daftari TK. Which disc as visualized by magnetic resonance imaging is actually a source of pain? A correlation between magnetic resonance imaging and discography. *Spine* 1992;17:S164–S171.

124. Panagiotacopulos ND, Pope MH, Krag MH, et al. Water content in human intervertebral discs. Part I. Measurements by magnetic resonance imaging. *Spine* 1987;12:912–917.

125. Aprill C, Bogduk N. High-intensity zone: a diagnostic sign of painful lumbar disc on magnetic resonance imaging. *Br J Radiol* 1992;65:361–369.

126. Colhoun E, McCall IW, Williams L, et al. Provocation discography as a guide to planning operations on the spine. *J Bone Joint Surg [Br]* 1988;70:267–271.

127. Collins HR. An evaluation of cervical and lumbar discography. *Clin Orthop* 1975;107:133–138.

128. Collis JS, Gardner WJ. Lumbar discography: analysis of 600 degenerated disks and diagnosis of degenerative disk disease. *JAMA* 1961;178:167–170.

129. Schwarzer AC, April CN, Derby R, et al. The relative contributions of the disc and zygapophyseal joint in chronic low back pain. *Spine* 1994;19:801–806.

130. Simmons EH, Segil CM. An evaluation of discography in the localization of symptomatic levels in discogenic disease of the spine. *Clin Orthop* 1975;108:57–69.

131. Windsor RE, Falco FJ, Dreyer SJ, et al. Lumbar discography, *Phys Med Rehab Clin N Am* 1995;6:743–770.

132. Heithoff KB. Magnetic resonance imaging of the lumbar spine. In: Kirklady-Willis WH, ed. *Managing low back pain*. New York: Churchill Livingstone, 1988:183–208.

133. Grenier N, Kressel HY, Schiebler ML, et al. Isthmic spondylolysis of the lumbar spine: MR imaging at 1.5T. *Radiology* 1989;170: 489.

134. Kibler BW, Chandler TJ, Pace BK. Principles of rehabilitation after chronic tendon injury. *Clin Sports Med* 1992;11:661–671.

135. Greenman F. Principles of soft tissue and articulatory (mobilization without impulse) technique. In: *Principles of manual medicine*. Baltimore: Williams & Wilkins, 1989:71–87.

136. McKenzie RA. *The lumbar spine: mechanical diagnosis and therapy*. Waikanae, New Zealand: Spinal Publications, 1981.

137. Travell JH, Simmons DG. *Myofascial pain and dysfunction: trigger point manual*. Baltimore: Williams & Wilkins, 1983.

138. Windsor R, Washington K. Clinical review of specific spinal injections. In: Windsor R, Lox D, eds. *Soft tissue injury—diagnosis and treatment*. Philadelphia: Hanley & Belfus, 1997.

139. Ferguson RJ, McMaster JH, et al. Low back pain in college football lineman. *J Sports Med* 1974;2:63.

140. Saal JA. Rehabilitation of football players with lumbar spine injury (part 1). *Phys Sports Med* 1988;16:61.

141. Cook T. The professional athlete. *Occup Med State Art Rev* 1992;7:87.

142. Semon RL, Spengler D. Significance of lumbar spondylolysis in college football players. *Spine* 1981;6:172.

143. Watkins R, Dennis S, et al. Dynamic EMG analysis of torque transfer in professional baseball pitchers. *Spine* 1989;14: 404–408.

Central Neurologic Disease and Injury

Chapter 72

Rehabilitation of Traumatic Brain Injury

Lawrence J. Horn
Mark Sherer

Interventions to treat traumatic brain injury (TBI) have been documented since prehistoric times. Boake (1) provided a detailed review of the modern history of TBI rehabilitation. However, current rehabilitative management strategies and indeed the "industry" of TBI rehabilitation have only existed for approximately the past two decades in the United States. One of the most prominent events was the establishment of the Head Injury Rehabilitation Project by the Rehabilitation Services Commission at Santa Clara Valley Medical Center in 1977 (2). At the time that project was initiated, many patients with TBI could not access intensive acute rehabilitative services because of their inability to consistently follow commands or because of severe behavioral disturbances. Since that report's publication, there has been a dramatic increase in the types of programs designed to specifically treat people with TBI and other residual deficits from the brain injury. Now there are specific Commission on Accreditation of Rehabilitation Facilities (CARF) accrediting criteria for acute rehabilitation programs, postacute rehabilitation programs, residential and vocational programs, and hospital-based and skilled nursing–based programs for this population. For the most part, people with TBI can now access rehabilitative services early (when it is purported to be most effective) and receive appropriate services to assist in the restitution to a functional lifestyle.

The purpose of this chapter is to review aspects of the epidemiology, pathophysiology, and rehabilitative strategies specific to TBI. Many of the interventions discussed, though often developed for traumatic causes of brain dysfunction, are equally applicable to other types of acquired brain disorders.

DEFINITIONS

The term *traumatic brain injury* is often used interchangeably in the literature with *head injury* or *head trauma*; TBI is preferred as it clearly indicates damage to the brain. For our purposes, TBI denotes an acquired injury to the brain secondary to an external force that results in impairment of cognitive, neurobehavioral, or physical functioning. *Closed* head injury implies integrity of the dura and usually the cranial vault itself. *Penetrating* head injury means that a foreign object has penetrated the skull and the dura; most typically these are missile (bullet) injuries, but may also include stab wounds. Nontraumatic brain injuries include hypoxic-ischemic encephalopathy, toxic brain injury, and infectious brain disorders. These are often optimally managed in TBI programs or systems.

Accurate classification of the severity of TBI is important because the initial severity of the injury is predictive of the duration of rehabilitation (3) and the eventual functional outcome (4,5). Injury severity has been classified by degree of impaired consciousness (6), duration of posttraumatic amnesia (7), and length of time before the patient can follow simple motor commands (4). Of these methods, degree of impaired consciousness as

Table 72-1: Glasgow Coma Scale	Score
Motor responses	
Obeys commands	6
Localizing response to pain	5
Generalized withdrawal to pain	4
Flexor posturing to pain	3
Extensor posturing to pain	2
No motor response to pain	1
Verbal responses	
Oriented	5
Confused conversation	4
Inappropriate speech	3
Incomprehensible speech	2
No speech	1
Eye opening	
Spontaneous eye opening	4
Eye opening to speech	3
Eye opening to pain	2
No eye opening	1

measured by the Glasgow Coma Scale (GCS) (6) is the most commonly used. The GCS score, as shown in Table 72-1, is obtained by assessing the patient's eye opening, motor responses, and verbal responses; assigning a value to each of these; and summing the values. GCS scores range from 3 to 15, with lower scores indicating greater impairment of consciousness. Patients with no eye opening and no purposeful verbal or motor responses are considered to be in a coma (8). The GCS score can be obtained quickly and extremely reliably (9). Many studies have shown GCS to be a valid predictor of patient outcome (10,11). Threats to the validity of GCS as a predictor of outcome include the score's susceptibility to the effects of intubation, intoxication, hypotension, and the postictal state (11,12).

Patients with postresuscitation GCS scores of 3 to 8 have had a severe TBI, those with scores 9 to 12 have had a moderate injury, and those with scores 13 to 15 have had a mild injury. Patients with mild TBI may have had no loss of consciousness, but show evidence of impaired consciousness by having some period of posttraumatic amnesia. Patients with mild TBI who have abnormalities on computed tomography (CT) scans of the brain or who have objective findings on neurologic examination may be classified as having a complicated mild injury. The functional outcome of patients with complicated mild TBI is poorer than that for patients with an uncomplicated injury and more closely resembles the outcome typically seen for patients with a moderate injury (13).

Severe TBI is associated with a morality rate of more than 50% (14) and those who survive are usually left with significant cognitive impairments and may have residual physical limitations (4,5). Only approximately 30% of severe TBI survivors recover to moderate disability or good recovery by 6 months after injury as measured by the Glasgow Outcome Scale (GOS) (8). Moderate TBI has a mortality rate of less than 10% (14) and many patients have only mild residual deficits (15). Approximately 70% of moderate TBI patients attain a GOS rating of moderate disability or good recovery by 6 months (8). Mild TBI rarely results in death and the majority of patients return to preinjury levels of functioning (16). Approximately 95% of mild TBI patients recover to a GOS rating of moderate disability or good recovery by 6 months (8).

EPIDEMIOLOGY

Current estimates would indicate that the annual incidence of TBI in the United States is over 2 million [200/100,000 (14)], with 500,000 hospitalized (17). According to the same report, there are estimated to be 100,000 deaths attributed to TBI; it is the leading cause of death and disability in children and young adults. It is believed that the annual costs of TBI now exceed the $25 billion in medical and rehabilitative care and lost income identified in 1989 by the Department of Health and Human Services (17). The male-female ratio is 2 to 3:1 (18); deaths from TBI account for somewhere between 26% and 52% of injury-related deaths (14,19); the highest rate of TBI-related *mortality*, however, is in those older than 75 (19). The risk factors for TBI include lower socioeconomic status, which has an inverse relationship with TBI incidence (20–22), and drug and alcohol abuse. Up to 70% to 75% of individuals who have sustained TBI are under the effects of alcohol or other drugs (20,23,24). There is also a relatively high recidivism rate. Rimel et al (20) indicated that 31% of patients had a previous history of TBI. Annegers et al (25) identified increasing risk for subsequent TBI as follows: a threefold increase for another TBI after one brain injury and an eightfold increase in risk for another TBI after more than one brain injury.

It is well established that the age group of 15 to 24 is most commonly afflicted by brain injury, of which motor vehicle crashes are the major cause. However, there is a smaller peak in age-related incidence in infants and young children, and another peak in the elderly, in whom falls are the major cause. In urban settings, violence is rapidly becoming a major (and most common) (26,27) cause of TBI in those 20 to 50 years old.

Nonetheless, the most common cause of TBI is still the motor vehicle accident, which is also responsible for the highest number of deaths (28). Motor vehicle accidents in this case include automobiles, motorcycles, and bicycles. Pedestrians are most likely to sustain TBI (28) and alcohol is a contributing factor in half of all pedestrian versus vehicle collisions.

Because of the human and financial cost of TBI, there has been a great deal of emphasis on primary prevention. This may take the form of vehicular equipment such as an airbag, which is estimated to prevent 25% of motor vehicle accident–related TBIs (29). Lap-shoulder belts decrease the incidence of fatality and moderate to critical injury from 45% to 50%; with an airbag this is improved to 55% to 60% (30,31). Unbelted individuals have more than eight times greater likelihood of TBI with loss of consciousness (32). The most dramatic impact of equipment-related interventions has been with the use of motorcycle helmets: without helmets, riders run a two to three times greater risk of TBI and three to nine times greater risk of fatality (33). It has been estimated that helmet use would decrease the risk of TBI by 41% and the acute care cost for motorcycle-related TBIs by 40% (34). In the case of bicycles, helmets will decrease the incidence of TBI by 74% to 85% (35). Unfortunately, some effective prevention strategies, such as speed limit reductions, have been repealed. It would seem that to be effective, our efforts at primary prevention need to target lawmakers as well as the general population.

PATHOPHYSIOLOGY

The pathophysiology of TBI is complex and has been categorized in a number of ways. For our purposes, *primary injury* refers to damage to the brain and neurons that is a direct consequence of the external forces applied to the head; the distribution and type of injury thus are governed by the pathomechanics of the event, which include both physiologic and anatomic damage to the brain. These primary injuries may be either closed or penetrating. Subsequent neurologic impairments in *penetrating* injury are somewhat focal in nature, in that they are confined to the track of the bullet and related to the volume of brain damage as well as the site of injury. Higher-velocity missile injuries are associated with greater severity since the percussion force of the bullet produces tissue damage as much as 30 times the diameter of the bullet (36). Fragments of bone and hair that enter the brain may also be a source of infection. The mortality and severity of disability are closely related to the neurologic status and presence of coma after a missile injury (37).

Conversely, *closed* head injuries do not involve direct penetration of the brain, although some depressed skull fractures may be included within this category. Pathomechanically, there may or may not be an impact injury to the head, but even so, the pathology is largely governed by the velocity, direction, and duration of an acceleration-deceleration inertial load. There is also an effect from the internal anatomy of the skull.

Cerebral contusions are hemorrhagic bruises on the surface of the brain over the crest of gyri that typically are distributed to the undersurfaces of the frontal and temporal lobes. These most typically occur as the result of acceleration in a sagittal plane, associated with a short-pulse duration (38) and directly related to the brain moving en masse over the rough base of the skull. Contusions may be seen as well beneath areas of blunt trauma, particularly in association with depressed skull fractures (which is the only time they are seen in the occipital lobe). Although the presence of contra coup contusions is largely overestimated, it has been suggested that when the head is in movement and strikes an object (as with a fall), the more severe brain injury is opposite the side of impact, whereas when the stationary head is struck by an object, the most severe injury is due to force waves conducted to the brain tissue immediately below the site of impact (8,39).

Intracranial hematomas are described in relationship to the dura. Extradural hematomas are almost always due to fracture of the skull with laceration of an artery, typically the middle meningeal, in the temporal parietal area. There may be no direct associated damage to the brain, but rather the damage is secondary to the expanding mass from arterial bleeding. Subdural hematomas are much more common and are caused by bleeding in the subdural space by "bridging veins." These are largely confined to the temporal areas, particularly the temporal tip, and may be associated with intracerebral hematomas. In animal studies (38), subdural and most intracerebral hematomas are seen with short-duration inertial loads and where the angular acceleration is sagittal as opposed to rotatory. This would be exemplified by a fall from a height of less than approximately 15 feet. The degree of permanent neurologic deficits from intracranial hematomas is related to the size and the location of the lesion. Small hemorrhagic areas in key areas such as the brain stem or basal ganglia may lead to severe neurologic deficits. However, even large masses, if they are evacuated rapidly, can leave relatively mild permanent disability.

A major cause of severe disability is diffuse axonal injury. Diffuse axonal injury is not correlated with skull fracture or impact but is seen almost exclusively in victims of motor vehicle accidents, although it may be a contributing factor in falls from great heights. The pathomechanics involve a long pulse duration with a rotatory component to the vector of the inertial load. These rotational forces shear brain tissue along the border between the gray matter and underlying white matter (since the gray matter has greater density). These density differences also result in lesions at the junction of the brain stem and in other deep gray nuclear structures (40). Diffuse axonal injury is characterized microscopically by axonal bulbs and microglial "stars." There may or may not be associated small punctate hemorrhages due to associated microvascular disruption. Larger hemorrhages in the basal ganglia are associated with diffuse axonal injury, as are "gliding contusions" located in the white matter at the base of sulci (38). Diffuse axonal injury is typically divided into three grades. The mildest, grade 1, is in the perisagittal white matter; grade 2 is in the corpus callosum; and grade 3 is in the dorsal lateral quadrants of the white matter of the midbrain and pons and is almost always seen in association with grades 1 and 2.

The common denominator among all of the

different types of brain injury is the associated chemical and molecular toxicity. Initiation of this cascade involves the massive release of excitatory amino acids, particularly glutamate and aspartate. This results in excessive activation of enzyme-linked calcium channels and then pathologic influx of calcium into the cell. This influx in turn increases enzymatic activity, which can set off a "self-destruct" program at the nuclear level, produce internal damage to the cell membrane, or significantly disrupt the microtubular system necessary for neuronal viability. There may be associated high levels of reactive oxygen (free radicals) that in turn cause additional damage to the cell membrane. Current focuses on acute management are mechanisms to interrupt this pathologic chemical cascade (41).

Secondary brain injury includes additional damage to neuronal tissues as a result of the primary insult. Secondary brain results include the release of inflammatory-mediated substances, free radicals as mentioned already, and the global cerebral physiologic response to the injury. There is often a significant disruption of the blood-brain barrier and the normal regulation of cerebral vasculature. This disruption can result in cerebral swelling, which is largely intravascular, or cerebral edema, which is extravascular but may be intracellular or extracellular. One management strategy for the cerebral swelling and raised intracranial pressure is hyperventilation, but this must be carefully regulated to avoid negative effects on regional cerebral blood flow (42,43). In addition, overzealous correction of hypertension that can accompany brain injury may also effect regional cerebral blood flow (44,45). Clearly, a consequence of cerebral edema, swelling, or expanding mass lesions is raised intracranial pressure, which can compromise delivery of fresh blood and oxygen to the injured brain. It also may produce herniation syndromes, first of the uncus and subsequently of the cerebellum on the brain stem. Efforts to control intracranial pressure should be instituted when it is above 20 mm Hg. In the event of tonsillar herniation of the cerebellum, there may be kinking of the brain stem with a resultant injury to the ventral tegmentum, particularly in the pons and mesencephalon.

Finally, as a consequence of difficulty in regulating regional blood flow or because of associated shock and hypovolemia or hypoxia, a secondary injury often seen with TBI is hypoxic-ischemic insult. Global hypoxic injury is present in one-third of subjects who have had fatal injuries (38); hypoxia preferentially affects the hippocampus, basal ganglia, and cerebellum. Boundary zone injuries are usually related to perfusion failures and the injury is confined to the overlapping territories of the major cerebral arteries (38). Hypoxic-ischemic encephalopathy accounts for significant disability, particularly in association with other kinds of acquired brain damage. Late complications of TBI include chronic subdural fluid collections, abscess, meningitis from unrecognized dural tears, traumatic fistulas, cavernous sinus thrombosis, and aneurysms.

THEORIES OF FUNCTIONAL RECOVERY AFTER BRAIN INJURY

Functional recovery from brain damage may or may not be directly related to physiologic responses of the brain to injury. Temporal factors heavily influence the recovery mechanisms. Clearly in the early phases of physiologic recovery in the first days to weeks after injury, stabilization of the intracranial milieu with the re-establishment of normal regional blood flow, and elimination of toxic by products may account for early evidence of neurologic improvement. Later changes include alterations (typically consisting of upregulation) of receptors that are further modified by axonal sprouting. The concept of *vicariation* whereby a remote area "takes over" for a damaged area of the cerebrum has been forwarded as a potential late mechanism of recovery; an example of this is seen in the plasticity of adjacent cortex and homotypical cortex near an injured cortical area. However, an effect resulting in functional restitution would require considerable reorganization from a more remote site.

Another theory includes *unmasking* of otherwise quiescent areas and this may not require significant cerebral reorganization. It is unclear how long a maturing central nervous system would maintain redundant pathways for this purpose, however. A related concept to vicariation is that of *diaschisis*. In this situation, the brain injury affects activity in a remote area of the central nervous system that is related or connected through neuronal systems. Recovery of these connecting neuronal systems permits normal functional restitution in the area of the brain that has not been affected directly by the trauma or injury. An example of this concept would be the branching noradrenergic systems from the locus ceruleus, which sends an axonal branch both to the ipsilateral cortex and to the contralateral cerebellar cortex. The branching noradrenergic system has been involved in some of the chemically mediated functional improvements seen after experimental cortical injury in the rodent and other animals.

Rerouting of damaged axonal sprouts may occur, but it is not genetically ordered as when a similar process occurs in the immature brain; it may not be a functional mechanism of late recovery due to vicissitudes in negotiating an appropriate path to the target neurons (there is no supporting architecture such as that in the peripheral nerve). There may also be some associated release of neurotrophic factors but this does not produce any target-specific growth. In the case of a sprouted axon, it may reach a location with no available receptive area, it may inappropriately synapse on a target that is unrelated functionally, or it could result in overinnervation of an area. Overall, regenerative sprouting seems to be an effective compensatory mechanism in the peripheral nervous system, but because the oligodendrocytes do not remyelinate axons, it is probably not very functional in the central nervous system. There are, however, opportunities for axons from intact fibers in a partially damaged system to branch amd supply vacant receptor sites in a homotypical functional system. On the other hand, fibers branching from a heterotypical functional system may have deleterious effects on recovery.

The momentum of the lesion also bears heavily on the recovery from brain injury. Larger areas of cerebral tissue may be lost with a slowly growing lesion or with a slow series of repetitive injuries than with one large lesion that involves a large volume of tissue (46).

The late phases of recovery may have some implications for pharmacotherapy; the timing of pharmacologic intervention is an extremely important variable, however. In the case of acetylcholine, treatment of animals with anticholinergics prior to experimental injury resulted in good outcomes, whereas treatment as soon as 30 or 60 minutes after injury was ineffective (47). Longer-term use of anticholinergic drugs after injury may have a detrimental effect on cognitive recovery. Benzodiazepines may also impede motor recovery, particularly when they are used chronically (48,49). The drugs that have the strongest evidence for efficacy in improving motor recovery in the experimental animal model, and to some degree in humans, are those that increase norepinephrine. Conversely, those that impede or block norepinephrine, and secondarily dopamine receptors, may retard motor recovery (50). This is true whether the drug is given systemically or as infusions into the contralateral cerebellum. In addition, drugs that do block noradrenergic activity may reinstate deficits from which the experimental animal has recovered (51). Serotonin agonists may cause brief retardations of motor recovery, as in a postacute setting. The motor effects seem to be related to task-relevant experience during the drug trial (52,53). In summary, substantial neural behavior recovery may occur in response to a variety of mechanisms. The clinical implications are that manipulation of neurochemistry may either enhance or retard certain aspects of neurologic recovery and this has been demonstrated particularly in the noradrenergic system.

EFFICACY OF REHABILITATION

While there are animal models to support the effectiveness of "rehabilitative" interventions for specific impairments from well-defined experimental lesions, there are relatively few studies devoted to the effectiveness of rehabilitation in global recovery from real-world brain injuries. Cope and Hall's study in 1982 (54) clearly demonstrated that timing of intervention is a relevant factor, with earlier rehabilitative service delivery resulting in better outcomes. Early admission to a rehabilitation hospital (<35 days) resulted in significant reductions in total duration of hospitalization, most notably in the rehabilitation hospital phase. While there is some reference to "plasticity," much of this effectiveness can be attributed to reductions in secondary complications and to the shifting of care emphasis from a medical/surgical focus to a functional focus sooner, especially since coordinated consulting trauma rehabilitation teams were essentially nonexistent at that time. Certainly most facilities can now easily achieve transfer to acute or subacute rehabilitation in less than 35 days after injury.

Of more contemporary relevance is the demonstrated effectiveness of formalized rehabilitation programs in the acute trauma setting: Length of rehabilitation hospitalization and the period of posttraumatic unawareness were reduced by one-half to two-thirds, length of acute hospitalization was also significantly reduced, and "long-term" cognitive outcomes were also better for the patients in the formalized program (55). While this study was compromised by the misuse of the Rancho Scale and by the apparent lack of physiatric and medical rehabilitative interventions, the implications for current practice in a health care system caught in the throws of managed care are obvious.

ASSESSMENT TOOLS

The focus of assessment after TBI changes during the course of recovery. Early assessment focuses on the patient's medical status and level of responsiveness. Initially, level of responsiveness is assessed with the GCS. For patients who remain in a nonresponsive or minimally responsive state for an extended period of time, several other scales have been developed. These include the Coma/Near Coma scale (56), the Coma Recovery Scale (57), and the Western Neuro Sensory Stimulation Profile (58). These scales provide a structured way to rate the patient's responses to a set of stimuli. A decline in responsiveness may indicate some medical complication such as sedating effects of mediation, urinary tract infection, or posttraumatic hydrocephalus. A pattern of improving scores indicates that the patient is becoming more responsive and may begin to respond purposefully. Additional research is needed to demonstrate whether early scores on these scales are predictive of eventual outcome.

Long-term survival in a nonresponsive state [persistent vegetative state (PVS)] is rare (59). Patients who become responsive and communicative are initially confused and disoriented (60). This state is called *posttraumatic amnesia* (PTA), and is the period of time after the injury in which the patient cannot acquire new information. The patient in severe PTA is acutely confused, oriented only to personal identity, and shows no ability to acquire new memories. As the patient improves, he or she becomes less distractible and shows evidence of new learning. Orientation to place and at least a superficial understanding of personal circumstances return first while orientation to time is last to recover (61). Patients with severe amnesia

Table 72-2: Traumatic Brain Injury Model Systems Neuropsychological Battery

Orientation
Galveston Orientation and Amnesia Test
Motor
Grooved Pegboard Test
Attention, speed of cognitive processing
Wechsler Memory Scale—Revised Digit Span
Symbol Digit Modalities Test
Visual scanning, analysis, and construction
Trailmaking Test
Benton Visual Discrimination Test
Wechsler Adult Intelligence Scale—Revised Block Design
Language
Controlled Oral Word Association Test
Multilingual Aphasia Examination Token Test
Memory
Wechsler Memory Scale—Revised Logical Memory
Rey Auditory Verbal Learning Test
Problem solving
Wisconsin Card Sorting Test

may never recover consistent orientation to day and date. The Galveston Orientation and Amnesia Test (GOAT) (62) provides a structured way to determine when the patient has emerged from PTA.

Neuropsychological assessment is useful to characterize the nature and severity of the patient's cognitive deficits (63) and to predict the patient's eventual functional recovery (10,64–66). The common standard of practice is to delay neuropsychological assessment until the patient has emerged from PTA. However, recent research has provided preliminary evidence that neuropsychological test results obtained prior to the resolution of PTA are predictive of long-term functional recovery (67).

The typical neuropsychological battery assesses simple motor and sensory functions, attention/concentration, speed of cognitive processing, visual analysis and scanning, construction praxis, receptive and expressive language, memory, reasoning, and cognitive flexibility. Most practitioners use a core battery of tests with modifications depending on the patient's need (68). The battery of tests used in the Traumatic Brain Injury Model Systems database is an example of a typical core battery. Tests included in this battery are shown in Table 72-2. In addition to cognitive abilities, neuropsychologists may also assess personality with such tests as the Minnesota Multiphasic Personality Inventory-2 (69) and behavioral competencies with such scales as the Neurobehavioral Rating Scale (70) and the Portland Adaptability Index (71).

As patients progress through the rehabilitation process, the focus of assessment shifts to measurement of the patient's ability to function in the home and community. Different scales may be used to rate the patient's global functioning, personal independence, or ability to fulfill social roles. The most commonly used measures of global outcome are the GOS (72), the Disability Rating Scale (DRS) (73), and the Levels of Cognitive Functioning Scale also known as the Rancho Scale (73a). All of these scales have been shown to have adequate reliability (74,75) and validity (74–79). They have been criticized for being insensitive to subtle changes in the patient's functional status and failing to distinguish different areas of patient functioning (79–81).

The Functional Independence Measure (FIM) (82) is the most commonly used measure of personal independence. The patient's motor and cognitive abilities are rated on a 7-point scale ranging from complete dependence to complete independence. The 18 FIM items assess such areas as dressing, toileting, locomotion, communication, and social interaction. The FIM has excellent reliability and validity (83,84). The FIM is useful for assessing a patient's progress during inpatient rehabilitation, but is insensitive to additional gains made in the postacute period of recovery and treatment (83). The Functional Assessment Measure (FAM) (83) consists of 12 items to be added to the FIM in an attempt to improve assessment of cognition, psychosocial adjustment, and communication. To date, findings do not indicate that FAM items make any additional contribution beyond the original FIM (83).

Two recently developed measures of social role functioning show promise as measures of long-term outcome after TBI. The Craig Handicap Assessment and Reporting Technique (CHART) (85) assesses functioning in the areas of physical independence, mobility, occupation, social integration, and economic self-sufficiency. The CHART was originally developed for spinal cord–injured patients, but it has also been shown to be appropriate for brain-injured persons (86). The Community Integration Questionnaire (CIQ) (87) assesses functioning in the areas of home integration, social integration, and productive activities. The CIQ was developed for TBI patients. Both the CHART and CIQ have good reliability (85,87) and scores from the two measures are significantly correlated with each other (87). Both the CHART and the CIQ have been shown to be sensitive to the treatment effects of postacute brain rehabilitation (88). While additional research is needed, these scales may prove to be useful for following patients long term as these scales may be more sensitive to subtle changes than the GOS, DRS, Rancho Scale, or FIM.

Medical Database

A medical database is necessary for both medical and rehabilitative treatment planning. A suggested database is outlined in Table 72-3.

Prognostic Factors

Preinjury

Preinjury patient characteristics that are predictive of eventual functional outcome include age at time of injury,

Table 72-3: Medical Database for Traumatic Brain Injury Rehabilitation

I. Historical data
   A. Date of injury
   B. Age
   C. Handedness
   D. Mechanism of injury
   E. Loss of consciousness and duration, if present
   F. Presence of seizures and when occurred
   G. GCS and specific findings at ER
   H. PTA estimate from patient recollection or records
   I. Duration of coma: if available from record as GCS score or when first eye opening and/or when first following commands
   J. CT scan or other imaging results relevant to nature of injuries
   K. Elevation of ICP and duration
   L. Presence of hypoxic/ischemic insult and severity estimate
   M. Presence and type of known associated injuries and procedures by body system
   N. Presence of agitation and how managed
   O. Presence of alcohol or drugs at time of injury
   P. Spinal column clearance (cervical spine especially) and how cleared
   Q. Current medications
   R. If seen in postacute period, nature of previous rehabilitative interventions
   S. Past medical Hx; any previous Hx of brain injury; psychiatric Hx
   T. Social and vocational Hx
   U. Drug and alcohol Hx
   V. What are patient's or significant other's expectations and desires of the rehabilitative process; goals
   W. Review of systems focused on neurologic and cognitive
      1. What does patient spontaneously complain about or identify?
      2. Memory, concentration, word finding?
      3. Sleep cycle or fatigue
      4. Behavior: initiation, aggression, anger control
      5. Headache: describe *c*haracter, *o*nset, *l*ocation, *d*uration, *e*xacerbation, *r*elief
      6. Vision: blurred, double, etc
      7. Hearing, tinnitus
      8. Balance, vertigo, light-headedness
      9. Smell, taste
      10. Swallowing or feeding system problems
      11. Weakness, movement, or coordination problems
      12. Pain or sensory changes
      13. Use of assistive device
      14. Bowel
      15. Bladder
      16. Sexual function and behaviors; menstrual irregularities

II. Relevant physical examination
   A. Neurologic, neuromuscular, and musculoskeletal examination with particular attention to:
      1. Cognition: arousal, attention, language, memory (verbal and visual stimuli; storage and retrieval), neglect
      2. Visual fields, extraocular movement, hearing
      3. Motor strength: patterns of weakness
      4. Patterns of reflex or tone abnormality: if it doesn't make sense, look for LMN problems, occult SCI
      5. Sensory abnormalities including DSS
      6. Coordination (cerebellar), balance (Romberg and sharpened Romberg, etc)
      7. Range of motion
      8. Swelling, heat, pain of an extremity
      9. Tenderness of cervical extensors, SCM, trapezius, or at egress of greater or lesser occipital nerves

III. Laboratory data
   A. Very important
      1. CT scan
      2. Neuropsychological assessment
      3. MRI in symptomatic MTBI
      4. Baseline bloodwork (in acute rehabilitation or if Rx is contemplated)
         a. Complete blood cell count
         b. Chem-20 or equivalent
         c. Urine analysis culture and sensitivity
         d. Drug levels
      5. Chest x-ray study
      6. Electrocardiography
      7. Radiographs of any known fractures, etc
      8. Venous Doppler studies if acute
      9. Videofluoroscopy for dysphagia
   B. Important in many cases
      1. MRI
      2. EEG
      3. Bone scan
   C. Important in specific circumstances
      1. Regional blood flow and SPECT
      2. Quantitative EEG
      3. Endocrine studies
      4. Balance Studies: ENG, rotary chair, Equitest
      5. Evoked potentials

GCS = Glasgow Coma Scale; ER = emergency room; PTA = posttraumatic amnesia; CT = computed tomography; ICP = intracranial pressure; Hx = history; LMN = lower motor neuron; SCI = spinal cord injury; DSS = double simultaneous stimulation; SCM = sternocleidomastoid; CT = computed tomography; MRI = magnetic resonance imaging; MTBI = mild traumatic brain injury; EEG = electroencephalography; ENG = electronystagmography; SPECT = single-photon emission computed tomography.

employment status, educational level, and history of substance abuse (10,66,89). Patients who were older at the time of injury, especially those older than 60, have higher mortality and morbidity (10,90). Patients with higher preinjury socioeconomic status as indicated by educational level and employment history have a more favorable outcome (91–93). Finally, a preinjury history of alcohol or drug abuse is associated with poorer long-term employment outcome (66).

Injury Related

Useful prognostic indicators are listed in Table 72-4. Even the most powerful prognostic indicators, when used as a group, are most effective for predicting death or good recovery and have less specificity for outcomes between these extremes. Generally, in the early acute phase, attempts at prognosticating long-term outcome are inappropriate, and indeed most indicators are far more relevant to predicting survival. Even with the most potent predictors or combination of predictors, a small, but individually meaningful percentage of patients may do considerably better or worse than predicted. The most useful functional information to be provided in the early phase of recovery relates to the pattern of impairments identified (memory, aphasia, hemiplegia, hemianopsia), which are likely to persist well into the postacute period or permanence. This kind of information can be used immediately by family members to understand the patient's responses or even to know they should approach the patient from one side or the other to be seen or heard. Long-term or "definitive" functional prognostication should best be held in abeyance until at least the end of acute rehabilitation, and probably delayed until several months after injury. Katz and Alexander (94) developed a prognostic set useful for predicting course of recovery and outcome based on the neuropathology of the injury. In essence, they group the pathologic substrates into diffuse axonal injury, which is stereotyped in terms of pattern of recovery; diffuse hypoxic-ischemic injury; focal cortical contusion; and focal hypoxic-ischemic injury or herniation syndromes. PTA duration is closely correlated with long-term outcome in patients with diffuse axonal injury and closely parallels the finding of Bond (96a) that a PTA duration of greater than 14 weeks indicates a poor prognosis for good recovery. With diffuse axonal injury, PTA is considerably lengthened by the presence of significant hypoxic-ischemic injury. The outcome of focal cortical contusion is correlated best with the location, bilaterality, and extent of injury.

Table 72-4: Prognostic Factors in Traumatic Brain Injury (TBI)

Indicator	Good Outcome	Poor Outcome
Age	<40	>50 or <2
Recurrent TBI	No	Yes
Coma duration	<2 wk	>4 wk
GCS (at 24 hours)	>5	≤5
Motor response on GCS		≤3
Pupillary reactivity	Bilateral reactive	Bilateral unreactive
PTA	≤2 wk	>12 wk
Mass lesions (+midline shift)		+
ICP	Normal	Increased
Hypertension		+
Hypoxia		+
Cerebral ischemia		+
Other system injury	None	>1 Organ
Evoked potentials	Grade I	Grade IV
Serum catecholamines	Normal	Increased
Serum glucose	Normal	Increased
Hydrocephalus ex vacuo		+
Early rehabilitation	+	

GCS = Glasgow Coma Scale; PTA = posttraumatic anesthesia; ICP = intracranial pressure.
Source: Adapted from Mysiw WJ, Fugate LP, Clinchot DM. Assessment, early rehabilitation intervention, and tertiary prevention. In: Horn LJ, Zasler ND, eds. Medical rehabilitation of traumatic brain injury. Philadelphia: Hanley & Belfus, 1996:53–76.

POSTINJURY FACTORS

Postinjury factors that are predictive of long-term functional outcome include severity of cognitive deficits, presence of behavioral problems, accuracy of patient self-awareness, adequacy of social support, and involvement in litigation. Patients with more severe cognitive deficits have poorer employment outcome (64,65,95,96). Patients who exhibit behavioral problems or who are reported by relatives to have a personality change due to TBI also have poorer employment outcome (97,98). Impaired self-awareness of deficits is a common effect of brain injury (99). Several studies showed that impaired self-awareness contributes to poor long-term employment outcome in TBI patients (100–102). Patient satisfaction with available family and social support is somewhat predictive of employment outcome (103). The relationship between involvement in litigation and employment outcome is complex. Taken together, results of previous studies suggest that involvement in litigation is a negative factor for return to work in patients with milder injuries, but has no effect on patients with more severe injuries (10).

TREATMENT PLANNING AND THE CONTINUUM OF CARE

Early Rehabilitation in the Trauma Setting

Ideally, rehabilitation services should be involved very early in the trauma management protocol. Members of the team should include a physiatrist, physical therapist, occupational therapist, speech pathologist, trauma nurses, social workers, and psychologists. The goals in the trauma setting are to

1. Prevent disabling consequences of the TBI and associated injuries
2. Manage medical complications unique to TBI
3. Identify patients who will require services after the acute trauma care (especially those with mild TBI) and assist in securing appropriate care
4. Provide early family education

The most notable preventative interventions are those pertaining to spasticity and contracture management, management of neurogenic bowel and bladder, correction of sleep disturbances, appropriate management of the neurobehavioral complications of TBI (agitation and the underaroused state), early mobilization when appropriate, skin care, and prevention of decubiti. Management of secondary medical problems includes those related to neuroendocrine problems, deep venous thrombosis, and central fever.

Acute Rehabilitation

Acute rehabilitation may be hospital based or located in another type of facility. The hallmarks of acute medical rehabilitation services are that there continue to be a significant need for ongoing medical care (with rapid access to diagnostic testing and consultations), rehabilitative nursing care, and intensive therapies. If the patient does not require a relatively high acuity of medical or nursing care, but still requires intensive therapy services, then a less medically oriented setting than a hospital-based unit may be appropriate, dependent on the expertise of those providing the services. The overall goals of "acute" rehabilitative care are

1. Medical stability
2. Clearing of PTA
3. Reduction of behavioral and physical dependence such that both are manageable by the next level of care or caregivers.

Depending on the environment and available resources, "subacute" care may be hardly distinguishable from "acute" rehabilitative care; this terminology may be superfluous with the maturation of managed care. It is no longer feasible or appropriate for the total rehabilitative care of the person with TBI to occur in a hospital-based rehabilitation unit. In the past, patients with TBI often "lived" in rehabilitation facilities for many months, to be discharged only after maximal functional recovery had occurred and all "loose ends" were addressed. Now there is considerable emphasis on completing intensive rehabilitation using less expensive resources in nonresidential or noninstitutional atmospheres, often on an outpatient basis with the patient living at home.

Postacute Brain Injury Rehabilitation

Many traumatically brain-injured patients continue to receive rehabilitation therapies after discharge from either the acute care hospital or the rehabilitation hospital or unit. This therapy may take the form of individual physical therapy, occupational therapy, or speech therapy, or a combination of therapies, with little coordination. Alternatively, this therapy may be provided in a coordinated day treatment or residential program with special emphasis on personal independence and community reintegration. This latter treatment model is referred to as postacute brain injury rehabilitation. In such programs, therapy is provided in a mixture of group and individual formats. Therapy activities include training in strategies to compensate for cognitive deficits, counseling regarding emotional response to injury and behavioral functioning, educational services to improve awareness of the effects of TBI, and supervised participation in community-based therapy activities designed to transition gains made in the clinic to the patient's real-world environments and activities (104). The goals of therapy are improved community integration as indicated by increased personal independence and participation in productive activities and improved psychosocial and emotional adjustment (105). Therapy is provided by neuropsychologists, speech therapists, occupational therapists, physical therapists, vocational specialists, and paraprofessionals such as job coaches.

As with other areas of rehabilitation, there is controversy regarding the effectiveness of postacute brain injury rehabilitation. Reviews of existing studies (105–107) generally concluded that postacute brain injury rehabilitation is effective in improving patients' independence and productivity outcome. These studies showed that patient improvement is not entirely accounted for by spontaneous recovery; however, no study used random assignment to treatment versus no-treatment conditions. Instead, these studies used historical controls (97,108), waiting-list controls (109), or comparison of different treatment protocols (110,111). Gains made during treatment are at least partially maintained at follow-up (105).

Studies of postacute brain injury rehabilitation that compared one mixture of treatment activities to another (110,111) found no advantage for one protocol over the other. This puzzling finding makes it impossible, at this point, to distinguish the elements of postacute brain injury rehabilitation that are helpful to patients from those that are not. There is particular controversy regarding whether the appropriate goal of postacute brain injury rehabilitation is restoration of cognitive function or compensation for cognitive deficits. Most programs include some therapy activities that could be restorative such as practice in improving response times and other interventions that are primarily compensatory such as training in use of a memory book or environmental alteration to decrease memory demands. Empirical investigations provided evidence that some cognitive abilities such as attention and response speed may respond to a restorative approach (112) while others such as memory do not (113). There is convincing evidence that functional improvement due to postacute brain injury rehabilitation is not primarily mediated by cognitive recovery, as patients who show substantial improvement in community functioning may show little or no improvement on tests of cognitive abilities (114). Additional research is needed to resolve this issue, but at this time it appears that therapy should focus primarily on compensation for deficits rather than on restoration of function. There is strong evidence that postacute brain injury rehabilitation is an effective treatment to increase patients' independence and productivity. The effectiveness of postacute brain injury rehabilitation appears to depend primarily on training in compensatory strategies, counseling, and education rather than on reacquisition of cognitive abilities.

MEDICAL PROBLEMS AFTER INJURY

Medical complications after TBI include those from associated injuries, iatrogenic problems, and those that are systemic manifestations of the brain injury. Extracranial injury does impact on outcome significantly, particularly mortality, and can add to the list of impairments addressed by trauma rehabilitation teams (115). The focus of this section is on the systemic manifestations of brain injury, however.

Remediable neurologic problems after TBI include posttraumatic epilepsy, posttraumatic hydrocephalus, neuroendocrine disorders, and other neurologic disorders that may or may not be remediable but that must be recognized as part of treatment planning (ocular disorders, anosmia, ageusia).

Posttraumatic epilepsy is present in roughly 5% of all TBI patients; the incidence rises with severity of injury and is highest for open or missile injuries, where it approaches 40%. The major types of posttraumatic epilepsy include simple partial, generalized, and partial complex seizures; the latter are part of the differential diagnosis for behavioral and cognitive problems after TBI. Historically, patients were placed on prophylactic anticonvulsants for extended periods of time after injury; this practice is currently being challenged. There is no cogent evidence to support the use of prophylactic anticonvulsants beyond the first 2 weeks after injury for patients with a closed head injury (116). If the patient has late seizures (after the first week), then anticonvulsants should be continued; similarly, clinicians may continue prophylactic anticonvulsants in patients with missile injury or open injury. Early seizures do increase the risk for late traumatic epilepsy, but even in a constellation of other risk factors, do not raise the risk above 40%. The preferred medications to manage posttraumatic epilepsy are carbamazepine and valproic acid, largely because of their side effect profile when compared to phenobarbital and phenytoin; gabapentin (Neurontin) may also be an appropriate first-line drug but is not approved for monotherapy in the United States (117). However, any of the anticonvulsants can produce significant cognitive impediments (118).

Hydrocephalus refers to the enlargement of the ventricular system. While it is feasible for posttraumatic hydrocephalus to be obstructive, generally it is nonobstructive in that the cerebrospinal fluid pathways are open. The ventriculomegaly may be related to true hydrocephalus, with a defect in absorption of cerebrospinal fluid at the level of the arachnoid villi, or hydrocephalus ex vacuo, which is related to the volume of cerebral tissue lost and exemplary of nature abhorring a vacuum. The classic triad of symptoms of idiopathic hydrocephalus (dementia, gait disturbance, incontinence) is typical of nearly every moderately to severely injured patient admitted to acute rehabilitation and hence cannot be relied on to be diagnostic of the disorder; indeed, some recovery from the acute head injury can occur in the setting of hydrocephalus, implying that waiting for some regression is not a valid clinical practice since the hydrocephalus may be far advanced. There is evidence that the reversibility of symptoms with shunting may be less the longer the process is present. The best approach may be to proactively evaluate patients for this problem, as suggested by Cope et al (119). Once hydrocephalus is identified, determination of whether it is an active process versus ex vacuo can be more challenging. Some authors advocate a "tap test" (120), whereas dynamic magnetic resonance imaging (MRI), nuclear medicine imaging, or computed tomography (CT) alone is also supportive. Ventricular shunting is the definitive treatment (121); infection, subdural hematoma, and shunt malfunction and obstruction are all potential complications from the procedure.

Neuroendocrine and autonomic disorders are most commonly encountered in the acute care and acute rehabilitation settings. These disorders include hypertension, hyperthermia, diencephalic "fits," hyperphagia, and hypothalamic-pituitary disorders (122,123). Hypertension after brain injury occurs as a new condition in 10% to 15% of patients (124), is related to specific neuroanatomic injury (to baso-orbital frontal area, hypothalamus, or brain stem regulatory structures), and is usually transient. Management is best undertaken with β-blockers given after the acute phase to avoid detrimental effects on regional cerebral blood flow; calcium channel blockers and other agents may also be effective. Care should be taken in the acute trauma setting as overzealous management of hypertension or tachycardia may have deleterious effects on regional cerebral blood flow. Hyperthermia, or central fever, is diagnosed after a detailed evaluation for infection. It may be related to anterior hypothalamic injury and is best treated with modalities (cooling blanket, or if severe, iced gastric lavage), nonsteroidal anti-inflammatory drugs

(NSAIDs) propranolol (125), or dopamine agonists. Diencephalic fits are episodes of hypertension, fever, and sweating that may respond to propranolol and dopamine agonists, but often require anticonvulsants. Hyperphagia is uncommon, and again is often related to hypothalamic or extrahypothalamic dysregulation; management is best undertaken with new classes of selective serotonin reuptake inhibitors (SSRIs) or possibly naltrexone (126). Pituitary dysfunction is most common in the acute setting and related to disorders of salt metabolism (127,128) (diabetes insipidus and syndrome of inappropriate secretion of antidiuretic hormone); in both cases the problem is usually transient and a careful evaluation of iatrogenic causes is relevant. Anterior pituitary disorders are rare, but are part of the differential diagnosis of sexual dysfunction.

Cranial neuropathies are another neurologic impairment common after TBI. Injury to cranial nerve I is relatively common (7.5% of blows to head or face), and is the most frequent cranial neuropathy in mild brain injury (129). Recovery is variable and may be incomplete; often, dysosmia produces dysgeusia as well, with a consequent loss of appetite in some patients. Visual deficits may be related to an injury to cranial nerve II, but are more often secondary to more proximal involvement in the optic tracts. Oculomotor palsy, with associated diplopia and ptosis, is seen in 17% of patients with TBI (130). Often, at least partial recovery will occur, although intervention with prism glasses or surgery may be necessary to help correct diplopia. Isolated cranial nerve IV and VI neuropathies are less common, but also produce characteristic diplopia; in some respects they are more easily correctable as only one extraocular muscle is served by each nerve. Trigeminal neuropathy could result in loss of tactile perception on the face and cornea (eye patches and lubricant), dysfunction of salivation (while there is synthetic saliva, sugarless gum and lozenges are better accepted), and some potential for disorders of mastication or even true trigeminal neuralgia. Peripheral facial neuropathy is typically associated (90%) with longitudinal or transverse temporal bone fractures affecting the labyrinthine segment of the facial nerve (131); this results in facial weakness of the lower motor neuron type and also has implications for ocular health given impediments to closing the eye, which may require tarsorrhaphy. Depending on the site of peripheral facial palsy, hearing and the sense of true taste may also be affected (as opposed to dysgeusia related to loss of smell). Vestibulocochlear nerve disorders are also related to temporal fractures, with nerve damage most common in the presence of transverse fractures. "Concussion" to the cranial nerve VIII or the auditory/vestibular end-organs may be associated with tinnitus, hearing loss, or true vertigo. Peripheral injury to the remaining cranial nerves is less common but may have the consequence of dysarthria, dysphagia, dysphonia, and weakness of the sternocleidomastoid or trapezius (XII). The Collet-Sicard syndrome is associated with fracture of the occipital bone and affects these last four cranial nerves given their egress through the base of the skull (132).

Gastrointestinal and Nutritional Needs

After TBI there is frequently a significant increase in metabolic demand, up to 5000 kcal/day in posturing patients. Sedation, paralysis, and the like in the acute care setting may limit this increased metabolism, whereas decubitus ulcers, fever, and so on may further increase it. Overall, it has been suggested that one can predict an increased energy need of 26% above that which is normally expected. Early and continuous attention to these nutritional needs has been associated with improved long-term outcome (133). While total parenteral nutrition may be necessary in the acute phase, if the gut works, it should be used. Gastrostomy tubes have the advantages of allowing bolus feeding and having a larger diameter when compared to jejunostomy tubes, and are best for chronic management; however, J-tubes may be preferable in the patient with stomach injury or recurrent and refractory reflux. Cisapride and possibly erythromycin are preferred medications for gastric motility over metoclopramide (Reglan), given a lower risk for side effects compared to this relative of major tranquilizers.

Although the evaluation and management of dysphagia are discussed elsewhere, factors pertinent to TBI are that 25% of TBI patients overall have dysphagia, with reduced cognition a more prominent cause than motor control problems (134). Eventual progression to safe oral feeding does occur in the vast majority of patients. Other gastrointestinal complications include gastritis and ulcers (stress related) (135), which are generally responsive to standard management techniques and drugs. Another common finding in patients with TBI is elevated liver enzyme levels. While this finding mandates screening for infectious causes, or serious problems secondary to local trauma, the most likely etiology is iatrogenic from anticonvulsants or antispasticity medications (136). Often the changes in liver enzymes reflect benign induction of the microsomal system (137) and do not necessarily mandate changing the drugs.

Orthopedic and Musculoskeletal Complications

Occult fractures are a serious problem in TBI, underdiagnosed in up to 30% (138). Peripheral nerve injuries are also commonly missed early in the acute management of TBI (11%–34%) (139,140). Heterotopic ossification is, perhaps, the most functionally devastating musculoskeletal complication of TBI, occurring in up to 76% of severely injured patients (141–143). Unlike spinal cord injury, the most common locations are relatively equally distributed between the hip, shoulder, and elbow (144). The incidence is higher in association with fractures and spasticity. Treatment can be challenging. While range of motion exercises are the hallmark in spinal cord injury, because of preserved sensation in the affected part, this may prove quite daunting in TBI. Etidronate, NSAIDs, and radiation treatments have been evaluated principally in association with disorders other than TBI (145–147). Ultimately, surgical intervention may be necessary, and is timed to coincide with a decrease in serum alkaline phosphatase and "cooling" of the bone scan (148). Finally, the incidence of deep venous thrombosis in TBI, although not well documented, is obviously part of the differential diagnosis of a swollen lower extremity, along with occult fracture and heterotopic ossification. Recently Meythaler et al (149) demonstrated the cost-effectiveness of screening for deep venous thrombosis. Low-dose heparin and pneumatic calf compression are recommended for prophylaxis.

Genitourinary System

Urinary incontinence after brain injury is extremely common; it is typically related to disinhibition and less commonly associated with a true "spastic" bladder. Instrumentation should be avoided and replaced with diapering and timed voiding programs. Rarely, bladder/external sphincter dyssynergia occurs in association with severe spasticity.

Sexual dysfunction is also common after brain injury. The most common abnormality is oligomenorrhea (150). Rarely, this is related to specific anterior pituitary dysfunction. Other complications include impotence, altered libido, and problems associated with the neurobehavioral consequences of TBI (151–153).

REHABILITATION ISSUES

Other Physical Impairments

Motor Disturbances

These include upper motor neuron (UMN) syndrome, spasticity, contractures, and movement disorders. While detailed discussion of these terms and problems is available elsewhere in this text, the major deficits encountered with TBI pertain to hyperactive deep tendon reflexes, increased tone, motor weakness, and decreased control and primitive patterns of movement dominating and impeding skilled functions. The consequences of spasticity and UMN syndrome to TBI is that in the acute setting, it may increase metabolic demand and potentially impact on intracranial pressure. It is also a significant etiology for early and severe contracture formation. Range of motion and stretching exercises and modalities play a role, but the principal medical rehabilitative interventions are the use of casting, tone-inhibiting orthotics, specific physical and occupational therapeutic techniques both to inhibit abnormal tone and movements and to facilitate normal skilled movement, and medications. Caution must be exercised with the medications since TBI patients may be more susceptible to cognitive side effects; hence, dantrolene is the preferred systemic medication. Increasingly, specific muscles and patterns are targeted, using clinical evaluation and motion analysis (154) for treatment with either phenol neurolysis/motor point blocks or botulinum toxin injection (155). These injections are temporary and may be employed in the trauma setting to specifically assist in the prevention of spastic contractures (e.g., heel cord). Another useful strategy in the acute setting is the use of intravenous dantrolene (156), which is subsequently given in enteral form; this can significantly reduce tone and posturing and the consequent risk for contracture formation. In the more chronic phase of recovery, consideration may be given to surgical intervention to control spasticity, such as placement of a baclofen pump, neurosurgical ablative interventions, or orthopedic tendon-lengthening procedures.

Other movement disorders after TBI include rigidity including a parkinsonian-like disorder, tremors, akathisia, ataxia, myoclonus (particularly palatal myoclonus), and dystonias including athetosis, ballism, and chorea (157). The relative incidence of these disorders after TBI is unknown; however, pugilistic parkinsonism, as part of dementia pugilistica, is well described, as are lesions in the basal ganglia (158). Pharmacologic intervention is with dopamine agonists and potentially anticholinergic agents, although the latter may impact on already dysfunctional memory. Essential tremors often respond to propranolol; clonazepam may also help but is variably tolerated, again because of sedation and cognitive side effects. Botulinum toxin has also been used with some success (159). Ataxia is an extremely difficult problem to treat with either therapies or medication; medications that have been tried include β-blockers, baclofen, clonazepam, acetazolamine, thyrotropin-releasing hormone, and serotonin agonists (160). Athetosis, ballism, and chorea are also difficult to treat; the armamentarium includes anticonvulsants (161) as well as potential surgical intervention. Botulinum toxin is commonly utilized for other dystonias including torticollis.

Sensory Disorders

Central and thalamic pain states may occur after brain injury. These are typically managed pharmacologically since the syndrome involves the hemicorpora; the typical medications include anticonvulsants, notably carbamazepine; antidepressants (both tricyclics and tetracyclics as well as newer SSRIs); and potentially mexiletine. If centrally mediated pain is more localized, it may be amenable to transcutaneous electrical nerve stimulation or desensitization techniques. Sympathetically medicated regional pain syndromes are also possible after TBI (reflex sympathetic dystrophy) and management is similar to that discussed elsewhere in this text.

As with cerebral vascular accident, a variety of modality-specific agnosias may occur after brain injury. Hemisensory neglect is possible with both failure to respond to stimuli in half a sensory "world" and failure to "explore" or initiate activity in that part of the world. In addition to therapeutic techniques to anchor and reorient the individual, some dopamine agonists have been purported to be effective for this disorder (162,163).

Cognitive Impairments

The cognitive and behavioral sequelae of TBI are more significant than motor or sensory deficits in determining a patient's long-term functional outcome and psychosocial adjustment (164,165). The residual pattern of cognitive and behavioral impairments after TBI depends on the initial severity of injury, the combination of diffuse and focal brain lesions, the occurrence of medical complications affecting brain function, the patient's preinjury level of functioning, and numerous other factors (166). Patients who have suffered blunt head trauma and have diffuse injuries with no large focal lesions show a typical pattern of cognitive deficits in the areas of arousal, attention, resistance to distraction, speed of cognitive processing, memory, abstract reasoning, cognitive flexibility, initiation, and self-awareness (167). Severe aphasia or visual/perceptual disorders are uncommon in such patients. Patients who have had penetrating head wounds may show aphasia, neglect, or other signs of focal brain lesions. Cognitive recovery continues for 6 to 18 months after moderate and severe TBI (168,169).

Behavioral deficits and psychosocial adjustment issues after TBI include depression, poor social awareness, impaired self-awareness, disorders of initiation, agitation, and aggressive behavior (170,171). These difficulties appear to be more severe in patients who have more damage to the frontal lobes (172), though similar problems are seen in patients with no evidence of focal frontal lesions (173). In contrast to the generally improving course for cognitive deficits during the period from 6 to 12 months after injury, behavioral and personality functioning, as judged by family member ratings, may decline over this period (174,175). These findings have led some clinicians to argue that the psychosocial consequences of TBI are more handicapping than the residual cognitive and physical deficits.

SPECIFIC REHABILITATIVE STRATEGIES IN THE CONTINUUM OF TRAUMATIC BRAIN INJURY

Coma and Minimally Responsive Patients

Up to 30% to 40% of survivors of severe TBI may demonstrate a profoundly limited behavioral repertoire. These individuals may consume a significant amount of health care resources, and the impact on the nuclear social system is every bit as devastating as the neurologic insult. The need to clarify the types of conditions responsible for posttraumatic "unawareness" is exemplified by the difficulties in accurately diagnosing the vegetative state (176). Coma, simply defined, is unarousable unconsciousness, with the eyes closed. The neuropathology is either widespread bilateral hemispheric dysfunction or more focal damage to brain stem reticular structures. There are no sustained visual pursuits and no ability to follow commands or to meaningfully interact with the environment or show appropriate responses to internal stimuli. Traumatic coma is associated with a GCS score of 8 or less, but this could be incorrectly interpreted in the setting of high cervical cord injury. True coma is a transient phenomenon, evolving into death or one of the following categories. The vegetative state is distinguished from coma by the presence of eye opening, intact basic autonomic functions, sleep-wake cycles, and possible responsiveness to optikokinetic stimulation. The additional adjective *persistent* has been the subject of considerable controversy. For nontraumatic brain injury, 3 months is the interval after which significant improvement is not expected; for trauma the interval is currently considered to be 12 months. It is currently believed that the pathology responsible for PVS, severe bilateral hemispheric damage with relative preservation of the brain stem, occurs in the peri-injury period. Whereas some individuals who present behaviorally as vegetative do have some reversible neuronal dysfunction, those destined to be in a PVS are not likely to respond to medical or therapeutic intervention to reverse or correct the process; it is, however, impossible to identify these individuals immediately at the time of injury. Locked-in syndrome is a specific condition secondary to injury in the pons or lower mesencephalon whereby eye opening is present, vertical eye movement is present volitionally, and there is severe quadriplegia, acutely involving bulbar musculature as well as the body (corporeal sensation may be preserved). Cognitive function may be intact. Akinetic mutism is a disorder classically related to a bilateral midline lesion in the area of the third ventricle (mesencephalon, cingulate gyrus, basal or mesial frontal lobe). Eye opening is present with spontaneous environmental tracking; patients follow commands inconsistently, initiation is profoundly impaired, and speech and movement are severely deficient. Finally, the minimally responsive patient resembles the patient with akinetic mutism but may have a slightly greater ability to follow commands, or their limitations can be explained by concomitant associated neurologic impairments (double hemiplegia). Latencies of response are often markedly prolonged, but a meaningful response is elicitable (177).

These differentiations are more than semantics; patients with akinetic mutism, minimally responsive patients, and even patients with locked-in syndrome have been shown to respond to dopamine agonists whereas patients who may superficially appear similar (those in a PVS) may not, lacking the neurologic substrate for such a response. In general, patients with prolonged posttraumatic unconsciousness who ultimately display meaningful behaviors are more likely to be younger. The "natural" time course of recovery indicates that the majority reach this milestone by 6 months (most within 3 months) after injury, and by 1 year, recovery is a reportable circumstance, although it *is* rarely reported (178–183).

The appropriate rehabilitation approach to minimally responsive patients involves a thorough search for any *correctable* medical etiology for their functional level. Specific problem areas include the presence of hydrocephalus or other intracranial space-occupying lesion, undiagnosed seizures, iatrogenic problems typically from medications, disorders related to other organ systems (hypoxemia), metabolic disorders (sodium balance), and fever. Rehabilitation strategies include efforts to minimize complications from bed rest and are largely passive, but valuable. These include appropriate attention to skin care, bowel and bladder dysfunction, nutrition and the securing of an appropriate route for chronic enteral feeding, pulmonary care, eye care, and management of neuroendocrine and autonomic dysfunction. The patients should be taken out of bed and placed in an appropriate wheelchair, which in part can be used as a "truncal orthosis" and can facilitate some prophylaxis from the effects of chronic bed rest. Spasticity should be managed aggressively and provision of appropriate orthotics and appliances to prevent or reverse contractures is fundamental to the care of the minimally responsive patient. Heterotopic ossification should also be addressed as appropriate.

To specifically "correct" the low level of responsiveness, there are two approaches. The first, and the one with the firmest scientific underpinning, is pharmacologic, principally using dopamine agonists, including L-dopa, amantadine, or bromocriptine (184–188), or psychostimulants such as methylphenidate (189). The psychostimulants may be particularly effective for patients who are not "minimally responsive" but who are at the higher end of the attention-arousal spectrum. Antidepressants have also been used to facilitate improved arousal and initiation after TBI (190). Animal studies indicate that pharmacologic intervention can facilitate recovery after experimental brain injury (48,191) and such intervention is rational, supporting the human data. The second approach involves structured sensory stimulation. There are animal data to suggest that enriched therapeutic environments, when contrasted to impoverished environments, facilitate neurologic recovery after experimental brain injury (191,192). However, the few reports on the use of therapeutic sensory stimulation do not corroborate its effectiveness in humans who are minimally responsive (193,194), although the data are complicated by small sample size, poor outcome measures, and inconsistencies in technique and causes of cerebral injury. This is not tantamount to discrediting the use of structured sensory stimulation or assessment as a "diagnostic" modality to assess the effectiveness of pharmacologic and other interventions. Indeed, given the severity of neurologic impairments, latencies of responses, and the like, this kind of structured interdisciplinary assessment is likely to be more sensitive to subtle changes in the minimally responsive patient than is a quick bedside check. A review of the utility of various types of assessment protocols is beyond the scope of this chapter but is available elsewhere in the literature (195).

Family counseling regarding the prognosis for the minimally responsive or vegetative patient is important to the family's adjustment and eventual ability to care for the patient. It is usually beneficial for the family to play a role in providing the patient's care as early as possible. This involvement gives family members the sense that they can make some contribution to the patient's comfort and provides an opportunity for rehabilitation staff to train family members in skills that they will need to care for the patient after discharge.

The "Agitated" Patient

As TBI patients progress from the nonresponsive state to resolution of PTA, many exhibit agitated and restless behavior. This agitation is characterized by confusion, emotional lability, excessive motor activity, and in some cases, aggression (196). The period of agitation is generally relatively brief, with resolution coming as the patient becomes better oriented and regains some ability to retain new memories. Nonetheless, agitation is a concern as it may be a manifestation of an underlying medical problem and agitated patients are often noncompliant with therapy. Possible medical complications such as electrolyte imbalance, seizure activity, sleep disturbance, discomfort due to musculoskeletal injury, or posttramautic hydrocephalus that may be exacerbating the patient's confusion should be searched for and treated (196).

The initial management of agitation involves ensuring that the patient does not injure himself or herself or others. Such patients may pull out tubes; strike out at staff during dressing, bathing, or therapy activities; or attempt to elope. If possible, physical restraints should be avoided as these frustrate the patient and result in increased agitation. Preferred management techniques include reducing stimulation and increasing the structure and familiarity of the patient's environment. Agitation will generally decrease if the patient is in a quiet room and primarily interacts with staff with whom he or she is familiar. Only one person should address the patient at a time and the tone of voice should be calm. Some patients respond to familiar music or pictures of family members. Craig beds or net beds that allow the patient to move but guard against self-injury may be helpful. Family members should be instructed regarding appropriate agitation management so that they do not inadvertently overstimulate the patient. Counseling regarding the recovering course of agitation is reassuring to family members, as the patient's physical and verbal outbursts can be quite upsetting. Sedating medicines such as neuroleptics and benzodiazepines may be necessary for the few patients who would otherwise injure themselves or others, but these should be avoided if at all possible as they will increase confusion and may have other adverse effects (197–199).

The Agitated Behavior Scale (200) provides a

reliable, easily obtained measure of patients' agitation. Structured assessment of agitation is highly recommended as subjective reports may be highly unreliable. Use of a measure such as the Agitated Behavior Scale increases the likelihood that patient improvement due to behavioral intervention, pharmacologic management, or spontaneous recovery will be detected.

As with the minimally responsive patient, it is incumbent on the clinician caring for the agitated patient to assess him or her for any correctable etiology for the neurobehavioral dysfunction. While epilepsy or space-occupying lesions are possible problems, particular attention should be paid to hypoxemia, fever, and iatrogenic causes from medication. The environment of most hospitals, especially the intensive care unit, is not typically conducive to orientation of confused and fearful individuals. Sleep disturbances should also be addressed; trazodone may be an effective agent for inducing sleep and nortriptyline for sustaining sleep. Ambien (zolpidem tartrate) may also be effective without the "hangover" associated with some benzodiazepine deriviatives, although rebound insomnia is still possible. Sources of pain should be evaluated and treated while guarding against impediments to cognition.

After correction of the medical problems contributing to "agitation," management strategies are pharmacologic and environmental. Medically, in acute settings when behavioral problems are most likely tied to impaired attention and PTA, dopamine agonists and psychostimulants, or antidepressants are the most rational choices for management (201–203). Other agents that may be effective include propranolol and anticonvulsants (204). Traditional major tranquilizers should be avoided because of increased risks of hyperthermia, extrapyramidal side effects, negative impact on cognition, and evidence that they may impede recovery (48); it is unclear whether the newer classes of major tranquilizers [risperidone (Risperdal)] mandate the same level of concern. Similarly, although benzodiazepines are medically safer, they do produce an anterograde memory dysfunction and state-dependent learning. Nonetheless, in an intensive care unit setting, when major sedation may be required, the use of benzodiazepines, narcotics, and other powerfully sedating drugs may be situationally appropriate; this is not as likely to be the case in a rehabilitation environment.

Certain individuals will experience chronic behavioral dysfunction after TBI related to disinhibition of premorbid personality or specific cerebral injury (e.g., frontal or temporal lobes). Often, psychostimulants or antidepressants, including the new SSRIs, will be helpful. The target remains correction of the behavioral disorder with (relative) preservation or enhancement of cognition and recovery. Anticonvulsants, particularly carbamazepine or valproic acid, are indicated in the management of episodic dyscontrol; β-blockers or buspirone (Buspar) may also be effective. In severely refractory individuals, lithium may be an appropriate agent, although patients must be monitored for a myriad of potential side effects including those affecting cardiac, renal, and thyroid functions. Aggressive hyperphagia may be managed with SSRIs or naltrexone (126). Rarely, aggression with a sexual resonance may require medroxyprogesterone acetate (Depo-Provera) or the equivalent of chemical castration.

Postconcussive Rehabilitation

Postconcussion syndrome is actually a "wastebasket" term for a constellation of symptoms that include characteristic physical complaints (e.g., headache, dizziness, photophobia, sonophobia) and neurobehavioral complaints (memory, concentration, irritability, fatigue). There may be several etiologic factors for these complaints: mild brain injury, injury to the musculoskeletal and soft-tissue structures of the head and neck, or injury to the so-called cerebral adnexa, the cranial nerves and associated peripheral cerebral structures.

Definition of Mild Traumatic Brain Injury

Approximately 80% of patients who sustain TBIs have had mild TBI as judged by GCS criteria, and of TBI patients who survive, 86% had mild injuries (14). The majority of these patients make excellent neurobehavioral recovery (16,205), but some have persistent and disabling symptoms. There has been a long-standing controversy regarding the relative contributions of neurologic and psychological factors to the symptoms of mild TBI patients with persisting disability (205,206). It has been argued that use of different definitions of mild TBI by different investigators has contributed to this controversy. In an attempt to increase consistency in the diagnosis of these patients, the Mild Traumatic Brain Injury Committee of the Head Injury Special Interest Group of the American Congress of Rehabilitation Medicine (206) developed detailed diagnostic criteria for mild TBI. These criteria are presented in Table 72-5.

Pathologically, the lesion in mild TBI patients may show little to no structural discontinuity, although in animal studies axonal disruption may be evident, especially in the hippocampus (207). The injury is likely to be largely due to the pathologic neurochemical cascade, but is insufficient to produce widespread neuronal dysfunction or the axonal disruption that characterizes more severe cerebral pathology. The pathology is centripetally distributed however, and may explain some of the characteristic postconcussive symptomatology: Surface lesions result in amnesia, impairments to short-term memory or attention, or other transient focal neurologic dysfunction; medullary injuries can result in nausea, vomiting, or respiratory or cardiac irregularities (all transient in the immediate postinjury period); pontine and mesencephalic involvement may produce the classic concussion with associated brief loss of consciousness. Nonclassic mild brain injury can occur without loss of consciousness; amnesia for the event and the peritraumatic period is, in our estimatation, a requisite

Table 72-5: Diagnostic Criteria for Mild Traumatic Brain Injury

I. Traumatically induced physiologic disruption of brain function as indicated by at least one of the following:
   A. Any period of loss of consciousness
   B. Any loss of memory for events immediately before or after the accident
   C. Any alteration in mental state at the time of the accident
   D. Focal neurologic deficits that may or may not be transient
II. Severity of the injury does not exceed:
   A. Loss of consciousness of 30 min
   B. Glasgow Coma Scale score of 13–15 after 30 min
   C. Posttraumatic amnesia of 24 h

for the diagnosis of mild brain injury. Other relevant pathology is demonstrated in the cervical spine and musculature, whereby whiplash injuries can lead to damage in the longus colli and anterior longitudinal ligament (208,209).

Diagnosis

Imaging

Diagnostic studies that may be useful in the documentation of mild TBI include MRI, which may show "unidentified bright objects" or early frontal and temporal abnormalities better than CT (210), electroencephalography, single-photon emission CT, brain electrical activity mapping, or multi-modality evoked potentials (211–216).

Neuropsychological Assessment and Cognitive and Behavioral Problems

The most common cognitive complaints after mild TBI are impaired memory, increased distractibility, and slowed speed of cognitive processing (217). These areas of cognitive function can be assessed quickly with a battery of tests such as the battery recommended by Ruff et al (218). In patients in whom malingering is suspected, additional tests that have been shown to be sensitive to malingering (219,220) should be added to the battery.

Emotional and behavioral symptoms reported after mild TBI include depression, anxiety, and irritability (221). Personality inventories such as the Minnesota Multiphasic Personality Inventory-2 (69) and behavioral rating scales such as the Neurobehavioral Rating Scale (16) and the Portland Adaptability Index (71) are useful in evaluating these complaints.

Effects of Litigation

There is much controversy regarding the possible impact of litigation on symptoms reported by mild TBI patients (222). Studies of groups of patients have produced conflicting findings on this issue, with some (223) finding a major impact of litigation on symptom presentation and others finding little or no impact (224). The findings of these studies notwithstanding, all clinicians must consider factors other than possible brain injury that can influence a patient's symptom picture. Litigation is just one of these factors. Careful review of patient information including initial medical records (GCS, CT or MRI findings, length of PTA, etc), premorbid medical history (previous head injury or other neurologic illness or injury, alcohol and substance abuse, etc), premorbid functioning (educational level, history of developmental or learning disability, employment history, psychiatric history, etc), postmorbid medical status (medications, possible seizures or other complications, etc), and postmorbid functional status (course of cognitive recovery, neuropsychological test findings, emotional and behavioral problems, interview with significant other, etc) will generally reveal whether the patient's symptoms are consistent with the expected course of recovery. When symptoms are not consistent, other explanations such as the possible impact of litigation must be considered.

Physical Complaints

Of the physical complaints reported from concussion, headache is the most common. Postconcussive headaches invariably have as the sole, or as a contributing etiology, a musculoskeletal component involving the head and neck and inclusive of craniomandibular or temporomandibular syndromes. Vascular etiologies are less common, although in children or those with a family history, trauma can precipitate "migraine" headache. Neuritic head pain may be due to local injury of a scalp nerve, or as a result of greater or lesser occipital neuralgia. Unusual postconcussive headaches include basilar artery migraine and those related to injury to the anterior or posterior cervical sympathetics. Management is specific to the type of headache (225).

Vestibular dysfunction and postconcussive dizziness may be related to a variety of factors including injury to the adnexa (cranial nerve VIII, semicircular canals, benign paroxysmal positional vertigo) or even cervicogenic factors (226–228). Detailed work-up may include electronystagmography, rotary chair, or stabilometry. Intervention includes specific physical therapy (229), but may require pharmacotherapy or surgery (230,231).

Medical Management of Postconcussive Neurobehavioral Problems

Of the cognitive complaints common to mild TBI, deficits related to memory and the attentional system are most evident. Again, the clinician must be circumspect to treatable medical causes related to these symptoms. Special attention should be paid to management of pain and improved sleep "hygiene." Psychostimulants such as methylphenidate and pemoline, stimulating antidepressants such as desipramine and protriptyline, and even SSRIs may have a beneficial effect on attention with a secondary improvement in other cognitive skills and memory. Irritability often responds to stabilization of the sleep cycle and the aforementioned pharmacotherapy for attention. If it does not, then consideration could be given to the use of other agents such as anticonvulsants, as discussed for the agitated patient.

TRAUMATIC BRAIN INJURY IN SOCIETY: CHANGES IN HEALTH CARE DELIVERY

It behooves providers of TBI rehabilitation services to become more effective in identifying and achieving realistic functional outcomes. The financial costs to society are astronomical in terms of medical dollars consumed, as well as lost productivity; not included in these estimates are the losses in productivity by members of the patient's nuclear social system. TBI rehabilitation has often led the way in the development of alternative service delivery models (as opposed to inpatient hospital-based rehabilitation); however, the effectiveness of specific interventions and the overall financial impacts are still under investigation (76,106,232). As managed care emerges as the major payor for services, people with chronic disability and TBI may be uniquely susceptible to some of the perverse incentives operational in a maturing environment: lack of coverage of needed services, inability to access specific components of care, abrogation of responsibility to other agencies, and the like. It is hoped that as the environment matures and capitation comes to include prospective care for all "lives," innovative approaches will be encouraged to grant a meaningful activity pattern to those surviving TBI and to assist and stabilize their nuclear social system, ensuring productive, functional lifestyles for all concerned.

REFERENCES

1. Boake C. A history of cognitive rehabilitation of head-injured patients, 1915 to 1980. *J Head Trauma Rehabil* 1989; 4(3):1–8.
2. *Head Injury Rehabilitation Project final report to the National Institute for Handicapped Research.* San Jose, CA: Santa Clara Valley Medical Center, 1982.
3. High WM, Hall KM, Rosenthal M, et al. Factors affecting hospital length of stay and charges following traumatic brain injury. *J Head Trauma Rehabil* 1996;11(5):85–96.
4. Levin HS, Gary HE, Eisenberg HM, et al. Neurobehavioral outcome one year after severe head injury: experience of the Traumatic Coma Data Bank. *J Neurosurg* 1990;73:699–709.
5. Ruff RM, Marshall LF, Crouch J, et al. Predictors of outcome following severe head trauma: follow-up data from the Traumatic Coma Data Bank. *Brain Inj* 1993;7:101–111.
6. Teasdale G, Jennett B. Assessment of coma and impaired consciousness: a practical scale. *Lancet* 1974;2:81–83.
7. Russell WR. Cerebral involvement in head injury: a study based on examination of two hundred cases. *Brain* 1932;55:549–603.
8. Jennett B, Teasdale G. *Management of head injuries.* Philadelphia: FA Davis, 1981.
9. Teasdale G, Jennett B. Assessment and prognosis of coma after head injury. *Acta Neurochir* 1976;34:45–55.
10. Crepeau F, Scherzer P. Predictors and indicators of work status after traumatic brain injury: a meta-analysis. *Neuropsychol Rehabil* 1993;3:5–35.
11. Vollmer DG. Prognosis and outcome of severe head injury. In: Cooper PR, ed. *Head injury.* Baltimore: Williams & Wilkins, 1993:553–581.
12. Eisenberg HM, Weiner RL. Input variable: how information from the acute injury can be used to characterize groups of patients for studies of outcome. In: Levin HS, Grafman J, Eisenberg HM, eds. *Neurobehavioral recovery from head injury.* New York: Oxford, 1987:13–29.
13. Williams DH, Levin HS, Eisenberg HM. Mild head injury classification. *Neurosurgery* 1990;27:422–428.
14. Kraus JF. Epidemiology of head injury. In: Cooper PR, ed. *Head injury.* Baltimore: Williams & Wilkins, 1993:1–25.
15. Dikmen S, Machamer J, Temkin N. Psychosocial outcome in patients with moderate to severe head injury: 2-year follow-up. *Brain Inj* 1993;7:113–124.
16. Levin HS, Mattis S, Ruff RM, et al. Neurobehavioral outcome following minor head injury: a three-center study. *J Neurosurg* 1987;66:234–243.
17. Department of Health and Human Services. *Interagency Head Injury Task Force report.* Washington, DC: Department of Health and Human Services, 1989.
18. Elovic E, Antoinette T. Epidemiology and primary prevention of traumatic brain injury. In: Horn L, Zasler N, eds. *Medical rehabilitation of traumatic brain injury.* Philadelphia: Hanley & Belfus, 1996:9.
19. Sosin DM, Sacks JJ, Smith S. Head injury associated deaths in the United States from 1979 to 1986. *JAMA* 1989;262:2251–2255.
20. Rimel RW, Jan JA, Bond MR. Characteristics of the head injured patient. In: Rosenthal M, Griffith ER, Bond MR, Miller JD, eds. *Rehabilitation of the adult*

and child with traumatic brain injury. Philadelphia: FA Davis, 1990:8–16.

21. Frankowski RF, Annegers J, Whitman S. *Epidemiological and descriptive studies: part 1. The descriptive epidemiology of head trauma in the United States. Central Nervous System Data report.* 1985:33–43.

22. Whitman S, Coonley-Hogason R, Desai B. Comparative head trauma experience in two socioeconomically different Chicago area communities: a population study. *Am J Epidemiol* 1984;119:570–580.

23. Lindenbaum GA, Carroll SF, Daskel I, et al. Patterns of alcohol and drug abuse in an urban trauma center: the increasing role of abuse. *J Trauma* 1989;29:1654–1658.

24. Sparadeo FR, Gill D. Effects of prior alcohol use on head injury recovery. *J Head Trauma Rehabil* 1989;4:72–82.

25. Annegers JF, Grabow JD, Kurland LT, et al. The incidence, causes and secular trends of head trauma in Olmsted County, Minnesota, 1935–1974. *Neurology* 1980;30:919–929.

26. Siccardi D, Cavaliere R, Pau A, et al. Penetrating craniocerebral missile injuries in civilians: a retrospective analysis of 314 cases. *Surg Neurol* 1991;35: 455–460.

27. Sosin DM, Sniezek JE, Waxweiler RJ. Trends in death associated with traumatic brain injury. *JAMA* 1995;273:1778–1780.

28. Gennarelli TA, Champion HR, Copes WS, Sarco WJ. Comparison of mortality, morbidity, and severity of 59,713 head injured patients with 114,447 patients with extracranial injuries. *J Trauma* 1994;37:962–968.

29. Jagger J, Vernber K, Jane J. Air bags reducing the toll of brain trauma. *Neurosurgery* 1987;20:815–817.

30. National Highway Traffic Safety Administration, National Center for Statistics and Analysis. *Traffic safety facts 1994: occupant protection.* Washington, DC: U.S. Department of Transportation, 1994.

31. National Highway Traffic Safety Administration, U.S. Department of Transportation. *Safety belt and motorcycle helmet use incentive grant program.* Washington, DC: U.S. Department of Transportation, 1993.

32. Centers for Disease Control and Prevention. Safety restraint assessment—Iowa, 1987–1988. *MMWR* 1989;38:735–738.

33. Watson GS, Zador PL, Wilks M. Helmet use, helmet use laws and motorcycle fatalities. *Am J Public Health* 1981;71:297–300.

34. Offner P, Rivara FP, Maier R. The impact of motorcycle helmet use. *J Trauma* 1992;32:636–642.

35. Thompson RS, Rivara FP, Thompson DL. A case control study of the effectiveness of bicycle safety helmets. *N Engl J Med* 1989;321:1194–1196.

36. DeMuth WE. Bullet velocity as applied to military rifle wounding capacity. *J Trauma* 1969;9:27–38.

37. Foulkes MA, Eisenberg HM, Jane JA, et al. The Traumatic Coma Data Bank: design, methods, and baseline characteristics. *J Neurosurg* 1991;75:S8–S13.

38. McLellan DR. The structural basis of coma and recovery: insights from brain injury in humans and experimental animals. *Phys Med Rehabil State Art Rev* 1990;4:389–407.

39. Gurdijian ES. Cerebral contusions: re-evaluation of the mechanisms of their development. *J Trauma* 1976;16:35–51.

40. Gennarelli TA, Thiboult LE, Adams JH, et al. Diffuse axonal injury and traumatic coma in the primate. *Ann Neurol* 1982;12: 564–574.

41. Lipton S, Rosenberg P. Excitatory amino acids as a final common pathway for neurologic disorders. *N Engl J Med* 1994;330:613–621.

42. Marion DW, Darby J, Yonas H. Acute regional cerebral blood flow changes caused by severe head injuries. *J Neurosurg* 1991;74:407–414.

43. Muizelaar JP, Marmarou A, Ward JD, et al. Adverse effects of prolonged hyperventilation in patients with severe head injury: a randomized clinical trial. *J Neurosurg* 1991;75: 731–739.

44. Bouma G, Muizelar JP, Bandoh K, Marmarou A. Blood pressure and intracranial pressure-volume dynamics in severe head injury: a relationship with cerebral blood flow. *J Neurosurg* 1992;77:15–19.

45. Rosner MJ. Intracranial pressure: a critical examination of its physiology and pathophysiology. In: Andrews B, ed. *Neurosurgical intensive care.* New York: McGraw-Hill, 1993:57–112.

46. Boyeson MG, Jones JL. Theoretical mechanisms of brain plasticity and therapeutic implications. In: Horn L, Zasler N, eds. *Medical rehabilitation of traumatic brain injury.* Philadelphia: Hanley & Belfus, 1996: 77–102.

47. Lyeth BG, Ray M, Hamm RJ, et al. Post-injury scopolamine administration in experimental traumatic brain injury. *Brain Res* 1992;569:281–286.

48. Sims JS, Jones TA, Fulton RL, et al. Benzodiazepine effects on recovery of function linked to trans-neuronal morphological events. *Soc Neurosci Abstr* 1990;16:342.

49. Schallert T, Hernandez TD, Barth TM. Recovery of function after brain damage: severe and chronic disruption by diazepam. *Brain Res* 1986;379:104–111.

50. Feeney DM, Gonzalez A, Law WA. Amphetamine, haloperidol, and experience interact to affect rate of recovery after motor cortex injury. *Science* 1982;217:855–857.

51. Stephens J, Goldberg G, Demopoulos JT. Clonidine reinstates deficits following recovery

from sensorimotor cortex lesion in rats. *Arch Phys Med Rehabil* 1986;67:666–667.

52. Chrisostomo EA, Duncan PW, Propst M, et al. Evidence that amphetamine with physical therapy promotes recovery of motor function in stroke patients. *Ann Neurol* 1988;23:94–97.

53. Walker-Batson D, Smith P, Curtis S, et al. Amphetamine paired with physical therapy accelerates motor recovery after stroke. *Stroke* 1995;26:2254–2259.

54. Cope N, Hall K. Head injury rehabilitation: benefit of early intervention. Arch Phys Med Rehabil 1982;63:433–437.

55. Mackay LE, Bernstein B, Chapman P, et al. Early intervention in severe head injury: long-term benefits of a formalized program. *Arch Phys Med Rehabil* 1992;73:635–641.

56. Rappaport M, Dougherty AM, Kelting DL. Evaluation of coma and vegetative states. *Arch Phys Med Rehabil* 1992;73:628–634.

57. Giacino JT, Kezmarsky MA, DeLuca J, Cicerone KD. Monitoring rate of recovery to predict outcome in minimally responsive patients. *Arch Phys Med Rehabil* 1991;72:897–901.

58. Ansell BJ, Keenan JE. The Western Neuro Sensory Stimulation Profile: a tool for assessing slow-to-recover head-injured patients. *Arch Phys Med Rehabil* 1989;70:104–108.

59. Multi-society Task Force on PVS. Medical aspects of the persistent vegetative state: statement of a multi-society task force. *N Engl J Med* 1994;330:1499–1508.

60. Levin HS, Benton AL, Grossman RG. *Neurobehavioral consequences of closed head injury.* New York: Oxford University Press, 1982.

61. High WM, Levin HS, Gary HE Jr. Recovery of orientation following closed head injury. *J Clin Neuropsychol* 1990;12:703–704.

62. Levin HS, O'Donnell VM, Grossman RG. The Galveston Orientation and Amnesia Test: a practical scale to assess cognition after head injury. *J Nerv Ment Dis* 1979;167:675–684.

63. Hannay HJ, Sherer M. Assessment of outcome from head injury. In: Narayan RK, Wilberger JE, Povlishock JT, eds. *Neurotrauma.* New York: McGraw-Hill, 1996:723–747.

64. Boake C, Millis SR, High WM, et al. Using early neuropsychological testing to predict long-term productivity outcome from traumatic brain injury. *J Int Neuropsychol Soc* 1997;3:12. Abstract.

65. Ryan TV, Sautter SW, Capps CF, et al. Utilizing neuropsychological measures to predict vocational outcome in a head trauma population. *Brain Inj* 1992;6:175–182.

66. Sherer M, Boake C. Prediction of return to productivity following traumatic brain injury. *J Int Neuropsychol Soc* 1984;1:55. Abstract.

67. Hannay HJ, Struchen MA, Contant CF, et al. Assessment of severely closed head injured patients and prediction of outcome. *J Int Neuropsychol Soc* 1994;1:73. Abstract.

68. Lezak MD. *Neuropsychological Assessment.* New York: Oxford, 1995.

69. Hathaway SR, McKinley JC. *Minnesota Multiphasic Personality Inventory-2: manual for administration and scoring.* Minneapolis: University of Minnesota Press, 1989.

70. Levin HS, High WM, Goethe K, et al. The Neurobehavioral Rating Scale: assessment of the behavioral sequelae of head injury by the clinician. *J Neurol Neurosurg Psychiatry* 1987;50:183–193.

71. Lezak MD. Relationships between personality disorders, social disturbances, and physical disability following rehabilitation for traumatic brain injury. *J Head Trauma Rehabil* 1987;2:57–69.

72. Jennett B, Bond MR. Assessment of outcome after severe brain damage: a practical scale. *Lancet* 1975;2:480–484.

73. Rappaport M, Hall KM, Hopkins K, et al. Disability Rating Scale for severe head trauma: coma to community. *Arch Phys Med Rehabil* 1982; 63:118–123.

73a. Hagen C. Language disorders in head trauma. In: Holland A, ed. *Language disorders in adults.* San Diego, CA: College-Hill, 1984.

74. Jennett B, Snoek J, Bond MR, et al. Disability after severe head injury: observations on the use of the Glasgow Outcome Scale. *J Neurol Neurosurg Psychiatry* 1981;44:285–293.

75. Gouvier WD, Blanton PD, LaPorte KK, Nepomuceno C. Reliability and validity of the Disability Rating Scale and the Levels of Cognitive Functioning Scale in monitoring recovery from severe head injury. *Arch Phys Med Rehabil* 1987;68:94–97.

76. Cope DN, Cole JR, Hall KM, Barkan H. Brain injury: analysis of outcome in a post-acute rehabilitation system. Part 1: general analysis. *Brain Inj* 1991;5:111-125.

77. Gennarelli TA, Spielman GM, Langfitt TW, et al. Influence of the type of intracranial lesion on outcome from severe head injury: a multicenter study using a new classification system. *J Neurosurg* 1982;56:26–32.

78. Spivack G, Spetell CM, Ellis DW, Ross SE. Effects of intensity of treatment and length of stay on rehabilitation outcomes. *Brain Inj* 1992;6:419–434.

79. Hall KM, Cope DN, Rappaport M. Glasgow Outcome Scale and Disability Rating Scale: comparative usefulness in following recovery in traumatic head injury. *Arch Phys Med Rehabil* 1985;66:35–37.

80. Hall KM. Overview of functional assessment scales in brain injury rehabilitation. *Neuro Rehabil* 1992;2:98–113.

81. Horn S, Shiel A, McLellan L, et al. A review of behavioral assess-

ment scales for monitoring recovery in and after coma with pilot data on a new scale of visual awareness. *NeuroRehabil* 1993;3:121–137.

82. Hamilton BB, Granger CV, Sherwin FS, et al. A uniform national data system for medical rehabilitation. In: Fuhrer MJ, ed. *Rehabilitation outcomes: analysis and measurement.* Baltimore: Brookes, 1987: 137–147.

83. Hall KM, Hamilton BB, Gordon WA, Zasler ND. Characteristics and comparisons of functional assessment indices: Disability Rating Scale, Functional Independence Measure, and Functional Measure. *J Head Trauma Rehabil* 1993;8(2): 60–74.

84. Dodds TA, Martin DP, Stolox WC, Deyo RA. A validation of the Functional Independence Measure and its performance among rehabilitation inpatients. *Arch Phys Med Rehabil* 1993;74:531–536.

85. Whiteneck GG, Charlifue SW, Gerhart KA, et al. Quantifying handicap: a new measure of long-term rehabilitation outcomes. *Arch Phys Med Rehabil* 1992;73:519–526.

86. Boake C, High WM. Functional outcome from traumatic brain injury: unidimensional or multidimensional. *Am J Phys Med Rehabil* 1996;75:1–10.

87. Willer B, Rosenthal M, Kreutzer JS, et al. Assessment of community integration following rehabilitation for traumatic brain injury. *J Head Trauma Rehabil* 1993;8:75–87.

88. High WM, Sherer M, Boake C, et al. Effect of postacute rehabilitation on social role functioning one to three years following traumatic brain injury. *J Int Neuropsychol Soc* 1997;3:59. Abstract.

89. Vollmer DG, Dacey TG. Prediction and assessment of outcome following closed head injury. In: Pitts LH, Wagner FC Jr, eds. *Craniospinal trauma.* New York: Thieme Medical, 1990:120–140.

90. Vollmer DG, Torner JC, Jane JA, et al. Age and outcome following traumatic coma: why do older patients fare worse? *J Neurosurg* 1991;75:S37–S49.

91. Brooks N, McKinlay W, Symington C, et al. Return to work within the first seven years of severe head injury. *Brain Inj* 1987;1:5–19.

92. Rimel RW, Giordani B, Barth JT, et al. Disability caused by minor head injury. *Neurosurgery* 1981;9:221–228.

93. Rimel RW, Giordani, B Barth JT, et al. Moderate head injury: completing the clinical spectrum of head trauma. *Neurosurgery* 1982;11:344–351.

94. Katz D, Alexander M. Traumatic brain injury: predicting course of recovery and outcome for patients admitted to rehabilitation. *Arch Neurol* 1994;51: 661–670.

95. Fraser R, Dikmen S, McLean A, et al. Employability of head injury survivors: first year post-injury. *Rehabil Couns Bull* 1988;31:276–288.

96. Najenson T, Groswasser Z, Mendelson L, Hackett P. Rehabilitation outcome of brain damaged patients after severe head injury. *Int Rehabil Med* 1980;2:17–22.

96a. Jennett B, Snoek J, Bond MR, Brooks N. Disability after severe head injury: observations on the use of the Glasgow Outcome Scale. *J Neurol Neurosurg Psychiat* 1981;44:285–293.

97. Prigatano GP, Fordyce DJ, Zeiner HK, et al. Neuropsychological rehabilitation after closed head injury in young adults. *J Neurol Neurosurg Psychiatry* 1984;47:505–513.

98. Rao N, Rosenthal M, Cronin-Stubbs D, et al. Return to work after rehabilitation following traumatic brain injury. *Brain Inj* 1990;4:49–56.

99. McGlynn SM, Schacter DL. Unawareness of deficits in neuropsychological syndromes. *J Clin Exp Neuropsychol* 1989;11:143–205.

100. Ezrachi O, Ben-Yishay Y, Kay T, et al. Predicting employment in traumatic brain injury following neuropsychological rehabilitation. *J Head Trauma Rehabil* 1991;6: 71–84.

101. Walker DE, Blankenship V, Ditty JA, Lynch KP. Prediction of recovery for closed-head-injured adults: an evaluation of the MMPI, the Adaptive Behavior Scale, and a "Quality of Life" rating scale. *J Clin Psychol* 1987;43:699–707.

102. Sherer M, Bergloff P, Levin E, et al. Impaired awareness and employment outcome after traumatic brain injury. *J Head Trauma Rehabil* 1998; 13(5):52–61.

103. Melamed S, Stern M, Rahmani L, et al. Attention capacity limitation, psychiatric parameters and their impact on work involvement following brain injury. *Scand J Rehabil Med* 1985;12:21–26.

104. Kreutzer JS, Wehman PH. *Cognitive rehabilitation for persons with traumatic brain injury: a functional approach.* Baltimore: Paul H. Brookes, 1991.

105. Malec JF, Basford JS. Postacute brain injury rehabilitation. *Arch Phys Med Rehabil* 1996;77:198–207.

106. Cope DN. The effectiveness of traumatic brain injury rehabilitation: a review. *Brain Inj* 1995;9:649–670.

107. Hall KM, Cope DN. The benefit of rehabilitation in traumatic brain injury: a literature review. *J Head Trauma Rehabil* 1995;10(5):1–13.

108. Prigatano GP, Klonoff PS, O'Brien KP, et al. Productivity after neuropsychologically oriented milieu rehabilitation. *J Head Trauma Rehabil* 1994; 9(1):91–102.

109. Blair DC, Lanyon RI. Retraining social and adaptive living skills in severely head injured adults. *Arch Clin Neuropsychol* 1987;2:33–43.

110. Rattok J, Ben-Yishay Y, Ezrachi O, et al. Outcome of different

treatment mixes in a multidimensional neuropsychological rehabilitation program. *Neuropsychology* 1992;6:395–415.

111. Ruff RM, Niemann H. Cognitive rehabilitation versus day treatment in head-injured adults: is there an impact on emotional and psychosocial adjustment? *Brain Inj* 1990;4:339–347.

112. Sohlberg MM, Mateer CA. Effectiveness of an attention training program. *J Clin Exp Neuropsychol* 1987;2:117–130.

113. Schacter DL, Glisky EL. Memory remediation: restoration, alleviation and the acquisition of domain-specific knowledge. In: Uzzell BP, Gross Y, eds. *Clinical neuropsychology of intervention.* Boston: Martinus Nijhoff, 1986:257–282.

114. Malec J, Schafer D, Jacket M. Comprehensive-integrated postacute outpatient brain injury rehabilitation. *NeuroRehabil* 1992;2:1–11.

115. Horn LJ, Garland D. Medical and orthopaedic problems associated with traumatic brain injury. In: Rosenthal M, Griffith ER, Bond MR, Miller JD, eds. *Rehabilitation of the adult and child with traumatic brain injury.* Philadelphia: FA Davis, 1990:107–126.

116. Temkin NR, Kikmen SS, Wilensky AJ, et al. A randomized, double-blind study of phenytoin for the prevention of post-traumatic seizures. *N Engl J Med* 1990;323:497–502.

117. Yablon S. Posttraumatic seizures. *Arch Phys Med Rehabil* 1993;74:983–1001.

118. Massagli TL. Neurobehavioral effects of phenytoin, carbamazepine and valproic acid: implications for use in traumatic brain injury. *Arch Phys Med Rehabil* 1991;72:219–226.

119. Cope DN, Date ES, Mar EY. Serial computed tomographic evaluations in traumatic head injury. *Arch Phys Med Rehabil* 1988;69:483–486.

120. Doherty D. Posttraumatic hydrocephalus. *Phys Med Rehabil Clin N Am* 1992;3:389–406.

121. Sheffler L, Ito V, Philip P, Sahgal V. Shunting in chronic posttraumatic hydrocephalus: demonstration of neurophysiologic improvement. *Arch Phys Med Rehabil* 1994;75:338–341.

122. Horn LJ. Pharmacologic interventions in neuroendocrine disorders following traumatic brain injury, part 1. *J Head Trauma Rehabil* 1988;3(2):87–90.

123. Horn LJ. Pharmacologic interventions in neuroendocrine disorders following traumatic brain injury, part 2. *J Head Trauma Rehabil,* 1988;3(3):86–96.

124. Labi MC, Horn LJ. Hypertension in traumatic brain injury. *Brain Inj* 1990;4:365–370.

125. Meythaler JM, Stinson AM. Fever of central origin in traumatic brain injury controlled with propranolol. *Arch Phys Med Rehabil* 1994;75:816–819.

126. Childs A. Naltrexone in organic bulemia: a preliminary report. *Brain Inj* 1987;1:49–55.

127. Chestnut RM. Medical complications of the head injured patient. In: Cooper PR, ed. *Head injury.* 3rd ed. Baltimore: Williams & Wilkins, 1993:459–501.

128. Hansen JR, Cook JS. Posttraumatic neuroendocrine disorders. *Phys Med Rehabil State Art Rev* 1993;7:569–580.

129. Sumner D. Post-traumatic anosmia. Brain 1964;87:107–120.

130. Sabates NR, Gonce MA, Farris BK. Neuro-ophthalmological findings in closed head trauma. *J Clin Neuroophthalmol* 1991;11:273–277.

131. Fisch U. Facial paralysis in fractures of the petrous bone. *Laryngoscope* 1974;84:2141–2154.

132. Wani MA, Tandon PN, Banerji AK, et al. Collet-Sicard syndrome resulting from closed head injury: case report. *J Trauma* 1991;31:1437–1439.

133. Young B, Ott L, Twyman D, et al. The effect of nutritional support on outcome from severe head injury. *J Neurosurg* 1987;67:668–676.

134. Winstein CJ. Neurogenic dysphagia. *Phys Ther* 1983;63:1992–1997.

135. Kamada T, Fusamoto H, Kawano S, et al. Gastrointestinal bleeding following head injury: a clinical study of 433 cases. *J Trauma* 1977;17:44–47.

136. Kalisky Z, Morrison DP, Meyers CA, Von Laufen A. Medical problems encountered during rehabilitation of patients with head injury. *Arch Phys Med Rehabil* 1985;66:25–29.

137. Aiges HW, Daum F, Olso M, et al. Effects of phenobarbital and diphenylhydantoin on liver function and morphology. *J Pediatr* 1980;97:22–26.

138. Sobus K, Alexander M, Harcke T. Undetected musculoskeletal trauma in children with traumatic brain injury or spinal cord injury. *Arch Phys Med Rehabil* 1993;74:902–904.

139. Garland D, Baily S. Undetected injuries in head injured adults. *Clin Orthop* 1981;155:162–165.

140. Stone L, Keenan M. Peripheral nerve injuries in the adult with traumatic brain injury. *Clin Orthop* 1988;233:136–144.

141. Garland DE, Blum CE, Waters RL. Periarticular heterotopic ossification in head-injured adults. *J Bone Joint Surg [Am]* 1980;62:1143–1146.

142. Sazbon L, Najenson T, Tartakovsky M, et al. Widespread periarticular new-bone formation in long term comatose patients. *J Bone Joint Surg [Br]* 1981;63:120.

143. Varghese G. Heterotopic ossification. *Phys Rehabil Clin N Am* 1992;3:407–415.

144. Garland D, Blum C, Waters R. Periarticular heterotopic ossification in head injured adults. *J Bone Joint Surg [Am]* 1980;62:1143–1146.

145. Mital MA, Garbar JE, Stinson JT. Ectopic bone formation in children and adolescents with head injury: its management. *J Pediatr Orthop* 1987;7:83–90.

146. Ritter MA, Gioe T. The effect of indomethacin on para-articular ectopic ossification following total hip arthroplasty. *Clin Orthop* 1982;167:113–117.

147. Gennarelli TA. Subject review: heterotopic ossification. *Brain Inj* 1988;2:175–178.

148. Garland D, Hanscom D, Keenan M, et al. Resection of heterotopic ossification in the adult with head trauma. *J Bone Joint Surg [Am]* 1985;67:1261–1269.

149. Meythaler JM, DeVivo MJ, Hayne JB. Cost-effectiveness of routine screening for proximal deep venous thrombosis in acquired brain injury patients admitted to rehabilitation. *Arch Phys Med Rehabil* 1996;77:1–5.

150. Garden F, Bontke C. Sexual functioning and marital adjustment after traumatic brain injury. *J Head Trauma Rehabil* 1990;5:(2)52–59.

151. Horn LJ, Zasler, N. Neuroanatomy and neurophysiology of sexual function. *J Head Trauma Rehabil* 1990:5(2):1–13.

152. Zasler N, Horn LJ. Rehabilitative management of sexual dysfunction. *J Head Trauma Rehabil* 1990;5(2):14–24.

153. Sandel ME. Sexuality and reproduction after traumatic brain injury. In: Horn LJ, Zasler N, eds. *Medical rehabilitation of traumatic brain injury.* Philadelphia: Hanley & Belfus, 1996:557–572.

154. Mayer NH, Exquenazi A, Keenan M. Analysis and management of spasticity, contracture, and impaired motor control. In: Horn L, Zasler N, eds. *Medical rehabilitation of traumatic brain injury.* Philadelphia: Hanley & Belfus, 1996:411–458.

155. Pierson SH, Katz DI, Tarsy D. Botulinum toxin A in the treatment of spasticity: functional implications and patient selection. *Arch Phys Med Rehabil* 1996;77:717–721.

156. Gittler M, Newman H. Intravenous dantrolene sodium for the treatment of spasticity in the trauma ICU. *Am J Phys Med Rehabil* 1996;75:163. Abstract.

157. Ivanhoe CB, Bontke CF. Movement disorders after traumatic brain injury. In: Horn L, Zasler N, eds. *Medical rehabilitation of traumatic brain injury.* Philadelphia: Hanley & Belfus, 1996: 395–410.

158. Maki Y, Akimoto H, Enomoto T. Injuries of basal ganglia following head trauma in children. *Childs Brain* 1980;7:113–123.

159. Jankovic J, Schwartz K. Botulinum toxin treatment of tremors. *Neurology* 1991;41:1185–1188.

160. Manyam BV. Recent advances in the treatment of cerebellar ataxia. *Clin Neuropharmacol* 1986;6:508–516.

161. Katz DI. Movement disorders following traumatic head injury. *J Head Trauma Rehabil* 1990;5(1):86–90.

162. Fleet WS, Valenstein E, Watson RT, et al. Dopamine agonist therapy for neglect in humans. *Neurology* 1987;37:1765–1771.

163. McNeny R, Zasler ND. Neuropharmacologic remediation of hemi-inattention following brain injury. *NeuroRehabil* 1991;1: 72–78.

164. Oddy M, Humphrey M, Uttley D. Subjective impairment and social recovery after closed head injury. *J Neurol Neurosurg Psychiatry* 1978;41:611–616.

165. Oddy M, Humphrey M. Social recovery during the year following severe head injury. *J Neurol Neurosurg Psychiatry* 1980;43: 798–802.

166. Levin HS. Neurobehavioral sequelae of closed head injury. In: Cooper PR, ed. *Head injury.* Baltimore: Williams & Wilkins, 1993;525–551.

167. Bleiberg J, Cope DN, Spector J. Cognitive assessment and therapy in traumatic brain injury. *Phys Med Rehabil State Art Rev* 1989;3:95–121.

168. Dikmen S, Reitan RM, Temkin NR. Neuropsychological recovery in head injury. *Arch Neurol* 1983;40:333–338.

169. Tabaddor K, Mattis S, Zazula T. Cognitive sequelae and recovery course after moderate and severe head injury. *Neurosurgery* 1984;14:701–708.

170. Prigatano GP. Personality disturbances associated with traumatic brain injury. *J Consult Clin Psychol* 1992;60:360–368.

171. Wood RLI. Neurobehavioural paradigm for brain injury rehabilitation. In: Wood RL, ed. *Neurobehavioral sequelae of traumatic brain injury.* New York: Taylor & Francis, 1990:3–17.

172. Mattson AJ, Levin HS. Frontal lobe dysfunction following closed head injury: a review of the literature. *J Nerv Ment Dis* 1990; 178:282–291.

173. Levin HS, Grossman RG. Behavioral sequelae of closed head injury: a quantitative study. *Arch Neurol* 1978;35:720–728.

174. Lezak MD. Psychological implications of traumatic brain damage for the patient's family. *Rehabil Psychol* 1986;31:241–250.

175. Brooks DN, McKinlay WW. Personality and behavioural change after severe blunt head injury—a relative's view. *J Neurol Neurosurg Psychiatry* 1983;46: 336–344.

176. Childs NL, Mercer WN, Childs HW. Accuracy of diagnosis of persistent vegetative state. *Neurology* 1993;43:1465–1467.

177. American Congress of Rehabilitation Medicine. Recommendations for use of uniform nomenclature pertinent to patients with severe alterations in consciousness. *Arch Phys Med Rehabil* 1995;76:205–209.

178. Ansell BJ. Slow to recover patients: improvement to rehabilitation readiness. *J Head Trauma Rehabil* 1993;8(3):88–98.

179. Braakman R, Jennett WB, Minderhoud JM. Prognosis of the post-traumatic vegetative state. *Acta Neurochir (Wien)* 1988;95: 49–52.

180. Bricolo A, Turazzi S, Feriotti G. Prolonged post-traumatic unconsciousness. *J Neurosurg* 1980; 52:625–634.

181. Bartokowski HM, Lovely MP. Prognosis in coma and the persistent vegetative state. *J Head Trauma Rehabil* 1986;1: 1–5.

182. Groswasser Z, Sazbon L. Outcome in 134 patients with prolonged posttraumatic unawareness. Part 2: functional outcome of 72 patients recovering consciousness. *J Neurosurg* 1990; 72:81–84.

183. Sazbon L, Groswasser Z. Outcome in 134 patients with prolonged posttraumatic unawareness. I: parameters determining late recovery of consciousness. *J Neurosurg* 1990;72:75–80.

184. Lal S, Merbitz CP, Grip JC. Modification of function in head-injured patients with Sinemet. *Brain Inj* 1988;2:225–233.

185. DiRicco C, Maira G, Meglio M, Rossi GF. L-Dopa treatment of comatose states due to cerebral lesions: preliminary findings. *J Neurosurg Sci* 1974;18:169–176.

186. Haig AJ, Ruess JM. Recovery from vegetative state of six months duration associated with Sinemet (levodopa/carbidopa). *Arch Phys Med Rehabil* 1990; 71:1081–1083.

187. Ross ED, Stewart MD. Akinetic mutism from hypothalamic damage: successful treatment with dopamine agonists. *Neurology* 1981;31:1435–1439.

188. Elovic E. Pharmacology of attention and arousal in the low level patient. *NeuroRehab* 1996;6: 57–68.

189. Kaelin DL, Cifu DX, Matthies B. Methylphenidate effect on attention deficit in the acutely brain-injured adult. *Arch Phys Med Rehabil* 1996;77:6–9.

190. Reinhard DL, Whyte J, Sandel ME. Improved arousal and initiation following tricyclic antidepressant use in severe brain injury. *Arch Phys Med Rehabil* 1996;77:80–83.

191. Goldstein LB, Davis JN. Post-lesion practice and amphetamine-facilitated recovery of beam-walking in the rat. *Res Neurol Neurosci* 1990;1: 311–314.

192. Rozenweig MR. Animal models for effects of brain lesions and for rehabilitation. In: Bach-y-Rita P, ed. *Recovery of function: theoretical considerations for brain injury rehabilitation.* Baltimore: University Park Press, 1980: 127–172.

193. Wood RL. Critical analysis of the concept of sensory stimulation for patients in vegetative states. *Brain Inj* 1991;5:401–409.

194. Giacino JT. Sensory stimulation: theoretical perspectives and the evidence for effectiveness. *NeuroRehabil* 1996;6:69–78.

195. O'Dell MW, Jasin P, Lyons N, et al. Standardized assessment instruments for minimally-responsive, brain injured patients. *NeuroRehabil* 1996;6:45–55.

196. Bontke CF, Boake C. Principles of brain injury rehabilitation. In: Braddom R, ed. *Textbook of physical medicine and rehabilitation.* Philadephia: WB Saunders, 1996:1027–1051.

197. Cope DN. Psychopharmacologic considerations in the treatment of traumatic brain injury. *J Head Trauma Rehabil* 1987;2(4)1–5.

198. Gualtieri CT. A review: pharmacotherapy and the neurobehavioral sequelae of traumatic brain injury. *Brain Inj* 1988;2:101–129.

199. Rose MJ. The place of drugs in the management of behavior disorders after traumatic brain injury. *J Head Trauma Rehabil* 1988;3(3):7–13.

200. Corrigan JD. Development of a scale for assessment of agitation following traumatic brain injury. *J Clin Exp Neuropsychol* 1989;11:261–277.

201. Gualtieri CT, Evans RW. Stimulant treatment for the neurobehavioral sequelae of traumatic brain injury. *Brain Inj* 1988;2: 273–290.

202. Chandler MC, Barnhill JL, Gualtieri CT. Amantadine for the agitated head-injury patient. *Brain Inj* 1988;2:309–311.

203. Mooney GF, Haas LJ. Effect of methylphenidate on brain injury-related anger. *Arch Phys Med Rehabil* 1993;74:153–160.

204. Horn LJ. "Atypical" medications for the treatment of disruptive aggressive behavior in the brain injured patient. *J Head Trauma Rehabil* 1987;2(4):18–28.

205. Dikmen SS, Levin HS. Methodological issues in the study of mild head injury. *J Head Trauma Rehabil* 1993;8(3):30–37.

206. Zasler ND. Mild traumatic brain injury: medical assessment and intervention. *J Head Trauma Rehabil* 1993;8(3):13–29.

207. Hicks RR, Smith DH, Lowenstein DH, et al. Mild experimental brain injury in the rat induces cognitive deficits associated with regional neuronal loss in the hippocampus. *J Neurotrauma* 1993;10:405–414.

208. MacNab I. Acceleration injuries of the cervical spine. *J Bone Joint Surg [Am]* 1962;46: 1797–1799.

209. MacNam J. The "whiplash syndrome." *Orthop Clin North Am* 1971;2:389–403.

210. Levin HS, Amparo E, Eisenberg HM, et al. Magnetic resonance imaging and computerized tomography in relation to the neurobehavioral sequela of mild and moderate head injuries. *J Neurosurg* 1987;66:706–713.

211. Bernard PG. Neurodiagnostic testing in patients with closed head injury. *Clin Electroencephalogr* 1991;22:203–210.

212. Sakas DE, Bullock MR, Patterson J, et al. Focal cerebral hyperemia

after focal head injury in humans: a benign phenomenon? *J Neurosurg* 1995;83:277–284.

213. Thatcher RW, Walker RA, Gerson I, Geisler FH. EEG discriminant analyses of mild head trauma. *Electroencephalogr Clin Neurophysiol* 1989;73:94–106.

214. Schoenhuber R, Gentilini M, Orlando A. Prognostic value of auditory brain-stem responses for late postconcussion symptoms following minor head injury. *J Neurosurg* 1988;68:742–744.

215. Ford MR, Khalil M. Evoked potential findings in mild traumatic brain injury. 1: middle latency component augmentation and cognitive component attenuation. *J Head Trauma Rehabil* 1996;11(6):1–15.

216. Epstein CM. Computerized EEG in the courtroom. *Neurology* 1994;44:1566–1569.

217. Gronwall D. Rehabilitation programs for patients with mild head injury: components, problems, and evaluation. *J Head Trauma Rehabil* 1986;1(21): 53–62.

218. Ruff RM, Levin HS, Marshall LF. Neurobehavioral methods of assessment and the study of outcome in minor head injury. *J Head Trauma Rehabil* 1986;1(21)43–52.

219. Binder LM. Assessment of malingering with the Portland Digit Recognition Test after mild head trauma. *J Clin Exp Neuropsychol* 1993;15:170–182.

220. Hiscock M, Hiscock CK. Refining the forced-choice method for the detection of malingering. *J Clin Exp Neuropsychol* 1989;11: 967–974.

221. Boake C, Bobetic KM, Bontke CF. Rehabilitation of the patient with mild traumatic brain injury. *NeuroRehab* 1991;1:70–78.

222. Ruff RM, Wylie T, Tennant W. Malingering and malingering-like aspects of mild closed head injury. *J head Trauma Rehabil* 1993;8(3):60–73.

223. Miller H. Accident neurosis. *BMJ* 1961;1:919–925.

224. Thompson MR. Post-traumatic psychoneurosis—a statistical study. *Am J Psychiatry* 1965;121:1043–1048.

225. Horn LJ. Post-concussive headache. *Phys Med Rehabil State Art Rev* 1992;6: 69–78.

226. Cytowic R, Stump DA, Larned DC. Closed head trauma: somatic, ophthalmic, and cognitive impairments in nonhospitalized patients. In: Whitaker HA, ed. *Neuropsychological studies of nonfocal brain damage.* New York: Springer, 1988: 226–264.

227. Davies RA, Luxon LM. Dizziness following head injury: a neuro-otological study. *J Neurol* 1995;242:222–230.

228. Zasler ND. Neuromedical diagnosis and management of postconcussive disorders. In: Horn L, Zasler N, eds. *Medical rehabilitation of traumatic brain injury.* Philadelphia: Hanley & Belfus, 1996:133–170.

229. Gizzi M. The efficacy of vestibular rehabilitation for patients with head trauma. *J Head Trauma Rehabil* 1995;10:60–77.

230. Chelen W, Kabrisky M, Hatsell C, et al. Use of phenytoin in the prevention of motion sickness. *Aviat Space Environ Med* 1990;61:1022–1025.

231. Olesen J. Calcium entry blockers in the treatment of vertigo. *Ann N Y Acad Sci* 1988; 522:690–697.

232. Johnston MV, Hall K, Carnevale G, Boake C. Functional assessment and outcome evaluation in traumatic brain injury rehabilitation. In: Horn L, Zasler N, eds. *Medical rehabilitation of traumatic brain injury.* Philadelphia: Hanley & Belfus, 1996: 197–221.

Chapter 73

Rehabilitation of Spinal Cord Injury

Diana D. Cardenas
Stephen P. Burns
Leighton Chan

EPIDEMIOLOGY

The incidence of spinal cord injury (SCI) in the United States has been estimated at 30 to 40 cases per million per year (1). The exact figure is difficult to determine because there is no mandatory national surveillance system in place. A few states have developed surveillance systems with the assistance of public health departments. The estimated prevalence is given as between 250,000 and 350,000 Americans, with approximately 10,000 new cases each year. Survival has continued to improve both for the acute period and in the long term. Recent data suggest that the age at onset of SCI is correlated to survival, with a markedly decreased life expectancy seen in older patients with cervical-level injuries and more neurologically complete injuries, in comparison to age-matched control subjects (2).

The national Model Systems program funded by the National Institute on Disability and Rehabilitation Research has provided a means to collect data from large SCI centers into a national data bank. The results of the first two decades of the Model Systems program are now available and provide useful information regarding the epidemiology, costs, and complications associated with SCI (3). The Veterans Administration also provides care for its patients at specialized SCI units.

CAUSES

The etiologies of SCI have changed over the last two decades. Motor vehicle accidents remain the number one cause of SCI, accounting for 44.5% of all injuries. Falls are the second leading cause (18.1%) and violence, the third leading cause of SCI (16.6%) over the last 20 years; however, if one examines the etiology for only the past 5 years, one finds that violence has surpassed falls as the second leading cause (1). Prevention continues to be a focus of much-needed research.

ECONOMIC CONSEQUENCES

Although SCI has a fairly low incidence (30/million/yr) compared to other diseases, its economic consequences are quite profound. These consequences include direct costs, which include acute, rehabilitative, and long-term medical care, as well as indirect costs such as lost wages.

Depending on the methodology used, the annual cost of SCI to society, including both direct and indirect costs, is somewhere between $7.3 and $8.3 billion (4,5) (all figures are adjusted to 1994 dollars using the Consumer Price Index for Hospital Services). By comparison, burns and drownings, both events that happen far more commonly than SCI, have annual costs to society of $5.9 billion and $3.7 billion, respectively (5).

While much has been written about the economic consequences of SCI (6–11), two landmark studies examined the issue closely, looking at both the direct and indirect costs. The first study was published in 1992 by Berkowitz et al (4) and was sponsored by the Paralyzed Veterans of America (PVA). They surveyed 758 patients with SCI. The second study was conducted in association with the Model Systems for SCI and enrolled 735 patients. Authored by DeVivo et al (5), it was published in 1995. The two studies were performed at different times and used different methodologies, and therefore their results vary. However, their conclusions are similar: SCI is a very expensive proposition, both for the patient and for society.

The Model Systems study found that the median charge for the medical care (within 1 year of injury) of an individual with SCI was $185,000. The higher the neurologic injury, the higher the charges. The median charges ranged from $464,000 for high cervical injuries, to $134,000 for those with Frankel grade D impairments. The PVA study looked at all medical care for 2 years after injury and found an average cost of $163,000. This ranged from $113,000 for incomplete paraplegia to $232,000 for complete quadriplegia.

In terms of the long-term costs of SCI, the studies found that after rehabilitation the average yearly costs were between $24,000 and $28,000. These costs represent all medical care, hospitalizations, institutionalization if any, and equipment required by the patient. In addition, the figures reflect the cost of personal assistance needed by the patient, which represented more than 40% of total long-term costs.

The PVA study estimated the average annual indirect cost (lost wages and benefits) to be $22,000 for an individual with SCI. Those with more severe deficits and those injured at an older age were less likely to be employed and thus had higher indirect costs. Unemployment was higher in the Model Systems study and therefore the mean annual indirect cost was higher ($43,000). Combining the direct and indirect costs, both studies calculated the lifetime cost of SCI. These calculations made some assumptions about the age of a patient at the time of injury and the present value of future costs (all figures calculated with 4% discount rate). According to the PVA study, a patient with complete quadriplegia injured at age 27 incurred lifetime costs totaling $2,130,000. A patient injured at age 43 with incomplete paraplegia had lifetime costs of $669,000. The Model Systems results were somewhat higher: A patient with a high cervical injury (C1–C4) at age 25 incurred lifetime costs of more than $3,000,000. Those injured at 50 with paraplegia had lifetime costs of $873,000.

CLASSIFICATION

The American Spinal Injury Association (ASIA) has developed and promulgated standards for neurologic classification of SCI based on the examination of key muscles and dermatome levels (12,13). Figure 73-1 describes the 10 key muscle groups to be tested and rated on a scale of 0 to 5, with 5 being normal. The motor level is determined as the most caudal level with at least a grade 3, provided the muscles above that level are normal. Clinical judgment is used to determine whether a muscle that is grade 4 is so because of pain or disuse rather than neurologic impairment. Figure 73-1 also shows the sensory points to be tested and rated, on a scale of 0 to 2. The sensory level is determined by the most caudal level that is normal, or grade 2. Sensation is graded as 0 if absent and 1 if present but impaired. The sensory modalities used to determine the sensory level are pinprick (pain sensation) and light touch. An inability to discriminate sharp from dull should be graded as 0 for pinprick, even if there is some perception of sensation at that sensory point. Using this system, one can determine the neurologic level for each side of the body. If there is a difference from side to side, each side's neurologic level should be described, for example, right (R)—C-6; left (L)—C-7. If the sensory (S) level is not the same as the motor (M) level, each can be described separately: R—C-6S, C-7M; L—C-7S, C-8M.

A lesion is incomplete if there is any preservation of sensory or motor function in the lowest sacral segment (14). Sacral sensation includes sensation at the anal mucocutaneous junction as well as deep anal sensation. The test for motor function determines the presence of voluntary contraction of the external anal sphincter upon digital examination, which should not be confused with passive protrusion as may occur with a Valsalva maneuver in patients with functioning abdominal muscles.

ASIA Impairment Scale

In 1992 the ASIA, in association with 11 other national and international professional organizations, modified the Frankel grading scale and published the ASIA Impairment Scale. The scale groups injuries into one of five broad categories based on whether some degree of sensory or motor function remains intact below the level of the lesion. The scale allows analysis of outcomes for each class of patients. For example, nearly all patients with ASIA grade D tetraplegia as the initial classification recover ambulation by the time of discharge from inpatient rehabilitation (15).

Classic Spinal Cord Injury Syndromes

Spinal cord injury frequently results in recognizable syndromes of neurologic dysfunction. These characteristic patterns of neurologic deficit are due to the anatomic distribution of the cord lesions, with interruption of normal function within certain parts of the cord. While they are named as distinct syndromes, there may be some overlap of features between syndromes and not all components of the syndrome may be present (16).

Central cord syndrome is the most common of the incomplete injury syndromes. It occurs with cervical-level lesions and is frequently seen in older patients with preexisting cervical spinal canal narrowing. The lesion produces sacral sensory sparing and greater weakness in the upper limbs than in the lower limbs. Initially the lesion was thought to be a central hemorrhage within the cord (17),

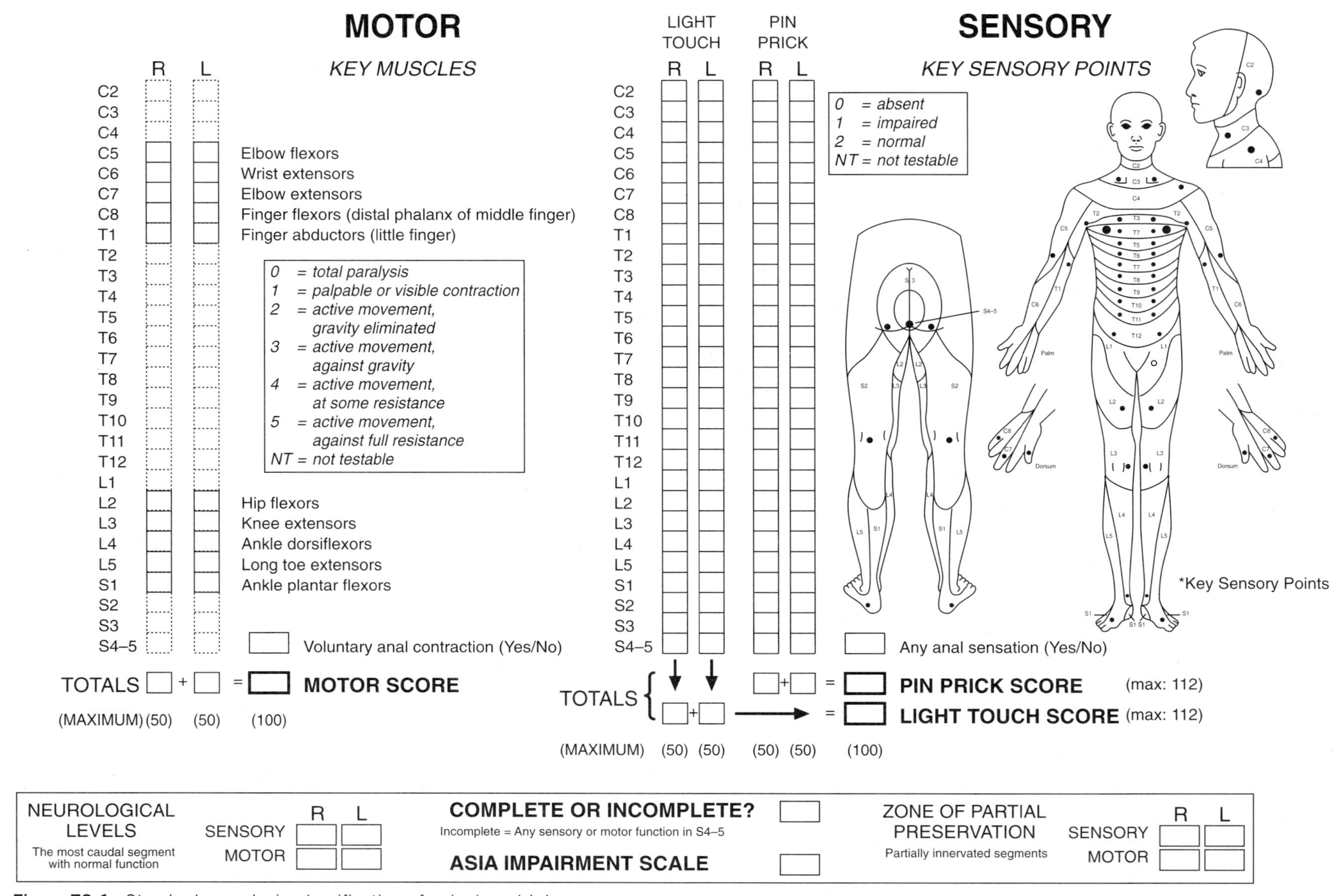

Figure 73-1. Standard neurologic classification of spinal cord injury.

but recently was shown to be essentially nonhemorrhagic, with disruption of axons of the lateral columns at the level of injury and with relative preservation of the gray matter (18).

Brown-Séquard syndrome results from an asymmetric cord lesion and is classically thought of as a cord hemisection, although a true hemisection is uncommon with traumatic injuries. The characteristic clinical features include greater ipsilateral motor and proprioceptive loss, with contralateral loss of pain and temperature sensation.

Anterior cord syndrome occurs as a result of interruption of the blood supply to the anterior portion of the spinal cord. It is characterized by motor paralysis with hypoesthesia, hypalgesia, and preservation of posterior column sensory function. Posterior cord syndrome results in motor paralysis with loss of posterior column sensory function. This very rare syndrome occurs with interruption of the blood supply to the posterior portion of the cord.

Injury at the terminal portion of the spinal cord can result in two syndromes with significant lower motor neuron components. The cauda equina syndrome involves disruption of the lumbosacral roots that continue below the end of the spinal cord. This is a purely lower motor neuron lesion. The conus medullaris syndrome results from injury at a slightly higher level, with damage to lumbar roots as well as the sacral portion of the cord. If a portion of the sacral cord is not entirely disrupted, then the muscles innervated by this most distal portion of the cord will show upper motor neuron features. Thus, the syndrome may involve a mix of upper and lower motor neuron findings.

ACUTE CARE MANAGEMENT

Comprehensive medical treatment for the patient with SCI begins at the scene of the injury. Increased recognition of the potential for further cord injury has led to use of immediate spine immobilization. This is the most likely explanation for the decreased percentage of complete SCIs seen by the early 1980s (19). However, 10% of patients with cervical spinal injuries are still transported without adequate spine immobilization (20). The ABCs of acute management are well described by many investigators and are beyond the scope of this text (21,22). High-dose intravenous methylprednisolone given within 8 hours of injury can improve motor recovery, as assessed at both 6 weeks and 1-year follow-up (23). A smaller study showed improvement in motor scores in patients receiving GM_1 ganglioside (24), and this agent and others are being evaluated in ongoing studies. The high frequency of multiple spinal fractures (25) necessitates radiographic examination of the entire spine including the C1–C2 and the C7–T1 junctions, areas that may require additional views to visualize. Extremity and pelvic fractures also occur commonly (26) and these are sometimes missed during the initial emergency room evaluation and only discovered when the patient arrives on a rehabilitation unit.

The role of the physiatrist in the acute management should begin with the admission of the patient to the hospital. Physiatrists frequently have the greatest skill in accurate documentation of the neurologic findings, and in certain patients, these skills may be of use in determining whether neurologic function is worsening or improving, or whether a cord injury does in fact exist. The presence of an incomplete versus complete injury, or a worsening of neurologic function, may influence the surgical management of the patient's spine, so clearly there is a need for the physiatrist to perform and document serial neurologic examinations on these patients and communicate with the surgical team. An accurate neurologic examination is also used to determine the prognosis for recovery of function (27–29), which is helpful in planning goals and length of stay for an inpatient rehabilitation program. Patient and family education should commence as early as possible during the hospitalization. Proper positioning, splinting, institution of range of motion exercises, and appropriate management of bladder, bowel, and skin care are best instituted early after injury with consultation of the physiatrist. Appropriate transfer to a specialized SCI rehabilitation service may ensure optimization of functional outcome.

Early mobilization of the acute SCI patient is desirable provided proper spine stabilization has been achieved by either surgical or nonsurgical means. The indications for surgery remain controversial and are being examined in a number of ongoing studies. One prospective study involving 269 patients showed no significant difference in motor score at 1-year follow-up after operative versus nonoperative management (30). About 50% of patients admitted to the Model Systems program undergo spine surgery, with the most common procedure being fusion and internal fixation without decompression (31). The use of surgical stabilization and spine orthoses allows patients to avoid months of bed rest and the resultant complications. The use of spinal orthoses is covered in detail elsewhere in the text. The notion that an acutely injured patient should go to a subacute facility or nursing home pending removal of a halo device is frought with the risk of serious complications, both physical and psychological, and we do not recommend this based on our experience with such patients. Furthermore, our data from the Northwest Regional Model SCI Care System indicate that there is no difference in the discharge Functional Independence Measure (FIM) score or length of stay in the patient with a halo as compared to the patient without a halo given the same neurologic level and an ASIA impairment score of A or B (32).

INITIAL REHABILITATION

The initial inpatient rehabilitation of a patient with a new SCI is critical to the future health and well-being of that patient. It is during initial rehabilitation that clinicians have the opportunity to use a systematic, intensive, coordinated team approach to all the bodily functions. Although outpatient and home care can provide necessary training, the optimal team is assembled in a hospital setting. The patient is able to learn and practice the skills necessary for daily living including learning to manage bladder and bowel function.

In the early stage homeostasis is developed. All new patients, particularly those with higher-level lesions (33), are at risk to develop orthostatic hypotension, which can both frighten the patient and lead to frank syncope if not counteracted with compression stockings and bandages, an abdominal binder, and in some patients, a sympathomimetic drug such as ephedrine.

Other concerns in the early phase are to reduce the risk of respiratory complications, especially pneumonia, and to optimize bladder and bowel function (see Chaps. 51 and 52). Intermittent catheterization reduces the incidence of bacteriuria and avoids the complications that occur from indwelling catheterization. Fluid restriction is generally necessary to avoid overdistention of the bladder and to maintain a reasonable intermittent catheterization schedule. During the early phase, excessive fluid mobilization at night may impact the intermittent catheterization schedule. A schedule of catheterization every 4 to 6 hours is a reasonable expectation during the initial stage. Even of patients with an upper motor neuron lesion, only 50% have any reflex detrusor activity at 4 months after injury (34). Thus, the patient may not develop a stable pattern of bladder function until after discharge from the initial inpatient rehabilitation.

Atelectasis and pneumonia are the most frequent pulmonary complications following acute SCI, and pulmonary complications remain the most common cause of death in the acute period as well as in the long term (35,36). With injuries at the thoracic level or higher, expiratory function is compromised, and with a neurologic level of C5 or higher, weakness of inspiration also results. Inadequate inspiratory muscle strength in patients with a high cervical lesion requires mechanical ventilatory support. Management issues regarding ventilatory failure, mechanical ventilation, and noninvasive ventilatory support are covered in Chapter 80. Inadequate expiratory muscle strength impairs the ability to generate an effective peak cough expiratory flow rate (37), and the ineffective cough does not adequately clear pulmonary secretions. Ineffective clearance of secretions is the primary alteration of pulmonary physiology that predisposes SCI patients to atelectasis and pneumonia. Restrictive changes are seen on pulmonary function testing, and mid to low cervical-level lesions typically result in vital capacities of 1000 to 1500 mL.

Patients are at greatest risk for pneumonia and atelectasis during the first 3 weeks following injury (38) and the risk of these complications is greater in patients with complete injuries (39). The incidence of atelectasis and pneumonia during the first 30 days is about 50%, and the 4:1 preponderance of left-versus right-sided involvement is hypothesized to be due to preferential direction of the suction catheter toward the right lung (40). Another factor contributing to pulmonary complications is a high incidence of dysphagia. Tetraplegic patients are at risk for dysphagia from the neck position produced by orthoses, and there is also a risk of nerve injury or edema as a result of surgical procedures performed on the anterior part of the neck. Vigorous pulmonary toilet, including early spine stabilization with facilitation of changes in bed position, deep breathing and incentive spirometry, chest percussion, and manually assisted cough, can decrease the risk of pulmonary complications (41). Bronchoscopy is frequently used for atelectasis unresponsive to these treatments, but it has not been shown to be superior to chest percussion and bronchodilators (42). Mechanical exsufflation can produce a peak cough expiratory force that is comparable to a normal cough and greater than a manually assisted cough, and thus is appropriate for management of pulmonary secretions (43).

POTENTIAL COMPLICATIONS

Deep Venous Thrombosis

Deep venous thrombosis (DVT) and pulmonary embolism (PE) are common complications of acute SCI. In prospective studies of patients with acute injuries, the incidence of DVT has ranged from 47% to 100% (44,45). The risk for DVT is highest in the first 2 weeks following injury, with as many as 62% of patients having positive venographic findings on days 6 to 8 after injury (46). Retrospective studies found an incidence of PE ranging from 3% to 15% (47,48), and the true frequency of PE is undoubtedly higher based on the greater than 50% prevalence of asymptomatic PE in patients with DVT (49).

Patients with acute SCI are predisposed to the development of DVT based on the presence of all three components of the Virchow triad for the development of thrombosis (50). Stasis of venous blood flow in the lower limbs occurs owing to the loss of pumping function normally provided by contracting limb muscles. Intimal injury may result from the release of vasoactive amines with trauma or surgery (51). Hypercoagulability in the acute period following SCI is due to an alteration in levels of clotting factors, with a resultant increase in platelet aggregation and adhesion (46).

Due to the high incidence of DVT and PE in acutely injured patients, a number of strategies for prophylaxis have been investigated. Standard-dose subcutaneous heparin appears to be no better than placebo for prophylaxis (44), while adjusted-dose heparin results in improved prophylaxis but increased bleeding (52). Combining external pneumatic compression with heparin results in a lower rate of DVT than does treatment with either modality alone (53). Low-molecular-weight heparin is awaiting approval from the Food and Drug Administration (FDA) for use as prophylaxis in SCI patients. Twelve weeks of prophylactic treatment is recommended, with some physicians choosing to use both pharmacologic and mechanical prophylaxis during the first 2 weeks (54).

In spite of the above measures, some SCI patients will fail prophylaxis and develop DVT. The clinical examination for DVT is unreliable in the neurologically intact population, and is likely to be more so in patients with SCI. Nevertheless, the lower-extremity examination should be performed carefully, and any swelling or asymmetry should be considered a DVT until proved otherwise. Duplex ultrasonography has become the diagnostic tool of choice at most centers, and venography generally is reserved for equivocal cases or as a gold standard for diagnosis in prospective studies of DVT. The differential diagnosis for lower-extremity swelling in a patient with SCI should also include heterotopic ossification (HO), infection, dependent edema, fracture or knee ligament disruption, and thigh hematoma (55). The diagnosis of PE should always be considered in SCI patients with symptoms such as shortness of breath, hypoxemia, chest pain, confusion, syncope, or cardiac arrest. Treatment of either DVT or PE in a patient with SCI is essentially the same as that for a neurologically intact patient.

Pressure Ulcers

Pressure ulcers are a significant problem in patients with SCI, both in acutely injured patients and in chronically injured patients. The annual incidence of pressure ulcers in this population is nearly 25% (56). Conservative and surgical treatments for this preventable complication make up a significant part of health care expenditures for patients with SCI. Identification of patients at risk combined with interventions to decrease risk factors and closely monitor patients has the potential to provide substantial cost savings.

The major risk factors for pressure ulcers in the SCI population include immobility, completeness of SCI, urinary incontinence, older age, cognitive impairment, anemia, and hypoalbuminemia. The majority of studies found an increased risk for skin breakdown in paraplegics versus tetraplegics (57). The incidence of pressure sores during initial hospitalization and rehabilitation is decreased in patients admitted to Model Systems facilities within 24 hours of injury (58). The most common site for breakdown during the initial hospitalization and rehabilitation is the sacrum, with the ischium becoming the most common site in long-term survivors of SCI (59). Other common sites include the trochanters and heels.

Prevention of pressure ulcers is critical during the acute phase, as care of even small wounds can prevent mobilization of the patient and add to the deleterious effects of immobilization. Grade 1 pressure ulcers may be present on the sacrum by the time the patient is taken off of the backboard, and the length of time spent on a backboard is significantly correlated with the development of pressure ulcers early in the hospitalization (60). Specialized beds are used for patients with potentially unstable spines to provide immobilization and limit the risk for skin breakdown. The most important treatment is removal of pressure from the ulcer the moment it is discovered, so as to limit the depth of the wound. Because nutrition is linked to wound formation and healing, it is important to maintain adequate caloric needs whether by tube feeding or orally. Details regarding the management of pressure ulcers are covered in Chapter 50.

Respiratory Complications

As noted earlier, pulmonary complications are a significant source of morbidity and mortality in both acutely injured and chronically injured patients. Patients with inadequate inspiratory muscle strength will require mechanical ventilation, most often delivered via tracheostomy and positive-pressure ventilation. The majority of patients requiring ventilatory support when initially admitted to rehabilitation, including 50% of patients with C3 tetraplegia (61), will eventually be weaned. There is an increased risk of pneumonia in both the acute and chronic periods, with an increased risk in patients with higher-level injuries. Immunization with pneumococcal vaccine polyvalent is recommended for patients with SCI.

Whether or not a patient is receiving mechanical ventilation, a tracheostomy can interfere with the ability to communicate vocally. In the earliest phase, communication usually involves lipreading or a system for yes and no responses. A number of devices can produce vibration of air within the oropharynx and allow production of speech. Once an inflated cuff on the tracheostomy tube is no longer required, vocalization can occur in a more normal way. A one-way valve on the tracheostomy tube will permit inspiration through the tube and will direct expiratory airflow past the vocal cords, allowing speech.

Late-onset chronic ventilatory failure is seen in some tetraplegic patients not previously requiring ventilatory assist. The pattern seen is a chronic alveolar hypoventilation, with the first blood gas abnormality being nocturnal hypercapnia. These patients develop more frequent pulmonary complications such as pneumonia and can go on to develop cor pulmonale. If they develop an upper respiratory tract infection, they may require mechanical ventilation due to acute respiratory failure (62). Chronic treatment may require nocturnal or continuous ventilatory support, which is best delivered through noninvasive means. Screening for chronic alveolar hypoventilation in the tetraplegic population may include nocturnal arterial blood gas analysis, nocturnal oximetry, and pulmonary function testing via spirometry.

The incidence of sleep apnea is increased in the SCI population. Potential predisposing factors include respiratory muscle weakness, obesity, and the use of antispasticity medications, which can be sedating and may cause decreased tone in upper airway muscles. Symptoms and signs may include daytime sleepiness, snoring, or hypertension, and longstanding cases can result in pulmonary hypertension and right ventricular failure. Significant episodes of nocturnal desaturation may be present in as many as 40% of patients with tetraplegia (63,64). Treatment for sleep apnea involves nocturnal use of continuous positive airway pressure, usually delivered by mask.

Autonomic Dysreflexia

Autonomic dysreflexia (AD) is a condition marked by paroxysmal hypertension, headache, sweating of the head and torso, piloerection, nasal congestion, and occasionally, reflex bradycardia. Owing to the hypertension, where systolic pressures may quickly reach as high as 300 mm Hg, AD should be considered an emergent condition requiring prompt medical attention.

In general, AD only affects patients whose lesions are at or above the T6 level (65), although AD has been observed in patients with lesions below this level. The prevalence estimates of AD for the patients at risk vary widely (66), but in general, about 50% of those at risk will experience at least one episode. AD usually occurs after a patient has recovered from spinal shock. Therefore, it is rare to see it until at least 2 to 6 months after acute injury (67).

The pathophysiology of AD is related to an alteration in the normal balance of sympathetic and parasympathetic nervous systems caused by the spinal cord lesion. When a patient experiences a noxious stimuli from below the level of the lesion, these impulses are transmitted to the sympathetic trunk, causing a reflex sympathetic discharge. Normally, this response is modulated by inhibitory signals from the brain; however, owing to the spinal cord lesion, these signals cannot get through. In addition to the physical blockage of autonomic signals, there are also changes at the neurotransmitter level that worsen symptoms, including an accumulation of substance P and impairment of γ-aminobutyric acid (GABA) release. The patient, therefore, experiences the symptoms of sympathetic overload, including headache, piloerection, and hypertension caused by vasoconstriction.

The increased blood pressure is detected at baroreceptors at the carotid sinus and aortic arch, which trigger a parasympathetic response above the level of the lesion. Reflex vasodilation leads to flushing and sweating of the face and trunk. Patients also complain of blurred vision. Bradycardia is often seen.

The elevation of blood pressure may produce significant complications including stroke, seizures, retinal hemorrhages, cardiac dysrhythmias, and rarely even death. Therefore, every effort should be made to begin treatment as soon as possible.

If AD is suspected in a patient, the blood pressure should be checked as soon as possible and should be rechecked every 2 to 3 minutes. If it is increased, the head of the bed should be elevated, and all tight clothing and restraints removed. A thorough search should then be performed for the noxious stimuli that started the episode. The most common causes of AD are bladder distention and fecal impaction, accounting for 90% of all episodes; however, AD can be triggered by almost any urologic or gastrointestinal complication, including bladder spasms, testicular torsion, renal calculi, acute appendicitis, and gastric or duodenal ulcers. Other causes of AD include decubitus ulcers, paronychia, ingrown nails, and chidbirth.

The treatment for AD is to remove the noxious stimuli that caused the episode. To avoid further exacerbating the symptoms, local anesthetics should be used during any maneuver that might cause an increase in the stimuli, such as fecal disimpaction or bladder catheterization. If no offending stimuli can be found, and if the patient's blood pressure gets critical, then medication to relieve the hypertension is necessary. Nifedipine and nitroglycerin are common oral agents. If the hypertension is severe and not responsive to oral agents, then intravenous medication may be required.

Since AD is likely to be a long-term complication for those who acquire it, patients and families should be well educated in its symptoms and initial management, as well as in its prevention.

Spasticity

SCI results in the development of abnormalities of muscle tone and reflexes, as well as abnormal motor function. *Spasticity* is an upper motor neuron disorder characterized by a velocity-dependent increase in resistance to passive movement. The term is also used by clinicians and patients to refer to clonus, spasms, and increased deep tendon reflexes (DTRs). Although these additional components of the clinical definition of spasticity are generally agreed on, they correlate poorly with each other in SCI patients when measured with clinical scales (68). In addition to spasticity, the upper motor neuron syndrome can also result in weakness, fatigability, muscle co-contraction, and loss of dexterity.

DTRs are depressed for a variable amount of time following SCI. This period, termed *spinal shock,* usually lasts for a few weeks and is frequently shorter in patients with incomplete injuries, although it can occasionally be as short as 2 days for patients with complete injuries (69). Velocity-dependent hypertonus begins after the return of DTRs, and usually it does not become severe until at least 6 to 12 weeks after injury. Noxious stimuli such as urinary tract infections and decubitus ulcers can cause an increase in spasticity, so any rapid increase in spasticity should trigger a search for treatable causes.

At 1-year follow-up, 78% of all patients with SCI and 91% of patients with tetraplegia, have findings of increased DTRs, spasticity, or involuntary muscle spasms (70). By the time of initial discharge from inpatient rehabilitation, 26% of patients are prescribed medications for the treatment of spasticity, and by 1 year after injury, 49% of patients are on antispasticity medications. During the initial hospitalization, patients with Frankel grade B or C are more likely to receive medications for spasticity treatment than are those with Frankel grade A or D.

The term *spasm* has been defined as involuntary movement of paralyzed muscles without provocative stimuli. Although spasms are not always included in the definition of spasticity, they are frequently present and problematic in patients with spasticity and are generally treated with the same medications. Over 95% of patients with chronic SCI report having experienced spasms (71). The majority of patients who develop spasms note the onset within 2 to 6 months of injury, which is similar to the time of onset for spasticity. Both baclofen and diazepam decrease the frequency and severity of spasms in SCI.

Spasticity in patients with SCI frequently does not require treatment. Some individuals are able to take advantage of spasticity to allow easier transfers or bed mobility. A number of theoretical medical advantages of spasticity including preservation of bone mineral density, preservation of muscle bulk, and prevention of DVT have been proposed in the past, but these effects remain unproved. Spasticity should be treated if it interferes with function, positioning, skin integrity, or sleep, or if it is painful for the patient. The specific goals of the treatment should be identified prior to starting medications, in order to assess the adequacy of the intervention.

Stretching and range of motion exercises are effective at temporarily decreasing spasticity in many SCI patients, and they should be the first-line therapy for all patients. Cryotherapy, involving the application of ice to a muscle for at least 20 minutes, can temporarily decrease spasticity in SCI patients (72), but there may be a rebound increase in spasticity after application, and it is not practical for generalized spasticity.

Oral baclofen is considered to be the best initial medication for the treatment of spasticity in SCI patients, as it is effective in many patients and avoids some of the negative side effects of other antispasticity medications. Some clinicians have noted beneficial effects on spasticity with doses exceeding the recommended total daily dose of 80 mg. The antispasticity effect of baclofen in SCI has been documented using the Ashworth scale as well as more quantitative measures (73).

Dantrolene sodium is used occasionally for the treatment of spasticity in SCI, but the drug carries the risk of hepatotoxicity, and there is concern that the drug, acting directly on both spastic and normal muscle, could interfere with strength. Diazepam is effective in decreasing spasticity for nearly all patients, but it can have significant side effects on mood and is overly sedating in many patients. The α_2-antagonist clonidine has been used in patients unresponsive to baclofen, with evidence of spasticity control. The use of clonidine in patients with SCI may be limited by the development of hypotension. Tizanidine, which also acts at the α_2 receptor, was recently approved by the FDA, and studies have shown it to be effective in reducing spasticity in SCI patients (74). Treatment options for problematic spasticity that is unresponsive to oral medications include intrathecal baclofen, percutaneous nerve blocks, and neurosurgical procedures. Patients showing favorable responses to test injections of intrathecal baclofen have been successfully treated with implantable pumps to deliver intrathecal baclofen, and the reported complications of this procedure have been minimal (75,76). Motor point blocks, with either phenol or alcohol, or botulinum toxin injections have been used successfully to treat spasticity in SCI. The duration of action of phenol blocks can be as short as 2 months or as long as 6 months (77).

Heterotopic Ossification

The term *heterotopic ossification* (HO) refers to the development of true bone tissue, and not solely calcification, in soft-tissue structures around a joint. It occurs with a wide range of disorders, including SCI, traumatic brain injury, and burns, and is also seen frequently following total hip replacement. There appears to be a combination of neurogenic and traumatic factors that influence its development; however, the exact pathogenesis of the disorder has not been determined. HO has been reported to occur in as few as 16% to as many as 53% of persons with SCI (78). The most common location is the hips, followed by the knees, shoulders, and elbows (79). Reported risk factors for HO in patients with SCI include complete neurologic injury, presence of pressure sores, and spasticity (80). HO occurs below the level of injury and causes loss of range of motion. When it occurs in the hip region, it can prevent sitting upright in a wheelchair because of a loss of hip flexion. Other potential complications of HO include nerve entrapment (81) and pressure sores (82,83).

HO is most frequently detected 1 to 3 months after injury, with most cases being diagnosed at about 2 months after injury (84). Presenting signs and symptoms include rapid loss of range of motion, pain in a patient with spared sensation, and swelling that when present at the knee may be indistinguishable from DVT on clinical examination. Triple-phase bone scanning can detect the presence of HO prior to the appearance of roentgenographic evidence of calcification (85). An elevation in serum alkaline phosphatase also occurs early in the course of disease, but the utility of this laboratory parameter can be limited by the frequent occurrence of elevated alkaline phosphatase levels secondary to fractures.

The optimal treatment of HO depends on early diagnosis and institution of treatment. Range of motion therapy of the affected joints should be continued to maintain as much joint range as possible (86). Disodium etidronate is found useful for prophylaxis in persons with motor complete SCI (87) and also may limit the extent of ossification when started early in the course of the disorder (88). Indomethacin is also of benefit once HO has developed, and has value as prophylaxis against HO in other patient populations (89). In patients in whom HO continues to grow despite medication, radiation therapy may be of value (90). Surgical resection is considered only in patients with severe joint range limitations interfering with function, or when HO results in increased skin pressure with risk for breakdown. Complications of the surgery include excessive bleeding, fractures, infections, and a significant risk of recurrence of HO (91). A normalization of the alkaline phosphatase level and of the appearance on bone scans as well as a mature appearance of HO on x-ray films, is sought prior to surgery. However, these are reported to be unreliable predictors for recurrence of HO (92). Surgical resection is typically delayed until at least 1 year after injury.

Gastrointestinal Complications

The problems associated with the bowel following SCI vary depending on the level and severity of the lesion. An upper motor neurogenic bowel results from a supraconal lesion whereas a lower motor neurogenic bowel is caused by any lesion that damages the related lower motor neurons or nerves. In either case, immediately after a spinal injury occurs, acute ileus is common. Acute ileus should resolve within a week as the bowel regains intrinsic activity; however, appropriate bowel management is necessary to promote evacuation and prevent chronic constipation. Gastrointestinal hemorrhage is an uncommon occurrence according to data compiled by the National Statistical SCI Center, perhaps owing to the routine use of ulcer prophylaxis (3). During the first 3 weeks of hospitalization, gastrointestinal complications develop in about 6% of patients, with the most common disorders being ileus, peptic ulcer disease, and gastritis (93). All of these complications are more common in cervical-level injuries than in thoracic- or lumbar-level injuries, and the increased risk of gastrointestinal hemorrhage and gastritis is thought to be due to a loss of sympathetic innervation and an unopposed parasympathetic stimulation of acid secretion. Other gastrointestinal complications occurring in the acute period include gastric dilatation, superior mesenteric artery syndrome, and pancreatitis. The superior mesenteric artery syndrome, although rare, deserves special consideration because it is preventable. This syndrome results from compression of the third portion of the duodenum by the superior mesenteric artery. It can occur in the patient who has lost the fat layer between the duodenum and the superior mesenteric artery such as after profound weight loss, or in a thin patient who is placed in a body cast in lordosis. In patients without a history of alcoholism or gallbladder disease, pancreatitis can result from spasm of the sphincter of Oddi; activation of trypsinogen by increased calcium; and the use of steroids causing increased viscosity of pancreatic secretions (93a).

Managing the neurogenic bowel with an appropriate bowel program is generally successful in preventing impactions or fecal incontinence. However, despite such routines, about a third of patients with SCI complain of significant bowel complications, usually impactions, at 5 years or more after injury even though early management was satisfactory (94). Other late complications include reflux, premature diverticulosis, and AD (95). Bloating and abdominal distention are other common complaints and their incidence can be reduced by increasing the frequency of the bowel program (96). Colostomy is seldom necessary to achieve continence and should not be used unless all other forms of management have failed.

Urinary Tract Infections

The Model Systems reported that urinary tract infection (UTI) is the most frequent medical complication during acute rehabilitation; however, the incidence of UTI among persons with SCI is unknown (96a). The risks of UTI may be divided into structural and physiologic, behavioral, and demographic. Much more is known about structural and physiologic risk factors such as outlet obstruction, vesicoureteral reflux, high-pressure voiding, bladder overdistention, and the presence of stones in the urinary tract. Less well understood are the effect of inadequate fluid intake, reduced host defenses, and pregnancy. Behavioral and demographic factors possibly associated with UTI include the patient's knowledge of the urinary system, adjustment to disability, personal hygiene, self-esteem, work or productivity, social support systems, age, gender, residence, and access to services (97).

The method of bladder management is also an important risk factor for UTI. Although no randomized trials have been done to determine the relative risks of indwelling catheterization, intermittent catheterization, and condom catheterization in predisposing the patient to UTI, it is likely that the greatest risk of bacteriuria is with the use of indwelling catheterization, which is associated with an increased risk for epididymitis, fistula formation, calculi, and carcinoma (98). This method is to be avoided when possible. Condom catheterization poses the least risk of UTI, but one study that defined bacteriuria as the presence of any organism in a catheter-collected urine specimen found it in more than 50% of patients using a condom catheter (99). Cardenas and Mayo (100) found that in patients using condom catheters, bacteriuria with fever was significantly reduced after sphincterotomy. Thus, eliminating outlet obstruction helped prevent recurrent UTIs.

A lack of consensus regarding the definitions of significant bacteriuria and the presence of asymptomatic bacteriuria makes comparisons of clinical studies difficult (98). Generally, treatment is not recommended for asymptomatic bacteriuria and prophylaxis is also not considered efficacious. The development of resistant bacteria has led to the opinion that it is better to treat recurrent infections rather than maintain the patient on an antimicrobial agent. However, exceptions may be appropriate in selected patients. The signs and symptoms suggestive of UTI in patients with SCI may include fever, increased spasticity, cloudy and foul-smelling urine, general malaise, onset of urinary incontinence, discomfort or pain over the kidney or bladder, and autonomic hyperreflexia (98).

Chronic Pain

Chronic pain is a common occurrence after SCI. Estimates of the prevalence of pain in persons with SCI, however, vary greatly across studies, owing to differences in the definitions of pain used by investigators, the pain type studied, and the populations sampled. Some estimates place the prevalence as high as 94% of all patients with SCI (101). Several studies (102–104) reported that one-third to one-half of all SCI patients describe some form of chronic, unpleasant sensations, but only about 10% are thought to have severe pain (105–107). Bonica (107a) reviewed 10 studies conducted over the past four decades and concluded that 69% of patients with SCI experienced pain, and in nearly one-third the pain was severe.

Investigators (101–104) have proposed several categories of chronic pain in SCI. *Central pain* is a term that has been applied to the diffuse SCI pain that occurs in anesthetic areas, usually the buttocks, legs, and perineum. Radicular pain, visceral pain, and pain in the sensory transition zone are other forms of pain found in patients with SCI.

Although some classification systems separate out a "psychogenic" cause of pain, our experience suggests that any form of pain may be associated with more or less psychological distress. None of the classification systems has been validated or generally accepted.

All current treatments of chronic pain in patients with SCI are empirical, that is, based on clinical judgment and experience. The approach relies on determining any organic treatable causes such as spine instability or intra-abdominal pathology, as well as identifying any psychological disorders such as depression. No single drug, modality, or behavioral strategy is uniformly successful in alleviating chronic pain in persons with SCI. The pharmacologic agents generally recommended are tricyclic antidepressants, anticonvulsants, local anesthetic antiarrhythmics, and nonsteroidal anti-inflammatory drugs. The use of opioids in our experience is of little value. Because some patients find that pain is worsened by or associated with muscle spasms, the use of antispasmodics may also be of value. Reducing all nociceptive inputs such as pressure sores, UTIs, and constipation may also help reduce pain.

Overuse Syndromes

Because of the mechanical alterations required in a patient with SCI, joints in the upper and lower extremities are subjected to stresses not seen in able-bodied individuals. The wrist and shoulder often become "weight-bearing joints" and over time can become the source of significant morbidity.

A common site of joint pain in both paraplegics and tetraplegics is the shoulder. While the true incidence of shoulder disorders is unknown, various studies have shown an incidence between 35% and 68% in those with an SCI (108–110). These numbers vary, depending on the survey methodology.

In general, increasing age and increasing time since injury predispose patients to shoulder problems, although newly injured patients and young patients are not immune. Heavy activity such as transfers, outdoor wheelchair ambulation, and moving a wheelchair in and out of a car often exacerbate shoulder symptoms. Both women and men suffer from shoulder problems (111).

Campbell and Koris (112), in a study of 24 tetraplegics with both acute and chronic shoulder pain, identified soft-tissue injuries as the most common source of pain. These injuries included adhesive capsulitis, rotator cuff tears or impingement, as well as anterior or multidirectional instability. A recent unpublished study of 24 consecutive patients with paraplegia revealed that 72% of those with shoulder pain and 28% of those without symptoms had evidence of a rotator cuff tear on magnetic resonance images (MRIs) (113). While soft-tissue injuries predominate, osteoarthritis, HO, and aseptic necrosis of the humeral head can also occur.

The pathophysiology of shoulder pain in the SCI patient is likely multifactorial. Some studies implicated high glenohumeral intra-articular pressures during strenuous activities (114), while others pointed out an imbalance in the shoulder musculature, with relatively weaker shoulder depressors and rotators, leading to a high-riding humerus (115).

These findings have led to several strategies for treating shoulder symptoms, including adaptive techniques for limiting shoulder stress during transfers and ambulation (108). In addition, others have begun exercise programs aimed at correcting muscle imbalance (115). In general, treatment should be tailored to individual patients. Some may require therapy, proper wheelchair positioning, or adaptive technology, and others may be better served by surgical correction.

Because shoulder pain in patients with SCI is so ubiquitous, it might seem inevitable. However, it is important to emphasize that shoulder pain in the SCI patient can be caused by many different factors, some of which can be altered with the appropriate intervention. Therefore, patients should be thoroughly evaluated for treatable causes of their pain.

The wrist is also a common site for overuse syndromes. One study put the incidence of wrist pain in SCI patients at 47% (110). Very often wrist pain in the SCI patient is due to carpal tunnel syndrome (CTS). Aljure et al (116) studied 47 patients with paraplegia and found that while 40% had clinical symptoms of CTS, 64% had electrodiagnostic evidence of it. In addition, ulnar neuropathy at the elbow was a common finding, being diagnosed in 45% of the patients by electromyographic (EMG) criteria. In general, findings were worse over time, and at 30 years after injury, 90% of patients had CTS diagnosed by nerve conduction studies.

As in able-bodied individuals, CTS should be treated quickly in the patient with SCI. Careful management is required because of the dependence of these patients on upper-extremity strength. In general, conservative management including splinting and wheelchair modification can help. However, in resistant or progressive cases, surgical release may be necessary.

Posttraumatic Syringomyelia

Syringomyelia, or posttraumatic cystic myelopathy, is an uncommon long-term complication of SCI. However, since its progression can lead to a significant loss of strength, sensation, and function, practitioners should have a high index of suspicion in regard to its diagnosis.

Prevalence estimates of syringomyelia range from 1% to 5%, depending on the study (117,118). It usually occurs within the first few years of an SCI; however, there have been reported cases occurring as early as 2 months (119) and as late as 30 years after injury. Syrinxes may develop at all levels of injury and in those with complete and incomplete lesions. The lesions may remain stable or extend in a rostral or caudal direction in the spinal cord. On rare occasions, they extend to the brain stem, causing cranial nerve symptoms.

Patients commonly present with new-onset pain and numbness. Occasionally, weakness can be the presenting complaint; however, this is usually associated with other symptoms including changes in spasticity, hyperhidrosis, Horner syndrome, and orthostatic hypotension. Frequently, symptoms are exacerbated by maneuvers that increase intra-abdominal or intrathoracic pressure such as coughing, sneezing, and defecation. The earliest clinical sign of syringomyelia is usually a change in DTRs. In addition, an ascending sensory level and changes in strength may also be noted.

The diagnosis of syringomyelia is usually made by MRI (120). Once the diagnosis is made, the patient should be followed closely for progression of the disorder (121). Efforts should be made to decrease activities that might worsen the condition (i.e., Valsalva maneuvers). Surgical treatment involves shunting the syrinx to the subarachnoid or intra-abdominal space and is usually reserved for those who have intractable pain and those who have progressive motor loss.

The etiology of syringomyelia is unclear. Pathogenic factors may include excessive cord compression and mobilization, ischemia, hematomas, edema, arachnoiditis, and kyphosis.

Sexuality and Reproduction

The area of sexuality and sexual behavior in SCI patients has engendered an increasing amount of research over the last two decades. The sum of this research supports the view that sexual adjustment is an integral factor in the individual's total psychological health. Sexual desire is unchanged after SCI. What seems to diminish in some patients is the feeling of sexual satisfaction. Providing information on the specifics of sexuality has a positive impact in many cases. Information must be extended to partners and families.

Several devices and medical interventions are now available to enhance both sex function and fertility in men with SCI. Erection may be enhanced by the use of vacuum constriction devices, intracorporeal injection of vasoactive agents, or penile prosthesis (122). Ejaculation may be induced by the use of vibrators or electrical stimulation. Microsurgical techniques allow retrieval of sperm directly from the vas deferens if other techniques fail (123). Since electroejaculation is not dependent on reflex activity, it may be used in men with upper motor neuron or lower motor neuron lesions. In one study, testicular biopsies revealed abnormalities such as maturation arrest, tubular atrophy, hypospermatogenesis, and interstitial fibrosis in more than 50% of patients (124).

Women with SCI may complain of inadequate vaginal lubrication or problems achieving orgasm. Recent data support the hypothesis that women with complete SCI are able to achieve reflex genital vasocongestion but not psychogenic genital vasocongestion (125). There are no data to support the loss of fertility in women with SCI, although during the initial few weeks to months menses may be interrupted temporarily. Pregnancy may be associated with increased medical problems such as UTIs, pressure sores, and increased spasticity (126). Although thromboembolic disease is a potential complication given the hypercoagulable state of pregnancy and the immobility of SCI patients, there have been few cases of DVT or PE reported. Pulmonary function in patients with high thoracic or cervical lesions may be impaired with the increased burden of pregnancy or the work of labor, and may cause a need for ventilatory support. Autonomic hyperreflexia is the most significant potential medical complication and may occur during any stage of pregnancy, labor, or delivery, and has even been reported in the early postpartum period. The risk of preterm delivery may be slightly increased. The mode of delivery is primarily determined by standard obstetric indications (126). Baker et al (127) reported a rate of cesarean delivery that is nearly identical to the rate in the general population (23%) and not greatly different from the current rate in the United States (about 25%).

Psychosocial Adjustment

SCI usually causes significant physical changes in the person that often result in changes in lifestyle and loss of economic status. Many acutely injured patients will go through a period of grief; however, others do not appear to develop clinical signs of depression. The impact of SCI is also felt by the family, including the spouse or significant other, who may have difficulties adjusting to the changes in their loved one. The family may also suffer economic losses as well as find it necessary to provide care on a daily basis. The family therefore needs psychological support as much as the patient does. Providing written educational materials on SCI is helpful for the patient as well as the family.

During the initial hospitalization, psychological service should be available to any person with SCI. In addition, psychiatric consultation may be useful, especially with regard to medication choices if clinical depression is present. It is known that suicide occurs somewhat more often in the SCI population than in the general population and its frequency is greatest during the first 5 years after injury. Recreational activities are important as are day passes, and near the end of the initial hospitalization, an overnight pass is highly recommended. As the person moves gradually back into the everyday world, he or she will gain more confidence. Body image is likely to be affected but each person is affected differently. Peer counseling is valuable in helping the newly injured patient learn what to expect during the next course of rehabilitation and after discharge.

Persons with chronic SCI may engage in various recreational and sports activities, but due to the paralysis, those who are sedentary are more prone to become obese. Psychosocial adjustment is a lifelong process and is helpful, as in those without SCI, by developing a sense of purpose through vocational or avocational activities. Developing a support system is also important. Although lifelong contact with health care providers is generally advocated, in this era of cost containment, mental health care may be difficult to secure. Peer support groups are also a valuable resource.

FUNCTIONAL OUTCOMES

The functional expectations for patients with complete injuries may be predicted based on the neurologic level of injury, summarized as follows:

1. Cervical (C1–C4) levels: The patient with a high-level SCI is dependent in self-care and transfers. Independence in a power wheelchair is achievable using switches operated and controlled by the mouth, chin, head, or even tongue. Computer interfaces using infrared devices, voice activation, or "sip-and-puff" devices open up opportunities for gainful employment as well as access to the Internet. Environmental control systems increase the possibilities to operate electronic devices at home. With SCI at the C1–C2 levels, the patient will be using mechanical ventilation. Those with complete lesions at the C1–C2 level may also be appropriate candidates for bilateral phrenic nerve stimulator implants and diaphragm pacing.
2. Cervical (C5) level: The patient at this level has added antigravity (grade 3/5) strength in the biceps muscle. This allows partial independence in eating skills using splints or other assistive devices such as a mobile arm support. Independence in power wheelchair ambulation is possible. Driving is also possible with specialized equipment and a modified van. Although tendon transfers are possible with lesions at this level, few patients with SCI at this level choose to undergo such surgery.
3. Cervical (C6) level: The patient at this level has added at least antigravity (grade 3/5) strength in the extensor carpi radialis (longus and brevis) and the pronator teres. For self-care, dressing requires partial physical assistance. A flexor hinge splint can increase self-care (eating, personal hygiene) and make writing possible. Transfers are now possible. Some patients require a frame over the bed with loops and a sliding board. Some are able to perform transfers with just a sliding board and others may even be able to perform transfers using a "hop-over" technique. With SCI at this level, a manual wheelchair with plastic rims or knobs can be used but a power wheelchair is needed for long distances. Some men are able to perform self-catheterization with a splint but are not able to apply a condom catheter. Women are generally not able to perform self-catheterization. The patient with C6 tetraplegia has the highest neurologic level at which driving with hand controls is possible. The following tendon transfers can provide some finger and thumb function and active elbow extension:
   A. Pronator teres to the flexor digitorum profundus
   B. Brachioradialis to the flexor pollicis longus
   C. Posterior deltoid to the triceps

   The reader is referred to an excellent review of tendon transfers by Waters et al (128).
4. Cervical (C7, C8) and thoracic (T1) levels: The major muscles added at each level are the triceps, the flexor digitorum profundus, and the interossei. Initially, personal hygiene, eating, dressing, writing, transfers, ambulation, and driving are impaired. With extensive treatment, almost all patients in this group become completely independent in all functions but may require assistive devices. Transfers, dressing, and personal hygiene may require partial or standby physical assistance. The patient may be able to live alone. Independent ambulation is with a manual wheelchair. The patient, male or female, with SCI at the C7 level is usually able to perform self-catheterization and male patients can apply

condom catheters. Clothing may need modification for bladder function.

5. Thoracic (T2–T5) levels: The muscles added are the intercostals. Independent in self-care including bladder and bowel function and in wheelchair ambulation can be achieved.
6. Thoracic (T6–T12) levels: The muscles added are the abdominals. Independent bipedal ambulation, if attempted, is usually achieved only for exercise. A walker and a swing-to-gait pattern is the typical mode of ambulation. Knee-ankle-foot orthoses (KAFOs) are required for bipedal ambulation unless functional electrical stimulation (FES) is used. FES requires appropriate responses to electrical current.
7. Lumbar (L1–L3) levels: The muscles added are the iliopsoas and the quadriceps. Independent bipedal ambulation with KAFOs is possible for short distances. A wheelchair is still needed. An isocentric reciprocating gait orthosis can allow free-standing balance and reduce energy expenditure during gait.
8. Lumbosacral (L4–S1) levels: The patient now has full quadriceps function. Usually ankle-foot orthoses are needed plus two canes or crutches. Although prolonged standing may be difficult, a wheelchair is not necessary for short-distance ambulation.

AGING WITH SPINAL CORD INJURY

Older patients with SCI differ from younger patients in a number of ways. The neurologic classification and mechanism of injury differ between the older and younger populations. Incomplete tetraplegia occurs in about 50% of SCI patients over age 65, versus 28% of those 16 to 30 years old (1). Falls are the cause of injury in the majority of patients over age 60, in contrast to the general population where falls account for less than 20% of injuries (1). There is a higher frequency of preexisting medical disease in this older population (129), which contributes to a higher incidence of medical complications during initial rehabilitation (130). Older patients are significantly less likely to achieve independence for self-care and more likely to reside in nursing homes than are younger patients (131).

The prevalence of patients injured at an older age and those injured at younger ages who have had long-term survival following injury is increasing, as the aged population grows and as long-term survival with SCI continues to improve. Until the middle of the twentieth century, survival of patients with SCI was a rare occurrence. Thus, there was only a limited population of patients with SCI who survived into a chronic state of disease and disability. As that population of SCI patients continues to grow, their unique medical needs are becoming clearer, and more research has been devoted to the subject.

The most frequent medical complications in patients who have survived 30 years with SCI include pressure sores, painful musculoskeletal conditions, gastrointestinal problems, cardiovascular problems, and UTIs (132). Each of these conditions affects about 15% of chronic SCI patients yearly. Both pneumonia and the development of contractures are more common in older patients (133). Osteoporosis predisposes patients to long-bone fractures, most frequently involving the supracondylar region of the femur (134). An additional complication with aging is loss of neurologic function secondary to syringomyelia and related disorders. The high frequency of complications involving multiple organ systems makes a comprehensive evaluation essential, and this evaluation is best done by a physiatrist and should be performed on a yearly basis (135).

Loss of independence for mobility and activities of daily living is a common occurrence in older patients with chronic SCI. Overuse syndromes of the upper extremity as well as a normal loss of strength with aging can impact on the ability to perform activities such as wheelchair propulsion. Frequently patients must change from a manual wheelchair to a power wheelchair, and when this is done a van with a lift becomes necessary to maintain community mobility. Some patients will require additional assistance for performing activities of daily living and transfers. A spouse who previously assisted the patient may lose the ability to assist, owing to the normal aging process or medical illness. The possibility of requiring power mobility and increased assistance in the future ideally should be discussed with all patients. Insurers who pay for durable medical equipment will usually require a detailed medical justification for such changes in wheelchair prescription, and it is the physiatrist's role to educate them regarding these expected changes with aging in SCI.

NEWER INTERVENTIONS

Functional Neuromuscular Stimulation

Functional neuromuscular stimulation (FNS) in the SCI population denotes the local application of electric current to cause contraction of a paralyzed muscle in order to enhance functional use of the muscle. The designation *FES* is frequently used to describe the same techniques. Most commonly, the stimulation is directed at limb muscles to improve functional use of the upper or lower limbs. Other applications, including phrenic nerve stimulation for the treatment of diaphragm paralysis and sacral nerve root stimulation to provide bladder emptying, are covered elsewhere in this text. FNS is generally believed to be practical only in patients with upper motor neuron injuries, since much larger currents are needed to stimulate denervated muscles, and these muscles also develop a greater degree of atrophy than do innervated, paralyzed muscles. FNS of extremity muscles has the potential to prevent some of the complications of chronic SCI as well as to improve function.

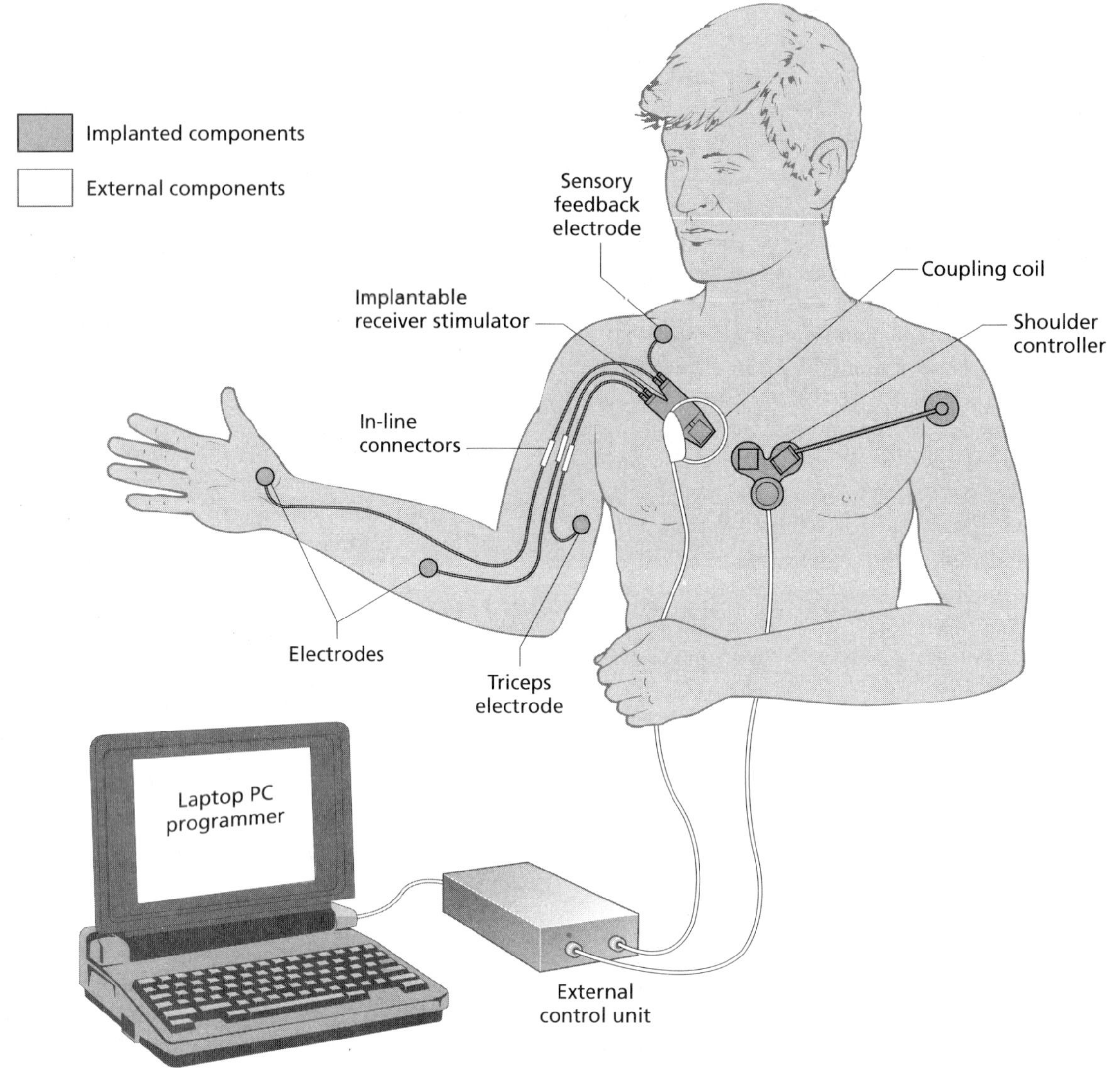

Figure 73-2. Functional electrical stimulation hand grasp system.

Systems for electrical stimulation to restore movement to the extremities are called *neuroprostheses*. Upper-extremity devices are generally used to provide grasp function in patients with C5- or C6-level tetraplegia, while lower-extremity devices are used to restore the ability to stand and walk. The essential components of a neuroprosthesis are a multichannel electrical stimulator, electrodes to deliver the current to localized areas, and some means to control the stimulator. Existing systems have an external stimulator with surface electrodes, an external stimulator with percutaneous intramuscular electrodes, or an implanted stimulator and intramuscular electrodes. The fully implanted stimulator system is controlled by radiofrequency link to an external control unit. Grasp and release function can be provided to individuals with C5 or C6 tetraplegia with devices such as the eight-channel implantable neuroprosthesis developed at Case Western Reserve University and the Cleveland Veterans Administration Medical Center (136,137) (Fig. 73-2). This device has been demonstrated to improve hand function for grasp and release tasks in patients with C5 tetraplegia (138). Lower-extremity applications of FNS include transfers, standing, and ambulation (139–141). The addition of conventional lower-extremity bracing or a reciprocating gate orthosis to FNS allows increased mechanical stability with potentially less muscle fatigue (142–144), but the combination has not been demonstrated to decrease energy expenditure (145). Another lower-extremity FNS application, bicycle ergometry, has no effect on the degree of lower-extremity osteoporosis in chronic SCI patients (146,147) but is able to increase the aerobic capacity of SCI patients (148). However, the increase in aerobic capacity is comparable to that which can be achieved with upper-extremity exercises. The majority of patients receiving FES ergometry note subjective benefits, including improved endurance, self-image, and perception of body appearance (149).

Restoration of Neurologic Function

Currently, medical and surgical treatment to maximize neurologic function after SCI is limited to interventions during the acute phase following injury. Optimal treatment includes immediate immobilization of the spine to prevent further injury, surgical spine stabilization and decompression when indicated, and the use of high-dose intravenous methylprednisolone within 8 hours of the injury (150). Advances in neurobiology in recent years have opened the possibility of treatment to improve neurologic function after the acute period. In animals with experimentally induced SCI, transplanted spinal cord tissue promotes neural regeneration on a cellular level and improves motor function (151,152).

It is unlikely that any single area of research by itself will provide practical restoration of neurologic function. Successful treatment will require combinations of strategies to minimize the degeneration of neural structures following injury, inhibit scar formation, stimulate regrowth of neural structures, and promote proper reinnervation (66). Studies currently in progress are likely to identify medications other than methylprednisolone that can be given at the time of injury to prevent further loss of neural elements. This may be followed by development of treatment strategies to promote regrowth and reinnervation, involving medications and possibly transplantation of spinal cord tissue. Once new neural connections are formed, facilitation of motor function and suppression of spasticity would be required. Treatment may include medications to minimize spasticity and promote the generation of impulses facilitating locomotion, use of partial body weight ambulation, and possibly FES to amplify the signals produced by the regenerating nervous system. Current treatment for SCI involves attaining a maximal degree of function given a fixed neurologic deficit, as well as minimizing numerous medical complications. Future treatment will undoubtedly involve significant restoration of neurologic function.

REFERENCES

1. Go BK, DeVivo MJ, Richards JS. The epidemiology of spinal cord injury. In: Stover SL, DeLisa JA, Whiteneck GG, eds. *Spinal cord injury: clinical outcomes from the Model Systems.* Gaithersburg, MD: Aspen, 1995:21–55.
2. DeVivo MJ, Stover SL. Long-term survival and causes of death. In: Stover SL, DeLisa JA, Whiteneck GG, eds. *Spinal cord injury: clinical outcomes from the Model Systems.* Gaithersburg, MD: Aspen, 1995:289–316.
3. Cardenas DD, Farrell-Roberts L, Sipski M, Rubner, D. Management of gastrointestinal, genitourinary, and sexual function. In: Stover SS, DeLisa JA, Whiteneck G, eds. *Spinal cord injury: clinical outcomes from the Model Systems.* Gaithersburg, MD: Aspen, 1995:120–144.
4. Berkowitz M, Harvey C, Greene CG, Wilson SE. The economic consequences of traumatic spinal cord injury. New York: Demos, 1992.
5. DeVivo MJ, Whiteneck GG, Charles ED. The economic impact of spinal cord injury. In: Stover SL, DeLisa JA, Whiteneck GG, eds. *Spinal cord injury: clinical outcomes from the Model Systems.* Gaithersburg, MD: Aspen, 1995:234–271.
6. Waters RL, Sie IH, Adkins RH. Rehabilitation of the patient with a spinal cord injury. *Orthop Clin North Am* 1995;26:117–122.
7. Menter RR, Whiteneck GG, Charlifue SW, et al. Impairment, disability, handicap and medical expenses of persons aging with spinal cord injury. *Paraplegia* 1991;29:613–619.
8. Tator CH, Duncan EG, Edmonds VE, et al. Complications and costs of management of acute spinal cord injury. *Paraplegia* 1993;31:700–714.
9. Cotler HB, Cotler JM, Alden ME, et al. The medical and economic impact of closed cervical spine dislocations. *Spine* 1990;15:448–452.
10. Richmond TS, Metcalf J, Daly M. Requirements for nursing care services and associated costs in acute spinal cord injury. *J Neurosci Nurs* 1995:27:47–52.
11. Price C, Makintubee S, Herndon W, Istrue GR. Epidemiology of traumatic spinal cord injury and acute hospitalization and rehabilitation charges for spinal cord injuries in Oklahoma, 1988–1990. *Am J Epidemiol* 1994;139:37–47.
12. American Spinal Injury Association and International Medical Society of Paraplegia. *Standards for neurological and functional classification of spinal cord injury, revised 1996.* Chicago: American Spinal Injury Association, 1996.
13. American Spinal Injury Association and International Medical Society of Paraplegia. *Reference manual for the standards for neurological and functional classification of spinal cord injury.* Chicago: American Spinal Injury Association, 1994.
14. Waters RL, Adkins RH, Yakura JS. Definition of complete spinal cord injury. *Paraplegia* 1991;9:573–581.
15. Penrod LE, Hegde SK, Ditunno JF. Age effect on prognosis for functional recovery in acute, traumatic central cord syndrome. *Arch Phys Med Rehabil* 1990;71:963–968.
16. Roth EJ, Park T, Pang T, et al. Traumatic cervical Brown-Séquard and Brown-Séquard-plus syndromes: the spectrum of presentations and outcomes. *Paraplegia* 1991;29:582–589.
17. Schneider RC, Cherry G, Pantek H. The syndrome of acute central cervical spinal cord injury: with

special reference to the mechanisms involved in hyperextension injuries of cervical spine. *J Neurosurg* 1954;11:546–577.

18. Quencer RM, Bunge RP, Egnor M, et al. Acute traumatic central cord syndrome: MRI-pathological correlations. *Neuroradiology* 1992;34:85–94.

19. Gunby I. New focus on spinal cord injury. *JAMA* 1981;245: 1201–1206.

20. Garfin SR, Marshall LF, Eisenberg HM, et al. Spinal cord injury in three regions in the United States. *Paraplegia* 1988;26:113. Abstract.

21. Chiles BW, Cooper PR. Acute spinal injury. *N Engl J Med* 1996;334:514–520.

22. Slucky AV, Eismont FJ. Treatment of acute injury of the cervical spine. *J Bone Joint Surg [Am]* 1994;76:1882–1896.

23. Bracken MB, Shepard MJ, Collins WF, et al. Methylprednisolone or naloxone treatment after acute spinal cord injury: 1-year follow-up data. *J Neurosurg* 1992;76:23–31.

24. Geisler FH, Dorsey FC, Coleman WP. Recovery of motor function after spinal-cord injury—a randomized, placebo-controlled trial with GM-1 ganglioside. *N Engl J Med* 1991;324:1829–1838.

25. Vaccaro AR, An JS, Lin SS, et al. Non-contiguous injuries of the spine. *J Spinal Disord* 1992;5:320–329.

26. Soderstrom CA, Brumback RJ. Early care of the patient with cervical spine injury. *Orthop Clin North Am* 1986;17:3–13.

27. Crozier KS, Graziani V, Ditunno JF, Herbison GJ. Spinal cord injury: prognosis for ambulation based on sensory examination in patients who are initially motor complete. *Arch Phys Med Rehabil* 1991;72:119–121.

28. Ditunno JF, Sipski ML, Posuniak EA. Wrist extensor recovery in traumatic quadriplegia. *Arch Phys Med Rehabil* 1987;68:287–290.

29. Weiss DJ, Fried GW, Chancellor MB, et al. Spinal cord injury and bladder recovery. *Arch Phys Med Rehabil* 1996;77:1133–1135.

30. Waters RL, Adkins RH, Yakura JS, Sie I. Effect of surgery on motor recovery following traumatic spinal cord injury. *Spinal Cord* 1996;34:188–192.

31. Waters RL, Apple DF, Meyer PR, et al. Emergency and acute management of spine trauma. In: Stover SL, DeLisa JA, Whiteneck GG, eds. *Spinal cord injury: clinical outcomes from the Model Systems.* Gaithersburg, MD: Aspen, 1995:56–78.

32. Standaert C, Cardenas DD. The effect of halo fixation on hospital length of stay for patients with acute spinal cord injury. *J Spinal Cord Med* 1996;19(2):166.

33. Gonzalez F, Chang JY, Banovac K, et al. Autoregulation of cerebral blood flow in patients with orthostatic hypotension after paraplegia. *Paraplegia* 1991;29:1–7.

34. Cardenas DD, Kelly E, Mayo ME. Manual stimulation of reflex voiding after spinal cord injury. *Arch Phys Med Rehabil* 1985;66:459–462.

35. Polatty RC, McElaney MA, Marcellino V. Pulmonary complications in the spinal cord injury patient. *Phys Med Rehabil State Art Rev* 1987;1:353–373.

36. Cheshire DJE. Respiratory management in acute traumatic tetraplegia. *Paraplegia* 1964;1:252–261.

37. Fugl-Meyer AR. The respiratory system. In: Vinken PJ, Bruyen GW, eds. *Handbook of clinical neurology.* New York: Elsevier, 1976:335–349.

38. Goetter WE, Stover SL, Kuhlemeier KV, Fine PR. Respiratory complications following spinal cord injury: a prospective study. *Arch Phys Med Rehabil* 1986;67:628.

39. Scher AT. The radiology of pulmonary complications associated with acute spinal cord injury. *S Afr Med J* 1982;62:321–324.

40. Fishburn MJ, Marino RJ, Ditunno JF. Atelectasis and pneumonia in acute spinal cord injury. *Arch Phys Med Rehabil* 1990;71:197–200.

41. McMichan JC, Michel L, Westbrook PR. Pulmonary dysfunction following traumatic quadriplegia. Recognition, prevention, and treatment. *JAMA* 1980;243:528–531.

42. Marini JJ, Pierson DJ, Hudson LD. Acute lobar atelectasis: a prospective comparison of fiberoptic bronchoscopy and respiratory therapy. *Am Rev Respir Dis* 1979;119:971–978.

43. Bach JR. Mechanical exsufflation, noninvasive ventilation, and new strategies for pulmonary rehabilitation and sleep disordered breathing. *Bull NY Acad Med* 1992;68:321–340.

44. Merli GJ, Herbison GJ, Ditunno JF. Deep vein thrombosis in acute spinal cord injured patients. *Arch Phys Med Rehabil* 1988;69:661–664.

45. Myllynen P, Kammonen M, Rokkanen P, et al. DVT and pulmonary embolism in patients with acute spinal cord injury: a comparison with nonparalyzed patients immobilized due to spinal fractures. *J Trauma* 1985;25:541–543.

46. Rossi E, Green D, Rosen J, et al. Sequential changes in factor VIII and platelets preceding deep vein thrombosis in patients with spinal cord injury. *Br J Haematol* 1980;45:143–151.

47. Walsh J, Tribe C. Phlebothrombosis and pulmonary embolism in paraplegia. *Paraplegia* 1965;3:209–213.

48. Naso F. Pulmonary embolism in acute spinal cord injury. *Arch Phys Med Rehabil* 1974;55:275–278.

49. Huisman MV, Buller HR, ten Cate JW, et al. Unexpected high prevalence of silent pulmonary embolism in patients with deep venous thrombosis. *Chest* 1989;95:498–502.

50. Virchow R. Neuer fall von todlichen. Embuli der lungenar-

terie. *Arch Pathol Anat* 1856;10: 225–228.

51. Stewart G, Schaub R, Niewiarowski S. Products of tissue injury: their induction of venous endothelial damage and blood cell adhesion in the dog. *Arch Pathol Lab Med* 1980;104:409–413.

52. Green D, Lee MY, Ito VA, et al. Fixed- vs. adjusted-dose heparin in the prophylaxis of thromboembolism in spinal cord injury. *JAMA* 1988;260:1255–1258.

53. Merli GJ, Crabbe S, Doyle L, et al. Mechanical plus pharmacological prophylaxis for deep vein thrombosis in acute spinal cord injury. *Paraplegia* 1992;30:558–562.

54. Merli GJ, Crabbe S, Paluzzi R, Fritz D. Etiology, incidence, and prevention of deep vein thrombosis in acute spinal cord injury. *Arch Phys Med Rehabil* 1993;74:1199–1205.

55. Yu DT, Odderson IR, Haeg JP. Thigh hematoma from car transfers in long-standing spinal cord injury. *Arch Phys Med Rehabil* 1995;76:1074–1075.

56. Whiteneck GG, Charlifue SW, Frankel HL, et al. Mortality, morbidity, and psychosocial outcomes of persons spinal cord injured more than 20 years ago. *Paraplegia* 1992;30:617–630.

57. Byrne DW, Salzberg CA. Major risk factors for pressure ulcers in the spinal cord disabled: a literature review. *Spinal Cord* 1996;34:255–263.

58. DeVivo MJ, Kartus PL, Stover SL, Fine PR. Benefits of early admission to an organized spinal cord injury care system. *Paraplegia* 1990;28:545–555.

59. Yarkony GM, Heinemann AW. Pressure ulcers. In: Stover SL, DeLisa JA, Whiteneck GG, eds. *Spinal cord injury: clinical outcomes from the Model Systems.* Gaithersburg, MD: Aspen, 1995:100–119.

60. Mawson AR, Biundo JJ, Neville P, et al. Risk factors for early occurring pressure ulcers following spinal cord injury. *Am J Phys Med Rehabil* 1988;67: 123–127.

61. Wicks AB, Menter RR. Long-term outlook in quadriplegic patients with initial ventilator dependency. *Chest* 1986;90:406–410.

62. Bach JR. Inappropriate weaning and late onset ventilatory failure of individuals with traumatic spinal cord injury. *Paraplegia* 1993;31:430–438.

63. Cahan C, Gothe B, Decker MJ, et al. Arterial oxygen saturation over time and sleep studies in quadriplegic patients. *Paraplegia* 1993;31:172–179.

64. Short DJ, Stradling JR, Williams SJ. Prevalence of sleep apnoea in patients over 40 years of age with spinal cord lesions. *J Neurol Neurosurg Psychiatry* 1992;55: 1032–1036.

65. Snow JC, Sideropoulos HP, Kripke BJ, et al. Autonomic hyperreflexia during cystoscopy in patients with high spinal cord injuries. *Paraplegia* 1978;15:327–332.

66. Harper GP, Banyard PC, Sharpe PC. The International Spinal Research Trust's strategic approach to the development of treatments for the repair of spinal cord injury. *Spinal Cord* 1996;34:449–459.

67. Lindan R, Joiner B, Freehafer AA, Hazel C. Incidence and clinical features of autonomic dysreflexia in patients with spinal cord injury. *Paraplegia* 1980;18:285–292.

68. Priebe MM, Sherwood AM, Thornby JI, et al. Clinical assessment of spasticity in spinal cord injury: a multidimensional problem. *Arch Phys Med Rehabil* 1996;77:713–716.

69. Leis AA, Kronenberg MF, Stetkarova I, et al. Spinal motoneuron excitability after acute spinal cord injury in humans. *Neurology* 1996;47:231–237.

70. Maynard FM, Karunas RS, Waring WP. Epidemiology of spasticity following traumatic spinal cord injury. *Arch Phys Med Rehabil* 1990;71:566–569.

71. Barolat G, Maiman DJ. Spasms in spinal cord injury: a study of 72 subjects. *J Am Paraplegia Soc* 1987;10(2):35–39.

72. Price R, Lehman JF, Boswell-Bessette S, et al. Influence of cryotherapy on spasticity at the human ankle. *Arch Phys Med Rehabil* 1993;74:300–304.

73. Nance PW. A comparison of clonidine, cyproheptadine and baclofen in spastic spinal cord injured patients. *J Am Paraplegia Soc* 1994;17(3):150–156.

74. Nance PW, Buggaresti J, Shellenberger K, et al. Efficacy and safety of tizanidine in the treatment of spasticity in patients with spinal cord injury. *Neurology* 1994;44(S9):S44–S51.

75. Coffey RJ, Cahill D, Steers W, et al. Intrathecal baclofen for intractable spasticity of spinal origin: results of a long-term multicenter study. *J Neurosurg* 1993;78:226–232.

76. Loubser PG, Narayan RK, Sandin KJ, et al. Continuous infusion of intrathecal baclofen: long-term effects on spasticity in spinal cord injury. *Paraplegia* 1991;29:48–64.

77. Garland DE, Menachem L, Keenan MA. Percutaneous phenol blocks to motor points of spastic forearm muscles in head-injured adults. *Arch Phys Med Rehabil* 1984;65:243–245.

78. Finerman GA, Stover SL. Heterotopic ossification following hip replacement or spinal cord injury: two clinical studies with EHDP. *Metab Bone Dis Relat Res* 1981;3:337–342.

79. Stover SL, Hathaway CJ, Zeiger HE. Heterotopic ossification in spinal cord injured patients. *Arch Phys Med Rehabil* 1975;56:199–204.

80. Bravo-Payno P, Esclarin A, Arzoz T, et al. Incidence and risk factors in the appearance of heterotopic ossification in spinal cord injury. *Paraplegia* 1992;30:740–745.

81. Brooke MM, Heard DL, de Lateur BJ, et al. Heterotopic ossification and peripheral nerve entrapment: early diagnosis and excision. *Arch Phys Med Rehabil* 1991;72:425–429.

82. Hassard GH. Heterotopic bone formation about the hip and unilateral decubitus ulcers in spinal cord injury. *Arch Phys Med Rehabil* 1975;56:355–358.

83. Damanski J. Heterotopic ossification in paraplegia. *J Bone Joint Surg [Br]* 1961;43:286–299.

84. Garland DE. A clinical perspective on common forms of acquired heterotopic ossification. *Clin Orthop* 1991;263:13–29.

85. Orzel JA, Rudd TG. Heterotopic bone formation. Clinical, laboratory and imaging correlation. *J Nucl Med* 1985;26: 125–132.

86. Hardy AG, Dickson JW. Pathological ossification in traumatic paraplegia. *J Bone Joint Surg [Br]* 1963;45:76–87.

87. Maynard FM, Karunas RS, Adkins RH, et al. Management of the neuromuscular systems. In: Stover SL, DeLisa JA, Whiteneck GG, eds. *Spinal cord injury: clinical outcomes from the Model Systems.* Gaithersburg, MD: Aspen 1995.

88. Stover SL, Neimann KM, Miller JM. Disodium etidronate in the prevention of post-operative recurrence of heterotopic ossification in spinal cord injury patients. *J Bone Joint Surg [Am]* 1976;58:683–688.

89. Schmidt SA, Kjaersgaard-Anderson P, Pederson NW, et al. The use of indomethacin to prevent the formation of heterotopic bone after total hip replacement. *J Bone Joint Surg [Am]* 1988;70:834–838.

90. Schaeffer MA, Sosner J. Heterotopic ossification: treatment of established bone with radiation therapy. *Arch Phys Med Rehabil* 1995;76:284–286.

91. Stover SL, Niemann KMW, Tuloss JR. Experience with surgical resection of heterotopic bone in spinal cord injury patients. *Clin Orthop* 1991;263:71–77.

92. Garland DE, Orwin JF. Resection of heterotopic ossification in patients with spinal cord injuries. *Clin Orthop* 1989;242:169–176.

93. Albert TJ, Levine MJ, Balderston RA, Cotler JM. Gastrointestinal complications in spinal cord injury. *Spine* 1991;16:S522–S525.

93a. Berczeller PH, Bezkor MF. Gastrointestinal complications. In: Berczeller PH, Bezkor MF, eds. *Medical complications of quadriplegia.* Chicago: Year Book, 1986:95–107.

94. Stone JM, Nino-Murcis M, Wolfe VA, Perkash I. Chronic gastrointestinal problems in spinal cord injury patients: a prospective analysis. *Am J Gastroenterol* 1990;85:1114–1119.

95. Gore RM, Mintzer RA, Calenoff L. Gastrointestinal complications of spinal cord injury. *Spine* 1981;6:538–544.

96. Cardenas DD, Mayo ME, King JC. Urinary tract and bowel management in the rehabilitation setting. In: Braddom RL, Buschbacher RM, Dumitru D, et al, eds. *Physical medicine and rehabilitation.* Philadelphia: WB Saunders, 1995:555–579.

96a. National Spinal Cord Injury Statistical Center. Annual reports 9 and 10 for the Model Spinal Cord Injury Care Systems. NSCISC, Birmingham, AL, June 1992.

97. The prevention and management of urinary tract infections among people with spinal cord injuries: National Institute on Disability and Rehabilitation Research consensus statement: January 27–29, 1992. *J Am Paraplegia Soc* 1992;15:194–204.

98. Cardenas DD, Hooton TM. Urinary tract infection in persons with spinal cord injury. *Arch Phys Med Rehabil* 1995;76:272–280.

99. Newman E, Price M. External catheters: hazards and benefits of their use by men with spinal cord lesions. *Arch Phys Med Rehabil* 1985;66:310–313.

100. Cardenas DD, Mayo ME. Bacteriuria with fever after spinal cord injury. *Arch Phys Med Rehabil* 1987;68:291–293.

101. Botterell EH, Callaghan JC, Jousse T. Pain in paraplegia: clinical management and surgical treatment. *Proc R Soc Med* 1953;7:281–288.

102. Kennedy RH. The new viewpoint toward spinal cord injuries. *Ann Surg* 1946;124:1057–1065.

103. Kaplan LI, Grynbaum BB, Lloyd KE, Rusk HA. Pain and spasticity in patients with spinal cord dysfunction: result of a follow-up study. *JAMA* 1962;182: 920–925.

104. Zankel HT, Sutton BB, Burney TE. A paraplegic program under physical medicine and rehabilitation: one year's experience. *Arch Phys Med Rehabil* 1954;35:296–302.

105. Tunks E. Pain in spinal cord injured patients. In: Bloch RF, Basbaum M, eds. *Management of spinal cord injuries.* Baltimore, MD: Williams & Wilkins, 1986:180–211.

106. Munro D. Two-year end results in the total rehabilitation of veterans with spinal-cord and cauda-equina injuries. *N Engl J Med* 1950;242:1–10.

107. Porter RW, Hohmann GW, Bors E, French JD. Cordotomy for pain following cauda equina injury. *Arch Surg* 1966;92:765–770.

107a. Bonica JJ. Introduction: semantic, epidemiologic, and educational issues. In: Casey KL, ed. *Pain and central nervous system disease: the central pain syndromes.* New York: Raven Press, 1991:13–29.

108. Nichols PJR, Norman PA, Ennis JR. Wheelchair user's shoulders? *Scand J Rehabil Med* 1979;11:29–32.

109. Gellman H, Sie I, Waters R. Late complications of the weight-bearing upper extremity in the paraplegic patient. *Clin Orthop* 1988;233:132–135.

110. Subbarao JV, Klopfstein J, Turpin R. Prevalence and impact of wrist and shoulder pain in patients with spinal cord injury. *J Spinal Cord Med* 1995; 18:9–13.

111. Pentland WE, Twomey LT. The weight-bearing upper extremity in women with long term paraplegia. *Paraplegia* 1991;29:521–530.

112. Campbell CC, Koris MJ. Etiologies of shoulder pain in cervical spinal cord injury. *Clin Orthop* 1996;322:140–145.

113. Escobedo E, Hunter J, Goldstein B. Prevalence of rotator cuff tears by MRI in individuals with paraplegia. *Radiology* (in press).

114. Bayley JC, Cochran TP, Sledge CB. The weight-bearing shoulder. *J Bone Joint Surg* [*Am*] 1987;69:676–678.

115. Burnham RS, May L, Nelson E, et al. Shoulder pain in wheelchair athletes. *Am J Sports Med* 1993;21:238–242.

116. Aljure J, Eltorai I, Bradley WE, et al. Carpal tunnel syndrome in paraplegic patients. *Paraplegia* 1985;23:182–186.

117. Rossier AB, Foo D, Shillito J, Dyro FM. Post-traumatic cervical syringomyelia. *Brain* 1985;108:439–461.

118. Schurch B, Wichmann W, Rossier AB. Post-traumatic syringomyelia (cystic myelopathy): a prospective study of 449 patients with spinal cord injury. *J Neurol Neurosurg Psychiatry* 1996;60:61–67.

119. Yarkony GM, Sheffler LR, Smith J, et al. Early onset posttraumatic cystic myelopathy complicating spinal cord injury. *Arch Phys Med Rehabil* 1994;75:102–105.

120. Hida K, Iwasaki Y, Imamura H, Abe H. Posttraumatic syringomyelia: its characteristic magnetic resonance imaging findings and surgical management. *Neurosurgery* 1994;35:886–891.

121. Little JW, Robinson LR, Goldstein B, et al. Electrophysiologic findings in post-traumatic syringomyelia: implications for clinical management. *J Am Paraplegia Soc* 1992;15:44–52.

122. Watanabe T, Chancellor MB, Rivas DA, et al. Epidemiology of current treatment for sexual dysfunction in spinal cord injured men in the USA model spinal cord injury centers. *J Spinal Cord Med* 1996;19:186–189.

123. Berger RE, Muller CH, Smith D, et al. Operative recovery of vasal sperm from anejaculatory men: preliminary report. *J Urol* 1986;135:948–950.

124. Leriche A, Berard E, Vauzell JL, et al. Histological and hormonal testicular changes in spinal cord patients. *Paraplegia* 1977–1978;15:274–279.

125. Sipski ML, Alexander CJ, Rosen RC. Physiological parameters associated with psychogenic sexual arousal in women with complete spinal cord injuries. *Arch Phys Med Rehabil* 1995;76:811–818.

126. Baker ER, Cardenas DD. Pregnancy in spinal cord injured women. *Arch Phys Med Rehabil* 1996;77:501–507.

127. Baker ER, Cardenas DD, Benedetti TJ. Risks associated with pregnancy in spinal cord-injured women. *Obstet Gynecol* 1992;80:425–428.

128. Waters RL, Sie IH, Gellman H, Tognella M. Functional hand surgery following tetraplegia. *Arch Phys Med Rehabil* 1996;77:86–94.

129. Roth EJ, Lovell L, Heinemann AW, et al. The older adult with a spinal cord injury. *Paraplegia* 1992;30:520–526.

130. DeVivo MJ, Kartus PL, Rutt RD, et al. The influence of age at time of spinal cord injury on rehabilitation outcome. *Arch Neurol* 1990;47:687–691.

131. DeVivo MJ, Shewchuk RM, Stover SL, et al. A cross-sectional study of the relationship between age and current health status for persons with spinal cord injuries. *Paraplegia* 1992;30:820–827.

132. Whiteneck GG, Charlifue SW, Frankel HL, et al. Mortality, morbidity, and psychosocial outcomes of persons spinal cord injured more than 20 years ago. *Paraplegia* 1992;30:617–630.

133. Mentor RR, Hudson LM. Effects of age at injury and the aging process. In: Stover SL, DeLisa JA, Whiteneck GG, eds. *Spinal cord injury: clinical outcomes from the Model Systems.* Gaithersburg, MD: Aspen, 1995:272–288.

134. Ragnarsson KT, Sell GH. Lower extremity fractures after spinal cord injury: a retrospective study. *Arch Phys Med Rehabil* 1981;62:418–423.

135. Ditunno JF, Formal CS. Chronic spinal cord injury. *N Engl J Med* 1994;330:550–556.

136. Smith B, Buckett JR, Peckham PH, et al. An externally powered, multichannel, implantable stimulator for versatile control of paralyzed muscle. *IEEE Trans Biomed Eng* 1983;4:499–508.

137. Keith MW, Peckham PH, Thrope GB, et al. Implantable functional FNS in the tetraplegic hand. *J Hand Surg* [*Am*] 1989;14:524–530.

138. Smith BT, Mulcahey MJ, Betz RR. Quantitative comparison of grasp and release abilities with and without functional neuromuscular stimulation in adolescents with tetraplegia. *Paraplegia* 1996;34:16–23.

139. Bajd T, Kralj A, Turk R, et al. The use of a four channel electrical stimulator as an ambulatory aid for paraplegic patients. *Phys Ther* 1983;63:1116–1120.

140. Marsolais EB, Kobetic R. Functional electrical stimulation for walking in paraplegia. *J Bone Joint Surg* [*Am*] 1987;69: 728–733.

141. Marsolais EB, Scheiner A, Miller PC, et al. Augmentation of transfers for a quadriplegic patient using an implanted FNS system. *Paraplegia* 1994;32:573–579.

142. Solomonow M, Baratta RV, Hirokawa S. The RGO generation

II: muscle stimulation powered orthosis as a practical walking system for paraplegics. *Orthopedics* 1989;12:1309–1315.

143. Marsolais EB, Kobetic R, Chizeck HJ, Jacobs JL. Orthoses and electrical stimulation for walking in complete paraplegia. *J Neurol Rehabil* 1991;5:13–22.

144. Thoumie P, Perrouin-Verbe B, Le Claire G, et al. Restoration of functional gait in paraplegic patients with the RGO-II hybrid orthosis. A multicentre controlled study. I. Clinical evaluation. *Paraplegia* 1995;33:647–653.

145. Sykes L, Campbell IG, Powell ES, et al. Energy expenditure of walking for adult patients with spinal cord lesions using the reciprocating gait orthosis and functional electrical stimulation. *Spinal Cord* 1996;34:659–665.

146. BeDell KK, Scremin AME, Perell KL, Kunkel CF. Effects of functional electrical stimulation-induced lower extremity cycling on bone density of spinal cord-injured patients. *Am J Phys Med Rehabil* 1996;75(1):29–34.

147. Leeds EM, Klose KJ, Ganz W, et al. Bone mineral density after bicycle ergometry training. *Arch Phys Med Rehabil* 1990;71:207–209.

148. Pollack SF, Axen K, Spielholz N, et al. Aerobic training effects of electrically induced lower extremity exercises in spinal cord injured people. *Arch Phys Med Rehabil* 1989;70:214–219.

149. Sipski ML, DeLisa JA, Schweer S. Functional electrical stimulation bicycle ergometry: patient perceptions. *Am J Phys Med Rehabil* 1989;68(3):147–149.

150. Bracken MB, Shepard MJ, Collins WF, et al. A randomized, controlled trial of methylprednisolone or naloxone in the treatment of acute spinal-cord injury. *N Engl J Med* 1990;322:1405–1411.

151. Cheng H, Cao Y, Olson L. Spinal cord repair in adult paraplegic rats: partial restoration of hind limb function. *Science* 1996;273:510–513.

152. Bregman BS, Kunkel-Bagden E, Reier PJ, et al. Recovery of function after spinal cord injury: mechanisms underlying transplant-mediated recovery of function differ after spinal cord injury in newborn and adult rats. *Exp Neurobiol* 1993;123:3–16.

Chapter 74

Stroke Rehabilitation

Mary L. Dombovy
Uma Aggarwal

EPIDEMIOLOGY

Cerebrovascular disease is the third leading cause of death in the United States in spite of the recent improvements in the management of acute stroke. It leaves the stroke survivors with significant physical and mental disability, thus creating a major social and economic burden.

The average age-adjusted incidence of first stroke has been reported to be 114 cases per 100,000 population, but ranges from 81 to 150 per 100,000 population in various studies depending on whether completed strokes as well as transient ischemic attacks (TIAs) are included (1). The incidence of stroke rises sharply with age and doubles with each decade after age 55. Men have a 30% to 80% higher rate than women (2). African-Americans have higher incidence rates than whites (3).

There is evidence that the incidence of stroke has decreased from 1945 to 1980, primarily owing to the reduction of modifiable risk factors, especially the treatment of hypertension (4–6). The decrease in stroke incidence coincides with decreased stroke mortality. The rate of decline has been similar for both men and women.

Kagan et al (7) reported a study of Hawaiian Japanese men from 1969 to 1988 and found a decline in the incidence and mortality of stroke. The decline was believed to be due to a combination of decreases in the risk factors (i.e., decline in blood pressure) and cigarette smoking as well as improvement in diagnosis and better care of acute stroke patients. In Australia and New Zealand, Bonita (8) also found a decrease in mortality arising out of declining case-fatality rates without a decreasing incidence. Similar findings were reported by Hong et al (9) from Shanghai, China.

Neissen et al (10) from Netherlands reported increased survival of stroke patients with a decrease in mortality and incidence rates. The study also hypothesized that an increase in cardiovascular survival leads to a further increase in stroke prevalence in older age groups.

There is evidence that the decline in stroke incidence may have slowed or even reversed. Broderick et al (2) found a 17% increase in stroke incidence from 1980 to 1984 compared to the period 1975 to 1979. This increase in incidence coincided with the availability of computed tomography (CT) in detecting less severe strokes.

Brown et al (11) from Rochester, Minnesota, also reported a 13% increase in stroke incidence for the same time period. The incidence rates remained essentially unchanged between 1985 and 1989. Similar trends were reported from East Germany (12). However, Feigin et al (13) reported a population-based study from Novosibirsk, Russia, showing a decline in the stroke incidence without any change in 30-day case-fatality rates during the period 1982 to 1992.

Stroke prevalence (the number of people who have had a stroke in a given population at a point in time) has been reported to be 500 to 800 cases per 100,000 population from Rochester, Minnesota (14,15). Stroke prevalence in the United States has increased by 20% in recent years, owing to the increased survival of stroke patients, although the incidence of stroke has decreased (5). Similar figures have been reported from other countries as well (1).

MORTALITY

Mortality from stroke is highest for the first 30 days after stroke. The average 30-day mortality ranges from 17% to 34% (2,5). Stroke mortality decreases over the next 18 months, and at this point approaches that of the general population matched for age and gender (16). Fifty percent of 30-day survivors will live at least another 5 years (16).

Mortality rates for intracerebral hemorrhage (ICH) are much higher than those for infarction. In Rochester, Minnesota, the 30-day case-fatality rate was 48% for ICH compared to 17% for all strokes (2). Stroke mortality has been declining steadily since the 1950s in all regions of the United States and in most Western European countries. The most rapid rates of decline were observed in the Southeast regions of the United States during the period 1970 to 1989 (17). Shahar et al (18) reported similar trends from Minneapolis, Minnesota. The 2-year survival rate following stroke improved by 40% in the 1980s, and the greatest improvement was found for patients with thrombotic strokes. The key elements in the decline of stroke mortality are thought to be the fall in stroke incidence, occurring mainly in the 1970s, and earlier accurate diagnosis and improved acute management (2).

Bounds et al (19) reported the common causes of early mortality in 100 stroke patients. The most frequent cause of death was transtentorial herniation, followed in frequency by pneumonia, cardiac causes, and pulmonary embolism. Cardiovascular disease is the most common comorbidity associated with stroke and has a negative impact on outcome (19–21).

RECURRENCE

Recurrent strokes account for 25% of all acute stroke events (1). The recurrence rate is 4% to 10% per year and is highest in the first year (approximately 13%) (22). The risk thereafter is 4% per year. In the study from Burn et al (22) the risk of recurrence was not related to age or the type of stroke. The Framingham study (23) reported higher recurrence rates among patients with thrombotic strokes. Secondary prevention with modification of risk factors should be started as soon as possible.

STROKE SYNDROMES

Middle Cerebral Artery Syndromes

The middle cerebral artery (MCA) is the largest branch of the internal carotid artery (ICA). Strokes in the MCA distribution are the most commonly seen in the rehabilitation setting. At the circle of Willis, the ICA bifurcates into the MCA and anterior cerebral artery (ACA). The main stem of the MCA turns laterally and gives off several small, deep perforating branches called *lenticulostriate arteries*, which penetrate into the brain to supply the basal ganglia and internal capsule. The main stem of the MCA then divides into the upper and lower divisions. Occlusion of the main stem of the MCA usually results in complete contralateral hemiplegia, associated with hemianesthesia and hemianopsia. Involvement of the dominant hemisphere results in global aphasia and apraxia. Involvement of the nondominant hemisphere results in visuospatial deficits and neglect syndrome.

Table 74-1: Middle Cerebral Artery Stroke

	Main Stem	Upper Division	Lower Division
Contralateral hemiparesis*	+++	++	+/–
Contralateral hemianesthesia	+++	++	+/–
Contralateral hemianopsia	+++	++	+++
Dominant hemisphere			
Aphasia	Global	Broca	Wernicke
Apraxia	++	+	–
Nondominant hemisphere			
Visuospatial deficits	++	+	–
Neglect syndrome	++	+	–
Dysphagia	++	+	–
Uninhibited neurogenic bladder	++	+	–

* Upper extremity weakness > lower extremity weakness.
+++ = almost always occurs; ++ = likely to occur; + = may occur; +/– = occasionally seen; – = never seen.

Occlusion of the upper division of the MCA usually gives almost the same picture as main stem infarction but the deficits are not as severe. Hemiparesis affects the face and arm more than the leg. Patients with a dominant hemispheric stroke have Broca (expressive) aphasia rather than global aphasia and those with nondominant hemispheric cerebrovascular accident (CVA) have hemineglect.

Strokes of the lower division are much less common. Motor and sensory functions are usually intact. Language dysfunction (i.e., Wernicke aphasia) is usually present, and hemianopsia may also be a prominent sign. The presence of visual and language impairment can result in significant functional disability, even in the presence of intact motor and sensory functions. Table 74-1 describes the MCA stroke syndromes. [See chapter by Mohr et al (24) for a review of MCA stroke.]

Anterior Cerebral Artery Syndromes

The ACA can be divided into proximal or A1 segment and a distal, A2 segment in relation to the anterior communicating artery. The distal segment has been further subdivided by different authors into four segments, A2 to A5. The ACA supplies the medial surfaces of the frontal and parietal lobes. The artery of Heubner arises from either the A1 segment or the proximal portion of the A2 segment. The artery of Heubner supplies the head of the caudate nucleus, anterior limb of the internal capsule, anterior portions of the globus pallidus, putamen, and hypothalamus. Infarction in the territory of the ACA is uncommon. Occlusion of the A1 segment is usually well tolerated because of the good collateral circulation from the opposite side.

The symptoms of occlusion of the ACA result in motor and sensory deficits in the contralateral leg, with more involvement seen distally. The face, forearm, and hand are usually spared. The sensory modalities most often affected are two-point discrimination, stereognosis, and proprioception. Pain and temperature sensation and gross touch may remain intact or mildly impaired. The head and eyes deviate to the side of the lesion. The patient also shows left ideomotor apraxia and agraphia because of collosal disconnection. A variety of emotional and intellectual disturbances have been reported with proximal ACA occlusion. Urinary incontinence can occur with unilateral or bilateral occlusion. Involvement of the artery of Heubner or anterior communicating artery can result in hemiparesis with weakness of the face and arm because of the involvement of the anterior limb of the internal capsule. Proximity of such a stroke to the supplementary motor area can also result in transcortical motor aphasia. Infarction in the bilateral ACA distribution can cause paraparesis with or without sensory loss, mimicking spinal cord pathology. [See the chapters by Burst (25) and Sawada and Kazul (26) for review of ACA stroke.]

Branches from the ACA anastomose with the internal branches of the MCA. These border zones or the watershed areas are of clinical importance, since hypoperfusion can result in infarction in this distribution. Anterior border-zone infarction may lead to bilateral upper-extremity weakness, greater in the proximal than in the distal regions, the so-called man in barrel syndrome. [See the work by Bogousslavsky et al (27) for review of border-zone infarction.]

Posterior Circulation Syndromes

Posterior Cerebral Artery Syndromes

The vertebral arteries (VAs) typically arise from the subclavian arteries. At the junction of the medulla and pons, the two VAs unite to form the basilar artery (BA), which again divides into posterior cerebral arteries (PCAs) near the top of the midbrain. The deep perforating branches of the PCA supply the midbrain and thalamus. The anterior and posterior inferior temporal arteries supply the undersurface of the temporal and occipital lobes and the calcarine artery supplies the visual cortex.

The occlusion of the perforating arteries of the PCA can cause *thalamic infarction* (28). Thalamic infarction may result in pure hemisensory deficits or sensory or motor deficits. Sensory impairment may be only slight, involving only a part of the body, or may be a severe hemisensory loss that includes hyperesthesias and dysesthesias. A central pain syndrome may develop weeks or months later. Memory may also be affected in patients with thalamic infarctions.

In *PAC territory unilateral infarcts*, visual disturbances are predominant and result from injury to the lateral geniculate body, optic radiations, and calcarine cortex of the occipital lobes. Patients may experience altered color discrimination and field cut disturbances. Impaired memory often results from infarction of the medical temporal lobes (visual memory on the right and verbal memory on the left).

Infarction in the *left PCA distribution* (left occipital cortex and posterior corpus callosum) can also result in visual agnosia associated with right hemianopsia. Alexia without agraphia may result from the disconnection between the right visual cortex and the primary language area of the left hemisphere.

Bilateral PCA infarction may result from occlusion of the top of the BA (top of the basilar syndrome). Bilateral PCA infarction results in bilateral occipital lobe infarctions leading to cortical blindness with denial of the deficits (Anton syndrome) and severe memory loss, which can be permanent. The rehabilitation potential for these patients is usually poor, because of their inability to form new memories or learn new tasks. [See the chapters by Caplan (29) and Ross Russell (30) for review.]

Vertebrobasilar Syndromes

The two (VAs) merge to form the BA at the pontomedullary junction. Each VA courses through and around many bony structures and ligaments and is relatively fixed in its course and is especially vulnerable to traumatic injury. There are four major branches of the VA and BA supplying the cerebellum and the brain stem. The posterior inferior cerebellar artery (PICA) is the largest branch of the vertebral artery. The PICA and anterior inferior cerebellar artery (AICA) supply most of the inferior surface of the cerebellum. The lateral part of the medulla is usually fed by the PICA. The superior part of the cerebellum receives its blood supply from the superior cerebellar artery (SCA), which is a branch from the BA. Throughout the course of the BA, there are many small, deep, perforating arteries supplying the medial, basilar, and lateral portions of the brain stem.

The *Wallenberg or lateral medullary syndrome* results from occlusion of the VA or PICA. This syndrome is characterized by a loss of pain and temperature sensation on the ipsilateral side of the face and contralateral side of the body, ipsilateral limb ataxia, Horner syndrome (myosis, ptosis, and anhydrosis), dysphagia, and dysarthria. Patients with lateral medullary syndrome are often seen in the rehabilitation setting, and the prognosis for functional recovery is excellent.

Cerebellar infarcts are common. Cerebellar strokes usually result in bilateral ataxia, with more involvement on one side. The large cerebellar infarct, where at least one-third of the cerebellar hemisphere is involved, may produce symptoms by causing the mass effect: The swollen cerebellar hemisphere may compress the fourth ventricle and lead to hydrocephalus. This is a neurosurgical emergency requiring decompression of the ventricles with ventriculostomy and removal of the necrotic cerebellar tissue. Patients will smaller cerebellar infarcts have an excellent prognosis.

The *locked-in syndrome* results from bilateral infarction of the basis pontis, resulting in quadriplegia, disruption of horizontal conjugate eye movements, and facial and laryngeal weakness. Vertical eye movements are spared since the upward gaze is controlled in the midbrain level. This may be the only means of communication left for the patient, in whom awareness is usually preserved.

There are many other brain stem syndromes. Two of the more common are 1) *Weber syndrome*, where contralateral hemiplegia and ipsilateral third cranial nerve palsy result from infarction in the medial portion of the midbrain; and 2) *Millard-Gubler syndrome*, where the patient has ipsilateral sixth and seventh cranial nerve palsy and contralateral hemiplegia, resulting from infarction in the lateral pons. [See chapter by Hachinski and Norris (31) for review of vascular syndromes.]

Lacunar Infarction

Lacunar strokes are caused by small-vessel disease. They are primarily seen in hypertensive and diabetic patients. Lacunar strokes are small areas of infarction in the brain occurring in the distribution of small penetrating arteries. Several classic syndromes have been described.

1. *Pure motor hemiplegia*: This is the most common lacunar syndrome encountered. It can be caused by lesions in the basal ganglia, internal capsule, thalamus, corona radiata, or pons. The patient has weakness in the face, arm, and leg of varying severity. The patient remains alert, without disturbances of sensory, visual, or language function. Rehabilitation prognosis is usually excellent.
2. *Pure hemisensory syndrome*: This usually results from lacunar infarction in the thalamus. The patient usually remains alert with normal motor strength. The degree of disability depends on which sensory modality is affected.
3. *Mixed motor-sensory syndrome*: This syndrome involves a combination of hemiparesis and hemisensory loss. The lesion is usually in the pons.
4. *Clumsy-hand dysarthria syndrome*: This syndrome usually results from a lacunar infarct in the pons. The patient has mild weakness and clumsiness of the arm, as well as slurred speech. Again, the prognosis is good.
5. *Ataxic hemiparesis*: The patient has mild weakness and ataxia on one leg or one side of the body. This is believed to be caused by lacunar infarcts in the pons and cerebellum.

Lacunar strokes are common and can present with a wide variety of other neurologic and functional deficits. Multiple lacunar infarcts often lead to dementia. [See the chapter by Hachinski and Norris (31) for review.]

STROKE IN YOUNG ADULTS

The definition of *young adults* varies in different studies. While most authors consider those 15 to 45 years old as young adults, others consider persons younger than 50 as young adults. One study further divided stroke patients into two groups: 16 to 30 year olds as very young adults and 31 to 45 year olds as young adults (32). Although stroke in young adults is uncommon, it is by no means rare to see a young patient with stroke. The financial impact of strokes on the lives of patients in this age group is substantial, since it strikes them during their most productive years. The rising incidence of ischemic infarction among young adults may be secondary to widespread use of alcohol and illicit drugs.

Most of the strokes in young adults are ischemic, but Mettinger et al (33) found a substantial incidence of hemorrhagic strokes in this age group. Just as in older age groups, the mortality rates were higher for hemorrhagic strokes in young adults. The discussion here is limited to ischemic strokes in young adults.

The incidence of stroke in the young adult varies from 10.4 to 47 per 100,000 population per year. In 1970, Schoenberg et al (34) reported an annual incidence rate from the Mayo Clinic to be 23.3 per 100,000 in women between 30 to 49 years old. Rates for the 15- to 29-year age group were lower, at 10.3 per 100,000. In Denmark, the stroke incidence was reported to be between 14.4 and 15.5 per 100,000 population for men and women, respectively (32). Women between 15 and 34 years old had higher incidence rates than did men. This was reversed in the 35- to 44-year age group. The higher incidence in younger women was believed to be secondary to the use of oral contraceptives. In Stockholm County, Sweden, Mettinger et al (33) found an annual incidence rate of 34 per 100,000 among young adults, which is slightly higher than the rates reported from other European countries.

Bogousslavsky and Pierre (35) in the Lausanne Stroke Registry found that 13.5% of all first strokes occur in persons 45 years old or younger. Leno et al (36) reported a prospective study of 81 young patients from Cantabria, Spain. The incidence rates of stroke for men and women were 17.3 and 10.4 per 100,000 population, respectively.

Thirty-day mortality was 22%. The prognosis among the survivors was favorable, with 79% of the survivors completely independent at follow-up.

Qureshi et al (37), in 1995, studied stroke in young black patients. Hypertension was more frequently seen in black patients. Cocaine use was frequent among both black and white patients. Mortality rates were similar as reported previously. ICH and lacunar infarctions were the most common subtypes of stroke seen in black patients. Seventy percent of all the patients were able to achieve independence in self-care.

Etiology and Risk Factors

Many of the causes are the same as those in older adults, but the distribution is different. Although in 65% to 70% of the patients the cause is either atherothrombotic or thromboembolic, in approximately 35% the cause of stroke is not identified (38). Table 74-2 lists the causes of stroke in young adults.

Atherosclerosis is a rather uncommon causative factor for stroke in people under the age of 40 without any predisposing factors. Hart and Miller (38) found that 18% of the patients in their series of young adult stroke had cerebrovascular atherosclerosis as the cause. All patients with artherosclerosis were either juvenile-onset diabetics or men over the age of 35 with one or more risk factors (e.g., hypertension, heavy tobacco use, or hyperlipidemia).

Cerebral embolism is one of the three most common causes of stroke in the young adult, accounting for approximately 20% of the strokes in this age group (38). Rheumatic valvular heart disease, prosthetic valves, PFO, infective endocarditis, and atrial fibrillation are some of the causes of embolic cerebral infarction. Valvular heart disease tends to show geographic variation. For instance, rheumatic heart disease is a much more frequent cause of stroke in India and developing countries, whereas mitral valve prolapse and patent foramen ovale (PFO) is seen more often in Europe and North America.

A high incidence of PFO has been reported in young adults. It ranges from 10% to 40% depending on the method of detection (39,40). To identify PFO as the risk factor for stroke, studies compared young stroke patients with control subjects (39,40). These studies consistently showed a higher rate of PFO in young patients with cryptogenic stroke as compared to the control group. Webster et al (39) found that 50% of the young stroke patients had right to left shunting as compared to 15% of the control group. Lachat et al (40) also showed a high prevalence of PFO in young patients with cryptogenic strokes as compared to the controls (54% versus 10%). In spite of the high prevalence of PFO, there is controversy in the literature. Some investigators (41) believe that PFO is an incidental finding and not responsible for paradoxical embolism. In a study, these investigators failed to show an association with history of Valsalva at onset, or any other evidence of paradoxical embolism. Of note, Stollberger et al (42), in 1993, found a high incidence of deep venous thrombosis (DVT) in young patients with cryptogenic stroke and PFO.

Table 74-2: Causes of Cerebral Infarction in Young Adults

Cause	%
Atherosclerosis	20%
Embolism	20%
Coagulopathy	10%
Arthropathy	10%
Peripartum	5%
Uncertain	35%

Source: Adapted from Hart RG, Miller VT. Cerebral infarction in young adults: a practical approach. *Stroke* 1983;14:110–114.

Homma et al (43), in 1994, reported that patients with cryptogenic stroke have larger PFOs with extensive right to left shunting as compared to patients with known causes of stroke. Cabanes et al (44) showed that atrial septal aneurysm and PFO have a synergistic effect and are independent risk factors for stroke. Atrial septal aneurysm with more than 10 mm of excursion is associated with a higher risk of stroke. No association between mitral valve prolapse and stroke was found in this study.

For the diagnosis of PFO and other cardiac abnormalities, various tests have been proposed and studies have evaluated the sensitivity and specificity of these tests (45). Transesophageal echocardiography with contrast enhancement is the most sensitive test and considered the gold standard (45). Stollberger et al (42) reported that when paradoxical embolism is suspected, Doppler studies of the lower extremities will often reveal clinically occult DVT.

The management of patients with PFO is controversial and there is no consensus regarding the treatment of patients with stroke and PFO. Available therapies include antiplatelet agents, anticoagulation, percutaneous closure with an umbrella, and surgical closure. Hanna et al (46) reported that aspirin therapy provides sufficient prophylaxis and results in low recurrence rates. Other interventions are reserved only for patients in whom aspirin is not effective. In patients with DVT, full anticoagulation or placement of an inferior vena cava filter is recommended.

Carotid and vertebral artery dissection can occur spontaneously or as a result of trauma. Vascular pathology also predisposes to dissection as well. There is evidence that fibromuscular dysplasia and Marfan syndrome are associated with an increased incidence of dissection. Diagnosis is made by angiography. Magnetic resonance imaging (MRI) and magnetic resonance angiography are complementary tools. Therapeutic approaches are controversial, and range from none to surgical intervention. Anticoagulation with warfarin, or antiplatelet therapy when anticoagulation is contraindicated, is recommended to avoid distal embolization. Surgery is reserved for only the patients in whom anticoagulation fails (47).

Table 74-3: Hypercoagulable States	
Primary Hypercoagulable States	**Secondary Hypercoagulable States**
Protein III deficiency	Antiphospholipid antibody syndrome
Protein C and S deficiency	Oral contraceptive use
Disorders in plasmin generation	Drug abuse
Dysfibrogenemias	Pregnancy
Homocystinuria	Cancer
Heparin cofactor II deficiency	

Source: Adapted from Nachman RL, Silverstein R. Hypercoagulable states. *Ann Intern Med* 1993;119:819–827.

Many disorders that promote thrombosis can cause stroke, especially in the young adult (48). Some of the causes of *primary and secondary hypercoagulable states* are listed in Table 74-3.

Antiphospholipid antibody syndrome (APAS) occurs because of the appearance of autoantibodies, especially to lupus anticoagulant or anticardiolipin. Clinical features include various manifestations of venous and arterial thrombosis. Stroke in young adults is one of the major manifestations of this syndrome. Many affected patients may have systemic lupus erythematosus or a lupus-like disorder, while others have a primary form of APAS without associated systemic disease. Young patients with stroke should be screened for the presence of lupus anticoagulant and anticardiolipin antibodies.

Recurrent thrombosis with APAS is a potentially serious problem. Rosove and Brewer (49), in a retrospective study, found a 53% recurrence rate during follow-up of 5.2 years. Khamashta et al (50) reported an even higher incidence of 60% for recurrent thrombosis during a 6-year follow-up. In both studies, site of the first event (arterial or venous) tended to predict the site of subsequent events. Recommended treatment is high-intensity warfarin [international normalized ratio (INR) >3]. In both studies, treatment with aspirin alone or low-intensity warfarin (INR < 3) with or without low-dose aspirin was not effective in preventing recurrent thrombosis. The rate of recurrent thrombosis was highest during the first 6 months after discontinuation of warfarin therapy. Bleeding complications were seen in 19.7% of the patients.

Several studies in the literature linked the use of *oral contraceptives* with stroke. Lidegaard (51) found a positive correlation between the dose of estrogen and the incidence of stroke. However, he found no synergistic interaction between smoking and contraceptive use. The risk of stroke from the use of oral contraceptives increases with age (51,52). In another study, oral contraceptive use was found to be a risk factor for cerebral venous thrombosis (53).

Elicit drug abuse is common among the young. Users of elicit drugs are at an increased risk for both hemorrhagic and ischemic strokes. Adrenergic stimulants, most importantly cocaine and amphetamines, cause vasospasm and vasoconstriction. Dara et al (54), in 1991, reported 18 cases of drug-related ischemic strokes in 15 men and 3 women between the ages of 21 and 47 years. Traditional risk factors were found only in 6 patients, suggesting that these factors are not necessary for the occurrence of cocaine-related infarcts. Multiple mechanisms—vasospasm, sudden-onset hypertension, myocardial infarction with cardiac arrhythmias, increased platelet aggregation, and vasculitis—were found to be responsible. Intravenous drug abusers are also at risk for developing endocarditis resulting in thromboembolic events. Cocaine abuse can also cause vasculitis resulting in cerebral infarction (55,56). Treatment with corticosteroids has been suggested for the management of vasculitis.

SUBARACHNOID HEMORRHAGE

Spontaneous subarachnoid hemorrhage (SAH) occurs at a rate of 10 to 20 per 100,000 population, at a mean age of 50 years. A ruptured aneurysm is the cause in 70% to 90% of patients (57–60). Aneurysms are most commonly located at the circle of Willis involving the anterior communicating artery complex, MCA trifurcation, carotid artery, and posterior communicating artery. Arteriovenous malformations and "unidentified" sources make up the remainder. SAH accounts for 5% to 10% of all strokes.

In North America, approximately 30,000 individuals are affected each year, of which 40% to 45% die within the first month, most from the initial bleed (58,61). Studies using global measures of outcome report that 45% to 75% of SAH survivors experience a "good outcome," having minimal to no neurologic deficit and becoming independent in basic activities of daily living (ADLs) (57,62,63). However, recent studies indicated that a high percentage of these patients continue to experience cognitive, behavioral, and social difficulties (64–66).

The type of cognitive deficits noted include impairments in short-term memory, attention and concentration, and executive functioning (65,66). Cognitive deficits relate not only to the severity of the initial bleed, but also to later complications, including delayed ischemia. Earlier studies suggested that cognitive outcome, particularly the formation of new memory, was worse following rupture of aneurysms of the anterior communicating artery complex, but a recent report suggested that this is not the case (66).

The management of SAH underwent a dramatic change in the mid-1980s. Prior to this time, surgical clipping of the aneurysm was delayed 10 to 14 days from the time of the bleed, owing to a fear of causing ischemia (i.e., "vasospasm"). However, evidence that rebleeding was the major cause of secondary mortality undoubtedly caused concern. The advent of calcium channel blockers, other ischemia-protective agents, and new microsurgical techniques led to a more aggressive approach toward immediate angiography and surgical management within hours to a few days, particularly for patients who had few neurologic deficits from the initial bleed. Current results indicate that this aggressive approach has marginally improved survival, but made a greater impact on functional outcome (62,63).

In addition to SAH, many patients will have an intracerebral component to the hemorrhage, an infarct as a result of delayed ischemia (a known complication of SAH), or intraventricular hemorrhage. Both SAH and intraventricular hemorrhage are risk factors for hydrocephalus, which occurs in 15% to 20% of patients with SAH. Patients with SAH should be monitored closely for the development of hydrocephalus, which in addition to occurring acutely, can present many months after SAH as a decline in function, gait, or cognition or simply as a failure to reach expected goals.

Most of the complications occurring in post-SAH patients are similar to those occurring in other stroke patients, with the exception of the much more common occurrence of the syndrome of inappropriate antidiuretic hormone.

SAH survivors tend to resemble more closely traumatic brain injury (TBI) patients rather than patients with cerebral infarction in terms of their cognitive, behavioral, and functional deficits. The general pattern of recovery following SAH is also similar to that of TBI, but in general, given the same deficit and same time after the event, the prognosis for SAH is not as good as for TBI, but better than for cerebral infarction.

This pattern of deficits and recovery after SAH, and the younger age often result in rehabilitation needs being best met in programs that also treat TBI and thus have the needed cognitive and behavioral services. At this time, there is no information about the rehabilitation outcomes for SAH.

RECOVERY

Motor Recovery

There is general agreement that the greatest neurologic recovery occurs during the first 3 months after the stroke, and remains statistically significant up to 6 months (67–69). Slow recovery may continue up to 1 year but does not reach statistical significance (68,70). Some authors (68) even reported functional recovery up to 2 years. The reasons for this are not entirely clear.

When seen within the first week after onset, 73% to 88% of stroke survivors have some degree of hemiparesis (67,69,71). Hemiparesis is present in 50% of stroke survivors at 6 months and in 30% at 1 year (67,69). The degree of neurologic recovery varies depending on the type of stroke. Patients with ICH may have a higher initial mortality and show greater initial weakness, but have greater potential for later recovery. These findings are due to at least a part of the dysfunction being secondary to tissue compression and edema rather than neuronal death.

Twitchell (72), in 1951, described a classic pattern for motor recovery and prognostic signs for improvement. In the initial stages, the paretic limb is flaccid, followed by a return of reflexes and development of spasticity. Return of voluntary movement follows in a sequential proximal to distal pattern. Movements are initially in a synergistic pattern (flexor synergies in the upper limb and extension synergies in the lower limb) followed by increased volitional control of individual movements and a decrease in spasticity. Motor recovery may plateau at any point, but usually by 8 to 12 weeks (69). The lower limb usually shows more recovery than the upper limb, owing to both greater involvement of the arm in the most common middle cerebral territory infarct, and the need for the recovery of more complex fine motor control for functional use of the arm.

Wade et al (73), in 1983, followed 56 stroke survivors with an initially nonfunctional arm. At 3 months, only 8 patients made a complete recovery, 14 showed partial recovery, and the remainder showed no recovery. Heller et al (74), in 1987, followed the recovery of arm function in 56 stroke survivors. They concluded that lack of measurable grip strength by 28 days was associated with a nonfunctional arm at 3 months. They also noticed that the maximum recovery of arm function occurs in the first 3 months.

Wade and Langton Hewer (69) reported that decreased sitting balance was found in nearly 50% of stroke survivors at 1 week. Sitting balance was associated with a poor prognostic for recovery. Truncal musculature weakness and control associated with extremity paresis are often overlooked as significant deficits that impact on functional outcome.

Sensory and Visuoperceptual Recovery

Proprioception is a key factor in executing and relearning motor function. Smith et al (75), in 1983, found that 1 week after stroke onset, approximately 44% of the patients had decreased proprioception. Proprioception recovered in 87% of the survivors by 8 weeks. Twelve percent to 49% of the patients with right-sided CVA experience a neglect syndrome. Gross neglect appears to resolve to a large extent in a majority of patients by 8 to 12 weeks, but subtle deficits impacting on function in a busy or distracting environment often remain.

Stroke patients who initially experience severe visuoperceptual deficits may continue to have the deficits for more than 1 year (76). Visual field defects are reported in 17% of stroke survivors (77), but recovery has not been studied extensively. Complete hemianopsia is a bad prognostic sign, and in one study (78) 49% of the patients with complete field defects did not survive to 28 days. Of the remaining survivors, persistent full field defects were seen in 39%, 27% improved to a partial visual field defect, and 34% made full recovery. Those who recovered completely did so within 2 to 10 days after stroke onset.

Language Function

Approximately 24% to 33% of stroke survivors have language dysfunction (79,80). Wade et al (80) performed a population-based study of 545 stroke patients and found that 24% were aphasic when seen within 1 week of onset. At 6 months, 12% of the survivors still had evidence of significant aphasia, but 44% of the patients and 54% of the caregivers thought that the speech was abnormal, probably representing mild impairment. The period of greatest language recovery is during the first 3 months, but the different types of aphasia have different recovery patterns. Global aphasia tends to show more functional recovery between 6 months and 1 year rather than during the first 6 months (i.e., improved ability to communicate, but not necessarily improved language) (81). The presence of aphasia has been variably associated with increased disability.

Bowel and Bladder Function

Bladder incontinence is commonly seen following stroke. It has been noted in approximately 30% to 70% of stroke survivors when seen at 1 week. Many patients will recover bladder function within 1 month. Barer (82) reported results of 362 stroke patients with bladder dysfunction; more than half were incontinent when first seen in the 24 hours after onset. Twenty-nine percent were still incontinent at 1 month. This percentage improved to 14% at 6 months. Bladder continence is a reliable positive prognostic indicator. Ninety-seven percent of stroke patients who were continent on day 1 survived. The majority of patients who were continent at 1 month were home within 6 months. Wade et al (83) reported that urinary incontinence 7 to 10 days after stroke onset is the most important adverse prognostic indicator of survival and functional recovery. Similarly, bowel incontinence is associated with a poor prognosis for recovery and return home.

Dysphagia

Dysphagia is a potentially life-threatening problem following stroke, because of the inherent risk for aspiration pneumonia. Dysphagia is present shortly after stroke onset in approximately 50% of stroke survivors, but the rate decreases to 4% by 1 year (84). Gordon et al (85) studied 91 stroke patients: 41 (45%) had dysphagia at onset, and 35 (86%) of these regained swallowing function within 14 days. Barer (86) assessed 357 patients within 48 hours. Twenty-nine percent had difficulty with swallowing water and 58% showed improvement within 1 week. At 1 and 6 months, swallowing dysfunction was associated with other complications that hamper functional recovery. Dysphagia is seen more frequently following brain stem strokes. Horner et al (87) studied 23 such patients and aspiration was seen in 15 (65%). However, the eventual outcome was good: 12 (80%) of the 15 resumed full oral nutrition at follow-up, at a mean of 3 months after stroke onset.

Depression

Poststroke depression is common, occurring in 25% to 60% of survivors, and often persists for at least 1 year (67,88–90). Poststroke depression is often underdiagnosed and is frequently thought to be reactive. Despite the evidence that antidepressant therapy may be effective, few receive pharmacologic treatment (90,91). There is evidence to suggest that depression is secondary to the disruption of physiologic pathways for neurotransmitters (92). Depression has some, but unclear, correlation with the severity of stroke (90). Some studies suggested that depression is more common in patients with left frontal lobe lesions while others found no correlation (89,90,93,94). Depression does not necessarily correlate with the presence of aphasia. However, Parikh et al (95) demonstrated poorer recovery in activities of daily living and language in depressed patients. Major depression is usually self-limiting and resolves by 2 years, whereas the prognosis for poststroke dysthymic depression is frequently unfavorable and often it persists for up to 2 years (96).

PREDICTION OF FUNCTIONAL RECOVERY

Functional outcome after stroke has been difficult to predict for two reasons:

1. Functional recovery is multifactorial, being dependent not only on the severity of stroke, but also on a host of other factors (e.g., patient motivation, family support, comorbidity, access to rehabilitation, and financial resources).
2. There has been a great deal of difficulty in drawing conclusions from the literature on functional recovery because of the differences in the stroke populations studied (community versus referral based), the variable timing of functional assessment, and the questionable validity and reliability of scales.

Course of Recovery

However, despite the difficulties in predicting outcome, a few general principles appear with some consistency. Most stroke survivors show significant recovery. One week after stroke onset, 68% to 88% of the patients are dependent in some aspect of self-care and mobility. The percentage decreases to between 40% and 62% by 6 months. At 1 year, only one-third of patients are dependent in self-care and mobility (67–69). The rate of recovery of function is fastest in the early weeks to 3 months following the stroke; however, statistically significant recovery continues to occur up to 6 months after stroke onset. Although some patients continue to show improvement up to 1 year following the stroke, this does not reach statistical significance for the group as a whole (68). Dombovy et al (68) found that 64% of patients maintained their level of function between 1 and 3 years following the stroke. Between 3 and 5 years, many patients experienced increasing disability rather than improvement, perhaps due to comorbidity and increasing age.

Reding and Potes (97) used the life-table analysis approach to study the recovery of function. Ninety-five percent of patients with unilateral strokes were divided into three groups: motor deficit only (M), motor and sensory deficits (MS), and motor sensory and visual deficits (MSV).

Each patient's ability to ambulate 150 feet independently, assisted ambulation of 150 feet, independence with self-care (Barthel >90), and achieving a Barthel index score of 60 (previously shown to predict home discharge) were assessed every 2 weeks until discharge from the rehabilitation unit. Independent ambulation was attained by more than 90% of the M group, but only 35% of the MS group and 3% of the MSV group. Assisted ambulation was attained by 90% in all groups, but at different time intervals (M group at 14 weeks, MS group at 22 weeks, MSV group at 26 weeks). Approximately 65% of the M and MS groups attained complete independence in ADLs, but the time necessary to achieve this goal was significantly longer in the MS group. Patients in the MSV group had a less than 10% chance of ever reaching this goal. However, all three groups were able to achieve a Barthel index score of 60, albeit over different time frames. This study illustrated the usefulness of predicting functional recovery based on clinical deficits, and the ability to incorporate assessments made at differing time frames after stroke using the life-table analysis approach.

Jorgensen et al (98) reported recovery of walking function in 804 stroke patients in a prospective community-based study. Initially 51% had no walking function, 12% could walk with assistance, and 37% were independent in walking. At the end of rehabilitation, 50% were independent in walking, 11% would walk with assistance, 18% had no walking function, and 21% had died. The time course and degree of recovery varied according to the severity of leg paresis and the initial impairment of walking function. Leg paresis of mild or moderate severity at 3 weeks was associated with a favorable prognosis. Overall, 95% of stroke survivors who were initially unable to walk regained walking function within the first 11 weeks. No further improvement was seen beyond this time.

Blower et al (99) studied the relationship between wheelchair propulsion and independent walking abilities. The ability to propel a wheelchair at 3 weeks was found to be a good predictor of walking potential in stroke patients.

Jorgensen et al (100) reported the outcome of 1197 stroke survivors. Patients were stratified according to the initial stroke severity (as measured by the Scandinavian Stroke Scale) and level of disability. Nineteen percent of the patients had very severe strokes, 14% had severe, 26% had moderate, and 41% of the patients had mild stroke. The percentage of the patients discharged to home increased gradually with decreasing initial stroke severity. After completing rehabilitation, 20% of the patients remained very severely or severely disabled in ADL function as measured by the Barthel index, 34% had mild to moderate disability, and 46% had no disability at all. In the second part of the same study (101), the authors noted that the time course of functional recovery was strongly related to initial stroke severity. Best ADL function was reached by 8.5 weeks in patients with mild strokes, versus 20 weeks in patients with very severe strokes. Overall, functional recovery was completed within 12.5 weeks from the onset of stroke in 95% of the patients.

Clinical Predictors

Clinical indicators applied 7 to 10 days after the onset of stroke that would allow the prediction of outcome and enable the selection of patients likely to benefit from rehabilitation would be of considerable clinical value. As mentioned earlier, prediction of recovery of function is a very difficult task and several factors can influence the outcome.

Factors reported to have an adverse effect on functional outcome include coma at onset, severity of the initial impairment, visuoperceptual deficits, poor cognitive function, incontinence 2 weeks after stroke onset, advanced age, and severe cardiovascular disease. Overall, the level of function on admission to a rehabilitation unit is one of the more reliable predictors of functional status at discharge (102–104). Alexander (105) reported the severity of stroke and age at the time of admission to be important variables in predicting outcome. Ninety-six percent of the patients with modest disability were discharged home, irrespective of age. All patients younger than 55 years were discharged home regardless of their initial stroke severity. Nakayama et al (106) also reported the influence of age on stroke outcome. Increasing age adversely influenced the ability to perform ADLs. These authors suggested that rehabilitation of the elderly stroke patient should be focused more on ADL training and compensation techniques rather than on neurologic recovery.

Upper-limb function at 4 weeks has been reported as a good indicator of functional prognosis (107). Visuoperceptual deficits and altered cognition play an important role in determining functional recovery. In general, stroke patients with decreased cognition have a worse outcome than do patients with pure visuoperceptual deficits, although most stroke patients have a combination of both. Rose et al (108) found that patients who extinguished to double simultaneous sensory stimulation (DSS) had lower Functional Independence Measure (FIM) scores on admission and at 6 months. Furthermore, patients who improved their performance on DSS had the greatest increase in FIM scores. This study demonstrated the efficacy of a simple bedside test in helping to predict the overall outcome.

Psychosocial factors have a significant impact on functional recovery, but are often underestimated. Lehman et al (109) found that financial resources and family support, in addition to the severity of the stroke, have a major impact on discharge outcome. Ahlsio et al (110) addressed the quality of life issue in stroke survivors. He followed the patients for 2 years. Most patients reported a decrease in function, particularly in ADLs, during this time. Depression and anxiety were found to be equally important factors affecting the quality of life as was the physical disability itself. A combination of decreased functional ability combined with decreased social support of family and friends appeared to produce the drop in life satisfaction. These studies make a very important point that greater emphasis should be placed on psychosocial issues in poststroke patients.

Imaging Predictors

In addition to the clinical predictors, several investigators have attempted to predict the outcome following stroke based on the size and location of the infarct (111,112). Chaudhuri et al (113) studied the functional gains and discharge outcome of 100 stroke patients and correlated these with findings on CT scans. Patients with bihemispheric infarcts were more likely to be discharged to an institution. Patients with small superficial infarcts achieved independence in function at discharge. Bushnell et al (114) studied acute stroke patients with single-photon emission computed tomography (SPECT) and correlated recovery with size of the infarct. Neurologic and language functions were assessed. Patients with smaller defects demonstrated significantly better recovery at 3 months when compared with patients with larger defects. Hanson et al (115) correlated the measured size of the ischemic infarct, using SPECT on admission, with neurologic deficits (determined on admission by the National Institutes of Health stroke scale) and functional outcome as measured by the Barthel index. Larger lesions on SPECT scans were associated with poor outcome. Saunders et al (116) reported that MCA infarct volume as measured by MRI is useful in assessing prognosis.

Many investigators have studied somatosensory evoked potentials (SSEPs) to predict the outcome in acute stroke patients, particularly in those who are in coma or have severe impairment of language or communication abilities. Pavot et al (117) evaluated SSEPs in 130 patients 2 weeks after stroke onset. The pattern of most impaired SSEPs was associated with abnormal gait and decreased hand function. Keren et al (118) also reported that upper-limb SSEPs have value in predicting the rehabilitation outcome in stroke patients.

ISCHEMIC INJURY, RECOVERY, AND EMERGING THERAPIES

The determinants of functional outcome following stroke are 1) *prelesion factors* such as age, educational level, intelligence, personality, socioeconomic situation, and associated medical problems; 2) *lesion factors* such as size and location; and 3) *postlesion factors* such as environment and training, medical complications, motivation, and family participation.

Our knowledge of the pathophysiology underlying ischemic injury and recovery has increased dramatically over the past 10 years. We now understand that the death of some ischemic neurons occurs in a delayed fashion, and that early thrombolytic or pharmacologic intervention has the potential to protect or "salvage" neurons that would otherwise not survive. We also know that at least part of the clinical deficit seen after stroke is related to neurotransmitter and synaptic alterations in areas of the brain that are remote from, but connected to the infarcted area.

It now appears that new interventions for acute cerebral ischemia, as well as rehabilitative and pharmacologic approaches that promote optimal reorganization of neuronal network days or weeks following stroke, are on the horizon. This section briefly reviews the pathophysiology of ischemic injury and recovery and identifies interventions aimed at limiting ischemia and facilitating recovery.

The potential to enhance neurologic recovery by salvaging ischemic but not yet infarcted neurons and by manipulating the biologic adaptability of the brain is now relevant to clinical practice. Both basic and clinical research suggests that physical and pharmacologic interventions, acting together with the brain's natural reaction to injury, may facilitate or conversely, hinder recovery of cognitive and motor functions. Table 74-4 outlines potential mechanisms underlying recovery. These mechanisms likely overlap and are interdependent over time.

Table 74-4: Mechanisms of Recovery from Stroke
Resolution of the ischemic penumbra
Resolution of edema
Resolution of diaschisis
Increased activity through partially spared pathways
Use of ipsilateral pathways
Recruitment of parallel systems and use of distributed networks
Cortical and subcortical reorganization, morphologic plasticity
Pharmacologic/neurotransmitter plasticity
Alternate behavioral strategies

Limiting Ischemic Injury

For many years, despite intense interest in laboratory models of cerebral ischemia, there were few clinical trials in humans. This lack of trials was likely the combined result of the advanced age of many patients and the spectrum of deficits, which meant that no therapy was required for some, and for others there seemed to be no useful therapy because of the apparent destruction of so much eloquent brain. The inordinate delay that occurs in these patients reaching the hospital obviates the 3- to 6-hour window of opportunity for therapeutic intervention. However, the development of the concept of a "brain attack," requiring emergent intervention, similar to that of a "heart attack" has served to educate physicians, emergency personnel, and the public that the nihilistic attitude that characterized stroke for so many years is no longer appropriate. In understanding new approaches to the acute treatment of stroke, it is useful to think of the observed clinical deficit as composed of three areas: an irreversible core of infarcted tissue, surrounded by a larger area of ischemic, nonfunctional, but salvageable neurons. Added to this are areas remote from the lesion that are rendered nonfunctional by transsynaptic deactivation (Fig. 74-1).

A particularly promising treatment for ischemic stroke is the intravascular infusion of tissue plasminogen activator (TPA) in an attempt to lyse the newly formed clot. A major TPA trial found improved clinical outcomes at what was deemed a reasonable risk in selected patients (119), and its use is likely to become more widespread.

The recognition that excitatory amino acid release exacerbates ischemic brain damage has led to considerable research on the effects of blockade of glutamate receptors (120,121). Ischemia results in uncontrolled glutamate-induced ionic depolarization of neurons, which then leads to calcium influx. There is substantial evidence in experimental models of both ischemic stroke and closed head injury that agents that interfere with glutamate-induced cellular depolarization and resultant calcium entry can significantly reduce ischemic brain damage (122–124). The most clearly studied glutamate receptors are the α-amino-3-hydroxy-5-methyl-4-isozole propionic acid (AMPA) and the *N*-methyl-D-aspartate (NMDA) receptors. A major problem with the glutamate antagonists has been side effects such as hallucinations, respiratory depression, and cardiac depression. New agents in this area are being developed and tested.

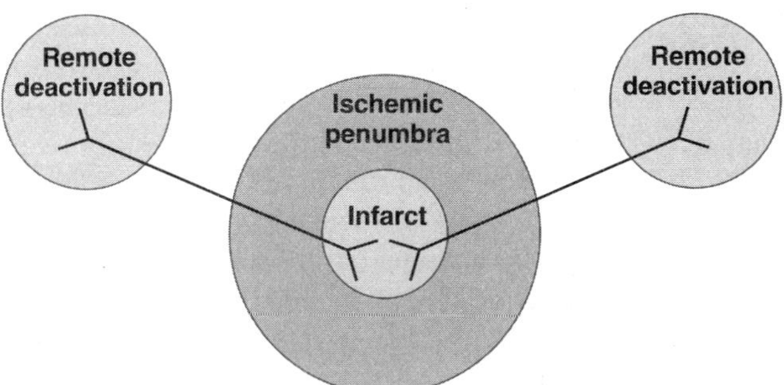

Figure 74-1. Diaschisis following stroke.

Tirilazad mesylate is a synthetic, nonglucocorticoid, 21-amino steroid that has shown some success in protecting the brain from ischemic insults following stroke, traumatic brain injury, and subarchnoid hemorrhage (125–128). The mechanism of action of this agent appears to be related to its localization within the lipid bilayer of the cell membrane where it scavenges lipid peroxyl radicals and reduces the formation of reactive oxygen, resulting in membrane stabilization. The results of clinical trials of tirilazad and other free-radical scavengers should soon emerge in the literature.

There has also been a major interest in the use of calcium channel–blocking agents to block calcium entry into the cell, thereby preventing irreversible changes. Clinical studies have reported results that are equivocal at this time (129).

Facilitating Recovery

The remote effects of an injury, due to a loss of transsynaptic activity along a neural pathway after one of its links has been damaged, or from a loss of noradrenergic, serotonergic, or cholinergic neurotransmission, could also contribute to the clinical deficit (diaschisis). Diaschisis has been demonstrated in positron emission tomography studies (130), and evidence exists that in some patients both the presence of diaschisis and the accompanying clinical deficit can be alleviated by pharmacologic intervention (131).

Partial sparing of some ascending and descending tracts, especially in the regions of the anterior and posterior limbs of the internal capsule and pontine corticospinal tract, may allow early gains. Denervation hypersensitivity occurs in the central as well as peripheral nervous system, and may underlie some of the recovery seen when there is partial sparing.

The ipsilateral motor cortex, via the uncrossed ventral corticospinal tract, has often been invoked as a pathway that might compensate for a contralateral cerebral injury. Studying recovering aphasics using an evoked potential technique, Papanicolaou et al (132) demonstrated greater activation in the right hemisphere when compared to controls.

Increasing evidence from neurophysiologic studies suggests that the primary motor cortex (M1) is not as somatotypically organized as once thought: Different spinal motor neuron pools receive input from broad overlapping cortical territories, and many M1 neurons have projections that diverge to more than one motor neuron pool. Hence, during movement of a particular body part, neurons distributed over a wide cortical region are active (133). Multiple overlapping representations are also found in nonprimary motor areas. These areas have independent inputs from adjacent and remote regions, and most have parallel but separate outputs to the brain and spinal cord. This organizational schema accounts for the clinical deficits in motor control that are seen following injury to motor areas, as well as provides a basis for recovery. Functional MRI and positron emission tomography studies recently demonstrated shifts in cortical activity to nonprimary motor areas in patients who recovered from internal capsule or M1 area strokes (134–137).

In addition, recent primate studies demonstrated cortical reorganization and the takeover of the function of ablated cortex by neighboring cortical areas following injury to the sensory cortex (138). The extent of this reorganization and the completeness of clinical recovery were dependent on differential use of the involved hand (139). This is an extremely important finding, as it demonstrates that use of the involved extremity is critical in directing cortical reorganization to occur in a fashion that is correlated with improved function.

Collateral sprouting of dendrites has been demonstrated in the brain, but its functional significance is not clear. When replaced synapses are from inappropriate sources, the effects could be malfunctional and contribute to the development of sequelae such as seizures and spasticity. However, in the setting of only partial damage to an afferent pathway, collateral sprouting of spared fibers from the same source might be beneficial just as it is at the neuromuscular junction.

Collateral sprouting of neurites from spared axons is limited to only very short distances (usually $< 250\,\mu m$), mainly within the gray matter. It is generally agreed that regeneration of injured axons occurs only to a very limited degree in the central nervous system of mammals. Failure of regeneration is not due to an intrinsic inability of the central nervous system axons to regenerate, but rather to inhibitory influences in their extracellular environment, including the mechanical effects of the astroglial scar, growth cone collapsing factors, and astrocyte-derived extracellular matrix molecules. Approaches to inducing regeneration in the central nervous system that have met with some success include placement of peripheral nerve bridges, transplantation of fetal cells, use of cells genetically engineered to produce specific neurotransmitters, and injection of antibodies to growth cone collapsing factors without or in combination with peripheral nerve grafts (140).

Drawing conclusions from research that supports the importance of activity in facilitating "neuronal reconnections," it is likely that rehabilitation will continue to play a role in optimizing the recovery from stroke as these regenerative techniques become a practical reality.

Solid evidence that pharmacologic enhancement of recovery is possible after focal cerebral injury has existed since the early 1980s (141). Amphetamine in combination with activity clearly enhances the ability of rats to perform a beam-walking task following a sensory-motor cortex injury (142). When given in conjunction with physical therapy, amphetamine may improve motor recovery in patients with stroke (143). One possible explanation is the activation of central noradrenergic pathways; another might be through enhancement of long-term potentiation (LTP), which is thought to underlie aspects of learning and memory.

Other transmitter systems may also play a role in recovery. GABAergic agents appear to suppress the induction of LTP. NMDA receptor antagonists also block the induction of LTP, thus disrupting learning and memory. Ironically, the same drugs that are effective as neuroprotective agents when given early after stroke may adversely affect later recovery.

The cholinergic system, based on work related to Alzheimer disease, is also important to learning and memory. Methylphenidate and amantadine may improve arousal, attention, and concentration following brain injury (144).

Thus, it is becoming increasingly clear that neurotransmitters and related drugs can profoundly influence the processes important to recovery. At this time, we have not yet defined which drugs, in which doses, given at what time after stroke will produce the optimal result. Of current practical concern is the potential that some medications commonly given after stroke may actually be detrimental to recovery. Examples include benzodiazepines, antipsychotics, some anticonvulsants, and α-blockers (145).

Therapy Approaches

Rehabilitation approaches train patients either to restore or approximate the lost motor function or to substitute for its absence (use the other arm, use a brace or device). Based on the previous discussion, substitution might be detrimental to recovery as it prevents the practice and activity-dependent reorganization of the nervous system that likely underlies the greater degree of clinical recovery. However, restitution strategies that may result in the most long-term improvement take time and practice, and thus are not always the quickest way to improve function. Economic (it costs too much to continue) and social (let's work on what has the quick payoff) concerns often dictate the therapies that get the patient out and home the fastest. This probably sacrifices the maximal level of recovery.

Rehabilitation strategies might also differ during "critical periods" when physical, cognitive, and pharmacologic interventions may interact to produce an optimal effector recovery. There are probably critical periods following stroke for relearning particular tasks, just as there are critical periods for learning during normal development (e.g., language acquisition).

An additional practical issue concerns the length of rehabilitation. It takes years of practice to become an accomplished pianist or a skilled craftsman or athlete. One also gains facility at playing the piano by practicing the piano and not by practicing the flute. Our clinical observations also tell us that determination and prolonged practice underlie the higher level of recovery seen in some patients. Yet, most poststroke patients receive only a few weeks or at most a few months of rehabilitation, much of which may not be specific to their deficits! Evolving approaches to therapy are combining what we now know about the neurophysiology of recovery with recent theories of motor control and motor learning as well as cognitive and attentional mechanisms. The retention and generalizability of performance may depend as much on how the patient is taught, as on what the patient is taught. Some of these strategies involve "forced use" of involved extremities, biofeedback, facilitation techniques, and other eclectic approaches.

At the current time, the following can be recommended:

1. Therapists and physicians need to recognize that underlying any program of rehabilitation is neuronal reorganization that occurs both at the site of the injury and distant from it, and that this reorganization begins early.
2. Clinicians should consider that "rote" or standardized approaches could be detrimental to functional recovery. Requiring the patient to use behavioral strategies that decrease input from the involved part(s) might inhibit optimal cortical reorganization.
3. Therapy (drug and rehabilitation) may need to change over time as the neurosystems and neurotransmitters involved change during the recovery process.
4. Whenever possible, rehabilitation should be behaviorally specific and involve repetition.
5. Physicians should carefully consider the potential impact of any medication on the recovery process.

Future research and functional neuroimaging should give us greater insights into the recovery process and facilitate the development of neurophysiologically based treatment programs.

RISK FACTORS AND STROKE PREVENTION

Table 74-5 identifies the major risk factors for stroke and separates them into categories: those that are modifiable, those that are treatable, and those that are not (146,147). Regarding the modifiable risk factors, the treatment of hypertension will have the greatest impact on stroke reduction, owing to its high relative risk (six times) and its high prevalence in the population (148). The risk of incurring a stroke is increased two to six times by the presence of heart disease (three times by atrial fibrillation), two times by tobacco smoking, two to four times by diabetes mellitus, ten times by a history of a prior stroke or TIA, and two times by heavy alcohol use (148). Age, gender, and race are unmodifiable risk factors. The incidence of stroke doubles in each successive decade for people over the age of 55, and is approximately 30% higher in men than in women (147). African-Americans have a risk of death and disability from stroke that is more than 60% higher than the risk for the white population (147).

Stroke is one of the most preventable medical catastrophes, with opportunity to intervene at every stage of the disease to forestall or minimize its effects. As new technology and treatment become available [e.g., diffusion-weighted MRI to differentiate infarcted tissue from ischemic tissue; TPA treatment of acute ischemic stroke (119)], each of these stages will become even more amenable to treatment. Public awareness of modifiable risk factors, medical management of risk factors, and promotion of lifestyle changes by physicians will have the greatest impact on reducing the incidence of new and recurrent stroke. Rehabilitation physicians are in an optimal position to address risk factor modification and treatment for both the patient (secondary prevention) and family members (primary prevention).

Two common conditions that are risk factors for stroke deserve additional mention: carotid artery stenosis and atrial fibrillation. If they are surgical candidates, patients with asymptomatic carotid artery stenosis of 60% or more should be considered for endarterectomy, as this procedure significantly reduces the risk of stroke over 5 years if the operative morbidity and mortality are less than 3% to 4% (149). Recommendations for symptomatic

Table 74-5: Risk Factors for Stroke

Modifiable Risk Factors	Potentially Treatable Risk Factors	Unmodifiable Risk Factors
Cigarette smoking	Atrial fibrillation	Age: risk doubles for each decade >55 yr
Diabetes mellitus	Carotid artery stenosis	Gender: incidence 30% higher in men
Heart disease	Myocardial infarction	
Heavy alcohol use	Previous stroke	Race: African-Americans with >60% higher risk than whites
Hypercholesterolemia	Transient ischemic attack	
Hypertension		

patients (TIA or nondisabling stroke) are similar (149). Antiplatelet therapy with aspirin, 650 mg twice a day, is recommended for those with nonoperable lesions and ischemic stroke or TIA.

The prevalence of atrial fibrillation increases with age, and the proportion of strokes attributed to atrial fibrillation also increases with age from 7% for those 50 to 59 years old to 36% for those over 80 years old (150). Patients with atrial fibrillation and additional risk factors (valvular heart disease, previous myocardial infarction, enlarged heart chambers, congestive heart failure) should be treated with warfarin anticoagulation regardless of age (151). Patients over the age of 75 should be monitored closely because of the potential risk of increased intracranial hemorrhage.

The time window for antithrombolytic therapy of acute ischemic stroke is very short (1.5–3.0 hours). Currently less than 20% of all stroke patients reach the hospital and are evaluated within that time frame. Massive public, physician, and other medical personnel education is needed to promote prompt recognition and management of stroke symptoms before these newly emerging acute treatments will have a measurable impact on stroke outcome.

MEDICAL COMPLICATIONS AND COMORBIDITIES

Most patients with stroke have other medical conditions that require monitoring, treatment, or both. These may be preexisting comorbidities such as hypertension and diabetes, or secondary complications of the stroke such as venous thromboembolism and aspiration pneumonia. Table 74-5 lists some of the more common medical conditions associated with stroke. A few of these are commented on.

Thromboembolism

DVT in the legs and the subsequent risk of pulmonary embolism is a major source of morbidity and mortality after stroke. The incidence is highest during the first week, but the risk persists thereafter. The incidence of DVT in the calf veins, within 1 week after stroke, has been reported to range between 50% and 75% (152). The incidence of proximal thrombi is 16% to 35% (153). The actual incidence can vary depending on the method of study. Although the incidence is more common in the hemiplegic leg, DVT has occurred in the uninvolved extremity (154). The incidence is higher in nonambulatory stroke patients (155).

The risk of pulmonary embolism due to DVT following stroke ranges from 9% to 15%. The risk of embolization is greatest 5 to 7 days after acute thrombus formation (154). Pulmonary embolism is the leading cause of death 2 to 4 weeks after stroke, and is the fourth leading cause of death overall in stroke patients (156).

Etiologic factors in the causation of DVT include venous stasis (as a result of immobilization and paralysis), hypercoagulability, and endothelial damage.

Edema, tenderness, palpable cords, and a positive Homan sign, although not very sensitive, serve as clinical indicators of DVT formation. While noninvasive tests such as fibrinogen scanning, impedance plethysmography, and Duplex ultrasound have been found to be helpful in establishing the diagnosis, each test has limitations (157). For a definitive diagnosis, contrast venography still remains the gold standard.

DVT prophylaxis is recommended for all stroke patients with significant lower-extremity weakness. A consensus development conference on the prevention of DVT convened by the National Institutes of Health (NIH Consensus Development Conference 1977–1978;1:1–43) recommended that all nonhemorrhagic stroke patients in the absence of contraindications should receive prophylaxis for DVT and pulmonary embolism.

DVT prophylaxis following stroke should be started as soon as possible. Pambianco et al (152), in 1995, reported that the greater amount of time a patient remains without DVT prophylaxis after stroke, the greater the risk of DVT development.

Various methods of prophylaxis include low-dose subcutaneous unfractionated heparin (5000 units two to three times a day), heparin compounds (low-molecular-weight heparin), and physical methods such as external pneumatic compression boots. Turpie et al (158) and Lensing et al (159) found that low-molecular-weight heparin is superior to unfractionated heparin, with less bleeding complications, for the prevention of DVT in patients with acute ischemic strokes. The optimal duration of prophylaxis is uncertain, but the patient's ambulatory status, muscle strength, and time interval from stroke onset can be used as guidelines for continuing prophylaxis.

Once the diagnosis of DVT is established, the patient should be on bed rest with elevation of the affected extremity for the first few days. Anticoagulation with intravenous heparin and oral warfarin should be started immediately. Treatment with warfarin is continued for 3 to 6 months, with frequent monitoring of the prothrombin time to keep it two to three times the control level. Shulman et al (160) reported that treatment with oral anticoagulation for 6 months following DVT is associated with a lower recurrence rate as compared to treatment lasting for only 6 weeks.

Nutrition and Swallowing

Many factors contribute to the often poor nutritional status after stroke. Decreased level of alertness, dysphagia, aphasia, hemiparesis, and concurrent infection may all interfere with adequate oral intake. Close monitoring of calorie and fluid intake, body weight, and laboratory parameters is an integral part of care.

Bedside assessment of swallowing should be performed shortly after admission, and appropriate recommendations made. The presence of a gag reflex is not indicative of a safe swallow. In any patient for whom there is a question of aspiration, the patient should not be fed orally until a videofluoroscopic swallow study can be performed. The videofluoroscopic assessment is also useful in guiding treatment. Swallowing therapy may include exercises to improve oral strength and control, thermal stimulation to trigger the swallowing reflex, and various compensatory strategies including positioning, reduced bolus size, modified consistency, and repetitive swallows with each bolus (161).

If oral intake is not thought to be safe or adequate, tube feedings via gastrostomy or nasogastric tube may be necessary on a temporary and in a few patients, a permanent basis.

Cardiac Disease and Deconditioning

Stroke and heart disease, most commonly ischemic heart disease, frequently coexist. In those who survive a stroke, coronary artery disease is the leading cause of late death (156). Manifestations of heart disease, such as congestive heart failure, angina, and arrhythmias, can complicate and limit rehabilitation. Activities such as dressing, bed mobility, and hemiplegic ambulation require more energy expenditure than before the stroke. The stroke patient usually compensates by performing these activities at a slower rate.

Cardiovascular and musculoskeletal deconditioning accompany acute medical illness and periods of bed rest. Of particular concern is that bed rest results in a higher resting heart rate and lower stroke volume. Since the two major determinants of myocardial oxygen consumption are heart rate and systemic vascular resistance, at any given level of activity the oxygen demand of the heart will be greater than it was prior to the period of bed rest. Thus, activities that may not have provoked angina prior to the stroke may now do so. Orthostatic hypotension is also a frequent problem.

Efforts should be made to optimize the medical evaluation and management and to monitor the patient's response to initial therapies (e.g., orthostatic blood pressures, heart rate and blood pressure response to exercise, and notation of symptoms such as dyspnea and chest pain). The program may need to include gradually increasing exercise to increase strength and endurance.

Seizures

The risk of seizures at the onset of stroke is 4% to 5% for patients with infarcts and 15% to 20% for those with intracerebral or subarachnoid hemorrhage (162). It is difficult to predict which patients who have early seizures will go on to develop recurrent seizures. Considering all types of stroke, the risk of developing recurrent seizures is 5% to 10% (162). This risk is substantially higher for those who have their first seizure more than 24 hours after onset (80%) and whose who have large frontal or temporal lobar hematomas. In general, anticonvulsants used simply for prophylaxis (i.e., no history of actual seizures) should be discontinued after 3 to 4 weeks after stroke onset.

Bowel and Bladder Dysfunction

Although continence is usually recovered in the majority of stroke patients, some initial management is often required. Urinary incontinence may result from urinary tract infection, neurogenic bladder, and cognitive and physical deficits. Initial management consists of discontinuing an indwelling catheter, if present, as soon as possible. This is followed by assessment for possible infection and monitoring bladder emptying and volumes (should be kept <500 mL, with residuals <100 mL). The neurogenic bladder pattern usually seen in suprapontine stroke is one in which the bladder fills and the detrusor autonomously contracts owing to a loss of central inhibition. At times there may be urinary retention secondary to peripheral nerve involvement (e.g., diabetes), outlet obstruction (e.g., enlarged prostate), previous bladder overdistention, or infection. If retention is not a problem, promoting awareness and subsequent control of voiding is done by offering a urinal, bedpan, or commode every few hours. Small amounts of oxybutynin may help with urgency and frequency.

Bowel regularity and continence can usually be maintained through adequate fluid intake, fiber or bulking agents, stool softeners, and occasional suppositories. If bowel incontinence continues, scheduled bowel evacuation using a suppository on a daily or every-other-day basis may be effective.

Spasticity

In general, spasticity should be treated only if it is interfering with function. In many patients, some extensor tone in the hemiparetic leg may increase weight-bearing stability, thus improving gait. Addressing spasticity begins with identifying the particular muscles or muscle groups that are functionally problematic, followed by a thorough search for any inciting factors that are removable or treatable with conservative measures.

Range of motion, stretching, and proper positioning are essential components of any spasticity program. Since most spasticity problems after stroke are focal or regional, approaches such as serial casting, motor point or nerve blocks, and botulinum toxin injections are used to manage problematic areas. Systemic pharmacotherapy for spasticity has a limited role in treating poststroke patients. The currently available agents tend to have side effects such as sedation, fatigue, and cognitive impairment that often limit their use.

The Hemiplegic Arm

Shoulder pain and dysfunction are common in the hemiparetic patient. The causes are not always clear, and there is general agreement that further research is needed (163,164). Glenohumeral subluxation is often associated with shoulder pain, but there is no conclusive evidence that it is causally related (163). There is also controversy about whether current methods of reducing subluxation are effective in preventing pain (165). Despite this uncertainty, attempts are usually made to support the hemiplegic upper extremity. Arm slings are usually used when the patient is standing or ambulating, and elevating arm boards or troughs when the patient is in a wheelchair.

Reflex sympathetic dystrophy (RSD), or shoulder-hand syndrome occurs in approximately 25% of hemiparetic stroke survivors (165). Common clinical features include swelling and pain in the hand and fingers, hyperpathia, vasomotor changes, and painful range of motion in the fingers, hand, wrist, and shoulder. Aggressive range of motion exercises are the cornerstone of therapy, and in combination with nonsteroidal anti-inflammatory drugs and ultrasound to the shoulder before the exercises, represent a first-line conservative approach. A short course of oral steroids is often the next step. Recent clinical experience suggests that tricyclic antidepressants may be helpful in managing the pain that accompanies this syndrome. Sympathetic blockade via stellate ganglion blocks or guanethidine Bier blocks may be necessary in some patients.

Over a period of time (usually several months) the pain and edema lessen and the hand takes on an atrophic appearance with thin, shiny skin, curved nails, and loss of hair. Osteoporosis may also be present, as well as varying degrees of loss of range of motion in the fingers, hand, and shoulder. In general, the prognosis for resolution with preserved range of motion is better in patients who regain some voluntary movement, who have less spasticity, and who do not have accompanying significant sensory loss.

Other conditions that contribute to shoulder pain and dysfunction include degenerative joint disease, rotator cuff inflammation and rupture, subacromial bursitis, and bicipital tendinitis (164). Brachial plexus injury should be suspected in any patient with an unusual pattern of return of motor function in the upper extremity (e.g., no shoulder movement in a patient with good return of function in the hand, or lack of finger flexion in a patient with good wrist and finger extension), absent or reduced reflexes, muscle atrophy, or patterns of sensory loss consistent with plexus injury (166). Brachial plexus stretch injury may occur during inappropriate transfer of the patient with a flaccid upper extremity (e.g., pulling on the arm, or moving the patient with the arm trapped in the bed rail), and is more common in patients with severe sensory loss or neglect.

Cognition and Behavior

The presence of cognitive impairments, whether due to the stroke itself or coexisting degenerative disease, will affect every facet of function, and is a key determinant in the patient's ultimate disability, irrespective of the degree of physical impairment. Deficits may occur in attention, memory, reasoning, judgment, visuoperceptual function, and language. Neuropsychological assessment is useful in identifying the presence and extent of these deficits, as well as in identifying areas of relative strength that will guide the development of appropriate restorative approaches and compensatory strategies.

The efficacy of rehabilitation for cognitive deficits after stroke is controversial. Studies generally support the efficacy of therapy for aphasia, although many have been criticized on methodologic grounds (167). Therapies for neglect and visuoperceptual disorders have shown some promise, particularly instruction in visual scanning techniques (168). There have been few studies of memory and learning dealing exclusively with stroke patients. In general, the more common techniques utilized in stroke patients include visual cues, imagery, or supplementation when verbal memory is impaired; using memory aides, such as alarm watches, calendars, posted schedules, and notebooks; and focusing on functional tasks and routines that may be critically important to the patient's ability to function at home (e.g., use of the telephone, morning routine). Drawers, doors, cupboards, and so on can also be labeled as to their contents. Fortunately, most stroke patients perform better than predicted by neuropsychological testing and by their performance on the rehabilitation unit, once they return home to a familiar setting.

Changes in affect, mood, and behavior occur commonly after stroke, and include lability, anxiety, anger, aggression, impulsivity, disinhibition, paranoia, delusional beliefs, mania, abulia, and depression. The most well described is depression, which negatively impacts on functional outcome and is undertreated (169). There is evidence that pharmacologic therapy is beneficial in treating poststroke depression (170,171), and the selective serotonin reuptake inhibitors are usually well tolerated in the elderly population.

Sexual Function

Sexuality continues to be an important aspect of life as people grow older. Despite this, sexual function after stroke is most often never addressed. A significant number of patients with stroke experience sexual dysfunction, including erectile and ejaculatory dysfunction in men; decreased vaginal lubrication and difficulty achieving orgasm in women; as well as decreased sexual satisfaction, decline in libido, and less frequent sexual activity in both (172). The causes of sexual dysfunction after stroke are multifactorial and include psychological factors, medication, lesion- and disability-related factors, and fear of causing another stroke. A good time to address sexual concerns is when the patient is making reasonable progress in therapies, by letting the patient and significant other know that the physician and team view sexuality as an important aspect of rehabilitation, and are able to help with any problems that may arise.

GENERAL PRINCIPLES OF STROKE REHABILITATION

Following stroke, the pattern of deficits and recovery, associated medical problems, and psychosocial factors vary among individuals and their families, and it becomes critical to individualize rehabilitation programs. The use of an interdisciplinary approach allows for the development of a comprehensive approach and coordination of care, thus facilitating communication between team members and avoiding fragmentation and duplication of services. This approach should occur regardless of the setting (i.e., acute rehabilitation, subacute, skilled nursing facility, home care, or outpatient).

Depending on the setting, the rehabilitation physician assumes a role as either an active team member or a team leader, guiding the team in the development of a realistic rehabilitation plan with achievable goals. In either setting, the physician must acknowledge the skills and competencies of the other rehabilitation professionals, and must be able to assess the effects of their proposed treatments on the patient's overall level of function.

The rehabilitation team generally follows a series of steps to ensure the accomplishment of rehabilitation goals (Table 74-6). Each team member actively participates in the goal-setting process, which should mesh the recommendations of professionals with the interests, values, and lifestyle of the patient and family. Goals are prioritized based on their importance to the patient and family, the degree of health risk to the patient, the likelihood of treatment response, and the initial steps required to reach larger overall goals. Rehabilitation goals must be appropriate (i.e., realistic and achievable) and measurable, so as to allow accurate documentation of progress and outcome. Discharge options and responsibilities are best initially discussed before admission to a rehabilitation unit, and updated and discussed frequently to ensure that the family is receiving essential education and has appropriate and realistic expectations. Counseling and case management services should be available to both patient and family. Coordinated discharge planning with appropriate services and follow-up will ease the transition home.

Outpatient or home-based rehabilitation often follows acute, subacute, or other facility-based rehabilitation, and focuses on improving community living skills. The issue of returning to driving often surfaces at this time. For many older individuals, driving is symbolic of independence. Fortunately, many stroke survivors are able to return to driving, as hemiparesis is often easily compensated for through vehicle modification and training. Cognitive, visuoperceptual deficits, and neglect are more significant barriers, and are often combined with denial or an inability to appreciate their functional impact. Driver's screening evaluations are often appropriate. In younger patients, return to work may be an important goal, and vocational services should be available.

The issues of when rehabilitation should begin, and what role rehabilitation should play acutely after stroke are changing rapidly. Based on studies demonstrating superior outcomes in programs that combine acute and rehabilitative care beginning immediately after stroke, many hospitals are developing practice protocols that require rehabilitation consultation and screening within 24 hours after stroke onset. Undoubtedly, economic pressures that encourage earlier discharge from acute care are also influencing this trend. Our therapeutic and rehabilitative approaches to stroke will also change as research identifies more about the neurobiology of the recovery process, and how we can best facilitate optimal function.

Table 74-6: Rehabilitation Team Process

1. *Evaluate*: impairments, disabilities, handicaps; baseline and treatment response
2. *Identify*: resources, interests, values, lifestyle
3. *Set goals*: initial, prioritize, reset
4. *Treat*: facilitate recovery, adapt, compensate, problem solve, train and educate, motivate
5. *Follow-up*: monitor patient status, problem solve, identify resources

EFFECTIVENESS OF STROKE REHABILITATION PROGRAMS

Stroke rehabilitation programs are not new. They have been around for several decades. Yet a basic question remains unanswered: Are the stroke units effective in reducing the disability after stroke and decreasing the long-term social and economic costs? According to Feldman et al (173), "formal rehabilitation was unnecessary if the attention was given to the ambulation and self care on the medical and neurological wards." Lind (174), upon review of several stroke studies, found conflicting results. He concluded that the functional improvement was from spontaneous recovery and not from rehabilitation. He made two important observations: 1) Although the functional improvement attributed to rehabilitation may be slight, it makes a difference between a patient returning home and a person being placed in an institution; 2) A subset of patients with marginal functional impairment may benefit from comprehensive rehabilitation.

Garraway et al (175,176) performed a population-based controlled prospective stroke rehabilitation study in Edinburgh, Scotland. Patients were randomized either to a stroke unit that provided both acute care and rehabilitation or to medical wards with later transfer to rehabilitation. Patients treated on the stroke unit showed more independence in ADLs at discharge and length of hospitalization was shorter, despite similar neurologic deficits in the two groups. These findings suggest that some aspect of the stroke unit, rather than spontaneous recovery alone, was responsible for the improvement.

Population-based studies from Umea, Sweden (177,178), and Finland (179) demonstrated similar findings. Patients treated on a stroke unit had improved independence in ambulation and self-care at discharge, and a shorter length of stay in the hospital than did patients admitted to medical wards. In a subset of patients with "mild" to "moderate" deficits or age less than 75 years, the stroke unit accelerated the rehabilitation process. For patients with "major" deficits and age 75 years or older, care in the stroke unit enhanced the proportion of patients able to return home.

Indredavik et al (180) randomized 220 patients either to a stroke unit providing acute and rehabilitation care or to the medical wards where rehabilitation was provided. At 6 weeks, 56.4% of the stroke unit patients had returned home, whereas only 32.7% of the medical unit patients were at home ($p = 0.0004$). At 1 year, 62.7% of the stroke unit patients were home, compared to 44.6% of medical unit patients ($p = 0.002$). Patients from the stroke unit had better functional status than did patients from the medical wards at 6 weeks and at 1 year as measured by the Barthel index. Patients on the stroke unit also had decreased mortality as compared to those on the medical wards (7.3% versus 17.3%). This is one of the first studies to show improved survival for patients treated on stroke units, in addition to the improved functional recovery.

Stevens et al (181) randomized 225 patients to receive treatment in a specialized stroke rehabilitation unit or in a conventional setting. The two groups were similar in demographic characteristics and stroke severity. Follow-up at 1 year showed a positive outcome in the patients treated in the stroke unit in terms of improved independence in self-care and an increased number of patients discharged to home.

Kalra et al (182) stratified 245 stroke patients into three prognostic groups. They were randomized to receive treatment either in a stroke unit or in the general medical ward. Functional outcome was similar for the poor- and good-prognosis groups in both units; however, there was a significant increase in mortality in the poor-prognosis group treated in the general medical ward. Patients in the general medical ward stayed longer and received more therapy. Patients with the intermediate prognosis had a better functional outcome when treated in the stroke units. A higher percentage of patients were discharged home from the stroke unit (75% versus 52%). Those on the stroke unit also had a shorter length of stay in the hospital. This study suggests that a stroke unit combining acute care with rehabilitation is beneficial for a subset of stroke patients with intermediate disability.

In a later study, Kalra et al (183) randomized 146 patients to receive treatment in either a stroke unit or general medical wards. Similar observations were made. The patients treated on the stroke unit showed significantly greater and more rapid functional recovery, as indicated by the higher Barthel score on discharge as well as a more rapid change in score. The length of stay was also significantly shorter in the patients treated in the stroke unit. More recently, Kalra and Eade (184) reported that even the severe stroke patients treated in the stroke unit had a significantly better outcome in terms of decreased mortality, increased number of home discharges, and shorter length of stay.

Jorgensen et al (185) reported on a community-based prospective study of 1241 unselected stroke patients. The patients in one community were treated in a stroke unit, while in the other they were treated in the neurologic and medical wards. The demographics for both communities were similar, and patients were admitted within 1 week after the onset of stroke. They found that the in-hospital mortality was 21% lower in the patients treated in the stroke unit and the case-fatality rate was 24% lower at 30 days, 20% lower at 6 months, and 18% lower at 1 year. There was a 16% increase in the home discharges for the patients treated in the stroke unit. The length of hospital stay was also reduced by 30%, resulting in significant cost savings. They made three very important observations: 1) This is the first study to report the effects of the stroke units on unselected patients, as compared to the traditional randomized stroke unit studies (i.e., the patients with severe strokes were not excluded from this study). 2) Previous studies that showed improved outcome were done on smaller number of patients (i.e., <300 patients). 3) This study found decreased mortality at 1 year after stroke as well as acutely.

CONCLUSIONS

Stroke remains a leading cause of death and disability. New acute and rehabilitative therapies and approaches hold the promise of reducing the dysfunction caused by stroke. Awareness of the pathophysiology and recovery patterns following stroke and attention to detail in medical and rehabilitative management enhance current functional outcome.

REFERENCES

1. Terent A. Stroke morbidity. In: Whisnant J, ed. *Populations, cohorts, and clinical trials. Stroke.* Boston: Butterworth-Heinemann, 1993:37–58.
2. Broderick JP, Philips SJ, Whisnant JP, et al. Incidence rates of stroke in the eighties:

the end of the decline in stroke? *Stroke* 1989;20:577–582.

3. Gillum RF. Stroke in black. *Stroke* 1988;19:1–9.

4. Garraway WM, Whisnant JP, Furlan AJ, et al. The declining incidence of stroke. *N Engl J Med* 1979;300:449–452.

5. Garraway WM, Whisnant JP, Drury I. The continuing decline in the incidence of stroke. *Mayo Clin Proc* 1983;58: 520–523.

6. Kotila M, Waltimo I, Biemi ML, et al. The profile of recovery from stroke and factors influencing outcome. *Stroke* 1984;15: 1039–1044.

7. Kagan A, Popper J, Reed DM, et al. Trends in stroke incidence and mortality in Hawaiian Japanese men. *Stroke* 1994;25:1170–1175.

8. Bonita R. Stroke trends in Australia and New Zealand: mortality, morbidity, and risk factors. *Ann Epidemiol* 1993;3: 529–533.

9. Hong Y, Bots MI, Pan X, et al. Stroke incidence and mortality in rural and urban Shanghai from 1984 through 1991. Findings from a community-based registry. *Stroke* 1994;25: 1165–1169.

10. Neissen LW, Barendregt JJ, Bonneux L, Koudsta PJ. Stroke trends in an aging population. *Stroke* 1993;24:931–939.

11. Brown RD, Whisnant JP, Sicks JD, et al. Stroke incidence, prevalence, and survival. Secular trends in Rochester, Minnesota, Through 1989.

12. Eissenblatter D, Heinemann I, Dipolocc BC. Community based stroke incidence. Trends from the 1970's through the 1980's in East Germany. *Stroke* 1995;26:919–923.

13. Feigin VI, Wiebers DO, Whisnant JP, O'Fallon WM. Stroke incidence and 30-day case fatality rates in Novosibirsk, Russia, 1992 through 1992. *Stroke* 1995;26:924–929.

14. Matsumoto N, Whisnant JP, Kurland LT, Okazaki H. Natural history of strokes in Rochester, Minnesota, 1995 through 1969; an extention of a previous study, 1945 through 1954. *Stroke* 1973;4:20–29.

15. Baum HM, Robins M. Survival and prevalence. *Stroke* 1981;12(suppl):59–68.

16. Dombovy MI, Basford JR, Whisnant JP, Bergstralh EJ. Disability and use of rehabilitation services following stroke in Rochester, Minnesota, 1975–1979. *Stroke* 1987;18: 830–836.

17. Lanska DI, Peterson PM. Geographic variation in the decline of stroke mortality in the United States. *Stroke* 1995;26: 1159–1165.

18. Shahar E, Mcgovern PG, Sprafka M, et al. Improved survival of stroke patients during the 1980's. *Stroke* 1995;26:1–6.

19. Bounds JV, Weibers DO, Whisnant JP, Okazaki H. Mechanism and timing of death from cerebral infarction. *Stroke* 1981;12:474–477.

20. Abu-Zeid HAH, Choi NW, Hsu PH, Maini KK. Prognostic factors in the survival of 1,484 stroke cases observed for 30 to 48 months. Diagnostic types and descriptive variables. *Arch Neurol* 1978;35:121–125.

21. Bamford J, Dennis M, Sandercock P, et al. The frequency, cause and timing of death within 30 days of a first stroke: the Oxfordshire Community Stroke Project. *J Neurol Neurosurg Psychiatry* 1990;53: 824–829.

22. Burn J, Dennis M, Bamford J, et al. Long term risk of recurrent stroke after a first ever stroke. The Oxfordshire Community Stroke Project. *Stroke* 1994;25:333–337.

23. Wolf PA. An overview of the epidemiology of stroke. *Stroke* 1992;21(suppl III):4–6.

24. Mohr JP, Gautier JC, Heir DB, Stein RW. Middle cerebral artery. In: Barnett HJM, Stein BM, Mohr JP, Yatsu FM, eds. *Stroke: pathophysiology, diagnosis, and management.* New York: Churchill Livingstone, 1986:377–450.

25. Burst JCM. Anterior cerebral artery. In: Barnett HJM, Stein BM, Mohr JP, Yatsu FM, eds. *Stroke: pathophysiology, diagnosis, and management.* New York: Churchill Livingstone, 1986:351–375.

26. Sawada T, Kazul S. Anterior cerebral artery. In: Bogousslavsky J, Caplan L, eds. *Stroke syndromes.* New York: Cambridge University Press, 1995:235–246.

27. Bogousslavsky J, Moulin T. Border-zone infarcts. In: Bogousslavsky J, Caplan L, eds. *Stroke syndromes.* New York: Cambridge University Press, 1995:358–365.

28. Barth A, Bogousslavsky J, Caplan LR. Thalamic infarcts and hemorrhages. In: Bogousslavsky J, Caplan L, eds. *Stroke syndromes.* New York: Cambridge University Press, 1995:276–283.

29. Mohr JP. Posterior cerebral artery. In: Barnett HJM, Stein BM, Mohr JP, Yatsu FM, eds. *Stroke: pathophysiology, diagnosis, and management.* New York: Churchill Livingstone, 1986:451–470.

30. Ross Russell RW. Clinical effects of posterior cerebral artery occlusion. In: Berguer R, Bauer RB, eds. *Vertebrobasilar arterial occlusive disease.* New York: Raven, 1984:77–83.

31. Hachinski V, Norris JW. Vascular syndromes. In: *The acute stroke.* Philadelphia: FA Davis, 1985:103–122.

32. Lidegaard O, Som, Anderson MVN. Cerebral thromboembolism among young women and men in Denmark 1977–1982. *Stroke* 1986;17:670–675.

33. Mettinger KL, Soderstrom CE, Allander E. Epidemiology of acute cerebrovascular disease before the age of 55 in the Stockholm County, 1973–1977: incidence and mortality rates. *Stroke* 1984;15:795–801.

34. Schoenberg BS, Whisnant JP, Taylor WF, Kempers RD. Strokes in women of childbearing age: a

population study. *Neurology* 1970;20:181–189.

35. Bogousslavsky J, Pierre P. Ischemic stroke in patients under age 45. *Neurol Clin North Am* 1992;10:113–124.

36. Leno C, Berciano J, Combarros O, et al. A prospective study of stroke in young adults in Cantabria, Spain. *Stroke* 1993;24:792–795.

37. Qureshi AI, Safdar K, Patel M, et al. Stroke in young black patients: risk factors, subtypes, and prognosis. *Stroke* 1995;26:1995–1998.

38. Hart RG, Miller VT. Cerebral infarction in young adults: a practical approach. *Stroke* 1983;14:110–114.

39. Webster MW, Chancellor AM, Smith HJ, et al. Patent foramen ovale in young stroke patients. *Lancet* 1988;2:11–12.

40. Lachat P, Mas JL, Lascault G, et al. Prevalence of patent foramen ovale in patients with stroke. *N Engl J Med* 1988;318: 1148–1152.

41. Ranous D, Cohen A, Cabanes L, et al. Patent foramen ovale: is stroke due to paradoxical embolism? *Stroke* 1993;24:31–34.

42. Stollberger C, Slany J, Schuster I, et al. The prevalence of deep venous thrombosis in patients with suspected paradoxical embolism. *Ann Intern Med* 1993;119:461–465.

43. Homma S, DiTullio MR, Sacco RL, et al. Characteristics of patent foramen ovale associated with cryptogenic stroke. A biplane transesophageal echocardiographic study. *Stroke* 1994;25:582–586.

44. Cabanes L, Mas JL, Cohen A, et al. Atrial septal aneurysm and patent foramen ovale as risk factors for cryptogenic stroke in patients less than 55 years of age. A study using transesophageal echocardiography. *Stroke* 1993;24:1865–1873.

45. DiTullio M, Sacco RL, Venketasubramanian N, et al. Comparison of diagnostic techniques for the detection of a patent foramen ovale in stroke patients. *Stroke* 1993;24:1020–1024.

46. Hanna JP, Sun JP, Furlan AJ, et al. Patent foramen ovale and brain infarct. Echocardiographic predictors, recurrence, and prevention. *Stroke* 1994;25: 782–786.

47. Bogousslavsky J, Piesse P. Ischemic stroke in patients under age 45. *Neurol Clin N Am* 1992;10:113–129.

48. Nachman RL, Silverstein R. Hypercoagulable states. *Ann Intern Med* 1993;119:819–827.

49. Rosove MH, Brewer PMC. Antiphospholipid thrombosis: clinical course after the first thrombotic event in 70 patients. *Ann Intern Med* 1992;117: 303–308.

50. Khamashta MA, Cuadrado MJ, Mujic F, et al. The management of thrombosis in the antiphospholipid antibody syndrome. *N Engl J Med* 1995;332: 993–997.

51. Lidegaard O. Oral contraception and risk of cerebral thromboembolic attack: results of a case-control study. *BMJ* 1993;306:956–963.

52. Vassey MP, Lawless M, Veates D. Oral contraceptives and stroke: findings in a large prospective study. *BMJ* 1984;289:530–531.

53. Bousser MG, Chiras J, Bories J, et al. Cerebral venous thrombosis: a review of 38 cases. *Stroke* 1985;16:199–212.

54. Dara M, Tuchman AJ, Marks S. Central nervous system infarction related to cocaine abuse. *Stroke* 1991;221:1320–1325.

55. Krendel DA, Ditter SM, Franel MR, Ross WK. Biopsy-proven cerebral vasculitis associated with cocaine abuse. *Neurology* 1990;40:1092–1094.

56. Fredericks RK, Lefkowitz DS, Challa VR, Troost BT. Cerebral vasculitis associated with cocaine abuse. *Stroke* 1991;221: 1437–1439.

57. Inagawa T, Ishikawa S, Hidenobu A, et al. Aneurysmal subarachnoid in Izumo City and Shimane Prefecture of Japan. *Stroke* 1988;19:170–175.

58. Phillips L, Whisnant J, O'Fallon M, Sundt T. The unchanging pattern of subarachnoid in a community. *Neurology* 1980;30:1034–1040.

59. Sivenius J, Heinonen O, Pyoala K, et al. The incidence of stroke in the Kuopio area of East Finland. *Stroke* 1985;16:188–192.

60. Bonita R, Thompson S. Subarachnoid hemorrhage: epidemiology diagnosis, management, and outcome. *Stroke* 1985;16:591–594.

61. Broderick JP, Brott JP, Duldner JE, et al. Initial and recurrent bleedings are the major causes of death following subarachnoid hemorrhage. *Stroke* 1994;25:1342–1347.

62. Kassel N, Torner J, Haley C, et al. The International Cooperative Study on the timing of aneurysm surgery. Part I: overall management results. *J Neurosurg* 1990;73:18–36.

63. Fogelhol R, Hernesniemi J, Vapalahti M. Impact of early surgery on outcome after aneurysmal subarchnoid hemorrhage, a population-based study. *Stroke* 1993;24:1649–1654.

64. Lungren B, Sonesson B, Saveland H, Brandt L. Cognition and adjustment after late and early operation for ruptured aneurysm. *Neurosurgery* 1987; 21:279–289.

65. Hutter BO, Gilsbach JM, Kreitschmann I. Quality of life and cognitive deficits after subarachnoid hemorrhage. *Br J Neurosurg* 1995;9:465–475.

66. Tidswell P, Dias PS, Sagar JH, et al. Cognitive outcome after aneurysm rupture: relationship to aneursym site and perioperative complications. *Neurology* 1995;45:875–882.

67. Kotila M, Waltimp I, Biemi ML, et al. The profile of recovery from stroke and factors influencing

outcome. *Stroke* 1994;15: 1039–1044.

68. Dombovy ML, Basford JR, Whisnant JP, Bergstralh EJ. Disability and use of rehabilitation services following stroke in Rochester, Minnesota, 1975–1979. *Stroke* 1987;18:830–836.

69. Wade DT, Langton Hewer R. Functional abilities after stroke: measurement, natural history and prognosis. *J Neurol Neurosurg Psychiatry* 1987;50: 177–182.

70. Andrews K, Brocklehurst JR, Richards B, Laycock PJ. The rate of recovery from stroke and its measurement. *Int Rehabil Med* 1981;3:155–161.

71. Bonita R, Beaglehole R. Recovery of motor function after stroke. *Stroke* 1988;19:1497–1500.

72. Twitchell T. The restoration of motor function following hemiplegia in man. *Brain* 1951;74:443–480.

73. Wade DT, Langton Hewer R, Wood VA, et al. The hemiplegic arm after stroke: measurement and recovery. *J Neurol Neurosurg Psychiatry* 1983;46: 521–524.

74. Heller A, Wade D, Wood VA, et al. Arm function after stroke: measurement and recovery over the first three months. *J Neurol Neurosurg Psychiatry* 1987;50:714–719.

75. Smith DL, Akhtar AJ, Garraway WM. Proprioception and spatial neglect after stroke. *Age Ageing* 1983;12:63–69.

76. Egelko S, Simon D, Riley E, et al. *Arch Phys Med Rehabil* 1989;70:297–302.

77. Isaeff W, Waller P, Duncan G. Ophthalmic findings in 332 patients with a cerebral vascular accident. *Ann Ophthalmol* 1974;6:1059–1069.

78. Gray C, French J, Bates D, et al. Recovery of visual fields in acute stroke: homonymous hemianopsia associated with adverse prognosis. *Age Ageing* 1989; 18:419–421.

79. Chapey R, ed. *Language intervention strategies in adult aphasia.* 2nd ed. Baltimore: Williams & Wilkins, 1986.

80. Wade DT, Langton Hewer R, David RM, Enderby PM. Aphasia after stroke: natural history and associated deficits. *J Neurol Neurosurg Psychiatry* 1986; 49:11–16.

81. Sarno M, Levita E. Recovery in treated aphasia in the first year post stroke. *Stroke* 1979;10:663–670.

82. Barer DH. Continence after stroke: useful predictor or goal of therapy. *Age Ageing* 1989;18:183–191.

83. Wade DT, Wood VA, Langton Hewer RL. Recovery after stroke—the first three months. *J Neurol Neurosurg Psychiatry* 1985;48:7–13.

84. Horner J, Massey EW, Riski JE, et al. Aspiration following stroke: clinical correlates and outcome. *Neurology* 1988;38:1359–1362.

85. Gordon C, Hewer RL, Wade DT. Dysphagia in acute stroke. *BMJ* 1987;295(6595):411–414.

86. Barer DH. The natural history and functional consequence of dysphagia after hemispheric stroke. *J Neurol Neurosurg Psychiatry* 1989;52:236–241.

87. Horner J, Buoyner FG, Alberts MS, Helms MJ. Dysphagia following brainstem stroke. *Arch Neurol* 1991;48:1170–1173.

88. Robinson RG, Price TR. Post stroke depressive disorders: a follow up study of 103 patients. *Stroke* 1982;13:635–640.

89. Sinyor D, Jacques P, Kaloupek DG, et al. Post-stroke depression and lesion location. An attempted replication. *Brain* 1986;109:537–546.

90. Wade DT, Leigh-Smith J, Langton Hewer R. Depressed mood after stroke: a community study of its frequency. *Br J Psychiatry* 1987;151:200–205.

91. Redding MJ, Orto LA, Winter SW, et al. Antidepressant therapy after stroke: a double blinded trial. *Arch Neurol* 1986;43: 763–765.

92. Robinson RG, Starr L, Price T. A two year longitudinal study of mood disorders following stroke. *Br J Psychiatry* 1984;144: 256–262.

93. Robinson RG, Starr LB, Lipsey JR, et al. A two-year longitudinal study of post-stroke mood disorders: in-hospital prognostic factors associated with six-month outcome. *J Nerv Ment Dis* 1985;173:221–226.

94. Starkstein SE, Robinson RG, Price TR. Comparison of cortical and subcortical lesions in the production of post-stroke mood disorders. *Brain* 1987;110: 1045–1059.

95. Parikh RM, Robinson RG, Lipsey JR, et al. The impact of post-stroke depression on recovery in activities of daily living over a two year follow up. *Arch Neurol* 1990;47:785–789.

96. Robinson RG, Bolduc PL, Price TR. Two year longitudinal study of post-stroke mood disorders: diagnosis and outcome at one and two years. *Stroke* 1987;18:837–843.

97. Reding MJ, Potes E. Rehabilitation outcome following initial unilateral hemispheric stroke. *Stroke* 1988;19:1354–1358.

98. Jorgensen HS, Nakayama H, Raaschou HO, Olsen TS. Recovery of walking function in stroke patients: the Copenhagen Stroke Study. *Arch Phys Med Rehabil* 1995;76:27–32.

99. Blower PW, Carter LC, Sulch DA. Rehabilitation between wheelchair propulsion and independent walking in hemiplegic stroke. *Stroke* 1995;26:606–608.

100. Jorgensen HS, Nakayama H, Raaschou HO, et al. Outcome and time course of recovery in stroke. Part I: outcome. The Copenhagen Stroke Study. *Arch Phys Med Rehabil* 1995;76:399–405.

101. Jorgensen HS, Nakayama H, Raaschou HO, et al. Outcome

and time course of recovery in stroke. Part II: outcome. The Copenhagen Stroke Study. *Arch Phys Med Rehabil* 1995;76:406–412.

102. Jongbloed L. Prediction of function after stroke: a critical review. *Stroke* 1986;17:765–776.

103. Shah S, Vanclay F, Cooper B. Predicting discharge status at commencement of stroke rehabilitation. *Stroke* 1989; 20:786.

104. Davidoff G, Keren O, Ring H, et al. Assessing candidates for inpatient stroke rehabilitation: predictors of outcome. *Phys Med Rehabil Clin N Am* 1991;2: 501–515.

105. Alexander MP. Stroke rehabilitation outcome: a potential use of predictive variables to establish levels of care. *Stroke* 1994;25:128–134.

106. Nakayama H, Jorgensen HS, Raaschou HO, Olsen TS. The influence of age on stroke outcome: the Copenhagen Stroke Study. *Stroke* 1994;25: 808–813.

107. Prescott RJ, Garraway WM, Akhtar AJ. Predicting functional outcome following acute stroke using a standard clinical examination. *Stroke* 1982;13: 641–647.

108. Rose L, Bakal DA, Fung TS, et al. Tactile extinction and functional status after stroke: a preliminary investigation. *Stroke* 1994;25:1973–1976.

109. Lehman J, Delateur B, Fowler R Jr, et al. Stroke: does rehabilitation affect outcome? *Arch Phys Med Rehabil* 1975;56: 375–382.

110. Ahlsio B, Britton M, Murray V, Theorell T. Disablement and quality of life after stroke. *Stroke* 1984;15:886–890.

111. Hertanu JS, Demopoulos JT, Yang WC, et al. Stroke rehabilitation: correlation and prognostic value of computerized tomography and sequential functional assessments. *Arch Phys Med Rehabil* 1984;65:505–508.

112. Valdimarsson E, Bergvall U, Samuelson K. Prognostic significance of cerebral computed tomography results in supratentorial infarction. *Acta Neurol Scand* 1982;65:133–145.

113. Chaudhuri G, Harvey RF, Sulton LD, Lamabert RW. Computerized tomography head scans as predictors of functional outcome of stroke patients. *Arch Phys Med Rehabil* 1988;69:496–498.

114. Bushnell DL, Gupta S, Mlcoch AG, Barnes E. Prediction of language and neurologic recovery after cerebral infarction with SPECT imaging using *N*-isopropyl-P (123) iodoamphetamine. *Arch Neurol* 1989;46:665–669.

115. Hanson SK, Grotta JC, Rhoades H, et al. Value of single-photon emission computed tomography in acute stroke therapeutic trials. *Stroke* 1993;24:1322–1329.

116. Saunders DE, Clifton AG, Brown MM. Measurement of infarct size using MRI predicts prognosis in middle cerebral artery infarction. *Stroke* 1995;26:2272–2276.

117. Pavot AP, Ignacio DR, Kuntavanish A, et al. The prognostic value of somatosensory evoked potentials in cerebrovascular accidents. *Electromyogr Clin Neurophysiol* 1986;26:333–340.

118. Keren O, Ring H, Solzi P, et al. Upper limb somatosensory evoked potentials as a predictor of rehabilitation progress in dominant hemisphere stroke patients. *Stroke* 1993;24:1789–1793.

119. The National Institute of Neurological Disorders and Stroke r-TPA Stroke Study Group. Tissue plasminogen activator for acute ischemic stroke. *N Engl J Med* 1995;333:1581–1587.

120. Meldrum B, Milliam MH, Obrenovitch TP. Excitatory amino acid release induced by injury. In: Globus MY-T, Dietrich WD, eds. *The role of neurotransmitters in brain injury.* New York: Plenum, 1992.

121. Choi D. Methods for antagonizing glutamate neurotoxicity. *Cerebrovasc Brain Metab Rev* 1990;2:105–147.

122. Chen M, Bullock R, Graham DI, et al. Evaluations of competitive NMDA antagonists (D-CPPene) in feline focal cerebral ischemia. *Ann Neurol* 1991;30:62–70.

123. Ginsberg MD, Busto R. Rodent models of cerebral ischemia. *Stroke* 1989;20:1627–1642.

124. Miller JD, Bullock R, Graham DI, et al. Ischemic brain damage in a model of acute subdural hematoma. *Neurosurgery* 1990;27:433–439.

125. Hall ED, Yonkers PA. Attenuation of post-ischemic cerebral hyperfusion by the twenty-one amino steroid U-74,006F. *Stroke* 1988;1930:340–344.

126. Hall ED, Yonkers PA, McCall JM, et al. Effects of the 21-aminosteroid U-74,006F on experimental head injury in mice. *J Neurosurg* 1988;68:456–461.

127. Hall ED, Pazara KE, Braughler J. 21-Aminosteroid lipid peroxidation inhibitor U-74,006F protects against cerebral ischemia in gerbils. *Stroke* 1988;19: 997–1002.

128. Kassell ND. Reduction in mortality in aneurysmal subarachnoid hemorrhage with tirilazad, a new antioxidant. In: *Proceedings of the World Congress of Neurosurgeons.* Acapulco, October 1993.

129. Pickard JD, Murray GD, Illingsworth R, et al. Effect of oral nimodipine on cerebral infarction and outcome after subarachnoid hemorrhage: British Aneurysm Nimodipine Trial. *BMJ* 1989;298:636–642.

130. Baron JC, Bousser MG, Comar D, et al. Crossed cerebellar diaschisis: a remote functional depression secondary to supratentorial infarction of man. *J Cereb Blood Flow Metab* 1981; 1(suppl):S500.

131. Feeney DM. Pharmacologic modulation of recovery after brain injury: a reconsideration of diaschisis. *J Neurol Rehabil* 1991;5:113–128.

132. Papanicolaou A, Moore B, Levin H, Eisenberg H. Evoked potential

correlates of right hemisphere involvement in language recovery following stroke. *Arch Neurol* 1987;47:521.

133. Schieber MH. Physiological bases for functional recovery. *J Neurol Rehabil* 1995;9:65–71.

134. Chollet F, DiPiero V, Wise RJS, et al. The functional anatomy of motor recovery after stroke in humans: a study with positron emission tomography. *Ann Neurol* 1991;29:63–71.

135. Knorr U, Schlaug G, Hefter H, et al. Activation of cortical motor areas: an individual PET analysis. *Soc Neurosci Abstr* 1993;19: 1209.

136. Weiller C, Ramsay St C, Wise RJS, et al. Individual patterns of functional reorganization in the human cerebral cortex after capsular infarction. *Ann Neurol* 1993;33:181–189.

137. Toole J, Good DC, eds. *Imaging in neurologic rehabilitation.* New York: Demos Vermande, 1996.

138. Jenkins WM, Merzenich MM, Fowler BC, Stuyker MP. The area 3b representation of the hand in owl monkeys reorganizes after induction of restricted cortical lesions. *Soc Neurosci Abstr* 1982;8:141.

139. Jenkins WM, Merzenick MM, Ochs MT. Behaviorally controlled differential use of restricted hand surfaces induce changes in cortical representation of the hand in area 3b of adult owl monkeys. *Soc Neurosci Abstr* 1984; 10:665.

140. Selzer ME. Mechanics of functional recovery in traumatic brain injury. *J Neurol Rehabil* 1995;9:73–84.

141. Goldstein LB. Pharmacological enhancement of recovery. In: Good DC, Couch JR, eds. *Handbook of neurorehabilitation.* New York: Marcel Dekker, 1994: 343–369.

142. Goldstein LB, Davis JN. Post-lesion practice and amphetamine-facilitated recovery of beam-walking in the rat. *Restor Neurol Neurosci* 1990;1: 311–314.

143. Cristoma EA, Duncan DW, Propst ME, et al. Evidence that amphetamine with physical therapy promotes recovery of motor function in stroke patients. *Ann Neurol* 1988;23:94–97.

144. Nickels J, Schneider W, Dombovy M, Wong T. Clinical use of amantadine in brain injury rehabilitation. *Brain Inj* 1994;8:708–718.

145. Goldstein LB, Matchar DB, Morgenlander JC, Davis JN. Influence of drugs on the recovery of sensorimotor function after stroke. *J Neurol Rehabil* 1990;4: 137–144.

146. Matchar DB, McCrory DC, Barnett HJM, Feussner JR. Medical treatment for stroke prevention. *Ann Intern Med* 1994;121:54–55.

147. *1991 Heart and stroke facts.* Dallas, TX: American Heart Association, 1991:1–48.

148. Smith D. Stroke prevention: the importance of risk factors. *Stroke Clin Updates* 1991;5:17–20.

149. National Institutes of Health National Institute of Neurologic Disorders and Stroke (NINDS). Major trial confirms benefit of stroke prevention surgery. *News Bull* September 30, 1994.

150. Wolf PA, Abbott RD, Kannel WB. Atrial fibrillation: a major contributor to stroke in the elderly. The Framingham study. *Arch Intern Med* 1987;147:1561–1564.

151. Atrial Fibrillation Investigators. Risk factors for stroke and efficacy of antithrombotic therapy in atrial fibrillation: analysis of pooled data from five randomized controlled trials. *Arch Intern Med* 1994;154:1449–1457.

152. Pambianco G, Orchard T, Landau P. Deep vein thrombosis: prevention in stroke patients during rehabilitation. *Arch Phys Med Rehabil* 1995;76:324–330.

153. Sioson ER, Crowe WE, Dawson NY. Occult proximal deep vein thrombosis: its prevalence among patients admitted to a rehabilitation hospital. *Arch Phys Med Rehabil* 1988;69:183–185.

154. Matzdorff AC, Green D. Deep vein thrombosis and pulmonary embolism: prevention, diagnosis and treatment. *Geriatrics* 1992;47:48–63.

155. Oczkowski WJ, Ginsberg JS, Shin A, Panju A. Venous thromboembolism in patients undergoing rehabilitation after stroke. *Arch Phys Med Rehabil* 1992;73: 712–716.

156. Bounds JY, Wiebers DO, Whisnant JP, Okazaki H. Mechanisms and timing of deaths from cerebral infarction. *Stroke* 1981;12: 474–477.

157. Izzo KL, Aquino E. Deep vein thrombosis in high risk hemiplegic patients: detection by impedance plethysmography. *Arch Phys Med Rehabil* 1986;67:799–802.

158. Turpie AGG, Gent M, Cote R, et al. A low-molecular-weight heparinoid compared with unfractionated heparin in the prevention of deep vein thrombosis in patients with acute ischemic stroke. *Ann Intern Med* 1992;117:353–357.

159. Lensing A, Prins M, Davidson B, Hirsch J. Treatment of deep venous thrombosis with low-molecular-weight heparin. *Arch Intern Med* 1995;155:601–607.

160. Schulman S, Rhedin A, Lindmarker P, et al. A comparison of six weeks with six months of oral anticoagulant therapy after a first episode of venous thromboembolism. *N Engl J Med* 1995;332:1661–1665.

161. Lazar RB, Rubin SM. Speech therapy and communicative disorders in neurological rehabilitation. In: Good DC, Courch JR, eds. *Handbook of neurorehabilitation.* New York: Marcel Dekker, 1994:219–239.

162. Dromerick A, Reding M. Medical and neurological complications during inpatient stroke rehabilitation. *Stroke* 1994;25:358–361.

163. Roy C. *Clin Rehabil* 1988;2: 35–44.

164. Griffin J. Hemiplegic shoulder pain. *Phys Ther* 1986;66: 1885–1893.

165. Hurd M, Farrell K, Waylonis G. Shoulder sling for hemiplegia: friend or foe? *Arch Phys Med Rehabil* 1974;55:519–523.

166. Meredith J, Taft G, Kaplan P. Diagnosis and treatment of the hemiplegic patient with brachial plexus injury. *Am J Occup Ther* 1981;35:656.

167. Wertz RT, Weiss J, Aten J, et al. Comparison of clinic, home, and deferred language treatment for aphasia. A Veterans Admin. Coop. Study. *Arch Neurol* 1986;43:653–658.

168. Schacter DL. Clinical neuropsychology of intervention. In: Uzzel BP, Gross Y, eds. Boston: Martinus Nijhoff, 1986:257–282.

169. Robinson R, Price T. Post stroke depressive disorders: a follow-up study of 103 patients. *Stroke* 1982;13:635–641.

170. Reding M, Orto L, Winter S, et al. The dexamethasone suppression test. An indicator of depression in stroke but not a predictor of rehabilitation outcome. *Arch Neurol* 1985;43:763.

171. Lipsey J, Robinson R. Nortriptyline treatment of post-stroke depression: a double-blind study. *Lancet* 1984;2:297.

172. Coslett HB, Heilmann KM. Male sexual function. Impairment after right hemisphere stroke. *Arch Neurol* 1986;43:1036–1039.

173. Feldman DJ, Lee PR, Unterecker J, et al. A comparison of functionally oriented medical care and formal rehabilitation in the management of patients with hemiplegia due to cerebrovascular disease. *J Chronic Dis* 1962;15:297–310.

174. Lind K. A synthesis of studies on stroke rehabilitation. *J Chronic Dis* 1982;35:133–149.

175. Garraway WM, Akhtar AJ, Prescott RJ, Hockey J. Management of acute stroke in the elderly: preliminary results of a controlled trial. *BMJ* 1980;280: 1040–1043.

176. Garraway WM, Akhtar AJ, Smith DL, Smith ME. The triage of stroke rehabilitation. *J Epidemiol Community Health* 1981;35: 39–44.

177. Strand T, Asplund K, Eriksson S, et al. A non-intensive stroke unit reduces functional disability and the need for long-term hospitalization. *Stroke* 1985;16:29–34.

178. Strand T, Asplund K, Erisson S, et al. Stroke unit care—who benefits? Comparisons with general medical care in relation to prognostic indicators on admission. *Stroke* 1986;17:377–381.

179. Sivenius J, Pyorala K, Heinonen OP, et al. The significance of intensity of rehabilitation of stroke—a controlled trial. *Stroke* 1985;16:928–931.

180. Indredavik B, Bakke F, Solberg R, et al. Benefit of a stroke unit: a randomized controlled trial. *Stroke* 1991;22:1026–1031.

181. Stevens RS, Ambler NR, Warren MD. A randomized controlled trial of a stroke rehabilitation ward. *Age Ageing* 1984;13: 65–75.

182. Kalra L, Dale P, Crome P. Improving stroke rehabilitation: a controlled study. *Stroke* 1993;24: 1462–1467.

183. Kalra L. The influence of stroke unit rehabilitation on functional recovery from stroke. *Stroke* 1994;25:821–825.

184. Kalra L, Eade J. Role of stroke rehabilitation units in managing severe disability after stroke. *Stroke* 1995;26:2031–2034.

185. Jorgensen HS, Nakayama H, Raaschou HO, et al. The effect of a stroke unit: reductions in mortality, discharge rate to nursing home, length of hospital stay, and cost savings. *Ugeskrift for Laeger* 1996;35:4894–4897.

Chapter 75

Parkinson Disease and Rehabilitation

Gary S. Friedman

Parkinson disease or paralysis agitans is a well-known movement disorder featuring a resting tremor, bradykinesia, and a stooped-forward or "simian" posture. Seborrhea and sialorrhea are also noted. Dementia develops in about 10% to 15% of this population. Other neuropsychological problems mostly concern visuospatial dyspraxia. Autonomic dysfunction may include orthostatic hypotension, dysphagia, esophageal dysmotility, and constipation. Bladder and erectile dysfunction can occur in men.

As managed care continues to influence medical practice, more and more ill and disabled patients will be leaving acute care hospitals prior to total recovery. They will likely go to non–diagnostic-related group (DRG) rehabilitation services and hospitals while still in need of some acute services and interventions.

Acute care physicians are learning more of what rehabilitation physicians can offer to their patients. Earlier and more frequent rehabilitation consultations can be anticipated, to help in patients' overall management. As such, physiatrists may become more active in treating Parkinson disease and its associated problems. It is therefore incumbent on rehabilitation professionals to be familiar with all of its manifestations and clinical features.

HISTORY

"Paralysis agitans" or the "shaking palsy" was first described by James Parkinson in 1817 (1). In his classic manuscript, he described six patients with the syndrome that bears his name. They had a resting tremor, "inability of motion," and facial hypomimia, or the mask-like facies with a paucity of emotional expressivity therein. There was difficulty in walking and difficulty initiating movement. Even some of the nonmotor problems, for example, "torpid" (2) or sluggish bowels and sialorrhea, "with the saliva . . . continually trickling from the mouth," were noted. Food is "difficultly swallowed." He also noted its progressive course to total debility, sphincter incontinence, and death.

Parkinson reported that "the intellect is preserved," although it is now known that Parkinson disease is associated with dementia and other cognitive and emotional problems.

Symptomatic treatment began with Charcot, who used atropine in the 1870s. Erb used scopolamine at the start of the twentieth century (2). In the 1950s, the centrally acting anticholinergic medications were introduced and replaced the two alkaloids (2). They helped the tremor and sialorrhea but did little or nothing for the debilitating bradykinesia (2).

In 1967 and 1969, Cotzias et al (3,4) reported that levodopa was effective in the treatment of Parkinson disease (5–8). The dose had to be very low initially and raised slowly, as vomiting was the major side effect. Therapeutic daily doses required at least 3 g.

In 1975, Sinemet, a combination pill of levodopa and carbidopa, was released. Carbidopa is a peripheral dopa decarboxylase inhibitor. It markedly decreased the side effects and the dosage of levodopa necessary to achieve a therapeutic effect.

Through the latter half of the 1970s, motor fluctuations were documented as one of the late effects of the disease. Dopamine receptor agonists were effective in helping to smooth out the response.

In 1991 controlled-release Sinemet was released to try to smooth out the therapeutic effect with the primary drug.

In 1987 Madrazo et al (9) reported two successful graftings of fetal adrenal cells to the caudate nucleus of two Parkinson patients that resulted in significant improvement. While many centers could not duplicate their results, in 1992 Spencer et al (10) published a series of four patients from Yale University and McGill University who had successful unilateral intracaudate grafts of fetal mesencephalic tissue that improved their parkinsonian status.

Ventrolateral thalamotomy (11,12) has become useful in the treatment of intractable tremor. Medial (11) pallidotomy is useful in treating bradykinesia and in improving "on" time in patients with dyskinesias (13). Ventral pallidotomy (14–16) decreases dyskinesias and "off" time. The above studies (and others) have noted contralateral and ipsilateral improvement after unilateral pallidotomy.

ASSESSMENT SCALES

The most widely used scale is the one by Hoehn and Yahr (17). It incorporates the clinical features of the disease and is generally easy to remember. It is also discrete, as the presence or absence of particular features absolutely designates the clinical stage. In drug studies, significant improvement was designated as a lowering of stage rather than improvement within a stage.

The best description and the one most relevant for rehabilitation is provided by Hoehn (18) in her 1992 article describing the natural history of Parkinson disease in the pre- and post-levodopa era. It is of note that her scale was devised in the 1960s before the widespread use of levodopa. It has withstood the test of time and is quoted below.

> *Stage I*: *Unilateral* tremor, rigidity, akinesia or postural abnormalities only.
>
> *Stage II*: *Bilateral tremor, rigidity, akinesia, or postural abnormalities*, with or without axial signs, such as bilateral facial masking; speech and swallowing abnormalities; axial rigidity, especially of the neck; stooped posture; slow and occasionally shuffling gait; and generalized stiffness.
>
> *Stage III*: This stage is little different from stage II. All of the above-mentioned signs may be somewhat worse. The delineating factor, however, is that *patients show the first signs of deteriorating balance*. Even now, as was true when the scale was devised, this earliest sign of disequilibrium seems to presage the onset of disability in performing activities of daily living. At this stage, however, the *patients still are fully independent*. The usual test of balance is to pull the patient backwards abruptly from a standing stable position; the normal person will take at the most two steps backwards before regaining equilibrium, usually none or one. The parkinsonian patient who is losing the sense of balance will take two or more, maintaining an upright stance with difficulty. The patient at Stage III, however, still is fully independent in all activities of daily living
>
> *Stage IV*: This stage is reached when *the patient requires help with some or all activities of daily living and, even with effort, would be unable to live alone without some assistance.*
>
> *Stage V*: *The patient is confined to wheelchair or bed unless assisted.*

While the Hoehn and Yahr scale is essentially a clinical scale, numerous attempts have been made to have a reliable and functional activities of daily living (ADL) scale. The first such attempt was from England and Schwab in 1956 (19). It later became the Schwab and England scale (20). Other ADL-oriented scales were developed by Canter et al (21) (Northwestern University Disability Score), Alba et al (22), Webster (23), Duvoisin et al (24,25) (the "Columbia" scale), and Lieberman (26). (New York University Scale).

The generally accepted scale in use today is the Unified Parkinson's Disease Rating Scale (27), the latest edition of which was published in 1987. It is based on the Columbia scale and includes six sections:

I. Mentation, behavior, and mood
II. ADLs with indications for "on/off"
III. Motor examination
IV. Complications of therapy with events that occurred in the past week
    A. Dyskinesias
    B. Clinical fluctuations
V. Modified Hoehn and Yahr scale
    Which adds: Stage 1.5—unilateral and axial involvement
    Stage 2.5—mild bilateral disease with recovery on pull test
VI. Schwab and England ADL scale which rates dependence to independence as percentages 0% to 100%, with 100% being essentially normal. It attempts to assess a percentage of normal activity.

ANATOMIC AND BIOCHEMICAL CONSIDERATIONS

The specific biochemical abnormality in Parkinson disease is the depletion of dopamine from the corpus striatum (the caudate and putamen). These nuclei receive dopamine from efferent fibers from the substantia nigra pars compacta. This structure contains cell bodies that synthesize dopa (L-dihydroxyphenylalanine) from tyrosine. In Parkinson disease there is drop-out of at least 80% of these cells to cause a significant depletion in striatal dopamine.

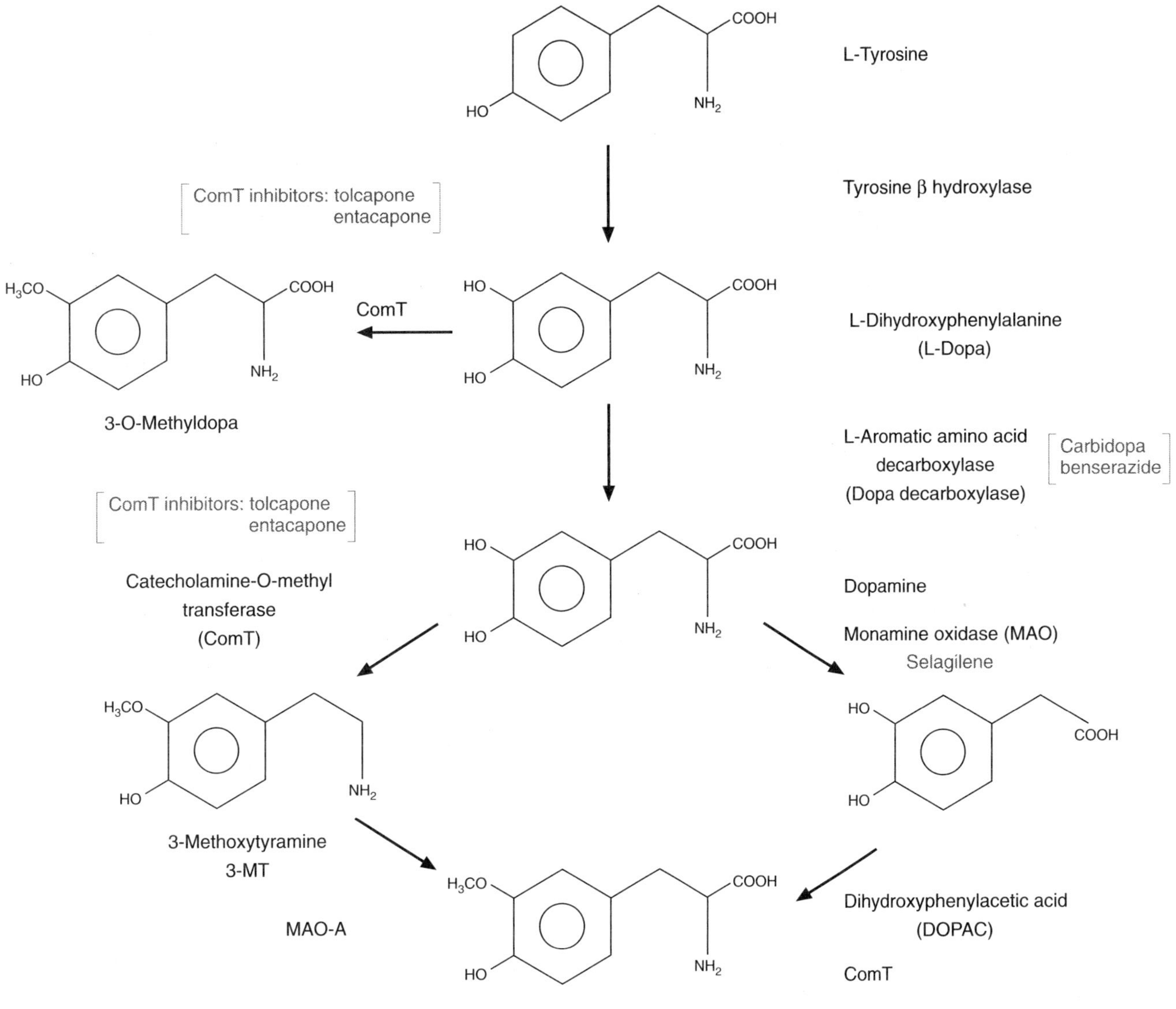

Figure 75-1. Biochemistry and sites of drug actions.

While dopamine is the major neurotransmitter, others are involved in the overall chemical balance within the basal ganglia (Fig. 75-1). The inhibitory neurotransmitters include gamma-amino-butyric acid (GABA), enkephalin, and substance P. The strictly stimulatory neurotransmitter is glutamate. Dopamine stimulates D_1 receptors and inhibits D_2 receptors.

The basal ganglia are a series of deep nuclei and their connections that comprise the seat of motor programming (Fig. 75-2). There are direct and indirect pathways to the major outflow nuclei: globus pallidus interna (GP_i) and substantia nigra pars reticulata (SN_r). They work in concert and will be discussed as a single functional unit: GP_i-SN_r.

GP_i-SN_r exerts an inhibitory influence on the ventrointerior and ventrolateral thalamic nuclei, which in turn stimulate the supplementary motor area prefrontal premotor, and primary motor cortex.

Under normal circumstances GP_i-SN_r is kept under inhibitory tone, which allows normal but not excessive movement. In hypokinetic disorders, e.g., Parkinson disease, GP_i-SN_r exerts relatively greater inhibitory tone, so that the VA/VL-cortical connections are relatively suppressed and the patient moves less. In hyperkinetic disorders, the GP_i-SN_r is itself inhibited, which allows increased activity of the thalamocortical connections, producing excessive movement.

CLINICAL FEATURES

The typical Parkinson patient likely to be seen in rehabilitation is moderately to severely disabled. As the syndrome

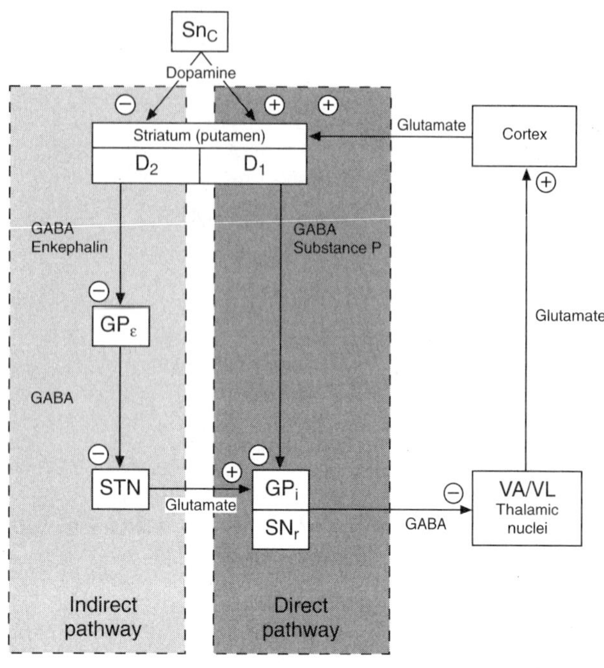

⊕ Stimulatory
⊖ Inhibitory
Sn$_C$ = substantia nigra pars compacta
GP$_\varepsilon$ = globus pallidus pars externa
GP$_i$ = globus pallidus pars interna
SN$_r$ = substantia nigra pars reticulata
VA/VL = ventroanterior/ ventrolateral thalamic nuclei
GABA = gamma aminobutyric acid

Figure 75-2. Basal ganglia circuits. The basal ganglia have direct and indirect pathways to the GP$_i$-SN$_r$. The direct system connects the putamen (D$_1$ receptor) to GP$_i$. In the intact individual, the putamen keeps GP$_i$-SN$_r$ relatively inhibited, thus allowing normal movement. The indirect pathway takes its origin from the putamen's D$_2$ receptors and exerts relative inhibition of the globus pallidus externa and the subthalamic nucleus. The latter stimulates the GP$_i$-SN$_r$ inhibitory complex. A lacunar stroke of the subthalamic nucleus produces hemiballismus, as a hyperkinetic dysinhibition. A more discrete surgical lesion has also been shown to help normalize movement in parkinsonism (167,168).

is well recognized, the physiatrist will not likely see any untreated patients in the virgin state. The physiatrist is more likely to see a patient with variable amounts of resting tremor, bradykinesia, flexed-forward ("simian") posture, impaired postural reflexes, and a festinating gait.

The classic resting tremor occurs at rest and is abolished by movement. It is often decreased by anticholinergic and dopaminergic medications and so is not reliably present or prominent in most treated patients. Many Parkinson patients also have an action tremor, which superimposes on any voluntary movement. Unlike cerebellar tremor, there is no overshoot of a target.

The resting tremor is generally not functionally disabling because it can be overcome with movement. However, many patients with early Parkinson disease find it cosmetically disturbing, especially if they are working and need to present a "perfect" picture at a job with a high public profile.

The major motor disabilities of Parkinson disease are bradykinesia and akinesia. This subtends the poverty of movement noted by Parkinson and other clinicians. The patient overall has difficulty initiating movement and decreased associated or secondary motions.

Bradykinesia most severely affects the initiation of movement and walking. The patient with moderately advanced disease has difficulty arising from a chair and often needs to use his or her arms to push himself or herself up. The patient does not have the usual associated movement of placing the feet under the chair to shift the center of gravity forward prior to lifting. Once standing, the patient has a flexed-forward or "simian" posture. He or she may or may not have difficulty initiating gait, but once started, it is a slow, cautious, moderately wide-based gait with small steps (marche à petits pas). The patient may suddenly stop at doorways but this is infrequent. More often, the patient may start out relatively slowly and then run with short steps, and may fall. With this festinating gait, the patient appears to be falling forward and then seems to race to catch up with his or her center of balance. It is a frequent cause of falls in the patient with advanced disease.

The patient's balance is easily disturbed due to the loss of postural reflexes. In the intact human, any postural perturbation or loss of balance causes a near-immediate correction to reorient the person over the center of gravity. Any step or misstep initiates the corrections that are believed to occur subconsciously through connections in the brain stem. Postural reflexes are defective in Parkinsonian patients, usually resulting in falls.

Turns are done en bloc. The intact person turns by leading with one leg and then turning the body to the new position. The Parkinson patient takes several small steps without any significant independent truncal motion. Falls can occur during turns.

Cogwheeling, a series of repetitive stops, may be elicited by passive flexion and extension of the muscles around the elbow joints. Cogwheeling is not disabling but is the defining feature of rigidity, the specific basal ganglia disorder of tone.

Patients with "motor fluctuations" demonstrate periods of decreased and increased unresponsiveness to their medications. There can be episodes of sudden transient freezing in which the patient approaches a threshold (e.g., a door) and stops in his or her tracks. Given the impaired postural reflexes, the patient may fall. Falls can be prevented by altering the environment. Parkinson patients seem better at stepping over floor markers, so high-contrast tape placed at appropriate intervals can help by altering the motor program.

While most patients may have periods of decreased responsiveness, others have periods of hyperkinesia that are choreoathetoid in nature. Some severely affected patients are nearly hemiballistic in their movements. These movements can usually be treated, but often not totally eradicated, with adjustments in the medication regimen (see Treatment).

Micrographia is another motor problem first noted by James Parkinson. The handwriting usually has a superimposed tremor and becomes progressively more illegible with poorly formed letters that get smaller and smaller. Facial hypomimia, as decreased facial expressivity referred to as the "mask-like facies," is another prominent motor feature.

Gait Studies

The Parkinson gait has been studied extensively (28). In a 1972 study, Knutsson (28) noted a decreased speed of forward progression due to decreased stride length and increased duration of each cycle. There was also an increased duration of double-limb support.

Knutsson also noted changes in joint excursions. The hip had decreased flexion but normal extension. The knee had both decreased flexion and extension. The ankle had decreased plantarflexion when it first touched the ground and decreased push off at the end of stance. There was also decreased to absent transverse motion of the pelvis (1).

Murray et al (29) reported short step lengths and wider strides. They found an overall slow velocity of gait in Parkinson patients but swing phases of about equal duration in normal and parkinsonian patients. In a later study, Blin et al (30) reported increased variability of stride duration and length in Parkinson patients.

In the normal walking cycle, the pelvis and thorax rotate in opposite directions in the horizontal plane. In the parkinsonian patient, the trunk and pelvis tend to rotate together (en bloc) as a single unit rather than in the thoracopelvic reciprocal pattern. However, the pattern tends to be normal in some, presumably less severely affected patients (29).

Parkinson patients have decreased hip flexion and excursion, which worsens as the disease progresses.

Falls

Patients with Parkinson disease fall. The simplest paradigm is due to the festinating gait in which patients with flexed posture run to keep up with their forwardly displaced center of gravity. This can result in a misstep or fall (31).

Koller et al (32) compared 100 patients with Parkinson gait disease to 5 patients with progressive supranuclear palsy. Thirty-eight Parkinson patients fell and 13% fell more than once a week. The incidence of serious fractures was 13%; hospitalization, 18%; and wheelchair confinement, 3%. The major predictive factor of falling in both groups was postural instability. Falling was also correlated with bradykinesia and rigidity but not tremor, sensory loss, dementia, heart disease, or antihypertensive medication. Pharmacotherapy had little if any effect. Physical therapy helped a few patients. Other significant features of patients who were more likely to fall were older age, longer disease duration (5.5 versus 10.1 years), higher Hoehn and Yahr stages (1.9 versus 3.03), worsened Schwab and England disability scores, worsened rigidity, worsened hand and foot agility, inability to arise from a chair, and gait impairment. The authors concluded that postural instability and falling are relatively resistant to levodopa treatment.

Orthostatic hypotension does occur with Parkinson disease. It is generally not as severe as in multisystem atrophy (Shy-Drager syndrome) but can still be clinically significant. In the study by Koller et al (32), while orthostatic hypotension was more frequent in the falling group, it was not believed to be a statistically significant factor.

A simple test for postural instability in elderly non-parkinsonian patients has been developed. It has obvious use among Parkinson patients. The subject is warned and given a modest thrust on the sternum. The number of steps the subject takes backward is counted, as a measure of retropulsion. Normal is considered one step backward. Two to four steps backward represents moderate impairment and more than four steps or a tendency to fall is rated as severe (33).

PHARMACOTHERAPY

The mainstay of treatment of Parkinson disease is pharmacotherapy. In the early stages of hemiparkinsonism with a resting tremor, one can use centrally acting anticholinergic medications. These are generally effective against tremor and sialorrhea as they decrease saliva production. However, a dry mouth may make speech more difficult and is uncomfortable for some patients. Nevertheless, many patients derive benefit from these medications.

Trihexyphenidyl (Artane) and benztropine (Cogentin) are used in the United States, with the former in more widespread use. Other medications in this class are procyclidine (Kemadrin) and biperiden (Akineton).

Trihexyphenidyl (34) is usually started at 0.5 to 1.0 mg orally twice daily and can be gradually increased to a dose of 2.0 mg orally twice a day. Other important side effects are memory impairment and confusion. Peripheral antimuscarinic side effects are tachycardia, blurred vision, nausea, urinary retention, decreased sweating, and temperature regulation. If these develop, the drug should be withdrawn gradually.

Amantadine can also be used for relatively mild Parkinson disease. The exact mechanism of action is not known, but it is believed to potentiate the action of dopamine. It appears to work on akinesia and rigidity but may not be as effective on tremor. The usual starting dose is 100 mg orally two times a day and usually goes up to 200 mg orally twice daily. The highest dose is 300 mg orally three times a day, although that would be unusual. Patients derive benefit from amantadine for about a year, after which time levodopa would be more effective (35).

Levodopa is much more helpful for bradykinesia, tremor, and rigidity. It is relatively less effective for axial motions, such as kneeling, turning around while supine (as in bed mobility), walking, and going from a supine to standing position. Lakke reported that bed mobility was relatively resistant to levodopa (36).

Selegiline (37,38) (Deprenyl, Eldepryl) is a monoamine oxidase B (MAOB) inhibitor and an antioxidant. In trials held through the late 1980s it was found to help in Parkinson disease and seemed to have a neuroprotective effect. It is dosed at 5 mg given orally at 8:00 AM and 12:00 PM, which generally inhibits MAOB for 24 hours at a time. The effect seems to work for about 1 to 2 years in patients in the early stages of Parkinson disease and may delay the onset of disability.

There is still some controversy as to when to start carbidopa-levodopa (Sinemet). Some start it early in the disease course. Most wait until stage II when bradykinesia and postural abnormalities begin. The usual starting dose is 25 mg of carbidopa with 100 mg of levodopa (sinemet 25/100) given orally three times a day. Carbidopa-levodopa works on the tremor but is more effective against the bradykinesia. It is best to give the medication while the patient is awake. Barring the need to use the bathroom at night, the patient does not need nighttime medication. As the short-acting combination takes 30 to 60 minutes to take effect, the caregiver may wish to give the medication about an hour prior to the patient's usual wake-up time. In the early stages of the disease, the effect of carbidopa/levodopa lasts about 4 to 6 hours. This duration progressively shortens and the interdose time may decrease to 2 to 3 hours.

Controlled-release carbidopa/levodopa was developed to try to make dosing easier and less frequent as the disease progressed. Its aim was to keep the dose schedule to every 4 hours or longer. The controlled-release formula is generally effective in keeping the blood levels of medication and neurologic function more even throughout the day. However, the generally slower release means a longer (60 minutes) time of onset of therapeutic effect. Many patients take controlled-release Sinemet 50/200 and regular Sinemet 25/100 so that they can be functional earlier before the longer-acting pill takes effect. If the patient goes to the bathroom within 4 to 6 hours of sleep, controlled-release Sinemet at bedtime is helpful. (Another approach is use of a bedside urinal or commode.)

Many practitioners prefer to start treatment with controlled-release Sinemet 25/100 orally twice a day. (Some older patients are very sensitive to side effects and may require lower initial doses.) Generally the long-acting preparation is less well absorbed and may require 20% to 30% more levodopa to achieve the same clinical response. Nevertheless, this preparation is easily titrated.

Motor fluctuations including on-off patterns, sudden transient freezing, and hyperkinesia may start to occur as early as 2 years and most often start at about 4 to 5 years. The easiest motor fluctuation to treat is the shortening of the therapeutic period. As already described, the length of time in which the medication works decreases. The usual treatment is to lower the dose slightly and decrease the interval of dosing. Another approach involves using a dopamine agonist.

Bromocriptine and pergolide are both alkaloids that directly stimulate dopamine receptors. Both also stimulate serotonin 1 and 2 receptors and α_1 adrenergic receptors about equally. They have relatively long periods of therapeutic effect and thereby can smooth out the clinical response. Bromocriptine with its 6- to 8-hour dosing schedule is also useful if the patient needs to walk at night. The usual starting dose is 1.25 or 2.5 mg orally every hour and additional 2.5 tablets are added every 3 to 7 days as tolerated. The usual effective total daily dose ranges from 5 to 15 mg. The maximum daily dose ranges from 30 to 50 mg divided into two or three doses. It can allow up to a 30% reduction of daily levodopa dose.

Pergolide (39) (Permax) is also dosed cautiously. (The usual catch phrase is low and slow.) It starts at 0.05 mg orally every day for the first 2 days and then can be increased by 0.1 to 0.15 mg/day every 3 days over the next 12 days. If it is tolerated well and the maximum therapeutic effect is not achieved, then the dose is raised by 0.25 mg orally every 3 days until the optimum therapeutic response is attained. Both bromocriptine and pergolide can produce hypotension and hallucinations. It is best to start the initial dose at bedtime.

Ropinirole (Requip), which was released in the United States in October 1997, stimulates D_3 more than D_2 receptors, but has no serotonergic or α-adrenergic effect. It is therefore much more specific. It is started at a low dose and raised over 4 weeks. The first week's dose is 0.25 mg orally 3 times a day. The second week is 0.50 mg 3 times a day, the third week is 0.75 mg 3 times a day and the fourth week is 1.0 mg 3 times a day. After the fourth week the dose is adjusted until the desired therapeutic response is achieved. The usual lower effective total daily dose is 4 mg, but many patients may require up to 24 mg a day (40). Once Ropinirole is up to therapeutic levels, the dose of carbidopa/levodopa can be reduced. Ropinirole can also be used as monotherapy.

Pramipexole (Mirapex), which was released on July 1997, also stimulates D_3 more than D_2 receptors with mild D_4 and α_2-adrenergic activity. It can be used with carbidopa/levodopa or as monotherapy. Pramipexole is started at 0.125 mg orally 3 times a day and is raised gradually over 7 weeks on a thrice-daily schedule. The recommended dosages are 0.25 mg 3 times a day for the second week, 0.5 mg 3 times a day for the third week 0.75 mg 3 times a day for the fourth week; 1.0 mg 3 times a day for the fifth week; 1.25 mg 3 times a day for the sixth week; and 1.5 mg 3 times a day for the 7th week. After that time, the medication is adjusted to achieve the desired therapeutic effect.

Generally, dopamine agonists are the preferred adjunctive medication for motor fluctuations. Later on carboxy-o-methyl transferase (COMT) inhibitors can be used. Their major effect is the peripheral inhibition of levodopa conversion to 3-o-methyldopa so that more gets into the brain. Tolcapone (Tasmar) (38,41) is dosed at 100 to 200 mg orally 3 times a day. Entacapone (Comtan) is usually dosed with each dose of levodopa. It is not yet released in the United States.

Levodopa is nearly totally absorbed in the gastrointestinal tract. If given alone, it must be converted to dopamine in the periphery. As dopamine does not cross the blood-brain barriers, only 30% of the original dose appears in the circulation and only 1% enters the brain.

Combination dosing of levodopa with a dopa decarboxylose inhibitor (e.g., Carbidopa or benserazide) allows 60% of levodopa to enter the circulation, but only 5% to 10% enters the brain. The major peripheral metabolite is 3-o-methyldopa by way of catechol-o-methyl transferase (COMT).

Further addition of a COMT inhibitor (tolcapone and entacapone) increases the amount of levodopa available to enter the striatum. Tolcapone works both peripherally and centrally in animal studies. However, it appears that the major pharmacologic effects are peripheral (42,43).

Cabergoline is a relatively new drug that is a direct dopamine receptor agonist. It is designed for once-a-day dosing. It is not used clinically in the United States.

In the late stages of Parkinson disease, great effort is directed to maintaining walking ability in the patient with progressively worsening disease who will ultimately become wheelchair bound. Motor fluctuations are the major problem that occurs in this period. The exact pathophysiology is not certain. Oral dopa crosses the blood-brain barrier and is converted to dopamine. In the intact human brain, native dopamine travels up axons directly to the target neurons and receptors in the caudate and putamen. In Parkinson disease, the exogenous dopa precursor is taken up by the target cells and other systems that contain the appropriate receptors. The exogenous dopamine may be stimulating other systems. Another theory postulates denervation hypersensitivity of the motor system neurons that overreact.

DIET

In the early stages, it is recommended that carbidopa-levodopa be taken with meals. Caloric intake should be relatively high at the upper limit of the age-related requirement (i.e., 30 mg/kg of ideal body weight). This is especially important if the patient is underweight. A daily calcium supplement of at least 800 mg is recommended, as are fiber supplements and fluids to prevent constipation (44).

In the later stage with motor fluctuations, it is more practical to restrict protein during the day and take levodopa at least 30 minutes prior to meals (1).

Mena and Cotzias (45) noted that a high-protein diet could produce the on-off effect. Protein restriction could improve this phenomenon. The authors found that the best response was in patients who consumed protein at 0.5 g/kg/day. It was considered adequate for adults over child-bearing age. Juncos et al (46) also documented that a high-protein meal blunted the effect of levodopa.

Further studies by Pincus with Barry (47,48) and Karstaedt (49) promulgated the protein redistribution diet. This diet entailed a severe restriction of dietary protein during the day to a total of 7 to 10 g. The evening meal was not restricted. This restriction restored "daytime sensitivity to levodopa"(5).

Levodopa is absorbed in the duodenum and proximal jejunum. Delayed gastric emptying can decrease the available amount of levodopa. Some types of dietary fiber can decrease gastric emptying. The gastric mucosa also contains dopa decarboxylase, which converts levodopa to dopamine, which cannot cross the blood-brain barrier. This conversion is significantly decreased with the use of dopa decarboxylase inhibitors (50). Nevertheless, in patients fed by nasoduodenal tubes, levodopa is very rapidly absorbed.

Levodopa absorption across the duodenal mucosa is accomplished by the L-neutral amino acid transport system. It is a stereospecific saturable active transport system that aids in the absorption of phenylalanine, tyrosine, tryptophan, leucine, isoleucine, valine, methionine, and histidine. High dietary protein intake produces increased competition for binding sites, which may decrease the absorption of levodopa. As stated earlier, this becomes especially important in the treatment of motor fluctuations.

Riley and Lang (51) also confirmed the efficacy of the low-protein diet. In order to achieve a restriction of 7 g during the day, one had to eliminate meat, dairy products, and foods with flour. The patients could have soup, fruits, vegetables, sweets, nondairy liquids, and nonprotein "bread"-type products made with wheat starch rather than wheat flour. The evening meals were not restricted. The diet overall was well tolerated and effective. Karstaedt and Pincus (49) reported that out of 43 patients, 30 (70%) were still on their diet for more than a year. Three patients with very severe disease had limited, if any, benefit. Ten patients stopped the diet but did have a positive therapeutic effect. Overall, the disability ratings improved and "on" time with a levodopa-mediated therapeutic effect increased. It is also of note that many patients developed chorea as an "overdose" effect of the diet (7,46,47). This effect was treated with reduction of the overall levodopa dosage.

In summary, management of late-stage motor fluctuations should include the following:

1. Give oral carbidopa-levodopa at least 30 minutes prior to each meal to avoid the effects of postprandial delayed gastric emptying.
2. Institute a generally decreased protein intake 0.8 to 1.6 g/kg/day (the lower the level, generally the better the response).
3. Try a protein redistribution diet, <7 g of protein for the period from awakening through the late afternoon. Supper is unrestricted.
4. Monitor weight and overall nutritional status. One may need to consult a nutritionist or dietitian.

REHABILITATIVE THERAPY

Prior to the advent of levodopa therapy for Parkinson disease, physical therapy was a major component of what could be offered to the patient. The dramatic improvement in most patients with levodopa replacement obviated a central role for physical therapy, although it is still believed to be useful.

A controlled trial of physical therapy for Parkinson disease by Comella et al (52) used a modification of the exercises by Wroe and Greer (53) that emphasized range of motion, balance, gait, and fine motor dexterity. The patients exercised 1 h/day, three times a week for 4 weeks. After 4 weeks, there were statistically significant improvements, but after the end of the program all of the patients stopped exercising. At 6-month follow-up they had lost all of their gains. The authors concluded that physical therapy was useful for moderately advanced Parkinson disease, but benefits were lost once the patients stopped exercising. Exercise seemed most helpful for rigidity and bradykinesia.

Most of the available sources emphasize essentially commonsense interventions to maintain muscle flexibility, range of motion, strength, and dexterity. Davis's Parkinson treatment protocols feature range of motion and flexibility exercises as well as balancing exercises that prepare for gait training (54).

As previous drug studies indicated that axial symptoms are relatively resistant to dopaminergic drug treatment, Davis's truncal exercises appear to be a significant complement to a complete approach. She also noted that members of her group had "particularly tight hip adductor and hamstring muscles."

Murray (55) in an article dated 1956 suggested a few therapeutic interventions that are still useful in gait training. The therapist asks the patient to walk a given distance and the therapist counts the number of steps. The therapist urges the patient to lengthen the stride to decrease the number of steps. Having the patient raise the knee and direct the heel forward helps. Placement of blocks for the patient to walk over is also suggested.

He also remarked on the flexed parkinsonian posture. In addition to trying to normalize gait, he suggested having the patient try to clasp the hands behind the back. This extends the thoracolumbar region of the spine and shifts the center of gravity posteriorly. It would reasonably facilitate an upright posture.

For bed mobility and going from a supine to sitting or standing position, he advised flexing the arms overhead and throwing them forward, having the trunk follow through to achieve sitting or upright posture.

A more recent post-levodopa study by Palmer et al (56) compared a United Parkinson's Disease Foundation exercise program to an upper-body karate program. Both groups of subjects showed improvement in all physical parameters, except for total body coordination.

Szekely et al (57) studied seven patients in Hoehn and Yahr stage II or III who participated in American Parkinson's Disease Association (APDA) exercise programs. They found statistical improvement in step length and average walking speed. The number of stand ups and sit downs they could do in 1 minute, as a measure of truncal mobility, was borderline significant. Arm and elbow reciprocation, finger flexion and extension, and the number of concentric circles drawn in 1 minute were improved but not at the statistically significant level. Balance, posture, and signature times did not improve. The authors also noted that group rather than individual exercises helped patients to motivate each other.

Kase and O'Riordan (58) spoke of a comprehensive approach including patients' families. They delineated seven major goals:

1. To maintain or increase active and passive range of motion, especially extension, and to prevent contractures by stretching tight muscles
2. To improve speed, flexibility, dexterity, and coordination of motor movements and repetitive tasks
3. To enhance awareness of posture and balance losses and correct where possible
4. To restore chest expansion/contraction not only as an end in itself, but to encourage relaxation and increase voice volume
5. To review gait with particular emphasis on increasing step length, widening the base of support, increasing the range of hip flexion, enhancing reciprocal arm movements, and improving stops, starts, and turns
6. To upgrade activities of daily living, teach simplification of tasks and conservation of energy techniques for the patient and caregiver
7. To function as a support, teacher, and information source for the patient, family, and medical team.

Schenkman et al (59) proposed a program comprising:

1. Relaxation
2. Breathing exercises
3. Passive muscle stretching positioning
4. Active range of motion and postural alignment
5. Weight shifting
6. Balance response
7. Gait activities
8. Patient home exercises

Stefaniwsky and Bilowit (60) in a 1973 study, showed that sensory stimuli and training could decrease the reaction time from stimulus onset to the initiation of movement. The tested motion was elbow extension. While this finding implied that training helps overcome bradykinesia, no studies have shown improvement generalized to the entire patient.

Knott (61) reported in 1957 a technique called *pumping up* in which the limb to be exercised is passively moved through the activity several times prior to the patient doing it on his or her own. The patient then does it as an active-assisted exercise and finally on his or her own. Knott reported that once the patient could do it on his or her own, the preparatory pumping up exercises could be stopped. Cold packs and compresses were also needed to help ease treatment by decreasing tone.

An English controlled trial of physical therapy completed in 1981 found that "remedial therapy" in a hospital outpatient department was not helpful for patients whose condition was stable and whose medications did not require an adjustment. The authors did allow that physical therapy "might help those who are rapidly deteriorating and in whom several factors might be leading to increasing disability" (62).

An early study of physical therapy for Parkinson disease by Bilowit (63) emphasized rhythmic motion. A punching bag was used in one exercise regimen to enhance flexion of the outstretched arms. Ultimately, the patients learned to jab the bag alternately to increase overall proximal, bilateral upper-extremity flexibility. Another exercise involving simultaneous shoulder flexion and elbow extension was catching a ball, which overall seemed easier for the patients rather than trying to do the specific motions.

For lower-extremity mobility, stair climbing (for those who could) and kicking a volleyball or soccer ball were helpful. Throwing and catching a large ball was similarly helpful for upper-extremity and truncal mobility.

According to Stelmach et al (64), Parkinson patients do not prepare movements as well as normal people and the problems are associated with controlling movement execution. Parkinsonian patients are not slower in judging distance or using the information for motor tasks.

Parkinson patients are sensitive to visual cues. Even back in 1956, placing blocks on the floor for the patient to step over was used in therapy. They helped normalize gait (63). Two reports described use of an inverted walking stick as a visual cue to enhance gait and overcome "freezing." Dunne et al (65) found it helpful in their two patients. Dietz et al (66) noted that only two of eight patients found the inverted walking stick helpful. The gait in six of the eight worsened. However, "initial success with the visual cue stick accurately predicted long-term benefit." Conversely if it did not help in the early phase, further training therewith was reasonably contraindicated.

Frozen shoulder is a significant musculoskeletal problem that occurs in Parkinson disease. Riley et al (67) studied 150 patients compared to 60 age-matched controls. Frozen shoulder occurred in 12.7% compared to 1.7% in the control group. It generally occurred in the arm more severely affected by rigidity and was more likely to develop in patients whose initial symptom was rigidity rather than tremor. Eight percent of patients developed a frozen shoulder in a 2-year period *prior* to the onset of Parkinson disease. While therapies were not discussed, it is assumed that they were treated with dopaminergic and other medications plus appropriate rehabilitative interventions.

SPEECH AND SPEECH THERAPY

The characteristic speech of Parkinson disease is a hypokinetic dysarthria in which the patient speaks in a low volume, at a rapid rate, and with diffuse articulatory imprecision. The voice may start out relatively strong at the beginning of a sentence and by the end may trail off into a low-volume jumble of sounds.

In a 1973 review article, Critchley (68) wrote a succinct overview of normal human speech and its parkinsonian deviations. In normal human speech, the vocal cords adduct and vibrate, either in segments or throughout their entire length. Tone is produced by expelling air in rapid puffs. Pitch varies with the duration of closed contact of the vocal cords.

In Parkinson disease, there is a breakdown of prosody and its component features. Vocal tone can be "breathy," harsh, and low pitched. There can also be incomplete glottal closure and faulty abduction and adduction of the vocal cords. In the early stages of the disease, with mild impairment, there is prompt abduction for inspiration and slow adduction for phonation. In the later severe stages, there is overall decreased vocal cord motion and associated tremor.

Logemann et al (69) in a study of 200 patients with Parkinson disease, noted that 178 (89%) had laryngeal disorders, including breathiness, hoarseness, roughness, and tremulousness of the voice. Ninety (45%) had articulation disorders involving coordination of tongue and lip movements, separately and together. Forty (20%) of the patients had abnormalities in the rate of speech. Hypernasality occurred in 20 (10%). Twenty-two (11%) of the sample patients had "no vocal tract disorders." Many of the patients had combinations of the above-mentioned disorders.

Another significant problem in Parkinson patients is dysprosody. Scott et al (70) reported that parkinsonian patients are unable to appreciate the prosodic features of speech in themselves or in others. This especially involves intonation and its affective import. They seem to have the greatest difficulty in recognizing and producing interrogative or angry statements. They also have difficulty recognizing and interpreting facial expression, which is believed to be an adjunctive component of their overall communication difficulty.

An early article on speech therapy by Sarno (71) in the pre-levodopa era concluded that speech therapy was not helpful overall. The patients could do well while in the therapeutic sessions but did not maintain their gains outside of therapy. Fortunately, things have improved.

With the advent of levodopa therapy, speech can improve as can all other motor functions. An early study by Rigrodsky and Morrison (72) noted a "trend in the direction of improved speech during L-dopa therapy," but this was less dramatic than the improvement in motor symptoms. In the early days of levodopa therapy, it was necessary to raise the medication gradually to avoid the major adverse effects of nausea and vomiting. As such, it was felt that speech might have further improved if the patients could have been followed to the point of maximal therapeutic dosing.

Nakano et al (73) reported that levodopa improved the intelligibility of speech, especially regarding labial sounds, and allowed faster and more natural lip movement.

Studies in the 1980s (74–77) showed that intensive 2-week speech therapy programs could produce sustained improvements in speech, especially prosody and its component parts (variation of intonation, pitch, volume, rate, and rhythm) for up to 3 months and sometimes up to 6 months.

A more recent study published in 1996 (78) compared two treatment regimens. One used breathing treatment and the other the Lee Silverman Voice Treatment (LSVT) program, which seeks to increase vocal intensity by increasing phonation and vocal volume. The patients attended 16 sessions over a 1-month period. The breathing treatment group had no sustained improvement. The LVST group had sustained benefit through 12 months after the end of the formal therapy.

AUTONOMIC DYSFUNCTION

Parkinson disease is typified by its peculiar motor dysfunction. However, it is not exclusively a motor disease. Various vegetative abnormalities affect blood pressure, gastrointestinal function, bladder function, sweating, and sexual function.

A survey of autonomic dysfunction by Singer et al (79) evaluated 48 patients with Parkinson disease and compared them with 32 healthy elderly non-Parkinson men. The mean age of the patients was 65.8 years, with a mean disease duration of 8 years. The mean age of the normal subjects was 70.4 years old.

The major statistically significant abnormalities are listed in Table 75-1.

Table 75-1: Statistically Significant Abnormalities in Autonomic Function

	Parkinson Patients	Controls
Erectile dysfunction	60.4%	37.5%
Sensation of incomplete bladder emptying	41.6%	15.6%
Urinary urgency	45.8%	31.25%
Constipation	43.9%	6.25%
Dysphagia	22.9%	6.25%
Orthostatic dizziness	21.95%	0%

Source: Singer C, Weiner WJ, Sanchez-Ramos JR. Autonomic dysfunction in men with Parkinson's disease. *Eur Neurol* 1992;32:134–140.

Sweating and Thermoregulation

Appenzeller and Goss (80) examined 25 patients and found that in 17, sweating was reduced in the body but increased in the face and armpits.

Goetz et al (81) also studied sweating. Before medication, patients had increased sweating on the head and neck and the general skin temperature was cooler. After medication, skin temperature alterations and sweating abnormalities resolved.

Blood Pressure Abnormalities

The results of studies are contradictory but it appears that Parkinson patients tend to have low blood pressure and the abnormalities therewith. Aminoff and Wilcox (82), in their 1971 study, found that parkinsonian patients have low resting blood pressure and 3 of 11 had "supersensitivity to intravenous norepinephrine," which implied a central adrenergic defect. In an earlier study, Barbeau et al (83) also reported low blood pressure in Parkinson disease, probably due to low renin activity and low serum aldosterone. They also noted that levodopa treatment lowered renin and aldosterone levels in patients. Patients taking daily doses of 3 to 5 g of levodopa had very low to virtually absent levels of these hormones. This was also believed to underlie the symptom of orthostatic hypotension.

Orthostatic hypotension does occur in Parkinson disease patients. It is not a primary feature and rarely is it disabling. (Orthostatic hypotension is a primary symptom of multisystem degeneration, a full discussion of which is beyond the scope of this chapter.)

Gross et al (84) examined the blood pressures of 20

Parkinson patients less than 63 years old. Supine blood pressure was normal but there was a great decrease in mean blood pressure on tilting when compared to the pressure in age-matched controls. The authors also believed that this implied a central adrenergic defect.

Levodopa treatment can also produce orthostatic hypotension. The earliest such study by McDowell and Lee (85) reported generally lower resting blood pressures in Parkinson patients compared to controls. In their series of 100 patients, 25 developed significant orthostasis with blood pressure drops ≥30 mm Hg or systolic blood pressure ≤80 mm Hg. Surprisingly, very few patients were symptomatic. Only 4 complained of orthostatic light-headedness and only 2 experienced syncope. Orthostatic hypotension occurred early in treatment and gradually resolved. The treatments originally suggested by McDowell and Lee (85) are still in current use: elastic stockings, ephedrine, increased sodium intake, and fludrocortisone.

Ballantyne (86) confirmed the above-cited findings. His 1973 study found a significantly decreased resting supine mean blood pressure and heart rate after 4 weeks of treatment with levodopa. By 6 months, the supine mean blood pressure had returned to normal despite a persistent mean decreased heart rate. There was no increase in the incidence of postural hypotension at 4 weeks or 6 months.

Postprandial hypotension has also been noted (87). This is believed to be due to shunting of blood to the splanchnic bed. The usual treatment is frequent smaller meals (88).

Goetz et al (80) studied 16 men and 16 women with Parkinson disease who had autonomic dysfunction, before and after medication. The mean age was 61 years (range, 44–80); the mean duration of symptoms, 10 years and 3 months (range, 14 years 8 months–18 years); and the mean Hoehr and Yahr stage, 3.1. Before medication, Parkinson patients compared to controls had elevated resting heart rates, greater orthostatic falls in blood pressure, and decreased responses to the Valsalva maneuver and cold pressure stimuli. After medication, the cardiovascular reflex abnormalities remained but were no worse.

A related study by Van Dijk et al (89) found that patients with early and mild disease who were on no medications had no evidence of autonomic dysfunction. Abnormal blood pressure responses were recorded in response to standing and hand grip. Worsened autonomic function correlated with higher Hoehn and Yahr stages and increased age.

In a relatively recent study, Irwin et al (90) evaluated blood pressure responses to levodopa in Parkinson patients. The higher the resting blood pressure, the greater were the hypotensive effects. The therapeutic effects of levodopa seemed to parallel its hypotensive effects. Phenylalanine, which competes with levodopa to cross the blood-brain barrier, decreased the therapeutic motor and hypotensive effect. (Both cross the blood-brain barrier through the L-neutral amino acid transport system.)

Gastrointestinal Disorders

Parkinson disease has significant gastrointestinal problems, the most common of which are dysphagia and constipation. A major study (91) listed the frequency of complaints (Table 74-2).

Oropharyngeal Disorders in Parkinson Disease

Dysphagia and sialorrhea together make oropharyngeal problems the most common gastrointestinal difficulties in Parkinson disease. Although the term sialorrhea implies excessive secretion of saliva, this is not the case. Impaired swallowing underlies the excessive oral pooling of saliva.

The earliest signs of sialorrhea are drooling at night, then daytime drooling. Anticholinergic medications work well on this symptom, but dry mouth can result, making swallowing more difficult. Sialorrhea has been reported in at least 70% of patients (92,93).

Dysphagia occurs in at least 50% of patients versus 6% of age-matched controls (91). The numbers vary among studies. In Parkinson disease, it also seems to affect solids more than liquids (94).

Swallowing comprises oral, pharyngeal, and esophageal phases. The oral phase has significant volitional and automatic component functions. The latter two phases are essentially involuntary and are felt to be under brainstem control.

The oral phase prepares the food bolus for digestion and transit to the pharynx. Normally the medial and posterior segments of the tongue blade elevate to "squeeze" the bolus posteriorly to the pharynx. In Parkinsonian patients, these tongue segments do not elevate sufficiently to move the bolus effectively to the back of the throat. Instead, there is a "rocking-like motion" (95). It usually takes two to five such motions to finally propel the food into the pharynx (95). When rocking propels small parts of the single bolus posteriorly, it produces a relatively inefficient "piece-meal deglutition (96). Repetitive tongue

Table 75-2: Frequency of Gastrointestinal Disorders

Disorder	Frequency
Abnormal salivation	70.2%
Defecatory dysfunction	65.9%
Dysphagia	52.1%
Bloating	50%
Heartburn	45%
Constipation	28.7%
Nausea	24.4%
Emesis	10%
Abdominal pain	29%

Source: Edwards LL, Pfeiffer RF, Quigley EMM, et al. Gastrointestinal symptoms in Parkinson's disease. *Mov Disord* 1991;6:151–154.

pumping describes abnormal tongue motion in progressing the bolus (95). The patient requires several lingual pumps to push portions of the food posteriorly, rather than one single efficient action transferring the entire bolus posteriorly. It is also understood that slow and overall abnormal tongue motion can result in poor bolus formation (94).

While dysphagia is quite common, a minority of patients complain about it. A study by Logemann et al (97) reported that 15% to 20% of her patients complained of difficulty swallowing while 95% had abnormalities by cineradiography. Overall there was slowed transit time in the oral, pharyngeal, and esophageal phase.

A study of 16 asymptomatic patients (98) reported 3 with aspiration and 14 with vallecular residue and therefore at risk for aspiration. Prolonged transit times and lingual dysmotility, especially pumping, were reported.

A later study by Bushmann et al (99) confirmed that patients without complaints of dysphagia frequently had abnormal swallows and silent aspiration. Most patients improved with levodopa.

Bedside swallowing evaluation was not absolutely predictive of swallowing abnormalities. Modified barium swallow is the standard. Johnston et al (94) recommended neck flexion to close off the trachea and prevent aspiration. Bushmann et al (99) taught her patients a modification of the supraglottic swallow to prevent aspiration. She advised her patients to hold their breath, tilt their chins to their chests, swallow, cough to clear material from the pharynx, then swallow again.

Logemann (100) had described supraglottic swallowing but used it to protect the airway in conditions in which there was impaired posterior propulsion of a food bolus. In her protocol of the patient with reduced tongue elevation, she advised the patient to take a breath, hold it, place the food in the mouth, tilt head backwards, swallow, then cough.

Thermal sensitization of the anterior faucial arches with a cold object might also be helpful. In a series of 25 patients with neurologic diseases, the single Parkinsonian patient had significantly improved pharyngeal transit time for paste, going from 12.7 seconds to 0.5 seconds (normal oral and pharyngeal transit times are typically ≤1 second) (101).

Esophageal Disorders

Esophageal dysmotility (102) occurs in Parkinson disease patients. Not all swallows produce effective primary peristaltic waves to conduct food to the stomach. Subcutaneous injection of 3 mg of apomorphine can improve esophageal efficiency. Most swallows can produce primary waves that empty barium into the stomach.

Gastroesophageal reflux (103) has also been reported, as has esophageal dilatation (104). Lewy bodies have been found in the esophagus. In the series of Qualman et al (105), Lewy bodies were found in the distal ganglion cells in the single patient who had them in the esophagus. Another parkinsonian patient had Lewy bodies in the colonic myenteric plexus. Lewy bodies have been found not only in the substantia nigra but also in the dorsal motor nucleus of the vagus nerve, among other locations (106,107). It is believed that most of the gastrointestinal problems in Parkinson disease have central and local defects underlying their dysmotility syndromes.

Gastric Dysfunction

Gastric emptying is delayed in Parkinson disease. There are conflicting reports on the effects of levodopa. Harada et al (108) reported improvement with dopaminergic agents, but Muller-Lissner et al (109) reported that dopamine slows gastric emptying. Regarding the latter, cisapride has been shown to be helpful. It increases the release of acetylcholine from the postganglionic nerve endings in the stomach wall. Metoclopramide (Reglan), a peripheral and central dopamine receptor antagonist should not be used because it can worsen parkinsonism.

Delayed or erratic gastric emptying has been implicated in the etiology of motor fluctuations (110,111) in patients. Kurlan et al (110) studied one patient with motor fluctuations. Standard oral therapy produced unpredictable motor function. When medication was delivered by nasoduodenal tube, the patient had predictable 60- to 90-minute periods of good motor function after each dose. Plasma levodopa concentrations were well correlated with the therapeutic effect.

A study by Djaldetti et al (112) reported that Cisapride decreased the latency from medication ingestion to onset of therapeutic effect ("on" time) from about an hour to about 45 minutes for both morning and evening doses of levodopa. Patients who suffered "no-on" type fluctuations in which a dose of levodopa produced no therapeutic effect, experienced fewer such dose failures.

In a subsequent study, Djaldetti et al (111) found delayed gastric emptying in 70% of their patients. Gastric retention and emptying were worse in the group with motor fluctuations. It was also thought that delayed or erratic gastric emptying contributed significantly to motor fluctuations.

Bowel Disorders

Constipation is another significant gastrointestinal complaint in Parkinson disease. Constipation is generally defined as ≤3 bowel movements per week (91). Transit time is generally increased and Lewy bodies have been found in nerve cells of the myenteric plexus (113). Given that the dorsal motor nucleus of the vagus nerve might be similarly affected, there may be local and central influences on bowel dysfunction.

Early reports (114,115) described the occurrence of megacolon and sigmoid volvulus in Parkinson disease. Both studies documented patient use of anticholinergic medications that can interfere with bowel motility. Both groups withdrew these medications as part of the treatment. A

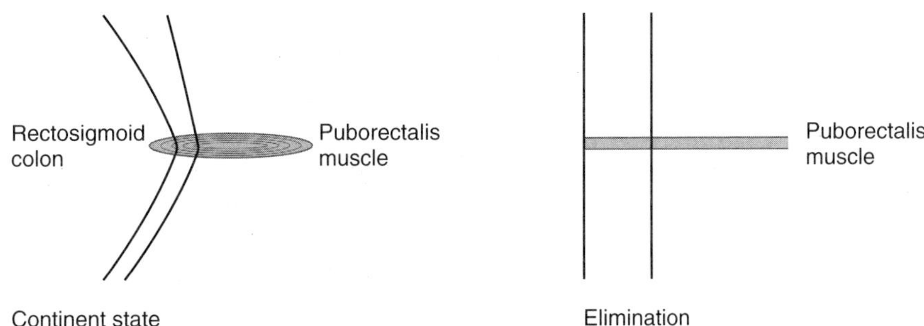

Figure 75-3. In the continent state the puborectalis muscle is contracted, increasing the rectosigmoid angle, which allows continence. In defecation, the puborectalis muscle relaxes, which allows straightening of the rectosigmoid angle. Gravity facilitates emptying of stool. In Parkinson disease, there can be a dystonic contraction of the puborectalis muscle, creating a functional obstruction.

1987 study of four patients with sigmoid volvulus indicated that parkinsonian patients are still at risk for it (116).

Jost and Schimrigk (117) documented prolonged colonic passage of 5 to 7 days in their study of colonic transit time. Most of their radiopaque pellets arrived in the colon by 24 hours, but were held up in the large bowel. This would be an example of "colonic inertia or slow transit constipation" (1) in which native colonic muscular dysfunction slows fecal transport.

Parkinsonian patients also have "outlet-type dysfunction" (1) in which transit time is essentially normal, but defecation is difficult (Fig. 75-3). They have a peculiar disorder of defecation in which there is a paradoxical contraction of the puborectal muscle (118,119). This usually occurs in patients with relatively advanced disease. The human external anal sphincter comprises the pelvic floor muscles, which can voluntarily contract to maintain continence. There is no anatomic internal sphincter, but there is a "functional" sphincter. The puborectal muscle is tonically contracted to maintain the rectoanal angle and therefore maintain continence. With volitional elimination, the pelvic floor musculature is relaxed and so is the puborectal muscle, which then allows straightening of the rectoanal angle and downward movement of the fecal contents. An inability to relax the puborectal muscle would create a functional obstruction. Mathers et al (119) treated affected patients with apomorphine.

Apomorphine has proven helpful in treatment of their problem (119,120). Mathus et al (119) used 3 to 10 mg of apomorphine. Subcutaneously, Edwards et al (120) used 6 mg by the same route. Both groups were pretreated with domperidone to prevent nausea and vomiting. Where domperidone cannot be used, Ligan can be substituted.

Urologic Problems

The major urologic abnormality in Parkinson disease is detrusor hyperreflexia (121–129). The usual symptoms are urgency incontinence, followed by hesitancy with a poor stream. Some patients may have both symptoms. Acute retention is relatively rare (3,9).

Fitzmaurice et al (123) studied 10 men with Parkinson disease. Eight had detrusor hyperreflexia. Five were worse during levodopa treatment and 3 were worse while off medications. Three patients had high residual volumes (incomplete emptying). Sphincter study results were normal. The retention was believed to be due to prostatic obstruction.

Urodynamic studies by Pavlakis et al (125) found detrusor hyperreflexia with external sphincter relaxation to occur in 75% of their patients. This combination is similar to an uninhibited bladder and sphincter, which could produce incontinence. The striated muscles of the pelvic floor demonstrated two types of EMG abnormalities. One was "pseudo-dyssynergia" (7%), which was a voluntary contraction to maintain continence against an overactive detrusor. The other was sphincter bradykinesia (11%), in which the skeletal muscle maintained tone during the initial phase of bladder contraction. It behaved like all other voluntary muscles in Parkinson disease, but here caused a physiologic type of outlet obstruction.

In patients with incomplete voiding, urinary tract infections may develop, and may worsen bladder irritability (126). Raz (127) found that levodopa helped coordinate bladder and sphincter function and reduced the urethral closing pressure, thus allowing bladder emptying. Treatment options varied. In patients with prostatic obstruction, surgery was recommended. However, not all patients became asymptomatic. Those with continued symptoms of urgency and leakage were given oxybutynin (Ditropan) or other anticholinergic medications. If these were not successful, condom catheter drainage was recommended (128). Biofeedback was helpful to a few who could learn to suppress involuntary detrusor contractions (128).

Christmas et al (129) reported that subcutaneous apomorphine as a dopamine receptor agonist was helpful in patients with difficulty voiding due to external sphincter bradykinesia. Apomorphine was believed to relax these muscles to allow passage of the urine stream. Its effects on the detrusor were variable: Some patients had improved detrusor function and others had worsened hyperreflexia.

If apomorphine produces a good urine flow rate,

then the patient has a physiologic obstruction and prostatectomy is not indicated. It is advised to use apomorphine at bedtime to accomplish, if possible, complete bladder emptying and avoid nocturia.

Detrusor areflexia is rare (8%–10%) (129) and is often of indeterminate etiology. It might cause a distended bladder with overflow incontinence. Multisystem degeneration is one cause that should be investigated. Sotolongo (126) reported that chronic outlet obstruction can also cause distention and areflexia. It is important to differentiate the two etiologies of neurogenic (denervation) areflexia and myogenic areflexia in which the innervated bladder becomes overstretched. A neurogenic areflexic bladder should be treated by intermittent catheterization. A myogenic areflexic bladder should recover its function once the chronic distention ceases (126); however, recovery can take several weeks and intermittent catheterization may be required in the interim.

Treatment of detrusor hyperreflexia without significant obstruction should respond to anticholinergics, for example, oxybutynin, 5 mg orally three times a day, or imipramine (Tofranil), 25 mg orally three times a day. They may produce dry mouth, which could help with sialorrhea or worsen problems with eating and speech.

Detrusor hyperreflexia with external sphincter bradykinesia and incomplete emptying may require bladder paralysis with anticholinergic medication and intermittent catheterization every 6 to 8 hours.

Sexual Disorders

As with any chronic neurologic disease, parkinsonism affects sexual function. A survey by Koller et al (130) evaluated 50 patients, 36 men and 14 women, at a mean age of 67.3 years. The mean duration of the disease was 6.96 years. Among the male respondents, 80% had decreased sexual frequency compared to the premorbid period; 44%, decreased sex drive and interest; 54% were impotent (described as a gradual decrease in function); 14% could maintain an erection; 60% denied nocturnal erection; 67% had an absence of morning erection; 50% (approximately) could not ejaculate; 70% had a more difficult time achieving arousal; 74% had a decreased frequency of arousal; and 19.4% had depression.

Among the women, 79% had decreased sexual frequency compared to the premorbid period; 71%, decreased sexual interest; 62%, reduction in sex drive; 38% could not achieve orgasm; 38% had vaginal dryness during intercourse; 67%, greater difficulty getting aroused; 75%, decreased frequency of arousal; and 7.17%, depression.

Thirty-five (70%) male patients had evidence of autonomic nervous system dysfunction and two-thirds of those patients had sexual problems. All patients were on medication.

These findings agree with those of other studies. Singer (131) reported that 60% of male patients had erectile dysfunction, compared to 38% of age-matched healthy control subjects. Previous alcohol use was also a significant risk factor in their study.

In a study of relatively young Parkinson patients, Wermuth and Stenager (132) evaluated 15 men and 10 women 36 to 56 years old. Overall 14 reported changed sexual function. Seven women (70%) versus 4 men (27%) noted reduced libido. Eight women (80%) versus 5 men (33.4%) reported decreased sexual activity after the onset of the disease. Three men (20%) reported erectile dysfunction. Depression did not seem to be a significant factor.

Lipe et al (133) compared married men with Parkinson disease to married men with arthritis. The types of arthritis included rheumatoid, psoriatic, and osteoarthritis involving more than two joints. The parkinsonian men were in Hoehn and Yahr stages I through IV. The average duration of the disease was 6 years. Most were on levodopa. As severity of illness for both groups increased, sexual function decreased. Age and depression were two other significant factors in decreasing sexual function. Lipe et al (133) concluded that the Parkinson disease group and arthritis group were more similar than not in their sexual dysfunction.

Brown et al (134) reported that both patients and nonaffected partners had sexual dissatisfaction and noted that noncommunication was a major issue. Men were still noted to have significant difficulties with impotence and premature ejaculation, but this report emphasized interpersonal relational issues.

According to a report by Golbe (135) on pregnancy in Parkinson disease. Women, the majority of those who completed pregnancies (10/17) had permanent worsening of their disease but their disability was not significantly worsened. Amantadine was used in four pregnancies and produced pre-eclampsia, vaginal bleeding, and two miscarriages. Nevertheless, in the entire series there was no significant increase in the rate of obstetric complications and fetal defects.

DEMENTIA AND COGNITIVE CHANGES

Dementia occurs in about 10% to 15% of patients with Parkinson disease. The incidence rises such that by the age of 85 years, the incidence of dementia in Parkinson disease is 65% (136). Several trends have been noted comparing demented versus nondemented parkinsonian patients. The demented group generally had later onset of symptoms, increased incidence of dystonic dyskinesia, and a worsened response to levodopa (137). Another study found that more severe bradykinesia, visuospatial dyspraxia, and psychomotor slowing were correlated with an increased risk of dementia (138).

While patients with early disease, usually of less than 2½ years' duration, are not generally demented, they do demonstrate cognitive defects (139–143). There is overall decreased cognitive flexibility and perseveration. Parkinsonian patients are unable to switch mental "sets," be they tasks or thinking styles. Therefore, they may continue a process from a previous task that is inappropriate for the new one at hand.

In the Modified Wisconsin Card-Sorting Test, which requires the patient to switch formats by suppressing previous right answers for new ones, Lees and Smith (140) found that parkinsonian patients completed fewer categories within the fixed number of cards for this test. Psychomotor skills are impaired (141). Reaction times are about 30% longer than control times. There are mild deficits in secondary memory, especially serial recall (142).

The above-mentioned cognitive findings and cluster of symptoms parallel work that implies two different subgroups of Parkinson disease (144–146). The group that was tremor dominant tended to have a better response to medication, younger age at onset, and better preservation of mental status. The other group has been referred to as having postural instability and gait difficulty (PIGD). This group has later onset, worse bradykinesia, and more often, cognitive decline.

Slowed acquisition of new material interferes with learning. This can be overcome with repetition of the information. Overall, language function is well preserved.

Visuospatial defects are also prominent in Parkinson disease. Proctor et al (147) noted that patients have impaired judgment of vertical postural orientation of their own bodies.

In later work, Bowen et al (148) found that patients with predominantly left-sided or symmetric motor involvement made more mistakes in identifying body parts. Patients who had more pronounced right-sided motor difficulties, and by extension, worsened left-sided brain function, did about as well as control subjects, except for identifying body parts in contralateral orientation to a presented test figure.

The above-mentioned deficits correlate with the general understanding of visuospatial or constructional apraxia being a right parietal lobe function. Bowen et al (149) also reported that parkinsonian patients with preferential left body or symmetric motor involvement had significant difficulties guiding themselves with a map. Patients with predominant right-sided motor symptoms did about as well as control subjects.

Parkinsonian patients also have difficulty tracking objects. In an experiment by Flowers (150), patients tracked a moving target across a screen in a ramp or sawtooth pattern. Tracking performance worsened during the period when the target disappeared. This was believed to indicate a failure to generate and use predictive strategies.

Other right-sided brain deficits are an inability to distinguish embedded figures in an overall design and difficulties with facial recognition (151).

A recommended neuropsychological testing battery for Parkinson patients would include examinations for dementia, immediate and delayed recall, verbal fluency, set (cognitive) shifting, spatial orientation, depression, and micrographia. Much of this information has practical application in driving, in which one needs to predict the direction of other cars and pedestrians and find one's way with or without a map. In a study of 150 Parkinson patients, 30 stopped driving because of their disease, although the precise reason was not given (152). While there was no increase of lifetime accidents in parkinsonian patients compared to normal subjects, it did appear that fewer patients drove less with a proportionately increased number of accidents. Most parkinsonian patients tended to drive larger vehicles, drive below the speed limit, avoid rush hour traffic, and do 90% of their driving in the daylight.

It is also understood that the average Parkinson patient has prolonged reaction and movement times. The difficulty changing cognitive sets would obviate quick decisions that could help avoid accidents.

DEPRESSION

Depression has been estimated to occur in 47% of the Parkinson population. While some authors felt that it may contribute to cognitive dysfunction (153), most other studies of parkinsonian dementia stated that depression appears to be an independent variable. The male-female ratio according to Dooneief et al (154) is 7:2.

The depression responds to the usual medications; however, there are reports of fluoxetine (155,156) (Prozac) and fluvoxamine (157) (Luvox) producing a worsening of parkinsonism. While these drugs are essentially serotonin reuptake inhibitors, a dopamine antagonistic mechanism is postulated.

In certain cases of intractable depression, electroconvulsive therapy (ECT) can be used. It has a fortuitous beneficial effect on the patients' Parkinson status. Fromm (158) found that rigidity, bradykinesia, and mental slowing improved in five of eight patients. The benefit lasted 2 to 3 months. One patient who had prominent tremor did not improve. Lebensohn and Jenkins (159) reported two patients who benefited from ECT in terms of rigidity and gait. The second patient had a decrease in tremor. The findings of Dysken et al (160) were similar to Fromm's (158). Bradykinesia and rigidity responded relatively well and tremor, the least. A recent review (161) recounted the history of ECT in Parkinson disease. As in psychiatry, it is a treatment of last resort when medications prove refractory.

PSYCHOSIS

Psychosis can occur in Parkinson disease patients, both as an aspect of mental deterioration and as a side effect of levodopa. The traditional phenothiazine and butyrophenone antipsychotic medications could worsen Parkinson disease. With the introduction of clozapine (162) (Clozaril), this is less likely to happen. Clozapine is a dibenzodiazepine with less avid binding to dopamine receptors. Few if any extrapyramidal side effects have been reported. The major concern is a 1% to 2% occurrence of agranulocytosis (163). This requires frequent hemograms and differential testing.

A relatively new antipsychotic drug, risperidone (164,165) (Risperdal) has also shown promise in treating psychosis in the Parkinson patient. It is a benzisoxazole derivative that moderately blocks dopamine D_2 receptors and strongly blocks serotonin $5HT_2$ receptors. In the study by Meco et al (154), relatively low doses, up to 1.25 mg/day, produced appropriate antipsychotic effects without worsening motor functions. It is believed that the combined dopaminergic and serotonergic blockage may protect against extrapyramidal side effects (166).

ACKNOWLEDGMENTS

This chapter could not have been done without the generous assistance of the following people: Carmen Garcia-Otero, Mark Fleetwood, and Barbara Michael at the Harry S. Truman VA Hospital medical library helped with research and article retrieval. Carolyn Gutierrez, librarian at the Jane Phillips Medical Center, continued to provide needed references. Neuropsychologist John W. Hickman, PhD, helped elucidate some of the neuropsychological aspects. Ronda Riden provided personal and administrative support at the Jane Phillips Medical Center. Elaine Vines, my secretary, did all the typing and arranged my schedule to allow time to do this. Lastly, I'd like to dedicate this chapter to my late father Joel Friedman, DDS, (1915–1994), former chief of prosthodontics at the old Jewish Chronic Disease Hospital, now Kingsbrook Jewish Medical Center in Brooklyn, New York, who first introduced me to Parkinson disease.

REFERENCES

1. Parkinson J. *An essay on the shaking palsy.* London: Sherwood, Neely and Jones, c.1817.
2. Fahn S. The history of parkinsonism. *Mov Disord* 1989;4:51–52.
3. Cotzias CG, Van Woert MH, Schaffer LM. Aromatic amino acids and modification of parkinsonism. *N Engl J Med* 1967;276:374–379.
4. Cotzias CG, Papvasiliou PS, Gellene R. Modification of parkinsonism—chronic treatment with L-dopa. *N Engl J Med* 1969;280:337–345.
5. Fahn S. "On-off" phenomenon with levodopa therapy in parkinsonism. *Neurology* 1974;24:431–441.
6. Shoulson I, Glaubiger GA, Chase TN. On-off response of clinical and biochemical correlations during oral and intravenous levodopa administration in Parkinson's patients. *Neurology* 1975;25:1144–1148.
7. Muenter MD, Sharpless NS, Tyce GM, Dailey FL. Patterns of dystonia ('I-D-I' and 'D-I-D') in response to L-dopa Therapy for Parkinson's disease. *Mayo Clinic Proc* 1977;52:163–174.
8. Lesser RP, Fahn S, Snider SR, et al. Analysis of clinical problems in parkinsonism and the complication of long-term levodopa therapy. *Neurology* 1979;29:1253–1260.
9. Madrazo I, Drucker-Colin R, Diaz V, et al. Open microsurgical autograft of adrenal medulla to the right caudate nucleus in to patients with intractable Parkinson's disease. *N Engl J Med* 1987;316:831–834.
10. Spencer DD, Robbins RJ, Naftolin F, et al. Unilateral transplantation of human fetal mesencephalic tissue into the caudate nucleus of patients with Parkinson's disease. *N Engl J Med* 1992;327:1541–1548.
11. Burchiel DJ. Thalamotomy for movement disorders. *Neurosurg Clin North Am* 1995;6:55–71.
12. Olanow CW, Marsden CD, Lang AE, Goetz CG. The role of surgery in Parkinson's disease management. *Neurology* 1994;44(suppl 1):517–520.
13. Samuel M, Caputo E, Brooks DJ, et al. A study of medial pallidotomy for Parkinson's disease: clinical outcome, MRI location and complications. *Brain* 1998;121:59–75.
14. Lang AE, Lozano AM, Montgomery E, et al. Posteroventral medial pallidotomy in advanced Parkinson's disease. *N Engl J Med* 1997;337: 1036–1042.
15. Fazzini E, Dogali M, Sterio D, et al. Steriotactic pallidotomy for Parkinson's disease: a long-term follow up of unilateral pallidotomy. *Neurology* 1997;48: 1273–1277.
16. Masterman D, DeSalles A, Baloh R. Motor cognitive and behavioral performance following unilateral ventroposterior pallidotomy for Parkinson's disease. *Arch Neurol* 1998;55:1201–1208.
17. Hoehn MM, Yahr MD. Parkinsonism: onset progression and mortality. *Neurology* 1967;17: 427–442.
18. Hoehn MMM. The natural history of Parkinson's disease in the pre-levodopa and post-levodopa era. *Neurol Clin North Am* 1992;10:331–339.
19. England AC Jr, Schwab RS. Postoperative medical evaluation of 26 selected patients with Parkinson's disease. *J Am Geriatr Soc* 1956;5:1219–1232.
20. Schwab RS, England AC Jr. Projection technique for evaluating

surgery in Parkinson's disease. In: Gillingham FJ, Donaldson IML, eds. *Third symposium on Parkinson's disease.* Edinburgh: Livingstone, 1969:152–157.

21. Canter CJ, de laTorre R, Mier M. A method of evaluating disability in patients with Parkinson's disease. *J Nerve Ment Dis* 1961;133:143–147.
22. Alba A, Trainor FS, Ritter W, Dacso MM. A clinical disability rating for Parkinson patients. *J Chron Dis* 1968;21:507–522.
23. Webster DD. Critical analysis of the disability in Parkinson's disease. *Med Treat* 1968;5:257–282.
24. Duvoisin RC. The evaluation of extrapyramidal disease. In: de Ajuriguerro J, ed. *Monoamines, noyaux gris centraux et syndrome de Parkinson.* Paris: Masson, 1970:313–325.
25. Yahr MD, Duvoisin RC, Shear MJ, et al. Treatment of parkinsonism with levodopa. *Arch Neurol* 1969;21:343–354.
26. Lieberman A. Parkinson's disease: a clinical review. *Am Med Sci* 1974;267:66–80.
27. Fahn S, Elton RC, members of the UPDRS Development Committee. Unified Parkinson's Disease Rating Scale. In: Fahn S, Marsden CD, Calne DB, Goldstein M, eds. *Recent developments in Parkinson's disease.* Vol. 2. Florahm Park, NJ: Macmillan Health Care Information, 1987:153–164.
28. Knutsson E. An analysis of parkinsonian gait. *Brain* 1972;95:475–486.
29. Murray MP, Sepic SB, Gardner GM, Downs WJ. Walking patterns of men with parkinsonism. *Am J Phys Med* 1978;57:278–294.
30. Blin O, Ferrandez AM, Serratrice G. Quantitative analysis of gait in Parkinson patients: increased variability of stride length. *Neurol Sci* 1990;98:91–97.
31. Aita JF. Why patients with Parkinson's disease fall. *JAMA* 1982;247:515–516.
32. Koller WC, Glatt S, Vetere-Overfield B, Hassanein R. Falls and Parkinson's disease. *Clin Neuropharmacol* 1989;12:98–105.
33. Weiner WJ, Nora LM, Glantz RH. Elderly inpatients postural reflex impairment. *Neurology* 1984;34:945–947.
34. Artane. In: *Physicians' desk reference.* 52nd ed. Montvale, NJ: Medical Economic, 1998:1388–1389.
35. Olanow CW, Koller WC. An algorithm (decision tree) for the management of Parkinson's disease: treatment guideline. *Neurology* 1998;50(suppl 3):551–557.
36. Lakke JPWF. Axial apraxia in Parkinson's disease. *J Neurol Sci* 1985;69:37–46.
37. The Parkinson Study Group. Effect of deprenyl on the progression of disability in early Parkinson's disease. *N Engl J Med* 1989;321:1364–1371.
38. The Parkinson Study Group. Effects of tocopherol and deprenyl on the progression of disability in early Parkinson's disease. *N Engl J Med* 1993;328:176–183.
39. Permax. In: *Physicians' desk reference.* 52nd ed. Montvale, NJ: Medical Economics, 1998:589–592.
40. Navsieda PA. Clinical observations on the use of Ropinirole in Parkinson's disease. *Parkinson Report* 1998;19:6–7.
41. Rajput AH, Martin W, Saint-Hilaire M-H, et al. Tolcapone improved motor function in parkinsonian patients with the "wearing off" phenomenon: a double-blind, placebo-controlled multicenter trial. *Neurology* 1997;49:1066–1071.
42. Männistö PR. Clinical potential of catechol-o-methyltransferase (COMT) inhibition as adjuvants in Parkinson's disease. *CNS Drugs* 1994;1:172–199.
43. Kaakkola S, Gordin A, Männistö P. General properties and clinical possibilities of new selective inhibition of catechol-o-methyltransferase. *Gen Pharmacol* 1994;25:813–824.
44. Kempster PA, Wahlqvist MD. Dietary factors in the management of Parkinson's disease. *Nutr Rev* 1994;52:51–58.
45. Mena I, Cotzias G. Protein intake and treatment of Parkinson's disease with levodopa. *N Engl J Med* 1975;292:181–184.
46. Juncos Jr JL, Fabbrini G, Mouradian MM, et al. Dietary influence on the antiparkinsonian response to levodopa. *Arch Neurol* 1987;44:1003–1005.
47. Pincus JH, Barry K. Influence of dietary protein on motor fluctuations in Parkinson's disease. *Arch Neurol* 1987;44: 270–272.
48. Pincus JH, Barry K. Protein redistribution diet restores motor function in patients with dopa resistant "off periods." *Neurology* 1988;38:481–483.
49. Karstaedt PJ, Pincus JH. Protein redistribution diet remains effective in patients with fluctuating parkinsonism. *Arch Neurol* 1992;49:149–151.
50. Rivera-Calimli M, Dujovne CA, Morgan JP, et al. Absorption and metabolism of L-dopa by the human stomach. *Eur J Clin Invest* 1971:313–320.
51. Riley D, Lang AE. Practical application of a low-protein diet for Parkinson's disease. *Neurology* 1988;38:1026–1031.
52. Comella CL, Stebbins GT, Brown-Toms N, Goetz CG. Physical therapy and Parkinson's disease: a controlled clinic trial. *Neurology* 1994;44:376–378.
53. Wroe M, Greer M. Parkinson's disease and physical therapy management. *Phys Ther* 1973;53:849–854.
54. Davis JC. Team management of Parkinson's disease. *Am J Occup Ther* 1977;31:300–308.
55. Murray W. Parkinson's disease, aspects of functional training. *Phys Ther Rev* 1956;36: 587–594.

56. Palmer SS, Mortimer JA, Webster DD, et al. Exercise therapy for Parkinson's disease. *Arch Phys Med Rehabil* 1986; 67:741–745.

57. Szekely BC, Neiberg-Kosanovish N, Sheppard W. Adjunctive treatment in Parkinson's disease: physical therapy and comprehensive group therapy. *Rehabil Literature* 1982; 43:42–76.

58. Kase SE, O'Riordan CA. Rehabilitation approach. In: Koller WC, ed. *Handbook of Parkinson's disease*. New York: Dekker, 1987:455–464.

59. Schenkman M, Donovan J, Tsubota J, et al. Management of individuals with Parkinson's disease: rational and case studies. *Phys Ther* 1989;69:944–955.

60. Stefaniwsky L, Bilowit DS. Parkinsonism: facilitation of motion by sensory stimulation. *Arch Phys Med Rehabil* 1973;54:75–77.

61. Knott M. Report of a case of Parkinson's treated with proprioceptive facilitator technics. *Phys Ther Rev* 1957;37:229.

62. Gibberd FB, Page NGR, Spencer KM, et al. Controlled trial of physiotherapy and occupational therapy for Parkinson's disease. *BMJ* 1981;282:1196.

63. Bilowit D. Establishing physical objectives in the rehabilitation of patients with Parkinson's disease (gymnastic activities). *Phys Ther Rev* 1956;36:176–178.

64. Stelmach GE, Phillips JG, Chau AW. Visuospatial processing in parkinsonians. *Neuropsychology* 1989;27:485–493.

65. Dunne JW, Hankey GJ, Edis RH. Parkinsonism: upturned walking stick as an aid to locomotion. *Arch Phys Med Rehabil* 1987;68:380–381.

66. Dietz MA, Goetz CG, Stebbins GT. Evaluation of a modified inverted walking stick as a treatment for Parkinson freezing episodes. *Mov Disord* 1990;5:243–247.

67. Riley D, Lang AE, Blair RDG, et al. Frozen shoulder and other shoulder disturbances in Parkinson's disease. *J Neurol Neurosurg Psychiatry* 1989;52: 63–66.

68. Critchley EMR. Speech disorders of parkinsonism: a review. *J Neurol Neurosurg Psychiatry* 1981;44:751–758.

69. Logemann J, Fisher HB, Boshes B, Blonsky ER. Frequency and cooccurrence of vocal tract dysfunctions in the speech of a large sample of Parkinson's patients. *J Speech Hear Disord* 1978;43:47–57.

70. Scott S, Caird F, Williams B. Evidence for an apparent sensory speech disorder in Parkinson's disease. *J Neurol Neurosurg Psychiatry* 1984;47:840–843.

71. Sarno MT. Speech impairment in Parkinson's disease. *Arch Phys Med Rehabil* 1968;49:269–275.

72. Rigrodsky S, Morrison EB. Speech changes in Parkinsonism during L-dopa therapy: preliminary findings. *J Am Geriatr Soc* 1970;18:142–151.

73. Nakano KK, Zubich H, Tyler HR. Speech defects of parkinsonian patients: effect of levodopa therapy on speech intelligibility. *Neurology* 1973;23:865–870.

74. Scott S, Caird FI. Speech therapy for patients with Parkinson's disease. *BMJ* 1981;283:1088.

75. Scott S, Caird FI. Speech therapy for Parkinson's disease. *J Neurol Neurosurg Psychiatry* 1983;46:140–144.

76. Scott S, Caird FI. The response of the apparent receptive speech disorders of Parkinson's disease to speech therapy. *J Neurol Neurosurg Psychiatry* 1984;47:302–304.

77. Robertson SJ, Thomson F. Speech therapy in Parkinson's disease: a study of the efficacy and long term effects in intensive treatment. *Br J Disord Commun* 1984;19:213–224.

78. Ramig LO, Contryman S, O'Brien C, et al. Intensive speech treatment for patients with Parkinson's disease: short and long-term comparison of two techniques. *Neurology* 1996;47: 1496–1504.

79. Singer C, Weiner WJ, Sanchez-Ramos JR. Autonomic dysfunction in men with Parkinson's disease. *Eur Neurol* 1992;32: 134–140.

80. Appenzellero, Goss JE. Autonomic defects in Parkinson's syndrome. *Arch Neurol* 1971;24: 50–57.

81. Goetz CG, Lutge W, Tanner CM. Autonomic dysfunction in Parkinson's disease. *Neurology* 1986;36:73–75.

82. Aminoff MJ, Wilcox CS, Assessment of autonomic function in patient with parkinsonian syndrome. *BMJ* 1971; 4:80–84.

83. Barbeau A, Gillo-Joffroy L, Boucher R, et al. Renin aldosterone system in Parkinson's disease. *Science* 1969;165: 291–292.

84. Gross M, Bannister R, Godwin-Austin R. Orthostatic hypotension in Parkinson's disease. *Lancet* 1972;1: 174–176.

85. McDowell FH, Lee JE. Levodopa, Parkinson's disease and hypotension. *Ann Intern Med* 1970;72: 751–752.

86. Ballantyne JP, Early and late effects of levodopa in the cardiovascular system in Parkinson's disease. *J Neurol Sci* 1973;9: 97–103.

87. Micieli G, Mortignoni E, Cavallni A, et al. Postprandial and orthostatic hypotension in Parkinson's disease. *Neurology* 1987;37:383–393.

88. Tanner CM, Goetz CG, Klawans HC. Autonomic nervous system disorders. In: Koller WC. *Handbook of Parkinson's disease*. New York: Marcel Dekker, 1987: 145–170.

89. Van Dijk JG, Hann J, Zwinderman K, et al. Autonomic nervous system dysfunction in Parkinson's disease: relationships with age, medication, duration, and

severity. *J Neurol Neurosurg Psychiatry* 1993;56:1090–1095.

90. Irwin RP, Nutt JG, Woodward WR, Gancher ST. Pharmacodynamics of the hypotensive effect of levodopa in Parkinson's patients. *Clin Neuropharmacol* 1992;15:365–374.

91. Edwards LL, Pfeiffer RF, Quigley EMM, et al. Gastrointestinal symptoms in Parkinson's disease. *Mov Dis* 1991;6:151–156.

92. Bateson MC, Gibberd FB, Wilson RSE. Salivary symptoms in Parkinson's disease. *Arch Neurol* 1973;29:274–275.

93. Edwards LL, Quigley EMM, Pfeiffer RF. Gastrointestinal dysfunction in Parkinson's disease: frequency and pathophysiology. *Neurology* 1992;42:725–732.

94. Johnston BT, Li Q, Castell JA, Castell DO. Swallowing and esophageal function in Parkinson's disease. *Am J Gastroenterol* 1995;90:1741–1746.

95. Logemann JA, Blonsky ER, Boshes B. Lingual control in Parkinson's disease. *Trans Am Neurol Assoc* 1973;98:276–278.

96. Robbins JA, Logemann JA, Kirshner JS. Swallowing and speech production in Parkinson's disease. *Ann Neurol* 1986;19:283–287.

97. Logemann JA, Blonsky ER, Boshes B. Dysphagia in Parkinsonism. *JAMA* 1975;321:69–70.

98. Bird MR, Woodward MC, Gibson EM, et al. Asymptomatic swallowing disorders in elderly patients with Parkinson's disease, a description of findings on clinical examination and video fluoroscopy in sixteen patients. *Age Aging* 1994;23:251–254.

99. Bushmann M, Dodmeyer SM, Leeker L, Perlmutter JS. Swallowing abnormalities and their response to treatment in Parkinson's disease. *Neurology* 1989;39:1309–1314.

100. Logemann J. *Evaluation and treatment of swallowing disorders.* Austin, TX: Pro Ed, 1983.

101. De Lama Lazzara G, Logemann JA. Impact of thermal stimulation on the triggering of the swallowing reflex. *Dysphagia* 1986;1:73–77.

102. Kempster PA, Lees AJ, Crichton P, et al. Off period belching due to a reversible disturbance of esophageal motility in Parkinson's disease and its treatment with apomorphine. *Mov Disord* 1989;4:47–52.

103. Byrne KG, Pfeiffer R, Quigley EMM. Gastrointestinal dysfunction in Parkinson's disease, a report of clinical experience at a single center. *Clin Gastroenterol* 1994;19:11–16.

104. Gibberd FB, Gleeson JA, Gossage AAR, Wilson RSE. Esophageal dilatation in Parkinson's disease. *J Neurol Neurosurg Psychiatry* 1974;37:938–940.

105. Qualman SJ, Haupt HM, Yang P, Hamiltor SR. Esophageal Lewy bodies associated with ganglion cell loss in achalasia: similarity to Parkinson's disease. *Gastroenterology* 1984;87: 848–856.

106. Den Hartog WA, Jager WA, Bethlem J. The distribution of Lewy bodies in the central and autonomic nervous systems in idiopathic paralysis agitans. *J Neurol Neurosurg Psychiatry* 1950;23:283–290.

107. Ohama E, Ikota F. Parkinson's disease: distribution of Lewy bodies and monoamine nervous system. *Acta Neuropathol (Berl)* 1976;34:311–315.

108. Harada T, Orita R, Hiwaki C, et al. Evaluation of gastric emptying in Parkinson's disease—Effect of L-dopa treatment. *Can J Neurol Sci* 1993;20:S119.

109. Muller-Lissner SA, Fraas C, Hartl A. Cisapride offset dopamine-induced slowing of fasting gastric emptying. *Dig Dis Sci* 1986;31:807–810.

110. Kurlan R, Rothfeld KP, Woodward WR, et al. Erratic gastric emptying of levodopa may cause random fluctuations of parkinsonian mobility. *Neurology* 1988;38:419–421.

111. Djaldetti R, Baron J, Ziv I, Melamed E. Gastric emptying in Parkinson's disease patients with and without response fluctuations. *Neurology* 1996;46:1051–1054.

112. Djaldetti R, Koren M, Ziv I, et al. Effect of cisapride on response fluctuations in Parkinson's disease. *Mov Dis* 1995;10:81–84.

113. Kupsky WJ, Grimes MM, Sweeting J, et al. Parkinson's disease and megacolon: concentric hyaline inclusion in enteric ganglion cells. *Neurology* 1987;37:1253–1255.

114. Lewitan A, Nathanson L, Slade WR. Megacolon and dilatation of the small bowel in Parkinsonism. *Gastroenterology* 1951;17: 367–374.

115. Caplan LH, Jacobson HG, Rubinstein BM, Rotman MZ. Megacolon and volvulus in Parkinson's disease. *Radiology* 1965;85:73–79.

116. Rosenthal MJ, Marshall CE. Sigmoid volvulus in association with parkinsonism, report of four cases. *J Am Geriatr Soc* 1987;35:683–684.

117. Jost WH, Schimrigk K. Constipation in Parkinson's disease. *Klin Wochenschr* 1991;69: 906–909.

118. Mathers SE, Kempster PA, Swash M, Lees AJ. Constipation and paradoxical puborectalis contraction in anismus and Parkinson's disease: a dystonic phenomenon? *J Neurol Neurosurg Psychiatry* 1988;51:1503–1507.

119. Mathers SE, Kempster PA, Law PJ, et al. Anal sphincter dysfunction in Parkinson's disease. *Arch Neurol* 1989;46: 1061–1064.

120. Edwards LL, Quigley EMM, Harned RK, et al. Defecatory function in Parkinson's disease: response to apomorphine. *Ann Neurol* 1993;33:490–493.

121. Murnaghan GF. Neurogenic disorders of the bladder in parkinsonism. *Br J Urol* 1961; 33:403–405.

122. Andersen JT, Bradley WE. Cystometric sphincter and electromyographic abnormalities in Parkinson's disease. *J Urol* 1976;116:75–78.

123. Fitzmaurice H, Fowler CJ, Rickards D, et al. Micturition disturbance in Parkinson's disease. *Br J Urol* 1985;57:652–656.

124. Chancellor MB, Blaivas JG, Diagnostic evaluation of incontinence in patients with neurological disorders. *Compr Ther* 1991;17(2):37–43.

125. Pavlakis AJ, Siroky MB, Goldstein I, Krane RJ. Neurologic findings in Parkinson's disease. *J Urol* 1983;129:80–83.

126. Sotolongo JR. Voiding function in Parkinson's disease. *Semin Neurol* 1988;8:166–169.

127. Raz S. Parkinsonism and neurogenic bladder: experimental and clinical observations. *Urol Res* 1976;4:133–138.

128. Berger Y, Blaivas JG, DeLaRoche ER, Salinas JM. Urodynamic findings in Parkinson's disease. *J Urol* 1987;138:836–838.

129. Christmas TJ, Kempster PA, Chapple CR, et al. Role of subcutaneous apomorphine in parkinsonian voiding dysfunction. *Lancet* 1988;2:1451–1453.

130. Koller WC, Vetere-Overfield B, Williamson A, et al. Sexual dysfunction in Parkinson's disease. *Clin Neuropharmacol* 1990;13:461–463.

131. Singer C, Weiner WJ, Sanchez-Ramos JR, Ackerman M. Sexual dysfunction in men with Parkinson's disease. *J Neurol Rehabil* 1989;3:199–204.

132. Wermuth L, Stenager E. Sexual problems in young patients with Parkinson's disease and their partners. *Acta Neurol Scand* 1995;91:453–455.

133. Lipe H, Longstreth WT, Bird TD, Linde M. Sexual function in married men with Parkinson's disease. *Neurology* 1990;40:1347–1349.

134. Brown RG, Jahanshahi M, Quinn N, Marsden CD. Sexual function in patients with Parkinson's disease and their partners. *J Neurol Neurosurg Psychiatry* 1990;53:480–486.

135. Golbe LI. Parkinson's disease and pregnancy. *Neurology* 1987;37:1245–1249.

136. Mayeux R, Chen J, Mirabello E, et al. An estimate of the incidence of dementia in idiopathic Parkinson's disease. *Neurology* 1990;40:1513–1517.

137. Caparro-Lefebvre D, Pecheux N, Petit V, et al. Which factors predict cognitive decline in Parkinson's disease? *J Neurol Neurosurg Psychiatry* 1995;58:51–55.

138. Mortimer JA, Pirozzolo FJ, Hansch EC, Webster DD. Relationship of motor symptoms to intellectual deficits in Parkinson's disease. *Neurology* 1982;32:133–137.

139. Cooper JA, Sagar HJ, Jordan N, et al. Cognitive impairment in early untreated Parkinson's disease and its relations to motor disability. *Brain* 1991;114:2095–2122.

140. Lees AJ, Smith E. Cognitive deficits in the early stages of Parkinson's disease. *Brain* 1983;106:257–270.

141. Hietanen M, Teravainen H. The effect of age of disease onset and neuropsychological performance in Parkinson's disease. *J Neurol Neurosurg Psychiatry* 1988;51:244–249.

142. La Rue A. *Aging and neuropsychological assessment.* New York: Plenum, 1992.

143. Soukup VM, Adams R. Parkinson's disease. In: Adams RL, Parsons OA, Culberston JL, Nixon SJ, eds. *Neuropsychology for clinical practice: etiology, assessment and treatment of common neurological disorders.* Washington, DC: American Psychological Association, 1996:243–267.

144. Zetusky WJ, Jankovic J, Pirozzolo FJ. The heterogeneity of Parkinson's disease. *Neurology* 1985;35:522–526.

145. Jankovic J, McDermott M, Carter J, et al. Variable expression of Parkinson's disease: a base-line analysis of the datatop cohort. *Neurology* 1990;40:1529–1534.

146. Rajput AH, Pahwa R, Pahwa P, Rajput A. Prognostic significance of the onset mode in parkinsonism. *Neurology* 1993;43:829–830.

147. Proctor F, Riklan M, Cooper IS, Teuber HL. Judgement of visual and postural vertical by parkinsonian patients. *Neurology* 1964;14:287–293.

148. Bowen FP, Burns MM, Brady EM, Yahr MD. A note on alterations of personal orientation in parkinsonism. *Neuropsychologia* 1976;14:425–429.

149. Bowen FP, Hoehn MM, Yahr MD. Parkinsonism: alterations in spatial orientation as determined by a route-walking test. *Neuropsychologia* 1972;10:355–361.

150. Flowers K. Lack of prediction in the motor behavior of Parkinsonism. *Brain* 1978;101:35–52.

151. Levin BE, Llabre MM, Weiner WJ. Cognitive impairments associated with early Parkinson's disease. *Neurology* 1989;39:557–561.

152. Dubinsky RM, Gray C, Husted D, et al. Driving and Parkinson's disease. *Neurology* 1991;41:517–520.

153. Mayeux R, Stern Y, Rosen J, Leventhal J. Depression, intellectual impairment and Parkinson's disease. *Neurology* 1981;31:645–650.

154. Dooneief G, Mirabello E, Bell K, et al. An estimate of incidence of depression in idiopathic Parkinson's disease. *Arch Neurol* 1952;49:305–307.

155. Bouchard RH, Pourcher E, Vincent P. Fluoxetine and extrapyramidal side effects. *Am J Psychiatry* 1989;146:1352–1353.

156. Jansen Steur ENH. Increase of Parkinson's disability often fluoxetine medication. *Neurology* 1993;63:211–213.

157. Wils V. Extrapyramidal symptoms in a patient treated with fluvoxamine. *J Neurol Neurosurg Psychiatry* 1992;55:330.

158. Fromm GH. Observations on the effect of electroshock treatment of patients with parkinsonism. *Bull Tulane Univ Med Faculty* 1959;8:71–73.

159. Lebensohn ZM, Jenkins RB. Improvement of parkinsonism in depressed patients treated with ECT. *Am J Psychiatry* 1975;132:283–285.

160. Dysken M, Evans HM, Char CH, Davis JM. Improvement of depression and parkinsonism during ECT: a case study. *Neuropsychobiology* 1976;2:81–86.

161. Rasmussen K, Abrams R. Treatment of Parkinson's disease with electroconvulsive therapy. *Psychiatr Clin North Am* 1991;14:925–933.

162. Friedman JH, Lannon MC. Clozapine in the treatment of psychosis in Parkinson's disease. *Neurology* 1989;39:1219–1221.

163. Alvir JMJ, Lieberman JA, Safferman AZ, et al. Clozapine-induced agranulocytosis: incidence and risk factors in the United States. *N Engl J Med* 1993;329:162–167.

164. Tavares AR. Risperidone in Parkinson's disease. *J Neurol Neurosurg Psychiatry* 1995;58:521.

165. Meco G, Alessandria A, Bonifati V, Giustini P. Risperidone for hallucinations in levodopa treated Parkinson's disease patients. *Lancet* 1994;343:1370–1371.

166. Livingston MG. Risperidone. *Lancet* 1994;343:457–460.

167. Lang AE, Lozano AM. Medical progress: Parkinson's disease [second of two parts]. *N Engl J Med* 1998;338:1130–1143.

168. Côté L, Crutcher MD. The basal ganglia. In: Kandel ER, Schwartz JH, Jessell TM, eds. *Principles of neural science.* 3rd ed. Norwalk, CT: Appleton & Lange 1991;647–659.

Chapter 76

Multiple Sclerosis

Michael Saffir
David Rosenblum

Multiple sclerosis (MS) is an inflammatory demyelinating disease of the central nervous system (CNS) creating focal lesions at multiple sites over time. It can cause a wide range of impairments and disability and is estimated to affect over 250,000 people in the United States alone. In many patients, MS has a progressive and unpredictable course. Recently, our knowledge and understanding of the disease have increased substantially. New interventions to alter the course of the disease as well as provide symptomatic treatment are available and many more potentially helpful interventions are undergoing clinical trials. The challenges faced by patients with MS cover a full spectrum including cognitive and psychological issues, weakness, fatigue and sensory disturbances, problems with mobility and self-care that may require assistive devices, vocational and avocational concerns, and even the fundamental ability to access appropriate medical treatment. A comprehensive treatment program with a dedicated interdisciplinary team including the patient is invaluable in addressing these issues, and maximizing the understanding of MS is essential for success in helping the patient.

EPIDEMIOLOGY

MS appears between the ages of 10 and 50, the average age being about 30 at the time of diagnosis (1,2). The risk of MS after the age of 60 is minimal (3). The incidence of MS is higher for women than for men (4–6). A longitudinal and comprehensive review of cases from Olmsted County in Rochester, Minnesota, found that over an 80-year period, the age-adjusted incidence rates were 3.0 and 7.0 per 100,000 population for males and females, respectively (5). In the United States, 250,000 to 300,000 people had MS diagnosed as of 1990 (7). The geographic distribution of MS has been well studied. Northern latitudes, such as those of the United States and Canada, have a higher prevalence, at 50 to 100 per 100,000 population, in comparison to southern latitudes such as in Asia and Africa, with a prevalence of 5 to 10 per 100,000 population (8,9) (Table 76-1). Migration is an important factor when considering incidence rates. If one migrates before adolescence, the risk characteristics of the new location apply. Migration later in life, however, does not appear to impact the risk of MS (5,10,11). This supports the hypothesis that environmental conditions play a part in the development of MS. MS prevalence also varies by race. Northern Europeans and their descendants have a much higher incidence than do Asians, African blacks, and Eskimos (3,4). Twin studies showed that concordance rates for monozygotic twin pairs are 25% to 28%, while for dizygotic twin pairs the concordance rates are 3% to 4% (12–14). Additional support for the significant role that genetics seems to have in MS comes from an adoption study which found that the risk of developing MS for nonbiologic family members is similar to that of the general population and less than the risk for biologic family members (15). The risk of MS for a child of a parent with

MS is estimated at 4%, and a person's risk of MS if their sibling has MS is 4% to 5% (13,16,17). While several genes may be responsible for susceptibility to MS, one susceptibility locus has been specifically linked to MS: HLA-DR2. This gene is found in many Northern Europeans and is also found in many people with MS (18). The presence of this gene does not guarantee the development of MS. Research in genome screening in MS revealed the presence of susceptibility loci, confirming that susceptibility to MS results from the activity of several genes (19–22). Chromosomal locations have been identified, which may lead to a discovery of specific genes. It does not appear that any single gene has a large effect. Evidence for nongene factors, such as environment, in the cause of MS is abundant: migration studies, geographic distribution studies, reported epidemics of MS (23), and twin and adoption studies. It is possible that MS is triggered by a viral infection that initiates an immune response. T-lymphocyte clones from MS patients that are specific for a myelin basic protein (MBP) peptide also recognize several common viruses (24). Viruses may cause demyelination directly, such as in postinfectious encephalomyelitis (4). However, specific viruses have not been consistently found in people with MS (25).

Table 76-1: Demographics of Multiple Sclerosis

Age: 10–50 yr, peak at 30 yr
Gender: female = male ratio, 2.3:1
Location: migration to a temperate climate before age 15
Race: white > black > Asian

NATURAL HISTORY

The definition of MS provides a framework for the findings in the disease. This definition encompasses multiple lesions in the CNS over time and emphasizes the spatial distribution of the lesions. Schumacher et al (26) characterized MS for research purposes as involving objective neurologic deficits in two or more areas, primarily reflecting white matter involvement. These deficits should occur at two or more points in time lasting longer than 24 hours and separated by more than 1 month, or in a slow progression of more than 6 months' duration. MS occurs between the ages of 10 and 50 years with a pattern of signs and symptoms that should not be better attributable to an alternative diagnosis (26). Owing to the significant degree of variability in the presentation of MS, the definition has evolved in terms of probability for the diagnosis given the findings. McAlpine et al (27) classified the diagnosis as definite, probable, and possible, based on clinical criteria. In 1983, Poser et al (28) updated this approach and defined MS as definite or probable (Table 76-2) in terms of clinical, paraclinical, and laboratory cerebrospinal fluid (CSF) findings.

Clinical Presentation

The typical areas affected and the distribution of the findings with their relative frequencies have been reviewed in a number of studies. Kurtzke (29) outlined this information as part of an ongoing study of several hundred Army veterans. A total of 762 were originally diagnosed as having MS but were subsequently reclassified: 476 had definite MS based on the Schumacher criteria and another 51 had probable MS, 45 had possible MS, 41 had an unknown disease, 146 had other diseases including 3 with primary lateral sclerosis (29). Kurtzke described these cases based

Table 76-2: Diagnostic Criteria for Multiple Sclerosis (MS)

Category	Attacks	Clinical Evidence		Paraclinical Evidence	CSF OB/IgG
Clinically definite (CD)					
CDMS A1	2	2			
CDMS A2	2	1	and	1	
Laboratory-supported definite (LSD)					
LSDMS B1	2	1	or	1	+
LSDMS B2	1	2			+
LSDMS B3	1	1	and	1	+
Clinically probable (CP)					
CPMS C1	2	1			
CPMS C2	1	2			
CPMS C3	1	1	and	1	
Laboratory-supported probable (LSP)					
LSPMS D1	2				+

Sources: Adapted with permission from Poser C, Paty DW, Scheinberg L, et al. New diagnostic criteria for multiple sclerosis: guidelines for research protocols. *Ann Neurol* 1983;13:229.
CSF = cerebrospinal fluid; OB = oligoclonal band.

Table 76-3: Frequency of Involvement by Functional Systems

Functional System	Percentage Involved
Pyramidal	85
Cerebellar	77
Brain stem	73
Sensory	55
Bladder and bowel	23
Visual	35
Cerebral	23
Other	15

Source: Adapted with permission from Kurtzke J. Rating neurologic impairment in multiple sclerosis: an Expanded Disability Status Scale (EDSS). *Neurology* 1983;33:1445.

on the percentage of patients with initial findings in eight different functional systems as part of his Disability Status Scale (DSS) rating. These systems include the pyramidal, cerebellar, brain stem, sensory, visual, cerebral, bladder and bowel, and other systems. Approximately three-fourths of patients had findings in the first three categories (Table 76-3) (30). Kraft et al (31) completed a survey of 656 individuals with MS and reported the frequency of symptoms along with the corresponding difficulties with activities in daily living (ADLs). Frequent problems included fatigue, difficulty with balance, weakness, paresthesias, bladder dysfunction, and spasticity, in decreasing order of frequency, although paresthesias were listed less frequently as a problem in terms of impact on ADLs (Table 76-4) (31). Vollmer and Waxman (32) described the findings in 55 patients at diagnosis and after 5 years (Table 76-5). Predominant findings were abnormal sensation and spastic paresis, with the percentage of patients having these findings roughly doubling over the 5 years, but more dramatic progression was seen for brain stem and cerebellar findings with ataxia, with the percentage of patients having these increasing approximately threefold and fourfold.

Table 76-4: Symptom Prevalence and Activities of Daily Living (ADLs) Impact

Symptoms	Difficulty in ADLs	No Difficulty in ADLs	Total
Fatigue	21	56	77
Balance problems	24	50	74
Weakness	18	45	63
Sensory disorder	39	24	63
Bladder problem	25	34	59
Spasticity	23	26	49
Bowel disorder	19	20	39
Memory problem	21	16	37
Depression	18	18	36
Pain	15	21	36
Lability of emotions	24	8	32
Visual problems	14	16	30
Tremor	14	13	27
Communication disorder	12	11	23
Problem-solving difficulty	12	9	21

Source: Adapted with permission from Kraft G, Freal JE, Coryell JK. Disability, disease duration and rehabilitation service needs in multiple sclerosis: patient perspectives. *Arch Phys Med Rehabil* 1986;67:165.

Table 76-5: Signs and Symptoms in Definite and Probable Multiple Sclerosis

Impairment/Problem	Percent at Diagnosis	Percent Within 5 Years
Spasticity/paresis	31	78
Sensory disorder	38	82
Visual loss	29	53
Diplopia	16	26
Brain stem signs	24	71
Ataxia	15	60
Sphincter dysfunction	9	42
Altered mental status	4	13

Source: Adapted with permission from Vollmer T, Waxman S. MS and other demyelinating disorders. In: Rosenberg R, ed. *Comprehensive neurology.* New York: Raven, 1991:498.

Patterns

In MS the development of active lesions may acutely cause new signs and symptoms, which can be termed an *exacerbation* or *relapse.* A period of clinical inactivity is a *remission,* which Charcot (33) described as early as 1875. By evaluating the clinical changes in patients at different points in time, one can reveal different patterns of MS exacerbations and remissions with varying degrees of residual impairments. These patterns have been characterized by McAlpine et al (27,34) and others, and have been recently updated to include: 1) benign MS with infrequent, mild exacerbations and extensive remissions with minimal residual impairments; 2) relapsing-remitting (R-R) MS, with a greater frequency (higher relapse rate) and extent of exacerbations with variable remissions and an increasing degree of impairment; 3) secondary progressive MS, with a relapsing-remitting course at first, followed by a gradual deterioration with or without relapses; 4) primary-progressive MS, with nearly continuous deterioration from the onset without distinct relapses; and 5) progressive-relapsing MS, with a gradual deterioration from the onset of symptoms but with superimposed relapses (Fig. 76-1). Primary-progressive disease may actually be a different variant of MS (35). In some patients the progression can

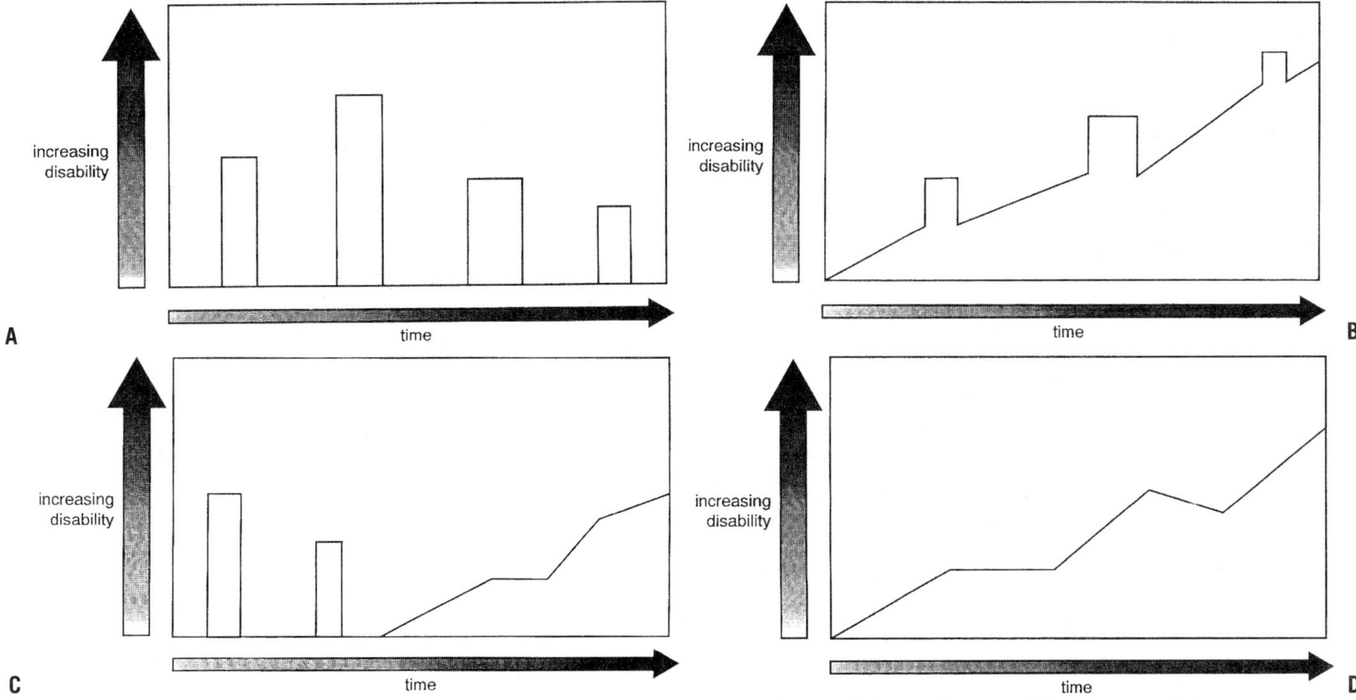

Figure 76-1. Clinical course definitions of multiple sclerosis. A. Relapsing-remitting: relapses with full or partial recovery. B. Progressive-relapsing progressive disease with acute relapses. C. Secondary-progressive: initially relapsing-remitting followed by progression with, or without, relapses. D. Primary progressive: disease progression. (Adapted with permission from Lubin F, Reingold F. Defining the clinical course of multiple sclerosis: results of an international survey. *Neurology* 1996;46:907–911.)

be rapid and severe, and has been characterized as a malignant form, distinct from the other types. This may be due to the localization of the lesions or may be a different variant along the spectrum of demyelinating disorders.

These different types describe the pattern of relapses, remissions, and progression often seen with MS (see Fig. 76-1). An important point is the conversion from the relapsing state to the progressive state, which is usually recognized over a period of time, often 2 years (36). The rate of conversion over the course of MS ranges from 30% to 50% after 5 years and increases in prevalence to 60% after 10 years (37,38). The incidence of conversion over time reaches a peak and then declines (39). The transition to a progressive course is related to the age at onset of MS where patients with a younger age at onset take longer to convert from the R-R form to progressive MS. Patients who develop MS at a later age account for a higher percentage in the primary progressive group and tend to do worse (29,34,37). Another important characteristic is the relapse frequency or rate, which can range from 0.1 to 1.0 per year (36). This rate is usually highest in the initial period after disease onset and then declines. Other significant factors include the duration and extent of each relapse and remission. There is a lower rate for relapse and for conversion to a progressive form in patients with longer and more complete remissions (40,41).

Progression and Assessment

The patterns describe disease activity over time, but the important issue to the patient is the impact it has on his or her life. The standard tool for assessing MS has been the Kurtzke DSS noted earlier, which was first introduced in 1955 with 10 levels of impairment ranging from normal to death. Functional systems with a scale for each were added in 1961 to represent more detailed neurophysiologic involvement relative to the functional status. The Expanded Disability Status Scale (EDSS) was developed in 1983 by dividing the original 10 levels in half, to increase the sensitivity for the functional status (Table 76-6) (30). Owing to variable interrater reliability, there has been some debate on the sensitivity of this tool for assessing significant changes, particularly for the cerebellar functional system (42). Additionally, it may be problematic in its focus on ambulation as the primary functional activity without considering other areas involving the upper extremities, fatigue, vision, and cognition (43). A review by Quick and Schapiro (44) of all the current published EDSS data indicated that additional data need to be collected.

The Minimal Record of Disability (MRD) was developed in 1985 to provide a comprehensive profile of patients with MS, covering the areas of impairment, disability, and handicap as outlined by the World Health Organization (45). The MRD started with the EDSS and

Table 76-6: Expanded Disability Status Scale (EDSS)

EDSS Score	Functional Status [with Functional Systems (FS) Grading (grade 0–5)]
0	Normal neurologic exam (FS all grade 0)
1.0	No disability (minimal signs in one FS)
1.5	No disability (minimal signs in more than one FS)
2.0	Minimal disability in one FS (grade 2)
2.5	Minimal disability in one FS (grade 2)
3.0	Moderate disability in one FS (grade 3) or mild in three or four; fully *ambulatory*
3.5	Moderate disability in one FS and mild (grade 2) in one or two FSs, or moderate in two FSs, or mild in five FSs
4.0	Severe disability with one FS (grade 4) or combinations of FS grades > prior levels; *fully ambulatory* >500 m without aid or rest
4.5	Severe disability with some limitations of regular activity with need for assistance and able to ambulate ~300 m without aid or rest
5.0	Severe disability with one FS (grade 5) or increasing combinations; unable to do full daily activities and can ambulate ~200 m without aid
5.5	Severe disability with one FS (grade 5) or two FSs ~(grade 3) with limited ambulation ~100 m without aid
6.0	Two or more FSs > (grade 3); assistance for ambulation with unilateral support and occasional resting to go ~100 m
6.5	As above with constant bilateral assists to ambulate 20 m without rest
7.0	Severe disability with two FSs > (grade 4) and limited ambulation < 5 m with assist; otherwise wheelchair dependent
7.5	Limited mobility for a few steps with assist; able to propel wheelchair short distances but cannot go long distances or manage independently a full day
8.0	Minimal mobility—essentially bed and chair restricted; can perform some self-care activities
8.5	Severe disability with several FSs > (grade 4); limited self-care activities
9.0	Bed bound requiring full assistance; able to communicate and eat
9.5	Totally dependent; unable to communicate or eat
10	Deceased

Source: Adapted with permission from Kurtzke J. Rating neurologic impairment in multiple sclerosis: an Expanded Disability Status Scale (EDSS). *Neurology* 1983;33:1444–1452.

DSS, which described the underlying impairment, and then included the Incapacity Status Scale (ISS) to assess functional disability and the Environmental Status Scale (ESS) to assess the handicap (45). Each scale has a range of 1 to 4 and 1 to 5, respectively. The ISS was developed by Kurtzke and Granger based on functional disabilities assessed in the original Kurtzke scales as well as other ADL assessments such as the Barthel scale. The Functional Independence Measure (FIM), which was also developed by Granger (46), is currently widely used and has good utility for assessing disability and need for assistance Granger et al (46) compared it with other scales for use in MS and revealed a good correlation between the FIM, Barthel index, ISS, ESS, and the Brief symptom inventory in assessing assistance needs and patient satisfaction. The FIM was found to be reliable with a good degree of precision, with the primary limitation being lack of assessment of visual problems (43). The quality of life (QOL) in MS was compared with that in patients with other chronic disorders such as rheumatoid arthritis and inflammatory bowel disease, using a QOL assessment tool that included four subscales for medical problems, functional and economic issues, social and recreational issues, and affect and life in general (47). The investigators found that primarily the visual functional system score by Kurtzke correlated with the overall QOL and subscales; the medical problems subscale correlated with the EDSS.

In monitoring the natural history of MS, measurements of impairment, disability, and handicap are fundamental elements. The correct use of appropriate scales is necessary to achieve valid and reliable results that describe effects and answer questions about MS. An evaluation of all MS patients in Olmsted County, Minnesota, utilized the MRD to describe their current status. There were 162 patients with a median duration of disease from onset of 15 years and a median age of 48 years, and 55% had an EDSS score of less than 6. The evaluation found that 50% were employed, 33% had severe paraparesis or paraplegia, and 25% needed catheterization for bladder management. It also showed bimodal EDSS distribution peaks at scores of 1 and 6.5 (48). Weinshenker et al (36,37,49) described the median time to reach an EDSS score of 6 as approximately 15 years, with 40% of the population having EDSS scores of 6 to 7 and 10% having scores higher than 8. Patients stayed at a score of 6 and 7 approximately 3 and 3.75 years, respectively. A more rapid progression with shorter time to reach EDSS score 6 was seen in association with certain risk factors such as cerebellar involvement, older age at onset, and insidious onset of motor deficits. Also noted were a higher relapse rate and shorter initial

Table 76-7: Prognostic Indicators: Survey of Multiple Sclerosis Clinic Directors

Indicators	Scale 1–4 [Not Useful–Very Useful]
Disability status	2.9
Pyramidal and cerebellar signs at 5 yr	2.7
Resolution of initial symptoms	2.5
Length of initial attack	2.4
Age at onset	2.3
Number of symptoms during first year	2.3
Onset: acute vs insidious	2.3
Duration of most recent attack	2.2
Cerebellar signs at initial presentation	2.0
Motor symptoms as initial presentation	1.7
Sensory symptoms as only presenting symptoms	1.5
Optic neuritis as only presenting symptom	1.5
Plantar extensor reflex at initial presentation	1.5

Source: Adapted with permission from Kraft G, Freal JE, Coryell JK, et al. Multiple Sclerosis: Early Prognostic Guidelines. *Arch Phys Med Rehabil* 1981;62:54–58.

remission. The average time from onset of MS to the progressive phase was approximately 6 years and then the subsequent time to reach an EDSS score of 6 and 8 was 4.5 and 24 years, respectively. The disability status can be used in this manner to characterize the natural history of MS and is highly relevant to both the patient and the clinician.

Prognostic factors can be considered in terms of disability levels as noted earlier and were identified in a survey of MS clinic directors by Kraft et al (34). Good factors included a lower current disability status, limited cerebellar and pyramidal findings at 5 years, no motor findings at onset, a rapid onset and resolution of the early flare-ups, and younger age at onset (Table 76-7). Another factor considered to be significant is trauma, which has been thought of as a risk factor but retrospective and prospective studies did not show any direct relationship (50). Pregnancy is also a concern; studies showed lower relapse rates during pregnancy and then significantly higher rates during the 3 to 6 months postpartum (51). However, the overall disability was not any different (52).

As Kraft et al (31) concluded, the use and need for medical and community support services are primarily a function of a patient's disability. Having an idea of what to expect with MS and a chance to adapt and learn can result in better outcomes.

PATHOPHYSIOLOGY

MS is characterized by recurrent and progressive episodes of inflammation in the spinal cord and brain. The myelin of the CNS is affected, with general sparing of axons. The passage of immune cells through the blood-brain barrier (BBB) is important in the pathogenesis of MS. BBB disruption may precede clinical signs of disease (53) and may be seen on gadolinium-enhanced magnetic resonance images (MRIs). CNS endothelial cells in the BBB may show persistent abnormalities, even in primary progressive MS (54). Lymphocytes, macrophages, and plasma cells access the CNS (55), and proinflammatory cytokines are released. A plaque is formed as myelin is destroyed. These plaques can be seen grossly at autopsy and with imaging studies such as MRI (see Diagnostic Approach). Active plaques are edematous, with leakage of plasma proteins from the capillary beds around the plaques (56). These lesions are infiltrated by inflammatory cells such as lymphocytes and macrophages (57). An old plaque is formed as oligodendrocytes become damaged and lost, and astrocytes proliferate (58). Loss of oligodendrocytes decreases the chance of remyelination. Multiple areas of gliosis form, which explains how MS was named.

The plaques of MS are often seen around the ventricles, optic tracts, and cerebellum. Other areas may include the basal ganglia, the gray matter, and the white matter of any lobe of the brain. The cervical region of the spinal cord is more affected than the thoracic area (59–61). The plaques and demyelination can cause disruption of nerve conduction. Myelin, composed of MBP and lipids, facilitates signal transmission in the axons by increasing the speed of conduction and allowing for saltatory conduction. Compromise of myelin causes decreased conduction velocity, conduction block, and the symptoms of MS (61). Sodium and potassium channels are important to the pathophysiology of demyelinated axons: "Unmasked" potassium channels interfere with conduction in demyelinated axons (62). This is the basis of clinical trials using potassium channel blockers such as 4-aminopyridine and 3,4 diaminopyridine (62–64). Factors that further decrease conduction velocity, such as elevated temperature, may make symptoms worse (59,65).

Immune Response

In the normal immune response, macrophages and other antigen-presenting cells present foreign antigens and self-antigens to helper T cells (66). These T cells recognize the antigen that is bound to a class II major histocompatibility complex (MHC). The MHC is on the surface of the antigen-presenting cell, or macrophage. This recognition causes the T cells to release cytokines such as interferons and interleukins. These substances are peptides that support the immune system response to a specific target. Suppression of the immune response may be mediated by many cell types, such as suppressor cytotoxic T cells

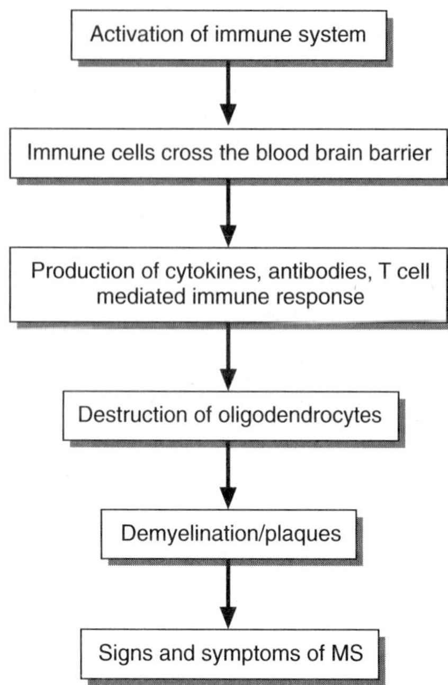

Figure 76-2. Pathophysiology of multiple sclerosis.

(CD8+) (67). If suppression is compromised, then T-cell activation may increase, which in turn releases more cytokines. Interestingly, the CD8+ suppressor cell function may be defective during MS attacks, and may be low in C-P MS (67). Interferon beta helps reverse this defect.

In MS, activated T cells may adhere to the endothelial wall of the BBB, cross the BBB, and invade the CNS (68,69). T cells are activated by cytokines secreted by macrophages and other cells (70). Proinflammatory cytokines may further contribute to a leaky BBB. Lymphocytes and macrophages are recruited, and myelin breakdown ensues. This T cell–mediated immune response destroys the oligodendrocytes (62) (Figs. 76-2 and 76-3). Exactly how this happens is not known. Antigen mimickry may be involved, where T cells respond to a foreign peptide but then mistakenly respond to a similar self-antigen such as a component of myelin (61). Alternatively, or additionally, there may be an autoimmune response to a self-antigen such as MBP. Cytotoxic T cells may directly kill oligodendrocytes (71). There may also be a direct action of cytokines on neurons unrelated to demyelination (67).

Additionally, plasma cells (B cells) are activated to produce antibodies against oligodendrocytes and myelin (57,68,72,73). Immunoglobulin synthesis increases, and oligoclonal bands are seen in the CSF of 90% of patients with MS (28). They may not be directed toward a specific antigen (59,60,74).

Experimental allergic encephalomyelitis (EAE) is an animal disease with similarities to MS. The features are inflammation, demyelination, and a fluctuating course. MBP, a constituent of myelin, can induce EAE following transfer of T-cell clones specific for the amino acid terminal of the MBP molecule (74,75). This further supports the concept of MS as an immune-mediated disease.

DIFFERENTIAL DIAGNOSIS

The diagnosis in patients with MS is challenging owing to the diverse presentation. The wide range of findings can be seen in a number of other conditions. The diagnosis is based on the overall pattern of clinical and laboratory findings as indicated by the criteria from Poser et al (28). The disease can present as a single symptom that can become relapsing and remitting, or progressive. It can also be multifocal with varying relapses and remissions. It may be progressive, and finally it can appear to be diffuse.

A monosymptomatic presentation often involves visual findings related to optic neuritis, which some experts believe is a precursor or mild variant along a spectrum of demyelinating disorders. Other causes of visual symptoms include retinopathies and CNS tumors. Funduscopic and ophthalmologic evaluation with a slit lamp can be helpful. Other visual symptoms including diplopia can be seen with MS as well as with myasthenia gravis and cerebrovascular disease, most often with diabetes. These diseases are often relapsing and remitting but can also be progressive. CNS tumors such as meningiomas and gliomas frequently present with cranial nerve, motor, and sensory findings in a progressive fashion, but early on these may fluctuate. This fluctuation can often be seen in conjunction with steroid therapy, which may be used with a presumptive diagnosis such as optic neuritis or transverse myelitis. A progressive course can be seen in other conditions such as myelopathy with cervical spondylosis and stenosis, or a Chiari malformation which may have bulbar and cerebellar findings. A progressive course can also be seen with intramedullary and extramedullary tumors and syringomyelia. The advent of MRI has facilitated the distinction of many of these diagnoses.

Multifocal findings that are common in MS are also seen with collagen vascular diseases (i.e., systemic lupus erythematosus, polyarteritis, Sjögren syndrome, sarcoidosis), encephalomyelitis secondary to Lyme disease, tropical spastic paraparesis, and human immunodeficiency virus (HIV) infection. These diseases are often identified by the various inflammatory and infectious markers with serology and other blood studies. These disorders can present in a relapsing and remitting pattern or become progressive. Other neurodegenerative disorders can similarly be multifocal in their presentation with a fluctuating or progressive course as with the spinocerebellar degenerations, leukodystrophies, vitamin B_{12} deficiency, subacute combined degenerative disorder, primary lateral sclerosis and amyotrophic lateral sclerosis (ALS), and postinfectious and acute disseminating encephalomyelitis.

The challenge is to make the best working diagnosis given the clinical context combined with the results of

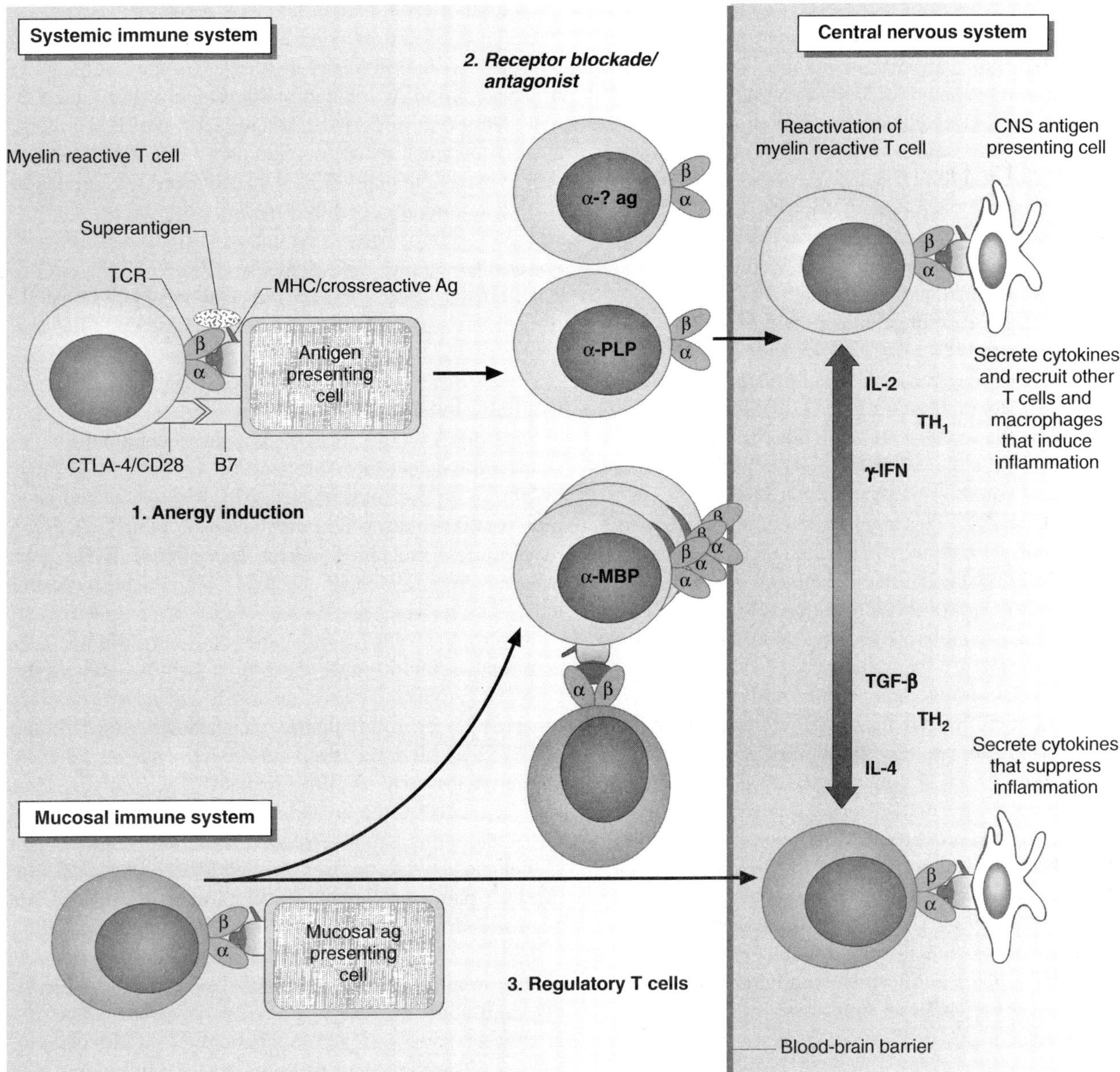

Figure 76-3. Immune mechanisms and strategies of immunotherapy in multiple sclerosis. Myelin-reactive T cells are activated in the periphery and migrate to the CNS where they initiate an autoimuune response against CNS myelin. Strategies of immunotherapy include 1) induction of anergy, or paralyzing myelin-reactive cells; 2) receptor blockade to interfere with the function or migration of myelin-reactive cells; and 3) generation of regulatory cells to inactivate myelin-reactive cells or secrete cytokines that suppress inflammation at the target organs. (Adapted with permission from Weiner HC, et al. *Neurology Clinics* 1995;13:182.)

diagnostic studies. The possibilities need to be discussed with the patient and then followed with further monitoring and education.

DIAGNOSTIC APPROACH

The diagnostic criteria for MS, prior to the availability of MRI and other ancillary tests, were based solely on the clinical history and physical examination. Disturbances of gait and vision and sensory symptoms are the most common symptoms at the time of initial presentation. The most common presenting signs in MS include abnormal reflexes, Babinski sign, ataxia, and decreased vibration sense (76,77). Schumaker et al (26) originally developed the most widely used clinical criteria. The development of computed tomography (CT), MRI, and CSF analysis led to the identification of previously undiagnosed lesions. Poser et al (28) (see Table 76-2) modified Schumacher's criteria to include laboratory-supported MS (76,78). The current diagnostic criteria define clinically definite and clinically probable MS as well using paraclinical evidence, which refers to CNS lesions found by examinations such as MRI or evoked potential (EP) testing. Attacks are defined as the occurrence of neurologic symptoms lasting 24 hours. By definition, each attack affects a different part of the CNS and is separated by at least 1 month (28).

Cerebrospinal Fluid Analysis

No CSF findings are diagnostic of MS (76), and the CSF may in fact be normal (77). CSF protein levels are elevated in approximately 25% of patients. CSF white blood cell counts may be elevated, although usually not beyond 25/µL (79). An increase in gamma globulin fraction of total CSF is seen in 60% to 70% of patients with definite MS, and may be seen even if the total protein CSF level is normal (79,80). The IgG index is the CSF globulin fraction divided by the serum gamma globulin fraction [IgG index = (CSF IgG/albumin)/(serum IgG/albumin)]. Values greater than or equal to 0.7 indicate that IgG is synthesized in the CNS (81). This abnormality is seen in 80% to 90% of patients with definite MS (79). The CSF gamma globulin in MS may form discrete bands on gel electrophoresis called *oligoclonal bands*. In normal CSF, IgG is polyclonal. Oligoclonal bands are present in 85% to 95% of MS patients (79,82,83) and therefore are very sensitive for MS (99). False positives may occur in 40% of patients with acute aseptic CNS inflammation, for example, and oligoclonal bands are not very specific (84). Oligoclonal bands may also be seen in viral encephalitis and meningitis (32). MBP is a sensitive marker for active demyelination, but is usually normal in chronic MS (79). It is elevated in 70% to 93% of patients with MS during an acute exacerbation, and quickly returns to normal usually within 2 weeks (79). The level of MBP relates to the size of the lesions (mass) and documents myelin damage (85). It is not a very specific finding, and may be seen in the setting of systemic lupus erythrematosus, transverse myelitis, and cerebral infarcts (32).

Evoked Potentials

EPs are electrical fields in the nervous system that occur in response to stimulation of the sensory system. The latency and waveform of the EPs are dependent on the conduction system and are very sensitive to demyelination. If transmission of the nerve impulse is slow, the latency is prolonged and the waveform altered. EPs may demonstrate subclinical lesions in the nerve pathways. Abnormal EPs are not specific for MS.

Visual evoked potentials (VEPs), obtained by stimulation with a checkerboard pattern or strobe, may be abnormal in 75% of patients with definite MS (76). VEPs can help establish abnormalities in the optic nerve and tract, and therefore are helpful diagnostically (86). While such abnormalities are common in MS, they also occur in other diseases such as compressive lesions of the visual pathways and spinocerebellar degeneration (32). Brain stem auditory evoked potentials (BAEPs) assess the pons and midbrain using auditory stimulation, and may be very effective in identifying subclinical lesions. Abnormality rates of 21% to 55% on BAEP testing may be seen in patients without a history of brain stem findings (86). One-third of patients with definite or suspected MS have abnormal BAEPs (86). BAEP abnormalities are not specific for MS. Somatosensory evoked potentials (SSEPs) are obtained by stimulation of the peripheral nerves. Forty-two percent of patients with MS without signs or symptoms may have SSEP abnormalities, and 75% of patients who do have signs or symptoms of sensory loss may have abnormalities on SSEP testing (85–87). SSEP abnormalities are related to the degree of sensory loss (88).

Magnetic Resonance Imaging

MRI is currently the preferred imaging technique to support the diagnosis of MS, and the findings are positive in 70% to 95% of patients with MS (76,89,90). MRI is more sensitive than CT in the diagnosis of MS (91), and it may visualize subclinical lesions. For example, MRI detected disseminated lesions in 61% of patients with isolated optic neuritis (92). Plaques are found characteristically in the periventricular location, but may also be commonly found in other areas of the white matter. Specific MRI criteria for the diagnosis of MS have been reported (93,94). Gadolinium-enhanced MRI may identify active disease and may distinguish new versus old lesions by identifying areas of BBB breakdown. The enhancement may be related to the breakdown of the BBB (76,94). Serial gadolinium-enhanced MRI is useful for detecting pathologic activity, and is advocated for use in clinical trials of new treatments (95–98). Quantitative assessment of MRI lesion load may also be effective in monitoring MS (99). Additionally, there may be a correlation between the change in number of MRI-detected lesions or total lesion load and disability (99–101). MRI may detect totally asymptomatic lesions (32). Refinements of MRI techniques such as fluid-attenuated inversion recovery, diffusion imaging, magnetization transfer imaging, and magnetic resonance spectroscopic imaging may prove to be more sensitive than conventional MRI (102).

Computed Tomography

CT may be useful to rule out diseases that present as an MS-like process. Cerebral atrophy is the most common finding, and may be observed early secondary to widespread lesions (91,103). Ten percent to 25% of patients with MS have contrast-enhanced lesions on CT scans (103). Low-density lesions on non-contrast-enhanced CT scans may be seen, especially in periventricular regions. CT is not very effective in showing lesions of the brain stem, cerebellum, and optic nerve (104).

Positron Emission Tomography

Cobalt-55 positron emission tomography (PET) was found to estimate disease activity in secondary progressive MS

(105). Cobalt uptake correlates with cellular calcium accumulation, and was used to trace calcium in MS patients. Calcium influx is found in both cell death and T-cell activation in MS (105). PET scanning may prove to be useful in the future to assess disease activity.

MEDICAL TREATMENT APPROACHES

For the treatment of MS, medications may be used to decrease inflammation and suppress the immune system. The goals of pharmacologic treatment may include improving recovery from exacerbations, decreasing the number of future exacerbations, decreasing disability, decreasing disease activity, and preventing the development of further disease and disability (106). The clinical treatment clearly needs to be individualized based on a patient's clinical course, medical history, and the pertinent signs and symptoms of MS. Risk and benefits must be considered and discussed.

Steroids

Steroids have been used to shorten the duration of acute exacerbations of MS due to their anti-inflammatory properties (107–108). Steroids may also impact the immune system by affecting T cells and interferon-γ release, decreasing IgG synthesis in the CNS, and reducing CSF antibodies to MBP and oligoclonal bands (106,107,109,110). High-dose steroids may also improve the integrity of the BBB (111). Short-term use of high-dose steroids suppress gadolinium enhancement in acute demyelinating lesions (112). The recovery from acute exacerbations of MS is hastened, but there does not appear to be any prevention of further attacks or progression of disease. Steroids also may be used to treat optic neuritis. Intravenous steroids such as methylprednisolone may decrease the rate of development of subsequently diagnosed MS in patients with optic neuritis (113). The risks of treatment with steroids may be significant, and careful clinical monitoring is essential. Depending on the duration of treatment, side effects may include hypokalemia, CNS effects such as psychosis, fluid retention, peptic ulcers, hyperglycemia, hypertension, aseptic necrosis, cataracts, adrenal insufficiency, opportunistic infections, and osteoporosis (107,114). Since chronic use of steroids may not slow progression of disease, and since it does have a significant risk of side effects, long-term use should be avoided (114).

Immune Modulating Therapy

It is widely believed that MS is an autoimmune disease (108,115). Agents that suppress the immune system have been used for many years to treat MS. The latest treatments for MS, such as interferon beta, actually modulate the immune system by enhancing and downregulating parts of the immune system. Therefore patients with MS may be considered for treatment with an immune altering agent.

Cyclophosphamide

Cyclophosphamide is an alkylating agent that was originally shown to reverse the course of EAE (117). Toxicity such as alopecia, nausea, hematuria, hemorrhagic cystitis, and malignancy may occur. Treatment with cyclophosphamide may be restricted for patients with aggressive progressive MS who are younger and who do not have other treatment options (108,116,117).

Azathioprine

This purine antimetabolite provides nonspecific immunosuppression (118) and may have modest benefit (119). It may be used for long periods of time, and in fact it is possible that the full effects may be underestimated by clinical trials, which are generally of short duration (117). It may take 2 years of treatment before an effect on disability is seen (119). Azathioprine is generally well tolerated, but careful medical follow-up is required to monitor for leukopenia and hepatotoxicity. There is a possible increased risk of cancer (117).

Cyclosporine

Cyclosporine is a fungal metabolite that has specific actions in the immune system such as inhibiting helper T cells (108,117). There may be modest benefit for patients with R-R or progressive MS (120), but significant toxicity such as hypertension and nephrotoxicity may limit its use (116,117,121). It may be considered in patients unable to take azathioprine, which is less toxic (108,122).

Cladribine

This antilymphocyte agent may slow the progression of disease in patients with primary progressive MS (123–125). The decrease in lymphocytes may decrease immune activation. It appears to be well tolerated, with monitoring necessary for possible bone marrow suppression. Further clinical trials are in progress to investigate this drug. It may reduce gadolinium-enhanced regions on MRI.

Glatiramer Acetate

This chain of four amino acids is immunologically cross reactive with MBP (126). It appears to inhibit T-cell responses to MBP. There are several theories on how glatiramer acetate may work, such as desensitization, suppressor T-cell production, and competition for MHC class II binding sites for MBP (116,117,127–129). Glatiramer acetate has been approved by the Food and Drug Administration (FDA) for use in treating R-R MS. It is given by subcutaneous injection each day. It could decrease the relapse rate of R-R MS by 32% after 2 years (116,117,126,130). Side effects include injection site reactions and postinjection reactions of flushing and chest tightness. The latter is self-limited and transient, with no long-term consequences reported.

Plasma Exchange

Plasma exchange has been considered in the treatment of MS, but needs further clinical research. Its cost and the limited benefits shown so far will probably prevent widespread use (131). It may prove to be a beneficial addition to immunosuppressive drug treatment for selected patients (132).

Methotrexate

Methotrexate has been used successfully for the treatment of rheumatoid arthritis, may provide global immunosuppression, and shows promise in helping control primary progressive MS (133,134). It also appears to be well tolerated. Further studies are necessary.

Interferon

This antiviral agent consists of three major types: alfa, beta, and gamma (135,136). Interferon gamma increases the exacerbation rate in MS (137). Interferon alfa may have the opposite effect in MS. Interferon beta clearly inhibits the effects of interferon-γ, and may also prevent the migration of lymphocytes into the brain by its effect on adhesion molecules on brain vascular endothelia (116). Interferon beta-1b (Betaseron), the first drug to be approved by the FDA, altered the course of the disease in a controlled clinical trial. Betaseron is made using recombinant technology in *Escherichia coli* bacteria and has an amino acid sequence that differs from the natural interferon by only one amino acid. It is typically given subcutaneously every other day. The precise mechanism of action is unclear. It may decrease T-cell production; block interferon-γ secretion; block the action of interferon-γ; decrease tumor necrosis factor, which has been shown to injure oligodendrocytes; and restore suppressor T-cell function (138). Interferon beta-1b reduced the exacerbation rate in MS patients by 35% compared with placebo (139). MRI showed a significant reduction in disease activity in treated patients (140). The most common adverse effects include flu-like symptoms and injection reactions (141). Antibodies may develop with continued use (142). In the one-third of patients estimated to develop antibodies after 1 year of treatment, the benefits of interferon beta may be lost.

Interferon beta-1a (Avonex) is also made by recombinant technology, is produced in mammalian cells, and has the same amino acid sequence and glycosylation that is found in naturally occurring interferon-β. It is administered intramuscularly once weekly, and has been approved by the FDA for relapsing forms of MS. Clinical trials demonstrated a 32% reduction in exacerbations, a decrease in the number and volume of MRI lesions, and an increase in time to sustained worsening of disability in those taking interferon beta-1a. The risk of progression of disability was reduced by 37% over 2 years. Side effects include flu-like symptoms such as fever, chills, muscle aches, and fatigue. Antibodies to interferon beta-1a may develop (143).

REHABILITATION MANAGEMENT

In rehabilitation, planning is based on a comprehensive evaluation done as early as possible. The findings can serve as a baseline to assess future changes. The evaluation requires a detailed history of signs and symptoms (see Tables 76-4 and 76-5), with a complete review of all systems and a physical examination for the findings of MS. The progression of findings should be identified and the patient's functional status determined, covering a number of areas such as in the FIM or MRD-ISS (Table 76-8). The patient's psychosocial situation must be evaluated to assess coping skills, support systems, and potential adaptive strategies including use of equipment to compensate and modification of activities. The MRD-ESS covers a number of these areas including problems with assistance, home, finances, work, socialization, transportation, and community resources. Overall, a complete list of problems should be developed and prioritized with appropriate goals. Scales such as the MRD provide a useful framework to identify the underlying impairments, the functional system deficits, and associated disabilities and handicaps (Table 76-9).

Problems can be treated at several levels, ranging from prevention to restorative and curative interventions that correct the underlying pathophysiology. Treatment may also help relieve problems by modifying their effects, and finally treatment can include managing a problem that cannot be changed. A comprehensive rehabilitation approach may involve prevention and restoration, where an impairment can be avoided or corrected such as with contracture and weakness. A compensatory technique with a prosthetic or orthotic device may be used. Adaptive strategies are also possible where a functional activity can

Table 76-8: Functional Domains (ISS/FIM)

Cognitive-behavioral	Expression, comprehension, memory and carryover, problem-solving skills, behavioral skills
Mobility	Transfers—bed/chair, toilet, tub Locomotion—level, uneven, stair
Activities of daily living	Toileting, bathing, grooming, dressing, eating, bladder and bowel, sexual function
Other	Visual functions, affect/mood, sleep

ISS = Incapacity Status Scale; FIM = Functional Independence Measure.

Table 76-9: Impairment Domains [Functional Systems (DSS/EDSS)]

Sensation [sensory]	Cognition [cerebral]
Vision [visual]	Affect/mood [cerebral]
Ataxia [cerebellar]	Weakness [pyramidal]
Dysarthria [cerebellar/ brain stem]	Spasticity [pyramidal]
Dysphagia [brain stem]	Contracture
Respiratory [brain stem]	Skin status
Bladder/bowel [brain stem]	Edema
Sexual function [brain stem]	Nutrition
Fatigue [other]	

DSS = Disability Status Scale; EDSS = Expanded Disability Status Scale.

Table 76-10: Treatment Team

Patient	Physicians
Nursing	Physical therapists
Occupational therapist	Speech-language therapists
Dietitian	Psychologist
Social worker	Spiritual counselor
Vocational counselor	Recreational therapist
Family	Aides and attendants
Consultants	Other

be restructured. A problem may have several dimensions and treatment may need to have multiple components. Spasticity, for example, can be treated by preventing irritation from urinary tract infection and bladder management, reducing postural stimulation and facilitating range of motion with stretching, modifying its severity using medications, compensating with bracing such as for ambulation, and finally using adaptive strategies such as an alternate mode of locomotion with a motorized scooter or changing to a desk job. The wide range of areas affected in MS can benefit most from a multidisciplinary approach.

Treatment by a dedicated interdisciplinary team can allow problems to be addressed in all areas (Table 76-10). Such an approach builds relationships that result in improved treatment, increased patient participation, and facilitated teaching. Treatment is better coordinated with effective resource management, and consistent follow-up can be provided. The team should be integrated with the community to identify the needs and resources available for patients with varying degrees of disability. The setting for appropriate services can range from an inpatient program to an outpatient center or clinic. A recent study by Aisen et al (144) reviewed 37 MS patients who underwent comprehensive inpatient rehabilitation 1 to 3 years previously. Two-thirds had primary progressive MS and the others were equally divided between having R-P and R-R MS. The results showed significant improvement based on scores using the FIM, EDSS, and functional systems at admission and discharge. Gains were maintained after discharge for the first 2 years. In the third year the functional system scores showed no significant change but the FIM scores, particularly for the locomotion subscale, decreased significantly. Feigenson et al (145) also showed that an intensive rehabilitation program can result in improvements that are maintained over a 1-year follow-up and thereby lower the overall costs of care including home care. The home care program should be an extension of the inpatient program and can be coordinated with an outpatient center or clinic for follow-up. Other studies identified patient needs in the community and treatment responses, noting, for example, that toileting and bladder care are areas where treatment can be very effective but may not have been well managed in the community (31,146). Counseling services were also noted to be less available (31). The ingredients of a successful team include having available resources, incorporating the right interests, maintaining morale, and having leadership for direction, growth, and stress management (147). This combination will improve the team dynamics and enhance synergies, with better professional skills and reduced burnout rates.

Paresthesias and Pain

Paresthesias represent a high percentage of the findings in MS, both early and late in the course (see Tables 76-4 and 76-5). Abnormal sensation may be bothersome to the patient but usually only becomes a functional problem when it is more severe with loss of proprioception or when there is a complete loss of sensation resulting in a loss of protective reflexes. There is no symptomatic treatment for this deficit and adaptive strategies must be utilized. Pain or dysesthesias can result in disability without physical impairments when the severity incapacitates a patient. In a study by Moulin et al (148), 159 patients in Ontario with MS were evaluated for pain syndromes. Fifty-seven percent had either an acute (9%) or chronic pain disorder (48%) as part of their history. The acute pain disorders typically involved paroxysmal symptoms, with half of them diagnosed as trigeminal neuralgia. These symptoms were noted to respond best to treatment with anticonvulsant medications such as carbamazepine and phenytoin. Side effects with increased weakness and ataxia were noted. Baclofen may also be useful as an alternative. Chronic symptoms were most often dysesthesias involving the extremities or back. Dysesthesias respond to treatment with tricyclic medications, with improvement noted by more than 50% of patients (149), although the results were more equivocal in the study by Foley. Additional measures considered in the treament of dysesthetic pain include the use of capsaicin cream and transcutaneous nerve stimulation (TENS). Electrical stimulation has been used with some success for the treatment of painful spasms (150). Newer treatments that are being tried include drugs such as mexiletine and gabapentin (Neurontin).

It is important to thoroughly evaluate patients with paresthesias and pain so that a correctable cause is not missed. Examples of correctable causes include carpal tunnel syndrome and postural low-back pain, both of which can be treated successfully.

Motor Disorders—Tremor, Ataxia, and Weakness

Motor dysfunction, including weakness and ataxia, is the major cause of disability in MS (31). The use of medications for motor problems is limited because of side effects such as sedation and increased fatigue. Drugs such as clonazepam (Klonopin) and hydroxyzine (Atarax) have been used for their damping effects with ataxia, while β-blockers such as propranolol (Inderal) have been used primarily for the treatment of tremors (151). Agents such as primidone (Mysoline) and isoniazid have also been used with limited success, but have greater side effects and a smaller therapeutic window (152). Neurosurgical procedures using stereotactic techniques for thalamotomies have been tried in patients with motor control disorders but can have limited benefits given the risk and subsequent recurrent difficulties (153). Apart from ataxia and tremor, movement disorders such as parkinsonism, dystonia, and myoclonus are relatively infrequent (154). Two studies (144,145) noted responses to treatment using rehabilitation therapies and medications. Motor training with biofeedback and Frenkel (155) exercises can be incorporated with weights to dampen the oscillation of ataxia. Orthotic intervention and bracing to improve motor control and stability may be helpful; for example, a soft cervical collar may increase head control. Training may be limited by an increased difficulty with weakness and fatigue so that resistive weights and equipment may not be tolerated. Active exercise in the past was avoided. However, current evaluations indicate that a generalized conditioning program can be used to optimize residual strength and endurance and improve function (156). A specific exercise prescription to minimize overexertion and limit increasing body temperatures such as with aquatic therapy in a cool pool can be helpful (157).

Electrical stimulation has also been used to treat paretic muscles in a number of conditions. An 8-week study by Kent-Braun et al (158) looked at fatigue for contractile tension force in the ankle dorsiflexors of six patients with MS. Twitch times, pH, phosphate-phosphocreatinine (Pi/PCr) ratio, and creatine phosphokinase levels were also assessed. Decreased fatigue with smaller reductions in contractile force was seen in four patients but fatigue and contractile force were increased in the other two. Some signs of muscle injury with increased Pi/PCr ratios and reduced contractions were seen transiently at the onset of treatment but returned to baseline within the first week.

Pharmacologic enhancement of depolarization may also be possible. Trials are currently underway evaluating medications that may improve motor function by facilitating nerve conduction through increased depolarization as a result of blocking potassium channels (159). A similar principle is the basis for which digitalis has been tried, owing to its block of the Na-K pump (160). Improving conduction will be a major area for neurotherapies in the future.

SPASTICITY

Spasticity is a frequent and significant problem for people with MS. It can limit comfort, function, level of independence, and QOL. Its characteristic spasms, involuntary muscle movement, muscle stiffness with movement, and increased reflexes are well known to many with MS. Both ambulation and dexterity can be greatly affected, and spasticity may increase the risk of decubiti and contractures. Hygiene may be impaired, and pain can be significant. Sleep disturbances are not unusual. Good use of remaining strength may be difficult because of increased tone and rigidity of movement (161). However, some individuals use the spasticity in their lower extremities for transfers, standing, or ambulation. This, in turn, may decrease osteopenia and help minimize atrophy. Without the stiffness associated with spasticity, functioning actually decreases in some individuals.

If an individual has progressive spasticity, or a recent change in the pattern or degree of spasticity, then a medical evaluation is appropriate to investigate possible causes. All potentially noxious stimuli such as an ingrown toenail, urinary tract infections, tight leg bags, and pressure should be addressed. A careful physical examination and history, which includes a review of bladder and bowel management, often identifies the culprit.

Treatment of spasticity in MS is indicated when its disadvantages outweigh any potential advantages (162). Good general care is the cornerstone of prevention and initial treatment: Proper skin care, pressure relief, early treatment of symptomatic bladder infections, good bowel programs, prevention of deep venous thrombosis, and avoidance of any noxious stimuli all help minimize spasticity. Proper posture and positioning, effective seating, and orthotics or splinting are also important. Active and passive range of motion exercises should be part of an active rehabilitation program, and may lead to relief of spasticity (163). Topical cold therapy may also be effective (164), and may have the added benefit of dissipating heat in MS patients who are heat intolerant.

MS is one of the best studied in regards to the pharmacologic treatment of spasticity, and almost all the usual medications used have efficacy in this disease (165). Baclofen is usually the first drug of choice for patients with MS. It is most useful in treating spasticity from spinal lesions such as those seen in spinal cord–injured patients and MS patients (166). It acts, in part, by interfering with the release of excitatory transmitters (167,168). Baclofen may be sedating and cause somnolence, especially at higher doses, and requires especially careful monitoring in MS patients with fatigue. However, some patients with MS can readily tolerate relatively large doses and therefore it may be appropriate to consider high doses when aggressive management is indicated (168,169). While some patients with MS report weakness as a side effect, the weakness may simply be the perception of less resistance to muscle contraction in patients with MS (170). Baclofen should be titrated with careful attention to efficacy, side effects, and function. It should not be discontinued abruptly.

Benzodiazepines also may be used to treat the spasticity of MS. Diazepam increases presynaptic inhibition and may be very effective (171). However, its sedative effect may make it intolerable to some, and its deleterious effects on attention and memory may be particularly problematic for patients with MS (164).

Dantrolene works as an antispasticity agent by reducing the release of calcium from the sarcoplasmic reticulum, which inhibits muscle contraction (164,173). It is effective in MS (174) and does not cause as much cognitive dysfunction as baclofen or diazepam (175). However, dantrolene may be a poor treatment option for patients with MS (165) because of its significant drug-induced weakness. Other potential side effects include hepatic injury, drowsiness, lethargy, and nausea.

Clonidine, a centrally acting α_2-adrenergic agonist, may be effective treatment for spinal spasticity in MS (176–180), and may be applied transdermally (172,175). Its use may be limited by hypotension and nausea. Tizanidine, an imidazoline derivative, also has α-adrenergic agonist activity. It has been approved by the FDA for the treatment of spasticity. Tizanidine shows promise in providing comparable or superior results to baclofen (165), and may be better tolerated in some patients (181). Its side effects include hypotension, sleepiness, dry mouth, and weakness (182). Tizanidine can reduce spasms and clonus in MS (183). Threonine has also been studied as treatment for MS (184), and other potential treatments include phenothiazines, glycine, progabide, phenytoin, and cannabis (162,164).

Nerve blocks and motor point blocks can be very effective in the selective treatment of spasticity in MS. Judicious use allows one to avoid systemic side effects while addressing localized spasticity. Intramuscular botulinum toxin can also be effective for MS patients.

Intrathecal morphine has been used to treat spasticity (185), but intrathecal baclofen is more commonly used. For patients with MS whose spasticity is poorly controlled with conservative treatment and oral medications, intrathecal baclofen should be considered before ablative surgical options. Intrathecal baclofen can control severe spinal spasticity and improve function (186–188). Computerized telemetry allows precise titration and treatment, since the pump can deliver different doses at various times of the day. Although intrathecal baclofen is not as effective for spasticity in the upper extremities as for the lower extremities, the low frequency of cognitive dysfunction associated with its use makes it a valuable option for the appropriate individual with MS. Additionally, it often allows a patient to take significantly less antispasticity medication, and in some cases may eliminate the need for oral agents. This reduced need is of particular benefit to MS patients who may enjoy improved function and QOL by avoiding the medications that can sedate and add cognitive dysfunction.

Surgical options for patients with MS who are not candidates for intrathecal baclofen include ablation of dorsal entry root zones, neurectomy, and myelotomy. (See Chap. 47 for a detailed discussion of spasticity.)

FATIGUE

Fatigue in MS may have a significant impact on QOL and function, and is the most common symptom of MS (189–192). It is also a common complaint in ambulatory patients in general, and may be seen with a variety of medical conditions (193). However, the fatigue of MS is believed to be unique and different from the normal fatigue that occurs from activities and the fatigue that resolves with simple rest (194). It must also be distinguished from chronic fatigue syndrome, which may have some findings that are similar to those in patients with the fatigue of MS (195,196). This fatigue is described as overwhelming or total exhaustion. The mechanism of fatigue is not known, but may have central components such as upper motor neuron dysfunction as well as peripheral components such as impaired muscular metabolism and excitation-contraction coupling (197). Many patients do better in the morning hours, but later become incapacitated by fatigue and sleepiness and experience decreased mobility and self-care (189,192). Cognitive dysfunction may be accentuated by fatigue. It can also contribute to social isolation. As a "silent symptom" that is not immediately obvious to a casual observer, the impact of the fatigue is often poorly understood by the patient's family, friends, and support system. Others may mistakenly believe that the patient is not trying or is poorly motivated. The fatigue can also interfere with attaining functional goals in rehabilitation. It increases lost days of employment and is a major contributor to unemployment in patients with MS (198,199).

The fatigue may be triggered by increased heat or any activity or energy expenditure, or may occur spontaneously. Other factors that may contribute to fatigue include depression, vigorous exercise, spasticity, ataxia, weakness, medications, stress and psychosocial factors, and exacerbations (Table 76-11). Early afternoon fatigue in MS patients may be related to an elevation in body core temperature (200).

Table 76-11: Factors Contributing to Fatigue in Multiple Sclerosis (MS)
Non-MS medical issues (i.e., medications, illness, disease)
Depression
Heat intolerance
Vigorous exercise
Spasticity
Ataxia
Weakness
Stress
Psychosocial factors
Vocational issues
Decreased mobility, need for orthotic management, etc
Decreased self-care, need for adaptive equipment, training, etc

Table 76-12: Fatigue in Multiple Sclerosis (MS)
Identify quality and quantity of fatigue
Obtain functional history of fatigue and its impact
Rule out non-MS causes (i.e., anemia, hypothyroidism, etc)
Identify contributing factors
Review medications and side effects
Treat identified contributing factors
Educate and provide treatment regarding work simplification, economy of efforts, pacing, and resting, to decrease energy consumption
Consider adjunctive pharmacologic therapy with amantadine or pemoline

The treatment of fatigue should be individualized and based on the patient's function and medical status (Table 76-12). Medications should be reviewed and streamlined. Other causes of fatigue such as anemia, hypothyroidism, and depression should be evaluated as appropriate. A detailed functional history can lead to specific interventions to conserve energy. Education regarding decreased energy consumption, economy of efforts, prioritization, work simplification, pacing, planning of activities, and rest periods should be provided by the rehabilitation team. Improving the efficiency of doing ADLs with a focus on technique and adaptive equipment is often helpful. Gait evaluation with appropriate use of orthotics and assistive devices is important. Often a home exercise program requires modification. Spasticity management should be emphasized, with careful attention to possible medication side effects. Psychological support for the responses to fatigue (194) may be necessary, as well as social support, peer support, and vocational intervention. Modification of the type of work, work environment, and temperature of the workplace can impact on the fatigue of MS. People who are able to have a sense of control or the ability to choose appropriate environments have less global fatigue and fatigue-related distress (201). Rehabilitation in the home as well as outpatient and inpatient rehabilitation should incorporate these principles, and should be provided at the patient's most active time of day. Shorter sessions with rest periods and avoiding back-to-back therapy sessions will improve tolerance to rehabilitation and may improve outcomes (200).

Current pharmacologic treatment options include pemoline (202), a CNS stimulant, and amantadine (203–206), which is an antiviral agent. The precise mechanisms of action are not clear. In a study comparing pemoline, amantadine, and placebo in patients with MS (207), amantadine was superior and there were fewer side effects. Neither of these medications compared with placebo appears to enhance cognitive performance in MS (208).

Table 76-13: Cognitive Impairments in MS
Attention
Memory
Visuospatial skills
Information processing
Less affected: recent memory, language, abstract reasoning

COGNITIVE DYSFUNCTION

Cognitive dysfunction in MS has been well documented. It was first reported in the 1870s by Charcot, who noted cognitive slowing in patients with MS. More recent studies suggested that 43% to 70% of MS patients may have impairment found on neuropsychological testing (209–214). Cognitive deficits may include decreased attention, memory, reasoning, visuospatial skills, information processing speed, and intelligence (Table 76-13). Each patient's cognition may be affected in various degrees with variable consequences. Cognitive changes may not correlate with the degree of physical disability (215). They may also be independent of illness duration (212). While these cognitive changes may also be unrelated to the severity of depression, they are associated with apathy and euphoria (214). Disease type is not a useful predictor of cognitive performance (216).

Overall, it appears that general intelligence in MS changes gradually over time, and verbal skills are affected less than performance skills (217). Language function is generally spared (218), which may relate to the characteristic pattern of brain lesions seen in MS. Retrieval of information is often delayed in patients with MS, and information processing is slowed (217–219). Conceptual reasoning may be impaired, and perseveration is not unusual (217,220,221). Recent memory and abstract reasoning are less affected than verbal intelligence, language, and memory span (211,212,218). The dementia seen in MS is often, but not always, "subcortical" in nature, with decreased insight, cognitive slowing, impaired memory, and dysarthria as the primary findings (215,217,222). Primary progressive MS often is associated with more severe cognitive impairment, independent of physical disability, in comparison to R-R MS (222).

The implications of cognitive dysfunction in MS are far reaching. Impairment of cognition may limit the ability to learn and to process information, and may challenge the rehabilitation professional's efforts to teach and improve functional independence. Social isolation may occur as relationships with family and friends are affected. Safety in the home and compliance with medications may be compromised, as well as follow-through with suggested medical interventions. Clearly, these disturbances can decrease function and the QOL of patients with MS. The impact of cognitive dysfunction on psychosocial functioning is impressive: Cognitively impaired patients with MS are less likely to be working, engage in fewer social and avocational activities, report more sexual dysfunction, and have greater difficulty with household tasks (223).

It is difficult to correlate specific anatomic lesions in MS with categories of cognitive dysfunction (223,224). Corpus callosum atrophy may be a significant finding (225,226). Clinical studies comparing cognitive test performance and imaging study findings such as brain lesion burden had mixed results, but it does appear that MRI findings do not consistently correlate strongly with functional scales (i.e., Kurtzke) (214,221,224–233). MRI findings are not a substitute for neuropsychological testing.

A complete evaluation of cognitive deficits cannot be done by brief interviewing. The Mini-Mental State Examination (MMSE) may predict cognitive impairment (234), but is insensitive to mild impairment (228). The neuropsychological screening battery designed by Franklin et al (228) may be more sensitive than the MMSE. Rao et al (212) developed a brief 20-minute screening battery that utilizes the most sensitive indicators from comprehensive batteries of tests. This instrument is sensitive (71%) and very specific (94%). Detailed testing allows clinicians to identify an individual's relative strengths and weaknesses.

Information from neuropsychological testing is helpful for clinical monitoring and has direct clinical value for rehabilitation. Specific findings may be utilized for patient and family counseling, vocational and avocational intervention, and rehabilitation designed to improve function, independence, and QOL. Detailed information on cognitive processes is invaluable to the treating rehabilitation team members, who can individualize treatment based on patient needs. Therapists may modify their remediation, compensation training, and adaptation techniques (213) based on a patient's skills and deficits. Psychologists and social workers find neuropsychological testing helpful in their treatment and support of the individual. For example, socialization, relations, depression and other affective disorders, defenses, and coping strategies are all impacted greatly by cognitive deficits. Home care professionals and rehabilitation nurses can use test results to identify the best techniques and tools to use for patient education and for teaching procedures such as catheterization and bowel programs. Compensatory measures and cognitive strategies can be designed to complement an individual's relative strengths.

VISION PROBLEMS

Vision problems can be characterized into four areas: loss of acuity, field deficits, loss of color or contrast sensitivity, and oculomotor dysfunction such as diplopia and nystagmus. The latter problems are typically seen with midbrain and brain stem lesions as with internuclear ophthalmoplegias. Treatment for diplopia and nystagmus includes the use of alternating eye patches or a trial with medication such as clonazepam or baclofen (235). Loss of acuity and reduced sensitivity for color and contrast are most frequently seen with optic neuritis. The findings are confirmed using VEPs (usually pattern shift visual evoked responses) and MRIs. When vision problems are the initial presentation, 50% to 60% of patients have additional white matter findings consistent with MS. Of patients with positive MRI findings, 25% to 50% go on to have definite MS, with the highest percentage being women (236). The association of optic neuritis with MS and the implications of treatment are significant. A detailed evaluation of treatment with corticosteroids revealed the unusual finding that oral prednisone alone was associated with a higher rate of recurrence and development of MS, almost double over the subsequent 2 years, compared with intravenous methylprednisolone and placebo (113). Compensatory treatment strategies involving equipment such as low-vision aids can also be helpful when persistent impairment exists (see Chap. 54).

BLADDER AND BOWEL DYSFUNCTION

The most common bladder problems include urinary tract infection, incontinence of urine, and retention. Bladder dysfunction is one of the main problems seen in hospitalized patients and has significant associated costs (146). Increasing severity of dysfunction has been related to hospitalization due to pyelonephritis and stone formation, but better management has reduced the morbidity and mortality from 50% to 5% over the last 30 years (237,238). The major difficulty is upper tract involvement, which can occur early or late in the disease course regardless of severity or degree of symptoms (239,240). The most common bladder symptoms are frequency and urgency (80%–90%), followed by hesistancy or actual incontinence (50%–70%) (239). The associated bladder disorders can be categorized into three types based on function and neurogenic status: disorders of storage, of emptying, and a combination, corresponding respectively to hyperreflexic, hyporeflexic, and dysynergic conditons. Over 50% of patients are hyperreflexic and as many as half of them have detrusor–external sphincter dysynergia (DSD) (240). The risk in these patients is from vesicoureteral reflux due to raised intravesicular pressures above 40 cm H_2O. The high bladder pressure and reflux can cause upper tract problems over time, including hydronephrosis and renal failure. In more severely involved patients, DSD is seen more often when they have hesistancy as a presenting problem (239). On clinical examination in one study, a finding of bilateral plantarreflexes was associated with findings of DSD in 70% of patients (241). Nonetheless, the history and physical examination alone cannot rule in or out DSD and elevated bladder pressures. The concern remains that the condition may be silent, and therefore thorough evaluation is indicated, including monitoring urinary volumes with routine measurement of postvoid residual (PVR) and regular urinalysis including culture and sensitivity tests and creatinine levels (240,242). PVR may be measured noninvasively by ultrasound, which reduces the risk of infection. The use of ultrasonography has become prevalent for both lower tract assessments and upper tract evaluation for stones and hydronephrosis. Detailed functional evaluation of urodynamics using cystometrics (cystometrography), voiding cystourethrography, and intravenous pyelography may be helpful in selected patients (242), and has been discussed in detail elsewhere (see Chap. 7).

Bladder management has been reviewed (see Chap. 51) and focuses on restoring function for storage and emptying while minimizing the risk for infection (242,243). If the patient is unable to store urine adequately, has low PVR volume, and has frequency due to hyperreflexia, then anticholinergics such as oxybutynin (Ditropan) or propantheline can be useful to reduce bladder tone. If there is difficulty voiding and elevated PVR volumes, then the risk of infection increases as a result of difficulty clearing the urine. Difficulty clearing the urine can be due to ineffective bladder emptying with hyporeflexia or due to obstruction with external sphincter spasticity resulting in dysynergia with a hyperreflexic bladder. In both cases assisted drainage using a catheter is necessary. Intermittent catheterization remains the best form of management along with regulation of fluid intake. An indwelling catheter may be necessary for some individuals who have difficulties with intermittent catheterization. Surgical treatment can include a suprapubic cystostomy, sphincteroplasty, and bladder augmentation. Sphincter problems can be managed with medications. Adrenergic agents or α-blockers can be utilized to reduce spasticity. α-Agonists can be used for sphincter insufficiency such as with stress incontinence if there is no hyperreflexia. The use of newer agents such as desmopressin acetate, an antidiuretic hormone, can effect urine production, which may help the timing of bladder management, facilitating nocturnal continence, for example.

Bowel dysfunction occurs in two-thirds of patients with MS (244). Bowel function is compromised by lesions affecting motor and autonomic pathways. The gastrocolic reflex may be compromised (245). Colonic transit time is decreased, and sensation may be decreased. Symptoms of bowel dysfunction include constipation, incontinence of bowel, and fecal urgency. A careful history should include fluid intake, current medications, and current bowel program. Physical examination should include a rectal examination to rule out impaction, tumors, and so on. The first step in treatment involves education. Adequate fluid intake is important. Having the patient use gravity as an assist, by sitting or using a commode, is helpful. Timing the bowel program after a meal utilizes the gastrocolic reflex as much as possible. The consistency of the stool can be managed with stool softeners, if necessary. Oral laxatives, such as senna (Senokot), may be taken at the appropriate time before the scheduled bowel program (i.e., at noon for an evening program). Fiber and exercise can also increase colonic motility. Enemas or suppositories such as bisacodyl (Dulcolax) may be used at the appropriate time. Some patients are able to use glycerin suppositories or digital stimulation. Therevac (minienema) may be an effective agent as well, but good hand dexterity is required to squeeze the medication into the rectal vault. The addition of a stimulant such as milk of magnesia or even magnesium citrate may also be necessary. Finally the use of anticholinergics—often needed for bladder management in patients with MS—should be minimized in those with constipation. A successful, coordinated bowel program can ensure timed voiding, minimize or eliminate incontinence, and give functional freedom and self-esteem to patients with MS and neurogenic bowels. Bowel disorders are easier to manage but require vigilance with the use of a regular routine specific to each patient. Developing routines that facilitate these aspects of self-care for the patient must be considered as part of the overall rehabilitation management.

SEXUAL DYSFUNCTION

Sexual dysfunction is very common in patients with MS and is a clear threat to QOL (246). It is therefore important for health care providers to address this important issue. Sexual dysfunction is associated with bladder dysfunction and spasticity but not with the loss of mobility or depression (247). It is also independent of age, duration of disease, and type of disease (248).

Sexual dysfunction may be tactfully addressed using the acronym PLISSIT model developed by Annon (249). *P* stands for permission to discuss the issues as a first step so patients are as comfortable as possible. Permission establishes that it is appropriate to discuss sexual dysfunction as much as one is comfortable doing so. *LI* stands for limited information that can be given regarding possible interventions. *SS* stands for specific suggestions, referring to individually based interventions such as devices. *IT*, or intensive therapy, is necessary when there are complex issues requiring a trained therapist.

A careful history is important because many of the symptoms of MS impact on sexual arousal and activity. For example, neurogenic bladder and bowel management and incontinence, weakness, pain, fatigue, ataxia, contractures, decubiti, and heat intolerance can all interfere with sexual function. A decreased libido has been described in patients with MS (247,250–252). Both libido and sexual dysfunction may fluctuate with disease activity (250). Medications can also be responsible. Corticosteroids may improve sexual functioning in some individuals with MS and sexual dysfunction (248). For the evaluation of sexual dysfunction, the physical examination should be complete and include, for example, an assessment of strength, sensation and sensory levels, spasticity, mobility, contractures, and anal and cremasteric reflexes.

Erectile dysfunction is a common complaint in up to 80% of men, and 10% have ejaculatory problems (253). Decreased penile sensation, inability to reach orgasm, premature ejaculation, inability to ejaculate, and trouble with achieving and maintaining erections have been reported (248). Neurophysiological testing indicates the presence of supra sacral spinal cord lesions in most men with sexual dysfunction (254,255). Treatment may include intracavernous injections of vasoactive agents (253,255), vacuum devices, penile prosthesis, and sexual counseling.

Sexual dysfunction is reported in up to 74% of women (250,251,280). It may also be a presenting symptom (256). In some individuals, the most common problem related to sexual function is fatigue (247). Decreased vaginal lubrication and decreased maintenance of lubrication, decreased vaginal sensation, and lack of orgasms are most commonly reported (248). Other findings include decreased libido, severe external dysesthesia, and vaginal dyspareunia (256). Changes in sexual function in women are related to weakness of the pelvic floor as well as bowel and bladder dysfunction (256). Pudendal-evoked potentials may be abnormal, as well as urodynamic studies, anal reflexes, and sensation (256–257). Treatment principles include correcting as many of the contributing factors as possible (i.e., spasticity, fatigue, etc). Sensory dysesthesia may be amenable to pharmacological intervention with low-dose tricyclic antidepressants. Water soluble vaginal lubricants may be helpful. Estrogen supplements may also help in post menopausal women.

Sexual dysfunction commonly causes marital problems (247,248). It is important for the treating health care professional to appreciate how common sexual dysfunction is, how difficult it is for some individuals to talk about it, and how factors associated with MS, such as spasticity, weakness, etc., impact sexual function. Appropriate interventions can make a significant impact on a patient and his or her significant other. Understanding sexuality will help facilitate treatment and adaptation.

Affective Disorders

Affective and psychiatric disorders are common in MS. Up to 30–40% of patients in the early stages of MS may have depression (258). As many as 75% of patients may experience depression at some time during their illness (78). Unfortunately, the suicide rate is 7.5 times higher in patients with MS than in the general population (259). The symptoms of depression, such as fatigue, sleep disturbance, lethargy, and cognitive deficits, may be similar to those seen frequently in MS. Fatigue can independently contribute to depression (260). These factors may lead to underdiagnosis of depression. Patients with cerebral involvement of disease are more likely to be depressed than those with cord involvement (261). Depression correlates with the degree of neurologic impairment (261). Although findings are mixed, it may also correlate with decreased functional capacity (262). Increased awareness of the signs and symptoms of depression will aid its early evaluation, diagnosis, and treatment to minimize the depression-related disability.

Emotional lability and euphoria may be observed in patients with MS (263). Pathological crying and laughing may be treated with amytriptyline (264). Euphoria may increase as the patient's condition worsens (265). Affective disorders may be related to lesions in the temporal lobes in patients with MS (266). Bipolar disease is estimated to be 13 times higher in MS (263). While psychosis may be seen in patients with MS, the incidence of schizophrenia is not increased (217,267).

It is not clear if psychiatric changes in MS are reactions to the disorder or are part of the disease process (217) caused by plaques and demyelination. Many patients respond to pharmacologic treatment and psychotherapy.

Patients with chronic progressive MS may have frontal lobe dysfunction resulting in behavior changes (211,220,268). Poor motivation, apathy, decreased initiation, inability to sustain goal-directed activities, and impulsivity may be seen. Inappropriate behavior and an apparent lack of direction are common (269). The activity of patients may become perseverative, or apparently aimless (270). Behavioral dyscontrol and disinhibition may be managed with provision of structure, supervision, cueing, and environmental changes (270). The rehabilitation team and health care professionals should be careful not to misinterpret the patient's actions and attitudes as necessarily deliberate and manipulative.

DYSARTHRIA, DYSPHONIA, DYSPHAGIA, AND RESPIRATORY DISORDERS

Poor oral-motor control, laryngeal and pharyngeal dysfunction, and respiratory disorders are frequent manifestations of brain stem dysfunction with weakness and spasticity. Brain stem findings as a whole are the third most common functional system to be affected as noted by Kurtzke (30). Treatment commonly centers on training exercises to improve breath control, pacing, and bolus control. The use of compensatory techniques such as head tilt and a modified diet can be incorporated with dietary counseling (271). Further adaptive techniques may include the use of a palatal lift, Teflon injections to stiffen the vocal cord, and the use of tubes for feeding.

Respiratory dysfunction due to complications such as pneumonia secondary to aspiration occurs more frequently than primary ventilatory dysfunction with weakness and/or medullary involvement. Respiratory weakness can be increased with increasing conduction block due to increased temperatures. Typically findings include decreased forced vital capacity (FVC) and maximal voluntary ventilation (MVV) with a normal forced expiratory ventilation in 1 second to FVC ratio, indicating minimal obstructive dysfunction. Bedside assessment of respiratory function can be done by evaluating cough and using single breath counting, with the ability to count up to 20 to 30 being fair to good. Checking for orthopnea should also be done, as both FVC and MVV decrease significantly in impaired patients from the seated to supine position. Ambulatory patients rarely show impairments (272).

MOBILITY

Disability due to functional limitations in mobility can arise from a number of underlying causes. This disability is most often secondary to impairments from paraparesis and spasticity. Fatigue and difficulty with balance and ataxia are also common. These problems progress as part of the natural history of the disease, where the majority of patients remain ambulatory with an EDSS score lower than 6 during the first 15 years of the disease and then progress to EDSS scores 6 and 7 over 3 to 4 years for each stage (see Table 76-6) (37). Rehabilitation should be initiated at the first sign of a problem, such as spastic paraparesis, for example, with the implementation of a stretching and exercise program to maintain range of motion, strength, and endurance. A recent study by Petajan et al (273) indicated that exercise three times a week improved work capacity 48%, with decreased fatigue and improved mood, although the EDSS score did not change. An independent program may be prescribed and aquatic therapy can also be helpful. Gait training for uneven surfaces and stairs may reduce the risk of falls. Compensatory techniques with assistive equipment such as canes (both regular straight canes and a quadripod cane), crutches (Lofstrand and Canadian), and walkers including rolling devices with brakes may be utilized with training for appropriate skills. Adaptive strategies may require substitution of some activities with alternatives, such as using a wheelchair or power scooter when ambulation is no longer an option. Such strategies may initially be necessary for traveling longer distances to allow energy conservation, but the patient should still be encouraged to walk for shorter distances as much as possible. The provision of a wheelchair or scooter is often arranged on an interdisciplinary basis, with physical therapy, occupational therapy, and possibly nursing input to address a number of concerns, including skin status as it pertains to seating pressure and position, and the use of appropriate control devices. Training with push-ups to relieve pressure and transfer training may be necessary. Removable armrests may be requested to allow the use of a sliding board for transfers. A hospital bed may also be necessary to facilitate bed mobility and care. Addressing these areas can have significant effects on the overall function of the individual and should be specified as part of the prescribed treatment.

Activities of Daily Living

These areas typically include self-care with eating, toileting, bathing, and dressing; instrumental ADLs (IADLs) such as shopping and preparing meals are also areas where functional problems and disabilities arise. The underlying impairments need to be addressed and a plan must be developed based on the patient's priorities, including a schedule that allows the patient to achieve his or her goals. A plan can help the patient compensate for fatigue by using pacing skills and energy conservation techniques. Activity simplification and adaptive equipment such as remote controls, reachers, Velcro closures, and bath benches can be used. A home or work site evaluation can provide additional ideas to facilitate functional activities and allow for accommodations.

VOCATIONAL EVALUATION

A vocational evaluation's purpose is to determine individual objectives for employment and to provide an assessment of employment potential. The latter is done by assessing specific and general skills and abilities. These include, for example, aptitude, interests, personality, values, attitudes, motivation, physical capacity, work tolerance and abilities, educability, social skills, work habits, and employment potential (274). The rehabilitation team has significant potential impact on employment, as issues such as functional independence, mobility, endurance, and self-care are addressed. Work site evaluations with review of the ergonomics and physical demands of the job may be needed. Patient and employer education is often useful. An assessment of barriers to employment may include investigation of cognitive function, neurogenic bladder and bowel issues, spasticity, visual and perceptual impairment, and heat intolerance.

Maintaining employment is related to employment in the public sector, having a sedentary job, and having the potential for specific improvements in the work environment (275). Additionally, mild disability and a high educational level are favorable (276). Risk factors for job loss include having a job requiring use of force, a rigid work schedule, need for manual precision, frequent moving, and a work day longer than 8 hours (275,277). Patients with cognitive impairment have less success in maintaining employment (223).

Patients with MS may require proactive assistance to maintain employment, to ensure that early intervention and changes at work are considered. The Americans with Disabilities Act of 1991, designed to extend civil rights to people with disabilities, prohibits employers from asking prospective employees about a disabling disease (278,279). Rather, the current impairment, not future health, should be used to make employment decisions (279). The Disabilities Act may also help patients with work accessibility.

The avocational and social needs of patients with MS are important. Social support is beneficial to both patients and their families. Family cohesiveness, supportive significant others, and social exchanges outside the family all contribute to good health and better stress management (280). The challenges of unemployment, family and financial stressors, and difficulty with household management are best met with support and comprehensive rehabilitation intervention (281). Therapists may have an impact on function, independence, and psychological health such as self-esteem. Psychologists can offer additional support and intervention to the patient and family. Social services can be used to provide education about community resources and reintegration. Therapeutic recreation can utilize and reinforce an individual's functional strengths while focusing on socialization and community reintegration.

SUPPORT SYSTEMS

It is clear that significant support is needed for individuals with MS. The National Multiple Sclerosis Society was founded in 1946 as a nonprofit organization and continues today to provide one of the largest support systems for people with MS and their significant others. There are now over 450,000 members and over 85 chapters offering a variety of services for people with MS and their families. Since its inception, the society has dedicated over $95 million for research grants and fellowships directed toward finding the cause and cure for MS. Additionally, on behalf of persons with disabilities and their families, the society advocates at the state and national level to work toward equal access to health care, employment, and public accommodations. The society's mission is to end the devastating effects of MS. The four components of the mission are research, service, education, and advocacy. There is a clear commitment to empower people with MS to live as independently as possible within their limits. It helps people with MS meet the challenges of life after the diagnosis is made, and focuses on their abilities rather than disabilities.

An individual chapter of the National Multiple Sclerosis Society may provide extensive information on MS and community resources for agencies and services. Public education and professional education help provide greater understanding of the issues of MS. Numerous publications covering a wide range of topics related to MS may be available for reference. Support groups are generally organized throughout a chapter area, and may include specifically designed groups for those recently diagnosed, those minimally disabled, and care partners. Chapters often recruit, train, and coordinate a network of dedicated volunteers to support members through phone calls and personal visits. Newsletters from chapters keep clients up-to-date. Some chapters are able to loan medical equipment on a short-term basis to individuals who are unable to obtain it from other resources, and financial assistance may be available. Even assistance in arranging and financing temporary respite care may be available. Fund-raising efforts on the chapter level help support all of these services and support systems, and also contribute to the national organization's support of research.

Local community agencies ranging from social services to home care services and disability action groups are also part of an extended network that can help people with MS manage with a wide array of problems.

OUTCOMES

In evaluating outcomes, one is considering the effects and end results of particular conditions. This evaluation is done by looking at measurable parameters or markers based on how a problem or condition is defined and what is considered important and valuable. Outcomes are often categorized using a patient-centered perspective into four domains: physical, psychological, social and role performance, and general health perception (282). Measurement scales or instruments that are used in this regard include the Rand Medical Outcomes Study (MOS) long- and short-form health status scales (283), the latter, also known as SF-36, being used more frequently; the Sickness Impact Profile (SIP); and the Minimal Record of Disability (MRD), which incorporates the domains of impairment, disability, and handicap as outlined by the World Health Organization (WHO). The MRD subscales are the Kurtzke EDSS, the ISS, and the ESS, and these areas can

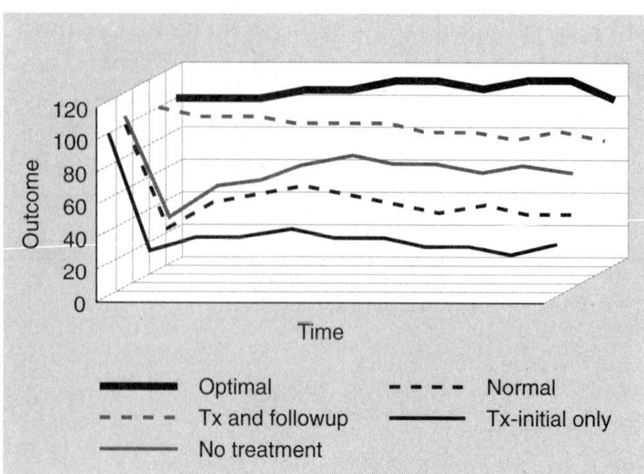

Figure 76-4. Outcomes over time. The upper curves represent optimal or normal status for a specific parameter of dimension over time. The lower curve represents the pattern of a particular disorder such as MS with no interventions. The middle curve represents the effect of a particular intervention. The second curve represents the possible effect of an intervention along with an ongoing influence such as a follow-up maintenance program.

be related to the four patient-centered domains. For example, the EDSS and ISS assess the physical and psychological domains, while the ISS and ESS cover the social and role performance and financial status areas. The Kurtzke scales can be correlated with QOL assessments to varying degrees in patients with chronic diseases (284). QOL studies indicate there is a specificity for the various scales, with different diseases showing different levels of impact for specific areas (283,285,286).

Time is another key parameter that must be taken into account when considering outcomes in conditions such as MS. Measurements are made at periodic intervals, often using 2 years and 5 years as end points. As outcomes are measured over time, they can generate a combined measure such as quality-adjusted life years (QALYs). This measure provides a more global assessement of the effects of different interventions at varying points over a life span. A similar measure called the Q-TWiST looks at quality-adjusted time without symptoms or toxicities (287). When one is looking at different effects, the natural history of any disease serves as a baseline for comparison. It represents the control group apart from any interventions. Figure 76-4 illustrates the relationships between treatments and outcomes over time. An example of the effects of rehabilitation on outcomes can be seen in terms of functional mobility where studies in patients with MS show a good outcome with durable improvement in independent function at discharge and 3 months after discharge (288).

Defining the problem, its context, and the process by which it will be analyzed are crucial steps. A useful study of MS patients in Olmstead County, Minnesota, looked at the overall MS population and described the general prevalence and impact of problems with MS (48). The MRD was used as the measurement instrument for a fairly detailed and specific assessment that included the work status and financial concerns. The authors indicated that this study was particularly significant as a baseline because it looked at the overall general MS population as opposed to more limited subgroups such as a clinic population, which had been the case in many of the prior studies. The issue is whether or not conclusions from a particular population can be extrapolated for comparison to other situations.

Several studies have identified a number of important areas in outcomes research. A national survey by the National Institutes of Health (NIH), done over 20 years ago, assessed concerns such as mobility, rate of employment, limitations on the average work status, and the financial impact that reflect disability and handicap as well as some primary symptoms, impairments, and demographics (289). Another early study, performed more than 15 years ago, looked at the cost and effectiveness of rehabilitation. Feigenson et al (145) found that significant and durable functional improvements could be achieved with rehabilitation, resulting in cost savings due to reduced needs for assistance a full year after discharge. Particular areas of focus for treatment such as bladder management training, transfers, and ADLs were indicated to be of high yield. The improvements were seen for functional performance while the underlying impairments with neurologic deficits were chronic and did not change. It is worth noting that treatment was on an inpatient basis after an outpatient treatment program had not been completely successful. A more recent study on veterans with MS (237) showed that significant cost benefits could be achieved by using proactive treatment to avoid hospitalization. The highest costs of care were Veterans Administration benefits including hospitalization and home care services. The primary reason for hospitalization was bladder problems, many of which could have been prevented with better outpatient training. Limiting disability was also important, as indicated by the finding that health care costs went up significantly for patients with an EDSS score above 5 and that any treatment that could delay a rise in EDSS above 5 would lower the overall cost of MS. Home care costs most closely correlated with the ISS results. The study also incorporated the SIP, which did correlate with costs but not as closely as the EDSS and ISS. In a study by Kraft et al (31), patients indicated that medical and rehabilitation needs were being adequately addressed except for bladder problems, where the need for assistance was seen to be greater than the services being provided. This concern was also seen for psychological, social, and vocational services as a whole. It seems reasonable that improvements in QOL could be

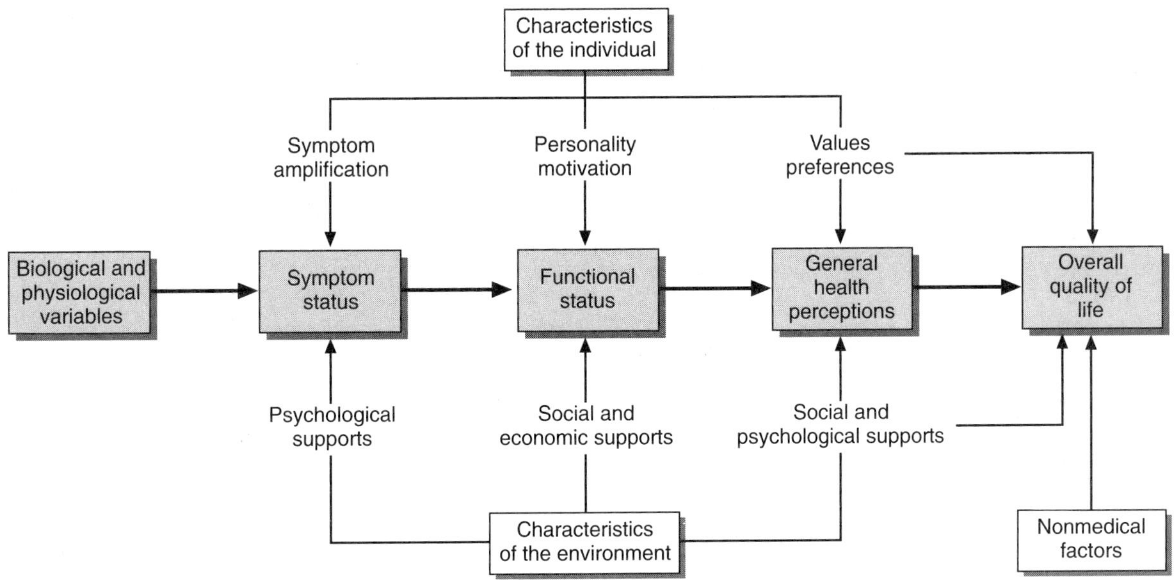

Figure 76-5. Outcome components. (Adapted with permission from Wilson IB, Cleary PD. Linking clinical variables with health related quality of life. *JAMA* 1995;273:59–65.)

achieved with these services and would facilitate community reintegration. Kottke (290) outlined these issues of QOL for an individual, and Figure 76-5 illustrates a recent model where functional status plays a central role (282). Studies on the effects and outcomes of rehabilitation, though limited thus far, clearly identify functional status as a key component of QOL and outcome.

The evaluation of outcomes in MS requires a good understanding of the disease in terms of its impairments, disabilities, and handicaps using appropriate measurement tools such as the MRD, EDSS, FIM, ISS, ESS, SIP, and SF-36, as well as specific cost-benefit analysis.

FUTURE DIRECTIONS

New advances in our understanding of MS have led to significant investigation into new pharmacologic treatments. The immune system's role is better understood, and clinical trials are underway to evaluate immune modulating drugs, or drugs designed to block immune activation. Additional work in progress is aimed at preventing the migration of cells across the BBB. Other trials are emphasizing the prevention or treatment of destruction of myelin in the CNS, as well as the role of cytokines. Preventing myelin destruction, repairing or replacing myelin, and improving conduction along demyelinated nerves are all areas of current investigation. Research on glial implantation and transplantation of myelin-forming cells has already provided insight into MS, and has provided hope for the future. There are currently more than 18 controlled clinical trials of potential therapies in the United States alone, and over 70 agents in various stages of testing around the world (291).

New technological advances have already made a significant impact on MS. Intrathecal baclofen now offers an effective treatment for severe spasticity. DNA testing has yielded genetic findings in MS that support the current belief that genes associated with the immune system correlate with susceptibility to MS. Advances in computer technology have improved environmental control units and general access. It is currently possible, for example, to use voice-activated units for environmental control and word processing. As new technology advances, we can expect it to positively impact on MS.

The delivery of health care and rehabilitation has changed significantly over the past few years. In general, length of stays for inpatient rehabilitation are shorter. Regular medical outpatient follow-up; coordinated, streamlined, comprehensive services; and home care delivery systems are becoming more common. In addition, there needs to be a focus on providing a continuum of care and placing more emphasis on the prevention of secondary illness. Outcomes must be monitored and care provided in a cost-effective way. The challenge, as the health care delivery system changes and moves forward, is to provide quality comprehensive lifelong care and rehabilitation.

ACKNOWLEDGMENTS

Heartfelt appreciation goes to our colleagues—Teal King, Meada Ebinger, and Lyn Crispino on the library staffs at St. Francis Hospital, Hartford, and Gaylord Hospital, Wallingford, Connecticut. Their efforts in helping us obtain information were invaluable.

REFERENCES

1. Noseworthy JH. Review: therapeutics of multiple sclerosis. *Clin Neuropharmacol* 1991;14:49–61.
2. Hansell R. The role of the general medical practitioner in the management of multiple sclerosis. *MS Manage* 1995;2(2):19–23.
3. Kurtzke JF. Epidemiology of multiple sclerosis. In: Hallpike JF, Adams CW, Tourtellote WW, eds. *Multiple sclerosis: pathology, diagnosis, and management.* London: Chapman & Hall, 1983:47–95.
4. Gorelick PB. Clues to the mystery of multiple sclerosis. *Postgrad Med* 1989;85: 125–134.
5. Wynn DR, Rodriguez M, O'Fallon WM, Kurland LT. Update on the epidemiology of multiple sclerosis. *Mayo Clin Proc* 1989; 64:808–817.
6. Duquette P, Pleines J, Girard M, et al. The increased susceptibility of women to multiple sclerosis. *Can J Neurol Sci* 1992; 19:466–471.
7. Anderson DW, Ellenberg JH, Leventhal CM, et al. Revised estimate of the prevalence of multiple sclerosis in the United States. *Ann Neurol* 1992;31: 333–336.
8. Kurtze JF. Epidemiologic contributions to multiple sclerosis: an overview. *Neurology* 1980;30: 61–79.
9. Cutler RW. Demyelinating disease. In: Rubinstien E, Federman DP, eds. *Scientific American medicine: neurology.* New York: Scientific American, 1987:Chapter 9.
10. Alter M, Kahana E, Lowenstron R. Migration and risk of multiple sclerosis. *Neurology* 1978;28: 1089–1093.
11. Detels R, Visscher BR, Haile RW, et al. Multiple sclerosis and age at migration. *Am J Epidemiol* 1978;108:380–393.
12. Mumford CJ, Wood NW, Kellar-Wood H, et al. The British Isles survey of multiple sclerosis in twins. *Neurology* 1994;44: 11–15.
13. Ebers GC, Bulman DE, Sadovnick AD, et al. A population-based study of multiple sclerosis in twins. *N Engl J Med* 1986;315:1638–1642.
14. Sadovnick AD, Armstrong H, Rice GPA, et al. A population-based study of multiple sclerosis in twins: update. *Ann Neurol* 1993;33:281–285.
15. Ebers GC, Sadovnick AD, Risch NJ, the Canadian Collaborative Study Group. A genetic basis for familial aggregation in multiple sclerosis. *Nature* 1995;377(14): 150–151.
16. Sadovnick AD, Baird PA, Ward RH. Multiple sclerosis: updated risks for relatives. *Am J Med Genet* 1988;29:533–535.
17. Sadovnick AD, Baird PA. The familial nature of multiple sclerosis: age corrected empiric recurrence risk for children and siblings of patients. *Neurology* 1988;38:990–991.
18. Compston DAS. Genetic susceptibility to multiple sclerosis. In: Matthews WB, Mc Alpine, D, eds., *McAlpine's multiple sclerosis.* 2nd ed. New York: Churchill Livingstone, 1991:301–320.
19. Sawcer S, Jones HB, Feakes R, et al. A genome screen in multiple sclerosis reveals susceptibility loci on chromosome 6p21 and 17q22. *Nat Genet* 1996;13:464–468.
20. Ebers GC, Kukay K, Bulman DE, et al. A full genome search in multiple sclerosis. *Nat Genet* 1996;13:472–476.
21. Haines JL, Ter-Minassian M, Bazyk A, et al. The Multiple Sclerosis Genetics Group. A complete genomic screen for multiple sclerosis underscores a role for the major histocompatibility complex. *Nat Genet* 1996;13:469–471.
22. Kuokkanen S, Sundvall M, Terwilliger JD, et al. A putative vulnerability locus to multiple sclerosis maps to 5p14-p12 in a region syntenic to the murine locus Eae2. *Nat Genet* 1996;13:477–480.
23. Kurtze JF, Hyllested K. Multiple sclerosis in the Faroe Islands. Clinical and epidemiological features. *Ann Neurol* 1979; 5:6–21.
24. Wucherpfennig KW, Strominger JL. Molecular mimicry in T cell-mediated autoimmunity: viral peptides activate human T cell clones specific for myelin basic protein. *Cell* 1995;80:695–705.
25. Booss J, Kim JH. Evidence for a viral etiology of multiple sclerosis. In: Cook SD, ed. *Handbook of multiple sclerosis.* New York: Marcel Dekker, 1990: 41–61.
26. Schumacher G, Beebe G, Kubler RF, et al. Problems of experimental trials of therapy in multiple sclerosis: report by the panel in the evaluation of experimental trials of therapy in MS. *Ann NY Acad Sci* 1965; 122:522–568.
27. McAlpine D, Compston ND, Acheson ED. *Multiple sclerosis: a reappraisal.* 2nd ed. London: Churchill Livingstone, 1972.
28. Poser CM, Paty DW, Scheinberg L, et al. New diagnostic criteria for multiple sclerosis: guidelines for research protocols. *Ann Neurol* 1983;13:227–231.
29. Kurtzke JF. Patterns of neurologic involvement in multiple sclerosis. *Neurology* 1989;39:1235–1238.
30. Kurtzke JF. Rating neurologic impairment in multiple sclerosis: an Expanded Disability Status Scale (EDSS). *Neurology* 1983;33:1444–1452.
31. Kraft G, Freal JE, Coryell JK. Disability, disease duration and rehabilitation service needs in multiple sclerosis: patient perspectives. *Arch Phys Med Rehabil* 1986;67:164–168.

32. Vollmer T, Waxman S. MS and other demyelinating disorders. In: Rosenberg R, ed. *Comprehensive neurology* New York: Raven, 1991:489–523.

33. Charcot JM. Lectures on the diseases of the nervous system. Second series. New York: Hafner, 1962. Facsimile of the London 1881 edition.

34. Kraft G, Freal JE, Coryell JK, et al. Multiple sclerosis: early prognostic guidelines. *Arch Phys Med Rehabil* 1981;62:54–58.

35. Thompson AJ, Kermode AG, Wicks D. Major differences in the dynamics of primary and secondary progressive multiple sclerosis. *Ann Neurol* 1991;29:53–62.

36. Weinshenker B, Sibley W. Natural history and treatment of multiple sclerosis. *Curr Opin Neurol Neurosurg* 1992;5: 203–211.

37. Weinshenker B, Bass B, Rice G, et al. The natural history of multiple sclerosis—clinical course and disability. *Brain* 1989;112: 133–146.

38. Confavreux C, Aimard G, Devic M. Course and prognosis of multiple sclerosis assessed by computerized data processing of 349 patients. *Brain* 1980;103: 281–300.

39. Runmarker B, Andersson C, Oden A, Andersen O. Prediction of outcome in MS based on multivariate models. *J Neurol* 1994;241:597–604.

40. Weinshenker B, Bass B, Rice G, et al. The natural history of multiple sclerosis—predictive value of the early course. *Brain* 1989;112:1419–1428.

41. Matthews WB, Compston A, Allen IV, Martyn CN. *McAlpine's multiple sclerosis.* London: Churchill Livingstone, 1991:143–149.

42. Noseworthy JH, Vandervoort MK, Wong CJ, et al. Interrater reliability with the EDSS and functional systems (FS) in a MS clinical trial. *Neurology* 1990;40:971–975.

43. Sharrack B, Hughes RAC. Clinical scales for multiple sclerosis. *J Neurol Sci* 1996;135:1–9.

44. Quick D, Schapiro R. Population dynamics of disability status scales for multiple sclerosis. *J Neurol Rehabil* 1996;10: 127–134.

45. International Federation of MS Societies. *Minimal record of disability.* New York: National MS Society, 1985.

46. Granger CV, Cotter AC, Hamilton BB, et al. Functional assessment scales: a study of persons with multiple sclerosis. *Arch Phys Med Rehabil* 1990;71:870–875.

47. Rudick RA, Miller D, Farmer RG, et al. Quality of life in multiple sclerosis: comparison with inflammatory bowel disease and rheumatoid arthritis. *Arch Neurol* 1992;49:1237–1242.

48. Rodriguez M, Siva A, Ward J, Stolp-Smith K, et al. Impairment, disability and handicap in multiple sclerosis. *Neurology* 1994;44:28–33.

49. Weinshenker BG, Rice GPA, Noseworthy JH, et al. The natural history of multiple sclerosis—multivariate analysis of predictive factors and models of outcome. *Brain* 1991;114:1045–1056.

50. Kurland LT. Trauma and multiple sclerosis. *Ann Neurol* 1994;36:S33–S37.

51. Weinreb H. Demyelinating and neoplastic diseases in pregnancy. *Neurol Clin* 1994; 12:511–514.

52. Thompson DS, Nelson LM, Burns A, et al. The effects of pregnancy in multiple sclerosis: a retrospective study. *Neurology* 1986;36:1097–1099.

53. Kermode AG, Thomson AJ, Tofts P, et al. Breakdown of the blood brain barrier precedes symptoms and other MRI signs of new lesions in multiple sclerosis. *Brain* 1990;113: 1477–1489.

54. Claudio L, Raine CS, Brosnan CF. Evidence of persistence of blood brain barrier abnormalities in chronic progressive multiple sclerosis. *Acta Neuropathol (Berl)* 1995;90:228–238.

55. Traugott U, Reinherz EL, Raine CS. Multiple sclerosis: distribution of T cells, T cell subsets with active chronic lesions. *Science* 1983;219:308–309.

56. Gay D, Esiri M. Blood brain barrier damage in acute multiple sclerosis plaques. *Brain* 1991;114:557–572.

57. Ffrench-Constant C. Pathogenesis of multiple sclerosis. *Lancet* 1994;342:271–275.

58. Gorelick P. Clues to the mystery of multiple sclerosis. *Postgrad Med* 1989;85:125–134.

59. Allen IV. Pathology of multiple sclerosis. In: Mathews WB, ed. *McAlpine's multiple sclerosis.* 2nd ed. New York: Churchill Livingstone, 1991:341–378.

60. Rodiguez M. Basic concepts and hypothesis in multiple sclerosis. *Mayo Clin Proc* 1989;64:570–575.

61. Waxman SG. Conduction in myelinated, unmyelinated, and demyelinated fibers. *Arch Neurol* 1977;34:585–589.

62. Waxman SG. Demyelination in spinal cord injury and multiple sclerosis: what can we do to enhance functional recovery? *J Neurotrauma* 1992;9: S105–S117.

63. Waxman SG, Utzsheider DA, Kocsis JD. Enhancement of action potential conduction following demyelination; experimental approaches to restoration of function in multiple sclerosis and spinal cord injury. *Prog Brain Res* 1994;100:233–243.

64. Bever CT. The current status of studies of aminopyridines in patients with multiple sclerosis. *Ann Neurol* 1994; 36(suppl):S118–S121.

65. Rasminsky M. The effects of temperature on conduction in demyelinated single nerve fibers. *Arch Neurol* 1973;28: 287–292.

66. Janeway CA Jr. How the immune system recognizes invaders. *Sci Am* 1993;269(3):73–79.

67. Arnason B. The role of cytokines in multiple sclerosis. *Neurology* 1995;45(suppl 6):S54–S55.

68. Steinman L. Autoimmune disease. *Sci Am* 1993;269(3):106–114.

69. Male D, Pyrce G, Kinke A, et al. Lymphocyte migration into the CNS modelled in vitro. *J Neuroimmunol* 1992;40: 167–172.

70. Agius MA. Multiple sclerosis. *West J Med* 1995;163:473.

71. Boos J, Kim JH. Evidence for a viral etiology of multiple sclerosis. In: Cook SD, ed. *Handbook of multiple sclerosis.* New York: Marcel Dekker, 1990: 41–61.

72. Hafler DA, Weiner HC. Multiple sclerosis: a CNS and systemic autoimmune disease. *Immunol Today* 1989;10:104–107.

73. Weiner HC, Hafler DA. Immunotherapy in multiple sclerosis. *Ann Neurol* 1988;23:211–222.

74. McFarland HF, Dhib-Jalbut S. Multiple sclerosis: possible immunological mechanisms. *Clin Immunol Immunopathol* 1989;50:S96–S105.

75. Zamuil SS, Nelson PA, Mitchell DJ, et al. Encephalitogenic T cell clones specific for myelin basic protein. An unusual bias in antigen recognition. *J Exp Med* 1985;162: 2107–2124.

76. Swanson JW. Multiple sclerosis: update in diagnosis and review of prognostic factors. *Mayo Clin Proc* 1989;64:577–586.

77. Ivers RR, Goldstein NP. Multiple sclerosis: a current appraisal of symptoms and signs. *Proc Staff Meet Mayo Clin* 1963;38: 457–466.

78. Miller AE. Clinical features. In: Cook SD, ed. *Handbook of multiple sclerosis.* New York: Marcel Dekker, 1990:169–181.

79. Hart RG, Sherman DG. The diagnosis of multiple sclerosis. *JAMA* 1982;247:498–503.

80. Kabat EA, Freedman DA, Murry JP, Knaub V. A study of crystalline albumin, gamma globulin and total protein in the cerebral spinal fluid of 100 cases of multiple sclerosis and in other diseases. *Am J Med Sci* 1950;219:55–64.

81. Hershey CA, Trotter JL. The use and abuse of the cerebral spinal fluid IgG profile in the adult: a practical evaluation. *Ann Neurol* 1980;8:426–434.

82. Lowenthal A, Van Sande M, Koucher D. The differential diagnosis of neurological disease by fractionating electrophoretically the cerebral spinal fluid gamma globulins. *J Neurochem* 1980;6:51–56.

83. Thompson EJ, Kaufmann P, Shortmann RC, et al. Oligoclonal immunoglobulins and plasma cells in spinal fluid of patients with multiple sclerosis. *BMJ* 1979;1:16–17.

84. Mathews WB, Compston A, Allen VI, Martin CN, eds. *McAlpine's multiple sclerosis.* 2nd ed. New York: Churchill Livingstone, 1991:321–339.

85. Whitaker JN, Benveniste EN, Zhou Z. Cerebral spinal fluid. In: Cook SD, ed. *Handbook of multiple sclerosis.* New York: Marcel Dekker, 1990:251–270.

86. Nuwer MR. Evoked potentials. In: Cook SD, ed. *Handbook of multiple sclerosis.* New York: Marcel Dekker, 1990:251–270.

87. Chiappa KH. Pattern-shift visual, brain stem auditory and short latency somatosensory evoked potentials in multiple sclerosis. *Ann NY Acad Sci* 1984;436: 315–326.

88. Namerow NS. Somatosensory evoked responses in multiple sclerosis patients with varying sensory loss. *Neurology* 1968;18:1197–1204.

89. Miller DH, McDonald WI, Blumhardt LD, et al. MRI in isolated noncompressive spinal cord syndromes. *Ann Neurol* 1987;22:714–723.

90. Wallace CJ, Seland TP, Fong TC. Multiple sclerosis: the impact of magnetic resonance imaging. *AJR* 1992;158:849–857.

91. Paty DW. Neuroimaging in multiple sclerosis. In: Cook SD, ed. *Handbook of multiplc sclerosis.* New York: Marcel Dekker, 1990:291–316.

92. Ormerod IEC, McDonald WI, du Boulay GH, et al. Disseminated lesions at presentation in patients with optic neuritis. *J Neurol Neurosurg Psychiatry* 1986;49:124–127.

93. Paty DW, Oger JJF, Kastrukoff LF, et al. MRI in the diagnosis of multiple sclerosis: a prospective study with comparison of clinical evaluation, evoked potentials, oligoclonal banding and computerised tomography. *Neurology* 1988;38:180–185.

94. Offenbacher H, Fazekas F, Schmidt R, Freidl W. Assessment of MRI criteria for a diagnosis of multiple sclerosis. *Neurology* 1993;43:905–909.

95. Gonzales-Scarano F, Grossman RI, Galetta S, et al. Multiple sclerosis disease activity correlates with gadolinium-enhanced MRI. *Ann Neurol* 1987;21: 300–306.

96. Miller DH, Albert DS, Barkhof F, et al. Guidelines for the use of magnetic resonance techniques in monitoring the treatment of multiple sclerosis. *Ann Neurol* 1996;39:6–16.

97. Guttman CG, Ahn SS, Hsu L, et al. The evolution of multiple sclerosis lesions in serial magnetic resonance. *AJNR* 1995;16:1481–1491.

98. Thompson AJ, Miller D, Youl B, et al. Serial gadolinium-enhanced MRI in relapsing/ remitting multiple sclerosis of varying disease duration. *Neurology* 1992;42:60–63.

99. Filippi M, Horsfield MA, Tofts PS, et al. Quantitative assessment of MRI lesion load in monitoring the evolution of multiple

sclerosis. *Brain* 1995;118:1601–1612.

100. Khoury SJ, Guttmann CRG, Orav EJ, et al. Longitudinal MRI in multiple sclerosis: correlation between disability and lesion burden. *Neurology* 1994;44:2120–2124.

101. Gass A, Barker GJ, Kudd D, et al. Correlation of magnetization transfer ratio with clinical disability in multiple sclerosis. *Ann Neurol* 1994;36:62–67.

102. Husted C. Contributions of neuroimaging to diagnosis and monitoring of multiple sclerosis. *Curr Opin Neurol* 1994;7: 234–241.

103. Noseworthy JH, Paty DW, Ebers GC. Neuroimaging in multiple sclerosis. *Neurol Clin* 1984;2:759–777.

104. Matthews WB, Compston A, Allen IV, Martin CN, eds. *McAlpine's multiple sclerosis.* 2nd ed. New York: Churchill Livingstone, 1991:189–229.

105. Jansen HMC, Willemsen ATM, Sinnige CGF, et al. Cobalt-55 positron emission tomography in relapsing-progressive multiple sclerosis. *J Neurol Sci* 1995;132:139–145.

106. Carter JL, Rodriguez M. Immunosuppressive treatment of multiple sclerosis. *Mayo Clin Proc* 1989;64:664–669.

107. Becker CC, Gidal BE, Fleming JO. Immunotherapy in multiple sclerosis. Part 1. *Am J Health Syst Pharm* 1995;52: 1985–2000.

108. Mitchell G. Update on multiple sclerosis therapy. *Med Clin North Am* 1993;77:231–249.

109. Durelli L, Cocito D, Riccio A, et al. High dose intravenous methylprednisolone in the treatment of multiple sclerosis: clinical-immunologic correlations. *Neurology* 1986;36: 238–243.

110. Weiner HL, Hohol MJ, Khoury SJ, et al. Therapy for multiple sclerosis. *Neurol Clin* 1995;13:173–196.

111. Toriano R, Cook SD. Corticosteroid therapy in acute multiple sclerosis. In: Cook SD, Dowling PC, eds. *Handbook of multiple sclerosis.* New York: Marcel Dekker, 1990:351–364.

112. Burnham JA, Wright RR, Dreisbach J, Murray RS. The effect of high dose steroids on MRI gadolinium enhancement in acute demyelinating lesions. *Neurology* 1991;41:1349–1354.

113. Beck RW, Cleary PA, Trobe JD, et al. The effect of corticosteroids for acute optic neuritis on the subsequent development of multiple sclerosis. *N Engl J Med* 1993;329:1764–1769.

114. Rudick RA, Goodkin DE, Ransohoff RM. Pharmacotherapy of multiple sclerosis: current status. *Cleve Clin J Med* 1992;59:269–277.

115. Weiner JC, Hafler DA. Immunotherapy of multiple sclerosis. *Ann Neurol* 1988;23: 211–222.

116. Vollmer TL. Multiple sclerosis: new approaches to immunotherapy. *Prog Clin Neurosci* 1996;2:127–136.

117. Becker CC, Gidal BE, Fleming JO. Immunotherapy in multiple sclerosis. Part 2. *Am J Health Syst Pharm* 1995;52: 2105–2120.

118. Goodkin DE, Bailly RC, Teetzen MC, et al. The efficacy of azathioprine in relapsing remitting multiple sclerosis. *Neurology* 1991;41:20–25.

119. Yudkin PL, Ellison GW, Ghezzi A, et al. Overview of azathioprine treatment in multiple sclerosis. *Lancet* 1991;338:1051–1055.

120. Scheinberg LC, Smith CR, Geisser BS, et al. Efficacy and toxicity of cyclosporin in chronic progressive multiple sclerosis: a randomized, double blinded, placebo-controlled clinical trial: the Multiple Sclerosis Study Group. *Ann Neurol* 1990; 27:591–605.

121. Rudge P, Koetsier JC, Mertin J, et al. Randomized double blind controlled trial of cyclosporin in multiple sclerosis. *J Neurol Neurosurg Psychiatry* 1989;52: 559–565.

122. Kappos L, Patzold U, Dommasch D, et al. Cyclosporin versus azathioprine in the long term treatment of multiple sclerosis—results of the German multicenter study. *Ann Neurol* 1988;23:56–63.

123. Sipe JC, Romine J, Koziol J, et al. Cladribine treatment of chronic progressive multiple sclerosis: a double blind, crossover study with 2 years observation. *Neurology* 1995;45(suppl 4):A418.

124. Sipe JC, Romine JS, Koziol JA, et al. Cladribine in the treatment of chronic progessive multiple sclerosis. *Lancet* 1994;344: 9–13.

125. Beutler E, Sipe J, Romine J, et al. Treatment of multiple sclerosis and other autoimmune diseases with cladribine. *Semin Hematol* 1996;33(N1): 45–52.

126. Bornstein MD, Miller A, Slagle S, et al. A placebo-controlled, double blind, randomized two center pilot trial of COP 1 in chronic progressive multiple sclerosis. *Neurology* 1991; 41:533–539.

127. Arnon R, Teitelbaum D, Sela M. Suppression of experimental allergic encephalomyelitis by COP 1—relevance to multiple sclerosis. *Isr J Med Sci* 1989;25:686–689.

128. Teitelbaum D, Aharoni R, Arnon R, et al. Specific inhibition of the T cell response to myelin basic protein by the synthetic copolymer COP 1. *Proc Natl Acad Sci USA* 1988;85: 9724–9728.

129. Fridig-Hareli M, Teitebaunt D, Gurevitch E, et al. Direct binding of myelin basic protein and synthetic copolymer I to class II major histocompatibility complex molecules on living antigen presenting cells—specificity and promiscuity. *Proc Natl Acad Sci USA* 1994;91: 4872–4876.

130. Bornstein MD, Miller A, Slagle S, et al. A pilot trial of COP 1 in exacerbating remitting multiple sclerosis. *N Engl J Med* 1987;317:408–414.

131. Goodkin DE, Ransohoft RM, Rudick RA. Experimental therapies for multiple sclerosis: current status. *Cleve Clin J Med* 1992;59:69–74.

132. Vamvakas EL, Pineda AA, Weinshenker BG. Meta-analysis of clinical studies of the efficacy of plasma exchange in the treatment of chronic progressive multiple sclerosis. *J Clin Apheresis* 1995;10:163–170.

133. Polman CH, Hartung HP. The treatment of multiple sclerosis current and future. *Curr Opin Neurol* 1995;8:200–209.

134. Goodkin DE, Rudick RA, Vanderburg MS, et al. Low dose (7.5 mg) oral methotrexate treatment reduces the rate of progression in chronic progressive multiple sclerosis. *Ann Neurol* 1995;37:30–40.

135. Bansil S, Troiano R, Dowling PC, et al. Advances in the pharmacological and neurological treatment of patients with multiple sclerosis. Neurorehabilitation 1993;3(4):1–8.

136. Alam JJ. Interferon B treatment of human disease. *Curr Opin Biotechnol* 1995;6:688–691.

137. Panitch MS, Hirsch RL, Schindler J, et al. Treatment of multiple sclerosis with gamma interferon: exacerbation associated with activation of the immune system. *Neurology* 1987;37:1097–1102.

138. Arnason BGW. Interferon beta in multiple sclerosis. *Neurology* 1993;43:641–643. Editorial.

139. IFNB Multiple Sclerosis Study Group. Interferon beta 1b is effective in relapsing remitting multiple sclerosis. I: clinical results of a multicenter, randomized, double blind, placebo controlled trial. *Neurology* 1993;43:655–661.

140. IFNB Multiple Sclerosis Study Group. Interferon beta 1b is effective in relapsing remitting multiple sclerosis. II: MRI analysis results of a multicenter, randomized, double blind, placebo controlled trial. *Neurology* 1993;43:662–667.

141. Lublin FD, Whitaker JN, Eidelman BH, et al. Management of patients receiving interferon beta 1b for multiple sclerosis: report of a consensus conference. *Neurology* 1996;46:12–18.

142. Interferon beta 1b in the treatment of multiple sclerosis: final outcome of the randomized controlled trial. The IFNB Multiple Sclerosis Study Group and The University of British Columbia MS/MRI Analysis Group. *Neurology* 1995;45:1277–1285.

143. Jacobs LD, Cookfair DL, Rudick RA, et al. Intramuscular interferon beta-1a for disease progression in relapsing remitting multiple sclerosis. The Multiple Sclerosis Collaborative Research Group (MSCRG). *Ann Neurol* 1996;39:285–294.

144. Aisen M, Sevilla D, Fox N. Inpatient rehabilitation for multiple sclerosis. *J Neurol Rehabil* 1996;10:43–46.

145. Feigneson JS, Scheinberg L, Catalano M, et al. The cost effectiveness of multiple sclerosis rehabilitation: a model. *Neurology* 1981;31:1316–1322.

146. Bourdette DN, Prochazka AV, Mitchell W, et al. Health care costs of veterans with multiple sclerosis: implications for the rehabilitation of MS. *Arch Phys Med Rehabil* 1993;74:26–30.

147. Burks J, Cobble N. The team approach to the management of multiple sclerosis. In: Maloney FP, Burks J, Ringel SP, eds. *Interdisciplinary rehabilitation of multiple sclerosis and neuromuscular disorders.* Philadelphia: JB Lippincott, 1985:11–31.

148. Moulin DE, Foley KM, Ebers GC. Pain syndromes in multiple sclerosis. *Neurology* 1988;38: 1830–1834.

149. Clifford DB, Trotter JL. Pain in multiple sclerosis. *Arch Neurol* 1984;41:1270–1272.

150. Mattisson PG. TENS in the management of painful muscle spasms in patients with MS. *Clin Rehabil* 1993;7:45–48.

151. Schapiro RT. Symptom management in multiple sclerosis. *Ann Neurol* 1994;36:S123–S129.

152. Hallet M, Lindsey JW, Adelstein BD, Riley PO. Controlled trial of INH for severe postural cerebellar tremor in multiple sclerosis. *Neurology* 1985;35: 1374–1377.

153. Goldman MS, Kelly PJ. Symptomatic and functional outcome of stereotactic thalamotomy. *J Neurosurg* 1993;78:223–229.

154. Tranchant C, Bhatia KP, Marsden CD. Review: movement disorders in multiple sclerosis. *Mov Disord* 1995;10:418–423.

155. Krebs MA. Degenerative disorders of the CNS. In: Halstead L, Grabois M, eds. *Medical rehabilitation.* New York: Raven, 1985: 251–263.

156. Kraft GH, Alquist AD, deLateur BJ. Effect of resistive exercise on physical function in multiple sclerosis. *Arch Phys Med Rehabil* 1996;77:984 and Veterans Affairs. *Rehabilitation Research and Development Progress Reports* 1996;33:328–329.

157. Ponichtera-Mulcare JA, Glaster JM. Evaluation of muscle performance and cardiopulmonary fitness in patients with MS: Implications for rehabilitation. Neurorehabilitation 1993;3(4): 17–29.

158. Kent-Braun JA, Sharma KR, Miller RG, Weiner MW. Effects of electrically stimulated exercise training on muscle function in MS. *J Neurol Rehabil* 1996;10: 143–153.

159. Schapiro RT, Langer SL. Symptomatic therapy of multiple sclerosis. *Curr Opin Neurol* 1994;7: 229–233.

160. Kaji R, Happel L, Sumner AJ. Effect of digitalis on clinical symptoms and conduction variables in patients with multiple sclerosis. *Ann Neurol* 1990; 28:582–584.

161. Mathews WB, Compston A, Allen IV, Martyn CN, eds. *McAlpine's multiple sclerosis.* 2nd ed. New York: Churchill Livingstone, 1991:251–298.

162. Parziale JR, Akelman E, Herz DA. Spasticity: pathophysiology and management. *Orthopedics* 1993;16:801–811.

163. Odeen I. Reduction of muscular hypertonus by long-term muscle stretch. *Scand J Rehabil Med* 1981;13:93–99.

164. Katz RT. Management of spasticity. *Am J Phys Med Rehabil* 1988;67:108–116.

165. Robinson KM, Whyte J. Pharmacological management. In: Glenn MB and Whyte J, eds. *The practical management of spasticity in children and adults.* Philadelphia: Lea & Febiger, 1990:1–26.

166. Young RR, Dewaine PJ. Drug therapy: spasticity. *N Engl J Med* 1981;304:96–99.

167. Davidoff RA. Antispasticity drugs: mechanism of action. *Ann Neurol* 1985;17:107–116.

168. Smith CR, LaRocca NG, Giessen BS, Scheinberg LC. High-dose oral baclofen: experience in patients with multiple sclerosis. *Neurology* 1991;41:1829–1831.

169. Aisen ML, Dietz MA, Rossi P, et al. Clinical and pharmacokinetic aspects of high dose oral baclofen therapy. *J Am Paraplegic Soc* 1992;15:211–216.

170. Smith MB, Brar SP, Nelson LM, et al. Baclofen effect on quadriceps strength in multiple sclerosis. *Arch Phys Med Rehabil* 1992;73:237–240.

171. Costa E, Guidott A. Molecular mechanisms in the receptor action of benzodiazepines. *Annu Rev Pharmacol Toxicol* 1979; 19:537–545.

172. Yablon SA, Sipski ML. Effect of transdermal clonidine on spinal spasticity. *Am J Phys Med Rehabil* 1993;72:154–157.

173. Ellis KO, Carpenter JF. Mechanism of control of skeletal muscle contraction by dantrolene sodium. *Arch Phys Med Rehabil* 1974;55:362–369.

174. Gelenberg AJ, Poskanzer DC. The effect of dantrolene sodium on spasticity in multiple sclerosis. *Neurology* 1973;23: 1313–1315.

175. Glenn MB. Antispasticity medications in the patient with traumatic brain injury. *J Head Trauma Rehabil* 1986;1:71–72.

176. Maynard FM. Early clinical experience with clonidine in spinal spasticity. *Paraplegia* 1986; 24:175–182.

177. Nance PW, Shears AH, Nance DM. Reflex changes induced by clonidine in spinal cord injury patients. *Paraplegia* 1989; 27:296–301.

178. Nance PW, Shears AH, Nance DM. Clonidine in spinal cord injury. *Can Med Assoc J* 1985;133:41–42.

179. Donovan WH, Carter RE, Rossi CD, Wilkerson MA. Clonidine effect on spasticity: a clinical trial. *Arch Phys Med Rehabil* 1988;69:193–194.

180. Khan OA, Olek MJ. Clonidine in the treatment of spasticity in patients with multiple sclerosis. *J Neurol* 1995;242: 712–713.

181. Katz R. Management of spastic hypertonia after stroke. *J Neurol Rehabil* 1991;5:S5–S12.

182. Stein R, Nordal HJ, Oftedal SI, Slettebo M. Treatment of spasticity in multiple sclerosis: a double blind clinical trial of a new anti-spasticity drug tizanidine compared with baclofen. *Acta Neurol Scand* 1987;75: 190–194.

183. Smith C, Birnhaum G, Carter JL, et al., the United States Tizanidine Group. Tizanidine treatment of spasticity caused by multiple sclerosis: results of a double-blind, placebo-controlled trial. *Neurology* 1994;44(suppl 9): S34–S43.

184. Hauser SL, Doolittle TH, Lopez-Bresnahn M, et al. An antispasticity effect of threonine in multiple sclerosis. *Arch Neurol* 1992;49:923–926.

185. Herman R, D'Luzanski SC. Pharmacologic management of spinal spasticity. *J Neurol Rehabil* 1991;5:S15–S20.

186. Azouvi P, Mane M, Thiebaut JB, et al. Intrathecal baclofen administration for control of severe spinal spasticity: functional improvement and long term follow up. *Arch Phys Med Rehabil* 1996;77(1):35–39.

187. Becker WJ, Harris CJ, Long ML, et al. Long term intrathecal baclofen therapy in patients with intractable spasticity. *Can J Neurol Sci* 1995;22:208–217.

188. Penn R, Kroin JS. Continuous intrathecal baclofen for severe spasticity. *Lancet* 1985;2: 125–127.

189. Freal JE, Kraft GH, Coryell JK. Symptomatic fatigue in multiple sclerosis. *Arch Phys Med Rehabil* 1984;65:135–138.

190. Packer TL, Sauriol A, Brovwer B. Fatigue secondary to chronic illness: postpolio syndrome, chronic fatigue syndrome, and multiple sclerosis. *Arch Phys Med* 1994;75:1122–1125.

191. Monks J. Experiencing symptoms in chronic illness: fatigue in multiple sclerosis. *Int Disabil Stud* 1989;11:78–83.

192. Krupp LB, Alvarez LA, LaRocca NG, Scheinberg LC. Fatigue in multiple sclerosis. *Arch Neurol* 1988;45:435–437.

193. Elnicki DM, Shockcor WT, Brick JE, Beyon DB. Evaluating the complaint of fatigue in primary care: diagnosis and outcomes. *Am J Med* 1992;93:303–306.

194. Hubsky EP, Sears JH. Fatigue in multiple sclerosis: guidelines for nursing care. *Rehabil Nurs* 1992;17(4):176–180.

195. Natelson BH, Johnson SK, DeLuca J, et al. Reducing heterogeneity in chronic fatigue syndrome: a comparison with depression and multiple sclerosis. *Clin Infect Dis* 1995; 21:1204–1210.

196. Johnson SK, DeLuca J, Natelson BH. Assessing somatization disorder in the chronic fatigue syndrome. *Psychosom Med* 1996; 58:50–57.

197. Sharma K, Kent-Braun J, Mynhier MA, et al. Evidence of an abnormal intramuscular component of fatigue in multiple sclerosis. *Muscle Nerve* 1995;18:1403–1411.

198. Edgley K, Sullivan M, Dehoux E. A survey of multiple sclerosis: II. Determinants of employment status. *Can J Rehabil* 1991;4: 127–132.

199. Jackson MF, Quaal L, Reeves MA. Effects of multiple sclerosis on occupational and career patterns. *Axone* 1991;13(1):16–22.

200. Brar SP, Wangaard L. Physical therapy for patients with multiple sclerosis. In: Maloney FP, Burkes JS, Ringel SP, eds. *Interdisciplinary rehabilitation of multiple sclerosis and neuromuscular disorders.* Philadelphia: JB Lippincott, 1985:83–102.

201. Schwartz C, Coulthard-Morris L, Zeng Q. Psychosocial correlates of fatigue in multiple sclerosis. *Arch Phys Med Rehabil* 1996; 77:165–170.

202. Weinshenker BG, Penman M, Bass B, et al. A double blind, randomized crossover trial of pemoline in fatigue associated with multiple sclerosis. *Neurology* 1992;42:1468–1471.

203. Murray TJ. Amantadine therapy for fatigue in multiple sclerosis. *Can J Neurol Sci* 1985;12: 251–254.

204. The Canadian Multiple Sclerosis Research Group. A randomized controlled trial of amantadine in fatigue associated with multiple sclerosis. *Can J Neurol Sci* 1987;14:273–278.

205. Cohn RA, Fisher M. Amantadine treatment of fatigue associated with multiple sclerosis. *Arch Neurol* 1989;46:667–680.

206. Rosenberg GA, Appenzeller O. Amantadine, fatigue, and multiple sclerosis. *Arch Neurol* 1988;45:1104–1106.

207. Krupp LB, Coyle KB, Doscher C, et al. Fatigue in multiple sclerosis: results of a double-blind, randomized, parallel trial of amantadine, pemoline and placebo. *Neurology* 1995;45: 1956–1961.

208. Geisler MW, Sliwinski M, Coyle K, et al. The effects of amantadine and pemoline on cognitive functioning in multiple sclerosis. *Arch Neurol* 1996;53: 185–188.

209. Jonsson A, Korfitzen EM, Heltberg A, et al. Effects of neuropsychological treatment in patients with multiple sclerosis. *Acta Neurol Scand* 1993;88: 394–400.

210. DeLuca J, Johnson S. Cognitive impairments in multiple sclerosis. Implications for rehabilitation. Neurorehabilitation 1993;3(4):9–16.

211. Rao SM. Neuropsychology of multiple sclerosis: a clinical review. *J Clin Exp Neuropsychol* 1986;5:503–542.

212. Rao SM, Leo GJ, Bernardin L, Unverzagt F. Cognitive dysfunction in multiple sclerosis. I: Frequency, patterns and prediction. *Neurology* 1991;41: 685–691.

213. Prosiegel M, Michael L. Neuropsychology and multiple sclerosis: diagnostic and rehabilitative approaches. *J Neurol Sci* 1993;115(suppl):S51–S54.

214. Rao SM. Neuropsychology of multiple sclerosis. *Curr Opin Neurol* 1995;8:216–220.

215. DeLisa JA, Miller RM, Mikulic MA, Hammond MC. Multiple sclerosis: part II. Common functional problems and rehabilitation. *Am Fam Physician* 1985; 32(5):127–132.

216. Beatty WW, Goodkind DE, Hertsgaurd D, Monson N. Clinical and demographic predictors of cognitive performance in multiple sclerosis. Do diagnostic type, disease duration, and disability matter? *Arch Neurol* 1990; 47:305–308.

217. Perterson R, Kokmen E. Cognitive and psychiatric abnormality in multiple sclerosis. *Mayo Clin Proc* 1989;64:657–663.

218. Staples D, Lincoln NB. Intellectual impairment in multiple sclerosis and its relation to functional abilities. *Rheumatol Rehabil* 1979;18:153–160.

219. Lituan I, Grafman J, Uendrell P, Martinez JM. Slowed information processing in multiple sclerosis. *Arch Neurol* 1988;45:281–285.

220. Rao SM, Hammeke TA. Hypothesis testing in patients with chronic progressive multiple sclerosis. *Brain Cogn* 1984;3: 94–104.

221. Peyser J, Edwards K, Posen C, Filskov S. Cognitive function in patients with multiple sclerosis. *Arch Neurol* 1980;37:577–579.

222. Comi G, Filippi M, Marinelli V, et al. Brain MRI correlates of cognitive impairment in primary and secondary progressive multiple sclerosis. *J Neurol Sci* 1995;132:222–227.

223. Rao SM, Leo GJ, Ellington L, et al. Cognitive dysfunction in multiple sclerosis. II: impact on employment and social function. *Neurology* 1991;41:692–696.

224. Matthews WB, Compston A, Allen IV, Martyn CN, eds. *McAlpine's multiple sclerosis.* 2nd ed. New York: Churchill Livingstone, 1991:43–77.

225. Huber SJ, Paulson GW, Shuttleworth EC, et al. MRI correlates of dementia in multiple sclerosis. *Arch Neurol* 1987;44:732–736.

226. Clark CM, James G, Li D, et al. Ventricular size, cognitive function and depression in patients with multiple sclerosis. *Can J Neurol Sci* 1992;19: 352–356.

227. Rao SM, Bernardin L, Leo GJ, et al. Cerebral disconnection in multiple sclerosis: relationship to atrophy of the corpus callosum. *Arch Neurol* 1989;46: 918–920.

228. Franklin GM, Heaton RK, Nelson LM, et al. Correlation of neuropsychological and MRI findings

in chronic progressive multiple sclerosis. *Neurology* 1988; 38:1826–1829.

229. Anzola GP, Bevilacqua L, Cappa SF, et al. Neuropsychological assessment in patients with relapsing-remitting multiple sclerosis and mild functional impairment: correlation with MRI. *J Neurol Neurosurg Psychiatry* 1990;53:142–145.

230. Rao SM, Leo GJ, Haughton VM, et al. Correlation to MRI with neuropsychological testing in multiple sclerosis. *Neurology* 1989;39:161–166.

231. Tsolaki M, Drevelegas A, Karachristianou S, et al. Correlation of dementia, neuropsychological and magnetic resonance imaging findings in multiple sclerosis. *Dementia* 1994; 5:48–52.

232. Pugnetti L, Mendozzi L, Motta A, et al. Magnetic resonance imaging and cognitive patterns in relapsing-remitting multiple sclerosis. *J Neurol Sci* 1993; 115:S59–S65.

233. Huber SJ, Bornstein RA, Rammohan KW, et al. Magnetic resonance imaging correlates of neuropsychological impairment in multiple sclerosis. *J Neuropsychiatry Clin Neurosci* 1992; 4:152–158.

234. Beatty WW, Goodkin DE. Screening for cognitive impairment in multiple sclerosis. An evaluation of the Mini-Mental State Examination. *Arch Neurol* 1990; 47:297–301.

235. Carlow TJ. Medical treatment of nystagmus and ocular motility disorders. *Int Ophthalmol Clin* 1986;26:251–264.

236. Beck RW, the Optic Neuritis Study Group. Optic neuritis treatment trial. *Arch Ophthalmol* 1993;111:773–775.

237. Blaivas JG. Management of bladder dysfunction in multiple sclerosis. *Neurology* 1980;30: 12–18.

238. Samellas W, Rubin B. Management of upper urinary tract complications in MS by urinary diversion to an ileal conduit. *J Urol* 1965;93:548–552.

239. Sliwa JA, Bell HK, Mason KD, et al. Upper urinary tract abnormalities in multiple sclerosis. *Arch Phys Med Rehabil* 1996;77: 247–251.

240. Chancellor MB, Blaivas JG. Urological and sexual problems in multiple sclerosis. *Clin Neurosci* 1994;2:189–195.

241. Goldstein I, Siroky MB, Sax DS, Krane RJ. The urodynamic characteristics of multiple sclerosis. *J Urol* 1982;128:541.

242. Blaivas JG, Holland NJ, Giesser B, et al. Multiple sclerosis bladder. *Ann NY Acad Sci* 1984; 436:329–345.

243. Beneton C, De Parisot O, Granjon M, Millet MF. Management of bladder disorders in multiple sclerosis. *Sex Disabil* 1996;14:21–31.

244. Nordenbo AM. Bowel dysfunction in MS. *Sex Disabil* 1996;19: 33–39.

245. Glick EM, Meshkinpour H, Haldeman S, et al. Colonic dysfunction in MS. *Gastroenterology* 1982;83:1002–1007.

246. Vermote R, Peuskens J. Sexual and micturition problems in multiple sclerosis patients: psychological issues. *Sex Disabil* 1996;14:73–82.

247. Valleroy M, Kraft G. Sexual dysfunction in multiple sclerosis. *Arch Phys Med Rehabil* 1984; 65:125–128.

248. Mattson D, Petrie M, Srivastava DK, McDermott M. Multiple sclerosis: sexual dysfunction and its response to medications. *Arch Neurol* 1995;52:862–868.

249. Annon J. The PLISSIT model: a proposed conceptual scheme for the behavioral treatment of sexual problems. *J Sex Educ Ther* 1976;2:1–15.

250. LiVius H, Valtones E, Wikstrom J. Sexual problems in patients suffering from multiple sclerosis. *J Chronic Dis* 1976;29:643–647.

251. Minderhoud J, Leemhius J, Kremer J, et al. Sexual disturbances arising from multiple sclerosis. *Acta Neurol Scand* 1984;70:299–306.

252. Lindberg P. Sexual dysfunction in patients with multiple sclerosis. *Sex Disabil* 1978;1: 218–222.

253. Opsomer RJ. Management of male sexual dysfunction in multiple sclerosis. *Sex Disabil* 1996; 14:57–63.

254. Betts CD. Pathophysiology of male sexual dysfunction in multiple sclerosis. *Sex Disabil* 1996; 14:41–55.

255. Vidal J, Curoll LI, Roig T, Bagunya J. Intracavernous pharmacotherapy for management of erectile dysfunction in multiple sclerosis patients. *Rev Neurol* 1995;24:269–271.

256. Lundberg PO, Hulter B. Female sexual dysfunction in multiple sclerosis: a review. *Sex Disabil* 1996;14:65–72.

257. Lundberg PO. Neurologic examination of patients with sexual dysfunction. *Med Aspects Hum Sex* 1977;11:59–60.

258. Sullivan MJL, Weinshenker B, Mikail S, Bishop SR. Screening for major depression in the early stages of multiple sclerosis. *Can J Neurol Sci* 1995;22: 228–231.

259. Sadovnik AD, Eisen K, Ebers GC, Paty DW. Cause of death in patients attending multiple sclerosis clinics. *Neurology* 1991;41:1193–1196.

260. Mainden SL, Schiffer RB. Depression and mood disorders in multiple sclerosis. *Neuropsychiatry Neuropsychol Behav Neurol* 1991;4:62–77.

261. Rabins PV, Brooks BR, O'Donnel P, et al. Structural brain correlates of emotional disorder in multiple sclerosis. *Brain* 1986;109:585–597.

262. Acorn S, Anderson S. Depression in multiple sclerosis; critique of the research literature. *J Neurosci Nurs* 1990;22: 209–214.

263. Joffe RT, Lippert GP, Gray TA, et al. Mood disorder and multiple sclerosis. *Arch Neurol* 1987; 44:376–378.

264. Schiffer RB, Herndon RM, Rudick RA. Treatment of pathological laughing and weeping with amytriptyline. *N Engl J Med* 1985;312:1480–1482.

265. Surridge D. An investigation into some psychiatric aspects of multiple sclerosis. *Br J Psychiatry* 1969;115(524):749–764.

266. Honer WG, Hurwitz T, Li DKB, et al. Temporal lobe involvement in multiple sclerosis patients with psychiatric disorders. *Arch Neurol* 1987;44:187–190.

267. Davison K, Bagley CR. Schizophrenia-like psychoses associated with organic disorders of the central nervous system: a review of the literature. *B J Psychiatry* 1969;4:113–184.

268. Rao SM, Hammeke TA, Speech TJ. Wisconsin Card sorting test performance in relapsing remitting and chronic progressive multiple sclerosis. *J Consult Clin Psychol* 1987;55:263–265.

269. Milner B, Petrides M. Behavioral effects of frontal-lobe lesions in man. *Trends Neurosci* 1984; 7:403–407.

270. Grigsby J, Kravcism N, Ayarbe SD, Busenbark D. Prediction of deficits in behavioral self-regulation among persons with multiple sclerosis. *Arch Phys Med* 1993;74:1350–1353.

271. Ruttenberg N. Assessment and treatment of speech and swallowing problems in multiple sclerosis. In: Maloney FP, Burks JS, Ringel SP, eds. *Interdisciplinary rehabilitation of multiple sclerosis and neuromuscular disorders.* Philadelphia: JB Lippincott, 1985:129–142.

272. Carter JL, Noseworthy JH. Ventilatory dysfunction in multiple sclerosis. *Clin Chest Med* 1994;15:693–703.

273. Petajan J, Grappmaier E, White AT, et al. Exercise recommended for MS patients. *Ann Neurol* 1996;39:432–441.

274. Litvin ME. Vocational rehabilitation and social security disability programs. In: Maloney FP, Burks JS, Ringel SP, eds. *Interdisciplinary rehabilitation of multiple sclerosis and neuromuscular disorders.* Philadelphia: JB Lippincott, 1985:413–425.

275. Verdier-Tallefer MH, Sazdovitch V, Boregl F, et al. Occupational environment as risk factor for unemployment in multiple sclerosis. *Acta Neurol Scand* 1995;92:59–62.

276. Larocca N, Kalb R, Scheinberg L, Kendall P. Factors associated with unemployment of patients with multiple sclerosis. *J Chron Dis* 1985;38:203–210.

277. Mitchell JN. Multiple sclerosis and the prospects for employment. *J Soc Occup Med* 1981;31:134–138.

278. Public Law 101-336 42 U.S.C. 1990.

279. Britell CW, Cooper LD. Medical, functional and legal aspects of vocational rehabilitation for people with multiple sclerosis. Neurorehabilitation 1993;3(4): 39–47.

280. O'Brien MT. Multiple sclerosis: the role of social support and disability. *Clin Nurs Res* 1993; 2(1):67–85.

281. Decker TW, Decker BB. Effects of multiple sclerosis on physical and psychosocial functioning. *Percept Mot Skills* 1994;79: 753–754.

282. Wilson I, Cleary P. Linking clinical variables with health-related quality of life. *JAMA* 1995; 273:59–65.

283. Stewart AL, Greenfield S, Hays RD, et al. Functional status and well being of patients with chronic conditions. *JAMA* 1989;262:907–930.

284. Brunet D, Hopman WM, Singer MA, et al. Assessment of HRQOL offers broader measure of disease burden than EDSS alone. *Can J Neurol Sci* 1996; 23:99–103.

285. Rudick R, Miller D, Clough JD, et al. Quality of life in multiple sclerosis. *Arch Neurol* 1992;49:1237–1242.

286. Lankhorst G, Jelles F, Smits RC, et al. A disability and impact profile to assess QOL in MS. *J Neurol* 1996;243:469–474.

287. Schwartz CE, Cole BF, Gelber RD. Measuring patient-centered outcomes in neurologic disease. *Arch Neurol* 1995;52: 7754–7762.

288. Greenspun B, Stineman M, Agri R. Multiple sclerosis and rehabilitation outcome. *Arch Phys Med Rehabil* 1987;68:434–437.

289. *Multiple sclerosis: a national survey.* National Institutes of Health publication no. 84-22479. Bethesda, MD: U.S. Department of Health and Human Services, Public Health Service, 1984.

290. Kottke FJ. Philosophic considerations of quality of life for the disabled. *Arch Phys Med Rehabil* 1982;63:60–62.

291. National Multiple Sclerosis Society. *Research highlights.* Winter/Spring 1996:1–8.

Chapter 77

Cerebral Palsy

Thomas E. Strax
Michael A. Alexander
Kerstin M. Sobus

Cerebral palsy is a term recognized in the medical and educational setting to describe a group of nonprogressive conditions that manifest as abnormalities of movement and posture. The etiology is thought to be static and related to injury to the central nervous system during the early period of brain development, generally defined as occurring prior to age 3 years (1). The designation *cerebral palsy* defines a group of individuals with similar needs for rehabilitation, educational, medical, and social services (2). Although the neurologic injury is static, the clinical signs and symptoms evolve and change with growth and development of the child, as do the specific medical, therapeutic, and educational needs. Periodic reassessment is necessary to provide current and preventive care to avoid secondary complications, and to plan for transition to adulthood.

PREVALENCE

The prevalence of cerebral palsy in the United States and industrial countries is 1.5 to 2.5 per 1000 live births. With improved obstetric care and advanced achievements in neonatal intensive care, more infants are surviving today compared to 1960 (3–5). Although there has been a slight increase in the prevalence of cerebral palsy, the failure of the rate to decline is probably secondary to congenital brain malformations that primarily cause abnormalities in development or place children at greater risk for central nervous system injury associated with perinatal asphyxia (6–8). There has been a decrease in the number of children in industrial countries with choreoathetoid cerebral palsy with the treatment of kernicterus and an increase in the presentation of spastic diplegia with increased survival rates for very-low-birth-weight infants (4).

ETIOLOGY

The underlying cause for the developmental abnormality of movement and posture in most children diagnosed with cerebral palsy remains unknown (6,9,10). Although the cause has been attributed to asphyxia, infection, genetic factors, metabolic disorders, trauma, or congenital malformation, in most infants the prenatal, perinatal, and postnatal courses are uncomplicated. It should not be implied that the etiology of an infant's disability is from severe anoxia or hypoxia at birth without evidence to support marked or prolonged intrapartum asphyxia in a newborn. Such a newborn would display signs of moderate or severe hypoxic-ischemic encephalopathy during the newborn period without evidence of other underlying conditions (6). In addition, clinical evaluation should include observation or review of the neonate's kidney, heart, and lung functions because birth asphyxia that is severe enough to damage the brain usually damages the kidneys, the lungs, and the heart. The usual outcome to anoxia severe enough to cause significant central nervous system injury is death

(6,11). Low birth weight increases the risk of cerebral palsy (5). Infants weighing less than 2500 g account for 33% of all children who later develop signs consistent with cerebral palsy. The rate of cerebral palsy is 25 to 30 times higher in infants whose birth weight is less than 1500 g than in full-size newborns (3,12).

The advancements in ultrasound techniques have enabled earlier identification of hypoxic-ischemic and hemorrhagic lesions in the neonatal brain. Serial ultrasound studies together with clinical assessment, electrophysiologic studies, computed tomography, and magnetic resonance imaging have enhanced understanding of the pathogenesis of early lesions in the preterm infant and prognostication of these lesions (13). Premature low-birth-weight infants are at greater risk for periventricular leukomalacia and periventricular hemorrhagic infarction than are full-term infants. The pathogenesis of both lesions is believed to be due to ischemia in the immature brain. The lesions of periventricular leukomalacia are generally symmetric and those of periventricular hemorrhage are asymmetric. The primary pathogenesis of periventricular hemorrhagic infarction appears to be secondary to germinal matrix–intraventricular hemorrhage. Through obstruction of the terminal veins, this may lead to periventricular venous congestion and ischemia (14).

With periventricular leukomalacia, the primary ischemia appears to affect the arterial circulation. The lesion is predominately seen in premature infants but can occur in the full-term infant. The primary site for periventricular leukomalacia is at the level of the cerebral white matter around the foramen of Monro. This is the "watershed" between the penetrating branches of the middle cerebral artery and the posterior choroidal branches of the posterior cerebral artery. The cerebral and periventricular vasculature to this area is related to gestational age, developing between 24 and 36 weeks. The premature infant is at greatest risk when this area is not mature, and thus is very susceptible to ischemia. With impairment of vascular autoregulation or major systemic hypotension, a fall in perfusion may occur, with ischemia following (14).

The rate of later development of cerebral palsy appears to be higher for infants whose images show hypoechoic areas than for those whose images show hyperechoic areas, and is greatest for infants with large, posterior, and bilateral lesions. The development of cystic periventricular leukomalacia also increases the risk for later development of cerebral palsy and its severity, especially if multiple cystic lesions are noted. Multiple cavities, particularly in the occipital regions, are associated with an extremely poor outcome. Long-term follow-up studies of preschool and kindergarten children with cerebral palsy revealed that those with a history of grade I or II (mild) hemorrhages are at risk for learning disabilities and impairment in visual motor, perceptual motor, and memory skills, although some do exhibit cognitive function in the normal range. Infants with ventricular dilatation, hydrocephalus, and cerebral atrophy are also at high risk for significant neurologic impairment (3,15–19).

ASSOCIATED CONDITIONS

The associated medical and developmental conditions seen in children with cerebral palsy reflect a continuum of the brain dysfunction. Intelligence is impaired in 50% to 70% of children. A large percentage of children have additional learning disabilities with or without intellectual impairment, which may adversely affect educational programming. Specific learning disabilities may include dyspraxia, disturbances of central perceptual sensory processing, and deficits of intersensory integration. Visual impairments include refractive errors, field defects, amblyopia, strabismus, nystagmus, and abnormalities of visual pursuit. Children with hemiparesis may have visual field deficits. The prevalence of hearing disturbances including deafness ranges from 6% to 16%, particularly in children with choreoathetoid cerebral palsy, and may impact developmental progression, particularly of speech and language skills. Communication and language disorders include expressive and receptive language delay, central processing problems, and dysarthria. Seizures may develop in 20% to 30%, with two-thirds of the seizures being seen in children with spasticity and 20% of seizures in children with athetosis. The usual onset is prior to age 2 years, with tonic-clonic and partial complex seizures being the most common (3–5,20–22). The incidence of urinary incontinence is thought to be higher in children with cerebral palsy. Although the data are limited, urinary incontinence may be secondary to detrusor hyperreflexia and reduced capacity. Urinary incontinence in many children with cerebral palsy may improve with treatment and thus one should not assume that incontinence is a feature of cerebral palsy and would be unresponsive to intervention (23). Other associated medical problems include dysphagia, gastroesophageal reflex, and hiatal hernia in patients with severe cerebral palsy, and may lead to poor nutrition, recurrent episodes of aspiration pneumonia, chronic lung disease, and delayed growth (24,25).

CLASSIFICATION

In general, clinical classification can be according to predominant neurologic signs and enhanced by adding functional and therapeutic divisions (20,26,27):

- Neurologic signs
  - Pyramidal (spastic)
  - Extrapyramidal (rigid, athetoid, or ataxic)
  - Mixed
  - Hypotonic/atonic
  - Dystonic
- Limb involvement

Diplegia—both lower extremities and the arms, to a lesser extent
Hemiplegia—an ipsilateral arm and leg
Double hemiplegia—both upper extremities and the lower extremities, to a lesser extent
Quadriplegia—all four limbs
Triplegia—one arm better than the other three limbs

Functional
Class I—no practical limitation
Class II—slight to moderate limitation
Class III—moderate to great limitation
Class IV—no useful activity

Therapeutic
Class A—no treatment required
Class B—minimal bracing and habilitation
Class C—extensive bracing or other apparatus; multidisciplinary team required for long-term habilitation
Class D—long-term care required

Patients in therapeutic class B, C, or D may require architectural or environmental barrier modification at home, school, or the workplace; psychosocial and vocational services; and sex education and counseling.

EVOLUTION OF PRESENTATION

The clinical presentation of cerebral palsy is not static but rather reflects a dynamic evolution influenced by developmental changes in growth, neuromotor organization, and function.

The newborn manifests a constellation of primitive reflexes controlled predominantly via brain stem responses. These movement patterns are stereotyped and predictable with no component of voluntary control. As higher cortical control develops, the primitive reflexes are suppressed and voluntary postural responses evolve, allowing a wide range of voluntary movement. The infant gradually matures and movement patterns expand. The key primitive reflexes include the Babinski, Galant (spinal incurvation), asymmetric and symmetric tonic neck, positive support, tonic labyrinthine, primitive neck righting, and foot placement reflexes. Thus, the clinical signs of persistent primitive reflexes, abnormal tone, and posture may not be present until after the first 4 to 5 months of life. It is not uncommon for the full-term infant to have had normal findings on two well-baby examinations prior to the clinical suspicion of cerebral palsy The premature infant may also have been discharged home prior to the evolution of signs and symptoms.

DIFFERENTIAL DIAGNOSIS

Two key points to the diagnosis of a child with probable cerebral palsy are that the underlying etiology is a neurologic injury that is static and nonprogressive, and that the diagnosis is one of exclusion. The clinician must be careful to rule out other neurologic conditions that can mimic cerebral palsy, including neurodegenerative disorders, spinal cord abnormalities, neuromuscular disorders, arthrogryposis, inborn errors of metabolism, mental retardation, and inherited syndromes such as familial spastic paraplegia, hereditary ataxia, and hereditary microcephaly (4,22,26).

Since young infants change rapidly over the first several weeks and months of life, the presenting motor impairment represents an evolutionary process. Some infants may display minor neurologic abnormalities in tone or movement in the first several weeks or months after birth that gradually disappear or change during the subsequent months (3,28–31).

The Collaborative Perinatal Project found that most children at 1 year of age who were considered to have a mild motor impairment age and even more of those who were only suspected to have mild motor impairment at age 1 year were free of cerebral palsy at 7 years old. The children who "outgrew" the diagnosis of mild motor impairment were more likely than children who never had the diagnosis to have nonfebrile seizures; residual language, attention, and learning deficits; or cognitive delay suggestive of persistence of cortical dysfunction (4,29).

Conversely, care should be exercised before prognosticating future outcome in a child under the age of 2 years who has mild signs of cerebral palsy, because subtle early motor abnormalities may evolve or change as the myelination of axons and maturation of neurons in the basal ganglia occur. It is believed that this maturation is necessary before spasticity, dystonia, and athetosis can become apparent (4). Therefore, in a young child whose central nervous system is maturing and evolving, the definitive diagnosis of cerebral palsy and a statement of likely prognosis should be deferred until the ages of 18 to 24 months. Before then, only a tentative diagnosis can be presented to the family, with an explanation as to the presentation and definition of cerebral palsy (4,30,32,33).

ORTHOPEDIC ISSUES

Children with cerebral palsy represent a diverse group with many variables influencing their orthopedic needs, including age, type and severity of cerebral palsy, previous treatment, parental desires, and access to treatment. Although cerebral palsy is defined as a static neurologic injury, as the child grows and develops, the abnormal movement, tone, and posture place him or her at risk for acquired orthopedic deformities. These deformities may be static or dynamic and may interfere with upper-extremity function, dressing, sitting, transfers, and gait. Children with spastic hemiplegia may have more distal impairment in the hand and wrist or foot and ankle, whereas those with

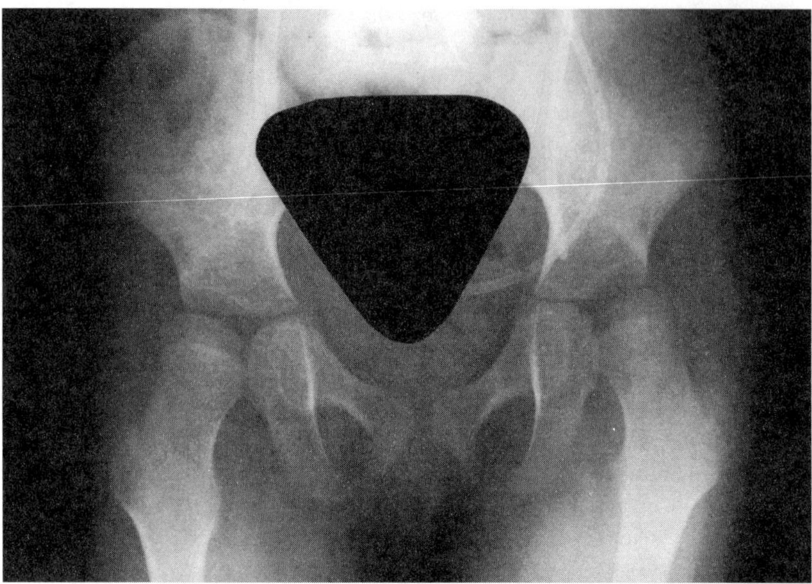

Figure 77-1. A patient with diplegic cerebral palsy, with 50% migration in the left hip and 25% on the right.

spastic diplegia may have more impairment with their hips. The child with severe spastic quadriplegia may have progressive deformities that lead to painful hip dislocation with or without scoliosis. These deformities may pose significant restrictions with hygiene and positioning in a bed or wheelchair.

Initially at birth, the child has normal bones and joints. The neurologic imbalance and chronic spasticity of the stronger muscle groups can progress to fixed musculotendinous contractures and acquired joint deformity (34–36). With involvement of a multidisciplinary team and a thorough understanding of the underlying injury that influences tone, movement, and posture, orthopedic management can assist and maximize outcome for both children and adults. The overall goal of orthopedic management includes the early detection of specific orthopedic problems and appropriate nonsurgical and surgical treatment.

Recent diagnostic and intervention planning includes gait analysis. Gait analysis has assisted with the planning of surgical intervention by identifying both static and dynamic contractures, evaluating muscle balance and function during the gait cycle, and allowing a differentiation between primary and compensatory abnormalities of posture and gait (37). The child or adult is evaluated dynamically with video cameras and simultaneous electromyographic (EMG) recording. Two video cameras are placed at specific locations, and markers are placed on the patient. The cameras simultaneously record the movements of the markers during gait, and specific software calculates the markers' positions and makes graphic records.

Dynamic EMG allows the patient to walk freely during simultaneous recordings by the video cameras. This study promotes accurate comparison of muscle activity at any phase of the gait cycle (38). Presurgical and postsurgical gait analyses can facilitate accurate evaluation, planning of appropriate surgical or nonsurgical intervention, and follow-up of outcome.

Detailed musculoskeletal examination is important to monitor orthopedic changes as the child grows. However, clinical examinations alone cannot assess hip stability. Hence, radiologic monitoring of the hips must be done regularly to detect early subluxation and prevent later dislocation, which can lead to a painful hip, pelvic obliquity, and scoliosis and predispose to difficulty with sitting and the potential development of pressure sores (35,36,39–43). Depending on the patient's strength, range of motion, control of motor system, and intellectual ability, radiographs of the hips should be taken at 6-month intervals during the crucial ages of 2 to 8 years to detect progressive subluxation (35). Several factors have been implicated as probable causes promoting subluxation or dislocation. The differential strength, the spasticity of the stronger hip adductors and flexors over the weak abductors and extensors, can cause the center of rotation of the hip joint to be shifted from the center of the femoral head to the lesser trochanter. Also, persistent coxa valgus, which may be perpetuated with delayed weight bearing, and femoral anteversion have been implicated (36,40,41,44). The risk of subluxation progressing to dislocation is higher in children of a younger age, with more severe cerebral palsy, and with a migration index greater than 50% (40) (Fig. 77-1). The reported incidence of advancement to hip dislocation, which is usually posterior, is 33% to 75% (40,42,43). The hips that dislocate are at significantly increased risk for degenerative changes and pain compared to those that are subluxed or reduced. The reported incidence of pain with hip dislocation in individuals with cerebral palsy ranges from 30% to 50% (40,42). The keys to the clinical management of hip dysplasia in children with cerebral palsy are diagnostic monitoring, early recognition with appropri-

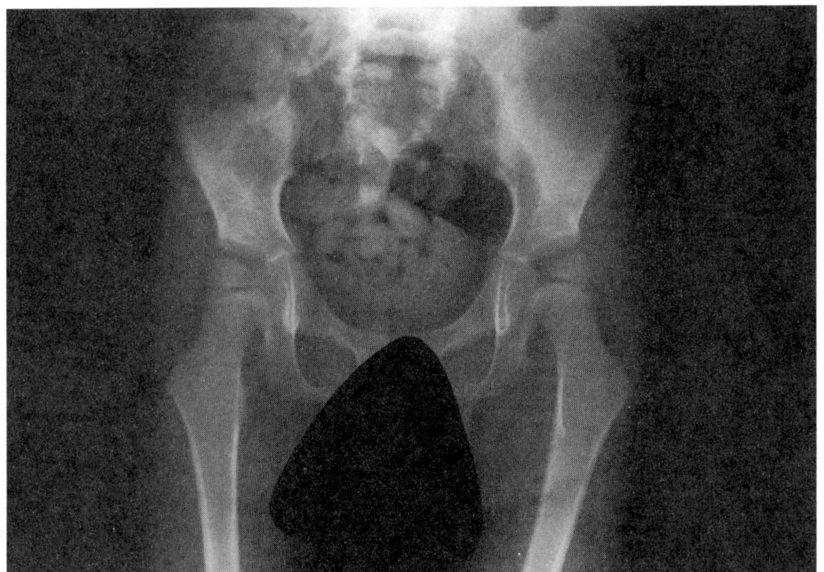

Figure 77-2. A 5-year-old patient, one of twins born at 32-week gestation. He is non-ambulatory. He underwent neurectomy of the anterior branch of the obturator nerve and adductor and hamstring releases.

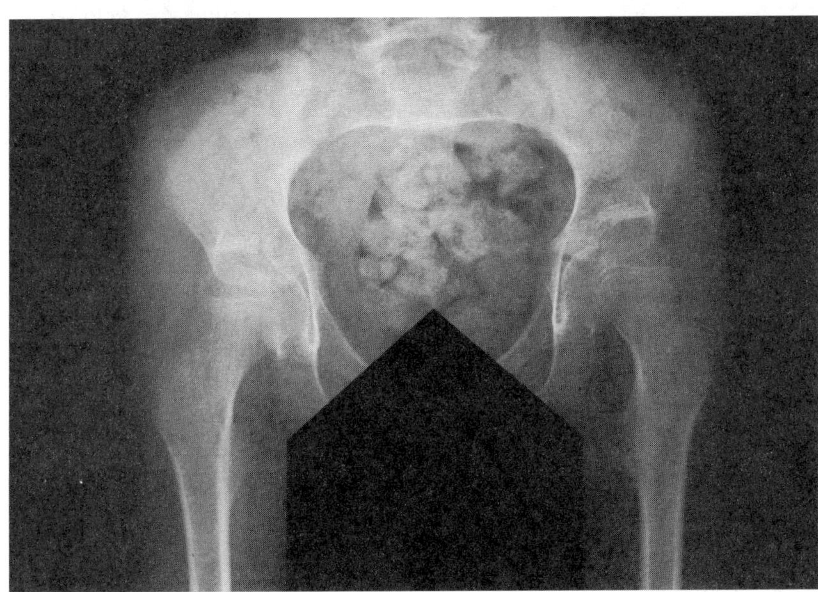

Figure 77-3. The same patient as in Figure 77-2, at age 14. No further hip surgery was needed since the surgery performed at age 5 years.

ate soft-tissue releases (Figs. 77-2 and 77-3), osteotomies when necessary, daily range of motion exercises, and good positioning in the wheelchair, stander, and bed.

The movement and position of the hips, knees, and ankles dynamically influence gait. Knee flexion deformities can place stress during ambulation and may lead to a non-ambulatory state. Ambulation with a knee flexion contracture greater than 30 degrees can result in a dramatic increase in the force that is transmitted through the patellar tendon, and necessitates increased muscle force of the quadriceps to maintain static and dynamic stability (35). With growth and the concomitant increase in body size and weight, combined with increasing contractures, the quadriceps musculature may be unable to provide sufficient force to support the growing individual, and a decline in functional ambulation may occur.

Gait analysis has proved beneficial for evaluating quadriceps and hamstring musculature in association with planning intervention. Surgical lengthening of the hamstrings may improve knee extension but has a limited effect on swing-phase knee flexion. Knee flexion may be augmented with distal rectus femoris transfer to a hamstring and hamstring lengthening. Knee flexion is most improved if the distal rectus femoris is transferred to the semitendinosus (45).

Equinus is the most common static and dynamic acquired deformity seen in children with cerebral palsy, seen secondary to muscle imbalance across the ankle. Children with hemiplegia are more likely to have equinovarus deformity with an associated varus, whereas children with diplegia or quadriplegia are more likely to have equinus or equinovalgus deformities (35).

Other orthopedic deformities seen in the lower extremities include patella alta, pes cavus, hallux valgus, and bunions. Treatment includes preventive daily stretching, fixed contractures, or surgical lengthening. Surgical intervention is indicated if the fixed contractures will not permit the foot to be passively dorsiflexed to a neutral position, with the foot in supination and the knee in full extension. Surgical interventions include distal Z-lengthening of the achilles tendon or the more proximal Strayer procedure.

The focus should include lower-extremity needs and also upper-extremity function. This focus is essentially important for children with fair to good intellectual ability and the potential for improved voluntary hand function. Selected surgical procedures by a skilled surgeon with experience and interest in upper-extremity function can reposition the sensory-intact deformed limb and enable the individual to function more effectively. Intervention has maximal results if it is accomplished in conjunction with an experienced therapist, motivated family, and patient with ability to follow through and understand the necessary postoperative therapeutic program (45–47).

NUTRITION

Fundamental to a child's health and well-being is good nutrition. Children with cerebral palsy are at significant risk for nutritional deficits. This problem is multifactorial and includes oral hypersensitivity, dysphagia, and postural abnormalities. Studies have demonstrated that children with cerebral palsy, including children with quadriplegia, hemiplegia, or diplegia, have decreased growth, abnormal laboratory values, and decreased caloric and nutritional intake (48).

Malnutrition can be associated with an increased risk for infection. In addition, depletion of specific proteins may place a child who has had orthopedic surgery at risk for impaired wound healing, sepsis, pneumonia, prolonged weakness, delayed physical recovery, and low energy to participate in therapy (48–50). The poorly nourished child may also be apathetic, with a decreased ability and interest to actively participate in social or educational activities (48).

Clinical nutritional evaluation should be part of the routine medical follow-up or scheduled well-child visits. A detailed history should be obtained to document clearly what food is being offered and consumed and to identify whether a child can communicate when he or she is hungry or what his or her food preferences are. The evaluation can determine if the child is being offered adequate calories, if the child is able to fully consume offered calories, whether the child is unable to consume all offered food secondary to dental problems, whether the child refuses food, and whether the child has oral-motor dysfunction (48,51). If inadequate caloric retention is suspected, it is important to rule out vomiting, malabsorption, or gastroesophageal reflux.

If nutritional supplementation is necessary, clinical judgment will require consideration of the safest route, oral versus tubal. Oral feeding is the natural selection but may not be a choice because of the presence of oral-motor dysfunction and aspiration. The potential risk of aspiration must be ruled out by videofluoroscopic evaluation using liquids and foods of all textures. The evaluation must also consider the time it takes the child to obtain the required nutrition, and the fatigue of the child or caregiver. Caloric adequacy can be facilitated with high-caloric food items and supplements such as Polycose. Feeding therapy using individualized positioning, handling, and swallowing techniques can assist with oral feeding and enhance a child's oral-motor skills to facilitate improved intake and to decrease the risk of aspiration.

The child should sit with his or her back and head supported by the feeder's chest and abdomen. With the child in this position, the individual feeding the child will have both hands free. With the nondominant hand, the feeder can bring the child's jaw forward, and with the free fingers, rub the cheek to stimulate the swallowing reflex. The dominant hand can be used to feed the child. This position allows the child's body and head to be controlled, permitting the feeder to flex his or her body forward, preventing extension of the child's neck and head. Stroking the cheek will also facilitate the sucking reflex.

If oral feeding cannot provide adequate nutritional or hydration support, then use of a nasogastric or gastrostomy tube should be considered. If the need for supplemental feeding is thought to be short term, then a simple nasogastric tube may suffice. However, if the need is for the long term, then elective placement of a gastrostomy tube may be beneficial to supplement oral feeding and hydration or to provide full support. If the patient has significant gastroesophageal reflux, surgical consideration for placement of a gastrostomy tube should include a Nissen fundoplication. Sucking and swallowing might be trained by utilizing a solid spoon coated with a food substance that can facilitate salivation, such as a thin layer of peanut butter. Allowing the individual to suck on this spoon while stimulating the sucking reflex may eventually train him or her to swallow the excess saliva. A spoon coated with peanut butter is perfectly safe to use, as there is nothing for the child to swallow and aspirate.

Consultation with a nutritionist may assist with selection of the appropriate formula for supplementation, selection of the appropriate high-caloric foods, and the choice of pureed food versus commercial formula. Recommendations can be made regarding the proper rate for nutritional supplementation of the malnourished child. A proper rate can avoid the complications of too rapid an infusion, which can include fluid overload, stool changes, temporary carbohydrate intolerance, and the most serious, congestive heart failure (48).

SPASTICITY

The functional and positional needs of children with cerebral palsy can be significantly impaired if moderate to severe spasticity is also present. Oral medications may assist children, particularly those with mild to moderate spasticity, but may also result in undesirable secondary side effects. The oral medications include baclofen, diazepam (Valium), and dantrolene (Dantrium).

Interventional options include selective dorsal rhizotomy, intrathecal administration of baclofen, and neuromuscular blockade. Selective dorsal rhizotomy is a good option for children with moderate to severe spastic diplegia without underlying athetosis, significant contracture, or muscle weakness. The primary purpose of the procedure is to improve the function or care of children whose primary handicap is the spasticity, through selective cutting of rootlets between L2 and S2 at the cauda equina. Careful selection of patients who are cooperative and for whom a nonsurgical approach failed, and extensive postoperative therapy improve the surgical outcome (52).

Intrathecal baclofen is a promising option in the management of spasticity. An infusion pump is surgically placed under the skin of the abdomen and is programmed to deliver a titrated dose of baclofen into the intrathecal space via a catheter. Since the baclofen is delivered directly to the spinal cord, much lower doses are required, compared to oral administration, and the systemic side effects seen with oral doses are greatly reduced. The benefits include significantly reduced spasticity in the upper and lower extremities and improved functional skills for transfers, ambulation, self-care, and positioning. Possible side effects include dose-related sleepiness, nausea, headache, excessive muscle weakness, and light-headedness. These symptoms are generally dose related and temporary and may be alleviated with a change in dose.

For a more specific, localized intervention of spasticity, intraneural or intramuscular neurolysis with alcohol, phenol, or botulinum toxin A may be of benefit. Botulinum toxin A has the advantage over phenol of being less caustic with less local discomfort, allowing for administration without general anesthesia and on an outpatient basis (53–58).

Functional electrical stimulation (FES) has many therapeutic benefits for individuals with cerebral palsy. For the child, FES can be used to facilitate specific muscle activation during gait or hand activities, to enhance the development of functional movements. Following botulinum toxin injection or tendon transfers, FES can be used to facilitate increased strength and contraction of a specific muscle or group. More recent studies revealed a positive gain in passive range of motion at the ankles among children receiving electrical stimulation (59).

THERAPY

Therapeutic intervention requires a transdisciplinary approach to facilitate the individual child to reach his or her maximum developmental potential. Therapeutic activities can begin early in the neonatal intensive care unit to assist with positioning and developmental stimulation. The Education of the Handicapped Act Amendments 1986 [Public Law (PL) 99–457 or Individuals with Disabilities Education Act] mandated early intervention for children 0 to 3 years old who are at developmental risk or are developmentally delayed. Public Law 94–142 mandates that all states must provide a free and appropriate public education to eligible school children (60,61).

Early intervention programs provide therapeutic activities in the home, at a center, or at day care for children. Therapeutic goals include training the parents or caregivers in range of motion exercises and proper positioning and handling techniques that can be incorporated into daily activities. Additional program goals include educating parents or caregivers as to their child's psychosocial needs, developmental activities, and associated medical needs. The therapist also tries to foster developmentally appropriate play activities with the child and parents to enhance language and cognitive development (20,62).

Most pediatric physical and occupational therapists in the United States use a combined approach in their treatment techniques, to allow flexibility and individualization to meet the child's and family's goals. These techniques are generally a combination of those developed by the Bobaths, Rood, and Ayres.

Karel and Berta Bobath developed the NDT neurodevelopmental treatment (NDT) approach in England in the 1940s. Their three main goals are to normalize tone, to inhibit the primitive or abnormal reflex patterns, and to facilitate automatic reactions and subsequent normal movement. The treatment goals are achieved through careful handling and positioning of the child. A key emphasis is placed on the family and other caregivers to utilize the handling techniques in the home environment (63–65). Margaret Rood developed the sensorimotor approach in the 1940s and 1950s. The overall goal is to activate movement and postural responses to an automatic level while following normal developmental sequences. Several specific sensory stimuli are utilized during treatment sessions (63,66,67). A. Jean Ayres developed the sensory integration theory to enhance the development of some preschool and school-age children with learning disabilities. The treatment techniques are designed to enhance the capacity of the child to organize and integrate sensory information by providing opportunities for specific, controlled sensory inputs that lead to an adaptive purposeful response (68,69).

Therapeutic intervention also includes speech and cognitive programming. The speech therapist provides a dynamic program to facilitate the child's receptive and expressive language, cognitive linguistic skills, and oral-motor development.

TECHNOLOGY

The world of technology assistance continues to grow rapidly, enhancing many beneficial opportunities for children and adults. The choices of power wheelchairs have grown tremendously, with many variations and styles now available to all ages. Children as young as 20 to 36 months can learn to master the power chair. The child or adult can control the chair through a variety of switch options (Fig. 77-4). These options include microswitch controls, joysticks, "sip 'n' puff" controls, head controls, and foot pedal controls. The control units can be designed to control the direction of the chair and the tilt or recline options. Additionally, environmental control options can be added. Ultrasonic detectors can be added to the wheelchair to assist visually impaired wheelchair users. Selected power chairs are foldable but generally have fewer control options for the patient. Others are heavy duty and require a lift. Some chairs can be used as a power mobility system or converted to a manual backup system. This manual chair, however, may not be as lightweight as other primary manual wheelchairs are. Independent mobility is very important not only for adults but also for young children, to offer the independence that is so important for psychosocial development.

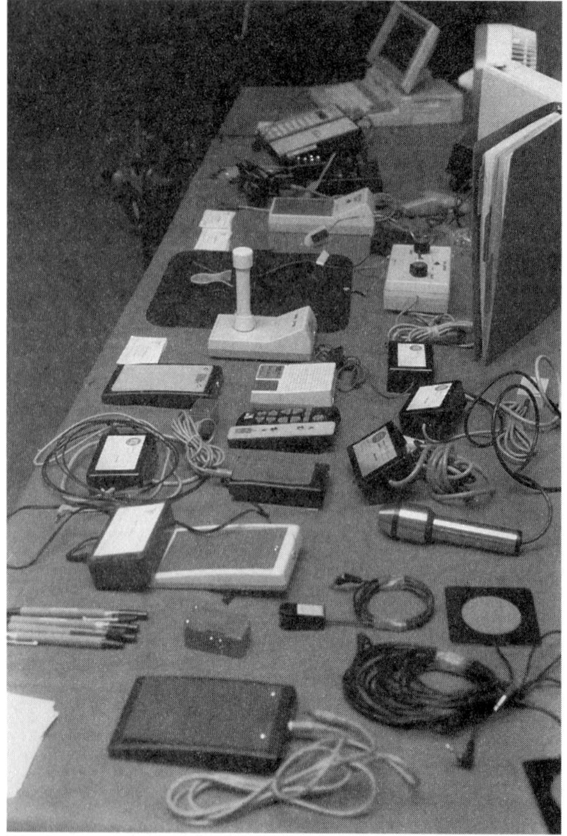

Figure 77-4. Array of switches and environmental control units.

Advances in computer technology have also enabled children and adults to communicate effectively through artificially spoken communication or written language (Fig. 77-5). Augmentative communication technology has expanded greatly from manual communication boards to electronic communication devices. The interface between the child and the augmentative communication device can involve a number of techniques including single switches, joysticks, expanded keyboards, and eye gaze. The primary goal is to select an input device that enables the child to take advantage of his or her best motor control capabilities (70). Output is based on the child's needs, cognitive ability, and environmental situation, for example, home, classroom, or community. Basic choices can range from yes or no to full complex sentences, depending on the system selected. The ability to communicate allows the child to develop and grow, indicate basic needs and wants, and interact socially with family and friends.

Computer technology has also enhanced the child's ability to participate with his or her peers in the classroom and learn to express himself or herself in written language. Additionally, many preacademic and academic activities can be learned through the computer. Keyboards, touch screens, and voice activators can be used to interface with the computer. The benefits of computer use include not only learning classroom academics but also participating in play and leisure activities.

Environmental control systems have also expanded and can provide independence to very physically challenged individuals. These control units provide multicommand access to allow an individual to turn on and off a number of electric items including lights, television, and stereo. As with all technology, the challenge is affordability. Many creative funding sources may be necessary to assist the family or adult in the purchase.

ADULT TRANSITION AND AGING

Ninety percent of children with cerebral palsy should be expected to live to adulthood. In children with severe involvement, the life expectancy is reduced (71). The most common cause of death in children with cerebral palsy is respiratory disease. This is most often seen in children with severe central nervous system deficits with accompanying severe mental retardation, profound delays in language development, and immobility. The primary and secondary causes of death in adults with cerebral palsy are cardiac

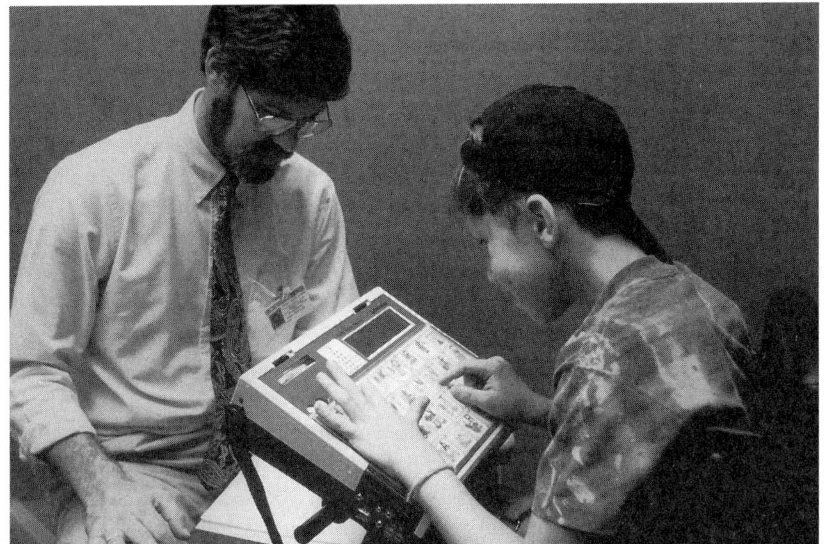

Figure 77-5. A 14-year-old patient with an augmentative communication device with speech output.

disease and cancer, the same as in the general population. The third leading cause of death in adults with cerebral palsy is respiratory disease. Factors contributing to respiratory disease include shallow respiration with decreased vital capacity, dysphagia with difficulty in swallowing and subsequent chronic aspiration of food and saliva, and ineffective coughing or clearance of secretions (72). Children with spastic diplegia or hemiplegia as well as those with mild choreoathetosis do better in general compared to children with quadriplegia or mild to severe choreoathetosis (73). Young children who sit independently by age 2 years are ambulatory. Generally, children who do not sit by age 2 years but whose reflexes are suppressed by 18 to 24 months ultimately achieve ambulation (33).

The transition from childhood to adulthood can be difficult for any teenager, but teenagers with cerebral palsy struggle with limited adult role models, society-imposed restrictions and options, and limited community resources. The nonambulatory young adult may find employment difficult if accessible public transportation for wheelchair users is not available or dependable.

To become a confident adult, the adolescent must consolidate his or her identity, separate from family, find a vocation, and find a significant other. Having a physical disability increases the stress and time it takes to achieve these developmental tasks. Cultural factors also influence the time it takes to achieve each of these tasks. Lack of experience and opportunity is a pervasive problem for individuals with physical disabilities.

Many studies have evaluated the attitudes of nondisabled individuals toward individuals with physical disabilities. Friedman (74), Tringo (75), and Yuker et al (76) researched this particular problem. Those with obvious deformities and movement disorders are most likely to be rejected by the able-bodied. Like their peers, people with physical disabilities will probably reject themselves. Working through this self-rejection is extremely important for individuals trying to find a place in society, find a job, as well as find a significant other. When adolescents with cerebral palsy finally enter the "outside" world, they are partially segregated and have problems with admission to peer groups. Without friends, they find life extremely lonely. In an attempt to cultivate friends and attract attention, the disabled sometimes turn toward inappropriate behavior such as loud talking and foolish demonstrations. The able-bodied individual who resorts to this type of activity usually gets instantaneous feedback from family, teachers, and peer group members. This is not the case with individuals with a physical disability.

Williams (77,78) discussed the alienation syndrome in adolescence. He pointed out that our society reinforces narcissistic, competitive individualism with an emphasis on performance, achievement, and productivity at the expense of relationships between young people. Unless individuals are successful in their relationships both in the family and with peer groups, they cannot establish a successful relationship later in adult life. A fast-moving, high-achievement society does not have a place for a slow individual. It is not fashionable to have disabled friends, or slow down for someone who needs extra help. Dorner (79), in studies of youngsters with spina bifida, found that the nonhandicapped friends of the patients during preadolescence were lost during adolescence. About half the children he studied were judged to be severely socially isolated. The more mobile the adolescent with spina bifida was, the less socially isolated the adolescent was.

Depression was extremely common in his study. Thirty-one percent of the girls and 15% of the boys had persistent periods of depression or suicide ideation. Anxiety about the future was extreme, with concerns primarily related to employment, independence from the family, and the possibility of marriage. Many adolescents with disabilities self-consciously worry and wonder if their defective bodies will function. A feeling of physical incompetence may lead to a feeling of genital incompetence. Individuals with a physical disability are less mobile and therefore have a lower chance of meeting and courting appropriate mates in the usual fashion available to their able-bodied peer group. Disabled persons who are emotionally mature and have self-esteem, confidence, and the need to find a mate must then deal with the problems of not being acceptable to people of the opposite sex.

Besides the social stigmata of a physical disability, there are practical problems. One study conducted by the Social Security Administration found that 40% of individuals with physical disabilities needed some help with their activities of daily life. This assistance was usually provided by an immediate member of the household. In half the cases, it was provided by a spouse or child. Only 10% of individuals had paid help and this was only for 1 day a week or less. Twenty-seven percent of those who needed help received none.

For the disabled population, finding a vocation, and with it economic independence, is extremely difficult, if not impossible. In spite of the Americans with Disabilities Act, many employees with disabilities are rejected simply because they have a physical disability. Two out of seven disabled individuals of employable age are employed. There are many myths about hiring the disabled, such as insurance rates will "skyrocket," or expensive workplace adjustments will have to be made, or able-bodied employees will feel that they are giving the disabled special privileges.

A large study performed by the National Association of Manufacturers found that 90% of 279 companies did not experience an increase in their insurance costs. The adjustments at the workplace had been minimal, usually consisting of simple changes such as lowered work space, a special desk, and occasional doorway modifications. DuPont found disabled workers to be safe workers; 96% of 1400 disabled employees had better safety records than their able-bodied counterparts. Individuals with a disability were competitive with the unimpaired workers in terms of productivity, attendance, safety, job stability, and the cost of employment. Seventy-nine percent of employees had better attendance records, and 93% had average or better turnover rates.

Community size may influence the employment options. Eventual employability is most influenced by intellectual ability and physical impairment. However, with improved adaptive equipment and computer technology, physical limitations can be reduced. The availability of quality education programs, community-based training, and technical support, along with a well-motivated family, can have a positive effect on outcome (80).

Adults with disabilities rank communication, activities of daily living, and mobility as more important issues in their daily function than ambulation (81).

The effects of aging may be more challenging than in the general population, secondary to the underlying spasticity, abnormal pressures, and posture imposed by the neurologic condition. Many musculoskeletal changes that occur naturally with age may need orthopedic intervention. Foot deformities including calcaneal valgus, severe pes planus, hallux valgus, and bunions may become symptomatic with pain or skin breakdown due to abnormal pressure. Joints placed at abnormal angles secondary to the contractures of spasticity may develop painful degenerative arthritis. A crouched gait in knee flexion greater than 15 degrees in an ambulatory adult places stress on the patella, which is displaced superiorly, causing degenerative changes in the knee joint. The hip joint can become problematic in both ambulatory and nonambulatory individuals. The subluxed hip may develop degenerative arthritis secondary to abnormal joint mechanical stress. In the nonambulatory adult, the subluxed or dislocated hip may alter the pressure distribution while sitting, leading to an increased risk of pressure sore development. In 33% of patients with dislocated hips, the hips will become painful. Salvage procedures are not without their problems. Of key importance is the prevention of dislocation in childhood (82).

Even after skeletal maturity, scoliosis with curves of more than 50 degrees will generally progress at 1 degree per year. Advanced curves of 90 to 150 degrees can present multiple problems for the adult. Not only are pulmonary and gastrointestinal problems present but also the associated pelvic obliquity will lead to unequal pressure on the ischial tuberosity during sitting and pressure on the ribs as they rest on the pelvic rim (82). Pressure sores may develop, limiting independence and severely restricting activities.

The health benefits of good balanced nutrition, regular exercise, and stretching are important to all adults with or without a disability. Many people with cerebral palsy would benefit if health clubs would expand the knowledge of their trainers to include physical fitness for individuals with a physical disability.

Many individuals will require assistance with activities of daily living, including homemaking and safety. Ongoing support and community assistance are vital to these individuals. Funding sources need to be expanded. Individuals with cerebral palsy need adequate funding in order to have a choice about where to live, daily activities, and recreational and leisure needs. For the disabled, adolescence and young adulthood are periods of self-examination and rejection. Hopefully this period will be followed by healthier and more realistic acceptance of themselves and their disability, their limitations, and their strengths. This usually happens with a good supportive family unit, and later with understanding peers as well as adequate medical, social, psychological, and vocational services.

REFERENCES

1. Galjaard H. *Early detection and management of cerebral palsy.* Zoetermeer, The Netherlands: Martinus-Nijhoff, 1987.
2. Nelson KB. In: Swarman K, ed. *Cerebral palsy in pediatric neurology, principles and practice.* CV Mosby, 1989:363–371.
3. Kubon K, Leviton A. Cerebral palsy. *N Engl J Med* 1994;330:188–195.
4. Eicher P, Batshaw M. Cerebral palsy. *Pediatr Clin North Am* 1993;40:537–551.
5. Bhushan V, Paneth N, Keily J. Impact of improved survival of very low birth weight infants on recent secular trends in the prevalence of cerebral palsy. *Pediatrics* 1993;91:1094–1100.
6. Freeman J, Nelson K. Intrapartum asphyxia and cerebral palsy. *Pediatrics* 1988;82:240–249.
7. Foley J. Dyskinetic and dystonic cerebral palsy and birth. *Acta Paediatr* 1992;81:57–60.
8. Hagberg B, Hagberg G, Zetterstrom R. Decreasing perinatal mortality: increase in cerebral palsy mortality. *Acta Paediatr Scand* 1989;78:664–670.
9. Nelson KB, Ellenberg JH. Antecedents of cerebral palsy: multivariate analysis of risk. *N Engl J Med* 1986;315:81–86.
10. Kitchen WH, Doyle LW, Ford GW, et al. Cerebral palsy in very low birthweight infants surviving to two years with modern perinatal intensive care. *Am J Perinatol* 1987;4:29–35.
11. Naeye R, Peters E, Bartholomew M, Landis R. Origin of cerebral palsy. *Am J Dis Child* 1989;143:1154–1161.
12. Stanley FJ. Survival and cerebral palsy in low birth weight infants: implications for perinatal care. *Paediatr Perinat Epidemiol* 1992;6:298–310.
13. de Vries L, Dubowitz L, Dubowitz V, Pennock J. *Color atlas of brain disorders in the newborn.* Chicago: Year Book Medical, 1990.
14. Volpe J. Brain injury in the preterm infant—current concepts of cerebral palsy following preterm birth. Lecture, St. Louis Children's Hospital, Washington School of Medicine, November 1993.
15. Costello AM, Hamilton PA, Baudin J, et al. Prediction of neurodevelopmental impairment at four years from brain ultrasound appearance of very preterm infants. *Dev Med Child Neurol* 1988;30:711–722.
16. Graham M, Levene M, Trounce J, et al. Prediction of cerebral palsy in very low birth weight infants: prospective ultrasound study. *Lancet* 1987;2:593–596.
17. Guzzetta F, Shackelford G, Volpe S, et al. Periventricular intraparenchymal echodensities in the premature newborn: critical determinant of neurologic outcome. *Pediatrics* 1986;78:995–1006.
18. Ford L, Han K, Steichen J, et al. Very low birth weight, preterm infants with or without intracranial hemorrhage. *Clin Pediatr* 1989;28:302–310.
19. Weisglas-Kuperus N, Uleman-Vleeschelrager M, Baerts W. Ventricular haemorrhages and hypoxic-ischaemic lesions in preterm infants: neurodevelopmental outcome at 3½ years. *Dev Med Child Neurol* 1987;29: 623–629.
20. Alexander MA, Bauer RE. *Handbook of developmental and physical disabilities.* New York: Pergamon Press, 1988:215–226.
21. Molnar G. Cerebral palsy: prognosis and how to judge it. *Pediatr Ann* 1979;8:596–605.
22. Barbabas G, Taft L. The early signs and differential diagnosis of cerebral palsy. *Pediatr Ann* 1986;15:203–214.
23. Borzyskowski RC. Lower urinary tract dysfunction in cerebral palsy. *Arch Dis Child* 1993;68:739–742.
24. Drvaric D, Roberts J, Burke SW, et al. Gastroesophageal evaluation in totally involved cerebral palsy patients. J Pediatr Orthop 1987;7:187–190.
25. Rogers B, Arvedson J. Hypoxemia during oral feeding of children with severe cerebral palsy. *Dev Med Child Neurol* 1993;35:3–10.
26. Vining E, Accardo P, Rubenstein J, et al. Cerebral palsy a pediatric developmentalist's overview. *Am J Dis Child* 1976;130:643–649.
27. Capute A, Accardo P. *Developmental disabilities in infancy and childhood.* Baltimore: Paul Brookes, 1991:335–348.
28. Barlow CF. Soft signs in children with learning disorders. *Am J Dis Child* 1974;128:605.
29. Nelson K, Ellenberg J. Childen who "outgrew" cerebral palsy. *Pediatrics* 1982;69:529–536.
30. Ford GW, Kitchen WH, Doyle LW, et al. Changing diagnoses of cerebral palsy in very low birth weight children. *Am J Perinatol* 1990;7:178–181.
31. Taudord K, Hansen FJ, Melchior JC, et al. Spontaneous remission of cerebral palsy. *Neuropediatrics* 1986;17:19–22.
32. Holt K. Medical examination of the child with cerebral palsy. *Pediatr Ann* 1979;8:581–588.
33. Molnar G, Gordon S. Cerebral palsy: predictive value of selected clinical signs for early prognostication of motor function. *Arch Phys Med Rehabil* 1976;57:153–158.
34. Dormans J. Orthopedic management of children with cerebral palsy. *Pediatr Clin North Am* 1993;40:645–657.
35. Jones E, Knapp D. Assessment and management of the lower extremity in cerebral palsy. *Orthop Clin North Am* 1987;18:725–738.
36. Hoffer M. Management of the hip in cerebral palsy. Current concepts review. *J Bone Joint Surg [Am]* 1986;68:629–631.
37. Gage J, Fabian D, Hick R, Tashman S. Pre- and postoperative

gait analysis in patients with spastic diplegia: a preliminary report. *J Pediatr Orthop* 1984;4:715–725.

38. Hoffinger S. Gait analysis in pediatric rehabilitation. *Phys Med Rehabil Clin N Am* 1991;2:817–845.

39. Scrutton D. Hip dysplasia in cerebral palsy. *Dev Med Child Neurol* 1993;35:1028–1030.

40. Bagg M, Farber J, Miller F. Long term follow-up of hip subluxation in cerebral palsy patients. *J Pediatr Orthop* 1993; 13:32–36.

41. Carr C, Gage J. The fate of the nonoperated hip in cerebral palsy. *J Pediatr Orthop* 1987;7: 262–267.

42. Cooperman D, Bartucci E, Dietrick E, Millar E. Hip dislocation in spastic cerebral palsy: long-term consequences. *J Pediatr Orthop* 1987;7:268–276.

43. Kalen V, Bleck E. Prevention of spastic paralytic dislocation of the hip. *Dev Med Child Neurol* 1985;25:17–24.

44. Eggers W, Evans B. Surgery in cerebral palsy. *J Bone Joint Surg [Am]* 1963;45:1275–1305.

45. Delp S, Ringwelski D, Carroll N. Transfer of the rectus femoris: effects of transfer site on movement arms about the knee and hip. *J Biomech* 1994;27: 1201–1211.

46. Beach W, Strecker W. Use of the green transfer in treatment of patients with spastic cerebral palsy: 17-year experience. *J Pediatr Orthop* 1991;11:731–736.

47. Manske P. Redirection of extensor pollicis longus in the treatment of spastic thumb-in-palm deformity. *J Hand Surg [Am]* 1985;10:553–560.

48. Fee M, Charney E, Robertson W. Nutritional assessment of the young child with cerebral palsy. *Infant Young Child* 1998;1(1): 33–40.

49. Stalling V, Charney E, Davies J, Cronk C. Nutritional status and growth of children with diplegia or hemiplegic cerebral palsy. *Dev Med Child Neurol* 1993;35:997–1006.

50. Jevsevar D, Karin L. The relationship between preoperative nutritional status and complications after an operation for scoliosis in patients who have cerebral palsy. *J Bone Joint Surg [Am]* 1993;75:880–884.

51. Campbell S. *Physical therapy for children.* Philadelphia: WB Saunders, 1995:489–523.

52. Boop F, Chaddrick W. Selective posterior rhizotomy for relief of spasticity. *J Ark Med Soc* 1991;512–514.

53. Calderon-Gonzales R, Calderon-Sepulveda R. Pathophysiology of spasticity and the role of botulinum toxin in its treatment. *Acta Neuropediatr* 1994;1:45–57.

54. Morrison J, Hertzberg D, Gourley S, et al. Motor point blocks in children: a technique to relieve spasticity using phenol injections. *AORN J* 1989;49: 1346–1354.

55. Chutorian A, Root L. Management of spasticity in children with botulinum A toxin. *Int Pediatr* 1994;9(suppl 1):35–43.

56. Cosgrove A, Corry I, Graham H. Botulinum toxin in the management of lower limb cerebral palsy. *Dev Med Child Neurol* 1994;36:386–396.

57. Carpenter E, Seitz D. Intramuscular alcohol as an aid in management of spastic cerebral palsy. *Dev Med Child Neurol* 1980;22: 497–500.

58. Calderon-Gonzales R, Calderon-Sepulveda R, Rincon-Reyes M, et al. Botulinum toxin A in management of cerebral palsy. *Pediatr Neurol* 1994;10:284–288.

59. Hazelwood M, Brown J, Rave P, Salter P. The use of therapeutic electrical stimulation in the treatment of hemiplegia cerebral palsy. *Dev Med Child Neurol* 1994;36:661–673.

60. Harris SR. Efficacy of early intervention in pediatric rehabilitation. *Phys Med Rehabil Clin N Am* 1991;2:725–742.

61. Healy A. Pediatrician's role in the development of implementation of an individual education plan (IEP) and/or individual family service plan (IFSP). *Pediatrics* 1992;89:340–342.

62. Haskins R, Finkelstein NW, Stedman DJ. Infant stimulation programs and their effects. *Pediatr Ann* 1978;7:99–128.

63. Harris S, Atwater S, Crowe T. Accepted and controversial neuromotor therapies for infants at high risk for cerebral palsy. *J Perinatol* 1985;8:3–13.

64. Bobath B. A neuro-developmental treatment of cerebral palsy. *Physiotherapy* 1963;49:242–244.

65. Bobath B, Bobath K. *Motor development in the different types of cerebral palsy.* London: Heinemann, 1977.

66. Rood M. Neurophysiological mechanism utilized in the treatment of neuromuscular dysfunction. *Am J Occup Ther* 1956;10:220–224.

67. Stockmeyer SA. An interpretation of the approach of Rood to the treatment of neuromuscular dysfunction. *Am J Phys Med* 1967;46:900–961.

68. Ayres AJ. *The development of sensory integration theory and practice.* Dubuque, IA: Kendall/Hunt, 1974.

69. Ayres AJ. *Sensory integration and learning disorders.* Los Angeles: Western Psychological Service, 1972.

70. Alexander M, Demasco P, Gilbert M, et al. Rehabilitation technology for disabled children. *Phys Med Rehabil State Art Rev* 1991;5:365–387.

71. Evans PM, Evans SJW, Alberman E. Cerebral palsy: why we must plan for survival. *Arch Dis Child* 1991;65:1329–1333.

72. Eymar R, Grossman H, Chaney R, Call T. The life expectancy of profoundly handicapped people with mental retardation. *N Engl J Med* 1990;323:584–589.

73. Urebrant P. Hemiplegic cerebral palsy. Aetiology and outcome. *Acta Paediatr* 1988;345:1–100.

74. Friedman RS. Modeling behavior of nondisabled and disabled adolescents based upon social preference for and similarity to nondisabled and disabled models. PhD dissertation. Hofstra University, Hempstead, Long Island, NY, 1974.

75. Tringo J. The hierarchy of preference toward disability groups. *J Special Educ* 1970;4:295–306.

76. Yuker HE, Block JR, Young JH. *The measurement of attitudes toward disabled persons.* New York: Albertson, 1970.

77. Schooler L, Centers R. Peer group attitudes toward the amputee child. *J Social Psychol* 1963;61:127–131.

78. Seidel UP, Chadwick OFD, Ruter M. Psychological disorders in crippled children. A comparative study of children with and without brain damage. *Dev Med Child Neurol* 1975;17:563–573.

79. Dorner S. Psychological and social problems of families of adolescent spinal bifida patients: a preliminary report. *Dev Med Child Neurol* 1973;29:24–26.

80. O'Grady R, Nishimura D, Kohn J, Bruvold W. Vocational predictions compared with present vocational status of 60 young adults with cerebral palsy. *Dev Med Child Neurol* 1985;27:775–784.

81. Bleck EE. *Orthopedic management of cerebral palsy.* Philadelphia: WB Saunders, 1982.

82. Bleck E. Where have all the CP children gone? The needs of adults. *Dev Med Child Neurol* 1984;26:669–676.

Chapter 78

Spina Bifida

Maureen R. Nelson
E. John Rott, III

Spina bifida is a common birth defect that has been with mankind since antiquity. The oldest skeleton found to have spina bifida was discovered in Morocco, and dated back over 12,000 years. Spina bifida was first written about in 1700 BC in ancient Babylonian tablets of priests' prophecies based on the birth of a child with spina bifida (1). Until the 1940s, when advances of modern neurosurgery made possible the closure of back lesions, virtually all infants with spina bifida died in infancy. Unfortunately, after closure most infants went on to die a year or two later from hydrocephalus or urologic complications. While the first valved shunt was introduced in 1957, it was not until 1960, with the successful introduction of the ventriculoatrial shunt, that the prospects for survival really began to improve (1,2). By 1965, 60% of aggressively treated children survived (1).

One of the primary goals in caring for children with myelomeningocele (MMC) is the prevention of secondary complications. A child's maximal cognitive, functional, and ambulation potential is set early on, but secondary acquired deficits can decrease this potential in all areas. Contractures are a secondary problem that can lead to decreased mobility, skin ulceration, and pain. Obesity can contribute to skin ulceration, to loss of mobility, and to social stress. Insufficient management of neurogenic bladder can lead to renal diseases. Improper school placement or assistance can lead to decreased social and vocational potential. All these secondary factors have the potential to increase stress in the child and in the entire family. It is the job of the health care team working with the family of a child with MMC to minimize any secondary acquired deficits in order to maximize functional capacity and growth.

Working toward independence must begin when children with MMC are young. The parents must be helped to understand the importance of a child's acquiring independence and be directed in age-appropriate ways for this to occur. As development progresses, a child needs to become aware of how his or her special needs, self-care activities, and mobility can be developed to prevent secondary problems. The way that the rehabilitation team, including the family and child, go about this undertaking varies with age and developmental stage (3).

DEFINITIONS AND EMBRYOLOGY

The term *spina bifida* was first used by Nicholas Tulpius in 1652 (4). It refers to a failure of closure of the posterior arch of the spine. This failure can occur without neurologic defects (spina bifida occulta) or with the meninges or spinal cord, or both, herniating out through the defect (meningocele and MMC). The types of spina bifida are graphically depicted in Figure 78-1. If the spinal cord is exposed on the surface of the back, the condition is called *myeloschisis*. Lesions most commonly occur in the lumbar and sacral regions, but can be found anywhere along the entire length of the spine. The distribution of lesions

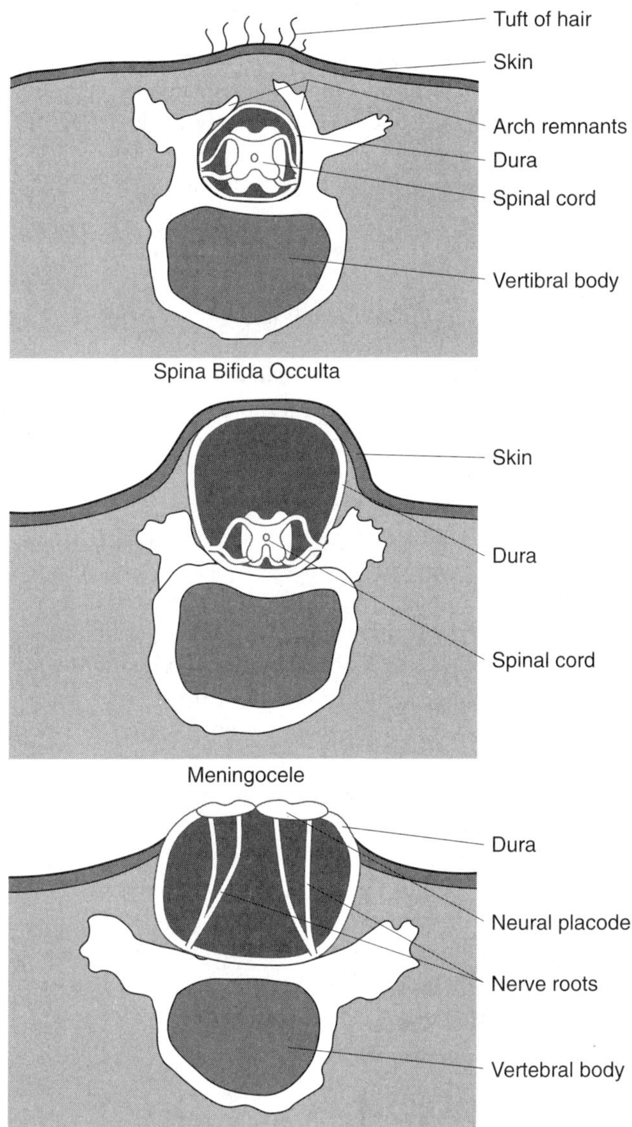

Figure 78-1. Types of spina bifida.

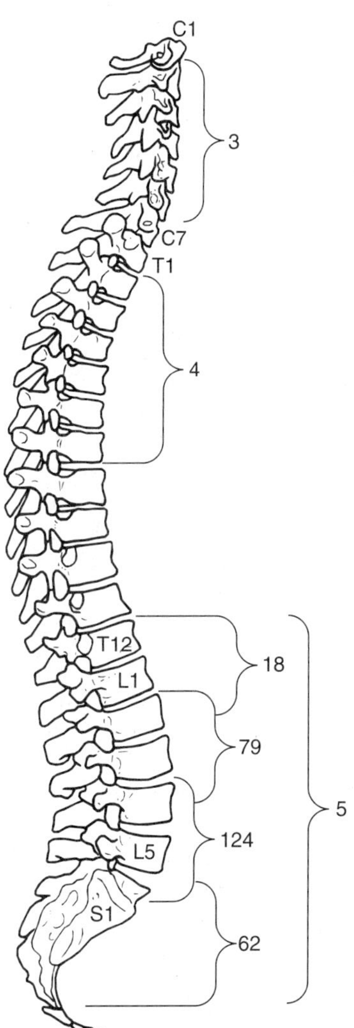

Figure 78-2. Distributions of meningomyeloceles from 295 patients, according to clinical level.

according to location in 295 patients is shown in Figure 78-2.

Between the twenty-second and twenty-fifth days of life, the neural folds on the surface of the embryo invaginate and fuse to form the neural tube that will develop into the brain and spinal cord (5). The neural tube is hollow and the caudal end closes on about the twenty-seventh day. Meningoceles and MMCs traditionally have been presumed to result from a failure of the closure of this tube. This defect then disrupts all of the overlying tissues, preventing the vertebral arch from closing. Some recent evidence suggests that if the posterior vertebral arch and overlying tissues do not form normally, the otherwise normal spinal cord and meninges may then herniate out through the defect and cause an MMC (6). If the vertebral arch fails to grow and fuse normally and the spinal cord and meninges are not disturbed, spina bifida occulta results. The important aspect of spina bifida clinically is not the involvement of the spine, but the degree of involvement of the spinal cord. For this reason, the more proper designation, *MMC,* will be used in place of *spina bifida.* Older terms for MMC include spina bifida cystica and spina bifida aperta.

There are several related malformations in patients with an MMC, the most important of which is the Arnold-Chiari type II deformity. This deformity is characterized by the herniation of the medulla oblongata and cerebellar vermis into the cervical spinal canal. Numerous other associated nervous system malformations include syringomyelia, diastematomyelia, and agenesis of the corpus callosum. Nonneurologic associations include spine malformations, hydronephrosis, cardiac defects, and gastrointestinal anomalies (7).

INCIDENCE

In 1916 Harrer reported the incidence of MMC in America to be 1.1 in 1000 births (8). This figure is identical to the current worldwide incidence. However, within specific populations there are significant variations. These range from a low incidence of 1 in 10,000 in Finland to a high of 5 in 1000 in Northern Ireland (9). The current incidence in America is about 0.6 per 1000, and there is good evidence that this has been steadily declining (10,11). This decrease may in part be due to the increasing practice of selectively aborting fetuses with MMC. There are also large variations in the incidence of MMC between some racial populations. The figures for African-Americans are often a third of those found for white Americans, while those for Hispanic-Americans are two to three times greater (12,13). Each year, at least 2000 children with MMC are born in the United States.

ETIOLOGY

There is clearly a strong genetic link in the development of neural tube defects. The risk of an adult with MMC having a child with a neural tube defect is 5%. The rate reduces to 2.5% for first-degree relatives, 1.25% for second-degree relatives, and 0.5% for third-degree relatives (9). This pattern suggests that inheritance is polygenic. The genes responsible have not yet been identified.

There is also evidence that environmental factors play a role. It is not clear if these factors act independently or function as triggers for an underlying genetic defect. Recently a great deal of work has evaluated the relationship of folic acid levels and neural tube defects. Women with low red blood cell folate levels during early pregnancy have up to a six times greater risk of having a child with a neural tube defect. In an elegant study from Ireland, Daly et al (14) showed that this relationship followed a predictable dose-response relationship. Multiple studies have now proved that maternal folic acid supplements dramatically reduce the incidence of neural tube defects (15–20). Currently the Centers for Disease Control and Prevention (CDC) recommend that women planning pregnancy take 0.4 mg of folic acid daily. It is estimated that if all women of childbearing age took the recommended folic acid, 50% of neural tube defects would be prevented (14). Unfortunately, less than half of pregnancies are planned and most mothers do not know they are pregnant before the critical first month has already passed. These factors coupled with low health care utilization by mothers of lower socioeconomic status make the potential impact of this approach limited.

There has been a great debate recently about fortification of the food supply with folic acid. Proponents believe that this would prevent at least 1000 cases of MMC a year in America. It also might have protective effects against cardiovascular disease for millions of Americans (21). Others worry about the effect of folate on a larger population of elderly Americans with pernicious anemia (22). Folic acid may mask the hematologic symptoms of this disease while permanent neurologic deterioration proceeds unnoticed. Interestingly, this problem would probably be eliminated if both folic acid and vitamin B_{12} were added.

The importance of other environmental factors has also been a source of debate. Two drugs have been shown to have a strong relationship with neural tube defects: aminopterin, a folate antagonist previously used to induce abortions, and valproic acid, a common anticonvulsant (9). Weak associations between neural tube defects and nuclear contamination, agricultural chemicals, and nitrate concentrations in drinking water have been found. There is a clear increase in risk with low socioeconomic status. While diet may explain some of this effect, detailed studies about occupational exposure to chemicals, which are also related to socioeconomic status, are lacking. There is preliminary evidence of increased risk in mothers working as dentists, hairdressers, farmers, and laborers and in occupations with solvent exposure. For fathers, an increased risk has been suggested for painters, printers, decorators, drivers, plastic production workers, farmers, food- and beverage-processing workers, textile workers, and workers exposed to low-level radiation (9).

A twofold increase in risk has been found in women exposed to heat during early pregnancy. This risk was defined as taking hot baths, using saunas or hot tubs, or having a febrile illness. While the mechanism for this effect is unknown, women in their first trimester are advised to avoid elevations of core body temperature (23,24).

PRENATAL DIAGNOSIS

Several techniques are currently used in conjunction to detect neural tube defects prenatally. Measurement of maternal serum α-fetoprotein (MSAFP) levels is a common screening test. If the level is elevated, indicating that any portion of the fetus is not covered by skin, this sensitive screening test is then followed by detailed ultrasonography. Initial ultrasound will diagnose 92% of neural tube defects. Mothers with elevated MSAFP levels and a normal-appearing ultrasound scan may be evaluated by amniocentesis for the presence of elevated acetylcholinesterase levels in the amniotic fluid (25). Elevated acetylcholinesterase is sensitive and specific for neural tube defects.

NEUROSURGERY

Management of the Newborn

In the delivery room the infant is placed in a prone position with a sterile dressing over the back defect. The exposed neural placode is quite fragile, so excessive handling or cleaning may result in additional loss of neurologic function (7). The child is started on intravenous antibiotics to cover exposure to vaginal and skin flora. Surgical closure of the defect can be delayed safely up to 72 hours (26,27). It may be advantageous to wait at least 24 hours so that the infant can be observed for any developing respiratory difficulties, and so that imaging of the head, heart, and kidneys can be performed. Postoperatively the infant should remain prone for at least a week. Because povidone-iodine (Betadine) is toxic to neural tissue, the fragile placode cannot be adequately cleaned. For this reason, wound infection rates range from 7% to 12% (7). Any infant showing early signs of sepsis in the first 3 days after surgery must have a ventricular tap performed immediately to rule out ventriculitis (26). Adhesive plastic dressings should be used to minimize the possibility of stool contaminating the wound. About 75% of infants with MMC will have significant hydrocephalus, which requires the placement of a ventriculoperitoneal (VP) shunt (28). This hydrocephalus is often exacerbated by the closure of the defect, which had been functioning as an outlet for cerebrospinal fluid (CSF). As pressure builds up behind the new closure, as many as 17% of patients may have small CSF leaks (7). Most of these resolve spontaneously without the need for shunt revision. VP shunts may be placed 1 to 2 weeks after primary closure has been performed. This delay in shunt placement is the result of concerns about possible increases in the risk of shunt infections due to contamination of the neural placode or dehiscence of the back wound. Two studies showed that simultaneous closure of the back and VP shunting can be performed without negative effects (27,29).

Early Neurosurgical Complications

The child with MMC is at greatest risk of serious morbidity and mortality in the first year of life. During the first 2 months following placement or revision of a VP shunt, the infant is at risk for ventriculitis. The presenting symptoms are usually nonspecific, including poor feeding, lethargy, temperature instability, and apnea. In the first 2 months the CSF will be immediately tested if any of these symptoms appear (26). Episodes of ventriculitis are related to a significant lowering of the child's subsequent IQ (30).

While symptoms of Chiari compression can occur at any time, presentation in the first year of life is associated with up to 50% mortality (31). Between 5% and 32% of infants with MMC will present with signs of Chiari compression, making it the most common cause of death in patients with MMC (26,28,31). In this syndrome, increasing pressure on the hindbrain causes dysfunction and ischemia of the hindbrain and lower cranial nerves. This often first manifests as poor feeding and regurgitation. Projectile vomiting and choking can occur but are usually inhibited by a weak or absent gag reflex. Partial paralysis of the vocal cords results in a weak cry or stridor. There may also be a "deadpan" expression from facial nerve involvement. Over the course of hours this may progress to a lethal stage of lethargy, obtundation, apnea, and bradycardia (26,31,32). The cause of death is usually central ventilatory dysfunction (CVD). The development of these symptoms is not related to the level of descent of the cerebellar vermis or size of the primary lesion. The only specific risk factor for a Chiari crisis is a high-level lesion (midthoracic or above) (26). It is unclear to what extent the Chiari crisis is due to compression versus brain stem hemorrhage (31–33). Infants with these symptoms need immediate decompression of the posterior fossa, as early intervention is crucial to achieving a good outcome.

A prominent kyphotic deformity may accompany high-level MMC. This presumably results from the loss of paraspinal muscle tone, which allows the normal functioning anterior abdominal muscles and intracostal muscles to buckle the spine (26). These malformations cause significant morbidity through problems in respiration, positioning, and skin breakdown. The merits of resecting kyphotic deformities are debated. If successful, the surgery will undoubtedly give the child an improved quality of life. Unfortunately, the mortality from this procedure is high.

Late Neurosurgical Complications

In general, the deficits associated with MMC are static. The current dictum is that "all deterioration in these children has a treatable cause" (34). Tethering of the spinal cord, shunt malfunction, Chiari compression, and syringomyelia are the most likely causes of any deterioration and all are treatable.

Tethering of the spinal cord is seen on the magnetic resonance images (MRIs) of 75% to 100% (31,35) of children with treated MMC (27). However, MRI findings do not correlate with clinical disease. Clinically significant tethering occurs in up to 27% of patients (26,34). Symptoms of this disorder include any of the following: progression of lower-extremity motor and sensory deficits, pain, new musculoskeletal deformities, or a change in bowel and bladder function (36). Patients with a tethered cord can have sudden irreversible neurologic damage if the cord is suddenly stretched by a blow or a fall (37). If promptly treated, most patients will show significant improvement after surgery (36). As tethering can present at any time, determination of motor and sensory levels should be a regular part of a patient's examinations. The incidence of a tethered cord peaks at the age of 6 years.

Shunt failure is another common late complication of MMC. The average patient requires three shunt revisions in his or her lifetime (38). Chronic headaches are the most frequently reported symptom. Prompt evaluation and revision are crucial, as sudden death from increased intracranial pressure may occur with little warning (38). During routine examinations patients should always be asked about headaches, and optic disks should be evaluated for papilledema. As changes in mental status occur relatively late, one should not wait on their occurrence before referral to a neurosurgeon.

Syringomyelia (also called *hydromyelia* and *hydrosyringomyelia*) is the dilation of a central portion of the spinal cord with CSF. This occurs in up to 40% of patients with a Chiari type II malformation (31). The true frequency may be even higher than this, given that lesions may collapse and become undetectable after the placement of a VP shunt. Lesions may be in communication with normal CSF channels or not. As there is no correlation between lesion size and clinical significance, surgical treatment is delayed until clinical symptoms appear. These symptoms include numbness (especially in the arms and hands), headache, neck pain, lower motor neuron weakness, atrophy of the muscles of the hands and arms, sensory loss, loss of fine motor coordination, and neurogenic arthropathies (Charcot joints). Rapidly progressing scoliosis is one of the most common symptoms of syringomyelia. The scoliosis is thought to be the result of damage by the asymmetrically expanding fluid cavity to the anterior horn cells that control the paravertebral muscles (39). Fortunately, surgical treatment of syringomyelia results in clinical improvement in the majority of patients (31). Although Chiari compression is most common in infancy, it may occur at any time. Symptoms in the older child and adult may be difficult to distinguish from syringomyelia. These include neck pain; arm numbness, weakness, or spasticity; "dancing" eyes; respiratory difficulties; and joint swelling (31,32). The majority of adults with this problem respond well to surgical intervention (31).

OBESITY

Management of body composition is one of the most challenging aspects of MMC care. Children with MMC have short stature. Short lower extremities as well as scoliosis and at times vertebral anomalies may contribute. Agre et al (40) found that height varied by neurologic motor level. Atencio et al (41) studied 100 children with MMC to evaluate growth. The children's heights were at or below the fifth percentile for age, and weights were at approximately the fiftieth percentile, with the weight-height ratio above the ninety-fifth percentile (41). At least 50% of MMC patients more than 3 years old are obese by strict body fat composition analysis (42–44). Traditionally, this has been assumed to be secondary to decreased energy expenditure among nonambulatory patients (42). Recent evidence suggests that hypothalamic-pituitary dysfunction may also play a role. Rotenstein and Breen (45) found that children with MMC had a decreased response to growth hormone stimulation. They found a significant effect on growth, obesity, and muscle strength in the growth hormone–treated group (45).

Typically, children with MMC reach their peak ambulatory abilities around the age of 10 years. They then experience a slow decline in function over the next 10 years. Asher and Olson (46) showed that in children with L1–L3 lesions, the effect of increasing obesity is a critical factor in the loss of ambulation. The children who ambulate more have a lower percentage of body fat. Those with higher-level lesions have a higher percentage of body fat (42).

The measurement of obesity in children with MMC is not a trivial matter. The traditional body mass index is not accurate in children with mid- to high-level lesions because of lower-extremity atrophy and deformities. Subjective assessments by clinicians have also been shown to be notoriously unreliable (42). The best practical measure of percent body fat seems to be a four-skinfold examination (biceps, triceps, subscapular, suprailiac) (43). Children with L3 or higher lesions should have this screening test done on a regular basis. One measure of linear growth in these children is arm span, which has been shown to not vary significantly with lesion level (43).

ALLERGIES

Two recent studies found that more than 70% of children with MMC have latex-specific IgE reactivity (47,48), as evidenced clinically by rhinitis, bronchospasm, urticaria, and anaphylactic shock. Kelly et al (48) reviewed perioperative anaphylaxis and found that children with MMC had a 500 times greater risk of anaphylaxis compared to other children. Almost 14% of children with MMC experienced an anaphylactic reaction characterized by a systolic blood pressure drop of at least 30 mm Hg, and either rash, angioedema, or bronchospasm (48). Konz et al (47) studied the latex reactivity of MMC patients compared with that of adults with spinal cord injury. Latex exposure was remarkably similar between these groups. Sixty-four percent of MMC patients had significant levels of latex-specific IgE, compared to only 4% of spinal cord injury patients (47). The authors speculated that either a defective "neuro-immune interaction" or exposure early in life might be responsible for this difference.

Children with MMC also have a high incidence of allergic reactions to ethylene oxide, a commonly used sterilizing agent. The clinical significance of this has yet to be determined (49).

REPRODUCTIVE FUNCTION

Precocious puberty occurs in approximately 16% of girls with MMC. The precocious puberty is believed to result from hydrocephalus (50). Jumper et al (51) reported a normal rate of progression through puberty in boys with MMC. There is a great deal of concern among people with MMC about reproductive functioning. Many assume that because of absent genital sensation or urinary diversions, they cannot have satisfying sex lives or bear normal children. Many adults with MMC enjoy sex and experience orgasms (52). Women with MMC have normal fertility rates. Previously it was believed that pregnant women with urinary diversions have problems with urinary tract infections, obstruction, and stomal changes. Fortunately, recent series showed these urinary complications to be rare (52,53). Among males, about 75% report being able to achieve erection and ejaculation, although when noctural erections were measured, many of these men had abnormal erectile function (52,54). Erection capability is related to lesion level and is often unrelated to the ability to ejaculate (54). For men with erection problems, a variety of interventions are available.

PSYCHOSOCIAL ISSUES

General long-term function of adults with MMC has not been well documented, owing to the fact that only recently have significant numbers of those with MMC lived to adulthood. A study published by Bomalski et al (55) in 1995 evaluated 38 patients with MMC who were over 18 years old (median age, 24 years), with regard to several factors. They found that education and living arrangements were comparable to those of age-matched individuals in the general population. Approximately 65% of them lived with their parents and one-third lived independently. Over 60% had a high school education and one-third had gone to college. Less than 20% had a full-time job and half were neither in school nor working. He found that women with MMC were more likely to be employed and to be involved in a sexual relationship than were men. Fifty-six percent of the men reported normal erections, with 13% having reported sexual intercourse. Just under half of the women were married, and about the same number reported being sexually active. Two-thirds of the men reported that they had no sexual interaction, compared to 20% of the women. The authors (55) found that approximately 20% of the patients had severe leakage of urine.

In the 1986 study by Cass et al (52) of 35 women and 12 men with MMC, 9 (75%) of the men reported having erections, 6 (50%) reported having had sexual intercourse, and 1 man reported paternity. In that study approximately half of the female patients reported sexual intercourse and one-third reported pregnancies. These numbers for women were similar to those in the Bomalski study while the males in this study reported more sexual activity than did those in the Bomalski study (55). The information in these studies was collected by self-report alone. Jumper et al (51) studied 25 boys by obtaining their history and performing extensive physical examinations. A majority reported erections, and erections were observed in 6 of the 23 patients during physical examination, with most occurring randomly without tactile stimulation. Erectile function and seminal emissions did not correlate with the level of MMC, the presence of bulbocavernosus reflex, rectal tone, or perianal sensation. Boys with an artificial sphincter device inserted surgically to correct incontinence showed no difference in sexual function from boys without the artificial sphincter (51).

In spite of the medical advances in the care of children with MMC, social outcomes are frequently poor. This was vividly shown by the Arkansas Spinal Commission survey of 380 MMC patients in 1993 (56). Of the subjects 17 years or older who were not in school, 66% graduated from high school and about 45% were ambulatory. Only 15% of these subjects held competitive jobs and another 12% held noncompetitive jobs in sheltered work environments. Just over 6% earned more than $10,000 per year, while 8% were attending or had completed college. Despite the fact that 45% were completely independent in self-care, only 10% lived independently or with a roommate. In a British series reported in a related article from Cambridge, England, 30% of 22- to 28-year-olds with MMC lived independently, and 61% of their cohorts reported no disability or moderate disability. Employment figures were not given (57).

The reason why so many people with MMC have difficulties as adults may be partially attributed to the "vulnerable child syndrome" described by Green and Solnit (58) in 1964. They used the term *vulnerable child* to describe the case of a person who developed behavioral and developmental problems after experiencing a life-threatening illness as a child (58). Their theory was that a mother's perception of a child as vulnerable leads to an overprotective parenting style in which the mother does not make sufficient demands on the child for normal development to occur. The child becomes overly dependent and lacks self-esteem, self-efficacy, and independence (59). Interestingly, in the Arkansas study, 56% of the people with MMC reported never having been left alone (56). Mothers of children with disabilities have been shown to have higher levels of depression, especially as the child passes the elementary school years (60). This may also contribute to a lack of effective parenting.

Several studies looked specifically at the predictors of good outcomes for people with MMC. Loomis et al (61) did extensive psychological testing of a cohort of 38 young adults with MMC (mean age, 28 years). They found employment to be related to five skills. Communication skills, socialization skills, and academic skills were highly correlated, while attention and verbal memory were more weakly correlated. The skill level of the job was highly related to intelligence. Interestingly, independent living was associated with intelligence, academic skills, and language skills and not with the person's ability to accomplish the basic tasks of daily living. In a separate study of adolescents by Goodwin and Shurtleff (62), independence was related to family and parenting factors, social acceptance, and cognitive performance. Parental achievement orientation, encouragement of independence, and family cohesion were especially important (62). We believe that a program designed to encourage appropriate parenting skills and to encourage communication and socialization skills should be a part of the care of every person with MMC.

NEUROGENIC BLADDER

The vast majority of children with MMC have a neurogenic bladder. Only 5.0% to 7.5% of the MMC population have normal urologic function (63). There are various types of neurogenic bladder, and these types require different forms of management and pose different risks. The bladder abnormalities can consist of 1) a hyperreflexic detrusor with hyperreflexic sphincter, 2) hyperreflexic detrusor with hyporeflexic sphincter, 3) areflexic detrusor with hyperreflexic sphincter, and 4) areflexic detrusor with areflexic sphincter (64) (see Chap. 51). Thirty percent to 40% of children with MMC will have a hyperreflexic bladder and sphincter (64). In this group the majority of children are able to become socially continent, most commonly with the use of clean intermittent catheterization (CIC) and with pharmacologic control (64). Approximately 19% of the children have a hyperreflexive detrusor with a hyporeflexic sphincter. The chances for continence with conservative therapy are approximately 10% in this group (64). An areflexic detrusor with hyperreflexic sphincter is found in 11% to 13% of patients (64). In this group continence may sometimes be achieved, but it depends on the sphincter pressure (64). Approximately one-third of the children have an areflexic detrusor and areflexic sphincter. Social continence again appears to depend on sphincter pressures and may be achieved through CIC (64). The type of bladder and sphincter pressure frequently decreases over time (65).

The goals in managing neurogenic bladder in MMC are protection of renal function and achievement of social continence. Specific interventions for each child are based on the type of neurogenic bladder found on urodynamic testing and radiographic imaging. Initial evaluation includes a renal ultrasound and measurements of blood urea nitrogen (BUN) and creatine.

Determination of renal size is commonly followed by ultrasound in patients with MMC, as a measure of kidney health. Sutherland et al (66) published a renal-size nomogram for patients with MMC and showed that renal size was smaller for all age groups than in the general population. Bladder capacity has also been studied and found to be approximately 25% less in children with MMC than in age-matched children who are neurologically intact. Bladder capacity for those with MMC is 24.5 times the age plus 64 mL (67).

Approximately 15% to 25% of babies with MMC have hydronephrosis initially; secondary to detrusor sphincter dysynergy, ureteral reflux, or a structural abnormality such as a horseshoe kidney; or transiently (68). Renal agenesis, horseshoe kidney, or fused kidney occurs in 3%, and cryptorchidism occurs in 5% of male infants with MMC (68). Infants should have a renal ultrasound every 6 months for the first 3 years, owing to frequent changes in urologic status. Bladder function may change over time from alteration of the central neurologic system or of the peripheral neurologic system, or from infection and fibrosis (65). Urodynamic examination must be undertaken since the specific detrusor and sphincter status cannot be predicted from neurologic examination (65).

Urodynamic testing includes evaluation of leak point pressure. When this pressure is 40 cm H_2O or more, there is a higher risk of upper tract deterioration and therefore more aggressive management is frequently carried out (69). With high leak point pressure as well as with evidence of hydronephrosis or vesicoureteral reflux (VUR), intermittent catheterization is begun (69). Plastic catheters are used because of the risk of latex allergy. Catheterization is generally done on infants three or four times a day in an attempt to decrease the upper tract pressure. Residual urine volume after CIC should be less than one-sixth of bladder capacity (65). Oxybutynin may also be begun at a dose of 1 to 2 mg twice a day (69). Parents must be advised of possible side effects.

Lapides was the first to use CIC for bladder management in 1972 (70). This was a turning point in the management of neurogenic bladder and in the protection of the upper tracts. To perform self-catheterization, a child must be able to follow multistep directions, must have the hand dexterity to manipulate the catheter and other equipment, and must have the balance to perform catheterization. Poor hand function, blindness, severe contractures, or severe obesity can make self-catheterization extremely difficult, though it is possible with these conditions (71).

CIC leads to improvement of dilatation and VUR in most patients with MMC (72). Urinary tract infections are decreased and incontinence is improved with CIC as well (70).

Oxybutynin is frequently used orally for MMC patients with bladder instability or poor compliance. Anticholinergic side effects however have been reported in 40% to 80% of patients, resulting in the dosage being reduced or discontinued (73). Because of this high rate, intravesical installation of oxybutynin as an alternative to oral administration is being studied. After intravesical administration, the plasma concentration of oxybutynin is higher than after oral administration.

Children with MMC using intravesical oxybutynin twice daily show a significant increase in bladder capacity and a decrease in intravesical pressure, with improved continence. However, patient compliance with this regimen has been shown to be poor (74).

Approximately 80% of children with MMC are able to achieve social continence with CIC and medication (75). If this is not effective, there are multiple procedures that can be performed, including augmentation cystoplasty, placement of an artificial urinary sphincter, continent diversion, or the nonsurgical possibility of a trial of electrical stimulation. One method of treatment for urinary incontinence is colonic urinary diversion, which results in an approximately 70% continence rate. However, approximately 45% of patients develop significant renal deterioration (75).

Treatment of neurogenic bladder by transurethral electrical bladder stimulation (TEBS) was recently described, first in Europe, then in the United States. TEBS has variable effects on bladder capacity. Some children show an improvement in the intravesical filling pressure and some who had not previously manifested bladder contractions do so after TEBS. The TEBS program is quite time-consuming and labor-intensive (76).

Several surgical options are available for bladder management if conservative management is unsuccessful. Vesicostomy involves forming a fistula between the bladder and the abdominal wall, with urine either draining into the diaper or through an opening that may be catheterized. Bladder augmentation may be performed to increase the bladder storage capacity (69). Augmentation is done using various tissues, including the appendix. The use of an artificial sphincter is another surgical option. The artificial sphincter provides improvement in continence; however, revisions are required frequently, secondary to mechanical and surgical failure (77). The artificial sphincter is reportedly removed from approximately 20% of patients. The sphincter has been described as having a mean operational life of 56 months (78). Muscular slings are also used to increase the function of the proximal urethral sphincter. Pubovaginal slings have been used in female patients, with a continence rate of approximately 90% (79). A strip of anterior bladder has also been used as a sling, with continence reported subsequently in females with MMC, but with variable continence in males (80).

Flood et al (81) examined voiding cystourethrograms in 209 patients with MMC and found VUR in 27%, of a high grade in 58% of that group. Conservative treatment with maintenance of the bladder pressure at less than 40 cm H_2O was associated with an increased resolution of VUR as well as less upper tract deterioration (81). VUR is found much more frequently in female than male patients with MMC (82).

Children with MMC with a leak point pressure at 40 cm H_2O or more who are treated with CIC, anticholinergic medications, and fluid restriction show a decrease of pressure approximately 70% of the time, along with resolution of VUR and hydronephrosis. Nonsurgical management in all patients studied by Hernandez et al (83) preserved the upper urinary tract in 90% and provided continence in 80%. The study by Merlini et al (84) of 641 children with MMC in Italy showed that half of the patients with reflux were cured by conservative treatment of CIC and medication.

One small, short-term study evaluated the use of selective dorsal rhizotomy (SDR) at the sacral level for management of high-pressure neurogenic bladder in children with MMC. SDR had a variable impact on bladder function but all children had increased bladder capacity (85). Currently there are no long-term studies looking at the efficacy or safety of SDR in bladder management.

A 1994 study from England of 72 patients in an MMC clinic showed 14 (19%) with renal parenchymal damage (86). There was a much higher incidence in the older patients, which may reflect both the effect of improving methods of bladder management and the effect of aging. Renal parenchymal damage was defined as persistent cortical defects seen on radiographs. Ottolini et al (87) studied 207 patients with MMC undergoing CIC to evaluate the clinical factors associated with renal scarring, and found that febrile infections, bladder trabeculation, VUR, or age over 20 years were associated with scarring. Asymptomatic bacteriuria was not associated with renal scarring and therefore does not require antibiotic therapy (87).

If bladder and renal management is not successful and renal failure occurs, there is no contraindication to renal transplantation in patients with MMC. A small study in Ireland found that patients had an improved perceived quality of life following renal transplantation (88).

NEUROGENIC BOWEL

Traditional bowel continence is present in approximately 10% of children with MMC (63,89). Several methods of training for the 90% of children with MMC with neurogenic bowel have been attempted. Timed daily toileting at specific times permits social continence in 50% to 75% of patients (89,90). Compliance has been a problem with some methods of bowel management (89,91). Instruction in the proper technique to use for a bowel training program is also critical and apparently lacking in many circumstances (89). Bowel training techniques include timing, use of a suppository, appropriate diet, use of an enema or minienema, biofeedback, behavioral management, and surgical treatment.

Initial intervention with the family may consist primarily of education about bowel function and changes in that general function in the patient with a neurogenic bowel. This teaching includes the concepts of gastrocolic reflex and the importance of both sensation and muscle control for neurologically intact bowel function, as well as manipulations available via diet. The goal of social bowel continence is discussed with the parents, being that the child empty the bowels at home at a socially convenient time, most frequently after the evening meal. To achieve this, the program must begin with a medium-sized, formed stool. The first step is generally the use of a pediatric glycerin suppository after the evening meal. The importance of proper insertion of the suppository so that it is placed past the internal sphincter is critical, as inadequate technique is the most common cause for failure (89,90). The child will then sit on a commode with the feet supported and balance maintained. The child will give abdominal pressure with a Valsalva maneuver. This maneuver can be achieved by having the child blow bubbles, laugh, or yell. If the suppository triggers a bowel movement less than 10 minutes after insertion, mechanical stimulation may be a critical factor. If that is the case, digital stimulation with a nonlatex glove and lubricant may be initiated without a suppository (89). If the glycerin suppository is insufficient, a bisacodyl (Dulcolax) suppository may be substituted after approximately a 2-week trial period. Elimination of bowel incontinence between times may be expected in 6 to 12 weeks after initiating the training program (89).

The presence of the anocutaneous reflex and bulbocavernosus reflex is associated with continence, as are compliance with the training program and initiation of the bowel training program before the age of 6 years. Neurologic level was not found to correlate with continence (89).

Microenemas are occasionally used for a bowel training program. The technique and action are similar to those of the glygerin suppository. The volume of traditional enema is generally 20 mL/kg but frequently the volume must be increased over time (89). Enemas are frequently dismissed as being messy or uncomfortable to use. Therefore, variations using enema continence catheters have been tried, to obtain the emptying effects of an enema in a neater fashion (91,92). Other methods involve using a Silastic balloon at the end of the tube to hold the enema contents until the child can be transferred onto a commode to expel the contents. Use of these devices is associated with some decrease in incontinence; however, patient compliance has been extremely low (91,92).

Potential problems with enema use include trauma to the rectum and bowel including perforation; electrolyte disturbances including hyponatremia; bacteremia; infection; and autonomic dysreflexia (91).

Constipation may cause stool incontinence around a blockage, abdominal discomfort, rectal prolapse, decreased urinary continence, decreased bladder capacity, and ureteral compression. Bowel incontinence causes odor, skin irritation, and social discomfort (91). Initiation of bowel training between the ages of 2 and 4 years, which coincides with the age of bowel training for neurologically intact peers, allows social continence prior to the child's beginning school. Beginning at this age, there is also increased compliance and therefore increased continence (89).

Of young people with MMC, approximately 80% become socially continent with a regimen including diet, stool softeners, and suppository or digital stimulation. This includes 60% of compliant people with no sensation, no reflexes, and no detectable voluntary sphincter activity (89).

Biofeedback has been attempted to deal with bowel management in individuals with MMC. These techniques are used to obtain control over voluntary muscle responses, including those of the external sphincter and gluteal muscles (63). In the small studies reported thus far, there was variability in the description of success, but it is clear that only a select group of patients may benefit. The patient must have rectal sensation for any possibility of success, and must have muscle strength in the abdominal and gluteal muscles, as well as coordination of these, to even have the potential for success. The child also must be able to understand and cooperate with the instructions, and be motivated (63). Some studies showed a decrease in episodes of fecal incontinence; however, there has not been proof of improvement of muscle strength (63). Neural stimulators for the sacral and pudendal nerves have also been initiated in some children with MMC (63). No large studies from which any recommendations may be generalized have been published.

SKIN

Children with myelodysplasia have insensate skin that correlates with their level of neurologic involvement. They will have sensory loss in the perineal region and generally in the feet, with various levels of involvement of the legs and trunk. This leads to an increased risk of skin ulceration. Neurogenic bowel and bladder may also contribute to skin ulceration if there is a problem with leaking, leading to macerated skin in the perineal region. Dampness, pressure, and shear forces are risks for skin ulceration in any individual with insensate skin. Therefore, parents and children must be taught how to protect the skin. These include touching bath water with the hand before getting into the tub, touching any playground equipment such as a slide or swing with the hand before sitting down, not leaning or sitting on any object without testing the temperature first with the hand, and careful daily inspection of the skin. A brace or a wheelchair that is too tight may cause pressure and skin problems. As children grow larger, they are taught methods of pressure relief for use when they are sitting.

Skin ulcerations are staged in the standard manner. The length, width, and depth of ulcers should be measured on photographs, to help monitor the progression of healing. Wound care includes débridement of the ulcer, along with cleaning, dressing, and removal of any factors that contributed to the formation of the wound.

There have been ulcers in patients with MMC that did not heal after 1 to 8 years of treatment but did heal after release of a tethered cord. This suggests the possibility of a neurotrophic factor in wound healing in patients with MMC (93). A study of 36 patients with MMC at a low lumbosacral level showed a relationship between skin breakdown and foot rigidity, surgical arthrodesis, and nonplantigrade positioning of the feet (94). Therefore, maintaining a supple foot in a plantigrade position may help minimize foot ulceration in patients with MMC. (See Chap. 50.)

THERAPY

Physical therapy and occupational therapy comprise one of the first educational processes for a parent of an infant with spina bifida. The rehabilitation team ideally sees the infant and parents during the initial hospitalization. At this time, instruction is begun in positioning and range of motion exercises. The goals of positioning are to promote development and to prevent contractures. Due to intrauterine positioning, decreased active movement, and unopposed muscle pull, the risk of contractures is high. In many cases contractures are also very predictable; for example, hip flexion contractures occur frequently in the setting of active hip flexors with minimal or no hip extensors. Positioning is thus encouraged to promote hip extension, and for development of the acetabulum by avoiding dislocation. Range of motion exercises are begun with the goal of maintaining functional joint range of motion. Exercises are begun in the hospital and are taught to the parents at that time. Parents are instructed to perform them one to several times a day.

As the infant grows, therapies advance to the promotion of equilibrium responses and righting reactions. Developmental stimulation is an important part of therapy. Therapy for the development of fine and gross motor skills, including coordination, is designed to assist with both general childhood activities of daily living as well as mobility. Children with MMC may have visual-perceptual, fine motor, sequencing, and perceptual motor dysfunction, as well as dyspraxia (95). This can lead to general developmental problems, as well as problems with training for mobility. Left-hand dominance is more frequent in patients with MMC who have progressive hydrocephalus. The failure to establish right-handedness is believed to reflect a disorder of lateralization due to hydrocephalus at an early age. Hand preference appears to be developed later in children with MMC and hydrocephalus (95). Mobility training includes crawling or scooting, depending on a child's motor abilities, and progresses to an upright mobility approach. Young children often start with a parapodium (Figs. 78-3 and 78-4) swivel walker to put them in a standing position, and then potentially advance to mobility using this device. As children become stronger in their upper extremities, and develop more coordination and an ability to follow commands, they may advance to other devices that lead to more independent mobility. If the neurologic level is above L3, a reciprocating gait orthosis (RGO) may be required, along with a walker or crutches (96). If the neurologic level is at L3–L4, a hip-knee-ankle-foot orthosis (HKAFO) and walker or crutches may be effective, with the hip portion sometimes discontinued with improvement of strength and coordination (97). With a neurologic level at L5, an ankle-foot orthosis (AFO) is frequently effective, and this is occasionally also indicated for involvement at an upper sacral level, for protection of the foot and ankle position along with the prevention of deformities. In the child with lower sacral involvement, a University of California Biomechanics Lab (UCBL) orthosis may be useful (97). (See Chap. 30.)

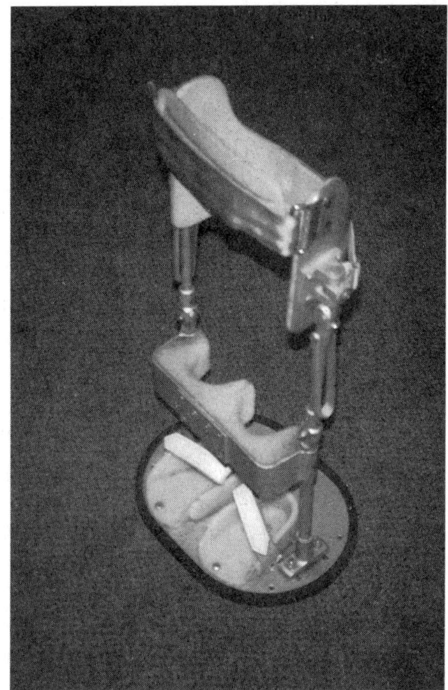

Figure 78-3. Parapodium.

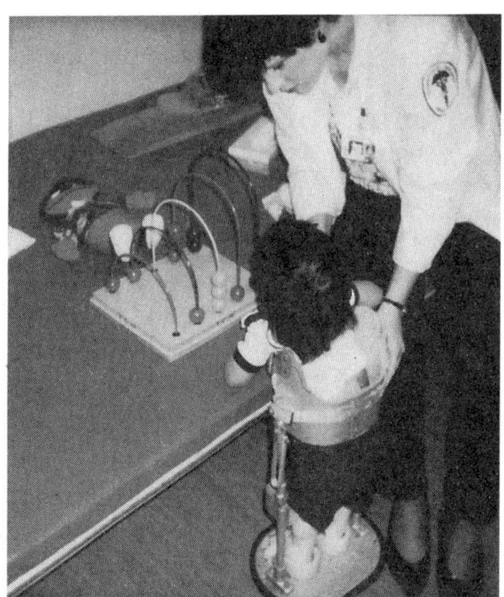

Figure 78-4. Mobility training with parapodium.

The ability of a child with MMC to walk is an important emotional, social, and functional issue for the entire family. Many studies have searched for the critical factor in determining ability to walk in a child with MMC. The neurologic level and active muscle activity, commonly the quadriceps, are two of the most frequently cited determining factors. Obesity, contractures, age, cognitive status, motivation, and other factors have important contributions

(46). Energy expenditure is involved in many of these factors. Energy expenditure for walking is defined as energy used per unit of time, or oxygen consumed per kilogram per minute (98). Children with MMC choose a slower gait, which consumes more oxygen per distance and is 218% less efficient than the gait of able-bodied children (99). A wheelchair is the most energy-efficient means of mobility for a child with MMC, but is only 38% as efficient as walking for a child without neurologic involvement. In a child using crutches, a swing-through gait pattern is 33% more efficient than a four-point gait (100).

Wheelchair mobility is another important area of training for children who will not be full-time ambulators. This can be started at the ages of approximately 18 months to 3 years and can be useful for sports activities, even for children who will use it minimally in day-to-day life. For some children, upper-extremity strengthening is an important prelude to learning wheelchair propulsion. Sequencing activities are important, in order for children to learn how to get in and out of the wheelchair safely, how to use the brakes and seatbelt, and how to effectively maneuver the wheelchair. This includes pushing the wheelchair forward and backward and turning. Training of the child and family in safe transfers in and out of the wheelchair is critical. Children must also learn weight-shifting pressure relief for the prevention of skin ulcerations.

A 1991 prospective study by Luthy et al (101) of 160 infants with MMC showed that infants delivered by cesarean section before labor had begun had a level of paralysis two segments below that of infants delivered vaginally or delivered via cesarean section after labor had begun. However, in a 3-year follow-up study published in 1994, a correction was done for the presence or absence of scoliosis or a gibbus. With this adaptation there was much less of a difference between the groups, with only a tendency to more severe paralysis in the infants delivered vaginally (102).

One study (103) compared children who use a parapodium for mobility and those who use a wheelchair. There was no difference in the incidence of urinary tract infections, reflux, or hydronephrosis. There was a similar rate of skin breakdown; however, the location of skin breakdown was in the gluteal region in those who used wheelchairs and in the lower extremities in those who used a parapodium; hip flexion contractures were no more common in those using a wheelchair, though knee flexion contractures were more common. Dislocation of the hip was more common in those who used a parapodium. The incidence of fractures was not significantly different between the two groups. Those who used a parapodium were actually more obese than those who used a wheelchair, although differences between the groups regarding a higher incidence of television watching may have been a more important factor. Children in wheelchairs had fewer bowel accidents, which was believed to be due to mechanical compression of the anus during sitting, whereas those who were upright in a parapodium had increased abdominal pressure. Wheelchairs were noted to be faster and more convenient for mobility, although parapodiums were viewed as having an emotional advantage by many families. The perceived advantage of being at the same eye level as their peers was dramatic for most families (103).

Agre et al (40) studied the capacity for physical activity in children with MMC. He evaluated 33 children between the ages of 10 and 15 years in regard to strength, ambulatory velocity, aerobic capacity, and energy cost and mobility. He divided the children into groups depending on motor function level: L2 and above, L3–L4, L5 to sacral, and those with no motor deficit but bladder involvement. Range of motion of the lower extremities was not dependent on neurologic level but on full-time ambulation, as those who walked had normal joint range of motion and those who never ambulated had more severe contractures. Walking and running speed correlated with motor function, especially hip extension and knee extension strength. The speed of walking in the L2-and-above group was 36% of normal values; in the L3–L4 group, 66% of normal; in the L5-to-sacral group, 74% of normal; and those without motor deficits had a speed 91% of normal values. In a quantitative evaluation of muscle strength, the group with no motor deficits on physical examination had hip extension strength 60% of normal values and knee extension strength 40% of normal values. Walking was twice as strenuous as wheelchair mobility for children with MMC who did both (40).

Research findings are quite variable as to the percentage of individuals with MMC who will be community ambulators or who will use wheelchairs only. The percentages vary depending on the level of neurologic involvement, as well as age and secondary associated conditions. Findley et al (104) studied 77 children, 11 to 15 years old, with MMC and found 22 not walking; 56 community ambulators, of whom 16 occasionally used wheelchairs; and 1 walking only in therapy. Five of this group had never walked, 16 stopped walking between the ages of 10 and 15, and 6 walked much less than previously. Many of the group who decreased or stopped walking associated this decline with a period of immobilization, due to equipment malfunction or unavailable bracing, surgical procedures, or weight gain. Fifty of the 77 did not have a decrease in walking. Only in those with no weakness or with paralysis at L2 or above was the ability to walk predicted well by neurologic level. For all others, mobility as a young child was a much better predictor of walking in adolescence. A child is predicted to walk as an adolescent if he or she is able to sit by 12 years, is able to walk outside by 4 years, and is not using a wheelchair by age 7. A child is predicted not to walk if he or she is not walking outside by age 6. Otherwise the child is predicted to both walk and use a wheelchair (104). Factors contributing to ambulation potential are neurologic level, mental ability, general health complications including shunt failure and urinary tract infections, ulceration of skin, contractures, and family support (104).

DeSouza and Carroll (94) found that children with MMC achieve their maximum walking ability by age 9, with 50% later stopping ambulation, most frequently between the ages of 10 and 20.

The use of crutches, and hence the upper extremities, for ambulation has been shown to help forward progression and gait, by reducing the compensatory pelvic rotation and hip abduction that children with lumbar-level MMC must use. By decreasing the demand on the weak musculature of the legs, crutches should help maintain functional ambulation and improve the gait pattern (105).

Asher and Olson's study (46) of 98 individuals with MMC found that neurologic level was the most important variable in determining ambulation. Patients with the neurologic level at L3 or above generally were nonambulators, while those with involvement at L4 or below were walking. Significant factors in limiting ambulation in individuals with MMC appeared to be hip deformity in patients with involvement at the L3 level, obesity with neurologic involvement at the L1 and L2 levels, and deformities of the knee, foot, and ankle in patients with neurologic involvement at the thoracic level. In this study, deterioration in mobility appeared to be due to lack of motivation, skin problems, obesity, and musculoskeletal deformity. Conversely, improvement in ambulatory function was noted most frequently in patients 5 to 10 years old, probably owing to orthotic use and motivation (46).

Stillwell and Menelaus's study (106) of 50 patients with MMC, all age 15 or older, revealed 36 ambulators. There were no household or nonfunctional ambulators. One-third with thoracic-level and upper-lumbar lesions walked, and almost all those with sacral and lower-lumbar levels did so. Those with high-level lesions with flexion contracture of the hip, severe pelvic obliquity, or severe scoliosis were likely not to walk (106).

Hoffer et al (107) reviewed 56 patients who had been followed for over 5 years and found that prolonged nonfunctional ambulation was very rare, particularly after age 9. All patients with sacral-level involvement were community ambulators and no one with thoracic-level involvement walked. Patients with lumbar-level involvement had other factors that were decisive in ambulation, including age, hydrocephalus, spasticity, deformities of the spinal column, fractures, mental retardation, contractures, and social factors (107). Brinker et al (108) studied 36 adults with sacral-level MMC at an average age of 29 years. Thirty-five (97%) of the patients had been community ambulators during childhood. However, 11 patients showed a decline in the ability to walk, from community ambulation to household ambulation (5 patients), nonfunctional ambulation (2), and nonambulation (4 patients). A decrease in the ability to plantarflex was also found in 14 patients and a decrease in plantar sensation in 15. There was a breakdown of skin over the plantar surface of the metatarsal heads and the heels in over half of the patients. Fifteen of the patients had had osteomyelitis and 11 had had amputations (108). Twenty-nine had some type of medical insurance (108). Thirty-five patients (97%) had intelligence in the normal range.

JOINT

The goals of the management of joints in children with MMC are to maintain a functional range of motion, maintain trunk balance and stability, and prevent or relieve contractures. There is a high rate of complications after surgical treatment of children with MMC, including urinary tract or other postoperative infections, wound healing problems secondary to vascular insufficiency, pressure ulceration underneath casts, and latex allergies (109).

SPINE

Spinal deformity is common in children with MMC. The two major types of deformities are scoliosis and severe kyphosis or gibbus. The former is very common and the latter is unusual.

The incidence of scoliosis depends on the level of neurologic involvement, with 85% to 98% of those with thoracic-level lesions, approximately half with L3–L4 involvement, and less than 10% of those with sacral-level involvement having scoliosis (97,109,110). Scoliosis in children with MMC progresses at approximately 5 degrees per year (111). There is a loss of stability of the spine leading to scoliosis due to muscle involvement at the level of paralysis, and absence of the posterior elements and intervening ligaments (110). Progression of scoliosis is faster in children with more severe curves (111). Children with MMC with asymmetric neurologic motor involvement have only a slightly higher incidence of scoliosis compared to those with symmetric involvement, and the muscle asymmetry does not lead to spinal curvature on a specific side (111). Scoliotic curves generally develop between the ages of 5 and 10 years, with the fastest rate of deterioration occurring between ages 10 and 15 (110).

The goals of spine treatment are maintenance of a balanced trunk and pelvis to help maintain a seating position and prevent skin problems, and preservation of respiratory function and maximal trunk height (109,110).

Treatment of scoliosis in children with MMC is with bracing or surgery. In Piggott's study (112) of 250 children with MMC, 90% had spinal deformity by the age of 10, with over 80% having scoliosis. Bracing may be undertaken in children with MMC with a curve of 20 degrees and progression of 5 degrees per year or more (111). Once a curve is 30 to 45 degrees or more, progression is almost inevitable (109,111). Bracing in this case is generally done to delay surgery as long as possible, to maintain spine

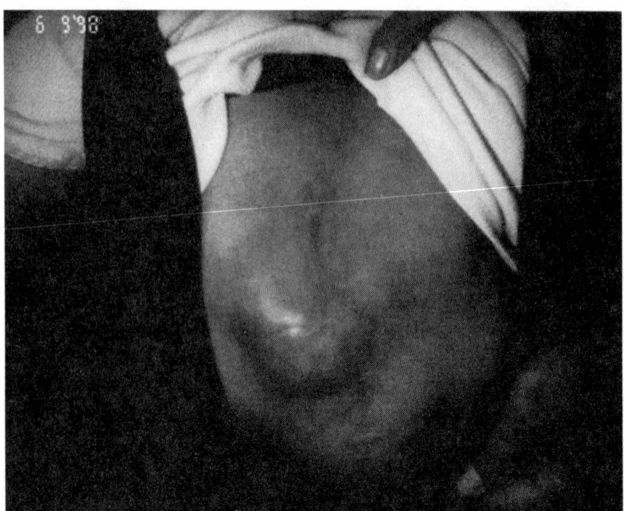

Figure 78-5. Kyphosis—abnormal veterbrae in severe anterior-posterior spinal deformity.

growth and to await resolution of any intervening medical problem. Potential problems with bracing include compromised pulmonary function, skin problems, and potential rib deformity (109). Spine orthotics are used for support during the time of growth as well as for protection postoperatively. A custom-molded thoracolumbosacral orthosis is used most commonly (97).

When scoliosis is noted in a child with MMC, one must determine whether there is a neurologic problem causing this, such as a tethered cord, hydrosyringomyelia, or hydrocephalus. MRI of the brain and spinal cord is used for evaluation (109). If neurologic causes are found, then neurosurgical intervention is undertaken.

Surgical care for children with scoliosis and MMC is spinal fusion. Most commonly, both anterior and posterior fusion is recommended. The entire curve is included and the fusion may extend distally to the lumbosacral joint when there is pelvic obliquity in a nonambulator. Sacral fusion is not frequently recommended in those who ambulate. Postoperatively two-person transfers are used to avoid any torque of the back that may disrupt the fixation (109).

A much less common problem is congenital kyphosis, also called gibbus. The incidence is approximately 10% in patients with MMC (113,114). Kyphosis may cause a very dramatic spinal deformity (Figs. 78-5 and 78-6). The mechanism for the sharp, rigid kyphotic segment is believed to be abnormal development of the vertebrae, which causes a shift of the weight-bearing axis to anterior to the spine with a resultant force of gravity in a posterior direction on the kyphotic segment. The posterior elements of the vertebrae are separated so that the paraspinal muscles are anterior to the apex and therefore act as flexors of the spine instead of their normal function as extensors (112,114). The angle and direction of force have been described as making the curve progression inevitable (113).

Problems caused by kyphosis are skin ulceration at the most prominent portion, respiratory difficulty due to decreased lung cavity size, compression of abdominal contents, seating problems, decreased urologic function, and decreased ability to use the hands well secondary to requiring increased use of the hands for balance (113,114). Bracing is impractical for long-term care because of skin ulceration and compression of abdominal structures (109,114). Surgical treatment has been shown to reduce the preoperative deformity and to maintain that position, or slow the progression, in long-term follow-up. Surgery is frequently delayed so that maximal spinal growth can be obtained, though there can be an increased height of the lumbar region of the spine postoperatively, which has been found to be greater in less skeletally mature patients (114). Surgical intervention consists of excision of the involved vertebrae. The remaining segments are then approximated and internal fixation is performed. Postoperatively patients are placed in a cast or in a custom-fit spinal orthosis that holds them supine. When they are allowed to be upright, it is only with use of a spinal orthosis for approximately 9 to 12 months postoperatively (109,113,114). The goals are skin protection, improved sitting posture, and increased upper-extremity use, along with preservation of pulmonary and abdominal cavity area.

HIP

Hip dislocation is frequent in children with MMC. Previously it was recommended that all dislocated hips be reduced, which led to many operations and long periods of immobilization. Unfortunately there is a high rate of failure in maintaining hip reduction and many hips are stiff after the procedure. Later recommendations evolved to surgical reduction of unilateral hip dislocation because of possible difficulties with pelvic obliquity and scoliosis. Keggi et al (115) examined 31 children over 10 years old with a neurologic level at L3 and L4, because they believed that involvement at these levels represented the greatest risk for hip instability. They found no causal relationship between hip instability and scoliosis, and no relationship between pelvic obliquity and unilateral hip instability (115). Broughton et al (116) studied hip x-ray films of 802 patients with MMC, finding that muscle imbalance is not a significant factor in producing hip flexion deformities or hip dislocation. In children with L4-level involvement who theoretically have maximum muscle imbalance across the hip, two-thirds of the hips were not dislocated. Hip dislocation and flexion contracture in children with higher-level lesions were thought to occur secondary to inactive muscle tone as well as prolonged sitting (116).

Dislocated hips are rarely painful in patients with MMC. Treatment of unilateral hip dislocation in the child with MMC remains controversial. If surgical correction is

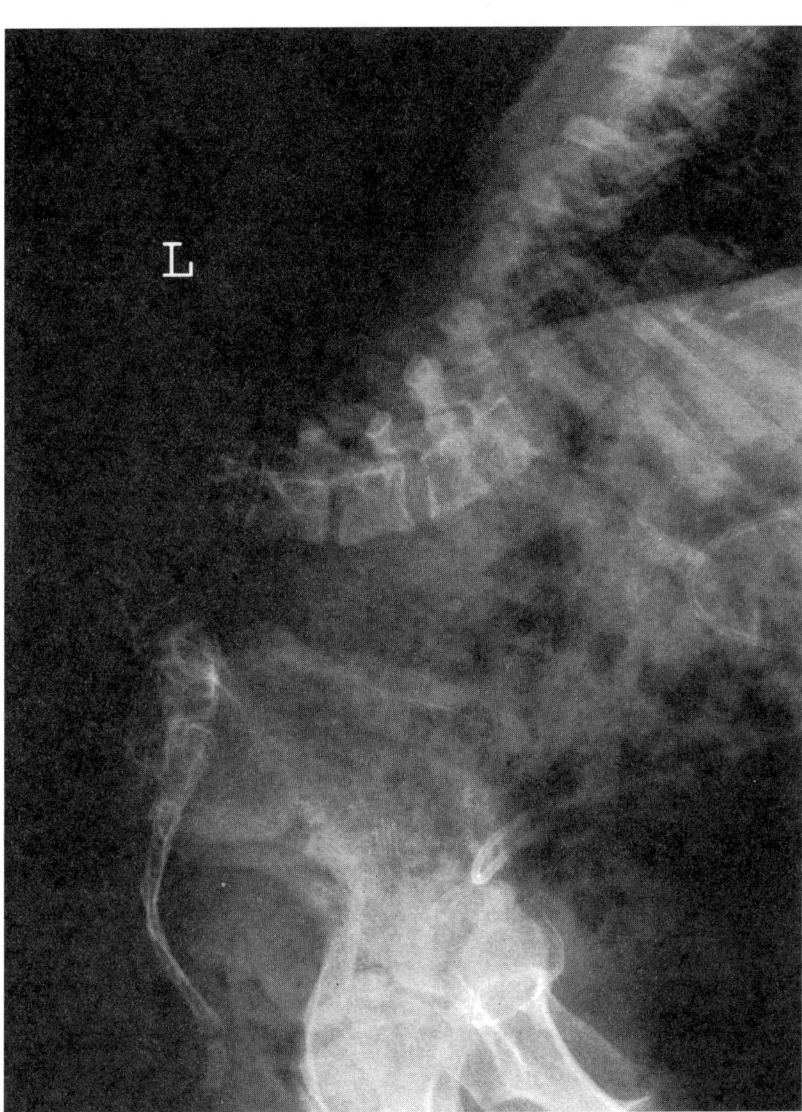

Figure 78-6. X-ray of kyphosis.

undertaken, it may include open reduction with proximal femoral varus osteotomy, and pelvic augmentation to repair acetabular dysplasia may be required. Muscle transfers including the classic Sharrard transfer of the iliopsoas to the posterior, greater trochanter, along with transfer of the external oblique muscle, may be performed simultaneously (109). Contractures of the hip muscles may be released to allow children to fit into orthoses. If the child uses a wheelchair instead of ambulating, the occurrence of flexion contractures is likely (109).

Stability of the hip during gait may be improved in some children with lumbar-level MMC by transfer of the external oblique adductors, and tensor fasciae latae muscles. These transfers are performed particularly when there is poor balance or hip control, or a crouched gait. They are also performed after surgery to reduce a dislocated hip (117).

KNEE

Knee flexion contractures may impede ambulation and interfere with brace use. Valgus deformity of the knee is common in ambulatory patients and is generally treated with orthotic modification (109). Williams et al (118) studied 72 community ambulators with MMC between the ages of 23 and 39 years, to evaluate knee problems. Seventeen (24%) of the patients had significant knee symptoms. Patients with pain had low-lumbar to sacral-level lesions. The symptomatic patients had a common gait pattern, an adductor lurch with knee valgus and a swivel push off with the foot pronated. This gait pattern was found in less than 10% of the ambulators who did not have knee problems. X-ray studies revealed arthritic changes in the patients with lumbar-level lesions who had painful knees. A knee-ankle-foot orthosis (KAFO) with a free knee joint may improve the alignment and slow the development of degenerative changes (118). The use of bilateral forearm crutches will decrease the force on the knees.

LEG

External tibial rotation is common in children with MMC. It can lead to out-turned feet bilaterally and subsequently a disturbance of gait. Treatment may be with orthotics or with distal osteotomy of the tibia. Varus deformity may also be noted at the ankle, with treatment also by orthotics or surgery. Flail ankle is treated with orthotics (109).

FEET

Sixty percent of children with MMC are born with rigid deformities of the feet, most commonly talipes equinovarus, or clubfeet. This may be treated with meticulous serial casting with particular care to avoid skin compromise, or surgically with plantar fascia release (109). Equinus contracture may also be present and may be treated with tenotomy and subsequent immobilization or casts. Calcaneovalgus deformity may also develop, particularly in children with involvement at the L4 or L5 level, due to activity of the anterior tibial or peroneal muscles without opposition. In patients with sacral-level lesions, cavus deformity or claw toes may be noted. Shoe inserts and soft-tissue releases may be effective. Claw toes lead to the risk of skin ulceration due to problems with shoe wear (109).

FRACTURES

Children with MMC have an increased risk of fractures in the legs secondary to a lack of sensation and to osteopenia. Fractures generally heal in the usual amount of time and soft casts may be sufficient owing to patients immobility. The fractured bones should be immobilized for a minimal period of time to avoid further demineralization (109).

CONCLUSIONS

Treatment of individuals with MMC begins prenatally and continues indefinitely, with attempts to maximize developmental progress and then adult function, and to minimize any complications that may limit these. Progress has been dramatic in the care of neurogenic bladder and of hydrocephalus, and continues in all areas, hopefully leading to continuing improvements in the health and functional status of individuals with MMC.

REFERENCES

1. Shurtleff D, Shurtleff H. Decision making for the treatment or nontreatment of congenitally malformed individuals. In: Shurtleff D, ed. *Myelodysplasias and extrophies: significance, prevention and treatment.* New York: Grune & Stratton, 1986:3–24.
2. Guthkelch A. Ethical considerations in management of spinal dysraphism. In: Park T, ed. *Spinal dysraphism.* Oxford: Blackwell Scientific, 1992:19–35.
3. Peterson PM, Rauen KK, Brown J, Cole J. Spina bifida: the transition into adulthood begins in infancy. *Rehabil Nurs* 1994;19:229–238.
4. Brockelhurst G. The nature of spina bifida. In: Brockelhurst G, ed. *Spina bifida for the clinician.* London: Spastics International, 1976:1–7.
5. Moore K. *The developing human.* Philadelphia: WB Saunders, 1988.
6. Meuli M, Meudi-Simmen C, Yingling C, et al. Creation of myelomeningocele in utero: a model of functional damage from spinal cord exposure in fetal sheep. *J Pediatr Surg* 1995;30:1028–1033.
7. Hahn S. Open myelomeningocele. *Neurosurg Clin North Am* 1995;6:231–241.
8. Smith E. *Spina bifida and the total care of spinal myelomeningocele.* Springfield: Thomas, 1965.
9. Blatter BM, van der Star M, Roeleveld N. Review of neural tube defects: risk factors in parental occupation and the environment. *Environ Health Perspect* 1994;102:140–145.
10. Yen I, Khoury M, Erickson J, et al. The changing epidemiology of neural tube defects. *Am J Dis Child* 1992;146:857–861.
11. Stein S, Feldman J, Friedlander M, Klein R. Is myelomeningocele a disappearing disease? *Pediatrics* 1982;69:511–514.
12. Feldman J, Stein S, Klein R, et al. The prevalence of neural tube defects among ethnic groups in Brooklyn, New York. *J Chronic Dis* 1982;35:53–60.
13. Shaw G, Jensvold N, Wasserman C, Lammer E. Epidemiologic characteristics of phenotypically neural tube defects among 0.7 million California births, 1983–1987. *Teratology* 1994;49:143–149.
14. Daly L, Kirke, Malloy A, et al. Folate levels and neural tube defects. *JAMA* 1995;274:1698–1702.
15. Wald W, Sneddon J, Densem J, et al. MRC Vitamin Study Research Group. Prevention of neural tube defects: results of the Medical Research Council Vitamin Study. *Lancet* 1991;338:131–137.

16. Czeizel A, Dudas I. Prevention of the first occurrence of neural tube defects by periconceptional vitamin supplementation. *N Engl J Med* 1992;327: 1832–1835.

17. Laurence K, James N, Miller M, et al. Double-blind randomized controlled trial of folate treatment before conception to prevent recurrence of neural tube defects. *BMJ* 1981;282: 1509–1511.

18. Allen WP. Folic acid in the prevention of birth defects. *Curr Opin Pediatr* 1996;8(6): 630–634.

19. Krike P, Daly L, Elwood J. A randomized trial of low dose folic acid to prevent neural tube defects. *Arch Dis Child* 1992;67:1442–1446.

20. Werler M, Shapiro S, Mitchell A. Preconceptional folic acid exposure and risk of occurrent neural tube defects. *JAMA* 1993;269: 1257–1261.

21. Oakley G, Adams M, Dickinson C. More folic acid for everyone, now. *J Nutr* 1996;126: 751S–755S.

22. Guall G, Testa C, Thomas P, Weinreich D. Fortification of the food supply with folic acid to prevent neural tube defects is not yet warranted. *J Nutr* 1996;126:773S–780S.

23. Sandford M, Kissling G, Joubert P. Neural tube defect etiology: new evidence concerning maternal hyperthermia, health, and diet. *Der Med Child Neurol* 1992;34:661–675.

24. Milunsky A, Ulcickas M, Rothman K, et al. Maternal heat exposure and neural tube defects. *JAMA* 1992;268: 882–885.

25. Budorick NE, Pretorius DH, Nelson TR. Sonography of the fetal spine technique, imaging findings, and clinical implications. *AJR* 1995;164:421–428.

26. Pang D. Surgical complications of open spinal dysraphism. *Neurosurg Clin North Am* 1995;6: 243–257.

27. Scott R, Moore M. Myelomeningocele repair. In: Park T, ed. *Spinal dysraphism.* Oxford: Blackwell Scientific 1992:48–58.

28. McCullough DC, Johnson DL. Myelomeningocele repair: technical considerations and complications. *Pediatr Neurosurg* 1994;21:83–90.

29. Parent AD, McMillan T. Contemporaneous shunting with repair of myelomeningocele. *Pediatr Neurosurg* 1995;22:132–136.

30. Mapstone TB, Rekate HL, Nulsen FE, et al. Relationship of cerebral spinal fluid shunting and IQ in children with myelomeningocele: a retrospective analysis. *Childs Brain* 1984;11:112–118.

31. Rauzzino M, Oakes WJ. Chiari II malformation and syringomyelia. *Neurosurg Clin North Am* 1995;6:293–309.

32. Oakes WJ, Gaskill S. Symptomatic Chiari malformations in childhood. In: Park T, ed. *Spinal dysraphism.* Oxford: Blackwell Scientific, 1992:104–125.

33. Nomura S, Akimura T, Eguchi Y, et al. Apnea associated with Chiari malformation: medullary hemorrhage revealed by MRI. *Childs Nerv Syst* 1993;9: 348–349.

34. McLone DG. Continuing concepts in the management of spina bifida. *Pediatr Neurosurg* 1992;18:254–256.

35. McEnery G. Borzyskowski M, Cox TC, Neville BG. The spinal cord in neurologically stable spina bifida: a clinical MRI study. *Dev Med Child Neurol* 1992;34: 342–347.

36. Yamada S. Tethered spinal cord: pathophysiology and management. In: Park T, ed. *Spinal dysraphism.* Oxford: Blackwell Scientific, 1992:74–90.

37. Yamada S, Iacono R, Andrade T, et al. Pathophysiology of tethered cord syndrome. *Neurosurg Clin North Am* 1995;6:311–323.

38. Tomlinson P, Sugarman ID. Complications with shunts in adults with spina bifida. *BMJ* 1995;311:286–287.

39. Isu T, Chono Y, Iwasaki Y, et al. Scoliosis associated with syringomyelia presenting in children. *Childs Nerv Syst* 1992;8:97–100.

40. Agre JC, Findley TW, McNally MC, et al. Physical activity capacity in children with myelomeningomyelocele. *Arch Phys Med Rehabil* 1987;68: 372–377.

41. Atencio PLF, Ekvall SW, Oppenheimer S, Grace E. Effect of level of lesion and quality of ambulation on growth chart measurements in children with myelomeningocele: a pilot study. *J Am Diet Assoc* 1992;92: 858–861.

42. Mita K, Akataki K, Itoh K, et al. Assessment of obesity of children with spina bifida. *Dev Med Child Neurol* 1993;35:305–311.

43. Roberts D, Shepherd RW, Shepherd K. Anthropometry and obesity in myelomeningocele. *J Paediatr Child Health* 1991;27(2):83–90 1991.

44. Shepard K, Roberts D, Golding S, et al. Body composition in myelomeningocele. *Am J Clin Nutr* 1991;53:1–6.

45. Rotenstein D, Breen TJ. Growth hormone treatment of children with myelomeningocele. *J Pediatr* 1996;128;S28–S31.

46. Asher M, Olson J. Factors affecting the ambulatory status of patients with spina bifida cystica. *J Bone Joint Surg [Am]* 1983; 65:350–356.

47. Konz KR, Chia JK, Kurup VP, et al. Comparison of latex hypersensitivity among patients with neurologic defects. *J Allergy Clin Immunol* 1995;95: 950–954.

48. Kelly KJ, Pearson ML, Kirup VP, et al. A cluster of anaphylactic reactions in children with spina bifida during general anesthesia: epidemiologic features, risk factors, and latex hypersensitivity. *J Allergy Clin Immunol* 1994;94:53–61.

49. Pittman T, Kiburz J, Steinhardt G, et al. Ethylene oxide allergy in children with spina bifida. *J Allergy Clin Immunol* 1995;96:486–488.

50. Elias ER. Precocious puberty in girls with myelodysplasia. *Pediatrics* 1994;93:521–522.

51. Jumper BM, McLorie GA, Churchill BM, et al. Effects of the artificial urinary sphincter on prostatic development and sexual function in pubertal boys with meningomyelocele. *J Urol* 1990;144:438–441.

52. Cass AS, Bloom BA, Luxenberg M. Sexual function in adults with myelomeningocele. *J Urol* 1986;136:425–426.

53. Greenberg R, Vaughan E Jr, Pitts W Jr. Normal pregnancy and delivery after ileal conduit urinary diversion. *J Urol* 1981;125:172.

54. Sandler A, Worley G, Leroy E, et al. Sexual knowledge and experience among young men and spina bifida. *Eur J Pediatr Surg* 1994;4:36–37.

55. Bomalski MD, Teague JL, Brooks B. The long-term impact of urological management on the quality of life of children with spina bifida. *J Urol* 1995;154:778–781.

56. Farley T, Vinwes C, McCluer S, et al. Secondary disabilities in Arkansana with spina bifida. *Eur J Pediatr Surg* 1994;4:39–40.

57. Hunt G. Open spina bifida: the Cambridge cohort in their twenties. *Eur J Pediatr Surg* 1992;2:39.

58. Green M, Solnit AJ. Reactions to the threatened loss of a child: a vulnerable child syndrome. *Pediatrics* 1964;34:58–66.

59. Wright L, Mullen T, West K, Wyatt P. The VCOP Scale: a measure of overprotection in parents of physically vulnerable children. *J Clin Psychol* 1993;49:790–798.

60. Miller AC, Gordon RM, Daniele RJ, Diller L. Stress, appraisal, and coping in mothers of disabled and non-disabled children. *J Pediatr Psychol* 1992;17:587–605.

61. Loomis JW, Linsey A, Javornisky JG, Monahan JJ. Measures of cognition and adaptive behavior as predictors of adjustment outcomes in young adults with spina bifida. *Eur J Pediatr Surg* 1994;4:35–36.

62. Goodwin Ma, Shurtleff DB. Biomedical and psychological factors predicting independence in activities of daily living (ADLs) and academic success of children with myelomeningocele. *Eur J Pediatr Surg* 1992;2(suppl 1):48.

63. Younoszai MK. Stooling problems in patients with myelomeningocele. *South Med J* 1992;85:718–724.

64. Knoll M, Madersbacher H. The chances of a spina bifida patient becoming continent/socially dry by conservative therapy. *Paraplegia* 1993;31:22–27.

65. Vereecken RL. Bladder pressure and kidney function in children with myelomeningocele: review article. *Paraplegia* 1992;30:153–159.

66. Sutherland RW, Wiener JS, Roth DR, Gonzales ET Jr. A renal size nomogram for the myelomeningocele patient. *J Urol* 1997;158:1265–1267.

67. Palmer LS, Richters I, Kaplan WE. Age related bladder capacity growth in children with myelodysplasia. *J Urol* 1997;158:1261–1264.

68. Selzman AA, Elder JS, Mapstone TB. Urologic consequences of myelodysplagia and other congenital abnormalities of the spinal cord. *Urol Clin North Am* 1993;20:485–500.

69. Stone AR. Neurourologic evaluation and urologic management of spinal dysraphism. *Neurosurg Clin North Am* 1995;6:269–277.

70. Lapides J, Diokno AC, Lowe BS, Kalish MD. Follow-up on unsterile, intermittent self-catheterization. *J Urol* 1974;111:184–187.

71. Lindehall B, Moller A, Hjalmas K, Jodal U. The long-term intermittent catheterization: the experience of teenagers and young adults with myelomeningocele. *J Urol* 1994;152:187–189.

72. Lindehall B, Claesson I, Hjalmas K, Jodal U. Effect of clean intermittent catheterization on radiological appearance of the upper urinary tract in children with myelomeningocele. *Br J Urol* 1991;67:415–419.

73. Moisey CU. The urodynamic and subjective results of detrusor instability with oxybutynin chloride. *Br J Urol* 1980;52:472–475.

74. Connor JP, Betrus G, Fleming P, et al. Early cystometrograms can predict the response to intravesical instillation of oxybutynin chloride in myelomeningocele patients. *J Urol* 1994;151:1045–1047.

75. Malone PS, Wheeler RA, Williams JE. Continence in patients with spina bifida: long-term results. *Arch Dis Child* 1994;70:107–110.

76. Decter RM, Snyder P, Laudermilch C. Transurethral electrical bladder stimulation: a follow-up report. *J Urol* 1994;152:812–814.

77. Belloli G, Campobasso P, Mercurella A. Neuropathic urinary incontinence in pediatric patients: management with artificial sphincter. *J Pediatr Surg* 1992;27:1461–1464.

78. Simeoni J, Guys JM, Mollard P, et al. Artificial urinary sphincter implantation for neurogenic bladder: a multi-institutional study of 107 children. *Br J Urol* 1996;78:287–293.

79. Gormley EA, Bloom DA, McGuire EJ, Ritchey ML. Pubovaginal slings for the management of urinary incontinence in female adolescents. *J Urol* 1994;152:822–825.

80. Kurtzrock EA, Lowe P, Hardy BE. Bladder wall pedicle wraparound sling for neurogenic urinary incontinence in children. *J Urol* 1996;155:305–308.

81. Flood HD, Ritchey ML, Bloom DA, et al. Outcome of reflux in children with myelodysplasia managed by bladder pressure monitoring. *J Urol* 1994;152: 1574–1577.

82. Kobayashi S, Shinno Y, Kakizaki H, et al. Relevance of detrusor hyper-reflexia vesical compliance and urethral pressure to the occurrence of vesicourethral reflux in myelodysplastic patients. *J Urol* 1992;147: 413–415.

83. Hernandez RD, Hurwitz RS, Foote JE, et al. Nonsurgical management of threatened upper urinary tracts and incontinence in children with myelomeningocele. *J Urol* 1994;152:1582–1585.

84. Merlini E, Beseghi U, De Castro R, et al. Treatment of vesicoureteric reflux in the neurogenic bladder. *Br J Urol* 1993;72:969–971.

85. Franco I, Storrs B, Firlit CF, et al. Selective sacral rhizotomy in children with high pressure neurogenic bladders; preliminary results. *J Urol* 1992;148: 648–650.

86. Lewis MA, Webb NJ, Gill R, et al. Investigative techniques in renal parenchymal damage in children with spina bifida. *Eur J Pediatr Surg* 1994;4(suppl 1):29–31.

87. Ottolini MC, Schaer CM, Rushton HG, et al. Relationship of asymptomatic bacteriuria and renal scarring in children with neuropathic bladders who are practicing clean intermittent catheterization. *J Pediatr* 1995;127:368–372.

88. Little DM, Gleeson MJ, Hickey DP, et al. Renal transplantation in patients with spina bifida. *Urology* 1994;44:319–321.

89. King JC, Currie DM, Wright E. Bowel training in spina bifida: importance of education, patient compliance, age, and anal reflexes. *Arch Phys Med Rehabil* 1993;75:243–247.

90. Gleeson RM. Bowel continence for the child with a neurogenic bowel. *Rehabil Nurs* 1990;15: 319–321.

91. Liptak GS, Revell GM. Management of bowel dysfunction in children with spinal cord disease or injury by means of the enema continence catheter. *J Pediatr* 1992;120:190–194.

92. Blair GK, Dgonlic K, Fraser GC, et al. The bowel management tube: an effective means for controlling fecal incontinence. *J Pediatr Surg* 1992;27:1269–1272.

93. Maynard MJ, Weiner LS, Burke SW. Neuropathic foot ulceration in patients with myelodysplasia. *J Pediatr Orthop* 1992;12:786–788.

94. DeSouza LJ, Carroll N. Ambulation of the braced myelomeningocele patient. *J Bone Joint Surg [Am]* 1976;76:1112–1118.

95. Wassing HE, Siebelink BM, Luyendijk W. Handedness in progressive hydrocephalus in spina bifida patients. *Der Med Child Neurol* 1993;35:788–797.

96. Patrick JH. Equipment evaluation. *Clin Rehabil* 1988;2: 333–337.

97. Banta JV, Lin R, Peterson M, Dagenais T. The team approach in the care of the child with myelomeningocele. *J Prosthet Orthot* 1989;2:365–375.

98. Waters RL, Lungford BR, Perry J, Byrd R. Energy-speed relationship of walking: standard tables. *J Orthop Res* 1988;6:215–222.

99. Williams LO, Anderson AD, Campbell J, et al. Energy cost of walking and of wheelchair propulsion by children with myelodysplasia: comparison with normal children. *Dev Med Child Neurol* 1983;25:617–624.

100. Flandery F, Burke S, Roberts JM, et al. Functional ambulation in myelodysplasia: the effect of orthotic selection of physical and physiologic performance. *J Pediatr Orthop* 1986;6:661–665.

101. Luthy DA, Wardinski T, Shurtleff DB, et al. Caesarian section before onset of labor and subsequent motor function in infants with myelomeningocele diagnosed antenatally. *N Engl J Med* 1991;324:662–666.

102. Shurtleff DB, Luthy DA, Nyberg DA, Mack LA. The outcome of fetal myelomeningocele brought to term. *Eur J Pediatr Surg* 1994;4:25–28.

103. Liptak GS, Shurtleff DB, Bloss JW, et al. Mobility aids for children with high-level myelomeningocele: parapodium versus wheelchair. *Dev Med Child Neurol* 1992;34:787–796.

104. Findley TW, Agre JC, Habeck RV, et al. Ambulation in the adolescent with myelomeningocele. I: early childhood predictors. *Arch Phys Med Rehabil* 1987;68: 518–522.

105. Vankoski SJ, Moore CA, Statler KD, et al. The influence of external support on pelvic and hip kinematic parameters in childhood community ambulators with low lumbar level myelomeningocele—don't throw away the crutches. *Dev Med Child Neurol Suppl* 1995;73:5–6.

106. Stillwell A, Menelaus MB. Walking ability in mature patients with spina bifida. *J Pediatr Orthop* 1983;3:184–190.

107. Hoffer MM, Feiwell E, Perry R, et al. Functional ambulation in patients with myelomeningocele. *J Bone Joint Surg [Am]* 1973;1:137–148.

108. Brinker MR, Rosenfeld SR, Feiwell E, et al. Myelomeningocele at the sacral level. Long-term outcomes in adults. *J Bone Joint Surg [Am]* 1994;76: 1293–1300.

109. Karol LA. Orthopedic management in myelomeningocele. *Neurosurg Clin North Am* 1995;6: 259–268.

110. Eysel P, Hopf C, Schwarz M, Voth D. Development of scoliosis in myelomeningocele. Differences in the history caused by idiopathic pattern. *Neurosurg Rev* 1993;16: 301–306.

111. Müller EB, Nordwall A, Oden A. Progression of scoliosis in chil-

dren with myelomeningocele. *Spine* 1994;19:147–150.

112. Piggott H. The natural history of scoliosis in myelodysplasia. *J Bone Joint Surg [Br]* 1980;62: 54–58.

113. Martin J Jr, Kumar SJ, Guille JT, et al. Congenital kyphosis of myelomeningocele: results following operative and nonoperative treatment. *J Pediatr Orthop* 1994;14:323–328.

114. Lintner SA, Lindseth RE. Kyphotic deformity in patients who have a myelomeningocele. Operative treatment and long-term follow-up. *J Bone Joint Surg [Am]* 1994;76:1301–1307.

115. Keggi JM, Banta JV, Walton C. The myelodysplastic hip and scoliosis. *Dev Med Child Neurol* 1992;34:240–246.

116. Broughton NS, Menelaus MB, Cole WG, Shurtleff DB. The natural history of hip deformity in myelomeningocele. *J Bone Joint Surg [Br]* 1993;75:760–763.

117. Phillips DP, Lindseth RE. Ambulation after transfer of adductors, external oblique, and tensor fascia lata in myelomeningocele. *J Pediatr Orthop* 1992;12:712–717.

118. Williams JJ, Graham GP, Dunne KB, Menelaus MB. Late knee problems in myelomeningocele. *J Pediatr Orthop* 1993;13:701–703.

Cardiopul-
monary and
Vascular
Problems

Chapter 79

Cardiac Rehabilitation

Matthew N. Bartels

EPIDEMIOLOGY OF HEART DISEASE

Cardiac disease is the leading cause of morbidity and mortality in the adult population in the United States. With increased public awareness of cardiac risk factors, better management of cardiac disease, and risk intervention by the medical community, these rates have been declining steadily. The death rate for coronary artery disease (CAD) declined by 22.4% between 1984 and 1994. The mortality rate for CAD was 228.1 per 100,000 population in 1970 and 94.9 per 100,000 in 1994 (1). CAD was the number one cause of mortality among men aged 45 years and older and women aged 75 years and older, and was the overall number one cause of death in the United States in 1994, accounting for 954,720 deaths. CAD is one of the largest causes of disability in the United States, representing approximately 19% of disabilities from all conditions. In 1991 to 1992, an estimated 7.9 million Americans aged 15 years and older had disabilities from cardiovascular conditions (1). In 1994, cardiovascular disease ranked number one among all disease categories in hospital discharges, accounting for more than 5.8 million discharges.

Cardiac disease accounts for a large portion of total health care expenditures. In 1992, cardiovascular disease was the single greatest cause of hospital admissions. It accounted for more than 3.9 million hospital admissions, more than 2.1 million for myocardial ischemia and more than 800,000 admissions for congestive heart failure (CHF). Nearly 550,000 admissions each year are for cardiac arrhythmias. Cardiac surgery accounts for the third largest number of surgical procedures for inpatients. In 1992, more than 1 million cardiac catheterizations were performed and more than 300,000 coronary artery bypass graft (CABG) procedures were performed (2).

With new technologies, patients with CHF are living longer, and more patients are surviving myocardial infarction (MI). For example, new abilities to allow patients to survive after transplantation have increased the number of cardiac transplant procedures performed. In 1992, there were more than 2100 heart transplantations and more than 2200 people were on the waiting list (3). The increasing numbers of procedures performed, the vast numbers of patients now living with cardiac disease, and the often pressing need to treat cardiac disease among the disabled indicate a need to address the problems of cardiac rehabilitation.

TYPES OF HEART DISEASE

The types of heart disease that are likely to be encountered by the physiatrist practicing cardiac rehabilitation have increased in recent years. Standard cardiac rehabilitation of the post-MI patient comprises the majority of the practice; however, increasing in recent years has been the referral of patients after CABG surgery, transplantation, or valvular surgery. The patient with severe CHF is now being referred for cardiac rehabilitation, and patients with life-threatening arrhythmias are also being seen. All of these different populations are discussed in later portions of this chapter.

As noted already, the incidence of cardiac disease has been lowered by the recognition of cardiac risk factors and interventions to prevent ischemic cardiac disease. In particular, decreased cigarette smoking, lower consumption of red meat, and increasing exercise have all contributed to a decrease in CAD.

AN OVERVIEW OF CARDIAC REHABILITATION

Currently, in the United States, only 10% to 15% of the 1 million survivors of acute MI go on to a cardiac rehabilitation program (4,5). These programs of cardiac rehabilitation cost an estimated $160 to $240 million annually (6). The goals of cardiac rehabilitation are simply to restore and improve cardiac function, reduce disability, identify and improve cardiac risk factors, and increase cardiac conditioning (7–9). These goals are achieved through the use of prescriptive exercise programs performed under the supervision of physicians and health professionals. For patients with cardiac disease, the purpose of a program of rehabilitation is to restore the ability to resume the activities of normal life without the occurrence of significant cardiac symptomatology. Each of the different types of cardiac disease lends itself to a different form of rehabilitation. The benefits, in terms of cardiac conditioning and improved survival, are well documented by numerous studies (10–13).

RISK FACTOR MODIFICATION

There are several facets to achieving a complete cardiac rehabilitation program. The first part of the program involves education of the patient regarding cardiac risk factors and the achievement of a healthier lifestyle through cardiac risk factor modification (7). Cardiac risk factors (Table 79-1) are divided into two major groups: reversible and irreversible risk factors. Irreversible risk factors include male gender, past history of vascular disease, age, and family history. It is important for the patient to be aware of the presence of these risks through family counseling. In situations where significant irreversible risk exists, early and aggressive attention to the reversible risk factors becomes even more crucial. Reversible risk factors for cardiac disease include obesity, sedentary lifestyle, hyperlipidemia, cigarette smoking, and conditions such as diabetes mellitus and hypertension (7,8,14–27). Modification of these risk factors can be readily achieved as part of a cardiac rehabilitation program, and should be part of the general routine care of all individuals. It is important that these principles also be applied to the disabled population, since disabled individuals often are at further increased risk through weight loss and deconditioning.

Table 79-1: Risk Factors for Coronary Artery Disease (CAD)

Irreversible Risks	Reversible Risks
Male gender	Cigarette smoking
Family history of premature CAD (before age 55 in a parent or sibling)	Hypertension
Past history of CAD	Low high-density-lipoprotein cholesterol [< 0.9 mmol/L (35 mg/dL)]
Past history of occlusive peripheral vascular disease	Hypercholesterolemia [> 5.20 mmol/L (200 mg/dL)]
Past history of cerebrovascular disease	High lipoprotein A
Age	Abdominal obesity
	Hypertriglyceridemia [> 2.8 mmol/L (250 mg/dL)]
	Hyperinsulinemia
	Diabetes mellitus
	Sedentary lifestyle

Modification of medical risks is done in conjunction with the patient's primary care physician. These efforts can include the physiatrist as well, especially in the care of disabled individuals. Each of them is discussed briefly.

Diabetes

Close control of diabetes is an important part of the care of individuals with heart disease. Good control of blood glucose levels decreases the risk of cardiac disease by slowing the development of atherosclerosis and secondary conditions such as nephrogenic hypertension (28,29). Exercise training can also help to improve diabetic control (22–24). The exact benefits of exercise training in combination with good glucose control are still being elucidated (30).

Hypertension

Control of hypertension is also important in the care of individuals with cardiac disease. Although control of hypertension is clearly beneficial in the prevention of stroke, the data for heart disease are more mixed (29). In patients with normal electrocardiograms, hypertensive control is especially useful (31,32). Two of the most important factors in the control of hypertension are reducing salt intake and increasing exercise to improve conditioning. Numerous pharmacologic agents are available for the control of hypertension, but a clear benefit with the use of one type of agent over another has not been demonstrated, except in some special situations (29). The major classes of agents for the control of hypertension are β-blockers, α-blockers, diuretics, calcium channel blockers, and angiotensin-converting enzyme (ACE) inhibitors. The agents that have been shown to be most beneficial are the β-blockers. In addition to their antihypertensive effects, these agents provide cardiac protection by decreasing the maximum cardiac oxygen consumption by decreasing inotropy and limiting the heart rate response. The studies demonstrating a reduction in heart disease only clearly showed a benefit in nonsmokers (33,34). Diuretics are the other agents that have been shown in large trials to have beneficial effects on decreasing mortality. The early data for ACE inhibitors show evidence for decreased mortality, although the effects may be decreased in black patients (35). The cardiac effects of calcium channel blockers are not clear, but some early data indicate an actual increase in the risk for MI with use of these agents (35). It is recommended that rehabilitation physicians seek the advice of the treating cardiologist or internist for assistance in the optimal management of each individual patient.

Hypercholesterolemia

Elevated level of serum cholesterol is another modifiable risk factor. Decreased cholesterol levels and increased high-density-lipoprotein (HDL) levels are associated with a decreased risk of cardiac disease (14,15,20). A decrease in the dietary intake of saturated fats and cholesterol can lower these serum levels and thereby decrease the cardiac risk. A risk factor modification program need not be extremely severe to have effect, and even moderate programs can help. Patients can decrease their lipid levels by adhering to a low-cholesterol, low-fat diet and reducing their weight, even without the addition of exercise (20). The American Heart Association (AHA) recommendations are that the total amount of calories from fat in the diet should not exceed 30% (36). Control of cholesterol can be achieved through a three-step program, as outlined in the National Cholesterol Education Program (NCEP) guidelines (37). Phase I is an adoption of nutritional guidelines, lifestyle changes, and general improvement in health habits. Phase II involves the addition of fiber supplements and possibly nicotinic acid. Phase III includes lipid-lowering drugs. Lipid-lowering programs can retard the progression of CAD (21,33,34). With the addition of physical activity, HDL cholesterol concentration can rise 5% to 16%, but the data on the lowering of low-density-lipoprotein (LDL) cholesterol are still controversial (7,38).

Obesity

Weight loss is an integral part of any cardiac rehabilitation program for individuals who are overweight. The benefits to the loss of weight include decreased blood pressure, improved lipid profile, and improved ability to perform exercise (7,22). The benefits of improved lipid profile and exercise have been discussed already.

Cigarette Smoking

Cigarette smoking is one of the greatest single modifiable risk factors for cardiac disease (18,38,39). The 10-year mortality in individuals with angiographically demonstrated CAD or MI who stopped smoking is decreased by more than 30% (40,41). Smoking causes accelerated atherosclerosis and is a contributor to hypertension. Exercising alone does not contribute to decreased smoking (18) and smokers tend to be less compliant in cardiac rehabilitation programs (42). However, a program of cardiac rehabilitation coupled with counseling for smoking cessation can decrease smoking (18,43). Because smoking cessation is important for survival, it is crucial to include counseling as part of a complete cardiac rehabilitation program.

CARDIAC ANATOMY

To participate effectively in the rehabilitation of patients with cardiac disease, the physiatrist or other health professional involved in cardiac rehabilitation must have a good understanding of the anatomy of the heart and its associated structures. Of particular importance is a familiarity with the normal distribution of the major arteries of the heart, valvular anatomy, and the structures at risk in the presence of ischemia or infarction in these distributions. Also, a good knowledge of the anatomy facilitates a more informed dialogue with the referring cardiologist and an ability to anticipate complications and problems associated with the specific patient's cardiac disease.

The heart consists of paired atria and ventricles. Deoxygenated venous blood enters the right atrium. Blood is then pumped by the right ventricle into the lungs, where it is oxygenated, returned to the left atrium, and pumped into the systemic arterial circulation by the left ventricle. The valves ensure a unidirectional flow of blood, and the atria act in coordination with the ventricles to augment cardiac output. The atrial contribution to the filling of the ventricles can add 15% to 20% to the total cardiac output, and is greater with increased heart rate and in conditions of decreased ventricular compliance (44). This contribution of atrial "kick" is especially important to consider in disease conditions involving atrial dysfunction such as atrial fibrillation.

The cardiac conduction system is a specialized system of muscle cells (myocytes) adapted to facilitate the appropriate sequencing of the contraction of the atria and ventricles at the physiologically appropriate rate (45,46) (Fig. 79-1). All of the muscle cells of the heart have the intrinsic ability to contract, and are able to conduct electrical activity to synchronize their contractions with other cells. The sinoatrial (SA) node is located in the right atrium

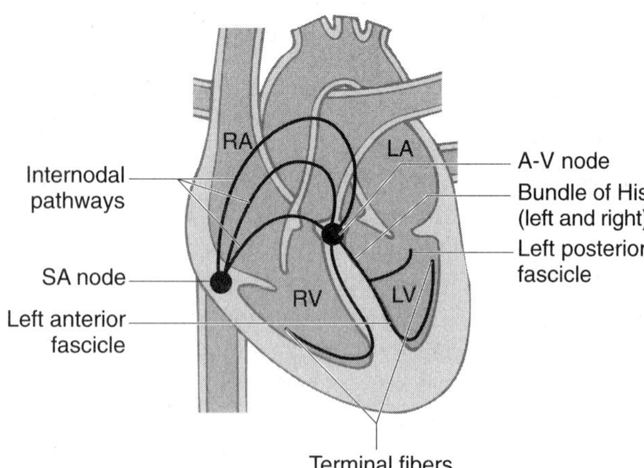

Figure 79-1. Conduction system of the heart. SA = sinoatrial; AV = atrioventricular; RA = right atrium; LA = left atrium; RV = right ventricle; LV = left ventricle.

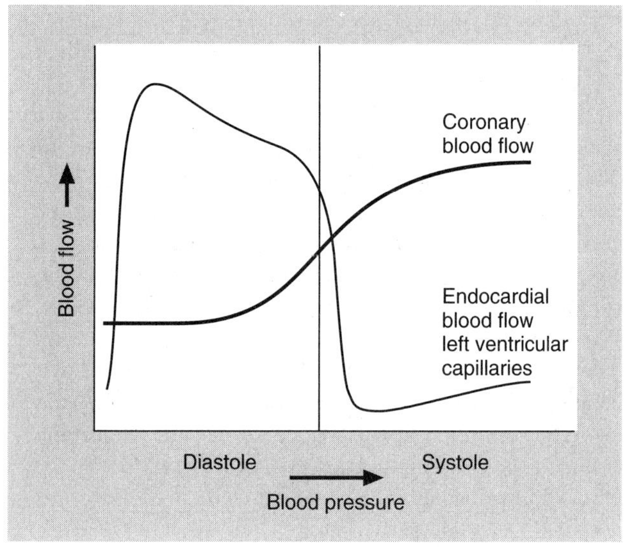

Figure 79-2. Coronary blood flow. (Adapted from Guyton AC. *Textbook of medical physiology*. 7th ed. Philadelphia: WB Saunders, 1986.)

and has the fastest intrinsic rate in the cardiac conduction system, making it the heart's natural pacemaker. The signal from the SA node travels through three atrial internodal pathways to the atrioventricular (AV) node and then via the bundle of His, located in the intraventricular septum, which divides further into left and right bundles. The left bundle divides into anterior and posterior fascicles. Terminal branches of the right and left conduction systems carry the signals that excite the myocytes. MI, aging, and other conditions can affect the conduction system, leading to a variety of conduction defects such as heart block and sick sinus syndrome. Congenital defects and accessory tracts can lead to life-threatening arrhythmias such as the Wolff-Parkinson-White (WPW) syndrome. The clinician practicing cardiac rehabilitation should have knowledge of the most common of these conditions in order to assess accurately the risks patients with these conditions face, prior to the initiation of cardiac conditioning programs.

Variation of Arteries

The usual anatomy of the cardiac arteries should be well known to the clinician practicing cardiac rehabilitation. Normally, there are left and right coronary arteries arising from the base of the aorta in the left and right aortic sinuses. The left main coronary artery divides into the left anterior descending and the circumflex arteries, while the right coronary artery continues on as a single vessel. The standard distributions of the vessels and their rates of occurrence are provided in Table 79-2 (47). The description of the anatomy of the coronary vessels in Table 79-2 reflects the most common situation, seen in approximately 60% of individuals, and is often termed *right dominant circulation*. In approximately 10% to 15% of individuals, the posterior descending artery arises from the left circumflex artery, in what is described as *left dominant circulation*. In approximately 30% of individuals, the posterior descending artery arises from the left circumflex and right coronary arteries, in what is described as *balanced circulation*. Table 79-3 lists the anatomy and the distributions of infarcts, with a description of associated cardiac syndromes.

CARDIAC PHYSIOLOGY

The myocytes of the heart are among the most metabolically active tissues in the body. Oxygen extraction is nearly maximal at all levels of activity and is nearly 65% (compared to 36% for brain and 26% for the rest of the body) (48). The heart is able to perform both anaerobic and aerobic metabolism, preferring aerobic metabolism, using a variety of substrates. Approximately 40% of the fuel is carbohydrates, with fatty acids making up most of the rest (49). Coronary blood flow is limited to diastole (Fig. 79-2), especially in the endocardium. Given the near maximum extraction of oxygen, there are only limited ways to increase the oxygen supply. One way the oxygen supply is increased, to meet the demands of exercise, for example, is by dilation of the coronary arteries. In addition, a number of substances secreted by the body increase coronary blood flow, with nitric oxide appearing to be the final agent of many pathways (50). The goal of many medical and surgical therapies is to restore the normal blood flow to the myocardium, and the efficiency of that effort is crucial to the ability of the patient to tolerate a cardiac rehabilitation program.

The ability of the heart to generate an increase in cardiac output is related to the increase in venous return,

Table 79-2: Coronary Artery Anatomy			
Arteries	**Main Branches**	**Distributions**	**Variations**
Right coronary artery	Nodal branch	Right atrium and SA node	—
	Right marginal branch	Right ventricle to apex	—
	Posterior intraventricular (descending) branch	AV node, posterior third of septum, right bundle of His	AV node in 85%–95% of individuals, distal anastomosis to the left circumflex artery
Left coronary artery	Anterior intraventricular (descending) branch	Anterior left and right ventricles, anterior two-thirds of septum, left bundle of His, AV node	AV node in 5%–15% of individuals, 40% with some contribution
	Circumflex artery	Left atrium, superior portions of left ventricle	—

SA = sinoatrial; AV = atrioventricular.

Table 79-3: Normal Anatomy and the Distributions of Infarcts		
Anatomy of Coronary Artery	**Area of Infarct**	**Syndrome**
Left anterior descending	Anterior wall and septum	Papillary muscle necrosis Left-sided heart failure Left ventricular aneurysm Anterior wall thrombus Conduction block
Left circumflex	Apex and lateral wall	Apical thrombus Left-sided heart failure
Left main coronary artery	Anterior and lateral wall, apex	Massive congestive heart failure Left ventricular aneurysm Anterior wall thrombus Conduction block
Right coronary artery	Inferior wall and right ventricle	Sinus node arrest Right ventricular failure Peripheral edema

which increases the length of the myocardial fibers in diastole prior to the initiation of cardiac contraction. With stretch, the overlap of the actin and myosin fibers is maximized and the strength of contraction is maximized. This is effective until, with further stretching, the overlap of myosin and actin begins to decrease, and the strength of contraction begins to decline again. The relationship between the length of the fibers and the filling of the ventricle, which leads to increased contractility, is described by the Frank-Starling curve (Fig. 79-3). It is useful to keep this relationship in mind when considering patients with constrictive heart disease (which limits the ability to move to the right on the Frank-Starling curve and increase output) as well as in patients with dilated cardiomyopathies (who are so far out on the curve that they can only increase cardiac output by decreasing the stretch of their ventricles) (51).

EXERCISE PHYSIOLOGY

In order to be able to discuss the basic principles of aerobic training and cardiac conditioning as they apply to cardiac rehabilitation, the basic vocabulary and basic concepts of exercise physiology must be appreciated.

Aerobic Capacity

Aerobic capacity ($\dot{V}O_2$ max) is often expressed in milliliters of oxygen per kilogram per minute, and is the work capacity of the individual. Oxygen consumption ($\dot{V}O_2$) has a linear relationship with workload, increasing up to a plateau that occurs at the $\dot{V}O_2$max. $\dot{V}O_2$ is measured through the analysis of expired gases, and for a given level of submaximal exercise, $\dot{V}O_2$ reaches steady state approximately 3 to 6 minutes of exercise. The slope of the line between $\dot{V}O_2$ and

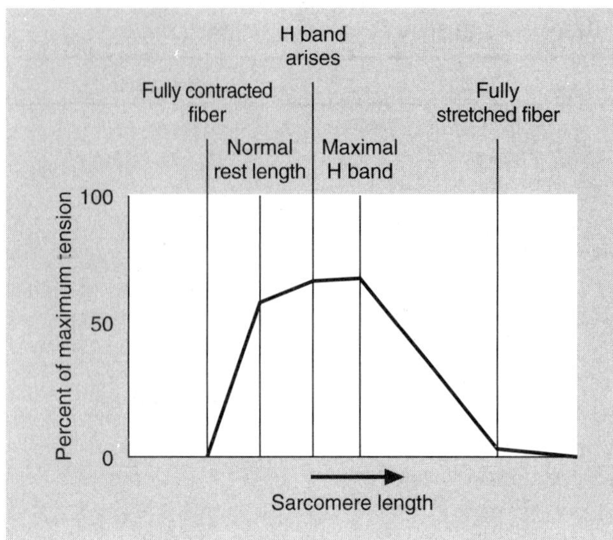

Figure 79-3. Frank-Starling mechanism. 1 = fully contracted fiber; 2 = normal rest length; 3 = H band arises; 4 = maximal H band; 5 = fully stretched fiber.

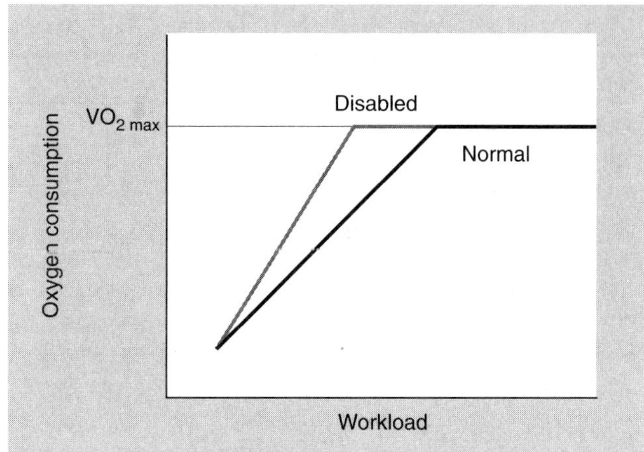

Figure 79-4. Aerobic capacity.

workload represents the mechanical efficiency of the activity being performed and in conditions such as spasticity, decreased efficiency is represented by an increase in the slope. Often the measure of work being done at submaximal effort is expressed as a percentage defined by $\dot{V}O_2$ divided by $\dot{V}O_2$max. The use of percent $\dot{V}O_2$max allows for normalization of data across individuals and for comparison of activities. $\dot{V}O_2$max was demonstrated to decrease with age in longitudinal studies such as the Baltimore Longitudinal Study of Aging (52) (Fig. 79-4).

Heart Rate

Heart rate has a linear increase in relation to $\dot{V}O_2$ or other measures of work. Maximum heart rate is determined by age and can be roughly estimated by subtracting the age of the individual in years from 220. The slope of the line between heart rate and $\dot{V}O_2$ is determined by physical conditioning and the maximum heart rate continues to decline with age even with ongoing exercise. The physiologic regulation of heart rate is mediated by the interaction of vagal and sympathetic tone and circulating catecholamines (Fig. 79-5).

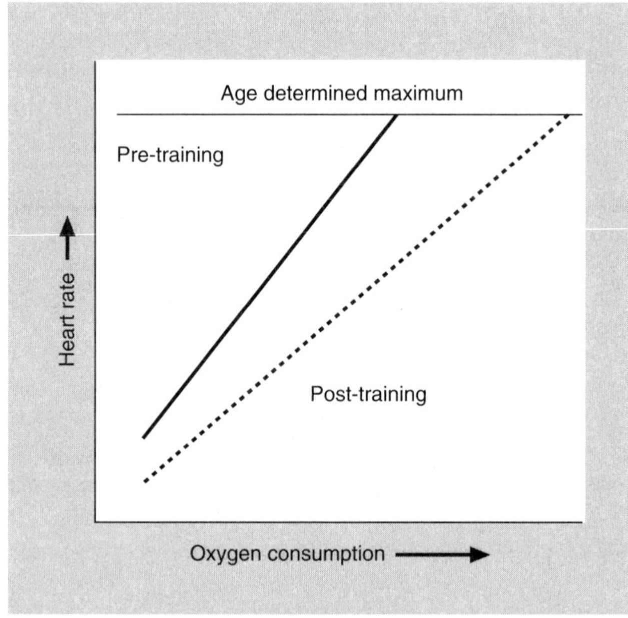

Figure 79-5. Heart rate and volume of oxygen consumption.

Stroke Volume

Stroke volume (SV) is the quantity of blood pumped with each heart beat. SV increases the most early in exercise, with the major determinant of SV being diastolic filling time. SV is sensitive to postural changes. It changes little during a supine position because it is near maximum at rest, while with an erect position, it increases in a curvilinear fashion until it reaches maximum at approximately 40% of $\dot{V}O_2$max (Fig. 79-6). There is also a decreased response of SV seen with advancing age and in cardiac conditions that result in decreased compliance, such as left ventricular hypertrophy.

Cardiac Output

Cardiac output is determined by the product of the heart rate and SV. Cardiac output increases linearly with work, and in early exercise the principal increase is via the Frank-Starling mechanism, while in late exercise it is solely determined by the increase in heart rate. In general, the relationship between cardiac output and $\dot{V}O_2$ is linear, with a break in the slope at the anaerobic threshold. The anaerobic threshold is the level of exercise at which the ability to deliver oxygen to the exercising muscles is below the demand, marking the transition from aerobic to anaer-

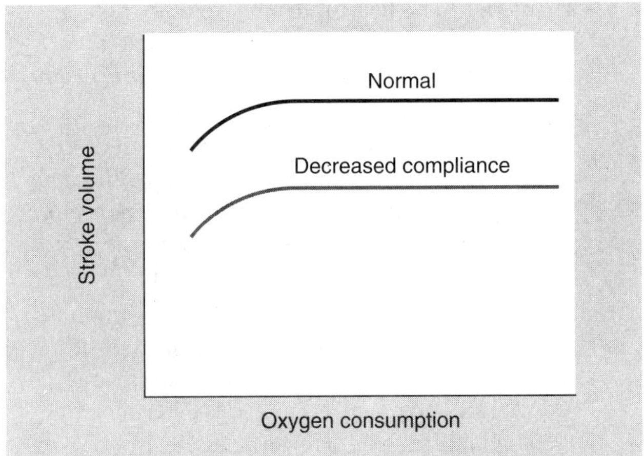

Figure 79-6. Stroke volume and oxygen consumption.

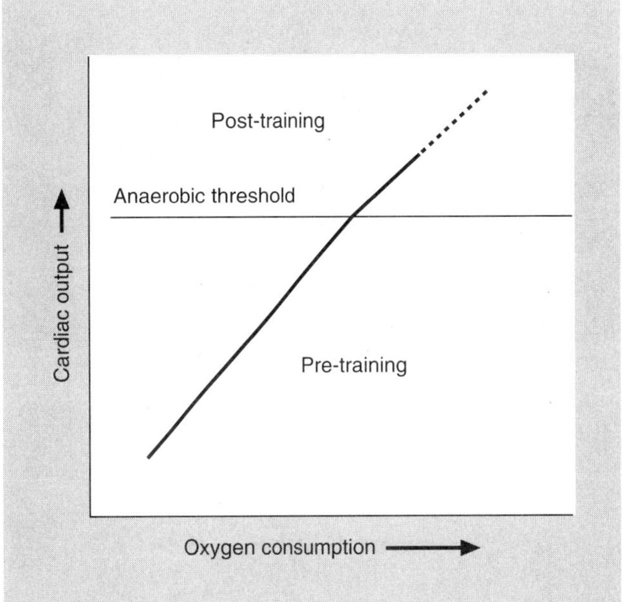

Figure 79-7. Cardiac output.

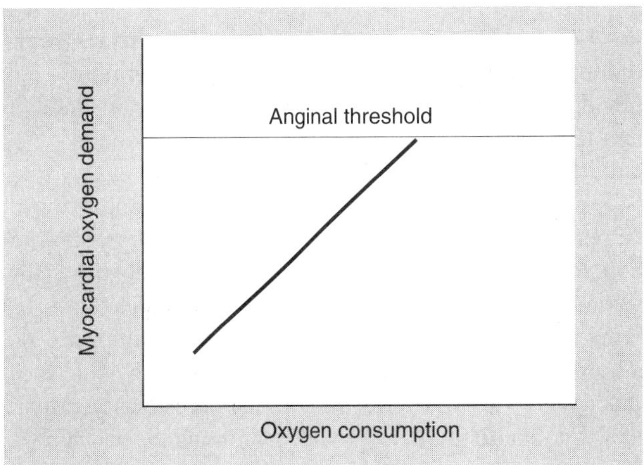

Figure 79-8. Myocardial oxygen demand.

obic metabolism. The maximum cardiac output is the primary determinant of $\dot{V}O_2max$, and it declines with age without any change in linearity or slope. The cardiac output seen with submaximal work is parallel, but it is lower during upright work compared to supine work, with $\dot{V}O_2max$ and maximal cardiac output lower during supine than erect positions (Fig. 79-7).

Myocardial Oxygen Consumption

Myocardial oxygen consumption ($M\dot{V}O_2$) is the actual oxygen consumption of the heart. It rises in a linear fashion with workload. $M\dot{V}O_2$ is limited by the anginal threshold, which represents maximum oxygen delivery to the coronary arteries. Although $M\dot{V}O_2$ can be determined directly with cardiac catheterization, this is not practical. The usual practice is to get an estimate of $M\dot{V}O_2$ by using the rate pressure product (RPP), which is the product of the heart rate and the systolic blood pressure divided by 100. In general, activities with the upper extremities and exercises with isometric components to them have a higher $M\dot{V}O_2$ for a given $\dot{V}O_2$. Activities performed in a supine position demonstrate a higher $M\dot{V}O_2$ at low intensity and a lower $M\dot{V}O_2$ at high intensity when compared to activities performed in the erect position. Finally, the $M\dot{V}O_2$ increases for any activity when performed in the cold, after smoking, or after eating (Fig. 79-8). $M\dot{V}O_2$ also is greater for a given level of $\dot{V}O_2$ with upper extremity exercises as compared to lower extremity exercises (Fig. 79-9).

Aerobic Training

Aerobic training is the term used to describe the physical exercises performed to increase cardiopulmonary capacity. The basic principles of aerobic training are divided into four areas: intensity, duration, frequency, and specificity.

Intensity of training is defined by either the physiologic response of the individual or the intensity of the exercise performed. For example, a program of exercises may be aimed at a target heart rate or RPP, or at a level of exercise intensity such as a speed and incline setting for a treadmill exercise. Usually, target heart rate is used for simplicity in writing exercise prescriptions for individuals. In a conditioning program, it can be set at 80% to 85% of the maximum heart rate determined on a baseline exercise tolerance test (ETT). It is usually accepted that exercises that evoke 60% or more of the maximal heart rate will have at least some training effect.

The *duration* of training in the usual exercise program is 20 to 30 minutes, excluding a 5- to 10-minute warm-up period before exercise and a similar cooldown period after exercising. In general, exercise at a lower intensity requires a longer duration to achieve a training effect than does exercise at a higher intensity.

Frequency of training is defined as the number of

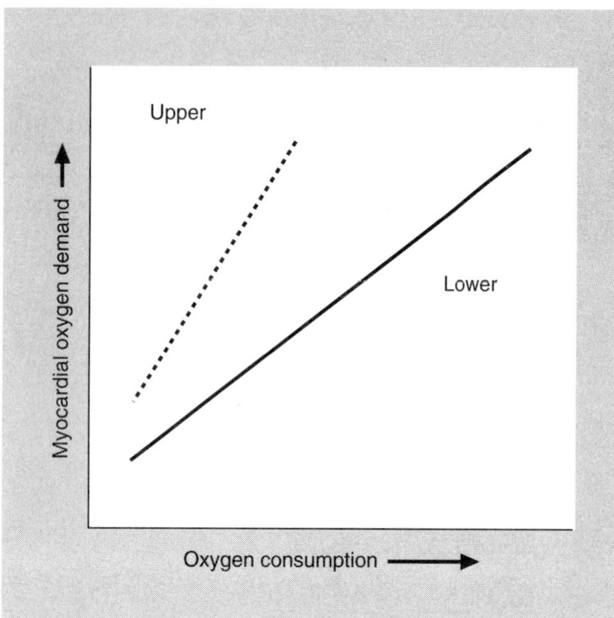

Figure 79-9. Myocardial oxygen demand for upper- and lower-extremity activity.

exercise periods in a given time, and is usually expressed in sessions per week. At a minimum, training programs should be done three times per week, and with low-intensity programs, five times per week may be required to offset the decreased intensity of training.

Specificity of training refers to the goal of improving the performance of functional activities through training in those targeted activities. It is essential to remember that the maximum training benefit in any activity is achieved through training in that specific activity. For example, to improve the efficiency and endurance of an individual for walking, it is best to train with ambulation exercises, rather than with arm ergometry or with swimming. Specifically, the exercises, activities and groups of muscles used in the design of a training program should be based on the vocational and recreational needs of each individual. This is also referred to as the law of the specificity of conditioning, and is commonly referred to in cardiac conditioning programs (53).

The effects of aerobic training are seen in a number of physiologic parameters (45):

1. Aerobic capacity. The aerobic capacity ($\dot{V}O_2$max) of the patient will increase with training. The resting $\dot{V}O_2$ does not change, and the $\dot{V}O_2$ at a given workload does not change. The changes are also specific to the muscle groups that are trained.
2. Cardiac output. The cardiac output is directly related to $\dot{V}O_2$ at rest and at a given workload, up to the anaerobic threshold. The maximum cardiac output increases with aerobic training. The direct relationship between $\dot{V}O_2$ and cardiac output does not change during training.
3. Heart rate. The heart rate after aerobic training is lower at rest and at any given workload. The maximum heart rate is not changed, as it is determined by age.
4. Stroke volume. The SV is increased at rest and at all levels of exercise after aerobic training. It is the increase in SV that allows for the maintenance of cardiac output at a given workload with the decrease in heart rate, described already.
5. Myocardial oxygen capacity. The $M\dot{V}O_2$ response to aerobic training is the most valuable part of training in cardiac rehabilitation. The maximum $M\dot{V}O_2$ does not change, since it is determined by the anginal threshold. However, at any given workload, the $M\dot{V}O_2$ decreases with training. This can allow individuals to markedly increase their exercise capacity and can lead to a marked improvement in function. After training they will be able to perform activities at $M\dot{V}O_2$ levels below the anginal threshold, levels that were above the anginal threshold before training. Pharmacologic interventions can affect the resting and submaximal $M\dot{V}O_2$, but only a revascularization procedure such as angioplasty or coronary bypass surgery can actually affect the maximum $M\dot{V}O_2$.
6. Peripheral resistance. The peripheral resistance (PR) decreases in response to exercise training. The PR is decreased at rest and at all levels of exercise. This response of the peripheral vasculature is due to the increased efficiency of oxygen extraction in the peripheral vascular beds, thus causing less shunting of the blood from visceral capillary beds. This results in a lower RPP and a lower $M\dot{V}O_2$ at a given workload and at rest.

Through an understanding of the physiology, the benefits of training can be seen clearly and are in two major areas: reduced cardiac risk and improved cardiac conditioning. The reduction of cardiac risk with a cardiac rehabilitation program and cardiac conditioning has been demonstrated in numerous studies. Pooled data from 22 randomized studies of 4554 patients following acute MI demonstrated a 20% to 25% reduction in all-cause mortality, fatal MI, and cardiac mortality at 3-year follow-up (54). This benefit has been seen in specific groups as well, including in the elderly (55–57), women (58), and bypass patients (59). In the evermore cost-conscious environment of modern medicine, there have also been analyses of the cost-effectiveness of cardiac rehabilitation programs, including a study by Oldridge et al (60) which demonstrated that in a cohort of patients with anxiety or mild depression after MI, there can be significant cost savings with cardiac rehabilitation in comparison with other therapies.

The benefits of the cardiac conditioning program can be more clearly understood, if a table of metabolic

Table 79-4: Sample Metabolic Equivalents (METs)			
Energy Costs	**METs**	**Energy Costs**	**METs**
Of activities of daily living		Running 12 min/mile	8–9
Sitting at rest	1	Running 11 min/mile	9–10
Dressing	2–3	Running 9 min/mile	10–11
Eating	1–2	Skiing, cross-country 3 mph	6–7
Hygiene (sitting)	1–2	Skiing, cross-country 5 mph	9–10
Hygiene (standing)	2–3	Skiing, downhill	5–9
Sexual intercourse	3–5	Skiing, water	5–7
Showering	4–5	Swimming (backstroke)	7–8
Tub bathing	2–3	Swimming (breaststroke)	8–9
Walking 1 mph	1–2	Swimming (crawl)	9–10
Walking 2 mph	2–3	Television	1–2
Walking 3 mph	3–3.5	Tennis (singles)	4–9
Walking 3.5 mph	3.5–4	Of vocational activities	
Walking 4 mph	5–6	Assembly line work	3–5
Climbing up stairs	4–7	Carpentry (light)	4–5
Bed making	2–6	Carry 20–44 lb	4–5
Carrying 18 lb upstairs	7–8	Carry 45–64 lb	5–6
Carrying suitcase	6–7	Carry 65–85 lb	7–8
Housework (general)	3–4	Chopping wood	7–8
Mowing lawn (push-power mower)	3–5	Desk work	1.5–2
Ironing	2–4	Digging ditches	7–8
Snow shoveling	6–7	Handyman	5–6
Of avocational activities		Janitorial (light)	2–3
Backpacking (45 lb)	6–11	Lift 100 lb	7–10
Baseball (competitive)	5–6	Painting	4–5
Baseball (noncompetitive)	4–5	Sawing hardwood	6–8
Basketball (competitive)	7–12	Sawing softwood	5–6
Basketball (noncompetitive)	3–9	Sawing (power)	3–4
Card playing	1–2	Shoveling 10 lb, 10/min	6–7
Cycling 5 mph	2–3	Shoveling 14 lb, 10/min	7–9
Cycling 8 mph	4–5	Shoveling 16 lb, 10/min	9–12
Cycling 10 mph	5–6	Tools (heavy)	5–6
Cycling 12 mph	7–8	Typing	1.5–2
Cycling 13 mph	8–9	Wood splitting	6–7
Karate	8–12		

Source: Adapted from Dafoe, WA. Table of energy requirements for activities of daily living, household tasks, recreational activities, and vocational activities. In: Pashkow FJ, Dafoe WA, eds. *Clinical cardiac rehabilitation*: a *cardiologist's guide*. Baltimore: Williams & Wilkins, 1993:359–376.

equivalents is used. A metabolic equivalent, or MET, is the amount of energy used by an individual at rest, and corresponds to the basal metabolic rate, which is approximately 1 kcal/min. At a given level of conditioning, the anginal threshold is not changed, but the workload that can be done before the threshold is reached is increased. This creates a greater margin of safety between the $M\dot{V}O_2$ demanded at routine activity and the anginal threshold. A sample of METs is shown in Table 79-4.

ABNORMAL PHYSIOLOGY

Cardiac disease can alter the normal physiology of the heart in several specific ways. MI will decrease the ejection fraction of the heart, and thus reduce the SV and cardiac output. Ischemic heart disease will cause the maximum heart rate to be lowered, and will lower the $M\dot{V}O_2$ and $\dot{V}O_2$max that can be achieved, and may decrease the SV if the ventricle becomes stiff during the ischemic episode. Valvular heart disease will decrease the maximum cardiac output, either through tight stenotic valves as in aortic stenosis, or through regurgitation as is seen in mitral insufficiency. The end result of the valve disease is a decreased $M\dot{V}O_2$ and $\dot{V}O_2$max and increased $\dot{V}O_2$ at any level of submaximal exercise. CHF leads to lower $\dot{V}O_2$max, lower SV, higher resting heart rates, and decreased cardiac output. Arrhythmias will decrease the cardiac output through decreased SV and increased heart rates. Cardiac transplantation will correct many of the abnormalities seen with CHF that usually precede the transplantation, but a persistently high heart rate and a limited ability to increase SV can limit the exercise response. The rehabilitation of

Table 79-5: Abnormal Physiology in Response to Exercise (as Compared to Normal Individuals)

	Aerobic Capacity ($\dot{V}O_2max$)	Cardiac Output	Heart Rate	Stroke Volume	Myocardial Oxygen Capacity ($M\dot{V}O_2$)	Peripheral Resistance
Myocardial infarction	↓	↓	↓, ↑, or ↔	↓ or ↔	↓	↑ or ↔
Ischemic heart disease	↓	↔ or ↓	↓, ↑, or ↔	↓ or ↔	↓	↓, ↑, or ↔
Valvular heart disease	↓	↓	↑ or ↔	↓, ↑, or ↔	↓ or ↔	↑ or ↔
Congestive heart failure	↓	↓	↑ or ↔	↓	↓	↑
Arrhythmias	↓ or ↔	↓ or ↔	↓, ↑, or ↔	↓ or ↔	↓ or ↔	↔
Cardiac transplant	↓	↓	↑ at submax ↓ at max	↓	↓	↑ or ↔

↔ = unchanged; ↓ = decreased; ↑ = increased.

these syndromes is discussed in detail later in the chapter. The effects of exercise on the standard physiologic parameters in patients with heart disease, as compared to normal individuals, are summarized in Table 79-5.

CARDIAC REHABILITATION PROGRAMS

Cardiac rehabilitation programs generally can be divided into two parts: primary prevention, which includes risk factor modification and education, and cardiac rehabilitation after the establishment of cardiac disease, including MI and other conditions.

Primary prevention programs focus on the reduction of cardiac risk factors. The education of patients and individuals at risk for cardiac disease can have a profound effect on the rate of cardiac disease (61,62). An increase in physical activity can decrease obesity (63), lower systolic blood pressure (64), and help modify lipid profiles. The education of individuals about risk factor modification should begin in childhood so that healthy behavior patterns can be established and then maintained through life. Programs can be started in schools and parental involvement is also appropriate (65).

Secondary risk factor modification programs also include all of the features of the primary prevention programs. There is clear benefit in the prevention of second cardiac events and in the reduction of mortality after MI with the initiation of risk factor modification programs (11). The lowering of blood cholesterol levels was shown to be advantageous in numerous studies performed since the 1960s, including the Oslo Study (66), the Western Electric Study (67), the Multiple Risk Factor Intervention Trial (68), Helsinki Heart Study (69), National Heart, Lung, and Blood Institute type II study (70), and others. Cessation of cigarette smoking is important, as the risk of heart disease returns to that of nonsmokers after 2 years of nonsmoking (71,72). The control of other risk factors such as hypertension and diabetes can also be affected by the secondary program.

CARDIAC REHABILITATION AFTER MYOCARDIAL INFARCTION

The actual cardiac rehabilitation of the post-MI patient usually follows the classic model as it was first described by Wenger et al (73). Cardiac rehabilitation is best viewed as being divided into four stages or phases. The first phase is the acute phase, which is the in-hospital period immediately following the MI and leading up to discharge. Rehabilitation during this phase includes early mobilization. The second phase is the convalescent phase, which is done at home and continues the program started in phase I, until the myocardial scar has matured. The third phase is the training phase initiated after healing is completed; the patient must be safe to begin the aerobic conditioning that is characteristic of phase III. the final phase is devoted to the maintenance of the aerobic conditioning gains made in phase III, through a program of regular exercise. Risk factor modifications are taught and re-emphasized throughout all phases.

Acute Phase (Phase I)

In the Wenger model (73) of cardiac rehabilitation, early mobilization is important. The basics of the original program of the early mobilization program are outlined in Table 79-6. This original program was designed to progress individuals from bed rest to climbing two flights of stairs in 14 days. Although this represents a marked increase in mobilization for its time, when hospitalizations as long as 6 weeks to 6 months were common, under the current drive to decrease the length of stay, clinicians have modified the classic program of cardiac rehabilitation to allow stays of 5 to 7 days. The steps of the 14-step program are now con-

Table 79-6: Wenger Protocol

Step	Activity
1	Passive ROM, ankle pumps, introduction to the program, self-feeding
2	As above, also dangle at side of bed
3	Active-assisted ROM, sitting upright in a chair, light recreation, use of bedside commode
4	Increased sitting time, light activities with minimal resistance, patient education
5	Light activities with moderate resistance, unlimited sitting, seated ADLs
6	Increased resistance, walking to bathroom, standing ADLs, up to 1-h-long group meetings
7	Walking up to 100 ft, standing warm-up exercises
8	Increased walking, walk down stairs (not up), continued education
9	Increased exercise program, review energy conservation and pacing techniques
10	Increase exercises with light weights and ambulation, begin education on home exercise program
11	Increased duration of activities
12	Walk down two flights of stairs, continue to increase resistance in exercises
13	Continue activities, education, and home exercise program teaching
14	Walk up and down two flights of stairs, complete instruction in home exercise program and in energy conservation and pacing techniques

ROM = range of motion; ADLs = activities of daily living.
Source: Wenger N, Gilbert C, Skoropa M. Cardiac Conditioning after myocardial infarction. An early intervention program. *J Cardiac Rehabil* 1971;2:17–22.

densed. As soon as medically stable, patients are encouraged to be sitting out of bed and in a chair, usually by day 1 or 2 (steps 1–5). By day 2 or 3, short-distance ambulation can be initiated, and bathroom privileges are full (steps 6–9). Around day 4 or 5, the patient is introduced to the home exercise program, and climbing stairs and increasing the duration of ambulation are encouraged (steps 10–13). After successful completion of a low-level ETT for risk stratification on day 5 or 6, the patient completes learning the home program and is discharged (step 14). The educational program relating to risk factor modification should be introduced at this time, especially as many patients are very ready to listen to advice during an acute hospitalization. During this mobilization program, it is usually recommended that cardiac monitoring be performed (73) under the supervision of a trained physical or occupational therapist or nurse (74). The post-MI heart rate rise with activity should be kept to within 20 bpm of baseline, and the systolic blood pressure rise within 20 mm Hg of baseline. Any decrease of systolic blood pressure of 10 mm Hg or more should be considered worrisome and the exercise halted (75). The major goal of phase I is to condition the patient to perform activities up to 4 METs, which is within the range of most daily activities at home after discharge (76).

Prolonged Acute Phase (Phase IB)

In patients with a prolonged hospitalization, or in whom secondary complications or other disabilities exist, a prolonged inpatient convalescent phase may be required. These individuals can often benefit from a stay on an acute inpatient rehabilitation service for either acute or a subacute inpatient rehabilitation. The goals and the precautions of phase I rehabilitation apply in this situation as well, and there should be trained staff, including nursing and physical therapy, as well as portable telemetry and close monitoring. The goal after the completion of this phase of rehabilitation is to achieve exercise tolerance up to 4 METs, as in standard phase I rehabilitation.

Convalescent Phase (Phase II)

During the convalescent phase the scar over the infarction is allowed to mature. Because there is vulnerability to myocardial rupture, arrhythmia, and sudden death if overexertion occurs during this time, the patient's exercise intensity is limited to a target heart rate that is known to be safe. The target heart rate is determined during a low-level ETT performed prior to discharge and at the end of phase I. This exercise test is usually performed to a level of approximately 70% of maximum heart rate or a MET level of 5 (77). For a person 40 years or older this generally represents a maximum heart rate of 130 bpm or 5 METs, and for an individual younger than 40 years, 140 bpm or 7 METs (78). A Borg rating of perceived exertion of 7 (modified scale) or 15 (old scale) can also be used to determine the maximum tolerated exercise (79). The Borg scale and modified Borg scale are shown in Table 79-7. The low-level ETT can also be used for cardiac risk stratification (80,81). The program can consist of six phase II monitored sessions of 1 hour each, with a home exercise program over 6 weeks for the uncomplicated patient (82). For patients at high risk, more closely monitored programs can be designed. A guideline for determining high risk during cardiac rehabilitation and the need for monitoring is included in Table 79-8. At the end of the 6-week healing period, a full-level ETT can be performed, and then the third, or training phase of cardiac rehabilitation can be started.

Training Phase (Phase III)

The training phase of the cardiac rehabilitation program is started after performance of the symptom-limited full-level ETT. The heart rate maximum obtained by this test is the one used to determine the maximum exertion to be performed by the patient during aerobic training. In patients who are low risk, a program designed to achieve 85% of the maximum heart rate is safe. Gradation of the program to lower target heart rates needs to be tailored to the indi-

Table 79-7: Borg Scale			
Borg Scale	**Perceived Exertion**	**Modified Borg Scale**	**Perceived Exertion**
—	—	0.0	Nothing at all
—	—	0.5	Very, very weak
—	—	1.0	Very weak
—	—	1.5	—
—	—	2.0	Weak (light)
6	—	2.5	—
7	Very, very light	3.0	Moderate
8	—	3.5	—
9	Very light	4.0	Somewhat strong
10	—	4.5	—
11	Fairly light	5.0	Strong (heavy effort)
12	—	5.5	—
13	Somewhat hard	6.0	—
14	—	6.5	—
15	Hard	7.0	Very strong
16	—	7.5	—
17	Very hard	8.0	—
18	—	8.5	—
19	Very, very hard	9.0	—
20	—	9.5	—
—	—	10	Very, very strong
—	—	>10	Maximal

Sources: Borg G. Psychopathological bases of perceived exertion. *Med Sci Sports Exerc* 1982;14:377–381; Blackburn GC, Dafoe WA, Horowitz LD, et al. Exercise prescription development and supervision. In: Pashkow FJ, Dafoe WA, eds. *Clinical cardiac rehabilitation: a cardiologist's guide.* Baltimore: Williams & Wilkins, 1993:115–140.

vidual patient based on the results of the ETT and the reason for cessation of exercise. For patients with life-threatening arrhythmias or chest pain, a lower target heart rate should be chosen. Even a target heart rate at 65% to 75% of maximum can be safe and effective in a regular program (83), and target rates as low as 60% can still yield a training benefit. For patients at higher risk, monitoring at each increase in activity level is appropriate. Some guidelines for activity classification and treatment are included in Table 79-9.

The classic duration of a cardiac training program is three sessions per week for 6 to 8 weeks. As limitations of availability, facilities, and financing imposed by managed care have arisen, creative new at-home programs for low-risk post-MI patients have been developed. These include community-based programs (84) and home programs (85). In all of these programs it is important that the patient be able to monitor himself or herself during the exercise program. Guidelines for self-monitoring are provided in Table 79-10. Each exercise session should begin with a stretching session, followed by a warm-up session, the training exercise, and a cooldown period. It is important to remember that the conditioning benefit is related to the specificity of training, and that the conditioning applies to the specific muscles exercised.

Table 79-8: Patients at High Risk During Cardiac Rehabilitation
Ischemic risk
Postoperative angina
LVEF < 35%
NYHA grade III or IV CHF
Ventricular tachycardia of fibrillation in the postoperative period
SBP drop of 10 points or more with exercise
Excessive ventricular ectopy with exercise
Incapable of self-monitoring
Myocardial ischemia with exercise
Arrhythmic risk
Acute infarction within 6 wk
Active ischemia by angina or exercise testing
Significant left ventricular dysfunction (LVEF < 30%)
History of sustained ventricular tachycardia
History of sustained life-threatening supraventricular arrhythmia
History of sudden death, not yet stabilized on medical therapy
Initial therapy of patient with automatic implantable cardioverter defibrillator (AICD)
Initial therapy of a patient with a rate-adaptive cardiac pacemaker

LVEF = left ventricular ejection fraction; NYHA = New York Heart Association; CHF = congestive heart failure; SBP = systolic blood pressure.

Maintenance Phase (Phase IV)

Although often the least discussed, the maintenance phase of a cardiac conditioning program is the most important part. If the patient stops exercising, the benefits gained from phase III can be lost in a few weeks. From the start of the cardiac rehabilitation program, the patient should be taught the importance of an ongoing exercise program and the concept should be re-emphasized throughout. The actual exercises need to be integrated into the patient's lifestyle and interests to ensure compliance. The secondary prevention measures also need to be integrated into the patient's lifestyle. The ongoing exercises should be performed at the target heart rate for at least 30 minutes three times a week, if at a moderate level of intensity. If at a low level of intensity, exercises need to be performed five times a week. During the maintenance phase, electrocardiographic monitoring is not necessary.

Table 79-9: Activity Classification				
Activity Class	**Clinical Characteristics**	**Activity Guidelines**	**ECG and BP Monitoring**	**Supervision Required**
Class A Healthy individuals No need for cardiac rehab program	< 40 yr old No known heart disease No symptoms of heart disease Normal ETT	No restrictions	None needed	None
Class B Known stable heart disease Low risk from cardiac exercise CAD Valvular heart disease Congenital heart disease Cardiomyopathy ETT abnormalities that are not class C and D	NYHA class 1 or 2 Exercise capacity > 6 METs No clinical heart failure No ischemia or angina at rest or on ETT at ≤ 6 METs Appropriate rise in BP with exercise No high-grade ventricular ectopy Ability to self-monitor activity	Individualized with exercise prescription by qualified personnel or restricted to walking	Only during prescriptive exercises, usually 6–12 sessions	Medical supervision during prescriptive sessions Nonmedical supervision for other exercise prescriptions
Class C Same as class B *and* Unable to self-regulate or -monitor activity Unable to understand prescribed activity levels	Same as class B *except* Unable to self-monitor activity	Individualized with exercise prescription by qualified personnel and supervised by nonmedical personnel trained in CPR	Only during prescriptive exercises, usually 6–12 sessions	Medical supervision during prescriptive sessions Nonmedical supervision for other exercise prescriptions
Class D Moderate to high risk for complications during exercise CAD Valvular heart disease Cardiomyopathy ETT abnormalities not directly related to ischemia Previous V-fib or sudden death not related to acute ischemia or cardiac procedure High-grade ventricular arrhythmias that	Two or more MIs NYHA class 3 or greater Exercise capacity < 6 METs Angina with exercise Downsloping or horizontal ST depression > 4 mm Fall in systolic BP with exercise Life-threatening medical problems Previous episodes of primary cardiac arrest Ventricular tachycardia at loads < 6 METs	Individualized with exercise prescription by qualified personnel	Continuous during rehab sessions until safety is established, usually 6–12 sessions	Medical supervision during all rehab sessions until safety is established

Table 79-9: Continued

Activity Class	Clinical Characteristics	Activity Guidelines	ECG and BP Monitoring	Supervision Required
are uncontrolled at mild to moderate work intensities Left mainartery disease or three-vessel disease EF < 30%				
Class E Unstable disease that restricts activity Unstable ischemia Uncontrolled heart failure Uncontrolled arrhythmia Severe symptomatic aortic stenosis Other conditions that can be aggravated by exercise	NYHA class 4 with uncontrolled heart failure Uncontrollable myocardial ischemia Refractory arrhythmias Irreparable valvular heart disease	No activity is recommended for conditioning purposes Try to achieve class D or better through medical management Daily activities as prescribed	No conditioning program	No conditioning program

ECG = electrocardiogram; BP = blood pressure; ETT = exercise tolerance test; CAD = coronary artery disease; NYHA = New York Heart Association; METs = metabolic equivalents; CPR = cardiopulmonary resuscitation; V-fib = ventricular fibrillation; EF = ejection fraction; MI = myocardial infarction.

Sources: Adapted from Juneau M, Rogers F, Desantos V, et al. Effectiveness of self monitored, home based, moderate intensity exercise training in sedentary middle aged men and women. *Am J Cardiol* 1987;60:66–70; and Juneau M, Geneau S, Marchand C, Brosseau R. Cardiac rehabilitation after coronary bypass surgery. *Cardiovasc Clin* 1991;21(2):25–42.

CARDIAC REHABILITATION PROGRAMS FOR SPECIAL CONDITIONS

With all the advances in medical technology over the last few decades, many new types of patients are being referred to cardiac rehabilitation programs. Patients with heart failure, valvular heart disease, or life-threatening arrhythmias are now entering rehabilitation programs. Surgical techniques have also created new groups of cardiac rehabilitation patients with diagnoses such as cardiac transplantation and coronary bypass grafting. This section deals briefly with each of these groups.

Angina Pectoris

For patients with a stable anginal syndrome, cardiac rehabilitation is appropriate. In these individuals, the training effect can be utilized to improve efficiency of performance below the anginal threshold (see Fig. 79-8). It is important to remember that the actual $M\dot{V}O_2$ (and thus the maximum heart rate) at which angina occurs will not change with conditioning. Before the initiation of the program of cardiac conditioning, a full-level ETT should be done to determine the maximum heart rate and rule out the potential occurrence of life-threatening events. Since these patients had no actual infarction, the program of rehabilitation can begin at phase III. Since the avoidance of MI is paramount in this group of patients, primary or secondary prevention, or both, is very important. The primary goal of rehabilitation in this group of patients is aimed at increasing work capacity. The increase in work capacity achieved will often lead to an increase in functional capacity that may significantly decrease the disability caused by the recurrent chest pain.

After Revascularization Procedures

Coronary Artery Bypass Grafting

A number of mechanisms account for the benefits of cardiac rehabilitation in the bypass patient (86). Because patients who undergo CABG often have not had a recent MI and have just been revascularized, they make excellent candidates for cardiac rehabilitation (87). Some patients

Table 79-10: Self-monitoring Guidelines	
Patient Guidelines	**Comments**
Wear proper clothing	Good shoes Loose-fitting garments Garments appropriate to the ambient temperature
Follow pacing guidelines	Follow exertional guidelines established by rehabilitation team Follow perceived exertional guidelines
Follow exercise guidelines	5–10-min low-intensity warm-up 20–30-min exercise at full intensity 5–10-min low-intensity cooldown
Stop exercising for adverse symptoms	Cardiac symptoms Chest pain Shortness of breath Light-headedness General symptoms Joint pains Faintness with exercise
No exercise while ill	Wait for 2 days after illness has passed
No exercise in environmental extremes	Avoid extreme cold Wear warm clothing Use a face mask Exercise indoors in winter Avoid extreme heat and humidity Lower pace Exercise in air-conditioned environment Exercise early in the morning or in the evening
No exercise after eating	Wait 2 hr after meals

have incomplete revascularization after CABG and can still be subject to ischemia. Also, with improvements in surgical technique, a larger number of patients with severe preexisting cardiac disease can now tolerate surgery, including patients with low ejection fractions and CHF. As a result, the rehabilitation program must be individualized to each patient's needs. A symptom-limited cardiac stress test can be useful in determining the level of exercise that a patient will tolerate, as the post-CABG patient often has a nondiagnostic thallium or electrocardiographic stress test. The exercise test can be safely performed at 3 to 4 weeks after surgery (88–90). The goal of the test is to determine the maximal functional capacity, the maximal heart rate, the blood pressure response to exercise, the presence of exercise-induced arrhythmias, and the anginal threshold. The initiation of a cardiac rehabilitation program also allows for the initiation of an education program to help

Table 79-11: Benefits of Cardiac Rehabilitation After Bypass Surgery
Increased ischemic threshold
Improved left ventricular function
Increased coronary collateral arteries
Ameliorated serum lipid levels
Decreased serum catecholamine levels
Decreased platelet aggregation and increased fibrinolysis
Improved psychological status

modify risk factors. Both supervised and unsupervised home programs are of benefit in preventing recurrent cardiac disease.

These improvements include improved cardiac conditioning, decreased immobility post surgery, improved sense of well being, and improved lipid status (Table 79-11).

Cardiac rehabilitation after CABG can be thought of in two stages: the immediate postoperative period and the later maintenance stage. The in-hospital first stage usually starts during the first week or so postoperatively, as patients are often sent home after that period of time. The initial period has three parts: 1) intensive mobilization in the immediate postoperative period, 2) progressive ambulation and daily exercises, and 3) discharge planning and exercise prescription for the maintenance stage (85).

Intensive mobilization in the intensive care unit on postoperative day 1 includes sitting upright, active leg exercises, and mobilization out of bed. Only an unstable postoperative course or severe CHF should interfere with this early mobilization. Aggressive early intervention has several benefits including decreasing the deleterious effects of bed rest such as deep venous thrombosis, pulmonary embolism, pulmonary complications, and cardiac deconditioning. The second through fifth days include progressive ambulation and daily exercise. Initial ambulation with supervision for distances of 150 to 200 feet is followed by gradually increasing the distance, with most patients beginning independent ambulation by the third day. In the last few days prior to discharge, the patient and physicians develop a program that can be self-monitored at home and allows for gradual progression to previous levels of activity.

The second stage of a program for a post-CABG patient is usually conducted at home or on an outpatient basis for most patients. High-risk patients or those who need other intensive interventions may require an inpatient rehabilitation setting. The home and outpatient rehabilitation patients are regularly supervised by their physicians. Patients can be stratified according to risk by the criteria shown in Table 79-9. Patients can be in one of three types of programs: low, moderate, or high intensity. A low-intensity program is a progressive walking program with energy expenditures in the area of 2 to 4 METs and a target heart rate at 65% to 75% of the maximum heart rate. A moderate-intensity program is a progressive walk to walk-jog program with energy expenditures of 3 to 6.5 METs and a target heart rate 70% to 80% of the maximum heart rate. A high-intensity program is a progression from walk-jog to jogging with expenditures of 5 to 8.5 METs and a target heart rate 75% to 85% of the maximum heart rate. In a patient taking a β-blocker, the target heart rate is 20 bpm above the resting heart rate, or can be determined through an ETT or exercise performed at a target MET level (91). The assignment of patients to a level of exercise is determined by both objective criteria and observation of the patient during the postoperative period. A submaximal stress test before discharge is an important way to evaluate the physiologic response to submaximal effort. A level of exercise that equals a rating of perceived exertion (RPE) of 13 is a level of training that can be prescribed safely for the outpatient setting (85). The inpatient program for high-risk patients has to be tailored to the specific needs of the patient, and is best designed in cooperation with the patient's cardiologist.

Percutaneous Transluminal Coronary Angioplasty

The rehabilitation of patients after percutaneous transluminal coronary angioplasty (PTCA) is essentially the same as that after CABG. PTCA patients tend to be younger and have disease limited to only one or two vessels (92). The exercise recommendations should be similar to those for the post-CABG patient population. In many ways, post-PTCA rehabilitation is more simple because there is not a significant postoperative recovery, and the patients can begin a conditioning and maintenance program right away. Some authors (93–95) believe that exercise testing performed before the PTCA for documentation of disease, followed by a sign- or symptom-limited exercise test immediately after PTCA, can document the improvement and set parameters for exercise prescription. Although ideal, this approach may not be practical in all settings and with all patients. As in the setting after CABG, some individuals may have incomplete revascularization or may develop restenosis. Risk factor modification training should be undertaken, and outpatient programs with both supervised and unsupervised home programs can be instituted. Since there is not a significant operative recovery period, the second-stage recommendations for CABG can be followed after PTCA. As after CABG, high-risk patients require closer monitoring and closer physician supervision. For low-risk post-PTCA patients, the recommendations in Table 79-9 can be followed.

Cardiac Transplant Surgery

As the techniques of orthotopic cardiac transplantation have improved, the numbers of patients with cardiac transplants have increased. Five-year and 10-year survival rates are now 82% and 74%, respectively (96). Typically, cardiac transplant patients are middle-aged, suffer from months of preoperative invalidism and general muscle weakness, and have depression and anxiety. The transplant itself usually resolves the cardiac disability, but a comprehensive approach to the patient is necessary.

The physiology of the transplant patient is somewhat different from that of the normal cardiac patient. Because of the loss of vagal inhibition to the SA node, the resting heart rate of the denervated heart is usually near 100 bpm (97). The resting tachycardia implies a small SV, and therefore, in response to light exercise, cardiac output can be increased via the Frank-Starling mechanism. With increased exercise, the circulating catecholamine-induced chronotropic and inotropic responses increase cardiac output (98–100). Therefore, because of loss of direct sympathetic innervation of the transplanted heart, patients have a blunted heart rate response to an incremental exercise test, with peak heart rates 20% to 25% lower than those seen in matched controls. Resting hypertension, thought to be due to the renal effects of cyclosporine, is common (101). Also seen after cardiac transplantation is a degree of diastolic dysfunction due to increased myocardial stiffness. Three possible factors lead to this: 1) myocardial ischemia from accelerated atherosclerosis, 2) side effects of immunosuppressive drugs, and 3) prolonged ischemic time for the donor heart (102). Transplant recipients also have a 10% to 50% loss of lean body mass from the lack of activity and the high-dose steroids given in the perioperative period. This means that maximum work output and maximum oxygen uptake are reduced to about two-thirds of those in the age-matched population (103). At submaximal exercise levels, perceived exertion, minute ventilation, and the ventilatory equivalent for oxygen are all higher than in normal individuals, while oxygen uptake is the same, implying an earlier onset of anaerobic metabolism. At maximum effort, transplant patients demonstrate lower work capacity, cardiac output, heart rate, systolic blood pressure, and oxygen uptake, while resting heart rate and systolic blood pressure are higher than those in normal individuals. Resting and exertional diastolic blood pressures are higher after cardiac transplantation than in normal individuals.

Exercise testing is usually done with a treadmill or a bicycle ergometer. Often a maximal exercise test cannot be performed because only about 50% of transplant patients can achieve an oxygen plateau ($M\dot{V}O_2$) at the initial test (103). When performing exercise testing, it is important to note that the denervated donor heart cannot demonstrate ischemia through anginal pain and that dyspnea, faintness, and electrocardiographic changes need to be followed vigilantly. Initial heart transplant patients have no electrocardiographic abnormalities, but in long-surviving transplant patients, accelerated atherosclerosis may develop and lead to cardiac ischemia.

The cardiac training regimen in transplant patients must address their overall conditioning as well as their cardiac function. Walking, jogging, cycling, and swimming are common exercises used in the program. In the initial postoperative period, sitting upright, lower-extremity exercises, and mobilization from the bed are encouraged. Patients are then encouraged to start ambulating, as with post-CABG patients. At the time of discharge, after patients have learned self-monitoring, they are encouraged to increase ambulation to 1 mile. The program then consists of progressively increasing distances for ambulation, with the pace designed to be at a level at 60% to 70% of peak effort for 30 to 60 minutes three to five times weekly (104). The RPE, using the old Borg scale, should be maintained at 13 or 14, with the level of activity increasing incrementally to stay at this level.

Other important aspects of the rehabilitation of the cardiac transplant patient include addressing the complicated medical regimen and the psychological needs of the patient. Patients will also need vocational rehabilitation before they can resume work. The physician will most likely need to prescribe a program of exercises to address generalized weakness.

The outcomes of rehabilitation in the cardiac transplant population have been generally favorable. Patients usually achieve increased work output and improved exercise tolerance (103). Some transplant patients can even resume competitive-level athletics (105). Regarding areas of general well-being and quality of life, in a recent survey transplant recipients reported a quality of life at the level of cardiac arrest survivors and post-MI patients, but less than that for normal individuals. There were also significant musculoskeletal complaints in this group of patients (106). It is hoped that the use of an exercise conditioning program in combination with reduction of other cardiac risk factors will help prevent accelerated atherosclerosis. The mechanism of this disease process is not known, but may be related to immunosuppressive drug therapy (107).

Valvular Heart Disease

In patients with valvular heart disease, the major problem is often deconditioning and CHF, as in the transplant population. Management of the valvular heart disease patient with CHF is essentially as outlined in the next section. After surgical correction, the patient's cardiac fitness improves as measured by improved $\dot{V}O_2$ (108). Training can increase physical work capacity by 60%, decrease the RPE, and decrease the RPP by 15% (109). A complicating feature in these patients is the fact that many of them are on anticoagulation therapy postoperatively, and need to be on low-impact exercises to avoid hemarthroses and bruising (Table 79-12). These patients also need special education to avoid injury (110). The training program is similar to that followed for the post-CABG patient.

Table 79-12: High- and Low-Impact Exercises

High-Impact Exercises	Low-Impact Exercises
Running	Swimming
Jogging	Cycling
High-impact aerobics	Walking
Rope skipping	Cross-country ski machine
Tennis/racquet sports	Stair climber
Contact sports	Low-impact aerobics
	Aquatic aerobics

Cardiomyopathy

With increasingly aggressive cardiac care, the number of patients with a left ventricular ejection fraction of less than 30% has increased, and this subset of the cardiac rehabilitation population is one of the fastest growing (110). These patients have different complications and expectations than the CABG or MI population, due to poor left ventricular function. They are at higher risk of sudden death and often are emotionally depressed owing to their chronic cardiac disability (111–113).

Patients with heart failure demonstrate inconsistent responses to exercise (114). Limited exercise capacity is one of the earliest findings in heart failure and can cause significant functional impairment. The hemodynamic alterations seen with exercise do not always correlate with the overall exercise capacity (115). The normal response to exercise is often absent. Exercise in heart failure patients can cause a drop in ejection fraction, a decrease in SV, exertional hypotension, and syncope. In the worst cases, cardiac output may not increase sufficiently to generate a dynamic exercise response at all. Low endurance and fatigue are also problems encountered with this population, with some experiencing fatigue for hours to days after achieving a high aerobic workload (116). In addition, there may be concomitant factors such as atrial fibrillation, fluid overload, or medication noncompliance that decrease exercise tolerance. Still, there is a documented benefit from exercise in this patient population (116,117). A gradual program of increasing the heart rate above the resting rate can be safe and increases oxygen extraction efficiency. Exercise duration can increase by as much as 18% to 34% (7,118,119) and peak oxygen uptake can increase by 18% to 25% (118,120). Patients who have participated in cardiac rehabilitation programs have lower heart rates at rest and during submaximal exercise, raised anaerobic thresholds, and increased maximal workloads (7,121). The improved ability to sustain activity at a low MET level can mean the difference between independent living and dependency for a patient with heart failure.

The evaluation of the CHF patient consists of a graded ETT and may include measurements of left ventricular ejection fraction by multiple gated acquisition scanning or echocardiography during exercise. Unstable angina, decompensated CHF, and unstable arrhythmias are contraindications to cardiac rehabilitation. In the design of the rehabilitation program, certain aspects specific to the CHF patient need to be kept in mind. Prolonged warm-up and cooldown periods are appropriate since these patients can increase the duration of exercise but are unable to tolerate more than a limited workload. Dynamic exercise is preferable to isometric exercise, and the target heart rate should be 10 bpm below any significant end point, such as exertional hypotension, significant dyspnea, or sustained arrhythmia seen in the pretraining exercise test (122). Isometric exercise should be avoided where possible, and limited to 2-minute intervals for those exercises performed. The exercise program is best done under supervision initially, until the patient is able to monitor himself or herself and prevent complications during exercise. Patients with severe left ventricular dysfunction will need to be followed by telemetry during the warm-up, exercise, and cooldown. Clinical status and progress can be monitored by measurements of body weight, blood pressure, and heart rate response to exercise.

Cardiac Arrhythmias

The risk of death from cardiac arrhythmia during rehabilitation exercises is very low. From 1980 to 1984, one arrest per 112,000 patient-hours of exercise was reported (123). This low risk means that it may be prudent to monitor continuously only those patients who are at high risk. Table 79-8 identifies patients at high risk of cardiac arrhythmias. For patients with life-threatening arrhythmias, the automatic implantable cardiac defibrillator is used increasingly (124). The modifications to the cardiac rehabilitation program in these patients are few. The devices are rate sensitive, so it is essential to ensure that during the exercise stress test this rate is not exceeded and that the heart rate achieved with exercise does not exceed this threshold. It is important to give support and reassurance to these patients during the exercise program, as anxiety about recurrent arrhythmia is a frequent concern (125).

CARDIAC REHABILITATION IN THE PHYSICALLY DISABLED

The disabled population with cardiac disease deserves some special considerations owing to the special challenges they present. Most of the challenges are due to limited mobility, which presents difficulties in testing and in exercise training. The difficulties presented in exercise testing are dealt with in Chapter 20. As the prognosis for patients with disability improves, more and more individuals are living to an age where cardiac disease becomes manifest. Disabled patients have several issues that place them at greater risk for cardiac disease than their nondisabled counterparts. They are usually more sedentary, which yields higher total cholesterol and lower HDL cholesterol levels (7,14,20,21). Obesity occurs frequently, and deconditioning is also often seen. In addition, the disabled usually require much higher energy expenditures for mobility, and thus need improved work capacity.

Exercise protocols need to be adapted to the individual patient. Those with lower-extremity impairment due to a neurologic or orthopedic condition can exercise using upper-extremity ergometry or alternatively, other exercise equipment that has been modified for them. Hemiplegic patients can use adapted bicycle ergometers or Airdynes (air-braked ergometers). Most exercise protocols for patients with a stroke or other conditions incorporate a large degree of upper-limb exercise, so the limitations of upper-extremity exercise that were mentioned earlier in the chapter should be considered when designing a cardiac rehabilitation program for these patients. Table 79-13 shows some of the relative cardiovascular responses to arm and leg exercises. Exercise training should follow the same basic principles of cardiac rehabilitation discussed earlier. It is essential that the training equipment be modified as necessary, and exercise should focus particularly on task-specific activities to improve aerobic conditioning and endurance. It is in the area of the design of cardiac rehabilitation programs for the disabled that the physiatrist is particularly suited to take a leadership role, as most cardiac rehabilitation programs have limited ability to accommodate physically disabled patients.

Table 79-13: Relative Cardiovascular Response to Upper-Extremity (UE) and Lower-Extremity (LE) Exercises

Parameter	Submaximal Exercise	Maximal Exercise
Work rate	UE = LE	UE < LE
Oxygen uptake	UE > LE	UE < LE
Cardiac output	UE > LE	UE < LE
Stroke volume	UE < LE	UE < LE
Heart rate	UE > LE	UE = LE
$M\dot{V}O_2$	UE > LE	
Systolic BP	UE > LE	UE = LE
Diastolic BP	UE > LE	UE > LE
Total peripheral resistance	UE > LE	UE > LE

BP = blood pressure; $M\dot{V}O_2$ = myocardial oxygen demand.

REFERENCES

1. *Statistical abstract of the United States: 1993.* 113th ed. Washington, DC. U.S. Bureau of the Census, 1993.

2. Graves EJ. *1992 Summary: National Hospital Discharge Survey. Advance data from vital and health statistics.* No. 249. Hyattsville, MD: National Center for Health Statistics, 1994.

3. *Statistical abstract of the United States: 1995.* 115th ed. Washington, DC: U.S. Bureau of the Census, 1995.

4. Wittels EH, Hay JW, Gotto AM. Medical costs of coronary artery disease in the United States. *Am J Cardiol* 1990;65:432–440.

5. American College of Chest Physicians. Cardiac rehabilitation services. *Ann Intern Med* 1988; 109:671–673.

6. Levin LA, Perk J, Hedback B. Cardiac rehabilitation—a cost analysis. *J Intern Med* 1991;230:427–434.

7. Balady GJ, Fletcher BJ, Froelicher ES, et al. Cardiac rehabilitation programs: a statement for healthcare professionals from the American Heart Association. *Circulation* 1994;90: 1602–1610.

8. Rehabilitation after cardiovascular diseases, with special emphasis on developing countries: report of a WHO Committee. *World Health Organ Tech Rep Ser* 1993;831:1–122.

9. Cannistra LB, Balady GJ, O'Malley CJ, et al. Comparison of the clinical profile and outcome of women and men in cardiac rehabilitation. *Am J Cardiol* 1992;69: 1274–1279.

10. Oldridge NB, Guyatt GH, Fischer ME, Rimm AA. Cardiac rehabilitation after myocardial infarction: combined experience of randomized clinical trials. *JAMA* 1988; 260:945–950.

11. O'Conner GT, Buring JE, Yusuf S, et al. An overview of randomized trials of rehabilitation with exercise after myocardial infarction. *Circulation* 1989;80:234–244.

12. Loen AS, Certo C, Comoss P, et al. Scientific evidence of the value of cardiac rehabilitation services with emphasis on patients following myocardial infarction. *J Cardiopulm Rehabil* 1990;10:79–87.

13. Thompson PD. The benefits and risks of exercise training in chronic coronary artery disease. *JAMA* 1988;259:1537–1540.

14. Brown G, Albers JJ, Fisher LD, et al. Regression of coronary artery disease as a result of intensive lipid lowering therapy in men with high levels of apolipoprotein B. *N Engl J Med* 1990;323: 1289–1298.

15. Watts GF, Lewis B, Brunt JN, et al. Effects on coronary disease of lipid lowering diet, or diet plus cholestyramine, in the St Thomas' Atherosclerosis Regression Study (STARS). *Lancet* 1992;339: 563–569.

16. *Report of the Joint National Committee on Detection, Evaluation, and Treatment of High Blood Pressure.* Department of Health, Education, and Welfare publication no. NIH 93–1088. Bethesda, MD: National Heart, Lung, and Blood Institute, 1993.

17. Smoking-attributable mortality and years of potential life lost—United States, 1988. *MMWR Morb Mortal Wkly Rep* 1991;40: 62–63, 69–71.

18. Jonas MA, Oates JA, Ockene JK, Hennekens CH. Statement on smoking and cardiovascular disease for healthcare professionals. *Circulation* 1992;86: 1664–1669.

19. Oldridge NB, Jones NL. Preventive use of exercise rehabilitation after myocardial infarction. *Acta Med Scand Suppl* 1986;711: 123–129.

20. Wood PD, Stefanick ML, Williams PT, Haskell WL. The effect on plasma lipoproteins of a prudent weight reducing diet, with or without exercise, in overweight men and women. *N Engl J Med* 1991;325:461–466.

21. Ornish D, Brown SE, Scherwitz LW, et al. Can lifestyle changes reverse coronary heart disease? The Lifestyle Heart Trial. *Lancet* 1990;336:129–133.

22. Bjorntorp P, Berchtold P, Grimby G, et al. Effects of physical training on glucose tolerance, plasma insulin and lipids and on body composition in men after myocardial infarction. *Acta Med Scand* 1972;192:439–443.

23. Loen AS. The role of exercise in the prevention and management of diabetes mellitus and blood lipid disorders. In: Shephard RJ, Miller HS, eds. *Exercise and the heart in health and disease.* New York: Marcel Dekker, 1992: 299–368.

24. Exercise and NIDDM. *Diabetes Care* 1990;13:785–789.

25. Hagberg JM, Seals DR. Exercise training and hypertension. *Acta Med Scand Suppl* 1986;711: 131–136.

26. American College of Sports Medicine position stand. The recommended quantity and quality of exercise for developing and maintaining cardiorespiratory and muscular fitness in healthy adults. *Med Sci Sports Exerc* 1990;22:265–274.

27. Fletcher GF, Froelicher VF, Hartley LH, et al. Exercise standards: a statement for health professionals from the American Heart Association. *Circulation* 1990;82:2286–2322.

28. Selwyn AP, Braunwald E. Ischemic heart disease. In: Isselbacher KJ, Braunwald E, Wilson JD, et al, eds. *Harrison's principles of internal medicine.* 13th ed. New York: McGraw-Hill, 1994:1077–1085.

29. Kaplan NM. Systemic hypertension: therapy. In: Braunwald E, ed. *Heart disease.* Philadelphia: WB Saunders, 1992:852–874.

30. Hiatt WR, Regensteiner JG, Wolfel EE. Special populations in cardiovascular rehabilitation. *Cardiol Clin* 1993;11:309–321.

31. Hypertension Detection and Follow-up Program Cooperative Research Group. The effect of antihypertensive drug treatment

on mortality in the presence of resting electrocardiographic abnormalities at baseline. The HDFP experience. *Circulation* 1984;70:996–1003.

32. Multiple Risk Factor Intervention Trial Research Group. Baseline rest electrocardiographic abnormalities, antihypertensive treatment, and mortality in the Multiple Risk Factor Intervention Trial. *Am J Cardiol* 1985;55: 1–15.

33. Schuler G, Hambrecht R, Schlierf G, et al. Myocardial perfusion and the regression of coronary artery disease in patient on a regimen of intensive physical exercise and low fat diet. *J Am Coll Cardiol* 1992;19:34–42.

34. Schuler G, Hambrecht R, Schlierf G, et al. Regular exercise and low fat diet: effects on progression of coronary artery disease. *Circulation* 1992;86:1–11.

35. Drugs for hypertension. *Med Lett* 1995;37:45–50.

36. Grundy SM, Brown WV, Dietschy JM, et al. AHA Conference Report on cholesterol: Workshop III: basis for dietary treatment. *Circulation* 1989;80:729–734.

37. The Expert Panel. Report of the National Cholesterol Education Program Expert Panel on the Detection, Evaluation, and Treatment of High Blood Cholesterol in Adults. *Arch Intern Med* 1988;148:36–39.

38. Bittner V, Oberman A. Efficacy studies in coronary rehabilitation. *Cardiol Clin* 1993;11:333–347.

39. Holbrook JH, Grundy SM, Hennekens CH, et al. Cigarette smoking and cardiovascular diseases: a statement for health professionals prepared by a task force appointed by the steering committee of the American Heart Association. *Circulation* 1984;70:1114A.

40. Sparrow D, Dauber TR, Colson T. The influence of cigarette smoking on prognosis after a first myocardial infarction. *J Chron Dis* 1978;38:425–432.

41. Vliestra RE, Kronmal RA, Oberman A, et al. Effect of cigarette smoking on survival of patients with angiographically documented coronary artery disease: a report from the CASS Registry. *JAMA* 1986;255: 1023–1027.

42. Oldridge NB, Donner AP, Buck CW, et al. Prediction of dropout from cardiac exercise rehabilitation: Ontario Exercise-Heart Collaborative Study. *Am J Cardiol* 1983;51:70–74.

43. Roman O, Gutierrez M, Luksic I, et al. Cardiac rehabilitation after acute myocardial infarction: 9 year controlled follow-up study. *Cardiology* 1983;70:223–231.

44. Ruskin J, McHale PA, Harley A, et al. Pressure-flow studies in man: effects of atrial systole on left ventricular function. *J Clin Invest* 1970;49:472–478.

45. Moldover JR, Stein J. Cardiopulmonary physiology. In: Downey JA, Myers S, Gonzalez E, et al, eds. *The physiological basis of rehabilitation medicine.* 2nd ed. Boston: Butterworth-Heinemann, 1994:127–147.

46. Moldover JR, Bartels MN. Cardiac rehabilitation. In: Braddom RL, ed. *Physical medicine and rehabilitation.* Philadelphia: WB Saunders, 1996:649–670.

47. April EW. *Anatomy*, Pennsylvania: John Wiley, 1984:143–161.

48. Guyton AC. *Textbook of medical physiology.* 7th ed. Philadelphia: WB Saunders, 1986.

49. Berne RB, Levy MN. *Cardiovascular physiology.* St Louis: CV Mosby, 1986.

50. Ignarro LJ. Endothelium derived nitric oxide: actions and properties. *FASEB J* 1989;3:31–36.

51. Braunwald E, Sonnenblick EH, Ross J. Normal and abnormal circulatory function. In: Braunwald E, ed. *Heart disease.* Philadelphia: WB Saunders, 1992: 351–392.

52. Vaitkevicius PV, Fleg JL, Engel JH, et al. Effects of age and aerobic capacity on arterial stiffness in healthy adults. *Circulation* 1993;88:1456–1462.

53. Blackburn GC, Dafoe WA, Horowitz LD, et al. Exercise prescription development and supervision. In: Pashkow FJ, Dafoe WA, eds. *Clinical cardiac rehabilitation: a cardiologist's guide.* Baltimore: Williams & Wilkins, 1993:115–140.

54. O'Conner GT, Burling JE, Yusuf S, et al. An overview of randomized trials of rehabilitation with exercise after myocardial infarction. *Circulation* 1989;80: 234–244.

55. Lavie CJ, Miliani RV. Effects of cardiac rehabilitation programs on exercise capacity, coronary risk factors, behavioral characteristics, and quality of life in a large elderly cohort. *Am J Cardiol* 1995;76:177–179.

56. Lavie CJ, Miliani RV, Littman AB. Benefits of cardiac rehabilitation and exercise training in secondary coronary conditioning in the elderly. *J Am Coll Cardiol* 1993;22:678–683.

57. Lavie CJ, Miliani RV, Boykin C. Marked benefits of cardiac rehabilitation and exercise training in an elderly cohort. *J Am Coll Cardiol* 1994;23:439. Abstract.

58. Cannistra LB, Balady GJ, O'Malley CJ, et al. Comparison of the clinical profile and outcome of women and men in cardiac rehabilitation. *Am J Cardiol* 1992;69:1274–1279.

59. Perk J, Hedback B, Engvall J. Effects of cardiac rehabilitation after coronary bypass grafting on readmissions, return to work, and physical fitness: a case control study. *Scand J Soc Med* 1990; 18:45–51.

60. Oldridge N, Furlong W, Feeny D, et al. Economic evaluation of cardiac rehabilitation soon after acute myocardial infarction. *Am J Cardiol* 1993;72:154–161.

61. Morris CK, Froelicher VF. Cardiovascular benefits of physical activity. *Herz* 1991;16:222–236.

62. Chandrasheckhar Y, Anand IS. Exercise as a coronary protective

factor. *Am Heart J* 1991;122: 1723–1739.

63. Tran ZW, Weltman A. Differential effects of exercise on serum lipid and lipoprotein levels seen with changes in body weight: a meta analysis. *JAMA* 1985;254: 919–924.

64. Martin JE, Dubbert PM, Cushman WC. Controlled trial of aerobic exercise in hypertension. *Circulation* 1990;81:1560–1567.

65. Fletcher GF, Blair SN, Blumenthal J, et al. Statement on exercise. Benefits and recommendations for physical activity programs for all Americans. A statement for health professionals by the Committee on Exercise and Cardiac Rehabilitation of the Council on Clinical Cardiology. American Heart Association. *Circulation* 1992;86(1): 76–84.

66. Leren P. The effect of plasma cholesterol lowering diet in male survivors of myocardial infarction. *Acta Med Scand* 1967;466: 1–92.

67. Shekelle RB, Shyrock AM, Paul O, et al. Diet, serum cholesterol, and death from coronary heart disease: the Western Electric Study. *N Engl J Med* 1981; 304:65–70.

68. Stamler J, Wentworth D, Neaton JD, for the MRFIT Research Group. Is relationship between serum cholesterol and risk of premature death from coronary heart disease continuous and graded? Findings in 356,222 primary screenees of the Multiple Risk Factor Intervention Trial (MRFIT). *JAMA* 1986;256: 2823–2828.

69. Frick MH, Elo O, Haapa K, et al. Helsinki Heart Study: primary prevention trial with gemfibrozil in middle aged men with dyslipidemia. *N Engl J Med* 1987;317:1237–1245.

70. Bresike JF, Levy RI, Kelsey SF, et al. Effects of therapy with cholestyramine on progression of coronary arteriosclerosis: results of the NHLBI type II coronary intervention study. *Circulation* 1984;69:313–324.

71. Gordon T, Kannel WB, McGee D. Death and coronary attacks in men after giving up cigarette smoking: a report from the Framingham study. *Lancet* 1974;2:1345–1348.

72. Salonen JT. Stopping smoking and long term mortality after acute myocardial infarction. *Br Heart J* 1980;43:463–469.

73. Wenger N, Gilbert C, Skoropa M. Cardiac conditioning after myocardial infarction. An early intervention program. *J Cardiac Rehabil* 1971;2:17–22.

74. Pashkow FJ, Pashkow PS, Schafer MN. *Successful cardiac rehabilitation: the complete guide for building cardiac rehab programs.* 1st ed. Loveland, CO: Heart Watchers Press, 1988:211–212.

75. Wenger N, Hellerstein H, Blackburn H, Castronova M. Uncomplicated myocardial infarction: current physician practice in patient management. *JAMA* 1973;224:511–514.

76. Froelicher VF. Exercise testing and training: clinical applications. *J Am Coll Cardiol* 1983;1: 114–125.

77. Sivarajan E, Lerman J, Mansfield L. Progressive ambulation and treadmill testing of patients with acute myocardial infarction during hospitalization: a feasibility study. *Arch Phys Med Rehabil* 1977;58:241–244.

78. Pashkow FJ. Issues in contemporary cardiac rehabilitation: a historical perspective. *J Am Coll Cardiol* 1993;21:822–824.

79. Borg G. Psychopathological bases of perceived exertion. *Med Sci Sports Exerc* 1982;14:377–381.

80. Krone RJ, Gillespie JA, Weld FM, et al. Low level exercise testing after myocardial infarction: usefulness in enhancing clinical risk stratification. *Circulation* 1985;71:80–89.

81. Krone RJ. The role of risk stratification in the early management of myocardial infarction. *Ann Intern Med* 1992;116: 223–237.

82. Fletcher BJ, Lloyd A, Fletcher GF. Outpatient rehabilitative training in patients with cardiovascular disease: emphasis on training method. *Heart Lung* 1988;17:199–205.

83. Juneau M, Rogers F, Desantos V, et al. Effectiveness of self monitored, home based, moderate intensity exercise training in sedentary middle aged men and women. *Am J Cardiol* 1987;60: 66–70.

84. Pashkow F, Schafer M, Pashkow P. Heart Watchers—low cost, community centered cardiac rehabilitation in Loveland, Colorado. *J Cardiopulm Rehabil* 1986;6:469–473.

85. DeBusk RF, Haskell WL, Miller NH. Medically directed at-home rehabilitation soon after clinically uncomplicated acute myocardial infarction: a new model for patient care. *Am J Cardiol* 1985;55:251–257.

86. Juneau M, Geneau S, Marchand C, Brosseau R. Cardiac rehabilitation after coronary bypass surgery. *Cardiovasc Clin* 1991;21(2):25–42.

87. Wenger NK. Rehabilitation of the coronary patient: status 1986. *Prog Cardiovasc Dis* 1986;29:181–204.

88. Pollock ML, Foster C, Anholm JD, et al. Diagnostic capabilities of exercise testing soon after myocardial revascularization surgery. *Cardiology* 1982;69:358.

89. Dubach P, Froelicher V, Klein J, et al. Use of the exercise test to predict prognosis after coronary artery bypass grafting. *Am J Cardiol* 1989;63:530.

90. Wainwright RJ, Brennand-Roper DA, Maisey MN, et al. Exercise thallium-201 myocardial scintigraphy in the follow-up of aortocoronary bypass graft surgery. *Br Heart J* 1980;43:56–66.

91. Hartley HL. Exercise for the cardiac patient. *Cardiol Clin* 1993;11:277–284.

92. Acinapura AJ, Jacobowitz IJ, Kramer MD, et al. Demographic changes in coronary artery bypass surgery and its effects on mortal-

ity. *Eur J Cardiotho-*
;4:175–181.

aitman BR. Role of
in relationship to
surgery and per-
luminal coronary
diology
1986;73:242–258.

94. Wijns W, Serruys PW, Reiber JH, et al. Early detection of restenosis after successful percutaneous transluminal coronary angioplasty by exercise-redistribution thallium scintigraphy. *Am J Cardiol* 1985;55:357–361.

95. Wijns W, Serruys PW, Simoons ML, et al. Predictive value of early maximal exercise test and thallium scintigraphy after successful percutaneous transluminal coronary angioplasty. *Br Heart J* 1985;53:194–200.

96. Heck CF, Shumway SJ, Kaye MP. The registry of the International Society for Heart Transplantation: sixth official report 1989. *J Heart Transplant* 1989;8:271–276.

97. de Marneffe M, Jacobs P, Haardt R, Englert M. Variations of normal sinus node function in relation to age: role of autonomic influence. *Eur Heart J* 1986;7:662.

98. Cannom DS, Rider AK, Stinson EB, et al. Electrophysiologic studies in the denervated transplanted human heart. *Am J Cardiol* 1975;36:859–866.

99. Yusuf S, Aikenhead J, Theodoropoulos S, et al. Mechanism of cardiac output during dynamic exercise in cardiac transplant patients. *J Am Coll Cardiol* 1986;7:225A. Abstract.

100. Yusuf S, Theodoropoulos S, Mathias CJ, et al. Increased sensitivity to the denervated transplanted human heart to isoprenaline both before and after beta-adrenergic blockade. *Circulation* 1987;75:696–704.

101. Starling RC, Cody RJ. Cardiac transplant hypertension. *Am J Cardiol* 1990;65:106–111.

102. Hausdorf G, Banner NR, Mitchell A, et al. Diastolic function after cardiac and heart lung transplantation. *Br Heart J* 1989;62: 123–132.

103. Kavanagh T, Yacoub M, Mertens DJ, et al. Cardiorespiratory responses to exercise training after orthotopic cardiac transplantation. *Circulation* 1988;77: 162–171.

104. Kavanagh T. Exercise training in patients after heart transplantation. Herz 1991;16:243–250.

105. Kavanaugh T, Yacoub MH, Campbell R, Mertens D. Marathon running after cardiac transplantation: a case history. *J Cardiac Rehab* 1986;6:16–20.

106. Rosenblum DS, Rosen ML, Pine ZM, et al. Health status and quality of life following cardiac transplantation. *Arch Phys Med Rehabil* 1993;74:490–493.

107. Billingham ME. Graft coronary disease: the lesions and the patients. *Transplant Proc* 1989; 21:3665–3666.

108. Newell JP, Kappagoda CT, Stoker JB, et al. Physical training after heart valve replacement. *Br Heart J* 1980;44:638–649.

109. Sire S. Physical training and occupational rehabilitation after aortic valve replacement. *Eur Heart J* 1987;8:1215–1220.

110. Pashkow F. Rehabilitation strategies for the complex cardiac patient. *Cleve Clin J Med* 1991;58:70–75.

111. Kannel WB, Plehn JF, Cupples LA. Cardiac failure and sudden death in the Framingham study. *Am Heart J* 1988;115:869–875.

112. Packer M. Sudden unexpected death in patients with congestive heart failure: a second frontier. *Circulation* 1985;72:681–685.

113. Christopherson LK. Cardiac transplantation: a psychological perspective. *Circulation* 1987;75: 57–62.

114. Sullivan MJ, Higginbotham MB, Cobb FR. Exercise training in patients with severe left ventricular dysfunction. *Circulation* 1990;81(suppl II):II-5–II-13.

115. McKirnan MD, Sullivan M, Jensen D, et al. Treadmill performance and cardiac function in selected patients with coronary heart disease. *J Am Coll Cardiol* 1984;3:253–261.

116. Dubach P, Froelicher VF. Cardiac rehabilitation for heart failure patients. *Cardiology* 1989;76:368–373.

117. Shabetai R. Beneficial effects of exercise training in compensated heart failure. *Circulation* 1988;78:775–776.

118. Coats AJ, Adamopoulos S, Radaelli A, et al. Controlled trial of physical training in chronic heart failure: exercise performance, hemodynamics, ventilation, and autonomic function. *Circulation* 1992;85: 2119–2131.

119. Koch M, Dougard H, Broustet JP. The benefit of graded physical exercise in chronic heart failure. *Chest* 1992;101(suppl 5): 231S–235S.

120. Coats AJ, Adamopoulos S, Meyer TE, et al. Effects of physical training in chronic heart failure. *Lancet* 1990;335:63–66.

121. Lee AP, Ice R, Blessey R, et al. Long-term effects of physical training in coronary patients with impaired ventricular function. *Circulation* 1979;60:1519–1526.

122. Pashkow FJ. Complicating conditions. In: Pashkow FJ, Pashkow P, Schafer M, eds. *Successful cardiac rehabilitation: the complete guide for building cardiac rehabilitation programs.* Loveland, CO: Heart Watchers Press, 1988:228–247.

123. Van Camp S, Peterson R, Cardiovascular complications of outpatient cardiac rehabilitation programs. *JAMA* 1986;256: 1160–1163.

124. Winkle RA, Mead RH, Ruder MA, et al. Long term outcome with the automatic implantable cardiac-defibrillator. *J Am Coll Cardiol* 1989;13:1353–1361.

125. Pycha C, Gulledge AD, Hutzler J, et al. Psychological response to the implantable defibrillator. *Psychosomatics* 1986;27: 841–845.

Chapter 80

Respiratory Dysfunction

Staci J. Schwartz
Stephen R. Gaspar

DEFINITION

"Pulmonary rehabilitation may be defined as an art of medical practice wherein an individually tailored, multidisciplinary program is formulated which through accurate diagnosis, therapy, emotional support, and education, stabilizes or reverses both the physio- and psychopathology of pulmonary diseases and attempts to return the patient to the highest possible functional capacity allowed by his pulmonary handicap and overall life situation" (1).

NORMAL PHYSIOLOGY OF RESPIRATION AND VENTILATION

The basic components contributing to the process of breathing include the lungs, chest wall, muscles of respiration, airways and supportive connective tissues, and the neurovascular lymphatic elements that supply these structures.

The lungs serve many functions, including the implementation of gas exchange between inspired air and the blood, the metabolism of various substances, the synthesis of surfactant, the production of immunoglobulins against inhaled antigens, and the filtration of small intravascular thrombi (2). Lung tissue exhibits varying degrees of compliance and elastance based on its elastic properties and intrinsic pressure-volume relationships, disease processes, and changes with aging.

The chest wall is composed of the ribs and bony thorax, the pleurae, and several groups of muscles. The primary muscles of inspiration include the intercostal muscles and the diaphragm. Shoulder girdle muscles can be used to lift the sternum when the distal end of the upper extremity is stabilized, and thus act as accessory muscles of inspiration. Accessory muscles of respiration include the sternocleidomastoid, scalene groups, trapezius, pectoral groups, serratus anterior, and latissimus dorsi (3). Accessory muscles, as well as the abdominal muscles and intercartilaginous muscles (4), come into play with increased ventilatory requirements.

Lung volumes at rest and during respiration depend on the elastance and compliance of the lungs and the chest wall. Lung elastance is conferred by a number of structural proteins, including reticulin and elastin, whose characteristics and quantity change with disease processes and aging. The chest wall compliance changes with diseases of the pleura, structural deformity or rigidity of the bony thorax, or obesity.

The airways can be considered as a series of progressively branching tubes with differing proportions of cartilage, smooth muscle, types of epithelial cells and glands, supportive connective tissue, and neurovascular elements. The trachea, bronchi, bronchioles, and terminal bronchioles constitute conducting airways, and serve as a passageway for air to reach the distal regions of gas exchange. These conducting airways are commonly referred to as *anatomic dead space*. The respiratory bronchi-

[illegible]lveolar ducts and sacs constitute the transitional [illegible]as exchange airways, respectively.

Cartilage is present only to the level of the bronchi and large bronchioles. Smooth muscle extends from the bronchi to the alveolar ducts (4); it can alter the diameter of the intraparenchymal airways, playing a key role in airway resistance. Smooth muscle is under the reactive influence of the autonomic nervous system (parasympathetic cholinergic stimulation causes bronchial constriction whereas adrenergic sympathetic stimulation causes bronchial dilatation), inhaled irritants, metabolic by-products [carbon dioxide (CO_2) decrease causes vasoconstriction], and mediators of inflammation. The bronchioles and alveolar ducts are held open by elastic and septal connective tissue elements. Alveoli are held open by these same elements and the effects of surfactant on surface tension forces.

Gas exchange occurs between the alveoli and the pulmonary capillaries over a potential estimated area of between 60 and 100 m^2 (4). Alveolar ventilation cannot be measured directly. Rather it is extrapolated from complicated equations. Oxygen (O_2) and CO_2 are the chief constituents that are exchanged to support the process of respiration and maintain the acid-base balance of the body. The process of diffusion involves multiple factors, including the partial pressures and volumes of gaseous elements, solubilities of the elements, tissue and blood cell properties, hemoglobin concentrations, surface area available for gas exchange, characteristics of the epithelial lining of the alveoli and the endothelial lining of the capillaries, interstitial elements and surfactant production, and the state of activity (rest versus exercise) of the individual (4,5). O_2 diffusion is slower than CO_2 diffusion, and O_2 pressure (pO_2) may fall as the individual's activity level increases, if the diffusing capacity is low. The CO_2 pressure (pCO_2) may rise with exercise if ventilatory mechanics are impaired.

The main vascular structures involved in pulmonary respiration include the pulmonary veins, arteries, capillaries, and pulmonary lymphatics. The pulmonary circulation has been described as a "high capacity, low resistance circuit" (6) under normal circumstances. Pulmonary vascular resistance has been estimated to be about one-tenth of systemic vascular resistance (4) and varies less with cardiac output and physiologic stress than the systemic circulation. The organization of the pulmonary arteries and veins is similar to the distribution of the branching airways. In addition to the pulmonary circulation, a separate bronchial circulation derives from the aorta and intercostal arteries; it supplies blood to the upper airways and other thoracic structures, and plays no role in gas exchange. The bronchial arteries carry a much higher blood pressure than the pulmonary arteries because they are part of the systemic arterial system.

Pulmonary lymphatics are scattered throughout various connective tissue spaces within and surrounding the lung parenchyma. The system forms channels with specialized valves that propel the lymph fluid toward the hilar regions of the lungs where it surrounds the lymph nodes. The pulmonary lymph then enters the systemic circulation via the thoracic duct.

Both ventilation and perfusion occur in nonuniform distributions within the lung, and will vary with the position of the individual, disease states, and age. In general, the basal portions of the lung receive more ventilation per unit of volume and more perfusion per unit of volume in the upright position than do the apical regions, owing to the differences in pressure, compliance, resistance, and gravity effects. The basal to apical perfusion gradient has been found to be more pronounced than the ventilation gradient (4), which leads to regional differences in ventilation-perfusion ratios among the alveoli. The degree of ventilation-perfusion mismatching correlates with arterial pO_2.

Once gas exchange occurs, O_2 and CO_2 are carried in their dissolved states in the blood. Both compounds are also carried in association with other proteins and molecular compounds. Hemoglobin molecules greatly increase the blood's capacity for O_2 transport to support metabolic and tissue demands. The oxyhemoglobin dissociation curve reflects the correlation between plasma pO_2 and percent saturation of hemoglobin with O_2 and is affected by many variables, including the affinity of hemoglobin for O_2, hypoxia, pH, temperature, pCO_2, 2,3-diphosphoglycerate levels, carbon monoxide levels, anemia, and myoglobin levels (4). The influence of these variables is such that knowing a patient's percent O_2 saturation is not a substitute for direct measurement of arterial pO_2 in critical clinical situations.

COUGH MECHANISM

Airway epithelial cells from the trachea through the terminal bronchioles contain cilia, which are responsible for the propulsion of the mucus produced by various glands and secretory cells toward the mouth and nose as an important part of the respiratory defense mechanism (4).

The cough mechanism, which is coordinated in the brain stem, is a very important part of routine airway cleaning; patients with impaired cough are prone to atelectasis. A cough includes a deep inhalation, closure of the glottis, contraction of abdominal and intercostal muscles to produce compression of the thorax and high intrathoracic pressure, and finally opening of the glottis and explosive exhalation through compressed upper airways. Airflow velocities of 250 to 300 m sec are measurable in normal people (7). The cough mechanism is usually stimulated by excess airway secretions, infections, certain inhaled agents or chemicals that irritate sensory nerve endings, or mechanical irritants that activate the stretch receptors in the lung or airways, or it is thought to be induced by certain drugs whose action is remote from the lungs [e.g., angiotensin-converting enzyme (ACE) inhibitors] (8).

PULMONARY FUNCTION TESTS

Pulmonary function tests are quite helpful for diagnostic evaluation, assessment of therapeutic efforts, and assessment of breathing techniques for patients with known or suspected pulmonary disease. The types of tests available include spirometry (vital capacity, FEV_1, forced vital capacity, total lung capacity, residual volume, etc); measurement of inspiratory and expiratory pressures; measurements of static and dynamic lung volumes; evaluations of respiratory muscle strength and diaphragm function, movement, and endurance; flow-volume loops; direct tests of airway resistance, lung compliance, and chest wall compliance; and indirect measurements of actual lung volumes, gas exchange parameters, and other cardiovascular parameters (9). Flow-volume loops are graphic representations that plot inspiratory and expiratory flow rates versus lung volumes. Electrodiagnostic assessment of phrenic nerve function may also prove helpful in the evaluation of lung function. Kelley (9) provided an excellent overview of the physiology on which these tests are based, as well as examples of normal and pathologic test results.

Spirogram

The spirogram plots volume against time; from it are derived several important values [adapted from Mines (5)]:

Total lung capacity—the amount of gas that fills the lung when the patient maximally inspires.

Vital capacity—the amount of gas that can be maximally exhaled after a maximum inspiration.

Residual volume—the amount of gas that is still present in the lung after maximum expiration.

Functional residual capacity—the amount of gas left in the lung after exhalation during normal quiet breathing.

Inspiratory capacity—the amount of gas that can be maximally inspired from the starting point of functional residual capacity.

Tidal volume—the amount of gas inspired during normal quiet breathing.

Inspiratory reserve volume—the amount of gas that can still be inspired starting at tidal volume to reach total lung capacity.

Expiratory reserve volume—the amount of gas that can still be expired starting at functional residual capacity and ending at residual volume.

RESPIRATORY CYCLE

The neurologic pathways that control respiration are both voluntary and involuntary. Respiration is controlled voluntarily by cortical centers and involuntarily by centers in the pons and medulla; the voluntary and involuntary pathways interact continually during various activities. There is a complex neural organization of components involved in the regulation of breathing. Control of respiration is influenced by stretch, chemical, and/or irritant and pH receptors in the lungs, airways, medulla, and several arterial vessels (including the carotid, pulmonary capillaries, and aorta); sympathetic and parasympathetic neurons and ganglia; sensory afferent neurons; C-fibers; and the vagus and phrenic nerves (5). States of arousal or relaxation affect the rate of respiration through brain centers, as well as the degree of relaxation of the airways via sympathetic or vagal activity.

The diaphragm is innervated by the phrenic nerve (C3, C4, C5); some authors (10) cite a contribution from C6. The intercostal muscles are innervated by the intercostal nerves (T1–T11) (10). The trapezius and sternocleidomastoid muscles are innervated from direct branches of the cervical plexus (C1–C4) and the eleventh cranial nerve. The scalenes are innervated by cervical segmental levels C4–C8 (10). Abdominal muscles of respiration receive innervation from the upper thoracic segments to L1, mostly from the lower thoracic spinal cord segments T6–T12 (11).

Inspiration

Sixty percent to 70% of tidal inspiration is performed by the diaphragm. The contraction of the diaphragm creates increased negative intrathoracic pressure; the lungs then expand passively. Forced inspiration calls other muscles into play, most importantly the muscles acting on the first rib and clavicle, predominantly the scalenes and the shoulder girdle muscles, which exert force on the thoracic wall when the upper extremities are stabilized.

As in all skeletal muscle, the force generated by the diaphragm is at its greatest when the diaphragm is stretched, and decreases as the muscle shortens. Thus, the diaphragm is more powerful at smaller than at larger lung volumes, and inspiration at expanded lung volumes may require accessory muscles in addition to the diaphragm.

The diaphragm is subject to all conditions that serve to weaken skeletal muscles in general. Serum potassium derangements weaken the diaphragm and potentially respond to therapy quickly. Protein malnutrition decreases the myosin content of all skeletal muscle and hence weakens the diaphragm; refeeding is a long-term project. Diaphragmatic protein loss also occurs with prolonged rest of the diaphragm, as happens when patients are mechanically ventilated for long periods; again, reconditioning of the diaphragm requires long-term treatment. Neuropathies, inflammatory and degenerative myopathies, anterior horn cell diseases, and diseases of the neuromuscular junction weaken the diaphragm. The effects of nondepolarizing paralytic drugs on the neuromuscular junction usually resolve in hours; in some individuals, these effects persist for many days.

The effect of position on inspiratory power is significant in the setting of diaphragm weakness. When the patient is erect, the work of the diaphragm consists of overcoming the tendency of the lungs to minimize intrathoracic volume; when the patient is recumbent, the diaphragm also has to move the abdominal contents, which press on it from below. In a normal state, this added work of inspiration is trivial, but it becomes significant if the diaphragm is weak.

Accessory muscles of inspiration are called into use in normal people for forceful breathing, such as during exercise. In patients with weak diaphragms, they may be responsible for a significant part of tidal inspiration. The shoulder girdle muscles ordinarily move the humerus; when the humerus is braced, these muscles act on their insertions, and their effect is to expand the rib cage. Therefore, the characteristic posture of patients with lung disease, the thorax bent forward and the elbows braced, is physiologically sound. All conditions that weaken proximal muscles also weaken the accessory muscles of respiration.

Expiration

Normal tidal expiration is passive. All the work is done by the diaphragm during inspiration; expiration happens when the lung is allowed to return to a smaller volume, owing to its elasticity. Forced expiration requires muscular contraction: The external intercostal muscles lower the rib cage, and the abdominal muscles force the contents of the abdomen up against the diaphragm.

PULMONARY FUNCTION CHANGES WITH AGING

Changes in pulmonary function that occur with aging can be the result of normal physiologic senescence or of deterioration due to pathologic lung disease. Some of the age-associated changes in pulmonary function in normal individuals that have been described include decreased lung elastic recoil, decreased maximal expiratory airflow rates, increased closing capacity, increased residual volume, and increased functional residual capacity (12), decreased lung volumes, increased work of breathing, decreased cough effectiveness and mucociliary clearance, increased ventilation-perfusion mismatch, decreased lung immunity, decreased sensitivity to the regulation of breathing by neural and chemical components (13), decreased chest wall compliance and muscle mass, decreased gas exchange (13), increased degenerative changes in the bony thorax, and increased kyphotic deformity of the spine. Maximum O_2 consumption ($\dot{V}O_2max$) decreases with age, but this is probably due to cardiovascular limitations in O_2 delivery (14). It is also interesting to note that the elderly may exhibit disordered breathing patterns during sleep with apneic and hypoxic periods (14).

PULMONARY FUNCTION CHANGES WITH BED REST

Pulmonary changes that occur as a result of prolonged bed rest and deconditioning can be summarized to include decreased $\dot{V}O_2max$, alterations in lung volumes and ventilation-perfusion parameters (15), increased work of breathing, ventilatory muscle weakness and decreased coordination, increased atelectasis, and decreased cough effectiveness.

ABNORMAL RESPIRATION AND VENTILATION

Restrictive Diseases

Restrictive diseases have as their hallmark a particular spirographic pattern, showing reduced total lung volume and residual volume. The flow-volume loops in restrictive disease show a small area within the loop, and a straight expiratory segment. The restriction can be due to abnormalities in the chest wall, leading to reduced compliance, or in the lung itself. Diseases characterized by weakness of the respiratory muscles without changes in compliance of the chest wall or lungs yield a restrictive spirographic pattern and hence are considered *restrictive disorders*.

A variety of conditions can act to decrease compliance of the chest wall. These include skeletal conditions, most notably severe kyphosis and scoliosis. Spasticity of the chest wall muscles and obesity also decrease compliance of the chest wall.

All causes of neuropathy or myopathy affecting proximal skeletal muscles may produce a restrictive ventilatory pattern.

Many conditions affecting the lung itself may produce restrictive ventilation. Fibrosis of the lung, either reactive, postinflammatory, or idiopathic, is a common cause of severe restrictive defects.

Obstructive Disease

Obstructive conditions are conditions of the airways, that have in common large total lung volumes, large reserve volumes, and a small flow-volume loop with a concave expiratory segment. Normal lung parenchyma is elastic; its protein matrix provides tension on the walls of the airways within it, keeping them open as the lung volumes shrink during expiration. This elasticity is destroyed in the patient with emphysema, because of processes still only partially understood; without the elasticity, small airways tend to collapse as intrathoracic pressure rises during expiration.

Airway goblet cells secrete mucus, which is moved by ciliary action toward the throat whence it is expectorated or swallowed. The normal response to airway inflammation is an increase in mucous production and a thickening of the airway wall; if the inflammation is chronic, constant secretion of copious amounts of mucus results. The smooth muscle of the airways can also become overreactive and hypertrophied as a result of chronic inflammation. The mucus, thick airway walls, and constriction of the smooth muscle obstruct expiratory flow.

Cystic fibrosis is a recessive disorder, caused by a "double dose" of an abnormal CFTR gene (16). Ciliary motion is impaired in persons with cystic fibrosis, and bronchial mucus is abnormally thick and tenacious; continual infection results, with progressive bronchiectasis. Over half of patients live into adulthood now. Most carriers of cystic fibrosis, and most fetuses destined to have the disease, can now be identified. Gene therapy shows great promise in animal models.

GOALS OF PULMONARY REHABILITATION

Most authors agree that pulmonary rehabilitation programs are not actually designed to reverse lung disease pathology or improve lung function. Most programs are designed with the major goal of improving quality of life, functional independence, and subjective symptomatology, primarily dyspnea (17,18). As Tiep (18) described, "The basic philosophy of training in the activities of daily living is for patients to be able to minimize the energy cost of such essential activities as grooming, hygiene, preparing meals, and maintaining environmental neatness and cleanliness, while leaving room for quality-of-life activities."

Table 80-1 is a list of goals of various pulmonary rehabilitation programs cited from multiple sources (18–20).

Table 80-1: Goals of Various Pulmonary Rehabilitation Programs
Decrease subjective dyspnea with activities (exertional dyspnea) (19)
Increase functional endurance (20) for activities of daily living and mobility and reverse as much disability as possible
Increase strength and endurance of respiratory muscles via a targeted muscle training program
Improve breathing patterns and coordination
Improve education regarding disease process, exacerbations, and early recognition of infection
Decrease or preferably eliminate smoking
Improve nutrition
Optimize medications and O_2 therapy
Decrease anxiety and depression
Increase energy
Improve quality of life and increase functional independence
Develop a safe exercise program to enhance function and prevent further deconditioning (18)
Effectively utilize activity pacing and prioritization of activities
Teach energy conservation, activity planning, and organization
Develop effective relaxation techniques
Improve body mechanics and decrease excessive body movements with activities (18)
Alter environmental contributors—i.e., minimize chemical exposure to lung pollutants, aerosols, powders, allergens, cigarette/cigar smoke (18)
Improve sleep patterns (18)

EVALUATION OF PULMONARY REHABILITATION CANDIDATES

Virtually any patient with respiratory or ventilatory impairment has potential goals for pulmonary rehabilitation. If serious contraindications to exercise are present, patient and family education may be the worthy goal. Patients with an extremely limited exercise capacity can often attain increased endurance for activities of daily living (ADLs) by an exercise program based on short intervals of functional activities (e.g., walking).

Every attempt should be made to evaluate the patient's motivation for improvement as fully as possible. The physician should discuss with the patient in detail what commitment of time and alterations in risk factors will be expected as part of the pulmonary rehabilitation program. If the patient believes he or she cannot fulfill the expectations, the program will have less likelihood of success. Some patients have unrealistic goals and cannot see the value of lesser, achievable goals; these patients are unlikely to feel they have benefited by a rehabilitation program. Patients who do not show sincere attempts to quit smoking are unlikely to benefit from a long course of pulmonary rehabilitation.

Detailed data on coexisting conditions; a history of heart, peripheral vascular, cerebrovascular, and orthopedic conditions; results of any relevant studies; and an accurate list of medications are necessary for the prerehabilitation evaluation. Patients may arrive for the first interview with inadequate documentation; every effort must be made at the time the appointment is made to get all relevant documentation in hand by the time the patient arrives.

Many aspects of the history and physical examination are of particular relevance with pulmonary patients, and may not routinely be a part of all physiatric examinations. At the preliminary interview, the physiatrist should find out how long the patient has been on supplemental O_2 (if applicable), how many times the patient has been intubated, the patient's steroid history for the past several months, the history of attempts at smoking cessation, and the history of exercise—both supervised and unsupervised.

The physical examination must make note of paradoxical breathing, an increase in rate, and the pattern of respiration during minimal exercise.

Functional assessment should include a 6-minute walk test or a similar integrated functional test, and serial capillary saturation checks (Pulsox) at rest and during and after exercise; neither spirometry nor analysis of resting blood gases can indicate in which patients O_2 desaturation will occur during exercise. A graded exercise test using a low-intensity protocol such as the McNaughton protocol is helpful to determine maximum O_2 usage and the presence of exercise-provoked arrhythmias, unsuspected cardiac ischemia, and unsuspected poor ventricular function, as well as to determine the maximal heart rate. The Bruce protocol, familiar to all cardiac stress laboratory personnel, is unsuited to most pulmonary rehabilitation candidates.

By considering the patient's background information as well as the results of selected tests as just mentioned, the physiatrist can arrive at a very exact notion of where the patient stands functionally with regard to the pulmonary disease, which will be much more exact than information gained solely by a general physiatric history and physical examination. This knowledge enables the physician to prescribe an individual, safe exercise program, and to monitor the patient's progress during and following the rehabilitation program.

The physiatrist also needs to inquire into the patient's nutritional history. If the patient is obese, the history should include information regarding attempts at weight loss and methods.

A significant number of pulmonary patients have psychological issues that will interfere with the best outcome of their rehabilitation. In addition, many pulmonary patients exhibit neuropsychiatric deficits that are not obvious during an interview or first examination. Such patients should be examined by a person or persons with expertise in both neuropsychiatric testing and clinical psychology.

MEMBERS OF THE PULMONARY REHABILITATION TEAM

The makeup of the pulmonary rehabilitation team depends on the type of program (inpatient, outpatient, home-based, or community-based program) and facility and the equipment available. Most programs include any or all of the team members listed in Table 80-2 (18,21).

Table 80-2: Pulmonary Rehabilitation Team Members
Pulmonologist/internist/family medicine practitioner/geriatrician
Physiatrist
Nurse
Respiratory therapist
Occupational therapist
Physical therapist
Social worker
Nutritionist
Psychologist (18)
Clinical pharmacist
Patient/family member
Recreational therapist
Exercise physiologist
Pastoral care representative
Psychiatrist
Vocational rehabilitation counselor
Speech therapist (especially for patient with tracheotomy, head/neck surgery, facial deformity, or neuromuscular weakness)
Biofeedback technician
Home care team
Program coordinator/medical director (21)
Thoracic surgeon
Prosthetist/orthotist (to fabricate and fit appropriate braces or custom interfaces for noninvasive ventilatory support)

TREATMENT ARMAMENTARIUM FOR PATIENTS WITH RESPIRATORY DYSFUNCTION

Pulmonary Medications

The major categories of medications used to treat various types of pulmonary diseases or conditions include the following (22–24):

- Bronchodilators. Oral, inhaled, intravenous, and mininebulizer. These preparations may have adrenergic or anticholinergic effects.
- β_2 selective or nonselective agents. Examples include albuterol and theophylline. These agents cause relaxation of bronchial smooth muscle, though the mechanism of action of theophylline is still unclear. The side effects generally include anxiety, arrhythmia, headache, nausea, vomiting, diarrhea, seizures, tremor, decreased peripheral vascular resistance with some agents, increased cardiac output, and insomnia. Theophylline has been reported to cause increased secretion of gastric acid (22) and may also act as a mild respiratory stimulant.
- Antibiotics.
- Steroids. These are available in oral, intravenous, and inhaled preparations. The mechanism of action is still largely unknown. The side effects include an increased susceptibility to infections, peptic ulcer disease exacerbation, osteoporosis, myopathy, blood glucose metabolism alterations, behavioral or psychiatric changes, congestive heart failure or exacerbation, cataracts (23), and appetite changes.
- Immunosuppressive agents and cytotoxic agents.
- Cough suppressants and expectorants.
- Mucolytic agents.
- Cromolyn sodium (disodium cromoglycate). This agent stabilizes mast cell membranes. It is used for prophylaxis only, not for acute attacks of bronchoconstriction.
- Psychotropic agents. These drugs reduce anxiety and promote relaxation.
- Vaccine (flu, pneumococcal). This is used for preventive purposes (24).

- Anticholinergic agents. These agents inhibit acetylcholine release from the intrapulmonary motor nerves that supply bronchial smooth muscle. Ipratropium bromide is the most commonly used of these agents. It is poorly absorbed and thus produces little to no systemic "atropine-like" effects (22).
- α_1-Antitrypsin replacement therapy for emphysema patients with known α_1-antitrypsin deficiency.

Most pharmacologic regimens for the patient with pulmonary disease involve some combination of the above-listed agents, and must be constantly monitored and adjusted for effective treatment.

Other Drugs That Affect Pulmonary Function

Medications taken for other conditions can affect pulmonary function. These may include various cardiac drugs, chemotherapeutic agents, antibiotics, anti-inflammatory drugs, oral hypoglycemics, antiepileptic agents, anticholinergic drugs including tricyclics (25), other drugs affecting the central nervous system, and other drugs [heroin, methadone, propoxyphene (Darvon), talc] (23).

Glucocorticosteroids

Congeners of cortisol commonly have toxicities that are significant in the patient's rehabilitation. Steroids are given over the short or long term for a variety of pulmonary diseases, because of their anti-inflammatory and immunosuppressive effects. A number of other drugs sharing steroidal, anti-inflammatory, and immunosuppressive properties, but with different toxicities, are now used instead of or in combination with steroids, so that smaller doses of steroids may be prescribed.

Steroid-induced myopathy initially affects the proximal skeletal muscles more than the distal muscles; as it advances, the distal muscles become more involved. The duration of steroid treatment seems more important than the dosage in the development of this disease. Unlike many other myopathies, it is not characterized by denervation on electromyograms (EMGs); accelerated recruitment of units and small units are typical, as in other myopathies. This condition is often suspected in patients who have suddenly accelerating weakness due to a number of potential causes in whom it is impossible to determine what percentage of a patient's weakness is due to a particular factor.

Treatment of this condition represents a formidable challenge: Stopping steroid therapy is desirable, but it cannot be done in most patients. Since stopping steroid usage is not an option, the physician must develop alternative management strategies. Treatment requires careful evaluation for other potential contributing factors, especially including malnutrition or other weakening drugs.

The effects of exercise therapy in the patient with steroid myopathy have not been well studied; a program of mild- to moderate-intensity exercise tailored to the patient's degree of weakness, in conjunction with correction of other weakening factors, strengthens the patient over time. Many months may be required, and often the patient is left with residual proximal weakness.

Steroids stimulate osteoclasts and inhibit osteoblasts; calcium loss from bone occurs in every patient taking steroids. If the steroids are continued for a long period of time, or if the patient previously had low bone density, clinically significant osteoporosis can occur. Painful vertebral compression fractures are common, but rarely lead to neurologic deficits. Rib fractures during coughing occur commonly. Administration of calcium, vitamin D, or sex hormones may slow but do not stop the calcium loss. Bisphosphonates and calcitonin are under evaluation (26).

Steroids interfere with the inflammatory and immune responses; common signs of local infection or of sepsis, including swelling, warmth, tenderness, erythema, fever, and malaise, may be absent. Cell-mediated immunity is depressed; fungal and other unusual infections occur. Even a short course of high-dose steroids may result in devastating infection. Steroids cause the demargination of polymorphonuclear leukocytes and hence white blood cell counts of 12,000 to 25,000/μL; the percentage of band cells is normal. Bandemia generally indicates infection.

Many patients on steroids experience changes in mood; a few patients experience psychotic mania or major depression. These effects are dose related; patients vary widely in their sensitivities to these drugs. The absence of a history of psychiatric diagnoses is no guarantee that a patient will not be very sensitive to the psychiatric effects of these drugs.

New or increased glucose intolerance caused by steroids often requires changes in insulin administration.

Cyclosporine

Cyclosporine is routinely used to prevent transplant rejection, and more recently has found use as an immunosuppressive agent for a variety of other diseases. In heart transplant patients, it causes calcium loss from bone (27); the same may hold true for lung transplant patients. The drug is nephrotoxic (28) and routinely causes hypertension, which is controllable by routine antihypertensive drugs (29). Sustension hand tremor is routinely seen, but rarely causes difficulty in ADLs; it may be ameliorated by β-blockers. Gum hyperplasia occurs often. Colchine causes myopathy in cyclosporine-treated patients.

PHYSICAL MEDICINE AND REHABILITATION MEASURES

Physical therapeutic measures for treating patients with pulmonary disease generally include positioning techniques, chest physical therapy maneuvers, assisted cough techniques, breathing exercises, and general conditioning exercises and respiratory muscle exercises. Additionally, strategies of energy conservation and work simplification, relaxation techniques and biofeedback, maximization of respiratory therapy (use of mini-nebulizers, metered-dose inhalators, O_2) with physical activity, psychological support for adjustment to disability, nutritional support, smoking cessation, vocational rehabilitation evaluations and treatment, and home assessments and family training also fall into the realm of the rehabilitation approach to the patient with pulmonary disease.

Positioning

Body position influences the length-tension relationships of the respiratory muscles and chest wall components, vascular volume shifts, changes in ventilation gradients, and O_2 transport to the body tissues. Positioning techniques are used with chest physical therapeutic programs to drain dislodged secretions. Position also plays a very important role in relaxation training; patients are taught positions that provide support of the body segments to promote relaxation of accessory, abdominal, neck, and shoulder girdle muscles (30). These positions can improve endurance for ADLs, sexual activities, and vocational and avocational interests; they can also be used to help patients regain control of their breathing if they become dyspneic with particular activities. In many patients with chronic obstructive pulmonary disease (COPD), breathing patterns are improved by the supine and leaning-forward positions, which tend to elevate the diaphragm, improve its excursion, and increase its efficiency of contraction (7). In patients with spinal cord injury (SCI), the level of injury can usually predict the degree of respiratory impairment that can be expected (combinations of altered ventilation volumes or cough dysfunction). In quadriplegic patients, "the vital capacity of these individuals improves when they are supine, because of the relative displacement of the diaphragm into the chest, resulting in improvement in the length-tension relation and in diaphragmatic function" (10). Abdominal binders are helpful for SCI patients for this same reason.

Chest Percussion and Physical Therapy

Chest physical therapy often refers to a venerable group of techniques aimed at loosening and clearing pulmonary secretions. The techniques include percussion, shaking, and vibration applied to a patient in specific body positions. The indications for their use for acute pneumonia or exacerbation of COPD remain controversial; they are still generally employed in patients with bronchiectasis or cystic fibrosis, and in select patients with neurologic diseases who have difficulty clearing secretions.

Percussion, or "clapping," is a technique in which the therapist uses cupped hands to deliver mild blows to designated areas of the chest wall to enhance postural drainage of secretions through the airways. Twelve basic positions for postural drainage have been described (31).

For the shaking technique, the therapist applies both hands to the designated area of the chest wall; the patient inhales deeply, and during exhalation the therapist shakes the chest wall rather vigorously to effect secretion clearance.

For the vibration technique, the therapist places his or her hands, one on top of the other, over the designated chest wall segment and tenses and relaxes the elbow extensors almost isometrically to deliver an in-and-out vibratory impulse.

Both shaking and vibration are most often utilized after percussion. These techniques, in addition to cough instruction and education, are employed to improve respiratory hygiene and can be administered manually or mechanically. A number of different protocols using these techniques have been developed through the years. In all, body position is the key so that secretions dislodged from the airway walls can drain toward the central airways and be cleared by cough or suctioning.

Relative contraindications to the use of chest physical therapy modalities include unstable cardiac disease or arrhythmias, traumatic or pathologic rib fractures, spinal instability, significant osteoporosis or other bone disease, coagulopathies or platelet dysfunction, any pulmonary or gastrointestinal condition that could lead to hemorrhage or bleeding in the upper thoracic structures, unstable neurologic disease or elevated intracranial pressure, or if chest physical therapy techniques exacerbate bronchospasm (32). Faling (7) also recommended that "percussion should not be applied to the spine, sternum, or soft tissues overlying the kidneys or other vital organs."

Recommendations for force, duration, and frequency of percussion therapy treatment sessions are variable throughout the literature.

Assisted Cough Techniques

Assisted cough techniques may be necessary to help patients with abdominal muscle weakness (e.g., SCI, neuromuscular disease, elderly, deconditioned, or trauma patients) generate enough expiratory force to clear their airways. Cough is facilitated by the therapist or patient by placing his or her first below the xiphoid process. The patient then takes a deep breath and during forced expiration against a closed glottis, the fist is thrust inward and upward in an attempt to increase diaphragm motion leading to increased expiratory pressure. Patients with weak upper extremities may bend their upper torso over their fist in the position just described during the expiratory phase of the cough. It is important to remember that coughing techniques are a precise discipline, and if they are performed incorrectly or uncontrollably, dyspnea and bronchospasm can actually worsen.

A mechanical device (In-Exsufflator, J. H. Emerson) is available to simulate steps in the cough mechanism for patients with inadequate cough. This machine delivers a maximal inspiration through a mask; it then develops an immediate negative pressure so that the lungs empty very rapidly. High flow velocities have been measured (33); no tracheostomy or tracheal suction is required.

When patients are unable to cough adequately even with the above-described methods, tracheal suctioning may be necessary to clear airways of secretions. Complications of suctioning include patient discomfort, hypoxemia, cardiac arrhythmias, alterations in blood pressure, tracheal injury, increased intracranial pressure, and infections (32).

Respiratory Muscle Exercises

According to Faling (7), "the intent of breathing training is to 1) restore the diaphragm to a more normal position and function, 2) control the respiratory rate and breathing pattern to diminish air trapping, 3) decrease the work of breathing, and 4) allay patient dyspnea and anxiety."

Breathing exercises include strengthening and endurance exercises for the ventilatory muscles, relaxation techniques, altered breathing patterns (breathing retraining and segmental breathing, glossopharyngeal breathing (GPB) in some limited circumstances), pursed-lip breathing, paced breathing, and chest wall mobilization techniques. The goals of breathing exercises are to increase tidal volumes and to improve oxygenation.

Muscles of inspiration can be strengthened by progressive resistance training. This is commonly accomplished by using one of a variety of inexpensive spring-loaded inspiratory resistance devices. The patient's maximum load is determined using the device, and he or she is then trained at about 30% of the maximum load daily. Progressive increases in maximum load occur over time. Clinical benefit has been more difficult to show for many patients, and factors predicting clinical benefit are under investigation.

Patients with moderately to severely advanced pulmonary disease show a variety of abnormalities in their pattern of breathing; a number of retraining techniques have been devised to correct the pattern. Breathing retraining techniques include diaphragmatic breathing exercises, pursed-lip breathing, paced breathing with exercise, and exhalation with exercise or activity (34).

In patients with neuromuscular disease, GPB is a distinctive method of respiration whereby air is moved to the trachea by pharyngeal muscles, a small amount at a time; the process is repeated until ultimately an adequate tidal volume is achieved. Most patients can be taught to perform GPB with greater or lesser success. Some patients can employ it for long ventilator-free periods. A sincere attempt should be made to teach GPB to all neuromuscular ventilated patients for emergency use, and for the convenience of at least short, ventilator-free intervals (see Glossopharyngeal Breathing section later in this chapter for a more detailed description of GPB).

Patients with obstructive lung disease with depressed diaphragms use accessory muscles of inspiration, while using their diaphragms less than normal people. With the technique of diaphragmatic breathing, many of these patients can be taught to make further use of their diaphragm by monitoring the motion of their hand on their abdomen as they inspire and expire. The technique involves slow controlled inspiration through the nose accompanied by increased abdominal contraction and protrusion of abdominal contents. These actions are followed by contraction of the abdominal muscles during exhalation. Once the patient has mastered the feeling of this type of respiration, it can be used in other activities, including walking and the performance of ADLs. A few patients report significant decreases in dyspnea by using this technique; most do not. Predictors of success are unknown.

Pursed-lip breathing is discovered by most severely involved COPD patients on their own. Pursed-lip breathing involves slow controlled inspiration followed by expiration through pursed lips with or without concomitant abdominal muscle contraction (7). In addition to slowing the respiratory rate, pursed-lip breathing apparently keeps small airways from closing too early in expiration (30). Many patients report that this technique helps them avert crises and get their breathing back in control.

Many patients with severe obstructive lung disease take fast, shallow breaths that barely suffice to ventilate dead space. Paced breathing is an attempt to give more time for expiration, and hence a larger tidal volume. The patient is taught to count during inspiration and expiration, and to allot a progressively longer time for expiration as training proceeds. In our experience, this method does work to slow breathing, especially in anxious COPD patients who get the benefit of relaxation as a result of concentrating on the technique.

Segmental lung expansion training is often mentioned, usually in the context of scoliotic or other bony deformities, or areas of atelectasis distal to a mucus plug. The theory is that the patient can learn to expand unaerated lung in the compromised areas of the chest, resulting in greater gas exchange. We have not observed much success with this type of training.

Relaxation training may involve respiratory counting, self-hypnosis, visual imagery, biofeedback, and position and posture retraining techniques to decrease dyspnea and tachypnea and improve respiratory efficiency.

Chest wall mobilization techniques are described as exercises designed to stretch the musculature of the thorax and improve rib excursion and thoracic posture.

General Conditioning Exercises

After obtaining an appropriate history, performing physical and office functional examinations, and reviewing the results of the pulmonary stress tests, the physician can write the exercise prescription. It behooves all health care clinicians who prescribe exercise for patients to become familiar with the guidelines for exercise stress testing including indications, precautions, and contraindications as described by the American College of Sports Medicine (35) and the American Heart Association (36). "An initial formal exercise test is useful for determining exercise capacity, for detecting oxygen desaturation, hypercapnia, and arrhythmias, and for helping to exclude coexistent ischemic heart disease" (37). The exercise prescription should include the type of exercise being recommended (including specification of aerobic versus anaerobic activity), the frequency with which it should be performed, the duration of the training sessions, the intensity of the activity, and appropriate warm-up and cooldown phases. Prescriptions should also include precautions with minima and maxima for vital signs, patient education regarding self-monitoring techniques (target heart rate, Borg scale, talk test, etc), and orders for the appropriate use of pulse oximetry monitoring, telemetry monitoring, and use and adjustment of supplemental O_2 during therapies. Blood gas and pulse oximetry measurements should be recorded both at rest and during exercise to obtain the most accurate assessment of supplemental O_2 requirements.

Patients with very severe COPD are usually restricted more by their ventilatory capacity than by their cardiovascular system, so teaching such patients to monitor their exercise intensity via use of a recommended target heart rate may not be feasible (38). The Borg scale may be a more practical index of intensity of activity for these patients.

A general conditioning program for the pulmonary patient usually includes appropriate warm-up and cooldown phases; strengthening and flexibility exercises for the legs (especially the hip extensors and muscles of mobility), arms, neck, trunk, abdomen, and shoulder girdle muscles; posture retraining; progressive functional training (stair climbing, walking on uneven surfaces, carrying objects, outdoor walking, managing supplementary O_2 canisters); and a progressive aerobic program involving walking (treadmill or routine) or cycling. For high-functioning patients, swimming provides a useful low-impact aerobic activity.

Upper-extremity activity at a given intensity of external work creates greater ventilatory demand than does lower-extremity activity (24). Since ADLs require much upper-extremity work, these extremities should be trained as well. Specific supported-arm strengthening and conditioning activities (e.g., arm ergometry, pulley work, and ball-throwing activities) are well tolerated and lead to greater strength and endurance for these activities. Whether these gains generalize to greater functionality and less dyspnea in ADLs has been questioned; we find that they do. A more specific discussion of particular exercises and activities for the pulmonary rehabilitation patient may be found in the section entitled Exercise Prescription later in this chapter.

Vocational Rehabilitation Evaluation and Treatment

Vocational rehabilitation evaluations involve assessment of the patient's occupational history and current appropriate vocational interests, and the development of a program that will result in the patient being able to return to gainful employment if possible. This end may be achieved by manipulation of current job hours, responsibilities, or environment (accessibility and adaptive equipment considerations), or training to develop other marketable skills with job placement services.

Home Assessments and Family Training

Home assessments should be performed by the treating therapists, when appropriate, to evaluate the home's layout to improve efficiency and decrease a patient's required energy expenditure during home tasks, evaluate the home environment for safety, assess for and design first-floor setups if necessary, and assess the need for specific durable medical equipment.

Before a patient is sent home for the first time with home ventilators or home O_2, the patient and family require much more instruction than do routine physical medicine and rehabilitation patients and their families. Early family meetings and education are imperative. (See Patient and Family Education section.)

Family training sessions may be of benefit in educating family members in the proper ways to safely assist the patient with ADLs and mobility and in the proper use of equipment, and in having them participate in all of the components of the rehabilitation process and provide encouragement to the patient.

Psychological Evaluation and Therapy

Like other disabilities, respiratory disease has all-encompassing effects on the patient's life; the patient's reactions to these effects are complex and often deserve evaluation by a psychologist or psychiatrist. Other psychological issues entirely unrelated to the pulmonary rehabilitation program, such as conflict with a spouse, may have bearing on a patient's ability to take advantage of the program; the psychologist is very helpful in sorting out such issues. Many patients with obstructive disease have subtle neuropsychological deficits, which can be evaluated by testing; these data can help the team formulate more realistic goals and plan the optimum way of presenting information to the patient.

By the time a patient seeks pulmonary rehabilitation, he or she often has anxiety, depression, or perception of decreased quality of life. The patient may be angry or hopeless, perceiving an erosion in his or her ability to perform as a spouse or provider and in other social roles. Psychotherapy with or without antidepressive or anxiolytic drugs may improve the patient's function and sense of well-being.

Some patients seem to sabotage their own progress, due to severe issues of control or to character disorders. An expert psychotherapist may be able to alter some of these behaviors sufficiently for program goals to be met; if not, the team may elect to end the patient's rehabilitation program.

Nutritional Considerations

Many patients with obstructive disease have decreased lean body mass at the time of evaluation for a rehabilitation program. Causes include decreased appetite due to drug toxicities or frequent infections, increased work of breathing causing increased basal metabolic rate, frequent tracheobronchitis, the physical demands of chewing and swallowing causing increased dyspnea, the necessity to stop breathing while swallowing, steroid therapy, and deconditioning. The muscles of respiration may be involved in the atrophy accompanying a loss of lean body mass. Estimation of the deficit in lean body mass and its correction through adequate nutrition are part of the pulmonary rehabilitation program.

Patients with ventilatory dysfunction due to neuropathies or myopathies also have atrophy because of their inherent disease, and in some cases due to superimposed deconditioning. Only the portion of atrophy due to deconditioning can be corrected by exercise and nutrition.

Despite having low lean body mass, patients may be obese because of lack of exercise. Obesity itself contributes to the ventilatory dysfunction by adding to the work of lifting an obese chest wall during each inspiration. It also adds to the physiologic work of ambulation and ADLs.

For patients found to be obese or atrophic, an individually constructed dietary plan is provided by the team nutritionist, who then follows the patient closely and reports progress or changes in the plan to the team.

Social Service Assessment

The social service evaluation of the pulmonary rehabilitation patient includes assessment of the home setup and accessibility, the family support structure, acquired and required durable medical equipment, an evaluation of financial resources and insurance coverage, and an appraisal of the patient's premorbid responsibilities in the home with a special emphasis on who performed the cooking, cleaning, shopping, child rearing (if applicable), and finance management. The social worker may also assess the patient's vocational and avocational interests, and help to plan for the patient's continued participation in these activities. The social worker may be instrumental in arranging for companions, skilled nursing services, or nursing home placement as needed. Additionally, he or she may arrange for transportation services, home meal delivery, home nursing services, as well as information on available support services (support groups, respite care, hospice) and community day programs for appropriate patients.

Environmental Manipulation

Patients with pulmonary disease should learn to make careful assessments of their environments to maximize conditions for comfortable breathing. Exposure to ambient factors such as smoke (both primary and secondhand), extreme humidity, extreme heat or cold, high pollen counts, and high smog counts should be avoided whenever possible. In many communities, an air conditioner is a necessity for these patients; some cities have ordinances prohibiting electric companies from stopping power to such patients if they cannot pay their bill. Strong perfumes, spray mists, powders, and cleaning chemicals with harsh fumes should also be minimized or avoided. Patients with pulmonary disease must also carefully plan long trips or vacations and make special arrangements for their necessary O_2 and other equipment on planes, buses, and ships. Airlines usually require request forms for in-flight O_2 and they can help to determine more accurate O_2 needs, taking into consideration the anticipated flying altitude and possible takeoff and landing delays (39). In addition, cabin pressure is never maintained at sea level during flight. Every effort should be made to ascertain beforehand the cabin pressure for the model of plane to be used, and to determine O_2 requirements appropriate for that pressure.

Smoking Cessation

Cigarette smoking is responsible for most cases of chronic obstructive lung disease. The smoke contains numerous toxins affecting many organs; in the lung they produce inflammation of the airways and destruction of the alveoli, as well as loss of elasticity.

Patients who smoke and have no clinical signs of obstructive disease can delay or prevent onset of the disease by stopping smoking, and patients with COPD can slow the rate of deterioration of lung function. In addition, mucus production, reactive bronchial constriction, and dyspnea may decrease perceptibly, so that patients feel noticeably better within days to weeks after cessation, even if they have been smoking only a few cigarettes a day.

Many techniques to aid smokers in quitting have been propounded, including aversive conditioning techniques, other behavioral programs, individual or group counseling, hypnosis, acupuncture (40), and combinations. Many studies reported the results of smoking cessation programs in persons without clinical disease, or with coronary artery disease; few have studied smoking cessation in pulmonary patients. The latter group of trials showed successful cessation rates of up to 40% one year after the study, with a few percent returning to smoking each year thereafter (41). The benefits to those who do succeed are significant enough to warrant sincere efforts on the part of the physician.

Certain subgroups of pulmonary patients are more likely to achieve lasting success. An older patient who is male and married, lives with a nonsmoker, is from a higher socioeconomic group, wants to quit, and predicts success in quitting belongs to all the groups. Some studies found that more severe pulmonary disease increases the likelihood of success (42); another did not (43).

Seriously couched advice from a physician in the office to a patient with chronic bronchitis resulted in a cessation rate almost double that of patients who received no such advice (44).

Some programs rely primarily on the physician and some rely on other members of the team, usually the psychologist. Among the former are programs that emphasize drugs or other specialized techniques, such as acupuncture. Among the latter are a host of behavior-oriented techniques.

Nicotine is a physiologically addictive drug for many smokers. On the other hand, some smokers are "chippers"; that is, for them smoking is not a physiologically reinforced behavior (45). Patients who smoke first thing in the morning and average more than one cigarette an hour throughout the day are most likely to be physiologic addicts (46).

Nicotine polacrilex gum or nicotine transdermal patches may be used to deliver nicotine to a smoker who is addicted, to produce a blood level lower than that obtained by smoking, yet tolerable; nicotine inhalers are being studied clinically. All three show benefit in cessation rates (47). None give the sharp increase in nicotine level produced by smoking a cigarette. The patient should be advised that cravings will persist, particularly in the first few days; a date should be set for total abstinence. Bupropion, originally developed as an antidepressant, can reduce craving and unpleasant sensations, and result in higher cessation rates (48).

Patients should be advised not to smoke during the duration of a gum or patch program. Smoking then can result in very high levels of nicotine, which obviates the gradual withdrawal effect one seeks with the program and potentiates the addiction, as well as being toxic in itself.

Patients must be instructed, repeatedly if necessary, in the proper way of chewing the gum; otherwise it will release too much nicotine into the saliva and nauseate the patient. Proper technique involves chewing a little and then tucking the gum into one's cheek, where the nicotine will be absorbed slowly transmucosally, with a tolerable toxicity. Patients differ widely in the blood level of nicotine required to decrease their craving, so the amount of gum required will vary. The amount of gum should be decreased gradually over time, finally stopping completely. It is important to set concrete goals, with dates, in advance.

More recently, transdermal nicotine patches have been available, and like gum, yield a relatively constant level of nicotine in the serum to reduce craving. Also like gum, a schedule of use is set at the start of the program, with concrete goals for gradual reduction of blood nicotine levels; the patches come in different strengths, which can aid in gradual lowering of levels.

Patients must be educated as to what to expect. They may have strong cravings many times a day; the intensity and frequency of the cravings will probably decrease after the first week or so. Boredom or drinking can weaken the patient's resistance to cravings.

Patients should be as active as they can, since inactivity is likely to lead to cravings. General anxiety accompanies the cravings, and physical activity helps to dissipate this anxiety. Recreational or sports activities, or a formal exercise program are helpful.

VENTILATORY AIDS AND OXYGEN

Electrophrenic Pacing

Electrophrenic pacing, in which one or both phrenic nerves are rhythmically stimulated by an implanted device, may allow some C1–C2 tetraplegics to be decannulated. In other patients it is not useful, because of cost, complications including sudden failure, and patient preferences (see Phrenic Nerve Disorders section later in chapter for more details).

Glossopharyngeal Breathing

GPB is a method by which patients with weak diaphragm and accessory muscles of ventilation can breathe using bulbar muscles of the pharynx and the tongue. It is also known as *frog breathing*. Frog breathing, easily demonstrable in practice but very difficult to describe, consists of trapping a bolus of air in the pharynx by raising the tongue, and then propelling the air by compression of the pharynx down the trachea. The patient repeats this maneuver many times as the amount of air in the lungs builds up to a sufficient tidal volume; exhalation is passive, as always. This method must be taught by somebody who knows the technique; training aids in book and video form are helpful (49,50). Around 30% of chronically ventilator-dependent patients in a large series mastered the method well enough to give themselves a little time off the ventilator, ranging from a few minutes to, in some causes, many hours (51,52). In appropriate patients, this technique can be a valuable safety measure.

Home Oxygen Therapy

Patients with chronic hypoxemia benefit from prolonged administration of an O_2-enriched gas mixture (53). Pulmonary hypertension and right-sided heart failure improve, and mortality declines. Patients who are hypoxemic at rest benefit from 24-hour-a-day O_2 therapy; patients who are hypoxemic only when sleeping or during exercise need only receive O_2 during those times.

O_2 concentrators are capable of delivering O_2 at 4 to 5 L/m within the home; they are the most inexpensive mode of delivery, but are not portable. Compressed O_2 in tanks is available for home use; small tanks are heavy, but portable. Liquid O_2 is the most expensive and the most readily portable, with a comparatively light shoulder-bag system. The prescribing physician must consider the patient's lifestyle, as well as limitations imposed by the payer.

Nasal cannulae are light and nonclaustrophobic, and interfere minimally with speaking or eating. They may produce discomfort or skin breakdown behind the ears or at the nostrils. They may not deliver the desired concentration of O_2 in mouth breathers with congested nasal passages, or patients with very high O_2 needs. Devices that restrict O_2 flow to inspiration are available; they may be more or less effective in a given patient. Masks cause claustrophobia in some patients, and interfere with speaking and eating. Less visually obtrusive methods exist for use outside the home. Eyeglass frames that incorporate an O_2 line are available. More invasively, a tracheocutaneous fistula can be made low in the neck; a narrow-gauge catheter can be inserted for low-flow O_2 that bypasses the upper-airway dead space. The catheter can be hidden with a handkerchief or cravat. These stomas may be difficult to maintain in some patients and may cause unacceptable amounts of mucous production.

The Health Care Financing Administration (HCFA) has published guidelines for physicians to use in selecting patients for O_2 therapy: arterial pO_2 of 55 mm Hg or less or arterial O_2 saturation of 88% or less on room air, or arterial pO_2 less than 60 mm Hg or O_2 saturation of 89% with hematocrit above 56% or cor pulmonale; measurement of arterial pO_2 or saturation by a hospital laboratory or other Medicare-qualified laboratory; optimal medical management before beginning long-term O_2 therapy; recertification following 60 to 90 days after hospital discharge, if the patient was not previously using O_2 at home; physician submission of Form HCVA-484; and annual recertification, with physician evaluation within 90 days. Most payors use the HCFA standards to determine for which patients they will pay for O_2 therapy.

To benefit from home O_2 therapy, either the patient or the family must be willing and able to learn to manage the equipment, emergency procedures, and fire-safety precautions. Residence in rural areas may not preclude home O_2 therapy, as vendor services are available in many such areas. The responsibilities of the vendor to provide O_2 and to maintain the equipment are so vital that the physician should select vendors with the highest standards.

Mechanical Ventilation

Many patients become candidates for chronic mechanical ventilation after emergency intubation for acute respiratory failure caused by exacerbation of chronic lung disease. In a smaller number of ventilated patients, progressive neuromuscular disease causes a gradual worsening of ventilation; in them, mechanical ventilation is instituted electively. In the latter group, it is a smoother process, allowing for patient and family education beforehand.

Positive-Pressure Ventilation

Positive-pressure ventilation, through an endotracheal tube or tracheostomy, is by far the most common means of emergent mechanical ventilation. It allows high inflation pressures and a high concentration of inhaled O_2. Suction is easily applied to the endotracheal tube or tracheostomy. Continuous positive airway pressure (CPAP) or other modes of pressure support are instituted easily. Positive pressure decreases the amount of blood returned to the heart and may lower blood pressure. Pneumothorax occurs, particularly with end-expiratory pressure support. Although devices have been designed to enable the patient to talk, in general they cannot be used for patients with stiff lungs or copious secretions. The inflated cuff interferes with swallowing and the tube creates tracheal secretions.

When the patient's condition has improved, it may be possible to abruptly discontinue mechanical ventilation. More commonly, a weaning procedure is necessary. No set of physiologic measurements accurately predicts successful weaning. The diaphragm is strengthened gradually, by decreasing the intermittent mandatory ventilation rate, increasing the trigger pressure, or increasing the amount of ventilator-free time; each method is successful at the centers where it is used.

Exercise training can start while patients receive mechanical ventilation. Sessions should be scheduled when the patient is not weaning, until the weaning process is well advanced.

Several causes may contribute to slow weaning or failure to wean. Severe obstructive disease, prolific production of thick mucus, heart failure, and low diffusing capacity are common. A weak diaphragm may also prolong the weaning process. Diaphragmatic weakness may be due to malnutrition, electrolyte disturbances, steroid therapy, neuropathy of critical illness, profound diaphragmatic deconditioning, and unsuspected motor neuron disease or other progressive neuromuscular disease; it should be considered in patients who fail to wean. Rarely, the diaphragm is weak following unsuspected SCI at the time of intubation or transfer in the presence of cervical stenosis, or owing to ischemia following hypotension or aortic cross-clamping.

Theophylline and progesterone may strengthen the drive to respiration in patients who plateau near the end of the weaning process. Carbohydrates produce more CO_2 per calorie; a diet poor in carbohydrates and rich in lipids may decrease the ventilatory requirements of such patients.

Negative-Pressure Ventilation

Inspiration can be produced by negative pressure on the chest wall with the mouth at atmospheric pressure; this is clinically useful primarily in patients with neuromuscular disease. Many of these patients can be maintained on negative-pressure systems without the need for a tracheostomy, thus eliminating the mucous production, decrease in blood return to the heart, and risk of pneumothorax that tracheostomy positive-pressure ventilation entails. These patients can also eat and talk. Negative-pressure devices generally do not allow the patient's position to be changed conveniently.

Tank ventilators ("iron lungs") are now produced with plastic tanks, thus eliminating much of the weight; they are quite durable and reliable. Many old ones are still in use; they are bulky and heavy and do not conveniently allow caretaker access to the patient.

The chest cuirass is an appliance fitting over the front of the chest and delivering cyclical negative pressure from a small ventilator. The cuirasses usually have to be custom cast, and they have to be replaced regularly if the patient is a growing child. In adults they also have to be replaced, although less frequently, as the shape of the chest wall changes in response to the asymmetric negative pressure.

The poncho ventilator is a garment of densely woven nylon that covers the patient and a grille around the patient's chest. The front of the poncho has a port for attachment to a negative-pressure hose. The ankles, wrists, and neck must be adequately sealed each time the garment is applied, which often is troublesome to achieve.

Rocker Bed Ventilator

A rocker bed tilts head-down, causing the abdominal contents to fall toward the chest, producing expiration, then it tilts head-up, producing inspiration. The beds allow very simple access to the patient. The beds are large. Patients and their families may not be able to accustom themselves to the noise and the motion. The inspiratory and expiratory pressures produced are small, and may not be adequate to ventilate patients with any lung, airway, or chest wall abnormalities.

Mouth Positive Pressure Ventilation

Positive pressure may be applied through a mouthpiece. For many patients with neuromuscular hypoventilation, this method provides physiologically adequate ventilation without the mobility restrictions of negative pressure or the medical complications of tracheostomy. The patient is free to change position in bed and be mobile in a wheelchair. The mouthpiece may be held close to the mouth by a wheelchair attachment, so that the patient can release it to speak or to eat. Some patients are able to hold the mouthpiece even while sleeping. For others, a special holder keeps the mouthpiece in position, or the pressure may be delivered through a nasal mask at night.

SURGERY

Lung Volume Reduction Surgery

The surgery aims to remove parts of the hyperinflated lungs of COPD patients that have little activity in gas exchange owing to disease, thereby reducing dead space ventilation and improving ventilatory mechanics. A variety of imaging methods are used to identify appropriate areas in each patient; the apices are most commonly chosen. Depending on the area chosen, a sternotomy or a small thoracotomy approach is used; many of the operations are done thoracoscopically, with visualization by video. Chest wall pain is often severe after minithoracotomy; cryoablation of intercostal nerves, or epidural catheter placement may be done in the operating room. The results of surgery vary widely; most patients need less supplemental O_2 and have less dyspnea and better endurance for activities after recovery. Benefits last for at least a year (54). The long-term effects are not yet known. The operation is under intensive study; it is still classified as "experimental" by many payors.

Lung Transplantation

Lung transplantations have been done since 1963; currently, about 1000 transplant operations are performed annually. The supply of donor lungs limits the number of transplantations; lungs are not hardy, and often are damaged by trauma or shock, which other transplantable organs survive.

The ABO blood type and size of the donor are matched to those of the recipient. When the recipient's lungs are infected, as in cystic fibrosis or bronchiectasis, both lungs must be transplanted; in most other patients, transplantation of a single lung is adequate, so that one donor can donate to two recipients. If the recipient has irreversible cor pulmonale, both the heart and lung(s) are used. COPD patients were at first thought to require double-lung transplantation, lest the remaining native lung expand and prevent proper function of the transplanted lung; more recently, single-lung transplants have been usual for COPD patients as well, sometimes with the addition of a volume-reduction procedure on the remaining native lung. Indications include severe COPD, pulmonary fibrosis, cystic fibrosis, and idiopathic pulmonary hypertension. Immunosuppression is accomplished with steroids, azathioprine, and cyclosporine; new agents are under investigation. Recent figures show survival rates after the operation approaching 90% at 1 year (55).

TREATMENT CONSIDERATIONS FOR SPECIFIC DIAGNOSTIC GROUPS

Patients with pulmonary pathology who may benefit from rehabilitation services include those with diseases or conditions that cause restrictive or obstructive pulmonary disease patterns, phrenic nerve disorders, or other types of disease with secondary lung involvement, and those who have undergone lung procedures (transplantation and lung reduction).

Restrictive Neuromuscular Diseases

Some of the more commonly described neuromuscular diseases that cause restrictive lung pathology include the myopathies (including the muscular dystrophies), generalized neuropathies, motor neuron diseases, Guillain-Barré syndrome, poliomyelitis and postpoliomyelitis, multiple sclerosis, myasthenia gravis (56), and cervical and thoracic SCIs. It is beyond the scope of this chapter to discuss all of the epidemiologies, proposed etiologies, or usual disease courses, and the reader is referred to more specialized texts for this information (57,58).

Physiatric Components

Physiatric evaluation and treatment modalities include a complete medical and functional history, a comprehensive physical examination, and a thorough assessment of the patient's impairment, disability, and handicap from physical and psychosocial perspectives while considering patient and family goals for realistic levels of functional independence. This assessment is best accomplished utilizing a multidisciplinary team. Additional physiatric measures include specific prescriptions for exercise (including upper- and lower-extremity activities); breathing exercises and chest physical therapy, with appropriate and specific precautions and instructions for monitoring; functional training for ADLs with or without assistive devices; mobility and ambulation training with or without walking aids; energy conservation techniques including training in biomechanics; relaxation training; home evaluations; family training; patient and family education; vocational and avocational assessments; stress management and psychological support for adjustment to disability; and assignment and fitting of appropriate orthotic devices, prosthetic devices, and adaptive and durable medical equipment.

Of particular importance is the prescription of a custom-fitted wheelchair and the appropriate timing of use, especially in children with neuromuscular diseases and spinal deformities. The wheelchair prescription should be individualized to maximize the patient's mobility, transfer capability, and trunk support and posture to facilitate performance of upper-extremity activities. The seating system should be designed to avoid pressure and shear forces on the skin. Proper seating can minimize contractures and skin breakdown, and make the patient comfortable; unfortunately, neither orthotic aids nor modular or custom wheelchair seating can actually prevent the progression of scoliotic deformities in patients with certain neuromuscular diseases such as Duchenne muscular dystrophy (59).

The speech pathologist plays an important role in the rehabilitation of neuromuscular, tracheostomized, or head and neck surgery patients. These specialists can perform evaluations of swallowing and aspiration risk, give advice regarding appropriate food consistencies for diets, and provide treatment strategies and adaptive equipment for patients with various communication disorders, tracheostomies, or oral prosthetic devices.

Nonphysiatric Components

Nonphysiatric measures in the evaluation and treatment of patients with ventilatory pathology as a consequence of neuromuscular disease include comprehensive physical examinations, evaluations and treatment for concomitant disease conditions, cardiac assessments if warranted, medication management and pharmacologic interventions, regulation of supplemental O_2 therapy, nutritional repletion, smoking cessation, and spinal and other corrective surgeries as indicated (tendon lengthenings and transfers, etc).

An additional, critically significant nonphysiatric intervention involves the prescription and management of invasive and noninvasive forms of ventilation. Invasive methods generally include endotracheal intubation [with or without intermittent positive-pressure ventilation (IPPV) or positive end-expiratory pressure (PEEP)] and electrophrenic respiration. Noninvasive methods include use of negative-pressure body ventilators (i.e., "iron lung"), CPAP (or BiPAP for bi-level positive airway pressure) via a nasal or oral interface, noninvasive IPPV, rocking beds, chest shell ventilators, wrap-style ventilators, mechanical insufflation-exsufflation devices, mechanical oscillation techniques, and thoracoabdominal binders and corsets (60). As mentioned previously, GPB techniques may be taught as a backup method in the case of invasive or noninvasive ventilatory failure.

Decisions to ventilate and the method of ventilation chosen are important considerations for each individual patient and the family. These questions often involve consideration of quality of life issues, financial situations, realistic choices regarding available equipment based on diagnosis and disease stage, family and caregiver support, patient age, ethical issues, and the number of hours of ventilatory support that are required each day.

Musculoskeletal Disorders

Musculoskeletal disorders such as kyphosis, scoliosis (or commonly the combination of the two, as often seen in the elderly), spinal fractures, spinal muscular injury, arthritic conditions, and infectious, metabolic, and endocrinologic diseases affecting the spine or the thoracic bony structures have various etiologies and epidemiologies. They can exist independently or as a consequence of neuromuscular or other disease. These disorders also tend to produce a restrictive pathology with regard to breathing mechanics with reduced lung volumes.

Specific evaluation involves comprehensive assessment of the musculoskeletal deformity, joint stability, range of motion, functional mobility, strength, skin integrity, and current pulmonary status (see Evaluation of Pulmonary Rehabilitation Candidates). Decisions regarding corrective spinal surgery or other surgical procedures for progressive conditions must be carefully timed for adequate lung function to be preserved, for the incidence of postoperative complications to be decreased, and especially for successful weaning from the ventilator if possible. "The goal of therapy is to maximize existing capabilities and prevent further loss of motion that may develop from contractures of joints and deformity" (61).

Therapy

Physiatric and nonphysiatric treatment strategies for musculoskeletal disease are basically similar to those mentioned for neuromuscular disease, and depend on the degree of associated lung dysfunction and whether the musculoskeletal deformity is progressive or static. Spinal deformity such as kyphosis and scoliosis can also lead to chronic bony pain syndromes (compression fractures, etc), severe mobility restriction, and gastrointestinal disorders such as constipation (especially in the elderly) due to displacement of abdominal contents.

Interstitial Lung Diseases

Interstitial lung diseases, usually chronic in nature, involve the constituents that comprise the lung parenchyma in the lower respiratory tract. Most of these disorders have inflammatory or immune-mediated etiologies (23,25). The estimated prevalence for interstitial lung diseases in the United States is approximately 20 to 40 per 100,000 population, and the etiologies are often unknown (25). Patients often present with the nonspecific symptoms of exertional dyspnea and fatigue. Patients with interstitial lung disease usually demonstrate a restrictive pattern of respiratory pathology, with a decreased vital capacity and expiratory flow rate (62). Physical examination initially may be remarkable for decreased chest wall excursion, fine rales, clubbing of the digits, and cyanosis. Later findings may include pulmonary hypertension, but right-sided heart failure is not common. Blood gases may be remarkable for mildly decreased pO_2 values (especially induced by exercise) but rarely reveal elevated CO_2 levels. Conditions often associated with severe interstitial lung pathology may represent contraindications to pulmonary rehabilitation (e.g., acute congestive heart failure, severe pulmonary hypertension); when the patient is stable, a low-intensity mobilization program is usually well tolerated and safe.

Therapy

Physiatric treatment measures include a comprehensive history and physical examination and functional assessment as previously mentioned. Prescriptions for exercises; breathing exercises; chest physical therapy if warranted; ADL training; mobility, flexibility, and endurance activities; relaxation training and energy conservation techniques are also important. Family training and patient and family education regarding the disease process are critical to treatment plans for patients with progressive disease. Finally, vocational rehabilitation efforts may play a significant role for the patient who must be removed from occupational exposures that may have precipitated the lung condition.

Nonphysiatric treatment measures are similar to those mentioned for the other restrictive diseases discussed earlier. Pharmacologic agents used in treatment depend on the isolation of a causative agent or the discovery of a coexistent systemic condition.

Chronic Obstructive Lung Diseases

Patients with chronic bronchitis and emphysema are at risk for coronary artery disease; a stress test will allow the physician to determine the need for electrocardiographic monitoring during exercise. All attempts must be made to help patients stop smoking. The patients are generally middle-aged or elderly; any musculoskeletal pathology should be sought out with a history and physical examination, and the exercise program written to accommodate it. Heat or cold modalities may be needed; injection into a joint or trigger point may allow much more activity in the program. Nonsteroidal anti-inflammatory drugs (NSAIDs) should be used only for very short courses if at all; the danger of gastrointestinal bleeding is great. These patients are often osteoporotic, and treatment should be started if not already done.

Cystic Fibrosis

Optimization of nutritional status is particularly important. Psychology and recreational therapy referrals can be very helpful in these young patients who are chronically ill from an early age.

Lung Transplantation

In the hospital, reverse isolation procedures should be used; at Temple University Hospital, the patients are not confined to their rooms and may exercise in the gym. Emphasis is placed on strengthening of proximal muscles, including the gluteals, as well as general conditioning. Sternotomy precautions are observed where appropriate. These patients weaken very quickly in bed, usually having a long history of exercise intolerance and steroid use; their exercise should begin as soon as they are awake with stable vital signs, even if still in the intensive care unit.

Lung Volume Reduction Surgery

Persistent postthoracotomy pain must be dealt with early, lest the shoulder become contracted due to splinting. Cold application or transcutaneous electrical nerve stimulation may help; blocking the intercostal nerve at the surgical level plus one level above and below almost always produces relief, and allows deep respiration and shoulder mobilization.

Spinal Cord Injury

Patients with SCI may suffer from several types of ventilatory insufficiency, depending on the level and degree of injury. Cell bodies of the phrenic nerve are located at C3–C5, with most at C4 according to most authorities. Cell bodies subserving the auxiliary muscles of inspiration are located in the cervical region of the cord; most axons travel through the brachial plexus, while those subserving the upper trapezius and sternocleidomastoid muscles travel rostrally in the spinal canal through the foramen magnum, joining the spinal accessory nerve. The cell bodies of intercostal nerves are distributed by level up and down the thoracic region of the cord. Lower thoracic segments contain cell bodies subserving the abdominal muscles as well.

If phrenic nerve dysfunction is slight, a patient may be able to accomplish tidal breathing, but not to sigh; atelectasis and mucous plugging result. GPB or mouth positive-pressure ventilation can give such patients additional tidal volume to accomplish sighing, to rest the diaphragm intermittently, or to increase volume before an assisted cough. Mouth positive-pressure ventilation or noninvasive negative-pressure ventilation may be necessary during bouts of respiratory illness.

More severe phrenic dysfunction causes denervation and atrophy of the diaphragm, and inspiratory failure. In injuries above C4, the phrenic nerve is intact, but inspiratory impulses from above are blocked; the phrenic nerve can be stimulated exogenously, producing inspiration, although this capability has thus far not been reliably implemented in practice. These patients will have to rely on mechanical ventilation most of the time. Some of the patients can use GPB for ventilator-free intervals, including times of ventilator malfunction. In most patients the chest wall is sufficiently stiff that negative-pressure ventilation is impractical.

The patient with thoracic or low cervical injuries will have more or less difficulty coughing effectively to clear secretions. Postural drainage and percussion help mobilize secretions, and several techniques exist for assisted coughing (see Assisted Cough Techniques). With a cervical or high thoracic level of injury, bronchoscopy may be needed from time to time to remove mucous plugs, especially during periods of tracheobronchitis.

Phrenic Nerve Disorders

The phrenic nerve consists of fibers from the anterior primary rami of C3–C5 cervical segments, plus varying contributions from C2 or C6 (63). The nerve courses through the neck and mediastinum to eventually innervate the diaphragm. Unilateral or bilateral phrenic nerve injuries have multiple etiologies, including direct traumatic injury to the nerve(s) during intrathoracic, neck, or high abdominal surgical procedures or from direct chest, neck, or abdominal trauma; high cervical spinal injury; neuralgic amyotrophy (64); open heart surgery performed with cold cardioplegia during bypass (65); generalized peripheral neuropathies; uremic neuropathy (66); critical illness neuropathy; and invasive neck or thoracic cancers.

Evaluation

Patients may present with complaints of dyspnea, exercise intolerance, other symptoms of peripheral neuropathy or neuromuscular junction disorder, failure to wean from a ventilator, or other signs or symptoms of respiratory insufficiency. Methods of evaluation always include a comprehensive history and physical examination. Chest computed tomography (67), chest radiographs, or diaphragmatic ultrasound or fluoroscopy can reveal abnormal diaphragm motion or position (68). Esophageal, gastric, and transdiaphragmatic pressure measurements can also provide information about diaphragmatic function (69). Phrenic nerve conduction studies and diaphragmatic electromyography may give even earlier indications of phrenic nerve dysfunction, as well as more useful prognostic information about recovery. Well-established and reliable methods for performing phrenic nerve conduction studies (63) and electromyographic evaluation of the diaphragm (70) have been described.

Patients with SCI at cervical level C1 or C2, above the segments that supply the diaphragm may be candidates for electrophrenic respiration "EPR requires the bilateral viability of the phrenic nerves" (10). "EPR involves the transmission of a radiowave signal by an antenna placed on the skin to an implanted receiver. The signal is converted to electrical impulses that are carried to electrodes in contact with the phrenic nerves. The impulses can be delivered in a manner that simulates the natural recruitment of phrenic nerve fibers to stimulate the diaphragm" (60). This requires the operative implantation of stimulating and receiving electrodes followed by an extensive training period for the patient, to ensure proper use and provide education regarding equipment management. The invasive nature of the procedure, limited population of appropriate candidates, extensive training requirements, high cost, and potential complications with this method make it one of the less commonly used treatment modalities.

Diseases with Secondary Lung Involvement

Various diseases without primary lung involvement may be associated with secondary lung pathology. Secondary lung pathology must always be considered in the prescription for rehabilitation for these patients. For example, patients with cardiac disease may have pulmonary congestion or effusions. Patients with some types of cancer may have metastatic involvement of the lung, postoperative atelectasis or phrenic nerve injury, or fibrotic lung changes from certain medications or radiation. Patients with any type of neuromuscular disease, musculoskeletal deformity, cerebrovascular disease, traumatic brain injury, cervical or thoracic SCI, multiple sclerosis, certain types of rheumatic disease, connective tissue or collagen vascular disease, or certain autoimmune diseases may be affected by secondary lung changes or respiratory compromise from diaphragmatic weakness. Appropriate precautions, monitoring, O_2 requirements, and exercise parameters should always be addressed in the exercise prescriptions for these patients.

EXERCISE PRESCRIPTION

The purpose of exercise in pulmonary patients is to strengthen the muscles of respiration if they are weak, increase endurance for mobility and other activities, lessen activity-associated dyspnea, lessen fatigue following activity, and aid in weight loss if needed.

Many pulmonary patients are incapable of even moderate-intensity exercise or prolonged exercise. They may be trained using short intervals of exercise interspersed with relatively long rest periods.

Both lower- and upper-extremity strengthening and endurance activities should be used. Higher-functioning patients need a few minutes for warm-up. Thirty minutes to an hour of exercise, including rest periods, is appropriate, depending on the patient. The intensity is low, and daily sessions seldom cause musculoskeletal problems; a home program should be included in the prescription for off days in patients who do not need electrocardiographic monitoring.

Ambulation is an important activity in pulmonary exercise programs. Treadmills can be altered to accommodate the slow walking speeds needed for the more involved patients who often cannot achieve the minimum speeds offered by many commercial treadmills. The patient walks at a tolerable speed until he or she can tolerate 15 to 20 minutes of activity; then the speed is increased by 5% to 10%, and this pattern is repeated as the patient's endurance increases. Grade rather than speed can be increased for more exercise of the plantarflexors if the patient must climb stairs or traverse hilly terrain.

Although ambulation is the preferred activity, because it uses more muscles and is more relevant to the patient's daily life, cycling is more comfortable for some patients. The same schedule of increasing intensity that is used for ambulation may be followed.

Due to the specificity of exercise training, upper-extremity exercise is necessary in addition to ambulation (71). Since severely involved patients use their shoulder girdle muscles for respiration, they tolerate exercises in which the upper extremities are supported better than when the upper extremity is free.

Arm ergometry is the most common form of upper-extremity exercise for these patients. In more severely involved patients, it should be started with no resistance and continued as tolerated. When the patient can continue for 10 to 15 minutes, resistance should be added.

Pulley exercise stretches the shoulder and rib cage and is a favorite among this group of patients. A simple pulley apparatus is available at many medical supply stores and can be hung over a door at the patient's home, where it can be used daily. The patient's muscles of shoulder extension and adduction can be progressively strengthened using an apparatus with several pulley positions and adjustable weights.

Unsupported arm exercise assimilates more closely ADLs. It is quite taxing for severely involved patients. Simple unilateral arm elevation, with the other arm braced, may be all that some patients can tolerate at first. As the patient becomes stronger, a 1-inch dowel grabbed with both hands provides an ideal resistance for a variety of movements. These movements may include elevations, curling motions, side-to-side, and pressing movements. When the patient can perform such movements 30 to 50 times, at a rate of 20 to 40 times a minute, ¼- to ½-lb wrist weights can be conveniently and progressively added to the dowel.

Higher-functioning patients will have a difference between resting heart rate and the maximal heart rate, determined by the exercise test given during the evaluation; a target heart rate for exercise can be set at the resting heart rate plus 60% of the reserve. Patients with more advanced disease will have essentially no heart rate reserve; onset of dyspnea or a form of the Borg perceived exertion scale must be used to gauge intensity.

The need for additional O_2 during exercise should be assessed during the evaluation period. In contrast to rest, the administration of extra O_2 during exercise almost never causes hypoventilation. Therefore, the administration during exercise of enough O_2 to keep the O_2 higher than 60 mm Hg, or the oxygen saturation higher than about 90%, is not to be feared; the rate of O_2 delivery should be returned to its basal level shortly after completion of exercise.

The need for electrocardiographic monitoring during exercise should be assessed during the evaluation for the program.

Few payors will support a pulmonary rehabilitation program lasting more than 8 to 12 weeks. The pulmonary rehabilitation program must always be designed to lead into a maintenance phase. Higher-functioning patients may choose to continue exercising at a local recreation center or a comparable exercise facility. Every effort should be made to evaluate the patient performing the activity that he or she will continue during maintenance. Many patients will have formed emotional ties to the staff or activities at the rehabilitation center, or are much more likely to continue exercising if they are occasionally supervised than if they are left on their own; many centers offer a self-pay maintenance program at a much reduced frequency, for a nominal fee.

RESULTS OF PULMONARY REHABILITATION PROGRAMS

The outcomes of pulmonary rehabilitation programs have been somewhat controversial and difficult to quantify. Most of the studies focused particularly on the large subpopulation of patients with COPD. Table 80-3 lists some of the documented results of pulmonary rehabilitation programs (17,19,20,21,24,72,73).

Patients have demonstrated improvements in exercise tolerance, improved performance on a 12-minute walk test, and subjective accounts of decreased dyspnea while performing work. Possible mechanisms of action for improved exercise tolerance may include "improved aerobic capacity

Table 80-3: Some of the Documented Results of Pulmonary Rehabilitation Programs
Improved exercise tolerance Enhanced quality of life Decreased number of hospitalizations and physician visits Improved functional capacity for ADLs and vocational and avocational interests Decreased subjective dyspnea with activity Decreased levels of anxiety Increased use of relaxation techniques Improvements in disease education for patients and their families

(an actual training response), increased motivation, desensitization to the sensation of dyspnea, and improved muscular efficiency during exercise (lower oxygen cost of exercise)" (37).

Improved disease education for patients and their families can result in the potential for more successful smoking cessation programs, earlier recognition of lung infection and disease decompensation, improved use of medications and metered-dose inhalers, and improved patient environmental manipulation to avoid exacerbation of symptoms (17,19,20,21,24,72,73).

Some papers have reported studies that suggested that there may be increased survival in some patients as a result of pulmonary rehabilitation programs (17); others did not. "Although oxygen therapy improves survival in selected patients with COPD, conclusive evidence that pulmonary rehabilitation decreases mortality is lacking (74). Interestingly, many studies indicated a substantial improvement in exercise performance and endurance even in patients with severe lung dysfunction (72), and in the elderly with multiple disabilities (73). Thus, these patient groups should not be restricted from participating in pulmonary rehabilitation programs. The literature still remains unclear with regard to the length of the training program necessary to obtain the above-mentioned benefits. A recent meta-analysis of multiple studies involving pulmonary rehabilitation programs for patients with COPD suggested that "at least 4 weeks of exercise training relieves dyspnea and improves control over chronic obstructive pulmonary disease" (75). The long-term effects of pulmonary rehabilitation programs also remain controversial.

In general, many authors agree that there are no consistent improvements in objective parameters such as pulmonary function values, arterial blood gas measurements, right-sided heart hemodynamics, or maximal exercise performance (17,72). Further research is required to better define the expected outcomes of pulmonary rehabilitation programs.

THE SETTING AND NECESSARY EQUIPMENT FOR PULMONARY REHABILITATION

There are many possible settings for pulmonary rehabilitation programs. Inpatient programs can be conducted in hospitals, rehabilitation facilities, nursing homes, or skilled nursing facilities, for example. Outpatient programs can be conducted in a variety of community facilities, physicians' offices, and rehabilitation centers or clinics. Prescriptions for pulmonary rehabilitation can also be carried out in the home with or without the supervision of the various rehabilitation team members. The determination of which type of setting is appropriate for each patient often depends on the number and type of essential treating specialists, the required amount of medical supervision, and the availability of emergency equipment necessary for each patient to perform the program safely. Equipment may include emergency resuscitation gear (fully stocked code carts, medications, O_2 delivery systems, electrocardiogram machines, tracheostomy kits), telemetry monitors, pulse oximeter machines, various types of exercise apparatus (e.g., cycles, ergometers, treadmills, weights or Nautilus-type equipment, rowing machines, swimming pools), and durable medical equipment (wheelchairs and assistive devices for ambulation and ADLs). Structural factors within the facility including ventilation and bathroom availability are dictated by state and federal safety codes for public facilities (21). Outpatient programs should be conducted at facilities with convenient parking and should be easily accessible for patients with disabilities (21).

PATIENT AND FAMILY EDUCATION

A critical part of the rehabilitation process for any disability involves patient and family education, and the patient with pulmonary disease is no exception. Information should be given regarding the patient's actual lung pathology, expected prognosis, and potentially reversible components, if known. It is helpful to review the patient's medications, including the purpose, dosages, and side effects, and encourage communication regarding these issues and questions about missed doses or drug interactions with other compounds. In addition, it is important to review the signs and symptoms of disease decompensation so that they can be recognized and treated as early as possible. Education about factors that could potentially exacerbate lung dysfunction (e.g., high altitudes, excessive heat or humidity, extreme cold, high levels of pollution, pollen, or other allergens or irritants) is important so that these could be avoided as possible. Smoking cessation efforts may be more successful with education and family support. Information about optimal nutrition, adequate sleep, and other healthy lifestyle changes should be discussed with the patient and the family.

Education about the psychological effects of disability can serve to encourage the patient to seek professional counseling if he or she feels overwhelmed and needs help managing anxiety, depression, changing family or vocational relationships, and other reactions to disability. Support groups can be made available to interested patients and family members as an alternative to individual counseling.

A very important and frequently overlooked area of education for the patient with pulmonary disease involves addressing the issue of sexual function. Medications, elements of the disease pathology itself, or multiple disabilities can have a profound effect on a patient's sexuality and intimate relationships. Though these issues may be a source for anxiety or depression, the patient may be reluctant to discuss them. Sexual counseling for these patients should include education regarding the safety of sexual activities based on their particular impairments and disabilities, methods to monitor their level of exertion (e.g., heart rate or Borg-type rating), modes of energy conservation (e.g., pacing, energy-efficient sexual positions), supplemental O_2 management and adjustment, and provision of at least one designated team member (e.g., physician, psychologist, therapist, or nurse) to be made available to answer questions or concerns regarding these issues (76). Appropriate patients should be educated about birth control and sexually transmitted diseases.

Finally, patient and family education plays a very important role in all aspects of physical, occupational, vocational, and recreational therapy activities. Patients and their family members should be taught safe and proper performance of all exercises including techniques of self-monitoring for vital signs or perceived effort. The purpose and proper use of all durable medical equipment and assistive devices, including education regarding equipment maintenance and service, should be explained to patients and their families.

REFERENCES

1. Official American Thoracic Society statement: pulmonary rehabilitation. *Am Rev Respir Dis* 1981;124:663.
2. Staub NC, Albertine KH. Anatomy and development of the respiratory tract. In: Murray JF, Nadel JA, eds. *Textbook of respiratory medicine.* Vol. 1. 2nd ed. Philadelphia: WB Saunders, 1994:3–35.
3. Crane LD. Functional anatomy and physiology in ventilation. In: Zadai CC, ed. *Pulmonary management in physical therapy. Clinics in physical therapy.* New York: Churchill Livingstone, 1992:1–21.
4. Levitzky MG. *Pulmonary physiology.* 3rd ed. New York: McGraw-Hill, 1991.
5. Mines AH. *Respiratory physiology.* 2nd ed. New York: Raven, 1986.
6. Palevsky HI. Pulmonary circulation. In: Grippi MA, ed. *Pulmonary pathophysiology.* Philadelphia: JB Lippincott 1995:179–194.
7. Faling JL. Pulmonary rehabilitation—physical modalities. *Clin Chest Med* 1986;7:599–618.
8. Fuller RW, Jackson DM. Physiology and treatment of cough. *Thorax* 1990;45:425–430.
9. Kelley MA. The physiologic basis of pulmonary function testing. In: Grippi MA, ed. *Pulmonary pathophysiology.* Philadelphia: JB Lippincott, 1995:53–76.
10. Lanig IS, Lammertse DP. The respiratory system in spinal cord injury. *Phys Med Rehabil Clin N Am* 1992;3:725–740.
11. Morgan MDL, Silver JR, Williams SJ. The respiratory system of the spinal cord patient. In: Bloch RF, Basbaum M, eds. *Management of spinal cord injuries.* Baltimore: Williams & Wilkins, 1986:78–116.
12. Grinton SF. Respiratory limitations in the aging population. *South Med J* 1994;87:S47–S49.
13. Webster JR, Kadah H. Unique aspects of respiratory disease in the aged. *Geriatrics* 1991;46:31–43.
14. Nelson P, Lefrak SS. The aging respiratory system. In: Felsenthal G, Garrison SJ, Steinberg FU, eds. *Rehabilitation of the aging and elderly patient.* Baltimore: Williams & Wilkins, 1994:23–34.
15. Dean E, Ross J. Mobilization and exercise conditioning. In: Zadai CC, ed. *Pulmonary management in physical therapy. Clinics in physical therapy.* New York: Churchill Livingstone, 1992:157–190.
16. Hilman BC. Genetic and immunologic aspects of cystic fibrosis. *Ann Allergy Asthma Immunol* 1997;79:379–390.
17. Ries AL. Position paper of the American Association of Cardiovascular and Pulmonary Rehabilitation: scientific basis of pulmonary rehabilitation. *J Cardiopulm Rehabil* 1990;10:418–441.
18. Tiep BL. Reversing disability of irreversible lung disease. In Rehabilitation medicine—adding life to years [special issue]. *West J Med* 1991;154:591–597.
19. Reardon J, Awad E, Normandin E, et al. The effect of comprehensive outpatient pulmonary rehabilitation on dyspnea. *Chest* 1994;105:1046–1052.
20. Celli BR. Pulmonary rehabilitation in patients with COPD. *Respir Crit Care Med* 1995;152:861–864.
21. Connors G, Hilling L, eds. *American Association of Cardiovascular and Pulmonary Rehabilitation: guidelines for pulmonary rehabilitation programs.* Champaign, IL: Human Kinetics, 1993.
22. Chapman KR. Pharmacologic interventions. In: Bach JR, ed. *Pulmonary rehabilitation: the obstructive and paralytic*

conditions. Philadelphia: Hanley & Belfus, 1996:53–63.

23. Wade JF, King TE. Infiltrative and interstitial lung disease in the elderly patient. *Clin Chest Med* 1993;14:501–521.

24. Rodrigues JC, Ilowite JS. Pulmonary rehabilitation in the elderly patient. *Clin Chest Med* 1993;14:429–436.

25. Crystal RG. Interstitial lung disease. In: Wyngaarden JB, Smith LH, Bennett JC, eds. *Cecil textbook of medicine*. 19th ed. Philadelphia: WB Saunders, 1992:396–409.

26. Reid IR. Glucocorticoid osteoporosis—mechanisms and management. *Eur J Endocrinol* 1997;137:209–217.

27. Epstein S, et al. The role of testosterone in cyclosporine-induced osteopenia. *J Bone Miner Res* 1997;12:607–615.

28. Goldstein DJ, Zuech N, Sehgal V, et al. Cyclosporine-associated end-stage nephropathy after cardiac transplantation: incidence and progression. *Transplantation* 1997;63:664–668.

29. Ventura HO, Mehra MR, Stapleton DD, Smart FW. Cyclosporine-induced hypertension in cardiac transplantation. *Med Clin North Am* 1997;81:1347–1357.

30. Garritan SL. Physical therapy interventions for persons with chronic obstructive pulmonary disease. In: Bach JR, ed. *Pulmonary rehabilitation: the obstructive and paralytic conditions*. Philadelphia: Hanley & Belfus, 1996:85–98.

31. Frownfelter D. Postural drainage. In: Frownfelter D, ed. *Chest physical therapy and pulmonary rehabilitation*. 2nd ed. Chicago: Year Book Medical, 1987:271–287.

32. Starr JA. Manual techniques of chest physical therapy and airway clearance techniques. In: Zadai CC, ed. *Pulmonary management in physical therapy. Clinics in physical therapy*. New York: Churchill Livingstone, 1992:99–133.

33. Siebens AA, Kirkby NA, Barnerias MJ. Cough following transection of the spinal cord at C-6. *Arch Phys Med Rehabil* 1964;45:1–8.

34. Levenson CR. Breathing exercises. In: Zadai CC, ed. *Pulmonary management in physical therapy. Clinics in physical therapy*. New York: Churchill Livingstone, 1992:135–155.

35. American College of Sports Medicine. *Guidelines for exercise testing and prescription*. 4th ed. Philadelphia: Lea & Febiger, 1991.

36. Fletcher GF, Balady G, Froelicher VF, et al. Exercise standards: a statement for healthcare professionals from the American Heart Association. *Circulation* 1995;91:580–615.

37. Olopade CO, Beck KC, Viggiano RW, Staats BA. Exercise limitation and pulmonary rehabilitation in chronic obstructive pulmonary disease. *Mayo Clin Proc* 1992;67:144–157.

38. Belman MJ. Exercise in chronic obstructive pulmonary disease. *Clin Chest Med* 1986;7:585–597.

39. Smeets F. Travel for technology-dependent patients with respiratory disease. In: Muir JF, Pierson DE, eds. Pulmonary rehabilitation in chronic respiratory insufficiency-6. *Thorax* 1994;49:77–81.

40. Berg JE, Hostmark AT. Effects of acupuncture on smoking cessation or reduction for motivated smokers. *Prev Med* 1997;26:208–214.

41. O'Hara P, Grill J, Ridgon MA, et al. Design and results of the initial intervention program for the Lung Health Study. *Prev Med* 1993;22:304–315.

42. Pederson LL, Baskerville JC, Wanklin JM. Multivariate statistical models for predicting change in smoking behavior following physician advice to quit smoking. *Prev Med* 1982;11:536–549.

43. Duncan CL, Cummings SR, Hudes ES, et al. Quitting smoking: reasons for quitting and predictors of cessation among medical patients. *J Gen Intern Med* 1992;7:398–404.

44. Foxman B, Sloss EM, Lohr KN, et al. Chronic bronchitis: prevalence, smoking habits, impact, and antismoking advice. *Prev Med* 1986;15:624–631.

45. Belafsky PC, Kissinger P, Amedee R. Nicotine addiction and smoking cessation. *J La State Med Soc* 1997;149:419–424.

46. Danis PG, Seaton TL. Helping your patients to quit smoking. *Am Family Phys* 1997;55:1207–1214, 1217–1218.

47. Blondal T, Franzon M, Westin A. A double-blind randomized trial of nicotine nasal spray as an aid in smoking cessation. *Eur Respir J* 1997;10:1585–1590.

48. Hurt RD, Sachs DP, Glover ED, et al. A comparison of sustained-release bupropion and placebo for smoking cessation. *N Engl J Med* 1997;337:1195–1202.

49. Dail CW, Affeldt JE. *Glossopharyngeal breathing*. College of Medical Evangelists, Los Angeles, CA. Video. 1954.

50. Dail CW, Rodgers M, Guess V, Adkins HV. *Glossopharyngeal breathing manual*. Downey, CA: Rancho Los Amigos Hospital, 1979.

51. Bach JR, Alba AS. Noninvasive options for ventilatory support of the traumatic high level quadriplegic. *Chest* 1990;98:613–619.

52. Bach JR. A comparison of long-term ventilatory support alternatives from the perspective of the patient and care giver. *Chest* 1993;104:1702–1706.

53. Kvale PA, Cugell DW, Anthonisen NR, et al. Continuous or nocturnal oxygen therapy in hypoxemic chronic obstructive lung disease. *Ann Intern Med* 1980;93:391–398.

54. Cordova F, O'Brien G, Furukawa S, et al. Stability of improvements in exercise performance and quality of life following bilateral lung volume reduction surgery in severe COPD. *Chest* 1997;112:907–915.

55. Grover FL, Fullerton DA, Zamora MR, et al. The past, present and future of lung transplantation. *Am J Surg* 1997;193:523–533.

56. Bach JR. Introduction to rehabilitation of neuromuscular disorders. *Semin Neurol* 1995;15:1–5.

57. Bach JR. Neuromuscular and skeletal disorders leading to global alveolar hypoventilation. In: Bach JR, ed. *Pulmonary rehabilitation: the obstructive and paralytic conditions.* Philadelphia: Hanley & Belfus, 1996: 257–273.

58. Bach JR. Conventional approaches to managing neuromuscular ventilatory failure. In: Bach JR, ed. *Pulmonary rehabilitation: the obstructive and paralytic conditions.* Philadelphia: Hanley & Belfus, 1996:285–301.

59. Duport G, Gayet E, Pries P, et al. Spinal deformities and wheelchair seating in Duchenne muscular dystrophy: twenty years of research and clinical experience. *Semin Neurol* 1995;15:29–37.

60. Bach JR. Prevention of morbidity and mortality with the use of physical medicine aids. In: Bach JR. *Pulmonary rehabilitation: the obstructive and paralytic conditions.* Philadelphia: Hanley & Belfus, 1996:303–329.

61. Simon DB, Ringel SP. Rehabilitation of neuromuscular disorders. In: Nickel VL, Botte MJ, eds. *Orthopaedic rehabilitation.* 2nd ed. New York: Churchill Livingstone, 1992:309–325.

62. Hillberg RE. Chronic obstructive pulmonary disease: Causes and clinicopathologic considerations. In: Bach JR, ed. *Pulmonary rehabilitation: the obstructive and paralytic conditions.* Philadelphia: Hanley & Belfus, 1996:27–38.

63. Dumitru D. *Electrodiagnostic medicine.* Philadelphia: Hanley & Belfus, 1995:111–176, 741–850.

64. Mulvey DA, Aquilina RJ, Elliott MW, et al. Diaphragmatic dysfunction in neuralgic amyotrophy: an electrophysiologic evaluation of 16 patients presenting with dyspnea. *Am Rev Respir Dis* 1993;147:66–71.

65. Mazzoni M, Solinas C, Sisillo E, et al. Intraoperative phrenic nerve monitoring in cardiac surgery. *Chest* 1996;109:1455–1460.

66. Zifko U, Auinger M, Albrecht G, et al. Phrenic neuropathy in chronic renal failure. *Thorax* 1995;50:793–794.

67. Harker CP, Stern EJ, Frank MS. Hemidiaphragm in paralysis: CT diagnosis. *J Thorac Imaging* 1994;9:166–168.

68. DeVita MA, Robinson LR, Rehder J, et al. Incidence and natural history of phrenic neuropathy occurring during open heart surgery. *Chest* 1993;103:850–856.

69. Diehl JL, Lofaso F, Deleuze P, et al. Clinically relevant diaphragmatic dysfunction after cardiac operations. *J Thorac Cardiovasc Surg* 1994;107:487–498.

70. Silverman JL, Rodriquez AA. Needle electromyographic evaluation of the diaphragm. *Electromyogr Clin Neurophysiol* 1994;34:509–511.

71. Ries AL, Ellis B, Hawkins RW. Upper extremity exercise training in chronic obstructive pulmonary disease. *Chest* 1988;93:688–692.

72. Niederman MS, Clemente PH, Fein AM, et al. Benefits of a multidisciplinary pulmonary rehabilitation program: improvements are independent of lung function. *Chest* 1991;99:798–804.

73. Couser JI Jr, Guthmann R, Hamadeh MA, Kane CS. Pulmonary rehabilitation improves exercise capacity in older elderly patients with COPD. *Chest* 1995;107:730–734.

74. Make BJ, Glenn K. Outcomes of pulmonary rehabilitation. In: Bach JR, ed. *Pulmonary rehabilitation: the obstructive and paralytic conditions.* Philadelphia: Hanley & Belfus, 1996: 173–192.

75. Lacasse Y, Wong E, Guyatt GH, et al. Meta-analysis of respiratory rehabilitation in chronic obstructive pulmonary disease. *Lancet* 1996;348:1115–1119.

76. Sipski M. Sexuality and individuals with respiratory impairment. In: Bach JR, ed. *Pulmonary rehabilitation: the obstructive and paralytic conditions.* Philadelphia: Hanley & Belfus, 1996:203–211.

Chapter 81

Peripheral Vascular Disease

Harvey Goldberg

Peripheral vascular disease, in its various forms, has been a major cause of disability in the general population.

Just as the properties and functional roles of each component of the peripheral vascular system are distinctive, so are the characteristics of the disorders that affect the peripheral arteries, veins, and lymphatic vessels. The common denominators relative to each are 1) the frequent occurrence of functional impairment or pain; 2) the frequent association with known underlying etiologies, risk factors, and comorbidities; and 3) the availability of treatment options, both conservative and surgical. Various restorative techniques have been applied to each of these in the form of exercise, physical modalities, and multidisciplinary rehabilitation.

The reported prevalence of intermittent claudication has been variable and somewhat dependent on the criteria used. Balkau et al (1) noted that prevalence ranges from 0.4% to 14.4% as diagnosed by the Rose questionnaire (2,3) and from 4.2% to 35% as diagnosed by the ankle-brachial pressure index, which is the current method of choice. Vogt et al (4) showed that prevalence increases sharply with age, from 3% in those under 60 years old to over 20% in those over 75. Four percent of the population over age 75 has limitations in mobility and level of functional independence due to lower-extremity peripheral arterial disease (4,5). Although claudication tends not to predict the occurrence of limb-threatening ischemia, it correlates significantly with generalized atherosclerotic vascular disease and cardiovascular mortality (6). The Framingham study reported a more than double increase in 10-year mortality in males and a quadruple increase in females. Most deaths were associated with myocardial infarction (7). The annual risk for amputation, however, was only 0.7%. In patients undergoing coronary artery bypass procedures, in-hospital mortality rates were 2.4-fold higher for those with indicators of peripheral vascular disease (8). Criqui et al (9) showed that the relative risk of dying among subjects with large-vessel peripheral arterial disease was 3.1 for deaths from all causes, 5.9 for all deaths from cardiovascular disease, and 6.6 for deaths from coronary heart disease. It has been estimated that approximately 40% of patients with intermittent claudication will die within 8 years (10).

BASIC VASCULAR ANATOMY AND ASSESSMENT

The circulatory system is composed of arteries, veins, and lymphatics designed to deliver oxygen and nutrients to the body's tissues and to eliminate waste products. The vascular conditions that most commonly affect the upper extremities are distinct from those prevalent in the lower extremities. Therefore, some of the particular characteristics of upper- and lower-extremity anatomy and clinical diagnosis are best considered separately.

Upper Extremities

In the upper extremities, the subclavian artery gives rise to the axillary and brachial arteries. The latter bifurcates at the elbow to form the radial and ulnar arteries. If either of these vessels is obstructed, circulation to the hand is protected by the interconnecting palmar arches (Fig. 81-1). Some of the more commonly encountered vascular conditions involving the upper extremity include thoracic outlet syndrome (neurovascular compression by cervical ribs or fibromuscular bands as the subclavian vessels and brachial plexus pass beneath the clavicle), vasospastic conditions (e.g., reflex sympathetic dystrophy, Raynaud phenomenon), and lymphedema.

The peripheral vascular examination of the upper extremities entails observation for color changes, edema, rash, scarring, hair distribution, and venous distention, with particular attention to side-to-side asymmetry. The examiner should determine asymmetry in temperature and should palpate the brachial, radial, and ulnar pulses, comparing amplitudes on each side. Brachial artery blood pressure in both arms is measured by auscultation for Korotkoff sounds in the antecubital fossa. If the findings are inconclusive, systolic blood pressure can be measured during deflation of the cuff on the arm by palpating the brachial artery pulse, or during deflation of the cuff on the forearm by palpating the radial or ulnar pulse.

The Allen test is a simple and reliable indicator of occlusion of the radial or ulnar artery, as well as competence of the palmar arch. The test is performed by compressing both the radial and ulnar arteries and having the patient clench his or her fist, evacuating blood from the hand. When the hand is opened, the palm appears pale. Pressure is then released from the radial artery, while keeping the ulnar artery compressed. In the presence of normal circulation, normal color should immediately return, along with possible hyperemia. If there is an occlusion of the radial artery, the hand remains pale and mottled until pressure is released from the ulnar artery. If there is an incomplete palmar arch, color returns to the radial side of the palm upon release of the radial artery, but the ulnar side of the hand remains pale. The test is then repeated with pressure applied to both arteries and clenching of the fist, after which pressure is released from the ulnar artery while it is maintained over the radial artery. Once again, color returns to the entire hand in the presence of normal circulation, but with an ulnar artery occlusion, the hand remains pale. If there is incompetence of the palmar arch, the radial side of the hand remains pale until pressure is released from the radial artery (Fig. 81-2).

Lower Extremities

Arterial circulation to the lower extremities originates in the abdominal aorta, which gives rise to the external iliac and in turn, the femoral and popliteal arteries. The latter bifurcates at the level of the knee to form the anterior

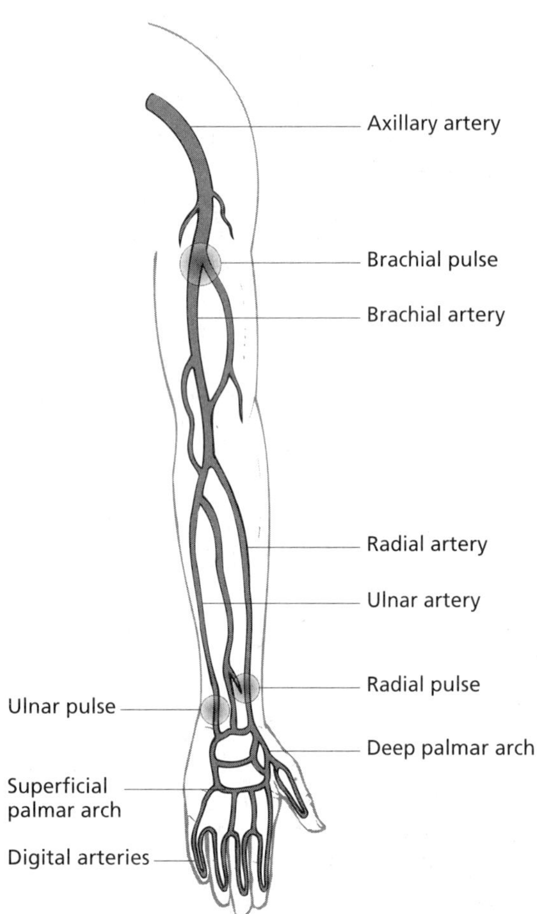

Figure 81-1. Major arteries of the upper extremity with sites for palpation of peripheral pulses.

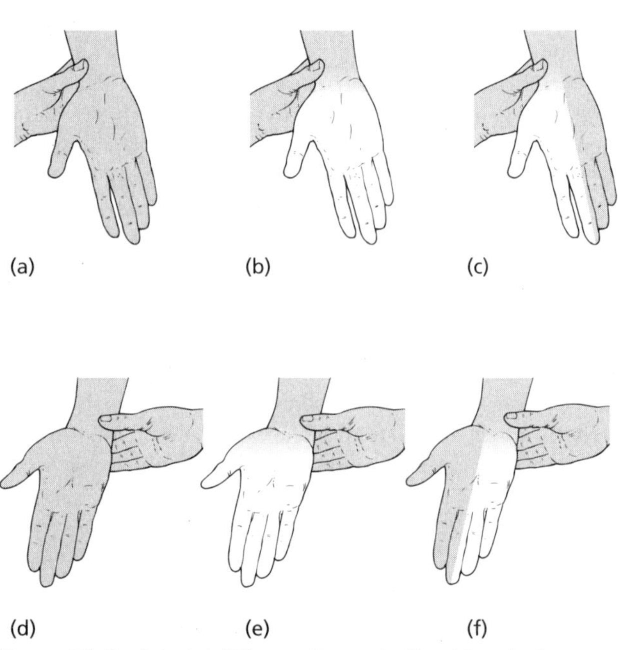

Figure 81-2. Arterial filling patterns in the Allen test. Retained radial artery compression (*top row*): *A.* Normal. B. Ulnar artery occlusion. C. Palmar arch incompetence. Retained ulnar artery compression (*bottom row*): *D.* Normal. E. Radial artery occlusion. F. Palmar arch incompetence.

tibial and posterior tibial arteries. In the foot, the anterior tibial artery bifurcates to form the dorsalis pedis and lateral tarsal arteries and the posterior tibial artery branches off into the medial and lateral plantar arteries. As in the upper extremities, interconnecting arches provide collateral circulation (Fig. 81-3).

The veins of the lower extremity are composed of deep (femoral) and superficial (saphenous) systems. The peroneal, anterior tibial, and posterior tibial veins empty into the femoral vein. The great saphenous vein runs from the dorsum of the foot to the groin and the small saphenous vein runs from the lateral side of the foot to the popliteal area. The femoral and greater saphenous veins flow into the external iliac vein and then to the inferior vena cava. Some of the common vascular conditions involving the lower extremities include arterial occlusive disease, deep vein thrombosis (DVT), and venous insufficiency (edema, stasis, ulceration).

Examination of the lower extremities should include observation for asymmetry in size, shape, color, texture, swelling, scarring, ulceration, and abnormal venous patterns. Particular attention should be paid to the distal regions of the legs and feet for ulceration, erythema, cyanosis, hyperpigmentation, hair distribution, and temperature. The toes should be separated to observe each interdigital space, as deep ulcers may be hidden in these areas. The examiner should palpate the femoral artery pulse half way between the anterior superior iliac spine and symphysis pubis (see Fig. 81-3). The femoral vein, which lies just medial, should be palpated for tenderness. Superficial lymph nodes (vertical and horizontal) should be palpated with observations of size, consistency, and tenderness. The popliteal pulse, generally found just lateral to the midline, should be palpated with the knee slightly flexed. Since the popliteal artery is relatively deep, palpation may be difficult. If necessary, the examiner can position the patient prone, flex the knee to 90 degrees, and press deeply. The dorsalis pedis, which is derived from the anterior tibial artery as it descends distal to the ankle joint, is located just lateral to the extensor hallucis longus tendon. In approximately 3.5% of limbs the anterior tibial artery does not reach the dorsum of the foot or is reduced to a very narrow diameter by this level (11). In 1.5% of feet, the anterior tibial artery takes a lateral course to the foot instead of running straight down anteriorly (11) such that the dorsalis pedis is, in some cases, congenitally absent. The posterior tibial pulse is palpable just behind the medial malleolus.

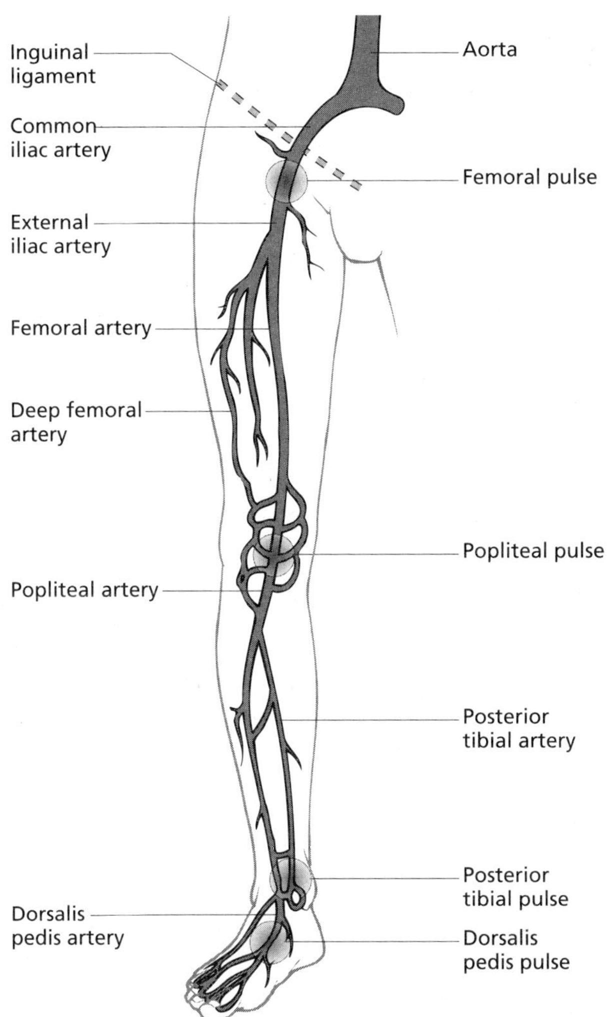

Figure 81-3. Major arteries of the lower extremity with sites for palpation of peripheral pulses.

The examiner should check for pitting edema and palpate calf muscles, observing for tenderness, firmness, and muscle tension. These findings may indicate DVT. With the patient in the supine position, both lower extremities should be elevated to approximately 60 degrees and observed for unusual pallor. The examiner should then sit the patient up, lower the feet into a dependent position, and observe for return of the usual color, which should occur within 10 seconds. The gradual appearance of rubor or dusky erythema suggests a compromise in arterial circulation. In the standing position, the examiner should inspect the saphenous system for varicosities, redness, or cords. Systolic blood pressure should be recorded in each arm and, using Doppler measurement, in each leg. From this, the ankle-arm index (AAI) can be calculated. The AAI is determined by dividing the ankle pressures on each side by the higher of the two brachial pressures (12). An assessment of the reliability of palpation of pulses found that the sensitivity was at least 95% for palpation over the femoral pulse; but ranged from 33% to 60% for observers of varying experience feeling for the posterior tibial pulse; the rate of false-positive observations was 20% (13). Therefore, it was suggested that pulse palpation alone is an unreliable physical sign and should be combined with other objective measurements to guide clinical management. An examination for suspected arterial disease should include auscultation of the abdomen for a bruit and palpation for an expansile pulsatile mass as signs of an abdominal aortic aneurysm (AAA). The absence of these findings, however, does not exclude an aneurysm and ancillary imaging studies need to be used in the work-up of persons at risk. Marcon et al (14) suggested that patients with normal findings on clinical examination and low risk factors can be considered free of arterial disease on clinical grounds alone, but patients with normal findings on clinical examination and high-risk factor scores should have an extensive noninvasive evaluation.

Finally, as noted below, the sensory neurologic examination is important. Pinprick sensation should be tested using a clean, preferably disposable pin or similar pointed object, and joint position and temperature sensation should be tested as well. Monofilament examination for cutaneous pressure sensation should be performed as an indicator for sensory loss and risk of injury.

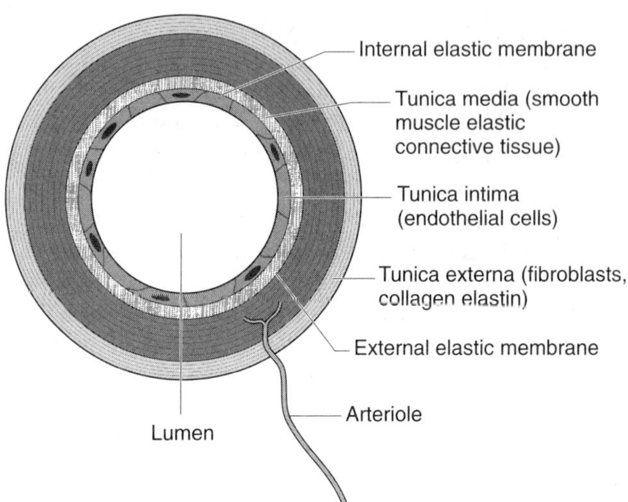

Figure 81-4. Cross-sectional structure of an artery. Note the three layers of the vascular wall (intima, media, externa) with penetrating arteriole.

ARTERIAL OBSTRUCTIVE DISEASE

Arterial Histology

The three histologic layers of an artery are the tunica intima, composed of endothelial cells; the tunica media, composed of smooth muscle cells and elastic connective tissue; and the tunica externa (or adventitia), containing fibroblasts, collagen, and elastin. These layers are separated by an internal elastic membrane (between the intima and media) and an external elastic membrane (between the media and adventitia) (Fig. 81-4). The major mechanisms of arterial disease are obstruction of the lumen and disruption of the vessel wall. Atherosclerotic disease begins with injury to the endothelial cells that comprise the intima. Established risk factors in the development of atherosclerotic disease include smoking, hypertension, hyperlipidemia, and diabetes. Platelets play an important role in the pathogenesis of atherosclerosis as well as in restenosis after vascular surgery (15). Endothelial damage that results from smoking stimulates the aggregation of platelets and in turn, the migration of cellular elements to the site of injury. In addition, smooth muscle proliferation results. These processes, as they occur in coronary and peripheral vessels, are potentially reversible, particularly with respect to the deposition of atheromatous plaques and intimal thickening or relaxation, when serum cholesterol levels are reduced (through diet or cholesterol-lowering drugs or both) in combination with smoking cessation and exercise (16–22). The more advanced changes of calcification and fibrosis are less likely to be reversed (17,19).

The overall distensibility of the arterial wall decreases with age. This decreased distensibility is partly caused by the complex and varied effects of atherosclerosis on the vessel. In addition, nonatherosclerotic effects of aging such as fragmentation of the elastic lamellae, deposition of collagen between the elastin fibers, and calcium deposits near the elastin fibers also contribute to age-related changes (23).

Antiplatelet Agents

Aspirin prevents platelet aggregation by interfering in the cyclooxygenase pathway of the platelet and preventing the production of thromboxane (a substance that produces platelet aggregation as well as vasoconstriction). However, aspirin also blocks the production of prostacycline analogues, which possess properties opposite to those of thromboxane in that they produce vasodilation and inhibition of platelet aggregation. Nevertheless, the net beneficial effect of aspirin is attributed to its ability to block the production of thromboxane in greater proportion than prostacycline. In addition, Yellin suggested that very low doses of aspirin (30 mg every other day) will block thromboxane production while exerting no blocking effect on the production of prostacycline. Various clinical trials have been carried out by investigators seeking to determine the efficacy of different doses of aspirin in relation to platelet inhibition (15,24,25). The results of the majority of the studies supported aspirin's role as an effective platelet inhibitor in peripheral vascular disease. Comparisons of outcomes resulting from higher and lower dosages generally found that there are no significant differences. Investigators thereby concluded that lower doses (50–100 mg daily) are preferable, since lower doses are accompanied by fewer side effects. An additional effect of aspirin that was demonstrated in an animal model involves a decrease in smooth muscle cell proliferation (26). More recent studies involving the use of ticlopidine (27–30) and naftidrofuryl (31) yielded promising results in controlling platelet aggregation in peripheral vascular disease.

Muscle Ischemia and Claudication

The normal peripheral vascular system provides sufficient blood flow to deliver oxygen in adequate amounts to satisfy the requirements of lower-extremity muscles during all activities. In the presence of peripheral vascular disease, the blood flow is compromised and the supply of oxygen to the muscles during exercise is not equal to the demand. Intermittent claudication is a result of muscle ischemia and in turn, can occur in response to any condition capable of compromising the arterial blood supply to muscles. While the most common cause of arterial obstruction is atherosclerosis and arteriosclerosis obliterans, other causes include emboli, thrombi, fibromuscular dysplasia, and external compression (23). Occlusions may occur at one or more points along the iliac, superficial femoral, popliteal, or distal arteries. In order for a reduction in blood flow to take place, a 75% narrowing of cross-sectional diameter of a vessel must be present. This serves to explain why slowly progressive atherosclerotic arterial disease does not usually manifest itself clinically until later in life when the critical threshold of 75% stenosis has been reached. It should be noted that the physiologic severity of a lesion depends on various factors including absolute vessel diameter and eccentricity, lesion length, presence of multiple lesions in the same vessel, and existence of collateral flow (32). Therefore, measurement of the reduction in the luminal diameter (in percent) caused by stenosis does not accurately predict blood flow. While lesser degrees of narrowing as measured on Doppler studies are often noted not to be "hemodynamically significant," this does not serve to exclude the possibility of acute embolization of distal vessels by atherosclerotic plaques resulting in obstruction and gangrene.

Hemodynamics and Blood Rheology

The total peripheral resistance in blood flow is partially determined by its rheologic properties (i.e., fluidity). Consequently, blood flow through diseased arteries can also be affected by factors impacting on rheology, which include viscosity, hematocrit, red blood cell deformability, and red blood cell aggregation (33). Energy losses in flowing blood occur as a result of friction (viscous losses) or changes in velocity or direction (inertial losses). Poiseuille law describes a flow model that can account for viscous energy losses in circulation. The principle states that flow along a tube is directly proportional to the pressure gradient along that tube and its radius, and inversely proportional to tube length and fluid viscosity (23). The following equation expresses Poiseuille law:

$$\text{flow} = P \times r^4/(v \times L)$$

where P, represents pressure; r, vessel radius; v, viscosity; and L, vessel length.

Various treatments have been instituted for the purpose of normalizing the viscosity of blood and have resulted in increased walking distances with a reduction in claudication symptoms. These interventions have included hemodilution (34–36), medication (37), and exercise (38).

Pentoxifylline (Trental)

Pentoxifylline has become a widely used hemorrheologically active agent in the treatment of intermittent claudication. The medication can improve abnormal erythrocyte deformability, reduce hyperviscosity, and diminish platelet hyperreactivity and plasma hypercoagulability. A significant segment of patients treated with the medication have shown improvement in pain-free walking distance and blood viscosity, particularly when it is used in conjunction with an exercise program (27,29). However, the drug has limitations because of its cost, delay in onset of symptom reduction (estimated at 4–6 weeks), and frequent gastrointestinal side effects.

Metabolic Considerations

The metabolic phenomena at the level of the muscle cell play an important role in the development of ischemic symptoms and in the response to interventions. When ischemia occurs and blood flow to the muscles diminishes, metabolic waste products accumulate. The local buildup of these substances produces pain and usually causes the patient to rest until the oxygen demand has again diminished and metabolic waste products are washed from the system. Immediately after treadmill testing, levels of lactate and hypoxanthine are noted to be significantly elevated in the bloodstream, returning to pre-exercise levels within 30 minutes (lactate) and 60 minutes (hypoxanthine) (39). Improved exercise tolerance can occur without changes in muscle blood flow during activity (38,40–43). This suggests that beneficial changes are occurring within the muscle itself, to adapt to a decreased blood flow. Results of animal studies suggested that the peripheral adaptations within active muscle cells include 1) a redistribution of blood flow, 2) enhanced capillary density, and 3) an increase in mitochondrial content (44,45). Despite limited blood flow, improvements in muscle metabolism may facilitate the extraction of oxygen and substrates and permit increased exercise capacity (46,47). Biopsy samples of ischemic muscles have shown a significant reduction in total plasma carnitine concentration, and treatment with carnitine supplements have restored normal levels along with improvements in exercise performance (46). Increases in maximum walking distance after training have been correlated to the enzyme activity of cytochrome-*c* oxidase in patients with peripheral arterial insufficiency. This metabolic adaptation reverses itself after arterial reconstructive surgery but the increased oxidative capacity can persist with a therapeutic program of surgery and training (48).

Diagnostic Testing for Peripheral Arterial Disease

Conventional contrast arteriography is extremely sensitive and specific in the diagnosis of vascular disease and has been considered the gold standard for determining the location and extent of arterial pathology. However, it has all the risks related to ionic contrast material, particularly in patients with renal compromise. For this reason, it is usually reserved for patients in whom revascularization procedures are planned (49).

Digital subtraction angiography (DSA) is a computer-enhanced angiographic study that employs a significantly lower volume of contrast medium and in turn, carries lower risk (49–51). Through the use of computerized digital subtraction techniques, small differences in density can be detected and amplified following intravenous injection of a contrast agent. The contrast and sensitivity are high but the spatial resolution is lower than that of conventional contrast arteriography (52). Nevertheless, in many patients DSA is sufficient to establish a diagnosis and plan therapy.

Magnetic resonance angiography (MRA) is another alternative to x-ray angiography, particularly for patients with impaired renal function or poor vascular access. MRA does not have the diagnostic accuracy to replace x-ray angiography but it can provide information that cannot be obtained with other modalities. It is particularly useful in the preoperative assessment of patients with advanced peripheral vascular disease. MRA sometimes increases the visualization of runoff vessels, unidentified stenoses, and vessels misidentified on contrast x-ray angiography (53,54). When a patient is evaluated for arterial reconstruction, an overlooked stenosis may result in placing a graft too distally, thereby necessitating revision of the graft. False-positive results may lead to graft placement more proximally than necessary, which can increase the risk for long-term graft failure.

Contrast angiography, DSA, and MRA provide anatomic information pertaining to large vessels but do not provide much information about the hemodynamic significance of borderline lesions, small-vessel disease, or the adequacy of collateral flow (32). Whole-body thallium scintigraphy can provide information about the hemodynamic significance of noncritical anatomic lesions and is 80% sensitive and 73% specific (32). Whole-body thallium exercise scintigraphy has been described as a valuable instrument in the detection of silent or subocclusive peripheral vascular disease and in the evaluation of multifocal atherosclerosis (55).

The AAI, or ankle-brachial index (ABI), is a quantitative technique widely used to determine the presence and severity of peripheral arterial disease. It is a prognostic indicator for mortality due to atherosclerotic disease in older men and women (1,56–58). Normally, systolic pressures should be higher in the lower extremities than in the upper extremities (59). When there is arterial occlusive disease in the lower extremities, pressures distal to the occlusion will be decreased. Some analyses proposed a stratification of severity, with mild disease corresponding to an AAI of 0.90 to 0.71, moderate disease having an AAI of 0.70 to 0.51, and severe disease corresponding to an AAI of 0.50 or less (56). High ankle pressures and a normal AAI sometimes occur despite advanced arterial disease, as a result of a loss of compressibility of lower-extremity arteries. This occurs particularly in diabetics with arteriosclerotic disease. Measurement of the AAI is useful in identifying those at high risk for mortality due to atherosclerotic heart disease who may benefit from aggressive therapy (56). Because AAI measurement is a simple procedure, it is suggested that it could be a useful component in geriatric screening programs (56).

Serial noninvasive testing is useful in assessing arterial obstructive disease and arterial bypass grafts and in diagnosing local vascular complications of arterial catheterization (60). Color-flow imaging combines high-resolution B-mode and Doppler imaging systems to provide simultaneous anatomic and physiologic information. B-mode ultrasonography provides a gray-scale image of the blood vessels while Doppler probes permit analysis of flow patterns and velocity (60). Color-flow Doppler and two-dimensional ultrasound have had an expanding role in the noninvasive evaluation of peripheral arterial diseases and can help to diagnose stenosis or occlusion by demonstrating absent, diminished, high-velocity, and collateral flow. They can also visualize atherosclerotic plaque or thrombus, calcified plaque or vessel wall (61), and aneurysms, pseudoaneurysms, perivascular masses, arteriovenous fistulae, and arterial conduit occlusions (62). Impedance plethysmography correlates well with known cardiovascular risk factors (63). Toe pressure measurements with digital volume plethysmography are simple and useful in screening patients with symptoms of coronary heart disease (64) (Fig. 81-5).

Management of Peripheral Arterial Disease

Since there is such a high correlation between peripheral arterial disease and cardiovascular morbidity and mortality, the management of associated cardiac disease, risk factors, and life expectancy must be integrated into the overall treatment scenario. The signs and symptoms of peripheral arterial disease are stable in the majority of patients and can often improve, but the occlusive process is progressive in approximately 20% of patients (56), in whom complications ranging from intermittent claudication to rest pain, skin ulcerations, and gangrene will develop. Most patients with intermittent claudication are not at immediate risk for limb loss; the primary goals of treatment in these individuals are to reduce risk factors and to improve exercise tolerance and functional capacity (65). These goals are generally achieved through education, exercise, and in some patients, drug therapy (66). Drug therapy has primarily consisted of treatment with hemorrheologic drugs (i.e., pentoxifylline) and antiplatelet agents (i.e., aspirin, ticlopidine), and there has been recent attention to the value of metabolism-enhancing agents (i.e., carnitine), as discussed earlier. No drug has been clearly proved to be effective in the treatment of limb-threatening ischemia (67). Various classes of vasodilators (adrenergic agents, direct-acting agents, calcium channel blockers, angiotensin-converting

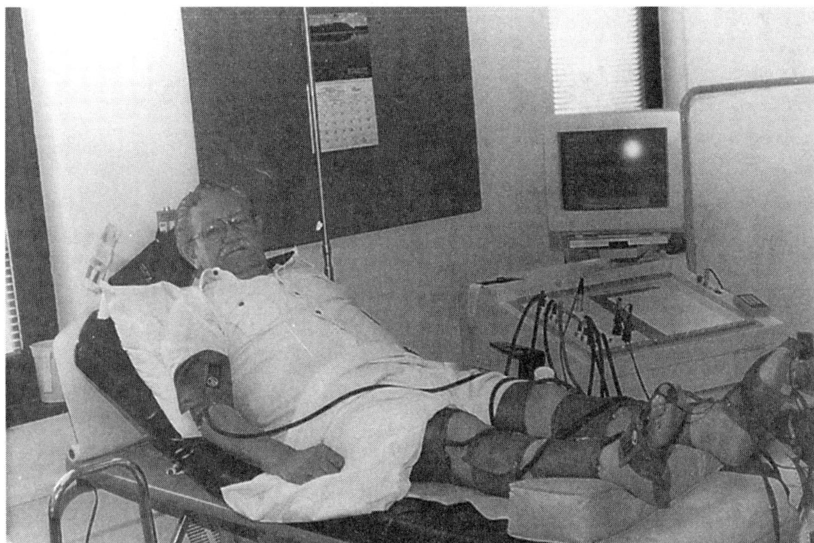

Figure 81-5. Noninvasive vascular testing with segmental limb pressure measurements and pulse volume recordings.

enzyme inhibitors, and prostaglandins) have been studied with respect to improvement of blood flow to ischemic areas and have been used in the treatment of obstructive arterial disease and vasospastic disorders (67). While heparin is used during vascular surgery or interventional radiologic procedures, the role of oral anticoagulants (i.e., warfarin) in the management of peripheral arterial disease has not been well established although they have been prescribed after distal bypass procedures (68,69). Other less widely utilized interventions include lumbar neurolytic sympathetic blockade (70), electrical spinal cord stimulation (71–74), ozone therapy (75,76), and hyperbaric oxygen (77). Patients with disabling claudication (inability to perform a job or normal daily life activities), rest pain, ulceration, gangrene, or Leriche syndrome (occlusion of the terminal aorta) should be considered for surgical revascularization (bypass) or angioplasty (65). Thrombolytic therapy, used for acute segmental arterial occlusion, has been successful in restoring distal pulses and improving the AAI in selected patients. The risk of complications, however, is significant and complications include thromboembolic events, arterial dissection, and major hemorrhage, with mortality rates as high as 25% (78).

Exercise in the Treatment of Intermittent Claudication

In 1898 Wilhelm Erb suggested that physical training in the form of walking could be used as a treatment for patients with intermittent claudication and this was based on the principle that muscle work increased blood flow to the ischemic limb (79). It was not until the 1950s and 1960s, however, that the concept of dynamic training for patients with ischemic peripheral arterial disease was reintroduced (40,79,80). Since that time, the role of exercise and physical training in the treatment of mild to moderate peripheral arterial disease of the lower extremities has been developed and studied extensively (33,38,40–42,46, 79,81–94). Exercise programs have been designed to be carried out both in supervised cardiovascular treatment settings (Fig. 81-6) using endurance training equipment and in unsupervised home and community settings, emphasizing walking and simple independently performed exercises. Various functional benefits have been established and include increased pain tolerance (1), increase in walking distance (41,82,90,94), increase in walking time (42,89), increase in duration of exercise tolerance (38,41), and improved motivation (38). Several possible mechanisms for increased walking ability that were proposed in earlier literature included development of increased collateral blood flow, redistribution of available flow, change in walking pattern, increased pain tolerance, and metabolic adaptation in leg muscles (79,89). While some later work continued to suggest enhanced blood flow to muscle resulting from physical training (46,86,91,93), studies have not provided consistent and significant evidence for these mechanisms (38,40–43). Some of the metabolic effects suggested in the literature were discussed earlier.

Exercise protocols published in the literature describe varying frequencies, durations, levels of supervision, and modes of exercise. A multitude of outcome measures have also been used to evaluate the results of these programs and have included walking distance, time to onset of claudication pain, hemodynamic parameters, and metabolic and biochemical factors (Table 81-1). Based on a meta-analysis of exercise rehabilitation programs aimed at reducing claudication pain in patients with peripheral arterial disease, Gardner and Poehlman (94) concluded that the optimal exercise program for improving claudication pain distances uses intermittent walking to near maximal pain during a program of at least 6 months' duration. Gardner et al (92) suggested that stair climbing might offer

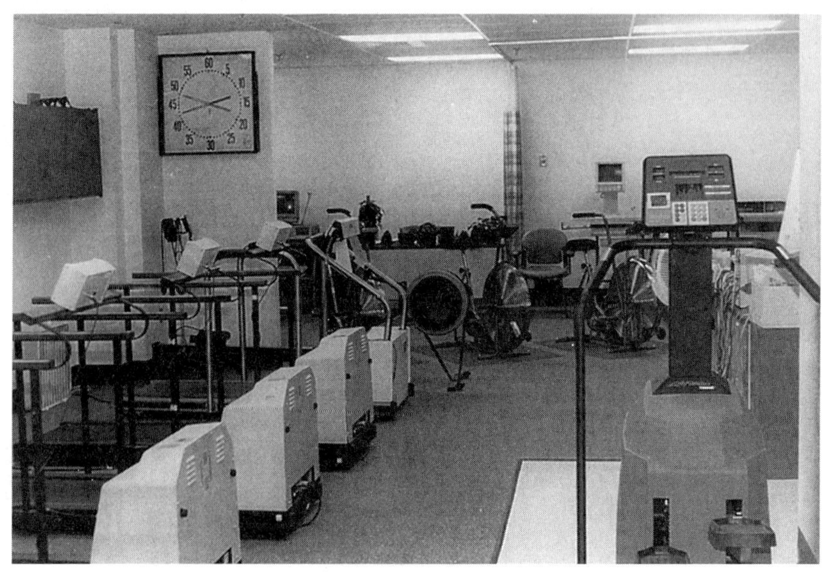

Figure 81-6. Cardiovascular training gym. Note the treadmills, bicycle ergometers, and stair climber.

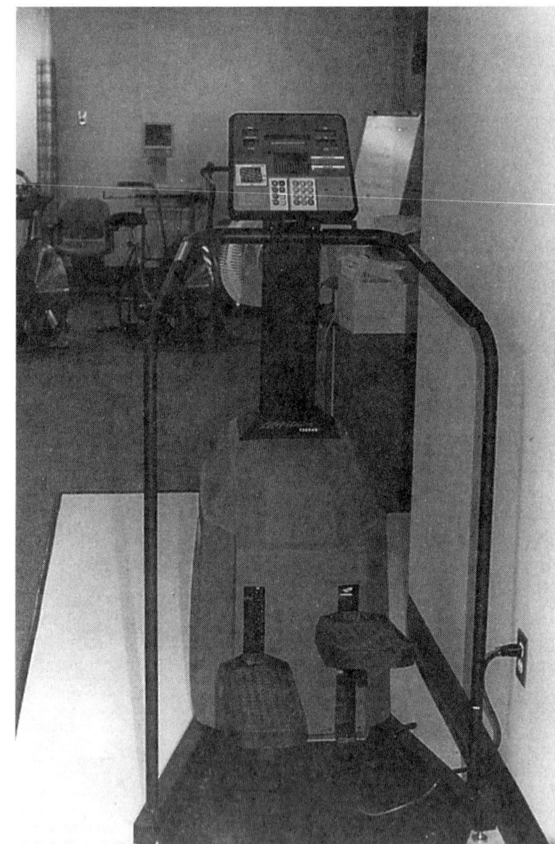

Figure 81-7. The stair climber yields metabolic and peripheral hemodynamic benefits with less demand on the cardiovascular system.

an advantage over treadmill walking for patients with claudication, noting that similar metabolic, claudication, and peripheral hemodynamic measurements are obtained with less demand on the cardiovascular system (Fig. 81-7).

Care of the Diabetic or Vascular Compromised Foot

The ischemic foot sustains damage usually from a combination of ischemia and neuropathy. Injury occurs from external forces that a person would normally avoid if warning pain were experienced (95,96). All patients with ischemia probably have some degree of neuropathy. Similarly, most patients with neuropathy also have some degree of ischemia (97). The coexistence of peripheral arterial disease and peripheral neuropathy has been well established in the literature (98–107). Evidence of peripheral neuropathy was found in 89% of patients with transmetatarsal amputation and diabetes (108,109). Most individuals with ischemic feet do well unless the foot is injured or ulcerated. The injuries or ulcerations that occur in ischemic feet, in turn, are often related to the prevailing neuropathic condition. Therefore, in caring for the ischemic foot, it is important not only to pay attention to the vascular compromise, but also to emphasize avoidance of the injury and infection that are so frequently associated with a sensory compromise. Early detection of sensory loss and implementation of prevention strategies, including routine examination, education in foot care, use of proper footwear, and careful management of ulcerations and infection, are key elements in avoiding amputation (110).

Breakdown in skin integrity requires mechanical or thermal injury. Direct trauma can result from a puncture (such as from a nail) or a high-pressure injury (such as from stepping on a small object). The pressure created on the bottom of a foot when stepping on a small pebble can be several hundred pounds per square inch. For these reasons, a patient with a vascular compromised foot should be instructed never to walk barefoot, even in the home. To avoid the possibility of traumatizing the foot on foreign bodies, shoes should be shaken out prior to donning. The presence of continuous low pressures, as low as 1 lb/inch^2,

Table 81-1: Exercise Protocols for Intermittent Claudication

Study	Frequency and Length of Session	Level of Supervision	Duration of Program	Exercise Type	Outcomes
Larsen and Lassen, 1966 (40)	Daily, 1 hr	Independent	6 mo	Walking to tolerance, rests as needed, pedometer monitoring	Increased walking time and walking distance, decreased anxiety and decreased use of nitroglycerin for angina
Skinner and Strandness, 1967 (89)	30 l-hr sessions	Supervised and individual	3–8 mo	Walking to 75% of maximal walking time alternating with rest	Increased time of onset of claudication pain (CPT), maximal walking time and resting ankle pressures
Ekroth et al, 1978 (41)	3×/wk, 30 min	Physical therapist supervised—in hospital—individual for first 2–3 sessions, then group plus daily home training	4–6 mo	Dynamic leg exercises, marking time, walking, running, dancing, playing ball	Increased walking ability, increased maximal calf blood flow in patients with femoropopliteal stenosis
Jonason et al, 1979 (85)	2×/wk, 30 min	Physical therapist supervised	3 mo	Simple movements of the feet and legs until near maximal pain (heel raising, jumping, dancing, rope skipping, bicycle)	Increased walking distance, decreased leg pain
Dahlloff et al, 1983 (79)	3×/wk, 30 min	Groups of 10–12 with physical therapist	Open ended	Walking, jogging, dynamic exercises	Increased walking distance
Ruell et al, 1984 (84)	3×/wk, 30 min	Groups under supervision	8 wk	Bicycle ergometer or treadmill	Increased pain-free walking distance and maximal walking tolerance, decreased venous lactate concentrations
Boyd et al, 1984 (38)	3×/wk, 25–40 min	Individually prescribed	12 wk	Treadmill, running track and/or bicycle ergometer	Increased walking distance, walking time, energy expenditure
Rosetzsky et al, 1985 (82)	3×/wk, 45 min	Groups with physical therapist	3 mo	Stretching, "general" exercise, conditioning to leg muscles (ascending and descending stairs)	Increased maximum walking distance
Ernst and Matrai, 1987 (33)	2×/day—5 days/wk on treadmill plus 2×/day independently	—	2 mo	Treadmill ergometer at 3 km/hr at angle of 13 degrees to maximal walking	Increase in maximal and pain-free walking distances; normalization of

Table 81-1: (*continued*)

Study	Frequency and Length of Session	Level of Supervision	Duration of Program	Exercise Type	Outcomes
	to onset of ischemic pain			distance	blood rheology (blood and plasma viscosity, blood cell filterability, red cell aggregation)
Jonason and Ringqvist, 1987 (83)	2×/wk, 45 min	Groups with physical therapist plus home exercise	3 mo	Walking, dancing, rope skipping, bicycle	Increase in maximum walking distance and pain-free walking distance
Mannarino et al, 1989 (42)	1 hr daily walking plus 2×/wk in outpatient department	Home training program plus supervised exercise sessions	6 mo	Daily walking plus twice-weekly slow walk, quick march, hopping, jogging, isometric and isotonic gymnastics, breathing exercises	Increased pain-free walking time
Rosfors et al, 1989 (214)	2×/wk, 30 min	Groups with physical therapist plus home exercise	6 mo	Dynamic and static leg exercises (heel raises, knee bends), walking	Increase in walking distance, lower serum fructosamine, variable change in serum insulin level, increase in serum growth hormone
Hiatt et al, 1990 (46)	3×/wk, 60 min	Groups 3×/wk plus independent walking at least 30 min 2×/wk	36 sessions—approx. 13 wk	Treadmill with progressive speed and grade increases	Increased peak walking time, peak oxygen consumption and pain-free walking time, decrease in plasma short-chain acylcarnitine concentration

as might occur with wearing shoes, can also aggravate ischemia, leading to ulceration. It is not uncommon for breakdown to occur, particularly when wearing a new pair of shoes for 4 or 5 hours or longer. A diabetic patient with sensory compromise might notice recent "changes" in shoe size and purchase shoes with narrower widths than previously. In reality, the patient's foot is probably not shrinking in size or width, but with progressing neuropathic sensory loss, the patient will not feel the usual snugness of the shoes unless they are tighter. Such overly tight shoes, however, can produce pressures sufficient to precipitate an ischemic ulceration, which usually develops on the edge of the foot (111) (Fig. 81-8).

Ulcerations that develop on the bottom of the foot over the metatarsal heads are often the result of the repetitive motion of walking. As the heel is raised higher, particularly with faster walking speeds, there is greater stress on the metatarsal heads. Footwear that spreads out weight-bearing pressures will counteract these forces. This is best achieved by molded shoes or custom orthotic inserts placed in extra-depth orthopedic Oxfords. The depth of the shoes should be sufficient to accommodate the orthotic inserts as well as any toe deformities, and soft thermoformable leather should be used (112). Leather can absorb foot perspiration while allowing evaporation of moisture from the foot and can also be stretched over bony prominences to reduce pressure (113). When high peaks of pressure exist under the metatarsal heads, a molded insert is more effective than a flat insert in reducing the pressure level (114). Rocker-bottom shoes also distribute concentrated weight-bearing pressure away from the metatarsal heads when the heel is raised (Fig. 81-9). The use of specially designed shoes is effective in preventing relapses in diabetic patients with previous ulceration (112).

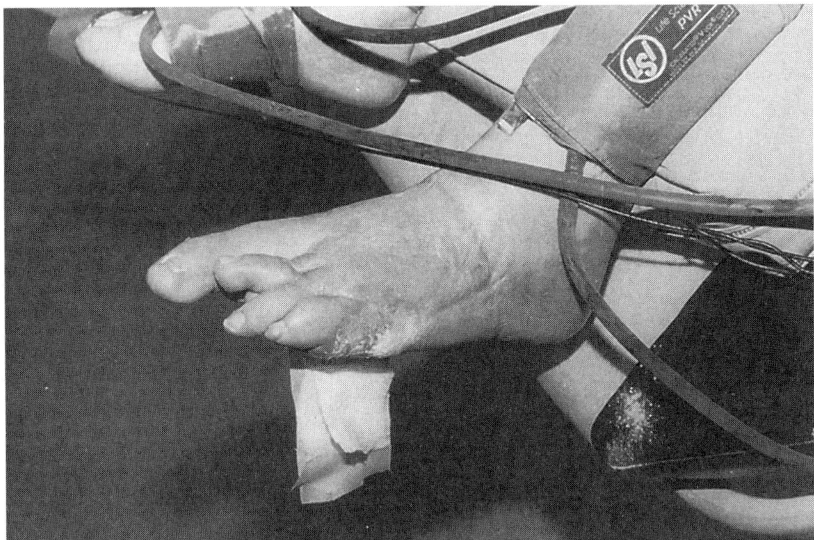

Figure 81-8. Healing ischemic ulcer on the lateral edge of the foot. Note the residual after second-toe amputation resulting from gangrene.

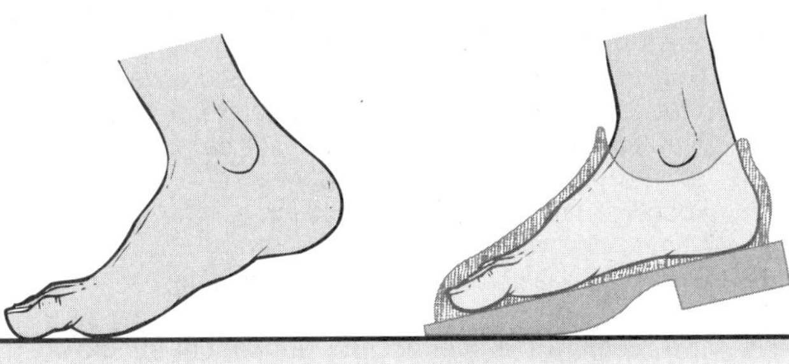

Figure 81-9. The rocker-bottom shoe decreases pressure on the metatarsal heads when the heel is raised. Without the shoe (*A*), weight is concentrated on the metatarsal heads. With the rocker-bottom shoe (*B*), distribution of weight is achieved over a larger area on the foot.

Thermography and aesthesiometry are objective techniques that can enhance assessment of the risk of breakdown. Bergtholdt and Brand (115,116) noted that early assessment of temperature changes over the feet by palpation and by thermography is a valuable method of detecting subclinical inflammatory changes of irritated tissue prior to skin breakdown and development of permanent injury. Use of the Semmes-Weinstein pressure aesthesiometer is a sensitive technique for screening for cutaneous pressure insensitivity of the diabetic foot (117,118). This instrument consists of a nylon monofilament (bristle) mounted on a plastic handle that exerts 10 g of pressure against the foot. If the patient is unable to feel the pressure of the monofilament over any 10 points located on the dorsal and plantar aspects of the foot, there is a loss of protective sensation, thereby signaling high risk for injury.

Wound Healing

When ulcers do occur, care consists of bed rest and antibiotics during the acute treatment phase. Mobilization while minimizing the risk of further trauma to the area is important. In some patients, the ulcers will not heal if there is weight bearing through the area. Total contact plaster casts can promote healing (119) while permitting some weight bearing.

Wound healing is more rapid in the upper extremities than in the lower extremities and significant delays in cutaneous wound healing occur in patients with peripheral vascular disease and diabetes (120–122). Histologically there are significantly reduced numbers of neutrophils and macrophages in 7-day-old wounds in patients with peripheral vascular disease. This also correlates with transcutaneous partial pressure of oxygen measurements of less than 20 mm Hg (122). A study of the healing of experimental wounds in hyperglycemic animals noted that tensile strength and the development of scar tissue were reduced. These changes were reversed when the animals were treated with insulin. These findings suggest that the diabetic state is associated with poor quality of wound healing, and this is partially responsive to treatment with insulin (121).

Risk Factor Modification

It is important to make every possible component of risk factor reduction available to the patient with peripheral arterial disease. This can be achieved through assessment, education of the patient and family, timely identification of problems, and early and effective intervention.

The assessment of risk should be part of every history and physical examination. In addition to addressing specific underlying medical and pathologic conditions, assessment should also focus closely on key areas, that in turn provide information needed to achieve the most effective risk management strategy. The history should include specific information relative to lower-extremity pain; numbness; coldness; claudication; walking distances; previous skin lesions (blisters, ulcerations, etc); medications; smoking; diet; vocational, avocational, and exercise activities; types of footwear used; general foot care and personal hygiene habits; home environment (e.g., stairs, ambulation distances, physical hazards); and family support. This information should be combined with the physical examination findings, with particular attention to any existing disabilities (e.g., visual loss, hemiparesis) that may impact on preparing the individual to carry out an active role in a preventive program. This information should serve as a baseline used to track progress and guide planning on follow-up visits. Various multidisciplinary clinic programs have been developed to provide patient education, preventive care, shoes, orthotics, and identification of candidates for prophylactic surgery aimed at improved pressure distribution or revascularization. In addition to preventing amputation, among patients who did require lower-extremity amputation, increased use of the multidisciplinary foot care clinic correlated with preservation of more residual limb (123).

Patients at risk for vascular foot complications should be given detailed preventive instructions (124) (Table 81-2).

Table 81-2: General Instructions to the Patient at Risk for Vascular Foot Complications

1. The feet should be washed on a daily basis with mild soap and warm water (hot water should be avoided to prevent burns), patting dry with a towel and drying between toes.
2. Lanolin should be applied for dryness and mild powder for excessive perspiration. Lamb's wool may be inserted between toes for added dryness. Do not use strong topical antiseptic agents.
3. Daily inspection of the feet should include the soles and between the toes with attention to redness, swelling, blisters, or openings in the skin.
4. Avoid any self-treatment of corns and calluses with a razor or knife. (Soaking is acceptable but if there is no improvement a podiatrist should be consulted.)
5. Toenails should be cut straight across after washing and filed to eliminate rough edges. (If they are too thick or brittle, they should be cut by a podiatrist.)
6. New shoes should be comfortable, and cover the feet completely. They should be made of soft leather or other natural materials. The patient should break them in gradually.
7. Footwear should be used at all times; the patient should not walk barefoot.
8. External heat or cold applications should be avoided.
9. If a break in the skin occurs, the patient should wash the area with soap and water, cover it with a dry sterile gauze, change the dressing daily, and inspect the area for redness, swelling, and drainage. The physician should be notified if there is no improvement within 2 or 3 days.
10. The patient should adhere closely to recommended treatment, including diet, and monitoring regimens for diabetes, hypertension, hyperlipidemia, and other medical conditions.
11. Smoking should be avoided.

VENOUS DISORDERS

Major rehabilitative concerns involving the venous system are largely related to the prevention of thromboembolic disease and control of chronic disorders that frequently cause edema, pain, and ulceration. Many of the conditions routinely treated in rehabilitation carry a high risk for the development of both acute and chronic venous conditions that must be recognized and managed concomitantly with the patient's primary disability.

Venous Thrombosis and Prophylaxis

Two of the most common and potentially life-threatening conditions associated with disability, surgery, and hospitalization are DVT and pulmonary thromboembolism. Most DVTs are asymptomatic. It is important to implement systematic screening for DVT in the proximal veins, because fatal pulmonary emboli are usually caused by thromboses at that level.

The pathophysiology of the development of DVT is based on the Virchow triad: 1) endothelial trauma, 2) venous stasis, and 3) increased blood coagulability. Prevention is based on addressing one or more of these. Prophylaxis in high-risk patients has traditionally consisted of "mini-dose" heparin in the form of 5000 units given subcutaneously every 8 or 12 hours. Intermittent pneumatic compression is an effective alternative to heparin. Other preventive methods have included antiplatelet medication such as aspirin or dipyridamole, electrical stimulation of the calves, graduated pressure stockings, and for long-term prophylaxis when anticoagulation is not feasible, vena caval filters. Prevention of venous stasis is an accepted measure for avoidance of DVT, and therefore, activity is encouraged wherever possible. There has been some controversy, however, concerning the benefits of early postoperative ambulation; it has been suggested that part of the process of early ambulation consists of having a patient walk to a chair and sit, thereby placing the legs in a dependent position, causing more stasis (125).

Deep Vein Thrombosis in Surgical Patients

Without prophylaxis, patients undergoing major orthopedic surgery have a 50% to 60% incidence of DVT, with 10% to 30% occurring in proximal veins, and after total hip replacement a 1% to 2% rate of fatal pulmonary embolism (126). The incidence of DVT following total knee arthroplasty is even higher, ranging from 55% to

70%. Low-molecular-weight heparins (LMWHs), derived by fragmentation of heparin, are mixtures of heparin molecules in the range of 3000 to 10,000 daltons (127). LMWHs are more effective and at least as safe as using standard heparin in the prevention of venous thrombosis following total hip replacement (126,128,129). They are also effective for prophylaxis of DVT associated with medical indications and for treatment of established DVT (127). Enoxaparin, a LMWH that is approved for use in the United States for prophylaxis against DVT following total hip replacement surgery, is more costly than unfractionated heparin or low-dose warfarin, but is cost-effective because it reduces the number of cases of DVT (130). The overall cost of warfarin may also be increased in relation to that of LMWHs, if the cost of measuring prothrombin times to monitor the intensity of anticoagulation is included (131). It has also been reported that enoxaparin has the potential to decrease the risk of DVT and the length of the hospital stay following hip replacement, as compared with unfractionated heparin (132). Similar benefits were reported for the use of LMWHs for prophylaxis of DVT in general surgery (133,134). While many reports note that LMWHs carry no higher risk of major bleeding, a series of 721 patients studied by Hull et al (132) revealed a higher incidence of major bleeding in the group treated with LMWH as compared to warfarin (2.8% and 1.2%, respectively). Thus, although the preponderance of studies supports the cost-effectiveness of LMWHs, controversy still exists regarding its use.

Deep Vein Thrombosis in Spinal Cord Injury and Stroke Rehabilitation

Patients with neurologic dysfunction are at increased risk for thromboembolic disorders. In a literature review by Merli et al (135), stasis and hypercoagulability were identified as the two major factors contributing to the development of DVT in persons with acute spinal cord injury. The incidence was noted to vary from 49% to 100% in the first 12 weeks, with the most frequent occurrence in the first 2 weeks. The incidence of DVT was reduced by 1) the combination of external pneumatic compression sleeves and either aspirin/dipyridamole or low-dose heparin, or 2) electrical stimulation plus low-dose heparin. The duration of prophylaxis varied between 8 and 12 weeks. Green et al (136) found LMWH to be safe and effective in the prevention of thromboembolism in selected patients with spinal cord injury and complete motor paralysis, with results superior to those obtained using standard heparin. Brandstater et al (137) noted an incidence of DVT in stroke patients without prophylaxis ranging from 23% to 75% and an incidence of pulmonary embolism of 10% to 20%, with mortality of up to 10%. In a series of 360 patients with stroke, Pambianco et al (138) noted time interval (from onset of stroke to admission) and lactic dehydrogenase (LDH) concentration to be significant risk factors and predictors for development of DVT. Patients were assigned randomly to four treatment groups: adjusted-dose heparin, intermittent pneumatic compression, functional electrical stimulation (FES), and control (below-knee stockings only). No significant difference was noted in the development of DVT among the three treatment groups and the control group. Suboptimal compliance with intermittent pneumatic compression prophylaxis associated with problems with patient tolerance was noted. Clagett et al (139) concluded that low-dose heparin (standard/unfractionated) and LMWH are preferable for DVT prophylaxis in stroke patients. Warfarin is effective in preventing DVT but is associated with a higher incidence of bleeding complications and has not been recommended for primary DVT prophylaxis in patients with stroke (137). When used as secondary prophylaxis (to prevent recurrence of DVT following an acute thrombosis) at therapeutic doses [international normalized ratio (INR) 2–3], the reported risk of intracranial hemorrhage ranges from 4% to 5% (137,140). To minimize the risk of DVT, stroke patients should be mobilized early, wear elastic stockings, and be treated by one of the accepted preventive treatment modalities (e.g., heparin, intermittent pneumatic compression) (141).

Diagnosis of Deep Vein Thrombosis

Clinical signs and symptoms have proved notoriously unreliable in diagnosing the presence of DVT (142,143). The traditional gold standard for the diagnosis of DVT has been the contrast venogram. This invasive procedure carries the risk of complications related to the use of radiopaque contrast material. Duplex scanning with B-mode ultrasound (143) has recently been the procedure of choice for screening, with a high degree of sensitivity to venous thrombi above the knee. Sensitivity is lower for calf thrombi. Impedance plethysmography measures maximal venous output and venous capacitance, which are lower in the presence of venous obstruction. While not sensitive to most calf thrombi or small nonoccluding proximal thrombi, impedance plethysmography was proved to be highly sensitive (approximately 95%) in various published trials (137). Impedance plethysmography is also less dependent on the technical skill of the operator than is Doppler. Color-flow Doppler ultrasound can diagnose calf DVT, with a sensitivity of 98% as compared with contrast venography (144). Iodine-125–labeled fibrinogen scanning is sensitive for detecting small calf thrombi and has been used in research. However, its clinical use has been very limited.

Treatment of Deep Vein Thrombosis

The mainstay of treatment for DVT is systemic heparin followed by warfarin. The duration of treatment with oral anticoagulation after the diagnosis of DVT has been variable. Tyrell et al (145) suggested that warfarin should be continued for 1 month for postoperative DVT and 3 months for spontaneous DVT. Shulman et al (146), however, demonstrated that prophylactic oral anticoagulation for 6 months after a first episode of venous thromboembolism led to a lower recurrence rate than did treatment lasting for 6 weeks. Once DVT is diagnosed, heparin is generally administered intravenously for at least 4 or 5 days, overlapped with initiation of warfarin. Status of anticoagulation is preferably followed with the INR, a reporting system proposed by the World Health Organization in collaboration with the International Committee on Thrombosis and Hemostasis and the International Council on the Standardization in Hematology, for the purpose of minimizing interlaboratory variability of coagulation instrument and reagent systems to monitor patients receiving warfarin therapy (147,148). Oral anticoagulant treatment is generally considered safe and effective if the INR is maintained at 2.0 to 3.0 (149). Recent clinical trials showed administration of standard heparin by the subcutaneous route to be as efficacious in the treatment of established DVT as when administered intravenously, with no significant differences in observed rates of clinically important events, thereby permitting safe treatment at home and avoiding the need for hospitalization (150). In a recent trial in the Netherlands comparing outcomes with in-hospital administered intravenous unfractionated heparin and fixed-dose LMWH administered subcutaneously at home, the latter was found to be feasible, effective, and safe (151).

Recurrent spontaneous occurrence of DVT has been suggested as an indication for lifelong anticoagulation. Some large thrombi require thrombolytic therapy (152) to lyse the clot and minimize damage to the valves, thereby possibly preventing postphlebitic syndrome. Complications of lytic therapy include severe bleeding, in addition to potential clot fragmentation and embolization.

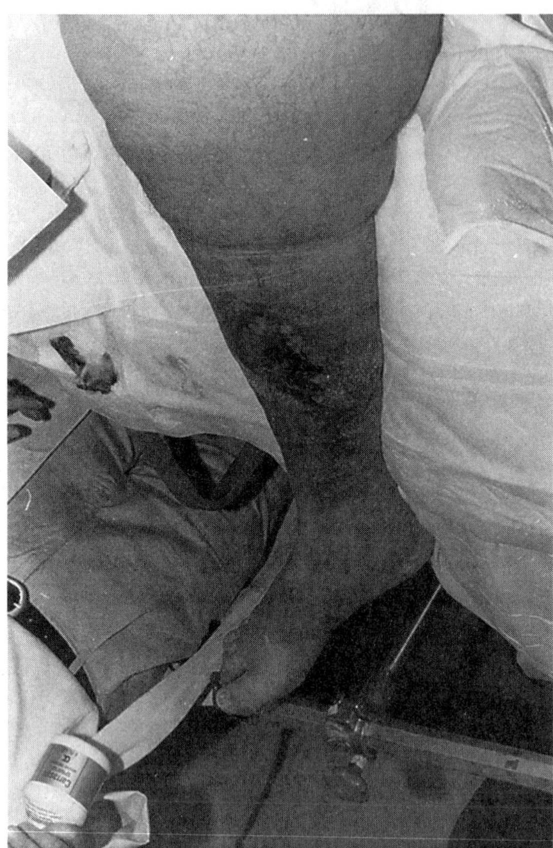

Figure 81-10. Venous ulcers account for the majority of leg ulcers and result from the edema associated with venous fluid backing up into the skin and subcutaneous tissue.

Venous Insufficiency

DVT is considered the most common cause of chronic insufficiency of the deep venous system in the lower extremities. This condition is frequently referred to as *postphlebitic syndrome* (153–156). Thrombosis and phlebitis in the deep venous system can result in destruction of the normal valvular mechanisms and lead to valvular incompetence, calf pump dysfunction, venous hypertension, and reflux (157,158). When there is incompetence of the perforating draining veins of the lower leg, blood flow from the deep venous system backs up into the skin and subcutaneous tissue, causing edema and, if persistent and severe enough, ulceration (Fig. 81-10). Hemosiderin deposits from stagnant blood result in the brown hyperpigmented appearance (Fig. 81-11).

The clinical manifestations of chronic venous insufficiency include swelling, pain, complaints of heaviness in the legs, dilated superficial veins, skin changes, and ulceration (159). The primary treatment for chronic venous insufficiency is compression therapy. Gradient compression hosiery was invented by Jobst in the 1950s to mimic the hydrostatic forces exerted by water in a swimming pool (160). Stockings exerting 40 mm Hg of pressure at the ankle are associated with a reduction in ambulatory venous pressure, which may in turn lead to clinical prevention or improvement of the various sequelae associated with chronic venous hypertension (161). A frequent pitfall in the use of elastic compression stockings is the difficulty many patients encounter in donning them, particularly patients who are older, debilitated, and arthritic. Such patients should be evaluated and supplied with appropriate assistive devices or the patient's caregiver should be instructed in assisting with the application of the stockings. Walking and gentle exercises are helpful in enlarging and maintaining venous collaterals. Tipping of the bed into a head-down position reduces edema and muscle compartment tension at night. Surgical treatment is indicated when severe stasis symptoms persist despite conservative therapy and also may be considered in younger patients and those requiring a rapid recovery and return to normal activities (162). Venous ligation and, when necessary, sclerotherapy have been used successfully in an outpatient setting in a young group of working patients who were able to return to work rapidly following treatment (163).

The majority of chronic leg ulcers are venous in origin (164,165) and tend to occur in older individuals with a history of DVT or an associated condition (165).

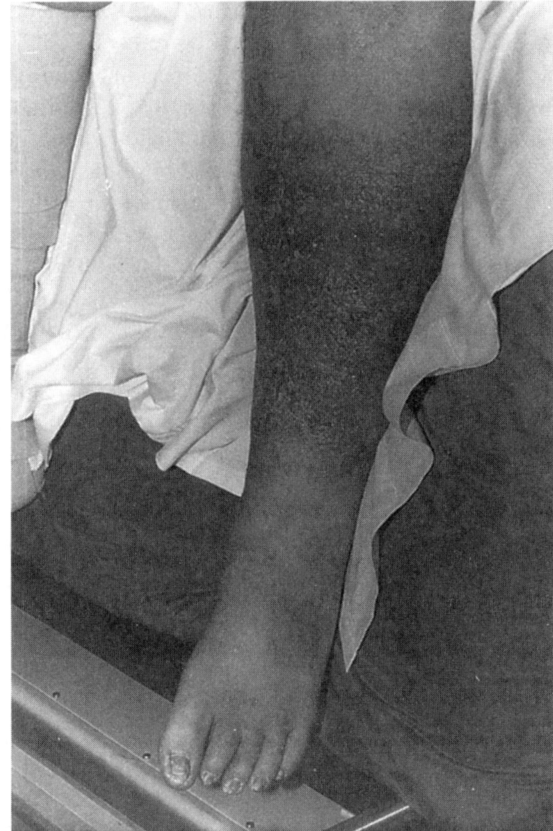

Figure 81-11. The brown discoloration associated with venous stasis results from hemosiderin deposits from stagnant blood.

The goal in treatment of a venous ulcer is rapid and permanent re-epithelialization of the ulcer bed (166). Early treatment will improve outcome. Management may be surgical or nonsurgical and can include wound débridement, electrical stimulation (159,167,168), compression therapy, exercise, leg elevation at rest, and paste gauze boots (Unna boot) (169,170). Moneta et al (160) indicated a protocol consisting of 1) assessment for infection and the extent of edema; 2) 5 to 7 days of bed rest, when necessary, to resolve the edema; 3) short-term intravenous or oral antibiotic treatment for cellulitis with dry gauze dressings changed every 12 hours; 4) avoidance of topical agents; 5) fitting with below-knee 30- to 40-mm Hg elastic compression stockings when edema or cellulitis has resolved (two pairs); 5) wound care throughout the course of therapy consisting of daily washing with soap and water and covering with a dry gauze dressing held in place with the compression stocking; 6) topical corticosteroids applied to the surrounding areas of significant stasis dermatitis but not to the ulcer itself; and 7) continued ambulatory compression therapy once the ulcer has healed. Skin should be clean and lubricated at all times. The need for hospitalization in the treatment of venous ulcers should be based on individual factors such as the specific interventions required (e.g., intravenous antibiotics), availability of home-based services, family support, and comorbidity.

Various other forms of elastic compression devices are available. The Circ-Aid is a compression orthosis that produces rigid compression, is easy to apply, and is adaptable to a reduction in edema (171). The orthosis is designed with multiple, pliable, rigid, adjustable compression bands that wrap around the leg from the ankle to the knee and are held in place with Velcro tape.

Hydrocolloid dressings (Duoderm) or zinc paste bandages (Unna boot) have been used as treatment for venous ulcers. These should be applied weekly and combined with compression bandages (169). Lippman et al (172) described the Unna boot as a "functional substitute for the failing muscle pump in chronic venous insufficiency"; it is a noninvasive ambulatory method of controlling edema and treating ulcers (Fig. 81-12). Duoderm CGF hydroactive (HD) dressing with compression has been reported to result in faster ulcer healing rates as compared with the Unna boot during initial therapy (the first 4 weeks), and possibly

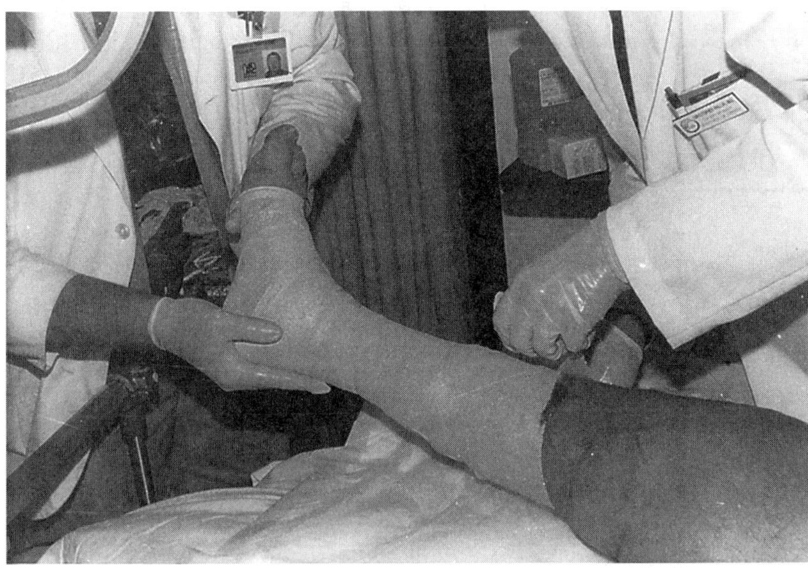

Figure 81-12. Unna boot, a medicated bandage impregnated with zinc oxide, should be applied weekly in the treatment of venous ulcers and followed by application of a compressive bandage.

over a 12-week treatment period (173). However, occlusive hydrocolloid dressings are also associated with an increased rate in infectious complications (174).

Silver sulfadiazine has antibacterial properties and can facilitate healing in wounds, possibly through keratinocyte replication and anti-inflammatory properties resulting in enhanced epithelialization (175).

Various medications have been investigated but are generally recognized to be of little benefit in the management of venous ulcerations (176,177). These drugs have included fibrinolytics, which were found to produce a relative decrease in area of lipodermatosclerosis (178); hydroxyrutosides, through slight reduction of edema (179); prostaglandins, through decreases in activation of white blood cells, platelet aggregation, and small-vessel vasodilation (180,181); pentoxifylline, with complete or increased ulcer healing compared to placebo controls (182); and flunarizine, through possible improvement in subcutaneous circulation in the lower legs (183). Venous ulcers have a recurrence rate of nearly 70% (159,175) and once healing is accomplished, compression stockings should be used on a permanent basis along with elevation and frequent lower-extremity motion (166).

LYMPHEDEMA

The function of the lymphatic system is to collect fluid as well as protein, red blood cells, bacteria, and other particles that are too large to drain through small venules. Lymph is transported from lymphatic capillaries through afferent vessels to regional lymph nodes, and then transported through the thoracic duct to the subclavian vein, or through other lymphovenous communications to the peripheral vessels (184). Lymph channels normally achieve central flow through the combined effect of lymphatic valves, muscular contractions, respiration, and arterial pulsation. Lymphedema results from an excessive accumulation of fluid associated with disruption or compromise of the lymph channels. The lymphatics normally protect against bacterial invasion; thus, limbs with lymphedema are at increased risk of infection.

Table 81-3: Classification of Lymphedema
Primary lymphedema
Lymphedema praecox
Lymphedema tarda
Secondary lymphedema
Malignancy
Radiation
Trauma
Surgical excision
Inflammation/infection
Parasitic (filiariasis)
Sarcoidosis
Paralysis
Acquired immunodeficiency syndrome

Lymphedema has been classified based on etiology, severity, time of onset, and anatomic features (185,186) (Table 81-3). Primary lymphedema is congenital and results from agenesis (complete failure to develop) or aplasia (poor development) of the lymphatic system. Primary lymphedema is typically noted in young females and characterized by diffuse swelling of the lower extremities (187). Lymphedema praecox generally occurs in females in the second or third decade of life (188) and lymphedema tarda is characterized by onset after age 35 (189). Hyperplasia can also result in a small percentage of cases of primary lymphedema (184). Secondary lymphedema is acquired and may occur in association with malignancy, radiation, trauma, surgical excision, inflammation or infection, parasitic invasion (filiariasis), sarcoidosis, paralysis, and acquired immuno deficiency syndrome (184,190,191).

Breast cancer affects one in nine women in the United States (192). Modified radical mastectomy with corresponding lymphadenectomy and radiation results in clinically symptomatic lymphedema in a significant portion of the postmastectomy patients, with reported incidence ranging from 5.5% to 80.0% (188,193,194). The diagnosis can usually be made 6 weeks after breast cancer surgery, when postsurgical swelling has subsided (195).

Treatment should be multidisciplinary and include both hygienic and mechanical components (187,196,197). Goals of treatment include relief of pain and discomfort, restoration of normal movement and body image, and psychosocial adjustment (192,198,199). Patient education, skin hygiene, and avoidance of injury are of primary importance. Elevation is recommended to reduce edema (88,187,200,201). Additionally, compression garments, elastic bandaging, massage, manual lymph drainage, and therapeutic exercises (202,203) can reduce edema and the feeling of heaviness in the arm. Pneumatic compression pumps have shown some evidence of success (199,204–206) but remain controversial (187). Subcontraction high-voltage electrical stimulation in the rat increased lymphatic uptake of labeled protein; it has been suggested that this modality has the potential to reduce edema (207). In one clinical trial, however, electrically stimulated lymphatic drainage did not demonstrate any benefit over treatment with an elastic sleeve (208). A combination of techniques to treat lymphedema has been referred to as "complex physical therapy" and "complex lymphedema therapy." This includes skin hygiene, a special lymphatic massage, compression bandaging, compression garments, and exercises (197,203).

Compression Therapy

Intermittent pneumatic compression is used in the treatment of lymphedema as well as the treatment of edema associated with venous insufficiency, venous ulceration, postoperative or posttraumatic edema, and prevention of

DVT (209). While devices that apply intermittent compression of uniform strength (single chamber) are available, those that produce sequential gradient compression (multichamber graded) have received the most attention (160). Theoretically, the disadvantage of a single-chamber device is related to high pressure exerted both proximally and distally, potentially forcing fluid into the distal portion of the extremity (210). In a comparison of multichamber to single-chamber devices in the treatment of lymphedema, the multichamber device decreased edema faster both in the upper and in the lower extremities, with treatment times of 2 hours with the multichamber device and 6 hours with the single-chamber device (211). In the treatment of venous ulcers, intermittent pneumatic compression administered in 45-minute sessions 5 days per week for 2 weeks, followed by treatment twice per week, was associated with a mean healing time of 5 weeks as compared with 13 weeks for patients treated with elastic compression bandages alone (212). Between treatments, elastic compression wraps and wet-to-dry dressings were used. In the treatment of lymphedema of the lower extremity, favorable outcomes were reported using a protocol consisting of 2 to 3 days of hospitalization with daily 6- to 8-hour treatment with sequential high-pressure intermittent pneumatic compression using the Lymphapress device, followed by the use of a custom two-way stretch elastic stocking (213).

Once reduction in limb size is achieved through pneumatic compression, elevation, and other methods, maintenance of limb size largely depends on the use of external support devices (210). Over-the-counter graduated elastic support stockings are sufficient in some patients but when there is severe edema or an unusual leg shape, custom-made stockings are necessary. Compression categories for elastic stockings include 20 to 30, 30 to 40, 40 to 50, and 50 to 60 mm Hg. Treatment of lymphedema generally requires a pressure of at least 40 to 50 mm Hg. Lower-pressure compression stockings can be useful in cases of venous insufficiency, particularly when the use of high-pressure compression stockings is limited by arthritis or arterial occlusive disease (210).

REFERENCES

1. Balkau B, Vray M, Eschwege E. Epidemiology of peripheral arterial disease. *J Cardiovasc Pharmacol* 1994;23(suppl 3): S8–S16.

2. Rose AG. The diagnosis of ischaemic heart pain and intermittent claudication in field surveys. *Bull Org Mond Sante* 1962;27:645–658.

3. Rose G, McCartney P, Reid DD. Self-administration of a questionnaire on chest pain and intermittent claudication. *Br J Prev Soc Med* 1977;31(1):42–48.

4. Vogt MT, Wolfson SK, Kuller LH. Lower extremity arterial disease and the aging process: a review. *J Clin Epidemiol* 1992;45: 529–542.

5. Fowkes FGR. *Epidemiology of peripheral vascular disease.* London: Springer 1991.

6. Radack K, Wyderski RJ. Conservative management of intermittent claudication. *Ann Intern Med* 1990;113:135–146.

7. Kannel WB, Skinner JJ Jr, Schwartz MG, Shurtleff D. Intermittent claudication. Incidence in the Framingham study. *Circulation* 1970;41:875–883.

8. Birkmeyer JD, O'Connor GT, Quinton HB, et al. The effect of peripheral vascular disease on in-hospital mortality rates with coronary artery bypass surgery: Northern New England Cardiovascular Disease Study Group. *J Vasc Surg* 1995;21:445–452.

9. Criqui MH, Langer RD, Fronek A, et al. Mortality over 10 years in patients with peripheral arterial disease. *N Engl J Med* 1992; 326:381–386.

10. O'Riordan DS, O'Donnell JA. Realistic expectations for the patient with intermittent claudication. *Br J Surg* 1991;78: 861–863.

11. Hollinshead WH. *Anatomy for surgeons: the back and limbs.* 3rd ed. Philadelphia: Harper & Row 1982:800.

12. Baker JD. The vascular laboratory. In: Moore WS, ed. *Vascular surgery: a comprehensive review.* 4th ed. Philadelphia: WB Saunders 1993.

13. Brearley S, Shearman CP, Simms MH. Peripheral pulse palpation: an unreliable physical sign. *Ann R Coll Surg Engl* 1992;74:1669–1671.

14. Marcon G, Barbato O, Scevola M, et al. Unnecessary arterial Doppler examination of the legs: clinical decision rules may help? *Qual Assur Health Care* 1991;3: 115–122.

15. Walters TK, Mitchell DC, Wood RFM. Low-dose aspirin fails to inhibit increased platelet reactivity in patients with peripheral vascular disease. *Br J Surg* 1993;80:1266–1268.

16. Harrison DG, Armstrong ML, Freiman PC, et al. Restoration of endothelium-dependent relaxation by dietary treatment of atherosclerosis. *J Clin Invest* 1987;80: 1808–1811.

17. Blankenhorn DH, Kramsch DM. Reversal of atherosis and sclerosis. The two components of atherosclerosis. *Circulation* 1989; 79:1–7.

18. Brown G, Albers JJ, Fisher LD, et al. Regression of coronary disease as a result of intensive lipid-lowering therapy in men with high levels of apolipoprotein B. *N Engl J Med* 1990;323: 1289–1298.

19. Kramsch DM, Blankenhorn DH. Regression of atherosclerosis: which components regress and

what influences their reversal. *Wein Klin Wochenschr* 1992; 104:2–9.

20. Blankenhorn DH, Hodis HN. Atherosclerosis—reversal with therapy. *West J Med* 1993;159: 172–179.

21. Bjelajac A, Goo AK, Weart CT. Prevention and regression of atherosclerosis: effects of HMG-CoA reductase inhibitors. *Ann Pharmacother* 1996;30: 1304–1315.

22. Schell Wd, Myers JN. Regression of atherosclerosis: a review. *Prog Cardiovasc Dis* 1997;39: 483–496.

23. Zierler E, Strandness DE Jr. Hemodynamics for the vascular surgeon. In: Moore WS, ed. *Vascular surgery: a comprehensive review.* 4th ed. Philadelphia: WB Saunders 1993.

24. Minar E, Ahmadi A, Koppensteiner R, et al. Comparison of effects of high-dose and low-dose aspirin on restenosis after femorpopliteal percutaneous transluminal angioplasty. *Circulation* 1995;91:2167–2173.

25. Ranke C, Creutzig A, Luska G, et al. Controlled trial of high- versus low-dose aspirin treatment after percutaneous transluminal angioplasty in patients with peripheral vascular disease. *Clin Invest* 1994;72:673–680.

26. Volker W, Faber V. Aspirin reduces the growth of medical and neointimal thickenings in balloon-injured rat carotid arteries. *Stroke* 1990;21(suppl 12): IV44–IV45.

27. Ernst E, Kollar L, Resch KL. Does pentoxifylline prolong the walking distance in exercised claudicants? A placebo-controlled double-blind trial. *Angiology* 1992;43:121–125.

28. Gonzalez ER, Liberto RB, Davidson HE, et al. Disease-based assessment of peripheral vascular disease in nursing facility patients. *Ann Pharmacother* 1995;29:671–675.

29. Frampton JE, Brogden RN. Pentoxiphylline (oxypentifylline): a review of its therapeutic efficacy in the management of peripheral vascular and cerebrovascular disorders. *Drugs Aging* 1995;7: 480–503.

30. Campbell RK. Clinical update on pentoxifylline therapy for diabetes-induced peripheral vascular disease. *Ann Pharmacother* 1993;27:1099–1105.

31. Drummond M, Davies L. Economic evaluation of drugs in peripheral vascular disease and stroke. *J Cardiovasc Pharmacol* 1994;23(suppl 3):S4–S7.

32. Segall GM, Lang EV, Lennon SE, Stevick CD. Functional imaging of peripheral vascular disease: a comparison between exercise whole body thallium perfusion imaging and contrast arteriography. *J Nucl Med* 1992;33: 1797–1800.

33. Ernst EEW, Matrai A. Intermittent claudication, exercise and rheology. *Circulation* 1987;76: 1110–1114.

34. Jonason T, Jonzon B, Rinqvist I, Oman-Rydberg A. Effect of physical training on different categories of patients with intermittent claudication. *Acta Med Scand* 1979;206:252–258.

35. Clifford PC, Davies PW, Hayne JA, Baird RN. Intermittent claudication: is a supervised exercise class worth while? *BMJ* 1980;280:1503–1505.

36. Winder WW. Adaptation of skeletal muscle to exercise. In: Lowenthal DT, Bharadwaja K, Okes WW, eds. *Therapeutics through exercise.* New York: Grune & Stratton 1979.

37. Zicot M. Claudication intermittents: introduction à la clinique. *Acta Cardiol* 1979;34:133–139.

38. Boyd CE, Bird PJ, Teates CD, et al. Pain free physical training in intermittent claudication *J Sports Med* 1984;24:112–122.

39. Duprez D, DeBuyzere M, Van Wassenhove A, Clement D. Evaluation of the metabolic compensation after treadmill test in patients with peripheral occlusive arterial disease. *Angiology* 1992; 43:126–133.

40. Larsen OA, Lassen NA. Effect of daily muscular exercise in patients with intermittent claudication. *Lancet* 1966;2: 1093–1096.

41. Ekroth R, Dahllof AG, Gundevall B, et al. Physical training of patients with intermittent claudication: indications, methods and results. *Surgery* 1978;84:640–643.

42. Mannarino E, Pasqualini L, Menna M, et al. Effects of physical training on peripheral vascular disease: a controlled study. *Angiology* 1989;40:5–10.

43. Lewis P, Psaila JV, Davies WT, et al. Nifedipine in patients with peripheral vascular disease. *Eur J Vasc Surg* 1989;3:159–164.

44. Terjung RL, Mathien GM, Erney TP, Ogilvie RW. Peripheral adaptations to low blood flow in muscle during exercise. *Am J Cardiol* 1988;62:15E–19E.

45. Nicholson CD, Angersbach D, Wilke R. The effect of physical training on rat calf muscle, oxygen tension, blood flow, metabolism and function in an animal model of chronic occlusive peripheral vascular disease. *Int J Sports Med* 1992;13:60–64.

46. Hiatt WR, Regensteiner JG, Hargarten ME, et al. Benefit of exercise conditioning for patients with peripheral arterial disease. *Circulation* 1990;81:602–609.

47. McCully KK, Halber C, Posner JD. Exercise-induced changes in oxygen saturation in the calf muscles of elderly subjects with peripheral vascular disease. *J Gerontol* 1994;49:B128–B134.

48. Lundgren F, Dahllof AG, Shersten T, Bylund-Fellenius AC. Muscle enzyme adaptation in patients with peripheral arterial insufficiency: spontaneous adaptation, effect of different treatments and consequences on walking performance. *Clin Sci* 1989;77:485–493.

49. Halperin JL, Creager MA. Arterial obstructive diseases of the

extremities. In: Loscalzo J, Creager MA, Dzau VJ, eds. *Vascular medicine: a textbook of vascular biology and diseases.* Boston: Little, Brown, 1992.

50. Wilson NM, Chan O, Thomal ML, Browse NL. Intravenous digital subtraction angiography in the management of peripheral vascular disease. *J Cardiovasc Surg* 1991;32:747–752.

51. Malden ES, Picus D, Vesely TM, et al. Peripheral vascular disease: evaluation with stepping DSA and conventional screen-film angiography. *Radiology* 1994;191: 149–153.

52. Gomes AS. Principles of angiography and interventional radiology. In: Moore WS, ed. *Vascular surgery: a comprehensive review.* 4th ed. Philadelphia: WB Saunders 1993.

53. Owen RS, Baum RA, Carpenter JP, et al. Symptomatic peripheral vascular disease: selection of imaging parameters and clinical evaluation with MR angiography. *Radiology* 1993;187:627–635.

54. Borello J. MR angiography versus conventional X-ray angiography in the lower extremities: everyone wins. *Radiology* 1993;187: 615–617.

55. Tellier P. Functional imaging of peripheral vascular disease. *J Nucl Med* 1993;34:865–866. Letter.

56. Vogt MT, McKenna M, Anderson SJ, et al. The relationship between ankle-arm index and mortality in older men and women. *J Am Geriatr Soc* 1993;41:523–530.

57. Duprez D. Natural history and evolution of peripheral obstructive arterial disease. *Int Angiol* 1992;11:165–168.

58. McDermott MM, Feinglass J, Slavensky R, Pearce WH. The ankle-brachial index as a predictor of survival in patients with peripheral vascular disease. *J Gen Intern Med* 1994;9: 445–449.

59. Winsor T. Influence of arterial disease on the systolic blood pressure gradients of the extremity. *Am J Med Sci* 1959;220: 117–126.

60. O'keefe ST, Persson AV. Use of noninvasive vascular laboratory in diagnosis of venous and arterial disease. *Cardiol Clin* 1991;9: 429–442.

61. Rosenfield K, Kelly SM, Fields CD, et al. Noninvasive assessment of peripheral vascular disease by color flow Doppler/ two-dimensional ultrasound. *Am J Cardiol* 1989;64:247–251.

62. Polak JF. Peripheral arterial disease: evaluation with color flow and duplex sonography. *Radiol Clin North Am* 1995;33: 71–90.

63. Shankar R. Noninvasive measurement of compliance of human leg arteries. *IIEEE Trans Biomed Eng* 1991;38:62–67.

64. Atmer B, Jogenstrand T, Laska J, Lund F. Peripheral artery disease in patients with coronary artery disease. *Int Angiol* 1995;14: 89–93.

65. Hiatt WR, Hirsch AT, Regensteiner JG, Brass EP. Clinical trials for claudication: assessment of exercise performance, functional status and clinical end points. *Circulation* 1995;92: 614–621.

66. Radack K, Wyderski RJ. Conservative management of intermittent claudication. *Ann Intern Med* 1990;113:135–146.

67. Kim YW, Taylor LM, Porter JM. Circulation-enhancing drugs. In: Rutherford RB, ed. *Vascular surgery.* 4th ed. Philadelphia: WB Saunders, 1995.

68. Lowe GD, Reid AW, Leiberman DP. Management of thrombosis in peripheral arterial disease. *Br Med Bull* 1994;50:923–935.

69. Wutschert R, Bounameaux H. [Use of antithrombotic agents in peripheral vascular diseases.] *Arch Mal Coeur Vaiss* 1966; 89(suppl 11):1551–1555.

70. Gleim M, Maier C, Melchert U. Lumbar neurolytic sympathetic blockades provide immediate and long-lasting improvement of painless walking distance and muscle metabolism in patients with severe peripheral vascular disease. *J Pain Symptom Manage* 1995;10:98–104.

71. Miles JB. Electrical stimulation of the spinal cord in peripheral vascular disease. *BMJ* 1992; 304:1313.

72. Talis RC, Illis LS, Sedgwick EM, et al. The effect of spinal cord stimulation upon peripheral blood flow in patients with chronic neurological disease. *Int Rehabil Med* 1982;5:4–9.

73. Augustinsson LE, Holm J, Carlsson CA, Fall M. Epidural electrical stimulation in severe ischemia: evidence of pain relief, increased blood flow and a possible limb-saving effect. *Ann Surg* 1985;202:104–111.

74. Talis R, Jacobs M, Miles JB. Spinal cord stimulation in peripheral vascular disease. *Br J Neurosurg* 1992;6:101–105.

75. Verazzo G, Coppola L, Luongo C, et al. Hyperbaric oxygen, oxygen-ozone therapy, and rheologic parameters of blood in patients with peripheral occlusive arterial disease. *Undersea Hyperb Med* 1995;22:17–22.

76. Coppola L,Giunta R, Verazzo G, et al. Influence of ozone on haemoglobin oxygen affinity in type-2 diabetic patients with peripheral vascular disease: in vitro studies. *Diabete Metab* 1995;21:252–255.

77. Vezzani G, Marziani L, Pizzola A, et al. [Non-surgical treatment of peripheral vascular diseases: diabetic foot and hyperbaric oxygenation.] *Minerva Anesthesiol* 1992;58: 1119–1120.

78. Smith CM, Yellen AE, Weaver FA, et al. Thrombolytic therapy for arterial occlusion: a mixed blessing. Am Surg 1994;60: 371–375.

79. Dahllof AG, Holm J, Schersten T. Exercise training of patients with intermittent claudication. *Scand J Rehabil Med* 1983; 15(suppl):20–26.

80. Foley WT. Treatment of gangrene of the feet and legs by walking. *Circulation* 1957;15:689.

81. Jonason T, Ringqvist I, Oman-Rydberg O. Home-training of patients with intermittent claudication. Scand J Rehabil Med 1981;13:137–141.

82. Rosetzsky J, Struckmann J, Mathiesen FR. Minimal walking distance following exercise in patients with arterial occlusive disease. Ann Chir Gynaecol 1985;74:261–264.

83. Jonason T, Ringqvist I. Prediction of the effect of training on the walking tolerance in patients with intermittent claudication. *Scand J Rehabil Med* 1987;19:47–50.

84. Ruell PA, Imperial ES, Bonar FJ, et al. Intermittent claudication: the effect of physical training on walking tolerance and venous lactate concentration. *Eur J Appl Physiol* 1984;52:420–425.

85. Jonason T, Jonzom B, Ringqvist I, Oman-Rydberg A. Effect of physical training on different categories of patients with intermittent claudication. *Acta Med Scand* 1979;206:253–258.

86. Hall JA, Dixson GH, Barnard RJ, Pritikin N. Effects of diet and exercise on peripheral vascular disease. *Phys Sports Med* 1982; 10:90–101.

87. Hiatt WR, Nawaz D, Regensteiner JG, Hossack KF. The evaluation of exercise performance in patients with peripheral vascular disease. *J Cardiopulm Rehabil* 1988;12:525–532.

88. Garden FH, Gillis TA. Principles of cancer rehabilitation. In: Braddom RL, ed. *Physical medicine and rehabilitation.* Philadelphia: WB Saunders, 1996.

89. Skinner JS, Strandness DE. Exercise and intermittent claudication: II. Effect of physical training. *Circulation* 1967;36: 23–29.

90. Spitzer S, Bach R, Schieffer H. Walk training and drug treatment in patients with peripheral arterial occlusive disease stage II: a review. *Int Angiol* 1992;11: 204–210.

91. Sidoti SP. Exercise and peripheral vascular disease. *Clin Podiatr* 1992;9:173–184.

92. Gardner AW, Skinner JS, Bryant CX, Smith LK. Stair climbing elicits a lower cardiovascular demand than walking in claudication patients. *J Cardiopulm Rehabil* 1995;15:134–142.

93. Regensteiner JG, Hiatt WR. Exercise rehabilitation for patients with peripheral arterial disease. *Exerc Sport Sci Rev* 1995;23: 1–24.

94. Gardner AW, Poehlman ET. Exercise rehabilitation programs for the treatment of claudication pain: a meta-analysis. *JAMA* 1995;274:975–980.

95. Brand PW. Management of the insensitive limb. *Phys Ther* 1979;59:8–12.

96. Boulton AJM, Betts RP, Franks CI, et al. Abnormalities of foot pressure in early diabetic neuropathy. *Diabet Med* 1987;4: 225–228.

97. Hall OC, Brand PW. The etiology of the neuropathic plantar ulcer: a review of the literature and a presentation of current concepts. *J Am Podiatr Assoc* 1979;69: 173–177.

98. England JD, Ferguson MA, Hiatt WR, Regensteiner JG. Progression of neuropathy in peripheral arterial disease. *Muscle Nerve* 1995; 18:380–387.

99. England JD, Regensteiner JG, Ringel SP, et al. Muscle denervation in peripheral arterial disease. *Neurology* 1992;42:994–999.

100. Regensteiner JG, Wolfel EE, Brass EP, et al. Chronic changes in skeletal muscle histology and function in peripheral arterial disease. *Circulation* 1993; 87:413–421.

101. Young MJ, Venes A, Smith JV, et al. Restoring lower limb blood flow improves conduction velocity in diabetic patients. *Diabetologia* 1995;38:1051–1054.

102. Rodriguez-Sanchez C, Medina Sanchez M, Malik RA, et al. Morphological abnormalities in the sural nerve from patients with peripheral vascular disease. *Histol Histopathol* 1991;6: 63–71.

103. Paradiso C, De Vito L, Rossi S, et al. Cervical and scalp recorded short latency somatosensory evoked potentials in response to epidural spinal cord stimulation in patients with peripheral vascular disease. *Electroencephalogr Clin Neurophysiol* 1995;96:105–113.

104. Migdalis IN, Dimakopoulos N, Kourti A, et al. The prevalence of peripheral vascular disease in type 2 diabetic patients with and without proteinuria. *Int Angiol* 1994;13:22–32.

105. Casale R, Buonocore M, De Massa A, Setacci C. Electromyographic signal frequency analysis in evaluating muscle fatigue of patients with peripheral arterial disease. *Arch Phys Med Rehabil* 1994;75:1118–1121.

106. Chopra JS. Electromyography in diabetes mellitus and chronic occlusive peripheral vascular disease. *Brain* 1969;92:97–108.

107. Chopra JS, Hurwitz LJ. A comparative study of peripheral nerve conduction in diabetes and non-diabetic chronic occlusive peripheral vascular disease. *Brain* 1969;92:83–96.

108. Sanders LJ, Dunlap G. Transmetatarsal amputation: a successful approach to limb salvage. *J AM Podiatr Med Assoc* 1992; 82:129–35.

109. Mueller MJ, Allen BT, Sinacore DR. Incidence of skin breakdown and higher amputation after transmetatarsal amputation: implications for rehabilitation. *Arch Phys Med Rehabil* 1995;76:50–54.

110. Caputo GM, Cavanagh PR, Ulbrecht JS, et al. Assessment and management of foot disease in patients with diabetes. *N Engl J Med* 1994;331:854–860.

111. Brand PW. The diabetic foot. In: Ellenberg M, Rifkin H, eds. *Diabetes mellitus: theory and prac-*

tice. 3rd ed. New Hyde Park: Medical Examination 1983.

112. Uccioli L, Faglia E, Monticone G, et al. Manufactured shoes in the prevention of diabetic foot ulcers. *Diabetes Care* 1995;18: 1376–1378.

113. Coleman WC. Footwear considerations. In: Frykberg RG, ed. *The high risk foot in diabetes mellitus.* New York: Churchill Livingstone, 1991.

114. Lord M, Hosein R. Pressure redistribution by molded inserts in diabetic footwear: a pilot study. *J Rehabil Res Dev* 1994; 31:214–221.

115. Bergtholdt HT, Brand PW. Thermography: an aid in the management of insensitive feet and stumps. *Arch Phys Med Rehabil* 1975;56:205–209.

116. Bergtholdt HT, Brand PW. Temperature assessment and plantar inflammation. *Lepr Rev* 1976;47: 211–219.

117. Holewski JJ, Stess RM, Graf PM, Grunfeld C. Aesthesiometry: quantification of cutaneous pressure sensation in diabetic peripheral neuropathy. *J Rehabil Res Dev* 1988;25:1–10.

118. Mueller MJ, Diamond JE, Delitto A, Sinacore DR. Insensitivity, limited joint mobility, and plantar ulcers in patients with diabetes mellitus. *Phys Ther* 1989;69:453–459.

119. Coleman WC, Brand PW, Birke JA. The total contact cast: a therapy for plantar ulceration on insensitive feet. *J Am Podiatr Assoc* 1984;74:548–552.

120. Bagdade JD, Neilson K, Root R, Bulger R. Host defense in diabetes mellitus: the feckless phagocyte during poor control and ketoacidosis. *Diabetes* 1970;19:364.

121. Goodson WH. Studies of wound healing in experimental diabetes mellitus. *J Surg Res* 1977;22: 221.

122. Olerud JE, Odland GF, Burgess EM, et al. A model for the study of wounds in normal elderly adults and patients with peripheral vascular disease or diabetes mellitus. *J Surg Res* 1995;59:349–360.

123. Weaver FM, Burdi MD, Pinzur MS. Outpatient foot care: correlation to amputation level. *Foot Ankle Int* 1994;15: 498–501.

124. Rusk HA. *Rehabilitation medicine.* 4th ed. New York: CV Mosby, 1977:599.

125. Greenfield LJ. Venous thromboembolic disease. In: Moore WS, ed. *Vascular surgery: a comprehensive review.* 4th ed. Philadelphia: WB Saunders 1993.

126. Turpie AG. Deep vein thrombosis prophylaxis in the outpatient setting: preventing complications following hospital discharge. *Orthopedics* 1995;18 (suppl): 15–17.

127. Wolf H. Low molecular weight heparin. *Med Clin North Am* 1994;78:733–743.

128. Colwell CW Jr. Recent advances in the use of low molecular weight heparins as prophylaxis for deep vein thrombosis. *Orthopedics* 1994;17(suppl):5–7.

129. Anderson DR, O'Brien BJ, Levine MN, et al. Efficacy and cost of low-molecular-weight heparin compared with standard heparin for the prevention of deep vein thrombosis after total hip arthroplasty. *Ann Intern Med* 1993;119:1105–1112.

130. Menzin J, Colditz GA, Regan MM, et al. Cost-effectiveness of enoxaparin vs low-dose warfarin in the prevention of deep-vein thrombosis after total hip replacement surgery. *Arch Intern Med* 1995;155:757–764.

131. Hull R, Raskob G, Pineo G, et al. A comparison of subcutaneous low-molecular-weight heparin with warfarin sodium for prophylaxis against deep-vein thrombosis after hip or knee implantation. *N Engl J Med* 1993;329:1370–1376.

132. Menzin J, Richner R, Huse D, et al. Prevention of deep-vein thrombosis following total hip replacement surgery with enoxaparin versus unfractionated heparin: a pharmacoeconomic evaluation. *Ann Pharmacother* 1994;28:271–275.

133. Nurmohamed MT, Verhaeghe R, Haas S, et al. A comparative trial of low molecular weight heparin (enoxaparin) versus standard heparin for the prophylaxis of postoperative deep vein thrombosis in general surgery. *Am J Surg* 1995;169:567–571.

134. Jorgensen LN, Wille-Jorgensen P, Hauch O. Prophylaxis of postoperative thromboembolism with low molecular weight heparins. *Br J Surg* 1993;80:689–704.

135. Merli GJ, Crabbe S, Paluzzi RG, Fritz D. *Arch Phys Med Rehabil* 1993;74:1199–1205.

136. Green D, Lee MY, Lim AC, et al. Prevention of thromboembolism after spinal cord injury using low-molecular-weight heparin. *Ann Intern Med* 1990; 113:571–574.

137. Brandstater ME, Roth EJ, Siebens HC. Venous thromboembolism in stroke: literature review and implications for clinical practice. *Arch Phys Med Rehabil* 1992;73:S379–S391.

138. Pambianco G, Orchard T, Landau P. Deep vein thrombosis: prevention in stroke patients during rehabilitation. *Arch Phys Med Rehabil* 1995;76:324–330.

139. Clagett GP, Anderson FA Jr, Levine MN, et al. Prevention of venous thromboembolism. *Chest* 1992;102(suppl 4):391S–407S.

140. Levine MN, Hirsh J. Hemorrhagic complications of anticoagulant therapy. *Semin Thromb Hemost* 1986;12:39–57.

141. Gresham GE, Duncan PW, Stason WB, et al. Post stroke rehabilitation. *Clinical practice guideline, no. 16.* AHCPR publication no. 95-0662 Rockville, MD: US Department of Health and Human Services, Public Health Service, Agency for Health Care Policy and Research, May 1995.

142. McLachlin J, Richards T, Paterson JC. An evaluation of clinical signs in the diagnosis of venous thrombosis. *Arch Surg* 1962;85:738–744.

143. Wheeler HB, Anderson FA Jr. Diagnostic methods for deep vein thrombosis. *Haemostasis* 1995; 25:6–26.

144. Bradley MJ, Spencer PA, Alexander L, Milner GR. Colour flow mapping in the diagnosis of the calf deep vein thrombosis. *Clin Radiol* 1993;47:399–402.

145. Tyrell MR, Birtle AJ, Taylor PR. Deep vein thrombosis. *Br J Clin Pract* 1995;49:252–256.

146. Schulman S, Rhedin AS, Lindmarker P, et al. A comparison of six weeks with six months of oral anticoagulant therapy after a first episode of venous thromboembolism: duration of Anticoagulation Trial Study Group. *N Engl J Med* 1995;332:1661–1665.

147. Habibzadeh F, Yadollahie M. A simple method for the derivation of the international normalized ratio for the reporting of prothrombin time results. *Am J Hematol* 1995;50:283–287.

148. Cunningham MT, Olson JD. Low interinstrument variability of the international normalized ratio with the coagamate X2/Simplastin excel system. *Am J Clin Pathol* 1996;105:301–304.

149. Cate JW, Koopman MM, Prins MH, Buller HR. Treatment of venous thromboembolism. *Thromb Haemost* 1995;74: 197–203.

150. Berkowitz SD. Treatment of established deep vein thrombosis: a review of the therapeutic armamentarium. *Orthopedics* 1995;18(suppl):18–20.

151. Koopman MM, Prandoni P, Piovella F, et al. Treatment of venous thrombosis with intravenous unfractionated heparin administered in the hospital as compared with low-molecular-weight heparin administered at home: the Tasman Study Group. *N Engl J Med* 1996;334: 682–687.

152. Levine MN. Thrombolytic therapy for venous thromboembolism: complications and contraindications. *Clin Chest Med* 1995;16: 321–328.

153. Donaldson MC. Chronic venous disorders. In: Loscalzo J, Creager MA, Dzau VJ, eds. *Vascular medicine: a textbook of vascular biology and diseases.* Boston: Little, Brown, 1992.

154. Lindner DJ. Long-term hemodynamic and clinical sequelae of lower extremity deep vein thrombosis. *J Vasc Surg* 1986;4:436.

155. Lawrence D, Kakkar VV. Post-phlebitic syndrome: a functional assessment. *Br J Surg* 1980;67: 686.

156. Strandness DE. Long-term sequelae of acute venous thrombosis. *JAMA* 1983;250:1289.

157. Miller WL. Chronic venous insufficiency. *Curr Opin Cardiol* 1995;10:543–548.

158. Araki CT, Back TL, Padberg FT, et al. The significance of calf muscle pump function in venous ulceration. *J Vasc Surg* 1994; 20:872–879.

159. Black SB. Venous stasis ulcers: a review. *Ostomy Wound Manage* 1995;41:20–30.

160. Moneta GL, Nehler MR, Chitwooed RW, et al. The natural history, pathophysiology, and nonoperative treatment of chronic venous insufficiency. In: Rutherford RB, ed. *Vascular surgery.* 4th ed. Philadelphia: WB Saunders 1995.

161. Noyes LD, Rice JC, Kerstein MD. Hemodynamic assessment of high-compression hosiery in chronic venous disease. *Surgery* 1987;102:813–815.

162. Raju S. Operative management of chronic venous insufficiency. In: Rutherford RB, ed. *Vascular surgery.* 4th ed. Philadelphia: WB Saunders, 1995.

163. Greason KL, Murray JD. Outpatient management of superficial venous insufficiency at a naval medical facility. *Ann Vasc Surg* 1996;10:524–529.

164. Nellzen O, Bergqvist D, Lindhagen A. Leg ulcer etiology: a cross sectional population study. *J Vasc Surg* 1991;14:557–564.

165. Baker SR, Stacey MC, Jopp-McKay AG, et al. Epidemiology of chronic venous ulcers. *Br J Surg* 1991;78:864–867.

166. Dickey JW Jr. Stasis ulcers: the role of compliance in healing. *South Med* J 1991;84:557–561.

167. Stiller MJ, Pak GH, Shupack JL, et al. A portable pulsed electromagnetic field (PEMF) device to enhance healing of recalcitrant venous ulcers: a double blind, placebo-controlled clinical trial. *Br J Dermatol* 1992:127: 147–154.

168. Ieran M, Zaffuto S, Bagnacani M, et al. Effect of low frequency pulsing electromagnetic fields on skin ulcers of venous origin in humans: a double-blind study. *J Orthop Res* 1990;8:276–282.

169. Hansson C. Optimal treatment of venous (stasis) ulcers in elderly patients. *Drugs Aging* 1994;5: 323–334.

170. Unna PG. Ueber Paraplase, eine neue Form medikamentoser Pfsaster. *Wien Med Wochenschr* 1896;43:1854.

171. Vernick SD, Shapiro D, Shaw FD. Legging orthosis for venous and lymphatic insufficiency. *Arch Phys Med Rehabil* 1987;68:459.

172. Lippmann H, Fishman LM, Farrar RH, et al. Edema control in the management of disabling chronic venous insufficiency. *Arch Phys Med Rehabil* 1994;75:436–441.

173. Cordts PR, Hanrahan LM, Rodriguez AA, et al. A prospective, randomized trial of Unna's boot versus Duoderm CGF hydroactive dressing plus compression in the management of venous leg ulcers. *J Vasc Surg* 1992;15:480–486.

174. Kitka MJ, Schuler JJ, Meyer JP, et al. A prospective, randomized trial of Unna's boots versus hydroactive dressings in the treatment of venous stasis ulcers. *J Vasc Surg* 1988;7:478.

175. Bishop JB, Phillips LG, Mustoe TA, et al. A prospective randomized evaluator-blinded trial of two potential wound healing agents for the treatment of venous stasis ulcers. *J Vasc Surg* 1992;16: 251–257.

176. Cheatle TR, Scurr JH, Smith PD. Drug treatment of chronic venous insufficiency and venous ulceration: a review. *J R Soc Med* 1991;84:354–358.

177. Colgan MP, Moore DJ, Shanik DG. New approaches in the medical management of venous ulceration. *Angiology* 1993;44: 138–142.

178. McMullin GM, Watkin GT, Coleridge GT, et al. The efficacy of fibrinolytic enhancement with stanozolol in the treatment of venous insufficiency. *Aust N Z J Surg* 1991;61:306.

179. Balmer A, Limoni C. A double-blind placebo-controlled trial of venorutin on the symptoms and signs of chronic venous insufficiency. *Vasa* 1980;9:36.

180. Sinzinger H, Virgolini I, Fitscha P. Pathomechanisms of atherosclerosis beneficially affected by prostaglandin $E_1(PGE_1)$—an update. *Vasa* 1989;28(suppl): 6.

181. Rudofsky G. Intravenous prostaglandin E_1 in the treatment of venous ulcers—a double blind, placebo controlled trial. *Vasa* 1989;28(suppl):39.

182. Barbarino C. Pentoxifylline in the treatment of venous leg ulcers. *Curr Med Res Opin* 1992;12: 547–551.

183. Nikolova K. Treatment of post-phlebitic syndrome and venous leg ulcers with flunarizine. *Methods Find Exp Clin Pharmacol* 1994;16:609–613.

184. Greenfield L. Venous and lymphatic disease. In: Schwartz SI, Shires GT, Spencer FT, eds. *Principles of surgery.* 6th ed. New York: McGraw-Hill, 1994.

185. Stillwell GK. Treatment of post-mastectomy lymphedema. *Mod Treatment* 1969;6:396–412.

186. Gloviczki P, Wahner HW. Clinical diagnosis and evaluation of lymphedema. In: Rutherford RB, ed. *Vascular surgery.* 4th ed. Philadelphia: WB Saunders, 1995.

187. Brennan MJ, DePompolo RW, Garden FH. Focused review: post-mastectomy lymphedema. *Arch Phys Med Rehabil* 1996; 77(suppl):S74–S80.

188. Allen EV. Lymphedema of the extremities: classification, etiology and differential diagnosis: a study of 300 cases. *Arch Intern Med* 1934;54:606–624.

189. Kinmonth JB, Taylor G, Tracy C, Marsh J. Primary lymphedema: clinical and lymphographic studies of a series of 107 patients in which the lower limbs were affected. *Br J Surg* 1957; 45:1.

190. Hammond MC, Merli GJ, Zierler RE. Rehabilitation of the patient with peripheral vascular disease of the lower extremity. In: DeLisa JA, Gans BM, eds. *Rehabilitation medicine: principles and practice.* 2nd ed. Philadelphia: JB Lippincott 1993.

191. Allen PJ, Gilllespie DL, Redfield RR, Gomez ER. Lower extremity lymphedema caused by acquired immune deficiency syndrome-related Kaposi's sarcoma: case report and review of the literature. *J Vasc Surg* 1995;22: 178–181.

192. Passik S, Newman M, Brennan M, Holland J. Psychiatric consultation for women undergoing rehabilitation for upper-extremity lymphedema following breast cancer treatment. *J Pain Symptom Manage* 1993;8: 226–233.

193. Logan V. Incidence and prevalence of lymphoedema: a literature review. *J Clin Nurs* 1995;4: 213–219.

194. Heytmanek G, Kubista E. [Therapy of postoperative lymphedema in breast cancer: lymph drainage.] *Geburtshilfe Frauenheilkd* 1988;48:433–435.

195. Whitman M, McDaniel RW. Preventing lymphedema: an unwelcome sequel to breast cancer. *Nursing* 1993;23:36.

196. Grabois M. Breast cancer: post-mastectomy lymphedema. *Phys Med Rehabil State Art Rev* 1994; 8:267–277.

197. Morgan RG, Casley-Smith JR, Mason MR. Complex physical therapy for the lymphedematous arm. *J Hand Surg [Br]* 1992;17: 437–441.

198. Kirshbaum M. Using massage in the relief of lymphedema. *Prof Nurse* 1996;11:230–232.

199. Mirolo BR, Bunce IH, Chapman M, et al. Psychosocial benefits of postmastectomy lymphedema therapy. *Cancer Nurs* 1995; 18:197–205.

200. Nelson PA. Rehabilitation of patients with lymphedema. In: Kottke FJ, Lehamann JF, eds. *Krusen's handbook of physical medicine and rehabilitation.* 4th ed. Philadelphia: WB Saunders, 1990.

201. Levinson SF. Rehabilitation of the patient with cancer or human immunodeficiency virus. In: DeLisa JA, Gans BM, eds. *Rehabilitation medicine: principles and practice.* 2nd ed. Philadelphia: JB Lippincott, 1993.

202. Farncombe M, Danniels G, Cross L. Lymphedema: the seemingly forgotten complication. *J Pain Symptom Manage* 1994;9: 269–276.

203. Boris M, Weindorf S, Lasinski B, Boris G. Lymphedema reduction by noninvasive complex lymphedema therapy. *Oncology (Huntingt)* 1994;8:95–106.

204. Airaksinen O, Kolari PJ, Pekanmaki K. Intermittent pneumatic compression therapy. *Crit Rev Phys Rehabil Med* 1992;3:219–237.

205. Bunce IH, Mirolo BR, Hennessy JM, et al. Post-mastectomy lymphoedema treatment and measurement. *Med J Aust* 1994;161:125–128.

206. Kim-Sing C, Basco VE. Postmastectomy lymphedema treated with

the Wright linear pump. *Can J Surg* 1987;30:368–370.

207. Cook HA, Morales M, La Rosa EM, et al. Effects of electrical stimulation on lymphatic flow and limb volume in the rat. *Phys Ther* 1994;74:1040–1046.

208. Bertelli G, Venturini M, Forno G, et al. Conservative treatment of postmastectomy lymphedema: a controlled randomized trial. *Ann Oncol* 1991;2:575–578.

209. Airaksinen O, Kolari PJ, Pekanmaki K. Intermittent pneumatic compression therapy. *Crit Rev Phys Med Rehabili Med* 1992;3:219–237.

210. Rooke TW, Gloviczki P. Nonoperative management of chronic lymphedema. In: Rutherford RB, ed. *Vascular surgery*. 4th ed. Philadelphia: WB Saunders, 1995.

211. Pohjola RT, Kolari PJ, Pekanmaki K. Intermittent pneumatic compression for lymphoedema: a comparison of two treatment modes. In: Partsch H, ed. *Progress in lymphology*. Amsterdam: Elsevier, 1988.

212. Pekanmaki K, Kolari PJ, Kiistala U. Intermittent pneumatic compression treatment for post-thrombotic leg ulcers. *Clin Exp Dermatol* 1987;12:350.

213. Pappas CJ, O'Donnell TF. Long-term results of compression treatment for lymphedema. *J Vasc Surg* 1992;16:555.

Musculo-skeletal Disease and Injury

Chapter 82

Arthritis and Connective Tissue Diseases

Victoria Anne Brander
Terry H. Oh
Neil Alpiner

RHEUMATOID ARTHRITIS

Rheumatoid arthritis (RA) is an inflammatory polyarthropathy typically affecting diarthrodial joints in a symmetric distribution. Women are affected three times more often than men; neither climate nor geography affect prevalence rates (about 1% for white adults). Genetic associations clearly exist, especially for patients with HLA-DR4 subtype Dw14 (1).

RA is a devastating illness. The mortality of RA may be comparable to that of diabetes (2). The typical outpatient has a one-in-four chance of moderate to severe functional disability, and approximately 50% of patients who were working at the onset of the disease are disabled and exit the work force within 5 years. People with RA who are still working earn between one-fourth and one-half as much income compared to their age-matched controls (3). RA is a chronic, often progressive, systemic joint disease and there is no cure. Aggressive treatment has not yet been shown to prevent the progressive destructive nature of the disease. Therefore, rehabilitative therapeutic approaches should be used early to help limit the severe physical impairments and functional limitations that occur from RA (4,5).

Etiology

RA is an autoimmune disorder characterized by synovitis. The inciting event may be a foreign antigen that invades a genetically susceptible host. A series of inflammatory events then lead to a host of pathologic changes in the structure and function of articular and system-wide structures.

Relatives of patients with seropositive RA have an increased risk of developing erosive arthritis (6). There is an association between class II HLA-DR genes and RA (7). Although various infectious organisms such as streptococci, rubella, Epstein-Barr virus, and parvovirus have been associated with arthritis, none has been shown to directly cause RA.

Several factors have been identified as instrumental to the profound systemic inflammation that occurs with RA. Vasoactive amines, prostaglandin, leukotrienes, complement tumor necrosis factor, and the interleukins are among the many mediators found to influence proliferation and degradation. A complete discussion of the roles of these mediators is beyond the scope of this chapter.

Normal Joint Structural Function

Synovial joints are composed of bone, articular soft tissue (joint capsule, articular cartilage, menisci), synovial fluid, and periarticular supporting structures (muscle tendon, ligament, and bursae) (Fig. 82-1). Synovium lines the joint at the peripheral margins. The joint is surrounded by a fibrous capsule, with muscular supporting structures either having their tendons attached to the fibrous capsule or having conjoined areas of attachment at more distal positions.

The articular cartilage is avascular and aneural,

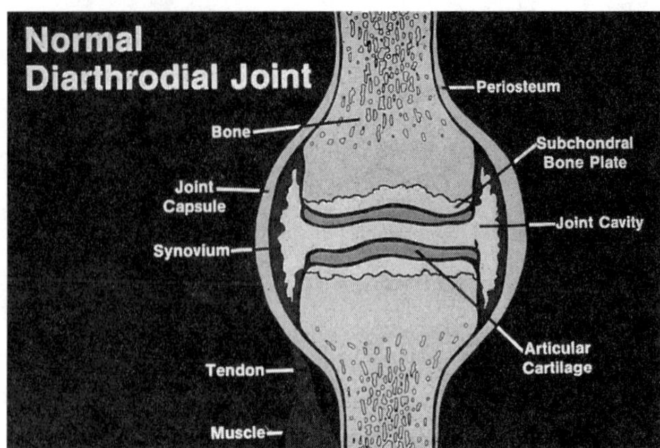

Figure 82-1. Normal joint structure.

composed of approximately 70% to 80% water and 20% to 30% type II collagen and proteoglycans. Collagen, produced by synovial fluid–nourished chondrocytes, is arranged in various nonconfluent configurations throughout the noncalcified articular cartilage; microscopically it is composed of tiny micropores and crevices. The proteoglycan is a complex monomer composed of a long protein core to which approximately 150 sulfated glycosaminoglycan chains are attached. At one of its ends there is a specific attachment for hyaluronic acid. Just beneath the cartilage lies a transitional calcified region adjoining to subchondral bone.

Synovium is only loose connective tissue, but is distinguished from other connective tissue by its many functions:

1. It produces nutrients for the avascular articular cartilage to flourish.
2. It metabolically controls passive diffusion of glucose in and out of the joint and active (probable) diffusion of protein molecules, and absorbs waste products produced by articular cartilage.
3. It is involved in the ingestion of free-floating joint debris.
4. It secretes a synovial fluid composed of hyaluronate, immunoglobins, and lysosomal enzymes.

The synovial fluid is typically less than 1 mL in small joints and up to 3 mL in larger joints. This fluid, a by-product of synovium, is the chief source of nutrition for chondrocytes, providing joint lubrication and altering resistance to shear. As the shearing forces across the joint increase, the ability of the synovial fluid to decrease resistance amplifies. Synovial fluid thus helps decrease the energy requirements necessary to produce movement.

Joints have adapted to maximally absorb the significant, repetitive loading forces (tensile, compressive, and shearing) to which they are exposed. The critical biomechanical properties of synovial joints provide passive and dynamic joint stability, distribute force, and lubricate the joints. Joint articulation is made nearly frictionless through synovial fluid lubrication. Cartilage matrix, while much too thin to contribute to shock absorption, dissipates tensile and compressive components through distributing weight (via its curvilinear structural geometry), deformation, and energy absorption. The periarticular muscles absorb most of the compressive forces distributed through the joint, through control of their acceleration and deceleration forces; they may absorb as much as 90% of the energy across the joint (2).

Pathophysiology

With inflammation (synovitis), the synovial lining of the joint may triple in size. This edematous synovium accumulates increased numbers of lymphocytes and macrophages, and creates extensive hypervascular networks (*angiogenesis*). Synovial hypertrophy at the joint margins creates the enlarged boggy joints identified on physical examination.

As synovial proliferation continues, the vascular supply is unable to keep pace with the tissue expansion, causing premature death to distal appendages. This results in fraying and amputation of debris into the synovial fluid, referred to as *rice bodies*. The synovium now begins to derange joint structures by progressive, interacting biochemical and mechanical insults that are a consequence of both proliferating and repair processes.

RA is not solely an articular disease. The systemic pathology that occurs is frequently a cause of the substantial morbidity and mortality (Table 82-1).

Clinical Presentation

RA is a clinical diagnosis, present when a patient has symmetric polyarthritis and morning stiffness for more than 60 days. There is no simple diagnostic test to establish the definitive diagnosis of RA. The diagnosis can be made based on a thorough clinical evaluation, referring to the revised 1988 American Rheumatism Association criteria (Table 82-2) (8). A baseline diagnostic work-up (Table 82-3) and radiographs assist in making the diagnosis (Table 82-4 and Fig. 82-2). There may be three subtypes of RA, each with its own natural history and prognosis. Type I RA is a self-limited process, usually postviral, rarely rheumatoid factor (RF) positive. Type II disease is persistent but minimally progressive. Type III disease is severe, progressive, and associated with rapid radiograph abnormalities and disability (9). Work disability has been reported after 5 years in more than 60% of patients with RA who are younger than 65 years at the time of diagnosis (9). RA is associated with premature mortality.

Treatment

The cornerstones to the management of RA are medications, splinting, and rest to suppress inflammation; exercise to maintain joint motion, strength, and cardiovascular endurance; functional training including the use of adaptive and assistive devices; education in joint protection,

Table 82-1: Systemic Manifestations of Rheumatoid Arthritis (RA): Disorders, Pathophysiology, Clinical Findings, Diagnosis, and Treatment

Disorder	Pathophysiology	Clinical Findings	Diagnosis	Treatment
1. Rheumatoid nodules	Necrotizing granulomas in subcutaneous tissue	Subcutaneous nodules at extensor tendon surfaces	Physical exam	None
2. Rheumatoid vasculitis	Small-vessel obliterative endarteritis	Nailbed and paronychial infarcts	Serologies: leukocytosis with eosinophilia, elevated complement, elevated WESR, confirmed by vessel biopsy	None
	Leukocytoclastic vasculitis	Palpable purpura, urticaria		Moderate-dose (20–40) mg/day) adrenocorticosteroids
	Necrotizing arteritis	Episcleritis, scleromalacia, serositis, fever, sensorimotor neuropathy, ulcerative skin lesions, rarely cerebral vasculitis		Cyclophosphamide, penicillamine, methotrexate, plasmapheresis, high-dose corticosteroids
3. Felty syndrome	Unusual (1%) with RA; secondary to margination of neutrophilia in spleen, decreased granulopoiesis, autoimmune destruction	Leukopenia and splenomegaly, leg ulcers, portal hypertension esophageal varices	Selective neutropenia (total white count < 2500/μL with no immature cells), anemia, thrombocytopenia, liver-spleen scan	(Consider toxic effects of drugs or concomitant SLE) Gold, penicillamine, cyclophosphamide, methotrexate, and corticosteroids, splenectomy
4. Cardiac disease	Myocarditis, pericarditis, conductive pathway disease, coronary arteritis, valvular disease	Chest pain, dyspnea, angina, arrhythmias, congestive failure, etc	Echocardiogram, thoracentesis, ECG, stress tests, and others as indicated	Medical management appropriate to specific diagnosis, cardiac rehabilitation, remittive therapy
5. Pulmonary abnormalities	Primary from inflammation/nodules or secondary to drugs; intestinal fibrosis, pneumonitis, Caplan syndrome, nodules, bronchiolitis, restrictive lung disease, pleuritis	Chest pain, cough, dyspnea, fatigue, exercise limitations, weight loss, etc	Radiographs, pulmonary function tests, bronchoscopy and biopsy	Medical management as appropriate to diagnosis, remittive therapy, pulmonary rehabilitation
6. Gastrointestinal and liver	Peptic ulcer disease secondary to NSAIDs, drug-induced liver disease, bowel vasculitis	Elevated hepatic enzymes, abdominal pain	Liver profile, blood count, stool occult blood, endoscopy, colonoscopy, biopsy	Change or reduce hepatotoxic agents; gastric protection via H_2 blockers, and misoprostol
7. Renal impairments	Drug induced—interstitial nephritis, Goodpasture syndrome, immune complex deposition, amyloidosis, vasculitis, infection, glomerulonephritis	Decreased creatinine clearance, elevated BUN or proteinuria, hyperkalemia, renal failure, pyuria, dysuria	Renal profile, urinalysis, creatinine clearance, renal biopsy, etc	Avoid offending agents
8. Sjögren syndrome	Xerostomia, keratoconjunctivitis sicca, and connective tissue disease (usually RA); lymphocytic infiltrates of glands; associated with HLA-DW4 tissue type	Dry eyes, dry mouth, arthritis, photophobia	Schirmer test to diagnose sicca syndrome	Methylcellulose tears, hydroxypropyl cellulose, ophthalmologic inserts, nighttime ointments, artificial saliva
9. Ocular involvement	Scleritis/episcleritis	Arching, increased tearing, reduced vision	Tender eye, conjunctival engorgement	If severe—systemic cytotoxic agent,

Table 82-1. (*Continued*)

Disorder	Pathophysiology	Clinical Findings	Diagnosis	Treatment
	Eye movement disorders secondary to nodules, vasculitis	Diplopia and painful eye movement	Cranial nerve evaluation for retinal angiography	NSAIDs, topical antibiotics Remittives for vasculitis
10. Neuropathies	Vasculitis; focal compression (such as carpal and tarsal tunnel syndrome)	Pain and other dysesthesia, sensory loss, weakness	Electrodiagnostic studies, laboratory tests to exclude other disorders and confirm vasculitis, sural nerve biopsy	If focal compression —injections, surgical excision
11. Myopathies, myalgias, proximal myopathy, myositis	Polymyositis secondary to lymphocytic infiltration, vasculitis; steroid myopathy	Weakness (proximal)	Electrodiagnostic studies, creatine kinase if myositis, ESR, biopsy	Oral corticosteroids and remittive agents if myositis, otherwise exercise
12. Osteoporosis	Diffuse inflammation, inactivity, corticosteroids	Asymptomatic, pain, fractures, kyphoscoliosis	Bone densitometry, laboratory tests to exclude other calcitonin systemic disease	Exercise, calcium, vitamin D, estrogen replacement therapy, alendronate, calcitonin

NSAIDs = nonsteroidal anti-inflammatory drugs; BUN = blood area nitrogen; WESR = Westgren erythrocyte sedimentation rate; ECG = electrocardiogram; SLE = systemic lupus erythematosus; ESR = erythrocyte sedimentation rate.

Table 82-2: 1988 Revised American Rheumatism Association Criteria for the Diagnosis of Rheumatoid Arthritis (RA)*

Criteria	Definition
1. Morning stiffness	Morning stiffness in and around the joints lasting at least 1 hr before maximal improvement.
2. Arthritis of three or more joint areas	At least three joint areas have simultaneously had soft-tissue swelling or fluid (not bony overgrowth alone) observed by a physician. The 14 possible joint areas are (right or left) PIP, MCP, wrist, elbow, knee, ankle, and MTP joints.
3. Arthritis of hand joints	At least one joint area swollen as above in wrist, MCP, or PIP joint.
4. Symmetric arthritis	Simultaneous involvement of the same joint (as in No. 2) on both sides of the body (bilateral involvement of PIP, MCP, or MTP joints is acceptable without absolute symmetry).
5. Rheumatoid nodules	Subcutaneous nodules over bony prominences or extensor surfaces, or in juxta-articular regions, observed by a physician.
6. Serum rheumatoid factor	Demonstration of abnormal amounts of serum rheumatoid factor by any method that has demonstrated positivity in less than 5% of control subjects.
7. Radiographic changes	Radiographic changes typical of RA on posteroanterior hand-wrist radiographs, which must include erosions or unequivocal bony decalcification localized to or most marked adjacent to the involved joints (osteoarthritis changes alone do not qualify).

PIP = proximal interphalangeal; MCP = metacarpophalangeal; MTP = metarsophalangeal.

* For classification purposes, a patient is said to have RA if he or she has satisfied at least four of the seven criteria. Criteria 1 through 4 must be present for at least 6 weeks.

Table 82-3: Baseline Diagnostic Work-up for Rheumatoid Arthritis
Blood
Complete blood cell count with differential and platelets. Exclude anemia of chronic disease, thrombocytosis, Felty syndrome.
Westgren erythrocyte sedimentation rate, C-reactive protein. Abnormal in up to 60% of patients.
Rheumatoid factor and titer. Present in 70%–90% of patients; may be false-positive.
Renal profile, liver function tests.
Other: complement, antinuclear antibody, etc, as indicated.
Urine
Urinalysis with microscopic analysis to exclude proteinuria.
Synovial fluid
Color, turbidity, and viscosity.
Cell count and differential. Synovial fluid in RA is inflammatory, translucent, 2000–20,000 white blood cells/mononuclear and polymorphonuclear cells.
Crystal analysis if gout, "pseudogout" suspected.
Radiographic studies
Baseline radiographs of selected joints—especially knees/hips, hands/feet, shoulders, cervical spine. Assess for erosive disease.
Bone densitometry. Assess for osteoporosis.
Functional status questionnaires
Health Assessment Questionnaire (HAQ).
Arthritis Impact Measurement Scales (AIMS).
Measures response to treatment, disease progression.

Source: Adapted from Pinkus T. Rheumatoid arthritis. In: Wegens ST, ed. *Clinical care in the rheumatic diseases.* American College of Rheumatology Press, 1996:147–155.

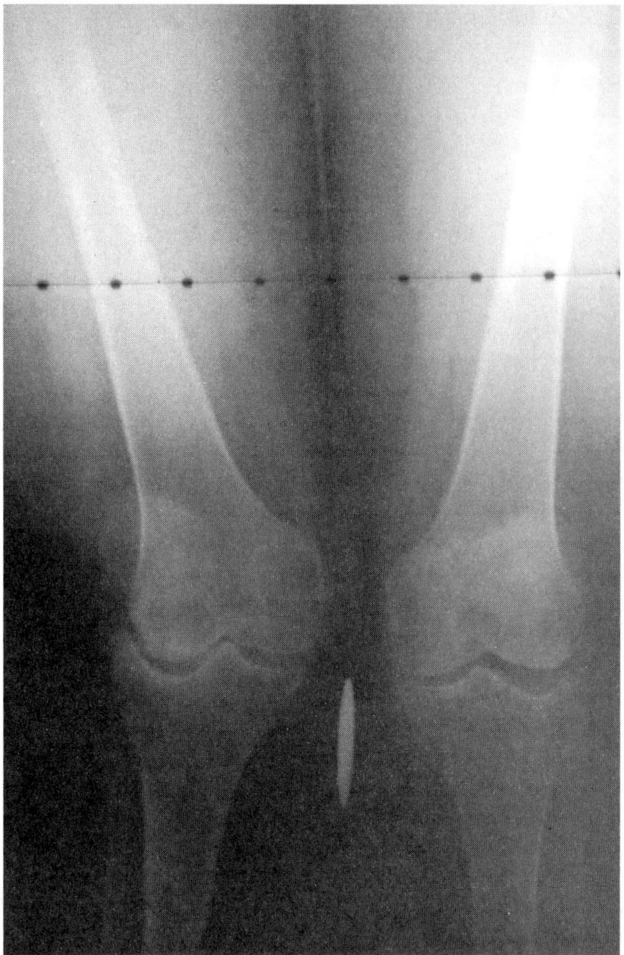

Figure 82-2. Radiograph of advanced rheumatoid arthritis of the knees.

Table 82-4: Radiographic Findings in Rheumatoid Arthritis
Soft-tissue swelling
Symmetric joint space narrowing
Juxta-articular osteoporosis
Bony erosions
Joint malalignment

energy conservation, and disease self-management; orthotics; environment modification; and psychosocial, vocational, and avocational interventions. First and primarily, inflammation must be suppressed, as this is the cause of joint and systemic deterioration. Then, rehabilitative measures will be useful. These concepts are described in the following sections.

Pharmacotherapy

Traditionally the pharmacotherapy of RA has been based on a pyramidal approach to treatment (4) (Fig. 82-3). Patients with milder disease and most patients when first diagnosed are treated with the drugs shown on the low end of the pyramid. However, patients whose disease is considered progressive, type III disease (such as those who present with radiographic erosions), should immediately begin second-line therapy with the drugs identified higher on the pyramid, including slow-acting antirheumatic drugs (SAARDs) (Tables 82-5 and 82-6). The decision as to whether a patient has self-limited or progressive RA usually can be made within 1 to 3 months, and aggressive treatment begun as soon as possible. Methotrexate is the most widely used SAARD, because of its fairly low toxicity and strong anti-inflammatory properties. Early combination chemotherapy, using two or more SAARDs, has come into favor for patients who present with aggressive disease and is probably superior to the traditional pyramidal approach (4). Steroids and surgery, on the lateral aspects of the pyramid, may be useful at many stages of intervention. Low-dose prednisone (7.5 mg/day or less) is an effective alternative to SAARD therapy for patients with refractory disease. This dose may be associated with much fewer steroid-induced side effects (diabetes, osteopenia, hyperten-

Figure 82-3. Traditional pyramid approach to rheumatoid arthritis therapy.

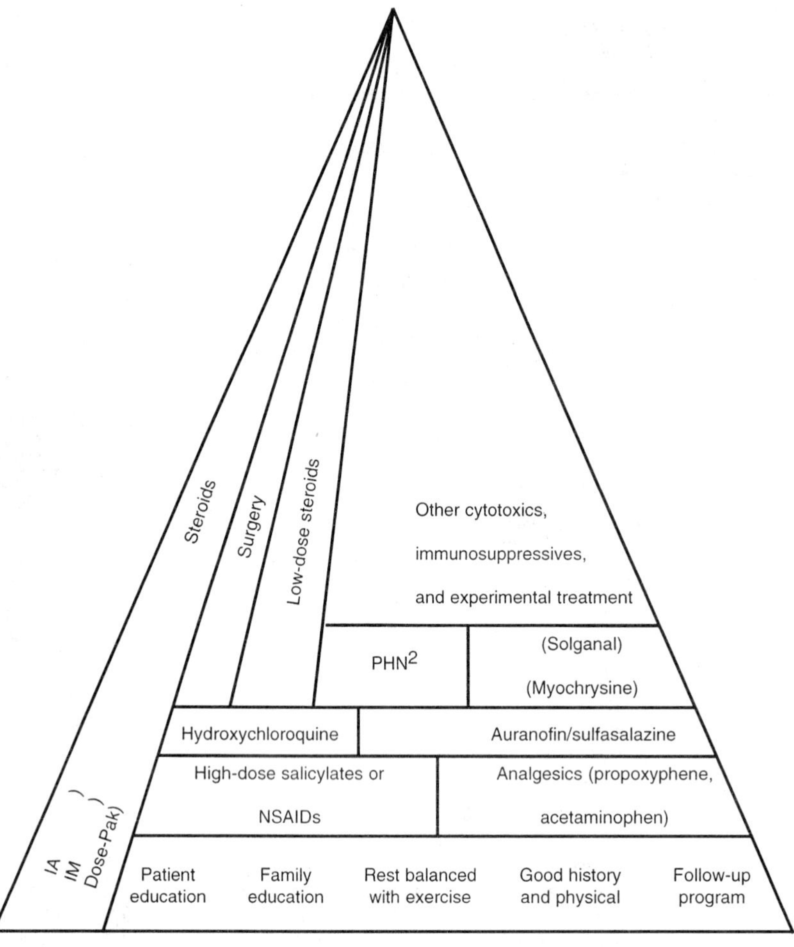

Table 82-5: Slow-Acting Antirheumatic Drugs (SAARDs)

Remittive Agent	Major Side Effects	Initial Monitoring Schedule	Stable Monitoring Schedule
Sulfasalazine	Gastrointestinal upset, nausea, leukopenia	CBC, platelet count, SMA at 3–4 wk	CBC, platelet count, SMA every 2–3 mo.
Hydroxychloroquine	Gastrointestinal upset, retinal degradation, corneal deposition	Baseline eye exam before or during the first month of therapy, CBC, SMA (baseline)	CBC, SMA, eye exam every 6 mo
Gold oralorinjectable	Diarrhea, rash, stomatitis, proteinuria, nephrotic syndrome, cytopenia	CBC, platelet count, urinalysis every 1–2 wk for first 6 months	Same as for oral gold
Penicillamine	Same as for gold; altered taste and smell, autoimmune reactions	Same as for injectable gold	CBC, platelet count, urinalysis every 4–6 wk; liver function tests every 4–6 mo

CBC = complete blood cell count; SMA = sequential multiple analyzer.

Table 82-6: Cytotoxic and Immunosuppressive Drugs Used for Rheumatoid Arthritis

	Side Effects		Monitoring Schedule	
Drug	**Common**	**Major**	**Initial**	**Stable**
Methotrexate	Stomatitis, abnormal liver function, gastrointestinal upset	Leukopenia, thrombocytopenia, anemia, intestinal pneumonitis, hepatic fibrosis, fetal toxicity	CBC, platelet count every 1–2 wk; liver function tests every 6–12 wk; creatinine every 3–12 mo; chest x-ray initially	CBC, platelet count every 1–3 mo; liver function tests every 1–3 mo; creatinine every 3–12 mo; creatinine every 3–12 mo; chest x-ray every 6–12 mo
Azathioprine (Imuran)	Gastrointestinal upset, rash	Leukopenia, thrombocytopenia, anemia, hepatitis, oncogenesis	CBC, platelet count every 1–2 wk; liver function tests every 3–6 mo	CBC, platelet count every 1–2 wk; liver function tests every 3–6 mo
Cyclophosphamide (Cytoxan)	Alopecia, sterility	Leukopenia, thrombocytopenia, anemia, hemorrhagic cystitis, oncogenesis	CBC, platelet count, urinalysis every 1–2 wk; chemistry screen initially	CBC, platelet count, urinalysis; chemistry screen every 3–6 mo

CBC = complete blood cell count.

sion, etc). Many newer immunoregulatory agents will be available in the near future, offering more hope for true disease modification and elimination.

Exercise

Exercise is one of the few interventional strategies available with proven efficacy. Exercise reverses many of the deteriorating effects of RA, increasing aerobic capacity, muscle strength, and force generation. Additional benefits that occur are decreased depression, reduced fatigue, resolution of sleep disturbances, less joint discomfort, and most importantly, increased activities of daily living and level of independence (10–16).

Traditionally, physicians and other health care professionals have discouraged patients with RA from exercising because of concern about accelerated joint damage. In the acute phases of inflammation, range of motion exercises and isotonic strengthening are believed to increase joint temperature and swelling and potentially accelerate joint deterioration. There is also concern about the deleterious effects of particular strengthening exercises on unstable joints. Unfortunately the overemphasis on these *theoretical* negatives by health care providers has greatly overshadowed the important benefits of exercise and arthritis. It is well known that those with RA have poorer muscle strength and endurance than the general population (10,17,18). Recent studies strongly indicated that aerobic and resistance exercises are significantly beneficial to RA patients, improving flexibility, strength, endurance, function, and cardiovascular fitness without aggravating symptoms (10,11,14,19,20). For example, one study included RA subjects with symptomatic weight-bearing joints in a 12-week graded aerobic exercise program. Significant gains in aerobic capacity, overall physical activity, 50-foot walk time, grip strength, and flexibility and in reducing anxiety and depression were demonstrated and maintained after 1 year (10). A combined dance-based aerobic exercise program and educational problem-solving skills-building program showed increases in quality of life measures and 50-foot walk time (11,14). Yet another study of RA subjects indicated that a program of muscle-strengthening exercises raised scores on physical fitness tests (19).

Table 82-7: Sample Exercise Prescription for Patients with Early-Stage Rheumatoid Arthritis

1. Begin with a 5-min warm-up of light aerobics and active range of motion exercises.
2. Follow warm-up with stretching program.
3. Perform vigorous aerobics and strengthening exercises after stretching. Begin by alternating days of aerobics and strengthening exercise.
4. Initially aerobic exercise should be low impact. Begin with 5–10-min duration and increase weekly. Attempt to reach 60%–80% of target heart rate (220 – age) during exercise.
5. Strength training should include balanced upper- and lower-body concentric and eccentric, open- and closed-chain exercises.
6. Complete exercise with a 15-min cooldown of active range of motion and light aerobic exercises.

Physicians should offer a specific exercise prescription that includes duration, intensity, and frequency for each RA patient (Table 82-7). Beforehand, assessment of joint instability and inflammation is critical so that potentially harmful exercises may be excluded. During acute joint inflammation it is important not to overstretch periarticular tissues, as their reduced tensile strength may lead to tears. Isometric exercise is recommended during inflammation; it is used in conjunction with dynamic resistive and aerobic exercise programs once inflammation subsides. Adequate warm-up and cooldown with gentle stretching and light aerobics ensures safety and comfort.

Aquatic exercise is highly recommended for RA patients. A heated pool with its warmth and buoyancy provides an almost pain-free environment in which to exercise. Regular pool therapy has been demonstrated to improve strength and conditioning. Other aerobic exercises such as low-impact aerobics, bicycling, and walking are recommended to improve cardiovascular conditioning without increasing pain or inflammation.

Patients with RA who have not exercised in a structured program before or those with identified physical impairments (such as joint contractures) should be referred to a physical therapist. This will best enable them to learn specifically which exercises are best for them and precisely how to perform them for the greatest benefit.

Regional and Anatomic Considerations

Ankle and Foot Impairments and Limitations

The sequelae of ankle and foot pathology relate more to capsular malfunction than to bony destruction. As synovial proliferation intensifies in the small intrinsic foot joints, capsular weakening and ligamentous laxity occur, resulting in intertarsal, metatarsal, and phalangeal bony creep. The forefoot initially undergoes changes at the metatarsal and proximal interphalangeal joint (PIP). Joint laxity and contracture or spasm of the intrinsic extensors create a deforming force that causes PIP flexion. Loss of fat pads, abnormal long tendon forces, and involvement of the intrinsic and lumbrical muscles and toe flexors lead to metatarsophalangeal hyperextension and "hammer toes." A laterally directed force at the great toe causes it to overlap the second, resulting in a medial outpouching of the proximal metatarsal head, pronation of the phalanx, plantar migration of the abductor hallucis muscle, and asymmetric capsule weakening medially. This disorder, *hallux valgus*, is a condition that can be excruciatingly painful and biomechanically disrupting. Callus formation with skin irritation occurs at the surface level, producing a bunion. The development of hallux valgus is associated with spreading of the metatarsal ligaments, which increases the vulnerability of interdigital nerves to pressure, particularly between the third and fourth metatarsal heads, resulting in metatarsalgia.

Ankle joint swelling, capsular weakness, and supporting muscle tenosynovitis (primarily the Achilles, but also the tibialis posterior tendon) results in ankle instability. A valgus position develops in the talocalcaneal joint, resulting in rotational and subluxing moments on the navicular head (also affected by tenosynovitis of the tibialis posterior muscle) and subtalar pronation. Because of this excessive pronation, the foot is less able to transform into the rigid structure necessary for proper push off. This makes the foot less capable of tolerating weight bearing and propulsion. In addition, increased stress on the plantar fascia during the push-off phase of gait results in pain from plantar fasciitis.

Tenosynovitis of the tibialis posterior, flexor digitorum longus, and flexor hallucis longus results in a narrowing of the tarsal canal, leading to tarsal tunnel syndrome. This is characterized by burning dysesthesia in the toes, sole of the foot, and possibly the heel. Intrinsic muscle wasting may also occur.

Therapeutic Interventions

Orthotics: Pain relief and the realignment of biomechanical disruptions are the goals of appropriate orthotic and footwear prescriptions. Ninety percent of RA patients have foot involvement during the course of the disease, the presenting symptom in 15% to 20% of them. For example, a well-designed orthotic can correct common calcaneal eversion and subtalar pronation. An ankle-foot orthosis can be used to immobilize an ankle with chronic effusion and structural pathology, reducing pain and improving gait.

Critical areas in shoe structure are those that can cause possible compression, specifically the toe box, heel counter, and vamp. A softer material for shoe fabrication is needed to accommodate abnormal foot anatomy. Shoes should have high and broad toe boxes, wide vamps, and nonconstraining heel counters to maximize inner shoe volumes and decrease metatarsal apposition. The sole of the shoe can be modified by the use of 1) a metatarsal bar to relieve pressure on the painful metatarsals; 2) a built-up lateral or medial undersurface to create a valgus or varus moment on the ankle; or 3) a rocker sole to alleviate metatarsal pressure, and make the push-off phase of gait more comfortable and efficient.

Thermal modalities: Superficial heat or cold penetrates the foot-ankle complex well. Deeper penetrating modalities are used to improve connective tissue elasticity prior to stretching, but are contraindicated in patients with acute inflammation or sensory loss. Cold is best tolerated if it is applied by stroking or rubbing instead of continuous application. All thermal modalities must be applied cautiously to a limb with arterial disease or reduced sensation.

Exercise: Exercise includes 1) passive stretching of the Achilles and the peronei tendons, 2) active range of motion exercises targeting the ankle and subtalar joints, 3) isometric exercises of the muscles of the anterior compartment, 4) concentric isotonic exercises of the posterior and anterior tibialis muscles from the elongated position, and 5) eccentric training of the gastrocnemius-soleus complex and peronei muscles from the shortened position.

Knee Impairments and Limitations

Once knee synovitis occurs, numerous problems arise:

1. Increased synovial fluid secretions cause a reflex capsular nociceptive response, with subsequent hamstring spasm and quadricep inhibition.
2. Collagen-degrading enzymes disrupt cartilage, limiting its ability to facilitate smooth joint motion. These enzymes also attack the menisci and cruciate ligaments, resulting in knee instability, locking or catching sensations as meniscal cartilage frays, decreased joint lubrication, and impaired gait.
3. Progressive, synovial hypertrophy (*pannus*) causes a physical impediment to motion and can progress to ankylosis.
4. Posterior joint capsule, gastrocnemius, and semi-membranosus tendon inflammation may erode the bursa until it is confluent with joint synovium, causing a *Baker's cyst.*
5. Mechanical malalignment occurs as a result of weakened articular capsule. Meniscal erosions lead to knee varus, valgus, and flexion deformities; abnormal hip and ankle pathology (such as pronated foot); protective flexor spasms; and tenosynovitis of these joints.

Therapeutic Interventions

Acute Inflammatory Phase

Orthotics: Weight bearing should be minimized. A resting splint, such as a soft knee immobilizer, may be used to provide maximal extension and facilitate local joint rest. Use of pillows under the knee should be avoided when the orthotic is removed during recumbency, to minimize the risk of knee flexion contracture.

Modalities: Brief applications of cold modalities are best tolerated during acute inflammation. Frozen vegetable packages are convenient. The use of superficial, moist heat can also provide patient comfort.

Exercise: Quadriceps strength must be maintained through isometric "quad sets." Isotonic or isokinetic exercises are not recommended in the acute phase.

Subacute or Chronic Inflammatory Phase

Orthotics and assistive devices: No specific orthotics are recommended as they are poorly tolerated by patients with long-standing arthritis. If knee flexion contractures persist, a soft knee immobilizer can be worn at night or in cases of pure hamstring tightness, an adjustable or spring-assisted knee extension orthosis can be used.

If a valgus knee deformity exists, an ankle-foot orthotic to decrease the pronation moment at the subtalar joint may be helpful. Additionally, building up the medial aspect of the foot creates a varus moment at the ankle and a varus moment at the knee. This orthotic intervention is most successful if the medial knee compartment is relatively intact.

Canes, walkers, and crutches decrease the force on the knee during gait and their use is encouraged.

Thermal modalities: In addition to the modalities listed for use in the acute phase, ultrasound may be used when inflammation is not active and stretching is desired. Transcutaneous electrical nerve stimulation (TENS) may be considered for patients with pain who are intolerant of or refractory to oral analgesic agents. Topical capsaicin is a pharmacologic alternative for pain management.

Exercise: Generalized limb strengthening with a focus on the quadriceps should be performed through isotonic open-chain exercises, progressing to closed-chain concentric and eccentric exercises. Stair exercises and inclined treadmill exercises may result in anterior knee pain syndromes and should be avoided. Aquatic exercises result in easier aerobic training, but less quadriceps-specific strengthening. For knee flexion contractures, slow hamstring stretching exercises are best tolerated, especially when preceded by superficial or deep heat.

Energy conservation and joint protection: Individuals may benefit from learning techniques for more efficient performance of activities of daily living (ADLs) and strategies to conserve energy and joint stress for their most important tasks. For example, repeated stair climbing (which increases force on the knee six to seven times normal) should be avoided; items can be stored on the stairs and then brought up all at once.

Hip Impairments and Limitations

The hip is involved in approximately 50% of patients with RA, characteristically bilaterally and symmetrically. Articular loss is present on both the femoral and acetabular sides, in contrast to the more focally superior articular deficits seen with osteoarthritis. As the disease progresses, clinical symptoms such as groin pain, joint stiffness, difficulty with ADLs, and antalgic gait become more apparent. Osseous erosions, joint narrowing, and cysts are seen on radiographs.

In the terminal stages of the disease, the femoral head may collapse, leading to bony ankylosis of the femur to the acetabulum. Avascular necrosis of the femoral head may occur in patients on long-term corticosteroid treatment.

Therapeutic Interventions

Ambulatory aids and orthotics: The hip joint is a structure not easily braced, owing to its proximal body position, difficulty with supporting belts, and significant force generation across the joint. However, the use of ambulatory aids such as a walker or cane can provide considerable relief during gait and reduce the forces acting on the joint. Platform walkers may be beneficial for patients with both upper- and lower-limb joint pathology.

Adaptive equipment: Elevated toilet seats, bath chairs, rails, and seat cushions assist patients with hip disease in performing ADLs while avoiding painful hip positions. In addition, use of long-handled devices to assist with lower-limb dressing and bathing helps to overcome limited hip motion and facilitate independence.

Thermal modalities: Superficial heat or cold, although not directly affecting intrinsic joint pathology, may relieve the pain of superficial structures (such as trochanteric bursitis). If inflammation is minimal, ultrasound may be used with stretching to alleviate joint capsular tightness.

Exercise (acute stages): Resting the joint while the patient is either prone or supine with pillows placed under the buttocks to extend the hip without flexing the knee is recommended. Simple isometric contraction of hip musculature can also be done by the patient.

Exercise (subacute and chronic stages): Aquatic therapy is an excellent medium for isotonic and aerobic exercises. Hip extensors and the abductor muscles should be targeted. The use of bicycle ergometry, treadmill exercises, and progressive walking are excellent for gaining strength and endurance. Pre-exercise and postexercise stretching is necessary.

Cervical Spine Impairments and Limitations

Biomechanical disruption of the cervical spine is caused from elongation and destruction of the ligamentous supporting structures. Of particular importance is the excessive motion and subsequent subluxation of the occiput-atlas-axis complex (Table 82-8 and Fig. 82-4). The early recognition of atlantoaxial subluxation is critical. The normal atlantoaxial distance should be less than 3.5 mm, the lateral masses of the atlas-axis should be less than 2 mm, and the posterior antlanto-ondontoid distance should be greater than 14 mm.

Table 82-8: Patterns of Atlantoaxial Subluxation in Rheumatoid Arthritis

1. Anterior—loss of integrity of the transverse and alar ligaments.
2. Posterior—principally because of erosion and fracture to bony elements, creating a backward directional force.
3. Lateral—abnormal rotational forces theoretically created by both ligamentous and bony destruction.
4. Vertical—when the occipitoaxial and atlantoaxial joints erode to the point of significant joint space narrowing, the occiput-atlax-axis complex may collapse, resulting in upward migration of the odontoid.

Therapeutic Interventions

Orthotics: Soft or semirigid cervical collars help the spinal muscles relax and decrease spasms. However, soft collars are ineffective in limiting neck range of motion. More aggressive immobilizing aids (occipital-cervical-thoracic) are indicated for patients with mild subluxation without spinal cord impingement and should be ordered after orthopedic consultation.

Thermal modalities and traction: The use of traction or high-force manipulation in patients with RA and neck pain is absolutely contraindicated, as involvement of the cervical spine frequently appears early in the course of the disease and occult ligamentous disruption may be present. Superficial heat or ultrasound or both often provide welcome relief to tightly bound cervical muscles.

Exercise: Optimizing cervical range of motion is best accomplished by regaining as much scapular and glenohumeral motion as possible. Soft-tissue mobilization, deep friction rub, and gentle myofacial relief methods may assist in attaining this motion. Isometric exercises can be performed by the patient by gently applying forward, backward, and lateral pressure with his or her hand to the forehead and scalp. Isotonic exercise should be used with caution.

Energy conservation and joint protection: Unloading the cervical spine can be accomplished by unweighing the upper limbs and using proper neck biomechanics. Suggested techniques are lifting lighter packages, lifting objects close to the body, and keeping the neck in neutral positions when bending or performing overhead activities.

Specific Hand and Wrist Impairments and Their Treatments

Swan-Neck Deformity

This condition is most commonly caused by metacarpophalangeal (MCP) synovitis and results in MCP joint flexion, PIP joint distal interphalangeal extension, and (DIP) joint flexion. Swelling of the MCP joint alters the extensor mechanism so that the pull of the extensor tendons is directed toward the palm, creating a flexion moment. This results in an unbalanced extensor moment on the PIP joint as the central slips of the extensor tendons become more taut. Subsequently, the DIP joints go passively into flexion.

If the PIP joint is the primary site, a different process

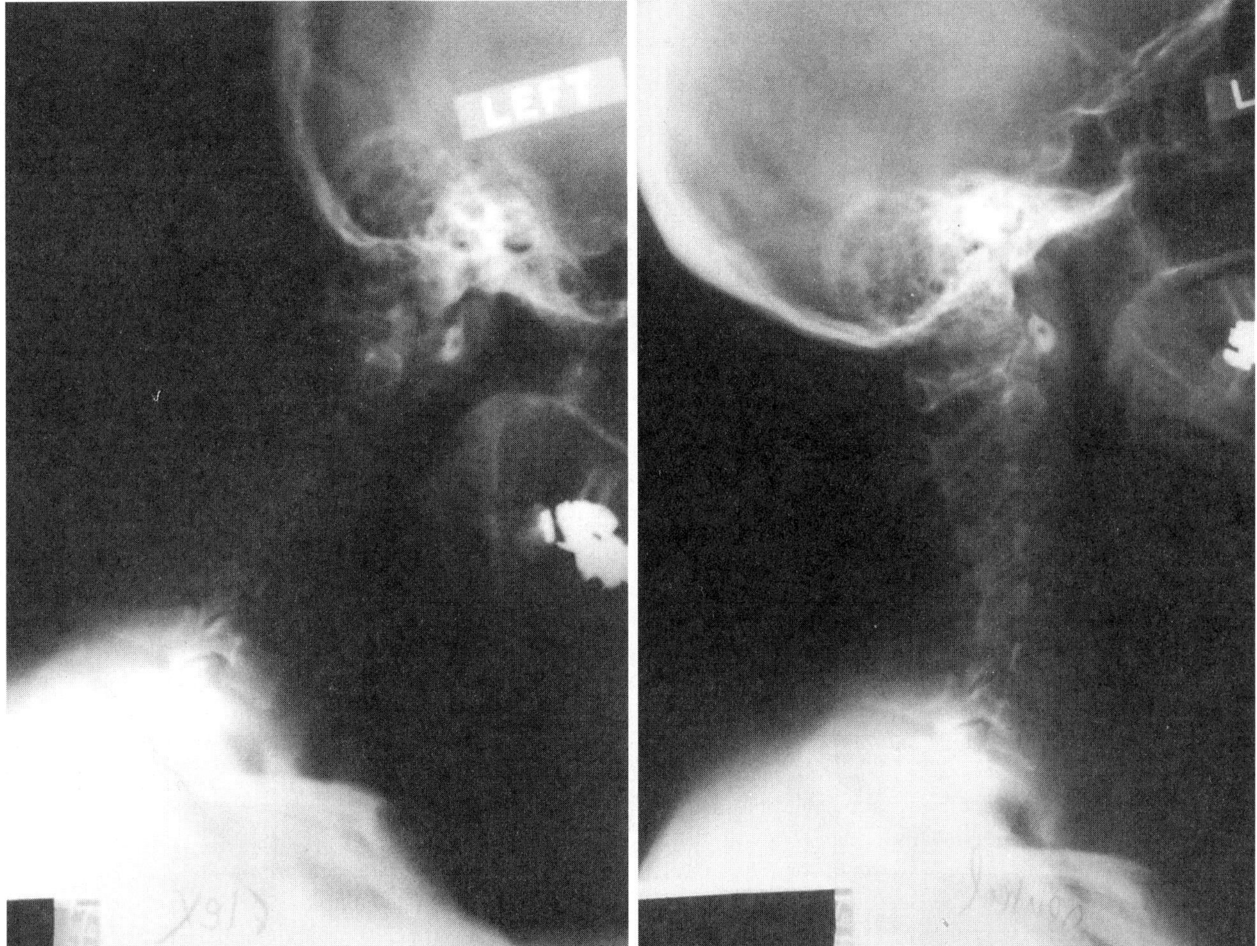

Figure 82-4. Radiographs of atlantoaxial subluxation.

causes the deformity. Expansion of the PIP joint capsule, secondary to inflammation, can cause asymmetric weakness on the volar aspect, creating a dorsally directed force on the extensor (lateral) tendon. This promotes an extension moment at the PIP joint and increased tension onto the centrally located flexor digitorum profundus tendon, resulting in a DIP joint flexion moment.

Regarding therapeutic interventions, the use of heated paraffin may loosen soft-tissue elements and provide analgesia. Digital massage may reduce edema and the risk of fibrous tissue development. "Ring splints," used principally over the PIP joint, are designed to create a flexion moment at the PIP joint, reversing the passive flexion moment at the DIP joint and offsetting MCP joint flexion deformity. Stretching should focus on elongation of the intrinsic muscles, promoting MCP extension and PIP flexion.

Boutonnière Deformity

This condition is caused by disturbance at the PIP joint resulting in PIP flexion, DIP extension, and MCP extension. Inflammation of the PIP joint causes joint expansion and damage to the extensor mechanism due to overstretching of the joint capsule. This elongation with subsequent weakening of the extensor (central) tendons creates a flexion moment on the PIP joint. Concurrently, the two long lateral extensors (destination, the distal phalanx) are displaced in a volar direction, creating an additional flexion moment at the PIP joint and a continual extension moment on the DIP joint.

Digital massage and paraffin may be useful therapy. Stretching exercises should encourage MCP flexion, PIP extension, and DIP flexion. Intrinsic muscle strengthening may provide some assistance with PIP extension and MCP flexion. Orthotics should promote an extension moment at the PIP joint to create a DIP flexion moment or attempt to provide a DIP flexion moment with three points of pressure and reversal of PIP joint flexion. The latter is more difficult because the forcing of the DIP joint into flexion strongly inhibits the extensor mechanism and PIP and MCP extension becomes limited.

Metacarpophalangeal Ulnar Deviation and Wrist Radial Deviation

Several factors are involved in the development of radial deviation of the wrist. First, wrist synovial inflammation causes weakness to the fibrous joint capsule, both the ulnar and radial sides. However, with selective damage to the triangular fibrocartilage, the ulnar side weakens further. Second, as inflammation increases and enzymatic destruction of the intrinsic ligaments progresses, the proximal-row carpal bones drift into a volar direction while the radius directs dorsally. These processes, in addition to other deforming forces, work destructively to cause an ulnar rotation of the proximal carpal bones, a radial rotation of the distal carpal bones, and a subsequent compensatory ulnar moment at the MCP joint—all in an attempt to realign the phalanx with the wrist. MCP ulnar deviation can also be created by synovitis affecting the MCP joint. When swelling at the MCP joint results in excessive capsular tension, the superficial flexor tendons drift into a volar position, creating an ulnar-directed force of pull, thus resulting in ulnar drift of the MCP and PIP joints.

The application of serial casting may prove beneficial by preventing ligamentous stretching and placing the joint at rest. This process is not intended to correct but to maintain. Casting an affected joint, however, may trigger more proximal or distal joint inflammation. Therefore, careful monitoring for MCP joint overuse must occur. Other physical modalities include paraffin, edema massage, and ultrasound.

Orthotics may be used to provide relief when the joint is at rest. However, functional splinting is often difficult to self-apply and can be quite bulky. In some cases, patients are aided by wrist or hand splints that focus on MCP radial return. The carpal tunnel splints are useful for patients who develop a compressive median neuropathy because of increased intracarpal canal pressures. Thumb dysfunction commonly seen at the carpometacarpal (CMC) joint responds to semirigid orthotics that rest the joint but allow distal interphalangeal and wrist joint motion.

Corticosteroids injected into intra-articular and tendon sheaths provide significant relief and may hasten functional recovery. The treatment of de Quervain syndrome, tenosynovitis of the abductor pollicis longus and extensor pollicis brevis, responds well to both orthotics, rest, and injections of corticosteroid into tendon sheaths.

Joint protection is especially important for wrist and metacarpal pathology. Occupational therapy consults can often assist in redesigning home and workplace activities to accomplish this.

Trigger Finger

Flexor and extensor tendons glide through narrow passages in the hands and wrists by way of long pulley mechanisms. If the tendons become inflamed or thickened, reducing the maneuvering capacity of these tendons within their "pseudocanals," leading to tendon serration and sticking. Clinically this presents as a catch or freezing of the finger, typically in flexion. This condition can be extremely painful and cause significant loss of grip strength and ADL function.

Conservative treatment consists of corticosteroid injections into the tendon sheaths. For more difficult cases, surgical release of the fibrous band is an option.

Intrinsic Tightness

The interossei, because of their unique insertion onto both the extensor mechanism dorsally and the proximal phalanx volarly, create a flexion moment at the MCP joint and an extension moment at the PIP joint. Shortening of these muscle fibers occurs because of reflex spasms to inflamed joint capsules, principally the MCP or PIP, or both, resulting in a hand that has decreased functional grip and intrinsic hand weakness.

The focus of therapeutic intervention is on stretching the shortened intrinsic muscles and the supportive connective tissue by providing MCP extension and PIP flexion. Use of paraffin and fluidotherapy may facilitate this stretching. Promoting functional skills that de-emphasize MCP flexion and PIP extension may impede the process of intrinsic tightening. This includes avoidance of habitual activities such as sitting on the palm of the hands and carrying draw strings or purse strings or grocery bags with the palmar surface of the hand.

Depression

Depression is a common comorbidity in patients with RA, a consequence of the complex psychosocial and physical manifestations of this chronic disease. Reported rates of depression in RA patients range from 10% to over 80%, with severe depression occurring in approximately 20% (21–23). Early investigators proposed an "arthritic personality," hypochondriacal, depressed and hysterical. However, these characteristics are common in a broad range of medical conditions, a consequence of chronic pain and illness.

Depression alone may be a significant predictor of disability and must be approached as aggressively as any other impairment affecting function (24). The diagnosis of depression requires a thorough history and physical and mental status examinations augmented by the use of psychological tests. Patients' initial complaints may be neurovegetative—poor appetite, impaired sleep, fatigue—easily confused with increased disease activity. Once diagnosed, major depression in RA appears to respond to aggressive treatment with antidepressants and psychotherapy; milder forms may also respond to antidepressants. As a consequence of their common neurochemical mechanisms, pain relief may accompany the pharmacologic, cognitive, and behavioral interventions used in the treatment of depression (21,25,26).

Work Disability

Work disability is a major problem for persons with RA. The prevalence ranges from 25% to 50% in persons when disease is present for more than 10 years, and over 90% when it is present longer (27,28). The most important risk factors for work disability are poor disease status, job physical demand, and older age (29).

Education, family and coworker support, depression, transportation difficulties and other societal factors, as well as employer disability management practices are contributing factors to the degree of work disability. Household disability is well known in women with RA, negatively impacting self-esteem and family dynamics. Prevention and early intervention are the best methods to reduce disability. Interventional strategies include patient and family counseling, worksite modification, energy conservation strategies, employer counseling, and vocational retraining. Termination of employment may be the only option for some persons with severe RA. They may need assistance obtaining disability benefits through Social Security. Those who are likely to be impaired for at least 12 months and have contributed adequately to Social Security currently qualify for Social Security disability income (SSDI). Those who have not contributed but who have severe financial need are eligible for Social Security income. Approval is based on medical disease criteria (such as x-rays and rheumatoid factor) or residual functional capacity when tests are inconclusive. Persons who receive SSDI are eligible for Medicare after 2 years; those receiving Social Security income are immediately eligible for Medicaid.

SPONDYLOARTHROPATHIES

The spondyloarthropathies are a group of rheumatic diseases sharing various clinical, radiographic, and genetic features (30). These diseases include ankylosing spondylitis (AS), Reiter syndrome, psoriatic arthritis, and arthritis of inflammatory bowel disease.

Clinical Presentation

The clinical and laboratory features of the spondyloarthropathies are spinal involvement with sacroiliitis; enthesopathy (inflammation at bony insertions of tendons and fascia); asymmetric peripheral arthritis of the lower limbs; familial occurrence; extra-articular manifestations of the skin, gut, urogenital system, and eyes; negative rheumatoid factor; and HLA-B27 association (31).

AS typically affects men younger than 35 years and targets the axial skeleton in 100%, in contrast to 20% to 40% involvement in Reiter syndrome and psoriatic arthritis and 10% in colitic arthritis. The predominant features are low-back pain that frequently awakens patients at night, is associated with morning stiffness of more than 30 minutes, and improves with exercise. A history of acute uveitis strengthens the diagnosis (31). Reiter syndrome and psoriatic arthritis are predominantly peripheral joint arthritis. Peripheral joint involvement is seen in 20% of patients with inflammatory bowel disease.

The physical findings of AS include pain on sacroiliac compression, paraspinal muscle spasm with vertebral tenderness, positive Schober test, and increased fingertip-to-floor and occiput-to-wall distances. Flattening of a normal lumbar lordosis, increased thoracic kyphosis with decreased expansion of the chest ligament, and cervical fixation in flexion are late findings.

Laboratory Findings

The laboratory findings are less remarkable in AS than in RA and include increased erythrocyte sedimentation rate with mild normocytic, normochromic anemia and negative results for rheumatoid factor and antinuclear antibodies. HLA-B27 is positive in more than 90% of AS patients, 63% to 75% of Reiter syndrome patients, 50% of patients with psoriatic arthritis with spinal involvement, and 50% of colitic spondylitis patients (30). The diagnostic value of HLA-B27 for AS is limited by low specificity. It may be most useful in early or atypical AS and Reiter syndrome.

Radiographic findings in AS (32) remain the most important diagnostic and monitoring tools; initial abnormalities occur in sacroiliac joints and thoracolumbar and lumbosacral junctions. All parts of the axial skeleton and sites of enthesopathy may develop characteristic abnormalities with advanced disease. Computed tomography shows detailed images of the sacroiliac joints and may be useful to clarify uncertain diagnoses. Magnetic resonance imaging is not superior to plain radiography or computed tomography for detecting sacroiliitis, but is helpful in the evaluation of cauda equina syndrome and medullary compression in atlantoaxial instability (31). The sacroiliitis of AS involves both sides of the sacroiliac joints, whereas osteitis condensans ilii involves only the iliac side and occurs more commonly in multiparous women. The sacroiliac joint is not usually involved in diffuse idiopathic skeletal hyperostosis. The vertical syndesmophytes and squaring of vertebrae in AS differentiate it from the large curved osteophytes and the paravertebral ossification of Reiter syndrome and psoriatic arthritis. Spotty involvement of the spine and absence of severe cervical spinal change are typical of Reiter syndrome and psoriatic arthritis. Spondylitis in inflammatory bowel disease resembles AS (33).

The current diagnostic criteria are listed in Table 82-9.

Etiology and Pathophysiology

Development of the spondyloarthropathies comprises triggering of inflammation, amplifying of the inflammation process, and injury to inflammatory tissue. Physical trauma and several microorganisms, including some gram-positive bacteria, may trigger the development of reactive arthritis. The degree of amplification contributes to the severity of tissue injury (34). HLA-B27 antigens are involved in the disease by acting as receptors for factors related to bacteria. A mechanism of molecular mimicry is implied by evidence of cross-reactivity between certain peptide

Table 82-9: Diagnostic Criteria for Ankylosing Spondylitis*

Low-back pain of at least 3-mo duration relieved by exercise but not by rest.
Limitation of motion of the lumbar spine in the sagittal and frontal planes.
Chest expansion decreased relative to normal values for age and sex.
Bilateral sacroiliitis of grades 2 to 4.
Unilateral sacroiliitis of grade 3 or 4.
Definite ankylosing spondylitis
Unilateral grade 3 or 4, or bilateral grade 2 to 4 sacroiliitis and at least one of the three clinical criteria.

* Modified New York criteria, 1984.
Source: Modified from Khan MA, van der Linden SM. Ankylosing spondylitis and other spondyloarthropathies. *Rheum Dis Clin North Am* 1990;16:551–579. By permission of WB Saunders Company.

sequences of HLA-B27 and one or more "arthritogenic" bacteria (35).

Prognosis

A predictable pattern of AS emerges within the first 10 years of the disease. Fewer than 20% of patients with adult-onset AS deteriorate to a condition of significant disability. The life span of patients with AS is nearly normal. Deaths are usually attributable to cardiac involvement, cervical spinal fractures or subluxation, or amyloidosis (36). Early peripheral joint disease, iritis, pulmonary fibrosis, and persistently high erythrocyte sedimentation rates indicate a poor prognosis (31).

Guillemin et al (37) found that patients with peripheral joint involvement performing heavy work tended to have prolonged sick leaves, whereas long-term disability was more frequent when work involved exposure to cold conditions and prolonged standing. Sedentary work and involvement in formal vocational rehabilitation programs lessened the incidence of long-term disability.

Many patients with Reiter syndrome experience relapses, often after many symptom-free years. Approximately 20% to 50% develop chronic peripheral arthritis or progressive spondylitis (30,38). Severe disability usually occurs from arthritis of the foot and the ankle, aggressive axial involvement, or blindness.

Therapeutic Interventions

Pharmacotherapy

Nonsteroidal anti-inflammatory drugs (NSAIDs), especially indomethacin, are effective in controlling the inflammation from AS (39,40). In contrast, systemic corticosteroids are minimally effective, and intra-articular corticosteroids are helpful but should be used sparingly. A multicenter study of sulfasalazine showed efficacy in the treatment of active spondyloarthropathy, especially in patients with psoriatic arthritis (41). A low percentage of patients (27%) with spondyloarthropathies have active disease requiring treatment with sulfasalazine in addition to NSAIDs (40). Methotrexate has been *beneficial* for psoriasis and psoriatic arthritis (30) and may help patients with refractory peripheral joint synovitis (42). No pharmaceutical agent, however, has yet been shown to alter the course of this disease.

Exercise

Therapeutic exercise is a critically important component of treatment. A lifelong, individualized, well-instructed exercise program may help to maintain maximal range of motion of the spine and costovertebral-girdle joints and potentially prevent flexion contractures and loss of height (43). The exercise prescription should include range of motion of the neck, shoulders, and hips; stretching of the pectoral, paraspinal, hip flexor, and hamstring muscles; deep breathing; and strengthening of the back and hip extensors and abdominal muscles. If peripheral joint involvement is not significant, the patient's lower extremities can be strengthened using a program of cardiovascular exercise with equipment such as a treadmill or stair-climbing device. The trunk and arms can be strengthened using a cross-country ski machine (40). Patients should be instructed in posture principles and the importance of recording key response variables, such as height and chest expansion. Regular medical follow-up helps promote compliance.

Before exercise, physical modalities such as heat, ice, massage, and TENS may be used to decrease pain and muscle spasm and to facilitate joint motion.

Physical fitness and sports activities assist in maintaining flexibility and strength, and patients should be encouraged to choose sports that promote good posture and back extension. In the early stages of spondylitis with primarily low-back pain, patients may be able to play basketball, volleyball, or tennis. In the advanced disease, bicycling with upright handlebars or swimming may be more suitable. Swimming may need adaptation because of these patients' limited cervical motion (44). These activities, however, do not take the place of therapeutic exercise. Contact sports are not advised because of the risk of spinal fracture.

Occupational Therapy, Physical Therapy, and Patient Education

Occupational therapy is frequently prescribed for evaluations of and retraining in ADLs as well as for work, avocational, or home adaptations. Assistive devices such as reachers, long-handled tools, and wide-angled panoramic rearview or spot mirrors may be useful to accommodate decreased spinal motion.

Patient education is essential. Instruction in the natural history of the disease, the rationale for each treatment modality, and orientation to community resources should be offered to all patients. The Spondylitis Association of America (P. O. Box 5872, Sherman Oaks, CA 91413), formerly the Ankylosing Spondylitis Association, is an excellent resource.

In a study by Kraag et al (45), a group of patients who received physiotherapy and disease education for 4 months had greater improvement in fingertip-to-floor distance and function (measured by a modified Toronto ADL questionnaire for AS) than did control subjects. There were no significant changes in pain, spinal alignment, or Schober test results. Improvement in fingertip-to-floor distance was thought to be related to stretching of the hamstrings or muscles about the shoulder girdle, increased hip flexion, and compensation of the restricted movement by unaffected or mildly affected segments of the spine that responded to exercise.

Fisher et al (46) reported that cardiovascular fitness helps to maintain work capacity in patients with AS. Components of their regimen targeted improving spinal mobility and increasing cardiorespiratory fitness. A randomized, controlled trial in 144 patients demonstrated that a program of group physical therapy was superior to home exercise in improving thoracolumbar mobility, fitness, and global effect on the health of AS patients. The program consisted of hydrotherapy, exercises, and sporting activities weekly for 3 hours per session (47).

Patients with severe deforming disease, especially involving the hips and knees, may benefit from total joint replacement. However, the outcome of total hip arthroplasty may be compromised by heterotopic ossification and reankylosis. Calin and Elswood (48) reported that 6% of patients with severe hip disease required total hip arthroplasty, with good or excellent results in more than two-thirds of patients.

Heel pain due to Achilles enthesopathy, Achilles bursitis, or plantar fasciitis frequently occurs with spondyloarthropathy (40). Inferior heel pain is most common and usually disappears spontaneously. Treatment includes heel pads, NSAIDs, orthotics, and local injections of steroids. Sulfasalazine may be prescribed for refractory heel pain.

Spinal Involvement and Complications

Impairments and Limitations

The ankylosed spine is frequently osteopenic and associated with ossification of spinal ligaments; therefore, the risk of fractures of the spine from even minor trauma is increased, especially in the cervical region (49). Because of the loss of ligamentous support, a fracture of an ankylosed spine is unstable. Spinal fractures should be considered in any patient with AS who experiences trauma. Unfortunately, plain film radiographs may not show the fracture. Tomography may be useful and radionuclide bone scanning is particularly useful in patients with chronic pseudarthrosis (50).

The inflammatory process initiated by synovial tissue in the occipital-atlantoaxial articulation causes ligamentous laxity and bony destruction and can lead to upper cervical instability. Symptoms of atlantoaxial instability may vary from radiating pain in the occipital region caused by compression of the greater occipital nerve to radiating arm pain, hyperreflexia, and various degrees of sensory and motor loss in the limbs caused by compression of the spinal cord. Clinicians should base decisions about surgery on the presence of significant neurologic deficit, vertebral artery symptoms, and intractable pain, and not solely on the degree of subluxation. The latter does not correlate with the degree of impairment (51).

Cauda equina syndrome begins late in the course of AS (50), even when the disease is inactive. The most frequent symptoms are cutaneous sensory loss in the lower lumbar and sacral dermatomes, disturbances in urinary and rectal sphincters of lower motor neuron type, mild to moderate weakness in the lumbosacral myotomes, and pain in the rectum or lower limbs. This syndrome is associated with enlarged dural sleeves and arachnoid diverticula that erode the lamina of the lumbosacral vertebrae. Radiographic evaluation by magnetic resonance imaging can establish the diagnosis and exclude a tumor (35).

Therapeutic Interventions

Conservative treatment for upper cervical instability that is satisfactory for most patients aims to relieve pain and discomfort, maintain or restore range of motion and muscle strength, and help patients modify the ADLs that aggravate neck pain. Cervical collars, commonly used to relieve discomfort and protect the neck, are often prescribed to prevent sudden neck flexion and extension that could result in neurologic impairment or death (52–54). Heat, ice, and TENS may relieve pain.

For fractures, nonoperative treatment with an emphasis on careful immobilization is often successful (55). Laminectomy is recommended for patients with progression of a neurologic lesion. Spinal fusion is recommended for fractures that cannot be externally stabilized (48).

Cardiopulmonary Involvement

Patients with AS rarely report respiratory symptoms or limitations. Despite diminished expansion of the chest ligament due to costovertebral joint fusion, patients with AS have only minor restrictive changes, with mildly reduced vital and total lung capacities on respiratory function tests (30). In order to compensate for the rigid chest wall, patients with AS rely on diaphragmatic movement in their respiratory function (46).

Aortic insufficiency and heart block are the most common cardiac complications and result from inflammation of the aortic valve and root as well as adjacent atrioventricular nodal tissue. Cardiac complications are more common in patients with long-standing disease (30).

Therapeutic Interventions

Patients should follow a therapeutic exercise program to maintain maximal range of motion of the spine, and costovertebral-girdle joints, as well as a cardiovascular fitness program. Patients who follow a modest amount of exercise regularly could maintain a satisfactory work capacity despite very restricted spinal and chest wall mobility (46). Patients' restrictive lung disease may be further compromised when the patient is immobilized owing to trauma, surgery, or other medical illnesses and vigorous pulmonary therapy is indicated. Patients with AS who have aortic insufficiency or any other cardiac abnormalities should have an exercise tolerance test before starting a fitness program.

INFLAMMATORY MYOPATHIES

Clinical Presentation

Inflammatory myopathies are acquired muscle diseases consisting of polymyositis (PM), dermatomyositis (DM), and inclusion body myositis (IBM). They are characterized by proximal and often symmetric muscle weakness of gradual onset. DM is accompanied by characteristic dermal changes, including a heliotrope rash on the eyelids and erythema over the knuckles (Gottron sign). IBM, known since 1978, is characterized by a poor response to steroid treatment, involvement of distal muscles, marked quadricep weakness and atrophy, and minimal increase in serum muscle enzyme levels (56,57).

Functional limitations relate to weakness of the pelvic and shoulder girdles. Patients may have difficulty in rising from a chair, going up stairs, getting in and out of the bathtub or car, lifting objects, dressing, combing, and eating. Those with advanced disease have difficulty holding the head up and lifting the head off a pillow.

DM and PM have been associated with an increased risk of malignancy. However, this association is controversial. Routine age-appropriate cancer screening is all that is required to exclude occult malignancies in most patients (58). When malignancy is present, the prognosis for recovery is poor (59).

Diagnostic Criteria

The five major diagnostic components are symmetric weakness of the limb girdle muscles and anterior neck flexors, muscle biopsy abnormalities, increase in skeletal muscle enzyme levels, myopathic electromyographic findings, and in DM, dermatologic features (60). Later, IBM diagnostic criteria were added (57). The diagnostic criteria are provided in Table 82-10 (61).

Etiology and Pathophysiology

Although the causes are unknown, inflammatory myopathies are thought to be caused by immune-mediated processes triggered by environmental factors in genetically susceptible individuals (62). Cellular and humoral immune mechanisms are central to these diseases. Frequent association with other autoimmune diseases and a high prevalence of circulatory antibodies support autoimmunity.

Table 82-10: Diagnostic Criteria for Inflammatory Myopathies

	Polymyositis		Dermatomyositis		
Criterion	Definite	Probable	Definite	Mild or Early	Definite Inclusion Body Myositis
Muscle strength	Myopathic muscle weakness	Myopathic muscle weakness	Myopathic muscle weakness	Seemingly normal strength	Myopathic muscle weakness with early distal muscle involvement
EMG findings	Myopathic	Myopathic	Myopathic	Myopathic or nonspecific	Myopathic with mixed potentials
Muscle enzyme levels	Increased (up to 50-fold)	Increased (up to 50-fold)	Increased (up to 50-fold) or normal	Increased (up to 10-fold) or normal	Increased (up to 10-fold) or normal
Muscle biopsy findings	Diagnostic for this type of inflammatory myopathy	Nonspecific myopathy without signs of primary inflammation	Diagnostic	Nonspecific or diagnostic	Diagnostic
Rash or calcinosis	Absent	Absent	Present	Present	Absent

EMG = electromyographic.
Source: Adapted by permission of the *New England Journal of Medicine*, from Dalakas MC. Polymyositis, dermatomyositis and inclusion-body myositis. *N Engl J Med* 1991;325:1487–1498.

Viruses have been suspected as the pathogens of the idiopathic inflammatory myopathies. The possibility of a genetic influence has been suggested on the basis of findings in studies of HLA associations, but this influence is not yet understood (63).

Therapeutic Interventions

Pharmacotherapy

Prednisone is the first-line drug used for treating inflammatory myopathies. An immunosuppressive drug (azathioprine or methotrexate) is indicated for serious complications of steroid use, repeated relapses with steroid taper, ineffective treatment, and rapidly progressive disease with severe weakness and respiratory failure (61).

IBM is generally refractory to therapy; an immunosuppressive drug may be added if no benefit from prednisone is apparent in 6 weeks (62). There is no specific test for steroid myopathy, which is often difficult to differentiate from the flare of inflammatory disease (62). A provocative challenge with higher doses of prednisone or rapid tapering of the dose is the only way to determine the cause of the clinical decline.

Intravenous gamma globulin therapy is a promising new treatment and is better tolerated by patients than are corticosteroids or the other immunosuppressive medications. However, this therapy is expensive and its efficacy is short-lived (mean duration of weeks). Patients require repeated treatments for long-term benefit (64). Gamma globulin may be considered for initial treatment in patients with contraindications for steroids, especially the elderly, to avoid steroid-induced side effects (65).

Patients treated early have the best clinical courses. In an outcome study of 65 patients with PM or DM who had an average follow-up of 2.5 years, those treated within 6 months or 1 year of disease onset with oral prednisone with or without other modalities including cytotoxic agents, plasmaphoresis, and intravenous bolus methylprednisolone had better outcomes than did those who received treatment later (66). Overall, the myopathy improved in 43.1%, did not change in 35.4%, and worsened in 21.5%. Patients with higher initial creatine phosphokinase levels (>5000 mU/mL) showed better improvement in strength than did those with lower levels.

Corticosteroid-related problems appear to contribute significantly to the functional disability reported by patients with PM or DM. Earlier use of immunosuppressive agents should be considered, particularly in older patients who are at increased risk for avascular necrosis and compression fractures (67).

Treatment programs for inflammatory myopathies require close follow-up and modification based on disease activity. Muscle strength and serum enzyme values should be monitored regularly during treatment. Of the two, muscle strength is a more important guide (50). The most critical clinical factor for therapeutic monitoring is improved function, as reflected in the patient's ADLs.

Modalities and Exercise

Heat modalities may be used to treat myalgias. A cervical collar often proves helpful for a patient with weakness of the neck muscles.

Bed rest with proper positioning is indicated in the acute phase. Passive range of motion exercises should be performed during periods of severe inflammation and progress to active-assisted and active range of motion exercises. Joint contractures can develop early, and are particularly severe in children with DM, who need ongoing, careful range of motion and stretching programs.

In the subacute phase, the rehabilitation program should include strengthening exercises and ambulatory and functional ADLs. Exercises of the trunk and lower extremities against resistance, which is applied depending on the strength of each muscle group, appear safe for the rehabilitation of PM and DM without causing a clinically significant increase in muscle enzyme levels (68). An isometric strengthening program is useful for strengthening affected muscles in inactive or stable inflammatory muscle disease (69).

Orthotics, Assistive Devices, and Patient Education

Gradually progressive mobility training including bed mobility, transfer training, and walking with gait aids as needed should be incorporated. Patients who have marked quadricep weakness may require ankle-foot orthoses. The use of a motorized scooter or wheelchair should be considered for patients with progressive weakness who are no longer able to walk. Seat lift chairs are useful for patients with proximal weakness who are able to ambulate but who are not able to stand up from a sitting position.

Patients' functional ADLs will expand during treatment as their strength improves. Patients should be instructed in the principles of energy conservation. Combinations of definite features of more than one connective tissue syndrome are called *overlap syndromes*. Overlap syndromes account for up to 20% of patients with inflammatory myopathies and are associated with rheumatoid arthritis, systemic sclerosis, systemic lupus erythematosus, Sjögren syndrome, and mixed connective tissue disease (64). The arthritis in overlap syndromes may require splints and joint protection techniques. Patients often need assistive devices for dressing and reaching and adaptive devices in the bathroom. Use of a mobile arm-support, ball-bearing orthosis allows a patient with weak proximal muscles to move more freely to perform progressive ADLs and avocational and vocational activities.

Dysphagia Training

Dysphagia, found in 12% to 38% of patients with PM or DM, predisposes the patient to aspiration (62,71). Patients with dysphagia need a swallowing evaluation and retraining to protect the airway and prevent aspiration pneumonia. The most common lung disease in PM and DM is pneumonia, generally due to aspiration (72). Pharyngeal weakness usually responds to corticosteroid therapy.

OSTEOARTHRITIS

Osteoarthritis (OA) is a degenerative disorder of joints, characterized by progressive loss of hyaline cartilage and overgrowth of subchondral bone. It is an extraordinarily common disorder, perhaps affecting up to 40 million persons in the United States alone. OA may be responsible for over 10% of physician visits per year.

Genetics, occupation, lifestyle, and longevity affect the prevalence of the disease worldwide. For example, an autosomal gene that is sex linked appears responsible for the development of primary "nodal" OA (characterized by Heberden and Bouchard nodes and degenerative hip and knee disease). Familial chondrocalcinosis and hereditary arthro-ophthalmopathy are inherited forms of premature OA. Epidemiologic studies describe a racial and geographic predominance in OA development (e.g., the high incidence of hip OA in Japanese), perhaps as a consequence of differences in the incidence of congenital hip disease.

The incidence of severe OA rises proportionately with age. Over the age of 65 years, 80% of individuals have radiographic evidence of OA. OA is the leading cause of impairment and disability in the older population. Repetitive activity does appear to be a risk factor for this disorder. There is a higher incidence of OA of the knees in heavy laborers. However, there is no established relationship between long-distance running and knee arthritis (73).

Trauma plays a distinct role in the development of OA by altering the biomechanics of articular and periarticular structures and inciting the repair and degradation cycle, which then leads to OA. For example, in both human and animal models, damage to the anterior cruciate ligament or meniscus, or both, leads to OA of the knee. This OA is particularly accelerated if there is a concomitant sensory deficit, suggesting a neurologic role in the process.

Etiology and Pathophysiology

OA develops as the end result of a variety of processes. The earliest step in OA involves an alteration in collagen composition and degradation of matrix proteoglycans. The decrease in proteoglycans results in an increase in water content and permeability, perhaps increasing the stiffness of the matrix. Chondrocytes sense the disruption and attempt repair through the release of mediators that stimulate a tissue response. Nitrous oxide is produced, stimulating interleukin-1, which then stimulates multiple degradative enzymes. Enzymatic degradation may in turn stimulate the production of proteoglycan and collagen. This initial repair may preserve the joint indefinitely. If the response is insufficient, however, the articular cartilage may repair with fibrocartilage, which is less able to tolerate mechanical stress. The overall result then is a joint that has lost mechanical integrity; less severe insults will engender inflammation or further degradation of cartilage matrix.

The subchondral bone is then subject to a greater translation of force and undergoes repeated microfracture and repair. New bone is formed through local fracture remodeling, seen as the characteristic osteophytes and subchondral sclerosis on radiographs. This new bone is stiffer and less likely to handle further stressors. Joint fluid is extruded from clefts in the damaged hyaline cartilage, reacting with osteoblasts and fibroblasts and leading to cysts in the subchondral bone. The chondrocyte proliferative response to cartilage damage declines over time, perhaps due to mechanical damage or a downregulation of the chondrocyte response to anabolic cytokines.

Secondary effects on the periarticular tissues contribute to the pain and disability of this disorder. Synovial tissue may respond with inflammation. Joint contractures occur, accompanied by atrophy of the surrounding musculature. Joint ligaments subject to repetitive mechanical insults may lose their integrity and joint instability ensues.

Clinical Presentation

OA is a gradual disorder involving one or more joints. The weight-bearing joints (hips, knees, and spine) are most commonly symptomatic, although radiographic evidence of OA of the hand is most common, present in over three-fourths of individuals over age 65. Pain is usually described as an aching, throbbing discomfort and its occurrence with motion is the earliest symptom. It is worsened by prolonged weight-bearing activity or immobilization and alleviated with brief periods of rest. Morning stiffness lasting less than 30 minutes relieved by activity is extremely common.

Patients with advanced disease experience pain at rest and may also report a grinding or grating sensation with joint motion. Their joints may feel unstable or lax, "giving way" during high-performance tasks. Joint effusions occasionally occur. Functional limitations are specific to the joint affected. For example, limitations in long-distance walking, stair climbing, kneeling, and lower-body dressing are common in individuals with hip or knee arthritis. Signs of the disorder on physical examination include localized tenderness, joint enlargement from proliferation of bone (such as Heberden nodes), and flexion contractures. Joint inflammation and effusion may occur. Periarticular muscle atrophy is common. As a consequence of the primary abnormal joint, secondary joint abnormalities above and below the joint can occur.

Table 82-11: Secondary Osteoarthritis	
Causes	**Mechansims**
Intra-articular fractures	Damage to articular cartilage or joint incongruity
Ligament and joint capsule	Joint instability
Meniscectomy or meniscal injury	Joint instability and altered joint loading
Joint dysplasias (developmental and hereditary joint and cartilage dysplasias)	Abnormal joint shape and/or abnormal articular cartilage
Aseptic necrosis	Bone necrosis leading to collapse of articular surface and joint incongruity
Hemophilia	Multiple joint hemorrhages
Stickler syndrome (progressive hereditary arthro-ophthalmopathy)	Abnormal joint and/or articular cartilage development
Gaucher disease (hereditary deficiency of enzyme glucocerebrosidase leading to accumulation of glucocerebroside)	Bone necrosis or pathologic bone fracture leading to joint incongruity
Hemochromatosis (excess iron deposition in multiple tissues)	Unknown
Ochronosis (hereditary deficiency of enzyme homogentisic acid oxide leads to accumulation of homogentisic acid)	Deposition of homogentisic acid polymers in articular cartilage
Acromegaly	Overgrowth of articular cartilage producing joint incongruity and/or abnormal cartilage
Ehlers-Danlos syndrome	Joint instability
Calcium pyrophosphate deposition disease	Accumulation of calcium pyrophosphate crystals in articular cartilage
Neuropathic arthropathy (Charcot joints, syphilis, diabetes mellitus, syringomyelia, meningomyelocele, leprosy, congenital insensitivity to pain)	Loss of proprioception and joint sensation and eventual joint instability
Paget disease	Distortion of incongruity of joints due to bone remodeling

Source: Reprinted with permission. *Clinical Symposia* Vol. 47, No. 2, 1995. Ciba-Geigy Corporation, Pharmaceuticals Division.

The diagnosis usually can be determined from the history and physical examination. Characteristic changes on radiographs include osteophytes, cysts, or sclerosis in the subchondral marrow, and joint space narrowing (Figs. 82-5 and 82-6). While more than 90% of patients over 40 years old have some of the radiographic changes of OA in weight-bearing joints, only 30% have clinical symptoms (74). No laboratory studies are diagnostic, yet they may be useful in excluding underlying causes of secondary OA (Table 82-11). Similarly, synovial fluid analysis is useful to exclude other causes of joint pain and inflammation. Use of bone scanning, computed tomography, and magnetic resonance imaging is limited by cost, availability, and resolution.

General Treatment

Pharmacotherapy

No pharmacologic agents have been shown to alter the course of OA. Pharmacotherapy is aimed at reducing pain and eliminating inflammation when present. Oral agents include pure analgesics (such as acetaminophen) and analgesic anti-inflammatories (such as NSAIDs). Currently acetaminophen is the recommended first-line agent prescribed for OA. Several recent prospective controlled trials in subjects with knee OA showed that it is as effective as the NSAIDs, which are more expensive and have more side effects (75,76). Because of the potential role of local inflammatory mediators in OA, some physicians contend that NSAIDs are more effective agents. Intra-articular or periarticular corticosteroid injections may provide significant temporary relief of symptoms but should not be repeated more than three times a year as they may contribute to deterioration of the cartilage, bone, and periarticular structures. A series of intra-articular hyaluronic acid (Hylan GF-20) injections in knees with OA may be at least as effective as a 6-month full-dose of NSAIDs (82). Topical capsaicin cream, which depletes sensory nerve endings of the peptide substance P, may reduce joint pain and tenderness when applied topically to treat OA of the knee and hand. Pharmacologic agents aimed at disease modification (such as doxycycline) offer treatment of OA and will be available in the near future. Selective prostaglandin-inhibiting NSAIDs (the "cox-2" inhibitor drugs) when available will offer anti-inflammatory treatment for patients who have been unable to use NSAIDs in the past because of NSAID side effects. Alternative therapies, such as glucosamine and chondroitin sulfate, are receiving significant media and patient attention. Early studies offer interesting potential for relief of pain and stiffness; however, more rigorous trials are necessary prior to widespread prescription of these compounds.

Figure 82-5. Stages of osteoarthritis of the knee. *A*. Stage I: mild osteoarthritis. *B*. Stage II: moderate osteoarthritis. *C*. Stage III: moderately severe osteoarthritis. *D*. Stage IV: severe osteoarthritis.

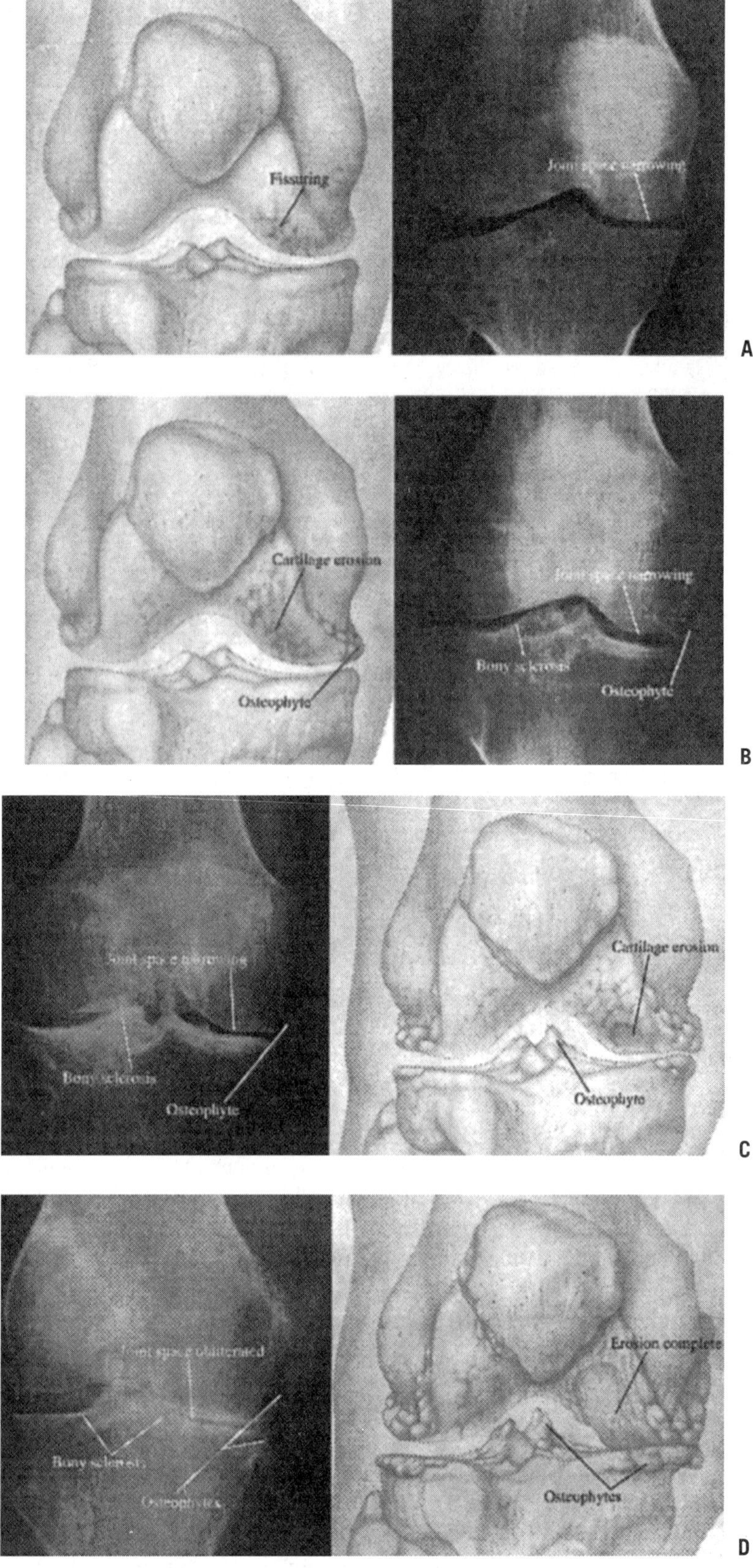

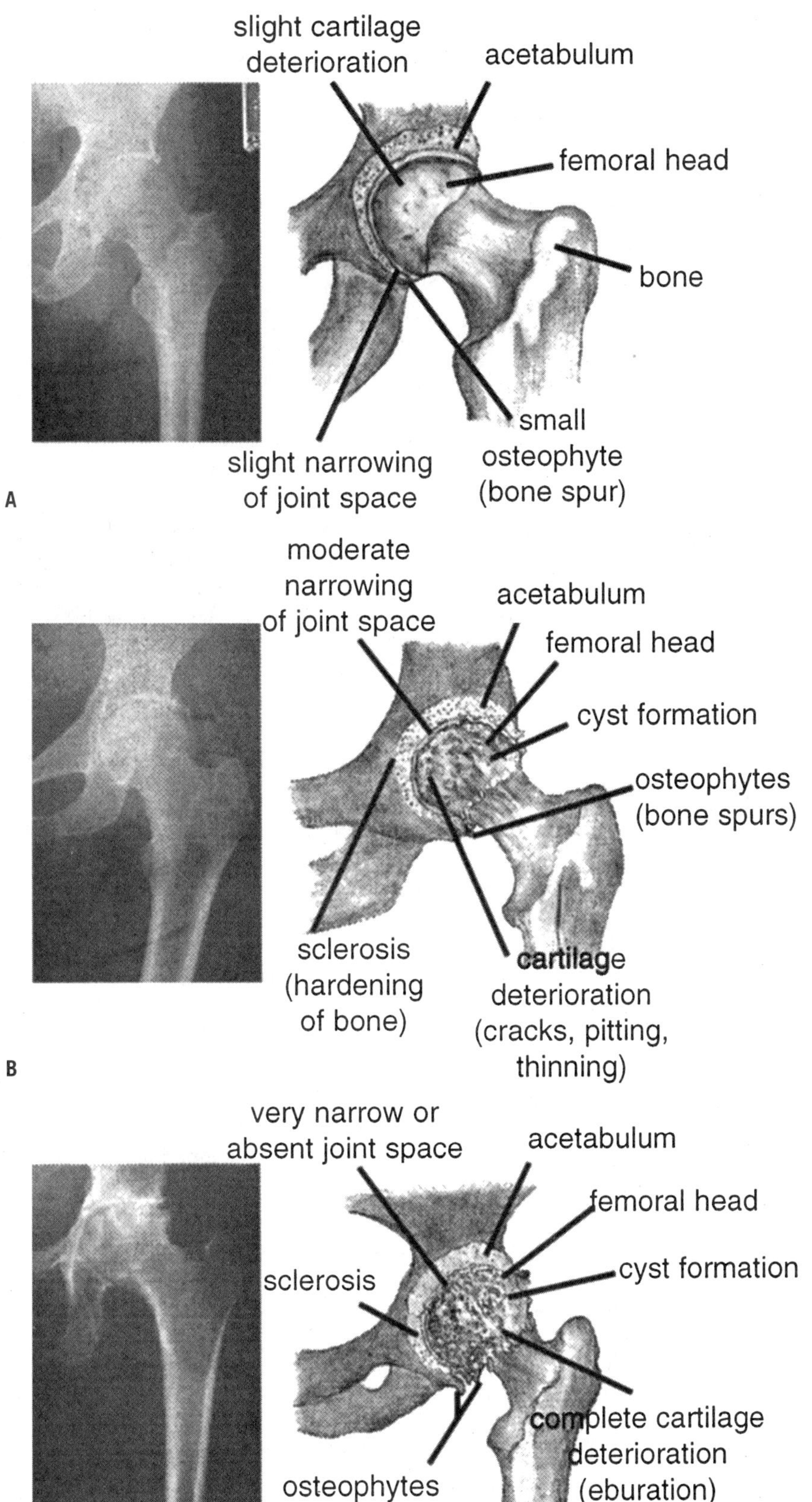

Figure 82-6. Stages of osteoarthritis of the hip. *A.* Stage I: mild osteoarthritis. *B.* Stage II: moderate osteoarthritis. *C.* Stage III: severe osteoarthritis.

Weight Loss

Obesity is a well-known risk factor for OA of the knee but not yet proven as a risk factor for hip OA. The Framingham study cohort data suggest that obese individuals, particularly women, are more likely to develop knee OA (78). Similarly, weight loss appears to reduce the incidence of symptomatic knee OA (79). Weight loss, like exercise, should be a standard recommendation of any arthritis treatment program.

Exercise

Patients commonly respond to their OA symptoms by limiting activity. The resulting restriction in motion leads to disuse atrophy, which promotes atrophy of the cartilage and thinning of the bone. This further compromises joint integrity and contributes to pain. Exercise is an extraordinarily promising avenue to use in managing the physical impairments and functional limitations in individuals with OA (77,80–84).

Surgery

When severe pain and functional limitations exist despite maximal nonoperative intervention, then joint reconstruction may be indicated. Osteotomy or fustion may provide temporary relief of pain in young patients with OA of the hip or knee who are not yet candidates for joint replacement because of their age. Osteotomy is of greatest benefit when disease is only moderately advanced. Arthroscopic removal of loose bodies and joint lavage may be useful in selected patients, particularly if focal acute pathology, such as meniscal tear, is suspected (Fig. 82-7). (85)

Total joint replacement is discussed in Chapter 84.

Clinical Presentation and Rehabilitation for Specific Joints

Rehabilitative techniques focus on exercise (to restore motion, strength, and endurance), superficial modalities, use of adaptive equipment and assistive devices, and education and counseling. Specific interventions are described for hip, knee, and shoulder OA.

Hip Impairments and Limitations

The accurate diagnosis of hip-region pain depends on a comprehensive history and careful musculoskeletal examination. The differential diagnosis includes articular hip pathology, bursitis and other soft-tissue disorders, lumbar spinal disease, abdominal tumors or infections involving the iliopsoas, and more unusually, pelvic bony tumors or infection.

OA pain originating from the hip is insidious in onset, described as an aching discomfort in the groin, buttock, or lateral part of the thigh and exacerbated by weight-bearing activities and movement of the hip. Physical findings include hip flexion contracture, revealed by a positive result on the Thomas test; painful and limited passive and active range of motion of the hip (particularly flexion and rotation); weakness of hip musculature, especially the hip abductors as shown by a positive finding on the Trendelenberg test; leg-length discrepancy; and frequently an antalgic gait with a shortened stance phase and stride length, limited active hip flexion, lumbar spine hyperlordosis, and the characteristic abductor lurch. Initial radiographic evaluation should include anterior-posterior and lateral views of the hip and standing anterior-posterior pelvic views to evaluate the opposite hip joint, pelvis, and sacroiliac joints. The earliest findings of OA of the hip represent the effect of localized mechanical overload of cartilage, with a thickening of the subchondral line. With loss of articular cartilage in the intermediate stages of the disease, radiographs reveal narrowing of the joint space in a distribution consistent with the underlying disease process. For example, narrowing of the superior or superolateral portion of the acetabulum is typical of a childhood acetabular insufficiency. In addition, femoral head flattening with proximal migration of the femur and osteophyte formation may occur. Advanced OA is characterized by near-complete obliteration of the joint space, femoral and acetabular cysts, osteophytes, and further flattening of the femoral head as a consequence of subchondral collapse (see Fig. 82-6).

Therapeutic Interventions

The rehabilitation program is specific to the impairments identified. The prescription includes aerobic conditioning, muscle strengthening, range of motion exercises, orthotics, functional training, and education about proper body mechanics and energy conservation.

Individuals with arthritis exhibit decreased aerobic conditioning compared with age-matched normal subjects. Aerobic conditioning programs improve aerobic capacity, 50-foot walking time, and scores for depression and anxiety in subjects with OA (81). In general, physical training programs aim for 30 to 40 minutes of aerobic exercise (with warm-up and cooldown periods) maintaining a target heart rate or perceived exertion level, three to four times weekly. Aerobic conditioning programs should include "low impact" activities such as swimming or walking.

Muscle strengthening exercises focus on the hip and lower back, particularly the hip abductors and extensors. Active hip abductor strengthening exercises include side-lying leg lifts, prone "skateboard" abduction exercises, and standing abduction exercises. Weights are added according to what the patient can tolerate. Exercise in the pool is an efficient method to increase strength, range of motion, and endurance in a pain-free environment. Hip extensors can be strengthened in the supine or standing position. Stretching exercises, particularly in abduction and extension, are exceedingly important. Patients should lie prone daily for a few minutes to stretch the hip flexors. Trunk strengthening and stretching exercises, use of shoe orthotics, and functional gait training are also important.

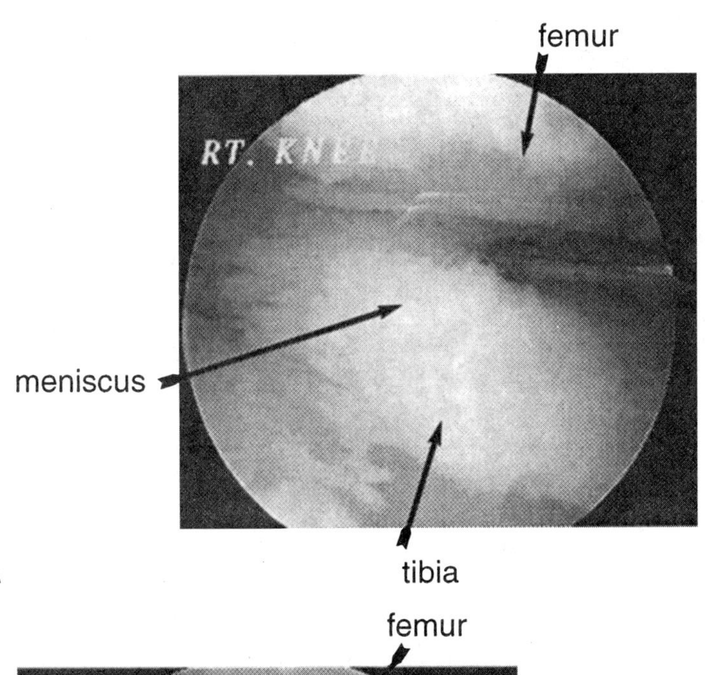

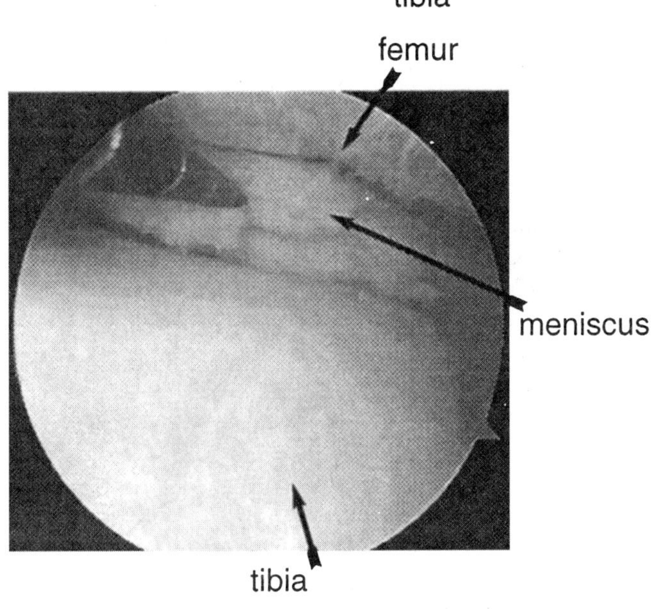

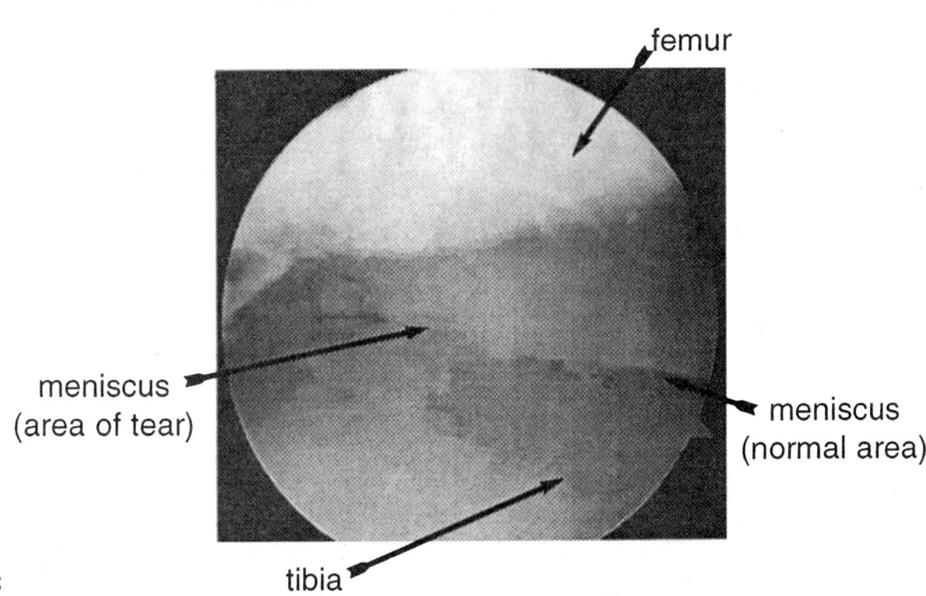

Figure 82-7. Arthroscopy in knee osteoarthritis. *A*. The medial (inside) femoral-tibial compartment of the right knee, viewed through an arthroscope. Both the femur and the tibia have severe arthritis. The meniscus has a degenerative tear related to the arthritis. *B*. The torn meniscal fragment has been partially removed from the right knee. *C*. The torn meniscal fragment has been removed from the right knee.

Adaptive equipment including long-handled sponges, reachers, sock donners, elevated toilet seats, grab bars, shower bench, and seat cushions may ease some functional tasks.

Educating the OA patient about energy conservation and joint protection completes the prescription. Understanding the hip joint as a simple lever system can direct the prescription of techniques to prevent abnormally high forces being distributed through the hip. For example, the loss of 1 lb of body weight translates to a 3-lb reduction in force distributed by the abductors. Use of a cane in the opposite hand acts to reduce the force generated by the abductors. Similarly, when reaching down to pick up an item, patients should support their weight on the contralateral hand (for instance, on a dresser) and lift with the ipsilateral hand. Heavy loads should be carried with two hands if possible, otherwise by the ipsilateral hand.

Knee Impairments and Limitations

The physical impairments common to individuals with knee OA include decreased aerobic capacity; muscle weakness, particularly of the hamstrings and quadriceps; decreased knee flexion and extension; gait disturbance; abnormal mechanical alignment with varus, valgus, and knee flexion deformities; other joint pathology such as OA of the hips, spine, or feet; and potentially, neurologic disturbances such as impaired sensation or proprioception.

The most common basic functional impairments in individuals with knee arthritis are difficulty walking for long distances or on uneven surfaces, climbing stairs, arising from low surfaces, kneeling, and performing lower-extremity dressing. Knee stiffness after sitting for prolonged periods is common; this usually improves with warm-up stretches before moving. Patients often have difficulties with higher-level tasks, such as housework, gardening, recreational sports, and carrying heavy objects.

Therapeutic Interventions

Rehabilitation is aimed at limiting physical and functional deficits. In a quantitative prospective study, physical therapy individualized to the subject's needs benefited those with severe OA of the knees, with improvements observed in strength, endurance, stair climbing, arising from a chair, pain relief, and walking ability (82). The following paragraphs describe the common components of a rehabilitation prescription for knee OA.

Active-assisted and active range of motion exercises are generally helpful. Since passive range of motion exercise induced inflammation in canine knee joints with crystal-induced synovitis, vigorous passive stretching is usually not prescribed for patients with warm, swollen joints in the acute stage. Modalities such as superficial or deep heat and cold help patients tolerate the discomfort of range of motion exercises.

Previous literature suggested that high-resistance exercises increase the strain on articular tissues and that certain types of exercise (particularly isotonic and isokinetic) are unsafe for individuals with arthritis or unstable joints. Consequently, initial muscle strengthening has traditionally been limited to isometric or isotonic programs with 1- to 2-lb weights. Recent findings seem to contradict that notion. In a rigorous, prospective randomized trial, Fisher et al (83) reported increased strength, endurance, and speed with no adverse effects after a 16-week muscle strengthening and endurance program in 15 subjects with advanced OA of the knee.

In contrast to the traditional "open-chain" isotonic and isometric exercises, kinetic closed-chain exercises are performed with the joint above (hip) and the joint below (ankle) "loaded." Standing and weight-shifting exercises that stress the various muscle groups around the knee are examples. These exercises are well tolerated by patients and may be quite beneficial.

When a varus or valgus deformity is present, selected medial or lateral quadricep strengthening may be prescribed. Patients are taught to isolate and strengthen their medial or lateral quadriceps using electrical stimulation or surface electromyography for biofeedback. This treatment is commonly prescribed for patients with disproportionately weakened medial quadriceps and patellar subluxation.

Therapy to ameliorate functional impairments includes gait training, centering on proper sequencing over level and uneven surfaces; transfer training, particularly from low chairs, bathtubs, and cars; stair climbing; ADLs focusing on lower-extremity dressing and bathing with equipment; and instruction in energy conservation and proper body mechanics.

Foot orthotics are frequently prescribed, but have not been well studied in patients with OA. For example, a medial sole wedge and total contact arch support may be appropriate for the patient with genu valgus and pronated feet. A heel lift may benefit a patient with a fixed knee contracture and apparent leg-length discrepancy. Orthotics must be "broken in." Patients are instructed to alternate wearing them and not wearing them every 2 hours so that gradually they build up tolerance. Without this gradual introduction, back, knee, or foot pain as a consequence of the orthotic may be so severe that the patient will abandon the orthotic. Knee orthotics may occasionally be prescribed for the purpose of correcting joint alignment, but rigid orthoses are poorly tolerated in individuals with varus or valgus deformities. Many patients report feeling increased knee stability when wearing an elastic bandage or gauntlet. Although these bandages do not provide true significant mechanical stability, the subjective improvement may justify its prescription.

Shoulder Impairments and Limitations

OA of the shoulder, though less common than hip or knee disease, can lead to significant impairment and disability. Pain and limitations from shoulder OA are usually a con-

Table 82-12: Common Causes of Shoulder Pain in Shoulder Osteoarthritis

Glenohumeral synovitis
- Swelling, warmth, and tenderness.
- Restricted active and passive ROM.
- Arm splinted in adduction and internal rotation.

Glenohumeral degeneration
- Muscle atrophy.
- Restricted ROM, particularly flexion, extension, abduction, and minimal to no rotation.
- Radiographic evidence of cartilage and bone destruction.

Acromioclavicular and sternoclavicular joint degeneration
- Shoulder arc painful, limited painful abduction.
- Tender joint, painful adduction with joint compression.

Rotator cuff atrophy/tear/tendinitis
- Impaired active abduction with better or full passive ROM.
- Painful active or restricted abduction, if acute night pain.
- Radiographs may reveal cephalad migration of humeral head.
- Arthrography reveals dye passed into bursae if cuff is torn.

Impingement syndrome
- "Catch" reported between 60–70 degrees is maximum at 100–120 degrees of abduction.
- Pain with compression of subacrominal tissue occurs at 90–100 degrees of flexion.
- Radiographic abnormalities such as osteophytes and acromial abnormalities are evident.

Subacromial/subdeltoid bursitis
- Impaired and painful abduction and external rotation.
- Tenderness over superior lateral part of shoulder.
- Swelling, warmth, and erythema.
- Radiographs usually normal.

Adhesive capsulitis
- Diffuse pain and stiffness.
- Glenohumeral tenderness.
- Reduced passive and active ROM in all planes.
- Arthrogram may be abnormal with reduced joint volume.

ROM = range of motion.

sequence of both articular and periarticular disease (Table 82-12). Often, the painful arthritic shoulder exhibits multiple, intermingled diagnoses that are not easily separated into distinct clinical entities.

Shoulder dysfunction is primarily related to glenohumeral and acromioclavicular disease. Sternoclavicular joint involvement only rarely causes disability. In an attempt to limit pain, the patient splints the arm in adduction and internal rotation, resulting in capsular and ligamentous adhesions. Joint effusions limit both motion and strength and occasional capsular ruptures can occur. Destruction of cartilage and subchondral bone causes pain and weakness as a result of reflex inhibition and biomechanical disadvantage. Weakness is exacerbated by the muscle atrophy that accompanies disuse and inflammation. Glenohumeral synovitis often coexists with rotator cuff inflammation. Rotator cuff dysfunction including tendinitis and tears may cause profound functional limitations. Pain is often worse at night. Subdeltoid bursitis is a common companion of glenohumeral arthritis and cuff tendinitis, further exacerbating pain and impairment. The end result is a patient with a painful shoulder that cannot forward flex, abduct, or rotate. The patient may complain of difficulty performing functional tasks such as hair styling and washing, upper-body dressing, orofacial hygiene, placing or retrieving items on shelves, and carrying heavy items.

The physical examination begins with visual inspection for muscle atrophy and bony deformities. Although unusual, glenohumeral synovitis may occur and is identified by direct tenderness over the joint line or as an effusion, which is easily identified as a bulge over the anterior part of the shoulder. Tenderness of the superior lateral aspect of the shoulder extending to the proximal part of the arm may signify subdeltoid bursitis. Bicipital tendinitis usually presents with tenderness over the bicipital groove and insertion site. When diffuse muscle tenderness is present, myopathic inflammation should be considered. Shoulder motion must be evaluated both actively and passively. Glenohumeral degeneration will manifest as crepitus, pain, weakness, and limited passive motion, primarily in abduction, flexion, and rotation. Pain or weakness on active movement, with preserved passive range of motion, suggests tendon or muscle pathology. For example, a patient with rotator cuff tendinitis presents with impaired active abduction, painful resisted abduction, and near-normal range of motion. Similarly, the Yergeson maneuver (resisted forearm supination and flexion referring pain to the biceps insertion site) is the classic test for bicipital tendinitis. Careful neurologic examination is essential to exclude a peripheral or central nervous system etiology of pain and weakness.

Conventional radiographs are essential for the evaluation of the painful or functionally impaired shoulder. Radiologic changes in the shoulder with OA are similar to those seen in other joints, including degenerative spurs, eburnation of bone, and flattening of the glenoid. Superior migration of the humeral head occurs as a result of thinning or tear of the rotator cuff. Distal clavicular tapering suggests advanced acromioclavicular erosion.

Arthroscopy, a well-established diagnostic and therapeutic tool, allows accurate imaging of mechanical derangements. Rotator cuff débridement, loose body removal, and repair of glenoid labrum tears are safe and effective arthroscopic procedures.

Therapeutic Interventions

Acute Phase

An acutely inflamed shoulder joint will benefit from local rest. (82) The shoulder can be immobilized in an arm sling for 2 or 3 days until inflammation subsides. Prolonged rest is not advised in light of the muscle atrophy and adhesions associated with immobility. Gentle range of motion exercises are important to minimize joint contractures during the acute inflammatory period. The critical amount of shoulder motion necessary for functional activities is 75 degrees of flexion, 75 degrees of abduction, 20 degrees of external rotation, and 45 degrees of internal rotation (86). Repetitive passive range of motion probably causes some significant joint inflammation (87). The risk of joint contracture and muscle atrophy must be weighed against this theoretical disadvantage. Many clinicians, however, will prescribe gentle passive or active-assisted range of motion in all planes of motions at least once daily. Icing is particularly effective if used for 15 to 20 minutes after therapy. Isometric exercise is often painful during the acute stage of shoulder inflammation, so it is not routinely prescribed.

Subacute and Chronic Phase

Active-assisted and active range of motion exercises can be performed twice daily after analgesics or modalities have minimized pain and inflammation is controlled. Movement should focus on forward flexion, abduction, and internal and external rotation. At this early stage, pendulum exercises are commonly prescribed (progressive shoulder circumduction performed with the patient leaning forward on a chair or table with the arm dangling).

Strengthening exercises, deferred through the acute phase, are now introduced. Isometric exercises can also begin. Isometric exercise is associated with the least amount of intra-articular pressure and joint stress (88,89). The patient is taught to contract the shoulder abductors, rotators, flexors, and extensors without limb movement. We prescribe one set of contractions one or two times daily during the subacute phase. "Wall walking" is a simple, common active-assisted range of motion and strengthening exercise used during this phase of recovery.

When pain is resolved or the shoulder reaches maximal resolution of inflammation, the clinician should prescribe a comprehensive shoulder rehabilitation program. This program should address range of motion, strength, endurance, functional tasks, equipment, and education. Range of motion exercises should be prescribed as isolated active abduction, forward flexion, extension, both internal and external rotation, and full shoulder circles. It is imperative to understand the degree of articular damage before prescribing range of motion or strengthening exercises. Aggressive stretching or vigorous isotonic strengthening exercises of the shoulder should not be performed when there is significant joint destruction. Ultrasound and other deep-heating methods may enhance stretching when it can be done.

When the joint is not too severely damaged, strengthening exercise should progress to more vigorous isometric or isotonic exercises. High-resistance, low-repetition isotonic exercises are probably not appropriate for arthritis patients because of the significant force distributed through the joints during these exercises (90). Lightweight repetitive exercises (using 1–2-1b cuff weights on the wrists) to the point of fatigue, through a limited arc of motion, are prescribed instead (90). This method of muscle strengthening probably produces comparable results without the consequent high levels of joint stress (91). Isokinetic exercises are usually not recommended for individuals with arthritis because of the high levels of joint stress. Isotonic exercise has been shown to be as effective as isokinetic exercise for muscle strengthening (92).

Endurance exercise should be prescribed to maximize overall health status, cardiovascular conditioning, and sense of well-being. Swimming is a particularly good endurance and strengthening exercise for arthritis patients with shoulder impairments. Aerobic exercise should be performed three times weekly.

Functional deficits must be addressed. Adaptive equipment, such as dressing sticks or button hooks, will help the individual perform simple ADLs that are affected by shoulder immobility. Also, compensatory techniques can be learned. Environmental modifications, such as lowered shelves and levers instead of knobs on doors, are helpful.

REFERENCES

1. Nepom GT, Nepom BS. Prediction of susceptibility to rheumatoid arthritis by human leukocyte antigen genotyping. *Rheum Dis Clinics North Am* 1992;18:785.
2. Spector TD. Rheumatoid arthritis. *Rheum Dis Clinics NA North Am* 1990;16:517.
3. Pincus T, Callahan LF. Reassessment of twelve traditional paradigms concerning the diagnosis, prevalence, morbidity, and mortality of rheumatoid arthritis. *Scand J Rheumatol Suppl* 1989; 79:67.
4. Wilske KR, Healy LA. Remodeling the pyramid; a concept whose time has come. *J Rheumatol* 1989;16:565.
5. Alpiner NM, Oh TN, Brander VA. Rehabilitation in joint and connective tissue diseases—SAE study guide. 1995;76(55):532.
6. Lawrence JS. Rheumatoid arthritis—nature or nurture? *Ann Rheum Dis* 1970;29:357–359.
7. Stastny P. Association of the B-cell alloantigen DRw4 with rheumatoid arthritis. *N Engl J Med* 1978;298: 869–871.
8. Shmerling RH, Liang MH. Evaluation of the patient. In: Schumacher HR, Klipper JH, Koopman WJ, eds. *Primer on the rheumatic diseases.* 10th ed.

Atlanta: Arthritis Foundation, 1993:60–62.

9. Pincus T. Rheumatoid arthritis. In: Wegener ST, ed. *Clinical care in the rheumatic diseases.* American College of Rheumatology 1996:147–155.

10. Minor MA, Hewitt JE, Webel RR, et al. Efficacy of physical conditioning exercise on inpatients with RA and OA. *Arthritis Rheum* 1989;32:1396–1405.

11. Perlman SG, Connel KG, Clark A, et al. Dance-based aerobiic exercise for rheumatoid arthritis. *Arthritis Care Res* 1990;3:29–35.

12. Nordemar R, Ekblom B, Zachrisson L, Lundquist K. Physical training in rheumatoid arthritis: a controlled long-term study. I. Functional capacity and general attitudes. *Scand J Rheumatol* 1981;10:17–23.

13. Nordemar R. Physical training in rheumatoid arthritis: a controlled long-term study. II. Functional capacity and general attitudes. *Scand J Rheumatol* 1981;10:25–30.

14. Gerber LH. Exercise and arthritis. *Bull Rheum Dis* 1990;39:1–9.

15. Perlman SG, Connell KJ, Clark A, et al. Dance-based aerobic exercise for rheumatoid arthritis. *Arthritis Care Res* 1990;3:29–55.

16. Hicks SE. Exercise in patients with inflammatory arthritis and connective tissue disease. *Rheum Dis Clinics North Am* 1990;16:845.

17. Clark SR, Burckhardt CS, Bennett RM. Exercise for prevention and Rx of illness. In: Goldberg L, Elliott DL, eds. *Exercise for prevention and treatment of illness.* Baltimore: FA Davis, 1994:83.

18. Basmajian JV, Wolf SL. In: Gerber LH, Hicks JE, eds. *Therapeutic exercise.* 5th ed. Baltimore: Williams & Wilkins, 1990:340.

19. Herbison GJ, Ditunno Jr, Jaweed MM. Muscle atrophy in rheumatoid arthritis. *J Rheumatol.* 1987;14(suppl 15):78–81.

20. Ekblom B, Lougren O, Alderin M. Physical performance in patients with rheumatoid arthritis. *Scand J Rheumatol* 1974;3:121–125.

21. Alarcon RD, Glover SG. Assessment and management of depression in rheumatoid arthritis. *Phys Med Rehabil Clin N Am* 1994;5:837–858.

22. Katz PP, Yelin EH. Prevalence and correlates of depressive symptoms among persons with rheumatoid arthritis. *J Rheumatol* 1993;20:790–796.

23. Frank RG, Beck NC, Parker JC, et al. Depression in rheumatoid arthritis. *J Rheumatol* 1988;15:920–925.

24. Beckham JC, Damico CJ, Rice JR, et al. Depression and level of functioning in patients with rheumatoid arthritis. *Can J Psychiatry* 1992;37:539–543.

25. Anderson KO, Bradley LA, Young LD, et al. Rheumatoid arthritis: review of psychological factors related to etiology, effects and treatment. *Psychol Bull* 1985;98:358–387.

26. Bradley LA. Psychosocial factors and arthritis. In: Schumacher HR, Klipper JH, Koopman WJ, eds. *Primer on rheumatic diseases.* 10th ed. Atlanta: Arthritis Foundation, 1993:319–322.

27. Yelin E, Henke C, Epstein W. The work dynamics of the person with rheumatoid arthritis. *Arthritis Rheum* 1987;30:507–512.

28. Reisine ST, Grady KE, Goodenow C, Fifield J. Work disability among women with rheumatoid arthritis: the relative importance of disease, social, work and family factors. *Arthritis Rheum* 1989;32:518–543.

29. Allaire SH, Anderson JJ, Meenan RF. Reducing work disability associated with rheumatoid arthritis: identification of additional risk factors with persons likely to benefit from intervention. *Arthritis Care Res* 1996;9:349–357.

30. Arnett F. Seronegative spondylarthropathies. *Bull Rheum Dis* 1987;37:1–12.

31. Wollheim FA. Ankylosing spondylitis. In: Kelley WN, Harris ED, Ruddy S, Sledge CB, eds. *Textbook of rheumatology.* Vol. 1. 4th ed. Philadelphia: WB Saunders, 1993:943–960.

32. Hicks JE, Sutin J. Rehabilitation in joint and connective tissue diseases. 2. Approach to the diagnosis of rheumatic diseases. *Arch Phys Med Rehabil* 1988;69:S-78–S-83.

33. Resnick D, Niwayama G. Ankylosing spondylitis. In: Resnick D, ed. *Diagnosis of bone and joint disorders.* 3rd ed. Philadelphia: WB Saunders, 1995:1008–1074.

34. Repo H, Ristola M, Leirisalo-Repo M. Enhanced inflammatory reactivity in the pathogenesis of spondyloarthropathies. *Autoimmunity* 1990;7:245–254.

35. Ball GV. Ankylosing spondylitis. In: McCarthy DJ, Koopman WJ, eds. *Arthritis and allied conditions: a textbook of rheumatology.* Vol. 1. 12th ed. Philadelphia: Lea & Febiger, 1993:1051–1060.

36. Carette S, Graham D, Little H, et al. The natural disease course of ankylosing spondylitis. *Arthritis Rheum* 1983;26:186–190.

37. Guillemin F, Briancon S, Pourel J, Gaucher A. Long-term disability and prolonged sick leaves as outcome measurements in ankylosing spondylitis. Possible predictive factors. *Arthritis Rheum* 1990;33:1001–1006.

38. Fox R, Calin A, Gerber RC, Gibson D. The chronicity of symptoms and disability in Reiter's syndrome. An analysis of 131 consecutive patients. *Ann Intern Med* 1979;91:190–193.

39. Godfrey RG, Calabro JJ, Mills D, Maltz BA. A double-blind crossover trial of aspirin, indomethacin and phenylbutazone in ankylosing spondylitis. *Arthritis Rheum* 1972;15:110. Abstract.

40. Amor B, Dougados M, Khan MA. Management of refractory ankylosing spondylitis and related spondyloarthropathies. *Rheum Dis Clin North Am* 1995;21:117–128.

41. Dougados M, van der Linden S, Leirisalo-Repo M, et al. Sulfasalazine in the treatment of

spondyloarthropathy. A randomized, multicenter, double-blind, placebo-controlled study. *Arthritis Rheum* 1995;38:618–627.

42. Pioro MH, Cash JM. Treatment of refractory psoriatic arthritis. *Rheum Dis Clin North Am* 1995;21:129–149.

43. Gall V. Exercise in the spondyloarthropathies. *Arthritis Care Res* 1994;7:215–220.

44. Swezey RL. *Straight talk on spondylitis.* 2nd ed. Sherman Oaks, CA: Spondylitis Association of America, 1992:30–32.

45. Kraag G, Stokes B, Groh J, et al. The effects of comprehensive home physiotherapy and supervision on patients with ankylosing spondylitis—a randomized controlled trial. *J Rheumatol* 1990;17:228–233.

46. Fisher LR, Cawley MI, Holgate ST. Relation between chest expansion, pulmonary function, and exercise tolerance in patients with ankylosing spondylitis. *Ann Rheum Dis* 1990;49:921–925.

47. Hidding A, van der Linden S, Boers M, et al. Is group physical therapy superior to individualized therapy in ankylosing spondylitis? A randomized controlled trial. *Arthritis Care Res* 1993; 6:117–125.

48. Calin A, Elswood J. The outcome of 138 total hip replacements and 12 revisions in ankylosing spondylitis: high success rate after a mean followup of 7.5 years. *J Rheumatol* 1989;16:955–958.

49. Wade W, Saltzstein R, Maiman D. Spinal fractures complicating ankylosing spondylitis. *Arch Phys Med Rehabil* 1989;70:398–401.

50. Hunter T. The spinal complications of ankylosing spondylitis. *Semin Arthritis Rheum* 1989;19: 172–182.

51. Fehring TK, Brooks AL. Upper cervical instability in rheumatoid arthritis. *Clin Orthop* 1987; 221:137–148.

52. Vanderschueren D, Decramer M, Van Den Daels P, Dequeker J. Pulmonary function and maximal transrespiratory pressure in ankylosing spondylitis. *Ann Rheum Dis* 1989;48:632–635.

53. Moncur C, Williams HJ. Cervical spine management in patients with rheumatoid arthritis. Review of the literature. *Phys Ther* 1988;68:509–515.

54. Rowed DW. Management of cervical spine cord injury in ankylosing spondylitis: the intervertebral disc as a cause of cord compression. *J Neurosurg* 1992; 77:241–246.

55. Haslock I. Ankylosing spondylitis. *Baillieres Clin Rheumatol* 1993;7:98–115.

56. Carpenter S, Karpati G, Heller I, Eisen A. Inclusion body myositis: a distinct variety of idiopathic inflammatory myopathy. *Neurology* 1978;28:8–17.

57. Calabrese LH, Mitsumoto H, Chou SM. Inclusion body myositis presenting as treatment-resistant polymyositis. *Arthritis Rheum* 1987;30:397–403.

58. Lakhanpal S, Bunch TW, Ilstrup DM, Melton LJ III. Polymyositis-dermatomyositis and malignant lesions: does an association exist? *Mayo Clin Proc* 1986;61:645–653.

59. Bohan A, Peter JB, Bowman RL, Pearson CM. Computer-assisted analysis of 153 patients with polymyositis and dermatomyositis. *Medicine (Baltimore)* 1977;56:255–286.

60. Bohan A, Peter JB. Polymyositis and dermatomyositis (first of two parts). *N Engl J Med* 1975;292: 344–347.

61. Dalakas MC. Polymyositis, dermatomyositis and inclusion-body myositis. *N Engl J Med* 1991;325:1487–1498.

62. Wortmann RL. Inflammatory diseases of muscle. In: Kelley WN, Harris ED Jr, Rudy S, Sledge CB, eds. *Textbook of rheumatology.* Vol. 2. 4th ed. Philadelphia: WB Saunders, 1993:1159–1188.

63. Kagen LJ. Polymyositis/dermatomyositis. In: McCarty DJ, Koopman WJ, eds. *Arthritis and allied conditions. A textbook of rheumatology.* Vol. 2. 12th ed. Philadelphia: Lea & Febiger, 1993:1225–1252.

64. Dalakas MC, Illa I, Dambrosia JM, et al. A controlled trial of high-dose intravenous immune globulin infusions as treatment for dermatomyositis. *N Engl J Med* 1993;329:1993–2000.

65. Cherin P, Piette JC, Wechsler B, et al. Intravenous gamma globulin as first line therapy in polymyositis and dermatomyositis: an open study in 11 adult patients. *J Rheumatol* 1994;21:1092–1097.

66. Fafalak RG, Peterson MG, Kagen LJ. Strength in polymyositis and dermatomyositis: best outcome in patients treated early. *J Rheumatol* 1994;21:643–648.

67. Clarke AE, Bloch DA, Medsger TA Jr, Oddis CV. A longitudinal study of functional disability in a national cohort of patients with polymyositis/dermatomyositis. *Arthritis Rheum* 1995;38: 1218–1224.

68. Escalante A, Miller L, Beardmore TD. Resistive exercise in the rehabilitation of polymyositis/dermatomyositis. *J Rheumatol* 1993;20: 1340–1344.

69. Hicks JE, Miller F, Plotz P, et al. Isometric exercise increases strength and does not produce sustained creatinine phosphokinase increases in a patient with polymyositis. *J Rheumatol* 1993;20:1399–1401.

70. Deshaies LD, Yasuda YL, Beardmore T. Occupational therapy management of a patient with severe polymyositis. *Arthritis Care Res* 1994;7:104–107.

71. Benbassat J, Gefel D, Larholt K, et al. Prognostic factors in polymyositis/dermatomyositis. A computer-assisted analysis of ninety-two cases. *Arthritis Rheum* 1985;28:249–255.

72. Dickey BF, Myers AR. Pulmonary disease in polymyositis/dermatomyositis. *Semin Arthritis Rheum* 1984;14:60–76.

73. Marti B, Knobloch M, Tschopp A, et al. Is excessive running pre-

dictive of degenerative hip disease? Controlled study of former elite athletes. *BMJ* 1989;299: 91–93.

74. Brandt KD. *Harrison's principle of internal medicine*. New York: McGraw-Hill, 1994;13: 1692–1698.

75. Bradley JD, Brandt KD, Katz BP, et al. Comparison of an antiinflammatory dose of ibuprofen, an analgesic dose of ibuprofen and acetaminophen in the treatment of patients with osteoarthritis of the knee. *N Engl J Med* 1991;325: 87–91.

76. Paakkari H. Epidemiological and financial aspects of use of nonsteroidal anti-inflammatory analgesics. *Pharmacol Toxicol* 1994;75(suppl 11):56–59.

77. Adams ME, Atkinson MH, Lussier AJ, et al. The role of viscosupplementation with Hylan GF-20 in the treatment of OA of the knee. *Osteoarthritis Cartilage* 1995;3:213–226.

78. Felson DT, Anderson JJ, Naimark A, et al. Obesity and knee osteoarthritis. The Framingham study. *Ann Intern Med* 1988;109:18–24.

79. Felson DT, Zhang Y, Anthony JM, et al. Weight loss reduces the risk for symptomatic knee osteoarthritis in women. The Framingham study. *Ann Intern Med* 1992;116: 535–539.

80. Kovar PA, Allegrante JP, MacKenzie CR, et al. Supervised fintness walking in patients with OA of the knee. *Ann Intern Med* 1992;116:529–534.

81. Minor MA, Hewett JE, Webel RR, et al. Efficacy of physical conditioning exercise in patients with RA and OA. *Arthritis Rheum* 1989;32:1396–1405.

82. Fisher NM, Gresham GE, Abrams M, et al. Quantitative effects of physical therapy on muscular and functional performance in subjects with osteoarthritis of the knees. *Arch Phys Med Rehabil* 1993;5: 229–223.

83. Fisher NM, Pendergast DR, Gresham GE, Calkins E. Muscle rehabilitation: its effect on muscular and functional performance in patients with knee osteoarthritis. *Arch Phys Med Rehabil* 1991;72:367–373.

84. Tan J, Baci N, Sepici V, Gener FA. Isokinetic and isometric stregth in OA of the knee. *Am J Phys Med Rehabil* 1995;74(5):364–369.

85. Chang RW, Falconer J, Stulberg SD, et al. A randomized controlled trial of arthroscopic sx vs. closed needle lavage for patients with OA of the knee. *Arthritis Rheum* 1993;36:289–296.

86. Hicks JE. Exercise in patients with inflammatory arthritis and connective tissue disease. *Rheum Dis Clin North Am* 1990;16(4):847–870.

87. Agudelo CA, Schumacher HR, Phelps P. Effect of exercise on urate crystal induced inflammation in canine joints. *Arthritis Rheum* 1972;15:609–616.

88. Jayson MIV, Dixon SJ. Intraarticular pressure in RA of the knee. Part III: pressure changes during joint use. *Ann Rheum Dis* 1972;29:401.

89. Warren CG, Lehman JF, Koblanski JN. Elongation of rat tail tendon: effect of load and temperature. *Arch Phys Med Rehabil* 1977;52:465.

90. DeLorme TL, Watkins AL. Techniques of progressive resistance exercise. *Arch Phys Med Rehabil* 1966;47:737.

91. DeLateur BJ, Lehmann JF. A test of the DeLorm axiom. *Arch Phys Med Rehabil* 1968;49:245.

92. DeLateur BJ, Lehman JF, Warren CG, et al. Comparison of effectiveness of isokinetic and isotonic exercise in quad strengthening. *Arch Phys Med Rehabil* 1982;53:60.

Chapter 83

Rehabilitation After Hip Fracture

David X. Cifu
Derek Burnett
J. Patrick McGowan

INCIDENCE

Hip fractures account for approximately 50% of fracture-care inpatient days. In the United States alone, the annual costs exceed $7 billion when all medical and rehabilitation costs are figured in (1). Morbidity and mortality significantly contribute to the total health care dollar expenditure (2). Ninety-five percent of hip fractures occur in patients 50 years or older, whereas hip dislocations are most common in individuals aged 30 to 40 years. The incidence of hip fractures in the United States is approximately 80 per 100,000 (3), and the incidence increases with age. After age 60 years, there is a doubling of incidence every 5 to 7 years (4). Hip fractures will take on an even greater importance as the population ages. Current estimates of hip fracture indicate that 250,000 fractures occur each year in people over 65 years old. The segment of the population aged 65 and older has gone from 3 million in 1900 to over 20 million by 1995, and is projected to increase to 28 million by 2000. The subgroup of people over age 85 is the fastest-growing segment, and it is projected there will be 5.6 million of these so-called "oldest-old" individuals by the year 2000 (5).

RISK FACTORS

The risk factors for hip fracture include increased age (6), increased incidence of falls (6), osteoporosis (7,8), female gender (3,7), white race (7), prior hip fracture (1), Alzheimer dementia (9), and low-calcium diet (10). Falls account for approximately 90% of hip fractures in the older adult (6). As more of the "vigorous" elders over 65 years old are staying active, they may be even more prone to falls, in addition to motor vehicle accidents. Medical advances have also allowed the "frail" elderly (i.e., older adults with multiple medical issues by age 70) to live longer. Thus, the number of both the "vigorous" and "frail" elderly at risk for hip fractures is increasing (11).

ANATOMY OF THE HIP

Joint

The hip joint is a "ball-and-socket" joint, with the femoral head aligning to the pelvic acetabulum (Fig. 83-1). Stability is achieved by ligaments that connect the femur to the pelvis, providing a capsule around the proximal end of the femur. This capsule has greater strength and stability anteriorly than posteriorly; thus, 85% to 90% of dislocations occur posteriorly (12). The iliofemoral ligament, or Y ligament of Bigelow, is the most important stabilizing ligament. This ligament is taut in full extension, thereby assisting in nonmuscular quiet standing, while it is slack in flexion.

Regions

The intracapsular or supratrochanteric portion of the femur consists of the femoral head and majority of the femoral neck. The architecture of the trabecular bone

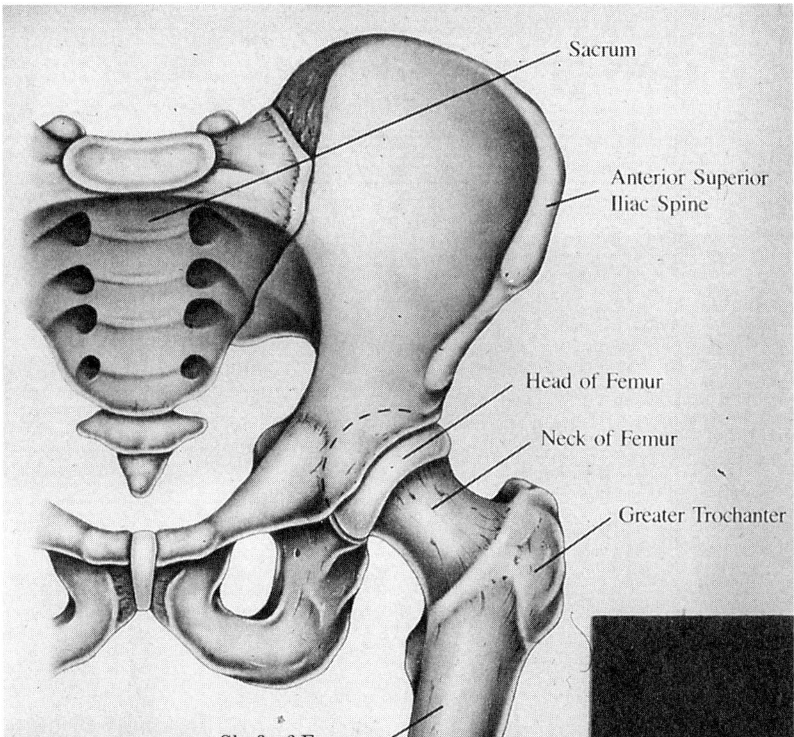

Figure 83-1. Bony anatomy of the hip.

allows for absorption and distribution of stresses from the body and pelvis to the cortical bone of the femoral neck and proximal end of the femoral shaft. The greater and lesser trochanters and the calcar femorale make up the intertrochanteric region, which is extracapsular. The gluteal musculature inserts on the trochanters, while the calcar femorale provides a conduit for stress transfer from the posterior portion of the neck to the posteromedial aspect of the shaft. The subtrochanteric region extends from the lesser trochanter to 5 cm distal (12).

Vasculature

The blood supply to the femoral head comes almost exclusively through the femoral neck. The medial and lateral circumflex arteries, which arise from the profunda femoris branch of the femoral artery, form an extracapsular arterial ring at the level of the trochanters, via ascending branches. Blood flows from this extracapsular ring via ascending arteries to join an intramedullary nutrient artery and form an intracapsular arterial ring. This intracapsular ring provides the primary (>90%) blood supply to the femoral head. A small artery within the ligamentum teres provides a secondary, although insignificant (<10%) supply. Therefore, disruption of the arterial blood supply in the femoral neck can prevent adequate perfusion of the femoral head, and lead to osteonecrosis. There is a greater than 20% incidence of osteonecrosis of the femoral head in a patient with a displaced femoral neck fracture (13).

Musculature

The hip musculature can be divided into functional groups, as shown in Table 83-1 (12).

Nervous Innervation

The nerve supply to the hip can be divided into muscular and sensory branches. Innervation to muscle groups is via five motor nerves: femoral (root level L2–L4 segments to hip flexors), obturator (root level L2–L4 segments to adductors), superior gluteal (root level L4 and L5 segment to abductors and internal rotators), inferior gluteal (root level L5–S2 segments to extensors and external rotators), tibial branch of the sciatic (root level L5–S2 segments to extensors), and small branches directly off the lumbosacral plexus (root level L4–S1 segments to external rotators). The hip joint receives sensory input from the femoral, obturator, and superior gluteal nerves and the nerve to the quadrator femoris (12). Pain from a hip fracture or joint abnormality may therefore be referred to any area supplied by these nerves. However, pain typically refers to the groin. Nerve injury occurs primarily by posterior dislocation and surgical implantation of the femoral endoprosthesis, which can cause contusion or traction injury to the sciatic nerve. The lateral branch of the sciatic nerve (which is called the common peroneal nerve by the midthigh) is more commonly affected in this situation. Additionally, an anterior dislocation can cause a contusion or traction injury to the femoral nerve.

Table 83-1: Musculature and Nervous Innervation of the Hip

Muscle Group	Muscles	Innervation
Adductors	Gracilis and adductor longus, brevis, and magnus	Obturator
Abductors	Tensor fasciae latae and gluteus medius and minimus	Superior gluteal
Extensors	Gluteus maximus	Inferior gluteal
	Adductor magnus (posterior head), semimembranosus	Tibial
	Semitendinosus, long head of biceps femoris	Tibial
Flexors	Rectus femoris, pectineus, sartorius	Femoral
	Iliopsoas	Lumbar plexus
External rotators	Gluteus maximus	Inferior gluteal
	Piriformis and obturator internus and externus	Lumbar plexus
	Gemellus superior and inferior and quadratus femoris	Lumbar plexus
Internal rotators	Gluteus medius and minimus and tensor fasciae latae	Superior gluteal

Table 83-2: Practical Classification of Fractures and Dislocations of the Hip

Injury	Classification
Dislocation	Anterior
	Stable, without fracture
	Unstable, without fracture
	Unstable, with fracture
	Posterior
	Stable, without fracture
	Unstable, without fracture
	Unstable, with fracture
Femoral neck fracture	Nondisplaced
	Displaced
Intertrochanteric fracture	Stable
	Unstable
Subtrochanteric fracture	Stable
	Unstable

Table 83-3: Garden Classification of Fractures of the Femoral Neck

Classification	Injury
I	Incomplete or impacted fracture
II	Complete fracture without displacement
III	Complete fracture with partial displacement (hip capsule partially intact)
IV	Complete fracture with full displacement (hip capsule usually completely disrupted)

CLASSIFICATION OF INJURY

Dislocations

Hip dislocations (Table 83-2) occur primarily in 30- to 40-year-olds, from high-speed or -intensity trauma (e.g., high-speed motor vehicle accident, fall from above ground level). Concomitant fractures of the acetabulum, femoral head, and femoral neck are not uncommon. Owing to the anterior stability of the hip joint capsule and the mechanism of injury, 85% to 90% of dislocations occur posteriorly.

Fractures

Femoral neck fractures occur mostly in older adults, owing to ground-level falls and low-velocity motor vehicle accidents. They more commonly affect women and the frail elderly (6) and occur with approximately the same incidence as intertrochanteric fractures (3,6,14). Femoral neck fractures are commonly classified according to the Garden classification (15), indicating the degree of fracture and fracture displacement (Table 83-3). Femoral neck fractures can also be more simply categorized as nondisplaced (including Garden type I and II fractures) or displaced (including Garden type 3 and 4 fractures) (11) (see Table 83-2). Intertrochanteric fractures are usually caused by significant trauma (non-ground-level falls and motor vehicle accidents), and are seen more commonly in males and the vigorous elderly (6,14). These fractures are typically grouped as stable or unstable (16) (see Table 83-2). Subtrochanteric fractures are generally caused by falls in older adults and motor vehicle accidents in younger adults. These fractures can be categorized by the number of parts or fragments present (one to four); however, they are more commonly grouped as stable or unstable (see Table 83-2). The subtrochanteric region is also the most common site of pathologic fracture from neoplastic disease.

SURGICAL MANAGEMENT

Acute surgical management should be instituted as soon as all necessary medical evaluations and treatments are completed. The majority of individuals with a hip fracture can and should have surgery within 24 hours after the fracture, with rehabilitation efforts begun as soon as possible thereafter. Dislocations require comprehensive evaluation of other organ systems because of the high-energy trauma necessary to cause them. In addition to other skeletal injuries, other systems are commonly involved in trauma and include the neurologic, vascular, and visceral.

Anterior Dislocations

Patients with an anterior dislocation without associated fractures treated by closed reduction are managed with 5 to 7 days of bed rest, with the hip in flexion, using mild skin traction or pillows. Initially passive and then active range of motion (ROM) exercises are started when tolerated, with limitations on extension past 180 degrees, abduction past 30 degrees, and external rotation past 0 degrees (neutral) for a minimum of 3 months. Ambulation with full weight bearing is begun on the fifth postoperative day. When stability (e.g., extensive damage to capsule, severe degenerative joint disease) and compliance (e.g., dementia) are in doubt, an orthosis that limits extension, abduction, and external rotation may be used for 6 to 8 weeks. Patients with an anterior dislocation without associated fractures treated by open reduction are managed similarly, but orthoses are always used. Small associated fractures of the femoral head or neck can be excised and treated similarly. Open reduction and internal fixation, primary prosthetic replacement, or total hip replacement is required if larger fragments are present. Postoperative management is the same as for these surgical interventions (see below), and includes use of an orthosis. The most common late complications are posttraumatic arthritis (30%–50%) and femoral head osteonecrosis (80%) (4).

Posterior Dislocations

Stable posterior dislocations without fracture are treated by closed reduction followed by 5 to 7 days of bed rest, with an abduction pillow for positioning. Pain tolerance dictates the initiation of initally passive and then active ROM exercises, with limitations on flexion past 90 degrees, adduction past 0 degrees (neutral), and internal rotation past 0 degrees (neutral) for a minimum of 3 months. Full weight-bearing ambulation is started by day 5. An orthosis to limit hip flexion, adduction, and internal rotation is used for 6 to 8 weeks in the poorly compliant patient. If fractures are present, open reduction and internal fixation, primary prosthetic replacement, or total hip replacement may be needed. Postoperative management is the same as for these surgical interventions, in addition to an orthosis. Unstable posterior dislocations that cannot be stabilized surgically (e.g., severe capsular disruption, severe degenerative joint disease, history of instability, medical condition precluding surgery) are treated with traction for 6 to 8 weeks. Patients who can be stabilized require the use of continuous passive motion (CPM) machines for hip flexion day and night, which is begun after traction is removed, on the first postoperative day. Isometric and active-assistive exercises are used in bed to maximize ROM, muscle bulk, strength, and cardiopulmonary endurance. Once stability is achieved (with or without an orthosis), touch-down or foot-flat weight bearing (<10% weight bearing) can be started, and is advanced over 4 to 6 weeks. When the limb is out of traction, an orthosis to limit adduction, flexion, and internal rotation is used. The most common late complication is posttraumatic arthritis (30%–100%) and femoral head osteonecrosis (10%–50%) (4).

Femoral Neck Fractures

Nondisplaced femoral neck fractures may be difficult to diagnose, initially, particularly Garden type I (incomplete or partial fracture with trabeculae intact) fractures (15). Often the only symptoms are groin pain, reluctance to fully bear weight, and increased comfort with external rotation of the leg. Once diagnosed, fractures are initially treated with bed rest and positioning the leg in slight hip flexion and external rotation. Surgical intervention is indicated in all patients except those who have severe or unstable medical conditions, who were nonambulatory premorbidly, or who are severely demented (17). Early aspiration or surgical decompression of a hemarthrosis is controversial and not commonly used. Individuals with nondisplaced fractures treated nonoperatively can be mobilized from bed to chair when tolerating pain. Displaced fractures can involve 6 to 8 weeks of traction if treated nonoperatively (4).

Nondisplaced, Garden type I or II (complete fracture, nondisplaced) fractures can be treated with internal fixation using multiple screws or pins. Patients should get out of bed on the first postoperative day and continue rapid mobilization. Weight-bearing-as-tolerated (WBAT) ambulation can begin on the second postoperative day. WBAT indicates that the individual may place as much of the full body weight on the affected hip as he or she can tolerate. Displaced Garden type III (partially displaced) or IV (total displacement of fracture fragments) fractures can be reduced (closed or open) and internally fixated, or treated with primary prosthetic replacement. If possible, reduction and fixation is used in the healthy active patient under 70 years old. Mobilization out of bed is encouraged starting the day after surgery. Weight-bearing restrictions are somewhat controversial for these fractures. Some clinicians recommend toe-touch (<5% body weight) to foot-flat (<10% body weight) weight bearing for 6 to 8 weeks, while others limit weight bearing to pain tolerance (same as WBAT), if there is good fixation (4). A compromise solution may be foot-flat weight bearing for 1 to 2 weeks, followed by partial (<50% body weight) weight bearing for 2

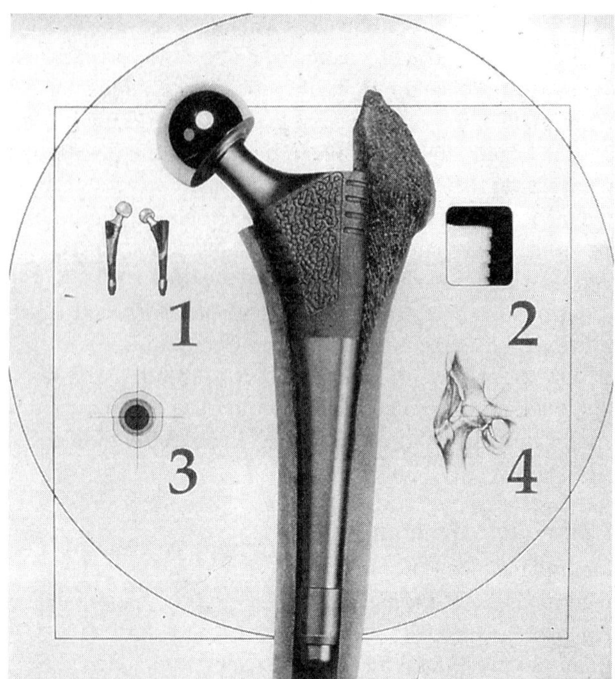

Figure 83-2. Femoral bipolar endoprosthesis.

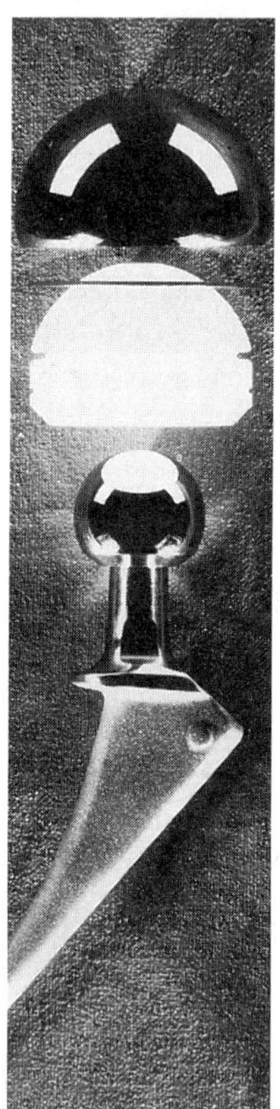

Figure 83-3. Bipolar endoprosthesis. Note the metal femoral head component that articulates via a polyethylene liner with a metal acetabular shell, which then articulates with the patient's acetabulum.

weeks. Orthoses are only indicated if there is a history of hip dislocation. For most patients, ROM restrictions, including avoidance of flexion beyond 90 degrees, internal rotation past neutral, and adduction past neutral (the so-called 90-90-90 rule), are recommended for at least the first month.

Femoral head osteonecrosis and failure of fixation are more common in the older patient and in those with displaced fractures. Patients with these risk factors are usually treated with a femoral prosthesis. The original "unipolar" endoprostheses used from the 1950s to the 1970s provided good fixation; however, their rigid design (a metal head rotating within the acetabulum) resulted in acetabular erosion and pain in approximately 5 years. "Bipolar" endoprostheses are designed to increase the surface area with the acetabulum, which reduces the chances of erosion. Additionally, bipolar prostheses have a metal femoral head that articulates via a polyethylene liner with a metal or ceramic acetabular shell (Figs. 83-2 and 83-3), which then articulates with the patient's acetabulum. This design allows for easy conversion to total hip replacement in the future, if needed. A lateral approach to the hip is the most commonly used, but anterior and posterior approaches are also employed. Theoretically, the specific surgical approach utilized should determine the specific ROM limitations necessary after femoral neck fracture repair. In most patients, however, an abduction pillow is used when in bed or sitting, to prevent adduction (i.e., crossing the legs). For most patients, ROM restrictions, including avoidance of flexion beyond 90 degrees, internal rotation past neutral, and adduction past neutral (the 90-90-90 rule), are strictly enforced for at least the first 3 months.

Endoprostheses are either cemented or uncemented. Bone cement was introduced in 1961 and greatly improved the short- and long-term fixation rates, especially in the older adult. The 10-year revision rate for endoprostheses is 10% for individuals over age 60 years, 25% for individuals under age 60 years, and 33% for individuals in their thirties. Bone cement also improved acute pain management, as solidly fixated prostheses reduced pain. Cemented prostheses are more common in older individuals, and offer the advantages of immediate stabilization and WBAT. Disadvantages include 1) difficulty revising the prosthesis, 2) greater difficulty eradicating hip joint infections, 3) potential restrictions using therapeutic ultrasound and other deep-heating modalities, 4) difficulties revising in the case of fractures below the prosthesis, 5) bone necrosis associated with the exothermic reaction of the cement setting, and 6) osteolysis due to the makeup of certain cements. Newer (i.e., second-generation) cements have reduced most of these potential side effects.

Uncemented endoprostheses are more commonly used in younger patients. The 5-year revision rate for uncemented, or porous-coated prosthetic hip implants is

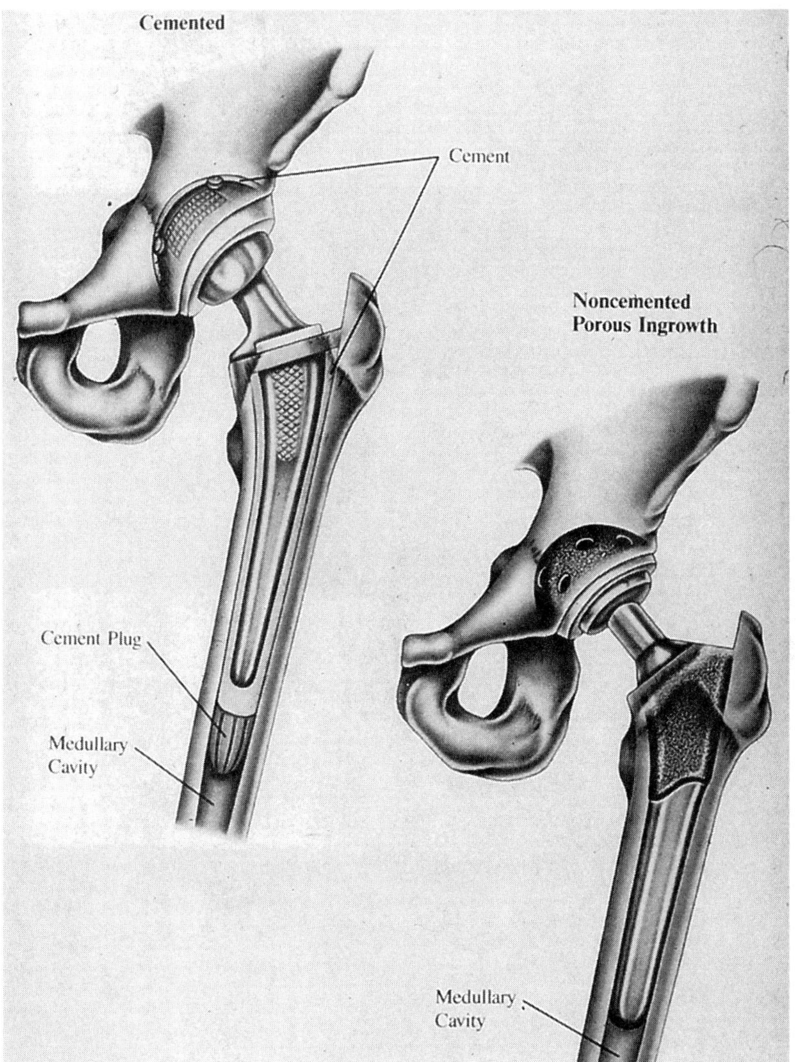

Figure 83-4. Total hip arthroplasty.

5%. These prostheses employ a more physiologic fixation by bony growth into the porous surface. Currently, bioactive ceramic sprays, composed of calcium and phosphorus and applied directly to the prosthesis, that stimulate bone binding are under investigation. Advantages include a longer life span and more secure fit of the prosthesis. The major disadvantage of uncemented prostheses is the non-weight-bearing status needed for 4 to 6 weeks (4).

Patients with femoral neck fractures with preexisting acetabular disease (including osteoarthritis, rheumatoid arthritis, and Paget disease) often receive primary total hip arthroplasty. The total hip arthroplasty involves both a bipolar endoprosthesis and an acetabular prosthetic component (Fig. 83-4). The majority of patients can be mobilized out of bed and ambulated by the first postoperative day. An abduction pillow is used whenever the patient is in bed or sitting up, and ROM restrictions by the 90-90-90 rule are strictly enforced for at least the first 3 months. An orthosis that prevents these movements may be utilized in patients with cognitive impairment, poor compliance, or repeated dislocation. Younger patients may receive an uncemented acetabular prosthesis, which offers a more physiologic fixation. The advantages and disadvantages are similar to those of an uncemented endoprosthesis (4).

Intertrochanteric Fractures

Intertrochanteric fractures occur in a proximal region of the femur that is well vascularized; therefore, nonunion and osteonecrosis are rare. Additionally, intertrochanteric fractures are extracapsular; thus, the joint capsule's integrity and stability are not affected. Surgical intervention is indicated unless severe or unstable medical conditions are present, the patient is nonambulatory, or the patient is severely demented (17). If treatment is nonoperative, 6 to 8 weeks of traction, followed by gradual weight bearing and ambulation, is typically recommended. In the severely demented patient, mobilization from bed to chair

Figure 83-5. Sliding compression screw for intertrochanteric fracture.

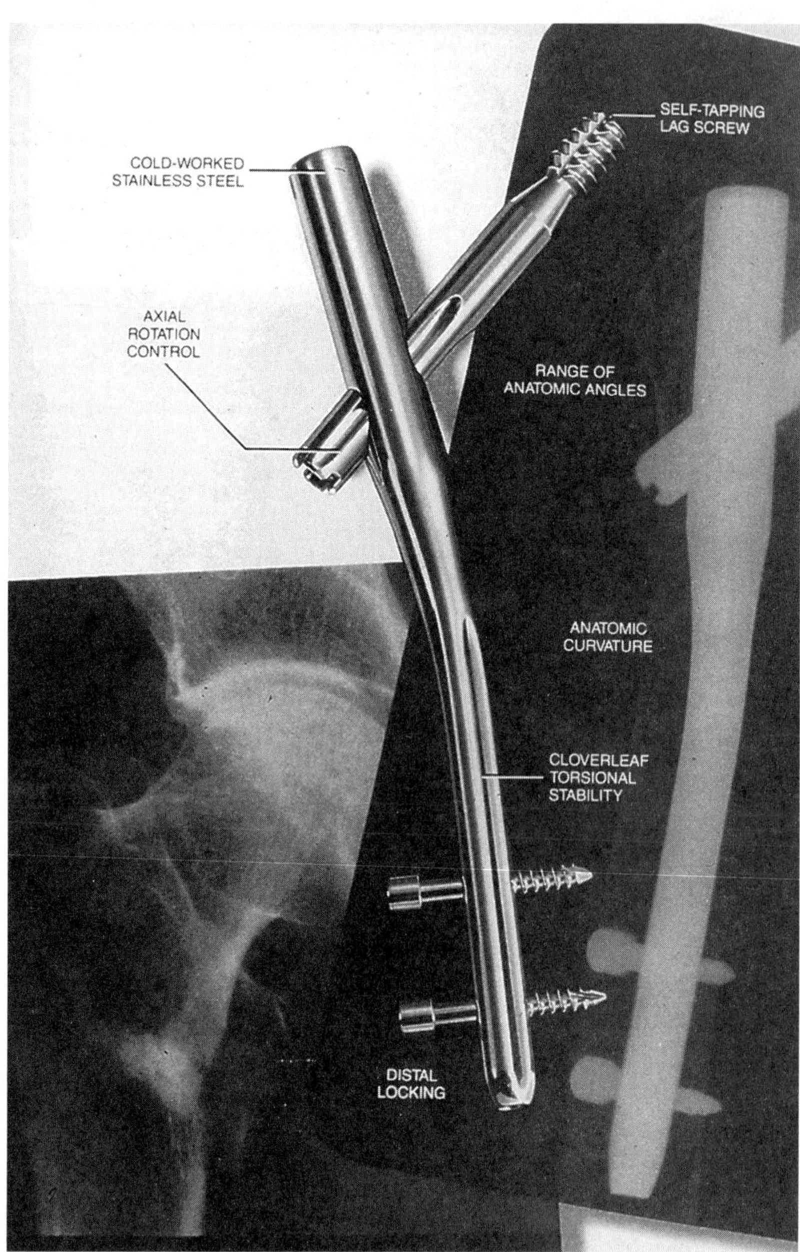

only may be indicated when pain is tolerated. Ambulation is not appropriate for 6 to 8 weeks (4).

Prior to the mid-1970s, fixation of intertrochanteric fractures included fixed-angle, nail-plate devices (e.g., Jewett nail, Holt nail). Unfortunately, these devices were limited by their inability to allow for impaction of the fracture fragments, which often resulted in device breakage or nail migration into the hip joint. The sliding hip screw (e.g., Richardson) provided an improvement by combining good static healing and physiologic healing, with dynamic impaction of the proximal and distal bone fragments (Fig. 83-5). Mobilization occurs on the first postoperative day; however, the degree of weight bearing remains controversial, ranging from toe touch for 6 to 8 weeks to immediate WBAT. A compromise solution employs 1 to 2 weeks of toe-touch weight bearing, followed by 2 to 3 weeks of partial weight bearing. ROM restrictions are not strictly enforced, as the joint capsule is not violated during surgery.

A second alternative for fixation includes the insertion of flexible intramedullary nails or rods. These devices are inserted distally, typically at the knee, and passed across the fracture site. This approach is advantageous if there are skin problems over the fracture area. Mobilization occurs on the first postoperative day, and weight bearing also varies between toe touch for 6 to 8 weeks to immediate WBAT. Endoprostheses are rarely used in the intertrochanteric region, as anchoring them is difficult.

They are occasionally used to allow full weight bearing in the frail or demented older adult.

Subtrochanteric Fractures

Subtrochanteric fractures are treated similarly to femoral neck and intertrochanteric fractures, with surgical fixation if possible. Intramedullary devices (i.e., nails, rods) are used most commonly. Prosthetic devices are not an option because of limitations in anchoring the device. Complications, including nonunion, malunion, and implant failure, are more common in this region than in the femoral neck or intertrochanteric regions. The subtrochanteric region is the most common site of pathologic femoral fractures; these fractures are also fixated if the patient has a life span of over 30 days or has significant pain. With all subtrochanteric fractures, mobilization varies from weight-bearing restrictions of toe touch for 6 to 8 weeks to immediate WBAT (4).

Table 83-4 summarizes the postoperative restrictions after treatment of hip fractures and dislocations.

Table 83-4: Postoperative Restrictions After Hip Fracture

Injury Type	Precautions
Dislocations without fracture	
Anterior	After hip is stabilized, WBAT with limited extension and abduction.
Posterior	After hip is stabilized, WBAT with limited flexion, adduction, and internal rotation.
Dislocations with fracture	Same as above, plus additional limitations based on fracture type.
Femoral neck fracture	
Nondisplaced	WBAT by postoperative day 2. No ROM limits.
Displaced	If internal fixation is used, then weight bearing is variable, but usually foot flat to partial for 4–6 wk. If cemented endoprosthesis is used, then WBAT immediately. No hip flexion, adduction, or internal rotation if endoprosthesis is used.
Intertrochanteric/ Subtrochanteric fracture	
Stable	If internal fixation is used, then weight bearing is variable, but usually WBAT by postoperative day 7–14. No ROM limits.
Unstable	If internal fixation is used, then weight bearing is variable, but usually foot flat to partial for 4–6 wk. No ROM limits.

WBAT = weight bearing as tolerated; ROM = range of motion.

COMMON COMPLICATIONS

The highest risk of mortality after hip fracture occurs in the first 4 to 6 months (4). The estimated overall mortality rate is 14% to 36% at 1 year (18–20) and remains as high at 2 years after injury (21). Increasing age (22,20,23), male gender (18,20), concomitant morbidity (20,23), fracture type and related systemic effects (24), pain (24), reversibility of trauma-induced pathophysiology (24), cognitive deficits (25), premorbid institutionalization (13), and limited premorbid function (22,26) contribute to increased morbidity and mortality after hip fracture. Incidence rates for complications after hip fracture are provided in Table 83-5 (22,27–39).

Orthopedic

The orthopedic complications after hip fracture include dislocation, subluxation, leg-length discrepancy, loosening of prosthetic components, nonunion, heterotopic ossification, nerve palsies, pain, hemorrhage, wound infections, and sepsis.

Dislocations

Following repair of dislocations and fractures, repeated posterior dislocations are usually the result of hip flexion, adduction, and internal rotation greater than 90 degrees, and may occur in approximately 3% to 5% of individuals. Individuals who have had a prior posterior dislocation or who require lateral or posterior surgical approaches are at greater risk for posterior dislocation than are individuals who require anterior incision approaches. Anterior dislocations usually are caused by hip extension or external rotation. Individuals who have had a prior anterior dislocation or who require anterior surgical approaches are at a greater risk for anterior dislocation. Hyperextension can also lead to dislocation following total hip arthroplasty using an anterior approach. Both types of dislocations can usually be treated conservatively, using closed reduction, with or without general anesthesia; however, occasionally reoperation is required (29).

Nonunion and Avascular Necrosis

In a review of long-term hip fracture complications in adults less than 50 years old, Dedrick et al (27) reported an incidence of nonunion of 20% and of avascular necrosis of 36%. In the elderly population, there is an incidence of nonunion of 15% and of avascular necrosis of 20% (28).

Table 83-5: The Incidence of Complications After Hip Fracture

Complication	Incidence
Dislocation	Highly variable
Pain	Highly variable (29,30)
Heterotopic ossification	Up to 70% (31)
Peroneal nerve injury	45% (32,33)
Avascular necrosis	20%–36% (27,28)
Nonunion	15%–20% (27,28)
Wound infection	5%–10% (22,34)
Sequential fractures	2.3% (35)
Major arterial injury	<0.5% (34)
Deep venous thrombosis	Up to 70% (36,37)
Decubitus ulcers	13%–66% (24,38)
Delirium	30%–50% (30,39)
Pulmonary embolism	Up to 16% (36,37)
Cardiovascular	12% (24,29)
Gastrointestinal	12% (29)
Pulmonary	12% (24)
Genitourinary	11% (29)
Neurologic	7% (29)

Leg-Length Discrepancy

Fracture healing, particularly of the lower extremity, is facilitated by compression of the affected bone, and thus small amounts of reduction in bone length are anticipated. Clinically significant leg-length discrepancies are not typical following uncomplicated hip fracture management. Patients with a femoral neck fracture are most likely to develop significant differences; therefore, side-to-side measurements should be performed 6 to 12 weeks after injury. Differences of more than ½ inch should be corrected, at least partially, with an orthosis (e.g., shoe inset, heel and/or sole lift).

Pain

Bernardini et al (29) reported musculoskeletal pain, including pain related to loosening of fixation, as an adverse clinical event with an incidence of 15%. Persistent hip or lower-extremity pain lasting longer than 6 weeks after injury is unusual unless nerve injury, preexisting painful disorders (e.g., arthritis), or acute joint pathology (e.g., refracture, prosthetic loosening, infection) are present. Intravenous or epidural pain medications are appropriate for 1 to 3 days after injury, followed by tapering doses of oral medications over a 2- to 4-week period. Use of narcotic medications should be avoided for longer than 2 weeks postoperatively, especially in the older adult. Scheduled-dose acetaminophen or nonsteroidal anti-inflammatory agents (NSAIDs) are more appropriate. Among surgical repair options (pinning, nail placement, open reduction with internal fixation, and arthroplasty), pinning has the lowest reported perioperative morbidity and mortality because it can be performed under regional anesthesia; however, it is also more commonly associated with chronic pain as a long-term complication. This is believed to be secondary to penetration of the pin into the femoral head (30).

Loosening of Prosthetic Components

The advent of newer prosthetic components, improved bone cement, and improved surgical techniques has decreased the incidence of prosthetic loosening, New onset of pain and radiolucency on x-ray films along the edge of the prosthesis are common indicators of loosening. Specifically, loosening is categorized as septic or aseptic. Aseptic loosening may be asymptomatic and only radiologic (i.e., 2 mm or more of lucency parallel to the bone-cement interface, any lucency parallel to the prosthesis-cement interface, or fracture of the cement) or symptomatic (i.e., painful). Decreased weight bearing for a 2- to 6-week period is typically recommended when loosening occurs, although the efficacy of this has not been well documented. Surgical revision is often necessary when prosthetic loosening occurs.

Heterotopic Ossification

Heterotopic ossification is the deposition of bone in aberrant locations, typically around the hip capsule, with resultant loss of motion. It has been reported to occur in as many as 70% of fractured hips, and is most frequently described in association with total hip arthroplasty (either elective or following hip fracture). It is also found after placement of an endoprosthesis or open reduction and internal fixation of the hip, but with less frequency. Recently, as locked intramedullary nailing has become the treatment of choice for proximal femoral fractures, heterotopic ossification has been observed at the head of the nail (usually near the greater trochanter) in 15% of patients (31). While the etiology of heterotopic ossification remains unclear, risk factors include a prior history of heterotopic ossification, age older than 60 years, hypertrophic osteoarthritis in males, ankylosing spondylitis, posttraumatic arthritis, diffuse idiopathic skeletal hyperostosis, Paget disease, and the use of noncemented prostheses. Irradiation of the hip (600–2000 rads) (40), use of NSAIDs, use of etidronate (EDTA), and controlled ROM are effective in the prophylaxis and treatment of heterotopic ossification developing after hip fracture; however, there are no universally accepted or utilized protocols.

Nerve Injury

The sciatic nerve (typically the peroneal component) is frequently injured in hips with dislocations or fracture dislocations. The injury is usually secondary to direct contusion, partial laceration, or traction. In the case of injury from dislocation, surgical reduction should be carried out emergently, as subsequent functional recovery has been reported in 60% to 70% of patients (32). Postreduction paresis has also been observed in association with unstable dislocations and persistently displaced posterior acetabular fragments. These patients typically complain of pain and paresthesia in the leg, prior to an onset of paralysis. Anterior dislocations may injure the femoral or obdurator nerve in a similar fashion. The peroneal division of the femoral nerve may also be injured during repair of fracture or placement of an endoprosthesis, most commonly for total hip replacement. Peroneal nerve injury was reported in 45% of patients with a subcapital fracture treated by insertion of an Austin Moore prosthesis (33). The mechanism of injury was believed to be placement of stretch on the sciatic nerve. Fortunately, 93% of the patients completely recovered within 60 days.

Wound Infection

In a review of 607 patients over a 6-year period, the incidence of wound infection for femoral neck or trochanteric fractures was 6.7% compared to 10% for subtrochanteric fractures (22). These observations were explained by the increased time required for more difficult procedures. Russin and Russin (24) reported a 5% incidence of postoperative infection in 1166 consecutive patients over a 20-year period. The most commonly reported organisms were coagulase-positive *Staphylococcus aureus*, *Escherichia coli*, and *Pseudomonas aeruginosa*.

Arterial Injury

During the process of hip fracture repair, major adjacent vessels in the immediate vicinity are occasionally injured, placing the patient at considerable risk for potential loss of limb or life. Nachbur and Meyer (34), based on an 8-year study, described five mechanisms of arterial injury involved in 15 reported patients requiring emergency vascular surgery: 1) major artery perforation with the tip of a retractor, which even after suturing can still lead to thrombosis and possible limb ischemia; 2) overextension of atherosclerotic arteries, causing intimal fracture and subsequent thrombus formation, involving the common femoral and external iliac arteries while attempting to expose the femoral head; 3) major artery laceration during total hip prosthesis placement secondary to strenuous mobilization or direct trauma, related to the use of an osteotome or protruding osteophyte and leading to hemorrhage or total limb ischemia; 4) thrombotic occlusion of a major artery related to the intense heat of polymerizing bone cement entering the pelvis through a defective acetabulum; and 5) false aneurysm and arteriovenous fistula formation secondary to repeated trauma by a projecting screw or excessive bone cement. Fortunately, these mishaps rarely occur, the incidence being less than 0.5%.

Sequential Fractures

In a prospective study of 1514 elderly hip fracture patients, Chiu and Pun (35) noted an incidence of subsequent fracture of the contralateral hip of 2.3% over 12 months. Significant factors found to correlate with the second event were institutionalization, concomitant neurologic disease (such as parkinsonism or stroke), and biochemical changes compatible with osteomalacia.

Medical

Medical complications after hip fracture include urinary tract infections, acute renal failure, myocardial infarction, cardiac failure, pneumonia, atelectasis, thrombophlebitis, gastrointestinal disorders, nerve palsies, and skin breakdown (see Table 83-5).

Deep Venous Thrombosis and Pulmonary Embolism

Deep venous thrombosis (DVT) may occur in up to 70% of patients after hip fracture. Concomitant pulmonary embolus occurs in up to 16% of patients. The majority of cases occur in the first week, and the risk for DVT declines significantly after the thirteenth to seventeenth postoperative day. Recent intraoperative transesophageal echocardiography studies suggested that many asymptomatic perioperative DVTs confined to the calf veins may be the source of microembolic showers, warranting some form of primary prophylaxis for all patients (36). The currently suggested prophylaxis for patients undergoing hip fracture surgery includes either preoperative, subcutaneous, fixed-dose, unmonitored low-molecular-weight heparin (e.g., enoxaparin) or oral anticoagulation therapy with warfarin [maintaining the international normalized ratio (INR) between 2.0 and 3.0] (37). For patients undergoing total hip replacement surgery, any one of the following prophylactic regimens may be used: 1) postoperative, subcutaneous, twice-daily, fixed-dose, unmonitored low-molecular-weight heparin (e.g., enoxaparin 30 mg every 12 hours); 2) preoperative or immediately postoperative low-intensity oral anticoagulation (INR between 2.0 and 3.0); or 3) adjusted-dose unfractionated heparin started preoperatively (37). Intermittent external compression devices and elastic stockings are still considered to be adjuvant therapy, while vena caval filters remain a last resort, unless pharmacologic anticoagulation is contraindicated (37). The duration of prophylaxis has not been well defined; however, it is usually continued until hospital discharge. While no research on the posthospitalization risk of DVT has been performed on individuals with hip fracture, recent studies examining individuals with elective total hip replacement revealed benefits from prophylaxis continued for at least 3 weeks after discharge (41). If anticoagulation therapy needs to be discontinued during acute or rehabilitation hospitalization, it should not be done until transfers and ambulation can be performed without significant assistance (usually 2–4 weeks after surgery).

Cardiovascular

In a review of 1166 community hospital hip fractures, 97.3% of patients with concomitant medical conditions had cardiovascular disease and 21.8% of deaths were attributed to cardiac causes (24). This is not an unexpected finding, as hip fracture is primarily a geriatric injury; however, it clearly illustrates the significant impact of associated disease. It is important to consider the effect this concomitant morbidity may have on the physiologic capacity of the patient to surmount the related systemic effects and pain. An analysis of adverse cardiovascular clinical events occurring during hip fracture rehabilitation of geriatric patients (29) reported an incidence of 12%. The complications most frequently observed were cardiogenic pulmonary edema, myocardial infarction, atrial fibrillation, and acute arterial occlusion.

Pulmonary

Pulmonary dysfunction (pulmonary edema, pneumonia, atelectasis) has been reported in 11.7% of patients (24). Patients' lack of motivation and pain related to immobility were believed to contribute significantly to complications of aspiration, thrombophlebitis, and fat emboli.

Genitourinary

Urinary tract infection is the most frequently encountered genitourinary problem seen after hip fracture, followed by hemorrhagic cystitis, acute renal failure, oliguria, hematuria, urinary retention, pyelonephritis, and stable incontinence (29). An 11% incidence of genitourinary abnormalities in geriatric hip fracture patients has been reported.

Gastrointestinal

Gastrointestinal abnormalities have been reported in 12% of older adults after hip fracture (29). In order of decreasing frequency, these disorders include adverse gastrointestinal morbidity (including nausea and vomiting), fecal impaction, diarrhea, abdominal pain, gastritis, and diverticulitis.

Decubitus Ulcers

Decubitus ulcers have been reported to occur in between 13% and 66% of hip fracture patients (24,38). Ulcers in various stages were related to the following factors: 1) prolonged waiting periods on high-pressure surfaces, in the emergency room and on the acute care units following traction placement; 2) preoperative dehydration- and sedation-related increased soft-tissue vulnerability to trauma; 3) waiting time for the surgical procedure; and 4) time spent on the operating table and in the recovery room. By the fifth hospital day, 83% of all patients who would eventually develop a pressure ulcer had at least one lesion. Common ulcer locations include bony prominences at the pelvic girdle, feet, sacrum, and heels. These occurrences can be minimized by placing patients on pressure-relieving mattresses, turning them according to schedule, maintaining adequate hydration and nutrition, and minimizing unnecessary delays in the emergency room, operating room, and postoperative recovery area.

Neurologic

Bernardini et al (29) reported a 7% incidence of neurologic complications following hip fracture, including confusion, stroke, delirium, headache, dizziness, herpes zoster, trigeminal neuralgia, dizziness, and transient ischemic attacks.

Delirium

Delirium, which develops in 30% to 50% of patients, usually occurs on postoperative days 1 to 5 and resolves by day 7 (39). Occurrence is not related to the type of anesthesia used or duration of surgery. Delirium and in-hospital mortality are strongly correlated; therefore, it is imperative to identify and correct its cause (30). Factors commonly associated with this syndrome include anticholinergic medications, hypoxia, infection, and urinary retention. Limiting the duration of narcotic pain medications (i.e., switching to nonnarcotic agents by 3–4 days after surgery), avoiding benzodiazepine and other sedating medications, early discontinuation of indwelling catheters and other potential sources of infection, and rapid mobilization will limit common iatrogenic causes of postsurgical delirium.

REHABILITATION

As the average age of the population continues to increase and older adults are remaining increasingly active, falls and associated hip fractures will continue as a major source of disability in the United States. While rehabilitation interventions to decrease the risk of falls, and thus prevent hip fractures, are of utmost importance (42), postfracture rehabilitation care is also crucial. These interventions should be initiated within the first postfixation day, and continued until the individual has maximized functional skills within the community. The increasing limits placed on health care resources are necessitating a shift in hip fracture rehabilitation care to lower-cost, alternative environments. In order to best serve the individual's needs, a thorough understanding of these newer treatment settings, available resources, and the appropriate medical and rehabilitation interventions necessary to minimize postfracture complications is crucial.

Assessment

A number of areas of physiatric assessment are unique to hip fracture patients, in particular the geriatric patient. Clearly, an understanding of the major acute and chronic medical issues is vital. This understanding assists in determining the degree of physiologic reserve remaining, which is a major factor in designing more specific strategies and precautions for the rehabilitation program. It also helps to focus the medical management of the individual, which is essential for successful participation. In general, a comprehensive assessment of physiologic functioning (e.g., cardiac stress testing, pulmonary function tests) of the individual prior to and after the hip fracture is not feasible or even recommended. Often it can be elucidated from premorbid activity levels or medications. Direct communication with the individual's primary care physician is also important, and if possible, integrating his or her management recommendations directly into the rehabilitation treatment program is suggested.

Of equal importance in the assessment of the older adult is a comprehensive review of the social rehabilitation plan. This involves understanding the formal and informal support systems available (5). Formal support systems include federal (Medicare, Social Security), state (Medicaid, disability, welfare), and local (physicians, Meals on Wheels, home health assistance) resources. Informal support systems include family and friends. Older adults sometimes have greater involvement of extended families in their systems of support, as they will often outlive spouses and even their children. Daughters and female caregivers are generally more likely to play a major support role than are sons (43,44). An understanding of the social supports available should be initiated during the acute care phase, often within the first 24 to 96 hours after injury. Early involvement of family and friends in the rehabilitation planning and then actual hands-on training are vital.

It is also important to understand a number of other aspects of the social makeup of the injured older adult. These areas include 1) the older adult's role in the family unit, 2) the role of the church and organized religion in the individual's life, 3) the patient and caregivers' conceptions about the medical process, 4) the patient and caregivers' ultimate goals, and 5) the patient and caregivers' views on advance directives. While an understanding of these components of an individual's life is important at any age, it becomes increasingly important in the older adult.

An awareness of the most common funding mechanisms available for hip fracture care of the older adult is vital. For example, 98% of the older adults in the United States are primarily funded by a single source, Medicare. Secondary or co-payment insurance ("MediGap") varies greatly in coverage, but will typically not pay for extensive rehabilitation services. Similarly, in Canada, Australia, and most European countries, the government funds the overwhelming majority of medical care for the elderly. Medicare is a federally sponsored program; therefore, its coverages are identical throughout the United States. With the recent advent of managed care of Medicare, certain benefits may vary. Any individual who has paid into the federal tax system for 40 quarters and meets one of the following three criteria will be covered for free by Medicare Part A: 1) age 65 or older, 2) disabled for longer than 2 years, or 3) end-stage renal disease. Medicare Part A reimburses for durable medical equipment and inpatient, nursing home, and home health services. Medicare Part B, which is available for a monthly fee, reimburses for outpatient and physician services. Medicaid (Medi-Cal in California) is a state-sponsored and therefore, a state-specific program that provides health insurance to the medically indigent. Medicaid pays for more than 85% of all nursing home care in the United States. Older adults who continue to work or who have been federal employees will typically have a private or managed care insurance as their primary funding source (45–47).

Settings

Older adults with acute physical impairments due to hip fracture should receive rehabilitation services in the least restrictive environment. While all patients may benefit from some type and intensity of therapy services, patients who are appropriate for intensive inpatient or day rehabilitation must demonstrate the following characteristics: 1) acute or new disability (i.e., significantly worse than baseline ability), 2) supportive family who can assist with return to home, 3) ability to participate in and improve in acute care therapies, and 4) appropriate funding source. A return to the prior living environment as soon as feasible is always the goal. Options include the following (48,49).

1. Acute care services (0.5–2.0 hr/day for 5–6 days/wk): These services are multidisciplinary in nature and usually include physician, nursing, physical therapy, occupational therapy, and social work services. They are reimbursed by Medicare under the diagnostic-related group (DRG) system (e.g., hip fracture with arthroplasty = 209, hip fracture with open reduction and internal fixation = 211) and by Medicaid, as long as medically necessary. Acute care services are useful acutely after injury to prevent complications and allow a comprehensive physiatric assessment of the individual during the early recovery period. The typical duration of services is 2 to 7 days.
2. Inpatient rehabilitation services (3.0–5.0 hr/day of therapy for 5–7 days/wk and 24 hr/day nursing): Inpatient rehabilitation units are interdisciplinary in nature with physician, nursing, physical therapy, occupational therapy, therapeutic recreation, social work, and psychology services available. They are reimbursed by Medicare and Medicaid to some degree, as long as demonstrable gains are being made in two or more therapies. Medicare reimbursement is institution specific. This is usually the most expensive of all the settings described here. These units are useful for moderately to severely impaired individuals with acute but limited medical needs and limited to good informal support systems. The typical duration of services is 2 to 5 weeks.
3. Geriatric evaluation and management (GEM) unit (3.0–5.0 hr/day of therapy for 5–7 days/wk and 24 hr/day nursing): GEM units are interdisciplinary in nature with physician (geriatrician), nursing, physical therapy, occupational therapy, therapeutic recre-

ation, and social work services available. These units only rehabilitate geriatric patients and therefore are better able to concentrate on issues commonly seen in this population. Outcomes have been shown to be superior to those of nongeriatric settings (50). Utilized in Europe primarily, these units are rare in the United States. This model has been adopted by the U.S. Veterans Administration medical system. GEM units are useful for moderately to severely impaired individuals with acute medical needs and limited to good informal support systems. The typical duration of services is 4 to 8 weeks (51–53).

4. Subacute rehabilitation services (1.5–2.5 hr/day for 5–7 days/wk): Subacute rehabilitation units are multidisciplinary or interdisciplinary in nature with physician, nursing, physical therapy, occupational therapy, and social work services available. They are located in acute care hospitals or skills nursing facilities. The services are reimbursed fully (80% of reasonable charges) by Medicare for 20 days and by Medicaid in most states. They are useful for severely impaired individuals who are expected to make very gradual recovery, may have significant medical issues, and have limited informal support systems. Individuals may progress to the level of inpatient rehabilitation services and then be transferred. In some areas, managed care insurers use subacute rehabilitation services in place of intensive inpatient rehabilitation services. The typical duration of services is 2 to 8 weeks (48).
5. Skilled nursing facilities (1.0–1.5 hr/day of therapy for 5 days/wk and 24 hr/day nursing availability): These facilities are multidisciplinary in nature, with nursing, physical therapy, occupational therapy, social work, and therapeutic recreation services. They are reimbursed by Medicare for a limited period of time and by Medicaid in most states. The facilities should be considered for patients who are medically stable, but too debilitated to participate in more intensive therapy programs, and who cannot be treated safely at home. Many patients eventually go home, while others progress to more intensive rehabilitation programs. Many others fail to progress, usually because of severe comorbidities, leading to placement in long-term custodial care facilities. The typical duration of services is 3 to 8 weeks.
6. Day rehabilitation services (3.0–5.0 hr/day for 5 days/wk): These services are interdisciplinary in nature with physician, nursing, physical therapy, occupational therapy, social work, and occasionally therapeutic recreation involvement. They are reimbursed by Medicare and Medicaid in some areas, as long as gains in two or more therapies are demonstrable. They are more often covered by private insurers. Transportation and occasionally housing (referred to as transitional living programs) may be provided, but are rarely directly funded by either Medicare or Medicaid. Day rehabilitation services are useful for moderately functioning individuals who have sufficient endurance to tolerate travel and fair to good informal support systems. Older adults may be limited by endurance issues. Use of these services is often a good way to shorten the length of stay in acute care hospitals or rehabilitation units. Individuals may enter the program after acute care hospital or inpatient rehabilitation services. Outpatient services are often used after day rehabilitation. The typical duration of services is 2 to 6 weeks.
7. Home health services (0.5–2.0 hr/day for 3 days/wk): Home health services are unidisciplinary in nature, usually including a nurse, physical therapist, and occupational therapist. They are reimbursed by Medicare, as long as medically necessary, and sometimes by Medicaid. Additionally, limited (at most 40 hr/wk) personal care services may be available through Medicaid; however, this is significantly affected by state or county spending limitations. These services are not reimbursable under Medicare. Home health services involve true supported living (full-time assistance at home is not generally reimbursable under Medicare and Medicaid). They are useful for severely physically or cognitively impaired, or oldest old (>85 years) individuals who are expected to make very gradual recovery, and have very strong informal support systems. Individuals may enter the program after receiving acute care hospital or inpatient rehabilitation services. The typical duration of services is 3 to 12 weeks.
8. Outpatient services (0.5–3.0 hr/day for 3 days/wk): Outpatient services are multidisciplinary in nature, usually including physical therapy and occupational therapy. They are reimbursed by Medicare and Medicaid, as long as medically necessary, usually as long as the patient is making documentable progress. No transportation is provided. These services are useful for high-functioning individuals who have very focused needs (e.g., balance deficits, gait endurance, community mobility). Outpatient services are not usually the preferred choice for the older adult, owing to transportation and endurance issues. Individuals may enter the program after receiving acute care hospital or inpatient rehabilitation services. The typical duration of services is 2 to 8 weeks.
9. Day care services (4.0–10.00 hr/day for 5 days/wk): These services are multidisciplinary in nature, with

nursing, physical therapy, occupational therapy, therapeutic recreation, and social work services sometimes available for limited periods of time. Primarily a setting for custodial care of community-dwelling older adults, day care services may be reimbursed in part by Medicaid only. They are useful for high-functioning individuals who require supervision or assistance for only minor functional skills (e.g., setup care for feeding or toileting). The typical duration of services is indefinite, usually long term.

Predictive Factors for Functional Outcome

The most clearly defined predictors of functional outcome, length of stay, and costs of rehabilitation after hip fracture include 1) age, 2) fracture type, 3) acute care complications, 4) discharge disposition from acute care, 5) functional status at admission to rehabilitation, 6) premorbid medical status, 7) premorbid emotional status, 8) premorbid functional abilities, 9) rehabilitation intervention used, and 10) premorbid social supports (17,54–57). Specifically, mobility and toileting items on the Functional Independence Measure (FIM) correlate with length of stay (i.e., individuals who score lower or are more dependent have longer lengths of stay); bladder, locomotion, and toileting items correlate with costs; and bladder, upper- and lower-extremity dressing, and cognition items correlate with discharge functional outcome (measured by the FIM) (54). Predictors of decreased functional abilities at 6 months after the fracture occurred include 1) increased age, 2) intertrochanteric fractures, 3) discharge to a nursing home, and 4) poor prefracture emotional status (57). One-year predictors of poor functional outcome include 1) poor premorbid functional abilities, 2) increased acute care complications, and 3) acute care discharge disposition to either a nursing home or rehabilitation unit (versus to home) (57). Finally, residing in a nursing home before the injury correlates with poor 1-year mobility skills (17).

There is limited research available to clearly identify the most appropriate rehabilitation interventions after hip fracture, specifically which treatment setting is most effective. Overall, when medically and socially feasible, home-based rehabilitation is more cost-effective than nursing home– or rehabilitation unit–based services (57–60). Recently, one study indicated that African-American individuals received less acute care therapy (both physical and occupational therapy) than did non-African-American individuals with similar fracture characteristics, suggesting that bias may impact interventions after hip fracture (61).

Interventions

All individuals with hip fracture should be mobilized out of bed as soon as medically and surgically possible. For the majority of patients, this can begin within 24 hours of surgical intervention. Early mobilization will assist in the prevention of complications (e.g., DVT, decubitus ulcer, atelectasis), facilitate healing, and initiate the process of remobilization. Early mobilization is best accomplished by nursing and therapy (physical and occupational therapy) staff. The length of postoperative acute care stay is clearly determined by the type of fracture, the operative procedure performed, and the medical status of the individual; however, 3 to 7 days is a typical course. While some advocated only a brief period of acute care physical and occupational therapy, followed by similar home-based therapy for 4 to 6 weeks (56–60), others recommended a more intensive 2- to 3-week inpatient rehabilitation unit stay (62). Recently, alternative approaches have included care in subacute rehabilitation units for 2 to 6 weeks (63,64), day rehabilitation services for 3 to 6 weeks, and interdisciplinary home rehabilitation (more interaction between therapists and sometimes more therapy than usually given at home) for 2 to 6 weeks. Each of these may need to be followed by lower-intensity outpatient or home care. Data comparing the cost-effectiveness and efficacy of these various treatment settings and intensities of therapy are not available for post–hip fracture rehabilitation.

Standard rehabilitation principles often are not effective for recovering self-care abilities in older adults with hip fracture. Older adults may have difficulty with attempts to utilize the concept of transfer of training skills (i.e., breaking down functional tasks into smaller components); therefore, very functional therapy is recommended. Automatic or overlearned activities often return rapidly, but new learning and significant adaptations may be more slowly integrated than in younger adults. A firm understanding of the individual's premorbid characteristics and habits is therefore vital.

Adaptive equipment may be extremely useful. However, patients may have difficulty accepting and effectively utilizing it. Typical equipment recommendations include 1) built-up assistive devices (e.g., canes, walkers) to accommodate for hand weakness, decreased dexterity, and joint limitations; 2) long-handled devices and reachers to accommodate for decreases in flexibility, surgical limitations to ROM, and poor truncal balance; and 3) bathroom safety aides (grab bars, tub benches, hand-held showers, raised commode chairs) to accommodate for ROM restrictions, balance deficits, and decreased strength. Home management skills must often be modified. Particular emphasis must be paid to the limited physical and cognitive endurance seen in the older adult.

Special considerations are also necessary to address mobility deficits in the older adult with hip fracture, including alterations in vision, decreased peripheral sensation, age-related imbalance, decreased strength, and limited physical endurance. Recovery of motor and balance function tends to occur more slowly in the older adult, owing to premorbid limitations, decreased tolerance for therapy, and joint or musculoskeletal pain. Household-level mobility may be facilitated by a home evaluation by members of the rehabilitation team assessing architectural barriers (e.g., doorways, stairs), spacing of furniture, appropriateness of floor coverings, adequacy of natural and artificial lighting, and available modifications. Gait and transfer assistive devices are almost always necessary during the initial period of healing (i.e., the first 6 weeks). The use and type of device are greatly influenced by fracture type, fixation used, postoperative medical course, and premorbid abilities.

Community mobility goals must take into account the ability to get to different areas in the community (driving, public transportation) and the ability to get around safely in different settings (malls, restaurants, golf courses, homes). The decision to permit an older adult to drive after hip fracture must take into account premorbid abilities and new limitations. Comprehensive driving evaluations may be helpful; however, funding for these programs is rarely available. Testing of ROM, muscle strength, proprioception, light touch, pathologic reflexes, vision, sitting balance, transfer skills, judgment, memory, attention, and reaction time is important, as is a behind-the-wheel evaluation (65). Available research data suggest that driving should be delayed a minimum of 8 weeks, to allow for return of lower-extremity coordination, reaction time, and endurance (66). Public transportation for the disabled is becoming increasingly available throughout the world; thus, physical limitations are becoming less important as barriers to community mobility. Specific transportation systems for the elderly are also becoming available, and these overcome both physical and cognitive barriers. Funding for these systems is often dependent on federal and local sources, which are becoming increasingly limited.

Treatment Protocols

Standardization of acute postoperative and rehabilitation treatment of individuals with hip fracture allows for efficient and comprehensive care. While all standardized protocols need to be capable of adjusting to the specialized needs of each individual, certain key elements of care are vital to all patients (Table 83-6). During the acute postoperative management, the following areas of care need to be addressed: 1) incision care, 2) pain management, 3) DVT prophylaxis, 4) bladder management, and 5) pulmonary toilet. Rehabilitation care must include the following key components: 1) social support assessment, 2) hip precaution education, 3) transfer skills, 4) ambulation skills, 5) ADL skills, and 6) adaptive equipment. Future research on outcomes will focus on the efficacy of these treatment protocols and the impact of modifications of these protocols on outcome.

Table 83-6: Treatment Protocol for Hip Fracture Rehabilitation

Time After Injury	Medical Issues	Rehabilitation Issues
	Phase I Acute care hospital	
0–1 days	DVT prophylaxis	Assess premorbid skills
	Pain management	Assess social supports
1–4 days	DVT prophylaxis	PT/OT evaluations
	Discontinue Foley catheter	Out of bed to chair/ ambulation
	Pain management	Basic ADLs
	Incision management	ROM precaution education
3–7 days	Finalize follow-up surgical care	D/C from acute care
	Phase II Rehabilitation setting (inpatient, subacute, day, outpatient)	
1–3 wk	DVT prophylaxis	Ambulation with supervision
	Pain management	Basic ADLs with adaptive aids
	Discontinue sutures or staples	LE strengthening
3–6 wk	Routine health maintenance	Community skills training
	Orthopedic follow-up	LE strengthening
6–8 wk		Rehabilitation medical follow-up
		Return to premorbid activities

DVT = deep venous thrombosis; D/C = discharge; PT/OT = physical therapy/occupational therapy; ADLs = activities of daily living; ROM = range of motion; LE = lower extremity.

REFERENCES

1. Holbrook TL, Grazier K, Kelsey JL, Stauffer RN. *The frequency of occurrence, impact and cost of selected musculoskeletal conditions in the United States.* Chicago: American Academy of Orthopaedic Surgeons, 1984.
2. Agarwal N, Reyes JD, Westerman DA, Cayten CG. Factors influencing DRG 210 (hip fracture) reimbursement. *J Trauma* 1986;26: 426–431.
3. Gallagher JC, Melton LJ, Riggs BC, Bergtrath E. Epidemiology of fractures of the proximal femur in Rochester, Minnesota. *Clin Orthop* 1980;150:163–167.
4. Zuckerman JD, Schon LC. Hip fractures. In: Zuckerman JD, ed. *Comprehensive care of orthopedic injuries in the elderly.* Baltimore: Urban & Schwarzenberg, 1990:23–111.
5. Gershkoff AM, Cifu DX, Means KM. Geriatric rehabilitation: social, attitudinal, and economic factors.

Arch Phys Med Rehabil 1993;74(suppl):402–405.

6. Means KM. Falls and fractures. *Phys Med Rehabil State Art Rev* 1990;4:39–48.
7. Farmer ME, White LR, Brody JA. Race and sex differences in hip fracture incidence. *Am J Public Health* 1984;74:1374–1380.
8. Riggs BL, Melton LJ III. Involutional osteoporosis. *N Engl J Med* 1986;314:1676–1686.
9. Buchner DM, Larson EB. Falls and fractures in patients with Alzheimer-type dementia. *JAMA* 1987;257:1492–1495.
10. Holbrook TL, Barret-Conner E, Wingard DL. Dietary calcium and risk of hip fracture: a 14 year prospective population study. *Lancet* 1988;2:1046–1049.
11. Cifu DX. Rehabilitation of fractures of the hip. *Phys Med Rehabil State Art Rev* 1995;9:125–139.
12. Williams P, Warwick R. *Gray's anatomy.* Philadelphia: WB Saunders, 1980:477–482, 727–728.
13. Nienman KMW, Martin HJ. Fractures about the hip in institutionalized patient population. *J Bone Joint Surg [Am]* 1968;50: 1327–1340.
14. Melton LJ, Ilstrup DM, Riggs BL, Beckenbaugh RD. Fifty year trend in hip fracture incidence. *Clin Orthop* 1982;162:144–149.
15. Garden RS. Low-angle fixation in fractures of the femoral neck. *J Bone Joint Surg [Br]* 1961;43:647–661.
16. Kyle RF, Gustilo RB, Premer RF. Analysis of 622 intertrochanteric hip fractures: a retrospective study. *J Bone Joint Surg [Am]* 1979;61:216–221.
17. Folman Y, Gepstein R, Assaraf A, Liberty S. Functional recovery after operative treatment of femoral neck fractures in an institutional elderly population. *Arch Phys Med Rehabil* 1994;75: 454–456.
18. Dahl E. Mortality and life expectancy after hip fractures. *Acta Orthop Scand* 1980;51: 163–170.
19. Jenson JS, Bagger J. Long term social prognosis after hip fractures. *Injury* 1984;15:411–414.
20. White BL, Fisher WD, Laurin CA. Rate of mortality for elderly patients after fracture of the hip in the 1980s. *J Bone Joint Surg [Am]* 1987;69:1335–1340.
21. Emerson S, Zetterberg CH, Anderson GJB. Ten year survival after fractures of the proximal end of the femur. *Gerontology* 1988;34: 186–191.
22. Beals RK. Survival following hip fracture: long follow-up of 607 patients. *J Chronic Dis* 1986;25: 235–244.
23. Kenzora JE, McCarthy R, Lowell JD, Sledge CB. Hip fracture mortality. *Clin Orthop* 1984;186: 45–56.
24. Russin LA, Russin MA. Hip fracture: a review of 1166 cases in a community hospital setting. *Orthopedics* 1981;4:23–34.
25. Miller CW. Survival and ambulation following hip fracture. *J Bone Joint Surg [Am]* 1978;60:930–934.
26. Ions GK, Stevens J. Prediction of survival in patients with femoral neck fracture. *J Bone Joint Surg [Br]* 1987;69:384–387.
27. Dedrick DK, Mackenzie JR, Burney RE. Complications of femoral neck fracture in young adults. *J Trauma* 1986;26:932–937.
28. Monoz E, Johanson H, Margolis I. DRG's, orthopedic surgery and age at an academic medical center. *Orthopedics* 1988;11:1645–1651.
29. Bernardini B, Meinecke C, Pagani M. Comorbidity and adverse clinical events in the rehabilitation of older adults after hip fracture. *J Am Geriatr Soc* 1995;43: 894–898.
30. Perez ED. Hip fracture: physicians take more active role in patient care. *Geriatrics* 1994;49:31–37.
31. Marks PH, Paley D, Kellam JF. Heterotopic ossification around the hip with intramedullary nailing of the femur. *J Trauma* 1988;28: 1207–1212.
32. Seddon H. *Surgical disorders of the peripheral nerves.* Baltimore: Williams & Wilkins, 1972.
33. Rodriguez MJ, Austin E, McBride EJ. Peroneal nerve damage following insertion of Austin-Moore prosthesis. *Arch Phys Med Rehabil* 1964;45:283–285.
34. Nachbur B, Meyer RP. The mechanisms of severe arterial injury in surgery of the hip joint. *Clin Orthop* 1979;141:122–133.
35. Chiu KY, Pun WK. Sequential fractures of both hip in elderly patients—a prospective study. *J Trauma* 1992;32:584–587.
36. Ereth M, Weber J, Abel M. Cemented versus noncemented total hip arthroplasty: embolism, hemodynamics and intrapulmonary shunting. *Mayo Clin Proc* 1992; 67:1066–1074.
37. Clagett GP, Anderson FA, Heit J. Prevention of venous thromboembolism. *Chest* 1995;108(suppl): 312s–334s.
38. Versluysen M. How elderly patients with femoral fracture develop pressure sores in hospital. *BMJ* 1986;292:1311–1313.
39. Berggren D, Gustafson Y, Eriksson B. Postoperative confusion after anesthesia in elderly patients with femoral neck fractures. *Anesth Analg* 1987;66: 497–504.
40. Ayes PC, McCollister E, Parkinson JR. The prevention of heterotopic ossification in high-risk patients by low-dose radiation after total hip arthroplasty. *J Bone Joint Surg [Am]* 1986;68:426–431.
41. Planes A, Vochelle N, Darmon J-Y. Risk of deep venous thrombosis after hospital discharge in patients having undergone total hip replacement: double blind randomised comparison of enoxaparin versus placebo. *Lancet* 1996;348: 224–228.
42. Rubenstein LZ, Robbins AS, Schulman BL, et al. Falls and instability in the elderly. *J Am Geriatr Soc* 1988;36:266–278.

43. Brody SJ, Paulson LG. *Aging and rehabilitation. II: the state of the practice.* New York: Springer, 1990:139–147.

44. Brody SJ, Ruff GE. *Aging and rehabilitation.* New York: Springer, 1986:36–46.

45. France AC, Schultz AK, Nanney MT. Medicare, geriatrics and the family physician. *Am Fam Physician* 1991;44:754–756.

46. Maloney FP, Means KM. *Rehabilitation and the aging population.* Philadelphia: Hanley & Belfus, 1990:143–166.

47. Sherman FT. Physician reimbursement for the care of the elderly: concerns of a practicing geriatrician. *Bull NY Acad Med* 1988;63:732–736.

48. Walker WC, Kreutzer JS, Witol AD. Level of care options for the low-functioning brain injury survivor. *Brain Inj* 1996;10:65–75.

49. Weber DC, Fleming KC, Evans JM. Rehabilitation of geriatric patients. *Mayo Clin Proc* 1995;70:1198–1204.

50. Applegate WB, Miller ST, Graney MJ. A randomized, controlled trial of a geriatric assessment unit in a community rehabilitation hospital. *N Engl J Med* 1990; 322:1572–1578.

51. Applegate WB, Deyo R, Kramer A. Geriatric evaluation and management: current status and future research directions. *J Am Geriatr Soc* 1991;39(suppl):25–75.

52. Rubenstein LZ, Stuck AE, Siu AL, et al. Impacts of geriatric evaluation and management programs on defined outcomes: overview of the evidence. *J Am Geriatr Soc* 1991;39(suppl):85–165.

53. Stewart DG, Cifu DX. Rehabilitation of the old, old stroke patient. *J Back Musculoskel Rehabil* 1994;4:135–140.

54. Grigsby J, Kooken R, Hershberger J. Simulated neural networks to predict outcomes, costs, and length of stay among orthopedic rehabilitation patients. *Arch Phys Med Rehabil* 1994;75:1077–1081.

55. Cedar L, Thorgen K, Walden B. Prognostic indicators and early home rehabilitation in elderly patients with hip fractures. *Clin Orthop* 1980;152:173–178.

56. Jette AM, Harris BA, Cleary PD, Campion EW. Functional recovery after hip fracture. *Arch Phys Med Rehabil* 1987;68:735–740.

57. Pryor G, Williams D. Rehabilitation after hip fractures: home and hospital management compared. *J Bone Joint Surg [Br]* 1989;71: 471–476.

58. Holmberg S, Ager E, Ersmark H. Rehabilitation at home after hip fracture. *Acta Orthop Scand* 1989;60:73–78.

59. Jarnlo G, Cedar L, Thorngen K. Early rehabilitation at home of elderly patients with hip fractures and consumption of resources in primary care. *Scand J Prim Health Care* 1984;2:105–110.

60. Tinetti ME, Baker DI, Gottschalk M, et al. Systematic home-based physical and functional therapy for older persons after hip fracture. *Arch Phys Med Rehabil* 1997;78:1237–1247.

61. Hoenig H, Rubenstein L, Kahn K. Rehabilitation after hip fracture—equal opportunity for all? *Arch Phys Med Rehabil* 1996;77: 58–63.

62. Cifu DX, Means KM, Currie DM, Gershkoff AM. Geriatric rehabilitation: diagnosis and management of acquired disabling disorders. *Arch Phys Med Rehabil* 1993;74: S406–S412.

63. Evans R, Halar E, Hendricks R. Effects of prospective payment financing on rehabilitation outcome. *Int J Rehabil Res* 1990; 13:27–32.

64. Fitzgerald J, Fagan L. Changing patterns of hip fracture care before and after implementation of the prospective payment system. *JAMA* 1987;258:218–225.

65. Hunt LA. Evaluation and retraining programs for older drivers. *Clin Geriatr Med* 1993;9:439–448.

66. Cifu DX. Rehabilitation of the elderly crash victim. *Clin Geriatr Med* 1993;9:473–483.

Chapter 84

Rehabilitation Following Arthroplasty

John J. Nicholas
Norman Aliga

During the last 20 years, the rehabilitation of rheumatic patients has increasingly consisted of rehabilitation following surgery for arthritic joints. The advent of successful medical treatment for rheumatic conditions, principally methotrexate for rheumatoid arthritis, and the decrease in hospitalization of rheumatic patients for rehabilitation because of the diagnostic-related groups of Medicare, have diminished the census of rheumatic patients in most rehabilitation centers. Improvements in the outcome of arthroplasty surgery, however, and its growing prevalence have increased the number of rheumatic patients requiring rehabilitation following arthroplasty. The experience at the Marianjoy Rehabilitation Hospital and Clinics and the Rush-Presbyterian-St. Luke's Medical Center, as well as a review of the literature, provides a background for this description of the techniques of rehabilitation of rheumatic patients following arthroplasty (1).

Every year approximately 800,000 arthroplasties are performed on rheumatic patients in the United States (2). These procedures have become increasingly successful (3–7). A study of 128 total knee arthroplasty patients and 211 total hip arthroplasty patients revealed that 69% and 83% reported satisfaction with activities of daily living (ADLs), and 81% and 88% reported satisfactory improvement from preoperative pain on the short form 36 (SF36) scale (8). Improvements in physical mobility and energy, compared to the preoperative status, have also been documented at 2 and 5 years after arthroplasty (9). Patients with both rheumatoid arthritis and osteoarthritis have shown improved movement and function and diminished pain for at least 3 years after surgery (10). Schulte et al (11) presented an additional study with a minimum of 20 years of follow-up after Charnley total hip arthroplasty was performed with cement in 98 hips in 83 patients and found 85% of hips to be pain free.

Many primary hip and knee arthroplasty patients are now able to recover from surgery and achieve sufficient function to be discharged promptly home within a few days. The average length of stay (LOS) at Rush-Presbyterian-St. Luke's Medical Center for primary hip and knee arthroplasties in 1995 was 4.9 (n = 202) and 4.9 (n = 190) days, respectively. Other patients, however, stay longer and require rehabilitation in a comprehensive rehabilitation unit or a skilled nursing/subacute rehabilitation unit. A list of causes for prolongation of the normal length of stay and treatment in a comprehensive rehabilitation facility derived from our experience is presented in Table 84-1. These causes are not obligatory reasons for comprehensive rehabilitation, but under most circumstances these comorbidities will slow the patient's progress and suggest the need for comprehensive rehabilitation services.

Zavadak et al (12) recently described 33 total hip arthroplasty patients and 48 total knee arthroplasty patients whose achievement of functional milestones varied widely, suggesting that arthroplasty patients frequently deviate from expected optimal recovery. Munin et al (13) further evaluated in a prospective study a series of arthroplasty patients discharged to home or to a comprehensive rehabilitation unit. The patients discharged from the acute hospital to a comprehensive inpatient rehabilitation unit were more likely to live alone, were older, had increased comorbid conditions, and had greater pain. Patients discharged to the rehabilitation center also tended to have diminished range of motion and less strength than did those discharged home. A model utilizing 1) age, 2) living alone, 3) supervision for sit-to-stand transfers after three physical therapy (PT) sessions, 4) walking 100 feet after three PT sessions, and 5) peak range of motion predicted on postoperative day 3, with 76% accuracy, which patients would likely be discharged to the rehabilitation unit. Patients discharged to the rehabilitation unit were older (6.3-year difference) and female, had more comorbidities, lived alone, were supported by Medicare, had fewer PT sessions, and had greater pain. Patients who had walkers, had fewer postoperative complications, and required only supervision for functional activities were more likely to be discharged home. The physiatrist should thus be able to predict fairly well which patients are likely to require further inpatient rehabilitation services.

Table 84-1: Indications for Comprehensive Inpatient Rehabilitation After Arthroplasty Procedures*
Complex medical problems
Multiple joint involvement
Severe contralateral joint disease
Stroke
Amputation
Congestive heart failure
Persistent pain
Bilateral arthroplasties
Revision arthroplasty
Bone grafting
Lack of knee flexion
Slow progress
Hemodialysis patients
Periprosthetic fractures
Possible infections
Anemia

* Reasons for prolonged hospitalization and/or treatment in a comprehensive rehabilitation unit, for arthroplasty patients at Rush-Presbyterian-St. Lukes Medical Center. Arthroplasty patients with these additional disorders should be strongly considered for admission to comprehensive inpatient intensive rehabilitation hospitals or units.

TOTAL HIP ARTHROPLASTY

Materials and Components

The total hip prosthesis commonly consists of a metal femoral stem component articulating with an ultra-high-molecular-weight polyethylene (UHMWPE) acetabular cup. The stem may be fixed to the head or, in the modular designs, stems and heads of different sizes may be interchanged (Fig. 84-1). The acetabular cup may be simply "press fit" into the acetabular cavity or secured with screws, cement, or both (Fig. 84-2). A screw-in device generally has not been found to be successful (Fig. 84-3). The earlier metal implants were made of stainless steel but they are inferior to other currently available materials in terms of corrosion, biocompatibility, and fatigue life. Cobalt-based alloys are most resistant to corrosion and fatigue fractures. Titanium and titanium-based alloys have relatively poor wear resistance and are not favored as articulat-

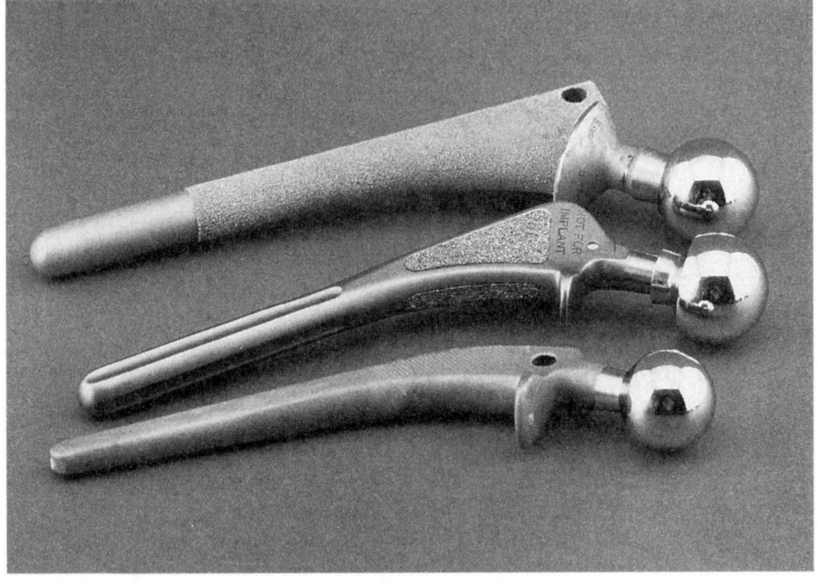

Figure 84-1. Examples of total hip arthroplasty femoral components. The stem and the heads are modular and therefore, interchangeable. The top two components have a porous coating that enables bone to grow in and form a union with the prosthesis. The bottom component is the more commonly used cemented total hip prosthesis.

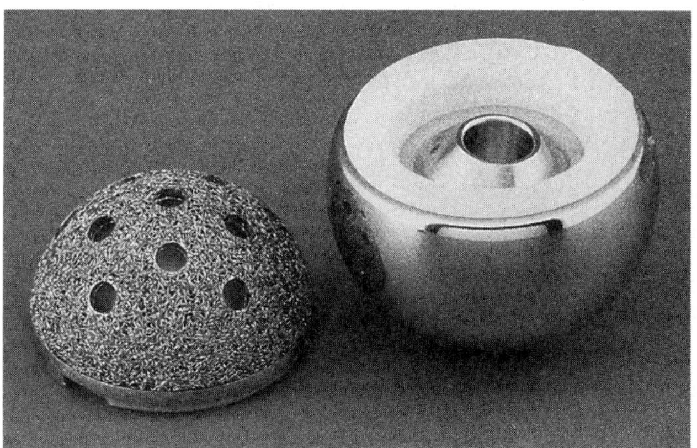

Figure 84-2. Acetabular components may have holes for screws used to secure the component and even a porous coating (*left*). The bipolar acetabular component (*right*) has an outer metal shell, an inner polyethylene liner, and a "captured" head. The head is attached to a stem and rotates within the polyethylene liner, and the shell rotates within the acetabulum. The rotation is thought to reduce wear, especially of an acetabulum free of disease (e.g., aseptic necrosis and hip fracture).

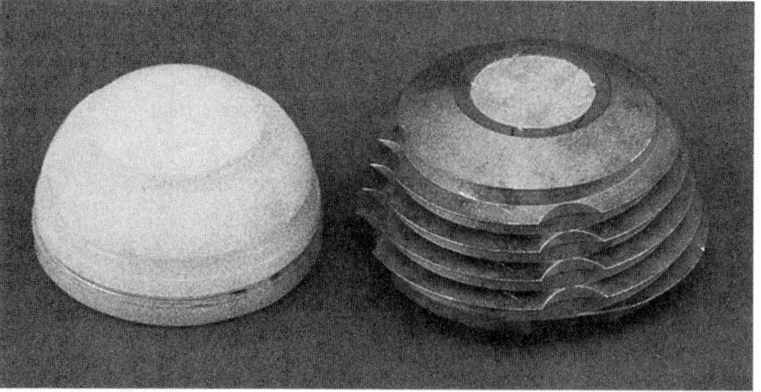

Figure 84-3. Acetabular components may be "screwed" into the acetabulum (*right*) or cemented (*left*) for stability.

ing components. Although titanium alloys are routinely used together with cobalt-based alloys, the use of different metals together is generally avoided, especially with stainless steel, because of the potential for galvanic corrosion. Ceramic femoral head components with a finer finish and harder surface, supported by metal stems, are now available (1).

The corresponding acetabular component is made of UHMWPE, which is tough and wear resistant. Since it is subject to deforming forces and potential loosening, it is usually provided with a metal backing, especially for arthroplasties in weight-bearing joints (14).

Fixation of the implants to bone is accomplished with or without the use of polymethylmethacrylate (PMMA) bone cement. The cement is prepared at surgery by mixing a powder containing prepolymerized PMMA, a catalyst, and liquid monomer with cross-linking agents and accelerators. When the cement is putty like, it is applied with a pressurized cement gun. The cement adheres to the prosthesis, but at the prosthesis-bone interface it fills in the interstices and crevices of the bone and distributes forces over a wider interface and eliminates motion between the implant and the bone. This allows a patient to bear weight as tolerated early in the postoperative period. Polymerization is an exothermic reaction, and so heat-stable powdered antibiotics may be added to treat infection if indicated.

Because bone cement is brittle and has the potential for breakage due to imperfections, newer methods of preparing and applying cement have been developed to reduce porosity or nonuniformity. Previously, bone cement was simply manually mixed and applied by finger packing, but this method has been associated with femoral loosening and lysis and an increased need for revisions (15,16). Results have improved with newer techniques, which include the use of an intramedullary femoral plug, application with a cement gun, pressurization, porosity reduction by mixing in a vacuum, precoating of metal surfaces with methylmethacrylate, and better-designed femoral stems with rounded and broader medial surfaces (17).

Uncemented techniques for fixation depend either on bony ingrowth into the porous coating of metal surfaces or on osseous integration with a surface coating of hydroxyapatite ceramic or tricalcium phosphate. With porous-coated hip implants, weight bearing is delayed for 6 weeks and progression to full weight bearing begins only at 12 weeks or later, to allow for enough bony interdigitation to avoid micromotion. The components are initially held rigidly to bone by being "press fit" or by the use of screws (18).

Harris and Sledge (18) asserted that after total hip arthroplasties, the 5-year clinical results with porous-coated uncemented and cemented acetabular components are equivalent. However, because of improved cementing techniques, there is less bony lysis with cemented femoral stems. Thus, more hip prostheses now include an uncemented acetabular cup with a cemented femoral components as a "hybrid" system.

Rehabilitation

Surgical procedures have been developed for diseases of the hip over many years. Girdlestone found that resection of the femoral head and neck for advanced septic arthritis of the hip provided successful pain relief and improved function in many patients (19). Hip fusion has been practiced for years, especially for granulomatous infectious diseases. The Austin Moore hemiarthroplasty prosthesis provided many successful outcomes for patients with displaced femoral neck fractures and an intact acetabula (Fig. 84-4).

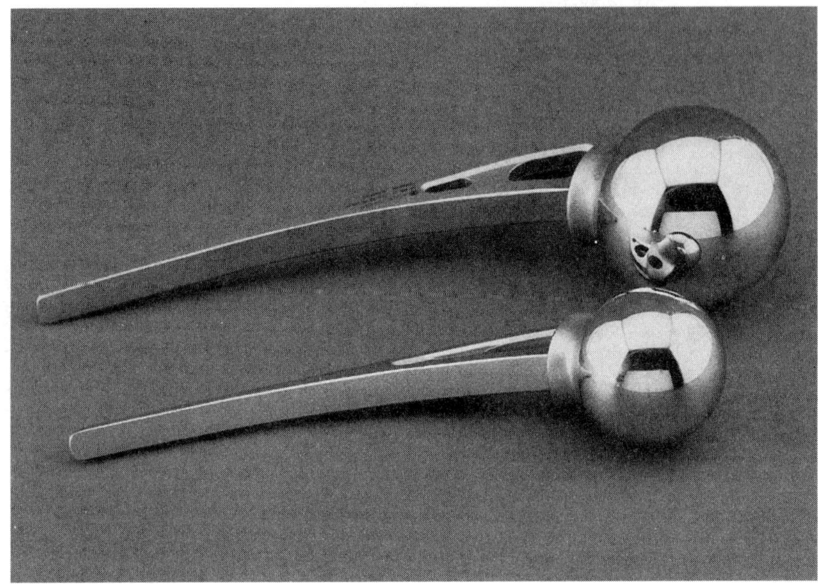

Figure 84-4. Unipolar endoprostheses used for hemiarthroplasties replace the femoral head only, not the acetabulum; the Austin Moore design is an example of this type of prosthesis. The larger head is required to fill the entire acetabulum.

Then, in 1961, Charnley (20) developed the cemented total hip arthroplasty. Various modifications of this procedure, including different surgical approaches, componentry, and modes of fixation, have added to the orthopedist's variety of techniques. Rehabilitation techniques following those procedures have been studied infrequently, however (21–23). The consensus for what constitutes medically necessary rehabilitation has varied over time and location and among procedures.

Preoperative education is helpful to prepare the patient for postoperative precautions and exercises. The consensus is to begin active physical rehabilitation on the first postoperative day with the patient being helped to sit up. Bed mobility and transfer training, if tolerated, are initiated. With cemented prostheses, weight bearing as tolerated is generally started immediately unless the quality of the bone stock was poor. With uncemented porous-coated femoral components, most orthopedists permit only minimal forces and limited weight bearing for approximately 6 to 8 weeks so bony ingrowth into the porous surface can occur. The term *non-weight bearing* should be avoided so that the patient is not led to think that he or she should lift the involved limb; this lifting may apply as much, if not more, force on the implants as does body weight (24). It is more accurate to specify "touch down weight-bearing" to obtain minimal stress across the hip. The patient should be fully weight bearing by 12 to 16 weeks. Hydroxyapatite-coated components are uncemented and the weight-bearing precautions are similar (25). The extent of weight bearing must be determined by communication with the orthopedic surgeon.

Longer, limited weight-bearing periods are required if bone grafts were used. The mean consolidation time is 4 months for morsellized cancellous grafts and 11 months for allografts that are larger than 3 cm (26).

Patients with cemented femoral components may experience pain in varying degrees initially, but usually will be able to bear weight with the aid of parallel bars or a walker. Safe walking with a walker or crutches outside the parallel bars is essential before the patient may be discharged home (27). A pair of crutches or a walker is used to regulate weight bearing during gait and for stability during standing activities. A rolling walker allows a reciprocal gait pattern in patients who are allowed full weight bearing. It also obviates the need to lift the device to advance it, which may be painful in patients with upper-extremity impairments. Also, a rolling walker requires 50% less energy than a standard walker to walk the same distance (28). However, a rolling walker is more difficult to use on carpet, particularly if the wheels are small. A standard walker is better for patients who 1) are not allowed full weight bearing, 2) cannot tolerate full weight bearing, or 3) tend to fall forward.

As balance, stability, strength, and weight-bearing tolerance improve, patients can progress to the use of a cane on the contralateral side. This allows a more rapid cadence and longer stride length and, therefore, increased gait velocity (29). It provides a wider than normal base of support and reduces the forces acting on the prosthetic femoral head at mid-stance.

Progressive active-assisted, active, and isometric exercises may be appropriate early, if begun gradually, but vigorous resistive strengthening exercises should not be performed for 2 to 3 months.

Most procedures are performed from a posterolateral surgical incision without disturbing the greater trochanter; mild isometric contractions of all hip extensors, flexors, and abductors will help such patients develop a sense of proprioception about the joint. Gentle passive and active-assisted range of motion exercises are begun immediately postoperatively to minimize joint contractions. Straight-leg raising should be avoided after use of the uncemented technique because it increases stress on the hip. A bolster may be placed under the knee or distal part of the thigh during isotonic quadriceps strengthening exercises.

Patients in whom a posterolateral approach was used must be carefully taught not to internally rotate, adduct, or flex their hips to more than 70 to 90 degrees. These motions force the head of the femur toward the weakened area of surgical exposure and capsulotomy and dislocation will more likely occur. Patients in whom an anterior or lateral approach with an anterior capsulotomy was used must avoid hyperextension as well as external rotation and adduction, especially when getting out of bed on the surgical side. Multidirectional instability, that is, the potential to dislocate in any direction, may be present when there is insufficient tension or strength in the surrounding soft tissues to keep the femoral head in the acetabular component. This may be seen following revision surgery where the exposure is wide, or when a prosthesis with a relatively short neck has been used. A lower extremity that is internally rotated and with a shortened femoral neck may lead to a posteriorly dislocating hip; a leg that is extremely externally rotated with the hip extended may lead to an anterior dislocation. If there is any question of a dislocation having occurred, an x-ray study of the hip, including an anteroposterior view and a crossed-leg lateral view (which does not require moving the affected limb between views), is mandatory.

The use of a direct lateral (Hardinge) or transtrochanteric incision with osteotomy of the greater trochanter requires that no active abduction exercises be performed.

Limited isometric contractions and gravity neutral exercise may be performed soon after surgery so that the patient can re-educate the muscles (including the gluteus medius) while undergoing ambulation. Vigorous strengthening exercises, however, cause too much stress on the components and soft tissues while healing is underway and should be avoided. There are no data to indicate whether or not vigorous strengthening exercises after 2 to 3 months contribute to the patient's strength and stability (1). However, it has been demonstrated that at 2 years there is often weakness in the hip muscles of the operated limb (30). Patients are instructed, therefore, not to walk without a cane until there is no limp present. Absence of a limp implies that the gluteus medius muscle is of sufficient strength to prevent a Trendelenburg gait upon weight bearing.

If range of motion exercises are necessary to avoid postoperative contractures, they must be limited so that dislocation does not occur. Patients are carefully warned about "hip precautions," which include reminders for those undergoing posterolateral incisions to avoid flexion, adduction, and internal rotation. ADL precautions are also taught to help the patient avoid hip dislocation. Elevated toilet seats and elevated chair seats are prescribed in order to avoid excessive hip flexion. Our patients are positioned in bed with an adductor splint or pillow between their knees to avoid excessive adduction. Postoperatively, selected patients should wear a knee immobilizer, which uses the weight of the leg to prevent flexion of the hip while supine. A small triangular cushion strapped between the knees may be used when the patient is in bed or sitting on a chair. This cushion may be preferred to the larger cushion that extends to the ankle because the larger cushion discourages movement of both legs, predisposing to heel and sacral pressure sores. It may be necessary for the patient following a revision hip arthroplasty to wear an abductor brace with an adjustable hip hinge (Newport brace) for 8 to 12 weeks, depending on the potential for dislocation (31). Patients with multidirectional instability and those with recurrent dislocations who are not suitable for revision may require a hip spica or a hip-knee-ankle-foot orthosis to control rotation as well as to allow a safe arc of hip motion.

Patients are cautioned to avoid adduction and internal rotation when rolling over in bed and getting in and out of bed. Although dislocations are uncommon, an incidence of approximately 3%, they usually occur early in the postoperative period. Dislocation precautions should however be observed for *at least* 8 to 12 weeks. Conditions frequently associated with dislocation are the use of a small femoral prosthetic head, previous surgery, use of a posterior rather than an anterolateral approach, component malposition, osteotomy of the greater trochanter, and use of a short femoral component (32–36). In addition, our experience suggests that organic brain disease or postoperative delirium is also associated with more frequent dislocations. If the acetabular component is too vertical, or too far in either anteversion or retroversion, dislocation is more likely. Large osteophytes may act as "levers" for the femoral component to impinge on and dislocate.

Studies of the efficacy of physical and occupational therapies have had mixed results. Occupational therapists are involved in teaching the patient how to avoid dislocation and how to perform essential ADLs by proper body positioning and the use of adaptive devices such as reachers and sock aids. Though it has been demonstrated that individual occupational therapy is essential to inculcate the principles of "hip precautions," group occupational therapy may well have a role and is more cost-effective (37).

Johnsson et al (38) failed to demonstrate whether organized PT after total hip arthroplasty could achieve greater functional results. Their study is flawed, however, in that so little PT was applied, it is not likely there would have been any difference.

Even when the patient is able to walk safely with a walker or crutches and has *demonstrated* a knowledge of "hip precautions," further training and advice are essential for other ADLs. Many patients will want to know just how vigorously they can stress their surgical result or "new hip." Kilgus et al (39) demonstrated that patients who were more active and performed "high-impact" activities in both sports and labor after hip arthroplasty performed for osteoarthritis had a greater incidence and an earlier need for revision. A survey of Mayo Clinic orthopedic surgeons and trainees provided a consensus tabulation listing surgeons' opinions regarding participation in sporting activities in patients after both hip and knee arthroplasties (40). Activities with relatively low impact and stress, including scuba diving, sailing, bowling, cycling, swimming, and golfing, were recommended by most surgeons. Several activities, including singles tennis, downhill skiing, doubles tennis, backpacking, and cross-country skiing, received an intermediate rating. More vigorous activities, including handball, racquet ball, jogging, hockey, water skiing, basketball, football, and baseball, were not recommended. While the success of participation in sporting activities will vary with the strength and skill of each individual, it should be the duty of the physiatrist to inform patients that clearly vigorous, high-impact use will hasten the necessity of revision of the procedure. There is just no way that a hip prosthesis can tolerate the wear and tear of vigorous activities the way a normal hip does (41).

Many patients will wish to know when they can resume driving an automobile. Macdonald and Owen (42) assessed the driving reaction speed of 25 patients compared to 15 normal patients before and after total hip arthroplasty. Arthroplasty patients took from 8 weeks to 8 months following surgery to recover normal reaction time on the side of the operation. If based solely on recovery of driver reaction times, the earliest that driving should be allowed is 8 weeks postoperatively. However, many surgeons, as a matter of personal preference, suggest waiting for the period of dislocation precautions (i.e., 8–12 weeks) before allowing their patients to drive. A practical rule may well be that patients cleared to ride in a car can be told to practice driving with a companion in a safe situation (such as a parking lot). If they feel they are successful, they should then obtain written consent from their auto insurance company or appropriate legal clearance before driving on public roads. In this way, both a functional trial will occur and the patient will have the full financial backing of his or her insurance carrier.

Sexual function following hip arthroplasty may be of interest to many patients. Stern et al (43) obtained information by questionnaire on patients' sexual activities. Inpatients felt that preoperative sexual difficulties were relieved following surgery. Sociologic data regarding sexual dysfunction, however, were not obtained. It is well known that up to 50% of normal patients complain of various sexual dysfunctions and these may well not be affected by hip arthroplasty (44). The highest preference of the postoperative subjects in Stern's study was for the position during sex to be supine. An alternative preference was the prone position for male patients and the side-lying position for female patients. Many requested a pamphlet regarding information, and so it can be presumed that many patients who might not otherwise request information would like to have it.

Complications

Physiatrists must be aware of the complications that occur in the postoperative period. Pai (45) described 264 primary arthroplasty procedures performed for osteoarthritis and found a 5% incidence of severe heterotopic ossification and a 42% prevalence of an insignificant amount. It has been noted that osteotomy of the trochanter is associated with a larger amount (46). Patients with previous occurrence of ectopic bone and ankylosing spondylitis have a more likely chance of severe ossification (32,35,47). Use of nonsteroidal anti-inflammatory agents and irradiation diminishes the amount and severity of postoperative heterotopic bone (47). Postoperative range of motion exercises should neither be eliminated nor decreased in intensity in the setting of heterotopic bone.

Nerve injury following hip arthroplasty has been well described by Nercessian et al (48). They reviewed total hip procedures performed from 1976 to 1989 at the New York Orthopedic Hospital and found an incidence of 0.63% of peripheral neuropathic injury. Such injury occurred more frequently with revision surgery, and there were 34 injuries in the leg (0.48%) and 11 injuries in the arms (0.64%). The common peroneal nerve in the leg and the ulnar nerve in the arm were the most commonly injured. Nerves in the lower extremity included the common peroneal (both ipsilaterally and contralaterally), femoral, obturator, and lateral femoral cutaneous. Upper-extremity injuries occurred to the brachial plexus and ulnar, axillary, and median nerves. Upper-extremity nerves recovered to a greater degree than did those in the lower extremity. Lower nerve injuries were not clearly related to leg lengthening, but were more common following procedures involving more than 2.0 cm of leg lengthening. Physiatrists must carefully examine the patient for evidence of sciatic nerve dysfunction also. In addition to stretching, compartment syndrome or hematomas may cause nerve dysfunction that requires urgent intervention.

A serious concern following arthroplasty is the development of significant deep venous thrombosis (49). Most authors recommend prophylactic anticoagulation following surgery. Warfarin or low-molecular-weight heparin may be given. Low-molecular-weight heparin has the advantage of not requiring any laboratory monitoring (50). The use of support hose or sequential compression devices by themselves is of questionable benefit, but they may be reasonable adjuncts for higher-risk patients and those unable to tolerate prophylactic anticoagulation (51). A recent meta-analysis by Imperiale and Speroff (52) suggested that low-molecular-weight heparin with compression stockings has the greatest relative efficacy in preventing venous thromboembolism following total hip replacement. There is no evidence at this time to show the benefit of continuing prophylaxis after hospital discharge (51). Even when anticoagulants are administered, the occurrence of persistent thigh swelling or calf swelling, without pain and inflammation, requires that ultrasound Doppler sonography be performed. Some physicians may wish to wrap the leg in a figure-eight technique with Ace bandages to diminish swelling.

Physiatrists should also watch for signs of superficial wound infections. The signs are persistent drainage, increased heat, redness of the wound area, induration, swelling, and pain. Superficial infections should be treated promptly with antibiotics in conjunction with the orthopedist and if necessary, an infectious disease consultant. Specimens for a Gram stain and culture should be obtained from any drainage and possibly the joint itself, especially when there are concomitant signs of infection. Infections elsewhere should also be treated aggressively because of the possibility of hematogenous seeding of the operative area. "Stitch abscesses" generally resolve after suture or staple removal.

Postoperative pain usually subsides gradually over several weeks. When pain persists, the physician should evaluate the patient closely. Pain after more than 5 or 6 days or any acute onset of pain should prompt an x-ray study, including anteroposterior and cross-leg lateral views. Patients should be evaluated for dislocation by estimating leg length, hip motion, and position of the foot and by x-ray study. Hip pain following exercise, but not with weight bearing or heel percussion, is probably from soft-tissue stretching and should not prompt discontinuation of therapy. Sometimes no cause for pain will be found.

Leg-length discrepancies occur commonly following arthroplasty (53). However, this may be of no concern to the patient if there is no pain or disequilibrium. In a study of 68 patients at a minimum of 2 years postoperatively (mean, 6.6 years), 22 (32%) were aware of a leg-length discrepancy. Those aware of the discrepancy had a mean discrepancy of 14.9 mm compared to 9.7 mm in those who were not aware. Of those aware of their discrepancy, 16 of the 22 were annoyed. Some leg-length discrepancies postoperatively are due to tightening of soft tissues and not true leg-length discrepancies and should not be corrected immediately. Annoying discrepancies may be corrected by having the patient walk with temporary cork soles of varying thickness taped to the shoe of the shorter limb. From this maneuver, the physician can estimate which height causes an improved subjective sense of well-being.

Rehabilitation patients who have undergone revision arthroplasty of a previously fused joint (arthrodesis) should be offered active muscle instruction, perhaps with biofeedback and functional electrical stimulation (FES), to activate the long unused muscles (54). This has been successful many times, but requires an alert participating patient. Martin et al (55) demonstrated an increase in the cross section and frequency of type II muscle fibers with FES 1 week following knee arthroplasty. The complication rate following revision is greatly increased (2).

Numerous scales have been developed to evaluate the outcome of hip arthroplasty surgery (56,57).

TOTAL KNEE ARTHROPLASTY

In the past, total knee arthroplasty has not been associated with as great success as total hip arthroplasty. However, longer and longer successful functional outcomes are being achieved. Initially, hemicompartmental and unicompartmental and constrained total knee replacements were performed (Fig. 84-5), but subsequently, unconstrained total knee arthroplasty has been found to be more effective (Fig. 84-6). Mintor and Door (58) demonstrated that *bilateral* total knee replacement is safe and followed by no greater functional deficits than *unilateral* knee arthroplasty. A meta-analysis revealed excellent outcomes following total knee arthroplasties in a very great number of patients (59). Rating scores improved 100%, and 89.3% of patients reported good or excellent outcomes.

Rehabilitation

The initial concern for the physiatrist is to determine how much weight the postoperative knee can bear. Ordinarily, all patients with cemented total knee prostheses, including those with uncemented femoral components with good bone stock, may undergo weight bearing as tolerated beginning on the first postoperative day. If there has been repair of a quadriceps tendon rupture, collateral ligament

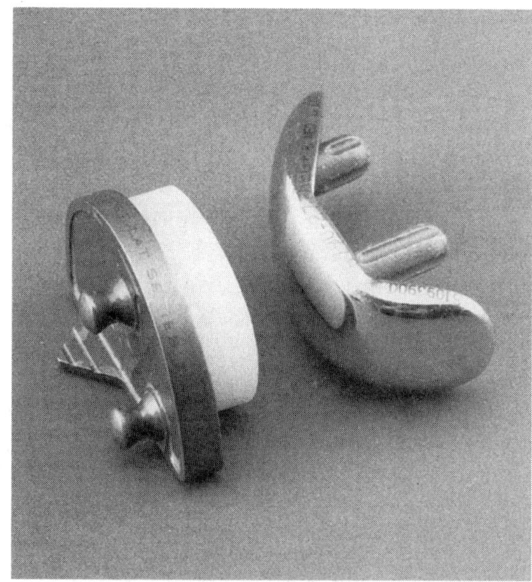

Figure 84-5. A unicompartmental total knee prosthesis replaces both the femoral and the tibial sides of the knee joint but *only* on the lateral or medial aspect. These particular components have short femoral and tibial stems.

Figure 84-6. Total knee arthroplasty replaces the femoral and tibial sides of the joint. They may have a short (*A*) or long stem (*B*).

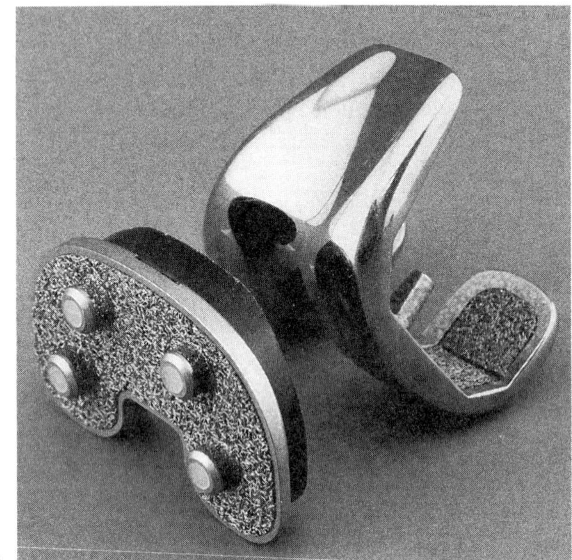

A

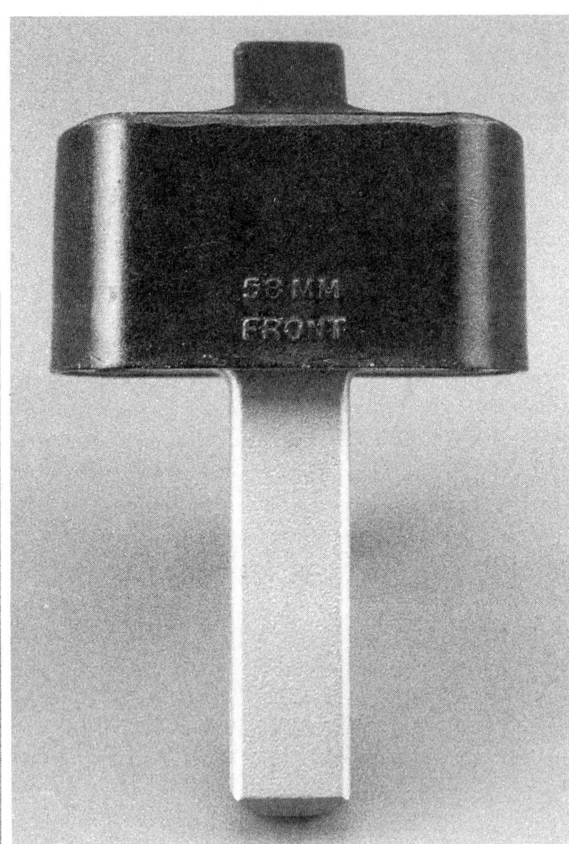

B

repair, or placement of bone grafts during revision surgery, full weight bearing must be delayed for 2 to 4 months.

The most common problems in rehabilitation of the total knee arthroplasty are pain with flexion and an extensor lag. On the first postoperative day, patients start active extension, while the therapist initiates passive flexion. Passive flexion must be performed in a controlled manner by the therapist, as partial quadriceps tendon rupture may occur. Flexion must also be limited following repair of a rupture of the quadriceps tendon or a collateral ligament. Cognitively intact patients may be trained to do the following exercise between therapy sessions: The ipsilateral foot is planted to the floor while the patient gently propels his or her wheelchair forward with the arms, causing passive knee flexion (for about two to three breaths' duration or 6–10 seconds). Then the patient actively raises the leg, extending the knee as much as tolerated, and this position is held for about 6 seconds. This cycle is repeated as often as the patient can tolerate. We have informally observed that these exercises give patients a sense of responsibility and investment in their rehabilitation and a more active participation in their therapies.

Patients must be encouraged to understand that the pain they are undergoing during exercise will in the long run allow them a straight, pain-free, quite flexible knee. Active quadriceps strengthening is initially difficult due to a painful inhibiting reflex. FES or biofeedback may increase the patient's ability to contract the painful muscle (54,55). However, vigorous strengthening isometric or resistive exercises should be delayed for 2 to 3 months, owing to excessive tension produced on the soft tissues. Ice is often applied after both strengthening and range of motion exercises. This reduces pain and swelling (60).

The use of a continuous passive motion (CPM) machine postoperatively is controversial. There have been numerous studies. Walker et al (61) demonstrated that CPM treatment slightly diminished knee pain but did not change the length of hospital stay. McInnes et al (62) demonstrated that CPM treatment did not decrease the pain or length of stay but was followed by a more rapid increase in flexion and a decrease in the necessity for postoperative manipulation, thus reducing the cost. Johnson and Eastwood (63) demonstrated that CPM treatment for 16 to 20 hours each day increased knee flexion and diminished the length of stay. Nadler et al (64) demonstrated that CPM treatment for 3 to 4 hours each day did not decrease the length of stay or pain or improve flexion after unilateral knee replacement, but there was a trend toward improvement if patients had undergone bilateral total knee arthroplasty. Wasilewski et al (65) demonstrated that CPM treatment 24 hours daily with the exception of toileting and exercise periods decreased wound infections, decreased analgesic use, decreased length of stay, and increased the rapidity of knee flexion. Maloney et al (66) demonstrated that 24-hour daily CPM treatment diminished length of stay and the incidence of pulmonary emboli, but there were a few more infections. It seems reasonable, therefore, to assume that the duration of CPM treatment should be as long as possible and that even 10 to 12 hours a day, if tolerated, is required to achieve better results. In our experience, most patients will not tolerate CPM treatment during the night. A compromise, therefore, is that as much CPM treatment as possible should be provided, and that a diminished length of stay and more rapid flexion may be achieved. Ultrasound diathermy applied over the quadriceps muscles may benefit patients who have difficulty gaining adequate range of flexion.

The use of walkers or crutches immediately following hip arthroplasties is common practice. Frequently the orthopedist recommends that patients maintain the use of a cane or crutches until no limp is present without one. Often, however, following *knee* surgery patients are able to use a cane alone. A four-patient study by Edwards (67) demonstrated that mean peak vertical floor reaction forces recorded with a foot transducer were greater with use of an ipsilateral cane than a contralateral cane, suggesting a cane in the contralateral hand will provide greater relief of weight bearing.

There have been no studies of sexual activity or dysfunction following total knee arthroplasty. Patients should be encouraged to resume presurgery activity *as tolerated* as soon as discharged home.

Participation in sports was well documented by the survey of McGrory et al (40). It was the consensus of their questionnaire of orthopedic surgeons that golfing, swimming, cycling, sailing, bowling, scuba diving, and cross-country skiing may be recommended as exercise activities, while handball, racquetball, hockey, water skiing, karate, soccer, baseball, running, basketball, and football are not recommended. Both doubles and singles tennis received an intermediate recommendation, as did volleyball, alpine skiing, ballet, and ice skating. Again, the surgeon, the physiatrist, and the patient must carefully weigh the effect of vigorous sports or vocational activities on the patient after a successful arthroplasty.

Driver reaction times have been studied following total knee arthroplasty. Spalding et al (68) demonstrated that it took 8 weeks for the patient's reaction time to return to normal following a right total knee arthroplasty. As with total hip arthroplasties, it is our recommendation that the patient attempt to measure his or her own functional capacity and then if the patient feels competent, obtain written approval from his or her auto insurance company.

Fast et al (69) presented a case and reviewed the literature for patients with Parkinson disease undergoing total knee arthroplasty. The conclusion from this small population is that patients who have Parkinson disease should be monitored carefully for achieving maximal medical treatment, and then undergo arthroplasty. In our experience, many Parkinson patients achieve successful outcomes following knee arthroplasty when treated in an intensive rehabilitation unit.

Complications

Ayers et al (70) published a splendid review of the common complications following total knee arthroplasty. They noted that the occurrence of perineal palsy is rare. Possible mechanisms of perineal palsy include ischemia due to stretching or direct compression. The factors associated with this complication are a preoperative flexion contracture or valgum deformity of more than 20 degrees. Treatment is directed at loosening the dressings and flexing the knee to 20 to 30 degrees. Surgical exploration should be limited to patients with good evidence of direct compression from a hematoma.

Direct injury to vessels may also occur, and palpation of pulses at the knee and the popliteal fossa for swelling or a decrease in force may demonstrate the need for further immediate vascular studies.

Reflex sympathetic dystrophy is rare. In our one patient in whom reflex sympathetic dystrophy developed (unpublished data), it was due to a lack of ability to flex the knee fully because of inappropriately sized components. Sympathetic blocks were successful in relieving the pain, and revision arthroplasty resulted in an increased range of motion with no extensor lag and 90 degrees of flexion.

Fractures also occur just proximal to total knee prosthesis. Any sudden and severe increase in pain during rehabilitation requires x-ray investigation. Anteroposterior and lateral views will show the full extent of the prosthetic components, including bone cement, as well as the surrounding bones. The patella should be carefully examined on the lateral view for signs of a fracture.

The postoperative occurrence of a deep infection is limited to about 2% of cases or less (70). Deep infection is more often associated with the use of constrained prostheses, previous surgery, open skin lesions, and rheumatoid arthritis. We suggest that the recommendations of the American Heart Association be followed during dental extractions in patients who have total joint arthroplasties. These recommendations were recently updated by an expert panel of the American Dental Association/American Academy of Orthopaedic Surgeons (71).

The diagnosis of a deep infection must be obtained by aspiration under surgically sterile conditions. Antibiotic treatment should be based on sensitivities. The removal or retention of the prosthesis subsequently depends on the overall assessment of the present and future function and health of each patient.

As with hip arthroplasties, the presence of tenderness, redness, induration, and discharge suggest infection. The physician should start antibiotics immediately in consultation with the orthopedic surgeon and if necessary, infectious disease consultant. Symptoms of infection need to be differentiated from simple irritation from exercise or CPM. The use of CPM may be irritating to a joint that is still undergoing postoperative inflammation. Although there may be warmth and redness, the hyperemia blanches and there is no significant induration; also the tenderness is minimal compared to the findings in cellulitis.

Dehiscence of the wound during rehabilitation can occur. Wound damage may be minor and inconsequential or an indication of deep infection. Conservative treatment or resuturing should be performed. Because the knee is a superficial joint with a potential for infection, any drainage material should be sent for culture and Gram stain, and if results are significant, then the physician should prescribe appropriate antibiotics. Only then can the patient resume minimal and carefully monitored motion.

We have seen a partial rupture of the quadriceps tendon during passive flexion exercises (unpublished case). Ace wrap stabilization resulted in healing.

Obesity was demonstrated not to have many adverse effects on patients undergoing total knee arthroplasty (72). A longer operative time was demonstrated, and the knee strength preoperatively was stronger. There were no other unusual complications.

The occurrence of deep venous thrombosis following total knee arthroplasty is quite high, but the occurrence of pulmonary embolism is quite low. Deep venous thrombosis in postoperative patients is usually confined to the calf. CPM machines have neither reduced nor increased the rate of deep venous thrombosis. Anticoagulation prophylaxis is appropriate, but so especially are the use of calf-high compression sleeves and a plantar impulse pad. The duration of prophylaxis or postoperative surveillance is not clear at this time, but it should be continued for days to weeks.

There are also problems associated with the extensor mechanism. The replaced patella may be unstable, it may fracture, or there may be loosening or "failure" of the component. There may be a patellar "klunk" or tendon rupture. Orthopedic consultation must be obtained when postoperative pain seems associated with the patella. Conservative treatment consists of quadriceps exercises, but tibial tubercle osteotomy or lateral retinacular release may be required.

Preventive Measures

Postoperatively, if the patient is slow achieving 90 degrees of flexion, surgical manipulation under anesthesia is sometimes performed. Some surgeons may do this if flexion of 90 degrees has not been achieved by 10 days. Others may temporize longer before considering manipulation.

The prophylaxis of deep venous thrombosis following total knee arthroplasty is also important. A study by Khaw et al (73) demonstrated that the incidence of fatal pulmonary embolism in 499 consecutive patients having 527 knee replacements—all of whom wore antithrombotic stockings only—was 0.19%. The investigators wondered if anticoagulation was necessary at all in this group of patients. A study by Faunø et al (74) of 185 patients following knee arthroplasty revealed deep venous thrombosis in 27% who received unfractionated heparin and in 23% who received low-molecular-weight heparin. There were no pulmonary emboli demonstrated on ventilation-perfusion scans. Orthopedists currently often prescribe low-molecular-weight heparin for 2 weeks postoperatively or warfarin anticoagulation for at least 4 to 6 weeks after surgery.

SHOULDER ARTHROPLASTY

Neer (75) is intimately associated with the development of the humeral head replacement arthroplasty. This procedure was developed at the Lennox Hill Hospital in New York City and characterized in large part by the surgeon's prolonged involvement in postoperative care.

The prosthesis may replace only the humeral head or both the head and the glenoid fossa surface. Modular systems provide the surgeon with the ability to match patient characteristics (Fig. 84-7).

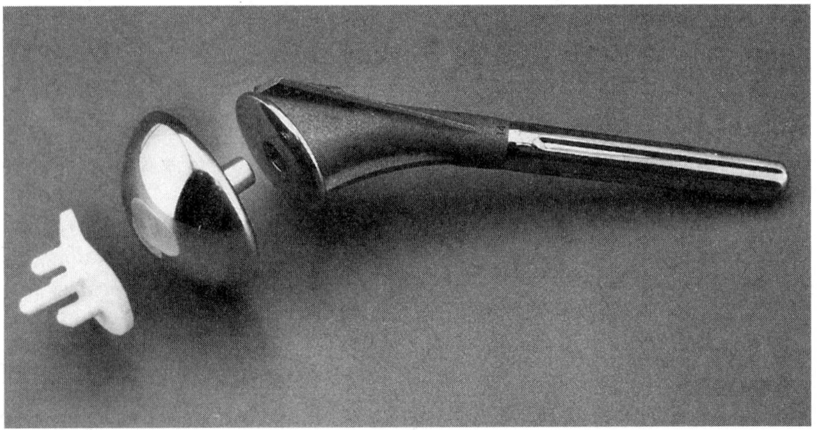

Figure 84-7. Shoulder arthroplasty components are preordered as one device consisting of the humeral head and shaft or as a modular system with multiple head and shaft sizes, as illustrated here. The glenoid is either replaced or left alone, depending on the integrity of the cartilaginous surface.

Cofield et al (76) recently described satisfactory relief of pain in 44 (66%) and improvement in 52 (78%) of 67 shoulders undergoing humeral head replacement for rheumatoid arthritis or osteoarthritis at 9.3 years. Deep infection occurs in less than 0.5% of patients (77) and loosening is common (50%) but requires revision in only 10% at 10 years (78). Noble and Bell (79) reviewed the causes of failure of total shoulder arthroplasty in detail. These include technical error, instability, rotator cuff tears, heterotopic ossification, loosening, modular component dislocation, sepsis, humeral fracture, and nerve injuries. Fewer complications have occurred with prostheses designed to have less constraint.

Rehabilitation

Even as recently as 1988, stability was more important than motion, and rehabilitation exercises were not begun for days to weeks following surgery (80,81). More recently, however, opinion has shifted, and rehabilitation is recommended to begin on the first postoperative day (82).

No human joint has so varied and complex a series of motions as the shoulder joint. Perhaps that is why postoperative rehabilitation requires such care and attention to detail. Brems (82) and Maybach and Schlegel (83) recommended preoperative strategy sessions between physicians, therapists, and patients, and then postoperative rehabilitation beginning the same day or the day following surgery. Recovery and healing of soft tissue is encouraged by resting, lack of motion, and careful avoidance of overstretching or overexercising the shoulder soft tissue. The only muscle divided for the current total shoulder arthroplasty procedure is the subscapularis; therefore, exercises can begin promptly.

Postoperatively, patients are placed in a compression dressing, and on the second postoperative day, after administration of analgesics, moist heat, or both, *several short* periods of stretching are begun. The patient is assisted in elevation and external rotation until reaching approximately 140 degrees of elevation (flexion) and 40 degrees of external rotation. This comprises phase I. Passive abduction may also be employed in phase I. If the rotator cuff has been damaged, patients may not proceed to phase II for 4 to 8 weeks (83).

Phase II usually begins at 10 to 14 days and active-assisted internal rotation exercises are started. It continues with active patient participation until 160 degrees of elevation and 60 degrees of external rotation are achieved. Isometric exercises, assistive exercises, and pulley exercises under supervision may all be employed during phase II.

Phase III begins anywhere from 3 to 6 weeks later. It begins with minimal weights, which are not changed until the patient can perform 10 repetitions. Phase III strengthening usually uses Therabands. The muscles to be strengthened include the anterior and posterior deltoids, and internal and external rotators. After 3 months, strengthening of the trapezius, rhomboid, latissimus dorsi, and pectoral muscles begins. A major consideration for treatment after shoulder arthroplasty is that passive and active range of motion exercises be performed during shorter but more frequent sessions, such as 5-minute sessions five times a day, to minimize shoulder stiffness.

The use of CPM machines after shoulder arthroplasty has not been universally successful and is controversial at this time.

Complications

Cofield et al (76) reported three complications: brachial plexus stretch, fracture of the humerus, and hematomas. Romeo (77) reported rotator cuff tear, instability, heterotopic ossification, glenoid component loosening, intraoperative fracture, nerve injury, infection, and humeral component loosening in decreasing order of frequency. Lack of motion may be caused by a humeral head that is too large, "overstuffing" the joint space.

Infection should be suspected and treated as described for hip and knee arthroplasty. Deep venous thrombosis appears not to be a problem. Heterotopic bone formation has not been reported.

ACKNOWLEDGMENT

We wish to acknowledge review of this manuscript by Dr. Joshua Jacobs, MD, Department of Orthopedic Surgery, Rush Medical Center, Chicago.

REFERENCES

1. NIH Consensus Conference. Total hip replacement. *JAMA* 1995;273:1950–1956.
2. Galante JO, Rosenberg AG, Callaghan JJ. *Total hip revision surgery.* New York: Raven, 1995:13.
3. Charnley J. Total hip replacement. *JAMA* 1974;230:1025.
4. Kavanaugh BF, Hassen AD, Coventry MB. Cemented hip replacement results. In: Morrey BF, ed. *Joint replacement arthroplasty.* New York: Churchill Livingstone, 1991: 639–646.
5. Martell JM, Pierson RH, Jacobs JJ, et al. Primary total hip reconstruction with a titanium fiber-coated prosthesis inserted without cement. *J Bone Joint Surg [Am]* 1993;75:554–571.
6. Salvati EA, Wilson PD, Jolley MN, et al. A ten-year follow-up study of our first one hundred consecutive Charnley total hip replacements. *J Bone Joint Surg [Am]* 1981;63: 753–767.
7. Scott WW Jr, Riley LH Jr, Dorfman HD. Focal lytic lesions associated

with femoral stem loosening in total hip prosthesis. *AJR* 1985;144:977–982.

8. Bayley KB, London MR, Grunkemeier GL, Lansky DJ. Measuring the success of treatment in patient terms. *Med Care* 1995;33:AS226–AS235.

9. Rissanen P, Aro S, Slätis P, et al. Health and quality of life before and after hip or knee arthroplasty. *J Arthroplasty* 1995;10:169–175.

10. Kirwan JR, Currey HL, Freeman MA, et al. Overall long-term impact of total hip and knee joint replacement surgery on patients with osteoarthritis and rheumatoid arthritis. *Br J Rheumatol* 1994;33:357–360.

11. Schulte KR, Callaghan JJ, Kelley SS, Johnston RC. The outcome of Charnley total hip arthroplasty with cement after a minimum twenty-year follow-up. *J Bone Joint Surg [Am]* 1993;75:961–975.

12. Zavadak KH, Gibson KR, Whitley DM, et al. Variability in the attainment of functional milestones during the acute care admission after total joint replacement. *J Rheumatol* 1995;22: 482–487.

13. Munin MC, Kwoh CK, Glynn N, et al. Predicting discharge outcome after elective hip and knee arthroplasty. *Am J Phys Med Rehabil* 1995;74:294–301.

14. Tooms RE, Harkess JW. Arthroplasty, introduction and overview. In: Crenshaw AH, ed. *Campbell's operative orthopedics.* Vol. 1. 8th ed. St. Louis: Mosby–Year Book, 1992:371–387.

15. Stauffer RN. Ten-year follow-up study of total hip replacement. *J Bone Joint Surg [Am]* 1982;64:983–990.

16. Sutherland CJ, Wilde AH, Border LS, et al. A ten-year follow up of one hundred consecutive Muller curved-stem total hip replacement arthroplasties. *J Bone Joint Surg [Am]* 1982;64:970–982.

17. Harris WH. The case for cementing all femoral components in total hip replacement. *Can J Surg* 1995;38(suppl 1):S55–S60.

18. Harris WH, Sledge CB. Total hip and total knee replacement. *N Engl J Med* 1990;323:725–731.

19. Ballard WT, Lowry DA, Brand RA. Resection arthroplasty of the hip. *J Arthroplasty* 1995;10:772–779.

20. Charnley J. Arthroplasty of the hip: a new operation. *Lancet* 1961;1:1129.

21. Garden FH. Rehabilitation following total hip arthroplasty. *J Back Musculoskel Rehabil* 1994;4: 185–192.

22. Foster RR, Khalifa S. Total knee replacement rehabilitation. *Sports Med Arthrosc Rev* 1996;4:83–91.

23. Nicholas JJ, Rosenberg AN. Arthritis and arthroplasties. In: Felsenthal G, Garrison SJ, Steinberg FU, eds. *Rehabilitation of the aging and elderly patient.* Baltimore: Williams & Wilkins, 1994:97–106.

24. Davy DT, Kotzar GM, Brown RH, et al. Telemetric force measurements across the hip after total arthroplasty. *J Bone Joint Surg [Am]* 1988;70:45–50.

25. Geesink RG, Hoefnagels NH. Six-year results of hydroxyapatite-coated total hip replacement. *J Bone Joint Surg [Br]* 1995;77:534–547.

26. Valenti JR, Leyes M, Schweitzer D. Allograft in revision total hip arthroplasty. Orthopedic proceedings. *J Bone Joint Surg [Br]* 1995;77(suppl II):165.

27. Haddad RJ, Cook SD, Thomas KA. Biological fixation of porous-coated implants. *J Bone Joint Surg [Am]* 1987;69:1459–1466.

28. Hamzeh MA, Bowker P, Sayegh A. The energy costs of ambulation using two types of walking frame. *Clin Rehabil* 1988;2:119.

29. Edwards BG. Contralateral and ipsilateral cane usage by patients with total knee or hip replacement. *Arch Phys Med Rehabil* 1986;67:734–740.

30. Loizeau J, Allard P, Eng P, et al. Bilateral gait patterns in subjects fitted with a total hip prosthesis. *Arch Phys Med Rehabil* 1995;76:552–557.

31. Lima D, Magnus R, Paprosky W. Team management of hip revision patients using a post-op hip orthosis. *J Prosth Orth* 1994;6: 20–24.

32. Beabout JW. Radiology of total hip arthroplasty. *Radiol Clin North Am* 1975;13:3–19.

33. Brien WW, Salvati EA, Wright TM, et al. Dissociation of acetabular components after total hip arthroplasty. Report of six cases. *J Bone Joint Surg [Am]* 1990;72: 1548–1550.

34. Coventry MB. Late dislocations in patients with Charnley total hip arthroplasty. *J Bone Joint Surg [Am]* 1985;67:832–841.

35. Morrey BF. Short stemmed uncemented femoral replacement component. In: *Joint replacement arthroplasty.* New York: Churchill Livingstone, 1991:667–672.

36. Wilson AJ, Monsees B, Blair VP III. Acetabular cup dislocation: a new complication of total joint arthroplasty. *AJR* 1988;151: 133–134.

37. Trahey PJ. A comparison of the cost-effectiveness of two types of occupational therapy services. *Am J Occup Ther* 1991;45:397–400.

38. Johnsson R, Melander A, Onnerfält R. Physiotherapy after total hip replacement for primary arthrosis. *Scand J Rehabil Med* 1988;20:43–45.

39. Kilgus DJ, Dorey FJ, Finerman GA, Amstutz HC. Patient activity, sports participation, and impact loading on the durability of cemented total hip replacements. *Clin Orthop* 1991;269:25–31.

40. McGrory BJ, Stuart MJ, Sim FH. Participation in sports after hip and knee arthroplasty: review of literature and survey of surgeon preferences. *Mayo Clin Proc* 1995;70:342–348.

41. Feller JA, Kay PR, Hodgkinson JP, Wroblewski BM. Activity and socket wear in the Charnley low-friction arthroplasty. *J Arthroplasty* 1994;9:341–345.

42. Macdonald W, Owen JW. The effect of total hip replacement on

driving reactions. *J Bone Joint Surg [Br]* 1988;70:202–205.

43. Stern SH, Fuchs MD, Ganz SB, et al. Sexual function after total hip arthroplasty. *Clin Orthop* 1991;269:228–235.

44. Frank E, Anderson C, Rubinstein D. Frequency of sexual dysfunction in "normal" couples. *N Engl J Med* 1978;299:111–115.

45. Pai VS. Heterotopic ossification in total hip arthroplasty. The influence of the approach. *J Arthroplasty* 1994;9:199–202.

46. Puzas JE, Reynolds PR. Basic science concepts related to the formation of heterotopic bone after total hip arthroplasty. *Semin Arthroplasty* 1996;7:3–11.

47. Seegenschmiedt MH, Goldmann AR, Martus P, et al. Prophylactic radiation therapy for prevention of heterotopic ossification after hip arthroplasty: results in 141 high-risk hips. *Radiology* 1993;188: 257–264.

48. Nercessian OA, Macaulay W, Stinchfield FE. Peripheral neuropathies following total hip arthroplasty. *J Arthroplasty* 1994;9: 645–651.

49. Warwick D, Williams MH, Bannister GC. Death and thromboembolic disease after total hip replacement: a series of 1162 cases with no routine chemical prophylaxis. *J Bone Joint Surg [Br]* 1995;77: 6–10.

50. Menzin J, Colditz GA, Regan MM, et al. Cost-effectiveness of enoxaparin vs low-dose warfarin in the prevention of deep vein thrombosis after total hip replacement surgery. *Arch Intern Med* 1995;155: 757–764.

51. Mohr EN, Silverstein MD, Ilstrup DM, et al. Venous thromboembolism associated with hip and knee arthroplasty: current prophylactic practices and outcomes. *Mayo Clin Proc* 1992;67: 861–870.

52. Imperiale TF, Speroff T. A meta-analysis of methods to prevent venous thromboembolism following total hip replacement. *JAMA* 1994;271:1780–1785.

53. Edeen J, Sharkey PF, Alexander AH. Clinical significance of leg-length inequality after total hip arthroplasty. *Am J Orthop* 1995;24:347–351.

54. Gotlin RS, Hershkowitz S, Juris PM, et al. Electrical stimulation effect on extensor lag and length of hospital stay after total knee arthroplasty. *Arch Phys Med Rehabil* 1994;75:957–959.

55. Martin TP, Gundersen LA, Blevins FT, Coutts RD. The influence of functional electrical stimulation on the properties of vastus lateralis fibres following total knee arthroplasty. *Scand J Rehabil Med* 1991;23:207–210.

56. Johanson NA, Charlson ME, Szatrowski TP, Ranawat CS. A self-administered hip-rating questionnaire for the assessment of outcome after total hip replacement. *J Bone Joint Surg [Am]* 1992;74:587–597.

57. Liang MH, Katz JN, Phillips C, et al. The total hip arthroplasty outcome evaluation form of the American Academy of Orthopaedic Surgeons. Results of a nominal group process. *J Bone Joint Surg [Am]* 1991;73:639–646.

58. Minter JE, Dorr LD. Indications for bilateral total knee replacement. *Contemp Orthop* 1995;31:108–111.

59. Callahan CM, Drake BG, Heck DA, Dittus RS. Patient outcomes following tricompartmental total knee replacement. A meta-analysis. *JAMA* 1994;271:1349–1357.

60. Ivey M, Johnston RV, Uchida T. Cryotherapy for postoperative pain relief following knee arthroplasty. *J Arthroplasty* 1994;9:285–290.

61. Walker RH, Morris BA, Angulo DL, et al. Postoperative use of continuous passive motion, transcutaneous electrical nerve stimulation, and continuous cooling pad following total knee arthroplasty. *J Arthroplasty* 1991;6:151–156.

62. McInnes J, Larson MG, Daltroy LH, et al. A controlled evaluation of continuous passive motion in patients undergoing total knee arthroplasty. *JAMA* 1992; 268:1423–1428.

63. Johnson DP, Eastwood DM. Beneficial effects of continuous passive motion after total condylar knee arthroplasty. *Ann R Coll Surg Engl* 1992;74:412–416.

64. Nadler SF, Malanga GA, Zimmerman JR. Continuous passive motion in the rehabilitation setting. A retrospective study. *Am J Phys Med Rehabil* 1993;72: 162–165.

65. Wasilewski SA, Woods LC, Torgerson WR, Healy WL. Value of continuous passive motion in total knee arthroplasty. *Orthopedics* 1990;13:291–295.

66. Maloney WJ, Schurman DJ, Hangen D, et al. The influence of continuous passive motion on outcome in total knee arthroplasty. *Clin Orthop* 1990;256: 162–168.

67. Edwards BG. Contralateral and ipsilateral cane usage by patients with total knee or hip replacement. *Arch Phys Med Rehabil* 1986;67: 734–740.

68. Spalding TJ, Kiss J, Kyberd P, et al. Driver reaction times after total knee replacement. *J Bone Joint Surg [Br]* 1994;76:754–756.

69. Fast A, Mendelsohn E, Sosner J. Total knee arthroplasty in Parkinson's disease. *Arch Phys Med Rehabil* 1994;75: 1269–1270.

70. Ayers DC, Dennis DA, Johanson NA, Pelligrini VD Jr. Common complications of total knee arthroplasty. *J Bone Joint Surg [Am]* 1997;79:278–311.

71. American Dental Association/American Academy of Orthopedic Surgeons Expert Panel. Antibiotic prophylaxis for dental patients with total joint replacements. *AAOS Bull* July 1997:9–11.

72. Smith BE, Askew MJ, Gradisar IA Jr. et al. The effect of patient weight on the functional outcome of total knee arthroplasty. *Clin Orthop* 1992;276:237–244.

73. Khaw FM, Moran CG, Pinder IM, Smith SR. The incidence of fatal pulmonary embolism after knee replacement with no prophylactic anticoagulation. *J Bone Joint Surg [Br]* 1993;75:940–941.

74. Faunø P, Suomalainen ÅO, Rehnberg V, et al. Prophylaxis for the prevention of venous thromboembolism after total knee arthroplasty. A comparison between unfractionated and low-molecular-weight heparin. *J Bone Joint Surg [Am]* 1994;76: 1814–1818.

75. Neer CS II. Articular replacement for the humeral head. *J Bone Joint Surg [Am]* 1955;37:215–228.

76. Cofield RH, Frankle MA, Zuckerman JD. Humeral head replacement for glenohumeral arthritis. *Semin Arthroplasty* 1995;6:214–221.

77. Romeo AA. Total shoulder arthroplasty: pearls and pitfalls in surgical technique. *Semin Arthroplasty* 1995;6:265–272.

78. Wilde AH. Shoulder arthroplasty. What is it good for and how good is it? In: Matsen FA III, Fu FH, Hawkins RJ, eds. *The shoulder: a balance of mobility and flexibility.* Rosemont, Ill: American Academy of Orthopaedic Surgeons, 1992:459–481.

79. Noble JS, Bell RH. Failure of total shoulder arthroplasty: why does it occur? *Semin Arthroplasty* 1995;6:280–288.

80. Craig EV. Total shoulder replacement. *Orthopedics* 1988;11:125–136.

81. Neer CS II. Unconstrained shoulder arthroplasty. *Instr Course Lect* 1985;34:278–286.

82. Brems JJ. Rehabilitation following total shoulder arthroplasty. *Clin Orthop* 1994;307:70–85.

83. Maybach A, Schlegel TF. Shoulder rehabilitation for the arthritic glenohumeral joint: preoperative and postoperative considerations. *Semin Arthroplasty* 1995;6: 297–304.

Chapter 85

Osteoporosis

Laurie A. Browngoehl

Osteoporosis, the most prevalent metabolic bone disease in the United States, is a major contributing cause of fractures, pain, and mobility dysfunction. As life expectancy increases, medical management and treatment of this disorder pose increasing challenges to health care providers. When osteoporosis results in significant disability, patients, families, and communities suffer. The economic and social burdens are high and appear to be increasing. Awareness of all available preventative measures and treatment options is essential for comprehensive management of osteoporosis.

DEFINITION

Osteoporosis was originally defined by Albright and Reifenstein in 1948 as "too little bone in the bone" (1). Since bone is both a tissue and an organ, a more exacting definition is a reduction in the amount of bone tissue in a given volume of bone organ. The bone present is normal, without any change in the amount or makeup of mineral components. This must be differentiated from osteomalacia in which there is a reduced mineral content but no reduction in bone tissue. Osteoporosis exists when the bone mass is more than 2 standard deviations below the mean mass in young adults of the same sex (2). Osteoporosis increases the risk of fracture because of decreases in bone density (3,4).

CLASSIFICATION

Albright and Reifenstein's original classification of osteoporosis included three types (1). Postmenopausal osteoporosis occurred in women less than 65 years old. Senile osteoporosis occurred in men and women over 65 years old. If there were no other identifiable causes, the osteoporosis was defined as idiopathic.

Osteoporosis is now classified into primary osteoporosis in which there is no associated disease and secondary osteoporosis, which occurs in association with a number of systemic and metabolic diseases, as well as from medications and immobilization.

Riggs and Melton (5) divided primary osteoporosis into types I and II. Type I, or postmenopausal osteoporosis, is primarily due to estrogen deficiency occurring in women after natural or surgical menopause. It is characterized both by increased bone turnover and by excessive bone resorption, primarily in trabecular bone. Although bone formation continues to occur, osteoclastic activity is increased, with a loss of osseous mass. Primary sites of bone loss and fracture are the spine and distal region of the forearm.

Type II or aging-associated osteoporosis, also labeled *senile osteoporosis*, is related directly to the aging process and affects both men and women. Reduced bone formation is the major contributing factor, with bone loss occurring at both trabecular and cortical sites. Primary complications are hip fractures and vertebral wedge fractures (6).

Metabolic diseases that can cause secondary osteoporosis include Cushing disease, hypogonadism, hyperthyroidism, and primary hyperparathyroidism. Corticosteroid-induced osteoporosis occurs because corticosteroids both decrease bone formation by reducing osteoblast function and increase bone resorption by increasing osteoclast function. Heparin, phenytoin, phenobarbital, and thyroid hormone are other medications that can cause secondary osteoporosis. Osteoporosis of immobilization can occur in patients immobilized due to quadriplegia, paraplegia, or hemiplegia (7) as well as immobilization from fracture or bed rest. Anorexia nervosa predisposes to osteoporosis through hypothalamic dysfunction (8).

EPIDEMIOLOGY

Osteoporosis is a major public health issue presenting increasing challenges as the population ages. The life expectancy of the aged in the United States is higher than that in other developed countries. For an 80-year-old white individual, the life expectancy is now 9.1 years for a woman and 7.0 years for a man (9). Increases in the incidence and prevalence of osteoporosis are to be expected.

The contribution of osteoporosis to loss of function, institutionalization, and death is considerable. The disease accounts for approximately 1.3 million fractures in the United States each year. One out of every three women over age 65 will have a vertebral fracture (5). The incidence of hip fracture increases rapidly with age (10). In a large population-based epidemiologic study of 18,214 hip fractures over a 12-month period, the increase in the age-adjusted rate for hip fracture was exponential (11). This was true for both men and women. Hip fractures have devastating effects on the lives of older individuals. Twenty-nine percent of people are institutionalized within 6 months after fracture (12). One year after hip fracture, the mortality rate ranges from 14% to 36% in elderly patients (13).

The direct medical costs associated with osteoporosis are estimated to range from $10 billion to $20 billion annually (14,15). It is clear that the physical, social, and economic burdens imposed by osteoporosis and osteoporosis-related fractures are tremendous.

PATHOGENESIS

The pathogenesis of osteoporosis is related to the interplay between peak bone mass, subsequent bone loss, and fracture risk. Peak bone mass, the highest level of bone achieved during normal growth, occurs between adolescence and as late as the age of 35 years (16). Although bones stop growing in length after puberty when growth plates close, bone mineral content increases with a resultant increase in strength. There may be a transient period of equilibrium after peak bone mass is reached, following which bone loss begins. This age-related bone loss occurs in both men and women and affects both trabecular and cortical bone. Because men have more bone mass than women, and blacks have more bone mass than whites, osteoporosis is less of a problem in men and in the black population (17).

After peak bone mass is reached, both men and women lose approximately 0.25% to 1.00% of bone yearly. In the years following menopause, bone loss is accelerated in women, with an average loss of 2% to 5% per year (18). After age 70 years, the rate of bone loss declines in both sexes and is approximately equal.

The increased bone loss in women after menopause reflects changes in ovarian function. Menopause is associated with a fall in the plasma levels of estradiol, the main estrogen secreted by the ovaries, and estrone, secreted by both the ovaries and the adrenal glands. After menopause, adrenal estrone becomes the primary estrogen secreted and overall plasma concentrations drop considerably.

Bone is constantly remodeling, with bone resorption mediated by osteoclasts and bone formation mediated by osteoblasts. During growth and development and up to late adolescence, bone remodeling is positive, with formation exceeding resorption. In adulthood, bone resorption and formation are "coupled" so that the bone mass remains essentially stable. When microdamage occurs with normal activity, bone remodeling allows skeletal repair. In osteoporosis, bone resorption is "negatively uncoupled"; bone resorption is increased and bone formation is unable to offset these losses. This results in a net loss of bone mass as well as an increased susceptibility to fracture.

RISK FACTORS

Multiple factors increase the risk for osteoporosis. As noted previously, different population groups have varying peak bone masses. Women as opposed to men, and whites and Orientals as compared to blacks are groups at increased risk for osteoporosis and subsequent fracture (19). Mother-daughter and twin studies support a genetic component for lower peak bone mass (20,21). A family history of osteoporosis is clearly seen as a risk factor and is an important part of a screening history. Smaller-bone individuals are more susceptible to osteoporosis. Those with heavier builds and increased body weights experience less osteoporosis. Risk factors for postmenopausal osteoporosis include lower peak bone mass at skeletal maturity, early menopause, inadequate calcium and vitamin D intake, and smoking (22,23). These factors may occur in varying degrees and act to accelerate bone loss and fracture risk.

Because of the effect of estrogen on bone mass, early menopause, either idiopathic or surgically induced, is an important risk factor. A woman who begins her menses later in life or who develops amenorrhea is also at increased risk. Amenorrhea or eumenorrhea due to heavy athletic activity decrease bone mineral content (24,25).

Nutritional factors that may increase the risk for osteoporosis include low calcium or vitamin D intake as well as high consumption of phosphate and caffeine. Heavy alcohol intake significantly decreases bone mass in both men and women (26). This appears to be secondary to defective osteoblastic function. Heavy cigarette smoking may depress estrogen levels and contribute to the development of osteoporosis (27).

Because bone loss occurs with reduced weight bearing, conditions that are associated with disuse increase the risk of osteoporosis. According to the Wolff law, bone remodeling is directly dependent on the mechanical load placed on it. Lack of muscle contraction, like reduced weight bearing, results in insufficient compressive force, making immobilization a significant contributor to osteoporosis.

CLINICAL FEATURES

Osteoporosis is often asymptomatic until a fracture occurs. The most common clinical presentation is back pain associated with a vertebral compression fracture. A compression fracture may occur suddenly following activity and result in acute pain, or may occur gradually, leading to a more insidious development of discomfort. A minor event such as a sneeze or cough can fracture an osteoporotic vertebra. Acute pain is usually localized over the affected vertebral body, although fractures at the midthoracic area may be perceived as pain in the lumbosacral region. Referred pain from the intercostal nerves may be experienced in the chest, flank, and abdomen. Frequently, pain is described as sharp and lancinating. It is exacerbated by back motion and relieved by rest. Pain may last days, weeks, or even months.

Fractures are most frequent at the middle to lower thoracic and upper lumbar areas. Cervical and upper thoracic fractures are unusual and in fact should lead the physician to rule out malignancy or other disorder.

Back pain may also be associated with postural abnormalities that slowly develop over time. Dorsal kyphosis, also known as *dowager's hump*, is caused by multiple compression fractures or vertebral body collapse producing anterior wedging (Fig. 85-1). This deformity causes stresses on the supporting structures of the spinal column and frequently results in muscle and ligamentous strain and discomfort. The intervertebral disks of many osteoporotic patients have undergone age-related changes such as decreased disk compliance, which may further exacerbate the deformity and subsequent pain.

Progressive spinal deformity also leads to a significant loss of height. Abdominal protuberance is common and may cause bloating and constipation. Iliocostal pain, often underrecognized, is caused by friction of the lower ribs against the iliac crest. The tenth, eleventh, and twelfth ribs may acutely irritate the tendons and the muscles inserting on the iliac crest, causing acute inflammation, bursitis, or both. Pain may be referred to the groin, buttocks, chest, and lower rib area.

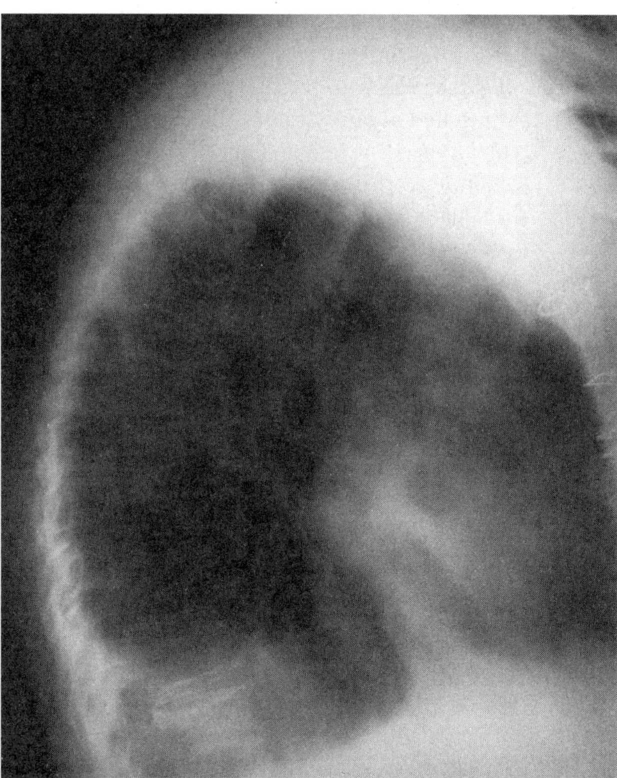

Figure 85-1. Lateral x-ray film of the spine in a patient with osteoporosis.

Hip fractures associated with osteoporosis are most commonly caused by falls, but in some cases the fracture precedes and then causes the fall. Hip fractures often occur in the home during the course of daily activity. In long-term-care facilities, hip fractures occur primarily in areas with significant activity and usually during ambulation (28). The most common fracture sites are the femoral neck and the intertrochanteric region. Treatment options usually include hip arthroplasty or open reduction with internal fixation.

Distal radial and other upper-extremity fractures are usually the result of more forceful falls and more frequently occur outside the home. In most cases, these fractures are treated with immobilization in casts or splints, which in turn can significantly impair the ability to perform self-care tasks.

DIAGNOSIS

History and Physical Examination

In the diagnostic work-up for osteoporosis, the history and physical examination are essential to guide the clinician to further evaluation and management. In reviewing a patient's history, the clinician must identify any risk factors, as discussed earlier. Previous fractures and the amount of trauma that resulted in injury must be elicited. The nature of any back pain needs to be carefully explored, identifying the location, intensity, and any exacerbating features. A nutritional evaluation will help determine if the patient is consuming adequate levels of calcium, vitamin D, and other essential nutrients.

The physical examination must include exact measurements of standing height and body weight. Sitting height can also be a useful assessment tool, as the ratio of sitting height to total height is decreased in the osteoporotic individual. Evaluation of posture must include identifying abnormalities such as thoracic kyphosis and increased lordosis. Paraspinal muscles should be assessed for spasm or tenderness. Palpation of the spinal processes may reveal point tenderness. Range of motion evaluation of the back, neck, and limbs is essential. Myelopathic signs such as hyperreflexia and upgoing plantar reflexes are rare but if present should alert the examiner to possible neoplasm.

Laboratory Studies

Blood and urine studies are primarily useful in identifying secondary causes of osteoporosis (29). A complete blood cell count is helpful in assessing for anemia associated with malignancy. Alkaline phosphatase can be increased in the setting of new fractures, osteomalacia, and bony metastases. Both erythrocyte sedimentation rate and serum protein electrophoresis can be useful in the diagnosis of multiple myeloma. Levels of plasma calcium, which is generally normal in the osteoporotic patient, can be abnormal with other metabolic bone diseases such as hyperparathyroidism and osteomalacia.

Serum and urine electrophoresis as well as studies for Bence-Jones proteins will help rule out multiple myeloma. A urinalysis may reveal proteinuria secondary to a nephrotic syndrome or a low pH secondary to renal tubular acidosis. Analysis of urine collected over 24 hours assesses the adequacy of intestinal calcium absorption and can exclude hypercalciuria.

Plain radiographs are helpful in assessing for fracture and excluding other conditions. However, they are not a sensitive measurement for bone mass and approximately 30% of bone loss is necessary before osteoporosis is visualized. A bone scan is a more sensitive measurement for vertebral fracture and is positive before plain radiography shows abnormalities. A bone scan will reveal increased uptake at the site of a recent fracture because of the increased metabolic activity from ongoing bone formation. Bone scans return to normal within 6 months after a fracture. A bone biopsy will help rule out metabolic bone disease and can also define high and low bone turnover but is not generally used in the work-up for osteoporosis.

Assays for pyridium cross-links of collagen, telopeptides of type I collagen, and bone-specific alkaline phosphatase are used primarily for investigational purposes at present. Potential uses include the prediction of bone loss rate and monitoring response to therapy (30).

Bone Densitometry

Bone densitometry is helpful both in the diagnosis of osteoporosis and in monitoring changes in individual patients. Dual-energy absorptiometry (DXA) (Fig. 85-2) is a

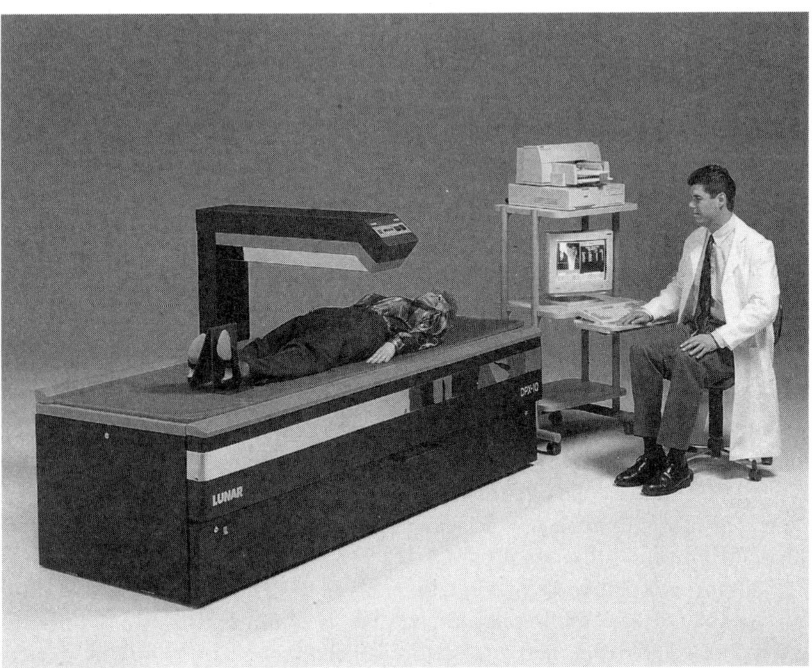

Figure 85-2. Dual-energy x-ray absorptiometry machine. (Courtesy of Lunar Corporation.)

widely accepted procedure that is both effective and safe (31–34). Bone mass can be measured at different skeletal sites including the lumbar region of the spine, the femoral neck, and the forearm and for the total skeleton. Measurement of femoral neck bone mineral density is an especially useful tool for diagnosis in elderly osteoporotic individuals; it is not significantly influenced by osteoarthritis, and is an excellent predictor of proximal femoral fracture (35). The amount of radiation administered in a test is 1 to 3 mrad. The short patient contact time of 10 to 20 minutes and an accuracy of 3% to 6% have helped DXA become increasingly accepted as the superior method of bone density measurement.

Single-energy absorptiometry was developed prior to dual-energy methods. Single-proton absorptiometry (SPA) and single-energy x-ray absorptiometry (SXA) assess bone mineral at peripheral sites such as the radius, ulna, and calcaneus. Low radiation exposure and low cost are advantages. As compared to single-energy absorptiometry, dual-energy methods are needed to measure axial sites where there are varying amounts of soft tissue. Dual-proton absorptiometry (DPA) measures the density of the lumbar region of the spine, the proximal end of the femur, and the entire skeleton. The accuracy and precision are less with DPA as compared to SPA. Scanning time is also long; a total skeletal scan can take up to 40 minutes. DXA, by improving the DPA technology, has allowed improved precision and shorter scanning time.

Quantitative computed tomography (QCT) is a technique in which cancellous and compact bone of the vertebral body is measured. A volumetric measurement in milligrams per cubic centimeter is calculated as opposed to the two-dimensional area derived from the DXA. The higher radiation dose with QCT compared to DXA and lower precision in measurement make QCT a less desirable measurement tool than DXA. The most useful indications for bone density studies involve prediction of fracture risk (36). As bone density declines, fracture risk increases (3,4). A decrease in bone mass of 1 standard deviation is associated with a 50% to 100% increase in fracture incidence (33). Fracture risk can be assessed globally or on a site-specific basis. For global fracture risk assessment, data from any one of the commonly measured skeletal sites are useful. Site-specific measurements, as in measurement of the proximal region of the femur for prediction of hip fractures (37), may be preferable for assessment of certain fracture locations (38).

Bone mass measurement is clinically useful in identifying estrogen-deficient women with low bone mass so that appropriate decisions can be made with regard to medication such as hormone replacement therapy (39). If bone mineral density is 1 standard deviation below the mean as compared to the density in premenopausal women, treatment can be recommended to decrease fracture risk. No intervention for fracture prevention is necessary if density is more than 1 standard deviation above the mean. For women with values 1 standard deviation above or below the mean, bone mass can be monitored periodically (33).

Measuring bone mass is clinically useful in premenopausal women with identifiable causes for bone loss such as premenopausal ovarian failure, glucocorticoid therapy, or multiple sclerosis (40). Both men and women on long-term glucocorticoids may rapidly lose bone. Therefore, knowledge of the extent of bone loss can influence the physician to alter medication dosage.

Patients with primary asymptomatic hyperparathyroidism may be considered stronger candidates for parathyroidectomy if bone mass is low and the patient is at high risk for fracture. This scenario presents a clear indication for bone mass studies.

Bone mass measurement is also useful for assessing efficacy of treatment. Because changes in bone mass can be detected over time, the response to therapy can be monitored. It usually takes several months to a year to see a significant change. As more information is obtained on rates of response, specific protocols can be used to monitor the effectiveness of interventions on bone mass.

Bone mass measurements may be useful as a screening tool in the general population (41). At this time, the expense of the procedures and the lack of clear treatment methods for all osteoporotic patients limit its utility (42). Further research in this area is needed to maximize the use of bone density screening in preventative care.

TREATMENT

The treatment of osteoporosis may include pharmacologic management and dietary manipulation as well as rehabilitative measures such as exercise prescription, bracing, and pain management.

Pharmacologic Management

Hormone Replacement Therapy

Hormone replacement therapy is often the treatment of choice for postmenopausal women with osteoporosis. Estrogen acts directly on estrogen receptors of bone cells to retard bone loss when prescribed soon after menopause. In the Framingham study, a retrospective study of 2873 postmenopausal women, estrogen supplementation clearly protected against hip fracture when taken within 4 years of menopause (43). An even larger cohort of 23,246 women indicated that treatment with estrogen reduced the risk of hip fracture within the first decade after menopause (44). Following menopause, estrogen therapy for at least 7 years is required for long-term preservation of bone mineral density (45).

The incidence of endometrial cancer may be increased when estrogens are given alone. However, when estrogen is given with progesterone, the incidence is lower than in women not receiving hormone replacement therapy (46).

The risk of breast cancer increases with long-term perimenopausal treatment with estrogens, even with the addition of progestins (47). Increased risk is most marked in women over 55 years old and those who have used hormone replacement therapy for more than 5 years (47,48). However, some of the data regarding breast cancer are conflicting, and unresolved issues remain and need to be studied further (49,50).

Postmenopausal women who take estrogens lower their rate of cardiovascular disease by 50%. Estrogen lowers the level of low-density lipoprotein and raises the level of high-density lipoprotein, which has a protective effect against cardiovascular disease (51). Other benefits of estrogen include a reduction in the vasomotor and urogenital symptoms of menopause.

Estrogen is currently used by less than one-third of all postmenopausal women in the United States. The chief determinants of whether or not hormone replacement is used are socioeconomic rather than medical (52). It is clear that the issue of hormone replacement therapy must be dealt with on an individual basis. Age as well as risk factors for heart disease and breast cancer should be evaluated with respect to the risks and benefits so that optimal health can be attained (53).

Biphosphonates

Biphosphonates are a class of synthetic compounds that are analogues of pyrophosphate, a physiologic inhibitor of bone mineralization. These compounds adhere to the hydroxyapatite content of bone and are important inhibitors of osteoclastic bone resorption. Etidronate, the first biphosphonate developed, has been used extensively to treat Paget disease and heterotopic ossification.

Biphosphonates increase the bone density in women with postmenopausal osteoporosis by about 5% to 10% over 1 year, after which bone density plateaus (54,55). Long-term continuous administration has been abandoned largely because of impairment of mineralization of new bone. Low-dose cyclical etidronate appears to increase bone density more effectively (56) and reduces the rate of vertebral fractures.

Alendronate sodium, approved by the Food and Drug Administration (FDA) for the treatment of postmenopausal osteoporosis in 1995, has a four-carbon amino side chain that conveys a high potency, permitting effective inhibition of osteoclast-mediated bone resorption at doses that do not impair mineralization. Daily treatment increases bone mass in the spine, hip, and total body (57) and decreases the incidence of vertebral fractures (58). Gastrointestinal irritation is the major complicating side effect of the biphosphonates (59), including alendronate (58). Chemical esophagitis with severe ulcerations can occur with alendronate use in some patients. Swallowing the medication with a full glass of water and remaining upright for at least 30 minutes afterward is recommended (60).

Raloxifene

Raloxifene, a nonsteroidal benzothiophene, is currently being evaluated for the treatment of osteoporosis. Daily therapy increases bone mineral density and decreases bone turnover. This medication does not stimulate the endometrium and therefore may not be associated with an increased risk of endometrial cancer (61).

Sodium Fluoride

Sodium fluoride stimulates bone formation and increases trabecular bone density, particularly in the vertebra. However, there is also histologic evidence of osteomalacia, which may be secondary to the toxic effects on osteoblasts. Several studies demonstrated unchanged vertebral fracture rates and possibly an increased risk of hip fracture (62,63).

One-third of patients on fluoride experience gastric intolerance including bloating, nausea, and abdominal pain. Pseudoarthritic pain in the joints of the lower limbs develops in another third of patients. This discomfort is experienced primarily in the heels and ankles and may be secondary to microfractures. Discontinuing the sodium fluoride reduces both gastrointestinal and lower-extremity pain complaints.

Using an intermittent slow-release fluoride preparation with continuous calcium citrate, recent studies demonstrated increased bone mass in the spine and inhibition of new vertebral fractures with significantly fewer side effects (64). This information has stimulated continuing interest in further trials using different dosage schedules and new preparations of sodium fluoride (65).

Calcitonin

Calcitonin is a polypeptide hormone synthesized and secreted by the thyroid gland that inhibits osteoclastic activity. Bone mass in postmenopausal osteoporosis increases with calcitonin (66,67). When given subcutaneously, the recommended dose is 100 IU (0.5 mL) daily or every other day.

Nasal administration has been approved more recently, and may improve patient compliance. Intranasal calcitonin at a dose of 50 IU/day can prevent trabecular bone loss and increase bone mass in nonobese, early postmenopausal women (68).

The major side effects include flushing and gastrointestinal symptoms. Both can be reduced by administering the medication at bedtime. Flushing is experienced as a warm feeling throughout the body associated with visible redness of the face, palms, and soles lasting 1 hour and occurring within minutes of subcutaneous injection. Calcitonin is a safe drug with excellent local tolerance to nasal administration.

Nutritional Considerations

Calcium and vitamin D, important components of the diet, are necessary to maintain bone tissue. The addition of both calcium and vitamin D to the diet can slow axial and appendicular bone loss in postmenopausal women (69,70). Calcium augmentation retards bone loss in the femoral neck and improves calcium balance (71). A reduced incidence of nonvertebral fractures is noted in men and women over age 65 who take supplemental calcium and vitamin D (72). The National Osteoporosis Foundation recommends 1500 mg of elemental calcium daily for postmenopausal women who are not taking estrogen. Unfortunately, many Americans, particularly the elderly, do not receive adequate dietary calcium. Calcium-enriched foods may be avoided due to real or perceived lactose intolerance, concern that milk and cheese contain too much cholesterol, or the belief that dairy products are constipating. The decline in taste and smell sensation often experienced by the elderly may lead to decreased food variety, which will also limit calcium consumption.

A dietary history is essential to determine whether adequate consumption of calcium exists. Approximately 300 mg of calcium is available in either 1 cup of milk, 8 oz of yogurt, or 1 cup of dark-green vegetables. Adding three of these servings daily may be sufficient to help achieve normal dietary requirements.

Medications such as laxatives and cholestyramine may adversely affect calcium status by binding dietary calcium and decreasing its availability. Aluminum-containing antacids can produce a reduction in phosphorus and decrease bone mineral content. Fiber supplements, often taken by the elderly, can decrease the amount of calcium absorption. Other medications may improve calcium status. By reducing urinary excretion of calcium, thiazide diuretics can actually reduce the incidence of hip fractures by about one-third (73).

Additional amounts of calcium beyond the recommended dose have not been demonstrated to prevent osteoporosis because as calcium consumption rises, absorption decreases. Supplements are not required if dietary history reveals an adequate calcium intake. Consumption of more than 2000 to 2500 mg of calcium per day can result in hypercalciuria and increase the risk of urinary calculi. Calcium supplements come in both nonprescription and prescription forms. An inexpensive calcium supplement available as an over-the-counter antacid is calcium carbonate, which includes 40% of calcium by weight. Other frequently used supplements include calcium citrate malate and calcium phosphate. Supplements should be consumed with milk or yogurt, as the vitamin D and lactose present in these products increases calcium absorption. In addition, supplements should be taken with food, as increased gastric content improves absorption.

Calcium is absorbed in the intestine through the actions of vitamin D, which is obtained through the diet and is manufactured in the skin with sunlight exposure. The recommended daily allowance (RDA) for vitamin D is 400 to 800 IU. Elderly who fail to consume vitamin D found in fortified dairy products or who are not exposed to the sunlight may experience a deficit of vitamin D. Most often, this occurs in patients who are home bound or reside in nursing homes. Calcitriol (1,25-dihydroxyvitamin D_3) increases the gastrointestinal absorption of calcium and stimulates both osteoblastic and osteoclastic activity in the skeleton. Although calcitriol was found to be ineffective in increasing bone mass with doses of 0.43 µg/day (74), 0.60 µg/day was associated with increased spinal bone density and total body calcium (75). Neither of these studies was large enough to evaluate fracture incidence. A large 3-year trial of 0.25 µg of calcitriol taken twice daily revealed a significantly reduced rate of new vertebral fractures without significant side effects (76). A study of 3270 ambulatory women in nursing homes treated with supplemental calcium and vitamin D noted a significant reduction in the risk of hip fractures and other nonvertebral fractures without significant side effects (77). Dietary intervention, including the use of calcium and vitamin D supplements as needed, is an essential component of treatment for osteoporosis.

Exercise

Exercise is an important therapeutic measure for osteoporosis because of its ability to decrease the rate of bone loss (78) and preserve bone density (79). Weight-bearing exercises promote bone growth by increasing mechanical load and stress on bone (80,81). Walking decreases bone loss in the trabecular bone of the spine (82). Strength training results in preservation of bone mineral density and increases muscle mass, strength, and balance (79,83).

Muscle weakness associated with osteoporosis may be generalized due to the deconditioning effect of decreased mobility or may be selective as in the case of loss of back extensor strength (84). Back extensor strengthening exercises have an important role in improving osteoporosis-impaired posture (85). Some types of exercises may be inappropriate for the osteoporotic individual. An increased number of vertebral fractures may occur with dynamic trunk flexion as compared to extension (86).

A recommended exercise program (Fig. 85-3) should include trunk extension and isometric exercises, upper- and lower-body resistance training, and postural and flexibility education (87). Stretching of the pectoral and intercostal muscles is helpful for improving chest expansion (88). Exercises should be performed at least two or three times per week. Walking, biking, and calisthenics are effective and often advised. Dancing, performed several times weekly, leads to increased spinal bone density and can also be considered (89).

One of the difficulties with exercise programs is that many patients are noncompliant and return to a sedentary lifestyle (82). Structured social support often encourages patients to continue active involvement in an exercise program (90).

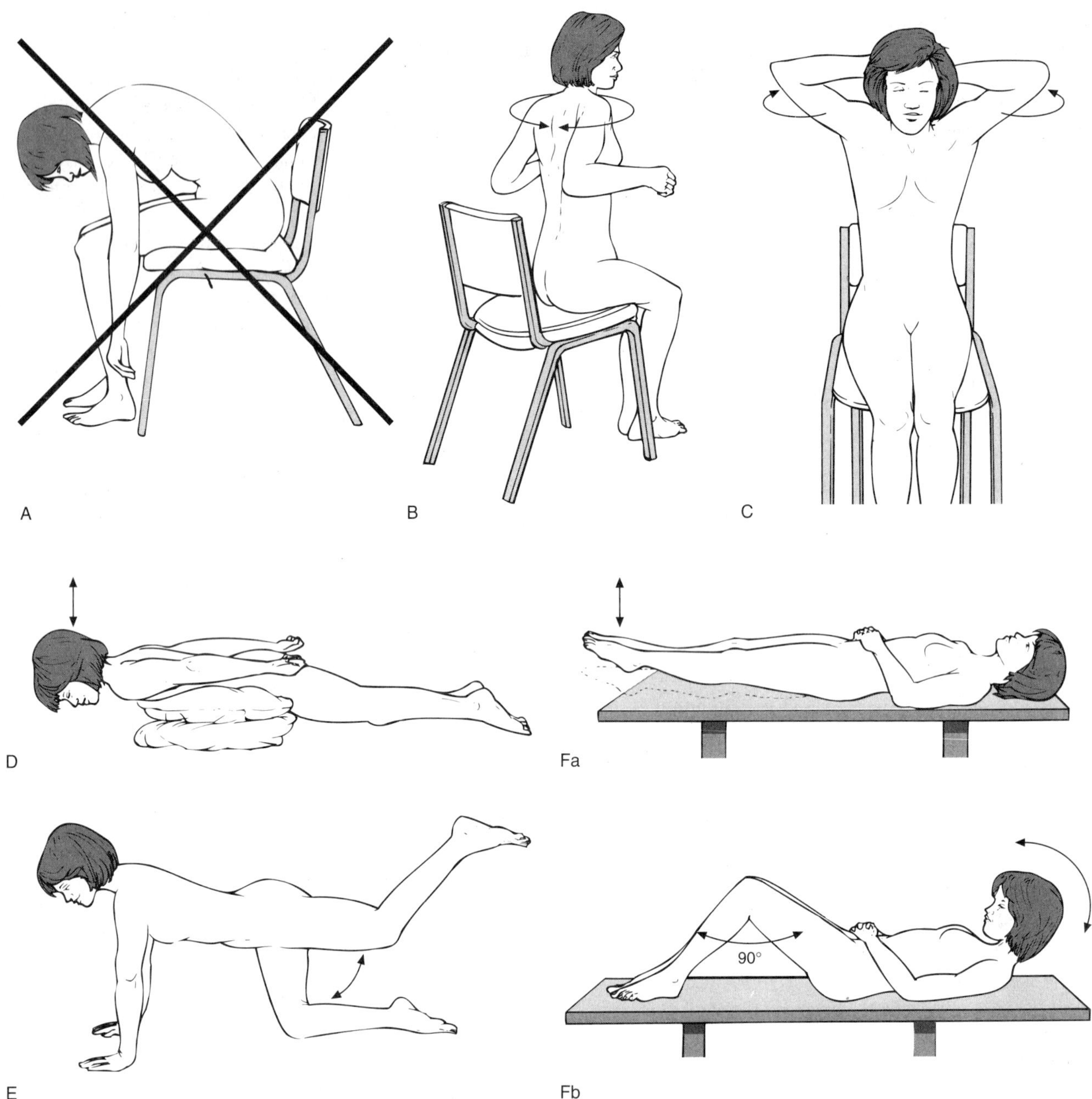

Figure 85-3. Exercises for patients with osteoporosis. *A.* Model demonstrates lumbar flexion exercise, which could contribute to a kyphotic posture and cause more compression of osteoporotic vertebrae. Patients should be advised *not* to perform these and other dynamic lumbar flexion exercises. *B.* Back extension exercise carried out in a sitting position. *C.* Deep-breathing exercises combined with pectoral stretching and back extension exercises. *D.* Back extension exercise performed in a prone position. In patients with severe osteoporosis, pain can be avoided or minimized by having the patient perform an extension exercise in a sitting position (*B*). *E.* Exercise for improving strength in the lumbar extensors and gluteus maximus muscles. *F.* Two techniques for strengthening abdominal muscles isometrically. (Reproduced by permission from Sinaki M. Postmenopausal spinal osteoporosis: physical therapy and rehabilitation principles. *Mayo Clin Proc* 1982;57:699–703.)

Orthoses

The use of a back orthosis is often advocated to improve mobility and prevent complications in osteoporosis. Symptomatic relief may be secondary to improved posture, restriction of spinal motion (91), or increased intra-abdominal pressure (92).

Jewett braces, often used following vertebral compression fractures, are lightweight and prevent thoracic and lumbar flexion. Designed to contact the base of the sternum and the pubic bone, they may be poorly tolerated by the elderly who may find them too cumbersome. Discomfort secondary to pressure can occur because the forces

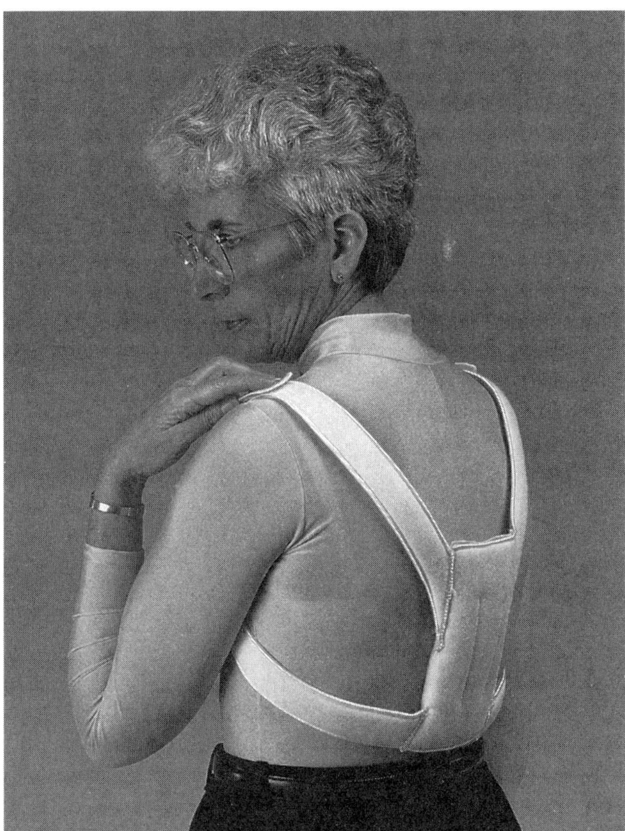

Figure 85-4. Postural training support (Camp PTS) orthosis. (Reproduced by permission of Camp International, Inc.)

are applied over small areas. Bivalved body jackets are custom fitted and evenly distribute pressure over the enclosed body surface. However, they are bulky under clothing, may cause the patient to be too warm, and can chafe the skin at the upper and lower contact points.

Flexible back supports constructed of cloth with rigid or semirigid stays may be more comfortable. Shoulder straps can be added to limit kyphotic posture. These corsets, however, can be difficult to don and doff. Abdominal binders without stays are generally comfortable and easier to apply. The lower edge may roll up, especially in patients with wide differences between their hip and waist circumferences.

A thoracolumbar orthosis used as a posture training support may also decrease pain and improve posture (93) (Fig. 85-4). A dependent weight hanging between the scapula decreases anterior compressive forces on the spine and acts as a proprioceptive reinforcer. Patients who wear this orthosis and are actively involved in a postural exercise program may develop increased back extensor strength (94).

For patients with severe kyphosis, a customized orthosis used while sitting can improve comfort. Sheepskin over the back of the wheelchair seat or other chair provides a cushion over the spinous processes and can reduce both pain and potential skin breakdown.

In general, compliance with many spinal orthoses is poor due to the difficulty of donning and doffing, discomfort, and bulkiness (95). However, with proper selection and careful physician supervision, back supports can be helpful in protecting the spine, providing pain relief, and improving posture.

Fall Prevention

Consequences of falls include not only fractures, resulting in significant morbidity and mortality, but also increased dependence in mobility and self-care, and psychological difficulties resulting from anxiety over falling. Prevention of falls, therefore, is a major treatment goal in the osteoporotic patient. Factors that contribute to falls include muscle weakness, decreased balance, physical inactivity, poor home safety, and cognitive impairment. Fall prevention programs that identify risk factors and implement strategies to reduce risk have been demonstrated to reduce the risk of falling (96–99). Tendency to fall rather than low bone mass may be the most important determinant of hip fracture (3).

Older adults frequently are taking multiple medications, which increases adverse drug reactions. Age-related changes in pharmacokinetics may also occur, including decreased hepatic and renal clearance, impaired metabolism, and increased drug sensitivity. Psychotropic agents and cardiovascular drugs that cause peripheral vasodilation are particularly associated with falls (100). For all these reasons, clinicians may need to modify medications to reduce the risk of falling.

Exercise, particularly balance training, may reduce the incidence of falls (101). Osteoporotic patients, especially those with kyphosis, have unique difficulties in maintaining balance (102). Dynamic and standing balance can often be improved with instruction in particular balance strategies, as well as the use of ambulatory devices. Home modifications such as improved lighting, removal of throw rugs, and installment of grab bars may improve safety. Visual impairment, if present, should be corrected. Because poor depth perception and reduced ability to perceive contrast appear to pose more of a risk than poor acuity (103), environmental adjustments may be most beneficial. Modification of the risk of falling should remain an essential component of treatment in the osteoporotic patient.

Pain Management

Effective pain management is an essential aspect of treatment and is an important consideration in improving basic functional activities. It is essential to identify the cause of pain, which may be due to vertebral compression fracture, postural abnormalities, iliocostal pain, or other sequelae of osteoporosis, so that proper treatment can be employed.

Modalities such as moist heat, cold packs, massage, and transcutaneous electrical nerve stimulation can be extremely beneficial in providing pain relief. Orthotic management of the spine may be an important component of pain management in selected individuals. Instruction in proper shoe wear is often neglected. Low-heeled shoes with soft inserts can decrease forces transmitted from the heel to the spine during ambulation. Assistive devices such as walkers or canes may further decrease these forces and lessen back pain.

In treating patients with iliocostal pain, lower rib compression with a strong elastic belt may be beneficial. By compressing the lower ribs and reducing contact with the iliac crest, the belt may decrease the friction that causes pain. The device may be necessary for a 4- to 6-week period and can then be discontinued. Injection into the osteotendinous junction and bursa may also provide relief (104).

Narcotic pain medication may be necessary, especially after acute compression fracture. Tramadol has a similar pain-relieving capacity as narcotics but has fewer central nervous system side effects and may be appropriate in certain individuals. Nonsteroidal anti-inflammatory drugs are very helpful in providing analgesia and decreasing inflammation. Muscle relaxants to reduce any associated paravertebral muscle spasm may be of significant benefit. If radicular pain is present, low-dose tricyclic antidepressants such as nortriptyline may be helpful in providing further analgesia. Calcitonin can reduce bone pain independent of its metabolic effect on bone turnover (105).

PSYCHOSOCIAL CONCERNS

Osteoporosis has significant effects on both psychological well-being and quality of life. Depression and anxiety are frequent, especially when patients must make major changes in their lifestyle. Because the associated disabilities may limit work and recreational activities, patients often become isolated from friends and family. Fear of falling is not limited to older persons who have fallen but includes all older adults with impaired mobility (106). This fear may lead to self-imposed activity restriction, which results in further dependence and anxiety.

The disfigurement often associated with osteoporosis may cause concern about body image. The use of braces, canes, or walkers may be viewed as a sign of failure and cause further erosion in self-image. The clinician must recognize psychosocial issues in managing the patient with osteoporosis. Initiating a discussion of emotional concerns, providing appropriate support to patients and families, and encouraging socialization and increased activity are all important aspects of treatment.

REFERENCES

1. Albright F, Reifenstein EC. *The parathyroid glands and metabolic disease*. Baltimore: Williams & Wilkins, 1948.
2. Kanis J. Treatment of symptomatic osteoporosis with fluoride. *Am J Med* 1993;95(suppl 5A): 535–615.
3. Cummings SR. Are patients with hip fractures more osteoporotic? *Am J Med* 1985; 78:487–494.
4. Melton LJ, Atkinson EJ, O'Fallen WM, et al. Long-term fracture prediction by bone mineral assessed at different skeletal sites. *J Bone Miner Res* 1993;8:1227–1233.
5. Riggs BL, Melton LJ. Evidence for two distinct syndromes of involutional osteoporosis. *Am J Med* 1983;75:899.
6. Riggs BL, Melton LF. Involutional osteoporosis. *N Engl J Med* 1986;314:1676–1677.
7. Hamdy RC, Moore SW, Cancellaro VA, Harvill LM. Long-term effects of strokes on bone mass. *AM J Med Rehabil* 1995;74: 351–356.
8. LaBan MM, Wilkins JC, Sackeyfio AH, Taylor RS. Osteoporotic stress fractures in anorexia nervosa: etiology, diagnosis, and review of four cases. *Arch Phys Med Rehabil* 1995;76: 884–887.
9. Manton KG, et al. Survival after the age of 80 in the United States, Sweden, France, England, and Japan. *N Engl J Med* 1995;333:1232–1235.
10. Obrant K, Bengren U, Johnell O, et al. Increasing age-adjusted risk of fragility fractures: a sign of increasing osteoporosis in successive generations? *Calcif Tissue Int* 1989;44:157–161.
11. Martin AD, Silverthorn KG, Houston CS, et al. The incidence of fracture of the proximal femur in two million Canadians from 1972 to 1974. *Clin Orthop* 1991;266:111–118.
12. Marottoli RA, Berkman LF, Leo-Summers L, Cooney LM. Predictors of mortality and institutionalization after hip fracture: the New Haven EPESE cohort. *Am J Public Health* 1994;84:1807–1812.
13. Zuckerman JD. Hip fracture. *N Engl J Med* 1996;334: 1519–1525.
14. Lindsay R. The burden of osteoporosis: cost. *Am J Med* 1995; 98(suppl 2A):9–11.
15. Barrett-Connor E. The economic and human costs of osteoporotic fracture. *Am J Med* 1995; 98(suppl 2A):3–8.
16. Rodin A, Murby B, Smith MA, et al. Premenopausal bone loss in the lumbar spine and neck of femur: a study of 225 Caucasian women. *Bone* 1990;211:1–5.

17. Pollitzer WS, Anderson JJB. Ethnic and genetic differences in bone mass: a review with a heredity vs. environmental perspective. *Am J Clin Nutr* 1989;50:1244–1259.

18. Thomsen K, Gotfredsen A, Christiansen C. Is post-menopausal bone loss an age-related phenomenon? *Calcif Tissue Int* 1986;39:123–127.

19. Farmer M, White L, Brody J, Bailey K. Race and sex differences in hip fracture incidence. *Am J Public Health* 1984;74:1374–1380.

20. Pocock NA, Eisman JA, Hopper JL, et al. Genetic determinants of bone mass in adults: a twin study. *J Clin Invest* 1987;80:706–710.

21. Seeman E, Isalamandris C, Formica C, et al. Reduced femoral neck bone density in the daughters of women with hip fracture: the role of low peak bone density in the pathogenesis of osteoporosis. *J Bone Miner Res* 1994;9:739–743.

22. Aloia JF, Cohn SH, Naswan AN, et al. Risk factors for post-menopausal osteoporosis. *Am J Med* 1985;78:95–100.

23. Paganini-Hill A, Ross R, Gerkins VR, et al. Menopausal estrogen therapy and hip fractures. *Ann Intern Med* 1981;95:28–31.

24. Drinkwater BL, Nilson K, Chestnut CH, et al. Bone mineral content of amenorrheic and eumenorrheic athletes. *N Engl J Med* 1984;311:277–281.

25. Rencken ML, Chestnut CH, Drinkwater BL. Bone density at multiple sites in amenorrheic athletes. *JAMA* 1996;276:238–240.

26. Heaney RP. Bone mass, nutrition and other lifestyle factors. *Am J Med* 1993;95(suppl SA): 295–335.

27. Jensen J, Christiansen C, Rodbro P. Cigarette smoking, serum estrogens and bone loss during hormone replacement therapy early after menopause. *N Engl J Med* 1985;313:973–975.

28. Cali CM, Kiel DP. An epidemiologic study of fall-related fractures among institutionalized older people. *J Am Geriatr Soc* 1995;43:1336–1340.

29. Binkley N. Assessment and management of the patient with osteoporosis. *Top Geriatr Rehabil* 1995;10(4):64–74.

30. Blumsohn A, Hannon R, Eastell R. Biochemical assessment of skeletal activity. *Phys Med Rehabil Clin N Am* 1995;6: 483–505.

31. Cole HM. Measurement of bone density with dual energy x-ray absorptiometry (DEXA). *JAMA* 1992;267:286–294.

32. Delmas P. Bone mass measurement: how, where, when and why? *Int J Fertil* 1993;38(suppl 2):70–76.

33. Johnston CC, Slemenda CW, Melton LJ. Clinical uses of bone densitometry. *N Engl J Med* 1991;324:1105–1109.

34. Mazess R. Dual-energy x-ray absorptiometry for the management of bone disease. *Phys Med Rehabil Clin N Am* 1995;6: 507–539.

35. Rizzoli R, Slosman D, Bonjour J. The role of dual energy x-ray absorptiometry of lumbar spine and proximal femur in the diagnosis and follow-up of osteoporosis. *Am J Med* 1995;98(suppl 2A):335–365.

36. Kellie SE. Diagnostic and therapeutic technology assessment: measurement of bone density with dual-energy x-ray absorptiometry. *JAMA* 1992;267: 286–294.

37. Cummings SR, Black DM, Nevitt MC, et al. Bone density at various sites for prediction of hip fractures. *Lancet* 1993;341: 72–75.

38. Bonnick S. Bone mass measurement techniques in clinical practice: methods and interpretation. *Top Geriatr Rehabil* 1995; 10(4):12–18.

39. Cummings SR, Browner WS, Grady D, Ettinger B. Should prescription of post menopausal hormone therapy be based on the results of bone densitometry? *Ann Intern Med* 1990;113:565–567.

40. Lindsay R. Bone mass measurements for premenopausal women. *Osteoporos Int* 1994;1(suppl):39–41.

41. Bachmann G. Prevention and treatment of osteoporosis. *Am J Managed Care* 1995;1:188–193.

42. Tosteson ANA, Rosenthal DI, Melton J, Milton MC. Cost effectiveness of screening perimenopausal white women for osteoporosis: bone densitometry and hormone replacement therapy. *Ann Intern Med* 1990;113:594–603.

43. Kiel D, Felson D, Anderson J, et al. Hip fracture and the use of estrogens in postmenopausal women. *N Engl J Med* 1987;317:1169–1174.

44. Naessen T, Persson I, Adami H, et al. Hormone replacement therapy and the risk for first fracture. *Ann Inter Med* 1990;113:95–103.

45. Felson D, Zhang Y, Hannan M, et al. The effect of postmenopausal estrogen therapy on bone density in elderly woman. *N Engl J Med* 1993;329:1142–1146.

46. Persson I, Adami HO, Bergvist L. Risk of endometrial cancer after treatment with estrogens alone or in conjunction with progestins; results of a prospective study. *BMJ* 1987;94:620–635.

47. Bergkvist L, Hans-Olov A, Persson I, et al. The risk of breast cancer after estrogen and estrogen-progestin replacement. *N Engl J Med* 1989;321: 293–297.

48. Colditz G, Hankinson S, Hunter D, et al. The use of estrogens and progestins and the risk of breast cancer in postmenopausal women. *N Engl J Med* 1995; 332:1589–1593.

49. Barrett-Connor E. Post-menopausal estrogen replacement and breast cancer. *N Engl J Med* 1989;321:319–320.

50. Davidson NE. Hormone replacement therapy—breast cancer versus heart versus bone. *N Engl J Med* 1995;332:1638–1639.

51. Walsh B, Schiff I, Rosner B. Effects of postmenopausal estrogen replacement on the concentrations and metabolism of plasma lipoproteins. *N Engl J Med* 1991;325:1196–1204.

52. Handa YL, Landerman R, Halan JT. Do older women use estrogen replacement? Data from the Duke Established Populations for Epidemiologic Studies of the Elderly (EPESE). *J Am Geriatr Soc* 1996;44:1–6.

53. AGS Clinical Practice Committee. Counseling postmenopausal women about preventive hormone therapy. *J Am Geriatr Soc* 1996;44:1120–1122.

54. Ott SM, Chestnut CH. Calcitriol treatment is not effective in postmenopausal osteoporosis. *Ann Inter Med* 1989;110:267–274.

55. Storm T, Thamsborg G, Steiniche T, et al. Effect of intermittent cyclical etidronate therapy on bone mass and fracture rate in women with post menopausal osteoporosis. *N Engl J Med* 1990;322:1265–1271.

56. Struys A, Snelder AA, Mulder H. Cyclical etidronate reverses bone loss of the spine and proximal femur in patients with established corticosteroid-induced osteoporosis. *Am J Med* 1995;99:235–242.

57. Chestnut CH, McClung MR, Ensrud KE, et al. Alendronate treatment of the postmenopausal osteoporotic woman: effect of multiple dosages on bone mass and bone remodeling. *Am J Med* 1995;99:144–151.

58. Liberman UA, Weiss SR, Broll J, et al. Effect of oral alendronate on bone mineral density and the incidence of fractures in postmenopausal osteoporosis. *N Engl J Med* 1995;333: 1437–1443.

59. Riggs BL, Melton LJ. The prevention and treatment of osteoporosis. *N Engl J Med* 1992;327:620–627.

60. DeGroen PC, Lubbe DF, Hirsch LJ, et al. Esophagitis associated with the use of alendronate. *N Engl J Med* 1996;335: 1016–1021.

61. Delmas PD, Bjornason NH, Mitlalc BM, et al. Effects of raloxifene on bone mineral density, serum cholesterol concentrations, and uterine endometrium in post-menopausal women. *N Engl J Med* 1997;337:1641–1647.

62. Kanis JA, Melton LJ, Christiansen C, et al. The diagnosis of osteoporosis. *J Bone Miner Res* 1994;9:1137–1141.

63. Riggs BL, Hodgson SF, O'Fallon WM, et al. Effect of fluoride treatment on the fracture rate in postmenopausal women with osteoporosis. *N Engl J Med* 1990;322:802–809.

64. Pak CY, Sakhaee K, Piziak V, et al. Slow-release sodium fluoride in the management of postmenopausal osteoporosis. *Ann Intern Med* 1994;120:625–632.

65. Heaney R. Fluoride and osteoporosis. *Ann Intern Med* 1994;120:689–690.

66. Aloi JF. Calcitonin and osteoporosis. *Geriatr Med Today* 1985;4:11.

67. Regnister J. Effect of calcitonin on bone mass and fracture rate. *Am J Med* 1991;91(suppl 5B):195–225.

68. Regnister JY, Deroisy R, Lecart M, et al. A double-blind, placebo-controlled, dose-finding trial of intermittent nasal salmon calcitonin for prevention of postmenopausal lumbar spine bone loss. *Am J Med* 1995;98: 452–457.

69. Reid IR, Ames RW, Evans MC, et al. Effect of calcium supplementation on bone loss in postmenopausal women. *N Engl J Med* 1993;328:460–464.

70. Dawson-Hughes B, Dallal GE, Krall EA, et al. A controlled trial of the effect of calcium supplementation on bone density in postmenopausal women. *N Engl J Med* 1990;323:878–883.

71. Aloia JF, Vaswania A, Yeh J, et al. Calcium supplementation with and without hormone replacement therapy to prevent postmenopausal bone loss. *Ann Intern Med* 1994;120:97–103.

72. Dawson-Hughes B, Harris SS, Krall EA, et al. Effect of calcium and vitamin D supplementation on bone density in men and women 65 years of age or older. *N Engl J Med* 1997;337: 670–702.

73. LaCroix A, Weinpahl J, White L, et al. Thiazide diuretic agents and the incidence of hip fracture. *N Engl J Med* 1990;322: 286–290.

74. Ott SM. Clinical effects of biphosphonates in involutional osteoporosis. *J Bone Miner Res* 1993;8:5597–5605.

75. Gallagher JC, Goldgar D. Treatment of postmenopausal osteoporosis with high doses of calcitriol. *Ann Intern Med* 1990;113:649–655.

76. Tilyard M, Spears GF, Thomson J, Dovey S. Treatment of postmenopausal osteoporosis with calcitriol or calcium. *N Engl J Med* 1992;326:357–362.

77. Chapuy MC, Arlot ME, Duboeuf F, et al. Vitamin D_3 and calcium to prevent hip fractures in elderly women. *N Engl J Med* 1992;327:1637–1642.

78. Inoue T, Kushida K, Kobayashi G, et al. Exercise therapy for osteoporosis. *Osteoporos Int* 1993;5(suppl 1):166–168.

79. Nelson ME, Fiatarone M, Morganti M, et al. Effects of high-intensity strength training on multiple risk factors for osteoporotic fractures. *JAMA* 1994;272:1909–1914.

80. Sinaki M. Exercise and osteoporosis. *Arch Phys Med Rehabil* 1989;70:220–229.

81. Smith EL. The role of exercise in the prevention and treatment of osteoporosis. *Top Geriatr Rehabil* 1995;10(4):55–63.

82. Nelson ME, Fisher EC, Dilmanian FA, et al. A1-y walking program

and increased dietary calcium in postmenopausal women: effects on bone. *Am J Clin Nutr* 1991;53:1304–1311.

83. Snow-Harter C, Whalen R, Myburgh K, et al. Bone mineral density, muscle strength, and recreational exercise in men. *J Bone Miner Res* 1992;7:1291–1296.

84. Sinaki M, Offord K. Physical activity in postmenopausal women: effect on back muscle strength and bone mineral density of the spine. *Arch Phys Med Rehabil* 1988;69:277–280.

85. Sinaki M, Wollen P, Scott RW, et al. Can strong back extensors prevent vertebral fractures in women with osteoporosis? *Mayo Clin Proc* 1996;71:951–956.

86. Sinaki M, Mikkelsen B. Postmenopausal spinal osteoporosis: flexion versus extension exercises. *Arch Phys Med Rehabil* 1984;65:593–596.

87. MacKinnon J. The role of physical therapy in the prevention and treatment of osteoporosis. *Top Geriatr Rehabil* 1995;10(4):48–54.

88. Sinaki M. Postmenopausal spinal osteoporosis; physical therapy and rehabilitation principles. *Mayo Clin Proc* 1982;57: 699–703.

89. Kudlacek S, Pietschmann F, Bernecker P, et al. The impact of a senior dancing program on spinal and peripheral bone mass. *Am J Phys Med Rehabil* 1997;76:477–481.

90. Harrison JE, Chow R, Dornan J, et al. Evaluation of a program for rehabilitation of osteoporotic patients (PRO): 4-year follow up. *Osteoporos Int* 1993;3:13–17.

91. Million R, Nilson K, Jayson MIV, Baker RD. Evaluation of low back pain and assessment of lumbar corsets with and without back supports. *Ann Rheum Dis* 1981;40:449–454.

92. Bartelink D. The role of abdominal pressure in relieving the pressure on the lumbar intervertebral discs. *J Bone Joint Surg [Br]* 1957;39:718–725.

93. Kaplan RS, Sinaki M. Posture training support: preliminary report on a series of patients with diminished symptomatic complications of osteoporosis. *Mayo Clin Proc* 1993;68:1171–1176.

94. Kaplan RS, Sinaki MS, Hameister MD. Effect of back supports on back strength in patients with osteoporosis: a pilot study. *Mayo Clin Proc* 1996;71:235–241.

95. Ahlgren S, Hansen T. The use of lumbosacral corsets prescribed for low back pain. *Prosthet Orthot Int* 1978;2:101–104.

96. Tinetti M, Baker D, McAvay G, et al. A multifactorial intervention to reduce the risk of falling among elderly people living in the community. *N Engl J Med* 1994;331:821–827.

97. Wagner E, LaCroix A, Grothaus L, et al. Preventing disability and falls in older adults: a population-based randomized trial. *Am J Public Health* 1991;84:1800–1806.

98. Wolter LL, Studenski SA. A clinical synthesis of falls intervention trials. *Top Geriatr Rehabil* 1996;11(3):9–19.

99. Rubenstein LZ, Robbins AS, Schulman BL, et al. Falls and instability in the elderly. *J Am Geriatr Soc* 1988;36:266–278.

100. Hanlon JT, Cotson T, Ruby CM, Drug-related falls in the older adult. *Top Geriatr Rehabil* 1995;11(3):38–54.

101. Province MA, Hadley EC, Hornbrook MC, et al. The effects of exercise on falls in elderly patients: a pre-planned meta-analysis of the FICSIT trials. *JAMA* 1995;273:1341–1347.

102. Lynn SG, Sinaki MA, Westerlind KC. Balance characteristics of persons with osteoporosis. *Am J Phys Med Rehabil* 1997;78:273–277.

103. Cummings SR, Nevitt MC, Browner WS. Risk factors for hip fracture in white women. *N Engl J Med* 1995;332:763–773.

104. Hirschberg GG, Williams KA, Byrd JG. Medical management of iliocostal pain. *Geriatrics* 1992;47(9):64–68.

105. Gennari C, Bocchi L, Orso CA, et al. The analgesic effect of calcitonin in active Paget's disease of bone and in metastatic bone disease. *Orthopedics* 1984;7:1449–1452.

106. Chandler JM, Duncan PW, Sanders L, Studenski S. The fear of falling syndrome: relationship to falls, physical performance, and activities of daily living in frail older persons. *Top Geriatr Rehabil* 1996;11(3):55–63.

Neuro-muscular Diseases

Chapter 86

Brachial Plexus Injury

Robert H. Meier, III

Closed injury to the brachial plexus (Fig. 86-1) most commonly occurs in young adult males and the cause is frequently a motorcycle accident (1). Hentz and Narakas (2) noted that 76% (87/114) of the complete brachial plexus injuries in their series were related to motorcycle accidents. Millesi (3) reported an incidence of 70% (173/247) of brachial plexus injuries related to motorcycle accidents. Other common causes for injuries of the brachial plexus include gunshot wounds, automobile accidents, and lacerations (4). The mechanisms of injury are usually related to stretching, compression, or penetration of the plexus components. In a motorcycle injury to the plexus, the biomechanical forces that result in stretch or avulsion injuries are produced with the arm down at the side or in the abducted position, with the head and neck tilted away from the side of the stretched plexus.

A brachial plexus injury is not commonplace but can result in a major alteration in function. Often, chronic pain is present. The complexity of this pathology often crosses many health care professional boundaries. Because few professionals see a sufficient quantity of patients with brachial plexus injuries to be very experienced in treatment, these patients frequently receive less than the standard of care for this disabling problem provided in centers of excellence. Imagine what it is like to experience difficulty in lifting a child, folding both hands in prayer, or performing simple activities of daily living with both hands? Evaluating a person with a brachial plexus injury requires detective work that should be a challenge for the physiatrist. The physician has to unravel the mystery of the location and the extent of the injury, usually without being able to see the injury. Attempting to solve this mystery and develop a long-range rehabilitation treatment plan requires a comprehensive knowledge of the basic, clinical, and psychosocial sciences.

This complex rehabilitation problem epitomizes the best of the unique features that physiatry has to contribute to contemporary health care and its cost-effectiveness. The pathophysiologic processes involved provide an odyssey for the physician through the areas of anatomy, kinesiology, neurophysiology, electrodiagnosis algology, orthotics, psychosocial science, surgery, occupational and physical therapy, and prosthetics. Comprehensive treatment of this problem requires an amalgam of professional opinions and approaches from an integrated team of experienced professionals.

LOCATION OF INJURY

A plexus injury can occur at any point from the takeoff of the spinal roots at the spinal cord level distally to the peripheral nerves as they arise from the cords of the plexus. The level of closed plexus injury can be classified as supraclavicular or infraclavicular. Supraclavicular injuries have poorer prognostic outcomes when it comes to neurologic recovery with the return of function in the arm and hand.

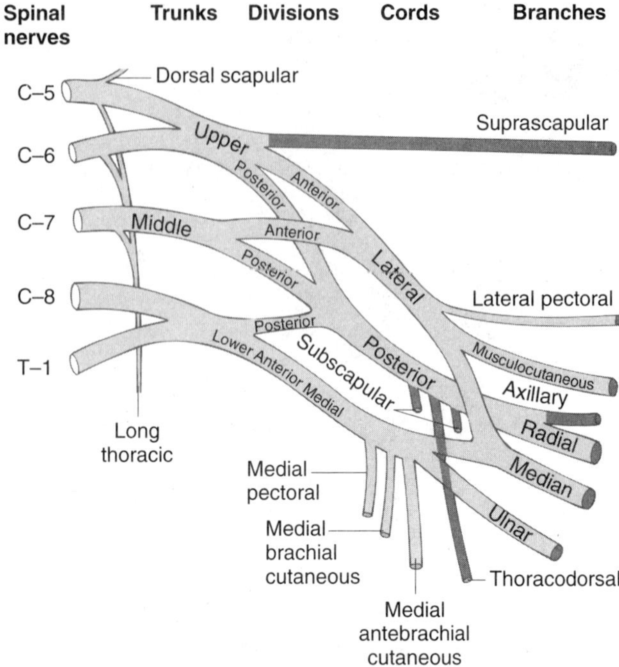

Figure 86-1. Diagram of the anatomic relationships of the component parts of the brachial plexus showing the spinal nerves, trunks, divisions, cords, and peripheral nerve branches.

Supraclavicular Injuries

Supraclavicular injury often results from motorcycle accident. The biker usually falls, striking the head and shoulder and stretching the neck. Without a helmet, the impact can damage the cranial contents, resulting in death or a closed head injury. If the tensile strength of the deep cervical fascia, scalene muscles, skeletal structures, and the meninges are exceeded, the nerves have little protection against elongation from traction. The cervical transverse processes may be avulsed or the first rib fractured. If these bony lesions are seen on x-ray films, then by inference, the corresponding nerve roots have been similarly avulsed from the spinal cord. The scalene muscles may also be torn, producing further scarring around the neuromas that form from the damaged nerves. If there is a complete nerve injury, the distal neurons are disassociated from their cell bodies and undergo wallerian degeneration. The portions of the neuron proximal to the lesion will attempt to regenerate and scar tissue forms around the regenerating axons forming a neuroma.

Neurapraxia, axonotmesis, and neurotmesis can be seen with brachial plexus injuries. Neurapraxia presents the best prognosis, and complete recovery should be anticipated within a short time (days to a few weeks) after injury. With axonotmesis, where the axonal sheath is intact, neural recovery is incomplete. Proximal muscles and sensation are more likely to recover than distal sensation and motor function. With neurotmesis, spontaneous recovery is unlikely and surgery will be required for the best opportunity of functional return.

The supraclavicular portion of the brachial plexus includes the plexus elements from the intradural spinal roots distally to the divisions. The infraclavicular portion includes the cords and terminal branches that are the individual peripheral nerves. The supraclavicular portion of the plexus is most consistently and severely damaged by the traction injuries described earlier (5). Supraclavicular lesions account for about 75% of brachial plexus injuries (6). In general, a neurapraxic injury is not as common in the setting of a supraclavicular plexus injury as in the setting of an infraclavicular injury.

Avulsion of one or more of the roots from the spinal cord carries the poorest chance for spontaneous recovery, whereas a stretch injury of the distal plexus following a neurapraxic insult often results in recovery. The injury should be viewed as a supraclavicular injury if the following findings are present (7):

1. Fracture of the clavicle or cervical transverse process
2. Evidence of injury to nerves arising from the supraclavicular portion (i.e., long thoracic or dorsal scapular nerves)
3. Horner syndrome
4. Swelling, induration, or tenderness in the supraclavicular fossa

Supraclavicular root injuries (75%) can be subdivided into upper, middle, lower, and total plexus palsies. The upper plexus (C5, C6, C7) is involved in 20% to 25% of patients while lower-plexus involvement (C8, T1) represents only 2% to 3%. Involvement of the middle plexus (C7) is associated with upper- or lower-plexus paralysis. Involvement of all plexus elements (C5–C8, T1) is most frequent, representing 75% to 80% of all plexus injuries.

Infraclavicular Injuries

Infraclavicular plexus lesions of the distal cords or peripheral nerves arising from the cords account for 25% of all brachial plexus injuries. These lesions usually involve the posterior cord (axillary and radial nerves), or with specific shoulder or humeral trauma, there may be individual radial or axillary damage. Common associated diagnoses include shoulder dislocation and humeral fracture.

A common infraclavicular injury to the axillary nerve occurs with shoulder dislocation. The nerve is rendered taut as it is stretched across the humeral head. Most of these lesions recover spontaneously, but more slowly than expected. Signs of recovery may be delayed for 3 to 6 months or longer.

The milder nature of the infraclavicular injury is due to the restricted excursion of the fractured or dislocated humerus. Also, since the traction occurs laterally at a point far removed from an anatomic point of anchorage, the normal elasticity of the nerve roots protects them from damage. The branch of the plexus nearest its anchorage is the axillary nerve.

PRESENTING SIGNS AND SYMPTOMS

The young patient presents with a variety of patterns of paralysis and sensory loss depending on the neural elements that have been damaged. In addition, because of the forces required to injure the plexus, there are frequently associated injuries involving the head, cervical region of the spine and cord, clavicle, scapula, arm bones, and the rib cage. Associated central nervous system (CNS) injuries often take precedence in the priority of treatment and the plexus injury may not be evident in the acute postinjury period because of the patient's altered level of consciousness, loss of sensation, or loss of motor function due to CNS damage.

For patients whose only findings are related to plexus damage, the loss of function is usually a catastrophic event in their life, especially since early prognostic assurance is difficult to provide, even for the experienced brachial plexus clinician. At this stage, the primary physician will hedge bets on the chance for recovery unless there is clear evidence that the injury is an incomplete one where some motor or sensory function of each portion of the plexus is maintained.

The initial evaluation of the person with brachial plexus injury includes obtaining a meticulous history and performing a physical examination. Exquisite attention to the early findings and changes in the motor and sensory patterns can lead to a clearer understanding of the prognosis. Whether the paralysis and sensory loss had an instantaneous onset or developed over a period of time is also useful information for prognostication. Associated loss of consciousness, swelling in the neck, or clavicular, humeral, or scapular fractures should be documented. If the patient is months from the onset of the plexopathy, the history should be searched for any change in motor and sensory function. Spontaneous sensory or motor recovery has important prognostic implications.

Physical examination of the muscles and sensory mapping may help differentiate a peripheral nerve injury from a cord, trunk, or root injury. A complete muscle examination should include the proximal shoulder girdle muscles as well as the arm and hand muscles. Function of the diaphragm, serratus anterior, levator scapulae, and rhomboideus muscles should be carefully documented. Also, the muscles that cross the glenohumeral, elbow, wrist, and finger joints must be tested. As this evaluation takes place, myotomal and peripheral nerve patterns of muscle innervation should be kept in mind to determine the level of the neurologic structure that has been damaged (Fig. 86-2 and Table 86-1). Likewise, mapping of altered sensation should be performed to determine a dermatomal or peripheral nerve pattern (Figs. 86-3 and 86-4). The presence of a Tinel sign and its measured location should be recorded. The use of brachial and peripheral nerve maps should be encouraged in the clinical setting. With each clinical visit, chronologic mapping of neurologic changes helps provide for consistency and continuity of patient care. The sequence of neurologic change, or its lack, is now essential in determining when and if surgical intervention should be considered.

In the case of distal rupture of a trunk, a positive Tinel sign gives strong evidence of the availability of proximal axons from which to graft. With axonotmesis and the nerve in continuity, repeated examinations over time will demonstrate distal migration along the nerves of the point from which the Tinel sign arises. A Tinel sign can be present before any testable muscle has been reinnervated.

TESTING

Laboratory evaluations have useful implications in establishing the level of plexus involvement but may still not provide enough information to provide a definitive diagnosis. Myelography is of use for evaluating the lesion caused by a stretch or contusion where there is a question of root avulsion (8). Both computed tomography (CT) and magnetic resonance imaging (MRI) have their proponents but as experience has been gained, neither study has been found to be conclusively better than the other (9).

Electrodiagnostic studies have long been useful in the diagnostic work-up of the brachial plexus injury. With the advent of evoked potentials and intraoperative monitoring, the ability to demonstrate complete and incomplete injuries has been enhanced. Electrodiagnostic studies are valuable for mapping out the many elements of the plexus, peripheral nerves, and arm muscles individually.

Kline and Hudson (10) advocate the use of nerve action potential or compound nerve action potential recordings for the evaluation of plexus lesions in continuity. There is good correlation between the absence of action potential recordings and the presence of neurotmesis. Electromyographic (EMG) changes in the affected muscles will occur within 21 days of the injury. About this time, a number of muscles should be sampled, especially in the patient with a seemingly complete supraclavicular injury.

Since serious traumatic injuries of the plexus produce axonal change, signs of denervation should be present on the EMG recording. In addition, small or absent M-waves and sensory nerve action potentials (SNAP) should occur. Little, if any, slowing in conduction velocity should be found. Persistence of SNAP implies a lesion proximal to the dorsal root ganglion (i.e., root avulsion). A combined lesion may also lead to small or absent SNAP, and concomitant pathology at the root level can be hard to recognize unless needle EMG indicates involvement of the paraspinal or other muscles innervated by proximal plexus elements (11). Loss of functional continuity of components of the plexus may be confirmed by F-wave responses or somatosensory-evoked potential (SEP) studies. SEPs may provide incomplete information if multi-

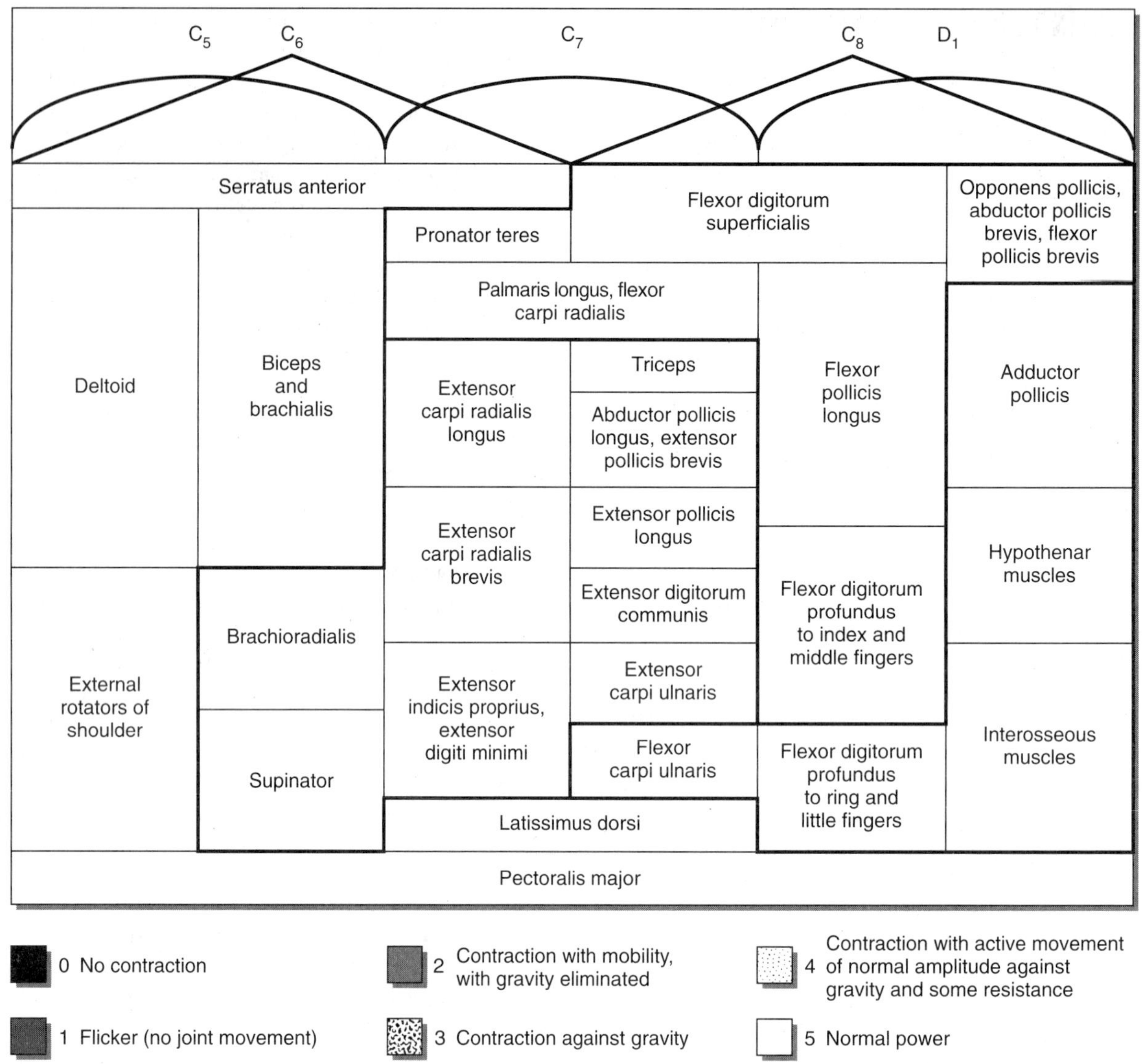

Figure 86-2. The C5-D1 spinal nerve contributions to the muscles of the upper extremity.

ple lesions are present. In addition, motor action potentials may be absent or show increased latency or latency asymmetry even without EMG signs of denervation in traumatic brachial plexus injuries. These electrical stimulation studies can complement EMG studies.

In patients with supraclavicular injuries, special EMG studies can answer how far proximally or medially the roots or spinal nerves are injured (11). A sampling of paravertebral muscles will help to establish if the posterior primary nerve has been involved, indicating a nerve root avulsion. In this case, signs of denervation will be present in paraspinal muscles as early as 10 days following the injury. Other proximal muscles may show spontaneous motor activity at 14 days and distal muscles should show positive signs by 21 days. The serratus anterior is another important muscle to study if the lesion is believed to be located at the root, trunk, or division level. Involvement of this muscle indicated a proximal level of nerve and plexus injury and has serious negative prognostic implications for neurologic recovery. Serratus anterior weakness also has negative implications for functional rehabilitation because of the proximal location of this muscle and its importance in arm stability. Other muscles whose involvement indicates proximal plexus problems include the levator scapulae, the diaphragm, the supraspinatus, and the infraspinatus. Patterns of muscle involvement become useful in determining the location of the plexus injury. Periodic re-evaluation by electrodiagnostic testing can

Table 86-1: Innervation of Muscles Responsible for Movements of the Shoulder Girdle and Upper Extremity

Muscle	Segmental Innervation	Peripheral Nerve
Trapezius	Cranial XI; C (2) 3–4	Spinal accessory nerve
Levator scapulae	C 3–4	Nerves to levator scapulae
	C 4–5	Dorsal scapular nerve
Rhomboideus major	C 4–5	Dorsal scapular nerve
Rhomboideus minor	C 4–5	Dorsal scapular nerve
Serratus anterior	C 5–7	Long thoracic nerve
Deltoid	C 5–6	Axillary nerve
Teres minor	C 5–6	Axillary nerve
Supraspinatus	C (4) 5–6	Suprascapular nerve
Infraspinatus	C (4) 5–6	Suprascapular nerve
Latissimus dorsi	C 6–8	Thoracodorsal nerve (long subscapular)
Pectoralis major	C 5–Th 1	Lateral and medial anterior thoracic
Pectoralis minor	C 7–Th 1	Medial anterior thoracic
Subscapularis	C 5–7	Subscapular nerves
Teres major	C 5–7	Lower subscapular nerve
Subclavius	C 5–6	Nerve to subclavius
Coracobrachialis	C 6–7	Musculocutaneous nerve
Biceps brachii	C 5–6	Musculocutaneous nerve
Brachialis	C 5–6	Musculocutaneous nerve
Brachioradialis	C 5–6	Radial nerve
Triceps brachii	C 6–8 (Th 1)	Radial nerve
Anconeus	C 7–8	Radial nerve
Supinator brevis	C 5–7	Radial nerve
Extensor carpi radialis longus	C (5) 6–7 (8)	Radial nerve
Extensor carpi radialis brevis	C (5) 6–7 (8)	Radial nerve
Extensor carpi ulnaris	C 6–8	Radial nerve
Extensor digitorum communis	C 6–8	Radial nerve
Extensor indicis proprius	C 6–8	Radial nerve
Extensor digiti minimi	C 6–8	Radial nerve
Extensor pollicis longus	C 6–8	Radial nerve
Extensor pollicis brevis	C 6–8	Radial nerve
Abductor pollicis longus	C 6–8	Radial nerve
Pronator teres	C 6–7	Median nerve
Flexor carpi radialis	C 6–7 (8)	Median nerve
Pronator quadratus	C 7–Th 1	Median nerve
Palmaris longus	C 7–Th 1	Median nerve
Flexor digitorum sublimis	C 7–Th 1	Median nerve
Flexor digitorum profundus (radial half)	C 7–Th 1	Median nerve
Lumbricales 1 and 2	C 7–Th 1	Median nerve
Flexor pollicis longus	C 8–Th 1	Median nerve
Flexor pollicis brevis (lateral head)	C 8–Th 1	Median nerve
Abductor pollicis brevis	C 8–Th 1	Median nerve
Opponens pollicis	C 8–Th 1	Median nerve
Flexor carpi ulnaris	C 7–Th 1	Ulnar nerve
Flexor digitorum profundus (ulnar half)	C 7–Th 1	Ulnar nerve
Interossei	C 8–Th 1	Ulnar nerve
Lumbricales 3 and 4	C 8–Th 1	Ulnar nerve
Flexor pollicis brevis (medial head)	C 8–Th 1	Ulnar nerve
Flexor digiti minimi brevis	C 8–Th 1	Ulnar nerve
Abductor digiti minimi	C 8–Th 1	Ulnar nerve
Opponens digiti minimi	C 8–Th 1	Ulnar nerve
Palmaris brevis	C 8–Th 1	Ulnar nerve
Adductor pollicis	C 8–Th 1	Ulnar nerve

Source: Reproduced by permission from De Jong R, Magee K. *The neurologic examination: incorporating the fundamentals of neuroanatomy and neurophysiology.* 4th ed. Hagerstown, MD: Harper & Row, 1979:342.

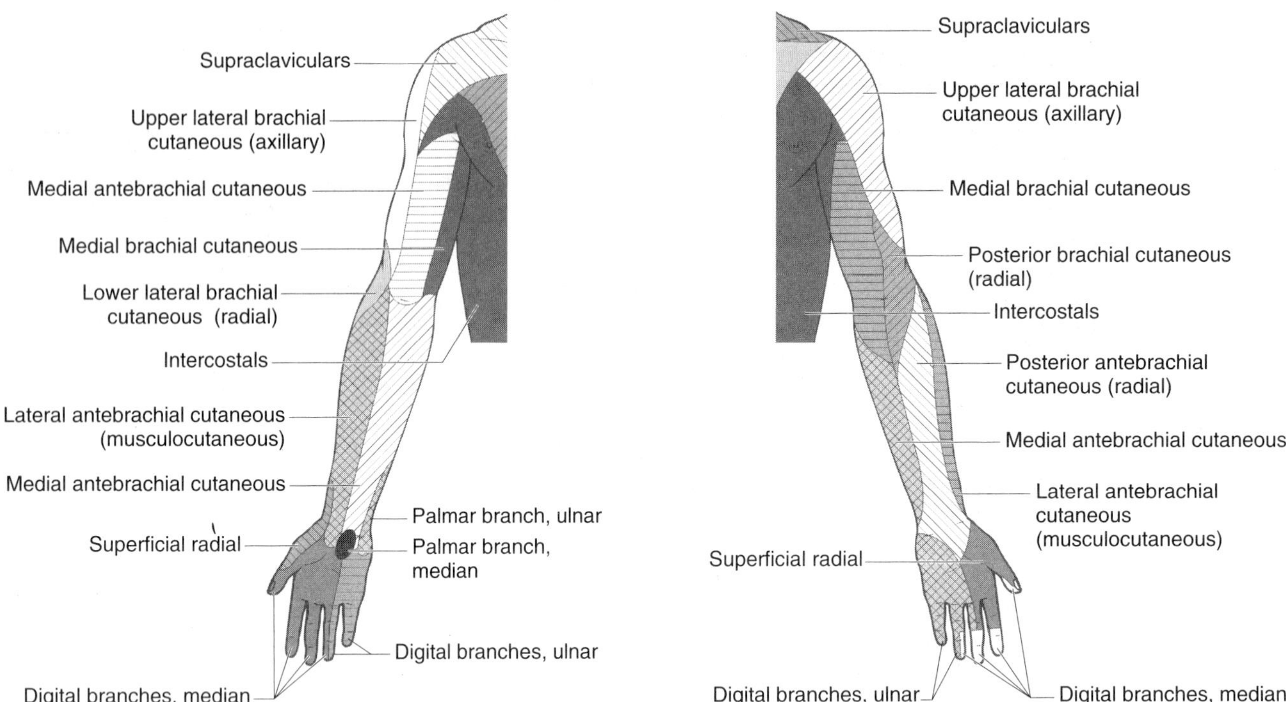

Figure 86-3. The sensory innervation of the upper extremity showing the peripheral nerve supply to the skin of the anterior and posterior surfaces. Left—anterior surface. Right—posterior surface. (From Flatau, E.: *Neurologische Schemata für die ärtzliche Praxis.* Berlin, Springer, 1915.)

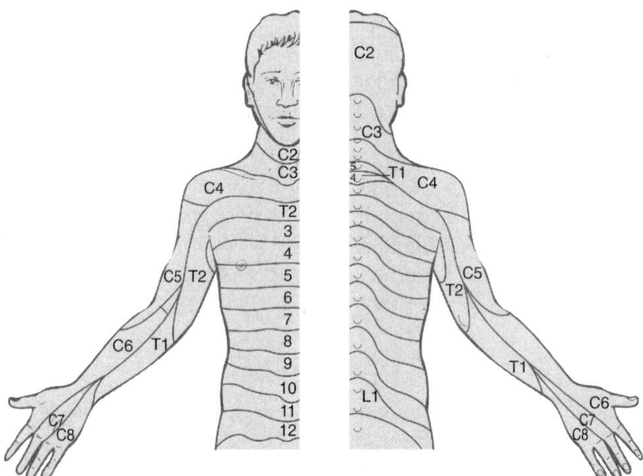

Figure 86-4. The sensory map of the upper extremity showing the dermatomal pattern of spinal segment innervation. (After Foerster, from Haymaker, W., and Woodhall, B.: *Peripheral Nerve Injuries* [ed. 2]. Philadelphia, Saunders, 1953.)

demonstrate neurologic improvement before signs of improved motor or sensory recovery will occur on physical examination.

Electrodiagnostic studies showing positive results should be repeated every 3 to 6 months, to aid in treatment planning and provide prognostic information.

PROGNOSTIC INFORMATION

Prognostic indicators, in addition to electrodiagnostic findings, include the history of the injury, early physical findings, and the mechanism of injury. Favorable prognostic factors include neurologic damage following a shoulder dislocation or an infraclavicular injury. The presence of incomplete paralysis in each myotome and a distally migrating Tinel sign are also favorable findings. Unfavorable prognostic indicators include severe initial trauma associated with other bodily injuries, involvement of the serratus anterior, and the presence of a Horner syndrome, indicating a severe proximal level of involvement at C8–T1. The Horner syndrome is present with a lesion at this level because there is disruption of the cervical sympathetic fibers. Sympathetic fibers at C8–T1 accompany the trigeminal nerve to the eye and innervate the dilator muscles of the iris, the tarsal muscles, and the orbital muscles. When these fibers are disrupted, a Horner syndrome including miosis, ptosis, and enophthalmos results.

REHABILITATION STAGING

In the first few months following a plexus injury, the rehabilitative philosophy is dual: prevention and maintenance. This phase focuses on educating patients about the injury they have sustained and which nerves and muscles have been affected. If there is extensive anesthesia in the hand and forearm, protective care is taught. An understanding of osteoporosis in the presence of paralysis should help prevent long-bone trauma. Additionally, passive range of motion exercises performed within the normal range are taught to patients and families so they can be accomplished at home at least twice daily. The paralyzed limb should be positioned so as to prevent edema and to provide support for the glenohumeral joint in an attempt to reduce subluxation. Some patients prefer to support the hand by putting it in the pants pocket rather than a sling. Placing the hand in the pants pocket also is a cosmetic way to disguise a flail arm.

If the affected limb is the dominant arm, then the teaching of one-handed activities of daily living and change-of-dominance activities should be instituted immediately after the injury. Special activities to concentrate on include writing (penmanship), food cutting (rocker knife), buttoning (button hook), and using one-handed methods to tie bows or knots. Other adaptive equipment may be useful based on the person's functional needs. Electrical stimulation of the muscles that show weak but volitional control may assist in strengthening them more quickly than do active-assistive range of motion exercises alone.

The emotional implications of the sudden loss of arm function are usually severe for a previously healthy, young adult. Additionally, there is often associated pain that may become chronic. The early acknowledgment of the tremendous physical loss and concomitant pain can overwhelm the emotional defenses of the injured person. An experienced rehabilitation psychologist should be consulted, to establish a psychotherapeutic relationship soon after the injury. This can help with the adjustment to disability and pain and in dealing with any issues suggestive of posttraumatic stress disorder. These rehabilitation therapeutic relationships are often long lasting since, for the patient with severe plexus injury, the outcome will not be known for many months.

For the patient who desperately hopes that upon awakening each morning there will be some sign of new sensation or a flicker of muscle movement, the waiting process is usually a period of emotional turmoil. This prolonged postinjury period requires regular medical reevaluation and honest communication regarding the likelihood of improvement. Clear and careful communication from the physician to the patient becomes essential in an attempt to keep the patient actively involved in the treatment plan. There can be a tendency to "doctor shop," but often a second opinion from a brachial plexus specialist is appropriate.

The previous philosophy of "watch and wait" to see if improvement occurs spontaneously is no longer appropriate. With increasing surgical knowledge and technique improvements, many more of these injuries will benefit from earlier surgical exploration, grafting, and reconstruction. The current axiom for brachial plexus surgery is that surgery should be performed if there is no recovery by 3 months or if the recovery has plateaued before 6 months following the injury. If surgery is performed more than 6 months following the injury, the chance for maximal recovery is reduced (12).

PAIN

Pain may become a chronic problem following injury to the brachial plexus. Wynn Parry (13) found that 90% of plexus injury patients in his series experienced pain, and at 3 years, a third still has significant pain. All attempts at conservative management should be made in the early postinjury phase. The cause of this pain is believed to be similar to that associated with other peripheral nerve injuries. Pain treatment should avoid the use of opioids or synthetic opioids. Contemporary pain medication options will include carbamazepine, gabapentin, phenytoin, clonidine, tricyclic antidepressants, baclofen, and mexiletine. The application of transcutaneous electrical nerve stimulation may also provide benefit in the alteration of pain. Relaxation and biofeedback techniques may also help diminish the pain, especially if there is secondary postural or myofascial pain.

For persons with pain not relieved by conservative techniques, surgical exploration of the injured plexus components and neurolysis may decrease the intensity of the pain. If there is a significant sympathetic component to the pain, stellate or Bier blocks may also diminish the level of pain. Other invasive techniques have been utilized to decrease the pain but studies are lacking. Techniques that have found some utility are dorsal root entry-zone rhizotomies (DREZs) (14,15), epidural stimulation, and thalamic stimulation. These techniques, in the hands of experienced surgeons, may improve the pain-disabled person's quality of life. The treatment algorithm should be developed and explained to the individual by members of an experienced pain treatment team.

ORTHOTIC APPLICATIONS

If the plexus injury predominately involves the C5 and C6 roots or the upper trunk carrying the C5 and C6 elements, then the proximal arm muscles that cross the glenohumeral joint are paralyzed. Loss of the C5 and C6 myotomal innervation also results in loss of normal elbow flexion. The loss of glenohumeral movement and stability, as well as the lack of elbow flexion, provides a challenge for orthotic and surgical restoration. If hand and forearm functions are preserved, then the functional challenge is to stabilize the glenohumeral joint and provide some force to produce elbow flexion. An orthosis with a shoulder piece (Fig. 86–5) and joint can assist to stabilize the shoulder, but it is quite bulky. The shoulder piece and joint can be attached to an elbow-locking mechanism that is manually activated. Alternatively, an axilla loop with a control cable can actively lock and unlock the elbow joint.

In the plexus-injured person with a C8–T1 injury, the hand is usually flail and assumes an intrinsic minus deformity in the claw position. A long opponens orthosis that positions the hand in a functional attitude can be worn to protect the hand from injury and to attempt to prevent a claw deformity. If C7 function is present, then the hand can provide gross grasp and release, which can be helpful in assisting the opposite hand in bimanual tasks. However, power grasp cannot be provided with orthotic or surgical interventions.

When C7, C8, and T1 roots are damaged, the hand and most of the forearm muscles, except for the radial wrist extensors, are nonfunctional. The radial wrist extensors will provide wrist dorsiflexion and a weak key pinch through a tenodesis effect. A stronger tenodesis pinch can be achieved orthotically with a wrist-driven flexor tenodesis orthosis. Surgically, improved pinch may be obtained using a variety of reconstructive procedures about the wrist and hand.

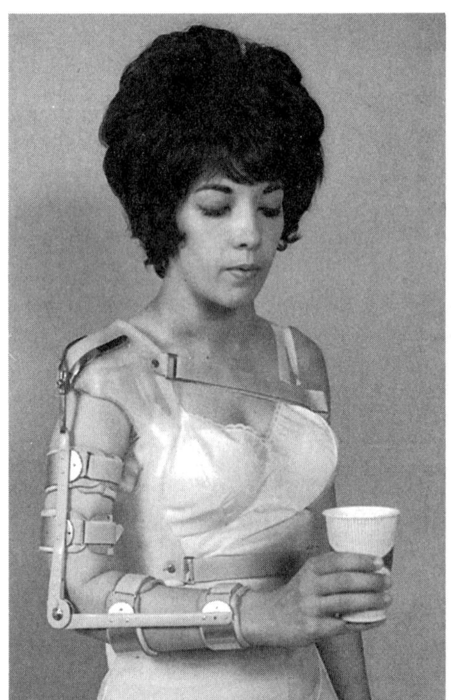

Figure 86-5. Orthotic option for a C5,6 brachial plexus injury with a functional hand. The unstable glenohumeral joint is supported and the elbow can be passively positioned and locked so that the hand can be placed in the desired position for function.

SURGICAL TECHNIQUES FOR INJURED NERVES

The surgical techniques for reconstruction of plexus elements include neurolysis, primary nerve repair, cable grafting, interfascicular grafting, neurotization (nerve transfers), and a combination of these procedures. Neurolysis is performed to remove the scar tissue from an injured nerve in continuity. Removal of the scar tissue is done to facilitate axon growth (16). Primary nerve repair has a limited place in the surgical management of these injuries because seldom are the nerves transected cleanly (17). The most commonly used technique for plexus repair is nerve grafting. These grafts are placed to facilitate return of muscle function in the shoulder girdle and across the elbow (18). Return of innervation to the distal region of the forearm and hand is much less likely to occur. Interfascicular grafts are used to repair the cords and branches and cable grafts are used for the repair of nerve roots and trunks (19). Nerve transfers are most commonly performed using the intercostal nerves, the cervical plexus nerves, the spinal accessory nerve, or a combination of these. Experienced surgeons have had improved functional outcomes in the properly selected patient with plexus injury. In general, surgical repair of the infraclavicular injury carries a better prognosis than that of the supraclavicular injury (20,21).

Intraoperative monitoring is useful to evaluate the presence of nerve action and sensory-evoked potentials. The use of nerve action potentials is applicable for an injured nerve in continuity at least 2 months following the injury (22). SEPs can be assessed at any interval following the injury. Electrical stimulation at the time of surgery can also help to identify nerves in continuity that could not be determined to contract clinically.

RECONSTRUCTIVE ORTHOPEDIC PROCEDURES

Upper-extremity reconstructive surgery in the individual with an incomplete brachial plexus injury may provide useful arm function, especially if the scapula and glenohumeral joints are stable and forearm flexion can be restored. If the serratus anterior is of normal strength, thereby stabilizing the scapula on the thorax, but there is significant weakness in the C5–C6-innervated muscles creating glenohumeral instability, a glenohumeral arthrodesis should be considered. If no active elbow flexion is present but there is residual C7–C8 muscle function, a tendon transfer to produce elbow flexion can be accomplished. Any muscle that has good to normal strength can be transferred; the pectoralis major, the triceps, or the latissimus dorsi muscle are used most frequently. The chosen muscle is tied into the biceps mechanism to achieve active elbow flexion against gravity. Often, electrodiagnostic and careful manual muscle testing will identify the muscles best suited for transfer.

Tendon transfers should be performed no sooner than 1 year after the injury occurred, to permit time for evidence of spontaneous return. An exception to this would be if there is documented evidence of neurotmesis, as seen at the time of surgical exploration.

If the shoulder is flail and arthrodesis is to be performed, Richard (23) suggested that the humerus be placed in 30 degrees of flexion and 30 degrees of internal rotation. Abduction at the shoulder should be in the 20- to 30-degree range.

AMPUTATION OF THE ARM IN THE PRESENCE OF A BRACHIAL PLEXUS INJURY

If the entire arm is flail and insensate but there is good scapular stability and scapular motion, a glenohumeral arthrodesis with an elective transhumeral amputation may be the starting point for prosthetic functional restoration. Proximal scapular and glenohumeral stability is essential if useful prosthetic function is to be an expected outcome. Successful prosthetic function also depends on the services of an experienced upper-limb prosthetist and a therapist who understands brachial plexus amputees, their residual muscle function, and the biomechanical changes present in the affected extremity. The person with a flail arm can expect a better functional outcome with the combination of a transhumeral amputation (Fig. 86–6), glenohumeral stability, appropriate prosthesis, and excellent prosthetic training.

If an amputation is considered and active elbow flexion can be obtained despite a flail, insensate hand, a transradial amputation could be considered. Even if the forearm lacks sensation, with active elbow flexion against gravity, a long transradial level should be chosen over a transhumeral level of amputation.

The plexus patient who has had a transradial amputation should be fitted with a body-powered transradial prosthesis. If there is insufficient residual elbow flexion strength to lift the terminal device, a forearm flexion lift assist can be added to the elbow hinge. This assist will counterbalance the weight of the residual forearm and prosthesis, making elbow flexion easier.

If there is significant anesthesia distal to the middle of the humerus and no chance for restoring active elbow flexion, a transhumeral amputation should be considered. The glenohumeral joint must be stabilized if there is insufficient intrinsic shoulder muscle strength. Glenohumeral stabilization can be performed at the time of the amputation. A distal transhumeral level of amputation should be chosen to provide the optimal lever arm to transmit forces to the prosthesis. If the scapular muscles do not have

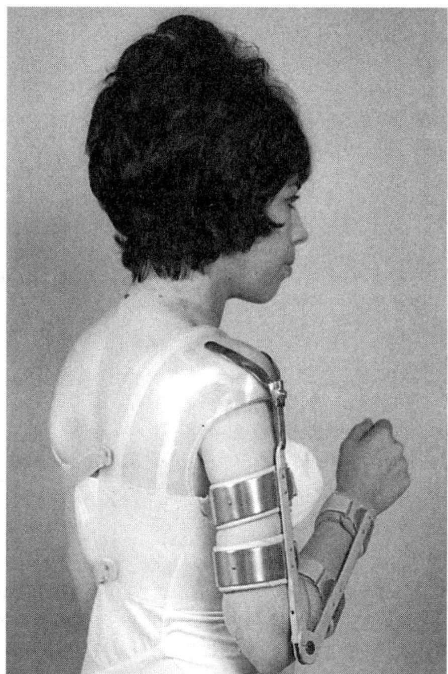

Figure 86-6. Posterior view of orthosis used in a C5,6 brachial plexus palsy showing the thoracic suspension component and the shoulder joint required to stabilize the glenohumeral joint.

nearly normal muscle strength, amputation and prosthetic replacement will not result in useful function.

The body-powered prosthesis for the plexus-injured patient who has had an amputation at a transhumeral level should contain the lightest-weight terminal device and wrist joint. Generally, there is not sufficient muscle signal remaining in the affected limb for an externally powered or myoelectric prosthesis to work in the brachial plexus–injured amputee. Proximal axial muscles may produce excellent EMG signals but their signals are difficult to isolate for prosthetic motor activation of the prosthesis.

CONCLUSIONS

The person with a brachial plexus injury presents a multifaceted challenge for the physiatrist who has an interest in the rehabilitation of peripheral nerve pathology and dysfunction. With the new surgical approaches available, surgical intervention has taken a new prominence in the rehabilitation management of these individuals. Thorough physical examination and electrodiagnostic evaluation are essential for developing a comprehensive interdisciplinary treatment plan. Diagramming the location and extent of the suspected lesion is important for this plan and for providing meaningful prognostic information for the person with the injury. Pain management and switch-of-dominance activities are important in the acute postinjury phase. Regular and periodic re-revaluations are essential for preventing disabling complications, developing patient rapport, keeping track of neural regeneration, and providing current rehabilitative interventions. A few individuals may elect to have a flail, insensate extremity amputated. Some of these individuals may find prosthetic restoration more useful than the arm segment that has been removed. Psychosocial assessment and follow-through are often useful during the period of unknown neurologic recovery.

REFERENCES

1. Wynn Parry CB. The management of injuries to the brachial plexus. *Proc R Soc Med* 1974;67:488.
2. Hentz VR, Narakas A. The results of microneurosurgical reconstruction in complete brachial plexus palsy. *Orthop Clin North Am* 1988;19:107–114.
3. Millesi H. Brachial plexus injuries. In: Chapman M, ed. *Operative orthopedics*. Philadelphia: JB Lippincott, 1988:1417.
4. Kline DG. Perspectives concerning brachial plexus injury and repair. *Neurosurg Clin North Am* 1991;2:151–164.
5. Leffert RD. *Brachial plexus injuries*. New York: Churchill Livingstone, 1985.
6. Alnot JY. Traumatic brachial plexus palsy in the adult. Retro- and infraclavicular lesions. *Clin Orthop* 1988;237:9–16.
7. Leffert RD, Seddon HJ. Infraclavicular brachial plexus injuries. *J Bone Joint Surg [Br]* 1965;47:9.
8. Campbell JB. Peripheral nerve repair. *Clin Neurosurg* 1970; 17:77–98.
9. Millesi H. Brachial plexus injuries. Management and results. *Clin Plast Surg* 1984;11:115–120.
10. Kline DG, Hudson AR. *Nerve injuries*. Philadelphia: WB Saunders, 1995.
11. Yiannikas L, Chahani B, Young R. The investigation of traumatic lesions of the brachial plexus by electromyography and short latency somatosensory potentials. *J Neurol Neurosurg Psychiatry* 1983;46:1014–1022.
12. Aminoff MJ, Olney RK, Parry GJ, Raskin NH. Relative utility of different electrophysiologic techniques in the evaluation of brachial plexopathies. *Neurology* 1988;38:546–550.
13. Wynn Parry CB. Pain in avulsion injuries of the brachial plexus. *Neurosurgery* 1984;15:960–965.
14. Thomas DGT, Jones SJ. Dorsal root entry zone lesions (Nashold's procedure) in brachial plexus avulsion. *Neurosurgery* 1984;15: 966–968.
15. Nashold BS, Ostdakl RH. Dorsal root entry zone lesions for pain relief. *J Neurosurg* 1979;51: 59–69.
16. Kline DG. Civilian gunshot wound to the brachial plexus. *J Neurosurg* 1989;70:166–174.
17. Kline DG, Judice DJ. Operative management of selected brachial plexus lesions. *J Neurosurg* 1983;58:631–649.
18. Millesi H. Brachial plexus injuries. Nerve grafting. *Clin Orthop* 1988;237:36–42.
19. Krakauer JD, Wood MB. Brachial plexus—adult injuries and salvage. In: Peimer CA, ed. *Surgery of the hand and upper extremity*. New York: McGraw-Hill, 1996: 1411–1442.
20. Leffert RD, Seddon H. Infraclavicular brachial plexus injuries. *J Bone Joint Surg [Br]* 1965; 47:9.
21. Bonney G. Prognosis in traction lesions of the brachial plexus. *J Bone Joint Surg [Br]* 1959; 41:4.
22. McGillicuddy JE. Clinical decision making in brachial plexus injuries. *Neurosurg Clin North Am* 1991;2:137–150.
23. Richard RR. Operative treatment for irreparable lesions of the brachial plexus. In: Gelberman R, ed. *Operative nerve repair and reconstruction*. Philadelphia: JB Lippincott, 1991.

Chapter 87

Poliomyelitis and Postpolio Syndrome

James C. Agre
Arthur A. Rodriquez

HISTORICAL PERSPECTIVE

As recently as 40 years ago, acute poliomyelitis was a major cause of death and paralysis and paresis in children and young adults in developed countries. Although the incidence of acute poliomyelitis dropped precipitously in developed countries after the introduction of the Salk vaccine, at the present time acute poliomyelitis remains a threat in many underdeveloped countries and will remain so for several years to come. There is great hope that poliomyelitis will be eradicated from the world by the year 2000; however, even if this occurs, individuals will still continue to have problems associated with the late effects of polio until well into the later half of the twenty-first century.

Although the first reports acknowledging the development of new weakness in polio survivors many years after the onset of acute poliomyelitis illness were over 120 years ago (1,2), only in the last two decades has this problem been more widely recognized by health care providers. The first descriptions of new weakness occurring years after the initial onset of polio were of young men who had poliomyelitis in infancy who developed new weakness after the performance of repetitive, physically demanding work. In 1962, Zilkha (3) reviewed the cases of several individuals who had developed new weakness 20 to 40 years after an acute poliomyelitis illness. He suggested that the new weakness in these individuals was related to their initial poliomyelitis illness.

Since these initial reports, a number of reports sporadically described similar findings, with complaints such as new weakness and fatigue occurring up to 71 years after the acute illness (4). These neurologic changes were commonly diagnosed as a form of progressive muscular atrophy, late progression of poliomyelitis, or a forme fruste amyotrophic lateral sclerosis (5,6). It was not until the mid-1980s, 30 to 40 years after the epidemics of the 1940s and 1950s, however, that the late effects of poliomyelitis began to become widely recognized by health care professionals. This was at the time of the first symposium on the late effects of poliomyelitis, held in Warm Springs, Georgia (7).

EPIDEMIOLOGY

The incidence of acute poliomyelitis in the United States was approximately 10 cases per 100,000 population during the epidemics of the 1940s. This incidence increased and peaked during the epidemic of 1952, when the incidence reached 15 cases per 100,000 population and over 57,800 new cases were reported (8). After the Salk vaccine was introduced in 1955 and the Sabin vaccine in 1961, the incidence of acute poliomyelitis dropped to 0.04 case per 100,000 population by 1963 and the last confirmed case of paralytic polio from domestic wild virus was in 1979 (8). Paralytic polio is now a very rare complication of the Sabin (oral, live, attenuated-virus) vaccine. In 1989, the incidence of paralytic polio from the Sabin vaccine was 0.23 case per 10 million doses (8).

The number of polio survivors in the United States at the present time is unknown; however, from a survey by the National Center for Health Statistics in 1987, it has been estimated that there are at least 640,000 survivors of paralytic poliomyelitis (9). Thus, although acute poliomyelitis has been virtually eliminated from the United States, paralytic polio is one of the most prevalent neuromuscular diseases.

The percentage of polio survivors in the United States experiencing new symptoms that may be related to their previous polio illness is unknown, but estimates have ranged from 25% to 60% (10–13). Thus, one might estimate that there are between 160,000 and 380,000 individuals in the United States at the present time who may be experiencing the late effects of polio. In all likelihood, this number will increase as polio survivors age.

PATHOPHYSIOLOGY OF ACUTE POLIOMYELITIS

Poliomyelitis occurs as a result of a generalized viral infection that has an affinity for motor neurons. The virus is a single-stranded RNA enterovirus belonging to the picornavirus group and has three antigenically distinguishable viruses (14). The wild polio virus usually enters the body through oral ingestion. It then replicates in the lymphoid tissues of the pharynx and ileum. It is an extremely infectious, but usually benign virus. Most individuals infected (approximately 90%–95%) are unaware of illness, while 4% to 8% of infected individuals are only aware of a nonspecific viral illness (such as fever, myalgia, upper respiratory tract or gastrointestinal symptoms), and only 1% to 2% of individuals develop paralysis (15). The spread to the central nervous system is thought to be by viremia. In these individuals, headache, nuchal rigidity, and backache usually develop, similar to individuals with a viral meningitis.

The rate of paralysis also varies with the strain of the virus and the individual's age. Paralysis occurs in 1 in 1000 infected children, while in adults the rate of paralysis is 1 in 75 (9). Paralysis is usually asymmetric and the legs are more commonly involved than the arms. Severe bulbar weakness occurs in 10% to 15% of paralytic patients (9). The pathologic findings of acute poliomyelitis consist of inflammation of the meninges and the motor neurons with loss of spinal and bulbar motor neurons (16). Other findings include abnormalities in the cerebellar nuclei, reticular formation, thalamus, hypothalamus, cortical neurons, and dorsal horn (16).

With death of the motor neurons, wallerian degeneration results, and the muscle fibers innervated by these neurons become "orphaned," resulting in motor weakness. In histologic studies of anterior horn cells of monkeys with paralytic poliomyelitis, Bodian (17) found that nearly all (97%) of the anterior horn cells of severely paralyzed limbs were affected by the virus during acute infection. About one-half of these motor neurons died during the early convalescent period, and the other half survived. A good correlation was noted between the proportion of destroyed motor neurons and the severity of paralysis (18).

The amount of recovery of strength and endurance following the acute poliomyelitis illness was determined by four major factors: 1) the number of motor neurons that recover and resume normal function, 2) the number of "orphaned" muscle fibers that are reinnervated by the surviving motor units through terminal axonal sprouting, 3) muscle hypertrophy resulting from increasing activity after the acute illness, and 4) improvement in muscle endurance capacity resulting from increasing activity after the acute illness.

It may have been difficult for the clinician to detect weakness in many polio patients unless most of the anterior horn cells of the particular muscle were destroyed. This concept is supported by three separate studies. Bodian and Howe (19) reported no observable paresis or paralysis in many muscle groups in patients with poliomyelitis, although postmortem histologic study showed that many of the motor neurons were destroyed. It was presumed that the anterior horn cell destruction was too scattered to involve one muscle group to the extent that clinically evident weakness would be noted. Sharrard (20) reported that manual muscle testing showed normal results in several muscle groups in a polio patient during his lifetime, although more than half of those muscle's anterior horn cells were shown to be destroyed at the time of a detailed postmortem study. Beasley (21) reported that the average postpolio patient, deemed to have normal strength of the quadriceps muscles by manual muscle testing, had a 50% reduction in strength when muscle strength was measured quantitatively. It is certainly plausible that a chronic deficit in strength in some muscle groups may be one contributing factor to the development of postpolio syndrome in some polio survivors at the present time (22).

PROPOSED ETIOLOGIES FOR LATE NEUROMUSCULAR DETERIORATION

A number of different etiologies have been proposed for the late deterioration reported by poliomyelitis survivors. These etiologies can be divided into pathophysiologic and functional etiologies.

Proposed Pathophysiologic Etiologies

A number of pathophysiologic etiologies for late neuromuscular deterioration in polio survivors have been proposed and reviewed in detail by Jubelt and Cashman (23). These possible etiologies are listed in Table 87-1. More recently, Gawne and Halstead (9) reviewed these factors and added an additional factor, the role of somatomedin C (SmC) or insulin-like growth factor type 1 (IGF-1). IGF-1

Table 87-1: Possible Etiology of Postpoliomyelitis Progressive Muscular Atrophy
Chronic poliovirus infection
Death of remaining motor neurons with normal aging, coupled with the previous loss from poliomyelitis
Premature aging of cells permanently damaged by poliovirus
Premature aging of remaining normal motor neurons due to an increased metabolic demand (increased motor unit size following poliomyelitis)
Loss of individual muscle fibers per reinnervated motor unit with advancing age in the large reinnervated motor units that developed after polio
Predisposition to motor neuron degeneration because of the glial, vascular, and lymphatic changes caused by poliovirus
Poliomyelitis-induced vulnerability of motor neurons to secondary insults
Genetic predisposition of motor neurons to both poliomyelitis and premature degeneration
An immune-mediated syndrome

Source: Reproduced by permission from Jubelt B, Cashman NR. Neurological manifestations of the postpolio syndrome. *Crit Rev Clin Neurobiol* 1987;3:199–220.

plays an important role in protein synthesis and aids in the proliferation of muscle satellite cells and the regeneration of peripheral nerve sprouts (24). The few reports on this topic are not consistent. In a small study of 12 stable postpolio and 10 unstable postpolio subjects, IGF-1 was markedly reduced in those with postpolio syndrome (25). In a much larger study, however, of 87 postpolio patients (with 57 of the subjects being unstable), serum IGF-1 levels were not different in the postpolio subjects compared to 392 nonpolio control subjects of similar age (26). For many of the proposed pathophysiologic factors, there has been a lack of consistent findings from study to study as well as a failure to uncover conclusive findings in all patients with postpolio syndrome. This certainly suggests that there is not a single pathophysiologic cause of new weakness, and this area could benefit from further research.

Proposed Functional Etiologies

A number of functional etiologic factors that could lead to apparent loss of neuromuscular function in the polio survivor have also been proposed (22). These factors, which include disuse weakness, overuse weakness, insidious weight gain, and chronic weakness, are briefly discussed.

Disuse Muscle Weakness

It is well known that disuse will lead to a decrease in muscle strength as well as in cardiorespiratory fitness. Müller (27) demonstrated that young, healthy individuals can lose over 20% of their strength with 1 week of immobilization. Saltin et al (28) demonstrated that young, healthy individuals can lose 25% of their cardiorespiratory fitness with 3 weeks of bed rest.

There is some indirect evidence suggesting that disuse may play a role in the loss of strength or endurance, at least in some postpolio individuals. In two studies, the concentration of citrate synthase, an aerobic enzyme, was very low in postpolio individuals and this was believed to be compatible with a reduced level of physical activity (29,30). And, a reduction in the concentration of aerobic enzymes within the muscle will reduce the muscle's ability to perform endurance activity. In a clinical report, 44% of postpolio patients seen in a postpolio clinic acknowledged that their decline in function began when they were hospitalized (31). It was suggested that the disuse brought on by bed rest led to strength loss from which the patient could not fully recover. In another clinical report (32), the concentration of high-density-lipoprotein (HDL) cholesterol was significantly reduced in postpolio men and it was thought that this reflected a reduced activity level in these individuals, as activity is known to increase the concentration of HDL cholesterol (33).

Overuse Muscle Weakness

Overuse of weakened muscles may be a cause for declining function in some polio survivors. Although the concept of overuse is not new, the mechanisms for it are not well understood. Several reports indirectly linked overuse to new weakness and problems in some polio survivors. The first reports of this kind were published over 120 years ago (1,2). Then in 1915, Lovett (34) reported that activity in some polio survivors led to deterioration rather than improvement in function. He noted that the level of activity correlated with the functional deterioration. In the 1950s, Bennett and Knowlton (35,36) cited five case reports in which postpolio individuals lost function with excessive activity. These anecdotal reports suggest that overuse may lead to decreasing strength, at least in some polio survivors.

A number of clinical studies also suggested that overuse may play a role in declining function in some polio survivors. Luna-Reyes et al (37) reported that the energy consumption of postpolio children was two to three times as great when a lower-limb orthosis was not used as compared to when an appropriate orthosis was utilized. And, many polio survivors are rather reluctant to use orthotic devices. In a kinesiologic study, Perry et al (38) evaluated 34 symptomatic postpolio individuals with dynamic electromyography. They reported that the average postpolio individual had excessive use of two muscle groups, suggesting that muscle overuse may have contributed to the subjects' complaints. In another kinesiologic study, Borg et al (39) noted that some polio survivors recruited all or nearly all of their tibialis anterior muscle motor units when simply walking. They postulated that this might lead to muscle overuse. In another study, we (40) reported that symptomatic postpolio subjects had a deficit in strength recovery after fatiguing exercise. We suggested that this deficit was related to greater metabolic muscle fatigue (41), which would be expected with muscle overuse. Two other studies reported that the concentration of creatine kinase was increased in symptomatic postpolio subjects (42,43). These data suggest that at least some postpolio individuals may be overusing their remaining musculature.

Weight Gain

An increase in body weight will result in greater energy expenditure in the performance of daily activities. It is well known in non-postpolio individuals that weight oftentimes increases with age. Increasing weight, as a result of deposition of adipose tissue, may be quite deleterious to the postpolio individual. There are few data concerning weight gain in postpolio individuals; however, the data available indicate that weight gain may very well be a problem. One clinical report indicated that 60% of patients seen in a postpolio clinic for evaluation acknowledged a recent gain in body weight (31). A 4-year longitudinal study of Swedish and American postpolio individuals found that American, but not Swedish, subjects gained a significant amount of weight. The average American subject gained 1 kg of body weight per year (44). Although body composition was not measured, it was thought that the gain in body weight reflected an increase in adiposity, as muscle strength was found to slightly decline over the same interval of time.

Chronic Muscle Weakness

It is most probable that most polio survivors are not specifically aware of the deficits in muscle strength that they may have had since their initial illness. As discussed already, it is likely that health care professionals may have had difficulty in identifying muscles weakened by acute poliomyelitis, and this appears to have been corroborated by Beasley's study (21), which demonstrated a 50% deficit in strength in postpolio subjects with supposedly "normal" strength.

Combination of Etiologies

Finally, it has been hypothesized that a number of different etiologies may lead to deteriorating function in polio survivors (9). The various suggested pathophysiologic and functional etiologies may interact with one another and multiply the effects of any single factor (Fig. 87-1). For instance, simple muscle overuse may result in pain, which may lead to the individual decreasing his or her level of activity. This may then result in disuse weakness and the decreasing level of activity may result in weight gain. With decreased activity, joint contracture may develop, leading to increasing joint or muscle pain, which may result in yet a further decrease in activity and further deterioration. Treatment of the postpolio individual needs to be based on the assessment of the individual and possible contributing factors leading to dysfunction and intervention whenever possible.

POSTPOLIO CHARACTERISTICS

Clinical Characteristics

A number of different studies over the past decade documented that many postpolio patients develop similar symptoms (Table 87-2) (11,13,31,45–47). Two of these studies were population based (11,13), one was questionnaire based (47), and the other three were clinically based (31,45,46), which may account for the differences in the prevalence of the various symptoms. Some functional problems are also commonly acknowledged by polio survivors (Table 87-3) (11,31,45,47,48).

The complaints are varied but generally can be divided into complaints of pain, fatigue, weakness, and other problems. Most prevalent of these complaints are complaints of musculoskeletal pain from muscle overuse or myofascial origin; pain from a progressive increase in skeletal deformity; pain in biomechanically disadvantaged, deformed, or marginally stable joints; fatigue; new muscle weakness or atrophy; respiratory impairment; cold intolerance; and a decline in activity of daily living (ADL) function. Most patients have a number of complaints when seen in a postpolio clinic.

Pain

General orthopedic problems leading to joint or muscle pain are very common in patients seen in postpolio clinics. In one study of 193 patients seen in a postpolio clinic, 58 (30%) had problems with their orthotic devices (49). Genu recurvatum was a problem for 54 (28%) of the patients and 40 of the 54 (75%) of these patients had knee pain as a significant concern. In another clinical report of 79 postpolio patients, joint pain was acknowledged by 61 (77%) and back pain by 55 (70%) (31). The most common diagnoses included degenerative arthritis or arthralgia [in 56 (71%) of patients] and muscle overuse pain or myofascial pain [in 56 (71%) of patients]. In another study of 183 patients, at the time of the evaluation only 25 patients (14%) used an orthosis and the average age of the orthosis was 15 years (50). A new orthosis was recommended for 57 of 183 (31%) of these patients and use of a cane or crutches, for an additional 15 of 183 (8%) of individuals. In another study of 103 patients, only 19 patients (18%) were using an orthosis at the time of the appointment. As a result of the evaluation, a new orthosis was recommended for 37 (36%) of the patients (51). In another study, a follow-up evaluation of 41 patients, orthopedic defects (including scoliosis, fracture sequelae, or joint pain) were noted in 24 patients (59%) (52).

Fatigue

Fatigue is a very difficult complaint to assess objectively, but is one of the two most common complaints acknowl-

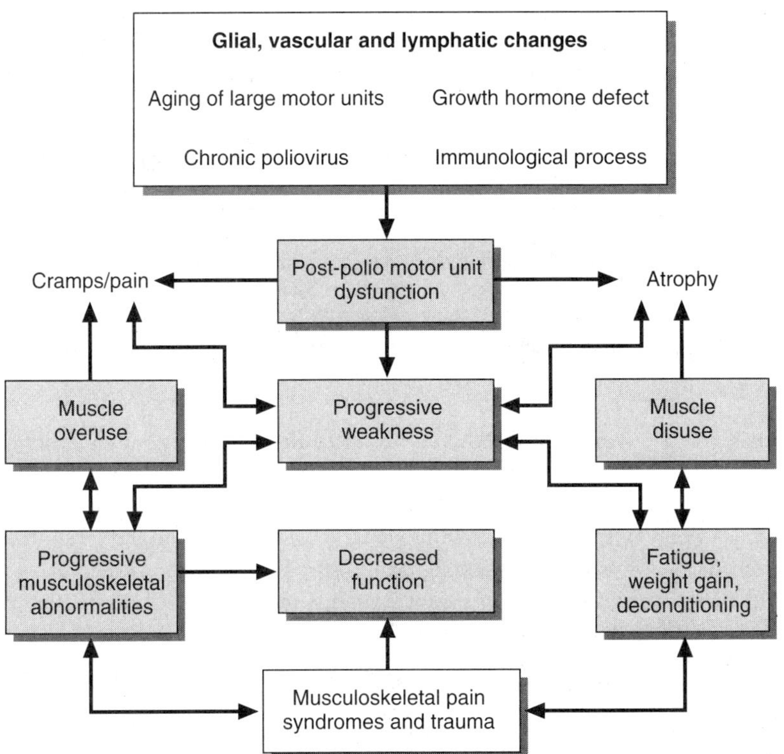

Figure 87-1. Schematic model showing possible etiologic factors for the late neuromuscular and musculoskeletal complaints of poliomyelitis and their interactions. (Reproduced by permission from Gawne AC, Halstead LS. Post-polio syndrome: pathophysiology and clinic management. *Crit Rev Phys Rehabil Med* 1995;7:147–188.)

Table 87-2: Comparison of Most Common New Symptoms in Subjects with a History of Paralytic Polio Reported in Six Studies

Symptom	Codd et al (11) (n = 28)	Halstead and Rossi (45) (n = 132)	Chetwynd and Hogan (46) (n = 694)	Agre et al (31) (n = 79)	Ramlow et al (13) (n = 474)	Halstead and Rossi (47) (n = 539)
Fatigue	59%	89%*	48%	86%*	34%	87%*
Joint pain	74%*	71%	60%*	77%	42%*	80%
Muscle pain	48%	71%	52%	86%	38%	79%
New weakness						
Affected muscle	66%	69%	N/A	80%	N/A	87%
Unaffected muscle	15%	50%	N/A	53%	N/A	77%
Cold sensitivity	46%	29%	N/A	N/A	26%	N/A

Source: Reproduced by permission from Gawne AC, Halstead LS. Post-polio syndrome: pathophysiology and clinic management. *Crit Rev Phys Rehabil Med* 1995;7:147–188.
* Most frequent symptom. n = number of subjects reported; N/A = not assessed.

edged by polio survivors. In most of the studies reporting on the prevalence of fatigue in the postpolio population, the term *fatigue* was not specifically defined. It is probable that the underlying basis for the acknowledgement of fatigue varies in different patients (53). Fatigue might be caused by a number of different factors, including emotional, "general," cardiovascular, or peripheral neuromuscular factors. Only after careful evaluation and interpretation of the fatigue complaint can proper therapeutic measures be taken for a postpolio patient with complaints of fatigue.

It is well known that many postpolio individuals are under a great deal of emotional distress or are depressed (54–57). And, it is well known clinically, as well as hypothesized for postpolio individuals, that emotional distress and depression can cause an individual to feel excessively fatigued (58).

A small study of 12 postpolio patients reported that

Table 87-3: Most Common New Functional Problems in Persons with a History of Paralytic Polio Reported in Five Studies (% of Patients Acknowledging the Problem)

Functional Problem	Codd et al (11) (n = 28)	Halstead and Rossi (45) (n = 132)	Agre et al (31) (n = 79)	Halstead and Rossi (47) (n = 539)	Grimby and Einarsson (48) (n = 41)
Difficulty walking	25%	63%	N/A	85%	66%
Difficulty climbing stairs	N/A	61%	67%	82%	N/A
Difficulty with ADLs	14%	17%	16%	62%	66%

n = number of subjects reported; N/A = not assessed; ADLs = activities of daily living.

the amount of fatigue experienced by these individuals, as measured by the Fatigue Severity Scale, was over twice that of the nondisabled population and was similar to levels in patients diagnosed with multiple sclerosis or systemic lupus erythematosus (59). It has also been reported that as a part of general fatigue, the postpolio individual may experience a pervasive sense of fatigue (such as "hitting the wall") (47). From this nationwide survey, 43% of individuals reported this phenomenon and in 68% this occurred on a daily basis. Most commonly, this polio "wall" was experienced in the mid to late afternoon.

Fatigue might also be caused by cardiovascular or local muscular factors. One study demonstrated that the aerobic power of the average postpolio individual was comparable to that of a non-postpolio individual shortly after the onset of acute myocardial infarction (60). One could speculate that many ADLs are then performed at close to maximal capacity, which can lead to fatigue. In another study, the single most common complaint of the postpolio patients was that of decreasing endurance (61). The investigators reported that 153 out of 154 unstable postpolio patients acknowledged progressive difficulty with endurance while performing their usual daily activities. In another clinical report, two-thirds of postpolio subjects complained of increasing loss of strength during activity or a heavy sensation of the muscles (62). These findings suggest that fatigue may be caused by cardiovascular or local muscle factors.

Weakness

Although new weakness is a very common complaint of postpolio individuals (11,31,45,47), and has been reported for well over 100 years (1,2), there is little evidence in the literature to indicate that the decline in strength in postpolio individuals is any greater than that which could be attributed to the aging process. Several of the early reports that substantiated new weakness in postpolio individuals were based on patient report and not longitudinal studies using valid and reliable techniques (63,64). Recent quantitative studies, however, showed that postpolio individuals do lose strength over time, at least in some muscle groups. In two studies (44,65), strength of the quadriceps femoris muscles declined by an average of 2% per year over a 4-year interval, while strength of the hamstring musculature over the same interval did not change. The rate of loss of quadriceps strength was twice that expected from normal aging studies and this may be evidence for an accelerated loss in muscle strength in postpolio individuals; however, neither study assessed a change in muscle strength in control, non-postpolio subjects.

Respiratory Dysfunction

New breathing difficulties occurring years after recovery from acute poliomyelitis are a great concern for many polio survivors, even those who apparently had no difficulties during the acute poliomyelitis illness. Approximately 10% to 20% of patients with acute paralytic polio during the epidemics of the 1950s required assisted ventilation (66–68), but most of these individuals could be weaned off ventilators during the convalescent stage (68,69). In a nationwide survey (70), 42% of respondents acknowledged new breathing difficulties. In other studies (31,47,71), the frequency of complaints of new breathing difficulties was less. A number of reports documented respiratory insufficiency in some polio survivors many years after the onset of acute illness. These problems included chronic hypoventilation (69,72–74), nocturnal rapid-eye-movement (REM) sleep–induced hypoxemia, and sleep apnea syndromes (75–78).

Symptoms of respiratory difficulty may develop insidiously and may often be related to nocturnal disturbances. Early recognition of symptoms (such as disturbed sleep, morning headache, daytime somnolence, and general fatigue) and examination of nocturnal blood gases are important because adequate treatment can reduce the symptoms, improve the quality of life, and prevent more serious cardiorespiratory complications such as cor pulmonale and life-threatening carbon dioxide retention (79).

Swallowing Dysfunction

The prevalence of swallowing dysfunction in polio survivors is not well known; however, for some patients dysphagia is one of the primary complaints, if not the primary complaint. A brief report from the National Institutes of Health (NIH) indicated that many patients referred there for a postpolio evaluation were unaware that they had any problem with swallowing, because they had learned to compensate for mild problems in transporting food or accepted that indigestion is a common mealtime sequela (80). Although no large-scale studies have been conducted on dysphagia in postpolio individuals, a few studies reported findings on small representative samples. In a study of 220 postpolio patients who responded to a swallowing function questionnaire, 40 (18%) acknowledged dysphagia (81). In another study, 20 patients underwent cinefluorography and all but 1 were found to exhibit some degree of pharyngeal abnormality as well as other structural problems that had contributed to dysphagia (82). In a random study of 32 of 72 patients with a diagnosis of postpolio progressive muscle atrophy, 24 patients acknowledged new swallowing difficulties and 18 had had a previous diagnosis of bulbar involvement (83). This last study suggested that new swallowing symptoms may merge as late effects regardless of whether the original polio affected bulbar musculature.

Activity of Daily Living Dysfunction

Most of the new symptoms acknowledged by postpolio individuals relate to mobility, as weakness appears to be more common in the lower- than the upper-limb musculature (84). In a detailed report by Einarsson and Grimby (85), independence in personal ADLs (such as bathing, dressing, toileting, transferring, and feeding) was reported by nearly 80% of postpolio patients. More difficulties were reported in instrumental ADLs. Difficulty with walking several blocks was acknowledged by 90% of patients, difficulty with walking one block or climbing one flight of stairs was acknowledged by 75% of patients, difficulty with light housework was acknowledged by 85% of patients, and difficulty with vigorous activities was acknowledged by 98% of patients. Only 12% of patients acknowledged no difficulty with using public transportation, while 40% were unable to use public transportation because of mobility difficulties. Only 30% of patients were independent in performing household activities, while 70% required varying levels of assistance.

Psychosocial Distress

A number of polio survivors may have psychological disturbances. In an early report by Halstead et al (70), 18% of patients acknowledged a change in personality after their maximal recovery from acute poliomyelitis. In another clinical report, the symptom profiles in a group of 93 postpolio individuals indicated psychological distress (86). In men, elevated scores on subscales of the Symptom Check List 90 Revised (SCL-90R) (87) were found for somatization, depression, anxiety, hostility, and phobia, while in women elevations were found for somatization, depression, anxiety, and psychoticism. Elevated scores were found in the subscales of the Psychosocial Adjustment to Illness Scale (PAIS-SR) (88) (pooling men and women) on health care orientation, social environment, and extended-family relationships. Other studies showed that type A behavior (89) or denial of limitations (90) may be precipitants of postpolio syndrome in some patients.

Features That Distinguish Unstable from Stable Postpolio Individuals

A number of studies attempted to differentiate between the postpolio patients acknowledging declining strength or function (unstable postpolio patients) and those denying declining strength or function (stable postpolio subjects). The results of these studies are summarized in Table 87-4 (40,41,43,44,47,91–97).

Table 87-4: Features from the Literature Delineating Similarities and Differences Between Stable and Unstable Postpolio Individuals

	References
Similarities	
1. Evidence of denervation/reinnervation of muscle fibers in motor units.	91–96
2. Incidence of elevated serum creatine kinase.	43
3. Muscular endurance (while performing exercise at a similar relative level of exertion).	40
4. Electrophysiologic evidence of local muscle fatigue (while performing exercise at a similar relative level of effort).	41
5. Rating of perceived exertion (while performing exercise at a similar relative level of effort).	40
6. Rate of loss in strength over time.	44
Differences	
1. Evidence of more widespread initial poliomyelitis illness in unstable postpolio individuals.	47,97
2. Unstable postpolio individuals had their acute illness at an older age.	40,47
3. Unstable postpolio individuals hospitalized longer at the time of their acute polio illness.	40,47
4. Unstable postpolio individuals acknowledge higher level of recent activity.	97
5. Unstable postpolio individuals have weaker muscles.	40
6. Unstable postpolio individuals have reduced capacity for muscular work.	40
7. Unstable postpolio individuals have a deficit in strength recovery after fatiguing exercise.	40

Source: Modified from Agre JC. Local muscle and total body fatigue. In: Halstead LS, Grimby G, eds. *Post-polio syndrome.* Philadelphia: Hanley & Belfus, 1995:35–67.

Neuromuscular Characteristics of Postpolio Patients

A detailed study was performed on the neuromuscular function of the quadriceps femoris muscles in 34 unstable postpolio (those acknowledging declining strength), 16 stable postpolio (those not acknowledging declining strength), and 41 control, non-postpolio subjects (40,41,98). All subjects were healthy and between 30 and 60 years old. All of the postpolio subjects had greater than antigravity strength of the quadriceps muscles evaluated. The strength, endurance, and isometric tension time index ("work capacity") after fatiguing exercise were determined in all subjects; the results are shown in Table 87-5. Muscle strength (expressed as torque) was significantly less in the unstable subjects as compared to the stable and control subjects. The isometric endurance time (the time the subject could maintain an isometric contraction at 40% of maximal torque), however, was not significantly different among the three groups. The isometric tension time index was significantly less in the unstable group as compared to the control group while no difference was found between the stable group and the control group.

During the isometric endurance test to failure, two electrophysiologic measures of local muscle fatigue (the median frequency of the power spectrum and root mean squared amplitude of the electromyographic signal, from which neuromuscular efficiency could be determined) were monitored, and at regular intervals throughout the test, subjects reported their rating of perceived exertion, which reflected their perception of exertion in the quadriceps muscle as a result of the exercise being performed. Figure 87-2 shows the results of the electrophysiologic testing and shows no difference among the three groups in either variable. Figure 87-3 shows the results of the rating of perceived exertion during the endurance test. Of significant clinical importance, the rating of perceived exertion did not differ among the three groups; that is, all groups similarly perceived the extent of local muscle fatigue within the muscle throughout the exercise period. In addition, the relationship between the rating of perceived exertion and the electrophysiologic variables of local muscle fatigue was examined. As the rating of perceived exertion increased in each of the three groups, the electrophysiologic variables of local muscle fatigue also showed that the muscle was

Table 87-5: Mean (±SD) Isometric Muscle Strength of the Quadriceps, Endurance Time (Time Subject Could Maintain an Isometric Contraction at 40% of Maximal Strength), and Isometric Tension Time Index ("Work Capacity") in Unstable Postpolio, Stable Postpolio, and Control Subjects

Variable	Unstable Postpolio (n + 34)	Stable Postpolio (n + 16)	Control (n + 41)
Isometric strength (nm)	113 ±75[a]	159 ± 87[b]	207 ± 61
Endurance time (sec)	102 ± 36	116 ± 52	119 ± 39
Tension time index (msec)	5024 ± 3213[a]	8221 ± 4140	9826 ± 4144

[a] Unstable subjects significantly ($p < 0.05$) less than stable and control subjects.

[b] Stable subjects significantly ($p < 0.05$) less than control subjects.

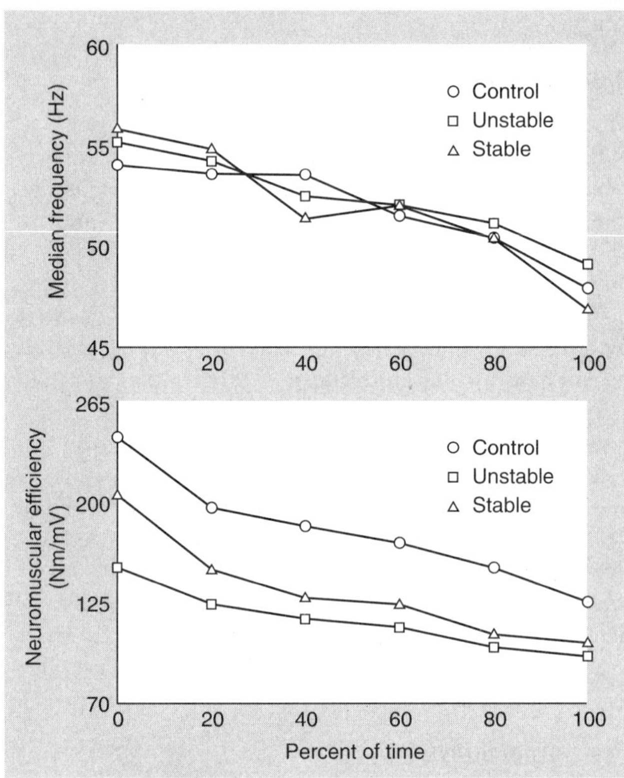

Figure 87-2. Mean change in neuromuscular efficiency (nm/mV) and median frequency of the power spectrum (Hz) during the endurance test from onset (0%) to failure (100%) in unstable postpolio, stable postpolio, and control subjects. No significant ($p > 0.05$) differences were found among groups for either variable. (Reproduced by permission from Rodriquez AA, Agre JC. Electrophysiologic study of the quadriceps muscles during fatiguing exercise and recovery: a comparison of symptomatic postpolios to asymptomatic postpolios and controls. *Arch Phys Med Rehabil* 1991;72:993–997.)

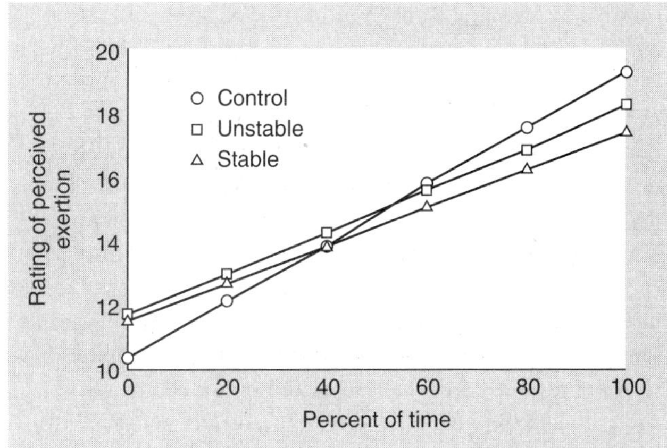

Figure 87-3. A comparison of the mean change in rating of perceived exertion during the endurance test from onset (0%) to failure (100%). No significant ($p > 0.05$) difference was found among groups. (Adapted by permission from Agre JC, Rodriquez AA. Neuromuscular function: comparison of symptomatic and asymptomatic polio subjects to control subjects. *Arch Phys Med Rehabil* 1990;71:545–551.)

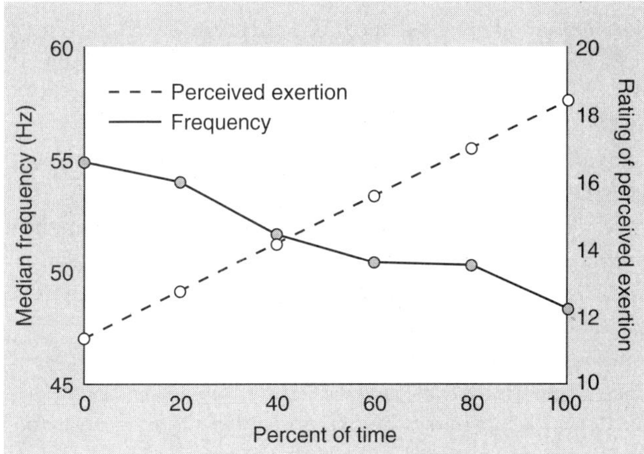

Figure 87-4. Interaction between rating of perceived exertion and median frequency of the power spectrum in the unstable postpolio group. Interaction is statistically ($p < 0.05$) significant. (Adapted by permission from Rodriquez AA, Agre JC. Physiologic parameters and perceived exertion with local muscle fatigue in postpolio subjects. *Arch Phys Med Rehabil* 1991;72:305–308.)

becoming more fatigued, and there was no difference among groups in this relationship. Figure 87-4 shows the relationship between the rating of perceived exertion and the change in median frequency of the power spectrum throughout the endurance test in the unstable postpolio group.

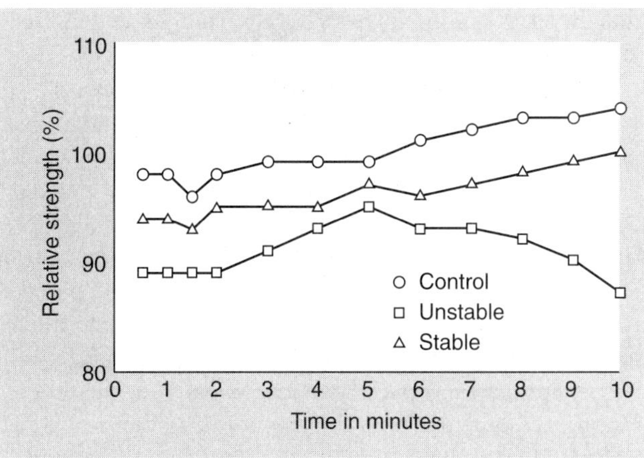

Figure 87-5. A comparison of recovery of mean relative isometric strength from 30 seconds to 10 minutes after failure to maintain isometric torque at 40% of maximal. Unstable subjects were significantly ($p < 0.05$) different from control subjects. Stable subjects were not significantly ($p > 0.05$) different from control subjects. (Adapted by permission from Agre JC, Rodriquez AA. Neuromuscular function: comparison of symptomatic and asymptomatic polio subjects to control subjects. *Arch Phys Med Rehabil* 1990;71;545–551.)

Muscle strength was also assessed after failure to maintain the isometric muscle contraction occurred. The results of this test are shown in Figure 87-5. Strength of the stable postpolio group recovered in a similar fashion to that of the control subjects. However, strength recovery of the unstable postpolio group was significantly less than that of the control group. This deficit in strength recovery did not appear to be due to lassitude or lack of volition, as the relative root mean squared electromyographic amplitude was the same in all three groups. The subjective time to recovery of strength after the testing was also significantly longer in the unstable postpolio group. The average time to subjective recovery of strength in the stable postpolio and control groups was within 1 day, while the average time to subjective recovery of strength in the unstable group was 2 to 3 days and this difference was statistically ($p < 0.05$) and clinically significant.

One laboratory study assessed whether rest breaks would result in the ability of unstable postpolio subjects to perform similar or more muscle work with less local muscle fatigue and greater strength recovery after the activity (99). Seven unstable postpolio subjects were assessed on 3 separate days at least 1 week apart. On the first test day, subjects performed an isometric endurance and strength recovery test as described earlier. On the second test day, subjects performed the same total amount of isometric activity; however, the activity was divided into four equal parts. Two minutes of rest was provided between each part. On the third test day, subjects performed a series of 20-second intervals of activity with 2-minute rest breaks until either the rating of perceived exertion exceeded "very hard" or they had performed 18 intervals of activity.

The results of this study showed that rest breaks were beneficial in reducing local muscle fatigue and enhancing recovery of muscle strength. At the completion of the exercise on each day, the measures of local muscle fatigue (both the rating of perceived exertion and the electrophysiologic assessment) showed a significant reduction in fatigue in both paradigms that included rest as compared to the paradigm that required the subject to work to the point of failure. Also, strength recovery was significantly better with both rest paradigms as compared to the other paradigm. Comparison of the amount of isometric "work" performed from the first day to the third day in these subjects showed that the average subject performed 237% more on average when taking rest breaks, and also that these subjects performed this with less local muscle fatigue. These findings certainly suggest that pacing (interspersing rest breaks during activity) can significantly reduce local muscle fatigue even when similar or greater amounts of total activity are actually performed.

POSTPOLIO MANAGEMENT

Corroborate Postpolio Diagnosis

When evaluating a patient's problems related to post-polio syndrome, it is important to rule out other medically treatable causes for the patient's complaints. The diagnosis of postpolio syndrome is really one of exclusion, exclusion of medical causes other than poliorelated causes for the patient's complaints. Adapted from previously published criteria (9,45), the following appear to be reasonable criteria for the diagnosis of postpolio syndrome:

1. A prior episode of paralytic polio confirmed by history and physical examination.
2. A period of neurologic recovery followed by an extended interval of neurologic and functional stability preceding the onset of new problems. The interval of stability usually lasts 20 years or more.
3. A gradual or abrupt onset of new weakness that may or may not be accompanied by other new health problems such as excessive fatigue, muscle pain, joint pain, decreased endurance, decreased function, and atrophy.
4. Exclusion of other medical or neurologic conditions other than polio-related conditions that might cause the health problems just listed.

The first criterion is documented by history and whenever possible, review of the patient's old medical records. It should also be noted that acute poliomyelitis was overdiagnosed during the acute polio epidemics of the 1940s and 1950s. We have seen several patients in our clinic who have carried the diagnosis of polio but who in all probability had a viral transverse myelitis (as upper motor neuron signs were found on physical examination and the patients acknowledged that such findings had been present since the time of the illness). The history should reveal an acute febrile illness producing motor but not sensory loss. One should inquire whether other family members, neighbors, or friends had a similar illness. The physical examination generally reveals evidence of an asymmetric lower motor neuron disease (focal asymmetric weakness, atrophy, and/or reduced muscle stretch reflexes on examination). Sensation is intact (unless the patient has a neuropathy from nerve compression or radiculopathy from nerve root compression) as the poliomyelitis virus rarely affects the afferent system. We do not recommend the routine performance of electromyographic evaluations on postpolio patients, but reserve this examination for the patients in whom a concern for some other pathology such as neuropathy or radiculopathy (both of which are common in postpolio patients) is present.

The second criterion is a characteristic pattern of recovery. Usually the individual recovers from the acute paralytic illness and tends to do rather well for a few decades thereafter. New problems tend to occur 20 to 30 years or later after the initial polio illness in most individuals.

The third criterion is the onset of new weakness. The new weakness is determined by history. In many cases the individual will have difficulty in precisely identifying the onset of new weakness, as it usually occurs gradually and only over time does it become perceptible to the patient. It is imperative that other medical causes for new weakness are excluded.

The fourth criterion is the exclusion of other medical and neurologic causes for the complaints of new weakness and the health-related problems other than polio-related conditions that might cause those problems. This may simply be a semantic argument, but there is some controversy concerning this criterion for the diagnosis. Some authors will not make the diagnosis of postpolio syndrome in the presence of such diagnoses as compression neuropathy, radiculopathy, arthritis, degenerative disk disease, or obesity. However, these diagnoses are very commonly found in postpolio individuals as well as non-postpolio middle-aged individuals. Also, most postpolio individuals are susceptible to these problems owing to their chronic weakness; use of biomechanically disadvantaged joints; use of assistive devices such as crutches, canes, and wheelchairs (leading to peripheral nerve compression); and reduced level of daily energy expenditure. We do not use these particular polio-related diagnoses as exclusionary criteria for the diagnosis of postpolio syndrome.

Treatment of Postpolio Problems

General Aspects

Each postpolio patient is unique and therefore, the need for treatment varies depending on the patient's unique set of circumstances and requirements. It is imperative to carefully identify the patient's primary concerns and identify the patient's functional problems, especially of new or of increasing dysfunction, and the attitude of the patient regarding his or her health condition. Patients are normally quite eager to obtain new information about the background and interpretation of their new health problems.

The functional sequelae of postpolio can be categorized by impairment, on the organic level, and disability, on the performance level. Patient management should be focused at reducing impairment, wherever possible, and avoiding the development of disability or reducing the level of disability if it is already present. The ultimate goal is to enhance the individual's function, independence, and well-being as much as possible so that the individual can fulfill his or her life role (48).

Treatment of Specific Problems

Pain

Joint pain, back pain, and muscle pain are common complaints of postpolio patients (31,45–47,70). Many subjects do not receive optimal support for their unstable joints from their lower-limb orthosis, which may lead to chronic joint pain. For instance, Perry and Fleming (100) reported that 54 (28%) of 193 patients had problems with genu recurvatum and fully 40 of the 54 (74%) of those patients had knee pain. This problem was essentially resolved with fitting of a proper orthosis. Other investigators also reported that many patients seen in postpolio clinics have problems with mobility or pain related to their not using an appropriate orthotic device (51,61). Waring et al (51) also noted that subjects receiving an orthosis reported, among other factors, a significant reduction in knee pain as well as overall pain while walking. Proper orthotic use may definitely reduce pain at multiple sites by altering the lurching gait pattern that is often used by the individual in the absence of a properly fitted orthosis. Common examples of orthotically correctable gait patterns are the forward weight shift to move the center of gravity anterior to the axis of the knee joint to assist with knee extension, and the side-to-side pattern, to circumduct the leg, in patients with footdrop (51).

Shoulder pain is also commonly reported in postpolio patients. In one clinical study, of 79 patients, nearly 30% of patients had shoulder pain (31). Shoulder pain is not uncommon in patients with significant lower-limb weakness who either ambulate using assistive devices such as canes or crutches or use a wheelchair and need to transfer in and out of the wheelchair. Over the years, these activities take their toll on the patient's shoulders, especially if the shoulder girdle musculature is somewhat weakened, and this can result in degenerative joint disease of the shoulders, rotator cuff problems, or myofascial pain of the shoulder girdle musculature. Careful assessment of the patient's specific problem is required, with the therapeutic intervention based on the results of the evaluation. In the patient who ambulates relatively long distances with crutches and has shoulder pain, the use of a wheelchair for long-distance mobility can be quite helpful in reducing the stress and subsequently the pain in the shoulders. In the patient who has shoulder pain related to transferring in and out of the wheelchair, assessment and appropriate modification of the transfer technique may be helpful. In some situations, the patient may need to use a lift device for safe transfer without excessively stressing the shoulder. For overweight patients, weight loss can also be helpful.

Back pain is a common complaint in postpolio patients. In one study 70% acknowledged this problem (31). The pain can be related to any number of factors including scoliosis and biomechanical stress placed on the back during ambulation or transfers, or can be aggravated by a poorly fitted seating system in the patient who primarily uses a wheelchair for mobility. A careful evaluation is needed to identify the causative factors, which can then be modified through an appropriate treatment plan.

Muscle pain is also quite common in postpolio patients and may be related either to muscle overuse pain or to myofascial pain. In one clinical study, 71% of patients had muscle pain related to these two factors (31). Muscle overuse pain can be diagnosed from the patient's history, wherein the patient complains of muscle pain that is exacerbated with activity and relieved by rest. Muscle overuse can be caused by a number of factors including the overuse of weakened muscles, but can also be found in relatively strong muscles. It is not uncommon for patients to complain of muscle overuse pain in the lower limb that was not involved or was minimally involved with polio initially. Owing to the weakness of the involved limb, patients place too much stress on the neurologically more intact limb, leading to muscle overuse pain. Many patients also have poor gait patterns, owing to lack of use of an orthosis, which could significantly benefit their gait pattern and reduce muscle stress and pain. Also, some postpolio patients continue to perform their daily activities until they can no longer do so and have to stop because of pain. Careful assessment is needed to identify the causative factors and implement appropriate treatment to reduce muscle stress and subsequent pain.

The use of nonsteroidal anti-inflammatory drugs can be helpful for managing joint and or muscle pain. However, these medications should not be used to simply mask the symptoms. Intervention should be implemented to modify the identified underlying causative factors. Also, some postpolio patients have difficulty sleeping due to their muscle, back, or joint pain. As with other pain patients who have difficulty with sleep, some of these patients benefit from the use of a tricyclic antidepressant.

Fatigue

As discussed earlier, fatigue can be due to a number of different factors in the postpolio patient. One needs to determine whether or not the fatigue might be related to local muscle fatigue, cardiovascular factors, general fatigue, or psychological distress. One also needs to rule out other possible medical causes for fatigue such as anemia, infection, collagen disorder, malignancy, diabetes mellitus, and hypothyroidism. Fatigue can also be associated with some medications such as β-blockers, sedatives, and antihistamines. Only after careful evaluation of the fatigue complaint can proper therapeutic endeavors be undertaken. When the medical causes for fatigue have been ruled out through proper evaluation, good clinical judgment is required to determine the most likely causes and institute the most appropriate treatment plan, because there is no objective laboratory test to precisely ascertain the cause for fatigue.

Studies have shown that many postpolio patients are very hard-working individuals, many have the type A personality trait (89), and a number tend to deny their limitations in their ability to function (90). This may cause individuals to exceed their physiologic capabilities to function, leading to local muscle, cardiovascular, or generalized overactivity fatigue. An early study reported that many postpolio individuals acknowledged "hitting the wall" on a daily basis, and most often in the mid-afternoon (47). The mechanism for this complaint of fatigue is unknown, but may be central in origin. Rest and reduction of activity are beneficial for most of these patients (47).

Pacing of activities (i.e., the interspersal of rest breaks during activity to avoid the development of excessive fatigue) also seems to be quite helpful for many postpolio patients with fatigue problems. As described earlier, in the research laboratory, the interspersal of rest breaks during an isometric muscle activity resulted in a significant reduction in local muscle fatigue (as measured by the subjective rating of perceived exertion and by the objective electrophysiologic correlates of local muscle fatigue) (99). In this study rest breaks allowed the postpolio individuals to perform the same or more activity with less local muscle fatigue and greater recovery of strength immediately after the activity. When our patients use this technique in their daily living situations, most acknowledge that it is quite helpful in reducing their fatigue.

Lifestyle adjustments and energy conservation techniques can also be useful in the reduction and control of fatigue (9,53). Some of the simple energy conservation techniques include using a handicap license plate (when appropriate), planning one's day and reducing the number of trips, balancing activity and rest, learning and then using techniques of work simplification as well as appropriate assistive devices in occupational therapy, and using a motorized scooter for long-distance mobility (when appropriate) (9,53,101–103).

It is quite probable that in many postpolio patients, as in other individuals as they age, adipose body mass gradually increases. Most patients seen in our clinic acknowledge this problem and we have found this in our research on postpolio syndrome (44). Weight gain increases the resistance against which the body must work to perform all of one's daily activities and will definitely make it more difficult for weakened muscles to complete most activities. In the situation where excessive adipose tissue is a part of the problem, weight loss through an appropriately prescribed weight loss diet can be helpful for the individual.

Many postpolio individuals also have deconditioning and disuse as a part of their particular problem. In fact in the same individual, overuse and disuse can be a problem, depending on the severity of the polio involvement (and its oftentimes scattered and asymmetric involvement). This makes the prescription of exercise somewhat difficult, but not impossible for most individuals. Exercise is discussed later.

A few studies investigated the effects of medications on postpolio fatigue. A placebo-controlled 6-week trial of the antiviral agent amantadine was performed on 25 patients with postpolio fatigue (104). Fatigue was measured by both a visual analog scale and the Fatigue Severity Scale. The results showed no significant difference between the amantadine and the placebo. Another study assessed the effect of prednisone on muscle strength as well as fatigue (105). Seventeen subjects participated in this randomized, placebo-controlled study. The treatment consisted of prednisone (80 mg) or placebo given once daily for 28 days. Thereafter, the medication was gradually decreased over a period of another 20 weeks. No difference was found between placebo and prednisone in muscle strength or in fatigue. A more promising study used the anticholinesterase inhibitor pyridostigmine in 17 postpolio patients (106). Oral pyridostigmine was initiated at 30 mg/day and the dose was increased every other day by 30 mg to a total dose of 180 mg/day given in three divided doses. One patient was maintained at 120 mg/day, owing to side effects at the higher dose. Treatment was maintained for 1 month. Fatigue was measured by the Hare Fatigue Scale at the beginning and end of the trial. A significant improvement with pyridostigmine treatment was defined as an improvement of at least 20% on the Hare Fatigue Scale. Nine (53%) of the 17 patients experienced a reduction in systemic fatigue by 20% to 88% while on the medication. At the present time, an international, multicenter, placebo-controlled trial is examining the effects of pyridostigmine on postpolio fatigue.

Weakness and Deconditioning

Muscle Strengthening Exercises

The effect of exercise on the postpolio patient was reviewed recently (107). The early studies on exercise in postpolio patients, performed in the 1940s, 1950s, and 1960s, yielded conflicting results. Some studies reported that strengthening exercises were beneficial (108–110), while other reports indicated that exercise or activity was detrimental (111–113). It appears that the key difference among these studies had to do with the intensity of the exercise program. The exercise programs that led to further dysfunction were performed at too vigorous a level for the individuals and probably led to overuse problems. The exercise programs in the more recent studies, performed within the last decade, appear to be beneficial for the patients.

Feldman and Soskolne (114) reported on the effect of a 6-month exercise program performed three times a week in six patients with postpolio syndrome. The exercise program involved a total of 32 muscle groups. The exercises consisted of nonfatiguing weight lifting. Patients began the program by lifting a weight five times, with the weight being 50% of the maximal amount of weight the subject could lift five times. The number of repetitions was gradually increased, being careful to avoid fatigue, until the patient could lift the weight 30 times. The weight was then increased and the number of repetitions decreased. Again, the number of repetitions was gradually increased. Strength was found to increase in 14 muscle groups, was maintained in 17 muscle groups, and decreased in 1 muscle group. In general, the authors believed that this result was favorable.

Einarsson and Grimby (115,116) reported the effect of a standardized, 6-week, thrice-weekly, maximal-effort isokinetic and isometric muscle strengthening exercise program on the quadriceps muscles in 12 postpolio patients (9 of whom had postpolio syndrome). All subjects had greater than antigravity strength at the onset of the study. Patients performed three sets of exercise, with rest breaks, for a total exercise duration of 96 seconds. Each exercise set consisted of eight 4-second bouts alternating between isokinetic and isometric exercise with 10-second rest breaks between each bout. Patients rested for 5 minutes between the exercise sets. Following the exercise program, muscle strength increased significantly, as measured both isokinetically and isometrically. Strength was not found to decline 6 to 12 months later and it was speculated that the increased amount of ordinary daily activity such as arising from a chair, climbing stairs, or walking maintained the strength gain. The exercise program did not appear to damage the muscle, as no histopathologic changes were seen. Most patients also acknowledged subjective improvements as a result of the exercise program.

Fillyaw et al (117) reported on the effect of long-term nonfatiguing exercise in a group of 17 patients with postpolio syndrome. All subjects had at least antigravity strength in the muscle group at the start of the study. Patients exercised every other day for 1 to 2 years. Initially, the amount of weight the patient could lift 10 times (10 RM) was determined. The exercise program consisted of three sets of 10 repetitions using weights 50%, 75%, and 100% of the 10 RM. Patients rested for 5 minutes between each set. Every 2 weeks the 10 RM was tested and the exercise program adjusted accordingly. At the completion of the study, the 10 RM increased in 16 of the 17 subjects and the average increase was 78%. Isometric strength increased by an average of 8.4% at the end of the exercise program.

We (118) recently reported on the effect of a closely supervised, 12-week, nonfatiguing, low-intensity exercise program on the quadriceps muscles in 12 patients with postpolio syndrome. All patients had at least antigravity strength in the muscle group prior to the exercise program. Exercise was performed every other day at home for 12 weeks. Individuals performed between 6 and 10 knee lifts with sandbag weights attached to the ankle. The exercise was to be performed until the rating of perceived exertion in the exercised muscle was "very hard" or 10 repetitions were performed. After 12 weeks of exercise, the amount of weight lifted significantly increased by an average of over 60%, although the isometrically measured strength did not significantly increase (only a 5% improvement). No patient experienced any problem with the exercise program and no apparent damage was done to the muscle or motor units, as creatine kinase level, jitter, blocking, and macroelectromyographic amplitude did not change after the exercise program as compared to beforehand. We concluded that such an exercise program may be able to improve muscle performance without adverse affects.

General and Cardiorespiratory Exercises

Jones et al (119) reported the response to a 16-week, thrice-weekly, aerobic exercise program in a total of 37 postpolio subjects. A total of 16 subjects performed the exercise program while 21 were nonexercise control subjects. Subjects exercised on a bicycle ergometer at an intensity of 70% of heart rate reserve plus resting heart rate. To avoid problems with excessive fatigue, subjects performed their exercise in periods lasting from 2 to 5 minutes with 1-minute rest breaks. Subjects exercised for 15 to 30 minutes per session. As compared to the control subjects, in whom no change was found, exercise subjects showed improvements in work capacity and aerobic power by 18% and 15%, respectively. Also, no untoward response to exercise was found in any exercise subject.

In a similar study, Kriz et al (120) examined the effect of an upper-extremity arm ergometry exercise program in 20 postpolio patients (10 control and 10 exercise subjects) who completed the study. Exercise was performed three times a week for 16 weeks at 70% to 75% of heart rate reserve plus resting heart rate for 20 minutes per session. Exercise was performed for 2- to 3-minute bouts interspersed with 1-minute rest breaks. As compared to the control group, in whom no change was found, the exercise group had significant improvements in aerobic power

(15%), maximum ventilation (16%), exercise time (10%), and power (14%). Also, no untoward response to exercise was found in any exercise subject.

Grimby and Einarsson (48) reported the effect of a 6-month, twice-weekly exercise program in 12 postpolio patients. All subjects were ambulatory, but 1 used a cane. The exercise program consisted of a 5-minute warm-up, followed by walking and bicycle exercise at submaximal levels for 5 to 10 minutes. Thereafter, mobility and stretching exercises were performed as were several different muscle strengthening exercises for individual muscle groups using body weight as the resistance. The subjects were also advised about home exercise programs and daily activities. At the end of the exercise program, the subjects reached peak exercise performance, as determined by bicycle ergometry testing. Muscle strength was also increased in some muscle groups undergoing exercise. Except for 1 subject, all showed improvement from the exercise program. In the 1 subject, deterioration in function was noted and was believed to be due to overwork. The objective tests showed reduced strength and endurance in this 1 subject. Although this subject acknowledged decreasing function and increasing fatigue as results of the exercise program, he continued on in the program, fully aware of the risk he was taking by continuing. During the subsequent ½ year, with a reduced level of activity, his muscle strength returned toward pretraining values and he noted a decrease in his level of fatigue. The authors of this study concluded that an exercise program that combined endurance training, stretching, and submaximal strengthening exercises can be conducted in postpolio subjects with positive effects, but that the cardiorespiratory condition effects of the program seemed to predominate. As this example demonstrated, such a program can also lead to overuse in some postpolio individuals and care must be taken in the exercise prescription of postpolio individuals.

Ambulatory Efficiency Improvement with Exercise

The effect of a modified aerobic exercise program on movement energetics was studied in a group of 20 postpolio subjects (121). Seven subjects performed a thrice-weekly exercise program on a treadmill while 13 were control subjects. The exercise subjects walked on a treadmill for 20 to 40 minutes per session at a speed and grade that were comfortable for the subject. The perception of exertion did not exceed "somewhat heavy" and pain never exceeded "light." As compared to the control subjects, at the end of the 6-week study period, the exercise subjects showed a significant improvement in movement economy (i.e., there was a significant reduction in the energy cost of walking). However, no change was found in cardiovascular fitness, a finding that was not unexpected given the low intensity and short duration of the program. The authors concluded that modified aerobic training does improve efficiency of movement. The authors also speculated that such training might enhance the postpolio individual's endurance capacity and reduce their level of fatigue in performing daily activities, although these variables were not measured.

Locomotor Function and Mobility

Many postpolio patients have difficulty with ambulation and mobility that is probably related to the greater involvement of lower-limb than upper-limb musculature at the time of the initial poliomyelitis illness. Use of ambulatory and mobility aids is common for postpolio patients. We (31) reported that 44% of patients used an orthosis, cane, or crutch at least part-time at the time of their clinic visit. An additional 18% of patients used a wheelchair at least part-time. These findings are fairly similar to those of a survey study by Einarsson and Grimby (85) in which 56% of patients used a cane or crutch and 20% were wheelchair bound.

Many patients seen in postpolio clinics can benefit from the prescription of new assistive devices for mobility. Perry and Fleming (100) reported problems with orthotic devices in 58 (30%) of the 193 patients they evaluated. They also reported that 54 patients (28%) had problems with genu recurvatum and 40 of the 54 (74%) of those patients had knee pain. This problem was essentially resolved with proper fitting of a orthosis. Cosgrove et al (61) found that only 26 (14%) of 183 patients seen in their postpolio clinic came into the clinic with an orthosis, whereas they had recommended orthoses for fully 57 (31%) of the patients they evaluated. Also, the average age of the orthosis worn into the clinic by patients was 15 years. Hence, most orthotic devices were quite old and certainly less than ideally functional. Waring et al (51) reported findings similar to Cosgrove et al (61) in that only 19 (18%) of 104 patients had an orthosis at the time of evaluation, but new lower-limb orthotics were recommended for 37 (36%) of the patients seen. In addition, 10 patients already using an orthosis at the time of evaluation were given a prescription for a new orthosis. Twenty-two of the 37 patients (nearly 60%) receiving a new orthosis reported daily use of the orthosis. In a follow-up questionnaire, individuals using their lower-limb orthotic devices reported improved ability to walk, perception of greater safety while walking, and a significant reduction in knee pain as well as overall pain. Proper orthotic management may definitely reduce pain at multiple sites by reducing the lurching gait pattern that is often used by the individual in the absence of a properly fitted orthosis. As stated earlier, the common orthotically correctable gait patterns are the forward weight shift to move the center of gravity anterior to the knee to assist with knee extension and the side-to-side pattern, to circumduct the leg, in patients with footdrop (51). Waring et al (51) also reported that the rehabilitation team approach helped improve compliance in the use of a lower-limb orthosis. This study clearly showed the necessity to actively identify patients who may benefit from the use of an orthotic device and the importance of follow-up on the patients. Many postpolio patients are still not aware of the benefit of an indicated orthosis and of modern orthotic design.

The need for new wheelchairs has also been reported. Waring et al (51) reported that 7% of patients not using a manual wheelchair when seen in a clinic required them for safe mobility. In a group of postpolio patients studied by Halstead and Rossi (45), 18% were prescribed new wheelchairs. In many postpolio individuals there is a period of time when both ambulation and wheelchair use are appropriate. For these individuals, ambulation is appropriate for short distances while wheelchair use is appropriate for longer distances. For many patients seen in our postpolio clinic, the reported longest distance they could ambulate at one time was one block. Obviously, for such patients, wheelchair usage for distance mobility is appropriate. Ambulation for short distances, however, may aid in mobility and help to maintain lower-limb strength so long as the patient does not overdo it.

For patients in whom ambulation is not possible or only short-distance ambulation is possible and arm strength is not adequate to use manual wheelchair, the use of a motorized wheelchair or scooter may be appropriate for mobility.

Respiratory Dysfunction

During acute poliomyelitis, respiratory compromise is one of the most feared complications. The prevalence of iron lung use was estimated to be 15% (68). The prevalence of new breathing problems in postpolio patients is quite high. The persons at greatest risk for serious late-onset pulmonary complications are those who had moderate to severe respiratory involvement during the acute poliomyelitis illness and who usually required ventilatory assistance at that time (9). The other group of patients at risk are those with severe spinal deformities such as scoliosis and kyphoscoliosis.

The pulmonary problems may include both obstructive and restrictive lung disease with symptoms of exertional dyspnea, reduced pulmonary endurance, and sleep apnea. These pulmonary problems are due to a number of factors, including respiratory musculature weakness, hypoventilation, decreased pulmonary compliance, increasing scoliosis, and the effects of other diseases such as asthma or of cigarette smoking.

Fischer (122), a pulmonary medicine specialist, found that sleep disorder breathing was common in the patients he evaluated. In a group of 155 patients, he found that 91 (59%) awoke frequently, 60 (39%) snored, and 64 (41%) reported daytime fatigue.

When a patient's pulmonary function status is questioned, a screening pulmonary function assessment is advised. This may include the determination of vital capacity, tidal volume, and forced expiratory volume in 1 second (FEV_1). Although there is no specific limitation in function that can be a standard criterion for further testing, if the initial vital capacity is less than 50% of predicted or less than 1.5 liters, further assessment is recommended. Clinical judgment is required and it is certainly better to erre on the cautious side. When nocturnal sleep disorder is suspected, overnight oxyhemoglobin saturation monitoring should be performed and in some patients polysomnography may be needed (123–125).

Both sleep disorder breathing and chronic hypoventilation can be reversed and symptoms markedly improved with the utilization of ventilatory assistance. Inspiratory positive-pressure ventilation (IPPV) can be delivered in a number of different ways including by continuous positive airway pressure (CPAP) or bilevel positive airway pressure (Bi-pap). Bi-pap independently varies the inspiratory and expiratory pressures. Both CPAP and Bi-pap can be delivered by an oral, nasal, or oral-nasal ventilator hose (126,127). Treatment for respiratory difficulties in postpolio patients is not different from that for patients with other neuromuscular disorders. This is discussed further in Chapter 80.

Dysphagia

Swallowing difficulties are a significant complaint in approximately 10% to 15% of patients with acute poliomyelitis (128) and in approximately 10% to 20% of postpolio patients (129). Dysphagia results from involvement of the bulbar musculature. For patients who present with dysphagia, videofluoroscopy supervised by a speech and language pathologist can oftentimes determine the causative factors for the problem and whether compensatory techniques may be helpful for the patient. Such compensatory techniques include 1) changing the consistency of the food or liquid, 2) turning the head to one side or leaning to one side so that the food travels down the patient's stronger side, 3) tucking the chin, 4) alternating food and liquid, 5) swallowing twice for each bolus, and 6) avoiding ingestion when fatigued. Further details on the treatment of dysphagia in patients with neuromuscular disorders are found in Chapter 14.

Activity of Daily Living Dysfunction

Dependence in personal ADLs is uncommon in postpolio patients; however, many patients are dependent in performing instrumental ADLs such as housekeeping and shopping (85). Each patient is unique and the patient's specific needs oftentimes can be met through a detailed evaluation in occupational therapy (101). The patient's abilities and difficulties in various ADLs can be assessed. The usefulness of assistive equipment can be determined. Modifications in activities at home and at work can be made. Education can be given regarding work simplification and energy conservation. The patient's own preferences can be taken into account by the therapist in making appropriate recommendations. Many of our postpolio patients stated that the assessment of ADL functions by occupational therapists was of great value to them.

Psychosocial Distress

Personality changes and emotional distress are common problems in postpolio patients. The emotional responses to the new problems related to polio can be just as troublesome and disabling as the physical problems. Some polio survivors may resist making lifestyle changes to accommodate their new problems because they had worked so very hard after the acute illness to overcome the initial paralysis and achieve a high level of function and personal fulfillment. Denial of limitations (90) is not uncommon in polio survivors and may play a role in the difficulties experienced by the patient. For some individuals the use of assistive devices is "giving in" to the polio, which is not acceptable to them. It should also be kept in mind that few polio survivors had received any psychological counseling or support at the time of the acute illness and convalescence thereafter. And the new health problems that they are now experiencing are bringing up issues that were never adequately dealt with in the past. To overcome the combination of denial and personal history of successful coping, which worked for the individual in the past, an interdisciplinary approach, including psychology, is recommended. Bruno and Frick (130) recommended psychosocial and psychological evaluation including administration of the Reinforcement Motivation Study and Beck Depression Inventory, the results of which can be utilized to develop the treatment plan for the patient. In treating postpolio patients, Conrady et al (86) stressed that physical functioning and psychological functioning need to be evaluated and treated in combination in order to maximize the patient's ability to cope and to achieve as high a level of function and fulfillment as possible. Postpolio support groups can also be helpful in assisting patients to achieve their highest level of functioning. These groups can provide appropriate information about resources within the community as well as support for the individual.

REFERENCES

1. Raymond M. Paralysie essentielle de l'enfance, atrophy musculaire consecutive. *CR Heb Seances Mem Soc Biol* 1875; 27:158–160.
2. Cornil V, Lepine R. Sur un cas de paralysie generale spinale anterieure subaigue, suivi d'autopsie. *Gaz Med Paris* 1875;4:127–129.
3. Zilkha KJ. Discussion on motor neuron disease. *Proc R Soc Med* 1962;55:1028–1029.
4. Weichers DO. Late effects of polio: historical perspectives. *Birth Defects* 1987;23(4):1–11.
5. Kayser-Gatchahan MC. Late muscular atrophy after poliomyelitis. *Eur Neuro* 1973;10:371.
6. Mulder DW, Rosembaum RA, Layton DD. Late progression of poliomyelitis or forme fruste amyotrophic lateral sclerosis. *Mayo Clin Proc* 1972;47:756–760.
7. Halstead LS, Weichers DO, eds. *Late effects of poliomyelitis.* Miami: Symposia Foundation, 1985:1–236.
8. Strebel PM, Sutter RW, Cochi SL, et al. Epidemiology of poliomyelitis in the United States one decade after the last reported case of indigenous wild virus associated disease. *Clin Infect Dis* 1992;14: 568–579.
9. Gawne AC, Halstead LS. Postpolio syndrome: pathophysiology and clinic management. *Crit Rev Phys Rehabil Med* 1995;7: 147–188.
10. Windebank AJ, Lichty WJ, Daube JR. Prospective cohort study of polio survivors in Olmstead County, Minnesota. *Ann NY Acad Sci* 1995;753:81–86.
11. Codd MB, Mulder DW, Kurland LT, et al. Poliomyelitis in Rochester, MN 1935–1955: epidemiology and long-term sequelae: a preliminary report. In: Halstead LS, Weichers DO, eds. *Late effects of poliomyelitis.* Miami: Symposia Foundation, 1985:121–134.
12. Speier JL, Owen RR, Knapp M, Canine JK. Occurrence of postpolio sequelae in an epidemic population. *Birth Defects* 1987;23:39–48.
13. Ramlow J, Alexander M, Laporte R, et al. Epidemiology of the post-polio syndrome. *Am J Epidemiol* 1992;136:769–784.
14. Melnick JL, Agol VI, Bachrach HL, et al. Picornaviridae. *Intervirology* 1974;4:303–316.
15. Horstmann DM. Epidemiology of poliomyelitis and allied diseases—1963. *Yale J Biol Med* 1963;36:5–26.
16. Bodian D. Poliomyelitis: pathological anatomy. In: *Poliomyelitis: papers and discussions presented at the first international poliomyelitis conference.* Philadelphia: JB Lippincott, 1949.
17. Bodian D. The virus, the nerve cell, and paralysis: study of experimental poliomyelitis in the spinal cord. *Bull Johns Hopkins Hosp* 1948;83:1–73.
18. Bodian D. Pathologic anatomy. In: *Poliomyelitis: transactions of the first international poliomyelitis conference.* Philadelphia: JB Lippincott, 1949.
19. Bodian D, Howe HA. The pathology of early arrested and nonparalytic poliomyelitis. *Bull Johns Hopkins Hosp* 1941;69: 135–147.
20. Sharrard WJW. Correlation between the changes in the

spinal cord and muscle paralysis in poliomyelitis: a preliminary report. *Proc R Soc Med* 1953;46:346–349.

21. Beasley WC. Quantitative muscle testing: principles and applications to research and clinic services. *Arch Phys Med Rehabil* 1961;42:398–425.

22. Agre JC, Rodriquez AA, Tafel JA. Late effects of polio: critical review of the literature on neuromuscular function. *Arch Phys Med Rehabil* 1991;72:923–931.

23. Jubelt B, Cashman NR. Neurological manifestations of the post-polio syndrome. *Crit Rev Clin Neurobiol* 1987;3:199–220.

24. Shetty KR, Matsson DE, Rudman IW, Rudman D. Hyposomatomedin in men with post-poliomyelitis syndrome. *J Am Geriatr Soc* 1991;39:185–191.

25. Rudman D, Shetty KR. Growth hormone and the post-poliomyelitis syndrome. Presentation at the American Academy of Physical Medicine and Rehabilitation Annual Meeting, Washington, DC, October 30, 1991.

26. Sunnerhagen KS, Bengtsson B-A, Lundberg P-A, et al. Normal concentrations of serum insulin-like growth factor-1 in late polio. *Arch Phys Med Rehabil* 1995;76:732–735.

27. Müller EA. Influence of training and of inactivity on muscle strength. *Arch Phys Med Rehabil* 1970;51:449–462.

28. Saltin B, Blomqvist G, Mitchell JH, et al. Response to exercise after bed rest and after training: longitudinal study of adaptive changes in oxygen transport and body composition. *Circulation* 1968;38(suppl 7):1–78.

29. Grimby G, Einarsson G, Hedberg M, Aniansson A. Muscle adaptive changes in post-polio subjects. *Scand J Rehabil Med* 1989;21: 19–26.

30. Borg K, Henriksson J. Prior poliomyelitis-reduced capillary supply and metabolic enzyme content in hypertrophic slow-twitch (type I) muscle fibres. *J Neurol Neurosurg Psychiatry* 1991;54:236–240.

31. Agre JC, Rodriquez AA, Sperling KB. Symptoms and clinic impressions of patients seen in a post-polio clinic. *Arch Phys Med Rehabil* 1989;70:367–370.

32. Agre JC, Rodriquez AA, Sperling KB. Plasma lipid and lipoprotein concentrations in symptomatic postpolio patients. *Arch Phys Med Rehabil* 1990;71:393–394.

33. Miller NE, Rao S, Lewis B, et al. High-density lipoprotein and physical activity. *Lancet* 1979;1:111.

34. Lovett RW. The treatment of infantile paralysis: preliminary report, based on a study of the Vermont epidemic of 1914. *JAMA* 1915;64:2118–2123.

35. Bennett RL, Knowlton GC. Overwork weakness in partially denervated skeletal muscle. *Clin Orthop* 1958;12:22–29.

36. Knowlton GC, Bennett RL. Overwork. *Arch Phys Med Rehabil* 1957;38:18–20.

37. Luna-Reyes OB, Reyes TM, So MLFY, et al. Energy cost of ambulation in healthy and disabled Filipino children. *Arch Phys Med Rehabil* 1988;69:946–949.

38. Perry J, Barnes G, Gronley JD. The postpolio syndrome: an overuse phenomenon. *Clin Orthop* 1988;233:145–162.

39. Borg K, Borg J, Edstrom L, Grimby L. Effects of excessive use of remaining muscle fibers in prior polio and LV lesion. *Muscle Nerve* 1988;11: 1219–1230.

40. Agre JC, Rodriquez AA. Neuromuscular function: comparison of symptomatic and asymptomatic polio subjects to control subjects. *Arch Phys Med Rehabil* 1990;71:545–551.

41. Rodriquez AA, Agre JC. Electrophysiologic study of the quadriceps muscles during fatiguing exercise and recovery: a comparison of symptomatic postpolios to asymptomatic postpolios and controls. *Arch Phys Med Rehabil* 1991;72:993–997.

42. Waring WP, Davidoff G, Werner R. Serum creatine kinase in the post-polio population. *Am J Phys Med Rehabil* 1989;68: 86–90.

43. Nelson KR. Creatine kinase and fibrillation potentials in patients with late sequelae of polio. *Muscle Nerve* 1990;13: 722–725.

44. Agre JC, Grimby G, Rodriquez AA, et al. A comparison of symptoms between Swedish and American post-polio individuals and assessment of lower limb strength—a four-year cohort study. *Scand J Rehabil Med* 1995;27:183–192.

45. Halstead LS, Rossi CD. Post-polio syndrome: clinical experience with 132 consecutive outpatients. *Birth Defects* 1987;23(4):13–26.

46. Chetwynd J, Hogan D. Post-polio syndrome in New Zealand: a survey of 700 polio survivors. *N Z Med J* 1993;106:406–408.

47. Halstead LS, Rossi CD. Post-polio syndrome: results of a survey of 539 survivors. *Orthopedics* 1985;8:845–850.

48. Grimby G, Einarsson G. Post-polio management. *CRC Crit Rev Phys Med Rehabil* 1991;2: 189–200.

49. Perry J, Fleming C. Polio: long-term problems. *Orthopedics* 1995;8:877.

50. Cosgrove JL, Alexander MA, Kitts EL, et al. Late effects of poliomyelitis. *Arch Phys Med Rehabil* 1987;68:4–7.

51. Waring WP, Maynard F, Grady W, et al. Influence of appropriate lower extremity orthotic management on ambulation, pain, and fatigue in a post-polio population. *Arch Phys Med Rehabil* 1989;70:371–375.

52. Einarsson G, Broberg C. Motor impairment in late poliomyelitis. In: *Muscle adaptation and disability in late poliomyelitis.* Department

of Rehabilitation Medicine, University of Göteborg, Sweden, PhD thesis. 1990.

53. Agre JC. Local muscle and total body fatigue. In: Halstead LS, Grimby G, eds. *Post-polio syndrome.* Philadelphia: Hanley & Belfus, 1995:35–67.

54. Frick NM. Post-polio sequelae and psychology of second disability. *Orthopedics* 1985;8: 851–853.

55. Kohl SJ. Emotional responses to the late effects of poliomyelitis. *Birth Defects* 1987;23(4): 137–145.

56. Conrady LJ, Wish JR, Agre JC, et al. Psychologic characteristics of polio survivors: a preliminary report. *Arch Phys Med Rehabil* 1989;70:458–463.

57. Bruno RL, Frick NM. The psychology of polio as prelude to post-polio sequelae: behavior modification and psychotherapy. *Orthopedics* 1991;14: 1185–1193.

58. Bruno RL, Frick NM, Cohen J. Polioencephalitis and the etiology of post-polio sequelae. *Orthopedics* 1991;14:1269–1276.

59. Packer TL, Martins I, Krefting L, Brouwer B. Activity and post-polio fatigue. *Orthopedics* 1991;14:1223–1226.

60. Owen RR, Jones D. Polio residuals clinic: conditioning exercise program. *Orthopedics* 1985;8:882–883.

61. Cosgrove JL, Alexander MA, Kitts EL, et al. Late effects of poliomyelitis. *Arch Phys Med Rehabil* 1987;68:4–7.

62. Berlly MH, Strauser WW, Hall KM. Fatigue in postpolio syndrome. *Arch Phys Med Rehabil* 1991;72:115–118.

63. Dalakas MC, Elder G, Hallett M, et al. A long-term follow-up of patients with post-poliomyelitis neuromuscular symptoms. *N Engl J Med* 1986;314:959–963.

64. Dalakas MC. New neuromuscular symptoms in patients with old poliomyelitis: a three-year follow-up study. *Eur Neurol* 1986;25: 381–387.

65. Grimby G, Hedberg M, Henning G-B. Changes in muscle morphology, strength, and enzymes in a four-five-year follow-up of subjects with poliomyelitis sequelae. *Scand J Rehabil Med* 1994; 26:121–130.

66. Hodes HL. Treatment of respiratory difficulty in poliomyelitis. In: *Papers and discussions presented at the third international poliomyelitis conference.* Philadelphia: JB Lippincott, 1955:91–113.

67. Kuafert PL, Kaufert JM. Methodological and conceptual issues in measuring the long term impact of disability: the experience of poliomyelitis patients in Manitoba. *Soc Sci Med* 1984; 19:609–618.

68. Lassen HCA. The epidemic of poliomyelitis in Copenhagen, 1952. *Proc R Soc Med* 1953;47:6–71.

69. Howard RS, Wiles CM, Spencer GT. The late sequelae of poliomyelitis. *Q J Med* 1988;66:219–232.

70. Halstead LS, Weichers DO, Rossi CD. Late effects of poliomyelitis: a national survey. In: Halstead LS, Weichers DO, eds. *Late effects of poliomyelitis.* Miami: Symposia Foundations, 1985:11–31.

71. Speier JL, Owen R, Knapp M, Canine JK. Occurrence of post-polio sequelae in an epidemic population. *Birth Defects* 1987;23(4):39–48.

72. Bach JR, Alba AS. Pulmonary dysfunction and sleep disordered breathing as post-polio sequelae: evaluation and management. *Orthopedics* 1991;14: 1329–1337.

73. Lane DJ, Hazleman B, Nichols PRJ. Late onset respiratory failure in patients with previous poliomyelitis. *Q J Med* 1974;172:551–568.

74. Newsom Davis J, Goldman M, Loh L, Casson M. Diaphragm function and alveolar hypoventilation. *Q J Med* 1976; 45:87–100.

75. Bye PTB, Ellis ER, Issa FG, et al. Respiratory failure and sleep in neuromuscular disease. *Thorax* 1990;45:241–247.

76. Fischer DA. Poliomyelitis: late respiratory complications and management. *Orthopedics* 1985;8:891–894.

77. Guilleminauls C, Motta J. Sleep apnea syndrome as a long term sequelae of poliomyelitis. In: Guilleminauls C, Dement WC, eds. *Sleep apnea syndromes.* New York: Alan R Liss, 1978:309–315.

78. Hill R, Robbins AW, Messing R, Arora NS. Sleep apnea syndrome after poliomyelitis. *Am Rev Respir Dis* 1983;127:129–131.

79. Borg J, Weinberg J. Respiratory management in late post-polio. In: Halstead LS, Grimby G, eds. *Post-polio syndrome.* Philadelphia: Hanley & Belfus, 1995:113–124.

80. Sonies BC. Long-term effects of post-polio on oral-motor and swallowing function. In: Halstead LS, Grimby G, eds. *Post-polio syndrome.* Philadelphia: Hanley & Belfus, 1995:125–137.

81. Coelho CA, Ferranti R. Incidence and nature of dysphagia in polio survivors. *Arch Phys Med Rehabil* 1991;72:1071–1075.

82. Jones B, Buchholz DW, Ravich WJ, Donner MW. Swallowing dysfunction in the post-polio syndrome: a cinefluorographic study. *AJR* 1992;158:283–286.

83. Sonies BC, Dalakas MC. Dysphagia in patients with the post-polio syndrome. *N Engl J Med* 1991;324:1162–1167.

84. Lonnberg F. Post-polio sequelae in Denmark: presentation and results of a nationwide survey of 3607 polio survivors. *Scand J Rehabil Med Suppl* 1993;28:1–32.

85. Einarsson G, Grimby G. Disability and handicap in late poliomyelitis. *Scand J Rehabil Med* 1990;22:113–121.

86. Conrady LJ, Wish JR, Agre JC, et al. Psychologic characteristics of polio survivors: a preliminary report. *Arch Phys Med Rehabil* 1989;70:458–463.

87. Derogatis LR, Rickels K, Roch AF. SCL-90 and MMPI: step in validation of new self-report scale. *Br J Psychiatry* 1976;128:280–289.

88. Derogatis LR, Lopez MC. *PAIS and PAIS-SR: administration, scoring and procedures manual.* Towson, MD: Psychometric Research, 1983.

89. Bruno RL, Frick NM. Stress and "type A" behaviour as precipitants of post-polio sequelae: the Felician/Columbia Survey. *Birth Defects* 1987;23(4):145–155.

90. Kohl SJ. Emotional responses to the late effects of poliomyelitis. *Birth Defects* 1987;23(4): 135–143.

91. Weichers DO, Hubbell SL. Late changes in the motor unit after acute poliomyelitis. *Muscle Nerve* 1981;4:524–528.

92. Cruz Martinez MA, Ferrer MT, Perez Conde MC. Electrophysiological features in patients with non-progressive and late progressive weakness after paralytic poliomyelitis: electromyogram and single fiber electromyography study. *Electromyogr Clin Neurophysiol* 1984;24:469–479.

93. Cashman NR, Maselli R, Wollmann RL, et al. Late denervation in patients with antecedent paralytic poliomyelitis. *N Engl J Med* 1987;317:7–12.

94. Einarsson G, Grimby G, Stalberg E. Electromyographic and morphological functional compensation in late poliomyelitis. *Muscle Nerve* 1990;13:165–171.

95. Ravits J, Hallett M, Baker M, et al. Clinical and electromyographic studies of post-poliomyelitis muscular atrophy. *Muscle Nerve* 1990;13: 667–674.

96. Maselli RA, Cashman NR, Wollman RL, et al. Neuromuscular transmission as a function of motor unit size in patients with prior poliomyelitis. *Muscle Nerve* 1992;15:648–655.

97. Klingman J, Chui H, Corgiat M, Perry J. Functional recovery: a major risk factor for development of postpoliomyelitis muscular atrophy. *Arch Neurol* 1988;45:645–647.

98. Rodriquez AA, Agre JC. Physiologic parameters and perceived exertion with local muscle fatigue in postpolio subjects. *Arch Phys Med Rehabil* 1991;72:305–308.

99. Agre JC, Rodriquez AA. Intermittent isometric activity: its effect on muscle fatigue in postpolio subjects. *Arch Phys Med Rehabil* 1991;72:971–975.

100. Perry J, Fleming C. Polio: long-term problems. *Orthopedics* 1985;8:877–881.

101. Young GR. Occupational therapy and the post-polio syndrome. *Am J Occup Ther* 1989;43:97–103.

102. McNellis A. Physical therapy management of post-polio syndrome. *Rehabil Manage* 1989:38–44.

103. Smith LK, Bonck J, Macrae A. Current issues in neurological rehabilitation. In: Umphred DA, ed. *Neurological rehabilitation.* 2nd ed. St. Louis: CV Mosby, 1990:509–528.

104. Stein DP, D'Ambrosia JM, Dalakas MC. A double-blind, placebo-controlled trial of amantidine for the treatment of fatigue in patients with the post-polio syndrome. *Ann NY Acad Sci* 1995;753:296–302.

105. Dinsmore ST, Dambrosia JM, Dalakas MC. A double-blind, placebo-controlled trial of high-dose prednisone for the treatment of post-poliomyelitis syndrome. *Ann NY Acad Sci* 1995;753:303–313.

106. Trojan DA, Cashman NR. Anticholinesterases, in post-poliomyelitis syndrome. *Ann NY Acad Sci* 1995;753:285–295.

107. Agre JC. The role of exercise on the patient with post-polio syndrome. *Ann NY Acad Sci* 1995;753:321–334.

108. DeLorme TL, Schwab RS, Watkins AL. The response of the quadriceps femoris to progressive resistance exercises in polio myelitic patients. *J Bone Joint [Am]* 1948;30:834–847.

109. Muller EA, Beckmann H. Die trainierbarkeit von kindern mit gelahmten muskeln durch isometrische kontraktionen. *Z Orthop* 1966;102:139–145.

110. Gurewitsch AD. Intensive graduated exercises in early infantile paralysis. *Arch Phys Med Rehabil* 1950;31:213–218.

111. Hyman G. Poliomyelitis. *Lancet* 1953;1:852.

112. Mitchell GP. Poliomyelitis and exercise. *Lancet* 1953;2:90–91.

113. Knowlton GC, Bennett RL. Overwork. *Arch Phys Med Rehabil* 1957;38:18–20.

114. Feldman RM, Soskolne CL. The use of nonfatiguing strengthening exercises in post-polio syndrome. *Birth Defects* 1987;23(4): 335–341.

115. Einarsson G, Grimby G. Strengthening exercise program in post-polio subjects. *Birth Defects* 1987;23(4):275–283.

116. Einarsson G. Muscle conditioning on late poliomyelitis. *Arch Phys Med Rehabil* 1991;72:11–14.

117. Fillyaw MJ, Badger GJ, Goodwin GD, et al. The effects of long-term non-fatiguing resistance exercise in subjects with post-polio syndrome. *Orthopedics* 1991;14:1253–1256.

118. Agre JC, Rodriquez AA, Franke TM, et al. Low-intensity, alternate-day exercise improves muscle performance without apparent adverse affect in post-polio patients. *Am J Phys Med Rehabil* 1996;75:50–58.

119. Jones DR, Speier J, Canine K, et al. Cardiorespiratory responses to aerobic training by patients with postpoliomyelitis sequelae. *JAMA* 1989;261:3255–3258.

120. Kriz JL, Jones DR, Speir JL, et al. Cardiorespiratory responses to upper extremity aerobic training

by post-polio subjects. *Arch Phys Med Rehabil* 1992;73:49–54.

121. Dean E, Ross J. Effect of modified aerobic training on movement energetics in polio survivors. *Orthopedics* 1991;14:1243–1246.

122. Fischer DA. Poliomyelitis: late respiratory complications and management. *Orthopedics* 1985;88:891–894.

123. Fischer DA. Sleep disordered breathing as a late effect of poliomyelitis. *Birth Defects* 1987;23(4):115–119.

124. Williams A, Santiago S, Stein M. Screening for sleep apnea. *Chest* 1989;96:451–453.

125. Saunders MH. Assessment of required nocturnal ventilatory assistance. *Eur Respir Rev* 1992;2:409–412.

126. Sanders MH, Kern N. Obstructive sleep apnea treated independently by adjusting inspiratory and expiratory pressures via nasal mask, physiological and clinical implications. *Chest* 1990;98:317–324.

127. Bach JR, Alba AS, Shin D. Management alternatives for post-polio respiratory insufficiency: assisted ventilation by nasal or oral nasal interface. *Am J Phys Med Rehabil* 1989;68:264–271.

128. Baker AB, Matzhe HA, Brown JR. Poliomyelitis III: a study of medullary function. *Arch Neurol* 1950;63:257.

129. Buckholtz DW, Jones B. Post-polio dysphagia: alarm or caution. *Orthopedics* 1991;14:1303–1304.

130. Bruno RL, Frick NM. The psychology of polio as prelude to post-polio sequelae: behavior modification and psychotherapy. *Orthopedics* 1991;14:1185–1193.

Chapter 88

Evaluation of Nonentrapment Neuropathies

James T. McDeavitt

Peripheral neuropathies are commonly encountered in physiatric practice. The peripheral nervous system (PNS) is an end organ that is damaged in a variety of disease states. To appropriately identify, diagnose, and treat neuropathies, the physician must understand both the basic pathophysiology of the PNS and the natural history of a variety of inherited and acquired diseases.

The following chapter provides a general overview of the evaluation of peripheral neuropathies, with an emphasis on the conditions that are common and potentially treatable. More exhaustive reviews are available (1,2).

DIAGNOSTIC APPROACH

History and Physical Examination

A good, basic history and physical examination are essential to establish the etiology of a peripheral neuropathy. The rapidity of symptom onset, distribution of symptoms, fiber-type predominance, and the presence or absence of pain provide valuable clues as to the etiology (Table 88-1) (3).

Abnormal sensations are commonly reported by patients with neuropathies. Neuropathic pain may be spontaneous or occur with stimulation of peripheral receptors. The nature of the abnormal sensation may provide clues as to the fiber type involved. Pain described as "dull" or "burning" is often mediated by nociceptors served by small-diameter C fibers, whereas a "sharp" or "prickling" sensation is due to the firing of larger A-delta fibers (4). Paresthesias are nonpainful but usually annoying sensations that occur spontaneously, and are often described as "tingling" or "pins and needles," while dysesthesias are subjectively similar but occur only with tactile stimulation (2). Both are common in the setting of ischemic and compressive neuropathies, and are probably generated by an ectopic source in the nerve trunk, not by the peripheral nociceptor (4).

Muscle cramps may also be the source of pain in neuropathies, and are caused by contraction of muscle due to the involuntary firing of the motor unit. Cramps are especially common in partially denervated muscle and with uremic neuropathy (4).

Involvement of the sympathetic nervous system may produce symptoms of minimal consequence, such as diminished sweating. Alternatively, autonomic nervous system involvement may cause a variety of disabling problems affecting the patient's general health and quality of life, including postural hypotension, problems with heart rate regulation, gastroparesis, urinary retention or incontinence, and impotence (5,6). Predominant autonomic involvement is also suggestive of certain disease states, such as diabetes or amyloidosis (Table 88-2).

Many findings on physical examination are nonspecific and merely indicative of lower motor neuron disease. These findings include weakness, atrophy, areflexia, and sensory loss. However, physical findings may provide clues

Table 88-1: Clinical Types of Peripheral Neuropathy

Acute onset
Guillain-Barré syndrome
Porphyria
Toxic (e.g., arsenic, nitrofurantoin)
Serum sickness
Diphtheria
Malignancy
Critical illness polyneuropathy
Diabetes, uremia (rarely)
Predominantly motor
Guillain-Barré syndrome
Porphyria
Diphtheria
Lead
Charcot-Marie-Tooth disease
Diabetes (diabetic amyotrophy)
Predominantly sensory
Leprosy
Diabetes (distal sensory polyneuropathy)
Vitamin B_{12} or thiamine deficiency
Malignancy
Hereditary sensory and autonomic neuropathy
Primary and familial amyloidosis
Uremia
Lyme disease
Sjögren syndrome
Radicular
Diabetic truncal neuropathy
Lyme disease
Sjögren syndrome
Painful neuropathies
Alcohol, nutritional deficiencies
Diabetes (acute painful neuropathy)
Hereditary sensory and autonomic neuropathy (HSAN type I)
Arsenic
Cryoglobulinemia
Lyme disease
Paraneoplastic sensory neuropathy
Vasculitic neuropathies

Source: Reproduced by permission from McLeod JG. Investigation of peripheral neuropathy. *J Neurol Neurosurg Psychiatry* 1995;58:381–382.

Table 88-2: Causes of Autonomic Dysfunction in Peripheral Nerve Disease

Autonomic dysfunction clinically important
Acute and subacute autonomic neuropathy
Diabetes
Primary amyloidosis and familial amyloid neuropathy type I (Portuguese)
Acute inflammatory neuropathy
Acute and intermittent variegate porphyria
HSAN type III (Riley-Day syndrome, familial dysautonomia)
HSAN type IV (Swanson)
Autonomic dysfunction usually clinically unimportant
Hereditary neuropathies
HMSN types I and II
Fabry disease
HSAN types I, II, and V
Amyloid disease (some familial amyloid polyneuropathies, secondary amyloidosis)
Navajo neuropathy type B
Chronic inflammatory demyelinating polyradiculopathy
Metabolic disorder
Chronic renal failure
Chronic liver disease
Vitamin B_{12} deficiency
Alcoholism and nutritional disorders
Malignancy
Toxic causes (vincristine, acrylamide, heavy metals, perhexiline maleate, organic solvents)
Connective tissue diseases
Rheumatoid arthritis
Systemic lupus erythematosus
Mixed connective tissue diseases
Infection
Leprosy
Human immunodeficiency virus
Chagas disease

HMSN = Hereditary motor and sensory neuropathy; HSAN = hereditary sensory and autonomic neuropathy.
Source: Reproduced by permission from McLeod JG. Autonomic dysfunction in peripheral nerve disorders. *Curr Opin Neurol Neurosurg* 1992;5:476–481.

to a specific diagnosis or a group of diagnoses. It is important to determine the distribution of neuropathic symptoms to distinguish between a diffuse and a multifocal process. In addition, the physical findings may suggest the predominant fiber type involved (motor, sensory, or mixed), which can aid in diagnosis (7,8). Sensory modalities of proprioception, position sense, and light touch are carried by large-diameter axons. Small-diameter, more slowly conducting fibers typically transmit information regarding pain and temperature sensation (9). Some authors (10,11) proposed use of quantitative sensory testing, which tests sensory thresholds for thermal or vibratory stimuli.

Laboratory Testing

Electrodiagnosis

Electrodiagnostic testing is often a useful extension of the history and physical examination (8), increasing the physician's ability to detect and quantify nerve disease. However, testing is subject to some significant limitation (6). Nerve conduction studies are insensitive to neuropathies that affect predominantly small fibers, such as amyloidosis. The latency obtained in a typical motor nerve conduction study reflects the fastest conducting axons within the nerve. Sensory latencies also reflect the fastest population of axons, if latency is measured from the onset of the sensory nerve action potential (SNAP). Fortunately, the majority of common diseases affecting the PNS involve large-diameter fibers (12).

Electrodiagnostic testing does have an important role in the evaluation of neuropathies. Although rarely diagnostic of a specific cause for neuropathy, the evaluation can help to limit the differential diagnosis by more accurately defining the pathologic changes. Nerve conduction studies and electromyography (EMG) can define whether a neuropathic process is predominantly axonal or demyelinating. In addition, the examination can determine whether the nerve damage is generalized, diffuse, and symmetric versus patchy and multifocal, a distinction that may not be apparent on physical examination.

Basic Laboratory Evaluation

The potential causes of peripheral neuropathy are myriad, and a "shotgun" diagnostic approach to ordering diagnostic tests is not appropriate. In many patients the etiology of the neuropathic process is obvious, and an extensive diagnostic evaluation is not warranted. For example, a known diabetic with a subacute onset of a distal, symmetric polyneuropathy may not require extensive diagnostic testing. The clinical picture painted by the history, physical examination, and electrodiagnostic evaluation should guide laboratory testing. A summary of a variety of diagnostic tests is outlined in Table 88-3 (3). A variety of diagnostic algorithms have been proposed (13,14), but none has been universally accepted.

Sural Nerve Biopsy

Sural nerve biopsy should be employed only when a specific diagnosis is suspected. Biopsy can aid in the evaluation of fiber type, size, and number; detection of alterations of axons and myelin; and the recognition of pathologic alterations of the interstitium (e.g., vasculitis, inflammation, edema, neoplasm, infiltrative diseases) (15). Selection of an appropriate nerve is important, as an electrodiagnostically normal nerve is unlikely to display pathologic changes. In addition, biopsy specimens should be prepared and the findings interpreted by an experienced neuropathologist. If a diagnosis is not strongly suspected prior to the biopsy, in almost half the patients the diagnosis will not be established by the procedure (16). It has been suggested that the diagnostic yield is greater in the individuals showing substantial slowing on nerve conduction testing (17).

Diagnostic Success

The physician's likelihood of successfully identifying the cause of a neuropathy has improved substantially over the past three decades. From 1960 to 1981, the percentage of patients who remained undiagnosed following extensive evaluation dropped progressively from 50% to 24% (18–20). Since that time, the nondiagnosis rate has dropped and stabilized between 10% and 14% (21–24). The improvement in diagnostic success is due to identification of new disease processes [e.g., chronic inflammatory demyelinating polyneuropathy (CIDP), monoclonal gammopathies] as well as improved diagnostic testing and classification of inherited peripheral neuropathies (24). Inherited neuropathies constitute up to 42% of the neuropathies for which the clinical cause is not readily apparent (20). A careful family history and electrodiagnostic evaluation of primary family members may be helpful.

ELECTRODIAGNOSTIC CLASSIFICATION

As stated earlier, electrodiagnostic evaluation of a peripheral neuropathy is an important step in determining etiology, although it is rarely the definitive diagnostic test. This is not surprising given the large number of diseases with PNS manifestations, and the limited manner in which the nervous system can respond to disease. The primary roles of electrodiagnostic testing are to 1) define the underlying neuropathophysiology and 2) establish the distribution of nerve involvement.

Damage to the PNS can result in one of two basic pathologies, axonopathy or demyelination, or a combination of the two (25). A process that is predominantly axonal in its effects will result in reduced compound motor unit action potentials (CMAPs) and SNAPs. Assuming the process has been present for more than 3 to 4 weeks, fibrillation potentials and positive sharp waves will be present on EMG analysis of the muscles served by the involved nerves. In contrast, a purely demyelinative process will result in significant prolongation of distal latencies and slowing of nerve conduction velocities. Amplitudes are generally preserved, reduced only by the effect of temporal dispersion, and in the absence of secondary axonopathic changes, EMG will display normal insertional activity (see Chap. 9). Therefore, electrodiagnostic analysis can help to define the underlying neuropathology. The results must be interpreted with regard to the remainder of the clinical picture, as many neuropathies are not "pure" in their pathologic effects. For example, Guillain-Barré syndrome (GBS) (26–28), CIDP (29,30), and multifocal motor neuropathy (MMN) (31) are known to be predominantly demyelinating processes, but frequently have an axonal component as well, resulting in fibrillation potentials and positive sharp waves on needle EMG.

The distribution of nerve damage is also of interest. Neuropathies can be broadly categorized as those that result in 1) diffuse, largely symmetric damage and 2) those with multifocal involvement.

When the distribution of nerve damage is considered with the neuropathologic type, all peripheral neuropathies can be grouped into four broad categories:

1. Predominant axonal damage with diffuse, symmetric involvement (axonal/diffuse). This is the largest single category and includes the majority of neuropathies induced by toxic and metabolic processes,

Table 88-3: Laboratory Investigation of Peripheral Neuropathies	
Condition	**Investigation**
Metabolic	
Diabetes	Urinalysis, fasting blood glucose, glucose tolerance test
Hypoglycemia	Fasting blood glucose, serum insulin, or C-peptide concentrations
Uremia	Blood urea, serum creatine, urinalysis
Porphyria	Urinary porphyrins, ALA, porphobilinogen; total fecal porphyrins; erythrocyte porphobilinogen deaminase
Hypothyroidism	Serum free thyroxine, serum TSH
Acromegaly	Serum growth hormone concentrations
Deficiencies	
B_1 (thiamine)	Erythrocyte transketolase activity plus enhancement with thiamine pyrophosphate
Vitamin B_6 (pyridoxine)	Erythrocyte aspartate amino transferase plus enhancement with pyridoxal-5 phosphate
Vitamin B_{12}	Serum B_{12}, Schilling test
Vitamin E	Serum vitamin E
Toxic	
Arsenic, lead, mercury, thallium	24-hour urinary heavy metals
Paraproteinemias, dysproteinemias	
Multiple myeloma, Waldenström macroglobulinemia, cryoglobulinemia, monoclonal gammopathy of uncertain significance	Hb, WCC, platelets, ESR, plasma immunoelectrophoresis, urinary Bence-Jones protein, radiologic skeletal survey, bone marrow biopsy, plasma cryoglobulins
Connective tissue disorders	
Systemic lupus erythematosus, mixed connective tissue disease, scleroderma, rheumatoid arthritis, polyarteritis nodosa, Sjögren syndrome, Wegener granulomatosis	Hb, WCC, platelets, ESR, serum immunoelectrophoresis, antinuclear antibodies, anti-double-stranded DNA antibodies, rheumatoid factor, serum complement (C3, C4, CH50), antineutrophil cytoplasmic antibodies
Sjögren syndrome	All of the above plus anti–Sjögren syndrome antibodies, Schirmer test, lip biopsy
Inflammatory neuropathies	
Acute inflammatory neuropathy	HIV, blood glucose, urinary porphyrins, Epstein-Barr virus, *Campylobacter*, cytomegalovirus, *Mycoplasma*
Chronic inflammatory demyelinating polyradiculoneuropathy	ESR, serum immunoelectrophoresis, antiganglioside GM_1 antibodies, antinuclear antibodies, antineutrophil cytoplasmic antibodies
Infections	
HIV	HIV serology
Lyme disease	Lyme serology
Leprosy	Lepromin test, skin and nasal scrapings, skin and nerve biopsy
Hereditary neuropathies with known biochemical abnormalities	
Primary amyloid neuropathy	Rectal, liver, renal, abdominal fat, and nerve biopsy; serum immunoelectrophoresis; urinary Bence-Jones protein
	Serum, tissue transthyretin
Familiar amyloid neuropathy	Blood leukocyte, skin fibroblast arylsulfatase
Metachromatic leukodystrophy	Blood leukocyte, skin fibroblast galactosylceramide
Krabbe disease (globoid cell leukodystrophy)	β-galactosidase
β-lipoproteinemia (Bassen-Kornzweig disease)	Acanthocytes in blood, serum cholesterol, plasma low-density and very-low-density lipoproteins
α-lipoproteinemia (Tangier disease)	Serum cholesterol
Refsum disease	Serum phytanic acid, α-oxidation of phytanic acid in skin fibroblasts

Source: Modified by permission from McLeod JG. Investigation of peripheral neuropathy. *J Neurol Neurosurg Psychiatry* 1995;58:381–382.

ALA = aminolevulenic acid; TSH = thyroid-stimulating hormone; Hb = hemoglobin; WCC = white cell count; ESR = erythrocyte sedimentation rate; HIV = human immunodeficiency virus.

Table 88-4: Classification of Peripheral Neuropathies Based on Primary Pathology and Predominant Fiber-Type Involved		
Demyelinating, uniform Mixed sensory/motor HMSN type I HMSN type III Most inherited neuropathies	Demyelinating, segmental Motor > sensory AIDP/GBS CIDP Most plasma cell dyscrasias Leprosy Arsenic poisoning (acute)	Axonal Motor > sensory Porphyria Axonal GBS Lead Vincristine Dapsone Hypoglycemia/ hyperinsulinemia HMSN type II Paraneoplastic
Axonal Mixed sensory/motor Most toxic neuropathies Most metabolic neuropathies Most nutritional neuropathies Most medication-induced neuropathies Connective tissue diseases Amyloidosis Sarcoidosis Lyme disease Multiple myeloma Paraneoplastic AIDS	Axonal Sensory Cisplatin Friedreich ataxia Paraneoplastic	Mixed axonal and demyelinating Mixed sensory/motor Diabetes mellitus Uremia

Source: Adapted from Donofrio PD, Albers JW. Polyneuropathy: classification by nerve conduction studies and electromyography. AAEM mininomograph #34. *Muscle Nerve* 1990;13:889–903.

HMSN = hereditary, motor and sensory neuropathy; AIDP = acute inflammatory demyelinating polyneuropathy; CIDP = chronic inflammatory demyelinating polyneuropathy; GBS = Guillain-Barré syndrome; AIDS = acquired immunodeficiency syndrome.

the archetype being the distal symmetric polyneuropathy associated with diabetes. The earliest and most severe damage usually involves the longest and therefore the most distal axons. This is presumably due to the distance of the damaged tissue from the cell body, from which the materials to repair the axon must be provided.

2. Predominant axonal damage with multifocal involvement (axonal/multifocal). This is the common pattern displayed in vasculitic and infiltrative neuropathies, and is likely due to regional nerve ischemia. Examples include the neuropathies associated with connective tissue diseases (32) and diabetic amyotrophy (33).
3. Predominant demyelination with diffuse, symmetric involvement (demyelinating/diffuse). The majority of inherited neuropathies, especially the multiple variants of the hereditary motor and sensory neuropathies (HMSNs) (34), fall into this category.
4. Predominant demyelination with multifocal involvement (demyelinating/multifocal). This category includes the acquired demyelinating neuropathies, especially GBS, CIDP, and MMN.

Along with the history and physical findings, categorization into one of these four groups is quite useful in helping to guide subsequent diagnostic testing. Donofrio and Albers (8) add additional refinement to this tool by incorporating the predominant fiber type involved, motor versus sensory (Table 88-4).

REPRESENTATIVE NEUROPATHIES

The following discussion reviews disease states that are commonly encountered in physiatric practice. For a more comprehensive review, the reader is referred to more exhaustive, comprehensive texts on this subject (1,2).

Axonal/Diffuse (Toxic/Metabolic)

Diabetes Mellitus

Diabetes mellitus is common, afflicting 5 million people in the United States. The sequelae of diabetes are well known, and affect a variety of organ systems. Peripheral neuropathy is the most common complication experienced by diabetics, and diabetes remains the most common cause of peripheral neuropathy in the developed world (35). Diabetes may result in mononeuropathies, mononeuropathy multiplex, or a diffuse, symmetric distal polyneuropathy, with the latter representing the most common form (36).

The exact incidence of peripheral neuropathy in diabetics varies from 5% to 100%, and has not been well defined (37). This variation is due in part to the definition of neuropathy used. For example, when neuropathy is defined symptomatically, 50% of individuals are considered affected. If electrodiagnostic criteria are applied, the incidence increases to 90% (38). The incidence increases with aging, with 4% of individuals affected 5 years following the diagnosis of diabetes and 15% after 20 years (39). In one study (40) of 4400 patients followed prospectively from the time of diagnosis, at diagnosis 7.5% exhibited neuropathic symptoms. After 25 years, 50% of the cohort had developed symptoms compatible with peripheral neuropathy. The incidence of peripheral neuropathy may be slightly lower in patients with non-insulin-dependent diabetes mellitus (NIDDM), but is still very high. In a large population-based study (n = 64,573), the incidence of neuropathy in patients with insulin-dependent diabetes mellitus (IDDM) was 66%, compared to 59% in individuals with NIDDM (1).

The metabolic culprit in diabetic neuropathy has not been definitively identified, although there are some strong suspects. Excess accumulation of intracellular sorbitol (41), glycosylation of cellular proteins, and metabolic derangement of cellular metabolism with resulting low levels of *myo*-inositol have all been suggested. In fact, high levels of sorbitol do correlate with the degree of loss of myelinated fibers. No such correlation exists with respect to *myo*-inositol levels (42).

In its diffuse form, the neuropathy of diabetes causes axonal damage of myelinated and unmyelinated fibers, resulting in wallerian degeneration (43). Incomplete but active nerve regeneration probably occurs throughout the course of the disease as documented by biopsy (44) and single-fiber EMG studies (45).

Uremia

Peripheral neuropathy associated with end-stage renal disease is common, affecting as many as 65% of patients at the time of initiation of dialysis (46). The involvement is usually distal and symmetric, including both sensory and motor fibers. Axonal damage predominates, although a degree of demyelination is usually present as well (47). An acute neuropathy similar to GBS has also been described (48).

Sensory symptoms, especially painful dysesthesias, are common. In addition, 42% of patients in one series (49) reported paradoxical heat sensation (a cool stimulus results in the subjective sensation of heat), perhaps due to involvement of A-delta fibers. The etiology of the damage has not been clearly defined, although it is presumed to be related to uremic toxins (50). Hemodialysis (51), peritoneal dialysis (52), and renal transplantation (53) have all resulted in a reduction of symptoms and improvement in electrophysiologic findings.

Hypothyroidism

Thyroid disease is common in the United States, with a prevalence of 1.0% to 1.5% if iatrogenic causes are excluded (54). Thyroid function tests are commonly performed as part of the evaluation of peripheral neuropathy. These tests are arguably overutilized given the low incidence of diffuse, symmetric peripheral polyneruropathy in patients with hypothyroidism.

A review of this topic reported the incidence of generalized peripheral neuropathy in hypothyroid patients to range from 20% to 70% (55). These rates are misleadingly high, as they are based on series of patients who were overtly myxedematous at presentation (56–60). Overt myxedema is a relatively infrequent phenomenon in the developed world, and consequently, the incidence of generalized peripheral neuropathy in a treated or recently diagnosed hypothyroid patient is probably quite low. According to one case series of two patients, peripheral neuropathy was the presenting symptom of hypothyroidism (61), but this is relatively unusual. When hypothyroidism is the cause of neuropathy, studies indicate predominately axonal involvement (62,63), although demyelination has been described as well (61). In summary, a generalized, diffuse polyneuropathy as a complication of hypothyroidism has been described, but is relatively rare in clinical practice.

Pernicious Anemia

A deficiency of vitamin B_{12} (cobalamin) classically produces a megaloblastic anemia with hypersegmented neutrophils. The most common cause is pernicious anemia, a disorder in which deficiency of gastric intrinsic factor prevents the absorption of vitamin B_{12} from the terminal ileum (64). Peripheral neuropathy is a common feature of the disease (65), with predominantly axonal pathology (66). Dysesthesias are a common presenting complaint (64) and studies confirm a disproportionate involvement of sensory fibers (67,68). The neuropathic process is reversible with treatment (69), especially if initiated early in the disease.

Alcoholism

The neuropathy of chronic alcoholism usually presents with sensory symptoms, and patients frequently describe "burning" paresthesias. The nerve damage is mainly axonal, with significant demyelination (70). Neurotoxicity may be due to the direct, toxic effects of alcohol or its metabolites, specifically acetaldehyde.

Nutritional and vitamin deficiencies, especially of niacin and thiamine, can cause a similar neuropathy and must be excluded. Abstinence from alcohol is essential to treatment, as the neuropathic process will likely progress in the alcoholic who continues to drink (71) and may improve in those who abstain (72).

Paraproteinemias

It is difficult to treat all the paraproteinemias as a single clinical entity because they represent a variety of disease states including multiple myeloma, amyloidosis, lymphoma, Waldenström macroglobulinemia, chronic lymphocytic leukemia, and nonmalignant gammopathies (73). A diffuse, distal symmetric pattern of involvement is most common, although the precise neuropathology is quite variable (74–76).

Multiple myeloma occurs with an incidence of 3 per 100,000 population per year, with a peak onset between the ages of 40 and 70 years (77). Symptomatic polyneuropathy occurs in about 5% of patients with multiple myeloma, usually with mild distal sensorimotor involvement (78). Radicular pain may occur as well, with or without vertebral fractures (79).

Amyloidosis may occur as a primary disease or in association with multiple myeloma. With amyloid neuropathy displaying a clear predilection for small-diameter fibers, suspicion should be heightened by loss of pain and temperature sensation or by a predominance of autonomic symptoms (78). Fully half of patients with primary amyloidosis will have some degree of PNS involvement, and in 40% of patients the symptoms on presentation will be attributable to a neurologic complaint (80). Sensory and autonomic symptoms predominate, and definitive diagnosis is made by fat aspiration, rectal mucosa biopsy, or nerve biopsy.

A peripheral neuropathy has also been associated with monoclonal serum proteins in the absence of any underlying disease state. The so-called polyneuropathy associated with monoclonal gammopathies of uncertain significance (MGUS) usually presents with predominantly sensory symptoms, and a mixed axonal and demyelinative picture (74).

When faced with an apparent MGUS-associated neuropathy, the clinician must be aware of three points. First, the incidence of monoclonal serum proteins in the general population is fairly high, especially in older patients (72). Therefore, the identification of a monoclonal protein in a patient with a neuropathy may be purely coincidental, and does not obviate the need for exploration into other causes of the neuropathy.

Second, identification of a monoclonal protein requires evaluation for malignant disease, often including referral to a hematologist, radiologic skeletal survey, and bone marrow biopsy. It is generally agreed (81) that patients with low serum levels of protein (<20 g of IgG per liter or <10 g of IgM or IgA per liter), normal peripheral hemogram and blood chemistry values, absence of Bence-Jones proteinuria, and no bone pain, may be observed without more invasive diagnostic testing.

Finally, it must be recognized that MGUS may be a harbinger of malignant disease. In one study of 241 patients with MGUS, 26 (11%) developed myeloma, macroglobulinemia, or amyloidosis within 5 years (82).

Axonal/Multifocal (Vasculitic)

Connective Tissue Diseases

Nerve injury due to vasculitis is common for most of the connective tissue diseases. The nerve damage is usually due to ischemia resulting from vasculitis of the epineurium and perineurium (83), and results in multiple mononeuropathies or mononeuritis multiplex (84,85). The one exception may be the neuropathy associated with Sjögren syndrome, which has been described as a symmetric sensorimotor neuropathy (86). Although experimentally small fibers are more susceptible to ischemic injury (87), clinically both large and small fibers may be involved (32). Dysesthetic pain is a common complaint, occurring in 70% to 80% of patients with a vasculitic neuropathy (88).

Rheumatoid arthritis (RA) is the most common connective tissue disease, and is frequently complicated by peripheral neuropathy. Systemic vasculitis occurs in 8% to 25% of patients with RA, and is predictive of the development of neuropathy. When vasculitis is present, a peripheral neuropathy will develop in 40% to 50% of patients (32). The presence of vasculitic peripheral neuropathy in RA patients may have some prognostic impact as well, as the 5-year survival rate is only 57% (83).

Demyelinating/Diffuse (Inherited)

Charcot-Marie-Tooth Disease

The majority of demyelinating neuropathies with a diffuse, symmetric pattern of involvement are inherited. The history and physical examination can point the examiner toward a genetic cause. Hereditary neuropathies occur in autosomal dominant, autosomal recessive, and X-linked forms, so a thorough family history is helpful. In addition, some physical features are relatively unique, owing to the long-standing nature of the neuropathy. Skeletal deformities, such as pes cavus and kyphoscoliosis, are common with some forms of inherited neuropathy.

HMSN type I usually presents in the first decade of life and is predominantly demyelinating. Nerve conduction velocities are therefore quite slow, usually less than 30 m/sec (89,90). Classic "onion bulbs" are visible by light microscopy and represent hypertrophy of the Schwann cells. Peripheral nerves may be palpable.

HMSN type II is generally less severe than, though often indistinguishable from, type I. The disease is primarily axonopathic, and conduction velocities are frequently normal or only mildly slowed, usually above 40 m/sec (89). HMSN type III (Dejerine-Sottas disease) is an amyelinative condition, with profound slowing of conduction velocities, usually to less than 6 m/sec (91).

Rapid advances in genetic testing are improving the

understanding of these syndromes. For example, it is clear that peripheral myelin protein 22 is abnormal in 90% of HMSN type I patients, and that this protein abnormality can be traced to a mutation on chromosome 17 in the majority of patients (92). Interested readers are referred to recent thorough reviews of the genetics of HMSNs (92–94).

Demyelinating/Multifocal

Guillain-Barré Syndrome and Chronic Inflammatory Demyelinating Polyneuropathy

GBS, also referred to as *acute inflammatory demyelinating polyneuropathy* (AIDP), is the most common disease producing an acute, generalized paralysis, with an annual incidence of 0.75 to 2.0 per 100,000 population (95). Despite advances in electrodiagnosis and immunochemistry, the diagnosis often relies on clinical features. Patients usually present with distal paresthesias, and generalized weakness subsequently develops over several days. Often there is an antecedent infection, although the syndrome may also be associated with immunizations or recent surgery (96). The weakness is generally, but not always symmetric, and is associated with a loss of deep tendon reflexes. Cranial nerve involvement is not uncommon. The facial nerve is affected most frequently, in one-third (95) to one-half (96) of patients. Although paresthesias are common, objective sensory loss is minimal. Proprioception and vibratory sense may be impaired (97).

Early mortality is generally related to respiratory failure, making meticulous respiratory therapy, monitoring, and support essential. Fully 30% of patients require mechanical ventilation (98). Autonomic nervous system involvement (99) is also seen, with resulting difficulties in regulating blood pressure, heart rate and rhythm, and body temperature. Dysautonomia also results in impairment of bowel and bladder function, although complete lower motor neuron denervation, with flaccid bowel and bladder, is rarely seen.

The pathology and electrodiagnosis of CIDP is very similar to those of GBS. The main difference is in the time course of the disease. Whereas GBS usually progresses and peaks within 2 to 3 weeks, CIDP may progress for 4 weeks or more. In addition, CIDP is more often associated with underlying disease, especially systemic lupus erythematosus, Hodgkin disease, sarcoidosis, and human immunodeficiency virus (HIV) infection (95).

GBS is clearly a demyelinative process, with documented invasion of the Schwann cell basal lamina by macrophages. Secondary axonal damage may occur, and is associated with a poorer prognosis. A pure axonal form has also been described in a single case series (100), although its existence as a distinct clinical entity with its own particular pathophysiology has been disputed (101).

Acquired demyelinative neuropathies almost certainly are related to an underlying autoimmune process. A variety of autoantibodies, including those with activity against myelin-associated glycoprotein and various gangliosides, have been isolated from the sera of involved individuals. Although these immunoglobulins help to strengthen the case for an autoimmune mechanism, they are of limited diagnostic utility for a variety of reasons. The antibodies do not occur consistently in all affected patients, and when present are usually in low titers. They may also be present in normal individuals, and in a variety of other disease states (102).

Effective treatment beyond pulmonary support and general rehabilitative care is directed toward modulating the immune response. Plasma exchange is a well-established and frequently successful treatment, shortening the course of the disease and improving functional outcomes. It is most effective when initiated within 2 weeks of the onset of the disease (95). Intravenous infusion of immunoglobulin has also proved effective (103). Treatment fails to impact the progression of the neuropathy in at least 30% of patients (104).

Electrodiagnostic findings are consistent with a multifocal, demyelinative process. Prolongation of distal latencies and lengthening of conduction velocities are typical findings, although about 20% of involved patients may have normal standard motor nerve conduction velocities. The F-wave is the most sensitive nerve conduction parameter, correctly identifying 92% and 95% of patients with GBS and CIDP, respectively. F-waves may exhibit diminished persistence (i.e., the failure to produce some waves with multiple stimulations) or prolonged minimum latencies. Chronodispersion (i.e., variability between the shortest and longest latency response) may also be increased, especially in patients with CIDP (105). The F-wave is more sensitive than somatosensory evoked responses (106). Given the frequency of involvement of the seventh cranial nerve, facial nerve conduction studies may also be useful, and help to distinguish the polyneuropathy from a more diffuse, symmetric distal process. Fibrillation potentials and positive sharp waves will be present after 3 to 4 weeks in patients with axonal involvement.

About 16% of patients with GBS will be left with a degree of permanent disability. The need for mechanical ventilation is associated with a poorer outcome (107). Electrically, the amplitude of the CMAP seems to have strong predictive power. In one study (27) of 60 patients, all individuals with a CMAP amplitude of the median, ulnar, or peroneal nerve greater than 10% of the lower limit of normal regained the ability to ambulate. Conversely, amplitudes of less than 10% of the lower limits of normal were frequently associated with inability to walk after 1 year, although very low amplitudes did not guarantee a poor outcome. Thus, in counseling patients regarding expectations for recovery of ambulation, preservation of the CMAP is very encouraging, while low amplitudes increase the likelihood of residual disability. The presence of fibrillation potentials has also been associated with poorer outcomes.

Children seem to have much greater propensity for recovery. In a small series (108), 23 children were identified as having definite GBS. Of these, 9 had electrical findings consistent with a poor prognosis, using similar criteria to those listed above. However, all 9 patients recovered without residual disability.

Variable Presentation

Some diseases cause PNS involvement in patterns that are too variable to be assigned to one of the four groups described earlier.

Human Immunodeficiency Virus Infection

Infection with HIV is commonly associated with involvement of the PNS. Peripheral neuropathy occurs in at least 50% of patients with acquired immunodeficiency syndrome (AIDS) (109). A diffuse, distal, symmetric, predominantly sensory pattern is most common (110) and usually involves painful dysesthesias of the feet. However, HIV infection may produce any pattern of neurologic involvement of the PNS. In one series of 14 patients (111), 8 displayed a painful sensorimotor neuropathy, while the remaining 6 had a clinical picture consistent with either CIDP, mononeuritis multiplex, or myopathy. HIV infection may produce a syndrome that is clinically indistinguishable from GBS or CIDP, and responds equally well to plasma exchange. Of note, demyelinative neuropathies commonly occur early in the course of HIV infection and may be the presenting problem in patients with previously undiagnosed HIV infection (110).

One condition bears special mention as it is potentially treatable if detected early, and is fatal if missed. A polyradicular pattern of neurologic involvement sometimes seen in HIV-infected patients may be due to cytomegalovirus (CMV) infection (112,113). Analysis of the cerebrospinal fluid is especially helpful in establishing the diagnosis, and usually reveals a marked pleocytosis with elevated protein and low glucose levels (113). Treatment with ganciclovir may be lifesaving if initiated early, and therapy should be initiated empirically while awaiting culture results.

The role of antiviral agents should also be considered in evaluating neuropathies in patients with HIV infection, as similar neuropathic syndromes can be produced by the drugs. Didanosine (2′,3′-dideoxyinosine), a reverse transcriptase inhibitor, produced a painful distal neuropathy in 8 of 37 patients (114), while high doses of 2′,3′-dideoxycytidine (ddC) produced similar symptoms in all patients treated. Of note, azidothymidine (AZT) does not commonly cause peripheral neuropathy.

Sarcoidosis

Sarcoidosis is associated with the deposition of noninflammatory epithelioid granuloma in a variety of body tissues. The nervous system is involved in about 5% of patients (115), and the PNS is involved in 6% to 18% of those with neurosarcoidosis (116). Cranial mononeuropathy is the most frequently reported pattern of involvement of the PNS. Facial nerve involvement is most common, although any cranial nerve can be affected.

Due to the low incidence of PNS involvement, information regarding the pattern of involvement of noncranial nerves is extracted from case reports and small case series. The peripheral neuropathy of sarcoidosis may present with practically any pattern of involvement, including mononeuritis multiplex; chronic sensorimotor, motor, or sensory neuropathy; or an acute GBS-like pattern (117–119). In one series of 10 patients, a chronic-onset, generalized pattern was most common (118). Predominant neuropathology is probably axonopathic, with secondary demyelination (117–119). One histologic study suggested that local compression by a granuloma may be a factor in producing axonal degeneration (117), although this has been disputed by others (120).

CONCLUSIONS

The PNS responds to systemic disease in a limited number of ways; hence, many neuropathic conditions produce similar clinical patterns. The timely and efficient evaluation of patients with disease of the peripheral nerve requires a complete history and physical examination. Electrodiagnostic examination may help to limit the differential diagnosis. Finally, the practitioner must have a thorough knowledge of the presentation of diseases that can affect the nerve.

REFERENCES

1. Dyck PJ, Thomas PK. *Peripheral neuropathy.* Vol. 2. 3rd ed. Philadelphia: WB Saunders, 1993.
2. Dumitru D. *Electrodiagnostic medicine.* Philadelphia: Hanley & Belfus, 1995:743.
3. McLeod JG. Investigation of peripheral neuropathy. *J Neurol Neurosurg Psychiatry* 1995;58: 381–382.
4. Thomas PK, Ochoa J. Clinical features and differential diagnosis. In: Dyck PJ, Thomas PK, eds. *Peripheral neuropathy.* Vol. 2. 3rd ed. Philadelphia: WB Saunders, 1993:754–755, 759, 760–761.
5. McLeod JG. Autonomic dysfunction in peripheral nerve disorders. *Curr Opin*

Neurol Neurosurg 1992;5: 476–481.

6. McDeavitt JT, Graziani V, Kowalske KJ, Hays RM. Neuromuscular disease: rehabilitation and electrodiagnosis: 2. Nerve disease. *Arch Phys Med Rehabil* 1995;76:510–520.

7. Thrush D. Investigation of peripheral neuropathy. *Br J Hosp Med* 1992;48:13–22.

8. Donofrio PD, Albers JW. Polyneuropathy: classification by nerve conduction studies and electromyography. AAEM minimonograph #34. *Muscle Nerve* 1990;13:889–903.

9. Kimura J. *Electrodiagnosis in diseases of nerve and muscle: principles and practice.* 2nd ed. Philadelphia: FA Davis, 1989:56–57.

10. Trojaborg W, Lange DJ. Neuropathies. *Curr Opin Neurol Neurosurg* 1992;5:659–665.

11. Arezzi J, Schaumburg H, Peterson C. Rapid screening for peripheral neuropathy: a field study with the Optacon. *Neurology* 1983;33:626–629.

12. Dyck PJ. Invited review: limitations in predicting pathologic abnormality of nerves from the EMG examination. *Muscle Nerve* 1990;13:371–375.

13. Asbury AK, Gilliatt RW. *Peripheral nerve disorders.* London: Butterworths, 1984:12.

14. Schaumburg HH, Berger AR, Thomas L. *Disorders of peripheral nerves.* 2nd ed. Philadelphia: FA Davis, 1992:25–32.

15. Dyck PJ, Giannini C, Lais A. Pathologic alterations of nerves. In: Dyck PJ, Thomas PK, eds. *Peripheral neuropathy.* Vol. 1. 3rd ed. Philadelphia: WB Saunders, 1993:515–516.

16. Rappaport WD, Valente J, Hunter GC, et al. Clinical utilization and complications of sural nerve biopsy. *Am J Surg* 1993;166: 252–256.

17. Argov Z, Steiner I, Soffer D. The diagnostic yield of sural nerve biopsy in the evaluation of peripheral neuropathies. *Acta Neurol Scand* 1989;79:243–245.

18. Ross FC. Discussion on neuropathies. *Proc R Soc Med* 1960;53:51–53.

19. Prineas JW. Polyneuropathies of undetermined causes. *Acta Neurol Scand Suppl* 1970;44: 1–72.

20. Dyck PJ, Oviatt KF, Lambert EH. Intensive evaluation of referred unclassified neuropathies yields improved diagnosis. *Ach Neurol* 1981;10:222–226.

21. McLeod JG, Tuck RR, Pollard JD, et al. Chronic polyneuropathy of undetermined cause. *J Neurol Neurosurg Psychiatry* 1984;47: 530–535.

22. Konig F, Neundorfer B, Kompf D. Polyneuropathien im hoheren Lebensalter. *Dtsch Med Wochenschr* 1984;109:735–773.

23. Corvisier N, Vallat JM, Hugon J, et al. Les polyneuropathies de cause indeterminee. *Rev Neurol (Paris)* 1987;143:279–283.

24. Notermans NC, Wokke JHJ, Franssen H, et al. Chronic idiopathic polyneuropathy presenting in middle or old age: a clinical and electrophysiological study of 75 patients. *J Neurol Neurosurg Psychiatry* 1993;56: 1066–1071.

25. McLeod JG, Prineas JW, Walsh JC. The relationship of conduction velocity to pathophysiology in peripheral nerves: a study of the sural nerve in 90 patients. In: Desmedt JE, ed. *New developments in electromyography and clinical neurophysiology.* Vol. 2. Basel: S Karger, 1973:248–258.

26. Miller RG. Electrophysiologic evidence of severe distal nerve segment pathology in the Guillain-Barré syndrome. *Muscle Nerve* 1987;10:524–529.

27. Miller RG, Peterson GW, Daube JR, Albers JW. Prognostic value of electrodiagnosis in Guillain-Barré syndrome. *Muscle Nerve* 1988;11:769–774.

28. Ropper AH, Wijdicks EF, Shahani BT. Electrodiagnostic abnormalities in 113 consecutive patients with Guillain-Barré syndrome. *Arch Neurol* 1990;47:881–887.

29. Bromberg MB, Feldman EL, Albers JW. Chronic inflammatory demyelinating polyradiculoneuropathy: comparison of patients with and without an associated monoclonal gammopathy. *Neurology* 1992;42:1157–1163.

30. Rostami AM. Pathogenesis of immune-mediated neuropathies. *Pediatr Res* 1993;33(1 suppl):S90–S94.

31. Parry GJ. Motorneuropathy with multifocal conduction block. *Semin Neurol* 1993;13:269–275.

32. Olney RK. Neuropathies in connective tissue disease. AAEM minimonograph #38. *Muscle Nerve* 1992;15:531–542.

33. Raff MC, Sangalang V, Asbury AK. Ischemic mononeuropathy multiplex associated with diabetes mellitus. *Arch Neurol* 1968;18:487–499.

34. Gabreels-Festen AA, Gabreels FJ, Jennekens FG. Hereditary motor and sensory neuropathies. Present status of types, I, II and III. *Clin Neurol Neurosurg* 1993;95:93–107.

35. Ross MA. Neuropathies associated with diabetes. *Med Clin North Am* 1993;77:111–124.

36. Dyck PJ, Kratz KM, Karnes JL, et al. The prevalence by staged severity of various types of diabetic neuropathy, retinopathy, and nephropathy in a population-based cohort: the Rochester Diabetic Neuropathy study. *Neurology* 1993;43:817–824.

37. Harati Y. Frequently asked questions about diabetic peripheral neuropathies. *Neurol Clin* 1992;10:783–807.

38. Horrobin DF. The effects of gamma-linolenic acid on breast pain and diabetic neuropathy: possible non-eicosanoids mechanisms. *Prostaglandins Leukot Essent Fatty Acids* 1993;48:101–104.

39. Palumbo PJ, Elveback LR, Whisnant SP. Neurologic complications of diabetes mellitus, transient ischemic attack, stroke, and peripheral neuropathy. *Adv Neurol* 1978;19:593.

40. Pirart J. Diabetes mellitus and its degenerative complications: a prospective study of 4,400 patients observed between 1947 and 1973. *Diabetes Care* 1978;1:168.

41. Nathan DM. The pathophysiology of diabetic complications: how much does the glucose hypothesis explain? *Ann Intern Med* 1996;124(1 Pt 2):86–89.

42. Dyck PJ, Zimmerman BR, Vilen TH, et al. Nerve glucose, fructose, sorbitol, myo-inositol, and fiber degeneration and regeneration in diabetic neuropathy. *N Engl J Med* 1988;319:542–548.

43. Clark CM Jr, Lee DA. Prevention and treatment of the complications of diabetes mellitus. *N Engl J Med* 1995;332:1210–1217.

44. Said G, Goulon-Goeau C, Slama G, et al. Severe early-onset polyneuropathy in insulin-dependent diabetes mellitus: a clinical and pathological study. *N Engl J Med* 1992;326: 1257–1263.

45. Bril V, Werb MR, Greene DA, Sima AA. Single-fiber electromyography in diabetic peripheral polyneuropathy. *Muscle Nerve* 1996;19:2–9.

46. Raskin NH, Fishman RA. Neurologic disorders in renal failure. *N Engl J Med* 1976;294: 143–148.

47. Fraser CL, Arieff AL. Nervous system complications in uremia. *Ann Intern Med* 1988;109: 143–153.

48. Ropper AH. Accelerated neuropathy of renal failure. *Arch Neurol* 1993;50:536–539.

49. Yosipovitch G, Yarnitsky D, Mermelstein V, et al. Paradoxical heat sensation in uremic polyneuropathy. *Muscle Nerve* 1995;18:768–771.

50. Tattersall JE, Cramp M, Shannon M, et al. Rapid high-flux dialysis can cure uraemic peripheral neuropathy. *Nephrol Dial Transplant* 1992;7:539–540.

51. D'Amour MI, Dufresne LR, Morin C, Slaughter D. Sensory nerve conduction in chronic uraemic patients during the first 6 months of dialysis. *Can J Neurol Sci* 1984;11:269–271.

52. Konoty-Ahulu FID, Baillod R, Comty CM, et al. The effect of periodic dialysis on the peripheral neuropathy of end-stage chronic renal failure. *BMJ* 1965;2:1211–1215.

53. Blonton CF, Balzn MA, Balzan RB. Effects of renal transplantation on uremic neuropathy. *N Engl J Med* 1971;284: 1170–1175.

54. Tunbridge WMG. The epidemiology of thyroid disease. In: Ingburn SH, Bravenman LE, eds. *The thyroid.* 5th ed. Philadelphia: JB Lippincott, 1986:622–625.

55. Laycock MF. The neuromuscular effects of hypothyroidism. *Semin Neurol* 1991;11:288–294.

56. Nickel SN, Frame B. Nervous and muscular systems in myxedema. *J Chronic Dis* 1961;14:570–581.

57. Crevasse LE, Logue RB. Peripheral neuropathy in myxedema. *Ann Intern Med* 1959;50: 1433–1437.

58. Beghi E, Delodovici ML, Bloglium G, et al. Hypothyroidism and polyneuropathy. *J Neurol Neurosurg Psychiatry* 1989;52: 1420–1423.

59. Meier C, Vischoff A. Polyneuropathy in hypothyroidism. Clinical and nerve biopsy study of four cases. *J Neurol* 1977;215; 103–114.

60. Neeck G, Riedel W, Schmidt KL. Neuropathy, myopathy and destructive arthropathy in primary hypothyroidism. *J Rheumatol* 1990;17:1697–1700.

61. Dyck PJ, Lambert EH. Polyneuropathy associated with hypothyroidism. *J Neuropathol Exp Neurol* 1970;29:631–658.

62. Nemni R, Bottacchi E, Fazio R, et al. Polyneuropathy in hypothyroidism: clinical, electrophysiologic and morphologic findings in four cases. *J Neurol Neurosurg Psychiatry* 1987;50: 1454–1460.

63. Pollard JD, McLeod JG, Honnibal TGA, Verheijden MA. Hypothyroid polyneuropathy clinical, electrophysiological and nerve biopsy findings in two cases. *J Neurol Sci* 1982;53:461–471.

64. Pruthi RK, Tefferi A. Pernicious anemia revisited. *Mayo Clin Proc* 1994;69:144–150.

65. Shorvon SD, Carney MWP, Chanarin I, Reynolds EH. The neuropsychiatry of megaloblastic anemia. *BMJ* 1980;281: 1036–1038.

66. McCombe PA, McLeod JG. The peripheral neuropathy of vitamin B-12 deficiency. *J Neurol Sci* 1984;106:117–126.

67. Fine EJ, Hallett M. Neurophysiological study of subacute combined degeneration. *J Neurol Soc* 1980;45:334–336.

68. Fine EJ, Soria E, Paroski MW, et al. The neurophysiological profile of vitamin B-12 deficiency. *Muscle Nerve* 1990;13: 158–164.

69. Shevell MI, Rosenblatt DS. The neurology of cobalamin. *Can J Neurol Sci* 1992;19: 472–486.

70. Charness ME, Sigmon RP, Geenberg DA. Ethanol and the nervous system. *N Engl J Med* 1989;321:442–454.

71. Kemppainen R, Juntunen J, Hillbom M. Drinking habits and peripheral alcoholic neuropathy. *Acta Neurol Scand* 1982;65: 11–18.

72. Hillborn M, Wennberg A. Prognosis of alcoholic peripheral neuropathy. *J Neurol Neurosurg Psychiatry* 1984;47:699–703.

73. Latov N. Evaluation and treatment of patients with neuropathy and monoclonal gammopathy. *Semin Neurol* 1994;14: 118–122.

74. Gosselin S, Kyle RA, Dyck PJ. Neuropathy associated with monoclonal gammopathies of undetermined significance. *Ann Neurol* 1991;30:54–61.

75. Simmons Z, Bromberg MB, Feldman EL, Blaivas M. Polyneuropathy associated with IgA monoclonal gammopathy of undetermined significance. *Muscle Nerve* 1993;16:77–83.

76. Glass JD, Cornblath DR. Chronic inflammatory demyelinating polyneuropathy and paraproteinemic neuropathies. *Curr Opin Neurol* 1994;7:393–397.

77. Kyle RA, Dyck PJ. Neuropathy associated with the monoclonal gammopathies. In: Dyck PJ, Thomas PK, eds. *Peripheral neuropathy.* Vol. 2. 3rd ed. Philadelphia: WB Saunders, 1993:1275–1287.

78. Bosch EP, Smith BE. Peripheral neuropathies associated with monoclonal proteins. *Med Clin North Am* 1993;77:125–139.

79. Silverstein A, Doniger DE. Neurologic complications of myelomatosis. *Arch Neurol* 1963;9:534–544.

80. Haan J, Peters WG. Amyloid and peripheral nervous system disease. *Clin Neurol Neurosurg* 1994;96:1–9.

81. Nemni R, Gerosa E, Piccolo G, Merlini G. Neuropathies associated with monoclonal gammopathies. *Haematologica* 1994;79:557–566.

82. Kyle RA. Monoclonal gammopathy of undetermined significance: natural history in 241 cases. *Am J Med* 1978;64:814–826.

83. Puechal Y, Said G, Hilliquin P, et al. Peripheral neuropathy with necrotizing vasculitis in rheumatoid arthritis. A clinicopathologic and prognostic study of thirty-two patients. *Arthritis Rheum* 1995;38:618–629.

84. Nishino H, Rubino FA, DeRemee RA, et al. Neurological involvement in Wegener's granulomatosis: an analysis of 324 consecutive patients at the Mayo Clinic. *Ann Neurol* 1993;33:4–9.

85. Kissel JT. Vasculitis of the peripheral nervous system. *Semin Neurol* 1994;14:361–369.

86. Mellgren SI, Conn DL, Stevens JC, Dyck PJ. Peripheral neuropathy in primary Sjögren's syndrome. *Neurology* 1989;39: 390–394.

87. Parry GJ, Brown MJ. Selective fiber vulnerability in acute ischemic neuropathy. *Ann Neurol* 1982;11:147–154.

88. Kissel JT, Mendell JR. Vasculitic neuropathy. *Neurol Clin* 1992; 10:761–781.

89. Bouche P, Gherardi R, Cathala HP, et al. Peroneal muscular atrophy. Part 1. Clinical and electrophysiological study. *J Neurol Sci* 1983;61:389–399.

90. Nicholson GA. Penetrance of the hereditary motor and sensory neuropathy Ia mutation: assessment by nerve conduction studies. *Neurology* 1991;41: 547–552.

91. Benstead TJ, Kuntz NL, Miller RG, Daube JR. The electrophysiologic profile of Dejerine-Sottas disease (HMSN III). *Muscle Nerve* 1990;13:586–592.

92. Harding AE. From the syndrome of Charcot, Marie and Tooth to disorders of peripheral myelin proteins. *Brain* 1995;118(Pt 3):809–818.

93. Ouvrier RA, Nicholson GA. Advances in the genetics of hereditary hypertrophic neuropathy in childhood. *Brain Dev* 1995;17(suppl):31–38.

94. Ionasescu VV. Charcot-Marie-Tooth neuropathies: from clinical description to molecular genetics. *Muscle Nerve* 1995;18: 267–275.

95. Ropper AH. The Guillain-Barré syndrome. *N Engl J Med* 1992;326:1130–1136.

96. Albers JW. Guillain-Barré syndrome. AAEE case report #4. *Muscle Nerve* 1989;12: 705–711.

97. Kanter ME, Nori SL. Sensory Guillain-Barré syndrome. *Arch Phys Med Rehabil* 1995;76: 882–883.

98. Anderson T, Siden A. A clinical study of the Guillain-Barré syndrome. *Acta Neurol Scand* 1982;66:316–317.

99. Tuck RR, McLeod JF. Autonomic dysfunction in Guillain-Barré syndrome. *J Neurol Neurosurg Psychiatry* 1981;44:983–990.

100. Feasby TE, Gilber JJ, Brown WF, et al. An acute axonal form of Guillain-Barré polyneuropathy. *Brain* 1986;109:115–126.

101. Cros D, Triggs WJ. There are no neurophysiologic features characteristic of "axonal" Guillain-Barré syndrome. *Muscle Nerve* 1994; 17:675–677.

102. Larner AJ. Recent advances in the understanding of the immunological basis of peripheral neuropathies. *Br J Clin Pract* 1993;47:262–265.

103. Van de Meche FGA, Schmitz PIM. The Dutch Guillain-Barré study group: a randomized trial comparing intravenous immune globulin and plasma exchange in Guillain-Barré syndrome. *N Engl J Med* 1992; 326:1123–1129.

104. Steck AJ. Inflammatory neuropathy: pathogenesis and clinical features. *Curr Opin Neurol Neurosurg* 1992;5:633–637.

105. Fraser JL, Olney RK. The relative diagnostic sensitivity of different F-wave parameters in various polyneuropathies. *Muscle Nerve* 1992;15:912–918.

106. Olney RK, Aminoff MJ. Electrodiagnostic features of the Guillain-Barré syndrome: the relative sensitivity of different techniques. *Neurology* 1990;40(3 Pt 1):471–475.

107. Winer JB, Greenwood RJ, Hughes RAC, et al. Prognosis in Guillain-Barré syndrome. *Lancet* 1;1985:1202–1203.

108. Bradshaw DY, Jones HR Jr. Guillain-Barré syndrome in children: clinical course, electrodiagnosis, and prognosis. *Muscle Nerve* 1992;15:500–506.

109. Comi G, Medaglini S, Galardi G, et al. Prognosis value of the nervous system involvement in HIV patients. *Acta Neurol Napoli* 1990;12:24–27.

110. Simpson DM, Wolfe DE. Neuromuscular complaints of HIV infection and its treatment. *AIDS* 1991;5:917–926.

111. Lange DJ, Britton CB, Younger DS, Hays AP. The neuromuscular manifestations of human immunodeficiency virus infections. *Arch Neurol* 1988;45:1084–1088.

112. de Gans J, Portegies P, Tiessers G, et al. Therapy for cytomegalovirus polyradiculopathy in patients with AIDS. Treatment with ganciclovir. *AIDS* 1990;4:421–425.

113. Miller RG, Storey JR, Greco CM. Ganciclovir in the treatment of progressive AIDS-related polyradiculopathy. *Neurology* 1990;40:569–574.

114. Lambert JS, Seidlin M, Reichmann RL, et al. 2′,3′-Dideoxyinosine (ddI) in patients with the acquired immunodeficiency syndrome of AIDS related complex—a phase I trial. *N Engl J Med* 1990;332:1333–1340.

115. Matthews WB. Sarcoid neuropathy. In: Dyck PJ, Thomas PK, eds. *Peripheral neuropathy*. Vol. 2. 3rd ed. Philadelphia: WB Saunders, 1993:1418–1423.

116. Scott TF. Neurosarcoidosis: progress and clinical aspects. *Neurology* 1993;43:8–12.

117. Gainsborough N, Hall SM, Hughes RA, Leibowitz S. Sarcoid neuropathy. *J Neurol* 1991;238:177–180.

118. Zuniga G, Ropper AH, Frank J. Sarcoid peripheral neuropathy. *Neurology* 1991;41:1558–1561.

119. Scott TS, Brillman J, Gross JA. Sarcoidosis of the peripheral nervous system. *Neurol Res* 1993;15:389–390.

120. Gallassi G, Gerbertoni M, Marcini A, et al. Sarcoidosis of the peripheral nerve: clinical, electrophysiological, and histologic study of two cases. *Eur Neurol* 1984;23:459–464.

Chapter 89

Neuromuscular Diseases

Andrew E. Kirsteins
Kat Kolaski

The neuromuscular diseases encompass a wide variety of illnesses that affect cells in the central nervous system (CNS), peripheral nervous system, and muscle. Neuromuscular diseases have been classified by location (e.g., neuromuscular junction, anterior horn cell), etiology (e.g., inflammatory, hereditary), clinical signs and symptoms (e.g., proximal weakness, bulbar signs), as well as other methods. The various modes of disease classification may be confusing at times and not always helpful from a clinical standpoint.

In this chapter, we narrow our focus to diseases affecting the α motor neuron, the neuromuscular junction, and the muscle itself. The one exception to this rule is amyotrophic lateral sclerosis (ALS), which may involve the cranial nerves and upper motor neurons. These diseases all have weakness, but not sensory changes. We discuss diseases that cannot be cured at this time, but that lend themselves to treatment via the physiatric approach. While we have included a variety of neuromuscular diseases, the text emphasizes the more common disorders. Keeping in line with World Health Organization definitions, we focus on disabilities, handicaps, and their underlying impairments rather than on the pathophysiology of the disease (1). Because ventilatory management is covered in another chapter, we do not address this. Similarly, diseases of peripheral nerves are covered in other chapters. The following chapter is organized by chronology of usual onset, that is, infancy, childhood, adolescence, and adulthood. This is to aid the reader in quick reference (Table 89-1).

ARTHROGRYPOSIS MULTIPLEX CONGENITA PRESENTATION: BIRTH OR EARLY INFANCY TYPE: ANTERIOR HORN CELL DISEASE

Classification, Incidence, and Clinical Features

Arthrogryposis multiplex congenita (AMC) is not a specific diagnosis but rather a general descriptive term for infants born with multiple joint contractures. The incidence is 1 in 3000 to 4000 live births (2). An exact etiology is unknown, but it is speculated that a congenital or acquired defect occurs in utero during the first trimester. This leads to the common pathogenesis of decreased intrauterine fetal movements that result in the abnormal development of joints and the formation of contractures (3). Various etiologic agents including chromosomal defects, viral or bacterial infection, chemical or drug agents, and environmental factors have been implicated (4). Many different congenital syndromes have been associated with AMC (5).

In some cases, the lesions that cause limitation of fetal movement in utero are related to an abnormal intrauterine environment (6) or may be the direct result of abnormal connective tissues or joints (3). Myopathic or neuropathic lesions that cause weakness in early fetal life may lead to decreased fetal movements and AMC. In a prospective study, Banker (7) classified AMC into either neuropathic or myopathic forms, based on pathologic and muscle biopsy data. The neurogenic type accounts for more than 90% of cases, the majority being related to CNS disorders and degeneration of the anterior horn cells,

Table 89-1: Neuromuscular Diseases				
	Birth–Early Infancy	Late Infancy–Early Childhood	Late Childhood–Adolescence	Adulthood
Anterior horn cell	Arthrogryposis multiplex congenita SMA type I	SMA type II	SMA type III	Amyotrophic lateral sclerosis SMA type IV
Neuromuscular junction	Congenital myasthenia gravis Transient neonatal myasthenia gravis Persistent neonatal myasthenia gravis Infantile botulism	—	Juvenile myasthenia gravis	Myasthenia gravis
Muscle	Central core disease Congenital muscular dystrophy Congenital myotonic dystrophy Glycogenoses	Duchenne muscular dystrophy Paramyotonia congenita Myotonia congenita Hyperkalemic periodic paralysis Mitochondrial myopathy Dermatomyositis	Hypokalemic periodic paralysis Limb girdle dystrophy Facioscapulohumeral dystrophy Emery-Dreifuss dystrophy Becker muscular dystrophy	Myotonic dystrophy Polymyositis/ dermatomyositis Inclusion body myositis Oculopharyngeal dystrophy Distal myopathy/distal muscular dystrophy

SMA = spinal muscular atrophy.

although more distal components of the peripheral nervous system may be responsible (8). The resultant syndromes associated with these neuropathic lesions are nonhereditary (9).

The recognized syndromes of multiple congenital contractures can be categorized into three groups: those with primarily limb involvement, those involving the limbs plus other body areas, and those with limb plus CNS involvement (10). The description of AMC is applied based on the typical clinical features. In addition to three or more, usually symmetric, joint contractures at birth, there is decreased or absent joint motion actively and passively; absent or atrophic muscle with shapeless, cylindrical limbs; absence of normal skin creases with dimpling of the skin; and normal sensation (11). The most common syndrome affects the limbs only and is referred to as "classic arthrogryposis" or amyoplasia (12). These infants are born with a typical positioning of the limbs giving them a "wooden doll"–like appearance (13). In the upper extremities, there is internal rotation of the shoulders, fixed extended elbows, and flexed wrists in ulnar deviation. In the lower extremities, the hips are flexed, externally rotated, and abducted, and there are severe equinovarus deformities of the feet. Amyoplasia is often referred to as AMC but it is distinct from the arthrogryposis seen in association with other syndromes (14).

AMC is nonprogressive, and the prognosis is good for those who survive the first 2 years of life (15,16). Pulmonary hypoplasia is the most common cause of death in children with AMC (7). In general, those with limb involvement only do well and those with extra-axial or CNS involvement tend to do worse.

Weakness

Weakness in AMC involves the limbs proximally and distally to varying degrees, and there is one form with distal involvement only. Weakness is often difficult to determine given the immobility of the major joints, but in general is moderate to severe, with significant associated atrophy. In most patients both the upper and lower extremities are involved, with relatively greater involvement of the lower extremities (16).

Self-Care

The ability to self-feed depends on hand function and elbow range of motion. Some children with AMC will use other body parts, such as their feet or mouth, to feed themselves and other fine motor skills requiring the manipulation of an object (17,18). If there is adequate range of motion but inadequate strength, the child may learn to support the arm on a leg or a table to assist in bringing the hand to the mouth. The height of the table or desktop may need to be adjusted so that the child can maneuver items by using a mouthstick or a wrist aid. Children with AMC, much like those with congenital limb deficiencies, will not use adaptive equipment if they can devise a compensatory strategy.

Mobility and Positioning

Positioning options are limited for infants with AMC. The infant may be assisted with positioning by towel rolls, wedges, and splinting. Affected infants learn to roll or scoot on their buttocks as their primary means of floor mobility. Standing should be facilitated around the ages of 6 months to 1 year, using a standing frame and splinting at the knee or ankle to address limitations in range of motion and strength. A standing program is beneficial for stretching and encourages children toward independent mobility, which becomes an important issue for the preschooler (18).

Because of intrinsic muscle weakness or weakness secondary to corrective orthopedic surgery, most children with AMC learn to ambulate with hip-knee-ankle-foot orthoses (HKAFOs) (18,19). A pelvic band may be necessary if there is significant hip weakness. Children with knee extension contractures tend to require less bracing than do those with knee flexion contractures. In a series of severely affected AMC patients, functional ambulation required a hip range to within 30 degrees of full extension and knee motion to within 20 degrees of full extension. Hip extensor strength of grade 4 and quadriceps strength of grade 3 were required for ambulation without orthotics or assistive devices (20), pointing out that arthrogrypotic children learning to walk may be limited in their independence if they do not have adequate strength or range of motion to manipulate an assistive device. Alternative modes of mobility may allow the children to participate more fully and efficiently in school and socially. Power mobility can be introduced to these children as early as age 4 or 5 years (21).

Contractures

The contractures of AMC can be in various directions, and the typically involved joints include, in decreasing order of incidence, the foot, knee, elbow, hip, hand, wrist, and shoulder (16,22). The contractures are characterized by the rigidity of the periarticular structures and are difficult to reduce manually. With growth, since these structures are fixed, contractures tend to progress (23).

Stretching is an essential part of the life of a child with AMC, especially during the first 2 years (14). A home program of stretching three to five times per day, usually conveniently done during diaper changes, dressing, or bathing times, is recommended (18). Splints or serial casts are used extensively to maintain a prolonged stretch in AMC patients (24). Efforts to maintain range of motion with splinting and stretching are interspersed with properly chosen and sequenced orthopedic procedures. Lower-extremity deformities are managed before the upper extremities, and surgeries are usually completed before the child is ready to walk (23).

Equinovarus deformities occur in up to 85% of patients (16) and the limb should be casted immediately after birth. Clubfoot surgery, most commonly a posteromediolateral release, is usually performed around the age of 1 year when the infant with AMC is interested in standing and walking (25,26). The goal is a plantigrade, shoeable, ambulatory foot. Recurrent deformities are common and require long-term bracing with ankle-foot orthoses (AFOs). Knee flexion contractures should be addressed early, with stretching and splinting beginning at the ages of 3 to 4 months. Flexion contractures of the knees are more common than extension contractures and usually require surgical correction with a radical posterior release (13,27). Hip deformities are usually flexion contractures with or without dislocations and tend to respond to conservative management. Open reduction is usually done for a unilateral dislocation or if it causes extreme stiffness and interferes with seating (28).

Splinting and surgery of the upper extremities should be done to improve function, so careful consideration needs to be given to the effect of a biomechanical change at a particular joint. The hand is the key to the decision regarding treatment of the upper extremity in AMC and determines what, if any, treatment is required at the elbow or shoulder (29). A typical goal is the ability to have one hand reach the perineum and one hand reach the mouth (18). Digit and thumb deformities should not be treated surgically if the hand has some functional grasp. Wrist splints are provided after the age of 3 months so that the infant can integrate the normal physiologic grasp reflex. Deformities of the wrist are addressed by fusion in an optimal position, a procedure that is done at maturity. Elbow flexion contractures are usually treated nonsurgically, but the more common elbow extension contractures can be managed surgically with a variety of procedures, usually when the child is more ambulatory and cooperative. Derotation osteotomy of the shoulder may achieve a more functional and biomechanical shoulder position (i.e., for crutch walking) (16,30).

Scoliosis

Scoliosis occurs commonly with AMC, affecting approximately 10% to 30% of patients (22,31,32). The most frequently reported pattern is the neuromuscular scoliosis, or long C curve, but congenital scoliosis is also seen. Scoliosis in AMC is present at birth or arises in the first decade of life and is usually associated with hip deformities and pelvic obliquity. Scoliosis frequently progresses and can be associated with considerable functional disability (20,31). Surgical fusion, typically fusion to the sacrum and posterior instrumentation, is recommended if the curve progresses to 50 degrees.

Psychosocial Issues

Early on in the affected child's development, caregivers should be educated about AMC and taught the appropriate exercise program. A successful splinting and exercise program depends on family participation. These children usually have normal to above average intelligence, but severe psychomotor delay may negatively influence social and emotional development (33). Children with AMC need to have developmental stimulation at an early age and therapists can work with families to adapt age-appropriate toys and activities. Children with AMC should be included in mainstream educational settings with the appropriate adaptations.

There is considerable dependence on the family; thus, it is important for the rehabilitation focus to shift to social and prevocational pursuits in adolescence (18). Higher education, along with computer skills, can allow adults with AMC to be competitive in the job market. Adapted driving and computer-based technology can further increase independence. Developmental guidance should continue into adulthood (33). In a study of adults with AMC, Carlson et al (16) found that independence with activities of daily living (ADLs) and mobility was not related to degree of physical impairment, but more to personality, education, and overall coping skills. This points out the importance of caregivers in providing encouragement for independence throughout the child's maturation.

SEVERE SPINAL MUSCULAR ATROPHY PRESENTATION: BIRTH OR EARLY INFANCY TYPE: ANTERIOR HORN CELL DISEASE

Classification, Incidence, and Clinical Features

The spinal muscular atrophies (SMAs) are the second most common autosomal recessive disease after cystic fibrosis (34,35). They are caused by selective destruction of the anterior horn cells of the spinal cord, and occasionally affect the motor nuclei of the brain stem. The SMAs are transmitted via an autosomal recessive trait that has been specifically mapped to chromosome 5q (36,37). The overall incidence of SMA has been reported as 1.4 new cases per million (38), and they represent the most common neuromuscular disorder affecting infants and children (39). The three well-recognized forms of the disease are commonly referred to as types I, II, and III.

The SMAs were originally separated into the different types on the basis of age at onset (40–42). Earlier age at onset was correlated with a worse prognosis. Currently, age at onset is regarded as an unreliable criterion for classification, given it is often difficult to define. In practical terms, prognosis is more related to clinical severity, and in particular to the extent of respiratory compromise (43–45). However, the correlation between the age at onset and severity is still generally accepted, although there are many exceptions. Dubowitz (46) makes the important point that there are not clear divisions between types, and that the "chaos" in classification is the result of a continuum of cases of SMA. The most recent clinical classification system (Table 89-2) was proposed by an international consortium and retains the three types of SMA, described by age at onset and two other criteria—course or maximal functional status, and age at death (47).

The natural course of the SMAs has traditionally

Table 89-2: Classification of Spinal Muscular Atrophy

Designation	Symptom (mo)	Course	Death (yr)
I (severe)	0–6	Never sit	< 2
II (intermediate)	< 18	Never stand	> 2
III (mild)	> 18	Stands alone	Adult

Source: Reprinted from *Neuromuscular disorders*, Vol 1, Munsat T; Workshop Report: International SMA Collaboration, page 81, 1991, with permission from Elsevier Science, Oxford, England.

been viewed as progressive (40,48,49), although some authors described a tendency for the SMAs to have a more benign course (50–55), especially after long periods of non-progression (56,57). Some investigators suggested that the congenital SMAs may not be a "degenerative" disease, but an inherited fetal defect of the anterior horn cell that has variable expression in onset and severity (58). This view, which is compatible with recent molecular genetic findings (59), explains the wide variation in clinical phenotypes, but is still not proved.

Severe SMA, also known as SMA type I or Werdnig-Hoffmann disease, accounts for 27.50% of all SMA cases (60,61). The incidence of type I is 1 per 15,000 to 1 per 20,000 live newborns and is higher in inbred communities (35,62,63). SMA type I is the most common inheritable cause of infant mortality (64). Some earlier investigators speculated that type I SMA was a unique disease entity as compared to types II and III, the more benign forms of SMA (40,65,66). However, recent advances in molecular genetics conclusively showed genetic homogeneity among the different forms, suggesting that different mutations—and not different alleles—at the same locus are responsible for the clinical heterogeneity (36,37,67–69). The gene has been identified and has been termed the *survival motor neuron (SMN) gene* (60). The SMN gene was found to be absent or truncated in nearly all types of SMA, with significant deletions being more commonly associated with the type I form (70).

Infants with type I SMA are affected by the disease in utero or during the first 6 months of life. The natural history of type I SMA is characterized by a failure to achieve any early motor milestones, and in functional terms comprises those who never sit alone (49,71,72). There is some disagreement among sources with regard to survival time that may relate to the large overlap among types and disagreements with regard to terminology. The majority of references on the infantile form of the disease report a markedly shortened life span, at most 3 to 4 years, with an average time of death at around 6 to 8 months (73–75). Some authors divided type I SMA into acute and chronic forms, with the recognition that many patients have onset at birth with similar clinical manifestations, but there is prolonged survival in the chronic SMA patients (48,50,52,53). In the most recent clinical classification schema (see Table 89-2), the age at death for type I SMA is defined rather loosely as "usually less than 2 years" (47).

Normal serum levels of muscle enzymes differentiate SMA from the primary myopathies. Examination of muscle biopsy specimens demonstrates groups of small, rounded, atrophic type I and II fibers intermingled with groups of hypertrophied, mainly type I, fibers. There are no degenerative muscle fiber changes and the nuclei are usually in the normal, peripheral position (76,77). Diminished muscle bulk and occasional "myopathic" features can make both the electromyographic (EMG) and muscle biopsy findings difficult to interpret (78–80).

Pulmonary toilet is a main focus of care in infants with SMA type I. They often require assisted ventilation, supplemental oxygen, or tracheostomy. Frequent suctioning, assisted coughing, and postural drainage can improve secretion management. This is especially important prior to and after feeding, as bulbar weakness increases the risk of aspiration of food and upper-airway secretions. Supported sitting can help with postural drainage, but external supports are poorly tolerated (see below under Mobility and Positioning). Respiratory infections require aggressive antibiotic treatment and supplemental oxygenation. The issue of assisted ventilation needs to be discussed early in the course of the disease. In the small series of Wang et al (81), those who became ventilator dependent in infancy had a high level of associated morbidity and required institutionalization.

The major role of rehabilitation for children with SMA type I has been to maximize the parent-child relationship and minimize physical discomfort. In addition, rehabilitation of these infants can potentially enhance the outcome of those who go on to have a less severe course. However, while there are reports of SMA type I children surviving long term (52,57), the prognosis should not be unrealistically optimistic, given the more typical trend for limited function and survival (82,83).

Weakness

There is often a history of relative lack of movement in utero, and some affected infants will have arthrogrypotic limbs. All of these infants are born floppy and on examination have profound weakness of the more proximal muscles of the extremities and the trunk. The lower limbs tend to be affected earlier and more severely than the upper limbs (73). These infants have a characteristic, gravity-dependent posture in a supine position, with the lower extremities externally rotated, abducted, and flexed at the hips and knees in a "frog leg" position, and the upper extremities partially abducted at the shoulders with flexion at the elbows in a "jug handle" position (84). There may be a pectus excavatum deformity of the chest because of intercostal muscle weakness. During inspiration, the unaffected diaphragm descends, and the abdomen protrudes, with paradoxical thoracic depression and intercostal space retraction. There is some movement of the hands and feet. There is a weak cry. The infants may make some whimpering sounds, but do not develop speech. There is a full head lag when the infant is pulled to sit up, as the neck flexors cannot resist gravity. With advanced disease, the head remains turned to one side because of weakness of the neck rotators. Despite their lack of movement, these infants typically appear bright and inquisitive as they respond appropriately with their eyes and faces. There are often fasciculations of the tongue (50,85), which if present can be used to separate SMA from a form of muscular dystrophy.

Feeding

Most infants with SMA type I require total or supplemental feeding via a nasogastric tube or gastrostomy. Tube feedings should be continuous rather than by bolus to prevent gastric distention, which can limit diaphragmatic excursion. An effective bowel program for regular and complete emptying should also be instituted for the same reason (86). A feeding program can be pursued if safe swallowing can be documented by a modified barium swallow study and if the infant's pulmonary status is stable. The airway should be suctioned prior to feeding. Fatigue and thus risk of aspiration can be decreased with special feeding techniques. Frequent, small feedings and jaw support with the infant in the semireclined position are recommended, along with the use of nipples with large openings that do not emit food without a suck (75).

Mobility and Positioning

Infants with SMA type I are limp and immobile and have no head control. Most early developmental postures are not possible and most standard seating devices are inadequate. Lying prone in particular is not well tolerated. These infants should be positioned supine or on their side, with their heads elevated with foam wedges, in an appropriate seating device fashioned from various plastics, foam rubber, or urethane foam (87). Spinal orthoses for sitting are not well tolerated because of increased abdominal pressure causing elevation of the diaphragm and skin problems due to decreased muscle bulk (88). Positioning with rolled towels or bolsters can be used to allow the hands to come together in the midline and to reach from the body. This gives infants the opportunity for exploration of and stimulation by lightweight toys or rattles that can be placed close to the hands or attached to the wrists with Velcro straps (89). The lower extremities should be supported in such a way as to prevent external rotation and abduction. Placing the infant in a hammock can allow for some independent movement with minimal muscular effort. Limited strengthening for improved head and trunk control can be performed against gravity on bolsters and wedges (89). Parents should be taught to move the children around as much as possible to give them some of the motor experiences they cannot gain on their own.

Contractures

Range of motion exercises should be carried out to maintain flexibility and comfort. Common deformities, such as contractures of the hip, knee, and elbow flexors, hip abductors, ankle plantarflexors, and positional torticollis, can be prevented by proper positioning and range of motion exercise (86,87,89).

Scoliosis

Infants with SMA type I should be monitored for spinal alignment in various positions and sitting devices. In children with SMA who survive infancy, scoliosis is common, with early onset and continuous progression (74), and is discussed later (see Scoliosis section under Intermediate Spinal Muscular Atrophy).

Psychosocial Issues

Supportive counseling and education for the families (parents and siblings) of these infants are extremely important. Decisions regarding assisted ventilation and resuscitation directives should be explored early on. As much as possible, the family members are encouraged to be involved in every aspect of the child's care so they can have the opportunity for bonding. Likewise, the families are encouraged to involve these babies in activities of family life as much as possible. Pediatric hospice services and home health nursing are good resources for these families if available, given the extremely high level of care required by affected infants. Contemporary genetic advances will greatly facilitate genetic counseling and allow a more precise estimation of recurrence risks and eventually allow for prenatal diagnosis (59).

CONGENITAL MYASTHENIA GRAVIS PRESENTATION: BIRTH OR EARLY INFANCY TYPE: NEUROMUSCULAR JUNCTION DISEASE

The congenital myasthenias are genetically transmitted and may result from a variety of defects in the neuromuscular junction that impair neuromuscular transmission directly or by secondary derangements (90). Most are transmitted by an autosomal recessive mechanism. Most congenital myasthenias are evident in the neonatal period or early infancy, although some patients do not present clinically until later childhood (91). The diagnosis is suspected clinically and by the absence of maternal disease as well as the absence of circulating anticholinesterase antibody. Precise characterization may require a comprehensive investigation including routine and single-fiber EMG and repetitive nerve stimulation studies, biopsy, and molecular genetic studies (92). These disorders respond variably to acetylcholinesterase inhibitors (44). Although there is considerable variability in clinical manifestations, children with postsynaptic defects are affected to a lesser degree than those with presynaptic defects and are more likely to benefit from anticholinesterase medications (93). Prednisone and thymectomy are not effective (92).

Ophthalmoplegia and facial and bulbar weakness may be present at birth or in the neonatal period, resulting in poor suck, impaired swallowing, weak cry, and respiratory problems. In some forms, episodic crises can be precipitated by fever, excitement, or vomiting and cause an acute exacerbation of symptoms. In other forms, the manifestations are less focal and occur later, with delayed motor development and generalized muscle weakness. There is a wide range of disability, and chronic rehabilitation issues are similar to those seen in classic adult myasthenia gravis (94).

TRANSIENT AND PERSISTENT NEONATAL MYASTHENIA PRESENTATION: BIRTH OR EARLY INFANCY TYPE: NEUROMUSCULAR JUNCTION DISEASES

Neonatal myasthenia may be a transient disorder of the newborn that occurs in 10% of offspring of mothers with myasthenia gravis (95). It is caused by the passive placental transfer of antibodies to the acetylcholine receptor from mother to infant and thus the disease is self-limited since the production of anticholinesterase antibodies does not occur in the infant. The degree of maternal involvement does not predict the severity of the neonatal condition (96). Clinical presentation may include feeding difficulty, generalized weakness and hypotonia, respiratory difficulties, weak cry, and facial weakness. Symptoms usually appear 4 to 24 hours after birth and may last up to 1 month, with the maternal antibodies and residual receptor defect persisting up to 2 to 3 months (91). Diagnosis is made by the demonstration of decrements on repetitive nerve stimulation or clinically by a prompt response to the administration of edrophonium. Care is supportive, and may involve ventilatory assistance and nasogastric feeding. Anticholinesterase medications may be required for 4 to 6 weeks or not at all if the infant does not have compromised swallowing or respiratory function. Maternal myasthenia gravis has been associated with recurrent cases of AMC and often results in fetal or neonatal death (97,98).

Neonatal myasthenia may also occur in the offspring of uninvolved mothers and be persistent as the result of an acquired autoimmune defect. Symptoms present in the first few days of life and are similar to those seen with transient myasthenia. The facial weakness and swallowing problems usually respond well to anticholinesterase therapy as with the transient form, but immunosuppressive therapy is sometimes required (91). In some cases, symptoms may be more subtle and develop insidiously, leading to a diagnosis in later childhood. Symptoms become more pronounced with disease progression, and chronic rehabilitation issues are similar to those for classic adult myasthenia gravis.

INFANTILE BOTULISM PRESENTATION: BIRTH OR EARLY INFANCY TYPE: NEUROMUSCULAR JUNCTION DISEASE

Incidence, Classification, and Clinical Features

Infantile botulism is seen exclusively in infants less than 1 year old, with the great majority of cases occurring in the first 4 months of life. Most cases have been diagnosed and reported in the United States (87,99). There is a heavier concentration of the disease in California, Utah, and Pennsylvania, a fact that has been related to the high levels of *Clostridium botulinum* spores in the soil (100). The spores are ingested and colonize the bowel where the toxin is synthesized and absorbed, causing irreversible blockade of the cholinergic synapses in the cranial, spinal, and peripheral nerves.

Honey and corn syrup have been implicated as offending foods, but a case-control study indicated that clearly defined food exposures account for a minority of cases (101). Other associated factors associated with infantile botulism are breast-feeding and decreased frequency of bowel movements. This suggests that preexisting host factors related to the intestinal flora or bowel motility may play a role in etiology (102).

The range of severity of infantile botulism is from asymptomatic carriers to varying degrees of paralysis to sudden death (100). In a case series review, the most common signs at presentation were weakness or floppiness, poor feeding, constipation, and lethargy (102,103). The child is usually afebrile. The diagnosis may be established by EMG (92) and later confirmed with identification of toxin and organisms in the stool (104).

Initial rapidly progressive weakness followed by some waxing and waning is the typical clinical course. Although the disease process is self-limited, affected infants require vigorous supportive care and the prognosis is excellent if intensive care facilities are available. In a case series review, the majority were intubated and mechanically ventilated, primarily for airway protection (103). An equine antitoxin is available, but has a high risk of anaphylaxis. Antibodies are not used for primary disease because of the concern that more toxin will be released from the gut, but are used to treat secondary infections (102).

Weakness

In infantile botulism, there is usually a predictable pattern of progressive weakness, starting with bulbar paralysis with facial weakness, ptosis, and decreased gag reflex (105). Impairment of the extraocular muscles and progression to the other cranial nerves then occur. The child goes on within a day or so to develop generalized weakness and hypotonia, and finally diaphragmatic weakness; autonomic instability may also develop. The diagnosis should be considered when an infant presents with acute hypotonia and reflexia (102). Recovery requires the regeneration of motor end-plates. Fortunately, most affected infants recover spontaneously after 1 to 5 months of illness (106).

Feeding

Nasogastric tubes are usually needed. With recovery, a modified barium swallow study should be performed to guide the safe transition to oral feeding.

Contractures

Affected infants typically have prolonged hospitalization, for an average of 104 days (103). Daily passive range of motion exercises and proper positioning will help to prevent any contractures developing as a result of severe weakness and the effects of gravity, particularly at the ankle joints. An air mattress and frequent repositioning will decrease the likelihood of skin breakdown, which commonly occurs in the occiput in this age group.

Mobility

With the return of muscle strength, these infants usually do not require any formal therapy interventions and are typically able to resume their developmental progress.

CONGENITAL MYOPATHIES PRESENTATION: BIRTH OR EARLY INFANCY TYPE: MYOPATHY

Classification, Incidence, and Clinical Features

These myopathies are inherited muscle disorders characterized by specific structural abnormalities of muscle. They tend to present in a similar, nonspecific way and there is also considerable overlap clinically with some of the metabolic myopathies (44). The definitive diagnosis is made with muscle biopsy. The different congenital myopathies also have some distinguishing, associated clinical features that can aid in diagnosis.

Central core disease is an autosomal dominant condition with variable penetrance carried on chromosome 19 (107). Its name is related to the pathology seen in the type I myofibrils, which contain a central core region that is deficient in mitochondria and the enzymes for oxidative metabolism (108). Affected infants have hypotonia and proximal weakness leading to delayed motor milestones. A typical pattern of mild to moderate weakness of the proximal muscles and face is usually apparent by ages 5 to 10 years (109,110). There is minimal muscle atrophy, but there may be associated skeletal deformities, including kyphoscoliosis, pes cavus, and congenital hip dislocation. The course is nonprogressive without increased mortality, although affected individuals are at risk for malignant hyperthermia (111,112).

Nemaline myopathy is an autosomal dominant condition that is named for the rod or thread-like structures that are found in muscle biopsy specimens (113). These nemaline bodies are believed to be a component of the sarcomere's Z band and can be seen in other myopathies and anterior horn cell diseases (114,115). There are several reported clinical presentations with earlier and later onsets (116). In the severe neonatal form, there is generalized along with bulbar weakness, and a high rate of pulmonary morbidity in the first year of life (117). The more common presentation is the floppy infant with proximal weakness and myopathic facies who may have difficulty feeding (44). There is typically an elongated face, open mouth, and high-arched, narrow palate. The weakness is relatively static or slowly progressive. Muscle atrophy is prominent and out of proportion to weakness (118). Skeletal deformities such as kyphosis, scoliosis, and pes cavus are frequently seen.

Myotubular myopathy is most often inherited as an autosomal recessive condition and can present at birth or in later childhood (119). Muscle biopsy evaluation reveals small type I muscle fiber cells that resemble the embryonic or myotube form of muscle (120). The fibers have centrally positioned nuclei, so this myopathy is also known as *centronuclear myopathy* (121). Affected infants are floppy, and severely weak and typically have significant respiratory compromise (122), which is more common in the X-linked recessive form of the disease (123). These infants have myopathic facies, a weak cry and suck, and extraocular muscle involvement with ptosis. Dysmorphic features such as elongated thin faces and high-arched palates are often present (115). Affected children tend to appear frail, with prominent muscle atrophy, which may be very obvious in the shoulder girdle. The disease tends to be slowly progressive up until around adolescence (124).

Congenital fiber-type disproportion is an autosomal recessive condition characterized by a reduction in the number and size of type I fibers (115). This muscle pathology can result in a variety of clinical conditions. A more severe form in infants has been recognized, with extremity, facial, and bulbar weakness that persists if the infant survives the neonatal period. The more typical presentation is that of the floppy infant with proximal weakness that tends to improve after the age of 2 years (44). Contractures and dysmorphic facial features can be seen along with a variety of orthopedic conditions.

Respiratory management, usually involving mechanical ventilation, is the major issue in the infants with congenital myopathy with a severe neonatal presentation. Infants with myotubular myopathy typically present with respiratory compromise, and later-onset problems such as nocturnal hypoventilation have been associated with nemaline rod myopathy (44). However, all the infants and children affected by weakness from congenital myopathy are susceptible to the problems of respiratory insufficiency. A preventative program including breathing exercises, postural drainage, and chest physical therapy should be pursued, especially in the context of respiratory infection. Later, symptoms of hypoventilation may respond to intermittent support with standard or positive-pressure ventilator devices (125).

Weakness

There is a similar presentation at birth or early infancy, with floppiness or hypotonia and weakness that is greater proximally than distally. With all types, there is a delay of motor milestones and, except for the severe neonatal forms, the progression of weakness is static to very slowly progressive.

In nemaline myopathy, progressive weakness and loss of function in adulthood have been related to complications of spinal deformity (118).

There have been no specific studies on the effect of strength training in patients with congenital myopathies. However, a number of studies documented the positive effects of submaximal resistance exercise in other slowly progressive myopathic diseases (126–130).

Feeding

Feeding may be an issue for infants with nemaline myopathy or myotubular myopathy because of palate or pharnygeal weakness and dysmorphia. A weak cry and suck may indicate the need for a modified barium swallow study to better assess the safety of swallowing and guide therapeutic feeding interventions.

Mobility and Positioning

While the motor milestones are slowly being achieved, infants and toddlers can be provided with a number of mobility options, including carts, wheeled floor mobility devices, standing frames, and the parapodium. A good stroller with proper postural support should be provided for transport. Affected children may have difficulty with stairs, running, and hopping. Some children may need a wheelchair for longer distances. Adolescents and adults with myotubular myopathy tend to have increasing difficulty with ambulation, which may be improved with assistive devices.

Contractures

Contracture prevention with range of motion exercises, splinting, and casting should begin when the myopathy is recognized, with particular attention to the hip flexors and ankle plantarflexors. Surgical releases are indicated to improve function.

Scoliosis

The progression of scoliosis in patients with congenital myopathy can be slowed with good trunk support in infancy and the use of a spinal orthosis in childhood.

Psychosocial Issues

Genetic counseling should be offered to families and affected individuals. The majority of the congenital myopathies have potentially good functional outcomes. Most affected children are able to attend regular school programs, but may need an adapted physical education program. Vocational counseling should be offered to the adolescent. Lifestyle modification such as energy conservation techniques can also help to maximize function.

CONGENITAL MUSCULAR DYSTROPHY PRESENTATION: BIRTH OR EARLY INFANCY TYPE: MYOPATHY/CONGENITAL

Congenital muscular dystrophy (CMD) is a term applied to several different muscle disorders with dystrophic muscle pathology that have a genetic etiology, usually autosomal recessive. The estimated prevalence is less than 5 per million (131). The clinical spectrum is broad, but most patients present with hypotonia and weakness at birth. Some infants may have arthrogryposis and musculoskeletal deformities related to prolonged intrauterine postures. Hip dislocations and equinus are most common. Later-onset CMD usually presents with delayed motor milestones.

Serum enzyme levels are usually normal or mildly elevated, but the dystrophic changes seen in muscle biopsy samples can help differentiate CMD from the congenital/structural myopathies or the SMAs (132). The muscle biopsy sample often appears worse than the clinical picture, with extensive replacement of muscle by adipose tissue (44) along with fiber-size variation. In some patients, the diaphragm and intercostal muscles become affected and can cause respiratory insufficiency and increased complications from infection in the neonatal period or in later childhood or adolescence (44). In the series from McMenamin et al (133), 6 of the 24 patients died of respiratory failure between the ages of 4 and 24 years.

The subtypes of CMD include types that involve muscle only, and those with muscle and brain involvement (134,135). The latter subtype is usually referred to as Fukuyama CMD, and this syndrome is second to Duchenne muscular dystrophy (DMD) in terms of neuromuscular disease prevalence in Japan, but extremely rare in other countries. Several other subtypes also have eye involvement (136). There has been a suggestion that the different subtypes are associated with alleles of the same gene (135,137), and progress in molecular genetics appears to be imminent. The gene locus for Fukuyama-type CMD has been identified on chromosome 9q31–33 (138). In addition, some patients with both "pure" CMD and the Fukuyama type have a reduction in merosin, a protein that is attached to the dystrophin-associated glycoproteins on the muscle membrane (139,140). An interesting recent finding was the correlation of deficient merosin with abnormal CNS myelination patterns in "pure" CMD (135).

Weakness

The weakness is greater proximally than distally and usually static to mildly progressive and may even improve (141). In a review of 24 patients, McMenamin et al (133) found that if progressive weakness becomes more generalized with age and affects the arms more than the legs. Weakness of the neck flexor muscles with head lag is a common problem (133). Facial muscles are usually involved as well, with sparing of the extraocular muscles.

Feeding and Activities of Daily Living

The general principles are the same as described for intermediate SMA.

Mobility

McMenamin et al (133) reported significant motor delay in all patients reviewed, with the average age for independent sitting 11.5 months and for walking 2.6 years. Most studies reported that approximately 50% to 75% of patients achieve independent ambulation (133,141). Lower-extremity bracing may be necessary for ambulation.

Contractures

Contractures at the ankles, knees, hips, and elbows are most common. Even though weakness tends to stabilize or be very slowly progressive, the tendency for contracture formation persists (142) and can interfere with ambulation more than the muscle weakness itself (44,141). Fixed, congenital contractures may need early surgical attention to maximize the potential for ambulation and independent ADL skills. Acquired contractures should be prevented with an aggressive home and outpatient program including range of motion exercises, positioning, and use of splints and serial casts. More severe contractures are found in children who have more severe weakness and who are wheelchair users, and patients who are diagnosed early and treated with regular stretching have a decreased incidence of contractures (141). If orthopedic procedures for contracture release and correction of bony deformity are eventually indicated, they should be delayed until the child is able to do some weight bearing on the lower extremities, since postoperative immobilization may promote contracture formation and limit ambulation (44,141).

Psychosocial Issues

The subtypes with structural brain involvement often are associated with seizure disorders or mental retardation, but most patients with "pure" CMD are of normal intelligence (44).

Long-term direct therapies are usually not indicated, as functional limitations tend to improve with maturity. Because of the expected slower rate of skill acquisition, families should be counseled to anticipate delays in development. Emphasis should be on contracture formation and keeping the child mobilized, including attending adapted physical education classes. Care must be taken in predicting functional outcomes since the course can vary widely (87).

CONGENITAL MYOTONIC DYSTROPHY PRESENTATION: BIRTH OR EARLY INFANCY TYPE: MYOPATHY/ION CHANNEL DISORDER

Myotonic dystrophy is a genetic disorder carried on the long arm of chromosome 19 (143). It is inherited as an autosomal dominant gene with incomplete penetrance and variable expression. The incidence has been estimated as 1 in 8000 (144). In typical congenital myotonic dystrophy, there may be a history of reduced fetal movement in utero and polyhydramnios. The latter may precipitate premature delivery, which is associated with more severe involvement (145). The infant presents with hypotonia that may result in severe or even fatal respiratory complications in the newborn period. There is no correlation between neonatal presentation and the severity of maternal disease. Other characteristic features in the neonate are equinovarus contractures and severe facial diplegia, usually presenting with an open, triangular "tented" mouth. Since the typical features of the adult disease are not present at this time and the disease may be asymptomatic or unrecognized in family members, diagnosis may be difficult in the infant and young child (146). EMG and muscle biopsy of the infant or young child are not helpful, but the diagnosis can be made by confirming the diagnosis in the mother (132).

Involvement of the intercostal muscles and diaphragm is responsible for a high incidence (>50%) of neonatal respiratory distress (146). In a series of 14 patients (147), most of whom were premature, 13 had birth asphyxia and 10 required mechanical ventilation from birth. The authors of this clinical series report suggested that the duration of mechanical ventilation is a good predictor of survival. Mortality in congenital myotonia dystrophy is usually caused by respiratory complications within the first year of life, but pulmonary problems tend not to be persistent (132).

In congenital myotonic dystrophy, myotonia does not present until after the ages of 2 to 3 years (44). In childhood-onset disease, it is usually present by the end of the first decade (148). As in adults, the myotonia in congenital disease tends to be more bothersome than disabling, except for articulation problems due to the myotonia that can affect the pharyngeal, tongue, and facial muscles. Pharmacologic management of myotonia and of the associated medical problems is discussed in the section on adult myotonic dystrophy.

Weakness

Affected newborns are floppy with poor head control. Hypotonia tends to improve in the first several years of life, but there is delayed motor development. A progressive increase in distal muscle weakness and wasting occurs in the second decade, along with the development of the other features of the adult form of myotonic dystrophy, including cataracts, cardiac arrhythmias, and gonadal atrophy. The weakness is slowly progressive, but tends to progress relatively more rapidly in the patients with earlier onset (148).

Feeding

The severe facial diplegia typically results in impaired sucking and swallowing, and feeding often requires the use of a nasogastric tube during the newborn period or early infancy. A swallowing study may be indicated to evaluate the potential for aspiration before an oral feeding program is initiated. If the newborn survives early respiratory problems, progressive improvement in both pulmonary and oromotor function is usually seen. This occurs at about 8 to 12 weeks in full-term infants, but may be longer in those born prematurely (44).

Mobility

In addition to a home stretching program, the family should be provided with a general program of activities to promote gross motor skill development. The patient usually attains independent ambulation (146), but it is often delayed by hip girdle weakness, and there may be associated gait abnormalities and a Gower sign (148). Safe ambulation may require an AFO, depending on the degree of anterior tibial weakness (39).

Contractures

Ankle equinus contractures should be managed aggressively in infancy with casting, splinting, and stretching, but may ultimately require surgical intervention.

Psychosocial Issues

Mental retardation is a common feature, usually mild to moderate in severity, and may exacerbate the delay in motor development. In one series (149), those with the most severe and earliest physical signs were found to be the most seriously affected intellectually. A structured individualized educational plan is important if mental retardation is present (39). Vocational counseling is important for affected adolescents because of speech impairments, weakness, and intellectual deficits. A longitudinal review of patients by O'Brien and Harper (150) suggested that the prognosis for gainful employment and "normal family life" is poor in this population.

GLYCOGENOSES PRESENTATION: BIRTH OR EARLY INFANCY TYPE: MYOPATHIES/METABOLIC

Classification, Incidence, and Clinical Features

There are several diseases characterized by glycogen abnormalities caused by specific enzyme defects in glycogen metabolism, both storage and utilization. Diagnosis is made by muscle biopsy. All of the metabolic myopathies have an autosomal recessive mode of inheritance. There is a wide clinical spectrum, and the muscle disease may be rapidly progressive and fatal or relatively benign. Affected infants present with weakness and hypotonia in the first 6 months of life. Failure to thrive is another typical feature and may be related to the abnormal glucose metabolism. Some of these disorders can be treated to some extent with dietary manipulations and enzyme replacements (44).

Infantile acid maltase deficiency or Pompe disease is characterized by the increased deposition of glycogen in skeletal and cardiac muscles resulting from the absence of the enzyme α-1,4-glucosidase. Examination of muscle biopsy specimens shows increased glycogen deposits in the muscle fibers. The gene has been localized to the long arm of chromosome 17, and the infantile and later-onset forms are considered to be allelic (44), with associated clinical and biochemical diversity. Severely affected infants are usually floppy at birth, but in some, there may be a period of apparently normal motor development with subsequent development of weakness and hypotonia. Both presentations are associated with a failure to thrive, poor feeding, difficulty swallowing, and a weak cry and can resemble the severe form of SMA. Distinguishing features of Pompe disease are facial weakness and enlargement of the tongue (44). The weakness progresses rapidly to death, which usually occurs by age 2, secondary to cardiopulmonary complications (151). There are also some patients who have later onset and are more mildly affected with proximal weakness, delayed milestones, and a clinical picture similar to that of limb girdle dystrophy (44). Chest radiographs reveal cardiomegaly and the electrocardiogram (ECG) demonstrates high-amplitude QRS complexes and other abnormalities. In general, the prognosis appears to be related to cardiac and respiratory muscle involvement.

Myophosphorylase deficiency or McArdle disease is an autosomal recessive disorder that is restricted to skeletal muscle (114). It can present as a severe, fatal infantile form along with other types characterized by early or late onset, but is usually not diagnosed until adult life (44). There may be a history of easy fatigability throughout childhood. Typical symptoms present in adolescence, with painful muscle cramps on exercise occasionally associated with myoglobinuria (152). Between attacks, patients are asymptomatic. Attacks can be prevented by modification of physical exertion (153). Older individuals with chronic symptoms may develop mild proximal weakness.

Debrancher enzyme deficiency or Forbes or Cori disease presents with hypotonia, weakness, and failure to thrive, along with mild hypoglycemia and hepatomegaly. The muscle and liver biopsy specimens show increased glycogen of an abnormal structure. A protuberant abdomen develops in early childhood. Growth failure is a problem, and the affected child typically is of short stature with little subcutaneous fat (148). Weakness and muscle wasting may be particularly obvious in the shoulder girdle muscles, but overall muscle weakness tends to be mild.

Brancher enzyme deficiency results primarily in liver disease, but there are some patients who have muscle weakness and wasting as well. The disease usually presents in the first 6 months of life with failure to thrive, hepatosplenomegaly, and liver failure with cirrhosis (148). Poor motor and social development, hypotonia, weakness, and muscle atrophy have been observed in these infants (154).

Glucose-6-phosphatase deficiency or von Gierke disease typically presents in infancy with seizures that are the consequence of hypoglycemia. The hypoglycemic effects on the developing brain can cause other neurologic problems such as spastic paralysis and cognitive impairment. These problems may be more prominent than the associated myopathy. Infants have enlarged liver and kidneys, increased subcutaneous fat, and xanthomas of the skin. The severity of the disease reaches a plateau around age 4 or 5 years, so vigorous early management, typically with various dietary manipulations, is indicated (148).

Rehabilitation Strategies

Rehabilitation strategies for Pompe disease are similar to those for the infant with SMA type I. In the others, contracture prevention with range of motion exercises and splinting is the basic intervention. Most affected children will have some degree of motor delay, but have a good prognosis for independent ambulation. There is usually normal intelligence. As with the other congenital myopathies, ongoing, formal therapy interventions are generally not indicated, as the motor delays can be addressed with home and school programs and because progression toward milestones occurs with time. More complicated rehabilitation issues may be presented by the child with von Gierke disease because of the associated neurologic problems.

INTERMEDIATE SPINAL MUSCULAR ATROPHY (SMA TYPE II) PRESENTATION: LATE INFANCY TO EARLY CHILDHOOD TYPE: ANTERIOR HORN CELL DISEASE

Classification, Incidence, and Clinical Features

Intermediate SMA is also known as SMA type II or chronic Werdnig-Hoffmann disease. In this group of patients, signs can be present as early as the age of 3 months, but are definitely apparent by 18 months (47). The creatine kinase (CK) level is normal to mildly elevated. Most children achieve the ability to sit unaided but then are unable to take weight on the legs and stand or ambulate independently (see Table 89-2). There is variable progression and survival is into adolescence or adulthood (40,50,52).

The majority of these patients develops restrictive lung disease, and this is the most important factor determining prognosis (44). Respiratory muscle weakness may be out of proportion to extremity weakness and result in chronic, alveolar hypoventilation and impaired secretion clearance. Such pulmonary compromise may be exacerbated by scoliosis. In a study that analyzed pulmonary function test data on 17 patients with SMA II (155), 12 patients (71%) met the criteria for mild, moderate, or severe restrictive lung disease. Respiratory complications were experienced by 15 of the 17 patients (88%) and were more common in those meeting criteria for severe restrictive lung disease. Four of the six patients with restrictive lung disease required mechanical ventilation. An aggressive maintenance program of chest physiotherapy (CPT), postural drainage, and deep-breathing exercises is indicated. The children with more severe weakness often require tracheostomy or negative- or positive-pressure ventilation. However, some may be able to be weaned once they survive into adolescence. SMA type II patients who required definitive ventilatory support later in childhood or as adults were found to benefit, with greatly prolonged survival and function in society (81).

Weakness

Clinical weakness is similar to that seen with SMA type I, with symmetric involvement, more proximally than distally, and more pronounced in the lower than the upper extremities with associated atrophy. In a sample of 10 children, Koch and Simenson (56) found upper-extremity strength to be 35% to 40% of normal. There is generalized hypotonia and joint extensibility, often striking in the hands (44). Tremors of the hands and fasciculations and atrophy of the tongue are often seen (156).

The progression of weakness is static to slowly progressive. In the study by Carter et al (155), the average decline per decade in muscle strength in SMA type II patients was similar to the decline per year in DMD patients (Table 89-3). Some children will attain, but then lose some of their early motor milestones such as independent sitting and standing. Some achieve limited ambulation, usually with orthoses. Weakness may be exacerbated by obesity and in situations that result in immobilization such as acute illness, fractures, and surgeries. Several studies that included limited numbers of SMA patients showed increases in strength with moderate resistance training, suggesting such exercise programs may be indicated for all SMA patients except those with the most severe and progressive weakness (127–130,157).

Self-Care

Independence with self-care can be facilitated with the use of adaptive clothing with Velcro fasteners, lightweight eating and writing utensils with built-up handles, balanced forearm orthoses, and toileting and bathing equipment. The ability to produce a measurable force for pinch or gross grasp was associated with independence in mobility, hand function, and ADLs in one study of this population (56).

Mobility

Transportation of the infant or toddler can be accomplished with an adapted stroller that provides adequate back and neck support. The child should be seated in a wheelchair when he or she outgrows or is not age appropriate for a stroller. The wheelchair should also have a firm seat and back and be able to grow with the child. However, the weaker child who does not sit or stand may require a spinal orthosis for support. Floor mobility devices such as scooters can help these children enjoy a variety of typical developmental motor experiences. Parents should be taught to move the children as much as possible to give them motor experiences they cannot gain on their own. In the child with adequate strength and respiratory reserve, mobility can be facilitated with the use of HKAFOs or reciprocating gait orthoses. Ambulatory children often show a hyperlordotic, Trendelenburg gait with shuffling feet (75).

In a 10-year retrospective review (48), SMA patients were classified by maximal motor function achieved. This study found that children who never walked became power chair dependent by age 14. In those who achieved ambulation with gait aids, walking ceased by age 14 and power mobility was needed by age 18.

Contractures

In the child who is nonambulatory, prevention of postural deformities is an essential aspect of care (75,158). In children who ambulate, prevention of contractures may prolong ambulation (49). Contractures were common in the longitudinal series by Carter et al (155), occurring most frequently at the shoulders, related to shoulder girdle weakness, and hips, knees, and feet, corresponding to prolonged sitting. Range of motion exercises must be performed at least daily (75). Torticollis and hip tightness are best controlled by proper positioning in supine and side-lying positions, often with the use of wedges and bolsters with attention to neutral spine and joint alignment. Lying prone is often not well tolerated because of the increased limitation of respiratory musculature. The feet should be plantigrade while seated, and this can be achieved with the footplate and straps or with a molded AFO. Night splints can also help to prevent contractures. Children with adequate head control can be stretched in the prone stander or parapodium, but may need external trunk support (87).

Scoliosis

In studies of combined SMA type II and III patients, the incidence of scoliosis was very common, estimated to be around 60% to 85% (54,82,159), and 90% for SMA type II children who are wheelchair dependent (160). Both

Table 89-3: Summary of Neuromuscular Disease Impairment and Disability Profiles

	Mean MMT	Decline in MMT Unit/Time	Contractures*	Scoliosis*	Abnormal* ECG	History of Cardiovascular Complications*	Severe* RLD	IQ
DMD (McDonald et al, 1995) (179)	<6 yr: 4.1 ± 0.7 13–15 yr: 2.1 ± 0.7	5–13 yr–0.25/yr ≥14 yr–0.06/yr	100% by 13 yr	>90% by 17 yr	Typical	Uncommon	100%	↓1 SD
BMD (McDonald et al, 1995) (291)	3.7+	–0.31/decade	Uncommon	Rare	Typical	Uncommon	Rare	N1
Noncongenital myotonic dystrophy (Johnson et al, 1995) (465)	4.0 ± 0.7	–0.36/decade	Rare	Rare	Typical	Common	Rare	Within 1 SD
Congenital myotonic dystrophy (Johnson et al, 1995c) (465)	3.8 ± 0.7	NP	Uncommon	Common	Typical	Uncommon	Uncommon	↓ By 1 SD
Late-onset and pelvifemoral types (McDonald et al, 1995) (324)	3.9 ± 0.7	NP	Rare	Rare	Typical	Uncommon	Rare	N1
Facioscapulohumoral muscular dystrophy (Kilmer et al, 1995) (332)	3.7 ± 0.8	–0.22/decade	Rare	Uncommon	Typical	Uncommon	Rare	N1
SMA type II (Carter et al, 1995) (155)	2.3 ± 0.6	–0.24/decade	Uncommon	Typical	Typical	Uncommon	Common	N1
SMA type III (Carter et al, 1995) (155)	3.8 ± 0.7	NP	Uncommon	Rare	Common	Uncommon	Rare	N1

Source: Data summarized from Fowler WM. Introduction: impairment and disability profiles of neuromuscular diseases. *Am J Phys Med Rehabil* 1995;74(suppl).

DMD = Duchenne muscular dystrophy; BMD = Becker muscular dystrophy; SMA = spinal muscular atrophy; MMT = manual muscle test; ECG = electrocardiogram; RLD = restrictive lung disease; IQ = intelligence quotient; SD = standard deviation; N1 = normal; NP = nonprogressive.

* Frequency of impairments scale (extrapolated from original authors' data): rare ≤20%; uncommon, 21%–34%; common, 35%–65%; typical, >66%.

ambulators and nonambulators can develop scoliosis, but the curves appear much earlier and are more severe in the latter, weaker group. A rigid, straight spine may result in loss of ambulation and decreased upper-extremity reach in some children, so the risks and benefits must be carefully considered prior to scoliosis surgery (161,162). Prolonged immobilization postoperatively should be avoided.

The clinical characteristics of SMA scoliosis were presented in Merlini et al's reviews of the literature (74,163). The deformity is a paralytic curve with early onset and continuous progression, even after spinal growth is completed, which may relate to the underlying joint hypermobility. The curve is typically throacolumbar and C shaped, progresses by 8 degrees per year from 4 to 21 years, and is often associated with marked kyphosis and pelvic obliquity. The literature does not support the use of spinal orthoses for the prevention of scoliosis or its progression (54,164).

Psychosocial Issues

These children have normal intelligence and from an early age, they should be encouraged to strive for social, emotional, and financial independence (75). Even if on a ventilator, they should be able to attend a regular school program with the appropriate accommodations and lack of barriers. If they are not healthy enough to attend school, either for short or long periods, a home program is necessary to provide early stimulation for the toddler and preschooler and quality educational programs for the school-age child. Computer skills are important to develop during the school years and can be incorporated into vocational planning. These children also benefit from participation in recreational activities such as wheelchair sports, swimming, and horseback riding to improve their endurance and self-esteem.

Families of these children will benefit from ongoing support and counseling with regard to parenting a child with a disability, and anticipation of medical needs. Families need to be prepared for any major changes in the child's status, such as need for gastrostomy placement, spine surgery, or ventilatory support. All of these issues should be addressed before a crisis situation occurs, particularly in regard to mechanical ventilation and "code" status (86). Families need to learn how to advocate for their child's needs with schools, insurance companies, and the community, and to keep current with the remarkable advances being made in the area of adaptive equipment. Established resources like the Muscular Dystrophy Association are available to these children and their families for education and support as well.

DUCHENNE MUSCULAR DYSTROPHY PRESENTATION: LATE INFANCY TO EARLY CHILDHOOD TYPE: MYOPATHY/DYSTROPHY

Incidence, Classification, and Clinical Features

DMD is inherited as an X-linked recessive gene that is passed to boys by mothers who are asymptomatic, except for a small percentage who are very mildly symptomatic (165). The prevalence is 63 per million, and the incidence is high, approximately 1 per 3500 live male births, of which one-third of cases are from spontaneous mutations (131). The DMD gene locus is responsible for this high mutation rate, as it includes over 2.5 million base pairs of human X chromosome, localized to the short arm of chromosome 21 (166). The gene codes for the dystrophin protein (167), which is a component of normal skeletal muscle sarcolemma and is involved in maintaining its structural integrity (168–170). Because of gene deletions (55%–65% of cases), duplications (5%–10% of cases), or point mutations (30%–40%) (171), dystrophin and its associated sarcolemmal glycoproteins are absent in the skeletal muscle fibers of DMD patients. The resultant structural deficiency is believed to render the sarcolemma vulnerable to physical stress, especially during contraction (172). This is the leading theory of the basic mechanism that leads to cell necrosis and the corresponding dystrophic changes in muscle that are characteristic of DMD muscle pathology (173,174).

A diagnosis of DMD is strongly suggested by the family history or clinical examination, or both, along with elevation of serum CK levels. Any male toddler who is not ambulating by 18 months should have serum CK levels measured (152). In DMD, the serum CK value is 50 to 100 times normal around the ages of 3 to 6 years and thereafter decreases approximately by 20% per year, reflecting a loss of muscle bulk (114). Confirmation of the diagnosis is made by muscle biopsy and histologic examination, which shows fibrosis with connective and adipose tissue replacement of muscle, variation in fiber size, and necrosis, with type I fiber predominance and a selective loss of type IIB fibers (114). Chromosome and dystrophin analysis may be necessary to confirm the diagnosis if the clinical and laboratory data are not conclusive (175).

Typically, clinical manifestations are not noted until around the ages of 2 to 3 years after a normal infancy and timely occurrence of early developmental milestones like sitting, crawling, and standing. At this time, there is usually obvious pseudohypertrophy of the calves, which also can be seen in the quadriceps, gluteal, deltoid, and infraspinous muscles. Around 3 to 5 years of age, there begins a well-described progression of weakness and gait abnormalities, which results in a rapid decline in mobility skills between the ages of 8 and 12 years. This progression is related to the adoption of specific postural adjustments to compensate for muscle weakness and imbalances at the hip and knee. Eventually, the limitations of the associated developing contractures and advancing weakness result in loss of upright balance and ambulation (84,176,177).

The pulmonary complications of DMD are the result of the severe, progressive restrictive lung disease present in all DMD boys, usually beginning in the second decade (see Table 89-3). Death from DMD usually occurs in the late teens and in approximately 70% of patients is related to the pulmonary complications associated with restrictive lung disease (178). Clinically, there may be no symptoms in younger boys, but changes in the mechanical properties of the thorax can be documented by early decreases in maximal static airway pressures (179). Decreased static airway pressures, particularly maximal inspiratory pressure, are considered more sensitive than vital capacity in the early stages of disease, since vital capacity increases with growth. Vital capacity, which reflects both thoracic wall compliance and respiratory muscle weakness, becomes a better indicator of pulmonary impairment later in the disease when mobility is lost (180).

The course of restrictive lung disease is directly correlated with the progression of weakness with age. Deterioration in pulmonary function was found to occur around the time a DMD boy cannot rise from a chair until the time when assistance is needed for walking (178). McDonald et al (179) found a linear decline in percent predicted FVC until the mean upper-extremity manual muscle test (MMT) score approaches a grade 2. The survival time for those with 35% or less of normal forced vital capacity was 3.2 years in one study (181). McDonald et al (179) also found that the rate of decline in percent predicted FVC related to the peak absolute FVC value obtained, so that this value may be used as a prognostic indicator of future disease progression.

Recent changes in the approach to the pulmonary care of DMD patients have been popularized (182–187). Early intervention is recommended to limit cardiopulmonary morbidity and to delay early death from respiratory failure. Several studies showed that advanced DMD patients on noninvasive or invasive ventilatory assistance have a longer life expectancy as well as a meaningful quality of life (188–192).

Degeneration of smooth muscle also occurs in DMD. There may be dystrophic and fibrotic changes in the myocardium, and 90% of ECGs are abnormal but most patients do not have cardiac symptomatology (179) (see Table 89-3). Similar muscle pathology can occur in the gastrointestinal tract, commonly causing esophageal and intestinal hypomotility, symptoms of reflux, and constipation (193,194), and in rare and potentially fatal cases, acute gastric dilatation (195).

Obesity may be seen in up to one-third of patients (196–198). This tendency is usually obvious in childhood and persists into adolescence. Loss of ambulation in early adolescence is not correlated with acute weight gain. In fact, in late adolescence, there is frequently weight loss, due to a state of relative hypercatabolism (199) along with the influences of worsening restrictive lung disease, dysphagia, and impaired self-feeding (200).

Several pharmacologic interventions have been advocated to slow the progression of DMD. Prednisone can improve strength and function in patients with DMD (201–204). Because of the potential risks of high-dose steroids, it is currently recommended as a short-term intervention while patients are still in the ambulatory phase (205). Other immunosuppressive therapies have been studied, but overall medical therapies do not appear to be effective (206–209).

Advancements in molecular genetics, such as cell and gene therapy, are more promising, but still experimental (210–212). Human myoblasts are donated from close male relatives, cultured, and injected into the affected boy's muscle (209,213,214). Success has been limited thus far by the low efficiency of transfer of the normal genetic material to the abnormal skeletal muscle cells. Gene therapy involves the direct implantation of a normal, cloned dystrophin gene, either directly or via some transfer agent such as a virus vector, liposome, or myoblast (215,216).

Weakness

Weakness progresses in a fairly linear fashion, without remissions or recovery (114,179,198,217). However, the course of loss of function is quite variable and progression of the disease in general as opposed to weakness per se may correspond better to time when function is lost than to chronologic age. Sutherland et al (177) described the early, transitional, and late stages of ambulation on the basis of a longitudinal gait analysis study of DMD boys and found considerable overlap in ages among groups, with a much shorter time interval between the transitional and late groups than between the early and transitional groups. Allsop and Ziter (218) described a trend of relatively slow decline in function despite progressive strength loss and then a relatively abrupt loss of function. Other studies timed the duration of functional activities to document progression of weakness (126,219–221). The findings in these studies suggest that the variability in function over time relates to both the progression of muscle weakness and the ability of DMD boys to use compensatory postures. The ability to compensate in order to maintain function may be influenced by many factors such as preservation of range of motion, scoliosis, obesity, medical illness, and psychological and emotional issues (176,222). Differences in the ability to compensate may explain some of the variability in function between DMD boys of similar age or extent of weakness, or both.

The steady progression of weakness in DMD occurs in a fairly predictable pattern. Quantitative strength measurements have been shown to be more sensitive than MMT, with differences between DMD boys and healthy control subjects evident as early as age 5 or 6 years (179,198). Before age 6 years, neck flexors are the muscle group with the most clinically apparent weakness on MMT, followed by trunk flexors, hip extensors, ankle dorsiflexors, and evertors. In the extremities, the proximal and extensor muscles are more affected than the distal and flexor muscles. Quantitative strength loss was found to occur at a mean rate of −0.25 MMT units per year between 5 and 13 years, and then decreased to a mean of −0.06 per year around 14 to 15 years (see Table 89-3) (179). Throughout the course of the disease, the upper-extremity muscles remain stronger than the lower-extremity muscles. Neck extensors are affected later in the disease, causing the head to assume a flexed posture.

In addition to muscle weakness, DMD boys have decreased cardiorespiratory capacity from restrictive lung disease and decreased peripheral oxygen utilization due to dystrophic muscle (223). Deconditioning can cause further decreases in cardiorespiratory capacity and strength that could limit exercise performance, which for DMD boys can be considered the endurance for daily functional activities. Thus, throughout the early and transitional phases of the disease, immobilization should be avoided. The criteria for reambulation after orthopedic surgery include a nonambulatory period of no longer than 3 to 4 weeks (224). When a wheelchair is first prescribed, it should be stored in the trunk of the family's motor vehicle so it is only used for longer distances. Ambulatory boys who go to camp should also be discouraged from unnecessary wheelchair use.

In DMD, there is greater involvement of type IIb or fast twitch fibers, which are more specifically trained with resistance exercise. Based on animal studies with dystrophic mice, the recommendations for strengthening in neuromuscular disease in general include initiation of resistance training early in the disease course, and increasing resistance gradually. Avoidance of eccentric contractions and overexertion is also suggested, based on the concern for overwork weakness and the potential for increased muscle damage (126,157).

If initiated early in the progression of DMD, the key muscles for strength training include the hip extensors and abductors, abdominals, and quadriceps (87). Unfortunately, studies of the benefits of strengthening exercise in DMD have been difficult to interpret as they usually include other forms of dystrophies, have been done on uncontrolled and small samples, and do not account for the effects of maturation. Vignos and Watkins (126) found less initial strength gains and an inability to stabilize weakness progression in DMD patients compared to other dystrophies. DeLateur and Giaconi (225) documented modest but not statistically significant increases in strength without overwork weakness with a program of submaximal exercise strengthening of the quadriceps in a small subject-controlled sample. Scott et al (217) demonstrated increased maximal voluntary contraction of the ankle dorsiflexors with electrical stimulation in younger DMD boys, while Milner-Brown and Miller (129,130) did not find increases in strength using electrical stimulation in a mixed sample with a majority of older, severely weak DMD subjects. Respiratory muscle training has not been found to improve strength but may influence endurance (226–228).

These results are consistent with the finding that greater improvements in strength are related to the pre-exercise strength of the muscle (126,129,130,157). Compared to the other muscular dystrophies (see Table 89-3), DMD is much more progressive throughout its course with greater absolute weakness. So while submaximal strengthening of key muscle groups early in the course of the disease is not harmful, more studies are needed to show functional gains in DMD patients who undergo resistance training programs.

Feeding

The bulbar and facial muscles are not affected in DMD, but patients, especially those who are nonambulatory, often experience dysphagia and reflux (194), so antireflux precautions and therapy may be indicated.

Self-care

Performance of ADLs involving fine motor skills is influenced primarily by decreased strength in the wrist extensors and decreased radial deviation (229,230), usually seen starting in early adolescence (231). Holding and picking up heavier objects become difficult, so lighter and smaller utensils and tools can be used. Dressing usually requires some physical assistance at this stage of the disease. A balanced forearm orthosis can allow hand-to-mouth function when hand function is intact, but there is poor proximal strength. Robotic arms mounted on the wheelchair tray can be used with only finger movements for wheelchair operation, feeding devices, and environmental controls (232). Mouthsticks can be used for turning pages, painting, buttoning, and maneuvering smaller objects. Voice-, eye-, and blink-operated environmental controls are available to give patients access to all appliances, computers, and telecommunication equipment (233).

Bathroom equipment, such as raised toilet seats, grab bars, bath seats, and roll-in showers, can assist in promoting safety and independence.

Mobility

Affected male toddlers may be slightly delayed in achieving ambulation and may be noted to be "clumsy." The affected child first develops a waddling-type gait and increased lumbar lordosis due to hip extensor weakness, representing the first postural compensation in DMD gait (177). A balanced stance in the setting of increasing weakness of the hips and knee extensors requires knee hyperextension and ankle plantarflexion, as well as further lumbar lordosis (84). The younger DMD boy does not require any assistance with mobility, but may have difficulty keeping up with peers, especially with running and hopping, and should be monitored for safety. Rising from the floor requires the Gower maneuver. Gradually, a wide-based gait develops to improve the instability caused by increasing hip and knee extensor weakness. At this time, stair climbing becomes more difficult and should be performed with a rail or contact guarding.

DMD boys experience a decrease in gait cadence and velocity as they progress from the early through the transitional to the late stages of gait. The early stage is characterized by progression of weakness and worsening contractures, resulting in a more vertical alignment of the centers of the hip, knee, and ankle joints. In the late stage, the gait of DMD boys requires significant energy expenditure and effort to maintain stability at the hips and knees. They begin to experience more falls and fatigue with ambulation, and safety outside the home becomes an issue. Prescription of a lightweight standard wheelchair with a solid cushion and back and footrests is appropriate. At this time, fit of the wheelchair must be evaluated regularly, with special attention given to alignment of the spine and pelvis. An alternative is the provision of early power mobility, either with a scooter or wheelchair (87). Both will allow for negotiation of uneven or inclined surfaces since proximal upper-extremity weakness is also compromised at this time. A disadvantage of the scooter is the lack of trunk support, which can be better addressed with a power chair. Sit-to-stand transfers can be aided with raised seats and grab bars and rails. Stand pivot transfers are usually indicated around the time when the child begins transitioning to the wheelchair.

Impairments in mobility and the termination of ambulation have been related to muscle strength, contractures, specific gait abnormalities, and loss of other mobility functions. A 50% loss in strength correlated most closely to loss of ability to stand from the supine position in one study (218). Other studies found that ambulation is discontinued specifically when the quadriceps and gluteal muscles lose more than 50% strength (176,217). In the longitudinal series by McDonald et al (179), all proximal lower-extremity and trunk muscle groups were less than antigravity at the time of transition to a wheelchair. Siegel (84) found that when knee extension lag while prone is more than 90 degrees, termination of ambulation is within a few months. Loss of ambulation occurred with an increased double-support phase in gait analysis. Sutherland et al's (177) classic study of gait biomechanics in DMD found quadriceps insufficiency to be the key deficit contributing to gait deterioration. Brooke et al (221) found that there was an average interval of 2.4 years between the time the child could no longer ascend four stairs in less than 5 seconds to the time of loss of independent standing and walking. The average interval between assisted ambulation and wheelchair reliance was 3.3 years.

Based on the fact that quadriceps insufficiency is a main contribution to gait deterioration, elastic knee supports have been used for a short interval in the early transitional phase, for help with knee stability mainly by sensory input and increasing confidence (234). AFOs are used for positioning, but not ambulation, since the fixation of the ankle interferes with the compensation for knee weakness achieved by the equinus posture (235). Prolongation of ambulation using long leg braces or knee-ankle-foot orthoses has been pursued in the late transitional or early nonambulatory phase of DMD, often in conjunction with surgical soft-tissue releases, which may be necessary for proper orthotic fitting (176,236–239). Several authors advocated earlier surgery, reporting increased time of brace-free ambulation by 1 to 2 years (158, 240–242). Lower-extremity soft-tissue surgery for prolongation of reambulation in DMD typically involves a combination of releases at the iliotibial band, hip flexors, Achilles tendon, or hamstrings (235). Manzur et al (243) showed no benefit of earlier surgery on strength or function in a randomized controlled study of 20 DMD boys aged 4 to 6 years. However, Rideau et al (220) reported multiple benefits of earlier surgery, including improvements in mean age of loss of ability to rise from the floor and decreased progression of lower-extremity weakness and contractures, but specified that successful surgery must be performed before a certain level of decline is reached in these areas.

Prevention of rapidly progressive scoliosis has also been regarded as a benefit of prolonged ambulation, given the frequently documented association between wheelchair reliance and scoliosis progression (244–246). However, this association seems to be more a secondary influence or coincidental. Other studies demonstrated that scoliosis is more strongly related to age and the timing of the adolescent growth spurt (247–249).

When patients begin to lose the ability to participate in transfers, equipment such as sliding boards and home lift devices may be safer than manual lifts, and decrease the physical burden on caregivers. Adequate head and trunk support should be taken into consideration with the use of any such devices. Caregivers should be instructed in proper safety and body mechanics with any type of transfer when the patient is more dependent. Adaptations for the wheelchair, such as lateral trunk supports, adductor pads, seat belt, chest strap, lap tray, and head support, should be added when indicated. A reclining back will allow for position changes and pressure relief. Pressure relief can also be accomplished with lateral weight shifts, with manual assistance if necessary. Power chairs may not be feasible in all environments and are subject to mechanical problems, so a "backup" manual chair is also recommended. Ramps for the home and a wheelchair accessible van with a lift allow teenagers to remain active outside the home. When bed mobility becomes more difficult, a hospital bed with electric controls may allow independent weight shifts as well as changes of position to promote comfort (39). Mattresses and pads that alternately deflate and inflate can promote pressure relief without manual repositioning.

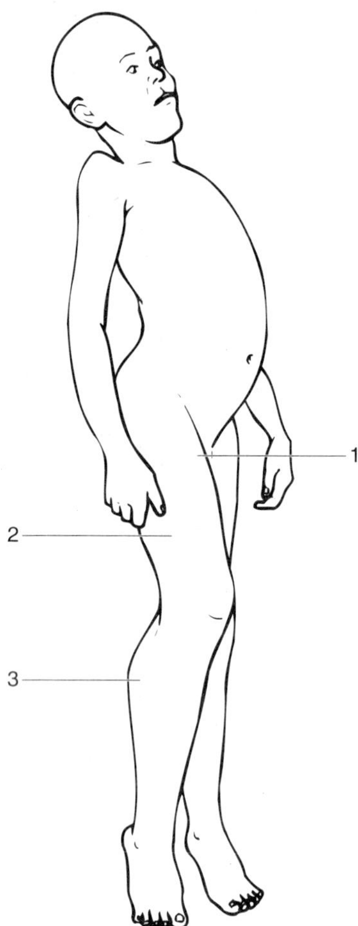

Figure 89-1. Contracted musculature contributing to myopathic stance and gait. (1) Hip flexors; (2) tensor fasciae latae; (3) triceps surae. (Adapted with permission from Siegel IM. Pathomechanics of stance in Duchenne muscular dystrophy. *Arch Phys Med Rehabil* 1991;543:405.)

Contractures

The typical sequence of contracture development in the lower extremities is related to progressive weakness and the biomechanical changes adopted in order to maintain stability in the setting of the competing demands of knee and hip stability (177). Early tightness of the iliotibial band, tensor fasciae latae, and gastrocnemius muscles occurs without significant muscle strength loss (Fig. 89-1). Contractures gradually develop in these muscles as well as in the hip flexors and hamstrings. In a longitudinal series, contractures were rare prior to age 9 years but were present in all patients by age 13 years, and thereafter increased in frequency and severity (179) (see Table 89-3). Lower-extremity contractures were strongly related to the onset of wheelchair reliance (235). In another longitudinal study, Brooke et al (221) found a significant correlation between the use of leg braces and the prevention of contractures in the gastrocnemius-soleus, hamstrings, and iliotibial band. These studies emphasized the importance of walking for active stretching and maintenance of range of motion.

In the upper extremities, contractures tend to develop from static positioning and the effects of gravity, and usually occur in the wrist and elbow flexors and ulnar deviators. Tightness in the fingers with various distal interphalangeal deformities also occurs (230). Maintenance of range of motion should be addressed early in the course of the disease with stretching, positioning, and strengthening of opposing muscle groups.

An initial stretching program works best if performed at home along with the use of night splints (250). Regular use of night splints for the ankles reduced severity of heel cords contractures (221,251). Prone positioning should be encouraged to slow the progression of hip and knee flexion contractures. A standing program with knee-ankle-foot orthoses, or standing frames or tilt tables or even swivel walkers (244) provides prolonged stretching as well as opportunities to participate in school and home activities in the upright position. With the loss of mobility skills, increased emphasis should be placed on maintenance of functional upper-extremity range of motion since hand and finger motion can allow significant independence with the use of adaptive equipment.

Maintenance of body alignment is an important factor in the prevention of musculoskeletal complications throughout the course of the disease. In the early course, this involves the use of good supportive seating and bedding, and, as much as possible, discouragement of abnormal postures (252). The minimal wheelchair prescription should include a solid back and seat, and footrests aligned in the neutral position. Joysticks on power wheelchairs should be placed in the midline to prevent the trunk from leaning toward one side (253).

Scoliosis

Scoliosis occurs in more than 90% of DMD boys (254). In a study of untreated scoliosis in DMD, the curves progressed to severe deformity (255,256) (see Fig. 89-6) Orthotic management of scoliosis in DMD with thoracolumbar supports does not prevent progression or decrease the rate of progression (160,249,257). The current treatment approach is aggressive, with most authors recommending fusion when the curve is 25 to 30 degrees with segmental-type instrumentation and fusion to the sacrum (160,258,259). Early correction of spinal deformity is done to avoid unacceptable operative risks due to restrictive lung disease, and permit maximal correction and balance of the spine (260,261). The major benefits of scoliosis correction are ease and comfort of seating and positioning (181,259,262,263).

Correction of spinal deformity has been associated with improvement in pulmonary function, although the literature offers conflicting opinions (88,264,265). In a retrospective study, Kurz et al (266) found that vital capacity is diminished by 4% with each 10-degree increase in scoliosis and each 1 year of age. Miller et al (181) found that DMD boys with a lower functional vital capacity had more advanced scoliotic curves. Galasko et al (259) reported slower deterioration in pulmonary function and prolonged survival in DMD patients undergoing spinal stabilization. No improvement or stabilization in pulmonary function was seen following scoliosis surgery in at least two well-designed studies (263,267). This has been supported by longitudinal data from McDonald et al (179), which showed that increasing age was primarily responsible for a reduction of pulmonary function, and scoliosis did not contribute a significant additive role. Miller et al (265) pointed out that scoliosis becomes more significant when there is already a significant decline in percent of functional vital capacity. Thus, the positive effects of scoliosis surgery and correction of the chest wall deformity on lung function are limited by the independent contribution of diminishing weakness with increasing age.

Psychosocial Issues

There is a relative mental retardation in the DMD population (268). Various studies have indicated an average IQ of around 85 or one standard deviation below normal for DMD boys, with approximately one-third of DMD boys having an IQ less than 75 (269). This subgroup is classified as mentally retarded and will need special classroom placements or tutoring. In a controlled study (270), significant cognitive deficits were found in certain DMD boys as compared to matched children with SMA. This suggests that the cognitive outcome in children with these two types of neuromuscular disorders is related to genetic factors and not environmental influences operative as a sequela to the physical handicap itself. In McDonald et al's study (179), neuropsychological testing revealed mild impairments of a global nature, but several studies detected specific problems in language abilities, reading, and memory (270–272). Billard et al (270) found that 40% of teenage DMD boys had not acquired reading fluency and had low educational achievement.

Dystrophin is found in the brain and has been localized to the neocortex, cerebellum, and hippocampus (273,274). It is not the same as muscle dystrophin (275). A general malfunction of the dystrophin gene as opposed to a specific deletion pattern is believed to be responsible for the variable reduction in intellectual function seen across the spectrum of Xp21 dystrophies (276,277). It has been shown that dystrophin-deficient mice are more susceptible to hypoxic brain injury. Hypoxic insults, possibly due to abnormalities in cerebral vasculature smooth muscle, may be the cause of the intellectual impairment in DMD boys (275,276).

DMD boys have not been found to have a higher rate of emotional disturbance or specific psychopathologies (278). Nevertheless, psychological and emotional issues figure prominently in the long-term rehabilitative management of DMD boys (39,279). In McDonald et al's study (179), 58% of DMD patients had psychological adjustment scale scores on standard personality testing that fell in the range for recommended psychological evaluation. Early in the course of DMD, children may experience anxiety from the fear of falling, resulting in self-imposed premature restrictions on activity (222). Older boys may display passive-aggressive or dependent personality traits (280). Fantasy and denial are often used as adjustment mechanisms because social contacts and role models may be limited. In addition, adolescents often display significant anxiety and withdrawal, which may relate to difficulties discussing issues such as death and dying with their families (281,282). This may be a period when referral for counseling can be particularly beneficial (283).

It is important for the medical caregivers to provide accurate information to the patient and family with regard to disease course and expected deteriorations in status so they are well prepared for such highly emotionally charged events such as first use of a wheelchair and decisions regarding ventilatory assistance. Counseling services should be available for patients and families, and the Muscular Dystrophy Association can be a resource for financial as well as emotional support.

BECKER MUSCULAR DYSTROPHY PRESENTATION: LATE CHILDHOOD TO ADOLESCENCE TYPE: MYOPATHY/DYSTROPHY

Incidence, Classification, and Clinical Features

Becker muscular dystrophy (BMD) is a more benign phenotype of DMD. There is involvement of both skeletal and cardiac muscle, but the course is more slowly progressive and the associated impairments and disabilities are less severe. BMD is less common than DMD, with an estimated incidence of 1 per 20,000 births (284). BMD is also inherited through an X-linked mechanism and is related to a mutation, typically a deletion, on the same gene as in DMD (175). This results in dystrophin of abnormal size or reduced amounts of normal dystrophin (284–286).

The initial clinical symptoms are typically not identified until late childhood or adolescence. There may be a protracted preclinical stage at which the only identifiable abnormality is calf pseudohypertrophy. At this stage, the serum CK level is grossly elevated, and is comparable with levels seen in much more clinically affected DMD boys (44). Thus, the diagnosis can be suggested by serum CK level and confirmed in young boys with a known family history. However, there may be some overlap in age at onset between DMD and BMD. In such cases, BMD is suggested by a milder weakness and ability to maintain ambulation through the early teen years. In a study by Emery and Skinner (287), 97% of adolescents with BMD were ambulatory as compared to adolescent DMD boys, of which 97% were using a wheelchair for mobility. Another differentiating feature in BMD is the frequent occurrence of muscle cramping with exercise (44,288). Other considerations in the differential diagnosis of BMD include limb girdle dystrophy and Emery-Dreifuss dystrophy. The diagnosis can be confirmed with chromosomal analysis or dystrophin analysis of muscle biopsy specimens (44,289).

Bushby and Gardner-Medwin (290) described two major patterns of progression in BMD, the typical slowly progressive and a more severe, rapidly progressive course. The patients with more severe BMD had earlier onset, more severe weakness and functional disability, and a higher incidence of ECG abnormalities. There has been no correlation between severity of disease and dystrophin analysis. In the review by Emery and Skinner (287), there was no correlation between age at onset and severity. Average age at onset has been reported to range from 8 to 12 years (287,290,291). In the slowly progressive types, there is typically survival to adulthood. The major risk of early death in BMD has been related to cardiac and not pulmonary complications (291).

A high percentage of BMD patients have ECG abnormalities related to cardiomyopathy (44,291,292). Cardiac involvement is usually a late manifestation. Several studies suggested that there is no correlation between skeletal muscle involvement, cardiac involvement, and extent of dystrophin abnormality (291,293). Thus, since even mildly weak BMD boys are at risk for life-threatening cardiac involvement, it is recommended that all BMD patients receive screening by ECG and echocardiography at regular intervals. Cardiac transplantation for BMD patients with end-stage cardiac failure has been reported (294). While some degree of restrictive lung disease may be present, pulmonary symptoms and complications are relatively rare in BMD (291).

Weakness

The weakness of BMD closely resembles that seen in DMD. The proximal lower extremities are involved early and are most severely affected. Proximal weakness in the upper extremities occurs 10 to 20 years after disease onset and is less severe than that in the lower extremities (290). The rate of progression in a longitudinal series over 10 years was less than one-half MMT unit per decade, with an average overall muscle score of 3.7 ± 0.8 MMT per decade (291) (see Table 89-2). In this series, neck flexor weakness was also seen early, but tended to stabilize around age 20 years, while early-onset hip and knee extensor weakness tended to progress with age and disease duration.

Successful muscle strengthening with resistance training in three BMD patients was reported in two studies by Milner-Brown and Miller (129,130).

Activities of Daily Living and Self-Care

Adaptive equipment may be necessary to maintain independence.

Mobility and Positioning

Ambulation is usually maintained until late adolescence or early adulthood, and in some, is never lost. Orthoses, or manual or power wheelchair mobility may be offered for the more severely affected who have an inefficient or unsafe gait.

Contractures

Early contractures are not a prominent feature of BMD (see Table 89-3), but do occur in the lower extremities, especially when ambulation is lost (44,291). Ambulatory patients tend to have heel cord tightness, which can be addressed by a range of motion program or splinting (87).

Scoliosis

The review by McDonald et al (291) demonstrated that spinal deformity is uncommon and usually mild in severity (see Table 89-3). No patient in this series required spinal stabilization, but the spine should be monitored routinely, especially during periods of growth and in the evaluation of mobility devices.

Psychosocial Issues

There is a mildly reduced intellectual function in a subset of BMD (44,290,291). Because longevity is the rule, affected boys should be provided with every opportunity for school and social participation. During adolescence, vocational rehabilitation evaluation may be helpful in making appropriate vocational choices. Support and resources may be provided through government benefits or the Muscular Dystrophy Association.

PARAMYOTONIA CONGENITA PRESENTATION: LATE INFANCY TO EARLY CHILDHOOD TYPE: METABOLIC MYOPATHY/ION CHANNEL DISORDER

Paramyotonia is sustained muscle contraction that worsens with increasing exertion. Paramyotonia congenita is considered to be allelic to hyperkalemic periodic paralysis and linked to the adult sodium channel gene on the long arm of chromosome 17 (295). There is myotonia of resting muscles on EMG, and examination of muscle biopsy specimens reveals myopathic changes. The myotonia in this syndrome is provoked by exposure to cold. There may be some associated mild weakness, but generally symptoms are mild, with a tendency to affect the face and hands, often with hypertrophy. Rewarming results in relief of the stiffness and return of strength in 30 minutes to several hours (44,296). Symptoms in this disorder also respond to cardiac antiarrhythmics (297).

MYOTONIA CONGENITA PRESENTATION: LATE INFANCY TO EARLY CHILDHOOD TYPE: METABOLIC MYOPATHY/ION CHANNEL DISORDER

There are two genetic forms of this primarily myotonic disorder: Thomsen disease, which is inherited as an autosomal dominant trait, and Becker disease, which is inherited recessively and is more common. In both diseases, EMG reveals classic myotonia and examination of muscle biopsy specimens shows absence of type IIB fibers. Thomsen disease is linked to the long arm of chromosome 7 and involves the voltage-dependent sodium channel controlled by chromosome 17 (298). Males may be more severely affected (296). The myotonia is the primary feature of the disorder and affected individuals usually experience stiffness in the hands, legs, and eyelids, but speech and chewing may also be affected. In addition, there is usually generalized muscle hypertrophy. Symptoms are aggravated by cold, rest, and emotional state and may increase during pregnancy. Symptoms can be relieved by ingestion of carbohydrates, or movement and exercise, and affected patients can often prevent symptoms by avoiding static positions (296). Thomsen disease usually presents at birth or in early childhood, and symptoms persist throughout life, but do not progress. The myotonia can be treated with drugs, usually the class I cardiac antiarrhythmics, but most patients learn to cope with the minimally disabling symptoms (44). Becker disease (299) is inherited recessively, and tends to have a later onset and more severe symptoms, including associated weakness (300).

HYPERKALEMIC PERIODIC PARALYSIS PRESENTATION: BIRTH OR EARLY INFANCY TYPE: METABOLIC MYOPATHY/ION CHANNEL DISORDER

The periodic paralyses are a group of disorders characterized by remitting and relapsing attacks of muscle weakness and flaccidity. They are transmitted as an autosomal dominant trait, with the defect being localized to the sarcoplasmic reticulum and T-tubule system of skeletal muscle. Hyperkalemic periodic paralysis is related to a defect in the sodium channel gene on the long arm of chromosome 17 and usually presents in infancy or childhood (295). Parents may note that the infant has spells during which they become floppy, have difficulty moving, or have a change in the sound of their cry. Attacks typically follow a period of rest after exercise, but may also be precipitated by cold, fasting, or potassium ingestion. Weakness progresses from the legs to the arms and may involve the extraocular and pharyngeal muscles. Attacks typically last from 30 minutes to several hours, but weakness may persist for days and in some patients is associated with myotonia, usually of the face, eyes, and tongue (296). The frequency and duration of attacks vary considerably in the affected patients, but tend to decrease with age, although some go on to develop a mild proximal weakness in adulthood. Affected individuals usually learn to adapt their activities to prevent severe attacks. When they occur, severe attacks can be treated with calcium gluconate and glucose infusion (44).

MITOCHONDRIAL MYOPATHIES PRESENTATION: LATE INFANCY TO EARLY CHILDHOOD TYPE: METABOLIC MYOPATHY

Mitochondrial myopathies are a group of extremely heterogeneous diseases that often have multisystem or nonmuscle tissue-specific involvement that is often characterized by various symptoms of CNS dysfunction. In addition, if symptomatic, the myopathy itself presents variably, and onset can be from infancy to adulthood, be severe or benign, generalized or focal, and may be associated with cramps and fatigue (301).

Mitochondrial abnormalities are related to a distinct morphology in muscle biopsy specimens, with strongly reacting, granular fibers with oxidative reactions and "ragged red" fibers seen with Gomori trichrome staining (302). Electron microscopy will demonstrate the abnormal mitochondria (303). Mitochondria, which are responsible for aerobic energy metabolism, have their own DNA, which primarily codes for proteins involved in the respiratory chain. The mitochondrial genome is subject to a high rate of spontaneous mutation, which can result in a wide range of phenotypes because of the fact that it exists as multiple copies within each cell, as compared to the single copy of nuclear DNA (44).

Mitochondrial disorders tend to affect the more highly oxidative tissues such as the CNS, heart, skeletal muscle, kidney, and liver (304). A large number of specific syndromes related to abnormal mitochondria have been described (305). A recent classification scheme divides mitochondrial diseases into three groups according to genetic etiology, including defects of nuclear DNA, those of mitochondrial DNA, and defects of communication between the two genomes (306). They can be further classified biochemically, according to the specific area of mitochondrial metabolism affected (defects of transport, substrate utilization, Kreb cycle, oxidative-phosphorylation coupling, or respiratory chain). The diseases caused by defects of nuclear DNA have mendelian inheritance and the clinical syndromes include fatal infantile multisystem disorders, encephalomyopathies, and myopathies (44).

Mitochondrial DNA defects may be caused by deletions and point mutations. Deletions are associated with several syndromes, of which Kearns-Sayre syndrome (KSS) is the best described. KSS is a sporadic disorder with ophthalmoplegia, retinal degeneration, heart block, weakness, ataxia, retardation, short stature, sensorineural hearing loss, and endocrine disturbances (307). Point mutations of mitochondrial DNA have been associated with at least five maternally inherited diseases, including myoclonus epilepsy with ragged red fibers (MERRF) and mitochondrial encephalomyopathy, lactic acidosis, and stroke-like episodes (MELAS). When fully expressed, MERRF is characterized by myoclonic seizures, weakness, ataxia, retardation, hearing loss, optic atrophy, and peripheral neuropathy (308). In MELAS, there is normal early development followed by severe, progressive encephalomyopathy characterized by stroke-like episodes (309). In both diseases, the symptoms typically present in childhood or adolescence, and tend to progress depending on the degree of expression.

The mitochondrial diseases have been treated with variable success with dietary manipulations, vitamin and cofactor supplementation, and corticosteroids (304,310). Many patients have a history of developmental delay and can often mimic other more common neuromuscular diseases (44). Once an accurate diagnosis is made, rehabilitation strategies relate to the specific presentation, and will be similar to those described for SMA type I in cases of severe infantile forms, limb girdle dystrophy for milder forms, and metabolic myopathies for those with exercise-related symptoms, along with attention to specific neurologic problems such as cognitive deficits, ophthalmoplegia, and spasticity.

JUVENILE DERMATOMYOSITIS PRESENTATION: LATE INFANCY–EARLY CHILDHOOD TYPE: MYOPATHY/INFLAMMATORY

Juvenile dermatomyositis is a multisystem inflammatory disorder of unknown cause. The main clinical features are proximal muscle weakness, general systemic symptoms, and skin lesions. Malaise, fatigue, or lethargy can be the main presenting complaint (311). In its classic presentation, there is a violaceous discoloration of the upper eyelids and a scaly, erythematous eruption over the malar area of the face with periorbital edema (44). There also may be erythema or a scaly rash over the interphalangeal and metacarpophalangeal joints, knees, elbows, and malleoli. The rash may precede or follow the onset of weakness. The serum creatinine phosphate level is usually elevated and there are myopathic features on the EMG. Inflammatory changes can be seen in muscle biopsy specimens from patients with chronic disease (312).

The course is extremely variable, from complete recovery to rapid death (313). Mortality has been reduced from about one-third of cases to less than 10% over the last two decades, primarily because of the use of steroid treatment. Gastrointestinal and respiratory disorders are the potentially life-threatening complications most commonly seen. Gastrointestinal tract vasculitis may result in mucosal ulceration or viscus perforation. Respiratory muscle weakness results in restrictive lung disease and possible failure. Such complications tend to occur in the patients who present with the most severe symptoms (314). Calcinosis can be another potentially, very debilitating complication that occurs with more chronic disease, but can occur even when weakness has resolved. These calcium deposits form in subcutaneous, interstitial, or muscle tissue, especially over pressure points, and can cause skin ulceration, discomfort, and decreased range of motion. There is no specific treatment for calcinosis, and it can resolve spontaneously (315).

The treatment mainstay of juvenile dermatomyositis has been high-dose steroids. In a review of 47 patients, the best predictor of both good functional outcome and minimal calcinosis was early steroid treatment after the onset of symptoms. A more severely affected subgroup that did poorly despite timely steroid intervention was identified, and it was recommended that these children be given combined immunosuppressive therapy early in the disease, usually methotrexate or azathioprine (316). The course can last for months to years, usually starts insidiously, and can be a single episode, relapsing and remitting, or chronic (313). In one study of outcome, approximately one-third of patients died, one-third had minimal sequelae, and one-third had moderate to severe impairment (317). There is an occasional association with connective tissue disease, but not to malignancy.

Weakness

The weakness is usually proximal and symmetric, but may present in a more generalized fashion in younger children (314). Signs may be frequent falls, difficulty with stairs, or the use of the Gower maneuver for rising from the floor. Muscle pain and tenderness may occur. More vigorous exercise is delayed until the serum CK level—as a measure of disease activity—begins to decrease toward the normal range (318).

Speech

Involvement of the soft palate may result in nasal speech. Involvement of the lower esophagus can cause difficulty swallowing and handling secretions, thus increasing the risk for aspiration. Modified barium swallow studies are useful to evaluate this and patients may need swallowing retraining with speech therapy.

Mobility and Positioning

As mentioned earlier, one-third of patients will go on to have moderate or severe impairments and may need special gait retraining. Toe walking, secondary to heel cord contractures, is often seen.

Contractures

Patients are prone to develop contractures, especially when immobilized during the acute stage of the disease. During this time, passive range of motion exercises and splinting should be pursued to prevent contractures. Later, it is important to remobilize as quickly as possible to avoid disuse atrophy and contractures.

MILD SPINAL MUSCULAR ATROPHY (SMA TYPE III) PRESENTATION: LATE CHILDHOOD TO EARLY ADOLESCENCE TYPE: ANTERIOR HORN CELL DISEASE

Mild SMA is also known as SMA type III or Kugelberg-Welander disease. In contrast to SMA types I and II in which there is significant morbidity and mortality, the impairments seen with SMA type III are relatively mild. Typical onset is late in the first decade or early adolescence, although weakness can be obvious in the early years of life (47). Children affected with SMA type III achieve early developmental milestones, although they may walk somewhat late and then begin to show evidence of mild proximal weakness (see Table 89-2). They may present with a complaint of difficulty keeping up with their peers, climbing stairs, and rising from the floor, which may require use of the Gower maneuver (319). Calf pseudohypertrophy is seen in 10% of patients, and thus SMA type III may resemble DMD (44). As seen in SMA type II, patients also may demonstrate fasciculations and hand tremors (156). As in the other SMAs, when the onset is earlier, there tends to be more pronounced weakness. Restrictive lung disease is rare (see Table 89-3).

The diagnosis may need to be supported with special investigations. CK levels may be elevated slightly to markedly. Examination of muscle biopsy specimens shows a histologic pattern of small-group atrophy versus the large-group atrophy seen in types I and II. In addition, a number of more "myopathic" changes have been described, such as central cores, target fibers, and internal nuclei, thought to be related to the chronicity of this type of SMA (44).

Weakness

In a longitudinal study (155), the degree of weakness was mild and essentially nonprogressive. Weakness is usually confined to the pelvic girdle muscles, and there is often atrophy. In some patients, there is improvement of function that may be the result of reinnervation. Some may show rapid deterioration that may be related to a growth spurt or other factors such as injuries, immobilization, and obesity. Specific strengthening of lower-extremity muscle groups may improve some functional skills.

Mobility

Trendelenburg gait and increased lumbar lordosis are common postural compensations for the pelvic girdle weakness. Stairs and higher gait activities may be difficult. Walking is generally maintained into adulthood. For patients with more severe disease, a wheelchair may be needed for longer distances.

Contractures

Contractures are generally not a major problem, given the mild degree of weakness. The Achilles tendon and shoulder are the most susceptible (155). Ankle range of motion should be monitored, and patients should be placed on a home stretching program for prevention.

Scoliosis

In the longitudinal study by Carter et al (155), spinal deformity was seen in only 7% of patients (see Table 89-3). Scoliosis is more likely to be of significance in the more severely affected patients associated with more wheelchair dependence. Nevertheless, all SMA type III patients should be monitored for scoliosis and its progression (163).

Psychosocial Issues

Affected individuals are of normal intelligence. These children may need an adapted physical education program at school. Since they are of normal intelligence but limited in their physical capacity, every effort should be made to explore appropriate vocational options. The physical impairments of SMA type III may limit participation in manual labor.

JUVENILE MYASTHENIA GRAVIS PRESENTATION: LATE CHILDHOOD TO ADOLESCENCE TYPE: NEUROMUSCULAR JUNCTION DISORDER

This form of myasthenia gravis presents with many clinical features that are similar to the adult form. Both have an autoimmune etiology. Presentation in childhood is usually after the age of 10 years, with about half of the cases presenting before puberty (91). Girls are affected five to six times as much as boys. Onset of the symptoms can be insidious or acute, and weakness can be focal or generalized. Extraocular muscles are invariably involved, with ptosis being the most common clinical finding. Weakness of the facial and bulbar muscles is also common. Limb weakness is proximal, affecting the upper more than the lower extremities, particularly the wrist extensors and neck flexors. Complaints of weakness are related to effort, so problems are typically experienced with reading, chewing, and speaking.

The degree and distribution of the weakness in each patient is extremely variable, even on a day-to-day basis, but the symptoms tend to be worse later in the day or when tired. The course is slowly progressive. There are intermittent exacerbations of severe weakness that may necessitate hospitalization and ventilatory support. The development of permanent weakness in the ocular or limb muscles is common. Anticholinesterase therapy, thymectomy, plasmapheresis, and immunosuppressive medications are used for treatment, and management is based on the extent of the weakness (91). There is a relatively high incidence of spontaneous remission in this form of the disease, especially after thymectomy (320,321). Thymoma is not a feature of the juvenile form, but there is a higher incidence of other autoimmune disorders (44).

HYPOKALEMIC PERIODIC PARALYSIS PRESENTATION: BIRTH OR EARLY INFANCY TYPE: METABOLIC MYOPATHY/ION CHANNEL DISORDER

Transient attacks of paralysis in this disorder are related to hypokalemia. Also inherited as an autosomal dominant trait, it affects males more frequently and more severely (44). Symptoms usually present in the first or second decade and reach a peak in early adult life. Attacks are precipitated by rest after exercise, heavy carbohydrate ingestion, alcohol, cold, and anxiety (44). Weakness can be focal or generalized, and in the latter instance, it typically ascends from the lower extremities and can result in total paralysis, but with sparing of the extraocular and respiratory muscles so that the patient is unable to move, but can still breathe, swallow, and speak. Attacks can last from hours to days and then subside abruptly, but may take 2 to 3 days to completely resolve. There occasionally may be persistent weakness after repeated attacks (296). Severe, acute attacks can be treated with potassium chloride, but the best treatment is prevention by avoiding the usual triggers.

LIMB GIRDLE DYSTROPHY PRESENTATION: LATE CHILDHOOD TO ADOLESCENCE TYPE: MYOPATHY/DYSTROPHY

Classification, Incidence, and Clinical Features

The limb girdle muscular dystrophy (LGMD) syndromes are an extremely heterogeneous group of myopathies with variability in inheritance, onset, and severity. Various reports have described affected kinships in particular geographic locations with variable autosomal inheritance and expression. Molecular genetic research using linkage analysis has led to the localization of several gene loci. These clinical and genetic studies support the clinical observation that LGMD is composed of a wide variety of muscle disorders and is not a distinct disease entity (322). Nevertheless, there currently exists considerable confusion in the literature, with regard to both nomenclature and classification (323).

The autosomal recessive form of the disease is associated with several syndromes. Autosomal recessive muscular dystrophy of childhood (ARMDC) was first described in and is still prevalent among certain inbred communities of North Africa (44). This syndrome, also known as severe childhood autosomal recessive muscular dystrophy (SCARMD), has been related to chromosomal defects localized to at least two sites (13q and 17q) that result in specific abnormalities in the dystrophin-associated glycoproteins (44,324,325). Yet there is considerable phenotypic hetereogeneity even within this relatively genetically homogeneous subtype of LGMD. The onset of symptoms is typically between 3 and 15 years, with a mean of 8.8 years reported in a recent study (324). Earlier age at onset is associated with more rapid progression and earlier loss of ambulation (326). In terms of clinical course of the myopathy, early-onset ARMDC tends to resemble DMD, and later-onset ARMDC tends to resemble BMD, but without calf hypertrophy. The other associated musculoskeletal and cardiopulmonary complications in ARMDC are more like those found in BMD (324). This high degree of clinical overlap highlights the importance and utility of chromosome and dystrophin analysis in the diagnostic evaluation.

Other recessive forms of the disease have been linked to chromosomes 15q and 2p, and are characterized by onset in late childhood or adolescence with moderate progression and primarily pelvifemoral muscle involvement (44).

Several forms of autosomal dominant disease have also been described, and in one form the defect has been localized to chromosome 5q. The most common phenotype is usually referred to as late-onset limb girdle syndrome (327). In this syndrome, the onset of mild weakness, greater in the hip than the shoulder, occurs in the later teens or adulthood and is slowly progressive. Another form of autosomal dominant LGMD, referred to as Bethlem myopathy, is characterized by the childhood onset of mild proximal weakness and atrophy with early flexion contractures of the elbows, ankles, and fingers (328,329).

Diagnosis is supported by a mildly elevated CK level, myopathic EMG findings, and dystrophic changes in muscle biopsy specimens. Intellectual function is normal in all forms. Pulmonary function studies in several subtypes of LGMD indicate a low incidence of severe restrictive lung disease. A higher percentage of respiratory complications and evidence of restrictive lung disease was found in the ARMDC group (324) (see Table 89-3). Such patients may benefit from ventilatory assistance, especially in the setting of infection (330).

Weakness

All forms have primary involvement of the shoulder or hip musculature. The forms with predominantly shoulder or hip involvement tend to have a milder course. Shoulder weakness has a classic clinical presentation, with depressed tips and webbed neck, downward sloping clavicles, and scapular winging. In contrast to facioscapulohumeral muscular dystrophy (FSHMD), the deltoid is involved, and there is selective weakness and often striking atrophy of the biceps (114). Pelvic girdle weakness may involve the paravertebral muscles, quadriceps, and hamstrings as well as the hip flexors and extensors.

Feeding and Self-care

Facial muscles are spared so these patients do not experience difficulties with feeding. In McDonald et al's (324) review of the three major subtypes, only 10% to 20% of patients had significant upper-extremity functional deficits and a higher proportion was seen in the ARMDC group. Such patients may benefit from mobile arm supports. Adaptive equipment and techniques for dressing, eating, and bathing may improve function in patients with less severe weakness who are likely to experience early fatigue.

Mobility

Very mildly affected patients may experience cramps during exercise (44). Most patients experience some difficulty with running, getting up from the floor, and climbing stairs. In the review by McDonald et al (324), 85% of ARMDC patients used a wheelchair part- or full-time, with a range in age of wheelchair reliance of 24 to 42 years. A lower percentage (34%–40%) of subjects using a wheelchair was found in the other later-onset subtypes. As with the other more slowly progressive myopathies, a monitored program of resistance training may improve strength and function. These patients should be encouraged to keep active and avoid prolonged periods of immobility, which might lead to more rapid progression of weakness and loss of function.

Contractures and Scoliosis

Contractures are not frequent, except in the early-onset autosomal dominant syndrome and occasionally in ARMDC (see Table 89-3). This may reflect the fact that there is more equal involvement of the flexor and extensor groups, thus limiting imbalances around joints.

In the review by McDonald et al (324), the ARMDC group had a prevalence and severity of scoliosis similar to those observed in BMD, while spinal deformity was infrequent in the other subtypes.

Psychosocial Issues

It is important to counsel patients and their families about the diagnosis and the difficulty in prognostication. Genetic counseling should be offered to parents of affected children, as there is a 25% chance of having another affected child.

As a group, the LGMD subjects in the profile by McDonald et al (324) did not exhibit symptoms indicative of psychopathology or personality alterations.

FACIOSCAPULOHUMERAL MUSCULAR DYSTROPHY PRESENTATION: LATE CHILDHOOD TO ADOLESCENCE TYPE: MYOPATHY/DYSTROPHY

Classification, Incidence, and Clinical Features

FSHMD has autosomal dominant inheritance and is related to a defect on chromosome 4 (331). The prevalence has been estimated at 3 to 20 per million (114).

In FSHMD, there is relatively less morbidity and no increased mortality compared to the other dystrophies. In addition, there are relatively minimal pathologic changes on muscle biopsy specimens, including fiber size variability, tiny fibers, and vacuoles (114).

The onset can be very insidious, and presentation is generally in the second decade, although it can present in later infancy or adulthood (311). Atrophy commonly occurs in FSHMD and may be out of proportion to weakness. Cardiac abnormalities are not associated and intellectual function is normal (see Table 89-3). While 50% of a series of patients had restrictive lung disease on pulmonary function tests, only 13% had severe involvement and only 22% experienced symptoms (332). Retinal vascular abnormalities (333) and sensorineural hearing loss (334) have been associated, but rarely symptomatic.

Weakness

The weakness first affects the facial muscles, especially the orbicularis oculi, zygomaticus, and orbicularis oris (335). Typically, although signs of facial weakness are present in childhood (incomplete eyelid closure, difficulty blowing up balloons and whistling), significant functional impairments do not usually present until adolescence (336). It may be noticed during school physical fitness screenings when affected youngsters are not able to perform push-ups or climb up a rope. Difficulty with overhead activities and carrying heavy objects are also common complaints on presentation. As in other myopathies, if significant weakness does present earlier in childhood, it is usually indicative of a more severe and progressive course (114,332).

Shoulder girdle weakness is first seen in the scapular fixators (latissimus dorsi, lower trapezius, rhomboids, and serratus anterior), resulting in problems with flexing and abducting the arm, despite relative sparing of deltoid function (114). Striking upriding of the scapula with attempted shoulder abduction is seen on physical examination. Asymmetry of the upper-extremity musculature is common (114), and appears to have a selective pattern, with greater weakness in the shoulder abductors, external rotators, and wrist extensors of the dominant limb (332,337). This may be related to overwork weakness. First described in a study of a three-generation FSHMD kinship that documented increased weakness and needle EMG changes in the dominant upper extremity (338), the overwork theory is controversial. More recent studies of exercise effects in neuromuscular disease in general, and FSHMD in particular, did not find any decrease in strength or evidence of increased muscle damage. In fact, studies of the effects of submaximal resistance training in FSHMD patients showed favorable results (126,127,129,130).

Progression is very slow and occurs in a descending manner from the face, to the shoulder, proximal arm, and then pelvic girdle, with the exception of the anterior tibial muscle, which in many patients becomes involved around the same time as symptomatic shoulder weakness (332,335) (see Table 89-3). Progression may arrest temporarily or permanently at any point, and in 50% of patients, the pelvic girdle muscles are not involved (335). Onset in the pelvic girdle muscles should suggest an alternative diagnosis (311).

Feeding

Chewing and swallowing are not problems, as the masseter and pharyngeal muscles are generally spared. These patients do have difficulty drinking from a straw.

Self-Care

Reaching and overhead activities become increasingly difficult with progression of shoulder weakness. To perform overhead activities, patients often learn to throw the dominant, usually more severely affected, arm overhead and hold it with the other less affected arm. Some benefit has been reported with orthopedic surgery to fix the scapula on the trunk (339). Patients should avoid heavy resistance and excessively repetitive upper-extremity activities to avoid overuse fatigue. However, gradually progressive, moderate- to high-resistance weight-training programs for selected upper-extremity muscles may be helpful (127,129,130).

Mobility and Positioning

Anterior tibial weakness may result in footdrop and the need for bracing at the ankle. Resistance weight training for lower-extremity muscles, especially the quadriceps, may help to maintain independence with transfers and ambulation. Bracing with a knee-ankle-foot orthosis may eventually be required. In the more severely affected patients with significant lower-extremity involvement, power mobility may also be indicated, as propulsion of a manual chair is limited by shoulder weakness.

Contractures

Contractures are not a significant problem (87,332), and this feature is part of the diagnostic criteria for this myopathy (see Table 89-3).

Scoliosis

Pelvic girdle weakness results in compensatory lumbar lordosis that can be extreme in childhood-onset disease (114). Hyperlordosis with and without scoliosis was found in over 50% of patients in one series (332). Scoliosis occurred in about a third of patients and was mild and nonprogressive.

Psychosocial Issues

The majority of patients with FSHMD are mildly affected and do not have significant disability. Even those with significant upper-extremity impairment are likely to be successful in well-chosen occupations (340). A diagnosis of FSHMD should be given, with reassurance about its generally benign course. Genetic counseling should be offered, since with dominant inheritance there is a 50% risk of a child being affected (341). Prenatal and presymptomatic diagnosis is now possible with a closely linked DNA marker (342).

More severely affected children may experience problems in social interactions as a result of facial weakness limiting their expressivity. The bony deformity and atrophy of the upper body may result in teasing and a poor body image, especially in the adolescent. Self-image may not necessarily correspond to the degree of disability (343). In the profile by Kilmer et al (332), FSHMD subjects did not exhibit increased neuropsychological symptoms other than those commonly found in all neuromuscular disease types.

EMERY-DREIFUSS MUSCULAR DYSTROPHY PRESENTATION: LATE CHILDHOOD OR EARLY ADOLESCENCE TYPE: MYOPATHY/DYSTROPHY

Emery-Dreifuss muscular dystrophy is a type of X-linked muscular dystrophy with unique genetics and clinical features (344). The defect has been localized to the long arm of chromosome 27 (345). Dystrophin is normal. There is a classic triad of symptoms: 1) early contractures, 2) slowly progressive myopathy in humeroperoneal distribution, and 3) cardiomyopathy (131). The incidence is estimated to be 1 in 100,000 (131). Although usually regarded as a benign disease, the myopathy can occasionally be severe, and the cardiomyopathy can cause conduction defects manifested as sinus bradycardia with or without syncope and is associated with a high incidence of heart block and sudden death (346) (see Table 89-3). Early evaluation with a Holter monitor and provision of cardiac pacemakers may be lifesaving interventions. The severity of the myopathy and the cardiomyopathy are not proportional (see Table 89-3).

Intellectual function is normal. Some patients may develop symptoms of nocturnal hypoventilation related to limited chest expansion because of a rigid spine. These patients may benefit from nocturnal mask ventilation devices (44).

Weakness

The weakness is mild and has a humeroperoneal distribution with dramatic atrophy of the calves and upper arms, and sparing of the deltoids and forearm muscles (346). With progression, the disease involves more of the shoulder and hip girdle musculature. Mild facial weakness may also be seen.

Feeding and Self-Care

Upper-extremity weakness and limited neck and trunk forward flexion may interfere with ADL performance, but most patients find compensatory strategies and remain functional. Adaptive equipment may be appropriate for some patients.

Mobility

Toe walking is commonly seen in affected children, and orthopedic release of the Achilles tendon may be indicated to improve gait (347). Bracing at the ankle before and after surgery can improve foot clearance and avoid falls. Ambulation is typically maintained into adulthood without significant disability.

Prolonged immobilization should be avoided and an active lifestyle encouraged. A supervised progressive strengthening program may help to maintain or improve strength and function.

Contractures

Contractures develop in childhood before there is any significant weakness, although presentation with tight muscles often does not occur until adolescence or early adulthood (348). Contractures usually involve the elbow flexors, spine extensors, and Achilles tendons (see Table 89-3). A program of frequent range of motion exercises and positioning, directed especially to the neck, elbows, and ankles, should be instituted early in the disease to prevent permanent shortening of the soft-tissue structures.

Psychosocial Issues

Affected children and adolescents may need an adapted physical education program. Depending on the degree of physical impairments and cardiac disease, there may be restrictions on vocational options.

AMYOTROPHIC LATERAL SCLEROSIS PRESENTATION: ADULTHOOD TYPE: ANTERIOR HORN CELL DISEASE

ALS, or Lou Gehrig disease, probably is the most well-known adult-onset neuromuscular disease. ALS is likely multifactorial in origin. Genetic predisposition, a cumulative environmental trigger, and loss of neural reserve have been postulated (349). The cascade of events may ultimately affect the corticomotor neuron, causing excessive glutamate release at the junction with the spinal anterior horn cell (349). Studies are focusing on blocking excessive glutamate release to prevent anterior horn cell death (350). The incidence increases with age from about 0.2 per 100,000 in the third decade to 7.4 per 100,000 in the eighth decade (351,352). There is a familial form that accounts for 5% to 10% of cases (114). The overall incidence is 1.6 to 2.4 per 100,000 and the prevalence is 4 to 6 per 100,000 (351,353). There are populations in geographic locations with much higher occurrence rates, such as W. New Guinea, Jakai, and Auyu tribes (incidence of 1.3%), as well as the Chamorro population on Guam (30 times higher than the average world incidence) (114). An

Table 89-4: Amyotrophic Lateral Sclerosis (ALS)–Related Syndromes					
Syndrome	**Incidence as a Percentage of Total ALS-Related Syndromes**	**Average Survival Time**	**Bulbar Signs**	**UMN Signs**	**LMN Signs**
Primary muscular atrophy	9%	90 mo	+	+	++
Progressive bulbar palsy	1%–2%	18–24 mo	++	+	+
Primary lateral sclerosis	4%	Years to decades	–	++	–
"Typical" ALS	85%	36 mo	+	+	+

Bulbar = involvement of oropharyngeal and facial musculature; UMN = Associated spasticity, lack of severe atrophy (upper motor neuron); LMN = no spasticity, severe atrophy (lower motor neuron).
Source: Adapted from Dumitru D. *Electrodiagnostic medicine.* Philadelphia: Hanley & Belfus, 1995.

association with the Parkinson dementia complex and environmental and genetic factors distinguishes these subsets from "classic" ALS (114).

Males outnumber females approximately two-to-one. The average age at onset is 62 years and the mean survival time is 2.5 years (351). It should be noted that survival times for ALS are much longer with earlier disease onset. Patients with disease onset before 40 years old survive an average of 8 years, whereas if onset is at 60 to 70 years old, survival is 2.5 years (353). Other related syndromes commonly associated with ALS are listed in Table 89-4. These factors should be considered when making treatment decisions.

Onset of focal asymmetric weakness that spreads over weeks to months is the most common complaint. In up to one-third of patients, bulbar weakness is the initial complaint, and heralds a poorer prognosis (354). The presence of upper motor neuron signs such as spasticity may add to disability and helps to distinguish ALS from other diseases. The cause of death is respiratory failure and aspiration (see Chap. 80 for further discussion).

While ALS patients supposedly have a "pure" motor neuronopathy, 80% of patients in one study had decreased thermal sensory thresholds (355). Patients may complain of vague sensory problems. Spasms and cramping of muscles at night, particularly in the legs, occur commonly (114). We saw one patient with cramping of the intercostal muscles resembling angina. Cardiac work-up was negative and the patient responded to phenytoin. Calcium gluconate, quinine, and diazepam may be helpful (114). Caution against using diazepam in patients with respiratory depression is advised. Phenytoin may also be useful and a normal therapeutic level is not always necessary.

Weakness

In the upper extremity, the wrist extensor, finger extensor, and hand intrinsic muscles tend to be weakest, with relative sparing of the wrist and finger flexors and elbow extensors. Other commonly affected muscles are the neck extensors, arm abductors, external rotators, and elbow flexors. In the lower extremities, the ankle dorsiflexor, invertor, and evertor muscles are weakest, with relative sparing of the ankle plantarflexors. Later, the knee extensors and hip girdle musculature become weak (355). Bulbar weakness tends to involve muscles innervated by cranial nerves X, XI, and XII more than V and VII and usually sparing the extraocular muscles (356).

The role of exercise in a rapidly progressive motor neuron disease is controversial. Regional ischemia of the forearm muscles during rest and exercise has been demonstrated (357). Based on this metabolic study, maximal exercise is not recommended. Muscular fatigue is a frequent complaint among ALS patients, which discourages some individuals from regular exercise to conserve strength for ADLs. A recent study demonstrated greater muscular fatigue (decreased maximal voluntary contraction and tetanic force) in ALS patients than control subjects after intermittent low-intensity isometric exercise (358). Excessive muscular fatigue was not due to diminished central activation or neuromuscular junction failure. Instead, decreased excitation-contraction coupling and calcium pump defects have been cited (358). Using prolonged (90-minute), progressive resistance bicycle ergometer exercise, ALS patients demonstrated decreased work capacity and decreased maximum oxygen consumption. These decreases correlated to a decline in functional score. There were increases in serum-free fatty acid, lactate, and β-hydroxybutyric acid levels in patients compared with control subjects (359).

In general, ALS patients show an abnormal response to exercise at the muscle level and systemic metabolic level, which decreases the tolerance to exercise. This is more pronounced in more severely involved patients. The recommendation that exercise above and beyond that provided by ADLs is warranted only in patients with mild difficulties and for slowly progressive disease appears to have support from metabolic studies.

Mobility

Approximately 20% of patients with ALS present with lower-extremity weakness, mainly footdrop, while most other patients develop it later. Because the plantarflexors and quadriceps are relatively spared, they may benefit from hinged AFOs to improve ambulation. ALS patients become wheelchair bound in 12 to 18 months on average (114). Whether patients require an electric or manual wheelchair depends on the distribution and degree of muscle weakness.

Patients with significant plantarflexor spasticity require regular heel cord stretching. The use of oral medications to control spasticity has not been well studied in ALS patients. One small study did not demonstrate a significant reduction in spasticity in patients (n = 9) taking 80 mg of baclofen per day over 5 weeks compared to placebo controls (n = 11) (360). The physiologic basis of spasticity differs in ALS patients versus spinal cord injury (SCI) patients. In ALS, there is a reduced recurrent inhibition via Renshaw cells, whereas with SCI this is increased (361). The use of oral medications may be limited by their side effects. Dantrolene sodium may cause muscle weakness, diazepam may cause sedation and respiratory depression, and baclofen may cause sedation as well as subjective weakness. Intramuscular injections of botulinum toxin are not recommended for ALS patients (362). The irreversible blockade of neuromuscular junctions causes collateral nerve sprouting to denervated muscle fibers. ALS patients already are having collateral sprouting due to α motor neuron loss. Phenol 5% solution causes a reversible axonotmesis of either the nerve trunk or motor point and can be used.

Contracture

Because of muscle imbalance, myotendinous contractures may occur in ALS patients. The most commonly involved are the finger and wrist flexors, shoulder internal rotators and adductors, as well as ankle plantarflexors. Intrinsic hand muscle weakness may cause a "claw hand" type of deformity (114). Twice-daily prolonged stretch to the affected muscles is primary treatment. Splinting with a static wrist-hand orthosis or AFO may be necessary. Management of underlying spasticity, if present, will also be of benefit.

Feeding

Swallowing problems occur in at least 73% of ALS patients before they require ventilatory support (363). The patients with severe bulbar involvement are at highest risk, as the laryngeal muscles innervated by cranial nerve X and the lingual muscles innervated by cranial nerve XIII are the most commonly affected. Most patients have more problems with solids than liquids, and a diet of pureed food or soft solids that stick together may be beneficial (364). Discoordinated contraction of the cricopharyngeal muscle can inhibit bolus passage so that cricopharyngeal myotomy may be necessary (364). Patients should be evaluated with videofluoroscopic swallowing studies if symptoms such as coughing after meals or food sticking in the back of the throat occur. Dietary modifications of food and liquid consistency as well as use of compensatory techniques may be helpful. For patients with pharyngeal constrictor weakness, clearing leafy vegetables may be particularly difficult. Severe cases may require gastrostomy tube feeding to prevent aspiration. Patients who aspirate their secretions may require surgical intervention (264). See Table 89-5 for a summary of swallowing interventions (364).

Psychosocial Issues

While cognitive dysfunction is not typical of ALS, several case series and small controlled studies demonstrated decreased memory and lower scores on selected neuropsychological tests (365). This may be more common with familial ALS (366). Emotional/lability occurs in about one-fourth of ALS patients (367). This should be differentiated from psychological dysfunction including depression.

Since ALS is a rapidly progressive, fatal disease, the issues of death and dying are prominent even early after diagnosis. Adjusting to the loss of body integrity has been compared to the stages presented by Kubler-Ross, namely denial, depression, anger, anxiety, and acceptance. Successful psychological adjustment involves focusing on the areas of life and self that are controllable and, after a period of mourning, accepting those areas that are not under the patient's control. Premorbid issues such as fear of trusting others need to be addressed as the patient becomes more dependent (368). Discussion regarding the use of respiratory aids or gastrostomy tube feedings should occur before there are severe problems with hypoventilation and dysphagia.

Special Considerations

Communication problems may result from dysarthria. Vocal quality may be harsh and strangled (spastic dysarthria) or breathy with audible inspirations (flaccid dysarthria), or may be a combination (364,369). Patients with bulbar ALS rarely have normal speech, progress to a more severe dysarthria, and may require an augmentative communication device (ACD). The rate of progression is quite variable, with some patients requiring an ACD within a year after diagnosis while others barely change over several years (370).

Compensatory strategies such as reducing the rate of speech, reducing the length of a phrase supported by one breath, and using a palatal lift (for patients with poor velopharyngeal function but adequate lip and tongue movement) may be helpful for mild to moderate dysarthria (364,371). In patients with moderate to severe dysarthria, an ACD may be needed. ACDs may range from a pen and writing pad, to voice amplifiers (for patients with reduced breath support), to voice synthesizers controlled by eye gaze (372,373). Appropriate selection of ACDs is based on residual speech function, upper-extremity function, and rate of progression and has been reviewed elsewhere (364,371–375). See Table 89-6 for a summary of speech interventions (364).

Table 89-5: Summary of Swallowing Intervention in Amyotrophic Lateral Sclerosis

	Early Swallowing Problems	Dietary Consistency Changes	Unable to Meet Needs Orally	Salivary Problems
Presenting features	Solid foods difficult to eat Longer mealtimes Need for smaller bites	Weight loss Chronic dehydration Loss of enjoyment	Decline in calorie intake Decline in fluid intake Food spillage from mouth Respiratory fatigue	Complaint of too much saliva Complaints of drooling
Intervention	Use chin tuck position Maintain liquid Try drinking through a straw Eliminate caffeine Use double swallow Learn choking first aid Avoid washing foods down with liquids	Change to soft diet Maintain liquid Eat calorie-dense foods Increase taste, temperature (colder), and texture sensations of liquids	Insert percutaneous endoscopic gastrostomy (PEG) or insert nasogastric tube	Maintain adequate hydration Use aspirator Use medication Surgically relocate salivary ducts

Source: Reproduced by permission from Yorkston KM, Miller RM, Strand EA. *Management of speech and swallowing in degenerative diseases.* Tucson: Communication Skill Builders, 1995.

ADULT-ONSET SPINAL MUSCULAR ATROPHY

A number of names (i.e., Aran Duchenne SMA type IV, progressive muscular atrophy) have been given to a slowly progressive disorder of the α motor neuron. Autosomal dominant, autosomal recessive, X-linked recessive, and sporadic cases have been described, raising the suspicion that the clinical syndrome is common to a number of diseases (355). The incidence has been reported as 0.02 to 0.5 per 100,000, with a male-female ratio of 6 or 7 to 1 (355). The incidence of the autosomal dominant form in England is reported to be 1 per 100,000, but is lower in the United States (376). Onset is between the ages 30 and 60 years, although the X-linked form may present between the ages 20 and 40 years (61,64,377–379). The mean survival time is 7 to 10 years, but sometimes longer than 15 years, and it improves with earlier age at onset (355,380). Lack of upper motor neuron signs and development of bulbar signs only very late in the disease process set this apart from ALS (355,381). Adult-onset SMA is very difficult to differentiate from the primary muscular atrophy variant of ALS and survival times, incidence, and male-female ratio are virtually identical. A pattern of inheritance may be the only differentiating factor. Aspiration pneumonia is a usual cause of death (382).

Weakness

Most patients present with asymmetric weakness and atrophy of the intrinsic hand muscles, causing difficulties with fine motor tasks. Cold will exacerbate weakness. Involvement spreads to the foot intrinsic and distal leg muscles. The shoulder girdle and proximal arm weakness is followed by pelvic girdle and proximal leg weakness. Trunk and bulbar muscles are affected last, with rare involvement of the diaphragm (64,355,381,382).

Although the literature does not specifically address adult-onset SMA, several patients have been included in studies of slowly progressive neuromuscular disease. One adult SMA patient with markedly weak (15%–25% of normal strength) knee extensors was able to double his/her strength after 12 months of light-resistance exercise using ankle weights. This patient worked up to five sets of 6 to 10 repetitions, four times a week. No detrimental effects were noted (383). A study combining electric stimulation and a low-resistance weight-training program in two adults (55 years old) and one adolescent (17 years old) demonstrated significant improvements in knee extensor strength. Patients doubled their isometric strength after 2 to 6 months of training. One-kilogram to 2.5-kg ankle weights were used in conjunction with femoral nerve stimulation of up to 2 hours, 5 days a week. No detrimental effects were recorded (129).

Mobility

While patients remain ambulatory until later stages of the disease, early involvement of distal leg muscles may require use of an AFO (64). Since quadriceps strength is preserved until later in the disease process, hinged AFOs may be used. Assistive devices such as canes and walkers may be useful, if hand function permits, to improve balance deficits due to weakness. Either a manual or electric wheelchair may be used later in the course of the illness, depending on the degree and distribution of weakness.

Contracture

Myotendinous contractures may occur due to muscle imbalance. Since spasticity is not present in adult SMA, contractures may not be as common as with ALS, but occur in similar muscles.

Feeding

While bulbar weakness is not typical of adult SMA, it may occur late in the disease process and can cause dysphagia (355). Truncal weakness may impair cough and increase aspiration risk. Diaphragmatic involvement is rare (130). Treatment of feeding problems is similar to that in ALS except that cricopharyngeal dysfunction is not reported. Gastrostomy tube feeding may be needed to prevent aspiration (see next section).

Psychosocial Issues

While adult SMA is a fatal disease, discussions of death and dying are not urgently needed, owing to the prolonged course of illness. Since respiratory failure may occur, discussions regarding use of respiratory muscle aids should occur prior to the development of signs of hypoventilation (see Chap. 80). Also, since aspiration pneumonia is the cause of death, discussion on the use of gastrostomy tubes for feeding is appropriate prior to the development of severe dysphagia. For patients with early-onset disease, establishment of the mode of inheritance and prognosis is important for family planning.

MYASTHENIA GRAVIS

Myasthenia gravis (MG) is an autoimmune disease associated with a decreased number of nicotinic acetylcholine (Ach) receptors at the motor end-plate, reduced postsynaptic membrane folds, and a widened synaptic cleft (355). Antibodies to Ach receptors are present in up to 53% to 80% of patients (383). While an annual incidence of 1 per 20,000 is commonly quoted, most studies reported incidences of 1.1 to 9.1 per 1,000,000 (384–393). Five percent of cases are "familial," although no pattern of inheritance is known (383). Untreated, the death rate is 35% to 50%, but MG is a rare cause of death in the appropriately treated patients (394,395). The female-male ratio before age 40 years is 7:3; after 40 years, it is 1:1. In both genders, there is a bimodal peak of age distribution, with one peak in young adulthood and the other peak after age 70 years (396).

Clinically the disease presents as a fluctuating weakness that worsens during the course of a day and with heat, and improves with rest (355,383,397–400). The majority of patients present with bulbar weakness (356). There is typically a course of exacerbation and remissions, which can be unpredictable. Spontaneous remission may occur in 5% to 10% of patients. The two main types of MG are ocular and generalized. Approximately half of the patients who present with ocular symptoms only develop generalized disease within a year (355,383).

Managed with medications, over 85% of patients show marked improvement, with about 30% showing complete remission (396,401). Prednisone has been used as a first-line agent and is effective in 70% to 80% of patients. Azathioprine is used both as a first- and second-line agent; cyclosporine and cyclophosphamide are third- and fourth-line agents, respectively. While cholinesterase inhibitors such as pyridostigmine and neostigmine improve weakness, they do not alter the disease course. Thymomas occur in approximately 10% of patients with MG and thymectomy is recommended. Improvement in disease course occurs in one-third of patients with thymoma, following thymectomy (402).

While respiratory failure and myasthenic crises are rare with current medication regimens, it is a danger in noncompliant patients and in severely affected individuals. Drowsiness, agitation, tachycardia, decreased alertness, and poor concentration are all signs of potential impending respiratory failure (355). Excessive use or an overdose of cholinesterase inhibitors can result in gastrointestinal hypermotility, vomiting, sialorrhea, and sweating, and anticholinergic reversal may become necessary (399).

The clinician should be aware of associated illnesses that may occur in MG patients. These may include polymyositis, systemic lupus erythematosus, rheumatoid arthritis, ulcerative colitis, and hyperthyroidism or hypothyroidism (114). Due to chronic use of corticosteroids, patients with MG are at risk for osteoporotic fractures and avascular necrosis.

Weakness

As noted earlier, weakness in MG increases with fatigue and heat. Also, the relapsing and remitting nature of the disease will cause variations in muscular strength. Approximately 20% to 30% of patients present with proximal limb and neck weakness (355). Over 70% of patients eventually have weakness in the neck, trunk, proximal limb, and bulbar musculature.

Strength training has not been extensively studied in MG patients. Since exercise, especially maximal, stresses

Table 89-6: Summary of Speech Intervention in Amyotrophic Lateral Sclerosis					
	Normal Speech Process	Detectable Speech Disturbance	Behavioral Modifications	Use of Augmentative Communication	Loss of Useful Speech
Presenting features	No changes or minimal changes are detected	Symptoms worsen with fatigue Changes are noticed by unfamiliar partners	Some reduction in speech intelligibility Need for repetition	Needs augmentative communication systems as primary or secondary system	No functional natural speech
Intervention	Confirm normalcy Answer questions	Minimize environmental adversity Establish context of message Maximize hearing of partners Teach strategies for copying with groups	Maintain slow speaking rate Conserve energy Fit with palatal life Develop breakdown resolution strategies Increase the precision of speech production	Begin alphabet supplement Suggest changing mode in different situations Set up alerting systems Teach strategies for telephone communication Introduce portable writing systems Introduce multipurpose communication systems	Develop adequate yes/no system Develop eye-gaze systems Enable communication for patients on ventilators

Source: Reproduced by permission from Yorkston KM, Miler RM, Strand EA. *Management of speech and swallowing in degenerative diseases*. Tucson: Communication Skill Builders, 1995.

the neuromuscular junction, it is theoretically inadvisable to recommend this to MG patients. A case report linked exacerbation of weakness in an MG patient to the use of therapeutic electric stimulation (402). In a small study of patients with mild to moderate MG, knee extensor strength improved after a 10-week training program using free weights in a sitting position. Patients performed two or three sets of 10 repetitions starting at 25% of maximum isometric force, working up to 40%. No adverse reactions were noted. For both elbow flexor and extensor strengthening, patients could not advance the amount of weight and number of sets on the same schedule just mentioned, and no improvements were seen in these areas (403). Based on this small study, moderate-intensity isometric strengthening in the lower limb appears safe in patients with mild disease.

Mobility

Patients with MG generally remain ambulatory unless they have severe disease. Gait may have a waddling quality due to hip abduction weakness. Fatigue may be a major limiting factor and afternoon rest periods may be beneficial. Air conditioning may help maintain mobility in a hot environment.

Feeding and Swallowing

While dysphagia is the presenting symptom in only 6% to 15% of patients with MG, it eventually occurs in 33% to 40% (355,383,404,405). In one survey, over 50% of respondents with MG had to exclude certain food items, owing to consistency. Both oral and pharyngeal phases are affected (406). Since MG affects striated muscle, only the upper portion of the esophagus typically shows decreased amplitude and increased duration of the peristaltic wave on manometric testing. The cricopharyngeal muscle shows reduced pressure, but relaxation and coordination are good, so that myotomy would be of no benefit (407). Oral mucosa dryness due to associated Sjögren syndrome or corticosteroids can interfere with the oral phase of swallowing. Depending on the specific complaint, dietary modification is often necessary but tube feeding is not needed.

Contracture

While any problems causing immobility may cause myotendinous contracture, this is not usually a problem in MG, because of the varying nature of the weakness.

Psychosocial Issues

Since stress may provoke exacerbation of disease activity, relaxation techniques may be useful. While family planning issues per se are not a factor in MG (i.e., not a hereditary disease), females with this disease should be advised of possible exacerbation of weakness, dysphagia, and respiratory difficulties with pregnancy (408–410). Transient neonatal MG is discussed elsewhere in this chapter.

The sometimes unpredictable nature of relapse makes coping with MG difficult. Patients may achieve some control over their illness by adjusting their cholinesterase inhibitors and corticosteroids in conjunction with their physician (402).

Myotonic Dystrophy

Myotonic dystrophy is the most common adult form of neuromuscular disease, with an incidence of 13 per 100,000 and a prevalence of 50 per 100,000 (131,355,411). Higher figures have been found in northern Quebec, Guam, and northern Transvaal (412–414). Inheritance is autosomal dominant, with genetic studies showing an increase in the CTG repeat sequence on chromosome 19q. The number of repeat sequences also separates the congenital versus the adult-onset ("noncongenital") forms of this disease, with more repeat sequences in the former (412,415,416). The adult form of this disease has a median onset at 21.2 years and a mean of 23 ± 13 years. The 10-year mortality in one study was 21%, with the mean age at death 55 ± 12 years (417). Myotonic dystrophy is truly a multiorgan system disease, as summarized in Table 89-7 (418).

Insulin receptor abnormalities may occur; however, clinical diabetes is uncommon. Early cataract formation is common; slit-lamp ophthalmoscopic examinations by an ophthalmologist can detect cataracts (114).

Patients with a "drawing" type of pain may be treated with carbamazepine, phenytoin, or quinidine. β-Blockers may worsen the myotonia while aminergic tricyclic antidepressants may improve it (419). Quinine, procainamide, and calcium channel blockers have been used to treat pain with myotonia but should be used with caution, as these patients already have a high incidence (33%) of P-R interval prolongation (114).

Table 89-7: Systematic Features of Myotonic Dystrophy

Heart	Conduction block* Atrial and ventricular arrhythmias* Increased incidence of sudden cardiac death* Dilating cardiomyopathy (rare) Mitral valve prolapse (common but benign)
Eye	Early lens opacities* Cataract* Ptosis* Poor rapid eye movements (saccades) Retinal pigmentary change
Central nervous system	Low average IQ* Hypersomnolence* Apathetic personality trait
Integument	Frontal balding (most marked in men) Association with multiple pilomatrixomas
Smooth muscle	Oesophagus (dysphagia) Colon (constipation, colic, faecal soiling) Gallbladder (higher incidence of stones at younger age) Uterus (tendency to poor labour)
Endocrine	Testicular tubular atrophy Secondary increase in FSH (±LH) Hyperresponsiveness of insulin to a glucose load Peripheral insulin resistance Clinical diabetes mellitus is uncommon
Skeletal	Cranial hyperostosis Small pituitary fossa Large paranasal sinuses

FSH = follicle-stimulating hormone; LH = luteinizing hormone.
Source: Reproduced by permission from Barnes PRJ. Clinical and genetic aspects of myotonic dystrophy. *Br J Hosp Med* 1993;50(1):22–30.

Weakness

Distal weakness and footdrop are frequently the presenting symptoms of myotonic dystrophy, although the trunk and neck flexors are the weakest overall, with an average MMT grade of 3/5. The limb muscles average in the 4/5 range, with greater involvement of the ankle dorsiflexors and plantarflexors, and invertor and evertors, and relative sparing of the quadriceps. Disease progression is slow. The average loss of strength is approximately 0.3 grade per decade (417). Due to the insensitivity of routine MMT, use of more quantitative measures such as dynamometry may document progression more accurately.

While there are no large studies demonstrating the effect of exercise training, there are small studies in which myotonic dystrophy patients made up a portion of the study subjects. Patients who had less than 5% to 10% of normal strength did not benefit from an isotonic strengthening program (129,420). Patients with more than 10% of normal strength were able to significantly increase strength in the knee extensors using ankle weights (130). Patients using a moderate-resistance program (up to 40% isometric maximum, three sets of four to eight repetitions, three times a week) showed similar improvement in knee extensor strength as those patients using a high-resistance program (five sets, four times a week) over a 12-week period (129,130). Elbow flexor strength did not improve in one study using high-resistance weight training, worsened in another study, and showed some improvement with moderate exercise (128–130). All studies gradually added one set per week during the first month of training. In one study, myotonic dystrophy patients showed no improvement in knee extensor or flexor strength after a 24-week training course using isotonic ankle weight exercises. This study used high-resistance exercises (60%–80% of maximum) but only 3 days a week (421). These results suggest that moderate-intensity (up to 40% isometric maximum) knee extensor exercises may be the most efficient way to increase quadriceps strength in myotonic dystrophy patients.

Exercise tolerance may be limited owing to cardiopulmonary factors. The mean oxygen uptake is only 42% of predicted values and the maximal heart rate is only 79% of predicted values; therefore, intensive aerobic exercise should be avoided (418). One small study using a moderate-intensity unsupervised walking program showed a significant ($p < 0.05$) improvement in aerobic capacity after 12 weeks of training. Patients ambulated without devices for 15 to 30 minutes per day, 3 or 4 days per week. The target heart rate (HR) was determined as follows: (maximum HR − resting HR) x + resting HR, where x = 50% to 60% (422). No adverse effects were reported. Based on cardiac conduction problems, atrial and ventricular arrhythmias, as well as an increased incidence of sudden cardiac death, any cardiac symptomatology should be thoroughly evaluated, particularly if one is considering an exercise program.

The symptoms of myotonia, a delay in the relaxation of a muscle once it contracts, is not a disabling condition in adult myotonic dystrophy patients. Myotonia occurs mainly in the hand, intrinsic, and forearm flexor muscles, but occasionally in the more proximal upper-extremity muscles. Myotonia is most pronounced early in the disease process and subsides with increasing weakness. It can be exacerbated by cold (355,420). It should be considered when prescribing exercise in the upper extremities, which involves tight gripping, but is not a factor for lower-extremity exercise.

Mobility

As mentioned, myotonic dystrophy patients generally remain ambulatory until very late in the disease course, but usually require bilateral AFOs once ankle dorsiflexor strength falls below 4/5. Since the quadriceps are generally spared, these patients can tolerate a hinged orthosis. They may also benefit from use of a cane to improve balance.

Contracture

Although contractures are not a significant problem in these patients, mild ankle plantarflexor and wrist flexor tightness may occur. These are myotendinous in nature and respond to prolonged stretching on a daily basis. Splinting is not necessary.

Feeding

While feeding itself is not a problem with myotonic dystrophy patients, swallowing may be, particularly late in the course of the disease. Facial weakness can impact the oral stage of swallowing and its severity is inversely related to disease onset. Esophageal dysmotility occurs with the smooth muscle effects of the disease. Patients may complain of food "sticking" in the sternal area. Cold liquids cause more problems than warm ones. Aspiration may occur at night. Diminished pulmonary muscle function may contribute to aspiration pneumonia (114,419).

Modified barium swallow studies will show oral stage problems, but not esophageal phase ones; therefore, a standard barium swallow study may be needed as well.

Psychosocial Issues

Of all muscular dystrophies, myotonia dystrophy produces the greatest and most consistent psychosocial adjustment problems. Thirty-five percent of patients fall in the clinically impaired range. Cognitive impairment overall is rated as mild, with particular problems relating to visuospatial constructional abilities. On the Minnesota Multiphasic Personality Inventory, 30% were found to be in the depressed range and 53% had hopelessness and hostility. Brooke (114) and others (418) observed that these patients tend to minimize the impact of their disease and not recognize its occurrence in family members.

Family Planning

Since this disease has an autosomal dominant mode of transmission, genetic counseling is important. With chromosome studies, both prenatal and postnatal screening is possible. Men may have infertility due to poor development of the seminiferous tubules. Females with this disease may have menstrual irregularities and infertility as well (114).

POLYMYOSITIS AND DERMATOMYOSITIS

Polymyositis (PM) and dermatomyositis (DM) are usually considered together as idiopathic inflammatory myopathies, owing to the similar clinical manifestations, except for the dermatologic findings seen in DM (355). Immunologic distinctions have become apparent. PM is believed to be T cell mediated with increased levels of J0-1 autoantibodies, while DM is B cell mediated with increased MI-2 autoantibodies (423,424). Histologically, PM has more muscle fiber inflammatory infiltrate while DM has more perivascular and perimysial infiltrates. While DM has both childhood and adult forms, PM presents almost exclusively in patients over 18 years old (425). The overall incidence is reported as 0.2 to 0.9 per 100,000; it is most common in black females (426–428). While mortality rates have been declining with appropriate medical management, these diseases are still potentially fatal, owing to cardiopulmonary involvement, with a mortality rate of 15% reported (429). Severe dysphagia with aspiration pneumonia can be fatal if not treated appropriately (see Feeding). High-dose prednisone results in complete improvement in 25% of patients and partial improvement in 61%, with DM showing a better response than PM (430). On the other hand, avascular necrosis and osteoporotic compression fractures resulting from steroid use contribute significantly to disability (431).

PM and DM are truly systemic diseases. Pulmonary function test results are abnormal in 50% of patients and show a restrictive pattern. Interstitial lung disease occurs in

5% to 10% of patients and may be fatal. Parenchymal lung disease occurs in 60% of patients with antisynthetase autoantibodies (e.g., J0-1) and may include interstitial pneumonia, diffuse alveolar damage, and bronchiolitis obliterans. Because of a high incidence of bronchogenic carcinoma in patients with PM or DM, any abnormal-appearing chest x-ray film may warrant further investigation such as chest computed tomography (432,433).

Arrhythmia and cardiomyopathy were seen in 33 of 55 patients with PM or DM studied retrospectively. Cardiac arrhythmias include atrioventricular block, premature ventricular contractions, and ventricular and supraventricular tachycardias. Congestive heart failure may result from myocardial inflammation (426). Adult DM is associated with a 10% to 20% incidence of neoplasia, most commonly breast, lung, ovarian, and stomach carcinomas (114). About 15% of patients with PM have a collagen vascular disease such as systemic lupus erythematosus, polyarteritis nodosa, or scleroderma (114). Up to 28% of patients have Raynaud phenomena (114,431).

Weakness

Hip extensor and quadriceps weakness is followed by shoulder abductor and flexor weakness as the most commonly involved muscles at onset (114,434). The pattern of weakness is usually symmetric, but occasionally PM or DM will present asymmetrically and become symmetric later (435). Progression may be acute (over weeks) or subacute to chronic (weeks to months). Proximal involvement is classic, but distal involvement in up to 25% of patients has been reported. The neck flexors show more weakness than the extensors. Muscle aching may occur in the buttocks, calves, and shoulders in 15% of patients, most often in those with concomitant connective tissue disease or arthritis (430).

Muscle strengthening exercise has not been well studied in PM or DM patients. One study using magnetic resonance spectroscopy found that weakness during leg lifts was secondary to poor utilization of energy substrates rather than muscle damage from inflammation. Counter to what is commonly believed, there was no connection between weakness and creatine phosphokinase values (436). Another study investigated cardiopulmonary response to cycle ergometry exercise. Although pulmonary hypertension was seen in 7 of 11 patients, it was asymptomatic. The testing was terminated early in 9 of 11 patients due to limb muscle weakness (436). During exacerbations, heat, massage, and passive range of motion exercises have been recommended. Isometric exercises can be added at the subacute phase, followed by active isotonic and resistive exercises (431). Differentiation of exacerbations of PM or DM from steroid myopathy may be aided by magnetic resonance imaging using Sher tau inversion recovery (431).

Contracture

Muscle inflammation and damage may result in myogenic (intrinsic) contractures, if range of motion exercises are not instituted. Susceptible joints include the wrist, elbow, and shoulder (426).

Mobility

Patients with PM or DM generally remain ambulatory but may require assistive devices such as manual wheelchairs during exacerbations.

Feeding

Dysphagia occurs in 20% to 50% of patients with PM or DM (437–440). Striated muscle weakness in the hypopharynx and upper esophagus causes decreased propulsion of the food bolus into the esophagus. Pressures generated in the hypopharynx may not be able to overcome a fibrotic cricopharyngeal muscle or the prolonged pharyngeal transit time may miss the relaxation of the cricopharyngeal muscle (441). There is evidence of smooth muscle involvement in the lower esophagus and delayed gastric emptying (441). Videofluoroscopic examination may show pharyngeal pooling and decreased contrast below the cricopharyngeal muscle (441). Solid dysphagia exceeds liquid dysphagia, and frequent small feedings, softer solid consistencies, frequent sips of liquids, and a slow feeding rate can improve symptoms (442). Upright positioning during and after meals can improve reflux symptoms (442). Cricopharyngeal myotomy may alleviate dysphagia in patients who fail to respond to conservative measures (442). Patients with very severe disease may require gastrostomy feedings to maintain nutrition. Unless they have more distal muscle involvement, most patients can feed themselves.

Psychosocial Issues

Since no hereditary factors have been identified, there are no family planning issues related to transmission. Although PM or DM has a relapsing-remitting course, exacerbations associated with pregnancy, such as those observed with MG, are not commonly seen. With appropriate medical care, mortality directly associated with PM or DM is limited to the most severely affected patients; however, PM is associated with collagen vascular diseases and DM is associated with neoplasms, both of which contribute to mortality.

INCLUSION BODY MYOSITIS

Once considered rare, inclusion body myositis (IBM) is recognized as a common form of idiopathic inflammatory myopathy. In one study, it accounted for 28% of diagnosed myopathies and was second only to PM (443). Like PM, IBM is thought to be a T cell–mediated disease but rare cases have shown an autosomal dominant or recessive pattern (424,425,444,445). The mean age at onset is 56 years, but it may present in the fifth, sixth, or seventh decade. The average duration from symptom onset to diagnosis is 6.3 years. A 3:1 male predominance has been reported. The clinical symptomatology and resistance to treatment with immunosuppressive agents set this disease apart from other inflammatory myopathies. Many patients are initially diagnosed with PM, but after lack of a response to medications, further investigations point to IBM. Systemic symptoms such as fever and myalgias are absent. Polyneuropathy is present in 15% to 20% of patients with IBM (431,443,446–449).

IBM is associated with other immune-mediated diseases such as systemic lupus erythematosus, Sjögren syndrome, interstitial lung disease, idiopathic thrombocytopenic purpura, and diabetes mellitus (443). Patients with IBM may have distal lower-extremity paresthesias that may or may not be associated with concomitant diabetic neuropathy.

Weakness

A slowly progressive but relentless pattern of weakness has been described. Patients progress to severe incapacitation over a decade or longer. In one large series, 30 of 40 patients presented with lower-extremity weakness only. The most severely affected lower-limb muscles included the quadriceps, iliopsoas, and anterior tibial muscles. In this same series, 29 of 30 patients had proximal onset of lower-extremity weakness (443). Anterior tibial weakness may be due to the peripheral neuropathy associated with IBM. Isolated upper-extremity weakness may be the presenting sign in about 15% of patients. The most severely affected upper-extremity muscles include the biceps and triceps. Patients may also present with various combinations of upper- and lower-extremity distal or proximal weakness (443). Rarely, patients may have facial weakness, mild in severity (355,426).

No studies have looked specifically at exercise in IBM patients. See Polymyositis and Dermatomyositis for guidelines.

Mobility

Patients with ankle dorsiflexor weakness may benefit from AFO, whereas those with more isolated quadriceps weakness may require a knee orthosis. A knee-ankle-foot orthosis is not usually needed. Most patients remain ambulatory but may need a cane for balance. Many patients need a motorized scooter or wheelchair for longer distances (426).

Feeding

If distal weakness is severe, built-up utensils or even a universal cuff may be needed for self-feeding. Dysphagia is present at onset in 10% of IBM patients and 40% of patients at the time of diagnosis (average duration from disease onset to diagnosis, 6.3 years). The mechanism of dysphagia is paresis of the pharyngeal wall with delayed emptying of the food bolus while the upper esophageal sphincter is open. Symptoms of repetitive swallows per bolus and choking with solids are common, and may improve with cricopharyngeal myotomy if pharyngeal weakness is not severe (426,450–452). (See Feeding section under Polymyositis and Dermatomyositis.)

Psychosocial Issues

Due to the later age at onset and rare genetic transmission, family planning is not an issue. IBM is slowly progressive but may be fatal, and patients with more advanced disease should be counseled accordingly. Patients should be prepared for progressive disability and perhaps loss of ambulation. Those with severe dysphagia may need gastrostomy feeding and this possibility should be discussed.

OCULOPHARYNGEAL DYSTROPHY

Oculopharyngeal muscular dystrophy is a relatively rare muscle disease, but has unique physical findings. It is more prevalent among French-Canadians in Quebec; Spanish-Americans in southern Colorado, northern New Mexico, and Arizona; and Jews from eastern Europe (453–455). Onset is in the fourth to sixth decade and transmission is autosomal dominant (354,426). Symptoms include progressive external ophthalmoplegia, prominent dysphagia during progressive ptosis, and sparing of pupillary responses (114,355,401,426,456,457). A normal life span may be preserved with appropriate management of dysphagia.

Weakness

While progressive weakness is most severe in extraocular and pharyngeal muscles (114,355,426), mild hip and shoulder girdle involvement may occur later in the disease process. A Japanese form of the disease may have distal limb weakness (458).

Mobility

Ambulation is typically not impaired, although step climbing and arising from low surfaces may be impaired with hip weakness.

Contractures

Patients with hip and shoulder girdle involvement would benefit from range of motion exercises; otherwise contractures are not a major issue.

Feeding

Dysphagia can be potentially life-threatening if not appropriately treated. Pharyngeal weakness may result in slow or diminished propulsion of the food bolus into the esophagus and a sensation of sticking in the throat. Solid dysphagia is more common than liquid dysphagia and repeated efforts at swallowing are the rule (114,426). In one study, 4 of 17 patients presented with a weight loss of over 5 kg.

Table 89-8: Distal Myopathies				
Type	**Inheritance**	**Musculoskeletal Features**	**Laboratory Studies**	**Other Systems**
Late-adult-onset Welander myopathy type I	Autosomal dominant (predominantly Scandinavian)	Onset in midlife; begins in hands, spreads to distal leg muscles; slowly progressive	CK level normal or slightly increased; biopsy—variable; vacuolar myopathy in some cases	None
Markesbery myopathy type II	Autosomal dominant (non-Scandinavian)	Onset in midlife; begins in distal leg muscles; spreads to hand muscles; slowly progressive	CK level normal or slightly increased; biopsy—vacuolar myopathy	Cardiomyopathy
Early-adult-onset type I (Nonaka)	Autosomal recessive or sporadic	Onset in legs (anterior compartment)	CK level increased, usually <10× normal; biopsy—vacuolar myopathy	None
Type II (Miyoshi)	Autosomal recessive or sporadic	Onset second–third decade; begins in distal leg muscles, spreads to hand muscles; slowly progressive	CK level increased, usually >10× normal; biopsy—dystrophy without vacuoles; gastrocnemius often "end stage"	None

Source: Reproduced by permission from Griggs RC, Mendell JR, Miller RG. *Evaluation and treatment of myopathies.* Philadelphia: FA Davis, 1995.
CK = creatine kinase.

Cricopharyngeal (upper esophageal sphincter) dysfunction was seen in 5 of 7 patients undergoing videofluoroscopy and 4 of 14 patients undergoing manometry (459). Both incomplete relaxation and reduced coordination of cricopharyngeal relaxation with the pharyngeal peristaltic wave appear to be the mechanisms of dysfunction. Myotomy of the cricopharyngeal muscle may reduce dysphagia provided that pharyngeal peristalsis is not severely impaired (356,426,459). Lower esophageal sphincter tone may be reduced as well and patients may benefit from treatment with metoclopramide or cisapride (426). Patients with pharyngeal aperistalsis may require gastrostomy (459).

Psychosocial Issues

Discussions regarding the possible need for gastrostomy tube feedings should take place before there is an urgent need for enteral feedings. Since the disease presents in the fourth decade in some patients, family planning should be discussed in regard to the autosomal dominant form of transmission.

DISTAL MYOPATHY/DISTAL MUSCULAR DYSTROPHY

A distal myopathy among 249 Scandinavian patients was described by Welander in 1951 (460). The mean age at onset is 47 years and the mode of transmission is autosomal dominant (355,460). Subsequently, other forms of distal myopathies have been reported (Table 89-8) (426). In general, the autosomal dominant forms have onset after age 40 and autosomal recessive forms have onset before age 40 (114,426). None of these diseases is responsive to medications. These rare diseases are nonfatal except for the late-onset type II myopathy, which may have cardiac involvement (426,461).

Weakness

The distal myopathy of Welander presents with hand weakness (particularly of the thumb and index finger), while other forms present with footdrop due to distal leg weakness (114,426,462,463). A case report of a 78-year-old man with distal myopathy demonstrated significant improvement using isometric exercises, therapeutic putty, and a Velcro hand exercise board for 20 minutes twice a day for 3 weeks (464). Congestive heart failure may occur due to myocardial fibrosis in the Markesbery form of distal myopathy and exercise intensity should be adjusted accordingly (426,461).

Mobility

Since distal leg weakness occurs early in these diseases, steppage gait may be a presenting symptom. Patients benefit from AFOs and may also need a cane for balance (426). While disease progression is slow, over decades it may eventually lead to a loss of ambulation.

Table 89-9: Disablement in Neuromuscular Diseases

Organ	Impairment (Usually Progressive)	Disability	Disadvantage (Handicap)
Skeletal muscle	Strength and endurance	Motor performance Mobility Upper-extremity function Fatigue	Quality of life Educational opportunities
Bone and joint	Joint contractures Spine deformity	Function Pain and deformity	Employment opportunities
Lungs	Pulmonary function	Restrictive lung disease (RLD)	Dependency and disadvantage
Heart	Cardiomyopathy Conduction defects	Fatigue Cardiopulmonary adaptations	—
Central nervous system	Intellectual capacity	Fatigue Learning ability Psychosocial adjustment	—

Table 89-10: Neuromuscular Diseases

- Motor neuron disease
  - Arthrogryposis multiplex congenita
  - Severe spinal muscular atrophy (SMA)
  - Intermediate SMA
  - Infantile neuroaxonal dystrophy
  - Mild SMA
  - Adult SMA
  - Amyotrophic lateral sclerosis
- Spinal nerve—see Chaps. 59 and 60
- Plexus—see Chap. 86
- Peripheral nerve—see Chap. 88
- Neuromuscular junction
  - Congenital myasthenia
  - Transient neonatal myasthenia gravis
  - Persistent neonatal myasthenia gravis
  - Infantile botulism
  - Juvenile myasthenia gravis
  - Myasthenia gravis
  - Lambert-Eaton syndrome
- Muscle
  - Central core disease
  - Nemaline rod myopathy, severe neonatal
  - Nemaline rod myopathy, infantile
  - Myotubular (centronuclear) myopathy
  - Congenital fiber-type disproportion
  - Congenital muscular dystrophy
  - Infantile acid maltase deficiency
  - Debrancher deficiency
  - Phosphorylase kinase deficiency
  - Myophosphorylase deficiency, neonatal
  - Hyperkalemic periodic paralysis
  - Congenital myotonic dystrophy
  - Duchenne muscular dystrophy
  - Becker muscular dystrophy
  - Childhood acid maltate deficiency
  - Paramyotonia congenita
  - Myotonia congenita
  - Mitochondrial myopathy
  - Dermatomyositis, childhood
  - Myophosphorylase deficiency (McArdle)
  - Phosphofructokinase deficiency
  - Limb girdle dystrophy
  - Facioscapulohumeral dystrophy
  - Emery-Dreifuss muscular dystrophy
  - Myotonic dystrophy (Steinert)
  - Oculopharyngeal dystrophy
  - Distal muscular dystrophy
  - Polymyositis/adult dermatomyositis
  - Inclusion body myositis

Feeding

Hand weakness may necessitate the use of devices such as a universal cuff or built-up utensil handles to allow self-feeding. Dysphagia is not an issue.

Contracture

Contractures may occur due to muscle imbalance and intrinsic fibrosis. Range of motion exercises and splinting may be indicated.

Psychosocial Issues

Family planning issues should be discussed as these diseases have well-defined inheritance patterns.

Table 89-11: Myopathies with Abnormalities of Deglutition

- Muscular dystrophy
  - Myotonic*
  - Oculopharyngeal*
  - Duchenne (rare)
- Inflammatory
  - Dermatomyositis
  - Polymyositis
  - Inclusion body myositis
- Metabolic
  - Mitochondrial

* Often presenting with dysphagia.
Source: Adapted from Griggs RC, Mendell JR, Miller RG. *Evaluation and treatment of myopathies.* Philadelphia: FA Davis, 1995.

REFERENCES

1. Fowler WM, Abresch RT, Aitkens BS, et al. Profiles of neuromuscular diseases. *Am J Phys Med Rehabil* 1995;5(suppl):562–569.

2. Goodman RM, Gorlin RJ. Arthrogryposis. In: Goodman RM, Gorlin RJ, eds. *The malformed infant and child.* New York: Oxford University Press, 1983:42–43.

3. Brown LM, Robson MJ, Sharrard WJW. The pathophysiology of AMC. *J Bone Joint Surg [Br]* 1980;62:291–295.

4. Swinyard CA, Bleck EE. The etiology of arthrogryposis. *Clin Orthop* 1985;194:15–29.

5. Hageman G, Willemse J. The pathogenesis of fetal hypokinesia—a neurological study of 75 cases of congenital contractures with emphasis on cerebral lesions. *Neuropediatrics* 1987;18:22–33.

6. Wynne-Davies R, Lloyd Roberts GC. Arthrogryposis multiplex congenita—search for prenatal factors in 66 sporadic cases. *Arch Dis Child* 1976;51:618–623.

7. Banker BQ. Neuropathologic aspects of arthrogryposis multiplex congenita. *Clin Orthop* 1985;194:30–43.

8. Strehl E, Vanasse M. Electromyographic and muscle biopsy studies in arthrogryposis multiplex congenita. *Neuropediatrics* 1985;16:25–227.

9. Hall JG. Genetic aspects of arthrogryposis. *Clin Orthop* 1985;194:44–53.

10. Hageman G, Ippel EP, Beemer FA, et al. The diagnostic management of newborns with congenital contractures and nosologic study of 75 cases. *Am J Med Genet* 1988;30:883–904.

11. Hageman G, Willemse J. Arthrogryposis multiplex congenita. *Neuropediatrics* 1983;14:6–11.

12. Hall JG, Reed SD, Driscoll EP. Amyoplasia. A common sporadic condition with congenital contractures. *Am J Med Genet* 1983;15:571–590.

13. Tachdjian MO. Arthrogryposis multiplex congenita. In: Tachdjian M, ed. *Pediatric orthopedics.* Philadelphia: WB Saunders, 1990:2086–2114.

14. Sarwark JF, MacEwen GD, Scott CI. Amyoplasia (a common form of arthrogryposis). *J Bone Joint Surg [Am]* 1990;72:465–469.

15. Jones LE, Schutt AH, Sawtell RR. Arthrogryposis multiplex congenita: a review of 40 cases seen at Mayo Clinic between 1966–1976. *Arch Phys Med Rehabil* 1977;58:506.

16. Carlson WO, Speck GJ, Vicari V, Wenger DR. Arthrogryposis multiplex congenita: a long term follow up study. *Clin Orthop* 1985;194:115–123.

17. Robinson RO. Arthrogryposis multiplex congenita: feeding, language and other health problems. *Neuropediatrics* 1990;21:177–178.

18. Donohoe M, Bleakney DA. Arthrogryposis multiplex congenita. In: Campbell SK, ed. *Physical therapy for children.* Philadelphia: WB Saunders, 1995:261–277.

19. Florence J. The orthotic management of arthrogryposis. *Prosthet Orthot Int* 1977;1:111–113.

20. Hoffer MM, Swank S, Eastman F, et al. Ambulation in severe arthrogryposis. *J Pediatr Orthop* 1983;3:293–296.

21. Schiulli C, Corradi Scalise D, Donatelli Schulthiss ML. Powered mobility vehicles as aids in independent locomotion for very young children. *Phys Ther* 1988;68:997–999.

22. Friedlander HL, Westin GW, Wood WC. Arthrogryposis multiplex congenita. *J Bone Joint Surg [Am]* 1968;50:89–112.

23. Thompson GH, Bilenker RM. Comprehensive management of arthrogryposis multiplex congenita. *Clin Orthop* 1985;194:6–14.

24. Palmer PM, MacEwen GD, Bowen JR, Matthews PA. Passive motion therapy for infants with arthrogryposis. *Clin Orthop* 1985;194:54–59.

25. Dias LS, Stern LS. Talectomy in the treatment of resistant talipes equinovarus deformity in myelomeningocele and arthrogryposis. *J Pediatr Orthop* 1987;7:39–41.

26. Williams PF. The management of arthrogryposis. *Orthop Clin North Am* 1978;9:67–88.

27. Sodergard J, Ryoppy S. The knee in arthrogryposis multiplex congenita. *J Pediatr Orthop* 1990;10:177–182.

28. Staheli LT, Chew DE, Elliott JS, Mosca VS. Management of hip dislocations in children with arthrogryposis. *J Pediatr Orthop* 1987;7:681–685.

29. Bayne LG. Hand assessment and management of arthrogryposis multiplex congenita. *Clin Orthop* 1985;194:68–73.

30. Williams PF. Management of upper limb problems in arthrogryposis. *Clin Orthop* 1985;194:60–67.

31. Drummond DS, MacKenzie DA. Scoliosis in arthrogryposis multiplex congenita. *Spine* 1978;3:146–151.

32. Daher YH, Lonstein JE, Winter RW, Moe JH. Spinal deformities in patients with arthrogryposis. A review of 16 patients. *Spine* 1985;10:609–613.

33. Sarwark JF, MacEwen GD, Scott CI. A multidisciplinary approach to amyoplasia congenita. *Orthop Trans* 1986;10:130.

34. Pearn J. Classification of the spinal muscular atrophies. *Lancet* 1980;1:919–921.

35. Czeizel A, Humula J. A Hungarian study on Werdnig Hoffmann disease. *J Med Genet* 1989;26:761–763.

36. Melki J, Sheth P, Abdelhak S, et al. Mapping of acute spinal

muscular atrophy to chromosome 5q12–q14. The French spinal muscular atrophy investigators. *Lancet* 1990;336:271–273.

37. Gilliam TC, Brzustowicz LM, Castilla LH, et al. Genetic homogeneity between acute and chronic forms of spinal muscular atrophy. *Nature* 1990;345: 823–825.

38. Winsor EJ, Murphy EG, Thompson W, Reed TE. Genetics of childhood spinal muscular atrophy. *J Med Genet* 1971;8:143–148.

39. Eng GD. Rehabilitation of children with neuromuscular diseases. In: Molnar GE, ed. *Pediatric rehabilitation*. 2nd ed. Baltimore: Williams & Wilkins, 1985:363–399.

40. Byers RK, Banker BQ. Infantile muscular atrophy. *Arch Neurol* 1961;5:140–164.

41. Fried K, Emery AEH. SMA type II. A separate genetic and clinical entity from type I and type III. *Clin Genet* 1971;2: 203–209.

42. Gordon N. The spinal muscular atrophies. *Dev Med Child Neurol* 1991;33:930–938.

43. Connolly MB, Roland EH, Hill A. Clinical features for prediction of survival in neonatal muscle disease. *Pediatr Neurol* 1992;8:285–288.

44. Dubowitz V. *Muscle disorders in childhood*. 2nd ed. Philadelphia: WB Saunders, 1995.

45. Ignatius J. The natural history of severe SMA—further evidence for clinical subtypes. *Neuromuscul Disord* 1994;4:527–528.

46. Dubowitz V. Chaos in the classification of the spinal muscular atrophies of childhood. *Neuromuscul Disord* 1991;1:77–80.

47. Munsat TL. Workshop report: international SMA collaboration. *Neuromuscul Disord* 1991;1:81.

48. Russman BS, Melchreif R, Drennzu JC. Spinal muscular atrophy: natural course of disease. *Muscle Nerve* 1983;6:179–181.

49. Evans GA, Drenann JC, Russman BS. Functional classification and orthopedic management of SMA. *J Bone Joint Surg [Br]* 1981;63:516–522.

50. Dubowitz V. Infantile muscular atrophy. A prospective study with particular reference to a slowly progressive variety. *Brain* 1964;87:707–718.

51. Benady SG. Spinal muscular atrophy in childhood: review of 50 cases. *Dev Med Child Neurol* 1978;20:746–757.

52. Munsat TL, Woods R, Fowler W, Pearson C. Neurogenic muscular atrophy of infancy with prolonged survival. *Brain* 1969;92:9–24.

53. Gardner Medwin D, Hudgson P, Walton JN. Benign spinal muscular atrophy arising in childhood and adolescence. *J Neurol Sci* 1967;5:121–158.

54. Schwentker EP, Gibson DA. The orthopedic aspects of spinal muscular atrophy. *J Bone Joint Surg [Am]* 1976;58:32–38.

55. Ignatius J. The natural history of severe spinal muscular atrophy—further evidence for clinical subtypes. *Neuromuscul Disord* 1994;4:527–528.

56. Koch BM, Simenson RL. Upper extremity strength and function in children with spinal muscular atrophy type II. *Arch Phys Med Rehabil* 1992;73:241–245.

57. Russman BS, Iannacone ST, Bunchez CR, et al. Spinal muscular atrophy: new thoughts on the pathogenesis and classification schema. *J Child Neurol* 1992;7:347–353.

58. Hausmanowa-Petrusewicz I, Fidzizaska A, Dobosz I, Strugalska MH. Is Kugelberg Welander spinal muscular atrophy a fetal defect? *Muscle Nerve* 1980;3:389–402.

59. Lefebvre S, Reboullet S, Burlet P, et al. Identification and characterization of a spinal muscular atrophy determining gene. *Cell* 1995;80:155–165.

60. Pearn JH, Gardner Medwin D, Wilson JA. A clinical study of chronic childhood spinal muscular atrophy. A review of 141 cases. *J Neurol Sci* 1978;38: 23–37.

61. Pearn JH, Hudgson P, Walton JN. A clinical and genetic study of spinal muscular atrophy of adult onset. *Brain* 1978;101: 591–606.

62. Pearn JH. The gene frequency of acute Werdnig Hoffmann disease (SMA type I). A total population survey in North-east England. *J Med Genet* 1973; 10:260–265.

63. Emery AEH. Review: nosology of the spinal muscular atrophies. *J Med Genet* 1971;8;481–495.

64. Munsat TL. The spinal muscular atrophies. In: Appeli SH, ed. *Current neurology*. Vol. 14. St. Louis: Mosby, 1996:55–69.

65. Pearn JH, Carter CO, Wilson J. The genetic identity of acute infantile spinal muscular atrophy. *Brain* 1973;96:463–470.

66. Hausmanowa-Petrusewicz I, Kaarwanska A. Electromyographic findings in different forms of infantile and juvenile proximal SMA. *Muscle Nerve* 1986;9:37–46.

67. Brzustowicz LM, Lehner T, Castilla LH, et al. Genetic mapping of chronic childhood onset SMA. *Nature* 1990; 344;540–541.

68. MacKenzie AE, Jacob P, Surh L, et al. Genetic heterogeneity in spinal muscular atrophy: a linkage analysis based assessment. *Neurology* 1994;44: 919–924.

69. Muller B, Melki J, Burlet P, Clerget Darpoux F. Proximal spinal muscular atrophy types II and III in the same sibship are not caused by different alleles at the SMA locus on 5q. *Am J Hum Genet* 1992;50: 892–895.

70. Melki J, Lefebvre S, Burglen L, et al. De novo and inherited deletions of the 5q13 region in spinal muscular atrophies. *Science* 1994;264:1474–1477.

71. Dubowitz V. *Color atlas of muscle disorders in childhood.* Chicago: Year Book Medical, 1989.

72. Dubowitz V. *The floppy infant.* 2nd ed. Clinics in developmental medicine, No. 31. Spastics international. Heinemann, 1980.

73. Pearn JH, Wilson J. Acute Werdnig Hoffmann disease, acute infantile spinal muscular atrophy. *Arch Dis Child* 1973;48: 425–430.

74. Merlini L, Granata C, Bonfiglioli S, et al. Scoliosis in spinal muscular atrophy: natural history and management. *Dev Med Child Neurol* 1989;31:501–508.

75. Eng G, Binder H, Koch B. Spinal muscular atrophy: experience in diagnosis and rehabilitation management of 60 patients. *Arch Phys Med Rehabil* 1984;65: 549–553.

76. Fenichel GM, Engle WK. Histochemistry of muscle in infantile spinal muscular atrophy. *Neurology* 1963;13:1059–1066.

77. Buchthal F, Olsen PZ. Electromyography and muscle biopsy in infantile spinal muscular atrophy. *Brain* 1970;93: 15–25.

78. Thompson CE. Pitfalls in muscle biopsies of hypotonic children. *Dev Med Child Neurol* 1985;27: 675–677.

79. Jones HER. EMG evaluation of the floppy infant: differential diagnosis and technical aspects. *Muscle Nerve* 1990;13: 338–347.

80. Eng GD. Electrodiagnosis. In: Molnar GE, ed. *Pediatric rehabilitation.* 2nd ed. Baltimore: Williams & Wilkins, 1985: 155–156.

81. Wang TG, Bach JR, Avilla C, et al. Survival of individuals with spinal muscular atrophy on ventilatory support. *Am J Phys Med Rehabil* 1994;3:207–211.

82. Granata C, Dubowitz V, eds. *Current concepts in childhood spinal muscular atrophy.* New York: Spinger-Verlag Wien, 1989:117–125.

83. Hausmanowa-Petrusewicz I, Zaremba J, Borkowska JJ, Chronic proximal muscular atrophy of childhood and adolescence: problem of classification and genetic counselling. *J Med Genet* 1985;22:350–353.

84. Siegel IM. Pathomechanics of stance in Duchenne muscular dystrophy. *Arch Phys Med Rehabil* 1972;53:403–406.

85. Munsat TL. Review of neuromuscular diseases. *Arch Phys Med Rehabil* 1988;2:467–480.

86. Binder H. New ideas in the rehabilitation of children with spinal muscular atrophy. In: Merlini L, Granata C, Dubowitz V, eds. *Current concepts in childhood spinal muscular atrophy.* New York: Spinger-Verlag Wien, 1989:117–125.

87. Stuberg WA. Muscular dystrophy and spinal muscular atrophy. In: Campbell SK, ed. *Physical therapy for children.* Philadelphia: WB Saunders, 1995: 295–321.

88. Noble Jamieson CM, Heckmatt JZ, Dubowitz V, et al. Effects of posture and bracing on respiratory function in neuromuscular diseases. *Arch Dis Child* 1986; 61;178–181.

89. Eng GD. Rehabilitation of the child with a severe form of spinal muscular atrophy (type I, infantile or Werdnig Hoffmann disease). In: Merlini L, Granata C, Dubowitz V, eds. *Current concepts in childhood spinal muscular atrophy.* New York: Springer-Verlag Wien, 1989: 113–115.

90. Engel AG. Myasthenic syndromes. In; Engel AG, Franzini-Armstrong C, eds. *Myology, basic and clinical.* 2nd ed. New York: McGraw-Hill, 1994: 1798–1835.

91. Swaiman KF. Diseases of the neuromuscular junction. In: Swaiman KF, ed. *Pediatric neurology: principles and practice.* 2nd ed. St. Louis: Mosby, 1994:1453–1476.

92. Cornblath DR. Disorders of NM transmission in infants and children. *Muscle Nerve* 1986;9: 606–611.

93. Misulis KE, Fenichel GM. Genetic forms of myasthenia gravis. *Pediatr Neurol* 1989;5: 205–210.

94. Engel AG. Congenital myasthenia syndromes. *J Child Neurol* 1988; 3:233–246.

95. Vernet-der Garabedian B, Lacokova M, Eymard B, et al. Association of neonatal myasthenia gravis with antibodies against the fetal acetylcholine receptor. *J Clin Invest* 1994;94:555–559.

96. Plauche WC. Myasthenia gravis in mothers and their newborns. *Clin Obstet Gynecol* 1991; 34:82–99.

97. Vincent A, Newland C, Brueton L, et al. Arthrogryposis multiplex congenita with maternal auto antibodies specific for a fetal antigen. *Lancet* 1995; 346:24–25.

98. Barnes PRJ, Kanabar DJ, Brueton L, et al. Recurrent congenital arthrogryposis leading to a diagnosis of myasthenia gravis in an initially asymptomatic mother. *Neuromuscul Disord* 1995;5: 59–65.

99. Dodds KL. Worldwide incidence and ecology of infant botulism. In: Hauschild AHW, Dodds KL, eds. *Clostridium botulinum: ecology and control in foods.* New York: Marcel Dekker, 1993:108–109.

100. Arnon SS, Damus K, Chin J. Infant botulism: epidemiology and relation to sudden infant death syndrome. *Epidemiol Rev* 1981;3:45–66.

101. Spika JS, Shaffer N, Hargrett-Bean N, et al. Risk factors for infant botulism in the US. *Am J Dis Child* 1989;143: 828–832.

102. Cochran DP, Appleton RE. Infant botulism—is it that rare? *Dev Med Child Neurol* 1995;37: 274–278.

103. Schreiner MS, Field E, Ruddy R. Infant botulism: a review of 12 years' experience at the

Children's Hospital of Philadelphia. *Pediatrics* 1991;87: 159–165.

104. Pickett J, Berg B, Chaplin E, Brunstetter-Shafer MA. Syndrome of botulism in infancy: clinical and electrophysiological study. *N Engl J Med* 1976;295:770–772.

105. Johnson RO, Clay SA, Arnon SS. Diagnosis and management of infant botulism. *Am J Dis Child* 1979;133:586–593.

106. Grover WD, Peckham GJ, Berman PH. Recovery following cranial nerve dysfunction and muscle weakness in infancy. *Dev Med Child Neurol* 1974;16:163–171.

107. Haan EA, Freemantle CJ, McCure JA, et al. Assignment of the gene for central core disease to chromosome 19. *Hum Genet* 1990;86:187–190.

108. Dubowitz V, Platts M. Central core disease of muscle: clinical, histochemical and electron microscopic studies of an affected mother and child. *Brain* 1970;93;133–146.

109. Dubowitz V, Roy S. Central core disease of muscle with focal wasting. *J Neurol Neurosurg Psychiatry* 1970;93;133–146.

110. Byrne E, Blumbergs PC, Hallpike JF. Central core disease. Study of a family with 5 affected generations. *J Neurol Sci* 1982;53: 7–83.

111. Eng GD, Epstein BS, Engel WK, et al. Malignant hyperthermia and central core disease in a child with congenital dislocating hips. *Arch Neurol* 1978;35: 189–197.

112. Frank JP, Harati Y, Butler IF, et al. Central core disease and malignant hyperthermia syndrome. *Ann Neurol* 1980;7: 11–17.

113. Wallgren Pettersson C, Kaariainen H, Rapola J, et al. Genetics of congenital nemaline myopathy: a study of 10 families. *J Med Genet* 1990;27:480–487.

114. Brooke MH. *A clinician's view of neuromuscular diseases.* 2nd ed. Baltimore: Williams & Wilkins, 1986.

115. Banker BQ. The congenital myopathies. In: Engel AG, Banker BQ, eds. *Myology.* New York: McGraw-Hill, 1986: 1527–1581.

116. Wallgren Pattterson C. Congenital nemaline myopathy: a clinical followup of 12 patients. *J Neurol Sci* 1989;89:1 14.

117. Norton P, Ellison P, Sulaiman AT, Harb J. Nemaline myopathy in the neonate. *Neurology* 1983;33;351–356.

118. Hopkins IJ, Lindsey JR, Ford FR. Nemaline myopathy: a long term clinicopathologic study of affected mother and daughter. *Brain* 1966;89:299–310.

119. Radu H, Killyen I, Ionescu V, Radu A. Myotubular (centronuclear) myopathy: clinical, genetic, and morphological studies. *J Neurol* 1977;15:285–300.

120. Munsat TL, Thompson LR, Colemen RF. Centronuclear ("myotubular") myopathy. *Arch Neurol* 1969;20:120–131.

121. DeAngelis MS, Palmucci L, Leone M, et al. Centronuclear myopathy: clinical, morphological and genetic characteristics. *J Neurol Sci* 1991;103:2–9.

122 Reitter B, Morrier W, Willie L. Neonatal respiratory insufficiency due to centronuclear myopathy. *Acta Paediatr Scand* 1979;68: 773–778.

123. Ambler MW, Neave C, Tutschka BG, et al. X linked chromosome recessive myotubular myopathy. I. Clinical and pathologic findings in a family. *Hum Pathol* 1984;15:566–574.

124. Wallgren Pettersson C, Thomas NST. Report on 20th ENMC-sponsored International Workshop: myotubular/centronuclear myopathy. *Neuromuscul Disord* 1994;4:71–74.

125. Heckmatt JZ, Loh L, Dubowitz V. Nocturnal hypoventilation in children with nonprogressive neuromuscular disease. *Pediatrics* 1989;83:250–255.

126. Vignos PJ, Watkins MP. Effect of exercise in muscular dystrophy. *JAMA* 1966;197: 843–848.

127. McCartney N, Moroz D, Garner SH, McComas AJ. The effects of strength training in patients with selected neuromuscular disorders. *Med Sci Sport Exerc* 1988;20:362–368.

128. Aitkens SG, McCrory MA, Kilmer DD, Bernauer EM. Moderate resistance exercise program: its effect in slowly progressive neuromuscular disease. *Arch Phys Med Rehabil* 1993;74:711–715.

129. Milner-Brown HS, Miller RG. Muscle strengthening through high resistance weight training in patients with neuromuscular disorders. *Arch Phys Med Rehabil* 1988;69:14–19.

130. Milner-Brown HS, Miller RG. Muscle strengthening through electrical stimulation combined with low resistance weights in patients with neuromuscular disorders. *Arch Phys Med Rehabil* 1988;69:20–24.

131. Emery AEH. Population frequencies of inherited neuromuscular diseases—a world survey. *Neuromuscul Disord* 1991;1:19–29.

132. Banker BQ. Congenital muscular dystrophy. In: Engel AG, Banker BQ, eds. *Myology* New York: McGraw-Hill, 1986:1367–1382.

133. McMenamin JB, Becker LE, Murphy EG. Congenital muscular dystrophy. *J Pediatr* 1982;100: 692–697.

134. Fukuyama Y, Osawa MM, Suzuki H. Congenital muscular dystrophy of the Fukuyama type. *Brain Dev* 1981;3:1–29.

135. Cook JD, Gascon GG, Haider A, et al. Congenital muscular dystrophy with abnormal radiographic myelin pattern. *J Child Neurol* 1992;7:S51–S63.

136. Santavuori P, Pihko H, Sainio K, et al. Muscle-eye-brain disease and Walker Warburg syndrome. *Am J Med Genet* 1990;36: 371–374.

137. Yoshioka M, Kuroki S, Nigami H, et al. Clinical variation within sibships in Fukuyama type con-

genital muscular dystrophy. *Brain Dev* 1992;14:334–337.

138. Toda T, Segawa M, Nomura Y, et al. Localization of a gene for Fukuyama type congenital muscular dystrophy to chromosome 9q31–33. *Nat Genet* 1993;5: 283–286.

139. Arahata K, Hayashi YK, Mizuno Y, et al. Dystrophin associated glycoprotein and dystrophin colocalization at sarcolemma in Fukuyama congenital muscular dystrophy. *Lancet* 1993;342: 623–624.

140. Tome FMS, Evangelista T, Leclerc A, et al. Congenital muscular dystrophy with merosin deficiency. *Life Sci* 1994;317: 351–357.

141. Jones R, Khan R, Hughes S, Dubowitz V. Congenital muscular dystrophy: the importance of early diagnosis and orthopedic management in the long term prognosis. *J Bone Joint Surg [Br]* 1979;61:13–17.

142. Lazaro RP, Fenichel GM, Kilroy AW. Congenital muscular dystrophy: case reports and reappraisal. *Muscle Nerve* 1979;2:349–355.

143. Harper PS. Myotonic disorders. In: Engel AG, Banker BQ, eds. *Myology.* New York: McGraw-Hill, 1986:1267–1296.

144. Harper PS. *Myotonic dystrophy.* 2nd edn. London: WB Saunders, 1989.

145. Pearse RG, Howeler CJ. Neonatal form of dystrophica myotonia: five cases in preterm babies and a review of earlier reports. *Arch Dis Child* 1979;54:331–338.

146. Harper PS. Congenital myotonic muscular dystrophy in Britain. Clinical aspects. *Arch Dis Child* 1975;50:505–513.

147. Rutherford MA, Heckmatt JZ, Dubowitz V. Congenital myotonic dystrophy: respiratory function at birth determines survival. *Arch Dis Child* 1989;64:191–195.

148. Swaiman KF, Smith SA. Progressive muscular dystrophies. In: Swaiman KF, ed. *Pediatric neurology: principles and practice.* 2nd ed. St. Louis: Mosby, 1994: 1477–1504.

149. Calderon R. Myotonic dystrophy: a neglected cause of mental retardation. *J Pediatr* 1966;68: 423–431.

150. O'Brien T, Harper PS. Course, prognosis and complications of childhood onset myotonic dystrophy. *Dev Med Child Neurol* 1984;26:62–67.

151. Engel AG. Acid maltase deficiency. In: Engel AG, Banker BQ, eds. *Myology* New York: McGraw-Hill, 1986:1629–1649.

152. Roper HP. Neuromuscular diseases in children. *Br J Hosp Med* 1993;49:537–545.

153. Puig JG, DeMiguel E, Mateos FA, et al. McArdle's disease and gout. *Muscle Nerve* 1992;15: 822–828.

154. Zellweger H, Mueller S, Ionasescu V, et al. Glycogenosis IV. A new cause of infantile hypotonia. *J Pediatr* 1972;80:842–844.

155. Carter GT, Abresch RT, Fowler WM, et al. Profiles of neuromuscular diseases: spinal muscular atrophy. *Am J Phys Med Rehabil* 1995;74(suppl):150–159.

156. Moosa A, Dubowitiz V. Spinal muscular atrophy in childhood: two clues to clinical diagnosis. *Arch Dis Child* 1973;48: 386–388.

157. Fowler WM. Management of musculoskeletal complications in neuromuscular diseases: weakness and the role of exercise. *Phys Med Rehabil: State Art Rev* 1988;2:484–504.

158. Hsu JD. Orthopedic approaches for the treatment of lower extremity contractures in Duchenne muscular dystrophy patient in the US and Canada. *Semin Neurol* 1995;15:6–8.

159. Phillips DP, Roye DP, Farcy JPC, et al. Surgical treatment of scoliosis in a SMA population. *Spine* 1990;15:942–945.

160. Hsu JD. The development of current approaches to the management of spinal deformity for patients with neuromuscular disease. *Semin Neurol* 1995;15: 24–28.

161. Furumasu J, Swank SM, Brown JC, et al. Activities in spinal muscular atrophy patients after spinal fusion. *Spine* 1989;14: 763–770.

162. Brown JC, Zeller JL, Swank SM, et al. Surgical and functional results of spine fusion in SMA. *Spine* 1989;14:771–775.

163. Granata C, Merlini L, Magni E, et al. Spinal muscular atrophy: natural history and orthopedic treatment of scoliosis. *Spine* 1989;14:760–762.

164. Riddick MF, Winter RB, Lutter LD. Spinal deformities in patients with spinal muscle atrophy. *Spine* 1982;7:476–483.

165. Moser H, Emery AEH. The manifesting carrier in Duchenne muscular dystrophy. *Clin Genet* 1974;5:271–284.

166. Koenig M, Hoffman EP, Bertelson CK, et al. Complete cloning of the Duchenne muscular dystrophy DNA and preliminary genomic organization of the Duchenne's muscular dystrophy gene in mouse and affected individuals. *Cell* 1987;50: 509–517.

167. Hoffman EP, Brown RH, Kunkel LM. Dystrophin: the protein product of the Duchenne muscular dystrophy locus. *Cell* 1987;51:919–928.

168. Bonilla E, Camitt CE, Miranda AF, et al. Duchenne muscular dystrophy: deficiency of dystrophin at the muscle cell surface. *Cell* 1988;54:447–452.

169. Arahata K, Ishiura S, Ishiguro T, et al. Immunostaining of skeletal and cardiac muscle surface membrane with antibody against Duchenne muscular dystrophy peptide. *Nature* 1988;333: 861–863.

170. Zubrzycka-Gaarn EE, Bulman DE, Karpati G. The Duchenne muscular gene product is localized in sarcolemma of human skeletal muscle. *Nature* 1988;33: 466–469.

171. Miller RG, Hoffman EP. Molecular diagnosis and modern management of Duchenne muscular dystrophy. *Neurol Clin* 1994;4: 699–725.

172. Moser H. Duchenne muscular dystrophy: pathogenetic aspects and genetic prevention. *Hum Genet* 1984;66:17–40.

173. Ohlendieck K, Matsummara K, Ionasescu VV, et al. Duchenne muscular dystrophy: deficiency of dystrophin associated proteins in the sarcolemma. *Neurology* 1993;43:795–800.

174. Matsumura K, Campbell KP. Dystrophin glycoprotein complex: its role in the molecular pathogenesis of muscular dystrophies. *Muscle Nerve* 1994;78: 625–633.

175. Kunkel LM. Analysis of deletions in the DNA of patients with Becker and Duchenne muscular dystrophy. *Nature* 1986;322: 73–77.

176. Vignos PJ, Archibald KC. Maintenance of ambulation in childhood muscular dystrophy. *J Chronic Dis* 1960;12:273–292.

177. Sutherland DH, Olshen R, Cooper L, et al. The pathomechanics of gait in Duchenne muscular dystrophy. *Dev Med Child Neurol* 1981;23:3–22.

178. Inkley SR, Oldenburg FC, Vignos PJ. Pulmonary function in Duchenne and muscular dystrophy related to stage of disease. *Am J Med* 1974;56:297–306.

179. McDonald CM, Abresch RT, Carter GT, et al. Profiles of neuromuscular diseases: Duchenne's muscular dystrophy. *Am J Phys Med Rehabil* 1995;74(suppl): 70–92.

180. Smith PFM, Calverley PMA, Edward RHT, et al. Practical problems in the respiratory care of patients with muscular dystrophy. *N Engl J Med* 1987;316: 1197–1205.

181. Miller F, Moseley CF, Koreska J, Levison H. Pulmonary function and scoliosis in Duchenne muscular dystrophy. *J Pediatr Orthop* 1988;8:133–137.

182. Bach JR. Standards of care in MDA clinics. *J Neurol Rehabil* 1992;6:67–73.

183. Bach JR. Pulmonary rehabilitation consideration for Duchenne's muscular dystrophy: the prolongation of life by respiratory aids. *Crit Rev Phys Rehabil Med* 1992;3:239–269.

184. Bach JR. Respiratory muscle aids for the prevention of pulmonary morbidity and mortality. *Semin Neurol* 1995;15:72–83.

185. Rideau Y, Gatin G, Bach J, Gines G. Prolongation of life in Duchenne muscular dystrophy. *Acta Neurol* 1983;5:118–124.

186. Segall D. Noninvasive nasal mask assisted ventilation in respiratory failure of Duchenne muscular dystrophy. *Chest* 1990;93: 1298–1300.

187. Splaingard ML, Frates RC, Harrison GM, et al. Home positive pressure ventilation. Twenty years' experience. *Chest* 1983; 84:376–382.

188. Alexander MA, Johnson EW, Petty J, Stauch D. Mechanical ventilation of patients with late stage Duchenne's muscular dystrophy: management in the home. *Arch Phys Med Rehabil* 1979;60: 289–292.

189. Baydur A, Gilgoff I, Prentice W, et al. Decline in respiratory function and experience with long term assisted ventilation in advanced Duchenne's MD. *Chest* 1990;97:884–889.

190. Bach JR, Campagnolo DL, Hoeman S. Life satisfaction of individuals with Duchenne's muscular dystrophy using long term mechanical ventilatory support. *Am J Phys Rehabil* 1991;70: 129–135.

191. Miller JR, Colbert AP, Osberg JS. Ventilator dependency: decision making, daily functioning and quality of life for patients with Duchenne muscular dystrophy. *Dev Med Child Neurology* 1990; 32:1078–1086.

192. Curran JF, Colbert AP. Ventilator management in Duchenne's muscular dystrophy and postpolio syndrome. *Arch Phys Med Rehabil* 1989;70:180–185.

193. Leon SH, Schuffler MD, Kettler M, Rohrman CA. Chronic intestinal pseudobstruction as a complication of Duchenne's muscular dystrophy. *Gastroenterology* 1986;90:455–459.

194. Jaffe KM, McDonald CM, Ingman E, Haas J. Symptoms of upper gastrointestinal dysfunction in Duchenne muscular dystrophy case control study. *Arch Phys Med Rehabil* 1990;71:742–744.

195. Barohn RJ, Levine EJ, Olson JD, Mendell JR. Gastric hypomotility in Duchenne muscular dystrophy. *N Engl J Med* 1988;319:15–18.

196. Edwards RHT, Round JM, Jackson MJ, et al. Weight reduction in boys with muscular dystrophy. *Dev Med Child Neurol* 1984;26:384–390.

197. Willing TN, Carlier L, Legrand M, et al. Nutritional assessment in Duchenne muscular dystrophy. *Dev Med Child Neurol* 1993;35: 1074–1085.

198. Fowler WM, Gardner GW. Quantitative strength measurements in muscular dystrophy. *Arch Phys Med Rehabil* 1967;49:554–565.

199. Okada K, Manabe S, Sakamoto S, et al. Protein and energy metabolism in patients with progressive muscular dystrophy. *J Nutr Sci Vitaminol (Tokyo)* 1992;38:141–154.

200. Willig TN, Bach JR, Venanace V, Navarro J. Nutritional rehabilitation in neuromuscular disorders. *Semin Neurol* 1995;15:18–23.

201. Brooke MH, Fenichel GM, Griggs RC, et al. Clinical investigation of Duchenne muscular dystrophy: interesting results in a trial of prednisone. *Arch Neurol* 1987;44:812–817.

202. Mendall JR, Moxley RT, Griggs RC, et al. Randomized double blind six-month trial of prednisone in Duchenne's muscular dystrophy. *N Engl J Med* 1989;20:1592–1597.

203. Fenichel GM, Florence JM, Pestronk A, et al. Long term benefit from prednisone therapy in Duchenne muscular dystrophy. *Neurology* 1991;41:1874–1877.

204. Griggs RC, Moxley RT, Mendell JR. Prednisone in Duchenne dystrophy. A randomized, controlled trial defining the time course and dose response. *Arch Neurol* 1991;48:383–388.

205. Khan MA. Corticosteroid therapy in Duchenne muscular dystrophy. *J Neurol Sci* 1993;120:8–14.

206. Fenichel GM, Brooke MH, Griggs RC, et al. Clinical investigation in Duchenne muscular dystrophy: penicillamine and vitamin E. *Muscle Nerve* 1988;11: 1164–1168.

207. Sharma KB, Mynhier MA, Miller RG. Cyclosporine increases muscular force generation in Duchenne's muscular dystrophy. *Neurology* 1993;43:527–532.

208. Griggs RC, Moxley RT, Mendell JR, et al. Duchenne dystrophy: randomized, controlled trial of prednisone (18 months) and azathioprine (12 months). *Neurology* 1993;43:520–527.

209. Karpati G, Ajdukovic D, Arnold D, et al. Myoblast transfer in Duchenne's muscular dystrophy. *Ann Neurol* 1993;34:8–17.

210. Partridge TA. Myoblast transfer: a possible therapy for inherited myopathies? *Muscle Nerve* 1991;14:197–212.

211. Coovert DD, Burghes AHM. Gene therapy for muscle diseases. *Curr Opin Neurol* 1994;7: 463–470.

212. Morgan JE. Cell and gene therapy in Duchenne muscular dystrophy. *Hum Gene Ther* 1994;5: 165–173.

213. Gussoni E, Pavlath GK, Lanctot AM, et al. Normal dystrophin transcripts detected in Duchenne muscular dystrophy patients after myoblast transplantation. *Nature* 1992;356:435–438.

214. Tremblay JP, Malouin F, Roy R, et al. Results of a double blind clinical study of myoblast transplantations without immunosuppressive treatment in young boys with Duchenne muscular dystrophy. *Cell Transplant* 1993;2: 99–112.

215. Clemens PR, Caskey CT. Gene therapy prospects for Duchenne muscular dystrophy. *Eur Neurol* 1994;34:181–185.

216. Wolff JA, Malone RW, Williams P, et al. Direct gene transfer into mouse muscle in vivo. *Science* 1990;247:1465–1468.

217. Scott OM, Hyde SA, Goddard C, Dubowitz V. Quantitation of muscle function in children: a prospective study in Duchenne muscular dystrophy. *Muscle Nerve* 1982;5:291–301.

218. Allsop KG, Ziter FA. Loss of strength and functional decline in Duchenne's dystrophy. *Arch Neurol* 1981;38:406–411.

219. Allsop KG, Ziter FA. Effectiveness of timed functional activities in Duchenne's muscular dystrophy. *Phys Ther* 1980;60:584.

220. Rideau Y, Duport G, Delaubier A, et al. Early treatment to preserve quality of locomotion for children with Duchenne muscular dystrophy. *Semin Neurol* 1995;15:9–17.

221. Brooke MH, Fenichel GM, Griggs RC, et al. Duchenne's muscular dystrophy: patterns of clinical progression and effects of supportive therapy. *Neurology* 1989;39:475–481.

222. Smith RA, Sibert JR, Harper PS. Early developments of boys with Duchenne's muscular dystrophy. *Dev Med Child Neurol* 1990;32:519–527.

223. Sockolow R, Irwin B, Dressendorfer RH, Bernauer EM, Exercise performance in 6–11 year old boys with Duchenne's muscular dystrophy. *Arch Phys Med Rehabil* 1977;58:195–201.

224. Bowker JH, Halpin PJ. Factors determining success in reambulation of the child with progressive muscular dystrophy. *Orthop Clin North Am* 1978;9:431–436.

225. DeLateur BJ, Giaconi RM. Effect on maximal strength of submaximal exercise in Duchenne muscular dystrophy. *Am J Phys Med* 1979;58:26–36.

226. Martin AJ, Steen L, Yeates J, et al. Respiratory muscle training in Duchenne muscular dystrophy. *Dev Med Child Neurol* 1986;28:314–318.

227. Stern LM, Martin AJ, Jones N, et al. Training inspiratory resistance in Duchenne dystrophy using adapted computer games. *Dev Med Child Neurol* 1989;31: 494–500.

228. Stern LM, Martin AJ, Jones N, et al. Respiratory training in Duchenne dystrophy. *Dev Med Child Neurol* 1991;33:648–649.

229. Wagner MB, Vignos PJ, Carlozzi C. Duchenne's muscular dystrophy: a study of wrist and hand function. *Muscle Nerve* 1989;12:236–244.

230. Wagner MB, Vignos PJ, Carlozzi C, et al. Assessment of hand function in Duchenne's muscular dystrophy. *Arch Phys Med Rehabil* 1993;74:801–804.

231. James WV, Orr JF. Upper limb weakness in children with Duchenne muscular dystrophy—a neglected problem. *Prosthet Orthot Int* 1984;8:11–13.

232. Bach JR, Zeelenberg A, Winter C. Wheelchair mounted robot manipulators: long term use by patients with Duchenne's muscular dystrophy. *Am J Phys Med Rehabil* 1990;69:59–69.

233. Bach JR. Therapeutic intervention and rehabilitation consideration—a historical perspective from tamplin to robotics for pseudohypertrophic muscular dystrophy. *Semin Neurol* 1995;15:38–45.

234. Mubarak SJ, Schultz P. Management of the child with Duchenne muscular dystrophy. AACPDM Instructional Course, San Diego, CA, October 1992:509–536.

235. Vignos PJ. Management of musculoskeletal complications in neuromuscular disease: limb contractures and the role of stretching, braces, and surgery. In: Fowler WM Jr, ed. *Advances in the Rehabilitation of Neuromuscular Diseases: State of the Art Reviews.* Philadelphia: Hanley & Belfus, 1988:509.

236. Spencer GE, Vignos PJ. Bracing for ambulation in childhood pro-

gressive MD. *J Bone Joint Surg [Am]* 1962;44:234–242.

237. Harris SE, Cherry DB. Childhood progressive muscular dystrophy and the role of physical therapy. *Phys Ther* 1974;54:4–12.

238. Heckmatt JZ, Dubowitz V, Hyde SA, et al. Prolongation of walking in Duchenne muscular dystrophy with lightweight orthoses—review of 57 cases. *Dev Med Child Neurol* 1985; 27:149–154.

239. Siegel IM, Miller JE, Ray RD. Subcutaneous lower limb tenotomy in the treatment of pseudohypertrophic MD. *Arch Phys Med Rehabil* 1972;53: 404–406.

240. Bach JR, McKeon J. Orthopedic surgery and rehab for the prolongation of brace free ambulation in patients with Duchenne's muscular dystrophy. *Am J Phys Med Rehabil* 1991; 70:323–331.

241. Rideau Y, Glorion B, Duport G. Prolongation of ambulation in the muscular dystrophies. *Acta Neurol* 1983;5:390–397.

242. Riccio V, Riccardi G, Cervone de Martino, M et al. Early treatment of lower limb deformities and preliminary muscular studies with ultrasound in Duchenne muscular dystrophy. *Acta Cardiomiol* 1991;3: 148–152.

243. Manzur AY, Hydes A, Rodill OE, et al. A randomized controlled study of early surgery in Duchenne's muscular dystrophy. *Neuromuscul Disord* 1992;2: 379–387.

244. Sibert JR, Williams V, Burkinshaw R, Sibert S. Swivel walkers in Duchenne's muscular dystrophy. *Arch Dis Child* 1987;62: 741–742.

245. Gardner Medwin D. Clinical features and classification of the muscular dystrophies. *Br Med Bull* 1980;36:109–115.

246. Galasko CS. Incidence of orthopedic problems in children with muscle disease. *Isr J Med Sci* 1977;13:165–176.

247. Rodillo EB, Fernandez E, Heckmatt JZ, Dubowitz V. Prevention of rapidly progressive scoliosis in Duchenne's muscular dystrophy by prolongation of walking with orthoses. *J Child Neurol* 1988;3:269–274.

248. Lord J, Behrman B, Varzos N, et al. Scoliosis associated with Duchenne's muscular dystrophy. *Arch Phys Med Rehabil* 1990;71:13–17.

249. Colbert AP, Craig C. Scoliosis management in Duchenne muscular dystrophy: prospective study of modified Jewett hyperextension brace. *Arch Phys Med Rehabil* 1987;68:302–304.

250. Scott OM, Hyde SA, Goddard C, Dubowitz V. Prevention of deformity in Duchenne muscular dystrophy. A prospective study of passive stretching and splinting. *Physiotherapy* 1981;67: 177–180.

251. Seeger BR, Caudrey DJ, Little JD. Progression of equinus deformity in Duchenne muscular dystrophy. *Arch Phys Med Rehabil* 1985;66:286–288.

252. Silverman M. Commercial options for positioning the client with muscular dystrophy. *Clin Prosthet Orthot* 1986;10:159–170.

253. Lehman M, Hsu AM, Hsu JD. The wheelchair dependent Duchenne's muscular dystrophy patient. A study of scoliosis, upper extremity use, function and dominance. *Dev Med Child Neurol* 1986;28:628–632.

254. Wilkins KE, Gibson DA. The patterns of spinal deformity in Duchenne muscular dystrophy. *J Bone Joint Surg [Am]* 1976;58: 24–32.

255. Hsu JD. The natural history of spine curvature progression in the nonambulatory Duchenne's muscular dystrophy patient. *Spine* 1983;7:771–775.

256. Smith AD, Koreska J, Moseley CF. Progression of scoliosis in Duchenne's muscular dystrophy. *J Bone Joint Surg [Am]* 1989; 71:1066–1074.

257. Seeger BR, Sutherland AD, Clark MA. Orthotic management of scoliosis in Duchenne muscular dystrophy. *Arch Phys Med Rehabil* 1984;65:83–86.

258. Duport G, Gayet E, Pries P, et al. Spinal deformities and wheelchair seating in Duchenne's muscular dystrophy: twenty years of research and clinical experience. *Semin Neurol* 1995;15:29–37.

259. Galasko CS, Delaney C, Morris P. Spinal stabilization in Duchenne muscular dystrophy. *J Bone Joint Surg [Br]* 1992;74:210–214.

260. Hsu JD. Spine care of the patient with Duchenne muscular dystrophy. *Spine* 1990;4:161–172.

261. LaPrade RF, Rowe DE. The operative treatment of scoliosis in Duchenne muscular dystrophy. *Orthop Rev* 1992;21:39–45.

262. Sussman MD. Advantage of early spinal stabilization and fusion in patients with Duchenne muscular dystrophy. *J Pediatr Orthop* 1984;4:532–537.

263. Shapiro F, Sethna N, Colan S, et al. Spinal fusion in Duchenne muscular dystrophy. A multidisciplinary approach. *Muscle Nerve* 1992;15:604–614.

264. Schulz P. Correlation of scoliosis and pulmonary function in Duchenne's muscular dystrophy. *J Pediatr Orthop* 1983;3: 347–353.

265. Miller RG, Chalmers AC, Dao H, et al. The effect of spinal fusion on respiratory function in Duchenne muscular dystrophy. *Neurology* 1991;41:38–40.

266. Kurz L, Mubarak S, Schultz, P et al. Correlation of scoliosis and pulmonary function in Duchenne's muscular dystrophy. *J Pediatr Orthop* 1983;3: 347–353.

267. Miller F, Moseley CF, Koreska J. Spinal fusion in Duchenne muscular dystrophy. *Dev Med Child Neurol* 1992;34:775–786.

268. Dubowitz V. Intellectual impairment in muscular dystrophy. *Arch Dis Child* 1977;40:296–301.

269. Emery AEH. *Duchenne muscular dystrophy*. Oxford: Oxford Medical, 1992.

270. Billard C, Gillet P, Signoret JL, et al. Cognitive function in Duchenne muscular dystrophy: a reappraisal and comparison with spinal muscular atrophy. *Neuromuscul Disord* 1992;2:371–378.

271. Leibowitz D, Dubowitz V. Intellect and behavior in Duchenne muscular dystrophy. *Dev Med Child Neurol* 1981;23:578–590.

272. Karagan N. Intellectual functioning in Duchenne's muscular dystrophy. *Dev Med Child Neurol* 1979;20:435–441.

273. Ahn AH, Kunkel LM. The structural and functional diversity of dystrophin. *Nat Genet* 1993;3:238–291.

274. Rosman N. The cerebral defect and myopathy in Duchenne's muscular dystrophy: a comparative clinicopathological study. *Neurology* 1970;20:329–335.

275. Nudel L, Zuk D, Einat P, et al. Duchenne's muscular dystrophy gene product is not identical in muscle and brain. *Nature* 1989;337:76–78.

276. Bushby KMD, Appleton R, Anderson LVB, et al. Deletion status and intellectual impairment in Duchenne muscular dystrophy. *Dev Med Child Neurol* 1995;37:260–269.

277. Rappaport D. Apparent association of mental retardation and specific patterns of deletions screened with probes is Duchenne's muscular dystrophy. *Am J Med Genet* 1991;39:437–441.

278. Fitzpatrick C, Barry C, Garvey C. Psychiatric disorder among boys with Duchenne MD. *Dev Med Child Neurol* 1986;28:589–595.

279. Harbor JL. Psychosocial aspects of MD and related diseases and their implications for patient care. *Adv Thanatol* 1986;5:15–22.

280. Siegal IM, Davidson H, Kornfeld M, et al. Coping with muscular dystrophy: psychological correlates of adaptation. *Muscle Nerve* 1983;10:607–609.

281. Bregman AM. Living with progressive childhood illness: parental management of neuromuscular disease. *Social Work Health Care* 1980;5:387–407.

282. Witte RA. The psychosocial impact of a progressive physical handicap and terminal illness (Duchenne muscular dystrophy) on adolescents and their families. *Br J Med Psychol* 1985;58:179–187.

283. Botvin-Madorsky JG, Raford LM, Neumann Em. Psychosocial aspects of death and dying in Duchenne muscular dystrophy. *Arch Phys Med Rehabil* 1984;65:79–82.

284. Bushby KM, Thambyayah M, Gardner Medwin D. Prevalence and incidence of Becker muscular dystrophy. *Lancet* 1991;337:1022–1024.

285. Monaco AP, Bertelson CJ, Liechti-Gallati S, et al. An explanation for the phenotype differences between patients bearing partial deletions of the Duchenne's muscular dystrophy locus. *Genomics* 1988;2:90–95.

286. Nicholson LVB, Johnson MA, Gardner Medwin D, et al. Heterogeneity of dystrophin expression in patients with Duchenne and Becker muscular dystrophy. *Acta Neuropathol (Berl)* 1991;80:239–250.

287. Emery AEH, Skinner R. Clinical studies in benign X linked MD. *Clin Genet* 1976;10:189–201.

288. Gospe SM, Lazaro RP, Lava NS, et al. Familial X linked myalgia and cramps: a nonprogressive myopathy associated with a deletion in the dystrophin gene. *Neurology* 1989;39:1277–1280.

289. Norman A, Thomas N, Coakley J, et al. Distinction of Becker from limb girdle muscular dystrophy by means of dystrophin DNA probes. *Lancet* 1989;1:466–468.

290. Bushby KM, Gardner Medwin D. The clinical, genetic, and dystrophin characteristics of Becker muscular dystrophy. 1. Natural history. *J Neurol* 1993;240:998–1004.

291. McDonald CM, Abresch RT, Carter GT, et al. Profiles of neuromuscular diseases: Becker's muscular dystrophy. *Am J Phys Med Rehabil* 1995;74(suppl):93–103.

292. Steare GE, Dubowitz V, Benatar A. Subclinical cardiomyopathy in Becker muscular dystrophy. *Br Heart J* 1992;68:304–308.

293. Melacini P, Fanin M, Danieli GA, et al. Cardiac involvement in Becker muscular dystrophy. *J Am Coll Cardiol* 1993;22:1927–1934.

294. Quinlivan RM, Dubowitz V. Cardiac transplantation in Becker muscular dystrophy. *Neuromuscul Disord* 1992;2:165–167.

295. Ebers GC, George AL, Barchi RL, et al. Paramyotonia congenita and nonmyotonic hyperkalemic periodic paralysis are linked to the adult muscle sodium channel gene. *Ann Neurol* 1991;30:810–816.

296. Smith SA. Congenital and metabolic myopathies. In: Swaiman KF, ed. *Pediatric neurology: principles and practice.* 2nd ed. St. Louis: Mosby, 1994:1505–1521.

297. Streib EW. Paramyotonia congenita: successful treatment with tocainide: clinical and electrophysiologic findings in seven patients. *Muscle Nerve* 1987;10:155–162.

298. Abdalla JA, Casley WL, Cousin HK, et al. Linkage of autosomal dominant myotonia congenita to the T-cell receptor beta gene locus on chromosome 7q35. *Am J Hum Genet* 1992;51:579–584.

299. Becker PE. Myotonia congenital and syndromes associated with myotonia: clinical-genetic strides of the mondystrophic myotonias. In: Becker PE, ed. *Topics in human genetics.* Stuttgart: Tricare, 1977.

300. Rudel R, Ricker K, Lehmann Horn F. Transient weakness and altered membrane characteristic in recessive generalized myotonia (Becker). *Muscle Nerve* 1988;1:202–211.

301. Petty RKH, Harding AE, Morgan Hughes JA. The clinical features

of mitochondrial myopathy. *Brain* 1986;109:915–938.

302. Egger J, Lake BD, Wilson J. Mitochondrial cytopathy: a multisystem disorder with ragged red fibers on muscle biopsy. *Arch Dis Child* 1981;56:741–752.

303. Morgan Hughes JA. The mitochondrial myopathies. In: Engel AG, Banker BQ, eds. *Myology,* New York: McGraw-Hill, 1986:1709–1743.

304. Schapira AH. Mitochondrial myopathies. BMJ 1989;298: 1127–1128.

305. Harding AE, Holt IF. Mitochondrial myopathies. Review article. *Prog Clin Biol Res* 1989;306: 117–128.

306. DiMauro S. Mitochondrial encephalomyopathies. In: Rosenberg RN, Prusiner SB, DiMauro S, et al, eds. *The molecular and genetic basis of neurological disease.* Boston: Butterworth-Heinemann, 1993:665–694.

307. DeVivo DC, DiMauro S. Mitochondrial diseases. In: Swaiman KF, ed. *Pediatric neurology: principles and practice.* 2nd ed. St. Louis: Mosby, 1994:1335–1356.

308. Wallace DC, Sing G, Lott MT, et al. Familial mitochondrial encephalopathy (MERFF): genetic, pathophysiological and biochemical characterization of a mitochondrial DNA disease. *Cell* 1988;55:601–610.

309. Hirano M, Ricci E, Koenigsberger MR, et al. MELAS: an original case and clinical criteria for diagnosis. *Neuromuscul Disord* 1992;2:125–135.

310. Calvani M, Koverech A, Caruso G. Treatment of mitochondrial diseases. In: Di Mauro S, Wallace DC, eds. *Mitochondrial DNA in human pathology.* New York: Raven, 1993.

311. Padberg GW, Lunt PW, Koach M, Fardeau M. Diagnostic criteria for facioscapulohumeral muscular dystrophy. *Neuromuscul Disord* 1991;1:231–234.

312. Bohan A, Peter J. Polymyositis and dermatomyositis. *N Engl J Med* 1975;292:344–347, 292:403–407.

313. Spencer CH, Hanson V, Singsen BH, et al. Course of treated juvenile dermatomyositis. *J Pediatr* 1984;105:399–408.

314. Pachman LM. Juvenile dermatomyositis. *Pediatr Clin North Am* 1986;33:1097–1117.

315. Kingston WJ, Moxley RT. Inflammatory myopathies. *Neurol Clin* 1988;6:545–561.

316. Bowyer SL, Blane CE, Sullivan DB, Cassidy JT. Childhood dermatomyositis: factors predicting functional outcome and development of dystrophic calcification. *J Pediatr* 1983;103:882–888.

317. Bitnum C, Dawschnor CW, Travis LB. Dermatomyositis. *J Pediatr* 1964;64:101–134.

318. Escalante A, Miller L, Beardmore TD. Resistive exercise in the rehabilitation of polymyositis/dermatomyositis. *J Rhematol* 1993;20:1340–1344.

319. Brett EM, Lake BD. Neuromuscular disorders: I. Primary muscle disease and anterior horn cell disorders. In: Brett EM, ed. *Pediatric neurology.* 2nd ed. New York: Churchill Livingstone, 1991:53–115.

320. Rodriguez M, Gomez MR, Howard FM. Myasthenia gravis in children: long term follow-up. *Ann Neurol* 1983;13:504–510.

321. Adams C, Theodorescu D, Murphy EG, et al. Thymectomy in juvenile myasthenia gravis. *J Child Neurol* 1990;5:215–218.

322. Jackson CE, Strehler PA. Limb girdle muscular dystrophy: clinical manifestation and deterioration of preclinical disease. *Pediatrics* 1968;41:495–502.

323. Bushby KM. Report on the 12th ENMC-sponsored international workshop on the "limb girdle" muscular dystrophies. *Neuromuscul Disord* 1992;2:3–5.

324. McDonald DM, Johnson ER, Abresch RT, et al. Profiles of neuromuscular diseases: limb girdle syndromes. *Am J Phys Med Rehabil* 1995; 74(suppl):117–130.

325. Romero NB, Tome FM, Leturcq F, et al. Genetic heterogeneity of severe childhood autosomal recessive muscular dystrophy with adhalin. *C R Acad Sci II* 1994;317:70–76.

326. Ben Hamida M, Fardeau M, Attia N. Severe childhood muscular dystrophy affecting both sexes and frequent in Tunisia. *Muscle Nerve* 1983;6:469–480.

327. Shields RW. Limb girdle syndromes. In: Engel AG, Banker BQ, eds. *Myology.* New York: McGraw-Hill, 1986:1349–1365.

328. Tachi N, Tachi M, Sasaki K, Inamijras S. Early onset benign autosomal dominant limb girdle myopathy with contractures. *Pediatr Neurol* 1989;5: 232–236.

329. Bethlem J, Van Wiingaarden GK. Benign myopathy with autosomal dominant inheritance. *Brain* 1976;99:91–100.

330. Edwards RHT. Management of muscular dystrophy in adults. *Br Med Bull* 1989;45:802–818.

331. Wijmenga C, Frants RR, Hewit JE, et al. Molecular genetics of facioscapulohumeral dystrophy. *Neuromuscul Disord* 1993;3: 487–491.

332. Kilmer DD, Abresch RT, McCrory MA, et al. Profiles of neuromuscular diseases: facioscapulohumeral dystrophy. *Am J Phys Med Rehabil* 1995;74(suppl): 131–139.

333. Fitzsimmons RB, Gurwin EB, Bird AC. Retinal vascular abnormalities in facioscapulohumeral muscular dystrophy: a general association with genetic and therapeutic implications. *Brain* 1987;110:631–648.

334. Korf BR, Bresnan MJ, Shapiro F, et al. Facioscapulohumeral dystrophy presenting in infancy with facial diplegia and sensorineural deafness. *Ann Neurol* 1985;17: 513–516.

335. Munsat TL. Facioscapulohumeral dystrophy and the scapuloper-

oneal syndrome. In: Engel AG, Banker BQ, eds. *Myology.* New York: McGraw-Hill, 1986: 1251–1266.

336. Workshop report: diagnostic criteria for FSH muscular dystrophy. *Neuromuscul Disord* 1991;1: 231–234.

337. Brouwer OF, Padberg GW, Vander Plueg JD, et al. The influence of handedness on the distribution of weakness of the arm in FSH muscular dystrophy. *Brain* 1992;115:1587–1598.

338. Johnson EW, Braddom R. Overwork weakness in facioscapulohumeral dystrophy. *Arch Phys Med Rehabil* 1971;53:333–336.

339. Bunch WH, Siegel IM. Scapulothoracic arthrodesis in facioscapulohumeral muscular dystrophy. *J Bone Joint Surg [Am]* 1993;75:372–376.

340. Wevers CWJ, Brouwer OF, Padbers GW, Nijboer ID. Job perspectives in facioscapulohumeral muscular dystrophy. *Disabil Rehabil* 1993;15:24–28.

341. Lunt PW, Compston DAS, Harper PS. Genetic counselling in facioscapulohumeral muscular dystrophy. *J Med Genet* 1991;28:655–664.

342. Upadhyaya M, Lunt PW, Sarfarazi M, et al. A closely linked DNA marker for facioscapulohumeral disease on chromosome 4q. *J Med Genet* 1991;28:665–671.

343. Ville I, Ravaud JF, Marchal F, et al. Social identity and the international classification of handicaps: an evaluation of the consequences of FSH dystrophy. *Disabil Rehabil* 1992;14: 168–175.

344. Emery AEH. Emery Dreifuss syndrome. *J Med Genet* 1989;26: 637–641.

345. Yates JRW, Affara NA, Jamieson DM, et al. Emery Dreifuss muscular dystrophy: localisation to Xq27 confirmed by linkage to the factor VIII gene. *J Med Genet* 1986;23:587–590.

346. Merlini L, Granata C, Dominici P, Bonfiglioli S. Emery Dreifuss MD. Report of 5 cases and review of the literature. *Muscle Nerve* 1986;9:481–485.

347. Shapiro F, Specht L. Orthopedic deformities in Emery Dreifuss muscular dystrophy. *J Pediatr Orthop* 1991;11: 336–340.

348. Voit T, Krogmann O, Lenard HG, et al. Emery Dreifuss muscular dystrophy: disease spectrum and differential diagnosis. *Neuropediatrics* 1988;19:62–71.

349. Eisen A. Amyotrophic lateral sclerosis is a multifactorial disease. *Muscle Nerve* 1995;18: 741–752.

350. Bensimon G, Lacombiez L, Meininger V. The ALS/Riluzole Study Group: a controlled trial of riluzole in amyotrophic lateral sclerosis. *N Engl J Med* 1994;330:585–591.

351. Hudson AJ. The motor neuron disease and related disorders. In: Joynt RJ, ed. *Clinical neurology.* Vol. 4. Philadelphia: JB Lippincott, 1991:7–35.

352. Hudson AJ, Davenport A, Hader WJ. The incidence of amyotrophic lateral sclerosis in Southwestern Ontario, Canada. Neurology 1986;36:1524–1528.

353. Eisen A, Schulzer M, MacNeil M, et al. Duration of amyotrophic lateral sclerosis is age dependent. *Muscle Nerve* 1993;16: 27–32.

354. Layzer R. Hereditary and acquired intrinsic motor neuron disease. In: *Cecil's textbook of medicine.* 20th ed. Philadelphia: WB Saunders, 1996:2052.

355. Dumitru D. *Electrodiagnostic medicine.* Philadelphia: Hanley & Belfus, 1995.

356. Harvey DG, Torack RM, Rosenbaum HE. Amyotrophic lateral sclerosis with ophthalmoplegia: a clinicopathologic study. *Arch Neurol* 1979;36:615–617.

357. Karpati G, Klassen G, Tanser P. Effects of chronic partial denervation on forearm metabolism. *Can J Neurol Sci* 1979;6: 105–112.

358. Sharma KR, Kent-Braun JA, Majumdar S, et al. Physiology of fatigue in amyotrophic lateral sclerosis. *Neurology* 1995;45:733–740.

359. Sanjak M, Paulson D, Sufit R, et al. Physiologic and metabolic response to progressive and prolonged exercise in amyotrophic lateral sclerosis. *Neurology* 1987;37:1217–1220.

360. Norris FH, Sang UK, Sachais B, Carey M. Trial of baclofen in amyotrophic lateral sclerosis. *Arch Neurol* 1979;36:715–716.

361. Raynor EM, Shefner JM. Recurrent inhibition is decreased in patients with amyotrophic lateral sclerosis. *Neurology* 1994;44:2148–2153.

362. Assessment: the clinical usefulness of botulinum toxin-A in treating neurologic disorders. Report of the Therapeutics and Technology Assessment subcommittee of the American Academy of Neurology. *Neurology* 1990;40:1332–1336.

363. Mayberry JF, Atkinson M. Swallowing problems in patients with motor neuron disease. *J Clin Gastroenterol* 1986;8:233–234.

364. Yorkston KM, Miller RM, Strand EA. *Management of speech and swallowing in degenerative disease.* Tucson: Communication Skill Builders, 1995:3–85.

365. Montgomery GK, Erickson LM. Neuropsychological perspectives in amyotrophic lateral sclerosis. *Neurol Clin* 1987; 5(1):61–81.

366. Hudson AJ. Amyotrophic lateral sclerosis and its association with dementia, parkinsonism, and other neurologic disorders; a review. *Brain* 1981;104: 217–247.

367. Gallagher JP. Pathologic laughter and crying in ALS: a search for their origin. *Acta Neurol Scand* 1989;80:114–117.

368. Barnett VA, Bach JR. Psychologic considerations in the treatment of individuals with generalized neuromuscular disorders. *Semin Neurol* 1995;15:58–64.

369. Darley FL, Aronson AE, Brown JR. *Motor speech disorders.* Philadelphia: WB Saunders, 1975.

370. Yorkston KM, Strand E, Miller R, et al. Speech deterioration in amyotrophic lateral sclerosis. Implications for the timing of intervention. *J Med Speech Lang Pathol* 1993;1:35–46.

371. Yorkston KM, Beukelman DR, Bell KR. *Clinical management of dysarthric speakers.* Austin, TX: Pro-Ed, 1988.

372. Kazandjian MS, Dikeman KJ, Bach JR. Assessment and management of communication impairment in neuro-muscular disease. *Semin Neurol* 1995;15:58–64.

373. Bach JR. Amyotrophic lateral sclerosis: communication status and survival with ventilatory support. *Am J Phys Med Rehabil* 1993;72:343–349.

374. Sitver MS, Kraat A. Augmentative communication for the person with amyotrophic lateral sclerosis. *ASHA* 1982;24:783.

375. Beukelman DR, Mireuda P. *Augmentative and alternative communication management of severe communication disorders in children and adults.* Baltimore: Paul H. Brookes, 1992.

376. Goossens C, Crain S. Overview of non-electronic eye-gaze communication techniques. *Augment Altern Commun* 1987;3(2): 77–89.

377. Norris FH. Adult spinal motor neuron disease; progressive muscular atrophy (Aran's disease) in relation to amyotrophic lateral sclerosis. In: Vinken PJ, Bruyn GW, DeJong JMBV, eds. *Handbook of clinical neurology.* Vol. 22. Amsterdam: North-Holland, 1975:1–56.

378. Norris FH. Adult progressive muscular atrophy and hereditary spinal muscular atrophies. In: Vinken PJ, Bruyn GW, Klawans HL, eds. *Handbook of clinical neurology.* Vol. 59. Amsterdam: North-Holland, 1991:13–34.

379. Rietschel M, Ruduik-Schoneborn S, Zerres K. Clinical variability of autosomal dominant spinal muscular atrophy. *J Neurol Sci* 1992;107:65–73.

380. Swash M, Schwartz MS. *Neuromuscular diseases.* London: Springer-Verlag, 1986.

381. Chio A, Brignolio F, Leone M, et al. A survival analysis of 155 cases of progressive muscular atrophy. *Acta Neurol Scand* 1985;72:407.

382. Adams RD, Victor M. *Principles of neurology.* 3rd ed. New York: McGraw-Hill, 1985.

383. Kimura J. *Electrodiagnosis in diseases of nerve and muscles.* Philadelphia: FA Davis, 1989.

384. Parhad IM, Clark WA, Barron KD, Staunton SB. Diaphragmatic paralysis in motor neuron disease: reports of 2 cases and a review of the literature. *Neurology* 1978;28:18–22.

385. Osserman KE, Genkins G. Studies in myasthenia gravis: a review of a 20 year old experience in over 1200 patients. *Mt. Sinai J Med* 1971; 38:497–537.

386. Alter M, Talbert OR, Kurland LT. Myasthenia gravis in a southern community. *Arch Neurol* 1960;3:65–69.

387. Cohen MS. Epidemiology of myasthenia gravis. *Monogr Allergy* 1987;21:246–251.

388. Garland H, Clark AN. Myasthenia gravis: a personal study of 60 cases. *BMJ* 1956;1:1259–1262.

389. Hokkanen E. Epidemiology of myasthenia gravis in Finland. *J Neurol Sci* 1969;9:463–478.

390. Kurland LT, Alter M. Current status of the epidemiology and genetics of myasthenia gravis. In: Viets HR, ed. *Myasthenia gravis.* Springfield, IL: Charles C Thomas, 1961:307–336.

391. Osserman KE, Genkins G. Clinical reappraisal of the use of edrophonium (Tensilon) chloride tests in myasthenia gravis and significance of clinical classification. *Ann NY Acad Sci* 1965;135:312–326.

392. Phillips LLt, Torner JC, Anderson MS, et al. The epidemiology of myasthenia gravis in central and western Virginia. *Neurology* 1992;42:1888–1893.

393. Storm-Mathisen A. Epidemiology of myasthenia gravis in Norway. *Acta Neurol Scand* 1976; 54:120.

394. Storm-Mathisen A. Epidemiology of myasthenia gravis in Norway. *Acta Neurol Scand* 1984;70:274–284.

395. Grob D, Brunner NG, Namba T. The natural course of myasthenia gravis and the effect of therapeutic measures. *Ann NY Acad Sci* 1981;377:606–613.

396. Cohen MS, Younger D. Aspects of the natural history of myasthenia gravis; crises and death. *Ann NY Acad Sci* 1981;377:670–677.

397. Somnier FE, Feidling N, Paulson OB. Epidemiology of myasthenia gravis. *Arch Neurol* 1991; 48:733–739.

398. Grob D, Brunner NG, Namba T. The natural course of myasthenia gravis and the effect of therapeutic measures. *Ann NY Acad Sci* 1971;38:497.

399. Lisaka RP, Barchi RL. *Myasthenia gravis.* Philadelphia: WB Saunders, 1982:157–184.

400. Lopate G, Pestronk A. Auto immune myasthenia gravis. *Hosp Pract* 1993;28:109–131.

401. Swash M, Schwartz MS. *Neuromuscular disease: a practical approach to diagnosis and management.* 2nd ed. London: Springer-Verlag, 1988.

402. Sanders DB, Scopetta C. The treatment of patients with myasthenia gravis. *Neurol Clin North Am* 1994;12:343–368.

403. Mann JD, Johns TR, Campa JF. Long-term administration of corticosteroids in myasthenia gravis. *Neurology* 1976;26:729–740.

404. Pease WS, Lagatutta FP. Exacerbation of a case of myasthenia gravis during therapeutic electric stimulation. *Arch Phys Med Rehabil* 1987;68:568–570.

405. Lohi EL, Linberg C, Anderson O. Physical training effects in myasthenia gravis. *Arch Phys Med Rehabil* 1993;74:1178–1180.

406. Khan OA, Campbell WW. Myasthenia gravis presenting as dysphagia: clinical considerations. *Am J Gastroenterol* 1994;89: 1083–1085.

407. Huang MH, King KL, Chien KY. Esophageal manometric studies in patients with myasthenia gravis. *J Thorac Cardiovasc Surg* 1988;95:281–285.

408. Willis TN, Paulus J, Lacau Saint Guily J, et al. Swallowing problems in neuromuscular disorders. *Arch Phys Med Rehabil* 1994;75:1175–1181.

409. Carr SR, Gilchrist JM, Abuelo DN, et al. Treatment of antenatal myasthenia gravis. *Obstet Gynecol* 1991;78:485–489.

410. Fennell DF, Ringle SP. Myasthenia gravis and pregnancy. *Gynecol Surv* 1987;41:414–421.

411. Mitchell P, Bebbington M. Myasthenia gravis pregnancy. *Obstet Gynecol* 1992;80:178–181.

412. Mahadevan M, Tsilfidis C, Sabourin L, et al. Myotonic dystrophy mutation; an unstable CTG repeat in the 3 untranslated regions of the gene. *Science* 1992;255:1253–1258.

413. Mathieu J, De Braekeleen M, Prevost C. Genealogical reconstruction of myotonic dystrophy in the Saguenay-Lac-Saint-Jean area (Quebec, Canada). *Neurology* 1990;40;839–842.

414. Chen KM, Brody JA, Kurland LT. Patterns of neurologic disease on Guam. *Arch Neurol* 1968;19: 573–578.

415. Lotz BP, van der Meyden CH. Myotonic dystrophy. Part I. A genealogical study in the northern Transvaal. *S Afr Med J* 1985;67:812–814.

416. Jennekens FGI, ten Kate LP, de Visser M, Wintzen AR. Myotonic dystrophy (Steinert's disease). In: Emery AEH, ed. *Diagnostic criteria for neuro muscular disorders.* Baarn, Netherlands: European Neuromuscular Centre, 1994: 35–38.

417. Fu YH, Friedman DL, Richard S, et al. Decreased expression of myotonic-protein kinase messenger RNA and protein in the adult form of myotonic dystrophy. *Science* 1993; 260:235–238.

418. Johnson ER, Abresch MS, Carter GT, et al. Profiles of neuromuscular disease: myotonic dystrophy. *Am J Phys Med Rehabil* 1995; 74(suppl):S104–S116.

419. Barnes PRJ. Clinical and genetic aspects of myotonic dystrophy. *Br J Hosp Med* 1993;50:22–30.

420. Milner-Brown HS, Miller RG. Myotonic dystrophy: quantification of muscle weakness and myotonia and the effect of amitriptyline and exercise. *Arch Phys Med Rehabil* 1990;71: 983–987.

421. Kilmer DD, McCrory MA, Wright NC, et al. The effect of a high resistance exercise program in slowly progressive neuromuscular disease. *Arch Phys Med Rehabil* 1994;75:560–567.

422. Lindeman E, Leffers P, Spaans F, et al. Strength training in patients with myotonic dystrophy and hereditary motor and sensory neuropathy: a randomized clinical trial. *Arch Phys Med Rehabil* 1995;76:612–620.

423. Wright NC, Kilmer DD, McCrory MA, et al. Aerobic walking in slowly progressive neuromuscular disease: effect of a 12-week program. *Arch Phys Med Rehabil* 1996;77:64–69.

424. Arahata K, Engel AG. Monoclonal antibody analysis of mononuclear cells in myopathies. I: quantitation of subsets according to diagnosis and sites of accumulation and demonstration and counts of muscle fibers invaded by T cells. *Ann Neurol* 1984;16:193.

425. Engel AG, Arahata K. Monoclonal antibody analysis of mononuclear cells in myopathies, II. Phenotypes of auto invasive cells in polymyositis and inclusion body myositis. *Ann Neurol* 1984;16:209.

426. Griggs RC, Mendell JR, Miller RG. *Evaluation and treatment of myopathies.* Philadelphia: FA Davis, 1995.

427. Benbassett J, Greffel D, Zlotnick A. Epidemiology of polymyositis dermatomyositis in Israel 1960–1976. *Isr J Med Sci* 1980;16:197–200.

428. Hockberg MC, Lopez-Acuna D, Giltelshon AM. Mortality from polymyositis and dermatomyositis in the United States, 1968–1978. *Arthritis Rheum* 1983;26:1465–1471.

429. Kurkland LT, Hauser WA, Ferguson RH, et al. Epidemiologic features of diffuse connective tissue disorders in Rochester, MN 1951–1967, with special reference to systemic lupus erythematosus. *Mayo Clin Proc* 1969;44:649–663.

430. Adams RD, Victor M. *Principles of neurology.* 5th ed. New York: McGraw-Hill, 1993:1202–1207.

431. Adams EM, Plotz PH. The treatment of myositis. *Rheum Dis Clin North Am* 1995;21:179–202.

432. Oddis CV, Hill P, Medser PA. Functional outcome in a national cohort of polymyositis dermatomyositis (PM-DM) patients. *Arthritis Rheum* 1992;35:588.

433. Rowland LP. Polymyositis. In: Rowland LP, ed. *Merritt's textbook of neurology.* 7th ed. Philadelphia: Lea & Febiger, 1984;582C–592D.

434. Stark RJ. Polymyositis presenting with severe weakness involving only one arm. *Aust N Z J Med* 1978;8:544–546.

435. Newman ED, Kurland RJ. P 31 Magnetic resonance spectroscopy in polymyositis and dermatomyositis. *Arthritis Rheum* 1992;35:199–202.

436. Hebert CA, Byrnes TJ, Baethge BA, et al. Exercise limitation in patients with polymyositis. *Chest* 1990;98:352–357.

437. Plotz PH, Leff RL, Miller FW. Inflammatory and metabolic myopathies. In: Schumacher HR, Klippel JH, Koopman WJ, eds.

Primer on the rheumatic diseases. 10th ed. Atlanta: Arthritis Foundation, 1993:127–131.

438. Dalakas MC. *Polymyositis and dermatomyositis.* Boston: Butterworths, 1988.

439. Plotz PH, Dalakas M, Leff RL, et al. Current concepts in the idiopathic inflammatory myopathies: polymyositis, dermatomyositis and related disorders. *Ann Intern Med* 1989;111:143–157.

440. Rowland RP, Clarke C, Olarte M. Therapy for dermatomyositis and polymyositis. *Adv Neurol* 1977;17:63–97.

441. Dietz F, Logeman JA, Sahgal V, Schmid FR. Cricopharyngeal muscle dysfunction in differential diagnosis of dysphagia in polymyositis. *Arthritis Rheum* 1980;23:491–495.

442. Pigg JS. Nursing care of the hospitalized patient with rheumatic disease. In: Ehrlich GE, ed. *Rehabilitation management of rheumatic conditions.* Baltimore: Williams & Wilkins, 1986:118.

443. Lotz BP, Engel AG, Nishono H, et al. Inclusion body myositis. *Brain* 1989;112:727–747.

444. Massa R, Wellen B, Karpati G, et al. Familial inclusion body myositis among Kurdish-Iranian Jews. *Arch Neurol* 1991;48:519–522.

445. Neville HE, Baumbach LL, Ringel SP, et al. Familial inclusion body myositis: evidence for autosomal dominant inheritance. *Neurology* 1992;42:897–902.

446. Joffe MM, Love LA, Leff RL, et al. Drug therapy of the idiopathic inflammatory myopathies. Predictors of response to prednisone, azathioprine, and methotrexate and a comparison of their efficacy. *Am J Med* 1993;94:379–387.

447. Love LA, Leff RL, Fraser DD, et al. A new approach to the classification of idiopathic inflammatory myopathy myositis specific auto-antibodies define useful homogeneous patient groups. *Medicine* 1991;70:360–374.

448. Calabrese LH, Mitsumoto H, Chou S-M. Inclusion body myositis presenting as treatment resistant polymyositis *Arthritis Rheum* 1987;30:397–340.

449. Danon MJ, Reyes MG, Demrena OH, et al. Inclusion body myositis: a corticosteroid-resistant idiopathic inflammatory myopathy. *Arch Neurol* 1982;39:760–764.

450. Wintzen AR, Bots GThAM, deBakker HM. et al. Dysphagia in inclusion body myositis. *J Neurol Neurosurg Psychiatry* 1988;51:1542–1545.

451. Verma A, Bradley WG, Adesina AM, et al. Inclusion body myositis with cricopharyngeus muscle involvement and severe dysphagia. *Muscle Nerve* 1991;14:470–473.

452. Danon MJ, Friedman M. Inclusion body myositis associated with progressive dysphagia: treatment with cricopharyngeal myotomy. *Can J Neurol Sci* 1989;16:436–438.

453. Barbeau A. The syndrome of late onset ptosis and dysphagia in French Canada. In: Kuhn E, ed. *Symposium Uber Progressive Muskeldystrophie, Myotonie Myasthenie.* Berlin: Springer-Verlag, 1966:102.

454. Barbeau A. Oculopharyngeal muscular dystrophy in French Canada. In: Burnette JT, Barbeau A, eds. *Progress in neuro-ophthalmology.* Amsterdam: Excerpta Medica, 1967:3.

455. Victor M, Hayes R, Adams RD. Oculopharyngeal muscular dystrophy: a familial disease of late life characterized by dysphagia and progressive ptosis of the eyelids. *N Engl J Med* 1962;267:1267.

456. Rowland LP. Progressive external ophthalmoplegia and ocular myopathies. In: Rowland LP, DiMauro S, eds. *Handbook of clinical neurology.* Vol. 18. Amsterdam: Elsevier, 1992: 287–329.

457. Tome FMS, Fardeau M. Ocular myopathies. In: Engel AG, Banker BQ, eds. *Myology.* New York: McGraw-Hill, 1986:1327–1347.

458. Satoyoshi E, Kimoshita M. Oculopharyngodistal myopathy. *Arch Neurol* 1977;34:89.

459. St. Giuily JL, Pe'rie' S, Willing T-N, et al. Swallowing disorders in muscular diseases: functional assessement and indications of cricopharyngeal myotomy. *Ear Nose Throat J* 1994;73:34–40.

460. Welander L. Myopathia distalis tarda hereditaria. *Acta Med Scand* 1951;141(suppl 265):1.

461. Markesbery WR, Griggs RC, Leach RP, Lapham LW. Late onset hereditary distal myopathy. *Neurology* 1974;24:127.

462. Buchman AS, Cochran EJ. Distal myopathies. In: Rowland LP, DiMauro S, eds. *Handbook of clinical neurology.* Vol. 18. Amsterdam: Elsevier, 1992: 197–208.

463. Markesbery WR, Griggs RC. Distal myopathies. In: Engel AG, Banker BQ, eds. *Myology.* New York: McGraw-Hill, 1986:1313–1325.

464. Erwin JH, Keller C, Anderson S, Costa J. Hand and wrist strengthening exercises during rehabilitation of a patient with hereditary distal myopathy. *Arch Phys Med Rehabil* 1991;72:701–702.

465. Johnson ER, Abresch RT, Carter T, et al. Profiles of neuromuscular disease: myotonic dystrophy. *Am J Phys Med Rehabil* 1995;74:S104–116.

Chapter 90

Respiratory Considerations for the Rehabilitation Patient

John R. Bach

ETIOLOGY OF RESPIRATORY COMPLICATIONS

All respiratory complications result from some combination of inspiratory, expiratory, and bulbar muscle dysfunction and intrinsic lung or airway disease. Most pulmonary morbidity and mortality in rehabilitation patients result from hypoventilation and difficulties in eliminating airway secretions. Hypoventilation is due to respiratory muscle dysfunction or mechanical factors that result in stiffening of the lung tissues and chest walls and in decreased pulmonary compliance. The greater the resulting hypercapnia, the greater the risk of pulmonary morbidity and mortality (1).

Clearance of airway secretions is adversely affected by any factors that increase secretion production, decrease mucociliary transport or peak cough flows (PCFs), or lend to aspiration of upper-airway secretions or food. Typically increases in the production of secretions occur and the mucociliary elevator is impaired by chronic exposure to cigarette smoke and by the bronchial mucosal denudation from tracheal suctioning and the chronic inflammation associated with the presence of an indwelling tracheostomy tube. Immobility and impaired consciousness also result in stasis and bronchial secretion retention.

Impaired ability to cough is probably the single most important factor leading to respiratory complications and acute respiratory failure in rehabilitation patients. Any combination of inspiratory, expiratory, and bulbar muscle dysfunction reduces PCFs. Bulbar muscle dysfunction can also result in swallowing impairment and in aspiration of food and secretions.

Although most rehabilitation patients develop respiratory complications from muscular dysfunction, much can be learned by considering patients who have intrinsic lung or airway disease. These patients have primarily an impaired ability to oxygenate the blood from an anatomically or functionally decreased respiratory exchange membrane and severe ventilation-perfusion mismatching. Typically, patients with chronic obstructive pulmonary disease (COPD) or restrictive lung disease from infiltrative processes such as pulmonary fibrosis fall into this category. These patients can be eucapnic or hypocapnic, often despite severe hypoxia, and they are susceptible to intercurrent exacerbations of lung disease that often result in pneumonia, hospitalization, and acute respiratory failure. Intercurrent morbidity and mortality are associated with chronic pathogenic bacterial colonization of the airways that impairs mucociliary transport and inspissates secretions (2), and from the inability to create sufficient transient PCFs throughout the airways to eliminate these inspissated secretions (3). While often chronically hypoxic, advanced and acutely ill patients can also become hypercapnic from failing to adequately ventilate sufficiently to maintain normal blood carbon dioxide tensions.

The primary strategy in treating acute exacerbations in COPD patients is to reverse any reversible bronchospasm with the use of bronchodilators; to ease trapped airway secretions up narrowed or chronically obstructed airways by applying chest percussion, mechanical vibration, or oscillation to the chest or directly to the airways in combination with postural drainage (4); and to reverse hypoxia by administering oxygen (4) and when necessary, by providing mechanical ventilatory support via translaryngeal or tracheostomy tubes. Weaning from the ventilator is usually attempted using some combination of synchronized intermittent mandatory ventilation (SIMV) or assist-control along with pressure support ventilation, positive end-expiratory pressure (PEEP), and supplemental oxygen, and patients' survival can be prolonged by long-term oxygen therapy (4). Rehabilitation strategies and programs for COPD patients have been described in this edition and elsewhere (5).

The majority of rehabilitation patients, on the other hand, have primarily ventilatory impairment. Hypoxia and decreases in oxyhemoglobin saturation (SaO_2) are secondary to the hypercapnia that results from global alveolar hypoventilation of the lung tissues. The application of therapeutic modalities designed for treating COPD or obstructive sleep apnea syndrome (OSAS) to patients with primarily ventilatory impairment is inappropriate and can be harmful. For example, bronchodilators have not been shown to be useful in the absence of reversible bronchospasm and they can augment anxiety and increase the tachycardia that is common in myopathic patients with cardiomyopathy. Nor is theophylline, often given to such individuals in an attempt to relieve diaphragm fatigue, apt to be effective (6). Indeed, in the presence of hypercapnia and hypoxia, theophylline was reported to increase or delay recovery from diaphragm fatigue (7). Low-flow oxygen in combination with protriptyline (8) has been used to treat sleep hypoxia in this patient population. This, however, appears to decrease sleep hypoxia by suppressing rapid-eye-movement (REM) sleep (8). This may only increase patient fatigue and lead to further hypoventilation, and the anticholinergic effects of protriptyline may be troublesome. Cardiac side effects should especially be considered because many of these patients have cardiomyopathies or decreased cardiac reserve due to scoliosis, cardiac conduction defects, or associated medical conditions. Medications such as doxapram hydrochloride, acetazolamide, medroxyprogesterone, and almitrine have also not been shown to benefit patients with primarily ventilatory dysfunction.

Oxygen therapy also poses serious problems. It is associated with a higher risk of pulmonary morbidity and rate of hospitalizations than is the use of ventilatory assistance or no treatment at all (9). By artificially maintaining normal SaO_2, it obscures the presence of bronchial mucous plugs that would otherwise be signaled by desaturations. Oxygen therapy also depresses ventilation by decreasing the hypoxic drive, thereby exacerbating hypercapnia. It has been shown to prolong hypopneas and apneas during REM sleep in individuals with Duchenne muscular dystrophy (DMD) (10) and it appears to suppress the reflex muscular activity mediated by the central nervous system (CNS) that is needed for successful nocturnal ventilatory assistance with the use of noninvasive intermittent positive-pressure ventilation (IPPV) (11).

Although episodes of acute respiratory failure are often preventable, most patients are not introduced to the necessary techniques and equipment, and as a result, respiratory failure results unnecessarily in translaryngeal intubation and often tracheostomy.

With the widespread use of endotracheal intubation and tracheostomy over the last 30 years, however, numerous complications have been reported. These include nosocomial pneumonia, and sudden death from cardiac arrhythmias, mucous plugging, accidental disconnections, and other causes. Gram-negative bacterial colonization is ubiquitous and commonly associated with fatal mucous plugging, chronic purulent bronchitis, granulation formation, and sepsis from stomal infection or paranasal sinusitis. Other complications include tracheomalacia and tracheal perforation, hemorrhage, stenosis, tracheoesophageal fistula, painful hemorrhagic tube changes, and psychosocial disturbances. These complications have been summarized and referenced elsewhere (12–14). A common complication of intubation and possibly tracheostomy is the presence of vocal cord and hypopharyngeal muscle dysfunction and airway collapse. The resulting chronic upper-airway obstruction can prevent the generation of adequate spontaneous or assisted PCFs through the upper airway and thus, cán preclude tracheostomy closure even in the presence of adequate autonomous ventilatory function.

The presence of a tracheostomy tube necessitates regular bronchial suctioning, tracheostomy site care, and tube and tubing changes. Supplemental humidification must be provided and attended to daily. Swallowing difficulties occur as the result of the restriction of upward laryngeal movement and rotation by anchoring of the trachea to the strap muscles and skin of the neck. This results in reduced glottic closure and increased laryngeal penetration, thus increasing the chances of aspiration. Interference with relaxation of the cricopharyngeal sphincter, compression of the esophagus, and changes in intratracheal pressure can add to the problem (15,16). In addition, a tracheostomy is an "open wound," which can prohibit community living and access to many institutions and places of education and employment, without prohibitively expensive nursing care for tracheal suctioning and wound care (17).

Tracheal suctioning causes irritation, increases secretions, may be accompanied by severe hypoxia (18), and is at best effective in clearing only superficial airway secretions. Routine tracheal suctioning misses mucous plugs adherent between the tube and the tracheal wall and misses the left main stem bronchus 54% to 92% of the time (19). This at least in part accounts for the fact that the majority of pneumonias occur in the left lung fields.

EPIDEMIOLOGY OF RESPIRATORY COMPLICATIONS

Spinal Cord Injury

Approximately 10,000 new spinal cord injuries occur annually in the United States, with the cervical region of the spinal cord involved in 60% of patients. Approximately 10% of spinal cord injuries result in complete tetraplegia (20). The respiratory complications of spinal cord injury depend on the level and extent of cord damage. The phrenic nerve outflow to the diaphragm originates from roots C3 to C5. Complete injuries above C3 produce immediate apnea and complete paralysis of both inspiratory and expiratory muscles. Unless prompt resuscitative measures are initiated, death ensues within minutes. Injury between levels C3 and C5 produces an immediate reduction in inspiratory and expiratory pressures, flow rates, and vital capacity (VC). Although sudden, intractable ventilatory muscle failure is seen in patients with acute spinal cord injury, more often spinal cord–injured individuals develop ventilatory failure and require ventilatory assistance from hours to up to 7 days after injury (21,22). This is often as a result of ascending spinal cord edema. Most patients are weaned from ventilator use before transfer to rehabilitation centers. Over a period of 27 years in one rehabilitation center, 109 (4.2%) of 2600 spinal cord–injured patients were admitted using ventilatory support but only 44 (40%) of them were discharged using ventilators (23). Based on an estimation of about 200,000 spinal cord–injured individuals in the United States (24), about 3400 spinal cord–injured ventilator users have been discharged to the community. Weaned patients can also develop late-onset chronic ventilatory insufficiency many years after acute injury (25).

Tetraplegic spinal cord–injured individuals demonstrate abnormalities of pulmonary mechanics, including paradoxical inward movement of the rib cage with inspiration due to intercostal muscle paralysis. With the use of accessory respiratory muscles, rib cage motion is altered further. Cranial displacement of the sternum and relatively greater anteroposterior expansion of the upper rib cage, compared to the lower rib cage occur. If motor function of the pectoralis major (innervated by C5–C7 levels) is preserved, contraction of the upper rib cage occurs, decreasing lung volume and assisting expiratory function.

Hypersecretion of bronchial mucus has been observed in 20% of tetraplegic patients (26). The chemical content of the mucus is also abnormal, suggesting disruption of neuronal control of bronchial mucous secretion. It has been suggested that the function of the cilia in the respiratory tract may be under adrenergic control and thus may also be adversely affected by injury (27).

Pulmonary embolism (PE) from a thrombus in the deep veins of the lower extremity is a leading cause of death in acutely spinal cord–injured individuals. The first 2 weeks after injury are the highest-risk period for deep venous thrombosis (DVT), with the incidence ranging from 10% to 100% depending on the method of evaluation (28). Prevention of DVT is obviously preferable to treatment of PE. A prospective study of 48 acutely spinal cord–injured patients found that the lowest rate of DVT resulted from treatment with low-dose heparin plus electrical stimulation to the calf muscles (1/15), compared to 8 of 17 in the placebo group and 8 of 16 treated with low-dose heparin alone (29).

Over time there is gradual improvement in pulmonary function after spinal cord injury. VC increases and often doubles by 3 months after injury. Much of the early dysfunction is related to airway closure and atelectasis. The improvement can also result from increases in accessory respiratory muscle strength and decreased thoracoabdominal distortion during inspiration as well as from partial neurologic recovery (20).

The incidence of ventilatory failure in patients with myelopathies of other etiologies is unknown; however, patients with severe spinal pathology of any etiology have the same abnormalities in pulmonary mechanics and are susceptible to intercurrent respiratory complications largely from airway secretion retention, and to acute or late-onset chronic ventilatory failure (30).

Multiple Sclerosis

Despite reports to the contrary (31,32), respiratory muscle weakness and pulmonary dysfunction are not uncommon in multiple sclerosis (MS), particularly in MS patients with severe limb or bulbar muscle paralysis, and especially during acute relapses (33). MS can affect almost any area of the CNS, but the areas that are involved with a higher frequency include the periventricular white matter, optic nerves, brain stem, and cervical region of the spinal cord. The various patterns of respiratory involvement in MS depend on the anatomic location and temporal course of the inflammatory demyelination that characterizes the disease.

Acute respiratory failure during acute exacerbations of MS is often due to plaque involvement of the upper cervical region of the spinal cord that results in unilateral or bilateral diaphragmatic paralysis. Quadriparesis and a high cervical level of sensory deficit can develop and the patient can exhibit paradoxic movements of the chest wall and abdomen, use of accessory muscles of respiration, and orthopnea. Localization of pathology to the upper cervical region of the spinal cord, brain stem, or both corticospinal tracts can result in paralysis of voluntary respiration, in which case the patient's clinical presentation can be that of an inability to voluntarily increase tidal volume or hold breath while automatic respirations remain intact. Central hypoventilation occurs particularly during sleep when conscious triggering of the nerves to respiratory muscles cannot occur via the corticospinal tract. Diaphragm paralysis occasionally occurs without concomitant bulbar or limb paralysis (34).

By contrast, lesions of the dorsomedial medulla, nucleus ambiguus, and medial lemniscus result in paralysis of automatic respiration, with normal voluntary control of respiration maintained while the patient is awake. MS plaques in the lower brain stem, reticular activating system, and reticulospinal tract have been reported to cause various patterns of respiratory dysfunction, including apneic pauses after hyperventilation, central hypoventilation, and episodes of inspiratory apneusis with preservation of voluntary control between episodes.

Bulbar involvement also commonly results in cough flows that are inadequate to clear airway secretions and in aspiration of upper-airway secretions and food. OSAS can also occur during brain stem exacerbation of MS (35). Neurogenic pulmonary edema has been correlated with magnetic resonance imaging areas of high signal intensity in the rostral medulla involving the floor of the fourth ventricle. It is believed that the area in and around the nucleus tractus solitarii is the effector site for neurogenic pulmonary edema (36).

Rapidly Developing Ventilatory Failure

Rapidly developing and often late-onset or recurrent ventilatory failure can also occur in patients with Guillain-Barré syndrome, myasthenia gravis, postpoliomyelitis, or basal ganglia or cerebellar disorders, and in any hypercapnic patients during intercurrent respiratory tract infections with bronchorrhea. All of these patients can develop ventilatory failure, especially when associated with bronchial mucous plugging, over a period of hours or days. Many patients who initially require the use of respiratory muscle aids only during intercurrent respiratory infections eventually require daily assistance.

Patients with myasthenia gravis often present with rapid shallow breathing, hypercapnia, a blunted ventilatory response to hypercapnia, and sleep apneas (37), often despite adequate VCs and inspiratory muscle strength. This occurs from some combination of impaired neuromuscular transmission (38), respiratory center depression, and attenuated respiratory muscle endurance. Obesity, intercurrent respiratory infections, bulbar muscle weakness, and surgical thymectomy can add to or trigger respiratory muscle compromise and ventilatory failure.

In Guillain-Barré syndrome, demyelinization affects the neural input to the respiratory and bulbar musculature. Twenty percent to 30% of patients require ventilatory support (39). The diaphragm is often more severely affected than other respiratory musculature. This often leads to disproportionate pulmonary dysfunction with the patient supine and results in severe orthopnea and the need for nocturnal ventilatory assistance. Bulbar muscles are usually, but not always, too severely involved to permit the use of noninvasive respiratory aids as alternatives to endotracheal intubation early on during the recovery process. An intractable 24-hour need for ventilatory support from the onset, and late-onset chronic failure can occur.

Muscular Dystrophy

Individuals with DMD develop dystrophic muscular deterioration of the diaphragm and other respiratory muscles. Their VCs plateau between the ages of 10 and 14 years (40) at 1000 to about 2800 mL. The magnitude of the VC plateau is an indication of the severity of the disorder and of life expectancy for those who are managed conventionally (41). Following the plateau, VC is then lost at a rate of 4% to 10% per year, with the rate of loss tapering off below 400 mL (42,43). Fifty-five percent (44) to 90% (45–47) of DMD patients who do not benefit from respiratory muscle aids die from pulmonary complications, most often between the ages of 16 and 19 years and rarely after age 25 (45,48). These patients inevitably have bouts of pneumonia and respiratory failure that lead to translaryngeal intubation and tracheostomy (48). Patients who die despite effective use of respiratory muscle aids most often die from complications of cardiomyopathy (43).

Patients with myotonic dystrophy, a disorder characterized by muscular dystrophy and numerous other systemic manifestations, usually present with slowly progressive generalized as well as respiratory and bulbar muscle weakness. Chronic hypercapnia often results from a combination of inspiratory muscle weakness, impaired ventilatory mechanics, and especially, altered central ventilatory control (49). The relatively reduced ventilatory response to carbon dioxide and hypoxemia (50,51) is likely due to CNS dysfunction (52). Many patients hypoventilate despite relatively normal VCs, and patients whose hypoventilation is corrected with assisted ventilation often experience no relief of symptoms. Narcolepsy-like excessive diurnal sleepiness appears characteristic of this disorder (53).

Patients with Becker, Emery-Dreifuss, or limb-girdle muscular dystrophy and many with nondystrophic myopathies also have variably progressive conditions with a high incidence of respiratory complications and often the need for ventilator use (54). Congenital muscular dystrophies are usually static conditions that result in intercurrent pulmonary complications and eventually the need for daily ventilator use. As for patients with myotonic dystrophy, patients with nemaline myopathy, mitochondrial myopathies, or myasthenia gravis often have ventilatory insufficiency that is out of proportion to the inspiratory muscle weakness or diminution in VC, suggesting a disturbance of the feedback required for normal control of breathing (55).

Anterior Horn Cell Disease

Patients with motor neuron disease are most often afflicted after their natural VC plateau is reached. Following onset of symptoms, there is often little change in VC for 2 to 4 years. Once the VC begins to decrease, however, the subsequent rate of loss can be 1 to 2 liters per year. Typically, patients who are able to walk but who have respiratory muscle weakness and relatively intact bulbar muscle function develop symptoms of chronic hypercapnia (56). Patients with predominantly bulbar muscle involvement have difficulty managing saliva and airway secretions and present with dyspnea or acute respiratory failure due to atelectasis or aspiration pneumonia, despite having VCs that are often greater than 50% of the predicted normal capacity. Although survival time can vary from less than a year to more than a decade with (57) or occasionally without ventilatory support, the average survival time without ventilator use is 3 to 4 years. Conventionally managed patients are typically hypercapnic during the last 20% of unaided survival (58).

Patients with spinal muscular atrophy patients with severe type 1 atrophy can present with ventilatory failure as neonates, but failure is most often triggered by an intercurrent respiratory tract infection after this period. Early spinal fusion to manage scoliosis stiffens the thoracic wall and along with early respiratory muscle weakness, results in severe restrictive pulmonary disease with inadequate growth and development of the bronchial tree and respiratory exchange membrane. These patients have paradoxical collapse of the chest wall during diaphragm activity, decreasing the efficiency of an already weakened diaphragm. Patients with mild type 2 or type 3 disease often tolerate mild hypercapnia for decades before ongoing ventilatory assistance becomes necessary (59).

Postpoliomyelitis patients have been reported to lose VC 70% faster than normal (56,60). Some required ventilatory assistance since the onset of polio, whereas others who were initially ventilator weaned developed late-onset chronic ventilatory insufficiency (61). Virtually none should require tracheostomy tubes.

Sleep Disordered Breathing

Sleep disordered breathing refers to the occurrence of central, obstructive, or mixed apneas, or hypopneas, or both during sleep. The obstructive apneas are most commonly due to hypopharyngeal collapse. Carskadon and Dement (62) found that 37.5% of men over age 62 had apneas or hypopneas, apneas being defined as the cessation of airflow for 10 seconds or more and hypopneas defined as reductions in normal tidal volumes by more than 30%. Many apneas and hypopneas are associated with decreases in SaO_2 of 4% or more (63). At least 3% of the general population is symptomatic for this condition (63). OSAS is diagnosed when such individuals are symptomatic and have 10 or more apneas and hypopneas per hour (63,64). Symptoms, which include hypersomnolence, morning headaches, fatigue, frequent nocturnal arousals with gasping or tachycardia, and nightmares, are similar to those of chronic alveolar hypoventilation (56). The risk of symptomatic sleep disordered breathing is higher in males and increases with age and in the setting of androgen therapy, obesity, brain stem and spinal cord lesions, hypothyroidism, generalized neuromuscular diseases, and any conditions that obstruct the airway (65,66).

Patients with neuromuscular disease may have a higher incidence of sleep disordered breathing because of a high incidence of bulbar muscle weakness and obesity (67,68), which can increase susceptibility to hypopharyngeal collapse during sleep (68,69). Sleep disordered breathing alone can result in chronic hypercapnia, hypoxia, right ventricular strain, and when severe, cardiopulmonary failure. It also occurs in most patients who use negative-pressure body ventilators (NPBVs) (70,71) or electrophrenic nerve pacing (72). Potentially serious cardiovascular and neuropsychiatric sequelae can result (73). Significant weight reduction can improve this condition for patients whose sleep disordered breathing is associated with obesity (71). However, obesity is rarely reversed indefinitely and even when weight gain does not recur, apneas and hypopneas can increase in frequency and symptoms often return (74).

The standard treatment is continuous positive airway pressure (CPAP). This acts as a pneumatic splint to maintain airway patency and permits inspiratory muscles to ventilate the lungs. Prone positioning in bed can be helpful. A convenient long-term solution can be the use of an orthodontic splint to bring the mandible and tongue forward (73,75). The use of nasopharyngeal tubes is poorly tolerated, and uvulopalatopharyngoplasty and mandibular advancement procedures are often ineffective and should be considered only as last resorts (71,76,77).

Although CPAP can maintain airway patency, the many hypercapnic, obese OSAS patients with VCs under 1000 mL require inspiratory muscle assistance. Conventionally, bilevel positive airway pressure (BPAP) is then used, but often at less than optimal inspiratory positive airway pressures (IPAPs) to normalize alveolar ventilation. An indwelling tracheostomy tube, which can be used to maintain airway patency as well as for the delivery of IPPV, is conventionally considered the ultimate solution for this problem. Instead of oxygen administration or tracheostomy for IPPV, however, these patients, too, can often benefit from the use of respiratory muscle aids to normalize alveolar ventilation and prevent respiratory complications.

Congenital central alveolar hypoventilation is a disorder of impaired control of ventilation of unknown etiology. Typically, these individuals maintain adequate ventilation when awake but hypoventilate severely during sleep and have absent or depressed ventilatory responses to hypercapnia and hypoxia at all times (78). A similar insensitivity to hypoxia and hypercapnia is seen in patients with familial dysautonomia and in some patients with diabetic microangiopathy (79).

Traumatic Brain Injury

Severe traumatic brain injury (defined by loss of consciousness for at least 6 hours) occurs with an annual incidence of 50,000 to 75,000 in the United States. Approximately one-third to one-half of these patients die, with the majority of deaths attributed to respiratory causes including pneumonia. Most closed head injuries due to falls, motor vehicle accidents, or motorcycle accidents coexist with other injuries that can affect respiratory function. Head injury severe enough to cause unconsciousness often results in apnea in both experimental animals and humans. Autoregulation of cerebral blood flow can be impaired by severe head injury, with the resulting hypovolemic hypotension exacerbating the traumatic and hypoxic cerebral insult.

Arterial hypoxemia is an early complication of traumatic brain injury. It is usually transient, but if progressive it correlates with poorer outcome. This hypoxemia, which is not induced by pulmonary edema, results from ventilation-perfusion mismatch and may be present despite mechanical ventilatory assistance. Hypoxemia may also be due to atelectasis, aspiration, venous thromboembolism or fat embolism, adult respiratory distress syndrome, or abnormal breathing patterns.

Because of disruption of central autonomic and voluntary control of respiration, abnormal breathing patterns may be seen in patients with traumatic brain injury. Cheyne-Stokes respiration, which is not unique to head injury, is a pattern of rhythmic periodic breaths with a regular oscillating pattern of tachypnea and hypopnea, ending in periods of apnea. It may occur as a result of an increased response to carbon dioxide resulting from interruption of normal cortical inhibition, and to abnormal functioning of central chemoreceptors. Other respiratory patterns described after brain injury include tachypnea, irregular breathing, and increased frequency of sighing (80).

The rapid onset of pulmonary edema after CNS injury is not well understood. It should be considered in any patient with severe head injury with a chest radiograph and clinical presentation suggestive of pulmonary edema. The mechanism for development of neurogenic pulmonary edema is thought to be a massive α-adrenergic discharge resulting from severe brain injury or other conditions that cause increased intracranial pressure. The result of this transient catecholamine release is generalized vasoconstriction. Pulmonary vasoconstriction causes a transient increase in pulmonary vascular pressure that disrupts pulmonary capillary function and leads to edema. The treatment of neurogenic pulmonary edema is supportive, but its rapid onset makes treatment difficult. α-Adrenergic blockade is probably ineffective because the pulmonary vascular bed is damaged at the capillary and alveolar epithelial cell level and is not capable of optimally responding to α-blocking agents.

Pneumonia is the most common cause of death related to the respiratory system in patients with severe head injury, with the incidence varying from 35% to 70% and mortality rates as high as 50%. Aspiration, tracheal suctioning, decreased cough reflex and PCF with resultant mucus retention, and use of neuromuscular blockade agents can all increase the risk of pneumonia. As with other patients in the intensive care setting, airway colonization is likely with *Pseudomonas*, *Staphylococcus*, or *Enterobacter* species.

After severe head injury compounded by hypoxia, it is imperative to maintain optimal ventilation and oxygenation to meet the increased metabolic demands of the injured brain and to minimize cerebral ischemia (81). Unlike for many other patients with primarily ventilatory impairment, for these patients intubation is often required for secretion clearance, ventilatory assistance, and oxygen administration.

Induced hypothermia is an emerging therapy in the early treatment of severe traumatic brain injury. Induction of a state of hypothermia to 32°C within 6 hours of injury may have a protective effect against such damaging factors as CNS glutamate release and ischemia. Pneumonia, however, may develop as a complication of hypothermic therapy (81).

Transtentorial herniation is the ultimate result of uncontrolled cerebral edema and is associated with a characteristic progression of respiratory dysfunction. As herniation proceeds, the respiratory pattern changes from normal breathing to Cheyne-Stokes respiration, to hyperventilation, and eventually to the irregular breathing that immediately precedes death. Hyperventilation, with its cerebral vasoconstrictive effects, has traditionally been advocated to reduce intracranial pressure (ICP). The recommendation has been to maintain an arterial oxygen tension of 80 mm Hg or higher and an arterial carbon dioxide tension of 20 to 30 mm Hg or lower for the first few days after head injury, with resultant respiratory alkalosis. There is concern, however, that hyperventilation may exacerbate ischemia, and some have advocated maintaining the arterial carbon dioxide tension at 35 mm Hg (81). PEEP can help maintain satisfactory oxygenation. Most patients tolerate pressures up to 10 mm Hg, but PEEP can decrease cardiac output and thus negatively impact on central perfusion pressure. Maintenance of proper hydration and mean arterial blood pressure is critical to avoid this effect.

Endotracheal suctioning is associated with a transient rise in mean ICP. Suctioning should be performed only as necessary, and be limited to two passes with the catheter after preoxygenation to minimize fluctuation in ICP (81). Mechanical insufflation-exsufflation (MI-E) via the tube may eventually be found to be an effective and safer alternative to tracheal suctioning. Patients with head injuries are usually positioned with the head of the bed elevated 30 degrees. If the brain is higher than the chest, the ICP is less affected by the increases in intrathoracic pressure induced by coughing or positive-pressure ventilation. In this position, there is also less likelihood of aspiration of stomach contents, reducing the risk of aspiration pneumonia.

Stroke

Following a cerebrovascular event, when bulbar involvement or a decreased level of consciousness or arousal affects swallowing, aspiration commonly occurs and is often subclinical. Prevention first requires a bedside evaluation of swallowing function with a videofluoroscopic swallowing study. Elevation of the head of the bed can be helpful in reducing the risk of aspiration and subsequent pneumonia.

The combined effects of immobility and lack of full motor power in the hemiplegic lower limb result in an increased risk of DVT and subsequent pulmonary embolization. This risk is even greater in the flaccid hemiplegic patient, who lacks the protective effect of increased lower-extremity tone for reducing the occurrence of DVT.

Hemispheric ischemic strokes exert only a modest influence on respiratory function. However both reduced chest wall movement and reduced diaphragmatic excursion contralateral to the stroke have been reported (82). Bilateral cortical strokes have been associated with Cheyne-Stokes respiration. This abnormal breathing pattern can persist for months to years following stroke, and has also been observed in the setting of unilateral lesions in the context of underlying pulmonary or cardiac disease. Another abnormal respiratory pattern reported in the presence of multiple bilateral hemispheric strokes is the inability to voluntarily take a deep breath. Ventral brainstem lesions can also inhibit voluntary deep breathing (83).

If a hemispheric stroke is severe enough to produce massive cerebral edema and increase ICP, brain stem herniation and progressive respiratory dysfunction can occur. Respiratory arrest by this mechanism represents the most common cause of mortality in the first days following acute hemispheric stroke. It has long been recognized that there are several interdependent brain stem centers acting on respiration. Any brain stem lesion that spares the dorsolateral medulla will not impair the normal rhythm of breathing. Thus, even patients with brain stem involvement so extensive as to leave them "locked in" may have physiologically effective breathing. By contrast, involvement of the dorsolateral medulla produces markedly abnormal regulation of breathing and a poor prognosis for survival.

Lateral medullary stroke (Wallenberg syndrome) may result in Ondine syndrome or central sleep apnea. In most such patients, unilateral infarctions have been identified, suggesting either lateralized control of respiration or interruption of decussating efferent pathways. In contrast with OSAS, this condition is position independent, and often requires assisted ventilation during sleep.

Parkinson Disease

In the past 20 years the spectrum of respiratory involvement in Parkinson disease has been recognized to be broader than impairment of ventilatory muscle function, and includes upper-airway obstruction, abnormalities in the control of respiration, and pulmonary sequelae of pharmacologic management (84). Pneumonia remains the most common cause of death in patients with Parkinson disease. Dementia and dysphagia put the patient at increased risk for the development of pneumonia, but the role of abnormal pulmonary function along with impaired cough and impaired clearance of secretions cannot be overlooked.

A number of studies on pulmonary function in Parkinson disease have been performed (85–88). In a group of 31 patients with severe Parkinson disease, those with spirometric evidence of obstruction had a significantly higher prevalence of asthma or chronic bronchitis, higher airway resistance, and decreased total lung elastic recoil. However, both Parkinson patients with and those without obstructive lung disease had an elevated residual volume and total lung capacity, decreased chest wall compliance, and normal lung compliance. The authors concluded that the most likely causes of obstruction in these patients were emphysema and airway disease independent of Parkinson disease, and that the elevated residual volume and total lung capacity were due to increased chest wall elastic forces (85).

Electromyographic studies of respiratory muscles in patients with Parkinson disease revealed essentially normal diaphragmatic function, while intercostal electromyography demonstrated continuous activity during expiration rather than the normal electrical silence (86). Electromyography of the accessory muscles of respiration showed an abnormal pattern of repetitive bursts of activity during both inspiration and expiration (89).

Even in patients with mild Parkinson disease with normal spirometry values, there is a reduced tolerance to inspiratory resistive loading and reduced respiratory muscle efficiency as assessed by the oxygen cost of breathing (87). Three possible mechanisms are suggested: alteration in neural drive, abnormal motor unit recruitment, and inappropriate activation of antagonist muscles. Any of these mechanisms could explain the restrictive neuromuscular pattern seen in more severely affected patients.

Upper-airway obstruction plays a role in respiratory dysfunction in some patients with Parkinson disease (88). Of 27 patients with extrapyramidal disorders (21 with Parkinson disease), 24 exhibited abnormalities of the flow-volume loop consistent with instability of upper-airway caliber. Laryngoscopy was performed in some of these patients and demonstrated either rhythmic or irregular adduction of the vocal cords and supraglottic structures. Videofluoroscopy of the diaphragm failed to reveal similar contractions.

Patients with Parkinson disease were compared to control subjects in terms of respiratory rates while awake and asleep (90). Awake, the rate averaged 4 respirations per minute more in the patients than in the controls. During REM sleep, respiratory rates were also increased in patients compared to controls, while during non-REM sleep respiratory rates were similar between the two groups. The authors suggested two possible etiologies: CNS dysfunction related to the disease or to therapy with L-dopamine (respiratory dyskinesia), or restrictive neuromuscular involvement, which commonly leads to a pattern of rapid, shallow respirations. In support of the latter mechanism, they noted that normalization of respiration during non-REM sleep parallels the improvement in tremor and rigidity during sleep.

PATIENT EVALUATION

A recent review found that specialized neuromuscular clinics are apt to resort to extensive pulmonary function testing that is not very useful because it is not directed at patients with primarily ventilatory impairment and the results are not used to guide treatment interventions (91). Simple spirometry, assessment of monitoring PCF, of end-tidal carbon dioxide, and oximetry are more important and are best performed in the clinic, home, or private office setting.

Patients with VCs under 55% of the predicted normal capacity are at risk for hypercapnia (92), and hypercapnia is generally worse during sleep when the patient is supine. Therefore, simple VC determination performed with the patient supine can provide a useful indication of the patient's ventilatory status and possible need for further testing. If a patient's lips are too weak to grab a mouthpiece for VC determination, the VC can be measured via an oral-nasal mask. The VC is determined via indwelling tracheostomy tubes when present. Forced expiratory flows, or at least a forced expiratory volume in 1 second, is determined when COPD or bronchospasm is suspected. Since patients with myasthenia gravis can experience subclinical airway collapse during inspiration, which can render them susceptible to hypoventilation and respiratory complications despite relatively normal VCs, flow-volume loops and assessment of forced inspiratory flow–forced expiratory flow ratios are indicated when these patients have chronic oxyhemoglobin desaturation, hypercapnia, or intercurrent respiratory difficulties (93).

The clinician is limited to blood gas testing for patients who cannot cooperate with pulmonary function testing. End-tidal carbon dioxide monitoring is reliable, is easy to perform for any patient, and can determine carbon dioxide levels day or night (9). It is accurate for patients with primarily ventilatory impairment without concomitant intrinsic lung disease that severely impairs blood gas diffusion. When diffusion abnormalities are severe, end-tidal carbon dioxide is correlated with carbon dioxide tension from an arterial blood gas sample.

Patients with VCs less than 40% of normal or daytime hypercapnia undergo nocturnal oximetry and possibly transcutaneous carbon dioxide monitoring (9). Although arterial carbon dioxide tensions can exceed 50 mm Hg in the presence of normal oximetry values, patients who maintain normal SaO_2 day and night are rarely symptomatic and therefore, will not need and rarely use nocturnal inspiratory muscle aids. Weaker patients, however, use respiratory muscle aids with oximetry as feedback. Since oxyhemoglobin desaturation can signal hypoventilation, by maintaining the SaO_2 within normal limits, these patients maintain adequate alveolar ventilation during waking hours (9). Oximetry can also document the benefit of nocturnal use of inspiratory muscle aids by demonstrating improvement in mean nocturnal SaO_2 with treatment. For patients with bulbar muscle dysfunction, SaO_2 levels below 95% in the presence of normal or low carbon dioxide tensions signal acute or ongoing aspiration of food or upper-airway secretions and significant risk for intercurrent pneumonias and atelectasis (94,95).

PCFs are decreased when the inspiratory muscles are unable to provide an inspiratory volume of 1.5 to 2.5 liters (3,96), when the expiratory muscles are unable to generate optimal thoracoabdominal pressures for an explosive decompression, and when bulbar muscle dysfunction prevents the patient from holding a deep breath with an adequately sealed glottus. Fixed upper-airway obstruction (e.g., with tracheal stenosis or a paralyzed vocal cord), or the irreversible lower-airway obstruction that typically occurs with COPD, reduces PCFs. PCFs are measured by asking patients to cough through peak flow meters. It has been shown that irrespective of the extent of respiratory muscle dysfunction, respiratory failure can be avoided in the long term without resorting to tracheal intubation or tracheostomy when PCFs can be generated to exceed about 3 L/sec (97). Further, the ability to generate PCFs of 3 L/sec or more indicates the possibility of safely removing a tracheostomy tube and allowing site closure irrespective of the extent of respiratory muscle dysfunction (98).

The deeper the breath or mechanically assisted insufflation that can be held, the greater the generation of PCFs with or without the application of a manual assist. Thus, since many patients do not have adequate VCs to attain the 1.5 liters necessary for an effective cough, patients can be taught to receive deep insufflations through a mouthpiece or facial interface before attempting to cough. Patients can also obtain deep insufflations by "air-stacking" breaths they receive from a manual resuscitator or volume-cycled ventilator. The greater this volume of air, the greater the PCF that can be achieved (96). The maximum volume of air that a patient can hold with a closed glottis is the maximum insufflation capacity (MIC).

Since many rehabilitation patients have neither fixed airway obstruction nor bulbar dysfunction sufficient to necessitate placement of a gastrostomy tube, most patients can generate adequate PCFs by using physical medicine aids to "air stack" and to assist coughing. Conditions for which patients have benefited from the use of physical medicine aids to prevent respiratory complications and as alternatives to tracheostomy for ventilatory support are listed in Table 90-1 (99).

THE RESPIRATORY MUSCLE AIDS

The respiratory muscles can be aided by manually or mechanically applying forces to the body or intermittent pressure changes to the airway. The devices that act on the body include the NPBVs, which assist respiratory muscles by creating atmospheric pressure changes around the thorax and abdomen; body ventilators and exsufflation devices, which apply force directly to the body to mechanically displace respiratory muscles; and devices that apply intermittent pressure changes directly to the airway.

It is generally unnecessary to attempt to treat chronic alveolar hypoventilation until there are symptoms in the presence of mean nocturnal SaO_2 levels below 95% or until intercurrent respiratory tract infections would otherwise result in acute respiratory failure. Patients are equipped and trained in the use of respiratory muscle aids to avoid intercurrent complications once the VC has decreased below 50% of predicted normal or the assisted PCFs have decreased below 4 L/sec. Training begins with the use of inspiratory muscle aids to provide regular deep insufflations to maintain pulmonary compliance and to maximize the MIC, and with the use of assisted coughing.

Inspiratory Muscle Aids

Negative-Pressure Body Ventilators

NPBVs intermittently create subatmospheric pressure around the thorax and abdomen to assist or support the inspiratory effort. Tank ventilators consist of a tank or cylinder (e.g., the iron lung) that envelopes the body up to the neck. Negative pressure is created in the tank by a motorized bellows. Negative pressure is created in the more portable tank-style PortaLung (Respironics, Pittsburgh, PA), as well as in chest shell and wrap-style NPBVs, by the action of a negative-pressure pump or ventilator.

NPBVs are generally less convenient and less effective than noninvasive IPPV methods. They are useful during transition from tracheostomy to noninvasive IPPV to expedite tracheostomy site closure; they are occasionally used as alternatives to nasal IPPV during colds when nasal congestion renders nasal IPPV problematic; and they can be used to support alveolar ventilation in small children who do not cooperate with noninvasive IPPV methods and for obtunded or comatose patients for whom noninvasive IPPV is ineffective. The reader is referred to other sources for more complete descriptions of these devices (14).

Table 90-1: Common Conditions for Which Physical Medicine Aids Have Been Reported to Prevent Ventilatory Failure

- Myopathies
  - Muscular dystrophies
    - Dystrophinopathies—Duchenne and Becker dystrophies
    - Other muscular dystrophies—limb-girdle, Emery-Dreifuss, facioscapulohumeral, congenital, childhood autosomal recessive, and myotonic dystrophy
  - Non-Duchenne myopathies
    - Congenital and metabolic myopathies like acid maltase deficiency
    - Inflammatory myopathies such as polymyositis
    - Diseases of the myoneural junction such as myasthenia gravis, mixed connective tissue disease
    - Myopathies of systemic disease such as carcinomatous myopathy, cachexia/anorexia nervosa, medication associated
- Neurologic disorders
  - Spinal muscular atrophies
  - Motor neuron diseases
  - Poliomyelitis
  - Neuropathies
    - Hereditary sensory motor neuropathies including familial hypertrophic interstitial polyneuropathy
    - Phrenic neuropathies—associated with cardiac hypothermia, surgical or other trauma, radiation, phrenic electrostimulation, familial, paraneoplastic or infectious etiology, and with lupus erythematosus, Guillain-Barré syndrome
  - Multiple sclerosis
  - Disorders of supraspinal tone such as Friedreich ataxia
  - Myelopathies of rheumatoid, infectious, spondylitic, vascular, traumatic, or idiopathic etiology
  - Tetraplegia associated with pancuronium bromide, botulism
- Sleep disordered breathing including obesity hypoventilation, central and congenital hypoventilation syndromes, and hypoventilation associated with diabetic microangiopathy, or familial dysautonomia
- Skeletal pathology such as kyphoscoliosis, osteogenesis imperfecta, and rigid spine syndrome
- After lung resection
- Chronic obstructive pulmonary disease

Source: Modified from Bach JR. Neuromuscular and skeletal disorders leading to global alveolar hypoventilation. In: Bach JR, ed. *Pulmonary rehabilitation: the obstructive and paralytic conditions.* Philadelphia: Hanley & Belfus, 1996:257–273.

Body Ventilators That Apply Pressure Directly to the Body

These ventilators include the rocking bed and the intermittent abdominal pressure ventilator (IAPV). The rocking bed (J. H. Emerson, Cambridge, MA) rocks the patient in an arc of 5 to 30 degrees. Gravity cyclically displaces the abdominal contents. This causes diaphragm excursion and assists ventilation. The rocking bed is generally less effective than NPBVs and noninvasive IPPV methods and is rarely used today (14).

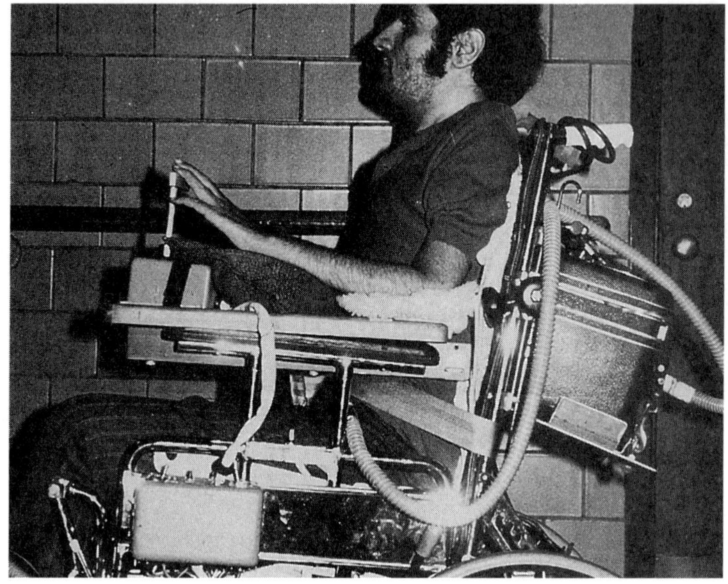

Figure 90-1. An individual with a high-level spinal cord injury who had his tracheostomy tube removed and the tracheostomy site closed 2 years after injury and was converted to 24-hour noninvasive ventilatory support. He used the intermittent abdominal pressure ventilator (seen here) during daytime hours and Lipseal intermittent positive-pressure ventilation overnight.

The IAPV involves the intermittent inflation of an air sac or bladder that is contained in a corset or belt. The sac is inflated by a positive-pressure ventilator (Exsufflation Belt, Respironics, Pittsburgh, PA) (Fig. 90-1). Bladder action moves the diaphragm upward, causing a forced exsufflation. During bladder deflation, the abdominal contents and diaphragm fall to the resting position and inspiration occurs passively. A trunk angle of 30 degrees or more from the horizontal is necessary for it to be effective. If the patient has any inspiratory capacity or is capable of glossopharyngeal breathing (GPB), he or she can add autonomous tidal volumes to the mechanically assisted inspiration. The IAPV generally augments tidal volumes by about 600 mL (100) but volumes as high as 1200 mL have been reported (101). Patients with less than 1 hour of ventilator-free breathing time usually prefer to use the IAPV when sitting rather than use noninvasive methods of IPPV (101). The IAPV is often inadequate in the presence of scoliosis or obesity.

Noninvasive Intermittent Positive-Pressure Ventilation

Positive-pressure ventilators became widely available in the United States in 1956. At that time many postpoliomyelitis iron lung users refused the advice of their physicians to undergo tracheostomy and continued to use body ventilators up to 24 hours a day. Many of these patients learned how to receive IPPV via a mouthpiece held between their lips and teeth or fixed near the mouth adjacent to the controls for a motorized wheelchair (Fig. 90-2). They grabbed the mouthpiece for IPPV as necessary (102). The Monaghan positive-pressure ventilator was placed on wheels and rolled behind the wheelchair. Patients were thus freed from their body ventilators during daytime hours.

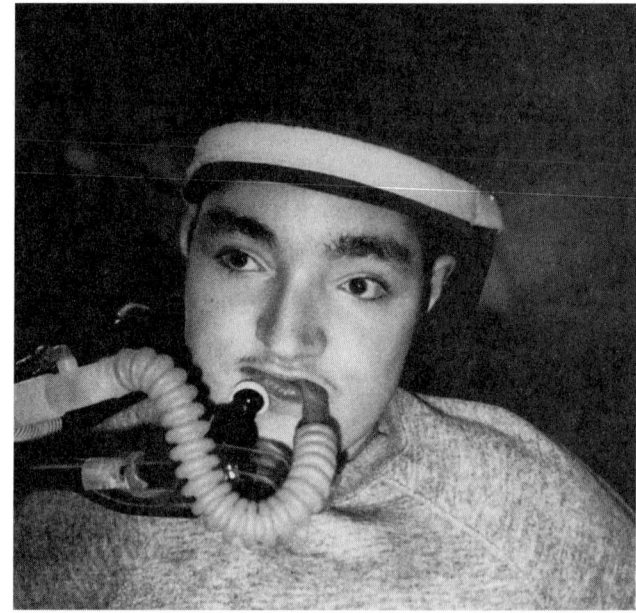

Figure 90-2. A 29-year-old patient with Duchenne muscular dystrophy who has been dependent on a ventilator 24 hours a day since age 14. He uses mouthpiece intermittent positive-pressure ventilation (IPPV) during the daytime with the mouthpiece fixed adjacent to the tongue control of his motorized wheelchair (seen here). He uses Lipseal IPPV overnight.

It was soon discovered that mouthpiece IPPV could be effective even while the patient slept (103). By 1964 a number of patients in 1 center had left their body ventilators to use mouthpiece IPPV up to 24 hours a day (103). Ultimately mouthpiece IPPV and IAPV use became the two patient-preferred methods of daytime ventilatory support (104). Orthodontic bite plates and shells can be

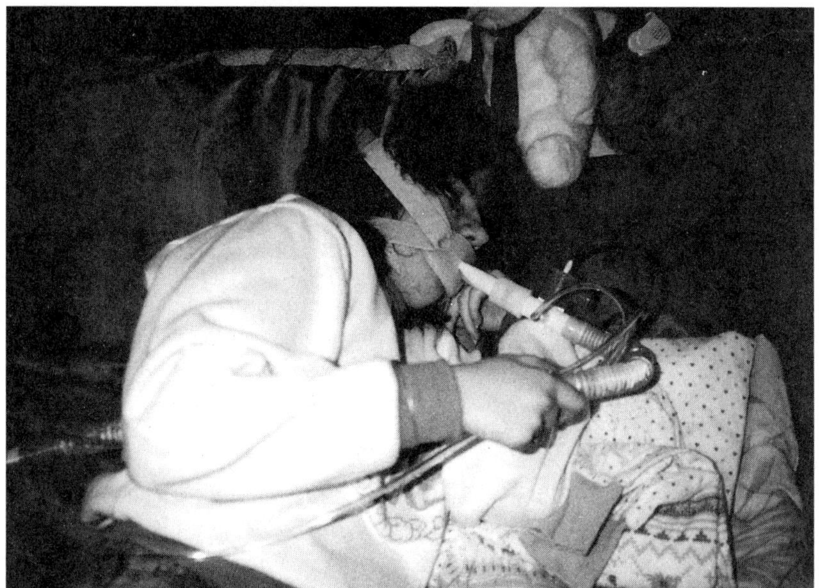

Figure 90-3. A 36-year-old woman with a congenital myopathy who has a severely impaired ability to ventilate her lungs when supine has used nocturnal Lipseal intermittent positive-pressure ventilation (seen here) since 1985.

fabricated to increase comfort and efficacy and eliminate the risk of orthodontic deformity with long-term use. The Puritan-Bennett Lipseal (Puritan-Bennett, Lanexa, KS) is used to optimize retention and minimize air leakage when mouthpiece IPPV is used during sleep (Fig. 90-3).

In 1982, as an alternative to the use of mouthpiece IPPV for "resting" the inspiratory muscles of French muscular dystrophy patients, DeLaubier, Rideau, and Bach delivered IPPV via urinary drainage catheters positioned into the nostrils (103,105). In 1984, nasal IPPV was first used for 24-hour ventilatory support for an MS patient with a VC of 100 mL and no ventilator-free breathing time, and it became clear that it could be used during sleep even for patients with little or no measurable VC (56,106).

Nasal IPPV is most often delivered via CPAP masks. There are now commercially available CPAP masks from Lifecare, Respironics (Murrysville, PA), Healthdyne (Minneapolis, MN), Puritan-Bennett, and Res Care (San Diego, CA). Each design applies pressure differently to the paranasal area. It is impossible to predict which model will best fit or be preferred by any particular patient. Many patients use different styles on alternate nights to vary skin contact pressure. Nasal bridge pressure and insufflation leakage into the eyes are common complaints with several generic models. Such difficulties resulted in the development of custom-molded nasal interfaces (107). Custom-molded nasal interfaces can now be obtained both commercially (SEFAM Company, distributed by Respironics, Pittsburgh, PA) and individually in New Jersey (107) (Fig. 90-4).

Nasal IPPV can be delivered by portable volume-cycled ventilators or by BPAP machines. The latter are pressure-limited blowers that do not deliver adequate volumes for effective coughing and therefore, should not be

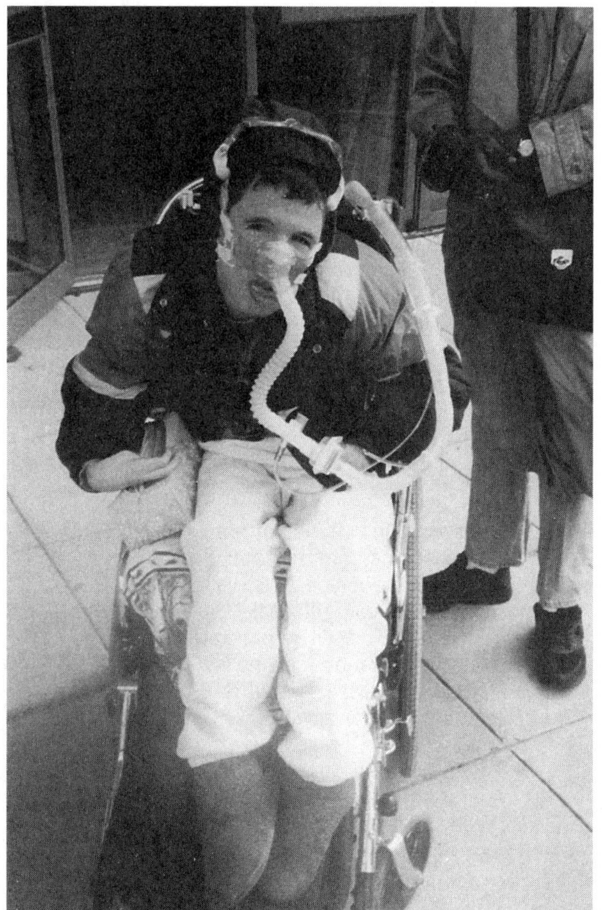

Figure 90-4. A patient with Duchenne muscular dystrophy who has required continuous ventilatory support since 1987. Since his lips are too weak to effectively use mouthpiece intermittent positive-pressure ventilation (IPPV), he has used up to 24-hour nasal IPPV since 1987.

used for long-term ventilatory assistance for patients with primarily ventilation impairment.

Since patients generally prefer to use mouthpiece IPPV or the IAPV for daytime use, nasal IPPV is most practical only for nocturnal use. Daytime nasal IPPV is indicated for those who cannot retain a mouthpiece because of oral muscle weakness or inadequate jaw opening or when there is insufficient neck movement to grab a mouthpiece (56). Nevertheless, 24-hour nasal IPPV can be a viable alternative to tracheostomy, even for some patients with severe lip and oropharyngeal muscle weakness. Although initially nasal IPPV was used almost exclusively for patients with neuromuscular ventilatory insufficiency, it is now being increasingly used as an alternative to intubation for patients with ventilatory insufficiency secondary to cystic fibrosis, COPD, and other lung diseases (108,109).

Strapless oral-nasal interfaces with bite-plate retention can also be used for the nocturnal delivery of IPPV (107,110). These interfaces provide an essentially airtight seal for the delivery of IPPV, and simple tongue thrust is adequate to expel them. The bite-plate retention is also important for patients living alone who are unable to independently don straps.

Glossopharyngeal Breathing

GPB is most commonly used as a method for providing maximal insufflations and as a noninvasive method for supporting ventilation. The patient is instructed to take a deep breath and then augment it by GPB. The tongue and pharyngeal muscles project boluses of air past the vocal cords. The vocal cords close with each "gulp." One breath usually consists of six to eight gulps of 60 to 200 mL each. During the training period, the efficiency of GPB is monitored by spirometrically measuring the number of milliliters of air per gulp, gulps per breath, and breaths per minute. An excellent training manual and video are available (111,112). GPB can provide patients who otherwise have little or no measurable VC with normal tidal volumes, minute ventilation, and hours of ventilator-free breathing time (113). Deep GPB is also useful for manually assisted coughing (114) and to prevent microatelectasis. GPB can normalize the volume and rhythm of speech and permit the patient to shout. It is a key reason for removal of a tracheostomy tube and transition to noninvasive methods of ventilatory support. A tracheostomy virtually precludes successful use of GPB, since even with the tube plugged, gulped air leaks around the tube and out the tracheostomy site.

Expiratory Muscle Aids

A normal cough requires a precough inspiration or insufflation to about 85% to 90% of total lung capacity (3). Glottic closure follows for about 0.2 second and sufficient intrathoracic pressures are generated to obtain transient PCFs exceeding 6 L/sec upon glottic opening (96,115). Total expiratory volume during normal coughing is about 2.3 ± 0.5 liters (3). Optimal PCFs and cough volumes can be provided by the use of inspiratory and expiratory muscle aids.

Manually Assisted Coughing

Techniques of manually assisted coughing involve different hand and arm placements for expiratory cycle thrusts (Fig. 90-5). For patients with less than 1.5 liters of VC, efficacy is enhanced by preceding the assisted exsufflation with a deep insufflation delivered via a manual resuscitator, intermittent positive-pressure breathing (IPPB) machine, or portable ventilator. Manually assisted coughing requires a cooperative patient, good coordination between the patient

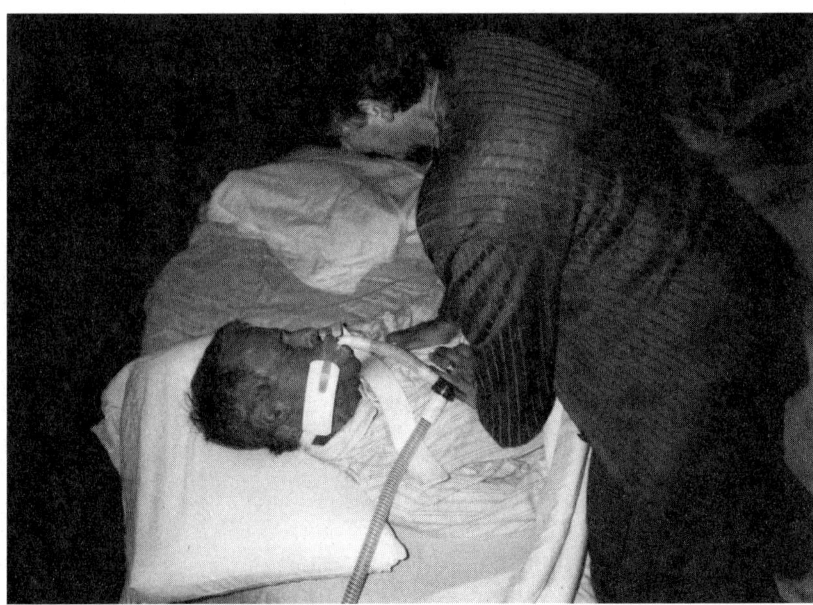

Figure 90-5. A postpoliomyelitis patient who has used a ventilator 24 hours a day since 1955 is seen here using lipseal intermittent positive-pressure ventilation and receiving a tussive squeeze to facilitate elimination of airway secretions. Tussive squeezes and abdominal thrusts are among the most commonly used and effective methods of manually assisted coughing.

and caregiver, and adequate physical effort and often frequent application by the caregiver. At least 12 methods of manually assisted coughing have been described (116). It is usually ineffective in the presence of significant scoliosis and certain techniques must be performed with caution in the presence of an osteoporotic rib cage. It should not be used after the patient has taken a meal. When manually assisted coughing is inadequate, the most effective alternative for generating optimal PCFs and clearing deep airway secretions is the use of MI-E.

Mechanical Insufflation-Exsufflation

In 1951 Barach et al (117) described an exsufflator attachment for iron lungs. The device used a vacuum cleaner motor with a 5-inch solenoid valve attachment to an iron lung portal. With the valve closed, the motor developed a negative intratank pressure to −40 mm Hg. At peak negative pressure the valve opened, triggering a return to atmospheric pressure in 0.06 second and causing passive exsufflation (117). This technique increased PCFs for six ventilator-supported poliomyelitis patients, An additional increase was obtained by timing an abdominal compression with valve opening (118).

In 1953 various portable devices were manufactured to deliver MI-E directly to the airway via a mouthpiece, facial interface, or endotracheal tube (103). Insufflation and exsufflation pressures were independently adjusted for comfort and efficacy. These devices typically inflated the lungs with positive pressures of 30 to 40 mm Hg over a 2-second period. The pressure in the upper respiratory passageway was then dropped to 30 to 40 mm Hg below atmosphere in 0.02 second and maintained for 1 to 3 seconds.

In February 1993, a MI-E (In-Exsufflator, J. H. Emerson Co., Cambridge, MA) essentially identical to the earlier models was approved by the Food and Drug Administration and released on the market. One treatment consists of about five cycles of MI-E followed by a period of normal breathing or ventilator use to avoid hyperventilation. The treatments are repeated until no further airway mucus is eliminated and VC and SaO_2 levels return to normal. An abdominal thrust applied during the exsufflation cycle further increases PCFs and airway secretion expulsion when the device is used via a facial interface or mouthpiece. Although no medications are usually required for effective MI-E, in neuromuscular ventilator users with respiratory infections, liquefaction of sputum using heated aerosol treatments can facilitate exsufflation when secretions are inspissated. MI-E can also be used effectively via a translaryngeal or tracheostomy tube. Use in this manner was effective in reversing acute atelectasis associated with productive airway secretions as far back as 1954 (119).

An increase in VC of 15% to 42% was noted immediately following treatment in 67 patients with "obstructive dyspnea" and a 55% increase in VC was noted following MI-E in patients with neuromuscular conditions (120). MI-E continues to be used to increase VC and SaO_2 (96) and to avert respiratory complications and the need for bronchoscopy (121). The physiologic basis for the effectiveness of MI-E has been reviewed elsewhere (122).

THERAPEUTIC STRATEGIES

Deteriorating Pulmonary Function

Patients with paralytic conditions who experience acute deterioration and impending ventilatory failure but who have assisted PCFs of 3 L/sec or more or for whom MI-E is documented to effectively reverse airway secretion–associated oxyhemoglobin desaturation are managed with the use of inspiratory and expiratory muscle aids and oximetry feedback. The goal is to maintain SaO_2 within normal limits and thus to avert respiratory failure with the use of these aids. If baseline SaO_2 decreases below 92% despite optimal use of noninvasive IPPV and assisted coughing, pneumonia is likely and conventional evaluation and management need to be undertaken.

Patients who are symptomatic for chronic alveolar hypoventilation undergo trials of nocturnal nasal and mouthpiece IPPV with lipseal IPPV. Trials of nocturnal nasal and lipseal IPPV are undertaken and oximetry monitoring documents treatment efficacy. The patient is trained to use oximetry feedback to guide daytime use of mouthpiece IPPV or use of the IAPV as inspiratory muscle weakness progresses and severe hypercapnia extends into daytime hours.

Ventilator Weaning

Intubated patients who require ventilatory support can be extubated while ventilation is supported by an NPBV. Once extubated, they are trained in the use of noninvasive IPPV and expiratory muscle aids (123). As noted, for tracheostomized patients, ventilator weaning attempts are most often made using a combination of concomitant SIMV or assist-control ventilation, with pressure support, PEEP, and supplemental oxygen administration. Occasionally, periods of ventilator-free breathing are tried with the patients receiving CPAP and oxygen by a T-piece. With these approaches, "weaning schedules" are imposed on the patient. Either this causes anxiety because the patient is not ready to breathe on his or her own, or the schedule is too conservative, delaying respiratory muscle reconditioning and function. An appropriate weaning strategy is to first wean the patient from oxygen administration by aggressively using MI-E to clear airway secretions and resolve atelectasis, then to wean the patient from the tracheostomy tube when assisted PCFs are adequate (9), and then when possible to wean from noninvasive IPPV. In addition, intubated patients and tracheostomy IPPV users often develop malnutrition and respiratory muscle reconditioning. Placing a fenestrated tracheostomy tube, capping it, and allowing the patient to take mouthpiece IPPV as needed with room air optimizes patient control and facilitates ventilator weaning (9). Once the patient is familiar with noninvasive IPPV, the tracheostomy tube can be removed and a tracheostomy button placed to keep the site open while the patient uses noninvasive IPPV for a few days before button removal and definitive site closure (123).

If the tracheostomy tube cannot be removed because of irreversible upper-airway obstruction, the cuff should nevertheless be deflated to facilitate swallowing and speech and to minimize tracheal damage. A methylene blue dye test or a swallow study in conjunction with oximetry can be done to ensure that aspiration of food and saliva is not excessive. Occasional nocturnal oximetry monitoring can document that alveolar ventilation continues to be adequate despite cuff deflation or removal (124).

Postsurgical Weaning Difficulties

Patients at risk for respiratory tract infection–associated respiratory failure are also at risk for failing to wean from ventilatory support following general anesthesia. If these patients are trained in the use of respiratory muscle aids prior to surgery, they can be extubated even when unable to support their own breathing, and supported by the use of respiratory muscle aids and oximetry feedback as described (9).

Comatose or uncooperative patients, whether from head injury, stroke, or other pathology, can have MI-E applied via their tracheostomy tubes as an alternative to or to complement tracheal suctioning. Once SaO_2 can be normalized by MI-E with the patient breathing room air, the tube can be capped, or for patients who breathe on their own, the tube can be removed and a button placed and MI-E applied through the upper airway. If mucous plug–associated oxyhemoglobin desaturations are not reversed by MI-E, an upper-airway-fiberoptic study is done to determine whether there are reversible causes of obstruction. It should be possible to maintain mean SaO_2 at or near-normal levels and to document assisted PCFs of 3 L/sec or more before attempting site closure.

Small Children

MI-E has been used safely at 30 cm of H_2O inspiratory and expiratory pressures in small children. However, because of a lack of ability to cooperate, the inspiratory and expiratory phases and abdominal thrusts must be timed to the child's crying and coughing. Alveolar ventilation can be supported by nasal or face-mask IPPV if the child cannot remove the interface, or else tank ventilators can be used (Baby-In-A-Bottle, J. H. Emerson, Cambridge, MA; Pediatric Iron Lung, Respironics, Pittsburgh, PA). Often these approaches fail because of an inability to effectively clear airway secretions and the child may require tracheal intubation with each cold that results in bronchorrhea until he or she is about 4 years old or old enough to cooperate with noninvasive methods.

Patients with Functionally Irreversible Airway Obstruction

Patients with irreversible upper-airway obstruction due to vocal cord adhesions or paralysis or upper-airway stenosis, patients with functionally irreversible lower-airway obstruction such as occurs with COPD and cystic fibrosis, and patients with neurologic disorders that impair glottic function or cooperation who have PCFs that cannot exceed at least 3 L/sec may benefit from mechanical percussion, vibration, or high-frequency oscillation applied to the chest wall or directly to the airway. Although there have been no studies on the use of these methods for patients with neurologic conditions or upper-airway obstruction, some information is available on their use for patients with chronic obstructive lung diseases.

Although it has never been shown that the use of chest physical therapy and postural drainage decreases the risk of pulmonary morbidity or the length of hospital stays, it is generally accepted that these methods can facilitate airway secretion elimination for patients with profuse secretions and obstructive pulmonary disease (125). The effects of mechanical chest percussion and vibration appear to be frequency dependent (126–129), with the most effective frequencies, between 10 and 15 Hz (126,128,130,131), not possible by strictly manual methods. With currently available technology, however, mechanical vibration is possible at frequencies up to 170 Hz (Hayek Oscillator, Breasy Medical Equipment, Stamford, CT). It can be delivered via chest shells, as with the Hayek Oscillator; via vests (ThAIRapy System, American Biosystems, St. Paul, MN); or via air column oscillators and percussors with the use of modified jet ventilators and intrapulmonary percussors, like the Percussionator (Percussionaire, Sandpoint, ID).

Warwick and Hansen (132) found long-term increases in forced VC and forced expiratory flows for cystic fibrosis patients treated with high-frequency chest wall compression as compared to those receiving manual chest percussion alone. The improved pulmonary function was thought to be related to improved mucus clearance. Two other studies reported improvement in gas exchange during high-frequency oscillation (133,134), and Sibuya et al (135) found that chest wall vibration decreased dyspnea. However, in another study of cystic fibrosis patients recovering from acute pulmonary exacerbations, no differences were found in pulmonary function or in the amount of expectorated mucus whether using conventional chest physical therapy or high-frequency chest wall compression (136). In fact, most studies on COPD and cystic fibrosis patients failed to demonstrate on objective benefit from percussion or vibration on mucus transport (137–140). The side effects of percussion and vibration can include increasing obstruction to airflow for some patients with COPD (4,141). In an animal model the application of vibration and percussion was also associated with the development of atelectasis (142).

Intrapulmonary percussive ventilation (IPV) was reported to be more effective than chest percussion and postural drainage in the treatment of postoperative atelectasis and secretion mobilization in COPD patients (143,144). These devices can deliver aerosolized medications while providing 2- to 7-Hz high-flow minibursts of air to the lungs as the patient is breathing. Although there have been no controlled studies, in one study the majority of patients using the technique felt that it was helpful (145).

Thus, although vibrators and percussors may facilitate secretion migration from the very periphery of the lungs to more proximal areas where assisted coughing can then more easily eliminate them, they do not appear to be necessary when PCFs are more than 3 L/sec with the use of manually assisted coughing or MI-E. When adequate PCFs cannot be generated by autonomous or assisted coughing methods, the use of mechanical oscillators, vibrators, and percussors may be considered, but it is reasonable to conclude that there is not enough evidence to justify their routine use at this time. Therefore, patients with functionally irreversible airflow obstruction or severe neurologic lesions for whom adequate PCFs cannot be generated are better managed by conventional translaryngeal intubation or tracheostomy. MI-E can always be performed via the indwelling tubes as an alternative to tracheal suctioning in these patients, provided that there is little risk of pneumothorax from severe lung disease. Once PCFs greater than 3 L/sec are documented, extubation can be attempted.

CONCLUSIONS

Respiratory complications are a major and often preventable source of morbidity and mortality for rehabilitation patients, Although these complications are caused by impairments in lung ventilation and in airway secretion elimination rather than lung disease and oxygenation impairment, they are often treated by interventions that are more appropriate for patients with intrinsic and obstructive airway diseases. This can be unnecessary at best, and harmful at worst. Fortunately, there are physical medicine interventions that can treat or prevent respiratory complications for most of these patients.

REFERENCES

1. Boushy SF, Thompson HK Jr, North LB, et al. Prognosis in chronic obstructive pulmonary disease. *Am Rev Respir Dis* 1973;108:1373–1383.
2. Niederman MS, Ferranti RD, Ziegler A, et al. Respiratory infection complicating long-term tracheostomy: the implication of persistent gram-negative tracheobronchial colonization. *Chest* 1984;85:39–44.
3. Leith DE. Cough. In: Brain JD, Proctor D, Reid L, eds. *Lung biology in health and disease: respiratory defense mechanisms.* Part 2. New York: Marcel Dekker, 1977:545–592.
4. Goldstein RS, van der Schans CP, Bach JR. Airway secretion management and oxygen therapy. *Phys Med Rehabil Clin N Am* 1996;7:101–122.
5. Bach JR, ed. *Pulmonary rehabilitation: the obstructive and paralytic conditions.* Philadelphia: Hanley & Belfus, 1996.
6. Moxham J. Aminophylline and the respiratory muscles: an alternative view. *Clin Chest Med* 1988;9:325–336.
7. Esau SA. The effect of theophylline on hypoxic, hypercapnic hamster diaphragm muscle in vitro. *Am Rev Respir Dis* 1991;143:954–959.
8. Smith PEM, Edwards RHT, Calverley PMA. Protriptyline treatment of sleep hypoxaemia in Duchenne muscular dystrophy. *Thorax* 1989;44:1002–1005.
9. Bach JR. Prevention of morbidity and mortality with the use of physical medicine aids. In: Bach JR, ed. *Pulmonary rehabilitation: the obstructive and paralytic conditions.* Philadelphia: Hanley & Belfus, 1996: 303–329.
10. Smith PEM, Edwards RHT, Calverley PMA. Oxygen treatment of sleep hypoxaemia in Duchenne muscular dystrophy. *Thorax* 1989;44:997–1001.
11. Bach JR, Robert D, Leger P, Langevin B. Sleep fragmentation in kyphoscoliotic individuals with alveolar hypoventilation treated by nasal IPPV. *Chest* 1995;107:1552–1558.
12. Bach JR, O'Connor K. Electrophrenic ventilation: a different perspective. *J Am Paraplegia Soc* 1991;14:9–17.
13. Bellamy R, Pitts FW, Stauffer S. Respiratory complications in traumatic quadriplegia. *J Neurosurg* 1973;39:596–600.
14. Bach JR. Update and perspectives on noninvasive respiratory muscle aids: part 1—the inspiratory muscle aids. *Chest* 1994;105:1230–1240.
15. Logemann JA. *Evaluation and treatment of swallowing disorders.* San Diego: College-Hill, 1983:119.
16. Bonanno P. Swallowing dysfunction after tracheostomy. *Ann Surg* 1971;174:29–33.
17. Bach JR, Intintola P, Alba AS, Holland I. The ventilator individual: cost analysis of institutionalization versus rehabilitation and in-home management. *Chest* 1992;101:26–30.
18. Bach JR, Sortor S, Sipski M. Sleep blood gas monitoring of high cervical quadriplegic patients with respiratory insufficiency by non-invasive techniques. In: *Abstracts Digest,*

14th Annual Scientific Meeting of the American Spinal Cord Injury Association. 1988:102. Abstract. Atlanta: American Spinal Cord Injury Association.

19. Fishburn MJ, Marino RJ, Ditunno JF. Atelectasis and pneumonia in acute spinal cord injury. *Arch Phys Med Rehabil* 1990;71: 197–200.

20. Slack RS, Shucart W. Respiratory dysfunction associated with traumatic injury to the central nervous system. *Clin Chest Med* 1994;15:739–749.

21. Jackson AB, Groomes TE. Incidence of respiratory complications following spinal cord injury. *Arch Phys Med Rehabil* 1994; 75:270–275.

22. Myllynen P, Kivioja A, Rokkanen P, Wilppula E. Cervical spinal cord injury: the correlations of initial clinical features and blood gas analyses with early prognosis. *Paraplegia* 1989;27: 19–26.

23. Carter RE, Donovan WH, Halstead L, Wilkerson MA. Comparative study of electrophrenic nerve stimulation and mechanical ventilatory support in traumatic spinal cord injury. *Paraplegia* 1987;25:86–91.

24. Bach JR. Inappropriate weaning and late onset ventilatory failure of individuals with traumatic quadriplegia. *Paraplegia* 1993;31:430–438.

25. Kraus JF. Epidemiological aspects of acute spinal cord injury: a review of incidence, prevalence, causes, and outcome. In: Becker DP, Povlishock JT, eds. *Central nervous system trauma status report—1985.* Bethesda, MD: National Institute of Neurological and Communicative Disorders and Stroke, National Institutes of Health, 1985:313–322.

26. Bhaskar KR, Brown R, O'Sullivan DD, et al. Bronchial mucus hypersecretion in acute quadriplegia: macromolecular yields and glycoconjugate composition. *Am Rev Respir Dis* 1991;143:640–648.

27. Foster WM, Bergofsky EH, Bohning DE, et al. Effect of adrenergic agents and their mode of action on mucociliary clearance in man. *J Appl Physiol* 1976;41:146–152.

28. Joffe SN. Incidence of postoperative deep vein thrombosis in neurosurgical patients. *J Neurosurg* 1975;42:201–211

29. Merli GJ, Herbison GJ, Ditunno JF, et al. Deep vein thrombosis: prophylaxis in acute spinal cord injured patients. *Arch Phys Med Rehabil* 1988;69:661–664.

30. Bach JR. Inappropriate weaning and late onset ventilatory failure of individuals with traumatic quadriplegia. *Paraplegia* 1993;31:430–438.

31. McAlpine D, Comston N. Some aspects of the natural history of disseminated sclerosis. *Q J Med* 1952;21:135–167.

32. McIntyre HD, McIntyre AP. Prognosis of multiple sclerosis. *Arch Neurol Neurosurg Psychiatry* 1943;50:431–439.

33. Tantucci C, Massucci M, Piperno R, et al. Control of breathing and respiratory muscle strength in patients with multiple sclerosis. *Chest* 1994;105: 1163–1170.

34. Aisen M, Arlt G, Foster S. Diaphragmatic paralysis without bulbar or limb paralysis in multiple sclerosis. *Chest* 1990;98: 499–501.

35. Carter J, Noseworthy JH. Ventilatory dysfunction in multiple sclerosis. *Clin Chest Med* 1994;15: 693–703.

36. Simon RP, Gean-Marton AD, Sander JE. Medullary lesion inducing pulmonary edema: a magnetic resonance imaging study. *Ann Neurol* 1991;30: 727–730.

37. Quera-Salra MA, Guilleminault C, Chevret S, et al. Breathing disorders during sleep in myasthenia gravis. *Ann Neurol* 1992;31: 86–92.

38. Bellemare F, Grassino A. Effect of pressure and timing of contraction on human diaphragm fatigue. *J Appl Physiol* 1982;53:1190–1195.

39. Gracey DR, McMichan JC, Divertie MB, Howard FM. Respiratory failure in Guillain-Barré syndrome. *Mayo Clin Proc* 1982;37:742–746.

40. Bach JR. Pulmonary assessment and management of the aging and older patient. In: Felsenthal G, Garrison SJ, Steinberg FU, eds. *Rehabilitation of the aging and elderly patient.* Baltimore: Williams & Wilkins, 1993:263–273.

41. Rideau Y, Jankowski LW, Grellet J. Respiratory function in the muscular dystrophies. *Muscle Nerve* 1981;4:155–164.

42. Bach J, Alba A, Pilkington LA, Lee M. Long-term rehabilitation in advanced stage of childhood onset, rapidly progressive muscular dystrophy. *Arch Phys Med Rehabil* 1981;62:328–331.

43. McDonald CM, Abresch RT, Carter GT, et al. Duchenne muscular dystrophy. *Am J Phys Med Rehabil* 1995;74:S70–S92.

44. Mukoyama M, Kondo K, Hizawa K, Nishitani H, the DMDR Group. Life spans of Duchenne muscular dystrophy patients in the hospital care program in Japan. *J Neurol Sci* 1987;81:155–158.

45. Rideau Y, Gatin G, Bach J, Gines G. Prolongation of life in Duchenne muscular dystrophy. *Acta Neurol* 1983;5:118–124.

46. Vignos PJ. Respiratory function and pulmonary infection in Duchenne muscular dystrophy. *Isr J Med Sci* 1977;13: 207–214.

47. Inkley SR, Oldenberg FC, Vignos PJ. Pulmonary function in Duchenne muscular dystrophy related to stage of disease. *Am J Med* 1974;56:297–306.

48. Gardner-Medwin D. Clinical features and classification of the muscular dystrophies. *Br Med Bull* 1980;36:109–115.

49. Begin R, Bureau MA, Lupien L, Lemieux B. Control and modula-

tion of respiration in Steinert's myotonic dystrophy. *Am Rev Respir Dis* 1980;121: 281–289.

50. Begin R, Bureau MA, Lupien L, et al. Pathogenesis of respiratory insufficiency in myotonic dystrophy. *Am Rev Respir Dis* 1982;125:312–318.

51. Begin R, Bureau MA, Lupien L, Lemieux B. Control and modulation of respiration in Steinert's myotonic dystrophy. *Am Rev Respir Dis* 1980;121: 281–289.

52. Rimmer KP, Golar S, Lee MA, Whitelaw WA. Myotonia of the respiratory muscles in myotonic dystrophy. *Am Rev Respir Dis* 1993;148:1018–1022.

53. Manni R, Zucca C, Martinetti M, et al. Hypersomnia in dystrophia myotonica: a neurophysiological and immunogenetic study. *Acta Neurol Scand* 1991;84: 498–502.

54. Lazzeroni E, Favaro L, Botti G. Dilated cardiomyopathy with regional myocardial hypoperfusion in Becker's muscular dystrophy. *Int J Cardiol* 1989;22: 126–129.

55. Maayan Ch, Springer C, Armon Y, et al. Nemaline myopathy as a cause of sleep hypoventilation. *Pediatrics* 1986;77:390–395.

56. Bach JR, Alba AS. Management of chronic alveolar hypoventilation by nasal ventilation. *Chest* 1990;97:52–57.

57. Gilgoff IS, Baydur A, Bach JR, et al. Tracheal intermittent positive pressure ventilation for patients with neuromuscular disease. *J Neurol Rehabil* 1992; 6:93–101.

58. Strong MJ, Ferguson KA, Ahmad D. The pulmonary function testing as a predictor of survival in amyotrophic lateral sclerosis. *Chest* 1992;102:180S.

59. Bach JR, Wang TG. Noninvasive long-term ventilatory support for individuals with spinal muscular atrophy and functional bulbar musculature. *Arch Phys Med Rehabil* 1995;76:213–217.

60. Bach JR, Alba AS, Bohatiuk G, et al. Mouth intermittent positive pressure ventilation in the management of post-polio respiratory insufficiency. *Chest* 1987; 91:859–864.

61. Bach JR. Management of post-polio respiratory sequelae. *Ann N Y Acad Sci* 1995;753: 96–102.

62. Carskadon M, Dement W. Respiration during sleep in the aged human. *J Gerontol* 1981;36: 420–425.

63. George CF, Millar TW, Kryger MH. Identification and quantification of apneas by computer-based analysis of oxygen saturation. *Am Rev Respir Dis* 1988;137: 1238–1240.

64. He J, Kryger MH, Zorick FJ, et al. Mortality and apnea index in obstructive sleep apnea. *Chest* 1988;94:9–14.

65. Bonekat HW, Andersen G, Squires J. Obstructive disorder breathing during sleep in patients with spinal cord injury. *Paraplegia* 1990;28:392–398.

66. Lombard R Jr, Zwillich CW. Medical therapy of obstructive sleep apnea. *Med Clin North Am* 1985;69:1317–1335.

67. Hodes HL. Treatment of respiratory difficulty in poliomyelitis. In: *Poliomyelitis: papers and discussions presented at the Third International Poliomyelitis Conference.* Philadelphia: JB Lippincott, 1955:91–113.

68. Bach JR, Tippett DC, McCrary MM. Bulbar dysfunction and associated cardiopulmonary considerations in polio and neuromuscular disease. *J Neurol Rehabil* 1992;6:121–128.

69. Guilleminault C, Motta J. Sleep apnea syndrome as a long-term sequela of poliomyelitis. In: Guilleminault C, ed. *Sleep apnea syndromes.* New York: KROC Foundation, 1978:309–315.

70. Katsantonis GP, Walsh JK, Schweitzer PK, Friedman WH. Further evaluation of uvulopalatopharyngoplasty in the treatment of obstructive sleep apnea syndrome. *Otolaryngol Head Neck Surg* 1985; 93:244–250.

71. Levy RD, Bradley TD, Newman SL, et al. Negative pressure ventilation: effects on ventilation during sleep in normal subjects. *Chest* 1989;65:95–99.

72. Bach JR, O'Connor K. Electrophrenic ventilation: a different perspective. *J Am Paraplegia Soc* 1991;14:9–17.

73. Bradley TD, Phillipson EA. Pathogenesis and pathophysiology of the obstructive sleep apnea syndrome. *Med Clin North Am* 1985;69:1169–1185.

74. Pillar G, Peled R, Lavie P. Recurrence of sleep apnea without concomitant weight increase 7.5 years after weight reduction surgery. *Chest* 1994;106:1702–1704.

75. Bonham PE, Currier GF, Orr WC, et al. The effect of a modified functional appliance on obstructive sleep apnea. *Am J Orthod Dentofacial Orthop* 1988;94: 384–392.

76. Bach JR, Penek J. Obstructive sleep apnea complicating negative pressure ventilatory support in patients with chronic paralytic/restrictive ventilatory dysfunction. *Chest* 1991;99: 1386–1391.

77. Riley RW, Powell NB, Guilleminault C, Mino-Murcia G. Maxillary, mandibular, and hyoid advancement: an alternative to tracheostomy in obstructive sleep apnea syndrome. *Otolaryngol Head Neck Surg* 1986; 94:584–588.

78. Oren J, Kelly DH, Shannon DC. Long-term follow-up of children with congenital central hypoventilation syndrome. *Pediatrics* 1987;80:375–380.

79. Silverstein D, Michlin B, Sobel HJ, Lavietes MH. Right ventricular failure in a patient with diabetic neuropathy (myopathy) and central alveolar hypoventilation. *Respiration* 1983;44: 460–465.

80. Plum F, Posner JB. *The diagnosis of stupor and coma.* 3rd ed. Philadelphia: FA Davis, 1980: 32–39.

81. Prendergast V. Current trends in research and treatment of intracranial hypertension. *Crit Care Nurs Q* 1994;17:1–8.

82. Vingerhoets F, Bogousslavsky J. Respiratory dysfunction in stroke. *Clin Chest Med* 1994;15: 729–737.

83. Plum F. Neurological integration of behavioural and metabolic control of breathing. In: Porter R, ed. *Ciba Foundation Hering Breuer Centenary Symposium: Breathing.* London: J. & A. Churchill, 1970:159.

84. Brown LK. Respiratory dysfunction in Parkinson's disease. *Clin Chest Med* 1994; 15:715–727.

85. Obenour WH, Stevens PM, Cohen AA, McCutchen JJ. The causes of abnormal pulmonary function in Parkinson's disease. *Am Rev Respir Dis* 1972; 105:382–387.

86. Petit JM, Delhez L. Activite electrique du diaphragme dans la maladie de Parkinson. *Arch Int Physiol Biochem* 1961;69: 413–419.

87. Tzelepis GE, McCool FD, Friedman JH, Hoppin FG. Respiratory muscle dysfunction in Parkinson's disease. *Am Rev Respir Dis* 1988;138: 266–271.

88. Vincken WG, Gauthier SG, Dollfuss RE, et al. Involvement of upper-airway muscles in extrapyramidal disorders. A cause of airflow limitation. *N Engl J Med* 1984;311:438–442.

89. Estenne M, Hubert M, De Troyer A. Respiratory muscle involvement in Parkinson's disease. *N Engl J Med* 1984;311: 1516–1521.

90. Apps MCP, Sheaff PC, Ingram DA, et al. Respiration and sleep in Parkinson's disease. *J Neurol Neurosurg Psychiatry* 1985;48: 1240–1246.

91. Bach JR. Ventilator use by muscular dystrophy association patients: an update. *Arch Phys Med Rehabil* 1992;73: 179–183.

92. Braun NMT, Arora MS, Rochester DF. Respiratory muscle and pulmonary function in polymyositis and other proximal myopathies. *Thorax* 1983;38: 616–623.

93. Putman MT, Wise RA. Myasthenia gravis and upper airway obstruction. *Chest* 1996;109: 400–404.

94. Rogers B, Msall M, Shucard D. Hypoxemia during oral feedings in adults with dysphagia and severe neurological disabilities. *Dysphagia* 1993;8:43–48.

95. Gilardeau C, Kazandjian MS, Bach JR, et al. The evaluation and management of dysphagia. *Semin Neurol* 1995; 15:46–51.

96. Bach JR. Mechanical insufflation-exsufflation: comparison of peak expiratory flows with manually assisted and unassisted coughing techniques. *Chest* 1993;104: 1553–1562.

97. Bach JR. Amyotrophic lateral sclerosis: predictors for prolongation of life by noninvasive respiratory aids. *Arch Phys Med Rehabil* 1995;76:828–832.

98. Bach JR, Saporito LR. Indications and criteria for decannulation and transition from invasive to noninvasive long-term ventilatory support. *Respir Care* 1994;39:515–531.

99. Bach JR. Neuromuscular and skeletal disorders leading to global alveolar hypoventilation. In: Bach JR, ed. *Pulmonary rehabilitation: the obstructive and paralytic conditions.* Philadelphia: Hanley & Belfus, 1996: 257–273.

100. Miller HJ, Thomas E, Wilmot CB. Pneumobelt use among high quadriplegic population. *Arch Phys Med Rehabil* 1988;69: 369–372.

101. Bach JR, Alba AS. Total ventilatory support by the intermittent abdominal pressure ventilator. *Chest* 1991;99:630–636.

102. Bach JR, Alba AS, Saporito LR. Intermittent positive pressure ventilation via the mouth as an alternative to tracheostomy for 257 ventilator users. *Chest* 1993;103:174–182.

103. Bach JR. A historical perspective on the use of noninvasive ventilatory support alternatives. *Respir Clin North Am* 1996;2: 161–181.

104. Bach JR. A comparison of long-term ventilatory support alternatives from the perspective of the patient and care giver. *Chest* 1993;104:1702–1706.

105. Delaubier A. Traitement de l'insuffisance respiratoire chronique dans les dystrophies musculaires. In: *Memoires de certificat d'etudes superieures de reeducation et readaptation fonctionnelles.* Paris: Universite R Descarte, 1984:1–124.

106. Bach JF, Alba A, Mosher R, Delaubier A. Intermittent positive pressure ventilation via nasal access in the management of respiratory insufficiency. *Chest* 1987;92:168–170.

107. McDermott I, Bach JR, Parker C, Sortor S. Custom-fabricated interfaces for intermittent positive pressure ventilation. *Int J Prosthodont* 1989;2:224–233.

108. Piper AJ, Parker S, Torzillo PJ, et al. Nocturnal nasal IPPV stabilizes patients with cystic fibrosis and hypercapnic respiratory failure. *Chest* 1992;102: 846–850.

109. Benhamou D, Girault C, Faure C, et al. Nasal mask ventilation in acute respiratory failure: experience in elderly patients. *Chest* 1992;102:912–917.

110. Bach JR, McDermott I. Strapless oral-nasal interfaces for positive pressure ventilation. *Arch Phys Med Rehabil* 1990; 71:908–911.

111. Dail CW, Affeldt JE. *Glossopharyngeal breathing* [videotape]. Los Angeles, CA: Los Angeles Department of Visual Education,

College of Medical Evangelists, 1954.

112. Dail C, Rodgers M, Guess V, Adkins HV. *Glossopharyngeal breathing manual.* Downey, CA: Professional Staff Association of Rancho Los Amigos Hospital, 1979.

113. Bach JR, Alba AS, Bodofsky E, et al. Glossopharyngeal breathing and non-invasive aids in the management of post-polio respiratory insufficiency. *Birth Defects* 1987;23:99–113.

114. Sortor S, McKenzie M. *Toward independence: assisted cough* [videotape]. Dallas, TX: BioScience Communications of Dallas, 1986.

115. Fugl-Meyer AR, Grimby G. Ventilatory function in tetraplegic patients. *Scand J Rehabil Med* 1971;3:151–160.

116. Massery M. Manual breathing and coughing aids. *Phys Med Rehabil Clin N Am* 1996;7: 407–422.

117. Barach AL, Beck GJ, Bickerman HA, Seanor HE. Mechanical coughing: studies on physical methods of producing high velocity flow rates during the expiratory cycle. *Trans Assoc Am Physicians* 1951;64: 360–363.

118. Barach AL, Beck GJ, Bickerman HA, et al. Physical methods simulating mechanisms of the human cough. *J Appl Physiol* 1952;5:85–91.

119. Beck GJ, Barach AL. Value of mechanical aids in the management of a patient with poliomyelitis. *Ann Intern Med* 1954;40:1081–1094.

120. Barach AL, Beck GJ. Exsufflation with negative pressure: physiologic and clinical studies in poliomyelitis, bronchial asthma, pulmonary emphysema and bronchiectasis. *Arch Intern Med* 1954;93:825–841.

121. Bach JR. Illustrative case studies of respiratory management. In: Back JR, ed. *Pulmonary rehabilitation: the obstructive and paralytic conditions.* Philadelphia: Hanley & Belfus, 1996: 331–346.

122. Bach JR. Update and perspectives on noninvasive respiratory muscle aids: part 2—the expiratory muscle aids. *Chest* 1994;105:1538–1544.

123. Viroslav J, Rosenblatt R, Morris-Tomazevic S. Respiratory management, survival, and quality of life for high level traumatic tetraplegics. *Respir Clin North Am* 1996;2:313–322.

124. Bach JR, Alba AS. Tracheostomy ventilation: a study of efficacy with deflated cuffs and cuffless tubes. *Chest* 1990;97:679–683.

125. Kirilloff LH, Owens GR, Rogers RM, Mazzocco MC. Does chest physical therapy work? *Chest* 1985;88:436–444.

126. King M, Phillips DM, Gross D, et al. Enhanced tracheal mucus clearance with high frequency chest wall compression. *Am Rev Respir Dis* 1983;128:511–515.

127. Radford R, Barutt J, Billingsley JG, et al. A rational basis for percussion augmented mucociliary clearance. *Respir Care* 1982;27:556–563.

128. Rubin EM, Scantlen GE, Chapman GA, et al. Effect of chest wall oscillation on mucus clearance: comparison of two vibrators. *Pediatr Pulmonol* 1989;6:123–127.

129. Richardson PS, Peatfield AC. The control of airway secretion. *Eur J Respir Dis* 1987;71(Suppl 153): 43–51.

130. Change HK, Weber ME, King M. Mucus transport by high frequency nonsymmetrical airflow. *J Appl Physiol* 1988;65: 1203–1209.

131. Flower KA, Eden RI, Lomax L, et al. New mechanical aid to physiotherapy in cystic fibrosis. *BMJ* 1979;2:630–631.

132. Warwick WJ, Hansen LG. The long-term effect of high-frequency chest compression therapy on pulmonary complications of cystic fibrosis. *Pediatr Pulmonol* 1991;11:265–271.

133. Holody B, Goldberg HS. The effect of mechanical vibration physiotherapy on arterial oxygenation in acutely ill patients with atelectasis or pneumonia. *Am Rev Respir Dis* 1981;124: 372–375.

134. Piquet J, Brochard L, Isabey D, et al. High frequency chest wall oscillation in patients with chronic air-flow obstruction. *Am Rev Respir Dis* 1987;136: 1355–1359.

135. Sibuya M, Yamada M, Kanamaru A, et al. Effect of chest wall vibration on dyspnea in patients with chronic respiratory disease. *Am J Respir Crit Care Med* 1994;149:1235–1240.

136. Arens R, Gozal D, Omlin KJ, et al. Comparison of high frequency chest compression and conventional chest physiotherapy in hospitalized patients with cystic fibrosis. *Am J Respir Crit Care Med* 1994;150: 1154–1157.

137. Pryor JA, Parker RA, Webber BA. A comparison of mechanical and manual percussion as adjuncts to postural drainage in the treatment of cystic fibrosis in adolescents and adults. *Physiotherapy* 1981;6:140–141.

138. Sutton PP, Parker RA, Webber BA, et al. Assessment of the forced expiration technique, postural drainage and directed coughing in chest physiotherapy. *Eur J Respir Dis* 1983;64: 62–68.

139. van der Schans CP, Piers DA, Postma DS. Effect of manual percussion on tracheobronchial clearance in patients with chronic airflow obstruction and excessive tracheobronchial secretion. *Thorax* 1986; 41:448–452.

140. van Hengstum M, Festen J, Beurskens C, et al. No effect of oral high frequency oscillation combined with forced expiration maneuvers on tracheobronchial clearance in chronic bronchitis. *Eur Respir J* 1990;3:14–18.

141. Campbell AH, O'Connell JM, Wilson F. The effect of chest physiotherapy upon the FEV1 in

chronic bronchitis. *Med J Aust* 1975;1:33–35.

142. Zidulka A, Chrome JF, Wight DW, et al. Clapping or percussion causes atelectasis in dogs and influences gas exchange. *J Appl Physiol* 1989;66:2833–2838.

143. Toussaint M, De Win H, Steens M, Soudon P. A new technique in secretion clearance by the percussionaire for patients with neuromuscular disease. In: *Programme des Journées Internationales de Ventilation à Domicile. Lyon, France: Hôpital de la Croix Rousse.* 1993:27. Abstract.

144. Thangathuria D, Holm AP, Mikhail M, et al. HFV in management of a patient with severe bronchorrhea. *Respir Manage* 1988;1:31–33.

145. McInturff SL, Shaw LI, Hodgkin JE, et al. Intrapulmonary percussive ventilation in the treatment of COPD. *Respir Care* 1985; 30:885.

Other Diseases and Problems

Chapter 91

Cancer

Richard S. Tunkel
Elisabeth Lachmann
Margaret L. Ho

According to National Cancer Institute data, almost 50% of males and almost 40% of females are likely to develop an invasive cancer at some time in their lives (1). The estimated incidence of new cancers in 1997 is almost 1.4 million. The relative 5-year survival rates for all cancers have significantly increased since 1960. This is especially true for children under the age of 15 years, for whom survival rates since 1960 have increased two-and-a-half-fold (1). This growing population of cancer patients and survivors has a broad spectrum of impairments, many of which would benefit from rehabilitative intervention.

Among the most prevalent problems seen in patients with cancer that can be addressed by appropriate rehabilitation care are functional impairments, pain, and psychological disturbances (2). Deconditioning and neurologic disorders are common underlying etiologies of these problems (3,4). As in most other populations requiring physiatric intervention, patients with cancer can benefit from treatment utilizing well-established rehabilitation techniques within an interdisciplinary framework (5,6). Management of the cancer patient may be more complicated, however, because of changes in the patient's oncologic condition producing a dynamic range of functional impairments, further challenging the rehabilitation team. For example, external-beam radiation treatments for epidural cord compression may provide substantial neurologic and thus functional improvement. Conversely, subsequent worsening paraparesis in such a patient may indicate recurrent cord compression at the same or a different level.

Dietz (7) categorized four levels of rehabilitation specifically for the patient with cancer.

1. Preventive rehabilitation is directed toward limiting impairments or disabilities that may arise from anticipated or continuing conditions or procedures. Patients isolated for prolonged periods because of bone marrow transplantation can easily become deconditioned. This may be prevented by an appropriate exercise program.
2. Restorative rehabilitation aims toward re-establishing the patient's previous level of function. Patients who develop proximal limb weakness following the use of high-dose corticosteroids would benefit from early therapeutic exercise and mobilization.
3. Supportive rehabilitation maximizes the function of the patient with new long-term impairments or disabilities, as in the prosthetic training of an amputee.
4. Palliative rehabilitation attempts to give comfort and support and decrease dependence in activities of daily living to patients with advanced or end-stage disease. Improving a patient's transfer skills may make home care a more viable option for caregivers.

Dietz (8) classified inpatients with a diagnosis of cancer according to rehabilitation treatment goals over a 3-year period. Thirty-two percent of the patients were classified as having a restorative rehabilitative goal; 39%, a supportive rehabilitation goal; and 23%, a palliative rehabilitation goal.

Few studies have evaluated the efficacy of rehabilitation of patients with cancer. In 1969 Dietz (8) reported the results of a cooperative rehabilitation project on cancer patients. Fifty-seven percent of patients showed moderate or marked functional improvement with some residual physical disability. Another 11% were fully independent with no residual disability. Marciniak et al (4) reported the functional outcomes following rehabilitation of patients with cancer in a free-standing rehabilitation hospital. They found that significant functional gains were made, with all subgroups of cancer patients making similar gains. Functional outcome was not affected by the presence of metastatic disease.

PHYSICAL IMPAIRMENTS IN CANCER PATIENTS

Direct Tumor Effects

Malignancy often gives rise to physical impairments through a mass effect, dependent on its location. Intracranial tumors may directly compress, and edema surrounding the tumor or a complicating hemorrhage may further compromise, local nerve tissue. Magnetic resonance imaging (MRI) is perhaps the most valuable diagnostic procedure for evaluation; MRI angiography may help distinguish vascular from nervous tissue (9). Hemiparesis, a common presentation of such tumors, may be accompanied by hemisensory deficit or neglect, homonymous hemianopia, aphasia, or dysphagia. The neurologic presentation and recovery may not resemble those of a cerebrovascular accident. In children, cancer involving the central nervous system is prevalent (10). In infants and toddlers, loss of hearing as a consequence of brain tumors may interfere with speech acquisition. Long-term or multiple hospital stays, regardless of what the primary tumor is, may result in reduced stimulation of the pediatric patient, leading to delayed or disordered development.

Epidural and other spinal malignancies can cause spinal cord injury and accompanying deficits. Metastatic epidural disease, most frequently seen in the thoracic region of the spine, often arises from lung, breast, or prostate primary tumors (11). Patients may initially present with back or radicular pain, even months prior to the onset of weakness (12). Rapid progression of neurologic impairment to paraparesis or tetraparesis may occur without prompt intervention (13). Treatment of epidural cord compression includes radiation therapy, high-dose corticosteroids, and cord decompression (11,12,14–16). In the nonemergent setting, chemotherapeutic treatment of the primary tumor may be considered (17).

Leptomeningeal disease of the spinal cord most commonly presents with paraparesis, with about one-third of patients presenting with cauda equina syndrome (18). Even with intervention, neurologic recovery may be limited (19). Involvement above the spinal cord may give rise to cranial neuropathies (20). Brachial plexopathy may arise from direct tumor invasion, often from breast or lung cancer. Limb weakness in the distribution of the lower brachial plexus, significant limb pain, and Horner syndrome suggest tumor invasion (21). Pelvic malignancy leading to compression of the lumbosacral plexus most commonly presents with low-back and leg pain and weakness (22). Three may be accompanying numbness, paresthesias, and edema in the ipsilateral leg, as well as rectal pain and hydronephrosis. Colorectal, breast, and cervical malignancies as well as sarcoma and lymphoma are frequently associated (23).

Most primary bone tumors are seen in young patients. The most common of these is osteogenic sarcoma, most frequently found at the knee. In contrast, bone marrow neoplasia occurs in adult patients, with multiple myeloma being the type most frequently encountered. However, metastatic carcinoma is the most common malignant tumor of bone. Bone metastases can give rise to pain, pathologic fracture, and hypercalcemia. Breast, prostate, thyroid, lung, and kidney carcinomas are the most common primary tumors to metastasize to bone (24). Metastases are usually found in the axial and proximal appendicular skeleton. Most cancers involve bone by hematogenous spread. Metastasis of tumor cells along the axial skeleton is facilitated by the Batson valveless venous plexus of the spine and pelvis (25). Tumor cells produce bone resorption by secreting factors that stimulate osteoclastic activity (26). Bone pain may arise because of these factors or from anatomic activation of nociceptors. Pain that is exacerbated by mechanical stress may represent an impending or occult fracture. Especially in patients with a history of an osteophilic primary tumor, bone pain must be considered secondary to metastasis until proved otherwise.

Skeletal radiographs are often used for initial evaluation. Most lesions are lytic in nature, but sclerotic (blastic) lesions are often seen with prostate cancer and sometimes with breast, gastrointestinal, and bladder cancer (27). A lytic lesion may be unifocal (geographic) or multifocal ("moth-eaten" or permeative). Lytic lesions, including permeative ones, sometimes difficult to see on plain radiographs, are more prone to pathologic fracture. As much as 50% of medullary bone must be destroyed in order to be visualized on plain radiographs (27). Guidelines for determining impending fractures of long bones, such as defects larger than 2.5 cm or more than 30% to 50% cortical destruction, have not been validated (27,28). Even smaller femoral neck lesions, avulsion fracture of the lesser trochanter, or lesion of the weight-bearing portion of the acetabulum may represent impending hip fracture. Mirels (29) described a scoring system for categorizing impending fractures of long bones in which peritrochanteric lesions are of greatest concern. The system assigned weighted scores depending on the site and size of the lesion, the

Table 91-1: Scoring System—Risk of Pathologic Fracture			
Variable	**1**	**2**	**3**
Site	Upper limb	Lower limb	Peritrochanter
Pain	Mild	Moderate	Functional
Lesion	Blastic	Mixed	Lytic
Size	$<^1/_3$	$^1/_3$–$^2/_3$	$>^2/_3$

Source: Reproduced by permission from Mirels H. Metastatic disease in long bones: a proposed scoring system for diagnosing impending pathologic fractures. *Clin Orthop* 1989;249:256–264.

blastic or lytic quality, and associated pain (Table 91-1). A score of 8 or more indicates that the lesion may be associated with an increased risk of fracture, therefore requiring prophylactic stabilization before irradiation.

The first radiographic evidence of bone metastasis may be loss of a pedicle from a vertebra ("winking owl" sign) (27). Radiographic criteria for determining thoracolumbar instability following spinal trauma have been applied to but not validated for malignancy. Denis (30) divided the spine into three columns. The anterior column consists of the anterior half of the vertebral body, intervertebral disk, and the anterior longitudinal ligament. The middle column is the posterior half of the vertebral body, intervertebral disk, and the posterior longitudinal ligament. The posterior column is made up of the remaining posterior elements and facets. When there is disruption of two of the three columns, the spine is considered to be unstable. A modified system of six columns, essentially dividing the Denis system into left and right columns, attempts to better define instability in the setting of spinal neoplasia (31). If three or more columns are destroyed, the spine is considered to be unstable. Angular deformity of more than 20 degrees is also suggestive of instability.

Radionuclide bone scanning can reveal bone lesions and nondisplaced fractures earlier than radiographs. However, bone scanning may miss lesions in multiple myeloma, lymphoma, highly aggressive tumors such as renal cell carcinoma, and very small lesions (27). Computed tomography (CT) and MRI may be more sensitive than plain radiographs in detecting bone lesions and fracture and help visualize soft-tissue and neurologic involvement (27,32). These imaging studies may be considered when plain radiographs are nondiagnostic and significant pain persists with use of the involved structure. With bone metastasis of the proximal end of the femur, there is often groin or deep buttock pain with weight bearing as well as pain reproduction with active straight-leg raising or passive rotation of the hip.

In the management of metastatic bone disease, the main emphasis is to diminish pain and maintain function. Hormonal or chemotherapy may be used to treat diffuse disease. Radiation therapy may be selected to treat focal bone lesions or to palliate pain. Indications for surgery include impending or actual pathologic fracture or spinal instability, persistent or recurrent pain or neurologic deficits in spite of irradiation, and rapidly progressing neurologic deficit (31,33). With the use of methylmethacrylate and modern orthopedic instrumentation, structural stability and early mobilization can often be achieved.

Remote Effects of Cancer

Cerebellar degeneration is the most common paraneoplastic disorder affecting the brain (34). Ataxic gait may progress to severe limb and truncal incoordination. Some patients may become wheelchair dependent (35). The most commonly associated malignancies are small-cell lung cancers, gynecologic cancers, and Hodgkin disease (36). Carcinomatous polyneuropathy is frequently a mixed sensorimotor axonal degeneration, most often associated with lung cancer. Bilateral footdrop and glove-and-stocking sensory deficit may be progressive and may precede diagnosis of the underlying malignancy (34,37). Paraneoplastic motor neuronopathy, seen in malignant lymphomas, may cause painless weakness in the legs.

Lambert-Eaton myasthenic syndrome (LEMS) produces proximal limb weakness due to a presynaptic deficit at the neuromuscular junction, usually sparing the neck, extraocular, and bulbar muscles. Small-cell lung cancer is the most common underlying malignancy, but it may be seen with kidney and rectal cancer, malignant thymoma, basal cell carcinoma, and leukemia (38). Nerve conduction studies show abnormally small compound muscle action potentials (CMAPs) that significantly increase following 10 to 20 seconds of voluntary muscle contraction or high rates of repetitive stimulation (39). Electrodiagnostic findings and weakness often improve after successful treatment of the underlying malignancy (40).

Polymyositis/dermatomyositis (PM/DM) type III is associated with underlying malignancy (41). Weakness precedes the diagnosis of cancer in the majority of patients (34). Tumors associated with PM/DM include breast, lung, ovary, stomach, colon, uterus, and prostate tumors (42). Electromyographic studies may reveal the classic triad of positive sharp waves and fibrillation potentials; complex repetitive discharges; and low-amplitude, short-duration, polyphasic potentials (38). Muscle pain and tenderness may interfere with rehabilitation. Symptomatic improvement may be seen not only with treatment of the underlying malignancy but also with the use of corticosteroids (43). Increasing weakness in patients may represent tumor progression, insufficient corticosteroid therapy, or steroid-induced myopathy.

Several malignancy-related conditions may provoke joint pain. Patients with hypertrophic osteoarthropathy (HOA) may present with a classic triad of digital clubbing, periostitis, and polyarthritis. Nearly 10% of adults with HOA will have an underlying pulmonary malignancy (44). Any of the manifestations of HOA may precede diagnosis of malignancy by more than 1 year (45). If treatment of the underlying malignancy is ineffective, symptomatic relief may be obtained with nonsteroidal anti-inflammatory drugs (NSAIDs) (44–46). Patients with carcinoma polyarthritis, most often associated with breast cancer, may have acute onset of asymmetric joint involvement, especially of the lower limbs (47). There is usually sparing of the wrists and small joints (48,49). Diagnosis of the underlying malignancy may follow the onset of symptoms. Again, symptoms may improve with successful cancer treatment and reappear with tumor recurrence. Asymmetric or migratory arthralgias or arthritis may be seen in patients with leukemias; amyloid arthropathy may be seen with multiple myeloma. In each, corticosteroids may be helpful (46). Arthralgias rarely arise in association with lymphomas (50).

Another remote effect of cancer can be a hypercoagulable state that may increase the risk of deep vein thrombosis (DVT) related to activation of clotting factors and platelets, endothelial damage, and inhibition of fibrinolysis (51). A severe anemia may be seen in patients with cancer. Weight loss and cachexia may also be considered as a paraneoplastic effect of malignancy contributing to decreased strength and endurance and the risk of pressure ulcers.

Chemotherapeutic Agents

The most common adverse effect of chemotherapeutic agents is myelosuppression. Patients are at increased risk of infection, owing to neutropenia. Anemias may lead to worsening fatigue and weakness. Thrombocytopenia is of great concern because of an increased risk of intracranial hemorrhage and may limit rehabilitative efforts.

Mucositis can cause painful ulcerations of the upper digestive tract mucous membranes, which can lead to odynophagia and reduced mobility of the oropharyngeal musculature (52). If mucositis is severe, patients may not be able to continue normal oral intake during chemotherapy. Patients may require a modified soft or liquid diet.

Neurotoxicity is also a well-known side effect of certain chemotherapeutic agents. The vinca alkaloids, especially vincristine, may produce a dose-limiting peripheral sensorimotor neuropathy. Asymptomatic areflexia may progress to numbness and paresthesias in a stocking-and-glove distribution as well as weakness, especially of the distal end of the lower limbs. Significant neuropathic pain may occur, further limiting functional mobility. Muscle cramps may begin up to 4 months after vincristine treatment is initiated (53). Equinovarus deformity has been observed in children receiving vincristine (54). Electrodiagnostic studies often reveal axonal degeneration (55). The majority of patients go on to full recovery, which may take many months (56).

Cisplatin has been associated with a sensory peripheral neuropathy (57). Dysesthesias and paresthesias of the hands and feet can progress to involve all sensory modalities (58). In severe cases a significant sensory gait ataxia can occur (59). Electrodiagnostic findings suggest both axonal and myelin degeneration (60). The most sensitive electrodiagnostic parameter may be somatosensory evoked potentials (61). Manifestations of cisplatin neuropathy usually resolve over time. Ototoxicity associated with the use of cisplatin may give rise to hearing loss (62,63). This can be deleterious in children who are still developing speech and language (64,65).

Other chemotherapeutic agents may have neurotoxic side effects. Paclitaxel (Taxol) may cause mild to moderate sensory peripheral neuropathies. With higher doses, severe sensory neuropathy with mild motor neuropathy may occur (66). Electrodiagnostic studies reveal axonal and myelin degeneration. The semisynthetic analogue of paclitaxel, docetaxel (Taxotere), may also cause mild peripheral neuropathy (67). Vinorelbine has been reported to cause peripheral neuropathy (68). Procarbazine can cause peripheral neuropathy with resultant paresthesias and gait ataxia, usually reversed with discontinuation of the drug (69). Suramin is known to cause a Guillain-Barré–like syndrome, with generalized limb weakness and distal sensory loss resulting from demyelination and axonal degeneration. Recovery may be incomplete (70). Cytarabine administration may produce clinical manifestations of cerebellar ataxia.

Pulmonary toxicity has been associated with bleomycin. Interstitial pneumonitis with dyspnea may present within 3 months of treatment (71). A later effect of bleomycin may be pulmonary fibrosis. A restrictive pattern is seen on pulmonary function testing. High doses of corticosteroids may be helpful, but 10% of those affected die from pulmonary fibrosis. Pulmonary toxicity may also occur with use of methotrexate, mitomycin, or alkylating agents including cyclophosphamide and BCNU (carmustine) (71).

Cardiac toxicity is associated with the use of the anthracyclines, doxorubicin, and daunorubicin. The effects range from transient electrocardiographic (ECG) changes to irreversible congestive heart failure (72). Radionuclide angiography is used to monitor patients to detect early myocardial damage. The anthracyclines may impair myocardial growth in pediatric patients (73).

Corticosteroids, especially in high doses, may produce proximal limb weakness and atrophy. Electrodiagnostic studies are typically unrevealing (38). Pseudorheumatism with diffuse joint and muscle pain may occur if high doses of corticosteroids are tapered too rapidly (74). Osteoporosis may occur with chronic use of glucocorticoids and is especially troublesome in postmenopausal women, immobilized patients, and those with metastatic disease to bone (75). The axial skeleton is the most common site of pathologic fracture. Aseptic necrosis, most commonly of the femoral head, may occur even with short-term glucocorticoid treatment. Once plain radiographic abnormalities are detected, progressive joint deterioration usually ensues. Adverse psychological effects may be seen with daily corticosteroid use, especially with higher doses. Affective symptoms may range from mild mood disturbances to hypomania or dysthymia. An organic psychosis with paranoid features can be seen.

Radiation Therapy

Nerve tissue is generally radioresistant, but over time and after high dose, postradiation changes may occur. Cranial irradiation may produce neuropsychological effects, most frequently in pediatric patients. The younger the patient, the more profound the effect can be (76). The vast majority of long-term survivors who received cranial irradiation before the age of 2 years have significant neurologic and psychological abnormalities (77). Adults receiving cranial irradiation for intracranial gliomas may also develop impairments, including short-term memory deficit and gait apraxia (78). However, some have found that long-term glioma survivors do not develop impaired neuropsychological function and maintain good performance levels while in remission (79).

Transient radiation myelopathy may occur several months following treatment. The Lhermitte sign, in which forward flexion of the neck produces an electric-like pain into the spine and limbs, is not accompanied by neurologic deficits and usually resolves within 6 months (80). Delayed radiation myelopathy occurs months to years following treatment. Initial sensory deficits progress to paresis of affected limbs and in some patients may become a complete transverse myelopathy (81). Corticosteroids or hyperbaric oxygen may provide temporary symptomatic relief (80). A transient postradiation plexopathy may occur and spontaneously resolve (82,83). Chronic postradiation plexopathy may occur months to years following treatment. With the brachial plexus there is a preponderance of upper plexus involvement and the ipsilateral limb may develop lymphedema. Pain is not a prominent symptom (21). Radiation-induced lumbosacral plexopathy often presents as painless leg weakness that progresses and often involves the opposite leg. In at least half of affected patients the legs do not become painful (22). Postradiation plexopathy generally progresses over time. Electromyography may demonstrate myokymic discharges, which have not been reported in neoplastic plexopathy (22,84). Isolated peripheral nerve injury has occurred following irradiation (85).

When the joints and periarticular tissues are exposed to high-dose radiation therapy, joint contracture may ensue (86). Irradiation of axillary or pelvic lymph nodes may predispose the limb to lymphedema. Radiation therapy for prostate cancer may produce sexual dysfunction with diminishing erectile potency over time (87). Radiation therapy when added to surgical treatment of cervical cancer may lead to a decreased quality of life and increased dyspareunia (88).

Radiotherapy for head and neck cancers may produce xerostomia (89). Changes in salivary flow can disrupt swallowing. Mucositis and edema may also occur during or after radiation therapy. Trismus, a reduction in mandibular excursion, can occur after the completion of radiation therapy, owing to fibrotic changes (90). Pharyngeal mobility may become reduced during and after radiation treatment, resulting in impairments of base of tongue retraction and laryngeal elevation (91). Up to 50% of lung cancer patients develop radiation-induced esophagitis and odynophagia and may require modified liquid diets (92).

Postradiation effects on the heart, though quite uncommon today because of proper shielding, have been described. Symptomatic pericarditis can develop following conservation surgery and adjuvant radiotherapy for breast cancer (93). Transient or chronic myocardial changes as well as coronary artery and valvular disease have also been seen following radiation therapy (94,95). Acute radiation pneumonitis may be seen 6 months after treatment (96) and can cause dyspnea and cough, which typically resolve within 3 months (97). Chronic progressive pulmonary fibrosis may develop even without preceding acute pneumonitis. Patients are often asymptomatic but may develop cough and dyspnea or uncommonly become disabled from the restrictive lung disease (96,98).

Bone Marrow Transplantation

Bone marrow transplantation has been used as a treatment for hematogenous neoplasia and solid tumor patients with advanced disease. Reverse isolation is required for myelosuppression. Thrombocytopenia may predispose to intracranial hemorrhage. Intramuscular and intra-articular hemorrhages are also a concern with increased bleeding time. There is controversy concerning minimum platelet count and safe levels of activity. Some have suggested avoiding resistive exercise with platelet counts less than 50,000/μL and avoiding all activity when counts are below 20,000/μL (99). Others have proposed the following guidelines after bone marrow transplantation: Patients with platelet counts greater than 10,000/μL may use a stationary bicycle, ambulate, and perform exercise; for those with platelet counts below this level, resistive exercises are completely avoided; patients with counts below 5000/μL are restricted to self-care activities only (100). Even in patients for whom resistive exercise is feasible, it is usually not necessary. The activity level permitted must also take into account other potential risk factors for hemorrhage. One study involving acute leukemia patients suggested that an acceptable threshold for prophylactic platelet transfusions for those without fever or manifestations of bleeding would be 5000/μL and would be 10,000/μL in those with these signs; the threshold should be at least 20,000/μL for those with coagulopathies, anatomic lesions, or on heparin (101).

Surgical Interventions

Because of surrounding edema, resection of tissues from the central nervous system may produce initial impairments greater than those observed prior to tumor resection, often with subsequent improvement. With large or multiple tumor resections, residual deficits can be expected.

Head and neck surgeries requiring neck dissection may sacrifice or damage the spinal accessory nerve (102–104). This nerve may also be damaged with resection of lymph nodes from the posterior cervical triangle (105). With spinal accessory nerve palsy the scapula is protracted and rotated inferiorly (lateral "winging") and there is deepening of the supraclavicular fossa. The shoulder may be painful when the limb is unsupported (106,107). Arm elevation is limited more with shoulder abduction than forward flexion. Electrodiagnostic studies may differentiate denervation from demyelination, the latter having a better prognosis (108,109).

Surgery for breast cancer has usually included axillary lymph node dissection, which predisposes the patient to subsequent lymphedema. During this procedure peripheral nerves including the axillary, pectoral, and long thoracic nerves may be damaged. Injury of the last nerve may present with medial scapular winging and greater difficulty forward flexing than abducting the arm at the shoulder. Pain may occur in the medial upper region of the arm, axilla, and lateral chest wall because of intercostobrachial nerve injury (110). Following radical or modified radical mastectomy, this pain can extend to the ipsilateral anterior chest wall due to injury of cutaneous branches of the region's intercostal nerves. If severe, postmastectomy pain syndrome may prove quite resistant to pain management.

Breast surgery for cancer may have a significant effect on sexuality and body image, especially in premenopausal women; this can be compounded by adjuvant treatment–induced premature menopause with vaginal atrophy and potential infertility (111). Total mastectomy may have a more profound psychosexual impact on body image and return to sexual activities than partial mastectomy and radiation therapy (112,113). Breast reconstruction following total mastectomy using implants or autogenous tissue may be elected to mitigate these negative psychosexual effects. The most commonly used autogenous tissue is the transverse rectus abdominis myocutaneous (TRAM) flap. Some patients following pedicled TRAM flap reconstruction demonstrate decreased abdominal strength (114). Patients generally return to their daily routine without difficulty, though they may encounter restrictions in more strenuous activities (115). Weakness is not as significant an issue when a free TRAM flap is used (116). Latissimus dorsi flap reconstruction may result in ipsilateral shoulder weakness and limited range of motion; use of a superior gluteal free flap may weaken hip abduction and use of an inferior gluteal free flap may weaken hip extension and external rotation (117).

Other reconstructive surgeries may also lead to functional deficits. Mandibular reconstruction may require a radial forearm fasciocutaneous free flap with bone, requiring a long arm cast postoperatively with a resultant impaired ability to perform activities of daily living (118). Weight bearing on full-thickness skin grafts involving the plantar aspect of the foot, as with melanoma resections, must initially be avoided. Reconstruction for soft-tissue sarcomas of the extremities using pedicled muscle flaps may result in further loss of function in an already impaired limb (119).

Patients after thoracotomy may experience temporary worsening of pulmonary symptoms. Postoperative pain and fluid accumulation may contribute. Worsening of a persistent postthoracotomy pain or recurrence of pain often signals the presence of underlying neoplasia. Subsequent diagnostic evaluation is mandatory (120). Patients who undergo resection for lung cancer may develop vocal cord paralysis due to recurrent laryngeal nerve injury, with resultant hoarseness and risk of aspiration (121–123).

Some degree of speech or swallowing dysfunction occurs in patients after head and neck surgery (121). Following total laryngectomy, loss of voice occurs after removal of the true vocal folds, whereas after supraglottic partial laryngectomy the true vocal folds are preserved and speech production is only mildly affected (122). A hemilaryngectomy involves the resection of one vertical half of the larynx including the ipsilateral true and false vocal folds; patients are able to produce a hoarse voice with the intact vocal fold against the reconstructed tissue (122). Following subtotal laryngectomy, most of the larynx is resected but low-pitched voice with pitch modulation may be achieved with the remaining arytenoid and vocal folds (124). Near-total laryngectomy involves resection of the larynx except for a narrow strip of tissue connecting the airway to the pharynx; the shunt that is formed allows vibration of the pharyngeal tissue for voice production (125,126).

Articulation deficits occur after base-of-tongue or floor-of-mouth resection, oral glossectomy, or mandibulectomy (127,128). If the oral glossectomy involves a total or a subtotal resection, the patient may not be able to articulate at all. Patients who have undergone maxillectomy and soft palate resection usually produce hypernasal speech; surgical flap reconstruction can minimize or eliminate the hypernasality (129).

Swallowing disorders may occur after oral cavity resection (122). Resection of the hard palate allows leakage into the maxillary sinus. Resection of the soft palate typically results in nasal regurgitation. After base-of-tongue resection, impaired propulsion of the bolus through the pharynx may occur (130). Supraglottic laryngectomy and hemilaryngectomy may increase the risk of aspiration (122). After total laryngectomy, reduced pharyngeal contraction, impaired esophageal peristalsis, and esophageal stricture may impair swallowing (130,131).

Regional pelvic adenectomy may predispose a

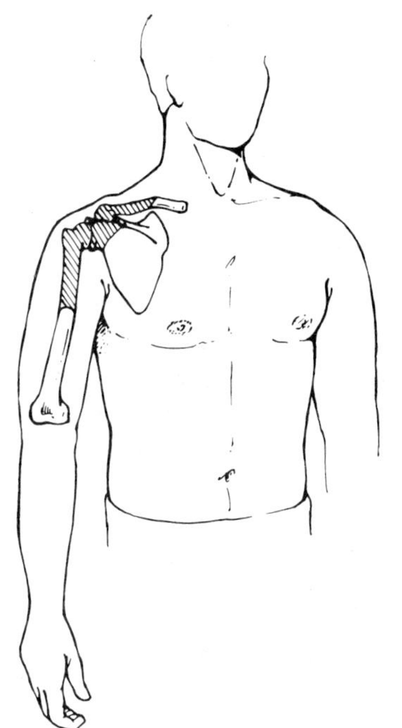

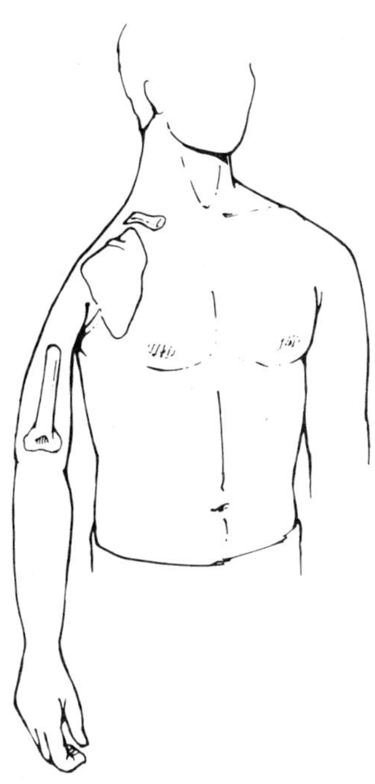

Figure 91-1. The Tikhoff-Linberg limb salvage procedure. The *shaded areas* in the *left diagram* represent the structures resected during the procedure, namely, the proximal end of the humerus, lateral end of the clavicle, and the lateral part of the scapula including the glenoid fossa. The *right diagram* demonstrates the altered contour of the shoulder when endoprosthetic reconstruction is not employed.

patient to lower-limb lymphedema. Radical prostatectomy may disrupt sexual function and produce loss of urinary continence, especially in those over age 70 (132,133). Peripheral nerves to the legs may be affected by pelvic surgery. Femoral nerve or lumbar plexus injury may result in knee extensor weakness. Patients will have difficulty walking up or down stairs and inclines. To compensate, patients may shorten the stride length on the affected side and move the center of gravity in front of the knee or push the knee into extension while bearing weight on that side (134). Other compensatory techniques include external rotation of the affected leg using the collateral ligaments to maintain knee extension and forcefully swinging the leg forward in a "goose step" fashion. Genu recurvatum may result from forceful knee hyperextension. Knee flexion contracture may develop owing to unopposed knee flexion (135). Electrodiagnostic studies may be helpful for prognosis.

Nerves may also be injured from patient positioning during surgical procedures (136). The two most commonly involved lower-limb nerves are the femoral and common peroneal nerves (137,138). Common peroneal compressive neuropathy is a frequent cause of footdrop, also seen with intermittent pneumatic compression devices and prolonged leg crossing, especially in conjunction with significant weight loss (139–141). Compensatory gait changes include a "steppage" gait, in which exaggerated hip and knee flexion allow foot clearance during the swing phase, and limb circumduction with hip hiking. Foot slap may be heard as the forefoot strikes the ground. Toe drag may predispose the patient to tripping and falling if the gait is not compensated. Weakness of ankle evertors may predispose the patient to inversion injuries of the ankle.

When tumor involves a limb, surgical limb salvage or amputation may be required. The goal of limb salvage procedures is to preserve the limb and its function without sacrificing effective cancer management (142). Soft-tissue sarcoma resections may result in minor functional deficits, but significant knee extensor weakness and resulting gait changes may occur after extensive quadriceps muscle resection. Primary bone tumors may require resection of bone and soft tissue. Bone may be replaced by an orthopedic endoprosthesis, or with bone allograft when large sections are to be replaced. Myodesis of the formerly attached limb musculature is important to maximize function. In the Tikhoff-Linberg and Girdlestone limb salvage procedures, the shoulder and hip joints, respectively, are removed (143). Distal limb function is preserved. In the former procedure, there is a flail shoulder (Fig. 91-1) but reconstruction using an endoprosthetic humerus and articulating custom-made scapula can allow very limited shoulder function (144). With the routine use of endoprosthetic arthroplasty, the Girdlestone procedure is rarely used as the procedure of choice. This procedure may be required should the proximal femoral endoprosthesis become involved with osteomyelitis (145). The patient will have difficulty regaining ambulation with a shortened limb.

When bone neoplasia affects the pelvis, internal hemipelvectomy may be used to salvage the lower limb. Enneking (146) described three main resections (Fig. 91-2). Type I internal hemipelvectomy involves resection of the ilium above the acetabulum. Maintaining or reconstructing the pelvic ring prevents limb shortening and gait impairment. Type II internal hemipelvectomy involves resection of the periacetabular region. To maintain limb length and functional gait, reconstruction may be accomplished with

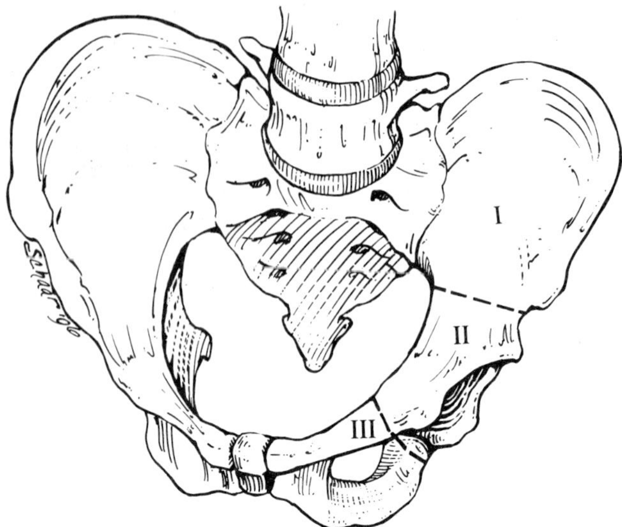

Figure 91-2. The three major types of internal hemipelvectomies: I—iliac; II—periacetabular; and III—ischiopubic. (Modified by permission from Enneking WF. *Musculoskeletal tumor surgery*. New York: Churchill Livingstone, 1983.)

arthrodesis or implantation of a prosthesis (147). Type III internal hemipelvectomy involves resection of the ischiopubic region, which in itself does not result in significant functional deficit, but with concurrent resection of the femoral neurovascular bundle, the femoral nerve is usually left unrepaired.

With the advent of limb salvage procedures, amputation has been less frequently employed in the treatment of limb tumors (142). Rehabilitation of the cancer amputee is similar to that for the nonmalignant amputee but consideration may be needed for concurrent sequelae. Two very uncommon amputations are sometimes selected for cancer patients. Scapulothoracic (forequarter) amputation involves resection of the limb and shoulder girdle (148). A major problem arises owing to loss of the normal shoulder contour. The modified Van Ness rotationplasty involves resection of the distal end of the femur and proximal end of the tibia. The distal limb is rotated 180 degrees and fused to the proximal end of the femur so the ankle may serve as a pseudoknee (149,150).

Surgical intervention for gynecologic cancers such as those of the vulva and cervix may have a profound impact on sexual function (151). Following ablative abdominal or pelvic procedures, disruption of the gastrointestinal or urinary tract may require creation of an artificial external opening. Cystectomy will require creation of a conduit, cutaneous ureterostomy or pyelostomy. With partial cystectomy, a vesicostomy can be performed (152). Colostomy, sometimes temporary, or ileostomy may be required, depending on the level and extent of bowel removed (153). With total pelvic exenteration or hemicorporectomy, urinary conduit and ileostomy are required.

Prolonged Immobilization and Deconditioning

The patient with cancer may be exposed to prolonged bed rest, owing to complications arising from the malignancy or treatment. Multiple organ system problems may arise related to prolonged immobilization (see Chap. 46). Generalized weakness, decreased endurance, and joint contractures may become apparent after short periods of immobility. Osteopenia and hypercalcemia resulting from immobility may compound problems with bone metastases. Orthostatic hypotension and decreased sitting tolerance from prolonged recumbency may further complicate any adverse effects of anemia or autonomic impairment. Decreased gastrointestinal mobility with bed rest can lead to significant constipation, which can be worsened with opioids. Venous stasis caused by prolonged immobility predisposes the patient to DVT. Other contributing factors for DVT include a hypercoagulable paraneoplastic state and limb paresis (51). Timely diagnosis is important to prevent life-threatening pulmonary embolism (154). Prevention is preferred to treatment once DVT occurs. In patients who have developed DVT and cannot be anticoagulated, an inferior vena cava filter may be used, but its use does not guarantee prevention of pulmonary embolism (155).

REHABILITATIVE INTERVENTIONS

Many of the rehabilitative interventions employed for patients with cancer are similar to those used in treating patients with other diagnoses. Some of the interventions are of particular importance to the cancer population.

Weakness and Decreased Endurance

Weakness and decreased endurance are common impairments seen in patients with a malignancy. An appropriate exercise program may prevent deconditioning in the room-isolated patient, and may retard skeletal muscle atrophy in those receiving glucocorticoid treatment (156). Modification of a proposed exercise program may be necessary in patients with significant thrombocytopenia, metastatic bone disease or impending fracture, significant cardiac or pulmonary impairment, or limb swelling. For spasticity, oral antispasticity agents may be helpful in management, but long-term intrathecal agents such as baclofen are usually not considered in those with metastatic disease to the spine because of their poor prognosis.

Several studies suggested an inverse relationship between history of exercise and incidence of certain cancers, including those of the colon, breast, prostate, testicle, and kidney (157–163). Others reported an enhanced immunologic response to exercise (164,165). Submaximal exercise has the potential of exerting an anabolic effect in the prevention of cancer cachexia (166). Fatigue in cancer patients is often multifactorial, and exercise may be an effective strategy against fatigue (167). The psychological benefits of exercise are also well documented (168,169).

Exercise may help mitigate the weight gain often seen in breast cancer patients during adjuvant chemotherapy (170). Aerobic exercise programs have included use of a cycle ergometer or walking. Some suggest caution when the patient, especially with a history of coronary artery disease, is severely anemic, or the patient has a platelet count less than 50,000/µL; this latter concern is certainly controversial (171,172).

Rehabilitation of Limb Impairments

Spinal accessory nerve palsy after neck dissection typically causes weakness of the ipsilateral trapezius muscle. Recovery time, even after traction injuries, may be quite prolonged or never occur if denervation has occurred (173). Even if the muscle is partially innervated, exercise and electrical stimulation may help to increase trapezius strength (174). Strengthening other shoulder girdle muscles may compensate in part for trapezius weakness (106,107). However, the upper trapezius remains the only muscle capable of elevating the tip of the shoulder. It is important to maintain full range of motion and prevent muscle shortening of the trapezius antagonists. Since shoulder pain usually arises when the shoulder is unsupported, limb positioning is important (174). A figure-eight harness or shoulder-elevating orthosis may therefore decrease pain and increase function (175). Glenohumeral range of motion must be maintained to prevent adhesive capsulitis (176).

Rehabilitation following orthopedic reconstruction may be complicated by other problems arising from the cancer itself or its treatment. After limb salvage procedures, functional recovery depends on the remaining musculature and its secure myodesis in a functional position. Terminal overgrowth of bone can penetrate the skin in pediatric patients, requiring surgical resection (177). In upper-limb amputees, the length of the residual limb tends to be directly related to the amount of functional recovery (178). Following scapulothoracic or forequarter amputation, patients are fitted with a simple shoulder filler prior to hospital discharge. This helps restore the shoulder contour, allowing regular clothes to be worn. A custom shoulder prosthesis is fabricated later, with or without a cosmetic arm (Fig. 91-3). A prosthesis with a functional mechanical or myoelectric arm is often heavy and impractical in these patients.

Specialized proximal lower-limb amputations may be performed in cancer patients. These patients tend to be younger and often healthier than are dysvascular patients. The Van Ness rotationplasty requires a unique type of prosthesis (149,150). The socket must accommodate the backward-turned foot, much as a below-knee prosthesis accommodates the residual foreleg (Fig. 91-4). The prosthesis must also provide mediolateral stability at the ankle, now functioning as a pseudoknee. This prosthesis gives a function equivalent to that of endoprosthetic replacement and is superior to the function of an above-knee residual limb with a prosthesis (179).

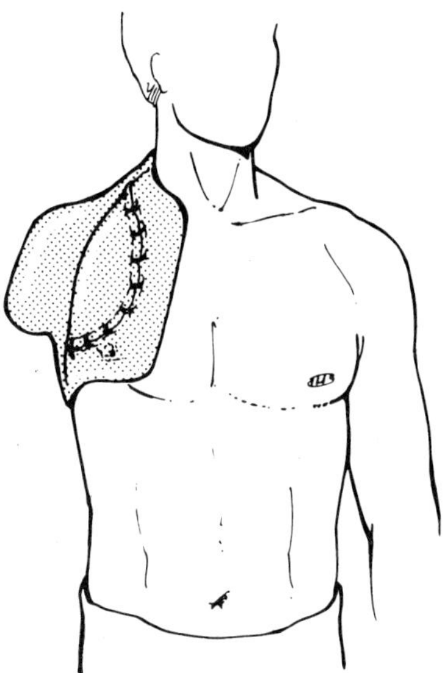

Figure 91-3. Illustration of a custom shoulder prosthesis without a cosmetic arm, restoring shoulder contour following a forequarter amputation.

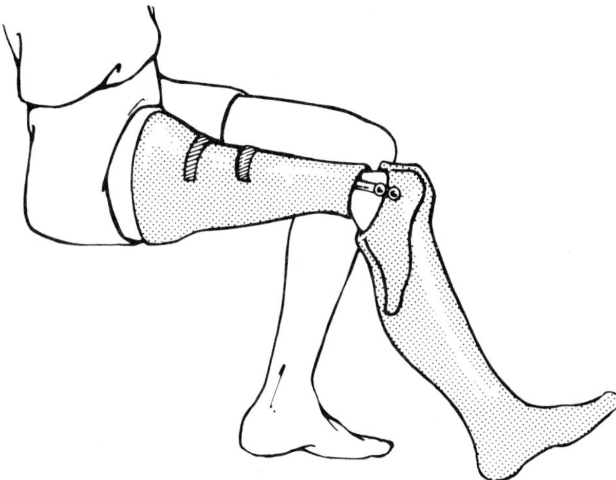

Figure 91-4. Illustration of a prosthesis being worn following a Van Ness rotationplasty. The rotated ankle joint serves as a pseudoknee.

Knee extensor weakness is often adequately compensated for without the use of an orthosis, especially when this is the only gait impairment. A locking-knee extension orthosis may be considered in patients with other gait deficits, patients with general debility, or those who walk on rough, uneven surfaces. The leg must be circumducted or the hip hiked to permit limb advancement. Knee extension also may be enhanced with the use of an ankle-foot orthosis in slight plantarflexion (135,180).

For the patient with significantly weak ankle dorsiflexion, an appropriate ankle-foot orthosis allows proper foot clearance during the swing phase of gait. For the patient with isolated dorsiflexion weakness without increased tone, a posterior leaf spring orthosis may be sufficient. With accompanying weakness of ankle eversion, a more rigid ankle-foot orthosis will provide greater ankle stability. An ankle-foot orthosis with an articulated ankle may be preferred when functional plantarflexion exists and mediolateral ankle stabilization is needed. If all ankle movements are significantly weak, a solid ankle-foot orthosis may be the best option.

Ataxia

Cerebellar ataxia is often resistant to rehabilitative intervention. Weights attached to the limb or the use of weighted utensils or a weighted walker may help by decreasing the amplitude of the tremor (181). Sensory ataxia can lead to functional problems, especially of gait. Assistive devices for gait may provide proprioceptive feedback through the upper limbs and widen the base of support. Safety precautions to help minimize the risk of falls include emphasis on visual feedback, adequate lighting, bathroom adaptations, and unobstructed walking areas (182).

Joint Contracture

The prevention of contracture is easier than treatment once contracture has occurred. Decreased shoulder range of motion can easily become a complication following axillary lymph node dissection, as in the treatment of breast cancer. In addition to restricted activities of daily living, adhesive capsulitis may impede positioning for breast irradiation, owing to limited shoulder abduction (183). Although all agree that therapeutic exercise will usually prevent adhesive capsulitis, there are conflicting reports on functional outcome when comparing an immediate versus a delayed program exercise (184–187). From a practical point of view, most use immediate shoulder mobilization because of today's short postoperative hospital stays (188). Ankle plantarflexion contracture may develop secondary to neurotoxicity from chemotherapeutic agents, especially in bedridden patients. The use of foot-positioning devices and early weight bearing may prevent this.

Metastatic Bone Disease

Activity modification may be necessary in the presence of bone metastases. Restriction of weight bearing through the affected limb may be required in the setting of impending or pathologic fracture. Bunting et al (189) found that those at higher risk of pathologic fracture are younger, have advanced disease, are female, and have lytic bone disease and a history of pathologic fracture. Radiation therapy for bone metastasis may decrease pain but also decrease bone strength (190,191). If weight-bearing restrictions are required in a lower limb, increased mechanical stress results in the contralateral lower limb. This may be problematic if there is bone neoplasia in that contralateral limb. Similarly, use of an assistive gait device requires weight bearing through one or both upper limbs. There may be cause for concern if metastatic disease to bone is present in the weight-bearing upper limb; modification of activities of daily living may be required. The incidence of pathologic fracture in patients being mobilized is relatively low (189). Cancer patients treated in a rehabilitation hospital for pathologic long-bone fractures require only slightly longer stays than do those with nonpathologic fractures, but hypercalcemia and the need for parenteral narcotics portend a poor rehabilitation outcome (192).

Many patients with spinal metastases are managed nonoperatively. Incident pain with spinal movement may be decreased by the patient's employing proper posture and body mechanics or with the use of a spinal orthosis. Patients are encouraged to avoid forward flexion and rotation to minimize stress on the anterior weight-bearing portion of the spine. Spinal orthoses may be required to prevent mechanically stressful spinal movement and provide added support. The location and extent of spinal metastases will determine the type of bracing that is appropriate. Ideally, the brace should extend several segments above and below the level to be supported. For example, painful metastatic bone lesions that involve the uppermost thoracic region of the spine may require a cervicothoracolumbosacral orthosis (CTLSO) (193). A custom-made bivalved body jacket with attached sterno-occipitomandibular immobilizer (SOMI) may provide adequate support. In the patient with multilevel thoracolumbar spinal disease who is asymptomatic but at risk for spinal compression deformities, a cruciform anterior-spine hyperextension (CASH) or Jewett hyperextension brace that prevents thoracolumbar flexion may be helpful. In patients needing prolonged immobilization of the cervical region, a thermoplastic Minerva body jacket [cervicothoracic orthosis (CTO)] may be considered instead of a halo vest (194).

When prescribing spinal orthoses, one must consider the presence of ostomies or postsurgical drains. This may require fabricating custom braces to allow openings for these sites. In patients with pulmonary compromise, restriction of abdominal movement may in turn impede diaphragmatic excursion, which may not be tolerated. A kyphus deformity, or any bony prominence may require a relief over or padding around that area to prevent skin irritation and breakdown.

Pulmonary Rehabilitation

Chest physical therapy can be very important in patients with restrictive lung disease, such as with pulmonary fibrosis. Preventing pooling of secretions may reduce the risk of pneumonia. Chest percussion or even vibration should be used cautiously and may be contraindicated in patients with known lytic lesions or pathologic fractures of the ribs. Caution regarding certain types of positioning should also be employed when using postural drainage for patients with spinal metastases. Increased stresses are applied to certain regions of the spine with these positions, which may increase the risk of pathologic compression fracture. Provocation of postresection incisional pain by coughing or other sudden movements can be minimized by splinting the chest or abdomen. Patients with cancer may also benefit from energy conservation techniques, including adequate periods of rest, use of proper posture and body mechanics, use of adaptive equipment such as a raised commode, and home modifications to increase energy efficiency (195).

Bowel, Bladder, and Ostomy Management

Bowel and bladder dysfunctions are usually approached and treated in a manner similar to those without cancer. A problem more specific to patients with cancer is the stoma and its care. With urostomy, a pouch for collection of urine is necessary. Most patients will resume a normal diet but may need acidification of the urine to decrease bacteremia (152,196). Patients receiving methotrexate cannot take urine acidification medication as this may provoke crystallization of the agent in the kidneys. Tight clothing may interfere with emptying of urine and should be avoided. Most patients may resume normal physical activity by 2 months following surgery. The aim of colostomy management is the production of a predictable daily evacuation through the manipulation of fluid and food intake as well as medication usage (197). A pouch is usually worn to prevent soiling. Colostomy irrigation may be used to control evacuation; by reducing odor and soiling, the stoma may require only a protective covering. Dietary monitoring is less important, but irrigation requires significant time and carries the added risk of colonic perforation (198). Special problems in the cancer population with stomas include chemotherapy producing constipation or diarrhea, mucosal ulceration, or stomal hemorrhage with thrombocytopenia. Radiation therapy may cause stomal ischemia, ulceration, atrophy, or thickening (196).

Speech and Language Rehabilitation

Patients who undergo total laryngectomy are offered one or more of the three alaryngeal speech methods. The battery-operated electrolarynx produces a vibratory tone transmitted into the oral cavity via the neck or an oral tube that has been placed. The tone is modulated into speech by moving the lips and tongue for articulation (121,199). This method is typically the first that is taught. Esophageal speech entails the intake of air through the mouth or nose into the esophagus. As a result of pressure changes, the esophageal walls vibrate to produce a voice (121,200). This method of speech typically takes 3 to 12 months to acquire. Tracheoesophageal puncture (TEP) is a surgically produced fistula between the trachea and esophagus, allowing pulmonary air to pass into the esophagus. With a TEP, the individual manually occludes the tracheostoma to divert the exhaled pulmonary air through the TEP into the esophagus during speech. The patient is fitted with a small voice prosthesis within the TEP tract

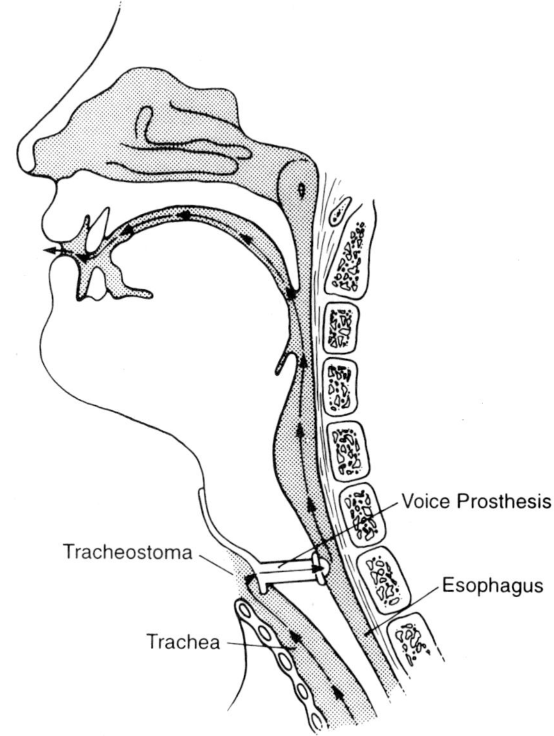

Figure 91-5. Diagram of a laryngectomized patient with a tracheoesophageal puncture and a voice prosthesis in place. The *arrows* represent the flow of air through the prosthesis when the tracheostoma is occluded. Air is directed into the esophagus and then the oral cavity.

that has a one-way valve to prevent aspiration and allow voicing (201–203) (Fig. 91-5). Tracheostoma breathing valves worn externally have been developed to enable hand-free tracheostoma occlusion during speech (204,205). Speech via the TEP is obtained almost immediately after placement of the voice prosthesis and may improve with speech therapy (202,205,206).

Speech therapy for patients with articulation deficits following head and neck surgery includes oral exercises to increase the range of motion and strength of the involved musculature. Specific problematic speech sounds are targeted. Patients who undergo glossectomy resecting 50% or more of the oral tongue may be candidates for a palatal augmentation (maxillary reshaping) prosthesis, which recontours and lowers the palatal vault to increase lingual-palatal contact (207,208) (Fig. 91-6). Patients often require speech therapy to improve articulation with the prosthesis in place. Patients who undergo soft palate resection or maxillectomy may benefit from a palatal obturator that extends into the defect (Fig. 91-7). Sometimes a prosthesis is not warranted following soft palate resection, owing to effective surgical reconstruction with a free flap to close a large defect.

Patients with dysphonia following hemilaryngectomy or unilateral vocal cord paralysis may benefit from voice

Figure 91-6. Palatal augmentation prosthesis. *A.* Open-mouth view of a patient following partial oral glossectomy. *B.* Custom-made palatal augmentation prosthesis. *C.* Patient with the appliance in place, allowing lingual contact with the prosthetic palate. (Courtesy of Ian Zlotolow, DMD, Chief of the Dental Service, Memorial Sloan-Kettering Cancer Center, New York.)

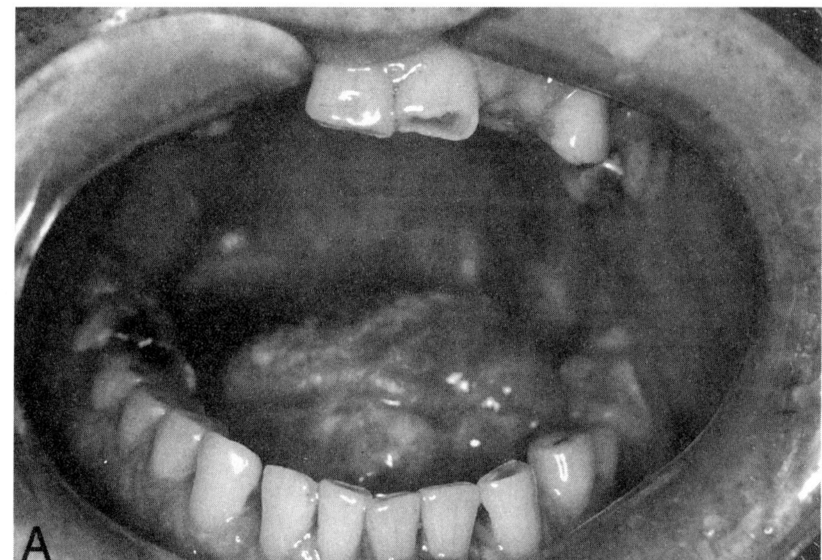

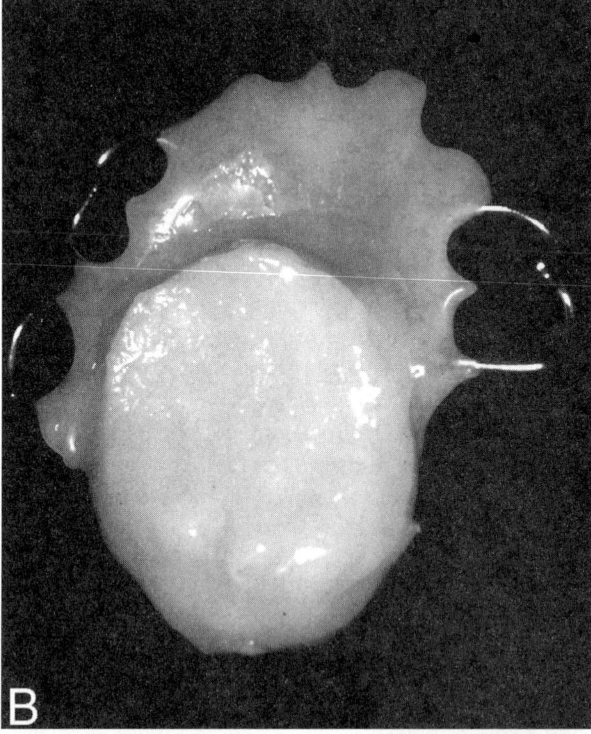

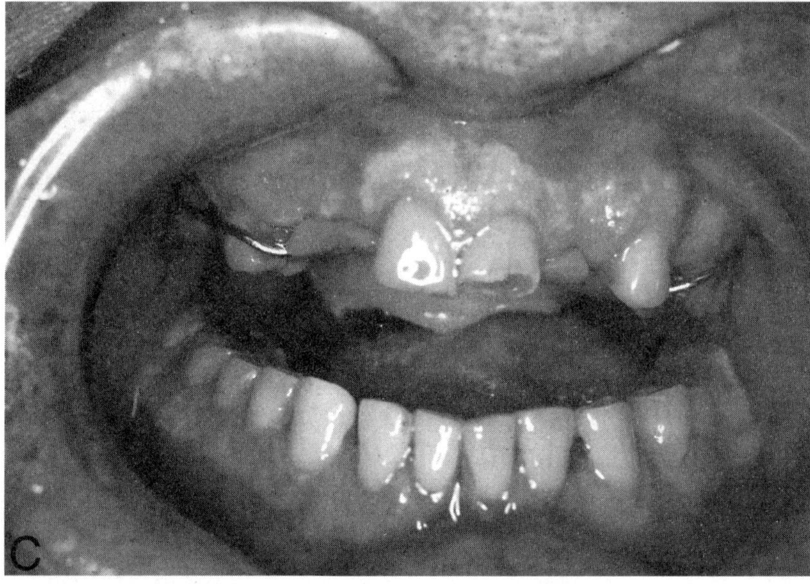

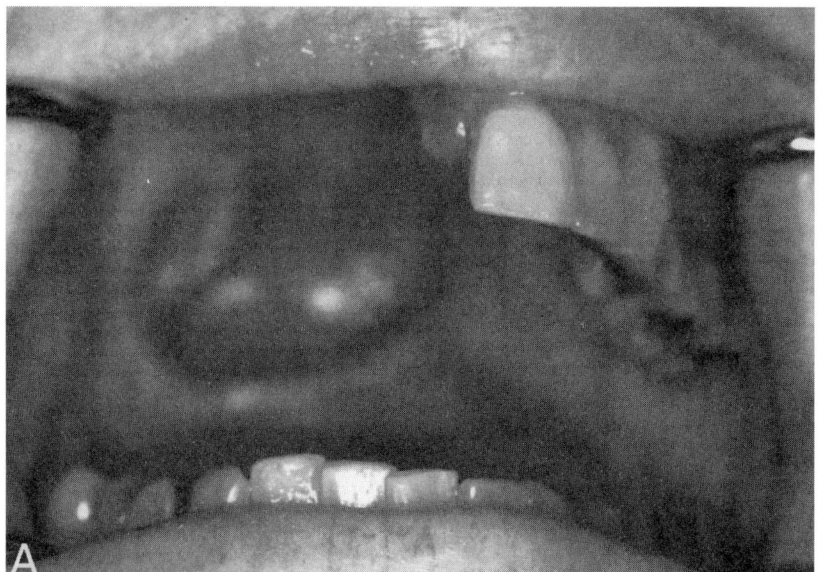

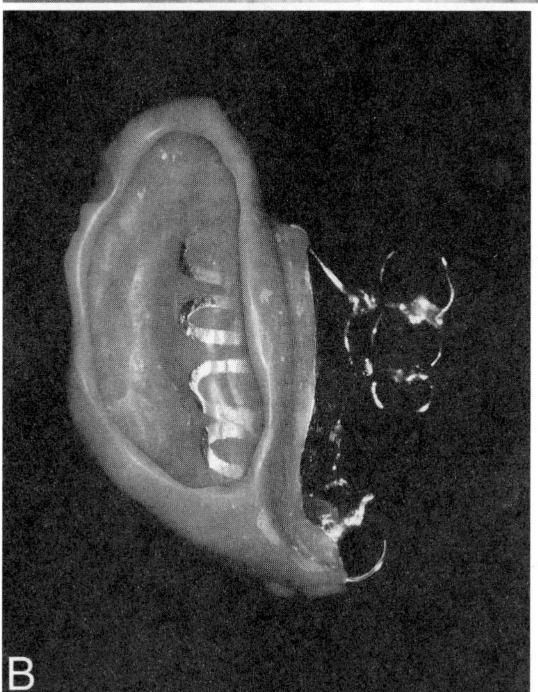

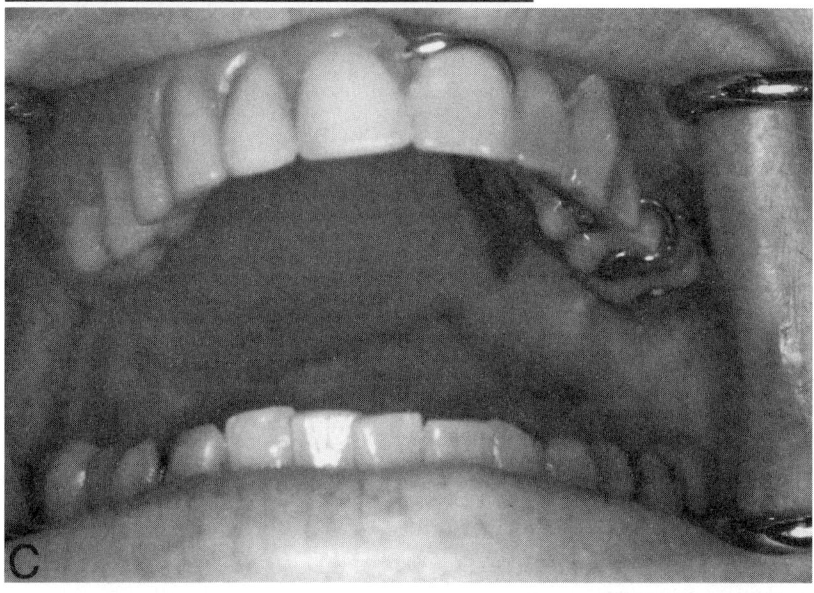

Figure 91-7. Palatal obturator. *A.* Open-mouth view of a patient following partial maxillectomy. *B.* Custom-made hard palate obturator. *C.* Patient with the prosthesis in place, filling the defect in the hard palate. (Courtesy of Ian Zlotolow, DMD, Chief of the Dental Service, Memorial Sloan-Kettering Cancer Center, New York.)

therapy involving vocal cord adduction exercises to improve approximation of the intact vocal cord to the opposing tissue or paralyzed vocal cord (121). Because these patients frequently develop maladaptive compensatory behaviors that result in increased vocal strain and hoarseness, approaches that aim to reduce laryngeal tension may be more successful (123). Some patients may also be advised to use a voice amplifier to increase vocal loudness. In patients with unilateral vocal cord paralysis, vocal cord medialization may be performed to improve vocal cord approximation (209,210).

A tracheostomy speaking valve attaches to the hub of the tracheostomy tube, allowing inhalation of air via the tube. With exhalation, the one-way valve closes and the air is redirected to the upper airway and through the vocal folds to produce voice. This may serve as an intermediate step prior to capping the tracheostomy tube. These valves enable the patient to occlude the tracheostomy tube without the use of the hands, and help reduce secretions and facilitate coughing and expectoration (211,212).

Following significant resections, such as total glossectomy with total laryngectomy, an augmentative communication system may be most appropriate. Depending on the patient's resources and communicative needs, an appropriate system could be as simple as a notebook or as sophisticated as a laptop computer with speech output (213–215).

Speech and language therapy for patients with brain tumors follows the same approach used with aphasic and dysarthric patients following stroke. Gestural and augmentative communication systems may be appropriate for the severely impaired (216–219). The palatal lift prosthesis is sometimes helpful in improving resonance for dysarthric patients with impaired velopharyngeal competence (213,218). In the pediatric cancer population, speech and language treatment approaches are as varied as in noncancer patients. The challenge is to provide regular and frequent speech therapy sessions. More often than not, children with cancer are too ill or busy with cancer treatment schedules to attend therapy regularly while they are hospitalized. Delivery of outpatient services may be more successful.

Swallowing Rehabilitation

Swallowing therapy is directed at specific deficits and the effectiveness of therapeutic techniques may be further assessed during the radiographic evaluation (see Chap. 14). Indirect swallowing techniques include compensatory maneuvers or activities that modify head or body posture or the manner of oral intake. The chin-down posture assists in reducing aspiration caused by delayed pharyngeal swallow. Turning the head to the side with pharyngeal weakness directs the bolus toward the stronger side (130,220–222). Sitting upright at 90 degrees reduces the risk of aspiration. Oral intake may be modified by presenting liquids with a spoon, using multiple swallows per bolus, decreasing bolus size, and decreasing the rate of intake (223,224). Direct techniques require specific instructions to and practice by the patient (130,225–230). The supraglottic swallow is taught to patients who exhibit reduced airway closure during swallowing. The breath is held before and during the swallow, closing the airway at the vocal folds. This is followed by a cough that clears the pharynx and laryngeal vestibule after the swallow. The super supraglottic swallow achieves airway closure at the level of the entrance to the laryngeal vestibule. Patients "bear down" while holding the breath and swallowing. The Mendelsohn maneuver helps maintain the larynx at its height during a swallow for several seconds in those with reduced laryngeal elevation. Patients with delayed or absent pharyngeal swallow may benefit from thermal stimulation performed regularly. Dysphagia due to reduced tongue base retraction is sometimes improved by the use of the effortful swallow technique, which involves "squeezing" the oral and pharyngeal musculature during the swallow. Vocal cord adduction exercises help with unilateral vocal cord paralysis.

Postirradiation xerostomia may further complicate dysphagia. Effective relief has been difficult to achieve, although some patients report partial benefit from the artificial saliva substitutes (89,90,231). In addition, a simple oral spray with plain water has been found to be helpful for many patients (89). Recent studies demonstrated the partial effectiveness of pilocarpine in relieving dryness (89,231,232).

Prosthodontic appliances may diminish dysphagia resulting from extensive oral cavity defects. A palatal augmentation prosthesis following partial or total glossectomy assists in achieving contact of the tongue to the hard palate for adequate oral preparation and improved transport of the bolus with decreased aspiration (207). Patients with surgical defects in the hard palate generally regain swallowing function with a palatal obturator (233). Improvement in swallowing function with prosthetic management of soft palate resections has been variable, depending on the size and location of the deficit (131,234).

Swallowing and feeding problems in infants and children typically are managed with therapy to increase oral motor and sensory functions. Behavior management, manipulation of environmental factors, and postural support are also utilized. Nonfood activities are introduced to develop oral motor function and reflexes prior to feeding situations (10,235,236).

Deep Vein Thrombosis

In patients with (DVT), there has been a concern about embolization caused by ambulation (237). Some recommended waiting as long as 7 days after anticoagulation therapy is started before initiating ambulation (238). Others suggest waiting until leg pain and swelling resolve, usually after 3 to 4 days of anticoagulation treatment (239). Hull et al (240) allowed patients to "move around as they wished" once they were anticoagulated with intravenous heparin. In a group of 199 subjects, only 1 was found to have developed pulmonary embolism, which occurred 17 days after starting anticoagulation (240).

Lymphedema

Lymphedema may arise in the patient with cancer following en bloc resection, neoplastic invasion, or irradiation of the lymph nodes draining the limb (241). Following surgery or irradiation, swelling may be acute and transient, or can become chronic, beginning months or years later (242,243). Once established, untreated chronic lymphedema gradually increases over time (244). Initially, lymphedema is pitting but may become brawny in nature. Generalized, achy pain associated with swelling is secondary to stretching of soft tissues (245). With severe lymphedema, limb function may become impaired because of increased weight and girth, and skin changes may occur. The skin may become hyperkeratotic, and vesicular and verrucous changes may produce elephantiasis (246). Rarely, lymphangiosarcoma (Stewart-Treves syndrome), which has a poor prognosis, occurs (247).

Several guidelines may be helpful in preventing the onset or exacerbation of lymphedema (241,248,249). Patients should avoid prolonged limb dependency, though this may only be helpful with soft, pitting edema (250). Moderate to heavy or sustained exercise or activity of the limb may initiate or increase swelling by increasing interstitial fluid production in response to muscle fatigue. Tight clothing or jewelry and blood pressure cuffs should not be applied to the limb, since these can cause a tourniquet-like effect, promoting local fluid collection. Trauma or burns of the affected limb may result in swelling from inflammation. The inflammation of greatest concern is infection, especially cellulitis and lymphangiitis; in such a case, appropriate antibiotic therapy should be administered promptly (251). For example, dicloxacillin or cephalexin at 500 mg may be given orally every 6 hours for 2 weeks in the absence of signs of systemic infection and when not otherwise contraindicated. For severe or systemic infection, intravenous antibiotics may be necessary. Patients with a history of infection have a risk of repeat infection that is greater than the risk of initial infection in those without such a history (252). Skin integrity must be maintained. Skin insults as minor as a fungal infection, a paper cut, or an insect bite may provide a portal of entry for gram-positive cocci, which can flourish in the lymphedematous fluids. Patients are encouraged to use skin moisturizers, since small cracks in dry skin may allow infection. Similarly, needle puncture should be avoided and cuticles should remain uncut on the affected limb. Heat and humidity as well as decreased atmospheric pressure (e.g., airplane travel) may also increase local lymph fluid production and thus provoke or promote lymphedema.

Several modalities are available for the treatment of lymphedema. Limb elevation and mild activity may be helpful (250). Static compression devices are used in most patients. They may help discourage local interstitial fluid production and may enhance the "muscle pump" effect in both venous and lymphatic vessels. Gradient pressure garments are most commonly employed; the pressure is greater distally than proximally. Upper-limb garments may require a hand piece if hand edema is present or if the use of a sleeve extending down to the wrist provokes hand or digital swelling (253). When possible, off-the-shelf garments are used instead of custom-made ones. In general, these garments lose their elasticity and therefore their function after several months. Bandaging is another way to apply static compression. Bandages are more time-consuming to apply than a gradient pressure garment and may require assistance for application. The materials used have little compliance compared to the gradient pressure garment and may better enhance the "muscle pumping" effect. An advantage of bandaging is the ability to conform to the changing shape of the limb with lymphedema (254). Lower-limb lymphedema may also benefit from use of a legging orthosis fabricated from a series of Velcro straps that extend up to the knee (255). It is easily adjusted while worn.

Dynamic compression may be applied to the limb using pneumatic pumping; its use is controversial. Intermittent pneumatic compression pumps were originally designed with a single chamber within the plastic sleeve applied to the affected limb. Various degrees of success in limb reduction have been reported (242,253,256–259). Subsequently, sleeves with multiple chambers were designed to sequentially compress the length of the limb in a distal to proximal direction, again with some reported success (249,260–263). A further modification is the gradient sequential pump, which applies more pressure distally than proximally while sequentially pumping the limb (264–266). Patients may undergo a trial using more than one pump to find which one is most effective in reducing edema and is most comfortable to use. A pump may be provided for home use. (Static compression garments are worn during the day, in between pumping sessions.) The optimal pump pressure is controversial, and some suggest that pressures exceeding 60 mm Hg may have a deleterious effect on lymphatic vessels (267). The optimal pump time is controversial. Many lymphedema specialists believe that the use of pneumatic pumping is at best controversial, and in the long run may be detrimental.

Medical massage treatments theoretically mobilize interstitial fluids, facilitating their uptake into lymphatic channels and their subsequent return to the bloodstream. Several forms of specialized massage have been practiced for many years in Europe and are referred to as *manual lymphedema treatment* (MLT) (268). Treatments often begin on the torso, theoretically encouraging lymphatic flow across the trunk via collateral lymph channels toward areas with undisturbed lymphatic drainage (269). In theory, deformation of subcutaneous tissue opens up terminal lymphangioles, allowing an inflow of interstitial fluid. This also may stimulate peristalsis in lymphatic channels. Treatments are best given on a daily or twice-daily basis, and are usually done for a minimum of 2 to 4 weeks or longer. Bandaging is applied to the limb in between treatment sessions and appropriate nonfatiguing therapeutic exercise is taught. Following these intensive treatments, the patient is instructed in a maintenance home program. This includes use of gradient pressure garments, limb bandaging at night, continued exercise, and sometimes self-massage. The benefits of this treatment can be significant and last for months or longer, potentially with further improvement over time (254,269).

Relative contraindications for the above physical treatments have been suggested. These include congestive heart failure, active malignancy, acute DVT, severe thrombocytopenia, and treatment over irradiated or inflamed tissues (268).

Benzopyrones have been used outside of the United States as a pharmacologic means to treat lymphedema. These medications were felt to promote macrophage aggregation and proteolysis (270). Presumably, this allowed smaller amino acids and polypeptides to reenter capillary walls to be removed by venous return, thus reducing interstitial oncotic pressure. Decreased edema and reduced incidence of infection had been reported (271). Edema reduction apparently required months of continuous treatment. A recent study has suggested that the benzopyrone, coumarin, was ineffective in treating lymphedema following treatment for breast cancer, and evidence of liver toxicity was seen in 6% of women in the study (272).

Some patients report exacerbation of edema with significantly increased salt or alcohol intake. Though advocated by some clinicians, diuretics have little effect in reducing chronic lymphedema (249,273). Re-establishing lymphatic drainage has been attempted by various surgical interventions (274–278). Suction curettage has been used to treat severe lymphedema (279,280).

Pain

When evaluating pain in the patient with a known history of cancer, the clinician should keep in mind that recurrence of malignancy may be its source. Such pain may be somatic or visceral nociceptive, neuropathic, or from deafferentation. For example, postthoracotomy pain syndrome with a recurrence or exacerbation of pain often arises because of neoplasia (120). The pain may be from somatic or visceral nociceptors or direct nerve injury. Even recurrence of a patient's chronic, intermittent back pain may represent a new malignancy. Pain may also arise from treatments for malignancy. Examples are the somatic shoulder pain following ipsilateral neck dissection and neuropathic postmastectomy pain syndrome (106,107,110).

The foundation for pharmacologic management of cancer pain is a stepwise approach using nonopioid, narcotic, and adjuvant analgesia, as illustrated by the World Health Organization analgesic ladder for the management of cancer pain (Fig. 91-8) (281). Nonopioid analgesics such as acetaminophen and nonsteroidal anti-inflammatory drugs (NSAIDs) may be prescribed initially. NSAIDs have several well-known adverse effects, potentially limiting their use for chronic pain. Of particular concern in cancer patients is the contraindication of NSAIDs in the setting of coagulopathy, such as in those receiving chemotherapy and developing thrombocytopenia. Although NSAIDs are usually prescribed in oral form, ketorolac is available in a parenteral form in the United States for short-term use (282). For mild to moderate pain, narcotics such as hydrocodone, codeine, and oxycodone may be required in addition to or instead of nonopioids. When provided in combination form with nonopioids, daily dosages of these narcotics may be limited by the maximum daily dose of the nonopioid, usually acetaminophen. Propoxyphene and meperidine have toxic metabolites, and especially the latter is typically contraindicated for chronic use, especially at higher doses (283).

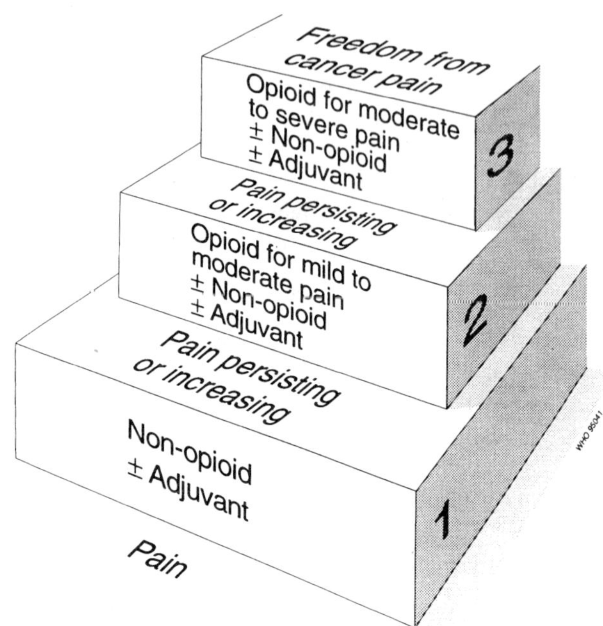

Figure 91-8. The World Health Organization three-step analgesic ladder for the management of cancer pain. (Reproduced by permission from World Health Organization. *Cancer pain relief.* 2nd ed. Geneva: World Health Organization, 1996:15.)

Various adjuvant analgesics may be added to improve analgesia when they are not contraindicated (284). Antidepressant medications have been useful for a number of chronic pain syndromes (285). They may be the first adjuvant tried in patients with neuropathic pain causing continuous dysesthesias. Amitriptyline is the best documented of the tricyclic antidepressants (TCAs). A secondary amine TCA (e.g., desipramine) may be tried to decrease anticholinergic effects. TCAs are often begun at very low bedtime doses and then the doses are incrementally increased, at times to antidepressant levels. Monoamine oxidase inhibitors (e.g., phenelzine) may have an analgesic effect but are contraindicated during simultaneous use of many other medications. The serotonin-selective reuptake inhibitor paroxetine has also been used as an adjuvant analgesic (286). Anticonvulsant medications have been used for various neuropathic pain syndromes, especially those with a sharp, lancinating quality. Carbamazepine had been used frequently. More recently, gabapentin has been employed increasingly for a diversity of neuropathic pain syndromes. Baclofen has also been reported to be helpful for lancinating pains (284). Topical agents including capsaicin, which reduces concentration of the nociceptive neurotransmitter substance P, and eutectic mixture of local anesthetics may also be used for local neuropathic pain (287,288). Oral and parenteral local anesthetics, corticosteroids, α_2-adrenergic agonists (e.g., clonidine), and neuroleptics (e.g., methotrimeprazine) have been used for a variety of cancer-related pain syndromes (289–292). Calcitonin, phenoxybenzamine, guanethidine, gabapentin, and other medications have been reported to be useful in some patients with reflex sympathetic dystrophy (284,293,294). Adjuvant pharmacologic therapy may be beneficial in the treatment of bone pain. Corticosteroids and NSAIDs may help by prostaglandin inhibition (295). Inhibitors of bone resorption such as calcitonin and bisphosphonates (e.g., pamidronate) have been useful adjuvants (296–298). Radionuclides such as strontium-89 may also decrease bone pain, but may be contraindicated because of bone marrow toxicity (299). All medications introduced for the treatment of pain must be monitored carefully.

Management of moderate to severe pain usually requires the use of narcotics. Short-acting opioids include morphine, oxycodone, hydromorphone, oxymorphone, and fentanyl (injectable). With moderate to severe cancer pain, a regular dosage schedule is preferred to taking narcotics on an "as needed" basis. Levorphanol and methadone have relatively long half-lives but usually require multiple daily doses for adequate analgesia. Long-term analgesia may be better accomplished by use of relatively long-acting opioid preparations such as controlled-release morphine, controlled-release oxycodone, or fentanyl patch (300,301). Along with these, as-needed "rescue doses" of shorter-acting opioids may be necessary for breakthrough pain. In addition to oral and transdermal delivery, portable infusion pumps allow outpatient subcutaneous and intravenous continuous basal narcotic delivery in combination with as-needed patient-controlled analgesia (PCA) for breakthrough pain (302). With continued narcotic use, increasing the dosage may be required to maintain adequate analgesia as tolerance develops.

Adequate management of the adverse effects arising from opioid use is necessary. Constipation is probably the most common side effect, especially in the older, debilitated patient with poor fluid intake. Treatment includes increasing mobility, modifying the diet, and using stool softeners and laxatives. Urinary retention is another potential adverse effect because of increased smooth muscle tone, especially in the elderly (303). Opioid-induced nausea and vomiting often resolve with continued treatment. Nonetheless, pharmacologic intervention may be needed to inhibit the brain stem chemoreceptor trigger zone with antidopaminergic agents (e.g., prochlorperazine), enhance gastric emptying with metoclopramide or cisapride, or treat the vestibular system with antivertiginous agents (e.g., meclizine) (303,304). As with nausea, tolerance to opioid-related somnolence and confusion usually develops, but may require the use of a psychostimulant such as methylphenidate or pemoline. Multifocal myoclonus is problematic in a minority of patients but may require clonazepam for treatment (305). For nausea, somnolence, pruritis, or myoclonus arising from opioid use, changing to a different narcotic may be an effective treatment. Medication delivered epidurally or intrathecally by infusion pump can also mitigate many adverse effects. Fortunately, both respiratory depression related to chronic opioid use and psychological addiction to narcotics when used for pain treatment are uncommon (306–309).

Regardless of the mode of delivery, when narcotic and adjuvant analgesia is inadequate, more invasive management may be required. For instance, nerve blocks may be of benefit for severe visceral, neuropathic, and complex regional pain syndromes. Neurosurgical interventions may be used to anatomically ablate a pain pathway or to implant epidural or peripheral nerve stimulators (310).

Myogenic pain is often overlooked and underdiagnosed in the patient with cancer (311). Therapeutic intervention is essentially the same as it is in the noncancer patient. Appropriate therapy would be one or more techniques to release spasm or tender or trigger points and the use of physical modalities and therapeutic exercises to recondition involved muscles (312,313). Several modalities including superficial heat and diathermy, vigorous electrical stimulation, and massage (or cold over irradiated tissues) have been considered contraindicated for use at or near malignancies or over irradiated tissues (314–317). Local ultrasound diathermy in mice enhances subcutaneous growth of malignancy (318). Hyperthermia inducing tumor temperatures above 42°C has been successfully used for tumoricidal effects, especially in conjunction with tumor irradiation (319). However, tumors may develop an increase in blood supply at temperatures of 40°C to 41°C (320). In theory, this may be a cause for concern regarding the use of local therapeutic heat over or near a tumor. Additionally, in patients with lymphedema, use of therapeutic heat is often withheld because of concern of increased production of interstitial fluid.

Transcutaneous electrical nerve stimulation (TENS) has been used to reduce myogenic pain, though it is not effective in reducing local tenderness or trigger point sensitivity (321). TENS may also be helpful for postsurgical pain syndromes, postherpetic neuralgia, and to a limited extent, phantom limb pain (322–324). Some have suggested a role for TENS in managing pain from metastatic bone disease and nerve root compression following vertebral collapse or mass effect from tumor; this is certainly controversial (325). At least some of the effectiveness might be attributed to the effect of TENS on the nonmalignant component of such pain. Acupuncture has also been suggested to be useful for managing cancer pain, especially hyperpathic pain and dysesthesias (326). When not otherwise contraindicated, therapeutic massage may reduce the level of perception of significant cancer pain and related anxiety while enhancing feelings of relaxation.

CONCLUSIONS

Both the incidence of invasive cancer and cancer survivorship have continued to increase over recent years. Timely rehabilitative intervention can help many patients maximize their level of function and quality of life. The services provided by the rehabilitation team can have a dramatic impact on this ever-increasing patient population and their families, regardless of the clinical setting.

REFERENCES

1. Parker SL, Tong T, Bolden S, Wingo PA. Cancer statistics, 1997. *CA Cancer J Clin* 1997;47(1):5–27.
2. Lehmann JF, DeLisa JA, Warren CG, et al. Cancer rehabilitation: assessment of need, development, and the evaluation of a model of care. *Arch Phys Med Rehabil* 1978;59: 410–419.
3. Brennan MJ, Warfel BS. Musculoskeletal complications of cancer. A survey of 50 patients. *J Back Musculoskel Rehabil* 1993;3(2):1–6.
4. Marciniak CM, Sliwa JA, Spill G, et al. Functional outcome following rehabilitation of the cancer patient. *Arch Phys Med Rehabil* 1996;77:54–57.
5. Warfel BS, Lachmann E, Nagler W. Physiatric evaluation of the cancer patient. *J Back Musculoskel Rehabil* 1993;3(2): 60–68.
6. Thorpe G. Introduction—rehabilitation in palliative care. In: Doyle D, Hanks GWC, MacDonald N, eds. *Oxford textbook of palliative* medicine. New York: Oxford University Press, 1993:527–562.
7. Dietz JH Jr. *Rehabilitation oncology.* New York: John Wiley, 1981.
8. Dietz JH. Rehabilitation of the cancer patient. *Med Clin North Am* 1969;53:607–624.
9. Black PMcL. Brain tumors (first of two parts). *N Engl J Med* 1991;324:1471–1476.
10. Arvedson JC, Rodgers BT. Pediatric swallowing and feeding disorders. *J Med Speech Lang Pathol* 1993;1:203–221.
11. Byrne TN. Spinal cord compression from epidural metastases. *N Engl J Med* 1992;327: 614–619.
12. Portenoy RK, Lipton RB, Foley KM. Back pain in the cancer patient: an algorithm for evaluation and management. Neurology 1987;37:134–138.
13. Rodichok LD, Harper GR, Ruckdeschel JC, et al. Early diagnosis of spinal epidural metastases. *Am J Med* 1981;70: 1181–1188.
14. Gilbert RW, Kim J-H, Posner JB. Epidural spinal cord compression from metastatic tumor: diagnosis and treatment. *Ann Neurol* 1978;3:40–51.
15. Young RF, Post FM, King GA. Treatment of spinal epidural metastases. Randomized prospective comparison of laminectomy and radiotherapy. *J Neurosurg* 1980;53:741–748.
16. Sundaresan N, Digiacinto GV, Hughes JE, et al. Treatment of neoplastic spinal cord compression: results of a prospective study. *Neurosurgery* 1991;29:645–650.
17. Slatkin NE, Posner JB. Management of spinal epidural metastases. *Clin Neurosurg* 1983;30:698–716.
18. Wasserstrom WR, Glass JP, Posner JB. Diagnosis and treatment of leptomeningeal metastases from solid tumors: experience with 90 patients. *Cancer* 1982;49:759–772.
19. Grossman SA, Moynihan TJ. Neoplastic meningitis. *Neurol Clin* 1991;9:843–856.
20. Chamberlain MC. A review of leptomeningeal metastases in pediatrics. *J Child Neurol* 1995;10:191–199.
21. Kori SH, Foley KM, Posner JB. Brachial plexus lesions in patients with cancer: 100 cases. Neurology 1981;31:45–50.
22. Thomas JE, Cascino TL, Earle JD. Differential diagnosis between radiation and tumor plexopathy of the pelvis. *Neurology* 1985;35:1–7.
23. Jaeckle KA, Young DF, Foley KM. The natural history of lumbosacral plexopathy in cancer. *Neurology* 1985;35: 8–15.
24. Orr FW, Sanchez-Sweatman OH, Kostenuik P, Singh G. Tumor-bone interactions in skeletal metastasis. *Clin Orthop* 1995; 312:19–33.
25. Batson OV. The function of the vertebral veins and their role in the spread of metastases. *Ann Surg* 1940;112:128–149.
26. Rubens RD, Coleman RE. Bone metastases. In: Abeloff MD, Armitage JO, Lichter AS, Niederhuber JE, eds. *Clinical oncology.* New York: Churchill Livingstone, 1995:643–665.

27. Galasko CSB. Diagnosis of skeletal metastases and assessment of response to treatment. *Clin Orthop* 1995;312: 64–75.

28. Hipp JA, Springfield DS, Hayes WC. Predicting pathologic fracture risk in the management of metastatic bone defects. *Clin Orthop* 1995;312:120–135.

29. Mirels H. Metastatic disease in long bones: a proposed scoring system for diagnosing impending pathologic fractures. *Clin Orthop* 1989;249:256–264.

30. Denis F. Spinal instability as defined by the three-column spine concept in acute spinal trauma. *Clin Orthop* 1984;189: 65–76.

31. Kostuik JP, Weinstein JN. Differential diagnosis and surgical treatment of metastatic spine tumors. In: Frymoyer JW, ed. *The adult spine: principles and practice.* New York: Raven, 1991:861–888.

32. Traill Z, Richards MA, Moore NR. Magnetic resonance imaging of metastatic bone disease. *Clin Orthop* 1995;312:76–88.

33. Hosono N, Yonenobu K, Fuji T, et al. Orthopaedic management of spinal metastases. *Clin Orthop* 1995;312:148–159.

34. Posner JB. Paraneoplastic syndromes. *Neurol Clin* 1991;9: 919–936.

35. Hammack J, Kotanides H, Rosenblum MK, Posner JB. Paraneoplastic cerebellar degeneration. II. Clinical and immunologic findings in 21 patients with Hodgkin's disease. *Neurology* 1992;42:1938–1943.

36. Posner JB. Paraneoplastic cerebellar degeneration. *Can J Neurol Sci* 1993;20(suppl 3): S117–S122.

37. Adams RD, Victor M. Principles of neurology. 4th ed. New York: McGraw-Hill, 1989.

38. Kimura J. Electrodiagnosis in *diseases of nerve and muscle: principles and practice.* 2nd ed. Philadelphia: FA Davis, 1989.

39. Jablecki CK. Lambert-Eaton myasthenic syndrome. AAEE case report #9. *Muscle Nerve* 1984; 7:250–257.

40. Rook JL, Green RF, Tunkel R, Lachmann E. Lower extremity weakness as the initial manifestation of lung cancer. *Arch Phys Med Rehabil* 1990; 71:995–999.

41. Cronin ME, Miller FW, Plotz PH. Polymyositis and dermatomyositis. In: Schumacher HR, ed. *Primer on the rheumatic diseases.* 9th ed. Atlanta: Arthritis Foundation, 1988: 120–123.

42. Joseph RR. Rheumatic manifestations of neoplastic disease. In: Katz WA, ed. *Diagnosis and management of rheumatic diseases.* 2nd ed. Philadelphia: JB Lippincott, 1988:692–698.

43. Henriksson KG, Lindvall B. Polymyositis and dermatomyositis 1990—diagnosis, treatment and prognosis. *Prog Neurobiol* 1990;35:181–193.

44. Altman RD, Gray RG. Bone disease. In: Katz WA, ed. *Diagnosis and management of rheumatic diseases.* 2nd ed. Philadelphia: JB Lippincott, 1988:620–630.

45. Martinez-Lavin M, Weisman MH, Pineda CJ. Hypertrophic osteoarthropathy. In: Schumacher HR Jr, ed. *Primer on the rheumatic disease.* 9th ed. Atlanta: Arthritis Foundation, 1988:240–242.

46. Caldwell DS, McCallum RM. Rheumatologic manifestations of cancer. *Med Clin North Am* 1986;70:385–415.

47. Sheon RP, Kirsner AB, Tangsintanapas P, et al. Malignancy in rheumatic disease: interrelationships. *J Am Geriatr Soc* 1977; 25:20–27.

48. Caldwell DS. Musculoskeletal syndromes associated with malignancy. *Semin Arthritis Rheum* 1981;10:198–223.

49. Caldwell DS. Carcinoma polyarthritis: manifestations and differential diagnosis. *Med Grand Rounds* 1982;1:378–385.

50. Krey PR. Arthropathies associated with hematologic disease and storage disorders. In: Schumacher HR Jr, ed. *Primer on the rheumatic diseases.* 9th ed. Atlanta: Arthritis Foundation, 1988:220–226.

51. Naschitz JE, Yerurun D, Lev LM. Thromboembolism in cancer. Changing trends. Cancer 1993; 71:1384–1390.

52. Grant M, Rhiner M, Padilla GV. Nutritional management in the head and neck cancer patient. *Semin Oncol Nurs* 1989;5: 195–204.

53. Hains N, Barron SA, Robinson E. Muscle cramps associated with vincristine therapy. *Acta Oncol* 1991:30:707–711.

54. Ryan JR, Emami A. Vincristine neurotoxicity with residual equinocavus deformity in children with acute leukemia. *Cancer* 1983;51:423–425.

55. Kraft GH. Peripheral neuropathies. In: Johnson EW, ed. Practical electromyography. 2nd ed. Baltimore: Williams & Wilkins, 1988:246–318.

56. Postma TJ, Benard BA, Huijgens PC, et al. Long term effects of vincristine on the peripheral nervous system. J Neurooncol 1993;15:23–27.

57. Daugaard G, Abildgaard U. Renal morbidity of chemotherapy. In: Plowman PN, McElwain TJ, Meadows AT, eds. *Complications of cancer management.* Oxford: Butterworth-Heinemann, 1991:213–231.

58. Kaplan RS, Wiernik PH. Neurotoxicity of antineoplastic drugs. Semin Oncol 1982;9: 103–130.

59. Mollman JE, Glover DJ, Hogan WM, Furman RE. Cisplatin neuropathy. Risk factors, prognosis, and protection by WR-2721. *Cancer* 1988;61: 2192–2195.

60. Riggs JE, Ashraf M, Snyder RD, Gutmann L. Prospective nerve conduction studies in cisplatin therapy. *Ann Neurol* 1988;23: 92–94.

61. Boogerd W, tenBookel Huinink WW, Dalesio O, et al. Cisplatin induced neuropathy: central, peripheral, and autonomic nerve involvement. *J Neurooncol* 1990; 9:255–263.

62. Kopelman J, Budnick AS, Sessions RB, et al. Ototoxicity of high-dose cisplatin by bolus administration in patients with advanced cancers and normal hearing. *Laryngoscope* 1988; 98(8 Pt 1):858–864.

63. Granowetter L, Rosenstock JG, Packer RJ. Enhanced cis-platinum neurotoxicity in pediatric patients with brain tumors. *J Neurooncol* 1983;1: 293–297.

64. Walker DA, Pillow J, Waters KD, Keir E. Enhanced cis-platinum ototoxicity in children with brain tumors who have received simultaneous or prior cranial irradiation. *Med Pediatr Oncol* 1989;17:48–52.

65. Brock PR, Bellman SC, Yeomans EC, et al. Cisplatin ototoxicity in children: a practical grading system. *Med Pediatr Oncol* 1991;19:295–300.

66. Rowinsky EK, Eisenhauer EA, Chaudry V, et al. Clinical toxicities encountered with paclitaxel (Taxol). Semin Oncol 1993; 20(4 suppl 3):1–15.

67. Bissett D, Setanoians A, Cassidy J, et al. Phase I and pharmacokinetic study of taxotere (RP 56976) administered as a 24-hour infusion. *Cancer Res* 1993;53:523–527.

68. Degardin M, Bonneterre J, Hecquet B, et al. Vinorelbine (Navelbine) as a salvage treatment for advanced breast cancer. *Ann Oncol* 1994;5: 423–426.

69. Kramer ED, Cohen BH, Packer RJ. Central nervous system morbidity secondary to chemotherapy. In: Plowman PN, McElwain T, Meadows A, eds. *Complications of cancer management.* Oxford: Butterworth-Heinemann, 1991:329–347.

70. LaRocca JV, Meer J, Gilliatt RW, et al. Suramin-induced polyneuropathy. *Neurology* 1990;40: 954–960.

71. Collis CH. Chemotherapy-related morbidity to the lungs. In: Plowman PN, McElwain TJ, Meadows AT, eds. Complications of cancer management. Oxford: Butterworth-Heinemann, 1991: 250–271.

72. McElwain TJ. Cardiac morbidity of chemotherapy. In: Plowman PN, McElwain TJ, Meadows AT, eds. *Complications of cancer management.* Oxford: Butterworth-Heinemann, 1991: 184–192.

73. Lipshultz SE, Colan SD, Gelber RD, et al. Late cardiac effects of doxorubicin therapy for acute lymphoblastic leukemia in childhood. *N Engl J Med* 1991;324: 808–815.

74. Dorwart BB. Arthropathies associated with endocrine diseases. In: Schumacher HR Jr, ed. *Primer on the rheumatic diseases.* 9th ed. Atlanta: Arthritis Foundation, 1988:217–219.

75. David DS, Grieco MH, Cushman P. Adrenal glucocorticoids after twenty years. A review of their clinically relevant consequences. *J Chronic Dis* 1970;22: 637–711.

76. Jannoun L, Bloom HJG. Long-term psychological effects in children treated for intracranial tumors. *Int J Radiat Oncol Biol Phys* 1990;18:747–753.

77. Spunberg JJ, Chang CH, Goldman M, et al. Quality of long-term survival following irradiation for intracranial tumors in children under the age of two. *Int J Radiat Oncol Biol Phys* 1981;7:727–736.

78. Imperato JP, Paleologos NA, Vick NA. Effects of treatment on long-term survivors with malignant astrocytomas. *Ann Neurol* 1990;28:818–822.

79. Kleinberg L, Wallner K, Malkin MG. Good performance status of long-term disease-free survivors of intracranial gliomas. Int J *Radiat Oncol* 1993;26:129–133.

80. Wara WM, Larson DA. Central nervous system manifestations of radiotherapy. In: Plowman PN, McElwain TJ, Meadows AT, eds. *Complications of cancer management.* Oxford: Butterworth-Heinemann, 1991;320–328.

81. Sutherland IA, Myers SJ. Radiation myelopathy. Arch Phys Med *Rehabil* 1976;57:81–84.

82. Salner AL, Botnick LE, Herzog AG, et al. Reversible brachial plexopathy following primary radiation therapy for breast cancer. *Cancer Treat Rep* 1981;65:797–802.

83. Enevoldson TP, Scadding JW, Rustin GJ, Senanayake LF. Spontaneous resolution of postirradiation lumbosacral plexopathy. *Neurology* 1992;42: 2224–2225.

84. Harper CM Jr, Thomas JE, Cascino TL, Litchy WJ. Distinction between neoplastic and radiation-induced brachial plexopathy with emphasis on the role of EMG. *Neurology* 1989;39: 502–506.

85. Pugliese GN, Green RF, Antonacci A. Radiation-induced long thoracic nerve palsy. Cancer 1987;60:1247–1248.

86. Hicks JE. Exercise for cancer patients. In: Basmajian JV, Wolf SL, eds. *Therapeutic exercise.* Baltimore: Williams & Wilkins, 1990:351–369.

87. Bagshaw MA. Organ and function preservation after X-irradiation for prostatic cancer. *Prog Clin Biol Res* 1991;370:257–268.

88. Schover LR, Fife M, Gershenson D. Sexual dysfunction and treatment for early stage cervical cancer. *Cancer* 1989;63: 204–212.

89. LeVeque FG, Montgomery M, Potter D, et al. A multicenter, randomized, double blind, placebo-controlled, dose titration study of oral pilocarpine for treatment of radiation-induced xerostomia in head and neck cancer patients. *J Clin Oncol* 1993;11: 1124–1131.

90. Groher ME. Management: general principles and guidelines. *Dysphagia* 1991;6:67–70.

91. Lazarus CL, Logemann JA, Pauloski BR, et al. Swallowing disorders in head and neck cancer patients treated with radiotherapy and adjuvant chemotherapy. *Laryngoscope* 1996;106:1157–1166.

92. Soffer EE, Mitros F, Doornbos JF, et al. Morphology and pathology of radiation-induced esophagitis. Double-blind study of naproxen vs. placebo for prevention of radiation injury. *Dig Dis Sci* 1994; 39:655–660.

93. Pierce SM, Recht A, Lingos TI, et al. Long-term radiation complications following conservative surgery (CS) and radiation therapy (RT) in patients with early stage breast cancer. *Int J Radiat Oncol Biol Phys* 1992; 23:915–923.

94. Trott, KR. Cardiovascular system morbidity of radiotherapy. In: Plowman PN, McElwain TJ, Meadows AT, eds. *Complications of cancer management.* Oxford: Butterworth-Heinemann, 1991: 177–183.

95. Carlson RG, Mayfield WR, Normann S, Alexander JA. Radiation-associated valvular disease. Chest 1991;99: 538–545.

96. Travis EL. Lung morbidity of radiotherapy. In: Plowman PN, McElwain TJ, Meadows AT, eds. *Complications of cancer management.* Oxford: Butterworth-Heinemann, 1991: 232–249.

97. Roberts CM, Foulcher E, Zaunders JJ, et al. Radiation pneumonitis: a possible lymphocytic-mediated hypersensitivity reaction. *Ann Intern Med* 1993;118:696–700.

98. Allavena C, Conroy T, Aletti P, et al. Late cardiopulmonary toxicity after treatment for Hodgkin's disease. *Br J Cancer* 1992;65:908–912.

99. Holtzman L, Chesney K. Rehabilitation of the leukemia/lymphoma patient. In: McGarvey CL, ed. *Physical therapy for the cancer patient.* New York: Churchill Livingstone, 1991:85–110.

100. Sayre RS, Marcoux BC. Exercise and autologous bone marrow transplants. *Clin Manage* 1992; 2(4):78–82.

101. Gmür J, Burger J, Schanz U, et al. Safety of stringent prophylactic platelet transfusion policy for patients with acute leukaemia. *Lancet* 1991;338: 1223–1226.

102. Ewing MR, Martin H. Disability following "radical neck dissection": an assessment based on postoperative evaluation of 100 patients. *Cancer* 1952;5: 873–883.

103. Schuller DE, Reiches NA, Hamaker RC, et al. Analysis of disability resulting from treatment including radical neck dissection or modified neck dissection. *Head Neck Surg* 1983;6:551–558.

104. Remmler D, Byers R, Scheetz J, et al. A prospective study of shoulder disability resulting from radical and modified neck dissections. *Head Neck Surg* 1986;8:280–286.

105. Olarte M, Adams D. Short report. Accessory nerve palsy. *J Neurol Neurosurg Psychiatry* 1977;40: 1113–1116.

106. Saunders WH, Johnson EW. Rehabilitation of the shoulder after radical neck dissection. *Ann Otol* 1975;84:812–816.

107. Fialka V, Vinzenz K. Investigations into shoulder function after radical neck dissection. *J Craniomaxillofac Surg* 1988;16: 143–147.

108. Petrera J, Trojaborg W. Conduction studies along the accessory nerve and follow up of patients with trapezius palsy. *J Neurol Neurosurg Psychiatry* 1984;47:630–636.

109. Green RF, Brien M. Accessory nerve latency to the middle and lower trapezius. *Arch Phys Med Rehabil* 1985;66: 23–24.

110. Granek I, Ashikari R, Foley KM. The post-mastectomy pain syndrome. Proc Am Soc Clin Oncol 1983;3:122.

111. Schover LR. Sexuality and body image in younger women with breast cancer. *Monogr Natl Cancer Inst* 1994;16:177–182.

112. Wellisch DK, DiMatteo R, Silverstein M, et al. Psychosocial outcome of breast cancer therapies: lumpectomy versus mastectomy. *Psychosomatics* 1989;30:365–373.

113. Kiebert GM, de Haes JCJM, van de Velde CJH. The impact of breast-conserving treatment and mastectomy on the quality of life of early-stage breast cancer patients: a review. *J Clin Oncol* 1991;9:1059–1070.

114. Mizgala CL, Hartrampf CR Jr, Bennett GK. Abdominal function after pedicled TRAM flap surgery. *Clin Plast Surg* 1994;21: 255–272.

115. Vásconez HC, Holley DT. Use of the TRAM and latissimus dorsi flaps in autogenous breast reconstruction. *Clin Plast Surg* 1995; 22:153–166.

116. Feller A-M. Free TRAM: results and abdominal wall function. Clin Plast Surg 1994;21: 223–232.

117. Murphy JB. Complications of breast reconstruction. In: Noone RB, ed. *Plastic and reconstructive surgery of the breast.* Philadelphia: BC Decker, 1991:448–454.

118. Cordeiro PG, Hidalgo DA. Conceptual considerations in mandibular reconstruction. *Clin Plast Surg* 1995;22:61–69.

119. Drake DB. Reconstruction for limb-sparing procedures in soft-tissue sarcomas of the extremities. *Clin Plast Surg* 1995;22:123–128.

120. Kanner RM, Martini N, Foley KM. The nature and incidence of post-thoracotomy pain. *Proc Am Soc Clin Oncol* 1982:1:152.

121. Prater RJ, Swift RW. *Manual of voice therapy.* Boston: Little, Brown, 1984.

122. Logemann JA. *Evaluation and treatment of swallowing disorders.* 2nd ed. Austin, TX: Pro-Ed, 1998.

123. Benninger MS, Crumley RL, Ford CN, et al. Evaluation and treatment of the unilateral paralyzed vocal fold. *Otolaryngol Head Neck Surg* 1994;111: 497–508.

124. Piquet JJ, Chevalier D. Subtotal laryngectomy with cricohyoid-epiglotto-pexy for the treatment of extended glottic carcinomas. Am J Surg 1991;162:357–361.

125. Levine PA, Debo RF, Reibel JF. Pearson near-total laryngectomy: a reproducible speaking shunt. *Head Neck* 1994;16: 323–325.

126. Zanaret M, Giovanni A, Gras R, Cannoni M. Near-total laryngectomy with epiglottic reconstruction: long-term results in 57 patients. *Am J Otolaryngol* 1993;14:419–425.

127. Imai S, Michi K. Articulatory function after resection of the tongue and floor of the mouth: palatometric and perceptual evaluation. *J Speech Hear Res* 1992;35:68–78.

128. Casper JK, Colton RH. *Clinical manual for laryngectomy and head and neck cancer rehabilitation.* San Diego: Singular Publishing Group, 1993.

129. Zlotolow IM, Huryn JM. Restoration of the acquired soft palate deformity with surgical resection and reconstruction. In: Zlotolow IM, Beumer J, Esposito S, eds. *Proceedings of the International Congress of Maxillofacial Prosthetics.* New York: Memorial Sloan-Kettering Cancer Center, 1995;49–55.

130. Logemann JA. *Manual for the videofluorographic study of swallowing.* 2nd ed. Austin, TX: Pro-Ed, 1993.

131. Kronenberger MB, Meyers AD. Dysphagia following head and neck cancer surgery. *Dysphagia* 1994;9:236–244.

132. Brendler CB, Walsh PC. The role of radical prostatectomy in the treatment of prostate cancer. *Cancer J Clin* 1992;42: 212–222.

133. Steiner MS, Morton RA, Walsh PC. Impact of anatomical radical prostatectomy on urinary continence. *J Urol* 1989;142: 1227–1229.

134. Soderberg GL. Gait and gait retraining. In: Basmajian JV, Wolf SL, eds. *Therapeutic exercise.* 5th ed. Baltimore: Williams & Wilkins, 1990:139–161.

135. Prosthetics and Orthotics Staff. *Lower-limb orthotics.* New York: New York University Medical Center, 1986:1–283.

136. Lincoln JR, Sawyer HP Jr. Complications related to body positions during surgical procedures. *Anesthesiology* 1961;12: 800–809.

137. Herrera-Ornelas L, Tolls RM, Petrelli NJ, et al. Common peroneal nerve palsy associated with pelvic surgery for cancer. An analysis of 11 cases. *Dis Colon Rectum* 1986;29:392–397.

138. Weber RJ. Motor and sensory conduction and entrapment syndromes. In: Johnson EW, ed. *Practical electromyography.* 2nd ed. Baltimore: Williams & Wilkins, 1988:92–186.

139. Lachmann EA, Rook JL, Tunkel R, Nagler W. Complications associated with intermittent pneumatic compression. *Arch Phys Med Rehabil* 1992;73: 482–485.

140. Sotaniemi K. Slimmer's paralysis-peroneal neuropathy during weight reduction. J Neurol Neurosurg Psychiatry 1984;47: 564–566.

141. Kaminsky F. Peroneal palsy by crossing the legs. JAMA 1947; 134:206.

142. Simon MA. Limb salvage for osteosarcoma in the 1980's. *Clin Orthop* 1991;270:264–270.

143. Marcove RC, Lewis MM, Huvos AG. En bloc upper humeral interscapulo thoracic resection. *Clin Orthop* 1977;124:219–228.

144. Shibata T. Reconstruction of skeletal defects after Tikhoff-Linberg procedure using alumina ceramic endoprosthesis and stabilization of the shoulder. In: Enneking WF, ed. *Limb salvage in musculoskeletal oncology.* New York: Churchill Livingstone, 1987:553–561.

145. Carnesale PG. Infectious arthritis. In: Crenshaw AH, ed. *Campbell's operative orthopaedics.* Vol. I. 7th ed. St. Louis: CV Mosby, 1987:677–697.

146. Enneking WF. The pelvis. In: Musculoskeletal tumor surgery. Vol. I. New York: Churchill Livingstone, 1983:483–529.

147. Enneking WF, Menendez LR. Functional evaluation of various reconstructions after periacetabular resection of iliac lesions. In: Enneking WF, ed. *Limb salvage in musculoskeletal oncology.* New York: Churchill Livingstone, 1987:117–135.

148. Tooms RE. Amputations of upper extremity. In: Crenshaw AH, ed. *Campbell's operative orthopaedics.* Vol. I. 7th ed. St. Louis: CV Mosby, 1987: 637–646.

149. Kotz R, Salzar M. Rotation-plasty for childhood osteosarcoma of the distal part of the femur. J *Bone Joint Surg [Am]* 1982;64: 959–969.

150. Markel KD, Gebhardt M, Springfield DS. Rotationplasty as a reconstructive operation after tumor resection. *Clin Orthop* 1991;270:231–236.

151. Corney RH, Everett H, Howells A, Crowther ME. Psychosocial adjustment following major gynaecological surgery for carcinoma of the cervix and vulva. J *Psychosomat Res* 1992;36: 561–568.

152. King AW. Nursing management of stomas of the genitourinary system. In: Broadwell DC, Jackson BS, eds. *Principles of ostomy care.* St. Louis: CV Mosby, 1982:290–320.

153. Goode PS. Nursing management of disorders of the gastrointestinal system. In: Broadwell DC, Jackson BS, eds. *Principles of ostomy care.* St. Louis: CV Mosby, 1982:257–289.

154. National Institutes of Health Consensus Development Conference.

Prevention of venous thrombosis and pulmonary embolism. *JAMA* 1986;256:744–749.

155. Schiff D, DeAngelis LM. Therapy of venous thromboembolism in patients with brain metastases. *Cancer* 1994;73:493–498.

156. Seene T. Turnover of skeletal muscle contractile proteins in glucocorticoid myopathy. *J Steroid Biochem Mol Biol* 1994;50:1–4.

157. Macfarlane GJ, Lowenfels AB. Physical activity and colon cancer. *Eur J Cancer Prevent* 1994;3:393–398.

158. Markowitz S, Morabia A, Garibaldi K, Wynder E. Effect of occupation and recreational activity on the risk of colorectal cancer among males: a case-control study. *Int J Epidemiol* 1992;21:1057–1062.

159. Friedenreich CM, Rohan TE. A review of physical activity and breast cancer. *Epidemiology* 1995;6:311–317.

160. Bernstein L, Henderson BE, Hanisch R, et al. Physical exercise and reduced risk of breast cancer in young women. *J Natl Cancer Inst* 1994;86: 1403–1408.

161. Andersson SO, Baron J, Wolk A, et al. Early life risk factors for prostate cancer: a population-based case-control study in Sweden. *Cancer Epidemiol, Biomarkers Prev* 1995;4:187–192.

162. United Kingdom Testicular Cancer Study Group. Aetiology of testicular cancer: association with congenital abnormalities, age at puberty, infertility, and exercise. *BJM* 1994;308: 1393–1399.

163. Lindblad P, Wolk A, Bergstrom R, et al. The role of obesity and weight fluctuations in the etiology of renal cell cancer: a population-based case-control study. *Cancer Epidemiol Biomarkers Prev* 1994;3:631–639.

164. Shephard RJ, Shek PN. Cancer, immune function, and physical activity. Can J Appl Physiol 1995;20:1–25.

165. Woods JA, Davis JM. Exercise, monocyte/macrophage function, and cancer. *Med Sci Sports Exerc* 1994;26:147–156.

166. Ng EH, Lowry SF. Nutritional support and cancer cachexia. Evolving concepts of mechanisms and adjunctive therapies. *Hematol Oncol Clin North Am* 1991;5:161–184.

167. Graydon JE, Bubela N, Irvine D, Vincent L. Fatigue-reducing strategies used by patients receiving treatment for cancer. *Cancer Nurs* 1995;18:23–28.

168. Morgan WP, Goldstein SE. *Exercise and mental health.* Washington, DC: Hemisphere Publishing, 1987.

169. Shephard RJ. Exercise in the prevention and treatment of cancer. An update. *Sports Med* 1993;15:258–280.

170. Levine EG, Raczynski JM, Carpenter JT. Weight gain with breast cancer adjuvant treatment. *Cancer* 1991;67:1954–1959.

171. Mock V, Burke MB, Sheehan P, et al. A nursing rehabilitation program for women with breast cancer receiving adjuvant chemotherapy. *Oncol Nurs Forum* 1994;21:899–907.

172. Winningham, ML, MacVicar MG, Burke CA. Exercise for cancer patients: guidelines and precautions. *Physician Sports Med* 1986;14:125–134.

173. Leipzig B, Suen JY, English JL, et al. Functional evaluation of the spinal accessory nerve after neck dissection. *Am J Surg* 1983;146:526–530.

174. Dudgeon BJ, DeLisa JA, Miller RM. Head and neck cancer, a rehabilitation approach. *Am J Occup Ther* 1980;34: 243–251.

175. Villanueva R, Ajmani C. The role of rehabilitation medicine in physical restoration of patients with head and neck cancer. *Cancer Bull* 1977;29:46–54.

176. Patten C, Hillel AD. The 11th nerve syndrome. Accessory nerve palsy or adhesive capsulitis? *Arch Otolaryngol Head Neck Surg* 1993;119:215–220.

177. Bernd L, Blasins K, Lohoscheck M. The autologous stump plasty: treatment for bony overgrowth in juvenile amputees. *J Bone Joint Surg [Br]* 1991;73:203–206.

178. Tooms RE Amputation surgery in the upper extremity. Orthop Clin North Am 1972;3:383–397.

179. Cammisa FP Jr, Glasser DB, Ortis JC, et al. The Van Ness rotation plasty. *J Bone Joint Surg [Am]* 1990;72:1541–1547.

180. Berger AR, Schaumburg HH. Rehabilitation of focal nerve injuries. *J Neurol Rehabil* 1988;2:65–91.

181. Hewer RL, Cooper R, Morgan MH. An investigation into the value of treating intention tremor by weighting the affected extremity. *Brain* 1972;95: 579–590.

182. Nance PW, Kirby RL. Rehabilitation of an adult with disabilities due to congenital sensory neuropathy. *Arch Phys Med Rehabil* 1985;66:123–124.

183. Dobbs J, Barrett A, Ash D. *Practical radiotherapy planning.* 2nd ed. London: Edward Arnold/Hodder and Stoughton, 1992:1–303.

184. Lotze MT, Duncan MA, Gerber LH, et al. Early versus delayed shoulder motion following axillary dissection. *Ann Surg* 1981;193: 288–295.

185. Van Der Horst CH, Kenter JAL, DeJong MT, Keeman JN. Shoulder function following early mobilization of the shoulder after mastectomy and axillary dissection. *Neth J Surg* 1985;37: 105–108.

186. Rodier JF, Gadonneix P, Dauplat J, et al. Influence of the timing of physiotherapy upon the lymphatic complications of axillary dissection for breast cancer. *Int Surg* 1987;72:166–169.

187. Wingate L, Croghan I, Natarajan N, et al. Rehabilitation of the mastectomy patient: a randomized, blind, prospective study.

Arch Phys Med Rehabil 1989; 70:21–24.

188. Konecne SM. Postsurgery breast cancer inpatient program. *Clin Manage* 1992;12:42–49.

189. Bunting R, Lamont-Havers W, Schweon D, Kliman A. Pathologic fracture risk in rehabilitation of patients with bony metastases. *Clin Orthop* 1985;192:222–227.

190. Hasselbacher P, Schumacher HR. Bilateral protrusion acetabulum following pelvic irradiation. *J Rheumatol* 1977;4:189–196.

191. Albrektsson T, Jacobsson M, Turesson I. Irradiation injury of bone tissue. A vital microscopic method. *Acta Radiol Oncol* 1980;19:235–239.

192. Bunting RW, Boublik M, Blevins FT, et al. Functional outcome of pathologic fracture secondary to malignant disease in a rehabilitation hospital. *Cancer* 1992;69: 98–102.

193. Stillo JV, Stein AB, Ragnarsson KT. Low-back orthoses. *Phys Med Rehabil Clin N Am* 1992;3:57–94.

194. Fisher SV. Cervical orthotics. *Phys Med Rehabil Clin N Am* 1992;3:29–43.

195. Kaszyk LK. Cardiac toxicity associated with cancer therapy. *Oncol Nurs Forum* 1986; 13(4):81–88.

196. Rodriquez DB. Special considerations: care of the ostomy patient receiving cancer therapy. In: Broadwell DC, Jackson BS, eds. *Principles of ostomy care.* St. Louis: CV Mosby, 1982:381–389.

197. Devlin HB. Management of a colostomy and its complications. In: Walker FC, ed. *Modern stoma care.* London: Churchill Livingstone, 1976:57–67.

198. Goode PS. Colostomy irrigation. In: Broadwell DC, Jackson BS, eds. *Principles of ostomy care.* St. Louis: CV Mosby, 1982:369–380.

199. Lerman JW. The artificial larynx. In: Salmon SJ, Mount KH, eds. *Alaryngeal speech rehabilitation for clinicians by clinicians.* Austin, TX: Pro-Ed, 1991:27–45.

200. Duguay MJ. Esophageal speech training: the initial phase. In: Salmon SJ, Mount KH, eds. *Alaryngeal speech rehabilitation for clinicians by clinicians.* Austin, TX: Pro-Ed, 1991:47–78.

201. Singer MI, Blom ED. An endoscopic technique for restoration of voice after laryngectomy. *Ann Otol Rhinol Laryngol* 1980;89:529–533.

202. Blom ED, Singer MI, Hamaker RC. A prospective study of tracheoesophageal speech. *Arch Otolaryngol Head Neck Surg* 1986;112:440–447.

203. Singer MI, Hamaker RC, Blom ED, Yoshida GY. Applications of the voice prosthesis during laryngectomy. *Ann Otol Rhinol Laryngol* 1989;98:(12 Pt 1):921–925.

204. Blom ED, Singer MI, Hamaker RC. Tracheostoma valve for postlaryngectomy voice rehabilitation. *Ann Otol Rhinol Laryngol* 1982;91:576–578.

205. Gerwin JM, Culton GL. Prosthetic voice restoration with the tracheostomal valve: a clinical experience. *Am J Otolaryngol* 1993;14:432–439.

206. Bosone ZT. Treatment following tracheoesophageal fistulization surgery. In: Salmon SJ, Mount KH, eds. *Alaryngeal speech rehabilitation for clinicians by clinicians.* Austin, TX: Pro-Ed, 1991:139–159.

207. Davis JW, Lazarus C, Logemann JA, Hurst PS. Effect of a maxillary glossectomy prosthesis on articulation and swallowing. *J Prosthet Dent* 1987;57: 715–719.

208. Wheeler RL, Logemann JA, Rosen MS. Maxillary reshaping prostheses: effectiveness in improving speech and swallowing of postsurgical oral cancer patients. J Prosthet Dent 1980; 43:313–319.

209. Netterville JL, Stone JE, Civantos FJ, et al. Silastic medialization and arytenoid adduction: the Vanderbilt experience. Ann Otol Rhinol Laryngol 1993;102: 413–424.

210. Tucker HM. Combined laryngeal framework medialization and reinnervation for unilateral vocal cord paralysis. *Ann Otol Rhinol Laryngol* 1990;99:778–781.

211. Mason MF. Vocal treatment strategies. In: Mason MF, ed. *Speech pathology for tracheostomized and ventilator dependent patients.* Newport Beach: Voicing, 1993:336–381.

212. Fornataro-Clerici L, Zajac DJ. Aerodynamic characteristics of tracheostomy speaking valves. *J Speech Hear Res* 1993;36: 529–532.

213. Yorkston KM, Beukelman DR, Bell KR. *Clinical management of dysarthric speakers.* Boston: College-Hill, 1988.

214. Bennet J. Talking about low technology. In: Enderby P, ed. *Assistive communication aids for the speech impaired.* Edinburgh: Churchill Livingstone, 1987:112–132.

215. Linebaugh CW, Baird JT, Baird CB, Armour RM. Special considerations for the development of microcomputer-based augmentative communication systems. In: Berry WR, ed. *Clinical dysarthria.* San Diego: College-Hill, 1983: 295–303.

216. Brookshire RH. Auditory comprehension and aphasia. In: Johns DF, ed. *Clinical management of neurogenic communicative disorders.* Boston: Little, Brown, 1978:103–128.

217. LaPointe LL. Aphasia therapy: some principles and strategies for treatment. In: Johns DF, ed. *Clinical management of neurogenic communicative disorders.* Boston: Little, Brown, 1978: 129–190.

218. Murray T. Treatment of ataxic dysarthria. In: Perkins WH, ed. *Dysarthria and apraxia.* New York: Thieme-Stratton, 1983:79–89.

219. Collins M. *Diagnosis and treatment of global aphasia.* San Diego: College-Hill, 1986.

220. Logemann JA, Rademaker AW, Pauloski BR, Kahrilas PJ. Effects of postural change on aspiration in head and neck surgical patients. *Otolaryngol Head Neck Surg* 1994;110:222–227.

221. Logemann JA, Kahrilas PJ, Kobara M, Vakil NB. The benefit of head rotation on pharyngoesophageal dysphagia. *Arch Phys Med Rehabil* 1989; 70:767–771.

222. Welch MV, Logemann JA, Rademaker AW, Kahrilas PJ. Changes in pharyngeal dimensions effected by chin tuck. *Arch Phys Med Rehabil* 1993;74: 178–181.

223. Aguilar NV, Olson ML, Shedd DP. Rehabilitation of deglutition problems in patients with head and neck cancer. *Am J Surg* 1979;138:501–507.

224. Linden-Castelli P. Treatment strategies for adult neurogenic dysphagia. *Semin Speech Lang* 1991;12:255–261.

225. Lazarus C, Logemann JA, Gibbons P. Effects of maneuvers on swallowing function in a dysphagic oral cancer patient. *Head Neck* 1993;15:419–424.

226. Kahrilas PJ, Logemann JA, Krugler C, Flanagan E. Volitional augmentation of upper esophageal sphincter opening during swallowing. *Am J Physiol* 1991;260(3 Pt 1):G450–G456.

227. Bartolome G, Neumann S. Swallowing therapy in patients with neurological disorders causing cricopharyngeal dysfunction. *Dysphagia* 1993;8: 146–149.

228. Logemann JA, Kahrilas PJ. Relearning to swallow after stroke—application of maneuvers and indirect biofeedback: a case study. *Neurology* 1990;40: 1136–1138.

229. Logemann JA. Treatment for aspiration related to dysphagia: an overview. *Dysphagia* 1986;1: 34–38.

230. Kaatzke-McDonald MN, App M, Post E, Davis PJ. The effects of cold, touch, and chemical stimulation of the anterior faucial pillar on human swallowing. *Dysphagia* 1996;11:198–206.

231. Johnson JT, Ferretti GA, Nethery WJ, et al. Oral pilocarpine for post-irradiation xerostomia in patients with head and neck cancer. *N Engl J Med* 1993; 329:390–395.

232. Wiseman LR, Faulds D. Oral pilocarpine: a review of its pharmacological properties and clinical potential in xerostomia. *Drugs* 1995;49:143–155.

233. DaBreo EL. Maxillofacial prosthetic rehabilitation of acquired defects. In: Cummings CW, ed. *Otolaryngology—head and neck surgery*. 2nd ed. St. Louis: Mosby Year Book, 1993: 1451–1477.

234. Davis JW. Prosthodontic management of swallowing disorders. *Dsyphagia* 1989;3:199–205.

235. Arvedson JC. Management of swallowing problems. In: Arvedson JC, Brodsky L, eds. *Pediatric swallowing and feeding: assessment and management.* San Diego: Singular Publishing Group, 1993:327–387.

236. Morris SE. Development of oral-motor skills in the neurologically impaired child receiving non-oral feedings. *Dysphagia* 1989;3:135–154.

237. Gibbs NM. Venous thrombosis of lower limbs with particular reference to bed-rest. Br J Surg 1957;45:209–236.

238. Hammond MC, Merli GJ, Zierler RE. Rehabilitation of the patient with peripheral vascular disease of the lower extremity. In: DeLisa JA, ed. *Rehabilitation medicine—principles and practice.* 2nd ed. Philadelphia: JB Lippincott, 1993:1082–1098.

239. Francis CW. Management of deep-vein thrombosis. *JAMA* 1994;271:556. Letter.

240. Hull RD, Raskob GF, Rosenbloom D, et al. Heparin for 5 days as compared with 10 days in the initial treatment of proximal venous thrombosis. *N Engl J Med* 1990;322:1260–1264.

241. Brennan MJ. Lymphedema following the surgical treatment of breast cancer: a review of pathophysiology and treatment. *J Pain Symptom Manage* 1992;7: 110–116.

242. Leis HP, Bowers WF, Dursi J. Postmastectomy edema of arm. *NY State J Med* 1966;66: 618–624.

243. Brennan MJ, Weitz J. Lymphedema 30 years after radical mastectomy. *Am J Phys Med Rehabil* 1992;71:12–14.

244. Casley-Smith JR. Alterations of untreated lymphedema and its grades over time. Lymphology 1995;28:174–185.

245. McGuire WL, Foley KM, Levy MH, Osborne CK. Pain control in breast cancer. *Breast Cancer Res Treat* 1989;13:5–15.

246. Mortimer P, Regnard C. Lymphostatic disorders. *BMJ* 1986;293:347–348.

247. Stewart FW, Treves N. Lymphangiosarcoma in postmastectomy lymphedema: a report of 6 cases in elephantiasis chirurgica. *Cancer* 1948;1:64–81.

248. Getz DH. The primary, secondary and tertiary nursing interventions of lymphedema. *Cancer Nurs* 1985;8:177–184.

249. Tish Knobf MK. Primary breast cancer: physical consequences and rehabilitation. *Semin Oncol Nurs* 1985;1:214–224.

250. Swedborg I, Norrefalk JR, Piller NB, Åsard C. Lymphoedema post-mastectomy: is elevation alone an effective treatment? *Scand J Rehabil Med* 1993;25: 79–82.

251. Mozes M, Papa MZ, Karasik A, et al. The role of infection in post-mastectomy lymphedema. *Surg Ann* 1982;14:73–83.

252. Benda K, Svestkova S. Incidence rate of recurrent erysipelas in our lymphedema patients. In: Witte MH, Witte CL, eds. *Progress in lymphology-XIV*. Zurich: International Society of Lymphology, 1994:519–522.

253. Swedborg I. Effects of treatment with an elastic sleeve and intermittent pneumatic compression in post-mastectomy patients with lymphoedema of the arm. *Scand J Rehabil Med* 1984;16:35–41.

254. Casley-Smith JR. Modern treatment of lymphedema. *Mod Med Austral* 1992;32:70–83.

255. Vernick SH, Shapiro D, Shaw FD. Leg orthosis for venous and lymphatic insufficiency. *Arch Phys Med Rehabil* 1987;68: 459–461.

256. Zeissler RH, Rose GB, Nelson PA. Postmastectomy lymphedema: late results of treatment in 385 patients. *Arch Phys Med Rehabil* 1972;53:159–166.

257. McNair TJ, Martin IJ, Orr JD. Intermittent compression for lymphoedema of arm. *Clin Oncol* 1976;2:339–342.

258. Zanolla R, Monzeglio C, Balzarini A, Martino G. Evaluation of the results of three different methods of postmastectomy lymphedema treatment. *J Surg Oncol* 1984;26:210–213.

259. Wood C, Gerber LH. Rehabilitation of the patient with breast cancer. In: Lippman ME, Lichter AS, Danforth DN, eds. *Diagnosis and management of breast cancer.* Philadelphia: WB Saunders, 1988:457–467.

260. Yamazaki Z, Idezuki Y, Nemoto T, Togawa T. Clinical experiences using pneumatic massage therapy for edematous limbs over the last 10 years. *Angiol J Vasc Dis* 1988;39:154–163.

261. Pappas DJ, O'Donnell TF. Long-term results of compression treatment for lymphedema. *J Vasc Surg* 1992;16:555–562.

262. Zelikovski A, Manoach M, Giler SH, Urca I. Lympha-Press: a new pneumatic device for the treatment of lymphedema of the limbs. *Lymphology* 1980;13: 68–73.

263. Zelikovski A, Haddad M, Reiss R. The "Lympha-Press" intermittent sequential pneumatic device for the treatment of lymphoedema: five years of clinical experience. *J Cardiovasc Surg* 1986;27: 288–290.

264. Alexander MA, Wright ES, Wright JB, Bikowski JB. Lymphedema treated with linear pump: pediatric case report. *Arch Phys Med Rehabil* 1983;64:132–133.

265. Kim-Sing C, Basco VE. Postmastectomy lymphedema treated with the Wright linear pump. *Can J Surg* 1987;30:368–370.

266. Klein MJ, Alexander MA, Wright JM, et al. Treatment of adult lower extremity lymphedema with Wright linear pump: statistical analysis of a clinical trial. *Arch Phys Med Rehabil* 1988;69: 202–206.

267. Eliska O, Eliskova M. Lymphedema: morphology of the lymphatics after manual massage. In: Witte MH, Witte CL, eds. *Progress in lymphology-XIV.* Zurich: International Society of Lymphology, 1994:132–135.

268. International Society of Lymphology Executive Committee. The diagnosis and treatment of peripheral lymphedema. *Lymphology* 1995;28:113–117.

269. Boris M, Weindorf S, Lasinski B. Persistence of lymphedema reduction after noninvasive complex lymphedema therapy. *Oncology* 1997;11:99–109.

270. Casley-Smith JR, Casley-Smith JR. Modern treatment of lymphoedema II. The benzopyrones. *Australas J Dermatol* 1992;3:69–74.

271. Casley-Smith JR, Casley-Smith JR. The pathophysiology of lymphedema and the action of benzo-pyrones in reducing it. *Lymphology* 1988;21:190–194.

272. Loprinz CL, Kugler JW, Sloan JA, et al. Lack of effect of coumarin in women with lymphedema after treatment for breast cancer. *N Engl J Med* 1999;340:346–350.

273. Foldi E, Foldi M, Clodius L. The lymphedema chaos: a lancet. *Ann Plast Surg* 1989;22: 505–515.

274. Degni M. Surgical management of selected patients with lymphedema of the extremities. *J Cardiovasc Surg* 1984;25: 481–488.

275. Chitale VR. Role of tensor fascia lata musculocutaneous flap in lymphedema of the lower extremity and external genitalia. *Ann Plast Surg* 1989;23:297–304.

276. Campisi C. A rational approach to the management of lymphedema. Lymphology 1991;24:48–53.

277. Egorov YS, Avalmasov KG, Ivanov VV, et al. Autotransplantation of the greater omentum in the treatment of chronic lymphedema. *Lymphology* 1994;27:137–143.

278. Campisi C. Lymphatic microsurgery: a potent weapon in the war on lymphedema. *Lymphology* 1995;28:110–112.

279. Louton RB, Terranova WA. The use of suction curettage as adjunct to the management of lymphedema. *Ann Plast Surg* 1989;22:354–357.

280. O'Brien BMcC, Khazanchi RK, Kumar PAV, et al. Liposuction in the treatment of lymphoedema: a preliminary report. *Br J Plast* Surg 1989;42:530–533.

281. World Health Organization. *Cancer pain relief.* 2nd ed. Geneva: World Health Organization, 1996:15.

282. Powell H, Smallman JM, Morgan M. Comparison of intramuscular ketorolac and morphine in pain control after laparotomy. *Anaesthesia* 1990;45:538–542.

283. Szeto HH, Inturrisi CE, Houde R, et al. Accumulation of normeperidine, an active metabolite of meperidine, in patients with renal failure or cancer. *Ann Intern Med* 1977;86:738–741.

284. Portenoy RK. Adjuvant analgesics in pain management. In: Doyle D, Hanks GWC, MacDonald N, eds. *Oxford textbook of palliative medicine.* New York: Oxford University Press, 1993:187–203.

285. Magni G. The use of antidepressants in the treatment of chronic pain: a review of the current evidence. *Drugs* 1991; 42:730–748.

286. Sindrup SH, Gram LF, Brosen K, et al. The selective serotonin reuptake inhibitor paroxetine is effective in the treatment of diabetic neuropathy symptoms. *Pain* 1990;42:135–144.

287. Watson CPN, Evans RJ. The postmastectomy pain syndrome and topical capsaicin: a randomized trial. *Pain* 1992;51: 375–379.

288. Stow PJ, Glynn CJ, Minor B. EMLA cream in the treatment of post herpetic neuralgia: efficacy and pharmacokinetic profile. *Pain* 1989;39:301–305.

289. Brose WG, Cousins MJ. Subcutaneous lidocaine for treatment of neuropathic cancer pain. Pain 1991;45:145–148.

290. Farr WC. The use of corticosteroids for symptom management in terminally ill patients. *Am J Hospice Care* 1990; 7:41–46.

291. Eisenach JC, Du Pen S, Dubois M, et al. Epidural clonidine analgesia for intractable cancer pain. Pain 1995;61:391–400.

292. Breivik H, Rennemo F. Clinical evaluation of combined treatment with methadone and psychotropic drugs in cancer patients. *Acta Anaesth Scand* 1982;74: 135–140.

293. Gobelet C, Waldburger M, Meier JL. The effect of adding calcitonin to physical treatment on reflex sympathetic dystrophy. *Pain* 1992;48:171–175.

294. Mellick GA, Mellick LB. Gabapentin in the management of reflex sympathetic dystrophy. J Pain Symptom Manage 1995; 10:265–266.

295. Payne R. Pharmacologic management of bone pain in the cancer patient. *Clin J Pain* 1989; 5(suppl 2):S43–S50.

296. Roth A, Kolaric K. Analgesic activity of calcitonin in patients with painful osteolytic metastases of breast cancer: results of a controlled randomized study. *Oncology* 1986;43:283–287.

297. Averbuch SD. New bisphosphonates in the treatment of bone metastases. *Cancer* 1993;72: 3443–3452.

298. Glover D, Lipton A, Keller A, et al. Intravenous pamidronate disodium treatment of bone metastases in patients with breast cancer. *Cancer* 1994;74: 2949–2955.

299. Robinson RG, Preston DF, Schiefelbein M, Baster KG. Strontium-89 therapy for the palliation of pain due to osseous metastases. *JAMA* 1995;274: 420–424.

300. Lapin J, Portenoy RK, Coyle N, et al. Guidelines for use of controlled-release oral morphine in cancer pain management. *Cancer Nurs* 1989;12:202–208.

301. Calis KA, Kohler DR, Corso DM. Transdermally administered fentanyl for pain management. *Clin Pharm* 1992;11:22–36.

302. Coyle N, Cherny NI, Portenoy RK, Subcutaneous opioid infusions at home. *Oncology* 1994; 8:21–27.

303. Inturrisi CE, Hanks G. Opioid analgesic therapy. In: Doyle D, Hanks GWC, MacDonald N, eds. *Oxford textbook of palliative medicine.* New York: Oxford University Press, 1993;166–182.

304. Allan SG. Nausea and vomiting. In: Doyle D, Hanks GWC, MacDonald N, eds. *Oxford textbook of palliative medicine.* New York: Oxford University Press, 1993: 282–290.

305. Eisele JH, Grigsby EJ, Dea G. Clonazepam treatment of myoclonic contractions associated with high dose opioids: a case report. *Pain* 1992;49: 231–232.

306. Porter J, Hick H. Addition rare in patients treated with narcotics. *N Engl J Med* 1980;302:123.

307. Kanner RM, Foley KM. Patterns of narcotic drug use in a cancer pain clinic. *Ann NY Acad Sci* 1981;362:161–172.

308. Perry S, Heidrich G. Management of pain during debridement: a survey of U.S. burn units. *Pain* 1982;13:267–280.

309. Morrison RA. Update on sickle cell disease: incidence of addiction and choice of opioid in pain management. *Pediatr Nurs* 1991; 10:7–8.

310. Tasker R. Neurostimulation and percutaneous neural destructive techniques. In: Cousins MJ, Bridenbaugh PO, eds. *Neural blockade in clinical anesthesia and management of pain.* 2nd ed. Philadelphia: JB Lippincott, 1988:1085–1118.

311. Patt RB. Classification of cancer pain and cancer pain syndromes. In: Patt RB, ed. *Cancer pain.* Philadelphia: JB Lippincott, 1993:3–22.

312. Travell JG, Simons DG. *Myofascial pain and dysfunction: the trigger point manual.* Vol. I. Baltimore: Williams & Wilkins, 1983:1–713.

313. Travell JG, Simons DG. *Myofascial pain and dysfunction: the trigger point manual.* Vol. II. Baltimore: Williams & Wilkins, 1991:1–607.

314. Basford JR. Physical agents and biofeedback. In: DeLisa JA, ed. *Rehabilitation medicine—principles and practice.* Philadelphia: JB Lippincott, 1988:404–424.

315. Lehmann JF, deLateur BJ. Diathermy and superficial heat, laser, and cold therapy. In: Kottke FJ, Lehmann JF, eds. *Krusen's handbook of physical medicine and rehabilitation.* 4th ed. Philadelphia: WB Saunders, 1990:283–367.

316. Knapp ME. Massage. In: Kottke FJ, Lehmann JF, eds. *Krusen's handbook of physical medicine and rehabilitation.* 4th ed. Philadelphia: WB Saunders, 1990:433–435.

317. Kloth L. Interference current. In: Nelson RM, Currier DP, eds. *Clinical electrotherapy.* Norwalk: Appleton & Lange, 1987: 183–207.

318. Sicard-Rosenbaum L, Lord D, Danoff JV, et al. Effects of continuous therapeutic ultrasound on growth and metastasis of subcutaneous murine tumors. *Phys Ther* 1995;75:3–13.

319. Hynynen K, Lulu BA. Hyperthermia in cancer treatment. *Investi Radiol* 1990;25:824–834.

320. Bicher HI, Wolfstein RS. Clinical use of regional hyperthermia. In: Bicher HI, McLaren JR, Pigliucci GM, eds. *Consensus on hyperthermia for the 1990's. Clinical practice in cancer treatment.* New York: Plenum 1990:1–36.

321. Graff-Radford SB, Reeves JL, Baker RL, Chiu D. Effects of transcutaneous electrical nerve stimulation on myofascial pain and trigger point sensitivity. *Pain* 1989;37:1–5.

322. Klein J, Pariser D. Transcutaneous electrical nerve stimulation. In: Nelson RM, Currier DP, eds. *Clinical electrotherapy.* Norwalk: Appleton & Lange, 1987:209–230.

323. Tyler E, Caldwell C, Ghia JN. Transcutaneous electrical nerve stimulation: an alternative approach to the management of postoperative pain. *Anesth Analg* 1982;61:449–456.

324. Cohen DJ. Overview of transcutaneous electrical nerve stimulation for treatment of acute postoperative pain. *Med Instrument* 1983;17:289–292.

325. Thompson JW, Filshie J. Transcutaneous electrical nerve stimulation (TENS) and acupuncture. In: Doyle D, Hanks GWC, MacDonald N, eds. *Oxford textbook of palliative medicine.* New York: Oxford University Press, 1993; 229–244.

326. Filshie J. The non-drug treatment of neuralgic and neuropathic pain of malignancy. *Cancer Surv* 1988;7:161–193.

327. Ferrell-Torry AT, Glick OJ. The use of therapeutic massage as a nursing intervention to modify anxiety and the perception of cancer pain. *Cancer Nurs* 1993;16:93–101.

Chapter 92

Rehabilitation and HIV Infection

Jay M. Meythaler

GENERAL OVERVIEW OF INFECTION

Biology and Natural History

Human immunodeficiency virus (HIV) is a member of the *Lenti virus* genus of the retrovirus family. Transmission of HIV is usually by intimate sexual contact, exposure to infected blood or blood products, or perinatally from mother to child (1,2). Retroviruses have a long latency period and mutate rapidly. They are noted for their ability to neutralize humoral immune response, which results in persistent viremia and leads to susceptibility of the host to secondary infections and diseases (cancers). HIV is a retrovirus infecting all cells with a CD4 receptor including CD4 lymphocytes, macrophages, and glial elements in the central nervous system (CNS) (2–4). Once the virus enters the CD4 cell, a DNA replica of viral RNA is synthesized utilizing the reverse transcriptase enzyme (5). Persons who are initially infected may experience a viral prodrome (6–8). The virus can also infect neurons and mucosal cells (5,9).

Acquired immunodeficiency syndrome (AIDS) is the final expression of the disease but the symptoms and sequelae can develop early in the disease course. The virus causes a selective deficit in the CD4 subset of lymphocytes (helper lymphocytes), resulting in a suppression of this subset. The Centers for Disease Control and Prevention (CDC) classification of HIV infection is based primarily on the history and clinical and laboratory findings (7). The diagnosis of AIDS is based on a defined set of clinical symptoms (Table 92-1) or a CD4 count of less than 200 cells/cm^3 (8). There appears to be a direct relationship between the CD4 helper cell count, which is the most important indicator of the degree of immunocompetence or dysfunction, and the development of AIDS (4,8). There can be latency periods of up to 12 years before there is an expression of the symptoms that can be diagnosed as AIDS. Many of the signs and symptoms that should lead one to suspect HIV infection are listed in Table 92-1.

Epidemiology and Demographics

During 1995 there were approximately 50,000 deaths related to HIV infection in the United States (10). However, the number fell in 1996 to a projected estimate of 44,000 for the first 6 months of 1996 (10). In 1993 AIDS became the leading cause of death for Americans between 25 and 44 years old (1). Among persons in this age group, HIV infection has remained the leading cause of death, accounting for 19% of the deaths in 1994 (11). The death rate was extremely high among non-Hispanic blacks, 41% for adults reported with AIDS (10). Women now constitute 20% of the deaths from AIDS, reflecting its increasingly heterosexual transmission (10). The actual number increased 5% and is estimated to have increased 10% in the last few years (11). Approximately 6000 births are to HIV-infected women annually. The largest yearly increases in the number of persons with AIDS occur in the 13- to 19-year and 20- to 29-year age group (11). While

Table 92-1: Physical Findings in HIV Disease

System	Signs and Symptoms	Possible Causes
General	Fever	HIV infection
	Weight loss	Opportunistic disease
	Fatigue	Malignant process
	Chronic pain	
Dermatologic	Rash	Seborrhea
	Dry skin	Kaposi sarcoma
	Papules	Molluscum contagiosum
	Macules	Herpes zoster
	Vesicles	Folliculitis
	Exfoliation	
Lymphatic	Swelling of cervical, axillary, or epitrochlear nodes	HIV infection
		Lymphoma
		MAI infection
		CMV infection
		Kaposi sarcoma
		Tuberculosis
Ocular	Peripheral field defects	CMV infection
	Cotton-wool spots	HIV infection
	Retinitis	Toxoplasmosis
Oral	White plaques	Candidiasis
	Ulceration	Oral hairy leukoplakia
	Purplish lesions	Kaposi sarcoma
	Periodontitis	Aphthous ulcer
		Herpes simplex
Cardiac	Third heart sound	Cardiomyopathy secondary to HIV infection
	Pericardial rub	CMV infection
	Cardiomegaly	Pericarditis
Pulmonary	Cough	*Pneumocystis carinii* pneumonia
	Rales	Bacterial pneumonia
	Rhonchi	Fungal infection
	Hypoxia	CMV pneumonia
		Tuberculosis
		Kaposi sarcoma
Gastrointestinal	Hepatomegaly	Hepatitis
	Splenomegaly	CMV infection
	Diarrhea	MAI infection
		Tuberculosis
		Toxoplasmosis
		Idiopathic thrombocytopenia purpura
		HIV infection
Genitourinary and perineal	Ulcerations	Herpes simplex
	Chancres	Chancroid
	Discharge	Syphilis
	Warts	Gonorrhea
	Fissures	Chlamydiosis
		Human papillomavirus infection
		Candidiasis
		Trichomoniasis
		Kaposi sarcoma
		Squamous cell carcinoma
Neurologic	Focal motor or sensory deficits	Central nervous system toxoplasmosis
	Spasticity	HIV infection
	Abnormal cognitive behavior	Lymphoma
	Incoordination	HIV-related myelopathy
	Ataxia	HIV-related dementia
	Loss of memory or concentration	Drug or metabolic delirium
	Decreased alertness	

MAI = *Mycobacterium avium-intracellulare*; CMV = cytomegalovirus.

almost 49,600 perished from AIDS in 1994, it is estimated that the death rate has leveled off (10,11).

The proportion of HIV-infected persons who will eventually go on to develop AIDS is high, almost 100% (12,13). With new medications and treatments it is expected that patients will survive longer after diagnosis. Once patients are exposed, they may or may not have a symptomatic viral prodrome a few weeks after infection. They will not seroconvert until 3 to 6 months later. Patients may be asymptomatic for varying time periods, but the average time to symptomatic infection is approximately 2 years (6,14).

Studies utilizing combination medications demonstrated that there will be a reduction in the morbidity of the disease and extended life after infection (15,16). The final result, however delayed, is a diminished immunologic system, with patients prone to opportunistic infections such as cytomegalovirus (CMV) infection, fungal infections such as candidiasis, and bacterial infections (*Pneumocystis carinii* is one of the most common pathogens). The median survival time of patients after the development of symptoms defined as "AIDS" can be over 20 months (14,17). Consequently, rehabilitation interventions can be of considerable benefit, improving the quality of life and reducing the cost of the illness.

Causes of Disability

The National Mortality Followback Survey suggested that 40% to 60% of AIDS patients require assistance or special equipment with activities of daily living (ADLs) and ambulation in the final year of life (18). Nine percent of HIV-infected individuals require assistance with ADLs and 22% of AIDS patients have difficulties with some ADLs at the time of first medical contact (18).

Various factors associated with HIV infection are related to the development of disability. Approximately 60% of AIDS patients require assistance in one area and 30% in 5 or more of the 18 areas evaluated by the Functional Independence Measure (FIM) (18). Rarely is one single impairment to blame. Urologic problems are rare, but infectious diarrhea is common (19). A lack of family support and the overwhelmed poorly staffed volunteer support systems are of considerable concern (20).

Rehabilitation Goals

Since the complications of HIV infection are as varied as those found in cancer, it is clear that rehabilitation intervention requires tailoring according to the manifestations and symptoms of the illness. The ultimate goals are to improve function and limit disability. Only in this way can clinicians improve the quality of life and limit the cost to society of the disease. For most patients this will involve an outpatient approach.

Rehabilitation physicians will need to present themselves to the directors of various outpatient AIDS clinics and make themselves available for consultation (17). Experience is the best teacher for both provider and patient as to how the physician may help combat the problem. This large area of medicine is essentially "untapped" by rehabilitation service providers in many areas of the United States. With the availability of research money there is potential for the development of more effective and significant rehabilitation interventions for this often devastating, disabling condition.

Social Consequences

One must consider the uncertainty of those infected with HIV. Generally the person has a fatal illness with no cure. The person is left to put his or her own affairs in order. If family and friends were unaware previously of an individual's HIV status, secrecy is now impossible once there is a manifestation of symptoms (21). Add to this the grim issues of guilt and possible rejection by family, and the health care provider is confronted by a patient more isolated than most any other one would encounter. Family and sexual counseling is required in most circumstances.

The National Association of People with AIDS has identified finances as the most important concern for persons with AIDS (22). While studies have identified that most persons infected with HIV were employed at the same rate as other Americans prior to the onset of symptoms, there is a rapid drop-off in employment after symptoms develop and a coincidental drop in coverage by private health care insurance (23). This results in many AIDS patients relying on the public sector for assistance. Vocational rehabilitation services are often necessary to keep these persons employed, involved in society, and less of a burden on society.

As treatment improves, so do morbidity and disability. However, the cost is staggering, with an estimated $10.3 billion spent just for medical treatment in the United States in 1992, and this amount was expected to rise by almost 50% by 1995 (24). In 1993 the lifetime costs for treating a person with HIV infection in the United States had been estimated retrospectively at $115,000 (25). This causes a significant strain on both the private and public medical insurance system.

NEUROLOGIC ISSUES

Autopsy findings have noted neurologic involvement in 80% to 90% of patients who have AIDS (26). Indeed, neurologic symptoms are reported in 40% of those diagnosed as having AIDS and are the first presenting symptoms in 10% to 20% (27,28).

Central Nervous System: Brain

HIV encephalopathy is also known as *AIDS dementia*, and has an estimated prevalence of 16% to 90% in AIDS patients (28–31). AIDS dementia complex typically presents after AIDS is diagnosed, but it can be the presenting symptom in many AIDS patients (30,32,33). Up to 65% of AIDS patients develop cognitive deficits during the course of their disease (34). Patients will typically present with forgetfulness, loss of concentration and spontaneity, apathy, and social withdrawal (9,27,31). One-third to one-half of AIDS patients will have late manifestations such as lower-extremity weakness, ataxia, hypertonia, incontinence, and an inability to perform complex ADLs (9,27). In most cases the dementia is progressive. Some patients exhibit a rapid decline, whereas others may follow a slower course, the rate probably being related to the underlying cause of the dementia (30,31). In the advanced stages, severe dementia and mutism may appear and can progress to a persistent vegetative state (9,18,27). Others may demonstrate frank psychosis (35).

HIV encephalopathy is believed to be caused in part by direct cortical invasion by the AIDS virus, and this form is thought to have a distinct clinical presentation (30,31,36). While HIV type-1 (HIV-1) has been directly linked to the development of dementia, many diffuse secondary infections and processes may also contribute. In most patients significant cognitive deficits probably do not occur before there is clinical evidence of immune system compromise (28,37). Severe dementia is seen in only 5% to 10% of patients with AIDS at end stage (28,38). Consequently, the prognosis of AIDS dementia complex is poor and survival can probably be measured in months (27,28,36).

Distinct from the dementia complexes are the encephalopathies and the meningitis that can develop. HIV itself causes aseptic meningitis in 5% to 10% of patients (31). Patients will typically present with fever, headache, meningeal signs, and cranial nerve involvement (31). Occasionally, aseptic meningitis due to HIV is the presenting symptom in the development of AIDS (29). The clinical course is usually self-limited or recurrent, rather than progressive in nature (29,31).

Cryptococcal meningitis patients present with the classic findings of chronic meningitis. Organisms (*Cryptococcus neoformans*) typically are seen in a cerebrospinal fluid (CSF) preparation with India ink (36,39). The onset is usually characterized by a subacute course characterized by headache, fever, and malaise, but with relatively normal findings on neuroimaging studies (27). Treatment usually consists of amphotericin B with concurrent use of flucytosine and fluconazole (39). The use of maintenance fluconazole after the initial induction of treatment can substantially decrease the relapse rate (40). However, survival time is still in the several-month range (27,41).

Toxoplasmosis is a common subclinical infection in most persons in the United States, with antibodies demonstrated in 40% to 90% of adults (17,28,42). Toxoplasmosis is the most common and a potentially reversible focal CNS lesion in AIDS patients, occurring in 3% to 40% of patients (17,28,36,43). Single or multiple ring enhancing lesions may be demonstrated on contrast-enhanced computed tomography (CT) scans or magnetic resonance images (MRIs). Definitive diagnosis is established by stereotactic biopsy. It usually responds to treatment with pyrimethamine and sulfonamides, and treatment is usually begun prophylactically in patients with a significantly elevated antibody titer (17,28,42).

Progressive multifocal leukoencephalopathy (PML) has been linked to papovavirus infection and typically appears as a late complication of chronic diseases that are associated with impaired cellular immunity (36). The usual presentation is focal to multifocal neurologic signs in the absence of fever and headache (27). PML has also been directly linked to HIV infection. It has a relatively poor prognosis and patients rarely survive more than 18 months (27,41).

The most common noninfectious, focal cerebral process in AIDS is CNS lymphoma (27,41). Lymphoma usually presents slowly. It occasionally will respond to palliative radiation therapy or chemotherapy (36,41,44). However, the long-term prognosis is relatively poor. Focal neurologic deficits may develop in patients whose lesions have been treated or resected, and the resulting syndromes are often associated with the anatomic area of the brain involved.

Herpesvirus encephalitis usually presents with the typical symptoms of encephalitis (45). High-dose oral or intravenous acyclovir appears to decrease the duration and severity of the infection. The emergence of resistant strains in HIV-infected patients has been reported. Herpes is well known to cause marked focal lesions, particularly in the frontal lobes and temporal lobes. Memory deficits are very common in these patients (45). As the swelling from the infection is controlled, some neurologic recovery can occur.

AIDS has also been linked to an increased risk for cerebrovascular accident (CVA). Thrombotic, embolic, and hemorrhagic strokes can occur in patients with HIV infection (27,28,36). Although the reported prevalence was as high as 34% of AIDS patients in one study, most CVAs are small and not clinically evident (26).

Cerebral toxoplasmosis infection is the most treatable cause of thrombotic CVAs associated with AIDS (41). These strokes generally carry a survival rate of 4 to 24 months; probably most present after the development of AIDS (27,28,41,46).

Rehabilitation Interventions

Patients may have global cognitive and neurologic issues that are similar to those seen with traumatic brain injury (28,47): The treatment program is often similar to an acquired brain injury program, with one major difference, however. The goal of the latter is to obtain a full potential recovery. For HIV-infected patients, the goal is to make the patient as functional as possible, or to return the patient home, if feasible, as soon as possible. Some of the rehabilitation issues to be confronted are motor weakness or paralysis, cognitive deficits, behavioral dyscontrol, attentional and memory problems, verbal aphasias, and spasticity (45,48).

In patients with CVA there are often hemiparesis and aphasia. For these patients a short acute, intensive inpatient stroke rehabilitation program should be provided (41). The focus should be on improving function to reduce the stress placed on home providers. In patients where the burden of care or the independence of the individual may result in a significant enhancement in the quality of life, a longer length of stay should be considered. Once home, the patient can continue the rehabilitation process on an outpatient basis.

Central Nervous System: Spinal Cord

Spinal cord involvement has been noted by autopsy in 20% or more of AIDS patients (28,49). Patients often present with symptoms of ataxia and spastic paraparesis, similar to the subacute degeneration noted with many other neurologic diseases (28,36). An isolated finding of spinal cord involvement, without other signs and symptoms of neurologic involvement, is rare. Most often the involvement is associated with AIDS dementia complex (28). There is no correlation between the severity of the dementia and the severity of myelopathy (31,50,51). Neuroimaging is useful to rule out mass effects on the spinal cord, such as an abscess or neoplastic tumor, which are the most treatable causes (36).

HIV-related myelopathy (vacuolar myelopathy) is noted in 11% to 22% of AIDS patients and is strongly associated with encephalopathy (9,34,52). It presents as a progressive motor and sensory paraparesis, often with symptoms of bowel and bladder dysfunction, gait ataxia, and spasticity (36). Brew (53) suggested that treatment with the antiretroviral agents commonly utilized to treat AIDS may be of benefit in reversing the course of neurologic deficits.

Varicella-zoster infection of the spinal cord may develop due to the immunocompromised condition of the patient (45). As with herpesvirus encephalitis, high-dose oral or intravenous acyclovir appears to decrease the duration and severity of the infection, but the emergence of resistant strains has been reported (45,54).

CMV infection has been linked to the development of HIV-related encephalitis and myelopathy (45). Recently, prophylaxis with ganciclovir when the CD4 count is less than $100/cm^3$ was found to be useful in preventing the development of symptoms (39).

More unusual presentations include an amyotrophic lateral sclerosis–like syndrome and a form of fulminant multiple sclerosis (55–57). All of these cases are an example of the diversity of neurologic conditions that can be associated with AIDS.

Rehabilitation Interventions

Patients with myelopathy present with problems similar to a patient with spinal cord injury including quadriparesis or paraparesis. Consequently, similar rehabilitation interventions are utilized. The clinician should focus particular attention on proper bowel and bladder care. Patients are usually immunocompromised and particularly prone to diarrhea and the complications of urinary tract infection. In many cases, rehabilitation providers need to be prepared for increased functional deficits from further neurologic deterioration.

Peripheral Nervous System

Subclinical evidence of peripheral neuropathy is found in 50% to 90% of patients with AIDS (36,56). This usually presents clinically and by electromyography (EMG) as a distal motor/sensory neuropathy (50,56,58,59). However, a symmetric sensory neuropathy occurs in 30% of patients with advanced disease (60). Pathologic studies indicate a primary axonal loss with associated patchy demyelination (61). The typical symptoms in both cases are painful dysesthesias, numbness, and paresthesias (28). Neurologic examination may demonstrate an absence of ankle jerks (9,36).

Distal peripheral neuropathies have been associated with some of the drugs used to treat AIDS, particularly didanosine and zalcitabine (62,63). Electrodiagnostic findings are consistent with a primary axonal polyneuropathy.

There have been increased reports of inflammatory demyelinating neuropathies associated with HIV infection (64,65). Both Guillain-Barré syndrome (GBS) and chronic inflammatory demyelinating polyneuropathy (CIDP) have been reported (36,64,65). Therefore it is recommended that any patient diagnosed with GBS be screened for HIV infection (66). Besides the classic EMG findings, CSF analysis may reveal pleocytosis and oligoclonal bands, and HIV may be found in culture (66). In some patients with GBS or CIDP, plasmapheresis or intravenous immunoglobulin (IVIg) are clinically helpful (66–68). Although some have suggested that the acute form of GBS associated with HIV infection carries a worse functional prognosis, over the short term the prognosis appears to be no different from that for idiopathic GBS (65).

Infection with CMV has been noted to result in a progressive ascending polyradicular syndrome that is distinct from the inflammatory demyelinating neuropathies associated with CMV infection (69,70). It presents as an ascending flaccid paresis. CMV infection that presents in this manner is usually fatal, although there has been some recent success with the use of ganciclovir (39,71,72).

Other peripheral neuropathies include compression neuropathies, the most common of which are ulnar and peroneal nerve neuropathies in bed-bound patients, secondary to immobilization (9,73). A vasculitic neuropathy has also been noted in immunocompromised patients. It presents as a mononeuropathy multiplex and is usually secondary to varicella-zoster infection (36,74).

Autonomic neuropathy is fairly common in patients with AIDS or HIV infection (36,75,76). It generally accompanies the more severe peripheral neuropathies and polyradiculoneuropathies and is clinically manifested by postural hypotension, hypertension and excessive sympathetic outflow, or bladder and bowel dysfunction. Severe postural hypotension frequently occurs in patients requiring inpatient rehabilitation (77,78). A recent review of the literature involving dysautonomia estimated that 19% to 50% of patients with an acute inflammatory polyradiculoneuropathy in a hospital setting will have evidence of postural hypotension (77). Patients with excessive sympathetic outflow and hypertension also appear to have extreme sensitivity to vasoactive drugs (77,79). With suctioning, such patients are prone to develop episodes of dysautonomia (80). Similarly, patients with acute demyelinating polyradiculoneuropathy are at risk for cardiac arrhythmia (81).

Rehabilitation Interventions

Beyond the usual acute treatment with steroids, plasmapheresis, or IVIg, rehabilitation is primarily directed toward strengthening and preserving remaining motor function, maintaining or increasing joint range of motion (ROM), and improving endurance (66).

There have been few studies of physical therapy in HIV-infected patients (28). Generally clinicians have adopted the approaches based on experience with other diseases. However, rehabilitation requires an organized program with defined end points. Clinical findings may be diverse, from quadriparesis to isolated weakness of the arm, leg, facial muscles, or oropharynx. It has been suggested that overfatiguing affected motor units in therapy may impede recovery (82,83). Overworking muscle groups in patients with peripheral nerve involvement has been clinically associated with paradoxical weakening (83).

Muscle weakness has been associated with muscle shortening and resultant joint contractures. These complications can be prevented by daily ROM exercises (73). Depending on the amount of weakness, the exercise can be passive, active-assistive, or active. Proper positioning of patients is necessary. Initial exercise even in the acutely ill can include a program of gradual strengthening involving isometric, low-resistive isotonic, isokinetic, and active nonresistive exercises carefully tailored to the clinical condition of the patient (73). Orthotics should be prescribed to aid in proper positioning of the joint and to aid residual motor function. The utilization of assistive devices for ambulation such as orthotics and gait aids may significantly improve function.

Some patients have decreased vibratory and joint position sensation. Proprioceptive losses can lead to ataxia and incoordination, resulting in increased functional deficits. Therapy directed toward improving balance and coordination can be useful.

Any suggestion that dysautonomia is clinically insignificant is incorrect. Treatment of dysautonomia should be directed toward physical modalities such as use of a compression hose, abdominal binders, and proper hydration. While most patients admitted to inpatient rehabilitation are not threatened by cardiac arrhythmias, they may still have problems with postural hypotension and other autonomic symptoms (77). Clinicians need to consider potential autonomic consequences when selecting medications for disease treatment or symptom control. Adverse autonomic effects are likely to complicate or slow the rehabilitation process.

Pain accounts for 17% to 34% of the referrals involving patients with AIDS to physiatrists (9). The types of pain include paresthesias, dysesthesias, axial and radicular pain, meningism, myalgia, joint pain, and visceral discomfort (9,84). Clearly, neuropathic pain is a significant contributor. Symptoms of mild depression, indicated by persistent mental fatigue, may be exacerbated by deafferent pain syndromes (66).

Treatment of pain has generally been directed by previous clinical experience, with the prominent use of modalities, tricyclic antidepressants, nonsteroidal anti-inflammatory drugs (NSAIDs), mexiletine, and in some patients, carbamazepine (9). More recently there have been verbal reports on the use of topical capsaicin and transcutaneous electrical stimulation to specific anatomic areas of well-localized deafferent pain (28,85). One report linked pain in the limbs and axial skeleton to impaired joint mobility in GBS (86). GBS patients with severe pain may have a poor tolerance for activity, which could result in a longer stay for inpatient rehabilitation.

Myopathies

Myopathies associated with HIV infection are often severe and disabling when they present (9,87–89). Autoimmune polymyositis is an early manifestation of HIV infection, generally preceding full-blown AIDS (90). It usually is steroid responsive (91,92). Late myopathies are much more serious and disabling (9,91).

A spectrum of pathologic changes in muscle has been observed in patients with HIV-associated myopathy. It includes noninflammatory infiltrates, nemaline rod bodies, and cytoplasmic bodies (91). EMG findings are consistent with myopathy (91). Patients can be advanced, as tolerated, to low-resistance strengthening exercises, in combination with strengthening using functional activities (transfers, ADLs, etc). Some subjects with myopathy have also been noted to have nerve conduction abnormalities such as reduced-amplitude sensory nerve action potentials and mildly prolonged distal nerve conduction velocities (91).

Steroids have been found to be clinically effective, leading to improvement in strength and reduction of creatinine kinase (CK) levels (91). Also, plasmapheresis has been reported to be useful (93). The treatment of HIV-infected patients with steroids must be carefully weighed against the possible side effects of steroids (9). While the use of steroids has not been fully evaluated, no significant acceleration in the course of HIV infection has been noted (91,94).

Myopathies have been associated with the use of

zidovudine (9,91). Patients usually present with disabling myalgias (67,91). These patients have muscle biopsy findings generally consistent with mitochondrial myopathy with prevalent ragged red fibers (91,92). Other histologic changes include inflammatory infiltrates and cytoplasmic bodies (91). The myopathy due to zidovudine use is usually seen after 9 months or more of drug use (67). These patients generally respond to a withdrawal of zidovudine (92). Patients also respond to prednisone and nonsteroidal anti-inflammatory agents (91).

Progressive weakness indicative of myopathy is also a feature of the ambiguously defined HIV wasting syndrome (91,95). Clinical, laboratory, and muscle biopsy findings have been consistent with myopathy (95). Corticosteroids are reportedly effective, but the withdrawal of zidovudine has had no effect on the course (91,95).

Rehabilitation Interventions

Similar to the peripheral neuropathies, there is a need for the clinician to avoid overwork or overfatigue of diseased muscles, as this can lead to increased muscle fiber necrosis (9,91). Patients with myopathy often present with progressive proximal weakness manifested by a difficulty with climbing stairs and rising from a chair (91). Joint protection techniques coupled with energy conservation methods are useful in the early symptomatic stages of illness.

Once the acute stage of myopathy has been medically treated, a gentle exercise program is useful (96). As noted with other myopathies, active ROM exercises can be initiated as soon as creatinine phosphokinase levels fall near normal (97). Adaptive equipment and physical therapy for the muscles of respiration have been reported to be of therapeutic value (9). This is extremely important since respiratory insufficiency combined with an immunocompromised state is the most common and disabling manifestation of AIDS (28,98).

ARTHRITIS AND RHEUMATOLOGIC DISORDERS

The arthritic conditions present as either a transient disorder or a chronic disorder (9). Fibromyalgias have been demonstrated in 11% to 29% of HIV-seropositive patients, and the incidence probably exceeds that seen in the general medical population (99). Arthralgias have a reported incidence of between 11% and 40% and may be associated with fibromyalgias (100–103). Generally they affect the lower limbs more than the upper limbs, particularly the ankles and knees (9). Both conditions probably contribute to complaints of pain and fatigue in AIDS patients.

Inflammatory arthritis such as Reiter syndrome, reactive arthritis, psoriatic arthritis, and an AIDS-associated arthritis have been reported (104,105). Occasionally, Sjögren syndrome, often associated with a lymphadenopathy, will appear. Treatment is symptomatic utilizing artificial tears, increased fluids, and careful dental hygiene (9). The mechanism by which HIV infection causes arthritis is multifactorial and may be related directly to the virus, to immunologic dysfunction secondary to the HIV infection, or to secondary infection by opportunistic agents (99,106).

Rehabilitation Interventions

Acutely swollen, hot, painful joints should be treated by rest and isometric exercises to strengthen muscles that improve joint stability. Treatment with NSAIDs, physical modalities, and analgesics is indicated at this stage (107). Orthotics can help protect and stabilize joints (9,99). They may also be necessary to correct or prevent the development of joint deformities.

Once the acute synovitis has resolved, active nonresistive ROM and gentle isotonic exercises may commence. Muscle strengthening should utilize isometric exercises to improve joint stability, often combined with splinting. Patient education in the use of energy conservation techniques, joint protection methods, and body mechanics by therapists can be quite useful.

VISION

Human CMV is an important pathogen in HIV-infected persons, and 90% of patients with AIDS have evidence of CMV infection at autopsy (71,108). CMV retinitis affects up to 25% to 40% of adult AIDS patients (71). Medical intervention may slow the course, but generally it only serves to delay the ultimate onset of blindness (9,109,110). It often is the first sign of CMV involvement, and systemic problems (particularly neurologic) may soon ensue (39,72,108). Both ganciclovir and foscarnet have been reported to be useful for treatment and prophylaxis (39,71,108,109).

Recently, the eye and head movements of HIV-infected patients have been noted to be reduced in accuracy, compared with those in normal subjects (110). In patients with CNS dysfunction, abnormalities in vertical eye movements and smooth pursuit gaze have been sensitive and consistent indicators of CNS dysfunction (110).

Rehabilitation Interventions

Appropriate rehabilitation interventions include referral to an appropriate low-vision clinic and education concerning ADL methods for the visually impaired. One must be sensitive to changes in the ability to track and focus the eyes, as these may be indicative of disease progression (110).

OTHER MEDICAL COMPLICATIONS

Fatigue

Fatigue is a multifactorial problem related to the various medical conditions that develop in association with HIV infection, and consequently, it is the most common symptom in AIDS (99,111). It may be related to the various secondary medical conditions associated with AIDS. However, 6% to 9% of patients with HIV infection who have not developed AIDS also have symptoms of fatigue (112,113). Some have suggested that psychological states such as depression, which may be related to the issue of facing a debilitating and ultimately fatal illness, are a primary cause (111,112,114).

Rehabilitation Interventions

Psychological counseling and antidepressants may be of particular use. In many patients, fatigue is due to medical causes that can be addressed. In others, conditions such as chronic pain, anemia, arthralgias, cardiopulmonary restrictions, or myopathies cause fatigue. In patients with CNS involvement and fatigue, amantadine and methylphenidate, which reduce fatigue in similar neurologic conditions, may be beneficial (115–119).

Cardiopulmonary

Pneumocystis carinii pneumonia (PCP) infects up to 85% of AIDS patients and is readily treatable (9,120). Patients may also have other pneumonias caused by bacteria (especially *Streptococcus pneumoniae* and *Haemophilus influenzae*), fungi (*Cryptococcus neoformans*, *Histoplasma capsulatum*, *Aspergillus fumigatus*), and viruses (CMV and herpes simplex) (121,122). *Mycobacterium tuberculosis* is also a common pathogen in AIDS patients (122). Appropriate treatment can limit the sequelae of these infections (39). Decisions regarding prophylaxis for opportunistic infections are based on illness staging (4,39,123). In particular, when CD4 counts are less than 200 cells/μL, the risk for PCP increases sharply (124). Many patients are placed on prophylactic antibiotics, which has decreased the incidence of pulmonary infections (39,124). In patients who present with pulmonary complications from malignancies such as non-Hodgkin lymphoma and Kaposi sarcoma, the prognosis is particularly grim (125).

The most frequent manifestations of cardiac involvement in HIV-infected persons are cardiomyopathy, followed by pericardial disease and valvular damage (126,127). However, cardiac disease is symptomatic in only 5% of those with HIV infection (127). In patients with pulmonary symptoms, the clinician should check for cardiomegaly in addition to lung findings on chest radiographs (127).

Rehabilitation Interventions

The principles of a pulmonary rehabilitation program should be employed. The goals should be to reverse the pathophysiologic processes, improve quality of life, and if appropriate, prolong life (128). Generally the best results are obtained when such a program is initiated early (28). Patients should be encouraged to stop smoking. All persons and their potential caregivers should be instructed on exercise methods, breathing techniques, chest physiotherapy, and proper nutrition. A "6-minute walking test" and use of a visual analog scale have been suggested for evaluation of outcome of a pulmonary rehabilitation program (126).

As with pulmonary manifestations, the first objective in a cardiac rehabilitation program should be reversal of the pathophysiologic processes. Digoxin, vasodilators, angiotensin-converting enzyme (ACE) inhibitors, and diuretics should be employed to improve cardiac function (126). These drugs will lower preload or afterload on the heart (129). Exercise can then be initiated utilizing frequent rest breaks, with fatigue and dyspnea as clinical indicators (129). A "long-duration, low-intensity" exercise program was in non-HIV-infected cardiac patients improved functional performance in a relatively short period of time (129). Similar results should be achievable utilizing these exercises to improve the quality of life in HIV-seropositive patients.

Oral and Gastrointestinal

The oral manifestations of HIV infection occur secondary to a variety of opportunistic infections and neoplasms (130). Most common are the oral form of candidiasis and hairy leukoplakia, which may be predictive of the development of AIDS (131). In AIDS patients, unusual forms of gingivitis and periodontal disease, as well as herpes simplex and herpes zoster lesions, are noted (130). In patients with dysphagia, CMV infection and various neoplastic diseases have been described (130).

Weight loss, cachexia, dysphagia, anorexia, and diarrhea are almost universally found at some point or other in the course of AIDS (19). Diarrhea is experienced by over 50% of patients with AIDS and specific pathogens may be isolated from 75% to 80% of patients (19). Most patients with wasting fail to meet minimal caloric consumption to support their metabolism (19). These gastrointestinal problems and reduced intake may affect drug absorption, particularly for those drugs whose absorption is dependent on being taken with food (132).

Rehabilitation Interventions

Regular dental care, an important part of ADL training, is vital because periodontal disease can be virulent in HIV-infected patients (133). For patients with a CD4 count of less than 500 cells/μL, an oral rinse with chlorhexidine gluconate twice daily is recommended (133). Dysphagia frequently results from infection of the oropharynx, often with esophageal extension, by *Candida* species, herpes simplex, or CMV. Therapy evaluation should include an oral examination, oral motor examination, and videofluoroscopy (9). Assuring appropriate nutrition will have a significant impact on endurance.

THE REHABILITATION PATIENT WITH CONCURRENT HIV INFECTION

It must be recognized that HIV-infected patients are at no less risk than the rest of the population for cardiovascular events, trauma, fractures, arthritis, and other disorders that benefit from rehabilitation services. The rehabilitation issues associated with these conditions often have no medical connection to the infection, and as such, the HIV infection is completely incidental to the disease processes that require treatment. It is important that rehabilitation physicians know the health and infection disease status of HIV-positive patients under their care. Concurrent HIV infection by itself should not contribute to the disability or change the goals for rehabilitation unless the patient has the symptoms of AIDS.

The clinician should be aware of the numerous specialities that deal with the complications of AIDS, such as infectious disease, pulmonary medicine, neurology, ophthalmology, gastroenterology, and oncology. All physicians who care for HIV-positive persons need to be aware of the various laboratory and clinical findings that predict the progression to AIDS (134). HIV-positive patients may present to rehabilitation for conditions other than those related to the infection, particularly trauma (135). It must be noted that trauma is an immunocompromising event and may result in the development of AIDS in the rehabilitation setting (135). Many of the conditions associated with major trauma such as weight loss, anemia, fevers of unknown origin, respiratory infections, urinary tract infections, and altered anergy panels develop in patients without HIV infection (135). It is not clear how the presence of trauma or these associated conditions should affect the decison of whether or not to initiate early antiretroviral therapy.

Table 92-2: Evaluation of Patients with New Diagnosis of HIV Infection

History
Including past immunizations
Physical examination
Including examination of ocular fundus and, in women, pelvic examination with Pap smear
Vaccinations
Polyvalent pneumococcal vaccine (Pneumovax 23, Pnu-Imune 23)
Influenza virus vaccine (Flu-Imune, Fluogen, Fluzone)
Consideration of hepatitis B vaccine (Engerix B, Heptavax-B, Recombivax HB)
Consideration of *Haemophilus influenzae* type b conjugate vaccine (HibTITER)
Laboratory studies
Complete blood cell count with differential
Platelet count
Chemistry panel, including creatinine kinase and liver enzyme levels
VDRL test
Hepatitis B surface antigen and antibody tests
Toxoplasmosis IgG serology
Glucose-6-phosphate dehydrogenase enzyme level
CD4+ T-lymphocyte count and percentage of total lymphocytes
Chest film
Tuberculin skin test with anergy battery including candidiasis and mumps
Pap smear

Medical Issues

When obtaining a past medical history, the clinician should note all previous diseases, especially tuberculosis, mononucleosis, varicella zoster, toxoplasmosis, histoplasmosis, coccidiomycosis, hepatitis, herpes simplex, candidiasis, and sexually transmitted diseases (133). These other "medical stresses" may increase the likelihood that AIDS has developed.

It was recently noted that many physicians miss the prominent clinical findings of HIV infection (136). Since asymptomatic carriers of HIV infection can also have a catastrophic illness such as trauma from a car accident, it is important for the rehabilitation physician to be familiar with the work-up and physical findings of HIV infection (133). The basic laboratory tests listed in Table 92-2 need to be performed on admission (133,137).

A number of clinical regimens can be useful in AIDS patients to prevent the development of opportunistic infections and treat their complications. Physicians treating these patients should be familiar with these regimens (Table 92-3).

The treatment of HIV infection and its complications can lead to significant medical complications that contribute to functional deficits (Tables 92-4 to 92-8). Zidovudine (AZT) has been noted to cause bone marrow suppression (133) (see Table 92-7). Another medication, didanosine, may improve morbidity and mortality but has been noted to produce peripheral neuropathy in up to 34% of those treated and pancreatitis in 9% (62) (see Table 82-7). Zalcitabine reportedly improves CD4 counts when used with zidovudine, but its use may also contribute to the development of peripheral neuropathy and occasionally pancreatitis (133) (see Table 92-7). The three medications zidovudine, saquinavir, and zalcitabine are associated with a 6% incidence of adverse effects when utilized in combination for improved efficacy against HIV-1 (15).

Recently, the protease inhibitors saquinavir, ritonavir, indinavir, and nelfinavir have emerged as critical drugs for patients with HIV-1 infection (132). These drugs have apparently unique safety and tolerability profiles (see Table 92-8). Saquinavir is the best tolerated but still causes nausea, diarrhea, abdominal discomfort, or rash and should be taken with a high fat–containing meal for best absorption (132). Ritonavir has convenient twice-a-day dosing but has been associated with considerable side effects including mild to moderate diarrhea, nausea, vomiting, anorexia, headaches, asthenia, fatigue, circumoral paresthesia, and taste disturbances (132). These side effects resulted in 17% of patients with advanced AIDS discontinuing this drug in one study (132). Indinavir is believed to

Table 92-3: Treatment of Infections Associated with AIDS			
Disease	**Primary Agents and Techniques**	**Alternatives**	**Comments**
Pneumocystis pneumonia	Trimethoprim-sulfamethoxazole Parenteral pentamidine isethionate (Pentam 300)	Trimethoprim (Proloprim, Trimpex) plus dapsone Clindamycin (Cleocin) plus primaquine phosphate BW566C80 Trimetrexate glucuronate, which must be given with leucovorin calcium (Wellcovorin)	Avoid aerosolized pentamidine isethionate (NebuPent) as sole therapy If $PaO_2 < 70\,mm\,Hg$ or $PAO_2 - PaO_2 > 35\,mm\,Hg$, concomitant corticosteroid therapy is indicated
Toxoplasmosis	Pyrimethamine (Daraprim) plus sulfadiazine with leucovorin	Pyrimethamine plus clindamycin BW566C80	—
Cryptosporidiosis, *Microsporidia* infection	Supportive therapy Octreotide acetate (Sandostatin) Hyperalimentation	—	No known effective antimicrobial agents Paromomycin sulfate (Humatin) and azithromycin (Zithromax) under study for cryptosporidiosis Albendazole (Zentel) under study for *Microsporidia* infection
Cytomegalovirus disease	Ganciclovir sodium (Cytovene) Foscarnet sodium (Foscavir)	Intravitreal ganciclovir (can be used in cases of retinitis if toxicity makes systemic therapy impossible)	—
Herpes simplex	Acyclovir (Zovirax)	Foscarnet (useful for acyclovir-resistant virus strains)	—
Cryptococcal disease	Amphotericin B (Fungizone)	Fluconazole (Diflucan) used to prevent recurrences and as primary therapy in selected cases	—
Candidiasis	Clotrimazole (Mycelex) Ketoconazole (Nizoral) Fluconazole	Amphotericin B (rarely necessary)	—
Histoplasmosis	Amphotericin B	Itraconazole (Sporanox) may prevent recurrence	Monitoring of *Histoplasma* antigen may be helpful
Mycobacterium avium-intracellulare infection	Combination of 4 or 5 of the following: ethambutol hydrochloride (Myambutol), clofazimine (Lamprene), ciprofloxacin (Cipro), amikacin sulfate (Amikin), clarithromycin (Biaxin Filmtabs), rifampin (Rifadin, Rimactane), rifabutin (Mycobutin)		Optimal regimen not defined
Tuberculosis	Isoniazid (Nydrazid) Rifampin (with pyrazinamide for first 2 mo)		Be alert for multiple drug-resistant viral isolates; alter regimen if drug resistance suspected Drug susceptibility testing and monitoring of compliance and response essential
Syphilis	Parenteral penicillin		Optimal management unclear Consider possibility of neurosyphilis

Table 92-4: Antibacterial Therapy

Drug	Major Adverse Reactions	Interactions
Trimethoprim-sulfamethoxazole	Rash Fever Transaminase elevation Neutropenia Nausea/vomiting Thrombocytopenia Hyperkalemia	Warfarin: increased prothrombin time Procainamide: decreased clearance by trimethoprim Phenytoin: increased half-life of phenytoin Dapsone: increased dapsone levels by trimethoprim
Dapsone	Rash Nausea/vomiting Anemia Methemoglobinemia Transaminase elevation Neutropenia Thrombocytopenia	Trimethoprim: increased trimethoprim levels by dapsone Rifampin: decreased half-life of dapsone ddI: decreased absorption of dapsone
Pentamidine	Nephrotoxicity Hypoglycemia* Hyperglycemia Transaminase elevation Hyperkalemia Neutropenia Thrombocytopenia Pancreatitis* Ventricular arrhythmia*	Foscarnet: severe hypocalcemia, increased risk of nephrotoxicity

* Potentially life-threatening.

be relatively safe and well tolerated (132). The most common adverse effects of indinavir have been nephrolithiasis, occurring in approximately 5% of patients, and a benign elevation of indirect bilirubin (132). The clinical experience with the protease inhibitor nelfinavir is limited and the most common side effect is diarrhea (132).

Various antibiotics can also lead to complications. Trimethoprim-sulfamethoxazole, which is utilized in the treatment and prophylaxis of *Pneumocystis carnii* infection, may affect glucose-6-phosphate dehydrogenase enzyme levels in those who may have a hereditary deficiency of this enzyme (133). A similar problem is noted in those who utilize oral dapsone (133).

Psychosocial and Psychiatric Issues

Life-threatenning and chronic diseases such as AIDS may be complicated by psychiatric symptoms and conditions (20). Neuropsychological impairment can precede a diagnosis of symptomatic AIDS (30). HIV-induced organic brain disease can cause symptoms indistinguishable from functional psychosis (138,139). For instance, many patients with HIV dementia may have disorders of mood and behavior rather than disorders of cognition. Consequently, the standard Mini-Mental Status Examination may not be sensitive for picking up all the neurocognitive disorders associated with AIDS (140).

Rehabilitation professionals need to recognize that many HIV-linked psychiatric syndromes may mimick purely functional disorders. In others, psychiatric conditions and mood disorders may be preexisting and exacerbated by the stressor of being HIV seropositive. The six major neuropsychiatric syndromes identified as complications of HIV infection are 1) depression, 2) dementia/organic brain disease, 3) anxiety/panic disorder, 4) delirium, 5) mania, and 6) psychosis (20). It is well established that depression is more common in medical patients, particularly those suffering from carcer and CNS disorders (141,142). The current prevalence of depression in HIV-seropositive persons is estimated to range between 4% and 14% (143). Dementia is a significant issue, with up to 70% of AIDS patients presenting with clinical signs of organic brain dysfunction (20). There is usually an underlying organic brain disorder in HIV patients with mania or psychosis (20).

Rehabilitation Intervention

Those confronted with the knowledge of HIV-seropositive status have a significant life stressor placed on them that will require psychological accommodation. The ability to cope with these changes and complications is dependent in part on their HIV psychological and social support networks. A good psychosocial history is important, and early involvement with social services and psychological counseling is necessary. Psychological intervention involves the process of "reframing," whereby the patient is encouraged to interpret the situation in a manner that is more psychologically empowering (20). Medical treatment options

Table 92-5: Antifungal Agents

Drug	Major Adverse Reactions	Interactions
Amphotericin B	Hyperkalemia Nephrotoxicity Fever Chills Nausea	Zidovudine: additive bone marrow toxicity Digitalis, carbenicillin, ticarcillin: enhanced hypokalemic effect of amphotericin B Nephrotoxic agents (aminoglycoside): additive nephrotoxicity
Flucytosine (5-FC)	Nausea/ vomiting Agranulocytosis Aplastic anemia	Amphotericin B, ganciclovir: additive hematologic toxicity Antacids: decreased 5-FC absorption
Fluconazole	Nausea Headache Skin rash Abdominal pain Vomiting/ diarrhea	Cyclosporine: increased cyclosporine levels Rifampin: decreased half-life of fluconazole Phenytoin, warfarin: decreased metabolism of phenytoin and warfarin Sulfonylureas: increased hypoglycemia

Table 92-6: Antiviral Agents

Drug	Major Adverse Reactions	Interactions
Acyclovir	Nausea Headache Nephrotoxicity Neurologic toxicity	Probenecid: decreased acyclovir clearance
Ganciclovir	Neutropenia Thrombocytopenia Anemia Fever Rash Transaminase elevation	Zidovudine: additive hematologic toxicity Imipenem-cilastatin: increased risk of seizures Amphotericin B, antineoplastic agents, flucytosine: increased bone marrow toxicity
Foscarnet	Nephrotoxicity Hypocalcemia Hypercalcemia Neurologic toxicity	Nephrotoxic agents: additive nephrotoxicity Pentamidine: additive hypocalcemia and nephrotoxicity

should be framed in the perspective of how much better the patient will be with successful medical and rehabilitation intervention.

The recommendations for pharmacologic management of depression in most studies have followed the same principles as for the general population (20). These should be tempered by the neurocognitive and physiologic side effects of the medications. Many of the same strategies associated with the treatment of depression in stroke or traumatic brain injury patients should be employed in patients with organic brain syndromes (144). In patients presenting initially with dementia or mania, treatment with zidovudine (or perhaps now with combination therapy) should be strongly considered, as it may reverse some of the symptoms (15,145). Lithium and the anticonvulsants valproic acid and carbamazepine have been useful for the treatment of mania, while neuroleptics are frequently employed for frank psychosis (20). For panic and anxiety disorders, buspirone and antidepressants have been useful (20). The β-blocker propranolol may be helpful to block some of the physiologic effects of anxiety or panic attacks.

Rehabilitation physicians should hold an educational meeting early on with the HIV-infected person and family members, much as they would with any rehabilitation patient. Advanced directives, durable power of attorney, and living wills should be discussed long before a patient's health declines in an effort to avoid controversy and confrontation later (146).

PEDIATRIC CONSIDERATIONS

The number of children infected with HIV in the United States is small when compared to the number of adults; children represent approximately 2% of all cases (147). Infants who have acquired HIV through vertical (maternal) transmission are typically asymptomatic at birth (147). These children have a very poor prognosis, with the average age of onset for severe immunodeficiency ranging from 5 to 10 months; 50% to 90% will be clinically symptomatic by their first birthday (147). Few survive until their third birthday (147). The clinical signs and symptoms of AIDS in infants are listed in Table 92-9. Neurologic involvement, usually encephalopathy, is a common and devastating clinical finding (148,149). Those with encephalopathy show impairment of language and cognition, ataxia, as well as spastic paraparesis and quadriparesis (147,149). Oppor-

Table 92-7: Antiretroviral Agents		
Drug	**Major Adverse Reactions**	**Interactions**
Zidovudine (AZT)	Anemia Neutropenia Myopathy Anorexia Nausea Fatigue Headache Malaise Myalgia Insomnia	Ganciclovir: increased hematologic toxicity Probenecid: increased zidovudine levels Trimethoprim-sulfamethoxazole: increased anemia and neutropenia; trimethoprim increased zidovudine levels Phenytoin: increased or decreased phenytoin levels Methadone: decreased zidovudine metabolism
Didanosine (ddI)	Pancreatitis Peripheral neuropathy Hyperamylasemia Diarrhea (due to antacid) Hyperuricemia Transaminase elevation	Dapsone, ketoconazole, quinolones, tetracycline: decreased absorption by ddI Sulfadiazine, pyrazinamide: increased urate levels Pentamidine: increased risk of pancreatitis
Zalcitabine (ddC)	Peripheral neuropathy Pancreatitis Vomiting Rash Stomatitis	Drugs that can cause peripheral neuropathy or pancreatitis: additive or synergistic toxicity with ddC

Table 92-8: Protease Inhibitors		
Drug	**Major Adverse Reactions**	**Interactions**
Saquinavir mesylate	Nausea Diarrhea Abdominal discomfort Rash	Bioavailability: high-fat meal increases absorption Rifampin, rifabutin: reduces saquinavir levels Terfenadine, astemizole, cisapride: increased risk for cardiac arrhythmia
Ritonavir	Nausea Vomiting Diarrhea Fatigue Abdominal pain Circumoral paresthesias Taste disturbances Anorexia Elevated triglycerides Elevated creatinine kinase Elevated liver transaminases	Terfenadine, astemizole, cisapride: increased risk for cardiac arrhythmias Benzodiazepines: oversedation Fentanyl citrate, hydrocodone, methadone hydrochloride, lidocaine, erythromycin, warfarin sodium, clonazepam, carbamazepine, trazodone, fluoxetine, dronabinol, ondansetron, ketoconazole, itraconazole, calcium channel blockers, neuroleptics, lovastatin, pravastatin sodium, ergotamine derivatives, corticosteroids: may have increased drug levels NSAIDs, phenytoin, glipizide, glyburide, omeprazole: may have reduced levels
Indinavir	Nephrolithiasis Abdominal discomfort Asymptomatic hyperbilirubinemia	Rifabutin: may have increased level Ketoconazole: increased levels of indinavir Rifampin, terfenadine, astemizole, cisapride, triazolam, midazolam: may have increased drug levels Didanosine: decreased levels of indinavir if taken together Bioavailability: high-fat meal decreases absorption
Nelfinavir mesylate	Diarrhea Loose stools	Terfenadine, astemizole, cisapride: increased risk for cardiac arrhythmias Ketoconazole, rifampin, rifabutin: increased levels of nelfinavir

NSAIDs = nonsteroidal anti-inflammatory drugs.

tunistic infections, *Mycobacterium avium-intracellulare* infection, candidal infections, and particularly PCP are common (147). The last of these occurs in approximately 50% of children with AIDS (147). Unlike adults, children are susceptible to frequent and serious bacterial infections involving common bacterial pathogens, particularly from encapsulated bacteria and salmonella (147).

Rehabilitation Intervention

Treatment with zidovudine may improve the encephalopathy seen in children as it does in adults (150). There is some concern about the exposure of these children to common pathogens if they are placed in day care (151,152). These children require diligent care and should be seen in consultation with a pediatric center capable of dealing with AIDS and its complications (147). Current recommendations call for routine immunizations, except the killed polio virus (Salk) is substituted for the live attenuated polio virus vaccine (Sabin) (147,153).

Rehabilitation approaches are similar to those for progressive neurologic diseases of children (151,154,155). They require experience in these protocols, as outlined in other chapters of this book. It is acknowledged that children who are school-age benefit by remaining in a normal classroom and do not pose a significant risk to their classmates (156).

Table 92-9: Clinical Signs and Symptoms of AIDS in Children

Failure to thrive	Neurologic involvement
Diarrhea	Developmental delay
Frequent otitis media	Loss of attained milestones
Frequent other common pediatric infections	Dementia
	Encephalopathy
Invasive or disseminated infections	Acquired or congenital microcephaly
Thrush	
Opportunistic infections	Cardiomyopathy
Lymphocytic interstitial pneumonia	Chronic eczematoid rash
Skin diseases (*Candida* and seborrhea)	Pneumonia
	Pneumocystis carinii
Parotid swellings	*Streptococcus* (B-hemolytic)
Lymphadenopathy	
Hepatosplenomegaly	*Haemophilus influenza*

FUTURE DIRECTIONS

In the last few years, considerable progress has been made in the medical management of AIDS (10,132). With the development of new treatment strategies, it is likely that AIDS and HIV infection will be classsified as a chronic medical disorder. While the end-stage management issues so well described recently will still be applicable (157), it is increasingly evident that the management of HIV- and AIDS-related complications will be more drawn out. This is where the use of appropriate rehabilitation techniques coupled with an appropriate understanding of the disease process and its complications will become so important.

REFERENCES

1. Stryker J, Coates TJ, Decarlo P, et al. Prevention of HIV infection. *JAMA* 1995;273:1143–1148.
2. Buehler JW, Petersen LR, Jaffe HW. Current trends in the epidemiology of HIV/AIDS. In: Sande MA, Volberding PA, eds. *The medical management of AIDS.* 4th ed. Philadelphia: WB Saunders, 1995:3–21.
3. Green WC. The molecular biology of human immunodeficiency virus type 1 infection. *N Engl J Med* 1991;324:308–317.
4. Davey RT Jr, Lane HC. Laboratory methods in the diagnosis and prognostic staging of infection with human immunodeficiency virus type 1. *Rev Infect Dis* 1990;12:912–930.
5. Greene WC. Molecular insights into HIV-1 infection. In: Sande MA, Volberding PA, eds. *The medical management of AIDS.* 4th ed. Philadelphia: WB Saunders, 1995:22–37.
6. Staprans SI, Feinberg MB. Natural history and immunopathogenesis of HIV-1 disease. In: Sande MA, Volberding PA, eds. *The medical management of AIDS.* 4th ed. Philadelphia: WB Saunders, 1995:38–64.
7. Centers for Disease Control. Revision of the CDC case definition for acquired immunodeficiency syndrome. *MMWR Morbid Mortal Wkly Rep* 1987;36:3S–15S.
8. Centers for Disease Control. 1993 Revised classification system for HIV infection and expanded surveillance case definition for AIDS among adolescents and adults. *MMWR Morbid Mortal Wkly Rep* 1993;41:1–5.
9. Levinson SF, O'Connell PG. Rehabilitation dimensions of AIDS: a review. *Arch Phys Med Rehabil* 1991;72:690–696.
10. Centers for Disease Control. Update: trends in AIDS incidence, deaths, and prevalence-United States, 1996. *MMWR Morb Mortal Wkly Rep* 1997;46:165–173.
11. Centers for Disease Control. Update: mortality attributable to HIV infection among persons aged 25–44 years-United States, 1994. *MMWR Morbid Mortal*

Wkly Rep 1996;45: 121–125.

12. Pederses C, Kolby P, Sindrup J, et al. The development of AIDS or AIDS-related conditions in a cohort of HIV antibody-positive homosexual men during a 3 year follow-up period. *J Intern Med* 1989;225: 405–409.

13. Schecter MT, Craib KJB, Le TN, et al. Progressing to AIDS and predictors of AIDS in seroprevalent and seroincident cohorts of homosexual men. *AIDS* 1989;3:347–353.

14. Tindall B, Carr A, Cooper DA. Primary HIV infection: clinical, immunologic, and serologic aspects. In: Sande MA, Volberding PA, eds. *The medical management of AIDS.* 4th ed. Philadelphia: WB Saunders, 1995:105–129.

15. Collier AC, Coombs RW, Schoenfeld DA, et al. Treatment of human immunodeficiency virus infection with saquinavir, zidovudine, and zalcitabine. *N Engl J Med* 1996;334: 1011–1017.

16. Stephenson J. New anti-HIV drugs and treatment strategies buoy AIDS researchers. *JAMA* 1996;275:579–580.

17. O'Dell MW, Levinson SF, Riggs RV. Focused review: physiatric management of HIV-related disability. *Arch Phys Med Rehabil* 1996;77:S66–S73.

18. O'Dell MW, Crawford A, Bohi ES, Bonner FJ. Disability in persons hospitalized with AIDS. *Am J Phys Med Rehabil* 1991;70: 91–95.

19. Cello JP. Gastrointestinal tract manifestations of AIDS. In: Sande MA, Volberding PA, eds. *The medical management of AIDS.* 4th ed. Philadelphia: WB Saunders, 1995:241–260.

20. Capaldini L. HIV disease: psychosocial issues and psychiatric complications. In: Sande MA, Volberding PA, eds. *The medical management of AIDS.* 4th ed. Philadelphia: WB Saunders, 1995:289–317.

21. Cassens BJ. Social consequences of the acquired immunodeficiency syndrome. *Ann Intern Med* 1985;103:768–771.

22. *HIV in America: a profile of challenges facing Americans living with HIV.* Washington, DC: National Association of People with AIDS 1992.

23. Vachon RA. Employment assistance and vocational rehabilitation for persons with HIV or AIDS: policy, practice and prospects. *Phys Med Rehabil State Art Rev* 1993;7(suppl): S203–S224.

24. Goldsmith MF. Costs of HIV/AIDS rise, care disparities increase. *JAMA* 1992;268:1246.

25. Hellinger FJ. The lifetime cost of treating a person with HIV. *JAMA* 1993;270:474–478.

26. Mizuswa H, Hirano A, Llena JF, Shintaku M. Cerebrovascular lesions in acquired immune deficiency syndrome (AIDS). *Acta Neuropathol (Berl)* 1988;76: 451–457.

27. Levy RM, Bredesen DE. Central nervous system dysfunction in acquired immunodeficiency syndrome. In: Rosenblum ML, Levy RM, Bredsen DE, eds. *AIDS and the nervous system.* New York: Raven, 1988:29–63.

28. O'Dell, Dillon ME. Rehabilitation in adults with human immunodeficiency virus-related diseases. *Am J Phys Med Rehabil* 1992;71:183–190.

29. Gabuzda DH, Hirsh MS. Neurological manifestations of infection with human immunodeficiency virus: clinical features and pathogenesis. *Ann Intern Med* 1987;107:383–891.

30. Navia BA, Price RW. The acquired immunodeficiency syndrome dementia complex as the presenting or sole manifestation of human immunodeficiency virus infection. *Arch Neurol* 1987;44:65–69.

31. Sliwa JA, Smith JC. Rehabilitation of neurological disability related to human immunodeficiency virus. *Arch Phys Med Rehabil* 1991;72: 759–762.

32. Levy RM, Bredesen DE. Central nervous system dysfunction in acquired immunodeficiency syndrome. *J Acquir Immune Defic Syndr Hum Retrovirol* 1988;1: 41–64.

33. Navia BA, Price RW. The AIDS dementia complex: I. Clinical features. *Ann Neurol* 1986;19: 517–524.

34. McArthur JC. Neurologic manifestations of AIDS. *Medicine* 1987; 66:407–437.

35. Perry S, Jacobsberg L, Fishman B, et al. Psychiatric diagnosis before serological testing for the human immunodeficiency virus. *Am J Psychiatry* 1990;147: 89–93.

36. Price RW, Worley JM. Management of neurologic complications of HIV-1 infection and AIDS. In: Sande MA, Volberding PA, eds. *The medical management of AIDS.* 4th ed. Philadelphia: WB Saunders, 1995:261–288.

37. Marotta R, Perry S. Early neuropsychological dysfunction caused by human immunodeficiency virus. *J Neuropsychiatry* 1989;1:225–235.

38. Auerbach V. Neuropsychological issues in HIV infection: implications for rehabilitation management. *Phys Med Rehabil State Art Rev* 1993;7(suppl): S119–S227.

39. Falloon J. Current therapy for HIV infection and its infections complications. *Postgrad Med* 1992;91:115–132.

40. Bozzette SA, Larsen RA, Chui J, et al. A placebo-controlled trial of maintenance therapy with fluconazole after treatment of cryptococcal meningitis in the acquired immunodeficiency syndrome. *N Engl J Med* 1990;324:580–584.

41. Engstrom JW, Lowenstein DH, Bredesen DE. Cerebral infarctions and transient neurologic deficits associated with acquired immun-

odeficiency syndrome. *Am J Med* 1989;86:528–532.

42. Simpson DM, Tagliati M. Neurological manifestations of HIV infection. *Ann Intern Med* 1994;121:769–785. [Published erratum appears in *Ann Intern Med* 1995;122:317.]

43. Israelski DM, Remington JS. Toxoplasmosis encephalitis in patients with AIDS. *Infect Dis Clin North Am* 1988;2:525–532.

44. Levine AM, Werz JC, Kaplan L, et al. Low dose chemotherapy with central nervous system prophylaxis and zidovudine maintenance in AIDS related lymphoma. *JAMA* 1991;266:84–88.

45. Drew WL, Buhles W, Erlich KS. Management of herpes virus infections (CMV, HSV, VZV). In: Sande MA, Volberding PA, eds. *The medical management of AIDS.* 4th ed. Philadelphia: WB Saunders, 1995:512–536.

46. Levy RM, Berger JR. Neurologic complications of HIV infection: diagnoses, therapy, and functional considerations. In: Mukand J, ed. *Rehabilitation for patients with HIV disease.* New York: McGraw-Hill, 1991: 55–76.

47. O'Dell MW. HIV-related disability: assessment and management. *Phys Med Rehabil State Art Rev* 1993;7(suppl):S1–S8.

48. Flower W, Sooy CD. AIDS: an introduction for speech-language pathologists and audiologists. *ASHA* 1987;29:25–30.

49. Berger JR, Levy RM. The neurologic complications of human immunodeficiency virus infection. *Med Clin North Am* 1993; 77:1–23.

50. Gabuzda DH, Hirsh MS. Neurologic manifestations of infection with human immunodeficiency virus: clinical features and pathogenesis. *Ann Intern Med* 1987; 107:383–391.

51. Petito CK, Navia BA, Cho ES, et al. Vacuolar myelopathy pathologically resembling subacute combined degeneration in patients with acquired immunodeficiency syndrome. *N Engl J Med* 1985;312: 874–879.

52. Grafe MR, Wiley CA. Spinal cord and peripheral nerve pathology in AIDS: the roles of cytomegalovirus and human immunodeficiency virus. *Ann Neurol* 1989;25:561–566.

53. Brew BJ. HIV-1 related neurological disease. *J Acquir Immune Defic Syndr Hum Retrovirol* 1993;6:S10–S15.

54. Jacobson MA, Berger TG, Fikrig S, et al. Acyclovir (ACV)-resistant varicella zoster virus (VCV) infection following chronic oral ACV therapy in patients with AIDS. *Ann Intern Med* 1990;112: 187–191.

55. Verma RK, Ziegler DK, Kepes JJ. HIV-related neuromuscular syndrome simulating motor neuron disease. *Neurology* 1990;40: 544–546.

56. Lange DJ. Neuromuscular diseases associated with HIV-1 infection. *Muscle Nerve* 1994; 17:16–30.

57. Gray F, Chimelli L, Mohr M, et al. Fulminating multiple sclerosis-like leukoencephalopathy revealing human immunodeficiency virus infection. *N Engl J Med* 1991;41:105–109.

58. So YT, Holtzman DM, Abrams DI, Olney RK. Peripheral neuropathy associated with acquired immunodeficiency syndrome: prevalence and clinical features from a population-based survey. *Arch Neurol* 1988;45:945–948.

59. Bailey RO, Baltch AL, Venkatash R, et al. Sensory motor neuropathy associated with AIDS. *Neurology* 1988;38:886–891.

60. Cornblath DR, McArthur JC. Predominantly sensory neuropathy in patients with AIDS and AIDS-related complex. *Neurology* 1988;38:794–796.

61. Mah V, Vartavarian LM, Akers MA, Vinters HV. Abnormalities of peripheral nerve in patients with human immunodeficiency virus infection. *Ann Neurol* 1988;24:713–717.

62. Lambert JS, Seidlin M, Reichman RC, et al. 2′,3′-Dideoxyinosine (ddi) in patients with the acquired immunodeficiency syndrome or AIDS-related complex. *N Engl J Med* 1990;322: 1333–1340.

63. Dubinsky RM, Yarchoan R, Dalakas M, Broder S. Reversible axonal neuropathy from the treatment of AIDS and related disorders with 2′,3′-dideoxycytidine (ddC). *Muscle Nerve* 1989;12: 856–860.

64. Cornblath DR. Treatment of the neuromuscular complications of human immunodeficiency virus infection. *Ann Neurol* 1988; 23(suppl):S88–S91.

65. Cornblath DR, McArthur JC, Kennedy PG, et al. Inflammatory demyelinating peripheral neuropathies associated with human T-cell lymphotrophic virus type III infection. *Ann Neurol* 1987; 21:32–40.

66. Ropper AH. The Guillain-Barré syndrome. *N Engl J Med* 1992;326:1130–1136.

67. Lange DJ. Neuromuscular diseases associated with HIV-1 infection. *Muscle Nerve* 1994; 17:16–30.

68. Simpson DM, Wolfe DE. Neuromuscular complication of HIV infection and its treatment. *AIDS* 1991;5:917–926.

69. Miller RG, Parry GJ, Pfaeffl W, et al. The spectrum of peripheral neuropathy associated with ARC and AIDS. *Muscle Nerve* 1988; 11:857–863.

70. Miller RG, Storey JR, Greco CM. Ganciclovir in the treatment of progressive AIDS-related polyradiculoneuropathy. *Neurology* 1990;40:569–574.

71. Spector SA, McKinley GF, Lalezari JP, et al. Oral ganciclovir for the prevention of cytomegalovirus disease in persons with AIDS. *N Engl J Med* 1996;334:1491–1497.

72. Studies of Ocular Complications of AIDS Research Group, in collaboration with the AIDS Clinical Trials Group. Mortality in patients

with the acquired immunodeficiency syndrome treated with either foscarnet or ganciclovir for cytomegalovirus retinitis. *N Engl J Med* 1992;326:213–220.

73. Bushbacher L. Rehabilitation of patients with peripheral neuropathies. In: Braddom RL, ed. *Physical medicine and rehabilitation.* Philadelphia: WB Saunders, 1995:972–989.

74. Dalakas MC, Pezeshkpour GH. Neuromuscular diseases associated with human immunodeficiency virus infection. *Ann Neurol* 1988;23(suppl): S49–S53.

75. Ruttiman S, Hilti P, Spinas GA, et al. High frequency of human immunodeficiency virus-associated autonomic neuropathy. *Arch Intern Med* 1991;152: 485–501.

76. Shahmanesh M, Bradbeer CS, Edwards A, et al. Autonomic dysfunction in patients with human immunodeficiency virus infection. *Int J STD AIDS* 1990;2: 419–423.

77. Zochodne DW. Autonomic involvement in Guillain-Barré syndrome: a review. *Muscle Nerve* 1994;17:1145–1155.

78. Meythaler JM, DeVivo MJ, Clausen GC, Braswell WC. Prediction of outcome in Guillain-Barré syndrome admitted to rehabilitation. *Arch Phys Med Rehabil* 1994;75:1027. Abstract.

79. Lichtenfield P. Autonomic dysfunction in the Guillain-Barré syndrome. *Am J Med* 1971;50:772–780.

80. Eiben RM, Gersony WM. Recognition, prognosis and treatment of the Guillain-Barré syndrome (acute idiopathic polyneuritis). *Med Clin North Am* 1963;47: 1371–1380.

81. Winer JB, Hughes RAC. Identification of patients at risk of arrhythmia in the Guillain-Barré syndrome. *Q J Med* 1988;68: 735–739.

82. Bensman A. Strenuous exercise may impair muscle function in Guillain-Barré patients. *JAMA* 1970;214:468–469.

83. Herbison GJ, Jaweed M, Ditunno JF. Exercise therapies in peripheral neuropathies. *Arch Phys Med Rehabil* 1983;64:201–205.

84. Pentland B, Daonald SM. Pain in the Guillain-Barré syndrome: a clinical review. *Pain* 1994;59:159–164.

85. Buck SH, Burks TF. The neuropharmacology of capsaicin: review of some recent observations. *Pharmacol Rev* 1986;38:179–226.

86. Soryal I, Sinclaire E, Hornby J, Pentland B. Impaired joint mobility in Guillain-Barré syndrome: a primary or a secondary phenomenon? *J Neurol Neurosurg Psychiatry* 1992;55:1014–1017.

87. Dalakas MC, Pezeshpour GH, Gravell M, Sever JL. Polymyositis associated with AIDS retrovirus. *JAMA* 1986;256:2381–2383.

88. Gorarad DA, Henry K, Guiloff RJ. Necrotizing myopathy and zidovudine. *Lancet* 1988;1:1050.

89. Simpson DM, Bender AN. Human immunodeficiency virus-associated myopathy: analysis of 11 patients. *Ann Neurol* 1988; 24:79–84.

90. Snider WD, Simpson DM, Nielson S, et al. Neurological complications of acquired immune deficiency syndrome: analysis of 50 patients. *Ann Neurol* 1983;14:403–418.

91. Simpson DM. Myopathies associated with human immunodeficiency virus infection and its treatment. *AAEM Course B: Neuromuscular complications of retroviral infections.* Rochester, MN: American Association of Electromyopathy and Electrodiagnosis, 1990:27–35.

92. Dalakas MC, Illa I, Pezehpour GH, et al. Mitochondrial myopathy caused by long-term zidovudine therapy. *N Engl J Med* 1990;322:1098–1105.

93. Gonzales MF, Olney RK, So YT, et al. Subacute structural myopathy associated with human immunodeficiency virus infection. *Arch Neurol* 1988;45:585–587.

94. Walsh C, Kriegel R, Lennett E, Karpatkin S. Thrombocytopenia in homosexual patients. *Ann Intern Med* 1985;103:542–545.

95. Simpson DM, Bender AN, Farraye J, et al. AIDS wasting syndrome may represent a treatable myopathy. *Neurology* 1990;40: 535–538.

96. Hicks JE. Comprehensive rehabilitative management of patients with polymyositis and dermatomyositis. In: Dalakas M, ed. *Polymyositis and dermatomyositis.* Boston: Butterworths, 1988:293–317.

97. Gerber LH, Hicks JE. Exercise in the rheumatic diseases. In: Basmajian JV, ed. *Therapeutic exercise.* Baltimore: Williams & Wilkins, 1990:333–350.

98. Rosen JM. Pulmonary complications of HIV infections. In: Mukand J, ed. *Rehabilitation for patients with HIV disease.* New York: McGraw-Hill, 1991: 119–129.

99. Lubeck DP, Nobunaga AI, Williams C, O'Dell MW. Rehabilitation of selected nonneurogenic HIV disability. *Phys Med Rehabil State Art Rev* 1993;7(suppl): S101–S108.

100. Kaye BR. Rheumatologic manifestations of infection with human immunodeficiency virus (HIV). *Ann Intern Med* 1989;111:158–167.

101. Berman A, Espinoza LR, Diaz JD, et al. Rheumatic manifestations of human immunodeficiency virus infection. *Am J Med* 1988;85: 59–64.

102. Buskila D, Gladman DD, Langevita P, et al. Rheumatologic manifestations of infection with human immunodeficiency virus (HIV). *Clin Exp Rheumatol* 1990;8:567–573.

103. Munoz-Fernandez S, Cardenal A, Balsa A, et al. Rheumatic manifestations in 556 patients with human immunodeficiency virus infection. *Semin Arthritis Rheum* 1991;21:30–39.

104. Espinoza LR, Aguilar JL, Berman A, et al. Rheumatic manifestations associated with human immunodeficiency virus infection. *Arthritis Rheum* 1989;32: 1615–1622.

105. Rynes RI, Goldenberg DL, DiGiacomo R, et al. Acquired immunodeficiency syndrome-associated arthritis. *Am J Med* 1988;84: 810–816.

106. Guiterrez VFJ, Martinez-Osuna P, Seleznick MJ, et al. Rheumatologic rehabilitation for patients with HIV. In: Mukand J, ed. *Rehabilitation in patients with HIV disease.* New York: McGraw-Hill, 1992:77–93.

107. Winchester R, Bernstein DH, Fisher HD, et al. The co-occurrence of Reiter's syndrome and acquired immunodeficiency. *Ann Intern Med* 1987;106: 19–26.

108. Lane HC, Laughon BE, Falloon J, et al. Recent advances in the management of AIDS-related opportunistic infections. *Ann Intern Med* 1994;120:945–955. [Erratum published in *Ann Intern Med* 1995;122:317.]

109. Bloom JN, Palestine AG. The diagnosis of cytomegalovirus retinitis. *Ann Intern Med* 1988;109:963–969.

110. Johnston JL, Miller JD, Nath A. Ocular motor dysfunction in HIV-1-infected subjects: a quantitative oculographic analysis. *Neurology* 1996;46:451–457.

111. Perdices M, Dunbar N, Grunseit A, et al. Anxiety, depression, and HIV-related symptomatology across the spectrum of HIV disease. *Aust N Z J Psychiatry* 1992;26:560–566.

112. Hoover DR, Saah AJ, Bacellar H, et al. Signs and symptoms of "asymptomatic" HIV-1-infected homosexual men. *J Acquir Immun Defic Syndr Hum Retrovirol* 1993;6:66–71.

113. O'Dell MW, Riggs RV. Correlates of HIV-related fatigue: a pilot study. *Arch Phys Med Rehabil* 1993;74:1243. Abstract.

114. Miller RG, Carson PJ, Moussavi RS, et al. Fatigue and myalgia in AIDS patients. *Neurology* 1991;41:1603–1607.

115. Gualtieri T, Chandler M, Coons TB, Brown LT. Amantadine: a clinical profile for traumatic brain injury. *Clin Neuropharmacol* 1989;12:258–270.

116. Muller HF, Dastoor DP, Klingner A, et al. Amantadine in senile dementia: electroencephalographic and clinical effects. *J Am Geriatr Soc* 1979;27:9–16.

117. Murray TJ. Amantadine therapy for fatigue in multiple sclerosis. *Can J Neurol Sci* 1985;12: 251–254.

118. Cohen RA, Fisher RS. Amantadine treatment of fatigue associated with multiple sclerosis. *Arch Neurol* 1989;46:676–680.

119. Fernandez F, Levy JK, Galizzi H. Response of HIV-related depression to psychostimulants: case reports. *Hosp Commun Psychiatry* 1988;39:628–631.

120. Davey RT, Masur H. Recent advances in the diagnosis, treatment, and prevention of *Pneumocystis carinii* pneumonia. *Antimicrob Agents Chemother* 1990;34:499–504.

121. Kovacs JA, Masur H. Opportunistic infections. In: DeVita VT Jr, Hellman S, Rosenberg SA, eds. *AIDS: etiology, diagnosis, treatment and prevention.* 2nd ed. Philadelphia: JB Lippincott, 1988:199–225.

122. Rosen MJ. Pulmonary complications of HIV infections. In: Mukand J, ed. *Rehabilitation for patients with HIV disease.* New York: McGraw-Hill, 1991: 119–129.

123. Centers for Disease Control. Purified protein derivative (PPD)-tuberculin anergy and HIV infection: guidelines for anergy testing and management of anergic persons at risk of tuberculosis. *MMWR Morbid Mortal Wkly Rep* 1991;40:27–33.

124. Centers for Disease Control. Guidelines for prophylaxis against *Pneumocystis carinii* pneumonia for persons infected with human immunodeficiency virus. *MMWR Morbid Mortal Wkly Rep* 1989;38:(S-5):1–9.

125. Krigel RL, Friedman-Kien AE. Kaposi's sarcoma in AIDS: diagnosis and treatment. In: DeVita VT, ed. *AIDS: etiology, diagnosis, treatment, and prevention.* Philadelphia: JB Lippincott, 1988:245–261.

126. Kaul S, Fishbein MC, Siegel RJ. Cardiac manifestations of acquired immunodeficiency syndrome; a 1991 update. *Am Heart J* 1991;122:535–544.

127. Monsuez JJ, Kinney EL, Vittwcoq D, et al. Comparison among acquired immunodeficiency syndrome patients with and without clinical evidence of cardiac disease. *Am J Cardiol* 1988;62: 1311–1313.

128. Celli BR. Pulmonary rehabilitation of the patient with AIDS. In: Mukand J, ed. *Rehabilitation for patients with HIV disease.* New York: McGraw-Hill, 1991: 131–139.

129. Wenger NK. Patients with left ventricular dysfunction and congestive heart failure. In: Wenger NK, ed. *Rehabilitation of the coronary patient.* New York: Churchill Livingstone, 1992: 403–431.

130. Greenspan JS, Greenspan D. Oral complications of HIV infection. In: Sande MA, Volberding PA, eds. *The medical management of AIDS.* 4th ed. Philadelphia: WB Saunders, 1995: 224–240.

131. Katz MH, Greenspan D, Westenhouse J, et al. Progression to AIDS in HIV-infected homosexual and bisexual men with hairy leukoplakia and oral candidiasis: results from three San Francisco epidemiologic cohorts. *AIDS* 1992; 6:95–100.

132. Deeks SG, Smith M, Holodniy M, Kahn JO. HIV-1 protease inhibitors: a review for clinicians. *JAMA* 1997;277:145–153.

133. Jewell ME, Sweet DE. Asymptomatic HIV infection: a primary care disease. *Postgrad Med* 1992;92:155–166.

134. O'Brien WA, Hartigan PM, Martin D, et al. Changes in plasma HIV-1 RNA and CD4+ lymphocyte counts and the risk or progression to AIDS. *N Engl J Med* 1996;334:426–431.

135. Meythaler JM, Cross LL. Traumatic spinal cord injury complicated by AIDS related complex. *Arch Phys Med Rehabil* 1988;69:219–222.

136. Paauw DS, Wenrich MD, Curtis JR, et al. Ability of primary care physicians to recognize physical findings associated with HIV infection. *JAMA* 1955;274: 1380–1382.

137. Saag MS. AIDS testing now and in the future. In: Sande MA, Volberding PA, eds. *The medical management of AIDS.* 4th ed. Philadelphia: WB Saunders, 1995:65–88.

138. Holland J, Tross S. The psychosocial and neuropsychiatric sequelae of the acquired immunodeficiency syndrome and related disorders. *Ann Intern Med* 1985;103:760–764.

139. Buhrich N, Cooper D, Freed E. HIV infections associated with symptoms indistinguishable from functional psychosis. *Br J Psychiatry* 1988;152:649–653.

140. Perry S. Organic mental disorders caused by HIV: update on early diagnosis and treatment. *Am J Psychiatry* 1990;147:696–710.

141. Cassem D. Anxiety and depression as secondary phenomena. *Psychiatr Clin North Am* 1990;13:597–612.

142. Katon W. Depression: relationship to somatization and chronic medical illness. *Clin Psychiatry* 1984;45:4–11.

143. Rabkin J, Gewirtz G. Depression and HIV. *GMHC Treatment Issues* 1992;6:1–7.

144. Cardenas DD, McLean A. Psychopharmacologic management of traumatic brain injury. *Phys Med Rehabil Clin N Amer* 1992;3:273–290.

145. Boccelari A, Dilley J, Shore M. Neuropsychiatric aspects of AIDS dementia complex: a report on a clinical series. *Neurotoxicology* 1988;9:381–390.

146. Schneiderman LJ. Who decides who decides? When disagreement occurs between the physician and the patient's appointed proxy about the patient's decision-making capacity. *Arch Intern Med* 1995;155:793–796.

147. Grossman M. Pediatric AIDS. In: Sande MA, Volberding PA, eds. *The medical management of AIDS.* 4th ed. Philadelphia: WB Saunders, 1995:632–647.

148. Belman A, Diamond G, Dickson D, et al. Pediatric acquired immunodeficiency syndrome: neurologic syndrome. *Am J Child* 1988;142:29–35.

149. Pizzo PA, Wilfert CM, eds. *Pediatric AIDS: the challenge of HIV infections in infants, children and adolescents.* Baltimore: Williams & Wilkins, 1993.

150. Pizzo PA, Eddy J, Falloon F, et al. Effect of continuous intravenous infusion of zidovudine (AZT) in children with symptomatic HIV infection. *N Engl J Med* 1988;319:889–896.

151. American Academy of Pediatrics. Committee on infectious disease: health guidelines for the attendance in day care and foster care settings of children infected with human immunodeficiency virus. *Pediatrics* 1987;79:466–471.

152. American Academy of Pediatrics. Guidelines for HIV-infected children and their foster families. *Pediatrics* 1992;89:681.

153. Centers for Disease Control. Immunization of children infected with human immunodeficiency virus: supplementary ACIP statement. *MMWR Morbid Mortal Wkly Rep* 1988;37:181–183.

154. Cohen LS, Kathirithamby R, Kaufman J. Rehabilitation needs in children with congenital AIDS. *Arch Phys Med Rehabil* 1987;68:666. Abstract.

155. Saturen P, Bartalos EP, Dhulipala V, et al. Pediatric acquired immune deficiency syndrome—a pilot intervention program. *Arch Phys Med Rehabil* 1988;69:775. Abstract.

156. Centers for Disease Control. Education and foster care of children infected with human T lymphocyte virus type III. *MMWR Morbid Mortal Wkly Rep* 1985;34:521.

157. Stansell JD, Follansbee SE. Management of late-stage AIDS. In: Sande MA, Volberding PA, eds. *The medical management of AIDS.* 4th ed. Philadelphia: WB Saunders, 1995:665–679.

Chapter 93

Amputation Rehabilitation

Alberto Esquenazi
Edward Wikoff
Maria Lucas

Amputation rehabilitation is not solely the provision of a prosthesis. Rather it is the restorative intervention necessary to return the patient who has had an amputation to the highest possible level of function and to minimize the impact of the amputation on his or her life. In the last two decades, with the advent of specialized treatment teams and new prosthetic devices, the outlook for the person who has had an amputation has improved. Outcomes that were never thought to be possible, such as exercising with a prosthesis or ambulation without the use of upper-limb support for the elderly, are now frequently achieved. We present our collective knowledge and understanding of the rehabilitation process, which represents the essential interventions necessary to optimize function for patients who are provided with a prosthesis and for those who are unable or choose not to use one.

CLASSIFICATION AND INCIDENCE OF AMPUTATION

Amputations are classified based on the anatomic level and site at which the amputation has taken place. For example, an amputation between the wrist and elbow is termed a *transradial amputation*. Other levels include transfemoral, transtibial, Syme, partial foot, hip disarticulation, and knee disarticulation for the lower limb. For the upper limb, transhumeral and partial hand amputations, and shoulder, elbow, and wrist disarticulations are the most common.

The congenital limb deficiencies are best classified following the International Organization of Standards and the International Society of Prosthetics and Orthotics classifications as modified from Frantz and O'Rahilly (1). The limb deficiencies can be transverse or longitudinal. The term *terminal* is used to describe the fact that the limb has developed normally to a particular level beyond which no skeletal element exists. With intercalary limb deficiency, there is a reduction or absence of one or more elements within the long axis of the limb, and there may be normal skeletal elements distal to the affected segments (2).

Amputation of the lower limb is performed significantly more frequently than amputation of the upper limb. Amputation of the distal segment of the limb is more common than that of the proximal segment. Amputations can occur at any age, but for lower extremities, the elderly are most commonly affected, with men more frequently affected than women. Upper-limb amputation affects men between the second and fourth decades most frequently, and the right upper extremity is more likely to be amputated than the left.

The most common reasons for lower-limb amputation are infection, arterial occlusive disease, and complications of diabetes mellitus. Less frequent but important causes are trauma, malignancy, and peripheral neuropathies. For the upper limb, trauma followed by malignancies and acute arterial insufficiency are the most common causes (Fig. 93-1).

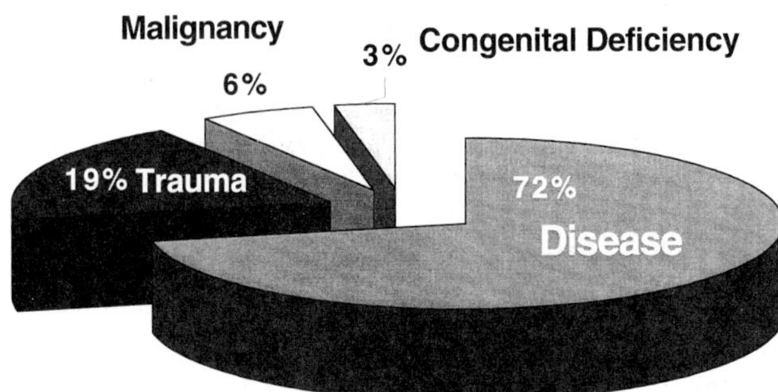

Figure 93-1. Distribution of the causes of amputation.

REHABILITATION TEAM

Limb loss is a condition that has physical, psychological, and social implications for the affected individual and the social support system. For treatment to be effective, it should include the care of the patient and his or her significant others. Expertise from various clinicians is required to accomplish this effectively. The development of a rehabilitation team working closely together to address each individual's needs is vital to the efficient and timely delivery of services. This approach will provide the patient a comprehensive treatment regimen.

A physician specializing in rehabilitation, or who has knowledge of biomechanics and prosthetics, assumes the role of team leader and coordinates the team's resources. The prosthetist fabricates the prosthetic appliance and works closely in the training stages with the therapist and patient to prevent complications, achieve appropriate alignment, and ensure proper fit of the prosthesis. The prosthetist also acts as a resource to other team members for information on the latest technologic advances in the field of prosthetics.

Physical and occupational therapists are critical members of the therapeutic team. The physical therapist participates in the care of the lower-extremity amputee by preparing him or her physically for using a prosthesis. This includes instructing the patient in management of the prosthesis, teaching functional mobility activities, and providing gait training to optimize the walking pattern. In the patient who has had a traumatic upper-extremity amputation, the intervention of the physical therapist is required only if there is a significant injury to joints or soft tissues. An occupational therapist will work closely with the team and the patient to incorporate use of the prosthesis during activities of daily living (ADLs) and for work simulation activities. For the upper-extremity amputee, the occupational therapist is frequently the primary therapist instructing the patient in the use of an upper-limb prosthesis.

Owing to the immense psychological impact that an amputation has on many patients and their families, each patient should have an assessment with a psychologist (3,4). A psychologist specializing in limb loss or disability is particularly suited in addressing feelings of depression and body image changes associated with amputation.

Along with these core members, the team should include other supporting clinicians. A social worker can assist patients with changes in family relationships and social status related to decreases in function or work abilities (5). Nurses can assist and instruct patients in medication management and with wound care. The recreational therapist provides information about community resources for recreational activities and support groups, and instructs patients in the adaptations necessary to participate in leisure activities. A vocational counselor, driving instructor, and when necessary, a school teacher may be involved in the care of the amputee as well.

The patient and team members should work together to set goals and develop an overall treatment plan. Subsequently, each team member participates in the patient's care as necessary to make the provision of services most efficient.

With so many clinicians contributing to the care of an individual, communication is an essential component of team interaction. Good communication will ensure that all team members are providing patients with quality care while avoiding duplication of services. Each team should develop some method of communication that is appropriate for the clinical setting, whether it be daily or weekly rounds, written documentation, computer linking, or team meetings (6–8).

PREAMPUTATION EDUCATION AND COUNSELING

The rehabilitation process for the individual with limb loss ideally should begin before any surgery occurs. The amputee can take better advantage of rehabilitation services once he or she has been educated regarding surgery, healing, exercise, future abilities and limitations, and the rehabilitation process. This education, as well as the actual multifaceted rehabilitation care, is best provided by a team of health care professionals with experience and expertise in the realm of amputation rehabilitation (9–11).

Patients facing amputation often know little about the disease process that threatens their limbs, or about what the future holds. Understanding that arterial insufficiency, infection, trauma, or tumor may necessitate amputation may enable the patient to accept the amputation as the appropriate treatment (12). Lacking this insight, patients may resist or delay amputation, risking sepsis, a contracted nonfunctional limb, analgesic abuse, deconditioning or other avoidable medical complications. Others may fear social isolation or stigmatization stemming from the amputation, and view the amputation as the end of their useful life. Most fear losing independence and work productivity, and becoming a burden on family and friends (2,12–19).

To fill these information gaps, the patient and family benefit from preamputation counseling from members of the rehabilitation team and from a prosthetic user who can provide firsthand information. The following topics should be covered, although with the apprehension of upcoming surgery, the patient may retain little of what is initially discussed.

1. Pain will certainly be present following surgery and its duration and intensity may not be predictable. The patient seeking pain relief as a result of amputation may not be satisfied, as the RL or phantom limb may also be painful (20).
2. Phantom sensation (and possibly pain) will likely be present following surgery (21).
3. Exercise and proper positioning in the early postoperative period will be very important to future rehabilitation.
4. A general time frame for acute hospitalization, wound healing, preprosthetic rehabilitation, and prosthetic use is very helpful to the patient.
5. The patient's expectations for future functional status are often unrealistic. Future activities will require equipment previously unfamiliar to the patient (e.g., wheelchair, crutches, prosthesis, etc). A discussion of this information with an amputee as closely matched demographically as possible will provide the patient with a more credible view of the future. Early contact with the patient also allows members of the rehabilitation team to evaluate the patient's premorbid status and current problems so that appropriate goals and plans can be made. The patient may also benefit from the continuity if the same members of the rehabilitation team are involved before and after the surgery.

EVALUATION OF THE AMPUTEE

Evaluation of the patient with upper- or lower-limb loss is indispensable to preparing the overall rehabilitation treatment plan, including the development of goals and objectives. It is also important in the prosthetic prescription process. Although the overall evaluation process for all amputees is similar, some important differences exist in the evaluation of patients with limb loss at different levels. These are reviewed later in this section.

A general physical examination that documents body weight, height, peripheral circulation, skin integrity, limb dominance, overall health, comorbidities, and mental status is necessary. The examination of the residual limb (RL) should include the soft-tissue length and shape, bone length and shape, and skin integrity, pliability, and mobility. Scar tissue is assessed as is the RL's tolerance to pressure, traction, and weight bearing. Sensation is also evaluated as well as the presence of neuroma or areas of hypersensitivity. The clinician should document the range of motion (ROM) and strength of the proximal joints. The status of the contralateral limb and the ROM, strength, and sensation of the other limbs are critical data in the planning of the rehabilitation program. Balance and coordination are also essential and should be tested.

Patients with peripheral neuropathy or skin grafts use vision as a compensatory mechanism for the lack of sensation in the prosthesis and the other limbs. Eye examination should be encouraged, as many patients need updated prescription eyeglasses and vision care.

In the patient whose amputation was caused by ischemia related to atherosclerosis or diabetes mellitus, similar arterial insufficiency involving the cardiac and cerebral vessels should be suspected. Knowledge of cardiopulmonary status and endurance is of primary importance. The use of sophisticated tests to assess these systems in patients with a cardiac history is usually unnecessary. Simple clinical indicators such as the ability to ambulate with a walker or crutches for 30 to 40 ft, while blood pressure and pulse rate are monitored, are adequate to determine whether the patient will be able to achieve the goal of limited household ambulation. Patients with a documented ejection fraction of 15% should be able to ambulate very short distances with an artificial limb. The cardiac risk in this population does not appear to be significantly increased when using a prosthesis or walking short distances. Therapeutic walking is an appropriate technique for cardiovascular training. In addition, the capacity for short-distance ambulation will often permit a patient to remain out of a long-term-care facility. This has additional psychosocial benefits that may outweigh the potential risks.

The patient's willingness and ability to learn new techniques and to participate in a variety of new activities are critical. Thus, cognitive and psychological evaluations are very important. The psychological impact of limb amputation is huge. Patients experience a variety of emotional and psychological responses, including anxiety, shame, depression, anger, and fear. The rehabilitation team must provide support, treatment, and guidance for the patient and his or her family (2,12–19). Nutritional status, which has a considerable impact on wound healing and strength, must not be neglected (22–24). The presence of a variety of other comorbidities such as diabetic retinopathy, peripheral polyneuropathy, nephropathy, and degenerative joint disease may also influence the rehabilitation of the amputee. In short, a thorough medical evaluation of the patient is necessary.

Other areas of importance that should be evaluated include the vocational and recreational activities that the patient performed in the past and wants to pursue in the future. Certain vocational or avocational activities may require alternative specialized prosthetic devices, training, or use of no prosthesis. Devices that may be exposed to extreme weather, water, or other elements that may be corrosive or destructive to the prosthesis should be made of special materials to protect the RL and the prosthesis.

Social support systems play an important role in the amputee's rehabilitation. The rehabilitation program for a person living with an able-bodied spouse in an elevator-accessible single-floor apartment is different from that of a person living alone in a third-story walk-up apartment.

Lastly, the rehabilitation team needs to evaluate and consider the patient's motivation, preferences, and desires, as well as the importance of cosmesis as a factor in prosthetic fabrication.

As previously mentioned, several important factors need to be considered during the evaluation of the patient with particular levels of limb loss. For the transfemoral level of amputation, assessing the length (short, mid, long) of the RL, ROM of the hip (particularly extension), and strength of the hip (particularly abduction, extension) is important. Knowledge of the type of surgical technique used for amputation is important; in particular, surgical reattachment of the adductor group (myodesis) has a significant impact on future function (25). The configuration of the distal end of the femur and the presence of heterotopic ossification or bone growth at the tip should be noted. Other characteristics of the RL that should be noted include location of surgical scars, position and type of grafts (skin or vascular), and ability to bear weight distally. These factors should be considered when the prosthetic socket is fabricated. Surgical revision should be considered when heterotopic bone, scars, grafts, or other features of the RL prevent adequate prosthetic fabrication.

Assessment of the transtibial RL involves similar considerations. The length is categorized as short, mid, or long. Strength and ROM of the hip and knee are evaluated. Assessment of hip and knee extension is particularly important. As with the transfemoral RL, location of scars, presence of skin or vascular grafts, and the nature of the surgical technique (myodesis or myoplasty) are also noted. The configuration of the distal end and its ability to bear weight are also important factors.

For the transradial level of amputation (short, mid, long), evaluation of the ROM and strength of the elbow, shoulder, and scapula and the quantification of pronation and supination are necessary. The position of surgical scars, configuration of the distal end, type of surgical closure carried out (myodesic or myoplastic), and the ability of the RL to receive distal pressure and weight bearing are assessed. Contractility of the underlying muscle is of particular importance if a myoelectric device is to be considered.

For the bilateral upper-limb amputee, the ROM and strength of shoulder and neck and trunk flexibility are important factors. One should assess the ability to use lower limbs for functional activities such as opening doors, stabilizing objects, feeding, and other essential functions. The ideal length of the limbs is determined by using a ratio of height; for very-proximal-level amputations, the forearm section is made shorter to improve elbow lift power by reducing the lever arm length. It is necessary to determine the optimal prosthetic control systems to be used (body power versus external power or both). For externally powered devices, myoelectric or switch control can be used. This decision also requires knowledge of the availability of appropriate funding sources and access to maintenance. Externally powered devices require more maintenance than body-powered devices. Projecting the patient's dependency on the prosthetic devices and the availability of help when the prosthesis fails will help to determine the need for a second set of artificial arms (usually of different control mechanism).

For patients who have had bilateral lower-limb amputation, the evaluation should focus on the strength, dexterity, and ROM of the upper limbs and the ability to use the upper limbs for support during walking. Assessment of the cardiopulmonary systems is essential in view of the expected increase in metabolic cost during walking. Limb-lengths should be determined based on the ability to transfer from sitting to standing (18 inches to the knee may be sufficient) while keeping a lower center of mass for improved balance and more efficient energy utilization during standing and walking. Choosing prosthetic components based on needs, desires, and available funding sources, as well as accessibility to maintenance, is critical. Projecting the patient's dependency on the prosthetic devices will permit determining the need for a wheelchair or a second set of artificial legs (maybe waterproof ones to be used also during showers).

When a myoelectric prosthesis is prescribed, the evaluation should begin with determination of the level of amputation (short, mid, long). ROM of the shoulder and scapula and strength of the shoulder muscles, primarily those of flexion and abduction, should be assessed. The presence of myodesic or myoplastic closure and the available control at the residual muscles for the wrist for transradial level and at the elbow for transhumeral level should be determined. Assessment of electromyographic (EMG) signal strength (>20 units on Myotester) of the muscles to be used to trigger the prosthesis is necessary. If the patient is not able to generate separate signals for flexors and extensors and co-contract them for full utilization of myoelectric controls, appropriate training with EMG feedback is to be implemented.

PREPROSTHETIC TRAINING

Preprosthetic training ideally focuses on the goals of functional independence without a prosthetic device. In addition, for individuals who will receive a prosthesis, the RL is prepared for prosthetic use.

The average age of the amputee population is 50 to 70 years old (26–28). Usually they will have several comorbidities and have lost strength and endurance in the weeks leading up to the amputation (29,30). A comprehensive supervised exercise program including ROM, strengthen-

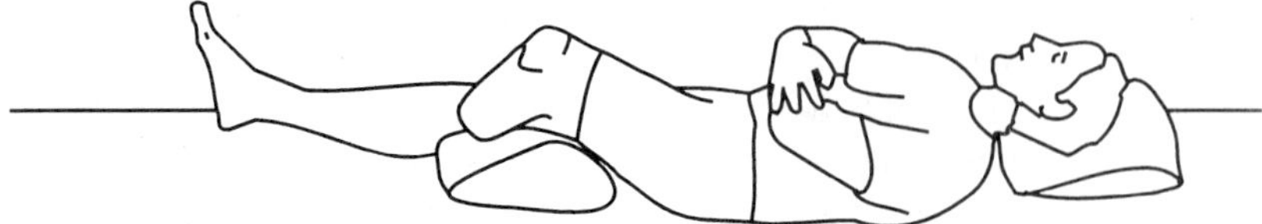

Figure 93-2. Inappropriate bed position of comfort that may promote contractures of the hip and knee.

ing, and endurance exercises, as well as functional activities, promotes improvement in these areas (31,32). Of course, precautions dictated by the patient's comorbidities are to be observed.

Patients are often eager to perform the upper-limb exercises that promote the strength and ROM required for self-care activities. However, most patients with recent limb loss are more concerned with mobility than bathing and dressing. Arms provide the power for wheelchair mobility and the use of walking aids. In particular, shoulder stabilizers, adductors, and depressors, elbow extensors, wrist stabilizers, and hand grasp strength are of prime importance for supporting the body for transfers and using the more common walking aids.

Trunk balance and strength must not be neglected. Strong flexible rotators, flexors, and extensors of the back and abdomen and the extensors of the hips facilitate sitting balance and bed mobility and transfers.

The importance of lower-limb exercise is obvious. The remaining limb for the unilateral amputee temporarily becomes the solitary support limb and frequently can develop symptoms consistent with overuse, particularly at the knee and ankle. Stance-phase stability requires adequate strength in the hip extensors, abductors, knee extensors, and plantarflexors. Swing-phase limb advancement and clearance require adequate hip flexor and ankle dorsiflexor strength.

Lower-limb contractures are distressingly common in the amputee population. Unfortunately, the position of comfort is often the position that can result in contractures. Patients often need continual reminders that contractures can significantly impair their future mobility and compromise the integrity of the nonamputated limb. The transfemoral-level amputee often develops contractures of the hip flexors, abductors, and external rotators. The transtibial-level amputee frequently develops hip and knee flexion contractures (Fig. 93-2). Contractures of the hip flexors, knee flexors, and plantarflexors of the intact limb of the unilateral amputee often result from prolonged bed rest in the comfortable semi-Fowler position. If soft-tissue contracture results in an equinus posture, the normal weight-bearing posture of the foot is compromised. Pressure distribution to the heel is lost and forces are focused on the forefoot. The increased pressure on the forefoot can lead to local pain and tissue breakdown of particular concern in the presence of peripheral neuropathy or arterial insufficiency.

The "ounce of prevention" approach certainly applies to limb contractures. Several factors can contribute to contractures: preoperative positioning, surgical technique, postoperative pain, deficient knowledge regarding ROM, and limited mobility related to ischemia, skin grafts, infection, or trauma that led to the amputation. Treatment of contractures may include heating modalities, prolonged passive stretch, spring-loaded orthoses, serial casting, nerve blocks, or further surgery. To avoid contractures, patients are instructed to move limbs through a full ROM frequently and to avoid postures of prolonged flexion. Periods of lying prone should be included in the lower-limb amputee's exercise program. A posterior splint may help prevent knee flexion contractures in the transtibial-level amputee. Frequent reminders and encouragement help the patient follow through on these instructions. Contractures are readily prevented through the use of an immediate postoperative rigid dressing (33,34). The rigid dressing extends proximally, enclosing the knee, preventing a flexion contracture.

The lower-limb amputee's outlook brightens considerably when he or she is allowed out of bed. Independence in transfers and functional mobility are of great importance. Bed mobility exercises include rolling from side to side and sitting up, to allow the patient to position himself or herself without calling for help. Transfer training allows the patient to expand his or her world beyond the bed and room. The patient may utilize sliding board, front-on/back-off, or stand (squat) pivot transfers to move from one surface to another.

Functional mobility for the amputee may take several forms. Most lower-limb amputees will use a wheelchair at some point and should learn proper wheelchair management, including using the leg rests and brakes. Safe techniques for propulsion and turns appear simple, but require teaching and practice. The wheelchair must be suitable for the individual. A person with limited strength or with significant cardiac impairment may be unable to safely propel a chair of normal weight. Removable armrests are needed for those who utilize a sliding board or squat pivot transfer to the chair (Fig. 93-3). The center of gravity of the person seated in a wheelchair shifts posteriorly if a lower limb is absent. Therefore, an off-set axle or antitippers are appropriate. These are of particular importance when going up a ramp or curb.

Ambulation training without the prosthesis is very important to the amputee. Initially, standing balance and standing tolerance are addressed. Once the patient can manage standing, then ambulation (hopping) using the parallel bars can begin. As strength and endurance improve, the patient may advance to a walker and to crutches. In

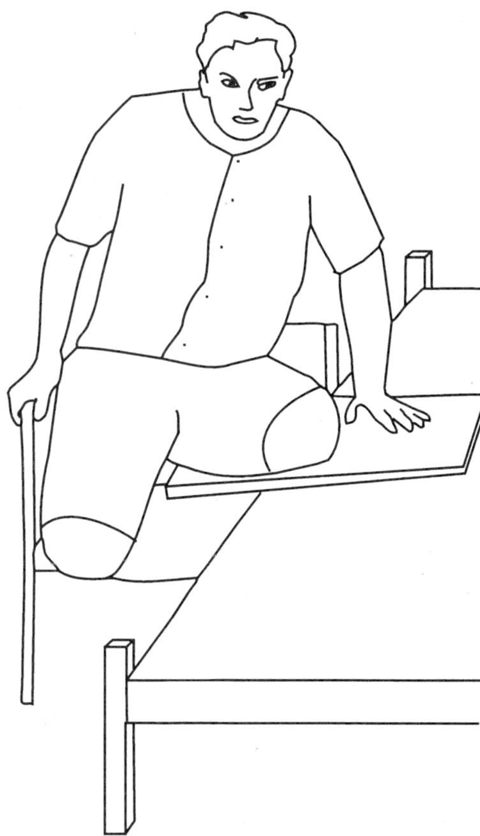

Figure 93-3. Sliding board transfer to a bed for the bilateral transfemoral amputee.

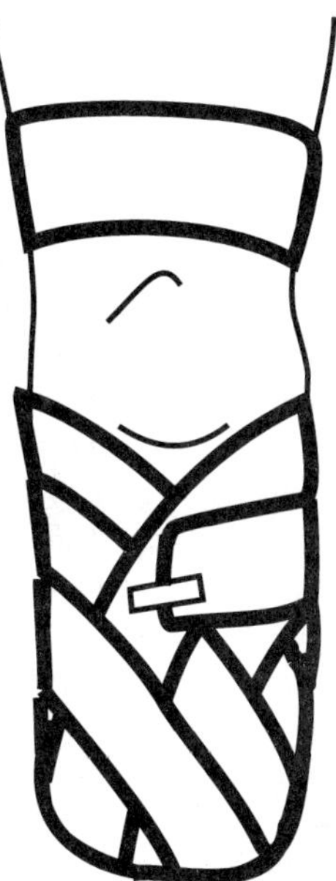

Figure 93-4. Elastic bandaging of the transtibial residual limb.

addition to allowing greater mobility, the activities improve lower-limb strength and ROM and serve to remind the patient that bipedal walking may soon be a reality.

Stairs are often a source of concern for the amputee. When walking up and down stairs is not yet possible, many individuals use a "bumping" technique to ascend or descend. The patient sits on the steps and uses the arms and remaining lower limb to propel himself or herself up or down. Of course, the floor transfer at the top or bottom of the stairs must also be addressed. Many amputees use a low box or stool as a "step" between the floor and the wheelchair or standing posture.

Not all patients can tolerate standing activities initially. For patients who cannot, because of orthostatic hypotension or other reasons, a more gradual approach is needed. Allowing the patient to press his or her foot against a foot board while in bed can simulate lower-limb weight bearing. Alternatively, the patient may hold a towel, a length of cloth, or a length of elastic tubing looped under the foot and apply pressure to the plantar surface of the foot. Gradual progression to a more erect posture may be achieved by elevating the head of the bed or using a tilt table.

While many amputees focus their attention on walking, their ability to perform self-care activities may be more important to their going home. As safe techniques for bathing and dressing and toileting are mastered, the amputee realizes that he or she need not fear being "a burden." Self-esteem and optimism are restored. In addition to self-care activities, many amputees must also perform homemaking activities to resume their life roles. Using a wheelchair, walker, or crutches, the amputee learns to prepare meals, do laundry, and perform other household chores.

Most of the preceding discussion is appropriate for the lower-limb amputee. For the upper-limb amputee, transfers and mobility are less problematic while self-care activities may be more difficult. Regardless of previous right- or left-handedness, the remaining limb becomes dominant for the upper-limb amputee. Thus, there may be considerable time spent on change of dominance. The patient will also learn various single-handed techniques for bathing, dressing, grooming, and other self-care activities (35).

Care of the RL focuses on several areas including wound healing, volume containment, optimization of strength and ROM, and desensitization. Needless to say, the healing wound should be kept clean and monitored for signs of infection. Volume containment can be achieved through several approaches. Ideally, the immediate postoperative rigid dressing, applied in the operating room, provides edema control as well as mechanical protection for the limb (33,34,36). As an alternative, the removable rigid dressing can be used, allowing the patient greater participation (37,38). The Unna boot also prevents swelling but requires no particular skill in its application (39–42). Ace bandages, tubular compression dressings, or stump shrinkers provide elastic compression and may be favored for their simplicity and neatness (Fig. 93-4) (43,44).

Because the RL is an end organ, responsible for the manipulation, positioning, control, and general operation of the prosthesis, exercises for the RL are crucial. Normal strength and ROM of the RL will help to optimize prosthetic use.

Many amputees will not receive a prosthesis. There may be cognitive, physical, psychological, financial, or other reasons for this. Other amputees may simply decline the option of using a prosthesis. For this group, therapies to optimize strength, endurance, and ROM and to achieve independence in mobility, self-care, and other life tasks without a prosthetic device are provided. There are also patients for whom functional independence is not a realistic goal. Some patients will always need some assistance for mobility and self-care. Therapies for these people will focus on caregivers as well as on the patient (18). Family members or other individuals involved in the care of the amputee are educated and trained in appropriate techniques for RL care, mobility, bathing, dressing, and hygiene.

REHABILITATION WITH PREPARATORY PROSTHESIS

Return to bipedal ambulation is the stated goal of most lower-limb amputees. Amputees often feel that only by returning to ambulation can they resume their previous lives, roles, activities, and socialization (12). Walking again is an enormously important transition for the amputee.

Starting with an accurate knowledge base is important for the patient and health care provider alike. A review of goals and expectations is appropriate at this point. Not all patients will recall the prior discussions regarding these topics, so reminders may be necessary. It is also appropriate for the therapist to review the patient's diagnosis and comorbidities as well as precautions, to minimize the complications that may develop as gait training proceeds.

Rehabilitation with the preparatory prosthesis begins by introducing the patient to the components of the preparatory prosthesis and its management. Explanations of how the prosthesis fits, where weight is borne, where and why discomfort may occur, and how adjustments can be made help put the patient at ease. It is useful to remind the patient that his or her weight must be supported by some pressure-tolerant portion of the RL, or walking would be impossible. Pressure is to be expected and this may be uncomfortable at first but should not be painful.

With experience and the teachings of the treatment team, the patient learns the appropriate fit of the prosthesis and the way to adjust the fit with stump socks when necessary. The patient needs to learn that the prosthetic fit is a dynamic entity and that he or she needs to be aware of subtle changes in socket fit or alignment that provide clues to necessary adjustments (43,45).

Gait training begins with weight bearing and weight shifting, using the parallel bars for upper-limb support. The patient gradually progresses to ambulation in the parallel bars. The therapist may find it difficult to focus the patient on proper technique including equal step length and appropriate weight shifting. Gait deviations frequently develop owing to the patient's eagerness to begin walking. As the patient establishes a consistent gait pattern and can maintain good form, he or she advances to use of a walker, crutches, and unilateral support devices. Once the patient is comfortable with level surfaces, he or she progresses to walking on stairs, curbs, and ramps, as well as uneven terrain. The patient also learns safe techniques for transfers, including to and from the floor (32).

Frequent monitoring of the skin allows for prompt corrections of socket-fit problems and avoids skin breakdown. Skin checks are done more frequently for the new prosthetic user and for the patient with delicate skin. Initially, checking the skin every 10 to 15 minutes or after every one or two walks may be necessary. Once the patient and therapist are comfortable with the socket fit, skin monitoring can occur less frequently.

Prosthetic wearing tolerance gradually increases over the first few weeks. Some patients can only wear the prosthesis for 2 to 3 hr/day during the first week of gait training. This gradually increases until it is worn all day (12–16 hours). Throughout the rehabilitation process, the patient should become well versed in skin care. The patient learns to monitor the skin of the RL, noting signs of appropriate weight bearing and watching for evidence of skin irritation or breakdown.

When the prosthesis is not worn, the patient wears a stump shrinker or an Ace bandage to prevent edema and provide volume containment (43,44).

As the amputee progresses with ambulation and management of the prosthesis, ambulatory self-care activities and homemaking activities can be addressed. Occupational therapy works with the patient to learn safe techniques for bathing, dressing, and toileting using the prosthesis. Some patients may find that initially, certain activities are more easily performed without the prosthesis. In these situations, it is important to remember that the primary goal of therapy is functional independence, not necessarily continuous prosthetic use. Many patients need to perform homemaking tasks as well. The therapist should include meal preparation, laundry, shopping, and other household chores in the training routine of these individuals, using the prosthesis if possible.

As the patient progresses through ambulation training, emotional and psychological needs must not be neglected. New anxieties or unfilled expectations may arise during training with the prosthesis and should be addressed by the psychologist and other members of the rehabilitation team. The patient is encouraged to express concerns and disappointments so that steps can be taken to rectify these problems. While some problems may not have solutions, the patient can be reassured that the rehabilitation team does not ignore the patient's perceived issues.

Few patients can proceed through ambulation training without experiencing problems with pain. Phantom discomfort has been extensively investigated (20,46–49). Approaches to treatment include biofeedback (50), imagery (51), relaxation techniques (52), massage, ultrasound (53), transcutaneous electrical nerve stimulation (TENS) (54), oral and injectable medications (20,46), and surgery (20,46). This topic is discussed in detail elsewhere in this text. RL pain is frequently related to socket fit and prosthetic alignment. By listening to the patient's complaint, examining the RL, and watching the patient use the prosthesis, the clinician can generally solve fit and alignment problems. Prosthetic component changes and alignment adjustments are more readily performed when modular, adjustable components are used. Because the RL and the patient's gait pattern are continually changing, it is common for pain problems to develop or recur without apparent provocation. Therefore, it is helpful for the members of the rehabilitation team to remind the patient that occasional difficulties and setbacks are common and are not reasons for despair.

REHABILITATION WITH PERMANENT PROSTHESIS

Ideally, rehabilitation of the amputee involves testing the definitive prosthetic componentry on the preparatory device. This allows the therapist and other team members to train the patient immediately in the appropriate use of the components that will be used in the definitive prosthesis. However, this is not always possible, because of reimbursement issues or various other factors, such as an inability to predict a patient's level of function early in the rehabilitation course. Therefore, a patient who receives different componentry in the definitive prosthesis than in the preparatory device will require retraining in the specifics of the new componentry. The socket and some components of a preparatory prosthesis are not as durable as those of the definitive prosthesis, thus limiting the patient's functional capabilities. Patients should refrain from using the pylon or preparatory prosthesis without an assistive device, even though they may eventually progress to this level when they receive their permanent prosthetic device. With more sophisticated componentry, patients may face higher functional expectations such as work simulation, ambulation on varied surfaces, and sports.

Concerning the socket, it is vital to allow the patient's RL to mature before fabrication of the permanent socket. The soft-tissue bulk of the RL decreases significantly, owing to resolution of edema as well as disuse atrophy of muscles and adipose tissue. These changes occur primarily during the first 2 to 5 months following the amputation. The definitive prosthesis frequently uses a suction suspension mechanism that is not usually recommended for a preparatory pylon because of fluctuations in RL girth (43). Patients often will require new instruction on donning techniques for the suction socket. Transfemoral-level amputees will have significant changes in their abilities depending on the knee unit prescribed, and instruction in mobility and gait should vary based on the type of mechanism used in the permanent prosthetic device. For example, patients ambulating with a cadence-responsive knee with swing and stance control will require a different gait pattern compared to patients using a weight-activated knee unit. They will also have different mechanisms for transferring from sitting to standing and ascending and descending stairs and inclines.

For the upper-limb amputee, early prosthetic fitting is vital to the acceptance of the prosthesis (36). Generally, the first prosthesis uses conventional or body-powered componentry. Myoelectric or externally powered prostheses are not usually recommended at this stage because of the fluctuation in girth as the RL matures. This fluctuation will make it difficult to achieve the intimate fit between the skin and socket needed for the myoelectric system to work properly. Additionally, one should verify that the patient will be a prosthetic user before incurring the higher cost of an externally powered prosthesis. Upper-limb amputees who are progressing from conventional to myoelectric prosthetics require a period of retraining, to instruct them in the proper use and care of the new prosthesis.

In conclusion, the transitions from a preparatory prosthesis to a permanent prosthesis will necessitate education of patients on any changes in the way that they don and doff their prostheses and the performance of their new componentry. Patients are made aware that whenever they receive a new socket, they must be vigilant about skin inspection, as there is potential for new areas of pressure or breakdown of the skin.

VOCATIONAL AND AVOCATIONAL TRAINING

It is important to note that a successful outcome for an amputee means returning as close as possible to the previous level of function. For the working-age patient, return to some gainful employment should be expected. Similarly, patients at any age should be able to return to previous or modified leisure activities including sports or hobbies. The patient should know early in rehabilitation that the long-range expectation is to return to work and play.

In the case of employment, work simulation activities should be incorporated into the patient's therapy programs early and should intensify in the latter part of the rehabilitation program. The rehabilitation team should make attempts to contact the patient's employer to establish the physical demand of the jobs. Wherever possible, employers should be informed and involved in the retraining. Work-site evaluations can be very helpful in understanding job

Table 93-1: Sport Organizations for the Amputee

American Amputee Foundation, Inc.	(501) 666-2523
Amputee Coalition of America	(708) 698-1628
Amputee Sports Association	(912) 927-5406
National Amputee Golf Association	(800) 633-NAGA
National Association of Disabled Swimmers	(813) 755-1078
National Association of Handicapped Outdoorsmen	(618) 532-4565
National Wheelchair Athletic Association	(719) 635-9300
Shake-A-Leg	(401) 849-8898

demands and making recommendations for work environment modifications or changes in the patient's job description. In some cases it is not feasible for the patient to meet the physical requirements of the previous job. Limiting factors often include heavy manual labor, prolonged standing periods, or jobs that require well-developed balance. For such situations it is very important to have the patient receive career counseling and job retraining (55). Contact with the local branch of the state office of vocational rehabilitation or its equivalent can be of great assistance as patients re-enter the workforce.

Similarly, the patient should be encouraged to return to his or her prior leisure activity. Participation in sports is often very important to younger amputees and sometimes older amputees. The patient should be provided with information on various sports groups, for example, the National Amputee Golf Association, amputee ski groups, and national disabled sports organizations (Table 93-1). Participation in some sports will require specific prosthetic componentry, and consideration of recreational goals should be given when one is formulating the prosthetic prescription (56). Efforts should be made to teach the patient specific sport skills.

A commonly stated desire for athletic ability is to be able to run again. This goal should be considered for all active amputees, even if it is to run just a short distance for a bus or to get out of danger. A good socket fit is crucial for running for both transtibial-level and transfemoral-level amputees. A good fit allows the patient to tolerate the tremendous amount of pressure and reaction forces translated to the limb without too much discomfort. For the healthy, active transtibial-level amputee, running is fairly easy to achieve (57,58). When the patient is ambulating independently without an assistive device, he or she is ready to begin training. Hopping and jumping activities will assist with building the patient's tolerance for increased force transmitted to the limb. A gradual progression from fast walking, to a trot and then a run is usually successful. The treadmill can be useful to progress the patient to higher speeds. The transfemoral-level amputee requires increased training to achieve running. For them the appropriate components such as cadence-responsive knees are vital to achieve a step-over-step running pattern.

Without a cadence-responsive knee unit, the patient has to wait for the shank of the prosthesis to come forward, resulting in an extra hop on the sound limb. Training techniques for the transfemoral running gait often begin with weight-bearing activities, balance activities, and exercise to improve pelvic and hip control. Initially there is an emphasis on hopping and jumping, to increase tolerance to increased forces translated to the residual limb. Fast walking and ambulating with an exaggerated step length and then a progression to jogging or running can occur. Again, once patients have achieved limited success at a step-over-step running pattern, running on a treadmill at gradually higher speeds can help to increase their cadence (59).

COMMUNITY REINTEGRATION

While many amputees simply say, "I want to walk again," ambulation is only a portion of comprehensive rehabilitation. The goals of a thorough rehabilitation program include helping the patient resume previous roles in the "family" and community. The entire rehabilitation team should help identify the patient's goals and roles. Each patient may not "open up" equally to all team members. The patient often has difficulty communicating because fear, anger, and depression dominate the thoughts in the days, weeks, and even months following amputation (3,12–17,19).

Several questions can help clarify the patient's previous role in the family or social network. What was the person's level of independence? Was the patient the primary homemaker or "breadwinner" in the family? If so, then who (if anyone) has taken on these roles during the patient's illness? Does the patient expect to return to these roles? Is the patient a spouse, parent, child, or other member of the family unit? Was the patient a caregiver or a care recipient prior to the amputation? Does the amputation change this role? If so, how?

It may be difficult to anticipate how the patient and the family will adapt to the amputee's return. There is often a confusing mixture of expectations on the part of each. The patient generally wants to get "back to normal" but may find it quite difficult. He or she may be expecting some assistance, but resenting assistance when it is provided. Members of the family may want to assist but not know how much or how little assistance is needed or welcomed. In general, an awkward situation frequently exists until communication, education, and experience occur. It is useful for members of the rehabilitation team to meet with the patient and family, individually and together, to facilitate resolution of these issues. Long-term counseling may be needed as the patient and family adjust. Discussing the importance of previous family roles and how the amputation may have changed these roles is helpful. This will help the patient and family reach decisions regarding which roles are most important and which may be abandoned or modified (18).

The new amputee's role in the community should be similarly examined. Was the patient an active participant in community events? Was he or she a passive spectator? Was he uninvolved? How does the amputation affect the person's participation in community outings such as shopping trips, trips to restaurants, or trips to the movies or theater? The previously active patient may find it difficult to resume these activities, for physical reasons or because of self-conscious feelings. Therapeutic outings with members of the rehabilitation team to restaurants, malls, or movie theaters can help desensitize the patient to these awkward feelings and facilitate resumption of these activities. Frequently, the patient must learn to be more aggressive or assertive to make use of programs or facilities not obviously available. This may be quite difficult for a person who is normally shy or passive. The patient should also be educated about community programs and resources that may facilitate participation by people with disabilities (60,61).

Returning to driving plays a significant role in many patients' resuming normal activities. Frequently, a minor modification or no modification to the vehicle is required for the amputee to resume driving. Without relying on others for mobility, the amputee's independence grows.

SPECIAL CONSIDERATIONS FOR THE COMPLEX AMPUTEE AND THE PATIENT WITH DUAL DISABILITY

It is increasingly common in the rehabilitation population to encounter patients with dual disability such as hemiplegia and limb loss, blindness and limb loss, and multiple limb loss. Each individual disability can be catastrophic on its own; the dual disability may be even more so, resulting in long-term placement of the patient in a nursing home. With the appropriate interventions and social support systems, many patients with dual disability can return to their home environment. A rehabilitated limb after amputation prior to the onset of hemiparesis from stroke has a better functional outcome than if the stroke had preceded the amputation (62). A right hemiparesis or an ipsilateral hemiplegia and limb loss also have a better prognosis, compared with a left hemiparesis or limb loss contralateral to the hemiplegia.

Clear simple step-by-step instructions and a modified prosthesis are very useful for these patients. For the blind patient, sensory input using raised markings, Velcro closures, and step-by-step sequencing is useful. A cane should be used whenever possible to provide protective auditory and tactile feedback to the patient. Appropriate home environment modifications should be carried out.

Fifty percent of patients who have had a lower-limb amputation due to disease are at risk for a second amputation within 3 years. If no other concurrent disabilities occur, the patient with a second transtibial amputation should achieve a level of independence similar to that attained prior to the second amputation. The heights of the prostheses are routinely decreased to improve balance and possibly decrease the energy required to maintain standing balance.

For patients with bilateral transfemoral amputation, there is a significant increase in energy consumption, estimated at over 100% (63), that may prevent long-distance ambulation. In general, most transfemoral bilateral amputees over 50 years old will find the wheelchair an easier and more practical means of locomotion. Ambulation should be attempted only when adequate cardiac function, strength, balance, and endurance exist; the use of multiaxis ankle-feet systems with lower height and weight-activated knee-locking mechanisms should facilitate the patient's ability to ambulate (64). The clinician can avoid unnecessary expenditures of resources in the geriatric population by careful selection of potentially functional ambulation candidates who have had bilateral transfemoral amputations (65).

Bilateral Amputation

Intuitively ambulation with bilateral lower-limb loss should be much more difficult than with single lower-limb loss. The limited data available support this thesis (65,66–69), but many bilateral amputees ambulate nonetheless, with varying degrees of proficiency. For all these individuals, there should be a long discussion on the difficulties they face, the risks (including falls and increased cardiac demand), and realistic goals before prosthetic fabrication commences.

Many bilateral transtibial-level amputees will achieve independence in ambulation with prostheses (Fig. 93-5). Several prosthetic modifications can be performed to make ambulation with bilateral transtibial prostheses less difficult. Although some patients may object, shortening the prostheses by 1 or 2 inches lowers the center of gravity and can improve balance and decrease energy consumption during standing and ambulation. Of course, the height can be restored later if the patient so chooses, and if walking skills have progressed satisfactorily. By out-setting the feet, the base of support is widened and balance is also enhanced (Fig. 93-6). Flexing the sockets or dorsiflexing the feet promotes a forward lean and slightly crouched posture, which also gives most bilateral transtibial-level amputees a sense of improved stability. Using articulated single-axis feet rather than fixed ankles may also improve balance and ambulation by reducing the knee flexion moment during the loading response. During normal gait, in the early-stance phase (initial contact and loading response), the ground reaction force falls behind the ankle, generating a plantarflexion moment (70). This plantarflexion is controlled by the activity of the pretibial muscles, allowing the foot to gradually descend to the floor. The ground reaction force lies behind the knee as well, requiring the knee extensors to prevent buckling of the knee. The magnitude of the knee flexion moment increases with the perpendicular distance between the ground reaction force and the knee joint center (71). For the transtibial-level amputee whose prosthesis has a fixed ankle, the ground reaction force is located farther behind the knee and remains there for a longer period of time. This generates a more significant flexion moment. When an articulated ankle is used, the prosthetic foot plantarflexes to a foot-flat posture promptly after initial contact. This moves the ground reaction force farther anterior, reducing the distance to the knee center and reducing the magnitude and duration of the flexion moment. Most patients will appreciate the flexibility of the articulated ankle, but others may find the ankle motion a source of instability and increased weight. Some patients report that the solid ankle of a SACH (solid-ankle cushion-heel) foot or most energy-storing feet feels more firm and stable, and therefore, more comfortable.

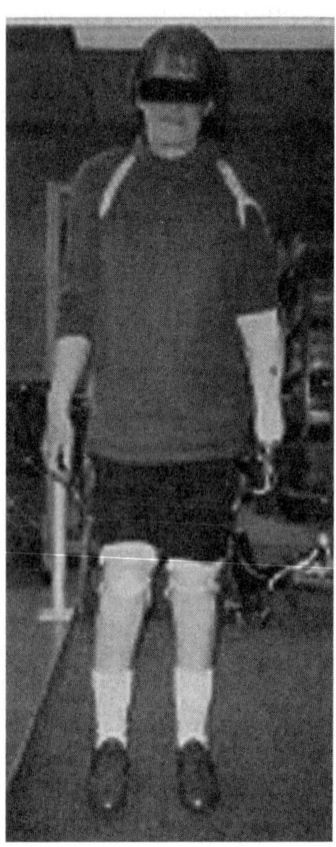

Figure 93-5. Bilateral transtibial amputee with prosthesis (digital image).

The bilateral amputee who has had one transtibial and one transfemoral amputation can benefit from some of the modifications indicated above. Widening the base of support, moving the center of mass forward, and lowering the center of mass can be helpful. Articulated ankles should also enhance standing and walking stability. The design of the knee on the transfemoral amputation side should be chosen carefully. If stability is a great concern, a simple lightweight manual-lock knee removes the risk of knee buckling. The data are limited, and studies have yielded conflicting conclusions about the energy costs of ambulation with a locked or swinging prosthetic knee. Traugh et al (72) found no significant difference in the energy cost of ambulation using a locked compared to an unlocked knee. Isakov et al (73) found that ambulation with a locked knee is more energy efficient. Meanwhile many patients prefer an unlocked knee because of the more natural-appearing gait and improved ability to transfer. A weight-activated or polycentric knee allows flexion during the swing phase but still resists knee flexion during stance. A hydraulic or pneumatic knee will provide a more

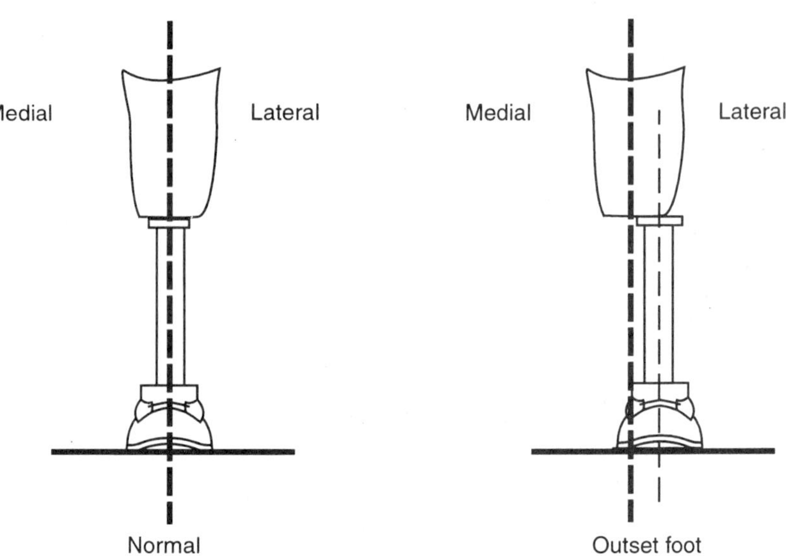

Figure 93-6. Alignment modifications to improve the base of support for bilateral amputees, outset foot.

physiologic function for the vigorous, high-activity-level patient, but its use in the geriatric population may be limited by weight and cost.

Many patients who have had transtibial and transfemoral amputations use the prosthesis on a limited basis, in the home or for social events, and may use alternative means of mobility such as a wheelchair most of the time. Other patients may use only a single prosthesis (usually the transtibial) for transfers, standing, and limited swing-through ambulation. For many individuals with significant cardiac or muscle strength limitations or contractures, no prostheses or only a transtibial prosthesis may be the best alternative for transfers.

Few bilateral transfemoral-level amputees will be functional long-distance ambulators, although many will achieve limited independence in ambulation with prostheses. The energy required for the bilateral transfemoral-level amputee to ambulate is simply too great (67,69). The modifications mentioned earlier can be utilized to make ambulation less difficult. Some patients may initially use "stubbies," short nonarticulated limbs with broad feet (74), and then graduate to taller limbs with knees. The choice of knees should be made after considering stability, safety, weight, cost, and activity level. As with the transtibial-transfemoral amputee population, many bilateral transfemoral-level amputees choose wheelchair mobility with no prostheses because of simplicity, energy efficiency, and comfort.

Several factors are relative contraindications to prescribing prostheses for the bilateral lower-limb amputee. These include lack of motivation, significant cognitive impairment, severe cardiac disease, severe contractures, and severe neurologic impairment (75). The degree of cardiac compromise a patient can tolerate while walking with bilateral prostheses is unclear. An ejection fraction of 20% may be chosen as an arbitrary cutoff, but no hard data exist to substantiate this. Prosthetic ambulation is possible in the setting of significant cardiac compromise because amputees adjust their walking speed to keep relative energy demands at a manageable level (76). Patients must participate in this decision-making process and should understand the rationale behind the decision. They should never feel that they were not given the opportunity to walk with prostheses "just because the doctor said I couldn't." When patients are presented with appropriate information regarding the risks and advantages of ambulation, and are provided with an accurate idea of what ambulation with bilateral prostheses will be like, they are generally able to reach rational decisions.

The sequence of amputations is thought to have an impact on future bilateral prosthetic ambulation (75). People who are able to ambulate with a transfemoral prosthesis are likely to be able to achieve bilateral prosthetic ambulation after a subsequent transtibial amputation. However, the transtibial prosthetic user who has a subsequent contralateral transfemoral amputation may have a more difficult time achieving ambulatory status following the second amputation.

The issue of rehabilitation for bilateral amputees has become increasingly important as the prevalence of bilateral lower-limb amputations rises and resources become scarcer. Kerstein et al (77) in 1974 noted that 23% of their amputee rehabilitation population were bilateral amputees. Esquenazi et al (26) in 1984 reported an increasing number of amputees readmitted for bilateral prosthetic training. Nondiabetic patients who undergo an amputation for ischemia have a 5% to 13% risk at 1 year and 28% risk at 5 years for contralateral amputation (78,79). For the diabetic population, the risk is higher, approximately 50% at 3 years (80).

The Blind Amputee

Since many amputees are diabetic with an increased incidence of retinopathy (81), they will frequently develop comorbidity of blindness or visual impairment. Patients who recently became blind should receive a program of instruction in compensatory techniques related to their new-onset blindness, to complement the amputation rehabilitation. More often, patients have had long-standing blindness. These patients should use tactile clues to allow them to manage their prostheses appropriately. Most people can identify sock ply simply by feeling the different thicknesses, so this is usually not an issue.

However, donning the prosthetic device with the correct orientation can be difficult. When this is a problem, tactile cues such as bumps or ridges should be placed on the socket or the insert to give the patient a reference point for donning. Also the suspension straps may require alternative fasteners such as those made of Velcro, to make them easier to manage. The blind patient should be instructed to inspect the skin of the RL and intact foot by feeling for wounds, abrasions, skin irregularities, or changes in temperature. If the patient has neuropathies that decrease the sensation in the hands, a caregiver should be instructed in assisting patient with skin inspection and prosthetic management (82).

The rehabilitation of the blind amputee should also address the environment. Ambulation with the appropriate cane for protective sensory and auditory feedback is taught. If the patient needs to use the upper limbs for support and balance, then it may be necessary to recommend walking with a companion who can serve as a guide. Of course, a home assessment should be performed before discharge of the person who is blind and has had an amputation. Modifications to the home environment can promote independence and improve safety.

Hemiplegic Amputee

As the elderly population increases and survival after stroke and amputation improve, we can expect to see more patients with generalized vasculopathy who have simultaneous vascular-related disabilities. In addition, many patients survive high-impact collisions with resulting head injuries and amputations. The dual disabilities of hemiparesis and limb loss present a spectrum of problems (62,83). The characteristics that complicate or simplify the rehabilitation process for a patient with these two disabilities are similar to the exacerbating and mitigating factors for the individual disabilities. For example, the rehabilitation of a patient after a transfemoral amputation would generally be more difficult than after a transtibial amputation, and the rehabilitation of a patient with severe hemiplegia with neglect and cognitive impairment would be more difficult than that of a patient with mild pure motor hemiparesis. The sequence of the onset of disabilities and the location (ipsilateral or contralateral) also influence the rehabilitation outcome. The individuals who first undergo an amputation and then later sustain a stroke generally achieve better functional status than do those who first are afflicted by the neurologic event (61). Ipsilateral involvement also suggests better outcome than contralateral involvement. In general, patients with right-sided hemiparesis tend to have a better functional outcome than do those with left-sided neurological residual. As one would expect, younger patients with these dual disabilities generally attain better functional outcomes than older patients.

The patient who is ambulatory after a lower-limb amputation and subsequently has a stroke with ipsilateral weakness can often regain independent ambulatory status, unless the stroke is very severe. The height and alignment of the prosthesis are adjusted to compensate for stroke-induced gait deviations where possible. Shortening the prosthesis may improve swing-phase clearance problems. Increased prosthetic ankle plantarflexion can assist weak knee extensors by providing mechanical stability to the knee joint during the stance phase. When flexor tone interferes with knee stability, the use of a thigh corset with external knee joints may be of benefit. The orthotic knee joints may be offset or single axis and equipped with drop locks to enhance stability during the stance phase. Widening the base of support by "outsetting" the prosthetic foot reduces balance problems. For the patient with severe hip adductor tone, the use of interventions to decrease spasticity focally, such as phenol block of the obturator nerve or surgical interventions (obturator neurectomy or adductor tenotomy), should be considered.

When necessary markings are placed on the prosthesis, the suspension straps, and even the socks, to make the task of donning the prosthesis a more structured process that can be made routine by a patient with cognitive deficits. Patients with significant upper-limb involvement will need to learn one-handed prosthetic management techniques. For the transtibial-level amputee, certain devices can be used to achieve one-handed donning, such as neoprene, spandex, or silicone sleeves, which can be rolled on with one hand. For the transfemoral-level amputee, the prosthesis, because of its size and weight, may be difficult to manage. In this situation, use of the TC-3 (84) socket, developed at the Tokyo Metropolitan Rehabilitation Center in Japan, permits the patient to handle the socket with the suspension system of choice, separate from the prosthesis. This option provides the patient with the advantage of handling a smaller section of the prosthesis, with decreased bulk and weight. Then the socket is inserted into a thin receptacle and attached with a Velcro strap. In addition, this system permits donning and doffing in the seating position.

Similar prosthetic adjustments improve the functional mobility of a person with a preexisting hemiplegia and new ipsilateral limb loss. Learning new concepts of prosthetic management such as donning and doffing the limb or adjusting the number of stump socks used may be difficult if the new amputee has preexisting cortical dysfunction. For the nonambulatory patient after a stroke and amputation, independence in transfers should still be possible, as the "intact" side should provide adequate strength and stability for standing and pivoting.

Contralateral hemiplegia and amputation pose more difficult problems. The severity of the stroke and the level of amputation determine which will be the patient's dominant leg and whether future ambulation is likely. For the transtibial-level amputee with contralateral hemiparesis, ambulation with an assistive device should be possible unless the stroke is very severe. Even with severe stroke sequelae, the patient will likely benefit from a prosthesis for standing and transfers. If the amputation is at the transfemoral level, then ambulation will be quite difficult or impossible unless the stroke is mild. For many such patients, prosthetic fabrication is not indicated.

LONG-TERM FOLLOW-UP

Long-term follow-up of the amputee involves not only prosthetic maintenance and skin checks, but also psychosocial rehabilitation and wellness behavior. For many amputees, the physiatrist is viewed as the primary physician, perhaps because the physiatrist sees the amputation as the most important health and medical issue in their lives. Thus, the physiatrist is likely to confront many health-related issues besides those associated with the RL or the prosthesis.

During a follow-up visit, the patient's prosthetic usage is discussed. Is the prosthesis worn daily? All day long? If not, are there problems with comfort that need to be addressed? If the prosthesis is not incorporated into the normal daily routine of the patient, it will always be viewed as heavy, clumsy, abnormal, and difficult to manage, despite hours of adjustments by the prosthetist and physician.

It is appropriate to review the patient's lifestyle. Does he or she leave the home for shopping, recreation, socialization, or work? People may choose to stay at home for different reasons. However, if architectural barriers or mobility dysfunction are the cause, then the patient may benefit from the physician's intervention. Further outpatient therapies to address mobility on stairs or other obstacles may be appropriate. Ramps, rails, stair glides, or other equipment may free the patient from unnecessary confinement. If the patient stays at home for medical or psychological reasons, then further evaluation and treatment of those specific problems may be necessary.

The fit and condition of the prosthesis warrant periodic evaluation. Over time, repairs to the components of the prosthesis are necessary. Changes in the size and shape of the RL require that a new socket be made periodically (85,86). Changes in the patient's condition will often dictate changes in the prosthetic prescription. For example, the transtibial-level amputee with a patellar tendon–bearing socket and elastic sleeve suspension may develop degenerative changes in the knee and may benefit from the addition of a thigh corset and mechanical knee joints for pressure relief and additional stability. While may amputees are resistant to changes in their prostheses, newer materials or components may prove advantageous. The physiatrist will need to educate the patient about the potential benefits of new technology.

Routine skin care needs to be reviewed. The patient is reminded of the importance of good hygiene. Skin irritation and breakdown may result from poor cleaning techniques. For the diabetic patient in particular, meticulous skin care is imperative. The patient is reminded to clean the skin gently with mild soap and warm water and to blot the skin dry, including between the toes of the intact foot. A skin moisturizer helps to keep the skin soft and supple, avoiding dryness, cracking, and fissures, which may lead to superficial infection. Lamb's wool placed between the toes helps avoid maceration and "kissing" ulcers. The patient is taught to avoid any potential trauma to the feet, including thermal injury. Cold feet deserve warm socks rather than a burn from a heating pad or hot water bottle. Socks should be worn with footwear, and walking barefoot is forbidden. The patient should check shoes before putting them on. At least one person required a transtibial amputation for a foot infection that began with an ulcer caused by walking with a coin in their shoe (87,88).

The routine follow-up visit is also the time to review health maintenance behavior. Cessation of smoking is an important topic for many amputees. Most people are aware that smoking leads to cardiac and pulmonary problems, but many are unaware that smoking increases the risk for limb ischemia and amputation. The patient with lower-limb ischemia and claudication would likely benefit from a regular exercise program (89). The follow-up visit is the time to introduce, clarify, or reinforce such an exercise regimen. The patient may also benefit from counseling regarding nutrition and proper body weight. While exercise and diet are important for all, it is beneficial to remind the diabetic patient that diet and exercise are the mainstays of therapy for diabetes. The patient may also need reminders regarding blood pressure checks, cholesterol monitoring, flu vaccinations, and general medical follow-up.

Finally, the routine check-up is a good time to remind the patient of his or her achievements and to discuss new goals. Absorbed in the daily routine, the amputee may lose sight of the fact that he or she overcame significant trauma. Positive feedback is very therapeutic. The clinician may want to suggest new activities such as cycling or swimming. Of course, rehabilitation professionals need not be reminded that the truly rehabilitated amputee does much more than simply walk.

CONCLUSIONS

Comprehensive rehabilitation of the amputee should be more than the provision of a prosthetic device. This is especially true for the geriatric amputee whose needs are greater because of comorbidity, fragile social supports, and limited resources. For the young, active patient, optimization of the prosthetic device and appropriate rehabilitation are necessary to preserve the patient in good health.

REFERENCES

1. Frantz CH, O'Rahilly R. Congenital skeletal limb deficiencies. *J Bone Joint Surg [AM].* 1961;43a: 1202–1224.
2. Kay H, Working Group, International Society of Prosthetics and Orthotics. A proposed international terminology for the classification of congenital limb deficiencies. *Orthot Prosthet* 1974;28(2): 33–48.
3. Dise-Lewis JE. Psychological adaptation to limb loss. In: Atkins D, Meier RH, eds. *Comprehensive management of the upper limb amputee.* New York: Springer, 1989:165–172.
4. Thompson DM, Haran D. Living with an amputation: what it means for patients and their helpers. *Int J Rehabil Res* 1984;7: 283–292.
5. Pohjolainen T, Alaranta H, Karkkainen M. Prosthetic use and functional and social outcomes following major lower limb amputation. *Prosthet Orthot Int* 1990;14:75–79.
6. Ham R, Regan JM, Roberts VC. Evaluation of introducing the team approach to the care of the amputee: the Dulwich study. *Prosthet Orthot Int* 1987;11: 25–30.
7. Kaplow M, Muroff F, Fish W, et al. The dysvascular amputee: multidisciplinary management. *Can J Surg* 1983;26:368–369.

8. Thompson RG, Kramer S. The amputee clinic team. In: *Atlas of limb prosthetics. American Academy of Orthopedic Surgeons.* St. Louis: CV Mosby, 1981:63–66.

9. Malone JM, Moore WS, Goldstone J, et al. Therapeutic and economic impact of a modern amputation program. *Ann Surg* 1979;189: 798–802.

10. Pinzur MS, Gottschalk F, Smith D, et al. Functional outcome of below-knee amputation in peripheral vascular insufficiency: a multicenter review. *Clin Orthop* 1993;286:247–249.

11. Stewart CPU, Jain AS. Dundee revisited—25 years of a total amputee service. *Prosthet Orthot Int* 1993;17:14–20.

12. Friedman LW. *The psychological rehabilitation of the amputee.* Springfield, IL: Charles C Thomas, 1978.

13. Bradway JK, Malone JM, Racy J, et al. Psychological adaptation to amputation: an overview. *Orthot Prosthet* 1984;38:46–50.

14. Kashani J, Frank R, Kashani S, et al. Depression among amputees. *J Clin Psychiatry* 1983;44: 256–258.

15. Malchow D, Clark J. Interviewing the amputee: a step toward rehabilitation. *Orthop Rev* 1984;13: 639–648.

16. Parkes CM. The psychological reaction to loss of a limb: the first year after amputation. In: Howells JG, ed. *Modern perspectives in the psychiatric aspects of surgery.* New York: Brunnel/Mazel, 1976:515–532.

17. Thompson D, Haran D. Living with an amputation: the patient. *Int Rehabil Med* 1983;5: 165–169.

18. Thompson D, Haran D. Living with an amputation: the helper. *Soc Sci Med* 1985;20:319–323.

19. Racy JC. Psychological aspects of amputation. In: Moore WS, Malone JM, eds. *Lower extremity amputation.* Philadelphia: WB Saunders, 1989:330–340.

20. Davis R. Phantom sensation, phantom pain, and stump pain. *Arch Phys Med Rehabil* 1993;74:79–91.

21. Melzak R. Phantom limbs and the concept of a neuromatrix. *Trends Neurosci* 1990;13:88–92.

22. Dickhaut S, DeLee J, Page C. Nutritional status: importance in predicting wound healing after amputation. *J Bone Joint Surg [AM]* 1984;66:71–75.

23. Hadley SA, Fitzsimmons L. Nutrition and wound healing. *Top Clin Nutr* 1990;5(4):72–81.

24. Kay S, Moreland J, Schmitter E. Nutritional status and wound healing in lower extremity amputations. *Clin Orthop* 1987;217: 253–256.

25. Gottschalk FA, Kourosh S, Stills M, et al. Does socket configuration influence the position of the femur in above-knee amputation? *J Prosthet Orthot* 1989;2:94–102.

26. Esquenazi A, Vachranukunkiet T, Torres M, Demopoulos JT. Characteristics of a current lower extremity amputee population: review of 919 cases. *Arch Phys Med Rehabil* 1984;65:623.

27. Glattly HW. A statistical study of 12,000 new amputees. *South Med J* 1964;57:1373–1378.

28. Kay HW, Newman JD. Relative incidences of new amputations: statistical comparisons of 6000 new amputees. *Orthot Prosthet* 1975;29:3–16.

29. Muller EA. Influence of training and inactivity on muscle strength. *Arch Phys Med Rehabil* 1970;51:449–462.

30. Saltin B, Blomqvist G, Mitchell JH, et al. Response to exercise after bedrest and training. *Circulation* 1968;38(suppl VII): 1–78.

31. Mensch G. Exercise for amputees. In: Basmajian JV, Wolf SL, eds. *Therapeutic exercise.* 5th ed. Baltimore: Williams & Wilkins, 1990:251–279.

32. Mensch G, Ellis P. *Physical therapy management of lower extremity amputations.* Rockville, MD: Aspen, 1986.

33. Berlemont M, Weber R, Willot JP. Ten years of experience with the immediate application of prosthetic devices to amputees of the lower extremities on the operating table. *Prosthet Int* 1969;3:8–18.

34. Burgess EM, Romano RL, Zettl JH. *The management of lower-extremity amputations.* Washington, DC: US Government Printing Office, 1969.

35. Atkins D. Postoperative and preprosthetic therapy programs. In: Atkins D, Meier RH, eds. *Comprehensive management of the upper limb amputee.* New York: Springer, 1989:11–15.

36. Malone JM; Fleming LL, Robenson J, et al. Immediate, early and late postsurgical management of upper-limb amputation. *J Rehabil Res Dev* 1984;21:33–41.

37. Wu Y, Keagy RD, Krick HJ, et al. An innovative removable rigid dressing technique for below-knee amputation. *J Bone Joint Surg [AM]* 1979;61:724–729.

38. Wu Y, Krick H. Removable rigid dressing for below-knee amputees. *Clin Prosthet Orthot* 1987; 11:33–44.

39. Fish S. Semirigid dressing for stump shrinkage. *Phys Ther* 1976;56:1376.

40. Ghiulamila R. Semirigid dressing for postoperative fitting of below knee prosthesis. *Arch Phys Med Rehabil* 1972;53:186–190.

41. MacLean N, Fick G. The effect of semirigid dressings on below knee amputations. *Phys Ther* 1994;74: 668–673.

42. Menzies H, Newnham J. Semirigid dressings: the best for lower extremity amputees. *Physiother Can* 1978;30:225.

43. Golbranson F, Wirta R, Kuncir E, et al. Volume changes occurring in postoperative below-knee residual limbs. *J Rehabil Res Dev* 1988; 25:11–18.

44. Manella K. Comparison of the effectiveness of elastic bandages and shrinker socks for lower

extremity amputees. *Phys Ther* 1981;61:334–337.

45. English RD, Hubbard WA. McElroy GK. Establishment of consistent gait after fitting of new components. *J Rehabil Res Dev* 1995; 32:32–35.

46. Kamen LB, Chapis GJ. Phantom limb sensation and phantom pain. *Phys Med Rehabil State Art Rev* 1994;8(1):73–88.

47. Sherman RA. Published treatments of phantom limb pain. *Am J Phys Med Rehabil* 1980;59:232–244.

48. Sherman RA, Sherman CJ, Gall NA. Survey of current phantom limb treatment in the United States. *Pain* 1980;8:85–99.

49. Sherman RA. Tippens JK. Suggested guidelines for treatment of phantom limb pain. *Orthopedics* 1982;5:1595–1600.

50. Sherman RA. Case reports of treatment of phantom pain with a combination of electromyographic biofeedback and verbal relaxation techniques. *Biofeedback Self Regul* 1976;1:353.

51. Siegel EF. Control of phantom pain by hypnosis. *Am J Clin Hypn* 1979;21:285–286.

52. Sherman R, Gall N, Gormly R. Treatment of phantom pain with muscular relaxation training to disrupt the pain-anxiety-tension cycle. *Pain* 1979;6:47–54.

53. Anderson M. Four cases of phantom limb treated with ultrasound. *Phys Ther Rev* 1958; 38:419–420.

54. Winnem M, Amundsen T. Treatment of phantom limb pain with TENS. *Pain* 1982;12: 299–300.

55. Millstein S, Bain D, Hunter GA. A review of employment patterns of industrial amputees—factors influencing rehabilitation. *Prosthet Orthot Int* 1985;9:69–78.

56. Michael JW, Gailey RS, Bowker JH. New developments in recreational prosthesis and adaptive devices for the amputee. *Clin Orthop* 1990;256:64–74.

57. Prince F, Allard P, Therrien RG, McFadyen BJ. Running gait impulse asymmetries in below knee amputees. *Prosthet Orthot Int* 1992;16:19–24.

58. Enoka RM, Millwer DI, Burgess EM. Below knee amputee running gait. *Am J Phys Med Rehabil* 1982;61:66–83.

59. Czerniecki JM, Gitter A. Insights into amputee running. A muscle work analysis. *Am J Phys Med Rehabil* 1992;71:209–219.

60. Mackenzie L, ed. *The complete directory for people with disabilities.* Lakeville, CT: Grey House Publishing, 1991.

61. Shrout RN. *Resource directory for the disabled.* New York: Facts on File, 1991.

62. Varghese G, Hinterbuchner C, Mondall P, Sakuma J. Rehabilitation outcome of patients with dual disability of hemiplegia and amputation. *Arch Phys Med Rehabil* 1978;59:121–123.

63. Friedman LW. *The surgical rehabilitation of the amputee.* Springfield, IL: Charles C Thomas, 1978: 205–209.

64. Torres MM, Esquenazi A. Bilateral lower limb amputee rehabilitation. A retrospective review. *West J Med* 1991;154:583–586.

65. Esquenazi A. Geriatric amputee rehabilitation. *Clin Geriatr Med* 1993;9:731–743.

66. Fisher SV, Gullickson G Jr. Energy cost of ambulation in health and disability: a literature review. *Arch Phys Med Rehabil* 1978;59: 124–133.

67. Waters RL, Perry J, Chambers R. Energy expenditure of amputee gait. In: Moore WS, Malone JM, eds. *Lower extremity amputation.* Philadelphia: WB Saunders, 1989:250–260.

68. DuBow LL, Witt PL, Kadaba MP, et al. Oxygen consumption of elderly persons with bilateral below knee amputations: ambulation vs. wheelchair propulsion. *Arch Phys Med Rehabil* 1983;64: 255–259.

69. Huang CT, Moore NB, [illegible] et al. Energy cost of am[illegible] for amputees: a study usi[illegible] mobile automatic metabolic [illegible]lyzer. *Arch Phys Med Rehabil* [illegible] 1977;58:521.

70. Hughes J, Jacobs N. Normal human locomotion. *Prosthet Orthot Int* 1979;3:4–12.

71. Lehman JF. Biomechanics of ankle-foot orthoses: prescription and design. *Arch Phys Med Rehabil* 1979;60:200–207.

72. Traugh GH, Corcoran PJ, Reyes RL. Energy expenditure of ambulation in patients with above knee amputations. *Arch Phys Med Rehabil* 1975;56:67–71.

73. Isakov E, Susak Z, Becker E. Energy expenditure and cardiac response in above knee amputees while using prostheses with open and locked knee mechanisms. *Scand J Rehabil Med Suppl* 1985;12:108–111.

74. Wainapel SF, March H, Steve L. Stubby prostheses: an alternative to conventional prosthetic devices. *Arch Phys Med Rehabil* 1985; 66:264–266.

75. Sakuma J, Hinterbucher C, Green RF, Silber M. Rehabilitation of geriatric patients having bilateral lower extremity amputations. *Arch Phys Med Rehabil* 1974;55: 101–111.

76. Waters RL, Perry J, Antonelli D, Hislop H. Energy cost of walking of amputees: the influence of level of amputation. *J Bone Joint Surg [Am]* 1976;58:42–46.

77. Kerstein MD, Zimmer H, Dugdale FE, Lerner E. Amputations of the lower extremity: a study of 194 cases. *Arch Phys Med Rehabil* 1974;55:454–459.

78. Mazat R, Schiller FJ, Dunn OJ, et al. *Influence of prosthesis wearing on health of geriatric amputee.* Washington, DC: Project 431. Office of Vocational Rehabilitation, March 1963.

79. Malone JM. Complications of lower extremity amputation. In: Moore WS, Malone JM, eds. *Lower extremity amputation.* Philadel-

989:

R. Amputa-
ulation:
treatment,
stom Ther

). Ocular
... of diabetes mellitus. In: Kahn CR, Weir GC, eds. *Joslin's diabetes mellitus.* 13th ed. Philadelphia: Lea & Febiger, 1994:772.

82. Altner PC, Rusin JJ, DeBoer A. Rehabilitation of blind patients with lower extremity amputations. *Arch Phys Med Rehabil* 1980; 61:82–85.

83. O'Connell PG, Gnatz S. Hemiplegia and amputation: rehabilitation in the dual disability. *Arch Phys Med Rehabil* 1989;70:451–454.

84. Koike K. Ishikura Y, Kakurai S, et al. The TC double socket above-knee prosthesis. *Prosthet Orthot Int* 1981;5:129–134.

85. Lowry R. Durability of lower extremity prostheses. *Arch Phys Med Rehabil* 1966;47:742–743.

86. Smith DG, Horn P, Malchow D, et al. Prosthetic history, prosthetic changes, and functional outcome of the isolated traumatic below-knee amputee. *J Trauma* 1995; 38:44–47.

87. Levin ME, O'Neal LW, Bowker JH, eds. *The diabetic foot.* St. Louis: CV Mosby, 1993.

88. Malone JM, Snyder M, Anderson G, et al. Prevention of amputation by diabetic education. *Am J Surg* 1989;158:520–524.

89. Jonason T, Jonzon B, Ringqvist I, Oman-Rydberg A. Effect of physical training on different categories of patients with intermittent claudication. *Acta Med Scand* 1979;206:253–258.

Chapter 94

Burn Rehabilitation

Lucretia Fitzpatrick
Patrick Murphy
Jill Androwick
Deborah Goldblum
Patricia Wardius
John Wijtyk

There are approximately 1.25 million burn injuries in the United States yearly, accounting for 51,000 acute hospital admissions and 5500 deaths (1). The cause and the risks of burn injury and death are influenced by age, economic circumstances, and occupation, with the greatest risk being economically disadvantaged. Seventy-five percent of all burn-related deaths are due to house fires, with young children and the elderly being most vulnerable. Flame burn is the predominant type of injury seen in patients admitted to burn centers, followed by scalding with hot liquids (2).

The majority of burns can be treated on an outpatient basis. However, the extent of the burn, or a complicating factor such as an associated injury or extreme age or youth, may warrant hospital admission. Inhalation injury, concomitant trauma, and significant preexisting medical conditions mandate burn center care for patients with burns of lesser extent (2).

Major burns are best cared for in a burn treatment center where the specialized skills of a multidisciplinary staff and burn-specific equipment ensure optimal survival. Major burns are classified as follows:

1. Greater than 10% of total body surface area (TBSA) at an age younger than 10 years or older than 50 years
2. Greater than 20% of TBSA in patients at an intervening age
3. Significant burns of the face, hands, feet, genitalia, perineum, or major joints
4. Full-thickness burns greater than 5% of TBSA
5. Significant electrical injury
6. Significant chemical injury

Burns are coagulative lesions involving surface layers of the body. They are usually caused by thermal agents but can also result from chemical agents, radiation, and electrical injury when electrical energy is transferred to thermal energy.

The skin is the largest organ of the human body and consists primarily of two layers, the epidermis and the dermis. The superficial cells of the epidermis are cells that arise from deeper germinal layers of keratinocytes. The underlying dermis consists of fibrous connective tissue, blood vessels, ataneous nerves, and the epithelial appendages (sweat glands and hair follicles). The epithelial cells that line these appendages can serve to repopulate lost epithelium when the entire epithelial layer is involved in a burn injury (3).

Clinically, burns are classified based on depth and extent of tissue damage (4). Burn depth classifications include superficial, partial thickness, and full thickness (Table 94-1). Superficial (or first-degree) burns, such as a sunburn, are painful. This type of burn is limited to the epidermis and heals spontaneously without scarring. Partial-thickness burns include the entire epidermis and variable portions of the dermis. They can be superficial or deep. Superficial partial-thickness burns are usually more painful but can heal spontaneously from the epidermal

Table 94-1: Type of Burn Wounds

Degree	Type	Layer of Involvement	Appearance	Healing
First	Superficial	Epidermis	Red Blanches with pressure Sensitive to air, light, touch	Spontaneous <>1 wk
Second	Partial-thickness superficial	Epidermis and upper layer of dermis	Red or pink skin color Blistered or mottled Blanches well Sensitive to touch	Spontaneous 5–21 days
Second	Deep	Destroys epidermis and deeper dermal structures	Soft elastic texture Eschar Wavy white to red color Sensitive to pressure, not to pinprick Large thick blisters	Occurs from dermal appendages May require grafting: if wounds are not healed within 21 days —potental for scarring
Third	Full thickness	Epidermis and entire dermis Subcutaneous tissue	White, tan, black charred No blanching Dry texture Leathery, thrombosed blood vessels visible Wound is anesthetic—nerve endings destroyed	Slowly from wound edges <>10–35 days Requires grafting
Fourth	Bone	All epidermis All dermis Subcutaneous fat Bone	Black Necrotic	Requires grafting or amputation May need a muscle flap for coverage

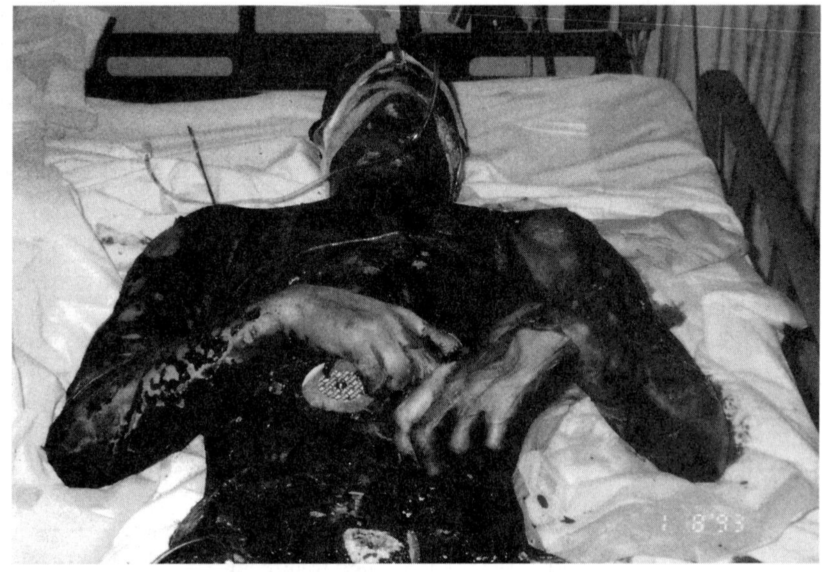

Figure 94-1. Full-thickness burns sustained from a flame injury. Eschar is white/brown and leather-like in appearance.

appendages anchored deep in the dermis. With deep partial-thickness injury, spontaneous healing is slow, as fewer epidermal cells remain and more scarring may occur. A full-thickness burn destroys both the epidermis and dermis; therefore, healing can only occur from the wound edges (Fig. 94-1). Skin grafting is needed to close the wound (3). Surgical intervention may be required for either a deep partial-thickness wound or full-thickness wound.

An inhalation injury is a chemical burn to the airways and can result in mucosal irritation, airway inflammation, interstitial edema, or in most severe injuries, mucosal necrosis and sloughing. Increased secretions can lead to distal airway obstruction, atelectasis, and bronchopneumonia. Ciliary function is impaired and risk for infection, such as tracheobronchitis, is high. Bronchospasms and bronchial edema can lead to hypoventilation. Coughing, pulmonary toilet, secretion management, bronchodilator therapy, ventilator assistance, and infection surveillance are crucial during the initial postinjury phase. Risk for infection can last for several weeks (5).

WOUND CARE

Wounds can be treated with an "open" or "closed" technique. An open technique is sometimes used for a small superficial burn, where serum dries to form a scab and serves as an adherent protective dressing. This treatment can be uncomfortable and unsightly (5).

Closed methods for wound care consist primarily of using 1) topical antimicrobial agents and dressings, 2) biologic dressings, and 3) synthetic dressings (Tables 94-2 and 94-3). Topical antimicrobial agents include silver nitrate, silver sulfadiazine, mafenide acetate (Sulfamylon), mupiricin (Bactroban), bacitracin, gentamicin sulfate (Garamycin) ointment, and Neosporin. One of the most common agents utilized is silver sulfadiazine (Silvadene), which provides broad antimicrobial coverage and assists in bringing eschar to the surface where it can be débrided. Once the eschar is débrided, the wound can then be covered with Xeroform, which assists in drying the tissue and promotes healing. The involved area can be wrapped in Kerlix or gauze dressing as needed. Fungal infections, which can occur, may respond to an equal-part mixture of nystatin, hydrocortisone, and mupiricin. With each dressing change, the old topical agent must be removed and the wound cleansed before reapplication. This method affords the opportunity for close surveillance of the wounds. The antimicrobial action lasts from 8 to 12 hours and the frequency of dressing changes will vary among institutions.

Biologic dressings consist of viable or frozen skin allografts and xenograft (pigskin). These can be used as a temporary skin covering until use of autografts is indicated. They are effective in promoting wound healing in all partial-thickness wounds. Biologic dressings may be used to test the readiness of a wound for autografting. Furthermore, these dressings reduce fluid and electrolyte losses, promote healing under grafted areas, minimize pain, and maintain sterile conditions (6).

Synthetic dressings include Opsite (semipermeable polyurethane film), Duoderm, Comfeel (hydrocolloid dressing), Elasto-gel (hydrogel dressing), and Biobrane (7,8). Biobrane is composed of knitted elastic nylon bonded to a Silastic semipermeable membrane coated with collagen polypeptides (Fig. 94-2). It will adhere to a viable wound surface, reduce fluid loss, and provide a wound vapor barrier. This minimizes fluid accumulation under the dressing while preventing the passage of bacteria from the environment to the wound surface. In selected wounds, this treatment may have some advantage over traditional antimicrobial dressings. Biobrane is usually placed on a wound under sterile conditions while using an anesthetic.

Wound infections can impede healing, delay wound closure, and cause skin graft loss. *Pseudomonas species*, *Staphylococcus aureus*, *Escherichia species*, *Proteus mirabilis*, and *Streptococcus faecalis* are the most common agents causing wound infections. Bacterial contamination leads to an increased inflammatory response and local release of cytokines and proteases, and can lead to local tissue damage. Local infection alters systemic metabolic activity and nutritional intake and can alter healing (7). Both local and systemic defenses against infection are impaired after a major burn. Sepsis is a leading cause of morbidity and mortality during the postburn period, owing to the loss of the skin barrier to microbial invasion, the decreased immunosuppressive state, and the presence of invasive

Table 94-2: Antimicrobial Agents

Dressing	Advantages	Disadvantages
Silver nitrate (solution)	Excellent antibacterial spectrum No allergic reactions, no pain	Ineffective treating established infections Causes staining or bleaching of chloride ions Messy, poor penetration
Sliver sulfadiazine cream (Silvadene SSD)	Broad antibacterial spectrum Minimal sensitivity, allergic reaction Eschar will dry after discontinuation Gram negative	Delays spontaneous separation of eschar, thus delaying wound closing Reported transient leukopenia Ineffective against establishment of wound sepsis Does not penetrate eschar well
Mafenide acetate (Sulfamylon)	Penetrates eschar well Excellent gram-negative coverage Good antimicrobial action	May cause pain (stinging) 10% allergic rate Inhibits carbonic anhydrase results in metabolic acidosis
Nitrofurazone	Dries wound well Good antibacterial spectrum	May cause rash
Mupiricin (Bactroban)	Effective against gram-positive organisms, especially streptococcus and staphylococcus	No effect on gram-negative bacteria

Table 94-3: Topical Dressings			
Agent	**Advantages**	**Disadvantages**	**Properties**
BioBrane	Transparent Inexpensive Available in variety of sizes Adheres to wound Barrier to pathogenic organisms	Wound must be débrided and cleaned in sterile environment Performed in operating room	Semipermeable Silcone membrane Bonded to nylon Fabric coated with collagen
OP-SITE	Inexpensive Transparent	Not permeable Depends on location Needs good 1-inch border	Semipermcable polyurethane film
Cadaver (graft)	Lower infection rates Temporary dressing	Availability Rejection Expensive Fragile Surgical procedure	Human skin
Xenograft	Lower infection rates Closely resembles human skin Temporary dressing	Rejection of tissue Fragile Not readily available	Pig skin
Duoderm	Barrier to pathogenic bacteria Higher absorption rate Infrequent dressing changes	Lower success with larger burns Unable to view progress of wound	Hydroactive occlusive dressing Water resistant Skin contact, adhesive inner layer
Xeroform	Direct application to wound surface Sterile prepackaged Dries wound	Minimal antibacterial effect when used alone	Fine-mesh absorbent gauze impregnated with 3% bismuth tribromophenate in nonmedicinal petrolatum blend
Adaptic	Can be combined with topical agents Will not stick to wound Sterile prepackaged	No antibacterial effects when used alone	Meshed open-knitted fabric made of cellular-acetate-rayon, petroleum based
Scarlet red	Applied directly to wound Sterile prepackaged Helps promote epithelial cell growth	Messy, stains Patient sensitive to azo dyes No antibacterial effects	Fine-mesh absorbent gauze impregnated with 5% scarlet red in nonmedicinal blend of lanolin, olive oil, and petrolatum
N-TERFACE Conformant 2	Can be combined with topical agent Will not stick to wound Allows wound to be observed	No antibacterial effects when used alone	Perforated high-density polyethylene sheeting Nonadherent
Vaseline gauze	Applied directly to wound Will not stick to wound	No antibacterial effect	Petroleum based

catheters. The most common sites of infection are the lungs, the burn wound, and vascular catheters (5). Cell-mediated immunity is impaired, as is macrocyte and phagocyte function. Complement, required for chemotaxis and phagocytosis, is depleted after a large burn. Central lines, endotracheal tubes, and urinary catheters all serve as sites for colonization and possible infection (5).

Systemic antibiotics should be used as indicated. Blood cultures should be obtained on admission and then as needed. Side effects as well as overall clinical response need to be monitored closely. It is not unusual for multiple antimicrobial agents to be used together for broad-spectrum coverage.

NUTRITION

Nutritional support can affect the outcome of a burn-injured patient. Providing the nutritional requirements of these patients is often difficult. The metabolic response to thermal injury can be greater than that seen with serious sepsis (9). Nutritional support is ideally managed by the enteral route. Parenteral or central nutrition may be necessary in the patient with a burn exceeding 50% of TBSA. Increased metabolic activity usually peaks between the seventh and tenth postburn days, and caloric requirements should be completely met by this time. The magnitude of increase is directly related to burn size and depth.

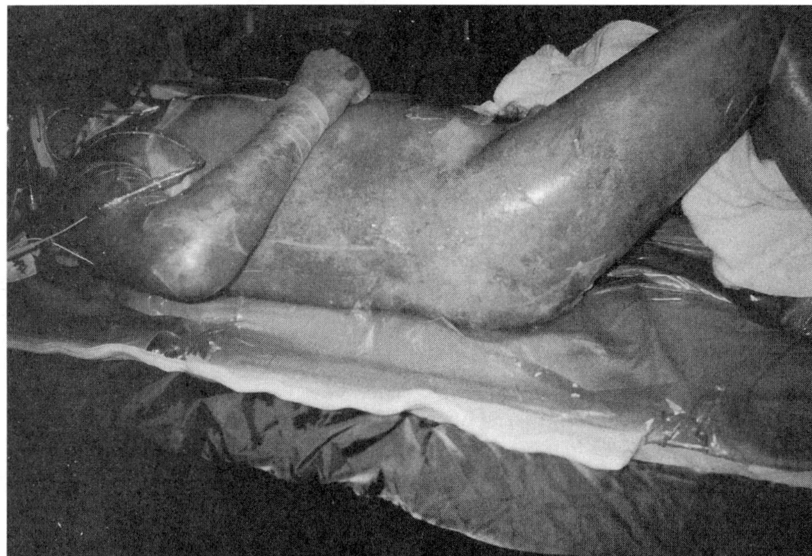

Figure 94-2. Biobrane utilized for pain control in a Stevens-Johnson syndrome patient.

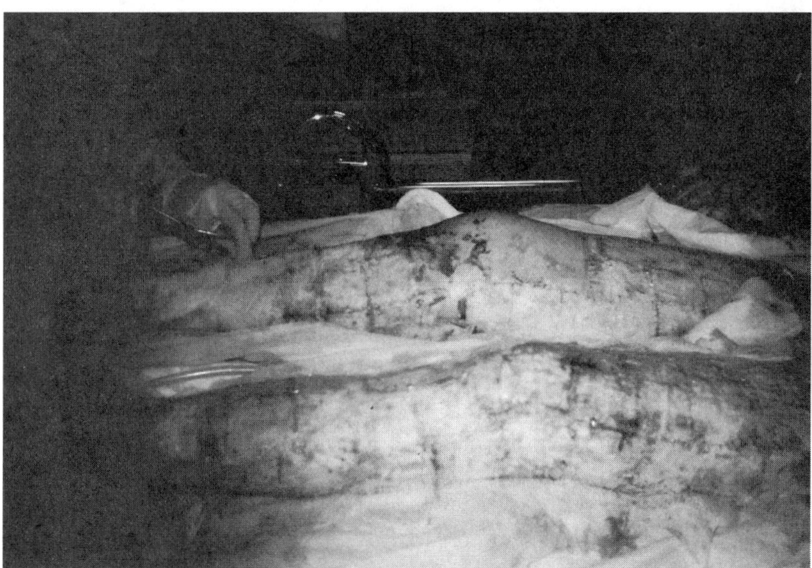

Figure 94-3. An example of cultured epithelial autografting. The epithelial cells are placed on a petroleum jelly gauze that resembles a "patch"-like configuration.

However, young patients appear to generate a higher post-burn metabolic rate than elderly patients (3). Continuous monitoring is needed to promote wound healing through the acute and rehabilitative phase.

GRAFTING

The goal of burn wound care is to permanently close the wound. For full-thickness burns, autografts provide ultimate wound closure. Allografts, xenografts, and artificial skin substitutes are temporary dressings used until they can be replaced by autografts. Mechanical dermatomes are used to harvest skin from the donor site and skin meshers are used to expand the size of the autograft and allow for coverage of wider areas (10). The skin at a donor site has a definite thickness, and is thinner in the very young and elderly. Each time a graft is harvested from a donor site, the skin becomes thinner or is replaced by scar tissue (11). With large burns, donor sites are limited; therefore, cultured epithelial autografting (CEA) may be employed (Fig. 94-3). With this technique, a skin fragment no larger than a postage stamp can be grown to a square meter in the course of a few weeks. This in vitro process is commercially available but costly, and time is needed to grow the grafts. Because only epithelial cells are utilized, CEA is fragile and nonadherence may occur (12). Periods of immobilization and bed rest may be significantly longer as compared to split-thickness grafting, leading to longer periods of rehabilitation. Despite its disadvantages, survival rates have increased and cosmetic outcomes are improved. A new development in wound management has been the creation of Integra artificial skin, which received Food and Drug Administration (FDA) approval in March 1996. Integra is a biologic, bilayer skin replacement system. The dermal layer is composed of fibers of bovine tendon collagen and glycosaminoglycan and serves as a template for fibroblasts and capillaries from the uninvolved dermis. As healing occurs, a neodermis is formed as new collagen replaces the bovine collagen. The temporary epidermal layer is composed of silicone and functions to control moisture loss from the wound. After 14 to 21 days, adequate vascularization of the dermal layer has occurred. The silicone layer is removed and a thin, meshed layer of epidermal autograft is placed over the neodermis. The advantage is immediate physiologic wound closure until donor skin is available, thus decreasing pain and the risk of infection. The epidermal autografts used also allow for thinner, quicker-healing donor sites and improved cosmetic and functional outcome (13).

Table 94-4: Common Short- and Long-Term Goals

Short-term goals
Control pain
Prevent contractures, deformity
Preserve joint mobility
Preserve strength, coordination, endurance
Promote ADL participation
Promote wound healing
Minimize edema
Patient and family education
Long-term goals
Minimize burn scar formation
Increase strength, coordination, endurance
Increase independence with ADLs
Compensate for physical impairment
Adjustment to disability
Reintegration into society
Education regarding skin care and scar management

ADL = activity of daily living.

ROLE OF REHABILITATION IN BURN CARE

Rehabilitation of a burned patient is a process that begins on arrival to the burn treatment center, continues throughout the hospital course, and often continues for years following injury. A team approach ensures a comprehensive and holistic perspective for each individual who is faced with this significant impairment. Team members can include general and plastic surgeons, pulmonary and critical care specialists, physiatrists, psychologists, nurses, social workers, occupational therapists, physical therapists, speech therapists, dietitians, orthotists, dysphagia services, vocational counselors, and aesthetic therapists. Rehabilitation professionals are an integral part of the acute phase in burn care and serve to complement other members of the team who provide critical care and surgical intervention. Survival among burn patients has improved dramatically, but equally important is for rehabilitation efforts to translate into returning survivors to the highest functional level and quality of life.

Rehabilitation should be viewed on a continuum with short- and long-term goals being established (Table 94-4). The ultimate goal is to heal the wound while maintaining and restoring maximal function. Acutely, life-threatening problems may hamper rehabilitation at times. In the setting of medical instability, restorative intervention may be passive in nature, with the patient becoming more active in the rehabilitative program as the condition permits.

Occupational and physical therapists may be involved in all stages of patient care and rehabilitation. Therapists begin their assessment of a patient during the acute phase of injury in conjunction with medical management. Patient evaluation begins with observation of the extent and location of the wound as well as its effects on joint range of motion (ROM), mobility, and activities of daily living (ADLs). In the case of electrical injury, muscle strength and sensation are assessed. A treatment plan is developed based on a comprehensive evaluation with ongoing assessment and modification.

Therapeutic exercise is a vital part of the burn patient's care because contractures and resultant loss of function can occur rapidly. Burn wound depth and location are determinants of the type and intensity of exercise. Deep partial- and full-thickness wounds have a higher incidence of decreased joint motion and scar contracture (Fig. 94-4). Therefore, the therapist must prioritize specific areas to exercise.

During the acute phase, ROM exercises are initiated with the goal of minimizing edema to ensure functional ROM. ROM may be passive, active-assisted, or active, depending on a patient's medical status (pain medications, affect, associated trauma) or wound status (thick eschar, tendon exposure). Although exercise will vary with patient status, there are circumstances that must be given special consideration. The clinical guidelines for starting ROM after excision and grafting vary among institutions (Table 94-5). Other conditions that may modify treatment include tendon, bone, or joint exposure; preexisting joint disease; periarticular calcification; deep venous thrombosis; and associated trauma.

Passive ROM (PROM) exercises are performed when the patient is unable to actively participate in the program. Guidelines to performing PROM exercises depend on a patient's physiologic status, placement of intravenous lines, eschar tightening or tearing, associated orthopedic or neurologic trauma, or preexisting joint conditions. Active ROM exercises are encouraged to ensure patient participation and assisted ROM exercises are especially effective in a multijoint stretch where the goal is to elongate the scar tissue over adjacent joints.

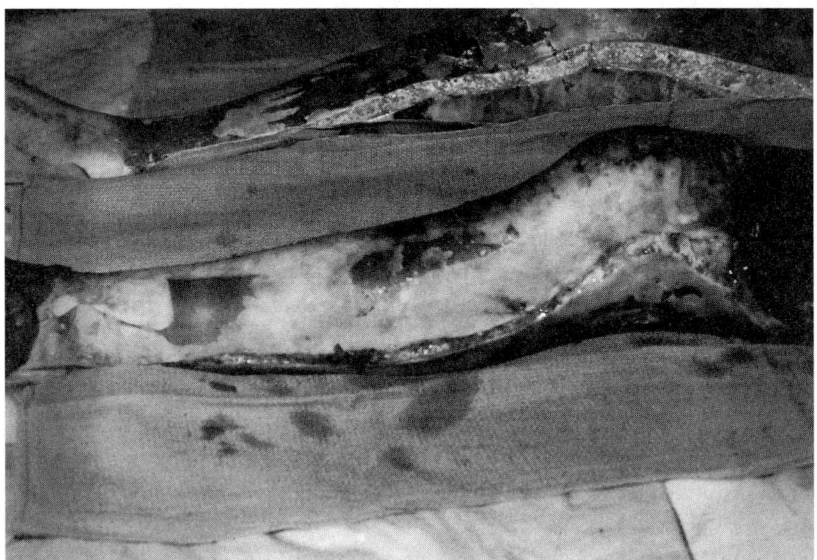

Figure 94-4. Circumferential full-thickness burns of both lower extremities, with the potential for decreased range of motion due to the location of the burns, crossing both knee joints.

Table 94-5: Clinical Guidelines for Starting Range of Motion (ROM) Exercise

Procedures	Clinical Guidelines
Autografting	Postop day 4—active ROM. Postop day 5—active-assisted ROM. Postop day 6—passive ROM.
Use of biobrane	Initiate ROM 24–48 hr after application. Aggressiveness depends on appearance.
Allografting	Same as for autografting.
Cultured epithelial autografting	Initiate active ROM after take down, which is 7–10 days after grafting. Aggressiveness depends on appearance.

ROM exercises can be implemented during a dressing change, giving the therapist the opportunity to continually assess the wound and make appropriate modifications to the program. Additional exercise sessions can occur at the bedside or in the clinic. A continuous passive motion (CPM) machine is often used to complement ROM exercises. Conditioning, coordination, and strengthening activities are also included in the rehabilitation program. Joint mobilization may also be part of a rehabilitation program, especially in the patient with prolonged immobility and soft-tissue contractures.

While ROM exercises are vital to maintaining joint motion, functional exercises should be emphasized to decrease progressive dependency, increase self-esteem, and promote independence. Functional exercises and ADLs should begin in the early phase of recovery as the patient's medical and surgical status allows. Treatment may include self-care activities such as feeding and personal hygiene. If possible, therapists should avoid the use of adaptive equipment for ADLs. It is better to increase the patient's joint motion through functional activities and prevent reliance on such devices.

Therapeutic intervention involves a balance between mobility and exercise versus positioning and splinting. Splints are used for a variety of purposes, including prevention of joint contracture and dysfunctional posturing, protection of an anatomic instability, postoperative immobilization, and scar control. If splints are used as positioning devices to prevent or minimize contractures, it is important that the splints be taken off multiple times per day for ROM exercises.

In the rehabilitative phase, the goals of therapy focus on preventing or minimizing joint contractures, controlling scars, and promoting return to functional independence. ROM exercises continue, especially for those areas predisposed to joint contractures. The use of reciprocal pulleys for upper-extremity stretching and prolonged positioning stretches over wedges and bolsters for the trunk and neck have been advocated. Therapeutic balls, foam bolsters, and wedges are useful in encouraging active motion. Given the physiology of scars and the development of additional soft-tissue tightness, therapeutic exercise in any form should be performed daily to four times a day.

Therapeutic exercises and functional activities are initiated during the acute phase and continued into the rehabilitative phase, which may extend for months after discharge from a burn or rehabilitation center. Outpatient treatment continues to focus on scar management, stretching, conditioning, and strengthening. Therapeutic exercise following surgical scar release is also essential and in most patients extends years after the burn occurred.

HAND BURNS

One of the most commonly involved and structurally vulnerable parts of the body in a burn injury is the hand (Fig. 94-5). Because of the natural human tendency to protect the face, dorsal hand burns are more common than palmar burns. In particular, the dorsum of the hand is at risk, owing to the superficial location of the extensor tendons and the minimal layers of subcutaneous fascia. Without early intervention, permanent damage to the hand can occur. Traumatic shedding of the extensor hood, ischemic changes secondary to edema, and increased tension at the proximal interphalangeal (PIP) joints are all too frequently present. In particular, with a burn trauma to the hands, the central slip and the lateral bands are jeopardized. In normal function, the lateral bands lie volar to the axis of flexion at the metaphalangeal (MP) joint and dorsal to the axis of flexion at the PIP joint. When injury occurs, the central slip is often disrupted, allowing the lateral bands to slip volarly, becoming flexors at the PIP joint and forcing the distal interphalangeal (DIP) joint into hyperextension. This is known as a *boutonnière deformity*. This and other deformities can be prevented by splinting, ROM, exercises and stretching, and proper positioning (14).

As with splinting in general, the hand should be splinted in a position opposite the expected deformity. The burn resting hand splint is one of the most common tools used to protect the hands. This splint varies slightly from other resting splints as it places the wrist in approximately 30 degrees of extension, the MP joints at approximately 70 degrees of flexion, the interphalangeal (IP) joints in full extension, and the thumb in opposition and maintains a good palmar arch (15). Straps are contraindicated for the acute stage of injury, for they may interfere with circulation and cause an increase in edema or edema "pocketing" (14). Instead, Ace wraps are used to secure most splints, wrapping in a distal to proximal manner. If the burn requires a skin graft, a modified hand splint is used during the operative procedure to position and immobilize the hand, allowing for optimum stretch and graft take (Fig. 94-6). These modifications include slits between the fingers, holes at the distal tip of each finger, notches around the side, and a "roll bar" attached to the thenar area of the splint. The digits are sutured, by a surgeon, into the holes at the top of the splint, while the slits allow for adequate drainage and the roll bar provides extra protection against damage to the graft. Other splints that are frequently indicated for the burned hand include, but are not limited to the following:

1. The gutter splint, which maintains or increases extension of one particular digit
2. The saddle splint, which prevents contracture of the thumb-index web space
3. The wrist cock-up splint to provide wrist extension, which aids in hand function

Splint requirements will change as the patient's medical status and functional needs change. Therefore, it is important to monitor a patient's splint on a daily basis to assess fit, reassess splinting needs, and check for pressure areas.

ROM exercises, another important aspect of burn therapy, are necessary not only to prevent skin contractures, but also to prevent joint stiffness and tendon adhesions. Active ROM exercises are always preferable, as they maintain muscle mass and strength. However, since this is not always feasible, PROM exercises may be performed. ROM exercises with burned joints need to be frequent and

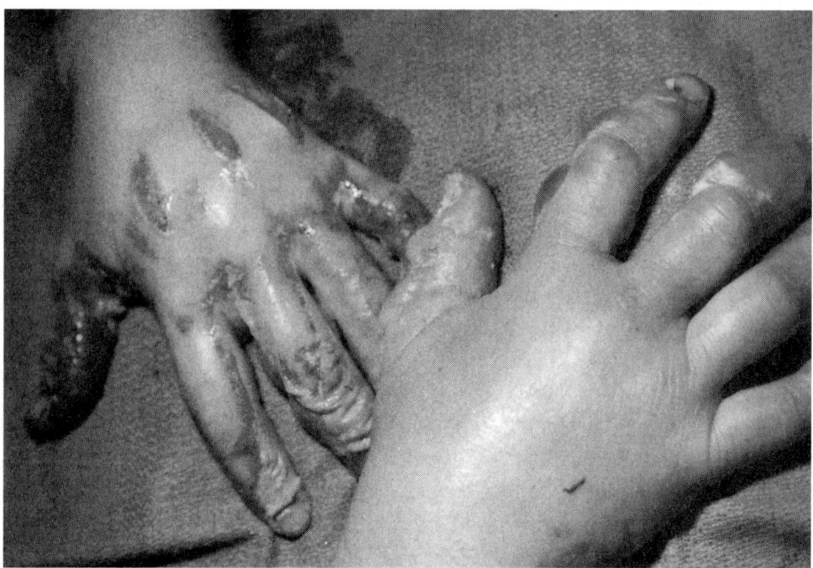

Figure 94-5. Partial degloving of the left hand to reveal a full-thickness burn injury.

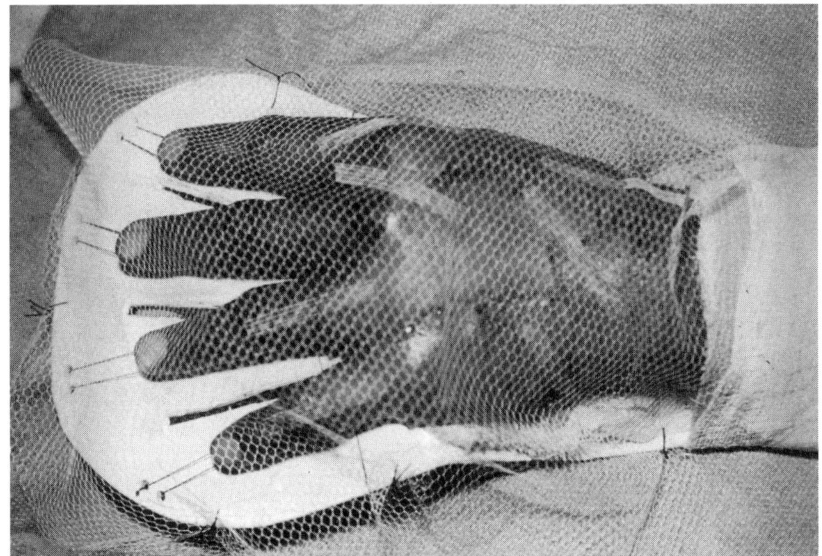

Figure 94-6. An example of a sheet graft placed on the dorsal aspect of a left hand. The fingertips are sutured and secured to the splint. The splint helps to maintain a functional position and keeps the hand immobilized to facilitate graft take.

aggressive but special attention must be paid to the delicate structures of the hand. With a full-thickness burn to the dorsum of the hand, a multijoint stretch is contraindicated. To maintain mobility while preserving tendon integrity, a modified flexion technique is performed. This involves achieving MP flexion with IP extension and then IP flexion with the MP joints extended. Patients should make a full fist only if the therapist is positive of the tendon status or if the wound has healed or been grafted. PROM is best completed while the patient's dressings are off. If possible, it is important to have the patient participate in active exercises and functional activities. This can be done in a gym or at the patient's bedside. Without daily exercise, muscle atrophy, tendon adherence, capsular shortening, and edema can be ongoing problems.

Proper positioning of the burned hand is essential for minimizing edema. When the body is subjected to thermal trauma, there is an immediate and rapid increase in capillary permeability. As a result, massive fluid accumulates in the area of trauma. This fluid can be very destructive to the fragile structures of the hand. One of the most common problems seen in the hand secondary to edema is the claw hand deformity. The result is that the MP joints are pulled into hyperextension; the IP joints, into flexion; and the thumb, into adduction (14). Elevation of the burned extremity and splinting will assist with the decrease of edema.

It must also be remembered that the hand functions as part of the upper extremity. Full hand motion is almost useless if significant contractures of the elbow or axilla prevent the patient from positioning the hand so that this motion can be utilized (16).

PAIN

Pain in burn patients must be managed carefully but aggressively. The patient's level of pain should not be underestimated. There is great variability in individual pain thresholds. Patients with "minor" surface area burns may report significant pain, while conversely a patient with a "major" surface area burn may have only minimal complaints.

Pain can occur with activity or at rest. Various approaches are used to measure pain. The most applicable to the burn patient appears to be the horizontal Visual Analog Scale (VAS) or the Verbal Descriptive Scale (VDS). In the pediatric population, the VAS and Pain Thermometers or the Procedural Behavior Checklist are useful. However, more research is indicated in this area.

Pain medications include opioids (morphine, meperidine, fentanyl, sufentanil), anti-inflammatories (ibuprofen, etc), local or general anesthetics (midazolam, nitrous oxide, lidocaine), and benzodiazepines (lorazepam). Each of these medications must be administered cautiously and the patient closely monitored for desired outcome and side effects. The response to opioids in particular can be significantly altered for months after burn injury. Administration of other medications, prior medical conditions, fluid volume status, and parenteral nutrition can affect the pharmacokinetics of drugs.

The route of medication delivery may include intravenous injections, patient-controlled epidural perfusion (PCA), oral route, or less preferable, intramuscular injections. Some patients will require opioids as well as behavioral modification, psychological supportive counseling, relaxation therapies, and in extreme cases, hypnosis.

Particularly with the pediatric population, the magnitude of pain must not be underestimated. Opiates, sedatives, behavioral modification, and even PCA have been used successfully with this population.

Aggressive pain management can lead to improved participation in burn rehabilitation as well as improved overall patient care. The most effective plan of care is tailored to the individual patient's needs.

COMPLICATIONS

Burn injuries can lead to significant compromise of the neurovascular system (Fig. 94-7). There are a number of neurologic complications seen after a burn injury. One such complication, burn encephalopathy, is a poorly defined clinical entity that may occur more frequently in children. Seen in about 30% of patients, it may be triggered by systemic factors, including fever. Peripheral neuropathies are seen more with burns of increased severity. They are commonly due to direct thermal, chemical, or electrical injury or secondary to treatment regimens (i.e., neurotoxic drugs, tight bandages, faulty positioning, or improper splinting). Mononeuritis multiplex is seen most frequently. Axonopathy of the critically ill is not uncommon. Burn injuries can be overwhelming and a prolonged recovery period can lead to generalized neural collapse. These patients may require mechanical ventilation, positioning, splinting, and a medical regimen.

Compartment syndrome can quickly develop as edema increases and compartment pressures rise. Eschar can contribute to the development of compartment syndrome because it lacks the compliance needed to accommodate a massive fluid shift. Compartment pressures may be monitored and decompressive surgery such as an escharotomy or fasciotomy of the involved area can be employed to reduce pressure and salvage tissue (Fig. 94-8).

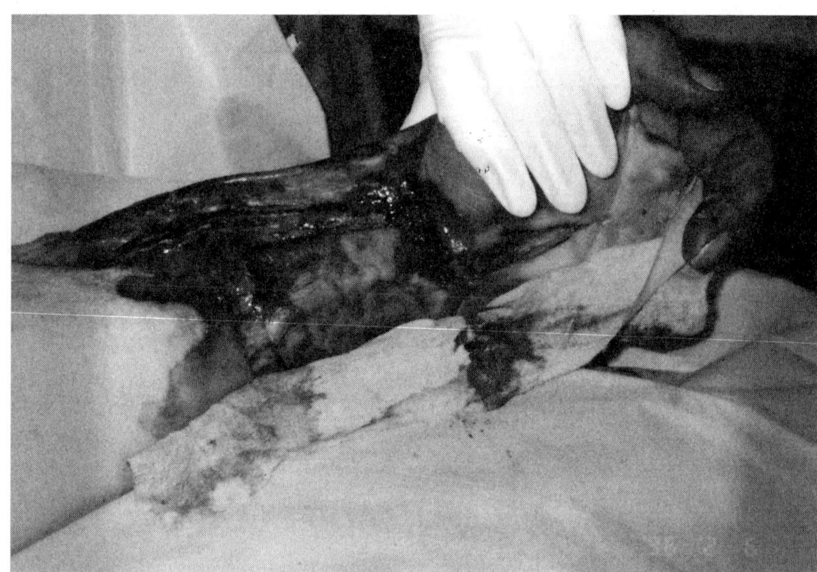

Figure 94-7. An exit site of a high-voltage electrical injury. An amputation was indicated secondary to neurovascular compromise.

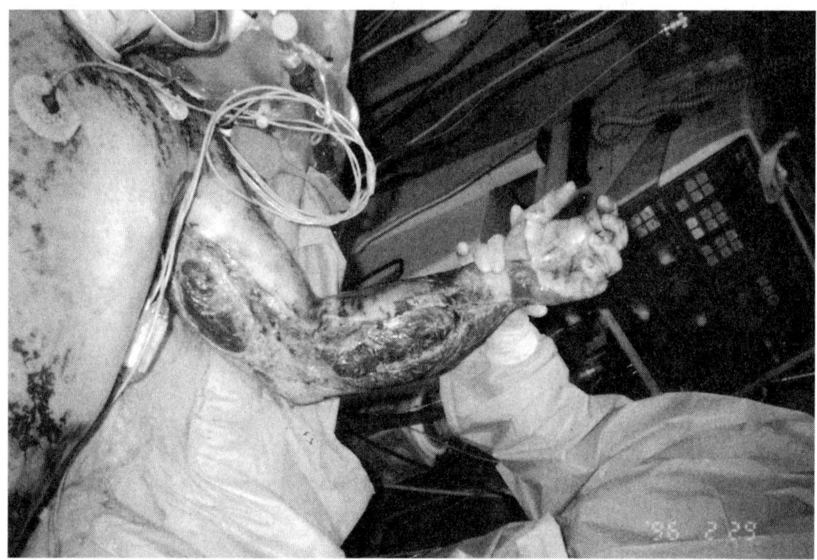

Figure 94-8. A fasciotomy allows deep tissues to expand, to prevent increased compartment pressures.

Heterotopic ossification is commonly found in burn patients who sustained deep burn wounds and have been immobile, particularly following grafting procedures over a joint. Diligent ROM exercises within surgical guidelines are optimal to reduce the risk of heterotopic ossification. Even with proper treatment, heterotopic ossification may still occur. Treatment for heterotopic ossification fluctuates from institution to institution.

HYPERTROPHIC SCARRING

The scarring process can limit ROM, cause contractures, and severely limit function. Most ongoing rehabilitation difficulties are secondary to the strong contractile properties of immature scars (17). Full scar maturation may take up to 12 to 18 months (18), with the most active scarring period being 4 to 6 months after injury (17). Early and aggressive treatment of the scars, via use of pressure, stretching, splinting, and positioning, is essential for good functional outcomes.

A healed wound is characterized by increased vascularity and an increased number of fibroblasts. Fibroblasts then synthesize excessive collagen, which redevelops in irregular shapes and whorl-like masses at four times the rate of normal skin (19). Early scar is readily influenced by external forces because cross-linking collagen bonds are weak and fewer in number in the early stages. Therefore, these bonds are likely to align themselves in a more organized parallel format. Pressure may also control collagen synthesis by producing ischemia in the scar (17) and decreasing wound vascularity.

The severity of scarring is affected by wound depth and the time needed for wound closure. If a wound requires skin grafting or takes longer than 14 days to heal, pressure therapy will be indicated (Fig. 94-9). Other factors influencing the severity of scarring include age, race, genetic disposition, anatomic location of the burn, and the type of grafting performed. Pediatric patients and patients with very fair or dark skin tend to be at higher risk for increased scarring. Burns of the hand, head, and axilla also tend to be more vulnerable to increased scar formation. Grafts placed on granulation tissue also tend to scar more than tangentially excised wounds (17).

Early pressure can be provided via Ace wrapping, tubular support bandages, interim garments, and prefabricated pressure gloves. These can be tolerated as early as 7 to 10 days after grafting or when open areas are no larger than the size of a dime (19). These methods of pressure are used while body weight and edema stabilize prior to having the patient measured for custom-fit pressure garments. Custom garments are made of a Dacron/spandex elastic fabric and provide capillary level pressures of at least 25 mm Hg (17). The wearing time may need to be increased gradually to 23 out of 24 hours per day, and the garments may need to be worn until full scar maturation has occurred. Proper fit is essential so the fit must be periodically examined and alterations or entire new garments may be needed.

The sustained use of capillary level pressure on the growing bones and tissues of small children has been controversial. However, it is now believed that if the fit is monitored closely to allow for growth, garment use is acceptable, with the exception of the head.

To maintain uniform pressure in concave areas of the body, inserts such as elastomer putty, Silastic elastomer with prosthetic foam, Plastizote, or thermoplastic conformers may be used. Silicone gel sheeting is another option for the treatment of hypertrophic or keloid scars. Although effective, the mechanism is not fully understood. The gel may promote hydration and the degree of occlusion may

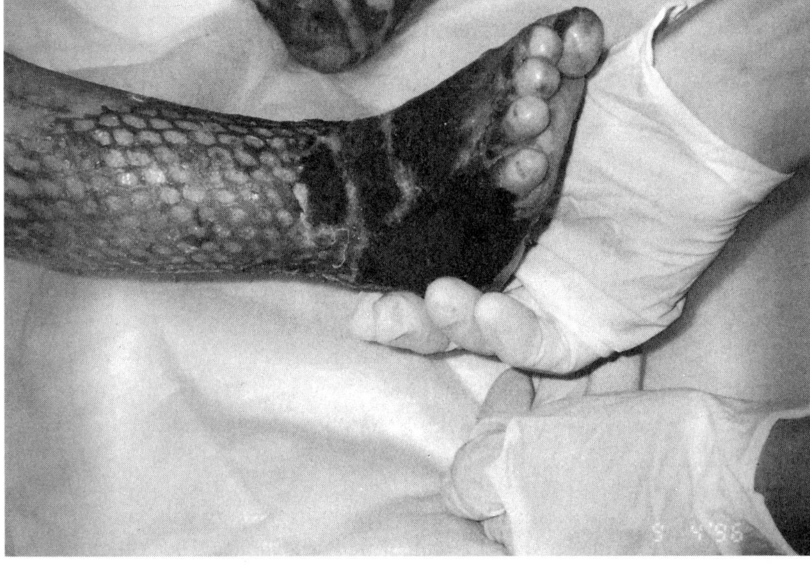

Figure 94-9. Scarring occurs along the margins of a meshed graft and between interstitial sites. This graft is ready for the initiation of pressure garments to help improve the cosmetic outcome.

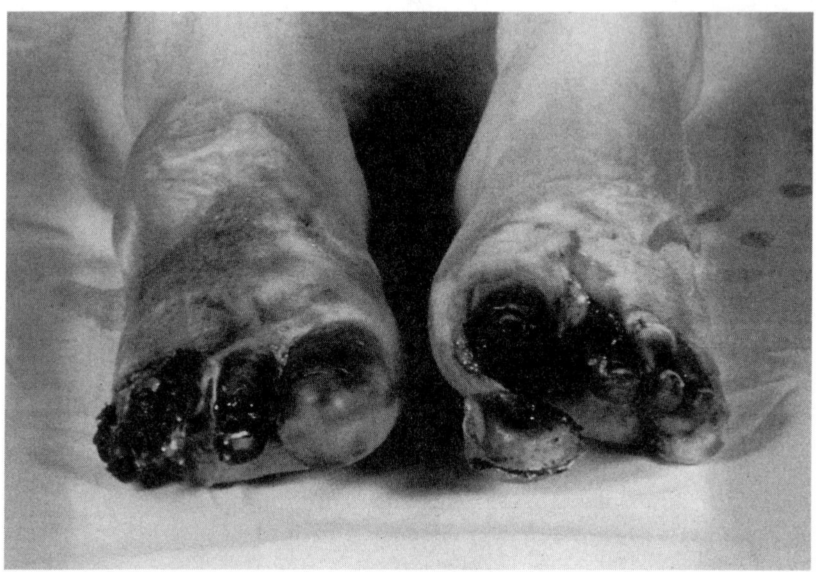

Figure 94-10. Exit site from a high-voltage electrical injury requiring bilateral transmetatarsal amputations.

also play a role (20). Silicone gel sheets may only be used on completely healed skin surfaces, as internal absorption remains controversial.

Proper pressure therapy can lead to favorable functional and cosmetic gains. Patient compliance is essential; otherwise, surgical intervention may be needed (Fig. 94-10).

COSMESIS

Following scar maturation, changes in the texture and color of the skin may still be present. The visible scarring may alter a patient's self-esteem. To minimize discoloration and disfigurement, cosmetics that camouflage these areas were developed. Paramedical camouflage is a process by which the appearance of scar or skin pigment alterations is normalized. This is achieved through the application of proper shades and placement of cosmetics. The makeup is specific for each individual. The patient is instructed in the proper use of these cosmetics so the desired effect can be achieved. Creams utilized usually contain a sunscreen and are waterproof.

DISABILITY

The evaluation of disability is an appraisal of the patient's present and future ability to engage in gainful activity as it is affected by factors such as age, sex, education, economics, and social relationships. These diverse and subjective factors are difficult to measure (7). For this reason, permanent impairment is the major criterion used in arriving at a permanent disability determination. Unlike disability, permanent impairment can be measured with a reasonable degree of accuracy and uniformity (21).

The American Medical Association's *Guides to the Evaluation of Permanent Impairment* is a widely accepted aid and provides a standard framework and method of analysis through which physicians can evaluate, report on, and communicate information about the impairments of any human organ system. Many state workers' compensation agencies mandate or recommend use of the *Guides*. Even though rating or estimating impairment cannot be totally objective, use of the *Guides* increases objectivity and enables physicians to report impairment in a standardized manner, so that reports from different observers are more likely to be comparable in content and completeness (22). The effects of a burn injury on the skin and its appendages are combined with the estimated impairment percentages of other body systems, including the musculoskeletal system, the nervous system, the respiratory system, the ears, the nose, the throat, and related structures. Additionally mental and behavioral disorders are discussed in the *Guides*.

PSYCHOLOGICAL ISSUES

Although the costs of burn treatment are tremendous in terms of health care dollars, time, effort, pain, suffering, and mental anguish to patients and families, it is rewarding if the patient emerges from this ordeal as a functioning member of society with self-respect and dignity intact. Certainly, some patients do emerge intact, and some resume their lives in a more productive and gratifying manner than before the injury. However, many patients, despite the best burn treatment, develop psychological complications that hinder their recovery. Healing on the outside may not always reflect healing on the inside.

Anxiety, denial, depression, grief, and mourning may be experienced. Depression may be transient and show improvement with the healing process or may intensify with time as the patient realizes what has been lost.

Many burn injuries are due to premorbid psychological problems. This includes a possible history of alcohol or drug abuse, violence, or fire starting. Depression, alcohol or drug abuse, and organic brain syndrome can be accompanied by poor concentration, impaired judgment, and slow motor response, all of which contribute to a high risk of burn trauma.

Symptoms of posttraumatic stress are expected in the postburn period. However, if they exacerbate, reintegration into society may be hindered.

Patients need to recover physically and psychologically after burn injury. All members of the team need to be aware of how these problems can impact on the patient's ultimate functional outcome. Emotional support is necessary, and patients may require additional assistance from mental health professionals.

FUTURE TRENDS

The changing health care milieu will affect burn care of the future. When feasible, outpatient management of burn injuries will replace more expensive inpatient services. Future trends also include new wound care technologies such as developments in artificial skin. A deeper understanding of new technology is required to keep pace with the frequent changes in burn care delivery.

REFERENCES

1. Brigham P, McLaughlin E. Burn incidence and medical care use in the U.S.: estimates, trends and data sources. *J Burn Care Rehabil* 1996;17:95–105.
2. Sabistan D, ed. *Textbook of surgery.* Philadelphia: WB Saunders, 1991:178.
3. Greenfield LJ. *Surgery—scientific principles and practice.* Philadelphia: JB Lippincott-Raven, 1997.
4. Clark JA. *Color atlas of burn injuries.* New York: Chapman & Hall Medical, 1992.
5. Demling R, LaLonde C. *Burn trauma.* New York: Thieme Medical, 1989.
6. Fitzpatrick T, et al. *Dermatology in general medicine.* Vol. I. New York: McGraw-Hill, 1993.
7. Richard R, Staley M. *Burn care & rehabilitation—Principles and practice.* Philadelphia: FA Davis, 1994.
8. Gerding RL, Emerman CL, Effron D, et al. Outpatient management of partial-thickness burns: Biobrane versus 1% silver sulfadiazine. *Ann Emerg Med* 1990;19: 121–124.
9. Lown D. Use and efficacy of nutritional protocol for patients with burns in intensive care. *J Burn Care Rehabil* 1991;12: 3371–3376.
10. Constable JD. The state of burn care past, present and future. *Burns* 1994;20:316–324.
11. Heimbach DM. A non-user's questions about cultured epidermal autograft. *J Burn Care Rehabil* 1992;13:127–129.
12. Cultured autologous keratinocytes suspended in fibrin glue to cover burn wounds. In: *Plastic surgery nerve repair burns.* Stark, et al. New York: 1995:143.
13. *Medical economics of Integra artificial skin.* Plainsboro, NJ: Integra Life Sciences, 1996.
14. Malick and Carr. *Manual on management of the burn patient* Pittsburgh: Harmarville Rehab Center, 1982.
15. Androwick, Goldblum, et al. "OT intervention for people with burns. *Advanced Magazine for Occupational Therapists* May 22, 1995.
16. Robson MC, Smith DJ Jr, VanderZee AJ, Roberts L. Making the burned hand functional. *Clin Plast Surg* 1992;19:663–671.
17. Ward RS. Pressure therapy for the control of hypertrophic scar formation after burn injury: a history and review. *J Burn Care Rehabil* 1991;12:257–262.
18. Trombly CA, ed. *OT for physical dysfunction.* 2nd ed. Baltimore: Williams & Wilkins, 1983.
19. *Willard & Spackman's OT.* 5th ed. Philadelphia: JB Lippincott, 1978.
20. Cica Care pamphlet. Smith & Nephew Rolyan, 1994.
21. Fisher S, Helm P. *Comprehensive rehabilitation of burns.* Baltimore: Williams & Wilkins, 1984.
22. Doege TC, ed. *Guides to the evaluation of permanent impairment.* 4th ed. Chicago: American Medical Association, 1993.

Part VI.

Specific Populations

Chapter 95

Pediatric Rehabilitation

Maureen R. Nelson
Kathryn A. Zidek

The goal of pediatric rehabilitation is to attain maximal functional ability for children with physical deficits within the limitations of their development. To accomplish this goal with pediatric patients, the same concepts essential to all rehabilitation are incorporated into patient care: a focus on the whole child and a team approach to rehabilitation. This chapter is a general overview of how pediatric physiatry is similar, but yet unique, in the rehabilitation spectrum. The developmental abilities and skills of the child must be embodied in the rehabilitation process. This overview highlights how therapy, adaptive equipment, mobility devices, seating systems, prosthetic devices, bowel and bladder management, and communication devices must be directed toward the child's developmental capabilities and growth potential. The importance of play as a tool in pediatric rehabilitation is stressed, as is the importance of addressing the complicated, yet inevitable, process of psychosocial and sexual development in children and adolescents with physical disabilities. The significant role of the family in the rehabilitation process is outlined, as well as the necessity of educating the family in facilitating the independence of the child with special needs. The incorporation of education into the rehabilitation process is discussed throughout the chapter, and the need for general well-child care recommended. Lastly, an approach to the special aspects of electrodiagnostics in children is offered to the reader.

TEAM ROLES

The physiatrist's role in rehabilitation is typically medical management and team coordination. The physiatrist designs the rehabilitation program, working with the therapists and nurses to set and work toward appropriate goals, as well as prevent secondary complications. The physician oversees respiratory care, including ventilator management, if required, and works with other physicians who remain or become involved in the patient's care.

The role of the pediatric physical therapist not only includes the traditional interventions of mobility training, transfer training, maintenance of range of motion, and therapeutic modalities, but also requires incorporation of knowledge about growth and development into these practices. Similarly, the pediatric occupational therapist instructs in activities of daily living (ADLs) and fine motor skills appropriate to the patient's developmental stage. For example, the pediatric patient may first need to be toilet trained, whereas the adult patient would be approached with retraining of previously learned skills. Improving different forms of fine motor skills in children may be accomplished through appropriate play activities such as coloring and use of scissors, puzzles, and other precision movement toys. Assistive devices for the pediatric patient can differ from the adult population and may include posterior walkers, parapodiums, prone scooters, arm-propelled carts, modified tricycles, manual or electric wheelchairs, upper- or lower-extremity orthoses including reciprocating gait orthoses, and spinal orthoses.

The role of the speech and language pathologist can be varied, from improving speech and language production to increasing oral-motor skills. What is unique in the pediatric population, however, is that the child's language skills are first developing, and that traditional interventions, for example, with the aphasic adult, are not appropriate. Feeding difficulties secondary to weakness or incoordination in oropharyngeal musculature may precede speech production delays as development continues. Speech therapists may also provide children with augmentative communication devices or train the child and their family in the use of sign language.

Nurses play a critical role in pediatric rehabilitation. Their role includes customary rehabilitation nursing interventions, as well as being the primary advocate for the child and parents. Nurses frequently interact with the patient's family and often relay information from other members of the team to them, especially with parents who are unable to be involved in rehabilitation during the day. They often include play in their daily activities with the patient.

Nutrition and dietary support are vital in pediatric rehabilitation. The child's changing needs according to his or her growth and the catabolic state following trauma must be considered during the recovery process. An age-appropriate diet including pediatric preferences should be offered on the rehabilitation unit. Additionally, some patients may require alternative methods of feeding, including use of nasogastric or gastrostomy tubes.

Social services have an expanded role on the pediatric rehabilitation team. They assist in facilitating communication with the patient and their family, and in obtaining funding for therapeutic services, equipment, and supplies. Social workers frequently assist with return to school and development of individualized education plans, and often follow the patient's progress in the educational system following discharge.

Respiratory therapists play an important role in the care of patients who are at risk for pulmonary insufficiency or infection. Rehabilitation engineers can be involved in obtaining the most appropriate mobility, seating, and environmental control devices for the patient in coordinated effort with other team members.

An orthotist will fabricate orthoses for the upper and lower extremities, as well as occasionally for the spine and skull. These devices can provide support, control, or assistance for particular body segments. The orthotist may also assist with seating and mobility, particularly for very small children who may not be easily or properly fit in traditional devices.

Behavior modification programs, developed with the input of a psychologist, may be an integral part of pediatric rehabilitation. They may be carried out by all the members of the team, including, most importantly, the family. Psychological or psychiatric services including counseling may also be needed to deal with reactive emotional responses and possible body image discomfort. Family counseling may also be of benefit, as siblings and parents are also affected by having a child with a disability in the family.

THE PEDIATRIC REHABILITATION SETTING

An inpatient pediatric rehabilitation unit is designed with adaptations for children such as a playroom where patients can go between therapy sessions with their siblings or other patients. It is here where patients can go about the work of childhood, play. For adolescents there is frequently a separate teen room where such patients may relax and socialize. Instead of toys, there are usually televisions, video games, telephones, a stereo, and a pool table or Ping-Pong table. Parents and younger children frequently are not allowed in this room. Medical procedures are also typically banned in these rooms, which creates a sense of security for patients. In addition, in some institutions the patient's room is also procedure free, with all necessary medical procedures, such as placing intravenous lines and drawing blood, occurring in a treatment room. The pediatric rehabilitation unit also will have a school or several small classrooms. Many are designed with computer access so patients with no or limited hand or finger function can write. A dayroom is also provided for parents so that they may relax or interact with other family members or other parents when they are not directly involved in their child's care. Some pediatric rehabilitation units have overnight rooms, including shower accommodations and beds. There is also a greater need for more direct observation of patient's rooms in a pediatric versus an adult unit, balancing the need to preserve a degree of privacy and maximum safety. There is frequently a separate therapy room on the unit for treatment of the inpatient children. This allows a more relaxed and comfortable therapeutic environment, as opposed to a larger gym with a variety of adult patients.

If there is an inpatient rehabilitation stay, the patient then ideally is transferred to an outpatient rehabilitation program, where appropriate therapies continue. Physician-to-therapist coordination is formalized in a written prescription, which should include the patient's diagnosis; a synopsis of the family's understanding and acceptance of the diagnosis, prognosis, and treatment plans; and a description of observed deficits, functional goals, precautions, and intensity of program desired (1). In addition, the physiatrist should continue to follow the patient as frequently as is needed to ensure close monitoring of his or her rehabilitative and medical status. The overall goals of outpatient and inpatient rehabilitation remain the same: the achievement of function at the greatest level possible within developmental boundaries. Returning to the family environment and society at large, including introduction or continuation of an educational or career path, is also a significant long-term goal for the pediatric patient moving into outpatient rehabilitation management. The ultimate level of independence depends on many things, including cognitive and motor deficits, age and developmental level, the existence of secondary complications such as skin ulcerations, and appropriate and well-fitting orthoses and methods of mobility.

Modifications of parts of a pediatric rehabilitation program are often necessary due to the fact that children are growing physically, emotionally, cognitively, socially, and spiritually. Therefore, the rehabilitation team has the added responsibility of being in tune with the special needs of the child at various levels of development, as well as their impact on the family. The specialized needs in rehabilitation vary from infancy through childhood to the teenage years and on into young adulthood. Included in the transition through these stages is the importance of general sex education, as well as sex education directed toward the child's specific disability and level of function.

CHILD DEVELOPMENT: IMPACT ON REHABILITATION APPROACH

Pediatric rehabilitation goals are developmentally oriented. The approaches used to attain goals, as well as the expected level of achievement, vary with age. To prepare a child with a physical disability for optimal functioning in adulthood, the rehabilitation process must consider the changing needs and concerns created by different stages of growth and development (2). The secondary complications that need to be avoided also change over childhood. It is important in all steps of development to promote growth in cognitive, social, and physical achievement.

Therapy in infancy varies with the diagnosis and needs, but is largely directed toward range of motion, positioning, premobility skills, and oftentimes oral-motor skills, and teaching the parents to perform these activities. These are performed with the goal of preventing secondary complications such as contractures and decubitus ulcers. Stimulation early in the life of infants with congenital disabilities such as cerebral palsy has been favored (3). There is, however, no definitive literature that specifies an ideal approach, and in fact, controversy over the efficacy of any therapies exists (3–6). Therapists instruct parents in home therapy programs in order that any activities learned for either active use by a child or passive performance by parents can be transferred to a functional skill in the child's home environment. Performance of a home program may help the family cope with their disabled child (7). A seating device allowing adequate support for infants with weakness in head and trunk control should be provided. Infants with upper-limb deficiencies should be fitted with a passive prosthetic device around the age of 4 to 5 months to promote bilateral upper-extremity use in play and assist with sitting (8). Infants with lower-limb deficiencies can usually be fitted with a prosthesis around 8 to 10 months to encourage pulling to a standing position. As the child grows into the early toddler years, therapy is then geared toward mobility skills. Play is used to attempt to teach a child a means of moving. Play is also used to increase upper-extremity function. In toddlers with upper-limb deficiencies, a functional terminal device that permits grasping and holding objects is added to the prosthesis around 12 to 18 months. Myoelectric prostheses are also successfully used by toddlers as young as 16 to 18 months (9). Assistive devices for standing are generally first used between the ages of 12 and 18 months. Devices such as scooter boards may be used for independent mobility. This is especially beneficial for skin protection in children who are insensate and would otherwise drag themselves along the floor, for example, children with paraplegia or those with thoracic to high-lumbar myelodysplasia. Many 2-year-olds can also independently manipulate a wheelchair. Some children at the same age are also able to independently and safely manipulate a power wheelchair (7). Children can attain independent wheelchair mobility after 1 to 3 weeks of training (10). They also can explore and move farther distances with power wheelchairs, but exploration is limited to objects that can be reached from the chair (11). Mobility devices are crucial for general development so that children can actively explore their environment and learn to interact with it. Prevention of contractures with range of motion exercises or orthotic devices, or both, to maintain correct joint positions is important at all ages.

Preschool children are developing more motor skills and are able to play games. As coordination improves, assistive devices for ambulation may be used. Crutches may be used by children ages 2 to 3 years who have good upper-extremity strength, balance, and coordination. Children with spinal cord injury neurologic levels higher than that which would allow an adult to walk are frequently able to ambulate. Wheelchairs are an important means of mobility during the preschool years, and adapted tricycles can also be beneficial. Children can use a standing table or frame both for the social benefits of being in an upright position along with other children and for possible musculoskeletal benefits from weight bearing and extending the hips and knees. Preschool children can also use adaptive equipment for age-appropriate ADLs, such as learning to dress or feed themselves with utensils. They are able to use simple tools and can begin to use modern technology to increase their ADL function or mobility and communication devices if needed. Bowel and bladder training can begin in the preschool years for children with neurogenic bowel and bladder. Children with a cognitive age of 5 or 6, good fine motor skills, and good sitting balance can learn to perform self-catheterization. Preschool age is an important time for learning social expectations. At this age children are learning to control their environment and how to interact with other children as well as adults. They are also learning how to play interactively with other children, to demonstrate control, to accept limits, and to follow guidelines.

In the school years, peer influence becomes significant. Social skills grow immensely, and children are able to advance their physical skills. Their verbal skills improve and they can increase their compensatory skills. They can manipulate more advanced technology to assist in their ADLs. The degree to which a child can move about and can communicate is critical in the ability to initiate social interaction (12). This is a critical time for education, and educational needs help to direct rehabilitation goals (7). In some cases, therapy can dominate a child's time to the point that it interferes with opportunities for socialization (13). This is a problem that both professionals and parents need to consider.

Adolescence can be a period of turmoil for any youngster and the stresses are accentuated by a disability. Biomechanically, this is typically a period of rapid growth; thereby, the tendency to develop scoliosis or contractures is increased. It is more difficult to ambulate with a larger, heavier body than a younger, smaller child's body. Social pressures are increased and this is the time when adolescents begin separating from their parents and striving for independence. Because of the physical needs of a disabled adolescent, there may be increased difficulty in achieving independence. Instruction in social skills is important for general social interactions, future job potential, as well as learning to instruct other individuals in assisting in daily care needs. Support groups of other teens with a similar disability can often be useful.

There may be an increased risk of secondary complications such as contractures, urinary tract infections, and pressure ulcers due to the rebellion commonly seen in the teenage years. Teens with disability may focus much of their behavior on feeling "normal" and being valued. Teens with spinal cord injury, for example, tend to formulate strategies in an attempt to promote these feelings, particularly in the areas of physical appearance, physical and emotional independence, and social skills (14).

PSYCHOSEXUAL DEVELOPMENT

The development of sexuality is a long-term process and is complicated in children or adolescents with a disability. A physical disability will impact total development, including sexual development. In infancy, children experience their first relationship with other individuals. These relationships provide a basis for their perception of all future relationships. Touch is a major factor that is believed to give children a feeling of security and bonding (15). In quadriplegia, and other conditions with motor and sensory loss, the inability for active movement of the extremities or insensate limbs may prevent the development of this feeling and may limit positive interactions that contribute to the development of trust of others and a healthy social and sexual development (16). By the time children are 2 years old, they generally have learned their gender identity and role, the things they do and say to indicate that they are male or female. Many experiences in childhood will contribute to children's concept of what being a boy or girl means. These experiences may be altered in children with a disability. With the extra demands placed on parents to take care of the disabled child's physical needs, they may not place as much emphasis on teaching about issues related to social skills and sexuality. The parents are the initial teachers and role models in sexuality for children. Children during the preschool period are continuing to learn their sexual role and by the time they enter school they have a fair idea of expectations for males and females. Generally, children in the 3- to 5-year-old range have an increased awareness of sexuality and the identification as a male or female is increased. Social isolation, however, may become a problem. Children with visible deficits often are rejected as playmates by healthy peers. There is frequently also a problem of not having a model of an adult with a similar disability to use as a standard for comparison (17). Privacy may be a problem for children with a disability as they may need to be more closely supervised by caretakers. The lack of privacy may affect children's perception of their own body and of personal boundaries in regard to touch. Some children with disabilities are frequently handled by many people for various medical procedures or care. This touch is very different from that of a family member's touch or a hug. Children may be partially or totally disrobed for the purpose of physical examination or other treatment. It may be very confusing for them to be touched so much by strangers and this may lead to confusion about public and private nudity, and appropriateness of touch (15).

Children in the elementary school years turn their focus from themselves to the outside world. They begin looking to their peer group for support, interaction, and information. This is where they develop their social skills and compare ideas, including those about sexuality. Children with disabilities may have limited opportunities for "practice" of basic social skills owing to social isolation, either due to lack of mobility and physical skills, or to overprotective family and other care providers. Having children participate in organized recreational and social activities such as sports, music, and hobbies can assist them in overcoming some of these obstacles. Children of this age are learning the cultural roles for each gender. This is also a common time when children may first develop a crush on an adult. This is an important time for children to find out there can be affection from someone outside their family and that they can find love in more than one place (18).

Lack of information about sexuality can include the knowledge of pubertal changes in the body. It is important that parents and others teach children about the changes that will occur in puberty prior to their occurrence, including menarche and nocturnal emissions. It is also important at this stage that children understand the difference between what is considered appropriate in private versus public situations. Children who are more isolated socially will need more information than other children because of fewer opportunities for spontaneous social learning, both by observing others and by interacting among themselves (19).

Adolescence is a tumultuous time for any youngster growing up. Puberty is a time when boys' and girls' bodies change and secondary sex characteristics develop. Girls begin to menstruate generally between the ages of 10 and 13 years, and boys begin to have nocturnal emissions between the ages of 13 and 15 years. Our cultural emphasis on a perfect body is learned by most children by this time. It places a good deal of stress on any adolescent and is magnified for someone with a physical disability. Looking or moving differently than one's peers is an exaggerated problem at this stage of development. Adolescents with a physical disability must adapt to a body image that frequently includes a wheelchair, braces, or a crutch (20). With the rapid changes seen in adolescence, the teen must find a balance between the positive and negative aspects of the body. This balance is made more difficult for teenagers with a physical disability. Adolescence is a time for moving toward independence, and that adjustment is made more difficult for persons who are dependent on their parents for physical care. Lack of experience in self-care and overprotection may add to this problem. To minimize the problem, it is helpful to have teens begin to participate in self-care activities within their abilities as early as possible and gradually increase this participation as their abilities allow. This may help minimize rebellion, which can lead to serious physical and emotional problems during adolescence. Experimentation and use of trial and error are common behaviors in teens attempting to gain independence, but these opportunities may be limited in adolescents with special needs. It is also reported that having a physical disability may lead to regression of personal development (21). Children who grow up being dependent in their activities and in their daily care may learn a pattern of "learned helplessness," which may make them overly compliant and make achieving independence more difficult (20). Independence from parents is not only emotional but financial. For teens with minimal opportunities to learn job skills and who have significant potential medical costs, the financial aspect is an added difficulty. Adolescence is a very helpful time to have a role model of another teen or adult, particularly one with a similar disability. Often one is not available in person but recently, positive disabled role models can be found in the mass media. The development of communication skills is of crucial importance for socialization.

Several trends are evident regarding social and sexual activity and knowledge of adolescents with disability, compared to others. The results vary but those of recent studies are more positive than those performed 10 or more years ago. Teens and young adults with physical disabilities, compared to other teenagers, much more frequently have not been on a date, and those who do date, do so less frequently than other teens (22). Additionally, a much higher percentage of disabled teens and young adults have not had sex, and more of those who are sexually active do not use birth control (22). Despite receiving sex education at school, knowledge of anatomy, sexual function, and reproduction was lower in several groups of teens with disabilities than other teens (22). It has been found that social interaction and success are more related to the environment and the family than they are to the severity of physical disability (22–24). Parental expectations are a significant factor in young women with disabilities having active social lives. Unfortunately, only a small percentage of parents of girls with disabilities ever expect their daughters to be sexually active (24,25). However, many parents do promote impressive educational goals (8,16). One study looking at disabled women and social and sexual experience showed that women with disabilities had dates, steady relationships, and sexual contact significantly later in life than their able-bodied counterparts. However, masturbation occurred at the same time for the two groups (23,26). This was interpreted to indicate that disabled young women had a similar awareness and interest in sexual feelings compared to their able-bodied peers, but fewer social opportunities for expression (27). Menarche is considered an important time for girls with disabilities, even more than in the general population. Some girls may perceive this as a positive occurrence in which the body finally does something it is supposed to do (25). Conversely, it may be unwelcome by the parents as a sign of their disabled daughter's emerging sexuality and possible independence (28). The girl may react to this with fear if she is unaware of menstruation.

Social skills, including the ability to relate to others in different situations and the ability to understand various levels of meaning, generally develop slowly throughout childhood and adolescence by both personal experience and observation. Similarly, the ability to learn the range of human emotions and how to control one's reaction to them occurs through many positive and negative experiences (28). With opportunities for spontaneous interactions limited because of physical constraints, efforts must be made by professionals and parents to supplement experiences and knowledge as appropriate as possible.

Sex education begins informally in very early life in

the family environment. It is important to acknowledge that each child is a sexual being, and to validate the child's or parent's concerns about sexuality (8,21). It is also important that developmentally appropriate social and sexual information be given to children to reduce the risk of sexual exploitation and abuse (16,29). Using language that is simple and appropriate, and using repetition, audiovisual material, and structured opportunities can be helpful in improving comfort with sexuality (30).

Prior to establishing and providing sex education programs, it is important to inform the patient's parents and to address any concerns they may have. Parents of disabled and nondisabled children alike have raised the concern that teaching sex education will prematurely interest children in sex and involve them in sexual activity. Research has shown that this is not the case (18). Additionally, parents of children with disabilities frequently fear that their children will be unable to establish a satisfactory relationship or that they will be used or hurt if they do become involved. Differing cultural and religious values also may be an area of concern for parents (19).

Sex education progresses along with a child's developmental status. It can go from a general gender identity program beginning in kindergarten along with socialization and communication skills, to addressing anatomy, physiology, responsible behavior, social consequences of behavior, sexually transmitted diseases, and contraception in an adolescent group. Sometimes sex education is included in a junior high or high school course, such as family life, which looks at other aspects including boy-girl differences, heredity, and dating (18).

People with and without physical disabilities make individual adjustments for their social and sexual needs. There are various ways to be sexually active and to express oneself sexually that vary with physical abilities as well as interest (31). It is particularly important for adolescents with a lack of genital sensation to understand this, and to understand that nongenital orgasms are possible.

Sexuality is a part of human personality that encompasses the physical, social, spiritual, and emotional realms. In children and adolescents with a disability, developing that aspect of the personality can be even more of a challenge than it is for children in general. By being aware of specific deficits and how to circumvent those areas, we can help children and their parents more readily develop a well-rounded personality and physical functioning. By modifying sex education to compensate for areas that may have been missed because of social isolation or physical deficits, particularly to include a larger social component, such as basic social skills, we can help children learn appropriate behavior, interactions, and responsibility. Additionally, by acknowledging specific problems in sexual function, including sexual development, actual sexual abilities, reproduction, and contraceptive needs, we can help parents to help their children become more knowledgeable adolescents and adults (19).

ROLE OF THE FAMILY IN PEDIATRIC REHABILITATION

The role of families in rehabilitation is particularly significant with pediatric patients. In the case of either congenital or acquired disabilities, it is common for parents to go through a series of reactions, including a period of grief in response to their feelings of loss of their "perfect child" (32). Support and empathy for parents and siblings through this period are important and can be provided effectively by the primary physician, social workers, nurses, psychologists, and support groups of parents of children with similar diagnoses. It has been shown that the physician's attitude about the child's disability contributes to the development of a supportive relationship with the family, as well as to the family's ability to participate in the rehabilitation program (33). It is vital that parents become enlisted as important members of the team, with support of their self-esteem vital for learning (34). The functioning of the family unit, parenting style, and ability to cope with having a disabled child must be evaluated by the pediatric rehabilitation team (7). Sibling support groups, if available, can also be helpful for the patient's siblings dealing with their own feelings, including possible feelings of jealousy over parental attention, guilt, concerns for the future of their injured sibling, or how their peers will react to the fact that their sibling has a disability (34). Self-esteem in children with disabilities has been described as positively correlated with organized and structured families who have activities and responsibilities clearly delineated, and negatively correlated with families in conflict (35).

PSYCHOSOCIAL ISSUES

Disabled children become disabled adults, and as adults, they need to be able to function in society to the best of their abilities. This involves the development of physical abilities, as well as intellectual, psychological, and social skills (36). Disabled children progress through the stages of development at varying rates and to different degrees. They may accomplish some milestones at the same time as other children, other milestones may be accomplished much later, and some developmental milestones may never be reached. Parents may react to this uncertainty by expecting too much while failing to accept or encourage what can be done; or by expecting too little and not encouraging performance that is possible (37,38).

Disabilities may interfere with learning by limiting peer exposure and social activities because of decreased mobility or time constraints due to extra care or therapies. Motor deficits may hinder physical separation from parents and delay emotional separation and individuation. This delay may have a lasting effect on personality development and secondarily on the family's style of child rearing (39,40). Motor deficits may also limit learning through trial and error. Visual, auditory, perceptual, and cognitive deficits may decrease the accuracy of observation and the interpretation of events. Social and psychological development can be neglected by families as they focus on physical accomplishments. Disabled children frequently are exposed to different social learning environments in the school system and as a result, their sense of self-identity may be affected. Their parents frequently give them fewer opportunities to learn independence, to make choices, and to learn from their mistakes.

Relationships within the family, including those between parents, siblings, and extended-family members, can be affected by the child's disability. Time demands on the primary caregiver can be extraordinary, with less energy available for siblings and spouse. Siblings may react either positively or negatively to their disabled brother or sister, with greater acceptance and altruism or with jealousy and anger. Parents may feel that their extended-family members are unable to understand or be supportive of the needs of their family.

Development of social skills including responsibility, acceptable behavior, and independence must be fostered by the family. Disabled children must be allowed to make choices if they are to learn responsibility, and must be encouraged to attempt new skills. Overprotection can interfere with the ultimate development of social, psychological, and cognitive abilities. Failing and trying again is part of learning for all children, disabled or able-bodied. Manners are necessary for social interaction and are best learned when taught early by the family. Appropriate expression of emotions can be taught within the child's abilities to comprehend and display feelings. Disabled children should be given opportunities to interact with peers at age-appropriate levels. Behavioral modification techniques can be helpful in dealing with egocentric or manipulative behavior.

EDUCATION

For hospitalized children, a school setting will be provided in the pediatric rehabilitation unit. When children with disabilities are in their home environment, they can fulfill their school requirements and attend a program at their relative age and ability level. Many times the same books and class plans are used in the home and hospital classroom. The teachers from the hospital ideally communicate with the children's regular school teachers both initially, to see how they were performing cognitively before the illness or injury, and through the rehabilitation stay. One of the most crucial roles of the rehabilitation team is to return children to the most appropriate school setting. Information regarding the lesson plans that were covered during the hospitalization, and any difficulties that were encountered, is passed to the school teachers. At discharge, the team helps to get the child into a school building that is accessible and safe for that child. Physical therapy, occupational therapy, and speech therapy are also frequently utilized at the school after return there. Public schools are required to provide appropriate education in the least restrictive environment, which includes providing therapies to help compensate for any deficits that interfere with educational performance. This includes speech therapy for a child who is unable to talk; occupational therapy for someone who is unable to write, including computer training to teach them to efficiently use a computer; and physical therapy for a child who is unable to sit or transfer independently at school. Some children may require an attendant for safe transfers or toileting. A nurse may also be required to assist with tube feedings, catheterizations, or other needs. Communication with the school throughout the rehabilitation stay, and extensive communication of the plan for return to school prior to the child's doing so, are very useful in easing the transition from rehabilitation to school. Early intervention programs for the first 3 years of life exist within each state to provide services based on each child's needs, including physical therapy, occupational therapy, speech and language pathology, early childhood intervention, adaptive technology, and diagnostic services. On the other end of the pediatric spectrum, it is important for the physiatrist to assist the teen with a disability with career planning after high school, whether it be college, technologic or vocational school, or job training and placement. Realistic evaluation of physical and cognitive abilities during high school can guide such activities. State rehabilitation commissions typically assist with such planning and training once appropriate referrals are made in the late teen years.

RECREATION

Recreation is important for all individuals and especially so for children. It is said that the work of children is to play and to go to school. The environment of the rehabilitation unit is such that opportunities for play are present during times outside of therapy, and during therapy play is used as much as possible. During rehabilitation, the opportunity for introduction to adaptive sports can beneficial. Pool therapy is often a great asset to rehabilitation. Water provides buoyancy to maintain the body weight, and allows increased mobility and a sense of freedom for many children.

Numerous opportunities exist for disabled children to participate in sporting and recreational events. With adaptations for individual needs, children can participate in activities including basketball, baseball, tennis, archery, skiing, fishing, and swimming, as well as others. The Special Olympics offers some children the opportunity to compete and improve their overall fitness level. Summer camps are available for children with similar disabilities and provide important opportunities for friendship, peer interaction, independence, and play, as well as family respite.

GENERAL WELL-CHILD CARE

Children with disabilities continue to require general pediatric care. In children with pulmonary compromise due to neuromuscular disease or high-level tetraplegia, respiratory care is even more significant. Vaccinations against influenza after age 6 months and *Haemophilus influenzae* and pneumococcus after age 2 are recommended (41). General immunizations following the regular pediatric schedule are also necessary. Visual and hearing deficits occur with greater frequency in disabled children and should be evaluated for early in life and reassessed periodically as they develop. Following nutritional status and weight is crucial during rehabilitation. Because of the initial period of catabolism following an injury, obtaining adequate nutrition may be an immediate problem, whereas once children are stabilized, eating patterns must be balanced to avoid obesity, particularly in children whose main mobility is the wheelchair. Conversely, children with severe swallowing difficulties, as well as children with significant spasticity, who have excess caloric expenditure due to this chronic muscular activity, may have problems maintaining sufficient weight.

The American Academy of Pediatrics recommends that all pediatricians ensure that every disabled child in their practice has access to the following: 1) conventional health care, 2) screening and surveillance for risk of a disabling condition or developmental delay, 3) participation in multidisciplinary assessment, 4) counsel and advice during the assessment process, 5) consultation during creation of an individualized education plan or individualized family service plan, 6) coordination of medical services, and 7) advocacy for improved community services for disabled children (42). Physiatrists assist pediatricians with these duties when involved in the care of disabled children, especially early on in their diagnosis.

APPROACH TO ELECTRODIAGNOSTICS IN CHILDREN

The pediatric electrodiagnostic examination can be challenging, but the efficiency of the study can be facilitated by careful planning based on findings from the history and physical examination. Electrodiagnostic results obtained during the course of the study should be used to modify the planned evaluation. The results of the history, physical examination, and electrodiagnostic evaluation should be interpreted as a whole, with regard for internal consistency and agreement.

Performing the pediatric electrodiagnostic evaluation is typically a skill with which the general physiatrist has had limited experience. Most practitioners who routinely perform pediatric electrodiagnostic examinations have gained their expertise through experience.

The study first should be carefully described to the parents, using nonthreatening terms to minimize the negative emotional impact. Parents can be given the choice of whether to be present for the evaluation; they can often be helpful in distracting and calming their child if they are present and can anticipate the progression of events. Parental anxiety can be somewhat allayed if parents first experience what their child will experience, a low-intensity nerve stimulus delivered to the wrist. Children should also have the procedure explained in nonthreatening terms that they can understand, such as using the terms *wire electrode* or *pin* rather than *needle*. Children can also be directed to "watch their muscle on the screen" as a distraction. Teenagers should be asked if they wish their parents to be present for the study, and should be directly given information regarding the procedure prior to its undertaking.

The physical examination should assess motor skills, through the use of play in children. The use of reflexes to accomplish active movement is helpful in infants, both during the physical examination and during needle electromyography (EMG) in the assessment of recruitment. Sedation is generally not needed for children; however, there are strong advocates for and against the use of sedation, analgesia, and general anesthesia in the pediatric population during the electrodiagnostic examination. These pharmacologic interventions have inherent risks and require appropriate support services for administration and monitoring, as well as equipment. Sedation interferes with assessing motor unit potential recruitment, though is occasionally used for repetitive nerve stimulation studies or other special circumstances (43). With proper planning, EMLA cream (lidocaine 2.5% and prilocaine 2.5%) can be used for local anesthesia of the skin in older infants or in children. Needle examination of a resting muscle can usually be performed accurately using distraction or muscle antagonist activity. Nerve conduction studies are typically well tolerated and should be performed first, with a subsequent selective needle evaluation.

Nerve conduction velocities in term infants are approximately one-half of normal adult values (44–46) and amplitudes are also smaller. Premature infants have nerve conduction velocities less than 20 m/sec, with the velocity matching their degree of maturation and myelination, which provides another method of evaluating gestational age (47). Median values for conduction velocities in children and adults equalize by age 5 years (48). Nerve conduction velocity is determined by a number of factors including axonal diameter and degree of myelination. Myelination occurs from 20 weeks' gestation, doubling from birth to the age of 1 year (49). Axonal diameter also continues to increase during the postnatal period up until the age of 1 year. In infants under age 1, upper- and lower-extremity conduction velocities are similar, whereas after age 1, conduction velocity increases relatively more quickly in the upper extremities than in the lower extremities, creating a gap in lower- versus upper-extremity velocities compared with adult values (43). Increases in nerve conduction velocity secondary to maturation are comparable with regard to rates in sensory and motor fibers. In addition to conduction velocity changes, by age 1, compound muscle action potentials (CMAPs) triple in size by both peripheral nerve and muscle maturation (50).

Temperature control is challenging and vital in evaluating an infant. Use of an incubator or warmer is sometimes helpful. Distance measurement error is a critical factor in nerve conduction studies in infants, as their arms and legs are short and the measurement error for a 1-cm difference is a 15% error in conduction velocity. Bony landmarks can also be difficult to determine, owing to baby fat (43). Shock artifact can be a potential problem due to short distances, which can be minimized by keeping the skin dry, thereby decreasing the skin impedance. Commercially available self-sticking electrodes also help minimize this problem because less electrode gel and tape are needed. In addition, adhesive self-sticking ring electrodes provide for a much better fit in comparison to standard ring electrodes. Either a standard or a small stimulator may be used.

During the study it may be wise to cup the needle electrode in one's hand so as not to allow the parents or child to see it, as it may appear more ominous than it is. A small concentric needle with less electrical noise may be used. Sensory nerve conduction studies are frequently described in the pediatric literature as being performed via an orthodromic technique assessing the median nerve (43,44,51). This can be performed using a ring electrode to stimulate from the second or third digit, with the recording electrode over the median nerve at the wrist. This study is preferred over the usual antidromic manner in infants, as the grasp reflex may cause movement artifact and obliterate the results. Motor nerve conduction studies in the infant and child are performed in a similar manner to that in the adult. Traditional distances for measurement cannot be used owing to the child's small size, so distances must always be documented. For both sensory and motor studies the reference electrode is typically placed on a separate digit to maintain appropriate interelectrode distance (44). F-waves may be evaluated with supramaximal stimulation, and H-reflexes with submaximal stimulation. The H-reflex can be obtained from any muscle during the first year of life (47).

EMG must be carefully planned and efficiently performed in children. EMG should include proximal and distal musculature in the upper and lower extremities. Frequently in an infant and young child, the discomfort of needle insertion will allow immediate evaluation of recruitment. If not, positive (reaching for a toy or candy) or negative (sharp) stimuli, as well as primitive reflexes, can be used to recruit motor units. Positioning the muscle is also helpful for evaluating both recruitment and spontaneous muscle activity. Due to the natural flexed positioning of infants, the biceps, iliopsoas, flexor digitorum superficialis, and anterior tibialis are frequently active and may be helpful in evaluating muscle recruitment. Conversely, extensor muscles may be good choices for evaluating insertional and spontaneous activity. These muscles include the vastus lateralis, gastrocnemius, first dorsal interosseus, and triceps (44).

Repetitive nerve stimulation results differ in infants than adults. At less than 5-Hz stimulation, the CMAP is stable in infants. At 5 to 10 Hz some normal infants show 10% or greater facilitation of CMAP. At 20 Hz most infants show a decrement of approximately 24%, with the decrement greatest in 34- to 36-week premature infants. After 50-Hz stimulation, virtually all infants show a decrement. It is believed that this demonstrates that infants have less normal neuromuscular junction reserve than do older individuals (51).

Muscle biopsies are often used as diagnostic tools in infants and children with neuromuscular diseases. As such, it is important that the electrodiagnostician identify the need for a potential biopsy site, and leave that site untouched during EMG procedures.

The electrodiagnostic examination is frequently requested for the evaluation of hypotonic infants, the most common etiology being a central nervous system disorder as a result of hypoxia, ischemia, or hemorrhage. Spinal cord damage by trauma, vascular compromise, or congenital anomaly may also present as hypotonia, extreme weakness, or absence of active movement below the level of the lesion or anomaly. Only 10% to 20% of hypotonic infants have a peripheral neuromuscular etiology (52,53). Spinal muscular atrophy is the most common peripheral neuromuscular etiology of a floppy baby (43,44,54,55). Congenital or acquired peripheral neuropathy may result in generalized hypotonia. Guillain-Barré syndrome has been observed as early as the first few months of life. Congenital peripheral neuropathies in infants include hereditary motor sensory neuropathies and more recently described congenital hypomyelination abnormalities (52). Neuromuscular junction abnormalities leading to floppy baby can arise from botulism or from a form of myasthenia gravis. Myopathies are the second most common peripheral neuromuscular cause of infantile hypotonia (44,45). These include congenital myotonic dystrophy, congenital muscular dystrophy, the many congenital myopathies, polymyositis, and abnormalities of mitochondrial function and of enzymes. A variety of systemic abnormalities may present as infantile hypotonia including Prader-Willi syndrome, Down syndrome, metachromatic leukodystrophy, Krabbe leukodystrophy, and Refsum disease. Lastly, benign congenital hypotonia presents as generalized infantile hypotonia.

Electrodiagnostic evaluations during childhood are most commonly conducted for symptoms of progressive weakness or for evaluation of gait dysfunction. Spinal muscular atrophy types II and III can present in this age group and the functional deficits associated with hereditary polyneuropathies can become evident as well. Myopathies such as Duchenne muscular dystrophy must be included in the differential diagnosis of weakness in boys ages 3 to 5 years, and other etiologies of weakness such as Guillain-Barré syndrome, dermatomyositis/polymyositis, and myasthenia gravis must be considered in the child or teenager. Peripheral neuropathies may be focal, such as those following trauma or compression, or more systemic, as seen in Lyme disease, juvenile-onset diabetes mellitus, and renal disease, and may be found in children and adolescents.

CONCLUSIONS

The goal of rehabilitation of the pediatric patient is to attain the maximal functional ability possible at each developmental stage. Adaptive equipment may be used to aid in this. The entire rehabilitation team works in conjunction with the individual and family in striving toward this goal. They work toward gaining maximal independence, while minimizing any secondary complications that may interfere. In dealing with pediatric patients, the same principles apply for working with adults with disability, with the added focus of physical, cognitive, and social development. The infant, child, or teen is growing physically, cognitively, and emotionally, and the team must consider this with each step of rehabilitation. The child is also developing socially and sexually, and the impact of a disability on social and sexual development and function must be acknowledged and addressed. Educational goals must continue to be addressed, along with recreation, as school and play are the work of children. Parents and siblings should be included and considered in all aspects of rehabilitation of a child. Electrodiagnostic examinations can provide useful diagnostic and prognostic information in the pediatric population when they are performed and interpreted by an experienced and skilled pediatric electromyographer.

REFERENCES

1. Levine M, Kleibhan L. Communication between physician and physical and occupational therapists: a neurodevelopmentally based prescription. *Pediatrics* 1991;68:208–214.
2. Molnar G. Intervention for physically handicapped children. In: Lewis M, Taft L, eds. *Developmental disabilities, theory, assessment and intervention.* New York: SP Medical and Scientific Books, 1982:149–174.
3. Palmer F, Shapiro B, Wachtel R, et al. The effects of physical therapy on cerebral palsy: a controlled trial in infants with spastic diplegia. *N Engl J Med* 1988;318:803–808.
4. Shonkoff JP, Hauser-Cram P. Early intervention for disabled infants and their families: a quantitative analysis. *Pediatrics* 1987;80:650–658.
5. Simeonsson RJ, Cooper DH, Scheiner AP. A review and analysis of the effectiveness of early intervention programs. *Pediatrics* 1982;69:635–641.
6. Tirosh E, Rabino S. Physiotherapy for children with cerebral palsy: evidence for its efficacy. *Am J Dis Child* 1989;143:552–555.
7. Challenor Y. Limb deficiencies in children. In: Molnar G, ed. *Pediatric rehabilitation.* 2nd ed. Baltimore: Williams & Wilkins, 1985:338–360.
8. Molnar G. A developmental perspective for the rehabilitation of children with physical disability. *Pediatr Ann* 1988;17:766–776.
9. Sorbye R. Myoelectric controlled hand prosthesis in children. *Int J Rehabil Res* 1977;1:15–25.
10. Butler C, Okamoto G, McKay T. Motorized wheelchair driving by disabled children. *Arch Phys Med Rehabil* 1984;65:95–97.
11. Butler C. Effects of power-based mobility on self-initiated behaviors of very young children with locomotor disability. *Dev Med Child Neurol* 1986;28:325–332.
12. Mulderij KJ. Peer relations and friendships in physically disabled children. *Child Care Health Dev* 1997;23:379–389.
13. Cogher L, Savage E, Smith MF, eds. *Cerebral palsy, the child and young person.* London: Chapman and Hall Medical, 1992.
14. Dewis M. Spinal cord injured adolescents and young adults: the meaning of body changes. *J Adv Nurs* 1989;14:389–396.
15. Cole S, Cole T. Sexuality, disability, and reproductive issues through the lifespan. *Sex Disabil* 1993;11:189–205.
16. Evans J, Conine T. Sexual habilitation of youngsters with chronic illness or disabling conditions. *J Allied Health* 1985;14:79–87.
17. Ziff S. The sexual concerns of the adolescent woman with cerebral palsy. *Issues Health Care Women* 1981;3:55–63.
18. Robinault IP. *Sex, society, and the disabled: a developmental inquiry into roles, reactions, and responsibilities.* New York: Harper & Row, 1978.
19. Nelson M. Sexuality in childhood disability. *Phys Med Rehabil State Art Rev* 1995;9:451–462.
20. Goldberg R. Toward an understanding of the rehabilitation of the disabled adolescent. *Rehabil Literature* 1981;42:66–74.
21. Greydanus D, Demarest D, Sears J. Sexuality of the chronically ill adolescent. *Med Aspects Hum Sexuality* 1985;19:36–52.
22. Cromer B, Enrile B, McCoy K, et al. Knowledge, attitudes, and behavior related to sexuality in adolescents with chronic disability. *Dev Med Child Neurol* 1990;32:602–610.
23. Kokkonen J, Saukkonen A, Timonen E, et al. Social outcome of handicapped children as adults. *Dev Med Child Neurol* 1991;33:1095–1100.

24. Rousso H. Daughters with disabilities: defective women or minority women? In: Fine M, Asch A, eds. *Women with disabilities: essays in psychology, culture, and politics.* Philadelphia: Temple University Press, 1988:139–171.

25. Rousso H. Affirming adolescent women's sexuality. *West J Med* 1991;154:629–630.

26. Blum R, Resnick M, Nelson R. Family and peer issues among adolescents with spina bifida and cerebral palsy. *Pediatrics* 1991;88:280–285.

27. Shaul S, Bogle J, Hale-Harbaugh J, et al. Toward intimacy: family planning and sexuality concerns of physically disabled women. In: Venables K, ed. *Task force on concerns of physically disabled women*, 2nd ed. New York: Human Sciences Press, 1978:34–57.

28. Winch R, Bengston L, McLaughlin J, et al. Neonatal status of infants born to women with cerebral palsy. *Dev Med Child Neurol* 1989;31(suppl):S37–S38.

29. Rousso H. Special considerations in counseling clients with cerebral palsy. *Sex Disabil* 1993;11:99–108.

30. Kreutner AL. Sexuality, fertility, and the problems of menstruation in mentally retarded adolescents. *Pediatr Clin North Am* 1981;28:475–480.

31. Thornton CE. Sex education for disabled children and adolescents. In: Bullard DG, Knight SE, eds. *Sexuality and physical disability: personal perspectives.* St. Louis: CV Mosby, 1991.

32. Hall D, Johnson S, Middleton J. Rehabilitation of head injured children. *Arch Dis Child* 1990;65:553–556.

33. Wolraich M. Communication between physicians and parents of handicapped children. *Except Child* 1982;48:316–327.

34. Klein S, Schliefer MJ, eds. *It isn't fair: siblings with disabilities.* Westport, CT: Bergin & Garvey, 1993.

35. Varni J, Rubenfield L, Talbot D, et al. Determinants of self-esteem in children with congenital/acquired limb deficiencies. *J Dev Behav Pediatr* 1989;10:13–16.

36. Easton J. Psychosocial issues. In: Molnar G, ed. *Pediatric rehabilitation.* 2nd ed. Baltimore: Williams & Wilkins, 1992:119–142.

37. Battle C. Disruptions in the socialization of a young severely handicapped child. *Rehabil Literature* 1974;35:130.

38. Furgang N, Yerxa E. Expectations of teachers for handicapped and normal first grade students. *Am J Occup Ther* 1979;33:697.

39. Mordock J. The separation individuation process and developmental disabilities. *Except Child* 1979;40:120–184.

40. Wasserman G, Allen R, Solomon C. At risk toddlers and their mothers: the special case of physical handicap. *Child Dev* 1985;56:73–83.

41. Eng G, Binder H. Rehabilitation of infants and children with neuromuscular disorders. *Pediatr Ann* 1988;17:745–755.

42. American Academy of Pediatrics. Pediatrician's role in the development and implementation of an individual education plan and/or an individual family service plan. *Pediatrics* 1992;89:340–342.

43. Turk M. Pediatric electrodiagnostic medicine. In: Dimitru D, ed. *Electrodiagnostic medicine.* Philadelphia: Hanley & Belfus, 1995;21:1133–1145.

44. Jones H. EMG evaluation of the floppy infant: differential diagnosis and technical aspects. *Muscle Nerve* 1990;13:338–347.

45. Miller RG, Kuntz NL. Nerve conduction studies in infants and children. *J Child Neurol* 1086;1:19–26.

46. Thomas JE, Lambert EH. Ulnar nerve conduction velocity and H-reflex in infants and children. *J Appl Physiol* 1960;51:1–9.

47. Miller G, Heckmatt JZ, Dubowitz LMS, Dubowitz V. Use of nerve conduction velocity to determine gestational age in infants at risk in very-low-weight infants. *J Pediatr* 1983;103:109–112.

48. Baer R, Johnson E. Motor nerve conduction velocities in normal children. *Arch Phys Med Rehabil* 1965;46:698–704.

49. Teixeira F, Aranda F, Becker L. Postnatal maturation of phrenic nerve in children. *Pediatr Neurol* 1992;8:450–454.

50. Thomas J, Lambert E. Ulnar nerve conduction velocity and H-reflex in infants and children. *J Appl Physiol* 1960;15:1–9.

51. Jablecki CK. Pediatric electrodiagnosis. *Phys Med Rehabil Clin N Am* 1991;2:917–929.

52. Kennedy WR, Sung JH, Berry JF. A case of hypomyelination neuropathy: clinical, morphological, and chemical studies. *Arch Neurol* 1977;34:337–345.

53. Pain R. The future of the "floppy infant": a followup study of 133 patients. *Dev Med Child Neurol* 1963;5:115–124.

54. David WS, Jones HR. Electromyography and biopsy correlation with suggested protocol for evaluation of the floppy infant. *Muscle Nerve* 1994;17:424–430.

55. Turk MA. Pediatric electrodiagnosis. *Phys Med Rehabil* 1989;3:791–808.

Chapter 96

Geriatric Rehabilitation: Caring for the Aged

Susan J. Garrison

All of us normally expect to live long lives, enjoying our health, our families, and daily activities. In spite of today's emphasis on retaining a youthful appearance, the wisdom that one acquires from simply experiencing life is in itself a reason for enjoying advancing years. However, one progresses in age on two different tracks, that is, both chronologically and physiologically. This fact makes geriatric care unique in comparison to the care of other age groups, particularly pediatrics, where specific developmental milestones are linked to certain time frames. The comparison is more appropriate for the period of puberty, which also has a time frame but with markedly individual differences. Therefore, one elderly adult may look, act, and feel years younger than another of the same age. When the consequences of various pathologic processes, such as diabetes, vascular insufficiencies, and degenerative joint disease, are added to the picture, even more differences begin to emerge. In addition, from a psychological standpoint, people tend to express exaggerations of their normal adult personalities as they age. Appropriate as well as less adaptive personality traits become more pronounced. Sheehy (1), writing about choosing how to age, stated that the effect of genes on health status and longevity is more pronounced prior to the age of 65 years. If we have not experienced catastrophic illnesses during the 20-year period from 45 to 65 years, the quality and length of the remainder of our lives are more determined by psychological attitude and behavior than genetics. It is easy to recognize how unique each geriatric patient's needs can be when all of the above-mentioned factors are considered. However, in order to do so, certain broad generalities can be identified and then addressed in caring for the aged patient.

GENERAL PERSPECTIVE

This chapter reflects my personal experiences acquired over 15 years of providing daily rehabilitative attending care to a variety of geriatric patients at a large, world-renowned, teaching medical-surgical hospital. The setting includes an acute inpatient rehabilitation center, a large physical medicine and rehabilitation inpatient consult service, a hospital-based skilled nursing facility (SNF), and an outpatient office for general physical medicine and rehabilitation as well as amputee clinics. In each of these areas, physical medicine and rehabilitation residents are taught rehabilitative patient management. There is a large geriatric population of independent community dwellers within 1 mile of the medical center, affording the medical community the opportunity to follow the well elderly in addition to the chronically and acutely ill.

The references for this chapter were chosen because they are specific, complete reviews, or are simply excellent in the manner in which they address the topic. The majority of the studies were conducted in the United States. Cultural influences regarding the provision of health care for the elderly can make studies from other nations difficult to appropriately utilize for these purposes.

Not surprisingly, the typical problems that lend themselves to rehabilitative efforts in the elderly are related to disuse, as well as a result of the cumulative effects of comorbidities over time. Typical examples are problems related to the cardiovascular system that may result in stroke or dysvascular amputation. Utilizing this general concept, this chapter explores geriatric rehabilitation in the main areas of disuse syndrome, osteoarthritis (OA), osteoporosis, hip fracture, amputation, and stroke. Other issues include falls, cognitive ability, motivation, and settings for rehabilitation. Specific adaptive devices, clothing, and equipment needs are addressed, as well as living situations. In each area, the reader is encouraged to refer to other chapters in this textbook for further information on these topics.

REHABILITATIVE CARE SETTINGS

Often the term *rehabilitation* is used by patients and health care providers to refer to "therapy." This may be confusing when the patient does not meet the criteria for the services of an acute, inpatient diagnostic-related group (DRG)–exempt rehabilitation unit. Geriatric patients who lack independence because of loss of functional abilities with respect to activities of daily living (ADLs), mobility, or communication may benefit from targeted therapies in a variety of settings. If a patient does not have the ability to learn, family or caregiver training may be more appropriate. Therapies may be prescribed in a variety of locations, depending on the patient's diagnosis, medical and surgical stability, endurance, service area, financial resources, available transportation, and personal preferences (Table 96-1).

Regardless of the setting, the exercise area for geriatric patients should be well lit, have a comfortable ambient air temperature, and include areas for privacy. The environment should be quiet enough for hearing-impaired patients to function. All equipment should be safe for use by those who may have decreased vision, hearing, or balance.

CANDIDATES FOR GERIATRIC REHABILITATION

Medical rehabilitation in the broadest sense involves learning to use new skills to compensate for abilities lost through the effects of disease or injury. Examples of this include learning to use a walker, incorporating a different way of getting into a bathtub, or utilizing special utensils for eating. Obviously, the patient must be mentally capable of learning the activity, as well as willing to do so. In this chapter, the term *rehabilitation* will be used to represent the use of therapies such as physical, occupational, and speech therapy to assist the patient in regaining abilities lost through disease or injury.

Discussing Care Options

During medical visits, the elderly individual may be accompanied by the spouse, an adult child, another family member, or someone else, perhaps even a friend who provides transportation. Greene et al (2) studied the effects of the presence of this third person in the initial medical interview in a primary care group practice. All interviews were recorded on audiotape. In the sample of 96 initial visits, 15 involved three people, rather than the customary two. These were then compared to 15 matched control visits that involved only two people. The investigators found that the presence of a third person in an interview changed the behaviors of the patients, but not that of the physicians. The patients asked fewer questions; were less responsive, assertive, and expressive; and participated less in joint decision making. Patients were frequently excluded from the conversation.

Therefore, the physician should talk directly to the individual being treated. Questions about proposed treatment plans should be encouraged and the patient asked to repeat what has been discussed, to ascertain any misconceptions. The bond that is established is important for current and future decision making about medical rehabilitation issues.

When caring for the elderly, it is important to keep the patient's goals as the focus. Banja and Bilsky (3) reviewed the complex topic of discussing cardiopulmonary resuscitation (CPR) with elderly rehabilitation patients. They reviewed outcome studies of patients who underwent CPR. These studies showed that among patients 70 years and older, the probability of survival to discharge was less than 1 in 10 following CPR. Considering this information, the authors (3) asserted that giving elderly patients information about CPR is necessary in order to assist them in making decisions about quality of life. They concluded that it is appropriate to rehabilitate individuals who have do-not-resuscitate (DNR) orders.

Motivation

Motivation to participate in rehabilitation plays a big role in the person's progress, often more so in the eyes of the rehabilitation team members than the individual. Lack of motivation is frequently cited by teams as a reason for "failure to progress" in a structured rehabilitation program. However, the patient may be motivated to stay in bed rather than leave the room. Labeling a patient as "not motivated" allows the team to give up and blame the lack of rehabilitative progress on the patient. Hesse and Campion (4) described multiple reasons why a geriatric patient may lack eagerness and enthusiasm to participate. Elderly individuals perform less well in the following three general types of tasks: those that appear less meaningful to them, those that are required to be performed rapidly, and those that involve risk taking and possible errors of omission. Specific reasons why the elderly may appear to be poorly motivated include decreased capacity, decreased

Table 96-1: Settings for Rehabilitative Therapies		
Location	**Advantages**	**Disadvantages**
Acute care hospital	All patients eligible for therapies Therapy can be bedside or in department	Not a comprehensive rehabilitation team approach Lacks rehabilitation milieu No peer group Uses acute Medicare days
DRG-exempt inpatient rehabilitation, hospital based or freestanding	Comprehensive team approach Therapeutic milieu Experienced nursing follow-through with activities Therapy can be bedside or in department	Not all patients are eligible for admission (must be able to participate in 3 hr of at least two different therapies daily) Uses acute Medicare days Most expensive per day
Skilled nursing facility, hospital or nursing home based	Serves patients with medical/surgical and/or PT, OT, or speech problems No requirement for 3 hr of therapy per day Does not use acute Medicare hospital days Length of stay typically longer than acute rehabilitation stay Therapy can be bedside or in department	Sometimes less goal oriented than acute rehabilitation Required by law to provide wheelchairs for use in the facility; patients cannot obtain their own until discharge Patients perceive a nursing home–like setting Nursing more likely to reinforce dependent patient behaviors Usual length of stay is 2–8 wk
Subacute care facility, hospital based or freestanding	Serves patients with medical/surgical and/or PT, OT, or speech problems No requirement for 3 hr of therapy per day Length of stay longer than SNF Therapy can be bedside or in department	Uses acute Medicare hospital days Usual length of stay is longer than SNF
Nursing home	Provides around-the-clock care Therapy available, but not required Therapy can be bedside or in department	Dependent role reinforced Patients become institutionalized Private pay or Medicaid
Home health care	Convenient Medicare and insurance allow Therapists can evaluate home setting for safety and support Eliminates transportation problems	Lacks equipment available in gym Only a certain number of visits allowed No peer group Family may interfere
Outpatient	Access to equipment and devices Covered by Medicare and most insurance Peer group More choices in locations, various therapists, and hours	Requires transportation

DRG = diagnostic-related group; PT = physical therapy; OT = occupational therapy; SNF = skilled nursing facility.

intensity, reset drive reduction, and age-specific changes. Decreased capacity may be secondary to cognitive dysfunction, communication disorders, or emotional states. Decreased intensity may occur as a result of a possible outcome of a compromised level of function despite rehabilitation efforts, in addition to the person's inability to envision achievement of the rehabilitation goals. Reset drive reduction, typified by the passive patient role during acute illness, involves acceptance of increasing levels of dependency, rather than independence. Finally, age-specific changes are related to cognition, stress, and avoidance of making errors (4).

With these factors in mind, one should search out reasons to explain why the geriatric patient appears to be unmotivated. Refuse to accept the label "not motivated" as an excuse. Make certain that the patient is not medically or psychiatrically ill. Anemia, electrolyte imbalances, medication effects, acute and chronic infections, pain, lack of sleep, and poor nutritional status may result in an apparent lack of motivation. Such problems should be actively pursued and corrected, if possible. Make certain that the patient understands the rehabilitative goals and believes that these goals are attainable. Involve the staff and family members in individualizing the program so that success is possible. Give appropriate positive feedback to promote active rather than passive behaviors. Simultaneously, recognize that several days to weeks of intensive contact with a patient will not significantly alter behaviors that have developed over a lifetime. Keep the focus on specific, directed behavioral goals related to the current deficits in ADLs, mobility, and communication. Place the patient in the most appropriate rehabilitative setting according to his or her abilities and endurance level so that the patient has an opportunity to progress at his or her own pace. Often acute inpatient rehabilitation programs are simply too fast-paced for these patients; their needs could be addressed more appropriately in another setting such as an SNF or subacute care facility.

Elderly patients may be subject to their own ageism. Their personal beliefs about aging may cause them to reject the need to be more independent. In a predominately agricultural society, hard physical labor was part of the normal day's activities. There was no need for physical exercise separate from work, other than as play. Those who did not enjoy physical sports at a younger age and throughout their lives are unlikely to change as they grow older. Unfortunately, they often do not recognize the need for continued physical activity to maintain good health. Generations differ, and as the so-called baby-boomers turn 50 years old in record numbers, there will be a continued emphasis on youth and fitness. Hopefully, this trend will positively influence their behaviors as future geriatric patients, as well as the generations who treat them.

COMMON ISSUES

Functional Decline

The current system of Medicare-financed geriatric care focuses on acute illness; there is little to no role for maintenance care, and it is difficult to treat functional decline unless it is related to an acute medical illness. It is well documented that Medicare expenditures increase at the time near death. In 1994, the 6.4% of Medicare enrollees who died used 20.6% of the total payments, costing $15,761 per person, compared to the survivors, who cost $4,131 each (5).

Even the elderly who are free from illness may be dependent in ADLs. Fried and Guralnik (6) discussed evidence about the significance, etiology, and risk of disability in older adults. They found that the predominant causes of physical disability are chronic diseases, including arthritis and cardiovascular diseases. They observed that certain combinations of conditions are risk factors for disability (Table 96-2). Obviously, an acute event, such as hip fracture or stroke, can be a factor.

Table 96-2: Chronic Diseases[a] Most Frequently Associated with Self-reported Moderate to Severe Disability[b] in Women 65 Years and Older
Visual impairment
Arthritis
Hypertension
Diabetes
Myocardial infarction
Angina
Lung disease
Cancer

[a] Self-report of physician diagnosis.
[b] Difficulty in at least one of the following areas: mobility, upper-limb function, basic activities of daily living, or household management tasks.
Source: Adapted from Fried LP, Furalnik JM. Disability in older adults: evidence regarding significance, etiology, and risk. *J Am Geriatr Soc* 1997;45:94.

Kiely et al (7) evaluated the differences in functional status over time between individuals with and those without specific medical conditions. This study involved a baseline assessment and two annual follow-up examinations of 1060 community dwellers, 65 years and older. All of them were totally functionally independent at baseline. Five medical conditions—heart problems, arthritis, diabetes, cancer, and stroke—were assessed. The investigators found that functional abilities declined over time, and that individuals with the listed conditions were initially more impaired than those without. Not surprisingly, additional medical conditions resulted in additional impairment. However, the rate of functional decline was not affected by the number of medical conditions present, and interestingly, did not significantly differ from that in individuals without any conditions. Stroke was found to be the most impairing condition. The authors suggested that efforts to prevent and treat these medical conditions will assist in maintaining functional independence in the elderly (7).

Hughes et al (8) performed a longitudinal study to ascertain factors predictive of decline in manual performance in 485 persons 60 years and older, including those in a continuing care retirement community, chronically home-bound adults, and ambulatory older adults. At baseline, the mean age was 78 years. The subjects performed a timed manual performance test. The authors found that for all age groups, the time increased slowly from baseline through the fourth year, but increased rapidly from the fourth to sixth years for the oldest group, consisting of individuals who were older than 85 years at baseline. The authors found that older age, less education, diminished grip strength, and psychological status with respect to anxiety and depression were predictors of decline over a 2-year period. They concluded that an important risk factor for the development of functional limitation is joint impairment (8).

Forrest et al (9) evaluated the impact of medical conditions and comorbidity on the self-reported driving patterns of 1768 women 71 years and older living in Pennsylvania. They found that 62.3% were driving, 19.1% had stopped, and 18.6% had never driven. Older women in the study drove less overall and proportionately stopped driving. Fractures, heart disease, diabetes, and poor vision or hearing, as well as comorbidity, were independently associated with decreased driving (9).

Self-report is the method typically utilized by health care professionals to evaluate ADLs in the aged population. However, reports and performance may differ. Sinoff and Ore (10) compared the Barthel activities of daily living index by self-report with observation of actual ADL performance scores in 126 patients 75 years and older in Haifa, Israel. They found that there were limitations in the use of the Barthel index in self-report form in the very old, those 85 years and older. They therefore suggested that this age group should be assessed by performance-based measures, or a different self-report test that is more reliable (10).

Functional Presentation of Disease

The aged patient may not respond to the onset of acute illness in the typical way that is represented in conventional medical models. Besdine (11) observed that a previously independent older adult who becomes acutely ill may quickly become dependent in areas of mobility, cognition, continence, or nutrition without development of the typical expected signs and symptoms. He termed these "functional presentations of disease" (Table 96-3). An unexplained decline in abilities should be noted and a medical explanation sought. Once a diagnosis has been established and appropriate treatment has begun, the patient's functional problem may resolve. As previously discussed, a patient who appears to be poorly motivated may simply be acutely ill.

Table 96-3: Besdine's Functional Presentations of Disease
Stopping eating or drinking
Falling
Urinary incontinence
Dizziness
Acute confusion
New onset or worsening of dementia
Weight loss
Failure to thrive

Source: Adapted from Besdine RW. The educational utility of comprehensive functional assessment in the elderly. *J Am Geriatr Soc* 1983;31:651–656.

Cognitive Performance

The ability to learn, and then incorporate and use the learned experiences is crucial to the rehabilitation effort. Issues and concerns about the population of the very old, those over 85 years old, continue to be of interest because this is the fastest-growing group of the population (12). Tombaugh and McIntyre (13) performed a comprehensive review of the literature over a 26-year period on use of the Mini-Mental State Examination (MMSE), which was originally designed to differentiate organic from functional hospitalized psychiatric patients. They found that scores were affected by age, education, and cultural issues, but not gender; and although the MMSE is sensitive for moderate to severe cognitive deficits, it is not helpful in identifying mild language deficits (13).

Sommers (14) reviewed the literature on aging and speech perception. He concluded that tests should be designed to assess both the sensory and cognitive abilities necessary for processing spoken language. There has been ongoing debate about the role of hearing loss with respect to cognitive deficits. Uhlmann et al (15) studied the relationship of hearing impairment to cognitive dysfunction in older adults. Communication is more difficult if the patient is unaware that he or she is not receiving necessary auditory information.

Perls et al (16) analyzed longitudinal data about the prevalence of cognitive disability from a sample of older nursing home residents (n = 1951) and a sample of older community dwellers (n = 2947) in three age groups of men and women (65–79, 80–89, and 90–99 years). They found that among elderly men, decreased cognitive performance is significantly associated with mortality. The population of men 90 to 99 years old had higher cognitive scores than did younger men or women of the same age. They concluded that there is less cognitive disability among very old men than has previously been assumed (16).

Schuman et al (17) studied patients over the age of 65 years with and without intellectual dysfunction who were referred to long-term care facilities. They found that standard rehabilitation techniques do not benefit patients with severe mental impairment, and concluded that severely demented patients should not be treated using traditional rehabilitation programs, but through the use of other treatment approaches specifically designed to meet their different needs.

Rentz (18) postulated that procedural memory is the element required for the older adult to benefit from rehabilitation. Procedural memory involves perceptual-motor learning as well as retaining skills and operations, whereas declarative memory, which is language dependent, involves recalling facts and specific episodes. This difference in memory types may account for the results of the study by Goldstein et al (19) of functional outcomes of cognitively impaired hip fracture patients who underwent traditional rehabilitation. The cognitively impaired and intact patients had similar overall motor improvements and functional gains, as measured by Functional Independence Measure (FIM) (19).

The effect of medications on cognition must be considered. Salzman et al (20) reviewed cognitive improvement in 13 elderly nursing home residents following discontinuation of chronic benzodiazepine therapy, compared to 12 control subjects in the same setting. Each patient who discontinued the drug showed improvement in all six memory tests utilized. Additionally, neither group showed changes in depression, anxiety, irritability, or sleep (20).

Medications

Polypharmacy is a well-recognized problem in the geriatric population. Studies showed that 30% of all medications prescribed are written for those over the age of 65 years (21). Many of these medications are for chronic diseases, so they must be taken day after day, and many of them require more than once-a-day dosing. Each forgotten dose represents an instance of noncompliance with the individual's medication regimen. The number of different drugs ingested increases the potential for drug interaction; this has been calculated to be 6% for two, 50% for five, and 100% for eight medications (22). Age-related metabolic changes are more likely in the older individual. In addition, alcohol reacts with approximately one-half of the most commonly prescribed medications, typically by increasing the desired effect of the drug (23).

Glickman et al (24) studied physicians' awareness of the costs of commonly used medications in the geriatric population and how this knowledge influenced their prescribing patterns. They surveyed 22 pharmacies for actual drug prices and then conducted in-person surveys of 132 primary care practitioners. They found that the physicians were likely to overestimate the cost of less expensive drugs and underestimate the cost of expensive drugs. Surprisingly, internists were less likely to make correct estimates than were those in other specialties. The authors concluded that physicians require more education about costs in order to prescribe more cost-effective medications (24).

Hanlon et al (25) performed a cohort study involving 167 older outpatients, each taking five or more scheduled medications, to assess the prevalence, types, and consequences of adverse drug effects (ADEs). The method utilized was self-report by interview. The information obtained was then analyzed by a research clinical pharmacist using standard texts to confirm known adverse outcomes. Thirty-five percent of the population reported ADEs involving 72 medications. Ninety-five percent of the ADEs were classified as predictable, most commonly involving medications in the cardiovascular and central nervous system classes. Gastrointestinal ADEs were also common, occurring in 30% of patients. Two-thirds of the patients with ADEs required physician management, 10% made visits to emergency rooms, and 11% were hospitalized. Unfortunately, these predictable ADEs created further health care utilization and cost, in addition to patient discomfort (25).

Stein (23) cited seven steps to writing safer prescriptions for this population (Table 96-4).

Nutritional Status

Geriatric patients must be adequately nourished and hydrated in order to participate in rehabilitative activities. Patients frequently do not drink enough liquids to maintain good hydration, and are less likely to adequately replace the increased fluids lost once they become more physically active. In a hospital or other institutional setting, access to favorite beverages may be limited. Patients initially hospitalized for acute illness may undergo prolonged periods of no intake by mouth during diagnostic evaluations, and are therefore nutritionally at risk when they begin rehabilitation. The diet ordered by the physician may differ substantially from the foods that patients typically prefer. These meals, as well as between-meal snacks, are typically served at standard times, rather than when patients may be hungry. The size of the portions is almost always a concern; patients frequently complain about being served too much to eat. A solution to this problem is to reduce the amounts of food served at mealtimes, while increasing the frequency and number of healthy snacks.

Poor dentition or improperly fitting dentures may cause individuals to avoid certain foods. Those who have been edentulous for long periods are usually able to chew food, even without dentures. Without dentures in place, gums typically change over a 3-week period; therefore, denture wearers should use them daily. Unfortunately, patients who have been ill for prolonged periods and therefore have not worn their dentures may require refitting.

The rehabilitation diagnosis, such as stroke, may indicate the potential for swallowing problems. If suspected and diagnosed, these problems can be managed through appropriate dietary modification, including the use of feeding tubes, if feeding by mouth creates a risk of aspiration. Patients who experience upper-limb problems may be unable to manipulate feeding utensils. Assistance at mealtimes can increase caloric intake when the problem is simply transporting the food from the plate to the mouth, although as in all rehabilitation efforts, individuals should be encouraged to be as independent as possible in feeding.

All of the above factors may contribute to poor nutritional intake, resulting in a less-than-optimal rehabilitative outcome. Refer to Chapters 14 and 15.

Failure to Thrive

The diagnosis "failure to thrive" has been used in various ways to describe older patients with functional decline or unexplained weight loss. Hildebrand et al (26) conducted a retrospective chart review of 132 veterans aged 65 years and older discharged from the Portland, Oregon Veterans

Table 96-4: Seven Steps to Writing Safer Medication Prescriptions for the Elderly	
Action	**Rationale**
1. Start at ½ of the lowest recommended amount and titrate up to the effect. "Start low and go slow."	The response in the elderly is at a lower dosage than that required in the younger population.
2. Use a simple dosing regimen, with the fewest medications possible; encourage lifestyle modifications rather than drugs.	Noncompliance and the incidence of adverse drug reactions decrease with fewer doses of less medications.
3. Whenever adding a new medication or changing the dosing of a current one, make certain that the instructions are well understood.	Detailed information can assist in preventing problems
4. Be aware of medication costs.	Patients are unlikely to be compliant with numerous expensive medications. They may continue to take a previously prescribed medication because "it's paid for." Note: Medicare does not pay for medications.
5. Review patient medications, including over-the-counter drugs, periodically; eliminate those not being taken, and attempt to keep the total number low. Dispose of them appropriately in your office.	This assists in preventing the possibility of drug-drug interactions, potentially reduces costs, and may prevent the accidental ingestion of medication. People are often hesitant to discard expensive medications, even when they are no longer using them. This also decreases the chances of "sharing" medications with another.
6. Create a written prescription record for the patient to keep in his or her possession.	Such a record is helpful to other physicians and pharmacists who may then review the list for possible drug problems. It is invaluable for the geriatric traveler and for emergency room visits.
7. Instruct home health nurses or aides to communicate directly with the physician about any medication problems.	The sooner a problem is recognized, the sooner action can be taken to correct the situation.

Source: Adapted from Stein BE. Avoiding drug reactions: seven steps to writing safe prescriptions. *Geriatrics* 1994;49:28–36.

Administration Medical Center over a 3-year period, in order to gain insight into the use of the term. The majority of patients, 83%, were admitted from home and 82% were dependent in at least one ADL. Over one-third of the patients were cognitively impaired. The most common diagnosis was cancer, followed by infection and dehydration. Less than half of the patients were discharged home; one-third went to nursing homes. Thirty-two percent of the study population died within 1 year following discharge from the hospital. The authors concluded that failure to thrive may be a discrete entity, much like in the pediatric population. However, there is still lack of consensus with regard to use of the term in the geriatric literature (26).

Disuse Phenomenon

Typically, adults in today's industrialized society have become more sedentary with age. It is now accepted that cardiovascular endurance and muscular strengthening exercise programs are as effective in the geriatric population as in the young. Sforzo et al (27) studied the effects of cardiac endurance and muscular strengthening in older adults, in addition to the consequences of lengthy training interruptions. They found training to be highly effective. After 10 weeks of no exercise, there were greater losses in muscular strength than in cardiovascular endurance. When the training programs were resumed, the functional benefits appeared additive. The authors concluded that older adults should be encouraged to exercise, but more importantly, to return to their fitness programs even after interruptions such as hospitalizations for acute illnesses (27).

Judge et al (28) compared the effects of resistive training of multiple lower-limb muscle groups to balance training in 110 healthy subjects over the age of 75 years. They found that resistive training increased lower-limb muscular strength, but balance training did not improve strength. Interestingly, neither type of training improved maximal gait velocity or chair rise time (28).

In a study designed to compare self-perceived and actual physical function in a population of 417 community dwellers and 200 nursing home residents aged 62 to 98 years, Cress et al (29) found significant differences in the two groups in all variables except age and gender. They concluded that self-selected gait speed is the greatest single predictor of self-perceived function. Therefore, gait speed can be easily used to clinically assess physical function (29).

Kohrt et al (30) evaluated common methods of prescribing exercise intensity in 112 healthy, sedentary, community-dwelling females 60 to 72 years old. They concluded that heart rate expressed as a percentage of maximal heart rate is an appropriate method of determining exercise intensity. The heart rate reserve method is not recommended in this age group (30). Refer to Chapter 79.

In a 5-year longitudinal study of 287 men and women, 75 years old, in Jyväsklä, Finland, Rantanen et al (31) found that strength alterations with age differed among muscle groups. They concluded that usual daily activities, such as housework and walking, may play an important role in maintaining strength in this population (31).

Falls

Falls must be included in the discussion of geriatric rehabilitative care because of the problems they represent. The patient who is a frequent faller may eventually sustain a fracture or other injury, such as a subdural hematoma, and subsequently require operative intervention, immobilization, and possible relocation to a different living situation. The elderly faller should be evaluated for a history of syncopal episodes; the possibility of diminished visual acuity; the presence of peripheral vascular disease, with resultant diminished sensation in the lower limbs; and type of footwear, as well as gait assistive devices. Kapoor (32) reviewed recent studies about syncope in older persons (Table 96-5).

In the Blue Mountains Eye Study, conducted in Sydney, Australia, Ivers et al (33) found that of 3299 individuals who answered questions about falls, 29.6% of those 65 years and older reported one fall or more in the preceding 12-month period. The authors reported independent relationships between recurrent falls and impaired visual function such as poor vision and reduced contrast sensitivity and visual field. Statistically significant variables for two or more falls included age, gender, psychotropic drug use, history of stroke, arthritis, and self-reported health status (33).

Norton et al (34) evaluated 911 individuals hospitalized in New Zealand for treatment of proximal femoral fractures. Data were obtained by a trained interviewer using a standardized questionnaire. At the time of the injury, 58% of the study population lived in private homes; 66% were 80 years or older. Women comprised 77% of the patients. Ninety-six percent of the fractures were related to a fall. Even though 85% of the falls occurred at home, only 25% of falls causing fractures were considered to be a result of environmental problems. The authors stated that few of these problems could have been altered to prevent falls. Therefore, to prevent falls, they concluded that further emphasis should be placed on balance and gait activities, rather than environmental modification (34).

Table 96-5: Major Etiologies of Syncope
Cardiac arrhythmias
Drugs
Organic cardiac diseases
Orthostatic hypotension
Situational
Cough
Defecation
Micturition
Swallow
Vasovagal

Source: Adapted from Kapoor WN. Syncope in older persons. *J Am Geriatr Soc* 1994:42:427.

To determine the incidence of and risk factors for falls within the first month after hospital discharge, Mahoney et al (35) performed a cohort study. They utilized a consecutive sample of 214 patients, 70 years and older, admitted to a community hospital for treatment of medical illness. Patients were not included in the study if they had been admitted from nursing homes, had been discharged to SNFs, or had terminal illnesses or neurologic diagnoses, or if their length of stay was less than 48 hours. The authors found that 13.6% of the patients fell during the specified period. Major risk factors at the time of discharge included decline in mobility, use of a gait assistive device, and cognitive impairment. Following discharge, self-reported confusion was found to be a risk factor. The authors concluded that patients who are functionally dependent are at high risk of falls following hospital discharge (35).

Maki (36) conducted a prospective cohort study of 75 ambulatory older adults, with a mean age of 82 years, to determine whether foot placement during gait is indicative of future falls, or whether this represents adaptation to a fear of falling. He found that decreased stride length and speed, as well as prolonged double support, may actually represent adaptations for stabilization related to a fear of falling. A wider stride, rather than serving to increase stability, appears to indicate that the individual is at risk for falls. The single best independent predictor of falling was stride-to-stride variability in speed (36).

There is no specific rehabilitation for falls. Even though individuals cannot be taught how to fall safely, they can be taught how to rise from the floor more easily. Alexander et al (37) studied the ability of older adults to rise from the floor. The subjects included young adult controls, older adult community dwellers, and elderly nursing home residents. The authors measured the time it took to rise from the floor from five initial positions—supine, on one side, prone, on all four limbs, and sitting—with and without the use of furniture support, while recording these activities on videotape. They found that the healthy older group required twice as much time to rise as did the young control group, but the group that lived in congregate housing took two to three times as long as the healthy old group. This apparently more-impaired group was best able to rise using a table for support when starting from a side-lying position. Good trunk balance appears to be a large factor in the ability to rise from the floor (37).

Home Sweet Home—or Somewhere Else?

The living situation of a geriatric patient is often in jeopardy when an acute illness, usually an exacerbation of a chronic problem, or a fall results in hospitalization. Several factors play a part in this phenomenon. Half of all women over the age of 65 years are widows (38). If she has been living alone, she may be unable to continue to do so. Even if this woman has children, they probably will not be home to care for her; in today's world, almost everyone works. The burden of elder care typically is assumed by the daughter of the patient. Ninety percent of adults who care for aging parents are women. More than one-third of these are over the age of 65 years. The typical American woman will devote more years to caring for her aging parents than she does to caring for her children (38). These duties may coincide for several years.

Typically, the patient's own home, if physically accessible and safe, is the most appropriate place to live. It is familiar and comforting for the patient to have possessions close at hand, as well as to easily locate light switches and the bathroom. However, if the patient needs physical assistance, requires 24-hour supervision for safety due to cognitive impairment, or has other special needs, alternative living arrangements must be considered. If the patient desires to remain at home, the option is expensive in-home care, which is paid for privately (Table 96-6).

Individual Choice and Values

Kane et al (39) studied issues of choice and control in 135 cognitively intact nursing home residents, three each from 45 nursing homes across the United States. They also surveyed 134 nursing home assistants, using semistructured interviews with fixed-choice and open-ended questions. The residents indicated that choice and control over issues such as times to wake up and to go to bed, food, roommates, trips out of the nursing home, use of money and the telephone, and contacting a physician are important to them. They were not satisfied with their control in these areas. While staff members viewed such areas as important for control, they did not rank them the same as the residents did, particularly in the areas of use of the telephone and personal money. The authors suggested that changes in nursing home routines, the roles of various health care practitioners, and public policies will be necessary to address these matters (39).

Chiou and Burnett (40) studied the similarity of values between young home care physical and occupational therapists and their elderly stroke clients. Twenty-eight of 29 therapist-patient pairs did not hold statistically significant views regarding the values of ADLs. Patient learning is enhanced when individual concerns and values, rather than those of the therapists, are addressed (40).

Equipment

Equipment to be used by the geriatric population should be thoughtfully prescribed to assist in restoration of function. This includes adaptive devices for mobility and ADLs. As with all equipment, safety and appropriate positioning of the device is paramount in its usage. Remember that any device, no matter how necessary, must be utilized by the patient or caregiver to be of benefit. Items that are

Table 96-6: Housing Options for the Elderly

Site	Advantages	Disadvantages	Financial Implications
House or apartment	Most independent Private Personal belongings Familiar area Pets	May not be accessible Lonely Upkeep Safety concerns	Mortgage or rent Utilities bills Paid caregivers "extra"
With relatives	Comforts of "home" Probably familiar Access to kitchen May have own room Companionship of siblings, children, or grandchildren May have supervision	Not "my" home May not be accessible Too much or too little activity Lack of privacy Implication of "burden" to family	Less expensive Paid caregivers "extra"
Personal care home	Allows some degree of independence Is a home setting Meals are prepared	Must live with strangers Must be able to take own medications Bathrooms shared	One price for room and board Medication costs not included
Assisted living	Allows some degree of independence	Must be able to ambulate to meals	Predominately private pay
Nursing home	Typically long-term placement Structured setting Therapies available	Signals inability for self-care Institutional regimen	Private pay Medicaid requires proof of indigence

uncomfortable, unsightly, or difficult to manipulate are likely to be used infrequently, if not totally abandoned.

Basic devices, though often overlooked, include glasses, hearing aids, dentures, and appropriate footwear. Unfortunately, although Medicare pays for evaluations of vision and hearing, it does not allow reimbursments for glasses or hearing aids. Similarly, certain dental work is covered, but not dentures. The same is true for footwear. Interestingly, although expensive prosthetic devices are covered, shoes, which may assist in the prevention of lower-limb amputation, are not.

Gait assistive devices include canes, crutches, and walkers. Each has its advantages and limitations for use in this population. As true for other equipment, individuals often become attached to use of a specific device, and are hesitant to change even when change is indicated from a safety standpoint. Straight canes should be used in the appropriate hand to provide stability or to unload weight on the opposite hip or knee. They should be the correct length. The cane tip should be checked routinely for signs of wear, and replaced whenever necessary. Use of a standard walker requires the ability to lift and to sequence placement of the walker during gait. Patients who are unable to do this must use wheeled walkers. Obviously, these walkers cannot be used on stairs.

Other mobility devices include wheelchairs and scooters. Wheelchairs are intended for mobility, not for years of daily sitting as is so often the case. They should be appropriately fitted for the individual with respect to seat width and depth. One size does not fit all. Scooters, now reimbursed by Medicare, should only be prescribed for those who cannot self-propel manual wheelchairs because of severe, chronic cardiopulmonary conditions that limit upper-extremity function.

Hospital beds are usually not required unless the patient is totally dependent for care. The use of overhead trapeze bars may result in debilitating shoulder muscular strain in the elderly; bed mobility without relying on the trapeze, if possible, should be taught.

Bedside commodes are more appropriate than bedpans from a rehabilitative standpoint. Bedpans, when left in place for long periods, can lead to pressure sores. Equipment such as raised toilet seats and grab bars that must be physically attached as bathroom fixtures are not reimbursable by Medicare. However, a drop-arm bedside commode, which is reimbursable, can be placed over the toilet, providing both a raised seat and arms for support. Unfortunately, neither shower chairs nor tub benches are reimbursable by Medicare.

There are numerous ADL adaptive devices such as reachers, built-up feeding utensils, swivel spoons, rocker knives, kitchen utensils, and walker baskets. Talking clocks can assist the visually impaired. Use of nightlights may help prevent falls at night. Patients should be encouraged to try these devices, but they should be prescribed in moderation; the use of too many items can be overwhelming. High-tech items, usually expensive, may be difficult to replace if lost or to repair if broken.

Other adaptive devices include telephones with larger numbers, amplified sound, and preprogrammed dialing. Use of portable phones and answering machines can eliminate the need to reach a ringing phone. Emergency response systems are helpful for those who live alone in the event that immediate assistance is required.

Clothing can be considered a type of equipment. Fortunately, a more casual appearance is acceptable today. T-shirts are easy to don and doff if an individual cannot manage buttons or zippers. Pants with elastic waists eliminate the need to manipulate zippers. Shoes can be fastened by Velcro or with elastic shoelaces.

Shoes should be the correct length and width. The toe box should be deep enough to clear the toes. The heel counter should be firm and grasp the foot so that the heel does not move like a piston during walking. Neither house slippers nor high-heeled shoes are appropriate for routine ambulation in this age group. Fortunately, athletic shoes are now worn by all ages. They are available in a variety of styles and price ranges. Again, the individual must be willing to wear them.

As current generations age, more and more technological advances will be incorporated into everyday life as a result of more people becoming computer literate. Even though these generations may be much more comfortable with using technology, they will probably be less tolerant of adaptive devices attached to the body. There will be more implantable devices, such as the current lens replacement following cataract removal. The result of the Americans with Disabilities Act (ADA) will ensure physical accessibility to public facilities such as parks, rest rooms, buildings, and transportation. The number of handicapped parking stickers issued will increase substantially as these individuals continue to be mobile. Refer to Part III, Therapeutic Interventions and Part IV, Specific Concerns for further information.

TYPICAL GERIATRIC REHABILITATIVE DIAGNOSES

Hip Fracture

A hip fracture is a life-altering event in many geriatric patients; the mortality rate in the year following hip fracture ranges from 14% to 36% (41). Twenty-five percent to 75% of those with a fracture experience prolonged functional impairment, such as the inability to walk well or dress their lower limbs. Many patients, especially those who are not bearing weight on the affected limb, are unable to return home immediately, requiring acute inpatient rehabilitation or admission to an SNF. Individuals who do not regain functional ambulation are at risk of becoming long-term nursing home residents.

Brainsky et al (42) evaluated the incremental cost in

the year following hip fracture. They found that it ranged from $16,322 to $18,727 (in 1993 dollars) in 759 community-dwelling older patients. These cost differences were due to hospitalizations, nursing home stays, and rehabilitation services (42).

Steiner et al (43) developed and validated a clinical prediction rule for nursing home residence 6 months after hip fracture. All patients were community dwellers at the time of fracture. The authors found four independent risk factors for nursing home residence: being unmarried, incontinent, dependent in ambulation, and cognitively impaired. In this study, 73.2% of patients who had all four risk factors were in nursing homes at 6 months. Not one patient without any risk factor was in a nursing home (43).

Young et al (44) prospectively studied predictors of functional recovery in 312 community-dwelling elders with subcapital hip fractures treated either by internal fixation or by hemiarthroplasty. They found that the type of surgical procedure was not significantly correlated with postoperative functional recovery. However, among those 85 years and older, patients who were disoriented after surgery had poorer functional recovery over time than did those who were oriented (44).

Fox et al (45) studied 306 community-dwelling hip fracture patients who were 65 years and older. Study subjects completed a gait and balance assessment at 2 months after fracture during a home interview. They were then followed for 2 years. Increased mortality was significantly associated with poor balance, as was an increase in hospitalizations up to 2 years after fracture. Poor gait and poor balance were associated with nursing home placement (45).

To study the incidence of hip dislocation following hip replacement, either total or hemiarthroplasty, Krotenberg et al (46) performed a retrospective chart review of 824 patients admitted to acute inpatient rehabilitation settings. The average age was 76 years; 19.7% were men; 80.5% were women. The authors found that the rate of hip dislocation in patients with a total hip replacement (THR) was not significantly higher in rehabilitation settings than in acute care settings. However, the dislocation rate was significantly lower for hemiarthroplasty patients in the rehabilitation settings than in those in an acute care setting. The reasons for this are unclear, though the authors speculated that the intrinsic healing process or the rehabilitative educational process could have been the cause (46) Refer to Chapter 83.

Osteoarthritis

There is considerable debate about whether OA is result of the aging process or a distinct disease. Ling and Bathon (47), in a comprehensive review, asserted that the relationship between aging and OA can be attributed to the decreased functional chondrocyte density that is typical of aging and makes cartilage susceptible to the degenerative process that distinguishes OA.

The role of medication in the treatment of OA is that of pain relief, since no medication slows disease progression. The initial drug of choice for elderly patients with symptomatic OA is acetaminophen, in doses up to 4000 mg/day (48,49). If further pain control is needed, nonsteroidal anti-inflammatory drugs (NSAIDs) are indicated. This population is at risk for gastric ulceration and renal impairment when NSAIDs are used; a low dosage should be considered and the patient monitored carefully. Topical medications such as capsaicin and methyl salicylate may be helpful for the knees or small joints of the hands. Intra-articular joint injections of glucocorticoids for patients with local inflammatory signs or effusions may be helpful, but should be limited. Surgical intervention is appropriate after four injections (47). Therapeutic modalities include local heat, such as from hot packs, heating pads, paraffin, and fluidotherapy; cold, such as from ice; and transcutaneous electrical nerve stimulation (TENS). Exercise is important in decreasing pain and improving physical function (50). Indications for total knee replacement (TKR) include presence of a varus angulation of more than 10 degrees, or ligamentous instability and any valgus deformity (51). Figure 96-1 indicates treatment options for OA. Refer to Chapter 82 for a detailed discussion of OA.

Rehabilitation of the geriatric patient with a TKR is relatively simple; the goals are to regain distance of ambulation and range of motion in the affected knee. The patient is full weight bearing on the affected limb and can typically use a standard or rolling walker to progressively increase distance of ambulation to over 100 feet within 3 to 5 days following surgery. The other area of rehabilitative focus is increasing the active range of motion of the affected knee. The goal, unless otherwise directed by the orthopedic surgeon, is full extension and flexion to at least 90 degrees.

THR is indicated for functional improvement and relief of pain after nonsurgical management strategies have failed. Two-thirds of THR are performed in patients over the age of 65 years. Based on preoperative function, it appears that women have more advanced disease than men at the time of surgery. The age-specific incidence rates for THR are highest for men between the ages of 65 and 74 years; for women they are highest almost a decade later, at ages between 75 and 84 years (52).

The postoperative rehabilitation of the arthritic geriatric patient with a THR includes teaching the patient to observe hip precautions while improving bed mobility, sitting to standing, and lower-limb dressing activities. This individual is usually weight bearing as tolerated on the affected limb. If the patient is severely arthritic, as a result of either OA or rheumatoid arthritis, joint protection techniques should be taught, in addition to careful nutritional

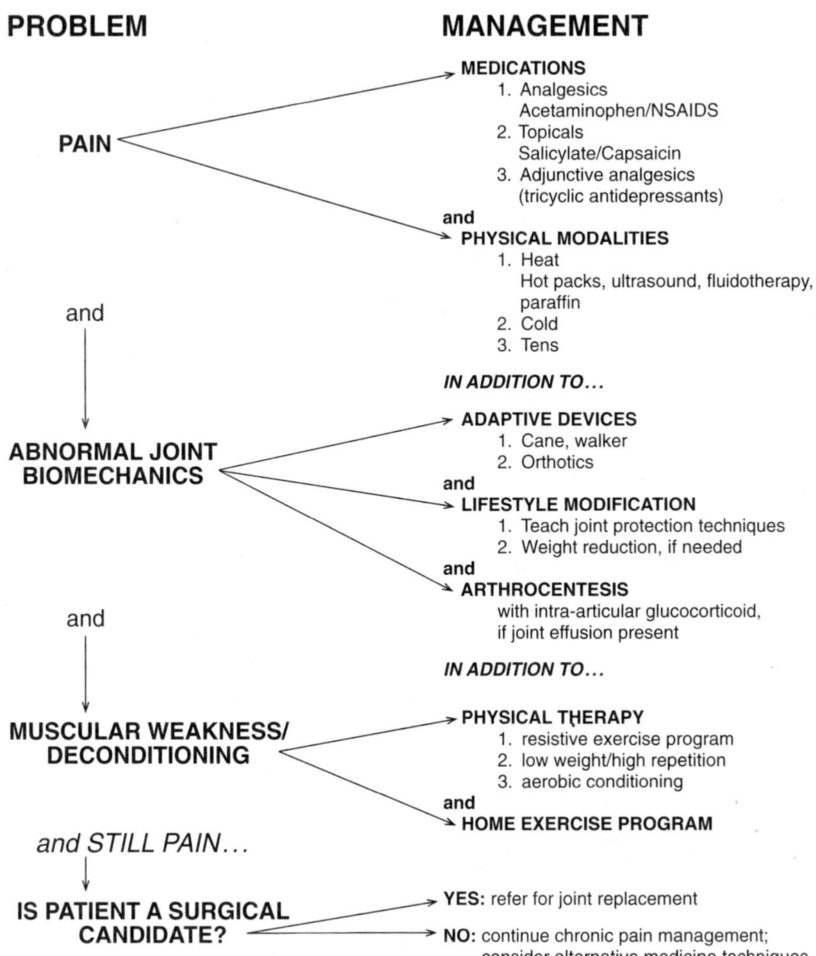

Figure 96-1. Management of osteoarthritis. NSAIDs = nonsteroidal anti-inflammatory drugs; TENS = transcutaneous electrical nerve stimulation. (Adapted from Ling SM, Bathon JM. Osteoarthritis in older adults. *J Am Geriatr Soc* 1998;46:222.)

assessment and follow-up. Pain medication should be scheduled frequently around the clock, alternating narcotics with NSAIDs or acetaminophen to provide enough pain relief so that the patient can participate in therapies postoperatively. Refer to Chapter 84.

Osteoporosis

Although generally considered a problem of postmenopausal women, osteoporosis is ubiquitous with aging. Small-framed men without large muscle mass who have experienced a sedentary lifestyle are also at risk as they age.

Kelley (53) performed a meta-analysis of 10 studies on osteoporosis that included postmenopausal women who had participated in aerobic exercise, compared to nonexercise groups, with measurement of changes in lumbar spinal bone mineral density. The change he found was primarily due to the loss of bone mineral density in the groups that did not exercise, rather than an increase in those who did (53).

Problems resulting from osteoporotic fractures include pain and complications directly related to immobility, such as severe deconditioning with muscular atrophy; lack of weight bearing, which increases the risk of further bone resorption; and overall loss of functional ability. As discussed previously, a hip fracture is a significant life event for the elderly patient, due to the issues of mobility and self-care that it entails.

The rehabilitative management of osteoporotic vertebral compression fractures in the geriatric patient involves gradual return to activities over time as allowed by pain. The individual may be unable to sit comfortably in an upright position for more than 5 to 10 minutes. The patient should be encouraged to rest in bed in a position of comfort; to use assistance for bed mobility, which may be impaired by pain; and to ambulate as much as possible. Over a period of 2 to 3 weeks, the pain will diminish as the fracture heals and there is less spasm in the surrounding paravertebral muscles. This spasm may be treated with local heat and oral muscle relaxants such as cyclobenzaprine hydrochloride (Flexeril), in addition to a trial of TENS to the affected areas. Frequent reassurance is also comforting.

Unfortunately, a vertebral compression fracture due

to osteoporosis simply requires time for healing. Unless she has help, the single, elderly woman who lives alone is typically unable to return home for several weeks after sustaining an acute osteoporotic vertebral compression fracture, due to her limited mobility secondary to pain. Such patients are not usually capable of participating in 3 hours of therapy a day, as required for admission to acute DRG-exempt rehabilitation units. Therefore, these patients may benefit from admission to an SNF, where they can participate in a limited amount of physical therapy and very gradually increase their sitting time as their pain allows. If this is not feasible, those who have the financial resources may temporarily enter a nursing facility where caregivers are available to assist with bed mobility, bathroom transfers, and meal preparation.

Finally, the role of educating family members must be emphasized. It may be too late to prevent bone loss in the postmenopausal 60-year-old daughter of an 80-year-old woman with an acute compression fracture. However, one can instruct the 40-year-old granddaughter and, in turn, her daughter that they should increase their weight-bearing exercises and their calcium intake. Refer to Chapter 85.

Stroke

Two-thirds of stroke patients are over the age of 65 years at the time of the stroke. All of those who sustain a unilateral stroke will eventually walk if they do not soon experience a second stroke or succumb to another problem. The primary risk factor for stroke is age; once a stroke has occurred, the primary risk factor is the previous stroke. Advanced age was once considered a poor prognostic indicator for a "good" outcome from stroke rehabilitation, but at that time discharge from rehabilitation to the previous home setting was considered a factor in outcome. In today's world where everyone works, there are simply no housewives who are available to care for invalids at home, contrary to the circumstances only a generation ago. Fortunately, use of standard outcome measures such as the FIM today allows comparison of functional gains in mobility, ADLs, and communication in order to demonstrate that elderly stroke patients do improve in traditional inpatient rehabilitation settings. They are therefore appropriate stroke rehabilitative candidates (54).

Proper rehabilitative management involves both the timing of and the settings for therapies. Regardless of age, a patient who has poor dynamic sitting balance and does not demonstrate improvement in this area over several days will probably not have the ability to participate in an acute inpatient rehabilitative setting, where the average length of stay after a stroke is now well under 21 days and continues to dramatically decrease as more rehabilitative care shifts to other treatment sites. The patient with poor dynamic sitting balance may be more appropriate for treatment in an SNF. The memory device "SNF—*s*lower, *n*ot *f*aster" is applicable in such a case. Elderly patients who are lethargic, are medically ill due to multiple comorbidities, or had a previous stroke, especially involving the contralateral hemisphere, may not be appropriate for SNF, but may require long-term-care placement for assistance (Fig. 96-2).

Typically, the adage "you're as good as you are" used for stroke patients applies to the geriatric individual as well. Those who progress quickly progress quickly, and those who improve slowly tend to do so throughout the entire course of their recovery. The goal of stroke rehabilitation is to teach the patient to use compensatory skills to substitute for lost functional abilities while muscular recovery occurs. All unilateral stroke patients demonstrate some degree of natural recovery over time. Therefore, almost any health care provider, anywhere, in any setting, can claim to provide stroke rehabilitation services. However, such rehabilitation may not be cost-effective or succcessful from the patients' or payors' standpoints.

As previously stated, teaching the patient to use compensatory strategies for lost functional abilities while natural recovery occurs over time is an integral concept of stroke rehabilitation. The ability to learn is therefore a key element. Table 96-7 lists the typical characteristics of a left hemiplegic as compared to right hemiplegic patient. Although the generalizations are broad, they serve to explain specific patient behaviors to both family and rehabilitation staff members. Frequently, the rehabilitation team can enhance the individual's learning process by taking these behaviors into account. The team should teach new skills in the manner that they are most readily learned by the individual stroke patient. For example, demonstration, rather than speech, can be used to show the aphasic right hemiplegic patient how to perform a wheelchair transfer (55). Use of a highly individualized program that emphasizes the strengths of the patient's

Table 96-7: Characteristics of Left and Right Hemiplegic Patients

Left Hemiplegic (Right Hemispheric Stroke)	Right Hemiplegic (Left Hemispheric Stroke)
Visual-motor-perceptual problems	Impaired communication
Left-side neglect	Learns from visual demonstration
Loss of visual-spatial memory	Follows gestural commands
Impulsive; lacks insight and judgment	Can learn from previous mistakes
Overestimates abilities; denies disabilities	Requires supervision if unable to speak

Source: Adapted from Garrison SJ: Learning after stroke: left versus right brain injury. *Top Geriatr Rehabil* 1991;6(3):48.

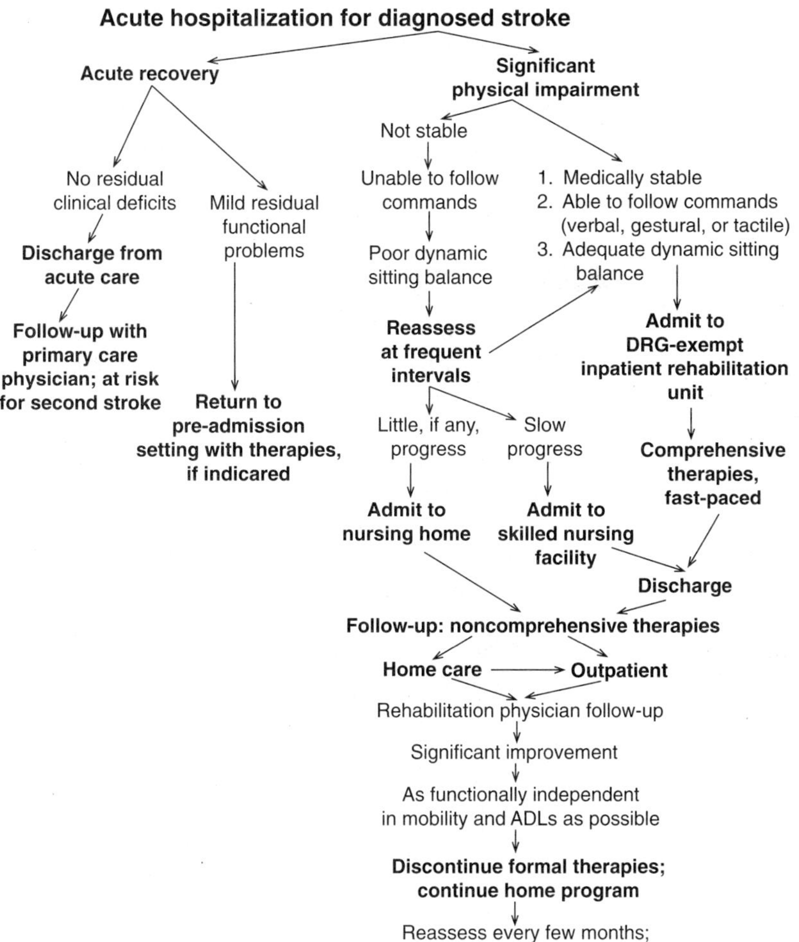

Figure 96-2. Stroke rehabilitation decision tree. DRG = diagnostic-related group; ADLs = activities of daily living. (Adapted from Garrison SJ. Geratric stroke rehabilitation. In: Felsenthal G, Garrison SJ, Steinberg FU, eds. *Rehabilitation of the aging and elderly patient.* Baltimore: Williams & Wilkins, 1994:176.)

uninvolved hemisphere, while acknowledging the potential problems related to the affected hemisphere, may yield a shorter length of stay, fewer complications, and higher functional outcome scores at the time of discharge from acute inpatient stroke rehabilitation.

Outpatient follow-up on a regular basis is essential for rehabilitative management of the poststroke geriatric patient. Depending on the individual's recovery from neurologic deficits and use of compensatory skills, the therapy program should emphasize mobility, ADLs, and speech. There is no simple cookbook approach; each stroke patient is unique. Some patients may require home care therapies prior to transitioning to an outpatient setting. Financial resources play a significant role in this as well; many payors, including Medicare, limit the number and timing of therapy sessions following acute illness, including stroke. Medicare does not reimburse therapies for a diagnosis that is over a year old, such as previous stroke. It is therefore important to educate patients and their caregivers to notify the physician if they experience acute illness or injury, such as a fall. Based on the assessment of their current functional status, patients may then be eligible for additional therapies to address problems related to mobility, ADLs, cognition, and communication.

Amputation

Amputation in the geriatric population is typically a result of dysvascular complications, from either ischemia or neuropathy related to hypertension, diabetes. or both. This section addresses only lower-limb amputees, both transfemoral and transtibial. Of these, the transtibial amputation is now the most common, since revascularization techniques and other surgical advances usually allow for preservation of the knee joint. This is of great significance with respect to the energy cost of ambulation in the geriatric population. For more information, refer to Chapter 30.

The emotional effect of limb loss, even when performed as an "elective" procedure, is significant. Patients and families need a supportive environment in which they can acknowledge and address their feelings. Previous methods of coping with loss are good indicators of current emotional strengths and weaknesses. Cultural roles and ethnic backgrounds often have much more of an influence in the adjustment to limb loss than is generally recognized. It is very helpful for amputees and their families to observe other amputees at various stages of prosthetic evaluation and restoration. This can be accomplished through formal, as well as informal, support groups. Scheduling outpatient amputee follow-up visits on a designated day allows opportunities for such informal interaction to occur in the waiting room.

Cutson and Bongiorni (56) reviewed the literature pertaining to outcomes of lower-limb prosthetic rehabilitation in the older patient. They concluded that age alone should not be a factor in making decisions about candidates for prosthetic restoration. To be considered for prosthetic restoration, an elderly patient must have enough upper-limb strength to push up in a wheelchair, and must be able to bear weight on the remaining limb. These requirements do not differ from those for younger amputees. Here, too, the rehabilitation concept of being able to learn and demonstrate new skills is paramount; the geriatric amputees cannot depend on caregivers to use the prostheses for them. Other factors that must be considered in the preprosthetic evaluation include the presence of preexisting neurologic deficits, such as hemiplegia due to stroke, poor endurance as a result of chronic cardiac or pulmonary problems, and hip or knee contractures.

At this time, any Medicare recipient is entitled to have a custom prosthesis fabricated. With the influx of managed care into the older adult market, it will be interesting to observe the way in which the prescription and fabrication of these very expensive custom devices are regulated. Unfortunately, this control may result in a sacrifice of quality for lower cost.

There are various ways in which the prosthesis can be modifed to better serve the needs of the older amputee. These modifications include suspension devices such as belts and lace-up corsets, padded socket inserts, safety-type knee mechanisms that lock when pressure is applied, more stable single-axis ankle joints, and energy-storing feet to assist in toe off. Ease of donning and doffing, comfortable fit, and the individual's perception of limb stability contribute to successful prosthetic usage in this population. Refer to Chapter 32.

The role of pure cosmesis has long been considered; the patient may choose to stay seated in a wheelchair, wearing a nonfunctional cosmetic artificial leg. This can be a very attractive idea for the elderly bilateral transfemoral amputee who is not a candidate for using articulated limbs due to the high energy cost of ambulation.

Contralateral limb loss is always a concern in the dysvascular geriatric amputee. Studies showed that 15% to 20% lose the contralateral limb within 2 years; this risk increases to 40% at 4 years. Despite advances in medical care, this risk has not decreased over the past 20 to 30 years (57). For these reasons, the clinician should limit the distance a dysvascular amputee without a prosthesis "ambulates" with a walker. The patient is actually hopping on the remaining limb, which is also affected by systemic vascular disease, thereby subjecting it to additional stress and risk of injury.

The patient and caregiver should be taught to protect the remaining leg and foot with appropriate skin care, a well-fitting shoe, treatment of fungal toenail infections, and proper toenail cutting, by a podiatrist, if necessary. Obviously, maintenance of normal muscular strength and full active range of motion of the joints in this limb is ideal.

RESEARCH IMPLICATIONS

Dychtwald (38) wrote in the *Age Wave* that "becoming more than we've ever been before is the point of extended life." Keeping the aging population healthy and mobile is a challenge that can be met. However, additional research is indicated. Kauffman (58) discussed the "generational conflict" over allocation of government medical financial resources between the young and the old. He observed that funding for research promoting healthy aging will benefit both the existing elderly population and the younger group as it ages. However, this is not always recognized by the young and middle-aged adult population.

Forbes and Hirdes (59) addressed the relationships of chronic disease and normal aging. They observed that it is incorrect to assume that research findings in a younger age group also apply to an elderly population. They also questioned whether research should be focused on disability, rather than mortality, due to quality of life issues. However, here, also, the degree of acceptable impairment should be considered. Priorities for research in the elderly population should be established with these points in mind (59).

USES OF HEALTH CARE FUNDING

As previously discussed, Medicare was developed with the concept of diagnosing and correcting acute illness. This funding source does not apply well to the geriatric population at the present time. It has been noted that 90% of the health care professionals are in the acute hospital setting, with 10% of the population requiring health care, while 90% of this population is located in the community, with only 10% of the health care workers. The entire system revolves around hospitalization for acute illnesses. This obviously creates limitations for the appropriate provision of health care that should emphasize prevention of health problems and maintenance of functional independence in this population.

Alternative health care delivery systems must be developed and assessed to meet the current needs more effectively. Tinetti et al (60) performed a demonstration study of a home-based protocol for the rehabilitation of hip fracture patients over the age of 65 years. The participants were 148 cognitively intact community dwellers. The program was over a 6-month period, much longer than the typical 2-month period generally allowed by Medicare. However, the costs were significantly less (60).

CONCLUSIONS

Care of the geriatric rehabilitation patient is both challenging and rewarding. It is easy to recognize the benefits of adding quality to life in the later years. Specific rehabilitative diagnoses related to the care of the aged population include disuse, falls, hip fracture, osteoarthritis, osteoporosis, stroke, and lower-limb dysvascular amputation. Issues that affect the rehabilitation process and outcome of these problems include cognitive ability, functional presentation of disease, nutritional status, functional decline, financial resources, and patient motivation. Various care settings may be utilized to best meet the individual rehabilitative needs of this population. Attitude is a significant factor as well. Since the current adult population values youthful appearance and physical fitness through regular exercise, it may prove to be a healthier geriatric population. Research is beginning to reveal differences in older individuals who are able to remain community dwellers, compared to those who live in long-term care facilities. Future areas for research, as well as funding, will be determined by health care policy created by people who have not yet personally experienced advanced age. It is our challenge, as health care professionals and future members of this population, to participate in areas that benefit the geriatric age group.

REFERENCES

1. Sheehy G. *New passages.* New York: Ballantine Books, 1995:419.
2. Greene MG, Majerovitz SD, Adelman RD, Rizzo C. The effects of the presence of a third person on the physician-older patient medical interview. *J Am Geriatr Soc* 1994;42:413–419.
3. Banja JD, Bilsky GS. Discussing cardiopulmonary resuscitation with elderly rehabilitation patients, ethical and clinical considerations toward the formation of policy. *Am J Phys Med Rehabil* 1995; 74(suppl I1):512–515.
4. Hesse KA, Campion EW. Motivating the geriatric patient for rehabilitation. *J Am Geriatr Soc* 1983;31:586–589.
5. Lubitz JD, Riley GF. Trends in Medicare payments in the last year of life. *N Engl J Med* 1993;3228: 1092–1096.
6. Fried LP, Guralnik JM. Disability in older adults: evidence regarding significance, etiology, and risk. *J Am Geriatr Soc* 1997;45:92–100.
7. Kiely DK, Morris JN, Morris SA, et al. The effect of specific medical conditions on functional decline. *J Am Geriatr Soc* 1997;45: 1459–1463.
8. Hughes S, Gibbs J, Dunlop D, et al. Predictors of decline in manual performance in older adults. *J Am Geriatr Soc* 1997;45: 905–910.
9. Forrest KY, Bunker CH, Songer TJ, et al. Driving patterns and medical conditions in older women. *J Am Geriatr Soc* 1997;45:1214–1218.
10. Sinoff G, Ore L. The Barthel activities of daily living index: self-reporting versus actual performance in the old-old (≥75 years). *J Am Geriatr Soc* 1997;45: 832–836.
11. Besdine RW. The educational utility of comprehensive functional assessment in the elderly. *J Am Geriatr Soc* 1983;31:651–656.
12. Verbrugge LM. The dynamics of population aging and health. In: Lewis SJ, ed. *Aging and health.* Chelsea, MI: Lewis, 1989: 23–40.
13. Tombaugh TN, McIntyre NJ. The Mini-Mental State Examination: a comprehensive review. *J Am Geriatr Soc* 1992;40:922–935.
14. Sommers MS. Speech perception in older adults: the importance of speech-specific cognitive abilities. *J Am Geriatr Soc* 1997;45: 633–637.
15. Uhlmann RD, Larson EB, Rees TS, et al. Relationship of hearing impairment to dementia and cognitive dysfunction in older adults. *JAMA* 1989;261:916–919.
16. Perls TT, Morris JN, Ooi WL, Lipsitz LA. The relationship between age, gender, and cognitive performance in the very old: the effect of selective survival. *J Am Geriatr Soc* 1993;41:1193–1201.
17. Schuman JE, Beattie EJ, Steed DA, et al. Geriatric patients with and without intellectual dysfunction: effectiveness of a standard rehabilitation program. *Arch Phys Med Rehabil* 1981;62: 612–618.
18. Rentz DM. The assessment of rehabilitation potential: cognitive factors. In: Hartke RJ, ed. *Psychological aspects of geriatric rehabilitation.* Gaithersburg, MD: Aspen, 1991:97–114.
19. Goldstein FC, Strasser DC, Woodard JL, Roberts VJ. Functional outcome of cognitively impaired hip fracture patients on a geriatric rehabilitation unit. *J Am Geriatr Soc* 1997;45:35–42.
20. Salzman C, Fisher J, Nobel K, et al. Cognitive improvement following benzodiazepine discontinuation in elderly nursing home residents. *Int J Geriatr Psychiatr* 1992;7:89–93.
21. United States Department of Health and Human Services. *Drug utilization review.* Washington, DC: Office of Inspector General, April 1989:5.
22. Sloan RW. *Practical geriatric therapeutics.* Oradel, NJ: Medical Economics Books, 1986:39–50.
23. Stein BE. Avoiding drug reactions: seven steps to writing safe pre-

scriptions. *Geriatrics* 1994;49: 28–36.

24. Glickman L, Bruce EA, Caro FG, Avorn J. Physicians' knowledge of drug costs for the elderly. *J Am Geriatr Soc* 1994;42: 992–996.

25. Hanlon JT, Schmader KE, Koronkowski MJ, et al. Adverse drug events in high risk older outpatients. *J Am Geriatr Soc* 1997;45:945–948.

26. Hildebrand JK, Joos SK, Lee MA. Use of diagnosis "failure to thrive" in older veterans. *J Am Geriatr Soc* 1997;45:1113–1117.

27. Sforzo GA, McManis BG, Black D, et al. Resilience to exercise detraining in healthy older adults. *J Am Geriatr Soc* 1995;43: 209–215.

28. Judge JO, Whipple RH, Wolfson LI. Effects of resistive and balance exercises on isokinetic strength in older persons. *J Am Geriatr Soc* 1994;42:937–946.

29. Cress ME, Schechtman KB, Mulrow CD, et al. Relationshp between physical performance and self-perceived physical function. *J Am Geriatr Soc* 1995;43: 93–101.

30. Kohrt WM, Spina RJ, Holloszy JO, Ehsani AA. Prescribing exercise intensity for older women. *J Am Geriatr Soc* 1998;46: 129–133.

31. Rantanen T, Era P, Heiikkinen E. Physical activity and the changes in maximal isometric strength in men and women from the age of 75 to 80 years. *J Am Geriatr Soc* 1997;45:1439–1445.

32. Kapoor WN. Syncope in older persons. *J Am Geriatr Soc* 1994;42:426–436.

33. Ivers RQ, Cumming RG, Mitchell P, Attebo K. Visual impairment and falls in older adults: the Blue Mountains Eye Study. *J Am Geriatr Soc* 1998;46:58–64.

34. Norton R, Campbell AJ, Lee-Joe T, et al. Circumstances of falls resulting in hip fractures among older people. *J Am Geriatr Soc* 1997; 45:1108–1112.

35. Mahoney J, Sager M, Dunham NC, Johnson J. Risk of falls after hospital discharge. *J Am Geriatr Soc* 1994;42:269–274.

36. Maki BE. Gait changes in older adults: predictors of falls or indicators of fear? *J Am Geriatr Soc* 1997;45:313–320.

37. Alexander NB, Ulbrich, J, Raheja A, Cham D. Rising from the floor in older adults. *J Am Geriatr Soc* 1997;45:564–569.

38. Dychtwald K. *Age wave.* Los Angeles: Jeremy P. Teacher, 1989.

39. Kane RA, Caplan AL, Urv-Wong EK, et al. Everyday matters in the lives of nursing home residents: wish for and perception of choice and control. *J Am Geriatr Soc* 1997;45:1086–1093.

40. Chiou IL, Burnett CN. Values of activities of daily living—a survey of stroke patients and their home therapies. *Phys Ther* 1985;65: 901–906.

41. Zuckerman JD. Hip fracture. *N Engl J Med* 1996;334: 1519–1525.

42. Brainsky A, Glick H, Lydick E, et al. The economic cost of hip fractures in community-dwelling older adults: a prospective study. *J Am Geriatr Soc* 1997;45: 281–287.

43. Steiner JF, Kramer AM, Eilertsen TB, Kowalsky JC. Development and validation of a clinical prediction rule for prolonged nursing home residence after hip fracture. *J Am Geriatr Soc* 1997;45: 1510–1514.

44. Young Y, Brant L, German P, et al. A longitudinal examination of functional recovery among older people with subcapital hip fractures. *J Am Geriatr Soc* 1997; 45:288–294.

45. Fox KM, Hawkes WG, Hebel JR, et al. Mobility after hip fracture predicts health outcomes. *J Am Geriatr Soc* 1998;46: 169–173.

46. Krotenberg R, Stitik T, Johnston MV. Incidence of dislocation following hip arthroplasty for patients in the rehabilitation setting. *Am J Phys Med Rehabil* 1995;74: 444–447.

47. Ling SM, Bathon JM. Osteoarthritis in older adults. *J Am Geriatr Soc* 1998;46:216–225.

48. Hochberg MC, Altman RD, Brandt KD, et al. Guidelines for the medical management of osteoarthritis. Part I. Osteoarthritis of the hip. *Arthritis Rheum* 1995;38:1535–1540.

49. Hochberg MC, Altman RD, Brandt KD, et al. Guidelines for the medical management of osteoarthritis. Part II. Osteoarthritis of the hip. *Arthritis Rheum* 1995;38:1541–1546.

50. Ettinger WH Jr, Burns R, Messier SP, et al. A randomized trial comparing aerobic exercise and resistance exercise with a health education program in older adults with knee osteoarthritis: The Fitness Arthritis and Seniors Trial (FAST). *JAMA* 1997;277:25–31.

51. Windsor A, Insall JN. The knee. In: Kelly WN, Harris ED, Ruddy S, Sledge CB, eds. *Textbook of rheumatology.* 5th ed. Philadelphia: WB Saunders, 1997: 1739–1758.

52. National Institutes of Health. *Total hip replacement, consensus statement.* 1994;September 12–14, vol 12,5.

53. Kelley G. Aerobic exercise and lumbar spine bone mineral density in postmenopausal women: a meta-analysis. *J Am Geriatr Soc* 1998;46:143–152.

54. Garrison SJ. Geriatric stroke rehabilitation. In: Felsenthal G, Garrison SJ, Steinberg FU, eds. *Rehabilitation of the aging and elderly patient.* Baltimore: Williams & Wilkins, 1994:175–186.

55. Garrison SJ. Learning after stroke: left versus right brain injury. *Top Geriatr Rehabil* 1991; 6(3):45–52.

56. Cutson TM, Bongiorni DR. Rehabilitation of the older lower limb amputee: a brief review. *J Am Geriatr Soc* 1996;44:1388–1393.

57. Weiss GN, Gorton TA, Read RC, Neal LA. Outcomes of lower

extremity amputations. *J Am Geriatr Soc* 1990;38:877–883.

58. Kauffman T. Research: a requisite for health care of the elderly. In: Lewis C, ed. *Aging: the health care challenge.* 2nd ed. Philadelphia: FA Davis, 1985:366–375.

59. Forbes WF, Hirdes JP. The relationship between aging and disease: geriatric ideology and myths of senility. *J Am Geriatr Soc* 1993;41:1267–1271.

60. Tinetti ME, Baker DI, Gottschalk M, et al. Systematic home-based physical and functional therapy for older persons after hip fracture. *Arch Phys Med Rehabil* 1987;78: 1237–1247.

Chapter 97

Performing Arts Medicine

Keith Bengtson
Clay Miller

Performing artists likely have had various performance-related medical problems for as long as such activities have been pursued. Poore (1) described "pianists' cramp" as early as 1887. Robert Schumann had an unknown ailment in his right ring finger, perhaps focal dystonia, that cut short his performing career (2). Reports of dancers experiencing leg ailments date back 300 years. However, only in the past 20 years have physicians responded to these problems with separate specialty clinics and informal specialization in the performing arts. This has been followed by the emergence of many organizations for the study and treatment of performing artists' medical problems. Some of these organizations include the Performing Arts Medical Association (PAMA), the International Alliance for Dance Medicine and Science (IADMS), and the International Arts Medicine Association (IAMA), all of which emerged in the late 1980s. In 1983 the first "Medical Problems of Musicians" conference was held in conjunction with the Aspen, Colorado Music Festival. This now occurs annually and includes medical problems of dancers as well as musicians. A quarterly journal, *Medical Problems of Performing Artists*, has also been published since 1986 to specifically address medical issues in the performing arts.

MUSCULOSKELETAL PROBLEMS OF MUSICIANS

Music medicine developed in a similar fashion to sports medicine—to meet the highly specialized needs of a specialized population. However, the musculoskeletal problems that musicians develop have more in common with industrial or clerical workers than with athletes. Musicians primarily have slowly progressive upper-extremity musculoskeletal ailments such as tendinitis, tenosynovitis, and nerve entrapment syndromes. In contrast, athletes have a wider variety of problems in the spine and upper and lower extremities related both to chronic overuse and to acute trauma.

The term *patient* will be used when referring to these musicians. However, it is sometimes popular to use the term *client* when speaking of musicians seen in an arts medicine clinic. This politically correct term is likely an attempt to make the setting less clinical and, therefore, less sterile or intimidating to the musician population.

Epidemiology

The prevalence of musculoskeletal problems among musicians has been investigated among many groups and in many different settings. Fry (3) interviewed 485 symphony orchestra members from Australia, England, and the United States and found a 64% incidence of what he broadly defined as "overuse syndrome." He also interviewed the students and staff of seven Australian music schools and found 116 of 1249 musicians to have some problems of overuse (4). Of the 900 students and professional musicians that he personally examined throughout his career, he found 379 (42%) with overuse syndrome (5).

Fishbein et al (6) in a survey of the International Conference of Symphony and Opera Musicians (ICSOM) reported an 82% incidence of medical problems among the 2122 respondents. In a questionnaire to 250 high-level musicians in northeastern Ohio, Caldron et al (7) found a 57% incidence of musculoskeletal problems related to playing. Revak (8) surveyed piano majors from seven music schools and reported that 30 (42%) of 71 respondents had "physical discomfort of hands or arms that persisted or recurred for more than one week and impaired their ability to practice the piano." Hiner et al (9) sent a questionnaire to violinists participating in an international competition and found (51%) of the 29 respondents to have performance-related problems. Newmark and Lederman (10) surveyed musicians at a musical conference and reported that 57 (72%) of the 79 musicians developed new playing-related problems while at the conference. In a survey of nonclassical musicians, Newmark and Salmon (11) detected a 44% incidence of "physical complaints related to playing" in 48 musicians. These studies clearly indicate that musculoskeletal problems plague musicians at all playing levels, whether they play classical or nonclassical music.

Music Medicine

One may see many types of musician-patients in the clinical setting. There is the 30-year-old professional orchestra musician who developed carpal tunnel syndrome on her recent concert tour. There is the 18-year-old music student who develops myofascial pain after practicing 12 hours per day for an upcoming audition. There is the 60-year-old piano teacher who complains of pain when playing scales because of basilar thumb degenerative arthritis. The uniting factor in these patients is the physical demands of making music. These demands include the need for strength as well as endurance of the small intrinsic muscles of the hand, the extrinsic muscles of the forearm, as well as the larger supporting muscles of the trunk and shoulders. Playing may also require excessively repetitive motions in often awkward postures. Any minor hindrance in physical ability is magnified because of the incredible neuromuscular control necessary to produce high-level music. Poore (1) described the situation quite well over 100 years ago:

> The machinery involved in the delicate manipulations necessary for a pianist is, indeed, so complicated that the wonder is break-down does not oftener occur. In playing the piano, all forms of sensation (cutaneous, articular, muscular) must be perfect; from peripheral nerve-endings to brain the sensory path must be free from all defects. The motor path must be equally free from defect from the cerebral cortex to the motor end plates on the muscles, and it must be borne in mind that a trouble affecting a fine nerve-twig supplying some little muscle of the fingers is as capable of upsetting the harmony of a delicate act like piano-playing as is damage to one of the chief cords of the brachial plexus. The muscles involved in the act must one and all be healthy.

Taking a Music Medicine History

In addition to a standard, thorough medical history, several items specific to musicians should be noted. Obviously the type of instrument(s) that the patient plays is important, as is the type of music that the patient plays. Each instrument has different physical demands, as does each type of music. Stringed orchestral instruments, for example, present different problems for the left (fingering) hand than for the right (bowing) hand. A flutist tends to have more problems with the left than the right hand because of the supinated and radially deviated posture of the left wrist. Larger and heavier instruments present more problems to the supporting structures of the shoulders and back.

One must also inquire about the patient's playing and practicing schedule, along with their level of training and expertise. Often a recent change in schedule, repertoire, or technique may trigger a musculoskeletal complaint. Typically a patient increases playing time in preparation for an upcoming performance. The added stress overloads the body's musculoskeletal capacity and the patient develops an injury. One must also consider how the patient's symptoms are temporally related to the playing schedule. Is the patient in pain immediately on picking up the instrument, or does discomfort develop only after a full day of playing?

Many musicians utilize the services of alternative medical care providers, either out of suspicion of allopathic medicine or because of peer recommendations. Therefore, it is important to inquire about previous nonallopathic treatments. Alexander and Feldenkrais techniques are two of the most popular alternative treatment methods used by musicians. Both teach relaxation and movement control through body awareness (12,13).

Table 97-1 provides a complete outline of the musicians' history as suggested by Newmark and Weinstein (14).

Physical Examination

The physical examination must include a complete examination of the upper extremities, shoulder, and neck in a standard fashion. X-rays films, electromyograms (EMGs), blood tests, and so on should be ordered as indicated. Beyond these basic procedures, the most important aspect of the examination is observing the patient playing his or her instrument. If the patient plays a nonportable instrument that cannot be brought into the physician's office, a videotape may have to suffice. While observing the patient perform, one should look for abnormal or stressful postures, co-contractions, dystonic movements, or unusual techniques. It is often helpful to be familiar with the particular instrument in order to recognize the latter. If one is unfamiliar with the instrument, the patient's instructor may be consulted. In general, the patient should appear relaxed and comfortable playing the instrument. If seated, the

Table 97-1: Musician's History

Dominant hand
Musical instrument
  Primary/secondary
Training/education (yr)
  Teacher
  Student
  Professional/semiprofessional
  Avocational
Practice schedule
  Consistent?
  Recent increases/decreases?
  Change of technique, repertoire, or instrument?
  Upcoming or changes in performances?
Type of music played
Exercises
  General (nonmusical)
  Specific
  Warm-up
  Cooldown
  How often?
  Other activities, i.e., hobbies/sports
Presenting complaint
Pain location
Dysfunction location
Factors/situations that increase or decrease pain
  Consider octaves, arpeggios, trills, etc
Neurologic complaints
  Numbness
  Weakness
  Incoordination
  Curling, drooping
  Paresthesias
  Cramping
  Bowel/bladder symptoms
Vegetative symptoms of depression/eating disorder
  Change of weight, appetite, sexual interest/activity
  Crying spells
  Fatigue
  Anhedonia
  Suicidal ideation
  Mood
  Sleep patterns
Medication
Allergies
Cigarette use—how much?
Alcohol use
Caffeine use
Illegal drug use
General medical history
Social history
Work (nonmusical)
Previous treatments
  Feldenkrais
  Alexander
  Modalities
  Occupational therapy
  Physical therapy exercise
  Biofeedback
  Chiropractic
  Other

Source: Newmark J, Weinstein MS. A proposed standardized medical history and physical form for musicians. *Med Probl Perform Art* 1995;10:137–139.

patient should have both feet flat on the floor, thighs horizontal, back straight, and shoulders relaxed. Standing posture should be relaxed but vertical. Having the patient play the most difficult passage he or she knows will often expose an abnormal technique or posture that is otherwise held in check. The goal is to find an abnormal stressor that may have resulted in the patient's injury.

Treatment

Naturally, treatment should be directed by the patient's specific ailment, many of which are discussed elsewhere in this book. However, the essence of treatment is elucidating the often multiple causative factors of the patient's ailment and then working to eliminate them. An error in technique, if not corrected with the initial treatment of the injury, could lead to frequently recurring problems. Once again, this emphasizes the need to observe the patient playing the instrument and to collaborate with the patient's instructor. The physician, therapist, and instructor should strive with the patient toward ideal ergonomics, relaxed posture, and fluid playing technique. Only then will the patient have the greatest chance of recovery and prevention of a recurrence.

Many times the most essential aspect of treatment is rest. Trying to convince the patient to stop playing the instrument is similar to convincing an athlete to take time off from training. Ideally the patient would rest until completely symptom free. However, a period of relative rest during which the patient decreases playing time and intensity may be sufficient to allow recovery. Then the patient would return to playing gradually in a symptom-free manner. Norris (15) proposed general guidelines for such a process (Table 97-2).

Aside from the well-described nerve entrapment syndromes, tendinitis, tenosynovitis, and degenerative joint dis-

Table 97-2: Return to Play Schedule

Level	Play	Rest	Play	Rest	Play	Rest	Play	Rest	Play
1	5	60	5						
2	10	50	10						
3	15	40	15	60	5				
4	20	30	20	50	10				
5	30	20	25	40	15	45	5		
6	35	15	35	30	20	35	10		
7	40	10	40	20	25	25	15	50	10
8	50	10	45	15	30	15	25	40	15
9	50	10	50	10	40	10	35	30	20
10	50	10	50	10	50	10	45	20	30

- Stay at each level for 3–7 days.
- Start with slow and easy pieces, progressing to faster, more difficult pieces.
- Warm up before playing.

Source: Norris RN. *The musician's survival guide: a guide to preventing and treating injuries in instrumentalists.* International conference of symphony and operal musicians. St. Louis: MMB Music, Inc., 1993:107.

eases, musicians often have other more diffuse and evasive upper-extremity pain problems. This is sometimes referred to as *overuse syndrome*. Rest is also a mainstay of treatment for overuse syndrome. Again, one must determine how much rest is reasonable given the severity of the illness. In patients with more limited overuse syndrome, regular breaks in playing (e.g., 5 minutes every 30 minutes) may be sufficient to calm the symptoms. In patients with more severe symptoms, discontinuing instrumental practice sessions is necessary for 1 to 2 weeks in order to reach a pain-free state. This again may be met with considerable resistance from the patient as well as the instructor or musical director.

Light aerobic exercise and regular stretching of upper-extremity muscles are recommended to maintain general fitness and flexibility. This approach is largely borrowed from the treatment protocols for fibromyalgia. However, it also stems from the observation that many of these patients are in poor physical condition and tend to have tight neck, shoulder girdle, and forearm muscles. The latter is likely secondary to prolonged co-contraction of upper-extremity muscles in response to painful tasks. Aerobic conditioning is most easily accomplished by a walking program consisting of 30 minutes or more three to four times a week at a moderate pace. This is usually well tolerated by the patients and requires minimal equipment or skills. Swimming or other pool exercise programs may be prescribed, depending on the patient's interests and means.

Physical modalities can be used as a means of pain control. Superficial heat or cold, ultrasound (with or without phonophoresis of cortisone), iontophoresis of lidocaine and cortisone, transcutaneous electrical nerve stimulation (TENS), massage, contrast baths, and fluidotherapy have been used with some success. Unfortunately their effects are inevitably temporary and the patient will have to be weaned from these modalities at some time. Physical modalities typically should be used during the peak of the symptoms in order to advance the exercise program in a supervised manner. If these modalities are used for a prolonged period, the patient may become addicted to them, and feel that passive modalities are continually required for a state of well-being.

Medications are inevitably used somewhere in the course of treatment for pain control, particularly in patients with prolonged symptoms. Nonsteroidal anti-inflammatory drugs (NSAIDs) are typically the first-line drugs used in treatment but usually have limited effect. More successful have been the tricyclic antidepressants used in low doses [e.g., amitriptyline (Elavil) 10–25 mg every night]. Pain control with these medications may be related to serotonin modulation of descending pain-inhibitory pathways in the spinal cord. Alternatively, increasing the amount of stage III and IV sleep may aid in muscle relaxation, thus decreasing pain. Another sleep-enhancing medication that has been effective for muscle pain is zolpidem (Ambien), 5 to 10 mg every night. Also, carbamazepine (Tegretol) and gabapentin (Neurontin) have been suggested as helpful for neuropathic pain. Carbamazepine acts as a membrane stabilizer and experimentally has been shown to be effective for neuroma pain.

Splinting has been used extensively in many overuse syndrome patients, often to their detriment. Ideally splinting should be used both to augment the resting portion of the patient's regimen and to aid in any ergonomic considerations. Splinting for an extended period will lead to atrophy of the splinted muscle groups, making them more susceptible to stresses, strains, and other painful conditions. As with the physical modalities, the patient will eventually have to be weaned from the splint. To make this task easier, splinting should be prescribed for a finite time period. If possible, the patient should only wear the splint 6 to 8 hours per day, with a tapering period planned and discussed with the patient ahead of time. When used properly, splints can speed up recovery time, but when used irresponsibly, they can become an addiction for the susceptible patient.

When the patient has significant pain-free intervals, or when the pain has reached a tolerable level, then a program of very gradual strengthening may be initiated, along with a gradual return to playing. The patient should be aware of the baseline pain level (i.e., the level of pain while at rest without the presence of any exacerbating factors). Any strengthening exercise should be undertaken with the understanding that it should not increase this baseline pain level for more than a 24-hour period. If the patient feels that the pain has increased from one day to the next, then the exercise level must decrease. A prolonged period of increased pain may be augmented by the next day's activities, thus continually increasing the patient's pain level. Experienced therapists are essential to help devise an exercise program both for general conditioning and for strengthening of specific muscle groups that are affected by the painful condition. The patient's progress may be excruciatingly slow and marked by frequent setbacks. However, if the patient remains motivated, and the treating physician resists the temptation to accelerate the program, the patient often obtains considerable relief from pain in the long term.

Musical instruments were not necessarily designed with the ergonomic needs of the musician in mind. Many instruments are actually quite awkward to play. Simple or complex modifications can help decrease the physical stress of playing an instrument. For example, in playing the clarinet, oboe, English horn, or soprano saxophone, the weight of the instrument is almost entirely supported by the right thumb. Chronic loading of the thumb has been implicated as the cause for many right thumb ailments (16). The use of a neck strap and abdominal post completely eliminates the weight-bearing function of the right thumb and may help with painful conditions in this area.

The most popular instrument modification is the violin shoulder rest. The violinist normally tucks the body of the violin between the chin and left shoulder where the instrument can be held hands-free. The shoulder rest, a small pad and post, fits onto the base of the violin. The effect of this device is to thicken the base of the instrument, resulting in less neck flexion and less shoulder elevation required to hold the violin in place. Surface EMG studies of violinists using this device show decreased tension on the left trapezius and right sternocleidomastoid muscles in some subjects (17).

Various flute modifications have been described. A thermoplastic splint, suggested for the left index finger, protects against compression of the index finger's radial digital nerve (18). Norris (19) described a right thumb guide to decrease the pressure on the thumb tip where it presses against the barrel of the flute. The same author designed a flute with an angled body. This decreases the tilt of the flutist's neck and the elevation of the musician's shoulders, thus preventing problems with the shoulder girdle and neck muscles (20).

The troubleshooting process involved in establishing an etiologic factor for the patient's ailment and organizing a treatment program requires close collaboration between the patient, the physician, the instructor, and the therapist. Alternative or complementary health care providers, such as Alexander (12) or Feldenkrais practitioners, may also aid in this endeavor. One must also consider the practice and performance demands on the musician and recognize the critical role that music making plays in his or her life.

DANCE MEDICINE

Dance medicine has grown exponentially over the past 10 to 15 years but remains a relatively new field of medicine. There are many different medical professionals involved in dance medicine, including physiatrists, orthopedists, internists, podiatrists, psychiatrists, psychologists, physical therapists, chiropractors, massage therapists, acupuncturists, dance therapists, and practitioners of Feldenkrais, Pilates, and Alexander techniques, to name a few.

Several arts medicine organizations exist to encompass these many different professionals. The PAMA is mainly a physician-organized group, the members of which specialize in treating dancers and musicians. The IADMS, the IAMA, and National Dance Association are other organizations combining memberships from all the professionals in the field of arts medicine.

The art of dance, particularly ballet, is one of the most physically demanding on the musculoskeletal system. Most of the dance medicine literature and medical treatments focus on classical ballet, probably because of the high injury rate [approximately 3%–10% of dancers per contract year (21–25)] and because classical ballet has the largest established professional companies.

The type of musculoskeletal problems that develop in dancers is based on their unique physical and anatomic qualities as well as their drive to excel in the field. The shear nature of their practice sets them up for numerous repetitive strain or overuse injuries of the lower extremities. Traumatic injuries can occur as well about the foot and ankle, knee, and back. The most common injuries of the repetitive strain type occur in the foot and ankle, followed by the knee, hip, and back (22,24–26).

Many factors including foot morphology, dance floor surfaces, training and technique errors, and poor nutrition contribute to the dancers' foot and ankle problems (27–29). Because many of these factors are not discussed in standard medical training, it is imperative that the health care provider for dancers have knowledge of their art form, technique, and working situation. Some health care providers who work with dancers were former dancers themselves; however, not all who will treat a dancer have this background. This section provides an overview of the areas of expertise needed to provide medical care to the dancer. This includes a specialized history and physical examination format, common injuries, common treatment approaches, and future considerations for dance medicine.

Overview

Dance medicine has developed into a multidisciplinary approach to preventing and treating the common medical problems of dancers. Many dancers will seek alternative medical approaches such as the Pilates, Feldenkrais, and Alexander techniques prior to seeking an allopathic physician. Traditionally, orthopedists have been the most common physicians to see dancers; however, physiatrists, internists, and family practice physicians are now also seeing increasing numbers of dancers as these areas subspecialize in arts medicine.

The most common injuries sustained by dancers are overuse injuries of the lower extremities (although traumatic injuries do occur) as has been well documented by several authors (22–24,26,30,31). Once the injury has been diagnosed, most physicians will exhaust conservative treatments to heal the injury. This usually includes activity modification, ice, NSAIDs, ultrasound, electrical stimulation, iontophoresis, stretching, and strengthening exercises. Chiropractic, acupuncture, Pilates, Feldenkrais, and Alexander therapies may also be included early or later in the course of treatment. Surgeries are then performed if the injury is persistent or traumatic (such as an anterior cruciate ligament tear), or if the dancer elects to forego conservative methods to possibly return to performance sooner.

Several important details are missing in the abovementioned standard approach. Studies showed that at least 3% to 5% of female dancers have eating disorders such as bulimia and anorexia (6). Poor nutrition in these dancers may result in poor healing and should not be overlooked.

Moreover, training and technique errors are not usually addressed, nor are footwear, dance surfaces, or psychological stresses, all of which can contribute to injuries. We recommend the following detailed history and physical examination to improve both the treatments and the outcomes of dancers' injuries.

The Dancer's History

As with any patient, a good history is essential to help the examiner obtain a definitive diagnosis. The usual information regarding the chief complaint, course, onset, duration, exacerbation, remission, and other associated symptoms should be obtained from the injured dancer as well as a complete past medical, family, and social history, information regarding current usage of medicines, and a review of systems. However, the dance performance history is where the expertise of arts medicine comes into play and is essential in formulating an accurate diagnosis and correct treatment plan (Table 97-3).

In addition to the standard physical examination of sensation, reflexes, range of motion, and strength, the dancer's examination should include a careful musculoskeletal evaluation: the Ely and Thomas tests for hip flexor tightness; the Ely and Ober tests for quadriceps and iliotibial band tightness; determination of the popliteal angle for hamstring tightness; and the straight-leg raise, Larsen and one-leg extension tests for the spine. The upper-extremity examination for common shoulder problems should include the Neer, Hawkins, and supraspinatus test and the 180-degree arc to check for rotator cuff problems, and Speed and Yergason tests for biceps tendon problems (Table 97-4). Skeletal abnormalities of the spine and lower extremities such as scoliosis, hyperlordosis, tibial torsion, pes planus, pes cavus, hallux valgus, and hallux rigidus should be looked for.

The clinician should also be familiar with the technique of dancers. For example, in ballet the dancer turn-out (externally rotating the hips, knees, and feet so that the feet lie close to a 180-degree line) places the dancers in a unique position for injury. For proper turn-out, the patella should be in line with the second metatarsal area and the medial arch of the feet should not invert. This basic alignment has to be maintained in all classical ballet positions and movements (i.e., first position, demi-plié, grande jeté, pirouette, etc) (Figs. 97-1 and 97-2). Dancers can try to force their turn-out to obtain the desired aesthetic quality; however, this can place abnormal forces on the feet, knees, hips, and back.

Dancers are hyperflexible but not necessarily hypermobile (23,32,33). Their flexibility is necessary for proper ballet technique. For example, in order for the female dancer to do pointe work (dancing on the toes with a supportive shoe) (Fig. 97-3) or demi-pointe work (dancing with the foot plantarflexed, toes dorsiflexed, and weight on the metatarsals) (Fig. 97-4), 90 degrees of plantarflexion and 45 degrees of great toe dorsiflexion are required

Table 97-3: Dancer's History

- Type of dance
- Training/years
  - Student (level)
  - Teacher
  - Preprofessional
  - Professional
  - College
  - Recreational
- Ballet pointe work
  - Age at onset
  - No. of years
- Practice/work schedule
  - Hours per week
  - Number of classes
  - Recent changes
  - Change in style
  - Auditions
  - Touring
  - Upcoming performance
  - Recent break/layoff
- Working conditions
  - Type of dance surface
  - Footwear used
- Current exercise program
  - Warm-up/cooldown
  - Other activities (sports)
  - Cross-training
  - Hobbies
  - Amount of time spent
- Previous dance injuries
- Previous treatments
  - Medical
  - Surgical
  - Alexander
  - Pilates
  - Feldenkrais
  - Physical therapy
  - Chiropractic
  - Acupuncture
  - Massage
  - Modalities
  - Other

Table 97-4: Lower and Upper Extremity Tests

Anatomic Part Tested	Test
Lower Extremity	
Hip flexors	Thomas, Ely
Quadriceps	Ely
Hamstrings	Popliteal angle (normal 0 degrees)
Iliotibial band	Ober
Lower spine	Larsen, one leg extension, straight-leg raise
Upper extremity	
Rotator cuff	Neer, Hawkins, supraspinatus, 180 degree arc
Biceps tendon	Speed, Yergason

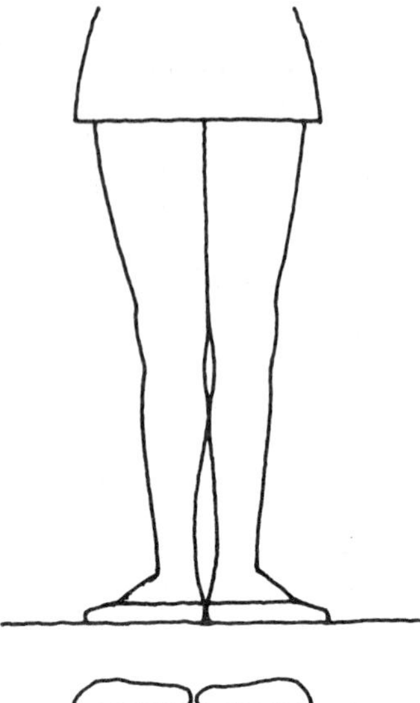

Figure 97-1. First position.

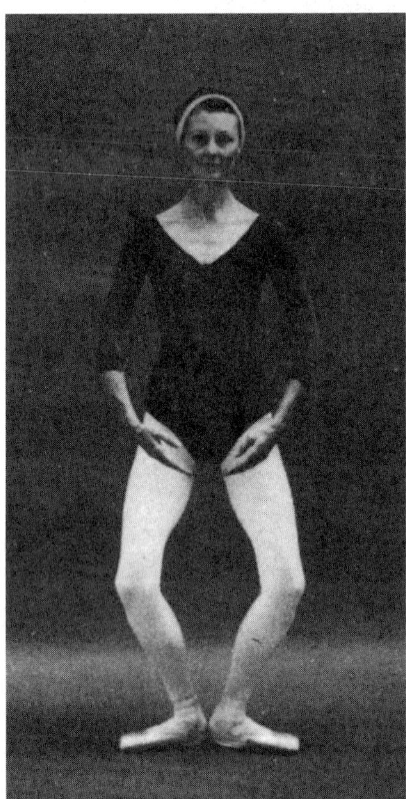

Figure 97-2. Demi-plié.

(21,23,34). Hip external rotation of more than 45 degrees is needed for adequate turn-out. Sixty percent of turn-out comes from the hips and 40% from the knees and feet (23,35). Dancers who are hypermobile are prone to injury (23,32,33,36). Their increased flexibility comes from years of stretching the hamstrings and the spine both in exten-

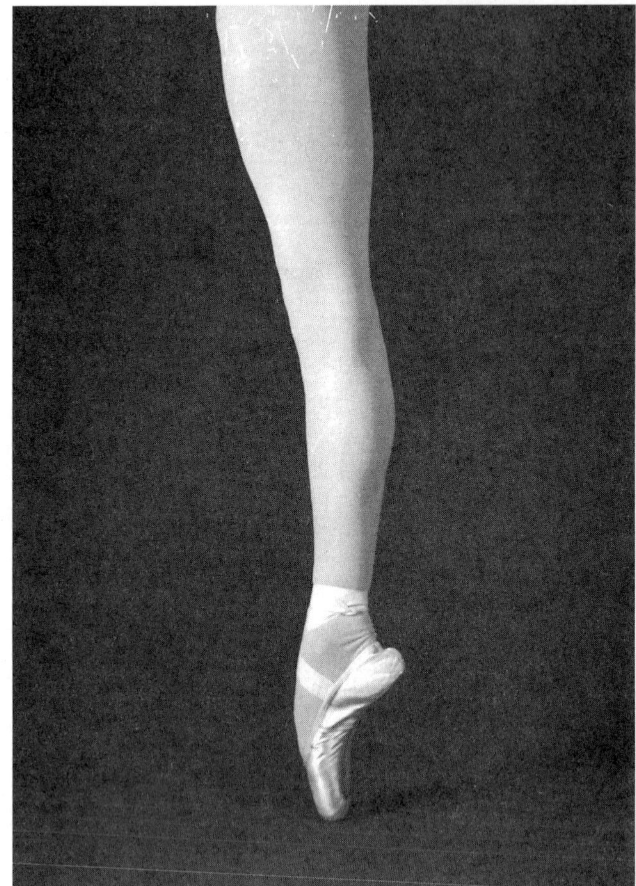

Figure 97-3. Pointe.

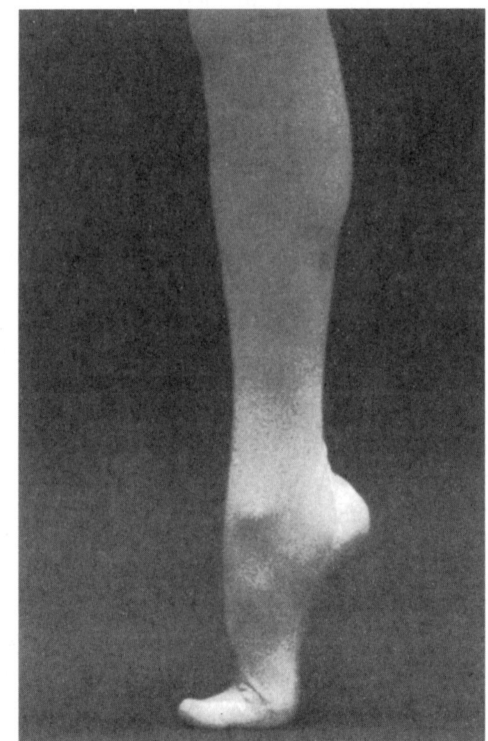

Figure 97-4. Demi-pointe.

sion and in flexion. They do not necessarily have increased range of motion in the hip as compared to nondancers, but do have increased flexibility in the knees and feet (23,32,33,35,36). All of these characteristics need careful attention during the dancer's examination. Once this detailed examination is completed, the clinician will be better equipped to accurately diagnose and treat the injured dancer.

Epidemiology

The most common injuries sustained by dancers are musculoskeletal overuse injuries to the lower extremities. These injuries account for 85% to 90% of all dance injuries. Female dancers sustain injuries more often than male dancers. In most professional ballet companies, approximately 10% of dancers are injured per contract year, with injury rates reported from 3.0 to 4.6 per dancer at all ages (21–23,25). The foot and ankle are the most commonly injured areas, followed by the knee, hip, and spine.

Several foot pathologies are seen, including hallux valgus, claw toes, hammer toes, bone spurs, stress fractures, corns, and calluses. These are mostly seen in female ballet dancers because of their pointe work. The most common foot injury is a stress fracture, usually involving the second metatarsal and occasionally the Lisfranc joint (37,38). The Lisfranc joint is formed by the medial and lateral cuneiforms around the base of the second metatarsal, which lock the second metatarsal into place, increasing stresses to this bone. Traumatic fractures including the Jones fracture and short oblique (dancer's) fracture also occur (39).

The least problematic foot morphology for the dancer is the peasant foot, where the first three toes are of equal length with a flat forefoot and sturdy arch. The Grecian (Morton) foot with the short first ray increases the dancer's risk of second metatarsal stress fractures because of the prominent second ray. Because of intense pressure to maintain an "ideal" lithe body, dancers have a higher rate of anorexia (3%), bulimia, amenorrhea, and late menarche (6), all of which can increase susceptibility to these stress fractures. Other foot and ankle problems include sprains, Achilles tendinitis, flexor hallucis tendinitis, plantar fasciitis, anterior and posterior impingement syndromes of the talus, and os trigonum (40,41).

The most common knee injuries are patellofemoral syndrome or anterior knee pain. Jumper's knee, shin splints, and subluxed patella follow in frequency. Traumatic injuries such as anterior cruciate ligament, medial collateral ligament, meniscal, and lateral collateral ligament tears do occur but less frequently (26).

In the hip, dancers often complain of pain and clicking while performing développé (lifting the leg to more than 90 degrees of flexion or abduction) (Fig. 97-5). This is usually caused by iliopsoas tendinitis or apophysitis, or less commonly by rectus femoris tendinitis or apophysitis. Thigh or groin strains are also common. Avulsion fractures of the sartorius and rectus femoris origins are seen less often (26).

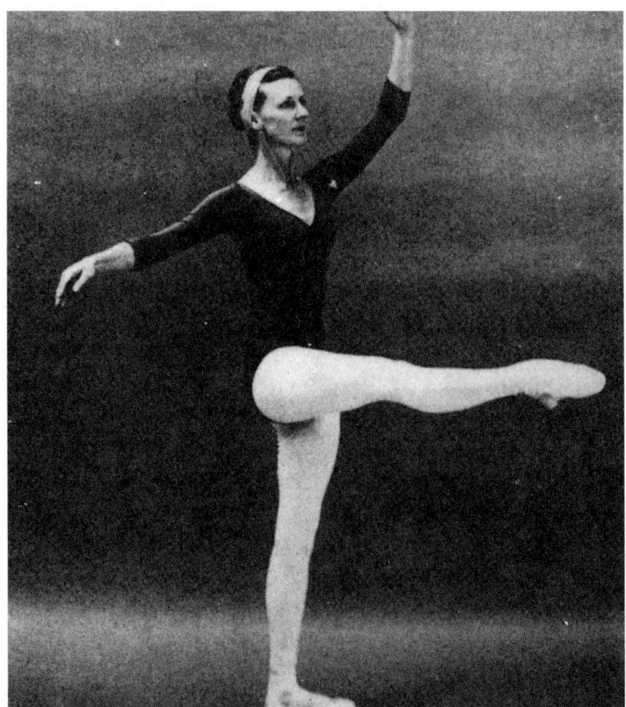

Figure 97-5. Développé.

Low-back pain in the dancer usually derives from muscular strains. However, because of the extreme hyperlordosis used to extend the spine, dancers do have an increased rate of stress fractures of the posterior elements, particularly pars defects or spondylolysis. Spondylolisthesis and disk herniations are rare (26).

Pathognomonics and Technique

Training and equipment errors can account for many of the overuse injuries in dancers. In addition to the great physical stressors of their work, dancers often have to put up with performing on hard surfaces using inadequate footwear. Ideally, dance surfaces should be a suspended floor of wood or marley surface since these special floors do reduce the risk of injuries (26). The ballet technique shoe (the soft shoe) can also be modified to reduce impact pressures without interfering with the dancer's feel for the floor (42). The pointe shoe—a hard toe box and wood shack that allows one to dance on the toes—forces the toes into a small area, predisposing the toes to deformities and injury. In contrast, the Gaynor Minden pointe shoe is form fitting and has some shock-absorbing qualities. Current research is pending on the actual functional benefits of this shoe.

Another area of concern is starting pointe work when a dancer is too young. Female dancers should not attempt pointe work until at least the age of 10 years, or until they have the strength and technical ability to perform pointe work. Dancers who are not strong enough

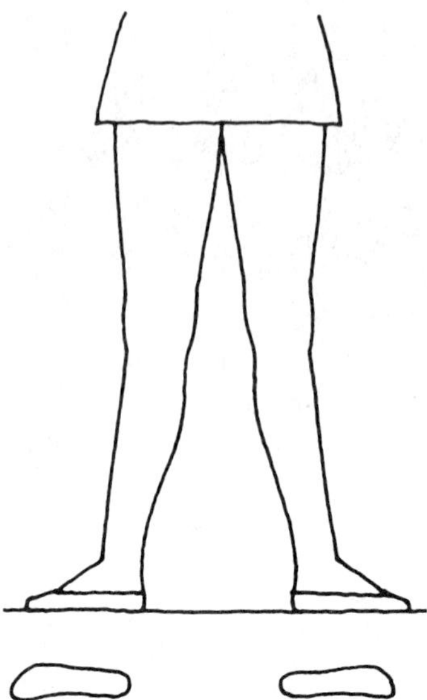

Figure 97-6. Second position.

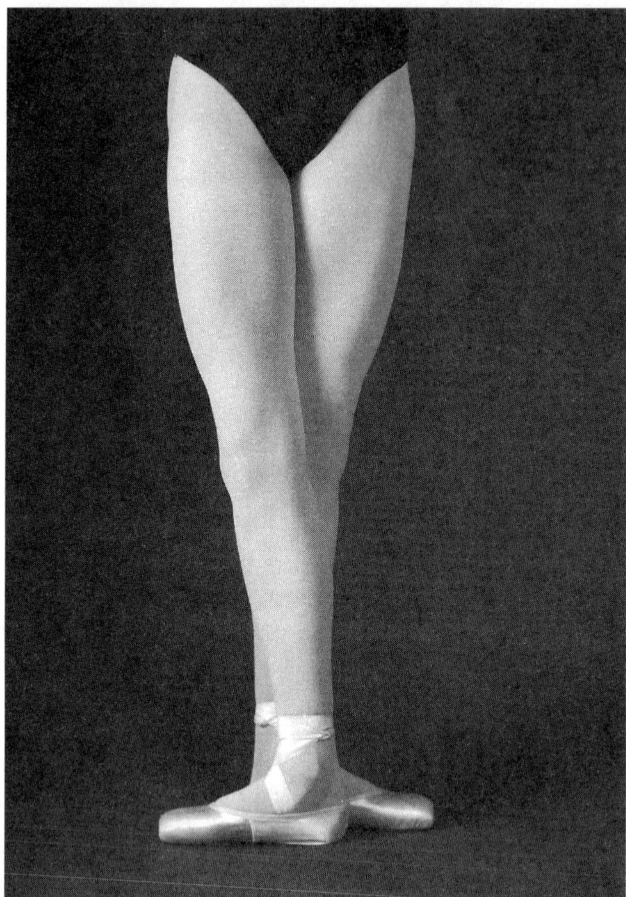

Figure 97-7. Third position.

to do pointe work tend to "knuckle down" or flex the toes inside the pointe shoe. This can lead to growth plate injury, stress fractures, joint deformities, and improper technical placement of the ankle, knees, hips, and spine along the kinetic chain.

Turn-out is the fundamental basis for ballet. There are five foot positions that dancers use in classical ballet—first, second, third, fourth, and fifth (see Figs. 97-1 and 97-6 to 97-9). Dancers need at least 45 degrees of external rotation at the hip to perform these positions. The amount of hip turn-out is determined by the femoral neck shaft angle, the anteversion angles, and the flexibility of the Y ligament of Bigelow. If dancers are lacking "perfect" turn-out, they have several ways of cheating, which leads to injury. One way of cheating is to tilt the pelvis back and hyperextend the spine. This can lead to hip problems as well as low-back injuries such as spondylolysis.

Another common cheating technique is to "screw the knee," "roll in" the foot, and excessively grip the floor. The dancer will place the feet in either of the five positions in 180-degree external rotation while the knees are half bent in a demi-plié. While doing this, the dancer allows the feet to invert on the floor, holding this position by gripping the floor with the flexor hallucis longus, flexor digitorum longus, and foot intrinsic musculature. The dancer then stands straight with an apparently perfect turned-out position. Unfortunately, this leads to great stresses on the knee, patellar, tibial, foot, and ankle structures, which predisposes the dancer to all the previously mentioned injuries of the lower extremity. The dancer should avoid this technique at all cost, and dance instructors should be correcting this training error. The clinician should also note the amount of tibial torsion that naturally occurs, because increased tibial torsion also increases a dancer's likelihood of injury to the knee and tibia (e.g., stress fractures, patellofemoral syndrome, and subluxing patella).

The final technique errors are sickling the foot (oversupinating) or winging the foot (overpronating). In order to have beautifully high-arched pointed feet, dancers may oversupinate the pointed or fully plantarflexed foot. This can lead to increased inversion sprains in the feet as well as impingement problems of the talonavicular articulation. Overpronating the foot also provides the dancer with a more beautiful line. The supinated foot is the most stable, yet most dancers hold the foot overpronated. This leads to overuse injuries. The foot biomechanics of dance are complex and have been well documented, but are beyond the scope of this chapter. For further information on this topic, the reader is referred to other works (28,38,43,44).

The aesthetic lines of the legs and feet are extremely important to ballet dancers. As long as they maintain a neutral pelvis with proper positioning of the lower extremity, the knees in a line over the second metatarsal, and the medial arch everting, they will develop fewer injuries. Their work requires a tremendous amount of loading to the tissues, so cumulative microtrauma occurs and some injuries may be unavoidable during a busy season.

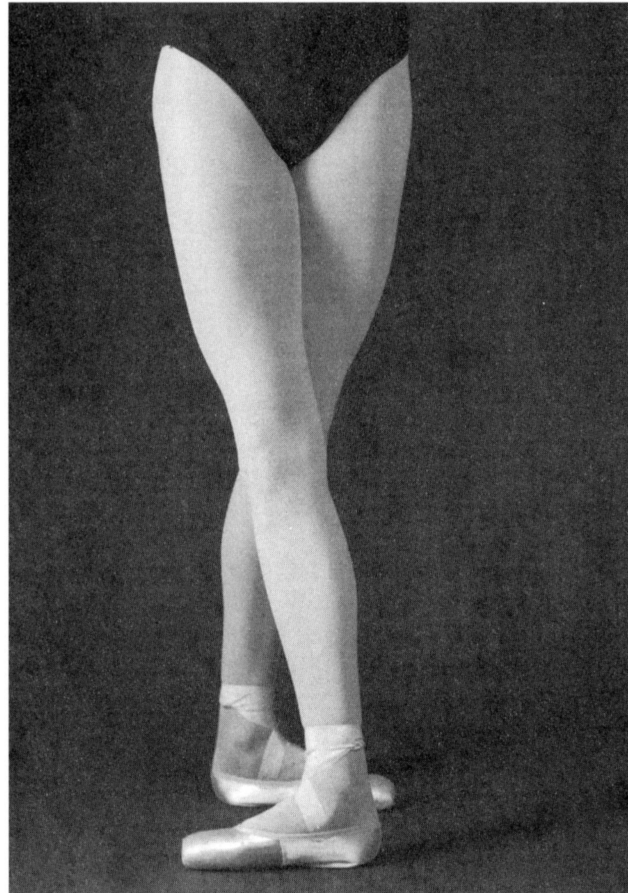

Figure 97-8. Fourth position.

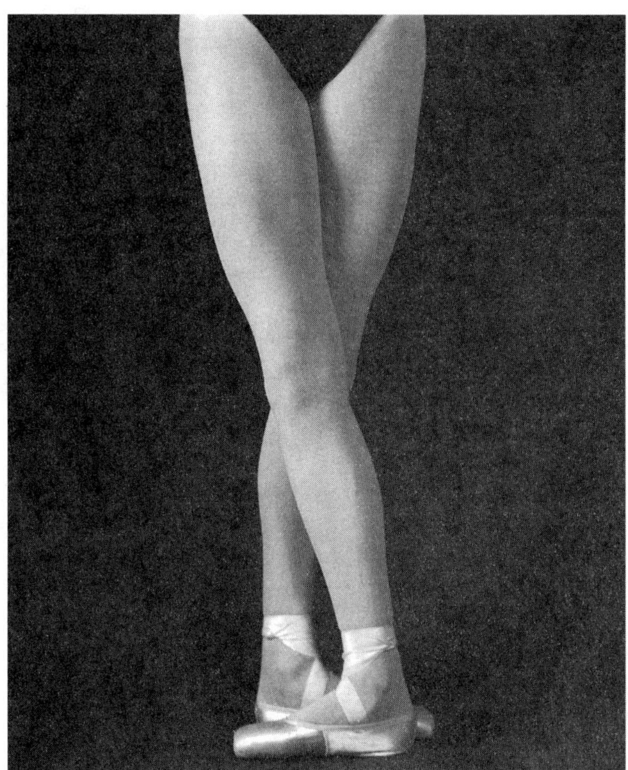

Figure 97-9. Fifth position.

Table 97-5: Lower-Extremity Flexibility Checks	
Site	**Degree**
Hips	>45 degrees of external rotation
Knee	Minimal tibial torsion
Ankle/foot	>90 degrees of plantarflexion; >10 degrees of dorsiflexion
Great toe	>45 degrees of dorsiflexion

Range of Motion

Dancers also develop tightness in their musculature, which then leads to injury and weakness. Maintaining proper flexibility and strength, therefore, is essential. Dancers in general have more flexibility in the feet, hips, and spine than do most people (Table 97-5). They are hyperflexible but not hypermobile; and dancers who are at the extreme ranges of flexibility are more prone to injuries (23,32,33,36). Several authors have documented range of motion characteristics of ballet dancers (21,23,34–36). Unfortunately, these studies were performed with different techniques so comparing the results is difficult. The reported mean ranges of motion of the hips, knee, and feet are listed in Table 97-6. These ranges can be used as guidelines only. A standard method for measuring the flexibility of dancers should be implemented for better clinical utility. Because dancers have numerous overuse injuries, maintaining their flexibility with a prolonged stretching program is extremely important.

Table 97-6: Range of Motion Data	
Site	**Mean (degrees)**
Hip	
Flexion/extension	107–135/29
Flexion + extension	198
Abduction	46–116
Abduction + adduction	80
External/internal rotation	43–54/22–54
Knee	
Flexion + extension	177
Hyperextension	7–10
Feet	
Plantarflexion/dorsiflexion	113–159/10–11
Ankle	
Inversion/eversion	23/15
Spine	
Flexion + extension	246
Lateral bending	110
Turn-out (feet measured on floor)	164

Figure 97-10. The reformer.

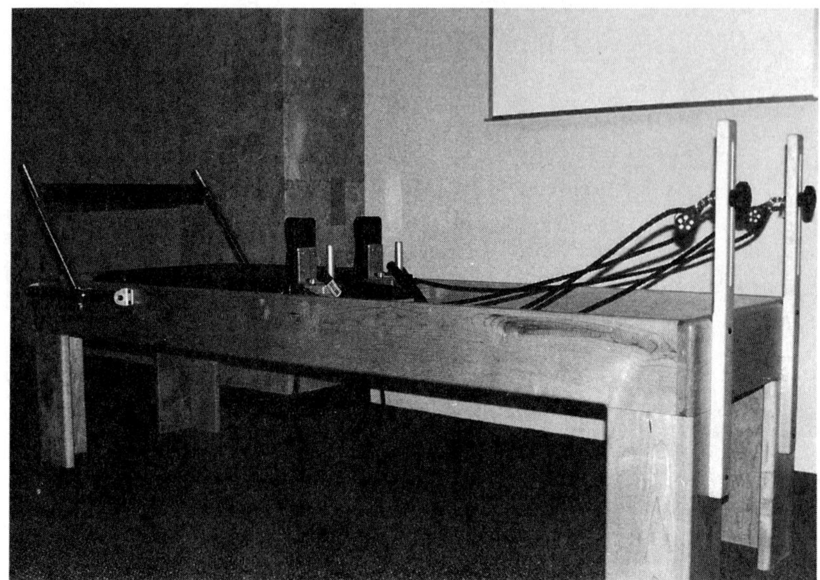

Strength

Dancers are extremely well-conditioned athletes, They have excellent muscle definition because of their low body fat (women typically have <15% of ideal body weight) and their acquired strength (23). Their art form demands anaerobic metabolism as well as aerobic capacity. The strength developed to perform ballet is highly exercise specific. There is some controversy in the literature as to whether dancers are stronger than other athletes. One study showed dancers' knee strength to fall between that of athletes and control subjects while another study showed no significant difference in knee and foot strength between dancers and controls (21,34).

Again, the methods for measuring strength are not standardized so drawing significant conclusions from this is difficult. One thing is certain: A female basketball player does not have the foot strength to do pointe work, and the female ballet dancer does not have the aerobic endurance to play a basketball game. This emphasizes the need for strengthening in an exercise-specific manner to achieve the desired physical ability. It is also important for the physician to recognize the dancer's normal strength to compare with the dancer's injured state.

Rehabilitation Principles

Treating dance injuries focuses on conservative measures while trying to avoid surgery at all costs. Most dancers will dance through injuries, which leads to chronic pain and sometimes even more severe injuries. The first general principle for all overuse injuries is to decrease pain. Relative rest or decrease in activity levels, medications (NSAIDs), modalities (ice, heat, ultrasound, iontophoresis, electrical stimulation, etc), and injections are standard. Early detection of technique and training errors is important to prevent injury recurrence. The next step is to restore or improve musculotendinous flexibility through pain-free stretches. Since dancers are more flexible than the average person, the stretches need to be challenging enough to adequately stretch the muscle and should be prolonged, more than 30 seconds, to break down the disulfide bonds that form in the myofibril unit.

As the injury improves, a progressive strengthening program is needed. Isometric strengthening is recommended intially during the acute stages of the injury. Later on, elastic tubing or isotonic exercises are commonly used for strengthening. Lifting low weights with multiple repetitions on pulley isotonic machines is also useful, as is aerobic conditioning in the pool or on a stationary bike. Isokinetic machines may be needed, depending on the injury or if the dancer is returning from surgery. The forms of strengthening exercises, however, should involve the ballet movements themselves.

The Pilates Method

Pilates therapy is a popular and effective strengthening method that is exercise specific for dance. Pilates therapy was developed in the 1930s from the teachings of Joseph H. Pilates, a boxer and weight lifter. This technique involves a series of floor exercises that focus on strengthening the abdominal musculature. In the Pilates method, these exercises are the basis for "finding the body's center." Ballet dancers benefit from this greatly because their technique requires excellent strength of their abdomen and control of their center of gravity. Pilates therapy also incorporates the use of several machines—the reformer, trap table, and chair. The reformer is more commonly used and is a plinth that slides horizontally on a wooden frame (Fig. 97-10). A series of springs attached to the platform increase the sliding resistance. The dancer pushes off from a footplate or bar for jumps or relevé work. At the other end are straps for use as an overhead pulley for the legs or arms. The dancer can essentially do a complete barré and some jumps on the reformer. They can rest the injured side and continue to keep the uninjured side in shape, as well as advance strengthening of the injured side in a non-weight-bearing manner. The reformer can also be used for stretching and strengthening eccentrically and concentrically in a closed-chain kinetic manner. Few studies are available on the use of the Pilates reformer, but one study by Henderson et al (45) showed that there is less impact pressure on the lower extremities when using the reformer.

Another nontraditional method of rehabilitating an injury is the Feldenkrais method (46). This form of therapy uses two principles. "Functional integration" is therapist-directed hands-on treatment to correct the patient's abnormal movement patterns. In "awareness through movement," the patient learns to correct abnormal patterns of muscle contraction by mentally imaging normal patterns with the help of a therapist's verbal cues. Feldenkrais therapy then is a form of neuromuscular relaxation, neuromuscular re-education, and biofeedback relaxation.

The Alexander technique is also a form of neuromuscular re-education and relaxation to restore normal movement patterns through the use of a therapist's verbal cuing. This technique is more popular with the musician.

Physical therapists can take courses on the Pilates, Feldenkrais, and Alexander techniques. Pilates certification requires a 6-week training course and 600 hours of clinical internship. The Feldenkrais method requires at least a year of training to incorporate this as a therapeutic method. Some physical therapists use the Feldenkrais method for arthritis rehabilitation and neuromuscular re-education. Further clinical studies are needed to help better define these treatment methods and outcomes in the current health care environment.

Surgical Considerations

Since most dance injuries are nontraumatic, surgery does not play a major role in dance medicine. The important consideration of any surgery is to make sure dancers do not lose the needed flexibility and strength to perform their art. Dancers have done well after meniscal repairs and reconstructive surgery for anterior cruciate ligament tears or internal derangements. There are no published reports on the best anterior cruciate ligament technique for dancers. However, the surgeon needs to consider how much flexibility and strength are required to return to dance. Some of the more common procedures performed are bone spur removal, os trigonum excision, flexor hallucis longus débridement, and patellar realignment. Achilles tendon rupture repair and disk herniation repairs usually signify career-ending injuries.

A complete and comprehensive conservative approach to all dance injuries should be pursued before surgery is considered. If surgery is needed, an aggressive postoperative rehabilitation program is required to restore the dancer's needed range of motion and strength. Pilates and pool therapies should be considered early, along with a carefully planned return to dance.

Future Considerations

The arts medicine field is still in its infancy. Many of the pressures of managed care and cost containment are just becoming an issue in this field. In the near future, arts medicine practitioners will be required to quantify and justify the results of their treatment programs. Therefore, it is essential that we develop adequate and accurate outcome measures for the practice of arts medicine. A yardstick for functional performance of an artist obviously would have to go beyond basic mobility and activities of daily living. The challenge will be to develop a tool that is specific enough to identify subtle functional deficits that could make or break a performer's career, yet general enough to apply to most performing artists. Once a standardized outcome measure is agreed upon, then clinical trials and multicentered studies may begin to test the worthiness of our traditional physical therapeutics. Only then can we legitimize our practice and justify the existence of this highly specialized field of medicine.

In addition to outcome studies, preventive techniques and education are needed in the areas of nutrition, substance abuse, human immunodeficiency virus, dance floors, protective footwear, ergonomics, and practice and training errors. The performing artists and their educators alike need to play active roles to help direct health care providers for their specific needs. Most of all, we as health care providers to the performing arts community must reach out to educate and learn from our patient population.

REFERENCES

1. Poore GV. Clinical lecture on certain conditions of the hand and arm which interfere with the performance of professional acts, especially piano playing. *BMJ* 1887;1:441–444.
2. Ostwald P. Historical perspectives on the treatment of performing and creative artists. *Med Probl Perform Art* 1994;9:113–118.
3. Fry HJH. Incidence of overuse syndrome in the symphony orchestra. *Med Probl Perform Art* 1986;1:51–55.

4. Fry HJH. Prevalence of overuse (injury) syndrome in Australian music schools. *Br J Ind Med* 1987;44:35–40.

5. Fry HJH. Overuse syndrome of the upper limb in musicians. *Med J Aust* 1986;144:182–183.

6. Fishbein M, Middlestadt SE, Ottati V, et al. Medical problems among ICSOM musicians: overview of a national survey. *Med Probl Perform Art* 1988;3:1–8.

7. Caldron PH, Calabrese LH, Clough JD, et al. A survey of musculoskeletal problems encountered in high-level musicians. *Med Probl Perform Art* 1986;1: 136–139.

8. Revak JM. Incidence of upper extremity discomfort among piano students. *Am J Occup Ther* 1988; 43:149–154.

9. Hiner WL, Brandt KD, Katz BP, et al. Performance-related medical problems among premier violinists. *Med Probl Perform Art* 1987;2: 67–71.

10. Newmark J, Lederman RJ. Practice doesn't necessarily make perfect: incidence of overuse syndromes in amateur instrumentalists. *Med Probl Perform Art* 1987;2: 142–144.

11. Newmark J, Salmon P. Playing-related complaints in nonclassical instrumentalists: a pilot questionnaire survey. *Med Probl Perform Art* 1990;5:106–108.

12. Batson G. Conscious use of the human body in movement: the peripheral neuroanatomic basis of Alexander technique. *Med Probl Perform Art* 1996;11:3–11.

13. Spire M. The Feldenkrais method: an interview with Anat Baniel. *Med Probl Perfom Art* 1989;4: 159–162.

14. Newmark J, Weinstein MS. A proposed standardized medical history and physical form for musicians. *Med Probl Perform Art* 1995;10: 137–139.

15. Norris RN. *The musician's survival guide: a guide to preventing and treating injuries in instrumentalists.* International Conference of Symphony and Opera Musicians. St. Louis: MMB Music, Inc., 1993:107.

16. Smutz WP, Bishop AT, Niblock H, et al. Load on the right thumb of the oboist. *Med Probl Perform Art* 1995;10:94–99.

17. Levy CE, Lee WA, Brandfonbrener AG, et al. Electromyographic analysis of muscular activity in the upper extremity generated by supporting a violin with and without a shoulder rest. *Med Probl Perform Art* 1992;7:103–109.

18. Andersen JI. Orthotic device for flutist's digital nerve compression. *Med Probl Perform Art* 1990;5: 91–93.

19. Norris RN. Design for a right thumb rest for the flute based on physical analysis. *Med Probl Perform Art* 1990;5:161–162.

20. Norris RN. Applied ergonomics: the angled-head flute. *Flutist Q* 1989;14:60–61.

21. Bejjani FJ. Performing artist's occupational disorders. In: Delisa JA, ed. *Rehabilitation medicine. Principles and practice.* 2nd ed. Philadelphia: JB Lippincott, 1993:1182–1190.

22. Garrick JG, Requa RK. Ballet injuries. An analysis of epidemiology and financial outcomes. *Am J Sports Med* 1993;21:586–590.

23. Hamilton WG, Hamilton LH, Marshall P, et al. A profile of the musculoskeletal characteristics of elite professional ballet dancers. *Am J Sports Med* 1992;20: 267–273.

24. Quirk R. Ballet injuries: the Australian experience. *Clin Sports Med* 1983;2:584.

25. Solomon R, Micheli LJ, Solomon J, et al. The cost of injuries in a professional ballet company: anatomy of a season. *Med Probl Perform Art* 1995;10:3–10.

26. Washington EL. Musculoskeletal injuries in theatrical dancers: site, frequency and severity. *Am J Sports Med* 1978;6:80–83.

27. Hamilton LH, Hamilton WG. Occupational stress in classical ballet dancers: the impact in different cultures. *Med Prob Perform Art* 1994;9:35–38.

28. Solomon RL, Trepman E, Micheli LJ. Foot morphology and injury patterns in ballet and modern dancers. *Kinet Med Dance* 1990;12:20–40.

29. Werter R. Dance floors: a causative factor in dance injuries. *J Am Podiatr Med Assoc* 1985;75: 355–358.

30. Hamilton WG. Tendinitis about the ankle joint in classical ballet dancers. *Am J Sports Med* 1977; 5:84–88.

31. Micheli LJ, Sohn RS, Solomon R. Stress fractures of the second metatarsal involving Lisfranc's joint in ballet dancers. *J Bone Joint Surg [Am]* 1985;76: 1372–1376.

32. Grahame R, Jenkins JM. Joint hypermobility—asset or liability? A study of joint mobility in ballet dancers. *Ann Rheum Dis* 1972; 31:109–111.

33. Klemp P, Stevens JE, LIsaacs S. A hypermobility study in ballet dancers. *J Rheumatol* 1984;11: 692–696.

34. Solomon R, Micheli LJ, Ireland ML. Physiological assessment to determine readiness for pointe work in ballet students. *Impulse* 1993;1:21–38.

35. Garrick JG, Requa RK. Turnout and training in ballet. *Med Prob Perform Art* 1994;9:43–49.

36. Miller CD, Gooch J, Haben M. Lower extremity range of motion in advanced level ballet dancers. *Kinet Med Dance* 1992;15:59–88.

37. Hamilton WG. Foot and ankle injuries in dancers. *Clin Sports Med* 1988;7:143–173.

38. Kravitz SR, Huber S, Ruziskey JA, et al. Biomechanical analysis of maximal pedal stress during ballet stance. *J Am Podiatr Med Assoc* 1987;77:484–489.

39. Zelko RR, Torg JS, Rachun A. Proximal diaphyseal fracture of the fifth metatarsal: treatment of fractures and their complications in

athletes. *Am J Sports Med* 1979;7:95–101.

40. Hamilton WG. Stenosing tenosynovitis of the flexor hallucis longus tendon and posterior impingement upon the os trigonum in ballet dancers. *Foot Ankle* 1982;3:74–80.

41. Marotta JJ, Micheli LJ. Os trigonum impringement in dancers. *Am J Sports Med* 1992;20: 533–536.

42. Miller CD, Paulos LE, Parker RD, et al. The ballet technique shoe: a preliminary study of eleven differently modified ballet technique shoes using force and pressure plates. *Foot Ankle* 1990;11: 97–100.

43. Hardaker WT. Foot and ankle injuries in classical ballet dancers. *Orthop Clin North Am* 1989;20: 621–627.

44. Marr SJ. The ballet foot. *J Am Podiatr Med Assoc* 1986;73: 124–132.

45. Henderson J, Brown SE, Price S, et al. Foot pressures during a common ballet jump in standing and supine positions. *Med Prob Perform Art* 1993;8:125–131.

46. Feldenkrais M. *Awareness through movement.* New York: HarperCollins, 1990.

RECOMMENDED READING

Journals

Medical problems of performing artists. Brandfonbrener A, ed. Philadelphia: Hanley & Belfus.

Journal of dance medicine and science. Clippinger KS, Brown SE. eds. Andover: J. Michael Ryan Publishing. Inc.

Books

Norris RN. *Musician's survival manual: a guide to preventing and treating injuries in instrumentalists.* St. Louis: MMB Music, Inc., 1993.

Samama A. *Muscle control for musicians: a series of exercises for daily practice.* Utrecht: Bohn, Scheltema & Holkema, 1981.

Sataloff RT, Brandfonbrener AG, Lederman RJ, eds. *Textbook of performing arts medicine.* New York: Raven, 1991.

Thomasen E. *Diseases and injuries of ballet dancers.* Copenhagen: Åarhuus Stiftbogtrykkerie, 1982.

Watkins A, Clarkson PM. *Dancing longer, dancing stronger: a dancer's guide to improving technique and preventing injury.* Princeton: Princeton Book, 1990.

Other

Internet access to Occupational Diseases of Performing Artists: Bibliography—http://www.sailor.lib.md.us/forms/music_bib.html, Maintained by Susan E. Harman, Associate Librarian, Clearinghouse Coordinator, Medical & Chirurgical Faculty Library, University of Maryland.

Chapter 98

Ethnic and Minority Issues

Timothy R. Elliott
Gitendra Uswatte

Multicultural issues have received great attention in recent years in the medical, behavioral, and social sciences. Unfortunately, researchers in physical medicine and rehabilitation have been conspicuously silent with regard to this topic, despite the fact that many racial and ethnic issues arise in the care of patients with chronic disease, injury, and disability. In the absence of meaningful conceptual models and rigorous empirical data, clinicians may inadvertently rely on anecdotal lore and subtle, if not blatant stereotypes of patients who are not members of the majority culture. The degree to which these practices can affect clinical care is generally unknown, although converging evidence suggests that the risk for insensitive and ineffectual treatment is high when cultural differences are ignored, minimized, or misconstrued. A rudimentary understanding and appreciation of ethnic and minority issues may help physicians enhance the care for and provide more efficacious treatments to members of the nonmajority cultures.

The multicultural issues addressed in the extant rehabilitation literature have been examined by specific service providers in vocational rehabilitation (1) or have been examined with respect to broader issues in the role of biopsychosocial mechanisms in behavioral health (2). More specialized and condition-specific issues have been studied in isolated research projects that have yet to be synthesized in any meaningful fashion for rehabilitation professionals. Thus, a rather disjointed literature speaks to ethnic and minority issues regarding spinal cord injury (SCI), pain, dementia, and other conditions typically seen by professionals in physical medicine and rehabilitation.

In this chapter, we first propose a definition of ethnic minorities in Western society and touch on some important general issues related to ethnicity. We then review specific social, behavioral, and environmental risk factors related to ethnic minority status that contribute to the onset of disabling conditions and secondary complications following rehabilitation. Ethnic and minority issues related to psychosocial reactions to disability and chronic disease are then discussed. These sections examine cultural differences in adjustment to disability, symptom expression, affective reactions, coping behaviors, family reactions, and societal and service perceptions of individuals of minority status with disability. Finally, implications for clinical practice and research are offered.

DEFINING ETHNIC MINORITIES IN WESTERN SOCIETIES

Ethnic groups are collections of individuals who identify themselves and who are identified by the larger society as sharing a common cultural heritage (3). This common history and experience can include country of origin, language, religion, values, art, cuisine, family structure, health beliefs, and other elements. In the United States, ethnic minority groups are generally considered to be those cultural groups with a non-European cultural heritage. The major categories of groups, in descending order of population, are African-Americans (31.1 million); Latinos, individuals whose ancestry lies in Mexico, Puerto Rico, Cuba, Central and South America, or Spain (22.3 million); Asian/Pacific Islanders (7.3 million); and Native Americans (1 million) (4–6). All of these groups are diverse and include subgroups with distinct cultures. The cultural groupings are often considered synonymous with race. The association, however, is not that close; for example, there are Latino persons with an African genetic heritage. The groupings are also associated with economic status. There are a disproportionate number of African-Americans (32.7%), Latinos (25%), and Native Americans (28%) with incomes below the poverty line (4,7).

An important difference identified by many researchers between the ethnic minority cultures and the majority culture in the United States is the emphasis on collectivistic versus individualistic behavior (8). In many minority cultures, the needs and desires of the family and the community hold much more weight than they do in the majority, European-American culture (9–11). This differential emphasis on collectivistic action and thought is related to a different conception of the self. In many minority cultures, the self is viewed as a function of one's social roles and environment or as a manifestation of some larger entity. This is in sharp contrast to the traditional European view of the self as located within one's person and as the creator and controller of thoughts and behavior (12). The implication of these contrasting world views for clinical practice is that patients and families from minority backgrounds may place very different values on independence as a goal for rehabilitation than patients and families from majority backgrounds do. In addition, persons from individualistic cultures are more apt to attribute behavior to individual characteristics (e.g., personality, motivation, abilities) while those from collectivistic cultures are more likely to attribute behavior to situational and environmental factors (8).

Another important difference for health care professionals between ethnic minority cultures and the majority involves beliefs about health care. Many ethnic minority individuals both espouse traditional forms of medicine native to their ethnic group and distrust modern medicine. A series of studies documented that Native Americans do not expect fair treatment from non-Native health care professionals (13), that less acculturated Asian-Americans sometimes view modern medicine as a last resort and may not value health insurance (14), and that African-Americans are skeptical of the opinions of physicians and rehabilitation professionals (15,16). Given this distrust of modern medicine, minority individuals may be more inclined to use herbs or potions, or seek the advice of a religious or spiritual community figure before seeking professional health care. Furthermore, research indicates that the interest in traditional forms of medicine among ethnic minority individuals is not mediated by level of education or income (17).

When an individual is identified as belonging to a certain ethnic group in the context of clinical practice or research, the assimilation and acculturation of the individual into the larger society and the majority culture are important factors to consider (18–20). *Assimilation* refers to the process of participating in the institutions of the society at large, while *acculturation* refers to the process of learning the manners and style of the dominant culture (3). Minority patients who are less assimilated and acculturated are more likely to hold to the cultural norms of their minority group exclusively and, therefore, require special attention. Minority patients who are more assimilated and acculturated can probably be treated using traditional assessment tools and intervention strategies (21). The Racial Attitudes and Identity Scale (RAIS) (22), the Acculturation Rating Scale for Mexican Americans II (ARSMA-II) (23), and the Suinn-Lew Asian Self-Identity Acculturation Scale (SL-ASIA) (24) are some research instruments that measure acculturation in African-American, Mexican-American, and Asian-American minority persons, respectively. In clinical practice, the age of entry to the United States and the English speech patterns of the patient can often be used to roughly gauge acculturation.

DISABILITY INCIDENCE AND RISK FACTORS RELATED TO ETHNIC MINORITY STATUS

A growing body of epidemiologic data indicates that the incidence of particular disabling diseases and injuries is higher among certain ethnic minority groups than in the majority population. The incidence of disability among African-Americans (14.8%) is substantially higher than among European-Americans (8.4%) (25), owing to higher rates of vascular disease, cancer, criminal assault, and diabetes (26). While the overall rate of disability in the Latino and Native American populations does not appear to diverge sharply from that in the majority population, the incidence of injuries and diabetes is higher in these groups than among European-Americans (26). This differential incidence of disability is probably driven by factors associated with ethnic minority status such as poverty, restricted occupational and educational opportunities, dangerous residential environments, limited access to health care, experience of discrimination, and culture-specific health behaviors (27).

The high rate of vascular disease among the African-American population is, among other factors, related to poor knowledge of health risks, limited access to health care, diet, and cognitive style. In a recent survey of African-Americans, one-fifth stated that they have no usual source of medical care and that they visit an emergency room or clinic when acute symptoms develop (26). Persons with this sort of access to health care are unlikely to receive screening for hypertensive problems and preventive treatment. African-Americans have a high fat-intake level in their diet compared to the majority population group. This bias toward fatty foods, which is largely due to a high consumption of fatty meats, is evident across all income levels (20) and is not common to other minority groups. The belief or cognitive style that one can control environmental stressors through hard work and determination, despite the lack of adequate socioeconomic resources, has been linked to hypertension among African-American men of low socioeconomic status (28,29). [This relationship has not been found among African-American college students (30).]

The relatively high incidence of certain types of cancer among African-Americans and some other ethnic minorities is, again among other factors, related to environmental and occupational hazards and health-related behaviors. Minority individuals are overrepresented in poor neighborhoods that are more likely than wealthy areas to contain or be located near environmental hazards (14). Similarly, research indicates that African-Americans who are employed in semiskilled, low-paying jobs are more likely than European-Americans to be exposed to carcinogens, even after controlling for job experience and education (31). In contrast to the exposure to environmental and occupational risk factors, minority groups traditionally have had lower rates of tobacco consumption than the majority population. However, recent Asian male immigrants exhibit very high rates of smoking (20). In addition, new smoking surveys show an increase in the rate of smoking among African-American men.

The disproportionate representation of certain minority groups among certain types of spinal cord and traumatic brain injury is, among other factors, related to occupational and environmental hazards and health and risk-taking behaviors. There is a disproportionately high representation of African-Americans and Latinos among patients with SCI of a violent origin (32). African-Americans and Latinos are more likely to live in high-crime areas, which have a greater preponderance of stores specializing in the sale of alcoholic beverages compared to European-American neighborhoods (33). However, the relatively high risk of suffering violent injury is also related to such subculture-specific risk-taking behaviors as establishing ranking in peer relations through aggression (34). Other minority groups are at high risk for other specific types of injury. For example, Native Americans have the highest rate of motor vehicle accidents of any ethnic group in America, which may be due to the relatively high prevalence of alcoholism among Native American persons.

PSYCHOSOCIAL REACTIONS TO DISABLING CONDITIONS

Cultural identity and processes are glaringly absent in contemporary models of stress appraisal and coping following the onset of severe illness and disability (35). Substantial evidence, however, demonstrates that 1) cultural identity mediates the presentation, reporting, and meaning of physical problems in the rehabilitation setting; 2) the role of family and significant others in the adjustment and caregiving process varies with ethnic identity; and 3) ethnic minority patients sometimes encounter discrimination from rehabilitation professionals.

Cultural values among less acculturated Latinos, for example, may directly affect emotional and behavioral reactions to disability (36,37). Latino persons often adhere to strong values of allocentrism and familialism, interdependence on others, and *simpatico* and *respecto* in working with rehabilitation service providers. They may cope within frameworks that emphasize *spiritual beliefs*, clearly defined gender roles, and a "*present-time*" orientation (38). Consequently, a less acculturated Latino family may exhibit strong nuclear family support that buffers the patient against affective disturbance, but inadvertently reinforces functional dependence. The patient may defer and acquiesce to professional advice (*respecto*) and avoid conflict with authority figures (*simpatico*), but may not internalize recommendations or display initiative in the rehabilitation program. Men may feel an acute loss of productivity within their defined roles (*machismo*), while women may endure (*aguantar*) in a prescribed manner that appears adaptive in terms of affective adjustment, but implies passive behavior in directive therapies. Spiritual beliefs, too, may foster affective acceptance of disability, but inadvertently promote passive involvement in rehabilitation. Finally, the "present-time" orientation may influence a preference for pragmatic and immediate solutions and a disinterest in long-term planning (38). Thus, values unique to a less acculturated individual from a collectivistic cultural background that have adaptive features may also present the rehabilitation provider with a special challenge.

Pain Behavior

Ethnicity affects the degree to which individuals experience and report painful sensations and conditions. The experimental study of laboratory-induced pain suggests that ethnicity does not moderate the ability to discriminate painful sensations (39), but that ethnicity influences pain complaints and pain-related behaviors (39,40). The effects of cultural identity appear to be most apparent in studies in which patients with a low degree of acculturation are compared to members of the majority culture. For example, Honeyman and Jacobs (41) demonstrated that cultural beliefs induce a substantially different pattern of disability-related behavior among Australian Aboriginals than typically observed in Europeans. Although many of the Aboriginal patients in this study had a clear medical diagnosis of spinal pain, public displays of pain and psychosocial impairment and avoidance of activities were rare. In this community, the value placed on performance of community functions by injured individuals clearly superseded that placed on public displays of pain and impairment. Johnson et al (14) wrote that less acculturated Asian-Americans tend to express negative feelings and physical complaints less frequently than European-Americans. This stoic attitude is thought to constitute "keeping face," a tradition in Asian culture of presenting an honorable image to society. Congruent with this hypothesis, available data suggest that Asian-Americans are more likely to somaticize their emotional distress and to report more physical symptoms than feelings of sadness or anxiety on self-report instruments (14,42,43). The influence of culture on pain behavior in more acculturated minority populations is less marked (16).

Recent research suggests that acculturation to Western society may be associated with more health complaints and pain behaviors (44). Lipton and Marbach (16) found that greater acceptance of Western medicine was associated with more pain complaints among African-Americans. This relationship, however, was moderated differently by locus of control within each ethnic group. A more internal locus of control was associated with greater pain intensity among European-Americans, while a more external locus of control was associated with greater pain intensity among Hispanics (44,45).

Affective Responses to Disability

The evidence concerning affective responses to disability is less clear. Results of a preliminary study suggest that minority women with SCI experience more emotional distress than other individuals with SCI (46). The results also indicate that minority patients with SCI report significantly more problems with financial issues and skill deficits than do European-American patients with SCI. In a 1993 study by Westbrook et al (47), health practitioners working in different ethnic communities in a Western country reported different reactions to and perceptions of their ethnic minority patients. Men with disabilities from a Chinese community were perceived by health practitioners as less likely to be emotionally communicative than a group of Europeans. Men of Greek and Arabic identity were perceived to be more likely to express grief than the Europeans in this study. The European men were perceived as more inclined to express anger, pessimism, shame, and depression than the other men. This finding is in contrast to a similar study which found ethnic minority patients to be significantly less optimistic about their future than European patients (48). This latter study also found that persons from minority groups were concerned that poverty, disability, and their ethnic identity would handicap them in society.

Adjustment to Disability

There is descriptive evidence of distinct relationships between ethnic minority status and adjustment among rehabilitation patients. In a survey of African-Americans with disabilities, Belgrave (49) found that social support, self-esteem, and perception of disability severity were significantly correlated with acceptance of disability. Davis et al (50) reported that African-Americans with SCI tend to have a less positive self-concept, a lower internal locus of control than European-Americans with SCI, and greater external expectancies of control than European-Americans. These expectancies for control over behavioral reinforcement are believed to be closely aligned with rates of reinforcement provided by the psychosocial environment. European-Americans may have more internal expectancies because they experience and perceive a greater correspondence between their behavior and actual rates of reinforcement for performance; African-Americans, in contrast, may experience and perceive *less* correspondence between their behavior and rates of reinforcement from the environment. Thus, many African-Americans may accurately perceive their behavior at times to be influenced more by external events outside the realm of personal volition than by controllable factors.

Data also suggest that persons of minority status may be at increased risk for secondary complications following disability. In the most comprehensive and thorough study to date, Furher et al (51) found that a greater proportion of African-Americans had severe pressure sores than did European-American patients. The reasons for this finding are unclear. The authors speculated that the dark skin pigmentation of African-Americans may make it more difficult to detect early skin breakdown. Poor access to preventive and routine health care relative to European-American patients may also hinder early detection (52).

Family Reactions and Caregiving

Social support, in particular family support, is an important factor in recovery and rehabilitation subsequent to a disabling injury. Cultural differences in family structures and dynamics, therefore, can be important considerations in the rehabilitation process.

The very constitution of family in minority ethnic groups can differ from that in the majority. Whereas in many European-American families the close family consists of mother, father, and children, in many minority families this can include grandparents, aunts, and uncles (18,53). African-American families often include members not related by blood or marriage, but by shared values, norms, and beliefs (54). This is exemplified by the findings of White-Means and Thornton (55) and Lawton et al (56) that caregivers in African-American families can be close or distant relatives or fictive kin and that the quality of care does not vary with the closeness of blood relationship.

The extended-family structure and the collectivistic spirit characteristic of many minority families suggest that these families might be able to cope better with a disabling injury to a family member than European-American families. Research comparing African-American and European-American families, in fact, indicates that African-American families may cope better with the challenge imposed by a disability than European-American families. Pickett et al (57) found that African-American parents of children with disabilities had higher feelings of self-worth and lower levels of depression than did European-American parents with disabled children. Haley et al (58) found that caregiving for Alzheimer dementia patients was associated with less depression and higher life satisfaction in African-American caregivers than in European-American caregivers. The diminished negative impact of caregiving in African-American families appears to be related to a view of caregiving as an expected family function (9,59) and a regard for elder family members independent of their cognitive and behavioral abilities (60). There is little research comparing other ethnic groups to the majority group or to each other on the impact of caregiving.

The limited amount of research on the relationship between minority status and marital status after a disabling injury suggests that cultural differences have a small or negligible impact on marriage and divorce rates. DeVivo and Richards (61), in a recent study of 6853 SCI persons, found that African-Americans and Latinos do not have significantly different marriage rates than European-Americans. The evidence on the relationship between minority status and divorce is mixed. In a 1985 study with 276 SCI persons, DeVivo and Fine (62) reported that African-American minority status is significantly associated with a higher divorce rate. In a more recent study with 662 SCI persons, African-Americans and Latinos displayed higher, but not significantly different, divorce rates than European-Americans (62,63). The higher rates of divorce reported correspond to higher rates of divorce for these minority groups in the general population. The number of Asian-Americans and Native Americans in these studies was too small to draw any statistical inferences. There is no research on the relationship between minority status and marital status in the traumatic brain injury and stroke populations.

Societal Reactions and Provision of Services to Ethnic Minorities

Researchers and activists have argued that ethnic minority persons with physical disabilities face "double discrimination." In fact, ethnic minority persons may experience "triple discrimination." They can face discrimination by the majority *and* minority cultures on the basis of their disability and in the majority culture on the basis of their ethnic identity (64).

Societal attitudes toward persons with disability vary across cultures (65,66). In Asian-American cultures, physical disability, and deviance in general, are often tolerated if the individual still contributes competently in some fashion to the greater good of the immediate community (65). Although traditional Asian-American communities can attach stigma and embarrassment to physical disability, the disabled person who maintains an inner strength and accepts suffering as a part of the natural order is treated with and conveys dignity (65).

The fact that minority individuals receive differential treatment from rehabilitation professionals and other service providers is of more immediate concern. Data suggest that physicians treat patients differently on the basis of ethnic identity. Researchers have found that Latinos presenting with fractures receive less pain analgesics than do European-Americans presenting with the same type of fractures. The tendency to prescribe fewer analgesics for Latino patients than for European-American patients did not appear to be due to differences in displays of pain or physician assessment of pain complaints (67,68). Data also suggest that certain service providers expend fewer resources toward the rehabilitation of minority individuals than European-American individuals. James et al (69) found that African-Americans with SCI treated by participating centers in the Model Systems Database received less sponsorship and vocational training than did European-Americans. This finding may partly explain the relatively high rate of unemployment among African-Americans with SCI (69–71). Descriptive research has found similar discrimination against Native American clients in certain state vocational rehabilitation services (72). In addition, some data suggest that Chinese-Canadian children with disabilities receive less benefits from Canadian rehabilitation services than do European-Canadian children (73).

Such differential treatment may be partly due to misattributions on the part of service providers about minority client behavior. For example, some service providers may view minority clients as unmotivated because they do not adhere to the prescribed regimen of outpatient visits. Minority clients, however, are more likely to rely on public transport than European-American clients (52,74). The poor compliance of some minority clients, therefore, may be a function of economic resources rather than personal characteristics (75).

IMPLICATIONS FOR CLINICAL PRACTICE

The review of the literature suggests many recommendations for improving rehabilitation practices regarding care for persons with an ethnic minority background. We delineate specific implications in terms of *service delivery* and *prevention of secondary complications.*

Service Delivery and Intervention

Cultural sensitivity will enhance the rehabilitation services. Preliminary evidence indicates that modern medical interventions can be enhanced with less acculturated individuals, by integrating modern forms of medicine and health care with more traditional practices and including individuals who are strongly identified with the patient's ethnic community in the treatment team (76). Attempts to provide more culturally congruent programs on a Navajo reservation were associated with a dramatic increase in employment of clients with disabilities in one study (76). In another study African-American clients appeared to be more responsive to African-American service providers and felt more comfortable with and continued longer in rehabilitation services when they perceived greater sensitivity and competence in the rehabilitation provider (77). These data indicate that culturally sensitive approaches can heighten cooperation and possibly circumvent mistrust among clientele.

In general, clinicians should be aware of their own cultural biases and stereotypes when working with persons of minority status. Clinicians should be aware that nonverbal behaviors play a substantial role in clinical diagnoses and decision making. Individuals who are less assimilated into the majority culture may exhibit nonverbal behaviors that may easily be misinterpreted by insensitive clinicians. For example, lack of eye contact with the clinician and displays of indifference from an African-American client may not signify disinterest or disdain for the clinician, but rather may be related to issues of cultural mistrust and attempts to preserve self-concept under duress. In addition, the client might be sensitive to clinician behaviors that could imply suspicion and lack of respect (e.g., being scolded or rebuked by the service provider, service provider being tardy for an appointment, service provider providing incomplete or inconsistent information, displays of condescending or contemptuous attitudes).

Nonverbal behaviors may also complicate clinical decision making in other realms. For example, less acculturated individuals from Hispanic and Asian communities may defer to clinical recommendations and opinion, when in fact they may be observing cultural norms for displaying respect for the professional without necessarily internalizing or understanding the nature of the recommended regimen. Similarly, a stoic demeanor may mislead a clinician in the assessment of pain and pain-related discomfort when considering possible prescriptions for pain relief. A thorough interview with the patient and significant others may assist the clinician in providing therapeutic advice to the patient and in determining the need for medication or other interventions.

Clinicians should be aware that minority individuals may place a different emphasis on independence and on the role of certain family members in the caregiving process, compared to majority individuals and families. Certain groups, such as African-Americans, may have an extended sense of family that will include persons who are not blood kin. These individuals may be comfortable with and skilled in their caregiving roles and should be incorporated into family training programs. In contrast, psychological interventions may be indicated for individuals of a majority culture, as white caregivers can have many difficulties with psychological adjustment. These individuals may also be more receptive to support groups and other community-based interventions. Other individuals, such as those from a less acculturated Asian background, may be less receptive to psychologically based interventions.

Clinicians should also pay attention to the role of minority individuals in the educational materials used by rehabilitation staff. Whenever possible, audiovisual and instructional materials should display individuals from minority backgrounds, with examples identifying patients of minority background to enhance receptivity and learning. Ideally, facilities treating patients of certain minority backgrounds will have professionals and clinicians on staff of that same background. This would certainly assist in lowering cultural mistrust and increasing receptivity to rehabilitation practices. Furthermore, it may be particularly helpful to identify individuals from the minority community who can work as "role models" or mentors, who might volunteer to visit and confer with current patients in inpatient and outpatient settings.

Finally, it behooves all the disciplines represented in rehabilitation to examine their resource allocation practices to identify possible areas of bias.

Prevention of Secondary Complications

When considering the prevention of secondary complications, issues germane to general primary prevention among ethnic minorities also apply to the rehabilitation setting. Among persons of minority status, access to appropriate health care appears to be a major concern (2). Many individuals of minority status do not have adequate access to health care facilities, which is vital to the prevention and early identification of secondary complications common to physical disability. As noted earlier in the chapter, this may be due to a variety of factors including lack of financial coverage and lack of transportation. Strategies that can increase the probability of outpatient visits and early diagnosis are needed. These may include greater use of home health services, routine telephone contact or mailings, and improved relations with the informal caregiver. Such strategies may also be helpful in improving adherence to self-care regimens.

Self-care can involve issues of diet, self-management, and performance of specific regimens such as range of motion exercises, stretching, and appropriate transfers. Individuals who are of minority status and who live below the poverty line may have particular difficulty in adhering to these practices for a variety of reasons. Thus, community-based interventions that provide regular "booster" sessions and enhance the salience and practicality of such activities in the home may be particularly effective. Research that identifies incentives for and barriers to adherence to home treatment regimens among minority populations is much needed. Problems with diet vary considerably across cultures and may require specific solutions for each ethnic group.

Certain individuals of minority status will be discharged into communities in which many environmental hazards exist. These hazards might include violence, crime, drug use, and unsafe structures. Although some of these hazards appear to be outside the realm of traditional rehabilitation medicine and psychology practice, rehabilitation professionals may desire and need to work with public health experts to combat these threats to health.

IMPLICATIONS FOR RESEARCH

Review of the literature suggests that culture plays a substantial role in the incidence of disabling conditions and injuries, in the responses of patients to disabling injuries and diseases, and in the reactions of families and service providers to persons with disabilities. Further empirical studies are called for on these issues and on issues where the implications of cultural differences are yet unclear. Research priorities might include 1) clinical studies that develop and evaluate culturally congruent treatment and follow-up programs for particular ethnic groups; 2) correlational and experimental studies that examine the relationship among physical injury, pain-related behaviors, affective reactions, and the response of care providers across ethnic groups; 3) correlational studies that examine the relationship between the value of independence and rehabilitation goals across ethnic groups; and 4) archival research that documents areas of ethnic and racial bias in resource allocation. During research, it will be important to include acculturation as a factor, as acculturation is likely to either mediate or moderate the relationship between minority status and other variables, and to study these issues within as well as between groups.

In addition, the involvement of minority persons in consumer advocacy groups will help clinicians to appreciate new ways of understanding the research to date and will help to develop more culturally sensitive and effective rehabilitation programs in the future. We can learn much by studying the differences and similarities between persons of different ethnic and cultural backgrounds. It is hoped that these lines of investigation result in better care for all patients.

REFERENCES

1. Leal A, Leung P, Martin WE, Harrison DK, ed. Multicultural aspects of rehabilitation counseling. *J Appl Rehabil Counsel* 1988;19(4).
2. Anderson MB, ed. Behavioral and sociocultural perspectives in ethnicity and health. [Special Issue.] *Health Psychol* 1995;14(7).
3. Dashefsky A, Shapiro H. Ethnicity and identity. In: Dashefsky A, ed. *Ethnic identity in society.* Chicago: Rand McNally, 1976:5–11.
4. U.S. Bureau of the Census. *The Hispanic population in the U.S.: March 1991.* Current population reports, series P-20, no. 445. Washington, DC: U.S. Government Printing Office, 1991.
5. U.S. Bureau of the Census. *Race and Hispanic origin, 1990.* Census profile no. 2. Washington, DC: U.S. Department of Commerce, 1991.
6. U.S. Bureau of the Census. *Marital status and living arrangements: March 1989.* Current population reports, series P-20, no. 445. Washington, DC: U.S. Government Printing Office, 1990.
7. Indian Health Service. *Trends in Indian health, 1990.* DHEW Publication no. 90-12009. Washington, DC: U.S. Department of Health and Human Services, 1990.
8. Basic Behavioral Science Task Force. Basic behavioral science research for mental health: sociocultural and environmental processes. *Am Psychol* 1996;51: 722–731.
9. Albert SM. Caregiving as a cultural system: conceptions of filial obligation and parental dependency in urban America. *Am Anthropol* 1990;92:319–331.
10. Durvasula RS, Mylvaganam GA. Mental health of Asian Indians: relevant issues and community implications. *J. Community Psychol* 1994;22:97–107.
11. Landrine H, Klonoff EA. Culture and health-related schemas: a review and proposal for interdisciplinary integration. *Health Psychol* 1992;11:267–276.
12. Landrine H. Clinical implications of cultural differences: the referential versus the indexical self. *Clin Psychol Rev* 1992;12: 401–415.
13. National Indian Council on Aging. *Access: a demonstration project entitlement program for Indian elders.* Albuquerque: National Indian Council on Aging, 1982.
14. Johnson KW, Anderson NV, Bastiba E, et al. Panel II: macrosocial and environmental influences on minority health. *Health Psychol* 1995;14:601–612.
15. Alston RJ, Bell TJ. Cultural mistrust and the rehabilitation enigma for African-Americans. *J Rehabil* 1996;52:16–20.
16. Lipton JA, Marbach JJ. Ethnicity and the pain experience. *Soc Sci Med* 1984;19:1279–1298.
17. Landrine H, Klonoff EA. Cultural diversity in causal attributions for illness: the role of the supernatural. *J Behav Med* 1994;17: 181–193.
18. Cavallo MM, Saucedo C. Traumatic brain injury in families from culturally diverse populations. *J Head Trauma Rehabil* 1995;10: 66–77.

19. Sue D, Sue S. Cultural factors in the clinical assessment of Asian Americans. *J Consult Clin Psychol* 1987;55:479–487.

20. Myers HF, Kagawa-Singer M, Kumanyika Sk, et al. Panel III: behavioral risk factors related to chronic diseases and ethnic minorities. *Health Psychol* 1995; 14:613–631.

21. National Institute on Disability and Rehabilitation Research, U.S. Department of Education. Culturally sensitive rehabilitation. *Rehabil Brief* 1993;15:1.

22. Parham TA, Helms JE. Attitudes of racial identity and self-esteem of black students: an exploratory investigation. *J College Student Personnel* 1985;26: 143–147.

23. Cuellar I, Arnold B, Maldonado R. Acculturation rating scale for Mexican Americans—II: A revision of the original ARSMA Scale. *Hispanic J Behav Sci* 1995;17: 275–304.

24. Suinn RM, Ahuna C, Khoo G. The Suinn-Lew Asian self-identity acculturation scale: concurrent and factorial validation. *Educa Psychol Meas* 1992;52: 1041–1046.

25. Bowe F. *Adults with disabilities: a portrait.* Washington, DC: President's Committee on Employment of People with Disabilities, U.S. Department of Labor, 1992.

26. Flack JM, Amaro H, Jenkins W, et al. Panel I: epidemiology of minority health. *Health Psychol* 1995;4:592–599.

27. Penn NE, Kar S, Kramer J, et al. Panel VI: ethnic minorities, health-care systems, and behavior. *Health Psychol* 1995;14:641–646.

28. James SA, Lacroix A, Kleinbaum D, Strogatz D. John Henryism and blood pressure differences among black men. II. The role of occupational stressors. *J Behav Med* 1984;7:259–274.

29. James SA, Hartnett SA, Kalsbeek WD. John Henryism and blood pressure differences among black men. *J Behav Med* 1983;6: 259–278.

30. Jackson LA, Adams-Campbell LL. John Henryism and blood pressure in black college students. *J Behav Med* 1994;17:69–79.

31. Robinson J. Racial inequality and the probability of occupation-related injury or illness. *Milbank Q* 1984;62:567–590.

32. Elliott TR, Richards JS, DeVivo MJ, et al. Spinal cord injury model systems of care: the legacy and the promise. *Neurol Rehabil* 1994;4:84–90.

33. Rabow J, Watts R. Alcohol availability, alcohol beverage sales, and alcohol-related problems. *J Stud Alcohol* 1984;43:767–801.

34. Yee BWK, Castro FG, Hammond WR, et al. Panel IV: risk-taking and abusive behavior among ethnic minorities. *Health Psychol* 1995;14:622–631.

35. Slavin L, Rainer K, McCreary M, Gowda K. Toward a multicultural model of the stress process. *J Counsel Dev* 1991;70:156–163.

36. Smart JS, Smart DW. Acceptance of disability in the Mexican-American culture. *Rehabil Counsel Bull* 1991;34:357–367.

37. Smart JS, Smart DW. Acculturation, biculturalism, and the rehabilitation of Mexican-Americans. *J Appl Rehabil Counsel* 1993;24:46–51.

38. Zea MC, Quezada T, Belgrave FZ. Latino cultural values: their role in adjustment to disability. *J Soc Behav Pers* 1994;9: 185–200.

39. Zatzick DS, Dimsdale JE. Cultural variations and response to painful stimuli. *Psychol Med* 1990;52: 554–557.

40. Greenwald HP. Interethnic differences in pain perceptions. *Pain* 1991;44:157–163.

41. Honeyman PT, Jacobs EA. Effects of culture on back pain in Australian Aboriginals. *Spine* 1996; 27:841–843.

42. Leong FT, Mallinckrodt B, Kralj M. Cross-cultural variations in stress and adjustment among Asian and Caucasian graduate students. *J Multicultural Counsel Dev* 1990; 18:19–28.

43. Leong FT, Tseung W, Wu DY. Cross-cultural variations in stressful life events: a preliminary study. *AMHCA J* 1985;7:72–77.

44. Bates MS, Edwards WT. Ethnic variations in the chronic pain experience. *Ethn Dis* 1992;2: 63–83.

45. Bates MS, Edwards WT, Anderson KO. Ethnocultural influences on variation in chronic pain perception. *Pain* 1993;52: 101–112.

46. Krause JS, Anson CA. Adjustment after spinal cord injury: relationship to gender and race. *Rehabil Psychol* 1997;42:31–46.

47. Westbrook MT, Legge V, Pennay M. Men's reactions to becoming disabled: a comparison of six communities in a multi-cultural society. *J Appl Rehabil Counsel* 1993;24:35–41.

48. Doyle Y, Moffatt P, Corlett S. Coping with disabilities: the perspective of young adults from different ethnic backgrounds in inner London. *Soc Sci Med* 1994;38:1491–1498.

49. Belgrave FC. Psychosocial predictors of adjustment to disability in African-Americans. *J Rehabil* 1991;57:37–40.

50. Davis M, Matthews B, Jackson WT, et al. Self-concept as an outcome of spinal cord injury: the relation of race, hardiness and locus of control. *SCI Psychosoc Process* 1995;8:95–100.

51. Fuhrer MJ, Garber SL, Rintala VH, et al. Pressure ulcers in community-resident persons with spinal cord injury: prevalence and risk factors. *Arch Phys Med Rehabil* 1993;74:1172–1177.

52. Belgrave FC, Walker S. Predictors of employment outcome of black persons with disabilities. *Rehabil Psychol* 1991;36:111–119.

53. Ramisetty-Mikler S. Asian Indian immigrants in America and sociocultural issues in counseling. *J Multicultural Counsel Dev* 1993; 21:36–49.

54. Belgrave FZ, Davis A, Vajada J. An examination of social support source, type, and satisfaction among African-American and Caucasians with disabilities. *J Soc Behav Pers* 1994;9: 307–320.

55. White-Means S, Thornton M. Ethnic differences in the production of informal home health care. *Gerontologist* 1990;30: 758–768.

56. Lawton MP, Rajgopal D, Brody E, Kleban MH. The dynamics of caregiving for a demented elder among black and white families. *J Gerontol B Psychol Sci Soc Sci* 1992;47:S156–S164.

57. Pickett SA, Vraniak DA, Cook JA, Bertram J. Strength in adversity: blacks bear burden better than whites. *Prof Psychol Res Pract* 1993;24:460–467.

58. Haley WE, West CAC, Wadley VG, et al. Psychological, social, and health impact of caregiving: a comparison of black and white dementia family caregivers and noncaregivers. *Psychol Aging* 1995;10:540–552.

59. Haley WE, Waff DL, Coleton MI, et al. Appraisal, coping, and social support as mediators of well-being in black and white family caregivers of patients with Alzheimer's disease. *J Consult Clin Psychol* 1996;64:121–129.

60. Dilworth-Anderson P, Anderson NB. Dementia caregiving in blacks: a contextual approach to research. In: Lebowitz B, Light E, Neiderehe G, eds. *Mental and physical health of Alzheimer's caregivers.* New York: Springer, 1994:385–409.

61. DeVivo MJ, Richards JS. Marriage rates among persons with spinal cord injuries. *Rehabil Psychol* 1996;41:321–339.

62. DeVivo MJ, Fine PR. Spinal cord injury: its short-term impact on marital status. *Arch Phys Med Rehabil* 1985;66:501–504.

63. DeVivo MJ, Hawkins LN, Richards S, Go BK. Outcomes of post-spinal cord injury marriages. *Arch Phys Med Rehabil* 1995;76: 130–138.

64. Jenkins AE, Amos OC. Being black and disabled. *J Rehabil* 1983; 49:54–60.

65. Lam CS. Cross-cultural rehabilitation: what Americans can learn from their foreign peers. *J Appl Rehabil Counsel* 1993;249: 26–30.

66. Arokiasamy C, Maria V, Rubin SE, Roessler RT. *Foundations of the vocational rehabilitation process.* 3rd ed., Austin, TX: Pro-Ed, 1987.

67. Todd KH, Lee T, Hoffman JR. The effect of ethnicity on physician estimates of pain severity in patients with isolated extremity trauma. *JAMA* 1994;271: 925–928.

68. Todd KH, Samaroo N, Hoffman JR. Ethnicity as a risk factor for inadequate emergency department analgesia. *JAMA* 1993;269: 1537–1539.

69. James M, DeVivo MJ, Richards JS. Post injury employment outcomes among African-American and white persons with spinal cord injury. *Rehabil Psychol* 1993;38: 151–164.

70. DeVivo MJ, Rutt RD, Stöver SL, Fine PR. Employment after spinal cord injury. *Arch Phys Med Rehabil* 1987;68:494–498.

71. Krause JS, Anson CA. Employment after spinal cord injury: relationship to selected participant characteristics. *Arch Phys Med Rehabil* 1996;77:737–743.

72. Fischer JM. A comparison between American Indian and non-Indian consumers of vocational rehabilitation services. *J Appl Rehabil Counsel* 1991;22: 43–45.

73. Anderson JM. Ethnicity and illness experience: ideological structures and the healthcare delivery system. *Soc Sci Med* 1986;22: 1277–1283.

74. Krause JS, Anson CA. Self-perceived reasons for unemployment cited by person with spinal cord injury: relationship to gender, race, age and level of injury. *Rehabil Counsel Bull* 1996;39: 217–227.

75. Alston RJ, McCowan CJ. Aptitude assessment in African-American clients: the interplay between cultural and psychometrics in rehabilitation. *J Rehabil* 1994;60:44–46.

76. Morgan CO, Guy E, Lee B, Cellini HR. Rehabilitation services for American Indians: The Navajo experience. *J Rehabil* 1986;52: 25–31.

77. Asbury CA, Walker S, Belgrave FZ, et al. Psychosocial, cultural and accessibility factors associated with participation of African-Americans in rehabilitation. *Rehabil Psychol* 1994;39: 113–121.

Chapter 99

Disability and the Health and Health Maintenance Behaviors of Women

Margaret A. Nosek
Carol A. Howland

Women experience disability very differently from men. Although the neurotrauma resulting from spinal cord injury (SCI), the pain and stiffness resulting from arthritis, and the cognitive deficits resulting from brain injury may be clinically indistinguishable by gender, the impact on overall health and ability to function in society is noticeably different. Acknowledgment of these differences is an important component of excellence in the practice of physiatry. This chapter offers information on the health and health maintenance practices of women with physical disabilities that can be used by physiatrists in assisting women to manage their disabling conditions and in serving as a resource for primary care physicians as they address the basic health needs of women with disabilities. After reviewing some of the literature on the health of women with physical disabilities, we present findings from a major national study of this population that was conducted by the Center for Research on Women with Disabilities (CROWD), at Baylor College of Medicine.

BACKGROUND

The proportion of women with physical disabilities in the U.S. population is substantial and growing. According to the 1992 census, 26 million women have disability-related work limitations, comprising 20% of the population of women as a whole (1). While very few empirical data are available on women with physical disabilities, we know from anecdotal resources (2,3) that they face significantly higher rates of unemployment and poverty, and are confronted with more serious barriers to obtaining education, Social Security benefits, and health insurance than are men with disabilities and women in general. Access to health services by persons with disabilities has not been well studied. One survey (4) revealed that 67% of people with disabilities are not receiving the health services needed to maintain optimal health. One of the objectives in Healthy People 2000 is to increase to at least 80% the proportion of people with disabilities who have received all of the health screening services at the appropriate intervals, and at least one of the counseling (information) services, appropriate for their age and gender as recommended by the U.S. Preventive Services Task Force (5). In 1991, a review of progress toward achieving this objective indicated that only 12% of people with disabilities had received the entire set of recommended services; this rate is reduced to 8% among those who have an annual income less than $10,000 (6).

The high incidence of preventable health problems such as decubitus ulcers, urinary tract infections, and respiratory infections in persons with severe physical disabilities compared to people without disabilities has been documented in numerous studies (7–17). The occurrence of excessive health problems in this population also can be inferred from frequent visits to emergency rooms, outpatient rehabilitation clinics, and primary care physicians (8,18,19). An abundance of studies documented that persons with disabilities are hospitalized more often than the general population (10,12,13,15,20–22). Surveillance activities conducted with independent living centers indicate that psychosocial problems such as depression and problems accessing the environment were the most problematic secondary conditions faced by adults with a variety of physical disabilities (23). Other secondary conditions frequently reported were chronic pain, isolation, fatigue, sleep disturbance, lack of weight control, lack of physical fitness, and limited mobility (23). Some resolution and prevention of these problems can result from effective self-management strategies (16). Frequent incidents of illness requiring confinement at home, extensive bed rest, or prolonged hospitalization can be expected to interrupt productive activities such as paid employment, homemaking, parenting, and education again and again, thereby thwarting goals for independent living.

The proceedings of a National Institutes of Health (NIH) conference on the health of women with physical disabilities (24) focused on applying the principles of wellness and health promotion to women with disabilities. Topics included health promotion for people with chronic neuromuscular disabilities (25), the impact of disability on fitness in women (26), adapted physical activity and sport (27), and coping with stress (28–30). Roller, a polio survivor herself, laments the inability to work out on local health club machines, lack of a wheelchair-accessible scale at weight loss centers, inaccessible swimming classes in water that is too cold, and lack of adapted coaching by the instructor (25). In a Canadian study reporting 40% of women with disabilities as being inactive, reported barriers to participation in physical activity were timing of programs, nature of programs, accessibility of facilities, transportation, lack of knowledgeable instructors, and lack of available information (31). Roller and Maynard (32) proposed an integrated community health promotion and wellness program offering a range of treatments in one location within driving distance of the participants, including nutrition, exercise, expansion of options for conducting daily activities, coping with stress, increasing self-acceptance and self-confidence, using assertive behavior to cope with anger, developing satisfying leisure-time activities, and establishing connections with available community service resources.

According to DePauw (27), few studies of health-related physical activity include significant numbers of girls and women with disabilities, but they are better represented in arthritis studies (26). DePauw and Sherrill (33) advocated adapted physical activity that identifies and solves motor problems throughout the life span. Results of intervention studies suggest that physiologic training effects can be achieved by individuals with disabilities and that integrating individuals with and without disabilities is effective in improving learning, motor performance, appropriate behavior, and social interaction (34,35). Turk (26) reviewed exercise programs that are appropriate for neuromuscular diseases (36–39), postpolio (40–44), SCI (45–49), brain injury (50–54), arthritis (55–62), and multiple sclerosis (63–66). She raised the issue of reconceptualizing fitness in the context of significant motor impairment.

Little has been published about how disability may produce stress. The presence of chronic physical disability has been postulated as a life strain (67), and both chronic strain and acute life events were significantly related to depression. Sources of stress related to life events and change for women with disabilities might include involuntary admission to a rehabilitation hospital, interruption of ordinary activities, inability to independently carry out self-care activities, changes in appearance, and search for a new personal assistant or accessible housing, while dealing with everyday unrelenting life hassles such as increased time, planning, and effort to do things (28). Other sources of stress are a paucity of positive events or uplifts (68) such as relationships, social support, achievements, and pleasures, poverty with resulting inadequate nutrition; lower levels of fitness; pain and illness; and vulnerability to abuse (69,70). In a study of persons with SCI, Rintala et al (30) found that women reported significantly more perceived stress than men, and that life satisfaction, depressive symptomatology, self-assessed health rating, and severity of pressure ulcers were all significantly related to perceived stress. They recommended identifying the causes of stress for women with disabilities and designing interventions to alleviate the causes. Patrick (29) described several techniques for stress management such as cognitive training, progressive relaxation (71–73), relaxation response meditative technique (74,75), autogenic training (76), Hatha yoga (77), meditation (74), vigorous physical activity (78), and leisure activity (79–83).

Information about the health and health maintenance practices of women with physical disabilities is restricted to very specific conditions within single groups of women with one disability diagnosis. In an effort to understand the issues faced by women who share the characteristic of impairment of mobility or self-care, the CROWD conducted a national study. The findings of that study that relate to health and health maintenance are now presented.

METHODOLOGY

In 1992, the CROWD was established at Baylor College of Medicine in Houston, Texas, to conduct research on issues of concern to women with disabilities and to disseminate the findings nationally. A grant was obtained from the NIH to study the broad range of issues facing women with physical disabilities. The research consisted of two phases. Phase I was a qualitative interview study of 31 women with physical disabilities that helped us understand various aspects of sexuality from the point of view of the woman with a disability. The themes we identified in these interviews fell into six basic domains: 1) sense of self, 2) relationship issues, 3) information about sexuality, 4) sexual functioning, 5) abuse, and 6) general and reproductive health. With the assistance of national and local advisors, including consumers, researchers, medical professionals, social workers, and educators, the research team developed a questionnaire that represented all the primary themes from the qualitative study and issues raised in the literature. In Phase II, we identified 1150 women with physical disabilities around the country who volunteered to participate in the study or who were recruited through independent living centers in each federal region. We sent each of them two copies of this questionnaire, one for her to complete and one for her to give to an able-bodied female friend to complete. We received responses from 45% of this sample, or a total of 946 women, 504 of whom had physical disabilities and 442 who did not have disabilities.

The final version of the questionnaire consisted of 311 items containing 1011 variables. Domains of inquiry reflected the six thematic groups identified in the qualitative study, as well as sexual functioning, disability status, psychological factors, social factors (demographics and social attitudes), and environmental factors related to sexuality. Special effort was made to use gender-neutral language in reference to romantic partners in order to accommodate women who were homosexual or bisexual.

A total of 946 surveys was returned; however, some were not completely filled out. Also, some were completed by women who did not meet all the eligibility criteria for the study; that is, they were not between the ages of 18 and 65, or they had a disability that was not mobility related, such as blindness or deafness. Analyses were conducted on 881 questionnaires received from 475 women with disabilities and 406 able-bodied women who made up the comparison group.

The women who participated in this study represented every part of the United States and a wide variety of personal, social, and demographic characteristics. The women with and those without disabilities in this sample were of similar racial background and socioeconomic status. The women without disabilities, however, were slightly younger, an average age of 39 years compared to 42 years for the sample of women with disabilities.

The most common primary disability type was SCI (26%), followed by polio (18%), muscular dystrophy (12%), cerebral palsy (10%), multiple sclerosis (10%), joint and connective tissue disorders (8%), and skeletal abnormality (5%). Nearly half of the sample (49%) had disabilities since childhood (0–11 years old); 10%, since adolescence (12–17 years old); and 41%, since adulthood (18 years and over). Twenty-two percent had severe functional limitations, 52% had moderate disabilities, and 26% had mild disabilities.

Eighty-two percent were white; 9%, African-American; 4%, Hispanic; 2%, Native American; and 2%, Asian. Those living in urban or suburban areas comprised 89% of the sample, with 11% living in small towns or rural areas.

The sample was well educated, with 53% of the women with disabilities and 42% of the women without disabilities having college degrees. Fifty-nine percent were working for a salary part-time or full-time, compared to 86% of women without disabilities. The median annual personal income of the sample of women with disabilities was $15,000, with a household income of $25,000, compared to a personal income for women without disabilities of $18,500 and household income of $32,000.

The remainder of this chapter draws on the findings from this study to illustrate issues related to the health and health maintenance practices of women with disabilities.

GYNECOLOGIC HEALTH ISSUES

Sexual Functioning

One of our investigators who has a severe physical disability was overheard saying, "I'm sure I could function just fine sexually, if I could only find a man!" This illustrates one of the main dilemmas facing women with disabilities. Social attitudes constitute a significant, if not insurmountable, barrier to realizing sexual potential. For this reason, many of the questionnaires that have been developed and validated for assessing sexual functioning for women in the general population are not relevant when applied to women with disabilities. They tend to focus on frequency of sexual activities of various sorts. For women with physical disabilities, frequency is more often a reflection of opportunity than interest or ability. To circumvent this problem, we let the assessment of sexual functioning in this study generate from the comments of the women themselves. In the interviews that preceded the national survey, the participants spoke about intimate touch as much as sexual intercourse. Sexual functioning for them included a broad range of activities. Throughout the survey, we were very careful to use the term *partner* as opposed to *boyfriend* or *husband* to allow accurate responses from homosexual or bisexual participants. We assessed sexual functioning in terms of desire, both fulfilled and unfulfilled; frequency of sexual activities; satisfaction with sexual activities; and physical problems encountered. We also examined the influence of various psychological, social, and environmental factors on level of sexual activity and degree of satisfaction with sex life.

Results

Almost all of the women with and without disabilities in this study reported having had sexual activity at some time in their lives. Only 3% of the able-bodied women and 6% of women with disabilities had never had sexual intercourse. About half of women with disabilities were sexually active at the time of the study, compared to about two-thirds of women without disabilities. However, women with disabilities had significantly lower rates of having intimate touch (58% versus 68%) and sexual intercourse (49% versus 61%) within the past month. Most problems with sexual activity reported by women with disabilities were different from those reported by women without disabilities. Women with disabilities reported that problems with sexual activity often related to weakness (40%), vaginal dryness (39%), lack of balance (38%), hip or knee pain (32%), and spasticity of legs (28%).

We first investigated whether or not there were differences between women with and those without disabilities on four dimensions of sexual functioning: desire, activity, response, and satisfaction with their sex lives. We found significant differences in level of sexual activity, response, and satisfaction, with women with disabilities reporting much lower levels. There were no differences, however, between the groups on sexual desire.

Next, we wanted to know if age at onset of disability made any difference in sexual functioning. There were no differences in levels of sexual activity, response, or overall satisfaction with sex life. Women who had childhood-onset disability reported higher levels of sexual desire than did women with adolescent or adult-onset disability.

Finally, we examined how psychological factors and factors related to disability, social status, social attitudes, or environmental barriers affected sexual functioning among women with physical disabilities. *Sexual desire* was most related to social status variables, including work status and age. Women who were younger expressed more sexual desire. Women who perceived more negative stereotypes in society's attitude toward sexuality and disability experienced higher levels of sexual desire.

The strongest predictor of *sexual activity* was, not surprisingly, whether or not the woman lived with a significant other. Secondary predictors were in the psychological domain. Women with disabilities who had a more positive sexual self-image and who perceived themselves to be approachable by potential romantic partners also had higher levels of sexual activity. It is very notable that severity of disability was not significantly related to level of sexual activity.

We were not successful in predicting *sexual response*. The only factors that had some predictive value were more positive attitudes toward the use of assistive devices, less concern about stereotypes, and higher household income. It is difficult to interpret the meaning of this finding. Women with SCI and stroke reported the lowest scores.

Social status and psychological variables were the best predictors of *sexual satisfaction*. Women with disabilities who lived together with a significant other, and therefore had a higher level of sexual activity, also reported greater sexual satisfaction. Interestingly, lower household income was positively associated with sexual satisfaction. Women who felt more positive about their use of assistive devices and who had never experienced sexual abuse reported higher levels of sexual satisfaction.

Most of the differences in sexual functioning between women with and those without disabilities can be accounted for by the difficulties women with disabilities experience in finding a romantic partner. Level of sexual desire was the same, but level of activity was less because significantly fewer women with disabilities had partners, and therefore, level of satisfaction was less. For women who had a partner, levels of sexual activity were about the same, regardless of disability, but level of satisfaction with sex life was still lower for women with disabilities. It was interesting to note that severity of disability was not related to level of sexual functioning or satisfaction with sex life. It must be acknowledged, however, that in some cases problems related to disability, such as weakness, pain, or spasticity, can affect the physical aspects of sexual functioning, and problems associated with certain types of disabilities, such as the neurologic effects of SCI, stroke, or multiple sclerosis, can affect sexual response. There is a need for more medical research and collaboration with physicians and physical therapists on ways that weakness, pain, and spasticity can be managed to allow for more satisfaction from sexual activity.

Pregnancy

Special concerns during pregnancy vary for women with different types of disabilities. We know from this study that women with disabilities are less likely to become pregnant than are women in general; therefore, it is difficult to find enough women with a particular type of disability to participate in a survey, even one as large as this, so that we can draw valid conclusions. We chose to examine the pregnancy experiences of the 120 women with SCI who participated in this study because it was the largest subgroup in the sample.

Few clinicians are informed about the pregnancy outcomes of women with SCI. Yet the majority of women who acquire an SCI are of childbearing age. Recent 10-year hospital studies indicated an increasing number of births among women with traumatic SCI. However, few clinicians have experience managing pregnancy, labor, and delivery in women with SCI. Therefore, clinical guidelines for this population are often based on case reports or small case series, which tend to report the most unusual and serious problems rather than uncomplicated cases. Unfounded assumptions of poor outcomes may influence clinicians to behave as though the risks are greater than they actually are for most women with SCI and to practice defensive medicine. If the chance for a positive pregnancy outcome is considered slim, or the threat to the mother's life too high, clinicians may encourage women who want to have their babies to have unnecessary or undesired therapeutic abortions.

In these analyses, we tried to determine whether women with SCI are at higher risk of specific pregnancy-related complications than are women without disabilities.

Results

Thirty-seven percent of the women with disabilities had natural (not adopted) children compared to half of the able-bodied comparison group. No significant difference was found between the groups in the rate of miscarriages, abortions, or stillbirths.

Among 120 women with SCI, 52 (43%) had been pregnant, and 21 had pregnancies diagnosed after the onset of injury. Pregnancy was impossible for 31% because of tubal ligation (11%), hysterectomy (15%), or other causes. Significantly more women without disabilities (50%) had live births, compared to 18% of women after SCI, a frequency that is consistent with the 10% to 20% rate of births found in other studies. Fewer women with SCI had miscarriages (11%), compared to women without disabilities (17%), whereas the number of reported induced abortions and stillbirths was about equal in both groups.

Certain prenatal complications were more prevalent among women with SCI than among women without disabilities. Ten percent of women with SCI, and 5.47% of women without disabilities, had gestational diabetes, but this difference was not significant. Significantly more women with SCI had bladder and kidney infections during pregnancy, with 52% and 29% of SCI women having had bladder and kidney infections, respectively, compared to 17% and 8% of nondisabled women.

Both autonomic hyperreflexia (32%) and preeclampsia (38%) were found at relatively high rates among women with SCI; only 13% of women without disabilities had preeclampsia. Yet there was no significant difference between the two groups for frequency of preterm labor (33% versus 22%), pre-term delivery (29% versus 18%), or low birth weight (14% versus 15%), despite a typical increased risk of these complications in association with autonomic hyperreflexia and preeclampsia. Frequency of failure to progress during labor was also similar between the two groups (24% versus 18%).

The lack of significant differences in complication frequency between our two groups may reflect limitations in the research design. The sample size of women with SCI who had been pregnant after injury is extremely small (21) compared to the size of the group of women without disabilities who had been pregnant (220). Objective hospital data to corroborate self-report data were not available with our written questionnaire method. Also, women who gave birth many years ago may not recall some details of their pregnancy and birth experience.

Physicians and women with SCI themselves often operate under the misconception that pregnancy following SCI should be avoided. Consequently, women with disabilities report difficulty in finding obstetricians or midwives willing to assist them with their "high-risk" pregnancies. However, the results of our study confirm findings from other studies that normal labor and delivery are possible, even routine, and generally pose little or no added risk to the mother or baby. Physicians do need to be alerted to the possible complications associated with SCI such as severe autonomic hyperreflexia in women with lesions at or above the T6 level, respiratory compromise, skin breakdown, increased risk of urinary tract infections, increased spasticity, and medications commonly used in SCI that could be toxic to the fetus.

Sexually Transmitted Diseases

Health care providers may mistakenly assume that women with disabilities are not sexually active, especially if their disability is disfiguring or severe, and neglect to screen for sexually transmitted diseases (STDs). Women with disabilities may be less likely to complain of symptoms suggesting an STD because mobility and sensory impairments may prevent them from noticing a rash or vaginal discharge, or from feeling pain and itching. Therefore, STDs are less likely to be detected and treated in women with disabilities, which could put them in jeopardy of getting pelvic inflammatory disease (PID) and increasing their risk of cervical cancer, infection with human immunodeficiency virus (HIV), ectopic pregnancy, and infertility. We asked women who participated in this study to indicate whether or not they had experienced an STD at any time in their lives, and if so, the type of STD.

Results

Our study dispelled the myth of asexuality in that most of the women with disabilities had been sexually active (94%), making them as susceptible as women without disabilities to getting STDs. In fact, the prevalence of STDs overall was similar in the two groups, slightly more than one-fifth of the sample. Women with and without disabilities were about equally likely to have had syphilis (0.4% versus 0.5%), gonorrhea (4% versus 5%), chlamydial infection (7% each), trichomoniasis (11% each), genital warts (8% versus 10%), or pubic lice (11% each). However, women with disabilities were significantly less likely to have had genital herpes (3% versus 7%) or a nonspecific STD (3% versus 5%). No one in either group reported being HIV positive. These rates may be higher in both groups, since STDs tend to be underreported and medical records were not available to corroborate the self-reported data. It is also possible that fewer cases have been detected among women with disabilities because they may be less likely to report symptoms, and physicians who perceive a lack of risk for STDs may not test for them.

Our findings indicate that getting information about STDs and safe sex practices is as important for women with disabilities as it is for any sexually active woman. Health care providers should not wait until the woman brings up the subject because some women with early-onset disabilities may have been sheltered from getting sexually related information, or may have grown up believing that their bodies are so different from those of able-bodied persons that they are not susceptible to getting the same diseases. Also, because of lack of sensation or the inability to notice unusual vaginal discharge or sores, women may not be prompted to seek medical attention until symptoms have reached an advanced stage, when complications are much more likely. Illustrations in consumer literature about STDs should include women with disabilities to help dispel misconceptions and lack of awareness.

Birth Control, Hysterectomy, and Cancer Screening

The default recommendation for women with severe physical disabilities seems to be to have a hysterectomy. We received many reports that physicians assume women with disabilities would never want, or be able to have, children safely, or that by removing the uterus they could save them years of trouble with menstruation. It is truly astounding how little information physicians are given about the effect of disability on reproductive capacity or the value women with disabilities ascribe to the ability to bear children. Few articles in the medical literature discuss the safety of oral contraceptives for women with various types of physical disabilities, alternative techniques for conducting pelvic examinations, or the importance of breast cancer screening for women who have difficulty accessing mammography equipment. Our study was the first to ask a large sample of women with a variety of physical disabilities about their experiences with gynecologic health care. The national survey included numerous items about types of contraception used and problems encountered, reasons for having a hysterectomy, frequency of going for pelvic examinations and mammograms, and reasons for not receiving cancer screening on a regular basis.

Results

Birth Control

Little is known about the safety or convenience of various methods of contraception for women with disabilities. Thirty percent of women with disabilities in our study believed that they had been given inaccurate information about birth control by their physicians, in contrast to only 9% of the able-bodied comparison group. More than one-third of women with disabilities were using no method of birth control, compared with nearly one-fourth of women without disabilities. Although failure to use birth control could reflect lack of sexual activity or desire to get pregnant, it is possible that some women with disabilities are dissatisfied with the safety or convenience of the methods available to them. Use of oral contraceptives was uncommon in both groups, although it was more common among women without disabilities (12%) than women with disabilities (7%). Clinicians often believe that oral contraceptives are contraindicated for women with mobility impairments due to an increased risk of blood clots, but recent studies demonstrated their safety (84–86). The relatively low rate of birth control pill use for able-bodied women may reflect the fact that nearly half of them were at least 40 years old; the age at which the risk of thrombosis rises is 35 years. Condoms were used by partners of 9% of women with disabilities and 15% of able-bodied women, but other barrier methods were rarely used by women with disabilities, probably due to limitations in manual dexterity. The most popular methods of birth control for both groups were surgical; 16% of women in both groups had a tubal ligation and 8% and 10% of the partners of women with and without disabilities, respectively, had a vasectomy.

Hysterectomy

Members of the disability community are concerned that some women with disabilities, particularly early-onset disabilities, are having medically unnecessary hysterectomies for the purpose of birth control. Some of the women interviewed in our qualitative study reported that a physician recommended they have a hysterectomy to make sure they would never get pregnant. Conversely, a woman with cerebral palsy reported pleading with her doctor to give her a hysterectomy because menstruation was so difficult for her to manage. Women with disabilities had a significantly higher rate of hysterectomy (22% versus 12%) than did able-bodied women. This difference mainly reflects the large difference in rates between young women with and those without disabilities, as there was no significant difference in hysterectomy rates between the two groups among women who were age 35 or older. Our findings indicate that women with disabilities are more likely to have a hysterectomy at a younger age than are women without disabilities. Women with disabilities were more likely than their able-bodied counterparts to have a hysterectomy for nonmedically necessary reasons such as birth control, personal convenience, or at the request of a parent or guardian (22% versus 12%). Menstrual management is typically inadequately addressed in the rehabilitation setting.

Cancer Screening

Women with disabilities are no less susceptible than any other woman to getting cervical cancer or breast cancer. Certain subpopulations of women, such as those with low income or low educational levels, Hispanics, and Asians, are less likely than other women to have regular pelvic examinations and mammograms to screen for cancer. We were concerned that access to pelvic examinations and mammograms may also be limited for women with disabilities, leading to a diagnosis of cancer at a later, less treatable stage.

There was a tendency for women with disabilities to be less likely to receive pelvic examinations within the recommended guidelines (once every 2 years) (67.1%) compared to women without disabilities (72.8%). It had been speculated that women with disabilities would be more likely never to have had a pelvic examination; however, that did not turn out to be the case. Women with more severe functional limitations were much less likely to have regular pelvic examinations. Minority women with disabilities were less likely to have regular pelvic examinations. Among the women with disabilities who did not have regular pelvic examinations, the most frequently selected reason was difficulty getting onto the examination table (37%), followed by being too busy (31%) and inability to find a physician that suited them (29%). Women with disabilities were significantly more likely than women without disabilities to select reasons of difficulty finding an accessible physician's office or clinic, difficulty finding transportation, difficulty getting onto an examination table, do not need them because of their disability, and cannot find a physician who is knowledgeable about their disability.

We found that women with disabilities who were at least age 40 received mammograms at about the same rate as women without disabilities (55% versus 50%). Women who had higher education levels were more likely to have a mammogram. Women who perceived that they had more control over their lives were less likely to have a mammogram; some believed they would be able to detect breast cancer by self-examination alone. Women with disabilities who had not had a mammogram cited different reasons for not going than did able-bodied women. Among women with disabilities who had not had a mammogram within the past 2 years, the most frequently given reason was inability to get into the required position (34%), followed by no physician recommendation for the screening (25%), then the belief that their cancer risk was too low to warrant getting a mammogram (24%).

Women with severe disabilities have reported that physicians are unable to give them a complete pelvic examination or that mammograms are unable to screen all of their breast tissue for abnormal masses. Further research is needed using registries of women with disabilities who have had breast cancer to see if inadequate or no cancer screening is leading to a diagnosis of cancer at a later, less treatable stage. There are also reports that treatment options for women with disabilities who get cancer are more limited.

The findings of this study led us to believe that women with physical disabilities, particularly those with more severe functional impairments, are not receiving the same quality of gynecologic health care as their able-bodied counterparts. It is more difficult for them to receive information about methods of birth control that would be safe and effective options in light of special considerations related to their disability. They are more likely to have hysterectomies for reasons that are not related to medical necessity. Though they may have intended to have regular pelvic examinations, they are discouraged by inaccessibility in physicians' offices. We have received reports from many physicians that they do not conduct a pelvic examination on a woman with a disability if having the staff lift her onto the examination table is perceived as being too difficult or is not allowed under the facility's policies, or if spasticity, contractures, or pain create positioning problems. In contrast, some women with disabilities were more likely to receive mammograms than were women without disabilities. Even so, positioning difficulties caused some women to believe that they were not receiving a complete examination. To remedy these inequities, we recommend education and training for both women with disabilities and clinicians. There is a need for programs and materials to inform women about how disability can affect their reproductive health, and how they can work with health care providers to ensure that they are receiving the same quality of service as all women. There is also a critical need for information to be available at undergraduate and postgraduate levels to physicians, physician assistants, nurse practitioners, nurse midwives, and nurses in general, about the reproductive health care needs of women with disabilities. The CROWD has begun developing materials and training curricula for these purposes.

GENERAL HEALTH ISSUES

Abuse

The issue of abuse emerged from this study with unexpected force. Although there has been a wealth of research on domestic violence and sexual assault against women, with clearly defined variables and strong scientific methodology, it almost never incorporates the element of disability. The literature in the disability arena has focused mostly on abuse of developmentally disabled children. A few studies have looked at the situation of women with disabilities; however, concepts are not well defined and the samples mix children and adults, and include the full spectrum of mental, sensory, and physical disabilities. Further, we found that the system of programs for battered women was only beginning to incorporate the need for accessibility for women with disabilities, and the system of disability-related services was almost totally unprepared to deal with issues of abuse. This is indeed new territory.

In the national survey we defined emotional abuse as being threatened, terrorized, corrupted, or severely rejected, isolated, ignored, or verbally attacked. Physical abuse is any form of violence against the body, such as being hit, kicked, restrained, or deprived of food or water. Sexual abuse was defined as being forced, threatened, or deceived into sexual activities ranging from looking or touching to intercourse or rape. In the survey, we included questions about which of these three types of abuse the women had experienced, and, for each experience, the age at which the abuse began and ended and their relationship to the perpetrator. Analyses we have conducted so far examined differences in the rates and types of abuse experienced by women with and without disabilities.

Results

Twenty-five of the 31 women with disabilities we interviewed in the first part of this study told us about 55 separate experiences of abuse. In many cases, these experiences strongly affected the way the women felt about themselves and their ability to engage in satisfying romantic relationships. Although most incidents of abuse were similar to those able-bodied women experience, such as verbally abusive parents or partners, battering, and rape, some types of abuse were specifically disability related, such as withholding needed orthotic equipment (wheelchairs, braces), medications, transportation, or essential assistance with personal tasks, such as dressing or getting out of bed. Some factors that increase the vulnerability to abuse among women with disabilities are their physical difficulty in escaping dangerous or abusive situations, a need for assistance with personal tasks from the perpetrator, their higher rate of exposure to institutional facilities (including hospitals), and the stereotype that they are dependent, passive, and easy prey.

The national survey showed, however, that overall, women with disabilities appear to be at risk for emotional, physical, and sexual abuse to the same extent as women without disabilities. The prevalence of any abuse (including emotional, physical, and sexual abuse) for women with and without disabilities was 62%. About the same proportion of women with disabilities compared to women without disabilities reported emotional abuse (52% versus 48%), physical abuse (36% for both), or sexual abuse (40% versus 37%). When the categories of physical and sexual abuse were combined, 52% of women with disabilities and 51% of women without disabilities responded positively. None of these types of abuse was significantly different for women with or without disabilities.

In the survey, husbands and live-in partners were included in the same category. More husbands abused women (both with and without disabilities) emotionally (26% for both) and physically (17% and 19%) than did other perpetrators. Parents were the next most common perpetrators of emotional and physical abuse for both groups of women. Strangers were the most often cited perpetrators of sexual abuse for both groups (11% for women with disabilities and 12% for women without disabilities).

Women with disabilities were significantly more likely to experience emotional abuse by attendants, strangers, or health care providers than were women without disabilities. There was a trend for more women with disabilities to experience emotional abuse by mothers, brothers, and other family members, as well. Two percent of women with disabilities were physically or sexually abused by attendants. There was a trend for women with disabilities to be more likely to experience sexual abuse by health care providers.

Women who had experienced abuse that lasted longer than a single incident were examined to determine differences in the duration of abuse. Women with disabilities experienced all types of abuse (emotional, physical, or sexual) for significantly longer periods of time than did women without disabilities.

Women with disabilities face the same risks of abuse that all women face, plus additional risks specifically related to their disability. Rates of abuse were extremely high in both groups of women in this study. It is notable that women with disabilities tended to experience abuse for longer periods of time, reflecting the reduced number of escape options open to them due to more severe economic dependence, the need for assistance with personal care, environmental barriers, and social isolation. It is difficult to separate the effect of disability from the effects of poverty, low self-esteem, and family background in identifying the precursors to violence against this population. There is much more that we need to know about how women with disabilities escape or resolve abusive situations. This study has shown the critical magnitude of this problem. Steps must be taken to train girls and women with disabilities to understand inappropriate touch, including that which occurs in medical settings, and to learn how to recognize and avoid or resolve abusive situations in the family and in the community. Important elements in this training are informing women that they do not need to tolerate abuse and linking them to community resources that could help them expand their options for removing violence from their lives. Consider this a loud call for advocacy to make all programs for battered women fully accessible, and all disability service programs equipped to identify abused women and refer them appropriately.

Chronic Conditions

The Centers for Disease Control and Prevention has funded a cadre of researchers to study the onset of new health problems among people with physical disabilities. These studies have begun to shed some light on the types of conditions people with disabilities experience as they age and on secondary prevention, that is, ways in which people with disabilities can get information on their options for medications, therapies, or lifestyle changes that could help them avoid acquiring new health problems that may or may not be directly related to their primary disability. Not much is known, however, about how the course of disability can lead to chronic conditions among women. In our survey, we gave a list of 15 chronic health problems that have been discussed in the literature and asked the participants to indicate which ones they have experienced. We analyzed the prevalence of each condition among the women with disabilities compared to the women without disabilities. For some of the conditions that were significantly more prevalent among women with disabilities, we examined factors that may distinguish those who have the condition from those who do not.

Results

Women with physical disabilities reported chronic conditions more often than did the comparison group without disabilities, and at younger ages. As women with disabilities age, a greater number of them report having chronic conditions compared to women without disabilities. Significantly more women with disabilities than women without reported having chronic urinary tract infections (18%), major depression (17%), osteoporosis (12%), restrictive lung disease (6%), inflammatory bowel disease (6%), heart disease (5%), seizure disorder (5%), and kidney disease (3%).

Urinary Tract Infection

Although chronic urinary tract infection was more prevalent among women with disabilities than women without disabilities, it was associated primarily with disorders characterized by neurogenic bladder, such as SCI (35%), multiple sclerosis (30%), and cerebral palsy (17%). However, 6% of women with polio had chronic urinary tract infection despite a presumably neurologically intact bladder. Factors that promote urinary tract infection in women with mobility impairment need further investigation, but may include difficulty in maintaining adequate cleanliness, restricting fluid intake to reduce the number of trips to the rest room or avoid searching for accessible rest rooms, contaminated catheterization, infrequent urination, and excess sweating with prolonged sitting in a wheelchair.

Depression

The rate of self-reported major depression that had been diagnosed by a health care professional was significantly higher for women with disabilities between the ages of 18 and 49 compared to younger women without disabilities. Among women age 50 or older, there was no difference between the two groups. The rate of depression was significantly different by disability type. The highest rate was in women with spina bifida (39%), with rates of 25% or more in women with limb loss, traumatic brain injury, and multiple sclerosis. The lowest rate was in women with SCI. There is a need for a more thorough investigation of depression in this population. Previous studies used measures of depression that contain questions about fatigue and weakness, symptoms that for women with physical disabilities, may be more reflective of the disability itself than of depression. We need to gain a better understanding of the role social support, social attitudes, and environmental barriers might play in engendering feelings of being devalued and overwhelmed by life that can lead to clinical depression.

Osteoporosis

Lack of weight bearing is a known risk factor for osteoporosis. Therefore, we predicted that women with mobility impairments would be at increased risk of getting osteoporosis at an earlier age. Most women are unaware that they have osteoporosis until spinal fractures are detected or they acquire fractures during a fall or while conducting ordinary daily activities. Therefore, it is remarkable that osteoporosis had already been diagnosed in women in their 30s with disabilities in our study. In this study, the women with disabilities had seven times the risk of getting osteoporosis as the women without disabilities. Research is needed on treatment that would delay the onset of osteoporosis among susceptible women with disabilities as well as on the most efficacious treatment to arrest its progress in the early stages in this population. Information on the osteoporosis experienced by younger women with mobility impairments may emerge from the medical experiments done by NASA's space program. Researchers have observed that immobilization produces a similar pattern of bone density loss as microgravity.

Heart Disease

The leading cause of death in women, like men, is coronary artery disease. Having a primary disability such as SCI, cerebral palsy, muscular dystrophy, or limb loss does not exempt women from also acquiring heart disease. However, physicians are more likely to attribute symptoms suggesting angina in women to noncardiac causes. When a woman also has a disability, the physician may be more likely to assume that chest pain and other symptoms are related to her underlying disabling condition. If the woman has impairment of sensation, she may experience silent ischemia, a phenomenon also noted in advanced diabetes. Other women with disabilities have atypical, nonspecific symptoms like indigestion. The disabling effects of heart disease may compound those from the primary disability, increasing total functional disability. The few studies of heart disease in people with disabilities used primarily male subjects. Is cardiovascular disease as rare in premenopausal women with disabilities as it is in premenopausal women without disabilities?

Among the 881 respondents, 33 women self-reported having heart disease, including 23 (5%) of the 475 women with physical disabilities and 10 (2.5%) of the 406 of those without disabilities. The difference in prevalence of heart disease between these two groups approached significance when examined for all age groups. As age increased, both groups experienced an increase in risk of having heart disease. There was no difference in prevalence of heart disease when postmenopausal women with and those without disabilities were compared. However, among premenopausal women aged 18 to 49 years, the number of cases of heart disease was significantly higher among women with disabilities; 17 (5%) of women with disabilities reported heart disease compared to 4 (1%) of the able-bodied comparison group.

Further studies are needed to investigate the association of known risk factors for heart disease among women with disabilities. Several factors are known to increase the risk for acquiring or accelerating the onset of coronary heart disease, but with worse outcomes in women. These risk factors include diabetes mellitus, smoking, hypertension, physical inactivity, obesity, high cholesterol, low levels of high-density lipoprotein (HDL), and postmenopausal status. Although these same risk factors can be expected to promote heart disease in women with disabilities, there has been no examination of the extent to which the additional presence of disability and limitations in the ability to exercise effectively may increase the degree of risk. Does having other chronic conditions also increase or change the risk profile of women with disabilities? Do women with disabilities have other risk factors for heart disease that are not found among women without disabilities?

Urinary tract infection, depression, osteoporosis, and heart disease are health problems that are faced more often by women with certain physical disabilities than by women without disabilities. It would not be fair to say that these conditions are entirely preventable; however, it is very possible that rates could be reduced by informing women with disabilities about their increased risk and offering suggestions on what they could do to reduce their risk or delay the onset of diseases of aging. When we presented our findings on chronic conditions to a group of physicians, the response was essentially a lack of surprise. For many years, the medical profession has understood that these conditions are an inevitable consequence of physical disability and not enough is known about how to alter the course. The message we received from our participants was that they are not content to live with such resignation. They want information and they want solutions. Much more research is needed before we can make specific recommendations on how chronic conditions can be prevented in women with physical disabilities. The CROWD was fortunate to receive new funding in 1996 from the NIH to pursue some of this research, particularly as it relates to strategies used by women with physical disabilities to avoid chronic conditions and maintain good health. It is our hope that other researchers, clinicians, and health educators will take an increased interest in some of these questions and assist in expanding the body of health information available to women with disabilities.

Health Maintenance Behaviors

Maintaining good health as a woman with a physical disability demands essentially the same precautions and proactive measures as for all women, with a few extra challenges. Keeping a diet that is low in fat is always advisable, but women with severe functional limitations may have to rely on attendants or friends to cook for them, making it harder to control the nutritional content of the meal. Others may be forced to skip meals to divide limited attendant hours among eating, bathing, and other essential activities. We all know to avoid carcinogens like cigarette smoke, but might there be an even greater negative effect for women who are less mobile or already have impaired breathing? Exercise seems to be a universal recommendation for maintaining good health, but for women with physical disabilities, options for exercise may be seriously limited by a lack of accessible equipment and facilities, a lack of information about what type of exercise is best for them, or the severity of their physical impairment itself. In the literature there has been considerable analysis of how an individual's beliefs about her health affect her health maintenance behaviors. We are concerned that the common stereotype that people with disabilities are sick may promote "sick role" behaviors, that is, passivity and exemption from the responsibilities of life. In the interview phase of this study, we analyzed factors that were associated with wellness. We found that women who led active, healthy lives had high self-esteem, and proactively sought out and followed information about how they could maximize their health. In the national survey, we included questions about whether or not participants followed a list of health maintenance behaviors, as well as questions about their height and weight to calculate their body mass index.

Results

We asked participants to indicate which health maintenance behaviors they practiced. No significant differences were found between women with disabilities and women without disabilities in eating a balanced diet (77% versus 73%), getting adequate rest (73% for both), maintaining a healthy weight (61% versus 56%), moderation in alcohol consumption (81% for both), not smoking (68% versus 66%), and not using recreational drugs (69% versus 72%). Significantly fewer women with disabilities, however, reported that they exercised regularly (46% versus 73%).

Our finding that women with and those without disabilities do not differ substantially on maintaining a healthy weight was based on a body mass index analysis (weight in kilograms divided by height in meters squared). The average body mass index of women with disabilities was 26 (the standard for normal is 20–25). About the same percentage of women with and without disabilities were in the various obesity categories (23% versus 28%); however, significantly more women with disabilities were in a lower body mass index category (20% versus 11%). Little exists in the literature about the appropriate body mass index goal for women with specific disabilities. In our sample, women with SCI or neuromuscular disorders were more likely to have a body mass index below 20 kg than were those with other disabilities, which is not surprising in light of the degree of loss of muscle mass in these disorders. More women with postpolio and multiple sclerosis were in the moderately obese category than were women with other disabilities. We wanted to know if whether or not a woman smoked, mantained a healthy diet, exercised, or had hypertension was associated with obesity. For women without disabilities, there was an association with diet, exercise, and hypertension. For women with SCI, obesity was associated with high blood pressure. For women with postpolio, obesity was associated with lack of exercise.

We now have evidence that women with disabilities practice about the same health maintenance behaviors as women without disabilities, with one important exception, exercise. Many factors may contribute to this difference: a lack of accessible exercise equipment and facilities; fatigue, pain, and weakness that may be related to the disability; a lack of time that may result from the increased effort needed to execute daily living tasks; warnings from physicians that exercise may aggravate the disability; or the assumption that there is little benefit to exercise for the person with a disability. We heard from many women who struggle to obtain information about what type of exercise could benefit them and what regimens they could follow to maintain optimal health. Research is needed on how to determine ideal body weight for women with physical disabilities, what the health and functional impact of increased body weight is, and whether some disabling conditions increase the risk of obesity or malnourishment. We have only begun our investigation of health maintenance for women with physical disabilities. In the next 3 years, we will be examining in more depth factors that are associated with wellness in this population and strategies that could help women with disabilities strengthen their belief in their capacity for good health and increase their health maintenance behaviors.

Health Care Utilization

According to the literature, persons with disabilities consume a larger share of health care services than the general population. We wanted to know more about the experience of women with disabilities in accessing health care services. In the interviews that began this study, we found our participants very eager to talk about these experiences; indeed, many used the opportunity to vent some very long-held frustrations. They complained bitterly about inaccessibility in health care settings, lack of knowledge among health care providers about their disability, and a perception that they were not getting the same quality of health care, particularly reproductive health care, as women in general. In the national survey, we focused our questions on the types of health care providers used within the past year, as well as the types of health care facilities used. We analyzed differences in utilization patterns between women with and those without disabilities. We also asked some general questions about how well their physicians were able to deal with their disability as it might affect an ordinary health problem.

Results

Women with physical disabilities who participated in this study were more likely to have used every major category of health care provider within the past 12 months than were women without disabilities. Significantly more women with disabilities had seen general practitioners, rehabilitation specialists, obstetricians/gynecologists, and other specialists. Ninety-one percent of women with disabilities had seen specialists of some type within the past year. Women with disabilities who lived alone were five times more likely to see specialists during the past year. Women who worked full- or part-time were less likely to see specialists. There was a slight trend for women with lower levels of functional impairment and women who work to less likely see specialists. Age, household income, duration of disability, self-esteem, perceived control of life, urban or rural residence, or education level did not increase the odds of seeing specialists. It is interesting to note that 24% of women with disabilities and 20% of women without disabilities used alternative health care providers, such as *curanderos*, homeopathists, and acupuncturists.

Women with physical disabilities were also more likely to have used every major category of health care facility within the past 12 months than were women without disabilities. Significantly more women with disabilities used public health clinics, rehabilitation hospitals, and emergency rooms. We were curious about the high rate of emergency room use, and tried to identify factors that were associated with it. Various disability and socioeconomic factors did not seem to be related; however, we found that women who perceived more control over their lives were less likely to use emergency rooms. Although more women with disabilities (54%) than women without disabilities (45%) reported seeing private physicians, this difference was not significant.

Five items in the national survey asked specifically about the ability of health care providers and facilities to accommodate disability-related needs. These items were grounded in statements made by women with disabilities who participated in the qualitative interviews that preceded the national survey. Thirty-nine percent reported that their physicians do not speak directly to them if a family member or other person accompanies them. Thirty-one percent have had a physician refuse to see them because of their disability. Twenty-six percent believed their physicians were not well informed about how their disability affects their reproductive health. Thirty-six percent had difficulty finding a physician who was willing or able to manage their pregnancy. More than half of women with SCI had this problem. Fifty-six percent reported that the hospital could not accommodate their disability-related needs when they gave birth.

Serious barriers exist that reduce the quality of health care available to women with physical disabilities. Architectural barriers in physicians' offices and hospitals still exist, despite the requirements of the Americans with Disabilities Act. There are invisible barriers as well, such as policies that deny service to women who cannot independently mount an examination table, and the refusal of physicians to see women solely on the basis of their disability, also in violation of the Americans with Disabilities Act. Advocacy is needed to inform persons in charge of medical facilities and clinical practices about their obligation to comply with legal requirements for physical and policy accessibility.

Our finding that women with disabilities make significantly greater use of services from specialists and emergency rooms has strong implications. With the advent of managed care, there are more stringent regulations on the use of specialists. For women whose health depends on timely access to physicians who have the specialized knowledge they need, these regulations could seriously affect their ability to maintain good health and prevent minor conditions from escalating into major ones that require more involved and more expensive treatment. Many of the complications of immobility and disability-related diagnoses are not taught in primary care training programs. A specialist may be the most appropriate primary care provider for some women with disabilities. This may also be an insight into the disproportionately high use of emergency rooms we found among women with disabilities. The many barriers to accessing health care, both within medical systems and in the community (such as lack of accessible transportation and attendant services), contribute to delayed treatment. When knowledgeable providers are not available or when systems barriers prevent them from delivering services in a timely manner, otherwise controllable health problems become ones that can only be handled in an emergency room. When we see the use of emergency room services declining, we will know that health care systems have made progress in removing some of these barriers to quality health care service.

RECOMMENDATIONS FOR PRACTICE

For the physiatrist who wishes to improve health care services for women with disabilities, we offer the following seven recommendations:

1. Give considerable weight to patients' own perceptions of deviations from what is normal for them. At the same time, be aware that disability and disability-related medications may mask or alter the perception of symptoms of serious health problems.
2. Acknowledge the sexuality of female patients. Inquire about menstrual history, sexual activity, and desire to bear children. Consider the possibility that nonspecific symptoms may result from STDs or pregnancy.
3. Be vigilant for the early onset of aging-related conditions, such as osteoporosis, heart disease, bladder dysfunction, and lung disease.
4. Identify and work to remove barriers to appropriate health care. Assist individuals to identify physicians knowledgeable about disability who are willing to approach each case creatively and establish linkages with specialists and other information resources. Establish collaborative relationships with the primary care physicians of your patients with disabilities.
5. Encourage maintenance of social activity level. Work to prevent onset of social isolation and depression resulting from reduced mobility and physical functioning, and loss of personal resources. Promote involvement in esteem-building activities.
6. Identify factors that could erode support systems, such as divorce, loss of earned income, and cutbacks in benefit programs; and investigate ways to compensate for their effects before the support is lost.
7. Be vigilant for signs of physical, sexual, and disability-related abuse. Advise individuals on how to protect themselves from such abuse and how to seek help when abuse occurs.

REFERENCES

1. McNeil JM. *Americans with disabilities: 1991–92.* Current population reports, P70-33. Washington, DC: Bureau of the Census, 1993.
2. Fine M, Asch A, eds. *Women with disabilities: essays in psychology, culture, and politics.* Philadelphia: Temple University Press, 1988.
3. Deegan MJ, Brooks NA, eds. *Women and disability: the double handicap.* New Brunswick, NJ: Transaction Books, 1984.
4. RWJ Foundation. Survey finds U.S. health care system not meeting needs of people with disabilities. *Advances* 1994;10:B11.
5. U.S. Preventive Services Task Force. Fisher M, Eckhart C, eds. *Guide to clinical preventive services: an assessment of the effectiveness of 169 interventions: report of the U.S. Preventive Services Task Force.* Baltimore: Williams & Wilkins, 1990.
6. *Healthy People 2000 review.* Hyattsville, MD: National Center for Health Statistics, 1993.
7. Batavia AI, DeJong G, Burns TJ, et al. *A managed care program for working-age persons with physical disabilities: a feasibility study.* Washington, DC: National Rehabilitation Hospital, Office of Research, 1989.
8. Batavia AI, DeJong G, Halstead L, Smith QW. Primary medical services for people with disabilities. *Am Rehabil* 1988;14(4):9–27.
9. DeJong G, Batavia AI. *Addressing the post-rehabilitation health care needs of persons with disabilities: a report of the SEAR Committee to the American Congress of Rehabilitation Medicine.* Washington, DC: National Rehabilitation Hospital, Office of Research, 1988.
10. DeJong G, Osberg JS, McGinnis GE, et al. Rehospitalization following rehabilitation: toward a demographic and functional profile. Presented at the annual session of American Congress of Rehabilitation Medicine, (forthcoming).
11. Garber SL, Rintala DH, Hart KA, et al. Prevalence of pressure sores in a cross-section of spinal cord injured men residing in the community. *Arch Phys Med Rehabil* 1990;71:797. Abstract.

12. Meyers AR, Feltin M, Master RJ, et al. Rehospitalization and spinal cord injury: cross sectional survey of adults living independently. *Arch Phys Med Rehabil* 1985;66: 704–708.

13. Shea JD, Sepulveda JA. Pressure sore profile. In: *Proceedings of the American Spinal Injury Association*, 1985.

14. Young JS, Burns PE, Bowen AM, et al. *Spinal cord injury statistics: experience of the regional spinal cord injury systems (WE 725 Spina 82)*. Phoenix: Good Samaritan Medical Center, 1982.

15. Young JS, Northup N. Rehospitalization in years two and three following spinal cord injury. *Spinal Cord Inj Dig* 1979;21:6.

16. Seekins T, Smith N, McCleary T, et al. Secondary disability prevention: involving consumers in the development of a public health surveillance instrument. *J Disabil Policy Stud* 1990;1(3):21–36.

17. Sugarman B. Infection and pressure sores. *Arch Phys Med Rehabil* 1985;66:177–179.

18. Meyers AR, Cupples A, Lederman RI. A prospective evaluation of the effect of managed care on medical care utilization among severely disabled independently living adults. *Med Care* 1987;25:1057–1068.

19. Nosek MA, Fuhrer MJ, Howland CA. Independence among people with disabilities: II. Personal Independence Profile. *Rehabil Counsel Bull* 1992;36(1):21–36.

20. Davidoff G, Schultz S, Lieb T, et al. Rehospitalization after initial rehabilitation for acute spinal cord injury: incidence and risk factors. *Arch Phys Med Rehabil* 1990; 71:121–124.

21. Turoff M. The policy Delphi. In: Linstone HA, Turoff M, eds. *The Delphi method: techniques and applications*. Reading, MA: Addison-Wesley, 1975:84–104.

22. Zook CJ, Savickis SF, Moore FD. Repeated hospitalization for the same disease: a multiplier of national health costs. *Milbank Mem Fund Q Health Soc* 1980;58(3).

23. Seekins T, Clay J, Ravesloot C. A descriptive study of secondary conditions reported by a population of adults with physical disabilities served by three independent living centers in a rural state. *J Rehabil* 1994;60:47–51.

24. Krotoski DM, Nosek MA, Turk MA, eds. *Women with physical disabilities: achieving and maintaining health and well-being.* Baltimore: Paul H. Brookes, 1996.

25. Roller S. Health promotion for people with chronic neuromuscular disabilities. In: Krotoski D, Nosek MA, Turk MA, eds. *Women with physical disabilities: achieving and maintaining health and well-being.* Baltimore: Paul H. Brookes, 1996:431–439.

26. Turk MA. The impact of disability on fitness in women: musculoskeletal issues. In: Krotoski D, Nosek MA, Turk MA, eds. *Women with physical disabilities: achieving and maintaining health and well-being.* Baltimore: Paul H. Brookes, 1996:391–405.

27. Depauw KP. Adapted physical activity and sport. In: Krotoski D, Nosek MA, Turk MA, eds. *Women with physical disabilities: achieving and maintaining health and well-being.* Baltimore: Paul H. Brookes, 1996:419–430.

28. Crewe NM, Clarke N. Stress and women with disabilities. In: Krotoski D, Nosek MA, Turk MA, eds. *Women with physical disabilities: Achieving and maintaining health and well-being.* Baltimore: Paul H. Brookes, 1996: 193–202.

29. Patrick GD. Traditional approaches to stress reduction through skills training. In: Krotoski D, Nosek MA, Turk MA, eds. *Women with physical disabilities: Achieving and maintaining health and well-being.* Baltimore: Paul H. Brookes, 1996: 259–271.

30. Rintala DH, Hart KA, Fuhrer MJ. Perceived stress in individuals with spinal cord injury. In: Krotoski D, Nosek MA, Turk MA, eds. *Women with physical disabilities: achieving and maintaining health and well-being.* Baltimore: Paul H. Brookes, 1996: 223–242.

31. Fitness Canada Women's Program. *Physical activity and women with disabilities: a national survey.* Ottawa, Ontario, Canada: Canada Women's Program, 1989.

32. Roller S, Maynard F. *Stay well! The Polio Network's manual for a health promotion program.* Ithaca, MI: Polio Network, 1991.

33. Depauw KP, Sherrill C. Adapted physical activity: present and future. *Phys Educ Revi* 1994; 17:6–13.

34. Rimmer JH. *Fitness and rehabilitation programs for special populations.* Dubuque, IA: Brown & Benchmark, 1994.

35. Shephard RJ. *Fitness in special populations.* Champaign, IL: Human Kinetics, 1990.

36. Milner-Brown HS, Miller RG. Muscle strengthening through electric stimulation combined with low-resistance weights in patients with neuromuscular disorders. *Arch Phys Med Rehabil* 1988; 69:20–24.

37. Milner-Brown HS, Miller RG. Muscle strengthening through high-resistance weight training in patients with neuromuscular disorders. *Arch Phys Med Rehabil* 1988;69:14–19.

38. Aitkens SG, McCrory MA, Kilmer DD, Bernauer EM. Moderate resistance exercise program: its effect in slowly progressive neuromuscular disease. *Arch Phys Med Rehabil* 1993;74:711–715.

39. Lohi EL, Lindberg C, Anderson O. Physical training effects in myasthenia gravis. *Arch Phys Med Rehabil* 1993;74:1178–1180.

40. Feldman RM, Soskolne CL. The use of non-fatiguing strengthening exercise in post-polio syndrome. *Birth Defects* 1987;23: 335–341.

41. Einarsson G. Muscle conditioning in late poliomyelitis. *Arch Phys Med Rehabil* 1991;72:11–14.

42. Kriz JL, Jones DR, Speirer JL, et al. Cardiorespiratory responses to upper extremity aerobic training by post-polio subjects. *Arch Phys Med Rehabil* 1992;73:49–54.

43. Milner-Brown HS. Muscle strengthening in a post polio subject through a high resistance weight training program. *Arch Phys Med Rehabil* 1993;74:1165–1167.

44. Perry J, Young S, Barnes G. *Strengthening exercise for post-polio sequela. Arch Phys Med Rehabil* 1987;68:660. Abstract.

45. Davis GM. Exercise capacity of individuals with paraplegia. *Medi Sci Sports Exerc* 1993;25: 423–432.

46. Klose KJ, Schmidt DL, Needham BM, et al. Rehabilitation therapy for patients with long-term spinal cord injuries. *Arch Phys Med Rehabil* 1990;71:659–662.

47. Roth EJ, Oken JE, Primack S, et al. Expiratory muscle training in spinal cord injury: preliminary results. *Arch Phys Med Rehabil* 1990;71:796. Abstract.

48. Weber RJ. Functional neuromuscular stimulation. In: DeLisa JA, eds. *Rehabilitation medicine: principles and practice.* 2nd ed. Philadelphia: JB Lippincott, 1993:463–476.

49. Whiting RB, Dreisinger TE, Dalton RB. Improved physical fitness and work capacity in quadriplegics by wheelchair exercise. *J Cardiac Rehabil* 1983;3:251–255.

50. Fernandez JE, Pitetti KH. Training of ambulatory individuals with cerebral palsy. *Arch Phys Med Rehabil* 1993;74:468–472.

51. Jankowski LW, Sullivan SJ. Aerobic and neuromuscular training: effect on the capacity, efficiency, and fatigability of patients with traumatic brain injuries. *Arch Phys Med Rehabil* 1990;71:500–504.

52. Laskowski ER. Rehabilitation of the physically challenged athlete. *Phys Med Rehabil Clin N Am* 1994;5(1):215–233.

53. Potempa K, Lopez M, Braun LT, et al. Physiologic outcomes of aerobic exercise training in hemiparetic stroke patients. *Stroke* 1995;26:101–105.

54. Schurrer R, Weltman A, Brammel H. Effects of physical training on cardiovascular fitness and behavior patterns of mentally retarded adults. *Am J Ment Defici* 1985; 90:167–170.

55. deLateur BJ, Lehmann JF. Therapeutic exercise to develop strength and endurance. In: Kottke FJ, Stilwell GK, Lehmann JF, eds. *Krusen's handbook of physical medicine and rehabilitation.* 4th ed. Philadelphia: WB Saunders, 1990:480 519.

56. Fisher NM, Pendergast DR. Two-year follow-up of the effects of muscle rehabilitation in patients with osteoarthritis of the knees. *Arch Phys Med Rehabil* 1992;73: 972. Abstract.

57. Fisher NM, Pendergast DR, Gresham GE. Progressive, quantitative rehabilitation of patients with osteoarthritis. *Arch Phys Med Rehabil* 1990;71:762. Abstract.

58. Hicks JE, Gerber LH. Rehabilitation of the patient with arthritis and connective tissue disease. In: DeLisa JA, ed. *Rehabilitation medicine: principles and practice.* 2nd ed. Philadelphia: WB Saunders, 1993:1047–1081.

59. Lynberg KK, Harreby M, Bentzen H, et al. Elderly rheumatoid arthritis patients on steroid treatment tolerate physical training without an increase in disease activity. *Arch Phys Med Rehabil* 1994; 75:1189–1195.

60. McNeal RL. Aquatic therapy for patients with rheumatic disease. *Rheumatol Dis Clin North Am* 1990;16:915–929.

61. Minor MA, Hewett JE, Webel RS, et al. Efficacy of physical conditioning exercise in patients with rheumatoid arthritis and osteoarthritis. *Arthritis Rheum* 1989;32:1396–1405.

62. Van Duesen J, Harlowe D. The efficacy of the ROM dance program for adults with rheumatoid arthritis. *Am J Occup Ther* 1987; 41(2):90–95.

63. Brar SP, Wangaard C. Physical therapy for patients with multiple sclerosis. In: Maloney FP, Burks JB, Ringel SP, eds. *Interdisciplinary rehabilitation of multiple sclerosis and neuromuscular disorders.* Philadelphia: JB Lippincott, 1985:364-391.

64. Cobble ND, Dietz MA, Grigsby J, et al. Rehabilitation of the patient with multiple sclerosis. In: DeLisa JA, ed. *Rehabilitation medicine: principles and practice.* 2nd ed. Philadelphia: WB Saunders, 1993:861–885.

65. Gehlsen GM, Grigsby SA, Winant DM. Effects of an aquatic fitness program on the muscular strength and endurance of patients with multiple sclerosis. *Phys Ther* 1984;64:653–657.

66. Shapiro RT, Petajan JH, Kosich D, et al. Role of cardiovascular fitness in multiple sclerosis. *J Neurol Rehabil* 1988;2:43–49.

67. Turner RJ, Wood DW. Depression and disability: the stress process in a chronically strained population. *Res Community Mental Health* 1985;5:77–109.

68. Lazarus RS. Puzzles in the study of daily hassles. *J Behav Med* 1984;7:375–389.

69. Finkelhor D. Current information on the scope and nature of child sexual abuse. *Future Child* 1994;4:31–53.

70. Nosek MA. Sexual abuse of women with physical disabilities. *Phys Med Rehabil State Art Rev* 1995; 9:487–502.

71. Jacobson E. *Progressive relaxation.* 2nd ed. Chicago, IL: University of Chicago Press, 1983.

72. Bernstein D, Borkovec T. *Progressive relaxation training: A manual for helping professions.* Champaign, IL: Research Press; 1963.

73. Bernstein D, Carlson C. Progressive relaxation: abbreviated methods. In: Lehrer P, Woolfolk R, eds. *Principles and practice of stress management.* 2nd ed. New York: Guilford Press, 1993:53–88.

74. Benson H. *The relaxation response.* New York: William Morrow, 1975.

75. Carrington P. *Clinically standardized meditation (CSM) instructor's kit.* Kendall Park, NJ: Pace Educational Systems, 1978.

76. Linden W. *Autogenic training: a clinical guide.* New York: Guilford, 1990.

77. Patel C. Yoga-based therapy. In: Lehrer P, Woolfolk R, eds. *Principles and practice of stress management.* 2nd ed. New York: Guilford, 1993:53–88.

78. Haskell W. Overview: health benefits of exercise. In: Matarazzo J, Weiss J, Heard J, Miller N, eds. *Behavioral health: a handbook of health enhancement and disease prevention.* New York: Wiley-Interscience, 1987:409–423.

79. Coleman D, Iso-Ahola S. Leisure and health: the role of social support and self-determination. *J Leisure Res* 1993;25:111–128.

80. Maranto C. Music therapy and stress management. In: Lehrer P, Woolfolk R, eds. *Principles and practice of stress management.* 2nd ed. New York: Guilford, 1993:407–442.

81. Ornstein R, Sobel D. *Healthy pleasures.* New York: Addison-Wesley, 1990.

82. Schriver M, Cutler-Riddick C. Effects of watching aquariums on elders' stress. *Anthrozoos* 1988;9(1):44–48.

83. Wankel L, Berger B. The psychological and social benefits of sport and physical activity. *J Leisure Res* 1990;22:167–182.

84. Rekers H, Norpoth T, Michaels MA. Oral contraceptive use and venous thromboembolism: a consideration of the impact of bias and confounding factors on epidemiological studies. *Eur J Contracept Reprod Health Care* 1996; 1:21–30.

85. Skouby SO. Oral contraceptives and venous thrombosis: end of the debate? *Eur J Contracept Reprod Health Care* 1998;3:59–64.

86. Westhoff CL. Oral contraceptives and thrombosis: an overview of study methods and recent results. *Am J Obstet Gynecol* 1998;179(3 Pt 2):S38–42.

Chapter 100

Rehabilitation in Developing Countries

Tyrone M. Reyes

On the international level, the ideal goal of medical rehabilitation is to promote effective measures for the prevention of disability and the provision of optimum rehabilitation treatments to all disabled persons who need them, with the aim of achieving full participation and equality in social life and economic development. This means that persons with a disability are entitled to the same rights and to equal opportunities as all other human beings. This principle should apply with the same scope and with the same urgency to all countries, regardless of their level of development.

However, the problems of disability in developing countries and in particular, the least developed countries need to be specially highlighted. The immensity of the task of improving the living conditions of the general population and the severe scarcity of resources make the rehabilitation of persons with disabilities much more difficult and challenging in these countries.

In such countries, the resources are not sufficient to detect and prevent disability or to treat and rehabilitate those with disabilities. The disability problem in these countries is further complicated by the population explosion that inexorably increases the number of disabled persons in both proportional and absolute terms (1).

It has been estimated that the world's population will grow by 60% from 1990 to 2025. This growth, however, will be uneven. In the more developed countries, the increase is projected at 12%, whereas in the less developed regions, it is forecast at 75%. Thus, the increase will be most pronounced in countries with the fewest resources to meet this increasing demand for rehabilitation services (2).

Studies on rehabilitation in developing countries are very limited. Few published reports have evaluated the problems, resources, and needs of the physically challenged in these countries. Fewer still are investigations on the efficacy of alternative rehabilitation treatments and delivery systems; the influence of socioeconomic, ethnic, and cultural factors; or the use of appropriate rehabilitation technologies to manage the unique needs of persons with disabilities in these countries.

STATISTICS ON DISABILITY IN DEVELOPING COUNTRIES

The United Nations estimates that more than 500 million persons in the world are disabled as a consequence of mental, physical, or sensory impairment. These data were apparently confirmed by surveys conducted on various segments of the world population and by observations reported by some experienced investigators. They cited a 10% to 25% prevalence worldwide of persons adversely affected by disability (1). While there may be general agreement on the rate of disability worldwide, there is a wide discrepancy in the reporting of the prevalence of disability in developing countries.

Whereas many developed countries like the United States and Canada have reported disability rates of 12.8%

to 17.0% (3,4), the developing countries of Central and South America have published an estimated disability prevalence of only 4% to 7% of their populations (5,6). This variability in the reported disability prevalence rates does not only occur between developed and developing nations but even within countries. In the Philippines, a disability survey reported on in 1983 by the National Commission Concerning Disabled Persons reported that 2.5 million Filipinos, or 5% of the population, had physical disabilities (7). In the 1990 population survey, the Philippine National Statistics Office reported that only 1 million of more than 60 million Filipinos had physical disabilities, a rate of less than 2% (8).

This possible underreporting of the true number of persons with disabilities in many developing countries may be due to confusion by either the enumerators or the families surveyed regarding their perception as to who should be considered disabled. This is borne out by experiences conducting disability surveys among children (9).

In 1990, the United Nations published the *Disability Statistics Compendium*, which contained data from 55 countries and showed that the percentages of the disabled population in these countries varied from 0.2% to 20.9% (10). It ascribed these significant discrepancies to two factors: the focus of the survey team on disabilities rather than impairments, which both enumerators and caretakers can identify much easier; and the marked differences in the populations surveyed as to age, sex, and even locality settings. There is a clear need to establish a more uniform database for developing countries that is understandable to all, with terms that can be translated easily to local dialects. The demographics of the populations sampled also need to be well described and made more uniform. Such information will be valuable in the long-term planning of services for persons with disabilities, primarily at the community level, for it is believed that as many as 80% of all persons with disabilities live in isolated rural communities in developing countries that are not reached by current rehabilitation facilities (1).

In 1990, it was estimated that 276 million people in the world had moderate or severe disabilities. Of these, 93 million lived in the more developed countries and 183 million lived in the less developed regions. The prevalence for developing countries in 1992 was estimated at 200 million. These figures do not include temporary or short-term disability caused by curable diseases or reversible conditions, or terminal disability associated with severe diseases (11).

Attempts have been made to estimate the prevalence and classify the functional limitations of persons with disabilities in developing countries. The estimates and classification used by the World Health Organization (WHO) are listed in Table 100-1. The actual prevalence of the types of limitations listed in Table 100-1 naturally vary from one area to another, depending on a multitude of factors. For example, in an area where trachoma is common, inevitably the number of persons with visual difficulty will be higher.

Table 100-1: Estimates and Classification Used by World Health Organization

Types of Limitations	Prevalence (%)
Moving difficulty	2.0–2.5
Seeing difficulty	0.5–0.8
Hearing/speech difficulty	0.5–0.8
Learning difficulty	0.2–0.4
Chronic fits	0.3–0.6
Strange behavior	0.1–0.3
Combinations of above	0.2–0.3
Total	4–5

Source: World Health Organization. *Draft to prepare curriculum on disability issues for doctors in PHC.* Geneva: World Health Organization, undated.

There is a greater strain on the families and communities where the prevalence of moderate and severe disability is high, perhaps even more so than in developed countries because persons with disabilities are quite often dependent on others physically, psychologically, socially, or economically. Therefore, the impact of disability on societies in developing countries can be significant.

SPECIAL GROUPS

The consequences of disability in developing countries are particularly serious for special groups, such as women, children, and the elderly. In many countries, women are subjected to social, cultural, and economic disadvantages that impede their access to rehabilitative care, making it more difficult for them to participate in community life. In families, tradition often dictates that women have the responsibility to care for a parent with disability, which further considerably limits their access to other activities.

For many children, an impairment bestows a stigma that can lead to rejection or isolation, and thus exclusion from the normal experiences of growing up. These developmental difficulties can be exacerbated further by a negative family attitude during the critical years when these children's personalities and self-images are developing.

The elderly, an increasing segment of the population in many developing countries, presents a multitude of special problems. Many have poor mobility from arthritis or strokes, with difficulty in communication due to poor hearing and vision, and a number are unable to participate in the decision-making process because of cognitive decline.

The problem is complicated further in these countries by the fact that most of these persons are usually very poor. There are presently about 200 million moderately and severely disabled people in developing countries where persons with disabilities are typically poverty ridden. Malnutrition, a by-product of poverty, by itself produces deficits in motor and perceptual skills in chronically malnourished children (12).

In other developing countries, significant causes of disability also include crime or torture, war (e.g., land mines), natural and man-made disasters, and foreign employment (migrant workers). There are over 10 million refugees and displaced persons in the world as a result of man-made disasters (1). Many of them are disabled physically and psychologically as a result of their sufferings from persecution and violence. Most live in third-world countries where rehabilitation facilities and services are extremely limited.

REHABILITATION MANPOWER NEEDS AND SUPPLY

Despite the dismal lack of accurate statistics on the number of disabled persons in developing countries, there is a general consensus that there is a critical lack of manpower supply and an even more severe maldistribution of trained rehabilitation caregivers in these countries (13). There are not enough physiatrists or allied rehabilitation professionals in the rural areas where the majority of the population of developing countries resides. In 1989, 91% of the population of Uganda lived in rural areas while only 24% of the country's physicians and 10% of its hospital beds were dedicated to their medical needs. In Thailand, the physician-patient ratio is 1:5000 population but the ratio in rural areas is much higher due to maldistribution (11). Based on a prevalence rate of 4% to 5% for moderate to severe disability in the general population, the disparity of the physiatrist-patient ratio has been noted to be as high as 1:2500 in Botswana to as low as 1:100 in Sweden (11).

Many physicians from developing countries in the 1950s and 1960s went to developed countries like the United States, England, and Canada to train in the specialty of physical medicine and rehabilitation. A significant number of these trained physicians did not return to their home countries, causing a "brain drain" in the physiatrist supply. In 1971, for example, the Philippines had only 10 trained physiatrists, all of whom were based in the capital city of Manila. The country experienced a paradoxical situation then when there were more Filipino physiatrists practicing in the state of New York than in the entire Philippines. This gave impetus to the establishment of a regional training center for Asia at the Santo Tomas University Hospital (STUH) in Manila for the developing countries in the Asia-Pacific region, with the goals of addressing the brain drain problem, the maldistribution of physiatrists, and the overly Western orientation of the training programs in the more advanced countries. The World Rehabilitation Fund (WRF), under Dr. Howard A. Rusk, fully supported this innovative training project, which subsequently became a model program in rehabilitation medicine for other developing regions in the world (14).

The physician trainees for the STUH program initially came from Indonesia and the Philippines, two countries with similar social and economic backgrounds. They were trained in patient care, research, administration, and public information, emphasizing local diseases and conditions while considering native cultural and psychological values.

Forty-eight physicians, 36 Filipinos and 12 Indonesians, were trained from 1977 to 1995. The 36 Filipino physiatrists are now situated in 10 of the country's 12 regions. The 12 Indonesian physiatrists have started their own in-country training program in Jakarta, Surabaya, and Bandung and are producing more than 50 graduates each year destined to serve the needs of its 200 million population (14).

More importantly, the WRF-supported program attained a 92% successful retention rate, with the graduates opting to permanently practice in their assigned localities! Analysis of the data showed that the factors important in ensuring a successful transition into a provincial assignment for the trained physiatrists included the availability of support from family and community in the area, the provision of equipment and personnel to start a clinical practice, patient networking, and regular updating in knowledge and skill from the mother program (14).

The training of allied rehabilitation professionals like physical, occupational, and speech therapists has also increased significantly in the past decades, especially in developing countries. Many schools have opened with the curricula patterned after those in Western countries and with English as the medium of instruction. Unfortunately, the impetus for these schools is not so much to meet the real manpower needs of these developing countries but to fill up clinical positions in developed countries where the compensation is far greater than what these individuals can expect to receive in their native countries (15).

Despite the progress just detailed, it is clear that there continues to be a significant lack of resources for the proper delivery of rehabilitation services in developing countries. Furthermore, many of the approaches in medical rehabilitation being utilized in developed countries cannot be applied effectively to developing countries where different socioeconomic conditions exist. Interestingly, some strategies that have evolved over the years have proved effective in serving the needs of the disabled in these communities, taking into account resource constraints, level of socioeconomic development, cultural traditions, and the capacity of local governments to formalize and implement specific programs for the rehabilitation of persons with disabilities.

COMMUNITY-BASED REHABILITATION

The WHO's major thrust of Health for All by the year 2000 and its related primary health care approach already include disability prevention and rehabilitation. In 1978, the International Conference in Primary Health Care, held in Alma-Ata, declared that the primary health care approach would best address the main health problems in the community through the provision of preventive, curative, and rehabilitation services (16). Following this declaration, WHO developed the strategy of community-based rehabilitation (CBR) as a means of integrating rehabilitation with health and development activities at the community level.

CBR is defined as a "strategy within community development for the rehabilitation, equalization of opportunities and social integration of all people with disabilities." It is implemented through the "combined efforts of disabled people themselves, their families and communities, and appropriate health, education, vocational and social services (17).

The WHO's Rehabilitation Unit officially introduced CBR through the use of simplified manuals in an international meeting in Mexico in 1979 (18). It gained considerable support worldwide during the United Nations–declared International Year of Disabled Persons in 1981 and the Decade of Disabled Persons in 1983–1992.

CBR is characterized by the active roles of people with disabilities, their families, and the community in the rehabilitation process. In CBR, Knowledge and skills for the basic training of people with disabilities are transferred to the adults with disabilities, to their families, and to community members. A community committee promotes the removal of physical and attitudinal barriers and ensures opportunities for people with disabilities to participate in school, work, leisure, social, and political activities within the community. A person is available in the community to work with persons with disabilities and their families in rehabilitation activities. Children with disabilities attend the local school. Community members provide local job training. Community groups assist the families of people with disabilities by providing physical care, transportation, or loans to initiate income-generating activities. Community resources are supported by referral services within the health, education, labor, and social service system. Personnel skilled in rehabilitation technology train and support community workers, and provide skilled intervention, as necessary (16).

The Pan American Health Organization (PAHO) has estimated that one-third of the 7% to 10% of persons with disabilities in Latin America can solve their own problems without specialized care. These are the people whose disabilities are minimal or moderate in their functional effects and social impact. Forty percent of the people are believed to be able to solve their problems through CBR, 20% would need further professional help, and 10% would require institutional rehabilitation (19).

The experiences of the WHO pilot projects in CBR in China and the Philippines have shown the following positive results:

1. Attitudinal changes: The public and families have more concern and sympathy for persons with disabilities, and are more willing to provide assistance.
2. Persons with disabilities develop a better outlook for their future. They became more confident and better motivated.
3. Motor function and ability to perform activities of daily living improve with an overall improvement in quality of life.
4. CBR has made rehabilitative treatments more accessible, convenient, and cost-effective, thus lessening the burden (economical and psychological) on the family (20,21).

Indeed, CBR appears to be a simple, low-cost, and effective strategy for the delivery of rehabilitation services in rural areas. A clear advantage is that CBR allows persons with disabilities to stay home with their families, thereby ensuring a more effective integration within that community.

REHABILITATION IN PRIMARY HEALTH CARE

Rehabilitation within the health care services traditionally has been thought to involve the provision of therapy—physical, occupational, and speech—as well as specialized equipment. Traditional rehabilitation services are provided in various settings such as special institutions, hospitals, and outpatient clinics. However, statistics show that in developing countries, such services only reach a small segment of those in need. The large service gap is created by the fact that most rehabilitation facilities are in large cities, leaving out the rural communities. Even among persons with disabilities in the urban centers where there are available rehabilitation services, many do not avail themselves of these services. The main reason for this is that the cost of such services is not within the reach of many persons with disabilities.

People with disabilities are socially and economically disadvantaged. The quality of their life is lower than that of the average population (22). Often, a low-priority program of many governments, the medical rehabilitation services available in developing countries cater to only a few of the total estimated number of persons with disabilities.

At the primary health care level, rehabilitation takes the form of measures to prevent disabilities. A strategy of prevention is essential for reducing the incidence of impairment and disability. Much disability can be prevented in developing countries through measures taken against malnutrition, environmental pollution, poor hygiene, inadequate prenatal and postnatal care, waterborne diseases, and accidents of all types. The international community could make a major breakthrough against disabilities caused by such diseases as poliomyelitis, diphtheria, and pertussis, through a worldwide expansion of programs of immunization. A more effective public health program for just two diseases—leprosy and malaria—would cut down drastically the disability rate in many developing countries.

The most important measures for prevention of impairment are avoidance of war; improvement of the educational, economic, and social status of the least privileged groups; identification of types of impairment and their causes within defined geographic areas; introduction of specific intervention measures through better nutritional practices; improvement of health services, including early detection and diagnosis; prenatal and postnatal care; proper health care instruction, including patient and physician education; family planning; legislation; modification of lifestyles; and education regarding environmental hazards.

The WHO has also adopted specific measures that should help in disability prevention, such as nutrition intervention programs directed at specific population groups most at risk for vitamin A and iodine deficiency; improved medical care for the aging; training and regulations to reduce the number of accidents in industry, in agriculture, on the roads, and in the homes; and control of environmental pollution and of the use and abuse of drugs and alcohol (1).

A model of a good disability prevention program is the one adopted by Singapore in 1988 (23). The program has three levels. The first level or primary prevention consists of measures to prevent diseases, injuries, or conditions that can result in impairment or disabilities. Such measures include genetic counseling; immunization against communicable diseases; health education to encourage better nutrition, hygiene, and physical fitness and discourage addiction and habituation; and programs to prevent or minimize accidents at work, on the road, at home, or during recreation.

The second level or secondary prevention consists of early intervention in the treatment of diseases, injuries, or conditions to prevent the development of impairments. In Singapore, this level involved neonatal screening (especially of low-birth-weight newborns), establishment of Developmental Assessment Clinics and School Psychological Services, and others.

The third level or tertiary prevention includes all measures to limit or reduce impairments and disabilities. Tertiary prevention includes the treatment of disabilities and may include training in self-care, communication, mobility, and even work skills. In the Singapore program, a National Aids and Appliances Centre for Disabled People was established to provide persons with disabilities artificial limbs, braces, and other self-help devices.

GENERAL HEALTH CARE FOR PEOPLE WITH DISABILITIES

It is not unusual for people with disabilities in developing countries to not receive health services that are routinely provided to able-bodied persons. Children with disabilities may not be immunized or may not receive care for common childhood illnesses. Adults with disabilities may also be deprived of health services. The reasons given to explain this situation include the following: health services may be inaccessible to people with disabilities; health professionals may not know how to judge the health status of a person with disabilities; persons with disabilities themselves may not expect to receive such services; and parents may hide their children because of the social stigma brought about by disability.

All health workers should be trained to work with people with disabilities. They need a basic understanding of rehabilitation principles and procedures to provide basic health services, and to advise people with disabilities and their families about prevention of deformities and their potential to lead as normal a life as possible. All health workers should also be aware of the resources available to people with disabilities through appropriate referral.

PRACTICE ISSUES IN DEVELOPING COUNTRIES

The primary causes of physical impairment in all age groups in many developing countries are still infectious in origin. Poliomyelitis, for example, is still the most prevalent reason for movement limitations in children and young adults (24,25) (Fig. 100-1). This situation is anticipated to drastically change, however, with the recent successful mass immunizations against polio conducted in many developing countries with the assistance of WHO, Rotary International, and other agencies (26). However, one must still deal with the present-day realities of the consequences of neglected, polio-ravaged children and young adults, and spend time, energy and resources in their surgical reconstruction and medical rehabilitation.

Tuberculosis of the spine (Pott disease) and falls from coconut trees are still responsible for a significant percentage of spinal cord injuries. However, acts of violence, rather than accidents, account for the majority of spinal cord injuries in many developing countries (27,28). In the course of performing electrodiagnostic procedures, practicing physiatrists may need to first rule out Hansen disease, parasitic neural invasion, or toxic reactions to heavy metals or banned insecticides, when faced with a conduction block or slowing (29,30).

In prescribing artificial limbs for persons with limb loss, physiatrists from the developing countries of Asia must cope with a low rate of prosthetic utilization because of the prohibitive price of the Western-style prostheses and their inadequacy for functional use in rural areas. The

1. **Exercises to keep full range of motion,** starting within days after paralysis appears and continuing throughout rehabilitation

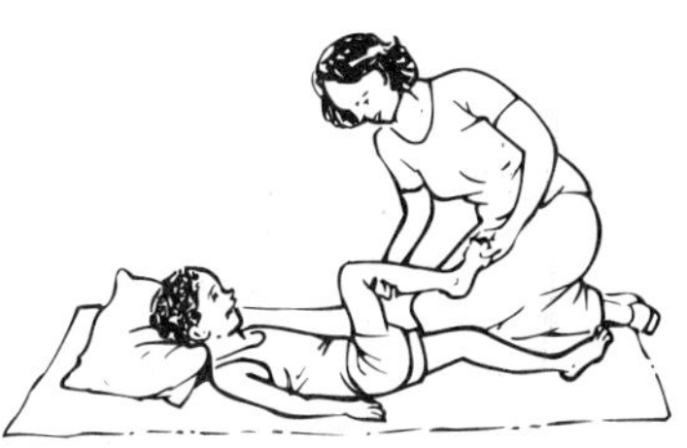

2. **Supported sitting in** positions that help prevent contractures

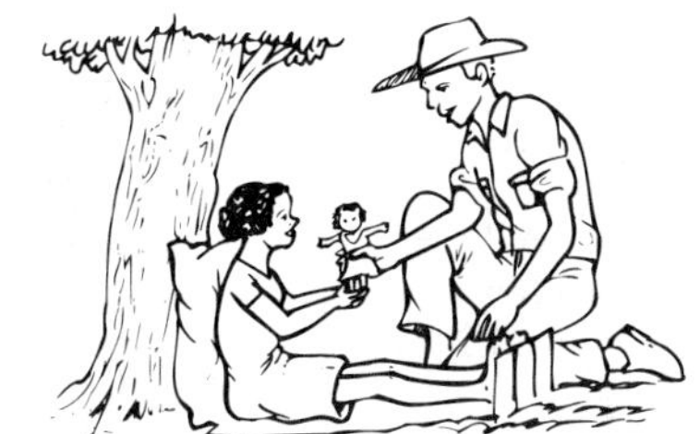

3. **Active exercises** with limbs supported, to gain strength and maintain full motion

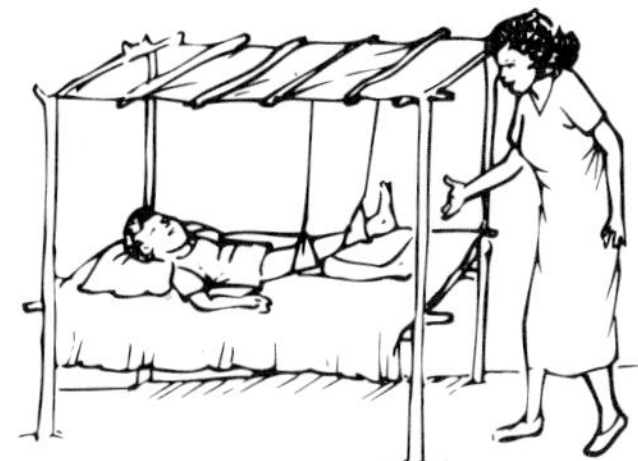

4. **Exercises in water –** walking, floating, and swimming, with the weight of the limbs supported by the water

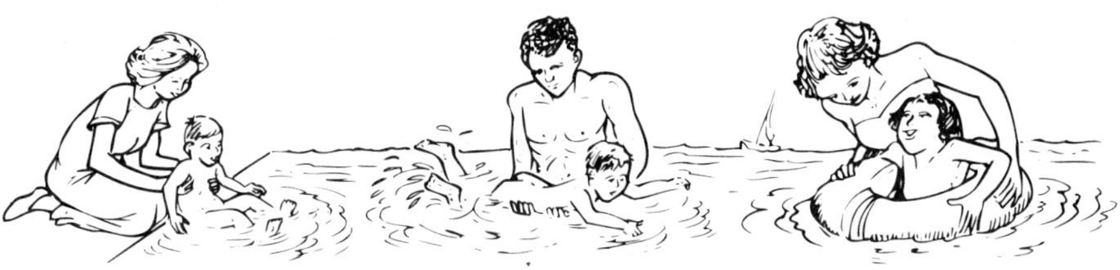

5. **Wheelchair or wheelboard** with supports to prevent or correct early contractures

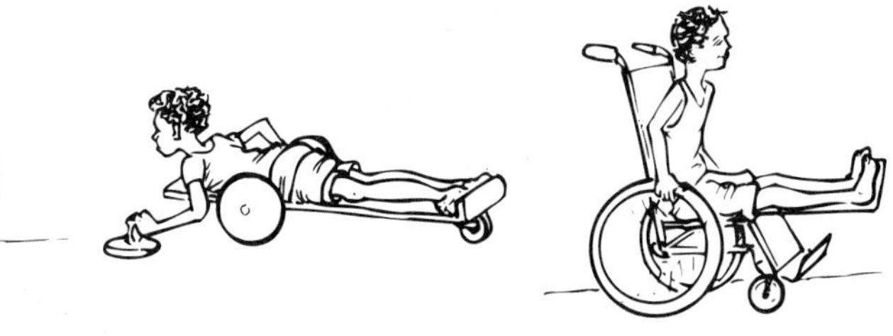

6. **Braces** to prevent contractures and prepare for walking

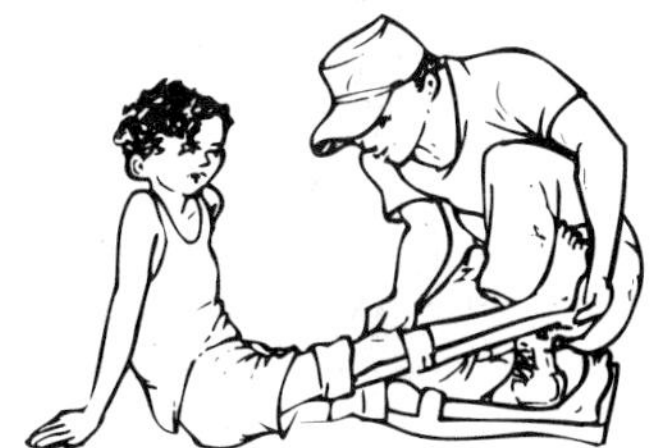

7. **Parallel bars** for beginning to balance and walk

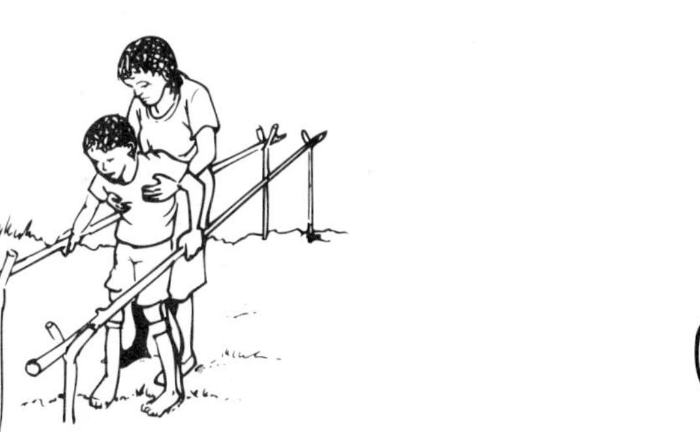

8. **Walking machine or 'walker'**

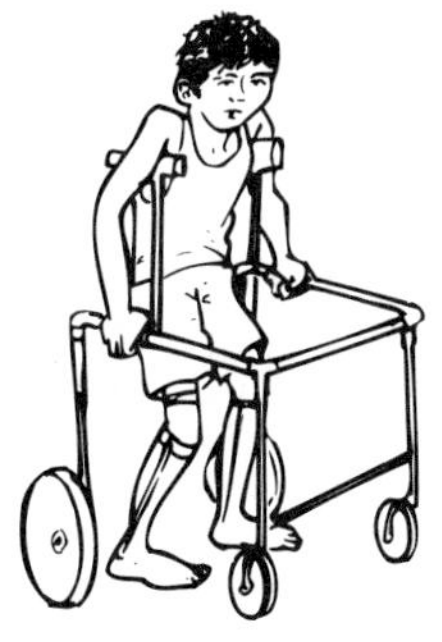

9. **Crutches modified as walker** for balance and extra support

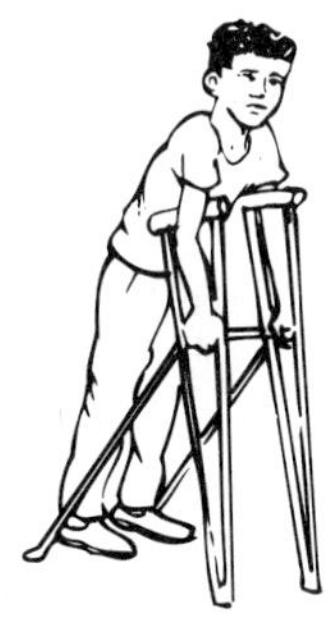

10. **Under arm crutches**

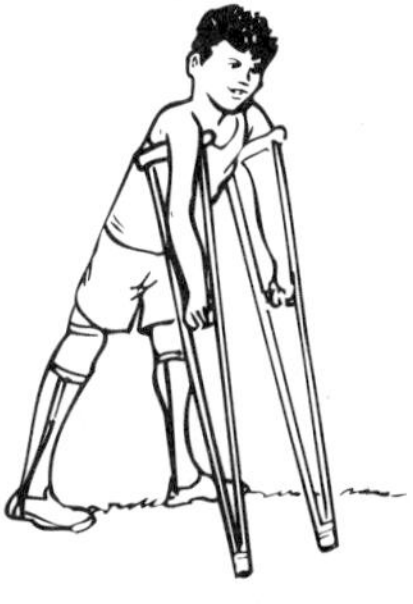

11. **Forearm crutches** and perhaps in time...

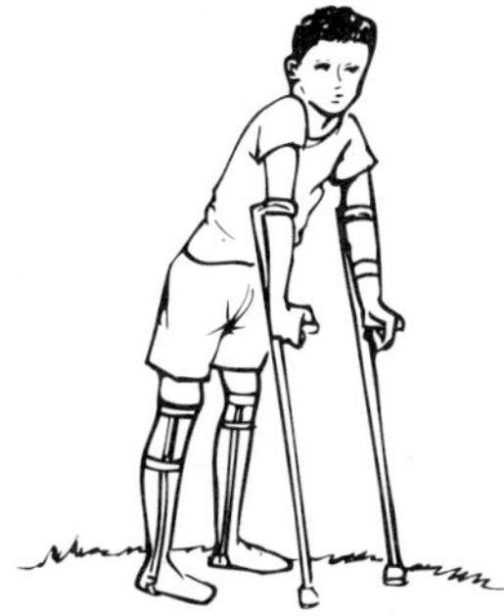

12. **A cane** or no arm supports at all

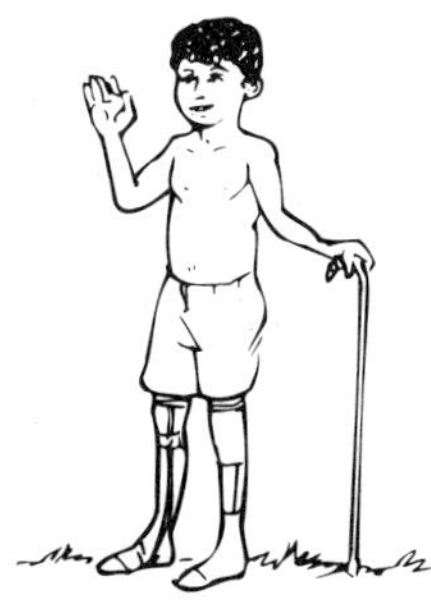

Figure 100-1. Simple treatment for children with poliomyelitis at the community level in developing countries. (Reproduced by permission from Werner DB. *Disabled village children.* Palo Alto, CA: The Hesperian Foundation, 1987.)

SACH foot could not be worn with sandals or thongs; the socket does not allow an amputee to squat; and the plastic laminate of the shaft disintegrates if used in rice paddies or sea water by farmers or fishermen. A significant milestone for persons with limb loss in Asia was the development of the Jaipur limb by Dr. Sethi in India (31) (Fig. 100-2) and the People's below-knee prosthesis in the Philippines (32), both of which answered the need for a cheap, lightweight, and versatile prosthesis with a short production time, low maintenance requirement, and high patient acceptability. Indigenous materials have also been used successfully in the fabrication of assistive devices for persons with disabilities due to limited resources in rural areas. An example is the use of bamboo for braces, parallel bars, and splints (Fig. 100-3).

Test batteries that are utilized to evaluate associated cognitive, motor-perceptual, or psychological problems were developed in the West and validated using Western norms. Oftentimes, physiatrists from Africa, Asia, or Latin America are perplexed by the findings of generally lower scores in the IQ test, Wechsler Adult Intelligence Scale–Revised (WAIS-R), or Bender-Gestalt. Many of these tests have not been validated for persons with disabilities in developing countries. To eliminate the bias imposed by language and culture, as well as the physical limitations of disability, there is a need to develop and validate tests locally in developing countries. An example of this is the Manila Motor-Perceptual Screening Test (MaMPS Test), which was developed and field tested in a nationwide screening of able-bodied and physically disabled 4- to 6-year-old children in 1986 (33,34).

The health care delivery system for persons with disabilities in many of the developing countries has been sponsored either partly or wholly by the government and delivered by its officials or by nongovernmental institutions like religious institutions, which subsidize charity hospitals for economically disadvantaged patients. Only a minority can afford to pay for the services rendered to persons with disabilities in developing countries.

Most physiatrists in these countries are either full-time or part-time government employees who are allowed limited private practice, or those who choose to devote a portion of their time to academic life and do private practice on a fee-for-service basis.

Delivery of care in many less developed countries is oftentimes supplemented by indigenous healers. Herbal medicines, acupuncture, and traditional healers like the bone-setters may be helpful but occasionally some of these practices may be detrimental to persons with disabilities (35,36). Okamoto et al (37–39) reported the beneficial impact of a rehabilitation technician project on the delivery of rehabilitation services in Micronesia and the other Pacific Basin countries.

There are minimal extended-care facilities or nursing homes for persons with disabilities or the elderly in many developing countries. Tradition dictates that family members must care for their sick and aged at home.

LIFE SATISFACTION

Three studies completed in the Philippines showed that 75% of subjects with disabilities interviewed expressed general satisfaction with their lives, compared to 69% of Americans with disabilities who were only somewhat satisfied with theirs (22,40,41). This higher life satisfaction score among a population with disabilities that is financially and educationally disadvantaged compared to its Western counterpart has been fascinating (21).The authors of the studies attributed the difference to the legendary cohesiveness of the Filipino family and its extended-family system, as well as the strength of the religious beliefs of persons with disabilities, which allowed them to be more accepting and less complaining of their disabilities (21).

CONCLUSIONS

The widespread nature of diseases in many countries, particularly preventable infectious disease in the developing countries, will continue to tax limited rehabilitation resources. The millions of individuals throughout the globe suffering from such avoidable diseases as poliomyelitis, meningitis, and leprosy add to the world's burden of disability. Conversely, if progress is made in reducing these infectious diseases (e.g., poliomyelitis) and if human nutrition is improved, the world's future burden of disability ultimately may be reduced. Similarly, as maternal and child health care services and occupational health and safety activities are increased, the burden of disability may be eased further. However, as life expectancy increases, higher percentages of persons with disabilities will survive to ages where chronic and degenerative diseases may take a higher toll. Thus, ironically, the demand for rehabilitation services will rise as overall health care improves.

It is essential in developing countries to make the fullest possible use of limited resources and trained personnel in rehabilitation programs for the disabled. It is evident, however, that despite limited resources, much can be done to improve the quality of life of persons with disabilities. Innovative and realistic approaches, such as CBR programs, have proved successful in improving the quality of life of persons with disabilities in developing countries. The WRF-STUH program to train physiatrists in Asia worked successfully in training physicians in rehabilitation medicine in that region, serving as a model for making available medical rehabilitation services to previously unserved urban and rural communities in some Asian countries.

Overall, despite limited resources, an expansion of rehabilitation services in developing countries has resulted

The foot is made of wood and sponge rubber and the 'vulcanized' (heat molded) with rubber, using a metal mold. The rubber gives the foot its life-like form and color and makes it strong and waterproof

Jaipur foot

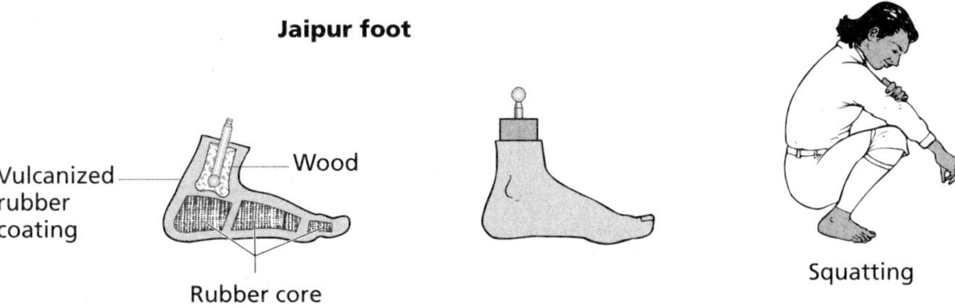

The limb is made of sheet aluminum

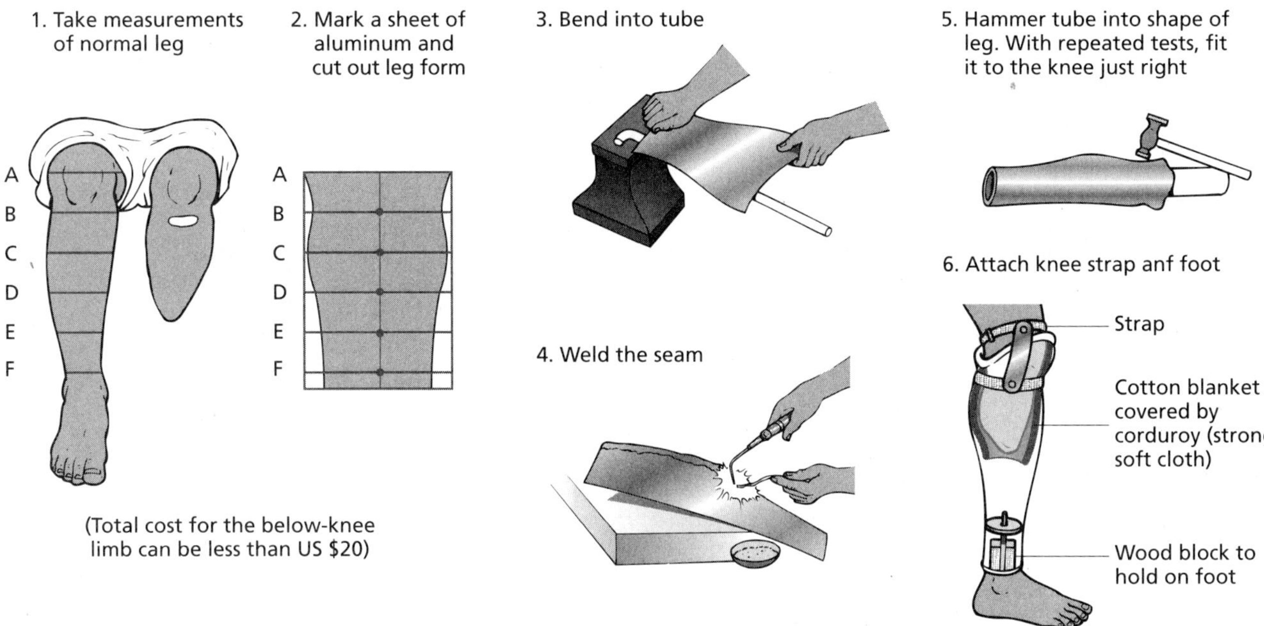

Jaipur above-knee design

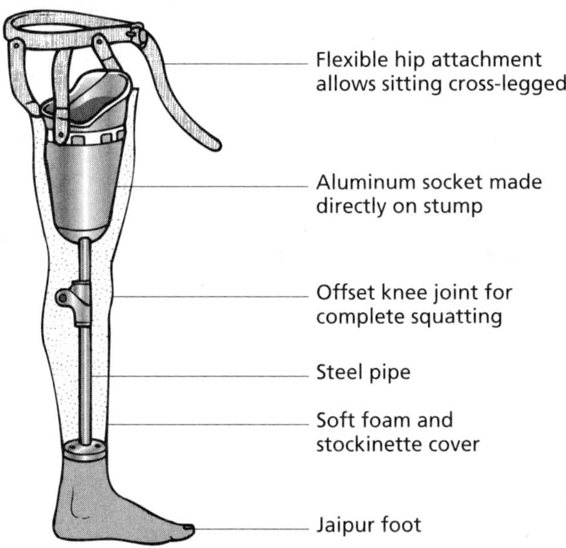

Figure 100-2. The Jaipur limb. (Reproduced by permission from Werner DB. *Disabled village children.* Palo Alto, CA: The Hesperian Foundation, 1987.)

A temporary leg splint of cardboard, folded paper, or the thick curved stem of a dried banana leaf, or palm leaf

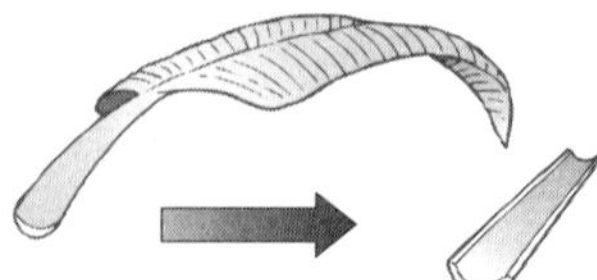

Aluminum tube finger splint

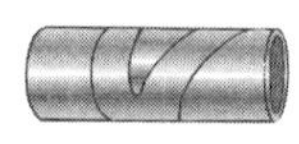

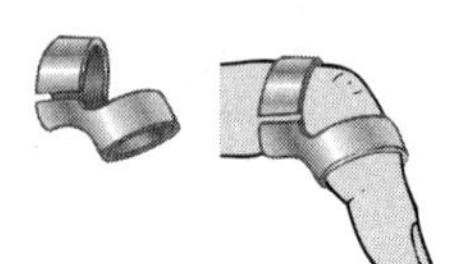

Mango seed finger splint

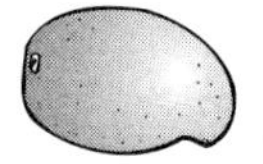

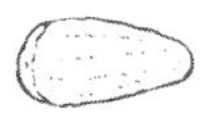

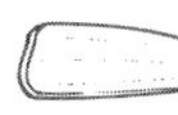

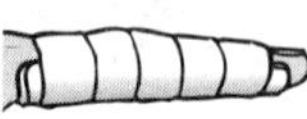

Remove the woody coat of a mango seed and wrap the coat firmly onto the finger. It will dry into a firm splint. To change its shape, first soak it in water

Bamboo ankle splint
A piece of seasoned bamboo can be heated and bent

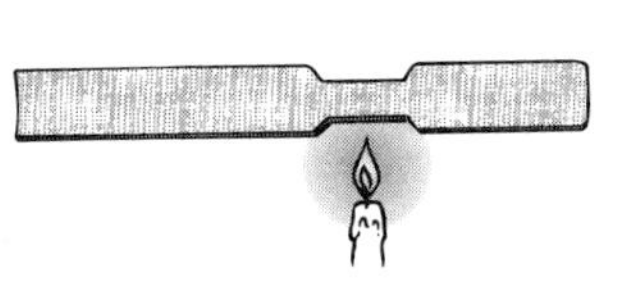

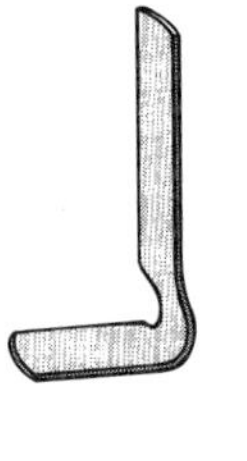

Plastic cup ankle braces for night or temporary use on a small child

For a small baby:

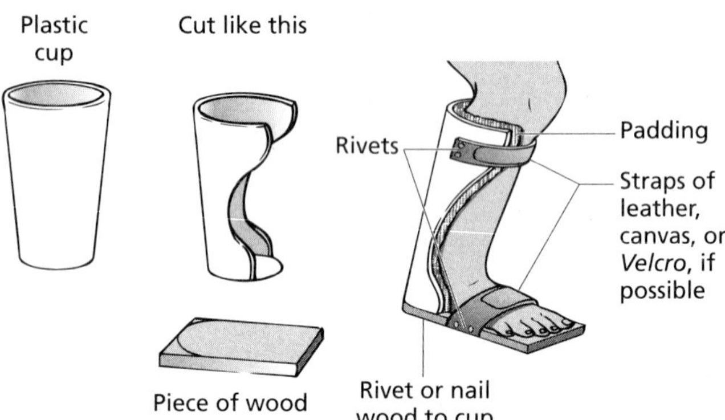

For a child:

3 cups cut and riveted together

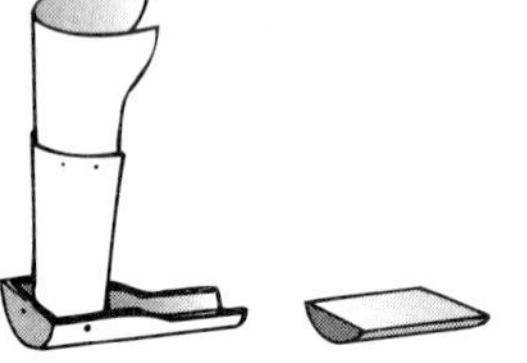

Make a flat inner sole out of cloth or wood

Or cut the foot piece from a flat plastic bottle

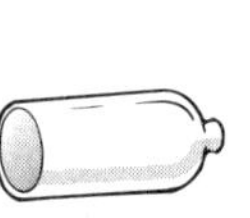

Add straps to fasten the brace around legs

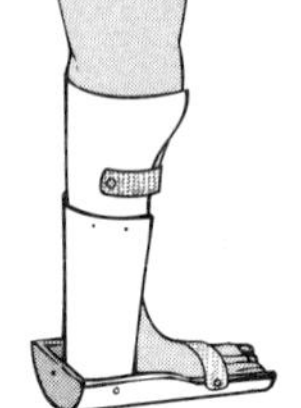

Figure 100-3. Simple, low-cost braces and splints made from indigenous materials. (Reproduced by permission from Werner DB. *Disabled village children.* Palo Alto, CA: The Hesperian Foundation, 1987.)

in a greater number of persons with disabilities being served, with more of them expressing satisfaction with the quality of their lives. However, the greatest asset of rehabilitation in developing countries continues to be the close family ties that survive in most of these societies. Support for a family member who is disabled continues to be strong, and respect and reverence for the elder members of the family remain a valued and valuable tradition. There is a greater awareness today that although much needs to be done, the problem is not insurmountable. At stake is the dignity, self-respect, and happiness of millions of people with disabilities all over the world.

REFERENCES

1. United Nations. *World programme of action concerning disabled persons.* New York: United Nations, 1983.
2. World Bank. *Investing in health. World development report.* Washington, DC: World Bank, 1993.
3. ICD-International Center for the Disabled. *The ICD survey of disabled Americans: bringing disabled Americans into the mainstream.* New York: Louis Harris and Associates, 1986.
4. Department of Secretary of State of Canada. *Report of the Canadian health and disability survey 1983–1984.* Toronto: Ministry of Supply and Services, 1986.
5. Pan American Health Organization. *Health condition in the Americas.* Washington, DC: Pan American Health Organization, 1986.
6. Pan American Health Organization. *Disability.* Washington, DC: Pan American Health Organization, 1990.
7. National Commission Concerning Disabled Persons (Philippines). *National disability survey.* Quezon

City: National Commission Concerning Disabled Persons, 1983.

8. National Statistics Office (Philippines). *The 1990 national census.* Manila: National Statistics Office, 1990.

9. Werner DB. *Disabled village children.* Palo Alto, CA: Hesperian Foundation, 1987.

10. United Nations. *Disability statistics compendium.* New York: UN Statistical Office, 1990.

11. World Health Organization. *Draft to prepare curriculum on disability issues for doctors in PHC.* Geneva: World Health Organization Rehabilitation Unit, undated.

12. Reyes MRL, Valdecanas CM, Reyes OR, Reyes TM. The effects of malnutrition on the motor, perceptual and cognitive functions of Filipino children. *J Disabil Stud* 1990;12: 131–136.

13. Reyes TM. Concepts in the rehabilitation of the Filipino handicapped. *Unitas* 1974;47:63–79.

14. Reyes TM, Reyes OL. A realistic approach to the training of Asian physiatrists. In: *Proceedings of the 16th Rehabilitation International World Congress.* Tokyo 1988:231–233.

15. Reyes TM, Reyes OL. Physical therapy—the profession. *Life Today* 1994;50:16–21.

16. World Health Organization. *Community-based rehabilitation and the health care referral services. A guide for programme managers.* Geneva: World Health Organization Rehabilitation Handbook 1, 1994.

17. ILO/UNESCO/WHO. *Joint position on community-based rehabilitation—for and with people with disabilities.* Geneva: International Labour Organization/United Nations Educational, Scientific, and Cultural Organization/World Health Organization, 1994.

18. World Health Organization. *Training the disabled in the community.* Geneva: World Health Organization, 1979.

19. Pan American Health Association. *Health of disabled persons.* Washington, DC: Pan American Health Association, 1984.

20. Zhuo D. An urban model of community based rehabilitation in China. In: *Proceedings of the 16th Rehabilitation International World Congress.* Tokyo, 1988:179–181.

21. Valdez L. *Community based rehabilitation: a development programme in Negros Occidental. Documentation report of Manila conference on the Asia Pacific decade of disabled persons.* Manila: National Council for the Welfare of Disabled Persons, 1994.

22. De Guzman RL, Reyes OL, Reyes TM. The AMRC study: bringing disabled Filipinos into the mainstream. *Santo Tomas J Med* 1994;43:20–32.

23. Singapore Advisory Council on the Disabled. *Opportunities for the disabled.* Singapore: Singapore National Printers, November 1988.

24. Oporto-Flordelis MJ, Reyes OL, Reyes TM. Paralytic poliomyelitis: a static disease? *Santo Tomas J Med* 1982;31:81–89.

25. Reyes OL, Reyes TM, So FY, et al. Energy cost of ambulation in healthy and disabled Filipino children. *Arch Phys Med Rehabil* 1988;69:946–949.

26. World Health Organization. *Eradication of polio in the region. In: Report of the Regional Committee* for the Western Pacific, Forty-Fourth Session. Manila: 1993:11.

27. Hart C, Williams E. Epidemiology of spinal cord injuries: a reflection of changes in South African society. *Paraplegia* 1994;32: 709–714.

28. Iwegbu CG. Traumatic paraplegia in Zaire and Nigeria: the case for a centre for injuries of the spine. *Paraplegia* 1983;21:81–85.

29. Soriano JY, Reyes TM, Reyes OL. Nerve conduction velocity studies in Filipinos with leprosy. *Phil J Leprosy* 1978:63–79.

30. Lorenzo SM, de Guzman RL, de Leon TR, et al. The effects of exposure to lead on peripheral nerves: a clinical and electrophysiological study. *Santo Tomas J Med* 1993;42:70–77.

31. Sethi PK, Udawat MP, Kasliwal SC, Chanda R. Vulcanized rubber foot for lower limb amputees. *J Prosthet Orthot Int* 1978;2:125–136.

32. Co-Albano CT, Reyes TM, Reyes OL. The People's below-knee prosthesis: its development and field investigation. *Santo Tomas J Med* 1986;35:150–167.

33. Buncio-Javier S, Reyes OL, Walter RT, et al. The Manila Motor-Perceptual Screening Test (MaMPS Test): its development and field investigation. *Santo Tomas J Med* 1988;137:126–169.

34. Reyes TM, Reyes OL, Manalang AM, et al. The motor-perceptual norms in Filipino children. *J Phil Med Assoc* 1990;66: 7–31.

35. Zhongwu C. Fighting back to good health. *Med China.* 1986; 2(Spring):70–71.

36. Suarez CG, Navarro JS, Valdecanas CM, et al. The treatment of musculoskeletal disorders by Filipino traditional healers. In: *Proceedings of the XVIth Southeast Asian Games Scientific Congress.* Manila: 1991.

37. Okamoto GA, Kelly SM, Brown M, Yee HFM. The training of rehabilitation technicians in Micronesia, Pacific Basin. In: *Proceedings of the 16th Rehabilitation International World Congress.* Tokyo, 1988:243–246.

38. Hartung GH, Kelly SM, Okamoto GA. Training rehabilitation technicians in the Pacific Basin. *J Disabil Stud* 1989;11: 103–107.

39. Yee HFM, Goebert DA, Okamoto GA. Rehabilitation technicians in the Pacific Basin. *World Health Forum* 1992;13:303–306.

40. Javier SB, Juan MF, Katigbak BC, et al. Chronic disability in Filipinos: its psychosocial impact. *Phil J Psychiatry* 1986;13:80–92.

41. Yu VL, Reyes OL, Reyes TM. Sexuality and the Filipino disabled. *Santo Tomas J Med* 1987;36: 162–184.

Part VII.

Other Issues

Chapter 101

Attitudinal Barriers Affecting Persons with Disabilities

Jean Cole Spencer

Society establishes the means of categorizing persons and the complement of attributes felt to be ordinary and natural for members of each of these categories. Social settings establish the categories of persons likely to be encountered there. The routines of social intercourse in established settings allow us to deal with anticipated others without special attention or thought. When a stranger comes into our presence, then, first appearances are likely to enable us to anticipate his category and attributes, his "social identity." . . . While the stranger is present before us, evidence can arise of his possessing an attribute that makes him different from others in the category of persons available for him to be, and of a less desirable kind. . . . He is thus reduced in our minds from a whole and usual person to a tainted, discounted one. Such an attribute is a stigma, especially when its discrediting effect is very extensive. . . . By definition, of course, we believe the person with a stigma is not quite human. On this assumption we exercise varieties of discrimination, through which we effectively, if often unthinkingly, reduce his life chances (1).

DISABILITY AS A SOCIAL CONSTRUCT

This chapter on attitudinal barriers is based on the premise that disability and its treatment occur within a physical, social, and cultural context that has a powerful effect on the lives of persons with disabilities and on the outcomes of the work of rehabilitation. In recent years, emphasis on context has been reflected in models of disablement that examine not only factors internal to the person (variously called *disease* or *pathology* and *impairments*), but also factors that reflect interactive processes between persons and environments (variously called *functional limitations*, *disabilities*, or *handicaps*) (2–4). Although use of terminology is inconsistent, current models of disablement include a level that addresses limitations in fulfillment of socially defined roles and tasks considered typical for a person of a given age, gender, and social position. This emphasis on performance of social roles and tasks in daily life settings leads to a view of outcomes of rehabilitation that emphasizes participation in community life rather than capacity to perform standardized tasks in a testing or clinic environment (5–7).

Attitudes have been defined as positive or negative reactions to an object (or in this case a social group), accompanied by specific beliefs that tend to impel the individual in a particular way toward an object (8). As commonly shared perceptions of various social categories or groups of persons, attitudes can be thought of as a fundamental aspect of the social and cultural context that shape expectations of how members of the particular social group will act and beliefs about the motivations that prompt their actions. Attitudes, in turn, powerfully affect how those who hold them behave in relation to others, based on their expectations about types of persons who are perceived as different from themselves. Although formal measures have been devised to study attitudes systematically, in general, attitudes are a tacit aspect of culture to which one does not consciously attend unless prompted to do so by some challenge to usual taken-for-granted ways of thinking.

In examining the significance of attitudes as a tacit and often unrecognized aspect of context, consider the following alternative statements about persons with disabilities (9):

1. Persons with disabilities have illnesses or impairments that interfere with their ability to participate in daily activities for which they come to health professionals for cures or treatment.
2. Persons with disabilities are socially disadvantaged and must look to the state or to society for support, which is provided as a charitable gift.
3. Persons with disabilities have extraordinary courage and tenacity, traits that allow them to perform accomplishments that are amazing for someone who has less-than-complete human capacities.
4. Persons with disabilities are costly to society because they require special accommodations that burden organizations that provide such accommodations.
5. Persons with disabilities are members of a community that has legitimate political grievances because their civil rights have been denied.
6. Persons with disabilities are a potential source of lawsuits based on charges of discrimination.
7. Persons with disabilities are multifaceted individuals who have strengths and weaknesses like all persons.
8. Persons with disabilities are an untapped consumer group that can make important contributions to society if jobs were available by which they could do productive work and earn income.

Each of these statements reflects a particular cultural lens or conceptual mindset through which persons with disabilities are viewed by health care personnel, business persons, public policy makers, neighbors, coworkers, and other persons with disabilities. [The statements are based on eight models by which persons with disability have been represented in the media such as newspapers or films; Haller (9) terms these the medical model, social pathology model, supercrip model, business model, minority/civil rights model, legal model, cultural pluralism model, and consumer model.] These contrasting perceptions illustrate that views of persons with disabilities are often partial and arbitrary constructions that are powerfully shaped by the social positions of those with whom they interact.

This examination of attitudinal barriers facing persons with disabilities is based on the notion of disability as a social construct. The disability studies movement emerged in an effort to study such phenomena, in contrast to an individual-centered view of disability that emphasizes impairments and functional limitations in the individual. Simi Linton, cited by Litvak (10), provided a definition of disability studies that captures this perspective:

> Disability Studies reframe the study of disability by focusing on it as a social phenomenon, social construct, metaphor, and cultural, utilizing a minority group model. It examines ideas related to disability in all forms of cultural representations throughout history, and examines the policies and practices of all societies to understand the social, rather than the physical or psychological, determinants of the experience of disability. . . . This focus shifts the emphasis away from a prevention/treatment/remediation paradigm to a social/cultural/political paradigm. This shift does not signify a denial of the presence of impairments, nor a rejection of the utility of intervention and treatment. Instead, Disability Studies has been developed to disentangle impairments from the myth, ideology, and stigma that influence social interaction and social policy. The scholarship challenges the idea that the economic and social status and assigned roles of people with disabilities are inevitable outcomes of their condition.

Existing knowledge about attitudes toward persons with disabilities is reflected in a substantial body of literature, with contributions from many disciplines based on alternative methods of study. In this chapter, attitudes are examined at three levels:

1. The first of these can be termed a *broad societal level* in which it is assumed that views about persons with disabilities are widely shared by large segments of the population, such as the health care community, the business community, blue collar laborers, or society at large.
2. The second is termed the *community level* in which individuals with disabilities lead their daily lives and in which they encounter attitudes about disability in the workplace, local restaurant, shopping mall, and residential or commercial neighborhood. Kleinman (11) coined the term *local worlds* to describe cultural environments at the scale of particular settings that have established patterns of activity and social interaction, as well as shared belief systems that give meaning to activities and interactions. Local worlds are the immediate contexts in which persons with disabilities enact the social roles and tasks referred to in models of disablement, and in which they have daily encounters with others whose attitudes shape both the opportunities and the limitations available in those settings.
3. The third level at which attitudes are examined is the level of personal experience of individuals with disabilities, which is reflected in a growing scholarly literature that examines disability as being simultaneously a personal and a social experience (12–14). Such studies allow us to understand commonly held attitudes toward persons with disabilities from an "insider's perspective" as they are encountered and managed by individuals with disabilities.

After examination of existing knowledge about attitudes toward disability at societal, community, and personal levels, the focus of the chapter then narrows to examine the special case of how attitudes concerning disability are reflected in health care personnel and institutions and how these attitudes shape our interactions and our therapeutic work with clients. Finally, the chapter explores a more reflective approach to conceptualization of disability by health care providers and its potential influence on rehabilitation practice.

ATTITUDES AT SOCIETAL, COMMUNITY, AND PERSONAL LEVELS

Societal Scale Manifestations of Attitudes Toward Disability

Some of the early work on attitudes about disability examined their manifestations historically and cross-culturally, as illustrated by the classic work of Safilios-Rothschild in *The Sociology and Social Psychology of Disability and Rehabilitation* (15). There have also been historical studies of the attitudes and social treatment of persons with particular illnesses and resulting disabilities such as tuberculosis (16), polio (17), and mental illness (18). With some notable exceptions, the themes of these historical reviews emphasize social isolation, exclusion from typical social roles, denial of goods and support available to others in society, and sometimes incarceration, physical stigmatization, or death for persons considered a threat to society. In recent work on cross-cultural comparison of attitudes toward persons with disabilities, Scheer and Groce (19) asserted that while the existence of impairments is a constant across all human societies, the social interpretations of the meaning of these phenomena are particular to specific cultures. According to these authors, in nonindustrialized societies, persons with disabilities are often integrated into families and other social groups where they play typical social roles. The social isolation and institutionalization of persons with disabilities in Western society are viewed as a result of processes of urbanization and industrialization that separated persons with disabilities from close-knit social groups.

The social sciences including sociology, anthropology, and psychology have developed various concepts and theories to describe social processes surrounding persons perceived as disabled and therefore different in important respects from those considered "normal." The sociologist Erving Goffman studied isolating social processes and the "spoiled identity" of persons with disabilities in his classic work on stigma (1), as well as the nature of settings in which such individuals often were placed in his work on asylums (20) as "total institutions" that controlled all aspects of an individual's life. Early work in the social sciences was predominantly based on the concept of deviance and its management (21–23). In more recent years, Murphy et al (24) conceptualized uncertain social relations between persons with disabilities and other members of society using the concept of liminality. [This emphasis on the uncertainty of social relations, in contrast to the emphasis on negative attitudes associated with stigma, was foreshadowed by Barker's (25) early statement that disabled persons "live on a social-psychological frontier" where they constantly face new and unknown situations.] The concept of liminality was developed in anthropology to describe persons undergoing rites of passage from one social status to another, such as puberty rites that initiate boys and girls into adult social roles as men and women. Borrowing from the work of Turner on such rituals of social transformation, Murphy et al (24) stated that "people in a liminal condition are without clear status, for their old position has been expunged and they have not yet been given a new one. . . . They are suspended in social space without firm identity or role definition, . . . making all interaction with them unpredictable and problematic." These authors described the onset of disability as an analogous process by which one's old social identity is lost without clearly defined new roles to enter, leaving persons with disabilities in a more or less permanent liminal state where they often remain in the "recesses of society." Other people typically deal with this indefinition "in the same way in which most ambivalent relations are handled: by setting up social distance through either hyperbole of conduct or by avoidance . . . and exclusion" (24).

Development of structured instruments to study attitudes toward persons with disabilities emerged in the 1960s and 1970s, based on classic methods for studying attitudes developed by Thurstone and Likert (8). Among the best known of these instruments is the Attitudes Toward Disabled Persons Scale devised by Yuker, Block, and Campbell in 1960, which has been used in a substantial body of research (26). This tool provides statements about the extent to which persons with disabilities are perceived as similar to or different from "normal" persons, to which respondents are asked to indicate the extent of their agreement. There are a number of tools based on similar methodology such as the Scale of Attitudes Toward Disabled Persons developed by Antonak (27). Another approach to the measurement of attitudes is based on the concept of social distance, or degree of intimacy an individual would allow to members of "out groups." The concept of social distance has been applied to the examination of attitudes toward persons with specific types of disabilities and "anomalous social conditions" such as having a prison record (28). Various studies found a hierarchy of preference that generally moves from persons with less visible impairments (such as diabetes) to those with potentially more visible impairments (such as cerebral palsy or strokes), with the least preferred groups being those with "disorders of the mind" such as mental retardation, alcoholism, or mental illness (28,29).

Literature and the media have been used as another source of evidence for the study of attitudes about disability at a societal scale. Various authors analyzed images of persons with disabilities as reflected in newspapers (30–32), television (33), comic books (34), books for children and for adults (35,36), and across various media (9,37). A variety of images were found in various media, as reflected in the eight models identified by Haller (9) and cited in the beginning of this chapter.

Societal scale attitudes are also reflected in social policy concerning persons with disabilities, an emerging formal field of study, although scholars in this field assert that it has a long undocumented and unacknowledged history, which may be due in part to a fragmentation of public programs intended to serve persons with disabilities. The scholarly domain of disability policy studies includes not only legislative acts, but also administrative acts, judicial and financial decisions, and the political context in which public policy decisions are made (10). The consolidation of this area of inquiry has been reflected in the establishment of the *Journal of Disability Policy Studies* in 1990 (38). Shriner (39) completed a review of literature documenting the history of this field in the areas of legal analyses, sociologic analyses, historical analyses, economic analyses, and political and policy development studies. In general, trends in disability policy can be said to reflect increasing inclusion of persons with disabilities in programs and services available to all citizens, and greater protection of the civil rights of individuals with disabilities in many domains. These trends have been spurred in large part during the past several decades by a number of social movements intended to change the way the situations of persons with disabilities are conceptualized and therefore how their needs can best be addressed, including the normalization movement (40), the independent living movement (41), the movement for mainstreaming children with disabilities in public schools (42), and the civil rights movement (43).

Community Scale Manifestations of Attitudes About Disability

In contrast to a broad societal perspective on attitudes that are thought to be widely shared in American culture, there is also a body of scholarship that examines attitudes as encountered by persons with disabilities in local-world contexts of daily life such as the home, workplace, and neighborhood. Several studies have been selected to represent this way of studying attitudes and their consequences, in which the neighborhood or community is the unit of study. Such studies examined social processes in depth as they unfold over time, in contrast to the synchronic perspective of most societal scale studies.

A focus on the local worlds of persons with disabilities is illustrated by a 3-year study by Kielhofner (44) of deinstitutionalized adults that investigated both their lives within the environments of several residential facilities and their experiences as they sought to participate in community settings such as grocery stores and restaurants. Notes made by a researcher on one such visit exemplify the attitudes commonly encountered in community settings. "In the coffee shop we stood out like a sore thumb. . . . We had a waitress who quite often remarked to the other waitress that she should 'Get a load of what's down there.' . . . Before we left I went to the rest room. When I returned I found all the heads turned in the restaurant to the four women who were huddled together. . . . We all left with everyone's eyes turned toward us" (44). The author concluded that the noticings, reactions, and curious or patronizing actions of others are the context within which persons with disabilities must always conduct themselves. "It means that settings that are normal in a commonsense way are not normal [for disabled persons] in a sociological sense" (44).

In another local-world study, McCuaig and Frank (45) used extensive interviews and participant observation to investigate how a 53-year-old woman with cerebral palsy managed independent living in a community apartment and local neighborhood in which she coordinated a complex array of personal assistance services. This woman, who used an electric wheelchair and an augmentative communication device, frequently encountered the attitude that because of difficulty moving and speaking she was assumed to lack competence in many areas. She developed various strategies, such as writing letters stating her concerns and questions prior to visiting physicians or other community resources, to ensure her active participation as a competent individual in social interactions. This study illustrates the commonly reported tendency of persons unfamiliar with disability to overgeneralize its effects (presuming in this case that because of difficulty speaking, the woman also lacked intelligence), leading to a felt need on the part of many disabled individuals to demonstrate their competence in ways that would not be expected of other persons.

Similar findings about social expectations were revealed in a study of persons with head injury living in the community conducted by Krefting (46) using ethnographic methods. As a result of perceived lack of public understanding of head injury and its significance, participants in the study went to considerable lengths to conceal their disabilities from persons they encountered in many community settings (including the offices of personnel providing disability-related services). In the words of one of the study participants, "I try to avoid telling anyone [about my disability]. I can not stand any more rejection" (46). Processes observed among individuals with head injury were interpreted as "recasting their social personhood" through strategies such as revising the meaning of work and independent living in order to define themselves in socially accepted ways. Krefting (46) stated that "the loss of person was universally experienced by the head injured persons that I knew. They were neither acknowledged nor valued by society."

A final study that illustrates attitudes toward persons with disabilities at the scale of local worlds of daily life was conducted by Groce (47) in a community on Martha's Vineyard where hereditary deafness was historically very prevalent. Using historical records and extensive interviews with residents old enough to remember the days when the community was largely a closed social system, Groce investigated the almost universal use of sign language that allowed individuals who were unable to hear to participate fully in common forms of work such as farming and fishing, in public education, in church activities, in social encounters in community locations such as stores and shops, in legal and political affairs of the community, and in family life. Groce attributed the taken-for-granted participation of individuals with hearing impairments in all aspects of community life to the fact that virtually all families had members and close friends who were hearing impaired and to the consequent social commitment to learn and maintain a shared form of communication that was usable by everyone. This striking illustration suggests that an attitude of "normalcy" concerning the occurrence of disability may lead to a social context in which methods for including individuals with disabilities can be readily devised and maintained.

Personal Scale Manifestations of Attitudes About Disability

Social attitudes and expectations have also been revealed through studies of the personal experience of individuals with disabilities that provide an "insider's perspective." A study by Scheer and Luborsky (14) of the biographies of persons who experienced both initial polio and later post-polio disabilities highlighted important differences in the cultural context of "early and late polio traditions" that were found in the prevaccine era (1990–1955) and the postvaccine era (1955–1990s). According to these authors, the early polio tradition emerged when disabilities were viewed largely as medical problems and in which polio survivors were expected to be "good patients," comply with treatment recommendations, and assimilate into the mainstream of American life. Important themes of this tradition included the "work ethic" and "forget your polio," which allowed polio survivors to use self-sufficiency, achievement, and productivity to counter stereotypical images of persons with disabilities as dependent, inactive, and unproductive. This value orientation, which was congruent with core American values of hard work in overcoming adversity and independence in being responsible for one's own life, allowed many polio survivors to achieve great success in "normal" social roles as workers, family members, and active participants in community life. In contrast, the late polio tradition emerged through changes prompted by the independent living and civil rights movements of the 1970s and 1980s, which consider disability to be the result of the interaction between impairments and the social environment and which view the goal of rehabilitation not as functional independence in performing daily activities but as self-direction in making life decisions. The incongruence between the earlier tradition and these attitudes and expectations about persons with disabilities have made it difficult for some polio survivors to give up their formerly successful ways of adapting in order to follow new advice to conserve remaining capabilities. This research illustrated the great power of cultural attitudes and social expectations to shape the adaptive strategies used by persons with disabilities, strategies that potentially may become less adaptive when both personal and contextual circumstances change.

In an account of his own experience with progressive paralysis due to a spinal cord tumor, Murphy (13) described his return as a wheelchair user to his teaching role at Columbia University where students and colleagues had previously known him as a nondisabled faculty member. Formerly familiar social situations, such as beginning a new course at the start of a semester, were now attended with great uncertainty on the part of all participants (including Murphy) as to how the teaching of the course would proceed. Although it was commonly recognized that his disability had no effects on his intellectual ability to teach, there were nonetheless many doubts and anxieties about his ability to manage the physical tasks of teaching, such as speaking loudly enough to be heard or writing on the board, and about the potential humiliation of not being able to manage these successfully. Murphy used the contrast between his experiences prior to the onset of his disability and those following his entry into the social world of persons with disabilities to analyze attitudes that powerfully shaped what he called "a journey that was as strange as any fieldtrip to remote cultures," similar to those where he had conducted anthropologic fieldwork on numerous occasions. Dealing with the uncertainties of his return to teaching as a person with a disability illustrates the liminal state described by Murphy et al (24). An attitude of uncertainty toward persons with disabilities may be as effortful and difficult to manage socially as either negative stigma or overly positive expectations for achievement and "forgetting your disability."

Frank, who reviewed the use of life histories or narratives as a way to study the experience of individuals with disabilities (48), conducted a study of a woman with congenital quadrilateral limb deficiencies (49). Her life history approach was based on the concept of "turnings," which she defined (based on earlier work of Mandelbaum) as "critical junctures in life in which the individual takes on a new set of roles, enters into fresh relationships with a new set of people, and acquires a new self-conception" (49). Turnings prompt a process of adaptation that involves changing some behaviors while also seeking to maintain continuity. In this form of research the turnings that mark periods in a person's life are identified by the individual whose life is being studied rather than by the researcher, thus articulating an insider's perspective on the meaning of life experiences. It is noteworthy that the turnings identified by Diane DeVries in this study seldom refer to major changes that might be thought significant by rehabilitation personnel (such as acquisition or discarding of prostheses or acquisition of an electric wheelchair), but rather center primarily on engagement in new social worlds such as involvement with a teenage drug subculture, graduation from high school, initiation to sexuality, moving to new living situations, living with a partner, going to college, and turning toward Christian spirituality and community. Major themes identified in her processes of adaptation involved seeking cultural normality (with an effort to do typical things and "not look like a crip"), finding institutional niches (with emphasis on use of mainstream support systems rather than affiliation with "a subculture of the disabled"), and orientation toward independent living (with greater autonomy in making decisions and "being able to function in society without having to rely on a whole stream of people and places"). Findings of this study suggest that in each period of her life, DeVries was able to find and establish relationships with individuals who were willing to see her as a typical young woman, rather than focusing on the physical limitations resulting from her disability. She sought to minimize negative or uncertain attitudes of others by purposefully looking and acting like a "normal" person. This reflects a view that disability experience is not a valued part of one's identity, a view that is increasingly challenged by some persons with disabilities but one that is perhaps socially advantageous in a society that typically does not value disability positively.

ATTITUDES IN HEALTH CARE PERSONNEL AND INSTITUTIONS

There is a body of literature that has used various structured attitude scales to examine the attitudes of health and social service personnel toward persons with disabilities, spanning the period from the initial development of these scales in the 1960s and 1970s to the present (50–55). There is also a history documenting the effects of various methods used to foster more positive attitudes among health personnel (56–58). Studies of factors that influence positive attitudes of health professionals emphasize the primary importance of contact with persons with disabilities, including its frequency, the settings in which contact occurs, and particularly the degree of equal status between the involved persons through role relationships such as friend, coworker, or teammate in contexts including school, employment, or social settings (59). Roush (60) suggested that contact with a person with a disability purely in a helper-caregiver role may not be conducive to the development of positive attitudes because the functional limitations and differences of such persons are highlighted rather than their strengths and similarities to persons without disabilities.

In addition to studies that examined attitudes toward persons with disabilities explicitly, there is also a body of literature that indicates various social distancing mechanisms between health care providers and patients. Medical sociologists frequently have examined power relationship in social interactions between physicians and their patients. The extensive literature on the concept of compliance by patients with treatment regimens prescribed by health personnel is an indicator of the nature of expectations between these groups, though there is some indication of a change in views of compliance in recent years (61,62). Another methodology used to examine relationships between health personnel and patients is analysis of patient narratives of their health care experience, through which Peloquin (63) found many examples of the "depersonalization" of patients. Studies of the cultures of treatment settings also indicated role expectations for staff and patients that tend to afford great influence to staff and little control to patients (64–66). In a recent qualitative study of one young man's rehabilitation experience following spinal cord injury, Spencer et al (67) found that staff were often so intent on teaching the patient new skills by referring him to standardized programs that they often failed to listen to this patient's attempts to draw on his past life experience in imaging his future and making plans to reach goals that he valued. This tendency may well be reinforced by current trends toward use of standardized critical pathways and treatment protocols. This study also revealed that staff and patients had very different views of major aspects of the rehabilitation process, such as introducing the patient to use of a wheelchair, with staff seeing this step as an opportunity for greater mobility whereas the patient saw the wheelchair as a dreaded symbol of disability and of his helplessness (68). A similar example of incongruence between staff emphasis on hard work and patient views of this expectation was recounted by Murphy (13), who found constant encouragement to work toward increasingly difficult goals during therapy to be demoralizing because accomplishments were never acknowledged and performance was never "good enough."

An additional perspective on the significance of attitudes of health care personnel toward persons with disabilities is suggested by literature that characterizes what might be called a "culture of rehabilitation." Scheer and Luborsky (14) described such a culture for the initial period of polio rehabilitation in which they identified themes of hard work to overcome adversity and expectations that persons will want to be as independent as possible in performing daily activities. Although Scheer and Luborsky (14) pointed to changes in the culture of postpolio management, there is evidence that the themes of hard work to control one's own fate and high value on physical independence are still very prominent in rehabilitation. The ubiquitous character of emphasis on independence is evidenced by the number of assessments used in rehabilitation that award high scores for performing physical tasks independently, with virtually no tools for assessing the ability of persons with disabilities to manage interdependent relationships or perform tasks collaboratively. This is true despite the fact that collaborative skills are likely to be extremely important for the large proportion of individuals who will need ongoing daily physical assistance following discharge from rehabilitation. One notable exception to the emphasis on physical task performance is the Personal Independence Profile developed by Nosek et al (69), which is based on the construct of independence as defined in the independent living movement. This tool includes subscales that measure perceived control, psychological self-reliance, and environmental resources as well as physical functioning. Research indicates that there is little relationship between an individual's physical capabilities and his or her "independent mindedness," a finding which suggests that the meaning of independence as performance of physical tasks in the culture of rehabilitation may be an inadequate indicator of the individual's ability to adapt later to life in the community (69). The taken-for-granted nature of expectations of patients associated with the "culture of rehabilitation" is also reflected by research on the processes by which treatment goals are established. Recent studies indicated that staff often assume that patients and families subscribe to the standard goals without serious question (70,71).

In reflecting on the culture of rehabilitation, one might argue that having an established shared set of beliefs and practices that guides this process is both desirable and inevitable in any social institution, and this is probably true. The point to be made here is that expecting all persons with disabilities to share these values fails to acknowledge the importance of individual differences and alternative backgrounds, which may lead patients to view the purposes and methods of rehabilitation very differently from staff and which may strongly shape long-term adaptive strategies such as those that value interdependence over independence. Differences between the values of persons with disabilities and the cultures of treatment settings are likely to become increasingly significant as patient populations become more ethnically diverse.

TOWARD MORE REFLECTIVE ATTITUDES ABOUT DISABILITY IN REHABILITATION PRACTICE

Existing research indicates that rehabilitation practitioners clearly have established expectations about persons with disabilities and how they should behave and interact in encounters. This research also suggests a tendency to focus heavily on the impairments and functional limitations that we know how to treat in established programs and to assume that patients with similar impairments share standard goals. There are certainly many pressures in today's health care environment to utilize resource utilization groups or other standardizing mechanisms to make treatment as efficient and cost-effective as possible. However, achieving great efficiency in reaching goals and teaching skills that are not relevant to patients' daily lives is a false economy if such knowledge and skills are not utilized in the community following discharge. Several authors suggested other views that may guide us to rethink our assumptions about persons with disabilities and our ways of collaborating with them.

One influential voice in urging new relationships between health care providers and patients, particularly those with chronic illnesses, is that of Arthur Kleinman whose book *The Illness Narratives* (72) examines the tendency of health care personnel to attend to disease rather than patients' illness experience. Kleinman used the term *illness* to refer to "how the sick person and members of the family or wider social network perceive, live with, and respond to symptoms and disability . . . including the patient's judgments about how best to cope with the distress and with the practical problems in daily living it creates" (72). In contrast, "disease . . . is what the practitioner creates in the recasting of illness in terms of theories of disorder. Disease is what practitioners have been trained to see through the theoretical lenses of their particular form of practice. . . . In the practitioner's act of recasting illness as disease, something essential to the experience of chronic illness is lost; it is not legitimated as a subject for clinical concern, nor does it receive an intervention" (72). Kleinman (72) advocated use of a method based on ethnography, originally developed in the discipline of anthropology to understand cultures different from those of the researcher through careful observation of activity and its context, interviews with members of the culture to learn the meanings they attach to experience, and interpretation of these findings from the perspective of both insiders who live in the culture and outsiders who bring alternative theories and points of view.

An analogous method, which Kleinman referred to as "ethnographic practice," can be applied to the problem of fostering translation and mutual understanding between the dual perspectives of patient and practitioner. The key elements of this process include 1) a mini-ethnography by which the practitioner comes to understand the daily life of the individual and the social context of the local world in which it occurs; 2) a brief life history, which allows an understanding of both continuity and change in the course of the person's life; 3) negotiation between explanatory models by which patient and practitioner understand the illness and its consequences and make decisions about treatment options; and 4) remoralization, which involves both attending to the emotional aspects of illness experience and collaborating with the patient to identify hope for the future. The essence of the method proposed by Kleinman is the ability to interpret and understand disability simultaneously from two perspectives, that of the patient's daily life and local world and that of the practitioner who has kinds of expertise that are potentially useful in solving problems, as well as the ability to translate understandings and negotiate as collaborators in managing both illness and disease.

Ways to incorporate these dual perspectives into the practice of rehabilitation have been suggested by Mattingly through a process which she termed "emplotment" (73). Emplotment refers to conceptualizing clinical interventions as aspects of the plot of the patient's evolving life story, which began before the person entered the health care system and will continue long after the person returns to his or her own local world. The concept of emplotment emerged from an extensive multiyear study of the clinical reasoning of occupational therapists that identified a narrative perspective on the patient's life story as one of three critical domains to which therapists attend (74). Emplotting therapy, or placing it within a context that makes sense from the point of view of the patient's life story and local world, offers two fundamental advantages over more standardized approaches to establishing goals and providing rehabilitation services. One is an increased commitment of patients to engage in the work of rehabilitation because they can see direct benefits for their daily lives. The second is increased likelihood that the knowledge and skills addressed during rehabilitation will actually be utilized when patients return home.

Jesse Peters is another voice that is advocating for a more reflective view of disability, one that incorporates subjective human experience and links it systematically to broader theory in models of disablement (75). Peters sees this perspective as crucial to understand and conduct research on the outcomes of rehabilitation in ways that address quality of life as the value that persons with disabilities place on their subjective life experiences, outcomes that are not necessarily closely related to health or functional status (76,77). This view is congruent with the current trend in health care research generally to consider quality of life and subjective well-being as crucial outcomes (6,78). Peters (79) thus argued both for a more comprehensive model of disablement that incorporates subjective experience along with other components, and for a broader repertoire of research approaches that can integrate qualitative understanding of subjective experience with quantitative measurement of objective factors. The studies cited in this chapter were chosen to reflect a range of research approaches, including those based on quantitative designs, tools, and analyses and those using qualitative methods such as ethnography and life history.

An important question to be raised about these ideas for a more reflective view of disability and for a practice of rehabilitation that incorporates understanding of the patient's perspective is whether they are practical and feasible in the current climate of health care. There are certainly many pressures to standardize both the provision of treatment and the documentation of outcomes, and efficiency when use of time is at a premium. One might envision the requirement of many hours of conversation with patients in order to appreciate their perspective, a luxury that health care facilities and practitioners cannot afford. However, I would argue that the fundamental requirement of the approach advocated here of anchoring rehabilitation in the patient's life story and local world is not more time but a new mindset, a commitment to integrating and reflecting on the knowledge of patients that we accumulate routinely during clinical encounters through casual conversation as bits and pieces of incidental information. In short, this approach requires an attitude about disability that sees it as a personal and social, as well as a physical experience. Incidents and stories about the patient's workplace, or leisure activities, or friends and family members are told routinely during therapy and other clinical encounters. Asking questions more systematically, listening more carefully to the significance of experiences in the patient's life, and considering the social and cultural contexts in which this experience has occurred contribute content which can be integrated to form an interpretation of the patient's life story and local world. This perspective can form the groundwork on which more collaborative goal setting and identification of hopes for the future can occur, and on which the emplotment of clinical practice in the life stories of patients can be based.

ACKNOWLEDGMENTS

My knowledge and views about attitudes concerning disability have been shaped by valued experiences with many colleagues and friends with disabilities going back to the early days of the independent living movement. They have also been shaped by long-term interactions with colleagues in anthropology and more recent ones with colleagues in occupational therapy through which I have sought to integrate ideas from social sciences and clinical practice. In preparing parts of this chapter I have drawn on a literature review ably completed by Megan Montgomery, and I am also grateful for the assistance with references provided by Colleen Rice. My greatest debt is to my husband and former mentor. Dr. William Spencer, whose holistic views of the lives of persons with disabilities and of the rehabilitation process have influenced those of numerous associates over many years.

REFERENCES

1. Goffman E. *Stigma: notes on the management of spoiled identity.* Englewood Cliffs, NJ: Prentice Hall, 1963.
2. World Health Organization. *International classification of impair-*

ments, disabilities, and handicaps. Geneva: World Health Organization, 1980.

3. Pope AM, Tarlov AR, eds. *Disability in America: toward a national agenda for prevention.* Washington, DC: National Academy Press, 1991.
4. Verbrugge, LM, Jette AM. The disablement process. *Soc Sci Med* 1994;38:1–14.
5. Whiteneck GG. Measuring what matters: key rehabilitation outcomes. *Arch Phys Med Rehabil* 1994;75:1073–1076.
6. Fuhrer MJ. Subjective well-being: implications for medical rehabilitation outcomes & models of disablement. *Am J Phys Med Rehabil* 1994;73:358–364.
7. DeJong G. Value perspectives and the challenge of managed care. In: Fuhrer MJ, ed. *Assessing medical rehabilitation practices: the promise of outcomes research.* Baltimore, MD: Paul H. Brookes, 1997:61–84.
8. Lemon N. *Attitudes and their measurement.* New York: Wiley, 1973.
9. Haller B. Rethinking models of media representation of disability. *Disabil Stud Q* 1995;15(2): 26–30.
10. Litvak S. Disability studies vs. disability policy studies. *Disabil Stud Q* 1994;14(2):23–26.
11. Kleinman A. Local worlds of suffering: an interpersonal focus for ethnographies of illness experience. *Qual Health Res* 1992;2: 127–134.
12. Zola IK. *Missing pieces.* Philadelphia: Temple University Press, 1982.
13. Murphy R. *The body silent.* New York: WW Norton, 1990.
14. Scheer J, Luborsky ML. The cultural context of polio biographies. *Orthopedics* 1991;14: 1173–1181.
15. Safilios-Rothschild C. *The sociology and social psychology of disability and rehabilitation.* New York: Random House, 1970.
16. Rothman S. *Living in the shadow of death.* New York: Basic Books, 1994.
17. Rogers N. *Dirt and disease.* New Jersey: Rutgers University Press, 1992.
18. Grob G. *The mad among us: a history of the care of America's mentally ill.* New York: The Free Press, 1994.
19. Scheer J, Groce N. Impairment as a human constant: cross cultural and historical perspectives on variation. *J Soc Issues* 1988; 44(1):23–37.
20. Goffman E. *Asylums: essays on the social situation of mental patients and other inmates.* Garden City, NJ: Anchor Books, 1961.
21. White RK, Wright BA, Dembo T. Studies in adjustment to physical injuries: evaluation of curiosity by the injured. *J Abnorm Soc Psychol* 1948;43:13–28.
22. Wright BA. *Physical disability: a psychological approach.* New York: Harper & Row, 1960.
23. Davis F. Deviance disavowal: the management of strained interaction by the visibly handicapped. *Soc Probl* 1961;9:120–124.
24. Murphy R, Scheer J, Murphy Y, Mack R. Physical disability and social liminality: a study in the rituals of adversity. *Soc Sci Med* 1988;26:235–242.
25. Barker R. The social psychology of physical disability. *J Soc Issues* 1948;4:31–36.
26. Yuker H, ed. *Attitudes toward persons with disabilities.* New York: Springer, 1988.
27. Antonak RF. Prediction of attitudes toward disabled persons: a multivariate analysis. *J Gen Psychol* 1981;104:119–123.
28. Tringo J. The hierarchy of preference toward disability groups. *J Special Educ* 1970;4: 295–305.
29. Lyons M, Hayes R. Student perceptions of persons with psychiatric and other disorders. *Am J Occup Ther* 1993;45:311–316.
30. Biklen D. Framed: journalism's treatment of disability. *Soc Policy* 1986;16(3):45–51.
31. Clogston J. *A content analysis of disability coverage in 16 newpapers Sept-Dec 1989.* Louisville, KY: Advocado Press, 1990.
32. Yoshida R, Wasilewski J, Friedman D. Recent newspaper coverage about persons with disabilities. *Except Child* 1990;56:418–423.
33. Donaldson J. The visibility and image of handicapped people on television. *Except Child* 1981;47: 413–416.
34. Weinberg N, Santana R. Comic books: champion of the disabled stereotype. *Rehabil Lit* 1978;39: 327–331.
35. Davidson I, Woodill G, Bredberg E. Images of disability in 19th century British children's literature. *Disabil Soc* 1994; 9(1):33–46.
36. Zola IK. "Any distinguishing features?"—the portrayal of disability in the crime-mystery genre. *Policy Stud J* 1987;15:485–513.
37. Zola IK. Depictions of disability—metaphor, message, and medium in the media: a research and political agenda. *Soc Sci J* 1985; 22(4):5–17.
38. Shriner KF. Why study disability policy? *J Disabil Policy Stud* 1990;1(1):1–7.
39. Shriner KF. Why study disability policy: a second look at disability policy studies. *Disabil Stud Q* 1994;14(2):26–33.
40. Wolfensberger W. *The principle of normalization in human services.* Toronto: National Institute on Mental Retardation, 1972.
41. DeJong G. Independent living: from social movement to analytic paradigm. *Arch Phys Med Rehabil* 1979;60:435–446.
42. Gliedman J, Roth W. *The unexpected minority: handicapped chil-*

dren in America. New York: Harcourt Brace Jovanovich, 1980.

43. Shapiro JP. *No pity: people with disabilities forging a new civil rights movement.* New York: Times Books, 1993.

44. Kielhofner G. An ethnographic study of deinstitutionalized adults: their community settings and daily life experiences. *Occup Ther J Res* 1981;1(2):125–142.

45. McCuaig M, Frank G. The able self: adaptive patterns and choices in independent living for a person with cerebral palsy. *Am J Occup Ther* 1991;45:224–234.

46. Krefting L. Reintegration into the community after head injury: the results of an ethnographic study. *Occup Ther J Res* 1989;9(2): 67–83.

47. Groce N. *Everyone here spoke sign language: hereditary deafness on Martha's Vineyard.* Cambridge: Harvard University Press, 1985.

48. Frank G. Life histories in occupational therapy clinical practice. *Am J Occup Ther* 1995;50:251–264.

49. Frank G. Life history model of adaptation to disability: the case of a "congenital amputee." *Soc Sci Med* 1984;19:639–645.

50. Wills TA. Perceptions of clients by professional helpers. *Psychol Bull* 1978;85:968–1000.

51. Chubon R. An analysis of research dealing with the attitudes of professionals toward disability. *J Rehabil* 1982;48:(1):25–30.

52. Potts M, Brandt K. Various health professional groups' beliefs about people with arthritis. *J Allied Health* 1986;15:245–256.

53. Benham P. Attitudes of occupational therapy personnel toward persons with disabilities. *Am J Occup Ther* 1988;42:305–311.

54. Short-DeGraff MA, Diamond KE, Rolker-Dolinsky B. Comparison of physical therapy majors and other college students' attitudes toward persons with disabilities. *J Postsecondary Educ Disabil* 1989; 7:27–36.

55. Biley AM. A handicap of negative attitudes and lack of choice: caring for inpatients with disabilities. *Prof Nurse* 1994;9:786–788.

56. Gelfand S, Ullman LP. Attitude change associated with psychiatric affiliation. *Nurs Res* 1961;10: 200–204.

57. Sadlick M, Penta FB. Changing nurse attitudes toward quadriplegics through the use of television. *Rehabil Lit* 1975;36:274–278.

58. Lee TMC, Paterson JG, Chan CCH. Effect of occupational therapy education on students' perceived attitudes toward persons with disabilities. *Am J Occup Ther* 1994; 48:633–638.

59. Donaldson J. Changing attitudes toward handicapped persons: a review and analysis of research. *Except Child* 1980;46:504–513.

60. Roush SE. Health professionals as contributors to attitudes toward persons with disabilities—a special communication. *Phys Ther* 1986; 66:1551–1554.

61. Gerber K, Nehemkis A, eds. *Compliance: the dilemma of the chronically ill.* New York: Springer, 1986.

62. Roberson J. The meaning of compliance: patient perspectives. *Qual Health Res* 1992;2:7–26.

63. Peloquin SM. The depersonalization of patients: a profile gleaned from narratives. *Am J Occup Ther* 1993;47:830–837.

64. Caudill W. *The psychiatric hospital as a small society.* Cambridge: Harvard University Press, 1953.

65. Moos R. *Evaluation of treatment environments: a sociological approach.* New York: Wiley, 1974.

66. Miller EJ, Gwynne GV. *A life apart.* London: Tavistock, 1972.

67. Spencer J, Young M, Rintala D, Bates S. Socialization to the culture of a rehabilitation hospital: an ethnographic study. *Am J Occup Ther* 1995;49:53–62.

68. Bates P, Spencer J, Young M, Rintala D. Assistive technology and the newly disabled adult: adaptation to wheelchair use. *Am J Occup Ther* 1993;47: 1014–1021.

69. Nosek MA, Fuhrer MJ, Howland CA. Independence among people with disabilities: II. Personal Independence Profile. *Rehabil Counsel Bull* 1992;36(1):21–36.

70. Northen JG, Rust DM, Nelson CE, Watts JH. Involvement of adult rehabilitation patients in setting occupational therapy goals. *Am J Occup Ther* 1995;49:214–220.

71. Neistadt M. Methods of assessing clients' priorities: a survey of adult physical dysfunction settings. *Am J Occup Ther* 1995;49:428–436.

72. Kleinman A. *The illness narratives: suffering, healing and the human condition.* New York: Basic Books, 1988.

73. Mattingly C. The concept of therapeutic "emplotment." *Soc Sci Med* 1994;38:811–822.

74. Mattingly C, Fleming M. *Clinical reasoning: forms of inquiry in a therapeutic practice.* Philadelphia: FA Davis, 1993.

75. Peters DJ. Human experience in disablement: the imperative of the ICIDH. *Disabil Rehabil* 1995;17: 135–144.

76. Weinberg N. Physically disabled persons assess the quality of their lives. *Rehabil Lit* 1984;45:12–15.

77. Bach JR, Tilton MC. Life satisfaction and well-being measures in ventilator assisted individuals with traumatic tetraplegia. *Arch Phys Med Rehabil* 1994;75:626–632.

78. Gill TM, Feinstein AR. A critical appraisal of the quality of quality-of-life measurements. *JAMA* 1994;272:619–626.

79. Peters DJ. Qualitative inquiry: expanding rehabilitation medicine's research repertoire. *Am J Phys Med Rehabil* 1996;75: 144–148.

Chapter 102

Advocating Disability Issues: Rethinking the Rehabilitation Professional's Role

Quentin Smith
Laura Smith
Jan Galvin
Lex Frieden
Wendy Wilkinson

When President George Bush signed the Americans with Disabilities Act (ADA) into law on July 26, 1990, it was hailed as ". . . an historical landmark and a milestone in America's commitment to full and equal opportunity for all its citizens" (1). At the ADA signing ceremony, attended by a number of leaders from the disability community, President Bush emphasized the significance of the ADA with the powerful statement, "Let the shameful walls of exclusion finally come tumbling down" (2). In many respects, the signing of the ADA into law represented the culmination of advocacy efforts on the part of millions of Americans with disabilities who had been disenfranchised through discriminatory beliefs and practices—including both overt and more subtle forms of discrimination—that often went unchallenged in America and in other parts of the world.

However, as important as the passage and implementation of the ADA may be, it represents only a partial victory for people with disabilities. Much work remains to be done if the promise of the ADA is to be realized. More effective advocacy is needed if people with disabilities are to access employment, health care, housing, social programs, and other aspects of living that bring quality to the lives that most of us take for granted. Following a brief review of the history of legislative actions that moved disability issues from a charity footing to a civil rights footing, this chapter explores the rationale for more proactive involvement of rehabilitation professionals in active advocacy efforts around disability rights. It also makes the case that addressing issues that deny people with disabilities opportunities to pursue meaningful lives will have a direct impact on outcomes realized from rehabilitation services. A new conceptual framework is proposed in which advocacy efforts begin early in the rehabilitation process and are sustained throughout toward the goals of empowerment, independence, and wellness, rather than simply absence of acute health problems.

Moving toward a more holistic approach to rehabilitative and other health services will require a change in mindset for many rehabilitation professionals. It will also require new tools and strategies for measuring outcomes that focus as much on quality-of-life issues as on measures of disease of functional deficit. At the time that this chapter was prepared, such tools and strategies were largely lacking, and it is not our intent to suggest how this lack should be addressed. It will take a good deal more research and development—with significant involvement of people with disabilities at every step of the way—before effective tools and strategies are available for use in examining rehabilitation outcomes from the holistic perspective suggested here. This chapter represents a call for action that will lead to better results for everyone—rehabilitation professionals and people with disabilities included.

A BRIEF OVERVIEW OF THE HISTORICAL ROOTS OF THE AMERICAN WITH DISABILITIES ACT

The factors that gave rise to the ADA have been documented in a number of excellent publications. Of the materials available on the ADA, two are perhaps most useful in gaining a clear perspective on the convergence of forces that made a legislative initiative like the ADA possible: *No Pity: People with Disabilities Forging a New Civil Rights Movement*; (3) and *Equality of Opportunity: The Making of the Americans with Disabilities Act* (4).

Efforts toward securing and protecting the rights of people with disabilities that reached fruition with passage of the ADA grew out of the race-related civil rights initiatives of the 1950s and 1960s (4). However, the legislation that emerged from the civil rights activism of the midtwentieth century made no reference to disability. It was not until passage of the Architectural Barriers Act of 1968—requiring physical access by people with disabilities to all buildings constructed, altered, or financed by the federal government—that any significant statute relating to disability rights was passed (5).

A watershed event in casting disability issues in a civil rights context occurred with reauthorization of the Vocational Rehabilitation Act in 1972. The legislative mandate was broadened by dropping of the term *vocational* and through inclusion of sections that added a civil rights flavor to disability issues. Section 502 established the Architectural and Transportation Barriers Compliance Board (ATBCB), designed to ensure compliance with the Architectural Barriers Act of 1968 in eliminating transportation barriers, as well as fostering access in housing stock. Section 503 required that parties contracting with the United States take affirmative action to employ persons with disabilities. Finally, and most importantly, Section 504 stated, "No otherwise qualified handicapped individual in the United States . . . shall, solely by reason of his handicap, be excluded from the participation in, be denied the benefits of, or be subjected to discrimination under any program or activity receiving Federal financial assistance" (6).

This portion of the law was modeled after Title VI of the Civil Rights Act of 1964 and Title IX of the Education Amendments Act of 1972, which prohibited discrimination in federally assisted programs on account of race, color, religion, national origin, or sex. However, unlike the Civil Rights Act of 1964, Section 504 did not emerge in response to public protest; it was simply inserted quietly by congressional staff members who were apparently concerned about the potential that persons who received vocational services might not benefit from such services because of discriminatory practices that denied them employment (4). There was no statement of congressional intent for Section 504, nor were there appropriations to finance it (4). As a matter of fact, later review of the legislative history of the Act did not reveal who had first suggested including this crucial civil rights language (3).

However, simply including civil rights language in the law provided no guarantee of federal support for such protections. Throughout the Nixon and Ford presidential administrations, development of regulations for implementing Section 504 were delayed. When implementation of the regulations was delayed further under the Carter Administration because of concerns by Health, Education, and Welfare (HEW) Secretary Joseph Califano about the costs associated with the statute, the failure to act on in-place legislation that offered much-needed protections to people who were experiencing discrimination in all facets of life provided a rallying point for the heretofore factional disability community. Protests were mounted in major cities around the country, including Atlanta, Boston, Chicago, Dallas, Denver, Philadelphia, New York, San Francisco, and Seattle, as well as in Washington, DC. The Washington protest at HEW offices forced Secretary Califano to meet with protesters, although no resolution of the issues emerged from those meetings. The San Francisco protest, the longest of all of the organized protests, involving 23 days of occupation of the HEW offices in that city, was perhaps the action that led to Secretary Califano's signing of Section 504 regulations on April 28, 1977—nearly 3½ years after the Rehabilitation Act of 1973 had become law. The protesters in San Francisco vacated the HEW offices 2 days after the regulations were signed.

The significance of the Section 504 experience was summarized in the National Council on Disability's 1997 report on the history of the ADA (4):

- Section 504 helped change the way in which people thought about disability; disability was elevated to the realm of civil rights and people with disabilities were given a new legal vehicle for asserting their place in American society;
- The battle over Section 504 regulations gave voice to the disability rights movement; the protests made it extremely difficult for the secretary to incorporate any changes that might have weakened the regulations;
- Section 504 established the legal standards for nondiscrimination tailored to the civil rights needs of persons with disabilities that would be later replicated in the ADA; ending discrimination for people with disabilities meant taking proactive steps to remove barriers and make reasonable accommodation.

While Section 504 of the Rehabilitation Act represented a major step forward for disability rights, retaining the rights promised through such initiatives required constant vigilance. Under the Reagan Administration, a deliberate effort was made, through the Task Force on Regulatory Relief, to significantly alter much of regulatory language for disability-related legislative programs, including Section 504, the Education for All Handicapped Children Act (P.L. 94–142), and the ATBCB. Through a combination of effective advocacy and skillful political negotiations, the regulations for these important programs remained intact, and changes that had "potentially staggering implications" were avoided (4).

Ironically, it was during the Reagan years, with *deregulation* as the buzzword, that one of the most far-reaching pieces of disability rights legislation enacted thus far—the ADA—was introduced. Actions taken during the Carter Administration had established an entity—then the National Council on the Handicapped, now the National Council on Disability—to bring order to the "incoherence and intrinsic tensions of various disability policies (4). The National Council on the Handicapped was initially housed within the Department of HEW. However, when the Council produced a report, entitled *National Policy on Disability*, on the state of persons with disabilities and policy recommendations to address disability issues, the Reagan Administration was not supportive and refused to provide funding for printing and distribution of the report. Effective advocacy efforts, again, brought about changes through the 1984 Amendments to the Rehabilitation Act that established the Council as an independent entity. In doing so, Congress noted that "the Council has not been able to meet congressional intent for an independent body to advise on all matters in the Government affecting handicapped individuals" (7).

In concert with establishing the Council as an independent agency, Congress issued a mandate that it produce a comprehensive analysis of federal disability programs and policy by February 1, 1986. In addition to providing a listing of programs based on the number of persons served, the mandate required that the Council evaluate the degree to which federal programs ". . . provide incentives or disincentives to the establishment of community-based services for handicapped individuals, promote the full integration of such individuals in the community, in schools, and in the workplace, and contribute to the independence and dignity of such individuals" (8). In response to this mandate, the Council produced *Toward Independence: An Assessment of Federal Laws and Programs Affecting Persons with Disabilities—with Legislative Recommendations* (9).

The landmark *Toward Independence* report contained over 40 recommendations dealing with issues ranging from transportation, to employment, to education, to housing. Perhaps most significant, however, was the recommendation for ". . . enactment of a comprehensive law requiring equal opportunity for individuals with disabilities, with broad coverage and setting clear, consistent, and enforceable standards prohibiting discrimination on the basis of handicap (9). Not only did the report provide the recommendation for preparing the legislation that was to become the ADA, for the first time, it provided a clear and documented rationale for why such legislation was needed. Although a few hurdles remained—including the stipulation that such a "liberal" report not bear the presidential seal—the report was provided to Congress and President Reagan on time. However, because of other demands on the President's time, it was Vice President George Bush who met with Council members and staff to receive and discuss the report. He demonstrated knowledge of its contents and an understanding of disability issues (4).

Drafted initially by staff of the National Council on the Handicapped, the first version of the ADA was introduced to Congress in 1988. For a variety of reasons, including attention to the 1988 elections that brought George Bush into the Oval Office, the ADA received little attention from Congress following its initial introduction. It would require two more years of struggle before the ADA made its way through the legislative labyrinth and was signed into law by President Bush on July 26, 1990. During this process, some key supporters, such as Senate sponsor Lowell Weicker, left the scene, but other champions, including Senator Tom Harkin, assumed leadership in the legislative process. All along the way, there were extraordinary advocacy efforts undertaken by an array of disability-related organizations, including American Disabled for Attendant Programs Today (ADAPT), the Consortium for Citizens with Disabilities (CCD), the Disability Rights Education and Defense Fund (DREDF), the National Council on Independent Living (NCIL), and others. As the recent report from the National Council on Disablity concluded, "There could have been no successful and meaningful ADA without a ground swell of people who demonstrated what happened in the absence of significant legal protections . . ." (4).

WHAT IS THE STATUS OF THE AMERICAN WITH DISABILITIES ACT TODAY?

As we prepare to enter the twenty-first century, few would argue that the ADA has had a profound impact on the lives of millions of Americans with disabilities. Unquestionably, the ADA has been a key to unlocking opportunities for many people with disabilities who had previously been denied access to employment, education, recreation, and a host of other activities taken for granted by people without disabilities. In fact, there are many people who believe that the ADA has solved the problems of discrimination and bias based on disability. If one reads the popular press, it might be assumed that thousands of ADA-related lawsuits are initiated monthly—some based on questionable claims and interpretations of the law never intended by the people who worked so hard for its enactment.

Notwithstanding some progress that has been made since enactment of the ADA, there is evidence that application of the law has not produced the hoped-for changes in opportunity for many people with disabilities. On the sixth anniversary of the enactment of the ADA—July 26,

1996—the National Council on Disability released a report entitled *Achieving Independence: The Challenge for the 21st Century—A Decade of Progress in Disability Policy/Setting an Agenda for the Future* (10). The report provided a comprehensive review of efforts to eliminate disability-based discrimination across key areas of life—education, employment, health insurance and health care, housing, and transportation. The three major conclusions included in the report (10) were:

- Disability policy has made steady progress in the last decade in empowering people with disabilities; however, this progress is threatened, compromised, and undermined by lack of understanding and support in Congress and among particular segments of society.
- Most public policy affecting people with disabilities does not yet promote the goals of the ADA—equality of opportunity, full participation, independent living, and economic self-sufficiency.
- Most Americans with disabilities remain outside the economic and social mainstream of American life.

The report's conclusions support what people with disabilities have been only too well aware of for some time—much more work is required by all segments of society if the promise of the ADA is to be realized. For each topical area covered in the report, a set of recommendations had been generated suggesting actions that should be pursued in addressing the issue(s) covered in that section. Although the full report should be required reading for all personnel in human service fields, the recommendations dealing with health insurance and health care should be integrated into training and professional development programs for entry-level rehabilitation professionals, as well as for rehabilitation professionals in practice. The two recommendations specific to education and training (10) were

- The federal government and the private sector should develop and implement education and training programs that will sensitize health care providers to the ongoing health care needs of people with disabilities, with the federal and state governments awarding grants to help develop such model educational programs.
- The federal government and state governments should provide training grants to consumer organizations, health care institutions, and educational organizations designed to enable people with disabilities to become more informed consumers of health plans.

These recommendations suggest an active role on the part of health care professionals in promoting the rights of people with disabilities. While some rehabilitation professionals may have viewed their roles as encompassing active advocacy on behalf of the people with disabilities whom they serve, this is a role that many health care professionals assume to only a limited degree, if at all.

A DIFFERENT PERSPECTIVE ON HEALTH, DISEASE, AND THE ROLE OF SERVICE PROVIDERS

The National Council on Disability report, cited previously, suggests an active and consumer-oriented role for health care providers in promoting equal rights for people with disabilities, including more aggressive efforts to foster ADA implementation. Such a role acknowledges the complexity of factors that come into play in determining one's relative health. An excellent illustration of the multiplicity of factors influencing health status can be found in Aday's discussion of populations that are most vulnerable to health problems (11).

As Figure 102-1 indicates, the likelihood that a person is at risk for health problems depends on more than his or her anatomy and physiology and on more than simply having access to adequate and appropriate health care services. The risk for health problems is related to education, employment, income, housing, social networks, and an array of other factors not typically perceived as being within the purview of the health care provider. It is worth taking a closer look at how these four domains—social status, social capital, human capital, and populations at risk—pertain to the notion of disability and the appropriate roles of service providers in advocating for changes that have the potential to reduce health risks in people with disabilities.

"*Social status* is associated with positions that individuals occupy in society as a function of age, sex, or race/ethnicity and the corollary socially defined opportunities and rewards, such as prestige and power, that they all have as a result" (12). Some segments of society (e.g., the elderly, poor people, members of minority groups) may have a combination of statuses that place them at higher risk for poor health and few material or nonmaterial resources to draw on in altering risk status. Individuals in these societal groups are highly vulnerable (13).

The question of the impact that severe disability has on social status has been examined by a number of authors. The nature of the relationship between disability and status is reflected in the observation by Heyman et al (14): "The class/handicap relationship is probably due to both handicapped people achieving lower socioeconomic status and lower status being associated with conditions which cause handicapping conditions" Nagler (15), likewise, discussed the notion of disability in the context of disadvantaged minorities with limited power. The minority perspective of disability is defensible in light of the definition of minority posited by Dworkin and Dworkin (16): ". . . identifiability, differential power, differential and pejorative treatment, and group awareness." The diminished social status typically accorded persons with disabilities is perhaps summed up most succinctly in five powerful conclusions reached by Fine and Asch (17) in their discussion

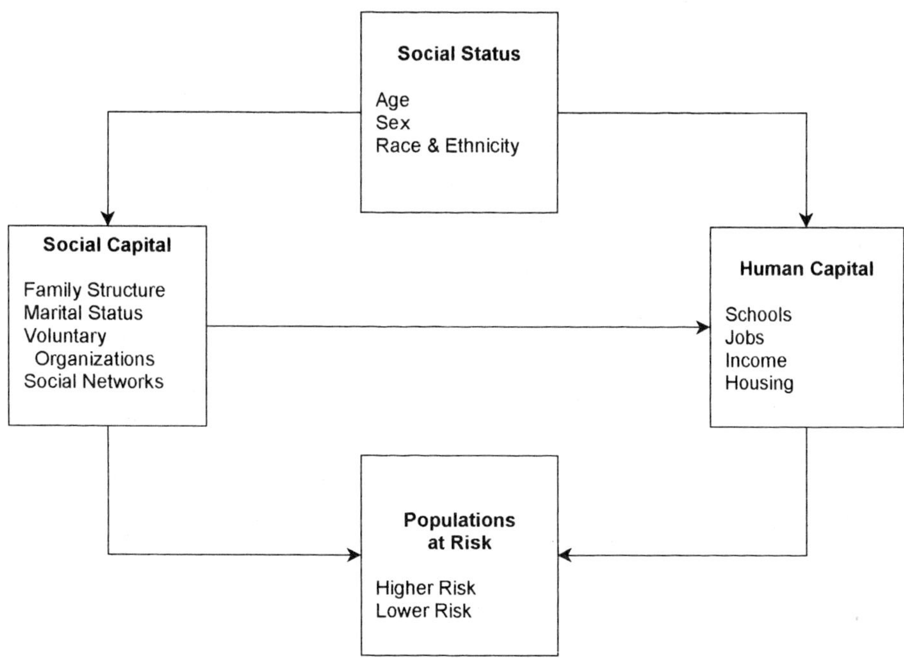

Figure 102-1. Predictors of populations at risk. (Aday LA. *At risk in America: the health and health care needs of vulnerable populations in the United States.* San Francisco: Jossey-Bass, 1993:7.)

of the "stigma" of disability and social interaction, discrimination, and activism:

- It is often assumed that disability is located solely in biology, and thus disability is accepted uncritically as an independent variable.
- When a disabled person faces problems, it is assumed that the impairment causes them.
- It is assumed that the disabled person is a "victim."
- It is assumed that disability is central to the disabled person's self-concept, self-definition, social comparison, and reference groups.
- It is assumed that having a disability is synonymous with needing help and social support.

Acceptance of the conclusions reached by Fine and Asch clearly places people with disabilities in a comparatively lower status than their nondisabled peers. It also offers the service provider—whether a health care provider or a provider of social, legal, or other services—an "out" in not assuming a more aggressive stance in advocating for equal rights and opportunities for people with disabilities.

"*Social capital* resides in the quantity and quality of interpersonal ties between people" (12). Aday (12) emphasized that communities constitute the "social reservoir" in which social capital resources are both generated and drawn on by individuals in the community. The importance of interpersonal relationships and family and community support in maintaining health is acknowledged by virtually everyone who has any knowledge of the complexities of health and disease. Notwithstanding this acknowledgment, it has taken decades—through enactment of legislation like the ADA, through more aggressive public education and community awareness efforts, and through commitment of public and private resources to the elimination of structural, attitudinal, and economic barriers to full participation—to begin to create opportunities for many people with disabilities and to develop the types of nurturing support systems that are essential in maintaining physical and mental health.

Extant conditions that limit opportunities for people with disabilities to draw upon the social capital resources essential to attainment of optimal health are not the result of happenstance. Hahn (18) summarized succinctly the role of public policy in reducing the opportunities for people with disabilities to engage in an array of social roles. In his analysis of the "socio-political view" of disability issues, Hahn (18) asserted:

> . . . this approach emphasizes that the functional demands exerted on human beings by the environment are fundamentally determined by public policy. The present forms of architectural structures and social institutions exist because statutes, ordinances, and codes either required or permitted them to be constructed in that manner. These public policies imply values, expectations, and assumptions about the physical and behavioral attributes that people possess in order to survive or to participate in community life. . . . These characteristics of the environment that have a discriminatory effect on disabled citizens cannot be considered simply coincidental, rather than reflecting immutable aspects of an environment decreed by natural law, they represent the consequences of prior policy decisions.

This more mutable view of the role of public policy as an instrument in denying opportunities to people with disabilities, whether or not so intended, suggests that the solution to correcting problems in the environment that foster intended or unintended discrimination lies in more concerted efforts to eliminate the sources of such discrimination. Such efforts can be accelerated if more people—including people (e.g., health care professionals, policy makers) who have higher social status and access to more extensive social and human capital resources—become active participants in efforts that foster opportunities for people with disabilities to live meaningful, productive, and rewarding lives.

"*Human capital* refers to investments in people's skills and capabilities (such as vocational or public education) that enable them to act in new ways (master a trade) or enhance their contributions to society (enter the labor force) (12). There is a lengthy history of resource commitment to programs and services designed to support Americans with disabilities in their pursuit of education and employment (19).

In a number of respects, the U.S. approach to investment in human capital as it relates to disability programs represents a more progressive perspective on disability than that seen in many developed countries of Europe and other parts of the world. In many of the industrial democracies of northern Europe, there is little expectation that people with disabilities will enter competitive employment. In a number of countries, people with severe disabilities are simply provided a living stipend that is fairly generous by U.S. standards. In contrast, the U.S. emphasis on vocational services designed to provide disabled adults with employment skills can be traced back to the 1920s, and programs designed to offer educational opportunities to disabled children have been in place since the 1960s (19).

However, it is only in the last quarter century that disability policy in the United States shifted from a ". . . long pattern of paternalistic and dehumanizing practices typified by institutionalization and segregation . . ." (19) to a civil rights–based perspective as reflected in the language of the ADA. The significance of this shift in policy as regards investment in human capital is very important; rather than providing for people who are the objects of pity and deserving of charity, the notion underlying the ADA and other disability rights legislation has to do with the right of every person to enjoy a reasonable quality of life and to participate in the full range of life activities—employment, recreation, social interaction—enjoyed by people without disabilities. As the previously cited recommendations from the National Council on Disability regarding training priorities suggest, health care professionals must become much more sensitive to the full range of needs of people with disabilities, including nonhealth factors (e.g., employment, recreation) that exert a powerful influence on health status.

At risk is a term used by Aday to refer to people for whom ". . . there is always a chance that an adverse health-related outcome will occur" (11). Aday included people with physical, psychological, and cognitive impairments among specific segments of the population she described as "vulnerable." As noted in the literature, many people with disabilities have a "narrow margin of health," making them more susceptible to health problems than many people without disabilities (20–22).

The higher risk for health care problems among people with disabilities is reflected in their disproportionate use of health services. One study found that Americans with disabilities spend more than four times as much on medical care, services, and equipment, on average, as their nondisabled counterparts (23). The findings indicated that noninstitutionalized persons with disabilities, while accounting for only 17% of the population, account for 47% of medical care expenditures (23). The higher level of risk suggests that greater attention should be given to the full constellation of factors that come into play in placing persons at risk. These factors include those identified by Aday in the paragraphs on *social status*, *social capital*, and *human capital* (11,12). They also include intrinsic health-related factors that have been the traditional domain of health care providers, including primary care providers and specialists in rehabilitation and other fields.

THE REASONABLENESS OF HOLISTIC HEALTH CARE IN A SERVICE SYSTEM UNDER SIEGE

During the last decade of the twentieth century, extraordinary change has been occurring in America's health care system. The benefits of a more holistic approach to health care—as reflected in Aday's model—have gained increasing credence in a health care system that for too long focused almost exclusively on resolving episodes of acute illness. Unfortunately, this recognition has come at a time when the health care system has been squeezed by socioeconomic forces offering little hope that a more comprehensive approach to medical management, as suggested by Aday's model, will be undertaken.

The impact of change in the health care service system is suggested by data from a study that examined changes in the health care market from 1985 to 1995. The study looked at two models of health maintenance organizations (HMOs)—the group-model HMO and the independent practice association (IPA) HMO. The rapid growth in both types of HMOs was emphasized, with enrollments going from about 6 million in 1976 to nearly 50 million in 1995 (24). The study found that the number of hospital days per 1000 non-Medicare enrollees in group-model HMOs had decreased from 353 in 1985 to 255 in 1995, a drop of roughly 28% in a 10-year period (24). An even greater decrease—nearly 35%, from 400 to 264 per 1000 non-Medicare enrollees—was documented for participants in IPA HMOs (24). The same study found that the number of ambulatory visits to service providers in the two service models studied had increased during the same time period, but the increase amounted to less than one additional visit per enrollee per year—4.4 in 1985 to 5.2 in 1995 for HMOs and 4.8 in 1985 to 5.5 in 1995 for IPAs. Notwithstanding the modest increase in ambulatory visits, these data suggest that late-twentieth-century changes in the nation's health care system have had a profound effect on health service utilization.

Unarguably, change was needed to control the rampant year-to-year escalation of health care costs that had characterized much of the latter half of the century. However, at least two questions come quickly to mind when considering these changes in light of their impact on persons who are atypical users of health care services, including many persons with disabilities.

1. How have these changes affected the scope and quality of health services available to people with disabilities?
2. What should service providers, including rehabilitation professionals, be doing to ensure access to services that enhance the likelihood of favorable rehabilitation outcomes for people with disabilities in a changing health care environment?

Providing adequate answers to these two questions poses something of a challenge, at least during the early months of 1998 when this publication was prepared. Data on the scope and quality of services available to people with disabilities who are enrolled in various health care plans, whether they are in managed care plans or more traditional fee-for-service or indemnity plans, were largely lacking during the first quarter of 1998. Perhaps the most thorough examination of the scope and quality of health care services available for people with disabilities was provided by the U.S. Government Accounting Office (GAO) in its 1996 assessment of services provided to persons with disabilities through state Medicaid programs (25). The GAO report suggested that people with disabilities enrolled under managed care plans are experiencing difficulties in receiving appropriate and timely health care services. Two points highlighted in the GAO report (25) with respect to the process that disabled enrollees may have to pursue in obtaining needed services are particularly striking: "... (1) the process requires a significant amount of self advocacy on the part of beneficiaries who may not be capable of it and (2) the process can be extremely time consuming." The first comprehensive study of disabled Medicare beneficiaries enrolled in HMOs revealed that "disabled Medicare enrollees are significantly more likely than non-disabled Medicare enrollees to experience access problems, and more report fair or poor satisfaction with various aspects of care" (26).

Data on how people with disabilities enrolled in public (i.e., Medicaid and Medicare) managed care programs are faring are scant, while data on the impact of managed care for people with disabilities in privately funded health care programs (e.g., employer-provided health care plans, individually purchased plans) were virtually nonexistent in early 1998. The lack of data on the scope and quality of services provided people with disabilities enrolled in nonpublic managed care programs was alluded to in the National Council on Disability's 1996 report on achieving independence (10): "All managed care plans, including those that service only privately insured persons, should be required to meet federal standards to ensure access to specialty care, adequate grievance and appeals procedures including ombudspersons, and equitable utilization review criteria."

Anecdotal data available on the experiences of persons with disabilities enrolled in privately funded managed care plans indicate that there are problems that have potentially significant implications for the long-term health and functional outcomes realized by these individuals. People with spinal cord injury who had experience with a managed care plan cited problems ranging from delays in obtaining approval to see urology specialists, to difficulty in obtaining pharmaceutical products, to routine denial of claims for services—even when prior approval of such services had been obtained from the individual's primary care provider (27). Clearly, there is a need for sound, objective data on the scope and quality of health care and related services being provided people with disabilities that can be used in developing appropriate public policy intended to address the problems in existing service programs.

IMPLICATIONS FOR SERVICE PROVIDERS—INCLUDING REHABILITATION PROFESSIONALS

Answering the second of the two questions posed previously—What should service providers, including rehabilitation professionals, be doing to ensure access to services that enhance the likelihood of favorable rehabilitation outcomes for people with disabilities in a changing health care environment?—represents the crux of this chapter. In answering this question, it is worth considering why a rehabilitation professional might become engaged in advocacy on behalf of persons with disabilities. At least one response to the "why" question has to do with moral imperatives that drive social programs. As Banja (28) noted, "A liberal democracy that prides itself on equal treatment for all cannot condone the unfairness of denying anyone access to social goods. What a society must do, within reasonable limits, is to eradicate those barriers and practices that create disadvantage among persons with disabilities."

However, there are those among us who might take issue, not without some justification, with the position

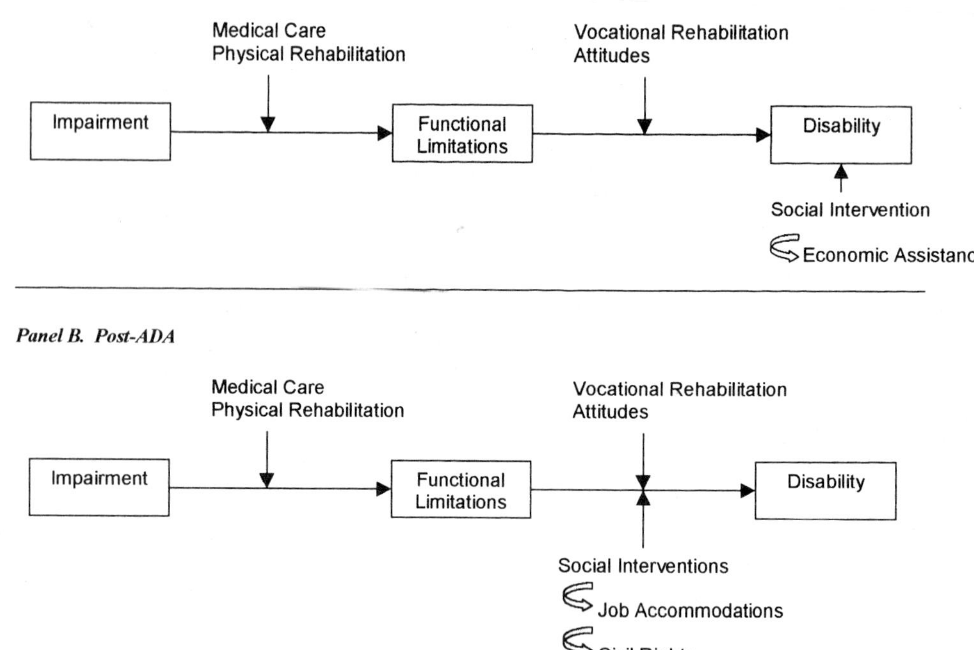

Figure 102-2. The process of disability. (Baldwin ML. Can the ADA achieve its employment goals? *Ann Am Acad Polit Soc Sci* 1997;549(January):37–52.)

couched in the moral imperative cited above—particularly in light of the inclusion of the caveat of "within reasonable limits." One could make the argument that much of the public expenditure on disability-related programs and services exceeds "reasonable limits." Extending this argument somewhat further, then, the case could be made that expecting rehabilitation professionals, who are already applying their clinical and technical skills to addressing the needs of people with disabilities, to become more substantively involved in advocacy efforts is exceeding reasonable limits. From the service provider's perspective, the question could be recast, What more do you want from us?

In framing an answer to this question, it is worth looking beyond the fairness-based moral imperative cited above. In this age of cost containment and accountability, those of us who are involved in service programs are increasingly expected to justify what we do and how we use available resources in terms of quantifiable outcomes realized from resource commitments. Rehabilitation professionals have long struggled with outcome-related issues that have been far simpler to address in clinical arenas that focus on cure—a goal often unattainable, at least for the present, in dealing with problems like spinal cord injury, stroke, and chronic neuromuscular disease. Rather, for the rehabilitation professional, outcomes often have to be measured in terms of incremental functional gains and often elusive measures of life quality.

Going back to the model for predictors of poor health proposed by Aday (11,12), one can make a valid argument that reductions of health risk among individuals in the population is a legitimate outcome for professionals engaged in the delivery of health-related services. One can then make a valid argument that commitment of capital resources, including efforts to secure adequate education, employment, and housing, to health risk reduction efforts is a legitimate role for the service provider. Indeed, a model (Fig. 102-2) suggesting the appropriateness of advocacy efforts on the part of people with disabilities was suggested by Baldwin (29) in her comparison of pre- and post-ADA employment-related efforts to intervene in the disability process. Figure 102-2 indicates the important role that accommodation and civil rights have in altering the nature of the resulting employment-related disability following an impairing event.

We would like to propose a somewhat different model for representing the need for more active and effective advocacy by rehabilitation professionals in support of the people with disabilities whom they serve. This model borrows from both Aday's conceptual framework for predictors of poor health and from Baldwin's model depicting the impact of the ADA as an intervening factor in the disability process. However, the proposed model (Fig. 102-3) departs from the referenced conceptual frameworks in its focus not on risk or on disability, but rather on positive outcomes to be gained from more active and effective efforts on the part of rehabilitation professionals, others in the community, and perhaps most importantly, people with disabilities themselves in advocating for fair and equal treatment.

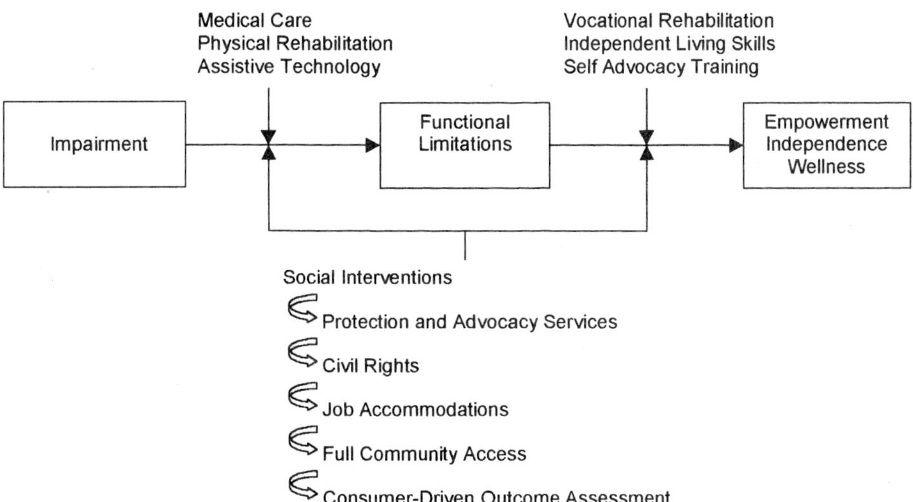

Figure 102-3. Conceptual model for advocacy inclusion in post–Americans with Disabilities Act rehabilitation service programs.

CONCLUDING REMARKS

This chapter provides a framework for rethinking the role that rehabilitation professionals should assume in advocating on the part of people with disabilities. For many rehabilitation professionals, the ideas contained within this chapter are ones that have already been embraced and that have been incorporated fully and effectively into their day-to-day service repertoires. However, for others in the rehabilitation professions, the role of active and assertive advocate on the part of people with disabilities is one with which they are not yet fully comfortable.

Some of the discomfort that professionals may experience in assuming a more active advocacy role with regard to disability issues may emanate from difficulties associated with documenting the benefits associated with such efforts. It may be hard for some professionals to justify advocacy efforts in terms of measurable benefits to the "patient." In fact, the prevailing methods of evaluating rehabilitation outcomes are grounded in what Fuhrer (30) termed "concepts of disablement." And as Fuhrer noted, while such concepts ". . . are crucial in evaluating the success of rehabilitation, they are not sufficient for that purpose." Fuhrer argued forcefully and cogently for inclusion of "quality-of-life" measures—including those targeted to health, income, and social activity—in evaluating rehabilitation outcomes. In calling for new approaches to studying subjective well-being, Fuhrer (30) emphasized that ". . . it would be unacceptable for us to feign indifference to people's happiness with their lives while we are providing rehabilitation services or evaluating their outcomes."

Simply evaluating the subjective well-being of the recipients of rehabilitation services, while contributing to an understanding of the relative effectiveness of rehabilitation in fostering desired outcomes, will not lead to the kinds of systemic changes that are likely to enhance the quality of life of people with disabilities. For significant change to result from rehabilitation efforts, rehabilitation professionals, other service providers, community leaders, families of people with disabilities, and most importantly, people with disabilities themselves must form partnerships to advocate effectively for full and effective implementation of the ADA and other civil rights protections. The model we propose suggests a much more proactive approach to advocacy than is typically assumed by most rehabilitation professionals.

In putting forth this model, we were guided by observations included in the National Council on Disability's 1996 report (10) on achieving independence: "The tenets of other civil rights perspectives apply to the disability rights perspective. The defining aspect of the perspective is that people with disabilities, as a group, have been subject to pervasive and persistent discriminatory treatment. The remedy for such treatment is a prohibition against discrimination, protection of civil rights, and empowerment of people with disabilities." The battle against discrimination is a battle that we must all continue to wage. So long as discrimination—whether it is based on race, gender, age, or disability status—is countenanced, then the quality of peoples' lives will be diminished. An avoidable diminishment in the quality of life for people with disabilities should be viewed as a less than desirable rehabilitation outcome. Effective advocacy on the part of all concerned parties, including rehabilitation professionals, can lead to enhanced rehabilitation outcomes as reflected in a better quality of life for people with disabilities.

REFERENCES

1. Equal Employment Opportunity Commission and the U.S. Department of Justice. *Americans with Disabilities Act handbook.* Washington, DC: Equal Employment Opportunity Commission and the U.S. Department of Justice, 1991:1.

2. Bush GHW. Remarks at ADA signing ceremony. Quoted in *Americans with Disabilities Act handbook.* Washington, DC: Equal Employment Opportunity Commission and the U.S. Department of Justice, 1991:1.

3. Shapiro JP. *No pity: people with disabilities forging a new civil rights movement.* New York: Times Books, 1993.

4. National Council on Disability. *Equality of opportunity: the making of the Americans with Disabilities Act.* Washington, DC: National Council on Disability, 1997.

5. Kaltenhauser S. Hugh Gallegher: ADA's hidden architect. *New Mobility* 1995;6:4–43.

6. *Rehabilitation Act of 1973.* Public law 93–112, 93rd Congress, 1st Session, September 26, 1973, §504.

7. U.S. Senate Committee on Labor and Human Resources. *Senate report no. 98–168, to accompany S. 1340,* May 23, 1983, reprinted in *1984 U.S. Code of Congressional and Administrative News,* p. 32.

8. *Rehabilitation Amendments of 1984.* Public law 98–221, 98th Congress, 2nd Session, 1984, §142(b).

9. National Council on the Handicapped. *Toward independence: an assessment of federal laws and programs affecting persons with disabilities—with legislative recommendations.* A Report to the President and to the Congress of the United States, February, 1986. Washington, DC: National Council on the Handicapped, 1986.

10. National Council on Disability. *Achieving independence: the challenge for the 21st century—a decade of progress in disability policy/setting an agenda for the future.* Washington, DC: National Council on Disability, 1996:3–4.

11. Aday LA. *At risk in America: the health and health care needs of vulnerable populations in the United States.* San Francisco: Jossey-Bass, 1993.

12. Aday LA. Equity, accessibility, and ethical issues: is the U.S. health care reform debate asking the right questions? *Am Behav Sci* 1993;36:724–740.

13. Kaplan HB. Health, disease, and social structure. In: Freeman HE, Levine S, eds. *Handbook of medical sociology.* 4th ed. Englewood Cliffs, NJ: Prentice-Hall, 1989:46–68.

14. Heyman B, Bell B, Kingham MR. Social class and the prevalence of handicapping conditions. *Disabil Handicap Soc* 1990;5:167–184.

15. Nagler M. The disabled: the acquisition of power. In: Nagler M, ed. *Perspectives on disability.* 2nd ed. Palo Alto, CA: Health Markets Research, 1993:33–36.

16. Dworkin A, Dworkin R, eds. *The minority report.* New York: Praeger, 1976.

17. Fine M, Asch A. Disability beyond stigma: social interaction, discrimination, and activism. *J Soc Issues* 1988;44(1):3–21.

18. Hahn H. The politics of physical differences: disability and discrimination. In: Nagler M, ed. *Perspectives on disability.* 2nd ed. Palo Alto, CA: Health Markets Research, 1993:37–42.

19. Shriner KF, Batavia AI. Disability law and social policy. In: Dell Orto AE, Martinelli R, eds. *Encyclopedia of disability and rehabilitation.* New York: Macmillan Library Reference USA, 1995.

20. Burns TJ, Batavia AI, Smith QW, DeJong G. Primary health care needs of persons with disabilities: what are research and service priorities? *Arch Phys Med Rehabil* 1990;71:138–143.

21. Batavia AI, DeJong G, Halstead LS, Smith QW. Primary medical services for people with disabilities. *Am Rehabil* 1988–89; 14(4):9–12, 26–27.

22. DeJong G, Batavia AI, Griss R. America's neglected health minority: working-age persons with disabilities. *Milbank Q* 1989; 67(suppl 2):311–351.

23. Max W, Rice DP, Trupin L. Medical expenditures for people with disabilities. *Disabil Stat Abstr* 1996;12:1–4.

24. Wholey DR, Christianson JB, Engberg J, Bryce C. HMO market structure and performance: 1985–1995. *Health Affairs* 1997;16(6):75–84.

25. U.S. Government Accounting Office. *Medicaid Managed Care: Serving the Disabled Challenges State Programs.* Washington, DC: U.S. Government Accounting Office, 1996.

26. Gold M, Nelson L, Brown R, et al. Disabled Medicare beneficiaries in HMOs. *Health Affairs* 1997;16(5): 149–162.

27. Frieden L, Smith L, Wilkinson W, Redd L, Smith QW. Spinal cord injury and managed care: a consumer perspective. *J Spinal Cord Inj Rehabil* 3(4):80–88.

28. Banja JD. Introduction. In: Banja JD, ed. *The persons served: ethical perspectives on CARF's accreditation standards and guidelines.* Tucson, AZ: CARF . . . The Rehabilitation Accreditation Commission, 1998:1–10.

29. Baldwin ML. Can the ADA achieve its employment goals? *Ann Am Acad Polit Soc Sci* 1997; 549(January):37–52.

30. Fuhrer MJ. Subjective well-being: implications for medical rehabilitation outcomes and models of disablement. *Am J Phys Med Rehabil* 1994;73:358–364.

Chapter 103

Reimbursement Issues Across the Continuum of Care

Rita M. Glass

REIMBURSEMENT TRENDS AND DIRECTIONS

The climate of reimbursement is shifting dramatically as the health care environment stresses cost containment. It is no longer business as usual in the acute care hospital. In both the acute and postacute settings, nonprofessional caregivers are replacing nurses and therapists to lower costs.

The need for specialists in the medical community is decreasing as we move to managed care. The new emphasis is on primary care. The American Medical Association (AMA) states that we are presently training too many physicians, 66% more specialists than we need, and is encouraging medical schools to reduce enrollments (1).

Therapists are being asked to do more with less. Professionals are being told to extend themselves through the increased use of assistants and aides to maintain market share. The role of the therapist is shifting dramatically. At the February 9, 1995 Combined Section Meeting of the American Physical Therapy Association in Reno, Nevada, Michael Burcham, in his presentation "Emerging Trends in the Delivery of Care," predicted that physical therapists in outpatient settings will be moving from supervising 1.5 extenders per physical therapist to supervising 3.5 extenders. Treatment times will be shifting from 60- to 90-minute sessions to 30-minute sessions (2).

The Health Care Financing Administration (HCFA) is capping the cost of therapy in skilled facilities, where rehabilitation costs have skyrocketed, and will not pay more than $60 for physical, occupational, or speech therapy. HCFA is further considering capping the Tax Equity and Fiscal Responsibility Act (TEFRA) rates of rehabilitation units and hospitals to between $17,000 and $18,000 (3).

The recent Balanced Budget Act of 1997 has changed reimbursement as we now know it. The primary purpose of this act was to reduce Medicare outlays by $115 billion. The implementation of the provisions of the Balanced Budget Act will take place over the next 5 years. Key provisions of the Act resulted in limitations on transfers to postacute care in select diagnosis-related groups (DRGs), major reimbursement adjustments, imposition of a $1500 beneficiary cap for outpatient settings, and the implementation of prospective payment rates for hospital outpatient services, skilled nursing facilities (SNFs), home health agencies, and rehabilitation hospitals. In January 1998, any provider wishing to participate in Medicare will have to post surety/compliance bonds of at least $50,000. Medicare appears to be trying to discourage small "mom and pop" rehabilitation.

The provisions start with placing a limit on the TEFRA target payments. For 1998 the TEFRA target payment for rehabilitation facilities was $19,250. The limit is set to the seventy-fifth percentile of similar facilities based on the 1997 cost report. The HCFA estimates that 23.2% of freestanding rehabilitation hospitals and 76.8% of hospital-based units will be over the new limits (4).

There are fundamental defects in the TEFRA system, which, when adopted, was to be temporary and replaced by a prospective payment system (PPS). To date, TEFRA remains in place. It discriminates against very acute and severely impaired patients because it assigns the same reimbursement value to all rehabilitation patients. Secondly, TEFRA limits vary widely among providers with similar costs and patient populations (5). The new TEFRA limit tries to address this as does the rehabilitation PPS system to be fully implemented by 2003. This is discussed further in the section on acute rehabilitation.

The days of therapy kings and queens are coming to an end. The era of a sign-on bonus of up to $6000, a $3000 bonus for bringing in a friend, or the enticement to "travel the world" with us is about over. Therapy recruiters and management companies are retrenching, the companies going into management consulting and software sales to make up the anticipated shortfalls.

In the new environment, therapists are moving away from a strictly hands-on approach to that of case management. Instead of 90% hands-on and 10% case management, therapists will be spending 50% of their time in hands-on activities and the remaining 50% of their time in supervision, education, training, and case management (2). Instead of doing it for the patient, the shift is to having the patient and family "do it for themselves." The role of training extenders is not new; it is, however, being dramatically broadened and accelerated. The term *complementary medicine* is being added to rehabilitation as more of the public demands massage therapy, acupuncture, and other nontraditional services as part of their rehabilitation treatments, with insurers paying for them. All of this is being done in the name of customer satisfaction and cost containment.

The new patient service delivery models demand that today's nurses, therapists, and physicians be trained in, and understand, reimbursement so they will be able to design programs and services that not only satisfy patients, and maximize their function, but are cost-effective.

It is my opinion that understanding reimbursement and containing costs are critical skills to today's patient care delivery systems. Reimbursement must be taught to all rehabilitation physicians, managers, and staff to assist them in designing integrated, effective, long-term programs across the continuum of care.

This chapter provides rehabilitation professionals with the basics in reimbursement trends and strategies as well as an understanding of how reimbursement can be applied across the continuum of care. This chapter discusses Medicare and Medicaid reimbursement and addresses the fundamental payment systems in place in the United States, moving the reader from a noncapitated to a capitated reimbursement environment and into managed care. As more organizations seek to provide coverage of coordinated care to Medicare beneficiaries and employees, the number of "O's" is getting confusing. We have gone from health maintenance organizations (HMOs), preferred provider organizations (PPOs), and physician-hospital organizations (PHOs), to physician/provider-sponsored coordinated care organizations (PCCOs), and provider-sponsored networks (PSNs). The latest acronym does not even have an "O" in it (6). It is all very confusing as systems are designed to become integrated networks providing everything to everyone. Therefore, I concentrate on the method of payment health care organizations receive, discussing noncapitated through capitated reimbursement.

REIMBURSEMENT TRENDS IN MEDICARE

We Never Know from Day to Day, or Is It State to State?

Medicare was created as a federal health care program in 1965 by Social Security. Medicare is composed of two separate and distinct parts: Part A and Part B. It is administered by the Secretary of the Department of Health and Human Services (HHS). The secretary has delegated the day-to-day operations for Medicare and Medicaid to HCFA. HCFA, in turn, uses fiscal intermediaries to administrate program operations at state and regional levels. The largest intermediaries are Blue Cross and Blue Shield, Aetna, Mutual of Omaha, and Travelers. Each Medicare provider has one intermediary to whom they are responsible. Providers submit annual cost reports, which are audited to determine the amount of program reimbursement. Part A provides traditional "hospital insurance" by reimbursing inpatient hospital, skilled nursing, hospice, and home health services. Generally it is "automatic" for most people over the age of 65.

Only certain identified entities, referred to as "providers of services," may provide Part A services to Medicare beneficiaries (7). Providers under the Medicare program include acute hospitals, skilled and long-term-care nursing facilities, home health agencies, hospices, and rural and primary care programs.

Part B is a voluntary insurance program for the aged and disabled, and provides "Supplementary Medicare Insurance" by paying physician and other medical and health services, as opposed to Part A, which generally is considered coverage for institutions.

Part B "suppliers" do not enter into provider agreements with HCFA. Their relationship is governed by statute and the Medicare regulations. A "supplier" is a physician or other practitioner, or entity, other than a provider, that furnishes health care services under Medicare (8). A supplier applies for and receives a Medicare provider number and then submits claims for payments to an intermediary or carrier (insurance company). Individuals in private practice and therapists who subcontract can obtain individual provider numbers. Payments are made from a fee schedule or on the basis of the charge (fee-for-service).

As Medicare is administered under more and more managed care systems, discounted fees and higher risk taking are being required of Medicare providers. It is important that providers know their state Medicare Part A and Part B administrators, as more and more often reimbursement rules, which are complex and fragmented, at times become contradictory. Providers will have to get more and more clarifications as health care is redesigned. This is true in new markets such as subacute programs, which can be accomplished in acute, skilled, and long-term care beds. Medicare surveys, and certifications of these new programs, continue to slow and providers wonder whether the strategy is to intentionally reduce Medicare funding by limiting surveys. Medicare administrators claim they do not have the funding to carry out the number of surveys being requested and providers in many states are presently unable to get initial surveys that initiate Medicare approval and funding (9).

Medicare rules and regulations for reimbursement are not consistent across the continuum of care. Interpretations of the regulations often vary by state. As health care systems attempt to integrate and provide Medicare services across their continua of care, they are having difficulty monitoring costs and the reimbursement system.

Medicare Reimbursement of Acute Care

Acute care is reimbursed under PPS utilizing DRGs. When a patient is admitted to a hospital, they are assigned a diagnosis that is related to a DRG. This controls payment by controlling the amount of services and length of stay (LOS). A code is assigned to the patient, depending on where in the human body the diagnosis is applicable. For example, number 1 starts at the top of the patient's body in the head, and is related to brain injury, while cerebral vascular accident (CVA) is number 14, 16, or 18, depending on whether it involves a right, left, or center site. LOS and payment are based on the DRG assigned to the patient. Outlier payments are possible for patients exceeding the DRG parameters. A patient can be assigned only one DRG number per acute hospital stay. DRG LOSs continue to shrink for certain diagnostic groups and payments are decreasing in most instances. With new regulations, TEFRA is being phased out and into a PPS by 2002.

HCFA appears to be shifting referral patterns away from sending patients being discharged from acute care hospitals to rehabilitation. Specifically, HCFA has implemented a regulation, referred to as the "transfer agreement," which provides financial incentives for hospitals to refer patients to SNFs, skilled unit and intermediate care facilities (ICF) outside the hospital, while providing a financial disincentive for use of rehabilitation units, rehabilitation hospitals, and long-term care hospitals (10). The purpose of this regulation was to impact referral patterns, shifting them away from PPS-excluded programs toward freestanding skilled facilities and their subacute and rehabilitation programs. Hospitals received a full DRG payment for patients transferred to a PPS-excluded program regardless of how long they were in the acute hospital prior to transfer. Hospitals were allowed to treat the transfer as a discharge. As of October 1, 1998, the Balanced Budget Act treats the movement of a patient from one PPS system acute hospital to another PPS system (e.g., SNF or Home Health) as a transfer rather than a discharge. Since rehabilitation is PPS exempt until 2002 (full PPS implementation of PPS for rehabilitation hospitals and units), the 10 most transferred patient DRGs will still be discharged and admitted to rehabilitation. Six of the ten recently announced transfer DRGs fall into the present 10 rehabilitation categories and include 14 CVAs, 113 amputations, 209, 210, 211, and 236 orthopedic (hip/femur fractures and procedures).

The transfer rule will have far-reaching impact on reimbursement by reducing the DRG payments to hospitals, especially those with high numbers of SNF beds or Home Health Programs. A blended DRG/per-diem rate will be paid when a patient with one of the 10 most frequently discharged DRGs is moved. This means hospitals have to treat movement of patients from acute PPS units to other PPS units or levels of care (SNF, ICF, Home Health Care) as transfers instead of discharges. The net effect of this change is to shift the economic incentives for transferring a patient.

Acute LOSs will, in all probability, increase and encourage more utilization of the acute rehabilitation unit (PPS exempt until 2001). This change argues against a fully integrated delivery system. The results of this change will restructure the market from a cost-plus market to a case-rate managed care market. Facilities will have to consider restructuring clinical protocols in conjunction with the acute unit and carefully analyzing the cost structure(s).

Medicare Reimbursement in Acute Rehabilitation Units/Hospitals

The Medicare payment for acute rehabilitation is the TEFRA rate (base year). The TEFRA rate is a flat rate paid for patients on the rehabilitation unit. The acute rehabilitation unit is cost based for the first year of operation. Total Medicare costs during the first year are calculated for the number of Medicare discharges, to determine the payment per patient that will be paid by Medicare for rehabilitation units in hospitals during the second year.

In freestanding rehabilitation hospitals, the third year is the base year. Costs are averaged during the third year of operations (base year) to determine the TEFRA limit. The TEFRA limit is established by the total allowable Medicare costs during the base year, divided by the number of Medicare discharges during the base year. The TEFRA limit is then applied during the fourth year of operations and every year thereafter. TEFRA limits are updated annually by the market basket update amount. The Balanced Budget Act is changing TEFRA to a rehabilitation PPS and it will begin to be implemented in a phase-in with cost reports beginning on and after October 1, 2000. In the first year, one-third of payments is to be controlled by the PPS, with two-thirds paid on cost (subject to the TEFRA limits modified by the Balanced Budget Act). In the second year, these percentages are reversed, with two-thirds of payments controlled by PPS and one-third paid on cost. Beginning in 2001, payment will be based 100% on PPS.

PPS does not appear to properly reflect the intensity and duration of rehabilitation services required by patients and will hurt providers and patients alike. In a December 5, 1997 transmittal from the American Rehabilitation Association, Carolyn Zollar noted that HCFA is mapping out its plan to utilize the minimum data set (MDS) with some alterations as the data assessment tool and the resource utilization groups (RUGS) as the patient classification system (11).

Ten diagnostic categories are included in acute rehabilitation. Seventy-five percent of the patients served in the acute rehabilitation unit/hospital must be in the following 10 diagnostic categories: amputations, arthritis, brain injury, burns, congenital deformity, CVA, multiple trauma, neurologic, orthopedic, and spinal cord. In other words, only 25% of the patients in a rehabilitation unit or hospital can have other than these 10 diagnoses. The Balanced Budget Act provides for additions to the 10 DRGs in years subsequent to fiscal year 2000.

The TEFRA limits for rehabilitation hospitals and units ranged dramatically from as low as $7000 to as high as $35,000 per patient. The range existed because the units and hospitals set up 15 years ago had lower costs. HCFA then determined that 1982 would be the base year for existing units in 1983. The existing facilities were not given notice, making it difficult to accelerate costs. HCFA recently became aware of these inequities and has offered the rehabilitation hospitals and units opened since 1990 the option of rebasing. The option was offered in September 1997 and had to be in by November 1, 1997 to be rebased.

There was no 3-hour rule in 1982. Patients had longer LOSs. Many patients are not being sent to acute rehabilitation today. They are bypassing acute rehabilitation, going directly from an acute care unit to a skilled unit, home health care, or an outpatient setting.

In the past, the acute hospital DRGs allowed longer LOSs before patients were transferred to rehabilitation. Today, the challenge is to manage the patient within the payment received for the DRG. Clinicians are getting patients with shorter LOSs who are still very sick and severely impaired when transferred to rehabilitation, requiring higher resource consumption on average. The increased rates of returns of rehabilitation patients to acute care are substantiated in national and regional data compiled by the Uniform Data Set (UDS) Functional Independence Measure (FIM) (12).

Because of the present inequities in TEFRA limits, today many older rehabilitation units and hospitals are operating above their TEFRA reimbursement and losing money. It is more cost-effective to keep acute rehabilitation beds empty than to lose $10,000 per patient. For example, if the TEFRA rate is $9000 and the caseload consists of high-level-care brain-injured patients with an average LOS of 22 days, spinal cord patients with an average LOS of 23 days, and patients recovering from severe strokes with an average LOS of 16 days and the coverage cost per day is $1000 for each patient, the costs are not covered. On the other hand, if the facility has patients who need only a short LOS such as those with mild stroke or simple orthopedic conditions (<9 days), the balance sheet will be positive.

All patients in acute rehabilitation hospitals or units, in order to receive Medicare reimbursement, must receive 3 hours of therapy a day. Therapy is documented in a cost center, and it can become too expensive, unless controlled. There is a belief among therapists, and some rehabilitation managers, that a patient in the hospital should receive individual therapy twice every day. Others maintain that patients should receive what they need to maximize their function. A study on stroke patients by Dr. Robert Keith (13), reported in 1995, showed that stroke patients receiving therapy improved if they received 2 hours of therapy as compared to 1; they progressed even more if they received 3 hours of therapy compared to 2, but therapy beyond 3 hours did not affect functional outcomes. It should be noted that the subjects studied were primarily elderly Medicare patients.

If one is paid a flat rate per discharge no matter what therapy is done or for how long (TEFRA), therapy managers must look carefully at therapy services exceeding 3 hours. Implementing a 3-hour protocol and having therapists or physicians justify any additional hours of service can improve efficiency without compromising patient outcomes. Orders for hourly treatments twice a day by an occupational therapist, a physical therapist, and a speech therapist for all patients on the rehabilitation unit are no longer reasonable (or possible). The use of extenders and groups must be considered for any order for twice-a-day therapy, as managers try to control costs with limited reimbursement availability. A rehabilitation unit is no longer a profit center. The question is no longer, Will we make money?; the question is, Can we afford this cost!? The TEFRA limit is forcing the direction for many health care facilities.

Another important issue is that patients presenting to rehabilitation are sicker and arriving sooner. The acute care LOS is being reduced and patients are being moved to acute rehabilitation sooner. If patients require high levels of medical and nursing intervention and are not physically able to tolerate 3 hours of therapy a day, placement in a skilled unit or facility may be worth considering. Patients in skilled units, where 3 hours of therapy is not required, can start off initially with 30 minutes or an hour of therapy, adding more therapy as their nursing and medical needs subside. Patients can then be transferred to acute rehabilitation when they are maximally able to benefit from the intensity of therapy required. In this way, patients' abilities to benefit from resources are maximized and reimbursement more nearly covers the costs. The key is not to lose patients to a skilled facility that cannot handle the nursing and therapy intensities.

If the TEFRA limit is exceeded, management may want to consider how many acute rehabilitation beds it can afford to keep open. One can decertify some of the acute care or rehabilitation beds and use them for managed care (private pay), providing less than 3 hours of therapy for patients in those beds. Having decertified beds, contiguous to acute rehabilitation, where less than 3 hours of therapy can occur, can enable one to take advantage of the rehabilitation team and their expertise.

Some acute care and severely impaired patients actually have trouble tolerating 3 hours of therapy. Several hospital systems have exchanged or closed acute rehabilitation beds in an attempt to reduce costs or to acquire lower-level-care beds (skilled and long-term care), where single rehabilitation service could be provided more cost-effectively.

Rehabilitation patient care is being shifted down to skilled beds. Many shorter-LOS stroke and orthopedic patients are being treated in skilled facilities, bypassing acute hospitals, or going to home health care directly from the acute units, making it even harder to keep rehabilitation beds filled. Rehabilitation unit administrators are bumping up against their TEFRA limits because lower-cost patients are going to SNFs.

Opening the rehabilitation units by granting admitting privileges to primary care physicians and internists to manage patients, solely or jointly, with a physiatrist is one strategy that is filling empty rehabilitation beds. The beds are being filled with less acute care patients who need a shorter LOS, thus improving the reimbursement picture for the rehabilitation unit cost center.

Another strategy is to implement a protocol for limiting therapy services on the skilled unit. Patients needing 3 hours of service are automatically transferred to rehabilitation (good strategy if the facility is not exceeding the TEFRA limit). The strategy can be reversed if the facility is exceeding the limit, to take advantage of being paid cost plus ancillary costs on skilled units, thus providing justifiable levels of therapy, even over 3 hours, if necessary and documented appropriately.

Physicians on acute rehabilitation units are being paid up to 7 days a week with proper documentation. There are many billable services per patient that need to be taken into account. Unless physicians are employed full-time by the hospital and the hospital is billing for the time they spend doing histories, physicals, rounds, conferences, and discharge summaries, the physicians are very likely to be billing for these services through their practices. It is no wonder physiatrists are unwilling to open their units to other physicians who want to directly manage short-term patients with mild strokes or orthopedic problems. Hospitals must be sure that the hours they are paying their medical directors are not the same hours being used to privately see and bill patients. Delineating administrative and clinic case hours is an important differentiation.

Medicare Reimbursement for Subacute Programs

A program called *subacute care* is emerging rapidly in rehabilitation. The Joint Commission on Accreditation of Healthcare Organizations (JCAHO) defines *subacute* as less than acute and more than skilled care. Subacute programs are being created primarily to replace skilled care beds in both acute hospitals and freestanding SNFs. A few subacute programs have been established in facilities with acute care and long-term care beds. Subacute programs can be provided within a skilled nursing unit or facility or within a certified distinct part of an existing acute rehabilitation hospital, thus allowing for higher reimbursement. Currently, there is no separate Medicare certification for subacute care. HCFA believes that the skilled level of care is adequate to meet the needs of subacute patients (less nursing and lower medical and therapy intensity). Subacute care can be provided within different licensure and certification settings, including acute care hospitals, SNFs, and long-term care hospitals. Funding sources of subacute care also vary and include insurance coverage: indemnity, managed care (PPO/HMO), property casualty, and Medicare.

Medicaid appears to be reimbursing subacute care on a state-by-state basis. California, Illinois, Maryland, New Jersey, New Hampshire, Vermont, Virginia, and Wisconsin have created special reimbursement rates or are allowing negotiated rates for subacute care. If Medicaid agencies in other states see subacute care as cost-effective, they will likely cover subacute care as well. Physician payment is increasing with the addition of patients requiring higher levels of medical and nursing services. Rehabilitation services are also increasing from the one visit per month to three to five visits per week, with supporting documentation of need. Some physicians are even being reimbursed for coverage of 7 days per week.

Medicare Reimbursement in Skilled Nursing Facility

In order for charges for patient care to be reimbursed under Medicare Part A in an SNF, firstly, the patient must need at least a 3-day hospital (inpatient) stay. Secondly, the patient must need a skilled level of medical and nursing intensity or 5 days of therapy, or both. The patient must be admitted to the SNF within 30 days after discharge from the acute care hospital. The patient's physician must certify the need for "skilled" care on a daily basis, and the admission must be medically justified. Ancillary services are reimbursed at cost. Ancillary services usually include pharmacy items, laboratory services, x-ray studies, physical therapy, occupational therapy, speech therapy, respiratory therapy, and orthotics and prosthetics. Respiratory therapy must be hospital based (billed from a hospital) for a skilled facility to receive the reimbursement.

The services provided to patients admitted to the skilled facility must be related to the patient's condition in the acute care hospital. Patients qualifying for Part A benefits in the SNF receive care for a maximum of 100 days per spell of illness. Twenty days are covered at full cost and 80 days require supplementation with coinsurance. Coinsurance in 1997 paid $89.50/day. If patients are discharged from the skilled facility and remain in the community for at least 60 days, they can start all over on their 100 days of reimbursement as long as they again need at least a 3-day acute care stay. Medicare Part B covers ancillary services and supplies but does not cover routine costs. All services must be medically justified and Medicare Part B requires both a deductible and coinsurance payments from the beneficiary. The deductible is usually $100.

Reimbursement for skilled facilities is cost based for the first 3 years: Direct cost + Indirect cost = Total cost. After year 3, SNF reimbursement is based on routine cost limitations plus ancillary service costs. Routine cost limitations include room, dietary needs, medical social services, psychiatric social services, all general nursing services, items furnished routinely and uniformly to all patients, items stocked at nursing stations or on the floor in gross supply, reusable items utilized by individual patients (i.e., ice bags, bed rails, etc), and special dietary supplements. Routine cost limitations are established differently, depending on whether the services are provided in a freestanding or a hospital-based SNF, and also on whether the institution is located in an urban or a rural area. Cost limitations are also adjusted by area wage index, market basket index (running 2%–3%), and administrative and general add-on costs for hospital-based SNFs. The lesser costs to charges (LCTC) rule applies to SNFs and units serving both Medicare and managed care patients. Care must be taken in pricing the services.

Discounted charges are reimbursed at the discounted rate. For example, if the facility's charge is $500/day and it discounts to $350/day to get the business, it will be reimbursed $350 even though the cost is $400/day. In some managed care markets, different groups are getting different rates. This is based on LOS and sometimes on resource intensities (level of care required). For example, services provided to a patient with a simple orthopedic problem might be reimbursed at a lower rate than those provided to a patient with spinal cord injury.

HCFA has set hourly caps for contract physical therapy services and will be establishing caps for occupational and speech therapy services as well. Rates are still being negotiated but are estimated to be between $42 and $50/hour, with a higher cap for physical therapy services. High therapy charges have prompted HCFA to set maximum amounts it will pay based on therapy salary equivalencies (14).

HCFA recently reviewed the ancillary services provided within a skilled environment and concluded that many services that were once considered part of routine care are now being billed as ancillary services, requiring additional payment. Most of these services are routine nursing and therapy services that HCFA states are "skilled" and not ancillary.

With regard to costs, HCFA states that everything not specified as being nonallowable is allowable, and these costs must be reasonable and related to patient care. Medicare pays for the portion of allowable costs related to Medicare patients. Examples of nonallowable costs include private duty personnel, luxury items (television and telephone services), fund raising, advertising, marketing, barber and beauty shop services, gift shop, meals served to guests and employees, and any unused or closed space.

HCFA is encouraging the use of skilled care and subacute programs rather than acute rehabilitation and other PPS-excluded programs by changing the regulations of SNFs, seeking adjustment to their limits, and making the process more expedient. With regard to physician participation and reimbursement, HCFA has relaxed its limitations of previously paying for one physician visit per patient per week. Physicians can now bill for attending the patient three to five times per week if supporting documentation is presented. This is encouraging physician participation and support of the lower-cost, alternative-care setting of a skilled unit or freestanding SNF.

Capital costs were not subject to the routine cost limit. With the Balanced Budget Act of 1997, HCFA has changed this and overall SNF reimbursement in two ways: first, by the transfer regulations described previously, and second, by the changes in the PPS. Transfers to SNFs from PPS hospitals are included in the same regulations as transfers to rehabilitation units and facilities. If a hospital has a subacute unit or a skilled unit/facility, then the hospital will have a decrease in DRG revenue. This will require systems to assess fully the costs and benefits of actually treating a patient in a subacute unit or skilled unit/facility. As mentioned already, SNFs were paid on a cost basis with nationally established limits on the routine portion of the payment. Ancillary services were paid on the basis of reasonable costs without limit. As of July 1998, the Balanced Budget Act phases in a PPS system over a 3-year period. A portion of the payment is based on the facility's specified costs encompassing both Part A SNF benefits as well as services billed under Part B. SNFs will then be reimbursed on the lesser of actual charges or "adjusted reasonable costs," which are defined as reasonable costs minus 10%. As of July 1998, the Balanced Budget Act also requires consolidated billing by SNFs. Service providers to SNF residents under Medicare Part B must be billed by the SNF and all nonphysician payments made to the SNF.

HCFA has also implemented the use of RUGs III to determine payment under PPS for SNF units/facilities. RUGS III is a 44-group classification system based on the amount of resources needed to care for patients. The top 14 are the rehabilitation RUGs. Categories are based on patient function score on the MDS and additional problems or services (rehabilitation therapy or nursing).

The end result will be that skilled nursing units/facilities will have decreased admissions and a shift from a cost-based system to a PPS. For the first 3 years, rates will be based on a blend of facility-specific and national average costs. Then rates will be based on federal per-diem figures. The Medicare reimbursement future looks lean!

Medicare Reimbursement in Long-Term Care Hospitals

A long-term care hospital, in order to be reimbursed by Medicare under TEFRA, must be licensed by the state and have an average patient LOS of 25 days. Long-term care is PPS exempt and is cost based for the first 3 years of operation. The third year, like that in the freestanding rehabilitation hospital, is the base year and establishes the TEFRA limit. Therefore, the TEFRA limit applies to the fourth year and every year thereafter with a small annual market basket adjustment. The LCTC rule does not apply after the base year. Rehabilitation services are being reimbursed at long-term care hospitals primarily with patients with debilitating illnesses and respirator-dependent patients. Long-term care hospitals will also be moved into a PPS.

Home Care

Home Health

One of the fastest-growing areas of health service delivery, home care, is the service of choice for most physicians and patients. Up to 40% of patients discharged from the hospitals receive home care (15). This is primarily due to early hospital discharge initiatives where patients can leave the hospital a day early. Managed care is forcing providers to look at home health care as a viable alternative in the continuum of care. It is predicted that the use of home care may eclipse the use of hospitals for the front end of care for many nonsurgical patients. Home care is judged to be more cost-effective than hospital care and the use and costs to HCFA are rising. A 166% increase in the use of home health care by the end of 1996 was predicted, with costs amounting to around $20 billion by the end of 1996 (16).

Reimbursement is covered through Medicare Parts A and B only if a physician certifies and recertifies (every 2 months) that the patient needs intermittent skilled nursing care, physical therapy, occupational therapy, or speech therapy and that home health services are required because the patient is confined to the home except when receiving outpatient services (17). Providers are reimbursed the actual costs incurred in patient care. No copayment is required for home health care, which accounts for its overutilization. Actual costs include both the direct and indirect costs of making the home visit, and the costs of coordinating the activities related to care delivery. Most home health care qualifies under Medicare and is based on a per-visit cost. A visit is a personal contact made in the place of residence of a patient for the purpose of providing a covered service by a home health agency worker, or a visit by a homebound patient on an outpatient basis to a hospital, SNF, rehabilitation center, or outpatient center affiliated with a medical school when it requires the use of equipment that cannot be made readily available in the home. There have been allegations of fraud in home health care and it is predicted that tighter scrutiny and regulation will be forthcoming. The cost of fraud has been predicted to be as high as 10% of total expenditures, forcing the entire system of reimbursement for home health care to be under review. President Clinton in the spring of 1997 actually put a moratorium on the granting of new home care licenses, stopping any new licenses from being processed, as the government attempts to get a handle on the fraud and abuse concerns that are being reported in home care service delivery. The Balanced Budget Act also affects home health care. Beginning October 1, 1999, the PPS for home health agencies is effective. The transfer agreement also applies to home health care. Discharges occurring on or after October 1, 1998, that fall within 10 DRGs, will be treated as transfers for payment purposes. The applicable DRGs are soon to be released by HCFA but should include orthopedics and stroke. Claims for services furnished on or after October 1, 1998, will have to contain an appropriate identifier for the physician prescribing home health services or certifying the need for care. Claims must also include information on the length of a service unit, in 15-minute increments. By tracking visits in units, HCFA hopes to reduce the poor therapy and nursing practices of stopping in for a 5-minute visit, since billing is per visit. Actual length of visits can be monitored by the unit-based recording requirement. The categories of services for which time information must be included on a claim are skilled nursing care; therapies (physical and occupational) and speech language pathology; medical and social services; and home health aide services. HCFA has stated that nurses and physical therapists can do respiratory visits.

Hospice

Since Congress passed the hospice Medicare benefit on a trial basis in 1982, and made that benefit permanent in 1986, the number of hospice programs has grown from 50 in 1977 to 2000 in 1994, of which 800 were hospital based. The average length of stay in 1994 was 62 days and the average cost per day was $101, or $6281 per admission. These numbers represent an increase of 17% from 1992 to 1994. When patients accept a Medicare hospice benefit, they must relinquish other Medicare benefits, except for the services of their attending physician and services unrelated to the terminal illness. The hospice in effect becomes the intermediary for all the care the patient requires for the terminal illness.

The benefit includes coverage for nursing care; medical and social services; home health aide and homemaker services; physical, occupational, and speech therapy services; volunteer and bereavement services; medical supplies and durable medical equipment; and medications for symptom control. Short-term inpatient care and short-term respite and continuous nursing care are reimbursed. The type and scope of services provided are determined by the hospice plan of care as developed by the hospice interdisciplinary team. The hospice interdisciplinary team is central to the delivery of hospice services. Most teams include a medical director, nurse, social worker, chaplain, personal care aides, and trained volunteers. The patient's eligibility for these services must be evaluated at the end of specific benefit periods (two 90-day intervals and one 30-day interval). When the patient lives longer than 210 days and is still determined to be eligible, the hospice continues to provide care. The reimbursement system, which reflects regional wage differences, is based on a per-diem payment for one of four levels of care:

1. Routine home care. The patient resides at home and receives care there. Hospice care provided as a part of routine home care services accounts for at least 80% of all hospice days.
2. Continuous home care. The patient resides at home and receives continuous care, primarily nursing, during periods of medical crisis.
3. General inpatient care. The patient is placed in an inpatient setting for acute pain or symptom management. The hospice must have a formal contract with the inpatient facility.
4. Inpatient respite care. The patient is placed in an inpatient setting to relieve the primary caregiver for up to five days (18).

The benefits available to Medicare-eligible hospice patients served by a Medicare-certified hospice are extensive. In addition, 36 states have developed hospice Medicaid benefits, which mirror the Medicare program in services and reimbursement. Clinicians should check with their state, as some states are beginning to reduce coverage for Medicaid, which may affect the hospice services that remain covered.

Outpatient Agencies

Medicare provides several outpatient rehabilitation facility certifications. The most common are the rehabilitation agency and CORF (comprehensive outpatient rehabilitation facility). A rehabilitation agency is primarily a single-service system, while a CORF is a license to serve comprehensive multiservice Medicare patients. Reimbursement was cost-related fee-for-service. Reimbursement is based on qualified staff performing the services. The agency can receive a Medicare license for either a CORF or rehabilitation agency. Personnel who do private therapy can be registered or licensed separately by Medicare to perform services.

Rehabilitation Agency

The rehabilitation agency is often referred to as the *physical therapy and speech agency.* It is primarily a single-service, non-complex service delivery and does not require a medical director. Other Medicare services include physician, psychology, social, and vocational services. Even though not specifically mentioned in the initial description of the rehabilitation agency certification, occupational therapy is covered in the regulations.

Comprehensive Outpatient Rehabilitation Facility

A CORF is established and operated exclusively for the purpose of providing diagnostic, therapeutic, and restorative services on an outpatient basis for the rehabilitation of injured, disabled, or sick persons at a single fixed location, by or under the supervision of a physician. The focus of the CORF is on providing medically supervised, multiservices to complex Medicare patients. A CORF requires a separate Medicare provider number and license. An on-site medical director is also required and may in fact assist in developing an integrated outpatient presence, generating new business and more multiservice referrals. Physical therapy and psychological services must also be available. Covered services in a CORF include physician services, physical therapy, occupational therapy, speech language pathology, respiratory therapy services, prosthetic and orthotic services and devices, social services, psychological services, nursing care, drugs and non-self-administered biological products, supplies and durable medical equipment, and other medically necessary items.

Services provided by a CORF were reimbursed under Medicare, on a reasonable cost basis. Outpatients paid 20% of the charges beyond the deductible. In other words, Medicare paid 80% and the patient or supplemental insurance paid 20%. As of January 1, 1998, payments are based on the lesser of the actual charges or "adjusted reasonable costs," which, as in the new SNF reimbursement, is defined as reasonable costs less 10%.

CORFs have been one of the fastest-growing new rehabilitation programs over the past few years. The Balanced Budget Act has put a screeching halt to this for hospitals and others as well. The Act established a PPS for hospital outpatient departments beginning January 1, 1999, using the UDS/RUGS classification system presently being determined by HCFA. The PPS will be based on 1996 cost data and will be budget neutral. Again, as if favoring larger integrated systems, HCFA is applying tougher conditions of participation for freestanding rehabilitation agencies, CORFs, and other providers to include a 10% reduction in operating and capital costs for 1998.

After 1998, payment will be based on 80% of the lesser of actual charges, or 80% of the applicable physician-fee-schedule amount; application of fee-schedule provisions for hospital outpatient would not apply. Effective January 1, 1999, per-beneficiary caps of $1500 for physical and speech therapy combined and $1500 for occupational therapy would apply.

There is a limit of 62.5% of customary charges on reimbursement for psychological services, except for diagnostic charges, which are set at 90% of the prevailing charges locally. For clinical social workers, the payment may not exceed 80% of the lesser of actual charges or 75% of the amount paid to a psychologist for the same service. Psychological and social services, not covered in a hospital's general Medicare license, are reimbursable in a CORF. Other advantages of a CORF include off-site service delivery capabilities for therapy services. Therapy services provided off-site can be billed as on site, through the CORF Medicare provider number. It is helpful to obtain approval and support from the intermediary to provide reimbursable alternative care delivery through the CORF license; for example, providing limited therapy visits to an assisted-living, skilled, or long-term care facility to improve function, or brief patient home visits, for continuity, before the orthopedic patient is ready for more specialized outpatient services. A *Tech Brief* published by the American Rehabilitation Association, after some clarification with HCFA, mentioned that CORFs could also provide off-site physical therapy, occupational therapy, and speech services, in an already established medical office buildings away from the approved CORF, and at a non-CORF "satellite" facility (19). The continuity of care offered by the same therapists with patients at various sites enhances community re-entry and outcomes and may get patients into an outpatient program sooner. A review of CORF regulations indicates that they appear to be consistent. However, the interpretation of the CORF regulations tends to vary by state, based on the interpretation of the regulations by the Medicare intermediary.

Alternative Care

Shifting from hospital-based care to care provided in the community, and emphasizing prevention of hospitalization or rehospitalization through prevention and wellness programs leads to better, lower-cost alternative care. Three of the most popular alternative care programs today are assisted living, day hospital, and day care. Home health services can enter an assisted-living center to provide care and be reimbursed, because the assisted-living center is the home for elderly persons needing some level of assistance. Day hospitals are more associated with a CORF where patients can come to spend the day and receive therapy services, support, and nursing care. When medically stable, patients may not need to be in rehabilitation. By shifting the therapy and training to a day treatment program, systems can further reduce costly inpatient LOSs. Day treatment programs can also prevent hospitalizations by increasing function and medical stability through daily treatment. Reimbursement systems will follow alternative care trends as private payers and Medicare continue to look for lower-cost solutions that keep people living as independently and self-managed as possible, within their communities.

MEDICAID REIMBURSEMENT

Medicaid reimbursement is determined on a state-by-state basis. Although current legislation is attempting to define funding, in most states, it remains inadequate.

As Medicaid funds are being distributed to the states, states are attempting to implement strategies that reduce their costs and risks. These strategies have a direct effect on the level of available reimbursement and therefore, services.

The most recent trend is a shift by states to place Medicaid under managed care. Under a plan about to be approved by HCFA, 1.1 million low-income Medicaid beneficiaries in Illinois will be shifted to managed care. The Illinois Department of Public Aid plans to move quickly to implement its "MediPlan Plus." The Pennsylvania state welfare department has also announced its plans to move 438,000 Medicaid beneficiaries to managed care (20).

California's innovative two-plan Medicaid managed care model received approval from HCFA in January 1996. State Medicaid beneficiaries will be able to choose between a plan offered by a commercial HMO and a "local initiative plan," which will include county hospitals and health care facilities, as well as other local providers. All Aid to Families with Dependent Children (AFDC) and AFDC-related Medicaid beneficiaries (about 3.3 million) will be able to enroll in the program (21).

The reimbursements are predicted to be far below those that are presently being paid. Indiana has set a daily Medicaid rate in SNFs at $90 and for intermediate care at $60.00. This flat rate of reimbursement is to include all therapies, durable medical equipment, and services. While some providers continue to raise questions about quality and availability of support services, initial cost appears to be the predominant factor in determining whether support and therapy services will continue to be provided to Medicaid recipients.

PAYMENT METHODS

The key to being successful in using any payment method is for each provider to know his or her costs and to negotiate from that knowledge. Numerous payment methods are being used today. I discuss the most frequently used as markets begin switching from a noncapitated to a capitated payment approach. With capitated payment, therapists and physicians will be moving to higher-risk methods of payment where survival depends on accurate information on costs, time frames, and volume. Payers utilize a variety of payment methods when compensating care providers directly or as part of an integrated delivery system or care continuum. Each method results in the transfer and assumption of varied amounts of risk to the provider. The following are payment methods by which health care facilities and providers are compensated, beginning with the lowest to the highest risk.

Managed Care

As managed care moves in and begins to change reimbursement, from a low-risk fee-for-service payment, to alternative higher-risk provider reimbursement methods, the whole area of reimbursement is shifting (managed care is any reimbursement method excluding nondiscounted fee-for-service). All the noncapitated reimbursements discussed below are commonly found in a managed care environment. Managed care administrators seek service providers who can provide the service for the least number of days at the lowest cost per day, and still achieve suitable outcomes. Some people jokingly refer to managed care as "managed payment." Reimbursement for managed care varies depending on the region of the country, the types of services, and levels of services included in the base contract rate. Reimbursement for pharmaceuticals and durable medical equipment is often negotiated separately and usually as an addition to the base rate.

Health Maintenance Organizations

An HMO is the most popular system being used to manage care. As insurance companies move to managed care environments, they are embracing affiliations with and ownership of HMOs. Several large corporations, like John Deere and Delta Airlines, have developed their own HMOs and are contracting directly with hospitals, physicians, and health care providers.

HMOs emphasize prevention and wellness and are initiating programs to teach patients to self-manage their illnesses in order to reduce the rate of rehospitalization and maintain the highest quality of life possible within the community.

Many employers led the charge to develop and use HMOs in the early 1990s, in an attempt to cut their spiraling health care costs. These same larger employers are decreasing the pressure on insurers to improve pricing; they are now aiming toward improved health care quality. They are also interested in measuring "outcomes" of various treatments, monitoring continuous quality improvement in hospitals, and even writing "practice guidelines to standardize doctors' practices" (22). Hospitals, too, are committed to quality and are attempting to reduce variation through use of "critical pathways" and "care maps," to keep procedures standardized. These processes will make it easier to predict costs, ensure quality, and document outcomes.

The major direction today from employers who use HMOs is to place their Medicare-eligible retirees into a managed care plan. According to a study by Foster Higgins & Co., for 35% of the large employers who supplement Medicare coverage for retirees, the Medicare-risk HMO is the route chosen to answer concerns about increased medical costs. The percentage of employers offering Medicare-risk HMOs tripled over the last 3 years (23).

The change is coming from employees asking their employers to choose HMOs to manage their Medicare. The employers are developing the means to determine the quality of the HMO and are regularly measuring it themselves or insisting on information regarding their employees' progress and outcomes. Employers are searching for accredited HMOs and for information on how these HMOs perform long term and on employee satisfaction. Several larger employers even visit the HMOs and keep data on the HMOs they utilize. The satisfaction of retired Medicare employees who use HMOs is higher than that of current employees (22). The formulas for setting Medicare HMO rates are complicated, with reimbursement varying up to 100% from one region of the country to another. According to the Governance Committee, Medicare-risk contracts are potentially the single most lucrative segment of the capitated business.

The Medicare market of 33 million persons is an enormous market for HMOs. HCFA is providing incentives to encourage Medicare beneficiaries to enroll in Medicare HMOs. As HCFA and employers move toward Medicare managed care, the number of participants in Medicare-risk HMOs will cause it to become the reimbursement system of choice. When the marketplace reaches 50% enrollment, Medicare will become managed care, an event that will occur soon.

Noncapitated Payment Method

Private insurance is considered primarily a fee-for-service reimbursement system. Reimbursement by commercial insurers is governed by the terms of the insurance contract. Terms of contracts may include rehabilitation services, which may be handled as an addition, a supplement, or exclusion. Coverage varies greatly among insurers. One trend is certain: The amount of money available for rehabilitation services through private insurers is shrinking.

Fee-for-Service

Payment is usually limited to the lesser of the provider's billed charges or the usual, customary, and reasonable amount as determined by the payer. This arrangement is the safest reimbursement method, as it involves the least amount of risk being shifted to the provider of services.

Characteristics of fee-for-service reimbursement include the following:

- Pricing is based on usual and customary charges.
- There are no discounts or specialized rates.
- Risk remains with the payer.

Discounted-Fee-for-Service

With this type of arrangement, the provider typically agrees to provide services at a discounted percentage of standard charges, or the reasonable and customary charges, whichever is less. Discounts are developed in various ways: a single percentage of the standard charge, various discount percentages for different services, or a reduced-fee schedule for services based on a multiplier or the market. There are risks in discounting: The care provider's profit margin may be reduced or the discounted rate will not cover the full costs of the service. A smart provider will negotiate a fair discounted rate based on accurate cost estimates, with scheduled increases to reflect rising costs.

Per Diem

Per diem means "per day." Under a per-diem arrangement, the provider receives a specified fixed amount per day for services provided to a patient. It does not matter what service is performed, how many times it is performed, or for how long, it is still a flat daily rate. This is referred to as an *all-inclusive per-diem* payment plan. All-inclusive per-diem plans work best with patients whose care is routine and basic, requiring few resources. They may not work well with patients needing high levels of resources and high-intensity medical and nursing care such as those hospitalized for trauma, severe brain injury, spinal cord injury, or acquired immunodeficiency syndrome (AIDS).

It is important to specifically state which services are included in the per-diem rate and which services will be reimbursed as additional (ancillary) charges. Commonly excluded ancillary charges in per-diem contracts include, but are not limited to drugs and pharmacy items, durable medical equipment, magnetic resonance imaging and computed tomography, dialysis, blood products, pulmonary services and oxygen, diagnostic procedures, and all services performed off the premises. This is usually referred to as *per-diem-plus-ancillary charges.*

Other providers may consider a *"stop-loss" threshold* in negotiating per-diem rates. A specific dollar amount, set in advance, is determined and if charges exceed that amount, reimbursement by the payer will shift to another method, such as fee-for-service or discounted-fee-for-service. Payers use stop-loss thresholds to prevent excessive LOSs, or to limit exposure to catastrophic, resource-intensive, high-intensity medical and nursing care patients. A *capitated per-diem* payment method is the payment of a daily rate for a specific number of days. This type of per-diem method is common in managed care where the payer authorizes the payment of $700 day up to 4 days. There are several *ways to structure per-diem payments* besides a flat daily rate:

- By diagnosis (paying $450 day for all patients with a diagnosis of CVA)
- By case mix (percentage of patients being treated for stroke, orthopedic problems, trauma, etc)
- By location (inpatient, skilled unit, acute rehabilitation)
- By level of care (level of nursing/medical intensity; ancillary care high, medium, or low)
- By risk of assignment (higher risk = higher rate)

It is important to remember that being paid on a per-diem basis precludes the payer from conducting a line-by-line audit. Services are billed as a single bundled charge. If items are analyzed one-by-one, the provider stands a greater chance of having some of them denied.

Per Case

A payment is negotiated based on the patient's level of functioning when services are initiated (as compared to a projected level of functioning to be attained at discharge). The LOS, resource allocation, level of care, place of service, and progress benchmarks are negotiated on a case-by-case basis. In some instances, in order to share risk, patients are reviewed within set time frames (weekly utilization review), with adjustments to the program and payment being made, throughout the course of treatment. The provider should be aware of several key issues when accepting a per-case reimbursement system:

- Pricing can be tailored to each patient's needs.
- Negotiations must take place, separately, for each patient.
- This system is used mostly for catastrophic injuries such as those of the brain or spinal cord.
- Risk is shared by payer and provider.
- Alternative, nonhospital care reduces cost.

Bundled Fee/Prospective Payment System

Integrated delivery systems providing continua of care can be paid under a bundled fee arrangement. A consortium of providers agrees to provide services at a pre-established rate per episode of treatment. One fee is negotiated for the several services involved. For example, evaluation and treatment charges from the primary care physician, hospital physiatrist, and physical therapist are bundled and covered by one fee. One of the providers receives the bundled fee and is then responsible for sharing it among the participants. If the integrated delivery system is separately incorporated, it would receive the bundled fee and distribute it to the various providers. PPS is the structure; exactly what the providers are paid for is the DRG. With the PPS the provider is paid per patient, if the provider sees the patient. Given the newly implemented Balanced Budget Act, Medicare is moving to the PPS. Many smart health care systems are beginning to extend their hospital-based clinical pathways across the continuum of care to ensure that alternative service deliveries are a large part of disease management, and are integrating both their clinical and financial data.

Capitated Payment System

Capitation is a method of receiving payment based on the number of individuals (enrollees) in a health plan who choose to receive services from the provider, whether or not each enrollee actually receives the service from the provider.

Capitation: Total $ = Number of enrollees in health plan × Charge (adjusted for copayment amount, if any)

Total payment is based on the number of enrollees rather than the utilization of services. More of the risk is thus shifted to the provider. The biggest risk to a provider receiving capitated payments is that the capitation revenues may not be adequate to cover expenses. There is no linkage between what the provider is paid per enrollee and the amount of enrollee utilization. Common reasons for problems in a capitated system include the following:

- The volume of capitated individuals is too low.
- The amount paid per enrollee is too low.
- Expenses exceed revenues (frequency of usage or cost of units is too high).
- Contract or state law does not allow direct billing of patients for additional expenses not covered.

The cost of an office visit of an enrollee per month is often referred to as the per-member per-month amount. Providers can take some steps to *minimize risk* when receiving capitated payment:

1. Know the characteristics of their patient population.
2. Specify each service through either a narrative description or a code.
3. List "carve-outs." (Services not included should be listed and detailed.)
4. Network and utilize other resources when possible.
5. Subcontract and outsource for additional services.
6. Use stop-loss and outlier protection clauses.
7. Purchase capitation insurance coverage.
8. Specifically state in the contract when payment is made.
9. In the contract, allow for inclusion and deletion of enrollees as it relates to capitation payments (e.g., if paid monthly, the provider will get paid for those enrolled or dropped in the middle of the month).
10. Allow for adjustments of the capitation rate in the capitation contract.

The ability to automatically adjust the capitation rate in a contract is important under certain circumstances. When the contract expires or is being renegotiated, based on cost data, the provider is in a good position to ask for a higher rate. At times the population the provider serves can shift, unexpectedly, and the actuarial assumptions under which the capitation rate was set are no longer valid. If cost data reflect effective expense management and profit margins, additional enrollees should be considered. At the time contracts are being negotiated, additional services or new technology should also be considered. Capitation can be expressed as a flat amount, as a percentage of premium with a guaranteed amount that is specified, or by another method. Moreover, it can be adjusted for age and sex of each enrollee, as well as the type of plan. Generally, capitation covers the provider's service as well as referral services. The provider has incentive to utilize the most cost-effective means of providing services to reduce overall expenses, which usually includes preventive care. It is less costly to keep patients out of the hospital through alternative and preventive care. Long-term data to demonstrate the actual cost savings are not yet available, but out-of-hospital costs are known to be significantly less.

Capitation is not an "all-or-nothing" arrangement. It is defined by the conditions of the contract between the payer and the provider. Sometimes it is used with other payment mechanisms. Some services can be contracted on a capitation basis while others are provided through a discounted-fee arrangement. Capitation can also be used up to a certain level of service and then switched to a per-diem or other method of payment. It is therefore important that providers initially negotiate the specific issues that regulate capitation, and that the agreed-upon arrangement be carefully documented and understood by both parties.

Something interesting occurs when the health care system shifts to capitation. The department and programs once known and loved as the *profit centers* become *cost centers.* The prestige of being a "high-revenue generator" is no longer apparent. Providers now justify and contain costs as they attempt to maximize billing. They are asking questions like, What are the most effective ways to allocate costs across the continuum of care in order to reduce inpatient LOS, maximize patient function, and limit resource consumption while maintaining patient and payer satisfaction? There is less "fighting" over patients among those representing the various levels of care because the number of patients treated is no longer the issue. The question now becomes, Can providers afford this cost?

The issue becomes the ability to access all levels of the continuum in order to utilize most appropriately the services available, in a timely manner, moving patients up and down the system as needed. The care units in the continuum of care must be flexible and responsive to ensure the best patient outcomes at the lowest costs. A case management approach—where someone is responsible for overseeing the patient's care throughout the entire illness, not episodic pieces and parts—often works best. A good case management system triages patients at the point of entry, often using strategic medical call centers as linkages to their care continua to appropriately serve patients in the least restrictive, lowest-cost settings where they can achieve and maintain the highest function possible. This is also being accomplished through the use of integrated care maps (a map of what happens to patients as they are treated, including when, where, and how), critical pathways (similar to care maps whereby the order and functions are sequenced and one step must occur before the next step), and service line case managers (service lines are major diagnostic groups that are managed across the continuum, e.g., CVA, orthopedics, cardiac, brain Injury, etc). Some service lines are narrow, while others include the whole spectrum of care including prevention and wellness at the beginning and end of the service line. Managers are asked, Are the costs being allocated to prevention and wellness worth it? Are the exercise, diet, physician follow-up, and other alternative care programs emptying beds? Is the program keeping patients in the community where they can be served more effectively? Are patients familiar with their disease states and are we aggressively educating them to self-manage out of the hospital setting? The thinking makes sense but the longitudinal data are not in yet. The jury is still out.

Global Capitation

An integrated delivery system can arrange for payments under a global capitation system. Under global capitation, a payer pays the integrated delivery system a set rate per month for each patient who elects to receive services from the providers affiliated with the system. Since the integrated delivery system is responsible for paying all the providers in the system, it assumes the financial risk of such services, incurring losses if the total payment to the provider exceeds the aggregated global capitation payments. This is a high-risk assumption for any integrated delivery system, which is why providers (cost centers) throughout the system must be effective at reducing costs and resource utilization. This effectiveness must be monitored vigilantly by the integrated delivery system.

Subcapitation

"Rehabilitation subcapitation agreements can be expected in the next 12 to 24 months" (24). Subcapitation can occur when providers negotiate capitated arrangements with subcontractors or vendors. Hospitals and physicians serve as subcontractors to provide services on a capitated basis to an integrated system of primary care physicians who actually hold and manage the capitation contract. If another provider holds the contract, then freestanding rehabilitation providers are quite vulnerable in the relationships. Russell Colie, president of the Health Forecasting Group, in his presentations on capitation strategies, speaks of ways "to sweeten the subcapitation deal" for rehabilitation hospitals as utilization drops. One way is to add a provision in the contract to share in the savings from reduced utilization through a risk pool or facilities budget. The HMO or physician's group that has the capitation contract may be charged on a per-diem basis as hospital services are rendered, with any surplus being shared 50/50 with the hospital, HMO, or physical organization (25).

Carve-Out Capitation

Rehabilitation is often considered a "carve-out" service and it is being pulled out of most hospital service agreements. Separate rehabilitation contracts can provide specialized hospital services in a defined clinical niche as "centers of excellence." This capitation strategy pays the hospital on a per-member per-month basis to provide a clearly defined range of specialty services. These specialty services are carved out of the comprehensive hospital services agreement. This has been a popular strategy for providers of home health, occupational health, and pharmacy services. HMOs and insurance companies have begun focusing this strategy on cardiology, oncology, ophthalmology, and orthopedics, which make up roughly 33% of a typical hospital's inpatient days.

Chronic Care Capitation

Chronic care capitation is a very costly area because chronic care niches are deeper and wider than the market for specialized procedures such as transplantations, coronary bypass grafting, and arterial grafting. The concept is rather simple. A hospital and its specialist contract with a capitated group or HMO to care for patients with specific chronic diseases, for example, spinal cord injury, brain injury, or AIDS. In most cases, chronic care capitation is paid on a case-by-case basis. The monthly payments are fixed but the amount may vary depending on the severity of the illness. The success under capitation depends on reducing hospital LOSs and substituting other lower-cost settings or ambulatory treatment. By rewarding lower-use patterns, providers hope to treat patients at cost-effective levels.

Risk Pooling and Withholds with Capitation

At times a portion of capitated payment may be set aside or "withheld" for patients needing certain types of care from specialists, for inpatient hospitalization, or for hospital or health care costs that were not anticipated. If the costs for special care exceed the budgeted amounts, the provider of service may be forced to give up the withheld money, or a portion of it. Risk is usually limited to the amount in the pool. Incentives involving the withhold pool are sometimes developed for providers: Any surplus that remains unused in a pool over a given time period can be returned to the providers who have not spent it. This is a way of rewarding control of utilization. Incentives are sometimes perceived as limiting patient access. Primary referrers have to be careful not to exclude needed consultations from specialists in order to obtain a share of the withheld money, at the cost of patient access to needed care.

Medicare Risk Taking

Medicare, too, is moving from fee-for-service to more risk-taking contracting and assuming the reimbursement characteristics of managed care. The Balanced Budget Act clearly directs payment to PPS. It is clear that providers who accept capitated payment face a greater risk of not covering their costs, although there is also an opportunity to profit under this arrangement. If the costs are known and expenditures are controlled, money can be made. By adding patient outcomes and satisfaction measures into an integrated health and reimbursement system, providers can even flourish.

THE REIMBURSEMENT DIFFERENTIATORS: COST, SATISFACTION, AND OUTCOMES

As the insurance industry, Medicare, and Medicaid shift from a noncapitated to a capitated environment of reimbursement, and embrace managed care, they are moving quickly to discounted-fee-for-service, PPPs, capitation, and other payment strategies. The big differentiator in this movement is costs. Decisions regarding choice of care providers are being made solely on costs.

Today the trend is finally shifting toward a demand for quality service. As data are analyzed, there is concern regarding the effects of years of cost cutting on quality. This transformation is being driven by large employers such as Xerox, GTE, Marriott, Pepsico, and USAir, the same companies who led the charge for lower-cost employee health care in the early 1990s. By the end of 1995, 71% of their workers had less-expensive managed care insurance plans. And although managed care plans have kept people as healthy as conventional insurance, employees were not satisfied. Companies have responded to employees' concerns and are beginning a quest to ensure quality.

As resources become limited and the systems of health care delivery shift to more prevention and wellness and out-of-hospital care, reimbursement coverage will continue to adjust to cover alternative care. The pendulum is beginning to swing back to concerns for quality. Employers, consumers, physicians, and hospitals have begun pushing insurers to make needed changes, insisting that improved health care quality will result in satisfied customers and maintain lower costs. The implied assumption must be true—effective patient care programs that produce the best outcomes are the most cost-efficient.

REFERENCES

1. McGrath S, Mitka M. Putting the brakes on physician supply. *American Medical News,* February 12, 1996, p. 1.
2. Burcham M. Emerging trends in the delivery of care. Presented at the Combined Section Meeting of the American Physical Therapy Association, Reno, NV, February 9, 1995.
3. Fleming J II. Current issues in rehabilitation. The Rand study. *Medical Rehabilitation Report* April 1996.
4. *Federal Register* (codified at 42 CFR §400, 409).
5. American Rehabilitation Association (ARA). Talking points for a Medicare prospective payment system for rehabilitation hospitals and units. *Tech Brief,* February 20, 1996.
6. Olsen GG. The coming wave: PSNs, PHOs, and PCCOs. *Rehab Management* October/November 1995.
7. Medicare Act §1861.
8. CFR §400.202.
9. American Rehabilitation Association (ARA). Medicare survey and certification. Off the Record No. 57, March 22, 1996.
10. American Rehabilitation Association (ARA). Transfer proposal. *Tech Brief* No. 11, October 25, 1994.
11. Off the Record, Late-breaking news for Medical Division, American Rehabilitation Association, December 5, 1997, Fax Transmittal.
12. Quarterly discharge data for all admissions, data summary of the uniform data system for medical rehabilitation, national and regional discharge to acute, 1993–1996. SUNY Research Foundation.
13. Keith RA, Wilson DB, Guitterrez P. Acute and subacute rehabilitation for stroke: a comparison. *Arch Phys Med Rehabil* 1995;76: 495–500.
14. Medicare hourly caps to replace "reasonable costs." *ASHA* 1995:18.
15. No place like home. *Hosp Health Care Networks,* October 5, 1994: 45.
16. Is fraud poisoning health care? *Business Week,* March 14, 1994: 70–73.
17. Medicare guidelines for home health §424.24. Requirements for Home Health. *Federal Register.*
18. Lerman D, Tehan C. Hospital-hospice management models, integration and collaboration. American Hospital Publishing Inc. *The Hospice Medicare Benefit* 1995:4–5.
19. American Rehabilitation Association (ARA). CORFs: delivery of offsite services. *Tech Brief* No. 37, April 5, 1996.
20. Ill., PA, plan for Medicaid managed care. *News at Deadline Hospitals & Healthcare Networks,* March 5, 1996:48.
21. Two-plan model for California Medicaid. *News at Deadline Hospitals & Healthcare Networks,* February 5, 1996:9.

22. Magnusson P, Hammonds K. Health care: the quest for quality. The industry is readjusting after years of cost cutting. *Business Week*, April 8, 1996:104–106.

23. McCaffery J. This isn't going to hurt a bit, Medicare-risk HMOs aim to win the retiree market. *CFO*, April 1996:81.

24. Colie R. Capitation strategies. *Rehab Management* 1995; 3(3):90.

25. Colie R. Capitation strategies. The Governance Committee Advisory Board Company 1994.

Chapter 104

Providing Testimony in Litigation

Wayne J. Miller

The legal process seeks expert testimony with the same thirst as a desert traveler coming upon an oasis. Modern litigation now features expert testimony in just about any area imaginable. Professionals in medical and related disciplines are particularly likely to be sought as expert witnesses in personal injury litigation.[1] In such cases, expert medical testimony typically is sought on questions of injury quantification, injury causation, standards of professional practice, and the mental states of persons involved in the injury-producing event.

The purpose of this chapter is to introduce the expert witness to the major issues, controversies, procedures, and practices that relate to expert testimony. The best way to learn is by doing. Therefore, this chapter should be viewed as a general introductory guide or orientation manual. Becoming an *expert* expert witness is a process of time and experience.

WHAT IS AN "EXPERT"?

Musings on "Experts"

Robert Frost once said that a jury consists of 12 persons chosen to decide who has the better lawyer.[2] Given the "battle of experts" so characteristic of modern litigation, lawyers know that jurors often make decisions based on who has the better expert. Therefore, the lawyer will want an expert who comes across better than the opponent in the various comparisons that will be drawn. These comparisons include matters such as credentials, logic of the opinion, and personal ethos.

What makes a good witness? There are as many theories on this topic as there are lawyers. Each lawyer has his or her own prejudices on the preferred expert. A recent commentator described the expert selection process as follows:

> This selection is not based upon the most knowledgeable or the most respected in the field, although lawyers certainly seek well-credentialed experts. Rather, lawyers shop for experts, ultimately choosing the one that talks right, looks right, has the right credentials, and will work with the lawyer in the development of opinions. "Thus, '[a] fool with a small flair for acting and mathematics might be a more successful witness than, say, Einstein.' In two recent studies almost half of the lawyers questioned admitted to shopping for experts. In one of the studies, eighty-six percent of the lawyers identified the adamancy of the expert's support for the party's position as important or very important in selecting an expert."[3]

[1] Samuel R. Gross, Expert Evidence, 1991 *Wis. L. Rev.* 1113.

[2] Robert Frost in *The Quotable Lawyer*, 153 (David Shrager & Elizabeth Frost eds., 1986).

[3] L. Timothy Perrin, Expert Witness Testimony: Back to the Future, 29 *U. Rich. L. Rev.* 1389, 1415–1416 (1995).

My own preferences are as follows. First, I want an expert who truly is expert; that is, I want somebody with consummate professional credentials. This generally means someone who has evaluated and treated a large number of patients, is board certified, is intimately familiar with the literature on the topic in question, and has contributed to the literature on the topic in question.

Second, of equal importance to expertise, is integrity.[4] Experts who may support just about any position can be found, for a price. I avoid these experts for several reasons. First, I avoid them for ethical reasons. Second, I avoid them for policy reasons: Whatever may happen in the individual case, I do not think that experts whose opinions are for sale advance the purposes for which we litigate (justice in individual cases, improved safety in all cases). Third, I avoid them for practical reasons: The paid prostitute is vulnerable to being revealed for what he or she is. After many years of practice, I have a number of experts with whom I have worked and in whom I place a great deal of trust. I use such experts as case "screeners." If they tell me I have a problem with my case, I listen.

Third, I want someone who can communicate to the jury. This means someone who is personable and who speaks in a polite, friendly, professional manner, and who will avoid jargon in favor of common language.

Fourth, I want someone who is concerned about my client, and about the legal issues involved. This means that the witness will not be indifferent to the consequences of his or her expert testimony, and will be an advocate for the truth as he or she understands it. I have never felt that this implies a compromise of professional objectivity. Rather, it implies that the witness will fight for the position he or she believes to be correct.

Finally, I want an expert who is meticulous by habit and temperament. This means that the expert will not simply rely on the exalted status of being an "expert," but will instead recognize that his or her expertise is tested continually by the work he or she does on all cases, including litigation cases.

Legal Definition of "Expert": Federal Rule of Evidence 702

Sources of Evidence Law

Expert testimony is a subject under the law of "evidence." "The law of Evidence is the system of rules and standards by which the admission of proof at the trial of a lawsuit is regulated."[5] Evidence rules developed over the centuries through the "common law."[6] The common law of evidence was codified in the federal system in 1975 with the advent of the *Federal Rules of Evidence* (FRE) (Table 104-1).[7] The FRE govern the federal court system. Each state has a distinct court system with a distinct body of evidence law. Many states have adopted their own codified rules of evidence that are patterned after the federal rules. Though many of the principles of the federal rules are applicable in state cases as well, the reader should be alert to differences in local practice and procedure.

Legal Definition of Expert

Historically, the law has been rigorous in the kinds of proofs that are deemed admissible as evidence in court. The law demands that a certain "foundation" be met by all witnesses who would offer testimony in court. Witnesses who testify to facts must have actually observed those facts.[8]

Distinctions between "fact" witnesses and "opinion" witnesses have been recognized. The law has historically expressed a hostility for opinion testimony.[9] Over time, the hostility has relaxed. The modern rule is to accept opinion testimony from laypersons if the opinions are: "(a) rationally based on the perception of the witness and (b) helpful to a clear understanding of his testimony of the determination of a fact in issue."[10] Under this modern view, laypersons can testify as to the kinds of things on which people commonly render opinions, such as the speed of a vehicle involved in an accident, or whether the defendant appeared drunk before he or she caused an injury. Expert opinion, however, historically remained the subject of more stringent foundational requirements.

FRE 702 governs testimony by experts and states: "If scientific, technical, or other specialized knowledge will assist the trier of fact to understand the evidence or to determine a fact in issue, a witness qualified as an expert by knowledge, skill, experience, training, or education, may testify thereto in the form of an opinion or otherwise."[11]

---

[4] The use of expert witnesses has been the subject of great criticism. The ethics of expert testimony is discussed in more detail in the final section.

[5] McCormick on Evidence 1 (Edward W. Cleary et al., eds., 2nd ed., 1972).

[6] The common law can be thought of as law made by judges, as opposed to law enacted by legislatures, which are called *statutes*. "'Common law' consists of those principles, usage and rules of action applicable to government and security of persons and property which do not rest for their authority upon any express and positive declaration of the will of the legislature." *Black's Law Dictionary* 251 (5th ed., 1979).

[7] The *Federal Rules of Evidence* may be obtained through the West Publishing Company of St. Paul, Minnesota. For ordering information, call 1-800-328-9352.

[8] *Fed. R. Evid.* 602.

[9] Determining that which is "fact" and that which is "opinion" has been problematic, and now is considered a distinction without significance. McCormick, *supra* note 5 at 21.

[10] *Fed. R. Evid.* 701.

[11] *Id.* This rule is perhaps the key rule of evidence for purposes of this chapter. Keep it in mind as a number of other rules will be cited.

Table 104-1: Rules of Evidence by State

State	FRE-Type Rules	Non-FRE-Type Rules
Alabama		X
Alaska	X	
Arizona	X	
Arkansas	X	
California	X	
Colorado	X	
Connecticut		X
Delaware	X	
Florida	X	
Georgia		X
Hawaii	X	
Idaho	X	
Illinois		X
Indiana		X
Iowa	X	
Kansas	X	
Kentucky		X
Louisiana	X	
Maine	X	
Maryland		X
Massachusetts		X
Michigan	X	
Minnesota	X	
Mississippi	X	
Missouri		X
Montana	X	
Nebraska	X	
Nevada	X	
New Hampshire	X	
New Jersey	X	
New Mexico	X	
New York		X
North Carolina	X	
North Dakota	X	
Ohio	X	
Oklahoma	X	
Oregon	X	
Pennsylvania		X
Rhode Island	X	
South Carolina		X
South Dakota	X	
Tennessee	X	
Texas	X	
Utah	X	
Vermont	X	
Virginia		X
Washington	X	
West Virginia	X	
Wisconsin	X	
Wyoming	X	

FRE = Federal Rules of Evidence.
Source: Kenneth W. Graham, State Adaptation of the Federal Rules: The Pros and Cons, 43 *Okla. L. Rev.* 293 (1990).

This rule and the cases interpreting it may surprise those who do not realize how easily this standard is met.[12] Expert testimony has been taken on subjects as diverse as burglars' tools, the effect on livestock of drinking salt water, carpentry, plumbing, and bricklaying.[13]

The focus of our rules on expert opinion evidence is whether the testimony will "assist the trier of fact." Special knowledge that does so can become "expert" opinion.

LIMITATIONS ON EXPERT OPINION TESTIMONY

Meeting the technical requirements of expertise does not confer a license to pontificate on every subject under the sun.[14] The law imposes additional limits on expert opinion. For example, experts cannot vouch for the credibility of another witness, because it is the jury's job to assess credibility.[15] Further, there has been controversy over the years as to whether experts can opine about the ultimate issue in the case.[16]

Perhaps the two most significant limitations on expert opinion are the rules pertaining to certainty of the experts' opinion and the rules pertaining to admission of "scientific" evidence. These are discussed in turn.

Requisite Level of Certainty Required of Expert Opinion

Experienced expert witnesses will be familiar with the question of whether their opinion is based on a "*reasonable degree of medical/professional certainty*." Experts are often asked questions that require them to employ a crystal ball: Will the impairment be permanent? How much income will the injured person lose over the course of his or her lifetime? Given the historical aversion to expert testimony in

---

[12] "Rule 702 is generous in its definition of an expert. . . . The standard is not difficult to satisfy. 'Almost everyone qualifies as an expert in one field or another.' It is rare for a trial court to exclude an expert witness because of a failure to qualify, and rarer yet for an appellate court to disturb the trial judge's decision." Perrin, *supra* note 3 at 1395.

[13] Graham C. Lilly, *An Introduction to the Law of Evidence* 484 (2nd ed., 1987).

[14] Some commentators disagree. For example, Perrin noted: "The Rules provide experts with powerful testimonial tools, such as a minimal standard of qualification, almost limitless permissible areas of testimony, the use of opinion testimony, the ability to state an opinion that encompasses the ultimate issue and to state it before giving the basis of the opinion, and the right to rely on inadmissible evidence in forming opinions." Perrin, *supra* note 3 at 1394–1395.

[15] *Johnson v. Corbet*, 377 N.W.2d 713 (Mich. 1985).

[16] FRE 704 now holds that testimony ". . . is not objectionable because it embraces an ultimate issue to be decided by the trier of fact." *Fed. R. Evid.* 704(a). Controversy remains, however. Some courts have held improper expert testimony that embraces the ultimate *legal* issue to be decided, as opposed to ultimate *factual* issues. See, e.g., *Berry v. City of Detroit*, 25 F.3d 1342 (6th Cir. 1994); *In Re Air Disaster at Lockerbie Scotland on December 21, 1988*, 37 F.3d 804, 826–827 (2nd Cir. 1994); and *McKnight v. Johnson Controls*, 36 F.3d 1396 (8th Cir. 1994).

general, it is not surprising that the law abhors guesswork in expert opinion.

By the same token, the law recognizes that questions may be asked of experts that are beyond the power of the expert to answer with scientific precision. Yet, expert answers to these kinds of questions are required for the smooth administration of justice. Accordingly, again it is not surprising that the law has fashioned a compromise. Expert testimony that is the product of pure speculation is not allowed. On the other hand, expert testimony with a "reasonable" level of certainty is allowed. Absolute certainty is neither possible nor required. The definition of reasonable certainty is elusive:

> "Expert witnesses should not be barred from expressing opinions merely because they are not willing to state their conclusions with absolute certainty. But expert opinions, if not stated in terms of the certain, must at least be stated in terms of the probable, and not merely of the possible. The test of whether an expert's testimony expresses a reasonable probability is not based upon the semantics of the expert or his or her use of any particular term or phrase, but rather, is determined by looking at the entire substance of the expert's testimony.[17]

Simply stated, an expert may not "speculate," but may testify as to a "reasonable degree of certainty."[18]

Limitations on Admissibility of "Scientific" Evidence: The *Frye/Daubert* Controversy

> The law looks to science for answers to factual questions that lie beyond the understanding and knowledge of nonscientists, but at the same time judges without scientific training must determine whether those answers are reliable enough to warrant their use at trial. This need to evaluate expertise while simultaneously depending on it creates a fundamental tension that permeates and shapes the way in which courts decide the admissibility of scientific evidence.[19]

The first case that applied a special rule for admissibility of "scientific" evidence was the 1923 decision of the Federal Court of Appeals in *Frye v. United States*.[20] Mr. Frye was a criminal defendant who sought to admit the results of a "lie detector" test. The court determined that lie detector technology was not sufficiently developed to have achieved "general acceptance" in its field. The court therefore excluded the lie detector evidence. The court offered the following important language in explanation:

> Just when a scientific principle or discovery crosses the line between the experimental and demonstrable stages is difficult to define. Somewhere in this twilight zone the evidential force of the principle must be recognized, and while courts will go a long way in admitting expert testimony deduced from a well-recognized scientific principle or discovery, the thing from which the deduction is made must be sufficiently established to have gained general acceptance in the particular field to which it belongs.[21]

The "general acceptance" test of *Frye* dominated legal thinking for many years. Starting in 1975, things began to change. The first development was the advent of the FRE in 1975. One consequence of this development was to raise the question as to whether the FRE, specifically Rule 702, overruled the "general acceptance" test of *Frye*. The second development was a broad tort reform movement that included vehement criticism of the use of "junk science" in the courts. Exemplary of this movement is the work of Peter Huber, the author of *Galileo's Revenge: Junk Science in the Courtroom*. Mr. Huber's criticisms have included the following comments:

> Maverick scientists shunned by their reputable colleagues have been embraced by lawyers. Eccentric theories that no respectable government agency would ever fund are rewarded munificently by the courts. Batteries of meaningless, high-tech tests that would amount to medical malpractice or insurance fraud if administered in a clinic for treatment are administered in court with complete impunity by fringe experts hired for litigation. The pursuit of truth, the whole truth and nothing but the truth has given way to reams of meaningless data, fearful speculation, and fantastic conjecture. Courts resound with elaborate, systematized, jargon-filled, serious sounding deceptions that fully deserve the contemptuous label used by trial lawyers themselves: *junk science*.[22]

Huber's assertions have been savaged by many critics, including Chesebro who noted:

> "Where are Huber's facts, statistics, hard evidence, and authorities? Huber cites none, and he does not attempt to build an empirical case of his own to demonstrate the significance of the problem on which he dwells. Not only are there no studies that support Huber's view, but a recent report by the authoritative Carnegie Commission . . . concluded that, as for the alleg[ations] that 'junk science' is flooding the courtroom, many of the concerns are greatly exaggerated and it does not appear that the federal courts are being inundated with fringe science."[23]

---

[17] 31A Am. Jur. 2d, *Expert and Opinion Evidence* §86 (1964).
[18] *Joy v. Bell Helicopter Textron, Inc.*, 999 F.2d 549 (D.C. Cir. 1993).
[19] Bert Black, Evolving Legal Standards for the Admissibility of Scientific Evidence, 239 *Science* 1508 (1988).
[20] 293 F. 1013 (1923).
[21] *Id.* at 1014.
[22] Peter W. Huber, *Galileo's Revenge: Junk Science in the Courtroom* 2 (1991).
[23] Kenneth J. Chesebro, Galileo's Retort: Peter Huber's Junk Scholarship, 42 *Am. U. L. Rev.* 1637 (1993). See also, Stephen Daniels and JoAnne Martin, *Civil Juries and the Politics of Reform* (1995); and Mark C. Rahdert, *Covering Accident Costs: Insurance, Liability, and Tort Reform* (1995).

It was in this atmosphere that the U.S. Supreme Court issued its opinion in the case of *Daubert v. Merrell Dow Pharmaceuticals*.[24] As *Daubert* clarifies the law on admissibility of scientific evidence, it merits further discussion. First, the facts of *Daubert*: Mrs. Daubert had taken Bendectin, a prescription antinausea drug, during her pregnancy. Two of her children were born with serious birth defects. The defendant presented expert testimony that no study has ever shown Bendectin to be capable of causing defects in human fetuses. The plaintiff responded with expert testimony to the contrary based on animal cell studies, live-animal studies, and chemical structure analyses, as well as reanalyses of previous and contrary epidemiologic studies. The trial court excluded this evidence, ruling that the methods of the plaintiff's experts were not generally accepted in the scientific community, as per the test in *Frye*.

The Supreme Court reversed, and overruled the 70-year-old precedent of *Frye*. The Court held that *Frye* had been displaced by FRE 702, which now governs the admissibility of purportedly scientific evidence. FRE 702 provides a two-part test for admissibility: relevance and reliability. As to reliability, the Court had the following preliminary comments:

> [Reliability] entails a preliminary assessment [by the trial judge] of whether the reasoning or methodology underlying the testimony is scientifically valid and of whether that reasoning or methodology properly can be applied to the facts in issue. We are confident that federal judges possess the capacity to undertake this review. Many factors will bear on the inquiry, and we do not presume to set out a definitive checklist or test.[25]

The Court held that a number of factors would be helpful in the determination of reliability, including whether the theory has been tested, whether it has been subjected to peer review and publication, and the known or potential rate of error. Even the old *Frye* test of general acceptance may be a factor.

The Court finally made some observations on the competing perspectives of the parties. To the defendant's concern that abandonment of the *Frye* test would result in a "free for all" in which jurors would be "confounded by absurd and irrational pseudoscientific assertions," the Court advised that conventional tools of advocacy coupled with the trial court as a gatekeeper are sufficient safeguards.[26] To the plaintiff's concern that exclusion of "invalid" evidence will sanction a stifling and repressive scientific orthodoxy and thereby impede the search for truth, the Court noted that "[c]onjectures that are probably wrong are of little use . . . in the project of reaching a quick, final, and binding legal judgment—often of great consequence—about a particular set of events in the past," and that this potential danger is part of the balance that must be struck.[27]

The Supreme Court in *Daubert* remanded the case back to the trial court. The trial court was instructed to reconsider the admissibility of the evidence in question according to the new standards announced in the Supreme Court decision.

As might be predicted, the aftermath of *Daubert* has been characterized by an onslaught of commentary. Peter Huber claimed victory for the champions of conservative science:

> Immediately after *Daubert*, both sides claimed victory. The plaintiffs' bar insisted that the opinion loosened the standards for scientific evidence. Anyone who read it, however, found only sensible guidelines for distinguishing serious science from junk—and a clear mandate to trial judges to screen evidence accordingly. In the year since, federal judges have had more than 40 occasions to apply the *Daubert* standard in other cases . . . [The results] are very reassuring . . . in criminal cases, judges are consistently admitting DNA evidence, excluding polygraphs and casting a dubious eye on the mushy scientific indisciplines of psychology and psychiatry.[28]

Law Professor Thomas Mack suggested that the practical implications of *Daubert* have been minimal: "The courts appear to have had little difficulty shifting from a general acceptance analysis [i.e., *Frye*] to a scientific validity analysis without any change in results."[29]

This may all prove to be a tempest in a teapot. First, *Daubert* is a federal decision and may not be adopted by state courts. Second, as Professor Mack suggested, courts applying *Daubert* may reach evidentiary decisions identical to *Frye*. Nevertheless, the implications could be significant. For example, at least one commentator suggested that psychiatric testimony formerly allowable under *Frye* will not meet *Daubert* standards of admissibility.[30]

In summary, those who contemplate giving expert testimony must be aware of the new standards announced in *Daubert* (relevance and reliability versus the *Frye* standard of general acceptance). Does the jurisdiction in which the expert will testify use the *Daubert* test, the old *Frye* test, or some variation or mixture thereof? Does the subject

---

[24] 509 U.S. 579 (1993).

[25] *Daubert*, 509 U.S. 579 at 592–593.

[26] *Id.* at 595–596.

[27] *Id.* at 597.

[28] Peter W. Huber, Fact Versus Quack, *Forbes*, July 4, 1994, at 132. See also, Lisa M. Agrimonti, Note, The Limitations of Daubert and Its Misapplication to Quasi-scientific Experts, 35 *Washburn L. J.* 134 (1995); and Edward J. Imwinkelreid, Evidence Law Visits Jurassic Park: The Far-reaching Implications of the Daubert Court's Recognition of the Uncertainty of the Scientific Enterprise, 81 *Iowa L. Rev.* 55 (1995).

[29] Thomas J. Mack, Scientific Testimony After *Daubert*: Some Early Returns from Lower Courts, *TRIAL*, August 1994 at 24.

[30] Ronald J. Allen, Expertise and the *Daubert* Decision, 84 *J. Crim. L. Criminology* 1157, 1172 (1994).

matter of the expert's testimony pose problems of admissibility under the standards of the jurisdiction?

RETENTION AS AN EXPERT WITNESS

The practical aspects of expert testimony, that is, the "how to," are discussed now.

When the expert is first contacted by the attorney, there are a number of matters that should be taken up in short order. The expert should not rely on the attorney to be thorough as to all of the following matters:

- Confidentiality. This generally is not an issue. The plaintiff's attorney will have received the client's authorization to inquire into medical information. The defendant's attorney will be able to review otherwise confidential information because the plaintiff waives claims of privilege for any injuries that are the subject of litigation.[31]
- Subject matter in dispute. Simply put, what is the fuss all about? What question is at issue and requires expert testimony? Attorneys may not be specific about this, and may request the expert simply to "review" a file. The expert may then be forced into the position of formulating the issue for the attorney.
- Expert witness fees. This is an area that can be fraught with problems for both attorney and expert. Many experts insist on an advance payment from the attorney to secure the first portion of work. This request is the result of bad experiences experts may have had with attorneys. My own practice is to set a limit on the amount of time to be expended by the expert, based on discussion with the expert on what a reasonable limit would be. The expert should make clear that the attorney, not the client, is responsible for payment. The expert should make clear that the bill is payable upon delivery, not at some uncertain future date, such as when the case is settled. In any event, the issue of fees should be discussed and agreed on in advance. Some experts now use a formal written contract to confirm their agreements with attorneys. Certainly, and at least, agreements should be confirmed in writing. Experts have a proprietary right to their opinions. As such, experts cannot be compelled to testify as to opinion matters.[32] Therefore, the attorney should want to avoid antagonizing the expert witness over a fee dispute.
- Timetable for completion of analysis. The expert should learn when an opinion will be required. An expert will want to make sure that there is sufficient time to obtain and analyze all relevant information and documents and to deliver an opinion. The expert should learn whether there are any trial dates or other relevant deadlines.
- Information gathering. The expert may find himself or herself working with attorneys of varying degrees of skill and experience. The attorneys may not have gathered information adequate for review. The attorneys may not even know what information should be obtained. It is not the expert's role to be the attorney. However, the expert must take some responsibility in getting information sufficient to make a proper analysis and decision.

By the time the expert has discussed these initial considerations with the attorney, the expert should be in a position to decide whether or not serving as an expert for the attorney is a matter of interest. The expert should feel free to decline the opportunity to participate.

PROCEDURE FOR GIVING EXPERT TESTIMONY: DISCOVERY DEPOSITIONS

Depositions in General

The popular notion of testimony comes from television: *Perry Mason* in the 1960s; *LA Law* in the 1980s; and the O. J. Simpson trial in 1995. The scenario is basically the same: an austere and intimidating courtroom; a taciturn judge; a large crowd; and a tense, hushed, and drama-laden ambience. This scenario may indeed occur, but the reality is most often quite different.

Since most civil cases are settled, very few such cases actually go to trial. In such cases, testimony is obtained without the witness ever visiting the courtroom. This is done by way of *deposition*. A deposition is a statement taken under oath but outside of court. The deposition is the most common manner of obtaining testimony. Typically, only the attorneys and the court reporter will be present, in addition to the witness.

There are two main kinds of deposition: a *discovery* deposition and a *de bene esse* deposition. The discovery deposition is taken for the purpose of learning what the witness has to say. The de bene esse deposition is taken in lieu of live testimony at trial. The de bene esse deposition is usually taken when there is concern over the witness's availability at the time of trial, due to physical infirmity or scheduling problems. De bene esse depositions of expert witnesses are often done by way of videotape. The remainder of this section focuses on the discovery deposition.

Deposition Procedure

There are two main bodies of rules that govern testimony. These are the rules of procedure and the rules of evi-

[31] For general status of rules on waiver of privilege, see Annotation, 21 A.L.R.3d *Commencing Action Involving Physical Condition of Plaintiff or Decedent as Waiving Physician-Patient Privilege as to Discovery Proceedings*, 912 (1968).

[32] Lilly, *supra* note 13 at 409–510; The Treating Physician as an Expert Witness, 83 *Tex. Med.* 74 (1987); *Klabunde v. Stanley*, 181 N.W.2d 918 (1970).

dence. I have already introduced the rules of evidence with the earlier discussion of the FRE, and in particular, Rule 702. Rules of evidence mainly govern the *substance* and *form* of the evidence to be admitted or excluded from evidence.[33] Procedural rules are distinct from the rules of evidence. In the federal courts, these rules are known as *The Federal Rules of Civil Procedure*, or FRCP.[34] Again, as with the FRE, the FRCP apply to the federal courts only; state courts are sure to have separate, though probably similar rules.

The FRCP consists of 86 separate and complex rules. Rules 26 to 37 govern discovery and depositions. Rules 38 to 53 govern trial procedures. A detailed review of these procedures is beyond the scope of this chapter. Here I attempt a more modest discussion of some of the specific provisions most likely to be encountered by expert witnesses. Rule 30 is the key rule governing deposition procedure. The following rules of deposition procedure can be derived from the several pages that comprise this rule:

1. Depositions are to be conducted as per the rules of evidence, with the obvious exception that no judge will supervise the deposition proceeding.[35]
2. Objections are to be noted, but the examination is to proceed subject to the objections. In other words, witnesses must answer questions even if there is an objection. The main exceptions are when a privilege is asserted or when the deposition is being conducted in bad faith (e.g., to harass the witness).[36] This rule is commonly violated as attorneys often improperly instruct witnesses not to answer questions.
3. The witness may review the transcript following the deposition and make changes in form or substance.[37] Some mistakenly believe that the opportunity to review the transcript exists only for the purpose of correcting typographical mistakes by the court reporter. To the contrary, FRCP 30 specifically authorizes changes to the substance of testimony.

Scope of Discovery Depositions

The main difference between trial (this includes de bene esse depositions taken in lieu of actual trial testimony) and deposition is that the scope of the trial is much more confined than that of the deposition. The deposition is used as a discovery tool, that is, to find out information for use at trial. As a result, the deposition will give the examining attorney the opportunity to explore all sorts of *potentially* relevant areas.[38] Questions must be answered even if they call for hearsay, or be of questionable relevance, or call for speculation, or otherwise violate the rules of evidence. While objections may be made during the deposition, the witness must answer most questions.[39]

Substance of Discovery Deposition Testimony

"Discovery" is just like it sounds: the opportunity for the attorney to discover important facts and theories of the opponent. Ultimately, the purpose of the discovery deposition is to help the attorney prepare for trial cross-examination. A discovery deposition may be formulaic, seeking only the experts' opinions and their bases. A well-prepared and thoughtful attorney may probe much more deeply.[40] The following areas are typical fodder for discovery depositions.

Credentials

The attorney will want to know what gives the witness the authority to testify as an expert, whether the expert meets the previously described standards of expertise, and how the expert will compare with the expert retained by the examining attorney. The expert should be aware that the

---

[33] Certainly, the evidence rules provide guidance on *procedure* as well as *substance*. For example, FRE 611 vests in the trial court substantial power of control over the mode and order of testimony: "(a) Control by court. The court shall exercise reasonable control over the mode and order of interrogating witnesses and presenting evidence so as to (1) make the interrogation and presentation effective for the ascertainment of truth, (2) avoid needless consumption of time, and (3) protect witnesses from harassment or undue embarrassment. . . ." *Fed. R. Evid.* 611(a).

[34] *The Federal Rules of Civil Procedure* is published by the West Publishing Company, of St. Paul, Minnesota, and may be ordered by calling 1-800-328-9352.

[35] *Fed. R. Civ. P.* 30(c).

[36] *Fed. R. Civ. P.* 30(c) and (d).

[37] *Fed. R. Civ. P.* 30(e).

[38] The scope of discovery in federal court is governed by FRCP 26. The general rule is FRCP 26(b)(1): "Parties may obtain discovery regarding any matter, not privileged, which is relevant to the subject matter involved in the pending action. . . . The information sought need not be admissible at the trial if the information sought appears reasonably calculated to lead to the discovery of admissible evidence." *Fed. R. Civ. P.* 26(b)(1).

[39] Objections *must* be made to certain kinds of questions, such as objections to the form of the question, or objections to the competence of the witness, or they are waived. *Fed. R. Civ. P.* 32. The purpose of this rule is to give the examining attorney an opportunity to cure whatever defect may exist in the question. If the opposing attorney does not object, the examining attorney cannot cure the defect.

[40] In the federal courts, certain discovery of basic information must be made even without a deposition. FRCP 26(a)(2) provides that expert witnesses are to prepare written reports containing

> ". . . a complete statement of all opinions to be expressed and the basis and reasons therefor; the data or other information considered by the witness in forming the opinions; any exhibits to be used as a summary of or support for the opinions; the qualifications of the witness, including a list of all publications authored by the witness within the preceding ten years; the compensation to be paid for the study and testimony; and a listing of any other cases in which the witness has testified as an expert or by deposition within the preceding four years." *Fed. R. Civ. P.* 26(a)(2)B.

attorney may already know a lot about him or her. A curriculum vita may already have been provided, expert witness interrogatories may have been answered, and lawyer organizations such as the Association of Trial Lawyers of America (ATLA) or the Defense Research Institute (DRI) may have the expert's vita on file from previous cases. Enterprising lawyers may also have done a great deal of background research on the expert before taking the deposition. In addition, an attorney may have reviewed the expert's publications, prior deposition testimony, and even interviewed past employers. This level of scrutiny may not be typical, but it certainly happens, and usually depends on the importance of the expert to the claim or defense of the attorney.

Materials Reviewed

The attorney will want to carefully review the expert's file to determine its contents, information contained therein, and information missing.

Opinions

This is among the most important aspects of the deposition. The attorney will probe for all opinions and will want to make sure that all opinions expressed are final. If opinions are not yet final, the attorney will want to know what further work is planned, and will insist on being informed of any supplemental opinions. If supplemental opinions emerge, the attorney may want to take an additional deposition.

Literature/Authorities

One of the important cross-examination techniques at trial (discussed under General Approaches, later) is the use of professional literature to impeach the witness. I typically spend a great deal of time at depositions in an effort to learn who the expert regards as authoritative, what he or she thinks about the peer-review process, and what books and magazines are held in high regard.[41]

Bias

This can be a significant area of deposition review. Billing rates, time spent, and total money received on the given case are reviewed. Much broader questions pertaining to the relationship of the expert to the retaining party, attorney, or even to the general opinions espoused can be reviewed in detail. The attorney may use information obtained from the deposition to seek a broader production of financial records of the witness, such as tax records, banking records, or even reports generated on other cases.

[41] I note that the American Medical Association (AMA) regards publication in a peer-reviewed journal as a good indicator of reliability. Charles Marwick, What Constitutes an Expert Witness?, 269 *JAMA* 2057 (1993).

TRIAL TESTIMONY: DIRECT EXAMINATION

The Context and Form of Direct Examination

Finally, the trial stage. Efforts to settle the case have failed. The parties, having assiduously taken discovery as just described, are ready for their day (more often a lot longer) in court. Following jury selection and opening statements, the plaintiff begins by presenting witnesses who are intended to sustain the plaintiff's burden of proof. Tactical decisions are made as to how many witnesses to put on, and in what order.

Expert testimony can be presented in three ways: written deposition that is read to the jury (usually by a member of the attorney's office, sometimes even by a hired actor); videotaped deposition; and live testimony. The reading of a deposition is the least expensive method of expert witness presentation. Because it is boring to have a jury sit while raw transcript is read, this method may not be used as much in modern practice.

The videotaped deposition is currently in vogue. It is certainly less expensive than having the expert testify live, because live testimony involves travel costs and the uncertainties of trial scheduling. Videotaped depositions are done at the expert's place of business, essentially at the convenience of the expert. Videotape also offers a very flexible medium for presentation of testimony. Charts, x-rays, models, anatomic drawings, and a host of demonstrative evidence can be conveyed effectively through the video medium. Attorneys and experts are well advised to make use of the demonstrative aids, as the mere presentation of a "talking head" can be terribly boring.

Leading Questions

Leading questions are those that suggest to the witness the answer desired by the examiner. Leading questions are typified by questions that begin with "Isn't it true that . . . ?" or "Don't you agree that . . . ?". Leading questions are ordinarily not permitted in direct examination.[42] For example, the question "Doctor, you examined the plaintiff on November 5, 1995, didn't you?" is improper as leading. A proper phrasing might be, "Doctor, when did you examine the plaintiff?"[43]

Typical Areas of Direct Examination of Experts

Direct examination can theoretically be very concise, following a very simple formula. The minimum requirement for obtaining an expert opinion is to obtain the expert's credentials, and the expert's opinions. Most direct examinations can be accomplished with only a few basic questions:

[42] *Fed. R. Evid.* 611(c).

[43] The leading question is permitted on *cross*-examination, and attorneys are typically instructed to ask only leading questions that can be answered yes or no.

1. What is your name?
2. Are you licensed to practice your profession in this state?
3. What do you know about this case?
4. Do you have an opinion on the issue in this case?
5. What is your opinion?

A direct examination will never be this brief. Important expert testimony will not be glossed over so glibly. These basic question areas will be expanded on as follows.

Credentials

Under FRE 702, the mere fact of licensure may be sufficient to establish the witness as an expert having ". . . scientific, technical, or other specialized knowledge . . ." However, the licensure alone is not sufficient to help the jury appreciate the authority with which the expert speaks. Therefore, the attorney ordinarily will go beyond the basic question of licensure. The attorney will ask about board certification, publications, research activities, the number of patients seen by the expert, and so on. The opposing attorney may offer to stipulate that the witness is an expert, ostensibly to expedite the examination process. The examining attorney ordinarily and politely will refuse such an offer. The attorney wants the jury to know the details that make the expert seem credible and authoritative.

Once the witness's credentials have been established, the witness is an "expert." The attorney may then proceed with questions seeking expert opinion. In the past, upon completion of the credentialing process, the examining attorney would offer the witness as an expert, and ask the court to certify the witness as an expert. Modern practice under the FRE is to simply continue with questioning once the witness's credentials have been established. The court will not "certify" an expert.[44] Rather, the examination will proceed subject to any objection from the opposing attorney as to whether a sufficient foundation has been established for further testimony to be taken.

The Expert's Discipline

As medicine becomes ever more specialized, one can expect juries to be unfamiliar with the subspecialties that are increasingly extant. The attorney will want the jury to know what a doctor of physical medicine and rehabilitation does, or what an otolaryngologist or a neuropsychologist is. With this in mind, the expert should work on how to present and describe his or her discipline in a simple and concise way that avoids the use of jargon. For example, the doctor of physical medicine and rehabilitation can be explained as the "captain of the rehabilitation ship" or the "quarterback of the rehabilitation team."

[44] *Berry v. City of Detroit*, 25 F.3d 1342 (6th Cir. 1994); *United States v. Kozminski*, 821 F.2d 1186 (6th Cir. 1987), *aff'd in part and remanded in part*, 487 U.S. 931 (1988).

Neuropsychological assessment can be described by comparison to a thermometer: Just like a thermometer is used to show normal and abnormal (higher than 98.6°F) temperatures, neuropsychological assessment is used to define normal for the many brain functions, and then to determine how far from "normal" a person's brain is functioning. Such definitions may lack technical precision. But they are quite helpful in explaining the arcane nature of technical disciplines.

The Basis for the Opinion

This section identifies another aspect of the "foundation" required for expert opinion. The first aspect, discussed in the previous section, is the expert's credentials, that is, the expertise that allows the expert to offer an opinion. This section goes to the information applied by the expert to reach an opinion. If the expert is a treating professional, the expert already knows the basis from firsthand knowledge, or from information obtained under his or her supervision. Retained experts may venture opinions based on personal examination, as well as review of the documents generated in the litigation.[45] Strangely enough, the FRE does not require that the expert disclose these bases for his or her opinion. FRE 705 provides: "The expert may testify in terms of opinion or inference and give reasons therefor without first testifying to the underlying facts or data, unless the court requires otherwise. The expert may in any event be required to disclose the underlying facts or data on cross-examination."

[45] In prior years, expert opinion was obtained largely on the basis of hypothetical questions posed to the experts. The bases for this practice and the problems in administering it are now only of historical interest. Modern practice expands the bases of expert opinion to reflect the actual practice of the experts in their own disciplines. FRE 703 provides as follows relative to the "Bases of Opinion Testimony By Experts":

> "The facts or data in the particular case upon which an expert bases an opinion or inference may be those perceived by or made known to the expert at or before the hearing. If of a type reasonable relied upon by experts in the particular field in forming opinions or inferences upon the subject, the facts or data need not be admissible in evidence." *Fed. R. Evid.* 703.

The comment to this rule is also instructive:

> ". . . the rule is designed to broaden the basis for expert opinions beyond that current in many jurisdictions and to bring the judicial practice into line with the practice of the experts themselves when not in court. Thus a physician in his own practice bases his diagnosis on information from numerous sources and of considerable variety, including statements by patients and relatives, reports and opinions from nurses, technicians and other doctors, hospital records and X rays. Most of them are admissible in evidence, but only with the expenditure of substantial time in producing and examining various authenticating witnesses. The physician makes life-and-death decisions in reliance upon them. His validation, expertly performed and subject to cross-examination, ought to suffice for judicial purposes." *Fed. R. Evid.* 703 advisory committee's note.

The decision to ask for the expert's bases of opinion will be a tactical decision of the attorney. In most cases, the attorney will initiate a detailed discussion of the bases of opinion; a simple opinion without any rationale, reasoning, or basis will lack the credibility required to prevail in the dispute.

Whether asked by the examining attorney, the court, or the opposing attorney, experts are well advised to be extremely well prepared on the factual basis supporting the opinion. One can be sure the opposing attorney will be. No other piece of advice is given so often, yet respected so little. La Rochefoucauld said it succinctly: "There is nothing more horrible than the murder of a beautiful theory by a brutal gang of facts."[46] Experts must make sure that they have been supplied with all of the salient facts, that they have reviewed them, that they understand them, and that they are facile with them. The section on cross-examination helps to explain how ignorance or an incomplete grasp of the facts can be calamitous.

The Opinion

This is the reason why the expert was called in the first place. Of central importance, it may involve only one or two questions. Some attorneys may go directly to the opinion, and leave the bases and other foundational matter for later, so that the jury is not kept waiting. Others may follow a methodical examination that ends at the opinion.

As discussed earlier, the opinion must not be speculative and must have a reasonable basis. As a result, experts will often be asked if their opinion is "based on a reasonable degree of professional certainty."

Miscellaneous

Other areas may be broached on direct examination. The attorney will want to disclose first any facts that may sound worse if the opposing attorney raised them first. This is known as"stealing their thunder." The witness may be asked if he or she is being compensated for time spent on the case. The witness may be asked if he or she has ever met or worked with the examining attorney previously, and so on.

TRIAL TESTIMONY: CROSS-EXAMINATION

Initial Thoughts

Unlike the many and highly technical rules of procedure and evidence, there are no rules governing the choice of what questions, techniques, and approaches are to be used by attorneys during the cross-examination. As might be expected, the variety to be encountered is virtually limitless. Still, there are some common aspects to cross-examination that can be explored.

Perhaps the earliest comment on cross-examination was issued by Cicero in ancient Rome: "When you have no basis for argument, abuse the plaintiff."[47] Cicero's advice, in theme and variation, is followed to this day. In fact, expert witnesses should take some comfort if they come under this kind of attack. It will be an indicator that the cross-examining attorney is in some trouble. The following section discusses more legitimate and substantive areas of examination.

General Approaches

Credentials

The "perfect" expert is a creature of myth, as the following progression of typical cross-examination approaches illustrates. Attorneys believe that the general public honors doctors, and views with suspicion those expert witnesses who are not doctors. Thus, an expert witness who is not a licensed osteopathic or allopathic physician can expect to be asked questions such as the following: "Sir, you are not a *medical* doctor, are you?" "You are not licensed to prescribe medications, are you?" "You are not licensed to give medical advice, are you?" A good reply might be, "No, I'm not a medical doctor; I'm a neuropsychologist, the person to whom the medical doctors look for answers when their standard diagnostic tests don't help."[48]

If the expert is a physician, the attorney will ask if he or she is board certified. If the expert has limited research or publication credentials, the attorney will point this out. If the expert has extensive research or publication credentials, the attorney will seek to suggest that the expert is confined to the "ivory tower" and has little expertise in actually helping patients. If the expert has outstanding practical, clinical, research, and publication credentials, the attorney, in the spirit of Cicero, may move along to other areas.

Learned Treatises

A powerful method of cross-examination employs the use of authoritative texts to contradict the testimony of the expert. Such material is hearsay, but there is a special exception to the hearsay rule that governs this technique:

> Learned Treatises. To the extent called to the attention of an expert witness upon cross-examination or relied upon by the expert witness in direct examination, statements contained in published treatises, periodicals, or pamphlets on a subject

---

[46] La Rochefoucauld. Francois in *The Quotable Lawyer, supra* note 2 at 109.

[47] Cicero in *The Quotable Lawyer, supra* note 2 at 74.

[48] See Stanley L. Brodsky, *Testifying in Court: Guidelines & Maxims for the Expert Witness* 58–59 (1991) for more examples of responses to the "you're not a doctor" line of questions. This work is also generally helpful to alert experts to the kinds of questions one might face, and suggested answers thereto.

of history, medicine, or other science or art, established as a reliable authority by the testimony or admission of the witness or by other expert testimony or by judicial notice. If admitted, the statements may be read into evidence but may not be received as exhibits.[49]

The purpose of this type of examination is to show that the expert is a "maverick" and that the weight of authority is against the expert's position.

In my experience, medical professionals often refuse to accept that there are any temporal "authorities," because medical professionals often view an "authority" as someone whose word or opinion cannot be questioned. It should be understood that the legal definition is much less stringent than this. Legally, authorities are deemed to be generally accepted sources of reliable information.[50]

Apart from the relatively lenient definition, an expert can be cross-examined on "authority" even if he or she does not admit the authority of a given text or author. FRE 803(18) allows authority to be established by direct examination of another expert, or even by judicial notice. Accordingly, the expert must be thoroughly familiar with the literature and current thought in his or her discipline, and on the disputed question in particular. While this is only common sense, it is surprising how often the personal and professional demands of the expert can prevent continuing education.

Prior Testimony/Remarks

This is somewhat related to the previous section. Instead of showing that the witness is a "maverick," inconsistent with prevailing professional thought, the attorney may try to show something even more damaging: that the expert is inconsistent with himself or herself. As an expert goes through professional life, a substantial "paper trail" may emerge. This will include forensic reports issued in previous cases, depositions, publications, and lectures or speeches. It is rare for an expert to have kept a file of his or her forensic activities, such as having forensic reports readily available, or depositions in a separate "bank." Nevertheless, the expert may be surprised to find that the opposing attorney has come up with a substantial amount of the expert's paper history. The plaintiff's and defendant's bar make an effort to compile reports and depositions of experts who often appear on the opposing side.

It is therefore advisable for experts to be aware of their past remarks, even if they do not want to go to the extent of maintaining a file of litigation materials, reports, and depositions. If experts are not familiar with their own prior works, they may find themselves confronted with an attorney who has accumulated a large amount of their past work product, and who is therefore more familiar with the experts' words than the experts! In one such case, I had the opportunity to obtain the audiotape of a speech the expert had given some years before. Perhaps because he was speaking to an audience of his colleagues, he felt that he could let his guard down. But, in any event, he made some rather injudicious remarks, and the following cross-examination resulted:

Q: Would you be more dramatic to a jury and try and score more points on cross examination when you have a jury trial than you would if you had a judge trial? Would you be different, in other words, in front of a jury than you would in front of a judge?

A: Yes, because most of the time a jury is not as well versed in rehabilitation or medical terms or techniques or services and, therefore, they need the education.

Q: Doctor, you remember what you said at this seminar regarding jury trials, don't you? You know what I'm about to play, don't you?

A: Again, what I said was that there are ways of presenting information so that the jury understands it well, and sometimes this needs to be done in a dramatic manner.

Q: Doctor, let me ask you if this is your lecture comments 3 years ago. (Whereupon a tape recording was played as follows):
The jury trial is a theater. In the administrative trials that I do, I'm certainly not as dramatic as I would be in a jury trial. I also don't try to score points in the same way on cross-examination. If you've got a judge there or an administrative law judge who's got, who's hearing the case and making the decisions, if you try to score points, you come across as an advocate and typically, they will dismiss part of your testimony. So I'm more dramatic in front of a jury because they don't know what the hell I'm talking about 90% of the time, and I'm trying to make an argument, where I will not do this in a nonjury trial.[51]

The lesson? Experts should be careful of what they say in public; someone might be listening. In addition, they should know their own personal literature as well as the professional literature.

Bias

Though contained in a discussion of cross-examination techniques, the issue of bias transcends this particular cate-

---

[49] *Fed. R. Evid.* 803(18).

[50] See, e.g., *Ward v. United States*, 838 F.2d 182 (6th Cir. 1988); *Ellis v. International Playtex, Inc.*, 745 F.2d 292 (4th Cir. 1984); *McCarty v. Sisters of Mercy*, 440 N.W.2d 417 (Mich. App. 1989), *lv app den* in 434 Mich. 862 (1990); and *Jacober v. St. Peter's Medical Center*, 608 A.2d 304 (N.J. Sup. Ct. 1992).

[51] This excerpt is from an actual case of mine. The name of the case and the expert will remain confidential. In the tape-recorded lecture, the expert made numerous other remarks about tricks that he had used in the course of his rather extensive litigation career. Any vestige of even-handed impartiality was blasted away when confronted with the actual audio recording of many of these remarks.

gory. Attorney and expert alike must always remember that the legal process is ideally a search for truth. Biased analysis and testimony corrupt this process. The ethics of expert testimony is discussed in a separate section later. At this point, it must be noted that the courts are particularly sensitive to the possibility of bias and wide latitude will be allowed in cross-examination on this issue.

Bias may occur by virtue of an expert's personal or philosophical predisposition to view a matter in a particular way. Or, the expert may be identified with a particular school of thought. More crassly, the expert may have a long history of providing testimony for a given party or of taking the same position in a wide variety of cases. A classic example of this is the Texas psychiatrist nicknamed "Dr. Death." "Dr. Death" testified at over 50 sentencing hearings in capital cases, and always found that the defendant would be violent in the future, whether or not he actually examined the defendant, and notwithstanding the position of the American Psychiatric Association that future violence could not be predicted. "Dr. Death" was, as one might imagine, an extremely popular expert witness for the prosecution.[52]

Bias by virtue of financial interests will be thoroughly explored. Financial incentives to slant one's testimony may come from the amount of money paid on a given case, or the amount of money paid on many cases by a particular "customer" or category of customer (e.g., plaintiff's attorneys, or insurance companies). Questions such as the following are commonly asked:

1. How often have you testified for the particular attorney or party?
2. How often do you participate in forensic activities?
3. How much of your income is derived from forensic activities?
4. How much of your forensic practice is devoted to plaintiffs/defendants?

It is not uncommon for the expert to answer, "Gee, I don't keep records or statistics, but I think maybe 10% of my income comes from doing IMEs and depositions for defendants." Often, the other attorney will simply let the matter drop. The expert should be aware that the attorney may follow up with a thorough investigation of matters relating to financial bias. The attorney may seek a court order compelling the expert to disclose intimate tax and business records and other documents from which precise answers to the above questions can be obtained.[53]

Substance of Opinion/Area of Expertise

Legendary trial attorney Francis Wellman suggested that attorneys should never take on experts, because the attorney will never be as expert as the expert.[54] In the century since the first edition of Wellman's book, lawyers have gotten dramatically more sophisticated and the advice has changed.[55] Specialization has increased to the point where the legal general practitioner is rare. There are specialists in particular varieties of tort law, and even subspecialties (e.g., birth trauma medical malpractice). There are numerous publications teaching attorneys about medicine and advising attorneys how to approach medical experts. One can and should expect lawyers to be far better prepared than those of a century ago. Moreover, the demands of modern medical practice may be such that the doctor is far less able to keep up with the lawyers, than vice versa. I often find doctors who are not familiar with the professional literature.

Substance of Opinion/Knowledge of Facts

In addition to cross-examination on the expert's general area of expertise, the expert can expect rigorous examination of the facts of the case. This generally takes two forms. First, the expert must know all the facts germane to the matters at issue in his or her testimony. I continue to be astounded at how poorly or incompletely a patient's history is documented. Apart from the importance in litigation, obtaining an accurate and complete history would seem to be of the utmost importance in treating the patient. Yet, it seems that important diagnostic and treatment decisions are made without aggressively pursuing and following up on historical matters. At the very least, this can give the appearance of sloppiness, as the expert is forced to testify, "The attorney did not supply this information to me," or "This wasn't important to my job on this case." Worse still, the omitted material may have a dramatic impact on the expert's testimony, entirely changing the thrust of the testimony.

Second, the expert must be thoroughly familiar with the information in his or her own file. Some years ago, I was involved in a case where the opposing expert clinical forensic psychologist had administered the Wechsler Adult Intelligence Scale-Revised (WAIS-R) as part of his assessment of my client. With the assistance of my own expert, I

---

[52] Perrin, *supra* note 3 at 1442.

[53] McCormick on *Evidence* 57 (John William Strong et al., eds., 4th ed., 1992); *United States v. Preciado-Gomez*, 529 F.2d 935, 942 (9th Cir. 1976), *cert. denied*, 425 U.S. 953 (1976); *Bissel Brothers Inc. v. Fares*, 611 So. 2d 620 (Fla. App. 2 Dist. 1993); *Dollar General, Inc. v. Fares*, 590 So. 2d 555 (Fla. App. 3 Dist. 1991); *Wood v. Tallahassee Memorial Medical Center, Inc.*, 593 So. 2d 1140 (Fla. App. 1 Dist. 1992); *Sears v. Rutishauser*, 466 N.E.2d 210 (Ill. App. 1984); *Trower v. Jones*, 520 N.E.2d 297, 300 (Ill. 1988); *Wilson v. Stilwell*, 309 N.W.2d 898 (Mich. 1981); *Fassahi v. St. Mary's Hospital*, 328 N.W.2d 132 (Mich. 1982); *McLaren v. Zeilinger*, 302 N.W.2d 583 (Mich. App. 1981); *Rappaport v. Rappaport*, 405 N.W.2d 165 (Mich. App. 1987); and *State ex rel. Lichtor v. Clark*, 845 S.W.2d 55, 64–65 (Mo. App. W.D. 1992).

[54] "As a general thing, it is unwise for the cross-examiner to attempt to cope with a specialist in his or her own field of inquiry. Lengthy cross-examinations along the lines of the expert's theory are usually disastrous and should rarely be attempted." Francis L. Wellman, *The Art of Cross-Examination* 95 (4th ed., 1936).

[55] Gross, *supra* note l at 1174.

carefully reviewed the data on which the expert's opinion was based, including the scoring of the WAIS-R. I learned that the expert had made a series of simple arithmetic mistakes, each of which was in the favor of my opponent. This led to the following cross-examination, where, after establishing the scoring, I asked:

Q: So, you erred then, didn't you, doctor?

A: Yes.

Q: You erred, in the favor of giving him a higher score; true?

A: Well, let me see. I mean, certainly, if I did, it was unintentional. But if—you know—as you point that out correctly, let me just see what it does.

Q: . . . My question was only did you make an error? Was your answer that you did? . . .

A: Yes.

Q: Is this an example of a subtle bias, induced by exorbitant fees paid?

A: No. I think it's an example, unfortunately, on my part, of carelessness.

Q: Okay.

A: Obviously, it's easy for you to catch an error like that, as embarrassingly you have pointed it out to me.

Q: It wasn't easy, let me tell you.

(After noting another calculation error, the following examination took place):

Q: And that error makes a 5-point difference then, in terms of the ultimate verbal score true?

A: That's correct. That's a—That's a significant error, on my part.

Q: Is that an example of error induced by an exorbitant fee paid?

A: No. I—again, I'm not making excuses for it. It was an error. It was an error—arithmetic error. I have no excuse, other than it was an error.[56]

Miscellaneous

Those who are often involved in the deposition process will be well advised to embrace their role as expert witness. Further study is appropriate. A very brief reading list is provided for those who want to hone their skills and receive some tips.[57]

[56] The case name and expert witness involved are from my personal files and will remain confidential.

[57] See, e.g., Thomas J. Vesper, Cross-examination of the Defendant's Medical Expert (or, Who's Afraid of the IME/NIME), 16 *Trial Diplomacy J.* 93 (1993); Brodsky, *supra* note 48; and A. Michael Barker, Tips for the Testifying Expert, *For the Defense*, March 1995, at 8.

ETHICS OF EXPERT TESTIMONY

A lengthy discussion of ethics in expert testimony is beyond the scope of this chapter. However, some general thoughts are offered. Specifically, I note a couple of aspects of the American Medical Association's (AMA's) guidelines for expert witness testimony. First:

> As a citizen and as a professional with special training and experience, the physician has an ethical obligation to assist in the administration of justice. If a patient who has a legal claim requests his physician's assistance, the physician should furnish medical evidence with the patient's consent in order to secure the patient's legal rights.[58]

I applaud this language. Too often, it seems that medical experts view lawyers and the legal process with suspicion and hostility. I view the legal process as an integral part of restoring a person to his or her optimal level of functioning. This is particularly true where lawyers obtain compensation from liability cases or entitlements to medical insurance benefits that are to pay for treatment. As such, lawyers and medical professionals are interdependent. It is therefore fair to view the lawyer as an adjunct to the treatment team, and to extend the assistance contemplated by the above-quoted ethical precept.

A second precept of the AMA's expert witness guidelines is that "the medical witness must not become an advocate or a partisan in the legal proceeding. The medical witness should be adequately prepared and should testify honestly and truthfully."[59]

Controversy over prostitution of and by expert witnesses now rages.[60] One cannot ignore the bias induced in expert witnesses by the "business" aspects of expert testimony.[61] These criticisms must be taken seriously by

[58] Committee on Medical Liability Guidelines for Expert Witness Testimony; 83 *Pediatrics* 2 (1989).

[59] *Pediatrics* Id.

[60] Robert L. Brent, The Irresponsible Expert Witness: A Failure of Biomedical Graduate Education and Professional Accountability, 70 *Pediatrics* 754 (1982); Committee on Medical Liability, Guidelines for Expert Witness Testimony, 83 *Pediatrics* 312–313 (1989); Richard A. Epstein, A New Regime For Expert Witnesses, 26 *Val. U. L. Rev.* 757 (1992); Gross, *supra* note 1; and Perrin, *supra* note 3.

[61] Professor Perrin presented a most interesting and astute discussion of the forces at play in litigation that tend to compromise the pristine nature of expert opinion. He noted:

> "The danger presented by expert witnesses, unlike the typical lay witness, is that experts have a financial interest in thorough preparation because they are paid for the time and they want to perform well so they will get hired again. Lawyers use their power of preparation to shape the expert's opinions. . . . Experts do shade their opinions, overstate the certainty of their opinions, use unreliable methodologies or rely on unproven theories, serve as conduits of inadmissible evidence and occasionally lie in the service of their clients. The financial incentive, when combined with the process of selection and preparation, is significant enough that even the most honorable expert is placed in a difficult dilemma." Perrin, *supra* note 3 at 1417–1420.

anyone who has an interest in the perhaps quaint notion that the product of the legal process is "truth."[62] Even so, the implication that honest and truthful testimony is necessarily inconsistent with advocacy is troubling. Consider the converse: Does indifference (both to the use put to testimony by the attorneys and to the ultimate result in the case) somehow enhance the truthfulness of the testimony? My belief is that an honest and truthful expert can have confidence in the strength of the opinion and the righteousness of the cause. If so, one should testify strongly and without fear that he or she is crossing any ethical line.

Accordingly, I think that the ethical admonition to avoid advocacy refers to improper influences on thinking as opposed to the ardency with which opinions are stated. In other words, *advocacy* implies that an expert has aligned himself or herself with a party or position for improper reasons such as financial incentives. Such influences on the bases for expert opinion therefore would be unethical. Ardent expressions of opinion that are not tainted by improper influence would not run afoul of the ethical precept. Obsequiousness does not suggest objectivity. Passion does not imply improper bias.[63]

Much more can be said about the ethics of expert testimony, and particularly about biases associated therewith. This chapter is confined to a description of the system as it exists and to suggest strategies for working therein. Temptations exist for lawyers and experts alike. Ethical and conscientious participants in the legal process must be aware of the temptations, be sensitive to their effects on judgment, and fight to retain their integrity. This process should improve the quality of expert participation in the legal process. However, sensitivity to ethical conflict should not obscure the importance of the expert's involvement in the legal process. Legal disputes are becoming ever more complex, and their resolution requires the involvement of experts. Honest and conscientious experts should not abandon the courtroom out of the fear of temptation.

---

[62] One of the frustrating aspects of this debate is the utter absence of data on the impact of expert witness practices on the fact finders. One would think that an issue of major significance is whether juries fall prey to unsavory practices, and whether "injustice" (i.e., inaccurate verdicts) is the result. Instead we get polemics who wail about the state of things without proving their point:

> "Remarkably the debate over expert witness testimony has been argued without much reference to reliable information about the jury. Instead, commentators have often relied on personal experience, intuition, and anecdotal evidence, rather than empirical research." *Id.* at 1426.

And:

> "The criticism of the use of expert witnesses in the courts as junk science has itself lacked scientific rigor. Attacks on expert witnesses in the popular press and recent books have relied upon anecdotal evidence." Daniel W. Shuman, Elizabeth Whitaker, & Anthony Champagne, An Empirical Examination of the Use of Expert Witnesses in the Courts—Part II: A Three City Study, 34 *Jurimetrics J.* 193, 194 (1994).

[63] The distinction between improper influences of the *formulation* of opinion, and appropriate passion in the *expression* of opinion is admittedly only one aspect of the ethics of expert testimony. Perhaps an even more common problem are the honest experts with a strong "philosophical bent" that influences their view of matters and of their testimony. "You can typically find people who will take reasonable and sometimes very unreasonable positions out of honest conviction." Michael Tigar et al., The Use and Misuse of Expert Evidence in the Courts, 77 *Judicature* 68, 73 (1993). This may be much more difficult to deal with on cross-examination than simple financial bias. Related to this is the problem of "seduction" of the expert through interaction with the attorney as part of the preparation process. John S. Applegate, Witness Preparation, 68 *Tex. L. Rev.* 277 (1989). See also, Gross, *supra* note 1.

Chapter 105

Injury Prevention: A Responsibility of All Health Care Professionals

L. Don Lehmkuhl

The numbers tell the tale—injury is the leading cause of death of persons younger than 25 years. More than 150,000 Americans are killed annually, over 500,000 become permanently disabled each year, and more than 10 million are temporarily disabled (1). The cost to society is about $500 million per day (2). That translates into a major public health problem!

Many health professionals are frustrated by the lack of public recognition of this problem and a lack of public support for attempts to address the problem. The very large numbers tend to cloud the ability to appreciate the significance of the issues. What is the significance of 42,000 deaths from automobile crashes every year (3)? When expressed on a daily basis, it is an average of 115 deaths a day (the crash of a major airliner with a full load of passengers—all of whom are killed—every day of the year!). Such a death toll occurring in the airline industry is unlikely to be written off as a series of "unavoidable accidents."

Perhaps the highway carnage has been so common for so long that the public is no longer sensitive to the issue. Would the societal impact of injury be any stronger if it were considered from a broader perspective, for example, the *years of life lost*? How does trauma stack up with other acknowledged major public health problems in terms of the cumulative years of life lost when the life expectancy of the deceased is calculated (Fig. 105-1)? Unintentional injury (the so-called accident) alone results in more years of life lost than any of the other major public health problems listed (last bar in the chart), and combining intentional (suicide, homicide) and unintentional injury results in a total for years of life lost that exceeds the total for all the other public health problems combined (1). Yet, the funding provided for research to study and alleviate these problems is grossly skewed in favor of problems other than those caused by trauma (Fig. 105-2). Given these data, only one conclusion is tenable: *Trauma is a major public health problem that has an impact on our society significantly greater than the impacts of other public health problems that receive significantly more recognition and resources.*

What is currently being done to address this major public health problem? The primary efforts appropriately have been directed at the treatment of the physical injury itself. In general, advances in the initial care and rehabilitation of injured persons have significantly reduced mortality and improved the outcome of those injured. The underlying cellular responses to injury are being studied so that the knowledge can be used to treat injured patients more effectively in the future. The recent emphasis on system development is contributing to improved early care of injured persons. Regional model system programs have been funded by the National Institute on Disability and Rehabilitation Research (U.S. Department of Education) to demonstrate improved care and rehabilitation of persons with spinal cord injury, brain injury, and burns. Members of the American Academy of Physical Medicine and Rehabilitation and the American Congress of Rehabilitation Medicine have played a major role in these

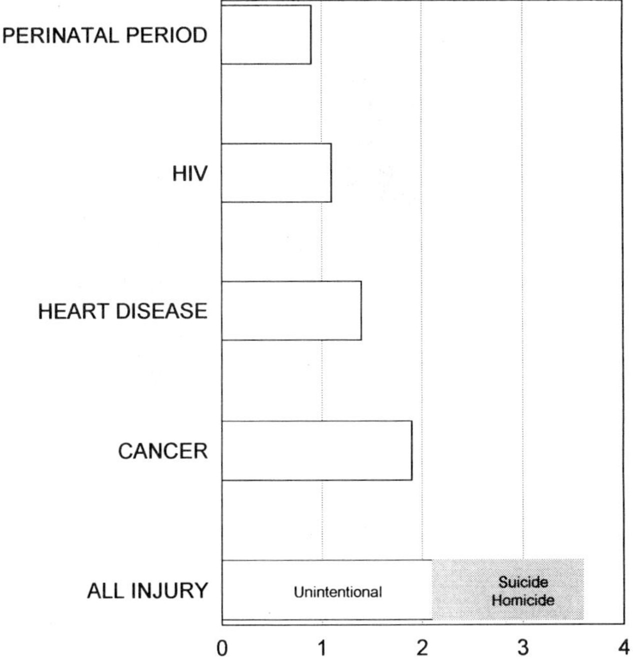

Figure 105-1. Comparison of estimated years of potential life lost following death by major causes of mortality in the United States during 1994. (Modified from National Center for Health Statistics. *Report of final mortality statistics.* MSVR 1995;45(Suppl. 2):1–80.)

advances through their direct involvement in education, system development, acute care, rehabilitation, and research. Additional improvements in the technology of trauma care, including improvements in the systemic support of injured patients ranging from prehospital care to extensive and sophisticated techniques in the intensive care unit, can be expected in the future.

Over the past 20 years, a small, but significant reduction in injury-related deaths has been achieved. That reduction has been comparable to the reduction in deaths from other public health problems, such as cancer, cerebrovascular disease, and heart disease (3). The absolute number of automobile deaths in this country declined from 19.2 deaths per 100,000 population in 1986 to 15.8 in 1996 (4).

Although there is good reason to be proud of the efforts and progress in reducing death rates from motor vehicular crashes, thus far, the reduction in the death rate has been less than 20% in 90 years (5). For deaths associated with traumatic brain injury, the rate declined from 24.6 per 100,000 U.S. residents in 1979 to 19.3 in 1992 (6). However, not all causes of death are declining. Firearm-related brain injuries leading to death increased 13% from 1984 through 1992, undermining a 25% decline in motor vehicle–related rates for the same period. This trend shown by the ascending slope of the line in Figure 105-3 is particularly alarming. Firearms surpassed motor vehicles as the largest single cause of death associated with traumatic brain injury in the United States (6). These data highlight the success of efforts to prevent traumatic brain injury due to motor vehicles and the failure to prevent such injuries due to firearms. A recent *60 Minutes* television program focused on guns in schools and the increasing use of guns. There is no question that violence is increasing and that it is a major public health problem. In addition, the incidence of *nonfatal* injuries is increasing. The local news in virtually every city in the country has stories of citizens being injured by "accidents" and violence of every sort. Thus, trauma is a major public health problem, but despite improvements in patient care and trauma systems, our impact on trauma is much less than desired. The question is, What can be done about it?

There are at least two aspects to addressing a major public health problem. First, the injured person must receive timely and appropriate treatment; but more importantly, the incidence of the problem must be reduced. The poliomyelitis epidemics of the 1940s and 1950s had a severe impact on young, healthy people in our society. The fear of death or muscle paralysis from the poliovirus was widespread. Although the treatment of those patients was crucial, this particular public health problem was controlled and largely eliminated by developing an effective vaccine. No vaccine can eliminate trauma, but changing the behaviors of persons at highest risk for encountering trauma can have a substantial impact on reducing the incidence of injury.

There is a growing national interest in injury prevention, and many professional groups are taking leadership roles. The question to be answered by the reader is whether those working in the field of physical medicine and rehabilitation should become more active in injury prevention, or leave it to others with more expertise. Perhaps the decision can be made more easily if certain information is supplied and pondered first. What is meant by *injury prevention*? How is it done? Does it work? These questions can be addressed by considering some of the misconceptions about injury prevention (Table 105-1).

Virtually all "accidents" are preventable; therefore, nearly all injuries that result from accidents are preventable. Many of the leaders in injury prevention have advocated not using the term *accident* in describing and reporting incidents that result in injury. For example, the term *motor vehicle accident* should become *motor vehicle crash* (a language change) to discourage the concept of inevitability. However, the prevention of injury goes far beyond chang-

Figure 105-2. Comparison of estimated Federal support from research into the leading causes of death and disability during 1984. (Adapted from Committee on Trauma Research, Commission on Life Sciences, National Research Council of the Institute of Medicine. *Injury in America.* Washington, DC, National Academy Press, 1985, p. 14.)

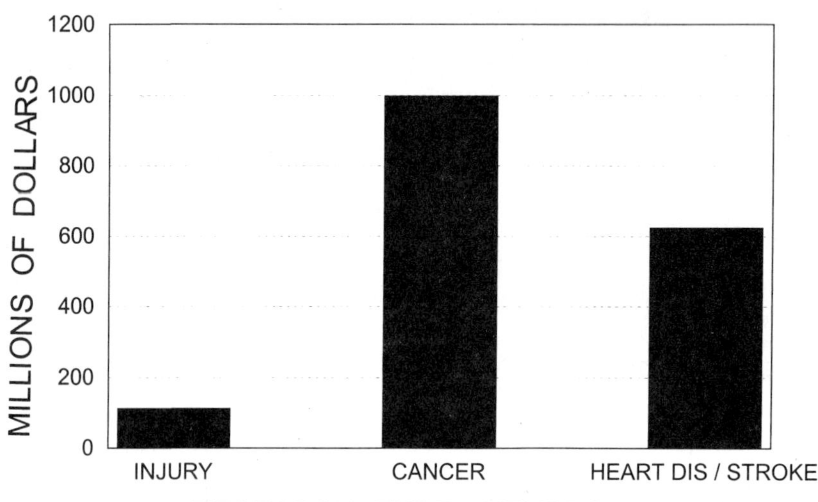

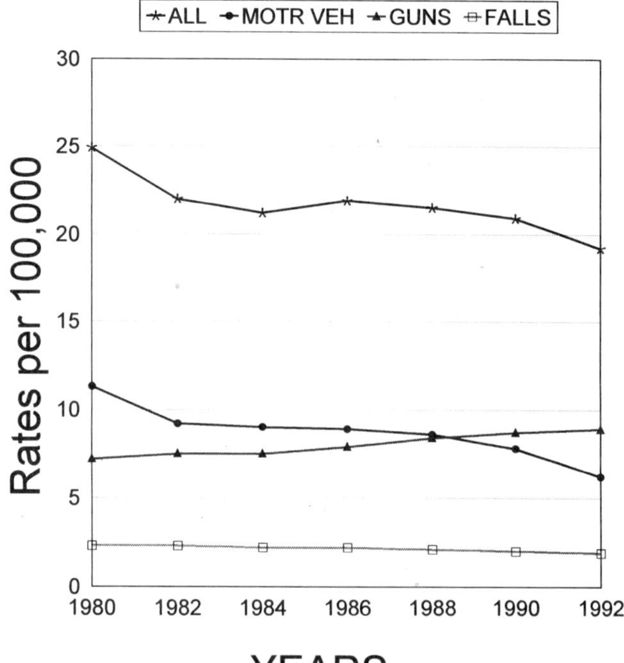

Figure 105-3. Trends of U.S. death rates from traumatic brain injury caused by different types of events. Note the increasing death rate from gunshot wounds to the head. (Source: Sosin DM, Sniezek JE, Waxweiler RJ. Trends in death associated with traumatic brain injury, 1979 through 1992: success and failure. JAMA 1995;273:1778–1780.)

Table 105-1: Misconceptions Regarding Injury Prevention
Accidents are not preventable.
Current efforts are not successful.
The paradigm to prevent injury is entirely different from traditional paradigms.
There are serious conflicts with civil rights.

ing the language used and prevention of the primary incident.

Primary prevention is directed at preventing the occurrence (of the incident), that is, prevention of the car crash, prevention of the burn, and prevention of the fall. A careful study of the factors that led up to the incident can identify antecedent behaviors that contributed to the person being in the particular situation that resulted in injury. The solution then is to help ensure that the environment and contributing behaviors are modified to preclude the incident. For example, erect stop signs at dangerous intersections; enforce speed limit laws; improve the design of tires to reduce stopping distance. If, despite these efforts the incident does occur, injury prevention does not end.

Secondary prevention consists of the steps taken to prevent further injury subsequent to the primary incident. Examples of this include using seat belts, helmets, car seats, sprinkler systems, and flame-retardant pajamas for children. When a crash occurs, the impact on the head of a cyclist is lessened by the presence of a helmet.

Tertiary prevention involves members of the health

Table 105-2: General Approach to Public Health

Define the problem
  Data collection
Identify the cause
  Risk factor identification
Develop and test interventions
  Evaluation research
Implement and monitor effectiveness
  Community intervention programs
  Training
  Public awareness

Source: Modified from Waxweiler RJ, Rosenberg ML, Fenley MA. *Injury control in the 1990's—a national action plan.* Atlanta: Centers for Disease Control and Prevention, 1993.

Table 105-3: Inclusive System Approach to Injury

Problem	Empiric Management	Establish Mechanisms	Specific Approaches
Societal	Evolving	Early attempts	Primary, secondary prevention
Physical injury	Usually successful (except heart, central nervous system)	Some information	Secondary, tertiary prevention
Organ system response	Physiologic support, intensive care unit	Ongoing	Total parenteral nutrition, cardiopulmonary support, dialysis
Cellular, molecular	Early attempts	Ongoing	Chemically binding free radicals released from injured cells

professions who use special techniques and interventions to prevent death and minimize disability when the injury does occur—precisely what trauma systems have focused on in recent years.

Integrating these primary, secondary, and tertiary approaches has the potential to prevent many of the injuries and to reduce their severity. Abundant evidence has been accumulated to refute the statement that current efforts are not successful. They have produced an absolute decrease as well as a relative decrease (deaths per 100,000 population) in motor vehicle mortality throughout the United States (4–7). A similar decrease in bicycle and motorcycle injuries has occurred (8,9). A decrease in deaths from burn injuries was recently documented, as was an impressive decrease in the number of burn injuries—resulting from a combination of public education, legislation, and environmental modification (10).

This brings us to the next concern: The traditional paradigms used in addressing infectious disease problems are difficult to apply to the problem of injury prevention. The principles, however, are still applicable and are listed in Table 105-2. Although injury prevention is a multifactorial problem, and although many of the approaches to injury prevention are more complex than the administration of a vaccine, the approach permits a progressive reduction of the problem to specific issues. The method permits interventions to be developed and tested, with ongoing assessment to identify other problems that can be subsequently evaluated. Throughout, the following criteria should be considered: 1) the problem being selected should be a significant one, 2) the approach used should be of proven effectiveness, 3) the approach should be appropriate to the population at risk, and 4) the outcome should be measurable.

In their proposal for injury control in the 1990s, the participants in the workshops of the Third National Injury Control Conference identified areas in which significant emphasis is appropriate (Table 105-3) (5). Many of these are problems for which progress has been made but for which there is a need to expand such efforts.

There are at least three ways to address injury prevention issues: education, legislation, and environmental modifications (or automation). Education (although slow, with some losing patience) is effective over the long term and helps to provide support for legislation. For example, educating the public on the advisability of using seat belts has been very successful. Youngsters, in particular, have been indoctrinated in the need to "buckle up" so that it becomes a habit each time they sit in a vehicle. Children are quick to remind their parents and grandparents to fasten their seat belts. Some of the recommendations regarding prevention of injury lead to the last concern—whether efforts directed at injury control will adversely affect the civil rights of some citizens. For example, some motorcycle riders contend that the government has no right to require them to wear a helmet—if they become injured, they are hurting no one but themselves. The counterargument is that a motorcyclist in a coma with serious brain injuries nearly always draws on the financial resources of the local government to obtain necessary medical and rehabilitation services (11). Wearing a helmet at the onset of the crash significantly reduces mortality and morbidity, thereby reducing the tax dollars needed to provide services (12).

When education is effective, legislatively required automation such as fire sprinklers, passenger restraints, helmets, and better automobile construction are no longer perceived as an invasion of civil rights. Rather, support of such legislation becomes an *expression* of our civil rights. Some problems are of such significance that we have to realize where our civil rights stop and where the good of society starts. The enforcement of speed limits, limits on how much a person can drink before driving, limits on whether a person can assault someone for saying something offensive—all of these have an impact on our civil rights, but they are crucial to society. In a healthy society the citizens relinquish some of their civil rights in order to protect their ability to live together safely.

Thus far, we have established that trauma is a major public health problem with appropriate means to promote injury prevention. Furthermore, injury prevention not only is a reasonable concept but also is *practical, applicable, and crucial.* The question is, What do we need to do as a profession and as an organization? Consider what might be gained for the public good if a fourth aspect were added to our thinking about the prevention of injury. In addition to treating the patient, *why not treat society? We need to address societal issues*! Until now, the efforts at dealing with societal issues have been empiric; the expertise of others is needed to gain understanding of the mechanisms operating to promote incidents that cause injuries. Health professionals must lend their support to efforts that focus on primary and secondary prevention as well as tertiary prevention.

It would be appropriate for members of the American Academy of Physical Medicine and Rehabilitation and the American Congress of Rehabilitation Medicine, and other health care professional societies, to play a major role in promoting and facilitating primary and secondary prevention of injury. As already indicated, some people may ask, Why should we become involved in an area where we have limited expertise? Why not leave that up to others with more expertise and continue to focus on treating patients and developing acute care systems and long-term care systems? The answers are multiple. The system now promoting injury prevention does not have sufficient manpower or resources to move at a satisfactory rate and needs a catalyst to move it forward. A few members are acquiring the necessary expertise in injury prevention centers in Seattle, Chicago, San Diego, Houston, and other communities across the country and need assistance in melding the knowledge of injuries with the knowledge of epidemiology. In addition, rehabilitation clinicians know perhaps more than anyone, except patients, the pain, the suffering, and the devastation that occur from this epidemic and as a result, have the energy and motivation to address it. Despite some erosion in the image of medicine in the past several years, health professionals have the credibility to serve as spokespersons and influence those responsible for education, legislation, and automation regarding injury control and prevention.

The concept of a trauma system needs to be expanded to emphasize injury prevention, community involvement, public education, and professional education. The organizations to which health professionals belong should give more than "lip service" to supporting injury prevention. They should be encouraged to establish a standing committee on injury prevention. A strong cadre of individuals needs to be appointed to serve on this committee, with a specific charge to increase the education and participation of physiatrists and other rehabilitation specialists in injury prevention efforts, to increase the expertise of others inside and outside of the field, to support and collaborate with established programs throughout the country, and to develop programs for preparing physiatrists and other rehabilitation specialists to bridge the gap between patient care and societal care.

While most health care professionals may not currently have expertise in this area, some do have expertise and others are capable of developing it. Toward this end, a number of fellowships should be created, specifically designed to prepare physiatrists and other rehabilitation specialists to earn a master's degree in public health and thus prepare them to participate actively in a societal approach to injury prevention.

In summary, trauma is a major public health problem in terms of cost, individual suffering, and societal damage. Acute care and rehabilitation are essential, and physiatrists and other rehabilitation specialists should continue their efforts in supporting acute care and rehabilitation research, but providing services only to the injured person is not sufficient. Work needs to continue toward an inclusive system in terms of geographic breadth, severity of injury, and the means to address both death and disability. Injury control and injury prevention are crucial to address this major public health problem. Professional organizations to which health professionals belong can play a major positive role in addressing this issue before injury consumes an even greater portion of the national economy. Health professionals in the field of physical medicine and rehabilitation have direct knowledge of the impact of the injury epidemic on individuals and families, as well as the motivation and energy to initiate change. They have a record of accomplishments and credibility that will allow them to be a major voice in addressing this major public health issue.

REFERENCES

1. Anderson RN, Kochanek K, Murphy SL. Report of final mortality statistics, 1995. *Monthly Vital Stat Rep* 1997;45(suppl 2, no. 11):7.
2. Rice DP, MacKenzie EJ. *Cost of injury in the United States: a report to Congress.* San Francisco: California Institute for Health and Aging, University of California Injury Prevention Center, The Johns Hopkins University, 1989:65–85.

3. Baker SP. Injuries in relation to other health problems. In: Baker SP, ed. *The injury fact book.* Lexington, MA: DC Heath, 1992: chapt 2:8–16.

4. National Highway Traffic Safety Administration, U.S. Department of Transportation. *Traffic safety facts, 1996.* Washington, D.C.: National Center for Statistics and Analysis, 1996:4

5. Waxweiler RJ, Rosenberg ML, Fenley MA. *Injury control in the 1990's—a national action plan.* Atlanta: Centers for Disease Control and Prevention, 1993.

6. Sosin DM, Sniezek JE, Waxweiler RJ. Trends in death associated with traumatic brain injury, 1978 through 1992: success and failure. *JAMA* 1995;273: 1778–1780.

7. Rutledge RR, Lalor A, Oller I, et al. The cost of not wearing seat belts: A comparison of outcomes in 3396 patients. *Ann Surg* 1992;217:122.

8. Fleming NS, Becker ER. The impact of the Texas 1989 Motorcycle Helmet Law on total and head-related fatalities, severe injuries and overall injuries. *Med Care* 1992:832–845.

9. Sacks J, Holmgreen P, Smith SM, et al. Bicycle-associated head injuries and deaths in the United States from 1984 through 1988: How many are preventable? *JAMA* 1991;266:3016–3018.

10. BurKe JF. From desperation to skin regeneration: Progress in burn treatment. *J Trauma* 1990; 30(suppl):S36–40.

11. Rivara FP, Dicker BG, Bergman AB, et al. The public cost of motorcycle trauma. *JAMA* 1988;260:221–223.

12. Kraus JS, Peek C, McArthur OL, Williams A. The effect of the 1992 Motorcycle Helmet Use Law on motorcycle crash fatalities and injuries. *JAMA* 1994;272: 1506–1511.

Chapter 106

Introduction to Clinical Research

Steven R. Hinderer
Kathleen A. Hinderer

The importance of clinical research for the field of medical rehabilitation has been emphasized by multiple authors (1–5). The recent Institute of Medicine report (6) provides an excellent comprehensive review of the current state of medical rehabilitation research and key areas that should be emphasized in the future to move the field foward. Fuhrer (7) provides further motivation to conduct research, regarding the potential of outcome research for supporting medical rehabilitation clinical practices.

The many reasons for conducting clinical research vary from proving and improving clinical care efficacy, determining the cost-effectiveness of interventions for marketing purposes as well as for making budget and staffing decisions, to promoting faculty and academic growth in departments and institutions. Regardless of the reasons why research is ultimately pursued, a critical issue is to determine why more medical rehabilitation professionals do not actively initiate or participate in clinical research studies. The most frequently cited obstacles to research are (in descending order) lack of funding, lack of nonfinancial research resources, lack of collaborators, lack of administrative support, lack of protected time, and limited knowledge of research techniques (8). An additional issue we observed and experienced is limited availability of participants from the specific disability populations of interest. The purpose of this chapter is to address each of these barriers to conducting clinical research with the hope that the discussion provided will assist you to better pursue your own research endeavors.

FUNDING OPPORTUNITIES

Finding Funding Sources

In many instances, conducting quality research without funding is impossible. The dilemma faced by investigators is that successful applications for external funding require preliminary data supporting the potential value of their proposed large-scale study; that is, often some of the research must already be done in order for it to get funded. Fortunately, there are some sources of seed funding available to generate pilot results as a basis for submitting a large external funding proposal to support the primary project.

Many universities and large health care institutions have seed grant funds that are available to their affiliated faculty and staff. Such grants typically offer a few to several thousand dollars to carry out pilot projects as a catalyst for generating larger competitive submissions for external funding. These funds are typically administrated through the office of the dean of the medical school or the chief administrator for grants and contracts of the institution. The advantage of applying for "internal" funding is that there is less competition for these funds than for external funds. The disadvantage is that the reviewers are often unfamiliar with the issues, importance, and potential for external funding of research pertaining to medical rehabilitation, and therefore may not recommend funding the proposal even though it has scientific merit.

The National Institute of Child Health and Human

Development (NICHD) recently developed a small grant program (RO3) to specifically support pilot research projects. Applications are submitted to, and directly reviewed by, the National Center for Medical Rehabilitation Research (NCMRR). These awards cannot exceed a total of $35,000 per year, and support immediate research costs only, that is, supplies, travel, small equipment up to $2000 per year, and "appropriate" other expenses. Salary support cannot be requested on RO3 applications (9).

Another source of start-up grant funds is the Young Physiatrist Award given through the American Academy of Physical Medicine and Rehabilitation. Applications are due each July lst and one person is awarded $5000. Applicants must be physical medicine and rehabilitation residents, fellows, or attendings, age 35 or younger. A similar program, the New Investigator Awards, is funded by the Physical Medicine and Rehabilitation Education and Research Fund administered through the American Academy of Physical Medicine and Rehabilitation. Applicants must be either a resident in an accredited physiatric training program or a physiatrist who is no more than 5 years beyond completion of postgraduate training. Two applicants per year are awarded $5000 for research activities with "no strings attached" (10).

Some medical rehabilitation facilities are fortunate enough to have internal endowment funds to support clinical research activities. Applications for these funds are typically limited to faculty and staff working at the facility, although outside collaborators can be enlisted as coinvestigators. The highest priority typically is given to projects with strong scientific merit and potential for leading to larger external funding applications.

Once an investigator has pilot data demonstrating the potential merit for conducting a larger-scale study, then target source(s) of external funding should be identified. The federal government has been a longstanding source of such funds through different agencies (5). The Centers for Disease Control and Prevention (CDC) has expanded its focus on injury prevention to include biomechanics, unintentional injury prevention, acute care, and prevention of secondary conditions in people with disabilities. The NCMRR, via the R, K, and T grant programs of the National Institutes of Health (NIH), prioritizes research on improving functional mobility, behavioral adaptation to disability, whole-body system responses to catastrophic injury/illnesses, adaptive technology, measurement and assessment methods, epidemiology, and treatment effectiveness. The National Institute on Disability and Rehabilitation Research (NIDRR), which is under the U.S. Department of Education, funds projects on engineering technology, promotion of employment, community integration, independent living initiatives, and policy issues, as well as the Model Systems institutional grants for burn injury, spinal cord injury, and traumatic brain injury. The Department of Veterans Affairs (VA) Rehabilitation Research and Development program funds a multitude of research initiatives with special emphasis on prosthetics and orthotics and assistive technologies. The VA also has an independent investigator program (Merit Review) available for individuals who hold at least a 60% appointment at a VA Medical Center. The grant and contracts office at most universities maintains a listing of these and other funding sources and can assist investigators with contacting specific agencies to find out about the nature of past projects funded, current funding priorities (and interest in your chosen topic), and acquisition of application materials. Often, this office also circulates a newsletter listing recent research funding announcements and deadlines. Consequently, it is worthwhile for medical rehabilitation researchers to be on this mailing list at their respective institutions.

An additional mechanism for identifying potential funding agencies is via the Internet. Most foundations and organizations that fund medical rehabilitation research have Web sites listing information regarding their research priorities and methods to obtain application materials. The Foundation Center (79 Fifth Avenue, New York, NY 10003-3076; Tel: (212) 620-4230; Fax: (212) 691-1828; Web site: http://www.fdncenter.org) is a resource organization for regional, national, and international directories of grantmakers, receivers of grants, funded topics, proposal writing courses, and so on. This organization offers electronic and printed publications as well as frequent updates on their Web site. It also offers free membership to an Internet list server, which includes the weekly publication *Philanthropy News Digest.*

Writing a Funding Proposal

Much has been written regarding the art and science of grant writing (11,12). The reader is encouraged to refer to available texts, to consult experienced grant writers, or to attend workshops to learn application preparation skills. A discussion of the basic content of a research grant proposal follows and is summarized in Table 106-1 (13).

The *title* should be short and attractive. Most importantly, it should be informative regarding the issues to be addressed by the project.

The *abstract* provides a succinct description of the background, significance, specific aims, methods, setting, and resources and capabilities of the investigators and the institution for carrying out the proposed research. The abstract is often the first part of the proposal read by reviewers; therefore, it is important to provide a positive initial impression as a basis for the rest of the review. Remember, the reviewers are reading multiple proposals, and yours must somehow stand out from the others.

The *background* section provides a generic statement of the practical or theoretical problems or issues that the proposed research will address. This statement must then be supported by a review of the literature that critically evaluates existing knowledge, and identifies missing information that the proposed project will provide.

Table 106-1: General Grant Proposal Outline

1. Cover page
2. Abstract
3. Table of contents
4. Introduction and review of the literature
   A. The problem
   B. Review of the literature (including ongoing work by other investigators)
   C. Review of the current practice in the field
   D. Background—earlier work done by the investigator(s) in this area
   E. Rationale for the proposed work (theoretical, underpinning/justification)
   F. Significance (contribution to knowledge, practical and applied benefits, meaning/impact of outcomes, limitations)
5. Specific aims (major issue/question/hypothesis to be pursued)
6. Method—project plan
   A. Overall design (groups, procedures, etc—overview)
   B. Instruments/techniques to be used (scientific basis, reliability/validity)
   C. Subjects (sample selection, sample size, etc)
   D. Data to be collected (format, quality, storage, error checking/correction, etc)
   E. Data analysis (statistical techniques) and interpretation
   F. Approach to control for potential pitfalls, biases, discrepant findings, measurement errors, sample losses, limitations, technical difficulties
   G. Time schedule, task list
   H. Facilities available (office/laboratory/clinical space, equipment, study population, consultants, computers, personnel)
   I. Applicant description
   J. Management and dissemination plan
7. Human subjects protection issues
8. Budget
   A. Direct costs
      (1) Salaries, percent functional time equivalent, fringes
      (2) Consultant fees, subject payments
      (3) Equipment
      (4) Supplies (copying, office, telephone, etc)
      (5) Travel (local to conduct research, national meetings to present results)
   B. Indirect costs
   C. Budget justification
9. Appendices
   A. Curricula vitae of investigators
   B. Letters of cooperation from other institutions and consultants
   C. Subcontracts (e.g., to pharmacy for drug studies)
   D. Details of measurement tools
   E. Details of facilities available
   F. Bibliography

The *significance* section is a description of the proposed work in terms of the benefit the knowledge to be acquired will provide for practice issues (e.g., improved treatment or epidemiologic data to support the causes of policy makers), or for better understanding of the underlying mechanisms of observed clinical phenomena (e.g., the relationship between strength changes and functional task performance). In the specific case where the research funding proposal is submitted in response to an agency-selected priority, this section should also include a discussion of how the project addresses this priority.

The *specific aims/hypotheses/research question* section gives a concise statement of the exact question(s) the research will answer, or the specific hypotheses that will be tested. Some or all of the aims, hypotheses, or research questions should relate to the broader long-term goals specified in the background and significance section.

The *work plan* is a description of how the investigative team will go about implementing the research. The work plan should include subject selection criteria; equipment and space requirements; research design; procedures for data collection; methods for data analysis and dissemination; a time table for key events; the staff needed to carry out tasks and assignment of responsibilities; the consultants, collaborators, or consortia needed to conduct the research; and the available resources at the institution that will be used to conduct the project.

A description of the *human subjects* who will participate in the research study needs to be provided (if not described previously) and to include recruitment plans, consent procedures, risks, procedures for protection against or minimizing risks/pain, procedures for providing care of injury that does occur, reimbursement (if any will be provided), and status of the Institutional Review Board (IRB) application (virtually all funding sources require IRB approval before funds will be disbursed for a project).

The *budget and budget justification* should give an overview of the anticipated research costs by major categories including personnel salaries/fringe benefits, equipment, supplies, travel, consultants/consortium, and indirect costs (if allowed by the funding agency). A detailed explanation should be provided for any cost items that are not completely self-explanatory.

Many funding agencies have a specific format for structuring funding applications that they expect to be followed and may include sections not described above. All required specifications, directions, forms, and so on should be carefully completed to ensure the proposal will be reviewed favorably.

Prior to submitting the proposal, you should have as many colleagues as possible read it and provide critical feedback. This requires you to have a "thick skin" since you will undoubtedly labor hard to pull together the proposal, and will find it challenging to accept someone else tearing it apart. Such feedback, however, is invaluable and serves to substantially strengthen the proposal and your chances of being funded. Seeking such feedback does not obligate you to incorporate all the suggestions made, but allows someone with a "fresh" perspective to react to your proposal, much as the reviewers will. It also has the side benefit of letting others know what your research interests are.

NONFINANCIAL RESOURCES REQUIRED FOR RESEARCH

Research Space

One of the most common constraints experienced by medical rehabilitation researchers is the lack of available space to conduct their studies without interruption, at times and locations that are convenient and accessible for the study participants and that allow for control of the study environment to limit the effect of other factors that can influence study results. The optimal situation is dedicated space in proximity to medical rehabilitation patient treatment areas, so that individuals who are already coming in for therapies can conveniently also participate in research protocols. Unfortunately, such space is often unavailable or is inconveniently located for access by study participants with physical disabilities. In most such situations, negotiating a compromise with the physical medicine and rehabilitation departmental administrator(s) responsible for space allocation and use is the best solution to the problem. Typically, physician outpatient clinic rooms have some "down time" during normal business hours on weekdays when research data collection can be scheduled. Depending on the size of the room and the equipment needed, it is often feasible to leave the room set up for data collection without interfering with its use for patient care, or at least research equipment can be stored nearby so that setup is quickly facilitated. An alternative venue for conducting research is to use therapy treatment areas, especially physical therapy booth space, during hours when such space is not being maximally utilized for clinical care (e.g., early morning, noon hour, or late afternoon). We have also observed situations where investigators have converted their own (or their chairperson's) office into a temporary research laboratory. Sometimes it is beneficial to seek a collaborator who has space available in his or her department (see discussion on finding collaborators). A less optimal, but occasionally workable solution is to schedule data collection during evenings or weekends when space availability is greatest. Unfortunately, this may limit the number of research participants who are available or willing to participate during "odd" hours. It has been our experience, however, that if there is sufficient potential benefit to the individual to participate, and especially if some sort of incentive is provided (e.g., donated prizes for children, or monetary reimbursement from grant funds for adults), people are often quite willing to avail themselves to less desirable times for research participation. Obviously, conducting research during evenings and weekends has implications and stresses for the investigators that must be contended with as well.

Equipment

A second important nonfinancial resource often required to conduct research is equipment. External funding agencies usually will not support laboratory development. With rare exception, it is expected that the investigator's institution will provide the facilities to conduct the proposed research. An example of an exception would be a submission for funding by an investigator with a strong track record in a given area of study, who could further advance his or her work with the addition of a new piece of hardware or software. Unfortunately, most medical rehabilitation researchers are not yet at this phase of their academic careers.

Investigators who are seeking a new faculty position should negotiate with the chairperson for both space and equipment needs. The chairperson often has access to "start-up" funds for laboratory development administered through the dean of the medical school or research office of the institution. For investigators who are already established at an institution, universities often conduct periodic initiatives to purchase new equipment for their faculty on a competitive submission basis. These initiatives are sometimes cost sharing or cost matching; that is, the university will share or match the cost with the department purchasing the equipment, which requires the investigator to negotiate with the chairperson or find alternative sources (e.g., donations, indirect account funds from a grant) to fund the balance not covered by the university equipment fund. The computer used to write this chapter was purchased under such a program. Internal institutional grant funding sources, as described earlier under Funding Opportunities, can be a partial or complete source for funding the purchase of equipment. During the start-up phase of a research project, it is often possible to borrow needed equipment from internal departmental sources or from collaborators, and then gradually purchase your own equipment as funding sources become available.

Personnel

Another key nonfinancial resource often required by investigators is personnel to assist with conducting research studies. The complexity of data collection will determine the credentials, level of training, and experience that a research assistant must have for a given project. The number, qualifications, specific role, and availability of research assistants needed for the project should be determined prior to recruiting study participants. If grant funding is being sought, the cost of these personnel positions should be included in the budget. Ideally, a specific person should be identified for each position, with his or her advanced consent, as well as agreement by his or her supervisor to provide release time (purchased from the grant funds), to participate in the research project.

If grant funds are not available to support research assistant time, then volunteer participation must be sought.

Practicing clinicians are often unavailable due to other demands on their time. Allied health students are frequently willing to volunteer their assistance with data collection for the benefit of gaining exposure to patient populations or to fulfill research requirements for their didactic course work. Allied health faculty, who are often on an academic tenure track, welcome the opportunity to collaborate if the outcome of their participation includes coauthorship on a national presentation or a manuscript submitted for publication, or availability of laboratory facilities or patient populations that would otherwise be difficult for them to access for their own independent investigations. Resident physicians similarly are often willing research assistants if their participation will lead to submission of an abstract that, if accepted, will result in the department paying their expenses to a national meeting or lead to a published manuscript. Medical students and undergraduate preprofessional students can also make excellent volunteer research assistants, if they meet appropriate qualifications for such a role, in return for being able to list the research activity on their curriculum vitae or for a letter of recommendation. Collaborating colleagues may also be able to share in the responsibility of data collection.

FINDING COLLABORATORS

There are different potential reasons for seeking collaborators in a research study. As discussed earlier, there may be a need to share the responsibility for the various tasks required to conduct a study. Collaborators from other departments or institutions are sometimes sought to access a larger number of study participants from the population of interest. More often, collaborators are sought to strengthen the science of a research project by their prior reputation for productive work in a content area or by offering additional expertise regarding such issues as population demographics, research design, tests and measures appropriate to the application, database management, or statistical analysis and interpretation. An additional reason for inviting someone to collaborate is to gain political support for the results of the study (e.g., inviting a skeptic of a specific treatment technique to participate in a study that examines the effectiveness of that treatment).

A more overarching reason for collaborating is to find basic and clinical scientists outside of medical rehabilitation who are skilled at taking the clinical "truths" on which we often base daily decisions to develop a more generalized theoretical basis for such observations, as well as a plan for conducting serial studies that will build on previous work as a basis for proof, disproof, or modification of medical rehabilitation theory. Theory building and testing, which is a basic component of the scientific method, is largely lacking from formal research training or the ultimate "line of study" of medical rehabilitation investigators. Enlisting collaborators with strength in theory building and testing is essential to develop the scientific foundation that the field of medical rehabilitation so desperately needs and to incorporate these methods as a standard part of research education and process. The importance of theory building is discussed further in the last section of this chapter.

The purpose for which a collaborator is needed will determine, in part, where you should look to identify co-investigators for a project. The most convenient place to begin such a search is in your own department. Informal discussions with colleagues from the same discipline will make them aware of your research interests, provide valuable input to the project, and may lead to discovering that someone shares a strong interest with you for the study topic and wishes to join the project. Colleagues often will know of other professionals within and outside of medical rehabilitation, at your own or nearby institutions, who can make valuable contributions to the study, and by virtue of their geographic proximity, are more likely to collaborate. Contacting department heads or supervisors of the rehabilitation disciplines at your institution and other local institutions or allied health schools may also lead you to potential collaborators.

It is common for a research topic to require input from disciplines outside of medical rehabilitation. Clinical disciplines commonly involved with medical rehabilitation research include neurology, neurosurgery, orthopedics, rheumatology, and less often cardiology and pulmonology. Basic scientists including anatomists, neurophysiologists, kinesiologists (motor control, biomechanics, exercise physiology), and bioengineers may also need to be involved. Calling departmental offices, reading institutional newsletters, reading announcements for continuing education programs and attending those pertinent to your research interest, reviewing annual summaries of various departmental publications and presentations, and informally consulting your colleagues from other medical disciplines can help to locate collaborators who are best suited to support your project. Recruiting graduate students from other departments to participate in your project can be a wonderful bridge to develop long-term relationships with basic science faculty, while simultaneously providing a forum for students to complete their graduate research requirements, and concurrently assist you with the tasks required to conduct your research.

Collaborating with individuals who are not at your institution or geographically too far away to meet with you periodically to discuss the project can be challenging and may delay its progress considerably. With the recent advancements in electronic media for communication and efficient, economic transfer of data and documents long distance, such collaboration is becoming increasingly feasible. A review of the literature for your topic of interest will reveal potential collaborators at other institutions. Many of these investigators have access to e-mail for ongoing discussion of potential collaborative projects. Additionally, an increasing number of medical rehabilitation–related list servers (electronic special interest groups) are available to query for potential collaborators and general input on your project from experts (and novices) in the field. Table 106-2 provides a listing of these list servers and other pertinent Internet Web sites.

ADMINISTRATIVE SUPPORT

Grant Coordinators

An academic department that is actively engaged in research activities often has an administrative staff member who is familiar with the process for submitting and administering grants and contracts. If the department has sufficient grant funding to justify it, the "grant coordinator" may have a full-time administrative position within the physical medicine and rehabilitation department. The grant coordinator is involved with the granting process from initial submission of the application to final closure of the account for a funded project. Specific duties of this person typically include acquiring grant application materials; completion of cover forms required by the funding agency and the investigator's institutional grant and contracts office; development of the grant budget and budget justification; acquiring the necessary signatures on grant submission forms (e.g., department chairperson) and letters of support from coinvestigators, consultants, and groups being contracted to provide services to support the project; delivering the completed application packet and copies to the institution's grant and contracts office sufficiently in advance of the grant deadline and tracking it through the various processes and sign-offs that must occur to ensure that the institution is committed to support the project as proposed (this latter process often requires 5 working days to complete, thereby requiring the investigator to finish his or her components of the application a week in advance of the deadline); making the number of copies of the application required by the funding agency to distribute to the grant review committee; and finally mailing the completed application packet to the agency to arrive in advance of the deadline.

Clearly, the assistance of a skilled grant coordinator is an enormous time saver for investigators and makes the task of submitting a grant application much less formidable. If such a skilled individual is not immediately available in your department, other larger clinical departments often have a grant coordinator whose assistance can be utilized if a coinvestigator from that department is involved with the project. If your department does not have sufficient funding to support a full-time position, sharing the cost of a grant coordinator with another department requiring only part-time support might be feasible. When none of these alternatives is available, the administrative staff at the institution's grant and contracts office are almost always willing to assist the investigator with many of these tasks, and investigators submitting a grant should not hesitate to request such assistance. The jobs of grant coordinators and institutional grant and contracts administrative staff depend on the success of funding applications by investigators, which provides a strong impetus for them to have a vested interest in your project!

In addition to assisting with grant submissions, a grant coordinator is an important support person for investigators to administer their grant funds when a funding application is successful. Accounts must initially be set up to pay research assistants, consultants, contracting agencies who will provide services supporting the project, and subjects who participate in the study. All equipment and supplies purchased with grant funds must be carefully monitored. Periodic forms and updated spreadsheets must be submitted to your institution's grant and contracts office and the funding agency. Requirements for progress reports and noncompetitive and competitive renewal applications for the funding organization must be met. The process of expending and accounting for grant funds is labor-intensive, going beyond the time constraints and experience of most medical rehabilitation researchers. This further underscores the need for a grant coordinator's support through your department, a collaborator's department, or the institution's grant and contracts office. It is essential for investigators who plan to seek grant funding to identify who will provide this support before the process of developing the proposal begins.

Directors/Coordinators of Research

Many academic medical rehabilitation departments have an appointed director or coordinator of research. In 1994, the Association of Academic Physiatrists Board of Directors created a Council of Research Coordinators and Directors to facilitate interactions among these individuals. In many instances, these people are experienced researchers from outside the field of medical rehabilitation who have been involved in collaborative efforts with medical rehabilitation professionals, and have ultimately developed a commitment to research within this field. Others are medical rehabilitation professionals who have pursued research fellowships or graduate school training in research methods. There are multiple ways that these people help to foster research within their departments and institutions. Their continuance as principal investigators on projects in their areas of interest or concentration and their awareness of ongoing projects being conducted by other investigators provide opportunities for them to guide students with limited experience, and professionals with limited time, to become involved in ongoing research activities. Coordinators/directors of research often help submit grant proposals for predoctoral and postdoctoral research fellowships funded through NIDRR and NCMRR and then help to recruit and mentor fellows once funding for such positions is acquired. They can serve as advisors,

Table 106-2: Medical Rehabilitation Research–Related Internet List Servers and Web Sites

Physical medicine and rehabilitation
1. LISTPROC@UWASHINGTON.EDU—request subscribe PHYSIATRY
2. The Association of Academic Physiatrists (AAP) is in the process of developing one or more list servers which should be on line by the end of 1998.

Neuropsychology
1. REHABPSYCH@LISTS.ACS.OHIO-STATE.EDU
2. MAILBASE@MAILBASE.AC.UK—neuropsychology discussion
3. APASD-L@VTVM1.CC.VT.EDU—APA research psychology network
4. LISTSERV@MIZZOU1.MISSOURI.EDU—subscribe SCR-L
   Study of Cognitive Rehabilitation

Physical therapy
1. MAILBASE@MAILBASE.AC.UK—subscribe PHYSIO (therapy)
2. LISTSERV@CMUVM.CSV.CMICH.EDU—subscribe MIPTR (Michigan PT Association Research Special Interest Group)

Orthotics and prosthetics
1. LISTSERV@NERVM.NERDC.UFL.EDU—subscribe OANDP-L

Kinesiology
1. BIOMCH-L@NIC.SURFNET.NL—biomechanics
2. MAJORDOMO@STONEBOW.OTAGO.AC.NZ—subscribe SPORTSCI
   Science to enhance performance in sports
3. GRADEXP@SJSUVM1.SJSU.EDU—graduate exercise physiology

Neuroscience
1. MAILSERV@AC.DAL.CA—subscribe NEURO1-L
2. NEUROMOTOR-REQUEST@AI.MIT.EDU
3. LISTSERV@MAELSTROM.STJOHNS.EDU—subscribe NEUROMUS
   Neuromuscular research and information list

Speech pathology
1. AUDITORY@MCGILL1.BITNET—research in auditory perception
2. AUDITORY@VM1.MCGILL.CA—research in auditory perception

Rehabilitation engineering/assistive technology
1. BIOREP-L@NIC.SURFNET.NL—biotechnology research in the European Union
2. LISTSERV@MAELSTROM.STJOHNS.EDU—subscribe RESNA
   Only RESNA members can join.
3. LISTSERV@AMERICAN.EDU—subscribe ADAPT-L

Traumatic brain injury
1. LISTSERV@MAELSTROM.STJOHNS.EDU—subscribe TBI-PROF

Stroke
1. LISTSERV@UKCC.UKY.EDU—subscribe STROKE-L

Back pain
1. BACKS-L@LIST.UVM.EDU—research on low-back pain

Geriatrics/gerontology
1. LISTERV@UBVM.CC.BUFFALO.EDU—subscribe GERINET

Rheumatoid arthritis
1. OMERACT@NIC.SURFNET.NL—outcome measures in rheumatoid arthritis clinical trials

Orthopedics
1. LISTSERV@GAIT2.GAIT.OHIO-STATE.EDU—subscribe ORTHO-L

Multiple sclerosis
1. LISTSERV@TECHNION.TECHNION.AC.IL—subscribe MSLIST-L

Brain tumor research
1. LISTSERV@MITVMA.MIT.EDU—subscribe BRAINTMR

Research administration
1. LISTSERV@LIST.NIH.GOV—subscribe NIHGDE-L
   NIH guide to grants and contracts
2. LISTSERV@LIST.NIH.GOV—subscribe NIHTOC-L
   Table of contents for NIH guide
3. AIR-L@LISTSERV.VT.EDU—institutional researchers/university planners
4. CRPGE-L@MAINE.MAINE.EDU—council on research policy and graduate education
5. CRC-LIST@TC.UMN.EDU—clinical research coordinators discussion group

Outcomes research and comprehensive quality indicators of health care
1. CECSTALK@LISTSERV.DARTMOUTH.EDU

Medical education research and development
1. DR-ED@MSU.EDU

Table 106-2: *(Continued)*

2. AERA-D@ASUVM.INRE.ASU.EDU—American Educational Research Association measurement and research methodology

Research methods

1. 201TALK@LIST.UVM.EDU—research methods
2. ED502S98@LISTSERV.UIC.EDU—qualitative research

Research and disability

1. DISL@RYEVM.RYERSON.EDU

Disability/rehabilitation list services

1. www.eskimo.com/˜jlubin/disabled/listserv.htm

Web sites of organizations promoting research

1. www.aap.org
2. www.acrm.org
3. www.apta.org
4. www.aota.org
5. www.asha.org (American Speech-Language Hearing Association)
6. www.naric.com/naric (National Rehabilitation Information Center)
7. www.ncdrr.org/ (National Center for the Dissemination of Disability Research)
8. www.resna.org
9. www.trace.wisc.edu (Trace Research and Development—assistive technology)
10. www.lcweb.loc.gov/ (Library of Congress)
11. www.nlm.nih.gov/ (National Library of Medicine—free access to literature databases)
12. www.cdc.gov/cdc.html (Centers for Disease Control and Prevention)
13. www.ed.gov/offices/OSERS/NIDRR
14. www.va.gov (Department of Veterans Affairs)
15. www.nih.gov (NIH)
16. www.os.dhhs.gov (Department of Health and Human Services)
17. www.rehabnet.com
18. www.kin.ucalgary.ca/isb/ (International Society of Biomechanics)
19. www.sfn.org (Society for Neuroscience)

Web sites covering disability topics

1. Amputee—www.portal.ca/˜igregson/index.html
2. Alternative medicine—www.pitt.edu/˜cbw/altm.html
3. Arthritis Foundation—www.arthritis.org
4. Assistive technology—www.abledata.com
5. Biomechanics—www.kin.ucalgary.ca/isb/biomech-l.html
6. Cancer—www.cancer.med.upenn.edu
7. Communication disorders and sciences—www.mankato.msus.edu/dept/comdis/kuster2/welcome.html
8. Ergonomics—www.ergoweb.com/
9. Families and disability—www.kuhttp.cc.ukans.edu/cwis/units/LSI/beachhp.html
10. Gerontology and aging—www.iog.wayne.edu/GeroWebd/GeroWeb.html
11. Hydrocephalus, syringomyelia, spina bifida, and allied disorders—www.neurosurgery.mgh.harvard.edu/hyd-rsrc.htm
12. Incontinence—www.IncontiNet.com
13. Multiple sclerosis—www.aguila.com/dean.sporlender/ms_home
14. Muscular dystrophy—www.mda.org.au
15. Musculoskeletal
    a. www.arcade.uiowa.edu/hardin-www/md-ortho.html
    b. www.uhrad.com/msiarc.htm
    c. www.ortho.hmc.psu.edu/MRL.html (Musculoskeletal Research Laboratory)
16. Neuromuscular control—www.activemed.com/neuromus
17. Orthopedics
    a. www.bonehome.com/
    b. www.worldortho.com/
18. Parkinson disease—www.rio.com/˜jskaye/pd/index.html
19. Performing arts medicine—www.ithaca.edu/hsph/pt/pt1/
20. Physical medicine and rehabilitation
    a. www.lib.uiowa.edu/hardin-www/md
    b. www.gen.emory.edu/medweb/medweb.rehab.html
21. Physical therapy—www.mailbase.ac.uk/lists/physio/archive.html
22. Polio
    a. www.eskimo.com/˜empt/polio.html
    b. www.zynet.co.uk/ott/polio/lincolnshire
23. Prosthetics and orthotics—www.pele.repoc.nwu.edu/nupoc/nupoc.html
24. Spinal cord injury
    a. www.cureparalysis.org

Table 106-2: (*Continued*)

	b. www.neurosurgery.mbh.harvard.edu/spine˜hp.htm
	c. www.ncddr.org/mscis (Model SCICS System)
25.	Spinal Manipulation Research Group—www.cchs.usyd.edu.au/ESS/smrg/smrg.html
26.	Sports and exercise science—www.sportsci.org
27.	Statistical computing on the Internet—www.biomed.nus.sg/MSTAT/welcome.html
28.	Stroke
	a. www.stroke.org
	b. www.reg.uci.edu/cardiology/prevention/facts/treatment.html
29.	Traumatic brain injury
	a. www.calamer.com/˜cns/rehab/refs/html
	b. www.tbi.pmr.vcu.edu
30.	Wound care—www.medicaledu.com/wndcover.htm

consultants, or collaborators to help other investigators to develop research questions, designs, analyses, and dissemination plans. They provide critical analysis to improve grant submissions, manuscripts for publication, and presentation of research outcomes. They help to coordinate support (personnel, equipment, supplies, etc) for the ongoing research activities in the department. Teaching and coordination interdepartmental research conferences that provide a forum for presenting current research activities and in-service workshops on research methods are other important roles of these individuals. They can serve as external monitors of the progress of projects and as a conscience (i.e., friendly nag) for other investigators to remind them of key steps that must be completed to fulfill obligations to funding agencies, and other participants in the research process. It is our contention that having a coordinator or director of research who is given the necessary resources of time, space, funding, personnel, and authority to carry out his or her charge is an essential component for success of a departmental or institutional research program.

Library Services/Computer Internet Access

Literature reviews are an essential component to the research process. A librarian who is skilled with accessing different medical literature databases outside of standard Medline searches (e.g., Index Medicus on CD-ROM) and with software that can enhance Medline searches (e.g., Grateful Med and Paper Chase) and who is familiar with publications containing research that is pertinent to medical rehabilitation as well as with the efficient use of keywords to focus the search can save an investigator both the time and the embarrassment of being unfamiliar with other investigators' work in their area of interest. The ability to acquire references in a timely fashion, especially those not immediately available in the home institution's library (via interlibrary loan), is also an extraordinarily helpful support to investigators. Knowledge of search engines for Internet access to Web sites with pertinent information regarding specific research topics is quickly becoming another indispensable library support service for clinical researchers. It behooves investigators to identify where these services are available at their or their collaborator's institution.

The following are tips to help researchers who conduct their own literature searches to efficiently identify pertinent articles. Find an article with an interesting and relevant title to the topic of interest. Look at the references cited in the article. Identify experts in the field whose names can be searched for further relevant work. Stick with articles from major peer-reviewed journals. Print abstracts of articles with titles that appear to be pertinent and review them. Screen out those publications that clearly do not fit. Finally acquire the "short" list of articles that are pertinent and critically review them for quality of research methods and conclusions drawn from the data. Retain only those studies that are of good quality to guide your work.

Biostatistics Support

Researchers often consult a biostatistician to assist with data analysis. Unfortunately, this is frequently done after the data are collected. The time to initially consult a statistician is during the process of developing the research methods, prior to any data collection. The reason for early consultation with a statistician is to avoid errors and pitfalls that can ultimately compromise the validity of the results of the project. Biostatisticians offer expertise in research design as well as data analysis. They can be helpful with selection of the dependent (outcome) variables to be measured, thereby increasing the likelihood that the statistics used will detect change if it has occurred (decreasing the probability of a type II error). They can also assist with sample size estimates to ensure that an adequate number of subjects are recruited for the study. Most large universities or institutions have biostatistics departments. Consultation is provided for faculty and students at no charge, or at a discounted charge. The fees that will potentially be incurred from consultation with a statistician can be determined in advance and budgeted in grant proposals submitted to fund the project.

Media Support Services

Another valuable administrative resource is access to a media department. As desktop publishing software and hardware become more sophisticated, developing graphics and slides to present research results, or submitting figures with manuscripts for publication, has become more practical. Yet, a professional touch is still often needed for more complex graphics, to develop poster presentations, and to edit and process slide and graphics files developed by the investigators. Additionally, media departments often employ professional photographers who can obtain or duplicate quality pictures or videotapes that may be needed for either data collection or documentation of results. Most institutions and universities have media departments that will provide services to faculty and students. It is important to know how much lead time they require to provide specific services and how any costs are handled. If media services are not free, then it may be important to include anticipated costs in the grant proposal budget submitted to fund the project, especially if your department does not have funds budgeted for this purpose or access to media department staff who can do the work at no cost to the investigator.

Protected Time

Perhaps the most precious administrative resource is protected time to engage in research activities. In the report from the 1996 Association of Academic Physiatrists Research Summit (5), the following statement was made:

> Presently most young faculty have little protected time unless and until they achieve substantial research funding, creating a vicious cycle in which the chances of achieving funding remain low because of inadequate time to consolidate a research direction. It was generally felt that 40% protected time is required, with the balance being devoted to clinical work, administration, and teaching. Up to five years of protected time may be ideal, but may not be achievable during the current fiscal climate, unless the individual candidate supplements the support through successful grant applications.

The challenge for young investigators is to find or negotiate employment positions with an adequate level of protected time, since department chairpersons and administrators have many other needs and constraints that work against such an arrangement.

LEARNING RESEARCH TECHNIQUES

Acquiring Research Training

In order for physiatrists and rehabilitation professionals to successfully conduct quality research projects and disseminate the findings, it is essential that they have formal training in research methods. Professional training programs in physiatry and many other rehabilitation disciplines contain minimal or no research content, unless the individual specifically seeks additional graduate (master of science or doctorate degree) or postgraduate fellowship experience. A subcommittee from the Research Committee of the Association of Academic Physiatrists developed a minimum curriculum in research that will hopefully be adopted as part of the requirements for accreditation of residency training programs by the American Board of Physical Medicine and Rehabilitation, making basic research skills a standard component of the program required of all physiatrists in training.

Many professional organizations (e.g., Association of Academic Physiatrists, American Physical Therapy Association, American Occupational Therapy Association, United Cerebral Palsy Foundation) now have internal or external programs to fund promising individuals, on a competitive basis, for fellowship training experiences. Federal agencies including the NCMRR in the NIH (e.g., T32, T35, RSA, KO8, K12, and R29 programs) and the NIDRR in the U.S. Department of Education (e.g., Switzer fellowship program) also offer individual competitive research fellowship training opportunities as well as institutional funding to develop fellowship programs. Information regarding these fellowship opportunities is available by mail and on Internet Web sites upon request from the respective organizations. Selected physiatric residency training programs offer optional graduate-level training in research methods, funded by the department, as part of residency training. Many universities offer graduate research training programs designed for clinicians where classes meet monthly, predominantly over a weekend, and self-paced learning occurs during the interim between classes. In locations where a formal funded fellowship program is unavailable, pseudofellowships can often be developed by offering a part-time faculty position to provide adequate support for living expenses, while leaving sufficient time uncommitted to pursue research training and participation. In summary, many opportunities are available to acquire the necessary training and experience to become an independent researcher for individuals who are committed to pursuing such experience.

References for Research Methods

Many excellent references are available to supplement formal research training. A recommended reading list with key references identified is provided at the end of this chapter. Issues covered in these references include developing a testable research question, study design, controls for confounding variables to maximize internal and external validity of results, selection of tests and measures to evaluate variables of interest, subject selection criteria and assignment to study protocol, data analysis, and interpretation.

Single-Subject Research Designs

At the beginning of this chapter, we identified a lack of available study participants as a specific barrier to research experienced by medical rehabilitation researchers. Ottenbacher and Barrett (14) evaluated 100 data-based studies exploring the effectiveness of rehabilitation procedures. They calculated the median power of the research designs for small, medium, and large possible treatment effects and found "the possibility of a high rate of type II experimental errors in the rehabilitation literature." The most important factor was insufficient sample size; that is, had more individuals been enrolled in these studies, it is possible that a treatment effect would have been found where none was reported. In a subsequent article, Ottenbacher (15) recommended single subject (idiographic model) research designs (SSRDs) to avoid this pitfall.

The "gold standard" for experimental studies in the medical sciences is purported to be the randomized clinical trial (4). There are, however, inherent problems that often preclude implementation of such trials in clinical settings. For instance, there are potential ethical problems of withholding treatment from control groups. There are practical problems including lack of availability of enough homogeneous subjects, the relatively high costs to implement such studies, inflexible design strategies that do not allow change to be implemented once the study commences, and difficulty with true random assignment to equivalent treatment and control groups, because of variability in age, gender, duration of symptoms, severity of disease, education level, and so on, of the available study populations. There are inherent statistical problems with randomized group designs in that statistical significance does not necessarily equate to clinical significance, and there is a high probability of a type II error with small sample sizes and heterogeneous patient groups, as mentioned already. There are also problems with external validity in such designs (the ability to generalize results to the study population as a whole). Group averages obscure individual outcomes. It is therefore difficult to determine which subject characteristics are correlated to improvement. Intrasubject variability and clinical course are ignored with only the pretest-posttest paradigm typically used in randomized clinical trials. SSRDs can overcome such problems.

There are a number of potential advantages of utilizing single-subject paradigms for studying clinical problems. Guyatt et al (16) stated that SSRD is the method of choice to evaluate the effect of two (or more) treatments for a given patient. Martin and Epstein (17) indicated that SSRD is the most optimal method to assess treatment effects in heterogeneous patient populations, such as those with traumatic brain injury or cerebral palsy. These designs permit individualized therapeutic approaches and can be systematically altered if the initial intervention is ineffective. The SSRD relies on within-individual variation as opposed to between-group differences as the level of data analysis, thus avoiding the potential pitfall of an insufficient number of subjects preventing detection of a true difference when one exists (type II error).

A perceived drawback of SSRD is that data analysis is performed using methods of visual and statistical analysis, which are less familiar than those used to analyze group design studies. This limited familiarity is often interpreted as a lack of scientific rigor, although many tenable arguments to the contrary have been documented and are cited in the Web site noted at the end of this section. Additionally, it is often feasible to enroll a sufficient number of study participants over time to be able to apply group design statistics, to further validate treatment effects beyond initial subject-level analyses. Repeated serial measurements, where the subjects serve as their own controls, are used with SSRD (hence the name "single-subject" as the unit of analysis, i.e., *not* the number of study participants). This is in contrast to single preintervention and postintervention measurements of group design. In situations where baseline performance varies greatly or timing and magnitude of the treatment effect are unknown, serial measurements with subjects serving as their own controls afford better control over issues of internal and external validity than do group designs (18). The findings of single-subject studies are directly relevant to the study participant, versus being relevant only to a certain "class" of subjects; that is, there is potentially more personal value received by subjects who participate in single-subject studies in return for that participation. Given that SSRD studies typically enroll a relatively small number of participants (often 3 to 12), these designs are practical and cost-effective to implement in clinical settings.

Internal validity (the study measures what it purports to) is established with SSRD by 1) randomly assigning participants to protocols that control for the effect of the order in which different treatments are administered; 2) using reliable measurement techniques (19); 3) employing nonreactive measurement strategies so that the process of collecting data does not affect subject performance; 4) extending assessment across both nontreatment (baseline) and treatment phases, making observed changes less likely due to chance; 5) sequentially applying and withdrawing treatment to replicate results within subjects (A-B-A-B-A and A-B-A-C-A designs), or using multiple baseline designs that compare untreated (baseline) and treated performance, where intervention is staggered in time across subjects to control for potential confounding factors to internal validity such as history (some external event rather than treatment causes change to occur) or maturation (inherent change occurs in the subject).

External validity (pertinence of results to individuals outside of those who participated in the study) is established using SSRD by direct replications of the specific intervention within a given clinical setting. Subjects are matched closely to original participants, to establish that a given intervention has an effect on a certain type of client within a specific setting. Systematic replications are then performed across various types of clients, settings, clinicians, or varying combinations of these factors. Ongoing clinical replication then supplies further evidence of external validity for observed treatment effects. This is especially noteworthy since replication of research results and consensus building are currently lacking in most areas of medical rehabilitation research and practice.

In summary, single-subject research paradigms embody the essential components of scientific investigation, are practical and cost-effective to implement in clinical settings, and exemplify evidence-based information gathering. Readers are strongly encouraged to learn more about these methods from our Internet Web site about SSRD, which includes a comprehensive reference list (www-personal.umich.edu/~hinderer/).

Medical Rehabilitation Science Theory Development

As noted earlier, an overview of the medical rehabilitation literature reveals a lack of direction or consensus on many topics. Studies are frequently performed in isolation of each other, rather than in series with a specific overarching plan and theoretical basis regarding how the work fits into the science of medical rehabilitation practice. In a classic article that should be mandatory reading for all medical scientists and their students, Platt (20) discussed the scientific thinking that tends to produce much more rapid progress in many scientific fields than do other methods of study. The reasoning method he recommended is inductive, rather than deductive. The latter infers cause from effect. The former requires a more rigorous process. Platt described four basic steps to inductive inference:

1. Devising alternative hypotheses to explain observed relationships between input (independent) and outcome (dependent) variables;
2. Devising a crucial experiment (or several of them), with alternative possible outcomes, each of which will, as nearly as possible, exclude one or more of the hypotheses;
3. Carrying out the experiments so as to get a clean result;
4. Recycling the procedure, making subhypotheses or sequential hypotheses to refine the possibilities that remain.

This theory-building method requires development of an inductive logic tree, stemming at each alternative hypothesis and leading to the final outcome. Each successive experiment excludes alternatives, with eventual adoption of what is left as an "axiom." "It offers a regular method for reaching firm inductive conclusions one after the other as rapidly as possible."

Given the extraordinarily busy schedules most medical rehabilitation scientists have, it is not surprising that many become "method oriented" rather than "problem oriented." The problem-oriented approach is more time-intensive and requires looking at the scope of the problem, then working backward toward possible causes. It is easy to fall into the trap of working on oversimplified questions and models or to become overly attached to a single hypothesis that seems satisfactory. The consequence is research that has little impact on clinical practice or moving the field forward—a common criticism by members of other medical and scientific disciplines regarding the quality of the current medical rehabilitation literature.

The challenge then is for medical rehabilitation scientists to come together to debate problems that need solutions, to probe possible causes for them, and to use optimal methods to test the causal hypotheses, so that the "scientific method" is fully employed in medical rehabilitation research. Consensus building has been pursued in the past (e.g., the Nagi, World Health Organization, and NIH models for the continuum from disease to disability). It is our contention, however, that such models, all of which describe a linear pathway, are still profoundly too simple relative to the interaction of factors we have observed in medical rehabilitation practice. The medical rehabilitation field must develop inductive theoretical trees with multiple branches of possible causes, then look at where we can most efficiently saw off the branches, leaving only the solid trunk, which is the scientific foundation for practice we so desperately seek. It is no longer enough for each of us to work in isolation, breaking off small twigs from the tree. This will not serve to move the field forward and may ultimately kill the tree.

CONCLUSIONS

The field of medical rehabilitation needs to step up substantially the rigor of its research and adopt an inductive, problem-solving approach to develop rehabilitation science theory and models. These theories and models can serve as the guide to a concentrated series of research studies, ultimately establishing the basic axioms underlying the solutions to problems encountered by the clients we serve. Such robust methods are required to unrefutably prove that rehabilitation does benefit our patients, and to permanently establish medical rehabilitation as a true medical science.

REFERENCES

1. Braddom RL. Why is physiatric research important? *Am J Phys Med Rehabil* 1991;70(suppl): S2–S3.
2. Kirby RL. Excellence in rehabilitation through research. *Am J Phys Med Rehabil* 1991;70(suppl): S7–S8. Commentary.
3. DeLisa J. Need for academic physiatry in the era of health care reform: a commentary. *Am J Phys Med Rehabil* 1995;74:234–236.

4. Katz RT, Campagnolo DI, Goldberg G, et al. Research in physical medicine and rehabilitation. In: Braddom RL, ed. *Physical medicine and rehabilitation.* Philadelphia: WB Saunders, 1996: 255–272.

5. Whyte J. Research summit final report and implementation issues. Association of Academic Physiatrists Communication, 1996.

6. Brandt EN, Pope AM, eds. *Enabling America: assessing the role of rehabilitation science and engineering.* Washington, DC: National Academy Press, 1997.

7. Fuhrer MJ, ed. *Assessing medical rehabilitation practice: the promise of outcomes research.* Baltimore: Paul H. Brookes, 1997.

8. Grabois M, Fuhrer MJ. Physiatrists' views on research. *Am J Phys Med Rehabil* 1988;67:171–174.

9. NCMRR announces new opportunity for funding medical rehabilitation research. *AAP Newsletter* Spring 1996:47.

10. *The Physiatrist* 1997;13(1):13. Official Membership Publication of the American Academy of Physical Medicine and Rehabilitation.

11. Ogden TE. *Research proposals: a guide to success.* New York: Raven, 1991.

12. Reif-Lehrer L. *Writing a successful grant application.* 2nd ed. Boston: Jones & Bartlett, 1989.

13. Dijkers MP. Fundamentals of research design. In: *Research in rehabilitation: design, methods and development of projects.* Detroit: Rehabilitation of Michigan, 1997.

14. Ottenbacher KJ, Barrett KA. Statistical conclusion validity of rehabilitation research: a quantitative analysis. *Am J Phys Med Rehabil* 1991;70(suppl):S138–S143.

15. Ottenbacher KJ. Clinically relevant designs for rehabilitation research: the idiographic model. *Am J Phys Med Rehabil* 1990;69:286–292.

16. Guyatt G, Sackett D, Taylor W, et al. Determining optimal therapy. *N Engl J Med* 1996;314:889–892.

17. Martin JE, Epstein L. Evaluating treatment of effectiveness in cerebral palsy. *Phys Ther* 1976;56: 285–294.

18. White OR. Selected issues in program evaluation: arguments for the individual. In: Keogh B, ed. *Advances in special education: documenting program impact.* Vol. 4. Greenwich, CT: JAI Press, 1984.

19. Hinderer SR, Hinderer KA. Principles and applications of measurement methods. In: DeLisa J, Gans BM, eds. *Rehabilitation medicine: principles and practice.* 3rd ed. 1998:109–136.

20. Platt JR. Strong inference. *Science* 1964;146:347–353.

READING LIST

Getting Started

Oxman AD, Sackett DL, Guyatt GH. How to get started. *JAMA* 1993;270: 2093–2095.

Findley TW. Research in physical medicine and rehabilitation. I. How to ask the question. *Am J Phys Med Rehabil* 1991;70(suppl):S11–S16.

Browne MN, Keeley SM. *Asking the right questions.* Englewood Cliffs, NJ: Prentice-Hall, 1981.

Reviewing the Literature

Findley TW. Research in physical medicine and rehabilitation. II. The conceptual review of the literature or how to read more articles than you ever want to see in your entire life. *Am J Phys Med Rehabil* 1991;70(suppl): S17–S22.

Cook DJ, Guyatt GH, Oxman AD, Sackett DL, the Evidence-Based Medicine Working Group. Users' guide to the medical literature. *JAMA* 1993;270:2093–2095, 2598–2601; 1994;271:59–63, 389–391, 703–707, 1615–1619.

Gehlbach SH. *Interpreting the medical literature.* 3rd ed. New York: McGraw-Hill, 1993.

Reigelman ME. *Studying a study and testing a test. How to read the medical literature.* Boston: Little, Brown, 1989.

Davis AM, Findley TW. Research in physical medicine and rehabilitation. X. Information resources. *Am J Phys Med Rehabil* 1991;70(suppl):S94–S106.

Research Designs

Isaac S, Michael WB. *Handbook in research and evaluation for education and the behavioral sciences.* 3rd ed, San Diego: Educational and Industrial Testing Services, 1997.

Payton OD. *Research: the validation of clinical practice.* 3rd ed. Philadelphia: FA Davis, 1994.

Reilly RP, Findley TW. Research in physical and rehabilitation. IV. Some practical research designs in applied research. *Am J Phys Med Rehabil* 1991;70(suppl):S31–S36.

Hulley SB, Cummings SR. *Designing clinical research. An epidemiologic approach.* Baltimore: Williams & Wilkins, 1988.

Hinderer KA, Hinderer SR. Single case research design reference Web site. http://www-personal.umich.edu/~hiderer/

Ottenbacher KJ. Clinically relevant designs for rehabilitation research: the idiographic model. *Am J Phys Med Rehabil* 1991;70(suppl): S144–S150.

Bass MJ, Dunn EV, Norton PG, et al. *Conducting research in the practice setting. Research methods for primary care.* Vol. 5. Newbury Park, CA: Sage, 1993.

Selwyn MR. *Principles of experimental design for the life sciences.* Boca Raton: CRC Press, 1996.

Andersen B. *Methodological errors in medical research.* Oxford: Blackwell Scientific, 1990.

Portney LG, Watkins MP. *Foundations of clinical research: applications to practice.* Norwalk, CT: Appleton & Lange, 1993.

Stein F, Cutler SK. *Clinical research in allied health and special education.* 3rd ed. San Diego: Singular Publishing Group, 1996.

Tests and Measures

Hinderer SR, Hinderer KA. Principles and applications of measurement methods. In: DeLisa J, Gans BM, eds. *Rehabilitation medicine: principles and practice.* 3rd ed. 1998:109–136.

Johnston MV, Keith RA, Hinderer SR. Measurement standards for interdisciplinary medical rehabilitation. *Arch Phys Med Rehabil* 1992;73(12S): S3–S23.

Rothstein JM, Echternach JL. *Primer on measurement: an introductory guide to measurement issues.* Alexandria, VA: American Physical Therapy Association, 1993.

Power Analysis

Ottenbacher KJ, Barrett KA. Statistical conclusion validity of rehabilitation research: a quantitative analysis. *Am J Phys Med Rehabil* 1991;70(suppl): S138–S143.

Ottenbacher KJ, Barrett KA. Measures of effect size in the reporting of rehabilitation research. *Am J Phys Med Rehabil* 1991;70(suppl): S131–S137.

Database Management

Shurtleff DB. Computer data bases for pediatric disability: clinical and research applications. *Phys Med Rehabil Clin N Am* 1991;2: 665–687.

Lehmann JF, Warren CG, Smith W, Larson J. Computerized data management as an aid to clinical decision making in rehabilitation medicine. *Arch Phys Med Rehabil* 1984;65:260–262.

Findley TW, Stineman MG. Research in physical medicine and rehabilitation. V. Data entry and early exploration data analysis. *Am J Phys Med Rehabil* 1991;70(suppl):S37–S48.

Statistical Analysis

Stevens JP. On seeing the statistician and some analysis caveats. *Am J Phys Med Rehabil* 1991;70(suppl): S151–S152.

Castle WM, North PM. *Statistics in small doses.* 3rd ed. London: Churchill Livingstone, 1995.

Hirsch RP, Riegelman PK. *Statistical first aid: interpretation of health research data.* Oxford: Blackwell Scientific, 1992.

Katz RT, Campagnolo DI, Goldberg G, et al. Research in physical medicine and rehabilitation. In: Braddom RL, ed. *Physical medicine and rehabilitation.* Philadelphia: WB Saunders, 1996: 255–272.

Bland M. *An introduction to medical statistics.* 2nd ed. London: Oxford Medical, 1995.

Glantz SA. *Primer of biostatistics.* 3rd ed. New York: McGraw-Hill, 1992.

Phillips JL Jr. *How to think about statistics.* Revised ed. New York: Freeman, 1992.

Bailar JC III, Mosteller F, eds. *Medical uses of statistics.* 2nd ed. Boston: NEJM Books, 1992.

Rovine MJ, von Eye A. *Applied statistics in longitudinal research.* Boston: Academic Press, 1991.

Edwards AL. *Multiple regression and the analysis of variance and covariance.* 2nd ed. New York: Freeman, 1985.

Krauth J. *Distribution-free statistics. An application-oriented approach.* Amsterdam: Elsevier, 1988.

Gouvier WD. *Methods of analysis for single subject research designs.* American Congress of Rehabilitation Medicine annual conference course book. 1989:138–160.

Scientific Writing

Braddom CL. A framework for writing and/or evaluating research papers. *Am J Phys Med Rehabil* 1991;70(suppl): S169–S171.

Huth EJ. Guidelines on authorship of medical papers. *Ann Intern Med* 1986;104:269–274.

Zeiger M. *Essentials of writing biomedical research papers.* New York: McGraw-Hill, 1991.

Day RA. *How to write and publish a scientific paper.* 2nd ed., Philadelphia: ISI Press, 1983.

Huth EJ. *How to write and publish papers in the medical sciences.* Philadelphia: ISI Press, 1983.

Troyka LQ. *Simon & Schuster handbook for writers.* 2nd ed. Englewood Cliffs, NJ: Prentice-Hall, 1990.

Chapter 107

The Business Aspects of Medical Practice

Charlotte Hoehne Smith

THE CHANGING ENVIRONMENT OF HEALTH CARE AND REHABILITATION

The current market for health care in the United States presents a multitude of challenges and opportunities for today's practicing physician. The ever-changing dynamics in the health care industry reflect a powerful and complex set of societal, technological, and economic factors that have developed in recent decades (Table 107-1). All physicians face pressures due to increased competition, decreasing reimbursements, limited resources to meet patient's needs, and increasing fragmentation of health care. Prioritization within the field of rehabilitation is especially challenging because of the continued lack of education of patients, payors, and health care providers about the benefits related to rehabilitation.

As cost containment becomes an increasingly powerful goal of health care reform, maintaining access for chronically ill, disabled, or catastrophically injured rehabilitation patients is often problematic. However, studies have documented the cost-effectiveness of rehabilitation. A 1995 study by the Health Insurance Association of America demonstrated that early rehabilitation leads to shorter overall hospitalization times, lower mortality rates, and fewer complications, resulting in savings of $30 for every $1 spent on rehabilitation (1). Optimal rehabilitation, which allows for return to a home setting rather than institutionalized management, ultimately results in both lower costs and improved quality of life. Managed care and other health care system initiatives are having an impact on the provision of rehabilitation services, resulting in the shifting from hospital-based units to other types of care to achieve cost savings. The long-term impact of these initiatives on quality of care and patient outcomes is unknown.

Today's health care consumer is increasingly sophisticated, better educated, and assertive about health care issues. Consumer concerns about the impact of managed care on access and quality of care have driven legislation at both national and state levels. Congress and state legislatures have debated legislation related to managed care regulation, comprehensive consumer rights bills, health maintenance organization (HMO) liability, and other health care–related bills that affect physicians (2,3).

Concurrently, the environment of medicine presents a multitude of opportunities for development of rehabilitation practices. New technologies have the potential to increase both the longevity and the quality of life of patients of all ages and diagnostic categories. This has resulted in a need for rehabilitation services for patients who are severely deconditioned from prolonged hospitalization due to severe medical illnesses, catastrophic trauma, or new procedures such as organ transplantation. The spectrum of such patients varies from the growing geriatric population to neonates surviving complications of prematurity. Increasing emphasis on the goal of shortened acute care and inpatient hospital stays, with early return home, has created an increasing need for rehabilitation services to

Table 107-1: Challenges Facing Health Care in the United States of America
Population increasing in number and age
Increasing sophistication of technology
Political and business pressures to control costs
Increasing number of uninsured and underinsured patients
Consumer demands and expectations

Table 107-2: Potential Practice Settings
Hospital based
Outpatient clinic
Consultation
Combination of the above three settings
Same-specialty group
Multiple-specialty group
Solo practice
Office/overhead-sharing arrangement

be implemented proactively as part of routine medical care.

Rehabilitation services are now provided in a variety of settings including inpatient, outpatient, subacute, day programs, skilled nursing, long-term care, home, and community settings. Demand for physicians with programmatic expertise in these areas continues to increase, creating many opportunities for professional growth. At the end of 1994, there were 4642 certified physiatrists, representing a 124% increase in volume over the past 10 years (4). It is anticipated that the need for physiatrists will continue to increase in the immediate future, as both the scope and number of patients treated by physical medicine and rehabilitation specialists continue to expand. A 1995 Physical Medicine and Rehabilitation Workforce Study concluded that if the profession is successful in informing the market of the efficacy and efficiency of physiatrists, a significant aggregate excess supply is not likely to emerge through the year 2015 (5).

PRACTICE OPTIONS AND SETTINGS

The large variety of practice settings and opportunities has created many choices for physicians embarking on a rehabilitation career or reconsidering their current practice setting (Table 107-2). Balancing individual interests and talents with the needs of the community requires evaluation, planning, coordination, and oftentimes, creativity. Consideration must be given to many factors in determining the optimal geographic location and setting for a practice.

Physicians may choose to provide generalized rehabilitation services or focus on a specialized area of rehabilitation (such as pediatric rehabilitation and spinal cord rehabilitation). In addition to the inpatient management of traditional rehabilitation patients (with diagnoses such as stroke, traumatic brain injury, orthopedic, and other diagnosis), there is a need for consultation and supervision of rehabilitation patients in subacute, skilled nursing, outpatient, and home services settings. The scope of the practice of physical medicine and rehabilitation continues to broaden as recognition of the role of physiatrists in the management of musculosketetal, spinal, occupational, and other areas of outpatient medicine increases. In many instances, physiatrists have become the primary treatment coordinators for a variety of selected patients with impairments or disabilities either directly or in collaboration with primary care physicians or other specialists. This is often done through the physiatrist's office or by interdisciplinary clinics specially designed for certain types of diagnoses or patient issues. Opportunities in these areas exist in both private practice and academic settings.

The percentage of physicians entering solo practice continues to decrease, as most physicians continue to enter single-specialty and multiple-specialty group practices (6). The balance between guaranteed initial remuneration and future opportunity for growth is usually a trade-off that must be negotiated when joining an existing practice. Starting an independent practice requires initial capitalization and increased financial risk, but allows maximal independence in decision making. As increasing market pressures due to managed care have impacted the health care system, more and more physicians are choosing to align themselves with other physicians or facilities. The percentage of primary care physicians and specialists being hired in salaried positions is increasing (7). Salaried positions are primarily seen in administrative roles, academic institutions, medium-size to larger groups, and HMOs. Increasing numbers of administrative positions are being created for physicians with interest and expertise in this area of medicine (6).

MANAGED CARE

Additional opportunities are being created by the development of newly formed networks in which providers and institutions are aligned to form integrated delivery systems. These types of alliances are becoming increasingly common as providers organize to allow a seamless delivery of health care services in an efficient and competitive manner consistent with the goals of managed care. Opportunities for alliance and sharing of overhead and risk are being developed through the use of preferred provider organizations (PPOs), independent practice associations, medical service organizations, and physician-hospital associations. These types of organizations have developed as a result of managed care.

Managed care has developed over the last two

decades as a controversial tool for health care reform. The American Academy of Physical Medicine and Rehabilitation defines managed care as follows: "Managed care entails market interventions to control the price, volume, delivery site and intensity of health services provided, the goal of which is to maximize the value of health benefits and the coordination of health care management for the covered population." The objectives of managed care are 1) to manage quality, 2) to maximize patient service, and 3) to minimize total costs per person per year. Nearly 80% of U.S. employers now offer a managed care plan and over 100 million consumers are now covered by an HMO or other form of managed care.

A physician's decision to participate in a managed care plan and the choice of organization to join can be facilitated by comparing the advantages and disadvantages of participation and considering this information in addition to other factors specific to that physician's individual practice situation. Advantages to participation include the following:

- Increase in patient base
- Potentially guaranteed capitated income based on number of covered lives
- Prevention of patient migration to other physicians who participate in this plan

Potential disadvantages to managed care include the following:

- Increase in practice expenses
- Decreased revenue per potential patient
- Prolonged accounts receivable days
- Potentially increased liability and malpractice costs
- Potential loss of large groups of patients with plan changes

These factors and other issues related to the impact of managed care on the physiatric practice are well outlined in a comprehensive practice management manual developed by the American Academy of Physical Medicine and Rehabilitation (8).

Collaborative arrangements between physicians, providers, and payors have become formalized, necessitating an understanding of a variety of definitions that are now common in managed care, including those defined in Tables 107-3 and 107-4. Currently, point-of-service plans are the fastest-growing form of managed care, while closed-panel HMOs and PPOs are the most common type of enrollment (9).

There are tremendous variations in payment models in managed care (Table 107-5). The manner in which managed care organizations reimburse for services varies by geographic region, specialty, type of services being reimbursed, setting in which care is delivered, the maturity of the market, and other factors. There is ongoing development of Medicare–managed care hybrid programs in which managed care is proposed as a tool for cost containment. This approach is also being used by many states in an effort to expand services for the Medicaid patient population. The long-term impact of these types of programs is being studied by many (10).

The Physical Medicine and Rehabilitation Workforce Study recommended that physiatrists evaluate opportunities to achieve contracting leverage and cost efficiencies through horizontal integration with larger physician groups, as well as through vertical integration with broad-based provider consortiums (5).

Table 107-3: Managed Care Definitions

Capitation (or cap rate): the expected health care costs consumed by an individual member of the covered group plan that form the basis of the payment amount transferred between the payor and provider.
Primary care physician (PCP): a physician who serves as the first point of contact and "gatekeeper" to more complex levels of care.
Point-of-service (POS): a plan in which the gatekeeper PCP assumes responsibilities for overseeing all referral activity within the contracted group utilizing in network and out-of-network processes.
Carve-outs: services in care areas presenting special challenges from an expense computation standpoint are separately designed and contracted to an exclusive, independent provider by a managed care plan.
Risk: a measure of variability of the return on investment; generally refers to the party who becomes responsible in the event that actual expenses exceed the anticipated expenses.

Table 107-4: Managed Care Alliances

Health maintenance organization (HMO): assumes financial risk to provide health services to an enrolled population for a fixed sum of money paid in advance for a specified period.
Independent practice association (IPA): an organization formed by a group of independent physicians for the purpose of contracting with a payor or group of payors.
Physician-hospital organization (PHO): similar to an IPA with the addition of a hospital to the provider mix; usually initiated by the hospital.
Preferred provider organization (PPO): a network of care providers who have agreed to perform services within the parameters defined by a contract with a payor source.
Medical service organization (MSO): a PHO or other group that coordinates all components of care delivery including insurance products so as to contract directly with employers or groups of employers.

Source: Becker BE. Fundamentals of medical practice economics. In: *Preparing yourself* for physiatric practice. Chicago: American Academy of Physical Medicine and Rehabilitation, 1997.

Table 107-5: How HMO Enrollment Breaks Down

Type of Enrollment	No. of Members (Jan. 96)	Percentage of Enrollees	95–96 Change
Closed-panel HMOs:	52,464,445	88.8%	18.6%
Commercial	39,678,728	67.1	8.8
Federal employees health benefits program	2,156,524	3.6	–0.7
Direct pay	1,381,660	2.3	71.1
Medicare	3,734,881	6.3	26.9
Medicaid	4,668,758	7.9	33.2
Other	843,894	1.4	N.A.
Open-ended HMOs (POS)	6,043,422	10.2	48.1
Supplemental Medicare	469,261	0.8	–6.3
Other HMO products	113,861	0.2	N.A.
Total HMO enrollment	59,090,989	100	16.7

NA = Not available.
Point-of-service or open-ended HMOs were growing much more rapidly than traditional, closed-panel HMOs, but had only 10% of HMO enrollees as of Jan. 1, 1996.
Source: Terry K. You can thrive under managed care. *Med Econ* April 7, 1997.

PREPARING FOR PRACTICE

The multitude of market factors impacting the practice of physical medicine and rehabilitation has directly affected the career choices made by both emerging and established physiatrists. Physicians today have a much more complex decision pathway for determining the optimal practice arrangement that fits their specific situation. A logical approach must be taken in initiating a job search for the ideal practice opportunity.

Extended periods of time may be required to obtain state licensing privileges and other credentials. Therefore, choosing the preferred geographic region to practice should be a priority when starting practice or relocating. Because of increasing numbers of applicants in many states, it is not unusual for the process of state licensing to require several months. Contacting local physiatrists, other physicians, rehabilitation centers, and other persons is helpful in evaluating opportunities. Job fair and networking opportunities also exist at the American Academy of Physical Medicine and Rehabilitation and other national meetings.

In addition to consideration of the geographic location for practice and the desired focus of a practice, lifestyle issues and the willingness to accept financial and other risks must be considered. Finding a good match for career and life goals within a specific practice opportunity may be an initial decision that has to be periodically revisited over time. The range of salaries and the final negotiated job packages are highly variable throughout the country. The factors impacting job opportunities ultimately are local market conditions, the demand for services offered, and the relationships that are developed.

Complete consideration of all issues related to obtaining a job or starting a practice are beyond the scope of this chapter; however, a variety of resources are available through national organizations, state and specialty medical organizations, and independent job placement services. The American Academy of Physical Medicine and Rehabilitation also holds an annual course for physiatrists preparing to enter medical practice. This course covers all aspects of job preparation from resume writing to evaluating practice opportunities, to contract negotiations, and is an excellent source of comprehensive information.

ESTABLISHED PHYSICIANS ARE CHANGING THEIR PRACTICES

Although the pace is slowing over the last few years, a recent study of established physicians indicated that 38% of randomly surveyed respondents had made a major change (such as merging, selling, joining another organization, relocating, or retiring) within the previous 12 months, or planned to do so within the following year (6). This same survey found that nearly as many physicians 50 years or older made practice changes as their younger colleagues did. The type of changes made varied by geographic region and specialty, but practice mergers were consistently the most common change made (6).

Other considerations in assessing job opportunities include lifestyle issues, such as the potential arrangements for sharing call coverage after office hours and on weekends. Both new and established physicians are re-evaluating the opportunities for improving the balance between professional and personal time. It is possible in the current market to carve out opportunities for nontraditional roles such as job sharing and part-time positions. With increasing numbers of female physicians entering the marketplace, this has become an accepted career path and can be feasible in the proper environment (11).

Even with the rapid changes occurring in most medical practices, most physicians are as happy with their professional lives today as they were at the beginning of the decade. About four out of five readers of the *Physician's Advisory* reported being satisfied to very satisfied with their professional lives (12).

MANAGING FINANCES AND OPERATIONS

As reimbursement for medical services continues to decrease as a result of managed care and other interventions, it becomes increasingly critical for physicians to maintain optimal practice finances and operations. Arranging to participate in managed care and other arrangements is a complex decision in which methods for measuring payment effectiveness and impact on the practice must be considered. Increasingly, practices are challenged to manage both fee-for-service patients and those in a capitated, bundled, or otherwise negotiated plan. Discounted-fee-for-service is outpacing the capitated growth rate, while the percentage of revenues received from indemnity plans continues to drop (9).

One progressive contracting approach involves risk sharing. Payors are drawn to providers who stand behind their cost-effectiveness claims by taking financial risk. When there are fixed-fee schedules, there is financial risk. As payment mechanisms such as capitation become more prevalent, physiatrists must learn to curb risk when negotiating such contracts (13).

Many physicians have enlisted the assistance of practice management companies to help with business aspects related to the practice of medicine. Smaller, single-specialty physician practice management companies appear to be performing better based on 1997 data (14).

Billing and Collection Systems

Creating optimal systems for billing and collections is increasingly difficult. Expertise and sophistication in billing and collections are mandatory as diversification of payment methods occurs. Developing dedicated staff to manage this business function is a complex process. There are numerous courses available through state and national organizations to assist with the training and development of staff in these positions. Increasingly, computer software and other data management systems are becoming commercially available to assist with this function. Many physicians choose to contract with external billing and collection companies. This may prove to be the most cost-effective approach, particularly for smaller practices, if appropriate supervision and controls are in place. Referral to providers of these types of services is usually obtained through local and regional organizations as well as through word of mouth from other physicians.

Physician Practice Expenses

Controlling the cost of overhead expenses is a powerful factor in the overall health and viability of a medical practice. Redefining the priorities for office spending and utilization of resources is imperative. Physician practice overhead varies widely by specialty, geographic location, group size, and other factors, ranging from \$174,800 to \$204,400 per physician annually (Table 107-6). The top spending areas for most practices continue to be personnel and office expenses (15). The demands of managed care, inflation, and other factors have caused all operating costs to increase in the face of stable or decreased revenues.

When focusing on cost containment, a balance between reduction of overhead expenses and optimal practice efficiency must be maintained (16). Expenses that directly help to generate patient revenues should not be compromised, particularly if they increase the profitability of the practice by allowing more patients to be seen. Optimal office space and staffing are two areas that must be carefully analyzed to ensure cost-effectiveness. The use of time-motion studies may be helpful in designing a practice environment with adequate space and staffing to enhance physician productivity (11). Use of qualified professionals specializing in medical office design is an expense that usually proves cost-effective in the long run.

Personnel Issues

Appropriate hiring and utilization of office personnel are critical for many reasons. In addition to accounting for the largest single overhead expense for most practices, physicians are responsible for the performances of their staff. A balance between practice efficiency and the quality of work performed must be achieved to allow optimal patient care and to minimize liability.

The use of health care "extenders" such as physician assistants and nurse practitioners in physician practices is becoming increasingly prevalent. Factors to consider when utilizing highly trained personnel include impact on physi-

Table 107-6: Physician Practice Expense Summary: National Averages, by Location Type

		Metropolitan Areas			
	Nonmetropolitan	Population < 1 Million		Population ≥ 1 Million	
Type of Expense	Areas Average	% Difference Average	% Difference from Nonmetropolitan	Average	from Nonmetropolitan
Personnel payroll	\$65,700	\$76,600	16.6%	\$69,800	6.2%
Office expense	45,900	53,600	16.8%	62,000	35.1%
Medical supplies	21,000	22,000	4.8%	18,900	−10.0%
Liability premiums	12,400	13,900	12.1%	16,300	31.5%
Medical equipment	9,500	9,600	1.1%	10,900	14.7%
Total practice expense	\$174,800	\$204,400	16.9%	\$202,600	15.9%

Source: All data are from the AMA's *Socioeconomic characteristics of medical practice.* Compiled by the Department of Health Care Financing, Division of Medical Economics, Texas Medical Association, 1997.

cian productivity, patient satisfaction, and relative cost (11,17).

An excellent staff consisting of motivated employees with good work relationships is an asset for any medical practice. Development of quality staff and appropriate work environment is a task that requires commitment and specific management skills. Many physicians utilize a practice administrator to manage personnel and other employment issues. If hiring a dedicated practice administrator is not financially feasible, other options exist to ensure that appropriate legal and business management practices are followed. Resources exist to assist physicians with the following:

- Development of office policy and procedure manuals
- Development of staff descriptions, hiring procedures, and performance appraisals
- Payroll and employment tax assistance
- Employee leasing and recruitment
- Development of salary and benefit programs
- Strategies for employee retention and team building.

A comprehensive section related to personnel issues is included in the American Academy of Physical Medicine and Rehabilitation practice management guide (8). There are also vendors throughout the country that specialize in physician practice support and provide materials or consultative services. National databases related to employee salaries and benefits are readily available (18). Recommendations for these types of vendors is best obtained from satisfied physician colleagues or professional physician societies (such as the American Academy of Physical Medicine and Rehabilitation, American Medical Association, or state medical societies).

DOCUMENTATION TRENDS

The demand for outcome data and completion of required documentation has made increased efficiency in medical information management a high priority for most practices. Reliance on technology and computer systems is mandatory when attempting to provide appropriate and timely documentation while limiting the number of personnel required to manage this task. Great strides have been made in the development of user-friendly, computer software systems that can guide documentation processes in a comprehensive manner promoting efficiency, quality improvement, and cost savings. Comparisons of computer systems typical for various practice situations are available to assist with decision making related to hardware, software, and consultant services (19).

Software products are now available for a variety of medical practice functions, including billing, scheduling, communications, and electronic patient records. New technology must be carefully evaluated to determine usability, practicality, cost-effectiveness, and whether use of the product will enhance office operations and facilitate optimal patient care. Global products are designed to meet practice needs utilizing a single product or vendor. In contrast is the plug-and-play approach to office automation in which a variety of programs are integrated to meet individual needs (8). Additional considerations related to office automation are outlined in Table 107-7.

Table 107-7: Considerations in Office Automation
Training
Technical support
Confidentiality and security
Coordination with existing charts
Backup and maintenance

Resources and vendors are also available to assist with the development of databases that can subsequently be used to generate electronic medical records and customized reports (Table 107-8). This approach can have many benefits, including lower transcription costs and a standardized approach that can improve quality of documentation and decrease liability. Formatted data can be used to generate user-defined reports that can assist the practice with outcome evaluations, quality assurance, cost evaluation, and referral development. Communication between involved parties can be improved through the use of computer networks, automated faxing, and electronic mail.

Table 107-8: Examples of Computer-Generated Medical Records
Hospital lists
Superbills
Narrative reports
Progress notes
Workers' compensation reports
Letters of necessity
Prescriptions
Patient instructions
Referral letters
Work limitations

PRACTICE MANAGEMENT AND PROMOTION

The Physical Medicine and Rehabilitation Workforce Study (5) concluded that "lack of understanding regarding who physiatrists are and what service they can deliver cost-effectively appears to be one of the most important factors relative to physiatric demand." It is critical that potential customers, including patients, payors, and referral sources, be informed of the benefits of physiatry. This information can be communicated in a variety of ways, the vast majority of which should be self-evident by the observed effectiveness of physiatric intervention. Customer satisfaction should be monitored closely, as reputation and word-of-mouth referrals are the single most effective marketing tool. As competition for referrals increases, customer satisfaction becomes critical. Each customer has unique needs and expectations.

Patients are becoming more sophisticated in their expectations of physicians. In addition to high-quality medical care, a well-managed practice that meets the needs of patients and provides added value is critical (3). Educating patients and families about the scope and benefits of physiatric consultation is a first step in meeting expectations. The accessibility and environment of the office as well as the attitudes and approach of the physician and staff impact the patient experience. Clear communication during all aspects of the patient encounter facilitates a positive patient-physician relationship. Surveys can clarify patient perceptions related to pricing, access, convenience, and other fundamental elements related to customer satisfaction. National polls continue to demonstrate that most patients' notion of quality in health care is based on their personal relationship with their physician rather than on his or her years of training or service. Patients envision a high-quality physician as someone who listens and takes the time to understand (20).

Payor sources such as employers or managed care providers are important customers with expectations that often differ from those of the patient. For payors, value is defined as achieving significantly improved outcomes at the lowest cost possible while maintaining high levels of patient satisfaction (8). Decreased future medical costs because of decreased utilization or lessened need for maintenance care are a tangible benefit of rehabilitation that must be demonstrated to payors. Providing specific and quantitative documentation related to proposed treatment plans along with clarification of expected outcome can facilitate approval of proposed services. Concise and timely communication assists the working relationship with payors.

Referring physicians also face challenges related to the changing environment of medicine. In order for referring physicians to justify physiatric consultation, they must be informed and aware of the benefits of referral. Frequently, physiatrists can assist with difficult clinical challenges that optimally can be managed within an interdisciplinary rehabilitation setting. Timely communication should be provided in a concise and convenient manner so that the referring physician's needs are met. The physiatrist must understand the expectations of the referring physician to optimally provide services.

CONCLUSIONS

Physical medicine and rehabilitation specialists face many challenges in today's health care environment. Market forces and the impact of managed care have the potential to adversely impact many facets of physiatric practice, including access to patients, clinical decision-making autonomy, reimbursement levels, and administrative burdens. However, physiatrists possess unique qualifications and skills that will serve patients well in a managed care setting. In fully integrated systems, physiatrists have a competitive advantage because of their holistic approach, care coordination skills, team orientation, and flexibility to perform a variety of clinical roles. The traditional specialist role of physiatrists most likely will expand to include roles as consultants, educators, coordinators of care, and primary care providers for persons with specially defined disabilities (5).

FUTURE OPPORTUNITIES

Physiatrists who successfully convince managed care entities and other payors of their cost-effectiveness will secure access to referral streams. Physiatrists should seek payment structures that reward them for what they save and value added rather than compensating them for care provided. Continued emphasis on outcome data, including the development of more exact and sophisticated outcome measures, is of utmost importance. Studies that demonstrate the impact of rehabilitation on both cost and improvement in quality of life must continue.

Physiatrists must be active in political and legislative processes that have the potential to impact patient care and the provision of rehabilitation. Adequate funding is often the largest barrier to access to rehabilitation services; therefore, political advocacy for provision of rehabilitative services is mandatory. Education of elected officials about the benefits of rehabilitation must occur at the local, state, and national levels. Physiatrists must also collaborate and build support within both the medical community and the general public.

Physiatrists must never lose sight of their primary purpose in medicine—serving patients by restoring function and promoting quality of life. In the midst of the many conflicting forces, the essential mission of helping patients and serving as patient advocate cannot be dismissed. Maintaining the sacred patient-physician bond while providing optimal value is tantamount to the success of health care reform. The future of physical medicine and rehabilitation depends on the specialty's ability to balance these forces.

REFERENCES

1. Health Insurance Association of America. *Survey of rehabilitation programs.* Research and statistical bulletin No. 2. Washington, DC: Health Insurance Association of America, 1995.
2. Tschida M. Whose agenda? *Mod Physician* Feb 1998:3.
3. Herzlinger R. *Market driven health care: who wins, who loses in the transformation of America's largest service industry.* Reading, MA: Addison-Wesley, 1997.
4. Brandstater ME. Physical medicine and rehabilitation. *JAMA* 1995; 273:1710–1712.
5. Hogan P, Dobson A, Haynie B. *Physical Medicine and Rehabilitation Workforce Study.* Chicago: American Academy of Physical Medicine and Rehabilitation, 1995.
6. Terry K. Doctors on the move. *Med Econ* Dec 8, 1997;74:144–155.
7. Moran M. More physicians are employees. *Am Med News* March 9, 1998:7.
8. Managing managed care. In: *The physiatrist's guide to practice management.* Chicago: American Academy of Physical Medicine and Rehabilitation, 1997.
9. John Erb, principal. Foster Higgins National Survey of Employer-Sponsored Health Plans, National highlights. Foster Higgins, New York City.
10. Terry K. Don't miss out on Medicare managed care. *Med Econ* April 7, 1997;74:58–70.
11. Beck L. *The Physician's Advisory* February 1998.
12. Practice beat—professional satisfaction. *Med Econ* Sept 22, 1997;74:36.
13. PM&R awareness initiative—curbing financial risk in the PM&R area. *Physiatrist* Dec 1997/Jan 1998:7.
14. Cook B. Size doesn't matter. *Mod Phys* March 1998;1997:18.
15. American Medical Associations. *Socioeconomic characteristics of medical practice.* Prepared by the Department of Health Care Financing, Division of Medical Economics, Texas Medical Association, 1997.
16. Lowes RL. How to deal with a stingy boss. *Med Econ* Jan 12, 1998;75:57–71.
17. Lowes RL. Making midlevel providers click with your group. *Med Econ* 1998;75:123–132.
18. Dolan KP. Are you paying your staff enough? *Med Econ* Jan 12, 1998;75:99–126.
19. Typical system: small group practice. ComputerTalk—Clinical and administrative systems for physician groups. 1998;16(1).
20. Pretzer M. Managed care is hurting your reputation. *Med Econ* Sept 22, 1997;74:47–50.

INDEX

Note: Page numbers followed by f indicate figures; those followed by t indicate tables.

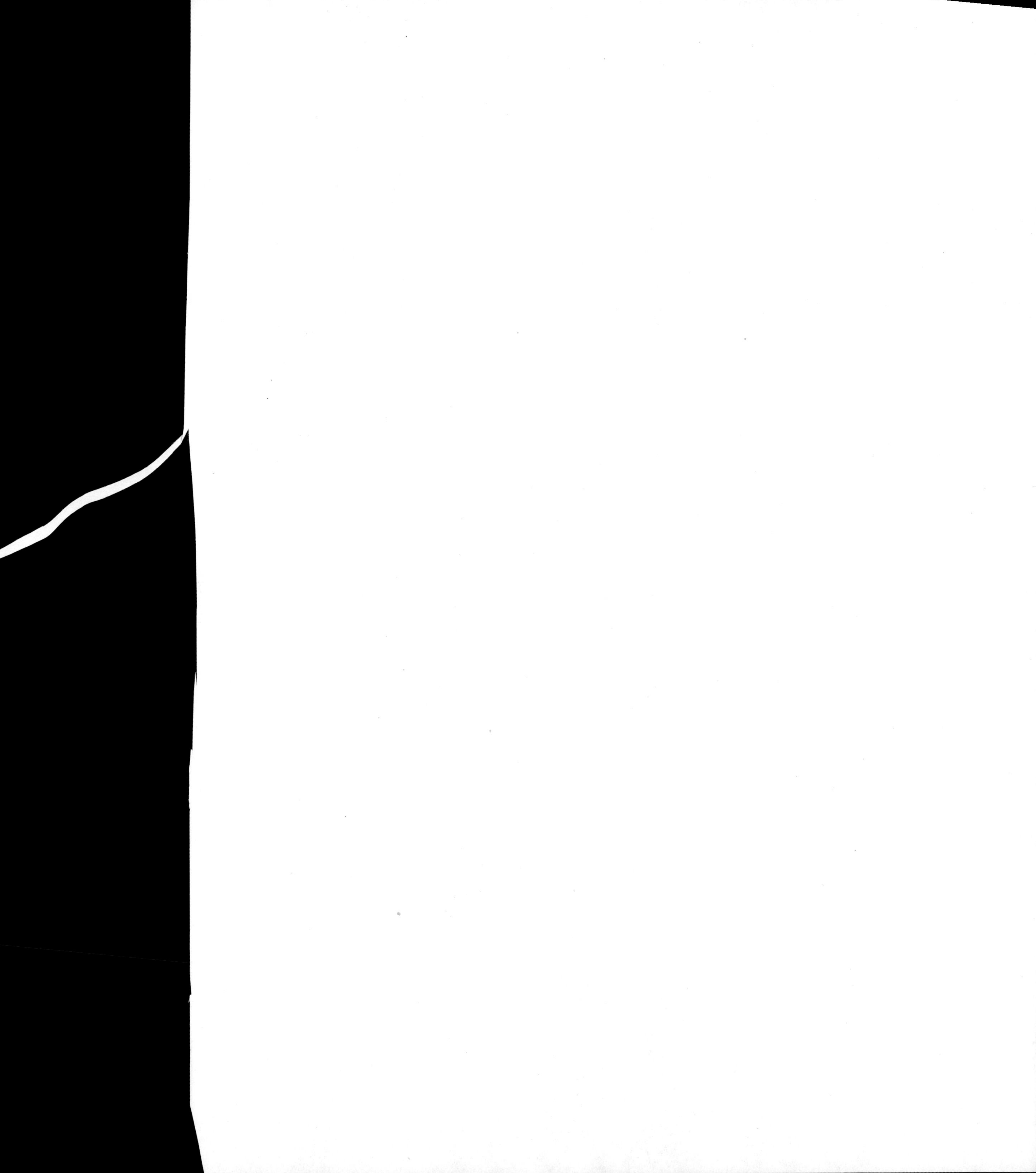